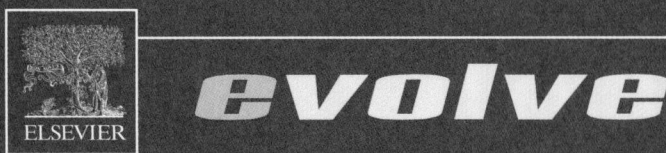

ELSEVIER

To access your Instructor Resources, visit:

http://evolve.elsevier.com/McCance/

Evolve® Student Learning Resources for *McCance and Huether: Pathophysiology: The Biologic Basis for Disease in Adults and Children,* **5th Edition**, offer the following features:

Student Resources

- **WebLinks**
  This useful resource links you to hundreds of websites carefully chosen to supplement the content of your textbook. The WebLinks are regularly updated, with new links added as they develop.

PATHOPHYSIOLOGY

The Biologic Basis for Disease in Adults and Children

PATHOPHYSIOLOGY

The Biologic Basis for Disease in Adults and Children

KATHRYN L. McCANCE, RN, PhD

Professor, College of Nursing
University of Utah
Salt Lake City, Utah

SUE E. HUETHER, RN, PhD

Professor, College of Nursing
University of Utah
Salt Lake City, Utah

FIFTH EDITION

with 1300 illustrations

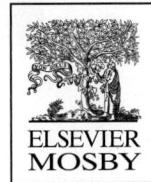

ELSEVIER
MOSBY

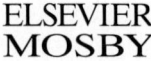

ELSEVIER
MOSBY

11830 Westline Industrial Drive
St. Louis, Missouri 63146

Pathophysiology: The Biologic Basis for Disease in Adults and Children   ISBN-13: 978-0-3230-3507-1
ISBN-10: 0-323-03507-8

NOTICE

ISBN-13: 978-0-323-03507-1
ISBN-10: 0-323-03507-8

Executive Publisher: Darlene Como
Managing Editor: Brian Dennison
Associate Developmental Editor: Betsy Stream
Publishing Services Manager: Jeffrey Patterson
Project Manager: Mary G. Stueck
Design Direction: Jyotika Shroff
Cover Designer: Jyotika Shroff
Text Designer: Jyotika Shroff
Cover Art: Barbara Cousins

Printed in the United States of America

Last digit is the print number: 9 8 7 6 5 4 3 2 1

CONTRIBUTORS

ROSE A. URDIALES BAKER, MSN, RN, CS
Burn Research Nurse
The Paul and Carol David Foundation Burn Institute
Clifford R. Boeckman, MD Regional Burn Center
Akron Children's Hospital
Akron, Ohio;
Instructor, College of Nursing
Kent State University
Kent, Ohio

KATHLEEN M. BALDWIN, PhD, RN, CNS, ANP, GNP
Associate Professor and Director of Graduate Studies
Harris School of Nursing
Texas Christian University
Fort Worth, Texas

PHILLIP BARNETTE, MD
Instructor
Pediatric Hematology/Oncology
University of Utah School of Medicine
Salt Lake City, Utah

BARBARA J. BOSS, RN, PhD, CFNP, CANP
Professor of Nursing
University of Mississippi Medical Center
Jackson, Mississippi

VALENTINA L. BRASHERS, MD
Professor of Nursing and Attending Physician in Internal Medicine
University of Virginia Health System
Charlottesville, Virginia

KRISTEN LEE CARROLL, MD
Associate Professor, Department of Orthopedics
University of Utah
Salt Lake City, Utah

DENNIS J. CHEEK, RN, PhD, FAHA
Abell-Hanger Professor of Gerontological Nursing
Texas Christian University
Harris School of Nursing and School of Nurse Anesthesia
Fort Worth, Texas

JEAN ANNE CONNOR, RN, DNSc, CPNP
Nurse Scientist, Cardiovascular Program
Faculty, Patient Safety and Quality
Children's Hospital Boston
Boston, Massachusetts

CHRISTY L. CROWTHER, RN, MS, CRNP
Adult Nurse Practitioner
Private Consultant
Millersville, Maryland

CURTIS B. DEFRIEZ, MD
Assistant Professor, Health Sciences
Weber State University
Ogden, Utah

ANGELA DENERIS, PhD, CNM
Associate Clinical Professor
Nurse-Midwifery and Women's Health
    Nurse Practitioners Programs
University of Utah College of Nursing
Salt Lake City, Utah

DEBORAH B. EVERS, DNS, RN, CPN
Professor, Parent-Child Nursing
Charity School of Nursing
Delgado Community College
New Orleans, Louisiana

BETH A. FORSHEE, PhD
Assistant Professor of Physiology
Lake Erie College of Osteopathic Medicine
Erie, Pennsylvania

DEBORAH K. FROH, MD
Associate Professor of Pediatrics
University of Virginia
Charlottesville, Virginia

MIKEL GRAY, PhD, FNP, CUNP, CCCN, FAAN
Nurse Practitioner and Professor
Department of Urology and School of Nursing
University of Virginia
Charlottesville, Virginia

TODD CAMERON GREY, MD
Chief Medical Examiner, State of Utah;
Associate Clinical Professor of Pathology
University of Utah School of Medicine
Salt Lake City, Utah

MARY FRAN HAZINSKI, RN, MSN, FAAN
Clinical Specialist, Pediatric Emergency and Critical Care
Vanderbilt Children's Hospital
Nashville, Tennessee

ROBERT E. JONES, MD, FACP, FACE
Adjunct Associate Professor of Medicine
University of Utah School of Medicine
Salt Lake City, Utah

LYNN B. JORDE, PhD
Professor and Associate Chair of Human Genetics
University of Utah School of Medicine
Salt Lake City, Utah

ELIZABETH KASSNER, MS, RN, CPNP, CPON
Pediatric Nurse Practitioner
Baylor College of Medicine
Texas Children's Hospital Center
Texas Children's Cancer Center
Houston, Texas

RENEE A. KLENKE, BSN, RN, CCRC
Certified Clinical Research Coordinator
Texas Children's Hospital
Texas Children's Cancer Center

NANCY E. KLINE, PhD, RN, CPNP, FAAN
Director, Research and Evidence-Based Practice
Department of Nursing
Memorial Sloan-Kettering Cancer Center
New York, New York

THOM J. MANSEN, PhD, RN
Associate Professor, College of Nursing
University of Utah
Salt Lake City, Utah

MARY A. MONDOZZI, MSN, RN, CS
Burn Center Education/Outreach Coordinator
Akron Children's Hospital
The Paul and Carol David Foundation Burn Institute
Clifford R. Boeckman, MD Regional Burn Center
Akron, Ohio

KATHERINE MORGAN, MSN, WHNP, ANP
Assistant Clinical Professor
University of Utah College of Nursing
Salt Lake City, Utah

STEPHEN E. MORRIS, MD, FACS
Trauma Medical Director
University of Utah School of Medicine
Department of Surgery
Salt Lake City, Utah

NOREEN HEER NICOL, MS, RN, FNP
Chief Clinical Officer
Dermatology Clinical Specialist/Nurse Practitioner
National Jewish Medical and Research Center;
Clinical Senior Instructor
University of Colorado School of Nursing
Denver, Colorado

KATHERINE PADGETT, RN, MN
Professor of Nursing
Delgado Community College/Charity School of Nursing
New Orleans, Louisiana

NEAL S. ROTE, PhD
Academic Vice Chair and Director of Research
Department of Obstetrics and Gynecology
University Hospitals of Cleveland;
Professor of Reproductive Biology and Pathology
Case School of Medicine
Case Western Reserve University
Cleveland, Ohio

JANE SHELBY, PhD
Associate Professor of Surgery
Department of Surgery
University of Utah
Salt Lake City, Utah

RICHARD A. SUGERMAN, PhD
Professor of Anatomy
Executive Assistant Dean for Basic Sciences and Research
Western University of Health Sciences
College of Osteopathic Medicine of the Pacific
Pomona, California

LOREY K. TAKAHASHI, PhD
Associate Professor
Department of Psychology
University of Hawaii
Honolulu, Hawaii

BARBARA CRIPPES TRASK, PhD
Assistant Professor
Weber State University
Ogden, Utah

DAVID M. VIRSHUP, MD
Willard Snow Hansen Professor of Cancer Research
Professor of Pediatrics
Huntsman Cancer Institute
University of Utah
Salt Lake City, Utah

ROBIN WEBER, MN, RN, FNP-C, DNC
Regional Clinical Coordinator, Dermatology
Genentech
Portland, Oregon

ROBIN R. WILKERSON, RN, PhD
Associate Professor
School of Nursing
University of Mississippi
Jackson, Mississippi

REVIEWERS

MARY K. BEARD, MD, FACOG
Clinical Professor, Department of Obstetrics and Gynecology
University of Utah;
Private Practice, LDS Hospital
Salt Lake City, Utah

KATHY GARDNER, MS(C)
Instructor, Pathophysiology
North Dakota State University
Fargo, North Dakota

KIRTLY PARKER JONES, MD
Associate Professor and Vicechair for Academic Affairs
Department of Obstetrics and Gynecology
University of Utah
Salt Lake City, Utah

MARY JO MATTOCKS, RN, MN, PhD
Clinical Nurse Educator
Benefis Healthcare
Great Falls, Montana

CHRISTINE MIASKOWSKI, RN, PhD, FAAN
Professor and Chair, Department of Physiological Nursing
University of California
San Francisco, California

SANDRA A. MITCHELL, CRNP, MSCN, AOCN
Oncology Nurse Practitioner
National Cancer Institute
Bethesda, Maryland

TIMOTHY J. PAGANA, MD, FACS
Medical Director
The Kathryn Candor Lundy Breast Health Center and
The SurgiCenter
Susquehanna Health System
Williamsport, Pennsylvania

PHYLLIS G. PETERSON, RN, MN, AOCN
Assistant Professor
Our Lady of Holy Cross College
New Orleans, Louisiana

PAMELA JOHNSON ROWSEY, PhD
Associate Professor
The University of North Carolina at Chapel Hill
Chapel Hill, North Carolina

CAMILLE A. SERVODIDIO, RN, MPH, CRNO
RN Coordinator
Cancer Clinical Research Office
Hartford Hospital
Hartford, Connecticut

KATHLEEN DORMAN WAGNER, RN, EDD (AED)
Lecturer
University of Kentucky College of Nursing
Lexington, Kentucky

SUSAN F. WILSON, RN, PhD, FNP
Associate Professor
Texas Christian University
College of Health and Human Sciences
Harris School of Nursing;
Staff Nurse
Harris Continued Care Hospital
Fort Worth, Texas

PREFACE

Pathophysiology is part of an emerging stream of incredible discoveries and advancing understandings in the biologic sciences. Although these advancements have created an ever-increasing state of excitement they have also created the problem of how students, teachers, and clinicians can cope with the expanding new information. Our approach in this book has been to emphasize this emergence by explaining new concepts in greater detail than perhaps is usual and by giving extra emphasis to important but difficult content. This information expansion involves a greater understanding of the behavior of individual cells, their surrounding environment, and of the molecules that not only make up those cells but also communicate with their surroundings. The many mechanisms that control important variables in individual cells are continually being elucidated in great detail. Thus in this edition are several major new chapters and extensively rewritten previous chapters with new art.

As in previous editions, our specific goals for the textbook are to:

- Draw attention to differences in etiology and epidemiology, pathophysiology, clinical manifestations, and treatment according to gender and age
- Integrate health promotion and disease prevention by updating risk factors, explaining the relationship between nutrition and disease, and noting screening recommendations and other therapeutic approaches
- Pay careful attention to presentations of emerging new data on controversial topics

ORGANIZATION AND CONTENT: WHAT'S NEW IN THE FIFTH EDITION

The book is organized into two parts. The application of the principles and concepts in Part One determines the learner's ability to grasp the cellular and tissue responses to the most common diseases presented in Part Two.

Part One: Central Concepts of Pathophysiology: Cells and Tissues

Part One begins with an in-depth study of the cell and progresses to cover the underlying processes of disease. Concepts covered include cell signaling and cell communication processes; genes and common genetic diseases; fluid electrolyte and acid–base balance; inflammation, cytokines and their biologic functions, normal and altered immunity; stress coping, and immunity, and tumor biology and metastasis.

Particularly important revisions and additions to Part One include the following:

- New content on the extracellular matrix, cell signaling pathways, and protein synthesis (Chapter 1)
- Updated content on oxidative stress, apoptosis, stem cells, and aging and frailty (Chapter 2)
- Completely rewritten chapters on normal innate and adaptive immunity (Chapters 6 and 7)
- Extensively revised chapter on alterations of immunity and inflammation (Chapter 8)
- Infection content reorganized into a separate chapter (Chapter 9)
- Extensive revisions on stress and disease (Chapter 10)
- Completely rewritten chapter on tumor biology and epidemiology of cancer (Chapter 11)
- New content on tumor invasion, the cellular microenvironment, and metastases (Chapter 12)

Part Two: Pathophysiologic Alterations: Organs and Systems

Part Two is a systematic survey of diseases within body systems. Each unit focuses on a specific body system and begins with an anatomy and physiology chapter to provide a basis of comparison for understanding the alterations brought about by disease. A brief summary of normal aging is included at the end of the section on anatomy and physiology. The discussion of each disease in the alterations chapters is developed in a logical manner that begins with an introductory paragraph on etiology and epidemiology, followed by pathophysiology, clinical manifestations, and evaluation and treatment. Separate chapters are dedicated to pediatric pathophysiology, and sensitivity is paid to gender and age. Especially significant revisions and additions to Part Two include the following:

- Completely rewritten section on pain (Chapter 15)
- Major revisions on mechanisms of brain injury and chronic neurologic disorders (Chapter 17)
- New content on schizophrenia, mood disorders, and anxiety (Chapter 18)
- Significant updates and reorganization of content on hormone signaling and regulation, including reproductive hormones (Chapter 20)
- Extensive updates on diabetes mellitus, thyroid disorders, and disorders of the pituitary and hypothalamus (Chapter 21)
- Extensively rewritten material on breast diseases and new section on breast cancer (Chapter 23)

- Extensively rewritten content on hemostasis, platelet function, and coagulation (Chapter 25)
- Rewritten content on leukemias, lymphoma, and myeloma (Chapter 27)
- Extensively updated coverage of atherosclerosis, endothelial injury and dysfunction, coronary artery disease, myocardial infarction, cardiomyopathies, and heart failure (Chapter 30)
- Reorganization of adult and pediatric respiratory disorders content including asthma, chronic obstructive diseases, infections, and cancer (Chapters 33 and 34)
- Major reorganization and updates on urinary tract and renal disorders including obstructive uropathies, glomerulopathies, and chronic renal failure (Chapter 36)
- Major revisions and new content on peptic ulcer disease, inflammatory bowel disease, intestinal obstruction, obesity, and liver disease (Chapter 39)
- Major revisions on bone remodeling, osteoporosis, rheumatoid arthritis, and osteoarthritis (Chapter 42)
- Updates on allergic and autoimmune diseases of the skin, skin infections, and skin cancer (Chapter 44)
- Major revisions on septic shock, multiple organ dysfunction syndrome, and burns for both adults and children (Chapters 46 and 47)

FEATURES TO PROMOTE LEARNING

Ease of learning has been enhanced by designing a number of features that guide and support understanding, including:

- *Chapter outlines* for each chapter, including page numbers
- *Special headings* to underscore the consistent treatment of each disease—Pathophysiology, Clinical Manifestations, and Evaluation and Treatment
- Ninety *What's New?* boxes review the most current research and clinical developments
- *Nutrition & Disease* boxes to emphasize nutrition as a health promotion strategy that may alter disease risk or pathogenesis
- End-of-chapter *Summary Review* sections summarize the content in each chapter and serve as built-in content review guides
- Boldface *key terms* with end-of-chapter term lists and page numbers for rapid access
- NEW! A comprehensive *Glossary* of approximately 1200 terms helps students with the often-difficult terminology related to pathophysiology

ART PROGRAM

The art program was given the same attention as the new and revised chapters. Over three hundred new full-color illustrations and photographs were created and strategically placed throughout the textbook. The art program, which is crucial for explaining pathophysiology, is spectacular! Also included are many new, high-quality, full-color photographs of clinical manifestations, pathologic specimens, and clinical imaging techniques. The combination of illustrations, algorithms, photographs and use of color for tables and boxes allow clarification for complex concepts and the emergence of easily recognized essential information.

ANCILLARIES

For Students

NEW! A **Companion CD** comes with every new copy of the book and includes over 750 review questions and answers presented in tutorial and test modes, and 20 animations to help students master the text content.

The **Study Guide and Workbook** includes learning objectives, special *Memory Check!* boxes, concise summaries of key concepts, and a practice examination for each chapter. Each of the disease chapters also includes a case study with a critical thinking question. Answers are found in the back.

In **Evolve,** students may register for free access to updated WebLinks, which are carefully chosen Internet sites related to each chapter in the text.

For Instructors

NEW! The **Instructor's Electronic Resource CD** for this textbook provides the following teaching aids:

- Instructor's Manual with teaching tips and case studies with critical thinking exercises and answers
- Computerized Test Bank in ExamView with over 2300 questions (in true/false, multiple choice, matching, and completion formats) with answers and textbook page references
- Image Collection with approximately 1000 key figures from the text
- NEW! Lecture Slides on PowerPoint for every chapter

This helpful resource is free to instructors with a qualified adoption. Contact your Elsevier sales representative for more information.

Evolve is an Internet-based learning environment that works in coordination with the text. The Evolve Instructor Resources for this book provide access to updated WebLinks plus everything on the *Instructor's Electronic Resource CD.* You can also take advantage of the Evolve Learning System and its helpful course management tools. These enable you to publish your class syllabus, outline, and lecture notes; set up "virtual office hours" and e-mail communication; share important dates and information through the online class calendar; and encourage student participation through chat rooms and discussion boards. Free with qualified adoption. Contact your sales representative or visit http://evolve.elsevier.com for more information about integrating Evolve into your curriculum.

ACKNOWLEDGMENTS

The arduous task of keeping this book current and readable greatly depends on our contributors. We thank them for tremendous labor of reviewing relevant literature, synthesizing it, and writing and revising chapters to make them highly readable for others. Several chapters were completely rewritten for this edition. To those contributors who spent enormous time and thought on this work we are deeply thankful. Notable are the chapters on inflammation and immunity that were rewritten for this edition by Dr. Neal Rote and Dr. Barbara Trask. New and complex material has been accumulating in the areas of inflammation and immunity for over a decade. This content is now becoming foundational for the understanding of numerous diseases and disorders, and requires expert hands to help students, faculty, and clinicians understand it! Tireless writing, editing, and the development of new illustrations were undertaken by Dr. Rote. We thank you Neal, so much, for your continued dedication to students, faculty, and clinicians, and to us.

We are also grateful to those who contributed to the book supplements. Textbook contributor Beth Forshee also wrote the glossary. Michelle McLean wrote the review questions for the companion CD. Kraig Chugg revised the instructor's manual and wrote the PowerPoint slides, and Susan Wilson revised and rewrote the test bank. Susan also provided very useful comments and suggestions while in the page proof stage. Thank you all for your help.

The process of completing this book is dependent on the "behind the scenes work" of numerous people. The initial preparation and management of the manuscript is a huge job and was done by Sue Meeks who has worked with us for 22 years. Her tireless dedication to excellence impacts all of us including the professional editorial team. If they did not quite know before—they now realize what she actually does—because during this edition Sue was unable to finish the project with us—she was needed elsewhere. Her best friend and husband Kent became very ill and Sue took care of him until he died this past Memorial Day. The whole team was profoundly affected by the loss of Kent. We are very grateful to two people who stepped in and did a heroic job to help us finish—Diane Ballard and Cathy Osborn.

Our managing editor at Elsevier is Brian Dennison. Brian deserves much credit for the quality of this textbook. Brian is a detail person—tenacious and hard-working with great ideas. Sometimes we are impatient with editorial suggestions but somehow Brian manages to skillfully keep us on track. Thank you Brian. Executive publisher Darlene Como is a steady reassuring presence. She provides wise counsel and continued encouragement. Thank you Darlene. Two Elsevier people new to this edition of the book proved to be invaluable: developmental editor Betsy Stream processed most of the manuscript and skillfully coordinated the instructor's resources and study guide, and editorial assistant Tina Sedor obtained the permissions for borrowed material and kept everything flowing smoothly. Thank you so much Betsy and Tina.

The copy editor for a book of this size and complexity of content has an enormous responsibility. We were fortunate because our copy editor was sent from heaven—Gail Brower is a tough critic, exacting, and easy to work with. She shares the same values we have and we cannot thank her enough. Despite numerous obstacles—shifting locations, a large cast of writers, vacations, and illnesses—Mary Stueck orchestrated the well-edited text and well-arranged pages. Not bothered for a nanosecond over changing pages if it meant better text, Mary got it done and did so promptly. Thank you Mary. Our book designer Jyotika Shroff did an outstanding job designing the interior portion of the book—we are especially pleased, though, with the wonderful cover. Thank you Jyotika.

Much of the new art program with spectacular renderings and colors was done by Gwen Gilbert of Graphic World Illustration Studio. We would also like to thank Barbara Cousins for carefully crafted and remarkably accurate drawings she created for this edition—and past editions—of the book. We would especially like to thank Barb for the outstanding illustration of a cell on the cover. We also thank the Department of Dermatology at the University of Utah School of Medicine, which provided numerous photos of skin lesions. And thanks to Dr. Arthur R. Brothman, University of Utah School of Medicine, for the *N-myc* gene amplification slides used to illustrate the discussion of neuroblastoma.

We are grateful to the many colleagues and friends at the University of Utah College of Nursing, School of Medicine, College of Pharmacy, and Eccles Medical Library for their assistance with references and consultation on content. In particular we would like to thank Lyn Pearse, Jean Geisler, and Mirela Milas for handling details related to submission of the manuscript.

Special thanks are given to students, particularly nursing and other health science students for the e-mails, letters, and phone calls we receive. Your questions and suggestions are inspiring and guide us in our efforts to prepare a manuscript that is clearly written and illustrated and easily understood.

As always we are grateful to our families for their enormous support, encouragement, and enduring sense of humor.

To some very supportive friends—the Wilson ladies, Dodie, Georgie, Inger, Nancy, Petie, Putzie, and Sue—an especially warm thank you and remember *upright and still breathing!*

Kathryn L McCance

Sue E Huether

CONTENTS

xiv   Contents

PART TWO   PATHOPHYSIOLOGIC ALTERATIONS: ORGANS AND SYSTEMS

Unit V   The Neurologic System

INTRODUCTION TO PATHOPHYSIOLOGY

The word root "patho" is derived from the Greek word *pathos,* which means suffering. The Greek word root *logos* means discourse or more commonly, system of formal study, and *physio-* pertains to functions of organisms. Generally, pathophysiology is the systematic study of the functional changes in cells, tissues, and organs altered by disease and/or injury. Important, however, is the inextricable component of suffering.

Knowledge of cellular biology as well as anatomy and physiology and the various organ systems of the body is an essential foundation for the study of pathophysiology. To understand pathophysiology, the student must also use principles, concepts, and basic knowledge from other fields of study, including pathology, genetics, immunology, and epidemiology. A number of terms are used to focus the discussion of pathophysiology; they may be used interchangeably at times, but that does not necessarily indicate that they have the same meaning. Those terms are reviewed in Table I-1.

Pathophysiology is one of the most important bridging sciences between preclinical and clinical courses for students in the health sciences and it requires in-depth study at an early stage in the curriculum. The definitions or conceptual models of pathophysiology that we carry in our minds influence what we do with our observations and what rationale we provide for our actions. Therefore the clinician must understand that while pathophysiology is a science, it also designates suffering in people; the clinician should never lose sight of this aspect of its definition.

As students study clinically related sciences, they learn to recognize and categorize disease. From the formulation of a differential diagnosis one understands the different *clinical manifestations,* the signs and symptoms of certain pathologies. These understandings structure further investigations, treatment plans, and evaluation. The interaction of these activities determines clinical outcomes and treatment success. Still, the concept of disease can be inherently ambiguous and elusive; many pathologies remain hidden and resist easy classification. One should appreciate that the naming and diagnosing of diseases involve evaluative judgments as well as scientific fact, and that the process is as much a social endeavor as it is a scientific one. Some diseases, such as tuberculosis, identify a highly specific causative or etiologic agent or process. Others, such as Alzheimer disease or arthritis, indicate pathologic changes of unclear cause. In addition, syndromes and functional disorders simply describe multiple symptoms and signs that frequently occur together. Does commonality exist in all of these labels?

The answer is both yes and no and depends on our conception of health and disease. In the strictest sense, objective scientific facts help us know if an individual is healthy or suffering from disease. However, the individual's conception of disease is based on personal beliefs and histories, professional and lay healers who interact with that individual, and society at large. Each idea or construct has the power to influence other ideas and constructs, and each relationship has the ability to shape the way disease is understood and experienced.[1] In short, defining and understanding disease is tremendously ambiguous. Perhaps the most important and desirable trait for the new student of pathophysiology is an open and toler-

Table I-1	Terms and Definitions Related to Pathophysiology
Pathology	Study of structural alterations in cells, tissues and organs which help to identify the cause of disease
Pathogenesis	Pattern of tissue changes associated with the development of disease
Etiology	Study of the cause(s) of disease and/or injury
Idiopathic	Diseases with no identifiable cause
Iatrogenic	Diseases and/or injury as a result of medical intervention
Clinical manifestations	Signs and symptoms
Nosocomial	Diseases acquired as a consequence of being in a hospital environment
Diagnosis	Naming or identification of disease
Prognosis	Expected outcome of a disease
Acute disease	Sudden appearance of signs and symptoms lasting a short time
Chronic disease	Develops more slowly lasting a longtime or a lifetime
Remissions	Periods when clinical manifestations disappear or diminish significantly
Exacerbations	Periods when clinical manifestations become worse or more severe
Sequelae	Any abnormal conditions that follow and are the result of a disease, treatment, or injury

ant mind. To believe that science alone can overcome ignorance and that clinical training and technology can overcome ineptitude only encourages arrogance and undermines the scientific purpose.

Pathophysiology has had great success in explaining the mechanisms and clinical manifestations associated with infectious diseases. Syndromes of unclear etiology such as headache and fibromyalgia have proven to be troublesome. Even more difficult are multifactorial conditions, such as atherosclerosis or type 2 diabetes mellitus, in which several interacting factors contribute to the etiology. Learning how interacting factors relate to one another to increase morbidity or actually cause disease contributes to an appreciation of how emerging concepts revolutionize current understandings. For example, for many years the bacterial forms seen in gastric biopsies were interpreted as contaminants. It took several decades to understand the bacterial origin of gastritis, peptic ulcer disease, and even gastric carcinoma. Such findings are a major revolution in thought. One current revolution in thought that has driven intensive research is that low levels of chronic inflammation cause or contribute to many diseases.

The language that clinicians use to discuss diseases and their manifestations is powerful. Lives are altered by a few words uttered by a clinician in a white coat or uniform. "AIDS," "cancer," and "heart attack" have become culturally ingrained symbols that portend an individual's future. Although some futures are determined by scientific evidence, others are determined by subjective experience.[2] For example, a person diagnosed with a familial disease may ask, "Will I suffer like my mother did?" This questioning influences the individuals' suffering.

In conclusion, pathophysiology—the understanding of disease—requires both descriptive evidence and an evaluative component regarding suffering and the language we use to describe it. Combining objective and subjective perspectives requires new conceptual models that take into account the complex interactions among the body, mind, culture, and spirit.

REFERENCES

1. Magid C: Developing tolerance for ambiguity, *JAMA* 285(1):88, 2001.
2. Goldstein J: In the twilight: life in the margins between sick and well, *JAMA* 285(1):92, 2001.

CELLULAR BIOLOGY

KATHRYN L. McCANCE

CHAPTER OUTLINE

All body functions depend on the integrity of cells. Therefore, an understanding of cellular biology is intrinsically necessary for an understanding of disease. An overwhelming amount of information is revealing how cells behave as a multicellular "social" organism. At the heart of cellular biology is cellular communication ("cellular crosstalk")—how messages originate and are transmitted, received, interpreted, and used by the cell. Fossil records suggest that unicellular organisms resembling bacteria were present on earth 3.5 billion years ago, yet it took another 2.5 billion years for the first multicellular organisms to appear. This delay was seemingly slow because elaborate signaling mechanisms had to evolve that would allow cells to crosstalk. This streamlined conversation between, among, and within cells maintains cellular function. Intercellular signals allow each cell to determine its position and specialized role. Cells must demonstrate a "chemical fondness" for other cells to maintain the integrity of the entire organism. When they no longer tolerate this fondness, the conversation breaks down and cells either adapt (sometimes altering function) or become vulnerable to isolation, injury, or disease.

PROKARYOTES AND EUKARYOTES

Living cells generally are divided into two major classes—eukaryotes and prokaryotes. The cells of higher animals and plants are eukaryotes, as are the single-celled organisms fungi, protozoa, and most algae. Prokaryotes include cyanobacteria (blue-green algae), bacteria, and rickettsiae. Prokaryotes traditionally were studied as core subjects of molecular biology. Current emphasis is on the eukaryotic cell; much of its structure and function has no counterpart in bacterial cells.

Eukaryotes (*eu* = good; *karyon* = nucleus) are larger and have more extensive intracellular anatomy and organization than do prokaryotes. Eukaryotic cells have a characteristic set of membrane-bound intracellular compartments, called *organelles*, that includes a well-defined nucleus. **Prokaryotes** contain no organelles, and their nuclear material is not encased by a nuclear membrane. Prokaryotic cells are characterized by lack of a distinct nucleus.

In addition to having structural differences, prokaryotic and eukaryotic cells differ in chemical composition and biochemical activity. The *nuclei* of prokaryotic cells carry genetic information in a single circular chromosome, and they lack a class of proteins called *histones,* which in eukaryotic cells bind with deoxyribonucleic acid (DNA) and are involved in the supercoiling of DNA (see Figure 1-2). Eukaryotic cells have several chromosomes. Protein production, or synthesis, in the two classes of cells also differs because of major structural differences in ribonucleic acid (RNA) protein complexes. Other distinctions include differences in mechanisms of transport across the outer cellular membrane and differences in enzyme content.

CELLULAR FUNCTIONS

Cells become specialized through the process of **differentiation,** or maturation, so that some cells eventually perform one kind of function and other cells perform other functions. Highly developed functions, such as movement, are often associated with the absence of some other property, such as hormone production, which is more highly developed in some other type of specialized cell. The eight chief cellular functions follow:

1. *Movement.* Muscle cells can generate forces that produce motion. Muscles that are attached to bones produce limb movements, whereas those that enclose hollow tubes or cavities move or empty contents when they contract. For example, the contraction of smooth muscle cells surrounding blood vessels changes the diameter of the vessels; the contraction of muscles in walls of the urinary bladder expels urine.
2. *Conductivity.* Conduction as a response to a stimulus is manifested by a wave of excitation, an electrical potential, that passes along the surface of the cell to reach its other parts. Conductivity is the chief function of nerve cells.
3. *Metabolic absorption.* All cells take in and use nutrients and other substances from their surroundings. Cells of the intestine and the kidney are specialized to carry out absorption. Cells of the kidney tubules reabsorb fluids and synthesize proteins. Intestinal epithelial cells reabsorb fluids and synthesize protein enzymes.
4. *Secretion.* Certain cells, such as mucous gland cells, can synthesize new substances from substances they absorb and then secrete the new substances to serve as needed elsewhere. Cells of the adrenal gland, testis, and ovary can secrete hormonal steroids.
5. *Excretion.* All cells can rid themselves of waste products resulting from the metabolic breakdown of nutrients. Membrane-bound sacs (lysosomes) within cells contain enzymes that break down, or digest, large molecules, turning them into waste products that are released from the cell.
6. *Respiration.* Cells absorb oxygen, which is used to transform nutrients into energy in the form of adenosine triphosphate (ATP). Cellular respiration, or oxidation, occurs in organelles called *mitochondria.*
7. *Reproduction.* Tissue growth occurs as cells enlarge and reproduce themselves. Even without growth, tissue

maintenance requires that new cells be produced to replace cells that are lost normally through cellular death. Not all cells are capable of continuous division, and some cells, such as nerve cells, cannot reproduce.
8. *Communication.* Communication is critical for all the other functions above that enable the survival of the society of cells. Pancreatic cells, for instance, secrete and release insulin to tell muscle cells to take up sugar from the blood for energy. Constant communication allows the maintenance of a dynamic steady state.

STRUCTURE AND FUNCTION OF CELLULAR COMPONENTS

Figure 1-1 shows a "typical" eukaryotic cell. It consists of three components: an outer membrane called the *plasma membrane,* or *plasmalemma;* a fluid filling called **cytoplasm;** and the "organs" of the cell-membrane–bound intracellular organelles, among them the nucleus.

Nucleus

The **nucleus,** which is surrounded by the cytoplasm and generally is located in the center of the cell, is the largest membrane-bound organelle. Two membranes compose the **nuclear envelope** (Figure 1-2, *A*). The outer membrane is continuous with membranes of the endoplasmic reticulum. The nucleus contains the **nucleolus,** a small dense structure composed largely of RNA; most of the cellular DNA; and the DNA-binding proteins, the histones, that regulate its activity. The DNA chain in eukaryotic cells is so extensive that the risk of breakage is high. Therefore the histones that bind to DNA cause the folding of DNA into chromosomes (Figure 1-2, *C*). The wrapping of DNA into tight packages of chromosomes is essential for cell division in eukaryotes.

The primary functions of the nucleus are cell division and control of genetic information. Other functions include the replication and repair of DNA and the transcription of the information stored in DNA. Genetic information is transcribed into RNA, which can be processed into messenger, transport, and ribosomal RNA and introduced into the cytoplasm, where it directs cellular activities. Most of the processing of RNA occurs in the nucleolus. (The role of DNA and RNA in protein synthesis is discussed in Chapter 4.)

Cytoplasmic Organelles

Cytoplasm is an aqueous solution (**cytosol**) that fills the **cytoplasmic matrix**—the space between the nuclear envelope and the plasma membrane. The cytosol represents about half the volume of a eukaryotic cell. It contains thousands of enzymes involved in intermediate metabolism and is crowded with ribosomes making proteins. Newly synthesized proteins remain in the cytosol if they lack a signal for transport to a cell organelle.[1] The organelles suspended in the cytoplasm are enclosed in biologic membranes, which enables them simultaneously to carry out functions that require different biochemical environments. These functions, many of which are

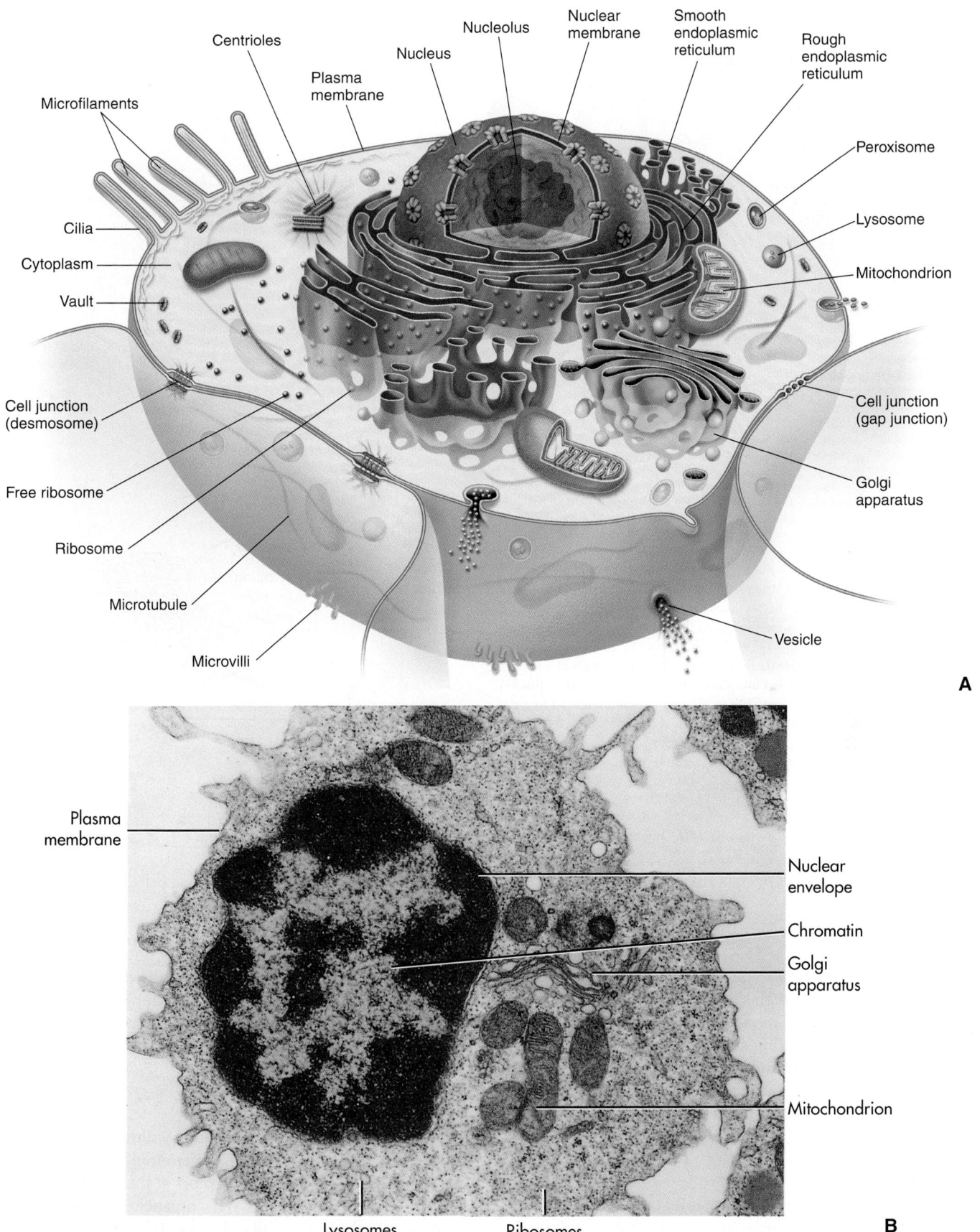

Figure 1-1 **Typical or composite cell. A,** Artist's interpretation of cell structure. **B,** Color-enhanced electron micrograph of a cell. Both show the many mitochondria known as the "power plants of the cell." Note, too, the innumerable dots bordering the endoplasmic reticulum. These are ribosomes, the cell's "protein factories." (**B** from Thibodeau GA, Patton KT: *Anatomy & physiology,* ed 5, St Louis, 2003, Mosby.)

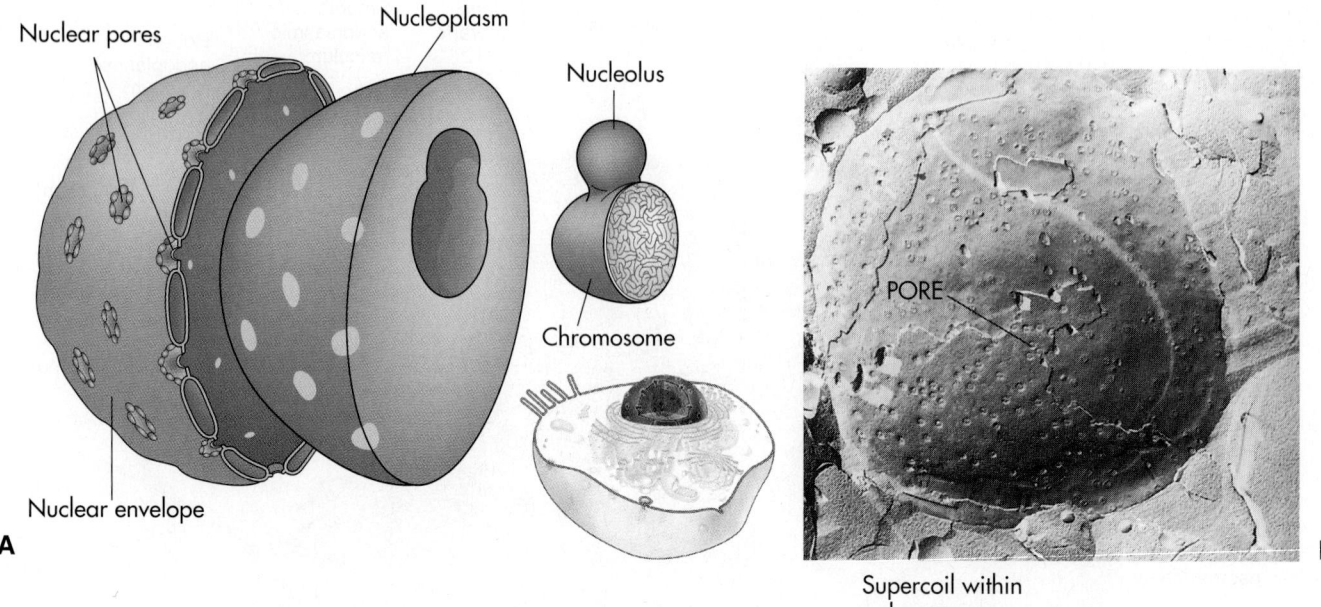

Figure 1-2 **The nucleus.** The nucleus is composed of a double membrane, called a *nuclear envelope,* that encloses the fluid-filled interior, called *nucleoplasm.* The chromosomes are suspended in the nucleoplasm (here shown much larger than real size to show the tightly packed DNA strands). **A,** Swelling at one or more points of the chromosome occurs at a nucleolus where genes are being copied into RNA. The nuclear envelope is studded with pores. **B,** The pores are visible as dimples in this freeze etch of a nuclear envelope. **C,** How DNA is coiled within a chromosome. (**B** from Raven PH, Johnson GB: *Biology,* St Louis, 1992, Mosby.)

directed by coded messages carried from the nucleus by RNA, include synthesis of proteins and hormones and their transport out of the cell, isolation and elimination of waste products from the cell, metabolic processes, breakdown and disposal of cellular debris and foreign proteins (antigens), and maintenance of cellular structure and motility. Also, the cytosol functions as a storage unit for fat, carbohydrate, and secretory vesicles.

Ribosomes

Ribosomes are RNA-protein complexes (nucleoproteins) that are synthesized in the nucleolus and secreted into the cytoplasm, possibly through pores in the nuclear envelope. These tiny organelles may float free in the cytoplasm or attach themselves to the outer membranes of the endoplasmic reticulum (see Figure 1-1). Their chief function is to provide sites for cellular protein synthesis. New information on how ribosomes are delivered to the endoplasmic reticulum is presented in the What's New? box on p. 5.

Endoplasmic Reticulum

The **endoplasmic reticulum** (*endo* = within; *plasma* = cytoplasm; *reticulum* = network) is a membrane factory that specializes in the synthesis and transport of the protein and lipid components of most of the cell's organelles. It consists of a network of tubular or saclike channels (cisternae) that extend throughout the cytoplasm and are continuous with the outer nuclear membrane (Figure 1-3). The folded membranes that

WHAT'S NEW? Delivery of Ribosomes to Rough Endoplasmic Reticulum

Newly formed ribosomes synthesize a "recognition sequence" that acts as a signal, similar to an address on a letter. Signal recognition particles (SRP), present in the cytosol, bind to the ribosome after recognizing the ribosome's signal or recognition sequence. The SRP, acting as a mail carrier, shuttles the ribosome to the "correct" address on the endoplasmic reticulum (ER) membrane. Receiver proteins, called *ribophorins,* found in the rough sections of the ER membrane act as the "address" on the membrane. The ribophorins serve as docking or binding sites on the ER. The SRP departs and the newly delivered ribosome directs synthesis of a specific protein. The developing protein threads its way through the ER membrane into the ER lumen. Here the recognition sequence is removed and the new protein chain is folded into its final conformation.

Data from Rosenblad M, Zwieb C, Samuelson T: *BMC Genomics* 5:5, 2004; Pool MR: *Biochem Soc Trans* 31(Pt 6):1232-1237, 2003; Sherwood L: *Human physiology: from cells to systems,* ed 3, Belmont, Calif, 1997, Wadsworth.

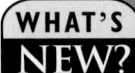

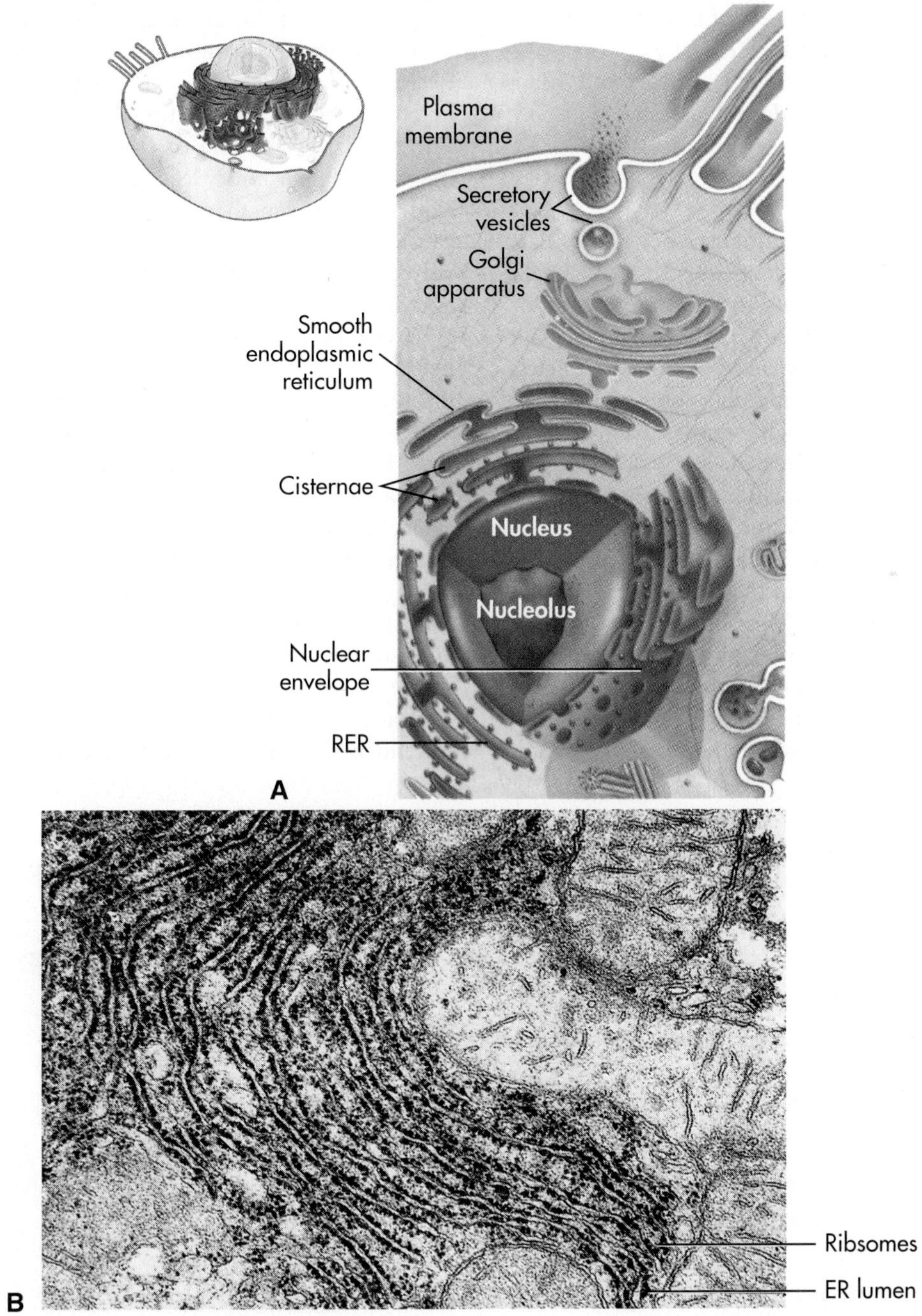

Figure 1-3 Endoplasmic reticulum (ER). **A,** The ER consists of rough endoplasmic reticulum (RER) arranged into ribosome-coated cisternae and vesicles of smooth endoplasmic reticulum (SER). **B,** Electron micrograph of rough and smooth ER. (**B** courtesy C. Kelloes and M. Farmer, Center for Advanced Ultrastructural Research, University of Georgia. From Lindsay DT: *Functional human anatomy*, St Louis, 1996, Mosby.)

form the cisternae of the endoplasmic reticulum may be *rough* (granular) or *smooth* (agranular). The **rough endoplasmic reticulum** is rough because ribosomes and ribonucleoprotein particles are attached to it (see Figure 1-3). Some of the proteins synthesized by these ribosomes remain in the endoplasmic reticulum, and others are used to construct membranes of other organelles (the Golgi complex, lysosomes, peroxisomes, nucleus) and of the cell itself.

Smooth endoplasmic reticulum does not contain ribosomes or ribonucleoprotein particles (see Figure 1-1). Rather, membranous surfaces of the smooth endoplasmic reticulum contain enzymes involved in the synthesis of steroid hormones and are responsible for a variety of reactions required to remove toxic substances from the cell. The endoplasmic reticulum communicates with the Golgi complex and interacts with other organelles, particularly lysosomes and peroxisomes.

Golgi Complex

The **Golgi complex** (or **Golgi apparatus**) is a network of flattened, smooth membranes and vesicles frequently located near the nucleus of the cell (Figure 1-4). Proteins from the endoplasmic reticulum are processed and packaged into small, membrane-bound sacs or vesicles called **secretory vesicles,** which collect at the end of the membranous folds of the Golgi bodies—called **cisternae.** The secretory vesicles then break off from the Golgi complex and migrate to a variety of intracellular and extracellular destinations, including the plasma membrane. The vesicles fuse with the plasma membrane, and their contents are released from the cell. The best known vesicles are those that have coats made largely of the protein **clathrin** and are called *clathrin-coated vesicles.* They bud from the Golgi complex on the outward secretory pathway and from the plasma membrane on the inward endocytotic pathway (see p. 30). Many molecules, including lipids, proteins, glycoproteins, and enzymes of lysosomes, pass through the Golgi complex at

some stage in their maturation. The Golgi complex is a refining plant and directs traffic (e.g., protein, polynucleotide, polysaccharide molecules) in the cell[1] (Figure 1-5).

Lysosomes

Lysosomes (*lyso* = dissolution; *soma* = body) are saclike structures that originate from the Golgi complex (see Figure 1-1). They contain more than 40 digestive enzymes called **hydrolases,** which catalyze bonds in proteins, lipids, nucleic acids, and carbohydrates. Lysosomes function as the intracellular digestive system (Figure 1-6). Lysosomal enzymes are capable of digesting most cellular constituents down to their basic forms, such as amino acids, fatty acids, and sugars.

The lysosomal membrane acts as a protective shield between the powerful digestive enzymes within the lysosome and the cytoplasm, preventing their leakage into the cytoplasmic matrix. Disruption of the membrane by various treatments or cellular injury leads to a release of the lysosomal enzymes, which can then react with their specific substrates, causing *cellular self-digestion.* Lysosomal abnormalities are involved in a number of conditions that involve cellular injury and death.

Lysosomal storage diseases may be the result of a genetic defect or lack of one or more lysosomal enzymes. For example, the lack of lysosomal α-1,4-glucosidase leads to an accumulation of glycogen in lysosomes known as *Pompe disease.* Tay-Sachs disease is characterized by an accumulation of GM2 ganglioside (a lipid) in lysosomes as a result of the deficiency or absence of lysosomal hexosaminidase A. In gout, undigested uric acid accumulates within lysosomes, damaging the lysosomal membrane. Subsequent enzyme leakage results in cell death and tissue injury.

Lysosomes are necessary for normal digestion of cellular nutrients, intracellular debris, and potentially harmful extracellular substances that must be removed from the body. Extracellular substances are taken into the cell and encapsulated

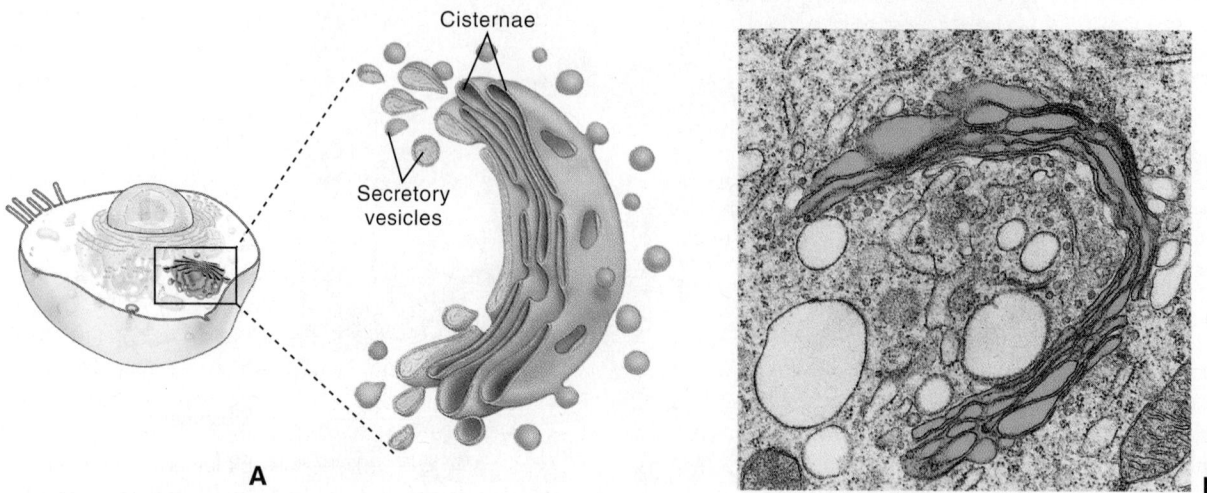

Figure 1-4 Golgi complex. **A,** Schematic representation of the Golgi complex showing a stack of flattened sacs, or cisternae, and numerous small membranous bubbles, or secretory vesicles. **B,** Transmission electron micrograph showing the Golgi complex highlighted with color. (From Thibodeau GA, Patton KT: *Anatomy & physiology,* ed 5, St Louis, 2003, Mosby.)

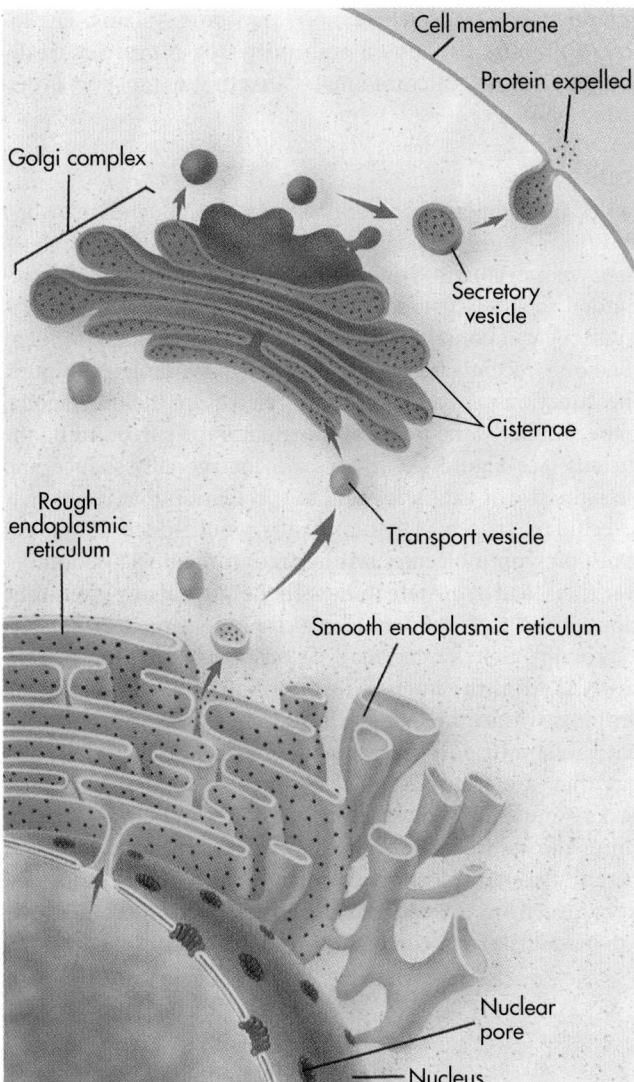

Figure 1-5 How the internal membrane system of a cell packages a protein for export. The instructions for making a protein that is destined for export from a cell, such as a digestive enzyme made by a pancreas cell, are first transcribed from DNA by RNA in the nucleus. The RNA then leaves the nucleus through a nuclear pore and proceeds to a ribosome located on the rough endoplasmic reticulum (ER). There it provides instructions for the correct sequence of amino acids for synthesizing that particular digestive enzyme. When enzyme synthesis is complete, the enzyme travels through the ER and is then encapsulated in a transport vesicle. The transport vesicle fuses with a Golgi body, releasing the enzyme. In the Golgi complex the enzyme is further modified and is then shunted to the ends of the Golgi complex, or cisternae. There the enzyme waits for a secretory vesicle, which will carry it to the perimeter of the cell, the cell membrane. The secretory vesicle membrane then fuses with the cell membrane, and the enzyme is released outside the cell. (From Raven PH, Johnson GB: *Understanding biology,* ed 3, Dubuque, Iowa, 1995, Brown.)

in a membrane-bound vesicle (see endocytosis, p. 30). Lysosomes merge with the vesicle to form a digestive vacuole. Lysosomes remain fully active by maintaining a low internal pH. They do this by pumping hydrogen ions into their interiors. The hydrolytic enzymes are only maximally active at acid pH values. Lysosomes that are not active do not maintain such an acid internal pH. Lysosomes in this "holding pattern"

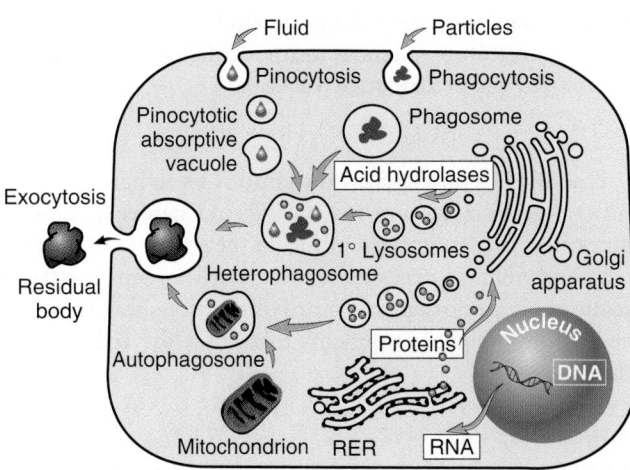

Figure 1-6 Lysosomes. Primary (1°) lysosomes, which originate from the Golgi apparatus, give rise to heterophagosomes and autophagosomes. Undigested material in phagosomes is extruded from the cell or remains in the cytoplasm as lipofuscin-rich residual bodies. *RER,* Rough endoplasmic reticulum. (From Damjanov I: *Pathology for the health-related professionals,* ed 2, Philadelphia, 2000, Saunders.)

are called **primary lysosomes.** When a primary lysosome fuses with a vacuole or other organelle, its pH falls and the hydrolytic enzymes become activated. When it becomes active, it is called a **secondary lysosome, or heterophagosome.**

As cells complete their life span and die, lysosomes digest the resultant cellular debris. Lysosomes involved in this process, which is called **autodigestion,** are called **autolysosomes,** or **autophagosomes.** In living cells, cellular debris is encapsulated within a vesicle that reacts with a lysosome to complete its degradation. This process is called **autophagy.** Autophagy also occurs during starvation, enabling the cell to use a part of its own substance for fuel without doing itself irreparable harm.

Products of autophagy (and of phagocytosis, the ingestion of harmful foreign substances; see Chapter 6) pass out of the lysosome and are reused by the cell. Indigestible material is stored in vesicles called **residual bodies,** whose contents are actively expelled from the cell (see Figure 1-6). High concentrations of lipids may accumulate within the residual bodies and remain there for a long time. The lipids are eventually oxidized, and a pigmented substance containing polyunsaturated fatty acids and proteins accumulates in the cell. This pigmented substance, termed *lipofuscin,* is often called "age pigment" and is noted in older individuals (see Chapter 2).

Peroxisomes

Peroxisomes (microbodies) are similar to lysosomes in microscopic appearance, but they are larger and oval or irregular in shape. Peroxisomes contain several oxidative enzymes, such as *catalase* and *urate oxidase.* Like mitochondria, peroxisomes are major sites of oxygen utilization. Peroxisomes are so named because they usually contain enzymes that use oxygen to remove hydrogen atoms from specific substrates in an oxidative reaction that produces hydrogen peroxide (H_2O_2). Hydrogen peroxide is a powerful oxidant, potentially destructive if it accumulates or escapes from peroxisomes. Catalase, an antioxidant enzyme, utilizes the H_2O_2 to oxidize a variety of other substrates—phenols, formic acid, formaldehyde, and alcohol—by the peroxidative reaction:

$$H_2O_2 + R^1H_2 \rightarrow R^1 + 2H_2O$$

Thus the reaction breaks down into H_2O_2 to harmless H_2O and O_2 (see discussion of free radicals in Chapter 2). Peroxisomes also have an important role in the synthesis of specialized phospholipids necessary for nerve cell myelination. Such reactions are important in detoxifying various wastes within the cell or foreign components that enter the cell, such as ethanol.

Mitochondria

Mitochondria (*mito* = thread; *chondros* = granule) are of much interest because of their role in cellular energy metabolism (see p. 22). These cytoplasmic organelles appear as spheres, rods, or filamentous bodies that are bound by a double membrane (Figure 1-7). The **outer membrane** is smooth and surrounds the mitochondrion itself; the inner membrane is convoluted in the mitochondrial matrix to form partitions called **cristae.** The **inner membrane** contains the enzymes of the respiratory chain—the name given to the electron transport chain. These enzymes are essential to the process of oxidative phosphorylation that generates most of the cell's ATP. Metabolic pathways involved in the metabolism of carbohydrates, lipids, and amino acids and special pathways involving urea and heme synthesis are located in the mitochondrial matrix.

The outer membrane is permeable (passable) to many substances, but the inner membrane is highly selective and contains many transmembranous transport systems. The inner membrane contains a transporter to move electrically charged calcium (calcium ions). (Membrane transport is discussed on p. 25.)

Vaults

Vaults are cytoplasmic ribonucleoproteins, much larger than ribosomes, and shaped like octagonal barrels (Figure 1-8). Their name comes from their multiple arches, which reminded their discoverers of vaulted or cathedral ceilings. A single cell can contain thousands of vaults. Vaults were identified only recently because of changes in staining techniques. The function of vaults may be related to their octagonal shape. Similarly, the pores in the membrane surrounding the nucleus (see Figure 1-2, *B*) are also octagonally shaped and the same size as vaults, leading to speculation that vaults may be cellular "trucks." Further, vaults would dock at nuclear pores, pick up molecules synthesized in the nucleus, and deliver their load elsewhere in the cell. Because at any given time about 5% of the vaults are localized near the nuclear pores, it is thought that vaults may be carrying messenger RNA (mRNA) from the nucleus to the ribosomal sites of protein synthesis within the cytoplasm. Recent observations suggest that vaults transport several copies of untranslated RNA and that they are transported along cytoskeletal-based cellular tracks—much like an assembly line.[2] Researchers are investigating the role of vaults in cancer cells' resistance to drug therapy. Perhaps transporting chemotherapy drugs to sites for exocytosis from the cancer cell increases the drugs' elimination or vaults may mediate multidrug resistance by transport-

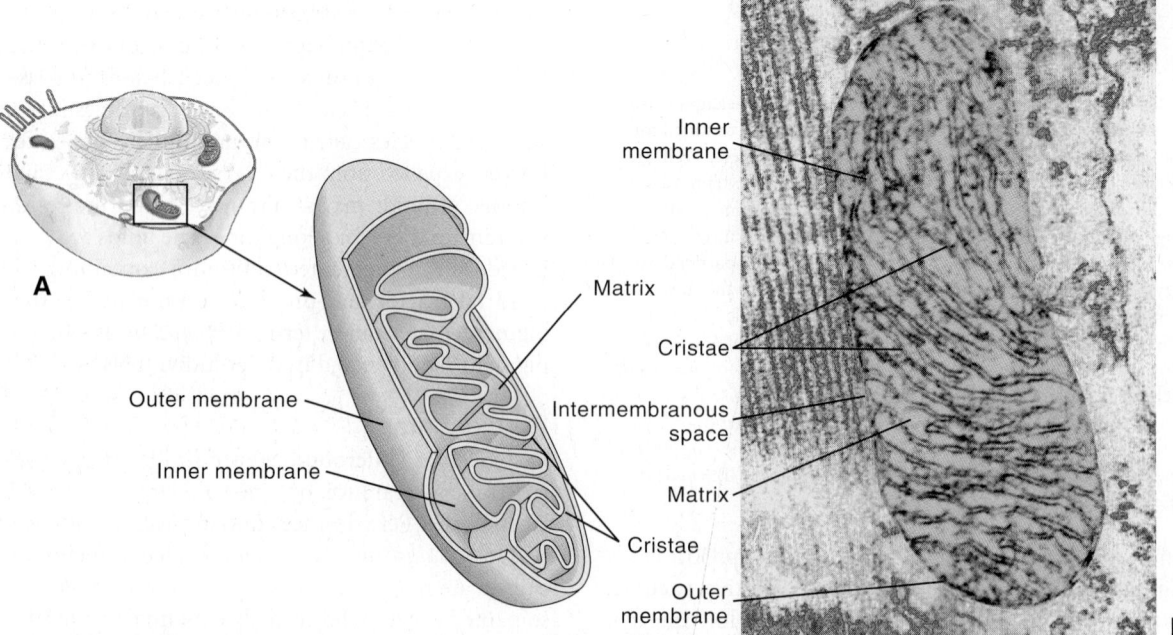

Figure 1-7 Mitochondrion. A, Cutaway sketch showing outer and inner membranes. Note the many folds (cristae) of the inner membrane. **B,** Transmission electron micrograph of a mitochondrion. Although some mitochondria have the capsule shape shown here, many are round or oval. (From Thibodeau GA, Patton KT: *Anatomy & physiology,* ed 5, St Louis, 2003, Mosby.)

ing drugs away from their intracellular targets, for example, the nucleous.[3] Although the normal cellular function of the vault is as yet undetermined, the structure of the vault is consistent with a role in either subcellular transport or sequestering large nuclear protein assemblies.[4]

Cytosol

Cytosol is the gelatinous, semiliquid portion of the cytoplasm accounting for about 55% of the total cell volume. Functions of the cytosol include intermediary metabolism involving enzymatic biochemical reactions; ribosomal protein synthesis; and storage of carbohydrates, fat, and secretory vesicles.

Intermediary metabolism refers to the intracellular chemical reactions that include synthesis, degradation, and transformation of small organic molecules (e.g., simple sugars, fatty acids, and amino acids). All intermediary metabolism occurs in the cytoplasm or that portion of the cell interior not occupied by the nucleus—with most of the metabolism being accomplished in the cytosol. These reactions enable energy to be used for cellular activities and for providing substrates to maintain cell integrity.

Ribosomal protein synthesis takes place in free ribosomes in the cytosol. Cytosolic ribosomes that synthesize identical proteins are collected together in "factories" known as **polyribosomes.**

Storage of excess nutrients not immediately used for ATP production are converted in the cytosol into storage forms, for example, excess glucose is stored as glycogen. These temporary masses are known as *inclusions* (see Chapter 2). Secretory vesicles that have been processed and packaged by the endoplasmic reticulum and Golgi complex also remain in the cytosol. By means of signaling, the vesicles transport and empty their contents to the outside.

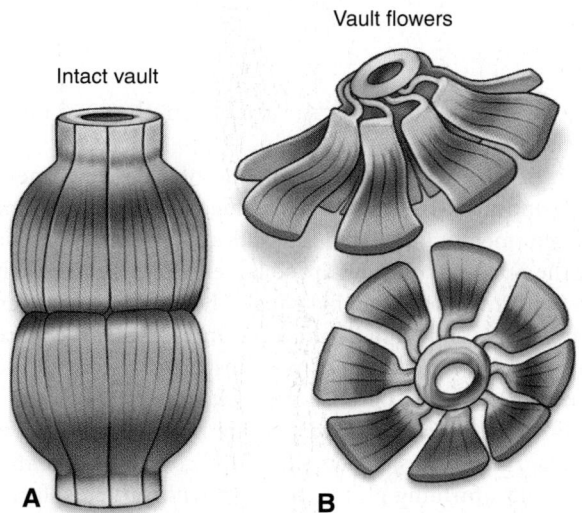

Figure 1-8 Vaults. A, Schematic three-dimensional representation of a vault, an octagonal barrel-shaped organelle believed to transport messenger RNA from the nucleus to the cytoplasmic ribosomes. **B,** Schematic representation of an opened vault, showing its octagonal structure.

Cytoskeleton

All eukaryotic cells contain elaborate and specialized internal structures in the cytosol that provide the "bones and muscles" of the cell—the **cytoskeleton.** The cytoskeleton maintains the cell's shape and internal organization, and it permits movement of substances within the cell and movement of external projections (cilia or microvilli; flagella in sperm) outside the plasma membrane. The internal skeleton is composed of a network of protein filaments; two of the most important are microtubules and actin filaments, or microfilaments.

Microtubules are small, hollow, cylindric, unbranched tubules made of protein. When found together, microtubules exhibit rigidity, unlike the rest of the cytoplasm. Microtubules thus add strength to the cell's structure (Figure 1-9, *A*). Within the cell, microtubules support and move organelles from one part of the cytoplasm to another, facilitate transport of impulses along nerve cells, and have roles in the inflammatory and immune responses and hormone secretion. Microtubules are also involved in external movement, or motility, of some cells.

Microtubules are arranged in the thickened base, or basal body, of a protrusion from the cell's plasma membrane. This arrangement occurs in the basal bodies of sperm flagella and the cilia of certain other cells. The long, whiplike flagella enable sperm cells to move. Cilia usually move substances past the cell, which remains stationary. For example, cilia on cells lining the respiratory tract move together to "beat" mucus toward the throat so it can be removed by coughing.

While the cell is not in the process of division, only a few microtubules are assembled; cellular division (mitosis) or defense (phagocytosis) does, however, induce a cycle of rapid assembly and disassembly. Microtubules involved in cellular division are arranged in a **centriole.** Centrioles always consist of nine bundles containing three microtubules each. During division the pairs of centrioles split and migrate to opposite poles of the cell (see p. 32).

Alterations of microtubular function are implicated in disease processes. For example, alterations in actin microfilament act as a driving force for cell extension during cancer spread.[5]

Actin filaments (microfilaments) are smaller fibrils that generally occur in bundles rather than singly (Figure 1-9, *C*). Like microtubules, actin filaments are associated with cellular locomotion and maintenance of cell and tissue shape.[5] In addition, microfilaments are necessary for regulating cell growth.[6] Cellular locomotion depends on contractile properties that involve both microtubules and actin filaments. Anesthetic drugs can affect both structures, disrupting intracellular movement and cellular motility.

Plasma Membranes

Whether they surround the cell or enclose an intracellular organelle, membranes are exceedingly important to normal physiologic function because they control the composition of the space, or compartment, they enclose. Membranes can include

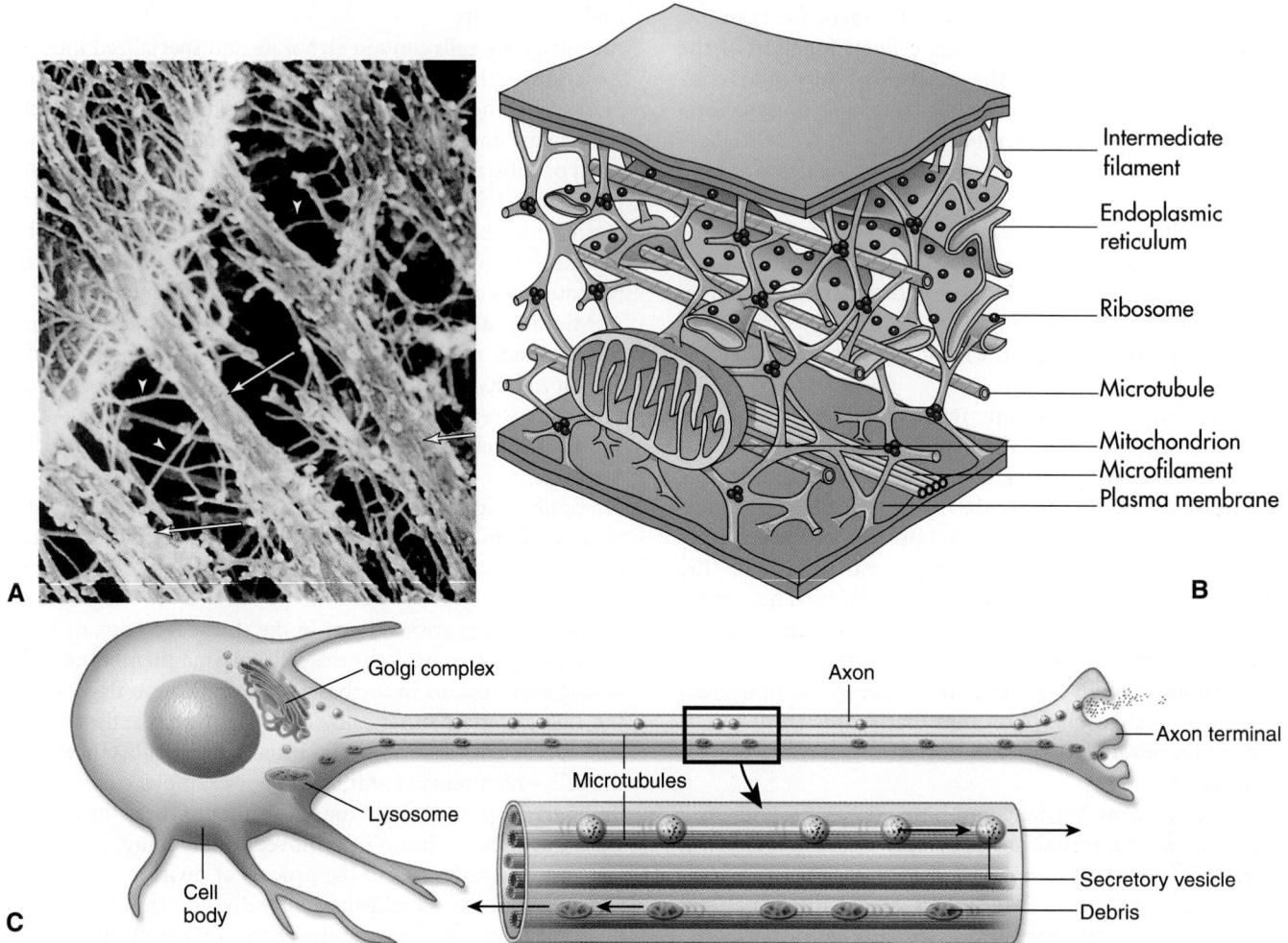

Figure 1-9 Cytoskeleton. A, Color-enhanced electron micrograph of a portion of the cell's internal framework. Arrowheads mark the intermediate filaments, and the complete arrows mark the microtubules. **B,** Artist's interpretation of the cell's internal framework. Note that the "free" ribosomes and other organelles are not really free at all. **C,** Microtubules are necessary for maintaining an asymmetrical cell shape, such as that of a nerve cell. In addition, specific chemicals are released from the terminal end of the axon to influence neural transmission. (**A** and **B** from Thibodeau GA, Patton KT: *Anatomy & physiology,* ed 5, St Louis, 2003, Mosby.)

or exclude various molecules, and because of selective transport systems, they can move molecules into or out of the space (Figure 1-10). By controlling the movement of substances from one compartment to another, membranes exert a powerful influence on metabolic pathways. In addition to these functions, the plasma membrane has an important role in cell-to-cell recognition. For example, protein receptors for hormones and for other chemical signals are associated with the membrane and act as markers that identify a cell to its neighbors. Other functions of the plasma membrane include cellular mobility and the maintenance of cellular shape (Table 1-1).

Membrane Composition

The outer surface of the plasma membrane is not smooth but dimpled with cavelike indentations known as **caveolae** ("tiny caves"). Caveolae were not thought to be functionally significant until the mid-1990s when evidence suggested that they (1) serve as a repository for some receptors, (2) provide a new route for transport into the cell, and (3) act as the initiator for

relaying signals from several extracellular chemical messengers into the cell's interior[7] (see p. 17).

The major chemical components of all membranes are lipids and proteins, but the percentage of each varies among different membranes. Lipid molecules are the most abundant, but the protein molecules are so large that in total mass these two constituents are roughly equal. The structure of a plasma membrane is shown in Figure 1-11. Intracellular membranes have a higher percentage of proteins than do plasma membranes, presumably because most enzymatic activity occurs within organelles. Carbohydrates are mainly associated with plasma membranes, where they are combined chemically with lipids, forming glycolipids, and with proteins, forming glycoproteins.

Lipids

The basic component of the plasma membrane is a bilayer of lipid molecules—phospholipids, glycolipids, and cholesterol (respective ratios 70:5:25). The lipids are responsible for the structural integrity of the membrane. Each lipid molecule

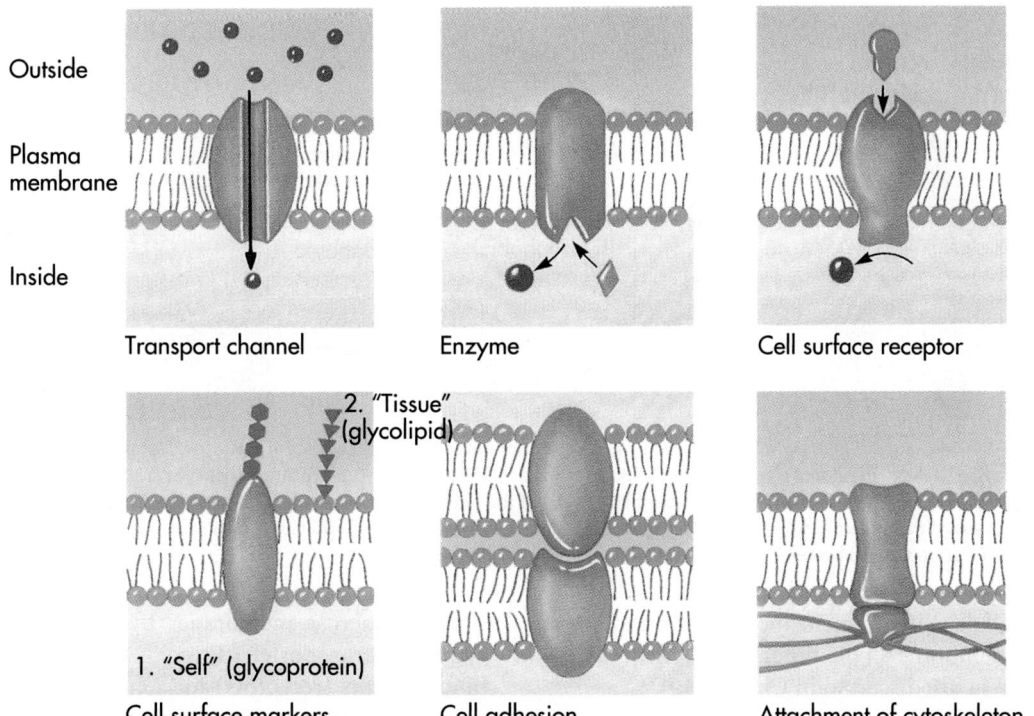

Figure 1-10 Functions of plasma membrane proteins. The plasma membrane proteins illustrated here show a variety of functions performed by the different types of plasma membranes. (From Raven PH, Johnson GB: *Understanding biology,* ed 3, Dubuque, Iowa, 1995, Brown.)

Table 1-1	Plasma Membrane Functions
Cellular Mechanism	**Membrane Functions**
Structure	Usually thicker than the membranes of intracellular organelles
	Containment of cellular organelles
	Maintenance of relationship with cytoskeleton, endoplasmic reticulum, and other organelles
	Outer surfaces in many cells are not smooth but are studded with cilia or even smaller cylindric projections called microvilli; both are capable of movement; caveolae are also outer indentations
	Maintenance of fluid and electrolyte balance
Protection	Barrier to toxic molecules and macromolecules (proteins, nucleic acid, polysaccharides)
	Barrier to foreign organisms and cells
Activation of cell	Hormones (regulation of cellular activity)
	Mitogens (cellular division, see Chapter 4)
	Antigens (antibody synthesis, see Chapter 7)
	Growth factors (proliferation and differentiation)
Transport	Diffusion and exchange diffusion
	Endocytosis (pinocytosis and phagocytosis); receptor-mediated endocytosis
	Exocytosis (secretion)
	Active transport
Cell-to-cell interaction	Communication and attachment at junctional complexes
	Symbiotic nutritive relationships
	Release of enzymes and antibodies to extracellular environment
	Relationships with extracellular matrix

Modified from King DW, Fenoglio CM, Lefkowitch JH: *General pathology: principles and dynamics,* Philadelphia, 1983, Lea & Febiger.

is said to be polar, or amphipathic. An **amphipathic molecule** is one in which one part is **hydrophobic** (uncharged, or "water hating") and another part is **hydrophilic** (charged, or "water loving") (see Figure 1-11). The membrane spontaneously organizes itself into a bilayer because of these two incompatible solubilities. The hydrophobic region (hydrophobic tail) of each lipid molecule is protected from water, whereas the hydrophilic region (hydrophilic head) is immersed in it. The bilayer's structure accounts for one of the essential functions of the plasma membrane: it is impermeable to most water-soluble molecules (molecules that dissolve in water) because they are insoluble in the oily core region. The bilayer serves as a barrier to the diffusion of water and hydrophilic substances while allowing lipid-soluble molecules, such as oxygen (O_2) and carbon dioxide (CO_2), to diffuse through it readily. Because the bilayer is fluid at temperatures above freezing, com-

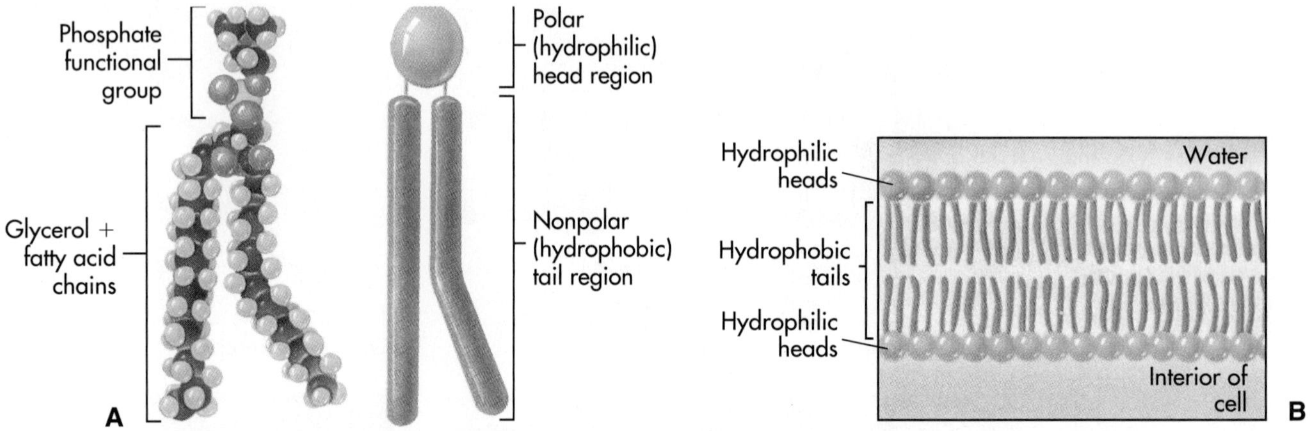

Figure 1-11 Structure of a phospholipid molecule. **A,** Each phospholipid molecule consists of a phosphate functional group and two fatty acid chains attached to a glycerol molecule. **B,** The fatty acid chains and glycerol form nonpolar, hydrophobic "tails," and the phosphate functional group forms the polar, hydrophilic "head" of the phospholipid molecule. **C,** When placed in water, the hydrophobic tails of the molecule face inward, away from the water, and the hydrophilic head faces outward, toward the water. (From Raven PH, Johnson GB: *Understanding biology,* ed 3, Dubuque, Iowa, 1995, Brown.)

ponents of the cellular environment move slowly and selectively across the membrane all the time. (Components of the cellular environment are discussed in Chapter 3.)

Proteins

Research suggests two ways to classify membrane proteins. One way is classification as peripheral or integral proteins. **Integral membrane proteins** are those embedded in the lipid bilayer linked to either *phosphatidylinositol,* a minor phospholipid, or a fatty acid chain. The integral proteins can be removed from the membrane only by detergents that solubilize (dissolve) the liquid. **Peripheral membrane proteins** are not embedded in the bilayer but reside at one surface or the other, bound to an integral protein.

Although the classification of membrane proteins as peripheral or integral is commonly used, it does not describe how proteins are associated with the bilayer. The second mode of classification does so by taking into account the membrane-spanning, or transmembranous, nature of membrane proteins[1] (see Figure 1-13). According to this classification, proteins are associated with the lipid bilayer in four ways:

1. Some proteins, called **transmembrane proteins,** extend across the bilayer and are exposed to an aqueous environment on both sides of it.
2. Some intracellular proteins extend their polypeptide chain partially through the bilayer by means of a fatty acid chain.
3. Some cell-surface proteins are attached to the bilayer by a covalent linkage (i.e., a specific oligosaccharide).
4. Some proteins do not extend even partially through the bilayer but are bound to the membrane by noncovalent linkages with other membrane proteins.

Proteins exist in densely folded molecular configurations rather than straight chains, so an excess of hydrophilic units is at the surface of the molecule and an excess of hydrophobic units is inside. Although membrane structure is determined by the lipid bilayer, membrane functions are determined largely by proteins. For example, proteins facilitate

transport across membranes by serving as receptors, enzymes, or transporters. Proteins act as (1) recognition and binding units (receptors) for substances moving in and out of the cell; (2) pores or transport channels for various electrically charged particles called *ions* or *electrolytes* and specific carriers for amino acids and monosaccharides; (3) specific enzymes that drive active pumps that promote concentration of certain ions, particularly potassium (K^+), within the cell while keeping concentrations of other ions, for example, sodium (Na^+), below concentrations found in the extracellular environment; (4) cell surface markers, such as **glycoproteins** (proteins attached to carbohydrates) that identify a cell to its neighbor; (5) **cell adhesion molecules (CAMs)** or proteins that allow cells to hook together and form attachments to the cytoskeleton for maintaining cellular shape; and (6) catalysts of chemical reactions, for example, conversion of lactose to glucose (see Figure 1-10). (Membrane transport is discussed on p. 25.)

The interaction of plasma membrane proteins with lipids is complex and is currently the subject of much research. The role of proteins in the onset and progression of disease is important because of their enzymatic, transport, and recognition-receptor functions in cellular physiology.

Proteolytic Cascades

About 500 human genes encode proteases.[8] Proteases are involved in the physiologic regulation of essential processes by participating in a tightly orchestrated sequence of events termed a **proteolytic cascade.** Four major proteolytic cascades with disease relevance are candidates for treatment modalities including (1) caspase-mediated apoptosis, (2) blood coagulation cascade, (3) matrix metalloproteinase cascade, and (4) the complement cascade. Some proteases within a proteolytic cascade act as initiators, others are involved in amplification and propagation and execution (Figure 1-12). Understanding the various steps involved is crucial for designing drug interventions. Dysregulation of proteases features prominently in many human diseases, including cancer, autoimmunity, and neurodegenerative disorders.[9,10]

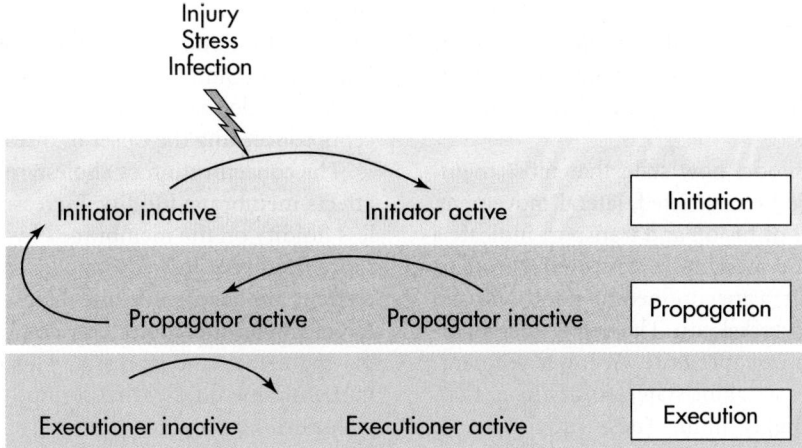

Figure 1-12 Schematic representation of a prototype proteolytic cascade. In the initiation phase, the cascade is triggered by an external stimulus, such as injury, stress, or infection. During the propagation phase, the initiator converts a downstream propagator into its active form by proteolysis. In the execution phase, the propagator will activate an executor. The process of coagulation is the best known proteolytic cascade. (Redrawn from Amour A et al: General considerations for proteolytic cascades, *Biochem Soc Trans* 32: 15-16, 2004.)

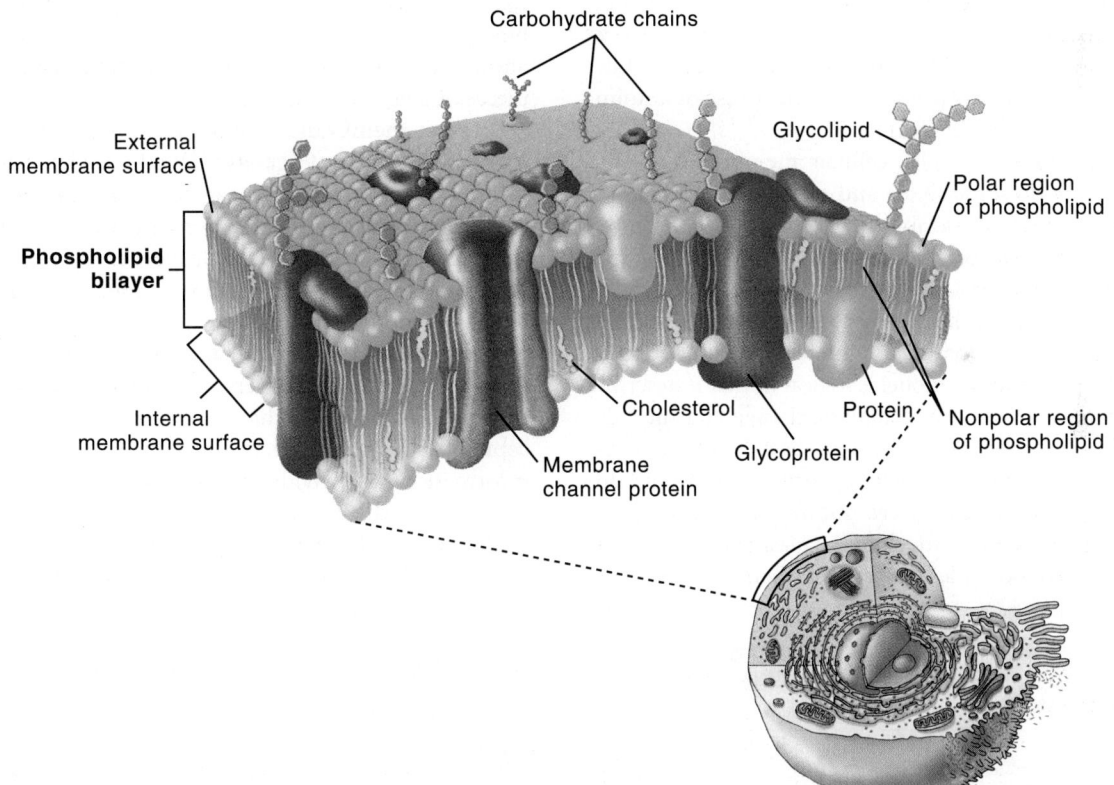

Figure 1-13 Fluid mosaic model. Schematic, three-dimensional view of the fluid mosaic model of membrane structure. The lipid bilayer provides the basic structure and serves as a relatively impermeable barrier to most water-soluble molecules. (Modified from Thibodeau GA, Patton KT: *Anatomy & physiology,* ed 5, St Louis, 2003, Mosby.)

Carbohydrates

A significant amount of carbohydrate is contained within the plasma membrane in the form of glycoprotein. Intercellular recognition, which is required for tissue formation, is an important function of membrane glycoproteins. Abnormal surface carbohydrate markers have been identified in certain tumor cells, leading investigators to claim that these markers are involved in tissue growth. Cells do not "trespass" their boundaries and overgrow their own territory.

Membrane Fluidity: The Fluid Mosaic Model

In the 1960s GL Nicholson and SJ Singer proposed the popular fluid mosaic model for biologic membranes (Figure 1-13). The model, which is continually being modified, presents integral proteins as pieces of a mosaic that float singly or as aggregates in the fluid lipid bilayer. The protein molecules serve to (1) transport other molecules into and out of the cell; (2) facilitate (catalyze) membrane reactions; (3) receive messages, thus acting as receptors for extracellular and intracellular signals; and (4) create structural linkages between the external and internal cellular environments. The fluid mosaic model accounts for the flexibility of cellular membranes, their self-sealing properties, and their impermeability to many substances.

New revisions of the model now state that most membrane proteins do not enjoy unrestricted, lateral movement. Instead, multiple modes of diffusion and transport indicate a mix or heterogeneity in the membrane. Thus *some* proteins may randomly diffuse, others are confined or static, and still others are tethered to the cytoskeleton. The degree of a membrane's fluidity depends on temperature. At lower temperatures the lipids are in a gel crystalline state, and at higher temperatures they become highly fluid. These properties are critical for cellular growth, division, and receptor function. Because some proteins are free to move within the plasma membranes (like floating icebergs), certain foreign proteins (antigens) may become buried in the bilayer, emerging at the surface only after injury and then attracting antibodies (proteins produced by the immune system), which attack host cells. Antigens and antibodies, which are the cause and effect of the immune response, are discussed in Chapter 7. The burial and reemergence of antigens may be one cause of autoimmune disease, described in Chapter 8.

In the fluid mosaic model, cellular membranes are dynamic. Not only do some lipids and proteins move laterally on the membrane, but also ions and other molecules move through it. Cells, however, do have ways of immobilizing specific membrane proteins in a specific region of the membrane. Confinement may be necessary for certain functions to occur, for example, formation of intercellular junctions by proteins. The fluid mosaic model is logical in that it describes the membrane as existing in a state of change and modulation, which allows the cell to protect itself actively against injurious agents. Hormones, bacteria, viruses, drugs, antibodies, chemicals that transmit nerve impulses (neurotransmitters), and other substances attach to the plasma membrane by means of receptor molecules on its outer layer. The number of

receptors present may vary at different times, and the cell is capable of modulating the effects of injurious agents by altering receptor number and pattern.[11] This aspect of the fluid mosaic model has drastically modified previously held concepts concerning the onset of disease.

The concentration of cholesterol in the plasma membrane affects membrane fluidity. Increased concentration results in less fluidity on the membrane's hydrophilic outer surface and more fluidity at its hydrophobic core. Changes in cholesterol content are factors in some diseases. In cirrhosis of the liver, for example, the cholesterol content of the red blood cell's plasma membrane increases. This causes an overall decrease in membrane fluidity that seriously affects the cell's ability to transport oxygen.

Cellular Receptors

Cellular receptors are protein molecules on the plasma membrane, in the cytoplasm, or in the nucleus that are capable of recognizing and binding with specific smaller molecules called **ligands.** Hormones, for example, are ligands. Recognition and binding depend on the chemical configuration of the receptor and its smaller ligand, which must fit together somewhat like pieces of a jigsaw puzzle (see Chapter 20).

Plasma membrane receptors are particularly important for cellular uptake of ligands (Table 1-2). They protrude from or are exposed at the external surface of the membrane and often are attached to integral proteins. Some of these recognition units have all the mobile properties related to membrane fluidity. The ligands that bind with membrane receptors include hormones, neurotransmitters, antigens, complement components, lipoproteins, infectious agents, drugs, and metabolites. The past several years have brought many new discoveries concerning the specific interactions of cellular receptors with their respective ligands. In many instances this information has provided a basis for understanding disease.

Although the chemical nature of both ligands and the receptors to which they bind differs, receptors are classified on the basis of their location and function (see Cellular Com-

Table 1-2	Classes of Plasma Membrane Receptors
Type of Receptor	**Description**
Channel linked	Also called ligand-gated channels; involve rapid synaptic signaling between electrically excitable cells. Channels open and close briefly in response to neurotransmitters changing ion permeability of plasma membrane of postsynaptic cell.
Catalytic	Once activated by ligands, function directly as enzymes. Composed of transmembrane proteins that function intracellularly as tyrosine-specific protein kinases.
G-protein linked	Indirectly activate or inactivate plasma membrane enzyme or ion channel; interaction mediated by guanosine triphosphate (GTP)–binding regulatory protein (G protein). When activated, a chain of reactions occurs that alters concentration of intracellular messengers, such as cyclic adenosine monophosphate (cAMP) and calcium, or signaling molecules. Other target proteins' behavior also altered. May also interact with inositol phospholipids, which are significant in cell signaling, and molecules involved in the inositol-phospholipid transduction pathway. A G protein–linked receptor activates the enzyme phosphoinositide-specific phospholipase, which in turn generates two intracellular messengers: (1) inositol triphosphate (InsP$_3$) releases Ca^{++}, and (2) diacylglycerol remains in the plasma membrane and activates protein kinase C. Protein kinase C further activates various cell proteins. Several different plasma membrane receptors are known to use the inositol-phospholipid transduction pathway.

Data from Alberts B et al: *Molecular biology of the cell,* ed 4, New York, 2001, Garland.

munication and Signal Transduction). Cellular type determines overall cellular function, but plasma membrane receptors determine which ligands a cell will bind with and how the cell will respond to binding with each. For example, the ability of a hormone or a neurotransmitter to stimulate a cell is regulated by the specificity and number of receptors present on the plasma membrane. Specific processes also control intracellular mechanisms. Hormone binding, for example, depends on special messenger molecules that regulate protein synthesis within the cell (see Chapter 20). Neurotransmitters (discussed in Chapter 14) also operate by causing special messengers to react with specific receptors.

Receptors for different drugs are found on the plasma membrane, in the cytoplasm, and in the nucleus. Membrane receptors have been found for certain anesthetics, opiates, endorphins, enkephalins, antibiotics, cancer chemotherapeutic agents, digitalis, and other drugs. Membrane receptors for endorphins, which are opiate-like peptides isolated from the pituitary gland, are found in large quantities in pain pathways of the nervous system (see Chapters 14 and 15). With binding, the endorphins (or drugs like morphine) change the cell's permeability to ions, increase the concentration of molecules that regulate intracellular protein synthesis, and initiate molecular events that modulate pain perception.

Receptors for infectious microorganisms, or antigen receptors, bind bacteria, viruses, and parasites. Antigen receptors on white blood cells (lymphocytes, monocytes, macro-

phages, granulocytes) recognize and bind with antigenic microorganisms and activate the immune and inflammatory responses (see Chapters 6 and 7).

CELL-TO-CELL ADHESIONS

Cells are small and squishy, not at all like bricks. They are enclosed only by a flimsy membrane, yet the cell depends on the integrity of this membrane for its survival. How can cells be formed together strongly, with their membranes intact, to form a muscle that can lift this textbook? Plasma membranes not only serve as the outer boundaries of all cells but also allow groups of cells to be held together robustly, in **cell-to-cell adhesions,** to form tissues and organs. Once arranged, cells are held together by three different means: the extracellular matrix, cell adhesion molecules in the cell's plasma membrane, and specialized cell junctions.

Extracellular Matrix

Cells can be bound together by attachment to one another or via the **extracellular matrix** (also including the **basement membrane**), which the cells secrete around themselves. The extracellular matrix is an intricate meshwork of fibrous proteins embedded in a watery, gel-like substance composed of complex carbohydrates (Figure 1-14). The matrix is like glue; however, it does provide a pathway for diffusion of nutrients, wastes, and other water-soluble traffic between the blood and

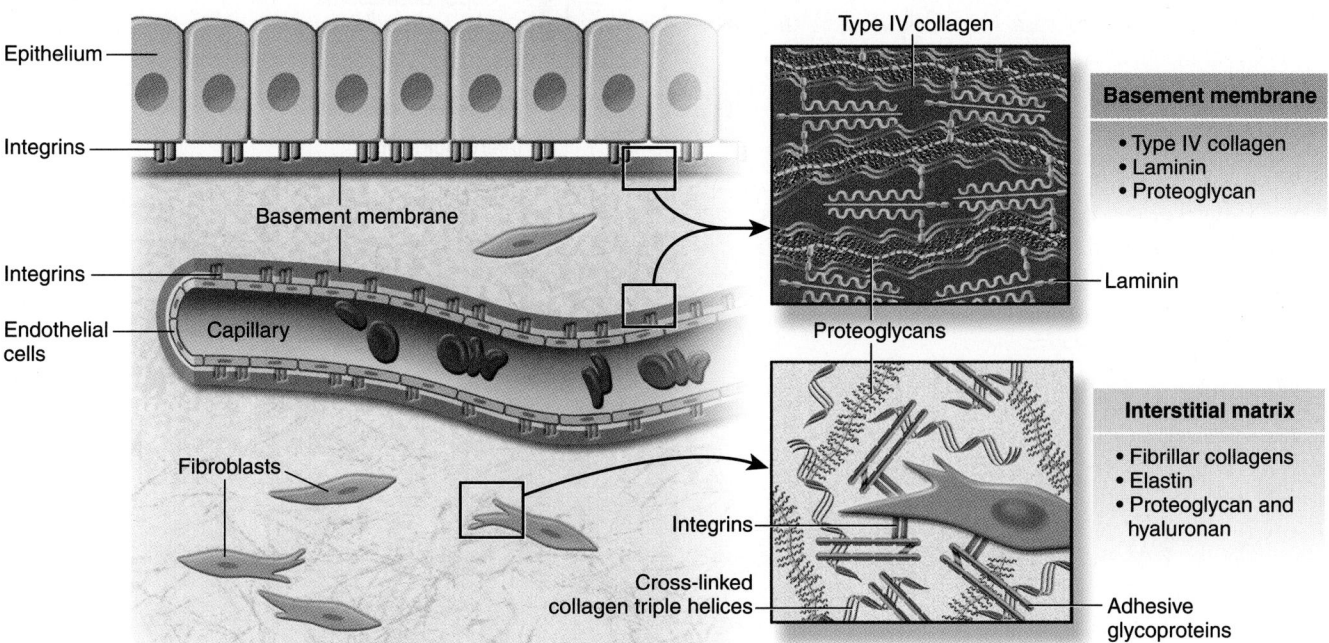

Figure 1-14 Extracellular matrix. Tissues are not just cells but also extracellular space. The extracellular space is an intricate network of macromolecules called the *extracellular matrix (ECM)*. The macromolecules that constitute the ECM are secreted locally (by mostly fibroblasts) and assembled into a meshwork in close association with the surface of the cell that produced them. Two main classes of macromolecules include proteoglycans, which are bound to polysaccharide chains called *glycosaminoglycans,* and fibrous proteins (e.g., collagen, elastin, fibronectin, and laminin), which have structural and adhesive properties. Together the proteogylcan molecules form a gel-like ground substance in which the fibrous proteins are embedded. The gel permits rapid diffusion of nutrients, metabolites, and hormones between the blood and the tissue cells. Matrix proteins modulate cell-matrix interactions including normal tissue remodeling (which can become abnormal, for example, with chronic inflammation), embryogenesis, wound healing, and angiogenesis. Disruptions of this balance results in serious diseases such as arthritis, tumor growth, and others. (Modified from Kumar V, Abbas A, Fausto N: *Robbins and Cotran pathologic basis of disease,* ed 7, Philadelphia, 2005, Saunders.)

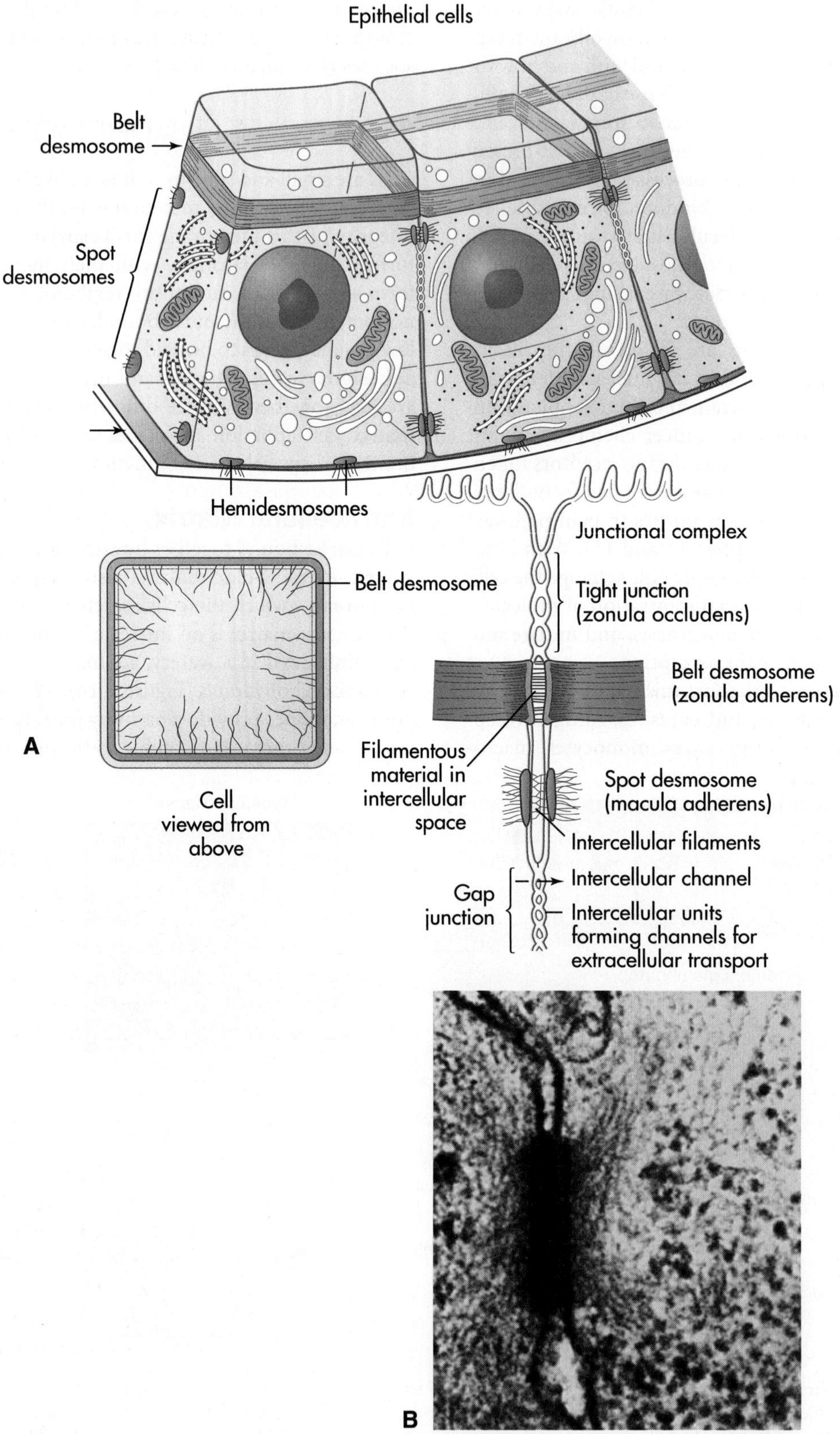

Epithelial cells

Belt desmosome →

Spot desmosomes

Hemidesmosomes

Junctional complex

Belt desmosome

A

Cell viewed from above

Tight junction (zonula occludens)

Belt desmosome (zonula adherens)

Filamentous material in intercellular space

Spot desmosome (macula adherens)

Intercellular filaments

Gap junction

Intercellular channel

Intercellular units forming channels for extracellular transport

B

Figure 1-15 Junctional complex. A, Schematic drawing of a belt desmosome between epithelial cells. This junction, also called *zonula adherens,* encircles each interacting cell. The spot desmosomes and hemidesmosomes, like the belt desmosomes, are adhering junctions. This tight junction is an impermeable junction that holds cells together but seals them in such a way that molecules cannot leak between them. The gap junction, as a communicating junction, mediates the passage of small molecules from one interacting cell to the other. **B,** Electron micrograph of desmosomes. (From Raven PH, Johnson GB: *Biology,* St Louis, 1992, Mosby.)

tissue cells. Interwoven within the matrix are three groups of **macromolecules:** (1) fibrous structural proteins, including collagen and elastin; (2) a diverse group of adhesive glyco-proteins, such as fibronectin; and (3) proteoglycans and hyaluronic acid.

Collagen forms cable-like fibers or sheets that provide ten-sile strength or resistance to longitudinal stress. Collagen breakdown, such as occurs in osteoarthritis, destroys the fi-brils that give cartilage its tensile strength.

Elastin is a rubber-like protein fiber most abundant in tis-sue that must be capable of stretching and recoiling, such as the lungs.

Fibronectin, a large glycoprotein, promotes cell adhesion and cell anchorage. Reduced amounts have been found in cer-tain types of cancerous cells; this allows cancer cells to travel or metastasize to other parts of the body.

All of these macromolecules occur in intracellular junc-tions and cell surfaces and may assemble into two different components: interstitial matrix and basement membrane (BM)[12] (see Figure 1-14, *A*).

The extracellular matrix is secreted by **fibroblasts** ("fiber formers"), local cells that are present in the matrix. The ma-trix and the cells within it are known collectively as *connective tissue* because they connect cells together to form tissue and organs. Human connective tissues are enormously varied. They can be hard and dense, like bone; flexible, like tendons or the dermis of the skin; resilient and shock-absorbing, like cartilage; or soft and transparent, like the jelly that fills the eye. In all these examples, the majority of the tissue is com-posed of extracellular matrix and the cells that produce the matrix are scattered within it like raisins in a pudding[13] (see Figure 1-14).

The matrix is not just a passive scaffolding for cellular at-tachment; it also helps regulate the functions of the cells within which it interacts. The matrix helps regulate cell growth, movement, and differentiation.

Specialized Cell Junctions

Cells in direct physical contact with neighboring cells are of-ten linked together at specialized regions of their plasma membranes called **cell junctions.** Cell junctions have two main functions: (1) to hold cells together and (2) to allow small molecules to pass from cell to cell, allowing coordina-tion of the activities of cells that form tissues. The three main types of cell junctions are (1) desmosomes (adhering junc-tions, or macula adherens), (2) tight junctions (impermeable junctions, or zonula occludens), and (3) gap junctions (ad-hering [communicating] junctions) (Figure 1-15). Together they form the **junctional complex. Desmosomes** hold cells together by forming either continuous bands or belts of ep-ithelial sheets or button-like points of contact. Desmosomes also act as a system of braces to maintain structural stability. **Tight junctions** serve as a barrier to diffusion, prevent the movement of substances through transport proteins in the plasma membrane, and prevent the leakage of small mole-cules between the plasma membranes of adjacent cells. **Gap**

junctions are clusters of communicating tunnels, **connexons,** that allow small ions and molecules to pass directly from the inside of one cell to the inside of another. Connexons are join-ing proteins that extend outward from each of the adjacent plasma membranes. Cells connected by gap junctions are considered ionically (electrically) and metabolically coupled. Gap junctions coordinate the activities of adjacent cells. They are important, for example, in synchronizing contractions of heart muscle cells through ionic coupling and in permitting action potentials to spread rapidly from cell to cell in neural tissues. The reason that gap junctions occur in tissues that are not electrically active is unknown. Although most gap junc-tions are associated with junctional complexes, they some-times exist as independent structures.

The junctional complex is a highly permeable part of the plasma membrane. Its permeability is controlled by a process called **gating,** which depends on concentrations of calcium ions in the cytoplasm. Increased cytoplasmic calcium causes decreased permeability at the junctional complex. Gating is an important cellular defense mechanism because it enables uninjured cells to seal themselves off from injured neighbors. As damaged cells release calcium, it travels through the junc-tional complex and increases calcium levels in neighboring cells. (The damaging effects of calcium influx are described in Chapter 2.) This decreases the permeability of the junctional complexes of the neighboring cells, which form a relatively impermeable wall around the injured area.

CELLULAR COMMUNICATION AND SIGNAL TRANSDUCTON

Cells need to communicate with each other to maintain a sta-ble internal environment, or **homeostasis;** to regulate their growth and division and their development and organization into tissues; and to coordinate their functions. Cells commu-nicate in three ways: (1) they form protein channels (gap junc-tions) that directly coordinate the activities of adjacent cells; (2) they display plasma membrane–bound signaling mole-cules (receptors) that affect the cell itself and other cells in di-rect physical contact; and (3) the most common means, they secrete chemicals that signal to cells some distance away (Fig-ure 1-16). Alterations in cellular communication affect disease onset and progression. In fact, if a cell is unable to perform gap junctional intercellular communication, it is hypothesized that normal growth control and cell differentiation are compro-mised, favoring cancerous tumor development (see Chapter 11). (Communication through gap junctions is discussed ear-lier, and contact signaling by plasma membrane–bound mole-cules is shown in Figure 1-16.) Secreted chemical signals in-volve communication at a distance. Primary modes of chemical signaling are hormonal, neurohormonal, paracrine, autocrine, and neurotransmitter (Figure 1-17).

Hormonal signaling involves specialized endocrine cells that secrete hormone chemicals released by one set of cells and travel through the tissue and through the bloodstream to produce a response in other sets of cells (see Chapter 20). In

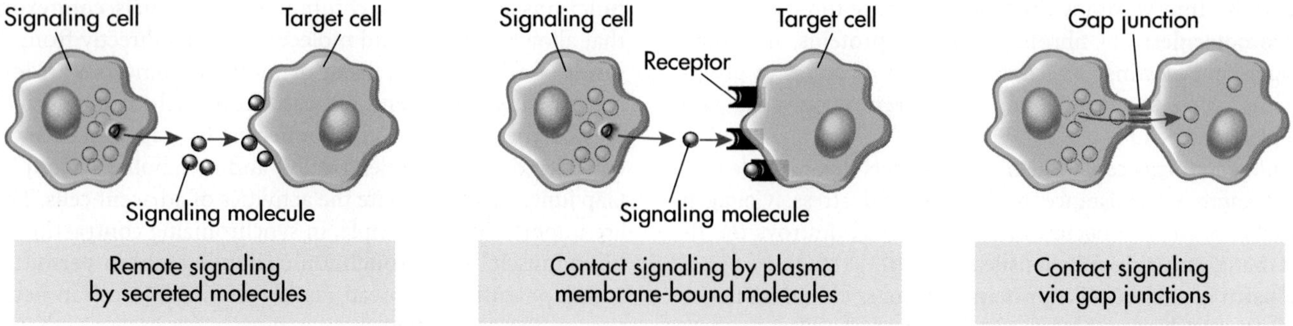

Figure 1-16 **Cellular communication.** Three ways in which cells communicate with one another.

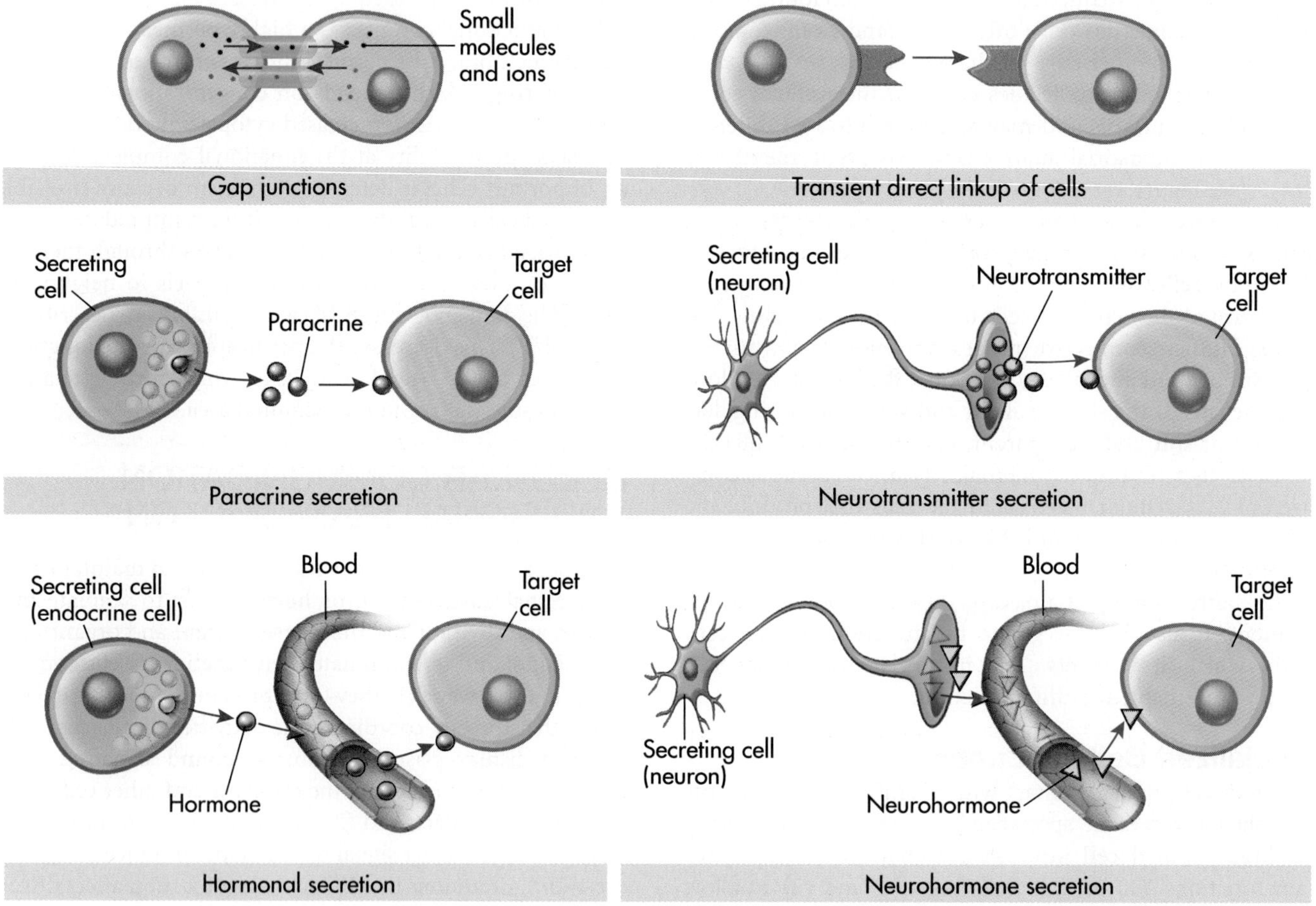

Figure 1-17 **Modes of chemical signaling and cell communication.** Paracrines, neurotransmitters, hormones, and neurohormones are all intercellular chemical messengers that accomplish communication between cells. Gap junctions provide the most intimate means of intercellular communication where small molecules and ions are exchanged between interacting cells without even entering the extracellular fluid. Autocrine stimulation (not illustrated) is when the secreting cell targets itself.

neurohormonal signaling hormones are released into the blood by neurosecretory neurons. Like endocrine cells, neurosecretory neurons release blood-borne chemical messengers, whereas ordinary neurons secrete short-range neurotransmitters into a small discrete space. In **paracrine signaling,** cells secrete local chemical mediators that are quickly taken up, destroyed, or immobilized. The mediators act only on nearby cells. In **autocrine signaling,** signaling molecules may act back on the cells of *origin* (i.e., *autostimulation*); autocrine circuits function as a component of normal growth-regulatory mechanisms in many adult tissue types.[14,15] Neurons communicate directly with the cells they innervate by releasing chemicals or **neurotransmitters** at specialized junctions called **chemical synapses;** the neutrotransmitter diffuses across the synaptic cleft and acts on the postsynaptic target cell (see Figure 1-18). In each type of chemical signaling, the target cell receives the signal by first attaching to its receptors. Many of these same signaling molecules are receptors used in hormonal, neurohormonal, paracrine, and autocrine signaling. The important differences lie in the speed and selectivity with which the signals are delivered to their targets.[1]

Plasma membrane receptors belong to one of three classes that are defined by the signaling (transduction) mechanism used. Table 1-2 summarizes these receptors.

Signal Transduction

Signal transduction involves incoming signals or instructions from extracellular chemical messengers (ligands) that are conveyed to the cell's interior for execution. Within the outer surface of the plasma membrane, specialized protein receptors bind with the selected chemical messengers. This combination of messenger with receptor triggers a cascade of cellular events important to the maintenance of homeostasis, such as membrane transport, cell division and differentiation, movement, secretion, and metabolism. Some types of altered cell behavior, such as increased cell growth and division, involve changes in gene expression and the synthesis of new proteins and therefore occur slowly. Others, such as changes in cell movement, secretion, or metabolism, do not involve the nuclear machinery and therefore occur more rapidly. If deprived of appropriate signals, most cells undergo a form of cell suicide known as *programmed cell death,* or *apoptosis* (see p. 81).

Signaling cascades, or relay chains, of intercellular signaling molecules have several important functions (Figure 1-18):

1. They physically *transfer* the signal from the place at which it is received to some other part of the cell where the response is expected.
2. They *amplify* the signal received, making it stronger; this is caused by a multiplying effect in the pathways; for example, binding of one ligand molecule to a receptor activates a number of adenylyl cyclase molecules.
3. They *distribute* the signal so that it influences several processes in parallel; at any step in the pathway, the signal can *diverge* and be relayed to several different intracellular targets, creating branches in the flow and causing a complex response (Figure 1-19).
4. Last, the signal can be *modulated* by other interfering factors prevailing inside or outside the cell.

Two general responses from binding of the extracellular chemical messenger, or **first messenger,** to the membrane receptors occur: (1) opening or closing specific channels in the membrane to regulate the movement of ions into or out of the cell and (2) transferring the signal to an intracellular messenger, or **second messenger,** which in turn triggers a cascade of biochemical events within the cell.

Extracellular Messengers and Channel Regulation

Membrane channels, or "gates," can open and close depending on the circumstances of the first messenger. Opening and closing occur because of conformational changes (shaping) of the proteins that form the channels—blocking the channel (closing) or permitting passage through it (opening). Channel opening and closing can be initiated in one of three ways:

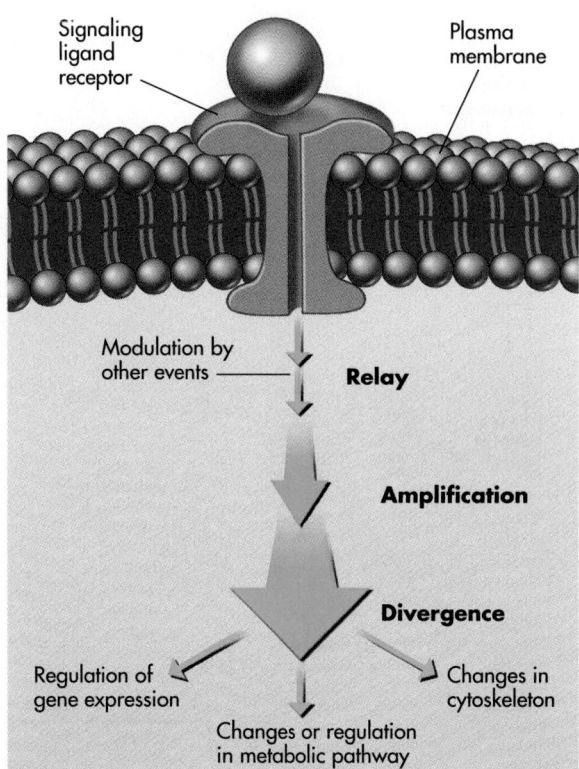

Figure 1-18 **An intracellular signaling cascade.** An extracellular chemical messenger (ligand) binds to a receptor protein located on the plasma membrane where it is transduced into an intracellular signal. This process initiates a signaling cascade that relays the signal into the cell interior, amplifying and distributing it en route. Steps in the cascade can be modulated by other events in the cell.

(1) by binding of a ligand to a specific membrane receptor that is closely associated with the channel, for example, G proteins; (2) by changes in electric current in the plasma membrane, altering flow of Na^+ and K^+; and (3) by stretching or other chemical deformation of the channel. Figure 1-19 summarizes ways by which extracellular messengers regulate channel function for the other two methods of controlling channels (see p. 21).

Second Messengers

Many ligands cannot enter their target cells to bring about the desired intracellular response. Instead, the first messengers, or ligands, issue orders by binding with receptors on the surface membrane, triggering a "pass it on" signal. Second messengers are generated in large numbers when the membrane-bound enzyme is activated, and they then rapidly diffuse away from their source, broadcasting the signal throughout the cell (Figure 1-20). Remember, most cell-surface receptor proteins belong to one of three large classes: ion-channel-linked receptors, G-protein-linked receptors, or enzyme-linked receptors.

The two major second messenger pathways are **cyclic adenosine monophosphate (cyclic AMP, cAMP)** and Ca^{++}. In the cAMP pathway, binding of the ligand to its surface receptor eventually activates the enzyme adenylyl cyclase on the inner surface of the membrane. A membrane-bound

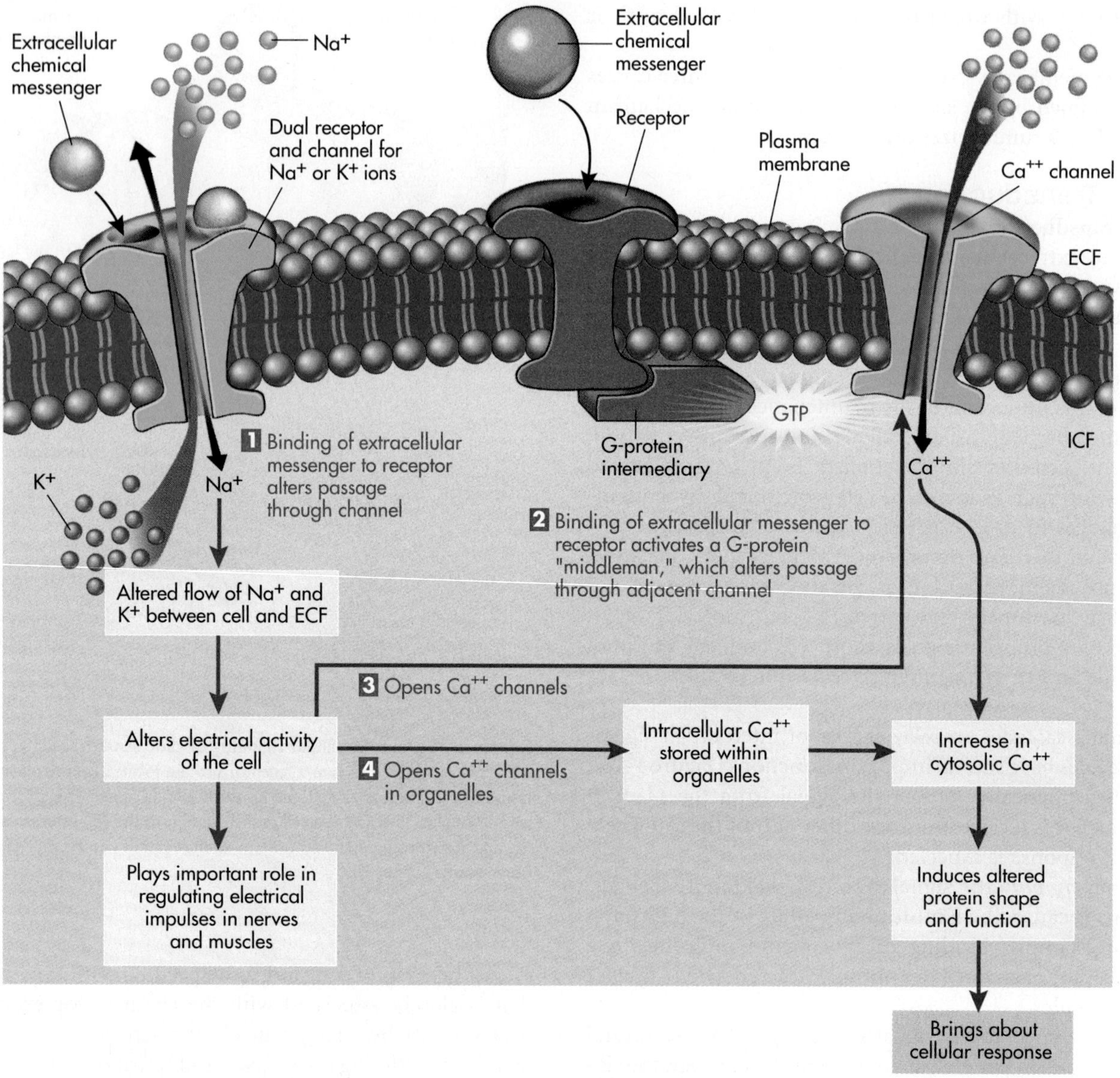

Figure 1-19 **How extracellular messengers regulate channel function.** Binding of an extracellular messenger to a dual receptor/
channel brings about a quick opening or closing of ion channels, such as Na^+ or K^+ channels, which generates electrical impulses
(1). A transient opening of membrane Ca^{++} channels occurs when binding of an extracellular messenger to a receptor activates a
G-protein intermediary, which alters a nearby ion channel, such as a Ca^{++} channel *(2)*. A transient opening of Ca^{++} channels also occurs indirectly in response to electrical impulses produced by extracellular messenger-induced changes in Na^+ and K^+ channels
(3). Release of Ca^{++} from intracellular stores results when Ca^{++} channels in organelles open in response to electrical impulses
(4). An increase in cytosolic Ca^{++} arising from pathways 2, 3, or 4 causes changes in the shape and function of specific intracellular
proteins to produce the desired cellular response. (Redrawn with permission from Sherwood L: *Human physiology: from cells to systems,* ed 3, Belmont, Calif, 1997, Wadsworth.)

"middleman," a **G protein,** acts as an intermediary between
the receptor and adenylyl cyclase. G proteins are named because they are bound to guanine nucleotides—**guanosine
triphosphate (GTP)** or **guanosine diphosphate (GDP).** An
unactivated G protein consists of a complex of alpha (α), beta
(β), and gamma (γ) subunits, with a GDP molecule bound to
the a subunit. The cAMP pathway with G proteins is summarized in Figure 1-20.

   Instead of cAMP, some cells use Ca^{++} as a second messenger. In this pathway, binding of the first messenger to the surface receptor eventually leads, by means of G proteins, to ac-

tivation of the enzyme phospholipase C, an enzyme protein
effector (an ion channel for an enzyme) that is bound to the
inner side of the membrane. Figure 1-21 summarizes the
Ca^{++} second messenger pathway. The cAMP and Ca^{++} pathways frequently overlap in bringing about a specific cellular
response. For example, cAMP and Ca^{++} can influence each
other. Calcium-activated calmodulin can regulate adenylyl
cyclase and thus influence cAMP; conversely, cAMP-dependent kinase may phosphorylate and thereby change the activity
of Ca^{++} channels or carriers. In some instances, both Ca^{++}
and cAMP regulate the same intracellular protein. In a few

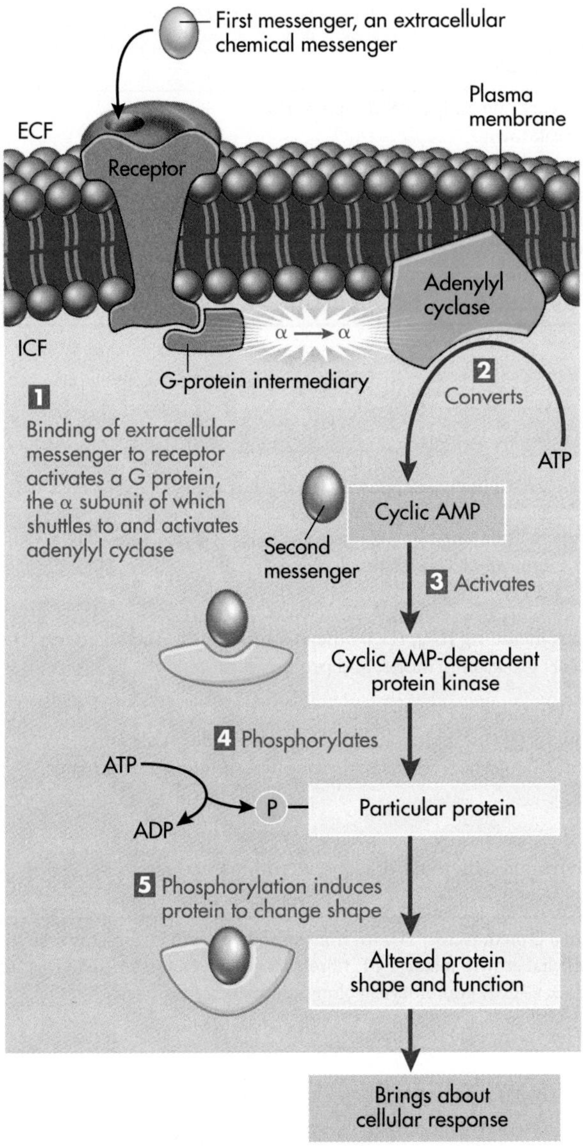

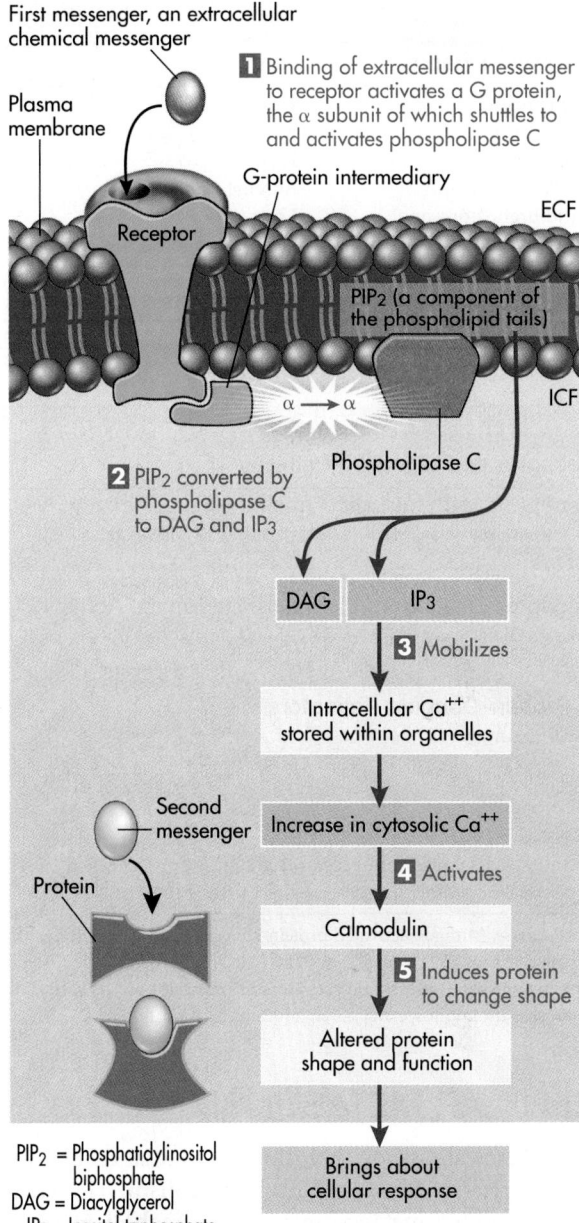

Figure 1-20 Extracellular messenger and activation of the cAMP second messenger system. The first messenger, or binding of an extracellular chemical messenger to a surface membrane receptor, activates the membrane-bound enzyme adenylyl cyclase by means of a G-protein intermediary *(1)*, which in turn converts intracellular ATP into cAMP *(2)*. cAMP is an intracellular second messenger, triggering the cellular response by activating the cAMP-dependent protein kinase *(3)*, which in turn phosphorylates *(4)* and therefore modifies *(5)* a specific intracellular protein. The altered protein then directs the cellular response dictated by the extracellular messenger. (Redrawn with permission from Sherwood L: *Human physiology: from cells to systems,* ed 3, Belmont, Calif, 1997, Wadsworth.)

Figure 1-21 Extracellular messenger and activation of the calcium second messenger system. Binding of an extracellular messenger to a membrane receptor activates the membrane-bound enzyme phospholipase C by means of a G-protein intermediary *(1)*. Phospholipase C converts phosphatidylinositol biphosphate (PIP$_2$) into diacylglycerol (DAG) and inositol triphosphate (IP$_3$) *(2)*. IP$_3$ then mobilizes Ca^{++} stored within organelles *(3)*. Ca^{++}, as a second messenger, activates calmodulin *(4)*, causing a change in the shape and function of a specific intracellular protein to produce the cellular response *(5)*. (Redrawn with permission from Sherwood L: *Human physiology: from cells to systems,* ed 3, Belmont, Calif, 1997, Wadsworth.)

cells, **cyclic guanosine monophosphate (cyclic GMP, cGMP)** serves as a second messenger similar to the cAMP pathway. For example, cGMP is the signal transduction pathway involved in vision. Some cellular responses mediated by cAMP and phospholipase C are summarized in Table 1-3. Major types of receptors and signal transduction pathways are contained in Table 1-4.

A large number of human disorders involve problematic signaling in cells. Cancer, for example, results from genetic mutations leading to the overactivity of proteins in signal relaying pathways that normally induce the cells to divide. Affected proteins cause cells to behave as if other cells were constantly telling them to reproduce, even when no such orders were sent.[16] Signal blockers are already in use against breast cancer.

Table 1-3	Hormone-Induced Cell Responses Mediated by cAMP	
Signaling Ligands	**Target Tissue**	**Major Response**
Epinephrine	Heart	Increase in heart rate and force of contraction
Epinephrine, ACTH	Muscle	Glycogen breakdown
Glucagon	Fat	Fat breakdown
ACTH	Adrenal gland	Cortisol secretion
Antidiuretic hormone	Liver	Glycogen breakdown
Acetylcholine	Pancreas; smooth muscle	Amylase secretion; contraction
Antigen	Mast cells	Histamine secretion
Thrombin	Blood platelets	Serotonin and platelet-derived growth factor secretion; platelet aggregation

cAMP, Cyclic adenosine monophosphate; *ACTH*, adrenocorticotropic hormone.

Table 1-4	Major Types of Receptors and Signaling Transduction Pathways
Receptor and Signaling Pathway	**Ligands**
Receptors with Intrinsic Tyrosine Kinase Activity	
P13 kinase pathway, MAP-kinase pathway, IP$_3$ pathway	Signaling ligands include most growth factors (EGF, TGF-α, HGF, PDGF, VEGF, FGF), stem cell factor, insulin
Receptor Lacking Intrinsic Tyrosine Kinase Activity	
JAK/STAT pathway	Several cytokines including IL-2, IL-3, others; interferons α, β, and γ; erythropoietin; G-CSF; growth hormone; and prolactin
G-Protein–Coupled Receptors	
cAMP pathway	ADH, serotonin, histamine, epinephrine, norepinephrine, calcitonin, glucagon, parathyroid hormone, corticotrophin, rhodopsin, and many drugs
Steroid Hormone Receptors	
Includes steroid hormone receptors and also a group called *peroxisome proliferator-activated receptors (PPARs)*	Many steroid hormones, thyroid hormone, vitamin D, and retinoids

MAP-kinase, Mitogen activated protein kinase; *IP$_3$*, inositol triphosphate; *EGF*, epidermal growth factor; *TGF-α*, transforming growth factor–alpha; *HGF*, hepatocyte growth factor; *PDGF*, platelet-derived growth factor; *VEGF*, vascular endothelial growth factor; *FGF*, fibroblast growth factor; *JAK-STAT*, Janus kinase-signal transducers and activators of transcription; *IL-2, IL-3*, Interleukin-2 and -3; *G-CSF*, granulocyte–colony stimulating factor; *cAMP*, cyclic adenosine monophosphate; *ADH*, antidiuretic hormone.

CELLULAR METABOLISM

All the chemical tasks of maintaining essential cellular functions are referred to as **cellular metabolism.** The energy-using process of metabolism is called **anabolism** (*ana* = upward), and the energy-releasing process is known as **catabolism** (*cata* = downward). Metabolism provides the cell with the energy it needs to synthesize (produce) cellular structures.

Dietary proteins, fats, and starches are hydrolyzed in the intestinal tract into amino acids, fatty acids, and glucose. These constituents are then absorbed, circulated, and taken up by the cell, where they may be used for various vital cellular processes, including the production of ATP. The process by which ATP is produced is one example of a series of reactions called a **metabolic pathway.** A metabolic pathway involves several intermediate steps whose end products are not always detectable. A key feature of cellular metabolism is the directing of biochemical reactions by protein catalysts, or enzymes. Most biochemical reactions in a pathway are catalyzed by a specific enzyme. Each enzyme has a high affinity for a **substrate**—a specific substance that is converted to a product of the reaction.

Role of Adenosine Triphosphate

For a cell to function, it must be able to extract and use the chemical energy contained within the structure of organic molecules. When 1 mole of glucose is metabolically broken down in the presence of oxygen into carbon dioxide (CO_2) and water (H_2O), 686 kilocalories (kcal) of energy are released. In a test tube this energy is released as heat. Because a cell cannot transform heat into work, chemical energy, rather than heat, is created by metabolism. The chemical energy lost by one molecule is transferred to the chemical structure of another molecule by an energy-carrying or transferring molecule, such as ATP. The energy stored in ATP can be used in a variety of energy-requiring reactions and in the process is generally converted to adenosine diphosphate (ADP) and inorganic phosphate (Pi). The energy available as a result of this reaction is about 7 kcal/mol of ATP. In addition to its use in synthesis (anabolism) of organic molecules, ATP is used by the cell for muscle contraction and active transport of molecules across cellular membranes. The function of ATP is not only to *store* energy but also to *transfer* it from one molecule to another. Energy is stored by molecules of carbohydrate, lipid, and protein, which, when catabolized, transfer energy to ATP.

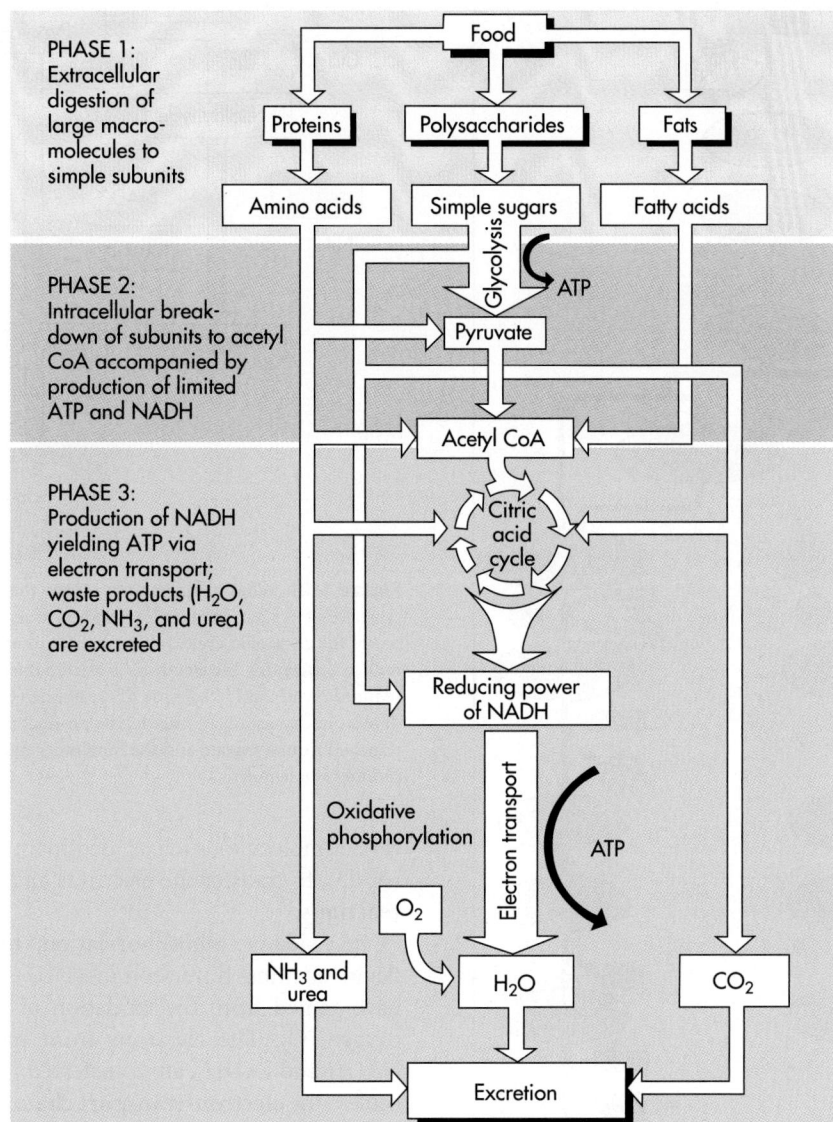

Figure 1-22 **Three phases of catabolism, which leads from food to waste products.** These reactions produce ATP, which is used to drive other processes in the cell.

Food and Production of Cellular Energy

The process of catabolism of the proteins, lipids, and polysaccharides found in food can be divided into three phases (Figure 1-22). In phase 1, large molecules are broken down into their smaller subunits—proteins into amino acids, polysaccharides into simple sugars, and fats into fatty acids and glycerol. These processes are called **digestion** and occur outside the cell by the action of secreted enzymes.

In phase 2 the small molecules enter cells and are further broken down in the cytoplasm. Most of the sugars are converted into pyruvate. Pyruvate then enters mitochondria and is converted to the acetyl groups of acetyl coenzyme A (acetyl CoA). Acetyl CoA, like ATP, releases energy when it is hydrolyzed. The most important part of phase 2 is the lysis (splitting) of glucose, known as **glycolysis** (Figure 1-23). Glycolysis produces a net of two molecules of ATP per glucose molecule through the process of **oxidation,** or the removal

and transfer of a pair of electrons. This process, often called **oxidative cellular metabolism,** involves 10 biochemical reactions. In reactions 1 through 5, glucose is converted to two, three-carbon aldehyde (glyceraldehyde-3-phosphate [G3P]), which requires energy in the form of ATP. The next five reactions convert G3P molecules into pyruvate molecules and generate four molecules of ATP for each two molecules of G3P. In addition, two molecules of NADH are further oxidized to produce four more molecules of ATP. After subtracting two molecules of ATP to drive the reactions, the net yield is six ATP molecules for each molecule of glucose.

Phase 3 occurs when the acetyl group of acetyl CoA is completely degraded to CO_2 and H_2O. It is in this final phase that most of the ATP is generated. Phase 3 begins with the **citric acid cycle** (also called the **Krebs cycle** or the **tricarboxylic acid cycle**) and ends with oxidative phosphorylation. The citric acid cycle accounts for approximately two thirds of the

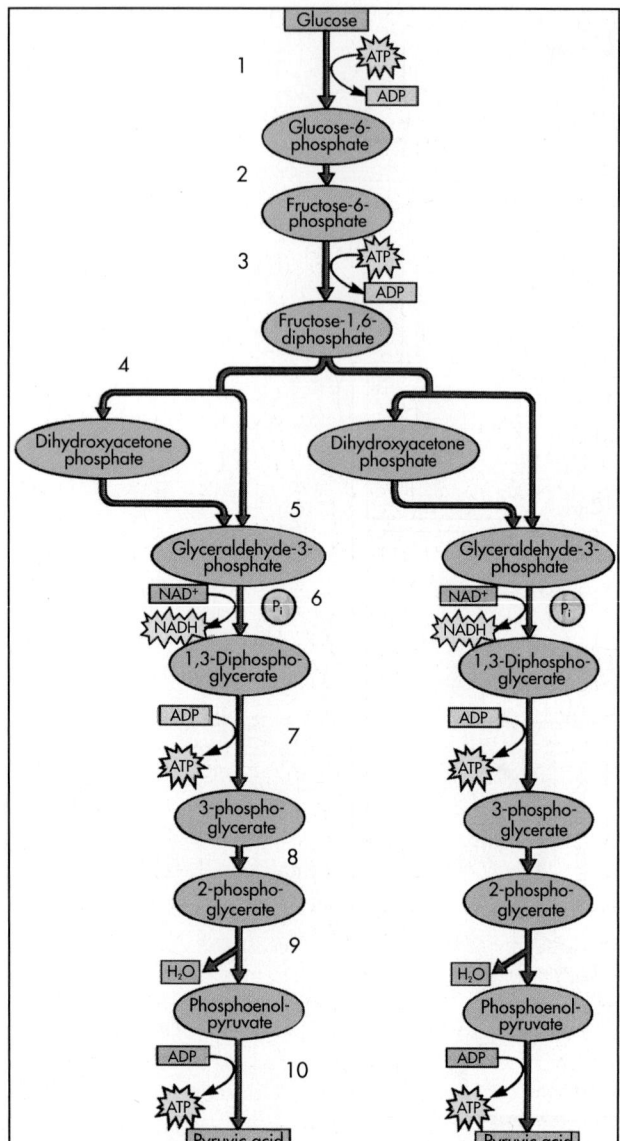

Figure 1-23 Glycolysis. Each of the numbered reactions is catalyzed by a different enzyme. At step 4, a six-carbon sugar is broken down to give two three-carbon sugars, so that the number of molecules at every step after this is doubled. Reactions 5 and 6 are the reactions responsible for the net synthesis of adenosine triphosphate (ATP) and reduced nicotinamide adenine dinucleotide (NADH) molecules. (Modified from Thibodeau GA, Patton KT: *Anatomy & physiology,* ed 5, St Louis, 2003, Mosby.)

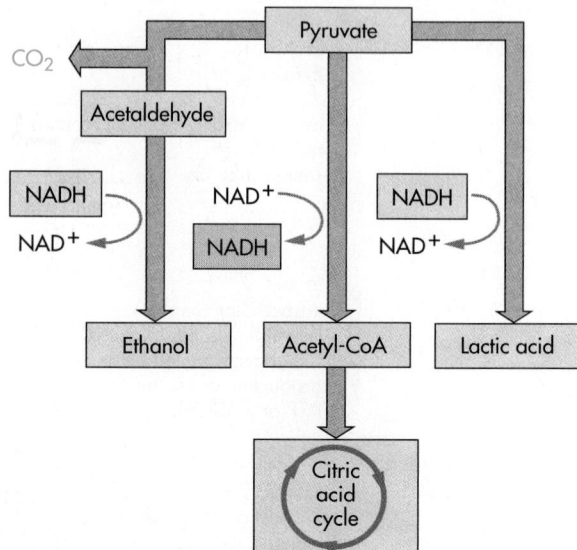

Figure 1-24 What happens to pyruvate, the product of glycolysis? In the presence of oxygen, pyruvate is oxidized to acetyl coenzyme A (CoA) and enters the citric acid cycle. In the absence of oxygen, pyruvate instead is reduced, accepting the electrons extracted during glycolysis and carried by reduced nicotinamide adenine dinucleotide (NADH). When pyruvate is reduced directly, as it is in muscle, the product is lactic acid. When CO_2 is first removed from pyruvate and the remainder reduced, as it is in yeasts, the product is ethanol.

total oxidation of carbon compounds in most cells. Its major end products are CO_2 and two dinucleotides, reduced nicotinamide adenine dinucleotide (NADH) and the reduced form of flavin adenine dinucleotide ($FADH_2$), which transfer their electrons into the electron-transport chain.

Oxidative Phosphorylation

Oxidative phosphorylation occurs in the mitochondria and is the mechanism by which the energy produced from carbohydrates, fats, and proteins is transferred to ATP. During the breakdown (catabolism) of foods, many of the reactions involve the removal of electrons from various intermediates. These reactions generally require a coenzyme (a nonprotein carrier molecule), such as nicotinamide adenine dinucleotide (NAD), to transfer the electrons and thus are called **transfer reactions.**

In oxidative phosphorylation, molecules of NAD and flavin adenine dinucleotide (FAD) transfer electrons they have gained from the oxidation of substrates to molecular oxygen, O_2. The electrons from reduced NAD and FAD, NADH and $FADH_2$, are transferred to a series of carrier molecules (the **electron-transport chain**) on the inner surfaces of the mitochondria with the release of hydrogen ions. Some of the carrier molecules are a group of brightly colored iron-containing proteins known as **cytochromes** that accept a pair of electrons. After passing through a sequence of different cytochromes, these electrons are eventually combined with molecular oxygen. If oxygen is not available to the electron-transport chain, ATP will not be formed by the mitochondria. Instead, an anaerobic (without oxygen) metabolic pathway synthesizes ATP. This process, called *substrate phosphorylation,* or **anaerobic glycolysis,** does not take place in the mitochondria and is linked to the breakdown (glycolysis) of carbohydrate (Figure 1-24).

Because glycolysis occurs in the cytoplasm of the cell, it provides energy for cells that lack mitochondria. However, as previously noted, glycolysis also provides energy to the cell when oxygen delivery is insufficient or delayed. The reactions in anaerobic glycolysis involve the conversion of glucose to pyruvic acid (pyruvate) with the simultaneous production of ATP. With the glycolysis of one molecule of glucose, two ATP molecules and two molecules of pyruvate are liberated. If oxygen is present, the two molecules of pyruvate move into the mitochondria, where they enter the citric acid cycle. If oxygen is absent, pyruvate is converted to lactic acid, and which is released into the extracellular fluid (see Figure 1-24). The conversion of pyruvic acid to lactic acid is reversible; therefore, once oxygen is restored, lactic acid is quickly converted back to either pyruvic acid or glucose. The anaerobic generation of ATP from glucose, through the reactions of glycolysis, is not as efficient as the aerobic generation of ATP. The addition of an oxygen-requiring stage to the catabolic process (stage 3) provides cells with a much more powerful method for extracting energy from food molecules.

MEMBRANE TRANSPORT: CELLULAR INTAKE AND OUTPUT

Cells continually take in nutrients, fluids, and chemical messengers from the extracellular environment and expel metabolites or the products of metabolism and end products of lysosomal digestion. Intake and output, or transport, occurs by different mechanisms, depending on the characteristics of the substance to be transported. Water and small, electrically uncharged molecules move easily through pores in the plasma membrane's lipid bilayer. This process, called **passive transport,** will occur naturally through any semipermeable barrier. It is driven by osmosis, hydrostatic pressure, and diffusion, all of which depend on the laws of physics and do not require life. The process is passive in that it does not require any expenditure of energy by the cell.

Other molecules cannot be driven across the plasma membrane solely by forces of diffusion, hydrostatic pressure, or osmosis because they are too large or are ligands that have bound with receptors on the cell's plasma membrane. Some of these molecules are moved into the cell by mechanisms of **active transport,** which requires life, biologic activity, and the expenditure of metabolic energy by the cell. Unlike passive transport, which can be duplicated across any semipermeable barrier in a laboratory, active transport occurs only across living membranes that (1) use energy generated by cellular metabolism and (2) have receptors that are capable of recognizing and binding with the substance to be transported. Large molecules (macromolecules), along with fluids, are transported by means of endocytosis (taking in) and exocytosis (expelling). Water and electrically charged molecules are transported by protein channels embedded in the plasma membrane. Ligands enter the cell by means of receptor-mediated endocytosis.

Movement of Water and Solutes

Cellular membranes are semipermeable and generally allow passage of water and small particles of dissolved substances called **solutes.** The movement of solute molecules through membranes is related to their size, solubility, electrical properties, and concentration on either side of the membrane. Small, lipid-soluble particles, such as oxygen, carbon dioxide, and urea, can readily pass the lipid bilayers of the plasma membrane. Larger, water-soluble particles may pass through pores in the membranes. Although large protein molecules, such as albumin and globulin, pass through membranes by

endocytosis, they influence the movement of water by exerting an osmotic effect (see p. 26).

Body fluids are composed of two types of solutes: **electrolytes,** which are electrically charged and dissociate into constituent **ions** when placed in solution; and nonelectrolytes, such as glucose, urea, and creatinine, which do not dissociate. Electrolytes account for approximately 95% of the solute molecules in body water. Electrolytes exhibit **polarity** by orienting themselves toward the positive or negative pole. Ions with a positive charge are known as **cations** and migrate toward the negative pole, or cathode, if an electrical current is passed through the electrolyte solution. **Anions** carry a negative charge and migrate toward the positive pole, or anode, in the presence of electrical current. Anions and cations are located in both the intracellular fluid (ICF) and extracellular fluid (ECF) compartments, although concentration of particular ions varies depending on their location. (Fluid and electrolyte balance between body compartments is discussed in Chapter 3.) For example, Na^+ is the predominant extracellular cation, and K^+ is the principal intracellular cation. The difference in ICF and ECF concentrations of these ions is important to the transmission of electrical impulses across the plasma membranes of nerve and muscle cells.

Electrolytes are measured in milliequivalents per liter (mEq/L) or milligrams per deciliter (mg/dl). Milliequivalents per liter indicate the number of electrical charges per unit volume of fluid. The term *milliequivalent* thus indicates the chemical-combining activity of an ion, which depends on the electrical charge, or valence, of its ions. In abbreviations, valence is indicated by the number of plus or minus signs. Monovalent ions, or ions with one charge, include sodium (Na^+), chloride (Cl^-), and potassium (K^+). Divalent ions, which have two charges, include calcium (Ca^{++}) and magnesium (Mg^{++}). One milliequivalent of any cation can combine chemically with 1 mEq of any anion: one monovalent anion will combine with one monovalent cation. Divalent ions combine more strongly than monovalent ions. To maintain electrochemical balance, one divalent ion will combine with two monovalent ions (e.g., $Ca^{++} + 2\,Cl^- = CaCl_2$).

Passive Transport: Diffusion, Filtration, and Osmosis

Diffusion

Diffusion is the movement of a solute molecule from an area of greater solute concentration to an area of lesser solute concentration. This difference in concentration is known as a **concentration gradient.** Particles in a solution move randomly in any direction. If the concentration of particles in one part of the solution is greater than in another part, the particles distribute themselves evenly throughout the solution. According to the same principle, if the concentration of particles is greater on one side of a *permeable membrane* than on the other side, the particles diffuse spontaneously from the area of greater concentration to the area of lesser concentration until equilibrium is reached. The higher the concentration on one side, the greater the diffusion rate. The overall effect of diffusion is the passive movement of particles "down" a concentration gradient, that is, from an area of high concentration to an area of low concentration.

The diffusion rate is influenced by differences of electrical potential across the membrane (see p. 31). Because the pores in the lipid bilayer are often linked with Ca^{++}, other cations (e.g., Na^+ and K^+) diffuse slowly because they are repelled by positive charges in the pores.

The rate of diffusion of a substance depends also on its size (diffusion coefficient) and its lipid solubility (Figure 1-25). Usually, the smaller the molecule and the more soluble it is in oil, the more hydrophobic or nonpolar it is and the more rapidly it will diffuse across the bilayer. Oxygen, carbon dioxide, and the steroid hormones are all examples of nonpolar molecules. Water-soluble substances, such as sugars and inorganic ions, diffuse very slowly, whereas uncharged lipophilic ("lipid-loving") molecules, such as fatty acids and steroids, diffuse rapidly. Ions and other polar molecules generally diffuse across cellular membranes more slowly than lipid-soluble substances.

Water readily diffuses through biologic membranes because water molecules are small and uncharged. Although the mechanism is not known with certainty, the dipolar structure of water allows it to cross rapidly the regions of the bilayer containing the lipid head groups. Lipid head groups constitute the two outer regions of the lipid bilayer.

Filtration: Hydrostatic Pressure

Filtration is the movement of water and solutes through a membrane because of a greater pushing pressure (force) on one side of the membrane than on the other side. **Hydrosta-**

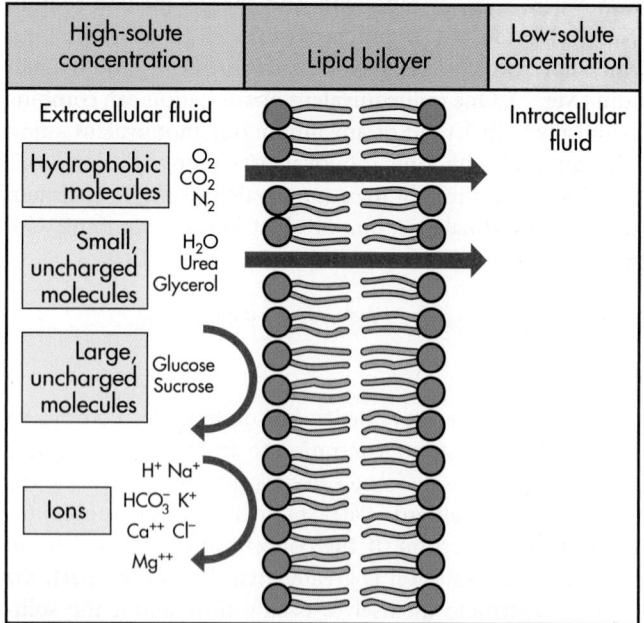

Figure 1-25 Passive diffusion of solute molecules across plasma membrane. Oxygen, nitrogen, water, urea, glycerol, and carbon dioxide can diffuse readily down the concentration gradient. Macromolecules are too large to diffuse through pores in the plasma membrane. Ions may be repelled if the pores contain substances with identical charges. If the pores are lined with cations, for example, other cations will have difficulty diffusing because the positive charges will repel one another. Diffusion can still occur, but it occurs more slowly.

tic pressure is the mechanical force of water pushing against cellular membranes. In the vascular system, hydrostatic pressure is the blood pressure generated in vessels by the contraction of the heart. Blood reaching the capillary bed has a hydrostatic pressure of 25 to 30 mm Hg, which is sufficient force to push water across the thin capillary membranes into the interstitial space. Hydrostatic pressure is partially balanced by osmotic pressure, whereby water moving *out* of the capillaries is partially balanced by osmotic forces that tend to *pull* water *into* the capillaries. Water that is not osmotically attracted back into the capillaries moves into the lymph system (see discussion of Starling forces in Chapter 3).

Osmosis

Osmosis is the movement of water "down" a concentration gradient, that is, across a semipermeable membrane from a region of higher water concentration to a lower water concentration. For osmosis to occur, the membrane must be more permeable to water than to solutes and the concentration of solutes must be greater so that water moves more easily. Osmosis is directly related to both hydrostatic pressure and solute concentration but *not* to particle size or weight. For example, particles of the plasma protein albumin are small but more concentrated in body fluids than the larger and heavier particles of globulin. Therefore albumin exerts a greater osmotic force than globulin.

Osmolality controls distribution and movement of water between body compartments. The terms *osmolality* and *osmolarity* are often used interchangeably in reference to osmotic activity, but they define different measurements. **Osmolality** is a measure of the number of milliosmoles per kilogram of water, or the concentration of molecules per *weight* of water. **Osmolarity** is a measure of the number of milliosmoles per liter of solution, or the concentration of molecules per *volume* of solution. When solute is added to water, the volume is expanded and includes the original liter of water plus the volume occupied by the solute particles. In measuring osmolarity, the volume of water is therefore reduced by an amount equal to the volume of added solute.

In solutions that contain only dissociable substances, such as Na^+ and Cl^-, the difference between the two measurements is negligible. In considering all the different solutes in plasma (e.g., proteins, glucose, lipids), however, the difference between osmolality and osmolarity becomes more significant. In plasma, less of the plasma weight is water and the overall concentration of particles is therefore greater. The osmolality will be greater than the osmolarity because of the smaller proportion of water. Osmolality is thus the preferred measure of osmotic activity in clinical assessment of individuals.

The normal osmolality of body fluids is 280 to 294 mOsm/kg (milliosmoles per kilogram). The osmolality of intracellular and extracellular fluid tends to equalize and so provides a measure of body fluid concentration and thus the body's hydration status (see Chapter 3). Hydration is also affected by hydrostatic pressure because the movement of water by osmosis can be opposed by an equal amount of hydrostatic pressure. The amount of hydrostatic pressure required to oppose the osmotic movement of water is called the **osmotic** pressure of the solution. Factors that determine osmotic pressure are the type and thickness of the plasma membrane, the size of the molecules, the concentration of molecules or the concentration gradient, and the solubility of molecules within the membrane. Examples of movement of water in relation to hydrostatic and osmotic forces occur in the glomerulus in the kidney (see Chapter 35) and in the capillaries of the microcirculation (see Chapter 29).

Effective osmolality is sustained osmotic activity and depends on the concentration of solutes remaining on one side of a permeable membrane. If the solutes penetrate the membrane and equilibrate with the solution on the other side of the membrane, the osmotic effect will be diminished or lost. For example, urea is a small solute that readily diffuses across cellular membranes. Solutions containing urea rapidly lose their effective osmolality because they rapidly equilibrate. Solutes too large to pass through the membrane thus sustain an effective osmolality, meaning that they enhance osmotic activity. Plasma proteins are examples of molecules that provide effective osmolality because they normally do not cross cellular membranes.

Plasma proteins also influence osmolality because they have a negative charge. The principle by which the plasma protein charge influences osmolality is known as *Gibbs-Donnan equilibrium,* and it affects the distribution of ions across cellular membranes. Gibbs-Donnan equilibrium occurs when fluid in one compartment contains small diffusible ions such as Na^+ and chloride Cl^-, together with large, nondiffusible charged particles, such as plasma proteins. Because the body tends to maintain an electrical equilibrium, the nondiffusible protein molecules cause asymmetry in the distribution of small ions. Anions such as Cl^- are thus driven out of the cell or plasma, and cations such as Na^+ are attracted. The protein-containing compartment will maintain a state of electroneutrality, but the osmolality will be higher. The overall osmotic effect of colloids, such as plasma proteins, is called the **oncotic pressure, or colloid osmotic pressure.**

Tonicity describes the effective osmolality of a solution. (The terms *osmolality* and *tonicity* may be used interchangeably; also see Chapter 3.) Solutions, then, have relative degrees of tonicity. An **isotonic solution** (or isoosmotic solution) has the same osmolality or concentration of particles (285 mOsm/kg) as the ICF or ECF. Diarrhea, for example, is loss of isoosmotic fluid from the gastrointestinal tract. As a result, ECF volume decreases but there is no change in ECF osmolarity. Examples of isotonic solutions include 5% dextrose in water and normal (0.9%) saline solution. A **hypotonic solution** has a lower concentration and is thus more dilute than body fluids. Water is a hypotonic solution. Consequently, water is osmotically pulled into the cells, causing them to swell or burst. A **hypertonic solution** has a concentration of more than 285 to 294 mOsm/kg. An example of a hypertonic solution is 3% saline solution. Water can be pulled out of the cells by a hypertonic solution, so the cells shrink. The concept of tonicity is important when correcting water and solute imbalances by administering different types of replacement solutions.

Mediated and Active Transport

Mediated Transport

Mediated transport (passive and active) involves integral or transmembrane proteins with receptors having a high degree of specificity for the substance being transported. Inorganic anions and cations (e.g., Na^+, K^+, Ca^{++}, Cl^-, HCO_3^-) and charged and uncharged organic compounds (e.g., amino acids, sugars) require specific transport systems to facilitate movement through different cellular membranes. Rates at which substances are moved by mediated transport mechanisms have often been measured, yet the specific membrane proteins involved have not been identified. Mediated transport is much faster than simple diffusion.

A **transport protein** (carrier protein) is a transmembrane or integral protein that binds with and transfers a specific solute molecule across the lipid bilayer. Each transport protein, or transporter, has receptors for a specific solute. When the transporter is saturated—that is, when all receptor sites are occupied by solute molecules—the rate of transport is maximal. Solute binding can be blocked by **competitive inhibitors** that compete for the same receptor site and may or may not be transported by the transport protein. Noncompetitive inhibitors bind elsewhere but can alter the structure of the transporter.

The transporter protein is a multipass, transmembrane protein; that is, its polypeptide chain crosses the lipid bilayer multiple times. This chain forms a continuous pathway enabling solutes to pass across the membrane without coming into direct contact with the hydrophobic interior of the lipid bilayer (Figure 1-26). (Transmembrane proteins are illustrated in Figure 1-13.)

Another mechanism of mediated transport is the channel protein. The protein transporter creates a water-filled pore or channel across the bilayer through which specific ions can diffuse. These channels are sometimes called *ion channels,* and because they are permeable mainly to K^+, they are also called K^+ *leak channels* (Figure 1-27). The channel is controlled by a gate mechanism that determines which receptor-bound solutes can move into the channel that is created after

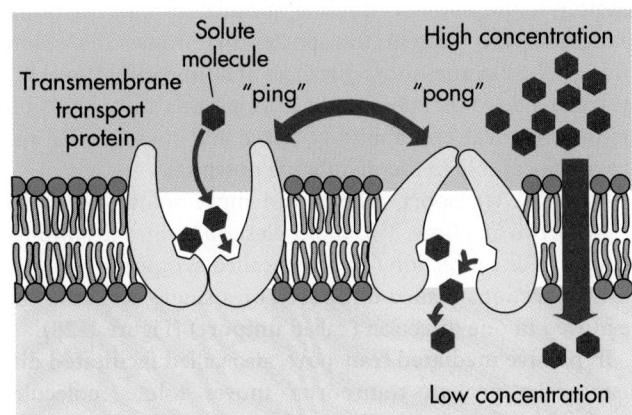

Figure 1-26 Conformational-change model of mediated transport (facilitated diffusion). The transporter protein has two states, "ping" and "pong." In the ping state, sites for molecules of a specific solute are exposed on the outside of the bilayer. In the pong state, the sites are exposed to the inner side of the bilayer.

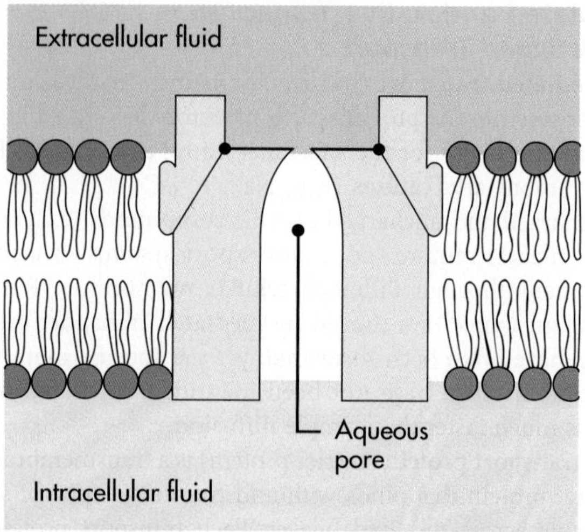

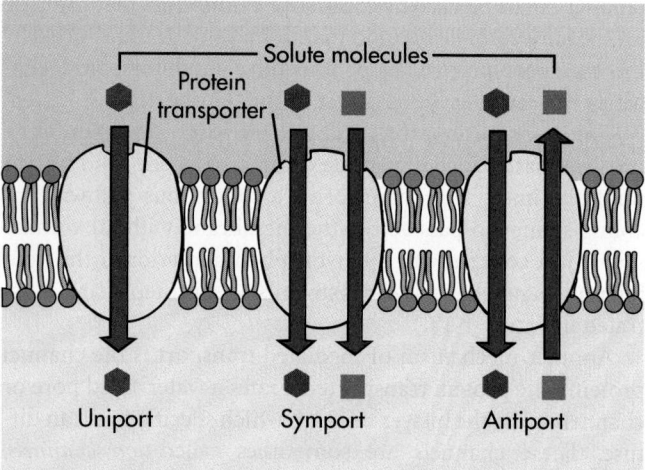

Figure 1-27 Channel mode of mediated transport (facilitated diffusion). A channel protein forms a water-filled pore across the bilayer through which specific ions can diffuse.

Figure 1-28 Mediated transport. Simultaneous movement of a single solute molecule in one direction (uniport), of two different solute molecules in one direction (symport), and of two different solute molecules in opposite directions (antiport).

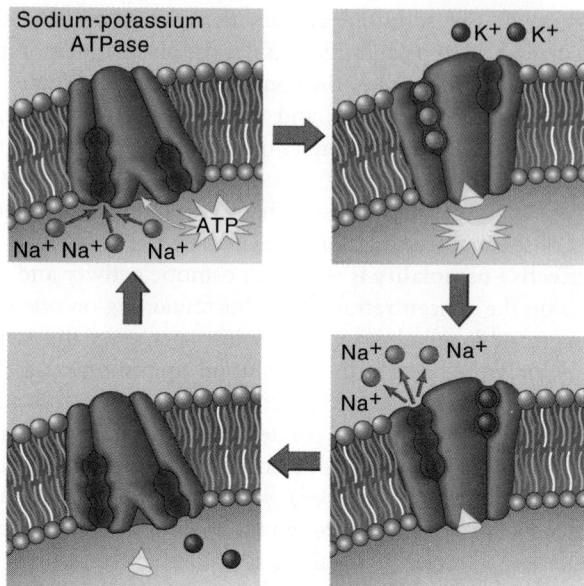

Figure 1-29 Active transport and the sodium-potassium pump. Three Na^+ ions bind to sodium-binding sites on the carrier's inner face. At the same time an energy-containing adenosine triphosphate (ATP) molecule produced by the cell's mitochondria binds to the carrier. The ATP breaks apart, transferring its stored energy to the carrier. The carrier then changes shape, releases the three Na^+ ions to the outside of the cell, and attracts two K^+ ions to its potassium-binding sites. The carrier then returns to its original shape, releasing the two K^+ ions and the remnant of the ATP molecule to the inside of the cell. The carrier is now ready for another pumping cycle. (From Thibodeau GA, Patton KT: *Anatomy & physiology*, ed 5, St Louis, 2003, Mosby.)

receptor-solute contact. Binding stimulates conformational changes in the protein transporter that move the solute through the channel short distances at a time until it reaches the other side of the membrane. Ion channels are responsible for the electrical excitability of nerve and muscle cells and play a critical role in the membrane potential.

Mediated transport systems can move solute molecules singly or two at a time. Two molecules can be moved simultaneously in one direction (a process called **symport**) or in opposite directions (called **antiport**), or a single molecule can be moved in one direction (called **uniport**) (Figure 1-28).

In **passive mediated transport,** also called **facilitated diffusion,** the protein transporter moves solute molecules through cellular membranes without expending metabolic energy. The direction of movement is the same as in simple diffusion—down the concentration gradient. Perhaps the most widely referred to passive transport system is that for glucose in erythrocytes (red blood cells). Glucose is trans-

ported by a uniport mechanism and demonstrates saturation kinetics; that is, the transport system is saturated when all the glucose-specific receptors on the membrane are occupied and operating at their maximal capacity.

The anions Cl^- and bicarbonate HCO_3^- also undergo passive mediated transport in the erythrocyte. This antiport mechanism allows Cl^- movement in one direction and simultaneous HCO_3^- movement in the opposite direction. The directions of movement depend on the concentration gradients of the ions across the membrane.

In **active mediated transport,** also called **active transport,** the protein transporter moves molecules against, or up, the concentration gradient. Unlike passive mediated transport, active mediated transport requires the expenditure of energy. Many active mediated transport systems, or pumps, have ATP as their primary energy source, but not all. Some use the electrochemical gradient of Na^+ across the membrane (Figure 1-29). Energy in the form of ATP, however, is required for activation of the Na^+ gradient.

A "carrier" mechanism in the plasma membrane mediates the transport of ions, such as Na^+, K^+, H^+, Cl^-, and HCO_3^-, and of nutrients, such as glucose and amino acids. Energy supplied by ATP is required to pump ions against a concentration gradient. The best-known pump is the Na^+-K^+–dependent ATPase pump. It continuously regulates the cells' volume by controlling leaks through pores or protein channels and maintains the ionic concentration gradient necessary for cellular excitation and membrane conductivity (see p. 32).

The maintenance of intracellular K^+ concentrations is also required for enzyme activity, including that of enzymes involved in protein synthesis.

Active Transport of Na⁺ and K⁺

The active transport system for Na^+ and K^+ is found in virtually all mammalian cells. The Na^+-K^+ antiport system (Na^+ moving out of and K^+ moving into the cell) uses the direct energy of ATP to move these cations. The transporter protein is an enzyme, ATPase. ATPase has a requirement for Na^+, K^+, and Mg^{++} ions. The concentration of ATPase in plasma membranes is directly related to Na^+-K^+ transport activity. Approximately 60% to 70% of the ATP synthesized by cells, especially muscle and nerve cells, is used to maintain the Na^+-K^+ transport system. Excitable tissues (e.g., muscle and nerve tissues) have a high concentration of Na^+-K^+ ATPase, as do other tissues that transport significant amounts of Na^+, for example, kidneys and salivary glands. For every ATP molecule hydrolyzed, three molecules of Na^+ are transported out of the cell, whereas only two molecules of K^+ move into the cell. The process leads to an electrical potential and is called *electrogenic,* with the inside of the cell more negative than the outside. The exact mechanism for transport of Na^+ and K^+ across the membrane is uncertain. One proposal is that ATPase induces the transporter protein to undergo several conformational changes, causing Na^+ and K^+ to move short distances (see Figure 1-29). The conformational change creates a lowering affinity for Na^+ and K^+ to the ATPase transporter, resulting in the release of the cations after transport.

The sarcoplasmic reticulum of heart muscle and skeletal muscle has an ATP-dependent Ca^{++} active transport system that regulates the Ca^{++} levels in the cell's cytoplasm, which in turn regulates muscle contraction and relaxation cycles (see Chapter 29). The Ca^{++} transport system depends on ATPase activity and is similar to that of Na^+-K^+ ATPase.

The transport of sugars and amino acids across the plasma membrane depends on the simultaneous movement (symport) of Na^+ or Na^+-dependent transport (see Figure 1-28). Na^+-dependent symport occurs primarily in the plasma membrane of epithelial cells of the kidney tubules and intestines. The transport of glucose is not directly dependent on the hydrolysis of ATP; however, the Na^+ gradient is ATP dependent, and thus ATP is indirectly involved in glucose transport.

The epithelial cells that line the intestines depend on Na^+ to transport various amino acids. Similarly, the uptake of Cl^- by the small intestine depends on Na^+ symport and antiport mechanisms for the secretion of Ca^{++} from the cell.

Table 1-5 summarizes the major mechanisms of transport through pores and protein transporters in the plasma membranes. Many disease states are caused or manifested by loss of these membrane transport systems.

Table 1-5	Major Transport Systems in Mammalian Cells	
Substance Transported	**Mechanism of Transport**	**Tissues**
Sugars		
Glucose	Passive protein channel	Most tissues
	Active: symport with Na^+	Small intestines and renal tubular cells
Fructose	Passive	Intestines and liver
Amino Acids	Coupled channels	
Amino acid specific transporters	Active: symport with Na^+	Intestines, kidney, and liver
All amino acids except proline	Active: group translocation	Liver
Specific amino acids	Passive	Small intestine
Other Organic Molecules		
Cholic acid, deoxycholic acid, and tauro-cholic acid	Active: symport with Na^+	Intestines
Organic anions, e.g., malate, α-ketoglutarate, glutamate	Antiport with counter-organic anion	Mitochondria of liver cells
ATP-ADP	Antiport transport of nucleotides; can be active	Mitochondria of liver cells
Inorganic Ions		
Na^+	Passive	Distal renal tubular cells
Na^+/H^+	Active antiport, proton pump	Proximal renal tubular cells and small intestines
Na^+/K^+	Active: ATP driven, protein channel	Plasma membrane of most cells
Ca^{++}	Active: ATP driven, antiport with Na^+	All cells, antiporter in red cells
H^+/K^+	Active	Parietal cells of gastric cells secreting H^+
Cl^-/HCO_3^- (perhaps other anions)	Mediated: antiport (anion transporter–band 3 protein)	Erythrocytes and many other cells
Water	Osmosis passive	All tissues

Data from Alberts B et al: *Molecular biology of the cell,* ed 4, New York, 2001, Garland; Devlin TM, editor: *Textbook of biochemistry: with clinical correlations,* ed 3, New York, 1992, Wiley; Raven PH, Johnson GB: *Understanding biology,* ed 3, Dubuque, Iowa, 1995, Brown.

NOTE: The known transport systems are listed here; others have been proposed. Most transport systems have been studied in only a few tissues, and their sites of activity may be more limited than indicated.

ATP, Adenosine triphosphate; *ADP,* adenosine diphosphate.

Transport by Vesicle Formation
Endocytosis and Exocytosis

The active transport mechanisms by which the cells move large proteins, polynucleotides, or polysaccharides (macromolecules) across the plasma membrane are very different from those that mediate small solute and ion transport. Transport of macromolecules involves the sequential formation and fusion of membrane-bound vesicles.

In **endocytosis** a section of the plasma membrane enfolds substances from outside the cell, invaginates (folds inward), and separates from the plasma membrane, forming a vesicle that moves into the inside of the cell (Figure 1-30, A). Two types of endocytosis are designated based on the size of the vesicle formed. **Pinocytosis** (cell drinking) involves the ingestion of fluids and solute molecules through formation of small vesicles, and **phagocytosis** (cell eating) involves the ingestion of large particles, such as bacteria, through formation of large vesicles (also called *vacuoles*).

Because most cells continually ingest fluid and solutes by pinocytosis, the terms *pinocytosis* and *endocytosis* are often used interchangeably. In pinocytosis the vesicle containing fluids, solutes, or both fuses with a lysosome, and lysosomal enzymes digest them for use by the cell. In phagocytosis the large molecular substances are engulfed by the plasma membrane and enter the cell so that they can be isolated and destroyed by lysosomal enzymes (see Chapter 6). Substances that are not degraded by lysosomes are isolated in residual bodies and released by the cell by exocytosis. Both pinocytosis and phagocytosis require metabolic energy and often involve binding of the substance with plasma membrane receptors before membrane invagination and fusion with lysosomes in the cell.

In eukaryotic cells, secretion of macromolecules almost always occurs by exocytosis (see Figure 1-30, B). For example, to secrete macromolecules of insulin across plasma membranes, insulin-producing cells store and package insulin molecules in intracellular vesicles, which fuse with the plasma membrane and open to the extracellular space, or matrix, releasing the insulin. Not all secreted substances are secreted into the extracellular matrix. Some adhere to the plasma membrane and are thought to replace segments of the membrane lost through endocytosis or diffuse into the blood to nourish or signal other cells. Recent findings suggest membrane lipids may be a regulator of exocytosis.[17] Exocytosis has two main functions: (1) replacement of portions of the plasma membrane that have been removed by endocytosis and (2) release of molecules synthesized by the cells into the extracellular matrix.

Receptor-Mediated Endocytosis

Ligand binding to *some* plasma membrane receptors leads to clustering, aggregation, and immobilization of the receptors in specialized areas of the membrane called **coated pits** (Figure 1-31). The pits, which are coated with bristle-like structures (clathrin), deepen and enfold (invaginate), internalizing ligand-receptor complexes and forming a coated vesicle. The clathrin coat or bristles are thought to be responsible for trapping membrane receptors in coated pits. This internalization process, called **receptor-mediated endocytosis (ligand internalization)**, is rapid and enables the cell to ingest large amounts of specific ligands without ingesting large volumes of extracellular fluid. Inside the cell, the ingested material is processed by lysosomal enzymes.

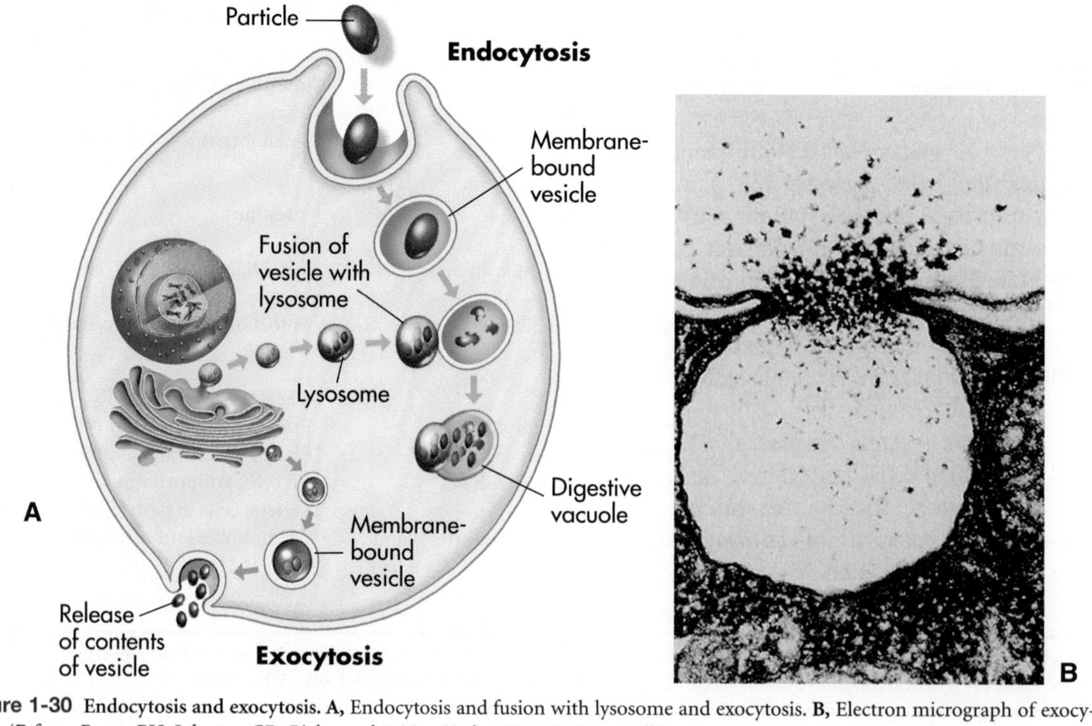

Figure 1-30 Endocytosis and exocytosis. A, Endocytosis and fusion with lysosome and exocytosis. **B,** Electron micrograph of exocytosis. (**B** from Raven PH, Johnson GB: *Biology,* ed 5, New York, 1999, McGraw-Hill.)

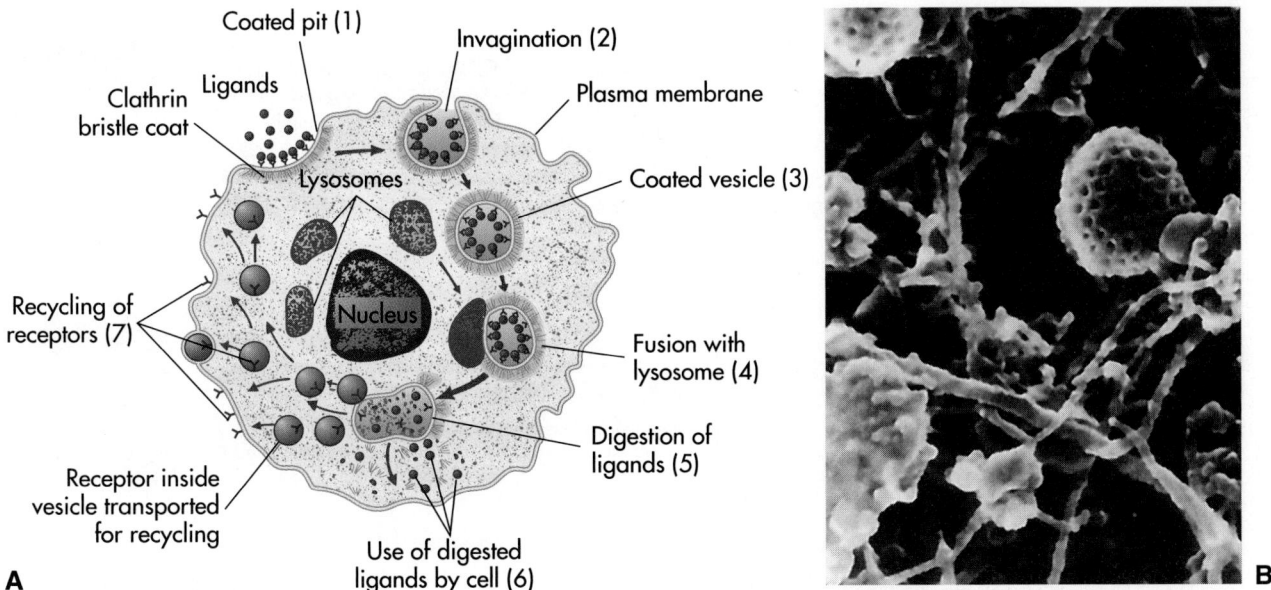

Figure 1-31 Ligand internalization by means of receptor-mediated endocytosis. **A,** The ligand attaches to its surface receptor (through the bristle coat or clathrin coat) and, through receptor-mediated endocytosis, enters the cell. The ingested material fuses with a lysosome and is processed by hydrolytic lysosomal enzymes. Processed molecules can then be transferred to other cellular components. **B,** Electron micrograph of a coated pit showing different sizes of filaments of the cytoskeleton (382,000). (**B** from Erlandsen SL, Magney JE: *Color atlas of histology,* St Louis, 1992, Mosby.)

The cellular uptake of cholesterol, for example, depends on receptor-mediated endocytosis. Cholesterol (a ligand) is carried primarily in blood plasma attached to an acceptor protein. This cholesterol-protein complex is called *low-density lipoprotein (LDL).* LDL receptors, which bind LDL to the plasma membrane, control the rate at which cholesterol is transferred into the cell (see Chapter 30).

Caveolae

The outer surface of the plasma membrane is dimpled with tiny flask-shaped pits (cavelike) called **caveolae** (see Figure 1-1). Caveolae are also called **microdomains.** Caveolae are cholesterol-rich domains where protein caveolin are involved in several processes, including clathrin-independent endocytosis, the regulation and transport of cellular cholesterol, and cell communication.[18] Many proteins, including a variety of receptors, cluster in these tiny chambers. Some of these receptors appear to be important in a new form of cellular uptake of small molecules and ions, for example, the cellular uptake of the B vitamin folic acid. When folic acid binds with its receptors, which are concentrated in the caveolae, the extracellular openings of these tiny caves close off. Closure of the caveolar indentation facilitates the movement of this vitamin across the caveolar membrane into the cytoplasm. Cellular uptake through the opening and closing of caveolae is called **potocytosis.** Potocytosis is thought to be an uptake mechanism for a variety of small molecules and ions, in contrast to receptor-mediated endocytosis, which transports selected large molecules into the cell. In potocytosis the caveolae are thought to *remain* attached to the plasma membrane and not form a membrane-enclosed vesicle such as occurs with endocytosis.

Caveolae not only function as uptake vesicles but also are important sites for signal transduction, a tedious process in which extracellular chemical messages or *signals* are communicated to the cell's interior for execution (see p. 17). For example, strong evidence now exists that plasma membrane estrogen receptors localize in caveolae and crosstalk with estradiol facilitates several intracellular functions, including cell growth and survival, migration, and new blood vessel formation.[19-21]

Movement of Electrical Impulses: Membrane Potentials

All body cells are electrically polarized, with the inside of the cell more negatively charged than the outside. The difference in electrical charge, or voltage, is known as the **resting membrane potential** and is about -70 to -85 millivolts. The difference in voltage across the plasma membrane is a result of the differences in ionic composition of ICF and ECF. Sodium ions have a greater concentration in the ECF, and potassium ions have a greater concentration in the ICF. The concentration difference is maintained by the active transport of Na^+ and K^+ (the sodium-potassium pump), which transports sodium outward and potassium inward (Figure 1-32). Because the resting plasma membrane is more permeable to K^+ than to Na^+, K^+ can diffuse easily from its area of higher concentration in the ICF to its area of lower concentration in the ECF. Because Na^+ and K^+ are both cations, the net result is an excess of anions inside the cell, resulting in the resting membrane potential.

Nerve and muscle cells are excitable and can change their resting membrane potential in response to electrochemical stimuli. Changes in resting membrane potential convey messages from cell to cell. When a nerve or muscle cell receives a stimulus that exceeds the membrane threshold value, there is

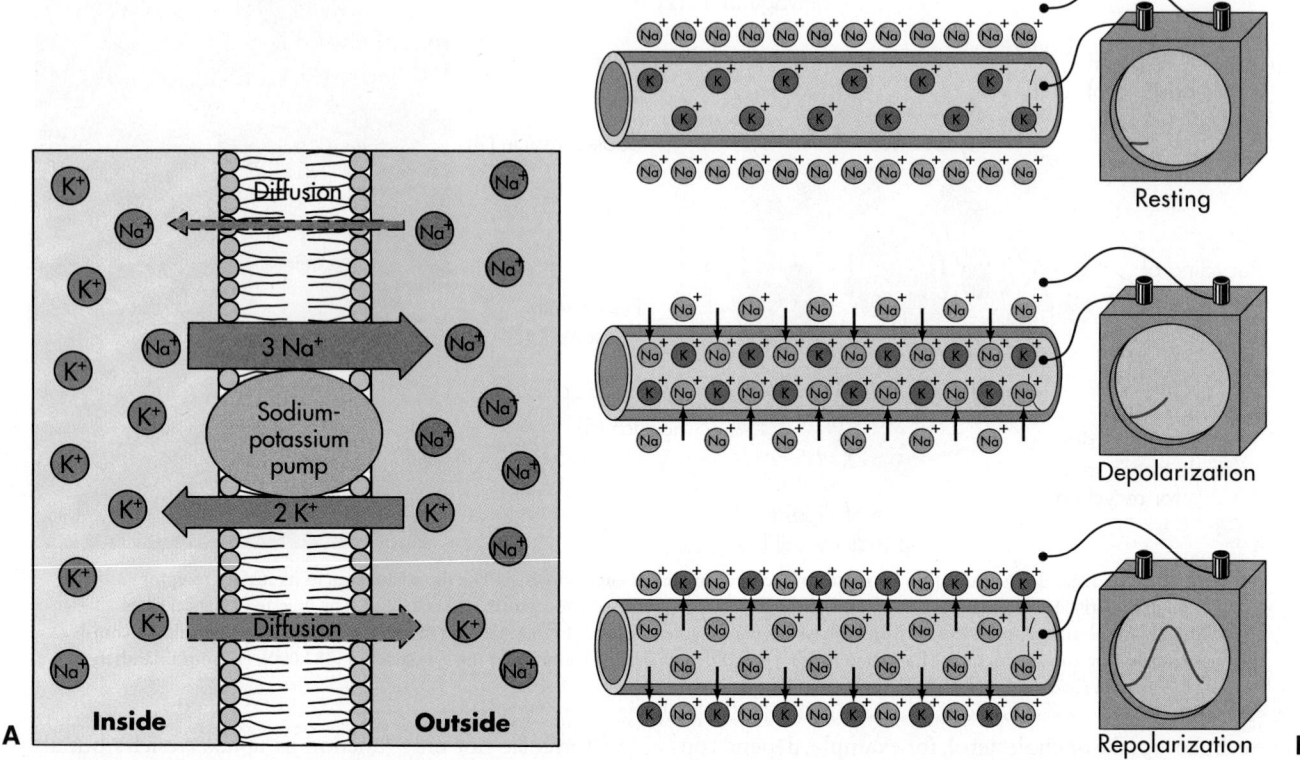

Figure 1-32 Sodium-potassium pump and propagation of an action potential. **A,** Concentration difference of Na$^+$ and K$^+$ intracellularly and extracellularly. The direction of active transport by the sodium-potassium pump is also shown. **B,** Top diagram represents the polarized state of a neuronal membrane when at rest. The lower diagrams represent changes in sodium and potassium membrane permeabilities with depolarization and repolarization. (From Thibodeau GA, Patton KT: *Anatomy & physiology*, ed 5, St Louis, 2003, Mosby.)

a rapid change in the resting membrane potential known as the **action potential.** The action potential carries signals along the nerve or muscle cell and conveys information from one cell to another. (Nerve impulses are described in Chapter 14.) When a resting cell is stimulated through voltage-regulated channels, the cell membranes become more permeable to sodium. There is a net movement of sodium into the cell, and the membrane potential decreases, or "moves forward," from a negative value (in millivolts) to zero. This decrease is known as **depolarization.** The depolarized cell is more positively charged, and its polarity is neutralized.

To generate an action potential and the resulting depolarization, a critical value known as the **threshold potential** must be reached. Generally this occurs when the cell has depolarized by 15 to 20 millivolts. When the threshold is reached, the cell will continue to depolarize with no further stimulation. The sodium gates open, and sodium rushes into the cell, causing the membrane potential to reduce to zero and then become positive (depolarization). The rapid reversal in polarity results in the action potential.

During **repolarization** the negative polarity of the resting membrane potential is reestablished. As the voltage-gated sodium channels begin to close, voltage-gated potassium channels open. Membrane permeability to sodium decreases, and potassium permeability increases, with an outward movement of potassium ions. The sodium gates close, and with the outward movement of potassium, the membrane

potential becomes more negative. The Na$^+$-K$^+$ pump then returns the membrane to the resting potential by pumping potassium back into the cell and sodium out of the cell.

During most of the action potential, the plasma membrane cannot respond to an additional stimulus. This time is known as the **absolute refractory period** and is related to changes in permeability to sodium. During the latter phase of the action potential, when permeability to potassium increases, a stronger-than-normal stimulus can evoke an action potential known as the **relative refractory period.**

When the membrane potential is more negative than normal, the cell is in a *hyperpolarized* (less excitable) state. A larger-than-normal stimulus is then required to reach the threshold potential and generate an action potential. When the membrane potential is more positive than normal, the cell is in a *hypopolarized* (more excitable than normal) state, and a smaller-than-normal stimulus is required to reach the threshold potential. Changes in the intracellular and extracellular concentration of ions or a change in membrane permeability can cause these alterations in membrane excitability.

CELLULAR REPRODUCTION: THE CELL CYCLE

Human cells are subject to wear and tear, and most do not last for the lifetime of the individual. In almost all tissues, new cells are created as fast as old ones die. Cellular reproduction is therefore necessary for the maintenance of life. Reproduction of gametes (sperm and egg cells) occurs through a process called *meiosis*, described in Chapter 4. The reproduction, or division, of other body cells (somatic cells) involves two sequential phases: **mitosis,** or nuclear division, and **cytokinesis,** or cytoplasmic division. These two phases occur in close succession, with cytokinesis beginning toward the end of mitosis. Before a cell can divide, however, it must double its mass and duplicate all its contents. Most of the work of preparing for division occurs during the growth phase, called **interphase.** The alternation between mitosis and interphase in all tissues with cellular turnover is known as the **cell cycle.**

Most of the early work on the cell cycle was limited to microscopic observation of mitosis and cytokinesis. Interphase was considered the "resting stage" of the cell. With recent technologic advances a considerable amount has been learned about the interphase part of the cell cycle. During interphase many important processes are taking place as the cell produces DNA, RNA, protein, lipids, and other substances, and

each pair of **chromosomes** (paired organelles that carry genetic information) also makes exact copies of themselves.

The four designated phases of the cell cycle are (1) the G_1 phase (G = gap), which is the period between the M phase and the start of DNA synthesis; (2) the S phase (S = synthesis), in which DNA is synthesized in the cell nucleus; (3) the G_2 phase, in which RNA and protein synthesis occurs, the period between the completion of DNA synthesis and the next phase (M); and (4) the M phase (M = mitosis), which includes both nuclear and cytoplasmic division (Figure 1-33).

Phases of Mitosis and Cytokinesis

Interphase (the G_1, S, and G_2 phases) is the longest phase of the cell cycle. During interphase the chromatin consists of very long, slender rods that are jumbled together in the nucleus. Late in interphase, strands of **chromatin** (the substance that gives the nucleus its granular appearance) begin to coil, causing them to shorten and thicken.

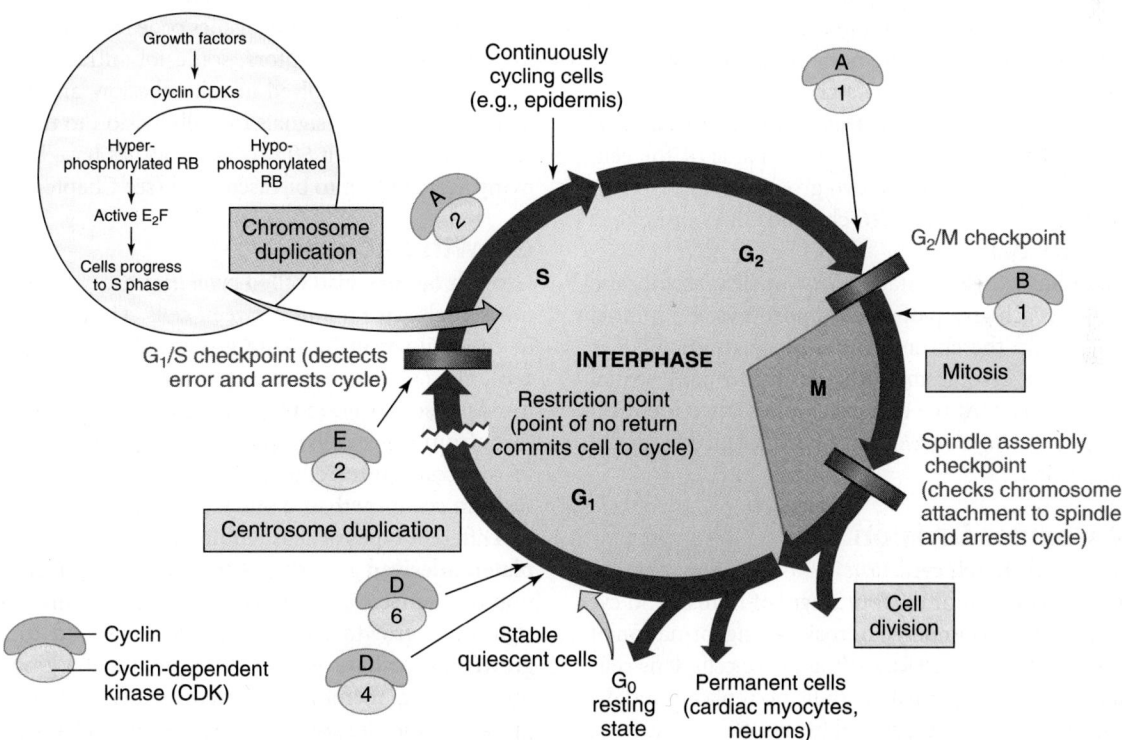

Figure 1-33 The cell cycle. The cell cycle consists of gap 1 (or G_1) (presynthesis), S (DNA synthesis), G_2 (premitotic) and M (mitotic) phases. Quiescent (quiet or resting state) are in the G_0 phase; however, most mature tissues have a combination of continuously dividing cells, terminally differentiated cells, stems cells, and some quiescent cells that infrequently enter the cell cycle. Continuously dividing cells replace those that are destroyed (e.g., epithelia of the oral cavity, skin). Quiescent or stable tissues exhibit a low level of replication; however, these cells can undergo rapid division in response to stimuli such as growth factors (e.g. EGF, TGF-α). Cyclins (see below) increase and activate cyclin-dependent protein kinase (CDK) complexes at the G_1/S restriction point causing phosphorylation (addition of phosphate group) of the molecular ON-OFF switch, the retinoblastoma susceptibility protein (RB). In its hypophosphorylated state, RB prevents cells from replicating by forming a tight inactive complex with the transcription factor E2F. Phosphorylation of RB eliminates the "brakes" to cell cycle progression and promotes cell replication. The orderly progression of cells through the phases of the cell cycle is regulated by cyclins, CDKs, and their inhibitors. Cyclin levels rise and fall (thus the name cyclin) during the cell cycle periodically activating CDKs. Unless CDKs are bound to cyclins, they have no protein kinase activity. Cyclin-CDK complexes trigger cell cycle events. Each complex phosphorylates a different set of proteins that then promote advancement to the next phase (G_1, S, G_2, M, G_0). After completion of the task, cyclin levels decline rapidly. The activity of cyclin-CDK complexes is regulated by CDK inhibitors including Cip/Kip and the 7NK4/ARF.

The M phase of the cell cycle, mitosis and cytokinesis, begins with **prophase,** the first appearance of chromosomes. As the phase proceeds, each chromosome is seen as two identical halves called **chromatids,** which lie together and are attached at some point by a spindle attachment site called a **centromere.** (The two chromatids of each chromosome, which are genetically identical, are sometimes called *sister chromatids.*) The nuclear membrane, which surrounds the nucleus, disappears. Spindle fibers are microtubules formed in the cytoplasm. **Spindle fibers** radiate from two centrioles located at opposite poles of the cell. The role of the spindle fibers is to pull the chromosomes to opposite sides of the cell.

During **metaphase,** the next phase of mitosis and cytokinesis, the spindle fibers begin to pull the centromeres of the chromosomes. The centromeres become aligned in the middle of the spindle, which is called the **equatorial plate** (or **metaphase plate**) of the cell. In this stage, chromosomes are easiest to observe microscopically because they are highly condensed and arranged in a relatively organized fashion in the two-dimensional equatorial plate.

Anaphase begins when the centromeres split and the sister chromatids are pulled apart. The spindle fibers shorten, causing the sister chromatids to be pulled, centromere first, toward opposite sides of the cell. When the sister chromatids are separated, each is considered to be a chromosome. Thus the cell has 92 chromosomes during this stage. By the end of anaphase, 46 chromosomes are lying at each side of the cell. Barring mitotic errors, each of the two groups of 46 chromosomes is identical to the original 46 chromosomes present at the start of the cell cycle.

During **telophase,** the final stage, a new nuclear membrane is formed around each group of 46 chromosomes, the spindle fibers disappear, and the chromosomes begin to uncoil. Cytokinesis causes the cytoplasm to divide into roughly equal parts during this phase. At the end of telophase, two identical diploid cells, called *daughter cells,* have been formed from the original cell.

Rates of Cellular Division

Although the complete cell cycle lasts 12 to 24 hours, about 1 hour is generally required for the four stages of mitosis and cytokinesis. All types of cells undergo mitosis during formation of the embryo, but many adult cells, such as nerve cells, lens cells of the eye, and muscle cells, lose their ability to replicate and divide. The cells of other tissues, particularly epithelial cells (e.g., of the intestine, lung, skin), divide continuously and rapidly, completing the entire cell cycle in less than 10 hours.

The difference between cells that divide slowly and cells that divide rapidly is the length of time spent in the G_1 phase of the cell cycle. Some cells that divide very slowly remain in the G_1 phase for days or even years. Once the S phase begins, however, progression through mitosis takes a relatively constant amount of time. Once a cell has progressed out of the G_1 phase, there is no turning back; it is committed to completing the S, G_2, and M phases. Times associated with the four successive phases differ.

The mechanisms that control cell division depend on "social control genes" and protein growth factors. Individual cells are members of a complex cellular society in which survival of the *entire organism* is key and not survival or proliferation of just the *individual cells.* To grow and divide, a cell must receive specific positive signals from other cells. Many of these signals *are* protein growth factors that act by overriding intracellular negative controls that block progress of the cell cycle.[1]

When a need arises for new cells, as in repair of injured cells, previously nondividing cells must be rapidly triggered to reenter the cell cycle. With continual wear and tear, the cell birth rate and the cell death rate must be kept in balance. Therefore cell-division controls must govern this balance. Protein growth factors governing the proliferation of different cell types and genes involved in the social control of cell division are currently being identified.[1]

The best model for understanding disruption of cell division and study of these so-called social control genes is tumor biology. Current emphasis in locating and identifying these genes is to study tumor cells that have presumably originated because of mutations to these genes, or proto-oncogenes. Proto-oncogenes are thought to encode key components of the normal system of social controls of cell division;[1] that is, the mechanisms by which signals from a cell's neighbors can impel it to divide, differentiate, or die. Some proto-oncogenes code for growth factors, some for growth factor receptors, some for intracellular regulatory proteins that are involved in cell adhesion, and some for proteins that help relay signals for cell division to the cell nucleus.[1] Although more than 50 proto-oncogenes have been identified, many more are yet to be discovered (see Chapter 11).

Growth Factors

Growth factors, also called *cytokines,* are peptides that transmit signals within and between cells. They have a major role in the regulation of tissue growth and development (Table 1-6). Having nutrients is not enough for a cell to proliferate, it must also receive stimulatory chemical signals (growth factors) from other cells, usually its neighbors. These signals act to overcome intracellular braking mechanisms that tend to restrain cell growth and block progress through the cell cycle.

Different types of cells require different factors; for example, **platelet-derived growth factor** (**PDGF**) stimulates the production of connective tissue cells. Table 1-6 summarizes the most significant growth factors. Cells that respond to a particular growth factor have specific receptors for the growth factor in their plasma membrane. Recent evidence shows that some growth factors are also regulators of other cell processes, such as cellular differentiation. In addition to growth factors that stimulate cellular processes, there are factors that inhibit functions; these factors are not well understood. Cells that are starved of growth factors come to a halt after mitosis and enter the **arrested,** or **G_0, state** of the cell cycle[1] (see p. 33 for cell cycle).

TISSUES

The body is made up of four levels of organization: cells, tissues, organs, and systems. Cells of common structure and function are organized into **tissues,** of which there are four primary types: *muscle, neural, epithelial,* and *connective* tissue.

Table 1-6	Examples of Growth Factors and Their Actions
Growth Factor	**Physiologic Actions**
Platelet-derived growth factor (PDGF)	Stimulates proliferation of connective tissue cells and neuroglial cells
Epidermal growth factor (EGF)	Stimulates proliferation of epidermal cells and other cell types
Insulin-like growth factor I (IGF-I)	Collaborates with PDGF and EGF; stimulates proliferation of fat cells and connective tissue cells
Insulin-like growth factor II (IGF-II)	Collaborates with PDGF and EGF; stimulates proliferation of fat cells and connective tissue cells
Transforming growth factor β (TGF-β)	Stimulates or inhibits response of most cells to other growth factors; regulates differentiation of some cell types (e.g., cartilage)
Fibroblast growth factor (FGF)	Stimulates proliferation of fibroblasts, endothelial cells, myoblasts, and other cell types
Interleukin-2 (IL-2)	Stimulates proliferation of T lymphocytes
Nerve growth factor (NGF)	Promotes axon growth and survival of sympathetic and some sensory and CNS neurons
Hemopoietic cell growth factors (IL-3, GM-CSF, M-CSF, G-CSF, erythropoietin)	See Chapter 24

CNS, Central nervous system; *GM,* granulocyte-macrophage; *CSF,* colony-stimulating factor; *M,* macrophage; *G,* granulocyte.

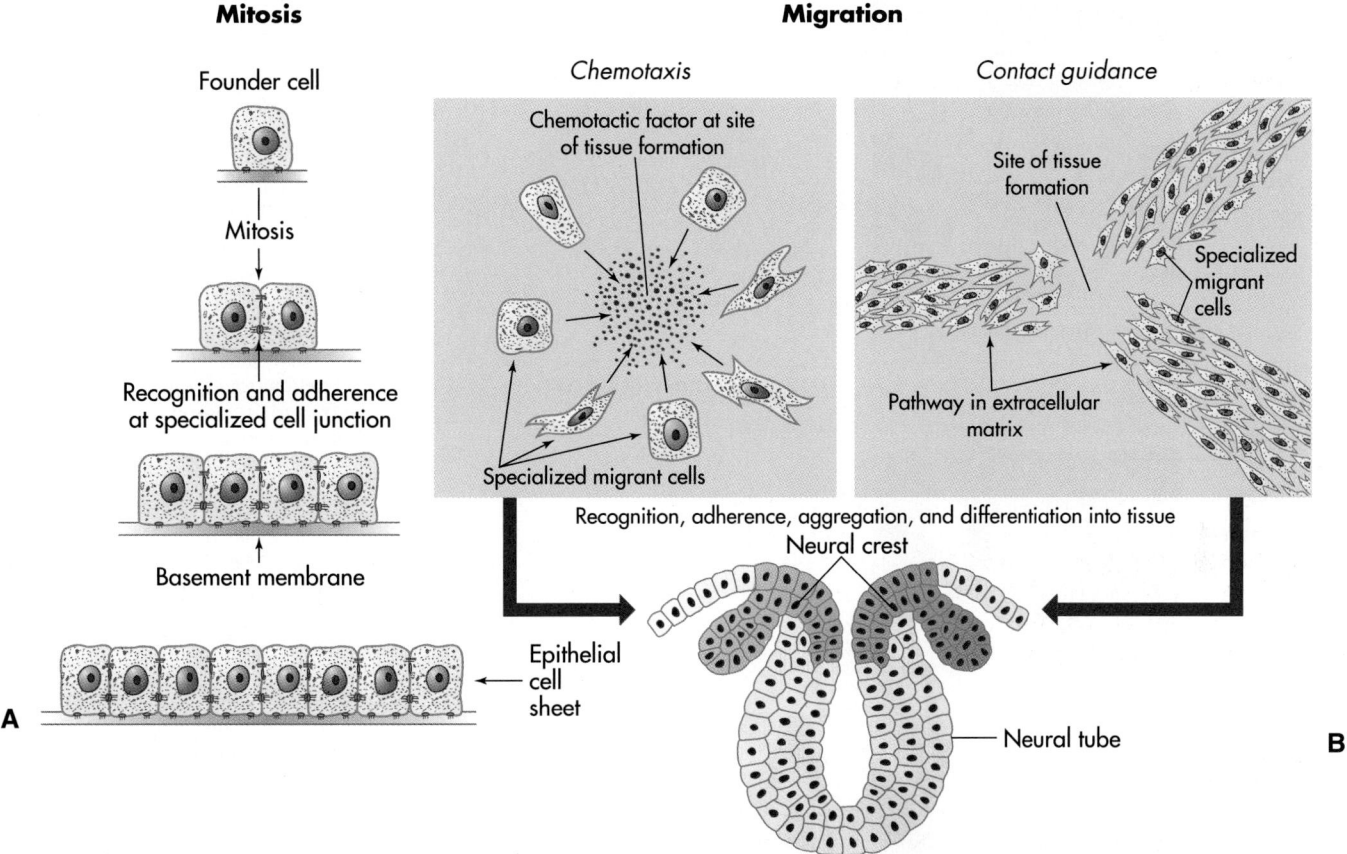

Figure 1-34 Tissue formation by mitosis and migration. A, Tissue formation by mitosis. Founder cells are kept in place by extracellular matrix and recognition and adherence at cell junctions. **B,** Tissue formation by migration. Specialized cells are attracted to the site of tissue formation by chemotaxis or contact guidance; then they aggregate and differentiate into organized tissue.

Tissue Formation

To form tissues, cells must exhibit intercellular recognition and adhesion. Specialized cells are thought to form a tissue in one of two ways. First and simplest is mitosis of one or more **founder cells** (the most basic precursor cell). Founder cells are prevented from "wandering away" by macromolecules in the extracellular matrix and by adherence to one another at specialized junctions on their plasma membranes. Mitosis of founder cells forms, for example, epithelial cell sheets (Figure 1-34).

The second way in which specialized cells form tissues involves their migration to and subsequent assembly at the site of tissue formation. During embryonic development, for example, cells from the neural crest migrate to several different regions, where they differentiate and assemble into a variety of tissues, including those of the peripheral nervous system. Migrant cells are thought to arrive at the site of tissue formation through chemotaxis or contact guidance. **Chemotaxis** is movement along a chemical gradient caused by chemical attraction (see Chapter 6). Cells at the migrant cells' destination secrete a chemical, called *chemotactic factor,* that attracts specific migrant cells. **Contact guidance** is movement along a pathway, or "pavement," in the extracellular matrix.[1]

Table 1-7   Some Types of Epithelial Tissue with Location and Function

Type of Epithelial Tissue	Location	Function
Cytoplasm — Nucleus — *Simple squamous*	Lines major organs (heart, air sacs of lungs, Bowman capsule of kidney); lines body cavity	Absorption, exchange of materials, filtration, secretion
Cytoplasm — Interior of kidney tubules — Nucleus — *Simple cuboidal*	Lines tubules and ducts of glands; covers surface of ovary; lines interior of eye	Absorption and secretion
Globular cell — Cytoplasm — Nucleus — *Simple columnar*	Lines gastrointestinal tract	Secretion from special goblet cells of materials, absorption
Stratified squamous	Lines interior of mouth, tongue, esophagus, vagina	Protection

Modified from Raven PH, Johnson GB: *Understanding biology,* ed 3, Dubuque, Iowa, 1995, Brown.

Table 1-7	Some Types of Epithelial Tissue with Location and Function—cont'd		
Type of Epithelial Tissue		**Location**	**Function**
Transitional		Lines urinary bladder	Permits stretching

Tissues are not randomly arranged into organs. No matter how tissue is formed, staying together in groups means that cells must recognize each other and remain distinct from the cells of surrounding tissues. Little is known about the mechanisms involved in these processes.

Types of Tissues

Epithelial Tissue

Epithelial tissue covers most internal and external surfaces of the body. Epithelial cells are closely joined and are attached to a basement membrane or lamina (extracellular matrix), which provides a supporting layer and separates the epithelium from underlying connective tissue (see Figure 1-14). Because of its variety of locations, epithelial tissue has several diverse functions, including protection, absorption, secretion, and excretion. For example, the epidermis provides a protective barrier between the host and the outside environment, and the linings of the internal body organs help absorb substances into the body, excrete waste products, and secrete substances into body cavities.

Epithelial cell surfaces differ according to their location and function. Epithelial cells that line body cavities and blood vessels are smooth, whereas other epithelial cells have tiny cytoplasmic projections called **microvilli** on their free surfaces. Microvilli considerably increase the cell's surface area and are found on cells whose main functions are absorption and secretion, such as the epithelial cells lining the digestive tract. **Cilia,** which are hairlike projections that propel mucus, pus, and dust particles out of the body, characterize cells lining the respiratory passages.

Epithelial tissue is classified in two ways: (1) according to the number and arrangement of cell layers and (2) according to cell shape. Epithelium that is formed by a single layer of cells, all of which are in contact with the basement membrane, is called **simple epithelium. Stratified epithelium** has two or more layers of cells, and only the deepest layer is in contact with the basement membrane. Tissue that appears to consist of several cellular layers but is actually a single layer with all cells contacting the basement membrane is called **pseudostratified epithelium.**

Three basic cell shapes are found in epithelium: squamous, cuboidal, and columnar. **Squamous cells** are flat and thin;

cuboidal cells are as high as they are wide and thus appear square in vertical sections; and **columnar cells** are taller than they are wide and appear rectangular in vertical sections. Overall classifications of epithelial tissue, which take into account both the number of cell layers and cell shape, are summarized in Table 1-7.

Connective Tissue

Connective tissue varies considerably in structure and function but is most common as the framework on which epithelial cells cluster to form organs. Other functions include binding various tissues and organs together, supporting them in their locations, and serving as storage sites for excess nutrients.

In contrast to epithelial tissue, connective tissue is characterized by an abundant extracellular matrix that surrounds few cells. The extracellular matrix is composed of ground substance and fibers. **Ground substance** is a homogeneous mass that varies in consistency from fluid to semisolid gel. Fibers are produced by connective tissue cells (fibroblasts) found within the ground substance. The three types of fibers are collagenous (white), elastic (yellow), and reticular. **Collagenous fibers** are formed of bundles of smaller fibers appearing as wavy bands under the microscope. These fibers are composed of the protein collagen and are strong and inelastic. (Collagen synthesis by fibroblasts is described with respect to tissue repair in Chapter 6.) **Elastic fibers** are long, branching fibers composed of a protein called *elastin* that enables the fibers to return to their original length after stretching. Elastin occurs not only as fibers but also as membranes, particularly the membranes of blood vessels. **Reticular fibers** are thin, short, branching fibers that form an inelastic network made from a collagen-like protein called *reticulum*. Reticular fibers form the internal framework (stroma) to which the epithelial cells of glands are attached. They are found in loose connective tissue, generally in bone marrow and in the **parenchyma** (i.e., the essential substance of an organ rather than its framework) of the liver, spleen, and lymph nodes.

Connective tissues are classified according to the consistency (e.g., loose, dense) of the ground substance and the type and organization of the fibers within it. Table 1-8 summarizes the characteristics of connective tissues.

Table 1-8   Types of Connective Tissue with Location and Function

Type of Connective Tissue	Location	Function
 Loose connective tissue	Deep layers of skin, blood vessels, nerves, body organs	Support, elasticity
 Dense connective tissue	Tendons, ligaments	Attaches structures to one another; provides great strength
 Elastic connective tissue	Lungs, arteries, trachea, vocal chords	Provides elasticity
 Reticular connective tissue	Spleen, liver, lymph nodes	Provides internal scaffold for soft organs

Modified from Raven PH, Johnson GB: *Understanding biology*, ed 3, Dubuque, Iowa, 1995, Brown.

Table 1-8	Types of Connective Tissue with Location and Function—cont'd	
Type of Connective Tissue	**Location**	**Function**
Chondrocyte — Matrix — Cartilage	Ends of long bones; tip of nose; parts of larynx, trachea	Provides flexibility and support
Haversian canal — Osteocyte — Bone	Bones	Protection, support, muscle attachment
Plasma cell — Leukocyte — Red blood cell — Vascular connective tissue	Within blood vessels	Transport oxygen and carbon dioxide; immune response; blood clotting
Adipocytes — Adipose tissue	Deep layers of skin; surrounds heart and kidneys; padding around joints; paracrine hormones	Support, protection, heat conservation, energy source

Table 1-9   Types of Muscle Tissue with Location and Function

Type of Connective Tissue	Location	Function
 Smooth muscle	Gastrointestinal tract, uterus, urinary bladder, blood vessels	Propulsion of materials
 Cardiac muscle	Heart	Contraction
 Skeletal muscle	Attached to bones	Movement

Modified from Raven PH, Johnson GB: *Understanding biology,* ed 3, Dubuque, Iowa, 1995, Brown.

Muscle Tissue

Muscle tissue is composed of long, thin cells or fibers called *myocytes*. Myocytes are highly contractile. The three types of muscle tissues are skeletal, cardiac, and smooth (Table 1-9). (Muscles are discussed in detail in Chapter 41.)

Neural Tissue

Neural tissue is composed of highly specialized cells called *neurons*, which receive and transmit electrical impulses very rapidly across junctions called synapses. **Synapses** are points of functional contact between neurons. At synapses, impulses pass from neuron to neuron or from a neuron to a muscle cell as chemical messengers called *neurotransmitters* are released (see Chapter 14). The total number of neurons is fixed at birth, and replacement is impossible thereafter.

Different types of neurons have special characteristics that depend on their distribution and function within the nervous system. All neurons, however, are composed of the following parts: (1) a cell body, (2) a single axon, and (3) one or more dendrites (see Figure 14-1 on p. 412). The cell body contains special cytoplasmic structures, as well as microtubules, actin filaments, Golgi complex, lysosomes, and lipofuscin. The axons and dendrites can be very long. Generally, the axon conducts nerve impulses away from the cell body, and dendrites conduct nerve impulses toward the cell body. (Neuronal transmission is discussed in Chapter 14.)

Cellular Functions

1. Cells become specialized through the process of differentiation, or maturation.
2. The eight specialized cellular functions are movement, conductivity, metabolic absorption, secretion, excretion, respiration, reproduction, and communication.

Structure and Function of Cellular Components

1. The eukaryotic cell consists of three general components: the plasma membrane, the cytoplasm, and the intracellular organelles.
2. The nucleus is the largest membrane-bound organelle and is usually found in the cell's center. The chief functions of the nucleus are cell division and control of genetic information.
3. Cytoplasm, or the cytoplasmic matrix, is an aqueous solution (cytosol) that fills the space between the nucleus and the plasma membrane.
4. The organelles are suspended in the cytoplasm and are enclosed in biologic membranes.
5. The endoplasmic reticulum is a network of tubular channels (cisternae) that extend throughout the outer nuclear membrane. It specializes in the synthesis and transport of protein and lipid components of most of the organelles.
6. The Golgi complex is a network of smooth membranes and vesicles located near the nucleus. The Golgi complex is responsible for processing and packaging proteins into secretory vesicles that break away from the Golgi complex and migrate to a variety of intracellular and extracellular destinations, including the plasma membrane.
7. Lysosomes are saclike structures that originate from the Golgi complex and contain digestive enzymes. These enzymes are responsible for digesting most cellular substances down to their basic form, such as amino acids, fatty acids, and sugars.
8. Cellular injury leads to a release of the lysosomal enzymes causing cellular self-digestion.
9. Peroxisomes are similar to lysosomes but contain several enzymes that either produce or use hydrogen peroxide.
10. Mitochondria contain the metabolic machinery necessary for cellular energy metabolism. The enzymes of the respiratory chain (electron transport chain), found in the inner membrane of the mitochondria, generate most of the cell's ATP.
11. Vaults are newly discovered ribonucleoproteins thought to function as cellular "trucks" carrying mRNA from the nucleus to the ribosomal sites of protein synthesis.
12. The cytoskeleton is the "bone and muscle" of the cell. The internal skeleton is composed of a network of protein filaments including microtubules and actin filaments (microfilaments).
13. The plasma membrane encloses the cell and, by controlling the movement of substances across it, exerts a powerful influence on metabolic pathways.
14. The plasma membrane is a bilayer of lipids (phospholipids, glycolipids) and cholesterol, which gives the membrane its structural integrity.
15. Membrane functions are determined largely by proteins. These functions include (a) recognition and binding units (receptors) for substances moving in and out of the cell; (b) pores or transport channels; (c) enzymes that drive active pumps; (d) cell surface markers, such as glycoproteins; (e) cell adhesion molecules; and (f) catalysts of chemical reactions.
16. The fluid mosaic model accounts for the fluidity of the lipid bilayer and the flexibility, self-sealing properties, and selective impermeability of the plasma membrane.
17. Cellular receptors are protein molecules on the plasma membrane, in the cytoplasm, or in the nucleus, capable of recognizing and binding smaller molecules, called *ligands*.
18. The dynamic nature of the fluid plasma membrane enables it to vary the number of receptors on its surface. The cell is therefore capable of "hiding" from injurious agents by altering receptor number and pattern.
19. The ligand-receptor complex initiates a series of protein interactions, causing adenylyl cyclase to catalyze the transformation of cellular ATP to messenger molecules that stimulate specific responses within the cell.

Cell-to-Cell Adhesions

1. Cell-to-cell adhesions are formed on plasma membranes thereby allowing the formation of tissues and organs. Cells are held together by three different means: (a) the extracellular membrane, (b) cell adhesion molecules in the cell's plasma membrane, and (c) specialized cell junctions.
2. The extracellular matrix includes three types of protein fibers: collagen, elastin, and fibronectin. The matrix helps regulate cell growth and differentiation.
3. The three main types of cell junctions are desmosomes, tight junctions, and gap junctions.

Cellular Communication and Signal Transduction

1. Cells communicate in three ways: (a) they form protein channels (gap junctions); (b) they display receptors that affect intracellular processes or other cells in direct physical contact; and (c) they secrete signals for long-distance communication.
2. Primary modes of chemical signaling include hormonal, neurohormonal, paracrine, autocrine, and neurotransmitter.
3. Signal transduction involves signals or instructions from extracellular chemical messengers that are conveyed to the cell's interior for execution.
4. Signaling cascades, or relay chains, have several important functions, including physically transferring the signal around the cell, amplifying the signal, distributing the signal, and modulating the signal.
5. Two important second messenger pathways are cAMP and Ca^{++}.
6. G protein is an intermediary between the receptor and adenylyl cyclase.
7. Phospholipase C, an enzyme protein effector, is bound to the inner side of the membrane.

Cellular Metabolism

1. The chemical tasks of maintaining essential cellular functions are referred to as *cellular metabolism*. Anabolism is the energy-using process of metabolism, whereas catabolism is the energy-releasing process.
2. Adenosine triphosphate (ATP) functions as an energy-transferring molecule. Energy is stored by molecules of carbohydrate, lipid, and protein, which, when catabolized, transfer energy to ATP.
3. Oxidative phosphorylation occurs in the mitochondria and is the mechanism by which the energy produced from carbohydrates, fats, and proteins is transferred to ATP.

Membrane Transport: Cellular Intake and Output

1. Water and small, electrically uncharged molecules move through pores in the plasma membrane's lipid bilayer in the process called *passive transport*.
2. Passive transport does not require the expenditure of energy; rather, it is driven by the physical effects of osmosis, hydrostatic pressure, and diffusion.
3. Larger molecules and molecular complexes (e.g., ligand-receptor complexes) are moved into the cell by active transport, which requires expenditure of energy (by means of ATP) by the cell.

Continued

SUMMARY REVIEW—cont'd

4. The largest molecules (macromolecules) and fluids are transported by the processes of endocytosis (ingestion) and exocytosis (expulsion).

5. Two types of solutes exist in body fluids: electrolytes and nonelectrolytes. Electrolytes are electrically charged and dissociate into constituent ions when placed in solution. Nonelectrolytes do not dissociate when placed in solution.

6. Diffusion is the passive movement of a solute from an area of higher solute concentration to an area of lower solute concentration.

7. Hydrostatic pressure is the mechanical force of water pushing against cellular membranes.

8. Osmosis is the movement of water across a semipermeable membrane from a region of lower solute concentration to a region of higher solute concentration.

9. The amount of hydrostatic pressure required to oppose the osmotic movement of water is called the *osmotic pressure* of the solution.

10. The overall osmotic effect of colloids, such as plasma proteins, is called the *oncotic pressure* or *colloid osmotic pressure*.

11. Mediated transport can be passive or active. Mediated transport includes the movement of two molecules simultaneously in one direction (symport) or in opposite directions (antiport) or the movement of a single molecule in one direction (uniport).

12. Passive mediated transport is also called *facilitated diffusion*. It does not require the expenditure of metabolic energy.

13. Active mediated transport requires metabolic energy (ATP) to move molecules against the concentration gradient.

14. Active transport also occurs by endocytosis, or vesicle formation, in which the substance to be transported is engulfed by a segment of the plasma membrane, forming a vesicle that moves into the cell.

15. Pinocytosis is a type of endocytosis in which fluids and solute molecules are ingested through formation of small vesicles.

16. Phagocytosis is a type of endocytosis in which large particles, such as bacteria, are ingested through formation of large vesicles, called *vacuoles*.

17. In receptor-mediated endocytosis, the plasma membrane receptors are clustered, along with bristle-like structures, in specialized areas called *coated pits*.

18. Endocytosis occurs when coated pits invaginate, internalizing ligand-receptor complexes in coated vesicles.

19. Inside the cell, material ingested by endocytosis is processed and digested by lysosomal enzymes.

20. Caveolae are tiny flask-shaped pits on the outer surface of the plasma membrane. Cellular uptake through the opening and closing of caveolae is called *potocytosis*.

21. All body cells are electrically polarized, with the inside of the cell more negatively charged than the outside. The difference in voltage across the plasma membrane is the resting membrane potential.

22. When an excitable (nerve or muscle) cell receives an electrochemical stimulus, cations enter the cell, causing a rapid change in the resting membrane potential known as the *action potential*. The action potential "moves" along the cell's plasma membrane and is transmitted to an adjacent cell. This is how electrochemical signals convey information from cell to cell.

Cellular Reproduction: The Cell Cycle

1. Cellular reproduction in body tissues involves mitosis (nuclear division) and cytokinesis (cytoplasmic division).

2. Only mature cells are capable of division. Maturation occurs during a stage of cellular life called *interphase* (growth phase).

3. The cell cycle is the reproductive process that begins after interphase in all tissues with cellular turnover. The four phases of the cell cycle are (a) the S phase, during which DNA synthesis takes place in the cell nucleus; (b) the G_2 phase, the period between the completion of DNA synthesis and the next phase (M); (c) the M phase, which involves both nuclear (mitotic) and cytoplasmic (cytokinetic) division; and (d) the G_1 phase (growth phase, or interphase), after which the cycle begins again.

4. The M phase (mitosis) involves four stages: prophase, metaphase, anaphase, and telophase.

5. The mechanisms that control cell division depend on "social control genes" and protein growth factors.

6. Cyclin-CDK complexes trigger cell cycle events.

Tissues

1. Cells of one or more types are organized into tissues, and different types of tissues compose organs. Organs are organized to function as tracts or systems.

2. Specialized cells are thought to form tissue by mitosis of one or more founder cells or by migration of founder cells and their subsequent assembly at the site of tissue formation.

3. The four basic types of tissues are epithelial, muscle, neural, and connective tissues.

4. Epithelial tissue covers most internal and external surfaces of the body. The functions of epithelial tissue include protection, absorption, secretion, and excretion.

5. Connective tissue binds various tissues and organs together, supporting them in their locations and serving as storage sites for excess nutrients.

6. Muscle tissue is composed of long, thin, highly contractile cells or fibers called *myocytes*. Muscle tissue that is attached to bones enables voluntary movement. Muscle tissues in internal organs enable involuntary movement, such as the heartbeat.

7. Neural tissue is composed of highly specialized cells called *neurons,* which receive and transmit electric impulses very rapidly across junctions called *synapses*.

KEY TERMS

Absolute refractory period, 32
Actin filaments (microfilaments), 9
Action potential, 32
Active mediated transport, 28
Active transport, 25
Amphipathic molecule, 11
Anabolism, 22
Anaerobic glycolysis, 24
Anaphase, 34

Anions, 25
Antiport, 28
Arrested (G_0) state, 34
Autocrine signaling, 18
Autodigestion, 7
Autolysosomes (autophagosomes), 7
Autophagy, 7
Catabolism, 22
Cations, 25

Caveolae, 10
Cell adhesion molecules (CAMs), 12
Cell cycle, 33
Cell junctions, 17
Cell-to-cell adhesions, 15
Cellular metabolism, 22
Cellular receptors, 14
Centriole, 9
Centromere, 34

KEY TERMS—cont'd

Chemical synapses, 18
Chemotaxis, 35
Chromatids, 34
Chromatin, 33
Chromosomes, 33
Cilia, 37
Cisternae, 6
Citric acid cycle (Krebs cycle, tricarboxylic acid cycle), 23
Clathrin, 6
Coated pits, 30
Collagen, 17
Collagenous fibers, 37
Columnar cells, 37
Competitive inhibitors, 27
Concentration gradient, 25
Connexons, 17
Contact guidance, 35
Cristae, 8
Cuboidal cells, 37
Cyclic adenosine monophosphate (cyclic AMP, cAMP), 19
Cyclic guanosine monophosphate (cyclic GMP, cGMP), 21
Cytochromes, 24
Cytokinesis, 33
Cytoplasm, 2
Cytoplasmic matrix, 2
Cytoskeleton, 9
Cytosol, 2
Depolarization, 32
Desmosomes, 17
Differentiation, 2
Diffusion, 25
Digestion, 23
Effective osmolality, 27
Elastic fibers, 37
Elastin, 17
Electrolytes, 25
Electron-transport chain, 24
Endocytosis, 30
Endoplasmic reticulum, 4
Equatorial plate (metaphase plate), 34
Eukaryotes, 1
Extracellular matrix (basement membrane), 15
Facilitated diffusion, 28
Fibroblasts, 17
Fibronectin, 17
Filtration, 26
First messenger, 19
Founder cells, 35

G protein, 20
Gap junctions, 17
Gating, 17
Glycolysis, 23
Glycoproteins, 12
Golgi complex (Golgi apparatus), 6
Ground substance, 37
Growth factors, 34
Guanosine diphosphate (GDP), 20
Guanosine triphosphate (GTP), 20
Homeostasis, 17
Hormonal signaling, 17
Hydrolases, 6
Hydrophilic, 11
Hydrophobic, 11
Hydrostatic pressure, 26
Hypertonic solution, 27
Hypotonic solution, 27
Inner membrane, 8
Integral membrane proteins, 12
Intermediary metabolism, 9
Interphase, 33
Ions, 25
Isotonic solution, 27
Junctional complex, 17
Ligands, 14
Lysosomes, 6
Macromolecules, 17
Mediated transport, 27
Metabolic pathway, 22
Metaphase, 34
Microdomains, 31
Microtubules, 9
Microvilli, 37
Mitochondria, 8
Mitosis, 33
Neurohormonal signaling, 18
Neurotransmitters, 18
Nuclear envelope, 2
Nucleolus, 2
Nucleus, 2
Oncotic pressure (colloid osmotic pressure), 27
Osmolality, 26
Osmolarity, 26
Osmosis, 26
Osmotic pressure, 26
Outer membrane, 8
Oxidation, 23
Oxidative cellular metabolism, 23
Oxidative phosphorylation, 24
Paracrine signaling, 18

Parenchyma, 37
Passive mediated transport (facilitated diffusion), 28
Passive transport, 25
Peripheral membrane proteins, 12
Peroxisomes (microbodies), 7
Phagocytosis, 30
Pinocytosis, 30
Plasma membrane receptors, 14
Platelet-derived growth factor (PDGF), 34
Polarity, 25
Polyribosomes, 9
Potocytosis, 31
Primary lysosomes, 7
Prokaryotes, 1
Prophase, 34
Proteolytic cascade, 12
Pseudostratified epithelium, 37
Receptor-mediated endocytosis (ligand internalization), 30
Relative refractory period, 32
Repolarization, 32
Residual bodies, 7
Resting membrane potential, 31
Reticular fibers, 37
Ribosomal protein synthesis, 9
Ribosomes, 4
Rough endoplasmic reticulum, 6
Second messenger, 19
Secondary lysosome (heterophagosome), 7
Secretory vesicles, 6
Signal transduction, 19
Simple epithelium, 37
Smooth endoplasmic reticulum, 6
Solutes, 25
Spindle fibers, 34
Squamous cells, 37
Stratified epithelium, 37
Substrate, 22
Symport, 28
Synapses, 40
Telophase, 34
Threshold potential, 32
Tight junctions, 17
Tissues, 34
Tonicity, 27
Transfer reactions, 24
Transmembrane proteins, 12
Transport protein, 27
Uniport, 28
Vaults, 8

MEDIA RESOURCES   *evolve*

Review questions and answers for this chapter are available in the *CD Companion* included with this book.

WebLinks—links to Internet sites pertaining to this chapter—are available on Evolve at http://evolve.elsevier.com/McCance/.

REFERENCES

1. Alberts B et al: *Molecular biology of the cell*, ed 4, New York, 2002, Garland.
2. Eichenmuller B et al: Vaults bind directly to microtubules via their caps and not their barrels, *Cell Motil Cytoskeleton* 56(4):225-236, 2003.
3. Mossink MH et al: Vaults: a ribonucleoprotein particle involved in drug resistance? *Oncogene* 22(47):7458-7467, 2003.
4. Kong LB et al: Structure of the vault, a ubiquitous cellular component, *Structure* 7(4):371-379, 1999.

5. Mooney DJ, Mikos AG: Growing new organs, *Sci Am* 280(4):60-65, 1999.

6. Fasshauer M, Iwig M, Glaesser D: Synthesis of proto-oncogene proteins and cyclins depends on intact microfilaments, *Eur J Cell Biol* 77(3): 188-195, 1998.

7. Lofthouse RA et al: Identification of caveolae and detection of caveolin in normal human osteoblasts, *J Bone Joint Surg Br* 83(1):124-129, 2001.

8. Southan C: Drug discovery, *Today* 6:681-8, 2001.

9. Amour A et al: General considerations for proteolytic cascades, *Biochem Soc Trans* 32(Pt 1):15-16, 2004.

10. Chang HY, Yang X: Proteases for cell suicide: functions and regulations of caspases, *Microbiol Mol Biol Rev* 64(4):821-846, 2000.

11. Catt KJ et al: Hormonal regulation of peptide receptors and target cell responses, *Nature* 280(5718):109-116, 1979.

12. Kumar V, Abbas A, Fausto N: *Robbins and Cotran pathologic basis of disease,* ed 7, Philadelphia, 2005, Saunders.

13. Alberts B et al: *Essential cell biology,* New York, 1998, Garland.

14. Baserga R, Morrione A: Differentiation and malignant transformation: two roads diverge in a wood, *J Cell Biochem Suppl* 32-33:68-75, 1999.

15. Gonzalez-Zulueta M et al: Requirement for nitric oxide activation of p21 (ras)/extracellular-regulated kinase in neuronal ischemic preconditioning, *Proc Natl Acad Sci U S A* 97(1):436-441, 2000.

16. Scott JD, Pawson T: Cell communication: the inside story, *Sci Am* 282(6):72-79, 2000.

17. Mizuno-Kamiya M et al: ATP-mediated activation of Ca^{2+}-independent phospholipase A2 in secretory granular membranes from rat parotid gland, *J Biochem* (Tokyo) 123(2):205-212, 1998.

18. Harris J et al: Caveolae and caveolin in immune cells: distribution and functions, *Trends Immunol* 23(3):158-164, 2002.

19. Levin ER: Cellular functions of plasma membrane estrogen receptors, *Steroids* 67(6):471-475, 2002.

20. Li L, Haynes MP, Bender JR: Plasma membrane localization and function of the estrogen receptor alpha variant (ER46) in human endothelial cells, *Proc Natl Acad Sci USA* 100(8):4807-4812, 2003.

21. Zhu W, Smart EJ: Caveolae, estrogen, and nitric oxide, *Trends Endocrinol Metab* 14(3):114-117, 2003.

ALTERED CELLULAR AND TISSUE BIOLOGY

KATHRYN L. McCANCE • TODD CAMERON GREY

CHAPTER OUTLINE

Knowledge of the structural and functional reactions of cells and tissues to injurious agents, including genetic defects, is key to understanding disease processes. Diseases are now defined and interpreted in molecular terms and not just in general descriptions of altered structure. Altered cellular and tissue biology can be the result of adaptation, injury, neoplasia, aging, or death. (Neoplasia is discussed in Chapters 11 through 13.) Adaptation occurs in response to both normal, or physiologic, conditions and adverse, or pathologic, conditions. For example, the uterus adapts to pregnancy—a normal physiologic state—by enlarging. Enlargement occurs because of an increase in the size and number of uterine cells. In an adverse condition, such as high blood pressure, myocardial cells are stimulated to enlarge by the increased work of pumping. Like most of the body's adaptive mechanisms, however, cellular adaptations to adverse conditions are usually only temporarily successful. Severe or long-term stressors overwhelm adaptive processes, and cellular injury or death ensues.

Cellular injury can be caused by any factor that disrupts cellular structures or deprives the cell of oxygen and nutrients required for survival. Injury may be reversible (sublethal) or irreversible (lethal) and is classified broadly as chemical, hypoxic (lack of sufficient oxygen), free radical, unintentional or intentional, and immunologic or inflammatory. Cellular injuries from various causes have different clinical and pathophysiologic manifestations.

Cellular death is confirmed by structural changes seen when cells are stained and examined with a microscope. The most important changes are nuclear changes; clearly, without a healthy nucleus, the cell cannot survive.

Cellular aging causes structural and functional changes that eventually lead to cellular death or a decreased capacity to recover from injury. Mechanisms explaining how and why cells age are not known, and distinguishing between pathologic changes and physiologic changes that occur with aging is often difficult. Aging clearly causes alterations in cellular structure and function, yet senescence is both inevitable and normal.

CELLULAR ADAPTATION

Cells adapt to their environment to escape and protect themselves from injury. An adapted cell is neither normal nor injured—its condition lies somewhere between these two states. Cellular adaptations, however, are a common and central part of many disease states. In the early stages of a successful adaptive response, cells may have enhanced function; thus it is hard to know what is a pathologic response vs. an extreme adaptation to an excessive functional demand. The most significant adaptive changes in cells include atrophy (decrease in cell size), hypertrophy (increase in cell size), hyperplasia (increase in cell number), and metaplasia (reversible replacement of one mature cell type by another less mature cell type). Dysplasia (deranged cellular growth) is not considered a true cellular adaptation but rather an atypical hyperplasia. These changes are shown in Figure 2-1.

Atrophy

Atrophy is a decrease or shrinkage in cellular size. If atrophy occurs in a sufficient number of an organ's cells, the entire organ shrinks or becomes atrophic. Atrophy can affect any organ, but it is most common in skeletal muscle, the heart, secondary sex organs, and the brain. Atrophy can be classified as *physiologic* or *pathologic*. **Physiologic atrophy** occurs with early development. For example, the thymus gland undergoes

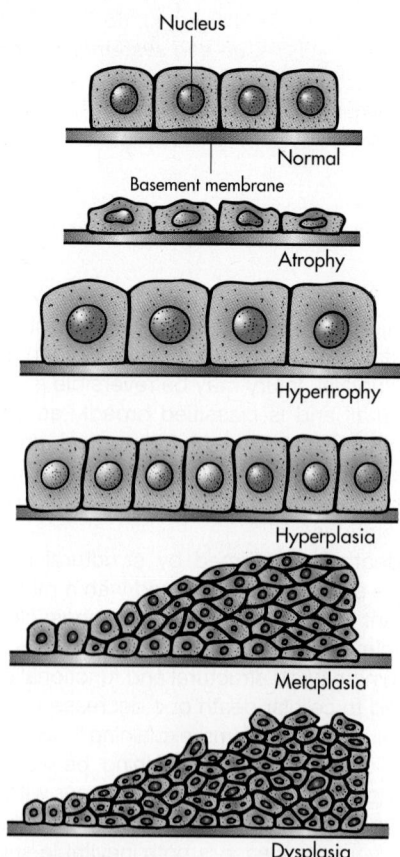

Figure 2-1 Adaptive alterations in simple cuboidal epithelial cells. (From Lewis SM, Heitkemper MM, Dirksen SR: *Medical-surgical nursing: assessment and management of clinical problems,* ed 6, St Louis, 2004, Mosby.)

physiologic atrophy during childhood. **Pathologic atrophy** occurs as a result of decreases in workload, use, pressure, blood supply, nutrition, hormonal stimulation, and nervous stimulation. Individuals immobilized in bed for a prolonged time exhibit a type of skeletal muscle atrophy called *disuse atrophy*. Aging causes brain cells to become atrophic and endocrine-dependent organs, such as the gonads, to shrink as hormonal stimulation decreases. Whether atrophy is caused by normal physiologic conditions or by pathologic conditions, atrophic cells exhibit the same basic changes.

The atrophic muscle cell contains less endoplasmic reticulum and fewer mitochondria and myofilaments (part of the muscle fiber that controls contraction) than does the normal cell. In muscular atrophy caused by nerve loss, oxygen consumption and amino acid uptake are rapidly reduced. The biochemical changes of atrophy are just beginning to be understood. The mechanisms probably include decreased protein synthesis, increased protein catabolism, or both. The primary pathway of protein catabolism is the **ubiquitin-proteosome pathway,** and signals activating this pathway include metabolic acidosis, glucocorticoids, and thyroid hormone.[1] Proteins degraded in this pathway are first conjugated to ubiquitin (another small protein) and then degraded within a large cytoplasmic proteolytic complex or proteosome.

Atrophy as a result of chronic malnutrition is often accompanied by an increase in the number of **autophagic vacuoles,** which are membrane-bound vesicles within the cell that contain cellular debris—small fragments of mitochondria and endoplasmic reticulum—and hydrolytic enzymes. Atrophic change causes a rapid increase in hydrolytic enzymes, which are isolated in autophagic vacuoles to prevent uncontrolled cellular destruction. Thus the vacuoles proliferate as needed to protect the uninjured organelles from the injured organelles and are eventually taken up and destroyed by lysosomes (a process described in Chapter 1). Certain contents of the autophagic vacuole may resist destruction by lysosomal enzymes and persist in membrane-bound residual bodies. An example of this is granules that contain **lipofuscin,** the yellow-brown age pigment. Lipofuscin accumulates primarily in liver cells, myocardial cells, and atrophic cells.

Hypertrophy

Hypertrophy is an increase in the size of cells and consequently in the size of the affected organ. The cells of the heart and kidneys are particularly responsive to enlargement. The increase in cellular size is associated with an increased accumulation of protein in the cellular components (plasma membrane, endoplasmic reticulum, myofilaments, mitochondria) and *not* with an increase in cellular fluid. Hypertrophy can be *physiologic* or *pathologic* and is caused by specific hormone stimulation or by increased functional demand. For example, physiologic hypertrophy during pregnancy is hormone induced and involves both hypertrophy and hyperplasia. Hypertrophy as an adaptive response—muscular enlargement—occurs in the striated muscle cells of both the heart and skeletal muscles. These cells cannot adapt to increased metabolic demands by mitotic division and production of new cells to share the work. Thus they enlarge and the stimulus appears to be an increased workload. In the heart, pathologic hypertrophy is secondary to hypertension or problem valves. In skeletal muscle, physiologic hypertrophy occurs in response to heavy work. Muscular hypertrophy tends to diminish if the excessive workload diminishes.

In myocardial hypertrophy, initial enlargement is caused by dilation of the cardiac chambers, but this is short lived and is followed by increased synthesis of cardiac muscle proteins, allowing muscle fibers to do more work. The nucleus is also hypertrophic and exhibits increased synthesis of deoxyri-

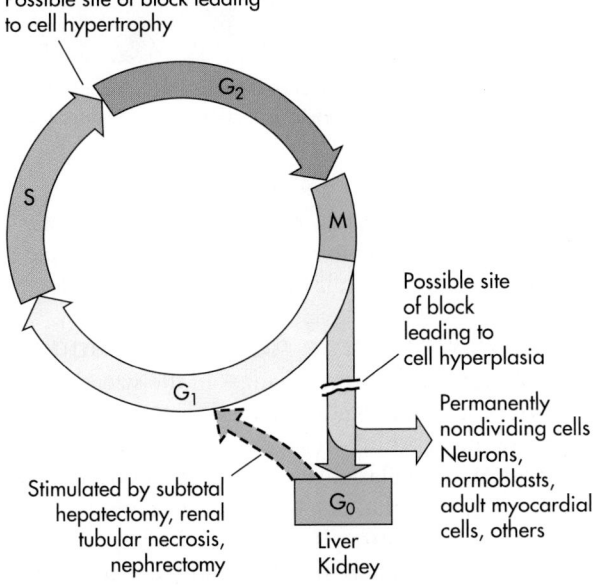

Figure 2-2 Cell cycle and possible sites of block.

bonucleic acid (DNA).[2] Although fully matured (e.g., terminally differentiated) muscle cells are unable to undergo further mitosis, they are capable of increased DNA synthesis. Why cardiac muscle cells are unable to progress through the cell cycle to mitosis is unclear; it may be because of a block that prevents them from entering G_2 of the cell cycle[3] (Figure 2-2) (see Chapters 1 and 11). Eventually, however, advanced hypertrophy can lead to myocardial failure (Figure 2-3) (see Chapter 30).

A number of genes are activated during hypertrophy, including the gene for atrial natriuretic factor (ANF). The ANF gene is usually expressed only during early development; however, with cardiac hypertrophy, it is reinduced and the ANF hormone causes salt secretion by the kidney, decreasing blood volume and pressure and reducing hemodynamic load. Other genes activated include regulatory factors (e.g., *c-fos, c-jun*), growth factors, vasoactive agents, certain components involved in receptor-mediated signaling pathways, and kinases. The triggers for hypertrophy include two types of signals: mechanical signals, such as stretch, and trophic signals, such as growth factors and vasoactive agents.

After removal of one kidney, the other kidney adapts to an increased demand for work with an increase in both the size and the number of cells. The major contribution to renal enlargement is hypertrophy.

Hyperplasia

Hyperplasia is an increase in the number of cells resulting from an increased rate of cellular division. Hyperplasia as a response to injury occurs when the injury has been severe and prolonged enough to have caused cell death.[2] Loss of epithelial cells and cells of the liver and kidney triggers DNA

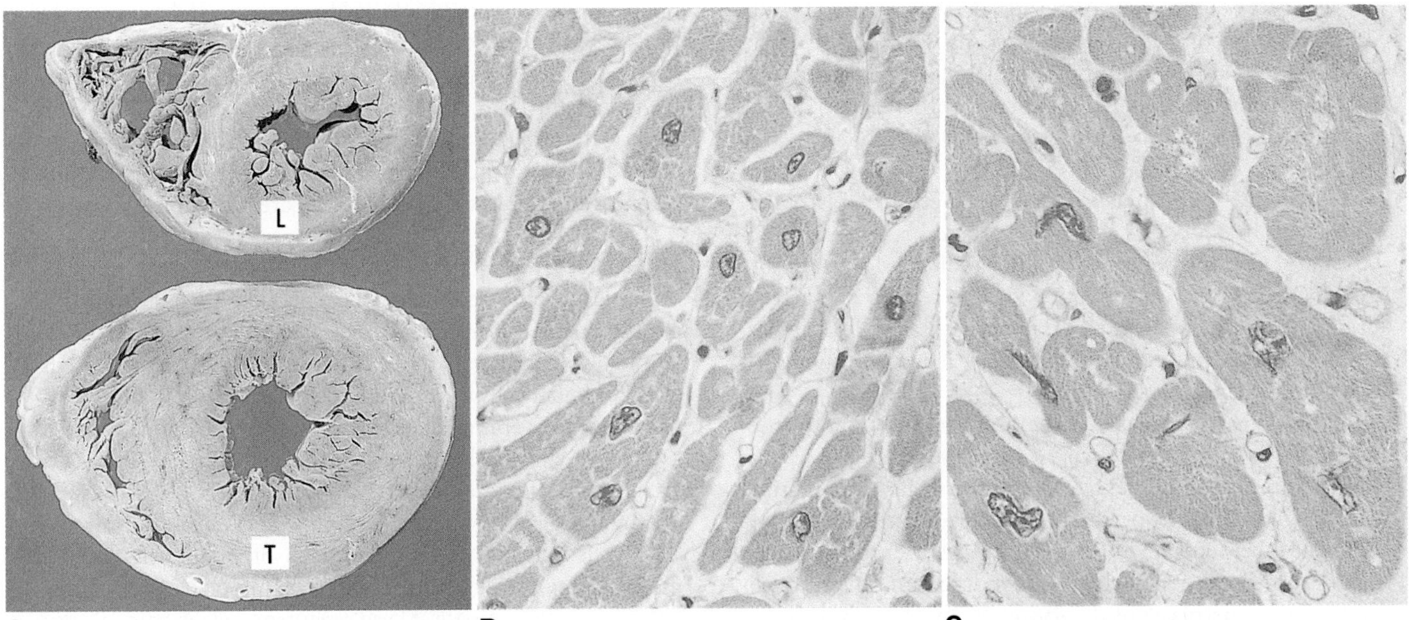

Figure 2-3 **Hypertrophy of cardiac muscle in response to valve disease. A,** Transverse slices of a normal heart and a heart with hypertrophy of the left ventricle. (*L,* Normal thickness of left ventricular wall; *T,* thickened wall from heart in which severe narrowing of aortic valve caused resistance to systolic ventricular emptying.) **B,** Histology of cardiac muscle from a normal heart. **C,** Histology of cardiac muscle from a hypertrophied heart. (From Stevens A, Lowe J: *Pathology,* London, 1995, Mosby.)

synthesis and mitotic division. Increased cell growth is a multistep process involving the production of growth factors, which stimulate the remaining cells to synthesize new cell components and, ultimately, to divide. Hyperplasia and hypertrophy often occur together, although the specific mechanism is unknown. Hyperplasia and hypertrophy both take place if the cells are capable of synthesizing DNA; however, in *nondividing cells* (e.g., myocardial fibers) only hypertrophy occurs.

Two types of normal, or physiologic, hyperplasia are compensatory hyperplasia and hormonal hyperplasia. **Compensatory hyperplasia** is an adaptive mechanism that enables certain organs to regenerate. For example, removal of part of the liver leads to hyperplasia of the remaining liver cells (hepatocytes) to compensate for the loss. Even with removal of 70% of the liver, regeneration is complete in about 2 weeks. The remarkable regenerating capacity of the liver was even noted by the ancient Greeks. According to one story, Prometheus was chained to a mountain and his liver was eaten daily by a vulture, only to regenerate every night. A new protein, **hepatocyte growth factor (HGF),** is thought to be a mediator in vitro of liver regeneration.[4] In addition, other in vitro growth factors and cytokines (cell-signaling proteins) that increase hepatic cell regeneration include transforming growth factor-α (TGF-α), epidermal growth factor (EGF), interleukin-6 (IL-6), and tumor necrosis factor–α (TNF-α).

Not all types of mature cells have the same capacity for compensatory hyperplastic growth. Some cells, such as nerve, skeletal muscle, and myocardial cells and the lens cells of the eye, do not regenerate. Skeletal muscle cells, however, can be made by the fusion of myoblasts.[5] Significant compensatory hyperplasia occurs in epidermal and intestinal epithelia, hepatocytes, bone marrow cells, and fibroblasts, and some hyperplasia is noted in bone, cartilage, and smooth muscle cells. An example of compensatory hyperplasia is a **callus,** or thickening, of the skin as a result of hyperplasia of epidermal cells in response to a mechanical stimulus. Another example is the response to wound healing as part of the inflammation process (see Chapter 6).

Hormonal hyperplasia occurs chiefly in estrogen-dependent organs, such as the uterus and breast. After ovulation, for example, estrogen stimulates the endometrium to grow and thicken for reception of the fertilized ovum. If pregnancy occurs, hormonal hyperplasia, as well as hypertrophy, enables the uterus to enlarge. (Hormone function is described in Chapters 20 and 21.)

Pathologic hyperplasia is the abnormal proliferation of normal cells and can occur as a response to excessive hormonal stimulation or the effects of growth factors on target cells (Figure 2-4). Hyperplastic cells are identified by pronounced nuclear enlargement, clumping of chromatin, and one or more enlarged nucleoli. The most common example is pathologic hyperplasia of the endometrium (which is caused by an imbalance between estrogen and progesterone secretion, with oversecretion of estrogen) (see Chapter 23). Pathologic endometrial hyperplasia, which causes excessive menstrual bleeding, is under the influence of regular growth

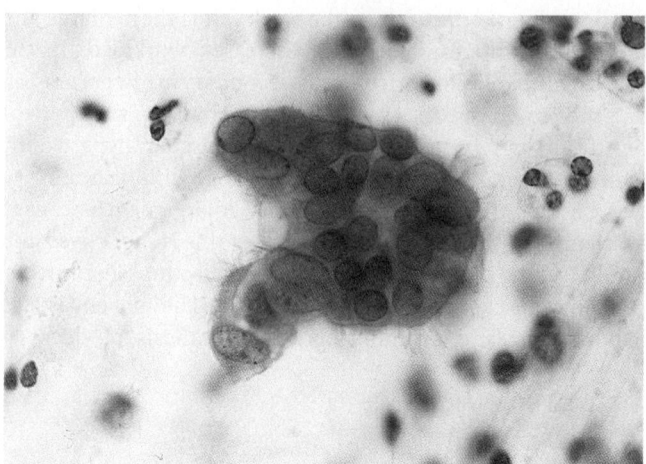

Figure 2-4 Hyperplasia of bronchial epithelium. (Bronchial brush.) (From Damjanov I, Linder J: *Anderson's pathology,* ed 10, St Louis, 1996, Mosby.)

inhibition controls. If these controls fail, hyperplastic endometrial cells can undergo malignant transformation. (Malignant cell transformation is discussed in Chapter 11.)

Dysplasia: Not a True Adaptive Change

Dysplasia refers to abnormal changes in the size, shape, and organization of mature cells. Dysplasia is not considered a true adaptive process but is related to hyperplasia and is often called **atypical hyperplasia.** Dysplastic changes frequently are encountered in epithelial tissue of the cervix and respiratory tract, where they are strongly associated with common neoplastic growths and often are found adjacent to cancerous cells.

Dysplasia is often classified as mild, moderate, or severe; however, this subjective scheme has prompted recommendations to use either "low grade" or "high grade." Grading of dysplasia, for example, of the female reproductive tract (i.e., Papanicolaou [Pap] test) is discussed in Chapter 23 (Figure 2-5). Data indicate that atypical hyperplasia is a strong predictor of breast cancer development.[6,7] If the inciting stimulus is removed, dysplastic changes often are reversible.

Metaplasia

Metaplasia is the reversible replacement of one mature cell by another, sometimes less differentiated, cell type. The best example of metaplasia is replacement of normal columnar ciliated epithelial cells of the bronchial (airway) lining by stratified squamous epithelial cells (Figure 2-6). The newly formed squamous epithelial cells do not secrete mucus or have cilia, causing loss of a vital protective mechanism.

Metaplasia is thought to develop from a reprogramming of stem cells existing in most epithelia or of undifferentiated mesenchymal (tissue from embryonic mesoderm) cells present in connective tissue. These precursor cells mature along a new pathway because of signals generated by cytokines and growth factors in the cell's environment.

Bronchial metaplasia can be reversed if the inducing stimulus, usually cigarette smoking, is removed. With prolonged

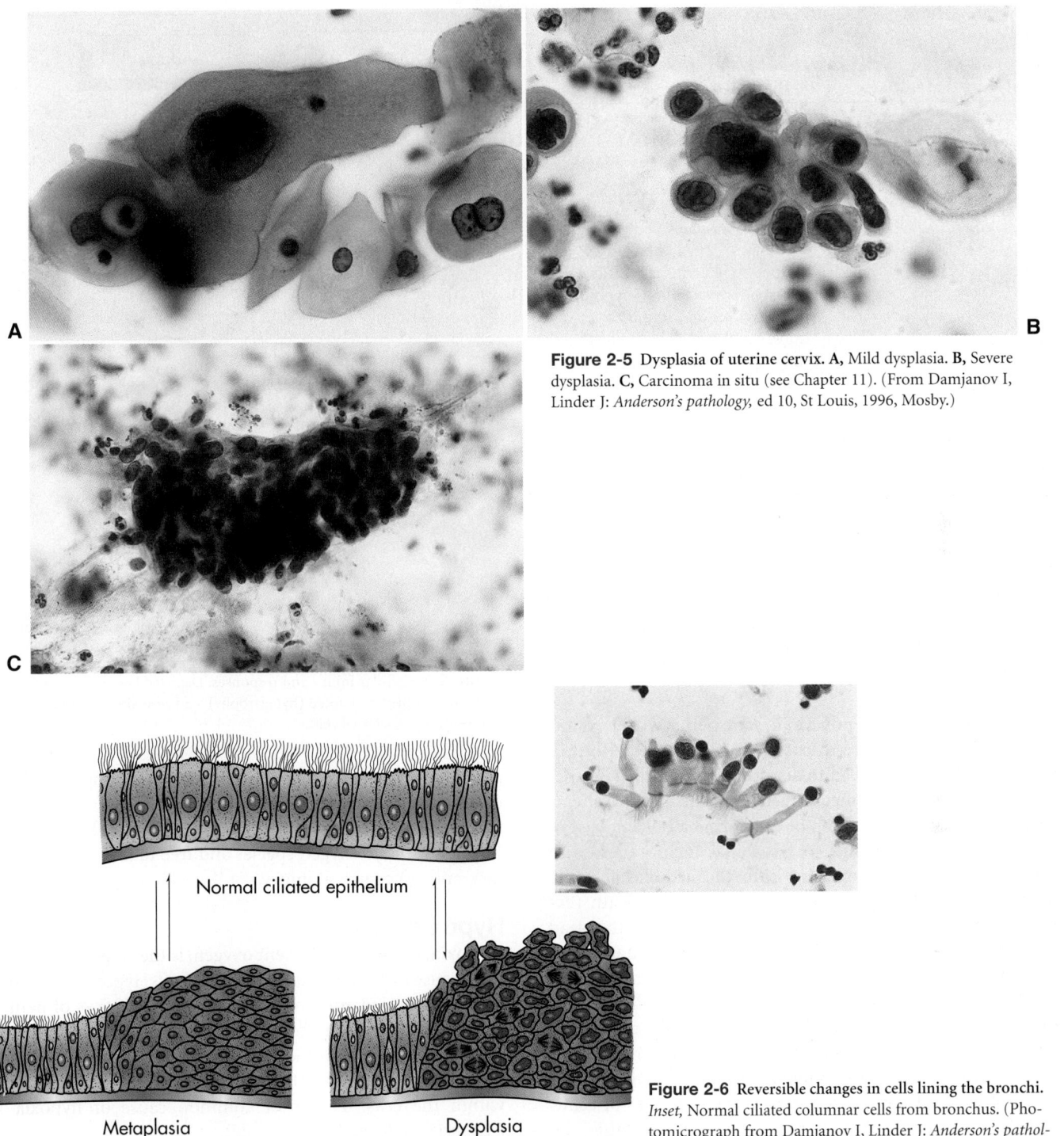

Figure 2-5 Dysplasia of uterine cervix. **A,** Mild dysplasia. **B,** Severe dysplasia. **C,** Carcinoma in situ (see Chapter 11). (From Damjanov I, Linder J: *Anderson's pathology,* ed 10, St Louis, 1996, Mosby.)

Normal ciliated epithelium

Metaplasia
Chronic injury or irritation

Dysplasia
Persistent severe injury or irritation

Figure 2-6 Reversible changes in cells lining the bronchi. *Inset,* Normal ciliated columnar cells from bronchus. (Photomicrograph from Damjanov I, Linder J: *Anderson's pathology,* ed 10, St Louis, 1996, Mosby.)

exposure to the inducing stimulus, however, cancerous transformation can occur.

CELLULAR INJURY

Most diseases begin with cell injury, and all forms of loss of function derive from cell injury and cell death. Cellular injury occurs if the cell is unable to maintain homeostasis—a normal or adaptive steady state—in the face of injurious stimuli.

Injured cells may recover (**reversible injury**) or die (**irreversible injury**). Injurious stimuli include chemical agents, lack of sufficient oxygen (hypoxia), free radicals, infectious agents, physical and mechanical factors, immunologic reactions, genetic factors, and nutritional imbalances. Types of cellular injury and their responses are summarized in Table 2-1 and Figure 2-7.

Cell injury and cell death often result from exposure to toxic chemicals, infections, and hypoxia. The mechanisms

Table 2-1	Progressive Types of Cell Injury and Responses
Type	**Responses**
Adaptation	Atrophy, hypertrophy, hyperplasia, metaplasia
Active cell injury	Immediate response of "entire" cell
Reversible	Loss of adenosine triphosphate (ATP), cellular swelling, detachment of ribosomes, autophagy of lysosomes
Irreversible	"Point of no return" structurally when severe vacuolization occurs of the mitochondria and Ca^{++} moves into the cell including the mitochondria membrane damage
Necrosis	Common type of cell death with severe cell swelling and breakdown of organelles
Apoptosis, or programmed cell death	Cellular self-destruction for elimination of unwanted cell populations
Chronic cell injury (subcellular alterations)	Persistent stimuli response may involve only specific organelles or cytoskeleton (e.g., phagocytosis of bacteria)
Accumulations or infiltrations	Water, pigments, lipids, glycogen, proteins
Pathologic calcification	Dystrophic and metastatic calcification

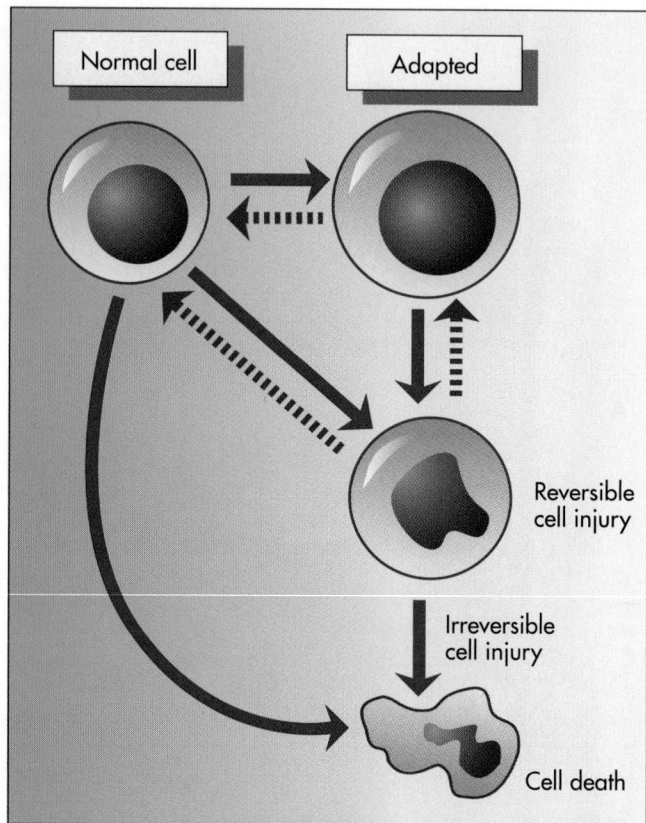

Figure 2-7 **Cellular injury and responses.** Depicted here is the relationship among normal, adapted (hypertrophy), and reversibly injured cells and cell death of myocardial cells.

causing chemical and hypoxic injury are perhaps the best understood. (Infections are discussed in Chapter 9.) Both of these mechanisms can lead to disruption of selective permeability (i.e., transport mechanisms) of the plasma membrane; reduction or cessation of cellular metabolism; lack of protein synthesis; damage to lysosomal membranes, with leakage of destructive enzymes into the cytoplasm; enzymatic destruction of cellular organelles; cellular death (exhibited by nuclear changes); and phagocytosis of the dead cell by cellular components of the acute inflammatory response (see Chapter 6). The extent of cellular injury depends on the type, state (including level of cell differentiation and increased susceptibility to fully differentiated cells), and adaptive processes of the cell, as well as the type, severity, and duration of the injurious stimulus. Two individuals exposed to an identical stimulus may incur varying degrees of cellular injury. Modifying factors, such as nutritional status, can profoundly influence the extent of injury. The precise "point of no return" that leads to cellular death is a biochemical puzzle, and the exact mechanisms responsible for the transition from reversible to irreversible cellular damage are currently being debated.

General Mechanisms of Cell Injury

Cells are complex units, and therefore the mechanisms responsible for cell injury leading to necrotic cell death are numerous and interrelated and depend on a delicate balance between intracellular and extracellular events. There are, however, four common biochemical themes important to cell injury and cell death regardless of the injuring agent (Table 2-2).

The three common forms of cell injury are (1) hypoxic injury, (2) reactive oxygen species and free radical–induced injury, and (3) chemical injury.

Hypoxic Injury

Hypoxia, or lack of sufficient oxygen, is the single most common cause of cellular injury (Figure 2-8). Hypoxia can result from a decreased amount of oxygen in the air, loss of hemoglobin or hemoglobin function, decreased production of red blood cells, diseases of the respiratory and cardiovascular systems, and poisoning of the oxidative enzymes (cytochromes) within the cells. The most common cause of hypoxia is **ischemia** (reduced blood supply).

Ischemic injury is often caused by gradual narrowing of arteries (arteriosclerosis) and complete blockage by blood clots (thrombosis). Progressive hypoxia caused by gradual arterial obstruction is better tolerated than the sudden acute **anoxia** (total lack of oxygen) caused by a sudden obstruction, such as can occur with an embolus (a blood clot or other plug in the circulation). An acute obstruction in a coronary artery can cause myocardial cell death (infarction) within minutes if the blood supply is not restored, whereas the gradual onset of ischemia usually results in myocardial adaptation. Myocardial infarction and stroke, which are common causes of death in

Table 2-2	Common Themes in Cell Injury and Cell Death
Theme	**Comments**
ATP depletion	Loss of mitochondrial ATP and decreased ATP synthesis; results include cellular swelling, decreased protein synthesis, decreased membrane transport, and lipogenesis, all changes that contribute to loss of integrity of plasma membrane (see text)
Oxygen and oxygen-derived free radicals	Lack of oxygen is key in progression of cell injury in ischemia (reduced blood supply); activated oxygen species (free radicals, O_2^-, H_2O_2, $OH\cdot$, NO) cause destruction of cell membranes and cell structure
Intracellular calcium and loss of calcium steady state	Normally intracellular cytosolic calcium concentrations are very low; ischemia and certain chemicals cause an increase in cytosolic Ca^{++} concentrations; sustained levels of Ca^{++} continue to increase with damage to plasma membrane; Ca^{++} causes intracellular damage by activating a number of enzymes (see text)
Defects in membrane permeability	Early loss of selective membrane permeability found in all forms of cell injury (see text)

ATP, Adenosine triphosphate.

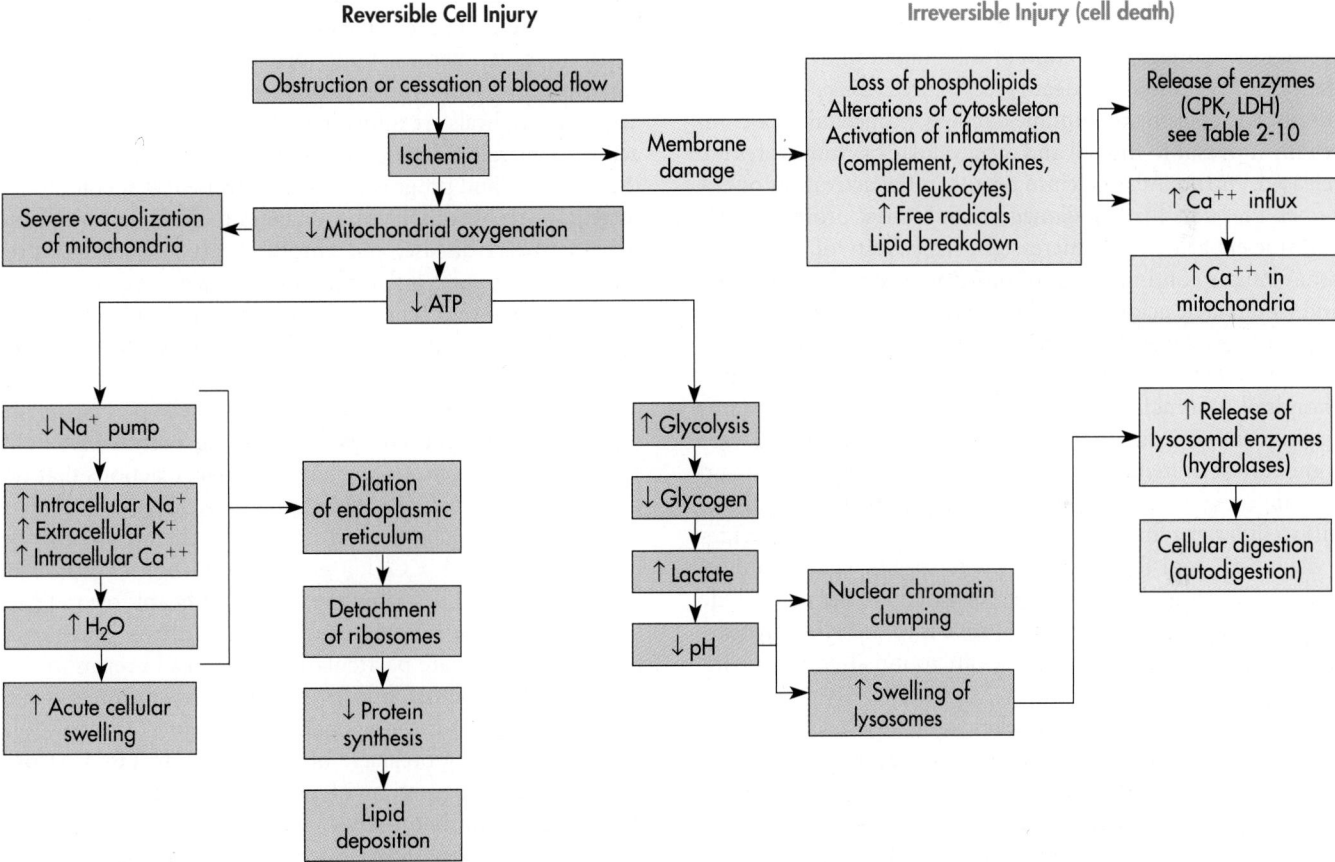

Figure 2-8 Hypoxic injury induced by ischemia. Purple boxes involve reversible cell injury, and light blue boxes involve irreversible cell death. Green boxes are clinical manifestations.

the United States, generally result from atherosclerosis (a type of arteriosclerosis) and consequent ischemic injury. (Vascular obstruction is discussed in Chapter 30.)

Cellular responses to hypoxic injury have been extensively studied in heart muscle. Within 1 minute after blood supply to the myocardium is interrupted, the heart becomes pale and has difficulty contracting normally. Within 3 to 5 minutes, the ischemic portion of the myocardium ceases to contract. The abrupt lack of contraction is caused by a rapid decrease in mitochondrial phosphorylation, which results in insufficient adenosine triphosphate (ATP) production. Lack

of ATP leads to an increase in anaerobic metabolism, which generates ATP from glycogen when there is insufficient oxygen. When glycogen stores are depleted, even anaerobic metabolism ceases.

A reduction in ATP levels causes the plasma membrane's sodium-potassium (Na^+-K^+) pump and sodium-calcium exchange to fail, which leads to an intracellular accumulation of sodium and calcium and diffusion of potassium out of the cell. (The Na^+-K^+ pump is discussed in Chapter 1.) Sodium and water then can enter the cell freely, and cellular swelling results. Since all cells are bathed in a fluid rich in calcium ions, cell membrane damage allows rapid movement of calcium intracellularly. The movement of water and ions into the cell causes early dilation of the endoplasmic reticulum. Dilation causes the ribosomes to detach from the rough endoplasmic reticulum, resulting in reduced protein synthesis. With continued hypoxia, the entire cell becomes markedly swollen, with increased concentrations of sodium, water, and chloride and decreased concentrations of potassium. These disruptions are reversible if oxygen is restored. If oxygen is not restored, however, there is vacuolation (formation of vacuoles) within the cytoplasm, swelling of lysosomes, and marked swelling of the mitochondria resulting from mitochondrial membrane damage. Continued hypoxic injury with accumulation of calcium subsequently activates multiple enzyme systems, including proteases, nitric oxide synthase, phospholipases, and endonuclease, resulting in cytoskeleton disruption, membrane damage, activation of inflammation, DNA degradation, and eventual cell death (see Figure 2-27, p. 77). Structurally, with plasma membrane damage, extracellular calcium readily moves into the cell and intracellular calcium stores are released. Intracellular calcium results in the activation of enzymes that can further damage membranes, proteins, ATP, and nucleic acids.[8] The increased permeability of the membrane causes continued loss of proteins, essential coenzymes, and ribonucleic acids. In addition, the substrates necessary to reconstitute ATP are lost. Irreversible damage is characterized by two events: (1) lack of ATP generation because of mitochondrial dysfunction and (2) major disturbances and damage in membrane function. Acid hydrolases from leaking lysosomes are activated in the reduced pH of the injured cell and they digest cytoplasmic and nuclear components. Leakage of intracellular enzymes into the peripheral circulation provides a diagnostic tool for detecting tissue-specific cellular injury and death using blood samples, for example, the contractile protein troponin from cardiac muscle is found after myocardial injury and liver transaminases are found after hepatic injury.

Restoration of oxygen, however, can cause additional injury called **reperfusion (reoxygenation) injury.** Reperfusion is a serious complication and an important mechanism of injury in instances of tissue transplantation and in myocardial, hepatic, intestinal, cerebral, renal, and other ischemic syndromes, including stroke.[9,10] Xanthine dehydrogenase, an enzyme which normally utilizes oxidized nicotinamide adenine dinucleotide (NAD^+) as an electron acceptor, is converted during reperfusion with oxygen to xanthine oxidase. During the ischemic period, excessive ATP consumption leads to the accumulation of the purine catabolites hypoxanthine and xanthine, which upon subsequent reperfusion and influx of oxygen are metabolized by xanthine oxidase to make *massive* amounts of superoxide and hydrogen peroxide. In addition, the highly reactive free radical nitric oxide is generated[11] (see Table 2-3). These radicals can all cause membrane damage and mitochondrial calcium overload.[11] Neutrophils are especially affected with reperfusion injury, and neutrophil adhe-

sion to the endothelium enhances the process. Antioxidant treatment reverses both neutrophil adhesion (leukocyte adhesion) and neutrophil (leukocyte) mediated heart injury in the postischemic period.[9] Other potential and current treatments may include blockage of inflammatory mediators and inhibition of apoptotic pathways.

Free Radicals and Reactive Oxygen Species

An important mechanism of membrane damage is injury induced by free radicals, especially by reactive oxygen species (ROS) called **oxidative stress.** Oxidative stress occurs when excess ROS overwhelms endogenous antioxidant systems. A **free radical** is an electrically uncharged atom or group of atoms having an unpaired electron. Having one unpaired electron makes the molecule unstable; thus to stabilize it gives up an electron to another molecule or steals one. Therefore it is capable of injurious chemical bond formation with proteins, lipids, carbohydrates—key molecules in membranes and nucleic acids. Free radicals are difficult to control and initiate chain reactions. Emerging data indicates that ROS play major roles in the initiation and progression of cardiovascular alterations associated with hyperlipidemia, diabetes mellitus, hypertension, ischemic heart disease, and chronic heart failure. ROS produced by migrating inflammatory cells (e.g., neutrophils), as well as vascular cells (endothelial cells, vascular smooth muscle cells, and adventitial fibroblasts) have distinct effects on each cell type.[12] These cell effects are shown in Figure 2-9.

Free radicals may be initiated within cells by (1) the absorption of extreme energy sources (e.g., ultraviolet light, x-rays); (2) endogenous, usually oxidative, reactions that occur during normal metabolic processes (Figure 2-10); or (3) enzymatic metabolism of exogenous chemicals or drugs (e.g., chloromethyl [CCl_3], a product of carbon tetrachloride [CCl_4]). Table 2-3 describes the most significant free radicals.

Although wide-ranging effects can occur from these reactive species, three are particularly important in regard to cell injury: (1) lipid peroxidation; (2) alterations of proteins causing fragmentation of polypeptide chains; and (3) alterations of DNA, including breakage of single strands. **Lipid peroxidation** is the destruction of unsaturated fatty acids. Fatty acids of lipids in membranes possess double bonds between some of the carbon atoms. Such bonds are vulnerable to attack by oxygen-derived free radicals, especially OH·. The lipid-radical interactions themselves yield peroxides. The peroxides set off a chain reaction resulting in membrane, organelle, and cellular destruction. Because of our understanding of free radicals, a growing number of diseases and disorders have been linked either directly or indirectly to these reactive species (Table 2-4).

It is fortunate that the body can sometimes rid itself of free radicals. Superoxide may spontaneously decay into oxygen and hydrogen peroxide. Table 2-5 and Figure 2-11 summarize other methods that contribute to inactivation or termination of free radicals. The toxicity of certain drugs and chemicals can be attributed to either conversion of these chemicals to

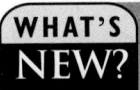

Figure 2-9 ROS can cause distinct functional effects depending on cell type. All cells are capable of making reactive oxygen species (ROS). Emphasis has been on inflammatory and vascular cells because of their widespread disease-causing impact. Some examples include angiotensin II, which can induce vascular smooth muscle cells (VSMC) to hypertrophy; NAD(P)H oxidase-derived ROS has been implicated in the growth response; H_2O_2 has been shown to induce proliferation and migration of endothelial cells; ROS act as mediators of vascular endothelial growth factor, thus modulating angiogenesis; endothelial injury or exposure to O_2^- and H_2O_2 induces apoptosis of endothelial cells. Activity of the extracellular matrix by matrix metalloproteinases (MMPs) can be modulated by ROS. Cytokines play a significant role in the progression of vascular lesions. An important mechanism by which cytokine gene expression is increased is the activation of nuclear factor-$_k\beta$ (NF-$_k\beta$). NF-$_k\beta$ is a ROS-sensitive transcription factor and has a role in the expression of proinflammatory genes. (Data from Dröge W: *Physiol Rev* 82:47-95, 2002; Duchen MR: *Diabetes* 53(Suppl 1): S96-S102, 2004; Buetler TM, Krauskopf A, Ruegg UT: *News Physiol Sci* 19:120-123, 2004.) (Also see What's New? on ROS and Proliferation, Apoptosis, and Necrosis below)

free radicals or the formation of oxygen-derived metabolites.[9] This process is discussed in Chemical Injury.

Chemical Injury

Mechanisms

Chemical injury begins with a biochemical interaction between a toxic substance and the cell's plasma membrane, which is ultimately damaged, leading to increased permeability. Not all the mechanisms causing chemically induced membrane destruction are known; however, the two general mechanisms include (1) direct toxicity by combining with a molecular component of the cell membrane or organelles and (2) reactive free radicals and lipid peroxidation.

Because it has been investigated extensively, carbon tetrachloride (CCl_4) injury is a useful example of chemical injury. Carbon tetrachloride, an agent formerly used in dry cleaning, harms cells because an enzyme system (P-450) in the smooth endoplasmic reticulum of liver cells converts it into chloromethyl (CCl_3), a highly toxic free radical.

In CCl_4 injury, newly formed CCl_3 rapidly destroys the endoplasmic reticulum of the liver cell by way of lipid peroxidation breaking down the reticulum's lipid component. The lipid molecules accumulate within the cytoplasm, starting within cisternae of the endoplasmic reticulum (Figure 2-12). Fatty liver develops because CCl_4 poisoning blocks the synthesis of **lipid-acceptor proteins (apoproteins)** that normally bind with triglycerides to form lipoproteins, which are transported out of the cell. Blockage of triglyceride (lipoprotein) secretion begins 10 to 15 minutes after CCl_4 exposure. Fat droplets that accumulate in cisternae of the endoplasmic

WHAT'S NEW? **ROS and Proliferation, Apoptosis, and Necrosis**

Cellular impact of reactive oxygen species (ROS) may depend on concentration levels. At low concentrations, ROS appear to exert a growth-stimulatory effect on a wide variety of cells and microorganisms. For example, bacteria such as *Escherichia coli* and *Salmonella typhimurium* need O_2^- for growth. Certain human cell lines also have shown this dependency in vitro. Yet when ROS levels increase, other signaling pathways may be activated that lead to apoptosis. When ROS levels rise even higher, a cell may die a sudden necrotic death. The apoptosis and necrosis modes are thought to be due to oxidative stress. Thus the signaling functions of ROS are now appreciated.

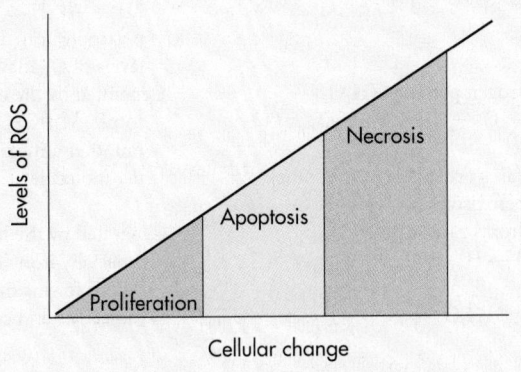

Data from Buetler TM, Krauskopf A, Ruegg UT: *News Physiol Sci* 19:120-123, 2004.

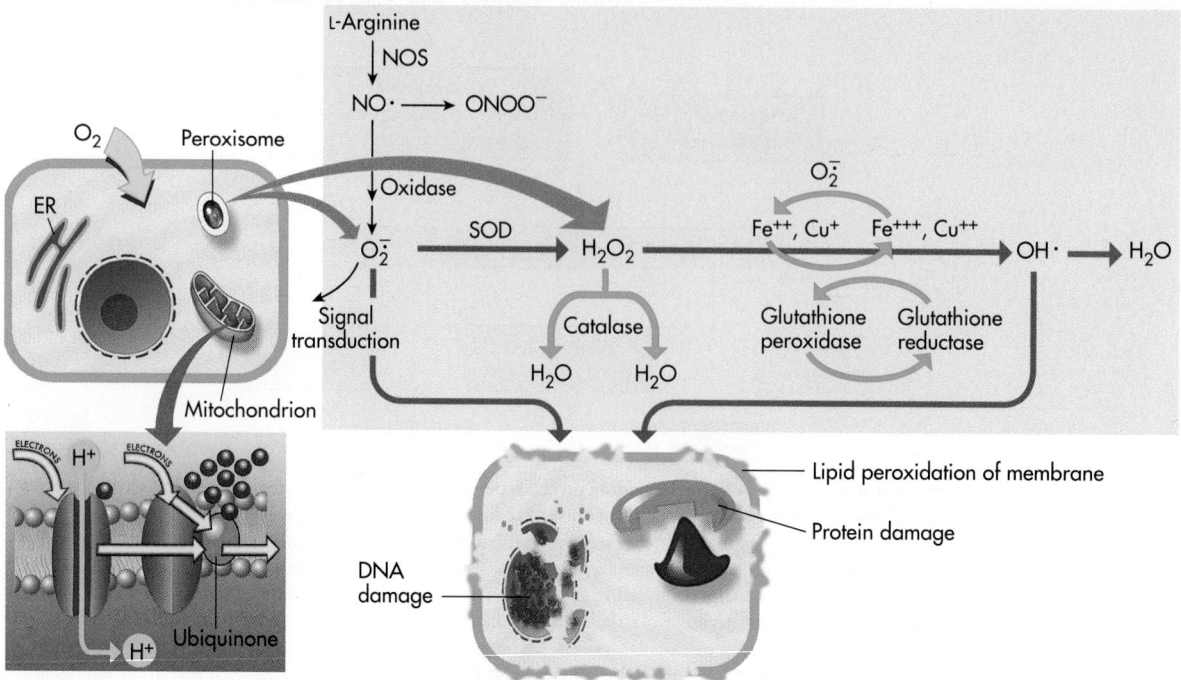

Figure 2-10 Generation of ROS and antioxidant mechanisms in biologic systems. Mitochondria have four sites of entry for electrons coming into the electron transport system: one for reduced nicotinamide adenine dinucleotide (NADH) and three for reduced form of flavin adenine dinucleotide ($FADH_2$). These pathways meet at the small, lipophilic molecule, ubiquinone (coenzyme Q), at the beginning of the common electron transport pathway. Ubiquinone transfers electrons in the inner membrane, ultimately enabling their interaction with O_2 and H_2 to yield H_2O. In so doing, the transport allows free energy change and the synthesis of one mole of ATP. With the transport of electrons, free radicals are generated within the mitochondria. Reactive oxygen species (ROS) (H_2O_2, OH·, and O_2^- and nitric oxide [NO]) act as physiologic modulators of some mitochondrial functions but also may cause cell damage. O_2 is converted to superoxide (O_2^-) by oxidative enzymes in the mitochondria, endoplasmic reticulum (ER), plasma membrane, peroxisomes, and cytosol. O_2 is converted to H_2O_2 by superoxide dismutase (SOD) and further to OH· by the Cu^{++}/Fe^{++} Fenton reaction. Superoxide catalyzes the reduction of Fe^{++} to Fe^{+++}, thus increasing OH· formation by the Fenton reaction. H_2O_2 is also derived from oxidases in peroxisomes. The NO· (radical) is produced by the oxidation of one of the terminal guanido-nitrogen atoms of L-arginine. Depending on the microenvironment, NO can be converted to other reactive nitrogen species including the highly reactive peroxynitrate ($ONOO-$). Both OH• and NOO^- are very reactive and can modify cellular macromolecules and cause toxicity. The less reactive molecules O_2^- and H_2O_2 can serve as cellular signaling molecules. The major antioxidant enzymes include SOD, catalase, and glutathione peroxidase. (Data from Dröge W: *Physiol Rev* 82:47-95, 2002; Buetler TM, Krauskopf A, Ruegg UT: *News Physiol Sci* 19: 120-123, 2004.)

Table 2-3	Biologically Relevant Free Radicals
Free Radical	**Comments**
Reactive oxygen species (ROS) Superoxide O_2^- $O_2 \xrightarrow{oxidase} O_2^-$	Generated either (1) directly during autooxidation in mitochondria or (2) enzymatically by enzymes in the cytoplasm, such as xanthine oxidase or cytochrome P-450; once produced, it can be inactivated spontaneously or more rapidly by the enzyme superoxide dismutase (SOD): $O_2^- + O_2^- + 2H^+ \xrightarrow{SOD} H_2O_2 + O_2$; O_2^-, a signaling molecule in growing or differentiating tissue, including hypertrophy, can alter cellular responses to growth factors and vasoconstrictor hormones; increasing levels of O_2^- may lead to apoptosis (see Figure 2-9)
Hydrogen peroxide (H_2O_2) $O_2^- + O_2^- + 2H \xrightarrow{SOD} H_2O_2 + O_2$ *or* oxidases present in peroxisomes O_2 peroxisome $O_2^- \xrightarrow{SOD} H_2O_2$	Generated by the enzyme superoxide dismutase (SOD) or directly by oxidases in intracellular peroxisomes; NOTE: SOD is considered an antioxidant because it converts superoxide to H_2O_2, catalase (another antioxidant) can then decompose H_2O_2 to $O_2 + H_2O$; H_2O_2 can serve as a cellular signaling molecule
Hydroxyl radicals (OH^-) $H_2O \rightarrow H· + OH·$ *or* $Fe^{++} + H_2O_2 \rightarrow Fe^{+++} + OH· + OH^-$ *or* $H_2O_2 + O_2^- \rightarrow OH· + OH^- + O_2$	Generated by the hydrolysis of water caused by ionizing radiation or by interaction with metals—especially iron (Fe) and copper (Cu); iron is important in toxic oxygen injury because it is required for maximal oxidative cell damage; OH· is highly reactive and can modify cellular macromolecules and cause toxicity
Nitric oxide (NO) $NO· + O_2^- \rightarrow ONOO^- + H^+$ $\uparrow\downarrow$ $OH· + NO_2 \rightleftharpoons ONOOH \rightarrow NO_3^-$	NO by itself is an important mediator that can act as a free radical; it can be converted to another radical—peroxynitrite anion ($ONOO^-$), as well as NO_2^- and NO_3^-; NO is formed in neuronal cells where it modulates neurotransmission, in endothelial cells as a modulator of vessel relaxation and in neutrophils and macrophages as a factor in vessel relaxation and inactivation of pathogens

Data from Kumar V, Abbas A, Fausto N: *Robbins and Cotran pathologic basis of disease*, ed 7, Philadelphia, 2005, Saunders; Buetler TM, Krauskopf A, Ruegg UT: *News Physiol Sci* 19:120-123, 2004.

Table 2-4	Diseases and Disorders Linked to Oxygen-Derived Free Radicals
Deterioration noted in aging	Iron overload
Atherosclerosis	Lung disorders
Heart disease	Asbestosis
Stroke	Oxygen toxicity
Brain disorders	Emphysema
Ischemic brain injury	Nutritional deficiencies
Aluminum toxicity	Radiation injury
Alzheimer disease	Reperfusion injury
Neurotoxins	Rheumatoid arthritis
Cancer	Skin disorders
Cardiac myopathy	Solar radiation
Chronic granulomatous disease	Burns
Diabetes mellitus	Contact dermatitis
Eye disorders	Bloom syndrome
Macular degeneration	Toxic states
Cataracts	Xenobiotics (CCl_4, paraquat, cigarette smoke, etc.)
Inflammatory disorders	Metal ions (Ni, Cu, Fe, etc.)

Data from Knight JA: *Ann Clin Lab Sci* 25(2):111, 1995; Bergendi L et al: *Life Sci* 65(18-19): 1865, 1999; Bergamini CM et al: *Curr Pharm Des* 10(14): 1611-1626, 2004.

Table 2-5	Methods Contributing to Inactivation or Termination of Free Radicals	
Method	**Process**	
Antioxidants	Endogenous or exogenous; either blocks synthesis or inactivates (e.g., scavenges) free radicals; includes vitamin E, vitamin C, cysteine, glutathione, albumin, ceruloplasmin, transferrin	
Enzymes	Superoxide dismutase,* which converts superoxide to H_2O_2; catalase* (in peroxisomes) decomposes H_2O_2; glutathione peroxidase* decomposes OH· and H_2O_2	

*These enzymes are important in modulating the cellular destructive effects of free radicals, also released in inflammation.

reticulum combine to form larger droplets and fill vacuoles, which in turn fill the entire cytoplasm. Approximately 10 to 12 hours later, the liver appears grossly enlarged and pale because of the accumulation of fat. (Accumulation of fat is discussed further on p. 75.)

In the meantime, cellular swelling progresses because of alterations in the selective permeability of the plasma membrane. Cellular swelling becomes severe when the plasma membrane loses its ability to prevent the passive inward diffusion of sodium ions, water, and calcium. The most serious consequence of plasma membrane damage is, as in hypoxic injury, to the mitochondria. An influx of calcium ions from the extracellular compartment activates multiple enzyme systems resulting in cytoskeleton disruption, membrane damage, activation of inflammation, and eventually DNA degradation. Calcium ion accumulation in the mitochondria cause the mitochondria to swell, an occurrence that is associated with irreversible cellular injury. The injured mitochondria can no longer generate ATP, but they do continue to accumulate calcium ions. The influx of calcium into the mitochondria interferes with oxidative metabolism (by uncoupling oxidative phosphorylation).

Decreasing cellular pH (caused by the loss of oxidative phosphorylation and ATP-stimulating glycolysis), together with fluid and electrolyte imbalances (increased sodium, calcium, and water and decreased potassium), leads to lysosomal membrane injury, causing a leakage of lysosomal enzymes into the cytoplasm. Enzymatic digestion of cellular organelles, including the nucleus and nucleolus, ensues, halting synthesis of DNA and ribonucleic acid (RNA). The leakage of lysosomal enzymes apparently occurs late in chemical injury, well after irreversible lipid accumulation, mitochondrial swelling, and ATP loss.

Chemical Agents

Many chemical agents cause cellular injury. Minute amounts of some, such as arsenic and cyanide, can rapidly destroy enough cells to cause death of the individual. Long-term exposure to air pollutants, insecticides, and herbicides can cause cellular injury. Carbon monoxide, carbon tetrachloride, and social drugs, such as alcohol, can significantly alter cellular function and injure cellular structures. Over-the-counter and prescribed drugs also may cause cellular injury, sometimes leading to death. Accidental or suicidal poisonings by chemical agents cause numerous deaths. The injurious effects of some of these agents—lead, carbon monoxide, ethyl alcohol, and mercury—exemplify common cellular injuries (see What's New? on Silent Neurotoxicity).

Lead. **Lead** is a heavy metal ubiquitous in the environment. Despite efforts to reduce exposure through government regulation, phasing-out production of leaded gasoline, and banning use of lead paint, excessive lead exposure still persists in the environment for many people and lead toxicity is still a primary hazard to children.[13] Particularly worrisome is lead exposure to the fetus during pregnancy because the developing nervous system is especially vulnerable. Developing

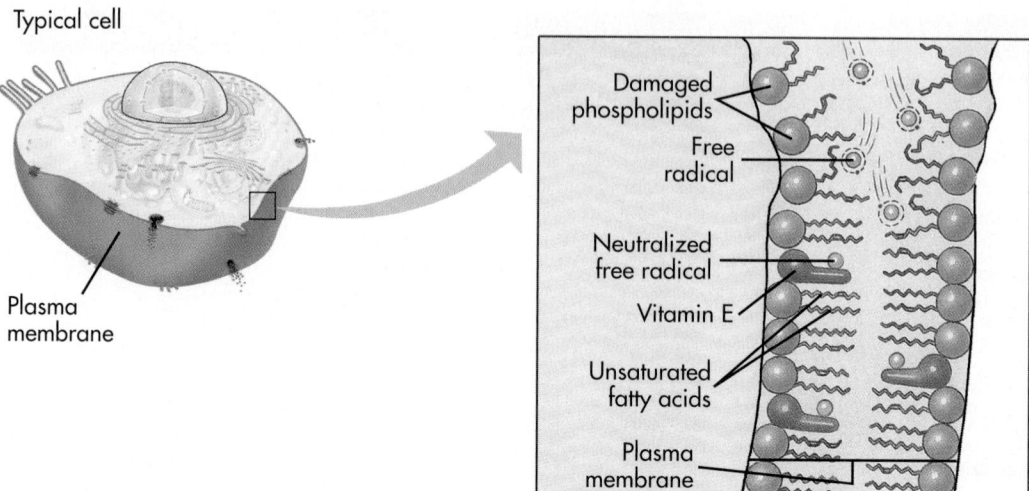

Typical cell

Plasma membrane

Damaged phospholipids

Free radical

Neutralized free radical

Vitamin E

Unsaturated fatty acids

Plasma membrane

Figure 2-11 Role of vitamin E. Vitamin E may act as an antioxidant, attracting and neutralizing molecules with unpaired electrons. (From Thibodeau GA, Patton KT: *Anatomy & physiology,* ed. 5, St Louis, 2003, Mosby.)

fetuses and young children absorb lead more easily than adults;[13] however, the exact transport mechanisms[14] have not yet been elucidated. Exposure to lead during neurologic development has significant effects on neurobehavioral and intellectual performance resulting in learning disorders, hyperactivity, and attention problems.[13]

Lead-based paint, which has a sweet taste, is often ingested by children when they have access to surfaces painted with it. Other sources of lead in daily life include the dust and soil found in inner-city urban and, possibly, rural areas, debris from household renovations, baby formula mixed with lead-contaminated tap water, newsprint, water that flows through lead water pipes, hair dyes, food stored in soldered tin cans or eaten off of pottery made with lead-based glazes, and contamination from leaded gasoline.[15] If nutrition is compromised, especially if dietary intake of iron, calcium, zinc, and vitamin D is insufficient, lead's toxic effects are enhanced.

The organ systems primarily affected by lead include the nervous system, the hematopoietic system (tissues that produce blood cells), and the kidneys. Lead affects many different biologic activities at the cellular and molecular levels, many of which may be related to its ability to interfere with the functions of calcium.[13] Lead is able to *increase* intracellular calcium concentrations and become a calcium substitute, and some calcium-binding proteins are capable of binding to lead.[13] Very tiny concentrations (subnanomolar) of lead activate protein kinase C (PKC) in a process that is partially dependent on calcium.[12,16] The PKC-mediated lead-induced rise in intracellular free calcium may be the cause of cellular disruption. Lead appears to have its greatest effects during the later stages of brain development, possibly by altering development of synaptic connections (i.e., trimming/pruning) and neuronal death (apoptosis).[13] Alterations in calcium may play a crucial role in the interference with neurotransmitters, which may cause hyperactive behavior and proliferation of capillaries of the white matter and intercerebral arteries.[2,13]

Lead inhibits several enzymes involved in hemoglobin synthesis. A significant manifestation of lead toxicity is anemia caused by lysis of red blood cells (hemolysis). Other manifestations of brain involvement include convulsions and delirium and, with peripheral nerve involvement, wrist, finger, and sometimes foot paralysis. Renal lesions can cause tubular dysfunction resulting in glycosuria (glucose in the urine), aminoaciduria (amino acids in the urine), and hyperphosphaturia (excess phosphate in the urine). Gastrointestinal symptoms are less severe and include nausea, loss of appetite, weight loss, and abdominal cramping.

Carbon Monoxide. Gaseous substances can be classified according to their ability to asphyxiate (interrupt respiration) or irritate. Toxic asphyxiants, such as carbon monoxide, hydrogen cyanide, and hydrogen sulfide, directly interfere with cellular respiration. Carbon monoxide is widely available.

Carbon monoxide (CO), a gas, is odorless, colorless, and undetectable unless it is mixed with a visible or odorous pollutant. It is produced by the incomplete combustion of such fuels as gasoline. In dense urban environments, CO produced by incomplete combustion from motor vehicles increases air pollution. Although CO is a chemical agent, the ultimate injury it produces is a hypoxic injury, namely, oxygen deprivation. Normally, oxygen molecules are carried to tissues bound to hemoglobin in red blood cells (see Chapter 29). Because CO's affinity for hemoglobin is 300 times greater than that of oxygen, it quickly binds with the hemoglobin, preventing oxygen molecules from doing so. Minute amounts of CO can produce significant percentages of **carboxyhemoglobin** (carbon monoxide bound with hemoglobin).

Symptoms related to CO poisoning include headache, giddiness, tinnitus (ringing in the ears), nausea, weakness, and vomiting. At risk for CO exposure are those who (1) breathe air polluted by gasoline engines or defective furnaces; (2) work in occupations such as coal mining, fire fighting, welding,[17] or engine repair; and (3) smoke cigarettes, cigars, or

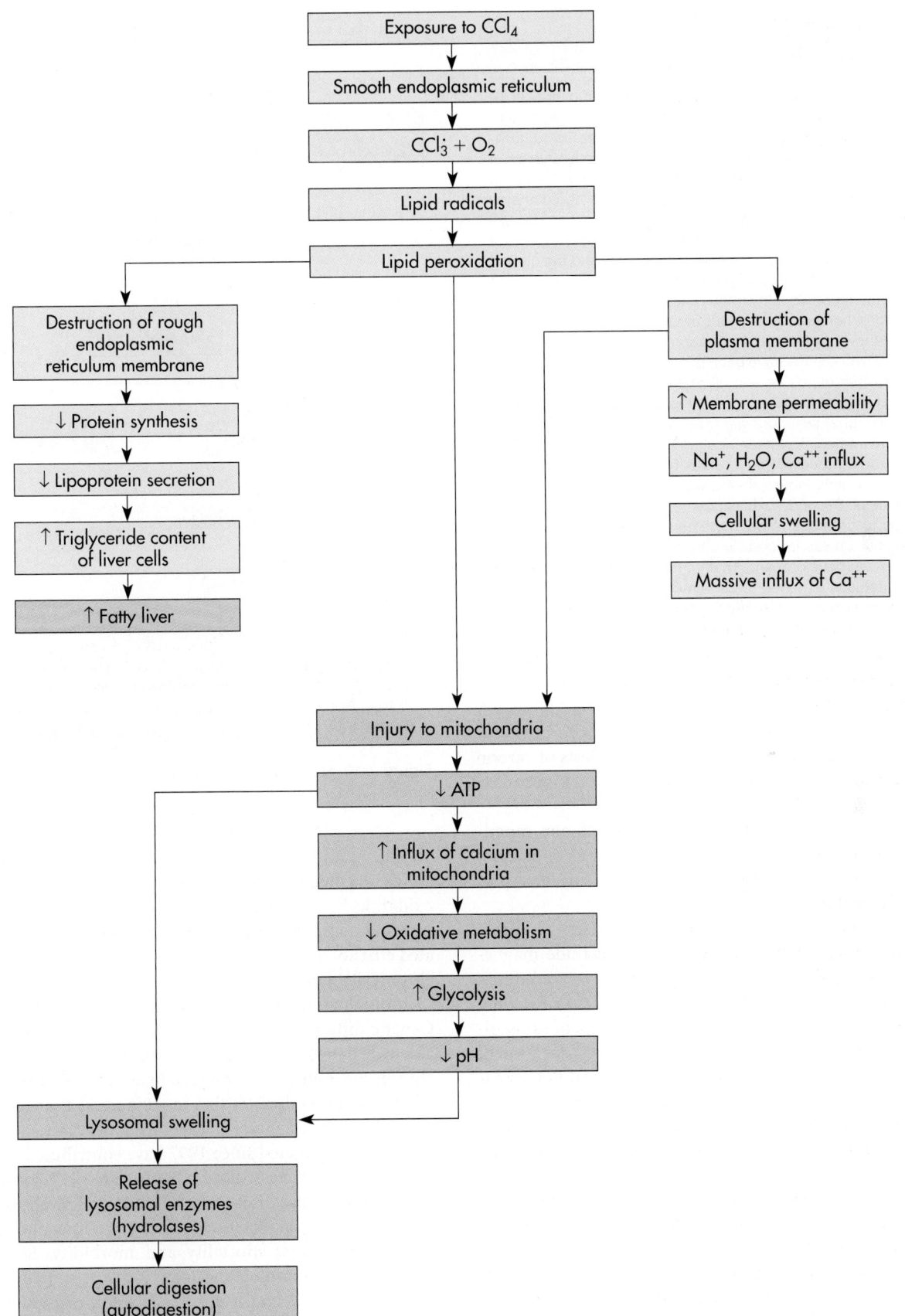

Figure 2-12 Chemical injury of liver cells induced by carbon tetrachloride (CCl_4) poisoning. Light blue boxes are mechanisms unique to chemical injury; purple boxes involve hypoxic injury. Green boxes are clinical manifestations.

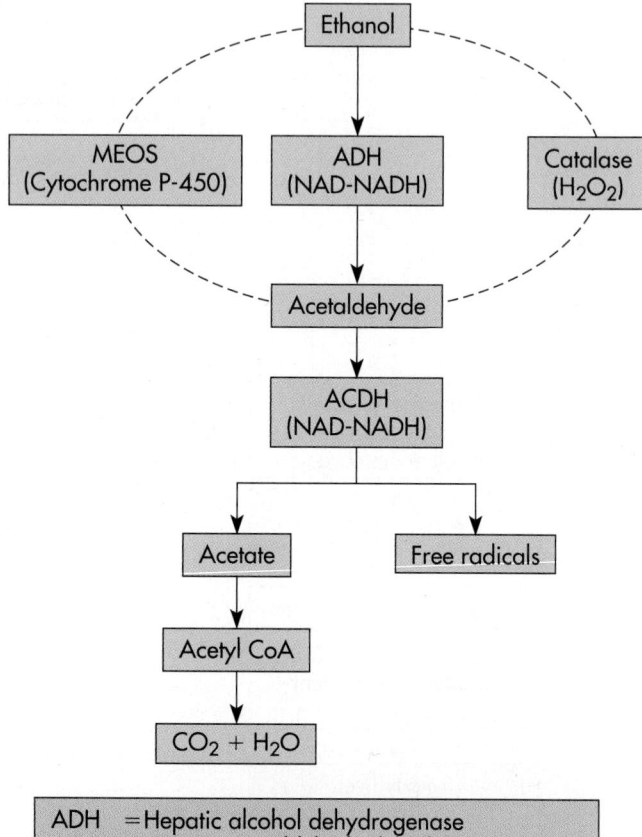

ADH = Hepatic alcohol dehydrogenase
ACDH = Hepatic acetaldehyde dehydrogenase
NAD = Nicotinamide adenine dinucleotide
NADH = Reduced nicotinamide adenine dinucleotide
MEOS = Microsomal ethanol oxidizing system

Figure 2-13 Major pathway of metabolism of alcohol in the liver through ADH.

pipes. The fetus is especially at risk from the effects of carbon monoxide because fetal carboxyhemoglobin levels are likely to be 10% to 15% greater than maternal levels.[18]

Ethanol. Alcohol (**ethanol**) is the number one mood-altering drug used in the United States. Because alcohol is not only a psychoactive drug but also a food, it is considered part of the basic food supply in many societies.

A large intake of alcohol has enormous effects on nutritional status. Major nutritional deficiencies include magnesium, vitamin B_6, thiamin, and phosphorus. Liver and nutritional disorders are the most serious consequences of alcohol abuse. New understandings of the mechanisms of ethanol-induced liver injury have emerged through the clarification of a pathway for ethanol oxidation, the microsomal P-450 oxidase pathway (see below).

The major effects of acute alcoholism involve the central nervous system (CNS). After ingestion, alcohol is absorbed, unaltered, into the stomach and small intestine. Fatty foods and milk slow absorption.[19] Alcohol then is distributed to all tissues and fluids of the body in direct proportion to the blood concentration.

Most of the alcohol in the blood is metabolized in the liver through one major and two accessory pathways. The major pathway involves hepatic alcohol dehydrogenase (ADH), an enzyme of the cytosol that catalyzes the conversion of ethanol to acetaldehyde (Figure 2-13).

The microsomal ethanol oxidizing system (MEOS) depends on cytochrome P-450, an enzyme necessary for cellular oxidation.[20] Activation of MEOS requires a high ethanol concentration and thus is thought to be important in the accelerated ethanol metabolism (i.e., tolerance) noted in people with chronic alcoholism.[20]

Individuals differ in their capability to metabolize alcohol. Genetic differences in metabolism of liver alcohol, including aldehyde dehydrogenases, have been identified.[21] Persons with chronic alcoholism develop certain levels of tolerance because of enzyme induction, leading to an increased rate of metabolism (e.g., P-450).

Studies conducted since 1997 have contributed to our understanding of the association between alcohol consumption and cardiovascular disease. Consistent results validate the so-called *J-shaped inverse association* between alcohol and cardiovascular disease mortality and morbidity. Surprisingly, consistent epidemiologic studies show that daily light-to-moderate alcohol intake reduces the risk of coronary heart disease (CHD) as compared with those who do not drink alcoholic beverages at all. Alcohol likely reduces the risk of CHD through increases in plasma high density lipoprotein-cholesterol (HDL-C) levels.[22] Limited data suggest that the level for optimal benefit may be slightly lower for women. Thus the American Heart Association recommends no more than two drinks per day for men and one drink per day for women.[22]

Acute alcoholism mainly affects the CNS but may induce reversible hepatic and gastric changes. The hepatic changes, initiated from acetaldehyde, include deposition in fat, enlargement of the liver, interruption of microtubular transport of proteins and their secretion, increase in intracellular water, depression of fatty acid oxidation in the mitochondria, increased membrane rigidity, and acute liver cell necrosis (see Chapter 39). In the CNS, alcohol is itself a depressant, initially affecting subcortical structures (probably the brain stem reticular formation).[23] Consequently, motor and intellectual activities become disoriented. Acute alcoholism contributes significantly to motor vehicle fatalities. At higher blood levels, medullary centers become depressed, affecting respiration. Much investigation is underway to determine the extent of the relationship between alcohol and snoring and obstructive sleep apnea (cessation of breathing).[24,25]

Chronic alcoholism causes structural alterations in practically all organs and tissues in the body, especially the liver and stomach. Much progress has been made in understanding the pathogenesis of alcoholic liver disease, which should increase the likelihood of prevention and successful therapy.[26] Cellular damage is increased by ROS and oxidative stress (see p. 52). Activation of proinflammatory cytokines from neutrophils and lymphocytes mediate liver damage.[27] Hepatoxic cytokines include tumor necrosis factor-alpha (TNF-α) and transforming growth factor–beta (TFG-β). Hepatic fibrosis is increased by TGF-β.[27] In addition, the activation of methionine, an essential amino acid, to S-adenosyl-L-methionine (SAMe) is decreased in those with alcoholism.[26] Replacement of SAMe in baboons decreased liver mitochondrial lesions, replenished the antioxidant glutathione, and reduced mortality from cirrhosis.[28] Oxidative stress is associated with phospholipid depletion. In baboons, replacement of polyenylphosphatidylcholine (PPC) corrected the phospholipid depletion.[28] Clinical trials with PPC involving individuals with alcoholic liver disease are ongoing. Chronic alcoholism is related to several disorders, including an increased tendency to hypertension, a higher incidence of acute and chronic pancreatitis, and regressive changes in skeletal muscle (see Chapter 39). Ethanol is implicated in the onset of a variety of immune defects, including effects on the production of cytokines involved in inflammatory responses. The deleterious effects of prenatal alcohol exposure (e.g., **fetal alcohol syndrome [FAS]**) also have been noted. FAS can lead to growth retardation, cognitive impairment, facial anomalies, and ocular disturbances.[29,30] In some cases, full-blown FAS may not be indicated but CNS defects may *still* be present and are classified as alcohol-related birth defects (ARBD) and alcohol-related neurodevelopmental disorders (ARND).[31]

Autopsies of children with FAS have revealed widespread severe damage, including failure of certain brain regions to

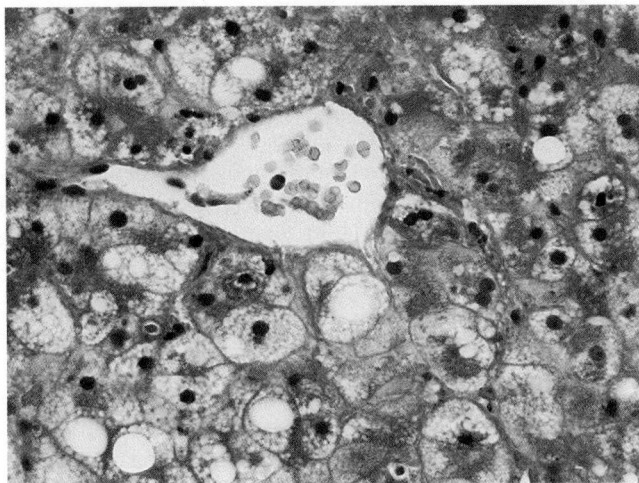

Figure 2-14 Alcoholic hepatitis. Chicken-wire fibrosis extending between hepatocytes. (Mallory trichrome stain.) (From Damjanov I, Linder J: *Anderson's pathology,* ed 10, St Louis, 1996, Mosby.)

develop, malformations of brain tissue, and failure of certain cells to migrate to their necessary location during development.[32] Imaging studies reveal that in addition to an overall reduction in brain size, the corpus callosum is reduced in size or missing, the cerebellum is significantly reduced, and the basal ganglia and caudate nucleus are significantly reduced.[13,33]

Animal studies have shown that ethanol at moderate concentrations inhibits epidermal growth factor–dependent replication of hepatocytes. This finding may account for the growth/development impairment associated with fetal alcohol syndrome and decreased liver regeneration in those with alcoholic liver disease.[34,35] The wide variety of cellular/biochemical effects of ethanol on fetal tissue is itself a puzzle reflecting a multifactorial problem. These effects are conceptually connected to membrane structure and function involving transport systems, membrane fluidity, Na⁺-K⁺ pump expression, and epidermal growth factor receptor expression.[35] Recent evidence points to oxidative stress as being potentially causative of these membrane-related events.[36] Additionally, ethanol has been shown to increase apoptotic cell death.[37]

Whatever the cause, people with chronic alcoholism have a significantly shortened life span related mainly to damage to the liver, stomach, brain, and heart. Alcohol is a well-known cause of hepatic injury, terminating in cirrhosis (see Chapter 39) (Figure 2-14).

Mercury. Mercury has been used medically and commercially for centuries.[38] In the past it was a common component in medications. Mercury is still present in some thermometers and blood pressure cuffs and in batteries, switches, and fluorescent light bulbs. Large amounts of mercury exist as part of the electrodes formed in the electrolytic production of chlorine and sodium hydroxide from saline. Today people are exposed to mercury from three major sources: fish consumption, dental amalgams, and vaccines.

All of these uses give rise to possible accidental and occupational exposures.[38]

Dental Amalgams. Dental amalgams have been used for over 150 years. They are believed to be more durable and easier to use than other types of fillings, as well as being relatively inexpensive. Amalgams consist of about 50% mercury amalgamated or combined with other metals, such as silver and copper. The controversies and heated debates concerning amalgams peaked in the 1970s with the discovery that amalgams can release mercury vapors into the mouth in concentrations that are higher than those deemed safe by occupational health guidelines.

Since then, it was realized that the actual inhaled dose was small because of the small volume of the oral cavity.[38] Yet, brain, blood, and urinary concentrations correlate with the number of amalgam surfaces present in a person. Removal of amalgam fillings also can cause temporary elevations in blood concentration—because the removal transiently increases the amount of mercury vapor inhaled.

Current health risk concerns arise from claims that long-term exposure to low concentrations of mercury vapor either causes or worsens degenerative diseases, such as amyotrophic lateral sclerosis, Alzheimer disease, multiple sclerosis, and Parkinson disease. Concern about the effect of mercury vapor in relation to Alzheimer disease was intensified for a time after a report that the brains of individuals with Alzheimer disease had elevated mercury concentrations. Several epidemiologic investigations, however, failed to provide evidence of a role of dental amalgams in these degenerative diseases; these include a long-term Swedish study,[39] an ongoing Swedish study,[40] and a study of 129 nuns 75 to 102 years of age.[41] A difficult problem is that mercury can inhibit various biochemical processes *in-vitro* without having the same effects *in vivo.* Thus, at present it is unknown whether removal of amalgams reduces risk of certain diseases, especially since removal itself effects blood concentrations of mercury vapor, which will rise before they eventually decline, thereby adding to the controversy.

Fish Consumption. The major source of exposure to methyl mercury is the consumption of fish and sea mammals. Clinical reports of mercury poisoning from fish consumption are those from Japan in the 1950s and 1960s. Environmental Protection Agency (EPA) guidelines are derived from reports of neuropsychologic changes noted in the Faeroe Islands study, in which subjects had been inadvertently exposed to methyl mercury mainly from whale consumption.[42] A similar study in the United States shows methyl mercury levels to be slightly higher than the EPA guideline for safe consumption.[38] The health risk posed by exposure to mercury from fish consumption is currently being debated. The Food and Drug Administration (FDA) has, however, recommended that pregnant women, nursing mothers, and young children avoid eating fish with a high mercury content (>1 parts per million [ppm]), such as shark, sword fish, tile fish, king mackerel, and whale meat.[38]

Vaccines. Thimerosal has been used as a preservative in many vaccines since the 1930s.[38] It contains the ethyl mercury radical ($CH_3CH_2Hg^+$). Earlier toxicology studies found no adverse effects; however, recently a re-evaluation of thimerosal performed by applying the revised EPA guideline for methyl mercury to ethyl mercury found the usual U.S. program of recommended vaccines caused patients to receive more ethyl mercury than the EPA guideline (i.e., >1 mcg of mercury per kilogram per day) deemed safe.[43,44] Steps were rapidly taken to remove thimerosal from vaccines by switching to single-dose vials that did not require a preservative. This removal process is now being completed in the United States. Recent findings indicate that the half-life of ethyl mercury compared to methyl mercury is shorter.[45] The half-life of methyl mercury in blood, which is used to indicate the total body burden, is assumed to be about 50 days.[46] For children receiving thimerosal in vaccines, however, the half-life of ethyl mercury in blood was 7 to 10 days, or $\frac{1}{7}$ to $\frac{1}{5}$ as long as that of methyl mercury.[44,45] Thus, in the 2-month periods between vaccinations (at birth and at 2, 4, and 6 months), all of the mercury should be excreted with no accumulation.[38]

Social or Street Drugs. The social or "recreational" use of psychoactive drugs is widespread in many parts of the world. Most popular are the drugs marijuana, cocaine, and heroin. The actual prevalence of marijuana and heroin use is unknown. Although evidence indicated cocaine use in the general population decreased beginning in 1986, morbidity and mortality related to cocaine increased sharply in the 1990s. Drug trafficking is a prevalent risk behavior among adolescents.[47] Table 2-6 summarizes the effects of these drugs.

Unintentional and Intentional Injuries

Unintentional and intentional injuries are an important health problem in the United States. In 2000 there were 148,209 deaths in this category, an injury death rate of 52.66/100,000.[48] Death due to injury is significantly more common for men than women; the overall rate for men is 74.79/100,000 vs. 31.36/100,000 for women. Significant racial differences exist in the death rate too: whites at 52.46/100,000, blacks at 62.54/100,000, and other racial groups at a combined rate of 31.29/100,000. A bimodal age distribution for injury-related deaths also has been noted, with peaks in the young adult and elderly groups. Unintentional injury is the leading cause of death for people between the ages of 1 and 34 years, with intentional injury (suicide, homicide) ranking between the second and fourth leading causes of death in this age group. Errors in health care are another leading cause of death in the United States.[49] Even using lower estimates from two studies (one in New York and one in Utah and Colorado) of large samples of hospital admissions and subsequent deaths in hospitals due to preventable adverse effects, the number of deaths exceed that attributed to the eighth leading cause of death (motor vehicle accidents, breast cancer, or AIDS)[50] (see What's New? on Errors in Health Care, p. 62). Statistics on nonfatal injuries are harder to document accurately, but they are known to be a significant cause of morbidity and disability and to cost society billions of dollars an-

Table 2-6	Social or Street Drugs
Type of Drug	**Comments**
Marijuana	Active substance: delta-9-tetrahydrocannabinol (THC) found in resin of the *Cannabis sativa* plant; with smoking (e.g., "joints"), about 50% is absorbed through the lungs; when ingested only 10% is absorbed; with heavy use the following adverse effects have been reported: alterations of sensory perceptions, cognitive and psychomotor impairment (e.g., inability to judge time, speed, and distance); smoking 3 or 4/day is similar to 20 cigarettes/day with frequency of chronic bronchitis; data from animal studies only indicate reproductive changes include reduced fertility, decreased sperm motility, and decreased circulatory testosterone; fetal abnormalities related to maternal use include low-birth-weight and increased frequency of childhood leukemia; increased frequency of infectious illnesses thought to be the result of depressed cell-mediated and humoral immunity.
Cocaine and crack	Extracted from the leaves of the coca plant and sold as a water-soluble powder (cocaine hydrochloride) liberally diluted with talcum powder or other white powders; extraction of pure alkaloid from cocaine hydrochloride is "free-base" called "crack" because it cracks when heated; crack is more potent than cocaine; cocaine is widely used as an anesthetic, usually in procedures of the oral cavity; it is a potent CNS stimulant blocking reuptake of neurotransmitters norepinephrine, dopamine, and serotonin; also increases synthesis of norepinephrine and dopamine; dopamine induces a sense of euphoria, and norepinephrine causes adrenergic potentiation including hypertension, tachycardia, and vasoconstriction; cocaine can therefore cause severe coronary artery narrowing and ischemia; increases thrombus formation; other cardiovascular effects include dysrhythmias, sudden death, dilated cardiomyopathy, rupture of descending aorta (i.e., secondary to hypertension), myocyte apoptosis; effects on the fetus include premature labor, retarded fetal development, stillbirth, hyperirritability.
Heroin	An opiate closely related to morphine, methadone, and codeine; highly addictive, and withdrawal causes intense fear ("I'll die without it"); sold "cut" with similar-looking white powder; dissolved in water it is often highly contaminated; feeling of tranquility and sedation lasts only a few hours and thus encourages repeated intravenous or subcutaneous injections; acts on the receptors enkephalins, endorphins, and dynorphins, which are widely distributed throughout the body with high affinity to the CNS; effects can include infectious complications, especially *Staphylococcus aureus*, granulomas of the lung, septic embolism, and pulmonary edema—in addition, viral infections from casual exchange of needles and HIV; sudden death is related to overdosage secondary to respiratory depression, cardiac output, and severe pulmonary edema.

Data from Kumar V, Abbas AK, Fausto N: *Robbins and Cotran pathologic basis of disease,* ed 7, Philadelphia, 2005, Saunders; Nahas G, Latour C: *Med J Australia* 156:495, 1992.

CNS, Central nervous system.

nually. The more common terms used to describe and classify unintentional and intentional injuries and brief descriptions of important features of these are discussed here.

Blunt Force Injuries

Blunt force injuries are the result of the application of mechanical energy to the body resulting in the tearing, shearing, or crushing of tissues. They are the most common type of injuries seen in most health care settings. Blunt force injury may be caused by blows (where a moving object strikes the body), impacts (where the moving body strikes a fixed object), or a combination of both. Motor vehicle accidents and falls are the most common causes of these injuries, accounting for 43,604 and 14,002 deaths, respectively, in 2000.

Contusion

A **contusion** (bruise) is bleeding into the skin or underlying tissues as a consequence of a blow that squeezes or crushes the soft tissues and consequently ruptures blood vessels without breaking the skin. It may take several hours after injury before any change in skin color is seen. A bruise will be red-purple initially, eventually becoming blue-black, and then gradually changing to yellow-brown or green before fully disappearing (Figure 2-15). These color changes reflect the progression of tissue damage and healing that develops in the area of underlying injury. The length of time depends on such factors as the extent and location of the injury and the degree of vascularization in the area. Small contusions may resolve in a matter of days, whereas larger ones can take weeks to completely heal. Bruising of soft tissues may sometimes be confined to deeper structures; thus no injury is visible externally. Blood in deeper structures may dissect along fascial planes so discoloration of the skin may be seen in areas not directly injured by the initiating blow or impact, such as bruising of the thigh occurring with a hip or pelvis fracture or "black eyes" with orbital plate fractures. Contusions also may be seen in internal organs in cases of severe injury.

A collection of blood in soft tissues or an enclosed space also may be referred to as a **hematoma** (see Figures 17-3 and 17-6). A **subdural hematoma** is a collection of blood between the inner surface of the dura mater and the surface of the brain, resulting from the shearing of small veins that bridge the subdural space. Subdural hematomas can result from blows, falls, or sudden acceleration/deceleration of the head, as occurs in *shaken baby syndrome.* An **epidural hematoma** is a collection of blood between the inner surface of the skull and the dura. It is caused by a torn artery and is almost always associated with a skull fracture.

Contusions of the brain may result from (1) a blow or (2) a fall or impact. In blows, when a moving object strikes the stationary head, a cerebral contusion grouped in the portions

Health care is not as safe as it should be. A notable body of evidence documents medical errors as a leading cause of injury and death. Two studies with sizable samples of hospital admissions, one in New York using 1984 data, and another involving Utah and Colorado using 1992 data, found that the proportion of hospital admissions experiencing an adverse event, defined as injuries caused by medical management, were 2.9% and 3.7%, respectively. The proportion of adverse events attributable to errors (i.e., preventable adverse events) was 58% in New York and 53% in Utah and Colorado. When extrapolated to the over 33.6 million admissions to U.S. hospitals in 1997, the implication was at least 44,000 to, possibly, 98,000 Americans die in hospitals each year as a result of medical errors. These deaths exceed the number of deaths attributable to motor vehicle accidents, breast cancer, and AIDS combined.

In terms of lives lost, patient safety is as important as worker safety. Although the literature about errors in health care has grown substantially over the last decade, we do not yet have a compelling analysis of the epidemiology of error. More is known about errors in hospitals than in other health care delivery settings.

Medication-related error has been extensively studied for several reasons: (1) it is the most common type of error, (2) substantial numbers of people are affected, and (3) it accounts for a large increase in health care costs. Medication errors are methodologically easier to study because the drug prescribing process provides documentation of medical decisions, administration of drugs is recorded, supplying drugs are documented, and deaths attributable to medication errors are recorded on death certificates.

Other errors, in addition to medication errors, occur during the course of providing health care. These include wrong-side surgery and surgical injuries; preventable suicides, restraint-related injuries, or death; hospital-acquired or other treatment-related infections; falls; burns; pressure ulcers; and mistaken identity.

Patient safety is one of the nation's most pressing health care challenges. Recommendations suggested to help achieve greater safety include the following:

What can you do? Be involved in your health care.

1. *The single most important way you can help prevent errors is to be an active member of your health care team*. That means taking part in every decision about your health care. Research shows that patients who are more involved with their care tend to get better results.

Medicines

2. Make sure your health care providers know about everything you are taking, including prescription and over-the-counter medicines and dietary supplements such as vitamins and herbs. At least once a year, bring all of your medications and supplements with you to your health care provider. "Brown bagging" your medications can help you and your provider talk about them and find out if there are any problems. This action also can help your provider keep your records up to date, which can help you get better quality care.

3. Make sure your health care providers know about any allergies and adverse reactions you have had to medication. This can help you avoid getting a medication that can harm you.

4. When your health care provider writes you a prescription, make sure you can read it. If you can't read your provider's handwriting, your pharmacist might not be able to either.

5. Ask for information about your medicines in terms you can understand—both when your medications are prescribed and when you receive them. What is the medicine for? How am I supposed to take it and for how long? What side effects are likely? What do I do if side effects occur? Is this medicine safe to take with other medicines or dietary supplements I am taking? What food, drink, or activities should I avoid while taking this medicine?

6. When you pick up your medicine from the pharmacy, ask, "Is this the medicine my provider prescribed?" A study in Massachusetts College of Pharmacy and Allied Health Sciences found that 88% of medicine errors involved the wrong drug or the wrong dose.

7. If you have any questions about the directions on your medicine label, ask. Medicine labels can be hard to understand. For example, ask if "four doses daily" means taking a dose every 6 hours around the clock or just during regular waking hours.

8. Ask your pharmacist for the best device to measure your liquid medicine. Also ask questions if you're not sure how to use it. Research shows that many people do not understand the right way to measure liquid medicines. For example, many use household teaspoons, which often do not hold a true teaspoon of liquid. Special devices, like marked syringes, help to measure the right dose. Being told how to use the devices helps even more.

9. Ask for written information about the side effects your medicine could cause. If you know what might happen, you will be better prepared if it does—or, if something unexpected happens instead, then you can report the problem right away and get help before it gets worse. A study found that written information about medicines can help patients recognize problem side effects and then give that information to their health care provider or pharmacist.

Hospital stays

10. *If you have a choice, choose a hospital in which many patients have the same procedure or surgery you need*. Research shows that patients tend to have better results when they are treated in hospitals that have a great deal of experience with their condition.

11. *If you are in a hospital, consider asking all health care workers who have direct contact with you whether they have washed their hands*. Handwashing is an important way to prevent the spread of infections in hospitals. Yet, it is not done regularly or thoroughly enough. A recent study found that when patients checked whether health care workers washed their hands, the workers washed their hands more often and used more soap.

12. *When you are being discharged from the hospital, ask your health care provider to explain the treatment plan you will use at home*. This includes learning about your medicines and finding out when you can get back to your regular activities. Recent studies show that at discharge time, health care providers think their patients understand more than they really do about what they should or should not do when they return home.

Data from Agency for Healthcare Research and Quality: *20 tips to help prevent medical errors* (pub no 00-PO30), Rockville, MD, 2000, Author; Bates DW et al: *JAMA* 274(1):29-34, 1995; Bates DW et al: *JAMA* 277(4):307-311, 1997; Centers for Disease Control and Prevention, National Center for Health Statistics: *Natl Vital Stats Rep 47* 191:27, 1999; Institute of Medicine: *To err is human: building a safer health system*, Washington, DC, 1999, National Academy Press.

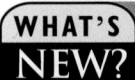

Surgery

13. *If you are having surgery, make sure you, your health care provider, and your surgeon all agree and are clear on exactly what will be done.* Performing surgery at the wrong site (for example, operating on the left knee instead of the right) is rare— but even once is too often. The good news is that wrong-site surgery is 100% preventable. The American Academy of Orthopaedic Surgeons urges its members to sign their initials directly on the site to be operated on before the surgery.

Other steps you can take

14. *Speak up if you have questions or concerns.* You have a right to question anyone who is involved with your care.

15. *Make sure that someone, such as your personal health care provider, is in charge of your care.* This is especially important if you have many health problems or are in a hospital.

16. *Make sure that all health professionals involved in your care have important health information about you.* Do not assume that everyone knows everything they need to.

17. *Ask a family member or friend to be there with you and to be your advocate (someone who can help get things done and speak up for you if you can't).* Even if you think you don't need help now, you might need it later.

18. *Know that "more" is not always better.* It is a good idea to find out why a test or treatment is needed and how it can help you. You could be better off without it.

19. *If you have a test, don't assume that no news is good news.* Ask about the results.

20. *Learn about your condition and treatments by asking your health care provider and nurse and by using other reliable sources.* For example, treatment recommendations based on the latest scientific evidence are available from the National Guidelines Clearinghouse at www.guideline.gov. Ask your provider if your treatment is based on the latest evidence.

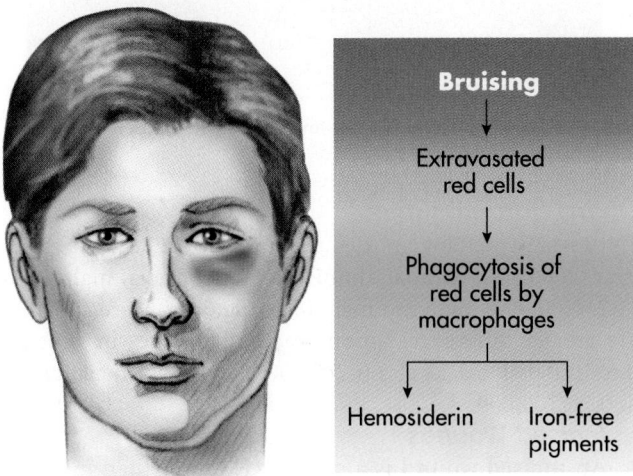

Figure 2-15 Hemosiderin accumulation is noted as the color changes in a "black eye."

of the brain underlying the area of scalp and skull injury is known as a *coup* pattern of injury. In falls or impacts, where the moving head strikes a fixed object, a cerebral contusion seen in the area of the brain opposite the external injury is known as a *contrecoup* pattern of injury (see Figure 17-1). Contrecoup injury results when the head accelerates and the brain lags behind and presses into the areas of the skull directly opposite the direction of motion. When the head suddenly stops, the areas of the brain pressing into the skull are injured. For example, a person who falls directly backward striking the occiput (back of the head) will have cerebral contusions of the frontal and temporal tips (these injuries are discussed further in Chapter 17).

Abrasion

An **abrasion** (scrape) results from removal of the superficial layers of the skin caused by friction between the skin and injuring object. Abrasions vary in size and severity from fine, thin scratches to large denuded areas (road rash). In cases where force is applied in a tangential, nonperpendicular direction to the skin surface, tags of tissue may be heaped up at the trailing or downstream edge of the abrasion. An abrasion will have a pale, moist, yellow-brown appearance at first. The color darkens to brown or even black as the injury dries. The injury may ooze fluid for 1 or 2 days until it is completely covered by a crust, or scab, which eventually flakes off of the underlying regenerated skin.

Abrasions and contusions may have a patterned appearance that mirrors the shape and features of an injuring object (Figure 2-16). Patterning of injuries can be of crucial importance in cases of automobile accidents, assaults, or homicides by documenting the connection between the victim's injuries and a suspect vehicle or weapon. Bite marks (usually a combination of abrasion and contusion) are another example of a patterned injury that can demonstrate a link between an assailant and victim.

Laceration

A **laceration** is a tear or rip resulting when the tensile strength of the skin or tissue is exceeded. Unlike an incision, where the tissue is cleanly divided by a sharp edge, a laceration is much more jagged and irregular, and the edges are abraded. The depths of the laceration are irregular, and often tissue "bridges" of small vessels or nerves that have been stretched but not broken are present, crossing from one side of the wound to the other. If the injuring force is applied perpendicularly to the skin, crushing of the surrounding tissue with associated abrasion and contusion will be noted. If force is applied tangentially, undermining of the wound also will occur, with tissues at the trailing edge of the wound being lifted away from the underlying structures, creating a pocket in the direction opposite from where the blow came. An extreme example is an **avulsion** (Figure 2-17), in which a wide area of tissue may be pulled away creating a large flap. Usually, the shallower the angle of incidence of the blow, the more extensive the undermining.

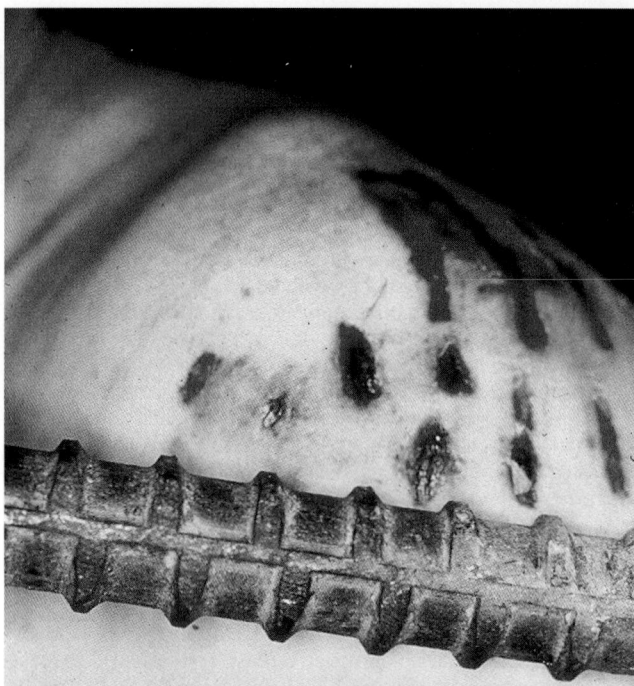

Figure 2-16 Patterned abrasion caused by a piece of rebar. Note the tissue tags at the inferior margins indicating the downward direction of the blow that caused this injury.

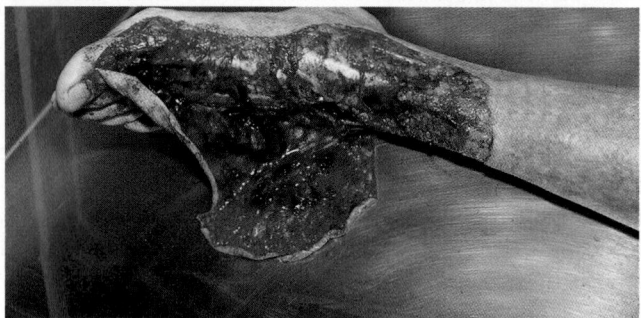

Figure 2-17 Avulsed laceration in motor vehicle accident victim. The victim was the driver and this injury most likely was caused by the brake pedal.

Lacerations of internal organs are not uncommon in blunt impact injuries. Lacerations of the liver, spleen, kidneys, and bowel may occur in cases of blows to the abdomen, often with no externally visible injury to the abdominal wall. The thoracic aorta may be lacerated in sudden deceleration accidents. This results from the arch of the aorta being freely mobile, whereas the descending portion is attached to the spinal column. Rapid deceleration causes horizontal shearing with either partial or complete transection just below the takeoff of the left subclavian artery. Severe blows or impacts to the chest also may cause rupturing of the heart with lacerations of the atria or ventricles.

Fractures

Blunt force blows or impacts also can cause bone to break or shatter. Fractures are extensively covered in Chapter 42 and are not discussed here.

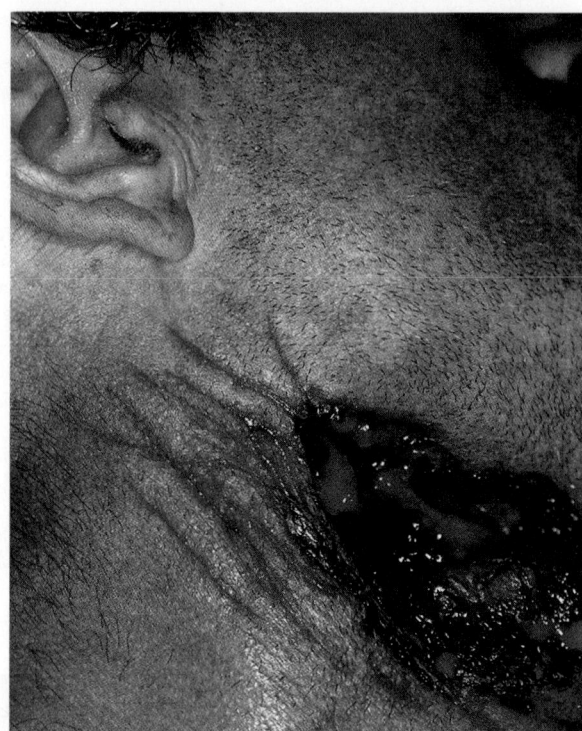

Figure 2-18 Self-inflicted incised wound of the neck with multiple hesitation marks.

Sharp Force Injuries

Cutting and piercing injuries accounted for 2288 deaths in the year 2000. As with all injuries, men have a higher rate (1.21/100,000) than women (0.43/100,000). Here too there are greater differences among races, with rates in whites at 0.63/100,000, blacks at 2.01/100,000, and other racial groups at 0.78/100,000.

Incised Wounds

An **incised wound** is a cut that is *longer* than it is *deep*. The wound may be straight or jagged, depending on the object used and how the injury occurred; sharp, distinct edges without abrasion. Because the wound is caused by a sharp edge, the tissues are cleanly divided and no tissue bridging or undermining occurs. An incised wound may be thin and narrow or more elliptic and gaping in appearance because of varying lines of tension in the skin, depending on the location and orientation of the wound. Incised wounds tend to produce significant external bleeding with minimal internal hemorrhage. These wounds are often seen in sharp force injury suicides. In most cases, in addition to a deep, lethal cut, multiple superficial incisions are grouped in the surrounding area; these are known as *hesitation marks* (Figure 2-18).

Stab Wounds

A **stab wound** is a penetrating sharp force injury that is *deeper* than it is *long*. Because a sharp instrument is used, the depths of the wound are clean and distinct with no underlying or associated crushing injury. The edges are usually clean but may be abraded if the object is inserted deeply with enough force so that a wider, blunter portion of the instru-

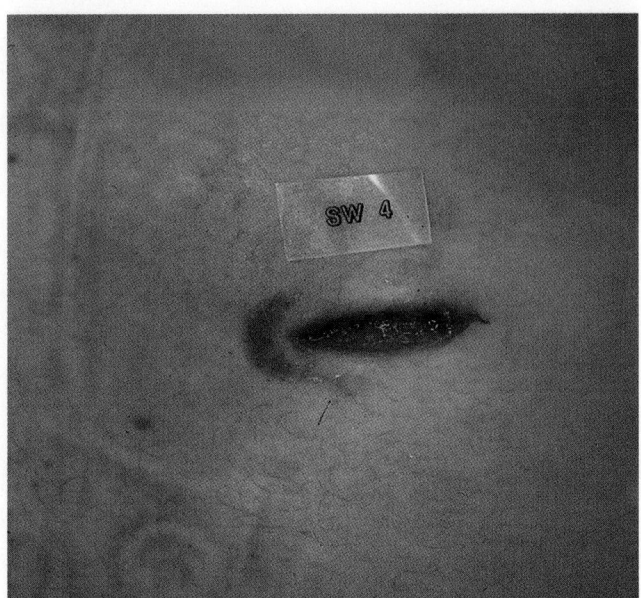

Figure 2-19 Stab wound with associated hilt mark. Note the sharp margin away from the hilt mark with the blunt margin toward it. This wound was caused by a single-edged knife.

ment (e.g., hilt of a knife) impacts the skin. Figure 2-19 illustrates this type of wound.

A number of the offending blade's characteristics may be determined from careful examination of the stab wound. If a *single-edge* blade is used, one margin of the wound will be sharp and the other blunt; if a *double-edge* blade causes the wound, both margins will have a sharp appearance. Stab wounds produced by a *serrated-edge* blade are often indistinguishable from those made by a *smooth-edge* blade. If any hesitation marks or scraping of the skin edges by the blade occur, an interrupted pattern of abrasion may be seen, but this is uncommon. As with incised wounds, skin tension may cause the wound to gape, giving it an elliptic appearance. The edges must be brought into opposition so there is no distortion before trying to determine whether the margins are sharp or blunt. The length of the stab wound may or may not correlate with the width of the blade, depending on whether there was any cutting or twisting when the blade was inserted or withdrawn. Once the edges are in opposition, the thickness of the blade may be estimated from the width of the wound. Depth of the wound may not correlate with the length of the blade because the blade may not have been inserted fully, or as a consequence of compression of tissues caused by a forceful thrust, the wound may be deeper than the length of the blade.

Depending on size and location of the stab wound, the amount of external bleeding may be surprisingly small. After an initial spurt, even if a major vessel or the heart is struck, the wound track may be almost completely closed by tissue pressure, allowing only a trickle of visible blood externally despite copious internal bleeding.

Puncture Wounds

Instruments or objects with sharp points but without sharp edges may produce penetrating **puncture wounds.** A classic example is a wound of the foot caused by stepping on a nail. These injuries often will have abrasion of the edges of the wound, are prone to infection, and also can be quite deep despite a sometimes innocuous external appearance.

Chopping Wounds

Heavy, edged instruments (axes, hatchets, propeller blades) will produce injuries—**chopping wounds**—with a combination of sharp and blunt force characteristics. In addition to cutting, there will usually be associated crushing of the wound edges and underlying tissues.

Gunshot Wounds

Injuries caused by gunfire accounted for 28,663 deaths in the United States in 2000. Of these, 16,586 were suicides, 11,071 homicides, 776 accidents, and 230 classified as undetermined. Men are much more likely to die from gunshot injury than women. The male death rate in 2000 was 17.81/100,000 vs. 2.85/100,000 for women. Black men between the ages of 15 and 24 years have the greatest gunfire injury death rate: 89.25/100,000. To put this statistic into perspective, if this was the rate for the United States as a whole, there would be more than 251,000 gunshot wound deaths per year.

Gunshot wounds may be either penetrating (bullet retained in the body) or perforating (bullet exits the body). In some cases, the bullet may fragment so pieces of the missile are retained even though there is an exit wound. The most important factors determining the appearance of a gunshot injury are whether it is an entrance or an exit wound and the range of fire.

Entrance Wounds

Although all **entrance wounds** share some common features, the overall appearance is most affected by the range of fire.

Contact range entrance wounds occur when the gun is held so the muzzle rests on or presses into the skin surface, causing a distinctive type of wound. In addition to the hole made by the bullet, there will be searing of the edges of the wound from the flame and hot gases exiting the barrel and soot or smoke deposited on the edges of and in the depths of the wound. In hard contact wounds, where the barrel is firmly pressed into the skin, there may be minimal soot and searing on the outside of the wound but deep penetration of smoke, burning gunpowder fragments, and hot gases into the depths of the injury. In hard contact wounds of the head, where there is only a thin layer of skin and muscle overlying bone, the large amount of gas and explosive energy sent into the wound may cause severe tearing and disruption of the tissues, giving the wound a large, gaping, and jagged appearance—a phenomenon known as **blow back.** In areas of the body with thicker layers of soft tissue, the blow back may not cause tearing but will forcefully drive the skin back onto the end of the barrel, producing a patterned abrasion that mirrors the features of the weapon, known as a **muzzle imprint** (Figure 2-20).

Intermediate range entrance wounds are surrounded by gunpowder tattooing or stippling (Figure 2-21). **Tattooing** results from fragments of burning or unburned pieces of

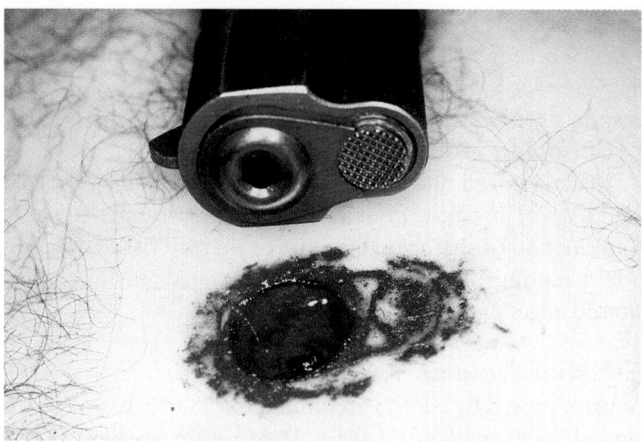

Figure 2-20 Contact range gunshot wound of the chest with a muzzle abrasion.

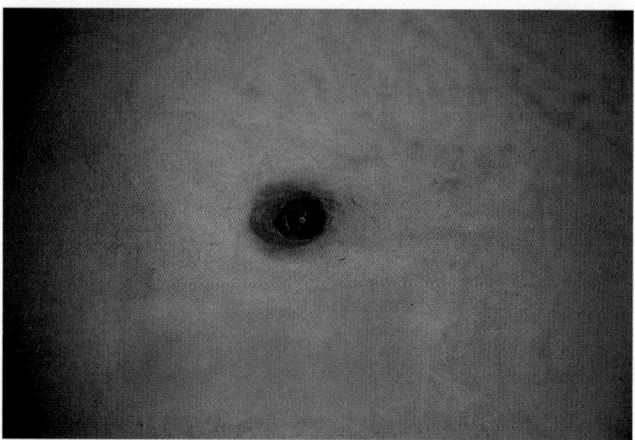

Figure 2-22 Indeterminate range entrance wound with eccentric collar of abrasion resulting from the bullet striking the skin at an angle.

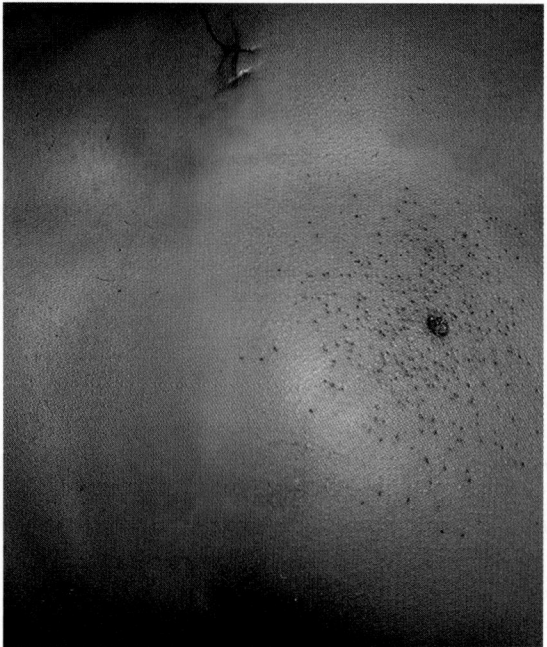

Figure 2-21 Intermediate range gunshot wound with stippling and tattooing.

gunpowder exiting the barrel and striking the skin surface with enough force to be driven into the epidermis or superficial dermis. **Stippling** results when fragments of powder strike with enough force to abrade the skin but not actually penetrate the surface. This phenomenon can be seen when the muzzle-to-target range of most handguns is less than 48 inches. Beyond this distance, pieces of gunpowder disperse and slow down so much that tattooing or stippling cannot occur. The closer the muzzle is to the skin, the tighter the distribution and greater the density of powder fragments will be around the actual entrance hole. Soot also may be deposited.

An **indeterminate (distant) range entrance wound** occurs when flame, soot, or gunpowder does not reach the skin surface and the only thing striking the body is the bullet. The term *indeterminate* is used rather than *distant* because it does not imply that one can actually determine the range of fire

from the appearance of the wound. For example, if an individual is shot through multiple layers of clothing, the entrance wound may have no sooting, searing, or stippling even though the actual range of fire is only a matter of inches; the wound would look the same as if the shot came from a range of 6 meters (20 feet) or more. Indeterminate wounds are characterized by a hole surrounded by a rim of abrasion. The size of the hole can vary according to a number of factors. It is important to remember that one cannot say what caliber of weapon inflicted the wound based solely on the size of the entrance wound. The collar of abrasion results from the fact that the bullet first causes stretching and scraping of the skin before it actually perforates. If the bullet strikes perpendicular to the skin, the margin of the abrasion collar is concentrically disturbed about the defect; if it strikes at an angle, the collar is eccentric, with the wider margin pointing in the direction from which the bullet came (Figure 2-22). If the bullet has struck an intermediary target before hitting the skin, it can be turning and tumbling, producing an irregular abrasion collar.

Exit Wounds

Exit wounds, or where the bullet comes out, have the same general appearance no matter what the range of fire. Their shape can vary from round to slitlike to completely irregular. As with entrance wounds, the size does not correlate very well with the caliber of the projectile making the wound. The most important factors affecting exit wounds are the speed of the projectile and the degree of deformation. A smaller, highly deformed bullet exiting at high speed can produce a large, irregular wound, whereas a larger, intact, slower-moving bullet may only make a small hole. Size *cannot* be used to determine whether the hole is an exit or entrance wound. In most cases, the margins of an exit wound will *not* have an abrasion collar. An exit wound will have clean edges that can often be reapproximated to cover the defect. The exception is when something is pressing against the skin surface at the exit site, such as tight clothing or the back of a chair. In that situation, the bullet will push the skin against the supporting surface causing rubbing and scraping around the exit defect as it comes out, a defect known as a **shored exit wound.**

It is important to remember that because the skin is so elastic and deformable, it is one of the toughest structures for a bullet to go through. It is not uncommon for a bullet to pass entirely through the body and be stopped just beneath the skin on the opposing side of the body. Often no visible injury of the overlying skin is seen; however, careful palpation of the area may allow one to locate the bullet.

Wounding Potential of Firearms

The amount of damage done by a bullet is a function of a number of variables. For the most part, the damage caused is a result of the amount of energy transferred to the tissues impacted. The energy a bullet has is determined by the following formula:

$$KE = \frac{1}{2}MV^2$$

where KE is the energy, M is the mass, and V is the speed.

Clearly, increasing the speed of a bullet has a much greater effect on its potential to cause damage than increasing its size. As the bullet passes through tissue and slows down, its energy is dissipated into the surrounding structures. This energy transfer causes tissue destruction in a zone that can be much larger than the actual size of the bullet; the zone of destruction may be several inches in diameter with very high powered bullets. This transfer of energy in head wounds may lead to orbital plate fractures and palpebral ecchymosis (black eyes) or blood draining from the ears even though the path of the bullet does not come near the base of the skull. The amount of damage caused may be exacerbated by the generation of secondary missiles of bone fragments when portions of the skeleton are struck. Some bullets are designed to expand or fragment when they strike an object, thereby increasing the cross-sectional area of the projectile, increasing drag, and enhancing the transfer of energy into the tissues. "Hollow-point" ammunition is an example of this kind of bullet.

Obviously the lethality of a gunshot injury depends on what structures are damaged. Depending on the extent of damage, even gunshot wounds of the brain may not be lethal; however, they are usually immediately incapacitating and lead to significant long-term disability. It is important to remember that a victim with a "lethal" injury (wound of the heart or aorta) may not be immediately incapacitated and may engage in varying degrees of physical activity after being injured. Just because the victim is active or even combative when first evaluated does not mean the individual may not have experienced a potentially lethal injury.

Asphyxial Injuries

Asphyxial injuries are caused by a failure of cells to receive or utilize oxygen. Deprivation of oxygen may be partial (hypoxia) or total (anoxia). Asphyxial injuries can be grouped into four general categories: suffocation, strangulation, chemical, and drowning.

Suffocation

Suffocation, or oxygen failing to reach the blood, can result from a lack of oxygen in the environment (entrapment in an enclosed space or filling the environment with a suffocating gas) or blockage of the external airways. Classic examples of these types of asphyxial injuries are a child who is trapped in an abandoned refrigerator or a person who commits suicide by putting a plastic bag over the head. A reduction in the ambient oxygen level to 16% (normal is 21%) is immediately dangerous. If the level is below 5%, death can ensue within a matter of minutes. The diagnosis of these types of asphyxial injuries depends on the history of what happened because there will be no specific physical findings.

Diagnosis and treatment in **choking asphyxiation** (obstruction of the internal airways) depend on locating and removing the obstructing material. Injury or disease also may cause swelling of the soft tissues of the airway, leading to partial or complete obstruction and subsequent asphyxiation. Suffocation also may result from compression of the chest or abdomen (mechanical or compressional asphyxia) preventing normal respiratory movements. Usual signs and symptoms include florid facial congestion and petechiae (pinpoint hemorrhages) of the eyes and face.

Strangulation

Strangulation is caused by compression and closure of the blood vessels and air passages resulting from external pressure on the neck. This causes cerebral hypoxia or anoxia secondary to the alteration or cessation of blood flow to and from the brain. It is important to remember that the amount of force needed to close the jugular veins (2 kg [4.5 lb]) or carotid arteries (5 kg [11 lb]) is significantly less than that required to crush the trachea (15 kg [33 lb]). It is the alteration of cerebral blood flow in most types of strangulation that causes injury or death—not the lack of air flow. With complete blockage of the carotid arteries, unconsciousness can occur within 10 to 15 seconds.

A noose is placed around the neck, and the weight of the body is used to cause constriction of the noose and compression of the neck in **hanging strangulations.** The body does not need to be completely suspended to produce severe injury or death. Depending on the type of ligature used, there will usually be a distinct mark on the neck, an inverted V with the base of the V pointing toward the point of suspension. Internal injuries of the neck are actually quite rare in hangings, and only in judicial hangings, where the body is weighted and dropped, will significant soft tissue or cervical spinal trauma be seen. Petechiae of the eyes or face may be seen, but they are rare.

In **ligature strangulation,** the mark on the neck is horizontal, without the inverted V pattern seen in hangings. Petechiae may be more common because intermittent opening and closure of the blood vessels may occur as a result of the victim's struggles. Internal injuries of the neck are rare.

Variable amounts of external trauma on the neck with contusions and abrasions are noted in **manual strangulation** caused either by the assailant or by the victim clawing at one's own neck in an attempt to remove the assailant's hands. Internal damage can be quite severe, with bruising of deep structures and even fractures of the hyoid bone and tracheal and cricoid cartilages. Petechiae are common.

Chemical Asphyxiants

Chemical asphyxiants either prevent the delivery of oxygen to the tissues or block its utilization. Carbon monoxide is the most common chemical asphyxiant (see p. 56). **Cyanide** acts as an asphyxiant by combining with the ferric iron atom in cytochrome oxidase, thereby blocking the intracellular utilization of oxygen. A victim of cyanide poisoning will have the same cherry-red appearance as a carbon monoxide intoxication victim because cyanide blocks the utilization of circulating oxyhemoglobin. An odor of bitter almonds also may be detected. (The ability to smell cyanide is a genetic trait that is absent in a significant portion of the general population.) **Hydrogen sulfide (sewer gas)** is a chemical asphyxiant in which victims of hydrogen cyanide poisoning may have brown-tinged blood in addition to the nonspecific signs of asphyxiation.

Drowning

Drowning is an alteration of oxygen delivery to tissues resulting from the breathing in of fluid, usually water. In 2000 there were 4073 drowning deaths in the United States. Although research done the 1940s and 1950s indicated that changes in blood electrolyte levels and volume as a result of absorption of fluid from the lungs may be an important factor in some drownings, the major mechanism of injury is hypoxemia (low blood oxygen levels). Even in freshwater drownings, where large amounts of water can pass through the alveolar-capillary interface, there is no evidence that increases in blood volume cause significant electrolyte disturbances or hemolysis, or that the amount of fluid loading is beyond the compensatory capabilities of the kidneys and heart. Airway obstruction is the more important pathologic abnormality, underscored by the fact that in up to 15% of drownings, little or no water enters the lungs because of vagal nerve–mediated laryngospasms. This phenomenon is called *dry-lung drowning.*

No matter what mechanism is involved, cerebral hypoxia will lead to unconsciousness in a matter of minutes. Whether this progresses to death depends on a number of factors, including age and health of the individual. One of the most important factors is the temperature of the water. Irreversible injury will develop much more rapidly in warm water than it will in cold water. Submersion times of up to 1 hour with subsequent survival have been reported in children retrieved from very cold water. Complete submersion is not necessary for a person to drown. An incapacitated or helpless individual (such as a person with epilepsy or alcoholism or an infant) may drown in only a few inches of water.

It is important to remember that there are no specific or diagnostic findings to *prove* that a person recovered from the water is actually a drowning victim. In cases where water has entered the lung, there may be large amounts of foam coming from the nose and mouth, although this also can be seen in certain types of drug overdoses. A body recovered from water with signs of prolonged immersion could just as easily be a victim of some other type of injury who has been put in the water to obscure the actual cause of death. When working with a living victim recovered from water, it is essential to keep in mind that an underlying condition may have led to the person's becoming incapacitated and submersed—a condition that also may need to be treated or corrected while correcting hypoxemia and dealing with its sequelae.

Infectious Injury

The pathogenicity (virulence) of microorganisms lies in their ability to survive and proliferate in the human body, where they injure cells and tissues. The disease-producing potential of a microorganism depends on its ability to (1) invade and destroy cells, (2) produce toxins, and (3) produce damaging hypersensitivity reactions (see Chapter 8 for further discussion).

Immunologic and Inflammatory Injury

Cellular membranes are injured by direct contact with cellular and chemical components of the immune and inflammatory responses, such as phagocytic cells (lymphocytes, macrophages) and substances such as histamine, antibodies, lymphokines, complement, and proteases (see Chapter 6). Complement is responsible for many of the membrane alterations that occur during immunologic injury.

Membrane alterations are associated with rapid leakage of potassium (K^+) out of the cell and rapid influx of water. Antibodies can interfere with membrane function by binding to and occupying receptor molecules on the plasma membrane. This type of injury is found in certain forms of diabetes mellitus and in myasthenia gravis. Antibodies also can block or destroy cellular junctions, interfering with intercellular communication (see Chapters 7 and 8).

Injurious Genetic Factors

Genetic disorders may be the result of genetic factors that alter the cell's nucleus and the plasma membrane's structure, shape, receptors, or transport mechanisms. For example, enzymatic genetic defects can lead to abnormalities in membrane transport. Genetic disorders that cause structural alterations of the red blood cell include sickle cell anemia, Huntington disease, muscular dystrophy, and abetalipoproteinemia. (Mechanisms causing genetic abnormalities are discussed in Unit II.)

Injurious Nutritional Imbalances

Essential nutrients—proteins, carbohydrates, lipids (fats), vitamins, and minerals—are required for cells to function normally. If these nutrients are not consumed in the diet and transported to the body's cells or if excessive amounts of nutrients are consumed and transported, pathophysiologic cellular effects develop.

Proteins, which consist of chains of amino acids, are the major structural units of the cell and participate in many enzymatic and hormonal functions. Protein deficiency causes a decrease in the intestinal mucosal mass, decreasing the absorptive function. The integrity of the pancreas is also affected, resulting in diminished exocrine secretion. With starvation or malnutrition, the lowered plasma proteins, particularly albumin, cause fluid to move into the interstitium (edema). Protein-calorie malnutrition (PCM) is the predominant worldwide type of malnutrition. Malnourished children are very susceptible to disease and often die of infectious diseases. Even with adequate protein intake, cellular injury can occur if amino acid transport mechanisms fail or are defective. In Fanconi syndrome, for example, renal tubular cells may contain accumulated protein droplets that have been absorbed but cannot be transported.

Glucose is the major carbohydrate obtained from the breakdown of starch (see Chapter 1). **Hyperglycemia** (excessive glucose in the blood) caused by excessive carbohydrate intake may lead to obesity. Deficiencies of glucose result from starvation or from lack of use, as in diabetes. In both conditions the body compensates by metabolizing fat (lipids). (For details on diabetes, see Chapter 21.)

In lipid deficiency, or **hypolipidemia,** the body compensates by mobilizing fatty acids from adipose tissue. This causes an increase in the production and circulation of ketone bodies, which are acidic by-products of lipid metabolism. The excretion of ketone bodies results in loss of water and electrolytes and causes dehydration and thirst. Severe increases in ketone bodies cause ketoacidosis, coma, and death. **Hyperlipidemia,** or an increase in lipoproteins in the blood, results in deposits of fat in the heart, liver, and muscle.

Vitamins are not sources of energy but are necessary for maintaining normal cellular functions. Adequate vitamin intake is necessary because most vitamins are not synthesized by the body. Research from the 1990s resulted in the identification of 13 vitamins as being essential for humans. These include 8 B vitamins (thiamin, niacin, riboflavin, folate, vitamin B_6, vitamin B_{12}, biotin, and pantothenic acid), vitamin C or ascorbic acid, and the fat soluble vitamins A, D, E, and K. Minerals are discussed in Chapter 3. Vitamins are involved in numerous reactions, including metabolism of visual pigments (vitamin A), calcium and phosphate metabolism (vitamin D), prothrombin synthesis (vitamin K), and antioxidation reactions (vitamins E and C). Pyridoxal (vitamin B_6) affects amino acid transfer reactions; flavin adenine dinucleotide (FAD), flavin mononucleotide (FMN), and nicotinamide adenine dinucleotide (NAD) help the reaction transfer of electrons (see Chapter 1). Table 2-7 presents vitamins and their association with deficiency-related diseases/disorders. New are the many diseases related to vitamin D deficiency, which may include many common cancers, type 1 diabetes, cardiovascular disease, osteoporosis, and fibromyalgia (see the Nutrition & Disease box on Vitamins and Disease Prevention).[51]

Injurious Physical Agents
Injurious physical agents include temperature extremes, changes in atmospheric pressure, radiation, illumination, mechanical factors, noise, and prolonged vibration. Physical injury can result from excessive exposure to many environmental agents, as well as to agents used for the diagnosis and treatment of illness.

Table 2-7	Vitamin Deficiencies and Associated Disorders and Diseases
Vitamin	**Associated Deficiency**
Niacin	Rough skin (pellagra) symptoms include lassitude, anorexia, dermatitis, diarrhea, inflammation of the mouth and other mucous membranes
Riboflavin (vitamin B_2)	Decreased growth; skin lesions; soreness and burning of the lips, mouth, and tongue; burning and itching of the eyes; stomatitis; photophobia; vascularization of the cornea; glossitis; anemia; neuropathy
Thiamin (vitamin B_1)	Beriberi; chronic alcoholism contributes to deficiency; megaloblastic anemia; lactate acidosis; subacute necrotizing encephalomyelopathy; individuals at risk include those undergoing long-term dialysis or intravenous feedings and those with chronic febrile infection
Folate	Defects in DNA synthesis (fast-growing tissue, embryo); megaloblastic anemia; vascular disease (e.g., hyperhomocysteinemia); cancers including colon cancer; malabsorption syndromes (tropical and nontropical sprue)
Vitamin B_{12}	Pernicious anemia; neurologic (demyelination and peripheral neuropathy); memory loss and dementia; hyperhomocysteinemia and vascular disease
Vitamin B_6	Seborrheic dermatitis; microcytic anemia; convulsions; depression; confusion
Pantothenic acid (vitamin B_5)	Listlessness, fatigue, and weakness; headaches; personality changes; sleep disturbances; impaired motor coordination; gastrointestinal disturbances
Biotin	Severe ketoacidosis, seizures, ataxia, lethargy, coma at birth; hair loss; skin rashes; hearing loss; optic atrophy
Vitamin C	Scurvy (bleeding under the skin, gums, joint pain, joint effusions, shortness of breath); fatigue; increased risk to infection (decreased immune function)
Vitamin K	Hemorrhagic disease of the newborn; depression of vitamin K–dependent coagulation factors; individuals at risk are those on antibiotic therapy (interferes with synthesis) and those who have osteoporosis
Vitamin E	Status may depend on selenium and sulfur-containing amino acids; necrotizing myopathy (skeletal, heart, smooth muscle); decreased life span of red blood cells and increased risk of hemolysis; neurologic abnormalities; increased susceptibility to effects of oxidizing agents in the environment; decreased immune function, possibly vascular disease and coronary heart disease; possibly certain cancers (head, neck, lung, colorectal)
Vitamin A	Possibly several types of cancer; decreased immune function; fetal malformations; vision abnormalities (including night blindness, cornea changes, drying)
Vitamin D	Rickets; type 1 diabetes; cardiovascular disease, some common cancers, osteoporosis; fibromyalgia; multiple sclerosis; parathyroid disorders

NUTRITION & DISEASE

Vitamins and Disease Prevention

Vitamins are essential to maintaining normal metabolic processes—growth, metabolism, and cellular integrity. The most common function of vitamins is as *essential* components of coenzymes. Coenzymes are small, organic molecules that are required by an enzyme as a coparticipant in the chemistry of catalysis. Other functions of some vitamins include the synthesis of hormones and acting as antioxidants. The amount of a specific vitamin required by an individual varies considerably and is influenced by several factors, including body size, growth rate, physical activity, and pregnancy. Most vitamins are stored in minimal amounts in human cells, but some (vitamins A and D) are stored in liver cells to a greater extent. A deficiency of B compounds , may be noticed within days, however, and a lack of vitamin C will take weeks to manifest. Table 2-7 lists specific vitamins and associated disorders/diseases.

Vitamin D and the role of vitamin D deficiency is currently a "hot topic." Vitamin D deficiency appears to increase the risk of many common and serious diseases, including some common cancers, type 1 diabetes, cardiovascular disease, osteoporosis, and fibromyalgia. Numerous epidemiologic studies suggest that exposure to sunlight, which increases the production of vitamin D(3) in the skin, is important in preventing many chronic diseases. Because very few foods naturally contain vitamin D (e.g., milk, some cereals, bread, some fish, etc.), sunlight supplies most of our vitamin D requirement. 25-Hydroxy vitamin D [25(OH)D] is the metabolite that should be measured in the blood to determine vitamin D status. Vitamin D deficiency can occur in infants who are solely breastfed and do not receive vitamin D supplementation, and in adults of all ages who have increased skin pigmentation or who always wear sun protection or limit their outdoor activities. A new source of dietary vitamin D is orange juice fortified with vitamin D. Studies in both human and animal models add compelling evidence to the hypothesis that the "unrecognized" epidemic of vitamin D deficiency worldwide is a contributing factor to many chronic debilitating diseases. The recommended adequate intakes for vitamin D are now thought to be inadequate. In the absence of exposure to sunlight, a minimum of 1000 IU of vitamin D is thought to be required to maintain a healthy concentration of 25(OH)D in the blood.

Data from Bsoul SA, Terezhalmy GT: *J Contemp Dent Pract* 5(2): 1-13, 2004; Holick MF: *Am J Clin Nutr* 79(3):362-371, 2004.

Temperature Extremes

Chilling or freezing of cells causes **hypothermic injury.** Hypothermia has proved to be strongly injurious to a variety of cells. Hypothermic injury has long been attributed to disturbances of cellular ion balance or homeostasis, especially of sodium balance (i.e., increased intracellular sodium levels). Hypothermia increases intracellular Ca^{++} by slowing the Na^{+}-K^{+}-ATPase pump activity, leading to Na^{+} accumulation intracellularly.[52] In recent years, however, a role for reactive oxygen species (ROS) has gained importance.[53] In animal studies, hypothermia resulted in cell damage caused by formation of ROS.[54-56] Hypothermic perfusion of the heart increased O_2^{-} (superoxide, see Table 2-3); in turn O_2^{-} reacted with nitric oxide (NO) to form another radical peroxynitrate anion ($ONOO^{-}$).[52]

Therapeutically, hypothermia is widely used to protect cells and tissues against injurious processes. In some cell types, however, such as hepatocytes and liver endothelial cells, hypothermia can cause pronounced cell injury mediated by ROS.[56] During the body's exposure to cold, incubation injury is inhibited by hypoxia and by a number of antioxidants, especially iron chelators.[56]

Indirect forms of injury occur because of changes in small blood vessels (the microcirculation). Slow chilling can cause vasoconstriction followed by paralysis of vasomotor control, resulting in vasodilation and increased membrane permeability causing cellular and tissue swelling. With an abrupt drop in temperature, vasoconstriction and increased viscosity of the blood cause ischemic injury—infarction and necrosis (cellular death) in affected tissues. With continued exposure to freezing temperatures, vasodilation produces severe swelling that causes degenerative changes in the myelin sheath that surrounds peripheral nerves, resulting in sensory and motor disturbances. Thrombosis also can occur and may lead to gangrene of the affected part. (Gangrene is discussed on p. 80.) These conditions often are called *frostbite*.

Hyperthermic injury (injury caused by excessive heat) is common and varies depending on the nature, intensity, and extent of the injury. Three types of hyperthermic injury include heat cramps, heat exhaustion (illness), and heat stroke. (For more detail see Chapter 15).

Heat cramps are cramping of voluntary muscles, usually as a result of vigorous exercise. Cramps are the result of salt and water loss as a consequence of sweat. Treatment is salt replacement.

Heat exhaustion occurs when sufficient salt and water loss results in hemoconcentration. Hypotension occurs secondary to fluid loss (hypovolemia), and the individual feels weak, nauseated, and can suddenly collapse. Collapsing results from a failure of the cardiovascular system to compensate for hypovolemia. Heat exhaustion is probably the most common heat-related injury.

Heat stroke is a life-threatening condition associated with high environmental temperatures and humidity. Core body temperature rises as a result of thermoregulatory failures. Clinically, a rectal temperature of 106° F is considered a life-threatening sign. Generalized peripheral vasodilation and decreased circulating blood volume are significant. At risk are the elderly, athletes, military recruits, and persons with cardiovascular disorders.

Burns are caused by local heat injury. A full-thickness burn is an open wound involving skin layers—epidermis, dermis, and subcutaneous layers—and causing extensive loss of fluids and plasma proteins. Cellular regeneration is not possible; therefore skin from a donor or from the host must be grafted to the site. Partial-thickness burns result in reddening of the area as a result of dilation of small blood vessels and increased permeability of cellular membranes, with loss of protein-rich fluid, resulting in the typical "burn blister." In surface epithelial cells, membrane permeability increases, causing both cytoplasmic and nuclear swelling. Temperature-sensitive enzymes within certain cells respond to heat by increasing cellular me-

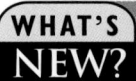

The summer of 2003 brought a region of high atmospheric pressure over western Europe and blocked the flow of rain-bearing, low pressure systems that arrive from the Atlantic Ocean. As a consequence the continent experienced a prolonged period of unusually hot, dry weather. Switzerland experienced the hottest June in 250 years, with the average temperatures in Basel around 29.5° C (85° F), about 5.9° C above normal. Temperatures in France soared to 40° C (104° F) and remained high for weeks.

France's National Institute of Health and Medical Research estimated that almost 15,000 people died in August 2003. In Italy it was estimated an excess death toll of more than 4000 residents occurred in the country's 21 largest cities. With estimates suggesting that Europe's 2003 heat wave claimed more than 30,000 lives, it became the continent's largest natural disaster in 50 years.

Since 1991, heat waves have killed an average of 235 U.S. residents each year, while floods claimed 86, tornadoes took 59, and lightening killed 53 people. Most often the victims of heat waves live in inner cities, are sick, isolated, or elderly. Heat waves take people by surprise and, thus, they are less prepared than with more dramatic weather changes. Heat-related deaths in July 1995 claimed an excess of at least 700 deaths. At greatest risk for heat-related deaths in Chicago were those (1) with known medical problems who were confined to bed or unable to care for themselves, (2) who did not leave home each day, and (3) who lived alone or on the top floor of a building. Having social contacts, such as group activities or friends, in the area was protective. The risk of death was reduced for people with working air conditioners and those with access to transportation. Deaths classified as due to cardiovascular causes had risk factors similar to those for heat-related death.

Data from Franklin CM: Lessons from a heat wave. In *Intensive care medicine*, 2003, Springer-Verlag, available at www.springer-link.com; Perkins S: *Sci News* 116:10-12, 2004; Semanza JC et al: *N Engl J Med* 335(2):84-90, 1996.

tabolism, with detrimental effects. Intense heat also damages the vascular endothelium and causes coagulation of the blood vessels. (Burns are discussed further in Chapter 46.)

Epidemiologic investigators have reported a relationship between overheating in infants, that is, overdressing infants in the winter, and sudden infant deaths. Studies suggest interactions between body temperature and respiratory responses to hypoxia or increased carbon dioxide (hypercapnia). The hypoxia/*hypo*thermia interaction depresses breathing, reducing the ventilatory response to hypercapnia. The effects of *hyper*thermia seem to be a significant problem only when it accompanies an infection and fever and alters or depresses the breathing responses. (Temperature changes are also discussed in Chapter 15.)

Changes in Atmospheric Pressure

Sudden increases or decreases in atmospheric pressure cause **blast injury,** which can be transmitted by either air (air blast) or water (immersion blast). With sudden increases in pressure, such as in air blast or explosive injuries, tissue injury is caused by compressive waves of air impinging on the body,

followed by a sudden wave of decreased pressure. The pressure changes may collapse the thorax, rupture internal solid organs, and cause widespread hemorrhage. In increased pressure caused by immersion blast, water pressure is applied suddenly to all sides of the body, forcing the body up out of water. The positive pressure compresses the abdomen and ruptures hollow internal organs, such as the spleen, kidneys, and liver.

With sudden decreases in pressure, carbon dioxide and nitrogen that are normally dissolved in the blood come out of solution and form tiny bubbles called *gas emboli.* At low atmospheric pressure, such as occurs at altitudes above 15,000 feet, there is a significant decrease in available oxygen. This causes hypoxic injury, and compensatory vasoconstriction shunts blood from the peripheral circulation (in the extremities) to the visceral organs, including the lungs. The combination of increases in pulmonary blood flow and systemic hypoxia causes "high-altitude pulmonary edema"[57] (see Chapter 33).

Deep sea divers and underwater construction workers who return to the surface too quickly develop a form of gas embolism called **decompression sickness** or **caisson disease** ("the bends"). If water pressure is reduced too rapidly, the gases dissolved in blood bubble out of solution, forming emboli. Oxygen is quickly redissolved, but nitrogen bubbles may persist and obstruct blood vessels. Ischemia resulting from gas emboli causes cellular hypoxia, particularly in the muscles, joints, and tendons, which are especially susceptible to changes in oxygen supply. Emboli and interstitial gas accumulate around the joints and skeletal muscles, causing the individual to double up in pain. Tissues of the heart and brain also may be affected by emboli, causing necrosis. The gases can be promptly redissolved in blood by raising the atmospheric pressure. This is accomplished by placing the individual in a decompression chamber. First, pressure is increased until it approximates pressure at the depth to which the diver had descended. This redissolves the gas bubbles in the blood. Then the pressure in the chamber is decreased gradually until it equals pressure at the surface of the water. The slow decrease in pressure slows the release of gas bubbles out of solution.

Ionizing Radiation

Ionizing radiation is any form of radiation capable of removing orbital electrons from atoms. Ionizing radiation is emitted by x-rays, gamma rays, and alpha and beta particles (which are emitted from atomic nuclei in the process of radioactive decay) and from neutrons, deuterons, protons, and pions (all of which are emitted from cobalt or linear accelerators). Occupational exposure to ionizing radiation is mostly limited to alpha- and beta-particle exposure and exposure to x-rays, gamma rays, and neutrons. Radiant energy from sunlight (solar radiation) also can injure cells.

The most abundant source of exposure to ionizing radiation is the environment. This source includes emission from radioactive material inside the body, cosmic rays from outer space, and radiation emitted from such substances as soil and building materials. Environmental radioactivity is emitted primarily by uranium, thorium, and potassium. Other

Table 2-8	Types of Ionizing Radiation and Their Tissue Penetration	
Type	**Tissue Penetration**
X-rays	High
Gamma (γ) rays	High
Beta (β) particles	Low
Alpha (α) particles	Very low
Protons	Intermediate between α and β
Neutrons	High

Data from Damjanov I, Linder J, editors: *Anderson's pathology*, ed 10, St Louis, 1996, Mosby.

sources are x-rays used for medical diagnosis and treatment, uranium and thorium mines, nuclear weapons, and nuclear reactors that generate electricity. Table 2-8 includes types of ionizing radiation and their magnitude of tissue penetration.

The mechanism by which ionizing radiation damages cells is shown in Figure 2-23. DNA is the most vulnerable target of radiation, particularly the bonds within the DNA molecule. All phases of the cell cycle can be affected by ionizing radiation. Sensitivity of the cell appears to be greatest in G_2, that gap of the cell just before mitosis; irradiation during this phase retards the onset of cell division. Irradiation during mitosis induces chromosomal aberrations. Chromosomal aberrations include breaks, deletions, translocations, and many other structural abnormalities. Membrane molecules and enzymes also are damaged by radiation (see Chapter 11). The intensity, duration, and cumulative effects of exposure to ionizing radiation determine the extent of injury.

Not all cells and tissues have the same sensitivity to radiation, although all cells can be affected. Radiosensitivity depends on rate of mitosis and cellular maturity. Because fetal cells are both immature and undergoing rapid cycling, the fetus is at great risk for injury caused by ionizing radiation. Particularly vulnerable are embryonic germ cells, which are precursors of ova and sperm. Throughout life, cells of the bone marrow, intestinal mucosa, testicular seminiferous epithelium, and ovarian follicles are susceptible to injury because they are always undergoing mitosis, which ensures the presence of vulnerable, immature daughter cells. A critical target for reactive free radicals, particularly O_2^-, is the DNA.

The effects of ionizing radiation may be acute or delayed. Acute effects of high doses, such as skin redness, skin damage, or chromosomal aberrations, occur within hours, days, or months. The delayed effects of low doses may not be evident for years. Effects are usually (1) somatic, involving the exposed individual's entire body (e.g., leukemia, other cancers); (2) genetic, involving offspring of the exposed individual; or (3) fetal, involving fetuses that are exposed in utero. Data suggest that low-dose exposures may affect apoptosis and epigenetic (a change in gene *expression* and not in the DNA sequence) processes.[58] According to the FDA uncertainty exists regarding the risk estimates for low levels of radiation exposure as commonly experienced in diagnostic radiology procedures.[59] (The carcinogenic effects of radiation are discussed in Chapter 11.)

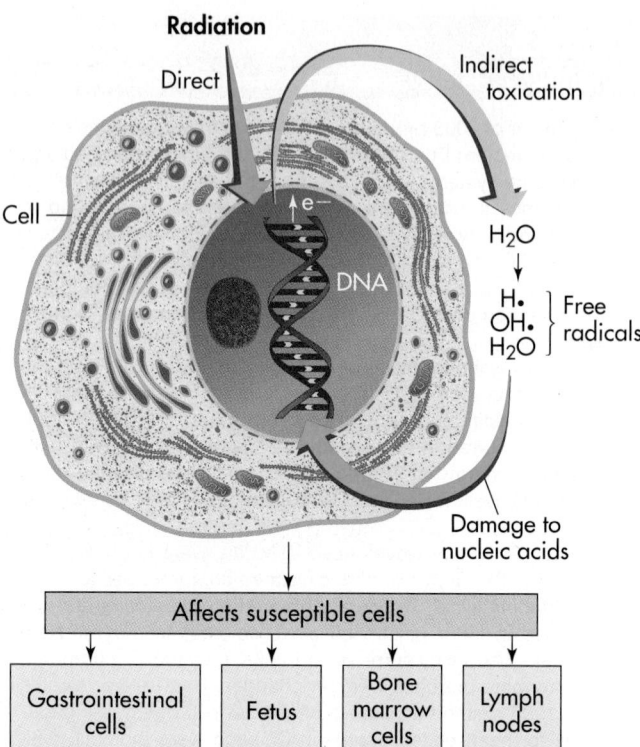

Figure 2-23 Cellular damage caused by ionizing radiation. Radiation can damage macromolecules in two ways: *(1)* directly, where the micromolecules are ionized; and *(2)* indirectly, where water is ionized and produces free radicals that in turn damage macromolecules. Cells that are particularly susceptible to damage are those of the gastrointestinal tract, bone marrow, lymph nodes, a fetus, and ovarian follicles. (Also see Chapter 18.)

Illumination

Illumination has biologic effects that are related to health.[60,61] The harmful effects of fluorescent lighting include eyestrain, obscured vision, and possibly cataract formation. The rapid modulation of light from fluorescent lamps is responsible for eyestrain and headaches.[62] The modulation can be reduced by wearing tinted glasses.[63] The shorter wavelengths in radiant energy in environmental lighting influence the absorption, scattering, and fluorescence, thus obscuring vision.[62]

Vision is obstructed at night by decreased illumination and by disabling glare from oncoming vehicle headlights. High intensity discharge (HID) headlamps project light farther down roads, thus improving the *owner's* driving safety. However, oncoming glare, which is proportional to headlamp brightness, is *not* good for any drivers of oncoming vehicles and even worse for older drivers. Older drivers experience more intraocular light scattering, glare sensitivity, and longer recovery time in reaction to photo stress.[64]

Studies have demonstrated the in vitro toxicity of halogen lamps.[65,66] A pilot study of 12 mice illuminated with varying intensities and durations of halogen exposure resulted in benign forms of skin cancer (papillomas) as well as malignant tumor growth. Emission of far-ultraviolet radiation from halogen lamps is thought to be in the range of wavelength responsible for inducing melanoma.[66] Fortunately, prevention is simple if commercial models are available with glass or plastic covers.

Mechanical Stresses

Mechanical injury is caused by physical impact or irritation. Injury may include damage to the nerves surrounding small blood vessels (perivascular) that mediate both vasodilation and vasoconstriction.[67] Recent interest in mechanical injury and blood vessel damage has lead investigators to study balloon catheterization or coronary angioplasty. Coronary angioplasty involves a catheter that is advanced along a blood vessel until it reaches the blocked region of the vessel. The balloon section of the catheter is then inflated, pushing the walls of the blocked vessel outward. Sometimes metal tubes, called *stents,* are inserted to keep the vessel open. Without the stents, however, vessel narrowing, or restenosis, often occurs at the balloon site. The injury causes an adaptive response of hypertrophy of the smooth muscle cells and an increase in macrophage activity. The macrophages release cytokines and growth factors causing intimal cell proliferation and subsequent renarrowing.

The major focus of occupational biomechanics is the response of tissue to mechanical stress, especially the prevention of overexertion disorders of the lower back and upper extremities. Many mechanical stresses can cause overt injuries (e.g., a head injury when a worker is struck in the head with a dropped object). Most stresses, however, are subtle and can cause *accumulative* injuries and disorders.[68] Table 2-9 summarizes common types of occupational mechanical stresses and associated types of injury.

Noise

Noise is sound that has the potential for inflicting bodily harm. The most common pathophysiologic effect of noise is hearing impairment. Noise trauma can be caused by acute loud noise, as well as by the cumulative effects of various intensities, frequencies, and durations of noise. Common irritating noise is caused by numerous sources, including lawn care machinery; high-decibel, low-frequency speakers; loud movies; roaring highways; and so on. According to the National Institutes of Health, more than 10 million Americans suffer some permanent noise-associated hearing loss.[69] The largest increase in hearing loss from noise occurs in people 45 to 64 years old. Noise pollution is now considered a public health threat.

Two types of hearing loss are associated with noise: (1) acoustic trauma, or instantaneous damage caused by a single sharply rising wave of sound (e.g., gunfire), and (2) noise-induced hearing loss, the more common type, which is the result of prolonged exposure to intense sound (e.g., noise associated with the workplace and leisure-time activities). Hearing loss can be a serious complication of critical illness. Individuals in intensive care units can experience hearing loss from mechanical or accidental trauma, ototoxic medications, infections, vascular disorders, autoimmune diseases, and environmental noise.[70] Acoustic trauma can rupture the eardrum, displace the ossicles of the middle ear, and damage the organ of Corti in the inner ear.

If the offending noise has not been too loud or the exposure to it too long, hearing will return to its original level, a

Table 2-9	Common Types of Occupational Mechanical Stresses and Associated Types of Injury	
Mechanical Stresses	**Type of Injury**
Forceful exertions (e.g., lifting, pushing, pulling of heavy loads)	Low back pain
Awkward trunk postures (e.g., flexion, lateral bending, axial twisting, prolonged sitting)	Low back pain
Whole body vibration (e.g., vibrating seat or platform)	Low back pain; bone deformities; alteration nerve conduction (carpal tunnel syndrome)
Repetitive or prolonged exposure (e.g., to any of the above)	Low back pain; numbness and tingling of wrists and hands
Extreme reaching	Trauma disorders of upper arms (synovitis, Raynaud phenomenon, bursitis, tendonitis)
Low temperatures (e.g., exposure to cold air, tools, materials)	
Vibration (segmental and whole)	
Forceful exertions (e.g., friction, balance, posture, pace, use of heavy objects)	
Ulnar deviation of the wrist	
Repetitive functions (e.g., walking, climbing stairs, carrying, shoveling, pushing, lifting objects, computer use)	Localized and/or whole body fatigue (shortness of breath, general weakness, hypoxic injury)

type of hearing loss called a *temporary threshold shift* (TTS). If the noise is louder than a certain value or the exposure time is long, the hearing threshold never returns to its original value, causing a *permanent threshold shift* (PTS). Structural changes associated with TTS, although not fully established, include intracellular changes in the sensory cells (hair cells) and swelling of the auditory nerve endings.[23] With PTS, cochlear blood flow may be impaired and hair cells are damaged with each exposure. Noise-induced hearing loss is gradual and painless. Symptoms of noise-induced hearing loss include loudness recruitment and tinnitus. In loudness recruitment, soft sounds are not heard but loud sounds are heard normally. Tinnitus is a constant, high-pitched ringing that annoys the individual and contributes to loss of sleep.

MANIFESTATIONS OF CELLULAR INJURY

Cellular Manifestations: Accumulations

Cellular accumulations, also known as **infiltrations,** occur not only as a result of sublethal injury sustained by cells but also as a result of normal (but inefficient) cell function. Common accumulations consist of substances that are normally present, such as fluids and electrolytes, triglycerides (lipids), glycogen, calcium, uric acid, proteins, melanin, and bilirubin. Abnormal accumulations of these substances can occur in the cytoplasm (frequently in the lysosomes) or in the nucleus if (1) the normal, endogenous substance is produced in excess or at an increased rate; (2) an endogenous substance (normal or abnormal) is not effectively catabolized, usually because of lack of a vital lysosomal enzyme; or (3) harmful exogenous materials, such as heavy metals, mineral dusts, or microorganisms, accumulate because of inhalation, ingestion, or infection.

In all storage diseases the cells attempt to digest, or catabolize, the "stored" substances. As a result, excessive amounts of metabolites (products of catabolism) accumulate in the cells and are expelled into the extracellular matrix, where they are taken up by phagocytic cells called *macrophages* (see Chapter 6). Some of these scavenger cells circulate throughout the body, whereas others remain fixed in certain tissues, such as the liver or spleen. As more and more macrophages and other phagocytes migrate to tissues that are producing excessive metabolites, the affected tissues begin to swell. This is the mechanism that causes enlargement of the liver (hepatomegaly) or the spleen (splenomegaly). Enlargement of one of these organs is a clinical manifestation of many of the storage diseases.

Water
Cellular swelling, the most common degenerative change, is caused by the shift of extracellular water into the cells. In hypoxic injury, movement of fluid and ions into the cell is asso-

ciated with acute failure of metabolism and loss of ATP production. Normally, the pump that transports sodium ions out of the cell is maintained by the presence of ATP and ATPase, the active-transport enzyme. In metabolic failure caused by hypoxia, reduced ATP and ATPase permit sodium to accumulate in the cell, whereas potassium diffuses outward. The increase of intracellular sodium increases osmotic pressure, which draws more water into the cell (transport mechanisms are described in Chapter 1). The cisternae of the endoplasmic reticulum become distended, rupture, and coalesce to form large vacuoles that isolate the water from the cytoplasm, a process called **vacuolation.** Progressive vacuolation results in **oncosis** (replaced old term hydropic degeneration) or **vacuolar degeneration** (degeneration by water) (Figure 2-24). If cellular swelling affects all cells in an organ, the organ increases in weight and becomes distended and pale.

Cellular swelling is reversible and is considered to be sublethal. It is, in fact, an early manifestation of almost all types of cellular injury, including severe or lethal cell injury. It is also associated with high fever, hypokalemia (abnormally low concentrations of potassium in the blood; see Chapter 3), and certain infections.

Lipids and Carbohydrates
Certain metabolic disorders result in the abnormal intracellular accumulation of carbohydrates and lipids. These substances may accumulate throughout the body but are found primarily in the cells of the spleen, liver, and CNS. Accumulations in cells of the CNS can cause neurologic dysfunction and

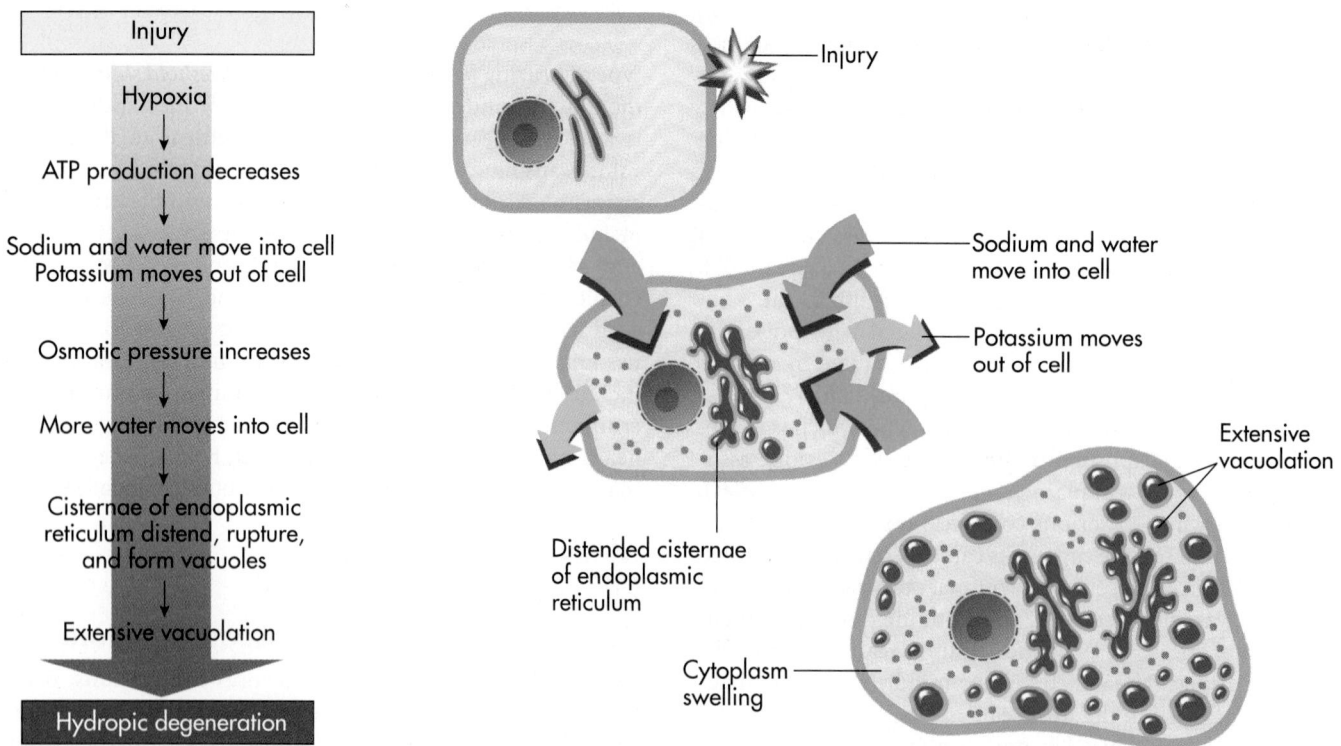

Figure 2-24 The process of oncosis (formerly known as hydropic degeneration). *ATP,* Adenosine triphosphate.

severe mental retardation. Lipids accumulate in Tay-Sachs, Neimann-Pick, and Gaucher diseases, whereas in the diseases known as mucopolysaccharidoses, carbohydrates are in excess. The mucopolysaccharidoses are progressive disorders that usually involve multiple organs, including liver, spleen, heart, and blood vessels. The accumulated mucopolysaccharides are found in reticuloendothelial cells, endothelial cells, intimal smooth muscle cells, and fibroblasts throughout the body. These carbohydrate accumulations can cause clouding of the cornea, joint stiffness, and mental retardation.[2]

Although lipids sometimes accumulate in heart and kidney cells, the most common site of intracellular lipid accumulation, or **fatty change,** is liver cells. Because hepatic metabolism and secretion of lipids are crucial to proper body function, imbalances and deficiencies in these processes lead to major pathologic changes. Lipid accumulation in liver cells causes an organic condition known as *fatty liver,* or *fatty change* (Figure 2-25). As lipids fill the cells, vacuolation pushes the nucleus and other organelles aside. Grossly, the liver looks yellowish and greasy.

Lipid accumulation in liver cells occurs after cellular injury sets one or more of the following mechanisms in motion:

1. Increased movement of free fatty acids into the liver (Starvation, for example, increases breakdown of triglycerides in adipose tissue, releasing fatty acids that subsequently enter liver cells.)
2. Failure of the metabolic process that converts fatty acids to phospholipids, resulting in the preferential conversion of the fatty acids to triglycerides
3. Increased synthesis of triglycerides from fatty acids (Increases in an enzyme, α-glycerophosphatase, can accelerate triglyceride synthesis.)
4. Decreased synthesis of apoproteins (lipid-acceptor proteins)
5. Failure of lipids to bind with apoproteins and form lipoproteins
6. Failure of mechanisms that transport lipoproteins out of the cell
7. Direct damage to the endoplasmic reticulum by free radicals released by alcohol's toxic effects

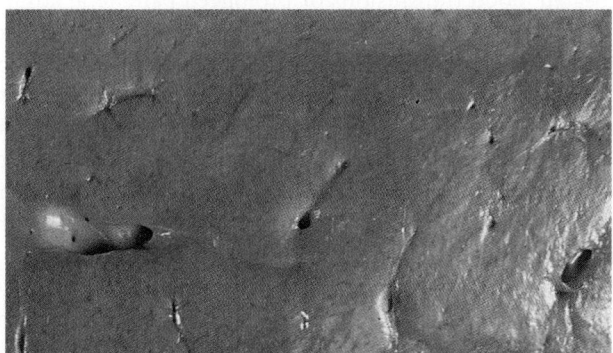

Figure 2-25 Fatty liver. The liver appears yellow. (From Damjanov I, Linder J: *Pathology: a color atlas,* St Louis, 2000, Mosby.)

Alcohol abuse is one of the most common causes of fatty liver (see Chapter 39). Fatty change caused by alcohol can lead to a form of liver fibrosis called *cirrhosis.* If alcohol intake ceases, the cirrhotic liver can return to a normal size and function. Fatty change from other causes, notably carbon tetrachloride poisoning, is often irreversible.

Glycogen

Intracellular accumulations of glycogen are seen in genetic disorders called *glycogen storage diseases* and in disorders of glucose and glycogen metabolism. Like water and lipid accumulation, glycogen accumulation results in excessive vacuolation of the cytoplasm. The most common cause of glycogen accumulation is diabetes mellitus, a disorder of glucose metabolism (see Chapter 21).

Proteins

Proteins provide cellular structure and constitute most of the cell's dry weight. They are synthesized on ribosomes in the cytoplasm from the essential amino acids lysine, threonine, leucine, isoleucine, methionine, tryptophan, valine, phenylalanine, and histidine. Protein accumulation probably damages cells in two ways. First, metabolites, produced when the cell attempts to digest some proteins, are enzymes that, when released from lysosomes, can damage cellular organelles. Second, excessive amounts of protein in the cytoplasm push against cellular organelles, disrupting organelle function and intracellular communication.

Protein excess accumulates primarily in the epithelial cells of the renal convoluted tubule and in the antibody-forming plasma cells (B lymphocytes) of the immune system. Several types of renal disorders cause excessive excretion of protein molecules in the urine (proteinuria). Normally, little or no protein is present in the urine, and its presence in significant amounts indicates cellular injury and altered cellular function.

Accumulations of protein in B lymphocytes can occur during active synthesis of antibodies during the immune response. The excess aggregates of protein are called *Russell bodies.* Russell bodies have been identified in multiple myeloma (plasma cell tumor) (see Chapters 27).

Pigments

Pigment accumulations may be normal or abnormal, endogenous (produced within the body) or exogenous (produced outside the body). Endogenous pigments are derived, for example, from amino acids (e.g., tyrosine, tryptophan). They include melanin and the blood proteins—porphyrins, hemoglobin, and hemosiderin (ferritin). Lipid-rich pigments such as lipofuscin (the aging pigment) give a yellow-brown color to cells undergoing slow, regressive, and often atrophic changes. Exogenous pigments include mineral dusts containing silica and iron particles, lead, silver salts, and dyes for tattoos.

Melanin

Melanin accumulates in epithelial cells (keratinocytes) of the skin and retina. It is an extremely important pigment because it protects the skin against long exposure to sunlight and is considered an essential factor in the prevention of skin cancer (see Chapters 12 and 44). Ultraviolet light (e.g., sunlight) stimulates the synthesis of melanin, which probably absorbs ultraviolet rays during subsequent exposure. Melanin also may protect the skin by trapping the injurious free radicals produced by the action of ultraviolet light on skin.

Melanin is a brown-black pigment derived from the amino acid tyrosine. It is synthesized by epidermal cells called *melanocytes* and is stored in membrane-bound cytoplasmic vesicles called *melanosomes.* Melanosomes are particularly abundant in projections of melanocytic cytoplasm, called *dendrites,* from which they are transmitted to neighboring keratinocytes, where melanin accumulation occurs.[10] (Keratinocytes, which constitute 95% of epidermal cells, are discussed with other skin components in Chapter 44.) The dendritic melanocytes form bridges between neighboring keratinocytes and inject melanosomes into the keratinocytes by an unknown mechanism.

Melanin also can accumulate in melanophores (melanin-containing pigment cells), macrophages, or other phagocytic cells in the dermis. Presumably these cells acquire the melanin from nearby melanocytes or from pigment that has been extruded from dying epidermal cells. This is the mechanism that causes freckles.

Although rare, melanin accumulation occurs in the skin of individuals with Addison disease (adrenocortical insufficiency resulting from disorders of the adrenal cortex; see Chapter 21). The increased melaninogenesis (melanin production) seen in Addison disease is caused by the loss of feedback control of adrenocorticotropic hormone (ACTH). Decreased hormonal secretion from the adrenal gland causes increased release of ACTH from the pituitary gland. In Addison disease the increase in melanin occurs presumably because a segment of the ACTH molecule contains the melanin-stimulating hormone (MSH).

An increase in melanin also occurs in the benign form of "pigmented moles" called *nevi* (Figure 2-26) (see Chapter 44).

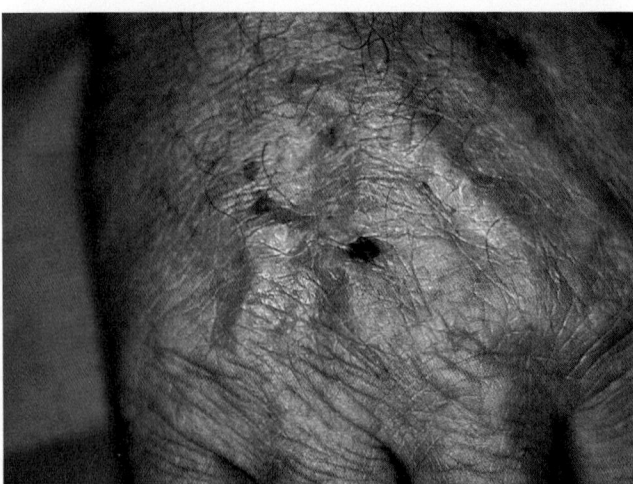

Figure 2-26 Blue nevus, common type. Nevus is a dark blue-black color and is small and symmetric. (From Damjanov I, Linder J: *Anderson's pathology,* ed 10, St Louis, 1996, Mosby.)

Malignant melanoma is a cancerous skin tumor that contains melanin and invades normal tissue early and widely and often leads to death.

A decrease in melanin production occurs in the inherited disorder of the melanin metabolism called *albinism.* Albinism is often diffuse, involving all the skin, the eyes, and the hair. Albinism is also related to phenylalanine metabolism. In classic types the person with albinism is unable to convert tyrosine to DOPA (3,4-dihydroxyphenylalanine), an intermediary in melanin biosynthesis. Melanin-producing cells are present in normal numbers, but they are unable to make melanin. Individuals with albinism are very sensitive to sunlight and quickly become sunburned. They are also at high risk for skin cancer.

Hemoproteins

Hemoproteins are among the most essential of the normal endogenous pigments. They include hemoglobin and the oxidative enzymes, the cytochromes. Central to an understanding of disorders involving these pigments is knowledge of iron uptake, metabolism, excretion, and storage (see Chapter 25). Hemoprotein accumulations in cells are caused by excessive storage of iron, which is transferred to the cells from the bloodstream. Iron enters the blood from three primary sources: (1) tissue stores, (2) the intestinal mucosa, and (3) macrophages that remove and destroy dead or defective red blood cells. The amount of iron in blood plasma also depends on the metabolism of the major iron-transport protein, *transferrin.*

Iron is stored in tissue cells in two forms: as ferritin and, when greater levels of iron are present, as hemosiderin. **Hemosiderin** is a yellow-brown pigment derived from hemoglobin. With pathologic states, excesses of iron cause hemosiderin to accumulate within cells. Accumulation of hemosiderin often occurs in areas of bruising and hemorrhage and in the lungs and spleen after congestion caused by heart failure. With a local hemorrhage, the skin first appears red-blue and then lysis of the escaped red blood cell occurs, causing the hemoglobin to be transformed to hemosiderin. The color changes noted in bruising reflect this transformation.

Hemosiderosis is a condition in which excess iron is stored as hemosiderin in the cells of many organs and tissues. This condition is common in individuals who have received repeated blood transfusions or prolonged parenteral administration of iron. Hemosiderosis is also associated with increased absorption of dietary iron, conditions in which iron storage and transport are impaired, and hemolytic anemia. Excessive alcohol ingestion also can lead to hemosiderosis. Normally, absorption of excessive dietary iron is prevented by an iron-absorption process in the intestines. Failure of this process can lead to total-body iron accumulations in the range of 60 to 80 g, compared with normal iron stores of 4.5 to 5 g. Excessive accumulations of iron, such as occur in hemochromatosis (a genetic disorder of iron metabolism and the most severe example of iron overload), are associated with liver and pancreatic cell damage.

It is debatable whether iron accumulation itself causes cellular injury or whether injury is the result of the basic defect that leads to iron storage. The finding that the extent of liver injury (cirrhosis) is related to the extent of iron accumulation[71] suggests that excessive iron accumulation does injure cells.

Bilirubin is a normal, yellow-to-green pigment of bile derived from the porphyrin structure of hemoglobin. Excesses of bilirubin within cells and tissues cause jaundice (icterus), or yellowing of the skin. Jaundice occurs when the bilirubin level exceeds 1.5 to 2 mg/dl of plasma, compared with the normal values of 0.4 to 1 mg/dl. Hyperbilirubinemia occurs with (1) destruction of red blood cells (erythrocytes), such as in hemolytic jaundice; (2) diseases affecting the metabolism and excretion of bilirubin in the liver; and (3) diseases that cause obstruction of the common bile duct, such as gallstones or pancreatic tumors. (For a detailed description of these diseases, see Chapter 39.) Certain drugs, specifically chlorpromazine and other phenothiazine derivatives, estrogenic hormones, and halothane (an anesthetic), can cause the obstruction of normal bile flow through the liver.

Because unconjugated bilirubin is lipid soluble, it can injure the lipid components of the plasma membrane. Albumin, a plasma protein, provides significant protection by binding unconjugated bilirubin in plasma. Unconjugated bilirubin causes two cellular effects: uncoupling of oxidative phosphorylation and a loss of cellular proteins. These two effects could cause structural injury to the various membranes of the cell.

Calcium

Calcium salts accumulate in both injured and dead tissues (Figure 2-27). An important mechanism of cellular calcification is the influx of extracellular calcium in injured mitochondria (see pp. 51 and 52). Another mechanism that causes calcium accumulation in alveoli (gas-exchange airways of the lungs), gastric epithelium, and renal tubules is the excretion of acid at these sites, leading to the local production of hydroxyl ions. Hydroxyl ions result in precipitation of calcium hydroxide ($Ca[OH]_2$) and hydroxyapatite ($3Ca_3[PO_4]_2Ca[OH]_2$), a mixed salt. Damage occurs when calcium salts clump and harden, interfering with normal cellular structure and function.

Pathologic calcification can be dystrophic or metastatic. **Dystrophic calcification** is the calcification of dying and dead tissues and occurs in chronic tuberculosis of the lungs and lymph nodes, in arteries with advanced atherosclerosis (narrowing as a result of plaque accumulation), and often in injured heart valves (Figure 2-28). Calcification of the heart valves interferes with opening and closing of the valves, causing heart murmurs (see Chapter 30). Calcification of the coronary arteries predisposes them to severe narrowing and thrombosis, which can lead to myocardial infarction. Another

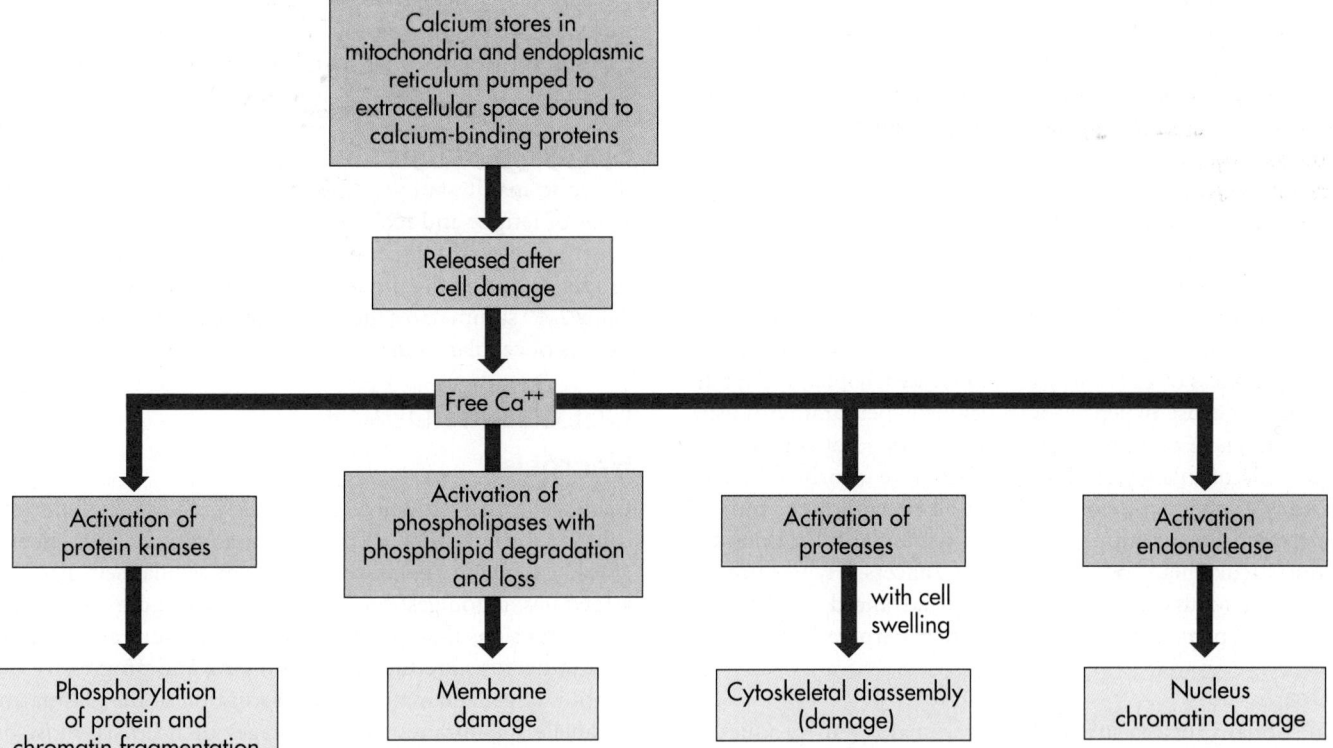

Figure 2-27 Free cytosolic calcium: a destructive agent. Normally, calcium is removed from the cytosol by ATP-dependent calcium pumps. In normal cells, calcium is bound to buffering proteins, such as calbindin or paralbumin, and is contained in the endoplasmic reticulum and the mitochondria. If there is abnormal permeability of calcium-ion channels, direct damage to membranes, or depletion of adenosine triphosphate (ATP) (i.e., hypoxic injury), calcium increases in the cytosol. If the free calcium cannot be buffered or pumped out of cells, uncontrolled enzyme activation takes place, causing further damage. Uncontrolled entry of calcium into the cytosol is an important final pathway in many causes of cell death.

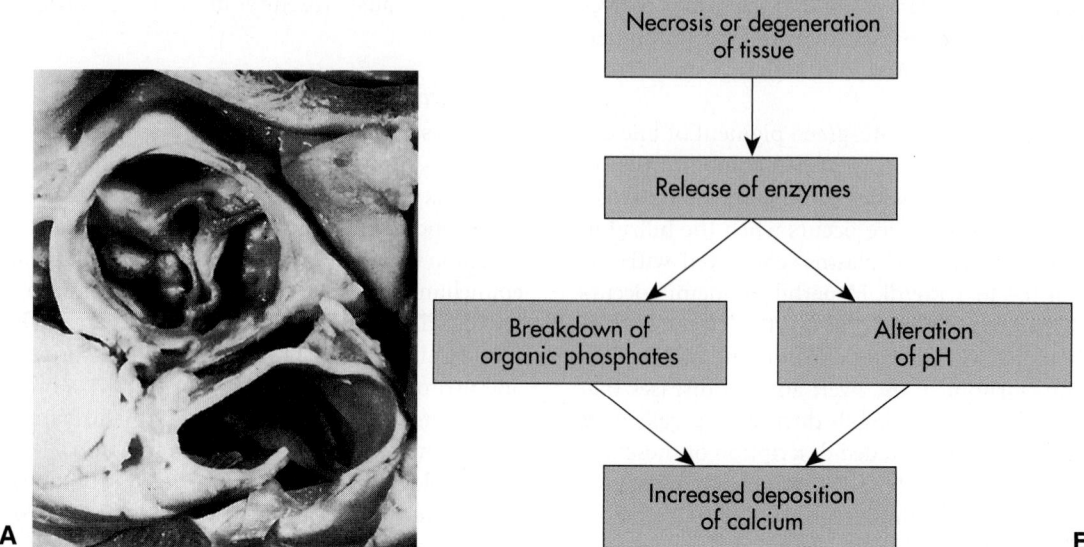

Figure 2-28 Aortic valve calcification. **A,** This aortic valve was unable to close because of calcification caused by rheumatic heart disease. **B,** Algorithm showing the dystrophic mechanism of calcification. (**A** from Damjanov I, Linder J, editors: *Anderson's pathology,* ed 10, St Louis, 1996, Mosby.)

site of dystrophic calcification is the center of tumors. Over time, the center is deprived of oxygen supply, dies, and becomes calcified. The calcium salts appear as gritty, clumped granules that can become hard as stone. When several layers clump together, they resemble grains of sand and are called **psammoma bodies.**

The exact pathogenic mechanisms responsible for dystrophic calcification are unknown. A popular hypothesis is that with progressive deterioration of dead cells, the exposed denatured (changed) proteins preferentially bind with phosphate ions. The phosphate ions then react with calcium ions to form deposits of phosphate carbonate precipitates and, sometimes, crystalline formations of calcium phosphate. Dystrophic calcification develops slowly and is an explicit marker for the site of dead cells.

Metastatic calcification consists of mineral deposits that occur in undamaged normal tissues as the result of hypercalcemia (excess of calcium in the blood; see Chapter 3). Conditions that cause hypercalcemia include hyperparathyroidism, toxic levels of vitamin D, hyperthyroidism, idiopathic hypercalcemia of infancy, Addison disease (adrenocortical insufficiency), systemic sarcoidosis, milk-alkali syndrome, and the increased bone demineralization that results from bone tumors, leukemia, and disseminated cancers. Hypercalcemia also can occur in some instances of advanced renal failure with phosphate retention, resulting in hyperparathyroidism.[10]

Urate

In humans, uric acid (**urate**) is the major end product of purine catabolism because of the absence of the enzyme urate oxidase. Serum urate concentration is, in general, stable: approximately 5 mg/dl in postpubertal males and 4.1 mg/dl in postpubertal females. Disturbances in maintaining serum urate levels result in hyperuricemia and deposition of sodium urate crystals in the tissues, leading to painful disorders collectively called *gout.* These disorders include acute arthritis, chronic gouty arthritis, tophus (firm nodular subcutaneous deposits of urate crystals surrounded by fibrosis), and nephritis (inflammation of the nephron).

Chronic hyperuricemia results in the deposition of urate in tissues, cell injury, and inflammation. Because urate crystals are not degraded by lysosomal enzymes, they persist in dead cells.

Systemic Manifestations

Systemic manifestations of cellular injury include a general sense of fatigue and malaise, a loss of well-being, and altered appetite. Fever is frequently present because of biochemicals produced during the inflammatory response (see Chapter 6). Table 2-10 summarizes the most significant systemic manifestations of cellular injury.

CELLULAR DEATH

Necrosis

Cellular death eventually leads to the process of cellular dissolution, or **necrosis.** Necrosis is the sum of cellular changes after local cell death and the process of cellular self-digestion known as autodigestion, or **autolysis** (Figure 2-29). The structural signs that indicate irreversible injury and progression to necrosis are the dense clumping and progressive disruption of genetic material and disruption of the plasma and organelle membranes. In later stages of necrosis, most organelles are disrupted, and **karyolysis** (nuclear dissolution and lysis of chromatin from the action of hydrolytic enzymes) is underway. In some cells the nucleus shrinks and becomes a small, dense mass of genetic material—a process called nuclear **pyknosis.** The pyknotic nucleus eventually dissolves (by

Table 2-10	Systemic Manifestations of Cellular Injury
Manifestation	**Cause**
Fever	Release of endogenous pyrogens (interleukin-1, tumor necrosis factor (TNF-α), prostaglandins) from bacteria or macrophages; acute inflammatory response
Increased heart rate	Increase in oxidative metabolic processes resulting from fever
Increase in leukocytes (leukocytosis)	Increase in total number of white blood cells because of infection; normal is 5000-9000/mm³ (increase is directly related to the severity of the infection)
Pain	Various mechanisms, such as release of bradykinins, obstruction, pressure
Presence of cellular enzymes in extracellular fluid	Release of enzymes from cells of tissue*
Lactate dehydrogenase (LDH) (LDH isoenzymes)	Release from red blood cells, liver, kidney, skeletal muscle
Creatine kinase (CK) (CK isoenzymes)	Release from skeletal muscle, brain, heart
Aspartate aminotransferase (AST; SGOT)	Release from heart, liver, skeletal muscle, kidney, pancreas
Alanine aminotransferase (ALT; SGPT)	Release from liver, kidney, heart
Alkaline phosphatase (ALP)	Release from liver, bone
Amylase	Release from pancreas
Aldolase	Release from skeletal muscle, heart

*The rapidity of enzyme transfer is a function of the weight of the enzyme and the concentration gradient across the cellular membrane. The specific metabolic and excretory rates of the enzymes determine how long levels of enzymes remain elevated.

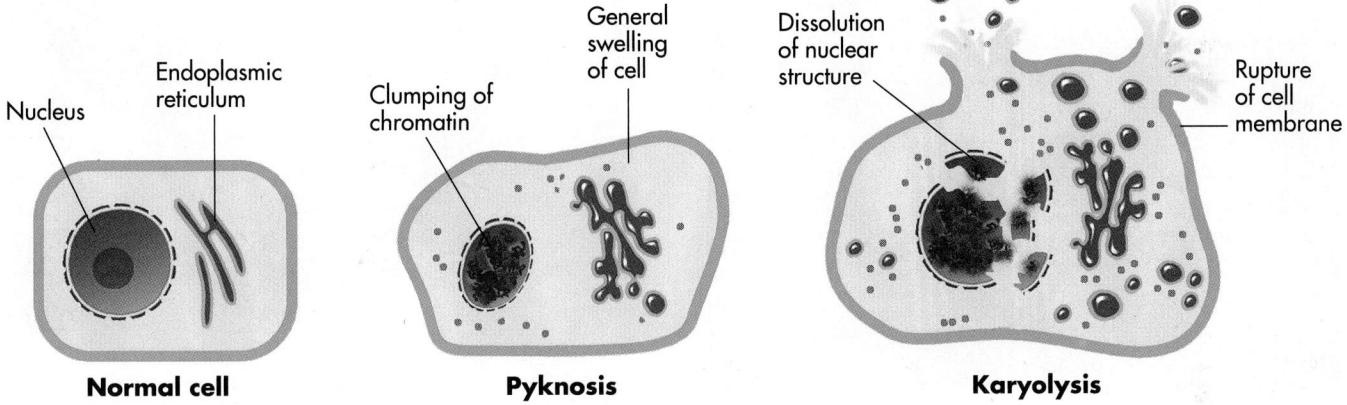

Figure 2-29 Stages of necrosis.

karyolysis) as a result of the action of hydrolytic lysosomal enzymes on DNA. **Karyorrhexis** means fragmentation of the nucleus into smaller particles or "nuclear dust."

Different types of necroses tend to occur in different organs or tissues and sometimes can indicate the mechanism or cause of cellular injury. The four major types of necroses are coagulative, liquefactive, caseous, and fatty. Another type, gangrenous necrosis, is *not* a distinctive type of cell death but refers to larger areas of tissue death.

Coagulative necrosis, which occurs primarily in the kidneys, heart, and adrenal glands, commonly results from hypoxia caused by severe ischemia or hypoxia caused by chemical injury, especially ingestion of mercuric chloride (Figure 2-30). Coagulation is caused by protein denaturation, which causes the protein albumin to change from a gelatinous, transparent state to a firm, opaque state, similar to that of a cooked egg white. The necrotic tissues appear firm and slightly swollen. Recent evidence indicates that an abnormality in intracellular levels of Ca^{++} (e.g., increased) may be a critical event in coagulation necrosis.[3]

Liquefactive necrosis commonly results from ischemic injury to neurons and glial cells in the brain (Figure 2-31). Dead brain tissue is readily affected by liquefactive necrosis because brain cells are rich in the digestive hydrolytic enzymes and lipids, and the brain contains little connective tissue. As the cells are digested by their own hydrolases, the tissue becomes soft, liquefies, and is walled off from healthy tissue, forming cysts. (Cyst formation is described in Chapter 6.)

Liquefactive necrosis can result also from bacterial infection, particularly by staphylococci, streptococci, and *Escherichia coli.* In this case the hydrolases are released from the lysosomes of neutrophils, which are phagocytes attracted to the infected area to kill the bacteria. Liquefaction of bacterial cells and neighboring tissue cells by neutrophilic hydrolases results in the accumulation of pus.

Caseous necrosis, which commonly results from tuberculous pulmonary infection, particularly by *Mycobacterium tuberculosis*, is a combination of coagulative and liquefactive necrosis (Figure 2-32). The dead cells disintegrate, but the debris is not digested completely by hydrolases. Tissues appear

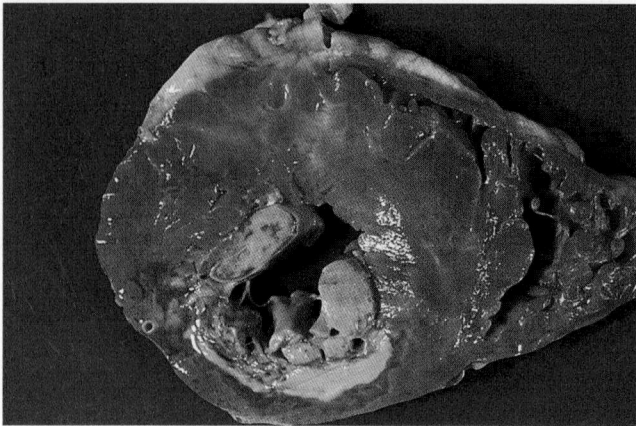

Figure 2-30 **Coagulative necrosis of myocardium of posterior wall of left ventricle of heart.** A large anemic (white) infarct is readily apparent; note also the necrosis of papillary muscle. (From Damjanov I, Linder J: *Anderson's pathology,* ed 10, St Louis, 1996, Mosby.)

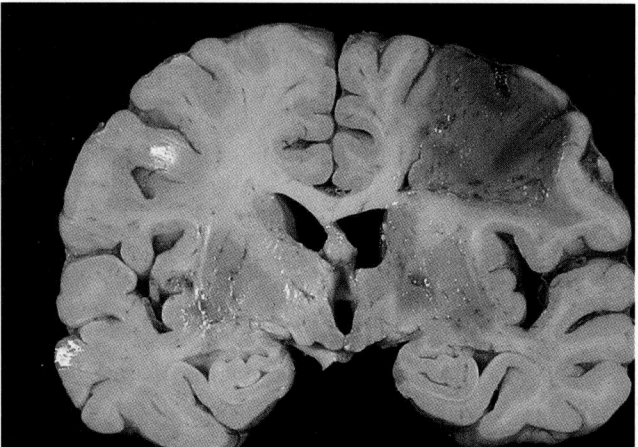

Figure 2-31 **Liquefactive necrosis.** Liquefactive necrosis of the brain developed at a large cerebral infarct caused by ischemia. (From Damjanov I, Linder J: *Anderson's pathology,* ed 10, St Louis, 1996, Mosby.)

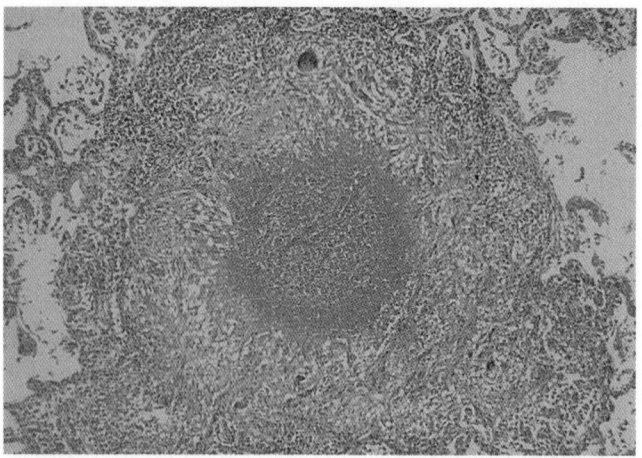

Fig, 2-32 Granuloma with central caseous necrosis typical of pulmonary tuberculosis. (From Damjanov I, Linder J: *Anderson's pathology,* ed 10, St Louis, 1996, Mosby.)

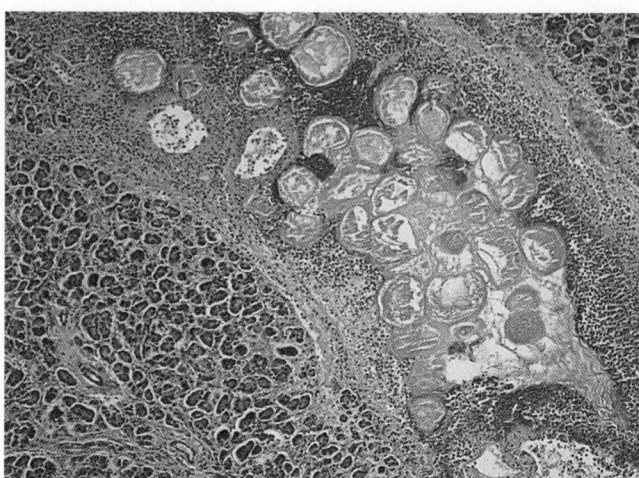

Figure 2-33 **Fat necrosis of pancreas.** Interlobular adipocytes are necrotic; these are surrounded by acute inflammatory cells. (From Damjanov I, Linder J: *Anderson's pathology,* ed 10, St Louis, 1996, Mosby.)

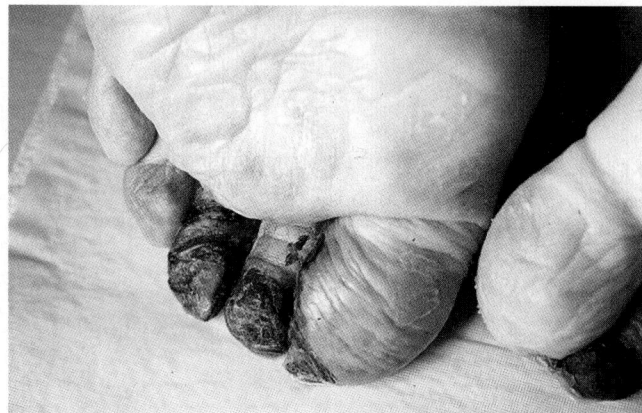

Figure 2-34 **Gangrene of toes.** Dry gangrene. (From Damjanov I: *Pathology for the health-related professions,* ed 2, Philadelphia, 2000, Saunders.)

soft and granular and resemble clumped cheese, which gives this type of necrosis its name. A granulomatous inflammatory wall encloses areas of caseous necrosis.

Fat necrosis, which occurs in the breast, pancreas, and other abdominal structures, is cellular dissolution caused by powerful enzymes called *lipases* (Figure 2-33). Lipases break down triglycerides, releasing free fatty acids, which then combine with calcium, magnesium, and sodium ions, creating soaps (a process known as *saponification*). The necrotic tissue appears opaque and chalk white.

Gangrenous necrosis, a term commonly used in surgical clinical practice, refers to death of tissue and results from severe hypoxic injury, commonly occurring because of arteriosclerosis, or blockage, of major arteries, especially in the lower leg. With hypoxia and subsequent bacterial invasion, the tissues can undergo necrosis. **Dry gangrene** is usually the result of coagulative necrosis. The skin becomes very dry and shrinks, resulting in wrinkles, and its color changes to dark brown or black (Figure 2-34). **Wet gangrene** develops when neutrophils invade the site, causing liquefactive necrosis. This usually occurs in in-

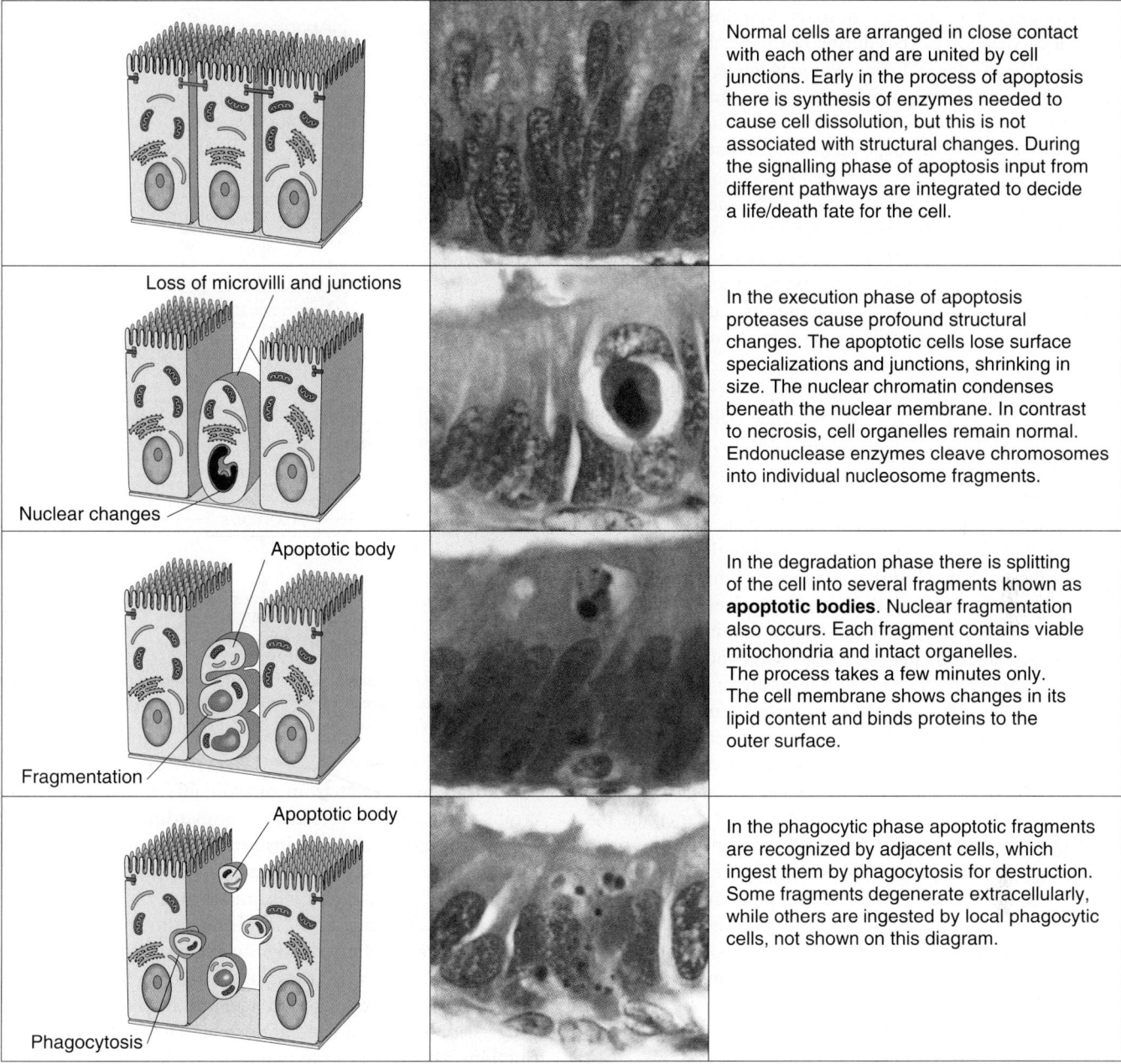

Figure 2-35 Apoptosis. Apoptosis of cells is a programmed and energy-dependent process designed specifically to switch cells off and eliminate them. This controlled pattern of cell death, termed *programmed cell death,* is very different from that which occurs as a direct result of a severe, damaging stimulus to cells. (From Stevens A, Lowe J: *Pathology,* ed 2, London, 2000, Mosby.)

ternal organs, causing the site to become cold, swollen, and black. A foul odor is present, produced by pus, and if systemic symptoms become severe, death can ensue.

Gas gangrene, a special type of gangrene, is caused by infection of injured tissue by one of many species of *Clostridium.* These anaerobic bacteria produce hydrolytic enzymes and toxins that destroy connective tissue and cellular membranes and cause bubbles of gas to form in muscle cells. Gas gangrene can be fatal if enzymes lyse the membranes of red blood cells, destroying their oxygen-carrying capacity. Death is the result of shock. The condition is treated with antitoxins and supplemental oxygen delivered in a hyperbaric (pressurized) chamber.

Apoptosis

Apoptosis (Greek for "dropping off") is an important, distinct type of cell death[72] that differs from necrosis in several respects (Figure 2-35). Apoptosis is an active process of cellular self-destruction, called *programmed cell death,* that is implicated in both normal and pathologic tissue changes.[73] Cells need to die, otherwise endless proliferation would lead to gigantic bodies. Every day an average adult may create 10 billion new cells and kill off the same number. Apoptosis is responsible for local deletion of cells during normal embryonic development, neurons dying during synaptogenesis, bone cells dying during turnover, lymphocytes dying during receptor repertoire selection, and so on. It has been shown to play a major role in endocrine-dependent tissues that are undergoing atrophic change and possibly following axonal injury and in neurodegenerative diseases, such as Alzheimer.[74-76] Apoptosis can occur spontaneously in malignant tumors and in normal, rapidly proliferating cells treated with cancer chemotherapeutic agents and ionizing radiation.[77] Defects in apoptosis can cause cancer.[78] Its significance in aging is unknown; however, apoptosis is required to maintain a balance between cell proliferation and cell death.[78]

Necrosis and apoptosis affect tissues differently. Unlike necrosis, apoptosis affects scattered, single cells. Apoptosis is nuclear and cytoplasmic shrinkage of a cell (i.e., unlike necrosis, in which cells swell and lyse) is followed by fragmentation into membrane-bound fragments and subsequent phagocytosis by neighboring, healthy cells.[10] Apoptosis depends on a tightly regulated cellular program for its initiation and execution.[77] Programmed cell death involves enzymes that cut up other proteins (proteases) that are, themselves, activated by proteolytic activity in response to signals that induce apoptosis.[79] The activated suicide proteases cleave, and thereby activate, other members of the family resulting in an amplifying "suicide" cascade. The activated proteases then cleave other key proteins in the cell, killing it quickly and neatly[79,80] (Figure 2-36). With necrosis, cell death is not neat because cells that die as a result of acute injury swell, burst, and spill their contents all over their neighbors causing a likely damaging inflammatory response.[79] Adjacent inflammation may be present in apoptosis. Molecular helpers in this program are present in different subcellular compartments, including the plasma membrane, cytosol, mitochondria, and nucleus. The progression of apoptosis depends on the interplay among these compartments and the exchange of specific signaling molecules.[77]

AGING AND ALTERED CELLULAR AND TISSUE BIOLOGY

Aging is usually defined as a normal physiologic process that is universal and inevitable. The basic mechanisms of aging depend on irreversible and universal processes at the cellular and molecular level. To understand aging requires the separation of irreversible processes from potentially reversible mechanisms (i.e., those that result from disease or age-related debilities)—a very difficult task.

Aging traditionally has not been considered a disease because it is "normal"; disease is usually considered "abnormal." Conceptually, this distinction seems clear until the concept of "injury" is introduced; disease has been defined by some pathologists as the result of injury. Aging has been defined as the time-dependent loss of structure and function that proceeds very slowly and in such small increments that it appears to be the result of the accumulation of small, imperceptible injuries—a gradual result of wear and tear.

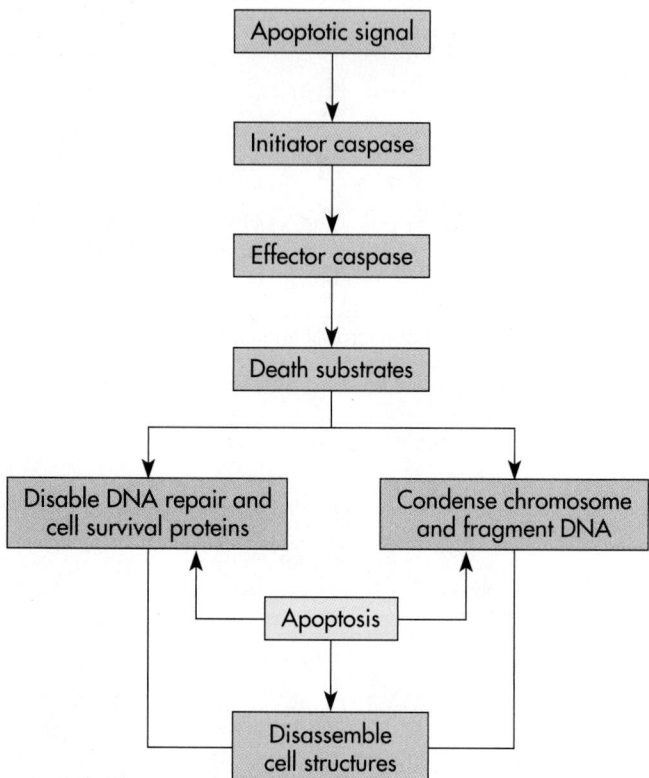

Figure 2-36 **Apoptosis via caspase cascade.** Apoptic signals trigger initiator caspases that activate the proteolytic cascade to eventually produce death substrates and apoptosis.

Injuries may result from unavoidable and universal microinsults caused by continuous bombardment by ultraviolet light, countless mechanical insults, and reactions to metabolites.[81,82] In this context the distinction between aging and disease is unclear. For example, some degree of atrophy of the brain is considered normal in old age until it proceeds far enough to cause clinically significant disability and is then called *disease*. Likewise, most humans have atherosclerosis, and the plaques progress with age, but at what point in this progression is it considered abnormal? These conceptual distinctions have given rise to two general categories of theories of aging. The first category proposes that aging is the result of the accumulation of random injuries and events. The second category proposes that aging is the result of a genetically controlled developmental program, or built-in self-destructive processes. (No matter what conceptual distinction is used as a basis, it seems clear that even in the absence of disease, the individual's frailty increases with age, and death inevitably results!) (See What's New? on Mitochondrial DNA.)

Normal Life Span

The **maximal life span** of humans is between 80 and 100 years and does not vary significantly among populations. However, in primitive societies, few individuals reach the maximal life span; most die in infancy and the early years.[83] In societies with improved sanitation, housing, nutrition, and health care, many persons attain the maximal life span. Al-

WHAT'S NEW?   Mitochondrial DNA, Diseases, and Aging

Mitochondria are the organelles responsible for the generation of most of the energy used by eukaryotic cells. Mitochondrial DNA (mtDNA) encodes some of the proteins of the electron transfer chain, the system necessary for the conversion of adenosine diphosphate (ADP) to adenosine triphosphate (ATP). Mutations in mtDNA can deprive the cell of ATP, and mutations are correlated with the aging process. The most common age-related mtDNA mutation in humans is a large rearrangement called the *4977 deletion*, or *common deletion,* and is found in humans over 40 years old. It is a deletion that removes all or part of 7 of the 13 protein-encoding mtDNA genes and 5 of the 22 tRNA genes. Individual cells containing this deletion have a condition known as *heteroplasmy*. Heteroplasmy levels rise with aging and are tissue-dependent.

The production of reactive oxygen species (ROS) under physiologic conditions is associated with activity of the respiratory chain in aerobic ATP production. Therefore, increased mitochondrial activity, per se, can be an "oxidative stress" to cells. The production of ROS is markedly increased in many pathologic conditions in which the respiratory chain is impaired. Because mtDNA, which is essential for normal oxidative phosphorylation, is located in close proximity to the ROS-generating respiratory chain, it is more oxidatively damaged than is nuclear DNA. Cumulative damage of mtDNA is implicated in the aging process as well as in the progression of such common diseases as diabetes, cancer, and heart failure.

Data from Butow RA, Avadhani NG: *Mol Cell* 14(1):1-15, 2004; Maasen JA et al: *Diabetes* 53(Suppl 1): S103-109, 2004; Samules DC: *Trends Genet* 20(5):226-229, 2004.

though the maximal life span has not changed significantly over time, the average life span, or **life expectancy,** has increased. Recently, the death rate for people 65 years of age and older has declined significantly, largely because of decreases in cardiovascular disease.[19] In each successive age group from 65 years and older, women outnumber men; thus women have a greater life expectancy than men. Increases in life expectancy have resulted in a large elderly population with inherent problems of disability, disease, and socioeconomic hardship.[84]

Life Expectancy and Gender Differences

The preliminary estimate of life expectancy at birth for the total population in 2001 was a record high of 77.2 years. These estimates, however, are based on mortality data only and, thus, differ substantially from the new World Health Organization (WHO) estimates that include years lost to disability. Life expectancy for females exceeds that for males (the gender gap) except in Bangladesh, Bhutan, India, Nepal, and Pakistan.[85] The preliminary estimate for the gender gap was 5.4 years in 2001.[86] The female advantage ranges from 4 to 8 years; however, the gender gap is continuing to decrease. Life expectancy for males increased 0.1 year, reaching a record 74.4 years. Female life expectancy also increased by 0.1 year, increasing from 79.7 years to 79.8 years between 2000 and 2001. Record high life expectancies were reached for white and black males (75.0 years and 68.6 years, respectively), as

well as for white and black females (80.2 years and 75.5 years, respectively).[86]

Traditionally, the causes of the gender gap have been divided into three very broad areas: biologic (genetic, hormonal), behavioral, and sociocultural. Investigators, however, challenge the explanation that women outlive men solely on hormonal and lifestyle differences.[87] For example, estrogen levels in postmenopausal women are similar to those in males. Furthermore, in many developed countries women are copying the so-called "unhealthy" lifestyle of men and men are adopting "healthier" lifestyles. A recent hypothesis that sexual size, with men generally being the larger sex, in conjunction with the limited replication potential of human somatic cells might account for higher mortality rates in males, especially at old age.[87] This hypothesis is based on the cellular mitotic clock discovered by Leonard Hayflick almost a century ago (discussed later). Recently an inverse correlation between mean telomere length (see Chapter 11) and mortality in people has been found.[88] In this study and two others, it was confirmed that males have shorter telomeres than females at the same age.[88] A larger body requires more cell doublings, especially because of regeneration of tissues over a lifetime. Thus, male cells may exhaust regeneration potential possibly contributing to early onset of age-associated diseases.[87] In addition, international variations in absolute and relative gender differences in mortality can, in part, be explained by smoking.[89]

Theories and Mechanisms of Aging

Relatively little "indisputable" knowledge exists on the subject of aging. Table 2-11 presents the historical development of aging research. Numerous theories exist about the causes of aging. Many of these theories overlap, interact, and are similar. Some of the theories have focused on a single mechanism—the so-called magic bullet approach to arrest aging. It is doubtful that a single theory will explain all the mechanisms of aging. As stated earlier, there are two general categories of theories of aging: (1) that aging is the result of the accumulation of injurious events, sometimes called *damage-accumulation theories;* or (2) that biologic changes of aging are the result of a genetically controlled developmental program. In the first category, random accumulation of errors in protein structure, mutations in somatic cells, the accumulation of metabolic waste products, and free radical–mediated damage (from highly reactive intermediates produced in the normal course of metabolism, such as hydroperoxides, aldehydes, and ketones) decrease the ability to maintain a physiologic steady state. The accumulation of these injuries increases one's susceptibility to disease. In the developmentally programmed theory of aging, aging is the result of certain genes that program senescence and cell death. Here supporters claim that because maximal life span is genetically determined, the aging process is also.

Evidence exists both for and against any particular theory of aging. However, three major areas of the mechanisms of aging have retained their appeal or have been extensively tested: (1) cellular changes produced by genetic, environmental, and

Table 2-11	Theories of Aging	
Theory	**Year**	**Proponent**
Waste product theory	1923	Carrell and Ebeling
Wear-and-tear theory	1924	Pearl
Rate of living theory[a]	1928	Pearl
Neuroendocrine theory (including DHEA and melatonin)	1947	Korenchevsky and Jones
Free-radical theory	1955	Harman
Collagen theory[b]	1957	Verzar
Metabolic theory[a]	1957; 1961	Carlson et al.; Johnson et al.
Somatic mutation theory	1959	Sziliard
Error-catastrophe theory	1963; 1970	Orgel
Cross-linking theory[b]	1968	Bjorksten
Programmed senescence theory	1969	Hayflick
Immunologic theory	1969	Walform
Evolution theory	1977	Kirkwood

Data from Schneider EL: Theories of aging: a perspective. In Warner HR et al, editors: *Modern biological theories of aging,* New York, 1987, Raven; Madison HE: Theories of Aging. In Lueckenotte A: *Gerontologic nursing,* ed 2, St Louis, 2000, Mosby; Hayflick L: *How and why we age,* New York, 1996, Ballantine Books.

NOTE: Theories with the same superscript may represent the same theory.

DHEA, Dehydroepiandosterone.

behavioral factors; (2) changes in cellular regulatory, or control, mechanisms, especially in cells of the neuroendocrine, immune, and central nervous systems; and (3) degenerative extracellular and vascular alterations.

Genetic and Environmental–Life-Style Factors

Cellular aging results from wear and tear that causes functional changes and eventual cellular death. Cellular damage may occur during replication as a result of factors within the cell, such as DNA and protein mechanisms, or factors outside the cell, such as ionizing radiation. Cells may already be programmed at birth or are injured during life so as to cause errors in mitotic division and in the replication of genetic material, eventually leading to either cellular atrophy or death. Atrophy is common in the thymus, testis, ovary, uterus, and breast of aged individuals, although these organs age differently.

One of the genetic mechanisms of aging is programmed aging. Regardless of damaging environmental factors, some investigators think that each normal cell may have a finite life span during which it can replicate. A classic experiment done by Hayflick[72] demonstrated that fibroblasts are limited to a finite number of generations (40 to 60 doublings). However, proponents do not propose that aging is the result of cells losing their ability to divide. Rather, they believe that an intrinsic program within the human genome progressively slows or shuts down certain physiologic mechanisms, including mitosis.[90]

The **somatic mutation hypothesis** proposes that aging is the result of DNA damage, inefficiency of repair, and loss of

integrity of DNA synthesis (i.e., mutations in somatic cells). Somatic mutations increase with age; however, it is not exactly known whether this occurs in a linear or exponential fashion, and this increase partly explains the age-related increase in cancer incidence. Somatic mutation of genes that regulate the cell cycle (e.g., *p53,* see Chapter 11) and apoptosis are likely to play a crucial role in cancer initiation. Data suggest that, with aging, life-style factors can contribute to an accumulation of genetic damage. An argument against the somatic mutation theory is that the frequency of mutations in various organs and tissues is thought to be low.[82]

The **catastrophic,** or **error-prone, theory,** initially proposed by Orgel in 1963, stated that the presence of errors in those enzymes involved in transcription and translation, and thus their own synthesis, lead to an increase in errors and eventually to the death of the cell. The theory was later modified by Orgel in 1970 by proposing the possibility that nongrowing cells may not be subject to error catastrophe if the rate of error production does not increase significantly during protein synthesis. Abnormal forms of some, but not all, cellular proteins do appear during senescence but not as a result of errors in protein synthesis as originally predicted.[91] Rather, the abnormal proteins appear to reflect several types of posttranslational modifications.[92] The error-catastrophe theory has attracted a great deal of interest. Most of the evidence, however, argues against this theory as originally formulated. The accumulation of altered proteins in aging may result from an increased production or decreased ability of aged cells to degrade their cellular proteins, or both.

Alterations of Cellular Control Mechanisms

The overall effects of aging may be caused by changes in certain cell populations that exert regulatory or control functions, such as cells of the central nervous system, neuroendocrine system, and immune system. The **neuroendocrine theory** of aging purports that a genetic program for aging is encoded in the brain and is controlled and relayed to peripheral tissues through hormonal and neural agents. Possible mechanisms include (1) increased hormonal degradation, (2) decreased rate of hormonal synthesis and secretion, and (3) decreased target-organ sensitivity related to the number of cellular receptors for hormonal ligands, ligand-receptor binding, or ligand internalization (see Chapter 1).

Proponents of immune theories of aging believe that the immune system is implicated in aging because (1) immune function declines with age; (2) the decline in immune function is related to certain diseases, such as cancer, and to many other secondary effects; and (3) the number of autoantibodies (antibodies that attack body tissues) increases with age. (Changes in the immune system with age are discussed in Chapter 7.)

Degenerative Extracellular Changes

Extracellular factors that affect the aging process include the binding of collagen; the increase in free radicals' effects on cells; the structural alterations of fascia, tendons, ligaments, bones, and joints; and peripheral vascular disease, particularly arteriosclerosis (see Chapter 30).

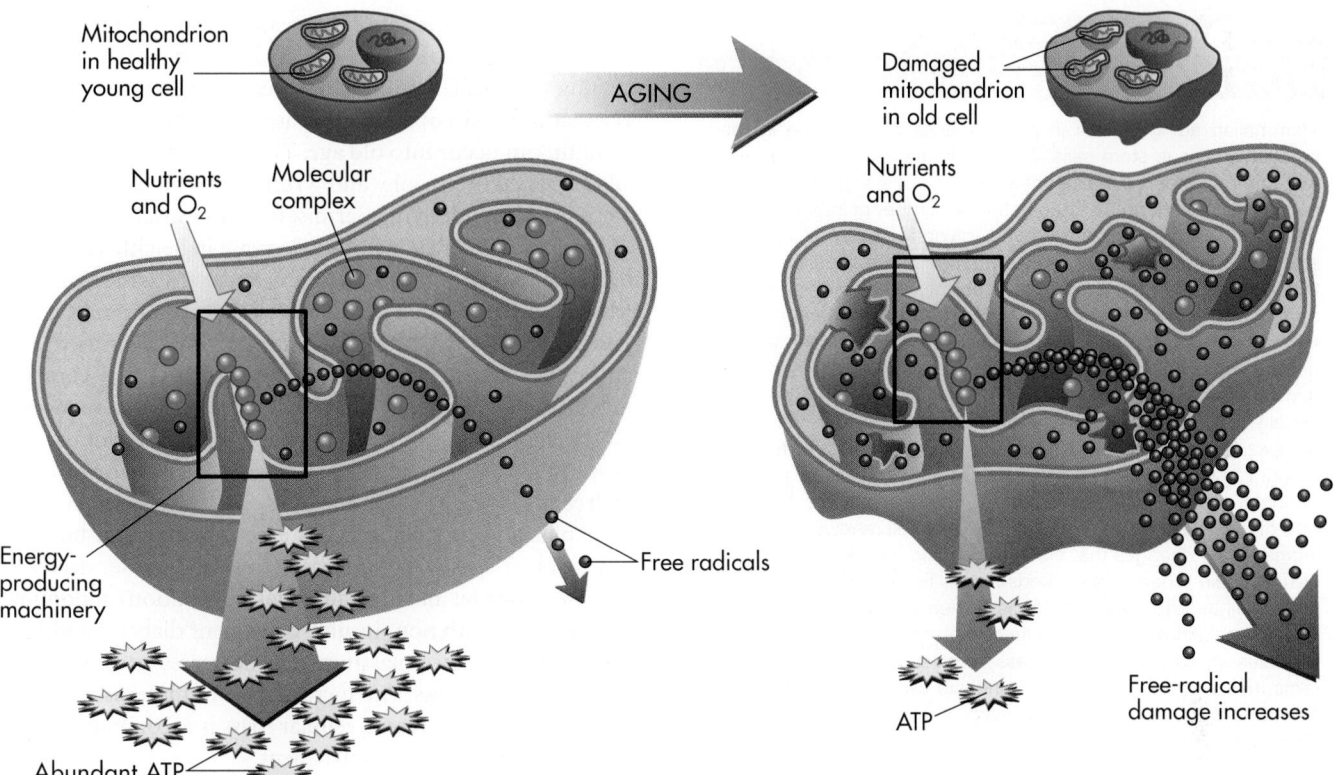

Figure 2-37 Theory of aging: destructive free radicals.

Aging affects the extracellular matrix with increased cross-linking (e.g., aging collagen becomes more insoluble, chemically stable, but rigid, resulting in a decrease of cell permeability), decreased synthesis, and increased degradation of collagen. These changes, together with the disappearance of elastin and changes in proteoglycans and plasma proteins, cause disorders of the ground substance that result in dehydration and wrinkling of the skin (see Chapter 44). Other age-related defects in the extracellular matrix include skeletal muscle alterations (e.g., atrophy, decreased tone, loss of contractility), cataracts, diverticula, hernias, and rupture of intervertebral disks.

Free radicals of oxygen that result from oxidative cellular metabolism (e.g., respiratory chain, phagocytosis, prostaglandin synthesis) are thought to damage tissues during the aging process (Figure 2-37). The oxygen radicals produced include superoxide radical, hydroxyl radical, and hydrogen peroxide (see p. 52). These oxygen products are extremely reactive and can damage nucleic acids, destroy polysaccharides, oxidize proteins, peroxidize unsaturated fatty acids, and kill and lyse cells. Oxidant effects on target cells can give rise to malignant transformation, presumably through DNA damage. That progressive and cumulative damage from oxygen radicals may lead to harmful alterations in cellular function is consistent with those alterations of aging. This hypothesis is founded on the wear-and-tear theory of aging, which states that damages accumulate with time, decreasing the organism's ability to maintain a steady state. Because these oxygen-reactive species not only can permanently damage cells but also may lead to

cell death, there is new support for their role in the aging process (see What's New? on p. 83).

Of much interest is the relationship between aging and the disappearance or alteration of extracellular substances important for vessel integrity. With aging, lipid, calcium, and plasma proteins are deposited in the walls of vessels. These depositions cause serious basement membrane thickening and alterations in smooth muscle functioning, resulting in arteriosclerosis. Arteriosclerosis is a progressive disease that causes serious problems in the aged individual, including stroke, myocardial infarction, renal disease, and peripheral vascular disease.

Cellular Aging

Cellular changes characteristic of aging include atrophy, decreased function, and loss of cells, possibly caused by apoptosis. Loss of cellular function from any of these causes initiates the compensatory mechanisms of hypertrophy and hyperplasia of remaining cells, which can lead to metaplasia, dysplasia, and neoplasia. All these changes can alter receptor placement and function, nutrient pathways, secretion of cellular products, and neuroendocrine control mechanisms. In the aged cell, DNA, RNA, cellular proteins, and membranes are most susceptible to injurious stimuli. DNA is particularly vulnerable to such injuries as breaks, deletions, and additions. Although DNA generally repairs itself with time, the aged cell's capacity for DNA repair is decreased. Lack of DNA repair increases the cell's susceptibility to mutations that may be lethal or may promote the development of neoplasia (see Chapter 11 and What's New? on Stem Cell, Aging, and Cancer).

Mammalian aging occurs in part because of a decline in the function of tissue stem cells. Stem cells are self-renewing cells that can be rendered malignant as a result of a small number of oncogenic mutations. To counter this, a number of integrated tumor prevention mechanisms have evolved to decrease the possibility of tumor development (e.g., *p16* ^{INK4a}* Rb, *ARF-p53*, and the telomere).† These beneficial antitumor pathways, however, appear to limit the stem cell life span, thereby contributing to aging. We constantly sacrifice many varied cell types, such as hepatocytes, keratinocytes, granulocytes, and erythrocytes, during homeostasis. For an individual to thrive, lost cells must be continually replaced. New information has identified significant capacities for repair and regeneration, even in organs mistakenly thought to no longer undergo mitosis, such as the brain and the pancreatic islet! Thus normal tissue function requires that the rate of cell loss be matched by the rate of cell renewal. Aging is increased by changes that either accelerate cellular loss or slow tissue repair. When loss exceeds repair, tissue and organ function declines and, ultimately, fails. When the condition occurs only in specific organs, it results in many chronic degenerative diseases. If, however, the process involves multiple organ systems, this progressive decline manifests clinically as frailty, accelerated aging, and eventually death.

Data from Sharplers NE, De Pinho RA: *J Clin Invest* 113:160-168, 2004.
p16 ^{INK4a} Rb: Retinoblastoma protein inhibits cell cycle progression; is frequently inactivated in cancer; *ARF-p53:* a regulator protein that induces cell cycle arrest or apoptosis in response to DNA damage or other cell stress.
†*Telomere:* Cells have special nucleotide sequences at the end of their chromosomes (tips) that are incorporated into telomeres; cells whereby chromosomes are defective and the tips not replicated completely withdraw, permanently, from the cell cycle and cease dividing; this function could be protective against cancer.

Tissue and Systemic Aging

It is probably safe to say that every physiologic process can be shown to function less efficiently with increasing age. The most characteristic tissue change with age is a progressive stiffness or rigidity that affects many systems, including the arterial, pulmonary, and musculoskeletal systems. A consequence of blood vessel and organ stiffness is a progressive increase in peripheral resistance to blood flow. The movement of intracellular and extracellular substances also usually decreases with age as does the diffusion capacity of the lung. Blood flow through organs decreases; for example, renal plasma flow decreases.

Changes in the endocrine and immune systems include thymus atrophy. Although this occurs at puberty, causing a decreased immune response to T-dependent antigens (foreign proteins), increased autoantibodies and immune complexes (antibodies bound to antigen) and an overall decrease in the immunologic tolerance for the host's own cells further diminish the effectiveness of the immune system later in life. The reproductive system loses ova in women, and spermatogenesis in men is decreased. Responsiveness to hormones decreases in the breast and endometrium.

The stomach experiences decreases in the rate of emptying and secretion of hormones and hydrochloric acid. Muscular atrophy diminishes mobility by decreasing motor tone and contractility. **Sarcopenia,** the loss of muscle mass and strength, can occur into old age. The skin of the aged individual is affected by atrophy and wrinkling of the epidermis and alterations in underlying dermis, fat, and muscle.

Total body changes include a decrease in height; a reduction in circumference of the neck, thighs, and arms; widening of the pelvis; and lengthening of the nose and ears. Several of these changes are the result of tissue atrophy and decreased bone mass caused by osteoporosis and osteoarthritis. Body composition changes with age.[93] With middle age there is an increase in body weight (men gain until 50 years of age and women until 70 years) and fat mass followed by a decrease in stature, weight, **fat-free mass (FFM)** (FFM includes all minerals, proteins, and water plus all other constituents except lipids), and body cell mass at older ages. As fat increases, total body water decreases. Increased body fat and centralized fat distribution (abdominal) are associated with non–insulin-dependent diabetes and heart disease. Total body potassium also decreases because of decreased cellular mass. An increased sodium/potassium ratio suggests that the decreased cellular mass is accompanied by an increased extracellular compartment.

Although some of these alterations are probably inherent in aging, others represent consequences of aging. Advanced age increases susceptibility to disease, and death occurs after an injury or insult because of diminished cellular, tissue, and organic function. To determine that an individual "died of old age" would be a monumental if not impossible task.

Frailty

Frailty is imprecisely defined as a wasting syndrome of aging leaving a person vulnerable to falls, functional decline, disease, and death.[94] The syndrome is complex, involving decreased protein synthesis, sarcopenia, neuroendocrine and muscular decline, and immune dysfunction. Several physiologic gender differences may explain differing levels of frailty: (1) higher baseline levels of muscle mass for men may be protective against frailty, (2) testosterone and growth hormone can provide advantages in muscle mass maintenance, (3) cortisol is more dysregulated in older women than older men, (4) alterations in immune function and immune responsiveness to sex steroids make men more vulnerable to sepsis and infection and women vulnerable to chronic inflammatory conditions and muscle mass loss, and (5) lower levels of activity and caloric intake may influence greater susceptibility to frailty in women.[95]

SOMATIC DEATH

Somatic death is death of the entire person. Unlike the changes that follow cellular death in a live body, **postmortem change** is diffuse and does not involve components of the inflammatory response. Within minutes of death, manifestations of postmortem change appear, eliminating any difficulty in determining that death has occurred. The most notable manifestations are complete cessation of respiration and circulation. The surface of the skin usually becomes pale and yellowish; however, the lifelike color of the cheeks and lips may persist after death from causes such as carbon monoxide poisoning, drowning, and chloroform poisoning.[96]

Body temperature falls gradually immediately after death and then more rapidly (approximately 1.0° to 1.5° F/hr) until, after 24 hours, body temperature equals that of the environment.[97] After death caused by certain infective diseases, body temperature may continue to rise for a short time. Postmortem reduction of body temperature is called **algor mortis.**

Blood pressure within the retinal vessels decreases, causing muscle tension to decrease and the pupils to become dilated. The face, nose, and chin begin to look "sharp" or "peaked" as blood and fluids drain away.[96] Gravity causes blood to settle in the most dependent, or lowest, tissues, which develop a purple discoloration called **livor mortis.** Incisions at this time usually fail to cause bleeding. The skin loses its elasticity and transparency.

Within 6 hours after death, acidic compounds accumulate within the muscles because of the breakdown of carbohydrate and depletion of ATP. This interferes with ATP-dependent detachment of myosin from actin (contractile proteins), and muscle stiffening, or **rigor mortis,** sets in. The smaller muscles are usually affected first, particularly the muscles of the jaw. Within 12 to 14 hours, rigor mortis usually affects the entire body.

Signs of putrefaction are generally obvious about 24 to 48 hours after death. Rigor mortis gradually diminishes, and the body becomes flaccid in 12 to 14 hours. Putrefactive changes vary depending on the temperature of the environment. The most visible is greenish discoloration of the skin, particularly on the abdomen. The discoloration is thought to be related to the diffusion of hemolyzed blood into the tissues and the production of sulfhemoglobin.[98] Slippage or loosening of the skin from underlying tissues occurs at the same time. After this, swelling or bloating of the body and liquefactive changes occur, sometimes causing opening of the body cavities. At a microscopic level, putrefactive changes are associated with the release of enzymes and lytic dissolution called **postmortem autolysis.**

SUMMARY REVIEW

Cellular Adaptation

1. Cellular adaptation is an alteration that enables the cell to maintain a steady state despite adverse conditions.
2. Atrophy is a decrease in cellular size. Amounts of endoplasmic reticulum, mitochondria, and microfilaments are decreased.
3. Physiologic atrophy occurs with early development; for example, the thymus gland involutes and atrophies. Pathologic atrophy occurs as a result of decreases in workload, use, pressure, blood supply, nutrition, hormonal stimulation, and nervous stimulation.
4. Aging causes brain cells and endocrine-dependent organs, such as the gonads, to become atrophic.
5. Hypertrophy is an increase in the size of cells by increased work demands or hormonal stimulation. Hypertrophy can be physiologic or pathologic. Amounts of protein in the plasma membrane, endoplasmic reticulum, microfilaments, and mitochondria are increased.
6. Hyperplasia is an increase in the number of cells caused by an increased rate of cellular division. Compensatory hyperplasia enables certain organs to regenerate. Hormonal hyperplasia is stimulated by hormones to replace lost tissue or support new growth, such as during pregnancy.
7. Pathologic hyperplasia is the abnormal proliferation of normal cells in response to excessive hormonal stimulation of growth factors on target cells.
8. Dysplasia, or atypical hyperplasia, is an abnormal change in the size, shape, and organization of mature tissue cells.
9. Metaplasia is the reversible replacement of one mature cell type by another less mature cell type. Metaplasia is thought to develop from a reprogramming of stem cells existing in most epithelia or of undifferentiated mesenchymal cells in connective tissue.

Cellular Injury

1. Most diseases begin with cell injury. Injured cells may recover (reversible injury) or die (irreversible injury).

2. Cellular injury is caused by a lack of oxygen (hypoxia), free radicals, caustic or toxic chemicals, infectious agents, unintentional and intentional injury, inflammatory and immune responses, genetic factors, insufficient nutrients, or physical trauma from many causes.
3. Cell injury can be acute or chronic, and it can be reversible or irreversible. It can involve necrosis, apoptosis, accumulation, or pathologic calcification.
4. Four biochemical themes are important to cell injury: (a) ATP depletion, (b) oxygen and oxygen-derived free radicals, (c) intracellular calcium and loss of calcium steady state, and (d) defects in membrane permeability.
5. The sequence of events leading to cell death is commonly decreased ATP production, failure of active transport mechanisms (the sodium-potassium pump), cellular swelling, detachment of ribosomes from the endoplasmic reticulum, cessation of protein synthesis, mitochondrial swelling as a result of calcium accumulation, vacuolation, leakage of digestive enzymes from lysosomes, autodigestion of intracellular structures, lysis of the plasma membrane, and death.
6. The initial insult in hypoxic injury is usually ischemia—the cessation of blood flow into vessels that supply the cell with oxygen and nutrients.
7. An important mechanism of membrane damage is injury caused by free radicals. Free radicals are difficult to control and initiate chain reactions.
8. Free radicals can cause (a) lipid peroxidation or the destruction of unsaturated fatty acids, (b) alterations of proteins, and (c) alterations in DNA.
9. The initial insult in chemical injury is damage or destruction of the plasma membrane. Examples of chemical agents that cause cellular injury include lead, carbon monoxide, ethanol, mercury, and social or street drugs.
10. Unintentional and intentional injuries are an important health problem in the United States. Death caused by injuries is more

Continued

SUMMARY REVIEW—cont'd

common for men than women and higher among blacks than whites and other racial groups.

11. Injuries by blunt force are the result of the application of mechanical energy to the body resulting in tearing, shearing, or crushing of tissues. The most common types of blunt force injuries include motor vehicle accidents and falls.

12. A contusion is bleeding into the skin or underlying tissues as a consequence of a blow. A collection of blood in soft tissues or an enclosed space may be referred to as a *hematoma*.

13. An abrasion (scrape) results from removal of the superficial layers of the skin caused by friction between the skin and injuring object. Abrasions and contusions may have a patterned appearance that mirrors the shape and features of an injuring object.

14. A laceration is a tear or rip resulting when the tensile strength of the skin or tissue is exceeded.

15. An incised wound is a cut that is longer than it is deep. A stab wound is a penetrating sharp force injury that is deeper than it is long.

16. Gunshot wounds may be either penetrating (bullet retained in the body) or perforating (bullet exits). The most important factors determining the appearance of a gunshot injury are whether it is an entrance or an exit wound and the range of fire.

17. Asphyxial injuries are caused by a failure of cells to receive or utilize oxygen. These injuries can be grouped into four general categories: suffocation, strangulation, chemical, and drowning.

18. Injury from microorganisms lies in their ability to survive and proliferate in the human body. Injury depends on the microorganisms' ability to invade and destroy cells, produce toxins, and produce damaging hypersensitivity reactions.

19. Activation of inflammation and immunity, which occurs after cellular injury or infection, involves powerful biochemicals and proteins capable of damaging normal (uninjured and uninfected) cells.

20. Genetic disorders injure cells by altering the nucleus and the plasma membrane's structure, shape, receptors, or transport mechanisms.

21. Deprivation of essential nutrients (proteins, carbohydrates, lipids, vitamins) can cause cellular injury by altering cellular structure and function, particularly of transport mechanisms, chromosomes, the nucleus, and DNA.

22. Injurious physical agents include temperature extremes, changes in atmospheric pressure, ionizing radiation, illumination, mechanical stresses (e.g., repetitive body movements), and noise.

Manifestations of Cellular Injury

1. Cellular manifestations of cellular injury include accumulations of water, lipids, carbohydrates, glycogen, proteins, pigments, hemosiderin, bilirubin, calcium, and urate.

2. Accumulations harm cells by "crowding" the organelles and by causing excessive (and sometimes harmful) metabolites to be produced during their catabolism. The metabolites are released into the cytoplasm or expelled into the extracellular matrix.

3. Cellular swelling, the accumulation of excessive water in the cell, is caused by the failure of transport mechanisms and is a sign of many types of cellular injury.

4. Accumulations of organic substances—lipids, carbohydrates, glycogen, proteins, and pigments—are caused by disorders in which (a) cellular uptake of the substance exceeds the cell's ca-

pacity to catabolize (digest) or use it or (b) cellular anabolism (synthesis) of the substance exceeds the cell's capacity to use or secrete it.

5. Dystrophic calcification (accumulation of calcium salts) is always a sign of pathologic change because it occurs only in injured or dead cells. Free calcium in the cytosol can cause activation of protein kinases, activation of phospholipases and membrane damage, and damage or disassembly of the cytoskeleton. Metastatic calcification, however, can occur in uninjured cells in individuals with hypercalcemia.

6. Disturbances in urate metabolism can result in hyperuricemia and deposition of sodium urate crystals in tissue, leading to painful disorders called *gout*.

7. Systemic manifestations of cellular injury include fever, leukocytosis, increased heart rate, pain, and serum elevations of enzymes in the plasma.

Cellular Death

1. Cellular death is manifested as cellular dissolution, or necrosis. Necrosis is the sum of the changes after local cell death and includes the process of autolysis, or cellular self-destruction.

2. The four major types of necrosis are coagulative, liquefactive, caseous, and fat. Different types of necrosis occur in different tissues.

3. Structural signs that indicate irreversible injury and progression to necrosis are the dense clumping and disruption of genetic material and the disruption of the plasma and organelle membranes.

4. Gangrenous necrosis, or gangrene, is tissue necrosis caused by hypoxia and subsequent bacterial invasion.

5. Apoptosis, a different type of cellular death, is a process of selective cellular self-destruction that occurs in both normal and pathologic tissue changes.

Aging

1. It is difficult to determine the physiologic (normal) from the pathologic changes of aging.

2. Humans have an inherent maximal life span (80 to 100 years) that is dictated by currently unknown intrinsic mechanisms.

3. Although the maximal life span has not changed significantly over time, the average life span, or life expectancy, has increased. Life expectancy for females exceeds that for males (gender gap) except in Bangladesh, Bhutan, India, Nepal, and Pakistan.

4. The physiologic mechanisms of aging are apparently associated with (a) cellular changes produced by genetic and environmental–life-style factors, (b) changes in cellular regulatory or control mechanisms, and (c) degenerative extracellular and vascular alterations.

5. Frailty is imprecisely defined as a wasting syndrome of aging that leaves a person vulnerable to falls, functional decline, disease, and death. Women have a higher risk of frailty then men.

Somatic Death

1. Somatic death is death of the entire organism. Postmortem change is diffuse and does not involve the inflammatory response.

2. Manifestations of somatic death include cessation of respiration and circulation, gradual lowering of body temperature, pupil dilation, loss of elasticity and transparency in the skin, muscle stiffening (rigor mortis), and skin discoloration (livor mortis). Signs of putrefaction are obvious about 24 to 48 hours after death.

KEY TERMS

Abrasion, 63
Algor mortis, 87
Anoxia, 50
Apoptosis, 81
Asphyxial injuries, 67
Atrophy, 46
Atypical hyperplasia, 48
Autolysis, 78
Autophagic vacuole, 46
Avulsion, 63
Bilirubin, 77
Blast injury, 71
Blow back, 65
Blunt force injuries, 61
Callus, 48
Carbon monoxide (CO), 56
Carboxyhemoglobin, 56
Caseous necrosis, 79
Catastrophic (error-prone) theory, 84
Cellular accumulations (infiltrations), 73
Cellular swelling, 74
Chemical asphyxiants, 68
Choking asphyxiation, 67
Chopping wounds, 65
Coagulative necrosis, 79
Compensatory hyperplasia, 48
Contact range entrance wounds, 65
Contusion, 61
Cyanide, 68
Decompression sickness
  (caisson disease), 71
Drowning, 68
Dry gangrene, 80
Dysplasia (atypical hyperplasia), 48
Dystrophic calcification, 77
Entrance wounds, 65
Epidural hematoma, 61
Ethanol, 58
Exit wounds, 66
Fat necrosis, 80

Fat-free mass (FFM), 86
Fatty change, 75
Fetal alcohol syndrome (FAS), 59
Frailty, 86
Free radical, 52
Gangrenous necrosis, 80
Gas gangrene, 81
Hanging strangulations, 67
Heat cramps, 70
Heat exhaustion, 70
Heat stroke, 70
Hematoma, 61
Hemoproteins, 76
Hemosiderin, 76
Hemosiderosis, 76
Hepatocyte growth factor (HGF), 48
Hormonal hyperplasia, 48
Hydrogen sulfide (sewer gas), 68
Hyperglycemia, 69
Hyperlipidemia, 69
Hyperplasia, 47
Hyperthermic injury, 70
Hypertrophy, 46
Hypolipidemia, 69
Hypothermic injury, 70
Hypoxia, 50
Incised wound, 64
Indeterminate (distant) range entrance
  wound, 66
Intermediate range entrance wounds, 65
Ionizing radiation, 71
Irreversible injury, 49
Ischemia, 50
Karyolysis, 78
Karyorrhexis, 79
Laceration, 63
Lead, 55
Life expectancy, 83
Ligature strangulation, 67
Lipid peroxidation, 52

Lipid-acceptor proteins (apoproteins), 53
Lipofuscin, 46
Liquefactive necrosis, 79
Livor mortis, 87
Manual strangulation, 67
Maximal life span, 82
Melanin, 75
Metaplasia, 48
Metastatic calcification, 78
Muzzle imprint, 65
Necrosis, 78
Neuroendocrine theory, 84
Noise, 73
Oncosis (vacuolar) degeneration, 74
Oxidative stress, 52
Pathologic atrophy, 46
Pathologic hyperplasia, 48
Physiologic atrophy, 46
Postmortem autolysis, 87
Postmortem change, 86
Psammoma body, 78
Puncture wound, 65
Pyknosis, 78
Reperfusion (reoxygenation) injury, 52
Reversible injury, 49
Rigor mortis, 87
Sarcopenia, 86
Shored exit wound, 66
Somatic death, 86
Somatic mutation hypothesis, 84
Stab wound, 64
Stippling, 66
Strangulation, 67
Subdural hematoma, 61
Suffocation, 67
Tattooing, 65
Ubiquitin-proteosome pathway, 46
Urate, 78
Vacuolation, 74
Wet gangrene, 80

MEDIA RESOURCES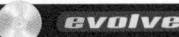

Review questions and answers for this chapter are available in the *CD Companion* included with this book.

WebLinks—links to Internet sites pertaining to this chapter—are available on Evolve at http://evolve.elsevier.com/McCance/.

REFERENCES

1. Kornitzer D, Ciechnover A: Modes of regulation of ubiquitin-mediated protein degradation, *J Cell Phys* 182(1):1, 2000.
2. Damjanov I, Linder J: *Anderson's pathology*, ed 10, St Louis, 1996, Mosby.
3. Yeldandi AU, Kaufman DE, Reddy JK: Cell injury and cellular adaptations. In Damjanov I, Linder J, editors: *Anderson's pathology*, ed 10, St Louis, 1996, Mosby.
4. Bottaro DP et al: Identification of the hepatocyte growth factor receptor as the c-met proto-oncogene product, *Science* 251(4995):802-804, 1991.
5. Alberts B et al: *Molecular biology of the cell*, ed 4, New York, 2002, Garland.
6. London SJ et al: A prospective study of benign breast disease and the risk of breast cancer, *JAMA* 267(7):941-944, 1992.
7. Reis-Filho JS, Lakhani SR: The diagnosis and management of pre-invasive breast disease: genetic alterations in pre-invasive lesions, *Breast Cancer Res* 5:313-319, 2004.
8. Kumar V, Abbas A, Fausto N: *Robbins and Cotran pathologic basis of disease*, ed 7, Philadelphia, 2005, Saunders.
9. Dröge W: Free radicals in the physiological control of cell function, *Physiol Rev* 82:47-95, 2002.
10. Li C, Jackson RM: Reactive species mechanisms of cellular hypoxia—reoxygenation injury, *Am J Physiol Cell Physiol* 282:C227-C241, 2002.
11. Duchen MR: Roles of mitochondria in health and disease, *Diabetes* 53(Suppl 1):S96-S102, 2004.
12. Taniyama Y, Griendling KK: Brief review. Reactive oxygen species in the vasculature: molecular and cellular mechanisms, *Hypertension* 42(6):1075-1081, 2003.
13. Costa LG, et al: Developmental neuropathy of environmental agents, *Annu Rev Pharmacol Toxicol* 44:87-110, 2004.
14. Davis JM, Svendsgaard DJ: Lead and child development, *Nature* 329:297-300, 1987.
15. Roberts JW et al: Reducing dust, lead, dust mites, bacteria, and fungi in carpets by vacuuming, *Arch Environ Contam Toxicol* 36(4):477-484, 1999.

16. Schanne FA, Long GJ, Rosen JF: Lead induced rise in intracellular free calcium is mediated through activation of protein kinase C in osteoblastic bone cells, *Biochem Biophys Acta* 1360(3):247-254, 1997.

17. Meo SA, Al-Khlawi T: Health hazards of welding fumes, *Saudi Med J* 24(11):1176-1182, 2003.

18. Holbrook J: Cigarette smoking. In Rom WH, editor: *Environmental and occupational medicine,* Boston, 1993, Little, Brown.

19. Cassel CK et al, editors: *Geriatric medicine,* ed 2, New York, 1990, Springer-Verlag.

20. Lieber CS: Microsomal ethanol-oxidizing system (MEOS): the first 30 years (1968-1998)—a review, *Alcohol Clin Exp Res* 23(6):991-1007, 1999. Review.

21. Agarwal DP: Genetic polymorphisms of alcohol metabolizing enzymes, *Pathol Biol (Paris)* 49(9):703-709, 2001. Review.

22. Sesso HD: Alcohol and cardiovascular health: recent findings, *Am J Cardiovacs Drugs* 1(3):167-172, 2001.

23. May JJ: Occupational hearing loss, *Am J Ind Med* 37(1):112-120, 2000.

24. Victor LD: Treatment of obstructive sleep apnea in primary care, *Am Fam Physician* 69(3):561-568, 2004.

25. Guilleminault A, Abad VC: Obstructive sleep apnea syndromes, *Med Clin North Am* 88(3):611-630, 2004.

26. Lieber CS: New concepts of the pathogenesis of alcoholic liver disease lead to novel treatments, *Curr Gastroenterol Rep* 6(1):60-65, 2004.

27. Song Z et al: Advances in alcoholic liver disease, *Curr Gastroenterol Rep* 6(1):71-76, 2004.

28. Lieber CS: Alcoholic liver disease: new insights in pathogenesis lead to new treatments, *J Hepatol* 32(1 Suppl):113-128, 2000.

29. Clark CM et al: Structural and functional brain integrity of fetal alcohol syndrome in nonretarded cases, *Pediatrics* 105(5):1096, 2000.

30. Ikonomidou C et al: Ethanol-induced apoptotic neurodegeneration and fetal alcohol syndrome, *Science* 287(5455):1056-1060, 2000.

31. Stratton K, Howe C, Battaglia F, eds: *Fetal alcohol syndrome: diagnosis, epidemiology, prevention and treatment,* Washington, DC, 1996, National Academy Press.

32. Mattson SN, Riley EP: Brain anomalies in fetal alcohol syndrome. In Abel EA, editor, *Fetal alcohol syndrome: from mechanism to prevention,* Boca Raton, FL, 1996, CRC Press.

33. Harris-Collazo MR et al: Quantitative magnetic resonance imaging analysis of fetal alcohol syndrome, *J Int Neuropsychol Sci* 4:48, 1998.

34. Boonstra J et al: The epidermal growth factor, *Cell Biol Int* 19(5):413-430, 1995.

35. Henderson GI et al: Ethanol, oxidative stress, reactive aldehydes, and the fetus, *Front Biosci* 15(4):D541, 1999.

36. Lieber CS: CYP2EI: from ASH to NASH, *Hepatol Res* 28(1):1-11, 2004.

37. Oberdoerster J, Rabin RA: Enhanced caspase activity during ethanol-induced apoptosis in rat cerebellar granule cells, *Eur J Pharmacol* 385(2-3):273-282, 1999.

38. Clarkson TW, Magos L, Myers GI: The toxicology of mercury—current exposures and clinical manifestations, *N Engl J Med* 349(18):1731-1737, 2003.

39. Ahlquist M et al: Serum mercury concentrations in relation to survival, symptoms, and disease: results from the prospective population study of women in Gothenbarg, Sweden, *Acta Odontol Scand* 57:168-174, 1999.

40. Bjorkman L, Pedersen NL, Lichtenstein P: Physical and mental health related to dental amalgam fillings in Swedish twins, *Community Dent Oral Epidemiol* 24(4):260-267, 1996.

41. Saxe SR et al: Dental amalgam and cognitive function in older women: findings from the Nun Study, *J Am Dent Assoc* 126(11):1495-1501, 1995.

42. Powell LW, Kerr JFR: Pathology of the liver in hemochromatosis, *Pathobiol Annu* 5:317-337, 1975.

43. Pichichero ME et al: Mercury concentrations and metabolism in infants receiving vaccines containing thimerosal: a descriptive study, *Lancet* 360(9347):1737-1741, 2002.

44. Smith JC, Farris FF: Methyl mercury pharmacokinetics in man: a reevaluation, *Toxicol Appl Pharmacol* 137(2):254-252, 1996.

45. Baumgartner RN et al: Age-related changes in sex hormones affect the sex difference in serum leptin independently of changes in body fat, *Metabolism* 48(3):378-384, 1999.

46. Fraker PJ, Lill-Elghanian DA: The many roles of apoptosis in immunity as modified by aging and nutritional status, *J Nutr Health Aging* 8(1):56-63, 2004.

47. Stanton B, Galbraith J: Drug trafficking among African-American early adolescents: prevalence, consequences, and associated behaviors and beliefs, *Pediatrics* 93(6, Pt 2):1039-1043, 1994.

48. Centers for Disease Control: *Injury statistics website,* Washington, DC, 2000, Centers for Disease Control.

49. Institute of Medicine: *To err is human: building a safer health system,* Washington, DC, 1999, National Academy Press.

50. Centers for Disease Control and Prevention, National Center for Health Statistics: Deaths final data for 1997, *Natl Vital Stats Rep* 47 191:27, 1999.

51. Holick MF: Vitamin D: importance in the prevention of cancers, type 1 diabetes, and osteoporosis, *Am J Clin Nutr* 79(3):362-372, 2004.

52. Camara AK et al: Hypothermia augments reactive oxygen species detected in the guinea pig isolated perfused heart, *Am J Physiol Heart Circ Physiol* 286(4):H1289-H1299, 2004.

53. Rauen U, de Groot H: Mammalian cell injury induced by hypothermia—the emerging role for reactive oxygen species, *Biol Chem* 383 (3-4):477-488, 2002.

54. Bartels-Stringer M et al: Preserved vascular reactivity of rat renal arteries after cold storage, *Cryobiology* 48(1):95-98, 2004.

55. Osorio RA et al: Reactive oxygen species in pregnant rats: effects of exercise and thermal stress, *Comp Biochem Physiol C Toxicol Pharmacol* 135(1):89-95, 2003.

56. Rauen U et al: Hypothermia: injury/cold-induced apoptosis—evidence of an increase in chelatable iron causing oxidative injury in spite of low O_2^-/H_2O_2 formation, *FASEB J,* 14(13):1953-1964, 2000.

57. Roy SB et al: Haemodynamic studies in high altitude pulmonary oedema, *Br Heart J* 31(1):52-58, 1969.

58. Trosko JE: Biomarkers for low-level exposure causing epigenetic responses in stem cells, *Stem Cells* 13(suppl 1):231-239, 1995.

59. Federal Drug Administration: *What are the radiation risks from CT?,* 2002. Available at www.fda.gov/edrh/et/risks.html

60. Koutz CA et al: Effect of dietary fat on the response of the rat retina to chronic and acute light stress, *Exp Eye Res* 60(3):307-316, 1995.

61. Weston HC: The effects of age and illumination upon visual performance with clore sights, *Br J Ophthalmol* 32:645, 1948.

62. Wilkins AJ, Wilkinson P: A tint to reduce eye-strain from fluorescent lighting? Preliminary observations, *Ophthalmic Physiol Opt* 11(2):172-175, 1991.

63. Zigman S, Sutliff G, Rounds M: Relationships between human cataracts and environmental radiant energy: cataract formation, light scattering, and fluorescence, *Lens Eye Toxic Res* 8(2-3):259-280, 1991.

64. Mainster MA, Timberlake GT: Why HID headlights bother older drivers, *Br J Opthalmol* 87(1):113-117, 2003.

65. De Flora S, D'Agostini F: Halogen lamp carcinogenicity, *Nature* 356(6370):569, 1992.

66. Bloom E et al: Halogen lamp phototoxicity, *Dermatology* 193(3):207-211, 1996.

67. Burnstock G, Ralevic V: New insights into the local regulation of blood flow by perivascular nerves and endothelium, *Br J Plast Surg* 47(8):527-543, 1994.

68. Keyserling WM, Armstrong TJ: Ergonomics. In Last JM, Wallace RB, editors: *Maxey-Roseneau-Last: public health and preventive medicine,* ed 13, Norwalk, Conn, 1992, Appleton & Lange.

69. NIDCD: *Statistics about hearing disorders, ear infections, and deafness,* Washington, DC, 2005, National Institutes of Health. Available at www.nidcd.nih.gov/health/statistics/nearing.asp.

70. Halpern NA et al: Hearing loss in critical care: an unappreciated phenomenon, *Crit Care Med* 27(1):211-219, 1999.

71. Powell LW, Kerr JFR: Pathology of the liver in hemochromatosis, *Pathobiol Annu* 5:317-337, 1975.

72. Hayflick L: The limited in vitro lifetime of human diploid cell strains, *Exp Cell Res* 37:614-636, 1965.

73. Kerr JFR, Searle J: Apoptosis: its nature and kinetic role. In Meyn RE, Withers HR, editors: *Radiation biology in cancer research,* New York, 1980, Raven.

74. Lo AC, Houenou LJ, Oppenheim RW: Apoptosis in the nervous system: morphological features, methods, pathology, and prevention, *Arch Histol Cytol* 58(2):139-149, 1995.

75. Sanders EJ, Wride MA: Programmed cell death in development, *Int Rev Cytol* 163:105, 1995.

76. Alenzi FQ: Links between apoptosis, proliferation, and the cell cycle, *Br J Biomed Sci* 61(2):99-102, 2004.

77. Wyllie AH, Kerr JFR, Currie AR: Cell death: the significance of apoptosis, *Int Rev Cytol* 68:251-306, 1980.

78. Basu A: Involvement of protein kinase C-delta in DNA damage-induced apoptosis, *J Cell Mol Med* 7(4):341-350, 2003.

79. Alberts B et al: *Essential cell biology: an introduction to the molecular biology of the cell,* ed 2, New York, 2004, Garland.

80. Amour A et al: General considerations for proteolytic cascades, *Biochem Soc Trans* 32(Pt 1):15-16, 2004.

81. Johnson HA, editor: Is aging physiological or pathological? In *Relations between normal aging and disease,* New York, 1985, Raven.

82. Vijg J: Somatic mutations and aging: a re-evaluation, *Mutat Res* 447(1):117-135, 2000.

83. Poehlman ET et al: Physiological predictors of increasing total and central adiposity in aging men and women, *Arch Intern Med* 155(22): 2443-2448, 1995.

84. Spillman BC, Lubitz J: The effect of longevity on spending for acute and long-term care, *N Engl J Med* 342(19):1409, 2000.

85. Trussel J: Women's longevity, *Science* 270(5237):719, 1995 (letter).

86. National Vital Statistics: Deaths: preliminary data for 2001, *Natl Vital Stats Rep* 52(3):1-115, 2003.

87. Stindl R: Tying it all together: telomeres, sexual size dimorphism, and the gender gap in life expectancy, *Med Hypotheses* 62(1):151-154, 2004.

88. Campbell K: Telomere length and mortality, *Lancet* 361(9364):1224, 2003.

89. Bobak M: Relative and absolute gender gap in all-cause mortality in Europe and the contribution of smoking, *Eur J Epidemiol* 18(1):15-18, 2003.

90. Russell RL: Evidence for and against the theory of developmentally programmed aging. In Warner HR et al, editors: *Modern biological theories of aging,* New York, 1987, Raven.

91. Cuervo AM, Dice JF: A receptor for the selective uptake and degradation of proteins by lysosomes, *Science* 273(5274):501-503, 1996.

92. Mera SL: Senescence and pathology of aging, *Med Lab Sci* 49(4): 271-282, 1992.

93. Baumgartner RN et al: Cross-sectional age differences in body composition in persons 60+ years of age, *J Gerontol A Biol Sci Med Sci* 50(6):M307-M316, 1995.

94. Muhlberg W, Sieber C: Sarcopenia and frailty in geriatric patients: implications for traning and prevention, *Z Gerontol Geriatr* 37(1):2-8, 2004.

95. Gillick M: Pinning down frailty, *J Gerontol A Biol Sci Med Sci* 56(3):M134-M135, 2001.

96. Shennan T: *Postmortems and morbid anatomy,* ed 3, Baltimore, 1935, William Wood.

97. Minckler J, Anstall HB, Minckler TM: *Pathobiology: an introduction,* St Louis, 1971, Mosby.

98. Richter C et al: Oxidants in mitochondria: from physiology to diseases, *Biochim Biophys Acta* 1271(1):67-74, 1995.

99. Buetler TM, Krauskopf A, Ruegg UT: Role of superoxide as a signaling molecule, *News Physiol Sci* 19:120-123, 2004.

THE CELLULAR ENVIRONMENT: FLUIDS AND ELECTROLYTES, ACIDS AND BASES

SUE E. HUETHER

CHAPTER OUTLINE

The cells of the body live in a fluid environment that requires an electrolyte concentration and pH value (measure of the acidity or alkalinity of a solution) that are regulated within a very narrow range. A balance is maintained by an integration of renal, hormonal, and neural functions. Changes in the composition of electrolytes affect electrical potentials of excitatory cells and cause shifts of fluid from one compartment to another. Alterations in pH disrupt the cellular function of enzyme systems. Fluid fluctuations affect blood volume and cellular function. Disturbances in these functions are common and can be life threatening. Understanding how alterations occur and the body's ability to compensate or correct the disturbance is important to understanding many pathophysiologic conditions.

DISTRIBUTION OF BODY FLUIDS

The fluids of the body are distributed among functional compartments, or spaces, and provide a transport medium for cellular and tissue function. Water moves freely among body compartments and is distributed by osmotic and hydrostatic forces. Two-thirds of the body's water is **intracellular fluid** (ICF) and one-third is in the **extracellular fluid** (ECF) compartments. The two main ECF compartments are the **interstitial fluid** and

the **intravascular fluid,** which is the blood plasma. Other ECF compartments include the lymph and the transcellular fluids, such as the synovial, intestinal, biliary, hepatic, pancreatic, and cerebrospinal fluids; sweat; urine; and pleural, synovial, peritoneal, pericardial, and intraocular fluids.

The sum of fluids within all compartments constitutes the **total body water (TBW)** (Table 3-1). The volume of TBW is usually expressed as a percentage of body weight in kilograms. The standard value for TBW is 60% of the weight of a 70-kg adult male, which is equivalent to 42 L of fluid (Table 3-2). The rest of the body weight is made up of fat and fat-free solids, particularly bone.

Although the amount of fluid within the various compartments is relatively constant, exchange of solutes and water occurs between compartments to maintain their unique compositions. The percentage of TBW varies with the amount of body fat and age. Because fat is water repelling (hydrophobic), very little water is contained in adipose cells. Individuals with more body fat have proportionately less TBW and tend to be more susceptible to fluid imbalances that cause dehydration.

AGING AND DISTRIBUTION OF BODY FLUIDS

The distribution and amount of TBW change with age (see Table 3-2). In newborn infants, TBW is about 75% to 80% of

Table 3-1	Distribution of Body Water	
	Percentage of Body Weight	Volume (L)
Intracellular fluid (ICF)	40	28
Extracellular fluid (ECF)	20	14
Interstitial	(15)	(11)
Intravascular	(5)	(3)
Total body water (TBW)	60	42

Table 3-2	Total Body Water in Relation to Body Weight		
Body Build	TBW (%) Adult Male	TBW (%) Adult Female	TBW (%) Infant
Normal	60	50	70
Lean	70	60	80
Obese	50	42	60

NOTE: TBW (total body water) is a percentage of body weight.

Table 3-3	Normal Water Gains and Losses (70-kg Man)		
	Daily Intake (ml)		Daily Output (ml)
Drinking	1400-1800	Urine	1400-1800
Water in food	700-1000	Stool	100
Water of oxidation	300-400	Skin	300-500
		Lungs	600-800
TOTAL	2400-3200		2400-3200

Normally, the largest amounts of water are lost through renal excretion. Lesser amounts are eliminated through the stool and through vaporization from the skin and lungs (insensible water loss) (Table 3-3).

Water Movement Between ICF and ECF

The movement of water between ICF and ECF compartments is primarily a function of osmotic forces. (Osmosis and other mechanisms of passive transport are discussed in Chapter 1.) Water moves freely across cell membranes, so the osmolality of TBW is normally at equilibrium. Sodium is the most abundant ECF ion and is responsible for the osmotic balance of the ECF space. Potassium maintains the osmotic balance of the ICF space. The osmotic force of ICF proteins and other nondiffusible substances is balanced by the active transport of ions out of the cell. Normally, the ICF is not subject to rapid changes in osmolality, but when there are changes in ECF osmolality, a net transfer of water from one compartment to another occurs until osmotic equilibrium is reestablished. Figure 3-1 shows a model of the maintenance of osmotic equilibrium.

Water Movement Between Plasma and Interstitial Fluid

The distribution of water and the movement of nutrients and waste products among the capillary, plasma, and interstitial spaces occur as a result of changes in hydrostatic pressure and osmotic forces at the arterial and venous ends of the capillary. **Aquaporins** are a family of water channel proteins that provide permeability to water at the capillary membrane.[2] Because water, sodium, and glucose readily move across the capillary membrane, the plasma proteins maintain the effective osmolality by generating plasma oncotic pressure. Osmotic forces within the capillary are balanced by the hydrostatic pressure, which arises from cardiac contraction. The movement of fluid back and forth across the capillary wall is called **net filtration** and is best described by the **Starling hypothesis**:

Net filtration = (Forces favoring filtration) −

(Forces opposing filtration)

The forces favoring filtration, or movement of water out of the capillary and into the interstitial space, include the capillary hydrostatic pressure and the interstitial oncotic pressure. The forces opposing filtration are the plasma oncotic pressure

body weight because infants store less fat. The percentage of TBW decreases to about 67% of body weight during the first year of life. In the immediate postnatal period, a physiologic loss of body water occurs, which amounts to 5% of body weight, as the infant adjusts to a new environment. Infants are particularly susceptible to significant changes in TBW because of their high metabolic rate and the accelerated turnover of body fluids in infants caused by their greater body surface area in proportion to total body size. Loss of fluids from diarrhea can represent a significant proportion of body weight. Renal mechanisms that regulate fluid and electrolyte conservation may not be mature enough to counter the losses, so dehydration may develop rapidly.

During childhood, TBW slowly decreases to 60% to 65% of body weight. At adolescence the percentage of TBW approaches adult proportions, and gender differences begin to appear. Males eventually have a greater percentage of body water as a function of increasing muscle mass. Females have more body fat and less muscle as a function of estrogens and therefore have less water.

With increasing age the percentage of TBW declines further still. The decrease is caused in part by an increased amount of fat and a decreased amount of muscle and by a reduced ability to regulate sodium and water balance. With older age the kidney becomes less efficient in producing concentrated urine, and the responses for conserving sodium become sluggish. Thirst perception may be impaired. The normal reduction of TBW in elderly people becomes clinically important when the body is under stress, such as development of fever or dehydration from any cause; loss of body fluids at such times can be severe and life threatening.[1]

Although daily fluid intake may fluctuate widely, the body regulates water volume within a relatively narrow range. The primary sources of body water are drinking, ingestion of water in food, and water derived from oxidative metabolism.

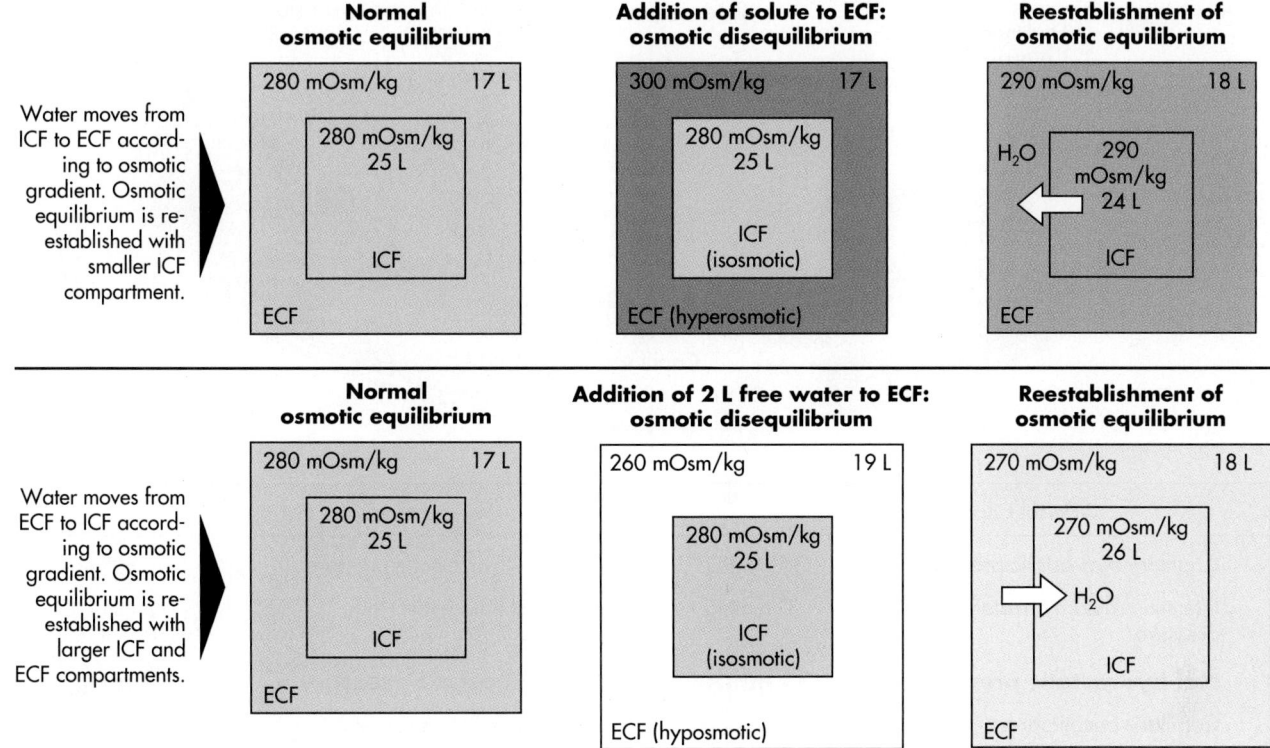

Figure 3-1 Model of osmotic equilibrium. *ICF,* Intracellular fluid; *ECF,* extracellular fluid.

and the interstitial hydrostatic pressure. Normally, the interstitial forces are negligible because only a very small percentage of plasma proteins crosses the capillary membrane and interstitial fluid moves into cells or is drawn back into the plasma. Thus the major forces for filtration are within the capillary.

As the plasma flows from the arterial to the venous end of the capillary, the force of hydrostatic pressure facilitates the movement of water across the capillary membrane. Oncotic pressure remains fairly constant because plasma proteins normally do not cross the capillary membrane. At the arterial end of the capillary, hydrostatic pressure is greater than capillary oncotic pressure and water filters into the interstitial space. Because of oncotic forces, some water moves back into the capillary, but the net effect is loss of water from the capillary. The movement of water from the plasma causes the hydrostatic pressure within the capillary to decrease. Thus at the venous end of the capillary, oncotic pressure exceeds hydrostatic pressure. Fluids then are attracted back into the circulation, balancing the movement of fluids between the plasma and the interstitial space. The overall effect is filtration at the arterial end and reabsorption at the venous end (Figure 3-2).

An important factor in capillary filtration of fluid is the integrity of the capillary membrane. Changes in membrane permeability may permit the escape of plasma proteins into the interstitial space. The normal relationship defined by the Starling hypothesis is altered with the osmotic movement of water into the interstitial space, causing tissue edema.

ALTERATIONS IN WATER MOVEMENT
Edema

Edema is the accumulation of fluid within the interstitial spaces. It is a problem of fluid distribution and does not necessarily indicate a fluid excess. In some conditions, sequestered fluids can cause both edema and dehydration. The pathophysiologic process is related to an increase in the forces favoring fluid filtration from the capillaries or lymphatic channels into the tissues. The four most common mechanisms are increased hydrostatic pressure, decreased plasma oncotic pressure, increased capillary membrane permeability, and lymphatic obstruction (Figure 3-3).

PATHOPHYSIOLOGY   An *increase in hydrostatic pressure* can result from venous obstruction or salt and water retention. *Venous obstruction* can increase the hydrostatic pressure of fluid within the capillaries enough to cause fluid to escape into the interstitial spaces. Thrombophlebitis, hepatic obstruction, tight clothing around the extremities, and prolonged standing are common causes of venous obstruction. Congestive heart failure and renal failure are both conditions associated with salt and water retention, which in turn cause volume overload, venous pressure, and edema.

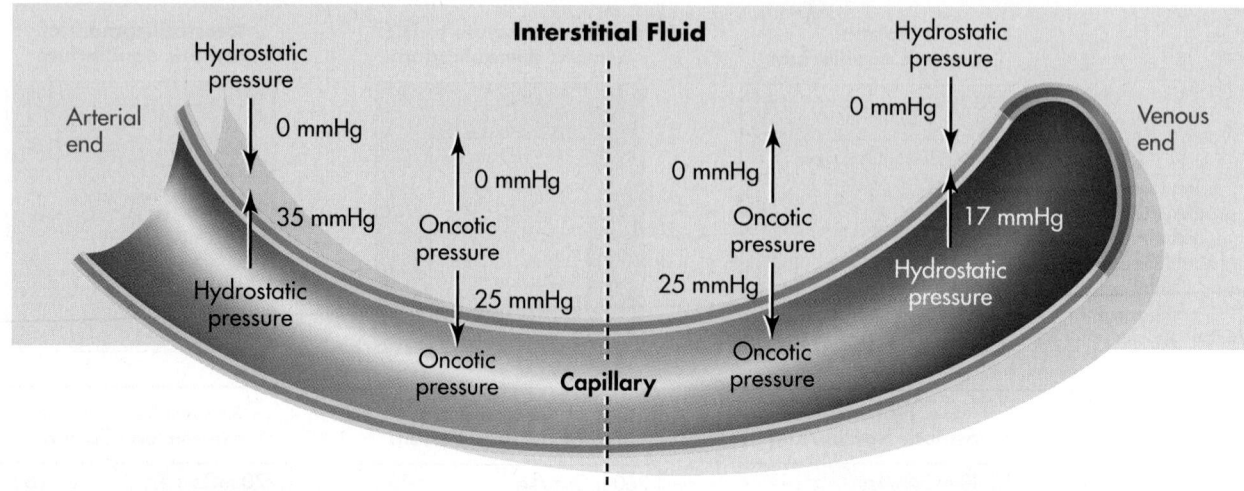

Arterial Capillary Pressures		Venous Capillary Pressures	
Capillary hydrostatic pressure	35 mmHg	Capillary hydrostatic pressure	17 mmHg
Interstitial fluid hydrostatic pressure	0 mmHg	Interstitial fluid hydrostatic pressure	0 mmHg
Net hydrostatic pressure	**35 mmHg**	**Net hydrostatic pressure**	**17 mmHg**
Capillary oncotic pressure	25 mmHg	Capillary oncotic pressure	25 mmHg
Interstitial fluid oncotic pressure	0 mmHg	Interstitial fluid oncotic pressure	0 mmHg
Net oncotic pressure	**25 mmHg**	**Net oncotic pressure**	**25 mmHg**
Net filtration pressure	**+10 mmHg**	Net filtration pressure	**−8 mmHg**

Figure 3-2 Capillary filtration forces. Water, electrolytes, and small molecules exchange freely between the vascular compartment and the interstitial space at the site of capillaries and small venules. The rate and amount of exchange is driven by the physical forces of hydrostatic and oncotic pressures and the permeability and surface area of the capillary membrane. The two opposing hydrostatic pressures are capillary hydrostatic pressure and interstitial hydrostatic pressure. The two opposing oncotic pressures are capillary oncotic pressure and interstitial oncotic pressure. The forces that favor filtration from the capillary are capillary hydrostatic pressure and interstitial oncotic pressure, and the forces that oppose filtration are capillary oncotic pressure and interstitial hydrostatic pressure. The sum of their effects is known as *net filtration pressure* (NFP). In the example of normal exchange above, a small amount of fluid moves to the lymph vessels, which accounts for the net filtration difference between the arterial and venous ends of the capillary.

Losses or diminished production of plasma albumin contributes to a decrease in plasma oncotic pressure. Decreased oncotic attraction of fluid within the capillary causes fluid to move into the interstitial space. Decreased production of plasma protein may occur with liver disease or protein malnutrition. Losses of plasma proteins occur with glomerular diseases of the kidney, serous drainage from open wounds, hemorrhage, burns, and cirrhosis of the liver.

Increases in capillary permeability are usually associated with inflammation and the immune response. (Immunity is discussed in Chapter 6; inflammation is discussed in Chapter 7.) These responses are often the result of trauma such as burns or crushing injuries, neoplastic disease, and allergic reactions. Proteins escape from the plasma and produce edema through a loss of capillary oncotic pressure and a gain in interstitial fluid proteins.

The lymphatic system normally absorbs interstitial fluid and the small amount of proteins that normally pass across the capillary membrane. When the lymphatic channels are blocked (because of infection) or are surgically removed, proteins and fluid accumulate in the interstitial space causing **lymphedema.** For example, lymphedema of the arm or leg will occur after surgical removal of axillary and femoral lymph nodes for treatment of carcinoma. Inflammation or tumors may be a cause of lymphatic obstruction leading to edema.

CLINICAL MANIFESTATIONS Edema may be localized or generalized. Some localized edema is limited to the site of trauma, as in a sprained finger or within particular organ systems. This includes cerebral edema, pulmonary edema, pleural effusion, pericardial effusion, and ascites (accumulation of fluid in the peritoneal space). Dependent edema, in which fluid accumulates in gravity-dependent areas of the body, might be a sign of more generalized edema. Dependent edema might appear in the feet and legs when standing and in the sacral area and buttocks when lying down. Dependent edema can be identified by using the fingers to press away

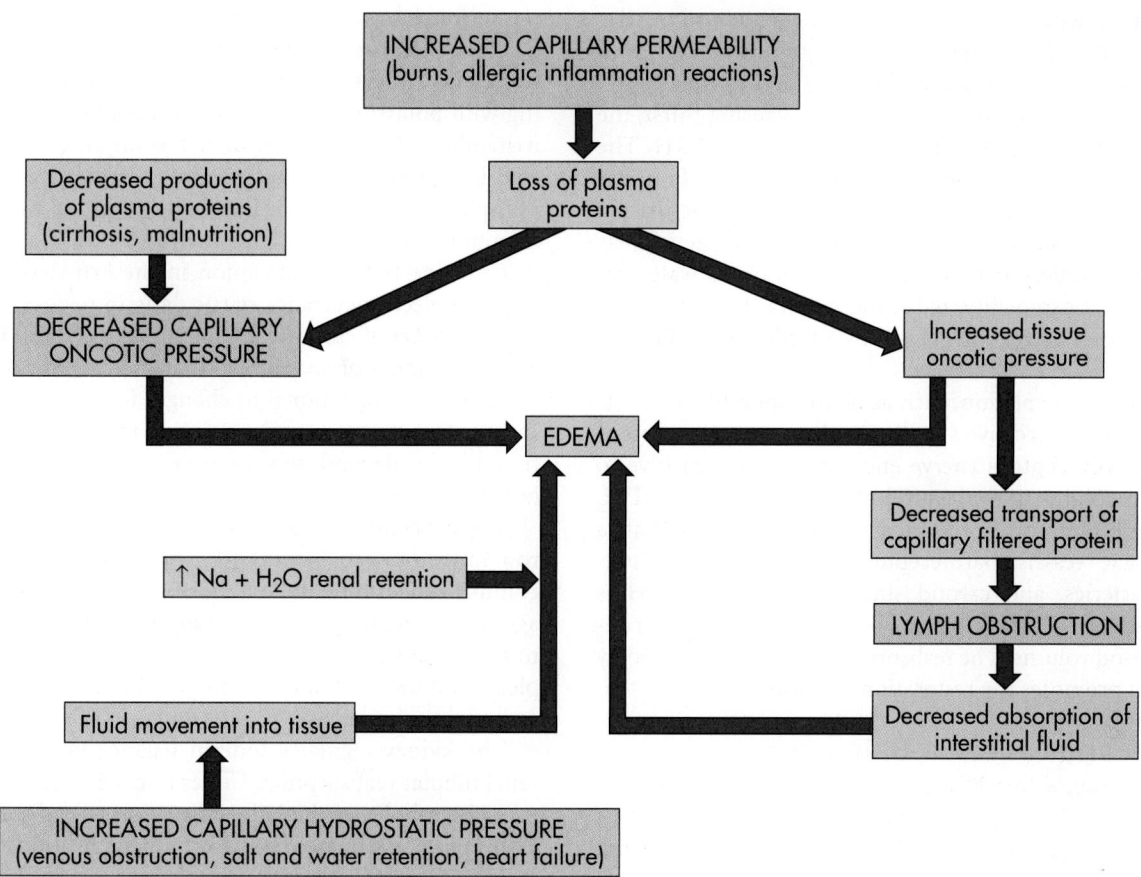

Figure 3-3 Mechanisms of edema formation.

edematous fluid in tissues overlying bony prominences. A pit will be left in the skin; hence the term *pitting edema.*

Edema is usually associated with weight gain, swelling and puffiness, tight-fitting clothes and shoes, limited movement of the affected area, and symptoms associated with the underlying pathologic condition. The accumulation of fluid increases the distance required for nutrients, oxygen, and wastes to move between capillaries and tissues. Increased tissue pressure may diminish capillary blood flow. Therefore wounds heal more slowly and the risks of infection and formation of pressure sores increase. Edema of specific organs, such as the brain, lung, or larynx, can be life threatening.

Although the accumulation of fluid is excessive, it is trapped in a "third space" and is not available for metabolic processes. Therefore a state of dehydration can develop as a result of the sequestering of the edematous fluid. An example of such sequestration occurs with severe burns, in which large amounts of vascular fluid are lost to the interstitial spaces, reducing plasma volume and causing shock (see Chapter 46).

EVALUATION AND TREATMENT   Specific conditions causing edema require diagnosis. Edema may be treated symptomatically until the underlying disorder is corrected. Supportive measures include elevating edematous limbs, using compression stockings, avoiding prolonged standing, restricting salt intake, and taking diuretics.

SODIUM, CHLORIDE, AND WATER BALANCE

The kidneys and hormones have a central role in maintaining sodium and water balance. Because water follows the osmotic gradients established by changes in salt concentration, sodium balance and water balance are intimately related. Water balance is primarily regulated by antidiuretic hormone (ADH; also known as *arginine-vasopressin*) from the posterior pituitary. Sodium is regulated by aldosterone from the adrenal cortex.

Water Balance

Secretion of ADH and perception of thirst are primary factors in the regulation of water balance. Thirst is a sensation that stimulates water-drinking behavior. Thirst is experienced when water loss equals 2% of an individual's body weight or when there is an increase in osmolality. Dry mouth, hyperosmolality, and plasma volume depletion activate **osmoreceptors** (neurons located in the hypothalamus that are stimulated by increased osmolality). The action of the osmoreceptors then causes thirst. Drinking water restores plasma volume and dilutes the ECF osmolality.

The secretion of ADH is initiated by an increase in plasma osmolality or a decrease in circulating blood volume and a lowered blood pressure. An increase in plasma osmolality occurs with a deficit of water or an excess of sodium in relation to water. The increased osmolality results in decreased extracellular and interstitial fluid volume and stimulates hypothalamic osmoreceptors. In addition to causing thirst, the stimulated osmoreceptors increase the release of ADH. The action of ADH is to increase the permeability of renal tubular cells to water, and water is then reabsorbed into the plasma from the distal tubules and collecting ducts of the kidney. Urine concentration increases, and the reabsorbed water decreases plasma osmolality, returning it toward normal. Like most hormones, ADH is regulated by a feedback mechanism (Figure 3-4).

With volume depletion, such as dehydration from vomiting, diarrhea, or excessive sweating, **volume-sensitive receptors** and **baroreceptors** (nerve endings that are sensitive to changes in volume and pressure) stimulate release of ADH. The volume receptors are located in the right and left atria and thoracic vessels; baroreceptors are in the aorta, pulmonary arteries, and carotid sinus. Secretion of ADH is caused also by a decrease in atrial pressure, as occurs with decreased blood volume. The reabsorption of water mediated by ADH then promotes the restoration of plasma volume.

Sodium and Chloride Balance

Sodium accounts for 90% of the ECF cations (positively charged ions). (The distribution of electrolytes in body compartments is summarized in Table 3-4.) As the most abundant ECF cation, along with its constituent anions (negatively charged ions) chloride and bicarbonate, sodium regulates osmotic forces and therefore regulates water balance. Sodium has many important body functions, including regulation of osmolality (interstitial and intravascular fluid volume), working with potassium and calcium to maintain neuromuscular irritability for conduction of nerve impulses, regulation of acid-base balance (through sodium bicarbonate and sodium phosphate), participation in cellular chemical reactions, and membrane transport.

Chloride is the major anion in the extracellular fluid. It provides electroneutrality, particularly in relation to sodium. The transport of chloride is generally passive and follows the active transport of sodium, so that increases or decreases in chloride are proportional to changes in sodium. Because bicarbonate is the other major anion in the ECF, the concentration of chloride tends to vary inversely with changes in bicarbonate concentration.

The concentration of sodium is maintained within a narrow range (136 to 145 mEq/L), primarily by the kidney in conjunction with neural and hormonal mediators. The average dietary intake of sodium ranges from 5 to 6 g/day; the minimal daily requirement of sodium is 500 mg. Sweating depletes sodium and water volume and increases the body's sodium requirement.

The kidney regulates sodium balance primarily through renal tubular reabsorption. Under normal rates of sodium intake, the tubules of the kidney function to reabsorb sodium. With an excess or deficit of sodium in relation to water, a combination of hormonal, neural, and renal mechanisms acts synergistically to control sodium balance.

The hormonal regulation of sodium balance is mediated by **aldosterone,** a mineralocorticoid synthesized and secreted from the adrenal cortex (see Chapter 20). The secretion of aldosterone is influenced by both circulating blood volume and plasma concentrations of sodium (Na^+) and potassium (K^+) (i.e., aldosterone is secreted when sodium levels are depressed, potassium levels are increased, or renal perfusion is decreased). The action of aldosterone is to in-

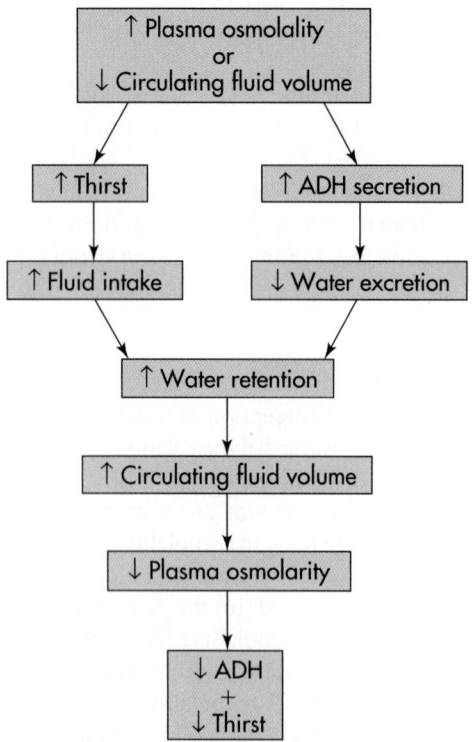

Figure 3-4 Regulation of thirst and antidiuretic hormone (ADH) secretion.

Table 3-4	Distribution of Electrolytes in Body Compartments	
	Extracellular Fluid (mEq/L)	Intracellular Fluid (mEq/L)
Cations		
Sodium	142	10
Potassium	5	156
Calcium	5	4
Magnesium	2	26
TOTAL	154	196
Anions		
Bicarbonate	24	12
Chloride	104	4
Phosphate	2	40-95
Proteins	16	54
Other anions	8	31-86
TOTAL	154	196 (average)

crease the reabsorption of sodium and secretion of potassium by the distal tubule of the kidney. As a result, sodium concentration of the ECF is enhanced and potassium is excreted with the urine.

When circulating blood volume is reduced, **renin,** an enzyme secreted by the juxtaglomerular cells of the kidney, is released in response to sympathetic nerve stimulation and decreased perfusion of the renal vasculature. Renin stimulates the formation of **angiotensin I,** an inactive polypeptide, which is then converted into **angiotensin II,** which acts as a hormone. Angiotensin II has two major functions: it stimulates the secretion of aldosterone, and it causes vasoconstriction. The aldosterone then promotes sodium and water reabsorption. The vasoconstriction elevates the systemic blood pressure and restores renal perfusion. The restoration of sodium levels, fluid volume, and renal perfusion then inhibits further release of renin. This sodium and water regulation mechanism is known as the **renin-angiotensin system** (see Chapter 35).

Natriuretic peptides are hormones produced by the heart (atrial natriuretic peptide [ANP]), brain (brain natriuretic peptide [BNP]), and kidney (urodilatin) and work to decrease blood pressure and increase sodium and water excretion. ANP is released when there is an increase in transmural atrial pressure (increased volume).[3] Natriuretic hormone is sometimes called a "third factor" in sodium regulation. (Increased glomerular filtration rate is thus the first factor and aldosterone the second factor.)

ALTERATIONS IN SODIUM, CHLORIDE, AND WATER BALANCE

Alterations in sodium and water balance are closely related. Water imbalances may develop because of changes in osmotic gradients caused by gain or loss of salt. Likewise, sodium imbalances occur with alterations in body water volume. Generally, the alterations can be classified as changes in tonicity, or the change in concentration of electrolytes in relation to water (see Chapter 1). Alterations can therefore be classified as isotonic, hypertonic, or hypotonic (Table 3-5).

Table 3-5	Water and Solute Imbalances
Tonicity	**Mechanism**
Isotonic (isoosmolar) imbalance	Gain or loss of extracellular fluid (ECF) resulting in a concentration equivalent to a 0.9% sodium chloride (salt) solution (normal saline); no shrinking or swelling of cells
Hypertonic (hyperosmolar) imbalance	Imbalances that result in an ECF concentration greater than 0.9% salt solution, i.e., water loss or solute gain; cells shrink in a hypertonic fluid
Hypotonic (hypoosmolar) imbalance	Imbalance that results in an ECF less than 0.9% salt solution, i.e., water gain or solute loss; cells swell in a hypotonic fluid

Isotonic Alterations

Isotonic alterations occur when changes in TBW are accompanied by proportional changes in electrolytes and water. For example, if an individual loses pure plasma or ECF, fluid volume is depleted but the number and type of electrolytes and the osmolality remain within a normal range. Excessive amounts of isotonic body fluids can result from excessive administration of intravenous normal saline or oversecretion of aldosterone with renal retention of both sodium and water. Losses of isotonic body fluids include hemorrhage, severe wound drainage, excessive diaphoresis, intestinal losses, and decreased fluid intake.

Isotonic volume depletion causes contraction of the ECF volume with resulting weight loss, dryness of skin and mucous membranes, decreased urine output, and symptoms of hypovolemia. Indicators of hypovolemia include a rapid heart rate, flattened neck veins, and normal or decreased blood pressure. In severe states, hypovolemic shock can occur (see Chapter 46).

Isotonic volume excesses are most commonly the result of excessive administration of intravenous fluids, hypersecretion of aldosterone, or the effects of drugs such as cortisone. As the plasma volume expands, symptoms of hypervolemia develop. Weight gain and a decrease in hematocrit and plasma protein concentration caused by the diluting effect of excess plasma volume will occur. The neck veins may distend, and the blood pressure increases. Increased capillary hydrostatic pressure leads to edema formation. If the plasma volume is great enough, pulmonary edema and heart failure develop.

Hypertonic Alterations

Hypertonic fluid alterations develop when the osmolality of the ECF is elevated above normal. The most common causes are an increased concentration of ECF sodium (hypernatremia) or a deficit of ECF free water. In both instances the hypertonicity of the ECF attracts water from the intracellular space, causing ICF dehydration. A primary increase in ECF sodium causes an osmotic attraction of water and symptoms of hypervolemia. In contrast, a hypertonic state caused primarily by free water loss leads to hypovolemia (Table 3-6).

Hypernatremia

PATHOPHYSIOLOGY **Hypernatremia** occurs when serum sodium levels exceed 147 mEq/L. Excessive serum sodium may be caused by an acute gain in sodium or a loss of water. Sodium gains cause intracellular dehydration; the movement of water to the ECF may cause hypervolemia. With an accompanying water loss, both ICF dehydration and ECF dehydration occur. Hyperosmolality is a common result of hypernatremia.

High amounts of dietary sodium rarely cause hypernatremia. More commonly, high sodium levels occur because of (1) inadequate free water intake, (2) inappropriate administration of hypertonic saline solution (e.g., as sodium bicarbonate for treatment of acidosis during cardiac arrest), (3) high sodium levels as a result of oversecretion of aldosterone (as in primary hyperaldosteronism), or (4) Cushing syndrome (caused by

Table 3-6	Causes and Consequences of Hypertonic Imbalances		
Causative Factor	**Mechanism**	**ECF Effects**	**ICF Effects**
Increased sodium (hypernatremia)	**Excessive hypertonic salt solutions** Intravenous hypertonic sodium Saline-induced abortions Selected infant formulas **Hyperaldosteronism** **Cushing syndrome**	**Hypervolemia** Weight gain Bounding pulse Increased blood pressure Edema Venous distention **Neuromuscular symptoms** Muscle weakness Seizures	**Intracellular dehydration** Thirst Fever Decreased urine output Shrinkage of brain cells Confusion Coma Cerebral hemorrhage
Water deficit	**Water deprivation** Confusion or coma Inability to communicate Loss of thirst **Water loss** Watery diarrhea Diabetes insipidus Excessive diuresis Excessive diaphoresis	**Hypovolemia** Weight loss Weak pulses Postural hypotension Tachycardia	**Intracellular dehydration** See above
Other factors	Hyperglycemia	Initial dilutional hyponatremia Polyuria Polydipsia Weight loss Hypovolemia Late hypernatremia	**Intracellular dehydration** See above

ECF, Extracellular fluid; *ICF,* intracellular fluid.

excess secretion of adrenocorticotropic hormone [ACTH], which also causes increased secretion of aldosterone).[4]

Increased sodium in relation to water loss is associated with fever or respiratory infections, which increase the respiratory rate and enhance water loss from the lungs. Diabetes insipidus (excess production of ADH), diabetes mellitus, polyuria, profuse sweating, and diarrhea cause water loss in relation to sodium concentration. Infants with severe diarrhea are particularly vulnerable. Insufficient water intake also can cause hypernatremia, particularly in individuals who are comatose, confused, or immobilized.

CLINICAL MANIFESTATIONS   Water is redistributed to the extracellular space, and intracellular dehydration ensues. Convulsions and pulmonary edema are the most serious symptoms. Thirst, fever, dry mucous membranes, hypotension, tachycardia, low jugular venous pressure, and restlessness are associated with hypernatremia as a result of water loss.

EVALUATION AND TREATMENT   The serum sodium level is usually more than 147 mEq/L. If there is water loss, urine specific gravity will be greater than 1.030 and hematocrit and plasma proteins will be elevated. The treatment of hypernatremia is to give an isotonic salt-free fluid (5% dextrose in water) until the serum sodium level returns to normal. Hypervolemia and edema require treatment of the underlying clinical condition.

Water Deficit

PATHOPHYSIOLOGY   **Dehydration** is an appropriate term to describe water deficit, but dehydration is also commonly used to indicate both sodium loss and water loss (isotonic or isoosmolar dehydration). Pure **water deficits** (hyperosmolar or hypertonic dehydration) are rare because most people have access to water. Individuals who are comatose or paralyzed will continue insensible water losses through the skin and lungs with a minimal obligatory formation of urine. Hyperventilation caused by fever also may precipitate water deficit. The most frequent cause of water loss is increased renal clearance of free water as a result of impaired tubular function or inability to concentrate the urine, as with diabetes insipidus (see Chapter 21).

CLINICAL MANIFESTATIONS   Marked water deficit is manifested by symptoms of dehydration: thirst, dry skin and mucous membranes, elevated temperature, weight loss, and concentrated urine (with the exception of diabetes insipidus). Skin turgor may be normal or decreased. Symptoms of hypovolemia, including tachycardia, weak pulses, and postural hypotension, may be present.

EVALUATION AND TREATMENT   An elevated hematocrit and serum sodium concentration are associated with moderate water loss in addition to clinical signs and symptoms.

Treatment is to give water. When intravenous replacement is required, 5% dextrose in water should be used because pure water lyses red blood cells.

Hyperchloremia

Hyperchloremia occurs clinically when there is an excess of sodium or a deficit of bicarbonate. Greater than normal amounts of chloride can be expected with hypernatremia or metabolic acidosis (see p. 113). Ingestion of excessive chloride infrequently accompanies the use of an ammonium chloride diuretic. No specific symptoms are associated with chloride excess.

Alterations in chloride levels are usually secondary to their pathophysiologic processes. Treatment therefore generally is related to management of the underlying disorder.

Hypotonic Alterations

Hypotonic fluid imbalances occur when the osmolality of the ECF is less than normal. The most common causes are sodium deficit (**hyponatremia**) or free water excess. Either of these causes leads to an intracellular overhydration (edema). When there is a sodium deficit, the osmotic pressure of the ECF decreases and water moves into the cell, where the osmotic pressure is greater. The plasma volume then decreases, leading to symptoms of hypovolemia. With free water excess, both the ICF volume and the ECF volume increase, causing symptoms of hypervolemia (Table 3-7) and water intoxication with cerebral and pulmonary edema.[5]

Hyponatremia

PATHOPHYSIOLOGY Hyponatremia develops when the serum sodium concentration decreases to less than 135 mEq/L. Sodium deficits usually cause hypoosmolality with movement of water into cells with cell swelling. Several clinical syndromes may cause hyponatremia. These syndromes may be caused by sodium loss, inadequate sodium intake, or dilution of the body's sodium level.

Pure sodium deficits usually are caused by diuretics[6] and extrarenal losses such as vomiting, diarrhea, gastrointestinal suctioning, or burns. **Inadequate intake** of dietary sodium is rare but can occur in individuals on low-sodium diets, particularly among those taking diuretics. **Dilutional hyponatremias** occur when there is an excess of TBW in relation to total body sodium or a shift of water from the ICF to ECF space (e.g., administration of mannitol). Replacement of fluid loss with intravenous 5% dextrose in water also can cause a dilutional hyponatremia once the glucose is metabolized, leaving a hypotonic solution with a diluting effect. In addition, excessive sweating may stimulate thirst and intake of large amounts of water, which dilute sodium.

Hyponatremia also may be hypoosmolar or hypertonic. During acute oliguric renal failure, severe congestive heart failure, or cirrhosis, renal excretion of water is impaired. Both TBW and sodium levels are increased, but TBW exceeds the increase in sodium, producing a **hypoosmolar hyponatremia.**

Table 3-7	Causes and Consequences of Hypotonic Imbalances		
Causative Factor	Mechanism	ECF Effects	ICF Effects

Decreased sodium (hyponatremia)	Inadequate intake
	Hypoaldosteronism
	Excessive diuretic therapy
	    Furosemide
	    Ethacrinic acid
	    Thiazides
		Extracellular volume contraction and hypovolemia (but may not be if there is water excess)	Increased intracellular water; edema
			Brain cell swelling, irritability, depression, confusion
			Systemic cellular edema, including weakness, anorexia, nausea, and diarrhea

Water excess	Excessive pure water intake
	    Excessive administration of hypotonic intravenous solutions
	Drinking water to replace isotonic fluid losses
	Tap water enemas
	    Psychogenic polydipsia
	    Renal water retention
	    Syndrome of inappropriate antidiuretic hormone (SIADH)
		Extracellular volume expands with hypervolemia (but may not be if fluid is trapped in intracellular space)	Edema (see above)

Other factors	Isotonic dehydration treated with intravenous D$_5$W; glucose in D$_5$W solution is metabolized to water, contributing to hyponatremia Nephrotic syndrome Cirrhosis Cardiac failure	Hypervolemia or hypovolemia	Edema (see above)

ECF, Extracellular fluid; *ICF,* intracellular fluid.

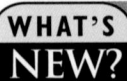

Hypertonic hyponatremia develops with hyperlipidemia, hyperproteinemia, and hyperglycemia. Increases in plasma lipids and proteins displace water volume and decrease sodium concentration. Hyperglycemia increases ECF osmolality and attracts water from the ICF compartment. The osmotic fluid shift to the ECF in turn dilutes the concentration of sodium and other electrolytes.

CLINICAL MANIFESTATIONS   Deficits of sodium alter the ability of cells to depolarize and repolarize normally (see Chapter 1). Behavioral and neurologic changes characteristic of hyponatremia include lethargy, headache, confusion, apprehension, seizures, and coma. Pure sodium losses may be accompanied by loss of ECF causing an isotonic **hypovolemia** with symptoms of hypotension, tachycardia, and decreased urine output. Weight gain, edema, ascites, and jugular vein distention are characteristic of dilutional hyponatremias.

EVALUATION AND TREATMENT   In hyponatremic states, serum sodium concentration falls to less than 135 mEq/L. With pure sodium deficits, the hematocrit and plasma protein levels may be elevated. Urine specific gravity is less than 1.010 when renal function is normal because sodium is maximally conserved.

Treatment of hyponatremia is related to the contributing disorder. Losses of sodium and water volume are calculated from the clinical evaluation, and appropriate solutions then are selected for replacement. Restriction of water intake is required in most cases of dilutional hyponatremia because body sodium levels may be normal or increased even though serum levels are low. Hypertonic saline solutions are used cautiously with severe symptoms, such as seizures.[7]

Water Excess

PATHOPHYSIOLOGY   When the body is functioning normally, it is almost impossible to produce an excess of TBW. However, some individuals with psychogenic disorders develop water intoxication from **compulsive water drinking.** Acute renal failure, severe congestive heart failure, and cirrhosis are clinical conditions that can precipitate water excess. **Decreased urine formation** from intrinsic renal disease or decreased renal blood flow contributes to water excess. The overall effect is dilution of the ECF with the movement of water to the intracellular space by osmosis. Water excess produces a hypotonic or hypoosmolar water imbalance.

The **syndrome of inappropriate secretion of ADH (SIADH)** is another circumstance contributing to excess water.[8] SIADH occurs when factors other than hyperosmolality or hypovolemia stimulate the secretion of or response to ADH. The amount of ADH is inappropriate in relation to sodium levels. Several clinical conditions associated with stress result in SIADH. These include fear, pain, acute infection, brain trauma, surgery, and drugs such as analgesics and anesthetics. The most common cause is cells that secrete ADH in bronchogenic cancer. SIADH is not caused by excess water intake but by decreased renal excretion of water. Therefore the presence of SIADH increases the risk of water excess if intravenous fluids are being administered. Serum sodium and osmolality are reduced. The kidney continues to excrete sodium and urine specific gravity is elevated, but urine volume is decreased or water is reabsorbed.

CLINICAL MANIFESTATIONS   The symptoms of water excess are related to the rate at which water loading has occurred. Acute excesses cause cerebral edema with confusion and convulsions. Weakness, nausea, muscle twitching, headache, and weight gain are common symptoms of chronic water accumulation.

EVALUATION AND TREATMENT   Serum sodium concentration can be decreased, but this also can occur with a pure sodium deficit. Serum osmolality is decreased because water will be in excess of sodium. The hematocrit therefore is reduced from the dilutional effect of water excess.

Withholding fluid for 24 hours is effective treatment if there are no convulsions. Small amounts of intravenous hypertonic sodium chloride can be given when symptoms are severe.

Hypochloremia

Loss of chloride, or **hypochloremia,** is usually the result of hyponatremia, or elevated bicarbonate concentration, as in metabolic alkalosis (see p. 115). Hypochloremia develops with vomiting and loss of hydrochloric acid. Sodium deficit related to restricted intake or use of diuretics is accompanied by chloride deficiency. Cystic fibrosis, for example, is also characterized by hypochloremia. As with hyperchloremia, treatment of the underlying condition is required.

ALTERATIONS IN POTASSIUM, CALCIUM, PHOSPHATE, AND MAGNESIUM BALANCE

Potassium

Potassium is the major intracellular electrolyte and contributes to many important cellular functions. Total body potassium content is about 4000 mEq, with most of it located in the cells. Daily dietary intake of potassium is 40 to 150 mEq/day, with an average of 1.5 mEq/kg body weight. The ICF concentration of K^+ is 150 to 160 mEq/L; the ECF concentration is 3.5 to 4.5 mEq/L. K^+ is found in most body fluids (Table 3-8).

The difference in the concentration is maintained by a sodium-potassium active transport system (Na^+, K^+ ATPase pump). The ratio of ECF K^+ to ICF K^+ is the major determinant of the resting membrane potential, which is necessary for the transmission of nerve impulses. (Membrane transport and membrane potentials are discussed in Chapter 1.) Changes in the ratio of ICF to ECF potassium are responsible for many of the symptoms associated with potassium imbalance.

Potassium is necessary for a variety of metabolic functions. As the predominant ICF ion, it exerts a major influence in the regulation of ICF osmolality and provides the balance for intracellular electrical neutrality in relation to hydrogen (H^+) and Na^+. Potassium is required for glycogen deposition in liver and skeletal muscle cells. The significant role of potassium in maintaining the resting membrane potential is reflected in transmission and conduction of nerve impulses, maintenance of normal cardiac rhythms, and skeletal and smooth muscle contraction.

The kidney provides the most efficient regulation of potassium balance. The amount of K^+ excreted varies in proportion to the dietary intake (40 to 120 mEq/day). Potassium is freely filtered by the renal glomerulus, and 90% is reabsorbed by the proximal tubule and loop of Henle. The principle cells in the collecting tubule secrete potassium. The reabsorption of K^+ occurs in the adjacent intercalated cell. Dietary potassium intake, aldosterone, and distal tubule urine flow determine the amount of K^+ excreted from the body. Unlike sodium, the renal mechanism for conserving K^+ is weak, even when total body potassium stores are depleted. A low K^+ intake also stimulates the protein tyrosine kinase dependent signal transduction pathway and suppresses renal K^+ excretion.[9]

Several factors related to passive transport and aldosterone contribute to renal regulation of potassium. These factors include the concentration gradients for potassium at the distal tubule and collecting duct, changes in pH (causing acidosis or alkalosis), changes in electrical potential differences across the distal tubule, and aldosterone levels. (Renal mechanisms are described in more detail in Chapter 35.)

The concentration of potassium in the distal tubular cell is determined primarily by the plasma concentration in the peritubular capillaries. When plasma K^+ concentration increases because of increased dietary intake or shifts from the ICF occur, potassium is secreted into the urine by the distal tubules. Decreases in plasma potassium result in decreased distal tubular secretion, although K^+ losses of approximately 5 to 15 mEq/day will continue. Changes in the rate of filtrate flow through the distal tubule also influence the concentration gradient for K^+ secretion. When the flow rate is high, as occurs with the administration of diuretics, the concentration of potassium in the distal tubular urine will be lower, favoring the secretion of potassium.[10]

Changes in pH and thus in hydrogen ion concentration also affect K^+ balance. Hydrogen ions move from the ECF to the ICF during states of acidosis. During acidosis, potassium shifts out of the cell to the ECF to maintain a balance of cations across the cell membrane. The decreased ICF K^+ results in decreased secretion of K^+ into the urine by the distal tubular cells, contributing to hyperkalemia. In contrast, intracellular fluid levels of hydrogen are diminished during states of alkalosis. Alkalosis causes potassium to shift into the cell, so the distal tubular cells increase their secretion of K^+ into the urine, contributing to hypokalemia.

Besides acting to conserve sodium, *aldosterone is a major factor in potassium regulation.* When potassium concentration is increased, aldosterone is released, stimulating secretion of potassium into the urine by the distal tubules of the kidney. Aldosterone also increases the secretion of K^+ from the sweat glands.

Insulin contributes to the regulation of plasma potassium levels by stimulating the Na^+, K^+-ATPase pump, thereby promoting the movement of potassium into liver and muscle cells simultaneously with glucose transport. Insulin therefore can be used to treat hyperkalemia, and dangerously low levels of plasma potassium can result from the administration of insulin when potassium levels are depressed. Potassium balance

Table 3-8	Approximate Concentration of Electrolytes in Body Fluids			
Fluid	Na^+ (mEq/L)	K^+ (mEq/L)	Cl^- (mEq/L)	HCO_3^- (mEq/L)
Saliva	33	20	34	0
Gastric juice*	60	9	84	0
Bile	149	5	101	45
Pancreatic juice	141	5	77	92
Ileal fluid	129	11	116	29
Cecal fluid	80	21	48	22
Cerebrospinal fluid	141	3	127	23
Sweat	45	5	58	0

From Smith LH, Thier SO: *Pathophysiology: the biological principles of disease*, Philadelphia, 1981, Saunders.
Na^+, Sodium; *K^+*, potassium; *Cl^-*, chloride; *HCO_3^-*, bicarbonate; *H^+*, hydrogen.
*The Cl^- concentration exceeds the Na^+, K^+ concentration by 15 mEq/L in gastric juice. This largely represents the secretions of H^+ by the parietal cells.

is especially significant in the treatment of conditions requiring insulin administration, such as insulin-dependent diabetes mellitus.

Catecholamines also influence K^+ concentration in ECF. β_2 adrenergics stimulate the movement of K^+ into cells, and α adrenergics shift K^+ out of cells.[11]

An interesting aspect of K^+ regulation is the ability of the body to adapt to increased levels of potassium intake over time. A sudden increase in potassium may be fatal, but if the intake of potassium is slowly increased by amounts no more than 120 mEq/day, the kidney is able to increase the urinary excretion of potassium and maintain potassium balance. This tolerance to increasing amounts of potassium is known as **potassium adaptation.**

Hypokalemia

PATHOPHYSIOLOGY   Potassium deficiency, or **hypokalemia,** develops when the serum potassium concentration decreases to less than 3.5 mEq/L. Because cellular and total body stores of potassium are difficult to measure, changes in potassium balance are described by the plasma concentration, although changes in total body potassium are not always reflected in the plasma potassium concentration. Generally, lowered serum potassium indicates a loss of total body potassium. Because potassium is lost from the ECF, the change in the concentration gradient favors movement of K^+ from the cell to the ECF. The ICF/ECF concentration ratio is maintained, but total body K^+ is depleted.

Extracellular fluid hypokalemia can develop, however, without losses of total body potassium, but only when potassium is redistributed between the ICF and ECF. For example, potassium shifts into the cell during states of respiratory or metabolic alkalosis or after administration of insulin. In the event of alkalosis, K^+ shifts into the cell in exchange for H^+ to maintain plasma acid-base balance. Insulin also promotes cellular uptake of K^+ and can cause a deficit in ECF potassium.

Plasma K^+ levels may be normal or elevated when total body potassium is depleted. In such instances, potassium shifts from the ICF to the ECF. One of the common causes of this problem is diabetic ketoacidosis, in which the increased hydrogen ion concentration in the ECF causes H^+ to shift into the cell in exchange for potassium. A normal level of potassium is maintained in the plasma, but potassium continues to be lost in the urine, causing a deficit in total body potassium. Severe, even fatal, hypokalemia may occur if insulin is administered without also providing potassium supplements. Thus total body potassium depletion becomes evident when insulin treatment is initiated.

Potassium loss also occurs through normal body functions, but without causing hypokalemia. Average daily losses of potassium are as follows:

Location	Daily Loss (mEq/L)
Stool	5-10
Sweat	0-20
Urine	40-120

Factors contributing to the development of hypokalemia include *reduced intake of potassium, increased entry of potassium into cells, and increased losses of body potassium.* Dietary deficiency of potassium is a rare cause of hypokalemia. It may occur in elderly individuals with both low protein intake and inadequate intake of fruits and vegetables and in persons with alcoholism or anorexia nervosa. Generally, reduced potassium intake becomes a problem when combined with other causes of potassium depletion.

Shifts of potassium from the extracellular to intracellular space cause apparent deficits in total body potassium. Alkalosis, particularly respiratory alkalosis, is the most common clinical problem. ECF potassium will exchange with ICF hydrogen and correct the alkalosis by decreasing the pH of the ECF. Treatment of pernicious anemia with vitamin B_{12} or folate also may precipitate hypokalemia if the formation of new red blood cells causes enough potassium uptake to effect an extracellular decrease in potassium. Catecholamines (β_2 adrenergics) promote intracellular uptake of K^+. Familial hypokalemic periodic paralysis is a rare genetically transmitted disease that also causes potassium to shift into the intracellular space.

Losses of potassium from body stores are most commonly caused by gastrointestinal and renal disorders. Diarrhea (from any cause), intestinal drainage tubes or fistulae, and laxative abuse also may result in hypokalemia. Normally, only 5 to 10 mEq of potassium and 100 to 150 ml of water are excreted in the stool each day. With diarrhea, fluid and electrolyte losses can be voluminous, with several liters of fluid and 100 to 200 mEq of potassium lost per day. Vomiting or continuous nasogastric suction frequently is associated with potassium depletion, partly because of the potassium lost from the gastric fluid but principally because of renal compensation for volume depletion and the metabolic alkalosis (elevated bicarbonate levels) that occurs from sodium, chloride, and hydrogen ion losses. The loss of fluid and sodium stimulates the secretion of aldosterone, which in turn causes renal losses of potassium. The elevated flow of bicarbonate at the distal tubule contributes to renal excretion of potassium because of increased tubular lumen electronegativity.

Renal losses of potassium are related to increased secretion of potassium by the distal tubule. Use of diuretics, excessive aldosterone secretion, increased distal tubular flow rate, and low plasma magnesium concentration all may contribute to urinary losses of potassium. Many diuretics, including thiazides, furosemide, ethacrynic acid, and osmotic diuretics, inhibit the reabsorption of sodium chloride, causing the diuretic effect. The distal tubular flow rate then increases, promoting potassium secretion. If sodium loss is severe, the compensating aldosterone secretion (which causes secondary hyperaldosteronism) may further deplete potassium stores. Primary hyperaldosteronism with excessive secretion of aldosterone from an adrenal adenoma also causes potassium wasting. Many kidney diseases result in a reduced ability to conserve sodium. The disordered sodium reabsorption produces a diuretic effect, and the increased distal tubule flow rate favors the secretion of potassium. Magnesium deficits stimulate renin release and hyperaldosteronism, causing hypokalemia. Several antibiotics, including amphotericin B, gentamicin, and carbenicillin, are known to cause hypokalemia.

CLINICAL MANIFESTATIONS   A wide range of metabolic dysfunctions may result from potassium deficiency. Carbohydrate metabolism is affected because hypokalemia depresses insulin secretion and alters hepatic and skeletal muscle glycogen synthesis. Renal function is impaired, with a decreased ability to concentrate urine. Polyuria (increased urine) and polydipsia (increased thirst) are associated with decreased responsiveness to ADH. Chronic potassium deficits lasting more than 1 month may damage renal tissue, with resulting interstitial fibrosis and tubular atrophy.

Neuromuscular and cardiac effects of hypokalemia produce the most common symptoms.[12] Neuromuscular excitability is decreased, causing skeletal muscle weakness, smooth muscle atony, and cardiac dysrhythmias. As Chapter 1 describes, the resting membrane potential (E_m) is determined by the *ratio* of extracellular to intracellular potassium ion concentration. Because the concentration of potassium in the ECF is small, only small changes in ECF potassium are required to influence the resting membrane potential and affect neuromuscular excitability. When extracellular potassium levels decrease rapidly and intracellular potassium concentration does not change, the resting membrane potential becomes more negative and the cell membrane is then **hyperpolarized.** If the threshold potential (E_t) remains stable, the difference between resting membrane potential and threshold

potential increases, requiring a stronger stimulus to initiate an action potential (Figure 3-5).

Factors such as calcium concentration and pH also contribute to the changes in neuromuscular excitability associated with hypokalemia. Increases in ECF calcium concentration tend to make the threshold potential less negative and decrease membrane excitability, potentiating the neuromuscular effects of hypokalemia.

The onset of symptoms is related to the rate of potassium depletion. Because the body can accommodate slow losses of potassium, the decrease in ECF concentration may be slow enough to allow potassium to shift from the intracellular space. The extracellular to intracellular potassium concentration gradient then is restored toward normal, with less severe neuromuscular changes. With acute losses of potassium, changes in neuromuscular excitability are more profound. Skeletal muscle weakness initially occurs in the larger muscles of the legs and arms and ultimately affects the diaphragm and depresses ventilation. Paralysis and respiratory arrest then can occur. Loss of smooth muscle tone is manifested by constipation, intestinal distention, anorexia, nausea, vomiting, and paralytic ileus.

The cardiac effects of hypokalemia are related also to changes in membrane excitability (see Figure 3-5). Because potassium contributes to the repolarization phase of the action potential, hypokalemia delays ventricular repolarization. A variety of dysrhythmias may occur, including sinus bradycardia, atrioventricular block, and paroxysmal atrial tachycardia. The characteristic changes in the electrocardiogram reflect delayed repolarization. For instance, the amplitude of the T wave is decreased; the amplitude of the U wave is increased; and the ST

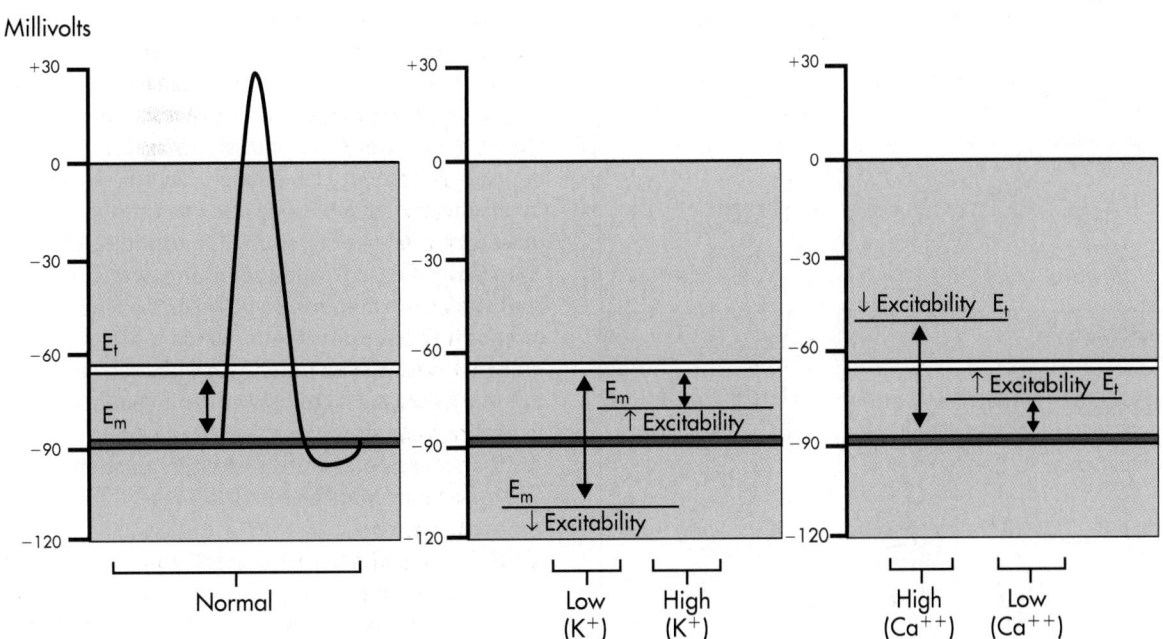

Figure 3-5 Effects of potassium (K^+) and calcium (Ca^{++}) on membrane excitability. Potassium affects resting membrane potential (Em), and calcium affects threshold potential (Et).

segment is depressed (Figure 3-6). In severe states of hypokalemia, P waves peak and the QRS complex is prolonged. Hypokalemia also increases the risk of digitalis toxicity.

EVALUATION AND TREATMENT   The diagnosis of hypokalemia is significantly related to the medical history and the identification of disorders associated with potassium loss. Treatment involves an estimation of total body potassium losses and correction of acid-base imbalances. Further losses of potassium should be prevented, and the individual should be encouraged to eat foods rich in potassium. The maximal rate of oral replacement is 40 to 80 mEq/day if renal function is normal. A maximal safe rate of intravenous replacement is 20 mEq/hr. Because potassium is irritating to blood vessels, a maximal concentration of 40 mEq/L should be used. Serum potassium values can be monitored until normokalemia is achieved.

Hyperkalemia

PATHOPHYSIOLOGY   An elevation of ECF potassium *above 5.5 mEq/L* constitutes **hyperkalemia.** Because of efficient renal excretion, increases in total body potassium are relatively rare. Acute increases in serum potassium are handled quickly through an increase in cellular uptake and renal excretion of body potassium excesses. Excretion is partially mediated by the secretion of aldosterone, because it facilitates losses of potassium in the urine.

Excesses of serum potassium may be caused by increased intake, a shift of potassium from cells to the ECF, or decreased renal excretion. If renal function is normal, slow, long-term increases in potassium intake are usually well tolerated through potassium adaptation, although acute potassium loading can exceed renal excretion rates. Use of stored whole blood and intravenous boluses of penicillin G or replacement potassium can precipitate hyperkalemia, particularly if renal function is impaired. Dietary excesses of potassium are uncommon, but accidental ingestion of potassium salt substitutes can cause toxicity.

Movement of potassium from the ICF to the ECF occurs with cell trauma or a change in cell membrane permeability, acidosis, insulin deficiency, or cell hypoxia. Burns, massive crushing injuries, and extensive surgeries can cause loss of potassium to the ECF. If renal function is sustained, potassium will be excreted. As cell repair begins, hypokalemia develops without an adequate intake of potassium.

In states of acidosis, hydrogen ions shift into the cells in exchange for ICF potassium and sodium; hyperkalemia and acidosis therefore often occur together. Because insulin promotes cellular entry of potassium, insulin deficits, which occur with conditions such as diabetic ketoacidosis, are accompanied by hyperkalemia. Hypoxia can lead to hyperkalemia by diminishing the efficiency of cell membrane active transport, resulting in the escape of potassium to the ECF. Digitalis overdose may cause hyperkalemia by inhibiting the Na^+, K^+ ATPase pump, which maintains high intracellular potassium and high extracellular sodium (see Chapter 1).

Decreased renal excretion of potassium commonly is associated with hyperkalemia. Renal failure that results in oliguria (urine output less than 30 ml/hr) is accompanied by elevations of serum potassium. The severity of hyperkalemia is related to the amount of potassium intake, the degree of acidosis, and the rate of cell damage. Decreases in the secretion or renal effects of aldosterone also can cause decreases in the urinary excretion of potassium. For example, Addison disease results in decreased production and secretion of aldosterone and thus contributes to hyperkalemia. Potassium-sparing diuretics (e.g., spironolactone, which inhibits sodium reabsorption and potassium and hydrogen secretion by the distal tubule) also may contribute to hyperkalemia. Frequently, however, these diuretics are used in combination with diuretics that cause potassium wasting in an attempt to balance renal potassium gains and losses.

CLINICAL MANIFESTATIONS   Symptoms of hyperkalemia vary, but common characteristics are muscle weakness or paralysis and changes in the electrocardiogram. During mild attacks, increased neuromuscular irritability may be manifested as tingling of lips and fingers, restlessness, intes-

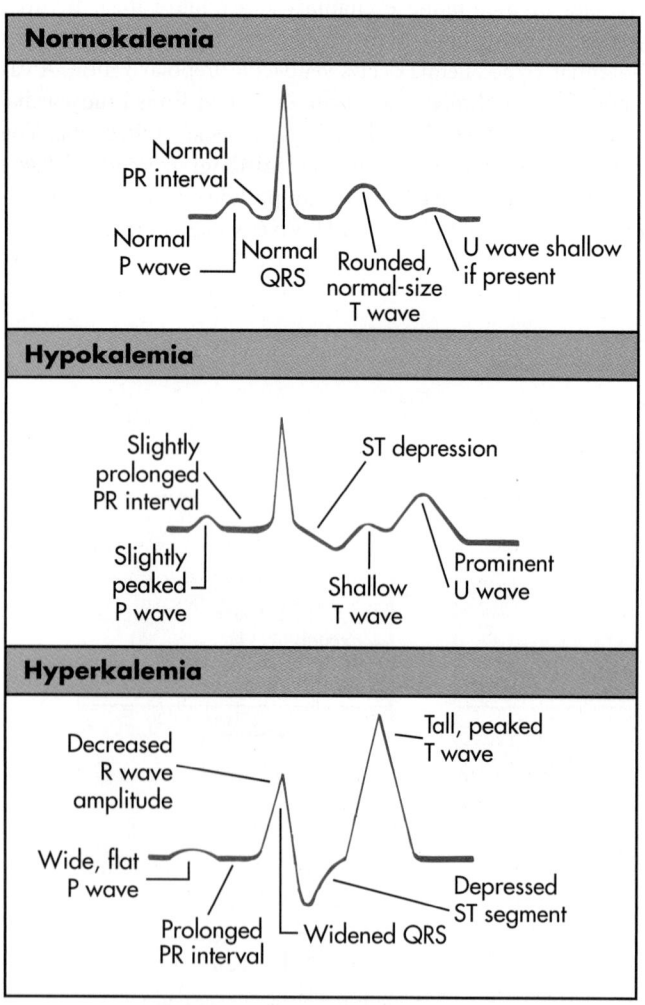

Figure 3-6 ECG changes with potassium imbalance.

tinal cramping, and diarrhea. Severe hyperkalemia causes muscle weakness, loss of muscle tone, and paralysis. In mild states of hyperkalemia, the more rapid repolarization is reflected in the electrocardiogram as narrow and taller T waves with a shortened QT interval. Severe hyperkalemia (serum levels ≥ 6.0 mEq/L) depresses the ST segment, prolongs the PR interval, and widens the QRS complex (see Figure 3-6). Bradydysrhythmias are common in hyperkalemia, with alterations in cardiac conduction causing ventricular fibrillation or cardiac arrest.

As with hypokalemia, changes in the ratio of intracellular to extracellular potassium concentration contribute to the symptoms of hyperkalemia. If extracellular potassium concentration increases without a significant change in intracellular potassium, the resting membrane potential becomes more positive and the cell membrane is **hypopolarized** (the inside of the cell becomes less negative or partially depolarized). (Electrical properties of cells are discussed in Chapter 1.) With relatively mild elevations in extracellular potassium, the cell more rapidly repolarizes and becomes more irritable (peaked T waves). An action potential then is initiated more rapidly because the distance between the resting membrane potential and the threshold potential has been shortened. With more severe hyperkalemia, the resting membrane potential approaches or exceeds the threshold potential (wide QRS merging with T wave). In this case the cell is not able to repolarize and therefore does not respond to excitation stimuli. The most serious consequence is cardiac standstill.

Like the effects of hypokalemia, the neuromuscular effects of hyperkalemia are related to the rate of increase in the ECF potassium concentration and the presence of other contributing factors, such as acidosis and calcium balance. Long-term increases in ECF potassium concentration result in shifts of potassium into the cell, because the tendency is to maintain a normal ratio of intracellular/extracellular potassium concentrations. Acute elevations of extracellular potassium affect neuromuscular irritability because this ratio is disrupted.

Because calcium influences the threshold potential, changes in extracellular fluid calcium concentration can augment or override the effects of hyperkalemia. With hypocalcemia the threshold potential becomes more negative, enhancing the neuromuscular effects of hyperkalemia. Hypercalcemia causes the threshold potential to become less negative, counteracting the effects of hyperkalemia on resting membrane potential (see Figure 3-5).

EVALUATION AND TREATMENT Hyperkalemia should be investigated when there is a history of renal disease, massive trauma, insulin deficiency, Addison disease, use of potassium salt substitutes, or metabolic acidosis. The acuity of the onset of symptoms may be related to the underlying cause.

Management of hyperkalemia is related to treating the contributing causes and correcting the potassium excess. Normalizing the extracellular potassium concentration can be achieved with a variety of methods; the treatment chosen is related to the cause and severity of the problem. Calcium gluconate can be administered to restore normal neuromuscular irritability when serum potassium levels are dangerously high. Administration of glucose, which readily stimulates insulin secretion, or administration of glucose and insulin for those with diabetes, facilitates cellular entry of potassium. Sodium bicarbonate corrects metabolic acidosis and lowers serum potassium. Oral or rectal administration of cation exchange resins, which exchange sodium for potassium in the intestine, can be effective. Dialysis effectively removes potassium when renal failure has occurred.

Calcium and Phosphate

The total body content of calcium is about 1200 g. Most calcium (99%) is located in bone as hydroxyapatite (an inorganic compound that contributes to bone rigidity), and the remainder is in the plasma and body cells. Of the calcium in the plasma, 50% is bound to plasma proteins (2.5 mEq/L), and about 40% is in the free or ionized form (2.4 mEq/L). The total fraction of calcium circulating in the blood is small (4.5 to 5.5 mEq/L, or 8.6 to 10.5 mg/dl). Ionized calcium has the most important physiologic functions.

Calcium is a necessary ion for many fundamental metabolic processes. It is the major cation for the structure of bones and teeth. It serves as an enzymatic cofactor for blood clotting and is required for hormone secretion and the function of cell receptors. Plasma membrane stability and permeability are directly related to calcium ions, as is the transmission of nerve impulses and the contraction of muscles. Intracellular calcium is located primarily in the mitochondria.

Phosphate is found primarily in bone (85%), with smaller amounts found within the intracellular and extracellular spaces. In the serum, phosphate exists in phospholipids and phosphate esters and as inorganic phosphate, which is the ionized form. The normal serum levels of inorganic phosphate range from 2.5 to 4.5 mg/dl and may be as high as 6.0 to 7.0 mg/dl in infants and young children. Intracellular phosphate has many metabolic forms, including the high-energy structures creatine phosphate and adenosine triphosphate (ATP). Phosphate acts as an intracellular and extracellular anion buffer in the regulation of acid-base balance; in the form of ATP it provides energy for muscle contraction.

Calcium and phosphate concentrations are rigidly controlled. They are related by the product of calcium (Ca^{++}) and phosphate ($HPO_4^=$), which is a constant ($Ca^{++} \times HPO_4^= = K^+$). Thus, if the concentration of one ion increases, that of the other decreases.

Calcium and phosphate balance is regulated by three hormones: parathyroid hormone (PTH), vitamin D, and calcitonin.[11] Acting together, these substances determine the amount of dietary calcium and phosphate absorbed from the intestine, the deposition and absorption of calcium and phosphate from the bone, and the renal reabsorption and excretion of calcium and phosphate by the kidney.

The parathyroid glands are sensitive to changes in serum calcium concentrations, and PTH controls ionized calcium in the blood and extracellular fluids. The parathyroid glands secrete PTH in response to low serum calcium. (The specific actions of PTH in relation to calcium and phosphorus are described in Chapter 20.) The renal regulation of calcium and phosphate balance requires PTH. As PTH secretion is stimulated by low levels of serum calcium, reabsorption of calcium along the distal part of the nephron increases and inhibition of phosphate resorption by the proximal segment of the nephron increases. The net result is an increase in serum calcium and urinary excretion of phosphate. Figure 3-7 summarizes hormonal regulation of calcium.

Another hormone important to calcium and phosphate regulation is vitamin D. Vitamin D (cholecalciferol) is a fat-soluble steroid ingested in food or synthesized in the skin in the presence of ultraviolet light. Several steps of activation are required before vitamin D can act on target tissues. The first step occurs in the liver; final activation is in the kidney. The renal activation of vitamin D begins when the serum calcium level decreases and stimulates secretion of PTH. PTH then acts to increase calcium reabsorption and enhance renal excretion of phosphate, producing decreased phosphate levels. The combination of low calcium, PTH secretion, and low phosphate thus causes the renal activation of vitamin D. The activated vitamin D then circulates in the plasma and acts to increase absorption of calcium in the small intestine, enhance bone absorption of calcium, and increase renal tubular reabsorption of calcium. When renal failure occurs, vitamin D is not activated; serum calcium levels decrease; and phosphate levels increase.

The exchange of calcium and phosphate between serum and bone is regulated also by hormones. When serum calcium levels are low, PTH increases and vitamin D stimulates intestinal calcium absorption and renal calcium reabsorption. Osteoclasts are stimulated to resorb bone and release calcium and phosphate into the plasma.

As calcium levels increase, an opposite adaptation occurs leading to suppression of PTH secretion, decreased renal vitamin D activation, and decreased intestinal calcium absorption and increased renal phosphate reabsorption.

The fractions of serum calcium that are freely ionized or bound to plasma proteins are influenced by pH. In states of acidosis, levels of ionized calcium increase. When alkalosis develops, with an increase in pH, protein-bound calcium increases and the physiologically active, ionized calcium decreases. The decreased concentration of ionized calcium may be great enough to cause symptoms of hypocalcemia, such as tetany.

Hypocalcemia

PATHOPHYSIOLOGY **Hypocalcemia** occurs when serum calcium concentrations are less than 8.5 mg/dl and ionized levels are less than 4.0 mg/dl. Deficits in calcium are related to inadequate intestinal absorption, deposition of ionized calcium into bone or soft tissue, blood administration, or decreases in PTH and vitamin D.

Nutritional deficiencies of calcium can occur in the instance of inadequate sources of dairy products or green, leafy vegetables. Excessive amounts of dietary phosphorus also bind with calcium, so neither mineral is absorbed when such as excess occurs. Blood transfusions are also a common cause of hypocalcemia because the citrate solution used in storing whole blood binds with calcium. Pancreatitis causes release of lipases into soft tissue spaces, so the free fatty acids that are formed bind calcium, causing a decrease in ionized calcium. Neoplastic bone metastases tend to inhibit bone resorption and increase calcium deposition into bone, thereby decreasing serum calcium levels.

Vitamin D deficiency, which can result from inadequate intake or avoidance of sunlight, causes decreased intestinal absorption of calcium. Malabsorption of fat, including fat-soluble vitamin D, may also contribute to calcium deficiency. Removal of the parathyroid glands with the resulting loss of PTH also causes hypocalcemia. Metabolic or respiratory alkalosis causes symptoms of hypocalcemia because the change in pH enhances protein binding of ionized calcium. Hypoalbuminemia lowers total serum calcium levels by decreasing the amount of bound calcium in the plasma.

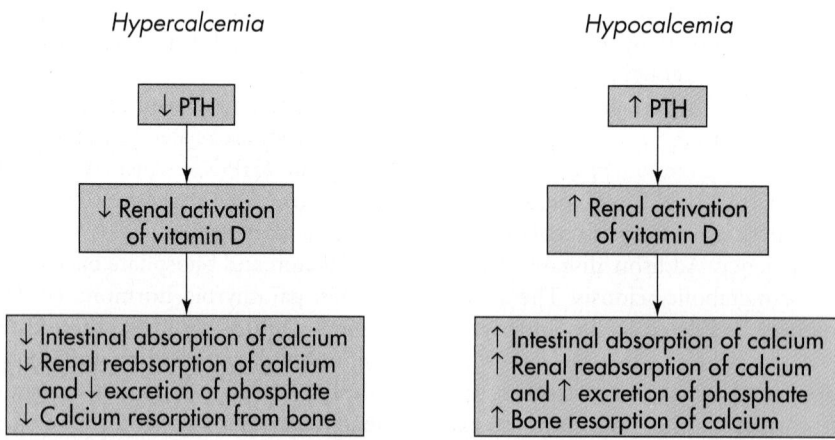

Figure 3-7 Hormonal regulation of calcium balance. *PTH,* Parathyroid hormone.

CLINICAL MANIFESTATIONS   The clinical manifestations of hypocalcemia are caused primarily by an increase in neuromuscular excitability. Calcium deficits cause partial depolarization of nerves and muscle as the threshold potential approaches the resting membrane potential (see Figure 3-5). Therefore a smaller stimulus is required for initiating the action potential. The symptoms include confusion, paresthesias around the mouth and in the digits, carpopedal spasm (muscle spasms in the hands and feet), and hyperreflexia.

Two clinical signs are Chvostek sign and Trousseau sign. Chvostek sign is elicited by tapping on the facial nerve just below the temple. A positive sign is a twitch of the nose or lip. Trousseau sign is contraction of the hand and fingers when the arterial blood flow in the arm is occluded for 5 minutes.

Severe symptoms include convulsions and tetany, a continuous severe muscle spasm that can interfere with breathing and cause death. The characteristic electrocardiogram (ECG) change is a prolonged QT interval, indicating prolonged ventricular depolarization and decreased cardiac contractility. Intestinal cramping and hyperactive bowel sounds also may be present because hypocalcemia affects the smooth muscles of the gastrointestinal tract.

EVALUATION AND TREATMENT   The health history may signify underlying pathologic conditions that require further evaluation and treatment. Severe symptoms of hypocalcemia require emergency treatment with intravenous 10% calcium gluconate. Oral calcium replacement should be initiated, and serum calcium levels should be monitored. Decreasing phosphate intake facilitates long-term management of hypocalcemia.

Hypercalcemia

PATHOPHYSIOLOGY   **Hypercalcemia** with serum calcium concentrations exceeding 12 mg/dl can be caused by a number of diseases. The most common among these are hyperparathyroidism; bone metastases with calcium resorption from breast, prostate, and cervical cancer; sarcoidosis; and excess vitamin D. Many tumors produce PTH and elevate the serum calcium levels. Sarcoidosis appears to increase vitamin D levels.

CLINICAL MANIFESTATIONS   Many symptoms of hypercalcemia are nonspecific. Because serum calcium levels are increased, a greater amount of calcium is also contained inside the cells. The threshold potential becomes more positive, and the cell membrane becomes refractory to depolarization (see Figure 3-5). Thus many of the symptoms are related to loss of cell membrane excitability. (Membrane potentials and membrane excitability are discussed in Chapter 1.) Fatigue, weakness, lethargy, anorexia, nausea, and constipation are common. Behavioral changes may occur. Impaired renal function frequently develops, and kidney stones form as precipitates of calcium salts. A shortened QT segment and depressed T waves also may be observed on the ECG, with bradycardia and varying degrees of heart block.

EVALUATION AND TREATMENT   With elevated serum calcium levels, often a reciprocal decrease in serum phosphate values occurs. Specific diagnostic procedures to identify the contributing pathologic condition are required.

Treatment is related to severity of symptoms and the underlying disease. When renal function is normal, oral phosphate administration is effective. When acute illness and high calcium levels are present, intravenous administration of large amounts of normal saline will enhance renal excretion of calcium. Corticosteroids and the cytotoxic drug mithramycin also are used to treat hypercalcemia. Ultimately, the underlying pathologic condition must be treated.

Hypophosphatemia

PATHOPHYSIOLOGY   **Hypophosphatemia** is a serum phosphate level less than 2.0 mg/dl and is usually an indication of phosphate deficiency. In some conditions, total body phosphate is normal but serum volumes are low. The most common causes are intestinal malabsorption and increased renal excretion of phosphate. Inadequate absorption is associated with vitamin D deficiency, use of magnesium- and aluminum-containing antacids (which bind with phosphorus), long-term alcohol abuse, and malabsorption syndromes. Respiratory alkalosis can cause severe hypophosphatemia because of cellular use of phosphorus for an accelerated glucose metabolism. Increased renal excretion of phosphorus is associated with hyperparathyroidism.

CLINICAL MANIFESTATIONS   The consequences of phosphate deficiency are related to reduced capacity for oxygen transport by red blood cells and to disturbed energy metabolism. Transport and release of oxygen are associated with 2,3-diphosphoglycerate (2,3-DPG) and ATP. When phosphate is depleted, 2,3-DPG and ATP levels become low and diminish release of oxygen to the tissues. The oxyhemoglobin curve shifts to the left (see Chapter 32), and hypoxia can occur with bradycardia and varying degrees of heart attack.

Leukocyte and platelet dysfunctions also are associated with hypophosphatemia. There is a greater risk of infection and blood-clotting impairment, with potential for hemorrhage. Nerve and muscle function can be affected because of derangement in energy metabolism. Irritability, confusion, numbness, coma, and convulsions develop with severe phosphate losses. Muscle weakness may become serious enough to cause respiratory failure, and cardiomyopathies also can develop. In response to low phosphate levels, bone resorption occurs and may lead to rickets or osteomalacia.

EVALUATION AND TREATMENT   To correct the condition, the underlying cause must be identified and treated. Although serum phosphate levels are below normal, the administration of phosphate salts is dangerous, and low phosphate levels are usually not considered life threatening.

Hyperphosphatemia

PATHOPHYSIOLOGY   **Hyperphosphatemia,** or an elevated serum phosphate level of more than 4.5 mg/dl, develops with exogenous or endogenous addition of phosphorus to the ECF or with significant loss of glomerular filtration.[13] Because most phosphate is located in cells, the cell destruction associated with treatment of metastatic tumors with chemotherapy can release large amounts of phosphate into the serum. Long-term use of phosphate-containing enemas or laxatives also may lead to hyperphosphatemia. Hypoparathyroidism can cause elevated phosphate by increasing renal tubular reabsorption of phosphate.

High levels of serum phosphate also lower serum calcium levels, and increased amounts of phosphate and calcium are deposited in bone and soft tissues. Serum calcium levels may become low enough to cause symptoms of hypocalcemia, including tetany.

CLINICAL MANIFESTATIONS   Symptoms of hyperphosphatemia are related primarily to low serum calcium levels and thus are comparable to symptoms of hypocalcemia. With prolonged hyperphosphatemia, calcification of soft tissues occurs in the lungs, kidneys, and joints.

EVALUATION AND TREATMENT   To correct the condition, the underlying pathologic condition must be identified and treated. Aluminum hydroxide may be administered because it binds phosphate in the gastrointestinal tract and is then eliminated. Dialysis is required for management of renal failure.

Magnesium

Magnesium (Mg^{++}) is a major intracellular cation. About 40% to 60% is stored in muscle and bone with 30% in the cells. A small amount (1%) is in the serum. Plasma concentration is 1.8 to 2.4 mEq/L with about one third bound to plasma proteins and the rest in ionized form. Regulation of magnesium metabolism is balanced by the small intestine and kidney. Low serum levels cause renal conservation of magnesium. Magnesium is a cofactor in intracellular enzymatic reactions, protein synthesis, nucleic acid stability, and neuromuscular excitability. Calcium and magnesium often interact in reactions at the cellular level.

Hypomagnesemia occurs when serum magnesium concentration is less than 1.5 mEq/L and increases in neuromuscular excitability and tetany are present. Malnutrition, malabsorption syndromes, alcoholism, renal tubular dysfunction, metabolic acidosis, and loop and thiazide diuretics can cause magnesium losses. Diabetes mellitus is associated with hypomagnesemia partly as a function of osmotic diuresis.[14] Signs and symptoms of hypomagnesemia are similar to those of hypocalcemia. Depression, confusion, irritability, increased reflexes, muscle weakness, ataxia, nystagmus, tetany, and convulsions may be observed.[14] Treatment is intramuscular or intravenous administration of magnesium sulfate.

Hypermagnesemia, in which magnesium concentration is greater than 2.5 mEq/L, is rare and usually is caused by renal failure. Magnesium-containing antacids (e.g., Gaviscon, Gelusil) can potentiate excess magnesium. Excess magnesium depresses skeletal muscle contraction and nerve function. Signs and symptoms include nausea and vomiting, muscle weakness, hypotension, bradycardia, and respiratory depression.[14] Treatment is avoidance of magnesium-containing substances and removal of magnesium by dialysis.

ACID-BASE BALANCE

Hydrogen ion concentration must be regulated within a narrow range for the body to function normally. Slight changes in amounts of hydrogen can significantly alter biologic processes in cells and tissues. Hydrogen ion is necessary to maintain membrane integrity and the speed of enzymatic reactions. Most pathologic conditions disturb acid-base balance, and the degree of severity may be more harmful than the disease process.

Hydrogen Ion and pH

The hydrogen ion concentration $[H^+]$ is commonly expressed as the pH, the negative logarithm of hydrogen ions in solution. The logarithmic value means that as the pH changes one unit (e.g., 7.0 to 6.0), the $[H^+]$ changes tenfold (i.e., 0.0000001 to 0.000001). The relationship is commonly expressed as follows:

$$pH = \log \frac{1}{[H^+]} \text{ or } pH = -\log_{10}[H^+]$$

As the $[H^+]$ increases, the pH decreases; likewise, as the $[H^+]$ decreases, the pH increases. The greater the $[H^+]$, the more acidic the solution and the lower the pH. The lower the $[H^+]$, the more basic the solution and the higher the pH. In biologic fluids, a pH of less than 7.4 is defined as acidic and a pH greater than 7.4 is defined as basic.

Different body fluids have different pH values as follows:

Body Fluid	pH
Gastric juices	1.0-3.0
Urine	5.0-6.0
Arterial blood	7.38-7.42
Venous blood	7.37
Cerebrospinal fluid	7.32
Pancreatic fluid	7.8-8.0

Body acids are formed as end products of cellular metabolism. The average person generates acid in the amount of 50 to 100 mEq/day from the metabolism of protein, carbohydrates, and fats and from loss of base in the stools. To maintain a normal pH, an equal amount of acid therefore must be neutralized or excreted. The lungs, kidneys, and bone are the major organs involved in the regulation of acid-base balance. The systems are interrelated and work together to regulate short- or long-term changes in acid-base status. Body acids exist in two forms: **volatile** (can be eliminated as carbon dioxide [CO_2] gas) and **nonvolatile**. The volatile acid is carbonic acid (H_2CO_3), which is formed from the hydration of carbon dioxide:

Regulated by lung   Regulated by kidney

$$CO_2 + H_2O \longleftrightarrow H_2CO_3 \longleftrightarrow HCO_3^- + H^+$$

Carbonic acid is a weak acid, and in the presence of carbonic anhydrase, it readily dissociates into carbon dioxide. Approximately 12,000 to 15,000 millimoles of CO_2 is produced in the human body per day.[15] The carbon dioxide is then eliminated by pulmonary ventilation. Sulfuric, phosphoric, and other organic acids are nonvolatile strong acids produced from the metabolism of proteins, carbohydrates, and fats. (Strong acids are those that readily give up their hydrogen; weak acids do not.) Nonvolatile acids are eliminated by the renal tubules with the regulation of HCO_3^-. Thus the lungs and kidneys, with the help of body buffer systems, are the prime regulators of acid-base balance.

Buffer Systems

Buffering occurs in response to changes in acid-base status. **Buffers** can absorb excessive H^+ (acid) or OH^- (base) without a significant change in pH. The buffer systems are located in both the ICF and ECF compartments, and they function at different rates. Buffer systems exist as buffer pairs, consisting of a weak acid and its conjugate base (Table 3-9). The most important plasma buffer systems are carbonic acid–bicarbonate and hemoglobin. Phosphate and protein are the most important intracellular buffers.

An important factor for effective buffering is a function known as the *pK value,* which represents the pH at which a buffer pair is half dissociated. Buffer pairs can associate and dissociate (see Table 3-9).

The pK provides a rate constant for the chemical reaction. A buffer system is most effective when the pK for the buffer is close to the pH of the fluid in which the buffer is acting. For the bicarbonate–carbonic acid buffer system, the pK is 6.1. This value is not as high as the pK for other buffer systems (see Table 3-9), but this buffer system is still very effective because carbon dioxide is rapidly removed from the blood by the lungs.

The pK value is also a term in the equation used to determine pH. The relationships among pH, pK, and the ratio of bicarbonate to carbonic acid can be expressed as follows by the *Henderson-Hasselbalch equation*:

$$pH = pK + \log \frac{[HCO_3^-]}{[H_2CO_3]}$$

The pH then can be determined when specific values are included in the equation:

$$pH = pK + \log \frac{[HCO_3^-]}{[H_2CO_3]}$$

$$= 6.1 + \log \frac{24}{1.2}$$

$$= 6.1 + \log \frac{20}{1}$$

$$= 6.1 + 1.3$$

$$= 7.40$$

Carbonic Acid–Bicarbonate Buffering

The carbonic acid–bicarbonate buffer pair operates in both the lung and the kidney. The greater the carbon dioxide partial pressure (Pco_2), the more carbonic acid is formed. The relationship that exists between carbonic acid (H_2CO_3) and carbon dioxide (Pco_2) can be expressed as follows:

$$H_2CO_3 = 0.03 \times Pco_2 \text{ (mmHg)}$$

The 0.03 represents the solubility coefficient for carbon dioxide in water. The Pco_2 of arterial blood is normally about 40 mmHg. Therefore the amount of H_2CO_3 is equal to about 1.2 mmol/L (0.03×40). As the amount of carbon dioxide increases or decreases, the amount of H_2CO_3 changes in the same direction.

The relationship between bicarbonate and carbonic acid is usually expressed as a ratio. When the pH is 7.40, this ratio is 20:1 (bicarbonate/carbonic acid). The ratio is defined by the amount of bicarbonate and carbon dioxide (carbonic acid) in the arterial blood. Bicarbonate concentration (HCO_3^-) is

Table 3-9	Buffer Systems			
Buffer Pairs	**Buffer System**	**pK Values**	**Reaction**	**Rate**
HCO_3^-/H_2CO_3	Bicarbonate	6.1	$H^+ + HCO_3^- \rightleftharpoons H_2O + CO_2$	Instantaneous
Hb^-/HHb	Hemoglobin	7.3	$HHb \rightleftharpoons H^+ + Hb^-$	Instantaneous
$HPO_4^-/H_2PO_4^-$	Phosphate	6.8	$H_2PO_4^- \rightleftharpoons H^+ + HPO_4^-$	Instantaneous
Pr^-/HPr	Plasma proteins	6.7	$HPr \rightleftharpoons H^+ + Pr^-$	Instantaneous
Organs	**Mechanism**			**Rate**
Lungs	Regulates retention or elimination of CO_2 and therefore H_2CO_3 concentration			Minutes-hours
Ionic shifts	Exchange of intracellular potassium and sodium for hydrogen			2-4 hours
Kidneys	Bicarbonate reabsorption and regeneration, ammonia formation, phosphate buffering			Hours-days
Bone	Exchanges of calcium, phosphate, and release of carbonate			Hours-days

HCO_3^-, Bicarbonate; *H_2CO_3,* carbonic acid; *Hb^-,* hemoglobin; *Pr^-,* protein; *$H_2PO_4^-$,* monobasic phosphate; *HPO_4^-,* dibasic phosphate; *HPr,* hydrogenated protein; *HHb,* hydrogenated hemoglobin.

normally about 24 mEq/L. Therefore the 20:1 ratio can be developed as follows:

$$\frac{[HCO_3^-] = 24 \text{ mEq/L}}{[H_2CO_3] = (0.03 \times 40 \text{ mmHg})} = \frac{24}{1.2} = \frac{20}{1}$$

The values for HCO_3^- and P_{CO_2} (H_2CO_3) can increase or decrease proportionately, but the 20:1 ratio is maintained.

The lungs can decrease the amount of carbonic acid by blowing off CO_2 and leaving water. The kidneys can reabsorb bicarbonate or regenerate new bicarbonate from CO_2 and water. The renal mechanism does not act as rapidly as the lungs, but the two systems are very effective together because acid concentration can be rapidly adjusted by the lungs and bicarbonate is easily reabsorbed or regenerated by the kidneys. The pH equation can be symbolically expressed as follows:

$$pH = \frac{Base}{Acid} \text{ or } pH = \frac{\text{Renal regulation (slow)}}{\text{Pulmonary regulation (fast)}}$$

or

$$pH = \frac{\text{Metabolic acid-base function}}{\text{Respiratory acid-base function}}$$

Changes in either the numerator or the denominator will change the pH. For example, if the amount of bicarbonate is decreased, the pH also decreases, causing a state of acidosis. The pH can be returned to a normal range if the value of the denominator or the amount of carbonic acid also decreases.

This type of adjustment in pH is known as **compensation**. With compensation, a 20:1 ratio may be achieved, but the actual values for HCO_3^- and H_2CO_3 are not normal. The respiratory system compensates for changes in pH by increasing or decreasing ventilation. The renal system compensates by producing more acidic or more alkaline urine. **Correction** occurs when the values for both components of the buffer pair return to normal (Figure 3-8).

Protein Buffering

Both intracellular and extracellular proteins have negative charges and can serve as buffers for H^+, but because most proteins are inside cells, they are primarily an intracellular buffer system. Hemoglobin (Hb) is an excellent intracellular buffer because of its ability to bind with H^+ (forming HHb) and carbon dioxide ($HHbCO_2$). Hemoglobin bound to H^+ becomes a weak acid. Unsaturated hemoglobin (venous blood) is a better buffer than hemoglobin saturated with oxygen (arterial blood). The hemoglobin buffer system is illustrated in Figure 3-9.

Renal Buffering

The distal tubule of the kidney regulates acid-base balance by secreting hydrogen into the urine and reabsorbing bicarbonate with a maximum acidity of about 4.4 to 4.7. Buffers in the tubular fluid combine with hydrogen ions, allowing more H^+ to be secreted before the limiting pH value is reached. Dibasic phosphate ($HPO_4^=$) and ammonia (NH_3) are two important renal buffers. Dibasic phosphate is filtered at the

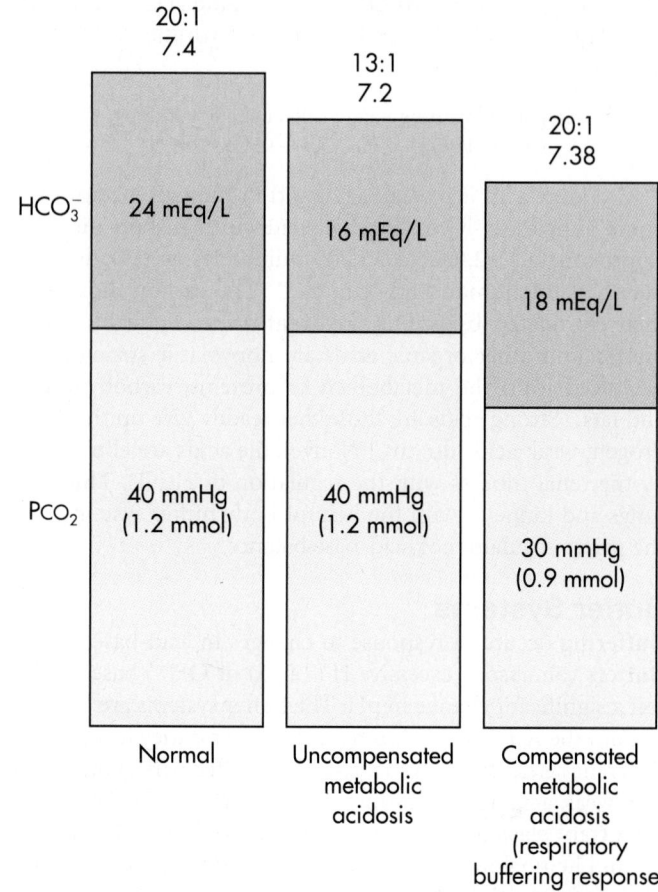

Figure 3-8 Maintenance of HCO_3^-/P_{CO_2} (H_2CO_3) ratio in metabolic acidosis.

glomerulus. About 75% is reabsorbed, and the remainder is available for buffering H^+. Secreted H^+ combines with $HPO_4^=$ to form monobasic phosphate ($H_2PO_4^-$). The remaining negative charge on the molecule makes it lipid insoluble, and it cannot diffuse back across the tubular cell and into the blood. Thus it is excreted in the urine (Figure 3-10).

Ammonia (NH_3) is an important renal buffer. Ammonia is not ionized (does not carry a charge), and therefore it is lipid soluble and can cross the cell membrane. The presence of NH_3 in the cell creates a concentration gradient, and it diffuses into the renal tubular fluid where it combines with hydrogen to form ammonium ion (NH_4^+), which is eliminated in the urine (see Figure 3-10). The renal buffering of hydrogen ions requires the use of CO_2 and H_2O to form H_2CO_3. The enzyme carbonic anhydrase catalyzes the formation of $H^+ + HCO_3^-$. The hydrogen is secreted from the tubular cell and buffered in the lumen by phosphate and ammonia. The bicarbonate is reabsorbed. The end effect is the addition of new bicarbonate, which contributes to the alkalinity of the plasma, because the hydrogen ion is excreted from the body (see Figure 3-10).

Other Buffers

A cellular ion exchange mechanism is also an important buffering system. The best example is the shift of potassium in exchange for hydrogen during states of acidosis or alkalo-

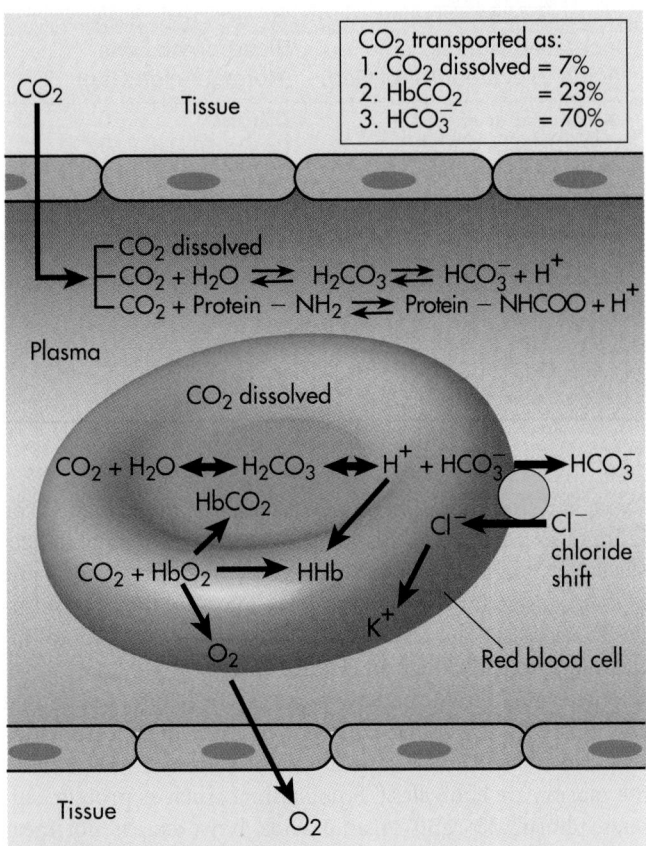

Figure 3-9 Buffering of hydrogen with hemoglobin and carbon dioxide (CO_2) transport. CO_2 is produced in tissue cells and diffuses to plasma, where it is transported as dissolved CO_2, or it combines with water to form carbonic acid (H_2CO_3), or it combines with protein from which hydrogen has been released. Most of the CO_2 diffuses into the red blood cell and combines with water to form H_2CO_3. The H_2CO_3 dissociates to form hydrogen (H^+) and bicarbonate (HCO_3^-). The HCO_3^- shifts into the plasma and chloride (Cl^-) shifts into the red blood cell to maintain electroneutrality. Hydrogen combines with hemoglobin that has released its oxygen to form HHb, which buffers the hydrogen and makes venous blood slightly more acidic than arterial blood.

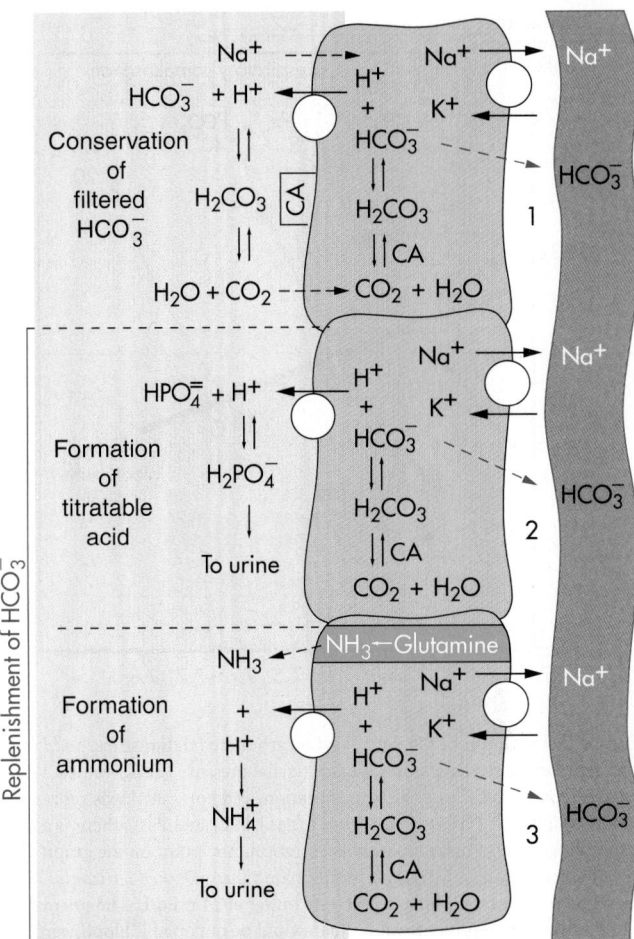

Figure 3-10 Renal excretion of acid. *1,* Conservation of filtered bicarbonate. Filtered bicarbonate combines with secreted hydrogen in the presence of carbon anhydrase (CA) to form carbonic acid (H_2CO_3), which then dissociates to water (H_2O) and carbon dioxide (CO_2); both diffuse into the epithelial cell. The CO_2 and H_2O combine to form H_2CO_3 in the presence of CA, and the resulting bicarbonate (HCO_3^-) is converted by reabsorption into the capillary. *2,* Formation of titratable acid. Hydrogen ion is secreted and combines with dibasic phosphate ($HPO_4^=$) to form monobasic phosphate ($H_2PO_4^-$). The secreted hydrogen is formed from the dissociation of H_2CO_3, and the remaining HCO_3^- is reabsorbed into the capillary. *3,* Formation of ammonium. Ammonia (NH_3) is produced from glutamine in the epithelial cell and diffused to the tubular lumen, where it combines with H^+ to form ammonium (NH_4^+). Once NH_4^+ has been formed, it cannot return to the epithelial cell (diffusional trapping), and the bicarbonate remaining in the epithelial cell is reabsorbed into the capillary.

sis. During acidosis, potassium tends to leave the intracellular space in exchange for hydrogen. The reverse occurs during alkalosis. Although the ionic shifts facilitate buffering, the changes in intracellular or extracellular potassium concentrations may have serious consequences.

Acid-Base Imbalances

Pathophysiologic changes in the concentration of hydrogen ion in the blood lead to acid-base imbalances. **Acidemia** is a state in which the pH of arterial blood is less than 7.35. A systemic increase in hydrogen ion concentration is termed **acidosis**. **Alkalemia** is a state in which the pH of arterial blood is greater than 7.45. A systemic decrease in hydrogen ion concentration is termed **alkalosis**. Acid-base imbalances may have a metabolic or respiratory etiology or may be of mixed etiology. Figure 3-11 summarizes the relationships among pH, P_{CO_2}, and bicarbonate during different acid-base alterations.

Metabolic Acidosis

PATHOPHYSIOLOGY In **metabolic acidosis,** noncarbonic acids increase or bicarbonate is lost from the extracellular fluid (Tables 3-10 and 3-11). This can occur quickly, as in lactic acidosis from poor perfusion, or more slowly, as in renal failure or diabetic ketoacidosis.

The buffer systems compensate for the excess acid and attempt to maintain the arterial pH within a normal range. Buffering by bicarbonate lowers the serum value of this ion. The respiratory system compensates for a metabolic acidosis as the reduced pH stimulates hyperventilation, lowering the

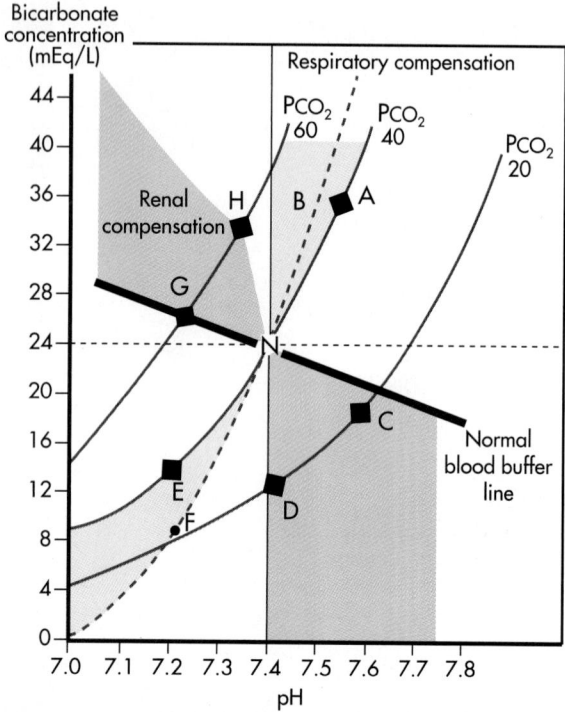

Figure 3-11 Graph of pH, Pco₂, and bicarbonate relationships. *Solid red lines* represent different carbon dioxide partial pressure (Pco₂) values. *Vertical axis* represents bicarbonate concentration, and horizontal axis represents acidity or alkalinity (pH) values. Thus for any indicated Pco₂, there is a corresponding pH and bicarbonate concentration. Any point on the graph predicts the required Pco₂, pH, and bicarbonate values. *Dashed horizontal line* shows behavior of bicarbonate as a pure buffer at 24 mEq/L. The normal blood buffer line represents values that would be obtained if blood were equilibrated at different CO₂ values. *Point N* represents normal values. *Point A* represents uncompensated metabolic alkalosis, indicated by a normal Pco₂ of 40 and pH greater than 7.4. Respiratory compensation is achieved by hypoventilation, which raises the Pco₂ to *point B* and decreases the pH. Uncompensated respiratory alkalosis is represented by point C and reflects hypocapnia (decreased Pco₂). Renal compensation for respiratory alkalosis is increased renal excretion of bicarbonate to normalize pH at *point D*. Uncompensated metabolic acidosis at *point E* represents normal Pco₂ and a decrease in bicarbonate and pH. Respiratory compensation by hyperventilation is indicated by *point F*. Uncompensated respiratory acidosis at *point G* indicates high Pco₂ and low pH values. Renal compensation for chronic high Pco₂ values is indicated by *point H*.

Table 3-10	**Primary and Compensatory Acid-Base Changes**					
	Primary Disturbance			**Compensations**		
	pH	Pco₂	HCO₃⁻	pH	Pco₂	HCO₃⁻
Metabolic acidosis	↓	N	↓	↑-N	↓	↓
Metabolic alkalosis	↑	N	↑	↓-N	↑	↑
Respiratory acidosis	↓	↑	N	↑-N	↑	↑
Respiratory alkalosis	↑	↓	N	↓-N	↓	↓

↑-*N*, Increase toward normal; ↓-*N*, decrease toward normal; *pH*, measure of the acidity or alkalinity of a solution; *Pco₂*, carbon dioxide partial pressure; *HCO₃⁻*, bicarbonate.

Table 3-11	Causes of Metabolic Acidosis
Increased Noncarbonic Acids (Elevated Anion Gap)	**Bicarbonate Loss (Normal Anion Gap)**
Increased H⁺ load	Diarrhea
Ketoacidosis (e.g., diabetes mellitus, starvation)	Ureterosigmoidoscopy
Lactic acidosis (e.g., shock)	Renal failure
Ingestions (e.g., ammonium chloride, ethylene glycol, methanol, salicylates, paraldehyde)	Proximal renal tubule acidosis
Decreased H⁺ excretion	
Uremia	
Distal renal tubule acidosis	

Paco₂ and the amount of H₂CO₃ circulating in the blood. The kidneys excrete the excess acid as NH₄⁺ and titratable acid (H₂PO₄⁻). When the acidosis is severe, the buffers are unable to compensate for the increasing H⁺ load and the pH continues to decrease. The result is a decrease in the 20:1 ratio of bicarbonate to carbonic acid (Figure 3-12).

The evaluation of the **anion gap** can be helpful when used cautiously to distinguish different types of metabolic acidosis.[16] Normally, the concentrations of cations and anions in the plasma are equivalent. Some anions, such as protein, sulfates, phosphates, and organic acids, however, are not measured in the common laboratory evaluations of the blood. Therefore the **normal anion gap** represents negative ions not usually measured (sulfate, phosphate, lactate, ketoacids, albumin). A convenient measure is the difference between the sum of Na⁺ and K⁺ and the sum of HCO₃⁻ and Cl⁻, or about 10 to 12 mEq:

$$\text{Anion gap} = [\text{Na}^+ (140) + \text{K}^+ (4.0)] - [\text{HCO}_3^- (24) + \text{Cl}^- (110)] = 10\text{-}12 \text{ mEq/L}$$

In metabolic acidosis a normal anion gap is characteristic of conditions related to bicarbonate loss with retention of chloride to maintain an ionic balance. This is called **hyperchloremic metabolic acidosis.** An elevated anion gap is characteristic of acidosis associated with accumulation of anions other than chloride (see Table 3-11).

CLINICAL MANIFESTATIONS Metabolic acidosis is manifested by changes in the neurologic, respiratory, gastrointestinal, and cardiovascular systems. Headache and lethargy are early symptoms, which progress to coma with severe acidosis. Deep, rapid respirations (Kussmaul respirations) are indicative of respiratory compensation. Anorexia, nausea, vomiting, diarrhea, and abdominal discomfort are common. Severe acidosis can compromise ventricular contraction and produce life-threatening dysrhythmias and hypotension.

EVALUATION AND TREATMENT The diagnosis of metabolic acidosis is established from the health history, clinical symptoms, and laboratory findings. Arterial blood

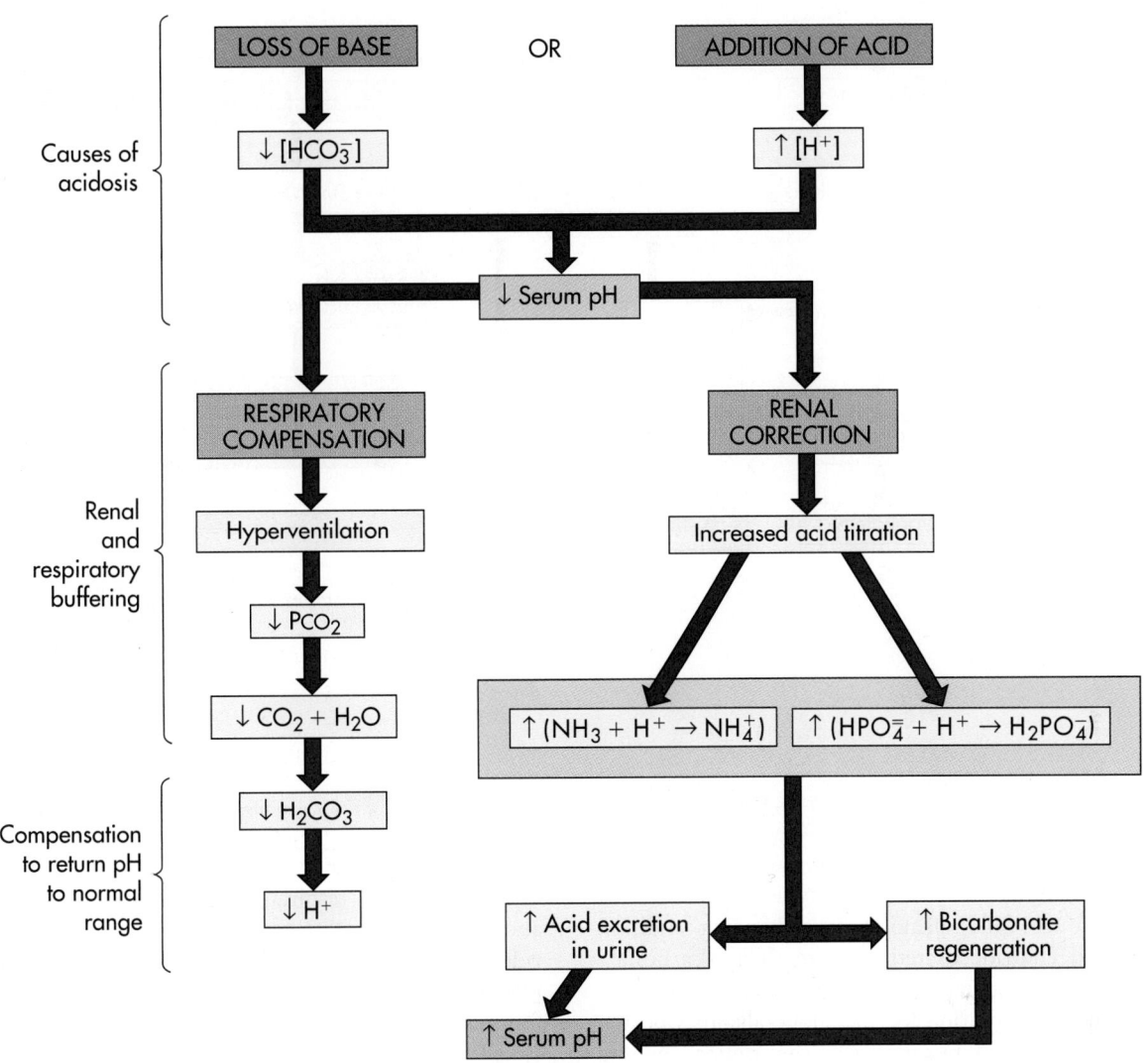

Figure 3-12 Metabolic acidosis with compensation and correction. See text for abbreviations.

pH is below 7.35, and bicarbonate concentration is less than 24 mEq/L. The anion gap can isolate the specific cause. The underlying condition must be diagnosed to establish effective treatment. During severe acidosis (pH ≤ 7.1), sodium bicarbonate administration is required to elevate the pH to a safe level, particularly if there is renal failure. Accompanying sodium and water deficits must also be corrected.[17]

Metabolic Alkalosis

PATHOPHYSIOLOGY   **Metabolic alkalosis** is common and occurs when bicarbonate is increased, usually caused by excessive loss of metabolic acids. Among the conditions that can result in metabolic alkalosis are prolonged vomiting, gastrointestinal suctioning, excessive bicarbonate intake, hyperaldosteronism, and diuretic therapy.[18]

When acid loss is caused by vomiting with depletion of ECF and chloride (**hypochloremic metabolic alkalosis**), renal compensation is not very effective because the volume depletion and loss of electrolytes (Na+, K+, H+, Cl−) stimulate a paradoxic response by the kidneys.[11] The kidneys increase sodium and bicarbonate reabsorption with excretion of hydrogen. Bicarbonate is reabsorbed because the ECF chloride concentration is decreased. When the potassium concentration is depleted, hydrogen moves to the intracellular space and is excreted to maintain an electrochemical balance. The urine is acidic, and the reabsorbed bicarbonate prevents correction of the alkalosis (Figure 3-13). Correction is achieved when the ECF is expanded with a solution of sodium chloride and potassium. The volume replacement decreases the renal stimulus to reabsorb Na+, and chloride as an anion is replaced. Bicarbonate then can be lost in the urine, and hydrogen ion excretion decreases, correcting the pH.

With hyperaldosteronism the excess aldosterone causes sodium retention and loss of hydrogen and potassium. Mild volume expansion ensues, and bicarbonate is retained along with the sodium, thereby causing alkalosis.

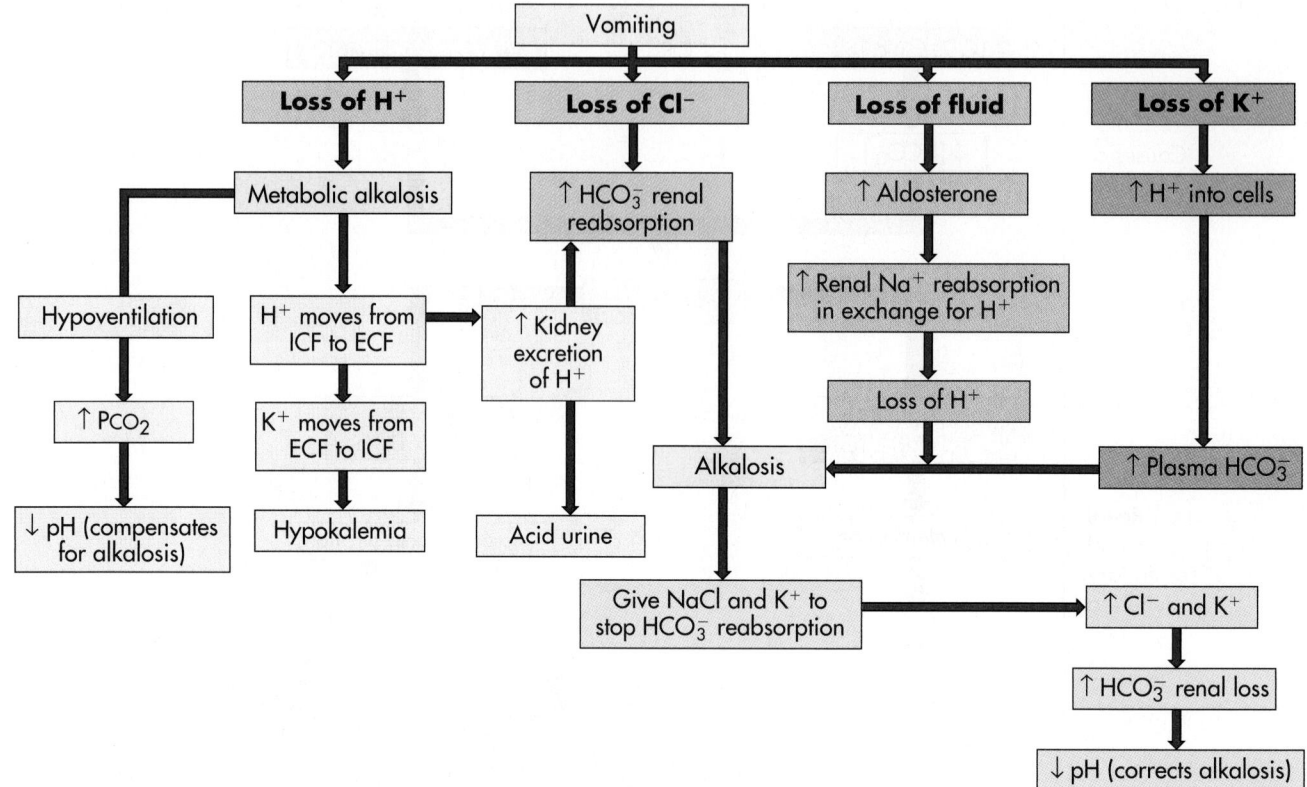

Figure 3-13 Hypochloremic metabolic alkalosis. See text for abbreviations.

Diuretics, such as thiazides, ethacrynic acid, and furosemide, produce mild alkalosis by enhancing sodium, potassium, and chloride excretion more than bicarbonate excretion.

Respiratory compensation for metabolic alkalosis occurs when the elevated pH inhibits the respiratory center. The rate and depth of ventilation are decreased, causing retention of carbon dioxide. The ratio of HCO_3^- to H_2CO_3 is reduced toward normal. Respiratory compensation is not very efficient, however, and chronic or severe metabolic alkalosis requires therapeutic intervention (Figure 3-14).

CLINICAL MANIFESTATIONS   Because of the many causes of metabolic alkalosis, the symptoms vary. Some common symptoms, such as weakness, muscle cramps, and hyperactive reflexes, are related to volume depletion and electrolyte losses. Because alkalosis causes a decrease in ionized calcium, tetany may develop.

Respirations are slow and shallow to increase carbon dioxide content. Confusion and convulsions occur with severe alkalosis. Atrial tachycardia is a potential problem. The oxyhemoglobin curve is shifted to the left (see Chapter 32), decreasing the dissociation of oxyhemoglobin and increasing the risk of dysrhythmias.

EVALUATION AND TREATMENT   The health history provides significant clues to the diagnosis of metabolic alkalosis. The arterial pH is above 7.45, and bicarbonate levels exceed 26 mEq/L. With respiratory compensation, the P_{CO_2} rises above 40 mmHg. With hypochloremic alkalosis, serum chloride values are below normal. Potassium levels are usually depleted because hydrogen is released from the cells in exchange for potassium to help regulate the pH level. The K^+ is then secreted from the distal tubule or kidney cells into the urine.

With hypochloremic alkalosis or contraction alkalosis with volume depletion, a sodium chloride solution is required for correction. The renal stimulus to increase ECF volume by retaining Na^+ is diminished, and HCO_3^- can be excreted as $NaHCO_3$ in the urine. The administration of potassium corrects alkalosis caused by hyperaldosteronism or hypokalemia. The potassium causes hydrogen to move back into the ECF and decreases loss of hydrogen from the distal tubule.

Respiratory Acidosis

PATHOPHYSIOLOGY   Respiratory disorders of acid-base balance are caused by increases or decreases of alveolar ventilation in relation to the metabolic production of carbon dioxide. **Respiratory acidosis** occurs when ventilation is depressed. Carbon dioxide is retained, increasing $[H^+]$ (as H_2CO_3) and producing acidosis. Carbon dioxide excess is called **hypercapnia.** The common causes include depression of the respiratory center (brain stem trauma, oversedation), respiratory muscle paralysis, disorders of the chest wall (kyphoscoliosis, pickwickian syndrome, flail chest), and disorders of the lung parenchyma (pneumonia, pulmonary edema, emphysema, asthma, bronchitis).

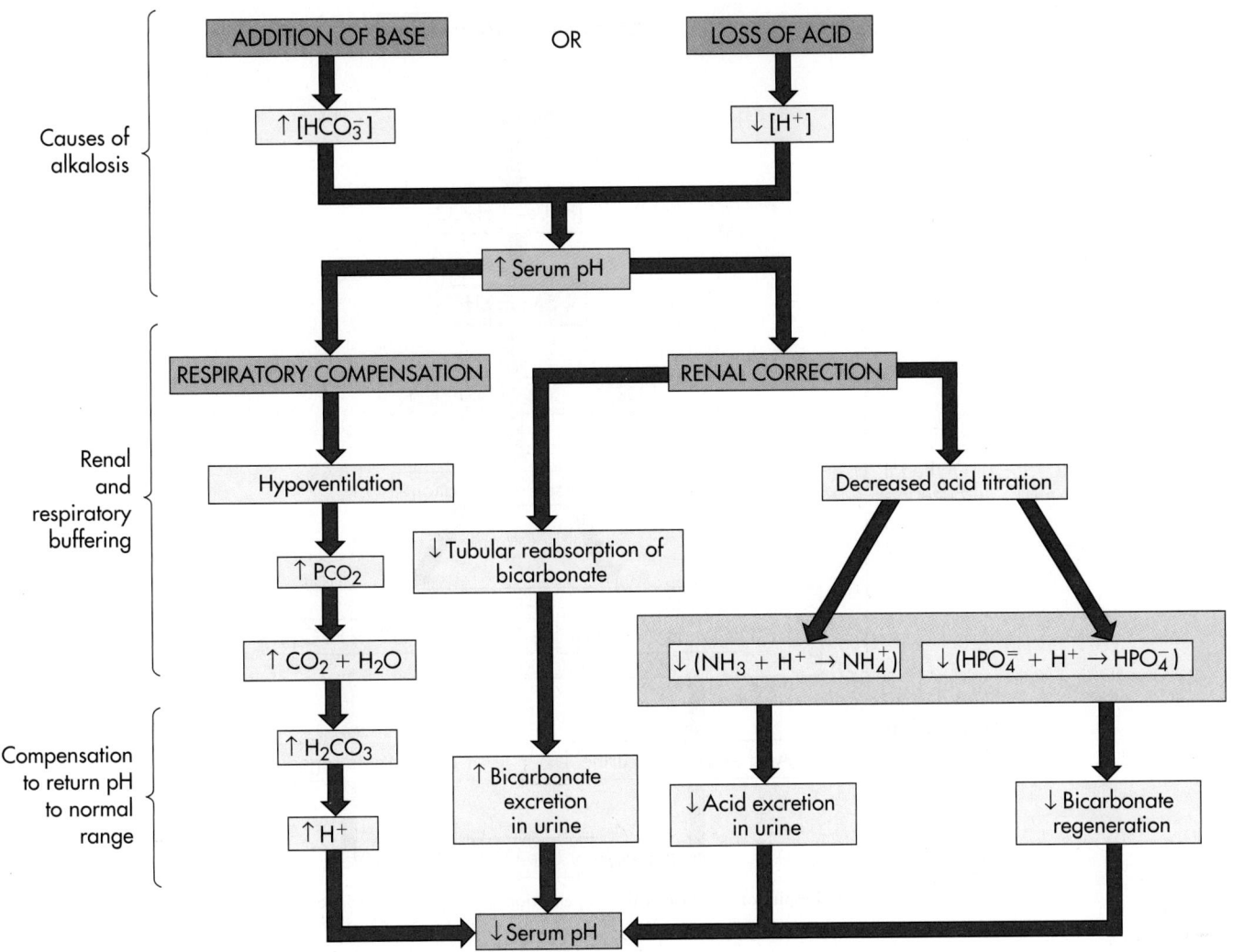

Figure 3-14 Metabolic alkalosis with compensation and correction. See text for abbreviations.

Respiratory acidosis may be acute or chronic. Airway obstruction is the most common cause of acute respiratory acidosis. Acute compensation for respiratory acidosis is not effective because the renal buffer mechanism takes time to function. Further, the protein buffers provide marginal compensation, and HCO_3^- is not a good buffer for CO_2. Acute uncompensated respiratory acidosis is characterized by a decreased pH, elevated PCO_2, and normal or slightly increased bicarbonate level.

Chronic respiratory acidosis is commonly associated with chronic obstructive pulmonary disease and deformities of the chest wall. Renal compensation is effective and is established over several days. The acidosis produced from CO_2 retention stimulates the kidney to secrete hydrogen ion and regenerate bicarbonate. Serum bicarbonate and arterial PCO_2 are elevated, and pH will be restored toward normal (Figure 3-15).

CLINICAL MANIFESTATIONS   The symptoms of respiratory acidosis are related to acuity of onset and severity of PCO_2 retention. Initial symptoms include headache, restlessness, blurred vision, and apprehension followed by lethargy, muscle twitching, tremors, convulsions, and coma. Neurologic symptoms are caused by a decrease in the pH of cerebrospinal fluid and vasodilation because CO_2 readily crosses the blood-brain barrier. The respiratory rate is rapid at first and gradually becomes depressed because, over time, the respiratory center adapts to increasing levels of CO_2. Cyanosis does not occur unless there is an accompanying hypoxemia, and the skin may instead be pink from vasodilation caused by the acidosis.

EVALUATION AND TREATMENT   The primary diagnostic indicators are an arterial pH less than 7.35 and hypercapnia. Acute respiratory acidosis must be distinguished from chronic acidosis; the health history and clinical laboratory data are therefore helpful. With renal compensation, bicarbonate levels are elevated and the pH is restored toward normal.

The restoration of adequate alveolar ventilation removes excess CO_2. If alveolar ventilation cannot be maintained spontaneously because of drug overdose or neuromuscular disorders, mechanical ventilation is required. The arterial pH, PCO_2, PO_2, and HCO_3^- must be carefully monitored. Rapid

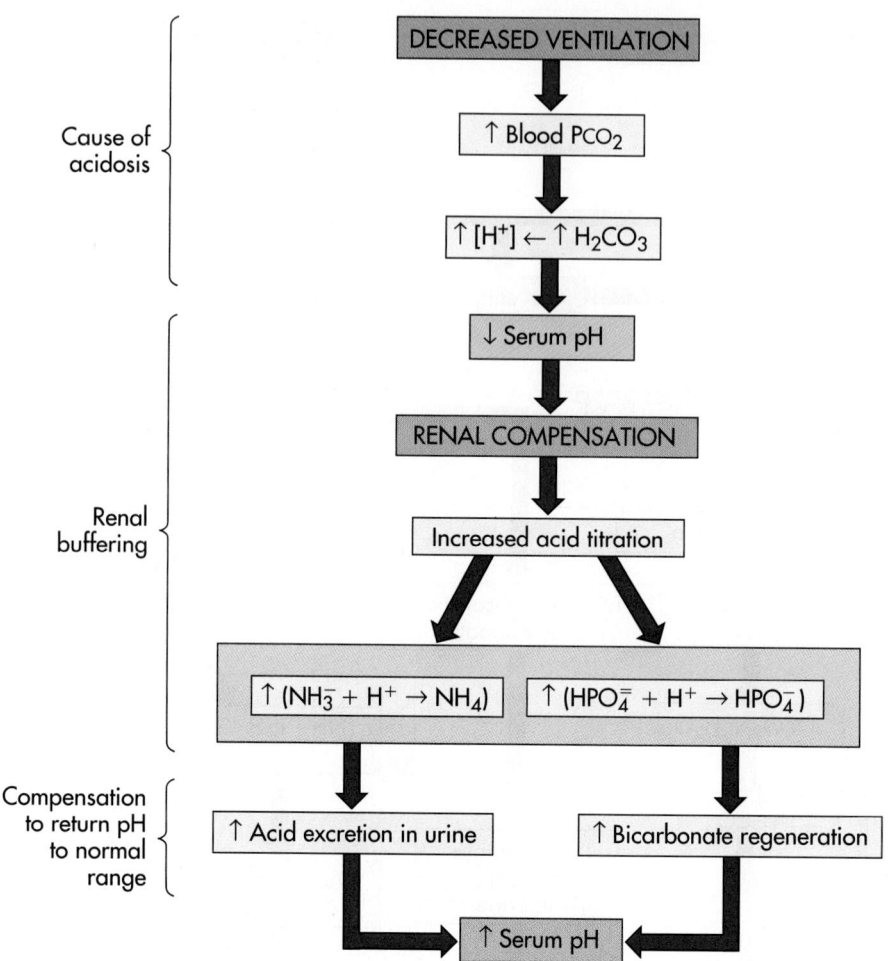

Figure 3-15 Respiratory acidosis with compensation. See text for abbreviations.

reduction of P_{CO_2} can cause respiratory alkalosis with seizures and death.

Renal buffering is usually effective in compensating for uncomplicated chronic respiratory acidosis. The underlying diseases are treated to achieve maximal ventilation. In the presence of hypoxemia and hypercapnia, oxygen can function as a respiratory depressant when the respiratory center is no longer stimulated by the lower pH and elevated P_{CO_2}. Therefore oxygen should be given cautiously.

Respiratory Alkalosis

PATHOPHYSIOLOGY   **Respiratory alkalosis** occurs when there is alveolar hyperventilation and excessive reduction of carbon dioxide (termed **hypocapnia**). Stimulation of ventilation is precipitated by hypoxemia, which may be caused by pulmonary disease, congestive heart failure, or high altitudes; hypermetabolic states such as fever, anemia, and thyrotoxicosis; early salicylate intoxication; hysteria; cirrhosis; and gram-negative sepsis. Improper use of mechanical ventilators can cause iatrogenic respiratory alkalosis. Secondary respiratory alkalosis may develop from hyperventilation stimulated by metabolic or respiratory acidosis.

The onset of respiratory alkalosis occurs within minutes of hyperventilation. Cellular buffers provide immediate compensation with shifts of H^+ from ICF to ECF. The H^+ shifts are not very effective, however, if P_{CO_2} is significantly decreased. When chronic respiratory alkalosis is present, renal compensation restores pH toward normal by decreasing H^+ excretion and bicarbonate absorption (Figure 3-16).

CLINICAL MANIFESTATIONS   Respiratory alkalosis, like metabolic alkalosis, is irritating to the central and peripheral nervous systems. Symptoms include dizziness, confusion, tingling of extremities (paresthesias), convulsions, and coma. Carpopedal spasm and other symptoms of hypocalcemia are similar to those of metabolic alkalosis. Deep and rapid respirations (tachypnea) are primary symptoms that cause respiratory alkalosis.

EVALUATION AND TREATMENT   The underlying disturbance must be identified. The arterial pH is above 7.45, and the P_{CO_2} is less than 38 mmHg. In acute states, bicarbonate levels are normal. With chronic respiratory alkalosis, a

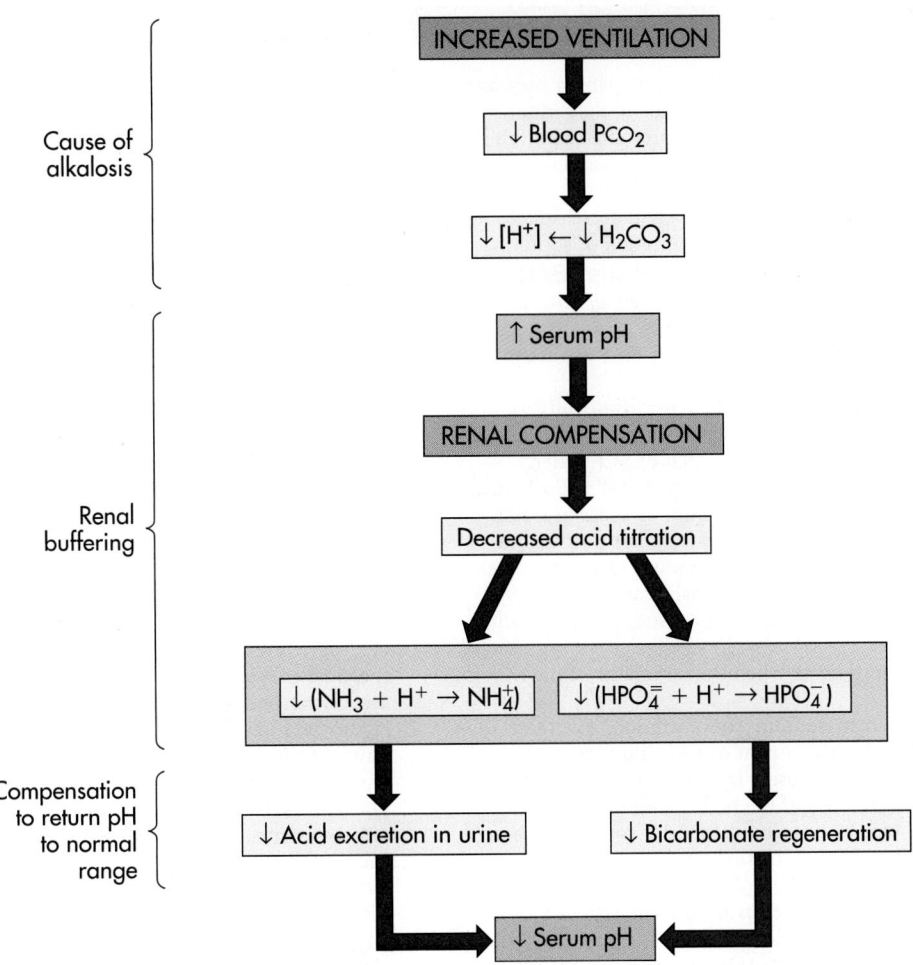

Figure 3-16 Respiratory alkalosis with compensation. See text for abbreviations.

compensatory decrease in the bicarbonate level occurs and the pH is closer to normal.

Treating the underlying disturbance is the most effective treatment. Hypoxemia must be corrected and hypermetabolic states reversed. Symptoms from hysterical hyperventilation can be corrected by rebreathing from a paper bag, which increases the concentration of inspired carbon dioxide and reverses the respiratory alkalosis.

SUMMARY REVIEW

Distribution of Body Fluids
1. Body fluids are distributed among functional compartments and are classified as intracellular fluid (ICF) or extracellular fluid (ECF).
2. The sum of all fluids is the total body water (TBW), which varies with age and amount of body fat.
3. Water moves between the ICF and ECF compartments principally by osmosis.
4. Water moves between the plasma and interstitial fluid by osmosis and hydrostatic pressure, which occur across the capillary membrane.
5. Movement across the capillary wall is called *net filtration* and is described according to the Starling law.

Alterations in Water Movement
1. Edema is a problem of fluid distribution that results in accumulation of fluid within the interstitial spaces.

2. Edema is caused by arterial dilation, venous or lymphatic obstruction, loss of plasma proteins, increased capillary permeability, and increased vascular volume.
3. The pathophysiologic process that leads to edema is related to an increase in forces favoring fluid filtration from the capillaries or lymphatic channels into the tissues.
4. Edema may be localized or generalized and usually is associated with weight gain, swelling and puffiness, tighter-fitting clothes and shoes, and limited movement of the affected area.

Sodium, Chloride, and Water Balance
1. Sodium and water balance are intimately related; chloride levels are generally proportional to changes in sodium levels.
2. Water balance is regulated by the sensation of thirst and by antidiuretic hormone, which is initiated by an increase in plasma osmolality or a decrease in circulating blood volume.

Continued

3. Sodium balance is regulated by aldosterone, which increases reabsorption of sodium by the distal tubule of the kidney.
4. Renin and angiotensin are enzymes that promote or inhibit secretion of aldosterone and thus regulate sodium and water balance.
5. Atrial natriuretic hormone is also involved in decreasing tubular resorption and promoting urinary excretion of sodium.

Alterations in Sodium, Chloride, and Water Balance

1. Alterations in water balance may be classified as isotonic, hypertonic, or hypotonic.
2. Isotonic alterations occur when changes in TBW are accompanied by proportional changes in electrolytes.
3. Hypertonic alterations develop when the osmolality of the ECF is elevated above normal, usually because of an increased concentration of ECF sodium or a deficit of ECF water.
4. Hypernatremia (sodium levels greater than 147 mEq/L) may be caused by an acute increase in sodium or a loss of water.
5. Water deficit, or hypertonic dehydration, is rare but can be caused by lack of access to water, pure water losses, hyperventilation, arid climates, or increased renal clearance.
6. Hyperchloremia is caused by an excess of sodium or a deficit of bicarbonate.
7. Hypotonic alterations occur when the osmolality of the ECF is less than normal.
8. Hyponatremia (serum sodium concentration less than 135 mEq/L) usually causes movement of water into cells.
9. Hyponatremia may be caused by sodium loss, inadequate sodium intake, or dilution of the body's sodium level.
10. Water excess is rare but can be caused by compulsive water drinking, decreased urine formation, or the syndrome of inappropriate secretion of ADH.
11. Hypochloremia is usually the result of hyponatremia or elevated bicarbonate concentrations.

Alterations in Potassium, Calcium, Phosphate, and Magnesium Balance

1. Potassium is the predominant ICF ion; it functions to regulate ICF osmolality, maintain the resting membrane potential, and deposit glycogen in liver and skeletal muscle cells.
2. Potassium balance is regulated by the kidney, by aldosterone and insulin secretion, and by changes in pH.
3. A mechanism known as *potassium adaptation* allows the body to accommodate slowly to increased levels of potassium intake.
4. Hypokalemia (serum potassium concentration less than 3.5 mEq/L) indicates loss of total body potassium, although ECF hypokalemia can develop without losses of total body potassium and plasma K^+ levels may be normal or elevated when total body potassium is depleted.
5. Hypokalemia may be caused by reduced potassium intake, increased ICF-to-ECF potassium concentration, loss of potassium from body stores, increased aldosterone secretion (e.g., caused by hypernatremia), and increased renal excretion.
6. Hyperkalemia (potassium levels greater than 5.5 mEq/L) may be caused by increased potassium intake, a shift from ICF to ECF potassium, or decreased renal excretion.
7. Calcium is a necessary ion in the structure of bones and teeth, in blood clotting, in hormone secretion and the function of cell receptors, and in membrane stability.
8. Phosphate acts as a buffer in acid-base regulation and provides energy for muscle contraction.
9. Calcium and phosphate concentrations are rigidly controlled by parathyroid hormone (PTH), vitamin D, and calcitonin.

10. Hypocalcemia (serum calcium concentration less than 8.5 mg/dl) is related to inadequate intestinal absorption, deposition of ionized calcium into bone or soft tissue, blood administration, or decreased PTH and vitamin D levels.
11. Hypercalcemia (serum calcium concentration greater than 12 mg/dl) can be caused by a number of diseases, including hyperparathyroidism, bone metastases, sarcoidosis, and excess vitamin D.
12. Hypophosphatemia is usually caused by intestinal malabsorption and increased renal excretion of phosphate.
13. Hyperphosphatemia develops with acute or chronic renal failure with significant loss of glomerular filtration.
14. Magnesium is a major intracellular cation and is principally regulated by PTH.
15. Magnesium functions in enzymatic reactions and often interacts with calcium at the cellular level.
16. Hypomagnesemia (serum magnesium concentrations less than 1.5 mEq/L) may be caused by malabsorption syndromes.
17. Hypermagnesemia (serum magnesium concentrations greater than 2.5 mEq/L) is rare and is usually caused by renal failure.

Acid-Base Balance

1. Hydrogen ions, which maintain membrane integrity and the speed of enzymatic reactions, must be concentrated within a narrow range if the body is to function normally.
2. Hydrogen ion concentration is expressed as pH, which represents the negative logarithm of hydrogen ions in solution.
3. Different body fluids have different pH values.
4. The renal and respiratory systems, together with the body's buffer systems, are the principal regulators of acid-base balance.
5. Buffers are substances that can absorb excessive acid or base without a significant change in pH.
6. Buffers exist as acid-base pairs; the principal plasma buffers are carbonic acid–bicarbonate, protein (hemoglobin), and phosphate.
7. Buffer pairs can associate and dissociate; the pK value is the pH at which a buffer pair is half dissociated.
8. The lungs and kidneys act to compensate for changes in pH by increasing or decreasing ventilation and by producing more acidic or more alkaline urine.
9. Correction is a process different from compensation; correction occurs when the values for both components of the buffer pair are returned to normal.
10. Acid-base imbalances are caused by changes in the concentration of H^+ in the blood; an increase causes acidosis, and a decrease causes alkalosis.
11. An abnormal increase or decrease in bicarbonate concentration causes metabolic acidosis or metabolic alkalosis; changes in the rate of alveolar ventilation produce respiratory acidosis or respiratory alkalosis.
12. Metabolic acidosis is caused by an increase in noncarbonic acids or loss of bicarbonate from the extracellular fluid.
13. Metabolic alkalosis occurs with an increase in bicarbonate usually caused by loss of metabolic acids from conditions such as vomiting, gastrointestinal suctioning, excessive bicarbonate intake, hyperaldosteronism, and diuretic therapy.
14. Respiratory acidosis occurs with a decrease of alveolar ventilation and an increase in levels of carbon dioxide, which in turn causes hypercapnia.
15. Respiratory alkalosis occurs with alveolar hyperventilation and excessive reduction of carbon dioxide, or hypocapnia.

KEY TERMS

MEDIA RESOURCES   evolve

Review questions and answers for this chapter are available in the *CD Companion* included with this book.

WebLinks—links to Internet sites pertaining to this chapter—are available on Evolve at http://evolve.elsevier.com/McCance/.

REFERENCES

1. Luckey AE, Parsa CJ: Fluid and electrolytes in the aged, *Arch Surg* 138(10):1055-1060, 2003.
2. Verkman AS: Aquaporin water channels and endothelial cell function, *J Anat* 200(6):617-627, 2002.
3. Baxter GF: The natriuretic peptides, *Basic Res Cardiol* 99(2):71-75, 2004.
4. Kang SK, Kim W, Oh MS: Pathogenesis and treatment of hypernatremia, *Nephron* 92(Suppl 1):14-17, 2002.
5. Montain SJ, Sawka MN, Wenger CB: Hyponatremia associated with exercise: risk factors and pathogenesis, *Execr Sport Sci Rev* 29(3):1131-1137, 2001.
6. Yeates KE, Singer M, Morton AR: Salt and water: a simple approach to hyponatremia, *CMAJ* 170(3):365-369, 2004.
7. Decaux G, Soupart A: Treatment of symptomatic hyponatremia, *Am J Med Sci* 326(1):25-30, 2003.
8. Baylis PH: The syndrome of inappropriate antidiuretic hormone secretion, *Int J Biochem Cell Biol* 35(11):1495-1499, 2003.
9. Wang W: Regulation of renal K transported by dietary K intake, *Annu Rev Physiol* 66:547-569, 2004.
10. Gennari FJ: Disorders of potassium homeostasis. Hypokalemia and hyperkalemia, *Crit Care Clin* 18(2):273-288, vi, 2002. Review.
11. Dubois D, Hamm LL: *Fluid and electrolyte disorders: a companion to Brenner and Rector's the kidney,* Philadelphia, 2002, Saunders.
12. Kim GH, Han JS: Therapeutic approach to hypokalemia, *Nephron* 92(Suppl 1):28-32, 2002.
13. Albaaj F, Hutchison A: Hyperphosphataemia in renal failure: causes, consequences and current management, *Drugs* 63(6):577-596, 2003.
14. Laires MH, Monteiro CP, Bicho M: Role of cellular magnesium in health and human disease, *Front Biosci* 9:262-276, 2004.
15. Rose DB, Post T: *Clinical physiology of acid-base and electrolyte disorders,* ed 5, New York, 2001, McGraw-Hill.
16. Lolekha PH, Vanavanan S, Lolekha S: Update on value of the anion gap in clinical diagnosis and laboratory evaluation, *Clin Chim Acta* 307 (1-2):33-36, 2001.
17. Levraut J, Grimaud D: Treatment of metabolic acidosis, *Curr Opin Crit Care* 9(4):260-265, 2003.
18. Galla JH: Metabolic alkalosis, *J Am Soc Nephrol* 11(2):369-375, 2000.

GENES AND GENETIC DISEASES

LYNN B. JORDE

CHAPTER OUTLINE

In the nineteenth century, microscopic studies of cells led scientists to suspect that the nucleus of the cell contained the important mechanisms of inheritance. Scientists found that chromatin, the substance that gives the nucleus a granular appearance, is observable in nondividing cells. Just before the cell divides, the chromatin condenses to form discrete, dark-staining organelles, which are called chromosomes. (Cell division is discussed in Chapter 1.) With the rediscovery of Gregor Mendel's important breeding experiments at the turn of the twentieth century, it soon became apparent that the chromosomes contained genes, the basic units of inheritance. Chromosomes were the subject of much study, but because of poorly developed laboratory techniques, progress was slow. Since the mid-1950s, however, technologic advances have permitted a rapid increase in scientific knowledge of the form, composition, and function of chromosomes.

The primary constituent of the chromatin is **deoxyribonucleic acid (DNA)**. Genes are composed of sequences of DNA. By serving as the blueprints of proteins in the body, genes ultimately influence all aspects of body structure and function. Estimates suggest that there are approximately 20,000 to 25,000 genes. An error in one of these genes can lead to a recognizable genetic disease.

To date, more than 15,000 genetic conditions have been identified and cataloged.[1] As infectious diseases come under increasingly effective control, the proportion of beds in pediatric hospitals occupied by children with genetic diseases has risen to one third.[2] In addition, many common diseases that affect primarily adults, such as hypertension, coronary heart disease, diabetes, and cancer, are now known to have important genetic components. (These diseases are also affected by environmental factors. The interaction between genetic and environmental components is discussed in Chapter 5.)

Great progress is being made in the diagnosis of genetic diseases and the understanding of genetic mechanisms underlying them. With the huge strides being made in molecular genetics, gene therapy—the direct alteration of genes in cells—has begun. Genetics is now one of the most rapidly advancing fields of medicine.

DNA, RNA, AND PROTEINS: HEREDITY AT THE MOLECULAR LEVEL

DNA

Composition and Structure

Genes are composed of DNA, which has three basic components: the pentose sugar molecule, deoxyribose; a phosphate molecule; and four types of nitrogenous bases. Two of the bases, **cytosine** and **thymine,** are single carbon-nitrogen rings called **pyrimidines.** The other two bases, **adenine** and **guanine,** are double carbon-nitrogen rings called **purines.** The four bases are commonly represented by their first letters: A, C, T, and G.

One of Watson and Crick's contributions was to demonstrate how these molecules are physically assembled together as DNA. They proposed the now-famous **double-helix** model, in which DNA can be envisioned as a twisted ladder with chemical bonds as its rungs (Figure 4-1). The two sides of the ladder are composed of the sugar and phosphate molecules, held together by strong phosphodiester bonds. Projecting from each side of the ladder, at regular intervals, are the nitrogenous bases. The base projecting from one side is bound to the base projecting from the other by a weak hydrogen bond. Therefore the nitrogenous bases form the rungs of the ladder; adenine pairs with thymine, and guanine pairs with cytosine. Each DNA subunit—consisting of one deoxyribose molecule, one phosphate group, and one base—is called a **nucleotide.**

DNA as the Genetic Code

To serve as the basis of genetic inheritance, DNA must be able to direct the synthesis of all the body's proteins. Proteins are composed of one or more **polypeptides** (intermediate pro-

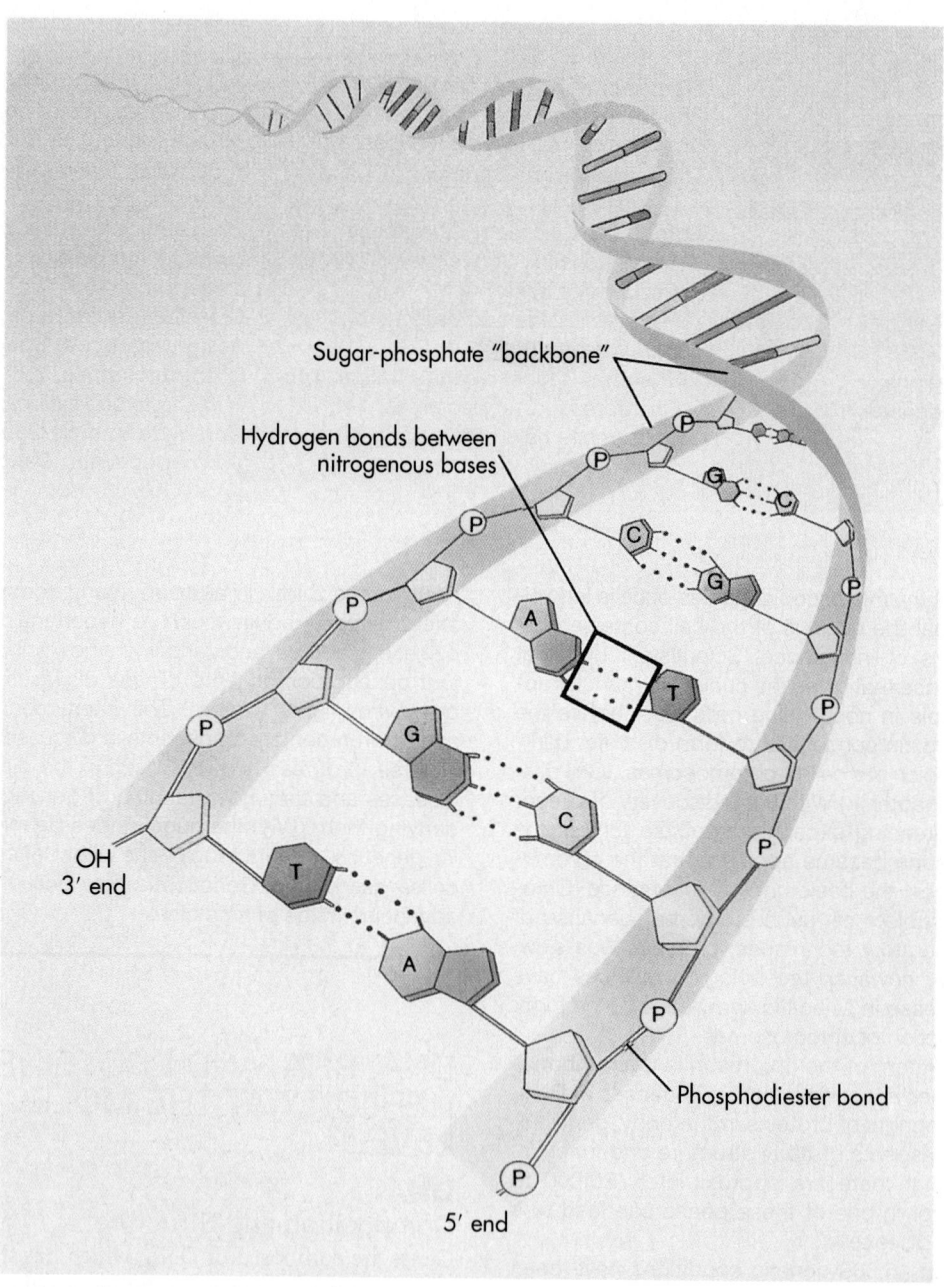

Figure 4-1 Structure of deoxyribonucleic acid (DNA). In a DNA double helix, only two nitrogenous base pairs are possible: adenine (A) with thymine (T); and guanine (G) with cytosine (C). The bases are linked in the middle of the molecule by hydrogen bonds. The "backbone" of the DNA molecule is composed of the deoxyribose sugars joined by phosphodiester bonds to phosphate groups (P). (From Raven PH, Johnson GB: *Understanding biology,* ed 3, Dubuque, Iowa, 1995, Brown.)

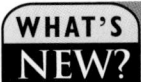

Genetic Engineering and Gene Therapy: The "New Genetics"

Terms such as *cloning, genetic engineering,* and *recombinant DNA* have received much exposure in the popular press during the past several years as the news media have recognized the potential importance of these techniques. Indeed they are part of the scientific revolution sometimes known as the *new genetics.*

Recombinant DNA

Genetic engineering refers to laboratory alteration of genes. Most alterations are accomplished by using recombinant DNA techniques, which involve combining the DNA of two or more different organisms. A number of sophisticated methods have been invented to do this; described here is a common approach that is similar in principle to most other approaches.

Among the key components of recombinant DNA research are bacterial plasmids—small, circular pieces of self-replicating DNA that reside in many bacteria but often are not essential to the growth or survival of the bacteria. Plasmids can therefore be extracted from or inserted into bacteria without seriously disrupting bacterial growth or reproduction. Once they are extracted from their bacterial hosts, the plasmids are exposed to restriction endonucleases, which are enzymes that cleave, or cut, the plasmid DNA at a specific nucleotide sequence, called a *restriction site.*

Different restriction endonucleases have different restriction sites. A commonly used restriction endonuclease is called *Eco*RI (from the bacteria that produce it, *Escherichia coli*). *Eco*RI cleaves DNA only when the sequence GAATTC is found on one DNA strand and the complementary sequence is found on the other strand. The DNA of another organism, such as a human, also can be exposed to *Eco*RI and can be cleaved at the same restriction sites. The resulting human restriction fragments, which are pieces of DNA, have exposed ends that have base sequences complementary to those of the cleaved plasmid DNA. The human DNA and plasmid DNA, if mixed together, undergo complementary base pairing (i.e., they recombine).

The result is that the human DNA is incorporated within the plasmid. The plasmids, which now contain human genes in addition to their own, are allowed to reenter bacteria. Selection processes can be applied to pick out the bacteria that contain the desired human genes. These are cultured and allowed to form clones (or genetically identical copies) through normal cell division. Through continued cell division, millions of bacterial clones are formed, all containing the same human gene. Like any other gene, the human gene directs protein synthesis in the bacteria, resulting in the production of human proteins by bacteria.

Because bacteria multiply rapidly, large amounts of a given human protein can be manufactured by using this procedure. It has already been used successfully to produce human insulin in mass quantities. Because the insulin produced this way is actually human insulin, it produces fewer allergic reactions than the insulin taken from animal pancreases. Interferon, a substance that may help the body fight cancer and viral infections, also has been produced this way, as has human growth hormone, a substance that can be used to cure pituitary dwarfism.

In trying to isolate a particular gene, it is often more convenient to begin work with the messenger ribonucleic acid (mRNA) that codes for the gene product. The mRNA can be purified from body cells, and then an enzyme called *reverse transcriptase* can be used to generate the DNA sequence that is complementary to the mRNA. This complementary DNA (cDNA) can be inserted into plasmids and cloned by using the same recombinant techniques, so that virtually unlimited quantities of the desired gene product can be manufactured.

Recombinant DNA methods have been applied toward the understanding of the single-gene disorder phenylketonuria (PKU), which is the result of a lack of the enzyme phenylalanine hydroxylase. First, mRNA coding for this enzyme was purified from rat liver cells. After attachment of a radioactive "label" to cDNA produced from this mRNA, the cDNA was used as a probe. The probe was exposed to a series of cells that had been manipulated in the laboratory so that each cell line contained only one or a few chromosomes. When the probe hybridized consistently with only the cells containing chromosome 12, it proved that the gene that produces phenylalanine hydroxylase and thus causes PKU is located on this chromosome. Knowing the chromosome location of a gene is a very important step in the diagnosis and understanding of a genetic disease. Ultimately, therapeutic techniques might be developed to correct such disorders by replacing or repairing the abnormal gene.

The use of recombinant DNA techniques to clone DNA sequences has been (and continues to be) of great importance in genetics. However, the cloning process can take a great deal of time, even for well-studied genes. When doing genetic diagnoses, it is often necessary to obtain results very quickly. A newer technique, the polymerase chain reaction (PCR), provides a very rapid means of making millions of copies of a DNA sequence in only a few hours (as opposed to 1 week or more using cloning techniques). PCR basically involves the artificial replication of a DNA sequence, achieved by exposing the DNA strand to alterations in temperature in the presence of free DNA bases. At lower temperatures the DNA undergoes complementary base pairing, and at higher temperatures the DNA strands separate to form new templates for another cycle of replication when the temperature is again lowered. By repeating this temperature cycling over and over, DNA copies can be produced rapidly. This technique is very useful for diagnostic purposes because it requires only a very small sample of blood or other tissue and because a large number of copies can be made in a very short time. In theory, even a single DNA molecule can be copied millions of times using PCR. It is also used extensively in forensic medicine (e.g., in identifying the DNA of criminal suspects by using blood, semen, or hair samples left at the scene of a crime).

The advent of this technology has led to fears that organisms that could pose grave threats to the human species might be created. In 1974 a group of molecular geneticists themselves called for a moratorium on recombinant DNA research when its implications began to be realized; however, after much study and the introduction of rules regarding laboratory containment, research was resumed. Because of the elaborate precautions taken to prevent inadvertent creation of harmful organisms and because of the very low probability that such organisms could survive outside the laboratory, the possibility that such organisms could survive outside the laboratory, the possibility of such an occurrence is now considered to be extremely remote.

Gene Therapy

An area in which recombinant DNA techniques have generated much interest is gene therapy, which essentially involves the insertion of normal genes. For example, by recombinant DNA methods, a normal gene might be inserted into a human chromosome to counteract the effects of an abnormal or missing gene.

Gene therapy can be applied in two ways. The less controversial approach is somatic cell therapy, which consists of inserting normal genes into the cells of an individual who has a genetic disease. Here a particular tissue, such as bone marrow cells that produce abnormal erythrocytes, would be treated. More controversial is the application of gene therapy very early in embryonic development. By inserting genes into the embryos, all body cells could be altered, including the germ cells. Thus not only would the

Continued

genetic constitution of the embryo and resulting individual be changed, but also all the descendants of that individual would have altered genetic constitutions. This procedure is sometimes referred to as *germ cell therapy.*

Somatic cell therapy has now been initiated for a number of human diseases, including hemophilia, cystic fibrosis, familial hypercholesterolemia, and several types of cancer.* More than 600 so-

matic cell gene therapy protocols are now being tested. Although significant setbacks have occurred, considerable technological progress is being made and somatic cell therapy is beginning to demonstrate therapeutic effects for some diseases. Because of several important technical and ethical considerations, germline therapy will not be attempted in humans in the foreseeable future.

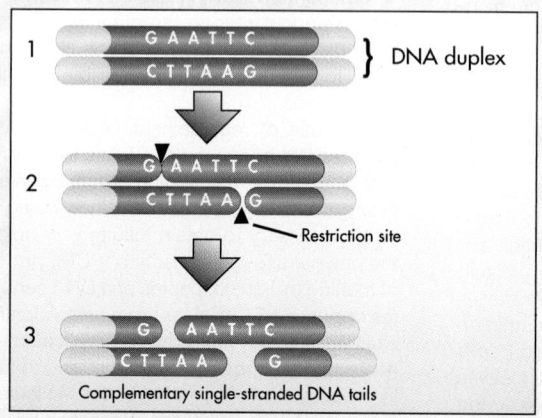

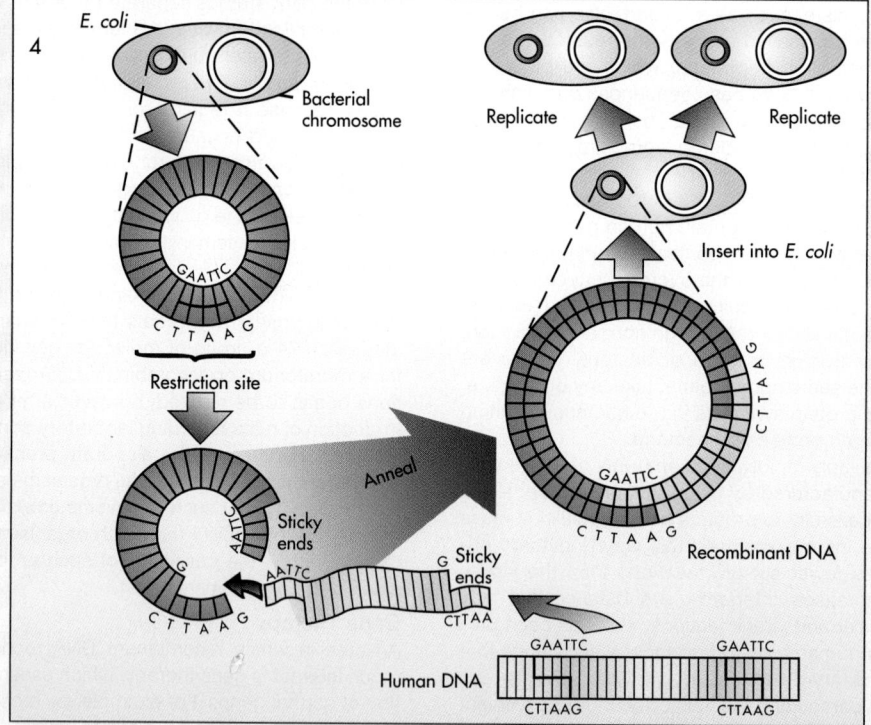

Recombinant DNA technology. Human DNA and circular plasmid DNA are both cleaved by a restriction enzyme, producing sticky ends *(1 to 3)*. This allows the human DNA to anneal and recombine with the plasmid DNA. Inserted into the plasmid DNA, the human DNA is now replicated when plasmid is inserted into the bacterium, such as *Escherichia coli (4)*. G, Guanine; A, adenine; T, thymine; C, cytosine. (From Jorde LB et al: *Medical genetics,* ed 3, St Louis, 2003, Mosby.)

*Kootstra NA, Verma IM: *Annu Rev Pharmacol Toxicol* 43:413-439, 2003; Thomas CE, Ehrhardt A, Kay MA: *Nat Rev Genet* 4:346-358, 2003.

tein compounds), which are in turn composed of sequences of **amino acids** (organic acids containing NH$_2$). The body contains 20 different types of amino acids, and the amino acid sequences that make up polypeptides must in some way be specified by the DNA molecule.

Because there are 20 possible amino acids and only four possible bases, each single nucleotide cannot specify an amino acid. Similarly, the amino acids cannot be specified by couplets of bases (e.g., adenine-guanine, thymine-guanine, guanine-cytosine) because there are only 4 × 4, or 16, possible couplets. If series of three bases are translated into amino acids, however, there are 4 × 4 × 4, or 64, possible combinations—more than enough to specify each different amino acid. By manufacturing synthetic nucleotide sequences and allowing them to direct the formation of amino acids in the laboratory, it was proved that amino acids were specified by these triplets of bases, or **codons.**

Of the 64 possible codons, three signal the end of a gene and are known as **termination,** or **nonsense, codons.** The remaining 61 all specify amino acids, which means that most amino acids can be specified by more than one codon. The genetic code is thus said to be redundant, although each codon can specify only one amino acid.

Another significant feature of the genetic code is that it is universal: all living organisms use precisely the same DNA codes to specify proteins. The one known exception to this rule occurs in mitochondria—cytoplasmic organelles that are the sites of cellular respiration (see Chapter 1). The mitochondria have their own extranuclear DNA. Several codons of mitochondrial DNA encode different amino acids than do the same nuclear DNA codons.

Replication

In addition to having the ability to specify amino acid sequences, DNA must be able to replicate itself accurately during cell division if it is to serve as the basic genetic material. DNA replication consists of the breaking of the weak hydrogen bonds between the bases, leaving a single strand with each base unpaired. The consistent pairing of adenine with thymine and of guanine with cytosine, known as **complementary base pairing,** is the key to accurate replication. The principle of complementary base pairing dictates that the unpaired base will attract a free nucleotide only if the nucleotide has the proper complementary base. Thus a portion of a single strand with a sequence of bases labeled ATTGCT will bond with a series of free nucleotides with the bases TAACGA. When replication is complete, a new double-stranded molecule identical to the original is formed (Figure 4-2). The single strand is said to be a **template,** or molecule on which a complementary molecule is built, and is the basis for synthesizing the new double strand.

Several different proteins are involved in DNA replication. One protein unwinds the double helix, one holds the strands apart, and others perform different distinct functions. The most important of these proteins is an enzyme known as **DNA polymerase.** This enzyme travels along the single DNA strand, adding the correct nucleotides to the free end of the new strand. Besides adding the new nucleotides, the DNA polymerase performs a proofreading procedure. After the new nucleotide has been added to the chain, the DNA polymerase checks to make sure that its base is actually complementary to the template base. If it is not, the incorrect nucleotide is excised and replaced with a correct one. This

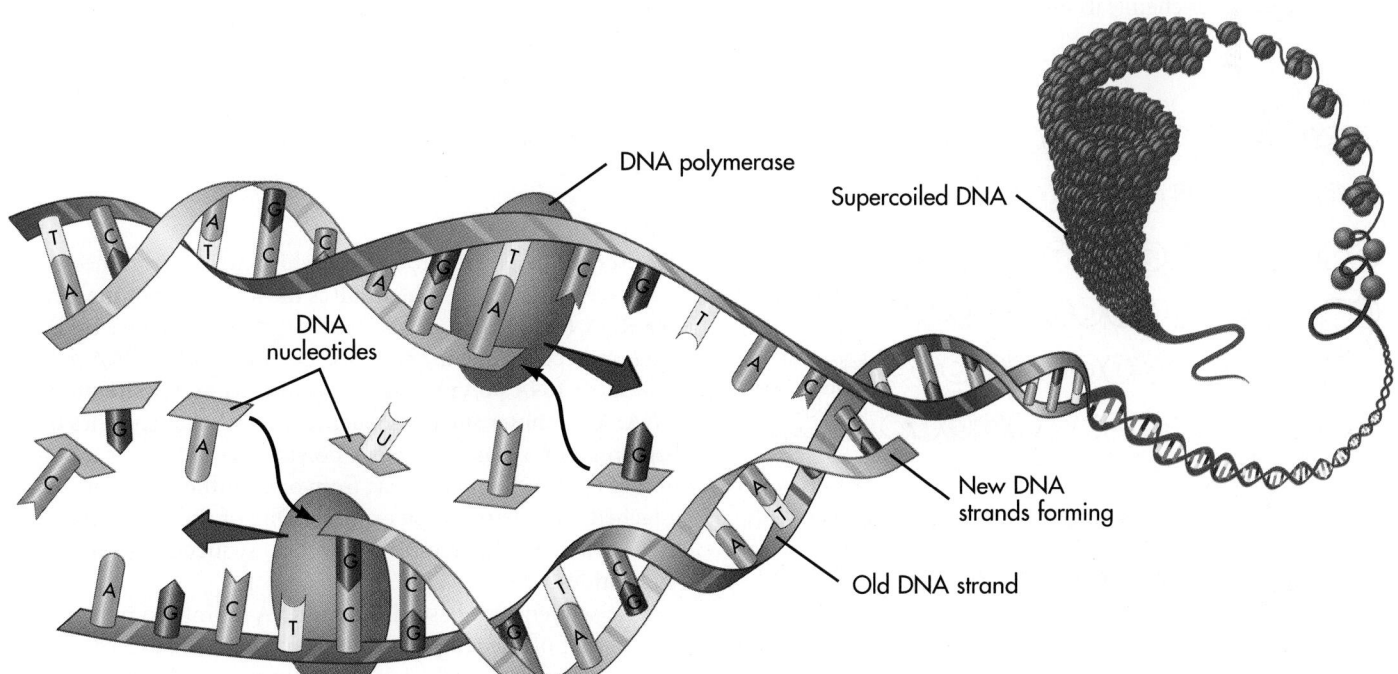

Figure 4-2 **Deoxyribonucleic acid (DNA) replication.** *A,* Adenine; *T,* thymine; *G,* guanine; *C,* cytosine. (From Thibodeau GA, Patton KT: *Anatomy & physiology,* ed 5, St Louis, 2003, Mosby.)

procedure, one of the mechanisms of DNA repair, substantially enhances the accuracy of DNA replication.

Mutation

A **mutation** is any inherited alteration of genetic material. Chromosome aberrations that cause congenital defects are examples of mutations. Other mutations are subtle and are not observable as chromosome aberrations. One such mutation is the **base pair substitution,** in which one base pair is replaced by another. This substitution sometimes results in a change in amino acid sequence, but because of the redundancy of the genetic code, it may have no consequence. If an amino acid change does not occur, the mutation is termed a **silent substitution.** Profound consequences can result, however, when an amino acid sequence is altered by a base pair substitution. (Many of the serious genetic diseases discussed later are the result of base pair substitutions.)

A second major type of mutation is the **frameshift mutation.** This alteration involves the insertion or deletion of one or more base pairs to the DNA molecule. As Figure 4-3 shows, these mutations can change the entire "reading frame" of the DNA sequence because codons consist of groups of three base pairs. A frameshift mutation thus can greatly alter the resulting amino acid sequence.

A large number of agents are known to increase the frequency of mutations. These agents are known collectively as **mutagens.** Radiation, such as that produced by x-rays and nuclear fallout, is an important mutagen and is known to cause cell damage (see Chapter 2). Radiation forms electrically charged ions that can produce chemical reactions, which in turn change DNA bases. A variety of chemicals also can induce mutations, often because they are chemically similar to DNA bases. Other chemicals mimic the effects of ionizing ra-

diation, and still others interfere with the process of base pairing. Hundreds of chemicals are now known to be mutagenic in humans or laboratory animals, such as nitrogen mustard, vinyl chloride, alkylating agents, formaldehyde, and sodium nitrite. Some of these chemicals, however, are much more potent mutagens than others. Nitrogen mustard, for example, is extremely mutagenic, whereas sodium nitrate is a weak mutagen.

Measurement of the mutation rate in humans is difficult, in part because mutations are very rare events. Current estimates are that the rate of **spontaneous mutation** (a mutation that occurs in the absence of exposure to known mutagens) in humans is about 10^{-4} to 10^{-7} per gene per generation. This rate appears to vary from one gene to another. Certain areas of some chromosomes have particularly high mutation rates and are known as **mutational hot spots.** In particular, sequences consisting of a cytosine base followed by a guanine base (CG) are highly susceptible to mutation and are known to account for a disproportionately large percentage of disease-causing mutations.[3]

From Genes to Proteins

Whereas DNA is formed and replicated in the cell nucleus, protein synthesis takes place in the cytoplasm. The transport of the DNA code from nucleus to cytoplasm and subsequent protein formation involves two basic processes: transcription and translation. Both of these processes are mediated by **ribonucleic acid (RNA)**, a type of nucleic acid that is chemically very similar to DNA. RNA is also composed of sugar molecules, phosphate groups, and nitrogenous bases. RNA differs from DNA in that the sugar molecule is ribose rather than deoxyribose and in that uracil rather than thymine is one of the four bases. The other bases of RNA, as in DNA, are adenine, cytosine, and guanine. Uracil is structurally very similar to thymine, so it also can pair with adenine. The final difference between RNA and DNA is that whereas DNA usually occurs as a double strand, RNA usually occurs as a single strand.

Transcription

Transcription is the process by which RNA is synthesized from a DNA template. The result is the formation of **messenger RNA (mRNA)** from the base sequence specified by the DNA molecule. An enzyme called *DNA-dependent RNA polymerase,* or **RNA polymerase,** binds to a **promoter site** on the DNA. A promoter site is a sequence of DNA that specifies the beginning of a gene. The RNA polymerase then pulls a portion of the DNA strands apart from one another, allowing unattached DNA bases to be exposed. One of the DNA strands then provides the template for the sequence of mRNA nucleotides.

The sequence of bases in the mRNA is thus complementary to that of the template strand, and with the exception of the presence of uracil instead of thymine, the mRNA sequence is identical to that of the other DNA strand. Tran-

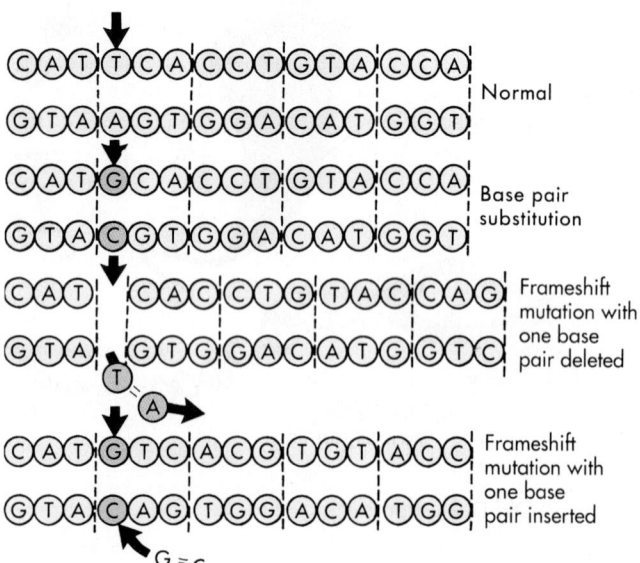

Figure 4-3 Different kinds of mutations. *A,* Adenine; *T,* thymine; *G,* guanine; *C,* cytosine.

scription continues until a DNA sequence called a **termination sequence** is reached. Then the RNA polymerase detaches from the DNA, and the transcribed mRNA is freed to move out of the nucleus and into the cytoplasm. Figure 4-4 summarizes the process of transcription.

Gene Splicing

After the mRNA first has been transcribed from the DNA template, it reflects exactly the base sequence of the DNA. The RNA in this state is sometimes called **heterogeneous nuclear RNA (hnRNA).** In eukaryotes an important step takes place before this RNA leaves the nucleus. Many of the RNA sequences are removed by nuclear enzymes, and the remaining sequences are spliced together to form the functional mRNA that will migrate to the cytoplasm.

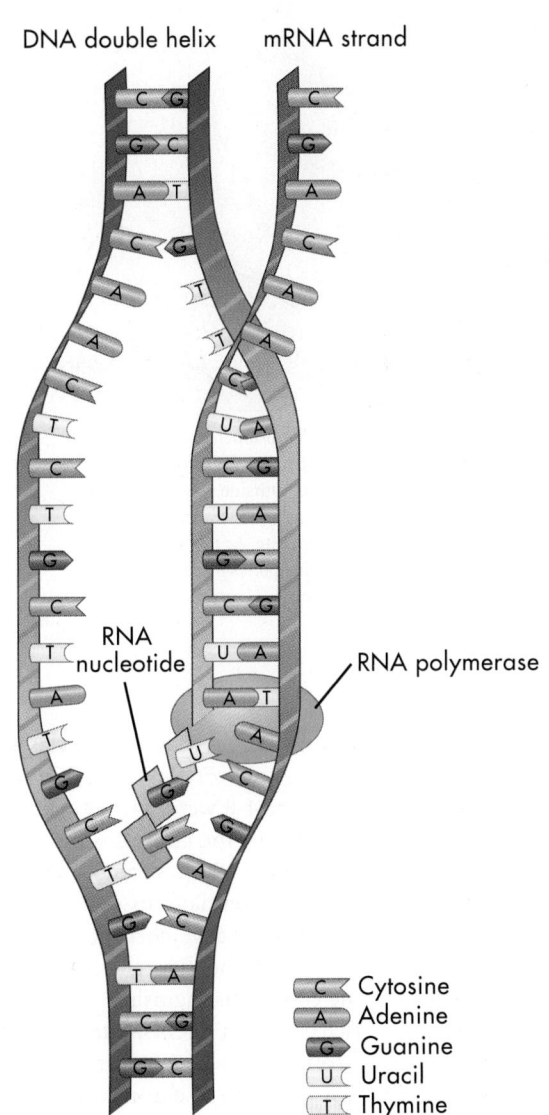

Figure 4-4 General scheme of ribonucleic acid (RNA) transcription. See text for explanation. (From Thibodeau GA, Patton KT: *Anatomy & physiology,* ed 5, St Louis, 2003, Mosby.)

The excised sequences are called **introns,** and the sequences that are left to code for proteins are called **exons.** The function, if any, of introns is not yet understood.

Translation

Translation is the process by which RNA directs the synthesis of a polypeptide (Figure 4-5). However, mRNA cannot code directly for amino acids. Instead, it interacts with **transfer RNA (tRNA),** a cloverleaf-shaped strand of about 80 nucleotides. The tRNA molecule has a site for the attachment of an amino acid. At the opposite side of the cloverleaf is a sequence of three nucleotides called the **anticodon.** The anticodon undergoes complementary base pairing with an appropriate codon in the mRNA. The mRNA thus specifies the sequence of amino acids by acting through the tRNA.

The site of actual protein synthesis is the **ribosome,** which consists of roughly equal parts of protein and **ribosomal RNA (rRNA).** During translation (Figure 4-6) the ribosome first binds to an initiation site on the mRNA sequence. The ribosome then binds the tRNA to its surface so that base pairing can occur between tRNA and mRNA. The ribosome then moves along the mRNA sequence, codon by codon. As each codon is processed, an amino acid is translated by the interaction of mRNA and tRNA.

In this process the ribosome provides an enzyme that catalyzes the formation of covalent peptide bonds between the adjacent amino acids, resulting in a growing polypeptide. When the ribosome arrives at a termination signal on the mRNA sequence, translation and polypeptide formation cease. The mRNA, ribosome, and polypeptide separate from one another, and the polypeptide is released into the cytoplasm to perform its required function.

CHROMOSOMES

Human cells can be categorized into two types: the **gametes** (sperm and egg cells) and the **somatic cells,** which include all cells other than gametes. Each somatic cell has 46 chromosomes in its nucleus. These are **diploid cells,** meaning that the chromosomes occur in pairs. Thus each cell actually contains 23 pairs of chromosomes. One member of each pair comes from the individual's mother, and one comes from the father. New somatic cells are formed through mitosis and cytokinesis, through which the cell nucleus and cytoplasm are replicated. (The division process that creates new copies of somatic cells is described in Chapter 1.) Gametes are **haploid cells:** they have only one member of each chromosome pair, giving them a total of 23 chromosomes. The process by which these haploid cells are formed from diploid cells is called **meiosis** (Figure 4-7).

In 22 of the 23 chromosome pairs, the two members of each pair are virtually identical in microscopic appearance and are thus said to be **homologous** to one another. These 22 chromosome pairs are homologous in both males and females and are termed **autosomes.** The remaining pair of

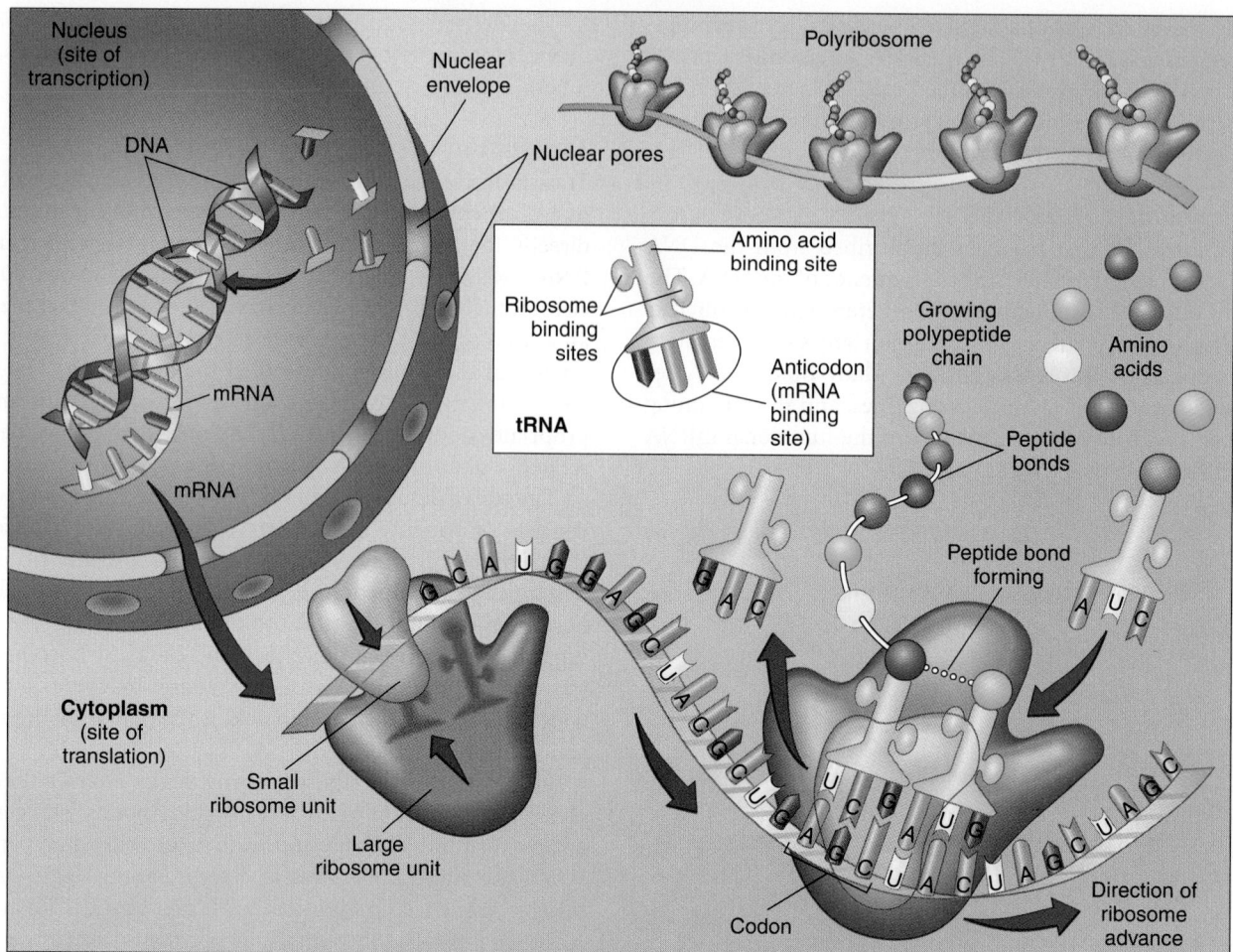

Figure 4-5 **Protein synthesis.** Protein synthesis begins with *transcription,* a process in which a messenger ribonucleic acid (mRNA) molecule forms along one gene sequence of a deoxyribonucleic acid (DNA) molecule within the cell's nucleus. As it is formed, the mRNA molecule separates from the DNA molecule and leaves the nucleus through the large nuclear pores. Outside the nucleus, ribosome subunits attach to the beginning of the mRNA molecule and begin the process of *translation.* In translation, transfer RNA (tRNA) molecules bring specific amino acids—encoded by each mRNA codon—into place at the ribosome site. As the amino acids are brought into the proper sequence, they are joined together by peptide bonds to form long strands called *polypeptides.* Several polypeptide chains may be needed to make a complete protein molecule. *A,* Adenine; *C,* cytosine; *G,* guanine; *U,* uracil. (From Thibodeau GA, Patton KT: *Anatomy & Physiology,* ed 5, St Louis, 2003, Mosby.)

chromosomes, the **sex chromosomes,** consists of two homologous X chromosomes in females and a nonhomologous pair, X and Y, in males.

Figure 4-8, *A,* illustrates a **metaphase spread,** which is a photograph of the chromosomes as they appear in the nucleus of a somatic cell during metaphase. (Chromosomes are easiest to visualize during this stage of mitosis.) A **karyotype** is an ordered display of chromosomes. In Figure 4-8, *B,* the chromosomes are cut out and arranged according to size, with the **homologous chromosomes** paired together. The 22 autosomes are numbered according to length, with chromosome 1 as the longest and chromosome 22 as the shortest. Some natural variation in relative chromosome length can be expected from person to person, however, so it is not always possible to distinguish each chromosome by its length. There-

fore the position of the centromere is also used to classify the chromosomes (Figure 4-9).

The chromosomes in Figure 4-8 were stained with a substance that penetrates all areas of the chromosome (a "solid stain"). In the late 1960s and early 1970s, several staining materials were found to bind preferentially to certain areas of chromosomes. The resulting distinctive **chromosome bands** are evident in various patterns in the different chromosomes so that each chromosome can be distinguished easily. One of the most commonly used stains is **Giemsa stain.** By using banding techniques, chromosomes can be unambiguously numbered, and individual variation in chromosome composition can be studied. Missing or duplicated portions of chromosomes, which often result in serious diseases, also can be readily identified.

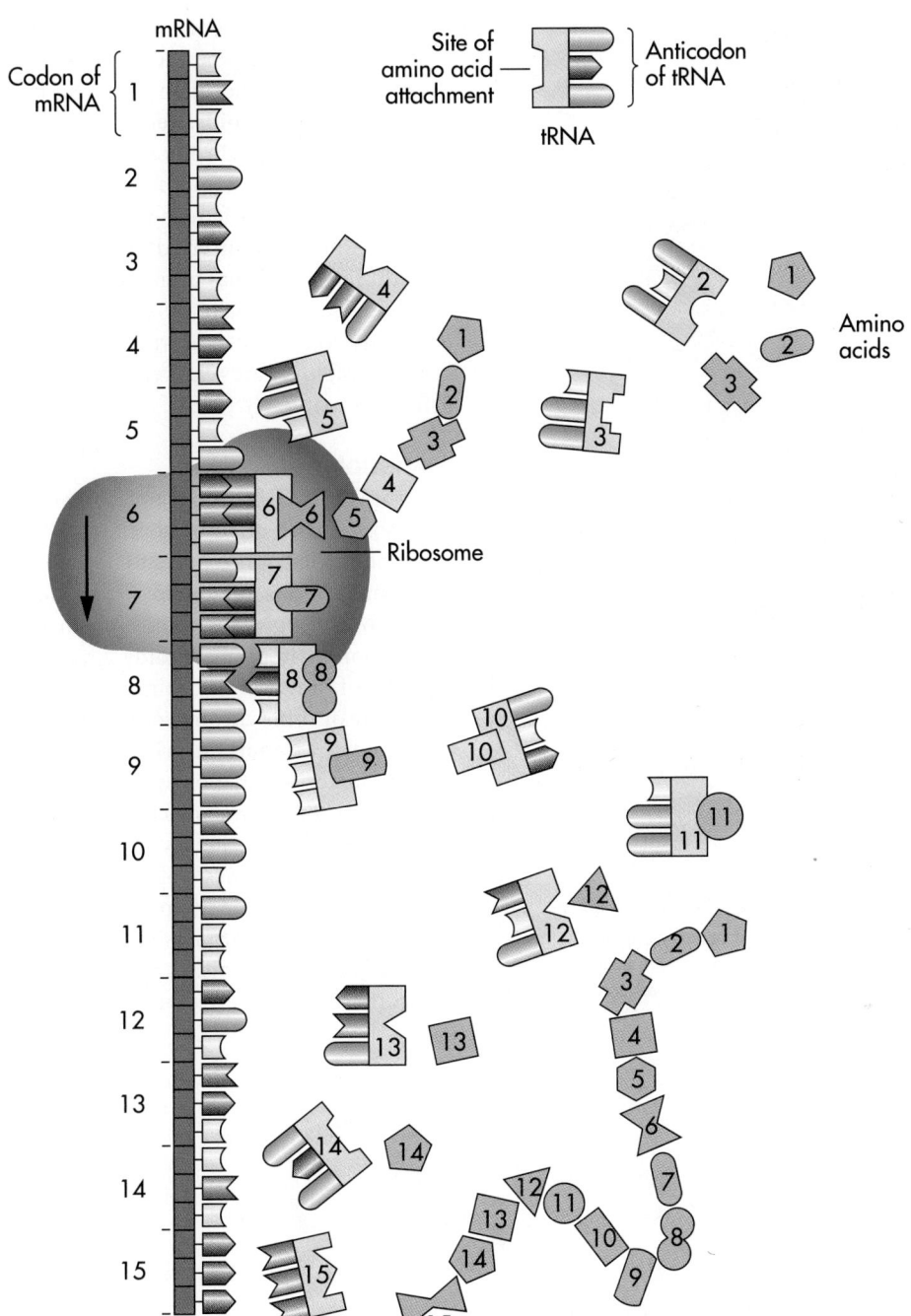

Figure 4-6 A ribosome "reading" the code of messenger ribonucleic acid (mRNA) and assembling a polypeptide chain.

Chromosome Aberrations and Associated Diseases

Chromosome abnormalities are the leading known cause of mental retardation and miscarriage. Estimates indicate that a major chromosome aberration occurs in at least 1 in 12 conceptions. Most of these fetuses do not survive to term; in fact, about 50% of all recovered first-trimester spontaneous abortuses have major chromosome aberrations.[4] The number of live births affected by these abnormalities is significant; about 1 in 150 has a major diagnosable chromosome abnormality[5] (see Box 4-1).

Polyploidy

Cells that have a multiple of the normal number of chromosomes are said to be **euploid cells** (Greek *eu* = good or true). Because normal gametes are haploid and most normal somatic cells are diploid, they are both euploid forms. When a euploid cell has more than the diploid number of chromosomes, it is said to be a **polyploid cell.** Several types of body

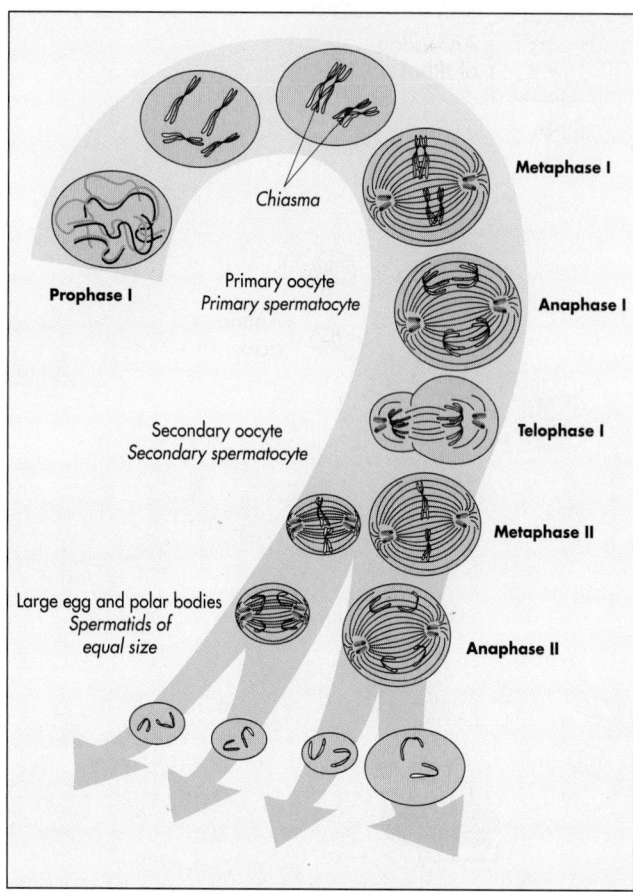

Figure 4-7 Stages of meiosis. Stages of meiosis, during which haploid gametes are formed from a diploid stem cell. For brevity, prophase II and telophase II are not shown. Note the relationship between meiosis and spermatogenesis and oogenesis. (From Jorde LB et al: *Medical genetics*, ed 3, St Louis, 2003, Mosby.)

tissues, including some liver, bronchial, and epithelial tissues, are normally polyploid. A zygote having three copies of each chromosome, rather than the usual two, has a form of polyploidy called **triploidy. Tetraploidy,** a condition in which euploid cells have 92 chromosomes, also has been observed. Both of these conditions are incompatible with postnatal survival. Nearly all triploid fetuses are spontaneously aborted or stillborn. A few have survived to term but have died shortly after birth. Tetraploidy has been found primarily in early abortuses, although occasionally affected infants have been born alive. Like triploid infants, however, they do not survive. Triploidy and tetraploidy are relatively common conditions, accounting for approximately 10% of all known miscarriages.[4]

Aneuploidy

A somatic cell that does not contain a multiple of 23 chromosomes is an **aneuploid cell.** A cell containing three copies of one chromosome is said to be trisomic (a condition termed **trisomy**) and is aneuploid. **Monosomy,** the presence of only one copy of a given chromosome in a diploid cell, is the other common form of aneuploidy. Among the autosomes, monosomy of any chromosome is lethal, but newborns with trisomy of some chromosomes can survive. This difference illustrates an important principle: in general, loss of chromosome material has more serious consequences than duplication of chromosome material.

Aneuploidy of the sex chromosomes is less serious than that of the autosomes. For the Y chromosome, this is true because very little genetic material is located on this chromosome. For the X chromosome, inactivation of extra chromosomes largely diminishes their effect. A zygote bearing *no* X chromosome, however, will not survive.

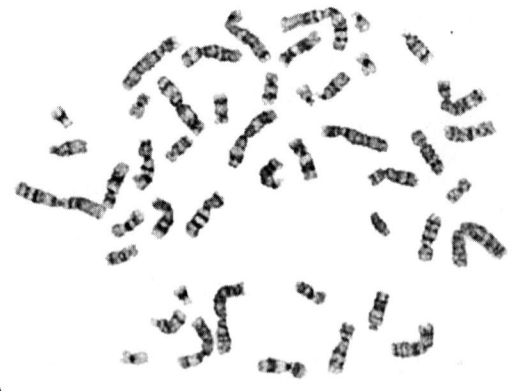

A

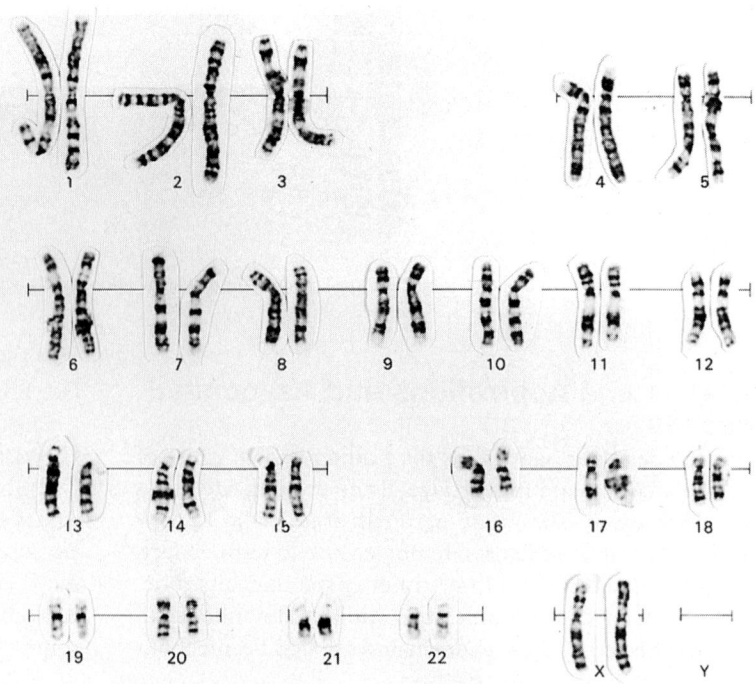

B

Figure 4-8 Karyotype of chromosomes. A, G-banded metaphase of a normal cell showing the bands of all normal chromosomes. **B,** G-banded karyotype of a normal female cell showing the banding patterns of the various chromosomes. Identical patterns characterize homologous chromosomes. The chromosomes are arranged from largest to smallest in size. (From Damjanov I, Linder J: *Anderson's pathology,* ed 10, St Louis, 1996, Mosby.)

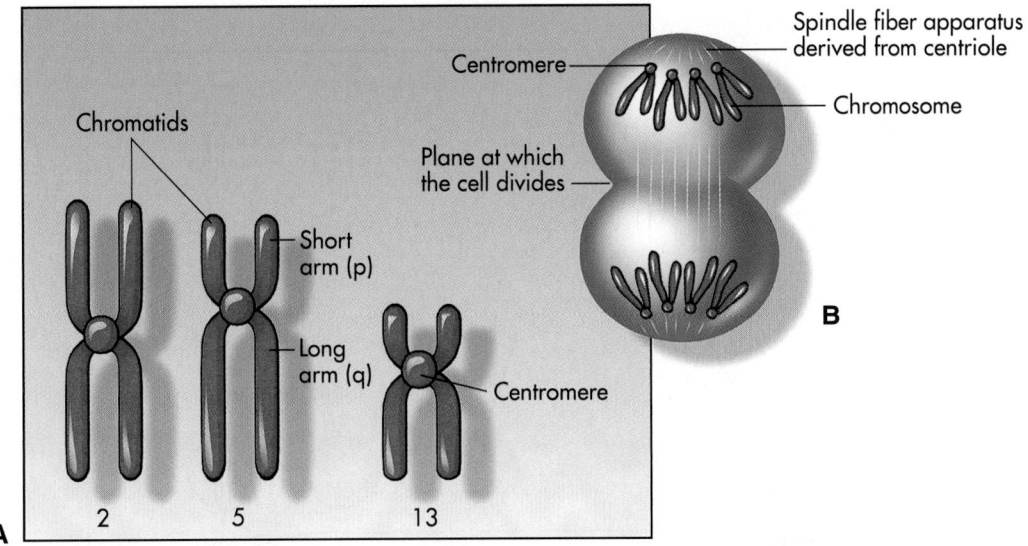

Figure 4-9 Structure of chromosomes. A, Human chromosomes 1, 5, and 13. Each is replicated and consists of two chromatids. Chromosome 1 is a metacentric chromosome because the centromere is close to middle; chromosome 5 is submetacentric because the centromere is set off from middle; chromosome 13 is acrocentric because the centromere is at or very near the end. **B,** During mitosis, the centromere divides and chromosomes move to opposite poles of cell. At the time of centromere division, the chromatids are designated chromosomes.

Box 4-1 Prenatal Diagnosis of Chromosome Abnormalities

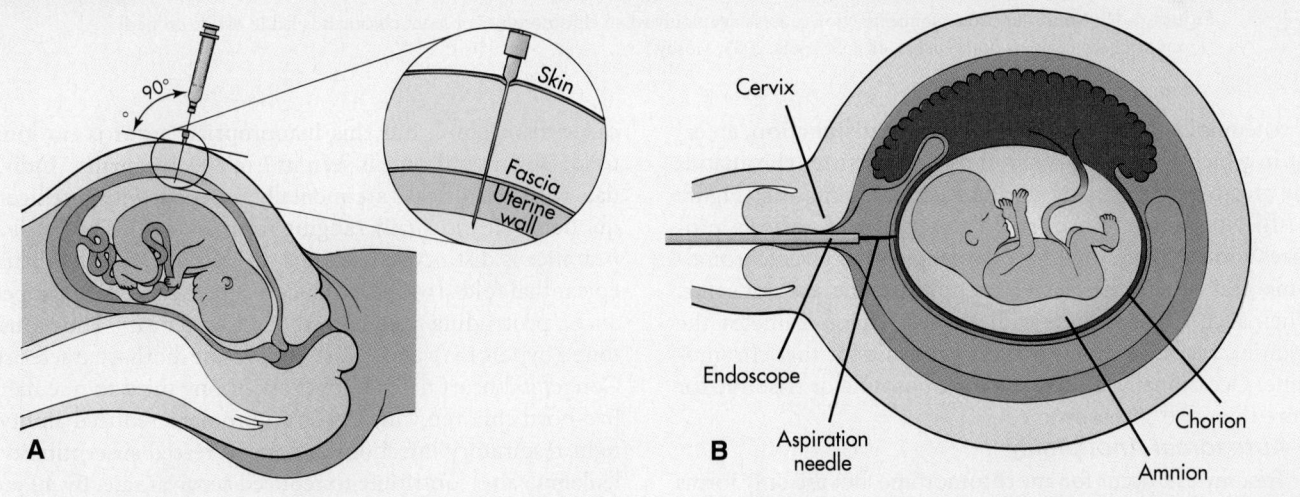

All the chromosome abnormalities discussed here can be detected prenatally, using a procedure called *amniocentesis (A)*. At about the sixteenth week of gestation, a sufficient amount of amniotic fluid is available to enable the withdrawal of a small amount of fluid (2 to 20 ml). This fluid contains live skin cells (fibroblasts) shed by the fetus. These cells can be cultured and karyotyped, and chromosome abnormalities can be detected.

Other disorders can be detected with this procedure. These include most neural tube defects, which cause an elevation of α-fetoprotein in the amniotic fluid, and several hundred diseases caused by mutations of single genes. The procedure involves a risk of losing the fetus, estimated to be about 0.5%. Thus amniocentesis is recommended only for pregnancies known to have an elevated risk for a genetic disease. These include pregnancies of women older than 35 years, in which the risk for Down syndrome and other aneuploidies is elevated, and pregnancies in which parents are known to carry translocations or certain disease genes.

One problem with prenatal diagnosis by amniocentesis is that by the time the sixteenth week of gestation is reached and another 2 or 3 weeks to culture the fibroblasts and test for genetic disease elapse, the mother is near the twentieth week of pregnancy. Pregnancy termination of an affected fetus at this stage can present serious emotional and personal dilemmas as well as some medical risk. For many parents, abortion would be more acceptable for a fetus at an earlier gestational age. A newer technique, *chorionic villus sampling (B)*, consists of extracting a small amount of villous tissue directly from the chorion. This procedure can be performed at 10 weeks' gestation and does not require in vitro culturing of cells because sufficient numbers are directly available in the extracted tissue. Thus the procedure allows prenatal diagnosis at about 2 months' gestation rather than at nearly 5 months' gestation. Chorionic villus sampling involves a slightly higher fetal loss rate than amniocentesis, approximately 1%.

Data from Wang BT et al: *Am J Med Genet* 53:307, 1994; illustrations from Pagana KD, Pagana TJ: *Mosby's manual of diagnostic and laboratory tests,* ed 2, St Louis, 2002, Mosby.

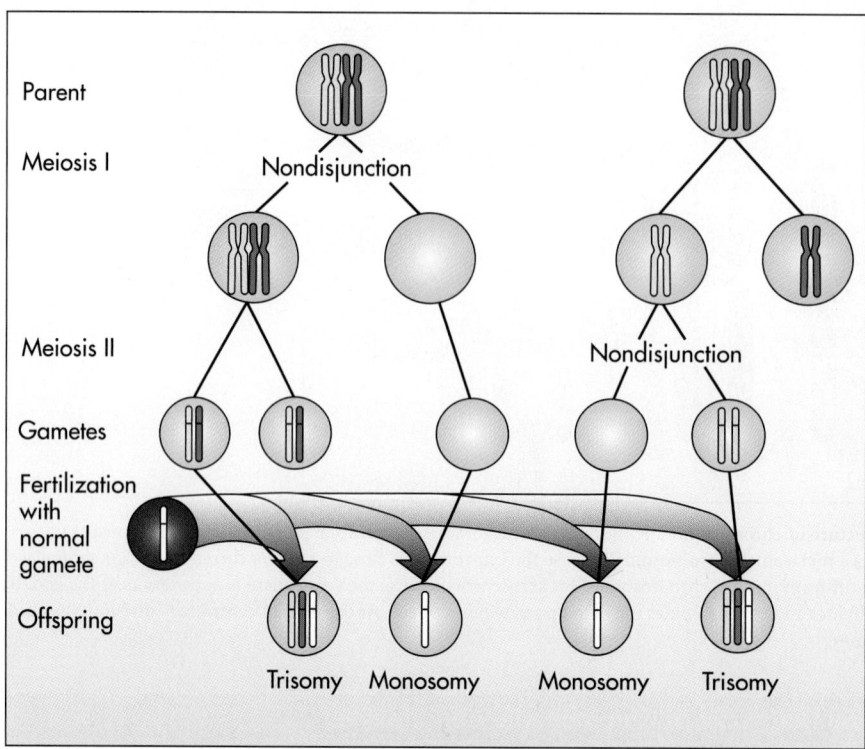

Figure 4-10 **Nondisjunction.** Nondisjunction causes aneuploidy when chromosomes or sister chromatids fail to divide properly. (From Jorde LB et al: *Medical genetics*, ed 3, St Louis, 2003, Mosby.)

Aneuploidy is usually the result of **nondisjunction,** an error in which homologous chromosomes or sister chromatids fail to separate normally during meiosis or mitosis (Figure 4-10). Nondisjunction during either stage of meiosis produces some gametes that have two copies of a given chromosome and others that have no copies of the chromosome. When such gametes unite with normal haploid gametes, the resulting zygote is monosomic or trisomic for that chromosome. Occasionally, a cell can be monosomic or trisomic for more than one chromosome.

Autosomal Aneuploidy

Trisomy can occur for any chromosome, but the only forms seen with an appreciable frequency in live births are trisomies of the thirteenth, eighteenth, or twenty-first chromosome. Fetuses with most other chromosomal trisomies do not survive to term. Trisomy 16, for example, is the most commonly known trisomy among abortuses, but it is not seen in live births.[4]

Partial trisomy, in which only an extra portion of a chromosome is present in each cell, also can occur. The consequences of partial trisomies are not as severe as those of complete trisomies. Trisomies also may occur in only some cells of the body. Individuals thus affected are said to be **chromosomal mosaics,** meaning that the body has two or more different cell lines, each of which has a different karyotype. Mosaics are usually formed by early mitotic nondisjunction occurring in one embryo cell but not in others.

The best-known example of aneuploidy in an autosome is trisomy of the twenty-first chromosome, which causes **Down syndrome** (named after J. Langdon Down, who first described the disease in 1866). Down syndrome was formerly called *mongolism,* but this inappropriate term is no longer used. Down syndrome is seen in 1 in 800 live births.[4] Individuals with this disease are mentally retarded, with intelligence quotients (IQs) usually ranging from 25 to 70. The facial appearance is distinctive (Figure 4-11), with a low nasal bridge, epicanthal folds (which produce a superficially Asian appearance), protruding tongue, and flat, low-set ears. Poor muscle tone (hypotonia) and short stature are both characteristic. Congenital heart defects affect about one third to one half of live-born children with Down syndrome; a reduced ability to fight respiratory infections and an increased susceptibility to leukemia also contribute to reduced survival rate. By 40 years of age, individuals with Down syndrome virtually always develop symptoms that are nearly identical to those of Alzheimer disease. About three fourths of fetuses known to have Down syndrome are spontaneously aborted or stillborn. About 20% of infants born with Down syndrome die during their first 10 years of life. For those who survive beyond 10 years, average life expectancy is now about 60 years.

About 97% of Down syndrome cases are caused by nondisjunction during the formation of one of the parent's gametes or during early embryonic development. The remaining 3% result from translocations (discussed later). In approximately 90% to 95% of cases, the nondisjunction occurs in the formation of the mother's egg cell. Paternal nondisjunction is responsible for the remaining cases. Among individuals with Down syndrome, about 1% are known to be mosaics. Because mosaics have a large number of normal cells, the effects of the trisomic cells are attenuated and symptoms are often less severe.

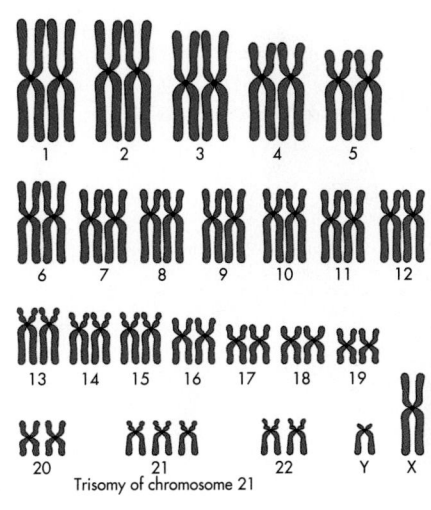

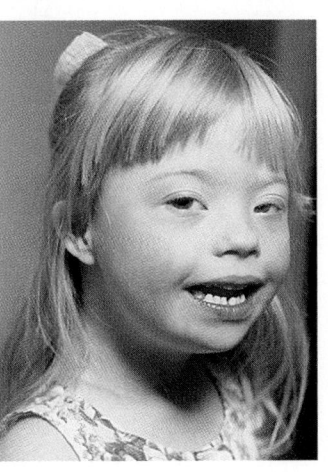

A   Trisomy of chromosome 21   **B**

Figure 4-11   **Down syndrome. A,** The karyotype of Down syndrome consists of 47 chromosomes and shows trisomy 21. **B,** A child with Down syndrome. (**A** from Damjanov I: *Pathology for the health-related professions,* ed 2, Philadelphia, 2000, Saunders; **B** courtesy A. Olney and M. MacDonald, University of Nebraska Medical Center, Omaha.)

The risk of having a child with Down syndrome increases greatly with maternal age. As Figure 4-12 demonstrates, women younger than 30 years have a risk ranging from about 1 in 1000 births to 1 in 2000 births. The risk begins to rise substantially after 35 years, and it reaches 3% to 5% for women older than 45 years. This dramatic increase in risk may be caused by the age of maternal egg cells, which are held in an arrested state of prophase I from the time they are formed in the female embryo until they are shed in ovulation. Thus an egg cell formed by a 45-year-old woman is itself 45 years old. This long suspended state may allow for the accumulation of errors leading to nondisjunction. The risk of Down syndrome, as well as other trisomies, does not appear to increase with paternal age.[6]

Sex Chromosome Aneuploidy

The incidence of sex chromosome aneuploidies is fairly high. Among live births, about 1 in 400 males and 1 in 650 females have a form of sex chromosome aneuploidy.[7] Because these conditions are generally less severe than autosomal aneuploidies, all forms except complete absence of an X chromosome allow at least some individuals to survive.

One of the most common sex chromosome aneuploidies, affecting about 1 in 1000 newborn females, is trisomy X. Instead of two X chromosomes, these females have three X chromosomes in each cell. Most of them have no overt physical abnormalities, although sterility, menstrual irregularity, or mental retardation is sometimes seen. Some females have four X chromosomes, and they are more often mentally retarded. Those with five or more X chromosomes generally have more severe mental retardation and various physical defects.

A condition that leads to somewhat more serious problems is the presence of a single X chromosome and no homologous X or Y chromosome, so the individual has a total of 45 chromosomes. The karyotype is designated 45,X, and it causes a set of symptoms known as **Turner syndrome** (Figure 4-13). Because they have no Y chromosomes, people with Turner syndrome are females. They are usually sterile, however, and have gonadal streaks rather than ovaries. These

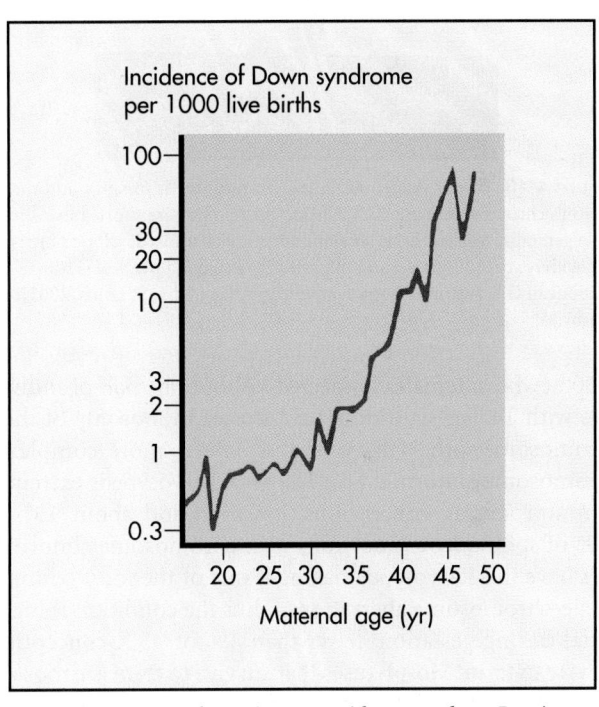

Figure 4-12   **Down syndrome increases with maternal age.** Rate is per 1000 live births related to maternal age.

streaks of connective tissue are susceptible to cancer in mosaics who have some cells containing a Y chromosome. Other features of the disorder include short stature, webbing of the neck in about half of cases, widely spaced nipples, coarctation (narrowing) of the aorta (in 15% to 20% of cases), edema of the feet in newborns, reduced carrying angle at the elbow (cubitus valgus), and sparse body hair. They are not considered retarded, although evidence indicates some impairment of spatial and mathematical reasoning ability. About three fourths of recognized 45,X conceptions inherit their X chromosome from the mother. Thus most cases are caused by a loss of the paternal X chromosome.

The frequency of Turner syndrome is low compared with that of other sex chromosome aneuploidies: only about 1 in

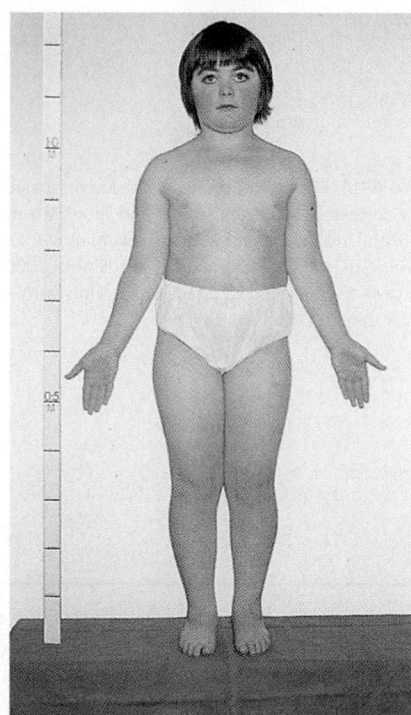

Figure 4-13 Turner syndrome. A sex chromosome is missing, and the person's chromosomes are 45,X. Characteristic signs are short stature, female genitalia, webbed neck, shieldlike chest with underdeveloped breasts and widely spaced nipples, and imperfectly developed ovaries. (From Thibodeau GA, Patton KT: *Anatomy & physiology,* ed 5, St Louis, 2003, Mosby.)

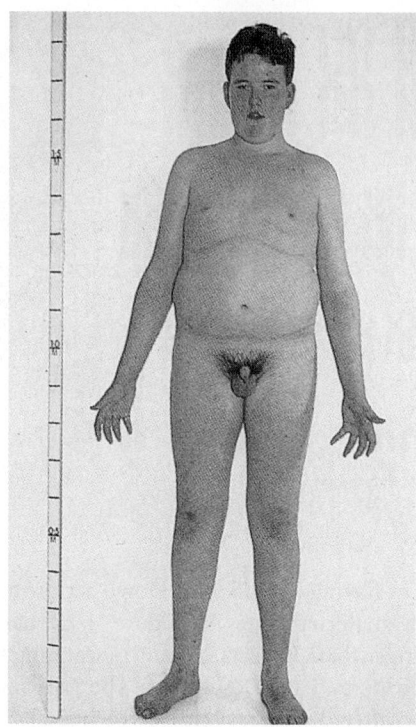

Figure 4-14 Klinefelter syndrome. This young man exhibits many characteristics of Klinefelter syndrome: small testes, some development of the breasts, sparse body hair, and long limbs. This syndrome results from the presence of two or more X chromosomes with one Y chromosome (genotypes XXY or XXXY, for example). (From Thibodeau GA, Patton KT: *Anatomy & physiology,* ed 5, St Louis, 2003, Mosby.)

3000 newborn females is affected.[8] About one half of individuals with Turner syndrome have simple monosomy of the X chromosome; others have one of several more complex X chromosome abnormalities. The 45,X karyotype is extremely common among conceptions, however, and about 15% to 20% of spontaneous abortions with chromosome abnormalities have this karyotype, making it one of the most common single-chromosome aberrations. Thus the condition is highly lethal during gestation: fewer than 1% of 45,X conceptions survive to term. Most fetuses that survive to term are mosaics, with combinations of 45,X cells and XX, XXX, or XY cells. It is likely that the presence of some normal cells in mosaic fetuses enhances fetal survival.

Teenagers with Turner syndrome are typically treated with estrogen to promote the development of secondary sexual characteristics. The dose is then continued at a reduced level to maintain these characteristics and to help avoid osteoporosis.

Individuals with at least two X chromosomes and a Y chromosome in each cell (47,XXY karyotype) have a disorder known as **Klinefelter syndrome** (Figure 4-14). Because of the presence of a Y chromosome, these individuals have a male appearance, but they are usually sterile, and about half develop female-like breasts (a condition called *gynecomastia*). The testes are small, body hair is sparse, the voice is often somewhat high pitched, stature is elevated, and a moderate degree of mental impairment may be present. Klinefelter syndrome is found in about 1 in 1000 male births. About two thirds of the cases are caused by nondisjunction of the X chromosomes in the

mother, and the frequency of the disorder rises with maternal age. Individuals with the XXXY and XXXXY karyotypes also are considered to have Klinefelter syndrome, and the degree of physical and mental impairment increases with each additional X chromosome. Regardless of the number of X chromosomes, however, these individuals have a male appearance. The presence of a single Y chromosome, which causes the undifferentiated gonads to become testes, always produces a male. Mosaicism is sometimes seen in Klinefelter syndrome; the most prevalent combination is XXY and XY cells.

The other sex chromosome aneuploidy that affects males is the 47,XYY karyotype. Individuals with this karyotype tend to be taller than average, and they have a 10- to 15-point reduction in average IQ. This condition, which causes few serious physical problems, achieved notoriety when it was found that its incidence in prison populations was about 1 in 30 (compared with 1 in 1000 in the general male population). This discovery led to the suggestion that this chromosome might predispose affected individuals to violent, criminal behavior. Several dozen studies have addressed this issue, and they have shown that XYY males are not inclined to commit violent crimes. However, even after adjusting for the effects of decreased IQ, some evidence exists for an increased incidence of behavioral disorders.

Abnormalities of Chromosome Structure

In addition to the loss or gain of whole chromosomes, parts of chromosomes can be lost or duplicated as gametes are formed, and the arrangement of genes on chromosomes can

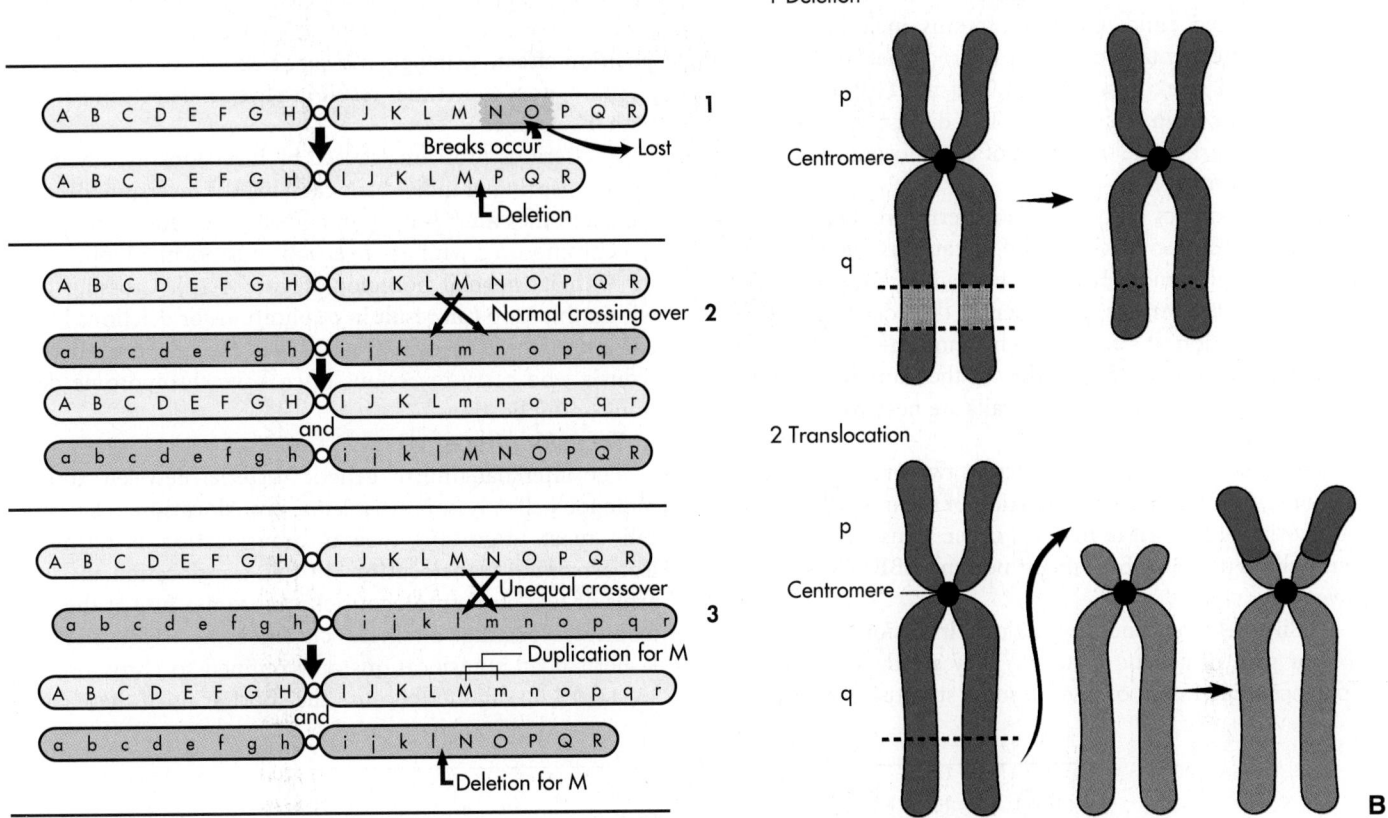

Figure 4-15 Abnormalities of chromosome structure. **A,** *(1)* Deletion occurs when a chromosome segment is lost; *(2)* normal crossing over; and *(3)* generation of duplication and deletion through unequal crossing over. **B,** Structural chromosomal abnormalities: *(1)* deletion and *(2)* translocation. (**B** from Damjanov I: *Pathology for the health-related professions,* ed 2, Philadelphia, 2000, Saunders.)

be altered. Unlike aneuploidy and polyploidy, these changes sometimes do not have serious consequences for an individual's health. Some of them can even go entirely unnoticed, especially when very small pieces of chromosomes are involved. Nevertheless, abnormalities of chromosome structure also can produce serious disease in individuals or their offspring.

During meiosis and mitosis, chromosomes usually maintain their structural integrity very well, but **chromosome breakage** occasionally does occur. Mechanisms exist to "heal" these breaks, and generally the break is repaired perfectly with no damage resulting to the daughter cell. Sometimes, however, the breaks remain, or they heal in a fashion that alters the structure of the chromosome. The extent of chromosome breakage is increased in the presence of certain harmful agents, called **clastogens.** Identified clastogens include ionizing radiation, some viral infections, and certain chemicals.

Deletions

Broken chromosomes and loss of DNA cause **deletions** (Figure 4-15). Usually a gamete with a deletion unites with a normal gamete to form a zygote. The zygote thus has one chromosome with the normal complement of genes and one with some missing genes. Because a fairly large number of genes can be lost in a deletion, serious consequences can result even though one chromosome is normal. The most often cited example of a disease caused by a chromosomal deletion is the **cri du chat syndrome** (Figure 4-16). The term, which

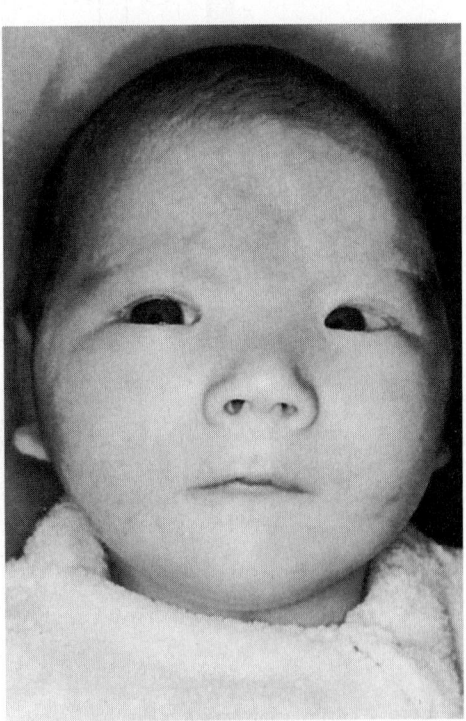

Figure 4-16 Infant with cri du chat syndrome. Syndrome is caused by deletion of part of the short arm of chromosome 5. (From Thompson MW, McInnes RR, Willard HF: *Genetics in medicine,* ed 5, Philadelphia, 1991, Saunders.)

literally means "cry of the cat," describes the characteristic cry of the affected child. Other symptoms include low birth weight, severe mental retardation, microcephaly (smaller than normal head size), heart defects, and the typical facial appearance shown in Figure 4-16. The disease is caused by a deletion of part of the short arm of chromosome 5.

Duplications

Duplications of chromosome material are, like deletions, a form of chromosome aberration. Because a deficiency of genetic material is more harmful than an excess, duplications usually have less serious consequences than deletions. For example, a deletion of a region of chromosome 5 causes cri du chat syndrome, but a duplication of the same region causes mental retardation but physical traits are nearly normal.

Inversions

An **inversion** is the occurrence of two breaks on a chromosome, followed by the reinsertion of the missing fragment at its original site but in inverted order. Thus a chromosome symbolized as ABCDEFG might become ABEDCFG after an inversion.

Unlike deletions and duplications, inversions result in no loss or gain of genetic material. They are thus said to be a "balanced" alteration of chromosome structure, and they of-

ten have no apparent physical effect. Genes are sometimes influenced by neighboring DNA sequences, however, and this **position effect,** a change in a gene's expression caused by its position, does sometimes result in physical defects in persons with inversions.

The serious problems caused by inversions usually occur in the offspring of individuals carrying the inversion. Because chromosomes must line up in perfect order during prophase I, a chromosome with an inversion must form a loop to line up with its normal homolog (Figure 4-17). Crossing over within this loop can result in duplications or deletions in the chromosomes of daughter cells. Thus the offspring of individuals who carry inversions often have chromosome deletions or duplications.

Translocations

The interchanging of genetic material between nonhomologous chromosomes is called **translocation.** The clinically most important type of translocation is termed a **Robertsonian translocation.** In this translocation the long arms of two nonhomologous chromosomes fuse at the centromere, forming a single chromosome (Figure 4-18). Robertsonian translocations are confined to chromosomes 13, 14, 15, 21, and 22 because the short arms of these chro-

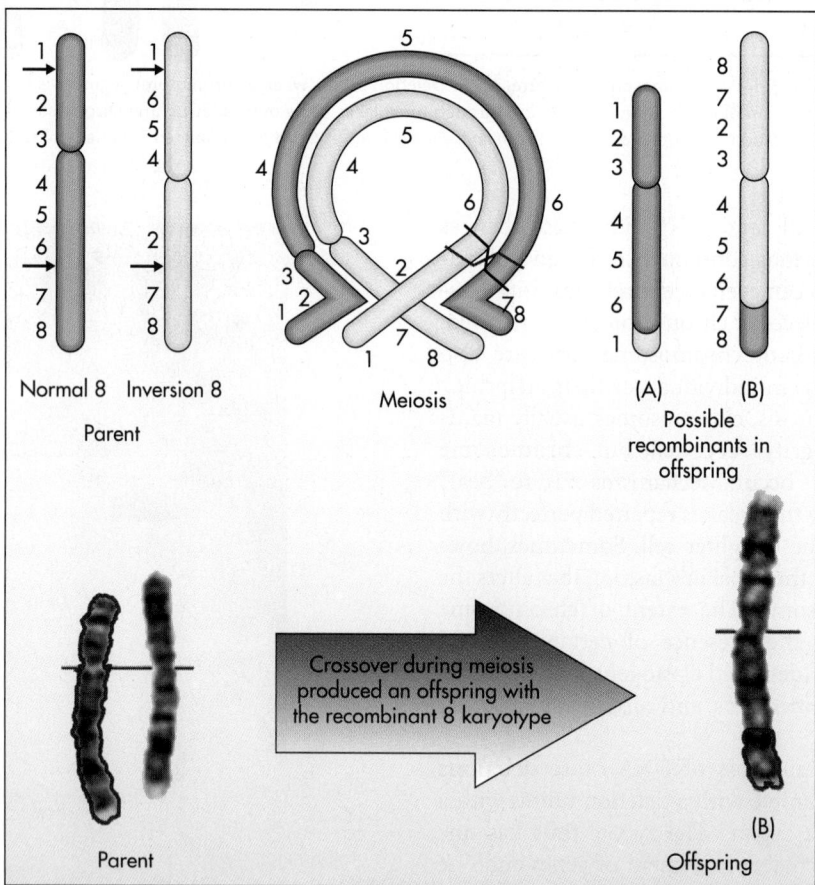

Figure 4-17 Inversion loop. A pericentric inversion (i.e., inversion does not involve centromere) in chromosome 8 causes the formation of a loop during the alignment of homologous chromosomes in meiosis Crossing over in this loop can produce duplications of deletions of chromosome material in the resulting gamete. The offspring in the lower panel received one of the recombinant 8 chromosomes from this parent. (From Jorde LB et al: *Medical genetics,* ed 3, St Louis, 2003, Mosby.)

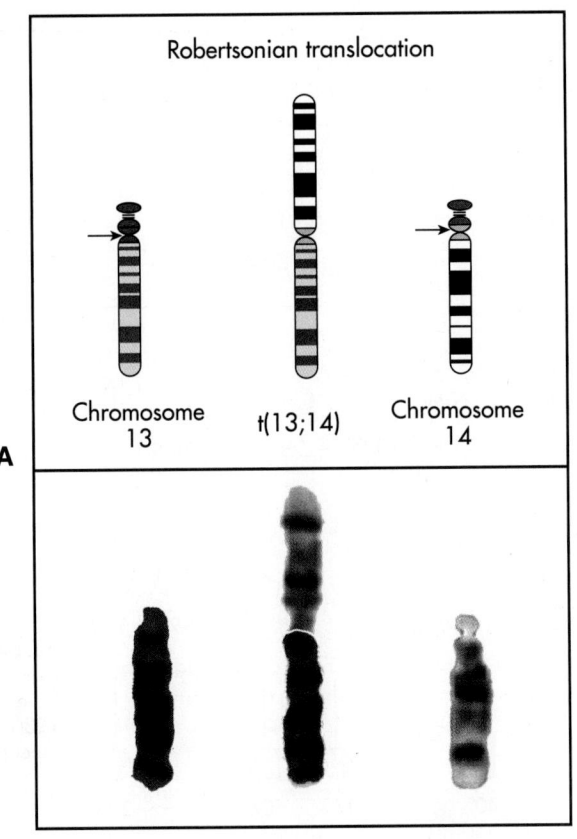

A

Figure 4-18 Translocation. **A,** In a Robertsonian translocation, shown here, the long arms of two acrocentric chromosomes (13 and 14) fuse, forming a single chromosome. **B,** The possible segregation patterns for gametes formed by a carrier of a Robertsonian translocation. Alternate segregation (quadrant a alone, or quadrant b with quadrant c) produces either a normal chromosome constitution or a translocation carrier with a normal phenotype. Adjacent segregation (quadrant a with c, quadrant c alone, quadrant a with b, or quadrant b alone) produces unbalanced gametes and results in conceptions with translocation Down syndrome, monosomy 21, trisomy 14, or monosomy 14, respectively. For example, monosomy 14 is produced when the parent who carries the translocation transmits a copy of chromosome 21 but does not transmit a copy of chromosome 14 (as in the lower right corner). (From Jorde LB et al: *Medical genetics*, ed 3, St. Louis, 2003, Mosby.)

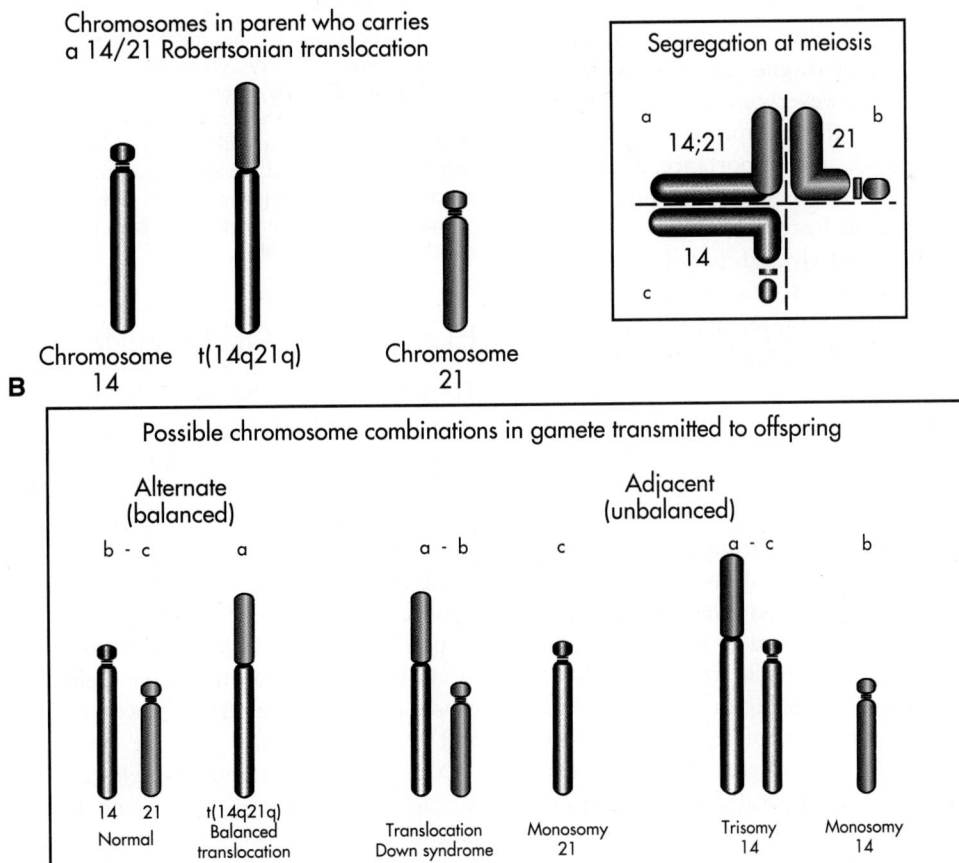

B

mosomes are very small and contain no essential genetic material. When a Robertsonian translocation takes place, the short arms are usually lost during subsequent cell divisions. Because the carriers of Robertsonian translocations lose no important genetic material, they are normal, although they have only 45 chromosomes in each cell. Their offspring, however, may have serious deletions or duplications (Figure 4-18). For example, a common Robertsonian translocation involves the fusion of the long arms of chromosomes 21 and 14. An offspring who inherits a gamete carrying the fused chromosome receives an extra copy of the long arm of chromosome 21 and thus develops Down syndrome. Robertsonian translocations are responsible for approximately 3% to 5% of Down syndrome cases. Parents who carry a Robertsonian translocation involving chromosome 21 have an increased risk for producing multiple offspring with Down syndrome.

A **reciprocal translocation** occurs when breaks take place in two different chromosomes and the material is exchanged. As with Robertsonian translocations, the carrier of a reciprocal translocation is usually normal because the individual has a normal complement of genetic material. However, the carrier's gametes can be normal, can carry the translocation, or can have duplications and deletions.

Fragile Sites

For reasons not yet fully understood, a number of areas on chromosomes develop distinctive breaks and gaps (observable microscopically) when the cells are cultured in a folate-deficient medium. Most of these **fragile sites** have no apparent relationship to disease. However, one particular fragile site, located on the long arm of the X chromosome, is associated with a disorder of considerable importance, both clinically and genetically. This disorder is known as the *fragile X syndrome*. The most important feature of this syndrome is mental retardation. With a relatively high population prevalence (affecting approximately 1 in 4000 males and 1 in 8000 females), the fragile X syndrome is the second most common genetic cause of mental retardation (after Down syndrome).

Fragile X syndrome involves a puzzling pattern of inheritance. In particular, males who inherit the mutation do not necessarily express the disease condition but they can pass it on to descendants who do express it. Ordinarily, a male who inherits a disease gene on the X chromosome expresses the condition because he has only one X chromosome. Another uncommon feature of this disease is that about one third of carrier females are affected, although less severely than males. Many mechanisms have been proposed to account for the complex mode of inheritance of the fragile X syndrome. It has been shown that unaffected transmitting males have an elevated number (more than about 50) of repeated DNA sequences in the first exon of the fragile X gene. These "repeats" consist of CGG sequences that are duplicated again and again. Affected males have a much larger number of these repeats—200 or more[9] (Figure 4-19). An increase in the number of these repeated sequences in successive generations can lead to expression of the fragile X syndrome. More than 20 other genetic diseases also are caused by this mechanism.[10,11]

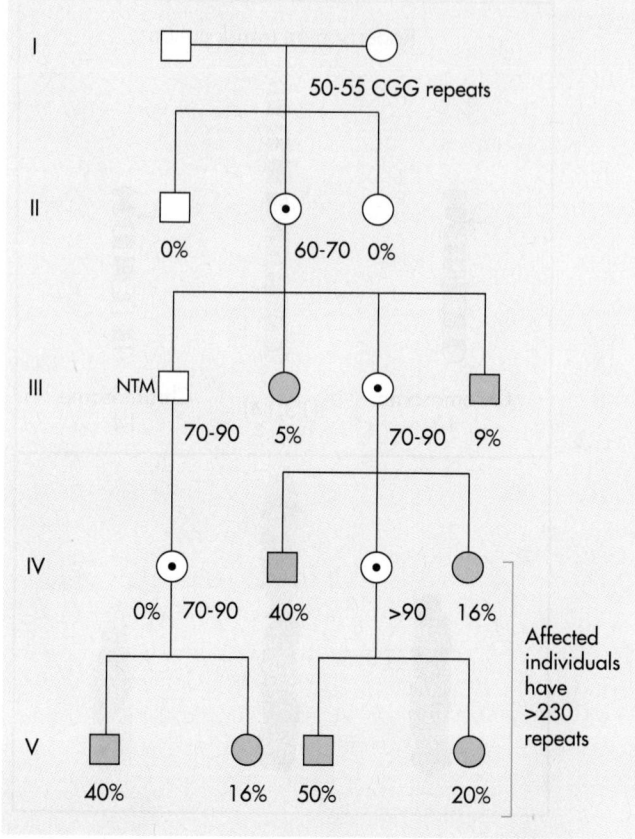

Figure 4-19 A pedigree showing the inheritance of the fragile X syndrome. Females who carry a premutation (50 to 320 CGG repeats) are dotted. Affected individuals are represented by solid symbols. A normal transmitting male (NTM), who carries a premutation of 70 to 90 repeats increases each time the mutation is passed through another female. Also, only 5% of the NTM's sisters are affected, and only 9% of his brothers are affected, but 40% of his grandsons and 16% of his granddaughters are affected. This is the Sherman paradox. (From Jorde LB et al: *Medical genetics*, ed 3, St Louis, 2003, Mosby.)

ELEMENTS OF FORMAL GENETICS

The mechanisms by which an individual's set of paired chromosomes produces traits are the principles of genetic inheritance. Mendel's work with garden peas first defined these principles. Later geneticists have refined Mendel's work to explain patterns of inheritance for traits and diseases that appear in families.

Analysis of traits that occur with defined, predictable patterns has helped geneticists link the pieces of the human gene map. Current research focuses on assigning genes to specific locations on chromosomes. Eventually, diseases and defects caused by single genes can be traced, and therapies to prevent and treat such diseases can be developed.

Many traits are caused by single genes and are often called *mendelian traits* (after Gregor Mendel). Each gene occupies a position along a chromosome known as a **locus.** The genes at a particular locus can take different forms (i.e., they can be composed of different nucleotide sequences). These different forms are called **alleles.** For example, most people have a type of hemoglobin known as *hemoglobin A.* A few individuals have an alternative form of hemoglobin, termed *hemoglobin S*, which differs from hemoglobin A by a single amino acid substitution in the beta-globin component of the molecule. The beta-globin locus thus has two different alleles, one that encodes hemoglobin A and another that encodes hemoglobin S. A locus that has two or more alleles that occur with an appreciable frequency in a population is said to be **polymorphic** or a **polymorphism.**

Because humans are diploid organisms, each chromosome is represented twice, with one member of the chromosome pair contributed by the father and one by the mother. At a given locus an individual has one gene whose origin is paternal and one whose origin is maternal. When the two genes are identical, the individual is **homozygous** at that locus. When the genes are not identical, the individual is **heterozygous** at the locus.

Phenotype and Genotype

The composition of genes at a given locus is known as the **genotype.** The outward appearance of an individual, which is the result of both genotype and environment, is the **phenotype.** For example, an infant who is born with an inability to metabolize the amino acid phenylalanine has the single-gene disorder known as *phenylketonuria (PKU)* and thus has the PKU genotype. If the condition is left untreated, abnormal metabolites of phenylalanine will begin to accumulate in the infant's brain and irreversible mental retardation will occur. Mental retardation is thus one aspect of the PKU phenotype. By imposing dietary restrictions to limit the intake of food containing phenylalanine, however, retardation can be prevented. Although the child still has the PKU genotype, a modification of the environment (in this case the child's diet) produces an outwardly normal phenotype.

Dominance and Recessiveness

In many loci the effects of one allele mask those of another when the two are found together in a **heterozygote.** The allele whose effects are observable is said to be **dominant.** The allele whose effects are hidden is said to be **recessive** (from the Latin root for "hiding"). Traditionally, for loci having two alleles, the dominant allele is denoted by an uppercase letter and the recessive allele is denoted by a lowercase letter. When one allele is dominant over another, the heterozygote genotype *Aa* has the same phenotype as the dominant homozygote *AA*. For the recessive allele to be expressed, it must exist in the **homozygote** form, *aa*.

When the heterozygote is distinguishable from both homozygotes, the locus is said to exhibit **codominance.** For example, in the MN blood group, both alleles, *M* and *N*, of the heterozygote are detectable and therefore codominant. Another example is the ABO blood group, in which heterozygotes having the *A* and *B* alleles express both of them as A and B antigens on their red cells (forming blood group AB).

A **carrier** is an individual who has a disease gene but is phenotypically normal. Most genes for recessive diseases occur in heterozygotes who carry one copy of the gene but do not express the disease. Because many recessive genes are lethal in the homozygous state, they are eliminated from the population when they occur in homozygotes. By "hiding" in carriers, however, most recessive genes for diseases survive to be passed on to the next generation.

TRANSMISSION OF GENETIC DISEASES

An important aspect of a genetic disease is the pattern in which it is inherited through the generations of a family, or its **mode of inheritance.** Once the mode of inheritance is known, much can be learned about the disease gene itself and reliable genetic counseling can be given to members of families in which the disease is present (see Chapter 5).

Modes of inheritance were systematically studied by Gregor Mendel, who formulated two basic laws of inheritance. His **principle of segregation** states that homologous genes separate from one another during reproduction and that each reproductive cell carries only one of the homologous genes. Mendel's second law, the **principle of independent assortment,** states that the hereditary transmission of one gene has no effect on the transmission of another. Mendel discovered these laws in the mid-nineteenth century by performing breeding experiments with garden peas. He had no knowledge of chromosomes. Early in the twentieth century geneticists found that the behavior of chromosomes does essentially correspond to Mendel's laws, which now form the basis for the **chromosome theory of inheritance.**

The known single-gene diseases can be classified into four major modes of inheritance: autosomal dominant, autosomal recessive, X-linked dominant, and X-linked recessive. The first two types involve genes known to occur on the 22 pairs of autosomes. The last two types occur on the X chromosome; no good documentation exists of disease genes occurring on the Y chromosome. The number of diseases assigned to each category is growing rapidly. Current catalogs of single-gene traits, which include disease-producing and nonclinical traits (e.g., attached earlobes), list 14,321 known autosomal traits and 856 X-linked traits.[1]

An important tool in the analysis of modes of inheritance is the **pedigree** chart. It summarizes family relationships and shows which members of a family are affected by a genetic disease (Figure 4-20). Generally, the pedigree begins with one individual in the family, the **proband,** also termed the **propositus** (male) or **proposita** (female). This individual is usually the first person in the family diagnosed or seen in a clinic.

Autosomal Dominant Inheritance
Characteristics of Pedigrees

Diseases caused by autosomal dominant genes are rare. The most common occur in fewer than 1 in 500 individuals, so it is uncommon for two individuals both affected by the same autosomal dominant disease to produce offspring together. Figure 4-21, *A*, illustrates this unusual pattern. More often, affected offspring are produced by the union of a normal

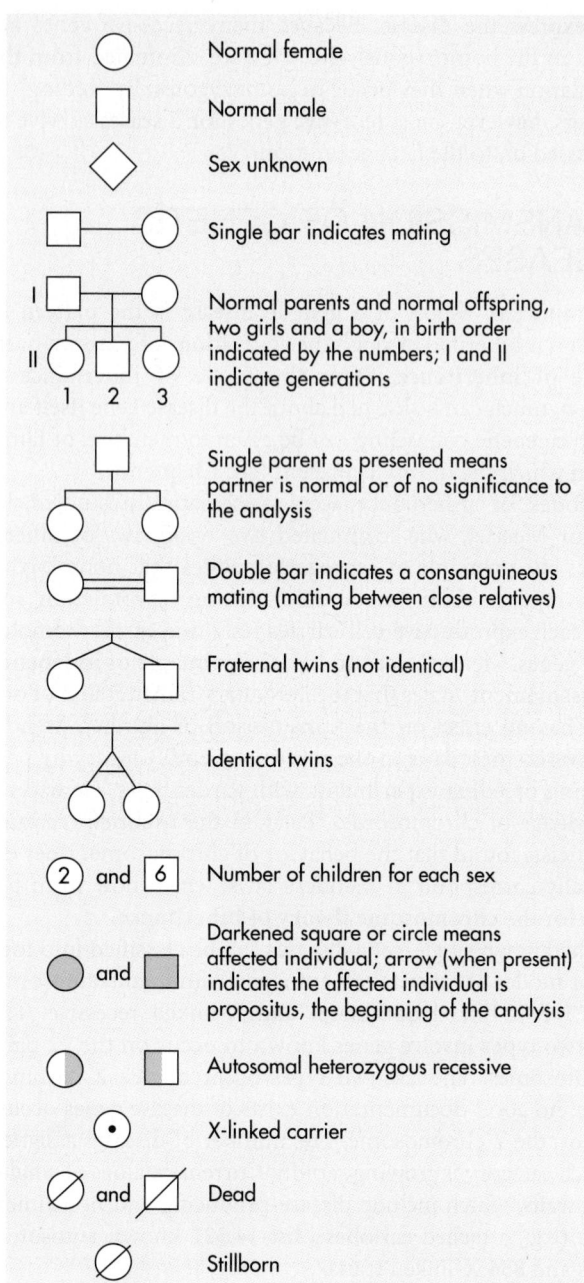

Figure 4-20 Symbols commonly used in pedigrees.

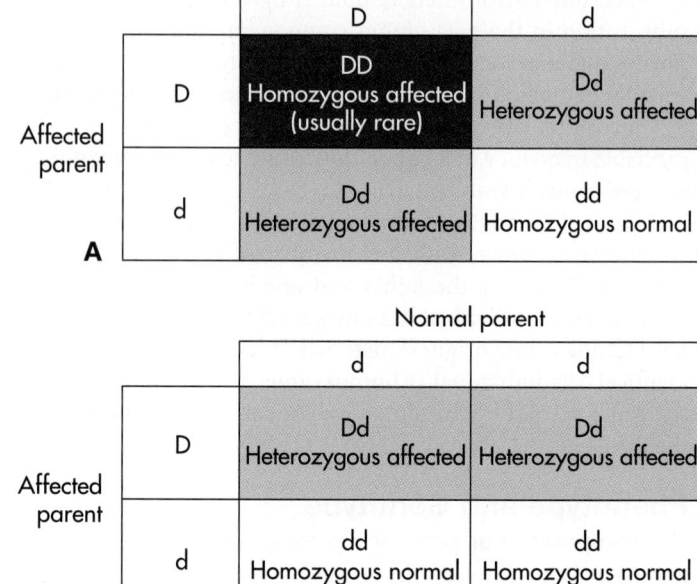

Figure 4-21 Punnett square and autosomal dominant traits. **A,** Punnett square for the mating of two individuals with an autosomal dominant gene. Here both parents are affected by the trait. **B,** Punnett square for the mating of a normal individual with a carrier for an autosomal dominant gene.

2. There is no skipping of generations. If an individual has achondroplasia, one parent must also have it. If neither parent has the trait, none of the children has it (with the exception of new mutations, as discussed later).
3. Affected heterozygous individuals transmit the trait to approximately half of their children, but because gamete transmission is subject to chance fluctuations, it is possible that all or none of the children of an affected parent may have the trait. When large numbers of matings of this type are studied, however, the proportion of affected children will closely approach one half.

Recurrence Risks

Parents at risk for producing children with a genetic disease nearly always ask the question, "What is the *chance* that our child will have this disease?" When one child has already been born with a genetic disease, the parents can be given a **recurrence risk,** which is the probability that subsequent children also will have the disease. If the parents have not yet had children but are known to be at risk for having children with a genetic disease, an **occurrence risk** (the probability that a child will have a specific disease) can be given. When one parent is affected by an autosomal dominant disease (and is a heterozygote) and the other is normal, the occurrence and recurrence risks for each child are one half.

An important principle is that each birth is an independent event, much like a coin toss. Thus, even though parents may already have had a child with the disease, their recurrence risk remains one half. Even if they have had several children, all affected (or all unaffected) by the disease, the law of independence dictates that the probability that their next child will have the disease is still one half. Parents' misunder-

parent with an affected heterozygous parent. The diagram (Punnett square) in Figure 4-21 illustrates this mating. The affected parent can pass either a disease gene or a normal gene to his or her children. Each event has a probability of 0.5; thus on the average, half of the children will be heterozygous and will express the disease and half will be normal.

Figure 4-22, *A*, is a typical pedigree showing the transmission of an autosomal dominant gene. The gene shown here causes achondroplasia (Figure 4-22, *B*). Several important characteristics of this pedigree support the conclusion that the trait is caused by an autosomal dominant gene:

1. The two sexes exhibit the trait in approximately equal proportions, and males and females are equally likely to transmit the trait to their offspring.

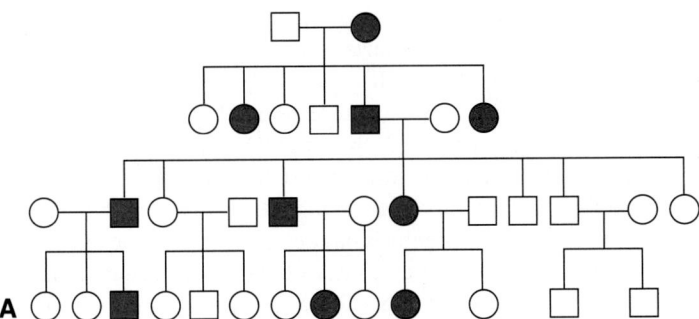

A

Figure 4-22 Pedigree for achondroplasia. **A,** Pedigree showing the transmission of an autosomal dominant disease. **B,** Achondroplasia. This girl has short limbs relative to trunk length. She also has a prominent forehead, low nasal root, and redundant skin folds in the arms and legs. (**B** from Jorde LB et al: *Medical genetics,* ed 3, St Louis, 2003, Mosby.)

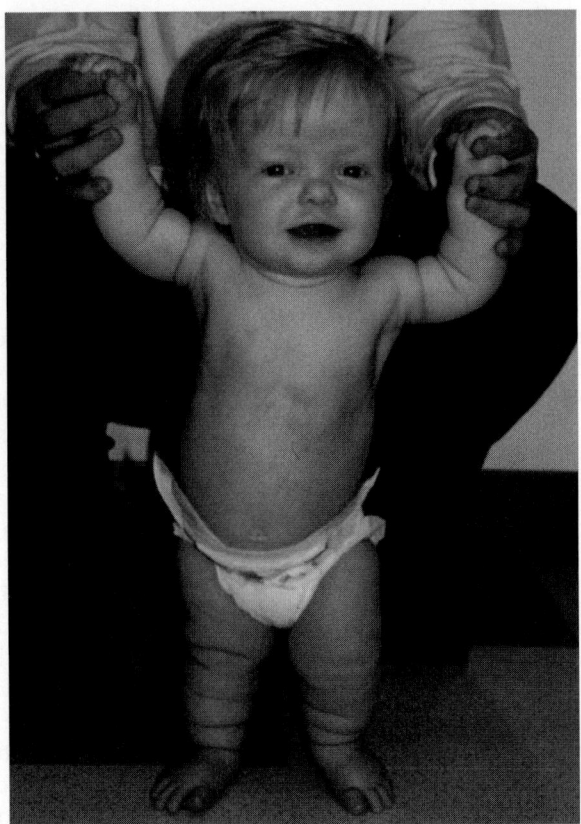

B

standing of this principle is a common problem encountered in genetic counseling.

If a child has been born with an autosomal dominant disease and there is no history of the disease in the family, the child is probably the product of a new mutation. The gene transmitted by one of the parents has thus undergone a mutation from a normal to a disease-causing allele. The genes at this locus in most of the parent's other germ cells would still be normal. In this situation the recurrence risk for the parent's subsequent offspring is not greater than that of the general population. The offspring of the affected child, however, will have an occurrence risk of one half. Because these diseases often reduce the potential for reproduction, a large proportion of the observed cases of many autosomal dominant diseases are the result of new mutations. For example, approximately seven eighths of all cases of achondroplasia are caused by new mutations.

Occasionally, two or more offspring will present symptoms of an autosomal dominant disease when there is no family history of the disease. Because mutation is a rare event, it is unlikely that this disease would be a result of multiple mutations in the same family. The mechanism most likely to be responsible is termed **germline mosaicism.** During the embryonic development of one of the parents, a mutation occurred that affected all or part of the germline but few or none of the somatic cells of the embryo. Thus the parent carries the mutation in his or her germline but does not actually express the disease. As a result, the unaffected parent can transmit the mutation to multiple offspring. This phenome-

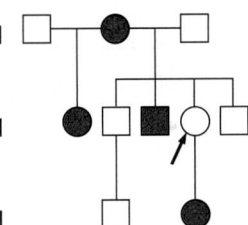

Figure 4-23 Pedigree for retinoblastoma showing incomplete penetrance. Female with marked arrow in line II must be heterozygous, but she does not express the trait.

non, although relatively rare, can have significant effects on recurrence risks.[12]

Penetrance and Expressivity

An important variation seen in some autosomal dominant diseases is incomplete penetrance. The **penetrance** of a trait is the percentage of individuals with a specific genotype who also exhibit the expected phenotype. Incomplete penetrance means that individuals who have the gene for a disease may not exhibit the disease phenotype at all, even though the gene and the associated disease may be transmitted to the next generation. A pedigree illustrating the transmission of an autosomal dominant gene with incomplete penetrance is given in Figure 4-23. Retinoblastoma, the most common malignant eye tumor affecting children, is one disease that typically exhibits incomplete penetrance. About 10% of the individuals who are **obligate carriers** of the gene (i.e., those who have an affected parent and affected children and therefore must themselves carry the gene) do not have the disease. The penetrance of the gene is then said to be 90%.

The gene responsible for retinoblastoma has been mapped to the long arm of chromosome 13, and its DNA sequence has been studied extensively. This gene is known as a **tumor-suppressor gene:** the normal function of its protein product is to regulate the cell cycle so that cells do not grow uncontrollably. When a mutation alters the protein, its tumor-suppressing capacity is lost and a tumor can form[13,14] (see Chapters 11 and 19).

Another well-known autosomal dominant diseases is Huntington disease, a neurologic disorder whose main features are progressive dementia and increasingly uncontrollable movements of the limbs (discussed further in Chapter 17). The latter is known as chorea (Greek *khoreia* = dance), and the disease was formerly called *Huntington chorea.*

One of the key features of this disease is that symptoms are not usually seen until age 40 years or later, a pattern known as **age-dependent** penetrance. Thus those persons who develop the disease often have had children before they are aware that they have the gene. If the disease were present at birth, nearly all affected persons would die before reaching reproductive age, and the occurrence of the gene in the population would be much lower. From the gene's "point of view," a delayed age of onset is quite advantageous. An individual whose parent has the disease has a 50% chance of developing it during middle age. He or she is thus confronted with a tortuous question: "Should I have children, knowing that there is a 50:50 chance that I may have this disease gene and pass it to half my children?" Age-dependent penetrance characterizes a number of important genetic diseases, including familial breast cancer, hemochromatosis, and polycystic kidney disease.

Most genetic diseases exhibit variable expressivity. **Expressivity** is the extent of variation in phenotype associated with a particular genotype. If expressivity of a disease is variable, the penetrance may be complete but the severity of the disease can vary greatly. A well-known example of variable expressivity in an autosomal dominant disease is type 1 neurofibromatosis, or von Recklinghausen disease. The gene that causes neurofibromatosis has been mapped to the long arm of chromosome 17, and studies of its DNA sequence indicate that it, like the retinoblastoma gene, is a tumor-suppressor gene.[15] This disease is sometimes called the *elephant man's disease.* However, Joseph Merrick, the man to whom this term was originally applied, probably had a rare disorder called *Proteus syndrome.* The expression of this gene can vary from a few harmless café-au-lait spots ("coffee with milk," describing the light-brown color) on the skin to numerous malignant neurofibromas, scoliosis, seizures, gliomas, neuromas, hypertension, and learning disabilities (Figure 4-24).

A parent with mild expression of the disease—so mild that he or she is not aware of it—can transmit the gene to a child, who can then exhibit severe expression of the disease. As with incomplete penetrance, variable expressivity provides a mechanism by which autosomal dominant genes can be maintained at higher prevalence rates in populations.

Several factors can cause variation in expressivity. Genes at other loci can sometimes modify the expression of a disease gene (these are termed *modifier genes*). Environmental factors also can influence the expression of a disease gene. Finally, different types of mutations at a locus can cause variation in severity. For example, a base substitution resulting in a single amino acid change usually produces a mild form of the clotting

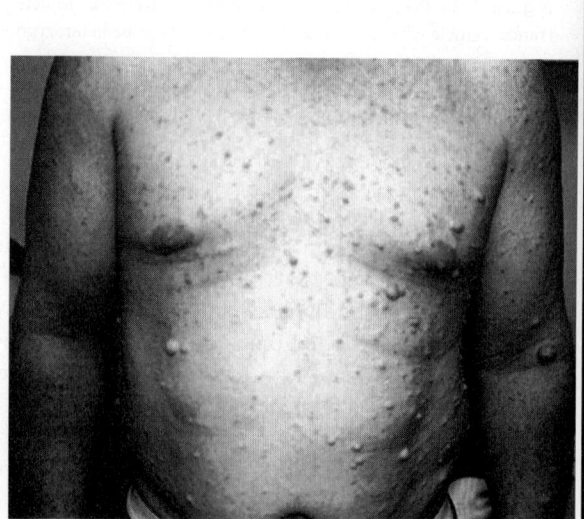
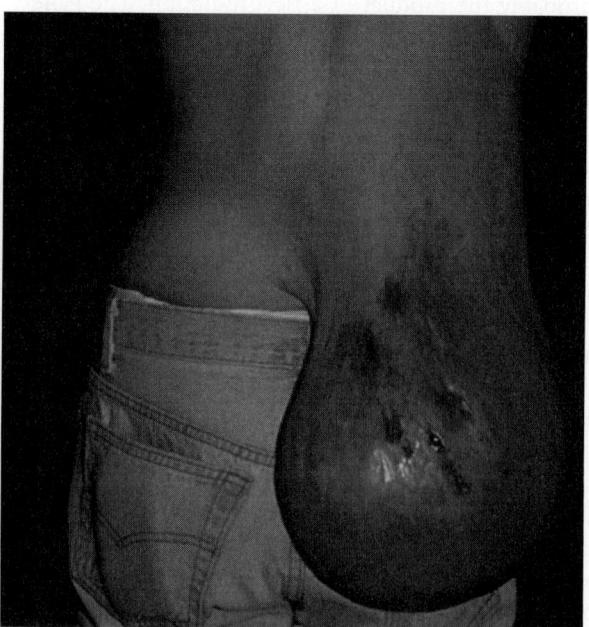

Figure 4-24 Neurofibromatosis. A, Young adult with multiple dermal neurofibromas of the trunk. Note also a café-au-lait spot in right upper abdomen. **B,** Individual has a large plexiform neurofibroma hanging from lower right back, causing considerable inconvenience and discomfort (substantially improved by surgical removal of tumor). (From Jorde LB et al: *Medical genetics,* ed 3, St Louis, 2003, Mosby. **B** courtesy Dr. D. Viskochil, University of Utah Health Sciences Center.)

disorder hemophilia A (Box 4-2). A base substitution resulting in a "stop" codon (and thus premature termination of translation) usually produces a more severe form of hemophilia A.

Genomic Imprinting

Mendel's experimental work with garden peas established that the phenotype is the same whether a given allele is inherited from the mother or the father. Indeed, this principle has been part of the central dogma of genetics. Recently, however, it has become increasingly apparent that this principle does

not always hold. A striking example is given by a deletion on the long arm of chromosome 15 (15q11-q13). When the deleted chromosome is inherited from the father, the offspring manifest a disease known as *Prader-Willi syndrome*. This disease phenotype includes short stature, obesity, and hypogonadism. When the deleted chromosome is inherited from the mother, the offspring develop *Angelman syndrome*, which is characterized by mental retardation, seizures, and an ataxic gait. The deletions inherited from the father and the mother are cytogenetically indistinguishable.

Box 4-2   Hemophilia A and the Russian Revolution

The figure (partial pedigree for descendants of Queen Victoria) is one of the best-known disease pedigrees in existence. It shows the transmission of hemophilia A in the European royal families. This disease, often called a *bleeder syndrome,* is caused by a defect in one of the blood-clotting factors, factor VIII, and can cause severe hemorrhages. In this pedigree Queen Victoria of England was the first known carrier of the disease, and several of her male descendants were affected by it. One of the most historically significant consequences of this pedigree involves the hemophiliac Czarevich Alexis, son of Czar Nicholas II of Russia. Gregori Rasputin, the "mad monk,"

was reputedly the only person able to prevent the young boy's bleeding episodes and was thus able to gain considerable power over the royal family. Rasputin's destabilizing influence is thought to have hastened the 1917 Bolshevik revolution.

The Russian royal family was again touched by genetics. Modern DNA "fingerprints" and mitochondrial DNA sequence were used to prove that a mass burial near Ekaterinburg, Russia, contained the remains of most of the executed members of the czar's family.

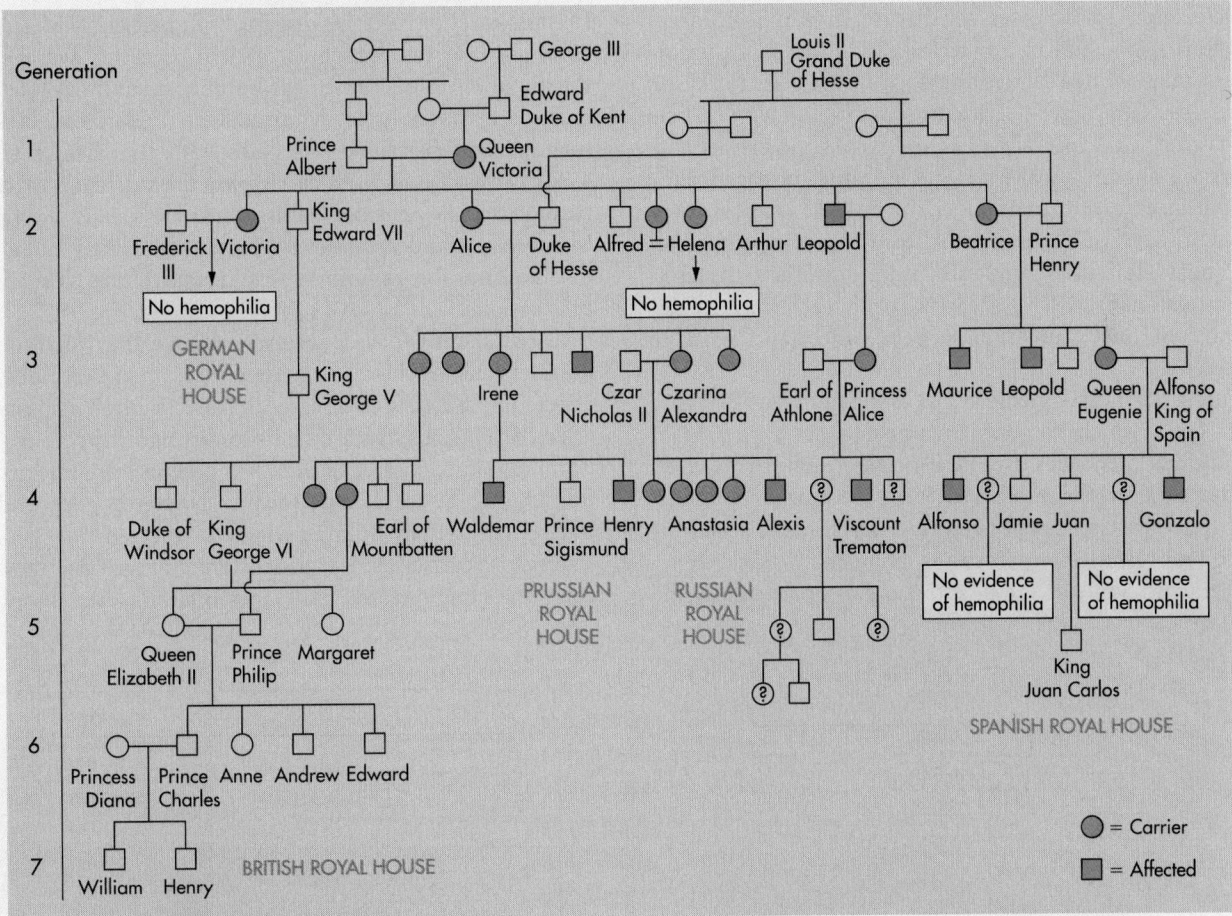

Partial pedigree for descendants of Queen Victoria, showing appearance of hemophilia A in one of her sons and in his descendants and in descendants of her daughters and granddaughters. Royal families of Prussia, Hesse, Battenberg (Mountbatten), Russia, and Spain were thus affected with the disease. The present royal family of England, however, is free of the disease, in spite of inbreeding.

What could cause these differences? The 3 to 4 Mb portion of chromosome 15 that is deleted in both syndromes is known as the "critical region." Within this region several genes are transcriptionally active only on the chromosome inherited from the father, and they are inactive on the chromosome inherited from the mother. Similarly, other genes are transcriptionally active only on the chromosome inherited from the mother and inactive on the chromosome inherited from the father. Thus several genes in the critical region are active on only one chromosome. If the single active copy of one of these genes is lost through a chromosome deletion, then no gene product is produced at all, and disease results. The differential activation of genes, depending on the parent from which they are inherited, is known as **genomic imprinting.** The transcriptionally inactive genes are said to be "imprinted" and their DNA is usually highly methylated. The activity level is associated with the degree of **methylation** of the gene (i.e., methyl groups are attached to the DNA sequences).

Autosomal Recessive Inheritance
Characteristics of Pedigrees

Like autosomal dominant diseases, those caused by autosomal recessive genes are rare in populations, although the number of carriers for recessive diseases can be high. The most common lethal recessive disease in white children, cystic fibrosis, occurs in about 1 in 2500 births. Approximately 1 in 25 whites carries one copy of the gene for cystic fibrosis (see Chapter 34). Because an individual must be homozygous for a recessive gene to express the disease, the carriers are phenotypically normal. Because most genes for recessive diseases are maintained in normal carriers, they are able to survive in the population from one generation to the next. As with many autosomal dominant diseases, many autosomal recessive diseases are characterized by delayed age of onset, incomplete penetrance, and variable expressivity.

Figure 4-25 shows a pedigree for cystic fibrosis. The cystic fibrosis gene, which has been mapped to the long arm of chromosome 7, encodes a protein product that forms chloride channels in the membranes of specialized epithelial cells.[17] Defective transport of chloride ions leads to a salt imbalance that results in secretions of abnormally thick, dehydrated mucus. Some of the digestive organs, particularly the pancreas, become obstructed, causing malnutrition, and the lungs become clogged with mucus, making them highly susceptible to bacterial infections (especially *Pseudomonas*). Death from lung disease or heart failure occurs on average by about 30 years of age. In the pedigree shown here, the two affected individuals are the offspring of the marriage of two first cousins. Marriage between related individuals, termed **consanguinity** (from the Latin root meaning "with blood"), is often a factor in producing children with recessive diseases because related individuals are more likely to share the same recessive genes. Consanguinity is seen most often in rare recessive diseases, because carriers of common recessive diseases have a fairly high probability of encountering one another just by chance.

Important criteria for discerning autosomal recessive inheritance include the following:

1. Males and females are affected in equal proportions.
2. Consanguinity is often present.
3. The disease is seen in siblings but usually not in their parents.
4. On the average, one fourth of the offspring of carrier parents will be affected.

Recurrence Risks

In most cases of recessive disease, both parents of affected individuals are heterozygous carriers. On the average, one fourth of their offspring will be normal homozygotes, one half will be phenotypically normal carrier heterozygotes, and one fourth will be homozygotes with the disease (Figure 4-26). Thus the recurrence risk for the offspring of carrier parents is 25%. As stated before, these are the *average* figures. In any given family, chance fluctuations are likely, but a study of a large number of families would yield figures close to these proportions.

If two parents have a recessive disease, they each must be homozygous for the disease. Therefore, when two parents are affected by a recessive disease, all their children also must be affected. This observation helps to distinguish recessive from dominant inheritance, because two parents both affected by a dominant gene are nearly always both heterozygotes and thus one fourth of their children will be unaffected.

Because carrier parents usually are unaware that they both carry the same recessive gene, they often produce an affected

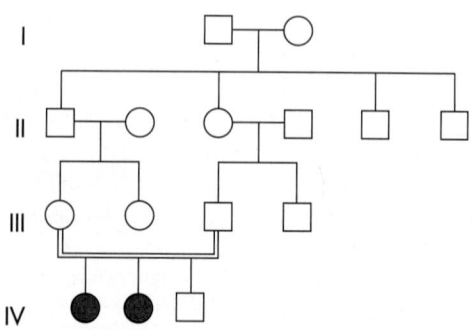

Figure 4-25 Pedigree for cystic fibrosis.

	D	d
D	DD Homozygous normal	Dd Heterozygous carrier
d	Dd Heterozygous carrier	dd Homozygous affected

Figure 4-26 Punnett square for the mating of heterozygous carriers. This is typical of most cases of recessive disease.

child before knowing of their condition. Increasingly, **carrier detection tests** that can identify heterozygotes by measuring the reduced amount of a critical enzyme are becoming available. The critical enzyme is totally lacking in a homozygous recessive individual, but an essentially normal phenotype is seen when it is present in a reduced quantity in the carrier. Often carriers also can be detected by direct examination of the disease locus for a mutation. Such testing is especially valuable for siblings of known carriers, who may themselves be carriers. Some recessive diseases for which carrier detection tests are now available are PKU, sickle cell disease, cystic fibrosis, Tay-Sachs disease, hemochromatosis, and galactosemia.

Consanguinity

Consanguinity and **inbreeding** are related concepts. *Consanguinity* refers to the mating of two related individuals, and the offspring of such matings are said to be *inbred.* Consanguinity is often an important characteristic of pedigrees for recessive diseases because relatives share a certain proportion of genes received from a common ancestor. The proportion of shared genes depends on the closeness of their biologic relationship. For example, siblings share one half of their genes on average. With each decreasing degree of relationship, this proportion is reduced by one half. Uncles share one fourth of their genes with nephews and nieces; first cousins share one eighth; first cousins once removed* share one sixteenth; second cousins share one thirty-second; and so on. With consanguineous matings, recessive disorders are significantly increased. Most empirical studies show that the proportion of offspring of marriages of first cousins who are affected by genetic diseases is approximately double that of the general population.[18] Marriages between first cousins are prohibited in most states of the United States. Marriages between closer relatives (except between double first cousins†) are prohibited throughout the United States.

X-Linked Inheritance

Not all genetic diseases are caused by genes located on the 22 autosomes. Some conditions are instead caused by genes located on the sex chromosomes, and that mode of inheritance is referred to as **sex-linked.** The Y chromosome contains only a few dozen genes, so most sex-linked traits are located on the X chromosome and are said to be X-linked. Only a few diseases are known to be inherited as X-linked dominant traits. Because these diseases are so seldom encountered, only the much more common X-linked recessive diseases are discussed here.

Because females receive two X chromosomes, one from the father and one from the mother, they can be homozygous for a disease allele at a given locus, homozygous for the normal allele at the locus, or heterozygous. Males, having only one X chromosome, are said to be **hemizygous** for genes on this chromosome. A male who inherits a recessive disease gene on the X chromosome will be affected by the disease because the Y chromosome does not carry a normal allele to counteract the effects of the disease gene. Males are always more frequently affected by X-linked recessive diseases, with the difference becoming more pronounced as the disease becomes rarer.

X Inactivation

In the late 1950s Mary Lyon proposed that one X chromosome in the somatic cells of females is permanently inactivated, a process termed *X inactivation.*[19] This proposal, known as the *Lyon hypothesis,* explains why most gene products coded by the X chromosome are present in equal amounts in males and females, even though males have only one X chromosome and females have two X chromosomes. This phenomenon is called **dosage compensation.** The inactivated X chromosomes are observable in many interphase cells as highly condensed intranuclear chromatin bodies, termed **Barr bodies** (after Barr and Bertram, who discovered them in the late 1940s). Normal females have one Barr body in each somatic cell, whereas normal males have no Barr bodies.

The actual process of inactivation occurs very early in embryonic development—approximately 7 to 14 days after fertilization. In each somatic cell one of the two X chromosomes is inactivated. In some cells the X chromosome contributed by the father is inactivated; in others the maternal X chromosome is inactivated. Because the inactivation process is random, the maternal X chromosome is inactivated in approximately half the cells and the paternal X chromosome is inactivated in approximately half the cells. Once the X chromosome has been inactivated in a cell, all the descendants of that cell have the same chromosome inactivated. Thus inactivation is said to be *random* but *fixed.*

Some individuals do not have the normal number of X chromosomes in their somatic cells. For example, males with Klinefelter syndrome typically have two X chromosomes and one Y chromosome. These males *do* have one Barr body in each cell. Females whose cell nuclei have three X chromosomes have two Barr bodies in each cell, and females whose cell nuclei have four X chromosomes have three Barr bodies in each cell. Females with Turner syndrome have only one X chromosome and no Barr bodies. Thus the number of Barr bodies is always one less than the number of X chromosomes in the cell. All but one X chromosome are always inactivated.

Persons with abnormal numbers of X chromosomes, such as those with Turner syndrome or Klinefelter syndrome, are not physically normal. This situation presents a puzzle because they presumably have only one active X chromosome, just as individuals with normal numbers of chromosomes do. However, the distal portions of the short and long arms of the X chromosome, as well as several other regions on the chromosome arm, are not inactivated. Thus X inactivation is also known to be *incomplete.*

The actual mechanism underlying X inactivation is still not well understood, although the gene responsible for initiating X inactivation has been located.[20] Methylation of X

---

*First cousins once removed are the offspring of one's own first cousins.
†Double first cousins share both sets of grandparents; ordinarily first cousins share just one set of grandparents.

chromosome DNA, a process in which DNA is inactivated when cytosine bases are enzymatically converted to 5-methylcytosine, appears to be involved. Inactive X chromosomes can be at least partially reactivated in vitro by administering 5-azacytidine, a demethylating agent.

Sex Determination

The process of sexual differentiation, in which the embryonic gonads become either testes or ovaries, begins during the sixth week of gestation. A key principle of sex determination in the human is that one copy of the Y chromosome is sufficient to initiate the process of gonadal differentiation that produces a male fetus. The number of X chromosomes does not alter this process. For example, an individual with two X chromosomes and one Y chromosome in each cell is still phenotypically a male. Thus it is logical that the Y chromosome must contain a gene that begins the process of male gonadal development.

This gene, termed *SRY* (for "sex-determining region on the Y") has been located on the short arm of the Y chromosome.[21,22] The *SRY* gene lies immediately proximal to the distal tip of the Y chromosome, known as the **pseudoautosomal** region (Figure 4-27). This portion of the Y chromosome is so

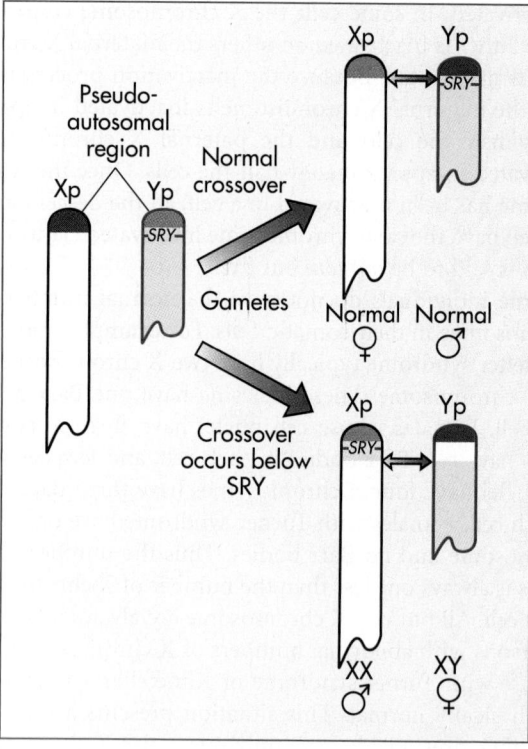

Figure 4-27 **The distal short arms of the X and Y chromosomes exchange material during meiosis in the male.** The region of the Y chromosome in which this crossover occurs is called the *pseudoautosomal region.* The *SRY* gene, which triggers the process leading to male gonadal differentiation, is located just outside the pseudoautosomal region. Occasionally, the crossover occurs on the centromeric side of the *SRY* gene, causing it to lie on an X chromosome instead of a Y chromosome. An offspring receiving this X chromosome will be an XX male, and an offspring receiving the Y chromosome will be an XY female. (From Jorde LB et al: *Medical genetics,* ed 3, St Louis, 2003, Mosby.)

named because it pairs with the distal tip of the short arm of the X chromosome during meiosis and exchanges genetic material with it (crossover), just as autosomes do. The DNA sequences of these regions on the X and Y chromosomes are highly similar. The remainder of the X and Y chromosomes, however, do not exchange material and are not similar in DNA sequence. An important piece of evidence that supports *SRY* as the male-determining gene is that female mouse embryos injected with this gene develop as phenotypic males.

Although the *SRY* gene is located on the Y chromosome, the other genes that contribute to male differentiation are located on other chromosomes. Thus *SRY* appears to act as a trigger that initiates the action of genes on other chromosomes (e.g., those that control Sertoli cell differentiation or secretion of müllerian-inhibiting substance). This concept is supported by the fact that the *SRY* gene is similar in sequence to other genes that are known to regulate the transcription of DNA (i.e., they turn other genes on and off).

Occasionally the crossover between X and Y occurs closer to the centromere than it should, placing the *SRY* gene on the X chromosome after crossover. This variation can result in offspring with an apparently normal XX karyotype but a male phenotype. Such XX males are seen in about 1 in 20,000 live births and closely resemble males with Klinefelter syndrome, although their stature is normal. Conversely, it is possible to inherit a Y chromosome that has lost the *SRY* gene (because of either a crossover error or a deletion of the gene). This situation produces an XY female. Such females have gonadal streaks rather than ovaries and have poorly developed secondary sex characteristics.

Characteristics of Pedigrees

X-linked pedigrees show distinctive modes of inheritance. The most striking characteristic is that females are seldom affected. To express an X-linked recessive trait, a female must be homozygous: either both her parents are affected or her father is affected and her mother is a carrier. Such matings are rare.

An important example of an X-linked recessive disease is hemophilia A. The pedigree shown in Box 4-2 demonstrates the following principles of X-linked recessive inheritance:

1. The trait is seen much more often in males than in females.
2. Because a father can give a son only a Y chromosome, the trait is never transmitted from father to son.
3. The gene can be transmitted through a series of carrier females, causing the appearance of a "skipped generation."
4. The gene is passed from an affected father to all his daughters, who, as phenotypically normal carriers, transmit it to approximately half their sons, who are affected.

The most common and severe of all X-linked recessive disorders is Duchenne muscular dystrophy (DMD), which affects approximately 1 in 3500 males. As its name suggests, this disorder is characterized by progressive muscle degeneration. Affected individuals are usually unable to walk by 10 to 12 years of age. The disease affects the heart and respiratory muscles, and death caused by respiratory or cardiac failure usually occurs before 20 years. Until recently, the underlying pathologic origin of this disorder was a mystery. However, mapping and cloning of the disease gene (on the short arm of the X chromosome) have greatly increased our understanding of the disorder.[23] The *DMD* gene is the largest gene ever found in the human, spanning over 2 million DNA bases. It encodes a previously undiscovered muscle protein, termed **dystrophin**. Extensive study of dystrophin indicates that it plays an essential role in maintaining the structural integrity of muscle cells: one end of the protein binds to actin filaments in the cytoplasm of the cell, and the other end binds to a group of membrane-spanning proteins known as the *dystrophin-associated glycoproteins*. When dystrophin is absent, as in individuals with DMD, the cell cannot survive and muscle deterioration ensues.

Most cases of Duchenne muscular dystrophy are caused by deletions of portions of the *DMD* gene. They generally involve frameshift deletions in which all the amino acids following the deletion are altered. It is interesting that an "in frame" deletion (in which a multiple of three bases is deleted, and the amino acids following the deletion are not altered) produces a milder form of muscular dystrophy, the Becker type. These two types of dystrophy are examples of a disease in which different types of mutations at the same locus produce variable expression of the disease.

Recurrence Risks

The most common mating type involving X-linked recessive genes is the combination of a carrier female and a normal male. On the average, the carrier mother will transmit the disease gene to half her sons and half her daughters. As Figure 4-28, *A*, shows, half the daughters in such a mating will be carriers, whereas half will be normal. Half the sons will be normal, whereas half will have the disease. These are probabilities that indicate what risks can be expected on the *average* (see Box 4-2).

The other common mating type is an affected father and a normal mother (Figure 4-28, *B*). In this situation all the sons must be normal because the father can transmit only his Y chromosome to them. Because all the daughters must receive the father's X chromosome, they will all be heterozygous carriers. Because the sons *must* receive the Y chromosome and the daughters *must* receive the X with the disease gene, these are predictions and not probabilities. None of the children will express the disease.

The final mating pattern, less common than the other two, involves an affected father and a carrier mother (Figure 4-28, *C*). With this pattern, on average, half the daughters will be heterozygous carriers and half will be homozygous for the disease gene and thus affected. Half the sons will be normal, and half will be affected. Some X-linked recessive diseases, such as DMD, are fatal or incapacitating before the affected individual reaches reproductive age, and therefore affected fathers are rare or nonexistent.

Sex-Limited and Sex-Influenced Traits

Confusion sometimes exists regarding the difference between traits that are sex-linked and those that are sex-limited or sex-influenced. A **sex-limited trait** is one that can occur in only one of the sexes, often because of anatomic differences. Inherited uterine and testicular defects are two obvious examples.

A **sex-influenced trait** is one that occurs much more often in one sex than in the other. A good example of a sex-influenced trait is male-pattern baldness, which occurs in both males and females but is much more common in males. In males it is inherited as a dominant trait, whereas in females it is inherited as a recessive trait. Because of their hormonal constitution, females need two copies of the gene to express male-pattern baldness. Another example is autosomal

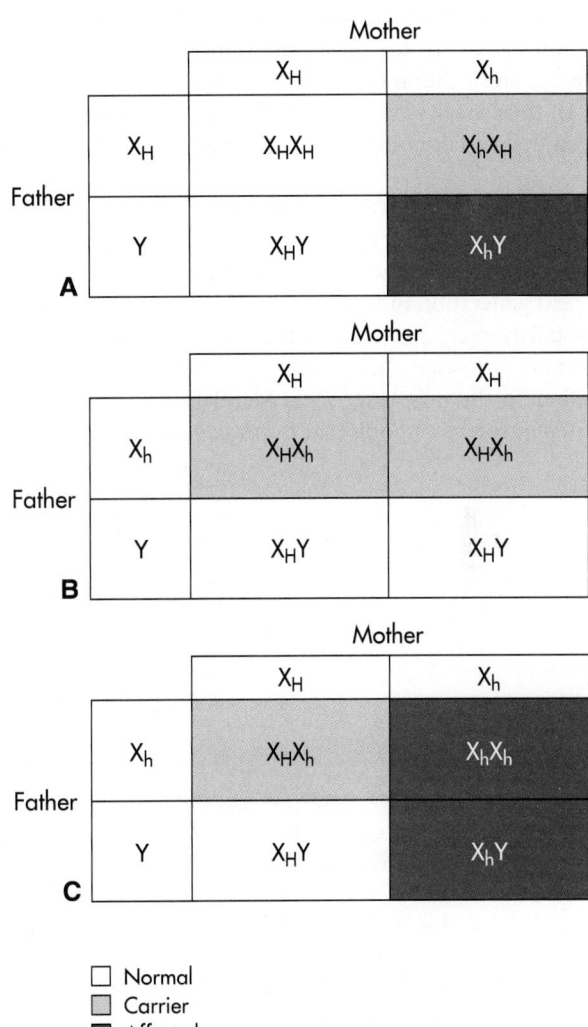

Figure 4-28 **Punnett square and X-linked recessive traits. A,** Punnett square for the mating of a normal male ($X_H Y$) and a female carrier of an X-linked recessive gene ($X_H X_h$). **B,** Punnett square for the mating of a normal female ($X_H X_H$) with a male affected by an X-linked recessive disease ($X_h Y$). **C,** Punnett square for the mating of a female who carries an X-linked recessive gene ($X_H X_h$) with a male who is affected with the disease caused by the gene ($X_h Y$).

dominant breast cancer, which is much more common in females than males.

Evaluation of Pedigrees

With complications such as incomplete penetrance, variable expressivity, delayed age of onset, and sex-influenced traits, it is not always possible simply to look at a disease pedigree and determine the mode of inheritance. A sophisticated statistical methodologic approach has evolved to deal with such complications. Incorporated into computer programs, these statistical techniques assess the probability of observing a certain pedigree if a particular mode of inheritance (e.g., autosomal dominant with incomplete penetrance) is in effect.

LINKAGE ANALYSIS AND GENE MAPPING

Locating genes on chromosomes and on specific areas of chromosomes is one of the most important endeavors in human genetics. The location of a gene can tell much about the function of the gene, its interaction with other genes, and the likelihood that certain individuals will develop a genetic disease.

Classical Pedigree Analysis

Mendel's second law, the principle of independent assortment, states that an individual's genes will be transmitted to the next generation independently of one another. This law is only partly true, however, because genes located close together on the same chromosome *do* tend to be transmitted together to the offspring. Thus Mendel's principle of independent assortment holds true for most pairs of genes but not those that occupy the same region of a chromosome. Such loci demonstrate **linkage** and are said to be linked.

During the first meiotic stage, the arms of homologous chromosome pairs intertwine and sometimes exchange portions of their DNA (Figure 4-29) in a process known as **crossing over.** During crossing over, new combinations of alleles can be formed. For example, two loci on a chromosome have alleles *A* and *a* and alleles *B* and *b*. Alleles *A* and *B* are located together on one chromosome arm, and alleles *a* and *b* are located on the other arm. The genotype of this individual is denoted as *AB/ab*.

As Figure 4-29, *A*, shows, the allele pairs *AB* and *ab* would be transmitted together when no crossing over occurs. However, when crossing over does occur (Figure 4-29, *B*), all four possible pairs of alleles can be transmitted to the offspring: *AB*, *aB*, *Ab*, and *ab*. The process of forming such new arrangements of alleles is called **recombination.** Crossing over does not necessarily lead to recombination, however, because double crossing over between two loci can result in no actual recombination of the alleles at the loci (Figure 4-29, *C*).

The rate of crossing over can be used to infer the distance between two loci on a chromosome because the probability of crossovers occurring between two loci increases as the loci become more distant. For example, if an individual with genotype *AB/ab* produces recombinant offspring gametes (composition of *Ab* and *aB*) 2% of the time, it is said that the two loci are two map units apart. One **map unit** equals a 1% recombination rate between two loci. When loci on the same chromosome are 50 or more map units apart, they are considered unlinked because their recombination frequency is just as great as it would be if they were on different chromosomes (where the probability of being transmitted together

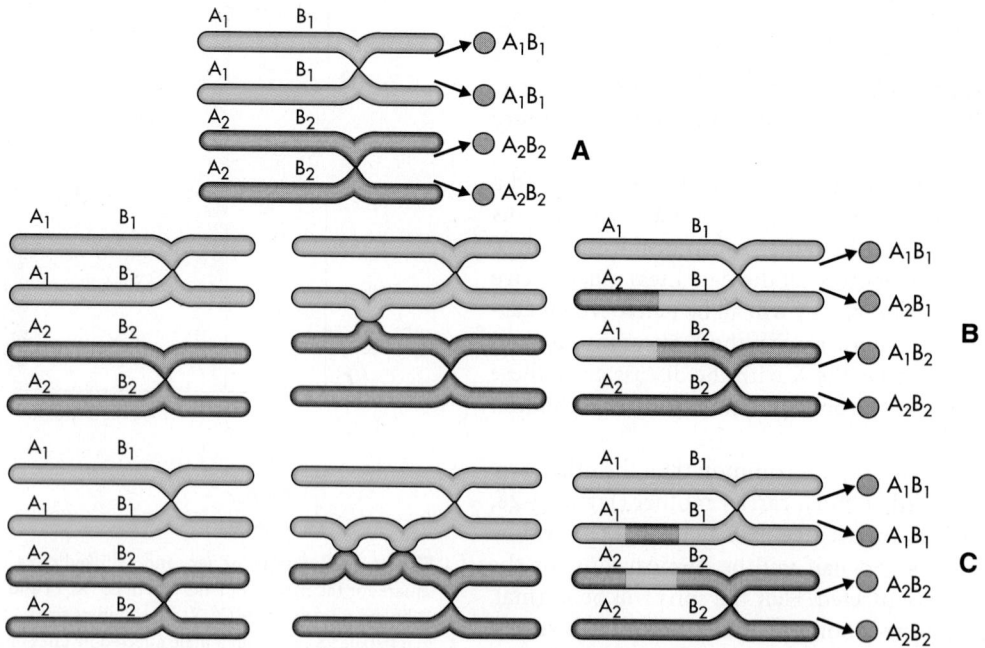

Figure 4-29 The genetic results of crossing over. **A,** No crossing over: A_1 and B_1 remain together after meiosis. **B,** Crossing over between A and B results in a recombination: A_1 and B_2 are inherited together on one chromosome, and A_2 and B_1 are inherited together on another chromosome. **C,** A double crossover between A and B results in no recombination of alleles.

must equal one half). Because they are on the same chromosome, they are said to be unlinked but **syntenic loci.** Recombination frequencies provide a good estimate of actual physical distance between loci at smaller distances, but because of double crossovers, they tend to yield underestimates at larger distances. On average, each map unit is equal to approximately 1 million DNA base pairs.

Pedigrees can be used to determine recombination rates between loci. Figure 4-30 shows a pedigree in which the rare disease *nail-patella syndrome* (an autosomal dominant disease consisting of malformed patellae and nails) is being transmitted. The individuals in this pedigree have been typed for the ABO blood group, whose locus is also located on chromosome 9. Examination of generations I and II shows that the nail-patella gene must be on the same chromosome arm as the gene for blood type A because the mother, whose blood type was B, was unaffected with the disease. The daughter's genotype would then be *AN/Bn*, where *N* indicates the disease allele and *n* indicates the normal allele. The daughter's husband (individual II-1) must have the genotype *On/On*. If the loci for nail-patella syndrome and the ABO blood group are linked, the children of this union who are affected with nail-patella syndrome should have blood type A; those who are unaffected should have blood type B. In six of seven cases we find this to be true. In one case a recombination occurred (individual III-6), indicating a recombination rate of 1 in 7, or 14%. The two loci are therefore 14 map units apart.

In practice, a much larger sample of families would be used to ensure against statistical artifacts. Also, as with the determination of mode of inheritance, the situation is not always as clear as that pictured in Figure 4-30. Elaborate statistical procedures have been devised to evaluate the probabilities that two loci are linked at a given map distance.

Once a close linkage has been established between a disease locus and a "marker" locus (e.g., a blood group) and once the alleles of the two loci that are inherited together within a family have been determined, reliable predictions of whether a member of a family will develop the disease can be made. If, for example, the recombination rate between a disease locus and a marker locus, such as the ABO blood group, is less than 1%, family members can simply have their ABO blood type assayed to find out, with 99% or greater certainty, whether each member carries the disease gene.

This capability is especially important for diseases with delayed age of onset. Linkage has been established between several DNA polymorphisms and the gene for Huntington disease. Determining this kind of linkage means that it is possible for offspring of an individual with Huntington disease to know whether they also carry the gene and thus could pass it on to their own children. The difficult decision of whether to have children will be made easier for these individuals, although some individuals may prefer to remain uninformed of their genotypes. Other delayed-onset diseases for which linked markers have been found include adult polycystic kidney disease, familial Alzheimer disease, and two forms of autosomal dominant breast cancer (about 5% of breast cancer cases are caused by an autosomal dominant gene). Pinpointing specific mutations in these genes also has made direct genetic diagnosis possible. The advantage of direct diagnosis is that it is more accurate because it tests for the disease-causing mutation itself.

For some genetic diseases, prophylactic treatment is available if the condition can be diagnosed in time. An example of this is hemochromatosis—a recessive genetic disease in which excess iron is retained, causing degeneration of the heart, liver, brain, and other vital organs. Diagnosis is usually made at about 40 years of age in males, after which most individuals survive only a few years. If earlier tests could determine whether an individual had the disease, preventive treatment, consisting of phlebotomies to remove blood and thus excess iron, could be administered before degeneration began. This has been made easier by mapping the hemochromatosis gene to a specific region of chromosome 6 and subsequently identifying the major disease-causing mutations. Individuals at risk for developing the disease can be identified by testing for presence of the mutations, and if necessary, preventive therapy can be given, ensuring an ordinary life span. This example is one instance in which genetics contributes to preventive medicine in its best sense.

Assigning Loci to Specific Chromosomes
In Situ Hybridization
In situ hybridization involves hybridizing a specific piece of radioactively labeled DNA or RNA (a probe) to fixed metaphase chromosomes that have been denatured so that their DNA is single structured. If the radioactive probe matches the DNA of a chromosome segment, it hybridizes and remains at a particular position on the chromosome (hence the term *in situ*). Its position can then be located by autoradiography—a procedure in which the radioactive emissions from the hybridized probe mark its location when exposed to x-ray film. The procedure is now performed most commonly with nonradioactive fluorescent probes (fluorescent in situ hybridization [FISH]).

With completion of the human DNA sequence (see below), computer analysis of the published sequence has become an effective and popular approach for identifying genes.

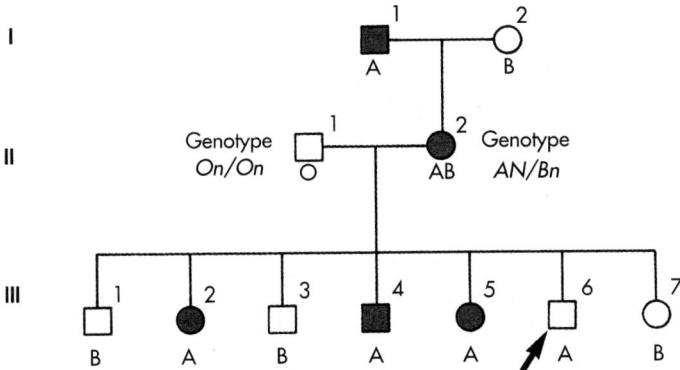

Figure 4-30 The ABO nail-patella linkage in three generations of a family. Letters below symbols indicate ABO blood groups. Individual III-6 shows recombination.

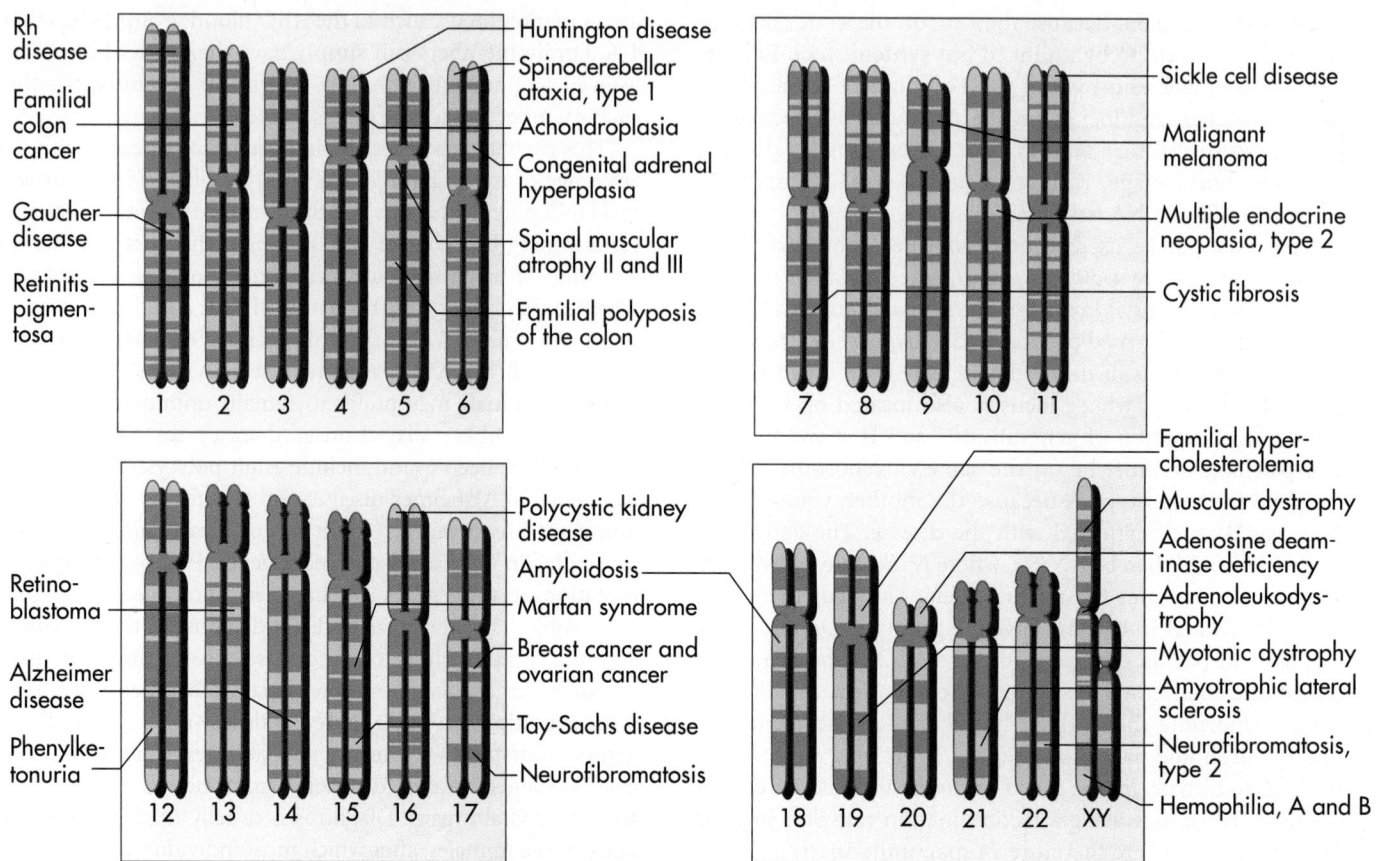

Figure 4-31 Example of diseases: gene map.

Computerized databases of known DNA sequences play an important role in gene identification. When studying a specific region of DNA to find a gene, it is common to search for similarity between DNA sequences from the region and DNA sequences in the database. The sequences in the database may derive from genes with known function or tissue-specific expression patterns. Suppose, for example, that we have used linkage analysis to identify a region containing a gene that causes a developmental disorder such as a limb malformation. As we evaluate DNA sequences in the region, we would look for similarity between a DNA sequence from this region and a plausible sequence from the database (e.g., sequence from a gene that encodes a protein involved in bone development, such as a fibroblast growth factor). Because genes that encode similar protein products usually have similar DNA sequences, a match between the sequence from our region and a sequence in the database could be a vital clue that this particular DNA sequence is actually part of the gene that causes the limb malformation.

Complete Human Gene Map: Prospects and Benefits

Rapid progress is currently being made in assigning genes to their chromosomal locations. A number of important genetic diseases have been located on specific areas of individual chromosomes: these include Huntington disease, retinoblastoma, DMD, hemophilia A, cystic fibrosis, PKU, neurofibromatosis, familial breast cancer, and familial Alzheimer disease[24] (Figure

4-31). Table 4-1 contains a partial list of mapped diseases. The development of thousands of new DNA markers is especially helpful in this effort. A marker map of the human genome has been completed, and completion of the entire sequence of the human genome was announced in April 2003. Achievement of this goal serves several purposes:

1. Marker genes are available to establish close linkages for genetic diseases. With the establishment of a comprehensive marker map, accurate predictions can be made for the inheritance of most genetic diseases.
2. Knowing the location of genes often yields valuable information about the way genes function and interact with one another. A number of genes with similar functions (e.g., some of the globin genes) are located close to one another on the same chromosome. This characteristic can have important implications for the diseases caused by these genes.
3. Mapping a disease gene is an important step toward isolating and **cloning** the gene (clones are identical copies of genes). Once a gene can be cloned, its DNA sequence can be studied to determine the nature and function of the protein encoded by the gene. Cloning the genes that cause diseases such as cystic fibrosis and DMD has contributed immensely to our understanding of the pathophysiologic aspect of these disorders. In addition, the ability to clone a gene opens up the possibility of gene therapy for the disorder.

Table 4-1   Examples of Disease Genes that Have Been Mapped and Cloned*

Disease	Chromosome Location	Gene Product
α-1-Antitrypsin deficiency	14q	Serine protease inhibitor
α-Thalassemia	16p	α-Globin component of hemoglobin
β-Thalassemia	11p	β-Globin component of hemoglobin
Achondroplasia	4p	Fibroblast growth factor receptor 3
Adult polycystic kidney disease	16p	Polycystin-1 membrane protein
Alzheimer disease*	14q	Presenilin 1
	1q	Presenilin 2
	19q	Apolipoprotein E
	21q	β-Amyloid precursor protein
Amyotrophic lateral sclerosis	21q	Superoxide dismutase 1
Ataxia telangiectasia	11q	Cell cycle control protein
Beckwith-Wiedemann syndrome	11p	Insulin-like growth factor II
Breast cancer (familial)	17q	BRCA1 tumor suppressor/DNA repair protein
	13q	BRCA2 tumor suppressor/DNA repair protein
	22q	CHEK2 DNA repair protein
Li-Fraumeni syndrome	17p	P53 tumor suppressor
Charcot-Marie-Tooth disease (type 1A)*	17p	Peripheral myelin protein 22
Cystic fibrosis	7q	Cystic fibrosis transmembrane regulator (CFTR)
Deafness, nonsyndromic (more than 75	13q	Connexin-26 gap junction protein
genes identified to date; representative	5q	Actin polymerization regulator
examples shown here)	7q	Pendrin (anion transporter; mutations also found in Pendred syndrome)
	11q	α-Tectorin
Diabetes		
(MODY1)	20q	Hepatocyte nuclear factor-4α
(MODY2)	7p	Glucokinase
(MODY3)	12q	Hepatocyte nuclear factor-1α
(MODY4)	13q	Insulin promoter factor-1
(MODY5)	17q	Hepatic transcription factor-2
(MODY6)	2q	NeuroD transcription factor
Duchenne/Becker muscular dystrophy	Xp	Dystrophin
Ehlers-Danlos syndrome*	2q	Collagen (COL3A1); numerous types of this disorder are known, most of which are produced by mutations in collagen genes
Ellis van Creveld syndrome	4p	Protein with possible leucine zipper domain
Familial polyposis coli	5q	APC tumor suppressor
Fragile X syndrome	Xq	FMR1 RNA-binding protein
Galactosemia	9p	Galactose-1-phosphate-uridyltransferase
Hemochromatosis	6p	Transferrin receptor binding protein
Hemophilia A	Xq	Clotting factor VIII
Hemophilia B	Xq	Clotting factor IX
Hereditary nonpolyposis colorectal cancer	3p	MLH1 DNA mismatch repair protein
Huntington disease	4p	Huntingtin
Hypercholesterolemia (familial)	19p	LDL receptor
Long QT syndrome (LQT1)*	11p	KVLQT1 cardiac potassium channel α subunit
Marfan syndrome	15q	Fibrillin-1
Melanoma (familial)*	9p	Cyclin-dependent kinase inhibitor tumor suppressor
	12q	Cyclin-dependent kinase 4
Myotonic dystrophy	19q	Protein kinase
	3q	Zinc finger protein
Myoclonus epilepsy (Unverricht-Lundborg)	21q	Cystatin B cysteine protease inhibitor
Neurofibromatosis type 1	17q	Neurofibromin tumor suppressor
Neurofibromatosis type 2	22q	Merlin (schwannomin) tumor suppressor
Parkinson disease		
(familial)	4q	α-Synuclein
(autosomal recessive early-onset)	6q	Parkin
Phenylketonuria	12q	Phenylalanine hydroxylase
Retinoblastoma	13q	pRB tumor suppressor
Sickle cell disease	11p	β-Globin component of hemoglobin
Tay-Sachs disease	15q	Hexosaminidase A
Wilms tumor*	11p	WT1 zinc finger protein tumor suppressor
Wilson disease	13q	Copper transporting ATPase
Von Willebrand disease	12q	von Willebrand clotting factor

Modified from Jorde LB et al: *Medical genetics,* ed 3, St Louis, 2003, Mosby.
*Additional disease-causing loci have been mapped and/or cloned.

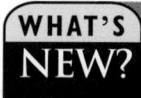

WHAT'S NEW?   Germline Therapy, Genetic Enhancement, and Human Cloning: Controversial New Issues in Medical Genetics

For a variety of reasons, germline gene therapy is not being undertaken in humans. Nevertheless, it has been noted that germline gene therapy is in many ways technically easier to perform than is somatic cell therapy. Germline therapy also offers (in theory) the possibility of "genetic enhancement," the introduction of favorable genes into the embryo. However, a gene that is favorable in one environment may be quite unfavorable in another (e.g., the sickle cell mutation, which is only advantageous for heterozygotes in a malarial environment). And, because of pleiotropy, the introduction of "favorable" genes may have completely unintended consequences (e.g., a gene thought to enhance one characteristic could negatively affect another). For these reasons, and because germline therapy usually destroys the targeted embryo, neither germline therapy nor genetic enhancement are advocated by the scientific community.

Controversy also surrounds the prospect of cloning humans. A number of species (e.g., sheep, pigs, cattle, goats, mice, and cats) have been successfully cloned by introducing a diploid nucleus from an adult cell into an egg cell from which the original haploid nucleus was removed. The cell is manipulated so that all of its genes can be expressed (recall that most genes in a typical adult cell are transcriptionally silent). This procedure, termed *reproductive cloning* when allowed to proceed through a full-term pregnancy, could likely be used to produce a human being. Some argue that human cloning offers childless couples the opportunity to produce children to whom they are biologically related or even to "replace" a child who has died. Others respond with the challenge that this method of creating life is too artificial. In any case, it is important to keep in mind that a clone is only a *genetic* copy. The environment of the individual, which also plays a large role in development, cannot be replicated. Furthermore, the great majority of cloning attempts in mammals fail: in most cases the embryo either dies or has gross malformations. Because the consequences of human cloning would almost certainly be similar, reproductive cloning to produce a human is condemned almost universally by scientists.

Recently, it became possible to derive embryonic stem cells from early-stage human embryos. These stem cells can potentially be treated to form many types of differentiated cells (e.g., neurons for individuals with Parkinson disease, myocytes for individuals with heart disease). The combination of embryonic stem cell technology and human cloning offers an interesting possibility: a pre-embryo could in theory be created from an individual's own cell, producing embryonic stem cells that would be immunologically a perfect match for the individual (creating a clone to provide embryonic stem cells has been termed *therapeutic cloning*).

Although these technologies offer the hope of effective treatment for some recalcitrant diseases, they also present thorny ethical issues. Clearly, decisions regarding their use must be guided by constructive input from scientists, legal scholars, philosophers, and others.

SUMMARY REVIEW

DNA, RNA, and Proteins: Heredity at the Molecular Level

1. Genes, the basic units of inheritance, are composed of deoxyribonucleic acid (DNA) and are located on the chromosomes.
2. DNA is composed of deoxyribose, a phosphate molecule, and four types of nitrogenous bases. The physical structure of DNA is a double helix.
3. The DNA bases code for amino acids, which in turn make up proteins. The amino acids are specified by triplet codons of nitrogenous bases.
4. DNA replication is based on complementary base pairing, in which a single strand of DNA serves as the template for attracting bases that form a new strand of DNA.
5. DNA polymerase is the primary enzyme involved in replication. It adds bases to the new DNA strand and performs "proofreading" functions.
6. A mutation is an inherited alteration of genetic material (i.e., DNA).
7. Substances that cause mutations are called *mutagens*.
8. The mutation rate in humans varies from locus to locus and ranges from 10^{-4} to 10^{-7} per gene per generation.
9. Transcription and translation, the two basic processes in which proteins are specified by DNA, both involve ribonucleic acid (RNA). RNA is chemically similar to DNA, but it is single stranded, has a ribose sugar molecule, and has uracil rather than thymine as one of its four nitrogenous bases.
10. Transcription is the process by which DNA specifies a sequence of messenger RNA (mRNA).
11. Much of the RNA sequence is spliced from the mRNA before the mRNA leaves the nucleus. The excised sequences are called *introns*, and those that remain to code for proteins are called *exons*.
12. Translation is the process by which RNA directs the synthesis of polypeptides. This process takes place in the ribosomes, which consist of proteins and ribosomal RNA (rRNA).
13. During translation, mRNA interacts with transfer RNA (tRNA), a molecule that has an attachment site for a specific amino acid.

Chromosomes

1. Human cells consist of diploid somatic cells (body cells) and haploid gametes (sperm and egg cells).
2. Humans have 23 pairs of chromosomes. Twenty-two of these pairs are autosomes. The remaining pair consists of the sex chromosomes. Females have two homologous X chromosomes as their sex chromosomes; males have an X and a Y chromosome.
3. A karyotype is an ordered display of chromosomes arranged according to length and the location of the centromere.
4. Various types of stains can be used to make chromosome bands more visible.
5. About 1 in 150 live births has a major diagnosable chromosome abnormality. Chromosome abnormalities are the leading known cause of mental retardation and miscarriage.
6. Polyploidy is a condition in which a euploid cell has some multiple of the normal number of chromosomes. Humans have been observed to have triploidy (three copies of each chromosome) and tetraploidy (four copies of each chromosome); both conditions are lethal.
7. Somatic cells that do not have a multiple of 23 chromosomes are aneuploid. Aneuploidy is usually the result of nondisjunction.
8. Trisomy is a type of aneuploidy in which one chromosome is present in three copies in somatic cells. A partial trisomy is one in which only part of a chromosome is present in three copies.

SUMMARY REVIEW—cont'd

9. Monosomy is a type of aneuploidy in which one chromosome is present in only one copy in somatic cells.
10. In general, monosomies cause more severe physical defects than do trisomies, illustrating the principle that the loss of chromosome material has more severe consequences than the duplication of chromosome material.
11. Down syndrome, a trisomy of chromosome 21, is the best-known disease caused by a chromosome aberration. It affects 1 in 800 live births and is much more likely to occur in women over 35 years of age.
12. Most aneuploidies of the sex chromosomes have less severe consequences than those of the autosomes.
13. The most commonly observed sex chromosome aneuploidies are the 47,XXX karyotype, 45,X karyotype (Turner syndrome), 47,XXY karyotype (Klinefelter syndrome), and 47,XYY karyotype.
14. Abnormalities of chromosome structure include deletions, duplications, inversions, and translocations.

Elements of Formal Genetics
1. Mendelian traits are caused by single genes, each of which occupies a position, or locus, on a chromosome.
2. Alleles are different forms of genes located at the same locus on the chromosome.
3. At any given locus in a somatic cell, an individual has two genes, one from each parent. An individual may be homozygous or heterozygous for a locus.
4. An individual's genotype is his or her genetic makeup, and the phenotype reflects the interaction of genotype and environment.
5. At a heterozygous locus, a dominant gene's effects mask those of a recessive gene. The recessive gene is expressed only when it is present in two copies.

Transmission of Genetic Diseases
1. Genetic diseases caused by single genes usually follow autosomal dominant, autosomal recessive, or X-linked recessive modes of inheritance.
2. Pedigree charts are an important tool in the analysis of modes of inheritance.
3. Recurrence risks specify the probability that future offspring will inherit a genetic disease. For single-gene diseases, recurrence risks remain the same for each offspring, regardless of the number of affected or unaffected offspring.
4. The recurrence risk for autosomal dominant diseases is usually 50%.
5. Germline mosaicism can alter recurrence risks for genetic diseases because unaffected parents can produce multiple affected offspring. This situation occurs because the germline of one parent is affected by a mutation but the parent's somatic cells are unaffected.
6. Skipped generations are not seen in classic autosomal dominant pedigrees.
7. Males and females are equally likely to exhibit autosomal dominant diseases and to pass them on to their offspring.
8. A gene that is not always expressed phenotypically is said to have incomplete penetrance.
9. Penetrance may be age-dependent, as in Huntington disease and familial breast cancer.
10. Variable expressivity is a characteristic of many genetic diseases.
11. Genomic imprinting, which may involve methylation, results in differing expressions of a disease gene, depending on which parent transmitted the gene.
12. Most commonly, parents of children with autosomal recessive diseases are both heterozygous carriers of the disease gene.
13. The recurrence risk for autosomal recessive diseases is 25%.
14. Males and females are equally likely to be affected by autosomal recessive diseases.
15. Consanguinity is often present in families with autosomal recessive diseases, and it becomes more prevalent with rarer recessive diseases.
16. Carrier detection tests for an increasing number of autosomal recessive diseases are available.
17. The frequency of genetic diseases approximately doubles in the offspring of first-cousin matings.
18. In each normal female somatic cell, one of the two X chromosomes is inactivated early in embryogenesis.
19. X inactivation is random, fixed, and incomplete (i.e., only part of the chromosome is actually inactivated). It may involve methylation.
20. Gender is determined embryonically by the presence of the *SRY* gene on the Y chromosome. Embryos that have a Y chromosome (and thus the *SRY* gene) become males, whereas those lacking the Y chromosome become females. When the Y chromosome lacks the *SRY* gene, an XY female can be produced. Similarly, an X chromosome that contains the *SRY* gene can produce an XX male.
21. X-linked genes are those that are located on the X chromosome. Nearly all known X-linked diseases are caused by X-linked recessive genes.
22. Males are hemizygous for genes on the X chromosome.
23. X-linked recessive diseases are seen much more often in males than in females because males need only one copy of the gene to express the disease.
24. Fathers cannot pass X-linked genes to their sons.
25. Skipped generations are often seen in X-linked recessive disease pedigrees because the gene can be transmitted through carrier females.
26. Recurrence risks for X-linked recessive diseases depend on the carrier and affected status of the mother and father.
27. A sex-limited trait is one that occurs in only one of the sexes.
28. A sex-influenced trait is one that occurs more often in one sex than in the other.

Linkage Analysis and Gene Mapping
1. During meiosis I, crossing over occurs and can cause recombinations of alleles located on the same chromosome.
2. The frequency of recombinations can be used to infer the map distance between loci on the same chromosome.
3. Loci that are on the same chromosome are syntenic.
4. A marker locus, when closely linked to a disease-gene locus, can be used to predict whether an individual will develop a genetic disease.
5. A more complete gene map will facilitate marker studies, studies of gene function and interaction, and gene therapy.

KEY TERMS

Adenine, 124
Age-dependent, 144
Alleles, 140
Amino acids, 127
Aneuploid cell, 132

Anticodon, 129
Autosomes, 129
Barr bodies, 147
Base pair substitution, 128
Carrier, 141

Carrier detection test, 147
Chromosomal mosaics, 134
Chromosome bands, 130
Chromosome breakage, 137
Chromosome theory of inheritance, 141

KEY TERMS—cont'd

MEDIA RESOURCES   evolve

Review questions and answers for this chapter are available in the *CD Companion* included with this book. Also see the CD for an animation of *gametogenesis*.

WebLinks—links to Internet sites pertaining to this chapter—are available on Evolve at http://evolve.elsevier.com/McCance/.

REFERENCES

1. Online: Mendelian inheritance in man, available at: www3.ncbi.nlm.nih.gov/entrez/
2. Hall JG et al: The frequency and financial burden of genetic disease in a pediatric hospital, *Am J Med Genet* 1(1):417-436, 1978.
3. Crow JF: The origins, patterns and implications of human spontaneous mutation, *Nat Rev Genet* 1:40-47, 2000.
4. Hassold T, Hunt P: To err (meiotically) is human: the genesis of human aneuploidy, *Nat Rev Genet* 2(4):280-291, 2001.
5. Tolmie JL: Down syndrome and other autosomal trisomies. In Rimoin DL, et al, editors: *Emery and Rimoin's principles and practice of medical genetics*, ed 4, vol 1, Churchill Livingstone, 2002, London.
6. Hassold T, Sherman S: Down syndrome: genetic recombination and the origin of the extra chromosome 21, *Clin Genet* 57(2):95-100, 2000.
7. Jorde LB et al: *Medical genetics*, ed 3, St Louis, 2003, Mosby.
8. Allanson JE, Graham GE (2002) Sex chromosome abnormalities. In: Rimoin DL et al., editors: *Emery and Rimoin's principles and practice of medical genetics*, ed 4, vol 1, Churchill Livingstone, 2002, London.

9. Jin P, Warren ST: New insights into fragile X syndrome: from molecules to neurobehaviors, *Trends Biochem Sci* 28(3):152-158, 2003.
10. Ranum LP, Day JW: Dominantly inherited, non-coding microsatellite expansion disorders. *Curr Opin Genet Dev* 12(3):266-271, 2002.
11. Sinden RR: Biological implications of the DNA structures associated with disease-causing triplet repeats, *Am J Hum Genet* 64(2):346-353, 1999.
12. Zlotogora J: Germ line mosaicism, *Hum Genet* 102(4):381-386, 1998.
13. Balmain A, Gray J, Ponder B: The genetics and genomics of cancer, *Nat Genet* 33:238-244, 2003.
14. Knudson AG: Cancer genetics, *Am J Med Genet* 111(1):96-102, 2002.
15. Reynolds RM et al: Von Recklinghausen's neurofibromatosis: neurofibromatosis type 1, *Lancet* 361(9368):1552-1554, 2003.
16. Reik W, Walter J: Genomic imprinting: parental influence on the genome, *Nat Rev Genet* 2(1):21-32, 2001.
17. Ratjen F, Doring G: Cystic fibrosis, *Lancet* 361(9358):681-689, 2003.
18. Jorde LB: Inbreeding in human populations. In Dulbecco R, editor: *Encyclopedia of human biology*, vol 5, New York, 1997, Academic Press.
19. Lyon MF: Sex chromatin and gene action in the mammalian X-chromosome, *Am J Hum Genet* 14:135-148, 1962.
20. Brockdorff N: X-chromosome inactivation: closing in on proteins that bind Xist RNA, *Trends Genet* 18(7):352-358, 2002.
21. Swain A, Lovell-Badge R: Mammalian sex determination: a molecular drama, *Genes Dev* 13(7):755-767, 1999.
22. Ostrer H: Sex determination: lessons from families and embryos, *Clin Genet* 59(4):207-215, 2001.
23. Dalkilic I, Kunkel LM: Muscular dystrophies: genes to pathogenesis. *Curr Opin Genet Dev* 13(3):231-238, 2003. Review.
24. Collins FS, Morgan M, Patrinos A: The Human Genome Project: lessons from large-scale biology, *Science* 300(5617):286-290, 2003.

GENES, ENVIRONMENT–LIFE-STYLE, AND COMMON DISEASES

LYNN B. JORDE

CHAPTER OUTLINE

Chapter 4 focuses on diseases that are caused by single genes or by abnormalities of single chromosomes. Much progress has been made in identifying specific mutations that cause these diseases, leading to better risk estimates and, in some cases, more effective treatment of the disease. However, these conditions form only a small portion of the total burden of human genetic disease. Most congenital malformations are not caused by single genes or chromosome defects. Many common adult diseases, such as cancer, heart disease, and diabetes, have genetic components, but again they are usually not caused by single genes or by chromosome abnormalities.[1] These diseases, whose treatment collectively occupies the attention of most health care practitioners, are the result of a complex interplay of multiple genetic and environmental factors.

FACTORS INFLUENCING INCIDENCE OF DISEASE IN POPULATIONS

Concepts of Incidence and Prevalence

How common is a given disease, such as diabetes, in a population? Well-established measures are used to answer this question.[2] The **incidence rate** is the number of new cases of a disease reported during a specific period (typically 1 year) divided by the number of individuals in the population. The denominator is often expressed as *person-years*. The incidence rate can be contrasted with the **prevalence rate,** which is the proportion of the population affected by a disease at a specific point in time. Prevalence is thus determined by both the incidence rate and the length of the survival period in affected individuals. For example, the prevalence rate of acquired immunodeficiency syndrome (AIDS) is larger than the yearly incidence rate because most people with AIDS survive for several years after diagnosis.

Many diseases vary in prevalence from one population to another. Cystic fibrosis is relatively common among Europeans, occurring about once in every 2500 births. In contrast, it is quite rare in Asians, occurring only once in every 90,000 births. Similarly, sickle cell disease affects approximately 1 in 600 American blacks, but it is rarely seen in whites. Both of these diseases are single-gene disorders, and they vary among populations because disease-causing mutations are more or less common in different populations. (This is in turn the result of differences in the evolutionary history of these populations.) Nongenetic (environmental) factors have little influence on the current prevalence of these diseases.

The picture often becomes more complex with the common diseases of adulthood. For example, colon cancer was, until recently, relatively rare in Japan, but it is the second most common cancer in the United States. Stomach cancer, on the other hand, is common in Japan but relatively rare in the United States. These statistics, in themselves, cannot distinguish environmental from genetic influences in the two populations. However, because large numbers of Japanese emigrated first to Hawaii and then to the U.S. mainland, we can observe what happens to the rates of stomach and colon cancer among the migrants. It is important that the Japanese émigrés have maintained a genetic identity, marrying largely among themselves. Among first-generation Japanese in Hawaii, the frequency of colon cancer rose several-fold—not yet as high as in the U.S. mainland but higher than in Japan. Among second-generation Japanese on the U.S. mainland, colon cancer rates rose to 5%, equal to the U.S. average. At the same time, stomach cancer has become relatively rare among Japanese-Americans.

These observations strongly indicate an important role for environmental or lifestyle factors in the etiology of cancers of the colon and stomach. In each case, diet is a likely culprit—a high-fat, low-fiber diet in the United States is thought to increase the risk of colon cancer, whereas techniques used to preserve and season the fish commonly eaten in Japan are thought to increase the risk of stomach cancer. It is interesting that the incidence of colon cancer in Japan has increased dramatically during the past several decades as the Japanese population has adopted a more "Western" diet. These results do not, however, rule out the potential contribution of genetic factors in common cancers. Genes also play a role in the etiology of colon and other cancers.

Analysis of Risk Factors

The comparison just discussed is one example of the analysis of risk factors (in this case, diet) and their influence on the prevalence of disease in populations. A common measure of the effect of a specific risk factor is the **relative risk.** This quantity is expressed as a ratio:

$$\frac{\text{Incidence rate of the disease among individuals exposed to a risk factor}}{\text{Incidence rate of the disease among individuals } \textit{not} \text{ exposed to a risk factor}}$$

A classic example of a relative risk analysis was carried out in a sample of more than 40,000 British physicians to determine the relationship between cigarette smoking and lung cancer. This study compared the incidence of death from lung cancer in physicians who smoked with those who did not. The incidence of death from lung cancer was 1.66 (per 1000 person-years) in heavy smokers (more than 25 cigarettes daily), but it was only 0.07 in the nonsmokers. The ratio of these two incidence rates is 1.66/0.07, which yields a relative risk of 23.7. We can thus conclude that the risk of dying from lung cancer increased by about 24-fold in heavy smokers compared with nonsmokers. Many other studies have obtained similar risk figures.

Although cigarette smoking clearly increases one's risk of developing lung cancer (as well as heart disease, as we will see below), it is equally clear that *most* smokers do not develop lung cancer. Other lifestyle factors are likely to contribute to one's risk of developing this disease (e.g., exposure to cancer-causing substances in the air, such as asbestos fibers). In addition, differences in genetic background may be involved. Some studies have suggested that mutations in a gene called *FHIT* may make some individuals more sensitive to the carcinogenic effects of tobacco smoke.

Many factors can influence the risk of acquiring a common disease such as cancer, diabetes, or high blood pressure.

These include age, gender, diet, exercise, and family history of the disease. Usually, complex interactions occur among these genetic and nongenetic factors. The effects of each factor can be quantified in terms of relative risks. The following discussion demonstrates how genetic and environmental factors contribute to the risk of developing common diseases.

PRINCIPLES OF MULTIFACTORIAL INHERITANCE

Basic Model

Traits in which variation is thought to be caused by the combined effects of multiple genes are **polygenic** ("many genes"). When environmental or lifestyle factors are also believed to cause variation in the trait, which is usually the case, the term **multifactorial trait** is used.[4] Many **quantitative traits** (those, such as blood pressure, that are measured on a continuous numeric scale) are multifactorial. Because they are caused by the additive effects of many genetic and environmental factors, these traits tend to follow a normal, or bell-shaped, distribution in populations.

An example illustrates this concept. To begin with the simplest case, suppose (unrealistically) that height is determined by a single gene with two alleles, A and a. Allele A tends to make people tall, whereas allele a tends to make them short. If there is no dominance at this locus, then the three possible genotypes (AA, Aa, aa) will produce three phenotypes: tall, intermediate, and short. Assume that the gene frequencies of A and a are each 0.50. If we look at a population of individuals, we will observe the height distribution depicted in Figure 5-1, A.

Now suppose, a bit more realistically, that height is determined by two loci instead of one. The second locus also has two alleles, B (tall) and b (short), and they affect height in exactly the same way as alleles A and a. There are now nine possible genotypes in our population: aabb, aaBb, aaBB, Aabb, AaBb, AaBB, AAbb, AABb, and AABB. An individual may have zero, one, two, three, or four "tall" alleles, so now five distinct phenotypes are possible (Figure 5-1, B). Although the height distribution in our fictional population is still not normal compared to an actual population, it approaches a normal distribution more closely than in the single-gene case just described.

We now extend our example so that *many* genes and environmental or lifestyle factors influence height, each having a small effect. Then many phenotypes are possible, each differing slightly from the others, and the height distribution of the population approaches the bell-shaped curve shown in Figure 5-1, C.

It should be emphasized that the individual genes underlying a multifactorial trait such as height follow the mendelian principles of segregation and independent assortment, just like any other gene. The only difference is that many of them *act together* to influence the trait.

Blood pressure is another example of a multifactorial trait. A correlation exists between parents' blood pressures (systolic

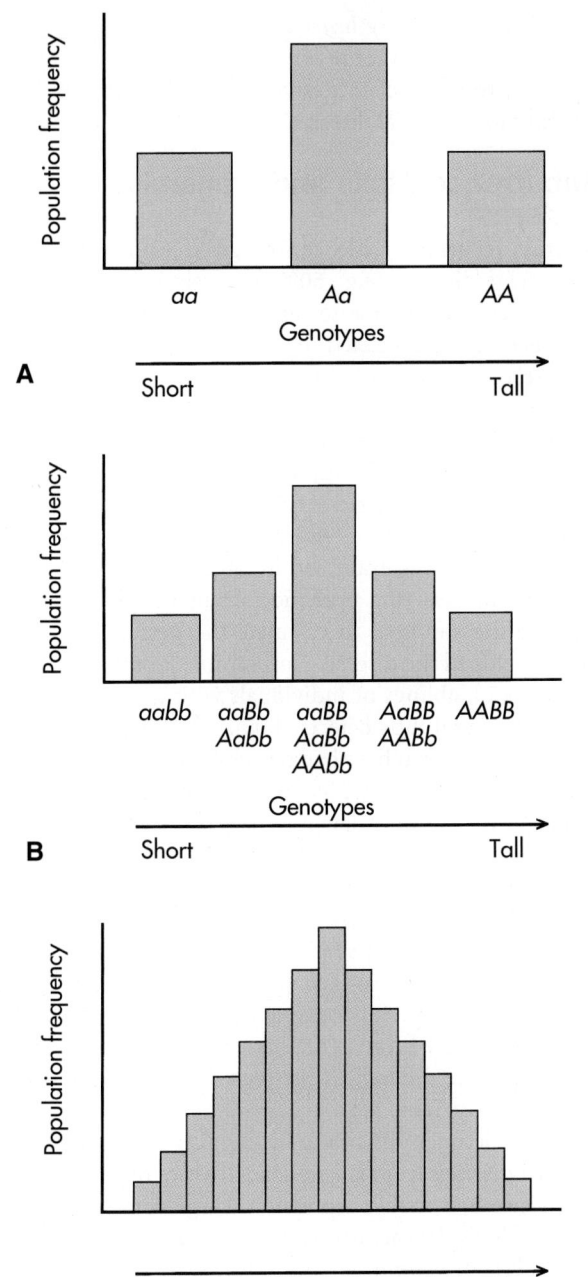

Figure 5-1 Distribution of height. A, Distribution of height in a population, assuming that height is controlled by a single locus with genotypes *AA, Aa,* and *aa.* **B,** Distribution of height, assuming that height is controlled by two loci. Five distinct genotypes are shown instead of three, and the distribution begins to look more like the normal distribution. **C,** Distribution of height, assuming that multiple factors, each with a small effect, contribute to the trait (multifactorial model). (From Jorde LB et al: *Medical genetics,* ed 3, St Louis, 2003, Mosby.)

and diastolic) and those of their children. The evidence is good that this correlation is partially caused by genes, but blood pressure is also influenced by environmental factors, such as diet, exercise, and stress. Two goals of genetic research are the identification and measurement of the relative roles of genes and environment in the causation of multifactorial diseases.

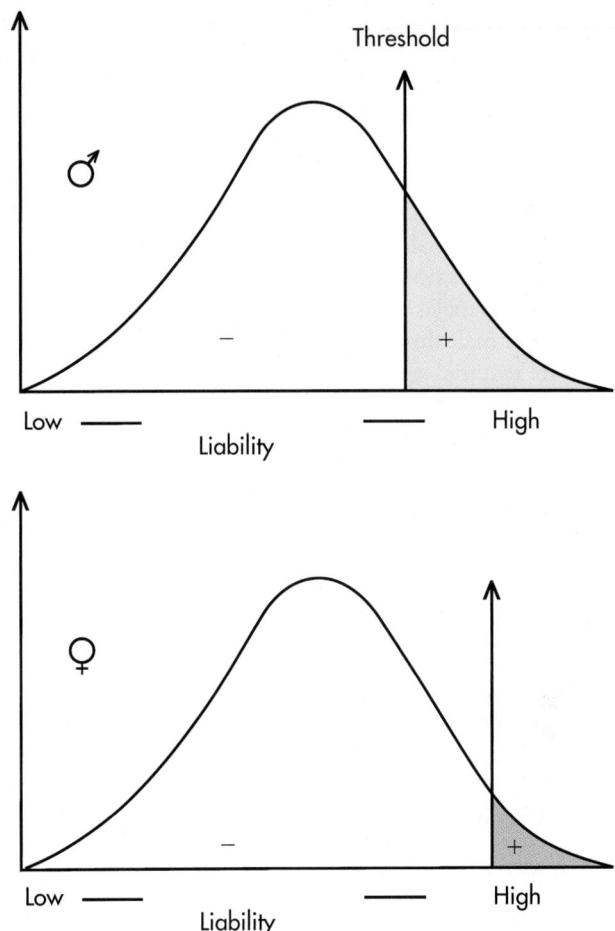

Figure 5-2 A liability distribution in a population for a multifactorial disease. To be affected with the disease, an individual must exceed the threshold on the liability distribution. This figure shows two thresholds, a lower one for males and a higher one for females (as in pyloric stenosis; see text). (From Jorde LB et al: *Medical genetics,* ed 3, St Louis, 2003, Mosby.)

Threshold Model

A number of diseases do not follow the bell-shaped distribution. Instead, they appear to be either present or absent in individuals; yet they do not follow the inheritance patterns expected of single-gene diseases. A commonly used explanation for such diseases is that there is an underlying **liability distribution** for the disease in a population (Figure 5-2). Those individuals who are on the "low" end of the distribution have little chance of developing the disease in question (i.e., they have few of the alleles or environmental factors that would cause the disease). Individuals who are closer to the "high" end of the distribution have more of the disease-causing genes and environmental factors and are more likely to develop the disease. For diseases that are either present or absent, it is thought that a **threshold of liability** must be crossed before the disease is expressed. Below the threshold, the individual appears normal; above it, he or she is affected by the disease.

A disease that is thought to correspond to this threshold model is *pyloric stenosis,* a disorder that presents shortly after birth and is caused by a narrowing or obstruction of the pylorus, the area between the stomach and intestine. Chronic vomiting, constipation, weight loss, and electrolyte imbalance result from the condition, but it sometimes resolves spontaneously or can be corrected by surgery. The prevalence of pyloric stenosis is about 3 per 1000 live births in whites. It is much more common in males than females, affecting 1 of 200 males and 1 of 1000 females. It is thought that this difference in prevalence reflects two thresholds in the liability distribution—a lower one in males and a higher one in females (see Figure 5-2). A lower male threshold implies that fewer disease-causing factors are required to generate the disorder in males.

The liability threshold concept may explain the pattern of recurrence risks for pyloric stenosis seen in Table 5-1. Note that males, having a lower threshold, always have a higher risk than females. However, the sibling risk also depends on the gender of the proband (i.e., the individual from which the pedigree begins). It is higher when the proband is female than when the proband is male. This reflects the concept that females, having a higher liability threshold, must be exposed to more disease-causing factors than males to develop the disease. Thus a family with an affected female must have more genetic and environmental risk factors, producing a higher recurrence risk for pyloric stenosis in future offspring. It would be expected that the highest risk category would be *male* relatives of *female* probands; Table 5-1 shows that this is the case.

A similar pattern has been observed in a study of *infantile autism*, a behavioral disorder in which the male/female ratio is approximately 4:1. As expected for a multifactorial disorder, the recurrence risks for siblings of male probands (3.5%) is substantially lower than that of siblings of female probands (7%). When the sex ratio for a disease is reversed (i.e., more affected females than males), one would expect a higher recurrence risk when the proband is male.

A number of other congenital malformations are thought to correspond to this model. They include *isolated cleft lip and/or cleft palate (CL/P), neural tube defects (anencephaly, spina bifida), clubfoot (talipes),* and some forms of *congenital heart disease.* In this context, *isolated* means that this is the only observed disease feature (i.e., the feature is not part of a larger constellation of findings, as in CL/P secondary to trisomy 13). In addition, many common adult diseases, such as

hypertension, coronary heart disease, stroke, diabetes mellitus (types 1 and 2), and some *cancers*, are caused by complex genetic, environmental, or lifestyle factors and can thus be considered multifactorial diseases.

Recurrence Risks and Transmission Patterns

Whereas recurrence risks can be given with confidence for single-gene diseases (e.g., 50% for typical autosomal dominant diseases, 25% for autosomal recessive diseases), the situation is more complicated for multifactorial diseases. This is because the number of genes contributing to the disease is usually not known, the precise allelic constitution of the parents is not known, and the extent of environmental or lifestyle effects can vary substantially. For most multifactorial diseases, **empirical risks** (i.e., risks based on direct observation of data) have been derived. To estimate empirical risks, a large series of families is examined in which one child has developed the disease (the proband). Then the siblings of each proband are surveyed to calculate the percentage who also have developed the disease. For example, in the United States about 3% of siblings of individuals with neural tube defects also have neural tube defects (Box 5-1). Thus the recurrence risk for parents who have had one child with a neural tube defect is 3% in the United States. For conditions such as cleft lip/palate that are not lethal or severely debilitating, recurrence risks also can be estimated for the offspring of affected parents. Empirical recurrence risks are, of course, specific for each multifactorial disease.

In contrast to most single-gene diseases, recurrence risks for multifactorial diseases can change substantially from one population to another because gene frequencies as well as environmental and lifestyle factors can differ among populations (note the differences between the London and Belfast populations in Table 5-1).

It is sometimes difficult to distinguish polygenic or multifactorial diseases from single-gene diseases that have reduced penetrance or variable expression. Large data sets and good epidemiologic data are necessary to make the distinction. Several criteria are commonly used to define multifactorial inheritance.

First, *the recurrence risk becomes higher if more than one family member is affected.* For example, the sibling recurrence risk for a *ventricular septal defect* (VSD), a type of congenital heart defect) is 3% if one sibling has had a VSD but increases to approximately 10% if two siblings have had VSDs.[5] In contrast, the recurrence risk for single-gene diseases remains the same regardless of the number of affected siblings. It should be emphasized that this increase does not mean that the family's risk has actually *changed*. Rather, it means that we now have more information about the family's true risk: because they have had two affected children, they are probably located higher on the liability distribution than a family with only one affected child. In other words, they have more risk factors (genetic or environmental) and are more likely to produce an affected child.

Table 5-1	Recurrence Risks (%) for Pyloric Stenosis, Subdivided by Genders of Affected Probands and Relatives*			
	Male Probands		Female Probands	
Relatives	London	Belfast	London	Belfast
Brothers	3.8	9.6	9.2	12.5
Sisters	2.7	3.0	3.8	3.8

Data from Carter CO: *Br Med Bull* 32(1):21-26, 1976.
*Note that the risks differ somewhat between the two populations.

Box 5-1 | Neural Tube Defects

Neural tube defects (NTDs), which include *anencephaly, spina bifida,* and *encephalocele* (as well as several other less common forms), are one of the most important classes of birth defects, with a birth prevalence of 1 to 3 per 1000.[25] The prevalence of NTDs among different populations varies considerably, with an especially high rate among some northern Chinese populations (as high as 6 or more per 1000 births). In the United States, NTDs are two to three times more common in the eastern than in the western parts of the country. For reasons that are not fully known, the prevalence of NTDs has been decreasing in many parts of the United States and Europe during the past 2½ decades.

Normally the neural tube closes at about the fourth week of gestation. A defect in closure, or a subsequent reopening of the neural tube, results in a neural tube defect. Spina bifida (Figure 5-3, *A*) is the most commonly observed NTD and consists of a protrusion of spinal tissue through the vertebral column (the tissue usually includes meninges, spinal cord, and nerve roots). About 75% of spina bifida patients have secondary hydrocephalus, which sometimes in turn produces mental retardation. Paralysis or muscle weakness, lack of sphincter control, and clubfeet are often observed. A study conducted in British Columbia showed that survival rates for spina bifida patients have improved dramatically over the past several decades. Fewer than 30% of patients born between 1952 and 1969 survived to 10 years of age, whereas 65% of those born between 1970 and 1986 survived to this age. Anencephaly (Figure 5-3, *B*) is characterized by partial or complete absence of the cranial vault and calvarium and partial or complete absence of the cerebral hemispheres. At least two thirds of newborns with anencephaly are stillborn; term deliveries do not survive more than a few hours or days.

NTDs are thought to arise from a combination of genetic environmental factors. In most populations surveyed thus far, empirical recurrence risks for siblings of affected patients range from 2% to 5%. Consistent with a multifactorial model, the recurrence risk increases with additional affected siblings. Studies conducted in Great Britain showed that the sibling recurrence risk was approximately 5% when one sibling was affected and 10% when two were affected. A Hungarian study showed that the overall prevalence of NTDs was 1 in 300 births and that the sibling recurrence risks were 3%, 12%, and 25% after one, two, and three affected offspring, respectively. Recurrence risks tend to be slightly lower in populations with lower NTD prevalence rates, as predicted by the multifactorial model. Recurrence risk data support the idea that the major forms of NTDs are caused by similar factors. An anencephalic conception increases the recurrence risk for subsequent spina bifida conceptions, and vice versa.

NTDs can usually be diagnosed prenatally, sometimes by ultrasound and usually by an elevation in α-fetoprotein (AFP) in the maternal serum or amniotic fluid (see Chapters 11 and 19). A spina bifida lesion can be either open or closed (i.e., covered with a layer of skin). Fetuses with open spina bifida are more likely to be detected by AFP assays.

A major epidemiologic finding is that mothers who supplement their diet with folic acid at the time of conception are less likely to produce children with NTDs. This result has been replicated in several different populations and thus appears to be well confirmed. It has been estimated that as many as 50% to 70% of NTDs can be avoided simply by dietary folic acid supplementation.[26] (Traditional prenatal vitamin supplements have little effect, since administration does not usually begin until well after the time that the neural tube closes.) Because mothers would be likely to ingest similar amounts of folic acid from one pregnancy to the next, folic acid deficiency could well account for at least part of the elevated sibling recurrence risk for NTDs. This is an important example of a *nongenetic* factor that contributes to familial clustering of a disease.

Second, *if the expression of the disease in the proband is more severe, the recurrence risk is higher.* This is again consistent with the liability model because a more severe expression indicates that the affected individual is at the extreme tail end of the liability distribution (see Figure 5-2). His or her relatives are thus at a higher risk for inheriting disease genes. For example, the occurrence of a bilateral (both sides) cleft lip/palate confers a higher recurrence risk on family members than does the occurrence of a unilateral (one side) cleft.

Third, *the recurrence risk is higher if the proband is of the less commonly affected sex* (see the preceding discussion of pyloric stenosis). This is because an affected individual of the less susceptible gender is usually at a more extreme position on the liability distribution.

Fourth, *the recurrence risk for the disease usually decreases rapidly in more remotely related relatives* (Table 5-2). Whereas the recurrence risk for single-gene diseases decreases by 50% with each degree of relationship (e.g., an autosomal dominant disease has a 50% recurrence risk for siblings, 25% for uncle-nephew relationships, 12.5% for first cousins), it decreases much more quickly for multifactorial diseases. This reflects the fact that many genes and environmental factors must combine to produce a trait. All the necessary risk factors are unlikely to be present in less closely related family members.

Table 5-2 | Recurrence Risks (%) for First-, Second-, and Third-Degree Relatives

	Risk			
Disease	First Degree	Second Degree	Third Degree	General Population
Cleft lip/palate	4.0	.7	.3	.1
Clubfoot	2.5	.5	.2	.1
Congenital hip dislocation	5.0	.6	.4	.2
Infantile autism	4.5	.1	.05	.04

Finally, *if the prevalence of the disease in a population is f, the risk for offspring and siblings of probands is approximately* $\sqrt{f}$. This does not hold true for single-gene traits because their recurrence risks are independent of population prevalence. It is not an absolute rule for multifactorial traits either, but many such diseases tend to conform to this prediction. Examination of the risks given in Table 5-2 shows that the first three diseases follow the prediction fairly well. However, the observed sibling risk for the fourth disease, infantile autism, is substantially higher than predicted by $\sqrt{f}$.

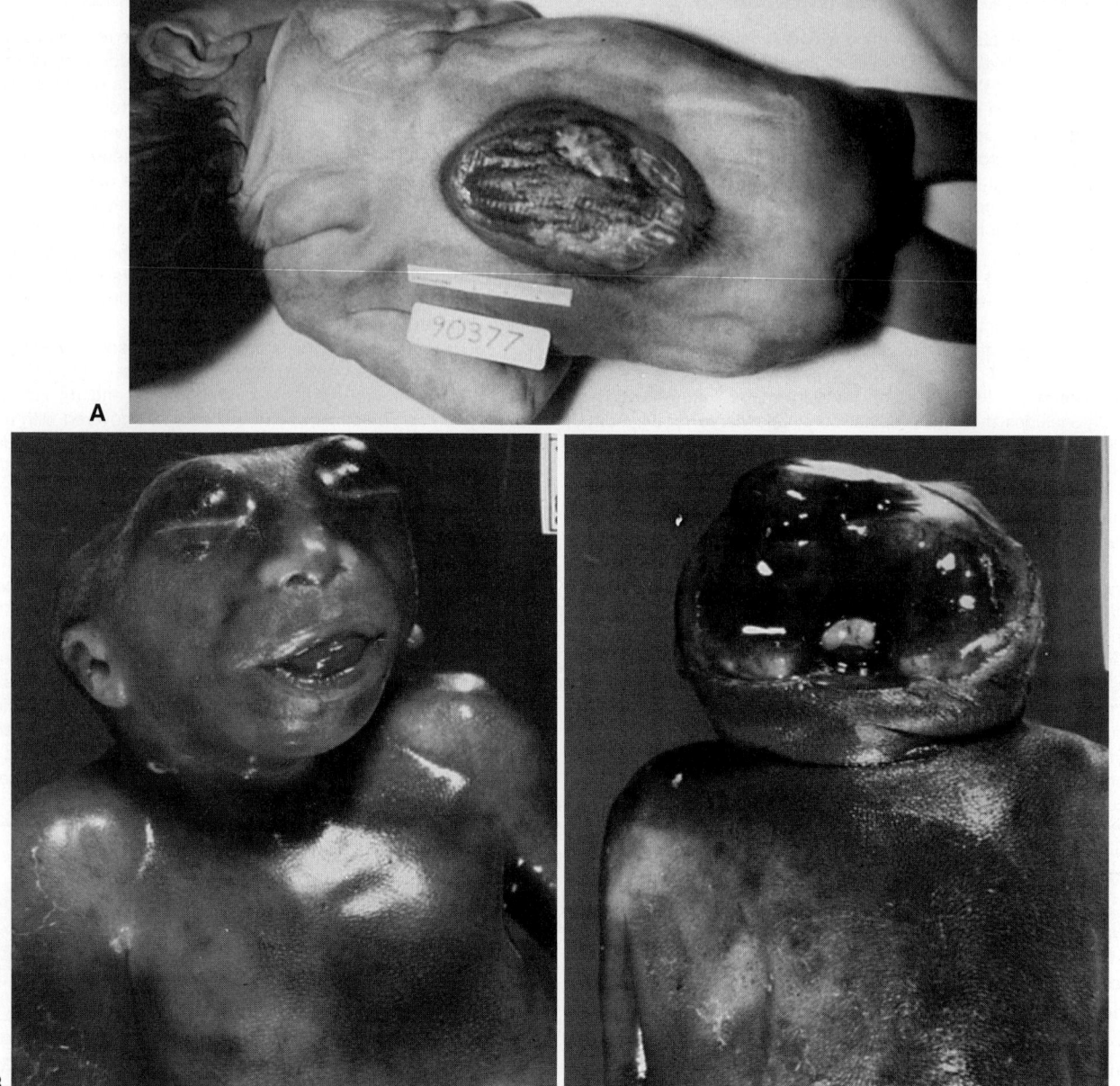

Figure 5-3 Spina bifida and anencephaly. **A,** Spina bifida in a newborn. **B** and **C,** Anencephaly, showing the absence of the cranial vault. (From Jorde LB et al: *Medical genetics,* ed 3, St Louis, 2003, Mosby.)

NATURE AND NURTURE: DISENTANGLING THE EFFECTS OF GENES AND ENVIRONMENT OR LIFE-STYLE

Family members share genes and a common environment. Family resemblance in traits such as blood pressure reflects both genetic and environmental–life-style commonality ("nature" and "nurture," respectively). For centuries people have debated the relative importance of these two types of factors. It is a mistake, of course, to view them as mutually exclusive. Few traits are influenced only by genes or only by environment or life-style factors. Most are influenced by both. It is

useful to try to determine the *relative* influence of genetic and environmental or life-style factors (Figure 5-4). This can lead to a better understanding of disease etiology. It can also help in planning public health strategies. A disease in which the genetic influence is relatively small, such as lung cancer, may be prevented most effectively through emphasis on life-style changes (avoidance of tobacco). When a disease has a relatively larger genetic component, as in breast cancer, examination of family history should be emphasized in addition to lifestyle modification.

Here, two research strategies are reviewed that often are used to estimate the relative influence of genes and environment: twin studies and adoption studies.

Twin Studies

Twins occur with a frequency of about 1 in 100 births in white populations. They are a bit more common in blacks and a bit less common among Asians. **Monozygotic** (MZ, or **"identical") twins** originate when, for unknown reasons, the developing embryo divides to form two separate but identical embryos. Because they are genetically identical, MZ twins are an example of natural clones. **Dizygotic** (DZ, or **"fraternal") twins** are the result of a double ovulation followed by the fertilization of each egg by a different sperm. Thus dizygotic twins are genetically no more similar than siblings. Because two different sperm cells are required to fertilize the two eggs, it is possible for each DZ twin to have a different father. Whereas MZ twinning rates are constant across populations,

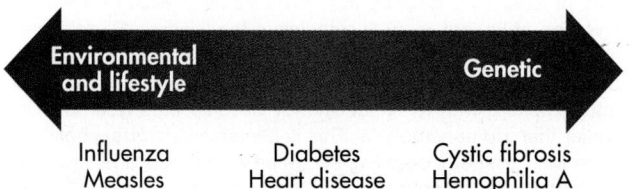

Figure 5-4 Continuum of genetic diseases. Some diseases (e.g., cystic fibrosis) are strongly determined by genes, whereas others (e.g., infectious diseases) are strongly determined by environment and lifestyle factors. (Adapted from Jorde LB et al: *Medical genetics,* ed 3, St Louis, 2003, Mosby.)

DZ twinning rates vary somewhat. DZ twinning increases with maternal age until about 40 years, after which it declines.

Because MZ twins are genetically identical, any differences between them should be caused only by environmental effects.[6] MZ twins should thus resemble one another very closely for traits that are strongly influenced by genes. DZ twins provide a convenient comparison because their environmental differences should be similar to those of MZ twins, but their genetic differences are as great as those between siblings. Twin studies thus usually consist of comparisons between MZ and DZ twins.[7] If both members of a twin pair share a trait (e.g., a cleft lip), it is said to be a **concordant trait.** If they do not share the trait, it is a **discordant trait.** For a trait determined totally by genes, MZ twins should always be concordant, whereas DZ twins should be concordant less often, because they, like siblings, share only 50% of their genes. Concordance rates may differ between opposite-sex DZ twin pairs and same-sex DZ pairs for some traits, such as those that have different frequencies in males and females. For such traits, only same-sex DZ twin pairs should be used when comparing MZ and DZ concordance rates, because MZ twins are necessarily of the same sex.

Table 5-3 gives concordance rates for a number of traits. Note that the concordance rates for contagious diseases such as measles are quite similar in MZ and DZ twins. This is

Table 5-3	Concordance Rates in MZ and DZ Twins for Selected Traits and Diseases*		
	Concordance Rate		
Trait or Disease	**MZ Twins**	**DZ Twins**	**Heritability**
Affective disorder (bipolar)	.79	.24	>1.00†
Affective disorder (unipolar)	.54	.19	.70
Alcoholism	>.60	<.30	.60
Autism	.92	.00	>1.00
Blood pressure (diastolic)‡	.58	.27	.62
Blood pressure (systolic)‡	.55	.25	.60
Body fat percentage‡	.73	.22	>1.00
Body mass index‡	.95	.53	.84
Cleft lip/palate	.38	.08	.60
Clubfoot	.32	.03	.58
Dermatoglyphics (finger ridge count)‡	.95	.49	.92
Diabetes mellitus	.45-.96	.03-.37	>1.00
Diabetes mellitus (type 1)	.55	—	—
Diabetes mellitus (type 2)	.90	—	—
Epilepsy (idiopathic)	.69	.14	>1.00
Height‡	.94	.44	1.00
Intelligence quotient (IQ)‡	.76	.51	.50
Measles	.95	.87	.16
Multiple sclerosis	.28	.03	.50
Myocardial infarction (males)	.39	.26	.26
Myocardial infarction (females)	.44	.14	.60
Schizophrenia	.47	.12	.70
Spina bifida	.72	.33	.78

NOTE: Heritability, which is defined as the proportion of the variation in a trait that is due to genetic factors, can be measured as $2(C_{MZ} - C_{DZ})$, where C_{MZ} and C_{DZ} are the concordance rates for MZ twins and DZ twins respectively.

*These figures were compiled from a large variety of sources and represent primarily European and U.S. populations.

†Several heritability estimates exceed 1.0. Because it is impossible for >100% of the variance of a trait to be genetically determined, these values indicate that other factors, such as shared environmental factors, must be operating.

‡Because these are quantitative traits, correlation coefficients are given rather than concordance rates.

expected, because a contagious disease is unlikely to be influenced markedly by genes. On the other hand, the concordance rates are quite dissimilar for *schizophrenia* and *bipolar affective disorder,* suggesting a sizable genetic component for these diseases. The MZ correlations for dermatoglyphics (fingerprints), which are determined almost entirely by genes, are close to 1.0.

At one time, twins were thought to provide a perfect "natural laboratory" in which to determine the relative influences of genetics and environment, but several difficulties arise. One of the most important is the assumption that the environments of MZ and DZ twins are equally similar. As one would expect, MZ twins are often treated more similarly than DZ twins. A greater similarity in environment can make MZ twins more concordant for a trait, inflating the apparent influence of genes. In addition, MZ twins may be more likely to seek the same type of environment, further reinforcing environmental similarity. On the other hand, it has been suggested that MZ twins tend to develop personality differences in an attempt to assert their individuality.

Adoption Studies

Studies of adopted children also are used to estimate the genetic contribution to a multifactorial trait. Children born to parents who have a disease but are then subsequently adopted by parents lacking the disease can be studied to find out whether these children develop the disease. In some cases such children develop the disease more often than a comparative control population (i.e., adopted children who were born to parents who do *not* have the disease). This provides some evidence that genes may be involved in the causation of the disease, because the adopted children do not share an environment with their affected natural parents. For example, about 8% to 10% of adopted children of a schizophrenic parent develop *schizophrenia,* whereas only 1% of adopted children of normal parents develop schizophrenia.

As with twin studies, several precautions must be exercised in interpreting the results of adoption studies. First, prenatal environmental influences could have long-lasting effects on an adopted child. Second, children are sometimes adopted after they are several years old, ensuring that some environmental influence would have been imparted by the natural parents. Finally, adoption agencies sometimes try to match the adoptive parents with the natural parents in terms of background, socioeconomic status, and so on. All of these factors could exaggerate the apparent influence of biologic inheritance.

These reservations, as well as those summarized for twin studies, underscore the need for caution in basing conclusions on twin and adoption studies. These approaches do not provide definitive measures of the role of genes in multifactorial disease nor can they identify specific genes responsible for disease. Instead, they serve a useful purpose in providing a preliminary indication of the extent to which a multifactorial disease may be caused by genetic factors. Currently, sophisticated molecular techniques are being used to identify the spe-

---

Box 5-2	α_1-Antitrypsin Deficiency: The Interaction of Genes and Environment–Life-style

α_1-Antitrypsin (α_1-AT) deficiency is one of the most common autosomal recessive disorders among whites, affecting approximately 1 in 2500 members of this ethnic group. α_1-AT, synthesized primarily in the liver, is a serine protease inhibitor. It does bind trypsin, as its name suggests. However, α_1-AT binds much more strongly to neutrophil elastase, a protease that is produced by neutrophils (a type of leukocyte) in response to infections and irritants. It carries out its binding and inhibitory role primarily in the lower respiratory tract, where it prevents elastase from digesting the alveolar septi of the lung.

Individuals with less than 10% to 15% of the normal level of α_1-AT activity will experience significant lung damage and typically develop emphysema during their 30s, 40s, or 50s. In addition, at least 10% develop liver cirrhosis as a result of the accumulation of variant α_1-AT molecules in the liver; α_1-AT deficiency accounts for nearly 20% of all nonalcoholic liver cirrhosis in the United States. An important feature of this disease is that cigarette smokers with α_1-AT deficiency develop emphysema much earlier than do nonsmokers. This is because cigarette smoke irritates lung tissue, increasing secretion of neutrophil elastase. At the same time it inactivates α_1-AT, so there is also less inhibition of elastase. One study showed that the median age of survival of nonsmokers with α_1-AT deficiency was 62 years, whereas it was only 40 years for smokers with this disease. Because the combination of cigarette smoking (an environmental–life-style factor) and the α_1-AT mutation (a genetic factor) produces more severe disease than either factor alone, it is an example of a gene-environment interaction.

---

cific genes that underlie predisposition to multifactorial diseases.

This discussion should make clear that most common diseases are not the result of either genetics *or* environment. Instead, genetic and nongenetic factors usually interact to influence one's likelihood of developing a common disease. In some cases a genetic predisposition may interact with an environmental factor to increase the risk of disease to a much higher level than would either factor acting alone. A good example of a **gene-environment–life-style interaction** is given by α_1-antitrypsin deficiency, a genetic condition that causes pulmonary emphysema and is greatly exacerbated by cigarette smoking (Box 5-2).

GENETICS OF COMMON DISEASES

Some common multifactorial disorders, the congenital malformations, are by definition present at birth. Others, including heart disease, cancer, diabetes, and most psychiatric disorders, are seen primarily in adolescents and adults. Because these disorders are complex, unraveling their genetics is a daunting task. Nonetheless, significant progress is now being made.

Congenital Malformations

Congenital diseases are present at birth. Approximately 2% of newborns present with a congenital malformation; most of these are multifactorial in etiology. Table 5-4 lists some more

Table 5-4	Prevalence Rates of Common Congenital Malformations in Whites
Disorder	**Prevalence per 1000 Births (Approximate)**
Cleft lip/palate	1
Clubfoot	1
Congenital heart defects	4-8
Hydrocephaly	0.5-2.5
Isolated cleft palate	0.4
Neural tube defects	1-3
Pyloric stenosis	3

Table 5-5	Prevalence of Common Adult Diseases in the United States
Disease	**Number Affected (Approximate)**
Alcoholism	14 million
Alzheimer disease	4 million
Arthritis	43 million
Asthma	17 million
Cancer	8 million
Cardiovascular disease (all forms)	
Coronary artery disease	13 million
Congestive heart failure	5 million
Congenital defects	1 million
Hypertension	50 million
Stroke	5 million
Depression and bipolar disorder	17 million
Diabetes (type 1)	1 million
Diabetes (type 2)	15 million
Epilepsy	2.5 million
Multiple sclerosis	350,000
Obesity*	60 million
Parkinson disease	500,000
Psoriasis	3–5 million
Schizophrenia	2 million

Data from National Center for Chronic Disease Prevention and Health Promotion; American Heart Association (2002 Heart and Stroke Statistical Update); National Institute on Alcohol Abuse and Alcoholism; Office of the U.S. Surgeon General; American Academy of Allergy, Asthma and Immunology; Cown WM, Kandel ER. *JAMA* 285:594-600, 2001; Flegal et al. *JAMA* 288:1723–1727, 2002.
*Body mass index >30.

common congenital malformations. In general, sibling recurrence risks for most of these disorders range from 1% to 5%.

Some congenital malformations, such as cleft lip/palate and pyloric stenosis, are relatively easy to repair and thus are not considered to be serious problems. Others, such as the neural tube defects, usually have more severe consequences. Although some cases of congenital malformations occur in the absence of any other problems, it is quite common for them to be associated with other disorders. For example, hydrocephaly and clubfoot are often seen secondary to spina bifida, cleft lip/palate is often seen in babies with trisomy 13, and congenital heart defects are seen in children with many other disorders, including Down syndrome.

Environmental factors also cause some congenital malformations. An example is thalidomide, a sedative used during pregnancy in the early 1960s. When ingested during early pregnancy this drug often caused **phocomelia** (severely shortened limbs) in babies. Maternal exposure to retinoic acid, which is used to treat acne, can cause congenital defects of the heart, ear, and central nervous system. Maternal rubella infection can cause congenital heart defects.

Multifactorial Disorders in the Adult Population

Until quite recently, very little was known about specific genes responsible for common adult diseases. With the more powerful laboratory and analytic techniques now available, this situation is changing. This section reviews recent progress in understanding the genetics of the major common adult diseases. Table 5-5 gives approximate prevalence figures for these disorders in the United States.

Coronary Heart Disease

It is well known that coronary heart disease (CHD) is the leading killer of Americans, accounting for approximately 25% of all deaths in the United States. It is caused by *atherosclerosis* (narrowing as a result of the formation of lipid-laden lesions) of the coronary arteries. This narrowing impedes blood flow to the heart and can eventually result in a *myocardial infarction* (destruction of heart tissue caused by an inadequate supply of oxygen). When atherosclerosis occurs in arteries supplying blood to the brain, a *stroke* can result. Many

risk factors for heart disease have been identified, including obesity, cigarette smoking, hypertension, elevated cholesterol level, and positive family history (usually defined as having one affected first-degree relative). Many studies have examined the role of family history in CHD, and they show that an individual with a positive family history is two to seven times more likely to have heart disease than is an individual with no family history (this would be the relative risk of heart disease as a result of a positive family history). Generally, these studies also show that the risk increases if (1) there are more affected relatives; (2) the affected relative or relatives are female (the less commonly affected sex) rather than male; and (3) age of onset in the affected relative is early (before 55 years). For example, one study showed that men between the ages of 20 and 39 years had a relative risk of 3.0 for CHD if they had one affected first-degree relative. The relative risk increased to 13 if two first-degree relatives were affected with CHD before 55 years of age.[8]

What part do genes play in the familial clustering of heart disease? Because of the key role of lipids in atherosclerosis, many current studies are focusing on the genetic determination of various lipoproteins.[9] Undoubtedly the most important advance in this area has been the isolation and cloning of the gene for the LDL (low-density lipoprotein) receptor

Box 5-3   Familial Hypercholesterolemia

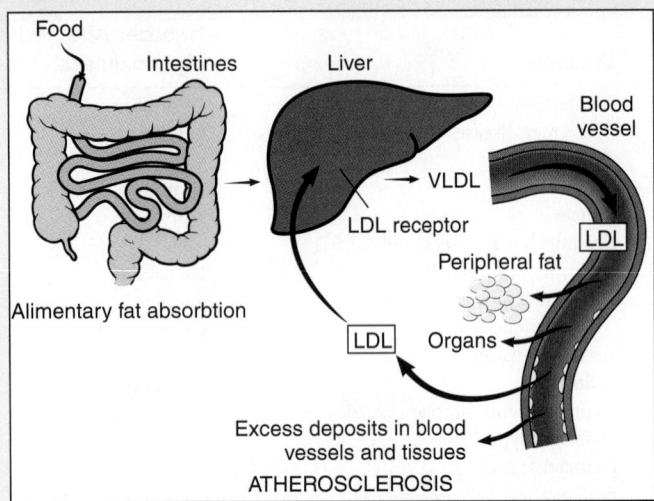

Autosomal dominant familial hypercholesterolemia (FH) is an important cause of heart disease, accounting for approximately 5% of myocardial infarctions in persons under 60 years of age.[27] FH is one of the most common autosomal dominant disorders: in most populations surveyed to date, about 1 in 500 persons is a heterozygote. Plasma cholesterol levels are approximately twice as high as normal (i.e., about 300 to 400 mg/dl), resulting in substantially accelerated atherosclerosis and distinctive cholesterol deposits in skin and tendons (xanthomas, Figure 5-5). Data compiled from five studies showed that approximately 75% of men with FH developed coronary disease and 50% had a fatal myocardial infarction by 60 years. The corresponding percentages for women were lower (45% and 15%) because women generally develop heart disease at a later age than men.

Consistent with Hardy-Weinberg predictions, about 1 in 1 million births is homozygous for the FH gene. Homozygotes are much more severely affected, with cholesterol levels ranging from 600 to 1200 mg/dl. Most experience myocardial infarctions before 20 years of age, and a myocardial infarction at 18 months of age has been reported. If untreated, most FH homozygotes die before 30 years of age.

All cells require cholesterol as a component of their plasma membrane. They can either synthesize their own cholesterol, or, preferably, obtain it from the extracellular environment, where it is carried primarily by low-density lipoprotein (LDL). In a process known as endocytosis, LDL-bound cholesterol is taken into the cell via LDL receptors on the cell's surface (Figure 5-6). FH is caused by a reduction in the number of functional LDL receptors on cell surfaces. Lacking the normal number of LDL receptors, cellular cholesterol uptake is reduced and circulating cholesterol levels increase.

Much of what we know about endocytosis has been learned through the study of LDL receptors. The process of endocytosis and the processing of LDL in the cell are described in detail in Figure 5-6 (endocytosis is discussed in Chapter 1). These processes result in a fine-tuned regulation of cholesterol levels within cells, and they influence the level of circulating cholesterol as well.

The isolation and cloning of the LDL receptor gene in 1984 were critical steps in understanding exactly how LDL receptor defects cause FH. This gene, located on chromosome 19, is 45 kb in length and consists of 18 exons and 17 introns. It encodes a 5.3-kb messenger ribonucleic acid (mRNA) transcript that ultimately produces a mature protein of 839 amino acids. More than 600 different muta-

tions, including missense and nonsense substitutions as well as insertions and deletions, have been identified in the LDL receptor gene. These can be grouped into five broad classes according to their effects on the activity of the receptor.[28] Class 1 mutations result in no detectable protein product. Thus heterozygotes would produce only half the normal number of LDL receptors. Class 2 mutations in the LDL receptor gene result in production of the LDL receptor, but it is altered such that it cannot leave the endoplasmic reticulum. It is eventually degraded. Class 3 mutations produce an LDL receptor that is capable of migrating to the cell surface but incapable of normal binding to LDL. Class 4 mutations, which are comparatively rare, produce receptors that are normal except that they do not migrate specifically to coated pits and thus cannot carry LDL into the cell. The final group of mutations, class 5, produces an LDL receptor that cannot dissociate from the LDL particle after entry into the cell. The receptor cannot return to the cell surface and is degraded. Each class of mutations reduces the number of effective LDL receptors, resulting in decreased LDL uptake and hence elevated levels of circulating cholesterol. The number of effective receptors is reduced by about half in FH heterozygotes, and homozygotes have virtually no functional LDL receptors.

Understanding the defects that lead to FH has helped to develop effective therapies for the disorder. Dietary reduction of cholesterol (primarily through the reduced intake of saturated fats) has only modest effects on cholesterol levels in FH heterozygotes. Because cholesterol is reabsorbed into the gut and then recycled through the liver (where most cholesterol synthesis takes place), serum cholesterol levels can be reduced by the administration of bile acid–absorbing resins, such as cholestyramine. The absorbed cholesterol is then excreted. It is interesting that reduced recirculation from the gut causes the liver cells to form additional LDL receptors, lowering circulating cholesterol levels. However, the decrease in intracellular cholesterol also stimulates cholesterol synthesis by liver cells, so the overall reduction in plasma LDL is only about 15% to 20%. This treatment is much more effective when combined with agents such as lovastatin that reduce cholesterol synthesis by inhibiting 3-hydroxy-3-methylglutaryl–coenzyme A (HMG-CoA) reductase. Decreased synthesis leads to further production of LDL receptors. When these therapies are used in combination, serum cholesterol levels in FH heterozygotes can be reduced to approximately normal levels.

The picture is less encouraging for FH homozygotes. The therapies just discussed can enhance cholesterol elimination and reduce its synthesis, but they are largely ineffective because homozygotes have few or no LDL receptors. Liver transplants, which provide hepatocytes that have normal LDL receptors, have been successful in some cases, but this option is often limited by a lack of donors. Plasma exchange, carried out every 1 to 2 weeks, in combination with drug therapy, can reduce cholesterol levels by about 50%. However, this therapy is difficult to continue for long periods. Somatic cell gene therapy, in which hepatocytes carrying normal LDL receptor genes are introduced into the portal circulation, is now being tested. It may eventually prove to be an effective treatment for FH homozygotes.

The FH story illustrates how medical research has made important contributions both to our understanding of basic cell biology and to advances in clinical therapy. The process of receptor-mediated endocytosis, elucidated largely by research on the LDL receptor defects, is of fundamental significance for cellular processes throughout the body. Equally important is that this research, by clarifying how cholesterol synthesis and uptake can be modified, has led to significant improvements in therapy for this important cause of heart disease.

Illustration from Damjanov I: Pathophysiology for the health-related professions, ed 2, Philadelphia, 2000, Saunders.

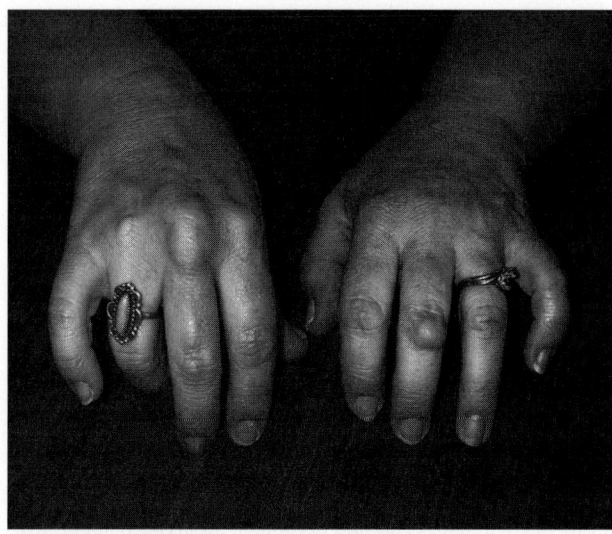

Figure 5-5 **Xanthoma.** Fatty deposits, referred to as xanthomas and seen here on the knuckles, are often noted in individuals with familial hypercholesterolemia. (From Jorde LB et al: *Medical genetics,* ed 3, St Louis, 2003, Mosby.)

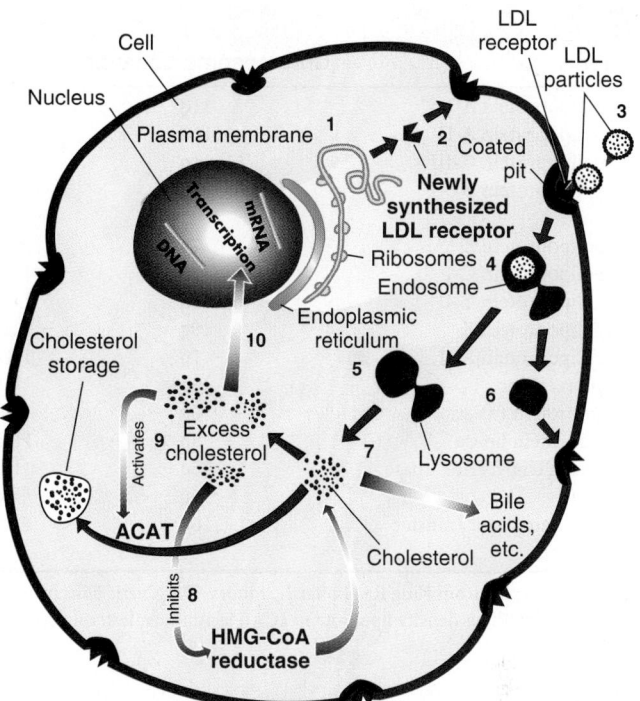

Figure 5-6 Process of receptor-mediated endocytosis. Numbers in parentheses correspond to numbers shown in the figure. *(1)* The low-density lipoprotein (LDL) receptors, which are glycoproteins, are synthesized in the endoplasmic reticulum of the cell. *(2)* From here, they pass through the Golgi apparatus to the cell surface, where part of the receptor protrudes outside the cell. *(3)* The circulating LDL particle is bound by the LDL receptor and localized in cell-surface depressions called *coated pits* (so named because they are coated with a protein called clathrin). *(4)* The coated pit invaginates, bringing the LDL particle inside the cell. *(5)* Once inside the cell, the LDL particle is separated from the receptor, taken into a lysosome, and broken down into its constituents by lysosomal enzymes. *(6)* The LDL receptor is recirculated to the cell surface to bind another LDL particle (each LDL receptor goes through this cycle approximately once every 10 minutes even if it is not occupied by an LDL particle). *(7)* Free cholesterol is released from the lysosome for incorporation into cell membranes or metabolism into bile acids or steroids. Excess cholesterol can be stored in the cell as a cholesterol ester or removed from the cell by associating with high-density lipoprotein (HDL). *(8)* As cholesterol levels in the cell rise, cellular cholesterol synthesis is reduced by inhibition of the rate-limiting enzyme HMG-CoA reductase (3-hydroxy-3-methylglutaryl-coenzyme A reductase). *(9)* Rising cholesterol levels also increase the activity of acyl coenzyme A (acyl-CoA): cholesterol acyltransferase (ACAT), an enzyme that modifies cholesterol for storage as cholesterol esters. *(10)* In addition, the number of LDL receptors is decreased by lowering the transcription rate of the LDL receptor gene itself. This decreases cholesterol uptake. (From Jorde LB et al: *Medical genetics,* ed 3, St Louis, 2003, Mosby.)

defects that cause *familial hypercholesterolemia* (Box 5-3). Nearly 20 other genes involved in lipid variation, coagulation, and hypertension have been identified, including several genes encoding apolipoproteins (the protein components of lipoproteins) (Table 5-6). Functional analysis of these genes is leading to an increased understanding, and eventually more effective treatment, of CHD.

Environmental and lifestyle factors, many of which are easily modified, are also important causes of CHD. Abundant epidemiologic evidence shows that cigarette smoking and obesity increase the risk of CHD, whereas exercise and a diet low in saturated fats decrease the risk. Indeed, the approximate 50% decline in CHD prevalence in the United States during the past 40 years is usually attributed to a decrease in the proportion of adults who smoke cigarettes, decreased consumption of saturated fats, and an increased emphasis on exercise and a generally healthier lifestyle.

Hypertension

Systemic hypertension, which is seen in at least 15% of the populations of most developed countries, is a key risk factor for heart disease, stroke, and kidney disease. Studies of blood pressure correlations within families indicate that about 20% to 40% of the variation in both systolic and diastolic blood pressure is caused by genetic factors. The fact that this figure is substantially less than 100% indicates that environmental and lifestyle factors also must be important causes of blood pressure variation. The most important environmental–lifestyle risk factors for hypertension are increased sodium intake, decreased physical activity, psychosocial stress, and obesity (but, as discussed below, the latter factor is itself influenced by both genes and environment).

Blood pressure regulation is a highly complex process that is influenced by many physiologic systems, including various aspects of kidney function, cellular ion transport, and heart function. Because of this complexity, it is unlikely that family studies of simple blood pressure will reveal much about genes responsible for hypertension. For this reason most research now focuses on specific components that may influence blood pressure variation, such as angiotensin, angiotensinogen, urinary kallikrein, and sodium-lithium countertransport[10] (Figure 5-7). These factors are more likely to be under the control of smaller numbers of genes. For example, studies have implicated the angiotensinogen gene in the causation of

Table 5-6	Lipoprotein Genes Known to Contribute to Coronary Heart Disease Risk	
Gene	**Chromosome Location**	**Function of Protein Product**
Apolipoprotein A-I	11q	HDL component; LCAT cofactor
Apolipoprotein A-IV	11q	Component of chylomicrons and HDL; may influence HDL metabolism
Apolipoprotein C-III	11q	Allelic variation associated with hypertriglyceridemia
Apolipoprotein B	2p	Ligand for LDL receptor; involved in formation of VLDL, LDL, IDL, and chylomicrons
Apolipoprotein D	2p	HDL component
Apolipoprotein C-I	19q	LCAT activation
Apolipoprotein C-II	19q	Lipoprotein lipase activation
Apolipoprotein E	19q	Ligand for LDL receptor
Apolipoprotein A-II	1p	HDL component
LDL receptor	19p	Uptake of circulating LDL particles
Lipoprotein (a)	6q	Cholesterol transport
Lipoprotein lipase	8p	Hydrolysis of lipoprotein lipids
Hepatic triglyceride lipase	15q	Hydrolysis of lipoprotein lipids
LCAT	16q	Cholesterol esterification
Cholesterol ester transfer protein	16q	Facilitates transfer of cholesterol esters and phospholipids between lipoproteins

Adapted in part from King RA, Rotter JI, editors: *The genetic basis of common diseases,* ed 2, New York, 2002, Oxford University Press.
IDL, Intermediate-density lipoprotein; *LCAT,* lecithin cholesterol acyltransferase; *VLDL,* very-low-density lipoprotein.

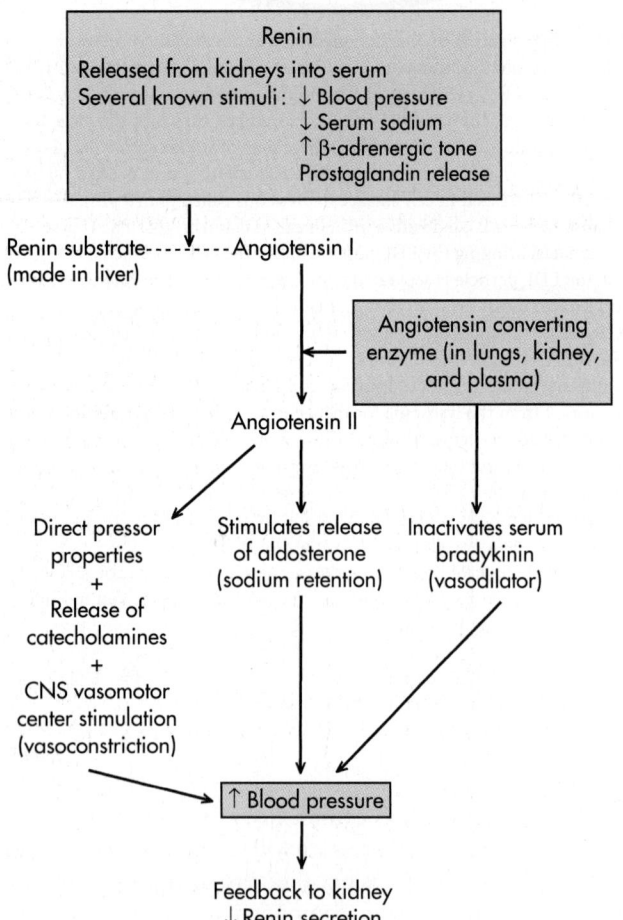

Figure 5-7 Renin-angiotensin-aldosterone system. *CNS,* Central nervous system. (From Jorde LB et al: *Medical genetics,* ed 3, St Louis, 2003, Mosby.)

both hypertension and preeclampsia (a form of pregnancy-induced hypertension).

Cancer

Cancer is the second leading cause of death in the United States. It is well established that many major types of cancer (e.g., breast, colon, prostate, ovarian) cluster strongly in families. This is caused by both shared genes and shared environmental–life-style factors. Although numerous cancer genes are being isolated,[11] environmental–life-style factors also play an important role in causing cancer. In particular, tobacco use is estimated to account for one third of all cancer cases in the United States, making it the most important known cause of cancer.[12]

Breast Cancer

Breast cancer is the most common cancer among women, affecting approximately 12% of American women who live to 85 years or more. Formerly the leading cause of cancer death among women, it has been surpassed by lung cancer. Breast cancer aggregates strongly in families. If a woman has one affected first-degree relative, her risk of developing breast cancer doubles. This risk increases if the age of onset in the affected relative is early and if the cancer is bilateral (tumors in both breasts).

An autosomal dominant form of breast cancer accounts for approximately 5% of breast cancer cases in the United States. Genes responsible for this form of breast cancer have been mapped to chromosomes 17 *(BRCA1)* and 13 *(BRCA2).* Each of these genes has now been cloned, and it is possible to test them for cancer-causing mutations.[13] Women who inherit a mutation in *BRCA1* or *BRCA2* experience a 50% to 80% lifetime risk of developing breast cancer. *BRCA1* mutations also increase the risk of ovarian cancer among women (20% to 50% lifetime risk), and they confer a modestly increased risk of prostate and colon cancers. *BRCA2* mutations also confer an increased risk of ovarian cancer (10% to 20% lifetime prevalence). Approximately 6% of males who inherit a *BRCA2* mutation will develop breast cancer; this represents a 100-fold increase over the risk in the general male population. The evaluation of the *BRCA1* and *BRCA2* gene products, which are both involved in deoxyribonucleic acid (DNA) repair, is yielding valuable evidence on the etiology of breast cancer in general.

Although *BRCA1* and *BRCA2* mutations are the most common known causes of inherited breast cancer, this disease also can be caused by inherited mutations in several other tumor suppressor genes (e.g., the *CHK2* and *TP53* genes). Germline mutations in a tumor suppressor gene called *PTEN* are responsible for Cowden disease, which is characterized by multiple benign tumors and an increased susceptibility to breast cancer. Some studies have suggested that heterozygous carriers of mutations in the *ATM* gene have an increased susceptibility for breast cancer, but these findings remain controversial.

Colorectal Cancer

Colorectal cancer is second only to lung cancer in the number of cases occurring annually in the United States, with 148,300 new cases in 2002.[3] Approximately 1 in 20 Americans will develop colorectal cancer. Like breast cancer, it clusters in families (in fact, familial clustering of this form of cancer was reported in the medical literature as early as 1881). The risk of colorectal cancer in people with one affected first-degree relative is two to three times higher than in the general population.

This familial aggregation is caused in part by subsets of colorectal cancer cases that are inherited as single-gene traits. *Familial adenomatous polyposis* occurs in approximately 1 in 8000 whites. The gene responsible for this disorder, *APC*, was mapped to chromosome 5, and the gene itself was subsequently cloned.[14] Cloning of this gene and its protein have provided has shown that it functions as a tumor suppressor. Importantly, somatic mutations of *APC* are found in at least 85% of all colon tumors. Thus although inherited *APC* mutations play a vital role in relatively rare familial adenomatous polyposis, somatic mutations are involved in the great majority of all common colon cancers.

Hereditary nonpolyposis colorectal cancer, which may account for as many as 5% of colorectal cancer cases, is caused by mutations in any of six genes.[15] Cloning of these genes has shown that all of them are involved in the vital process of DNA repair. When this function is compromised, cancer-causing mutations can persist in cells, leading eventually to growth of a tumor.

Other colorectal cancer cases are likely to be caused by a complex interaction of multiple genes. In addition, environmental factors, such as a high-fat, low-fiber diet, are thought to increase the risk of colorectal cancer.

Other Cancers

The genetic basis of various other cancers, including retinoblastoma, has been discussed. Although each of these cancers is relatively rare, study of the causative genes has provided many important insights into the nature of carcinogenesis in general. This will lead to more effective treatment and prevention of all cancers.

Diabetes Mellitus

Like the other disorders discussed in this chapter, the etiology of diabetes mellitus is complex and not fully understood. Nevertheless, progress is being made in understanding the genetic basis of this disorder, which is a leading cause of blindness, heart disease, and kidney failure.[16,17] An important advance has been the recognition that diabetes is actually a heterogeneous group of disorders, all characterized by elevated blood sugar. The focus here is on the two major types of diabetes—type 1 (insulin-dependent diabetes mellitus [IDDM]) and type 2 (non–insulin-dependent diabetes mellitus [NIDDM]).

Type 1 Diabetes

Type 1 diabetes, which is characterized by T cell infiltration of the pancreas and destruction of the insulin-producing beta cells, usually (but not always) presents before age 40 years. Individuals with type 1 diabetes must receive exogenous insulin to survive. The pathologic manifestations of the disorder, together with the common finding of antibodies against pancreatic beta cells and a very strong association with several human leukocyte antigen (HLA) class II alleles, suggest that type 1 diabetes is an autoimmune disorder. Siblings of individuals with type 1 diabetes face a substantial elevation in risk: approximately 6%, as opposed to a risk of about 0.3% to 0.5% in the general population. Although the sexes are affected in almost equal proportions (there is a slight excess of males), recurrence risks for offspring vary substantially with the sex of the parent. The risk to offspring of diabetic mothers is only 1% to 3%, but it is 4% to 6% for the offspring of diabetic fathers (note that this is inconsistent with the sex-specific threshold model for multifactorial traits). Twin studies show that the empirical risks for identical twins of individuals with type 1 diabetes range from 30% to 50%. The fact that type 1 diabetes is not 100% concordant among identical twins indicates that genetic factors are not solely responsible for the disorder. Good evidence indicates that viral infections, for example, contribute to the causation of type 1 diabetes in at least some individuals.

The association of specific HLA class II alleles (see Chapter 21) and type 1 diabetes has been studied intensively. Ninety-five percent of whites with type 1 diabetes have the HLA *DR3* and/or *DR4* allele, whereas only about 50% of the general white population has either of these alleles. If an affected proband and a sibling are both heterozygous for the *DR3* and *DR4* alleles, the sibling's risk of developing type 1 diabetes is nearly 20% (i.e., about 40 times higher than the risk in the general population). In addition, the presence of aspartic acid at position 57 of the HLA DQβ chain is strongly associated with resistance to type 1 diabetes. In fact, those who have this amino acid at position 57 are 100 times less likely to develop the disease than are individuals homozygous for other amino acids (alanine, serine, valine). It is probable that this particular amino acid is involved in T cell recognition and that those who lack it are more likely to experience an autoimmune episode.

The insulin gene itself, which is located on chromosome 11p, is another logical candidate for type 1 diabetes susceptibility. Polymorphisms in and around the insulin gene have been studied extensively, and alleles of some of these polymorphisms are associated with susceptibility to type 1 diabetes. These associations are not strict: not everybody who carries a given allele will develop type 1 diabetes. This is expected, given the many other factors, both genetic and nongenetic, that appear to be involved in causing type 1 diabetes.

Type 2 Diabetes

Type 2 diabetes accounts for more than 90% of all diabetes cases in the United States. A number of features distinguish it from type 1 diabetes. Unlike type 1 diabetes, some endogenous insulin production in persons with type 2 diabetes is nearly always present, and thus it can often be treated successfully with dietary modification and/or oral drugs. Individuals with type 2 diabetes also experience insulin resistance (i.e., their bodies have difficulty using the insulin they produce). This disease typically occurs among people over 40 years of age and, in contrast to type 1 diabetes, is seen more commonly among obese persons. Neither HLA associations nor autoantibodies are seen commonly in this form of diabetes. Monozygotic twin concordance rates are substantially higher than in type 1 diabetes, often exceeding 90% (because of age dependence, the concordance rate increases if older subjects are studied). The empirical recurrence risks for first-degree relatives of type 2 diabetes cases are higher than those for type 1, generally ranging from 10% to 15%. The differences between type 1 and type 2 diabetes are summarized in Table 5-7.

Genetic studies suggest that mutations in a gene that encodes calpain-10 (a cysteine protease) are associated with type 2 diabetes susceptibility. This association has been replicated in some populations but not in others. A significant association also has been observed between type 2 diabetes and a common allele of the gene that encodes peroxisome prolifer-ator-activated receptor-γ (PPAR-γ), a transcription factor that is involved in adipocyte differentiation and glucose metabolism. Although this allele confers only a 25% increase in the risk of developing type 2 diabetes, it is found in more than 75% of individuals of European descent. Thus it may help to account for a significant proportion of type 2 diabetes cases.

The two most important risk factors for type 2 diabetes are positive family history and obesity (the latter increases insulin resistance). The disease tends to rise in prevalence when populations adopt a more Western diet and exercise pattern. Increases have been seen, for example, among Japanese immigrants to the United States and among some native populations of the South Pacific, Australia, and the Americas. Several studies, conducted on both male and female subjects, have shown that regular exercise can substantially lower one's risk of developing type 2 diabetes, even among individuals with a family history of the disease. This is partly because exercise reduces obesity. However, even in the absence of weight loss, exercise increases insulin sensitivity and improves glucose tolerance.

Because of the dramatic increase in obesity in the United States and other developed countries, the prevalence of type 2 diabetes is also rising rapidly, and the average age of onset is decreasing. A small proportion of type 2 diabetes cases occurs early in life, typically before 25 years of age, and typically exhibits autosomal dominant inheritance (unlike most type 2 diabetes). This subset is termed *maturity-onset diabetes of the young* (MODY). Studies of MODY pedigrees have shown that about half of cases of the disease are caused by mutations in the glucokinase gene. Glucokinase converts glucose to glucose-6-phosphate in the pancreas. In addition to the glucokinase gene, five other genes, all of which are involved in pancreatic development or insulin regulation, have now been shown to be causes of MODY.

Obesity

Obesity is most commonly defined as a body mass index (BMI) greater than 30.* Using this criterion, a survey published in 2002 showed that approximately 30% of American adults are obese, and an additional 35% are overweight (BMI greater than 25 but less than 30). The proportion of obese adults and children continues to increase rapidly. Although obesity itself is not a "disease," it is an important risk factor for several common diseases, including heart disease, stroke, hypertension, and type 2 diabetes.

As one might expect, a strong correlation exists between obesity in parents and their children. This could easily be ascribed to common environmental–life-style effects: parents and children usually share similar dietary and exercise habits. Indeed, it may seem that obesity should be influenced almost exclusively by environmental–life-style factors. However, good evidence exists for genetic components as well. Four different adoption studies each showed that the body weights of adopted individuals correlated significantly with their natural

Table 5-7	Comparison of Major Features of Types 1 and 2 Diabetes Mellitus	
Feature	**Type 1 Diabetes**	**Type 2 Diabetes**
Age of onset	Usually <40 yr	Usually >40 yr (except maturity-onset diabetes of the young [MODY])
Insulin production	None	Partial
Insulin resistance	No	Yes
Autoimmunity	Yes	No
Obesity	Not common	Common
Monozygotic (MZ) twin concordance	.55	.90
Sibling recurrence risk	1%-6%	10%-15%

*W/H², where W is weight in kilograms and H is height in meters.

parents' body weights but not with those of their adoptive parents. Twin studies also provide evidence for a genetic effect on body weight, with most studies showing significantly higher concordance in MZ twins than in DZ twins. Statistical analyses of family data have shown that major genes, as well as polygenic effects, may be associated with obesity. A gene that encodes leptin, a protein involved in appetite regulation, has been cloned in mice and humans.[18] Leptin injections can reduce obesity in some mice; unfortunately, they do not have a substantial effect in humans. Genetic studies have shown that several additional genes, including those encoding neuropeptide Y and the melanocortin-4 receptor, play important roles in appetite regulation.

Alzheimer Disease

Alzheimer disease (AD), which is responsible for 60% to 70% of cases of progressive cognitive impairment among the elderly, affects approximately 10% of the population older than 65 years of age and 40% of the population older than 85 years of age. Because of the aging of the population, the number of Americans with AD is predicted to increase from the current figure of 4 million to a total of 10 million by the year 2010. AD is characterized by progressive dementia and memory loss and by the formation of amyloid plaques and neurofibrillary tangles in the brain, particularly in the cerebral cortex and hippocampus. The plaques and tangles lead to progressive neuronal loss, and death usually occurs within 7 to 10 years after the first appearance of symptoms.

The risk of developing AD doubles in individuals who have an affected first-degree relative. Although most cases do not appear to be caused by single loci, approximately 10% follow an autosomal dominant mode of transmission. About 3% to 5% of AD cases occur before age 65 and are considered early onset; these are much more likely to be inherited in autosomal dominant fashion.[19]

AD is a genetically heterogeneous disorder. Approximately half of early-onset cases can be attributed to mutations in any of three genes, all of which affect amyloid-β deposition.[20] Two of the genes, presenilin 1 (PS1) and presenilin 2 (PS2), are very similar to one another, and their protein products are involved in cleavage of the amyloid-β precursor protein (APP). When APP is not cleaved normally, a long form of it accumulates excessively and is deposited in the brain. This is thought to be a primary cause of AD. Mutations in PS1 typically result in especially early onset of AD, with the first occurrence of symptoms in the fifth decade of life.

A small number of cases of early-onset AD are caused by mutations of the gene that encodes APP itself, which is located on chromosome 21. These mutations disrupt normal cleavage sites in APP, again leading to the accumulation of the longer protein product. It is interesting that this gene is present in three copies in trisomy 21 individuals, where the extra gene copy leads to amyloid deposition and the occurrence of AD in Down syndrome patients (see Chapter 4).

An important risk factor for the more common late-onset form of AD is allelic variation in the apolipoprotein E (APOE) locus, which has three major alleles: ϵ2, ϵ3, and ϵ4. Studies conducted in diverse populations have shown that persons who have one copy of the ϵ4 allele are at least 2 to 5 times more likely to develop AD, whereas those with two copies of this allele are at least 5 to 10 times more likely to develop AD. The risk varies somewhat by population, with higher ϵ4-associated risks in Europeans and Japanese and relatively lower risks in Hispanics and African-Americans. Despite the strong association between ϵ4 and AD, approximately half of individuals who develop late-onset AD do not have a copy of the ϵ4 allele, and many who are homozygous for ϵ4 remain free of AD even at advanced age. The apolipoprotein E protein product is not involved in cleavage of APP but instead appears to be associated with clearance of amyloid from the brain.

Alcoholism

At some point, alcoholism is diagnosed in approximately 10% of adult males and 3% to 5% of adult females in the United States. The national cost of alcoholism, in terms of lost productivity and direct medical costs, exceeds $165 billion per year. More than 100 studies have shown that this disease clusters in families.[21] The risk of developing alcoholism among individuals with one affected parent is three to five times higher than for those with unaffected parents.

Most twin studies have yielded concordance rates for DZ twins less than 30% and concordance rates for MZ twins in excess of 60%. Adoption studies have shown that the offspring of an alcoholic parent, even when raised by nonalcoholic parents, have a fourfold increased risk of developing the disorder. To control for possible prenatal effects in an alcoholic mother, some studies have included only the offspring of alcoholic fathers. The results have remained the same. One study showed that the offspring of nonalcoholic parents, when reared by alcoholics, did *not* have an increased risk of developing alcoholism. These data argue that there may be genes that predispose some people to alcoholism.

It has long been known that an individual's physiologic response to alcohol can be influenced by variation in the key enzymes responsible for alcohol metabolism (alcohol dehydrogenases [ADH]), which convert ethanol to acetaldehyde, and aldehyde dehydrogenases (ALDH), which convert acetaldehyde to acetate. In particular, an allele of the ALDH2 gene (ALDH2*2) results in excessive accumulation of acetaldehyde and thus in facial flushing, nausea, palpitations, and light-headedness. Because of these unpleasant effects, individuals who have the ALDH2*2 allele are much less likely to become alcoholics. This "protective" allele is common in some Asian populations but is rare in other populations.

Currently less reliable evidence regarding genes that may predispose individuals to become addicted to alcohol has come to light. Evidence has been published for an association between alcoholism and a DNA polymorphism linked to the dopamine D2 receptor gene on chromosome 11q. Because the dopamine receptors are part of the brain's reward pathway, this association has some intuitive appeal. However, many additional studies in other populations have failed to replicate this evidence. It now appears unlikely that this polymorphism contributes importantly to alcoholism susceptibility.[21] Nevertheless, the twin and adoption studies just mentioned are compelling, and it is possible that further studies may reveal genes that do in fact influence susceptibility to this important disease.

It should be underscored that genes may increase one's *susceptibility* to alcoholism. Obviously, this is a disease that requires an environmental component, regardless of genetic constitution.

Psychiatric Disorders

The major psychiatric diseases, schizophrenia and affective disorder, have been the subjects of numerous genetic studies.[22] Twin, adoption, and family studies have shown that both disorders aggregate in families.

Schizophrenia

Schizophrenia is a severe emotional disorder characterized by delusions, hallucinations, retreat from reality, and bizarre, withdrawn, or inappropriate behavior. (Contrary to popular belief, schizophrenia is not a "split personality" disorder.) The lifetime recurrence risk for schizophrenia among the offspring of one affected parent is approximately 8% to 10%, which is about 10 times higher than the risk in the general population.[23] As one might expect, the empirical risks increase when more relatives are affected. For example, an individual with an affected sibling and an affected parent has a risk of about 17%, and an individual with two affected parents has a risk of 46%. The risks decrease when the affected family member is a second- or third-degree relative. Details are given in Table 5-8. On inspection of Table 5-8, it may seem puzzling that the proportion of schizophrenic probands who have a schizophrenic parent is only about 5%, which is substantially lower than the risk for other first-degree relatives (e.g., siblings, affected parents, their offspring). This can be explained by the fact that people with schizophrenia are less likely to marry and produce children than are other individuals. Thus substantial selection against schizophrenia occurs in the population.

Twin and adoption studies also indicate that genetic factors are likely to be involved in schizophrenia. Data pooled from five different twin studies show a 47% concordance rate

Table 5-8	Recurrence Risks for Relatives of Schizophrenic Probands*
Relationship to Proband	Recurrence Risk (%)
Monozygotic twin	44.3
Dizygotic twin	12.1
Offspring	9.4
Sibling	7.3
Niece/nephew	2.7
Grandchild	2.8
First cousin	1.6
Spouse	1.0

Data from McGue M, Gottesman II, Rao DC: *Behav Genet* 16(1):75-87, 1986.

*Figures are based on multiple studies of Western European populations.

for MZ twins, compared with a concordance rate of only 12% for DZ twins. When the offspring of a schizophrenic parent are adopted by normal parents, their risk of developing the disease is about 10%, which is approximately the same as the risk when raised by a schizophrenic biologic parent. Although no schizophrenia gene has yet been conclusively identified, promising associations have been uncovered between schizophrenia and several brain-expressed genes whose products interact with glutamate receptors. These include dysbindin 1 (chromosome 6p), neuregulin 1 (chromosome 8p), and G72 (chromosome 13q). Each of these associations has been identified in a specific population, and further studies in other populations will be needed to replicate these findings.

Bipolar Affective Disorder

Bipolar affective disorder, also known as *manic-depressive disorder,* is a form of psychosis with extreme mood swings and emotional instability. The incidence of the disorder in the general population is approximately 0.5%, but it rises to 5% to 10% among those with an affected first-degree relative. A study using the Danish twin registry yielded concordance rates of 79% and 24% for MZ and DZ twins, respectively.[24] The corresponding concordance rates for unipolar disorder (major depression) were 54% and 19%. In general, it appears that bipolar disorder is more strongly influenced by genetic factors than is unipolar disorder.

Comments on Psychiatric Disorders

Large-scale linkage studies involving hundreds of polymorphisms throughout the genome have now been carried out for both schizophrenia and bipolar affective disorder. Most of these studies have produced negative results, although a few recent large-scale studies have yielded promising findings. A number of candidate genes have been tested for linkage or association with both diseases. Most of these candidates were chosen on the basis of the known involvement of certain neurotransmitters, receptors, or neurotransmitter-related enzymes in each disease (e.g., schizophrenia can be treated by drugs that block dopamine receptors, and bipolar affective disorder is sometimes treated with lithium). None of the candidate genes tested thus far, including those for sodium-lithium countertransport, various components of the dopaminergic system, and several neurotransmitter-related enzymes (e.g., monoamine oxidase, dopamine-β-hydroxylase, tyrosine hydroxylase), has been shown unequivocally to be linked or associated with either disease.

These results reflect some of the difficulties encountered in doing genetic studies of psychiatric disorders. These disorders are undoubtedly heterogeneous, reflecting the influence of numerous genetic and environmental factors. Also, definition of the phenotype is not always straightforward and it may change through time, significantly complicating genetic analysis.

Other Complex Disorders

The disorders discussed in this chapter represent some of the most common multifactorial disorders and those for which significant progress has been made in identifying genes. Many other multifactorial disorders are being studied as well, and in some cases specific susceptibility genes have been identified.

These include, for example, Parkinson disease, hearing loss, multiple sclerosis, amyotrophic lateral sclerosis, epilepsy, asthma, inflammatory bowel disease, and some forms of blindness.

Some General Principles and Conclusions

Some general principles can be deduced from the results obtained thus far on the genetics of complex disorders. First, the more strongly inherited forms of complex disorders generally have an earlier age of onset (e.g., breast cancer, Alzheimer disease, heart disease). Often these represent subsets of cases in which there is single-gene inheritance. Second, when laterality is a component, the bilateral forms are more likely to cluster strongly in families (e.g., breast cancer, cleft lip/palate). Third, although the sex-specific threshold model fits some of the complex disorders (e.g., pyloric stenosis, cleft lip/palate, autism, heart disease), it fails to fit others (e.g., type 1 diabetes).

A tendency exists, particularly among the lay public, to assume that the presence of a genetic component means that the course of a disease cannot be altered. *This is incorrect.* Most of the diseases discussed in this chapter have both genetic and environmental–lifestyle components. Thus environmental–lifestyle modification (e.g., diet, exercise, stress reduction) often can reduce risk significantly. Such modification may be especially important for individuals with a family history of a disease, because they are likely to develop the disease earlier in life. Those with a family history of heart disease, for example, can often add many years of productive living with relatively minor lifestyle alterations. By targeting those who can benefit most from intervention, genetics helps to serve the goal of preventive medicine.

In addition, it should be stressed that the identification of a specific genetic lesion can lead to more effective prevention and treatment of the disease. Identification of mutations that cause autosomal dominant breast cancer may enable early screening and prevention of metastasis. Pinpointing a gene responsible for a neurotransmitter defect in a behavioral disorder such as schizophrenia could lead to the development of more effective drug treatments. In some cases, such as those with familial hypercholesterolemia, gene therapy may prove to be useful in treating the disease. It is important for health care practitioners to help individuals understand these facts.

Although the genetics of common disorders is complex and often confusing, the community health impact of these diseases, together with the evidence for hereditary factors in their etiology, demands that genetic studies be pursued. Substantial progress is already being made. The next decade will undoubtedly witness many further advances in the understanding and treatment of these disorders.

SUMMARY REVIEW

Factors Influencing Incidence of Disease in Populations

1. The incidence rate is the number of new cases of a disease reported during a specific period (typically 1 year) divided by the number of individuals in the population.
2. The prevalence rate is the proportion of the population affected by a disease at a specific point in time.
3. Diseases vary in prevalence from one population to another.
4. Relative risk is a common measure of the effect of a specific risk factor. It is expressed as a ratio of the incidence rate of the disease among individuals exposed to a risk factor divided by the incidence of the disease among individuals *not* exposed to a risk factor.
5. Many factors can influence the risk of acquiring a common disease, such as cancer, diabetes, or hypertension. The factors can include age, gender, diet, exercise, and family history of the disease.

Principles of Multifactorial Inheritance

1. Traits in which variation is thought to be caused by the combined effects of multiple genes are polygenic.
2. The term *multifactorial* is used when environmental–life-style factors also are believed to cause variation in the trait.
3. Many quantitative traits (e.g., blood pressure) are multifactorial.
4. Because traits are caused by the additive effects of many genetic and environmental–life-style factors, they tend to follow a normal or bell-shaped distribution in populations.
5. Those diseases, however, that do not follow a bell-shaped distribution appear to be either present or absent in individuals. They do not follow the inheritance patterns of single-gene disease. Instead, such diseases may follow an underlying liability distribution. It is thought that a threshold of liability must be crossed before the disease is expressed.
6. Examples of diseases that correspond to the liability model include pyloric stenosis, infantile autism, neural tube defects, cleft lip/palate, and some forms of congenital heart disease.
7. Many of the common adult diseases, such as hypertension, coronary heart disease, stroke, diabetes mellitus (types 1 and 2), and some cancers, are caused by complex genetic and environmental–life-style factors and are thus multifactorial diseases.
8. For most multifactorial diseases, empirical risks, risks based on direct observation of data, have been derived.
9. In contrast to most single-gene diseases, recurrence risks for multifactorial diseases can change significantly from one population to another because gene frequencies, as well as environmental–life-style factors, can differ among populations.
10. Several criteria are used to define multifactorial inheritance: (a) the recurrence risk becomes higher if more than one family member is affected; (b) if the expression of the disease in a proband is more severe, the recurrence risk is higher; (c) the recurrence risk is higher if the proband is of the less commonly affected gender; (d) the recurrence risk for the disease usually decreases rapidly in more remotely related relatives; and (e) if the prevalence of the disease in a population is f, the risk for offspring and siblings of probands is approximately $\sqrt{f}$.

Nature and Nurture: Disentangling the Effects of Genes and Environment or Life-Style

1. Family members share genes and a common environment; therefore resemblance in traits, such as high blood pressure, reflects both genetic and environmental–life-style commonality (nature and nurture, respectively).

SUMMARY REVIEW—cont'd

2. Few traits are influenced *only* by genes or *only* by environment–life-style. Most are influenced by both.
3. When a disease has a relatively larger genetic component, as in breast cancer, examination of family history should be emphasized in addition to lifestyle modification.
4. Two research strategies often are used to estimate the relative influence of genes and environment–life-style: twin studies and adoption studies.
5. Monozygotic twins originate when the developing embryo divides to form two separate but identical embryos.
6. Dizygotic twins are the result of a double ovulation followed by the fertilization of each egg by a different sperm.
7. If both members of a twin pair share a trait, they are said to be *concordant*. If they do not share the same trait, they are *discordant*.

8. Studies of adopted children also are used to estimate the genetic contribution to a multifactorial trait.
9. A genetic predisposition may interact with an environmental–life-style factor to increase the risk of disease; this is called a *gene-environment interaction*.

Genetics of Common Diseases

1. Congenital diseases are those present at birth. Most of these diseases are multifactorial in etiology.
2. Multifactorial diseases in adults include coronary heart disease, hypertension, breast cancer, colon cancer, diabetes mellitus, obesity, Alzheimer disease, alcoholism, schizophrenia, and bipolar affective disorder.
3. It is incorrect to assume that the presence of a genetic component means that the course of a disease cannot be altered—most diseases have *both* genetic and environmental–lifestyle aspects.

KEY TERMS

Concordant trait, 163
Congenital diseases, 164
Discordant trait, 163
Dizygotic (fraternal) twins, 163
Empirical risks, 160

Gene-environment–life-style
  interaction, 164
Incidence rate, 157
Liability distribution, 159
Monozygotic (identical) twins, 163
Multifactorial trait, 158

Phocomelia, 165
Polygenic, 158
Prevalence rate, 157
Quantitative traits, 158
Relative risk, 158
Threshold of liability, 159

MEDIA RESOURCES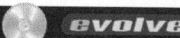

Review questions and answers for this chapter are available in the *CD Companion* included with this book.

WebLinks—links to Internet sites pertaining to this chapter—are available on Evolve at http://evolve.elsevier.com/McCance/.

REFERENCES

1. King RA, Rotter JI, Motulsky AG: *The genetic basis of common diseases,* ed 2, Oxford, 2002, Oxford University Press.
2. Rothman KJ: *Modern epidemiology,* New York, 1998, Lippincott.
3. American Cancer Society: Cancer statistics, website: www.cancer.org/docroot/STT/stt_0.asp.
4. Anderson NH, Dominiczak AF: Genetic analysis of complex traits. In Rimoin DL, Connor JM, Pyeritz RE, Kork BR, editors: *Emery and Rimoin's principles and practice of medical genetics,* ed 4, vol 1, pp 410-424, London, 2002, Churchill Livingstone.
5. Harper PS: *Practical genetic counseling,* ed 5, Oxford, 1998, Butterworth Heineman.
6. Boomsma D, Busjahn A, Peltonen L: Classical twin studies and beyond, *Nat Rev Genet* 3(11):872-882, 2002.
7. Neale MC, Cardon LR: *Methodology for genetic studies of twins and families,* Dordrecht, The Netherlands, 1992, Kluwer Academic Publishers.
8. Hunt SC, Williams RR, Barlow GK: A comparison of positive family history definitions for defining risk of future disease, *J Chron Dis* 39(10): 809-821, 1986.
9. Breslow JL: Genetics of lipoprotein abnormalities associated with coronary artery disease susceptibility, *Annu Rev Genet* 34:233-254, 2000.
10. Hunt SC, Hopkins PN, Lalouel J-M: Hypertension. In King RA, Rotter JI, Motulsky AG, editors: *The genetic basis of common diseases,* ed 2, Oxford, 2002, Oxford University Press, pp 127-154.
11. Vogelstein B, Kinzler KW: *The genetic basis of human cancer,* New York, 1998, McGraw-Hill.

12. Peto J: Cancer epidemiology in the last century and the next decade, *Nature* 411(6835):390-395, 2001.
13. Wooster R, Weber BL: Breast and ovarian cancer, *N Engl J Med* 348(23):2339-2347, 2003.
14. Fodde R, Smits R, Clevers H: APC, signal transduction, and genetic instability in colorectal cancer, *Nat Rev Cancer* 1(1):55-67, 2001.
15. Lynch HT, de la Chapelle A: Hereditary colorectal cancer, *N Engl J Med* 348(10):919-932, 2003.
16. Busch CP, Hegele RA: Genetic determinants of type 2 diabetes mellitus, *Clin Genet* 60(4):243-254, 2001.
17. Florez JC, Hirschhorn J, Altshuler D: The inherited basis of diabetes mellitus: implications for the genetic analysis of complex traits, *Annu Rev Genomics Hum Genet* 4:257-291, 2003.
18. Cummings DE, Schwartz MW: Genetics and pathophysiology of human obesity, *Annu Rev Med* 54:453-471, 2003.
19. Selkoe DJ, Podlismy MB: Deciphering the genetic basis of Alzheimer's disease, *Annu Rev Genomics Hum Genet* 3:67-99, 2002.
20. Nussbaum RL, Ellis CE: Alzheimer's disease and Parkinson's disease, *N Engl J Med* 348(14):1356-1364, 2003.
21. Reich T et al: Genetic studies of alcoholism and substance dependence, *Am J Hum Genet* 65(3):599-605, 1999.
22. Evans KL et al: Nuts and bolts of pshychiatric genetic: building on the Human Genome Project, *Trends Genet* 17(1):35-40, 2001.
23. Freedman R: Schizophrenia, *N Engl J Med* 349(18):1738-1749, 2003.
24. Bertelsen A, Harvald B, Hauge M: a Danish twin study of manic-depressive disorders, *Br J Psychiatry* 130:330-351, 1977.
25. Melvin EC et al: Genetic studies in neural tube defects. NTD Collaborative Group, *Pediatr Neurosurg* 32(1):1-9, 2000.
26. Daly LE et al: Folate levels and neural tube defects: implications for prevention, *JAMA* 274(21):1698-1702, 1995.
27. Marks D et al: A review on the diagnosis, natural history, and treatment of familial hypercholesterolaemia, *Atherosclerosis* 168(1):1-14, 2003.
28. Jansen AC et al: Phenotypic variability in familial hypercholesterolaemia: an update, *Curr Opin Lipidol* 13(2):165-171, 2002.

INNATE IMMUNITY: INFLAMMATION

BARBARA CRIPPES TRASK • NEAL S. ROTE • SUE E. HUETHER

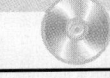

CHAPTER OUTLINE

New and significant discoveries being made in the study of immunity and inflammation are greatly advancing the knowledge and understanding of these processes, and have precipitated changes in the concepts and nomenclature used to describe the immune systems and their processes. The information presented in this chapter introduces the components and processes of innate immunity and sets the stage for Chapter 7, which discusses adaptive immunity. Knowledge of innate resistance (innate immunity) is crucial to understanding how tissue damage can be contained, how infection can be prevented, and how best to treat injuries to promote healing. Although these bodily responses are thought of as protective, they also have the potential to cause disease or harm when the responses are either inadequate or excessive and uncontrolled. Here too, new understanding of how and why the body responds to such threats is helping researchers devise treatments that will aid the body in thwarting the onset of disease. This chapter is designed to render an overview of innate mechanisms of protection. It is not intended to be all-inclusive. The currently known numbers of soluble factors and cellular receptors that mediate the innate response are extremely large and would require many more pages to discuss in adequate detail. Throughout the chapter, we will present different classes or groups of participants in innate resistance, but only a few examples will be described in detail in order to illustrate the finely designed and complex network of components and interactions that make up innate resistance. Some components of innate resistance are designed to limit and contain tissue injury, regardless of the cause, whereas others are focused more on prevention of infection by environmental microorganisms. In most cases, specific components have dual activities of preventing both further injury and infection.

HUMAN DEFENSE MECHANISMS

The human body has developed several means of protecting itself from injury and infection. **Innate resistance** or **immunity,** also known as *natural* or *native immunity,* includes natural barriers (physical, mechanical, and biochemical) and inflammation (Table 6-1). A variety of innate barriers form the first line of defense at the body's surfaces and are in place at birth to prevent damage by substances in the environment and thwart infection by pathogenic microorganisms. If the surface barriers are breached, the second line of defense, the **inflammatory response,** is activated to protect the body from further injury, prevent infection of the injured tissue, and promote healing. The inflammatory response is a rapid

Table 6-1   Overview of Human Defenses

Characteristics	Innate Immunity		Adaptive (Acquired) Immunity
	Barriers	Inflammatory Response	
Level of defense	First line of defense against infection and tissue injury	Second line of defense; occurs as a response to tissue injury or infection	Third line of defense; becomes active when innate immune system signals the cells of adaptive immunity
Timing of defense	Constant	Immediate response	There is a delay between exposure to antigen and maximum response
Specificity	Broadly specific	Broadly specific	Response is very specific towards "antigen"
Receptors	Pattern recognition receptors	Pattern recognition receptors	T-cell receptor and B-cell receptor
Cells	Epithelial cells	Mast cells, granulocytes (neutrophils, eosinophils, basophils), monocytes/macrophages, NK cells, platelets, endothelial cells	T lymphocytes, B lymphocytes, macrophages, dendritic cells
Memory	No memory involved	No memory involved	Specific immunologic memory by T and B lymphocytes
Peptides	Defensins, cathelicidins, lactoferrin, bacterial toxins	Complement, clotting factors, kinins	Antibodies, complement
Cytokines and chemokines	Few	Many *Examples:* TNF, IL, GF, CSFs, IFs, PAF, chemokines (CC and CXC)	Many *Examples:* TNF, IL, GF, CSFs, IFs, PAF, chemokines (CC and CXC)
Protection	Protection includes anatomic barriers (i.e., skin and mucous membranes), cells and secretory molecules or cytokines (i.e., lysozymes, low pH of stomach and urine) and ciliary activity	Protection includes vascular responses, cellular components (mast cells, neutrophils, macrophages), secretory molecules or cytokines, and activation of plasma protein systems	Protection includes activated T and B lymphocytes, chemical mediators, and memory

TNF, Tumor necrosis factor; *IL,* interleukins; *GR,* growth factor; *CSFs,* colony-stimulating factors; *IFs,* interferons; *PAF,* platelet-activating factor.

activation of biochemical and cellular mechanisms that is relatively nonspecific, with similar responses being initiated against a wide variety of causes of tissue damage. An additional third line of defense, **adaptive immunity** (also known as *acquired* or *specific immunity*) is a relatively slower and more specific process. It is able to target particular invading microorganisms for the purpose of eradicating them. Adaptive immunity also involves "memory," which facilitates more rapid responses during future exposure to the same microorganism.

FIRST LINE OF DEFENSE: PHYSICAL, MECHANICAL, AND BIOCHEMICAL BARRIERS

Physical and Mechanical Barriers

The physical barriers that protect against pathogenic invasion are easily defined as a relatively impenetrable "cellular roadblock" to microorganisms. This barricade is comprised of tightly associated epithelial cells including those of the skin and those of the membranous sheets lining the gastrointestinal, genitourinary, and respiratory tracts. When pathogens attempt to penetrate this physical barrier, they may be prevented from doing so simply by means of mechanical clearance—a consequence of being sloughed off with dead skin cells as they are routinely replaced, being expelled by coughing or sneezing, being vomited from the stomach, or being flushed from the urinary tract by urine. Epithelial cells of the upper respiratory tract also produce mucus that traps pathogens and have hairlike cilia that mechanically move the entrapped pathogens upwards to be expelled by coughing or sneezing. Additionally, the low temperature on the body's surface generally inhibits microorganisms, most of which routinely require temperatures near 37° C for more efficient growth.

Biochemical Barriers

Epithelial surfaces provide biochemical barriers, as well as physical barriers, by synthesizing and secreting substances meant to trap or destroy pathogens. Mucus, perspiration (or sweat), saliva, tears, and earwax are all examples of biochemical secretions that can trap potential invaders and contain substances that will kill the microorganisms. Sebaceous glands in the skin also secrete antibacterial and antifungal fatty acids and lactic acid. Perspiration, tears, and saliva contain an enzyme (lysozyme) that attacks the cell walls of gram-positive bacteria. These glandular secretions result in the surface of the skin being acidic (pH 3 to 5), making it an inhospitable environment for most bacteria.

In addition, the body has a complex array of proteins that function to destroy pathogens before they can colonize a human host. Some of these proteins function on the surface of the same epithelial sheets that provide the physical barrier. Others, however, are meant to defeat microorganisms that have already crossed the physical barrier.

Epithelial-Derived Chemicals

The small molecular weight proteins secreted by the epithelial cells, generically termed **antimicrobial peptides,** generally are positively charged strings of approximately 15 to 95 amino acids. Antimicrobial peptides can be divided into two classes—**cathelicidins** and **defensins**—based upon their three-dimensional structures. Both classes are in very high local concentrations and are toxic to certain bacteria, fungi, and viruses.[1-3] Cathelicidins have a linear α-helical shape, and only one (LL-37) is currently known to function in humans. In contrast, at least eight different defensins have been identified thus far in humans. All are triple-stranded β-sheet structures. Defensin molecules contain three intrachain disulfide bonds and can be further subdivided into α and β types, depending on how the cysteine residues are connected during formation of the disulfide linkages.[3] The α defensins often require activation by proteolytic enzymes, whereas the β defensins are synthesized in active forms.[2] Bacteria have cholesterol-free cell membranes, which may allow cathelicidins to insert into and disrupt their membranes.[2] Given the similarity in their chemical charges, defensins may kill bacteria in the same way. These same chemicals also may contribute to other means of protection because they are also produced by monocytes, macrophages, and neutrophils, which are components of the inflammatory response. The α-defensins are particularly rich in the granules of neutrophils and may contribute to the killing of bacteria by those cells. Both classes of antimicrobial peptides also can activate cells of innate and acquired immunity. Some of the important characteristics of these antimicrobial peptides are summarized in Table 6-2.[1,2]

The lung also produces **collectins,** known as surfactant proteins A through D. Surfactant proteins A and D are hydrophilic, whereas B and C are hydrophobic. Only surfactant A and D appear to participate in innate resistance by promoting phagocytosis and interacting with the acquired immune system.[4,5]

Bacteria-Derived Chemicals

Many of the body's surfaces are colonized with a spectrum of nonpathogenic bacteria, which is collectively referred to as the **normal bacterial flora.** Some bacteria in the lower gastrointestinal tract benefit us by helping digest our food, releasing nutrients that are taken up by the body. The normal flora also contributes to our innate protection against pathogenic microorganisms. For instance, the intestine contains hundreds of different species of bacteria. Colonization of the lower gut begins very quickly after birth, and the number and concentration of microorganisms increases progressively during the first year of life. Many of these microorganisms help digest fatty acids, large polysaccharides, and other dietary substances, produce vitamin K, and assist in the absorption of various ions, such as calcium, iron, and magnesium. They also produce several chemicals (ammonia, phenols, indols, and other toxic chemicals) that inhibit colonization by pathogenic microorganisms. Prolonged

Table 6-2	Summary of Important Characteristics of Antimicrobial Peptides		
Antimicrobial Peptide	Secondary Structure	Cellular Expression	Activation
Cathelicidin	Linear α-helix conformation	Epithelial cells, granulocytes, lymphocytes, monocytes, mast cells, keratinocytes	Synthesized as an inactive precursor; activated by microbial components and cytokines such as TNF-α and IL-1β
α-Defensins	Triple-stranded β sheet conformation	Intestinal epithelial cells, granulocytes, alveolar macrophages, monocytes, T lymphocytes	Synthesized as inactive propeptide; activated by microbial components and cytokines, such as TNF-α and IL-1β
β-Defensins	Triple-stranded β sheet conformation	Skin, respiratory, and intestinal epithelial cells; keratinocytes; urinary epithelial cells; mast cells; monocytes; dendritic cells	Synthesized as active peptide

TNF-α, Tumor necrosis factor–alpha; IL-1β, interleukin-1 beta.

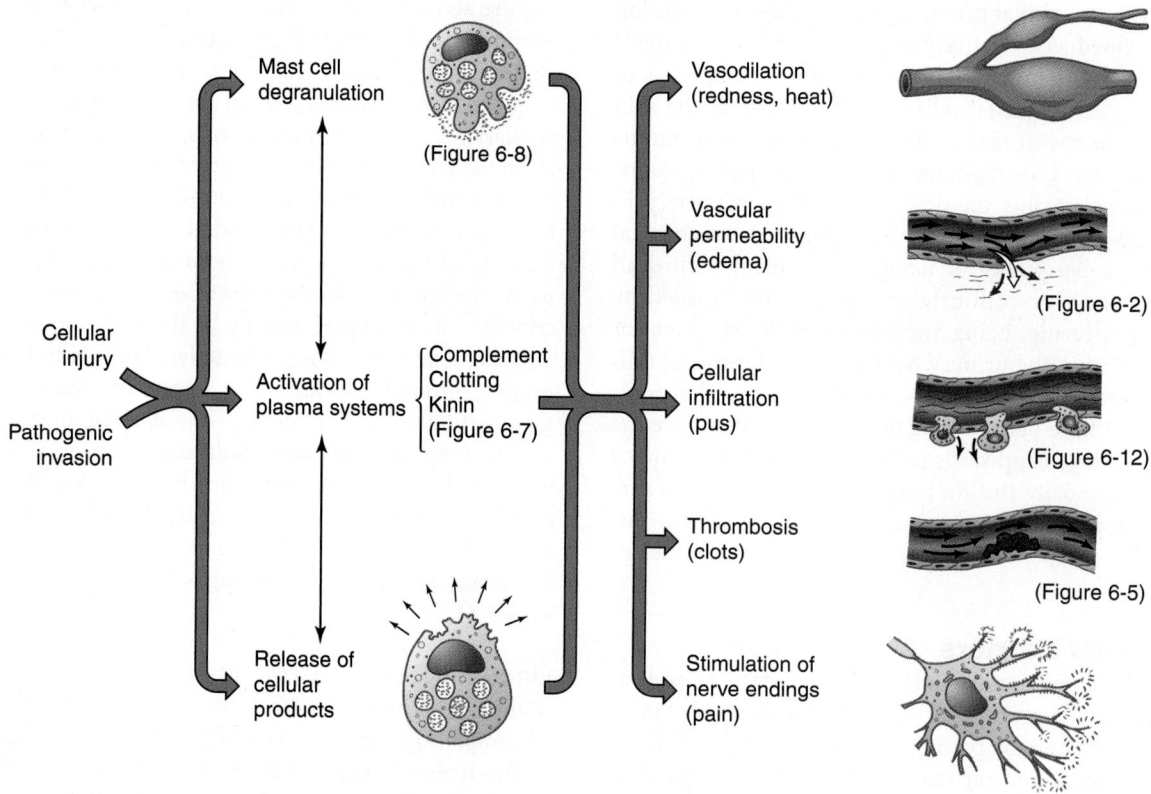

Figure 6-1 Acute inflammatory response. Inflammation is usually initiated by cellular injury. Mast cell degranulation, the activation of three plasma systems, and the release of subcellular components from the damaged cells occur as a consequence of cellular injury. These systems are interdependent, so that induction of one (e.g., mast cell degranulation) can result in the induction of the other two. The result is the development of microscopic changes in the inflamed site, as well as characteristic clinical manifestations. The figure numbers refer to those in which more detailed information may be found on that portion of the response.

antibiotic treatment can alter the normal intestinal flora, decreasing its protective activity, and lead to overgrowth of pathogenic microorganisms, such as the yeast *Candida albicans* or the bacteria *Clostridium difficile*. For another example, the bacteria *Lactobacillus* is a major constituent of the normal vaginal flora in healthy women. This microorganism produces a variety of chemicals (hydrogen peroxide, lactic acid, bacteriocins, and other molecules) that help prevent infections of the vagina and urinary tract by other bacteria and yeast. Diminished colonization with lactobacillus (e.g.,

as a result of prolonged antibiotic treatment) increases the risk for urologic or vaginal infections, such as toxic shock syndrome.

SECOND LINE OF DEFENSE: THE INFLAMMATORY RESPONSE

Activation of the inflammatory response occurs at sites of tissue injury caused by a variety of materials, including infection, mechanical damage, oxygen deprivation (ischemia), nu-

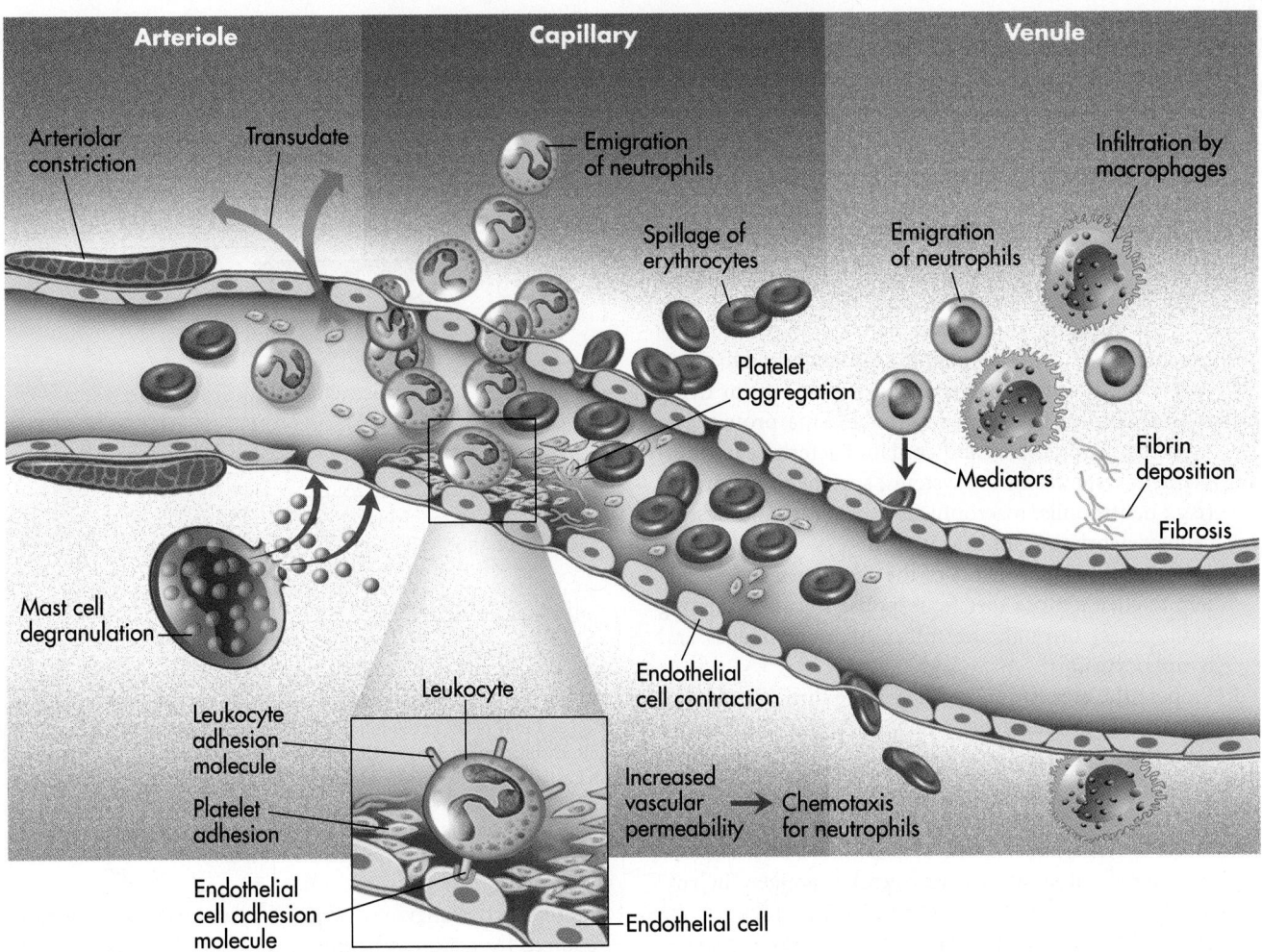

Figure 6-2 Sequence of events in the process of inflammation. See text for details.

trient deprivation, genetic or immune defects, chemical agents, temperature extremes, or ionizing radiation (Figure 6-1). This response is similar to the protection afforded by barriers in two ways: (1) it depends on the activity of both cellular and chemical components and (2) it is nonspecific, meaning that it takes place in approximately the same way regardless of the type of stimulus or whether exposure to the same stimulus has occurred in the past. This nonspecificity is relative to the third line of defense, the adaptive immune system, in that the latter is extremely specific and has memory (see Chapter 7).

Vascular Response

Inflammation occurs in vascularized tissue and results in a group of classic and superficially observable characteristics: *redness, heat, swelling,* and *pain.* Microscopically, inflammatory changes occur at the vascular level (Figure 6-2). The three characteristic changes in the microcirculation (arterioles, capillaries, and venules) near the site of an injury include the following:

1. Blood vessel dilation
2. Increased vascular permeability and leakage of fluid out of the vessel

3. White blood cell adherence to the inner walls of vessels and their migration through vessel walls to the site of injury

The effects of inflammation on the vasculature are visible within seconds. First, arterioles near the site of infection or injury constrict briefly. Vasodilation then causes slower blood velocity and increases local blood flow to the injured site. The increased flow and capillary permeability result in leakage of plasma from the vessels, causing swelling (edema) at the site of injury. As plasma moves outward, blood remaining in the microcirculation flows more slowly and becomes more viscous. The increased blood flow and increasing concentration of red cells at the site of inflammation cause locally increased warmth and redness. Leukocytes adhere to vessel walls. At the same time, biochemical mediators (e.g., histamine, bradykinin, leukotrienes, substance P, and prostaglandins) stimulate the endothelial cells that line capillaries and venules to retract, creating spaces at junctions between the cells, allowing leukocytes and plasma to enter the surrounding tissue (intercellular junctions are described in Chapter 1).

Each of the characteristic superficial and microscopic changes associated with inflammation is the direct result of the activities and interactions of a host of chemicals and cellular components found in the blood and tissues. The vascular changes deliver leukocytes, plasma proteins, and other biochemical mediators to the site of injury. Once in the tissues, the cells and chemicals associated with the inflammatory response act in concert to do the following:

1. Limit and control the inflammatory process through the influx of plasma protein systems (e.g., clotting system), plasma enzymes, and cells (e.g., eosinophils) that prevent the inflammatory response from spreading to areas of healthy tissue

2. Prevent infection and further damage by contaminating microorganisms through the influx of fluid to dilute toxins produced by bacteria and released from dying cells, the influx and activation of plasma protein systems that help destroy and contain bacteria (e.g., complement system, clotting system), and the influx of cells (e.g., neutrophils, macrophages) that "eat" and destroy cellular debris and infectious agents

3. Interact with components of the adaptive immune system to elicit a more specific response to contaminating pathogen(s) through the influx of macrophages and lymphocytes[10]

4. Prepare the area of injury for healing through removal of bacterial products, dead cells, and other products of inflammation (e.g., by way of channels through the epithelium or drainage by lymphatic vessels) and initiation of mechanisms of healing and repair

Drainage by lymphatic vessels also facilitates the development of acquired immunity because microbial antigens in lymphatic fluid pass through the lymph nodes, where they activate both B and T lymphocytes. (This process is discussed in Chapter 7, and the lymphatic system is described in Chapter 27.)

Inflammation and repair can be divided into several phases (Figure 6-3). The characteristics of the early (i.e., acute) inflammatory response differ from those of the later (i.e., chronic) response, and each phase involves different biochemical mediators and cells that function together to (1) destroy injurious agents and remove them from the inflammatory site, (2) wall off and confine these agents so as to limit their effects on the host, (3) stimulate and enhance the adaptive immune response, and (4) promote healing.

The acute inflammatory response is self-limiting; that is, it continues only until the threat to the host is eliminated. This usually takes 8 to 10 days from onset to healing. The acute inflammatory response begins immediately after cellular injury or infection (see Figure 6-3) and involves a vascular response, activation of plasma protein systems, and activation of a variety of cells. (Mechanisms of cellular injury are described in Chapter 2.)

Plasma Protein Systems

The inflammatory response includes activation of three key **plasma protein systems:** the complement system, the clotting system, and the kinin system. Although each of these systems functions differently from the others to provide protection, they have highly similar characteristics. Each consists of a se-

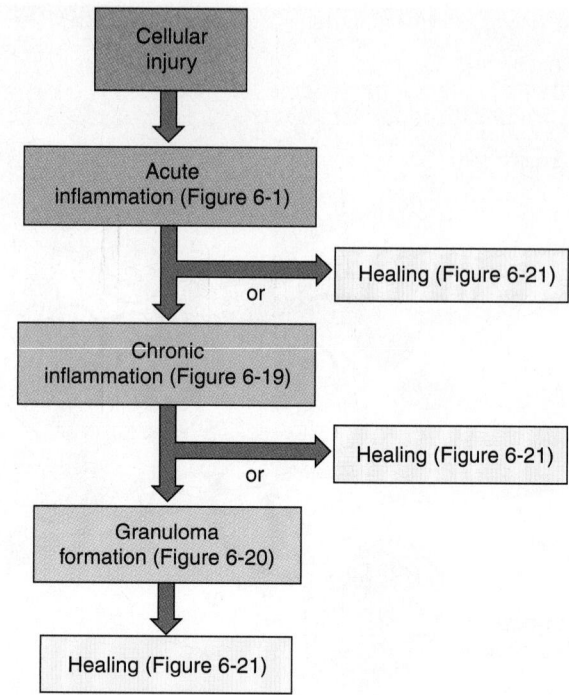

Figure 6-3 Inflammatory phases. Cellular injury leads to acute inflammation and may result in resolution and healing of the injured site or progress into chronic inflammation. Chronic inflammation in turn may either result in healing or progress to development of a granuloma. The final step of the inflammatory process is usually healing and reconstruction of the damaged tissue. The figure numbers refer to those in which more detailed information on that portion of the process may be found.

ries of inactive enzymes, or **proenzymes,** whose activation is required for action to be initiated. When the first proenzyme in the series is converted to an active enzyme, it initiates a cascade in which the substrate of the activated enzyme becomes the next component in the series. Therefore, activation of the entire cascade is initiated simply by activation of the first component. This activation usually involves the proteolytic cleavage of the proenzyme into two (or more) products. The larger product is an active enzyme whose substrate is the next proenzyme in the series; the smaller product also may be functional, usually serving as a potent biochemical mediator of the inflammatory response.

Complement System

The complement system consists of several plasma proteins (sometimes called *complement components*) that together constitute about 10% of the total circulating serum protein. The complement system is extremely important because activated components of the **complement cascade** may destroy pathogens directly and can activate or collaborate with virtually every other component of the inflammatory response.[6,7] For these reasons, proteins of the complement system are among the body's most potent defenders against bacterial infection.

Like the other plasma protein systems, the complement system is activated when the first protein in the complement cascade is proteolytically cleaved into fragments that are active themselves. Complement activation can be accomplished in three different ways, all of which converge at the third component (C3) of the pathway:

1. **Classical pathway:** activated by proteins of the acquired immune system (antibodies) bound to their specific targets (antigen)
2. **Lectin pathway:** activated by certain bacterial carbohydrates
3. **Alternative pathway:** activated by gram-negative bacterial and fungal cell wall polysaccharides

The principle routes by which the complement cascade may be activated are shown in Figure 6-4.

Activation of the *classical pathway* begins with the activation of protein C1 and is preceded by formation of a complex between an antigen and an antibody to form an **antigen-**

antibody complex (immune complex) (discussed in Chapter 7). The antigen(s) may be a unique chemical component(s) of the surface of a bacteria or other microorganism. Most pathogens express multiple antigens, therefore multiple antibodies are usually bound in the complex. Complement activation through the classical pathway occurs as a result of antibody clustering with these antigens. The first component of the classical complement cascade, C1, has six sites that can bind to antibodies, and efficient activation of the complement cascade usually requires concurrent binding of at least two of those sites to antibody. The complex formed by antigen-antibody-complement binding is shown in Figure 6-4. C1 is a macromolecular complex consisting of C1q and two molecules each of C1r and C1s. After binding simultaneously to two antibodies, C1q undergoes a conformational change

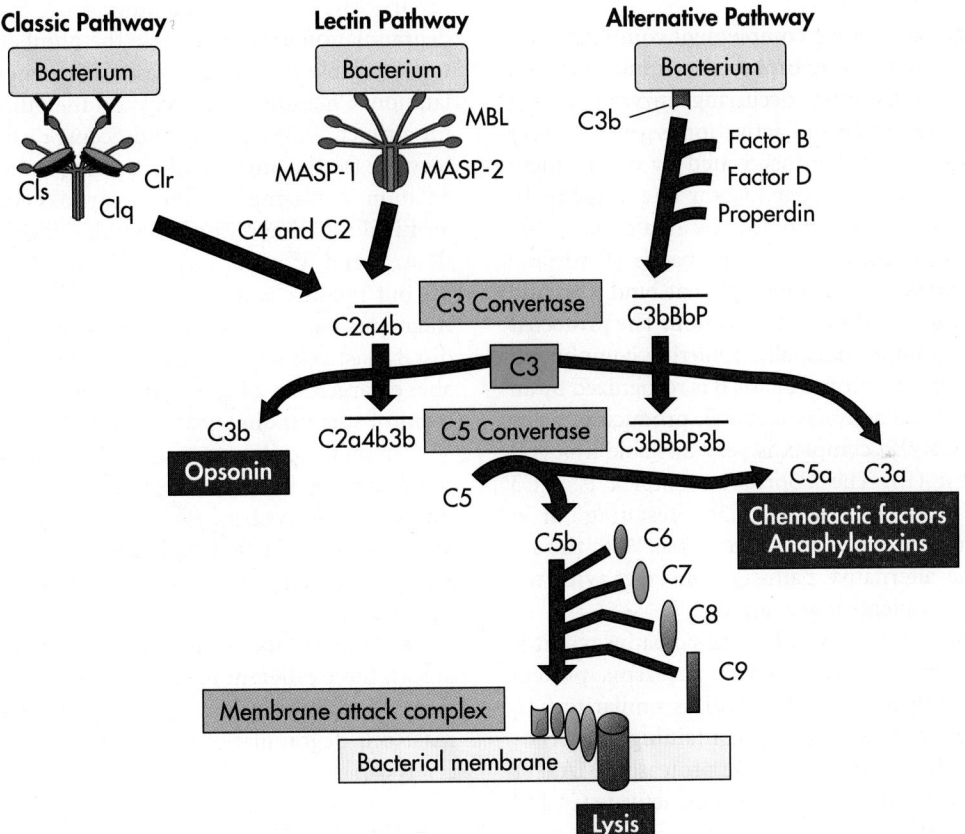

Figure 6-4 Pathways of complement cascade activation. The complement system is activated by three pathways: the classic pathway, the lectin pathway, or the alternative pathway. During activation, many complement components are cleaved into fragments (denoted by *lowercase letters*). The smaller fragments frequently have potent biologic activities. The larger activated fragment is usually converted into an active enzyme (indicated by the bar above the fragment) and forms a complex with the preceding components in the cascade. The classic pathway is usually activated by antigen-antibody complexes through component C1, which consists of C1q and two C1r and C1s molecules. As indicated, the C1q must simultaneously bind to two antibody molecules (indicated by Y-shaped structures). The lectin pathway is activated by mannose-binding lectin (MBL), which binds to two mannose-rich pathogen-associated molecular patterns on the surface of a bacterium. MBL contains two associated enzymes, MASP-1 and MASP-2, and functions in a manner similar to C1. C1 and MBL each activate complement components C4 and C2 (the resultant fragments C4a and C2b are not shown). The alternative pathway is activated by many agents, such as bacterial polysaccharides, which bind and stabilize C3b, which is produced by normal breakdown of C3 in the blood. The C3b forms the site of binding of factor B (activated by factor D into Bb and the fragment Ba [not shown]) and properdin. Each pathway produces C3 and C5 convertases, which are enzymatically active complexes that activate C3 and C5, respectively. C5b initiates assemblage of the membrane attack complex (MAC), which results in multiple C9 molecules forming a pore in the bacterial membrane.

resulting in the enzymatically active C1r coming into proximity with C1s so that C1s is activated to become an enzyme (C1 esterase) whose substrates are C4 and C2. The resultant complex formed by the interaction of C1, C4, and C2 uses C3 as a substrate resulting in the production of C3a and C3b. A complex that has C3 as a substrate is generally referred to as a **C3 convertase.** The complex formed by the activation of C3 then has C5 as a substrate, resulting in the conversion of C5 to C5a and C5b. A complex that has C5 as a substrate is generally called a **C5 convertase.** Thus activation of C1 initiates the sequential enzymatic activation of all other components of the classic pathway, ultimately resulting in the activation of C5, at which point each of the complement pathways converge. The classical pathway also can be activated to a lesser degree by biologic molecules other than antibody, including heparin (a charged molecule that prevents clotting), DNA or RNA, and C-reactive protein, which is increased in the blood during inflammation.

Small amounts of circulating complement component C3 are naturally and spontaneously broken down into C3b and C3a by a number of naturally occurring enzymes in the blood. The rate of C3 spontaneous activation is generally very low, and C3b is usually readily inactivated by complement regulator proteins in the blood (e.g., factor H and factor I). The *alternative pathway* is initiated by materials (e.g., lipopolysaccharides [endotoxin] on the bacterial surface, yeast cell wall carbohydrates [zymosan]) that bind C3b and protect it from factor H and from destruction. The protected C3b can react with another normally occurring component, factor B. The complex of C3b and factor B is recognized by an enzyme, factor D, which activates factor B, producing factor Bb. The resultant C3b/Bb complex is very unstable unless it binds to properdin (P). The C3b/Bb/P complex is a C3 convertase that produces further C3b, resulting in a C3b/Bb/P/C3b complex that is a C5 convertase. With the activation of C5, the alternative pathway converges with the classic pathway of complement activation.

The *lectin pathway* is similar to the classic pathway but is antibody-independent. It is activated by a plasma protein called *mannose-binding lectin (MBL).* MBL is similar to C1q and binds to bacterial polysaccharides containing the carbohydrate mannose. MBL-associated serine proteases (MASP-1 and MASP-2) substitute for C1r and C1s and activate C4 and C2 to create a C3 convertase.

After activation of C5, the cascade continues through the terminal components C6, C7, C8, and C9. Components C5b through C9 assemble to form complexes *(membrane attack complex or MAC)* capable of creating pores in bacterial cell membranes and permitting the influx of water and ions and may ultimately result in **cell lysis** and in destruction of the pathogen.

Probably the most important aspect of the complement system is the activities of the small fragments generated during the activation of C4, C2, C3, and C5. C3b adheres to the surface of a pathogenic microorganism and serves as an efficient **opsonin.** Opsonins are molecules that 'tag' pathogenic

microorganisms for destruction by cells of the inflammatory system (primarily neutrophils and macrophages). C4a, C2b, C3a, and C5a are soluble, low-molecular-weight fragments that contribute in other ways to the inflammatory response. C2b affects smooth muscle causing vasodilation and increased vascular permeability. C3a, C5a, and to a limited extent, C4a are **anaphylatoxins;** that is, they induce the rapid **degranulation** (i.e., release of granular contents) and the release of histamine from mast cells (see Figure 6-8, p. 187) causing vasodilation and increased capillary permeability.

C5a is the major chemotactic factor for neutrophils. C3a is approximately 100 times less potent in chemotactic and anaphylatoxic activity. A **chemotactic factor** is a biochemical substance that attracts leukocytes to the site of inflammation. The dual functions, as a chemotactic factor and an anaphylatoxin, are not needed simultaneously or to the same degree. Anaphylatoxic activity is necessary early in inflammation and occurs close to the inflammatory site to induce local mast cell degranulation and to increase the number of soluble mediators available to enhance vascular permeability and vasodilatation. Chemotactic activity, on the other hand, is required for a much longer period and occurs distal to the inflammatory site for the purpose of attracting leukocytes from the circulation. A plasma enzyme, a **carboxypeptidase,** removes a terminal arginine on both peptides, thereby producing "C3a desArg" and "C5a desArg," which are inactive as anaphylatoxins but retain chemotactic activity. Thus these complement fragments can have chemotactic activity, while not inducing distal mast cell degranulation that would result in considerable enlargement of the inflammatory response to the detriment of surrounding healthy tissue.

C3b on the cell surface also can be broken down into inactive fragments by several enzymes in the blood. The inactivation is progressive because a sequence of proteolytic cleavages are made leading first to inactive C3b (iC3b) and then to smaller fragments with diminishing biologic activity (e.g., C3d, C3dg).

In summary, the complement cascades can be activated by at least three different means and its products have four functions: (1) opsonization, (2) anaphylatoxic activity resulting in mast cell degranulation, (3) leukocyte chemotaxis, and (4) cell lysis.

Clotting System

The clotting (coagulation) system is a group of plasma proteins that form a fibrinous meshwork at an injured or inflamed site. This (1) prevents the spread of infection to adjacent tissues, (2) keeps microorganisms and foreign bodies at the site of greatest inflammatory cell activity, (3) forms a clot that stops bleeding, and (4) provides a framework for future repair and healing. The main substance in this fibrinous mesh is an insoluble protein called *fibrin* that is the end product of the **coagulation cascade.**

Like the complement cascade, the coagulation cascade can be activated through different pathways that converge at the point where each pathway produces the same substance (Figure 6-5). In the complement cascade the classic and alternative pathways converge when each has activated C5; in the coagulation cascade the **extrinsic pathway** and the **intrinsic pathway** converge at factor X. From that point on, the cascade proceeds on a common pathway until fibrin is formed. The coagulation cascade is discussed further and illustrated again in Chapter 25.

The clotting system can be activated by many substances that are released during tissue destruction and infection, including collagen, proteinases, kallikrein, and plasmin, as well as by bacterial products such as endotoxins. As with the complement cascade, activation of the clotting cascade produces fragments that enhance the inflammatory response. Two low-molecular-weight fibrinopeptides, A and B, are released when fibrinogen is cleaved to produce fibrin. Both fibrinopeptides (especially fibrinopeptide B) are chemotactic for neutrophils and increase vascular permeability by enhancing the effects of bradykinin (formed from the kinin system).

Kinin System

The third plasma protein system, the **kinin system,** interacts closely with the coagulation system and therefore also functions to compartmentalize and trap invading pathogens, although its primary role is to activate and assist inflammatory cells. The primary kinin is **bradykinin,** which, at low doses, causes dilation of blood vessels, acts with prostaglandins to induce pain, causes smooth muscle cell contraction, increases vascular permeability, and may increase leukocyte chemotaxis (see Figure 6-1). Bradykinin induces smooth muscle contraction more slowly than histamine and may be more important during the prolonged phases of inflammation because it,

along with prostaglandins of the E series, is probably responsible for endothelial cell retraction and increased vascular permeability in the later phases of inflammation (endothelial cell retraction is shown in Figure 6-12, p. 192).

The kinin system is activated by stimulation of the **plasma kinin cascade** (Figure 6-6). The conversion of plasma prekallikrein to kallikrein is induced by *prekallikrein activator,* which is identical to factor XIIa (the product that results from activation of Hageman factor—factor XII) of the clotting cascade. Kallikrein then converts kininogen to bradykinin. Although the plasma kinin cascade is one pathway that leads to the production of bradykinin, tissue kalikreins in saliva, sweat, tears, urine and feces provide another source for

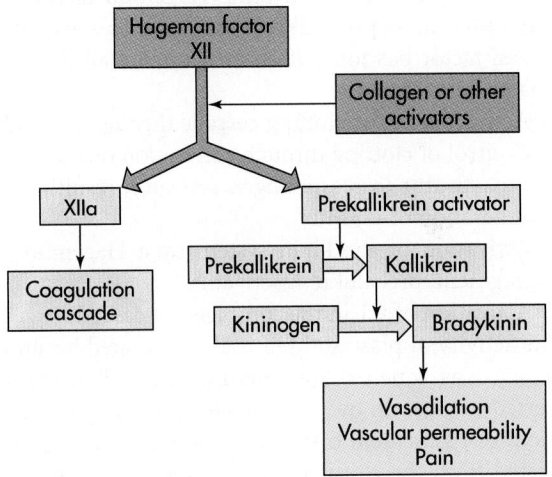

Figure 6-6 Plasma kinin cascade.

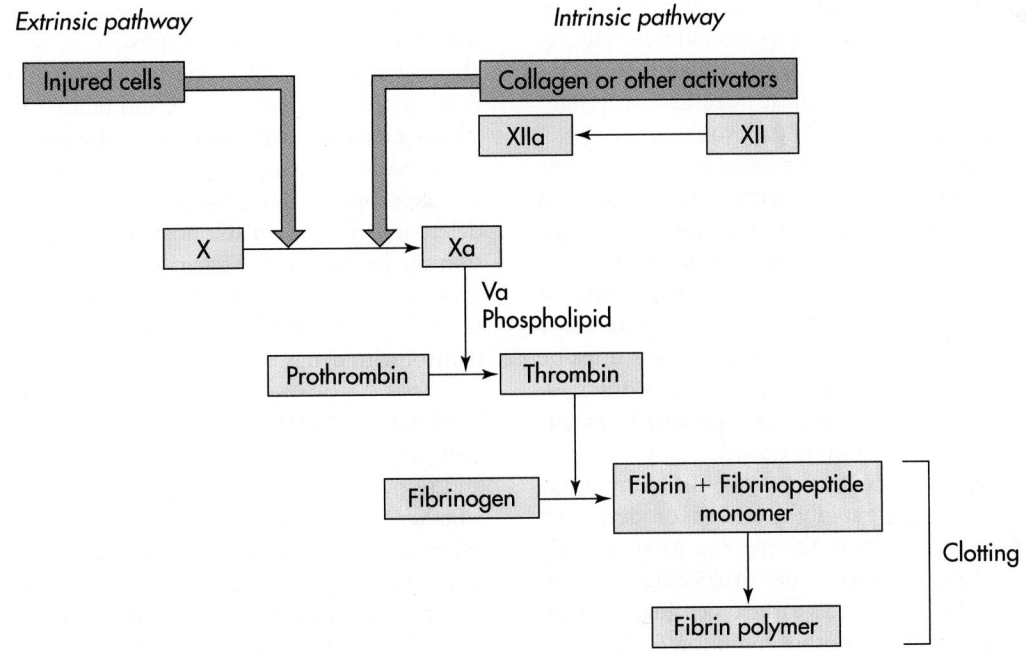

Figure 6-5 **Coagulation cascade.** During activation of the coagulation cascade, several components are converted from inactive to active forms. The active components are designated with an "a."

this inflammatory mediator. These tissue kallikreins convert serum kininogens to kallidin, also known as *Lys-bradykinin*, which may be converted to bradykinin by plasma aminopeptidase. Kinins are rapidly degraded and therefore controlled by **kininases,** enzymes present in plasma and tissues.

Interactions Among the Plasma Protein Systems

Interaction between the three plasma protein systems is such that activation or control of one system results in a similar effect on the others (Figure 6-7). As an example, **plasmin** functions in clot formation by degrading fibrin and fibrinogen, and it also can activate the complement cascade through components C1, C3, and C5. Plasmin can activate the plasma kinin cascade as well by activating **Hageman factor (factor XII)** and producing prekallikrein activator. This activation of Hageman factor has four effects that impact all three of the plasma protein systems:

1. Activation of the clotting cascade through factor XI
2. Control of clotting through conversion of plasminogen proactivator to plasminogen activator, resulting in the generation of plasmin
3. Activation of the kinin system by a Hageman factor fragment, prekallikrein activator
4. Activation of C1 in the complement cascade

The activity of plasmin itself is also regulated because it is synthesized as a proenzyme, plasminogen. Plasminogen is converted to plasmin by several factors, including plasminogen activator generated from the kallikrein system, thrombin generated from the clotting system, bacterial factors such as streptokinase produced by hemolytic streptococci, plasminogen activators produced by endothelial cells, and several cellular enzymes released during tissue destruction.

Activation of any of the plasma protein systems results in production of a large number of very potent, biologically active substances that further activate the inflammatory response and assist in protection against infection. Very tight control of these processes is essential for two reasons:

1. The inflammatory processes mediated by these systems are so critical for protection against infection that its activation must be guaranteed, and consequentially, multiple means of initiating them must be in place.
2. The activities of the biochemical mediators generated during these processes are so potent and potentially detrimental to the host itself that their actions must be strictly confined to injured or infected tissues only.

Therefore, multiple mechanisms are also available to *inactivate* or *regulate* the products of these cascades.

This tight control is apparent at many levels. Many products of these pathways are rapidly modified or destroyed within seconds by enzymes from the plasma. As previously mentioned, the anaphylatoxic activities of C3a and C5a are inactivated by the plasma enzyme carboxypeptidase, which removes a terminal arginine. Another inhibitor, **C1 esterase inhibitor (C1 inh)** binds to C1r and C1s to inhibit from further activation of the classic complement cascade. It also

binds to elements of the kinin (e.g., kallikrein, activated Hageman factor), plasmin, and clotting systems (e.g., activated factor XI) to prevent limit their activation.[8] Many other natural inhibitors are present, including enzymes that degrade histamine (histaminase), kinins (kinases), activated complement components, kallikrein, and plasmin.

Cellular Mediators of Inflammation

The cellular components of the inflammatory response consist primarily of cells of the granulocytic or monocytic lines of leukocytes. Most are generally found in the blood, but several are also found in the tissues. The primary circulating white blood cells are granulocytes, so-called because of the many enzyme-containing granules in their cytoplasm, which include neutrophils, eosinophils, and basophils. Other blood components include platelets, agranular monocytes (probable precursors of tissue macrophages), and various forms of lymphocytes. Circulating cells continually contact endothelial cells lining the blood vessels. Changes in the interactions of endothelium with circulating leukocytes and platelets occur during inflammation and account for several of the characteristic changes observed during the inflammatory response. Other cellular members of the inflammatory system are found in various tissues and organs. These include mast cells and cells derived from the monocytes/macrophage lineage. Lymphoid-derived natural killer cells (NK cells) are found both in the circulation and tissues and can recognize and destroy cells that have been altered by viral infection or malignancy.

The cells of the inflammatory system both secrete and respond to biochemical mediators. Thus most of these cells are recruited and activated by products of activation of the plasma protein systems and by biochemicals released during cell destruction, secreted by other inflammatory cells, or produced by microbes. All of these inflammatory cells and protein systems, along with the substances they produce, preferably act at the site of tissue injury to confine the extent of damage, kill microorganisms, and remove the debris of "battle" in preparation for healing: tissue regeneration or repair (processes known as *resolution*).

Inappropriate or exaggerated inflammatory processes have deleterious effects on the host. Even appropriate inflammation can be painful and harm healthy tissues. Because inflammation is complex, is nonspecific, and can be triggered and maintained by a great variety of stimuli, it is often difficult to control with drugs.

Cellular Receptors

Cells of both innate and acquired immunity must recognize and respond to abnormal components of their environment, whether products of damaged cells or potential pathogenic microorganisms. Recognition is usually through the binding of these materials to receptors on the cell surface, resulting in activation of an intracellular signaling pathway and activation of the cell itself. As will be discussed in Chapter 7, B and T lymphocytes of the acquired immune system have evolved surface receptors (i.e., the T-cell receptor, or TCR, and the

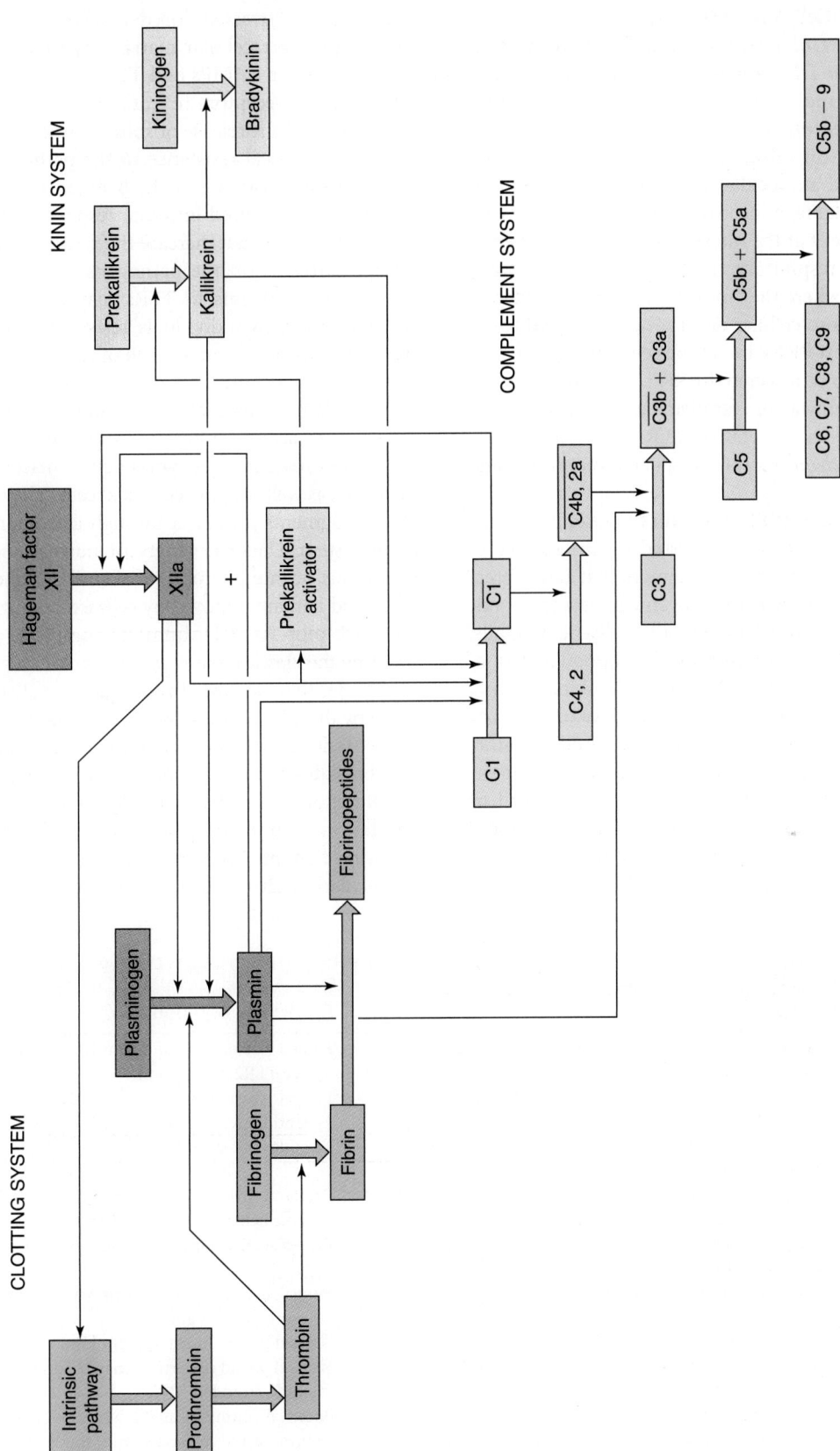

Figure 6-7 Interactions between the complement, clotting, kinin, and fibrinolytic (plasmin) systems. *Thick arrows* denote the activation of factors within a system. *Thin arrows* denote where a particular factor activates another system.

B-cell receptor, or BCR) that bind antigen, are developed during somatic rearrangement of DNA and span a large spectrum of specificities. Cells involved in innate resistance have evolved a different set of receptors, which are already contained in the germ line DNA and recognize a much more limited array of specific molecules. These are referred to as **pattern recognition receptors (PRRs)**, and they recognize molecular "patterns" on infectious agents or their products (**pathogen-associated molecular patterns, or PAMPs)**, or products of cellular damage (necrosis or apoptosis). PRRs are generally found on cells at the interface of the host and environment (i.e., skin, respiratory tract, gastrointestinal tract, genitourinary tract) where they monitor for flaws in external barriers that result from cellular damage and may lead to infection. Although most PRRs are on the cell surface, some are secreted. An example of a secreted PRR is mannose-binding lectin of the lectin pathway of complement activation. Cellular PRRs include Toll-like receptors (TLRs), complement receptors (CRs), scavenger receptors, glucan receptors, and mannose receptors.

At least 10 different **Toll-like receptors (TLRs)** have been described in humans. They are expressed on the surface of many cells as homodimers or heterodimers that have direct and early contact with potential pathogenic microorganisms. These include mucosal epithelial cells, mast cells, neutrophils, macrophages, dendritic cells, and some subpopulations of lymphocytes. (Dendritic cells are found in the skin, mucosa, and lymphoid tissues, where they have developed from Langerhans cells and function as highly specialized initiators of the acquired immune response.) TLRs recognize a large variety of PAMPs located on the microorganism's cell wall or surface (e.g., bacterial lipopolysaccharide [LPS], peptidoglycans, and lipoproteins, yeast zymosan, viral coat proteins), other surface structures (e.g., bacterial flagellin), or microbial

nucleic acid (e.g., bacterial unmethylated DNA, viral double-stranded RNA). Some TLRs recognize host factors that are produced by "stressed" or damaged cells (e.g., breakdown products of extracellular matrix proteins, chromatin). Interactions between PAMPs and TLRs, with the collaboration of other cellular receptors (e.g., CD14), can result in activation of the cell and the release of soluble products (e.g., cytokines) that increase local resistance to the pathogenic microorganism. TLRs are also one of the bridges between innate resistance and the acquired immune response through the induction of cytokines that increase the response of lymphocytes to foreign antigens on the pathogens. Recently discovered genetic polymorphisms in TLRs may explain some observed differences among individuals' resistance and susceptibility to infections. Information on each of the TLRs found in humans is shown in Table 6-3.[9,11]

Complement receptors are found on many cells of the innate and acquire immune responses (e.g., granulocytes, monocytes/macrophages, lymphocytes, mast cells, erythrocytes, platelets), as well as some epithelial cells. They recognize a variety of fragments produced through activation of the complement system. Under a variety of normal and disease-related conditions, immune complexes of antibody and antigen form in the blood and are removed by cells expressing surface complement receptor-1 (CR1). Immune complexes activate complement by the classical pathway and contain a great deal of C4b, C3b, and C3b breakdown products (e.g., iC3b) which are recognized by the CR1 binding site. CR2 is found on B lymphocytes, as well as dendritic cells and some epithelial cells, and recognizes C3b breakdown products (particularly iC3b and C3dg), as well as interferon-alpha (INF-α). CR2 appears to facilitate B-cell function and antibody production. Both CR3 and CR4 are integrins that primarily recognize C3b breakdown products (particularly iC3b). CR3 (integrin αMβ2, also called CD11b/

Table 6-3	Cellular Source and Microbial Target for Each Toll-like Receptor (TLR)	
Receptor	Cellular Expression Pattern	PAMP Recognition
TLR1	Cell surface (ubiquitous): neutrophils, monocytes/macrophages, dendritic cells, T cells, B cells, NK cells	Fungal, bacterial, viral; forms heterodimer with TLR2 (see TLR2 recognition)
TLR2	Cell surface: neutrophils, monocytes/macrophages, dendritic cells	Fungal (yeast zymosan), bacterial (gram-positive bacterial peptidoglycan, lipoproteins), viral (lipoproteins)
TLR3	Intracellular: monocytes/macrophages, dendritic cells, T cells, NK cells, epithelial cells	Viral double-stranded DNA
TLR4	Cell surface: granulocytes, monocytes/macrophages, dendritic cells, T cells, B cells, epithelial cells	Bacterial (primarily gram-negative bacterial LPS, lipoteichoic acids), viral (RSV F protein, hepatitis C)
TLR5	Cell surface: granulocytes, monocytes/macrophages, dendritic cells, NK cells, epithelial cells	Bacterial (flagellin); forms heterodimer with TLR4
TLR6	Cell surface: monocytes/macrophages, dendritic cells, B cells, NK cells	Fungal, bacterial, viral; forms heterodimer with TLR2 (see TLR2 recognition)
TLR7	Intracellular: monocytes/macrophages, dendritic cells, B cells	Natural ligand uncertain; may bind viral single-strand RNA
TLR8	Cell surface: monocytes/macrophages, dendritic cells, NK cells	Natural ligand uncertain; may bind fungal PAMPs or viral single-stranded RNA
TLR9	Intracellular: monocytes/macrophages, dendritic cells, B cells	Bacterial (unmethylated DNA [CpG dinucleotides])
TLR10	Cell surface: monocytes/macrophages, dendritic cells, B cells	Natural ligand uncertain; may form heterodimers with TLR2

NK cells, Natural killer cells; *LPS,* lipopolysaccharide; *RSV,* respiratory syncytial virus; *PAMPs,* pathogen-associated molecular patterns.

CD18) facilitates phagocytosis by neutrophils and monocytes/macrophages. CR4 (αXβ2, also called CD11c/CD18) is found primarily on platelets. (Integrins are discussed in more detail below.) Other complement receptors include those for C3a, C4a, C5a (recognizes C5a and C5a desArg), and C1q.[12,13]

Scavenger receptors are primarily expressed on macrophages and facilitate recognition and phagocytosis of bacterial pathogens, as well as damaged cells and altered soluble lipoproteins associated with vascular damage (e.g., HDL, acetylated LDL, oxidized LDL). More than eight receptors have been identified. Some scavenger receptors (e.g., SR-PSOX) recognize the cell membrane phospholipid phosphatidyl serine (PS). PS is normally sequestered on the cytoplasmic surface of the cell membrane, but is externalized under a very limited variety of conditions, including erythrocyte senescence and cellular apoptosis. Thus macrophages, through this receptor, can identify and remove old red blood cells and cells undergoing apoptosis. Another important scavenger receptor is CD14, which recognizes the complex of LPS and LPS-binding protein. LPS-binding protein is up-regulated during inflammation by the cytokines IL-6 and IL-1 and helps remove bacterial lipopolysaccharide (endotoxin) from the circulation.[14-16]

Mast Cells

A central cell in inflammation is the mast cell. **Mast cells,** first described by Paul Ehrlich[17] in 1877, are cellular bags of granules located in the loose connective tissues close to blood vessels (Figure 6-8). They are found in large numbers in the skin and lining the gastrointestinal and respiratory tracts. A great number of stimuli cause mast cells to become activated, resulting in initiation of the inflammatory response. Typical causes of mast cell activation include (1) physical injury (e.g., heat, mechanical trauma, ultraviolet light, and x-rays); (2)

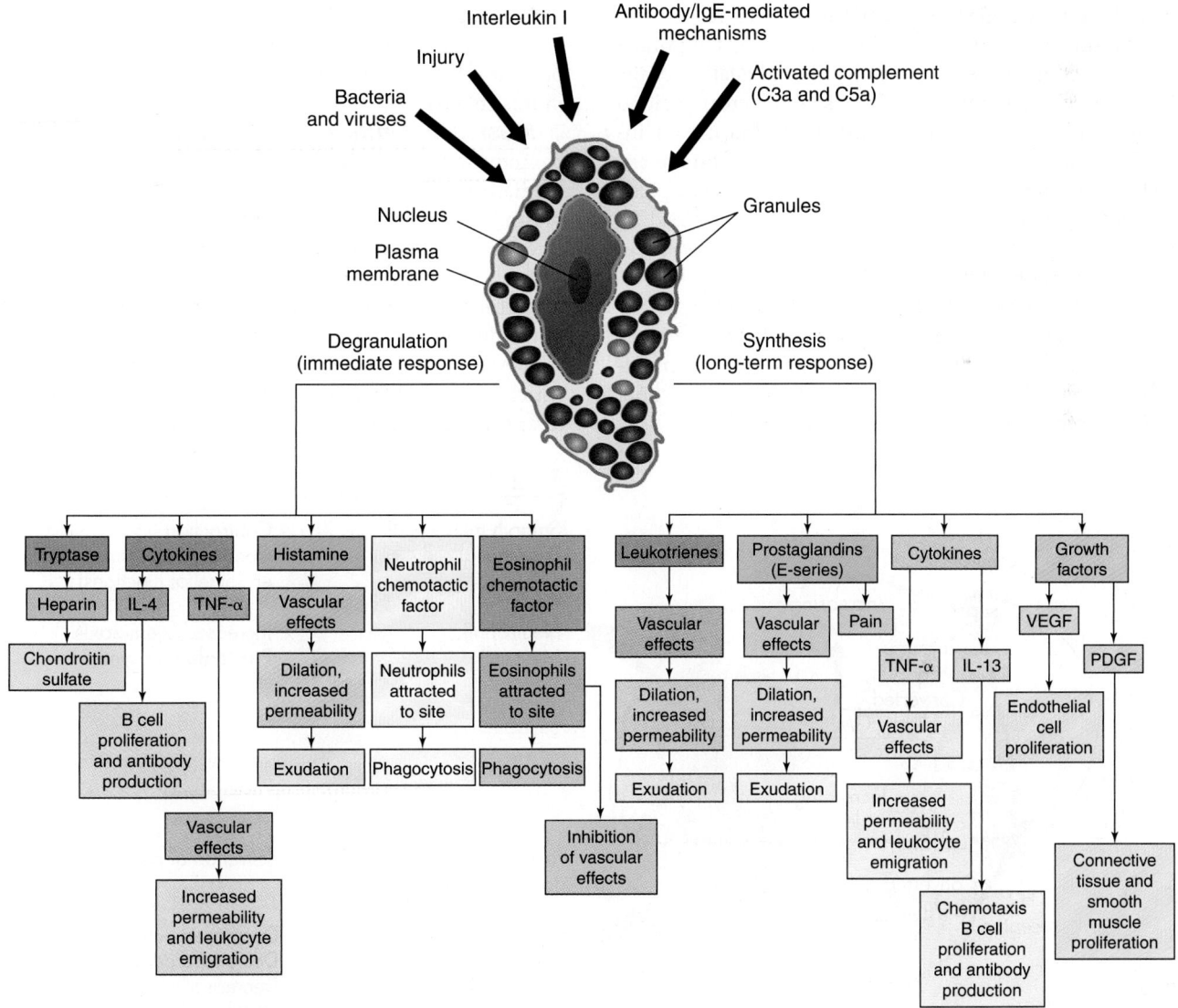

Figure 6-8 Effects of degranulation *(left)* and synthesis *(right)* by mast cells. The depiction of a tissue mast cell shows darkly stained granules in the cytoplasm. *VEGF,* Vascular endothelial growth factor; *PDGF,* platelet derived growth factor.

chemical agents (e.g., toxins, snake and bee venoms, proteolytic enzymes, and antimicrobial peptides); (3) immunologic means (e.g., anaphylatoxins released during activation of complement components or particular types of antibody produced by cells of the acquired immune response, see Chapter 7); and (4) activation of Toll-like receptors by bacteria and viruses.[18-20] Soluble and extremely potent chemicals from the mast cell are responsible for its effects on inflammation. These are released in two ways: by release of the contents of their preformed granules (*degranulation*) and by new synthesis of lipid-derived inflammatory mediators. Mast cells are also involved in initiating many allergic responses (discussed in Chapters 7 and 8).

Mast Cell Degranulation

In response to a stimulus, biochemical mediators in the mast cell granules, including histamine, chemotactic factors (e.g., neutrophil chemotactic factor, **eosinophil chemotactic factor of anaphylaxis** or **ECF-A**), and cytokines (e.g., tumor necrosis factor–alpha [TNF-α], IL-4) are released within seconds and exert their effects immediately (see Figure 6-8).

Histamine is a vasoactive amine that causes temporary, rapid constriction of the large vessel walls and dilation of the postcapillary venules, both of which result in increased blood flow into the microcirculation. Histamine also causes increased vascular permeability resulting from retraction of endothelial cells lining the capillaries (see Figure 6-2). The pharmacologic effects of histamine are partially determined by histamine receptors on the host's target cells.[21,22] Two main histamine receptors are the H1 and H2 receptors (Figure 6-9). Binding of histamine to the *H1 receptor* is essentially proinflammatory; that is it promotes inflammation. On the other hand, binding to the *H2 receptor* is generally anti-inflammatory because it results in suppression of leukocyte function. The H1 receptor is present on smooth muscle cells, especially those of the bronchi, and causes bronchial smooth muscle to contract (bronchoconstriction) when stimulated. Both types of receptors are distributed among many different cells and are often present on the same cells and may act in an antagonistic fashion. For instance, neutrophils express both types of receptors, with stimulation of H1 receptors resulting in the augmentation of neutrophil chemotaxis, and H2 stimulation resulting in its inhibition. The H2 receptor is especially abundant on parietal cells of the stomach mucosa and induces the secretion of gastric acid as part of the normal physiology of the stomach. The role of H1 and H2 receptors is discussed further in Chapter 8.

Two chemotactic factors, neutrophil chemotactic factor and ECF-A, are also released during mast cell degranulation. **Chemotaxis** is directional movement of cells along a chemical gradient formed by a chemotactic factor (Figure 6-10). Neutrophil chemotactic factor attracts neutrophils, and ECF-A attracts eosinophils to the site of inflammation. Neutrophils are the predominant leukocytes at work during the early phases of acute inflammation, and eosinophils have several functions in the inflammatory process; both of these important inflammatory cells are discussed in more detail later in this chapter.

Mast Cell Synthesis of Mediators

Activated mast cells begin new synthesis of other mediators of inflammation, including those derived from plasma membrane lipids, cytokines (TNF-α, various interleukins), and factors that stimulate cell growth and angiogenesis). Leukotrienes, prostaglandins, and platelet-activating factor are lipid-derived products that are synthesized during mast cell activation (Figure 6-11). Leukotrienes are a product of another lipid, arachidonic acid, which is released from mast cell membranes by an intracellular phospholipase that acts on membrane phospholipids.

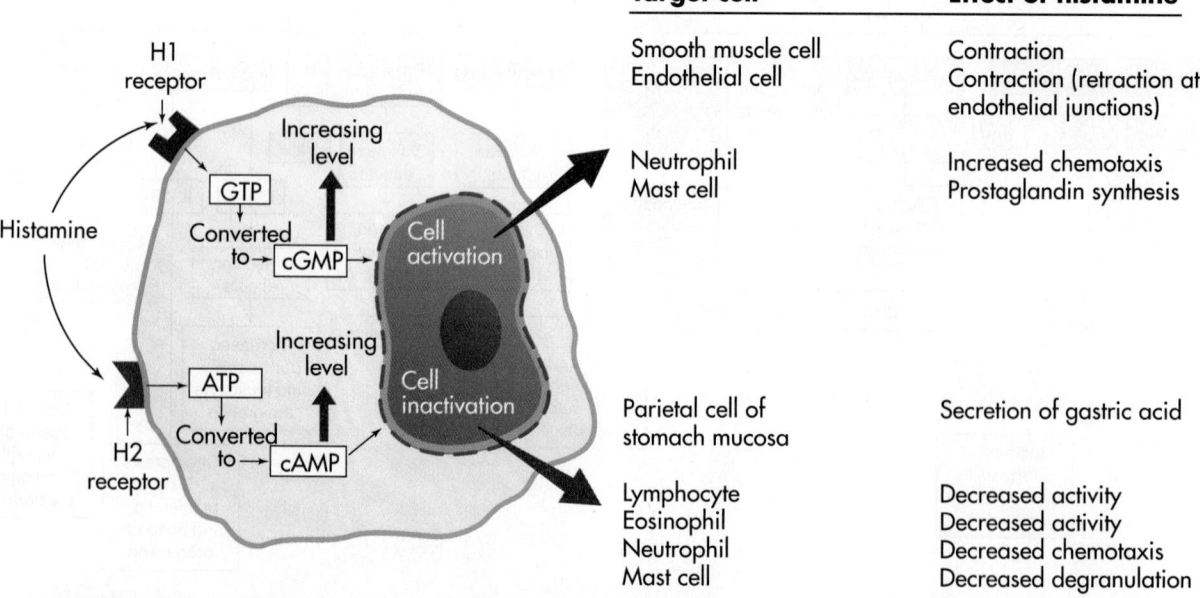

Target cell	Effect of histamine
Smooth muscle cell	Contraction
Endothelial cell	Contraction (retraction at endothelial junctions)
Neutrophil	Increased chemotaxis
Mast cell	Prostaglandin synthesis
Parietal cell of stomach mucosa	Secretion of gastric acid
Lymphocyte	Decreased activity
Eosinophil	Decreased activity
Neutrophil	Decreased chemotaxis
Mast cell	Decreased degranulation

Figure 6-9 Effects of histamine through H1 and H2 receptors. Effects depend on (*1*) density and affinity of H1 or H2 receptors on the target cell and (*2*) the identity of the target cell. *GTP*, Guanosine triphosphate; *cGMP*, cyclic guanosine monophosphate; *ATP*, adenosine triphosphate; *cAMP*, cyclic adenosine monophosphate.

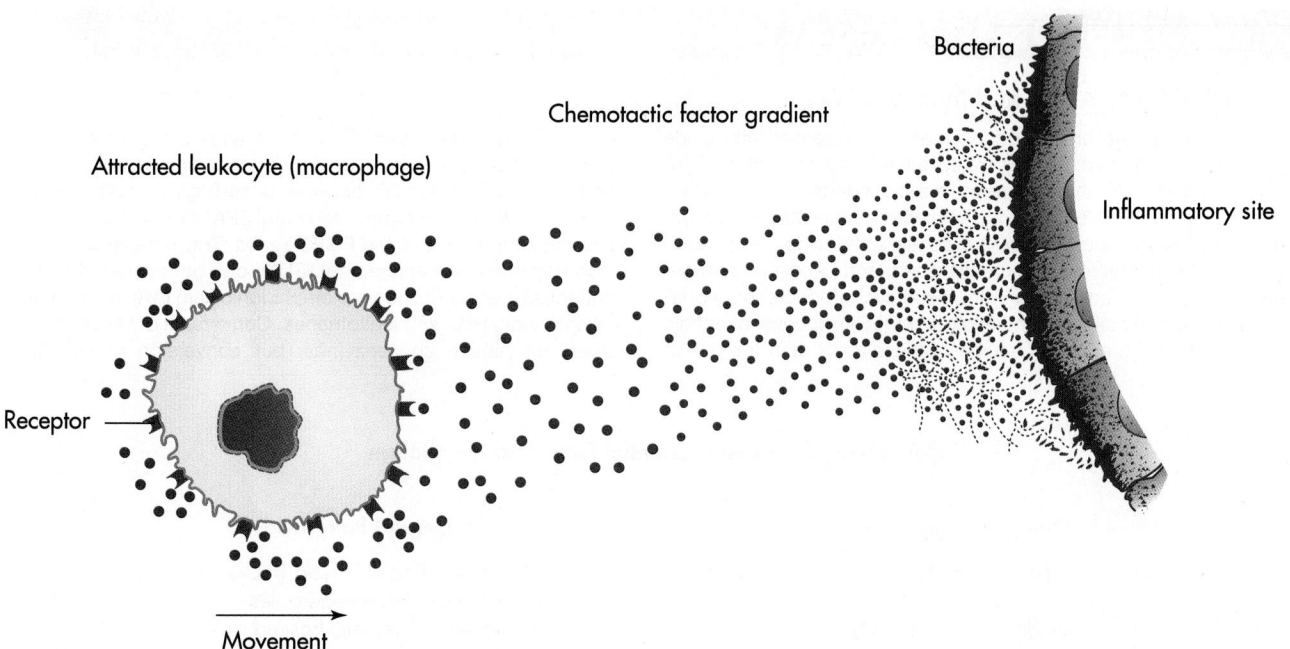

Figure 6-10 Chemotaxis. Multiple receptors on the leukocyte's plasma membrane sense the area of highest concentration of a chemotactic factor *(dots)*, and the leukocyte (usually a phagocyte) moves toward this area.

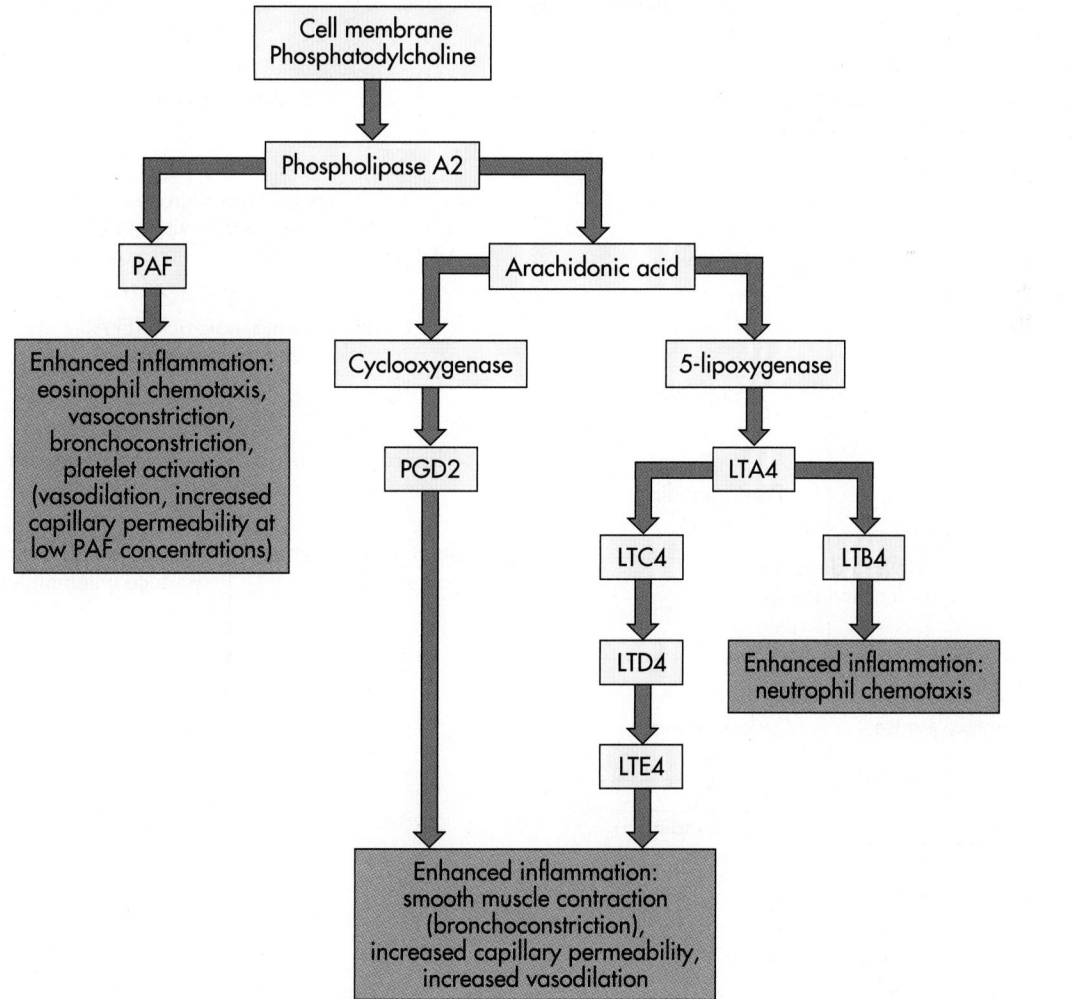

Figure 6-11 Production of lipid vasoactive substances by mast cells. *PAF,* Platelet-activating factor; *LTA4, LTC4, LTD4, LTE4, LTB4,* various leukotriene molecules; *PGD2,* prostaglandin D2.

Essential Fatty Acids and Inflammation

Both omega-3 and omega-6 fatty acids are essential fatty acids available only in the diet. They are essential because human physiology cannot add the necessary double bonds to the carbon chains. Omega-6 fatty acids are contained in vegetable oils and most are linoleic acid. Omega-3 essential fatty acids are found in green leafy vegetables, walnuts, flaxseed, and canola oil and are mostly alpha-linolenic acid. The metabolic products of alpha-linolenic acid are eicosapentaenoic acid (EPA) docosahexaenoic acid (DHA) and the richest source of these acids is in the oils of

deep-sea cold-water fish. Both the omega-3 and omega-6 fatty acids use the same enzymes to produce their metabolic products and they compete for this enzyme, delta-5-desaturase (see figure below). *Delta-5-desaturase* converts EPA into anti-inflammatory prostaglandins (PG) of the PGE3 series. The omega-6 fatty acid, dihomogamma-linolenic acid (DGLA), can be converted to either anti-inflammatory PG1 or into arachidonic acid (AA), a precursor of inflammatory PG2 and leukotrienes. Conversion of DGLA into PG1 does not require any enzymes, but conversion of DGLA into

Inflammatory Products of Essential Fatty Acid Metabolism

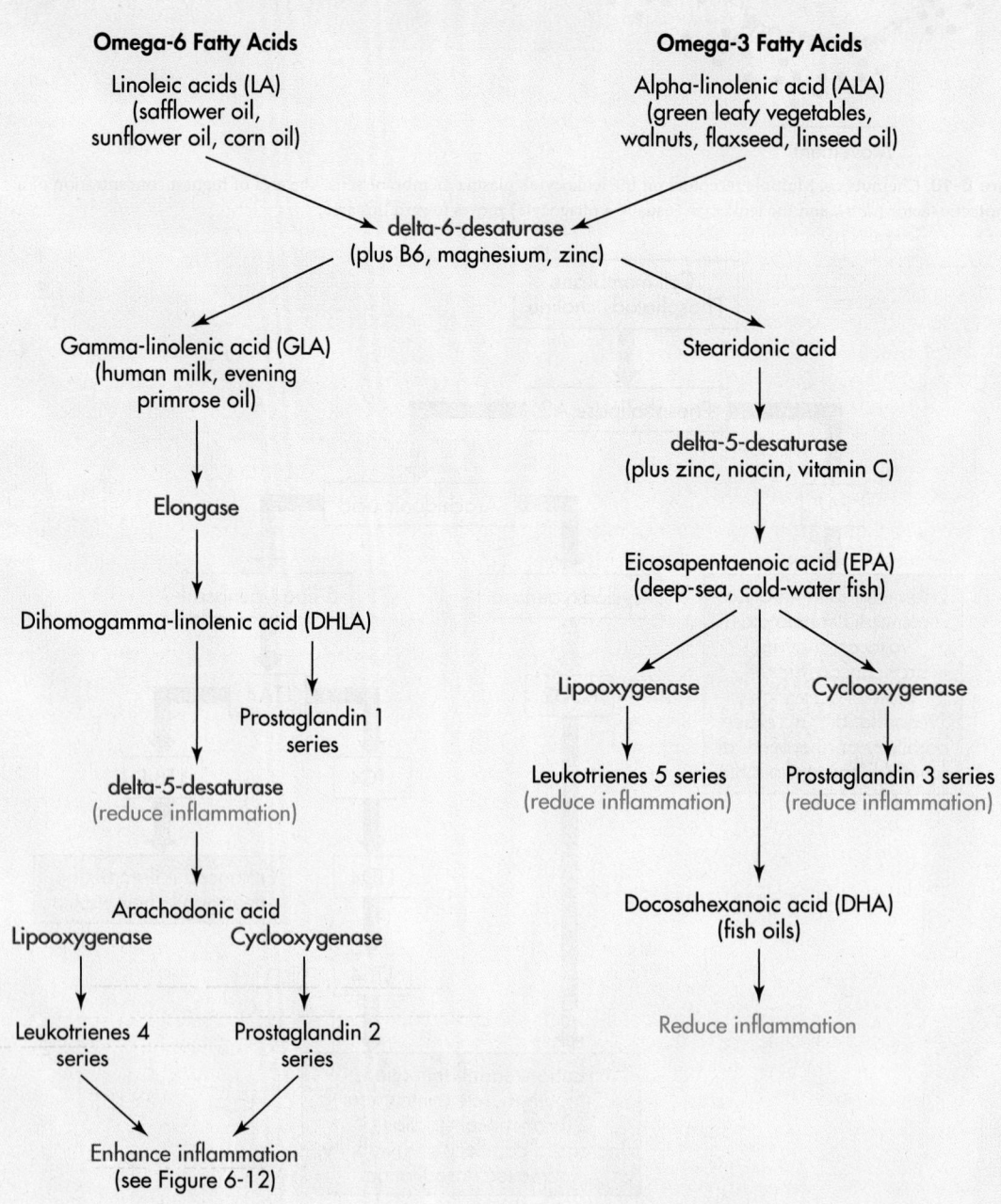

AA requires the enzyme delta-6 and -5 desaturase. When the diet is high in omega-3 fatty acids, most of the delta-5-desaturase will be used in the omega-3 pathway and the production of anti-inflammatory prostaglandins. Little delta-5-desaturase will be available to convert DGLA into arachidonic acid, and subsequently inflammatory mediators. DGLA ends up being converted into the anti-inflammatory PG1 and overall, inflammation is decreased. The resulting anti-inflammatory effects of omega-3 essential fatty acids decreases the risk for cardiovascular disease, cancer and other conditions associated with inflammation. Omega-3 fatty acids have been shown to decrease blood triglyceride concentrations; decrease production of chemoattractants, growth factors, and ad-

hesion molecules; lower blood pressure, increase nitric oxide production and endothelial relaxation and vascular compliance; decrease thrombosis and cardiac arrhythmias, and stabilize atherosclerotic plaque. The American diet tends to be high in saturated and omega-6 fatty acids and deficient in omega-3 fatty acids with a ratio estimated at about 15:1. The Mediterranean-style diet has more whole grains, fish, olive oil, fresh fruits and vegetables and a more balanced ratio of omega-6 to omega-3 fatty acids estimated at about 3-4:1. Increasing omega-3 fatty acids in the diet may significantly improve health and reduce the risk of cardiovascular disease and cancer.

Data from Calder PC: *Clin Sci (Lond)* 107(1):1-11, 2004; Chrysohoou C et al: *J Am Coll Cardiol* 44(1):152-158, 2004; Covington MB: *Am Fam Physician* 70(1):133-140, 2004; Esposito K et al: *JAMA* 292(12):1440-1446, 2004; Larsson SC et al: *Am J Clin Nutr* 79(6):935-945, 2004; Oddy WH et al: *J Asthma* 41(3):319-326, 2004; Stark KD, Holub BJ: *Am J Clin Nutr* 79(5):765-773, 2004.

Leukotrienes are acidic, sulfur-containing lipids that produce effects similar to those of histamine, namely, smooth muscle contraction, increased vascular permeability, and perhaps neutrophil and eosinophil chemotaxis. Leukotrienes appear to be important in the later stages of the inflammatory response because they stimulate slower and more prolonged responses than do histamines.

The mast cell also synthesizes **prostaglandins,** which, like leukotrienes, are a product of arachidonic acid and cause increased vascular permeability and neutrophil chemotaxis. Prostaglandins also induce pain. They are long-chain, unsaturated fatty acids produced by the action of the enzyme *cyclooxygenase* and are classified into groups (E, D, A, F, and B) according to their structure. Prostaglandins E_1 and E_2 cause increased vascular permeability and smooth muscle contraction, apparently acting directly on postcapillary venules. They can inhibit some aspects of inflammation by suppressing both the release of histamine from mast cells and the release of lysosomal enzymes (enzymes responsible for killing and digesting microorganisms) from neutrophils. Enhancement or suppression of the inflammatory response may be related to the concentration of prostaglandins. Aspirin and some other nonsteroidal anti-inflammatory drugs (NSAIDs) block the synthesis of prostaglandins of the E series and other arachidonic acid derivatives, thereby inhibiting inflammation.

Platelet-activating factor (PAF), another mast cell–derived lipid, is produced by removal of a fatty acid from the plasma membrane phospholipid phosphatidlycholine by phospholipase A_2. Although mast cells are a major source of PAF, this molecule also can be produced during inflammation by neutrophils, monocytes, endothelial cells, and platelets. The biologic activity of PAF is virtually identical to that of leukotrienes, namely causing endothelial cell retraction to increase vascular permeability, leukocyte adhesion to endothelial cells, and platelet activation.

Phagocytosis

Phagocytosis describes the process by which a cell ingests and disposes of foreign material, including microorganisms.[23] Because most phagocytes are circulating in the blood, they must leave the blood stream and migrate to the site of inflammation before initiating phagocytosis. Under normal conditions, the circulation in the capillaries and venules is rapidly moving with red blood cells in the main stream and neutrophils and other leukocytes tending to flow more slowly along the vessel's periphery. Many of the biochemical products produced early at inflammatory sites (e.g., histamine, TNF-α bradykinin, leukotrienes, prostaglandins) diffuse to the vessels and affect both leukocytes and endothelial cells.[24] Both cell populations respond by producing new **adhesion molecules** on their surfaces[25,26] (Table 6-4). (For information on selectins and integrins; see Chapter 1.) The reciprocal change in adhesion molecules on leukocytes, as well as platelets, promote their interaction with the endothelial cells. The initial change of surface molecules increases the adhesion, or stickiness, between leukocytes and endothelial cells, causing the leukocytes to adhere more avidly to the walls of the capillaries and venules in a process called **margination,** or **pavementing.** Adhesion molecules that are expressed later lead to **diapedesis,** or emigration of the cells through the endothelial junctions that have retracted in response to the same mediators (Figure 6-12). The leukocytes digest the basement membrane and migrate into the surrounding tissues.

Additionally, **endothelial cells** release nitric oxide (NO), a gas that has at least two inflammatory effects. First, NO causes vasodilation by inducing relaxation of vascular smooth muscle, a response that is local and short-lived. Secondly, NO also may suppress mast cell function and decrease platelet adhesion and aggregation.[27]

Once inside the connective tissue in the perivascular space, leukocytes are attracted to the inflammatory site by means of chemotaxis. They detect chemotactic factors in the

Table 6-4	Examples of Cellular Adhesion Molecules (CAMs) Involved in Leukocyte Interaction with Endothelial Cells		
	Activity of Leukocyte		
	"Rolling" Low Affinity	"Margination" Firm Attachment	"Diapedesis"
Leukocyte adhesion molecule	L-selectin	Integrin α4β1 (VLA-4) Integrin α4β7	Integrin αLβ2 (LFA-1) Integrin αMβ2 (MAC-1) PCAM-1
Endothelial adhesion molecule	P-selectin E-selectin	VCAM-1	ICAM-1 ICAM-2 PCAM-1

Selectins (lectin-like molecules): *L-selectin*, leukocyte selectin; *P-selectin*, platelet selectin; *E-selectin*, endothelial selectin.
Integrins (noncovalent heterodimers of alpha [α] and beta [β] subunits): *VLA-4*, very late antigen-4; *LFA-1*, lymphocyte function antigen-1; *MAC-1*, macrophage antigen-1.
Immunoglobulin-like molecules: *VCAM-1*, vascular cell adhesion molecule-1; *ICAM-1, ICAM-2*, immunoglobulin-like molecules-1 and 2; *PCAM-1*, platelet-endothelial cell adhesion molecule-1.

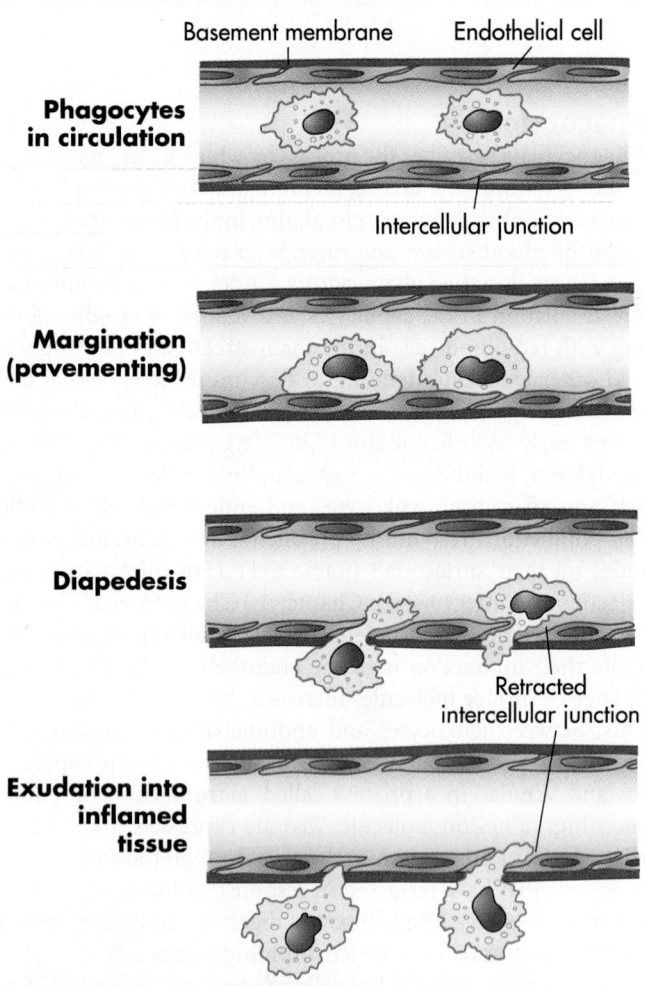

Figure 6-12 Diapedesis of a phagocyte. Phagocytes are capable of ameboid movement, which allows them to squeeze through intercellular junctions and migrate to inflammatory lesions.

environment through chemoreceptors at multiple locations on their plasma membranes and migrate in the direction of highest concentration (see Figure 6-10). The primary chemotactic factors include many bacterial products, complement fragments C3a and C5a, kallikrein, plasminogen activator, products of fibrin degradation, and chemokines. Eosinophils and neutrophils also respond to chemotactic factors released from mast cells. Monocytes are attracted toward a factor that has been released by neutrophils already at the site of injury. And although histamine is not itself chemotactic, it may facilitate the chemotactic effects of other factors.

Once the phagocytic cell enters the inflammatory site, the process of phagocytosis involves four steps: (1) *opsonization, recognition* of the target and *adherence* of the phagocyte to it, (2) *engulfment* (ingestion or endocytosis), (3) formation of *phagosome*, (4) *fusion* with lysosomal granules within the phagocyte, and (5) *destruction* of the target (Figure 6-13) (lysosomes are described in Chapter 1). Throughout the process, both the target and digestive enzymes are isolated within membrane-bound vesicles. Isolation protects the phagocyte itself from the harmful effects of the target microorganisms, as well as its own enzymes.

Most phagocytes can trap and engulf bacteria that have not been coated with an opsonin, but the process is slow and inefficient. Opsonization, usually by antibody or complement component C3b, greatly enhances both recognition and adherence. Phagocytosis of an opsonized (antibody and/or complement-protein coated) red blood cell is illustrated in Figure 6-14. Opsonins function as "glue" between the phagocyte and the target cell because receptors on the phagocyte are specific for sites on the opsonin (Fc receptors for antibody, C3b receptors for C3b). This enables the phagocyte to bind an opsonized target very tightly to its surface. Antibody forms a stronger attachment, but C3b facilitates phagocytosis to a greater extent.

Although the inflammatory response is considered to be nonspecific, opsonins and other recognition molecules add a degree of specificity to efficient phagocytosis. Antibodies on

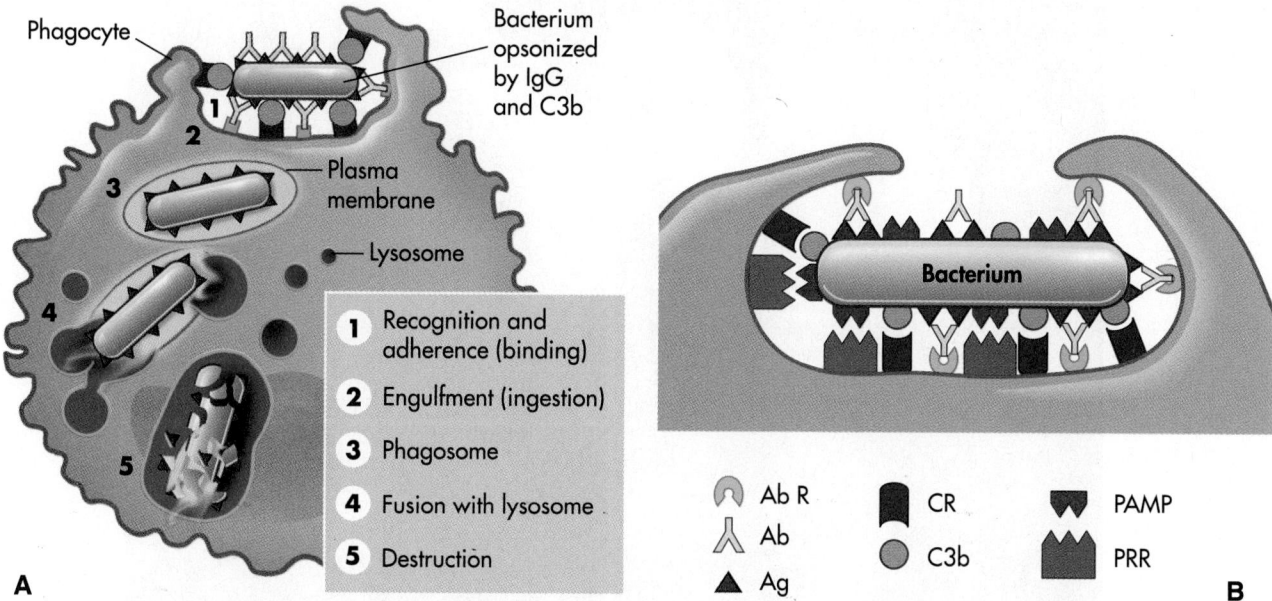

Figure 6-13 Phases of phagocytosis. **A,** Opsonized microorganisms bind to the surface of a phagocyte *(1)* and are ingested *(2)* into a phagocytic vacuole, or phagosome *(3)*. Lysosomes fuse with the phagosome *(4)*, releasing their digestive enzymes into the vacuole, resulting in the formation of a phagolysosome *(5)*, within which the microorganism is killed and digested. **B,** Enlargement showing an opsonized bacterium. *Ab R,* Antibody receptor; *Ab,* antibody; *CR,* complement receptor; *C3b,* complement component; *PAMP,* pathogen-associated molecular patterns; *PRR,* pattern recognition receptors.

the surface of bacteria are directed against antigens that are highly specific to that particular microorganism. If the complement fragment C3b serves as an opsonin, those bacteria with certain polysaccharide coatings are particularly sensitive to activation of the alternative and lectin pathways of complement activation.

Engulfment (endocytosis) is carried out by small pseudopods that extend from the plasma membrane and surround the adherent microorganism (see Figure 6-14) forming an intracellular phagocytic vacuole, or **phagosome.** The membrane that surrounds the phagosome consists of inverted plasma membrane. After the formation of the phagosome, lysosomes converge, fuse with the phagosome, and discharge their contents, creating a **phagolysosome.** Destruction of the bacterium takes place within the phagolysosome (see Figure 6-13) and is accomplished by both oxygen-dependent and oxygen-independent mechanisms.

Phagocytosis is accompanied by a burst of oxygen uptake by the phagocyte; this is termed the "respiratory burst" and results from a shift in much of the cell's glucose metabolism to the hexose-monophosphate shunt. The nicotinamide adenine dinucleotide phosphate (NADPH) that is produced because of this shift is used by a membrane-associated enzyme, NADPH oxidase, to generate superoxide, a reactive oxygen intermediate that is converted to hydrogen peroxide and other reactive oxygen species that can be highly damaging to cells. These steps comprise what is known as an *oxygen-dependent killing mechanism.* Many of the reactive oxygen species are directly toxic to the microorganism. Hy-

drogen peroxide also can collaborate with the lysosomal enzyme *myeloperoxidase* and halide anions (Cl^-, and Br^-) to form acids, such as hypochlorous (HClO) and hypobromous (HBrO) acids. These acids probably kill bacteria and fungi by adding Cl^- or Br^- to the surface of these cells.[28] *Oxygen-independent mechanisms* of microbial killing are likely the result of (1) the acidic pH (3.5 to 4.0) of the phagolysosome caused by lactic acid production; (2) cationic proteins, such as defensins and cathelicidins, that bind to and damage target cell membranes; (3) enzymatic attack of the mucopeptides in the target cell wall by lysozyme and elastase; and (4) inhibition of bacterial growth by lactoferrin binding of iron.

When a phagocyte dies at an inflammatory site, it frequently lyses (breaks open) and releases its cytoplasmic contents, including the lysosomal enzymes, into the tissue. Enzymes released from lysosomes can digest the connective tissue matrix, causing much of the tissue destruction associated with inflammation. The destructive effects of many enzymes released by dying phagocytes are minimized by natural inhibitors found in the blood, such as **α₁-antitrypsin,** a plasma protein produced by the liver. An inherited deficiency of α₁-antitrypsin often results in chronic lung damage and emphysema as a result of inflammation. (The pulmonary effects of α₁-antitrypsin deficiency are described in Chapter 33.) Released lysosomal products also may contribute to inflammation by increasing vascular permeability, attracting additional monocytes, and activating the complement and kinin systems.

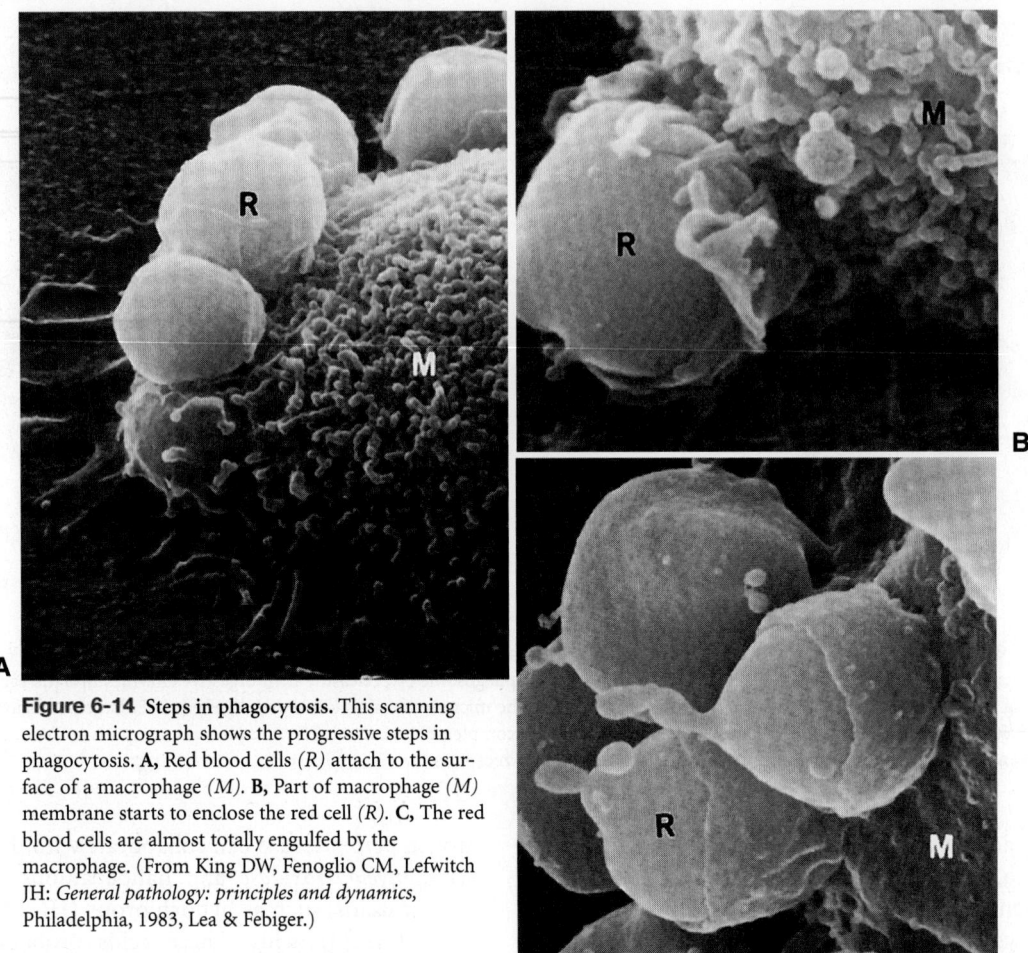

Figure 6-14 Steps in phagocytosis. This scanning electron micrograph shows the progressive steps in phagocytosis. **A,** Red blood cells *(R)* attach to the surface of a macrophage *(M).* **B,** Part of macrophage *(M)* membrane starts to enclose the red cell *(R).* **C,** The red blood cells are almost totally engulfed by the macrophage. (From King DW, Fenoglio CM, Lefwitch JH: *General pathology: principles and dynamics,* Philadelphia, 1983, Lea & Febiger.)

Neutrophils

The **neutrophil,** or **polymorphonuclear neutrophil (PMN),** is a member of the granulocytic series and is named for the characteristic staining pattern of its granules as well as its multilobed nucleus. Neutrophils are the predominant **phagocytes** in the early inflammatory site, arriving within 6 to 12 hours after the initial injury, where they ingest (phagocytose) bacteria, dead cells, and cellular debris. Several inflammatory mediators (e.g., some bacterial proteins, complement fragments C3a and C5a, and mast cell neutrophil chemotactic factor) specifically attract neutrophils from the circulation and activate them. Macrophages and lymphocytes, on the other hand, enter the site later, usually after 24 hours, and gradually replace the neutrophils.

Because the neutrophil is a mature cell incapable of division and sensitive to the acidic environment of inflammatory lesions, it is short lived at the inflammatory site and becomes a component of the purulent exudate, or *pus,* which is removed from the body through the epithelium or via the lymphatic system. (The lymphatic system is described in Chapter 29.) The primary roles of the neutrophil are removal of debris in sterile lesions, such as burns, and phagocytosis of bacteria in nonsterile lesions.

Monocytes and Macrophages

The next phagocytes on the scene are monocytes and macrophages, which perform many of the same functions as neutrophils but for a longer time and in a later stage of the inflammatory response. **Monocytes** are the largest normal blood cells (14 to 20 μm in diameter) and have a nucleus that is often indented or horseshoe shaped. Monocytes are produced in the bone marrow, enter the circulation, and migrate to the inflammatory site, where they develop into macrophages. Monocytes also appear to be the precursors of macrophages that are fixed in tissues (tissue macrophages, discussed in Chapter 7), including Kupffer cells in the liver, alveolar macrophages in the lungs, and microglia in the brain.

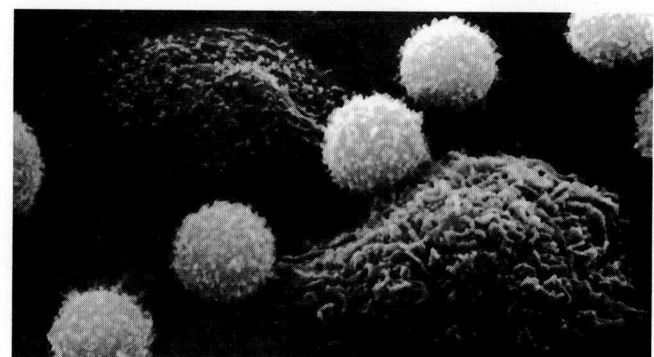

Figure 6-15 Scanning electron micrograph of lymphocytes and macrophages. The lymphocytes are small and spherical; the macrophages are larger and more irregular in shape. (From Raven PH, Johnson GB: *Biology*, St Louis, 1992, Mosby.)

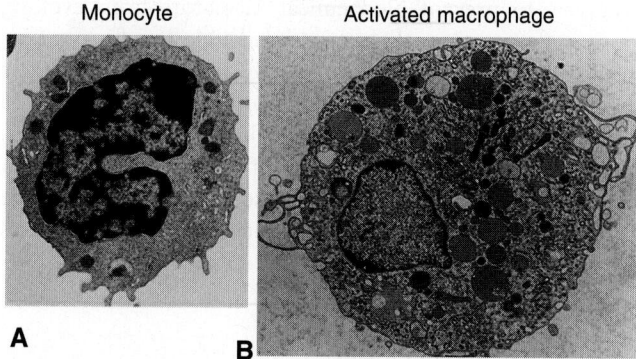

Figure 6-16 Macrophage activation. **A,** Electron micrograph of a peripheral blood monocyte. **B,** Electron micrograph of an activated tissue macrophage showing numerous phagocytic vacuoles and cytoplasmic organelles. (**A,** from Abbas AK, Lichtman AH: *Cellular and molecular immunology*, ed 5, Philadelphia, 2003, Saunders; **B,** From Bloom W, Fawcett DW: *A textbook of histology*, ed 11, Philadelphia, 1986; Saunders.)

Macrophages are generally larger (20 to 40 μm) and are more active as phagocytes than their monocytic precursors. Macrophages, particularly those residing in the tissues, are often important cellular initiators of the inflammatory response (Figures 6-15 and 6-16).

Monocyte-derived macrophages from the circulation may appear at the inflammatory site as soon as 24 hours after the initial neutrophil infiltration, but usually arrive 3 to 7 days later. They migrate to the site more slowly than neutrophils because they move more sluggishly and also because many of the chemotactic factors that attract them, such as macrophage chemotactic factor, must first be released by neutrophils. Macrophages are better suited than neutrophils to long-term defense against infectious agents because macrophages can survive and divide in the acidic inflammatory site.

Neutrophils and monocytes/macrophages differ chiefly in the following ways:

1. *Speed:* Neutrophils arrive at the injury site first
2. *Active life span:* Macrophages survive and divide in the inflammatory site, whereas neutrophils cannot.
3. *Chemotactic factors:* Neutrophils and macrophages are not attracted by the same factors
4. *Enzymatic content of their lysosomes, or digestive vacuoles*
5. *Role in the immune response:* Macrophages, but not neutrophils, are involved in activation of the adaptive immune system

Macrophage Activation

Several bacteria are resistant to killing by granulocytes and can even survive inside macrophages. Microorganisms such as *Mycobacterium tuberculosis, Mycobacterium leprae, Salmonella typhi, Brucella abortus,* and *Listeria monocytogenes* can remain dormant or even multiply inside the phagolysosomes of macrophages. However, the bactericidal activity of macrophages can be markedly increased with the help of inflammatory **cytokines** produced by cells of the acquired immune system (subsets of T lymphocytes) or cells activated through Toll-like receptors. (Cytokines are discussed in detail later in this chapter.) Macrophages have cell surface receptors for these cytokines and are further activated to become more effective killers of infectious microorganisms.

Macrophage activation results in increased (1) phagocytic activity, (2) size, (3) plasma membrane area, (4) glucose metabolism, and (5) number of lysosomes.[29] Activated macrophages also secrete factors that stimulate the growth, differentiation, and activation of additional inflammatory cells, as well as control the initiation of healing processes. These include granulocyte-colony stimulating factor (G-CSF), gamma interferon (IFN-γ), interleukin-1 (IL-1β), angiogenic factor, fibroblast activating factor, and growth factors that promote regrowth of damaged tissues. In some cases, inadequate macrophage activation results from defects in acquired immune responses and deficits in the production of appropriate cytokines. For example, a form of leprosy called *lepromatous leprosy* is characterized by the survival of phagocytosed *M. leprae* bacteria in macrophage phagolysosomes. In individuals with lepromatous leprosy, cells of the acquired immune system have failed to secrete the cytokines necessary to transform macrophages into highly efficient killing cells.

Eosinophils

Although **eosinophils** are only mildly phagocytic, they have two specific functions: (1) they serve as the body's primary defense against parasites and (2) they help regulate vascular mediators released from mast cells. Their role in resistance to parasites occurs in collaboration with specific antibodies produced by the acquired immune system and will be discussed in Chapter 7.

The second function, regulation of mast cell-derived inflammatory mediators, is a critical function of eosinophils. As with most defense systems of the body, the acute inflammatory response is usually needed only in a circumscribed area and for a limited time. Therefore, control mechanisms are necessary to prevent biochemical mediators from evoking more inflammation than is needed. Mast cells produce eosinophil chemotactic factor-A (ECF-A), which attracts eosinophils to the site of inflammation. Eosinophil lysosomes contain several enzymes that degrade vasoactive molecules, thereby controlling the vascular effects of inflammation. These enzymes include histaminase, which mediates the degradation of histamine, and arylsulfatase B, which mediates the degradation of some of the lipid-derived mediators produced by mast cells.

Natural Killer (NK) Cells

The main function of **natural killer (NK) cells** is recognition and elimination of cells infected with viruses, although they are also somewhat effective at elimination of other abnormal host cells, specifically cancer cells. NK cells seem to be more efficient in this role when they encounter an infected cell within the circulatory system as opposed to within tissues.[30] Along with Toll-like receptors (TLR), NK cells have additional inhibitory and activating receptors that allow differentiation between infected or tumor cells and normal cells. If the NK cell binds to a target cell through activating receptors, it produces several cytokines and toxic molecules that can kill the target. (Mechanisms of cell to cell killing by NK cells and T cells will be discussed further in Chapter 7.)

Platelets

Platelets are cellular fragments formed from megakaryocytes. They circulate in the bloodstream until vascular injury occurs. After injury, platelets can be activated by many products of both the innate and adaptive immune responses, including collagen, thrombin, thromboxane, platelet-activating factor (PAF), and antigen-antibody complexes. Activation results in (1) their interaction with components of the coagulation cascade to stop bleeding and (2) degranulation. Platelets contain several types of granules; alpha (α)-granules, dense granules, and lysosomal granules. Alpha-granules generally contain polypeptides that affect inflammation, including coagulation proteins (e.g., fibrinogen, factor V), soluble adhesion molecules (e.g., von Willebrand factor, vitronectin), growth factors (e.g., platelet-derived growth factor, epidermal growth factor), protease inhibitors (e.g., plasminogen activator inhibitor-1, α2-antiplasmin), and membrane adhesion molecules (e.g., P-selectin, αIIbβ3). Dense granules contain several small molecules, including adenosine diphosphate (ADP), serotonin, calcium, and magnesium. Serotonin is a vasoactive amine with vascular effects similar to those of histamine. (Platelet function is described in detail in Chapter 25.)

Cellular Products

To elicit an effective inflammatory (or acquired immune) response, it is necessary that many different kinds of cells cooperate. Many host cells secrete soluble factors that contribute to the regulation of innate or acquired resistance by affecting other neighboring host cells (Figure 6-17). These factors are referred to as *chemokines* or *cytokines* and are either *pro-inflammatory* or *anti-inflammatory* in nature, depending on whether they tend to induce or inhibit the inflammatory response. These molecules usually diffuse over short distances, bind to the appropriate target cells, and affect the function of the target cell. Some effects occur over long distances, such as the systemic induction of fever by some cytokines (i.e., endogenous pyrogens) that are produced at an inflammatory site. The binding of chemokines or cytokines to a target cell often induces synthesis of additional cellular products. For example, binding of the cytokine tumor necrosis factor–alpha (TNF-α) to a cell may result in synthesis and release of IL-1. Chemokine and cytokine binding is mediated through specific cell-surface receptors that are themselves sometimes under the regulation of secreted cellular products.

The actions of chemokines and cytokines are *pleiotropic*, indicating that the same molecule may have a large variety of different biologic activities depending on the particular target cell to which it binds. In addition, the same molecule may be produced by a large spectrum of cells, many of which are not part of inflammation or the immune system. These molecules may be *synergistic*, so that their combined activity exceeds the sum of their individual activities, or have *antagonistic* properties, which causes them to inhibit each other. A partial list of relevant cytokines is provided in Chapter 7 (Table 7-7).

Cytokines

The majority of important cytokines are classified as interleukins (ILs) or interferons (IFNs). Other critical cytokines, however, are not classified as either. Many of these same cytokines are produced by cells of the acquired immune system in response to specific antigens and will be discussed further in Chapter 7.

Interleukins

The **interleukins (IL)** are biochemical messengers produced predominantly by macrophages and lymphocytes in response to their recognition of a pathogen or stimulation by other products of inflammation. One important function of this class of cytokines is enhancement of the acquired immune response against pathogens and other foreign substances. Interleukins, however, are both produced by and have effects on a large variety of cells, often independent of infection.

IL-1 is a pro-inflammatory cytokine produced mainly by macrophages that have been stimulated by substances associated with infection, including many of the PAMPs discussed earlier in this chapter, as well as by other cytokines. IL-1 is synthesized in two forms, α and β that often elicit the same biologic responses. IL-1 is an endogenous pyrogen (i.e., fever-causing cytokine), which reacts with receptors on cells of the hypothalamus and affects the body's thermostat. It also activates phagocytes and lymphocytes, thereby enhancing both the innate and acquired immunity, and acts as a growth factor for many cells. It has several effects on neutrophils, including induction of proliferation (resulting in an increase in the number of circulating neutrophils), chemotaxis, increased cellular respiration, and increased lysosomal enzyme activity.

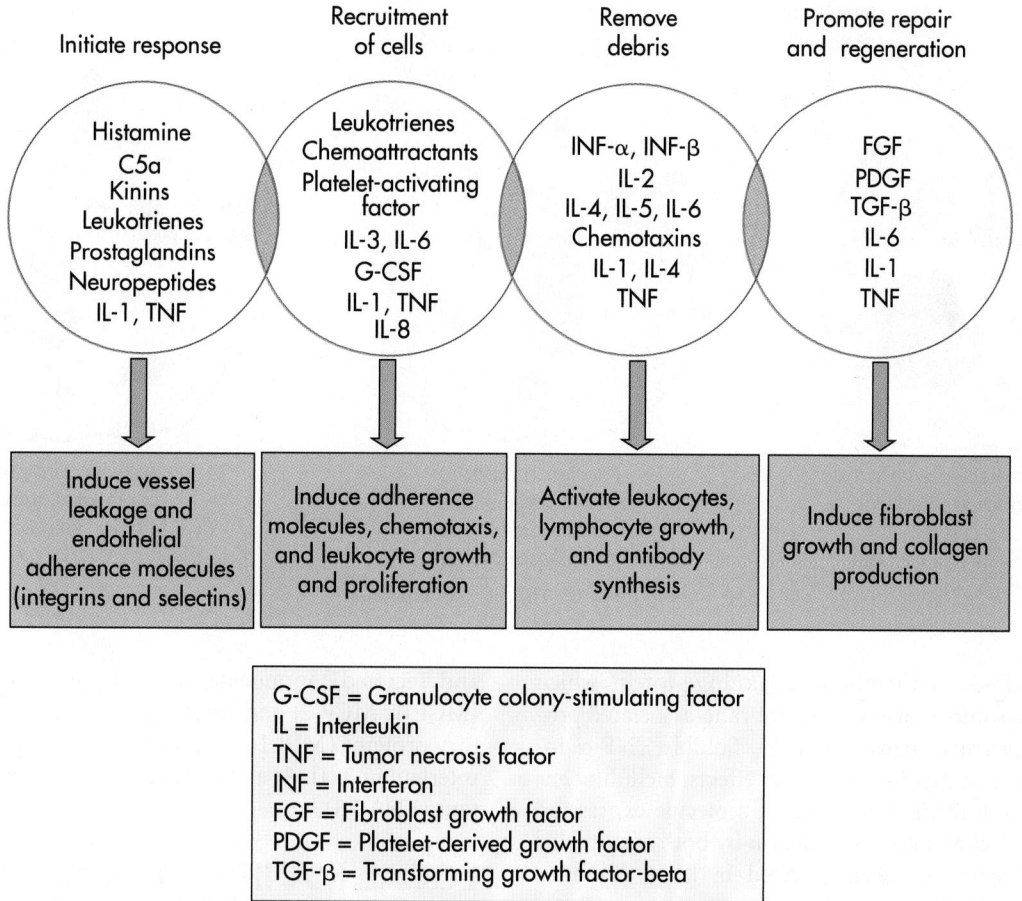

Figure 6-17 Cytokines associated with stages of inflammation. The stages of inflammation overlap and can be concurrent.

IL-10 is an example of an anti-inflammatory cytokine and is primarily produced by lymphocytes to down-regulate both the inflammatory and acquired immune responses. IL-10 suppresses growth of lymphocyte and production of pro-inflammatory cytokines by macrophages.

At least 30 human interleukins have been identified, although the function of several have not yet been defined. Their varied effects include the following:

1. Alteration of adhesion molecule expression on many types of cells
2. Induction of leukocyte chemotaxis
3. Induction of proliferation and maturation of leukocytes in the bone marrow
4. General enhancement or suppression of inflammation (see Table 7-7)

Interferons

Interferons (INFs) are low-molecular-weight proteins that protect against viral infections.[31] (Mechanisms of viral infection are described in Chapter 2.) INFs are produced and released by virally infected host cells in response to viral double-stranded RNA. Different kinds of INFs are produced by different types of cells; macrophages are the primary producers of both IFN-α and IFN-β, whereas T lymphocytes release IFN-γ. These INFs do not kill viruses directly but instead prevent them from infecting additional healthy cells.

Interferons also enhance the efficiency of developing an acquired immune response.

IFN-α and IFN-β induce production of antiviral proteins, thereby conferring protection on uninfected cells. IFN-α or IFN-β is released from virally infected cells, attaches to a receptor on a neighboring host cell, and if the neighboring cell is uninfected, stimulates the production of antiviral proteins that will interfere with transcription of viral nucleic acids or with viral replication (Figure 6-18). These interferons have no effect on cells that have already been virally infected. IFN-γ enhances the inflammatory response by increasing the microbiocidal activity of macrophages. This cytokine also facilitates development of the acquired immune response against viral antigens on infected cells. Interferons are host specific, meaning that human interferon is effective only in humans; however, these cytokines are not virus specific, meaning that they are effective against almost all viruses.

Other Cytokines

Despite the numerous interleukins and interferons, other essential cytokines are needed to mount an efficient inflammatory response. One of the most important of these is **tumor necrosis factor–alpha (TNF-α)**. Macrophages secrete TNF-α in response to recognition of PAMPs by Toll-like receptors. Other cells, such as mast cells, are additional and crucial sources of this pro-inflammatory cytokine.[32] TNF-α is

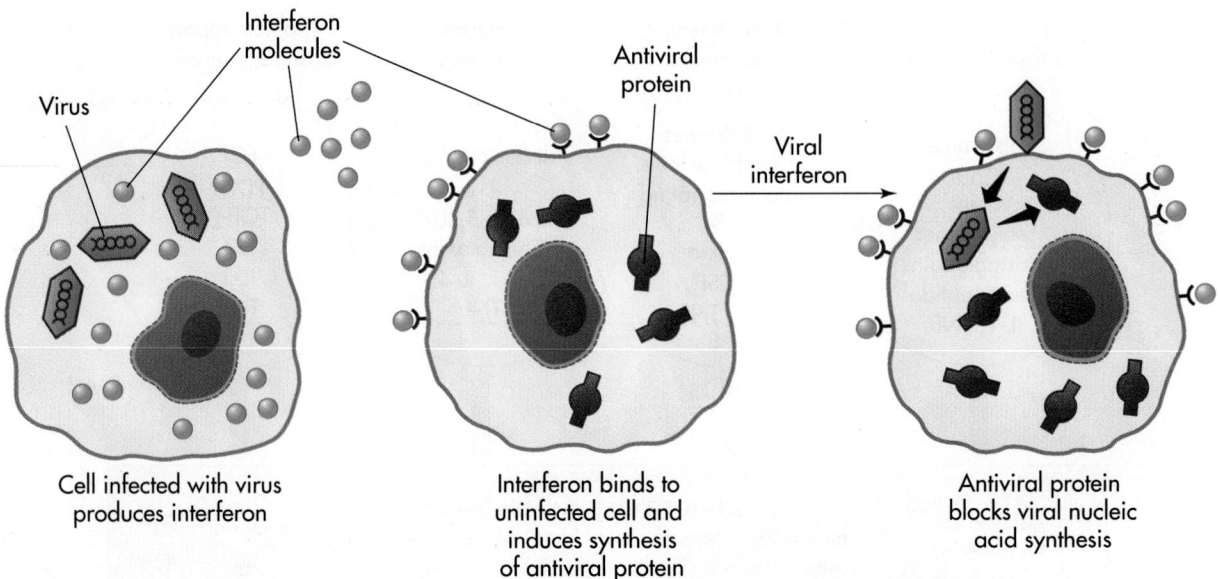

Figure 6-18 The action of interferon.

initially synthesized as a membrane-spanning protein, which is cleaved into a soluble form by a membrane-associated protease, TNF-converting enzyme (TACE). Soluble TNF-α induces a multitude of pro-inflammatory effects, including enhancement of endothelial cell adhesion molecule expression and induction of chemokine production by both endothelial cells and macrophages. When secreted in large amounts, TNF-α has systemic effects as well:

1. Induces fever by acting as an endogenous pyrogen
2. Causes increased synthesis of inflammatory serum proteins by the liver
3. Causes muscle wasting (cachexia) and intravascular thrombosis as a consequence of prolonged exposure in cases of severe infection

Chemokines

Chemokines are a family of low-molecular-weight (8 to 10 kDa) peptides that function primarily to induce leukocyte chemotaxis. This response can be elicited either by soluble chemokines or by chemokines that are bound to extracellular glycosaminoglycan carbohydrates. Chemokines can be synthesized by multiple cell types, including macrophages, fibroblasts, and endothelial cells, in response to pro-inflammatory cytokines. Macrophages can be stimulated to produce chemokines by recognition of either infectious microorganisms or a β-defensin (both through TLR-4). To date, more than 40 different human chemokines have been described, the vast majority of which are classified as either CC-chemokines or CXC-chemokines, depending on the arrangement of cysteine amino acids in the protein.[33] This amino acid arrangement also determines which target cell(s) will respond to a given chemokine. CC-chemokines affect mainly monocytes, lymphocytes, and eosinophils, whereas CXC-chemokines generally affect neutrophils. Examples of CXC-chemokines include RANTES (regulated on activation, normal T expressed

and secreted), monocyte/macrophage chemotactic proteins (MCP-1, MCP-2, and MCP-3), and macrophage inflammatory proteins (MIP-1α and MIP-1β). CC-chemokines include interleukin 8 (IL-8) and epithelial-dermoid neutrophil attractant (ENA-78).

LOCAL MANIFESTATIONS OF INFLAMMATION

The cells and plasma protein systems described above interact to produce all the characteristics of inflammation, whether local or systemic, as well as determine the duration of inflammation, either acute or chronic. Local inflammation accompanies all types of cellular and tissue injury, whether infected or sterile, from fractures or strains of the musculoskeletal system to burn injuries (see Chapter 2) and is responsible for initiating healing.

All the *local* manifestations of acute inflammation (i.e., swelling, pain, heat, and redness) result from vascular changes and the subsequent leakage of circulating components into the tissue. **Heat** and **redness** are the result of vasodilation and increased blood flow through the injured site. **Swelling** occurs as exudate (fluid and cells) accumulates. Swelling is usually accompanied by **pain** caused by pressure exerted by exudate accumulation, as well as the presence of soluble biochemical mediators such as prostaglandins and bradykinin.

Exudate varies in composition, depending on the stage of the inflammatory response and, to some extent, the injurious stimulus. In early or mild inflammation, the exudate is watery (**serous**) with very few plasma proteins or leukocytes. An example of serous exudate is the fluid in a blister. In more severe or advanced inflammation, the exudate may be thick and clotted (**fibrinous exudate**), such as in the lungs of individuals with pneumonia. If a large number of leukocytes accumulate, as in persistent bacterial infections, the exudate consists of pus and is called a **purulent (suppurative) exudate.** Purulent exudate is characteristic of walled-off lesions (**cysts or abscesses**). If bleeding occurs, the exudate is filled with erythrocytes and is described as a **hemorrhagic exudate.**

Although the local manifestations of inflammation can affect all vascularized tissues, lesions vary depending on the organ or tissue involved. The lesion resulting from widespread cellular death (necrosis), for example, differs in myocardial (heart muscle), brain, and hepatic (liver) tissues. Cellular death resulting from myocardial infarction (deprivation of oxygen caused by cessation of blood flow) causes a response that proceeds to replacement of the dead tissue with a fibrinous scar. The same injury to brain tissue is more likely to result in the formation of an abscess filled with necrotic tissue (types of necrosis are described in Chapter 2). Destruction of liver tissue stimulates the regrowth, or regeneration, of liver cells.

SYSTEMIC MANIFESTATIONS OF ACUTE INFLAMMATION

The three primary *systemic* changes associated with the acute inflammatory response are fever, leukocytosis (a transient increase in circulating leukocytes), and increased levels in circulating plasma proteins.[34]

Fever

An early systemic response is **fever,** which is partially induced by specific cytokines, for example, IL-1 released from neutrophils and macrophages. These fever-causing cytokines are known as **endogenous pyrogens** to differentiate them from pathogen-produced *exogenous pyrogens.* Pyrogens act directly on the hypothalamus, the portion of the brain that controls the body's thermostat. The release of endogenous pyrogens by inflammatory cells occurs after phagocytosis, after exposure to bacterial endotoxin, or after exposure to antigen-antibody complexes. (Mechanisms of temperature regulation are discussed in Chapter 14.)

The generation of a febrile response can be beneficial because the microorganisms that cause some conditions (e.g., syphilis, gonococcal urethritis) are highly sensitive to small increases in body temperature. On the other hand, fever may have some harmful side effects because it may enhance the host's susceptibility to the effects of endotoxins associated with gram-negative bacterial infections (bacterial toxins are described in Chapter 2).

Leukocytosis

Another systemic change associated with acute inflammation is **leukocytosis.** During many infections, numbers of circulating leukocytes, primarily neutrophils, increase. This increase is usually accompanied by a 'left shift' in the ratio of immature to mature neutrophils, so that the more immature forms of neutrophils, such as band cells, metamyelocytes, and occasionally myelocytes, are present in relatively greater than normal proportions. (Chapter 25 discusses the development and maturation of blood cells.) Production of immature leukocytes increases primarily because proliferation and release of granulocyte and monocyte precursors in the bone marrow is stimulated by several products of inflammation, including complement product C3a and G-CSF.

Plasma Protein Synthesis

The synthesis of many plasma proteins, most of which are products of the liver, is increased during the primary stages of inflammation. These proteins, which can be either pro- or antiinflammatory in nature, are referred to as **acute-phase reactants**[35,36] (Table 6-5). Acute-phase reactants reach maximal circulating levels within 10 to 40 hours of initial infection. In addition to inducing fever, IL-1 also indirectly induces the synthesis of acute-phase reactants. IL-1 up-regulates release of IL-6, which then increases synthesis of acute-phase reactants directly by stimulating liver cells. Administration of IL-1 into animals leads to both fever and elevation of most acute-phase reactants, including fibrinogen, C-reactive protein, haptoglobin, amyloid A, α_1-antitrypsin, and ceruloplasmin.[36]

Table 6-5	Circulating Levels of Acute-Phase Reactants During Inflammation		
Function	**Increased**		**Decreased**
Coagulation components	Fibrinogen		None
	Prothrombin		
	Factor VIII		
	Plasminogen		
Protease inhibitors	α_1-Antitrypsin		Inter-α-antitrypsin
	α_1-Antichymotrypsin		
Transport proteins	Haptoglobin		Transferrin
	Hemopexin		
	Ceruloplasmin		
	Ferritin		
Complement components	C1s, C2, C3, C4, C5, C9, factor B, C1 inhibitor		Properdin
Miscellaneous proteins	α_1-Acid glycoprotein		Albumin
	Fibronectin		Prealbumin
	Serum amyloid A (SAA)		α_1-Lipoprotein
	C-reactive protein (CRP)		β-Lipoprotein

Acute inflammation can be verified by a series of hematologic tests, which are described in detail in Chapter 25. For example, an increase in blood levels of acute-phase reactants, primarily fibrinogen, is usually associated with an increased erythrocyte sedimentation rate. The alteration in plasma proteins probably leads to an enhanced erythrocyte rouleaux formation (stacking of erythrocytes, as in a stack of coins) and thereby an increased rate of sedimentation. Although increased erythrocyte sedimentation is a nonspecific reaction, it is considered a good indicator of an acute inflammatory response. The symptoms of acute inflammation also include somnolence, malaise, anorexia, and muscle aching.

CHRONIC INFLAMMATION

Superficially, the difference between acute and chronic inflammation is purely one of duration, in that chronic inflammation lasts 2 weeks or longer, regardless of cause. Characteristic histologic and mechanistic differences also may be present (Figure 6-19). Chronic inflammation is sometimes preceded by an unsuccessful acute inflammatory response. For example, if bacterial contamination or foreign objects (e.g., dirt, wood splinter, glass) persist in a traumatic wound, an acute response may be prolonged beyond 2 weeks. Pus formation, suppuration (purulent discharge), and incomplete wound healing may characterize this type of chronic inflammation.

Chronic inflammation can occur also as a distinct process without much previous acute inflammation. Some microorganisms (e.g., mycobacteria that cause tuberculosis) have cell walls with a very high lipid and wax content, making them relatively insensitive to degradation by phagocytes and therefore relatively resistant to clearance in an acute inflammatory response. Other microorganisms, such as those that cause leprosy, syphilis, and brucellosis, can survive within the macrophage and thereby also avoid clearance by the acute inflammatory response. In addition, some microorganisms produce toxins that stimulate tissue-damaging reactions even after they themselves are killed. Persistent inflammation can result from prolonged irritation by these toxins. Finally, chemicals, particulate matter, or physical irritants (e.g., inhaled dusts, wood splinters, and suture material) also can cause an inflammatory response that lasts longer than 2 weeks in duration.

Chronic inflammation is characterized by a dense infiltration of lymphocytes and macrophages. If macrophages are unable to protect the host from tissue damage, the body attempts to wall off and isolate the infected area, thus forming a **granuloma** (Figure 6-20). Granulomas may form if neutrophils and macrophages are unable to destroy microorganisms during the acute inflammatory response.[37] For example, infections caused by some bacteria (*Listeria* sp., *Brucella* sp.), fungi (histoplasmosis, coccidioidomycosis) and parasites (leishmaniasis, schistosomiasis, toxoplasmosis) can result in

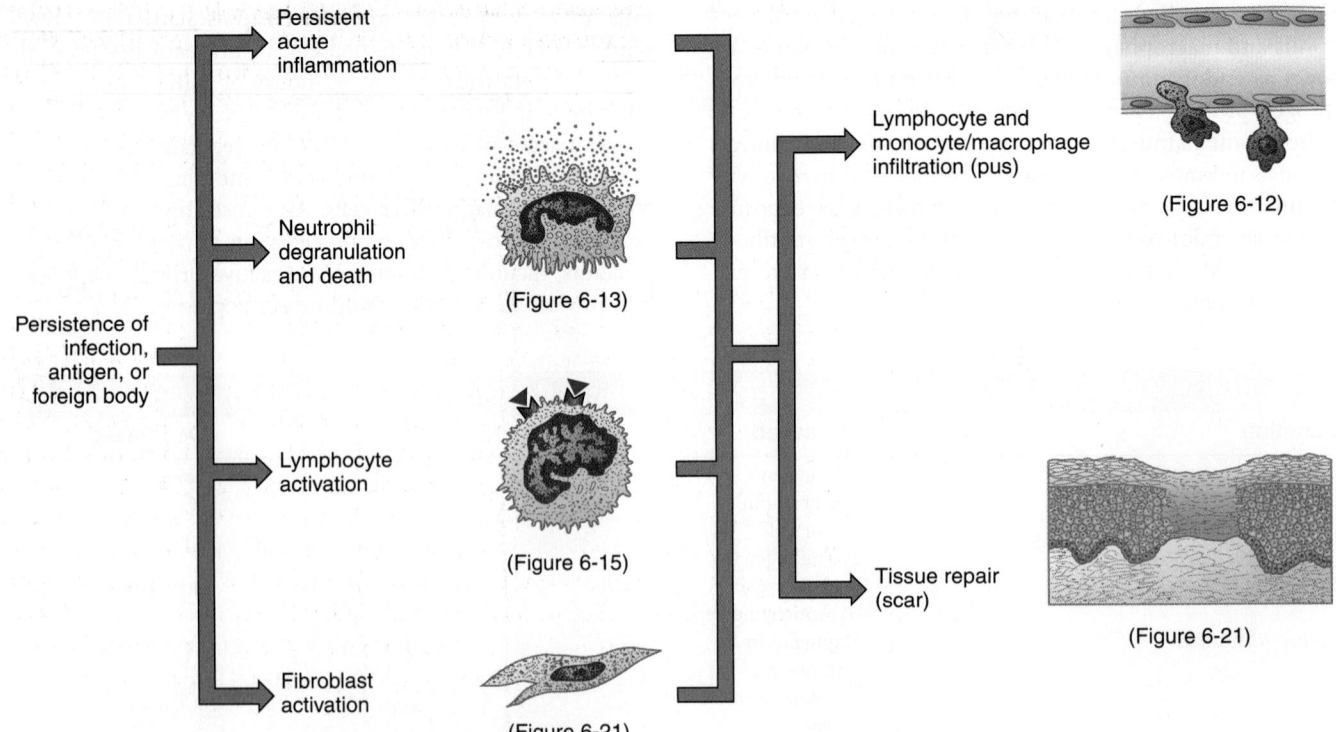

Figure 6-19 The chronic inflammatory response. Inflammation usually becomes chronic because of the persistence of an infection, an antibody, or a foreign body in the wound. Chronic inflammation is characterized by the persistence of many of the processes of acute inflammation. In addition, large amounts of neutrophil degranulation and death, the activation of lymphocytes, and the concurrent activation of fibroblasts result in the release of mediators that induce the infiltration of more lymphocytes and monocytes/macrophages and the beginning of wound healing and tissue repair. The figure numbers refer to those in which more detailed information may be found on that portion of the response.

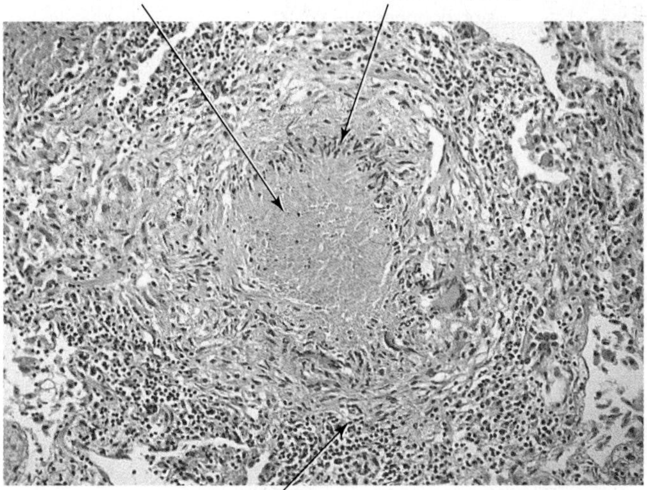

Caseous necrosis　　Activated macrophages

Lymphocytes

Figure 6-20 **Tuberculous granuloma.** A central area of amorphous caseous necrosis is surrounded by a zone of activated macrophages, in which multinucleate macrophages (Langerhans giant cells) are present. There are outer layers of lymphocytes and fibroblasts. (From Stevens A, Lowe J: *Pathology*, ed 2, London, 2000, Mosby.)

granuloma formation. Large antigen-antibody complexes such as those present in rheumatoid arthritis also can result in the formation of these structures. The process of granuloma formation begins when some of the macrophages differentiate into large **epithelioid cells,** cells that are incapable of phagocytosing large bacteria but are capable of taking up debris and other small particles. Other macrophages fuse into multinucleated **giant cells,** which are active phagocytes that can engulf very large particles—larger than can be engulfed by a single macrophage. These two types of differentiated macrophages form the center of the granuloma, which is surrounded by a wall of lymphocytes. The granuloma itself is also often encapsulated by fibrous deposits of collagen and may become cartilaginous or possibly calcified by deposits of calcium carbonate and calcium phosphate.

The classic granuloma associated with tuberculosis is characterized by a wall of epithelioid cells surrounding a center of dead and decaying tissue (caseous necrosis; see Chapter 2) and mycobacteria. Decay of cells within the granuloma results in the release of acids and the enzymatic contents of lysosomes from dead phagocytes. In this inhospitable environment, the cellular debris is broken down into its basic constituents and a clear fluid remains (liquefaction necrosis; see Chapter 2). Eventually, this fluid diffuses out and leaves a hollow, thick-walled structure in the tissue that may remain for the life of the individual.

RESOLUTION AND REPAIR

Destruction of tissue is followed by a period of healing that begins during acute inflammation and may not be complete for as long as 2 years. The most favorable outcome of healing is complete return to normal structure and function. This is an ideal that is often not possible, particularly in adults. However, if damage is minor, no complications occur, and destroyed tissues are capable of **regeneration,** it is possible to return injured tissues to an approximation of their original structure and physiologic function. This restoration is called **resolution.** On the other hand, if extensive damage is present, if injury occurs in tissues not capable of regeneration, if infection results in abscess or granuloma formation, or if fibrin persists in the lesion, resolution is not possible and repair takes place instead. **Repair** is the replacement of destroyed tissue with scar tissue. **Scar tissue** is composed primarily of collagen that fills in the lesion and restores tensile strength but cannot carry out the physiologic functions of destroyed tissue.

Both regeneration and repair actually begin with phagocytosis of the particulate matter found at the site of injury (fibrin from dissolved clots, microorganisms, erythrocytes, and dead tissue cells). This cleanup of the lesion, which also involves dissolution of fibrin clots (or scabs) by fibrinolytic enzymes, is called **débridement.** After débridement, the remaining debris is drained away and the vascular dilation and permeability associated with inflammation are reversed, thus preparing the lesion for either regeneration or repair.

Healing always involves processes that (1) fill in, (2) seal, and (3) shrink the wound. These common denominators of healing vary in importance and duration among different types of wounds. A clean incision, such as a paper cut or a sutured surgical wound, heals primarily through the process of collagen synthesis. Because sealing of this type of wound has already been facilitated by minimal tissue loss and close apposition of the wound edges, very little sealing (**epithelialization**) and shrinkage (**contraction**) are required for healing. Wounds that heal under conditions of minimal tissue loss are said to heal by **primary intention** (Figure 6-21).

Other wounds do not heal so neatly and easily. Healing of an open wound, such as a stage IV pressure sore (decubitus ulcer), requires a great deal more tissue replacement than healing of a surgical incision. With an open wound, epithelialization, scar formation, and contraction take longer and healing occurs through **secondary intention** (see Figure 6-21). Healing by either primary or secondary intention may occur at different rates for different types of tissue injury.

Both resolution and repair occur in two overlapping phases. The first phase, called the **reconstructive phase,** begins 3 to 4 days after the initial injury and continues for as long as 2 weeks. During this phase the lesion is characterized by fibroblast (connective tissue cell) proliferation, followed by collagen synthesis by the fibroblasts, epithelialization, contraction of the wound, and cellular differentiation. The second phase, the **maturation phase,** begins several weeks after injury and is normally complete within 2 years. During this phase, there is continuation of cellular differentiation, scar formation, and scar remodeling.

Reconstructive Phase

Because surgical wounds exhibit both the reconstructive and maturation phases, they are useful models of both normal and abnormal (dysfunctional) healing. Such wounds are

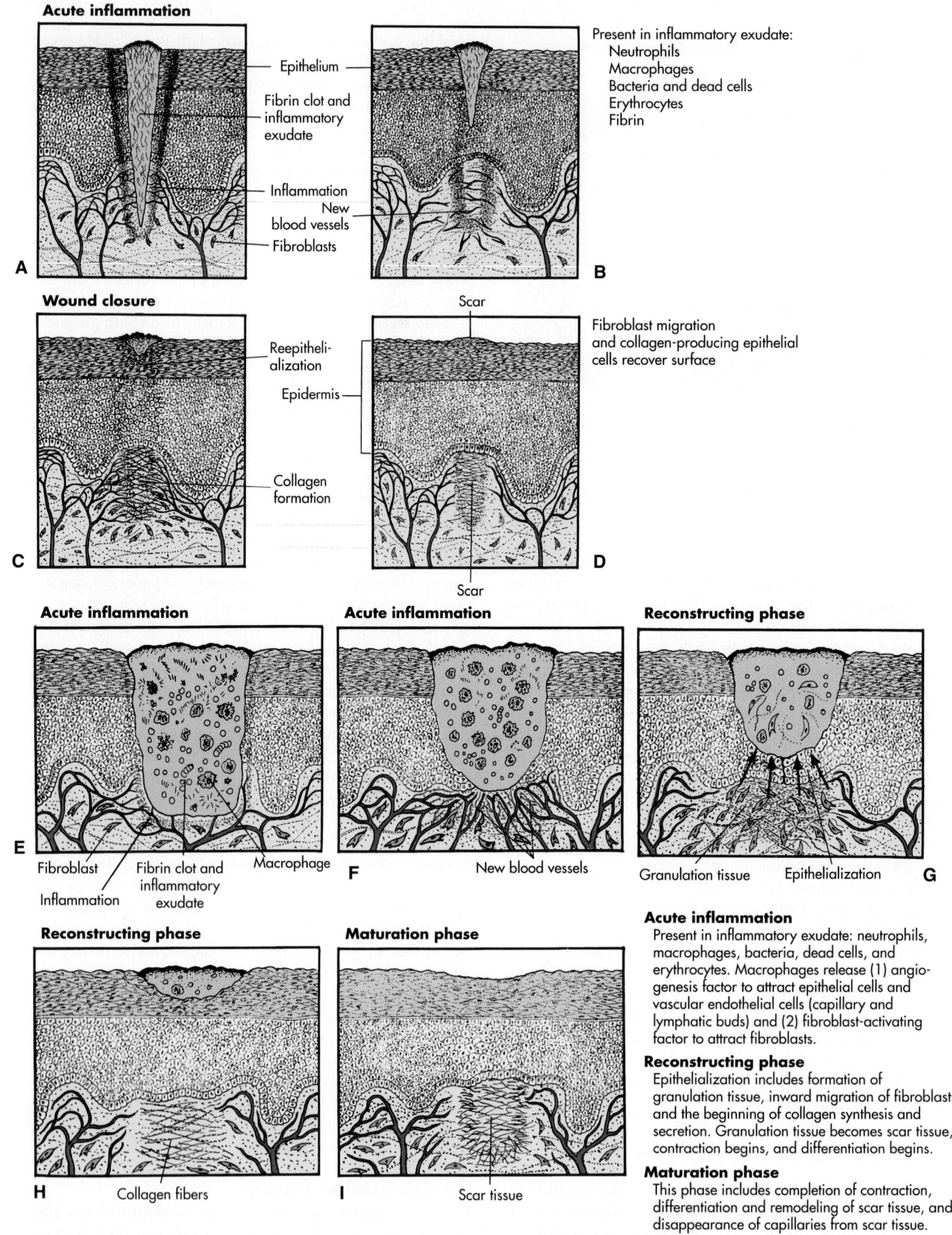

Acute inflammation

Epithelium

Fibrin clot and inflammatory exudate

Inflammation
New blood vessels
Fibroblasts

A

B

Present in inflammatory exudate:
Neutrophils
Macrophages
Bacteria and dead cells
Erythrocytes
Fibrin

Wound closure

Scar

Reepithelialization

Epidermis

Collagen formation

C

Scar

D

Fibroblast migration and collagen-producing epithelial cells recover surface

Acute inflammation

E

Fibroblast   Fibrin clot and inflammatory exudate   Macrophage

Inflammation

Acute inflammation

F

New blood vessels

Reconstructing phase

Granulation tissue   Epithelialization

G

Reconstructing phase

H

Collagen fibers

Maturation phase

I

Scar tissue

Acute inflammation
Present in inflammatory exudate: neutrophils, macrophages, bacteria, dead cells, and erythrocytes. Macrophages release (1) angiogenesis factor to attract epithelial cells and vascular endothelial cells (capillary and lymphatic buds) and (2) fibroblast-activating factor to attract fibroblasts.

Reconstructing phase
Epithelialization includes formation of granulation tissue, inward migration of fibroblasts, and the beginning of collagen synthesis and secretion. Granulation tissue becomes scar tissue, contraction begins, and differentiation begins.

Maturation phase
This phase includes completion of contraction, differentiation and remodeling of scar tissue, and disappearance of capillaries from scar tissue.

Figure 6-21 Wound repair by primary or secondary intention. **A** to **D**, Healing by primary intention. **E** to **I**, Healing by secondary intention.

initially sealed off by a blood clot containing fibrin and trapped cells. The cross-linked mesh of fibrin is created by activation of the coagulation cascade and initially traps platelets to form a platelet plug that further seals damaged vessels (see Chapter 25). Most surgical wounds are completely sealed with platelet plugs within hours after closure. This sealing helps unite the wound edges and also acts to create a physical barrier to bacterial invasion, although pathogenic invasion is not always prevented. The fibrin mesh ultimately acts as a scaffold for the collagen or regenerated tissue cells that ultimately will fill the wound.

For healing to proceed, the fibrin clot must be dissolved and then replaced by normal tissue (for resolution) or scar tissue (for repair). Enzymatic digestion of the clot usually occurs after activation of the plasma fibrinolytic system (plasmin generation; see Chapter 25) or release of lysosomal enzymes from dead neutrophils. Macrophages invade the dissolving clot and, by phagocytosis, clear away debris and dead cells. Débridement by macrophages and remaining neutrophils is then simply followed by regeneration of destroyed cells (resolution) or, if regeneration is not possible, by repair (see Figure 6-21).

The process of healing begins as **granulation tissue** grows inward from surrounding healthy connective tissue. Granulation tissue is filled with new capillaries (angiogenesis) that give it a red, granular appearance and is surrounded by fibroblasts and macrophages. First, capillary buds sprout from vascular endothelial cells around the wound and extend into the débrided areas. Loops form when the young capillaries join (anastomose). The loops are more fragile and permeable than mature vessels, resulting in leakage of erythrocytes and neutrophils. The erythrocytes are phagocytosed by macrophages and the neutrophils assist in further débridement of the inflammatory lesion. Many of the new capillaries differentiate into larger vessels as repair continues. New lymphatic vessels also grow into the granulation tissue by a similar process.

In addition to their role in débriding, macrophages at the site of injury secrete several biochemical mediators that promote healing:

1. **Transforming growth factor–beta (TGF-β),** which stimulates fibroblasts entering the lesion to synthesize and secrete the collagen precursor **procollagen**
2. **Angiogenesis factors** such as vascular endothelial growth factor (VEGF) and fibroblast growth factor-2 (FGF-2), which stimulate vascular endothelial cells to form capillary buds that grow into the lesion
3. **Matrix metalloproteinases (MMPs),** which may function in the degradation and remodeling of extracellular matrix proteins (e.g., collagen and fibrin) at the site of injury

As the clot or scab is being dissolved and granulation tissue is being formed, the healing wound must be protected. This is accomplished by epithelialization, the process by which epithelial cells grow into the wound from surrounding healthy tissue. Inching along the exposed collagenous matrix,

epithelial cells migrate under the clot or scab using MMPs to unravel collagen as they travel. Unraveling the collagen enables the epithelial cells to move rather than remain immobile (see Figure 6-21); the intact collagen ahead of them provides a pathway on which they can maneuver forward.[38] Eventually the migrating epithelial cells contact similar cells from all sides of the wound and seal it, thereby halting migration and proliferation. The epithelial cells do remain active, however, undergoing differentiation to give rise to the various epidermal layers (see Chapter 44). Epithelialization of a skin wound can be hastened if the wound is kept moist, preventing the fibrin clot from becoming a scab.

Fibroblasts are the most important cells during the reconstructive phase of wound healing because they synthesize and secrete collagen and other connective tissue proteins. Fibroblasts are stimulated by macrophage-derived TGF-β to proliferate, enter the lesion, and produce these proteins. The collagen and connective tissue proteins produced by fibroblasts are deposited in débrided areas about 6 days after the fibroblasts have entered the lesion.[39] **Collagen** is the most abundant protein in the body. It contains high concentrations of the amino acids glycine, proline, and lysine, although many of the proline and lysine amino acids are enzymatically modified as the protein is being synthesized. Modification of these amino acids requires several cofactors and is absolutely necessary for proper collagen polymerization and function. The cofactors required include iron, ascorbic acid (vitamin C), and molecular oxygen (O_2); absence of any of these results in incomplete or impaired wound healing.

Immature collagen (i.e., procollagen) is secreted by fibroblasts as a complex of three polypeptide chains cross-linked by intermolecular bonds. Procollagen is converted to mature collagen by the proteolytic removal of small polypeptide sequences at both ends of the trimer. As healing progresses, collagen molecules are cross-linked by intramolecular covalent bonds to form collagen fibrils that are further cross-linked to form collagen fibers. The process of complete collagen matrix assembly takes several months because collagen is initially deposited randomly but then is remodeled by repeated dissolution (by MMPs) and re-assembly. During this remodeling period, collagen fibers orient along the lines of mechanical stress; further cross-linking adds strength to the final collagen matrix.

Wound contraction is the final process of the reconstructive phase of healing. It is necessary for closure of all wounds, but especially those that heal by secondary intention. Contraction is noticeable 6 to 12 days after injury and may amount to inward movement of the wound edge by approximately 0.5 mm/day in normal healing. The granulation tissue of a healing wound contains **myofibroblasts**—specialized cells that are likely responsible for wound contraction. As their name implies, myofibroblasts have features of both smooth muscle cells and fibroblasts. They appear microscopically similar to fibroblasts, but differ in that their cytoplasm contains bundles of parallel fibers similar to those found in smooth muscle cells. Wound contraction occurs as extensions from the plasma membrane of myofibroblasts establish connections between neighboring cells, contract their fibers, and exert tension on the neighboring cells while anchoring themselves to the wound bed.

Maturation Phase

Collagen matrix assembly, tissue regeneration, and wound contraction all *begin* during the reconstructive phase but are not yet completed when the reconstructive phase ends, about 2 weeks after injury. Therefore, these processes continue into the maturation phase—a phase that can persist for years. During the maturation phase, scar tissue is remodeled and capillaries disappear, leaving the scar avascular. Within 2 to 3 weeks after maturation has begun, the scar tissue has gained about two thirds of its eventual maximum strength.

Neither epidermal wounds that heal by secondary intention nor unsutured internal lesions are completely restored by healing. At best, repaired tissue regains 80% of its original tensile strength. Only epithelial, hepatic (liver), and bone marrow cells are capable of the complete mitotic regeneration known as *compensatory hyperplasia* (hyperplasia is described in Chapter 2). In fibrous connective tissue such as joints and ligaments, normal healing results in replacement of the original tissue with new tissue that does not have exactly the same structure or function as that of the original. Some tissues heal without replacement of cells. For example, damage resulting from myocardial infarction heals with a scar composed of fibrous tissue rather than with cardiac muscle cell replacement. Although the composition of various healed tissues may differ, the healing process—reconstruction followed by wound maturation—is essentially the same for all wounds.

Dysfunctional Wound Healing

Dysfunctional wound healing may occur if any of the involved processes occurs abnormally. This can include abnormalities in the inflammatory response itself, insufficient or excessive repair, or if a wound is re-infected. Abnormalities may result from a predisposing disease, such as diabetes mellitus, or from an acquired condition, such as hypoxemia (insufficient oxygen in arterial blood). Numerous drugs and nutrients can affect wound healing as well.

Dysfunction During Inflammatory Response

Healing may be prolonged if bleeding is not stopped during acute inflammation. *Hemorrhage* in a damaged area delays healing for several reasons. Initially, the excess blood cells that accumulate at the site of injury must be cleared—a process that requires additional time. In addition to the cellular accumulation caused by excessive bleeding, formation of a clot increases the amount of space that granulation tissue has to fill and serves as a mechanical barrier to oxygen diffusion. The great amount of fibrin that is released during hemorrhage also must eventually be reabsorbed in order to prevent its organization into *fibrous adhesions*. Once formed, these adhesions can bind organs together by fibrous bands; with time, shrinkage of these bands can distort or strangulate nearby or-

gans. This is clinically significant, particularly if they form within the pleural, pericardial, or abdominal cavities.

Accumulated blood as a result of hemorrhage also serves as an excellent culture medium for bacteria, promoting continued *infection* and prolonging inflammation by increasing purulent exudate formation. Prolonged infection can promote *excess scar formation* or even prevent healing completely. Continued infection of a wound, termed *wound sepsis*, can be clinically treated in several ways. Most important is the débridement of necrotic tissue and foreign bodies. This removal is accomplished either through surgery or through the use of absorbent dressings. Wound irrigation and antibiotic therapy also may assist in combating continued infection.

Although local hemorrhage during the inflammatory process can pose a huge impediment to healing, many additional factors, both physiologic and pharmacologic, also may adversely affect the healing of an inflamed tissue. *Hypovolemia*—decreased blood volume—hinders inflammation. The physiologic response to hypovolemia is vessel constriction rather than the dilation required to deliver inflammatory cells to the site of injury. Optimal nutrition is important during all phases of healing because metabolic needs are increased. The nutrients most essential for healing are glucose, oxygen, and amino acids. Because leukocytes need glucose to produce the energy needed for chemotaxis, phagocytosis, and intercellular killing, the wounds of persons with diabetes who receive insufficient insulin heal poorly, mainly due to a prolonging of infection. Persons with diabetes are also at risk for ischemic wounds because they are likely to have both small-vessel diseases that impair the microcirculation and altered (glycosylated) hemoglobin, which has an increased affinity for oxygen and thus does not readily release oxygen in tissues. (Hemoglobin's function as the oxygen-carrying component of blood is described in Chapter 25.) Oxygen delivery is also compromised by hypoxemic states because ischemic tissue is susceptible to infection. *Hypoproteinemia* prolongs inflammation because the associated decrease in available amino acids is an impediment to fibroblast proliferation. Finally, anti-inflammatory steroids can have an impact upon wound healing. These drugs prevent macrophages from migrating to the site of injury and inhibit their release of collagenase and plasminogen activator.[40] *Anti-inflammatory steroids* also inhibit fibroblast migration into the wound during the reconstructive phase of healing and impair angiogenesis, wound contraction, and reepithelialization.[41]

Dysfunction During Reconstructive Phase of Healing

Three of the essential processes that occur during the reconstructive phase are assembly and remodeling of the collagen matrix, epithelialization of the wound bed, and contraction of the wound. Dysfunctional wound healing can result from the impairment of any of these processes.

Impaired Collagen Matrix Assembly

A number of factors may interfere with the production of collagen in healing tissues, most being nutritional. Scurvy, for example, is a condition caused by a deficiency in ascorbic acid, one of the cofactors required for the amino acid modification that is necessary for proper collagen matrix assembly. The implication of scurvy, then, is a poorly formed collagen matrix and, therefore, greatly impaired wound healing. Other nutrients, including iron, copper, and calcium, play additional roles in the enzymatic reactions required for collagen modification and assembly. Usually, however, such minute amounts of these substances are required that deficiencies are not clinically significant. Nutritionally, appropriate protein intake is also essential for collagen synthesis. The amino acid methionine that is found in proteins is converted to cysteine, the role of which in collagen synthesis is twofold: (1) it functions as an important cofactor in the enzymatic reactions required for collagen synthesis; and (2) it contains sulfur, which contributes to formation of the strong covalent bonds in cross-linked collagen fibrils.

In addition to improper collagen assembly, dysfunctional healing also may result from excessive production of collagen. Overproduction of collagen causes surface overhealing, which is manifested in the skin by formation of a keloid or a hypertrophic scar (Figure 6-22). A **keloid** is a raised scar that extends beyond the original boundaries of the wound. It invades surrounding tissue and is likely to recur after surgical removal. A familial tendency toward keloid formation has been observed, with a greater incidence in blacks relative to whites. Similar to a keloid, a **hypertrophic scar** is also raised but differs in that it remains within the original boundaries of the wound. Hypertrophic scars tend to regress over time whereas keloids do not. Both keloids and hypertrophic scars are caused by an imbalance between collagen synthesis and collagen degradation in which synthesis is increased relative to degradation. Although the precise mechanism of this imbalance is unknown, recent evidence suggests that communication between two cell types, keratinocytes and fibroblasts, is aberrant.[42]

Impaired Epithelialization

Like inflammation, the process of epithelialization is suppressed by anti-inflammatory steroids, hypoxemia, and nutritional deficiencies. Anti-inflammatory steroids inhibit phagocyte production of the biochemical mediators required for epithelialization, hypoxemia deprives cells of the energy required for the process, and dietary zinc is necessary for the MMP activity that is crucial to cellular migration.

Wound care techniques also may greatly influence epithelial cell migration. External wounds that are draining or healing by secondary intention often are clinically débrided and protected with dressings. The ideal dressing is one that absorbs some drainage without being incorporated into the clot or granulation tissue. Because epithelial cells must migrate across the wound during healing, dressings that débride healthy epithelial cells along with necrotic tissue prolong epithelialization. Many solutions that traditionally have been used to clean or irrigate wounds are now known to be deleterious to the fragile new cells in the wound bed. Normal saline is the most innocuous solution that can be used to cleanse or

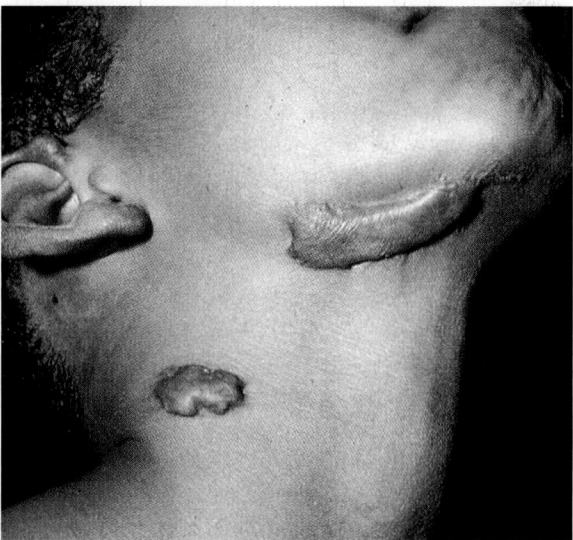

Figure 6-22 Keloids. (From Damjanov I, Linder J: *Anderson's pathology,* ed 10, St Louis, 1996, Mosby.)

irrigate a wound that is healing primarily by epithelialization. Solutions such as povidone-iodine and hydrogen peroxide are desiccating (drying) and, as such, inhibit rather than promote epithelial cell migration.

Impaired Contraction

Wound contraction may become pathologic when contraction is excessive, resulting in a deformity or **contracture.** Burn wounds are especially susceptible to the development of contractures. Internal contractures may occur as well, and are common in cirrhosis of the liver. Internally, scar tissue that becomes contracted constricts blood flow that may contribute to the development of portal hypertension and esophageal varices. Other types of internal contraction deformity include duodenal strictures caused by dysfunctional healing of an ulcer and esophageal strictures caused by chemical burns.

Proper positioning and range-of-motion exercises, as well as surgery, are among the physical means used to overcome the excessive myofibroblast-derived tension that results in contractures. Clinical use of pharmacologic methods for control of wound contracture is still largely experimental, however, attempts have been made. These attempted methods include control of myofibroblast contraction by the administration of smooth muscle cell inhibitors such as colchicine and inhibition of proper collagen matrix assembly with drugs that prevent either collagen cross-linking or MMP activity. These latter treatments are based on the knowledge that myofibroblast binding to collagen can 'lock' contracted cells into position.

Wound Disruption

Finally, a potential complication in the healing of wounds that are sutured closed is **dehiscence,** in which the wound pulls apart at the suture line. The greatest incidence of dehiscence occurs 5 to 12 days after suturing, paradoxically at the time when collagen synthesis is at its peak. Approximately

50% of dehiscence occurrences are associated with wound sepsis, although dehiscence also may occur when sutures break as a result of excessive strain. Obesity increases the risk of suture breakage because adipose tissue is difficult to suture. Wound dehiscence usually is heralded by an increase in serous drainage from the wound. In addition, patients may report a feeling that "something gave way." Prompt surgical attention is required.

PEDIATRICS AND MECHANISMS OF SELF-DEFENSE

Neonates commonly have transiently depressed inflammatory and immune function. For example, neutrophils and perhaps monocytes may not be capable of efficient chemotaxis. Insufficient response to chemotactic factors appears to be caused by lack of fluidity in the phagocyte's plasma membrane, so that pseudopod formation and migration are impaired. Neonates are prone to infections associated with chemotactic defects, including cutaneous abscesses caused by staphylococci and cutaneous candidiasis. Further, neutrophils in neonates who were stressed by *in utero* infection or respiratory insufficiency have diminished oxidative and bacterial responses. (Acquired phagocytic defects, which may be induced by a variety of infections, metabolic disorders, nutrition deficiencies, or drugs, are described in Chapter 8.)

Neonates also are partially deficient in complement, especially components of the alternative pathway. They tend to have a relative deficiency of factor B and to develop severe, overwhelming sepsis and meningitis when infected with bacteria against which there is no transferred maternal antibody. They also may be deficient in some of the collectins and collectin-like proteins (see What's New: Collectins). This is especially true of preterm neonates.[43] Some preterm infants with respiratory distress syndrome are deficient in at least one collectin, which provide innate defense against respiratory infections.[43-45]

AGING AND MECHANISMS OF SELF-DEFENSE

The elderly population is also at risk for impaired inflammation and wound healing. In some cases, impaired healing is not directly associated with aging in general but can instead be linked to a chronic illness such as cardiovascular disease or diabetes mellitus. In addition, many elderly persons require medications such as anti-inflammatory steroids that can interfere with the healing process.

The elderly have increased susceptibility to bacterial infections of the lungs, urinary tract, and skin. Because of im-

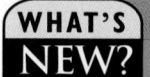

WHAT'S NEW?   Collectins

Collectins are a small family of secreted glycoproteins that have an important function in innate immunity. Each collectin glycoprotein contains two distinctive domains: a collagen-like region and a carbohydrate recognition/binding domain (CRD). Collectins function in innate immunity by recognizing different patterns of monosaccharide distribution on microbial surfaces and binding to these carbohydrates through their CRD. The CRD of each collectin binds with different affinities to a range of monosaccharides, enabling collectins to recognize a wide array of pathogenic microorganisms. Collectin "tagging" of the microorganism facilitates recognition by macrophages, enhancing macrophage attachment, phagocytosis, and killing. The mechanism by which macrophages recognize collectin-tagged pathogens, however, remains a matter of dispute because receptors for these molecules have not been clearly identified. Three different collectins, including surfactant proteins A and D (SP-A and SP-D) and mannose-binding lectin (MBL), have been identified as playing a major role in protection against respiratory infections.

Data from Gadjeva M, Takahaski K, Thiel, S: *Mol Immunol* 41(2):113-121, 2004; Gold JA et al: *Infect Immun* 72(2):645-650, 2004; Hickling TP et al:, *J Leukoc Biol* 75:27-33, 2004; Leth-Larsen R et al: *Mol Hum Reprod* 10(3):149-154, 2004.

paired sensation or mobility and physiologic changes in the skin, the elderly are at increased risk for sustaining various wounds. With aging, subcutaneous fat is lost, diminishing a layer of protection. Collagen fibers become thicker and a certain percentage of elastin is lost, thus further contributing to loss of protection. The regenerative capability of the skin is maintained with aging, but the epidermis undergoes age-associated changes that include atrophy of the underlying capillaries. The consequent decrease of perfusion makes the elderly more susceptible than others to the adverse effects of hypoxia in the wound bed. In addition, aging fibroblasts may have a slower rate of proliferation and therefore wound healing is attenuated.[46]

Infections of other organ systems in the elderly may be due to a diminished natural ability to ward off infection. Several cellular components of innate resistance are deficient in number (e.g., alveolar macrophages) or have diminished activity (e.g., neutrophil chemotaxis, degranulation, and phagocytosis).[47] One explanation for this diminished inflammatory cellular activity is an age-related decrease in expression and function of several, if not all, TLRs.[47]

SUMMARY REVIEW

Human Defense Mechanisms

1. There are two types of human defense: innate resistance or immunity conferred by natural barriers and the inflammatory response, and the adaptive (acquired) immune system.

First Line of Defense: Physical, Mechanical, and Biochemical Barriers

1. Physical and mechanical barriers are the first lines of defense encountered by invading pathogens; these include the skin and mucous membranes.

2. Antibacterial peptides in mucous secretions, perspiration, saliva, tears, and other secretions provide a biochemical barrier against invading pathogens in the extracellular space.

3. Cathelicidins and defensins are two classes of antimicrobial peptides produced by epithelial cells.

4. The normal bacterial flora provide protection by inhibiting colonization by pathogens and by releasing chemicals that prevent infection.

Second Line of Defense: The Inflammatory Response

1. The inflammatory response, our body's second line of defense against invading microorganisms, is nonspecific, rapidly initiated, and has no memory cells.
2. The vascular response in acute inflammation includes vasodilation, increased capillary permeability, and white blood cell adherence to inner vessel walls and their migration through vessel walls.
3. Three plasma protein systems provide a biochemical barrier against invading pathogens in the circulation. These include the complement system, the clotting system, and the kinin system.
4. The plasma protein systems work together with each other as well as with antimicrobial peptides and the cellular component of the innate immune system to prevent microbial infection.
5. The complement proteins can be activated in three pathways: the classical pathway, the alternative pathway, and the lectin pathway.
6. Activation of the complement pathways results in opsonization, activation of anaphylatoxins, cell lysis, and leukocyte chemotaxis.
7. The clotting (coagulation) cascade prevents spread of microorganisms, contains microorganisms and foreign bodies at site of greatest inflammatory cell activity, and provides a framework for repair and healing.
8. The kinin system proteins promote vasodilation and increased capillary permeability and induce pain.
9. Plasmin and Hageman factor (factor XII) interact to activate the clotting cascade, the complement system, and the kinin proteins.
10. The plasma proteins are finely regulated to prevent injury to host tissue and to guarantee activation when needed; some of the inhibitors in the plasma protein systems include carboxypeptidase, histaminases, kinases, and C_1 esterase inhibitor.
11. Many different types of cells are involved in the inflammatory process including mast cells, neutrophils, monocytes and macrophages, eosinophils, natural killer (NK) cells, platelets, and nonleukocytic cells.
12. The cells of the innate immune system secrete many biochemical mediators that are responsible for the vascular changes associated with inflammation and for modulating the localization and activities of other inflammatory cells. The mediators include histamine, chemotactic factors, leukotrienes, prostaglandins, and platelet-activating factor.
13. The inflammatory response is initiated upon tissue injury or when pathogen-associated molecular patterns (PAMPs) are recognized by pattern recognition receptors (PRRs) on cells of the innate immune system.
14. The PRRs include Toll-like receptors (TLRs), complement, scavenger, glycan, and mannose receptors.
15. TLRs recognize PAMPs; complement receptors recognize complement fragments; and scavenger receptors promote phagocytosis.
16. Most cells are central cells of inflammation and release histamine chemotactic factors, cytokines, leukotrienes, prostaglandins, growth factors, and other mediators.
17. H1 histamine receptors promote inflammation, and H2 histamine receptors inhibit the inflammatory response.
18. Phagocytosis is the destruction of microorganisms and cellular debris.
19. The stages of phagocytosis include recognition and adherence, engulfment, lysosomal fusion, and destruction.
20. Phagocytic killing can be oxygen-dependent with the production of reactive oxygen intermediates or oxygen-independent with lysosomal enzymes.
21. Neutrophils are the predominant phagocyte of early inflammation. They are attracted to the inflammatory site by chemotoxins.
22. Monocytes and macrophages arrive at the inflammatory site later than neutrophils and remain longer to clean up debris and promote wound healing.
23. Eosinophils help control mast cell vascular mediators and defend against parasite infection.
24. Natural killer cells recognize and eliminate viruses, cancer cells, and other abnormal cells.
25. Platelets interact with the coagulation cascade to stop bleeding and release a number of mediators that promote and control inflammation.
26. Cytokines are soluble factors that regulate the inflammatory response and include interleukins, interferons, and tumor necrosis factor.
27. Interleukins (IL) are biochemical messengers primarily produced by macrophages and lymphocytes and significantly help regulate the inflammatory response.
28. Interferons (INFs) provide protection from viral infection in uninfected cells.
29. Tumor necrosis factor is primarily produced by macrophages and promotes inflammation with both local and systemic effects.
30. Chemokines are synthesized by a number of different cells and induce leukocytes chemotaxis, and are classified as either CC or CXC, depending on their amino acid arrangement. CC chemokines affect monocytes, lymphocytes, and eosinophils. CXC chemokines generally affect neutrophils.

Local Manifestations of Inflammation

1. Local manifestations of inflammation are the result of the vascular changes associated with the inflammatory process, including vasodilation and increased capillary permeability. The symptoms include redness, heat, swelling, and pain.
2. The functions of the vascular changes are to dilute toxins, carry plasma proteins and leukocytes to the injury site, and carry bacterial toxins and debris away from the site.

Systemic Manifestations of Acute Inflammation

1. The three primary systemic effects of inflammation are fever, leukocytosis, and increase in levels of circulating plasma proteins.
2. Acute phase reactants are proteins produced by the liver during acute inflammation and include fibrinogen, C-reactive protein, haptoglobin, amyloid A, α_1-antitrypsin, and ceruloplasmin.

Chronic Inflammation

1. Chronic inflammation can be a continuation of acute inflammation that lasts 2 weeks or longer. It also can occur as a distinct process without much preceding acute inflammation.
2. Chronic inflammation is characterized by a dense infiltration of lymphocytes and macrophages. The body may wall off and isolate the infection to protect against tissue damage by formation of a granuloma.

Resolution and Repair

1. Resolution (regeneration) is the return of tissue to nearly normal structure and function. Repair is healing by scar tissue formation.
2. Inflammatory lesions proceed to resolution, meaning that original tissue structure and function have been restored, if little tissue has been lost or injured tissue is capable of regeneration. This is called *healing by primary intention*.

Continued

SUMMARY REVIEW—cont'd

3. Inflammatory lesions that involve extensive damage or tissues incapable of regeneration heal by the process of repair that results in the formation of a scar. This is called *healing by secondary intention*.
4. Resolution and repair occur in two separate phases, the *reconstructive phase* in which the wound begins to heal and the *maturation phase* in which the healed wound is remodeled.
5. Dysfunctional wound healing can occur as a result of abnormalities in either the inflammatory response or in the reconstructive phase of resolution and repair.

PEDIATRICS AND MECHANISMS OF SELF-DEFENSE

1. Neonates commonly have transiently depressed inflammatory function.
2. Infants often have deficiencies in complement and in a number of collectins, making them more susceptible to bacterial infection.

AGING AND MECHANISMS OF SELF-DEFENSE

1. The elderly are at risk for impaired wound healing, often because of underlying illnesses.
2. Diminished immune function may interfere with the elderly person's natural ability to ward off infection.

KEY TERMS

α₁-antitrypsin, 193
Abscesses, 199
Acute-phase reactants, 199
Adaptive immunity (acquired or specific immunity), 177
Adhesion molecules, 191
Alternative pathway, 181
Anaphylatoxins, 182
Angiogenesis factors, 203
Antigen-antibody complex (immune complex), 181
Antimicrobial peptide, 177
Bradykinin, 183
C1 esterase inhibitor (C1 inh), 184
C3 convertase, 182
C5 convertase, 182
Carboxypeptidase, 182
Cathelicidins, 177
Cell lysis, 182
Chemokines, 198
Chemotactic factor, 182
Chemotaxis, 188
Classical pathway, 181
Coagulation cascade, 182
Collagen, 203
Collectins, 177
Complement cascade, 180
Complement receptors, 186
Contraction, 201
Contracture, 205
Cysts, 199
Cytokines, 195
Débridement, 201
Defensins, 177
Degranulation, 182
Dehiscence, 205
Diapedesis, 191
Endogenous pyrogens, 199

Endothelial cells, 191
Eosinophil chemotactic factor of anaphylaxis (ECF-A), 188
Eosinophils, 195
Epithelialization, 201
Epithelioid cells, 201
Extrinsic pathway, 183
Exudate, 198
Fever, 199
Fibrinous exudate, 198
Fibroblasts, 203
Giant cells, 201
Granulation tissue, 203
Granuloma, 200
Hageman factor (factor XII), 184
Heat, 198
Hemorrhagic exudate, 199
Histamine, 188
Hypertrophic scar, 205
Immunity, 175
Inflammatory response, 175
Innate resistance, 175
Interferons (INFs), 197
Interleukins (IL), 196
Intrinsic pathway, 183
Keloid, 205
Kinin system, 183
Kininases, 184
Lectin pathway, 181
Leukocytosis, 199
Leukotrienes, 191
Macrophages, 195
Margination (pavementing), 191
Mast cells, 187
Matrix metalloproteinases (MMPs), 203
Maturation phase, 201
Monocytes, 194
Myofibroblasts, 203

Natural killer (NK) cells, 196
Neutrophil, 194
Normal bacterial flora, 177
Opsonin, 182
Pain, 198
Pathogen-associated molecular patterns (PAMPs), 186
Pattern recognition receptors (PRRs), 186
Phagocytes, 194
Phagocytosis, 191
Phagolysosome, 193
Phagosome, 193
Plasma kinin cascade, 183
Plasma protein systems, 180
Plasmin, 184
Platelets, 196
Platelet-activating factor (PAF), 191
Polymorphonuclear neutrophil (PMN), 194
Primary intention, 201
Procollagen, 203
Proenzymes, 180
Prostaglandins, 191
Purulent (suppurative) exudate, 199
Reconstructive phase, 201
Redness, 198
Regeneration, 201
Repair, 201
Resolution, 201
Scar tissue, 201
Scavenger receptors, 187
Secondary intention, 201
Serous, 198
Swelling, 198
Toll-like receptors (TLRs), 186
Transforming growth factor–beta (TGF-β), 203
Tumor necrosis factor–alpha (TNF-α), 197
Wound contraction, 203

MEDIA RESOURCES   evolve

Review questions and answers for this chapter are available in the *CD Companion* included with this book. Also see the CD for an animation of the *inflammatory response*.

WebLinks—links to Internet sites pertaining to this chapter—are available on Evolve at http://evolve.elsevier.com/McCance/.

REFERENCES

1. Ganz T: Defensins: antimicrobial peptides of innate immunity, *Nat Rev* 3:710, 2003.
2. Boman HG: Antibacterial peptides: basic facts and emerging concepts, *J Intern Med* 254(3):197-215, 2003.
3. Oppenheim JJ, Biragyn A, Kwak LW et al: Roles of antimicrobial peptides such as defensins in innate and adaptive immunity, *Ann Rheum Dis* 62(Suppl 2):ii17-21, 2003.
4. Hickling TP, Clark H, Malhotra R, Sim RB: Collectins and their role in lung immunity, *J Leukoc Biol* 75(1):27-33, 2004.
5. Holmskov U, Theil S, Jensenius JC: Collections and ficolins: humoral lectins of the innate immune defense, *Annu Rev Immunol* 21:547-578, 2004.
6. Morgan BP: Physiology and pathophysiology of complement: progress and trends, *Crit Rev Clin Lab Sci* 32(3):265-298, 1995.
7. Czermak BJ, Friedl HP, Ward PA: Complement, cytokines, and adhesion molecule expression in inflammatory reactions, *Proc Assoc Am Physicians* 110(4):306-312, 1998.
8. Roitt I, Brostoff J, Male D: *Immunology,* ed 6, Edinburgh, 2001, Mosby.
9. Janssens S, Beyaert R: Role of Toll-like receptors in pathogen recognition, *Clin Microbiol Rev* 16(4):637-646, 2003.
10. Dempsey PW, Vaidya SA, Cheng G: The art of war: innate and adaptive immune responses, *Cell Mol Life Sci* 60(12):2604-2621, 2003.
11. Beutler B, Hoebe K, Du X et al: How we detect microbes and respond to them: the Toll-like receptors and their transducers, *J Leukoc Biol* 74(4):479-485, 2003.
12. Bohana-Kashtan O, Ziporen L, Donin N et al: Cell signals transduced by complement, *Mol Immunol* 41(6-7):583-597, 2004.
13. Carroll MC: The complement system in regulation of adaptive immunity, *Nat Immunol* 5(10):981-986, 2004.
14. Azhar S, Leers-Sucheta S, Reaven E: Cholesterol update in adrenal and gonadal tissues: the SR-B1 and "selective" pathway connection, *Front Biosci* 8:s998-1029, 2003. Review.
15. Horiuchi S, Sakamoto Y, Sakai M: Scavenger receptors for oxidized and glycated proteins, *Amino Acids* 25(3-4):283-292, 2003.
16. Rhainds D, Brissette L: The role of scavenger receptor class B type I (SR-B1) in lipid trafficking: defining the rules for lipid traders, *Int J Biochem Cell Biol* 36(1):39-77, 2004.
17. Ehrlich P: Dietbage zur Kenntnis der Anilinsfarb und Ihrer Verwendung nin ungen der Mikroskopichen technik, *Arch Mikr Anat* 13:263, 1877.
18. Bellou A, Schaub B, Ting L et al: Toll receptors modulate allergic responses: interaction with dendritic cells, T cells and mast cells, *Curr Opin Allergy Clin Immunol* 3(6):487-494, 2003.
19. Kulka M, Alexopoulou L, Flavell RA et al: Activation of mast cells by double-stranded RNA: evidence for activation through Toll-like receptor 3, *J Allergy Clin Immunol* 114(1):174-182, 2004.
20. Marshall JS, King CA, McCurdy JD: Mast cell cytokine and chemokine responses to bacterial and viral infection, *Curr Pharm Des* 9(1):11-24, 2003.
21. Arrang JM: Molecular and functional diversity of histamine receptor subtypes, *Ann N Y Acad Sci* 757:314-323, 1995.
22. Leurs R, Smit MJ, Timmerman H: Molecular pharmacological aspects of histamine receptors, *Pharmacol Therap* 66(3):413-463, 1995.
23. Brown EJ: Phagocytosis, *Bioessays* 17(2):109-117, 1995.
24. Vestweber D: Molecular mechanisms that control endothelial cell contacts, *J Pathol* 190(3):281-291, 2000.
25. Crockett-Torabi E: Selectins and mechanisms of signal transduction, *J Leukoc Biol* 63(1):1-14, 1998.
26. Repo H, Harlan JM: Mechanisms and consequences of phagocyte adhesion to endothelium, *Ann Med* 31(3):156-165, 1999.
27. Pearson JD: Normal endothelial cell function, *Lupus* 9(3):183-188, 2000. Review.
28. Babior BM: NADPH oxidase, *Curr Opin Immunol* 16(1):42-47, 2004.
29. Ma J, Chen T, Mandelin J et al: Regulation of macrophage activation, *Cell Mol Life Sci* 60(11):2334-2346, 2003.
30. Yokoyama WM, Kim S, French AR: The dynamic life of natural killer cells, *Annu Rev Immunol* 22:405-429, 2004.
31. Kalvakolanu DV, Borden EC: An overview of the interferon system: signal transduction and mechanisms of action, *Cancer Invest* 14(1):25-53, 1996.
32. Galli SJ, Nakae S: Mast cells to the defense, *Nat Immunol* 4(12):1160-1162, 2003.
33. Rot A, vonAndrian UH: Chemokines in innate and adaptive host defense: basic chemokinese grammar for immune cells, *Annu Rev Immunol* 22:891-928, 2004.
34. Dinarello CA: Cytokines as endogenous pyrogens, *J Infect Dis* 179(Suppl 2):S294-304, 1999.
35. Jakab L, Kalabay L: The acute phase reaction syndrome: the acute reactants (a survey), *Acta Microbiol Immunol Hung* 45(3-4):409, 1998.
36. Suffredini AF et al: New insights into the biology of the acute phase response, *J Clin Immunol* 19(4):203-214, 1999.
37. Munk ME, Emoto M: Functions of T-cell subsets and cytokines in mycobacterial infections, *Eur Respir J* 20:668s-675s, 1995. Review.
38. Parks WC: Matrix metalloproteinases in repair, *Wound Repair Regen* 7(6):423-432, 1999.
39. Kosir MA et al: Matrix glycosaminoglycans in the growth phase of fibroblasts: more of the story in wound healing, *J Surg Res* 92(1):45-52, 2000.
40. Alvarez OM, Levendorf KD, Smerbeck RV et al: Effect of topically applied steroidal and nonsteroidal anti-inflammatory agents on skin repair and regeneration, *Fed Proc* 43(13): 2793-2798, 1984.
41. Anstead GM: Steroids, retinoids, and wound healing, *Adv Wound Care* 11(6):277-285, 1998.
42. Yang GP, Lim IJ, Phan TT et al: From scarless fetal wounds to keloids: molecular studies in wound healing, *Wound Repair Regen* 11(6):411-418, 2003.
43. Awasthi S, Coalson JJ, Yoder BA et al: Deficiencies in lung surfactant proteins A and D are associated with lung infection in very premature neonatal baboons, *Am J Respir Crit Care Med* 163(2):389-397, 2001.
44. Koch A, Melbye M, Sorensen P et al: Acute respiratory tract infections and mannose-binding lectin insufficiency in small children, *Ugeskr Laeger* 164(48):5635, 2002.
45. Khubchandani KR, Snyder JM: Surfactant protein A (SP-A): the alveolus and beyond, *FASEB J* 15(1):59-69, 2001.
46. Khorramizadeh MR, Tredget EE, Telasky C et al: Aging differentially modulates the expression of collagen and collagenase in dermal fibroblasts, *Mol Cell Biochem* 194(1-2):99-108, 1999.
47. Renshaw M, Rockwel J, Engleman C et al: Cutting edge: impaired toll-like receptor expression and function in aging, *J Immunol* 169(9):4697-4701, 2002.

ADAPTIVE IMMUNITY

NEAL S. ROTE • BARBARA CRIPPES TRASK

CHAPTER OUTLINE

The third line of defense in the human body is **adaptive (acquired) immunity,** often called the **immune response,** or **immunity.** Once external barriers have been compromised and inflammation (see Chapter 6) has been activated, the adaptive immune response is called into action. The molecules and cells of the immune response are closely integrated with those of the innate response. Many components of the innate response facilitate the development of the adaptive immune response. Conversely, products of the adaptive immune response use many components of the inflammatory response. Thus both systems are essential for complete protection against infectious disease: inflammation is relatively rapid, nonspecific, and short-lived, whereas adaptive immunity is slower-acting, specific, and very long-lived. Because many inflammatory processes are triggered or affected by immune processes and vice versa, an understanding of both systems is necessary for a complete appreciation of how pathogenic infections are combated. Chapter 8 discusses medically relevant aberrations in both inflammation and immunity, including allergies, diseases that involve unwanted immunologic destruction of healthy tissue, and diseases that

are caused by a deficiency in the normal immune or inflammatory responses. Chapter 9 presents an overview of infection and Chapter 10 discusses the connection between stress and disease and the interrelatedness of the immune, nervous, and endocrine systems.

GENERAL CHARACTERISTICS OF ADAPTIVE IMMUNITY

The immune system of the normal adult is continually challenged by a spectrum of substances that it may recognize as foreign, or "non-self." These substances, called **antigens,** are often associated with pathogens such as viruses, bacteria, fungi, or parasites, although they are also found on noninfectious environmental agents such as pollens, foods, and bee venom, and still others are associated with clinically derived drugs, vaccines, transfusions, and transplanted tissues (Table

Table 7-1	Clinical Use of Antigen or Antibody			
	Use of Antigen or Antibody			
Antigen Source	Protection: Combat Active Disease	Protection: Vaccination	Diagnosis	Therapy
Infectious agents	Neutralize or destroy pathogenic microorganisms (e.g., antibody response against viral infections)	Induce safe and protective immune response (e.g., recommended childhood vaccines)	Measure circulating antigen from infectious agent or antibody (e.g., diagnosis of hepatitis B infection)	Passive treatment with antibody to treat or prevent infection (e.g., administration of antibody against hepatitis A)
Cancers	Prevent tumor growth or spread (e.g., immune surveillance to prevent early cancers)	Prevent cancer growth or spread (e.g., vaccination with cancer antigens)	Measure circulating antigen (e.g., circulating PSA for diagnosis of prostate cancer)	Immunotherapy (e.g., treatment of cancer with antibodies against cancer antigens)
Environmental substances	Prevent entrance into body (e.g., secretory IgA limits systemic exposure to potential allergens)	No clear example	Measure circulating antigen or antibody (e.g., diagnosis of allergy by measuring circulating IgE)	Immunotherapy (e.g., administration of antigen for desensitization of individuals with severe allergies)
Self-antigens	Immune system tolerance to self-antigens, which may be altered by an infectious agent leading to autoimmune disease (see Chapter 8)	Some cases of vaccination alter tolerance to self-antigens leading to autoimmune disease	Measure circulating antibody against self-antigen for diagnosis of autoimmune disease (see Chapter 8)	No clear example

PSA, Prostate-specific antigen.

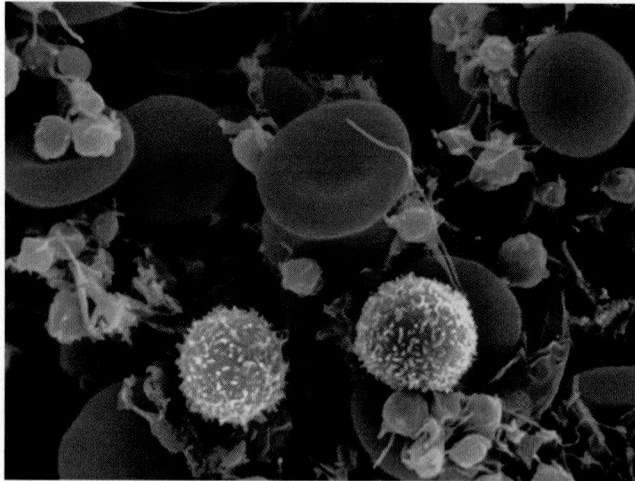

Figure 7-1 Scanning electron micrograph showing lymphocytes (yellow), red blood cells, and platelets. (Copyright Dennis Kunkel Microscopy, Inc.)

7-1). Unlike inflammation, which is nonspecifically activated by cellular damage as well as pathogenic microorganisms, the immune response is primarily designed to afford long-term specific protection (i.e., immunity) against particular invading microorganisms, that is, it has a "memory" function. The products of the adaptive immune responses include a type of serum protein—**immunoglobulins,** or **antibodies**—and a type of blood cell—**lymphocytes** (Figure 7-1).

Specificity and memory are the primary characteristics that differentiate the immune response from other protective mechanisms. This chapter first discusses the nature of that specificity by defining the various types of antigens that may be seen by the immune system, how they are recognized by antibodies and lymphocytes, and the specific intercellular recognition molecules that are necessary for effective immune responses. After the recognition molecules are defined, the development of the immune response is discussed. An immune response can be divided into two phases (Figure 7-2). Before birth, humans produce a large population of **T lymphocytes (T cells)** and **B lymphocytes (B cells)** that have the capacity to recognize almost any foreign antigen found in the environment. Each individual T or B cell, however, specifically recognizes only one particular antigen, but the sum of the population of lymphocyte specificities may recognize millions of foreign antigens. This process is called the *generation of clonal diversity* and occurs in specialized (primary) lymphoid organs; the thymus for T cells and the bone marrow for B cells. While passing through these tissues, the lymphocytes mature and undergo changes that commit them to becoming either B or T cells. Lymphocytes are released from these organs into the circulation as immature cells that have the capacity to react with antigen (**immunocompetent**). These cells migrate to other (secondary) lymphoid organs in the body in preparation for future exposure to antigen (Figure 7-3).

Antigen initiates the second phase of the immune response, *clonal selection.* This process involves a complex interaction among cells. To initiate an effective immune response, most antigens must be "processed," in that they

**GENERATION OF
CLONAL DIVERSITY**

Production of T and B cells
with all possible receptors
for antigen

CLONAL SELECTION

Selection, proliferation, and differentiation of
individual T and B cells with receptors for a
specific antigen

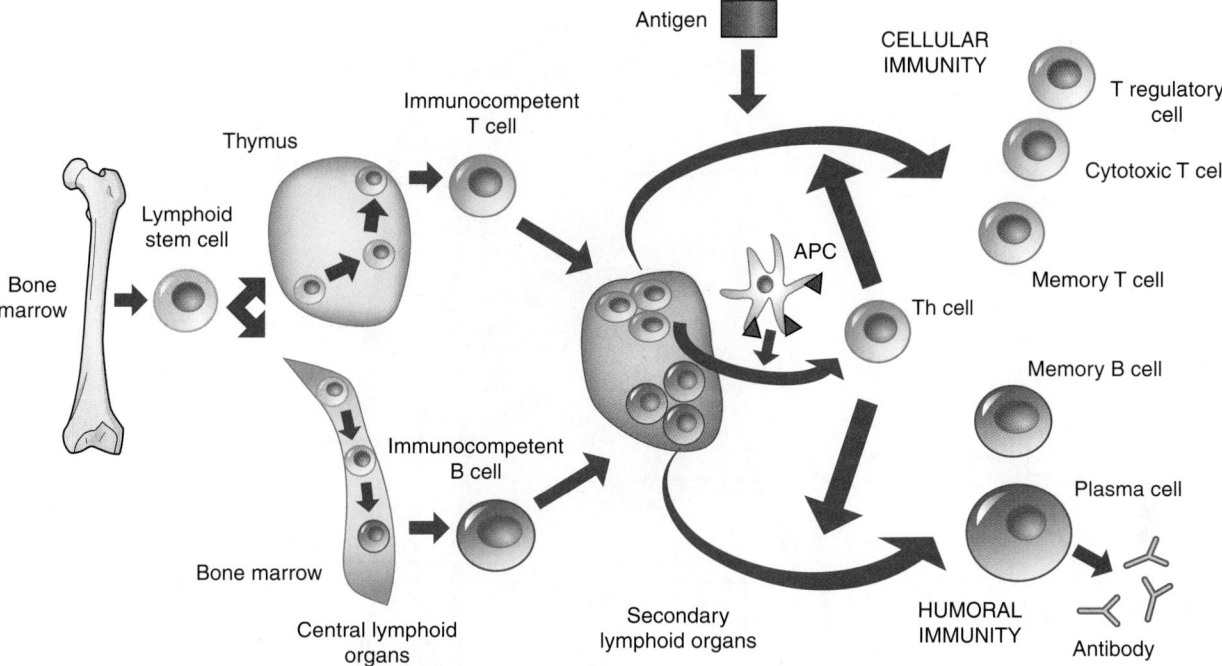

Figure 7-2 Overview of immune response. The immune response can be separated into two phases: the *generation of clonal diversity* and *clonal selection.* During the generation of clonal diversity, lymphoid stem cells from the bone marrow migrate to the central lymphoid organs (the thymus or regions of the bone marrow) where they undergo a series of cellular division and differentiation stages resulting in either immunocompetent T cells from the thymus or immunocompetent B cells from the bone marrow. (This process is outlined in more detail in Figures 7-9 and 7-11.) These cells are still naïve, in that they have never encountered foreign antigen. The immunocompetent cells enter the circulation and migrate to the secondary lymphoid organs (e.g., spleen and lymph nodes), where they take up residence in B- and T-cell–rich areas. The clonal selection phase is initiated by exposure to foreign antigen. The antigen is usually processed by antigen-presenting cells (APCs) for presentation to helper T cells (Th cells) (more detail in Figure 7-15). The intercellular cooperation among APCs, Th cells, and immunocompetent T and B cells results in a second stage of cellular proliferation and differentiation (more details in Figures 7-18 and 7-21). Because antigen has "selected" those T and B cells with compatible antigen receptors, only a small population of T and B cells undergo this process at one time. The end result is an active cellular immunity or humoral immunity, or both. Cellular immunity is mediated by a population of "effector" T cells that can kill targets (cytotoxic T cells) or regulate the immune response (T regulatory cells), as well as a population of memory cells (memory T cells) that can respond more quickly to a second challenge with the same antigen. Humoral immunity is mediated by a population of soluble proteins (antibodies) produced by plasma cells and by a population of memory B cells that can produce more antibody rapidly to a second challenge with the same antigen.

cannot react directly with cells of the immune system but must be shown or "presented" to the immune cells in a very specific manner. This is the job of antigen-processing (antigen-presenting) cells, generally referred to as APCs. The interaction among APCs, subpopulations of T cells that facilitate immune responses (**helper T cells**), and immunocompetent B or T cells results in differentiation of B cells into active antibody-producing cells (plasma cells) and T cells into effector cells, such as cytotoxic T cells. The last portion of this chapter discusses how these products (antibody and T cells) protect against infection, including how they interact with components of the inflammatory process.

Humoral and Cell-Mediated Immunity

The immune response has two arms: antibody and T cells, both of which protect against infection. Antibody circulates in the blood and binds to antigens on infectious agents. This interaction can result in direct inactivation of the microorganism or activation of a variety of inflammatory mediators that will destroy the pathogen. Antibody is primarily responsible for protection against many bacteria and viruses. This arm of the immune response is termed **humoral immunity.**

T cells also undergo differentiation during an immune response and develop into several subpopulations of cells that react directly with antigen on the surface of infectious agents. Some develop into T cells that can stimulate the activities of

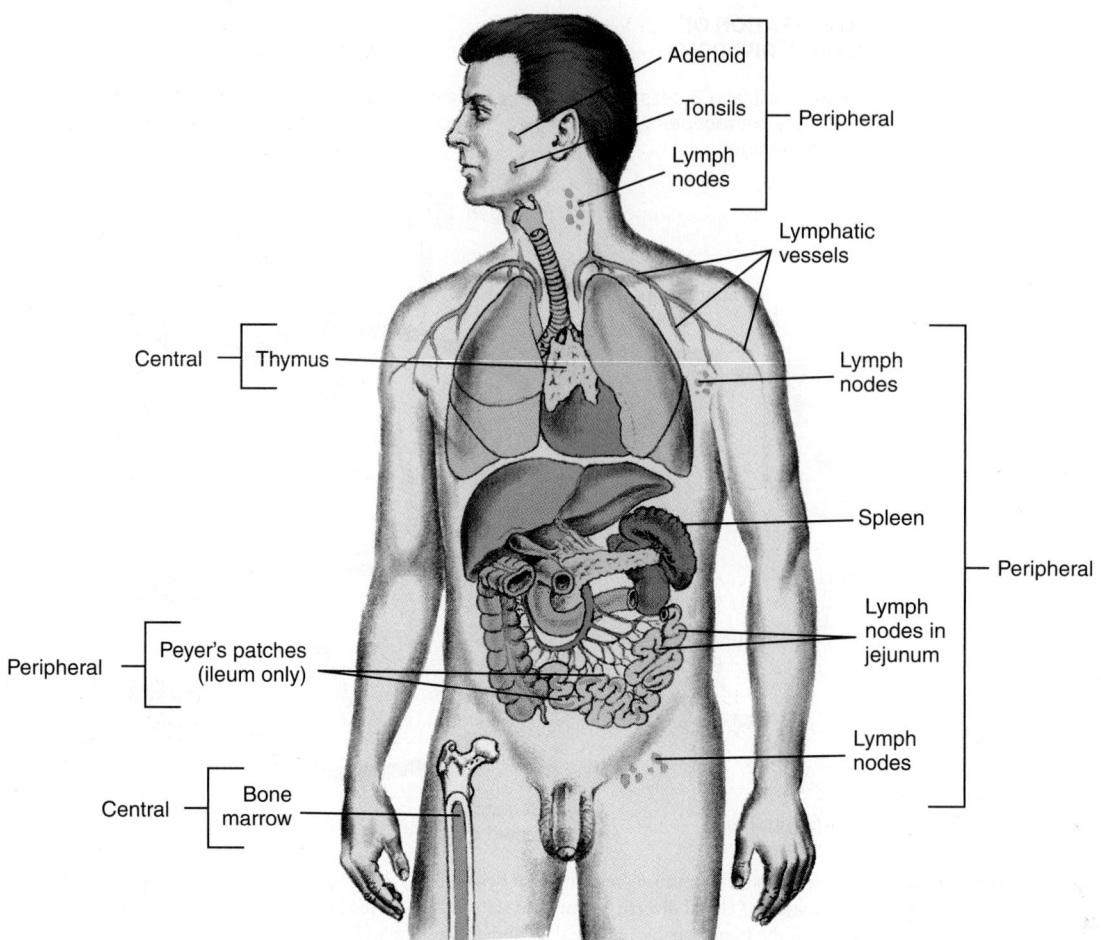

Figure 7-3 **Lymphoid tissues: sites of B cell and T cell differentiation.** Immature lymphocytes migrate through central (primary) lymphoid tissues: the bone marrow (central lymphoid tissue for B lymphocytes) and the thymus (central lymphoid tissue for T lymphocytes). Mature lymphocytes later reside in the T- and B-lymphocyte–rich areas of the peripheral (secondary) lymphoid tissues.

other leukocytes via cell-to-cell contact or through the secretion of cytokines. Others develop into **cytotoxic T cells (Tc cells)** that attack and kill targets directly. Targets for Tc cells include cells infected by a variety of viruses, as well as cells that have become cancerous. This arm of the immune response is termed **cellular immunity.** As discussed in this chapter, the humoral and cellular immune responses are not independent of each other, but instead are interdependent at many levels. In the end, the success of an acquired immune response depends on the functions of both the humoral and cellular responses, as well as the appropriate interactions between them. Additionally, both arms produce specialized subpopulations of **memory cells,** which are capable of "remembering" the antigen and responding more rapidly and efficiently if the associated pathogen invades again.

Active vs. Passive Immunity

Adaptive immunity can be either active or passive, depending on whether the antibodies or T cells are produced by the individual in response to antigen or are administered directly. **Active acquired immunity (active immunity)** is produced by an individual after either natural exposure to an antigen or after immunization, whereas **passive acquired immunity (pas-**

sive immunity) does not involve the host's immune response at all. Rather, passive immunity occurs when preformed antibodies or T lymphocytes are transferred from a donor to the recipient. This can occur naturally, as in the passage of maternal antibodies across the placenta to the fetus, or artificially, as in a clinical immunotherapy for a specific disease.[1] Unvaccinated individuals who are exposed to particular infectious agents (e.g., hepatitis A virus, rabies virus) often will be given immune globulins, which are prepared from individuals who already have antibodies against that particular pathogen. Whereas active acquired immunity is long-lived, passive immunity is only temporary because the donor's antibodies or T cells are eventually destroyed.

RECOGNITION AND RESPONSE

The foundation of any successful immune response is the specific recognition of antigen by antibody or receptors on the surface of B or T cells, followed by a set of complex intercellular communications among a variety of antigen-presenting cells and lymphocytes. To fully understand the immune response, it is necessary to initially understand the basis for that recognition. Many of the molecules discussed in this chapter are part of a nomenclature that uses the prefix "CD" followed by a number (e.g., CD1 or CD2) (Table 7-2). The definition of the **CD (cluster of differentiation)** format has changed over time. It was originally used to describe proteins found on the surface of lymphocytes. Currently, CD is the accepted format for labeling a very large family of proteins found on the surface of many cells. Many have alternative names, which may be used in this chapter. The list of identified molecules is constantly increasing (the number of molecules with a CD designation is probably in excess of 250). In a similar fashion, the list of known cytokines is continually growing, with more than 100 having been identified so far. A large number of CD molecules and cytokines contribute to the acquired immune response. We have attempted here to focus on a small number of highly important examples to illustrate the immensely complicated, but highly effective, interactions that take place to produce a protective immune response.

Antigens and Immunogens

An **antigen** is a molecule that can *react with* antibodies or antigen receptors on B and T cells. Most, but not all, antigens are also **immunogens.** An antigen that is **immunogenic** will induce an immune response resulting in the production of antibodies or functional T cells. Although the terms *antigen* and *immunogen* commonly are used as synonyms, there are some differences between the two, so a substance may be antigenic and yet not be immunogenic.

To function as an antigen, at least a portion of a molecule's chemical structure must be recognized by and bound to an antibody and/or to specific receptors on a lymphocyte. The precise portion of the antigen that is configured for recognition and binding is called its **antigenic determinant,** or **epitope.** The matching portion on the antibody or the lymphocyte receptor is sometimes referred to as the *antigen-binding site,* or **paratope.** The size of an antigenic determinant is relatively small, perhaps just a few amino acids or sugar residues. Therefore, large macromolecules (e.g., proteins, polysaccharides, nucleic acids) usually contain multiple and diverse antigenic determinants, and the immune response against the macromolecule will usually consist of a mixture of specific antibodies against several of these determinants.

Certain criteria influence the degree to which an antigen is immunogenic. These include (1) foreignness to the host, (2) appropriateness in size, (3) having an adequate chemical complexity, and (4) being present in a sufficient quantity.

Foremost among the criteria for immunogenicity is the antigen's foreignness. A **self-antigen** that fulfills all the criteria listed above *except* foreignness does not normally elicit an immune response. Thus most individuals are tolerant to their own antigens. The immune system has an exquisite ability to distinguish self (self-antigens) from non-self (foreign antigens). **Tolerance,** once thought to be a state of nonresponsiveness in which the immune system passively allowed self-antigens to persist, is now known to have a variety of mechanisms. In some cases, a state of **central tolerance** exists, in which lymphocytes with receptors against self-antigens have been eliminated. In other cases, tolerance is **peripheral tolerance** and part of the adaptive immune response. Rather than merely tolerating some self-antigens, the immune system actively prevents their recognition by lymphocytes and antibodies. The response to self-antigens may be actively regulated by specialized T lymphocytes called *T regulatory (Treg) cells,* previously called *T suppressor cells* (see Figure 7-2). Some pathogens have a survival advantage endowed by means of their capacity to mimic self-antigens and avoid inducing an immune response.

Molecular size also contributes to an antigen's immunogenicity. In general, large molecules (those bigger than 10,000 daltons), such as proteins, polysaccharides, and nucleic acids, are most immunogenic. Low-molecular-weight molecules such as amino acids, monosaccharides, fatty acids, and the purine and pyrimidine bases, tend to be unable to induce an immune response. Many molecules in this size range can function as **haptens:** antigens that are too small to be im-

Table 7-2	Select CD Molecules and Their Functions	
CD Molecules	**Primary Location**	**Functions**
CD1	APCs	Presents lipid antigens
CD2	All T cells, NK cells	T-cell marker; adhesion molecule that binds to CD58 (LFA-3) and provides a co-stimulatory signal
CD3	All T cells	Associated with TCR and provides intracellular signaling
CD4	Th cells	Binds to MHC class II as co-receptor with the TCR
CD8	Tc cells	Binds to MHC class I as co-receptor with the TCR
CD19	B cells	Complexes with CD21 to form a co-receptor for B cells
CD20	B cells	Major regulator of B-cell function
CD21	B cells	A receptor for complement that complexes with CD19 to form a co-receptor for B cells
CD25	Activated T cells	IL-2 receptor
CD28	T cells	Adhesion molecule that binds to CD80 to provide co-stimulatory signal for Tc cells
CD40	B cells, macrophages	Adhesion molecule that binds to CD154 to provide co-stimulatory signal for B cells
CD45	All lymphocytes	Has multiple types; augments antigen signal
CD58 (LFA-3)	Most cells	Adhesion molecule that binds to CD2 to provide a co-stimulatory signal
CD80 (B7-1)	APCs	Adhesion molecule that binds to CD28 to provide a co-stimulatory signal
CD154 (CD40L)	Th2 cells	Adhesion molecule that binds to CD40 to provide a co-stimulatory signal

APCs, Antigen-presenting cells; *NK cell,* natural killer cell; *TCR,* T-cell receptor; *Th cell,* helper T cell; *MHC,* major histocompatibility complex; *Tc cell,* cytotoxic T cell.

munogens by themselves but become immunogenic in combination with larger molecules that function as **carriers** for the hapten. For example, the antigens of penicillin and poison ivy are haptens, but they initiate allergic responses only after binding to large-molecular-weight proteins in the allergic individual's blood or skin. Antigens that induce an allergic response are also called **allergens.**

Chemical complexity affects immunogenicity. The best immunogens contain a diversity of chemically different components. For instance, a large synthetic protein consisting only of alanine amino acids would not be very immunogenic, despite its size and foreignness. However, if other amino acids, such as tyrosine, tryptophan, or phenylalanine, were inserted into the structure, the degree of immunogenicity would increase greatly.

Finally, antigens that are present in extremely small or large quantities may be unable to elicit an immune response and therefore by definition are also nonimmunogenic. In many cases, high or low extremes of antigen quantities may induce a state of tolerance rather than immunity.

Even if an antigen fulfills all these criteria, the quality and intensity of the immune response may still be affected by a variety of additional factors. For example, the route and vehicle of antigenic entry or administration are critical to the immunogenicity of some antigens. This has important clinical implications. The most common routes for clinical administration of antigen are intravenous, intraperitoneal, subcutaneous, intranasal, and oral. Each route preferentially stimulates a different set of lymphocyte-containing (lymphoid) tissues and therefore results in the induction of different types of cell-mediated or humoral immune responses. For some vaccines, the route may affect the protectiveness of the immune response so that the individual is protected if immu-

nized by one route, but may remain susceptible to infection if administered through a different route. Immunogenicity of an antigen also may be altered by being delivered along with substances that stimulate the immune response; these substances are known as *adjuvants.* Finally, the genetic makeup of a host can play a critical role in the immune system's ability to respond to many antigens; some individuals appear to be unable to respond to immunization with a particular antigen, whereas they respond well to other antigens. For instance, a small percentage of the population fails to produce a measurable immune response to the most common vaccines, despite multiple injections. Many other factors can modulate the immune response. These include the individual's age, nutritional status, genetic background, and reproductive status, as well as exposure to traumatic injury, concurrent disease, or the use of immunosuppressive medications.

Molecules that Present Antigen

For an effective immune response, most antigens must be processed within cells and expressed on the surface of those cells in a very specific manner. Some types of antigen are managed only by highly specialized cells: **antigen-presenting cells,** or **APCs.** Other types of antigens can be processed and presented by almost any type of cell. Several sets of cell-surface molecules have the responsibility for appropriately presenting antigen. These molecules are described below.

Major Histocompatibility Complex

An essential set of recognition molecules are members of the **major histocompatibility complex (MHC).** Most antibody and cellular immune responses are dependent on antigen presentation by APCs. Additionally, the role of cytotoxic T cells in killing virally infected cells depends on presentation of

Table 7-3	Molecules that Present Antigen		
	MHC Class I	**MHC Class II**	**CD1**
Gene Products	HLA-A HLA-B HLA-C	HLA-DR HLA-DQ HLA-DP	CD1a CD1b CD1c CD1d CD1E (not transcribed)
Characteristics	Single transmembrane polypeptide (α-chain) complexed with β2-microglobulin	Two transmembrane polypeptides (α and β chains)	Single transmembrane polypeptide (α-chain) complexed with β2-microglobulin
	Found on all nucleated cells and platelets	Found on B cells, APCs, and some epithelial cells	Found on APCs
	Presents endogenous antigens derived from intracellular peptides	Presents exogenous antigens derived from phagocytosed and digested extracellular pathogens	Presents exogenous antigens derived from phagocytosed and digested extracellular pathogens
	Presents very small peptide antigens (8-10 amino acids)	Presents larger peptide antigens of variable length	Presents lipid antigens
	Recognized by CD8	Recognized by CD4	Unknown recognition by CD4 or CD8

APCs, Antigen-presenting cells.

the viral antigen on the infected cell's surface. **Antigen presentation** is the primary role of molecules of the MHC.[2]

MHC molecules are glycoproteins found on the surface of all human cells except red blood cells. They are divided into two general classes, class I and class II, based on their molecular structure, distribution among cell populations, and function in antigen presentation. MHC class I molecules are heterodimers composed of a heavy α-chain along with a light chain called β_2 *microglobulin.* MHC class II molecules are also heterodimers with both α- and β-chains. The general properties of each of the MHC classes are summarized in Table 7-3.

Molecules of the two MHC classes are encoded from different genetic loci that are located as a large complex of genes on the short arm of human chromosome 6 (Figure 7-4). The MHC also contains other genes that control the quality and quantity of an immune response, which are commonly referred to as class III MHC genes. The primary **MHC class I**

genes consist of three closely linked loci on this chromosome labeled A, B, and C. The major **MHC class II genes** are located within the D region, which actually consists of three separate and independent loci, DR, DP, and DQ.

The class I and class II MHC loci are the most genetically diverse (polymorphic) of any human genetic loci. Within the human population, the numbers of possible different alleles (i.e., forms of the gene) expressed by each locus is astounding: 303 at the A locus, 559 at the B locus, 150 at the C locus, 439 at the DR locus, 56 at the DQ locus, and 107 at the DP locus. These numbers are based on the polymorphism of observed DNA sequences and may not reflect differences in function. Clearly, not every allele is expressed in the same individual. Humans have two copies of each MHC locus (one inherited from each parent) that are co-dominant so that molecules encoded by each parent's genes are expressed on the cell surface. Within an individual, each locus will be expressing only one

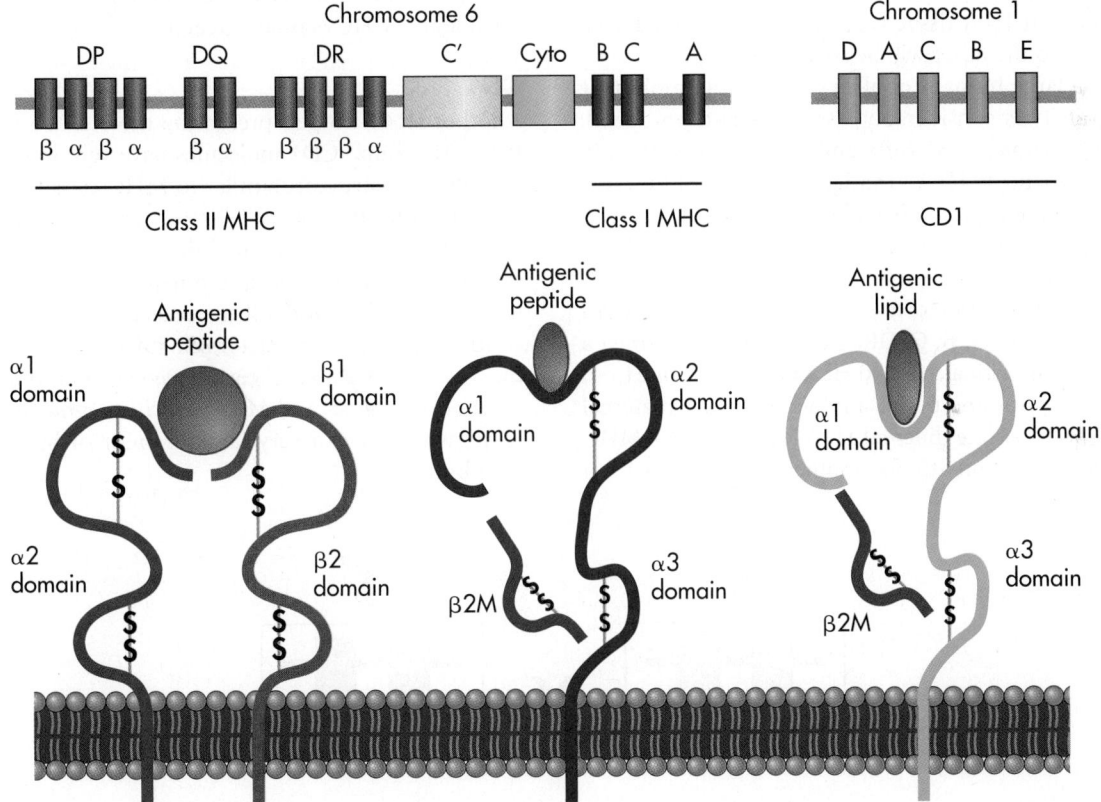

Figure 7-4 **Genetics and structure of antigen-presenting molecules.** Three sets of molecules are primarily responsible for antigen presentation: MHC class I, MHC class II, and CD1. The MHC molecules are encoded from the MHC region on chromosome 6, which contains information for class I and class II molecules, as well as for several other molecules that participate in the innate or immune responses. These include several complement proteins *(C')* and cytokines *(cyto)*, which are referred to as MHC class III molecules. Three principal class I molecules are presented here, HLA-A, HLA-B, and HLA-C, but this region contains information for the α-chains of several other molecules, including HLA-E, HLA-F, and HLA-G. The MHC class I products complex with β2-microglobulin, which is encoded by a gene on chromosome 15. The MHC class I molecules present small peptide antigens in a pocket formed by the α1 and α2 domains of the α-chain. The conformation of the molecule is stabilized by β2-microglobulin as well as by intrachain disulfide bonds *(-S-S-)*. The α- and β-chains of class II molecules are also encoded in this region: HLA-DR, HLA-DP, and HLA-DQ. In some cases, multiple genes for α- and β-chains are available. The MHC class II molecules present peptide antigens in a pocket formed by the α1 domain of the α-chain and β1 domain of the β-chain. The genes for CD1 molecules are encoded on chromosome 1, which contains genes for five α-chains. Only four (CD1A, CD1B, CD1C, and CD1D) are transcribed, and the α-chains complex with β2-microglobulin to present lipid antigens in a pocket formed by the α1 and α2 domains. All three sets of antigen-presenting molecules are anchored to the plasma membrane by hydrophobic regions on the ends of the α and β chains.

allele. For instance, each person will have only two different A proteins (one from each parent). However, with the tremendous number of possible alleles that can be expressed, it is likely that any two unrelated individuals will have different sets of MHC molecules on their cell surfaces.

Transplantation

The diversity of MHC molecules becomes clinically relevant during organ transplantation. Cells in transplanted tissue or organs from one individual will have a different set of MHC surface antigens than those of the recipient, therefore the recipient can mount an immune response against the foreign MHC antigens, resulting in rejection of the transplanted tissue. As a result of studies of transplantation, the human MHC molecules are also referred to as **human leukocyte antigens (HLA)** and the different MHC genetic loci are commonly called HLA-A, HLA-B, HLA-C, HLA-DR, HLA-DQ, and HLA-DP. To minimize the chance of tissue rejection, the donor and recipient are often *tissue typed* beforehand to identify differences in HLA antigens.[3] The more similar two individuals are in their HLA tissue type, the more likely a transplant from one to the other will be successful.

Although a large number of alleles exist at the molecular level, the diversity is considerably less at the antigenic level: there are approximately 67 different HLA-A antigens, 149 HLA-B antigens, and 39 HLA-C antigens. Because of the large number of different alleles, it is highly unlikely that a perfect "match" can be found in the general population between a potential donor and the recipient.

The specific combination of alleles at the six major HLA loci on one chromosome (A, B, C, DR, DQ, and DP) is termed a **haplotype.** Each individual, has two HLA haplotypes, one from the paternal chromosome 6 and another from the maternal chromosome. Because the different HLA loci within the MHC are in such close proximity to one another, haplotypes are not

usually disrupted by recombination and are thus inherited intact. Each parent passes on one HLA haplotype to each of his or her offspring, meaning that children usually share one haplotype with each parent (Figure 7-5). Odds dictate that children will share one haplotype with half of their siblings and either no haplotypes or both haplotypes with a quarter of their siblings. Thus the chance of finding a match among siblings is much higher (25%) than the general population.

It should be noted, however, that although HLA alleles are the primary contributor to rejection of a transplant, a number of other antigens also have a role in determining tissue compatibility. Some of these are encoded on other chromosomes and are inherited independently of HLA antigens. This means that although two people have the same HLA makeup, a graft or transplant still may be rejected because of differences between other antigens. It is preferable to obtain a graft or transplant from a closely related individual, such as a sibling, because the chance of sharing both the same HLA antigens and other undetermined antigenic differences encoded outside the MHC is much greater.

CD1

Another set of antigen-presenting molecules are members of the CD1 group.[4] CD1 molecules have very low genetic polymorphism, a structure similar to MHC class I, and are found primarily on APCs and cells in the thymus. Unlike MHC molecules that present proteins, the CD1 molecules appear to specialize in presenting lipid antigens contained in lipoproteins, glycolipids, and other molecules. These antigens are commonly important factors in infections with bacteria of the *Mycobacterium* spp. (e.g., *Mycobacterium tuberculosis* that causes tuberculosis and *Mycobacterium leprae* that causes leprosy), which have a very large amount of lipid in their cell membranes.

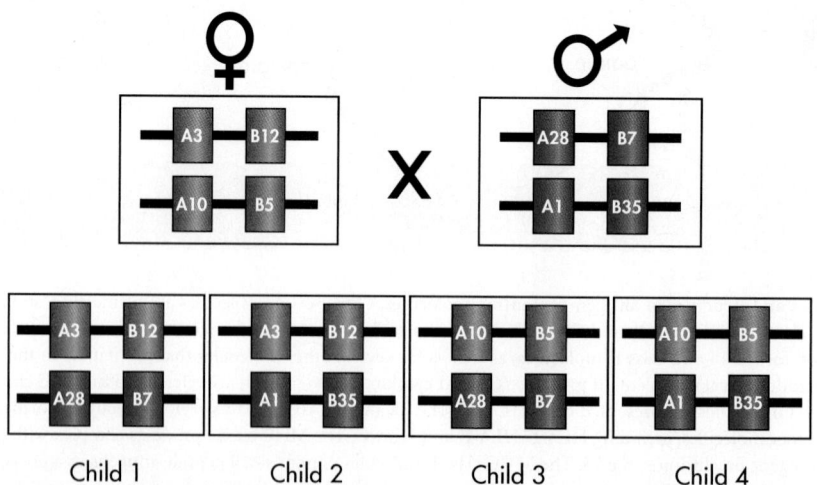

Figure 7-5 Inheritance of HLA. HLA alleles are inherited in a co-dominant fashion so that both maternal and paternal antigens are expressed. Specific HLA alleles are commonly given numbers to indicate different antigens. In this example, the mother has linked genes for HLA-A3 and HLA-B12 on one chromosome 6 and genes for HLA-A10 and HLA-B5 on the second chromosome 6. The father has HLA-A28 and HLA-B7 on one chromosome and HLA-A1 and HLA-B35 on the second chromosome. On one particular chromosome, the HLA antigens are firmly linked, with crossovers occurring in only 1% of individuals. The children from this pairing may have one of four possible combinations of maternal and paternal HLA.

Molecules that Recognize Antigen

Antigen is directly recognized by three molecules: circulating antibody and antigen receptors on the surface of B lymphocytes (**B-cell receptor**, or **BCR**) and T lymphocytes (**T-cell receptor**, or **TCR**) (Figure 7-6).

Antibody

An **antibody,** or immunoglobulin, is a serum glycoprotein produced by plasma cells in response to a challenge by an immunogen. The term *immunoglobulin* is used to denote all molecules that are known to have specificity for antigen,

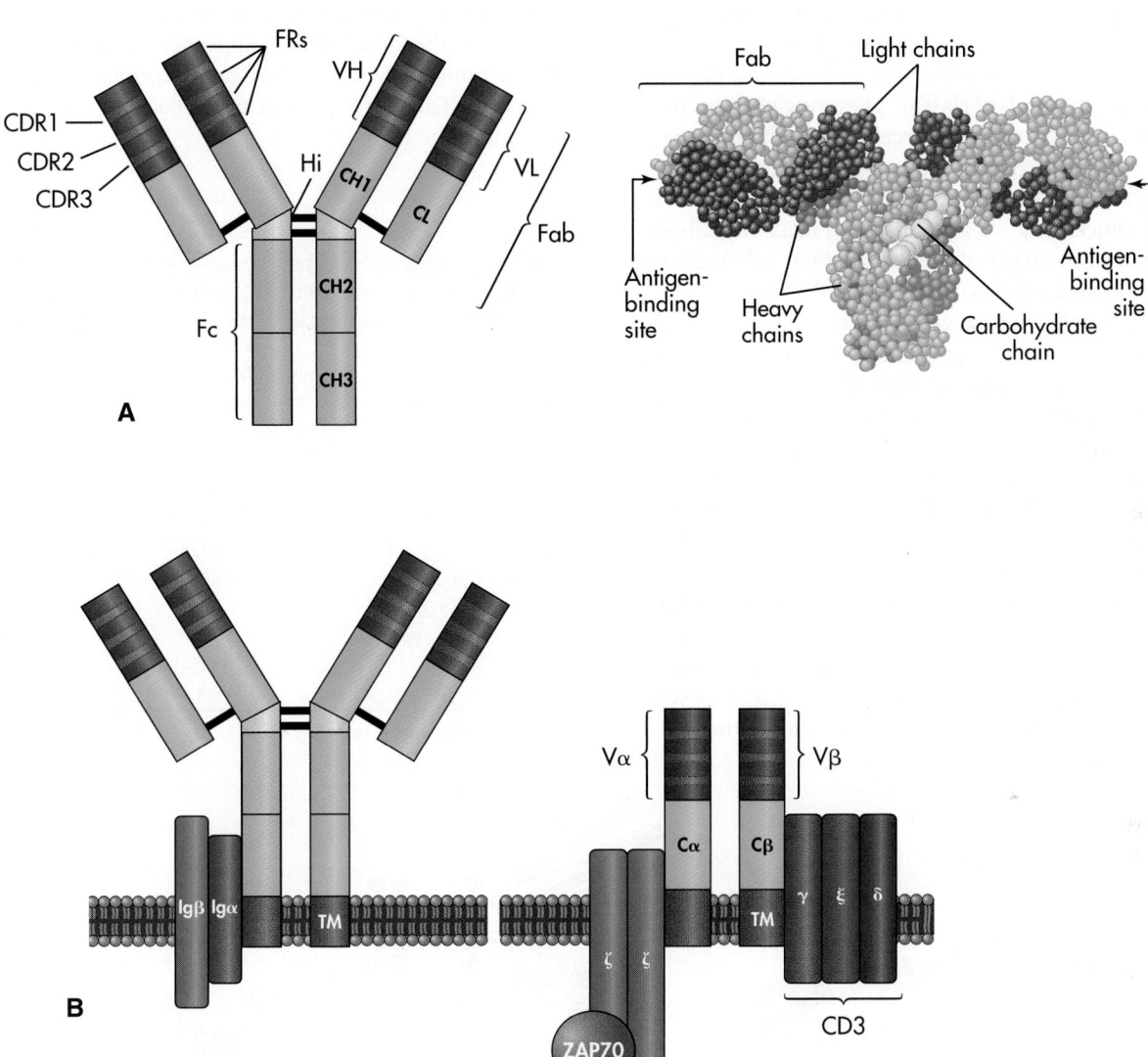

Figure 7-6 Antigen-binding molecules. Antigen-binding molecules include soluble antibody (**A**) and cell-surface receptors (**B**). The typical antibody molecule consists of two identical heavy chains and two identical light chains connected by interchain disulfide bonds (— between chains in the figure). Each heavy chain is divided into three regions with relatively constant amino acid sequences *(CH1, CH2,* and *CH3)* and a region with a variable amino acid sequence *(VH)*. Each light chain is divided into a constant region (CL) and a variable region (VL). The molecule itself has different regions that include an *Fc* and two *Fab* portions. The hinge region *(Hi)* provides flexibility in some classes of antibody. Within each variable region are three highly variable complementary-determining regions *(CDR1, CDR2, CDR3)* separated by relatively constant framework regions *(FRs)*. As the antibody folds (**A** on right), the CDRs are placed in close proximity to form the antigen-binding site. The antigen receptor on the surface of B cells (BCR complex) is a monomeric antibody with a structure similar to circulating antibody, with an additional hydrophobic transmembrane region *(TM)* that anchors the molecule to the cell surface. The active BCR complex contains molecules (Igα and Igβ) that are responsible for intracellular signaling after the receptor has bound antigen. The T-cell receptor (TCR) consists of an α- and a β-chain joined by a disulfide bond. Each chain consists of a constant region *(Cα* and *Cβ)* and a variable region *(Vα* and *Vβ)*. Each variable region contains CDRs and FRs in a structure similar to that of antibody. The active TCR is associated with several molecules that are responsible for intracellular signaling. These include CD3, which is a complex of γ (gamma), ε (epsilon), and δ (delta) subunits and a complex of two ζ (zeta) molecules. The ζ molecules are attached to a cytoplasmic protein kinase *(ZAP70)* that is critical to intracellular signaling. (Insert in **A** from Thibodeau GA, Patton KT: *Anatomy & physiology,* ed 5, St Louis, 2003, Mosby.)

whereas the term *antibody* is generally used to denote one particular set of immunoglobulins with known antigenic specificity. There are five molecular classes of immunoglobulins (IgG, IgA, IgM, IgE, and IgD) that are characterized by antigenic, structural, and functional differences (Figure 7-7). Within two of the immunoglobulin classes are several distinct subclasses including four subclasses of IgG and two subclasses of IgA.

Classes

IgG is the most abundant class of immunoglobulins; they constitute 80% to 85% of those circulating in the body and account for most of the protective activity against infections (Tables 7-4 and 7-5). As a result of selective transport across the placenta, maternal IgG is also the major class of antibody found in blood of the fetus and newborn. Four subclasses of IgG have been described: IgG1, IgG2, IgG3, and IgG4.

IgA can be divided into two subclasses, IgA1 and IgA2. IgA1 molecules are found predominantly in the blood, whereas IgA2 is the predominant class of antibody found in normal body secretions. The IgA molecules found in bodily secretions are dimers anchored together through a J chain and "secretory piece." This secretory piece is attached to the IgAs inside mucosal epithelial cells and may function to protect these immunoglobulins against degradation by enzymes also found in the secretions.

IgM is the largest of the immunoglobulins and usually exists as a pentamer that is stabilized by a J chain. It is the first antibody produced during the initial, or primary, response to antigen. IgM is synthesized early in neonatal life, and its synthesis may be increased as a response to infection *in utero*.

Information on the role of IgD is very limited. This class of immunoglobulins is found in very low concentrations in the blood, where they do not appear to have a known function. IgD is located primarily on the surface of developing B lymphocytes, where they function as one type of B-cell antigen receptors.

IgE is the least concentrated of any of the immunoglobulin classes in the circulation. It appears to have very specialized functions as a mediator of many common allergic responses (see Chapter 8) and in the defense against parasitic infections.

Table 7-4	Physicochemical Properties of Immunoglobulins			
Class	**Subclass**	**Heavy Chain**	**Molecular Weight (daltons)**	**Adult Serum Levels (mg/dl)**
IgG	IgG1	(γ_1)	146,000	800-900
	IgG2	(γ_2)	146,000	280-300
	IgG3	(γ_3)	165,000	90-100
IgG4	(γ_4)	146,000	50	
IgM	IgM	(μ)	970,000	120-150
IgA	IgA1	(α_1)	160,000	280-300
IgA2	(α_2)	50		
sIgA	(α_1, α_2)	385,000	5	
IgD	IgD	(δ)	184,000	3
IgE	IgE	(ϵ)	190,000	0.03

Ig, Immunoglobulin; *s,* secretory.

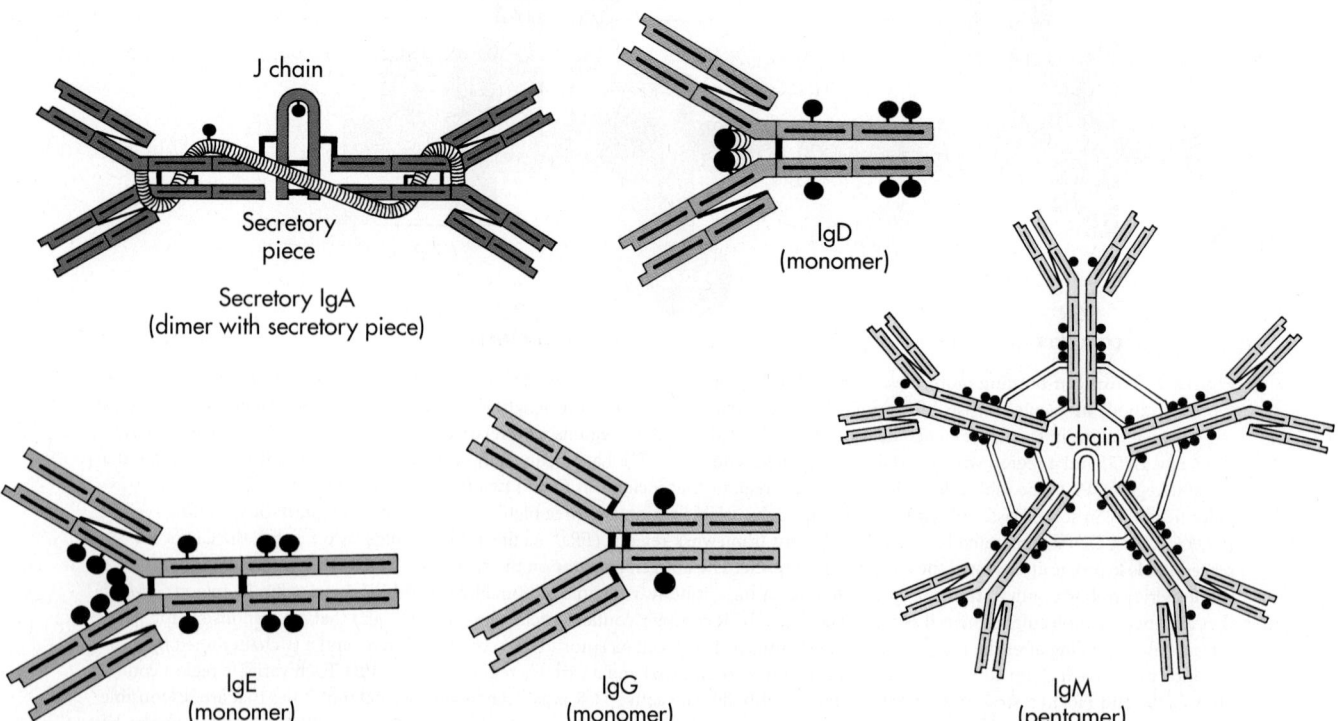

Figure 7-7 **Structure of different immunoglobulins.** Secretory IgA, IgD, IgE, IgG, and IgM. The black circles attached to each molecule represent carbohydrate residues.

Table 7-5	Biologic Properties of Immunoglobulins

Subclass	Complement Activation		Binding to Fc Receptors on				Placental Transfer	Presence in Secretions	Induction of Agglutination
	Classic	Alternate	Macrophages	PMNs	Mast Cells	Platelets			
IgG1	++	−	+	+	−	+	+++	±	+
IgG2	+	−	−	−	−	+	+	±	+
IgG3	+++	−	+	+	−	+	+++	±	+
IgG4	−	−	−	±	+	+	++	±	+
IgM	++++	−	−	−	−	−	−	+	+++
IgA1	−	+	−	±	−	−	−	+	+
IgA2	−	+	−	±	−	−	−	+	−
sIgA	−	−	−	−	−	−	−	++++	−
IgD	−	±	−	−	−	−	−	−	−
IgE	−	±	?	−	+++	−	−	+	−

Fc, Crystalline fragment; *PMN*, polymorphonuclear neutrophil; *Ig*, immunoglobulin; −, lack of activity; +, relative degree of activity; *sIgA*, secretory immunoglobulin A.

Molecular Structure

Structural analysis of immunoglobulins began with Porter's early studies on the effects of the enzyme papain on IgG.[5] The commonly used nomenclature of antibody structure originated from that work. Limited papain digestion cleaved IgG into three fragments, two of which were identical. The two identical fragments were found to retain the ability to bind antigen, and each was termed an **antigen-binding fragment (Fab)**. The third fragment crystallized when separated from the Fab portions and was termed the **crystalline fragment (Fc)** (see Figure 7-6).

What Porter learned about the structure of IgG still applies not only to this class of immunoglobulin but also to each of the other classes. The Fab portions of an immunoglobulin contain the recognition sites (receptors) for antigenic determinants and confer the molecule's specificity towards a particular antigen. The Fc portion is responsible for most of the biologic functions of antibodies, including activation of the complement cascade (see p. 180) and binding to the surface of the cells of the innate immune system to induce phagocytosis.

The basic structure of the antibody molecule consists of four polypeptide chains—two identical light (L) chains and two identical heavy (H) chains (see Figure 7-6). Within the same molecule, the two heavy chains are identical and the two light chains are identical. The class of antibody is determined by which heavy chain is used: gamma (IgG), mu (IgM), alpha (IgA), epsilon (IgE), or delta (IgD). The light chains of an antibody molecule are of either the kappa (κ) or lambda (λ) type. The light and heavy chains are held together by two major forces: noncovalent bonds and disulfide linkages. A set of disulfide linkages between the heavy chains occurs in the **hinge region** and, in some instances, lends a degree of molecular flexibility at that site.

Both light and heavy chains are further subdivided into constant (C) and variable (V) regions. The constant regions have relatively stable amino acid sequences within a particular immunoglobulin class or subclass. Thus the amino acid sequence of the constant region of one IgG1 should be almost identical with the sequence of the same region of another IgG1, even if they react with different antigens. Conversely, among different antibodies, the sequences of the variable regions are characterized by a large number of amino acid differences. Therefore, two IgG1 molecules against different antigens may have many differences in the amino acid sequence of their variable regions. The variable region can be further subdivided because most of the region's viability in amino acid sequence is localized into three areas of the variable region. These three areas were once called *hypervariable regions,* but are now called **complementary-determining regions (CDRs)**. The four regions surrounding the CDRs have relatively stable amino acid sequences and are called **framework regions (FRs)**.

Antigen Binding

The combined amino acid sequences of the variable regions of both the heavy (V_H) and light (V_L) chains determine the conformation of the antigen-binding site and therefore the antigenic specificity of the immunoglobulin molecule.[6] Most proteins will naturally fold and take on secondary or tertiary structures. As the immunoglobulin molecules fold, the FRs control the accuracy of folding, and the CDRs in both variable regions are moved into close proximity, resulting in a antigen-binding site that is lined by the three CDRs of the heavy chain and the three CDRs of the light chain. The chemical nature of the particular amino acids in those sites, as well as the topography of the site, determine specificity towards a particular antigen. The antigen that will bind most strongly must have complementary chemistry and topography with the binding site formed by the antibody. The antigen fits into this binding site with the specificity of a key into a lock and is held there by noncovalent chemical interactions (Figure 7-8). In some cases the substitution of a single critical amino acid may have a significant effect on the shape of the binding site and thus the specificity of the antibody molecule.

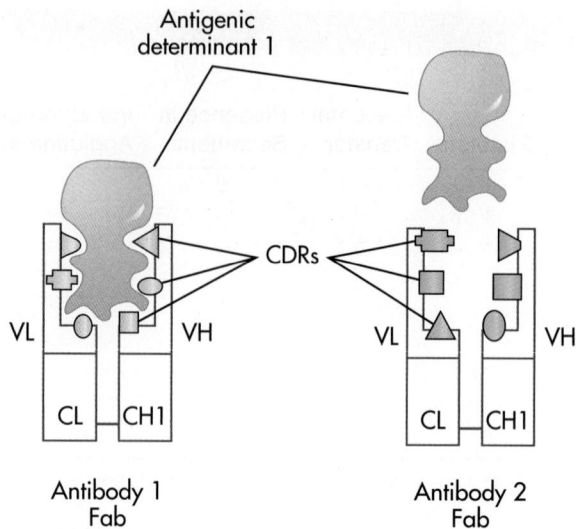

Figure 7-8 Antigen-antibody binding. The specificity required for antibody binding with an antigen is determined by the shape and chemistry of the six complementary-determining regions (*CDRs*) in the combining site on the variable region of the antibody. This figure indicates two different antibodies (Fab portions of antibody 1 and antibody 2), which have different sets of CDRs and, therefore, different specificities. As indicated, the antigenic determinant that reacts well with antibody 1 is unable to react with antibody 2 because of differences in the antibody combining site. *Fab,* Antigen-binding fragment.

Because the heavy and light chains are identical within the same antibody molecule, the two binding sites are also identical and have specificity for the same antigen. The number of functional binding sites is called the antibody's **valence.** Most antibody classes (i.e., IgG, IgE, IgD, and circulating IgA) have a valence of two, but secretory IgA has a valence of four. IgM, being a pentamer, has a theoretical valence of 10, but can simultaneously use only about five binding sites because a large antigen binding to one site blocks antigen binding to another site.

B-Cell Receptor Complex
The **B-cell receptor (BCR) complex** is located on the surface of B lymphocytes (see Figure 7-6). Its role is to recognize antigen, but unlike circulating antibody, the receptor must communicate that information to the cell's nucleus.[7] Therefore, the BCR complex consists of antigen-recognition molecules (antibody of the IgM or IgD classes) and accessory molecules involved in intracellular signaling (Igα and Igβ). BCRs on the surface of immunocompetent B cells are membrane-associated IgM and IgD immunoglobulins that are produced from the same genes that are used by plasma cells to produce soluble antibodies. As a BCR, however, IgM is a monomer rather than the pentamer primarily found in the blood.

The BCR signaling complex consists of two Igα and Igβ heterodimers, which are closely associated with the BCR and contain tyrosine kinase signaling activity. The antibody portion of the BCR complex is responsible for recognition and binding to an antigen, but by itself cannot provide the intracellular signals required to activate the B cell, resulting in its

complete maturation and the production of antibodies. That message is conveyed by the Igα and Igβ heterodimers.

T-Cell Receptor Complex
T lymphocytes use a similar but distinct array of proteins in their recognition and response to antigens. The **T-cell receptor (TCR) complex** is composed of an antibody-like transmembrane protein (*TCR*) and a group of accessory proteins (collectively referred to as *CD3*) that are involved in intracellular signaling[8] (see Figure 7-6). Similar to activation of the B lymphocyte, the TCR is responsible for recognition and binding to the antigen, whereas the accessory proteins are responsible for the intracellular signaling necessary for activation and differentiation of the T cell. Each of the individual components of the TCR complex is important, and several severe defects in the T-cell immune response have been related to mutations in individual components of the complex (see Chapter 8).

Molecules that Hold Cells Together
The efficient development of an immune response requires several antigen-independent interactions between cells. The interactions between specific cellular receptors and their ligands result in intracellular signaling events that are independent of the TCR or BCR complexes but are necessary complements to the antigen-specific signal. Several of these molecules are listed in Box 7-1.

Cytokines and Their Receptors
As discussed in Chapter 6, cytokines are low-molecular-weight proteins, or glycoproteins, that function as chemical signals between cells. Cytokines are produced by a wide variety of cells and play important roles not only in inflammation but also in the acquired immune response. A large number of cytokines secreted by APCs and lymphocytes provide both positive and negative regulation of the response. The effects of particular cytokines depend on binding to specific cellular receptors, which are linked to intracellular signaling pathways. The target cell may respond in many ways. One of the most common responses is an increase in the production of proteins, many of which are other cytokines or cytokine receptors. Many cytokines also cause a target cell to proliferate and differentiate. Many are growth factors that induce the proliferation and differentiation of cells other than lymphocytes,

including cells of the inflammatory response and hematopoietic blood cells (see Chapter 25). Because these effects are shared among cytokines, the system has a great deal of redundancy in that different cytokines have similar effects on the same targets. On the other hand, some cytokines are antagonistic, in that two different cytokines induce opposite effects on the same cell. The participation of cytokines is essential to the development of an adequate immune response, and in general, the precise combination of cytokines influences the ultimate response of a given cell. Specific deficiencies in the immune response that result from genetic mutations that lead to defective cytokine production or defective cytokine receptors are discussed in Chapter 8. Table 7-6 provides information about key cytokines and receptors that are known to influence the immune response.

GENERATION OF CLONAL DIVERSITY

It has been suggested that more than 10^8 different antigenic determinants may be recognized by receptors on an individual's immunocompetent B cells. A similar number may be recognized by T-cell receptors. However, each T or B cell has only a single receptor specificity that recognizes only one antigen, and each is present before that individual is ever exposed to foreign antigen. Thus before the individual is exposed to any foreign antigen, millions of different T- and B-cell antigen receptors must be constructed to recognize *any* potential antigenic determinant.

Several theories were proposed to explain how such a great diversity of recognition could be produced. The process occurs in two phases: the **generation of clonal diversity,** during

Table 7-6　Key Cytokines and Receptors that Influence the Immune Response

Cytokine	Primary Source	Primary Function
Interleukins (IL)		
IL-1	APCs	Stimulates T cells to proliferation and differentiation; induces acute phase proteins in inflammatory response; endogenous pyrogen
IL-2	Th1 cells, NK cells	Stimulates proliferation and differentiation of T cells and NK cells
IL-4	Th2 cells, mast cells	Induces B-cell proliferation and differentiation; up-regulates MHC class II expression; induces class-switch to IgE
IL-5	Th2 cells, mast cells	Induces eosinophil proliferation and differentiation; induces B-cell proliferation and differentiation
IL-6	Th2 cells, APCs	Induces B-cell proliferation and differentiation; induces acute phase proteins in inflammatory response
IL-7	Thymic epithelial cells, bone marrow stromal cells	Major cytokine for induction of B- and T-cell proliferation and differentiation in the central lymphoid organs
IL-8	Macrophages	Chemotactic factor for neutrophils and T cells
IL-10	Th cells, B cells	Inhibits cytokine production; activator of B cells
IL-12	B cells, APCs	Induces NK-cell proliferation; increases production of IFN-γ
IL-13	Th2 cells	IL-4–like properties; decreases inflammatory responses
Interferons (INF)		
IFN-α, IFN-β	Macrophages, some virally infected cells	Antiviral; increases expression of MHC class I; activates NK cells
IFN-γ	Th1 cells, NK cells, Tc cells	Increases expression of MHC class II; activates macrophages and NK cells
Tumor Necrosis Factors (TNF)		
TNF-α (cachectin)	Macrophages	IL-1–like properties; induces cellular proliferation
TNF-β (lymphotoxin)	Tc cells	Kills some cells; increases phagocytosis by macrophages and neutrophils
Transforming Growth Factor (TGF)		
TGF-β	Lymphocytes, Macrophages, fibroblasts	Chemotactic for macrophages; increases macrophage IL-1 production; stimulates wound healing

Cytokine Receptors

Type of Receptor	Ligand	Additional Information
Class I receptors		
Dimers (α and β chains)	IL-3, IL-5, IL-6, IL-11, IL-12, IL-13	IL-3 and IL-5 share a common β chain; IL-6 and IL-11 share a common β chain
Trimers (α, β, and γ chains)	IL-2, IL-4, IL-7, IL-9, IL-15	All share a common γ chain
Class II receptors	IFNα, β, and γ	Two chains
TNF receptors	TNF-α, TNF-β, CD40, Fas	Single chain
Immunoglobulin-like receptors	IL-1	Single chain with immunoglobulin-like characteristics

APCs, Antigen-presenting cells; *Th cells,* helper T cells; *NK cells,* natural killer cells; *Tc cells;* cytotoxic T cells; *MHC,* major histocompatibility complex.

which all the necessary receptor specificities are produced, and **clonal selection,** during which antigen selects those lymphocytes with compatible receptors, expands their population, and causes differentiation into antibody-secreting plasma cells or mature T cells[9,10] (Table 7-7). The generation of clonal diversity takes place in the **primary (central) lymphoid organs** (i.e., thymus and bone marrow), is driven by hormones, does not require foreign antigen, and results in the generation of immature but immunocompetent T and B cells with receptors that can recognize virtually any antigenic molecule. Both T and B cells are derived from common precursor cells (**lymphoid stem cells**) that arise in either the liver (in the fetus) or in the bone marrow (of a child or adult). These precursor cells are distinct from the precursor cells that give rise to cells of the innate immune system. The immunocompetent T and B cells migrate from the primary lymphoid organs to **secondary (peripheral) lymphoid organs** (e.g., spleen, lymph nodes, adenoids, tonsils, Peyer's patches), where they await antigen. Clonal selection is initiated by antigen and results in a mature and specific immune response against that antigen.

Although generation of clonal diversity primarily occurs in the fetus, it probably continues to a low degree throughout most of adult life. Clonal selection can begin at about the eighth week of gestation in humans and proceeds throughout the life of the individual as new antigens are encountered.

As a result of this process, T and B lymphocytes have the capacity to react against virtually any antigen found in nature. This endless array of possible antibodies and TCRs certainly cannot be constructed from the amount of DNA that is in the nucleus of a human lymphocyte. The enormous repertoire of specificities is instead made possible by rearrangement of existing DNA during T and B cell development in the primary lymphoid organs. Loci in the DNA that encode for the variable regions of immunoglobulins and TCRs are recombined in a unique way to generate receptors that collectively can recognize and bind to any possible antigen. The DNA in the nucleus of a developing T and B cell is actually cut and spliced

(repaired), a process known as **somatic recombination,** so that after this manipulation, the progeny of a single lymphocyte will synthesize identical immunoglobulins or TCRs. Those variable regions, however, are cut and spliced differently from those of another lymphocyte, making each cell unique and therefore able to react with different antigens. The particular process for B and T cells is discussed below.

T-Cell Maturation
Central Lymphoid Organ
The central lymphoid organ for T-cell development is the thymus, which is an organ located near the heart. Precursor cells (lymphoid stem cells) arise in early embryonic life from the yolk sac and fetal liver and later from the bone marrow. They migrate to the thymus and enter in the subcapsular region.[11-13] As the cells move through the thymic cortex to the medulla, they are instructed by interactions with various thymic cells (epithelial cells, macrophages, and dendritic cells) and thymic hormones to undergo proliferation and progressive development of the characteristics of immunocompetent T cells (Figure 7-9). Changes include the development of the T-cell receptor complex and expression of characteristic surface molecules. Many developing T cells randomly develop TCRs against self-antigens and undergo negative selection resulting in the deletion of a large number of self-reactive T cells. The final antigen-reactive T cells are released into the blood and take up residence in the secondary lymphoid organs to await antigen.

Production of the T-Cell Receptor
Like antibody, the **T-cell receptor (TCR)** reacts with antigen (see Figure 7-6). The TCR structure closely resembles a Fab portion of antibody, with two protein chains held together by a disulfide linkage. However, the TCR uses different protein chains than are used for antibody. The most common TCR contains α- and β-chains, each of which has a variable region and a constant region. Within each variable region are three CDR regions separated by FR regions.

Table 7-7	Generation of Clonal Diversity vs. Clonal Selection	
	Generation of Clonal Diversity	**Clonal Selection**
Purpose?	To produce large numbers of T and B lymphocytes with the maximum diversity of antigen receptors	Select, expand, and differentiate clones of T and B cells against a specific antigen
When does it occur?	Primarily in the fetus	Primarily after birth and throughout life
Where does it occur?	Central lymphoid organs: thymus for T cells, bone marrow for B cells	Peripheral lymphoid organs, including lymph nodes, spleen, and other lymphoid tissues
Is foreign antigen involved?	No	Yes, antigen determines which clones of cells will be selected
What hormones/cytokines are involved?	Thymic hormones, IL-7, others	Many cytokines produced by Th cells and APCs
Is tolerance induced?	Central tolerance induced as autoreactive cells are deleted	Peripheral tolerance induced as autoreactive cells are regulated
Final product?	Immunocompetent T and B cells that can react with antigen, but have not seen antigen, and migrate to the secondary lymphoid organs	Plasma cells that produce antibody, effector T cells that help (Th), kill targets (Tc), or regulate immune responses (Treg); memory B and T cells

Th cells, Helper T cells; *APCs,* antigen-presenting cells; *Tc cells,* cytotoxic T cells; *Treg cells,* regulatory T cells.

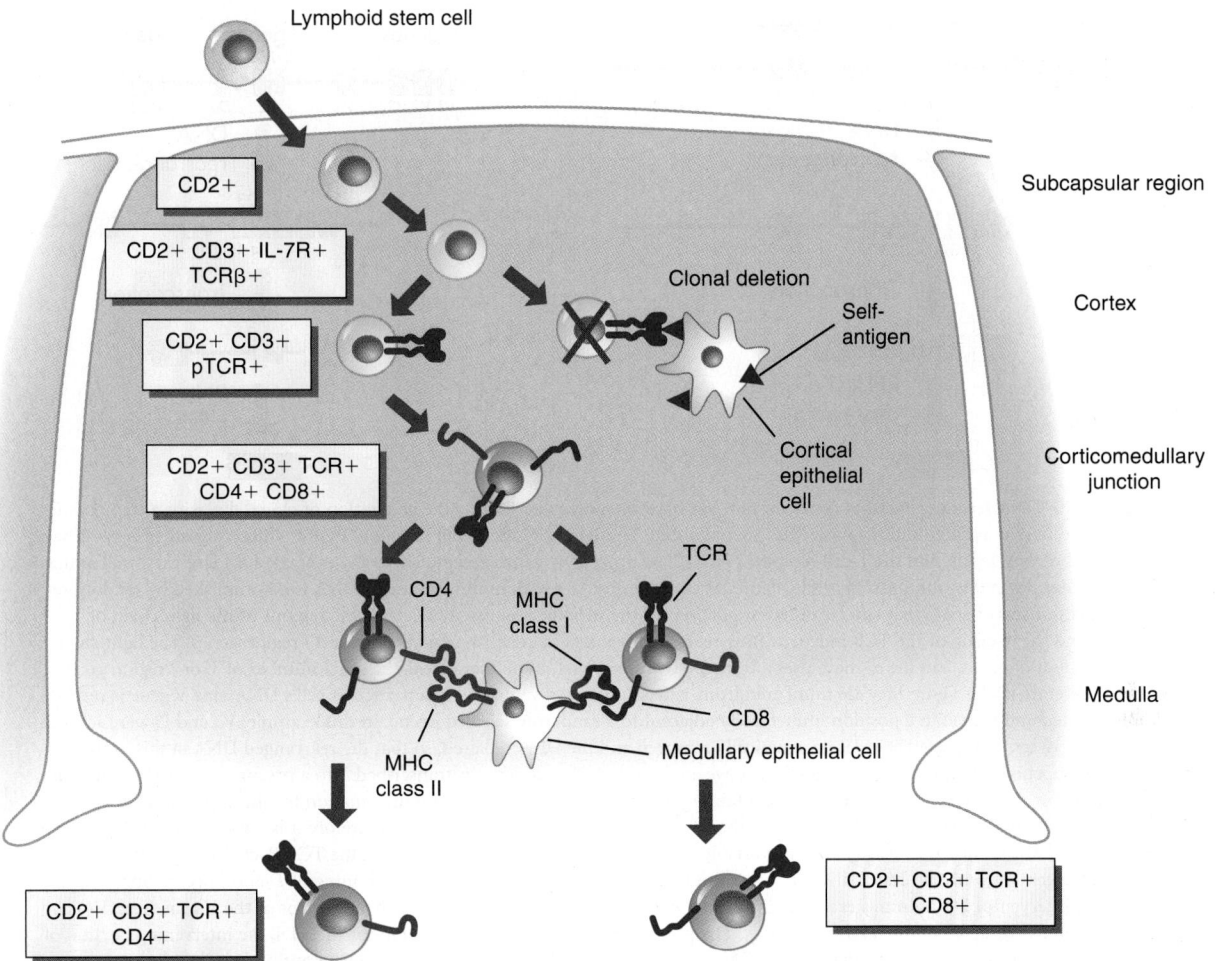

Figure 7-9 T-cell development in the thymus. During the generation of clonal diversity in the fetus, lymphoid stem cells undergo several stages of cellular division and differentiation in a central lymphoid organ (the thymus) under the control of hormones but without the influence of foreign antigen. A simplified scheme for that process is presented here. The differentiation process is characterized by the up-regulation of many important surface molecules (only some of which are shown) and the random development of a huge number of different T-cell receptors against all possible antigens that the adult may encounter. The lymphoid stem cell enters the subcapsular region of the thymus where it begins to undergo differentiation. One of the first surface changes is the appearance of the molecule CD2, which is a marker for all T cells. In the cortex of the thymus, the developing cell encounters epithelial cells that guide most of the early differentiation process. The pre–T cell begins expressing the surface receptor for the cytokine IL-7, which is produced by the epithelial cell along with other thymic hormones to drive the T-cell differentiation process. At this stage the T cell begins constructing the T-cell receptor (TCR) by first rearranging and expressing the TCR β-chain (more detail is provided in Figure 7-10) and expressing CD3 molecules. Although the TCR α-chain has not yet been produced, the β-chain is expressed on the surface as a pre-TCR (pTCR) using a protein that acts as a surrogate for the α-chain. Because of the randomness of the process, some pTCRs are produced with specificities towards self-antigens. Many of these undergo negative selection and are deleted (clonal deletion) by apoptosis induced through interactions with self-antigens presented by the epithelial cells. Survivors of negative selection move towards the thymic cortex and begin expressing the TCR α-chain, the normal TCR, and both CD4 and CD8 on their surfaces. These CD4+, CD8+ "double-positive" cells encounter medullary epithelial cells that express both MHC class I and class II molecules. The phenotype of the developing T cell is positively selected so that interaction between CD4 and MHC class II selects for retention of CD4 expression, whereas interaction between CD8 and MHC class I favors the CD8 phenotype. Thus two populations of "single-positive" immunocompetent T cells leave the thymus: one cell is CD4+, CD8− (destined to be a helper T [Th] cell) and the other is CD4−, CD8+ (destined to be a cytotoxic T [Tc] cell).

The great amount of variable region diversity necessary for identifying the huge number of antigens found in nature is produced by random recombination of multiple genes to encode the variable regions of both the α- and β-chains. In the germ line genes, the information for the amino acid sequence of the α-chain variable region is found on chromosome 14 in two separated, but closely associated, locations: a set of V re-

gion genes and a set of J region genes (Figure 7-10). The TCR α-chain locus has multiple (at least 50) V genes and multiple (at least 50) J genes. During somatic recombination in a developing T cell, one of the possible V genes is randomly selected and spliced to one of the J genes, with the intervening DNA being removed. This DNA rearrangement process is controlled by two enzymes produced by the genes RAG-1 and

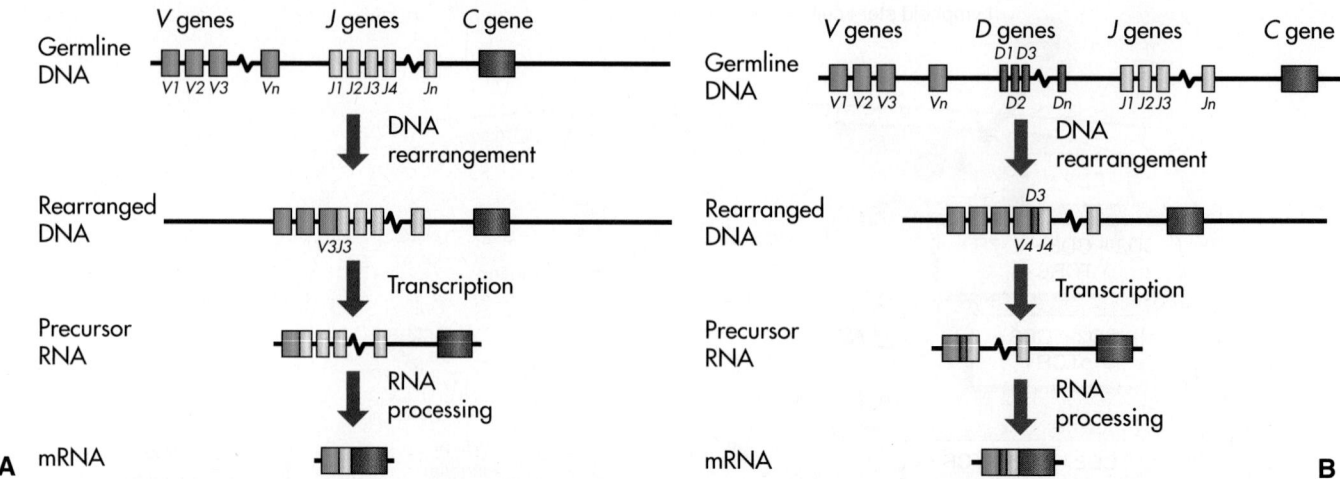

Figure 7-10 DNA rearrangement of genes for antigen-binding molecules. During the generation of clonal diversity, a tremendous number of different antigen-binding molecules are produced. These include the B-cell receptor (BCR), which consists of a membrane-bound antibody molecule, and the T-cell receptor (TCR). The process by which receptor diversity is created is identical for all antigen-binding molecules and is summarized in this figure. Maximum diversity with minimum use of DNA is accomplished by random rearrangement of sets of genes that encode different portions of the variable regions. **A,** The variable regions of the light chain of antibody and the α-chain of the TCR independently rearrange two sets of genes: V region genes and J region genes. The light chain uses its own set of genes, and the α-chain uses a completely different set. In neither case is the exact number of V or J region genes known; therefore in this figure they are numbered from 1 to an unknown value (*n*). In a particular cell's DNA, one V gene is randomly selected and moved to a position immediately adjacent to a randomly selected J gene. In this example, V3 and J3 were selected. The DNA between the selected genes is enzymatically removed and the DNA repaired, so that the rearranged DNA in this example is missing the portion found in the germline DNA between V3 and J3. This product is transcribed into a precursor RNA that contains information for the rearranged VJ pair, a span containing other unselected J regions, and information for the appropriate constant region (C gene) of the molecule. The RNA between the VJ and the C regions is *not* translated, therefore it is removed by RNA processing to produce an mRNA that *is* translated. **B,** The variable region of the antibody heavy chain and the TCR β-chain results from a similar DNA rearrangement, with the added diversity contributed by a group of D region genes. The joining of D and J occurs first, with the removal of intervening DNA. In this example, D3 and J4 were chosen. This is followed by rearrangement of the V gene (e.g., V4) and formation of a VDJ region in the rearranged DNA. The precursor RNA contains information for the VDJ, the intervening portion of DNA, and the appropriate constant region. After RNA processing, an mRNA is formed for the intact antibody heavy chain or the TCR β-chain. Once the DNA is rearranged and spliced in a given B or T cell, all of the antigen receptors produced by that cell employ the same V, D, and J segments and have the same specificity.

RAG-2 (recombination activating genes). These enzymes cut double-stranded DNA at specific recognition sites (recombinant signal sequences), then repair the break resulting in excision of the DNA between the selected V and J genes. At transcription, the genetic information for the α-chain variable region is still separated from the gene for the α-chain constant region. This product is transcribed into messenger RNA (mRNA) that contains information for the variable region (VJ) separated by a span of RNA from the information for the α-chain constant region. An RNA processing step removes the intervening span, bringing the message for the variable and constant regions together into a final mRNA product that is translated into the intact α-chain protein. The random selection and pairing of 50 V and 50 J genes by a large number of developing T cells can potentially result in more than 2500 possible α-chains.

In a similar fashion, the TCR β-chain locus on chromosome 7 has three sets of multiple genes that rearrange to encode the variable region of that chain: at least 20 V genes, 13 J genes, and 2 intervening and relatively short D genes that add further diversity. Using the RAG-1 and RAG-2 enzymes, a developing T cell randomly selects a set of V, D, and J genes

for DNA recombination. The VDJ rearranged segment is transcribed with a β-chain constant region, the intervening RNA is removed during processing, and the final mRNA is translated into an intact β chain.

The α- and β-chains are joined by that cell and inserted into the membrane to make an antigen-specific TCR. The enormous number of possible combinations of α-chain V and J regions along with the β-chain V, D, and J regions enables the generation of a population of T cells with a large diversity of TCRs. For both chains, the V region genes encode the amino acid sequences that include CDR1 and CDR2 and their appropriate FR regions. The J regions contain information for CDR3 and FR4. The TCR β-chain D regions encode a short amino acid sequence found in the CDR3 and greatly increases the diversity of the β-chain CDR3. Imprecise joining increases the diversity of the CDR3 regions of both the α- and β-chains even further. For example, the sites of VJ and VDJ joining may shift slightly resulting in an amino acid being inserted or deleted from the protein.

Although the αβ TCR is the preferred antigen receptor, some T cells use alternative genes: gamma (γ) (chromosome 7) and delta (δ) (chromosome 14, in middle of α-chain genes). T cells with γδ TCRs appear to migrate to unique areas of the body (the epithelial areas in the skin, reproductive tract, intestine, respiratory tract) and have different and less well understood functions than the T cells with αβ TCRs.

Changes in Characteristic Surface Markers

Differentiation of T cells in the thymus also results in changes in a variety of important surface molecules. As the developing T cells move through the thymic cortex, they initiate the expression of the molecule CD2 on the cell surface. CD2 is a marker for T cells and is expressed on virtually every subpopulation of cells that have undergone development in the thymus. Within the cortex, the cells begin rearranging the variable region genes necessary for forming a functional T-cell receptor. The T-cell receptor undergoes several stepwise changes until the final αβ TCR is formed. Concurrently, the TCR accessory molecules that make up CD3 are expressed. The cell also begins making two important surface proteins, CD4 and CD8, which are concurrently expressed on the developing cell's surface at this stage. These CD4+, CD8+ cells are often called "double-positive" cells. Much of T-cell development is controlled by hormones and cytokines in the thymus, and an early step in maturation is expression of the receptor for IL-7 (IL-7R), which is a major cytokine that drives the differentiation process. After entering the medulla of the thymus, the double-positive cells become "single-positive." That is, some of the cells suppress production of the CD8 molecule and remain only CD4+, whereas others suppress CD4 production and remain CD8+. This branch in the differentiation pathway leads to two groups of cells with different functional characteristics: CD4 cells tend to recognize antigen presented by MHC class II molecules and develop into helpers in the later clonal selection process (helper T cells), whereas CD8 cells recognize antigen presented by MHC class I molecules and become mediators of cell-mediated immunity and kill other cells directly (cytotoxic T cells).

Central Tolerance

During the random rearrangement of *VJ* and *VDJ* genes to produce the T-cell receptor, some combinations result in specificities that recognize self-antigens. A severe immunologic reaction against the individual's own tissues could result if some of these *autoreactive* T cells were allowed to progress further in development and leave the thymus. One stage at which tolerance for self-antigens is maintained is the deletion of autoreactive T cells in the thymus, which is referred to as central tolerance.

A variety of self-antigens are expressed by thymic cells. Many cells express MHC class I or MHC class II molecules. During the T cell's double-positive stage, if a TCR strongly reacts with MHC class I or class II, the T cell will undergo apoptosis, referred to as *clonal deletion*. A large spectrum of other self-antigens are expressed on the surface of thymic macrophages, dendritic cells, and especially epithelial cells. If a developing T cell's TCR binds strongly with a self-antigen, it is deleted. Although this process of *negative selection* induces more than 95% of T cells to undergo apoptosis in the thymus,

a limited number of autoreactive clones persist and must be controlled by other means in the peripheral lymphoid organs (**peripheral tolerance**).

The destiny of the double-positive cells with TCRs specific for foreign antigens (which are not expressed in the thymus) is determined by their interaction in the thymus with MHC antigens. If their surface CD4 molecules bind to MHC class II molecules on the thymic cells, the T cell will become CD4 single-positive. However, if their surface CD8 reacts with MHC class I molecules, the cells will become CD8 single-positive. This *positive selection* process results in about 60% of immunocompetent T cells being CD4+ and 40% being CD8+ when they leave the thymus.

B-Cell Maturation
Central Lymphoid Organ

Although the thymus is the central lymphoid organ for T-cell development, humans do not appear to have a discrete organ for B-cell development. In chickens, B lymphocytes undergo differentiation in an organ called the *bursa of Fabricius*. In humans, portions of the bone marrow function as a bursal-equivalent tissue for B-cell development.[14]

Regardless of the lack of a discrete organ, B-cell differentiation undergoes a very similar process to that described above for T cells. Lymphoid stem cells in the bone marrow interact with stromal cells through a variety of intercellular adhesion molecules (Figure 7-11). As the stem cell begins to mature, it progressively develops a variety of necessary surface markers, the earliest being CD45R and the IL-7 receptor. IL-7, produced by the stromal cells, is critical in driving the further differentiation and proliferation of the B cell. The next stage in development is formation of the B-cell receptor.

Production of the B-Cell Receptor

The **B-cell receptor (BCR)** is an antibody that is anchored to the plasma membrane. The process by which BCR diversity is generated is virtually identical to the process in T cells and also requires the genetic rearrangement of V, D, and J genes.[15] The segments of DNA that encode either kappa (κ) (chromosome 2) or lambda (λ) (chromosome 22) light chains contain about 70 V and 5 J segments, whereas the heavy chain locus on chromosome 14 contains about 80 V, 30 D, and 6 J regions. The locus for the antibody heavy chain also contains multiple sequential regions for different constant regions, with the gene for the mu (μ) constant region being closest to the VDJ region, and the delta (δ) constant region gene being next in sequence (Figure 7-12). These are followed by the constant region genes for other classes and subclasses. In the developing B cell, the initial RNA transcript contains information for the *VDJ* recombination, the μ constant region, and the δ constant region. Transcription is signaled to stop immediately after the δ constant region. During the following RNA processing step to form a final mRNA product, the cell can alternatively process one mRNA to retain the μ constant region only or process another mRNA molecule to remove the μ constant region and retain the δ constant region. Thus one cell can use multiple

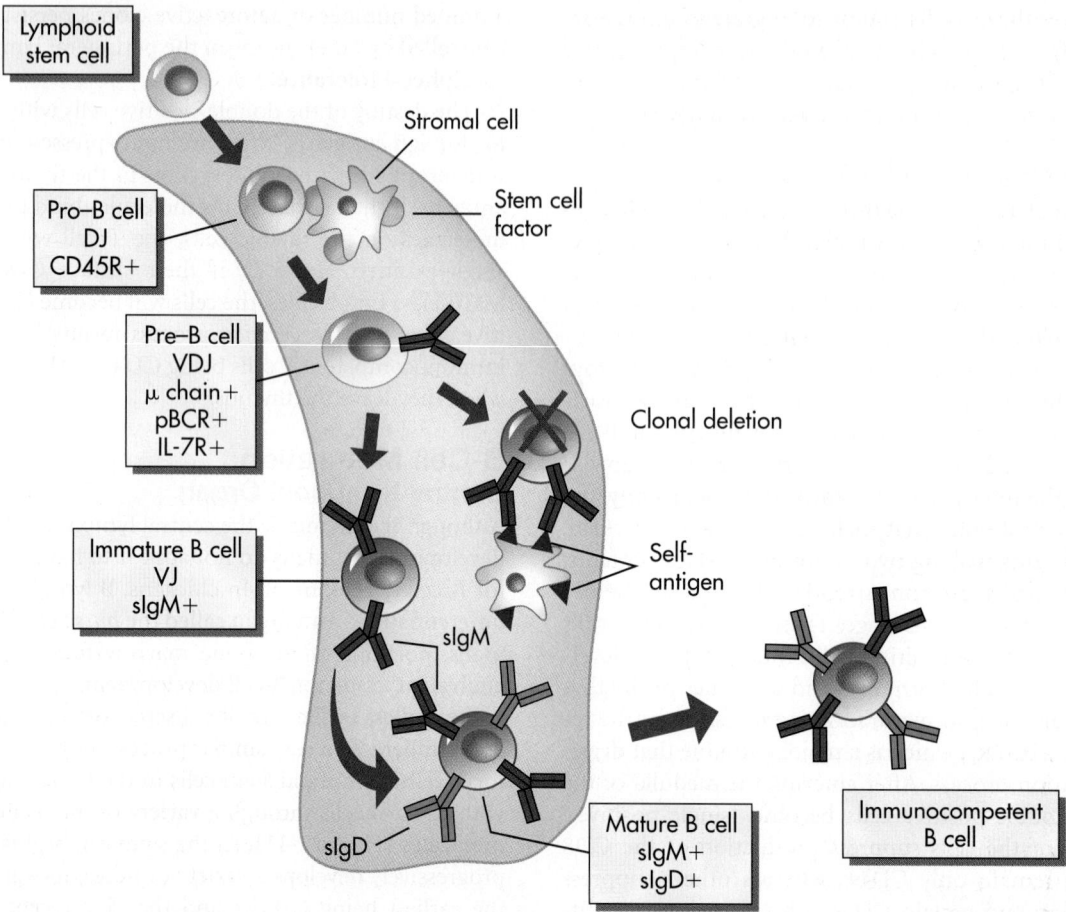

Figure 7-11 B-cell development in the bone marrow. During the generation of clonal diversity, lymphoid stem cells enter portions of the bone marrow that serve as the central lymph organ for B-cell development. Interactions with a series of bone marrow stromal cells guide the proliferation and differentiation process through direct cell-to-cell contact and the production of cytokines and hormones by the stromal cells, but without the presence of foreign antigen. A simplified scheme for that process is presented here. As with T-cell development, the differentiation process of B cells is characterized by the up-regulation of many important surface molecules (only some of which are shown) and the random development of a huge number of different B-cell receptors. The early B cell (pro–B cell) binds to a membrane-bound cytokine (stem cell factor) on the stromal cell and initiates expression of the surface molecule CD45R and begins to rearrange the *DJ* regions of the antibody heavy chain gene. As the cell progresses to the pre–B-cell stage, it concludes DNA rearrangement of the heavy chain *(VDJ)* and begins expressing cytoplasmic mu (μ) heavy chain. The μ chain is incorporated into a pre-B-cell receptor (pBCR) using a surrogate protein in place of the light chain. The cell also up-regulates the IL-7 receptor (IL-7R), which interacts with IL-7 produced by the stromal cells to drive the remaining steps in differentiation. Some pBCRs have specificities towards self-antigen. Many of these encounter self-antigen expressed on the stromal cells and undergo negative selection (clonal deletion). The surviving cells (immature B cells) rearrange the light chain DNA *(VJ)* and express a BCR consisting of light chain and the μ heavy chain (surface IgM [sIgM]). In the mature B cell, changes in processing of the heavy chain precursor RNA results in co-expression of surface IgM and IgD (sIgD) (see Figure 7-12 for more details).

Figure 7-12 Genetics of the B-cell receptor. Most mature immunocompetent B cells express both surface IgM and IgD as the B-cell receptor. In the germline DNA, the heavy chain gene complex consists of a series of *V, D, J,* and constant region genes. In humans, each class and subclass of antibody has a unique constant region gene arranged in the indicated order. Switch regions occur preceding every constant region gene, except mu (μ)(IgM) and delta (δ) (IgD). After successful DNA rearrangement of the *VDJ* regions, an RNA molecule is transcribed that contains the information from the *VDJ*, intervening DNA, the μ constant region, and the δ constant region. Precursor RNA molecules are alternatively processed to produce mRNAs containing either μ or δ. Initially, RNA processing favors the μ chain and production of surface IgM (see Figure 7-11), but as the B cell matures, both mRNA molecules are produced.

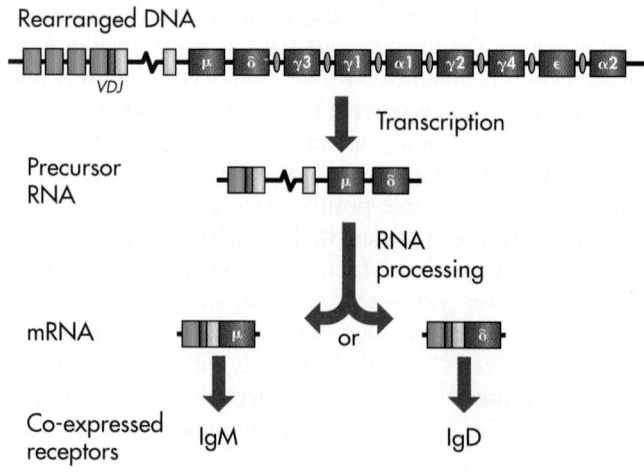

mRNA molecules and alternative RNA processing to simultaneously produce two different heavy chains, μ and δ, both of which have the same variable region.

The developing B cell rearranges and expresses the heavy chain, which is followed by the rearrangement of either the κ or λ light chain so that only one type is produced. The light chains are assembled with two μ heavy chains to form a monomeric IgM antibody or with two δ chains to form an IgD antibody. Because each heavy chain used the same VDJ rearrangement and the same light chain, the variable regions and therefore the specificities of the IgM and IgD are identical. At this stage of B-cell development, both antibodies have hydrophobic, or sticky, "tails" attached that results in insertion into the plasma membrane and the coexpression of IgM and IgD receptors on the cell surface.

Changes in Characteristic Surface Markers
As with T cells, B-cell differentiation is also characterized by the development of a variety of important surface molecules. These include CD21 (a complement receptor) and CD40 (adhesion molecule required for later interactions with Th).

Central Tolerance
During formation of the BCR in the bone marrow, a large number of autoreactive B cells are eliminated if exposed to self-antigen.[16] However unlike T cells, the B cell has the opportunity of changing the specificity of its BCR away from reactivity to a self-antigen. If the B cell encounters a self-antigen that crosslinks its B-cell receptors, it may attempt to reprogram itself by *receptor editing* to change the specificity of its BCR. Editing appears to be accomplished by reexpressing the RAG enzymes and attempting to rearrange a different light chain gene. Replacement of the light chain in the BCR would provide three new CDRs in the light chain variable region and potentially change the antigenic specificity of the BCR. If editing is unsuccessful or if additional self-antigens are encountered, the B cell will undergo apoptosis. It is estimated that more than 90% of developing B cells are induced to undergo apoptosis.

INDUCTION OF AN IMMUNE RESPONSE: CLONAL SELECTION

As described in the previous chapter, successful invasion by a pathogen will initially elicit an inflammatory response as a host attempts to destroy and clear the invading microorganism. In addition to carrying out their roles as inflammatory effector cells, some of the cells involved in innate immunity are responsible for communicating with immature B and T lymphocytes to initiate specific and longer-acting acquired immunity. This intercellular communication occurs via direct cellular contact in peripheral lymphoid tissues and is essential for the specificity of the adaptive immune response.

Secondary Lymphoid Organs
The secondary lymphoid organs include the spleen, lymph nodes, adenoids, tonsils, Peyer's patches (intestines), and the appendix (see Figure 7-3). Immunocompetent lymphocytes enter the secondary lymphoid organs through the blood and enter specialized small veins, called **high endothelial venules (HEV),** where they bind to the endothelium through a family of adhesion molecules.[17] The lymphocytes migrate from the vessels into the lymphoid tissues, which contain B- and T-cell–rich areas. B lymphocytes that encounter antigen in the secondary lymph organs usually undergo a process of differentiation and proliferation that results in the formation of specialized germinal centers in these organs (Figure 7-13).

Antigen Processing and Presentation
Most antigens do not react directly with T or B cells, but require processing and presentation in the appropriate fashion. This is the duty of antigen-presenting cells (APCs).

Pathogens that penetrate the external barriers and enter the tissues or blood stream encounter a variety of phagocytic cells and are therefore likely to be ingested and destroyed. If the infectious agent is in the tissues, they may elicit an inflammatory response that results in the infiltration of macrophages into the site. Additionally, the infectious agent or fragments of the microorganism may be removed by the lymphatics, which drain to the lymph nodes. The lymph nodes are extremely rich in dendritic cells and macrophages, which phagocytose the material and function as APCs for T and B lymphocytes in the lymph nodes. Pathogens entering through the blood stream may be removed by phagocytic cells in the spleen and other lymphoid tissues. In either case, the phagocytic cells that digest invading pathogens are also responsible for processing antigens from the pathogen and displaying or presenting those antigens on the phagocyte's surface to neighboring lymphocytes in order to initiate the adaptive immune response against that specific pathogen.

Many cells have the capacity to present antigen to some degree, but dendritic cells, macrophages, and B lymphocytes are so efficient at antigen presentation that they are considered "professional" APCs. Each of these three APCs is responsible for the presentation of antigens of different types and from different sources. B cells present antigen to Th cells that facilitate development of the humoral immune response. Macrophages are very effective in presenting antigen to memory Th cells in order to initiate a rapid response to antigens (i.e., secondary immune response). The dendritic cells are perhaps the most effective in presenting antigen to naïve immunocompetent Th cells. Dendritic cells develop from bone marrow precursor cells, either of myeloid or lymphoid lineage (at least two populations of dendritic cells have been described). They migrate to the peripheral tissues (e.g., skin, intestinal tract) and to the secondary lymphoid organs. Immature dendritic cells at a site of inflammation function as phagocytes, and the process of phagocytosis can initiate differentiation and directed migration to the secondary lymphoid organs, particularly the lymph nodes (Figure 7-14). Thus dendritic cells can carry processed antigen from a site of inflammation to the T-cell–rich areas of the lymph nodes.

Both antigen processing and presentation are necessary for an adaptive immune response to occur. Although B and T

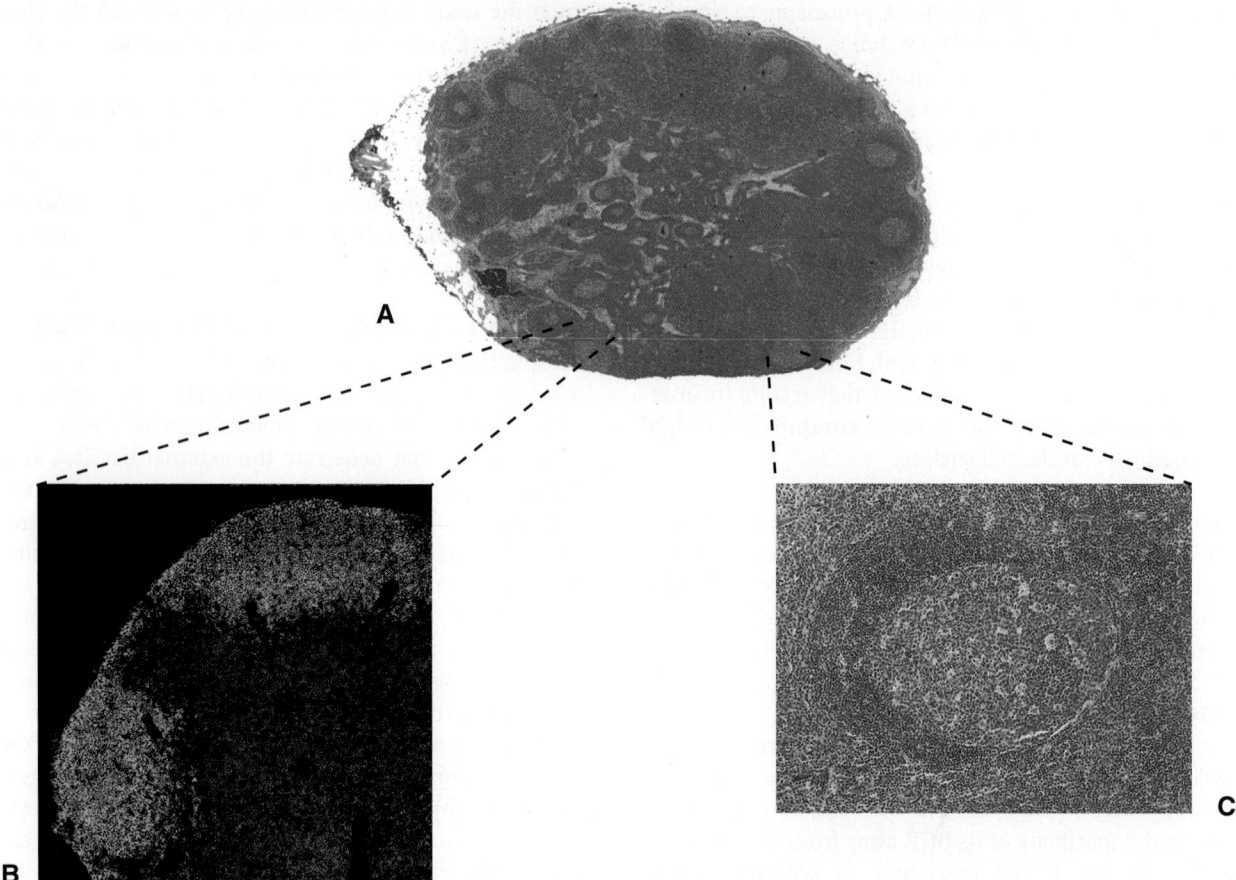

Figure 7-13 Histology of a secondary lymphoid organ. A, A lymph node is organized into an outer cortex and an inner medulla.
B, The lymph node contains areas that are rich in immunocompetent B cells (stained green), and T cells (stained red). **C,** In response
to antigen, B cells undergo proliferation resulting in the formation of germinal centers. (From Kumar V, Abbas A, Fausto N: *Robbins
and Cotran pathologic basis of disease,* ed 7, Philadelphia, 2005, Saunders.)

lymphocytes are immunocompetent before they have "seen" an antigen on the surface of an APC, they are considered "naïve" until they have actually done so. The processing and presentation of antigens to naïve lymphocytes results in activation of an acquired immune response only if (1) the antigen is of the appropriate type; (2) the lymphocytes are prepared to recognize the presented antigen; and (3) the antigen is presented appropriately.

Pathways of Antigen Processing

In general, the immune system responses to two types of antigens: exogenous and endogenous.[18] Using infection as a model, exogenous antigens are carried on microorganisms that are trapped and killed by phagocytic cells, therefore they come from outside the cell. Endogenous antigens are synthesized within a cell. These include viral antigens because viruses infect cells and use the normal cellular protein-synthesizing machinery to translate the viral genes into viral proteins. Endogenous antigens also may include those uniquely produced by cancerous cells. When many cells undergo malignant change, they begin producing unique proteins that are specific to cancer cells and are presented as foreign antigens on the cell surface.

Exogenous and endogenous antigens are preferentially presented by different classes of MHC molecules: class I MHC molecules generally present endogenous antigens, and class II molecules prefer exogenous antigens (Figure 7-15). Because class I MHC molecules are expressed on all cells, except red blood cells, any change in that cell due to viral infection or malignancy may result in foreign antigen being presented by MHC class I on that cell's surface. Class II MHC molecules are coexpressed with MHC class I on a more limited number of cells that have APC function, including macrophages, dendritic cells, B lymphocytes, activated T lymphocytes, and some endothelial cells.

Thus the term **antigen processing** relates to the process by which exogenous and endogenous antigens are linked with the appropriate MHC molecules. Endogenous antigens are usually components of proteins synthesized in the cytosol. They are degraded in the cytosol by proteosomes into small peptides and transported by TAP (transporter associated with antigen processing) proteins (TAP-1 and TAP-2) into the en-

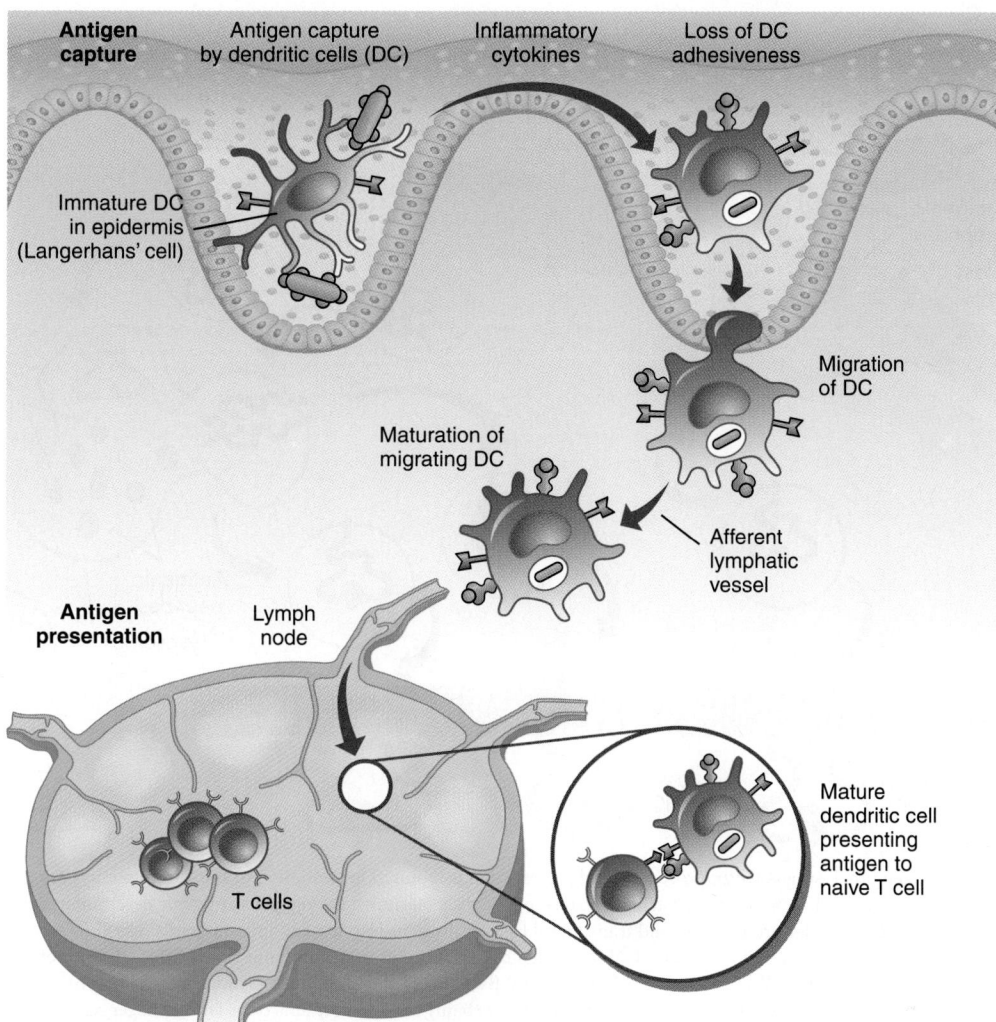

Figure 7-14 **The role of the dendritic cell in capturing antigen.** Immature dendritic cells in the tissues encounter and phagocytose antigen, which results in the production of inflammatory cytokines and a loss of adhesive interactions with neighboring cells. The maturing dendritic cell migrates through the lymphatic vessels to a regional lymph node, where it presents the antigen to immunocompetent T cells to initiate the clonal selection process. (Redrawn from Kumar V, Abbas A, Fausto N: *Robbins and Cotran pathologic basis of disease,* ed 7, Philadelphia, 2005, Saunders.)

doplasmic reticulum where MHC class I and class II molecules are assembled. The class I MHC molecules have open antigen-binding sites so that antigen, the class I MHC α-chain, and a β2 microglobulin molecule form a stable complex that is transported through the Golgi apparatus to the plasma membrane. The antigenic peptides presented by class I MHC are usually very small, 8 to 10 amino acids in length.

MHC class II molecules are also assembled in the endoplasmic reticulum, but do not bind with endogenous antigen because the antigen-binding site is blocked by a small protein called **invariant chain**. Exogenous antigens are internalized by phagocytosis and small antigenic molecules produced by digestion in the lysosomes. The MHC class II complex of the class II α- and β-chains, with invariant chain, are transported to the lysosomes containing exogenous antigens. In the lysosomal environment, the invariant chain is digested and replaced by antigenic molecules that are usually slightly larger (in excess of 12 amino acids in length) than those presented by MHC class I.

CD1 presents a variety of lipid-containing antigens that are usually derived from phagocytosis and digestion of infectious microorganisms with very high lipid content in their cell membranes. Therefore, CD1 complexes with antigen in the lysosomes, in a fashion similar to MHC class II. The "pocket" that holds antigen for presentation by CD1 is generally more narrow and deeper than described for MHC molecules, and it is lined with many hydrophobic amino acids that interact with lipid.

Helper T Lymphocytes

Regardless of whether an antigen primarily induces a cellular or humoral immune response, a subpopulation of T lymphocytes, **helper T cells (Th cells),** are usually necessary for the process.[19,20] As indicated by the name, this group of T cells *helps* the antigen-driven maturation of both B and T cells. They perform this task by facilitating and magnifying the interaction between APCs and the immunocompetent lympho-

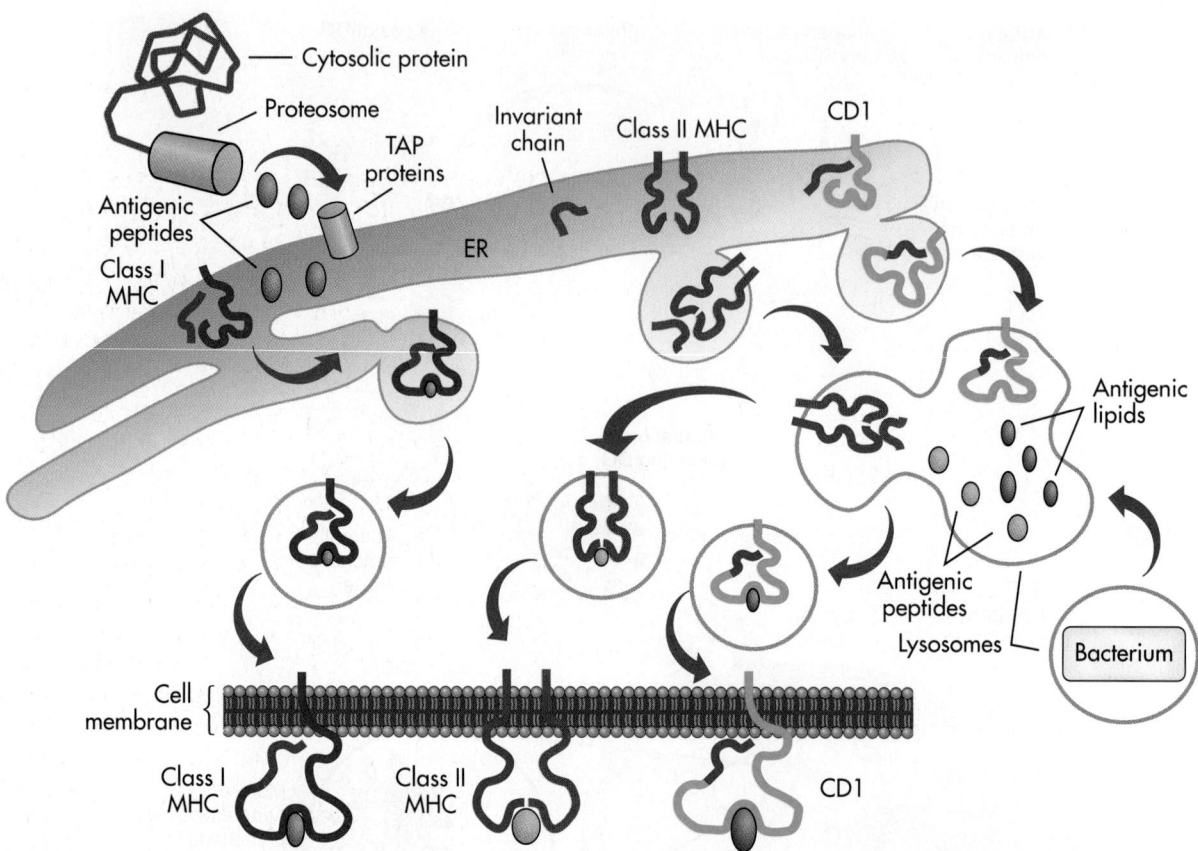

Figure 7-15 Antigen processing. Antigen processing and presentation is required for initiation of most immune responses. Foreign antigen may be either endogenous (cytosolic protein) or exogenous (e.g., bacterium). Endogenous antigenic determinants (antigenic peptides) are produced by cellular proteosomes and transported by TAP proteins into the endoplasmic reticulum *(ER)* where the MHC and CD1 molecules are being assembled. In the ER, antigenic peptides bind to the α-chains of the MHC class I molecule, and the complex is transported to the cell surface. In the ER, the α- and β-chains of the MHC class II molecules are also being assembled, but the antigen-binding site is blocked by a small molecule (invariant chain) to prevent interactions with endogenous antigenic peptides. The MHC class II–invariant chain complex is transported to lysosomes where exogenous antigenic fragments have been generated as a result of phagocytosis. In the lysosomes, the invariant chain is digested and replaced by exogenous antigenic peptides, after which the MHC class II–antigen complex is inserted into the cell membrane. CD1 is also assembled in the ER, but its antigen-binding site is specific for lipid antigenic determinants and does not bind endogenous antigenic peptides. The CD1 molecule is transported to the lysosomes and may encounter and bind antigenic lipids produced by phagocytic digestion of engulfed bacteria. The CD1-antigen complex is transported to the cell membrane and presents lipid antigens.

cytes. This extremely important role involves three distinct steps: (1) the Th cell directly interacts with the APC through a variety of antigen-specific and antigen-independent mechanisms; (2) the Th cell undergoes a differentiation process during which a variety of cytokine genes are activated; and (3) depending on the pattern of cytokines expressed, the mature Th cell interacts with either immunocompetent B or T cells to enhance their response to antigen, which results in differentiation into either plasma cells or effector T cells, such as cytotoxic T cells. Th cells are critical to most immune responses, and a variety of major Th-cell defects that lead to severely diminished immune responses are discussed in later chapters.

APC-Th Cooperation

Cells that are destined to become Th cells emerge from the thymus with characteristic cell surface markers. They have a functional αβ TCR complex and express the surface molecule CD4 and lack CD8. These are generally referred to as precur-

sor Th cells, or sometimes Thp cells (Figure 7-16). As described previously, the TCR recognizes antigen, and the CD4 molecule confines antigen presentation to MHC class II molecules, thus CD4+ cells are *class II restricted*. In order to undergo maturation, the Th cell must receive three independent signals; antigen binding through the combined interaction of the TCR complex and CD4, costimulatory signals through a variety of intercellular adhesion molecules, and activation of specific cytokine receptors. If the appropriate signaling pathways are activated, the cell will differentiate through multiple intermediate stages into functional Th cells.

The complex of an antigenic peptide presented by an MHC class II molecule is recognized by multiple molecules on the Th-cell surface. The TCR binds directly to the antigen, whereas CD4 independently binds to a different site on the MHC class II β-chain. This co-recognition of the MHC/antigen complex by the TCR and CD4 brings CD4 into close proximity with the CD3 components of the TCR complex,

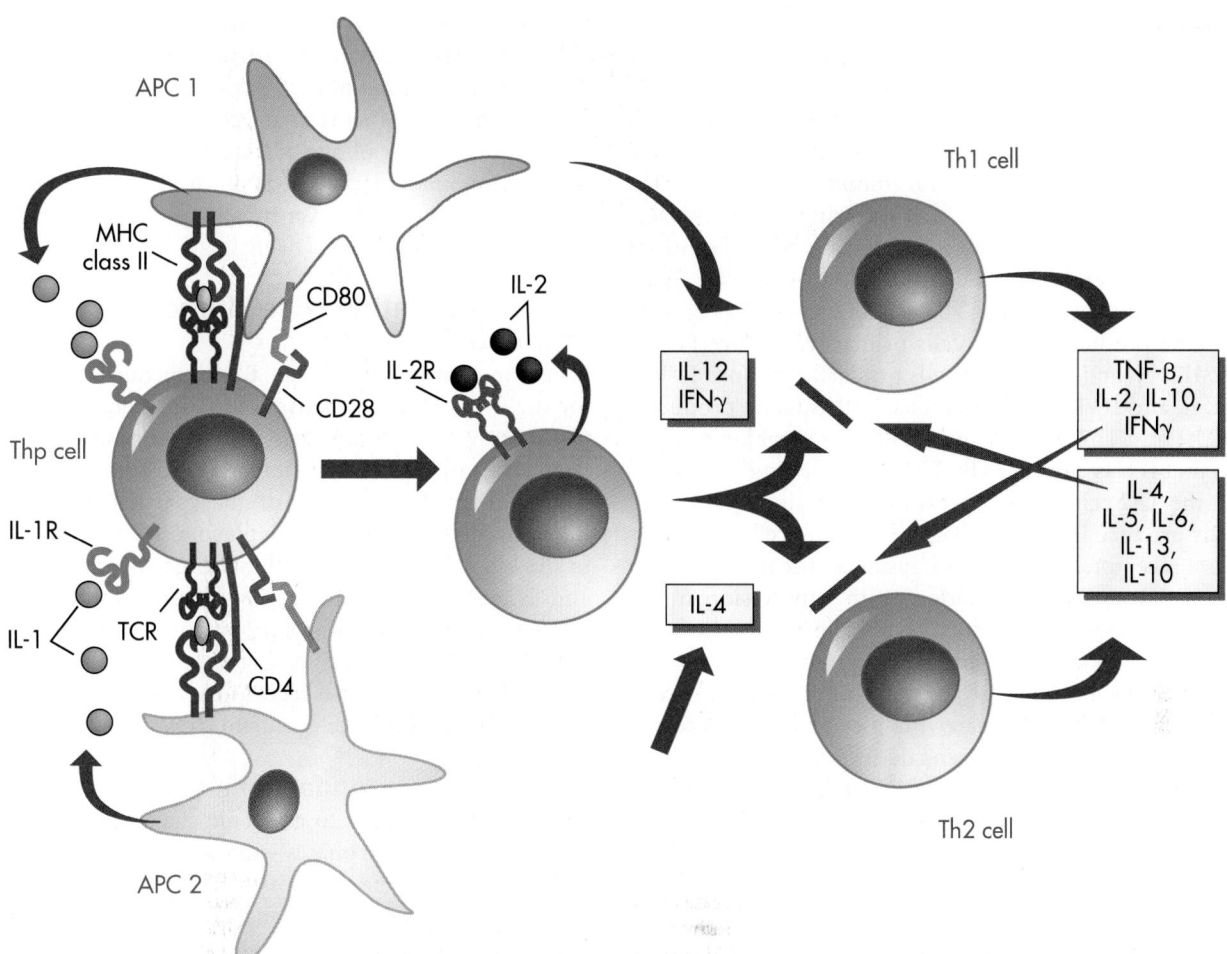

Figure 7-16 Development of Th1 and Th2 cells. The most important step in clonal selection is the production of two populations of helper T (Th) cells (Th1 and Th2) that are necessary for the development of both cellular and humoral immune responses. In this model, different populations of APC cells (APC 1 and APC 2) may influence whether a precursor Th cell (Thp cell) will differentiate into a Th1 or Th2 cell. Differentiation of the Thp cell is initiated by three signaling events. The antigen signal is produced by the interaction of the T-cell receptor (TCR) and CD4 with antigen presented by MHC class II molecules. A set of co-stimulatory signals is produced from interactions between adhesion molecules (e.g., CD80 and CD28). A third signal is produced by the interactions of cytokines (particularly IL-1) with appropriate cytokine receptors (IL-1R) on the Thp cell. The Thp cell up-regulates IL-2 production and expression of the IL-2 receptor (IL-2R), which act in an autocrine fashion to accelerate Thp-cell differentiation and proliferation. Commitment to a Th1 or Th2 phenotype results from the relative concentrations of cytokines. IL-12 and IFN-γ produced by some populations of APCs favor differentiation into the Th1-cell phenotype, whereas IL-4, which is produced by a variety of cells, favors differentiation into the Th2-cell phenotype. The Th1 cell is characterized by the production of cytokines that assist in the differentiation of cytotoxic T (Tc) cells, whereas the Th2 cell produces cytokines that favor B-cell differentiation. Th1 and Th2 cells affect each other through the production of inhibitory cytokines: IFN-γ will inhibit development of Th2 cells, and IL-4 will inhibit the development of Th1 cells.

which initiates a series of enzymatic interactions among other molecules associated with the cytoplasmic portions of CD3 and CD4, such as the protein kinases p56^{lck} and ZAP-70. These molecules activate a signaling pathway from the TCR to the Th-cell nucleus.

The antigenic signal alone is inadequate and may even inactivate the Th cell if co-stimulatory signals are not present. Co-stimulatory molecules are necessary for proper differentiation to occur. A variety of molecular interactions have been described, but the most critical appears to involve B7 on the APC and CD28 on the Th cell. Other interactions occur between CD48 on the APC and CD2 on the Th cell and between a variety of other adhesion molecules. In each case, the Th-

cell molecule sends an activation signal to the nucleus. An additional signal is provided by cytokine. At this early stage of Th-cell differentiation, IL-1 secreted by the APC provides this signal through interaction with the IL-1 receptor on the Th cell.

The initial differentiation response by the Th cell includes the production of the cytokine IL-2 and up-regulation of IL-2 receptors. IL-2 is secreted and acts in an autocrine (self-stimulating) fashion to induce further maturation and proliferation of the Th cell. Without IL-2 production, the Th cell cannot efficiently mature into a functional helper cell. At this point, Th cells undergo one of several different differentiation pathways into Th subsets.

Th Subsets

The most clearly characterized Th-cell subsets are **Th1** and **Th2 cells** (see Figure 7-16). These subsets have different functions: Th1 cells appear to provide more help in developing cell-mediated immunity, whereas Th2 cells provide more help for developing humoral immunity. The two Th subsets differ considerably in the spectrum of cytokines produced by each, as well as the expression of surface cytokine receptors and intercellular adhesion molecules. The initial description of Th1 and Th2 cell differences was based on cytokine production: Th1 cells primarily produce IL-2, TNF-β, IFN-γ, and IL-12. Th2 cells primarily produce IL-4, IL-5, IL-6, and IL-13.[19,20] In humans, both subsets produce IL-10. Th1 and Th2 cells also have different cytokine receptors, so that IFN-γ produced by Th1 cells will bind to receptors on the Th2 cells and suppress their function. Likewise, Th2 cells produce IL-4, which suppresses Th1 cells through their IL-4 receptors. Thus in some instances the immune response favors antibody formation, with suppression of a cell-mediated response, whereas in other instances the opposite is true. For example, antigens derived from viral or bacterial pathogens and those derived from cancer cells are hypothesized to induce a greater number of Th1 cells relative to Th2 cells, whereas antigens derived from multicellular parasites and allergens are hypothesized to result in production of more Th2 cells.[20] Many antigens (e.g., tetanus vaccine), however, will produce excellent humoral and cell-mediated responses simultaneously.

How a Th cell is guided into becoming a Th1 or Th2 cell is not fully known. Some evidence indicates that different subpopulations of APCs influence the choice by secreting different profiles of cytokines that may favor one route of differentiation over another. Nutrition or other environmental variables may favor one pathway over another. For example, local concentrations of the nutritional supplements zinc and selenium or hormones such as progesterone may result in the production of more of one or the other subset.[20] Other nutritional components such as probiotic bacteria (e.g., *Lactobacillus* spp. found in yogurt) can enhance production of Th2 cells relative to Th1 cells.[20]

B-Cell Activation: The Humoral Immune Response

When an immunocompetent B cell encounters an antigen for the first time, only those cells with specific BCRs complementary to that antigen's determinant sites are stimulated to proliferate and differentiate (clonal selection), resulting in multiple copies of that particular B cell. The differentiated B cell becomes a **plasma cell** and can be found in the blood, secondary lymphoid organs (primarily spleen and lymph nodes), and some inflammatory sites. Each plasma cell is a factory for antibody production and is dedicated to the secretion of a single class or subclass of antibody with one variable region and, therefore, specificity against one antigenic determinant.

Primary and Secondary Immune Responses

The immune response to antigenic challenge has classically been divided into two phases—the primary and secondary responses—that can be most easily demonstrated by serologic tests that measure plasma concentrations of antibody over time (Figure 7-17). Upon initial exposure to most antigens, there is a latent period, or lag phase, during which B-cell differentiation and proliferation occurs. After approximately 5

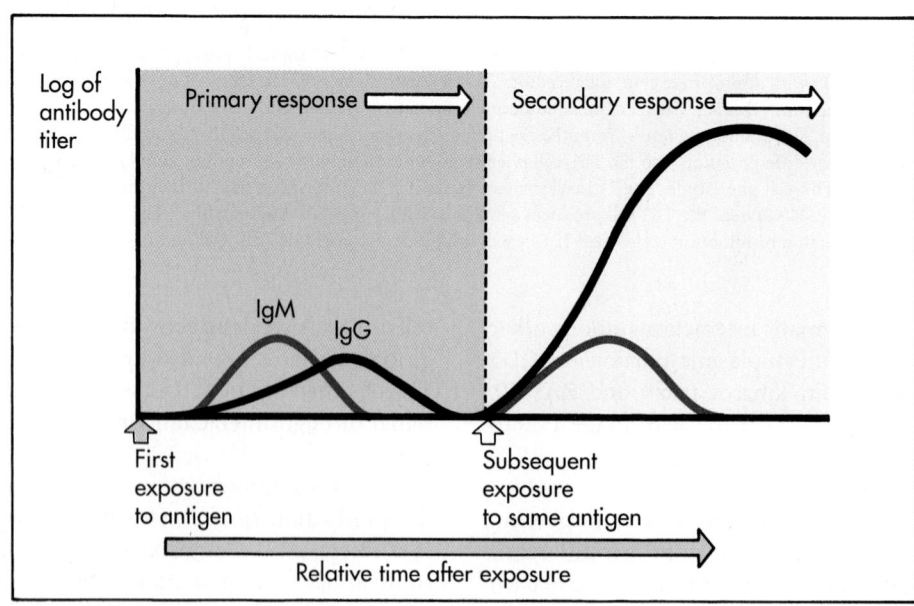

Figure 7-17 Primary and secondary immune responses. Antigen responses are dominated by two classes of immunoglobulins, IgM and IgG. IgM predominates upon initial exposure to the antigen in the primary response, with IgG appearing later. After the host's immune system is primed, another challenge by the same antigen induces the secondary response in which some IgM and larger amounts of IgG are produced.

to 7 days, IgM antibody specific for that antigen can be detected in the circulation. The lag phase is a result of the time necessary for clonal selection, including antigen processing and presentation, induction of Th cells, interactions between immunocompetent B cells and Th cells, and the maturation and proliferation of the B cells into plasma cells and memory cells.

This is the initial response, or **primary immune response.** Typically, IgM will be produced first, followed by IgG against the same antigen. The quantity of IgG may be about equal to or less than the amount of IgM production. If no further exposure to the antigen occurs, the circulating antibody is catabolized (broken down) and measurable quantities fall. The individual's immune system, however, has been primed. A second challenge by the same antigen results in the **secondary (anamnestic) immune response,** which is characterized by the more rapid production of a larger amount of antibody than the primary response. The rapidity of the secondary immune response is the result of the presence of memory cells that do not require further differentiation. IgM may be transiently produced in the secondary response and the quantity may be about the same as that produced in the primary response. IgG production is increased considerably, making it the predominant antibody class of the secondary response. It is often present in concentrations several times larger than those of IgM, and levels of circulating IgG specific for that antigen may remain elevated for an extended period of time. If the antigenic challenge is in the form of a vaccine or occurs through natural infection, the level of protective IgG may remain elevated for decades.

The existence of a prolonged and protective secondary immune response explains how vaccinations are able to provide protection against certain pathogenic microorganisms. Edward Jenner, an English physician of the late eighteenth century, performed the first well-documented vaccine trial.[21,22] Although some of the stories about Jenner's experiments are fanciful, it is known that Jenner recognized that milkmaids were protected from the deadly smallpox virus if they had previously developed cowpox, a bovine equivalent of smallpox that causes only mild disease in humans. Jenner took material from a cowpox pustule on the hand of an infected milkmaid and injected it into the arm of an 8-year-old boy. After the boy's initial inflammatory reaction to the injection subsided, Jenner injected him again, this time with material from a smallpox pustule. Fortunately, the experiment was a success because Jenner is reported to have re-injected smallpox virus into the boy at least 20 times without the child becoming ill. In Jenner's experiment, the antigens on the cowpox virus and the smallpox virus were sufficiently similar that the cowpox antigen functioned as an altered or attenuated smallpox antigen. The antibodies and lymphocytes that recognized and destroyed cowpox also were able to recognize the smallpox virus, thereby protecting the immunized child against smallpox. In 1798, Jenner used the term *vaccination* (*vacca* = cow) to describe his technique.

Cellular Interactions

As with most aspects of immunity, a sequence of cellular interactions is required to produce an effective antibody response (Figure 7-18). The immunocompetent B cell is also an APC and expresses surface IgM and IgD B-cell receptors (BCRs). Unlike the T-cell receptor that can only "see" processed and presented antigen, the BCR can react with soluble antigen. Antigen binding to the BCR complex activates intracellular kinases, in a fashion similar to the TCR receptor complex. In many instances, circulating antigen, either on macromolecules or the surface of a pathogen, will have activated the complement system through the alternative or lectin pathways. Thus complement receptors on the B cell, such as CD19 and CD21, act as co-receptors to bind antigen. As a result of signaling from the BCR complex and other surface co-receptors, the macromolecule-bearing antigen is internalized, broken down in the lysosomes, and complexes with MHC class II molecules for presentation on the cell surface where it is recognized by a Th2 cell through the TCR and CD4. The intercellular bridge created through antigen induces the Th2 cell to up-regulate additional surface receptors and secrete cytokines. Direct interaction between CD40 on the B-cell surface and the CD40 ligand (CD40L, also called *CD154*) on the Th2 cell, as well as the interaction of B7 on the B cell and CD28 on the Th cell and exposure of the B cell to Th2-cell cytokines (particularly IL-4) induces proliferation of the B cell and maturation into a plasma cell. A major component of maturation is class switch.

Class-Switch

The immunocompetent B cell uses IgM and IgD as receptors. During the clonal selection process, however, each B cell has the option of changing the class of antibody to a secreted form of one of the four IgG subclasses, one of the two IgA subclasses, or IgE, or continuing to produce IgM but changing to a secreted form, usually a pentamer. This process is called **class-** or **isotype-switch.** During this process the variable region of the antibody heavy chain is conserved, and the light chain remains unchanged from that used in the BCR, therefore the antigenic specificity also remains unchanged.

The mechanism of class-switch involves another DNA rearrangement, during which the *VDJ* region encoding the heavy chain's variable region is moved to another site on the DNA that is adjacent to the gene for a different constant region[23] (Figure 7-19). Using yet to be identified enzymes, the DNA is cut and mended with removal of the DNA that was between the *VDJ* site and the new constant region. Specific recognition sites (switch regions) precede each constant region gene, and the particular constant region chosen for class-switch appears to be, at least partially, under the control of specific Th2 cytokines. IL-4, IL-5, and transforming growth factor-β (TGF-β) are among the cytokines that affect class switch. For instance, IL-4 and IL-13 appear to preferentially stimulate switch to IgE, and TGF-β and IL-5 appear to play major roles in class-switch to IgA.

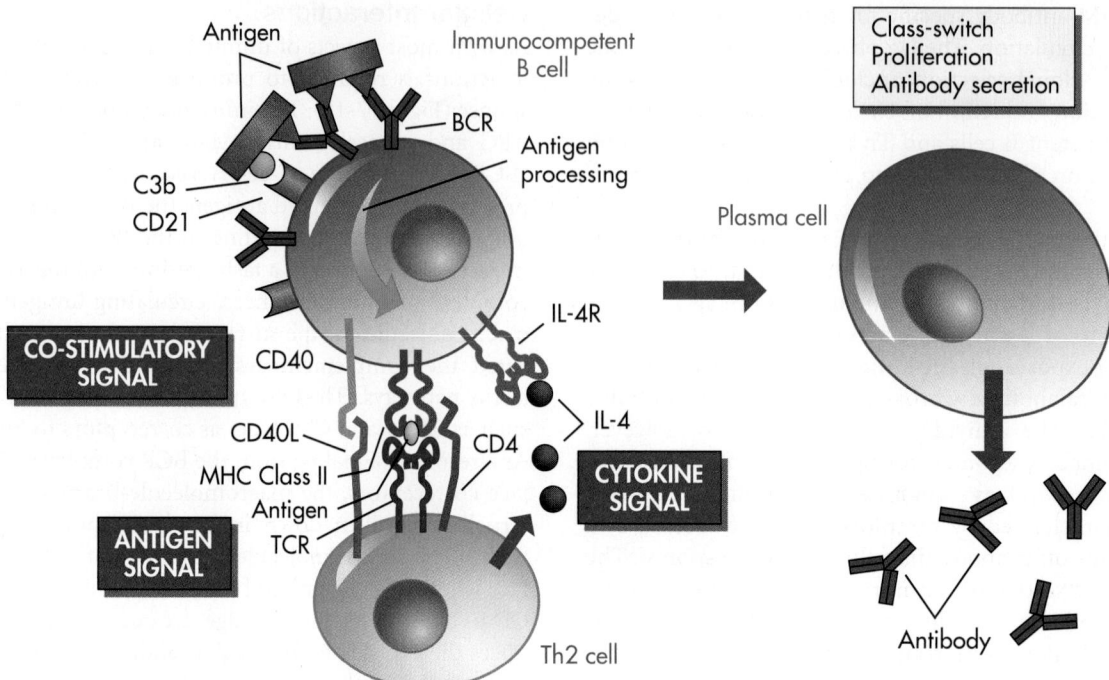

Figure 7-18 **B-cell clonal selection.** Immunocompetent B cells undergo proliferation and differentiation into antibody-secreting plasma cells. Three signals are necessary. The antigen signal is provided by the B cell itself. A B cell can recognize soluble antigen directly through the B-cell receptor and co-receptors, such as complement receptors (CD21), which usually involve accessory molecules such as CD19 (not shown). Antigen is internalized and processed for presentation by MHC class II molecules, which interact with the T-cell receptor (TCR) and CD4 on Th2 cells. Co-stimulatory signals are provided through adhesion molecules, particularly CD40 and CD40L (CD154). The cytokine signal is provided by Th2 cytokines (particularly IL-4) binding to appropriate cytokine receptors (IL-4R) on the B cell. Additional cytokines influence switch to particular classes or subclasses of antibody.

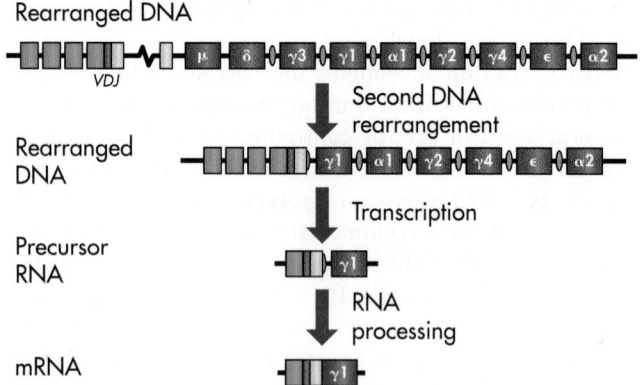

Figure 7-19 **Genetics of class-switch.** During clonal selection, most B cells switch from expression of surface IgM and IgD to a different class or subclass of antibody. A first set of DNA rearrangements during the generation of clonal diversity resulted in formation of the *VDJ* region. The class-switch process involves a second DNA rearrangement during which the *VDJ* region is moved to a switch region (*orange ovals*) immediately preceding the new class/subclass of antibody. In this example, the B cell undergoes class-switch to a γ1 heavy chain and secretion of an IgG1 antibody. The intervening DNA between the *VDJ* and the selected switch region is excised, and the DNA is repaired (DNA after second rearrangement) and transcribed into a precursor RNA. The RNA is processed to a mRNA with information for the new heavy chain.

A few antigens can bypass the need for Th cells and can directly stimulate B-cell maturation and proliferation. These are called *T-independent antigens* (Figure 7-20). They are mostly bacterial products that are large and are likely to have repeating antigenic determinants (multiple identical antigenic determinant sites) that bind and crosslink several B-cell receptors. The accumulated intracellular signal is adequate to induce differentiation to a plasma cell but is not adequate to induce class-switch. The CD40-CD40L interaction is a necessary component of the signal that leads to class-switch. Therefore, T-independent antigens usually induce a relatively pure IgM primary and secondary immune response.

Cellular Differentiation

During the clonal selection process, B cells differentiate into antibody-producing plasma cells and into a set of long-lived memory cells. During B cells differentiation into plasma cells, the CDR portions of the antibody variable region are prone to somatic point mutations that lead to changes in single amino acids. Some of these changes produce better antibodies that bind more strongly (higher affinity) to the antigen. The presence of antigen creates a positive selective pressure towards the developing B cells that express the higher-affinity antibody, which results in a process called *affinity maturation*, in which the quality of the circulating antibody improves over time.

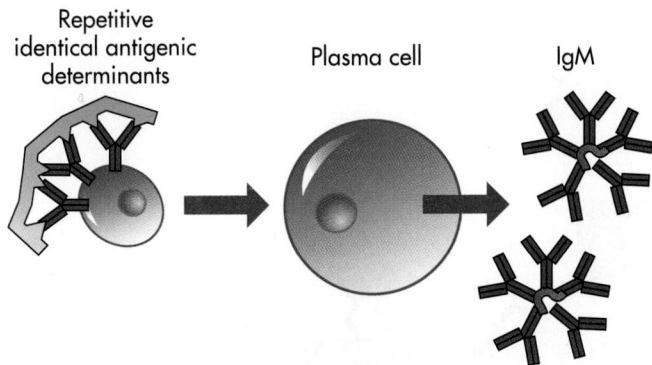

Figure 7-20 Activation of a B cell by a T cell–independent antigen. Molecules containing repeating identical antigenic determinants may interact simultaneously with several receptors on the surface of the B cell and induce the proliferation and production of immunoglobulins, mainly IgM.

The memory cells remain inactive until subsequent exposure to the same antigen. Upon re-exposure, these memory cells do not require much further differentiation and will therefore differentiate rapidly into new plasma cells.

T-Cell Activation: The Cellular Immune Response

Activation of the cell-mediated arm of the immune response begins with the binding of antigen to specific T-cell receptors. Through a variety of intercellular collaborations that are mediated by specific cellular receptors and cytokines, the naïve T cell proliferates and differentiates into a functional (effector) T cell. The two main effector functions of activated T cells are (1) direct killing of foreign and/or abnormal cells and (2) assistance and/or activation of other cells, such as macrophages. The first function is carried out by a subclass of T cells termed cytotoxic T lymphocytes (Tc cells, or CTLs). Activation of macrophages is performed by a special subset of Th cells. Additional T cells develop into cells that regulate the immune response in order to avoid inadvertently attacking self-antigens or to avoid overactivation of the immune response. This mixed population of cells is termed **T regulatory (Treg) cells.** Finally, **memory T cells** are also produced to help induce secondary cell-mediated immune responses.

Cellular Interactions

During the clonal selection phase of the cell-mediated immune response, immunocompetent T cells in the peripheral lymphoid organs must recognize antigen that has been processed and presented by MHC class I molecules[24] (Figure 7-21). The antigen is usually an endogenous antigen expressed on the surface of cells infected with a virus or that have become malignant. The T cells have a functional αβ TCR complex and express the surface molecule CD8, rather than CD4. The presence of the CD8 molecule confines antigen recognition to MHC class I molecules, therefore CD8+ T cells are *class I restricted*. The TCR binds directly to the antigenic peptide, whereas CD8 independently binds to a different site on the MHC class I α-chain. This co-recognition of

the MHC/antigen complex by the TCR and CD8 brings CD8 into close proximity with the CD3 components of the TCR complex, which initiates a series of enzymatic interactions among other molecules associated with the cytoplasmic portions of CD3 and CD4, as was described for Th-cell activation. These molecules activate a signaling pathway from the TCR to the T-cell nucleus.

To undergo maturation, the T cell must receive independent signals from a variety of co-stimulatory intercellular adhesion molecules and specific cytokine receptors. If the appropriate signaling pathways are activated, the cell will proliferate and differentiate through multiple intermediate stages into functional Tc cells. The co-stimulatory signals for Tc-cell maturation are virtually the same as has been described for Th-cell maturation: B7 on the cell-presenting antigen and CD28 on the T cell, CD48 on the antigen-presenting cell and CD2 on the T cell, and a variety of other adhesion molecules. Development of Tc cells also requires cytokines, especially IL-2, produced by the Th1 cell.

Cellular Differentiation

The result of the cellular interactions described above is the production of active Tc cells with the capacity to identify antigens on the surface of infected or malignant cells and then to destroy those cells. As with B cells, some of the T cells that become activated in response to antigen presentation will not become effectors that destroy infected targets, but instead will develop into a population of memory T cells. These cells have the capacity to rapidly respond to further exposure to the same antigen.

Superantigens

A recently recognized group of molecules has the ability to bind the variable portion of the TCR β-chain outside of its normal antigen-specific binding site, as well as the α-chain of MHC class II molecules outside of their antigen-presentation sites (Figure 7-22). Thus these molecules are not digested and processed by an APC to be presented to an immune cell. This binding results in adherence of the TCR and MHC class II molecules, independent of antigen-recognition, and provides an activation signal for Th-cell activation and proliferation. The normal antigen-specific recognition between Th cells and APCs results in activation of a relatively few cells: only those cells with specific TCRs against that antigen. The type of binding described here results in activation of large populations of T lymphocytes, regardless of antigen specificity.[25,26] Thus these molecules have been referred to as **superantigens (SAGs).**

SAGs induce an excessive production of cytokines, including IL-2, IFN-γ and TNF-α.[25,26] The overproduction of inflammatory cytokines results in symptoms of a systemic inflammatory reaction, including fever, low blood pressure, and potentially, fatal shock.[26] Some examples of SAGs are the bacterial toxins produced by *Staphylococcus aureus* and *Streptococcus pyogenes* (including the superantigens that cause toxic shock syndrome and food poisoning). Some viruses are also

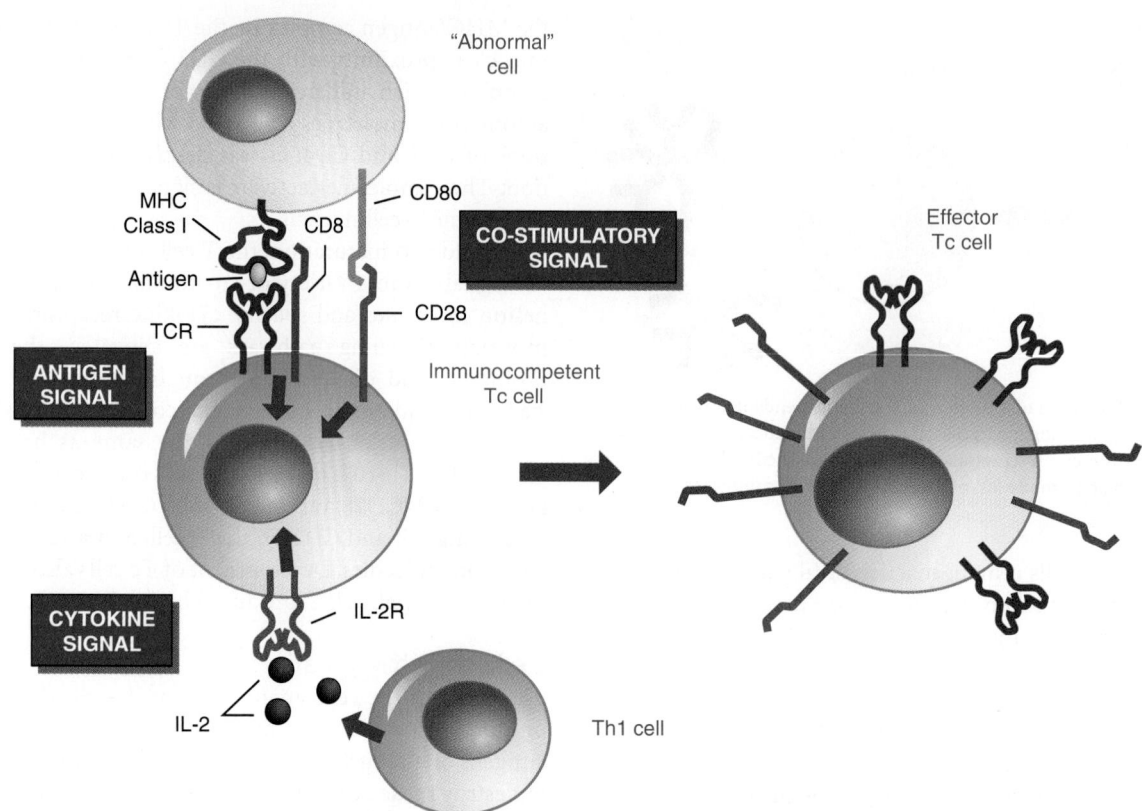

Figure 7-21 Tc-cell clonal selection. The development of effector cytotoxic T (Tc) cells during clonal selection results from three co-operative signaling events provided by antigen, co-stimulatory adhesion molecules, and cytokines. The immunocompetent Tc cell "sees" antigen presented by MHC class I molecules on the surface of a virally infected or cancerous "abnormal" cell. The antigen–MHC class I complex is recognized simultaneously by the T-cell receptor (TCR), which binds to antigen, and CD8, which binds to the MHC class I molecule. The proximity of signaling molecules associated with the cytoplasmic portions of CD8 and the TCR result in intracellular signaling. A separate signal results from the interaction of several groups of adhesion molecules (e.g., CD80 and CD28 in this example). The third signal is provided by the interaction of cytokine, particularly IL-2 from Th1 cells, and the appropriate receptor.

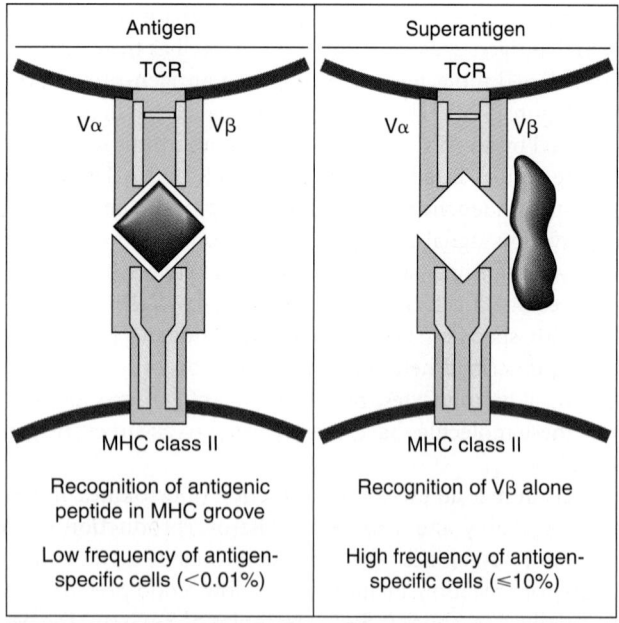

Figure 7-22 Superantigens. The T-cell receptor (TCR) and an MHC class II molecule normally simultaneously interact with a processed antigen to induce T-cell differentiation. Superantigens, such as some bacterial toxins, bind directly to the TCR and the MHC class II molecules. Superantigens activate Th cells independently of TCR antigen specificity.

able to produce superantigens, although the exact nature of these antigens is unclear.

EFFECTOR MECHANISMS

Antibody Function

Protection Against Infection

The chief function of circulating antibodies is to protect the host from infection. Protection can be afforded by antibody in several ways, either directly or indirectly (Figure 7-23). Directly, antibody can cause **neutralization** (inactivating or blocking the binding of an antigen to a receptor), **agglutination** (clumping insoluble particles that are in suspension), or **precipitation** (making a soluble antigen into an insoluble precipitate) of infectious agents or their toxic products. Indirectly, antibodies activate several components of innate immunity, including complement and phagocytes.

Direct Effects

To cause infection, many pathogens must attach to specific receptors on the host's cells. For instance, viruses that cause the common cold or the influenza virus must attach to specific receptors on epithelial cells. Some bacteria, such as *Neisseria gonorrhoeae* that causes gonorrhea, must attach to specific sites on epithelial cells. Antibodies may protect the host

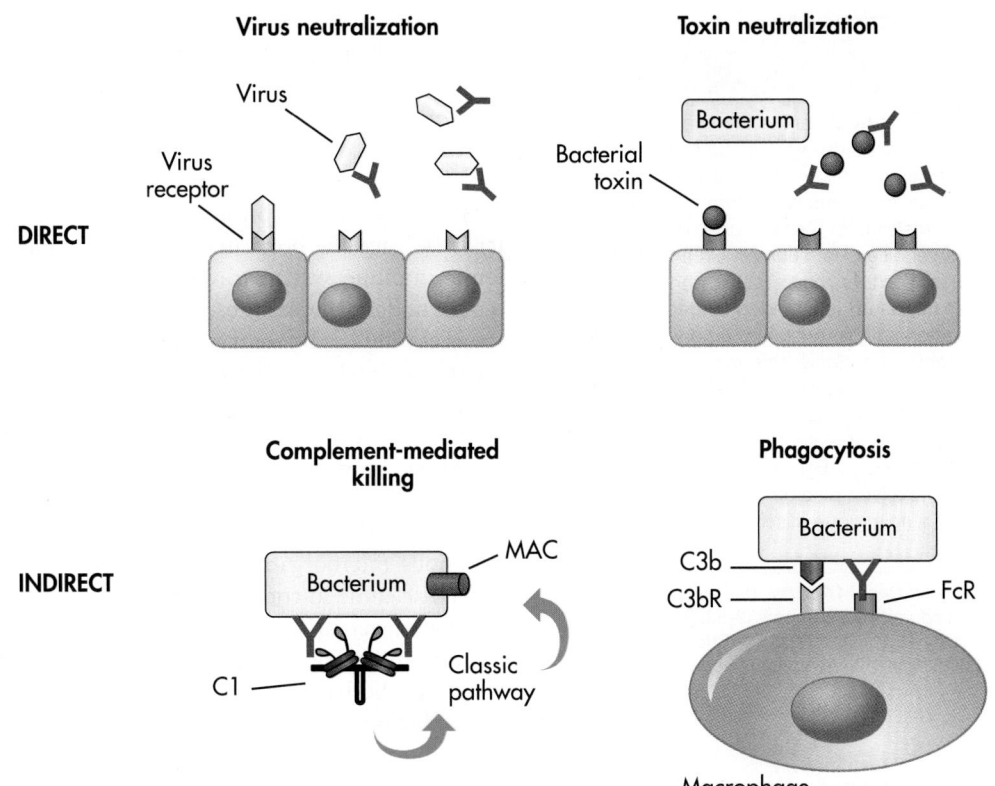

Figure 7-23 Direct and indirect functions of antibody. Protective activities of antibodies can be direct (through the action of antibody alone) or indirect (requiring activation of other components of the innate immune response, usually through the Fc region). Direct means include neutralization of viruses or bacterial toxins before they bind to receptors on the surface of the host's cells. Indirect means include activation of the classical complement pathway through C1 resulting in formation of the membrane-attack complex (MAC) or by increased phagocytosis of bacteria opsonized with antibody and complement components bound to appropriate surface receptors (FcR and C3bR).

against infection by covering the portions of the microorganism that it needs to bind to the host cell. Neutralization, or prevention of attachment to the host cell, thereby prevents infection of the host.

Protection against many viral infections can be elicited effectively by vaccination with inactivated or **attenuated** (weakened) **viruses** to induce neutralizing antibody production at the site of typical viral entrance into the body. A good indication of the degree of protection against viral infection is the level of circulating antibodies found in the blood. The level of circulating antibodies is referred to as an **antibody titer.** However, many viruses (e.g., measles, herpes) are inaccessible to antibodies after initial infection because they do not circulate in the bloodstream but instead remain inside infected cells, spreading by direct cell-to-cell contact. Neutralizing antibodies against this type of virus are most effective in preventing the initial infection. Other viruses, such as polio and influenza, spread through the blood, are more susceptible to the effects of circulating antibodies and can be controlled by antibodies even after the initial infection.

The symptoms of some infectious diseases result directly from toxins produced by infecting bacteria. For instance, the symptoms of tetanus or diphtheria are mediated by specific toxins. To cause disease, most toxins must bind to surface

molecules on the host's cells. Protective antibodies can bind to the toxins, prevent their interaction with host cells, and neutralize their biologic effects. Detection of the presence of an antibody response against a specific toxin (antibodies referred to as *antitoxins*) can aid in the diagnosis of diseases. For example, laboratory tests that detect anti-streptolysin O can be very useful in diagnosing group A streptococcal infections. Antibodies that neutralize bacterial toxins can be induced to confer immunity against bacterial pathogens by means of immunization. To prevent harming the recipient of immunization, bacterial toxins are chemically inactivated so that they have lost most of their harmful properties but still retain their immunogenicity. These are referred to as *toxoids*. Examples of bacterial pathogens for which immunization with toxoids can provide immunologic protection include those that cause diphtheria and tetanus.

A new therapeutic application of antibodies uses their normal properties to treat human disease (see What's New? Antibodies as Drugs).

Indirect Effects

Antibody can be protective by interacting with or activating components of nonspecific inflammation. Indirect effects are mediated by the Fc portion of the antibody molecule and include opsonic activity leading to enhanced phagocytosis

WHAT'S NEW? Antibodies as Drugs

A recent development in clinical treatment is the use of laboratory-produced immunoglobulins as drugs. Two such drugs currently commercially available are infliximab (Remicade) and Rituximab (Rituxan). Infliximab, a recombinant chimeric antibody directed against tumor necrosis factor (TNF), is used in the treatment of inflammatory bowel diseases, such as Crohn disease, and autoimmune diseases, such as rheumatoid arthritis. Intravenous administration of Infliximab is intended to decrease inflammation by neutralization of the proinflammatory cytokine TNF. Rituximab is a recombinant antibody that recognizes a glycoprotein on the surface of B lymphocytes (CD20). Administration of Rituximab results in antibody CD20–binding and subsequent immunoglobulin- and complement-mediated killing of CD20-positive B cells. Depletion of B cells is effective in the treatment of lymphoproliferative disorders, such as non-Hodgkin lymphoma, and autoimmune diseases, such as hemolytic anemia.

Data from Joyce RM et al: *Ann Oncol* 14(Suppl 1):i21-27, 2003; Moreland LW: *Pharmacoeconomics* 22(2 Suppl):39-53, 2004; Nagajothi N et al: *Leuk Lymphoma* 45(4):795-799, 2004; Stio M et al: *Dig Dis Sci* 49(2):328-335, 2004; Wakim M et al: *Am J Hematol* 76(2):152-155, 2004.

and activation of the complement system that may lead to complement-mediated destruction of the pathogen or increased opsonic activity through deposition of C3b.[27,28]

In their role as **opsonins,** antibody and C3b make the pathogen more susceptible to phagocytosis through binding to Fc or C3b receptors on the phagocyte's surface. **Opsonization** is often necessary for efficient bacterial clearance because many bacteria have an outer capsule that deters recognition by phagocytes unless it is coated with an antibody or complement protein. Bacterial surface molecules are usually complex and have multiple accessible antigenic determinants, enabling them to bind several different antibodies simultaneously. When an antigen reacts with the Fab regions of antibody, the Fc portion of that antibody is held in close proximity to the Fc regions of the multiple other antibodies that are associated with the same pathogen. The clustering of Fc regions results in recognition and binding of the opsonized pathogen to Fc receptors on the surfaces of inflammatory cells. Engagement of Fc receptors results in their activation, making phagocytosis of the opsonized bacterium more efficient. The clustering of Fc regions has the added effect of more efficient complement activation.

Secretory Immune Response

The immune response that protects the entire body is produced by the **systemic immune system.** A distinct set of lymphoid tissues makes up another, partially independent, immune system at the external surfaces of the body. This system is called the **secretory (mucosal) immune system** (Figure 7-24). Most humoral immune responses occur when antibodies or B cells encounter antigens in the blood, but sometimes this encounter occurs in other body fluids. Antibodies are present in bodily secretions such as tears, sweat, saliva, mucus, and breast milk, where they can protect the body against antigens that have not yet penetrated the skin or mucous membranes.

Antibodies in secretions are produced by plasma cells of the secretory (mucosal) immune system.[29] The B cells of these two systems follow a different pattern of migration after they leave the bone marrow. B lymphocytes of the systemic immune system travel through the spleen and most lymph nodes, whereas those of the secretory immune system travel through a different group of lymphoid tissues including the lacrimal and salivary glands and the lymphoid tissues of the breasts, bronchi, intestines, and genitourinary tract. Immunoglobulins that are secreted at these sites are called **secretory immunoglobulins** and act locally rather than systemically.

Local protection is necessary to combat antigens (chiefly infectious microorganisms) that are inhaled, swallowed, or otherwise come in contact with external body surfaces. Once they have taken up residence in the external layers of the body, harmful microorganisms can cause local disease or possibly penetrate the barriers described in Chapter 6 to cause systemic disease. Alternatively, the microorganisms may fail to cause disease in the individual, either because the microorganisms are passed out of the body without any ill effects or because the infection is thwarted by the systemic immune system. In the latter case, the individual may continue to "carry" the infectious agent in the mucosal areas thereby enabling its spread to other individuals. The major function of the secretory immune system is to halt viral and bacterial invasion before local or systemic disease can develop and to prevent a carrier state that may result in spread of the infection to others. When secretory immunoglobulins bind to microorganisms, the pathogenic surface antigens are blocked, preventing the microorganism from attaching to and invading mucosal tissue.

IgA is the dominant secretory immunoglobulin, although IgM and IgG also are present in secretions. The primary role of IgA is to prevent the attachment and invasion of pathogens through mucosal membranes, such as those of the gastrointestinal, pulmonary, and genitourinary tracts. To induce protective immunity against some pathogens that enter through these routes, local immunization seems to be preferable to inducing only systemic immunity. For instance, the Sabin vaccine against polio is administered orally as an attenuated (i.e., inactivated so as to render relatively harmless) live virus. This route causes a transient, limited infection and induces effective systemic immunity and secretory immunity, preventing both the disease and the establishment of a carrier state. The Salk vaccine, on the other hand, consists of killed viruses that are administered intradermally. It induces adequate systemic protection but does not generally prevent an intestinal carrier state.

Because B lymphocytes of the secretory/mucosal immune system travel through breast-associated lymphoid tissue, most antigens to which the mother has been exposed gas-

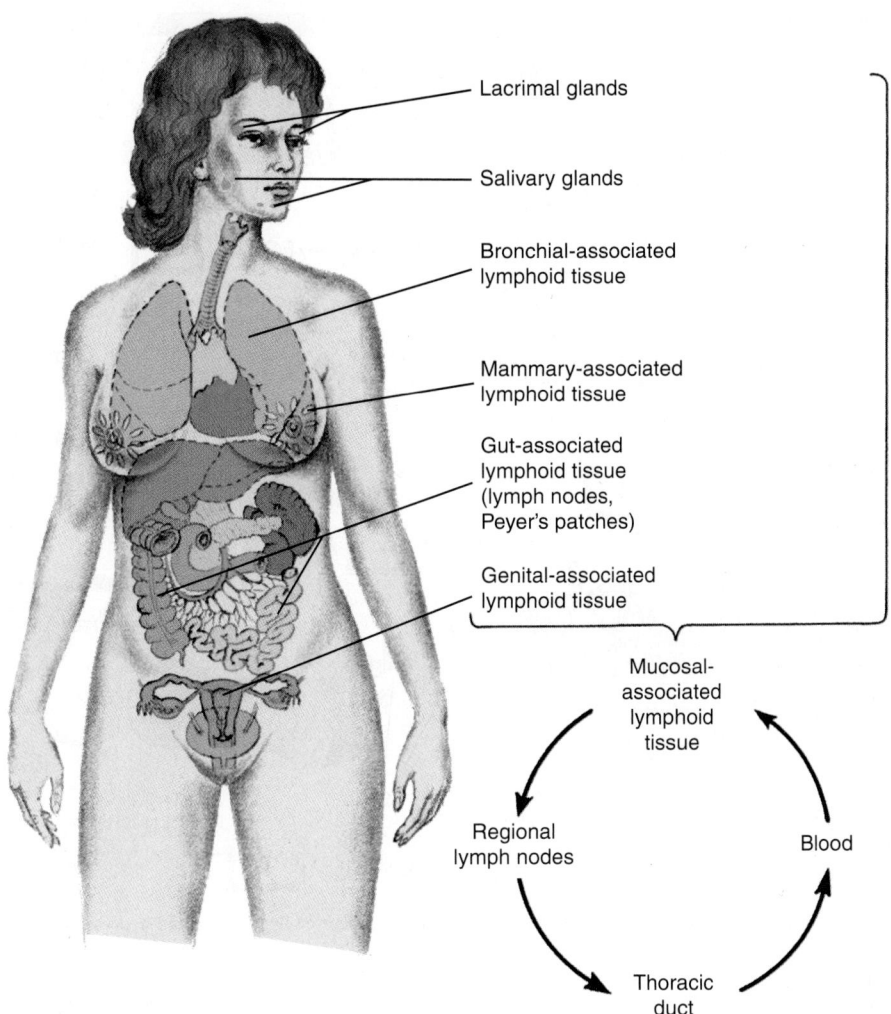

Lacrimal glands

Salivary glands

Bronchial-associated
lymphoid tissue

Mammary-associated
lymphoid tissue

Gut-associated
lymphoid tissue
(lymph nodes,
Peyer's patches)

Genital-associated
lymphoid tissue

Mucosal-
associated
lymphoid
tissue

Regional
lymph nodes

Blood

Thoracic
duct

Figure 7-24 Secretory immune system. Lymphocytes from the mucosal-associated lymphoid tissues circulate throughout the body in a pattern separate from other lymphocytes. For example, lymphocytes from the gut-associated lymphoid tissue circulate through the regional lymph nodes, the thoracic duct, and the blood and return to other mucosal-associated lymphoid tissues rather than to lymphoid tissue of the systemic immune system.

trointestinally (e.g., polio virus) induce secretion of specific IgAs, IgMs, and IgGs into the breast milk. Antibodies in the milk may provide protection against these infectious disease agents to the nursing newborn. Although colostral antibodies (i.e., found in colostrum of breast milk) provide the newborn with passive immunity against gastrointestinal infections, they do not provide systemic immunity because they do not cross the newborn's gut into the blood stream after the first 24 hours of life. Passive systemic immunity is provided by maternal antibodies that passed across the placenta into the fetus before birth.

The mechanisms and functions of antigen-antibody binding are the same in the secretory immune system as they are in the systemic immune systems; that is, binding neutralizes or opsonizes the antigen, preventing it from harming the host. The major differences between the two systems include (1) the order of utilization—the secretory immune response is part of the body's first-line defense, whereas the systemic response is the body's final defense; (2) the lymphocytes of each system follow different paths of migration and pass through different secondary lymphoid tissues; and (3) the secretory response occurs locally and externally (in body secretions), whereas the systemic response occurs systemically and internally (in blood and tissues).

IgE

IgE is a special class of antibody that is designed to protect the host from infection with large parasites.[30] However, when IgE is produced against relatively innocuous environmental antigens, it is also the primary cause of common allergies (e.g., hay fever, dust allergies, bee stings). The role of IgE in allergies is discussed in Chapter 8.

Large multicellular parasites usually invade mucosal tissues (Figure 7-25). Many antigens from the parasites induce a considerable amount of IgE, as well as other antibody classes. IgG, IgM, and IgA bind to the surface of parasites, activate complement, generate chemotactic factors for neutrophils and macrophages, and serve as opsonins for those phagocytic cells.

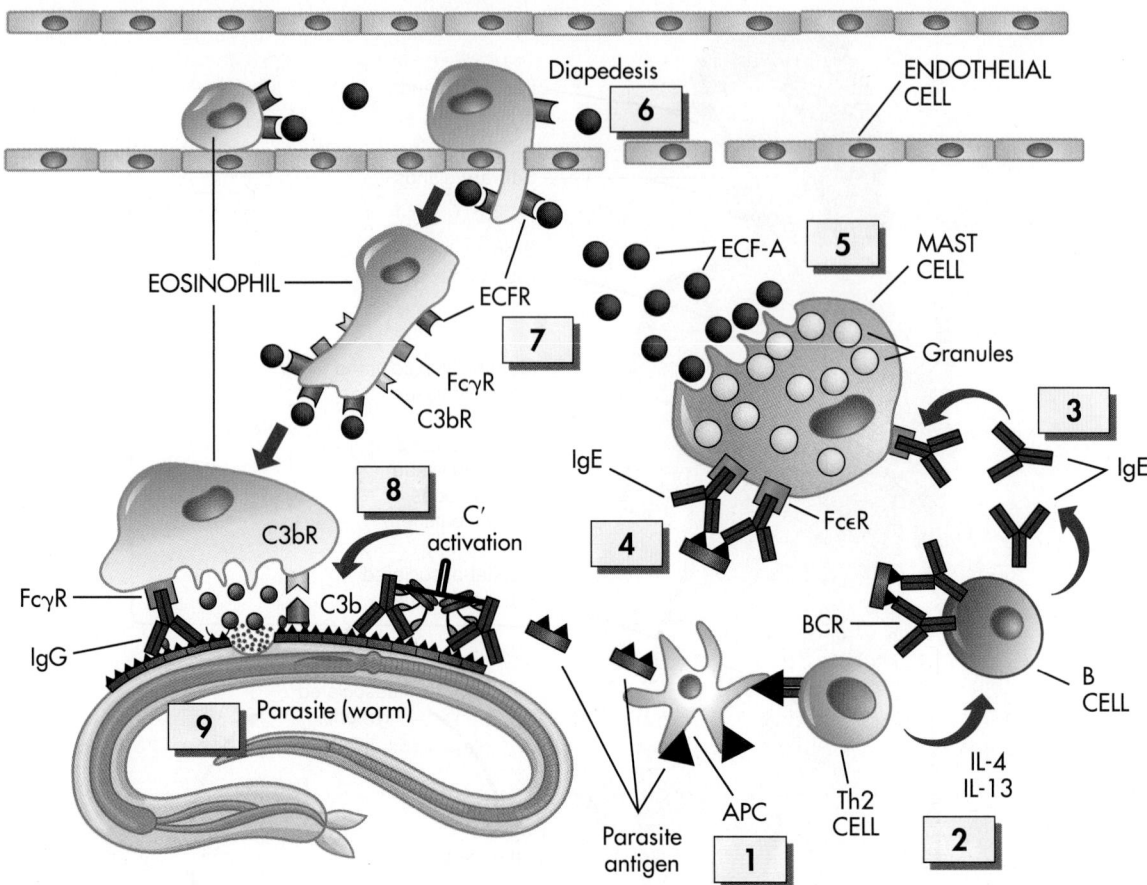

Figure 7-25 IgE function. Soluble antigens from a parasitic infection are processed by local antigen-processing cells *(APCs)* and presented to Th2 cells **(1)**, which respond by producing cytokines that favor class-switch to IgE production **(2)**. B cells bind soluble parasite antigen, and some switch to producing IgG, whereas others switch to IgE. The secreted IgE molecules bind to IgE-specific receptors (FcεR) on the mast cell surface **(3)**. Additional soluble parasite antigen crosslinks IgE-FcεR complexes on the mast cell surface **(4)** leading to mast cell degranulation and release of many pro-inflammatory products, including eosinophil chemotactic factor of anaphylaxis *(ECF-A)* **(5)**. Eosinophils have receptors for ECF-A *(ECFR)* and are stimulated to increase adherence to the vessel walls and initiate diapedesis **(6)** and invasion of the surrounding tissue. The eosinophil also responds by increasing the density of surface receptors for IgG (FcγR) and complement component C3b (C3bR) **(7)**. IgG had previously attached to the antigens on the parasite's surface and activated the complement cascade *(C' activation)* in a failed attempt to damage the parasite. The eosinophil attaches to the parasite's surface through Fc and C3b receptors **(8)**. Once bound to the parasite, the eosinophil releases its lysosomal enzymes onto the parasite, damaging its outer membrane **(9)**.

This response, however, does not greatly damage parasites. The only inflammatory cell that can adequately damage a parasite is the eosinophil because of the special contents of its granules, particularly *major basic protein*. Thus IgE is designed to specifically initiate an inflammatory reaction that preferentially attracts eosinophils to the site of parasitic infection.

Mast cells in the tissues have Fc receptors that specifically and with very high affinity react with IgE. In response to parasitic antigens, many B cells class-switch to IgE-secreting plasma cells. Because of the high affinity of the mast cell Fc receptor, IgE molecules are rapidly bound to the mast cell surface. Soluble macromolecules with multiple antigenic determinants are released from the parasite and will diffuse to neighboring mast cells, where they bind simultaneously to multiple IgE molecules. The crosslinking of IgE-Fc receptor complexes on the mast cell surface produces a strong intracellular signal leading to mast cell degranulation (see Chapter

6). One preformed component of the mast cell granules is eosinophil chemotactic factor of anaphylaxis (ECF-A). As the name implies, ECF-A is highly chemotactic for eosinophils, resulting in eosinophil migration from the circulation into the tissues as well as up-regulation of surface receptors for IgG and complement component C3b. The eosinophil attaches to the surface of the parasite through these receptors and attempts phagocytosis. Because of the extremely large size of typical parasites, engulfment is unsuccessful. The eosinophilic granules move to the cell membrane in contact with the parasite and undergo normal degranulation releasing the granular contents, including major basic protein and other antimicrobial peptides, onto the parasite's surface. Being highly cationic, major basic protein acts almost like sodium hydroxide and causes extensive damage to the parasite. The parasite will die if an adequate number of eosinophils are involved. The tight fit between the eosinophil

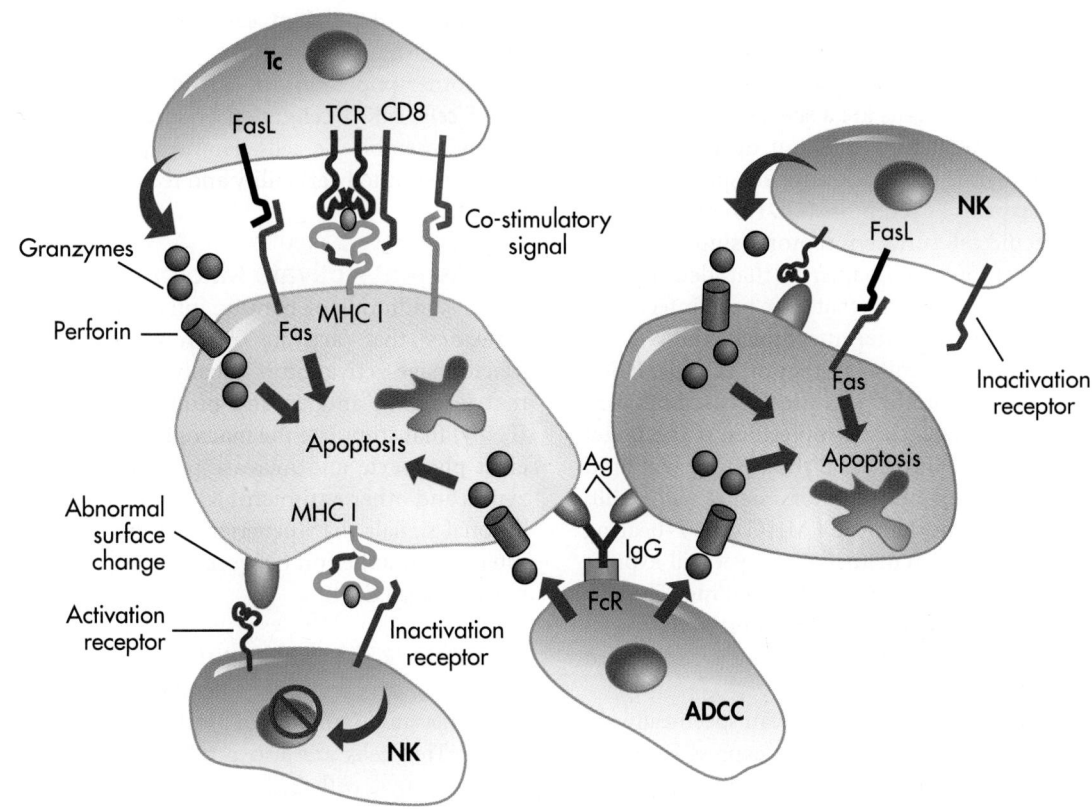

Figure 7-26 Cell killing mechanisms. Several cells have the capacity to kill abnormal (e.g., virally infected, cancerous) target cells. Cytotoxic T (Tc) cells recognized endogenous antigen presented by MHC class I molecules *(cell on upper left)*. The intercellular interaction is enhanced through a variety of co-stimulatory adhesion molecules. The Tc cell mobilizes multiple killing mechanisms that induce apoptosis of the target cell, including the secretion of perforin that creates pores for the entrance of granzymes into the target cell and stimulation of Fas molecules on the target cell surface by Fas ligand *(FasL)* on the Tc cell. Natural killer (NK) cells *(cell on upper right)* use the same mechanisms to kill target cells through activation receptors that recognize "abnormal surface changes." NK cells specifically kill targets that have down-regulated expression of surface MHC class I molecules. Targets expressing MHC class I molecules inactivate NK cells through a variety of inactivation receptors *(cell on lower left)*. Several cells, including macrophages and NK cells, can kill by antibody-dependent cellular cytotoxicity *(ADCC)*. IgG antibody binds to foreign antigen on the target cell. Cells involved in ADCC *(cell on lower right)* bind IgG through Fc receptors *(FcR)* and initiate killing.

and the parasite usually minimizes damage to the surrounding host tissues.

T-Lymphocyte Function
Killing Abnormal Cells
Cytotoxic T Lymphocytes

Cytotoxic T lymphocytes (Tc cells or CTLs) are responsible for the cell-mediated destruction of such targets as tumor cells or cells infected with viruses.[31] To perform this function, the Tc cell must directly adhere to the target cell through antigen presentation in association with MHC class I molecules and appropriate adhesion molecules (Figure 7-26). Most Tc-cell killing requires the αβ TCR complex and CD8. Tc-cell–mediated killing is therefore *class I restricted*. Because of the cellular distribution of MHC class I molecules, Tc cells can recognize antigen on the surface of almost any type of cell that has been infected by a virus or has become cancerous.

After attachment to a target cell, killing can occur by at least two different mechanisms that induce apoptosis: through the actions of perforin and granzyme or direct receptor interactions. Perforins and granzymes are contained in the Tc-cell lysosomal granules, which are released onto the surface of the target cell. Perforin acts in a fashion similar to C9 of the complement cascade and penetrates, polymerizes, and forms pores in the target cell's plasma membrane. The granzymes enter the target cell through the perforin-lined pores and activate cellular enzymes (caspases) that are involved in apoptosis, resulting in death of the target. Additionally, target cell apoptosis can be induced directly through the stimulation of specific receptors on the cell surface. For instance, Tc cells express a surface molecule called *Fas ligand*, which is very similar to TNF-α and reacts with a protein called *Fas* (CD95) on the target cell surface. Activation of Fas signals the target cell to undergo apoptosis.

Other Cells that Kill Abnormal Cells

A variety of other cells kill targets in a fashion similar to Tc lymphocytes. Prominent among these cells are NK (natural killer) cells (see Chapter 6). In many ways, NK cells complement the effects of Tc cells.[32] In some instances, a virally infected or cancerous cell will "protect" itself by down-regulating MHC class I molecule expression. Without surface MHC class I molecules, a cell becomes resistant to Tc-cell recognition and killing. NK cells are a special group of lymphoid cells that are similar to T cells but do not undergo maturation in the thymus and lack antigen-specific receptors. Instead, they express Fc receptors (CD16) for IgG and a variety of NK-specific cell surface receptors (similar to pattern recognition receptors, see Chapter 6) that identify protein changes on the surface of cells that have been infected or are in other ways abnormal. After attachment, the NK cell kills its target in a manner similar to that of Tc cells. However, NK cells also express another set of receptors, inhibitory receptors, that bind to MHC class I molecules. If the target cell continues to express MHC class I, the NK cell will bind to the class I molecule, and an inhibitory signal will result. Thus NK cells do not inadvertently kill MHC class I–bearing cells. If these cells are infected or malignant, yet still express MHC class I, they remain sensitive to Tc cell killing. Thus Tc cells kill abnormal cells that continue to express MHC class I, whereas NK cells kill abnormal cells that have suppressed MHC class I expression.

NK cells, as well as some macrophages, can specifically kill targets through use of antibody. These cells express Fc receptors on their surface. If a pathogen or abnormal cell expresses a foreign antigen that elicits IgG antibody, which binds to the antigen, the NK cell can attach to the IgG through Fc receptors and activate its normal killing mechanisms. This is referred to as **antibody-dependent cellular cytotoxicity (ADCC)** (see Figure 7-26).

Another population of NK-like cells has been identified, NK-T cells. NK-T cells are produced in the thymus and more closely resemble Tc cells. However, they express TCRs that have very limited variability and recognize antigens presented by CD1.

T Cells that Activate Macrophages

Under conditions of chronic inflammation, T cells produce cytokines that activate macrophages (see Chapter 6). Macrophage activation is usually accomplished by Th1 cells that recognize antigen and produce cytokines (particularly IFN-γ) that stimulate the macrophage to become a more efficient phagocyte and increase production of proteolytic enzymes and other antimicrobial substances (Figure 7-27). Additional signals that increase macrophage activation include intercellular adhesion between the Th1 cell (CD40L) and the macrophage (CD40).

Regulatory T Lymphocytes

One form of peripheral tolerance to self-antigens occurs through a subpopulation of T cells called **regulatory T (Treg) cells.**[33] Treg cells are also produced in response to antigen recognition. As with CTLs, Treg cells are activated when antigen is presented in a complex with class I MHC molecules. The role of Treg cells is to control or limit the immune response to protect the host's own tissues against autoimmune

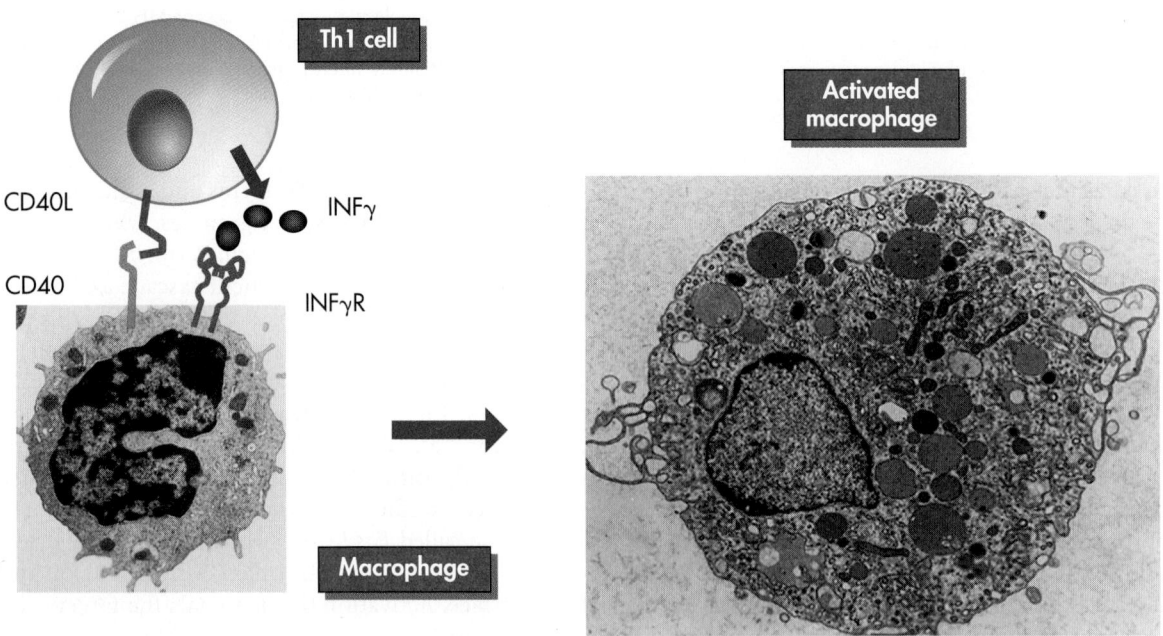

Figure 7-27 Activation of a macrophage by a T cell. A population of T cells that helps immune and inflammatory responses (helper T cells or Th1 cells) produces cytokines that activate macrophages. Optimal macrophage activation also requires close contact between the cells, which is mediated by a variety of adhesion molecules expressed on the surface of each cell (CD40L and CD40 shown here). *CD40L*, CD40 ligand; *INFγ*, interferon-gamma; *INFγR*, receptor for interferon-gamma. (Micrograph in **A** from Abbas AK, Lichtman AH: *Cellular and molecular immunology,* ed 5, Philadelphia, 2003, Saunders; **B** from Bloom W, Fawcett DW: *A textbook of histology,* ed 11, Philadelphia, 1986, Saunders.)

reactions. Treg cells exert their effects in multiple ways. Some Treg cells affect the recognition of antigen, and others suppress the proliferative steps that follow antigen recognition. The role of Treg cells is currently under intense investigation to determine the degree of their heterogeneity of derivation, function, and specificity.

FETAL AND NEONATAL IMMUNE FUNCTION
The normal human infant is immunologically immature at birth. Although cell-mediated immunologic capabilities begin developing early in gestation and probably are completely functional at birth, antibody production is clearly deficient. In the last trimester, the fetus appears capable of producing a primary immune response (almost entirely IgM) to antigenic challenge *in utero* but is unable to produce a significant IgG response. Although some IgA can be detected, the capacity to produce IgA is underdeveloped.

To protect the child against infectious agents both *in utero* and during the first few postnatal months, a system of active transport facilitates the passage of maternal antibodies into the fetal circulation[34] (Figure 7-28). In the placenta, maternal and fetal blood is separated by a layer of specialized cells termed *trophoblasts.* Immunoglobulins are too large to diffuse across this cellular layer so the trophoblastic cells actively transport immunoglobulins from the maternal to the fetal circulation. Active transport of maternal IgG is mediated by surface receptors that are specific for the Fc portion of free IgG but not for IgM, IgE, or IgA. Active transport sometimes results in higher antibody titers in umbilical cord blood than in maternal blood. (Active transport mechanisms are discussed in Chapter 1.)

At birth, total IgG levels in the umbilical cord are near adult levels (Figure 7-29). When the source of maternal anti-

bodies is severed at birth, antibody titers in the newborn begin to drop as maternal antibody is catabolized. Thus antibody titers drop rapidly as the neonate's production of IgG is beginning to rise. The rate of catabolism is usually more rapid than the rate of production so that the total immunoglobulin levels reach a minimum at 5 to 6 months in the normal child, occasionally causing transient hypogammaglobulinemia (insufficient quantities of circulating immunoglobulins). Many normal infants experience recurrent mild respiratory tract infections at this age.

AGING AND IMMUNE FUNCTION
Immune function decreases in old age as a result of changes in both lymphocyte function and relative lymphocyte populations. Individuals over 60 years of age generally exhibit decreased T cell activity as demonstrated by laboratory assays of T-cell function,[35] as well as *in vivo* reductions in cell-mediated responses to infections. The thymus, where T cells begin their development, reaches its maximum size at sexual maturity and then begins involuting until thymic size is only 15% of its maximum by middle age. Thymic capacity to mediate T-cell differentiation decreases with this atrophy. Although the total number of circulating T cells does not decrease with age, there is a shift in the populations of T-cell subtypes.

B-cell function is also altered with age as shown by decreases in specific antibody production in response to antigenic challenge, with concomitant increases in circulating immune complexes and in circulating autoantibodies (antibodies against self-antigens). A decrease in the number of circulating memory B cells is also observed.

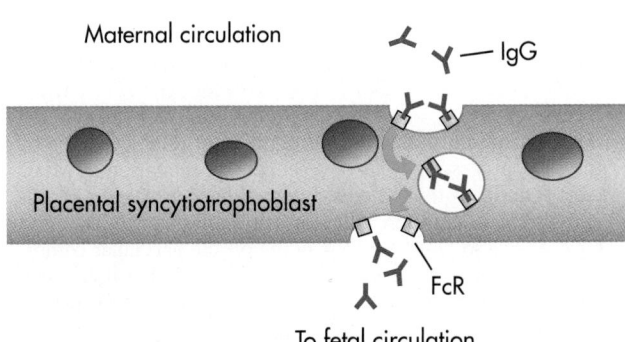

Figure 7-28 Transport of IgG across the syncytiotrophoblast. The human placenta is covered with a specialized multinucleate cell, the syncytiotrophoblast. Transport of maternal IgG across the syncytiotrophoblast and into the fetal circulation is an active process. Maternal IgG binds to Fc receptors on the surface of the syncytiotrophoblast and is internalized by the process of endocytosis. Receptors on the syncytiotrophoblast are specific for the Fc portion of IgG and do not bind other classes of immunoglobulins. Interaction of IgG with Fc receptors protects the antibody from lysosomal digestion during transport of the vacuole across the cell (i.e., transcytosis). On the fetal side of the syncytiotrophoblast, IgG is released by exocytosis (see Chapter 1).

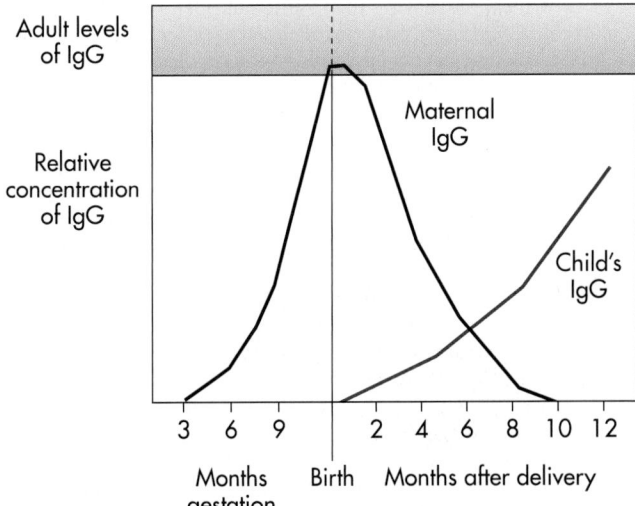

Figure 7-29 Antibody levels in umbilical cord blood and in neonatal circulation. Early in gestation, maternal IgG begins crossing the placenta and enters the fetal circulation as shown in Figure 7-28. At birth, the fetal circulation may contain nearly adult levels of IgG, which is almost exclusively from the maternal source. The fetal immune system has the capacity to produce IgM and small amounts of IgA before birth (not shown). After delivery, maternal IgG is rapidly catabolized and neonatal IgG production increases.

General Characteristics of Adaptive Immunity

1. Compared with the innate inflammatory response, the adaptive immune response is slower, specific rather than nonspecific or general, and has "memory" that makes it much longer lived.
2. The adaptive immune response is most often initiated by cells of the innate system. These cells process and present portions of invading pathogens (i.e., antigens) to lymphocytes in peripheral lymphoid tissue.
3. The adaptive immune response is mediated by two different types of lymphocytes—B lymphocytes and T lymphocytes. Each has distinct functions. B cells are responsible for humoral immunity that is mediated by circulating antibodies, whereas T cells are responsible for cell-mediated immunity, in which they kill targets directly or stimulate the activity of other leukocytes.
4. Adaptive immunity can be either active or passive depending on whether immune response components originated in the host or came from a donor.

Recognition and Response

1. Antigens are the molecules that can react with components of the adaptive immune system, including antibodies and lymphocyte surface receptors. Immunogens are antigens that can initiate the adaptive immune response. To be immunogenic, an antigen must be of the correct type, size, and complexity and be present in sufficient quantities. Haptens are small molecular weight antigens that are not themselves immunogenic.
2. For most antigens to elicit an immune response, they must be presented to lymphocytes by molecules on the surface of antigen-presenting cells. Endogenous protein antigens are presented by Class I molecules of major histocompatibility complex (MHC). Exogenous protein antigens are presented by Class II MHC molecules. Lipid antigens are presented by CD1.
3. The major histocompatibility complex (MHC) is a cluster of genes found on human chromosome 6. The products of these genes are also called *HLA antigens*. The MHC genes are highly polymorphic, having many different possible alleles. An individual will carry only two alleles at each locus, one from each parent. The particular combination of alleles a given individual carries defines his or her MHC haplotype.
4. Both B and T lymphocytes bind antigen through cognate receptor complexes on their surfaces. These receptor complexes (i.e., the BCR and TCR complexes, respectively) work in conjunction with accessory proteins to produce lymphocyte activation.
5. The antigen-binding molecule of the BCR is antibody. Antibodies are comprised of four polypeptide chains, two identical heavy chains and two identical light chains, that are held together by disulfide bonds. Each heavy chain has a variable region and a large constant region. Each light chain has a variable region and a short constant region. The class of antibody is determined by which constant regions make up their heavy chains, giving each class a slightly different molecular structure. The classes include IgG (the most prevalent), IgA (mostly in secretions), IgE (the most rare), IgD, and IgM (the first and largest immunoglobulin produced). The parts of antibody that bind antigen are called the *Fab,* and the part that reacts with cells and molecules of the innate system is called the *Fc.* Antigen binds to hypervariable regions (complementary determining regions, or CDRs) of both the heavy and light chain.
6. For an immune response to develop, a variety of cells must interact through surface adhesion molecules.
7. During their interactions, cells must communicate with each other through soluble cytokines. In addition to their roles in the innate immune response, cytokines have multiple functions in the adaptive immune response including both positive and negative regulation of B cell and T cell maturation. In general, it is the precise combination of cytokines influencing a given cell that ultimately determines that cell's response.

Generation of Clonal Diversity

1. The generation of clonal diversity occurs in the primary lymphoid organs (thymus for T cells, bone marrow for B cells) in the fetus.
2. An individual's population of T cells and B cells have the collective ability to respond to virtually any antigen. This ability results from genetic rearrangement of various genes to form the variable regions for the TCR and BCR. Rearrangement of *V* and *J* genes result in the variable regions of the TCR α chain and the BCR light chain, and rearrangement of *V, D,* and *J* genes result in the variable regions of the TCR β chain and the BCR heavy chain.
3. Differentiation of B cells and T cells in the primary lymphoid organs results in expression of several characteristic surface markers, such as CD4 on helper T cells, CD8 on cytotoxic T cells, and CD21 and CD40 on B cells.
4. During generation of clonal diversity, B cells and T cells that produce receptors against self-antigens are eliminated by a process of central tolerance.
5. Cells leaving the primary lymphoid organs are immunocompetent (capable of reacting to antigen) and enter the circulation and secondary lymphoid organs.

Induction of an Immune Response: Clonal Selection

1. Clonal selection is the process by which antigen selects lymphocytes with complementary TCRs or BCRs and induces an immune response with the production of specific antibody or cytotoxic T cells, or both.
2. For lymphocyte activation, most antigens must be processed and presented by an antigen presenting cell (APC) in the context of the appropriate molecule, either MHC class I, MHC class II, or CD1 molecules.
3. Most immune responses require helper T cells (Th cells). Precursor Th cells interact with APCs through the TCR/CD4 complex, a variety of adhesion molecules, and cytokines, especially IL-1, and develop into either Th1 or Th2 subsets. Th1 cells are responsible for helping to activate macrophages and cytotoxic T cells, whereas Th2 cells are responsible for helping to activate B cells.
4. B cell activation results from recognition of soluble antigen by the BCR, processing of the antigen, and presentation by MHC class II antigens to Th2 cells. Interactions between the B cells and Th2 cells through adhesion molecules (e.g., CD40 and CD40L) is also required. Depending on the particular combination of cytokines produced by the Th2 cell, the B cells can undergo class-switch from making IgM antibody to making and secreting either IgA, IgE, or IgG.
5. The humoral immune response is divided into two phases, primary and secondary. These differ in the relative amounts of IgG produced—the secondary response having a much higher proportion of IgG relative to IgM. The two responses also differ in the speed with which each occurs after antigen challenge—the secondary response being much more rapid than the primary response because of the presence of memory cells in the secondary phase.
6. B cells become activated upon recognition of a particular antigen to proliferate and differentiate into plasma cells that function as factories for the synthesis of large amounts of antibody

that is specific for the recognized antigen or into memory B cells.

7. T cell activation results from recognition by the TCR and CD8 of antigen presented by MHC class I. Appropriate intercellular adhesion molecules and cytokines, such as IL-2 from Th1 cells, are also necessary for efficient differentiation. T cells become cytotoxic T lymphocytes (CTLs) or memory T cells.

8. Superantigens are molecules produced by infectious agents that can bind to the Th cell's TCR outside the normal antigen-binding site and to Class II MHC on the APCs, resulting in activation of a large number of Th cells and excessive production of pro-inflammatory cytokines that may cause shock and death of the patient. Examples of these antigens, called *superantigens,* include the bacterial toxins that can cause toxic shock syndrome and food poisoning.

Effector Mechanisms

1. The antibodies that are produced by B cells affect antigens by several different mechanisms that can be categorized as either direct or indirect. Direct mechanisms are mediated by the antigen-binding portions of antibodies (the Fab portions containing the variable regions). This binding results in neutralization of the biologic activity of antigens and possibly removal of the antigen by agglutination or precipitation. Indirect mechanisms depend on both the Fab and the nonantigen-binding portion of antibodies (the Fc portions containing the constant regions), which interact with components of innate immunity.

2. Antibodies of the systemic immune system function throughout the body whereas antibodies of the secretory (mucosal) immune system—primarily immunoglobulins of the IgA class—are associated with bodily secretions and function to prevent pathogenic infection on epithelial surfaces.

3. Cytotoxic T cells (Tc cells) adhere directly to antigen presented by MHC Class I on target cells (virus-infected cells or cancer cells) through the TCR, CD8, and a variety of adhesion proteins. This contact results in killing of the target by apoptosis through the release of perforin and granzymes and/or direct stimulation of apoptotic receptors on the target (e.g., Fas).

4. Natural killer cells (NK cells) kill targets in a fashion similar to that of Tc cells. However, NK cells recognize target cells that do not express MHC Class I.

5. With infections that are resistant to cells of innate immunity, some Th1 cells produce cytokines that activate macrophages to become more efficient phagocytes.

Fetal and Neonatal Immune Function

1. The human neonate has a poorly developed immune response, particularly in the production of IgG. The fetus and neonate are protected in utero and during the first few postnatal months by maternal antibody that was actively transported across the placenta.

2. The maternal antibodies are slowly catabolized after birth until they disappear altogether by about 10 months of age. The neonate begins producing IgG at birth, and the child's antibodies reach protective levels after about 6 months of age.

Aging and Immune Function

1. T cell activity is deficient in the elderly and a shift in the balance of T cell subsets is observed. These changes may result in increased susceptibility to infection.

2. Antibody production to specific antigens is inferior, although elderly people tend to have increased levels of circulating autoantibodies.

KEY TERMS

Adaptive (acquired) immunity (immune response), 211
Active acquired immunity (active immunity), 214
Agglutination, 238
Allergens, 216
Antibodies, 212, 219
Antibody-dependent cellular cytotoxicity (ADCC), 244
Antibody titer, 239
Antigens, 211, 215
Antigen-binding fragment (Fab), 221
Antigenic determinant, 215
Antigen presentation, 217
Antigen-presenting cells (APCs), 216
Antigen processing, 230
Attenuated virus, 239
B lymphocytes (B cells), 212
B-cell receptor (BCR), 219, 227
B-cell receptor (BCR) complex, 222
Carrier, 216
CD (cluster of differentiation), 215
Cellular immunity, 214
Central tolerance, 215
Class-switch, 235
Clonal selection, 224
Complementary-determining regions (CDRs), 221
Crystalline fragment (Fc), 221

Cytotoxic T lymphocytes (Tc cells or CTL), 214
Epitope, 215
Framework regions (FRs), 221
Generation of clonal diversity, 223
Haplotype, 218
Haptens, 215
Helper T cells (Th cells), 213, 231
Hinge region, 221
High endothelial venule (HEV), 229
Human leukocyte antigens (HLA), 218
Humoral immunity, 213
Immunity, 211
Immunocompetent, 212
Immunogens, 215
Immunogenic, 215
Immunoglobulins, 212
Invariant chain, 231
Isotype-switch, 235
Lymphocytes, 212
Lymphoid stem cells, 224
Major histocompatibility complex (MHC), 216
MHC class I genes, 217
MHC class II genes, 217
Memory cells, 214
Memory T cells, 237
Neutralization, 238
Opsonins, 240

Opsonization, 240
Paratope, 215
Passive acquired immunity (passive immunity), 214
Peripheral tolerance, 215, 227
Plasma cell, 234
Precipitation, 238
Primary (central) lymphoid organ, 224
Primary immune response, 235
Regulatory T (Treg) cell, 244
Secondary (anamnestic) immune response, 235
Secondary (peripheral) lymphoid organs, 224
Secretory (mucosal) immune system, 240
Secretory immunoglobulins, 240
Self-antigen, 215
Somatic recombination, 224
Superantigens (SAGs), 237
Systemic immune system, 240
T-cell receptor (TCR), 219, 224
T-cell receptor (TCR) complex, 222
Th1 cell, 234
Th2 cell, 234
T lymphocytes (T cells), 212
Tolerance, 215
T regulatory (Treg) cells, 237
Valence, 222

MEDIA RESOURCES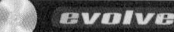

Review questions and answers for this chapter are available in the *CD Companion* included with this book. Also see the CD for animations of *immunity* and *antibody functions.*

WebLinks—links to Internet sites pertaining to this chapter—are available on Evolve at http://evolve.elsevier.com/McCance/.

REFERENCES

1. Casadevall A, Dadachova E, Pirofski LA: Passive antibody therapy for infectious diseases, *Nat Rev Microbiol* 2(9):695-703, 2004.
2. Morris CR et al: Association of intracellular proteins with folded major histocompatibility complex class I molecules, *Immunol Res* 30(2):171-179, 2004.
3. *Immunogenetics database,* accessed March 24, 2004, available at www.ebi.ac.uk/imgt/hla/stats.html.
4. Lawton AP, Kronenberg M: The third way: progress on pathways of antigen processing and presentation by CD1, *Immunol Cell Biol* 82(3):295-306, 2004.
5. Porter RR: The hydrolysis of rabbit γ-globulin and antibodies with crystalline papain, *Biochem J* 73:119-126, 1959.
6. Vargas-Madrazo E, Paz-Garcia E: An improved model of association for VH-VL immunoglobulin domains: asymmetries between VH and VL in the packing of some interface residues, *J Mol Recognit* 16(3):113-120, 2003.
7. Dal Porto JM et al: B cell antigen receptor signaling 101, *Mol Immunol* 41(6-7):599-613, 2004.
8. Krogsgaard M, Davis MM: How T cells 'see' antigen, *Nat Immunol* 6(3):239-245, 2005.
9. Burnet FM: *The clonal selection theory of acquired immunity,* London, 1959, Cambridge University Press.
10. Jerne NK: The natural-selection theory of antibody formation, *Proc Natl Acad Sci U S A* 41:849-857, 1955.
11. Kyewski B, Derbinski J: Self-representation in the thymus: an extended view, *Nat Rev Immunol* 4(9):688-698, 2004.
12. von Boehmer H: Selection of the T-cell repertoire: receptor-controlled checkpoints in T-cell development, *Adv Immunol* 84:201-238, 2004.
13. Bosselut R: CD4/CD8-lineage differentiation in the thymus: from nuclear effectors to membrane signals, *Nat Rev Immunol* 4(7):529-540, 2004.
14. Fuentes-Panana EM, Bannish G, Monroe JG: Basal B-cell receptor signaling in B lymphocytes: mechanisms of regulation and role in positive selection, differentiation, and peripheral survival, *Immunol Rev* 197:26-40, 2004.
15. Chowdhury D, Sen R: Regulation of immunoglobulin heavy-chain gene rearrangements, *Immunol Rev* 200:182-196, 2004.
16. Verkoczy LK, Martensson AS, Nemazee D: The scope of receptor editing and its association with autoimmunity, *Curr Opin Immunol* 16(6):808-814, 2004.
17. Pabst O, Herbrand H, Bernhardt G, Forster R: Elucidating the functional anatomy of secondary lymphoid organs, *Curr Opin Immunol* 16(4):394-399, 2004.
18. Watts C: The exogenous pathway for antigen presentation on major histocompatibility complex class II and CD1 molecules, *Nat Immunol* 5(7):685-692, 2004.
19. Romagnani S et al: TH1 and TH2 cells, *Res Immunol* 149(9):871-873, 1998.
20. Kidd P: Th1/Th2 balance: the hypothesis, its limitations, and implications for health and disease, *Altern Med Rev* 8(3):223-246, 2003.
21. Eyler JM: Smallpox in history: the birth, death, and impact of a dread disease, *J Lab Clin Med* 142(4):216-220, 2003.
22. Jenner E: *An inquiry into the causes and effects of the variolae vaccinae: a disease discovered in some of the western counties of England, particularly Gloucestershire, and known by the name of the cow pox,* London, 1798, Sampson Low.
23. Chaudhuri J, Alt FW: Class-switch recombination: interplay of transcription, DNA deamination and DNA repair, *Nat Rev Immunol* 4(7):541-552, 2004.
24. van der Merwe PA, Davis SJ: Molecular interactions mediating T cell antigen recognition, *Annu Rev Immunol* 21:659-684, 2003.
25. Petersson K, Forsberg G, Walse B: Interplay between superantigens and immunoreceptors, *Scand J Immunol* 59(4):345-355, 2004.
26. Baker MD, Acharya KR: Superantigens: structure-function relationships, *Int J Med Microbiol* 293(7-8):529-537, 2004.
27. Delves PJ, Roitt IM: The immune system. I, *N Engl J Med* 343(1):37-49, 2000.
28. Delves PJ, Roitt IM: The immune system. II, *N Engl J Med* 343(1):108-117, 2000.
29. Brandtzaeg P: Role of secretory antibodies in the defence against infections, *Int J Med Microbiol* 293(1):3-15, 2003.
30. Zacharia B, Sherman P: Atopy, helminths, and cancer, *Med Hypotheses* 60(1):1-5, 2003.
31. Waterhouse NJ et al: Cytotoxic lymphocytes; instigators of dramatic target cell death, *Biochem Pharmacol* 15;68(6):1033-1040, 2004.
32. Bottino C et al: Learning how to discriminate between friends and enemies, a lesson from natural killer cells, *Mol Immunol* 41(6-7):569-575, 2004.
33. TretJiang H, Chess L: An integrated view of suppressor T cell subsets in immunoregulation, *J Clin Invest* 114(9):1198-1208, 2004.
34. Simister NE: Placental transport of immunoglobulin G, *Vaccine* 21(24):3365-3369, 2003.
35. Hakim FT et al: Aging, immunity and cancer, *Curr Opin Immunol* 16(2):151-156, 2004.

ALTERATIONS IN IMMUNITY AND INFLAMMATION

NEAL S. ROTE

CHAPTER OUTLINE

The immune system is a finely tuned network that protects the host against foreign antigens, particularly infectious agents. Sometimes this network breaks down, causing the immune system to react inappropriately. Inappropriate immune responses may be (1) exaggerated against environmental antigens (allergy); (2) misdirected against the host's own cells (autoimmunity); (3) directed against beneficial foreign tissues, such as transfusions or transplants (alloimmunity); or (4) insufficient to protect the host (immune deficiency). All of these can be serious or life threatening. Exaggerated immune responses (allergy) are the most common, but usually the least life threatening.

HYPERSENSITIVITY: ALLERGY, AUTOIMMUNITY, AND ALLOIMMUNITY

Allergy, autoimmunity, and alloimmunity can be collectively classified as *hypersensitivity reactions*. **Hypersensitivity** is an altered immunologic response to an antigen that

results in disease or damage to the host. Allergy, autoimmunity, and alloimmunity (also termed *isoimmunity*) can be most easily understood in relationship to the source of the antigen against which the hypersensitivity response is directed (Table 8-1). The term **allergy** originally denoted both facets of the immune response: immunity, which is beneficial, and hypersensitivity, which is harmful. Allergy has now come to mean the deleterious effects of hypersensitivity to environmental (exogenous) antigens, and immunity means the protective responses to antigens expressed by disease-causing agents.

Autoimmunity is a disturbance in the immunologic tolerance of self-antigens. The immune system normally does not strongly recognize the individual's own antigens. Healthy individuals of all ages, but particularly the elderly, may produce low quantities of antibodies against their own antigens (*autoantibodies*), without development of overt autoimmune disease. Therefore the presence of low quantities of autoantibodies does not necessarily indicate a disease state. Autoimmune diseases occur when the immune system reacts against self-antigens to such a degree that host tissues are damaged by autoantibodies or autoreactive T cells. Many clinical disorders are associated with autoim-

Table 8-1	Relative Incidences and Examples of Hypersensitivity Reactions*			
	Mechanism			
Target Antigen	Type I (Immunoglobulin E– [IgE] Mediated)	Type II (Tissue Specific)	Type III (Immune Complex)	Type IV (Cell Mediated)
Allergy Environmental antigens	++++ Hay fever	+ Hemolysis in drug allergies	+ Gluten (wheat) allergy	++ Poison ivy allergy
Autoimmunity Self-antigens	± May contribute to some type III reactions	++ Autoimmune thrombo-cytopenia	+++ Systemic lupus erythe-matosus	+ Hashimoto thyroiditis
Alloimmunity Another person's antigens	± May contribute to some type III reactions	++ Hemolytic disease of the newborn	+ Anaphylaxis to IgA in IV γ-globulin	++ Graft rejection

*The frequency of each reaction is indicated in a range from rare (±) to very common (++++). An example of each reaction is given.

munity and are generally referred to as **autoimmune diseases** (Table 8-2).

Alloimmune diseases occur when the immune system of one individual produces an immunologic reaction against tissues of another individual. Alloimmunity can be observed during immunologic reactions against transfusions, transplanted tissue, or the fetus during pregnancy.

The mechanism that initiates the onset of hypersensitivity, whether it consists of allergy, autoimmunity, or alloimmunity, is not completely understood. It is generally accepted that genetic, infectious, and possibly environmental factors contribute to hypersensitivity. Most diseases caused by hypersensitivity develop because of the interactions of at least three variables: (1) an original "insult," which alters **immunologic homeostasis** (a steady state of tolerance to self-antigens or lack of immune reaction against environmental antigens); (2) the individual's genetic makeup, which determines the degree of the resultant immune response from the effects of the insult; and (3) an immunologic process that causes the symptoms of the disease.

Mechanisms of Hypersensitivity

Diseases caused by hypersensitivity reactions can be characterized also by the particular immune mechanism that results in the disease (see Table 8-1). These mechanisms are apparent in most hypersensitivity reactions and have been divided into four distinct types: *type I* (IgE-mediated reactions), *type II* (tissue-specific reactions), *type III* (immune complex–mediated reactions), and *type IV* (cell-mediated reactions)[1] (Table 8-3). This classification is artificial and seldom is a particular disease associated with only a single mechanism. The four mechanisms are interrelated, and in most hypersensitivity reactions, several mechanisms can be at work simultaneously or sequentially. Some of the mechanisms are secondary to the disease and not directly involved in the pathologic process, whereas others are the primary cause of tissue destruction.

As with all immune responses, hypersensitivity reactions require sensitization against a particular antigen that results in a primary immune response. Symptoms appear after an adequate secondary immune response occurs. Hypersensitivity reactions are immediate or delayed, depending on the time required to elicit clinical symptoms after reexposure to the antigen. Reactions that occur within minutes to a few hours after exposure to antigen are termed **immediate hypersensitivity reactions**. **Delayed hypersensitivity reactions** may take several hours to appear and are at maximum severity days after reexposure to the antigen.

The most rapid and severe immediate hypersensitivity reaction is **anaphylaxis.** Anaphylaxis occurs within minutes of reexposure to the antigen and can be either systemic (generalized) or cutaneous (localized).[2] Symptoms of systemic anaphylaxis include itching, erythema, vomiting, abdominal cramps, diarrhea, and breathing difficulties. In severe cases, contraction of bronchial smooth muscle, laryngeal edema, and vascular collapse may result in respiratory distress, decreased blood pressure, shock, and death. An example of systemic anaphylaxis is an allergic reaction to bee stings. Cutaneous anaphylaxis causes the less severe symptoms of local inflammation.

Type I: IgE-Mediated Hypersensitivity Reactions

Type I reactions are mediated by antigen-specific IgE and the products of tissue mast cells (Figure 8-1). Most common allergic reactions are type I reactions. In addition, most type I reactions occur against environmental antigens and are therefore allergic. Because of this strong association, many healthcare professionals use the term *allergy* to indicate only IgE-mediated reactions. However, IgE can contribute to some autoimmune and alloimmune diseases, and many common allergies (e.g., poison ivy) are not mediated by IgE. Antigens that cause allergic responses are called **allergens.** It is not known why some antigens are allergens and others are not, but most allergens appear to be foreign proteins that enter the host from the environment.

Role of IgE

In some individuals, exposure to an allergen causes primarily IgE production.[3] Repeated exposure to relatively large doses of allergen usually is required to elicit enough IgE so

Table 8-2   Disorders Associated with Autoimmunity

System Disease	Organ or Tissue	Probable Self-Antigen
Endocrine System		
Hyperthyroidism (Graves disease)	Thyroid gland	Receptors for thyroid-stimulating hormone on plasma membrane of thyroid cells
Autoimmune thyroiditis	Thyroid gland	Thyroglobulin; microsomes
Primary myxedema	Thyroid gland	Microsomes
Insulin-dependent diabetes	Pancreas	Islet cells, insulin, insulin receptors on pancreatic cells
Addison disease	Adrenal gland	Surface antigens on steroid-producing cells; microsomes of adrenal cortex
Premature gonadal failure	Ovary	Interstitial cells; corpus luteum
Male infertility	Testis	Surface antigens on spermatozoa
Orchitis	Testis	Germinal epithelium
Female infertility	Ovary	Zona pellucida
Idiopathic hypoparathyroidism	Parathyroid gland	Surface antigens on chief cells (epithelial cells of gland)
Partial pituitary deficiency	Pituitary gland	Prolactin-producing cells; growth hormone–producing cells
Skin		
Pemphigus vulgaris	Skin	Intercellular substances in stratified squamous epithelium
Bullous pemphigoid	Skin	Basement membrane
Dermatitis herpetiformis	Skin	Basement membrane (immunoglobulin A[IgA])
Vitiligo	Skin	Surface antigens on melanocytes (melanin-producing cells)
Neuromuscular Tissue		
Polymyositis (dermatomyositis)	Muscle	Nuclear materials; myosin
Multiple sclerosis	Neural tissue	Unknown
Myasthenia gravis	Neuromuscular junction	Acetylcholine receptors; striations of skeletal and cardiac muscle
Polyneuritis	Nerve cell	Peripheral myelin
Rheumatic fever	Heart	Cardiac tissue (subsarcolemmal membrane); cross reaction with group A streptococcal antigen
Cardiomyopathy	Heart	Cardiac muscle
Postvaccinal or postinfectious encephalitis	Central nervous system	Central nervous system myelin or basic protein
Gastrointestinal System		
Celiac disease (gluten-sensitive enteropathy)	Intestine	Gluten
Ulcerative colitis	Colon	Mucosal cells
Crohn disease	Ileum	Unknown
Pernicious anemia	Stomach	Surface antigens of parietal cells; intrinsic factor
Atrophic gastritis	Stomach	Parietal cells
Primary biliary cirrhosis	Liver	Mitochondria; cells of bile duct
Chronic active hepatitis	Liver	Surface antigens, nuclei, microsomes, mitochondria or hepatocytes; smooth muscle
Eye		
Sjögren syndrome	Lacrimal gland	Antigens of lacrimal gland, salivary gland, thyroid, and nuclei of cells; immunoglobulin G (IgG)
Uveitis	Uveal structures	Antigens of the iris, ciliary body, and choroid
Connective Tissue		
Ankylosing spondylitis	Joints	Sacroiliac and spinal apophyseal joint
Rheumatoid arthritis	Joints	IgG, collagen
Systemic lupus erythematosus	Multiple sites	Numerous antigens in nuclei, organelles, and extracellular matrix
Mixed connective tissue disease	Multiple sites	Ribonucleoprotein and numerous other nucleoproteins
Polyarteritis nodosa (nercotizing vasculitis)	Arterioles (small arteries)	Unknown
Scleroderma (progressive systemic sclerosis)	Multiple organs	Nuclear antigens; IgG
Felty syndrome	Joints	IgG
Antiphospholipid antibody syndrome	Platelets, endothelial cells, trophoblast of placenta	Membrane phospholipids, especially phosphatidylserine
Renal System		
Immune complex glomerulonephritis	Kidney	Numerous immune complexes
Goodpasture disease	Kidney	Glomerular basement membrane
Hematologic System		
Idiopathic neutropenia	Neutrophil	Surface antigens on polymorphonuclear neutrophils
Idiopathic lymphopenia	Lymphocytes	Surface antigens on lymphocytes
Autoimmune hemolytic anemia	Erythrocytes	Surface antigens on erythrocytes
Autoimmune thrombocytopenic purpura	Platelets	Surface antigens on platelets
Respiratory System		
Goodpasture disease	Lung	Septal membrane of alveolus

Table 8-3   Immunologic Mechanisms of Tissue Destruction

Type	Name	Rate of Development	Class of Antibody Involved	Principal Effector Cells Involved	Complement Participation	Examples of Disorders
I	IgE-mediated reaction	Immediate	IgE	Mast cells	No	Seasonal allergic rhinitis
II	Tissue-specific reaction	Immediate	IgG IgM	Macrophages in tissues	Frequently	Autoimmune thrombocytopenic purpura, Graves disease, autoimmune hemolytic anemia
III	Immune complex–mediated reaction	Immediate	IgG IgM	Neutrophils	Yes	Systemic lupus erythematosus
IV	Cell-mediated reaction	Delayed	None	Lymphocytes Macrophages	No	Contact sensitivity to poison ivy and metals (jewelry)

Ig, Immunoglobulin.

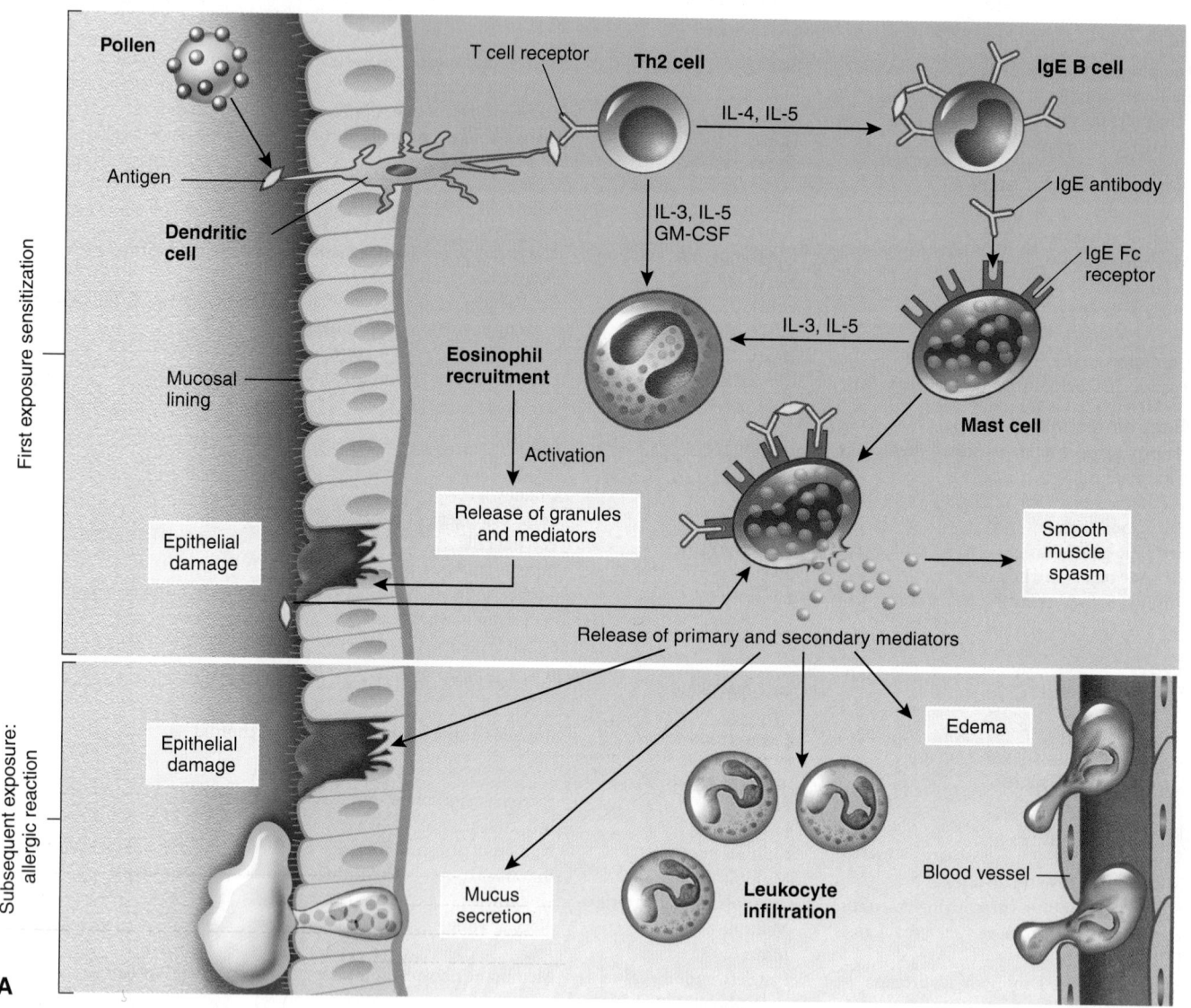

Figure 8-1 **Mechanism of type I IgE–mediated reactions. A,** Th2 cells are activated by antigen-presenting dendritic cells to produce cytokines, including IL-3, IL-4, IL-5, and granulocyte-macrophage colony-stimulating factor (GM-CSF). IL-3, IL-5, and GM-CSF attract and promote the survival of eosinophils. Other cytokines (e.g., IL-4) induce B cells to class-switch to IgE-producing plasma cells. The IgE coats the surface of the mast cell by binding with IgE-specific Fc receptors on the mast cell's plasma membrane (sensitization). Further exposure to the same allergen cross-links the surface-bound IgE and activates signals from the cytoplasmic portion of the IgE Fc receptors. These signals initiate two parallel and interdependent processes: mast cell degranulation and discharge of preformed mediators (e.g., histamine, eosinophil-chemotactic factor of anaphylaxis) and production of newly formed mediators such as arachidonic metabolites (leukotrienes, prostaglandins). Many local type I hypersensitivity reactions have two well-defined phases. The *initial phase* is characterized by vasodilation, vascular leakage, and depending on the location, smooth muscle spasm or glandular secretions. These changes usually become evident within 5 to 30 minutes after exposure to the antigen. The *late phase* occurs 2 to 8 hours later without additional exposure to the antigen. The late phase has more intense infiltration of tissues with eosinophils, neutrophils, basophils, monocytes, and Th cells and tissue destruction in the form of mucosal epithelial cell damage.

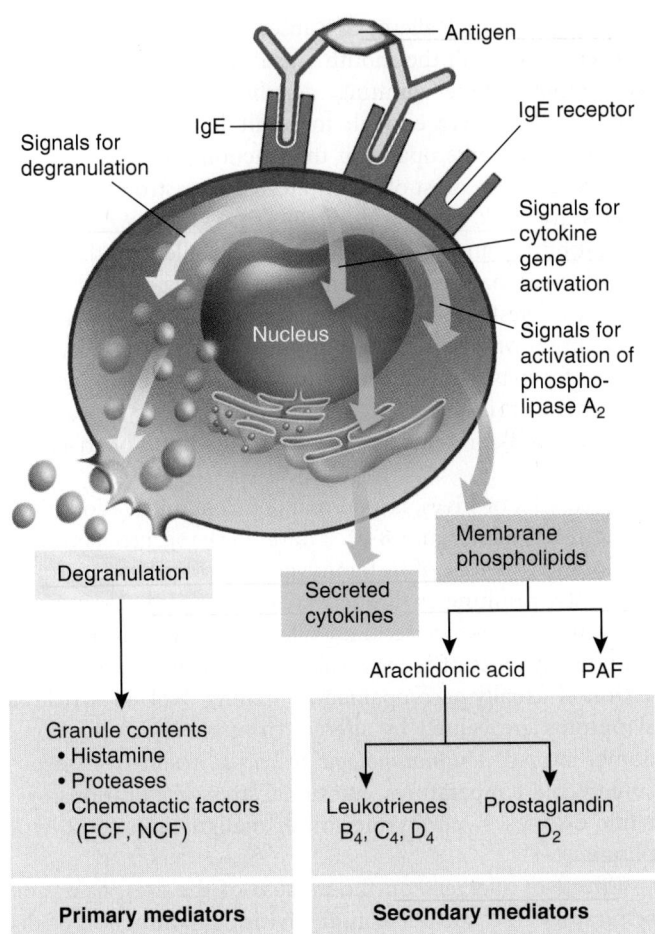

Figure 8-1, cont'd Mechanism of type I IgE–mediated reactions. **B,** Activation of mast cells leading to degranulation of preformed mediators (primary mediators) and synthesis of newly formed *(de novo)* mediators (secondary mediators). *PAF,* Platelet-activating factor; *ECF,* eosinophilic chemotactic factor; *NCF,* neutrophil chemotactic factor.

that the person becomes "sensitized." IgE has a relatively short lifespan in the blood because it rapidly binds to Fc receptors on the plasma membranes of mast cells (see Figure 8-1). The Fc region of IgE and the subclass IgG4 have binding sites specific for receptors on the mast cell. Antibody that binds to mast cells is termed **cytotropic antibody** (able to bind to cell surfaces). **Reagin,** or skin-sensitizing antibody, has been used interchangeably with the term *cytotropic antibody.* Unlike Fc receptors on phagocytes, which bind IgG that has reacted with antigen, the Fc receptors on mast cells bind with IgE that has not previously interacted with antigen.

Further exposure of a sensitized individual to the allergen results in the allergen's antigenic determinants binding to IgE on the mast cell's surface. An allergen must have at least two antigenic determinants on the same molecule in order to interact simultaneously (cross-link) with two IgE-Fc receptor complexes. This reaction initiates degranulation of the mast cell and the release of a plethora of mast cell products (see Figure 8-1, *B,* and Chapter 6). Sometimes an IgE-mediated response is beneficial to the host, as is the case of some immune

reactions against parasites. (This mechanism is described in Chapter 7 and illustrated in Figure 7-25.)

Mechanisms of IgE-Mediated Hypersensitivity

The products of mast cell degranulation can modulate almost all aspects of an acute inflammatory response.[4] (The effects of biochemical mediators released by mast cells are illustrated in Figure 6-8). The most potent mediator of IgE-mediated hypersensitivity is histamine, which affects several key target cells.[5] Acting through certain histamine receptors (H1 receptors), histamine contracts bronchial smooth muscles, causing bronchial constriction; increases vascular permeability, causing edema; and causes vasodilation, increasing blood flow into the affected area (see Figures 6-2 and 6-9). The interaction of histamine with H2 receptors results in increased gastric acid secretion and a decrease of histamine released from mast cells and basophils. (Basophils are granulocytes in the blood that are thought to be similar to mast cells.) The action of histamine through H2 receptors suggests an important negative-feedback mechanism that stops degranulation. That is, the released histamine inhibits release of additional histamine by interacting with H2 receptors on the mast cells. Histamine also may affect control of the immune response through H2 receptors on most cells of the immune system.[6] Another important activity of histamine is that of enhancing the chemotactic activity of other factors, such as eosinophil chemotactic factor of anaphylaxis (ECF-A), which attracts eosinophils into sites of allergic inflammatory reactions and also prevents them from migrating out of the inflammatory site. (The role of the eosinophil in inflammation is discussed in Chapter 6.)

Although some type I allergic responses can be controlled by blocking histamine receptors with antihistamines, the primary mechanism of control is the autonomic nervous system. The autonomic nervous system includes biochemical mediators (e.g., epinephrine, acetylcholine) that, like the mediators of the inflammatory response, have profound effects on the behavior of specific target cells in the host tissue. These mediators bind to appropriate receptors on both mast cells and the target cells of inflammation, thereby controlling (1) release of inflammatory mediators from mast cells and (2) the degree to which target cells respond to inflammatory mediators (see Chapter 6). For example, if an individual develops an anaphylactic reaction to a bee sting, the administration of antihistamines will have little effect because histamine has already bound H1 receptors and initiated severe bronchial smooth muscle contraction. The effects of histamine can be reversed by the immediate injection of epinephrine.

CLINICAL MANIFESTATIONS   The clinical manifestations of type I reactions are attributable mostly to the biologic effects of histamine.[7] The tissues most commonly affected by type I responses contain large numbers of mast cells and are sensitive to the effects of histamine released from them. These tissues are found in the gastrointestinal tract, the skin, and the respiratory tract (Figure 8-2 and Table 8-4).

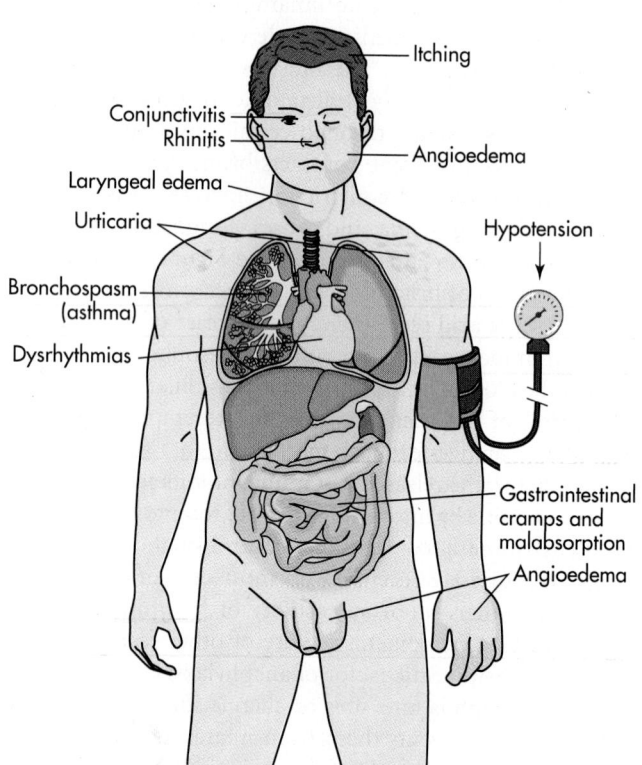

Figure 8-2 Type I hypersensitivity reactions. Manifestations of allergic reactions as a result of type I hypersensitivity include itching, angioedema (swelling caused by exudation), edema of the larynx, urticaria (hives), bronchospasm (constriction of airways in the lungs), hypotension (low blood pressure) and dysrhythmias (irregular heartbeat) because of anaphylactic shock, and gastrointestinal cramping caused by inflammation of the gastrointestinal mucosa.

Gastrointestinal allergy is caused primarily by allergens that enter through the mouth—usually foods or medicines. Symptoms include vomiting, diarrhea, or abdominal pain and may be severe enough to result in malabsorption or protein-losing enteropathy, if the reactions are prolonged or recurrent. Foods most often implicated in gastrointestinal allergies are milk, chocolate, citrus fruits, eggs, wheat, nuts, peanut butter, and fish. When food is the allergen, the active immunogen may be an unidentifiable product of food breakdown by digestive enzymes. Sometimes the allergen is a drug, an additive, or a preservative in the food. For example, cows treated for mastitis with penicillin yield milk containing trace amounts of this antibiotic. Thus hypersensitivity apparently caused by milk proteins may instead be the result of an allergy to penicillin.

Urticaria, or **hives,** is a dermal (skin) manifestation of allergic reactions (Figure 8-3). The underlying mechanism is the localized release of histamine and increased vascular permeability, resulting in limited areas of edema. Urticaria is characterized by white fluid-filled blisters (wheals) surrounded by areas of redness (flares). The **wheal and flare reaction** is usually accompanied by itching. Not all urticarial symptoms are caused by allergic (immunologic) reactions. Some, termed *nonimmunologic urticaria,* result from exposure to cold temperatures, emotional stress, medications, systemic diseases, hyperthyroidism, or malignancies (e.g., lymphomas).

Effects of allergens on the mucosa of the eyes, nose, and respiratory tract include conjunctivitis (inflammation of the membranes lining the eyelids), rhinitis (inflammation of the mucous membranes of the nose), and asthma (constriction of the bronchi). Symptoms are caused by vasodilation, hypersecretion of mucus, edema, and swelling of the respiratory mucosa. Because the mucous membranes lining the respiratory tract (accessory sinuses, nasopharynx, and upper and

Table 8-4	Causes of Clinical Manifestations of Allergy	
Typical Allergen	**Mechanism of Hypersensitivity**	**Clinical Manifestation**
Ingestants		
Foods	Type I	Gastrointestinal allergy
Drugs	Types I, II, III	Urticaria, immediate drug reaction, hemolytic anemia, serum sickness
Inhalants		
Pollens, dust, molds	Type I	Allergic rhinitis, bronchial asthma
Aspergillus fumigatus	Types, I, III	Allergic bronchopulmonary aspergillosis
Thermophilic actinomycetes*	Types III, IV	Extrinsic allergic alveolitis
Injectants		
Drugs	Types, I, II, III	Immediate drug reaction, hemolytic anemia, serum sickness
Bee venom	Type I	Anaphylaxis
Vaccines	Type III	Localized Arthus reaction
Serum	Types I, III	Anaphylaxis, serum sickness
Contactants		
Poison ivy, metals	Type IV	Contact dermatitis

Modified from Bellanti JA: *Immunology III,* Philadelphia, 1985, Saunders.
*An order of fungi that is stimulated by warmth to grow and proliferate.

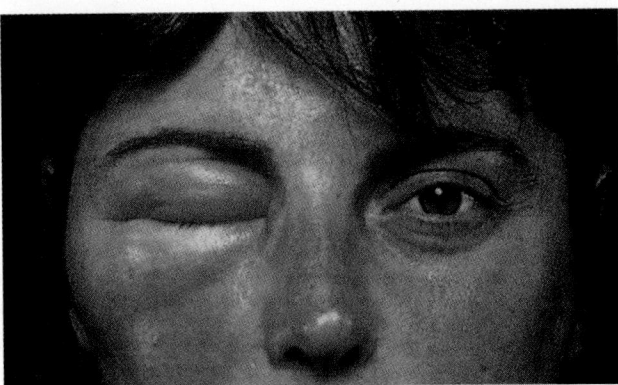

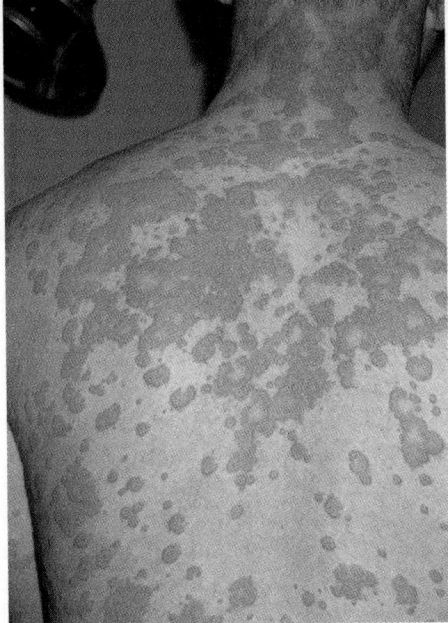

Figure 8-3 Allergic urticaria. This photo shows a diffuse allergic-like eye and skin reaction on an individual. The lesions have raised edges and develop within minutes or hours, with resolution occurring after about 12 hours. (From Roitt I, Brostoff J, Male D: *Immunology,* ed 6, St. Louis, 2001, Mosby.)

lower respiratory tract) are continuous, they are all adversely affected. The degree to which each is affected determines the symptoms of the disease.

The central defect in allergic diseases of the lung, such as asthma, is obstruction of the lumen of the large and small airways (bronchi) of the lower respiratory tract by bronchospasm (constriction of smooth muscle in airway walls), edema, thick secretions, and hyperplasia of smooth muscle and mucus-secreting glands. This leads to ventilatory insufficiency, wheezing, and difficult or labored breathing. Asthma is acute, intermittent, and reversible. Extrinsic asthma is an allergic reaction caused by a known exogenous allergen, whereas intrinsic asthma has no known cause. (Asthma is described further in Chapter 32.)

Genetic Predisposition

Certain individuals are genetically predisposed to develop allergies and are called *atopic.*[8,9] In families in which one parent has an allergy, allergies develop in about 40% of the offspring. If both parents have allergies, the incidence in the offspring may be as high as 80%. (Principles of genetic inheritance are discussed in Chapter 4.)

Atopic individuals tend to produce higher quantities of IgE and to have more Fc receptors for IgE on their mast cells. The airways and the skin of atopic individuals are also more responsive to a wide variety of both specific and nonspecific stimuli than are the airways and skin of individuals who are not atopic. Multiple genes have been associated with the atopic state, including polymorphisms in a large variety of cytokines and cellular receptors.

Tests of IgE-Mediated Hypersensitivity

Allergic reactions can be life threatening; therefore it is essential that severely allergic individuals be made aware of the specific allergen against which they are sensitized and instructed to avoid contact with that material. Several tests are available to evaluate allergic individuals. These include food challenges, skin tests with allergens, and laboratory tests for total IgE and allergen-specific IgE.

Reactivity to a particular food allergen may be tested by controlled administration of small doses of the suspected allergen in order to evoke a mild allergic response. This approach can be dangerous if the individual has a history of anaphylactic responses. A safer approach is injection of an allergen into (intradermal) or onto (epicutaneous or prick test) the skin of a sensitized individual. If the individual is allergic to a particular allergen, a local reaction may occur within a few minutes at the site of injection. The reaction consists of a localized pale area of swelling and a surrounding area of redness (a wheal and flare reaction). The diameter of the flare reaction is usually indicative of the individual's degree of sensitivity to that allergen. In the most severely allergic individuals, even the extremely small amounts of allergen used for the skin test may evoke a systemic anaphylaxis.

A variety of laboratory tests can detect IgE antibodies. These assays have various commercial acronyms, depending on whether they are radioimmunoassays (RIA; reactivity detected by measuring a radioactive reagent) or enzyme immunoassays (EIA or ELISA [enzyme-linked immunosorbent assay]; reactivity detected by measuring a color change caused by an enzyme-labeled reagent). One set of assays measures circulating levels of total IgE, with atopic individuals usually having elevated levels. Other assays are capable of measuring circulating levels of specific IgE antibodies against selected allergens. The amount of IgE against a specific allergen correlates well with the degree of skin test reactivity and the severity of clinical symptoms related to the same allergen.

Desensitization

Clinical desensitization to allergens can be achieved in some individuals.[10] Minute quantities of the allergen to which the person is sensitive are injected in increasing doses over a prolonged period. This procedure may reduce the severity of the allergic reaction in the treated individual. However, this form of therapy is associated with a risk of systemic anaphylaxis, which can be severe and life threatening.[11] Desensitization may work by inducing the production of large amounts of so-called blocking antibodies. A **blocking antibody** presumably competes in the tissues or in the circulation for binding with antigenic determinants on the allergen. Thus neutralized, the antigen is unable to bind with IgE on mast cells. In serum, blocking antibodies are predominantly IgG. Alternatively, some IgG may bind to IgG Fc receptors on mast cells and decrease their sensitivity to IgE-mediated degranulation. The role of blocking antibodies has not been firmly established. Desensitization injections also may stimulate the generation of clones of regulatory T lymphocytes, which inhibit hypersensitivity by suppressing the production of IgE or modifying the Th1/Th2 interactions in favor of production of anti-inflammatory cytokines.

Recently, other approaches to suppressing type I allergic responses have been tested with some preliminary success. An example is injection of anti-IgE antibody directed against the Fc portion of the molecule in order to decrease binding of IgE to mast cells.

Type II: Tissue-Specific Hypersensitivity Reactions

Type II hypersensitivity reactions are generally characterized by a specific cell or tissue being the target of an immune response. In addition to major histocompatibility locus antigens (HLAs), most cells have other antigens on their surfaces. Some of these other antigens are called **tissue-specific antigens,** because they are expressed on the plasma membranes of only certain cells in specific tissues. Platelets, for example, have groups of antigens that are found on no other cells of the body. The symptoms of many type II diseases are determined by which tissue or organ expresses the particular antigen. Environmental antigens (e.g., drugs or their metabolites) may bind to the plasma membranes of specific cells (especially erythrocytes and platelets) and function as targets of type II reactions.

The five general mechanisms by which type II hypersensitivity reactions can affect cells are shown in Figure 8-4. All of these mechanisms begin with antibody binding to tissue-specific antigens or antigens that have attached to particular tissues. First, the cell is destroyed by antibody and complement. The antibody (IgM or IgG) reacts with an antigen present on the surface of the cell, causing activation of the complement cascade through the classical pathway. Formation of the membrane attack complex (C5-9) damages the membrane and may result in lysis of the cell (see Figure 8-4, *A*). For example, erythrocytes are destroyed by complement-mediated lysis in individuals with autoimmune hemolytic anemia (see Chapter 25) or as a result of an alloimmune reaction to ABO-mismatched transfused blood cells.

Second, antibody may cause cell destruction through phagocytosis by macrophages of the mononuclear phagocyte system. The antibody binds to antigens on the cell and activates the complement cascade, resulting in the deposition of C3b on the cell surface. Receptors on the macrophage recognize and bind opsonins on the cell surface (e.g., antibody or C3b) (see Figure 8-4, *B*). Phagocytosis of the target cell follows. (Phagocytosis is illustrated in Figures 6-13 and 6-14.) For example, an-

tibodies against platelet-specific antigens or against red blood cell antigens of the Rh system coat those cells at low density, resulting in their preferential removal by phagocytosis in the spleen, rather than by complement-mediated lysis.

Third, soluble antigen may enter the circulation, by way of being released from cells within the body or from infectious agents or by way of drugs or medications. In some instances, the antigens are deposited on the surface of tissues, where they bind antibody (see Figure 8-4, *C*). The antibody may initiate the complement cascade, resulting in the release of C3a and C5a, which are chemotactic for neutrophils, and deposition of complement component C3b. Neutrophils are attracted, bind to the tissues through receptors for the Fc portion of antibody (Fc receptor) or for C3b and then attempt to phagocytose the tissue. Because the tissue is large, phagocytosis cannot be completed; even so, neutrophils release their granules onto the healthy tissue. The components of neutrophil granules, as well as the several toxic oxygen products produced by these cells, will damage the tissue.

The fourth mechanism is **antibody-dependent cell-mediated cytotoxicity (ADCC)** (see Figure 8-4, *D*). This mechanism involves a subpopulation of cytotoxic cells that are not antigen specific (natural killer [NK] cells). Antibody on the target cell is recognized by Fc receptors on the NK cells, which release toxic substances that destroy the target cell.

The fifth mechanism does not destroy the target cell, but rather causes it to malfunction. In this mechanism of type II injury, the antibody is usually directed against antigenic determinants associated with specific cell-surface receptors, and the symptoms of the disease are a result of a direct effect of antibody binding alone (see Figure 8-4, *E*). The antibody reacts with the receptors on the target cell surface and modulates the function of the receptor by preventing interactions with their normal ligands, replacing the ligand and inappropriately stimulating the receptor, or destroying the receptor. For example, in the hyperthyroidism (excessive thyroid activity) of Graves disease, autoantibody binds to and activates receptors for thyroid-stimulating hormone (TSH) (a pituitary hormone that controls the production of the hormone *thyroxine* by the thyroid). In this way, the antibody stimulates the thyroid cells to produce thyroxine. Under normal conditions, the increasing levels of thyroxine in the blood would signal the pituitary to decrease TSH production, which would result in less stimulation of the TSH receptor in the thyroid and a concomitant decrease in thyroxine production. Because the level of anti-TSH receptor antibody is not controlled by the pituitary, increasing amounts of thyroxine in the blood have no effect on antibody levels, and thyroxine production continues to increase despite decreasing amounts of TSH (see Chapter 21).

Type III: Immune Complex–Mediated Hypersensitivity Reactions

Mechanisms of Type III Hypersensitivity

Most type III hypersensitivity diseases are caused by antigen-antibody (immune) complexes that are formed in the circulation and deposited later in vessel walls or extravascular tissues (Figure 8-5). The primary difference between type II and

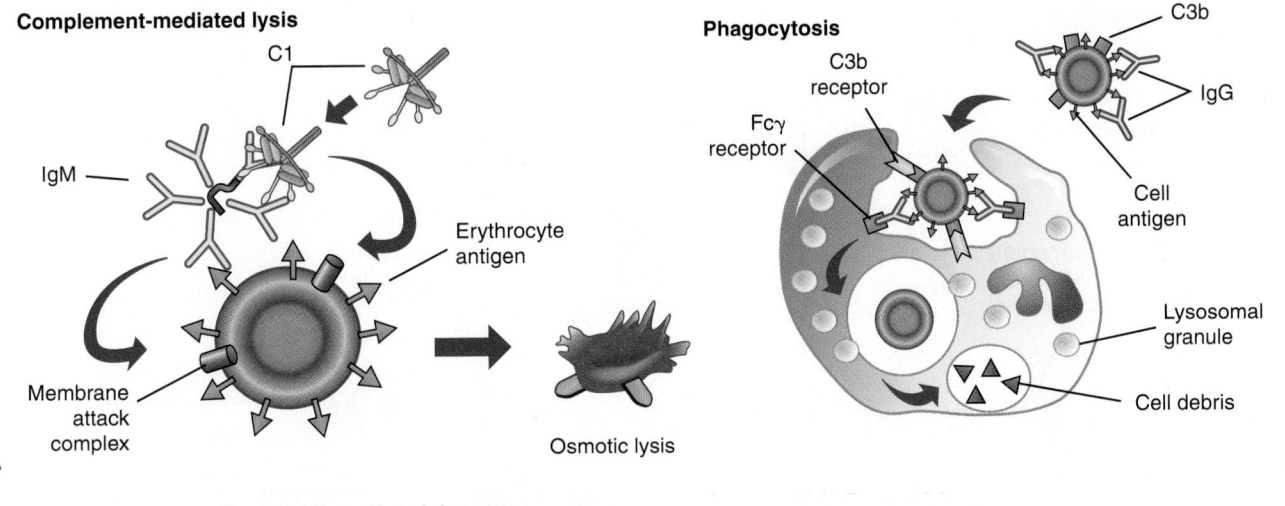

Complement-mediated lysis

C1

IgM

Erythrocyte antigen

Membrane attack complex

Osmotic lysis

A

Phagocytosis

C3b

C3b receptor

Fcγ receptor

IgG

Cell antigen

Lysosomal granule

Cell debris

B

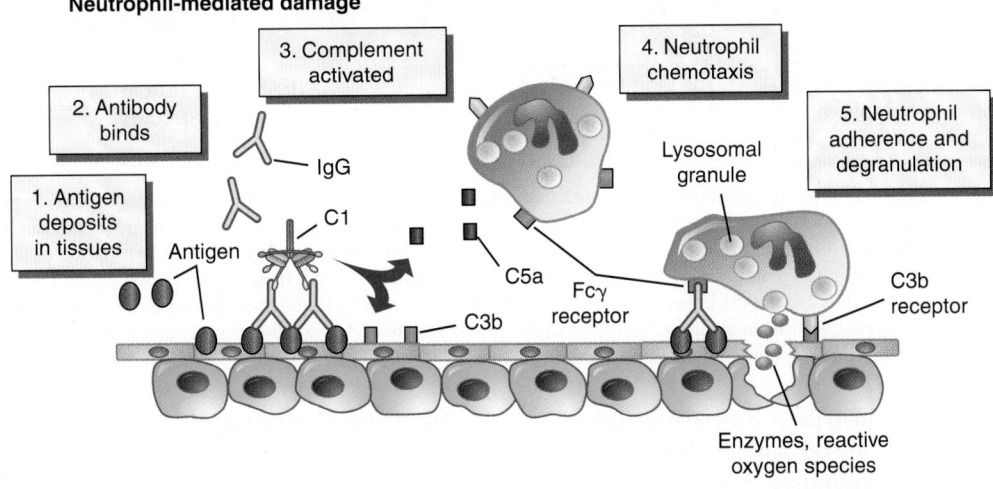

Neutrophil-mediated damage

2. Antibody binds

3. Complement activated

4. Neutrophil chemotaxis

5. Neutrophil adherence and degranulation

1. Antigen deposits in tissues

IgG

C1

Antigen

C5a

C3b

Fcγ receptor

Lysosomal granule

C3b receptor

Enzymes, reactive oxygen species

C

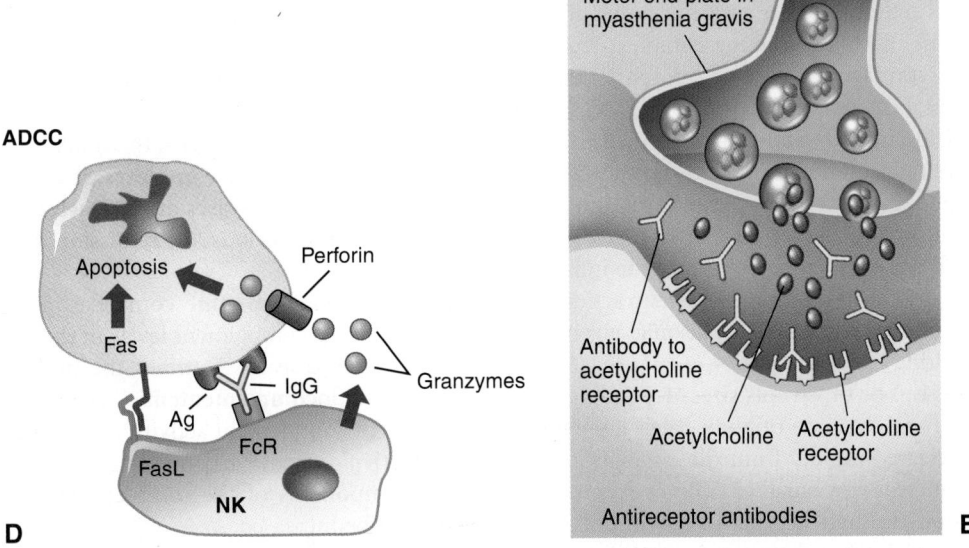

ADCC

Apoptosis

Fas

Perforin

IgG

Ag

FcR

Granzymes

FasL

NK

D

Motor end-plate in myasthenia gravis

Antibody to acetylcholine receptor

Acetylcholine

Acetylcholine receptor

Antireceptor antibodies

E

Figure 8-4 Mechanisms of type II, tissue-specific, reactions. Antigens on the target cell bind with antibody and are destroyed or prevented from functioning by **A,** complement-mediated lysis (an erythrocyte target is illustrated here); **B,** clearance (phagocytosis) by macrophages in the tissue; **C,** neutrophil-mediated immune destruction; **D,** antibody-dependent cell-mediated cytotoxicity (ADCC) (apoptosis of target cells is induced by granzymes and perforin produced by natural killer [NK] cells and interactions of Fas ligand [FasL] on the surface of NK cells with Fas on the surface of target cells); or **E,** modulation or blocking the normal function of receptors by antireceptor antibody. This example of mechanism E depicts myasthenia gravis in which acetylcholine receptor antibodies block acetylcholine from attaching to its receptors on the motor end plates of skeletal muscle, thereby impairing neuromuscular transmission and causing muscle weakness. *C1,* Complement component C1; *C3b,* complement fragment produced from C3, which acts as an opsonin; *C5a,* complement fragment produced from C5, which acts as a chemotactic factor for neutrophils; *Fcγ receptor,* cellular receptor for the Fc portion of IgG; *FcR,* Fc receptor.

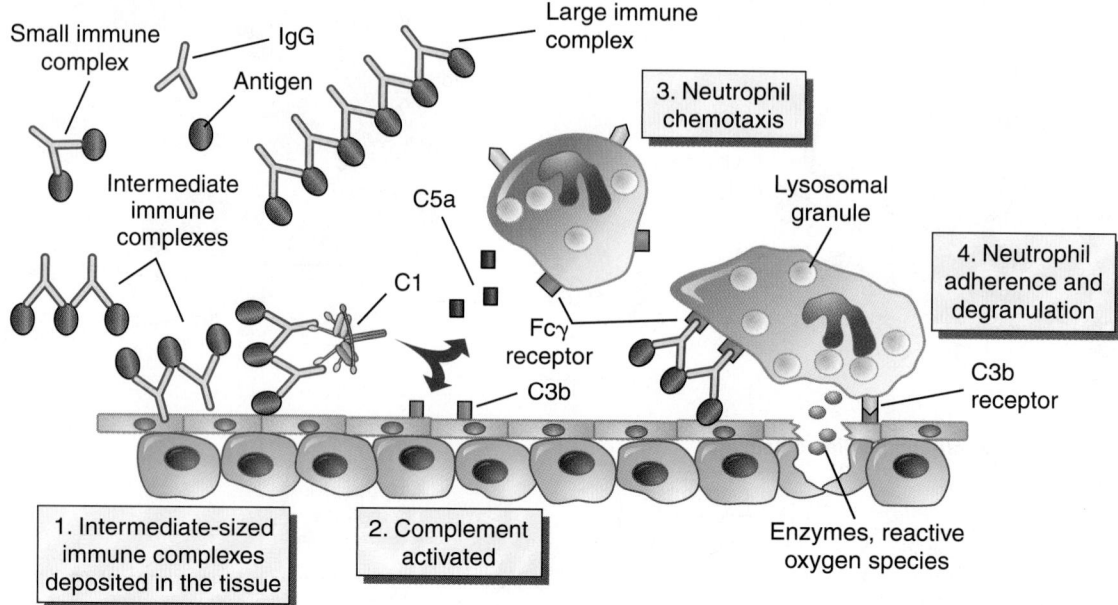

Figure 8-5 Mechanism of type III, immune complex–mediated reactions. Immune complexes form in the blood from circulating antigen and antibody. Both small and large immune complexes are removed successfully from the circulation and do not cause tissue damage. Intermediate-sized complexes are deposited in certain target tissues in which the circulation is slow or filtration of the blood occurs. The complexes activate the complement cascade through C1 and generate fragments including C5a and C3b. C5a is chemotactic for neutrophils, which migrate into the inflamed area and attach to the IgG and C3b in the immune complexes. The neutrophils attempt unsuccessfully to phagocytose the tissue and in the process release a variety of degradative enzymes that destroy the healthy tissues. Fcγ receptor is the cellular receptor for the Fc portion of IgG.

type III mechanisms is that in type II hypersensitivity antibody binds to the antigen on the cell surface, whereas in type III the antibody binds to soluble antigen that was released into the blood or body fluids, and the complex is then deposited in the tissues. Type III reactions are not organ specific, and symptoms have little to do with the particular antigenic target of the antibody.[12] The harmful effects of immune complex deposition are caused by complement activation, particularly through the generation of chemotactic factors for neutrophils. The neutrophils bind to antibody and C3b contained in the complexes and attempt to ingest the immune complexes. They are often unsuccessful because the complexes are bound to large areas of tissue. During the attempted phagocytosis, large quantities of lysosomal enzymes are released into the inflammatory site instead of into phagolysosomes. The attraction of neutrophils and the subsequent release of lysosomal enzymes cause most of the resulting tissue damage.

Immune complexes can be of various sizes, depending on the relative amounts of antigen and antibody. Fairly large immune complexes are cleared rapidly from the circulation by tissue macrophages, whereas very small complexes eventually are filtered from blood through the kidneys, without any pathologic consequences. Intermediate-sized immune complexes (formed at a ratio of antigen to antibody that has a slight excess of antigen) are likely to be deposited in certain target tissues, where they have severe pathologic consequences, such as inflammation in the kidneys (glomerulonephritis), the vessels (vasculitis), or the joints (arthritis or degenerative joint disease).

Immune Complex Disease

The nature of the immune complexes may change during the progression of the disease, with resultant changes in the severity of the symptoms. Immune complex formation is dynamic as variations in the ratio of antigen to antibody, the class and subclass of antibody, and the quantity and quality of circulating antigen occur. Thus complexes formed early in a disease process may differ from those formed later, and at any one time, several types of immune complexes may be present simultaneously. With the tremendous potential heterogeneity of immune complexes, it is not surprising that immune-complex diseases are characterized by a variety of symptoms and periods of remission or exacerbation of symptoms.

Because many immune complexes activate complement very effectively, complement levels in the blood may decrease during active disease. At times the individual's blood may become **hypocomplementemic** (i.e., contains decreased amounts of complement activity). During type I, II, or IV hypersensitivity reactions, complement levels are unaffected, or some components of the complement cascade, such as C3, may even be increased.

Two prototypic models of type III hypersensitivity help explain the variety of diseases in this category. Serum sickness is a model of systemic type III hypersensitivities, and the Arthus reaction is a model of localized or cutaneous reactions.

Serum sickness. The systemic prototype of immune complex–mediated disease is called **serum sickness** because it was initially described as being caused by the therapeutic administration of foreign serum, such as horse serum that contained antibody against tetanus toxin.[13] Foreign serum generally is not administered to individuals today, although serum sickness reactions can be caused by the repeated intravenous administration of other antigens, such as drugs, and the characteristics of serum sickness are observed in systemic type III autoimmune diseases. Serum sickness–type reactions are caused by the formation of immune complexes in the blood and their subsequent generalized deposition in target tissues. Typically affected tissues are the blood vessels, joints, and kidneys. Other symptoms include fever, enlarged lymph nodes, rash, and pain at sites of inflammation.

A form of serum sickness is **Raynaud phenomenon,** a condition caused by the temperature-dependent deposition of immune complexes in the capillary beds of the peripheral circulation. Certain immune complexes precipitate at temperatures below normal body temperature, particularly in the tips of the fingers, toes, and nose and are called **cryoglobulins.** The precipitates block the circulation and cause localized pallor and numbness, followed by cyanosis (a bluish tinge resulting from oxygen deprivation) and eventually gangrene if the circulation is not restored.

Arthus reaction. An **Arthus reaction** is the prototypic example of a localized immune complex–mediated inflammatory response.[14] It is caused by repeated local exposure to an antigen that reacts with preformed antibody and forms immune complexes in the walls of the local blood vessels. Symptoms of an Arthus reaction begin within 1 hour of exposure and peak 6 to 12 hours later. The lesions are characterized by a typical inflammatory reaction, with increased vascular permeability, an accumulation of neutrophils, edema, hemorrhage, clotting, and tissue damage.

Arthus reactions may be observed after injection, ingestion, or inhalation of allergens. Skin reactions can follow subcutaneous or intradermal inoculation with drugs, fungal extracts, or antigens used in skin tests. Gastrointestinal reactions, such as gluten-sensitive enteropathy (celiac disease), follow ingestion of antigen, usually gluten from wheat products (see Chapter 39). Allergic alveolitis (farmer's lung; pigeon breeder's disease) is an Arthus-like acute hemorrhagic inflammation of the air sacs (alveoli) of the lungs resulting from inhalation of fungal antigens, usually particles from moldy hay or pigeon feces (see Chapter 33).

Type IV: Cell-Mediated Hypersensitivity Reactions

Whereas types I, II, and III hypersensitivity reactions are mediated by antibody, type IV reactions are mediated by T lymphocytes and do not involve antibody (Figure 8-6). Type IV mechanisms occur through either cytotoxic T lymphocytes (Tc cells) or lymphokine-producing Th1 cells. Tc cells attack and destroy cellular targets directly. Th1 cells produce cytokines that recruit and activate phagocytic cells, especially macrophages. Destruction of the tissue is usually caused by direct killing by toxins from Tc cells or the release of soluble

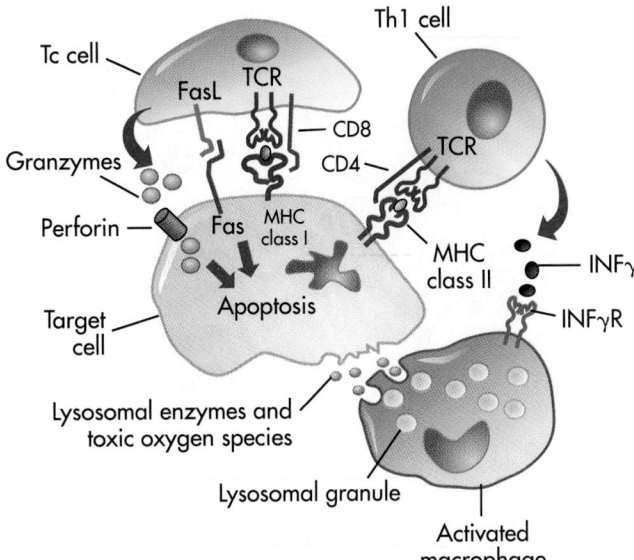

Figure 8-6 Mechanism of type IV, cell-mediated, reactions. Antigens from target cells stimulate T cells to differentiate into cytotoxic T cells (*Tc cells*), which have direct cytotoxic activity, and helper T cells (*Th1 cells*) involved in delayed hypersensitivity. The Th1 cells produce lymphokines (especially interferon-γ [IFNγ]) that activate the macrophage through specific receptors (e.g. IFNγ receptor [IFNγR]). The macrophages can attach to targets and release enzymes and reactive oxygen species that are responsible for most of the tissue destruction.

factors, such as lysosomal enzymes and toxic reactive oxygen species (ROS), from activated macrophages.

Clinical examples of type IV hypersensitivity reactions include graft rejection, the skin test for tuberculosis, and allergic reactions resulting from contact with such substances as poison ivy and metals. A type IV component also may be present in many autoimmune diseases. For example, T cells against type II collagen (a protein present in joint tissues) contribute to the destruction of joints in rheumatoid arthritis; T cells against a thyroid cell surface antigen contribute to the destruction of the thyroid in autoimmune thyroiditis (Hashimoto disease); and T cells against an antigen on the surface of pancreatic beta cells (the cell that normally produces insulin) are responsible for beta-cell destruction in insulin-dependent (type 1) diabetes mellitus.

A type IV hypersensitivity reaction in the skin was thoroughly described first by Ehrlich in 1891 and led to the development of a diagnostic skin test for tuberculosis.[15] The reaction follows an intradermal injection of tuberculin antigen into a suitably sensitized individual and is called a *delayed hypersensitivity skin test* because of its slow onset—24 to 72 hours to reach maximum intensity. The reaction site is infiltrated with T lymphocytes and macrophages, resulting in a clear hard center (induration) and a reddish surrounding area (erythema). One of the characteristics of delayed hypersensitivity is that it can be transferred to an unreactive recipient by cells but not by serum, confirming that type IV hypersensitivity reactions are mediated by lymphocytes rather than by antibody.

Allergic type IV reactions are elicited by some environmental antigens that are too small to be immunogenic by

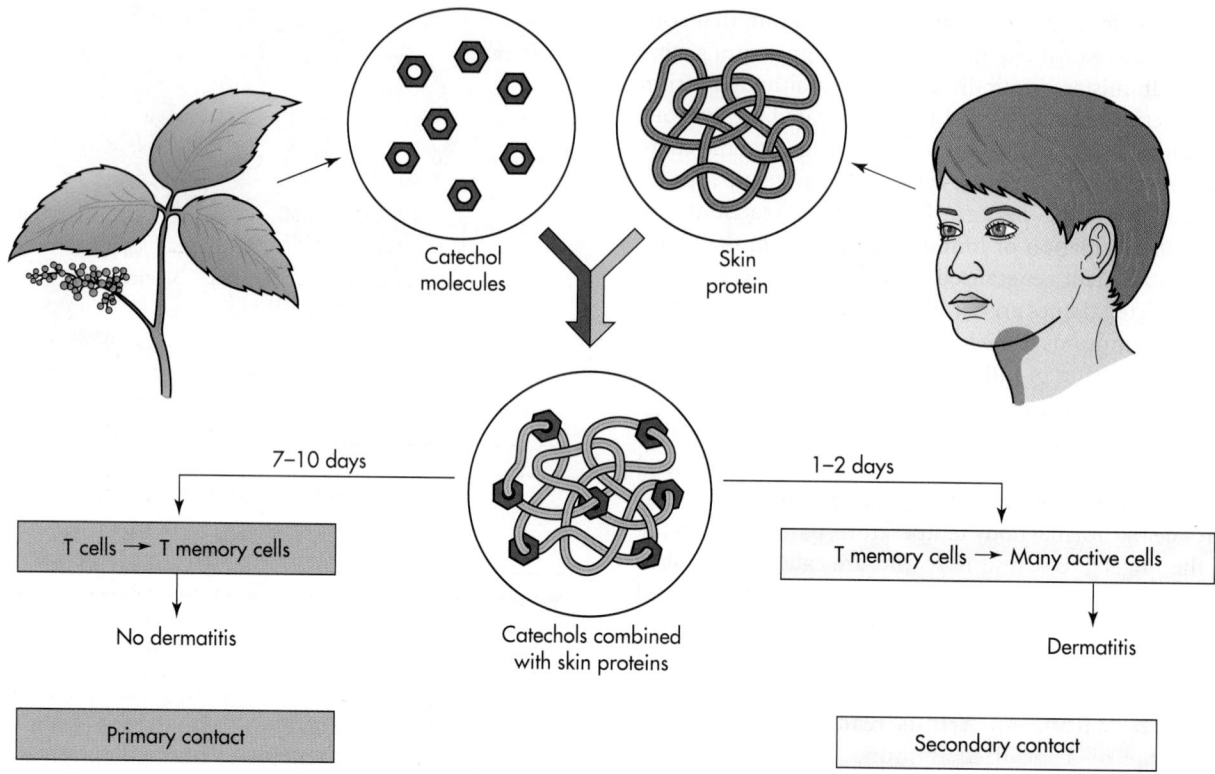

Figure 8-7 Development of allergic contact dermatitis, a delayed hypersensitivity reaction. Shown here is the development of allergy to catechols from poison ivy. No dermatitis results from the primary contact because the antigens (catechols) are sensitizing the immune response and producing memory T cells. Secondary contact, however, quickly activates a type IV, cell-mediated, reaction that causes dermatitis.

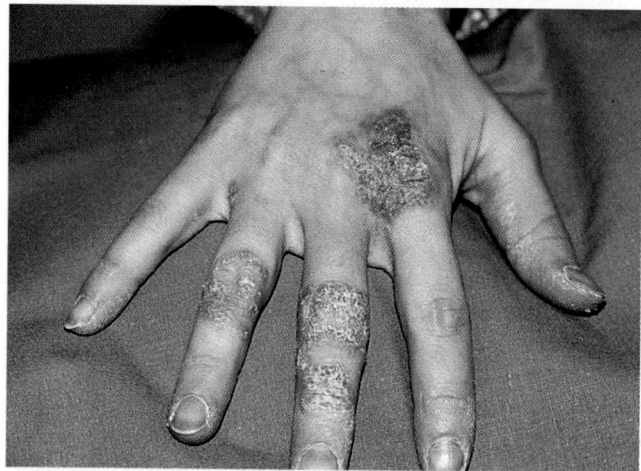

Figure 8-8 Contact dermatitis. This contact dermatitis was caused by a delayed hypersensitivity reaction that lead to vesicles and scaling at the sites of contact. (From Damjanov I, Linder J: *Anderson's pathology,* ed 10, St Louis, 1996, Mosby.)

themselves (haptens).[16] (Immunogenicity is described in Chapter 7.) Antigens with a molecular weight of less than 1000 daltons are not usually immunogenic but become so after binding with a carrier protein in the host. In cases of allergic **contact dermatitis,** the carrier protein is in the skin. The best-known example of allergic contact dermatitis is poison ivy (Figure 8-7). The antigen in that instance is a plant catechol, *urushiol,* that reacts with normal skin proteins and evokes a cell-mediated immune response. Skin reactions to industrial chemicals, cosmetics, detergents, clothing, food, metals, and topical medicines (such as penicillin) are elicited by the same mechanism.

Skin reactions are also a symptom of some immediate hypersensitivity reactions (e.g., hives formed during an allergic reaction to a particular food). The distribution of the lesions may suggest whether the reaction is caused by immediate or delayed hypersensitivity mechanisms. Immediate hypersensitivity reactions, termed **atopic dermatitis,** are usually characterized by widely distributed lesions, whereas contact dermatitis consists of lesions only at the site of contact with the allergen, such as a metal allergy to jewelry (Figure 8-8).

Antigenic Targets of Hypersensitivity Reactions
Allergy

Allergens are environmental antigens that cause atypical immunologic responses in genetically predisposed individuals. Typical allergens include pollens (e.g., ragweed), molds and fungi (e.g., *Penicillium notatum*), foods (e.g., milk, eggs, fish), animals (e.g., cat dander, dog dander), cigarette smoke, and components of house dust (e.g., fecal pellets of house mites).Often the allergen is contained within a particle that is too large to be phagocytosed or is surrounded by a protective nonallergenic coat. The actual allergen is released after enzymatic breakdown (e.g., by lysozyme in secretions) of the larger particle. Most allergens are either haptens that have the capacity to react with proteins or low-molecular-weight immunogenic proteins.

Haptenic allergens complex with proteins of the host tissue and elicit an immune response. For instance, allergic reactions to many drugs (e.g., penicillin, sulfonamides) occur after the drug binds to proteins on the plasma membranes of host cells and becomes immunogenic. The immune system attacks the allergen on the host cell's membrane and destroys the cell as well. In allergic reactions to penicillin, the immunogenic antigen is a metabolite of penicillin catabolism that binds to the plasma membranes of erythrocytes and induces an antibody response that destroys the cells, causing anemia.

The allergens that induce contact hypersensitivity, a type IV allergic reaction, are also haptens (e.g., metals such as nickel, acetylates and chemicals in rubber, resins in poison ivy and poison oak), which react with normal self-proteins in the skin. When presented in this fashion, these antigens induce a cell-mediated response.

Original Insult

The initiating factor of allergic diseases is apparent. For example, in drug-induced anemia or thrombocytopenia (decreased numbers of circulating platelets), immunologic destruction of erythrocytes or platelets follows the integration of a drug or its metabolite into the plasma membranes of the host cells. Allergic reactions also can occur against antigens of infectious diseases. For instance, rubella virus infects cells of the nervous system and expresses a viral antigen on the cell's plasma membrane. The viral antigen may elicit an immune response that also damages the infected cell, resulting in encephalitis.

Autoimmunity

Breakdown of Tolerance

Self-antigens are usually in a state of tolerance, or immunologic homeostasis, with the host's own immune system.[17] *Central tolerance* develops in humans during the embryonic period as autoreactive lymphocytes are either eliminated or suppressed in the primary lymphoid organs during differentiation and proliferation of immature T or B lymphocytes (see Figs. 7-9 and 7-11). Clones of cells with antigen receptors for self-antigens are deleted. *Peripheral tolerance* is maintained in the secondary lymphoid organs through the action of regulatory T lymphocytes or antigen-presenting dendritic cells. **Autoimmunity** is a breakdown of tolerance in which the body's immune system begins to recognize self-antigens as foreign.[18] In most autoimmune conditions the mechanism of tolerance breakdown is unknown, although several potential mechanisms have been suggested.

Sequestered Antigen. The induction of central tolerance requires that the self-antigen be present in the fetus and exposed to the developing fetal immune system. Some self-antigens may not normally encounter the immune system in either fetal or adult life. For example, areas of the cornea of the eye and the testicles are not drained by the lymphatics and actively suppress the function of any T lymphocyte that may enter the tissue. Self-antigens in these sites are not normally seen by the immune system and are, therefore, not immunogenic. They are sequestered or hidden from the immune system in **immunologically privileged sites,** so named because foreign tissues can be transplanted into these sites without danger of immunologic rejection. Immunologically privileged sites are vascular, so that if an immunologic reaction should occur, the resultant antibodies and lymphocytes can enter the site and cause immunologic damage to the tissue. For instance, physical trauma to one eye may result in release of sequestered antigen into the blood or lymphatics, resulting in immunologic injury to the other eye (sympathetic uveitis).

Infectious Disease. A longstanding hypothesis is that foreign antigens from infectious microorganisms can initiate autoimmune disease through a process of **molecular mimicry.**[19] Some antigens of infectious agents so closely resemble (mimic) a particular self-antigen that antibodies or T cells produced to protect against the infection also recognize the self-antigen as foreign (**cross-reactive antibody** or T cell). Although the relationship between many autoimmune diseases and predisposing infections is being investigated, the only clearly defined example so far is acute rheumatic fever that may occur after a Group A streptococcal sore throat (see below).

Neoantigen. In certain situations a neoantigen that induces an allergic reaction may lead also to autoimmunity. Many **neoantigens** (new antigens) are haptens, which become immunogenic after binding to host proteins. The immune reaction against the neoantigen may lead to an immunologic reaction against the unaltered host protein. Many experimental autoimmune diseases (e.g., experimental autoimmune thyroiditis) can be initiated by this mechanism.

Forbidden Clone. During differentiation and proliferation of lymphoid stem cells into immature T and B lymphocytes (see Figures 7-9 and 7-11), some lymphocytes produce receptors that react with self-antigens. Many autoreactive lymphocytes interact with self-antigens and other co-stimulatory molecules on the surface of thymic epithelial cells and are induced to undergo clonal deletion by a process of apoptosis.[20] Thus lymphocytes reactive against self-antigen are prevented, or "forbidden," from maturing. Autoimmunity may result from the survival of a **forbidden clone** and its proliferation later in life.

Ineffective Peripheral Tolerance. Tolerance to some self-antigens is controlled in the secondary lymphoid organs. This process is controlled by a variety of cells, including antigen-presenting dendritic cells and members of a family of regulatory T lymphocytes. Some of these regulatory T lymphocytes have been called *suppressor cells.* Defects in particular regulatory cells may result in expansion of clones of autoreactive cells and the development of autoimmune disease. Systemic lupus erythematosus (SLE), which is characterized by the production of a large array of autoantibodies, may be caused by a general breakdown in the regulatory network.

Original Insult

Although many theories exist, the initial cause of most autoimmune diseases is unknown. It is suspected that some autoimmune diseases are initiated by infections that have resolved without leaving evidence that would lead to identification of the particular infectious agent. The evidence for an infectious causation is clear for only one autoimmune disease: acute rheumatic fever. In a small number of individuals with Group A streptococcal sore throats, the M proteins in the bacterial capsule induce antibodies that also react with proteins in the heart valve, damaging the valve.

Additionally, some streptococcal skin or throat infections result in the release of bacterial antigens into the blood and the formation of circulating immune complexes. The complexes may deposit in the kidneys and initiate an immune complex glomerulonephritis (inflammation of the kidney). Thus capsular antigens of the Group A *Streptococcus* may mimic (*antigenic mimicry*) normal heart antigens resulting in a type II autoimmune hypersensitivity (rheumatic fever), whereas in another person this infection may release bacterial antigen (an environmental antigen) into the blood, resulting in a type III allergic hypersensitivity (post-streptococcal glomerulonephritis).

Genetic Factors

Genetic factors that contribute to autoimmunity are easier to identify than the original insult that initiates the disease.[21] It is fairly well established that autoimmune diseases can be familial. Affected family members may not all develop the same disease, but several members may have different disorders characterized by a variety of hypersensitivity reactions, including autoimmune and allergic.

Associations with particular autoimmune diseases have been identified for a variety of major histocompatibility complex (MHC) alleles (see Chapter 7) or non-MHC genes. The specific HLA alleles of susceptible and resistant individuals have been analyzed for almost every known disease, and almost universally, individuals with certain diseases are more likely than the general population to have a specific HLA allele or set of alleles. Some associations are strong; others are more tenuous (Table 8-5). The reason some HLA alleles are associated with inappropriate immune function is unclear, but it may directly involve the ability of particular HLA molecules to present antigen or the use of particular HLAs as receptors for disease-causing microorganisms. These genes may determine an individual's susceptibility to specific infectious agents or the capacity of that individual to mount an immune response against specific antigens. Therefore an individual of a specific HLA type may have inappropriate or exaggerated immune responses against a microorganism, resulting in a hypersensitivity reaction.

A large variety of non-MHC genes also have been identified as risk factors for the development of specific autoimmune diseases. Most of these genes encode for inflammatory cytokines or co-stimulatory molecules found on the cell surface.

Table 8-5	Examples of Associations Between Specific HLA Alleles and Disease	
Disease	**HLA Allele**	**RR**
Acute anterior uveitis	B27	14
Addison disease	DR3	6
Ankylosing spondylitis	B27	90
Behçet syndrome	B51	4
Celiac disease	DR3	11
Chronic active hepatitis	DR3	13
Dermatitis herpetiformis	DR3	16
Diabetes (type I)	DR3	5
	DR4	6
	DR3/DR4	20
Goodpasture syndrome	DR2	16
Graves disease	DR3	4
Hashimoto disease	DR11	3
Multiple sclerosis	DR2	4
Myasthenia gravis	DR3	3
Pemphigus vulgaris	DR4	13
Post-gonococcal arthritis	B27	14
Reiter syndrome	B27	37
Rheumatoid arthritis	DR4	4
Sjögren syndrome	DR3	9
Systemic lupus erythematosus	DR3	6

HLA, Human leukocyte antigen; *RR,* the approximate relative risk, which is the frequency of a disease in individuals with the particular HLA allele compared with individuals without that allele.

Alloimmunity

Alloimmunity occurs when an individual's immune system reacts against antigens on the tissues of other members of the same species. The two clinically relevant examples of this reactivity are (1) several transient neonatal diseases (in which the maternal immune system becomes sensitized against antigens expressed by the fetus) and (2) transplant rejection and transfusion reactions (in which the immune system of a recipient of an organ transplant or blood transfusion reacts against antigens on the donor cells).

Transient Neonatal Alloimmunity

Because the fetus is a hybrid between the mother and father, it expresses paternal antigens that are not found in the mother. Occasionally, these fetal antigens cross the placenta and elicit an immune response in the mother (e.g., production of alloantibodies against the fetal antigens). The maternal alloantibody may be transported across the placenta into the fetal circulation, bind to the fetal cells, and produce alloimmune disease in the fetus and neonate. The mother's immune system produces the antibody, but because her cells do not express the target antigen, she has no symptoms of the disease.

Neonatal alloimmune disease may be secondary to maternal autoimmune diseases in which the mother produces an IgG autoantibody specific for maternal self-antigens that are found on fetal cells as well. Therefore symptoms of the same autoimmune disease may affect both mother and child, even though the autoantibody is being produced only by the mother's immune system. This form of disease usually occurs only in association with type II (tissue-specific) hypersensitivity reactions. It does not occur in association with IgE-mediated (type I) reactions, immune complex–mediated (type III) reactions, or cell-mediated (type IV) reactions, because the immunologic products of these reactions do not readily cross the placenta and enter the fetal circulation in sufficient quantity.

At birth, maternal circulating antibody can no longer enter the child. Symptoms of the alloimmune disease may be present in utero or immediately after birth and may be fatal to the fetus or neonate. If symptoms are successfully treated at birth, the disease will disappear as the maternal antibody is catabolized.

At least one alloimmune disease is transported through breast milk. Human breast milk contains antibodies of the secretory immune system, primarily IgA. The gut of the human newborn will not transport antibody from the ingested milk into the circulation after about 24 hours after delivery, therefore the antibody in breast milk protects the newborn against gastrointestinal infections. In some mothers with pernicious anemia, the breast milk contains IgA against intrinsic factor, which is normally secreted into the gut to bind and transport dietary vitamin B_{12} into the child. The presence of IgA anti-intrinsic factor may prevent its interaction with B_{12} leading to symptoms of B_{12} deficiency from an alloimmune pernicious anemia in the child.

Examples of maternal immunologic hypersensitivity diseases in which the child can be affected include the following antibody-mediated diseases:

1. *Graves disease*—an autoimmune disease in which maternal antibody against the receptor for thyroid-stimulating hormone (TSH) causes neonatal hyperthyroidism
2. *Myasthenia gravis*—an autoimmune disease in which maternal antibody binds with receptors for neural transmitters on muscle cells (acetylcholine receptors), causing neonatal muscular weakness (see Chapter 17)
3. *Immune thrombocytopenic purpura*—both autoimmune and alloimmune variants in which maternal antiplatelet antibody destroys platelets in the fetus and neonate (see Chapter 27)
4. *Alloimmune neutropenia*—in which maternal antibody against neutrophils destroys neutrophils in the neonate
5. *Systemic lupus erythematosus*—autoimmune disease in which diverse maternal autoantibodies induce anomalies (e.g., congenital heart defects) in the fetus or cause pregnancy loss
6. *Rh and ABO alloimmunization (e.g., erythroblastosis fetalis)*—in which maternal antibody against erythrocyte antigens induces anemia in the child (see Chapter 28)
7. *Alloimmune pernicious anemia*—anemia in the newborn resulting from maternal IgA anti-intrinsic factor in the breast milk

Autoimmune and Alloimmune Diseases

Many examples of autoimmune or alloimmune diseases have been described. Several basic principles are exemplified by two examples, systemic lupus erythematosus (SLE) (an autoimmune disease) and tissue rejection (i.e., transplant rejection or transfusion reaction) (an alloimmune phenomenon). Most of the classic autoimmune diseases, including disorders of the endocrine system (autoimmune thyroiditis and Graves disease), hematologic system (the hemolytic and pernicious anemias), nervous system (myasthenia gravis), and connective tissue in joints (rheumatoid arthritis), are discussed in Unit II of this book.

Systemic Lupus Erythematosus

Systemic lupus erythematosus (SLE) is a chronic, multisystem, inflammatory disease and is one of the most common, complex, and serious of the autoimmune disorders.[22,23] SLE is characterized by the production of a large variety of autoantibodies against nucleic acids, erythrocytes, coagulation proteins, phospholipids, lymphocytes, platelets, and many other self-components. The most characteristic autoantibodies produced in SLE are against nucleic acids (e.g., single-stranded DNA, double-stranded DNA), histones, ribonucleoproteins, and other nuclear materials.

Deposition of circulating immune complexes containing antibody against host DNA produces tissue damage in individuals with SLE. DNA and DNA-containing immune complexes have a high affinity for glomerular basement membranes and therefore may be selectively deposited in the glomerulus (Figure 8-9). (Kidney structures are described in Chapter 35.) The presence of DNA in the circulation increases from cellular damage in response to trauma, drugs, or infections and is usually removed in the liver. Removal of circulating DNA is slowed in the presence of immune complexes, thereby increasing the potential for deposition in the kidney. (The liver's role in removing waste products from the blood is discussed in Chapter 35.) Deposition of immune complexes composed of DNA and antibody also causes inflammatory lesions in the renal tubular basement membranes, brain (choroid plexus), heart, spleen, lung, gastrointestinal tract, skin (see Figure 8-9), and peritoneum.

SLE, as with most autoimmune diseases, occurs more often in women (approximately a 10:1 predominance of females), especially in the 20- to 40-year-old age group. Blacks are affected more often than whites (about an eightfold increased risk). A genetic predisposition for the disease has been implicated on the basis of increased incidence in twins and the existence of autoimmune disease in the families of individuals with SLE.[24]

A transient lupus-like syndrome that is indistinguishable both clinically and in the laboratory from spontaneously occurring SLE can develop from the prolonged use of drugs. The drugs most often implicated are hydralazine (an antihypertensive agent) and procainamide (an antidysrhythmic drug). In genetically susceptible individuals, certain environmental agents, such as ultraviolet light, and several infectious agents may trigger lupus-like immune reactions.

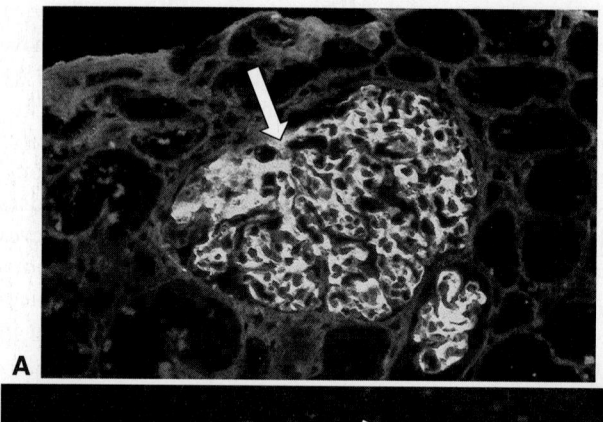

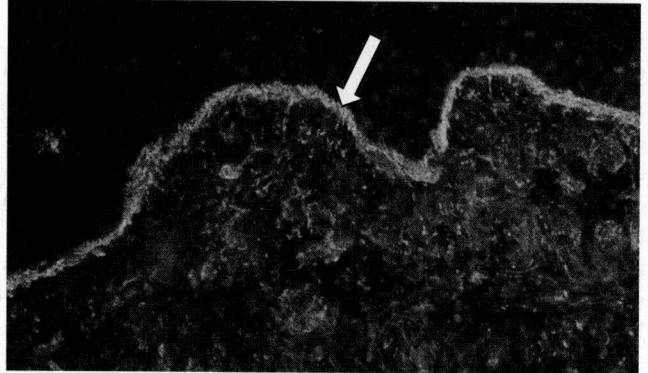

Figure 8-9 Deposition of IgG in the kidney and skin of persons with lupus. These photographs of tissue were obtained from persons with lupus and stained with fluorescent anti-IgG. **A,** Section from a kidney showing a glomerulus with deposits of IgG (*arrow* indicating bright areas of staining). **B,** Section of the skin showing deposition of IgG along the dermal-epidermal junction (*arrow* indicating bright green staining). (**A** courtesy of Dr. Helmut Rennke, Department of Pathology, Brigham and Women's Hospital, Boston, Mass; **B** courtesy of Dr. Richard Sontheimer, Department of Dermatology, University of Texas Southwestern Medical School, Dallas, Tex. Modified from Kumar V, Abbas A, Fausto N: *Robbins and Cotran pathologic basis of disease,* ed 7, Philadelphia, 2005, Saunders.)

Clinical manifestations of SLE include arthralgias or arthritis (90% of individuals), vasculitis and rash (70% to 80% of individuals), renal disease (40% to 50% of individuals), hematologic abnormalities (50% of individuals, with anemia being the most common complication), and cardiovascular diseases (30% to 50% of individuals). As with most autoimmune diseases, SLE is characterized by frequent remissions and exacerbations. Because the signs and symptoms affect almost every body system and tend to come and go, SLE is extremely difficult to diagnose. This has led to the development of a list of 11 common clinical findings. The serial or simultaneous presence of at least four of them indicates that the individual has SLE. The findings are as follows[25]:

1. Facial rash confined to the cheeks (malar rash)
2. Discoid rash (raised patches, scaling)
3. Photosensitivity (skin rash developed as a result of exposure to sunlight)
4. Oral or nasopharyngeal ulcers
5. Nonerosive arthritis of at least two peripheral joints
6. Serositis (pleurisy, pericarditis)
7. Renal disorder (proteinuria of 0.5 g/day or cellular casts)
8. Neurologic disorders (seizures or psychosis)
9. Hematologic disorders (hemolytic anemia, leukopenia, lymphopenia, or thrombocytopenia)
10. Immunologic disorders (positive lupus erythematosus [LE] cell preparation, anti–double stranded DNA, anti-Smith [Sm] antigen, false-positive serologic test for syphilis, or antiphospholipid antibodies [anticardiolipin antibody or lupus anticoagulant])
11. Presence of antinuclear antibody (ANA)

Graft Rejection

Transplantation of organs commonly is complicated by an immune response against antigens—primarily HLA—on the donated tissue. Most of our knowledge on the transplantation of organs is based on renal transplant studies. The primary mechanism of the rejection of transplanted organs is a type IV, cell-mediated reaction. Two randomly chosen individuals are almost certainly antigenically different to some degree. Organ transplants between them could be rejected in approximately 2 weeks without the extensive use of immunosuppressive drugs.

Because HLAs are the principal targets of the rejection reaction, HLA matching of donor and recipient enhances the probability of acceptance of the graft. Not all HLA loci are equally important; matching at the HLA-DR locus appears to be the most critical for graft acceptance, and matching at HLA-A and HLA-B of slightly lesser importance. (These loci are discussed in Chapter 7.)

Transplant rejection may be classified as hyperacute, acute, or chronic, depending on the amount of time that elapses between transplantation and rejection. **Hyperacute rejection** is immediate and rare. When the circulation is reestablished to the grafted area, the graft may immediately turn white (the so-called *white graft*) instead of a normal pink color. Hyperacute rejection usually occurs in recipients with preexisting antibody to antigens in the graft. The antibodies may have resulted from rejection of a previous graft or from prior blood transfusions that contained platelets and white blood cells with foreign HLA. Additionally, about half of women who have had multiple pregnancies will have circulating antibodies against their husband's HLA antigens. As the circulation to the graft is established, antibodies bind to the vascular endothelial cells in the grafted tissue and activate the inflammatory response, including the coagulation cascade, which results in stasis of blood flow into the tissue (Figure 8-10). (Coagulation is described in Chapters 6 and 25.) Biopsies of the graft often show deposits of antibody (IgG and IgM), complement, and neutrophils. This condition is rare because of effective pretransplantation cross-matching during which a recipient is tested for antibodies against the HLA antigens of the potential donor.

Acute rejection is a cell-mediated immune response that occurs within days to months after transplantation. This type of rejection occurs when the recipient develops an immune

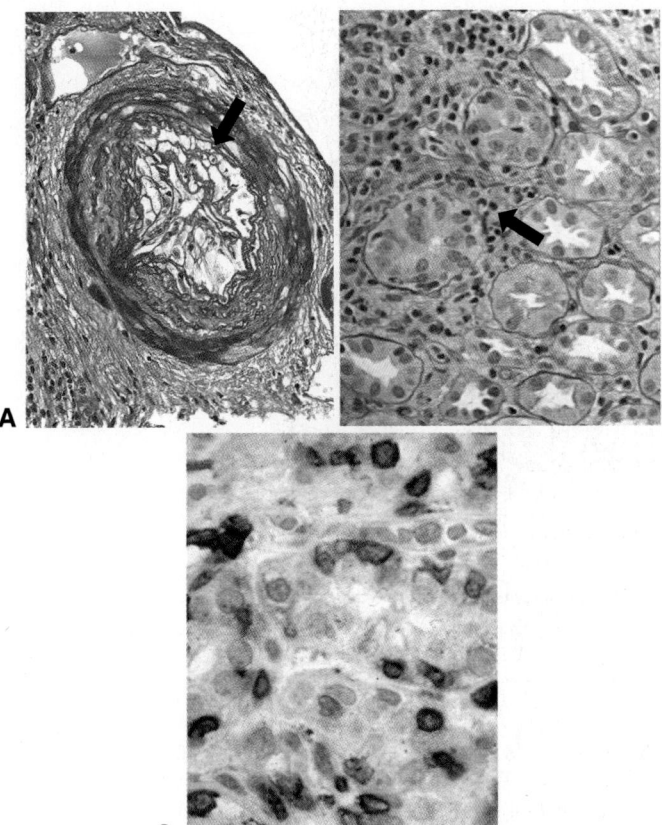

Figure 8-10 Examples of hyperacute and acute rejection of renal allografts. **A,** Hyperacute antibody-mediated damage to the blood vessel of a renal allograft. The blood vessel is thickened, and the lumen *(arrow)* is obstructed by proliferating fibroblasts and macrophages. **B,** Acute cellular rejection of a renal allograft with intense mononuclear cell infiltrate *(arrow)*. **C,** Acute cellular rejection stained with immunoperoxidase reagent (brown color) against T cells, which are infiltrating the tissue. (**A** courtesy of Dr. Ihsan Housini, Department of Pathology, University of Texas Southwestern Medical School, Dallas, Tex; **B** and **C** courtesy of Dr. Robert Colvin, Department of Pathology, Massachusetts General Hospital, Boston, Mass. Modified from Kumar V, Abbas A, Fausto N: *Robbins and Cotran pathologic basis of disease,* ed 7, Philadelphia, 2005, Saunders.)

response against unmatched HLAs after transplantation. Sensitization is usually initiated by the recipient's lymphocytes interacting with the donor's dendritic cells within the transplanted tissue, resulting in induction of recipient Th1 and Tc cells against the donor's antigens. The Th1 cells release cytokines that activate infiltrating macrophages, and the Tc cells directly attack the endothelial cells in the transplanted tissue. A biopsy of the rejected organ usually shows an infiltration of lymphocytes and macrophages characteristic of a type IV reaction. Immunosuppressive drugs may delay or lessen the intensity of acute rejection.

Chronic rejection may occur after a period of months or years of normal function. It is characterized by slow, progressive organ failure. Chronic rejection may be caused by inflammatory damage to endothelial cells lining blood vessels as a result of a weak cell-mediated immunologic reaction against minor histocompatibility antigens on the grafted tissue.

Transfusion Reactions

Red blood cells (erythrocytes) express several important surface antigens, known collectively as the **blood group antigens,** which can be targets of alloimmune reactions. More than 80 different red cell antigens are grouped into several dozen blood group systems, each determined by a different locus or set of loci. The most important of these, because they provoke the strongest humoral alloimmune response, are the ABO and Rh systems.

ABO System

Human blood transfusions were carried out as early as 1818, but they were often unsuccessful. Sometimes after a transfusion, the recipient's red blood cells would clump together, thereby blocking the capillaries and causing death in some instances. In 1901, Karl Landsteiner reported that this reaction was related to the ABO antigens located on the surface of erythrocytes.

The **ABO blood group** consists of two major carbohydrate antigens, labeled A and B (Figure 8-11). These two carbohydrate antigens are co-dominant, which means that both A and B can be simultaneously expressed, resulting in an individual having any one of four different blood types. The erythrocytes of persons with blood type A have the type A carbohydrate antigen (i.e., carry the A antigen), those with blood type B carry the B antigen, those with blood type AB carry both A and B antigens, and those of blood type O carry neither the A nor the B antigen. A person with type A blood also has circulating antibodies to the B carbohydrate antigen. If this person receives blood containing B antigens (i.e., blood from a type AB or B individual), a severe transfusion reaction occurs and the transfused erythrocytes are destroyed by agglutination (Figure 8-12) or complement-mediated lysis. Similarly, a type B individual (whose blood contains anti-A antibodies) cannot receive blood from a type A or AB donor. Type O individuals, who have neither antigen but have both anti-A and anti-B antibodies, cannot accept blood from any of the other three types. These naturally occurring antibodies, called **isohemagglutinins,** are immunoglobulins of the IgM class and are induced by similar antigens expressed on naturally occurring bacteria in the intestinal tract.

Because individuals with type O blood lack both types of antigens, they are considered **universal donors,** meaning that anyone can accept their red blood cells. Similarly, type AB individuals are considered **universal recipients** because they lack both anti-A and anti-B antibodies and can be transfused with any ABO blood type. When large volumes of *whole blood* (i.e., cells plus plasma) are transfused, however, antibodies in the *donor's* blood can bind to antigenic determinants on the *recipient's* erythrocytes, causing agglutination of the recipient's own cells. Agglutination and lysis cause harmful transfusion reactions that can be prevented only by complete and careful ABO matching between donor and recipient.

Rh System

The **Rh blood group** (inaccurately named after the Rhesus monkey in which a similar antigen system was first de-

Blood Type

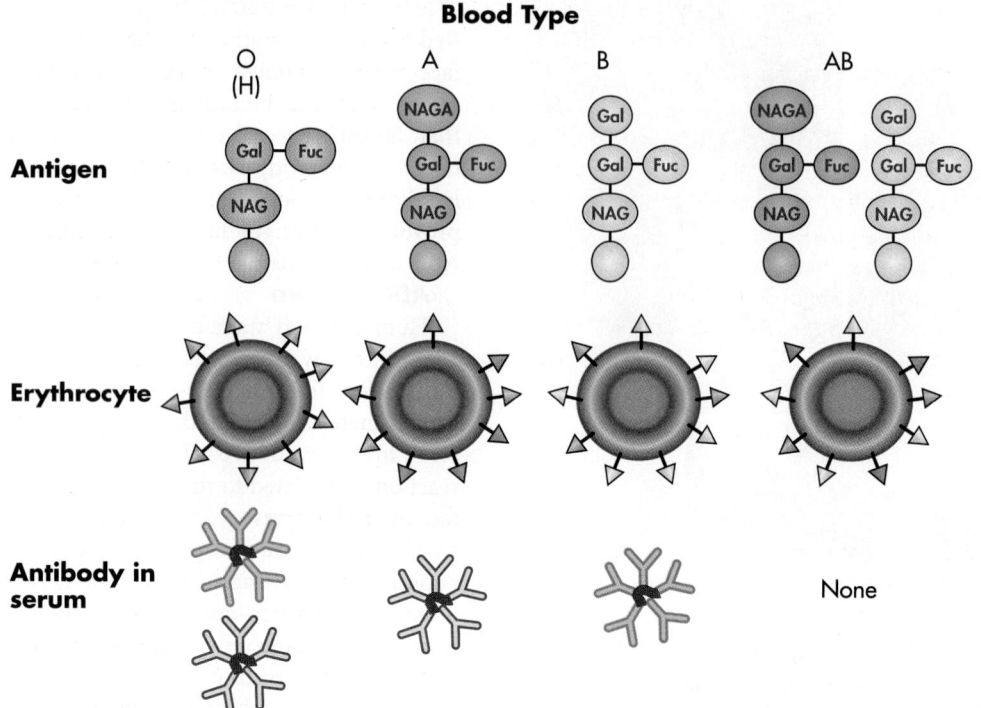

Figure 8-11 ABO blood types. This figure shows the antigens and antibodies associated with the ABO blood groups. The surfaces of erythrocytes of individuals with blood group O have the core H antigenic carbohydrate. Their sera contain IgM antibodies against both A and B carbohydrates. In individuals of the blood group A, some of the H antigens have been modified into A antigens by the addition of N-acetylgalactosamine (NAGA). The sera of these individuals have IgM antibodies against the B antigen. In individuals with blood group B, some of the H antigens have been modified into B antigens by the addition of galactose (Gal). These individuals have IgM antibodies against the A antigen in their sera. In individuals of the blood group AB, some of the H antigens have been modified into both the A and B antigens. These individuals do not have antibody to either A or B antigens. *NAG*, N-acetylglucosamine; *Fuc*, fucose.

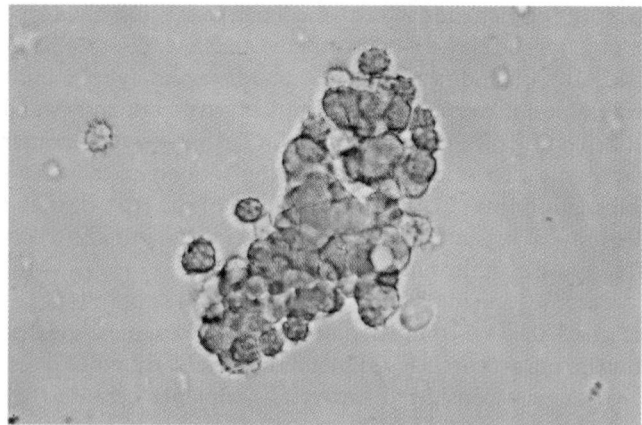

Figure 8-12 Mismatched transfused blood cells. Agglutination of erythrocytes caused by anti-A blood typing serum. (Copyright Ed Reschke.)

scribed), is the most polymorphic system of red cell antigens, consisting of at least 45 separate antigens. At least five major antigens and a large number of rare variants have been identified and are expressed only on erythrocytes.[26] The major antigens are contained on two proteins. The RhD protein expresses the dominant antigen, which determines whether an individual is Rh-positive or Rh-negative. Individuals who express the D antigen on the RhD protein are Rh-positive,

whereas individuals who do not express the D antigen are Rh-negative. The letter *d* is used to indicate lack of D. Rh-positive individuals can have either a *DD* or *Dd* genotype, whereas Rh-negative individuals have the *dd* genotype. About 85% of North Americans are Rh positive. Rh-negative individuals can make anti-D if exposed to Rh-positive erythrocytes, but because the letter *d* is used to indicate the lack of the D antigen and does not represent a different antigen, Rh-positive individuals do not produce an antibody against *d*. The second protein, RhCE, expresses two different antigens, C and E, each of which have two different alleles (C or c, E or e). Therefore, four potential haplotypes of C and E antigens are commonly observed: *CE, Ce, cE,* and *ce*).

IgG anti-D alloantibody produced by Rh-negative mothers against erythrocytes of their Rh-positive fetuses was the primary cause of Rh maternal-fetal incompatibility and the resulting hemolytic disease of the newborn (see Chapter 28). However, over the last several decades, the incidence of mothers with high titers of anti-D antibody has decreased dramatically because of the use of prophylactic anti-D immunoglobulin. By mechanisms that are still not completely understood, administration of anti-D antibody within a few days of exposure to RhD-positive erythrocytes completely prevents sensitization against the D antigen. Because hemolytic disease of the newborn related to the D antigen has been controlled, alloantibodies against the other Rh antigens (usually C, c, or E) have become more important. In general, these alloantibodies are associated with a less severe hemolytic disease.

One form of autoimmune hemolytic anemia is often caused by autoantibodies against Rh antigens, especially e. This variant is caused by IgG antibodies that react with erythrocytes at normal body temperature (thus called *warm autoimmune hemolytic anemia*) and increase phagocytic destruction of the red cell. This characteristic differentiates the warm variant from another form of autoimmune hemolytic anemia, which is caused by IgM autoantibodies that react optimally with erythrocytes in the cooler portions of the body (e.g., fingers, toes) and is referred to as *cold autoimmune hemolytic anemia.*

DEFICIENCIES IN IMMUNITY

Disorders resulting from immune deficiency are the clinical sequelae (results) of impaired function of one or more components of the immune or inflammatory response, including B cells, T cells, phagocytes, and complement (Table 8-6). An **immune deficiency** is the failure of these mechanisms of self-defense to function at their normal capacity, resulting in increased susceptibility to infections. **Primary (congenital) immune deficiency** is caused by a genetic anomaly, whereas **secondary (acquired) immune deficiency** is caused by another illness, such as cancer or viral infection, or by normal physiologic changes, such as aging. Acquired forms of immune deficiency are far more common than the congenital forms.

Initial Clinical Presentation

The clinical hallmark of immune deficiency is a tendency to develop unusual or recurrent, severe infections. Preschool and school-age children normally may have 6 to 12 infections per year, of which three to four are ear infections, and adults may have two to four infections per year. Most of these are not severe and are limited to viral infections of the upper respiratory tract, recurrent streptococcal pharyngitis, or mild otitis media.

Potential immune deficiencies are considered if the individual has had severe, documented bouts of pneumonia, otitis media, sinusitis, bronchitis, septicemia, or meningitis or infections with opportunistic microorganisms that normally are not pathogenic (e.g., *Pneumocystis carinii*). Infections are generally recurrent with only short intervals of relative health, and multiple simultaneous infections are common. Individuals with immune deficiencies often have eight or more ear infections, two or more serious sinus infections, and two or more pneumonias, recurrent abscesses, or persistent fungal infections (particularly thrush) within a year. Recurrent internal infections, such as meningitis, osetomyelitis, or sepsis, are common. Prolonged antibiotic use is commonly ineffective by oral or injected routes and may necessitate intravenous administration. A familial history of immune deficiency may be found in some types of primary deficiency.

The type of recurrent infections that manifest may indicate the type of immune defect. Deficiencies in T-cell immune responses are suggested when recurrent infections are caused by certain viruses (e.g., varicella, vaccinia, herpes, cytomegalovirus), fungi and yeasts (e.g., *Candida, Histoplasma*), or certain atypical microorganisms (e.g., *P. carinii*). B-cell deficiencies and phagocyte deficiencies, however, are suggested if the individual has documented, recurrent infections with microorganisms that require opsonization (e.g., encapsulated bacteria) or viruses against which humoral immunity is normally effective (e.g., rubella). Some complement deficiencies resemble defects in antibody or phagocyte function, but others are commonly associated with disseminated infections with bacteria of the genus *Neisseria* (*Neisseria meningitides* and *Neisseria gonorrhoeae*).

Much of our current understanding of the development of the immune system and the interactions of the cells in the immune response was developed by studying congenital and acquired immune deficiencies or, as they have been called, "experiments of nature." Many immune deficiencies result from selective altering or removal of one component of the immune system. Our understanding of the importance of that component is arrived at by observing the effect of its removal on the remainder of the immune response.

Primary Immune Deficiencies

Most primary immune deficiencies are the result of a single gene defect[27,28] (Figure 8-13). Generally, the mutations are sporadic and not inherited: a family history exists in only about 25% of individuals. The sporadic mutations occur before birth, but the onset of symptoms may be early or later, depending on the particular syndrome. In some instances, symptoms of immune deficiency appear within the first 2 years of life. Other immune deficiencies are progressive, with the onset of symptoms appearing in the second or third decade of life. The most common symptoms include sinusitis (68% of individuals), pneumonia (51%), ear infections (51%), diarrhea (30%), and bronchitis (55%), with the incidence varying depending on the specific syndrome.

Many immune deficiencies also are associated with other characteristic defects; some of which appear to be unrelated to the immune system yet may be life threatening by themselves. Examples include eczema and thrombocytopenia (in Wiskott-Aldrich syndrome); cardiac anomalies, low levels of calcium in the blood, and structural anomalies of the face (in DiGeorge syndrome); or a severe lack of muscular coordination and dilation of the small blood vessels (in ataxia-telangiectasia). These associated symptoms can be useful diagnostically and can clarify the pathophysiology of the disease. For instance, the principal immunologic defect in **DiGeorge syndrome** is the partial or complete absence of T-cell immunity. However, this syndrome is also characterized by severe congenital structural defects of the heart and low levels of calcium, which may result in seizures.

Individually, primary immune deficiencies are very rare. For instance, only 30 to 50 new cases of severe combined im-

Table 8-6	Classes of Primary Immune Deficiencies		
Classification*	**Example**	**Mutation**	**Immune Deficiency**
B-Cell Defects			
B-cell receptor signaling	Bruton/X-linked agammaglobulinemia	Btk	Little or no B-cell maturation or antibody
	Autosomal agammaglobulinemia	IgMμ chain	
Class-switch: Hyper-IgM	X-linked hyper-IgM syndrome	CD40 ligand	Little or no class-switch to IgG or IgA, with overproduction of IgM
	Autosomal hyper-IgM syndrome	CD40	
	AICD deficiency	AICD	
Class-switch: Selective	IgG subclass deficiency	Unknown	Defective switch to an IgG subclass
	Selective IgA deficiency	Unknown	Defective switch to IgA
	Common variable immune deficiency	Unknown	Defective switch to ≥1 antibody class
T-Cell Defects			
Defective primary lymphoid organ for T-cell development	DiGeorge syndrome	Development of 3rd and 4th pharyngeal pouches	Little or no T-cell maturation
Antigen specific response	Chronic mucocutaneous candidiasis	Unknown	Little or no response to *Candida*
Combined T- and B-Cell Defects			
SCID: No wbc stem cells	Reticular dysgenesis	Unknown	Complete; lack of white blood cells
SCID: Purine metabolism defects	Adenosine deaminase deficiency	ADA	Complete; few or no T, B, or NK cells
	Purine nucleoside phosphorylase deficiency	PNP	Partial; few T or NK cells
SCID: Cytokine receptor defects	X-linked SCID	IL-2Rγ	Partial; little or no maturation of Th or NK cells
	IL-7 receptor deficiency	IL-7Rα	
	JAK3 deficiency	JAK3	
SCID: TCR/BCR defects	RAG-1 or RAG-2 deficiency	RAG-1/RAG-2	Complete; little or no maturation of T or B cells; normal NK cells
SCID: TCR defects S	CD45 deficiency	CD45	Partial; incomplete T-cell maturation, normal B and NK cells
	CD3 deficiency	CD3 γ, δ, or ε chains	
	ZAP-70 deficiency	ZAP-70	
Antigen presentation defects	MHC class I deficiency	TAP1 or TAP2	Abnormal cytotoxic T cell activity
	MHC class II deficiency	Multiple	Abnormal helper T cell activity
Cytoskeletal defect	Wiskott-Aldrich syndrome	WASP	Altered T and B cells; decreased IgM
DNA repair defect	Ataxia-telangiectasia	AT	Altered T and B cells; absent IgA
Complement Defects			
Classical pathway	C1q,r,s, C4, or C2 deficiency	C1q,r, or s, C4, or C2	Defective classical pathway, intact alternative pathway
Lectin pathway	Mannose-binding lectin deficiency	MBL	Defective lectin pathway
Alternative pathway	Properdin, factor D deficiency	Properdin, factor D	Defective alternative pathway
	Factor H, Factor I	Factor H, Factor I	Secondary C3 deficiency
C3	C3 deficiency	C3	Entire complement cascade blocked
Terminal pathway	C5, C6, C7, C8, or C9 deficiency	C5, C6, C7, C8, or C9	Membrane attack complex blocked, normal opsonization and chemotaxis
Phagocyte Defects			
Quantitative defects	Severe congenital neutropenia	Unknown	Inadequate numbers of neutrophils
	Cyclic neutropenia	ELA2	
Adhesion defects	Leukocyte adhesion defect (LAD)-1	CD18	Decreased phagocyte adhesion to endothelium
	LAD-2	Transport enzymes for fucose	
Phagocytosis defects	C3 receptor deficiency	C3R	Defective opsonization
Bacterial killing defects	Chédiak-Higashi syndrome	CHS1	Defective lysosomal granules
	Myeloperoxidase deficiency	MPO	Lack of myeloperoxidase
	Chronic granulomatous disease	NADPH oxidase	Defective production of H_2O_2

AICD, Activation-induced cytidine deaminase; *SCID*, severe combined immune deficiency; *TCB/BCR*, T-cell receptor/B-cell receptor; *MHC*, major histocompatibility complex; *NADPH*, nicotinamide adenine dinucleotide phosphate.

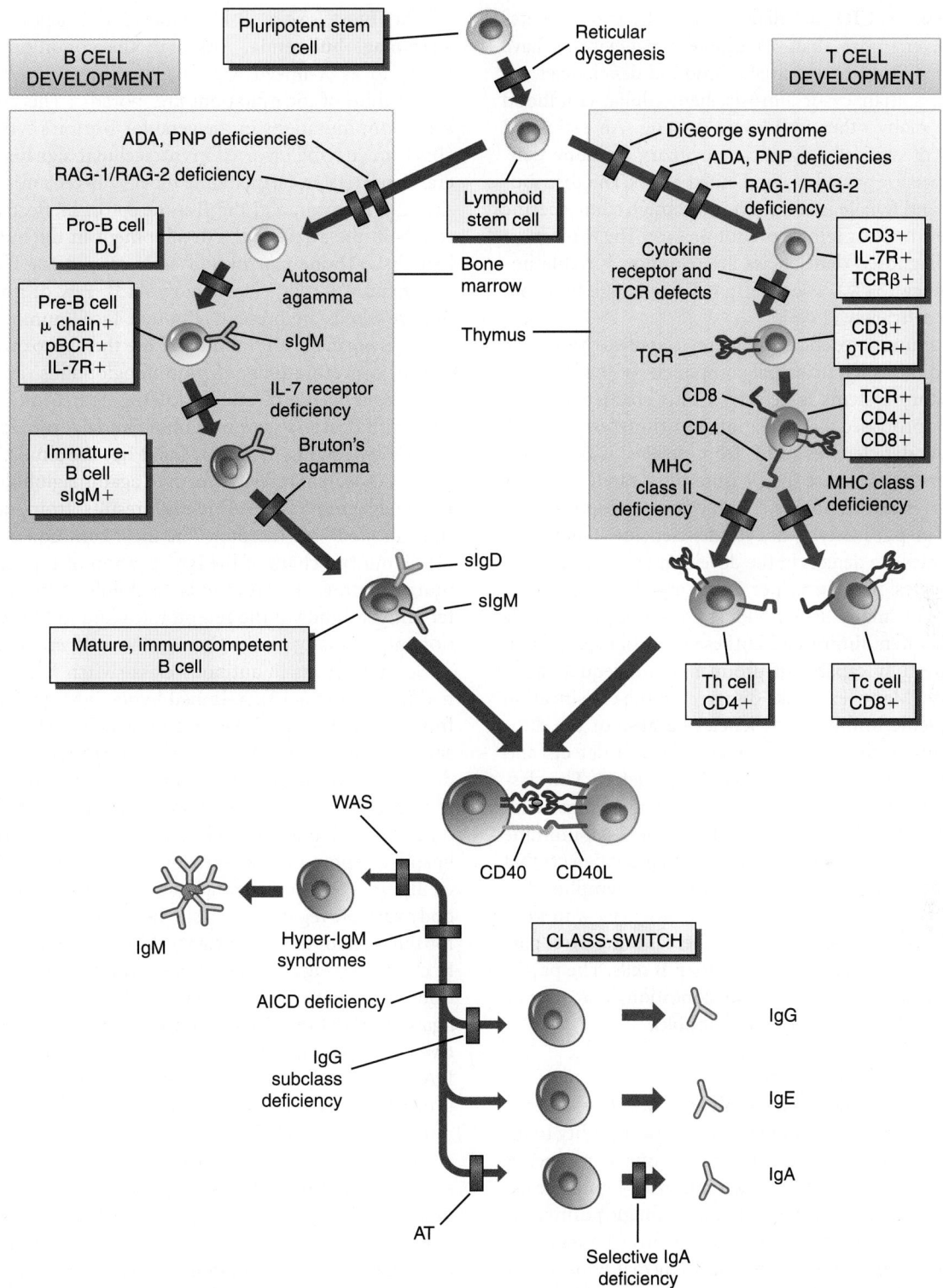

Figure 8-13 Lymphocyte development defects. This diagram shows defects in lymphocyte development that may account for congenital (primary) immune deficiencies. See the text and refer to Figures 7-9 through 7-13 for more detailed information. Pluripotent stem cell indicates the common stem cells for lymphocytic, granulocytic, and monocytic lineages. Cytokine receptor defects include X-linked severe combined immunodeficiency (SCID) (IL-2 receptor defect), JAK3 defects, and IL-7 receptor defects. T-cell receptor (TCR) defects include defects in CD3, CD45, and ZAP-70. Neither common variable immune deficiency nor chronic mucocutaneous candidiasis is included in this figure because the cause of these defects remains unknown. *Agamma,* Agammaglobulinemia; *WAS,* Wiskott-Aldrich syndrome; *AT,* ataxia-telangiectasia; *AICD* deficiency, a deficiency in the DNA editing enzyme activation-induced cytidine deaminase. Hyper-IgM syndromes include X-linked (C40L defect) and autosomal (CD40 defect) variants. *sIgM* and *sIgD,* Surface immunoglobulin as a component of the B-cell receptor (BCR). *ADA,* Adenosine deaminase deficiency; *PNP,* purine nucleoside phosphorylase deficiency.

mune deficiency (SCID) are diagnosed in the United States yearly. However, more than 70 different deficiencies have been identified. Together, primary immune deficiencies are more common than cystic fibrosis, hemophilia, childhood leukemia, or many other well-know diseases. An estimated 50,000 cases of clinically significant primary immune deficiency have been reported in the United States The distribution of male and female is about even, although some specific diseases have a male or female predominance. The three most commonly diagnosed deficiencies are common variable immune deficiency (34%), selective IgA deficiency (24%), and IgG subclass deficiency (17%).

Primary immune deficiencies are classified into five groups, based on which principal component of the immune or inflammatory systems is defective. This chapter uses the classifications proposed by the National Institutes of Health.[29] **B-lymphocyte deficiencies** result from defects in B-cell immune responses.[30] Because T-cell immunity rarely depends on competent B-cell responses, T-cell immune responses are not affected in pure B-lymphocyte deficiencies. **T-lymphocyte deficiencies** are defects in the development and function of T lymphocytes. Because helper T cells are obligatory in the development of many B-lymphocyte responses, antibody production is often diminished in these conditions, although the B cells are fully capable of producing an adequate antibody response. Many textbooks disagree on the classification of several specific immune deficiencies because of the difficulty in distinguishing between primary B-cell defects and those that are secondary to a primary T-cell defect. The classifications described below define T-cell defects as those with a clear defect in T-cell immunity, with normal B-cell immune responses. Combined defects result from inherent defects that directly affect the development of both T and B lymphocytes. Some combined deficiencies result in major defects in both the T- and B-cell immune responses, whereas others are "partial" and more adversely affect T cells than B cells. The partial combined deficiencies include many conditions that may be classified as T-cell defects in other textbooks.

B-Lymphocyte Deficiencies

A defect in B-cell development results in lower levels of circulating immunoglobulins and increased susceptibility to infections in which antibodies are the primary protective mechanism. The condition in which immunoglobulin levels are lower than normal is termed **hypogammaglobulinemia.** The condition in which they are totally or nearly totally absent is termed **agammaglobulinemia.** (Normal lymphocyte development is discussed in Chapter 7.) Recurrent infections range from life-threatening to mild, depending on the severity of the deficiency. Characteristic infections are caused by microorganisms that are particularly sensitive to antibody-mediated immunity. These include encapsulated bacteria (e.g., *Streptococcus pneumoniae* or *Hemophilus influenzae*) that may cause pneumonia or sepsis and other microorganisms that cause infections of the sinuses, ears, and gastrointestinal tract.

The most severe B-lymphocyte deficiency is **Bruton's agammaglobulinemia.** Although the condition is also referred to as X-linked agammaglobulinemia, somewhat less than a third of the mutations are sporadic. This condition results from mutations in the gene for Bruton's tyrosine kinase (Btk), an enzyme involved in intracellular signaling from several B-cell receptors, including the IgM B-cell antigen receptor, the IL-5 receptor, and the IL-6 receptor. Ineffective signaling results in the arrest of the development in the bursal-equivalent tissue (bone marrow) of early cells in the B-cell lineage into mature B cells[31] (see Figure 8-13). Few or no circulating mature B cells are present, although T-cell number and function are normal. At 6 months of life the approximate normal serum concentrations of immunoglobulins are IgG, 400 mg/dl; IgM, 40 mg/dl; and IgA, 30 mg/dl. In 6-month-old children with Bruton's agammaglobulinemia, serum IgG levels are well below 100 mg/dl and IgM and IgA are almost absent.

An autosomal recessive form of agammaglobulinemia (**autosomal agammaglobulinemia**) results from other mutations in the B-cell receptor. The most common is a mutation of the mu (μ) chain of the IgM portion of the receptor. This mutation prevents intracellular signaling in the pre–B cell after antigen binds to the receptor, leading to blocked maturation, no antibody production, and very severe infections.

Several defects in antibody class-switch have been identified (see Figure 8-13). **X-linked hyper-IgM syndrome** results from a mutation in CD40 ligand, which is expressed on the surface of helper T (Th) cells. Th cells stimulate B cells to undergo a switch in the class of antibody they produce through multiple Th–B cell interactions involving ligands expressed on one cell binding to specific receptors on the other cell. The ligand-receptor interaction results in an intracellular signal facilitating genetic rearrangement of the genes for the antibody variable region from a site near the constant region gene for the μ chain to the constant region for a different antibody H chain (see Figure 7-19). A critical ligand-receptor interaction occurs between the receptor CD40 on the B cell and its ligand (CD154 or CD40L) on the Th cell. The result is **defective class-switch,** decreased or absent production of IgG and IgA, poor development of memory B cells, and overproduction of IgM, which does not require class-switch. T-cell immunity is not affected.

Defects in other components of Th–B-cell interaction result in **autosomal hyper-IgM syndrome.** Mutations in CD40 on B cells results in a similar effect to that described above. A defect in a DNA editing enzyme (activation-induced cytidine deaminase; AICD) also inhibits class-switch. During class-switch and movement of the H chain genetic information for the variable region to a different constant region gene, the double-stranded DNA must be cut and mended. This enzyme is responsible for cutting and mending the DNA.

Deficiencies in particular subclasses of antibody (**IgG subclass deficiency**), particularly IgG2, may reflect a defect in switch to a particular subclass constant region (see Figure 8-13). The IgG2 subclass is often increased in response to polysaccharide antigens such as those on the surface of encapsulated bacteria. Low levels of IgG2 may be responsible for recurrent risk for pneumonias caused by these bacteria. Whether IgG subclass deficiencies are unique immune deficiency conditions is unclear because many are apparently early indications of the development of common variable immune deficiency (see below) or are secondary to selective IgA deficiency.

One of the most common primary immune deficiency is a **selective IgA deficiency.** Because many affected individuals are asymptomatic, the true incidence is uncertain, although estimates of 1 person in 300 to 1 in 3000 have been made. Individuals with selective IgA deficiency are able to produce other classes of immunoglobulins but fail to produce IgA (see Figure 8-13). Many will have B cells that have undergone class-switch to IgA, but for unknown reasons, cannot undergo the terminal steps of differentiation to IgA-secreting plasma cells. Although many individuals are asymptomatic, others present with a history of severe recurring sinus, lung, and gastrointestinal infections. They commonly also have chronic intestinal candidiasis (infection with *C. albicans*). (The secretory, or mucosal, immune system is described in Chapter 7.)

Complications of IgA deficiency include severe atopic disease and autoimmune diseases; selective IgA deficiency is two or three times more common in atopic individuals than in others. Secretory IgA normally may prevent the uptake of allergens from the environment so that IgA deficiency may lead to increased allergen uptake and a more intense challenge to the immune system because of prolonged exposure to environmental antigens. One of the most severe complications of IgA deficiency is an anaphylactic reaction that can follow administration of blood products that contain IgA. Serious anaphylactic reactions can occur in individuals totally lacking IgA because the immune system recognizes donor IgA as a foreign antigen. Initial sensitization can occur in fetal life through exposure to maternal IgA or later through the ingestion of maternal IgA in breast milk or bovine IgA in cow's milk. Sensitization also can occur with initial administration of blood products containing IgA. The individual's primed immune system then acts against donor IgA on subsequent exposure.

The most commonly diagnosed immune deficiency because of recurrent clinically relevant infections is **common variable immune deficiency.** As the name implies, the presentation is very heterogeneous. It is characterized by hypogammaglobulinemia, but the particular class of antibody that is decreased varies: most have low amounts of IgG, which may or may not be accompanied by decreased levels of IgA or IgM, or both, with normal numbers of B cells. Some may have accompanying T-cell defects. Several defects in terminal differentiation may account for this condition, although no specific one has been identified. The age of onset of symptoms, such as recurrent bacterial respiratory tract infections, is generally later than most primary immune deficiencies (late 20s). Secondary complications include arthritis (infectious and non-infectious), autoimmune disease (anemia, thrombocy-topenia, endocrine diseases), and cancer (of the lymphoid system, skin, and gastrointestinal tract).

T-Lymphocyte Deficiencies

Two well-studied examples of T-lymphocyte defects that represent different ends of the T-cell differentiation process include DiGeorge syndrome and chronic mucocutaneous candidiasis. Lymphoid stem cells begin maturing into functional T lymphocytes in the thymus. DiGeorge syndrome (congenital thymic aplasia or hypoplasia) is caused by the lack, or more commonly partial lack, of the thymus, resulting in greatly decreased T-cell numbers and function and in life-threatening viral, fungal, and intracellular bacterial infections[32,33] (see Figure 8-13). The defect is attributed usually to deletions on chromosome 22 (some deletions also have been identified on chromosome 10); about 25% of which are inherited. The deleted region encodes information for formation of organs that originate from the third and fourth pharyngeal pouches during the twelfth week of gestation. In addition to the lack of thymus development, the individual may present with a partial or complete absence of the parathyroid gland (resulting in decreased blood calcium levels), major structural defects in the heart and the aorta (resulting in inadequate blood flow and inadequate oxygenation of the tissues), and abnormal facial characteristics (e.g., underdeveloped chin, low-set ears, shortened structure of the upper lip) (Figure 8-14).

Chronic mucocutaneous candidiasis is a primary defect of T lymphocytes in response to a specific infectious agent, the yeast *Candida albicans*. At least seven variants of this condition have been described. All are characterized by mild to extremely severe chronic mucocutaneous candidiasis: *Candida* infections that involve the mucous membranes, nails, and skin. Invasive candidiasis is extremely rare. Although most B- and T-cell immune responses may be normal, most individuals with this defect cannot react to antigens from *Candida*. The cause of this defect is unknown.

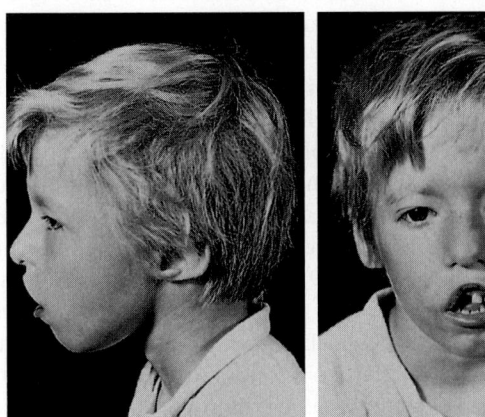

Figure 8-14 Facial anomalies associated with DiGeorge syndrome. Note the wide-set eyes, low-set ears, and shortened structure of the upper lip. (From Roitt I, Brostoff J, Male D: *Immunology*, ed 6, St Louis, 2001, Mosby.)

Combined T- and B-Lymphocyte Deficiencies

The most severe deficiencies usually occur when both the B- and T-cell immune responses are affected. A great deal of knowledge about the evolution of bone marrow stem cells into functional B- and T-cell effectors came from studying children with the most severe immune deficiency, **severe combined immune deficiency (SCID)**.[34] The most severe form of SCID is **reticular dysgenesis** (failure of blood cells to develop), in which a common stem cell for all white blood cells is absent; therefore T cells, B cells, and phagocytic cells never develop (see Figure 8-13). Most children with reticular dysgenesis die in utero or very soon after birth. More typically, a defect occurs after some stem cells become committed to developing into lymphocytes (lymphoid stem cells); therefore most individuals with SCID are deficient in lymphocyte development, but have normal numbers of all other white blood cells. SCID often results in few or absent T and B lymphocytes in the circulation and secondary lymphoid organs (spleen, lymph nodes). The thymus is usually hypoplastic (underdeveloped) because of the absence of T cells. Immunoglobulin levels, especially of IgM and IgA, are absent or greatly reduced, although IgG levels may be almost normal in the first months of life because of the presence of maternal antibodies. In the most severe defects, death occurs at about 1 year of life.

At least 20 different forms of SCID have been identified. Depending on the specific genetic mutation, the defect may involve T cells, B cells, and NK cells or may suppress more severely the function of one cell type, with relatively minor effects on the others. All three cells are adversely affected (T−, B−, NK−) in SCID resulting from a deficiency of adenosine deaminase (**adenosine deaminase [ADA] deficiency),** which is an enzyme involved in purine metabolism[34] (see Figure 8-13). This defect is autosomal recessive and results in the accumulation of toxic purine metabolites to which rapidly dividing cells, such as lymphocytes, are especially sensitive. ADA deficiency accounts for about 16% of all persons with SCID. The development of T cells, B cells, and NK cells is arrested very early, and very few lymphocytic cells are found in the blood. In some forms of SCID, the defect resides in receptors for cytokines that are necessary for maturation of lymphocytes (see Figure 8-13). T cells and NK cells are preferentially affected (T−, B+, NK−), but often the defect results in the production of immature B cells that cannot respond well to antigen because of the lack of Th cells. The most common (44% of those with SCID) is an **X-linked SCID** resulting from a defect in the IL-2 receptor gamma (γ) chain (IL-2Rγ). This protein is a component of several receptors for cytokines, including IL-2, IL-4, IL-7, IL-9, IL-15, and IL-21. These cytokines participate in the early development of immunocytes, particularly T and NK cells. Defective IL-2Rγ results in arrested maturation of T and NK cells and the production of immature B cells. A similar deficiency occurs with mutation in JAK3 (**JAK3 deficiency),** which is an enzyme (a tyrosine kinase) that associates with IL-2Rγ in normal cells and communicates information from the receptor to the nucleus.

Thus cells with defects in JAK3 cannot respond to cytokines that bind to these receptors on the cell surface. An autosomal form results from mutations of one of the protein chains (α chain) of the IL-7 receptor (**IL-7 receptor deficiency**). IL-7 appears to be necessary for the maturation of T cells, so that this deficiency has relatively normal levels of B cells and NK cells.

Mutations in another purine metabolism enzyme, purine nucleoside phosphorylase (**purine nucleoside phosphorylase [PNP] deficiency**) is less severe than ADA deficiency (see Figure 8-13). T cells and NK cells appear to be more susceptible to mutations in PNP so that B-cell function can be relatively normal.

Another form of SCID preferentially affects T cells and B cells (T−, B−, NK+). T and B lymphocytes possess receptors for antigen, whereas NK cells do not. Those receptors result from a process of genetic rearrangement of *V* and *J* genes to form the variable regions of the L chain (B-cell receptor, BCR) and the α chain (T-cell receptor, TCR) and the *V, D,* and *J* genes to form the variable regions of the H chain (BCR) and β chain (TCR). Successful rearrangement is controlled by two recombination activating enzymes (RAG-1 and RAG-2). RAG enzymes cut and repair double-stranded breaks in DNA that are necessary for genetic rearrangement. **RAG-1** or **RAG-2 deficiencies** are autosomal recessive and result in arrested lymphocyte development from blocked recombination of variable regions of B-cell and T-cell receptors (see Figure 8-13).

Forms of partial SCID, with the defect being primarily of T cells, arise from mutations in several components of the TCR complex (see Figure 8-13). Defects in the TCR result in inadequate maturation of T cells, with normal B and NK cells. Antibody production may be depressed because of the lack of Th cells. The TCR is a complex organization of proteins that react with antigen (α and β chains), then provide an intracellular signal to the nucleus (γ, δ, and ε chains and the associated molecules CD45 and ZAP-70). Examples of these deficiencies include mutations in CD3, CD45, or ZAP-70. The T-cell defect in each can range from mild to severe in nature, with normal B lymphocytes.

Even if nearly adequate numbers of B and T cells are produced, their ability to process and present antigen may be defective. The **bare lymphocyte syndrome** is a group of immune deficiencies characterized by an inability of lymphocytes and macrophages to present antigen because of defects in class I or class II major histocompatibility complex (MHC) antigen expression (see Figure 8-13). **MHC class I deficiency** results from mutations in the genes for TAP1 or TAP2, which control the transport of antigenic protein fragments across the endoplasmic reticulum and the formation of MHC class I/antigen complexes for transportation to the cell surface (see Figure 7-15). Because MHC class I molecules preferentially present antigen to CD8+ Tc cells, the resultant deficiency is of CD8+ cytotoxic cells, with normal levels of CD4+ helper cells and normal antibody production. **MHC class II deficiency** is more severe. A variety of mutations prevent normal production of MHC class II molecules, which present antigen to CD4+ helper cells. Because of defective recruitment of helper T cells, normal antibody responses are greatly suppressed. Children with this deficiency develop life-threatening infections and usually die before age 5 years.

Some combined immune deficiencies are secondary to mutations that affect a variety of cells other than immunocytes. For instance, **Wiskott-Aldrich syndrome** (WAS; an X-linked recessive disorder) results from sporadic mutations in the WAS protein (WASP), which is involved in intracellular signaling and regulation of the organization of the cell's actin cytoskeleton (see Figure 8-13). The defects in the cytoskeleton lead to the classic symptoms of thrombocytopenia (with resultant bleeding disorders), scaly eczema, and defective T and B cells. IgA and IgG levels are usually normal, but IgM responses are highly depressed. Antibody responses against antigens that elicit primarily an IgM response, such as polysaccharide antigens from bacterial cell walls (e.g., of *P. aeruginosa, S. pneumoniae, H. influenzae*, and other microorganisms with polysaccharide outer capsules), are deficient.[35] Persons with WAS have a very high risk of lymphoid malignancies (leukemias and lymphomas).

Ataxia-telangiectasia (AT) is an autosomal recessive disorder resulting from a large variety of sporadic mutations in the *AT* gene, which encodes a protein involved in repair of double-stranded breaks in DNA. Affected infants often develop ataxia (unsteady gait), which usually becomes apparent when the child is learning to walk. The neurologic defect may eventually lead to confinement in a wheel chair. Telangiectasia (dilation of capillaries) can occur in the eyes and skin, especially on the ears, neck, and extremities. Both B and T cells are variably affected and unrepaired double stranded DNA breaks are commonly observed in the regions encoding the T-cell and B-cell receptors. About 70% of those with AT are IgA deficient, occasionally accompanied by deficiencies in IgG (see Figure 8-13). Individuals with AT are at high risk for developing leukemias and lymphomas.

Complement Deficiencies

Protection against many infectious agents is mediated by antibody that activates the complement cascade. As a result, some defects in the complement cascade often resemble antibody deficiencies, with recurrent infections with encapsulated bacteria (e.g., *Hemophilus influenzae* and *Streptococcus pneumoniaea*). Additionally, the Fc portion of IgG and some activated complement components, such as C3b, function as opsonins and facilitate phagocytosis by neutrophils and macrophages. As previously noted, excessive levels of circulating complexes of antibody, antigen, and complement may lead to type III hypersensitivity diseases (immune complex diseases). Healthy individuals release small amounts of soluble intracellular antigens into the blood during normal cell turnover. Clearance of that antigen appears to be helped by low levels of naturally occurring autoantibodies, without any overt disease. The classical pathway of the complement system through C3 may assist in removal of these complexes by cells of the phagocytic system. Deficiencies in the classical pathway commonly lead to a SLE-like syndrome, which may result from decreased clearance of natural immune complexes from the blood. **C2 deficiency,** more so than **C1** or **C4 deficiencies,** has an increased risk for recurrent respiratory infections with encapsulated bacteria. C2 deficiencies are found primarily in whites (Figure 8-15).

C3 deficiency is the most severe complement defect. C3 is the component that unites all pathways of complement activation, and complement component C3b is a major opsonin. Persons with C3 deficiency are at risk for recurrent life-threatening infections with encapsulated bacteria at an early age, as well as a SLE-like syndrome that may be complicated by kidney disease (glomerulonephritis).

Mannose-binding lectin (MBL) deficiency is the primary defect of the lectin pathway of complement activation. The defect results in increased risk of infection with microorganisms that have polysaccharide capsules that are rich in mannose, particularly the yeast Saccharomyces cerevisiae and encapsulated bacteria such as *Neisseria meningitides* and *Streptococcus pneumoniae.*

Deficiencies in the alternative pathway also result in recurrent infections with encapsulated bacteria. **Properdin deficiency** is X-linked, whereas all other complement deficiencies are autosomal recessive. Symptoms generally appear in the second decade of life. Factor I and factor H are major regulators of the complement cascade and control the level of spontaneous activation of C3. **Factor I deficiency** or **factor H deficiency** can be severe because they lead to increased spontaneous destruction of C3 and a secondary C3 deficiency.

Deficiencies of components of the terminal portion of the complement cascade (C5, C6, C7, C8, or C9 deficiencies) are associated with increased infections with only one group of bacteria; those of the genus *Neisseria (Neisseria meningitides or N. gonorrhoeae). Neisseria* usually cause localized infections (meningitis or gonorrhea), but those with terminal pathway defects have more than an 8000-fold increased risk for systemic infections with atypical strains of these microorganisms. **C9 deficiency** is the most common terminal pathway defect, appears primarily in Japanese populations, and is generally asymptomatic. The other deficiencies of the terminal pathway are extremely rare, but are characterized by more aggressive infections. The risk for systemic infections with *Neisseria* is also increased in those with deficiencies of C2, factor D, and properdin.

Phagocytic Deficiencies

Phagocytosis and bacterial killing are generally aided by bacterial opsonization with IgG or C3b, therefore defects in phagocytic killing usually result in recurrent infections with the same group of microorganisms (encapsulated bacteria) associated with antibody and complement deficiencies.[36] Phagocytosis and bacterial killing is a multistep process that involves initial adhesion between circulating phagocytes and the endothelial cells lining the circulation (see Figure 6-12). The phagocytes exit the circulation and move to a site of infection by a chemotactic process in response to soluble

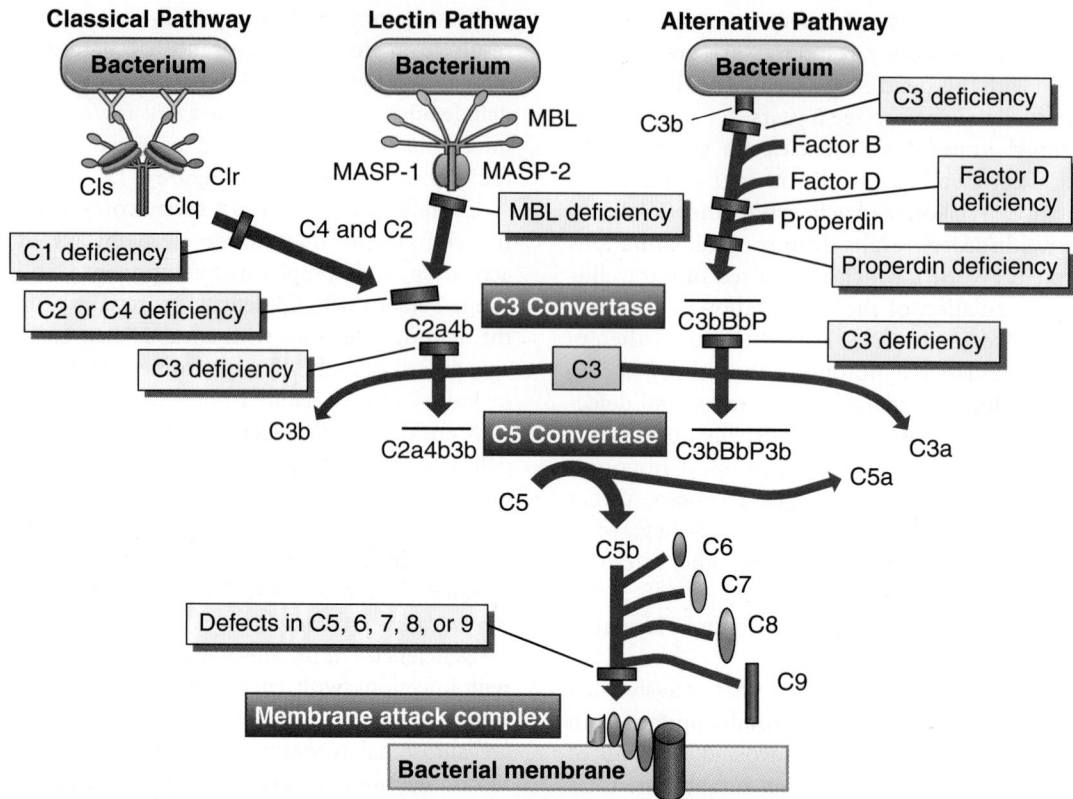

Figure 8-15 **Complement defects.** The complement cascade is initiated through three pathways: the classical pathway, the lectin pathway, and the alternative pathway. Each of the three pathways produces a C3 convertase, which activates C3 leading to the formation of a C5 convertase. The activation of C5 initiates formation of the membrane attack complex (MAC). For more details, see the text and Figure 6-4. The most severe defect is a C3 deficiency because it blocks all three pathways. *MBL,* Mannose-binding lectin; *MASP,* MBL-associated serine protease.

chemotactic factors released by the infection. The process of phagocytosis itself begins with attachment of the phagocyte to the targeted bacteria through the interaction of opsonins on the microorganism and matched receptors on the phagocyte's surface. Phagocytic engulfment results in internalization of the infectious agent and activation of a variety of oxygen-dependent and oxygen-independent killing mechanisms. Deficiencies can arise from mutations that affect one or more of these steps (Figure 8-16).

Inadequate numbers of phagocytes, particularly neutrophils (**severe congenital neutropenias**), result in a variety of recurrent and severe bacterial infections beginning early in life. The underlying mutation causing this disease is unknown. Cells of the entire myeloid series fail to mature, which may indicate a defect in receptors for cytokines or other factors or in intracellular signaling pathways from those receptors. A milder form, **cyclic neutropenia,** is autosomal dominant and arises from a mutation in the neutrophil elastase gene (ELA2). Neutrophil levels are cyclic and may remain at or near normal for 2 to 3 weeks, followed by periods of neutropenia lasting a few days to weeks. During the neutropenia, the individual has increased susceptibility to recurrent bacterial infections.

Near sites of inflammation, soluble mediators diffuse into the circulation and induce expression of a variety of adhesion molecules on the phagocyte surface. These interact with complementary molecules on the endothelial cells to increase adherence between the phagocyte and the vessel wall and allow for margination and diapedesis to occur. **Leukocyte adhesion deficiencies (LAD)** result from mutations in various phagocyte adhesion molecules (see Table 6-4). Leukocyte adhesion deficiency, type 1 (LAD-1) results from an autosomal recessive mutation in CD18, which is a β_2 integrin chain that is shared by several different receptors. LAD-2 results from a defect in adding the monosaccharide fucose to carbohydrates on the phagocyte surface. Surface carbohydrates with fucose are ligands for selectins on the endothelial and leukocyte. These and other defects in leukocyte adhesion molecules usually result in increased levels of neutrophils in the blood (leukocytosis) because they cannot leave the circulation and in recurrent bacterial and fungal infections.

Additional deficiencies diminish the leukocyte's recognition of opsonins of the complement cascade. C3b serves as an opsonin by interacting with complement receptors on phagocytes. Deficiencies in the complement receptor for C3 (**C3 receptor deficiency**) result in recurrent bacterial infections, particularly of the skin.

A variety of defects in killing of microorganisms have been described. **Chédiak-Higashi syndrome** results from a defect in cytoplasmic granules from an autosomal recessive muta-

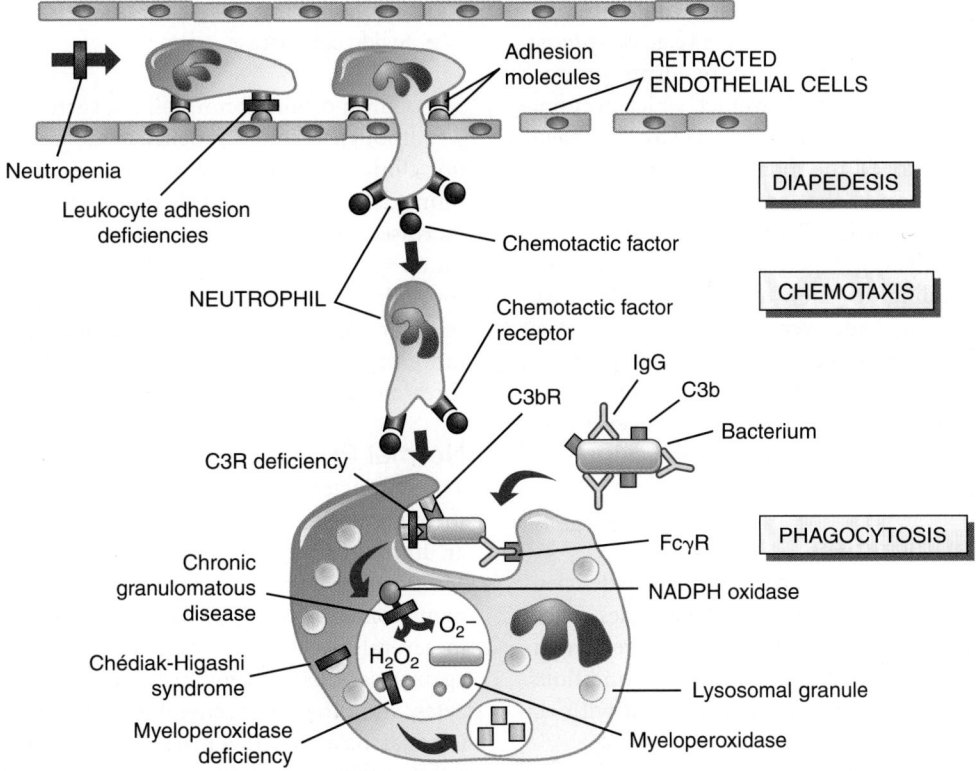

Figure 8-16 Phagocytic defects. Several genetic defects in the process leading up to and including phagocytosis result in increased susceptibility to bacterial infections. See the text and refer to Figures 6-12 through 6-14 and Table 6-4 for more detailed information. The phagocyte leaves the blood stream and enters the tissue through interactions between leukocyte and endothelial adhesion molecules and the process of diapedesis. The cell is attracted to the inflammatory site by chemotaxis, where it encounters opsonized bacteria, and attaches to and engulfs the microorganism. Inside the phagocyte, the bacteria is killed and broken down by the combination of lysosomal granule constituents and reactive oxygen products of the hexose-monophosphate shunt and nicotinamide adenine dinucleotide phosphate (NADPH) oxidase. *C3R,* C3 receptor, which includes the C3b receptor (C3bR); *FcγR,* receptor for the Fc portion of IgG; H_2O_2, hydrogen peroxide; O_2^-, reactive oxygen.

tion in the lysosomal trafficking regulator gene *(CHS1).* The CHS1 protein helps control movement of granules to cellular membranes in preparation for degranulation. As a result of these mutations, the granules remain in the cytoplasm and form large aggregates that are readily apparent microscopically. Leukocytes from individuals with Chédiak-Higashi syndrome have decreased chemotaxis, granular fusion, and bacterial killing. Platelet granules also may be affected resulting in prolonged bleeding, and partial albinism can occur because of defects in melanocyte granules. Affected children develop recurrent infections of the skin, respiratory tract, and mucous membranes, especially with gram-positive bacteria.

The enzyme myeloperoxidase participates in a major mechanism of bacterial killing in phagocytes. Myeloperoxidase is found in primary granules and catalyzes the formation of acids from halides (e.g., chloride ion) and hydrogen peroxide (H_2O_2). As a result of phagocytosis, neutrophils and other phagocytes switch much of their glucose metabolism to the hexose-monophosphate shunt. A byproduct of this pathway is the conversion of molecular oxygen by nicotinamide adenine dinucleotide phosphate (NADPH) oxidase and other enzymes into highly reactive and toxic oxygen derivatives, including hydrogen peroxide. Two deficiencies in the myeloperoxidase–

hydrogen peroxide killing process have been extensively studied. **Myeloperoxidase deficiency** is a relatively mild disorder characterized by a complete or partial deficiency in myeloperoxidase. Individuals do not have severe recurrent infections because most infectious bacteria are sensitive to direct killing by many of the toxic oxygen molecules produced by NADPH oxidase. The exception is the person with concurrent diabetes, who may have recurrent disseminated candidiasis.

Chronic granulomatous disease (CGD) is a more severe defect in the myeloperoxidase-hydrogen peroxide system. Several forms of the disease have been characterized, both X-linked (about 70% of the individuals) and autosomal recessive, with the X-linked being the more severe. CGD results from a variety of mutations (at least four have been identified) in portions of the NADPH oxidase complex, resulting in deficiencies in the production of hydrogen peroxide and other oxygen products. Thus individuals have adequate myeloperoxidase and chloride but lack the necessary hydrogen peroxide. Individuals with CGD have recurrent severe pneumonias, tumor-like granulomas in lungs, skin, and bones, and other infections with some normal, relatively innocuous microorganisms, such as *Staphylococcus aureus, Serratia marcescens, Aspergillus spp.,* and others. These are catalase-positive microorganisms. Infections with more virulent, but catalase-negative, microorganisms (e.g., *Streptococcus pneumoniae*) are rare. Most microorganisms produce their own hydrogen peroxide as a byproduct, which accumulates in the phagocytic vacuole and can be used by the phagocyte's myeloperoxidase to kill the microorganism. Some microorganisms also produce the enzyme catalase, which breaks down hydrogen peroxide. Thus catalase-negative microorganisms donate hydrogen peroxide to the phagocyte's myeloperoxidase, leading to their own death. Catalase-positive microorganisms, however, destroy the bacterial hydrogen peroxide, but are killed if the phagocyte produces adequate levels of hydrogen peroxide for use by the myeloperoxidase. In CGD, the phagocyte's hydrogen peroxide is missing, and the catalase-positive microorganisms survive and cause infection.

Secondary Deficiencies

Secondary, or acquired, immune and inflammatory deficiencies are far more common than primary deficiencies. These deficiencies are not related to genetic defects, but are complications of other physiologic or pathophysiologic conditions. Some conditions that are known to be associated with acquired deficiencies include:

Normal physiologic conditions
- Pregnancy
- Infancy
- Aging

Psychologic stress
- Emotional trauma
- Eating disorders

Dietary insufficiencies
- Malnutrition caused by insufficient intake of large categories of nutrients, such as protein or calories
- Insufficient intake of specific nutrients, such as vitamins, iron, or zinc

Infections
- Congenital infections, such as rubella, cytomegalovirus, hepatitis B
- Acquired infections, such as AIDS

Malignancies
- Malignancies of lymphoid tissues, such as Hodgkin disease, acute or chronic leukemia, or myeloma
- Malignancies of nonlymphoid tissues, such as sarcomas and carcinomas

Physical trauma
- Burns

Medical treatments
- Stress caused by surgery
- Anesthesia
- Immunosuppressive treatment with corticosteroids or antilymphocyte antibodies
- Splenectomy
- Cancer treatment with cytotoxic drugs or ionizing radiation

Other diseases or genetic syndromes
- Diabetes
- Alcoholic cirrhosis
- Sickle cell disease
- SLE
- Chromosome abnormalities, such as Down syndrome

Although secondary deficiencies are common, many are not clinically relevant. In many cases, the degree of the immune deficiency is relatively minor and without any apparent increased susceptibility to infection. Alternatively, the immune system may be substantially suppressed, but only for a short duration, thus minimizing the incidence of clinically relevant infections. Some secondary immune deficiencies, however, are extremely severe and may result in recurrent life-threatening infections.

Normal Physiologic Conditions

The competence of an individual's immune system varies throughout life. Pregnancy itself is considered by many to be an immunocompromised condition (see What's New? box: Maternal Microchimerism and Autoimmune Disease). Pregnant women may have decreased reactivity or altered results in several tests of the immune system, including skin tests against various antigens, circulating numbers of T lymphocytes, and other very general tests. Pregnancy itself, however, is not associated with a marked change in infections, suggesting that the mother's immune system is not severely altered.

The newborn child is immunologically immature. Although T-cell immune responses may be normal or near normal, other components of the immune system (especially antibody production) are just beginning to mature. During pregnancy, the placenta has transported maternal antibodies into the fetal blood to protect the child during the first months of life (see Figure 7-28). After the delivery, the level of the mother's antibodies slowly decreases in the newborn so that maternal antibodies no longer protect the child by about 6 months of life. By 6 to 8 months, the newborn is efficiently protected by antibodies produced by its own B cells. In some infants, the development of antibody production is delayed, and a transient low level of antibody may persist for several months (**transient hypogammaglobulinemia of infancy**), during which the child has increased susceptibility to infections.

Aging is also associated with a progressive depression in immune responses.[43,44] The elderly generally have more severe bacterial and fungal infections, greater difficulty resolving those infections, and lower responses to vaccination. Several meaningful changes occur during aging, although variations in the degree of change and a corresponding increased susceptibility to infection can be considerable among individuals. The thymus involutes over time, resulting in decreased production of fresh T cells. A concurrent depletion of memory T cells results in depressed responses to both new and "recall" antigens. A shift towards Th2 cells also may occur with a resultant decrease in Th1 cytokines. Total numbers of B cells may decrease. Numbers of NK cells may remain normal, although their activity is decreased. Similarly, neutrophil numbers may remain normal, with decreased phagocytosis and killing.

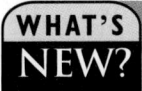

WHAT'S NEW? Maternal Microchimerism and Autoimmune Disease

Half of the genes of a child are from its father. Therefore, fetal cells express antigens that are foreign to the mother. The placenta was once considered an immunologic "barrier" that protected the fetus from the mother's immune rejection. New understandings, however, reveal the barrier is porous. Both maternal and fetal cells routinely cross the placenta so that fetal cells can be found in the mother's blood, and maternal cells can be found in the child's blood. The possible long-term implications of that exchange have only recently been described. It now seems that the child's cells can take up long-term residence in the mother's tissues and develop a state of **microchimerism** (mixing of cells of different origins).

Microchimerism is documented usually by the presence of male (Y-chromosome) DNA or male cells in the mother's blood or tissues. Using fluorescent probes that are specific for markers on the X or Y chromosome, male cells can be detected in the woman's blood and tissues for decades after the woman's last pregnancy with a male child.[37] Maternal cells also cross the placenta and can persist in the child into adulthood.[38] Because the techniques used in these studies differentiate between cells with or without the Y chromosome, there is no clear information on the degree of microchimerism resulting from carrying a female child.

Increased amounts of male DNA or cells is linked to several autoimmune diseases, such as scleroderma, dermatomyositis, Sjögren's syndrome, thyroiditis, primary biliary cirrhosis, and systemic lupus erythematosus. Healthy individuals have low levels of fetal microchimerism. In a study of systemic sclerosis, the level of male DNA in the circulation was much higher in patients with sclerosis than in healthy controls.[39] Elevated levels of male DNA was also found in skin lesions in patients with this disease.[40]

Maternal microchimerism in the offspring also may increase their risk for autoimmune disease. Increased levels of maternal cells in the child's blood have been reported in cases of juvenile inflammatory myopathy and neonatal lupus syndrome.[41]

Both maternal and fetal microchimerism involve lymphocytes and other cells. Several cell types have been detected, including liver cells, epithelial cells, lymphocytes, and others.[42] Many of these cell types may originate from stem cells that cross the placenta, take up residence in various organs, and differentiate into cells characteristic of that organ.

The primary question is the significance of microchimerism. To date, increased indications of microchimerism have been associated with autoimmune disease in the mother and the child. However, it cannot yet be determined whether the foreign cells are initiators of autoimmune damage or whether injury to the tissue results in their increased proliferation. Thus these observations remain intriguing, but of unknown significance.

Psychologic Stress

The relationship between emotional stress and depressed immune function has become an area of intense clinical and research interest.[45] For many decades anecdotal reports have suggested that increased incidence of infection and malignancy are associated with periods of both intense stress (e.g., the loss of a loved one, divorce) and relatively minor stress (e.g., final examination periods at colleges and universities). In addition, early studies showed that immune function, as demonstrated by delayed hypersensitivity skin test results, could be depressed through posthypnotic suggestion.

We are now beginning to understand the mechanisms of the relationship between emotional stress and the immune system. Many lymphoid organs are innervated and can be affected by nerve stimulation. In addition, lymphocytes have receptors for many hormones (e.g., sex hormones, neurotransmitters, and neuropeptides) and can respond to changing levels of these chemicals with increased or decreased function. For instance, stress-induced catecholamines affect the expression of adhesion molecules and movement of lymphocytes among lymphoid organs. (Further discussion of the effects of stress on susceptibility to disease is the subject of Chapter 10.)

Dietary Insufficiencies

Nutritional status can have a profound effect on immune function. Severe deficits in calorie or protein intake lead to deficiencies in T-cell function and numbers. The humoral immune response is less affected by starvation, although complement activity, neutrophil chemotaxis, and bacterial killing within neutrophils often are depressed, resulting in infections with microorganisms that are normally disabled by opsonization and phagocytosis.

Deficient zinc intake can profoundly depress both T- and B-cell function. Zinc is required as a cofactor for at least 70 different enzymes, some of which are found in lymphocytes and are necessary for their function. Secondary zinc deficiencies may be associated with malabsorption syndrome (failure to absorb zinc), chronic renal disease (loss of zinc in the urine), chronic diarrhea (loss of zinc through the gut), or burns or severe psoriasis (loss of zinc through the skin). Deficiencies of other enzyme cofactors, such as vitamins (e.g., pyridoxine, pantothenic acid, folic acid, vitamins A, C, E, and B_{12}), also may result in severe depressions of B- and T-cell function, phagocytosis, and complement activity.

Malignancies

A very close relationship exists between the immune system and the development of malignancies. It is generally accepted that successful malignancies have developed mechanisms that make it possible for them to avoid rejection by the individual's immune system. Persons with primary immune deficiencies are usually at greater risk for developing malignancies, particularly malignancies of lymphoid tissues, such as leukemias or lymphomas. In those with healthy immune systems, malignancies aggressively depress the individual's immune system. The effect is commonly nonspecific, resulting in a generalized deficiency of the immune response and a greatly increased susceptibility to developing life-threatening infections. In fact, many people with malignancies die from infection rather than from direct effects of the tumor.

Malignancies of lymphoid tissues, such as Hodgkin disease, acute or chronic leukemia, or myeloma, result in depletion of normal lymphocytes and their replacement by the malignant cells. Thus the number of B or T cells capable of responding to infections is depleted. Many malignancies, even those of nonlymphoid tissues, produce cytokines (e.g., transforming growth factor–β [TGFβ], vascular endothelial growth factor [VEGF]) that nonspecifically suppress the immune responses.

Physical Trauma

Burn victims are susceptible to severe bacterial infections. Thermal burns appear to be associated with decreased neutrophil function (especially chemotaxis), decreased complement levels, decreased cell-mediated immunity, and decreased primary humoral responses, although secondary humoral responses are normal. The mechanism of this immunosuppression may be twofold. Blood from burned individuals contains nonspecific immunosuppressive factors (all immune responses are suppressed, regardless of the antigen involved). In addition, burn victims also have increased regulatory T-cell function, which may increase antigen-specific suppression.

Medical Treatments

Medical treatments themselves may produce suppression of immune responses. Depression of B- and T-cell formation is manifested as a progressive increase in infections with opportunistic microorganisms (especially *P. carinii*, cytomegalovirus, *C. albicans*, and other fungi), the extent and location of which are unusual.

Many drugs that are used to fight cancer (e.g., cancer chemotherapeutic agents) are not specific for cancer cells, but are designed to attack cells in susceptible stages in their cell cycles or rapidly proliferating cells, which includes cells of the immune system as well as malignant cells. The immunosuppressive effects of chemotherapeutic drugs are exacerbated by concurrent treatment with ionizing radiation (x rays), which also affect cells that are rapidly making new DNA. Therefore, the person's immune response can be profoundly depressed as a result of the therapy. Other drugs, such as corticosteroids, are intentionally used to suppress the immune system and control hypersensitivity diseases (especially autoimmune disease) or prevent rejection of transplants. Because of their nonspecific activity, however, immune responses against infectious agents also can be suppressed, increasing the individual's susceptibility to infection. The list of drugs that affect the immune response is ever increasing and includes analgesics, antithyroid medications, anticonvulsants, antihistamines, antimicrobial agents, antilymphocyte antibodies, and tranquilizers.

Surgery and anesthesia also can suppress both T- and B-cell function. Transient, severe lymphopenia is a common postoperative condition that can last as long as 1 month. Surgery to remove the spleen (splenectomy) can result in a depressed humoral response against encapsulated bacteria (especially *S. pneumoniae, H. influenzae, S. aureus,* the group A streptococci, and *N. meningitidis*), depressed serum IgM levels, and decreased levels of opsonins.

Infections

Many infectious microorganisms are successful at invading the human body because they have evolved mechanisms for fighting off specific immune/inflammatory responses against themselves. However, some infectious agents (e.g., HIV, Epstein-Barr virus [EBV], cytomegalovirus [CMV], herpes simplex virus type 6) can generally suppress the immune response. HIV is one of the few microorganisms that directly attacks the central processes involved in the development of an immune response. It infects and destroys the helper T cell, which is necessary to provide help for the maturation of both plasma cells and cytotoxic T cells. Therefore HIV suppresses the immune response against itself and, secondarily, creates a generalized immune deficiency by suppressing the development of immune responses against other pathogens and opportunistic microorganisms (see p. 285).

Several viruses (e.g., hepatitis B, rubella, CMV) can establish congenital infections through transmission from an infected mother to her child at birth when the child's immune system is immature. These children may have suppressed immune responses, although the degree of the deficiency is not usually severe.

Acquired Immunodeficiency Syndrome (AIDS)

The most notable form of secondary or acquired immune deficiency caused by an infection is **acquired immunodeficiency syndrome (AIDS)**. AIDS is a viral disease caused by the human immunodeficiency virus (HIV). HIV infects and depletes a portion of the immune system (Th cells), making individuals extremely susceptible to life-threatening infections and malignancies.

Despite major efforts by healthcare agencies around the world, the number of cases and deaths from HIV infection and AIDS (HIV/AIDS) continues to increase rapidly. According to a 2004 report by the United Nations (UNAIDS) and World Health Organization (WHO), the number of people living with HIV/AIDS worldwide is estimated at 40 million, of which 2.5 million are under the age of 15.[46] The rate of spread of the disease is still out of control: the number of people newly infected with HIV in 2003 is estimated at 5 million, with 700,000 being under the age of 15. Deaths from AIDS in 2003 alone were about 3 million, of which 500,000 were under 15. Since the end of 1998, an estimated 13 million people have died of HIV/AIDS.

The majority of cases are still in sub-Saharan Africa, but the epidemic is worldwide, and the number of new cases is increasing rapidly, particularly in Asia. As an example of the prevalence of HIV/AIDS, in the African country of Zambia it is estimated that 30% of the women age 30 to 34 years are HIV infected. In South Africa, about 35% of the pregnant women age 25 to 29 are HIV infected.

In the United States, the spread of HIV/AIDS remains somewhat stable. The Centers for Disease Control and Prevention (CDC) surveillance report for 2003 estimates that since the year 2000 the rate of new cases of HIV/AIDS has remained at about 31,000 per year.[47] The number of new cases in children under the age of 13 has dropped dramatically from 952 in 1992 to 59 in 2003. The number of deaths related to HIV/AIDS continues at about 18,000 per year (Figure 8-17). The total number of HIV/AIDS-related deaths in the United States through 2003 is 524,060, and more than 400,000 individuals are currently living with AIDS.

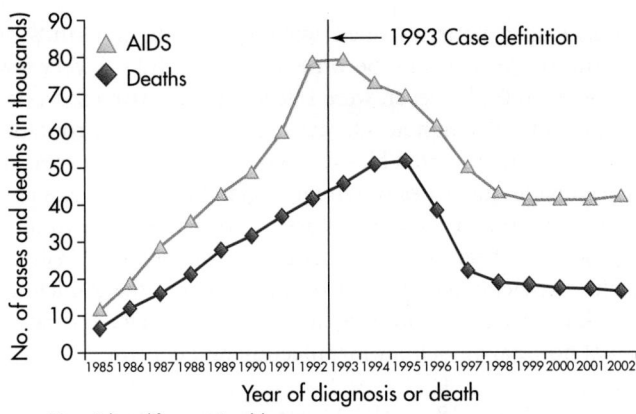

Figure 8-17 Estimated incidence of AIDS and deaths among adults and adolescents with AIDS in the United States (1985-2002). The incidence of acquired immune deficiency syndrome (AIDS) and deaths related to AIDS rose almost linearly until about 1994. The introduction of highly active antiviral therapy (HAART) antiviral protocols in the mid-1990s slowed the progression of the disease from HIV infection to AIDS and has maintained the number of AIDS-related deaths at about 18,000 per year. *HAART,* Highly active antiviral therapy. (Redrawn from Centers for Disease Control website, 2005. Available at www.cdc.gov/nchstp/od/nchstp.html.)

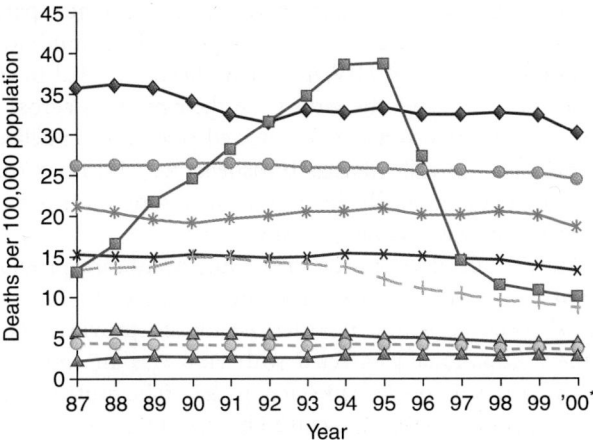

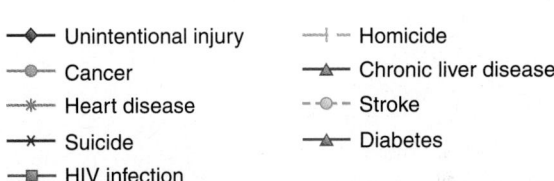

Figure 8-18 Trends in annual rates of leading causes of death among persons 25 to 44 years old in the United States (1987-2000). In 1995, HIV/AIDS caused about 20% of deaths in this age group. After implementation of HAART protocols, HIV/AIDS-related deaths dropped to 6% of the total in 2000. Of all HIV/AIDS-related deaths, 70% occurred in the 25 to 44 age group. In males, HIV/AIDS was the leading cause of death from 1992 through 1995 (24% of total) (data not shown). In women, HIV/AIDS was at most the third leading cause (1995) behind cancer and unintentional injury (11% of total), but dropped to 5% in 2000 (data not shown). *HIV/AIDS,* Human immunodeficiency virus/acquired immune deficiency syndrome; *HAART,* highly active antiviral therapy. (Redrawn from Centers for Disease Control website, 2005. Available at www.cdc.gov/nchstp/od/nchstp.html.)

Before the implementation of massive public health campaigns and the use of antiviral drugs in the United States, the progression from HIV infection to AIDS and death was unrelenting. In 1995, AIDS became the number one killer of individuals between the ages of 25 and 44 years of age (Figure 8-18). With the advent of effective therapy in the mid 1990s, HIV infection has become a chronic disease in the United States, with many fewer deaths.

The origins of HIV and AIDS remain uncertain. The best evidence suggests that HIV arose from a simian immunodeficiency virus (SIV) and was transmitted to humans from chimpanzees or other primates, which are routinely kept as pets or used as food in parts of Africa. Based on comparative genetic sequencing, the main variant of HIV (the M group) began diversifying in about 1931 and produced the large number of viral variants we observe today.[48] The earliest documented case of HIV infection in humans was obtained from testing a serum sample that was stored in 1959 in Democratic Republic of Congo. The disease drew attention in the United States following two reports from the CDC on young, homosexual men who were dying of unusual infections and cancers.

EPIDEMIOLOGY HIV is a blood-borne pathogen with the typical routes of transmission: blood or blood products, intravenous drug abuse, both heterosexual and homosexual activity, and maternal-child transmission before or during birth. Although the disease first gained attention in the United States as being related to sexual transmission between males, the most common route worldwide is through heterosexual activity, which is becoming the trend in the United States (Figure 8-19). Worldwide, women make up more than half of those living with HIV/AIDS. In the United States, as in the rest of the world, the predominant means of transmission is through heterosexual contact (Figure 8-20), and the incidence

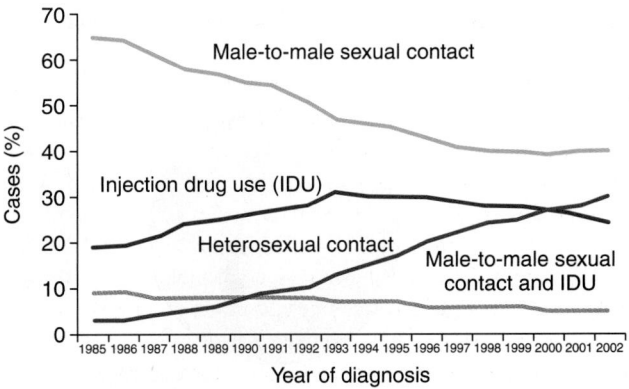

Figure 8-19 Proportion of AIDS cases among adults and adolescents, by exposure category and year of diagnosis, in the United States (1985-2002). Worldwide, acquired immune deficiency syndrome (AIDS) is primarily spread by heterosexual transmission. In the United States, the predominant route was by male-to-male sexual contact. The trend, however, is towards increasing heterosexual transmission. Transmission by injected drug use has remained relatively stable. (Redrawn from Centers for Disease Control website, 2005. Available at www.cdc.gov/nchstp/od/nchstp.html.)

of HIV/AIDS is increasing faster in women than men, particularly in the adolescent age groups (Figure 8-21). Hundreds of thousands of cases of HIV/AIDS have been reported in children who contracted the virus from their mothers across the placenta, through contact with infected blood during delivery, or through the milk during breastfeeding.[49] Without treatment, symptoms usually develop within 6 months of life, and life expectancy is generally less than 3 years.

As with all blood-borne infections, healthcare providers are at increased risk of contracting the infection from patients' blood. The first reported healthcare provider to become occupationally infected with HIV was an emergency room nurse who became infected in 1986. The route of infection was probably through cuts in her hand that came in contact with contaminated blood through a gauze pad she was

holding on a patient's open wound. Tens of thousands of healthcare workers have become infected with HIV. Very few (less than 100), however, were infected while caring for a patient, mostly through accidental sticks with needles containing virus-contaminated blood or exposure of broken areas of skin to large quantities of contaminated blood.[50] Nurses and clinical laboratory technicians are by far the most commonly exposed healthcare workers. Because of the potential risk, all healthcare personnel should routinely follow the guidelines for Universal Precautions published by the CDC and additional hospital guidelines for infection and control.[50]

PATHOGENESIS   HIV-1 was initially isolated by researchers at the Pasteur Institute as the lymphadenopathy/AIDS virus (LAV).[51] A second major variant, HIV-2, was identified later. Viruses in general are very simple microorganisms consisting of nucleic acid (the viral genome) protected from the environment by a layer or layers of proteins. They are sensitive to many environmental factors and cannot survive for long outside a cell. Viruses usually have surface molecules that act as receptors for molecules found on the surface of target cells. The specificity of the receptors provides a degree of tropism so that most viruses infect selected target cells, which determines the symptoms of that particular infection. For instance, viruses that cause upper respiratory tract infections are generally tropic for respiratory epithelial cells. A virus will attach to the target cell, insert its genome into the cell, utilize the cell's protein synthesizing capacity to translate viral proteins, increase the number of copies of its genome, and package the viral proteins and nucleic acid into new viral particles (virions) that are then released from the cell in order to infect other cells.

A large diversity of differences occurs among viruses. HIV is a member of a family of viruses called *retroviruses,* which carry genetic information in the form of RNA rather than DNA (Figure 8-22). Retroviruses use a viral enzyme, **reverse transcriptase,** to convert RNA into double-stranded DNA (Figure 8-23). Using a second viral enzyme, an **integrase,** the new DNA is inserted into the infected cell's genetic material,

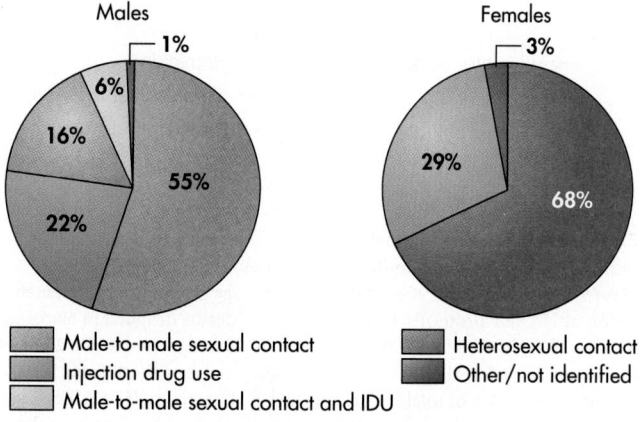

Figure 8-20 Proportion of AIDS cases diagnosed in 2002 among adults and adolescents in the United States, by gender and exposure category. In the most recent data, about half of the new cases of acquired immune deficiency syndrome (AIDS) in males were contracted by male-to-male sexual contact, whereas about 16% were contracted by heterosexual contact. In females newly diagnosed with AIDS, two thirds were infected by heterosexual contact. *IDU,* Injection drug use. (Redrawn from Centers for Disease Control web site, 2005. Available at www.cdc.gov/nchstp/od/nchstp.html.)

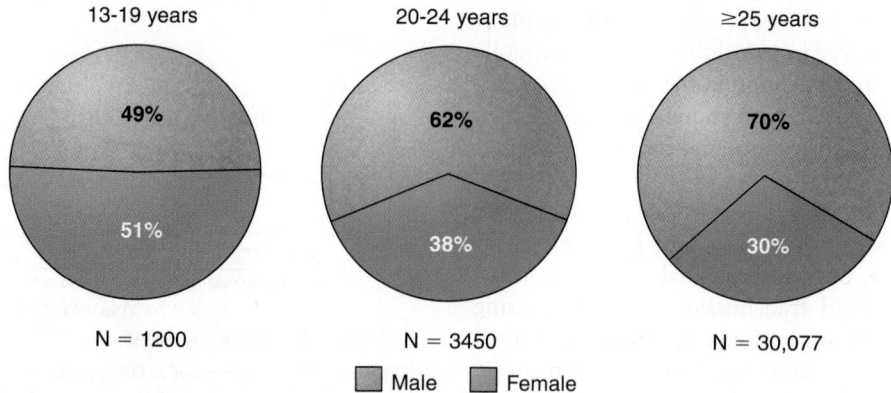

Figure 8-21 Proportion of cases of HIV infection (not AIDS) reported in 2002 among adults and adolescents in the United States, by gender and age group. The route of contracting human immunodeficiency virus (HIV) infection varies among age groups. These data illustrate the evolution of HIV infection in the United States from a preponderance of males who were infected by male-to-male sexual contact to equal incidence of males and females who were infected by heterosexual contact. *AIDS,* acquired immune deficiency syndrome. (Redrawn from Centers for Disease Control website, 2005. Available at www.cdc.gov/nchstp/od/nchstp.html.)

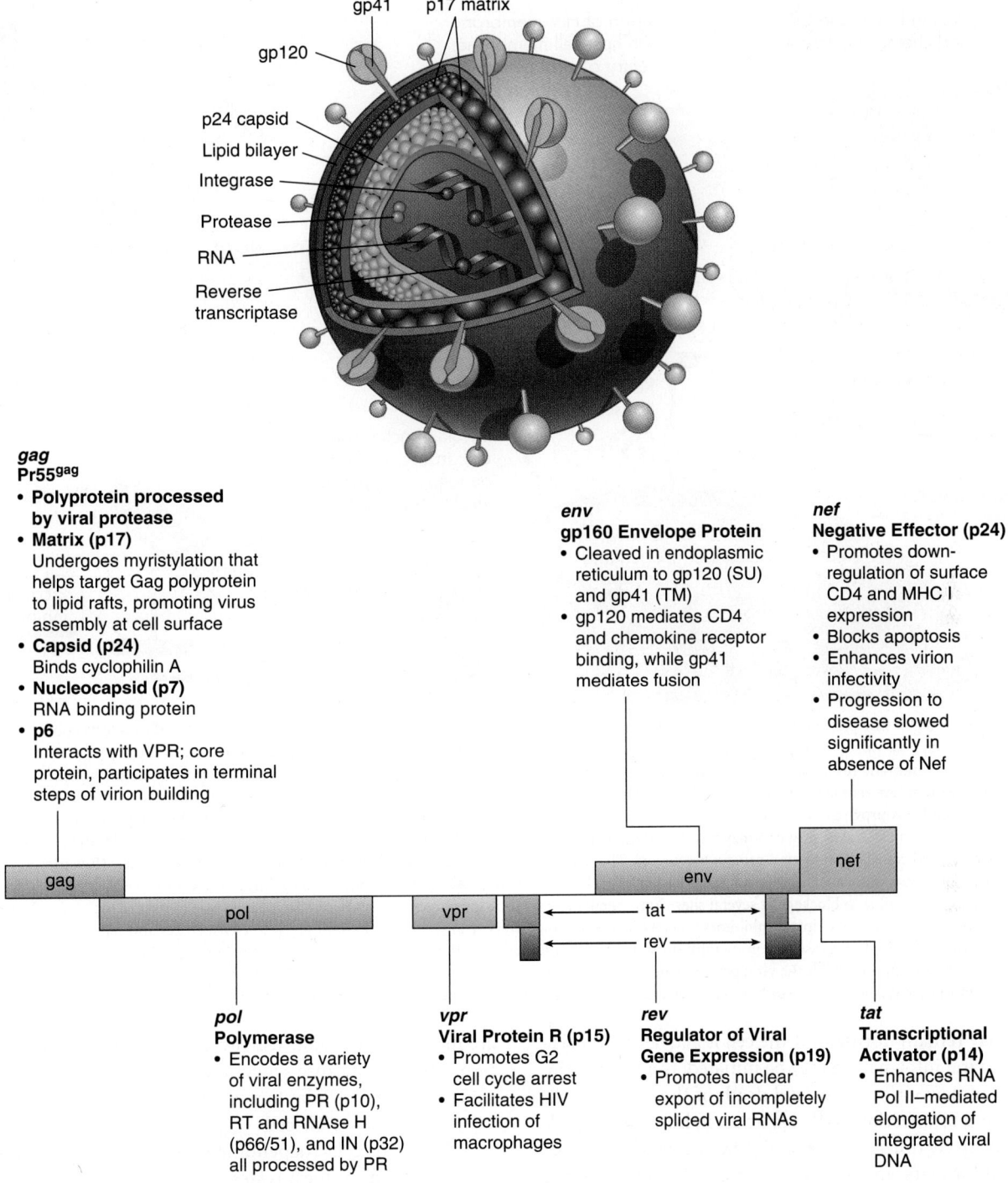

gag
Pr55^gag

- **Polyprotein processed by viral protease**
- **Matrix (p17)**
  Undergoes myristylation that helps target Gag polyprotein to lipid rafts, promoting virus assembly at cell surface
- **Capsid (p24)**
  Binds cyclophilin A
- **Nucleocapsid (p7)**
  RNA binding protein
- **p6**
  Interacts with VPR; core protein, participates in terminal steps of virion building

env
gp160 Envelope Protein
- Cleaved in endoplasmic reticulum to gp120 (SU) and gp41 (TM)
- gp120 mediates CD4 and chemokine receptor binding, while gp41 mediates fusion

nef
Negative Effector (p24)
- Promotes down-regulation of surface CD4 and MHC I expression
- Blocks apoptosis
- Enhances virion infectivity
- Progression to disease slowed significantly in absence of Nef

pol
Polymerase
- Encodes a variety of viral enzymes, including PR (p10), RT and RNAse H (p66/51), and IN (p32) all processed by PR

vpr
Viral Protein R (p15)
- Promotes G2 cell cycle arrest
- Facilitates HIV infection of macrophages

rev
Regulator of Viral Gene Expression (p19)
- Promotes nuclear export of incompletely spliced viral RNAs

tat
Transcriptional Activator (p14)
- Enhances RNA Pol II–mediated elongation of integrated viral DNA

Figure 8-22 The structure and genetic map of HIV-1. The human immunodeficiency virus-1 (HIV-1) virion consists of a core of two identical strands of viral ribonucleic acid (RNA) molecules of viral enzymes (reverse transcriptase [RT], protease [PR], integrase [IN]), encoated in a core capsid structure consisting primarily of the structural viral protein p24. The capsid is further encased in a matrix consisting primarily of a viral protein, p17. The outer surface is an envelope consisting of the plasma membrane of the cell from which the virus budded (lipid bilayer) and two viral glycoproteins: a transmembrane gp41 and a noncovalently attached surface protein, gp120. The HIV-1 genome contains regions that encode the structural proteins *(gag)*, the viral enzymes *(pol)*, and the envelope proteins *(env)*. The *gag* region is translated into a large precursor (Pr55^gag) that is cut by the HIV protease into smaller proteins that construct the capsid and matrix. The *env* region is translated into a gp160 precursor protein that is cut by a host-cell protease into the gp120 and gp41 envelope proteins. The genome of complex retroviruses, like HIV-1, often contain a variety of small regions that regulate expression of the virus. (Modified from Kumar V, Abbas A, Fausto N: *Robbins and Cotran pathologic basis of disease,* ed 7, Philadelphia, 2005, Saunders.)

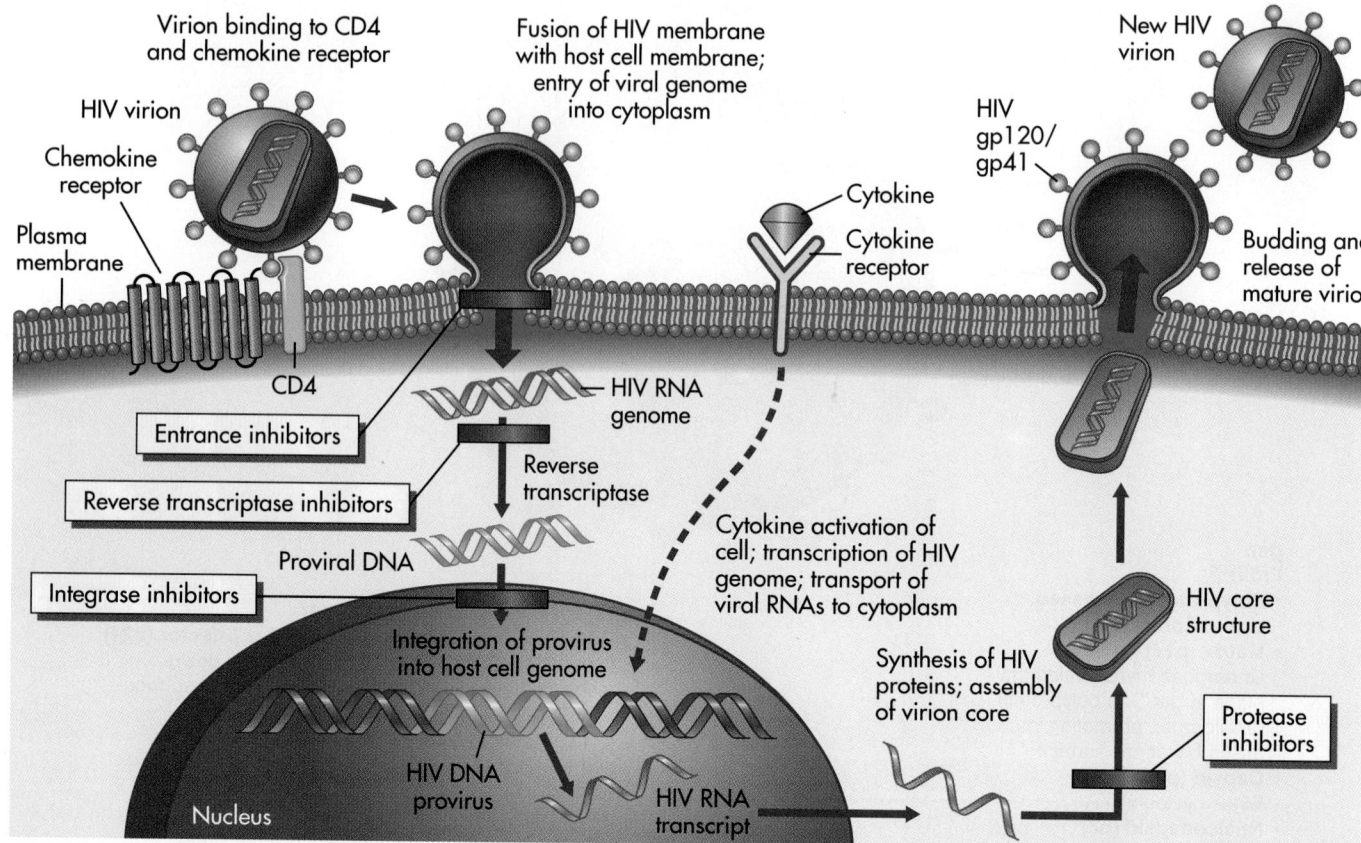

Figure 8-23 Life cycle and possible sites of therapeutic intervention of HIV-1. Human immunodeficiency virus (HIV) infection begins when a virion, or virus particle, binds to CD4 and chemokine co-receptors on a susceptible cell, and the viral envelope and the plasma membrane fuse, and the core of the virus is injected into the cytoplasm. Uncoating occurs in the cytoplasm, during which the core proteins are removed, and the viral RNA is released into the infected cell's cytoplasm. The viral RNA is converted to a double-stranded DNA provirus by the action of the viral reverse transcriptase. The provirus migrates into the nucleus and is integrated into the cell's own DNA. The provirus may remain latent. If the infected cell is activated (e.g., by cytokines), the provirus may be transcribed and translated into viral protein precursors. The precursor proteins are modified by viral (Gag proteins) and cellular (Env proteins) proteases into smaller proteins that are used to package the viral RNA into new virions that bud from the cell. The HIV-1 life cycle is susceptible to blockage at several sites. Some agents could block the attachment and entrance of the virus (entrance inhibitors). Reverse transcriptase inhibitors (e.g., AZT) prevent the reverse transcription of viral RNA into DNA. Drugs also may be able to inhibit the viral integrase (integrase inhibitors) and prevent insertion of the provirus into the host's chromosomes. Protease inhibitors specifically inhibit the viral protease and prevent the processing of the gp160 into viral capsid and matrix proteins. (Modified from Kumar V, Abbas A, Fausto N: *Robbins and Cotran pathologic basis of disease,* ed 7, Philadelphia, 2005, Saunders.)

where it may remain dormant. If the cell is activated, translation of the viral information may be initiated, resulting in the formation of new virions, lysis and death of the infected cell, and shedding of infectious HIV particles. If, however, the cell remains relatively dormant, the viral genetic material may remain latent for years, and is probably present for the life of the individual.[52]

The primary surface receptor on HIV is the envelope protein gp120, which binds to the molecule CD4, found primarily on the surface of helper T cells (Figure 8-24). Several other necessary co-receptors have been identified on the target cells, particularly the chemokine receptors CXCR4 and CCR5. Different strains of HIV-1 are selective for the CXCR4 or CCR5 co-receptors, which influences the tropism for different target cells. Strains that prefer the CXCR4 co-receptor tend to be T-cell tropic, usually found later in an infection, and cause infected cells to fuse and form a multinucleate **syncytium.** Strains that react better with the co-receptor CCR5

are macrophage-tropic, usually cause the primary HIV infection, and do not cause syncytium formation.

The primary cellular targets for HIV include the following:
- CD4-positive Th-cells
- Dendritic cells (depending on the level of chemokine receptors the cell expresses)
- Macrophages (express low levels of CD4, but high amounts of heparin sulfate proteoglycans [syndecan] and other molecules that bind to gp120 and adsorbs HIV)
- CD8-positive Tc cells (low rate of infection, but CD4 can be expressed by activated CD8-cells)
- Double positive thymic cells (express both CD4 and CD8 simultaneously)
- NK cells (some are CD4+, CCR5+)
- Neural cells of monocyte origin (macrophages and microglial cells)

Initially, the lymphoid areas of the mucosal surfaces are the primary sites of infection[53] (Figure 8-25). Dendritic cells and

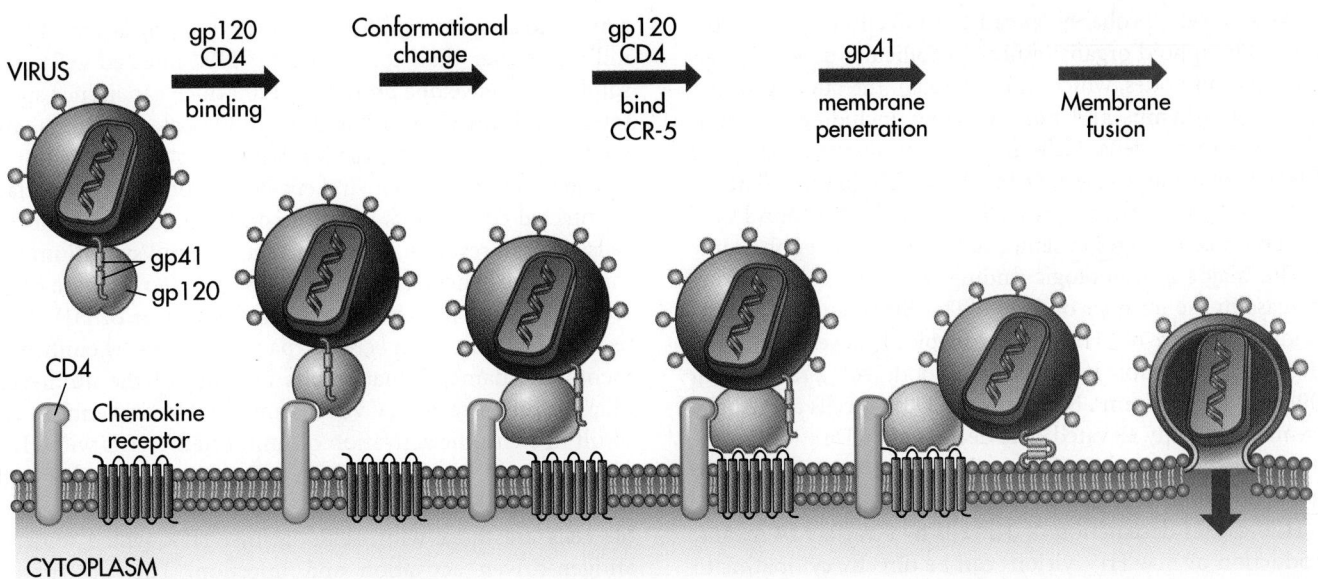

Figure 8-24 **Mechanism of HIV entry into host cells.** Interactions with CD4 and the CCR5 co-receptor are illustrated. (Original art from Wain-Hobson S: HIV: one on one meets two, *Nature* 384:117, 1996. Copyright 1996, Macmillam Magazines Limited. Redrawn from adapted figure in Kumar V, Abbas A, Fausto N: *Robbins and Cotran pathologic basis of disease,* ed 7, Philadelphia, 2005, Saunders.)

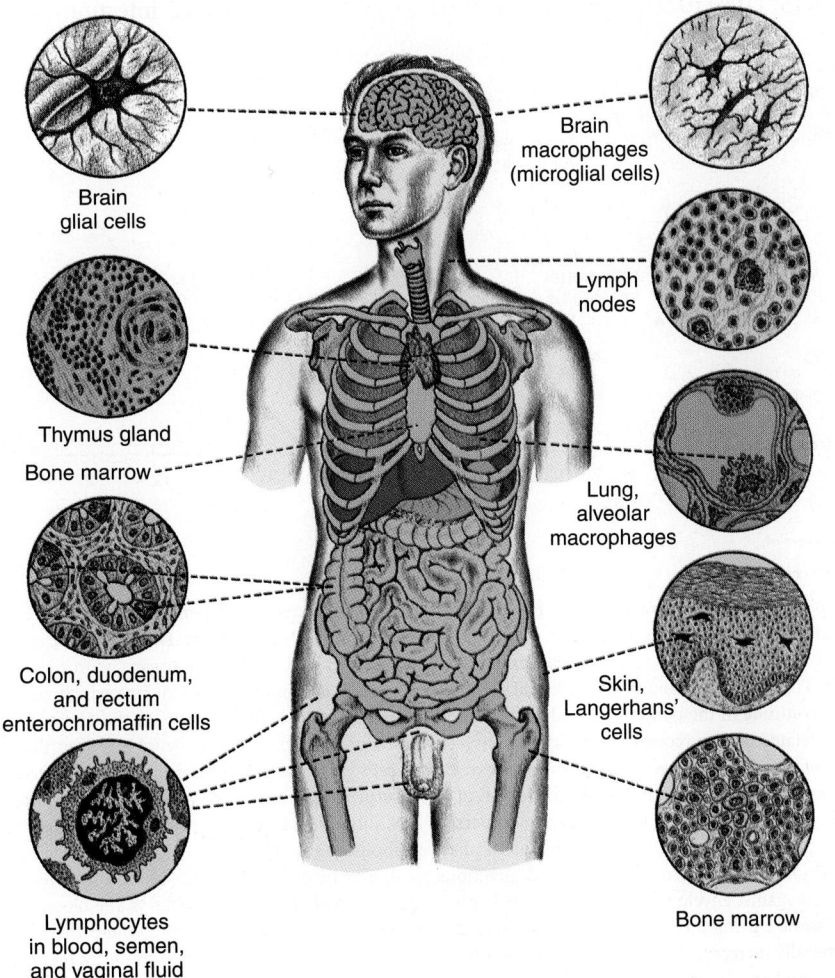

Figure 8-25 **Distribution of tissues that can be infected by the HIV.** Infection is closely linked to the presence of CD4 receptors or chemokine co-receptors on host tissue, particularly T cells and macrophages. (Modified from Weber JN, Weiss RA: HIV infection: the cellular picture, in the science of AIDS: readings from *Scientific American,* New York, 1989, Freeman.)

mucosal T cells probably spread the infection to other peripheral lymphoid organs (especially follicular dendritic cells in the lymph nodes, which infect T cells). Infection also may involve the thymus and bone marrow, including the bone marrow stromal cells. Cells in the central nervous system (CNS) may act as a reservoir in which HIV can be relatively protected from antiviral drugs. The virus is also found in T cells and macrophages in semen and in the renal epithelium.

The major immunologic finding in AIDS is the striking decrease in the number of CD4+ Th cells (Figure 8-26). Individuals who are not HIV-infected typically have 800 to 1000 CD4+ cells per cubic millimeter of blood, with a range from 600/mm³ to 1200/mm³. Numbers of CD8+ T cells are usually normal or slightly elevated. The decrease in CD4+ cell numbers results in a reversal of the normal CD4/CD8 T-cell ratio (normally about 1.9) to lower than 0.9 and often near zero.

HIV causes destruction of Th cells by a variety of means. Production of new HIV virions can be directly cytopathic to the infected cell, causing lysis (breakdown of the cell) or inducing apoptosis. Additionally, HIV infected cells express new surface antigens and are targets for Tc-mediated lysis.

However, it is not unusual for a large majority (>98%) of peripheral CD4+ T cells to *not* be infected with HIV-1, although a significant amount (10% to 50%) show signs or are primed to apoptosis.[54] Therefore, HIV-1 killing is probably an indirect rather than direct effect.[55] HIV-infected cells shed soluble viral envelope protein, gp120, which can induce apoptotic cell death of uninfected T lymphocytes, neurons, and monocytes through interaction with cell surface receptors.[56] The interaction between viral envelope protein on the surface of infected cells and its receptors on neighboring uninfected cells also can result in intercellular fusion and syncytium formation. The syncytia undergo apoptosis after a phase of latency. Envelope protein present on the surface of HIV-1 infected cells also can create partial fusion (hemifusion, membrane damage) that results in death of the uninfected cell. The presence of HIV virions and soluble viral antigen can result in a chronic activation of uninfected T cells with HIV-specific T-cell receptors (TCRs). Because activated T cells more efficiently support HIV replication, the most susceptible cells are those with TCRs against HIV, which undergo antigen-driven activation and infection. This observation may not bode well for successful vaccine development if the induced and supposedly protective CD4+ cells are also the most susceptible targets for HIV.

As a result of the processes described above, the level of T cells decreases (particularly memory T cells, which seem more susceptible to HIV infection), thymic production of new T

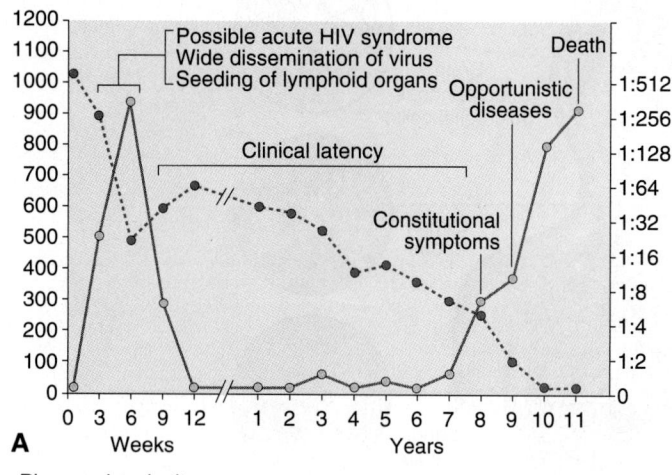

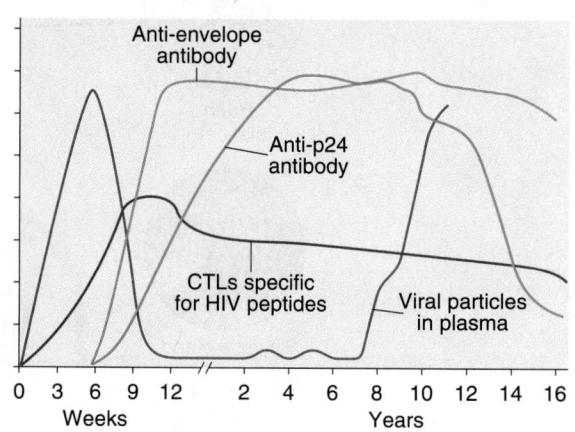

Plasma viremia titer ○——○
CD4 T cells/mm³ ●------●

Figure 8-26 Typical course of progression from HIV infection to AIDS in untreated patients. **A,** Within weeks after infection, the patient may experience symptoms of acute human immunodeficiency virus (HIV) syndrome. During this early period, the virus progressively infects mucosal T cells and dendritic cells, propagates, and spreads to the lymphoid organs, with a sharp decrease in circulating CD4+ T cells. The resulting immune response usually induces a period of clinical latency, during which viral replication and T-cell destruction continue in the lymph nodes, although the patient is generally asymptomatic. As the disease progresses, the person may develop HIV-related disease (constitutional symptoms)—a variety of symptoms of acute viral infection that do not involve opportunistic infections or malignancies. When the number of CD4+ cells is critically suppressed, the patient becomes susceptible to a variety of opportunistic infections and cancers. The length of time for progression from HIV infection to acquired immune deficiency syndrome (AIDS) may vary considerably from person to person. **B,** Antibody and Tc cell (cytotoxic T lymphocytes [CTLs]) levels change during the progression to AIDS. During the initial phase antibodies against HIV-1 are not yet detectable (window period), but viral products, including p24 antigen, viral RNA, and infectious virus, may be detectable in the blood a few weeks after infection. Most antibodies produced against envelope proteins in the early phase are absorbed onto viral particles in the blood and are not detectable by most routine assays. During the latent phase of infection antibody levels against p24 and other viral proteins, as well as HIV-specific CTLs, generally increase, then remain constant until the development of AIDS. As the immune system becomes severely depressed and excess viral antigen is released into the blood, measurable antibody levels decrease. Disease progression usually ends in the death of the untreated individual. (**A** redrawn from Fauci AS, Lane HC: Human immunodeficiency virus disease: AIDS and related conditions. In Fauci AS, et al, editors: *Harrison's principles of internal medicine,* ed 14, New York, 1997, McGraw-Hill. **B** from Kumar V, Abbas A, Fausto N: *Robbins and Cotran pathologic basis of disease,* ed 7, Philadelphia, 2005, Saunders.)

cells is decreased, and the secondary lymphoid organs (particularly the lymph nodes) are damaged.

CLINICAL MANIFESTATIONS Depletion of CD4+ cells has a profound effect on the immune system, causing a severely diminished response to a wide array of infectious pathogens and malignant tumors (Box 8-1).

At the time of diagnosis, the individual may manifest one of several different conditions: serologically negative (no detectable antibody), serologically positive (positive for antibody against HIV) but asymptomatic, early stages of HIV disease, or AIDS (see Figure 8-26).

The presence of circulating antibody against the HIV indicates infection by the virus, although many of these individuals are asymptomatic. Antibody appears rather rapidly after infection through blood products, usually within 4 to 7 weeks. After sexual transmission, however, the individual can be infected yet seronegative for 6 to 14 months or, in at least one case, for years. In addition, in the late stages of the disease, some individuals become seronegative because of a deficient immune system.

The period between infection and the appearance of antibody is referred to as the **window period** (see Figure 8-26).

Although the patient may not have antibody, he or she may have virus growing, have virus in the blood and body fluids, and be infectious to others.

Patients with the early stages of HIV disease *(early-stage disease)* usually present with relatively mild symptoms resembling influenza, such as night sweats, swollen lymph glands, diarrhea, or fatigue. The early stage may last as long as 10 years. Although individuals appear to be in clinical latency, the virus is actively proliferating in lymph nodes.[57]

The currently accepted definition of AIDS relies on both laboratory tests and clinical symptoms. The most common

---

Box 8-1	AIDS-Defining Opportunistic Infections and Neoplasms Found in Individuals with HIV Infection

Infections

Protozoal and helminthic infections
Cryptosporidiosis or isosporiasis (enteritis)
Pneumocystosis (pneumonia or disseminated infection)
Toxoplasmosis (pneumonia or CNS infection)

Fungal infections
Candidiasis (esophageal, tracheal, or pulmonary)
Cryptococcosis (CNS infection)
Coccidioidomycosis (disseminated)
Histoplasmosis (disseminated)

Bacterial infections
Mycobacteriosis (atypical, e.g., *M. avium-intracellulare*, disseminated or extrapulmonary; *M. tuberculosis*, pulmonary or extrapulmonary)
Nocardiosis (pneumonia, meningitis, disseminated)
Salmonella infections (disseminated)

Viral infections
Cytomegalovirus (pulmonary, intestinal, retinitis, or CNS infections)
Herpes simplex virus (localized or disseminated)
Varicella-zoster virus (localized or disseminated)
Progressive multifocal (leukoencephalopathy

Neoplasms
Kaposi sarcoma
B-cell non-Hodgkin lymphomas
Primary lymphoma of the brain
Invasive cancer of the uterine cervix

CNS, Central nervous system.
(From Kumar V, Abbas A, Fausto N: *Robbins and Cotran pathologic basis of disease*, ed 7, Philadelphia, 2005, Saunders.)

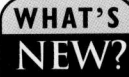

WHAT'S NEW?   Kaposi Sarcoma Regression

Kaposi sarcoma continues to reach epidemic proportions in parts of Africa and in the Western world. Emerging is new and important information regarding its epidemiology, biology, and management. Seropositivity to Kaposi sarcoma herpes virus/human herpes virus 8 (HHV8) exceeds the incidence of Kaposi sarcoma. Therefore other cofactors have been implicated in its progression including blood-sucking arthropods, angiotensin-converting enzyme inhibitors, hemodialysis, and iron. The detection of HHV8 in Kaposi sarcoma lesions has provided a new diagnostic tool for confirmation of the disease. Kaposi sarcoma is now confirmed to be of lymphatic origin and to express several chemokine receptors that help explain its preference for skin. For the first time Kaposi sarcoma has been reported to regress with the highly active antiviral therapy (HAART) regimens (see p. 286). Some Kaposi tumor cells, even in completely regressed lesions, remain in an atropic state, thus they have the potential to recur.

Data from Pananowitz L, Dezube BJ: *Curr Opin Oncol* 16(5):443-449, 2004.

WHAT'S NEW?   AIDS-Related Insulin Resistance/ Lipodystrophy Syndrome

Recent advances in highly active antiviral therapy (HAART) and the development of three different types of antiviral drugs, the nucleotide and non-nucleotide reverse transcriptase inhibitors (NRTIs) and the nonpeptide viral protease inhibitors (PI), have improved the clinical course and life expectancy in individuals with AIDS. These drugs, however, present new complications. AIDS-related insulin resistance and lipodystrophy syndrome is characterized by a significant phenotype and striking metabolic consequences. HIV-1 accessory proteins, V_{Pr}, have multiple functions, including viron incorporation, nuclear translocation of the HIV-1, nucleocytoplasmic movement, transcriptional activation, and induction of apoptosis. Therefore V_{Pr} may act as a hormone that is secreted into the extracellular space and affects distant organs. V_{Pr} is a coactivator of the glucocorticoid receptor and enhances the action of glycocorticoid hormones. V_{Pr} also suppresses transcription factors for insulin; thus it may cause resistance of tissues to insulin. Through these two functions, coactivator of glucocorticoid receptor activity and inhibition of insulin, V_{Pr} may participate in AIDS-related insulin resistance/ lipodystrophy syndrome.

Data from Kino T, Chrousos GF: *Ann NY Acad Sci* 1024:153-167, 2004.

laboratory test is for antibodies against HIV. If the patient is seropositive, the diagnosis of AIDS is made in association with various clinical symptoms (see Box 8-1). The symptoms include atypical or opportunistic infections and cancers, as well as indications of debilitating chronic disease (e.g., wasting syndrome, recurrent fevers) (Figure 8-27). In 1993, the CDC included CD4+ T-cell counts at or below 200 cells/mm^3. Most commonly, new cases of AIDS are diagnosed initially by decreased CD4+ T-cell numbers.

The average time from infection to development of AIDS has been estimated at just over 10 years. Some estimates are that approximately 99% of untreated HIV-infected individuals would eventually progress to AIDS.

TREATMENT AND PREVENTION   The current regimen for treatment of HIV infection is a combination of drugs,

termed **highly active antiretroviral therapy (HAART).** The combination includes inhibitors of reverse transcriptase (**reverse transcriptase inhibitors**) and of the viral protease (**protease inhibitors**)[58,59] (see Figure 8-23). The clinical benefits of HAART are profound and durable. Death from AIDS-related diseases has been reduced significantly since the introduction of HAART. However, resistant variants to these drugs have been identified. Drug therapy for AIDS is difficult because, like most retroviruses, the AIDS virus incorporates into the genetic material of the host and may never be removed by antimicrobial therapy. Therefore drug administration to control the virus may have to continue for the lifetime of the individual. Additionally, HIV may persist in regions where the antiviral drugs are not as effective, such as the CNS. Recently inhibitors of the initial viral entrance into the target cell (**entrance inhibitors**) and inhibitors of the viral integrase (**integrase in-**

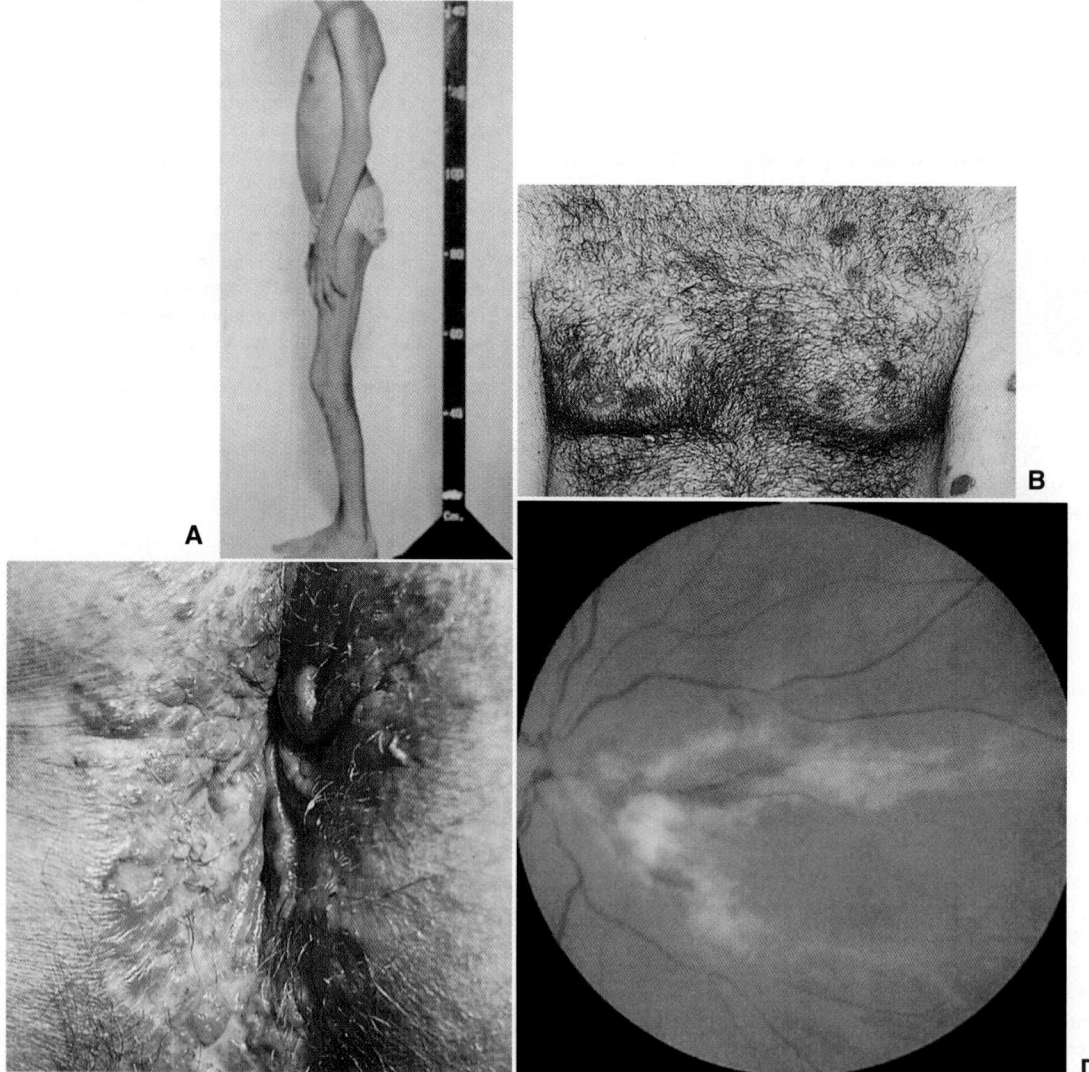

Figure 8-27 Clinical symptoms of acquired immunodeficiency syndrome (AIDS). **A,** Severe weight loss and anorexia. **B,** Biopsy-proven Kaposi sarcoma lesions. **C,** Perianal vesicular and ulcerative lesions of herpes simplex infection. **D,** Deterioration of vision from cytomegalovirus retinitis leading to areas of infection; unless treated the progressive impairment will lead to blindness. (**A** and **D,** from Taylor PK: *Diagnostic picture tests in sexually transmitted diseases,* London, 1995, Mosby; **B** and **C,** from Morse SA, Ballard RC, Holmes KK, et al editors: *Atlas of sexually transmitted diseases and AIDS,* ed 3, London, 2003, Mosby.)

hibitors) have undergone clinical trials and eventually may be added to the combination.[60-63] Entrance inhibitors include the natural or modified ligands for the co-receptors (CXCR4 and CCR5) and can block infection and inhibit cell membrane fusion.

Vaccine development is probably the most effective means of preventing HIV infection and may be useful in treating preexisting infection. Most common viral vaccines (e.g., rubella, mumps, influenza) induce protective antibodies that block the initial infection. Only one vaccine (rabies) is used after the infection has occurred. That approach is successful because the rabies virus proliferates and spreads very slowly. Whether an HIV vaccine would be effective in either preventing or treating HIV infection is problematic for several reasons. *First,* the AIDS virus is genetically and antigenically variable, like the influenza virus, so that a vaccine created against one variant may not provide protection against another variant. *Second,* although individuals with AIDS have high levels of circulating antibodies against the virus, these antibodies do not appear to be protective. Therefore even if a circulating antibody response can be induced by vaccination, that response might not be effective. A vaccine may have to induce both circulating and secretory (to prevent initial infection of the mucosal T cell) antibody and Tc cells.[64] *Third,* the AIDS virus is transmitted from cell-to-cell and initially may enter the body in an infected cell. Microorganisms that spread by cell-to-cell contact usually are not susceptible to circulating antibody. HIV-infected cells also tend to fuse with other cells, so that infection can spread to uninfected cells without viral particles being produced. It is unknown whether antibodies against HIV prevent intercellular fusion between infected and uninfected cells. *Fourth,* good animal models for AIDS experimentation are not available, therefore the efficacy and toxicity of candidate vaccines cannot easily be evaluated.

Clinical Evaluation of Immunity

Evaluation and Care of Those with Immune Deficiency

Routine care of individuals with immune deficiencies must be tempered with the knowledge that the immune system may be totally ineffective. It may be unsafe to administer conventional immunizing agents or blood products to many of these individuals because of the risk that the immunizing agent will cause an uncontrolled infection. Uncontrolled infection is a problem when attenuated vaccines that contain live but weakened microorganisms are used (e.g., live polio vaccine, vaccines against measles, mumps, and rubella). Although the vaccine virus is attenuated enough to be destroyed by a normal immune system, it can survive, multiply, and cause severe disease in an immune-deficient recipient. Additionally, even healthy recipients of vaccines containing live microorganisms can shed those microorganisms for a short period of time. Individuals with some severe immune deficiencies may be susceptible to those microorganisms. Thus individuals who are immune deficient should be isolated from recently vaccinated family members. Further, even simple procedures, such as penetrating the skin for routine blood tests, may lead to fatal septicemia (bacterial infection of the blood) in the immune-deficient person.

Individuals with immune deficiencies are also at risk for **graft-versus-host disease (GVHD)**.[65] This occurs if T cells in a transplanted graft (e.g., transfused blood) are mature and are therefore capable of the cell-mediated destruction of tissues in the graft recipient. GVHD may develop if the recipient's cells express histocompatibility antigens not found on the donor's cells. GVHD occurs when immunocompetent T lymphocytes in the grafted material recognize foreign antigens in the recipient, initiating a type IV hypersensitivity reaction against the recipient's tissues. Symptoms of an acute GVH reaction usually appear within 10 to 30 days after the transplant. The primary targets for GVHD are the skin (e.g., rash, loss or increase of pigment, thickening of skin), liver (e.g., damage to bile duct, hepatomegaly), mouth (e.g., dry mouth, ulcers, infections), eyes (e.g., burning, irritation, dryness), and gastrointestinal tract (e.g., severe diarrhea) and may lead to death from infections.

GVHD is not a problem when the recipient is immunocompetent, that is, has an immune system that can control the donor's lymphocytes. If, however, the recipient's immune system is deficient, the grafted T cells remain unchecked and attack the recipient's tissues. Most GVHD should be prevented by the current practices of treating blood with irradiation to kill white blood cells before transfusion.

The most common presenting symptom of immune deficiencies is recurrent severe infections.[66] Significant information on the specific immune deficiency can be obtained by noting certain characteristics of the individual, including the presence of any associated anomalies, age, gender, the types of infections (bacterial, viral, or fungal, and the specific microorganisms involved), family history, and risk factors associated with secondary immune deficiencies. A variety of laboratory tests are available to evaluate specific immune deficiencies (Table 8-7). The choice of which particular tests to perform is determined on the characteristics described above. A basic screening test is a **complete blood count (CBC)** with a differential. The CBC provides information on the numbers of red cells, white cells, and platelets, and the differential indicates the quantities of lymphocytes, granulocytes, and monocytes in the blood. Quantitative determination of immunoglobulins (IgG, IgM, IgA) is a screening test for antibody production, and an assay for total complement (total hemolytic complement, CH_{50}) is useful if a complement defect is suspected.

If the nature of the immune deficiency remains uncertain after the screening tests described above are performed, additional relatively common tests can be performed. For instance, subpopulations of lymphocytes or antibodies can be quantified. The proportion of B and T lymphocytes can be determined using characteristic surface markers, such as surface immunoglobulin for B cells and CD3 for T cells. T-cell populations can be further subdivided using additional sur-

Table 8-7	Laboratory Evaluation of Immunodeficiencies	
Function Tested	**Laboratory Test**	**Interpretation of Test**
Tests of Humoral Immune Function		
Antibody production	Total immunoglobulin levels	Presence of antibody-producing B cells
	Levels of isohemagglutinins	Capacity to produce specific IgM antibodies
	Levels of antibodies against vaccines—especially diphtheria and tetanus toxoids	Capacity to produce specific IgG antibodies
B-cell numbers	Numbers of lymphocytes with surface immunoglobulin	Presence of circulating B cells
Tests of Cellular Immune Function		
Delayed hypersensitivity skin test	Skin test reaction against previously encountered antigens—especially *Candida albicans* or tetanus toxoid	Presence of antigen-responsive T cells and cellular interactions (e.g., lymphokine activity and macrophage function)
T-cell numbers	Numbers of T cells forming rosettes with sheep erythrocytes or expressing membrane CD3 or CD11 antigen	Presence of circulating T cells
T-cell proliferation in vitro	Proliferative response to nonspecific mitogens (e.g., phytohemagglutinin)	Capacity of all T cells to divide in response to nonspecific stimulation (mitogens)
	Proliferative response to antigens (e.g., tetanus toxoid)	Capacity of antigen-reactive T cells to respond to antigen

face markers, such as CD4 (helper T cells) or CD8 (cytotoxic T cells). For antibodies, routine assays are available to quantify subclasses of IgG, such as IgG2.

An additional level of testing would include determination of immune responses against specific antigens. Determination of isohemagglutinins is informative about antigen-specific IgM production, if the person is of the appropriate blood type. Those who are blood type AB do not have measurable amounts of isohemagglutinins. Antibody responses to vaccines (e.g., tetanus, pertussis, measles, diphtheria, hepatitis B) are usually indicative of IgG responses. T-cell immunity against specific antigens can be measured by skin tests against "recall antigens." These include antigens from vaccines (e.g., mumps, tetanus) or from microorganisms with which the person had a previous active infection (e.g., *Candida*). An adequate T-cell immunity results in a positive delayed hypersensitivity skin test reaction.

If the tests described above do not identify the immune deficiency, more esoteric tests are offered by reference laboratories or research laboratories. These include quantification of individual complement components, in vitro proliferation (mitogenic response) of T or B cells to antigens or nonspecific mitogens, and a variety of tests of phagocyte function (e.g., nitroblue tetrazolium test [NBT] for hexose-monophosphate shunt activity, specific tests for phagocytosis, chemotaxis, or bacterial killing).

Replacement Therapies for Immune Deficiencies

Gamma-Globulin Therapy

Individuals with B-cell deficiencies that cause hypogammaglobulinemia or agammaglobulinemia usually can be treated successfully with administration of gamma-globulins, which are antibody-rich fractions prepared from plasma pooled from large numbers of donors. Administration of gamma-globulin temporarily replaces the individual's antibodies. An-

tibodies from these preparations are removed slowly from the person's blood, with half of the antibodies being removed by 3 to 4 weeks. Thus individuals must be treated repeatedly to maintain a protective level of antibodies in the blood.

Commercial gamma-globulin preparations are usually administered intramuscularly (IM) or by intravenous (IV) infusion. The dosage varies among individuals and is primarily determined by body weight. The schedule and dosage are also determined according to titers of circulating immunoglobulins and the incidence of infections in the individual. Commercial gamma-globulin preparations usually contain small amounts of IgM and IgA. Individuals with selective IgA deficiency occasionally develop allergic reactions to IgA in gamma-globulin preparations.

Individuals who need larger amounts of IgM or IgA can be given fresh-frozen plasma in monthly IV infusions. Complications associated with plasma therapy include the potential transmission of hepatitis or AIDS. The plasma is irradiated to destroy immunocompetent T cells and to avoid GVHD in individuals with accompanying T-cell deficiencies. Administration of fresh-frozen plasma is successful in individuals with Wiskott-Aldrich syndrome (IgM deficient), ataxia-telangiectasia (IgA deficient), or complement component deficiencies.

Transplantation and Transfusion

Several primary immune deficiencies originate from defects in lymphoid stem cells that interfere with their development in the primary lymphoid organs. Some of these (e.g., SCID, Wiskott-Aldrich syndrome, leukocyte adhesion defect) have benefited from replacement of stem cells through transplantation of bone marrow, umbilical cord cells, or other cell populations that are rich in stem cells.

The source of donor cells, particularly bone marrow, may contain a mixed population of stem cells and more mature T lymphocytes. In order to avoid GVHD, the preferred donor would be matched with the recipient for HLA antigens. Several other diseases involving depletion of the bone marrow (i.e., aplastic anemia, leukemia requiring eradication of tumor cells in the marrow) also are treated by bone marrow transplantation.[67] At least 75% of bone marrow transplants between individuals who are matched for HLA-A, HLA-B, HLA-C, and HLA-DR are accepted. In immunocompetent recipients, most rejections of HLA-matched transplants occur because of recognition of minor histocompatibility antigens by individuals who have received multiple blood transfusions and are, as a result, sensitized against those antigens, which are not evaluated in tissue typing. For stem cell transplants, differences in minor histocompatibility antigens may lead to GVHD. Because HLA antigens are inherited in a co-dominant fashion, the preferred donor would be a relative, especially a sibling. Although the donor is not tested for minor histocompatibility antigens, the use of a close relative also would minimize differences at those loci.

Chronic GVHD appears in 30% to 50% of transplants between HLA-matched siblings and 60% to 70% of transplants between unrelated donors. Symptoms may appear about 4 to 7 months after the transplant, but may begin much earlier or later. Depletion of T cells from bone marrow before transplantation significantly lowers the incidence of both acute and chronic GVHD. One method of doing this is to infuse the graft with monoclonal antibody against plasma membrane antigens found only on mature T cells. Another is to use fetal tissue as the graft. For example, fetal liver, which contains stem cells but not immunocompetent lymphocytes, is sometimes grafted in place of bone marrow if an HLA-matched donor cannot be found.

One therapy for deficiency diseases in which the individual lacks a thymus or thymic function (e.g., DiGeorge syndrome, ataxia-telangiectasia, or chronic mucocutaneous candidiasis) is reconstitution of thymic function. The procedure is to transplant fetal thymus tissue, which lacks immunocompetent T cells, or thymic epithelial cells (the cells that produce the thymic hormones) from which mature T cells have been removed. In some individuals transplantation increases the number of circulating mature T cells, but in most cases improvement is only temporary.

Enzymatic defects that cause SCID (e.g., adenosine deaminase deficiency) have been treated successfully with transfusions of glycerol frozen-packed erythrocytes. The donor erythrocytes contain the needed enzyme and can, at least temporarily, provide sufficient enzyme for normal lymphocyte function. An alternative method is administration of purified adenosine deaminase that has been stabilized with polyethylene glycol (PEG).

Treatment with Soluble Immune Modulators

The administration of soluble materials that affect lymphocyte function can restore T-cell function, especially in individuals with Wiskott-Aldrich syndrome or chronic mucocutaneous candidiasis. Successful for some individuals is the use of transfer factor, a low-molecular-weight nucleoprotein prepared from lymphocyte lysates, which can confer specific reactivity against certain antigens. Thymosin, a thymic hormone, also has been used, although with limited success. Cytokine therapy also has been effective in some cases of chronic granulomatous disease.

Gene Therapy

The first successful therapeutic replacement of defective genes was performed in two girls with SCID caused by an ADA deficiency.[68,69] The normal gene for ADA had been cloned and inserted into a retroviral vector. The gene for ADA had replaced some retroviral genes, resulting in a virus that carried the normal human gene but did not cause disease. The virus was used to infect bone marrow stem cells from these children. The retrovirus inserted the normal ADA gene into the individuals' genetic material. The genetically altered stem cells were infused into the children, resulting in reconstitution of their immune systems.

SUMMARY REVIEW

Hypersensitivity: Allergy, Autoimmunity, and Alloimmunity

1. Inappropriate immune responses are misdirected against the host's own tissues (autoimmunity); directed against beneficial foreign tissues, such as transfusions or transplants (alloimmunity); exaggerated responses against environmental antigens (allergy); or insufficient to protect the host (immune deficiency).
2. Allergy, autoimmunity, and alloimmunity are collectively know as *hypersensitivity reactions.*
3. Mechanisms of hypersensitivity are classified as type I (IgE-mediated) reactions, type II (tissue-specific) reactions, type III (immune complex–mediated) reactions, and type IV (cell-mediated) reactions.
4. Hypersensitivity reactions can be immediate (developing within minutes to a few hours) or delayed (developing within several hours or days).
5. Anaphylaxis, the most rapid immediate hypersensitivity reaction, is an explosive reaction that occurs within minutes of re-exposure to the antigen and can lead to cardiovascular shock.
6. Allergens are antigens that cause allergic responses.
7. Type I (IgE-mediated) reactions are mediated through the binding of IgE to Fc receptors on mast cells and cross-linking of IgE by antigens that bind to the Fab portions of IgE. Cross-linking causes mast cell degranulation and the release of histamine (the most potent mediator) and other inflammatory substances.
8. Histamine enhances the chemotaxis of eosinophils into sites of type I allergic reactions
9. Atopic individuals tend to produce higher quantities of IgE and to have more Fc receptors for IgE on their mast cells.
10. Type II (tissue-specific) reactions are caused by five possible mechanisms: complement-mediated lysis, opsonization and phagocytosis, neutrophil-mediated tissue damage, antibody-

dependent cell-mediated cytotoxicity, and modulation of cellular function.

11. Type III (immune complex–mediated) reactions are caused by the formation of immune complexes that are deposited in target tissues, where they activate the complement cascade, generating chemotactic fragments that attract neutrophils into the inflammatory site. Neutrophils release lysosomal enzymes that result in tissue damage.

12. Intermediate-sized immune complexes are the most likely to have severe pathologic consequences.

13. Immune complex disease can be a systemic reaction, such as serum sickness, or localized, such as the Arthus reaction.

14. Type IV (cell-mediated) reactions are caused by either cytotoxic T lymphocytes (Tc cells) or lymphokine-producing Th1 cells.

15. Typical allergens include pollen, molds and fungi, certain foods (milk, eggs, fish), animals, certain drugs, cigarette smoke, and house dust.

16. Clinical manifestations of allergic reactions usually are confined to the areas of initial intake or contact with the allergen. Ingested allergens induce gastrointestinal symptoms, airborne allergens induce respiratory or skin manifestations, and contact allergens induce allergic responses at the site of contact.

17. Autoimmunity is a breakdown of immunologic homeostasis, the immune system's tolerance of self-antigens. Central tolerance develops during the embryonic period. Peripheral tolerance is maintained in secondary lymphoid organs by regulatory T lymphocytes or antigen-presenting dendritic cells.

18. Autoimmune disease can be caused by the exposure of a previously sequestered antigen, the development of a neoantigen, the complications of infectious disease, the emergence of a forbidden clone of lymphocytes, or ineffective peripheral tolerance.

19. Alloimmunity is the immune system's reaction against antigens on the tissues of other members of the same species.

20. Alloimmune disorders include transient neonatal disease, in which the maternal immune system becomes sensitized against antigens expressed by the fetus, transplant rejection, and transfusion reactions, in which the immune system of the recipient of an organ transplant or blood transfusion reacts against foreign antigens on the donor's cells.

21. Systemic lupus erythematosus (SLE) is a chronic, multisystem, inflammatory disease and is one of the most serious of the autoimmune disorders. SLE is characterized by the production of a large variety of autoantibodies.

22. Hyperacute graft rejection (preexisting antibody) is immediate and rare, acute rejection is cell-mediated and occurs days to months after transplantation, and chronic rejection is caused by inflammatory damage to endothelial cells as a result of a weak cell-mediated reaction.

23. Red blood cell antigens may be the targets of autoimmune or alloimmune reactions. The most important of these, because they provoke the strongest humoral immune response, are the ABO and Rh systems.

Deficiencies in Immunity

1. Disorders resulting from immune deficiency are the clinical sequelae of impaired function of components of the immune or inflammatory response, phagocytes, or complement.

2. Immune deficiency is the failure of mechanisms of self-defense to function in their normal capacity.

3. Immune deficiencies are either congenital (primary) or acquired (secondary). Primary immune deficiencies are caused by genetic defects that disrupt lymphocyte development, whereas secondary immune deficiencies are secondary to disease or other physiologic alterations.

4. The clinical hallmark of immune deficiency is a propensity to unusual or recurrent severe infections. The type of infection usually reflects the immune system defect.

5. The most common infections in individuals with defects of cell-mediated immune response are fungal and viral, whereas infections in individuals with defects of the humoral immune response or complement function are primarily bacterial.

6. Defects in B-cell function are diverse, ranging from a complete lack of the human bursal equivalent function, the lymphoid organs required for B-cell maturation (as in Bruton's agammaglobulinemia), to deficiencies in a single class of immunoglobulins (e.g., selective IgA deficiency).

7. DiGeorge syndrome (congenital thymic aplasia or hypoplasia) is characterized by complete or partial lack of the thymus (resulting in depressed T-cell immunity) and the parathyroid glands (resulting in hypocalcemia) and the presence of cardiac anomalies.

8. Severe combined immune deficiency (SCID) is a total lack of T-cell function and a severe (either partial or total) lack of B-cell function. SCID can result from mutations in critical enzymes (adenosine deaminase [ADA] deficiency, purine nucleoside phosphorylase [PNP] deficiency), in cytokine receptors (X-linked SCID, JAK3 deficiency, IL-7 receptor deficiency), or in antigen receptors (RAG-1/RAG-2 deficiencies, CD45 deficiency, CD3 deficiency, ZAP-70 deficiency). Other combined defects may result from deficiencies in antigen presenting molecules (bare lymphocyte syndrome), cytoskeletal proteins (Wiskott-Aldrich syndrome), or DNA repair (ataxia-telangiectasia).

9. Almost any portion of the complement cascade may be defective. The most severe defect is C3 deficiency, which results in recurrent life-threatening bacterial infections. Defects in proteins of the membrane-attack complex usually result in unusual disseminated infections with bacteria of the species *Neisseria*.

10. Defects in phagocyte function, which include insufficient numbers of phagocytes or defects of chemotaxis, phagocytosis, or killing, can result in recurrent, life-threatening infections, such as septicemia and disseminated pyogenic lesions.

11. Acquired immunodeficiencies are caused by superimposed conditions, such as aging, malnutrition, infections, malignancies, physical or psychologic trauma, some medical treatments, or other diseases.

12. AIDS is an acquired dysfunction of the immune system caused by a retrovirus (HIV) that mostly infects and destroys CD4+ lymphocytes (helper T cells). The disease is progressive, developing from HIV infection to AIDS in about 10 years in untreated individuals. Therapy with combined drug regiments usually controls progression so that AIDS in the United States is now a chronic disease.

13. Deficiencies in immunity usually are treated by replacement therapy. Deficient antibody production is treated by replacement of missing immunoglobulins with commercial γ-globulin preparations. Lymphocyte deficiencies are treated with the replacement of host lymphocytes with transplants of bone marrow, fetal liver, or fetal thymus from a donor.

KEY TERMS

MEDIA RESOURCES 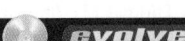 *evolve*

Review questions and answers for this chapter are available in the *CD Companion* included with this book. Also see the CD for an animation on the *HIV life cycle.*

WebLinks—links to Internet sites pertaining to this chapter—are available on Evolve at http://evolve.elsevier.com/McCance/.

REFERENCES

1. Gell PGH, Coombs RRA, Lachman PT: *Clinical aspects of immunology,* Oxford, England, 1975, Blackwell Scientific.
2. Portier P, Richet C: De l'action anaphylactique de certains venins, *Comptes Rendus Societie Biologie (Paris)* 54:170, 1902.
3. Saini SS, MacGlashan D: How IgE upregulates the allergic response, *Curr Opin Immunol* 14(6):694-697, 2002.
4. Robbie-Ryan M, Brown MA, The role of the mast cells in allergy and autoimmunity, *Curr Opin Immunol* 14(6):728-733, 2002.
5. Galli SJ: Mast cells and basophils, *Curr Opin Hematol* 7(1):32-39, 2000.
6. Jutel M et al.: Immune regulation by histamine, *Curr Opin Immunol* 14(6):735-740, 2002.
7. Kinet J-P: Allergy and hypersensitivity, *Curr Opin Immunol* 14:685-687, 2002.
8. Geha RS: Allergy and hypersensitivity: nature versus nurture in allergy and hypersensitivity, *Curr Opin Immunol* 15(6):603-608, 2003.
9. Akbari O et al: Role of regulatory T cells in allergy and asthma, *Curr Opin Immunol* 15(6):627-633, 2003.
10. Akdis CA, Blaser K: Immunologic mechanisms of specific immunotherapy, *Allergy* 54(suppl 56):31-32, 1999.
11. Haselden BM, Kay AB, Larche M: Peptide-mediated immune responses in specific immunotherapy, *Int Arch Allergy Immunol* 122(4):229-237, 2000.
12. Abramson SB, Belmont HM: SLE: mechanisms of vascular injury, *Hosp Pract* 33(4):107110, 113-114, 119-122, 1998.
13. Pirquet C, Schick B: *Serum sickness,* Leipzig, Germany, 1905, Franz Denticke.
14. Arthus M, Breton M: Lésions cutanées produites par les injections de sérum, *Comptes Rendus Societe de Biologie* 55:817, 1903.
15. Koch R: Fortsetzung der mitteilungen, ber ein heilmittel gegen tuberkulose, *Deutsche Med Wochenschr* 9:101, 1891.
16. Belsito DV: The diagnostic evaluation, treatment, and prevention of allergic contact dermatitis in the new millennium, *J Allergy Clin Immunol* 105:409-420, 2000.
17. Schwartz RS: Shattuck lecture: diversity of the immune repertoire and immunoregulation, *N Engl J Med* 348(11):1017-1026, 2003.
18. Ohashi PS, DeFranco AL: Making and breaking tolerance, *Curr Opin Immunol* 14(6):744-759, 2002.
19. Fourneau JM et al.: The elusive case for a role of mimicry in autoimmune diseases, *Mol Immunol* 40(14-15):1095-1102, 2004.
20. Venanzi ES, Benoist C, Mathis D: Good riddance: thymocyte clonal deletion prevents autoimmunity, *Curr Opin Immunol* 16(2):197-202, 2004.

21. Morahan G, Morel L: Genetics of autoimmune diseases in humans and in animal models, *Curr Opin Immunol* 14(6):803-811, 2002.

22. Kuper BC, Failla S: Systemic lupus erythematosus: a multisystem autoimmune disorder, *Nurs Clin North Am* 35(6):253-265, 2000.

23. Shmerling RH: Autoantibodies in systemic lupus erythematosus—there before you know it, *N Engl J Med* 349(16):1499-1500, 2003.

24. Perdriger A, Werner-Leyval S, Rollot-Elamrani K: The genetic basis for systemic lupus erythematosus, *Joint Bone Spine* 70(2):103-108, 2003.

25. Tan EM et al: A critical evaluation of enzyme immunoassays for detection of antinuclear autoantibodies of defined specificities. I. Precision, sensitivity, and specificity, *Arthritis Rheum* 42(3):455-464, 1999.

26. Avent ND, Reid ME: The Rh blood group system: a review, *Blood* 95(2):375-387, 2000.

27. Jones AM, Gaspar HB: Immunogenetics: changing the face of immunodeficiency, *J Clin Pathol* 53(1):60-65, 2000.

28. Cooper MA, Pommering TL, Koranyi K: Primary immunodeficiencies, *Am Fam Physician* 68(10):2001-2008, 2003.

29. *Primary immunodeficiency NICHD*. Available at www.nichd.nih.gov/publications/pubs/PrimaryImmuoBooklet.htm, accessed 2004.

30. Simonte SJ, Cunningham-Rundles C: Update on primary immunodeficiency: defects of lymphocytes, *Clin Immunol* 109(2):109-118, 2003.

31. Bruton OC: Agammaglobulinemia, *Pediatrics* 9(6):722-728, 1952.

32. Demczuk S, Aurias A: DiGeorge syndrome and related syndromes associated with 22q11.2 deletions, *Annales Genetique* 38:59, 1995.

33. DiGeorge AM: Congenital absence of the thymus and its immunologic consequences. In Bergsma D, McKusick FA, editors: *Immunologic deficiency diseases in man, National Foundation—March of Dimes Original Article Series*, Baltimore, 1968, Williams & Wilkins.

34. Fischer A: Have we seen the last variant of severe combined immunodeficiency? *N Engl J Med* 349(19):1789-1792, 2003.

35. Thrasher AJ, Kinnon C: The Wiskott-Aldrich syndrome, *Clin Exp Immunol* 120(1):2-9, 2000.

36. Lekstrom-Himes JA, Gallin JI: Immunodeficiency diseases caused by defects in phagocytes, *N Engl J Med* 343(23):1703-1714, 2000.

37. Adams KM, Nelson JL: Microchimerism: an investigative frontier in autoimmunity and transplantation, *JAMA* 291(9):1127-1131, 2004.

38. Maloney S et al: Microchimerism of maternal origin persists into adult life, *J Clin Invest* 104(1):41-47, 1999.

39. Nelson JL et al: Microchimerism and HLA-compatible relationships of pregnancy in scleroderma, *Lancet* 351(9102):559-562, 1998.

40. Ohtsuka T et al: Quantitative analysis of microchimerism in systemic sclerosis skin tissue, *Arch Dermatol Res* 293(8):387-391, 2001.

41. Artlett CM et al: Chimeric cells of maternal origin in juvenile idiopathic inflammatory myopathies, *Lancet* 356(9248):2155-2156, 2000.

42. Khosrotehrani K et al: Transfer of fetal cells with multilineage potential to maternal tissue, *JAMA* 292(1):75-80, 2004.

43. Schroder AK, Rink L: Neutrophil immunity of the elderly, *Mech Ageing Dev* 124(4):419-425, 2003.

44. Hakim FT, et al: Aging, immunity and cancer, *Curr Opin Immunol* 16(2):151-156, 2004.

45. Masek K et al: Past, present and future of psychoneuroimmunology, *Toxicology* 142(3):179-188, 2000.

46. UNAIDS/WHO: *AIDS Epidemic Update: 2003*. Geneva, Switzerland: UNAIDS; 2004:1-48. Also available at www.unaids.org

47. Centers for Disease Control and Prevention: *HIV/AIDS Surveillance Report*, 2003 (Vol 15). Atlanta: US Department of Health and Human Services, Centers for Disease Control and Prevention; 2004:1-46. Also available at www.cdc.gov/hiv/stats/hasrlink.htm

48. Takeb EY, Kusagawa S, Motomura K: Molecular epidemiology of HIV: tracking AIDS pandemic, *Pediatr Int* 46(2):236-244, 2004.

49. Thorne C, Newell ML: Mother-to-child transmission of HIV infection and its prevention, *Curr HIV Res* 1(4):447-462, 2003.

50. Centers for Disease Control and Prevention: Updated U.S. Public Health Service guidelines for the management of occupational exposures to HBV, HCV, and HIV and recommendations for postexposure prophylaxis, *MMWR* 50:1-67, 2001.

51. Barre-Sinoussi F et al: Isolation of a T-lymphotropic retrovirus from a patient at risk for acquired immune deficiency syndrome (AIDS), *Science* 220(4599):868-871, 1983.

52. Ho DD, Pomerantz RJ, Kaplan JC: Pathogenesis of infection with human immunodeficiency virus, *N Engl J Med* 317(5):278-286, 1987.

53. Stebbing J, Gazzard B, Douek DC: Where does HIV live? *N Eng J Med* 350(18):1872-1880, 2004.

54. Badley AD et al: Mechanisms of HIV-associated lymphocyte apoptosis, *Blood* 96(9):2951-2964, 2000.

55. Castedo M et al: Mitochondrial apoptosis induced by the HIV-1 envelope, *Ann NY Acad Sci* 1010:19-28, 2003.

56. Becker Y: HIV-1 induced AIDS is an allergy and the allergen is the shed gp120 – a review, hypothesis, and implications, *Virus Genes* 28(3):319-331, 2004.

57. Pantaleo G, Graziosi C, Fauci AS: The role of lymphoid organs and the pathogenesis of HIV infection, *Semin Immunol* 5(3):157-163, 1993.

58. De Clercq E: Antiviral drugs in current clinical use, *J Clin Virol* 30(2):115-133, 2004.

59. Wynn GH et al: Antiretrovirals, part 1: overview, history, and focus on protease inhibitors, *Psychosomatics* 45(3):262-270, 2004.

60. Schols D: HIV co-receptors as targets for antiviral therapy, *Curr Top Med Chem* 4(9):883-893, 2004.

61. Menendez-Arias L, Este JA: HIV-resistance to viral entry inhibitors, *Curr Pharm Des* 10(15):1845-1860, 2004.

62. Anthony NJ: HIV-1 integrase: a target for new AIDS chemotherapeutics, *Curr Top Med Chem* 4(9):979-990, 2004.

63. Johnson AA, Marchand C, Pommier Y: HIV-1 integrase inhibitors: a decade of research and two drugs in clinical trial, *Curr Top Med Chem* 4(10):1059-1077, 2004.

64. Stevceva L, Strober W: Mucosal HIV vaccines: where are we now?, *Curr HIV Res* 2(1):1-10, 2004.

65. Bhushan V, Collins RH Jr: Chronic graft-vs-host disease, *JAMA* 290(19):2599-2603, 2003.

66. Conley ME, Notarangelo LD, Etzioni A: Diagnostic criteria for primary immunodeficiencies, *Clin Immunol* 93(3):190-197, 1999.

67. Thomas ED: Bone marrow transplantation: a review, *Semin Hematol* 36(suppl 7):95-103, 1999.

68. Blaese RM: Development of gene therapy for immunodeficiency: adenosine deaminase deficiency, *Pediatr Res* 33:S49-S59, 1993.

69. Onodera M et al: Gene therapy for severe combined immunodeficiency caused by adenosine deaminase deficiency: improved retroviral vectors for clinical trials, *Acta Haematol* 101(2):89-96, 1999.

INFECTION

NEAL S. ROTE • SUE E. HUETHER

CHAPTER OUTLINE

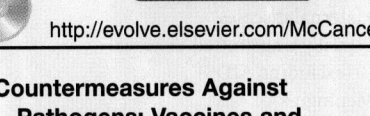

Modern health care has shown great progress in preventing and treating infectious diseases. In developed countries the advent of sanitary living conditions, clean water, uncontaminated food, vaccinations, and antimicrobials have improved the health of many and made death from infectious disease most common among those with debilitating diseases, nutritional deficiencies, or immunosuppression. Infectious disease remains a significant threat to life in many parts of the world, including India, Africa, and Southeast Asia. The recent emergence of new infectious agents and of common agents that have developed resistance to most antimicrobial drugs, however, has greatly increased the risk of severe infection and mortality in all parts of the world.

INFECTIOUS AGENTS

Infectious diseases are the number one cause of death worldwide (Table 9-1). Dense populations in developing countries with poor sanitation are victims of plague, cholera, malaria, tuberculosis, leprosy, and schistosomiasis. Only smallpox has been eradicated from the world by vaccination. Vaccination also has eradicated polio from the Western Hemisphere. In the United States, heart disease and malignancies greatly surpass infectious disease as major causes of death (Table 9-2). Although vaccines and antimicrobials have altered the prevalence of infectious disease, mutant strains of bacteria have emerged that have resistance to protection previously provided by antimicrobial drug therapy. New diseases, such as West Nile virus, severe acute respiratory syndrome (SARS), Lyme disease, *Hantavirus,* the global spread of human immunodeficiency virus (HIV), and drug-resistant tuberculosis

are examples of the current intense challenge being faced in the struggle to prevent and control infectious disease.

Microorganisms and Humans: A Dynamic Relationship

Many microorganisms find human bodies to be hospitable sites in which to grow and flourish; there they are provided with nutrients and the appropriate conditions of temperature and humidity. In many cases a mutual relationship exists, in which both humans and microorganisms benefit (Box 9-1). These microorganisms are called the *normal flora;* they are found in different parts of the body, including the skin, mouth, gastrointestinal tract, respiratory tract, and genital tract. For instance, the human gut is colonized by a large variety of microorganisms that make up the normal human flora. These bacteria are provided with nutrients from food ingested by their human host and in exchange produce enzymes that facilitate the digestion and use of many of the more complex molecules found in the human diet, produce antibacterial factors (e.g., bacteriocins, colicins) that prevent colonization by pathogenic microorganisms, and produce usable metabolites (e.g., vitamin K, B vitamins). This beneficial homeostasis is normally maintained through the physical integrity of the gut and other mechanisms that guarantee that the immune and inflammatory systems do not attack these symbiotes. In return they remain in the gut and do not attempt to invade other parts of the body. This relationship can be breached as a result of injury that releases intestinal bacteria into the bloodstream, potentially leading to sepsis, shock, and death.

Much of the symbiotic relationship is maintained by the immune and inflammatory systems. If those systems are com-

Table 9-1	Estimated Annual Number of Deaths by Cause Worldwide		
Cause of Death		**Number**	**%**
Communicable Diseases		18,324,000	22.1
Respiratory infections		3,963,000	
HIV/AIDS*		2,777,000	
Perinatal diseases		2,462,000	
Diarrheal diseases		1,798,000	
Tuberculosis		1,566,000	
Childhood diseases		1,124,000	
Malaria		1,272,000	
Maternal diseases		510,000	
Sexually transmitted diseases (excluding AIDS)		180,000	
Meningitis		173,000	
Tropical diseases		129,000	
Hepatitis		157,000	
Noncommunicable Diseases		33,537,000	58.8
Cardiovascular diseases		16,733,000	
Malignant neoplasms		7,121,000	
Respiratory diseases		3,702,000	
Digestive system disorders		1,968,000	
Genitourinary disorders		848,000	
Diabetes mellitus		988,000	
Nutritional diseases		243,000	
External Causes (e.g., accidents, suicide)		5,168,000	9.1

From World Health Organization. The World Health Report 2004. Annex Table 2; Death by cause, sex, and mortality stratum in WHO regions, estimates for 2002, The Organization.
*Global data for acquired immunodeficiency syndrome (AIDS) cases reported remain highly distorted for three reasons: (1) wide intercountry and interregional differences in the completeness of AIDS case detection and reporting, (2) reporting of AIDS cases to public health authorities and recognition of its importance have occurred in different countries at different times, and (3) pediatric AIDS remains substantially underrecognized and underreported.

promised, many microorganisms will leave their normal sites and cause infection elsewhere in the body. Individuals with deficiencies in their immune systems easily become infected with *opportunistic microorganisms,* which are microorganisms that normally would not cause disease but seize the opportunity to do so when a person's immune or inflammatory responses are decreased (see Chapter 8).

Four separate stages are associated with pathologic infection: colonization, invasion, multiplication, and spread. These stages are summarized in Table 9-3. Infection by a pathogen is influenced by several factors as listed below:

- *Mechanism of action:* direct damage of cells, interference with cellular metabolism, and rendering a cell dysfunctional because of the accumulation of pathogenic substances and toxin production (see p. 296).
- *Infectivity:* ability of the pathogen to invade and multiply in the host—for example, coagulase, an enzymatic product of some pathogens that causes coagulation and allows some microorganisms, such as staphylococci, to clot and form a sticky layer around themselves, protects the pathogens against host defenses.
- *Pathogenicity:* ability of an agent to produce disease—success depends on speed of pathogen reproduction, extent of tissue damage, and production of toxins (see p. 299).
- *Virulence:* potency of a pathogen measured in terms of the number of microorganisms or micrograms of toxin required to kill a host—for example, measles virus is of low virulence; rabies virus is highly virulent.
- *Immunogenicity:* ability of pathogens to induce an immune response.
- *Toxigenicity:* a factor important in determining a pathogen's degree of virulence, that is, the ability to produce disease by production of a soluble toxin, such as hemolysin, leucocidin, other exotoxins, and endotoxins—for example, hemolysin

Table 9-2	Death Rates and Percent of Total Deaths for the 15 Leading Causes of Death in the United States (2001)		
Rank Order*	**Cause of Death**	**Rate†**	**Percent of Total Deaths**
1	Diseases of heart	245.8	29.0
2	Malignant neoplasms	194.4	22.9
3	Cardiovascular diseases	157.5	6.8
4	Chronic lower respiratory diseases	43.2	5.1
5	Accidents (unintentional injuries)	35.7	4.2
6	Diabetes mellitus	25.1	3.0
7	Influenza and pneumonia	21.8	2.6
8	Alzheimer disease	18.9	2.2
9	Nephritis, nephrotic syndrome, and nephrosis	13.9	1.6
10	Septicemia	11.3	1.3
11	Intentional self harm (suicide)	10.8	1.3
12	Chronic liver disease and cirrhosis	9.5	1.1
13	Assault (homicide)	7.1	0.8
14	Essential hypertension and hypertensive disease	6.8	0.8
15	Pneumonitis due to solids and liquids	6.1	0.7

Data from *National Vital Statistics Report* 51, No 5, 2003; National Center for Health Statistics, www.cdc.gov/nchs.
*Rank based on number of deaths.
†Rates per 100,000 population.

destroys erythrocytes, and leukocidin destroys leukocytes; both are products of streptococci and staphylococci.

• *Portal of entry:* route by which a pathogenic microorganism infects the host: direct contact, inhalation, ingestion, or bites of an animal or insect—spread of infection is facilitated by the ability of pathogens to spread through lymph and blood and into tissues and organs, where they multiply and cause disease.

Classes of Infectious Microorganisms

Infectious disease can be caused by microorganisms that range in size from 20 nm (poliovirus) to 10 m (tapeworm). Classes of pathogenic microorganisms and their characteristics are summarized in Table 9-4.

Box 9-1	The Many Relationships Between Humans and Organisms

Symbiosis: Benefits only the human; no harm to the organism
Mutualism: Benefits the human and the organism
Commensalism: Benefits only the organism; no harm to the human
Pathogenicity: Benefits the organism; harms the human (*opportunism* is a situation in which benign human organisms become pathogenic because of decreased human host resistance)

PATHOGEN SURVIVAL MECHANISMS
Innate Host Defense Mechanisms

The first lines of defense against infectious microorganisms are external barriers, including the skin and mucous membranes and the cells and biochemicals of innate immunity (see Chapter 6). The digestive, respiratory, and genitourinary tracts form a closed barrier between the internal organs and the environment (Figure 9-1). Cells of innate immunity express Toll-like receptors that recognize pathogens and activate inflammation and adaptive immunity, the second and third lines of defense (see Chapters 6 and 7).

Once a microorganism penetrates the first lines of defense and invades the body, the inflammatory response is initiated, especially the phagocytes. The neutrophils actively attack bacteria, engulf them, and destroy the microorganism (phagocytosis). Natural killer cells (NK cells) attack virus-infected cells.

The adaptation of the immune system actively neutralizes bacterial defense mechanisms (Figure 9-2). The complement system, through the alternative and lectin pathways, produces C3b, which attaches itself to the surface of the bacterium with carbohydrate capsules. C3b functions as a highly effective opsonin that allows adherence between the bacterium and C3b receptors on the phagocyte's surface, thus facilitating phagocytosis. The C5b-C9 membrane lytic complex kills bacteria.

Table 9-3	Stages of Infection	
Stage	Mechanism	Consequences
Colonization	Pathogens present on or in body without tissue invasion	Source of cross infection to others
Invasion	Resists host defenses; attaches to host cells through adhesion molecules and receptors	Opportunity for cell injury, alterations in function, or cell death
Multiplication	Uses host nutrients and environment, or cell organelles, for reproduction	Tissue damage, cell alterations, or cell death and disease symptoms
Spread	Migrates locally or through bloodstream and lymphatics	Local or systemic manifestations of disease through cell injury or effect of toxins

Table 9-4	Classes of Organisms Infectious to Humans		
Class	Size	Site of Reproduction	Example
Virus	20-30 nm	Intracellular	Poliomyelitis
Chlamydia	200-1000 nm	Intracellular	Trachoma
Rickettsiae	300-1200 nm	Intracellular	Rocky Mountain spotted fever
Mycoplasma	125-350 nm	Extracellular	Mycoplasma pneumonia
Bacteria	0.8-15 mcg	Skin	Staphylococcal wound infection
		Mucous membranes	Cholera
		Intracellular	Streptococcal pneumonia
		Extracellular	Tuberculosis
Fungi	2-200 mcg	Skin	Tinea pedis (athlete's foot)
		Mucous membranes	Candida (i.e., thrush)
		Intracellular	Sporotrichosis
		Extracellular	Histoplasmosis
Protozoa	1-50 mm	Mucosal	Giardiasis
		Extracellular	Sleeping sickness
Helminths	3 mm to 10 m	Intracellular	Trichinosis
		Extracellular	Filariasis

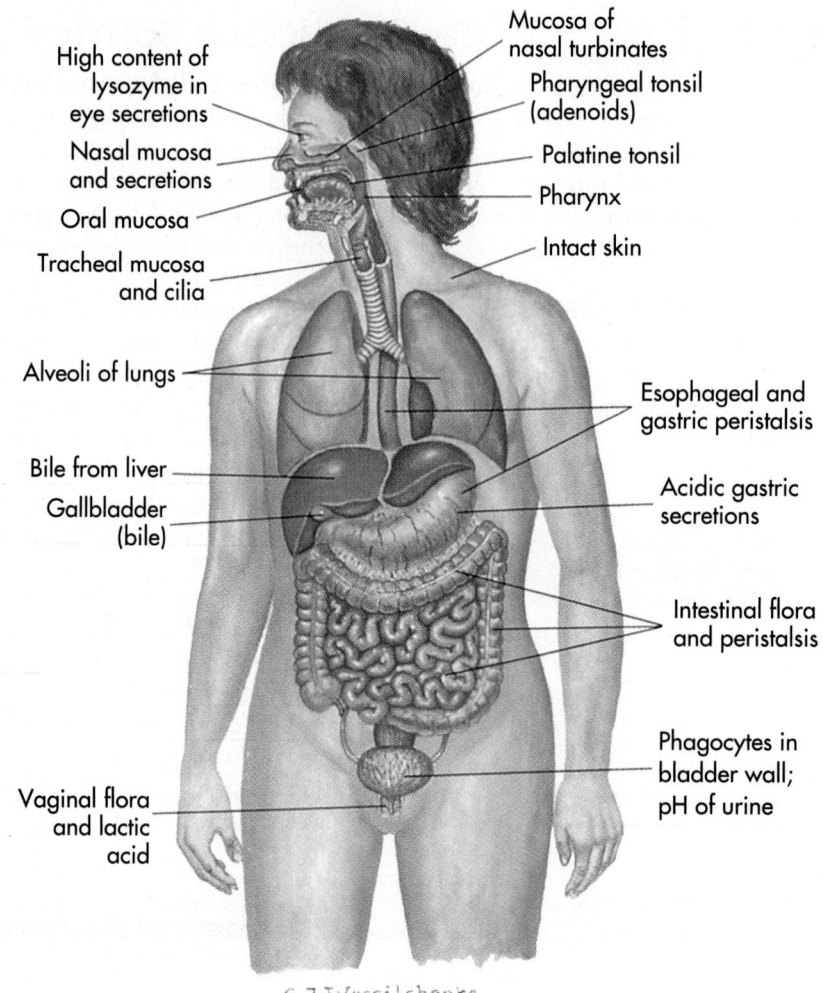

High content of
lysozyme in
eye secretions

Nasal mucosa
and secretions

Oral mucosa

Tracheal mucosa
and cilia

Mucosa of
nasal turbinates

Pharyngeal tonsil
(adenoids)

Palatine tonsil

Pharynx

Intact skin

Alveoli of lungs

Esophageal and
gastric peristalsis

Bile from liver

Gallbladder
(bile)

Acidic gastric
secretions

Intestinal flora
and peristalsis

Phagocytes in
bladder wall;
pH of urine

Vaginal flora
and lactic
acid

G.J.Wassilchenko

Figure 9-1 **The closed barrier.** The digestive, respiratory, and genitourinary tracts form closed barriers between the internal organs and the environment. (From Grimes DE: *Infectious diseases,* St Louis, 1991, Mosby.)

Antibodies bind to the surface of bacteria, act as opsonins, and activate complement. Antibodies are produced against most of the bacterial toxins, thereby neutralizing their effects. Figure 9-3 summarizes the role of antibodies in defense against bacteria.

Pathogenic Defense Mechanisms

True pathogens have devised means to circumvent the host's defenses. Examples of these adaptations include surface coats that inhibit phagocytosis, surface receptors that bind to host cells, and toxins that damage cells or alter their function.

If the immune system is compromised, infections cannot be regulated. As a result, a normally limited and clinically mild viral or bacterial infection becomes systemic and potentially fatal to the individual. Table 9-5 gives examples of microorganisms that fight off or alter the human inflammatory response or resist immune defenses.

Another mechanism successfully used by pathogens to escape recognition by host defenses is **antigenic variation.**[1] Antigenic variation allows the pathogen to change appear-

ances by altering surface molecules (antigens), thus challenging the specificity of the immune system. The three primary mechanisms are *mutation, recombination,* and *gene switching.* Antigenic variation can occur during the course of an infection in the host or during the spread of infection through the environment. Influenza infection provides an example of how this occurs. **Antigenic drift** is the change that results from **mutations** allowing, for example, the emergence of new strains of influenza virus, and thus creating the need for new vaccines every year. **Antigenic shifts** are major changes in antigenicity that occur from **recombination** of genomes ("jumping genes") from different strains of pathogens and can result in pandemics. For example, influenza A virus developed from recombination of avian and human virus strains. Other pathogens use **gene switching** to avoid the immune response. Pathogens carry thousands of genes for different surface molecules that they can switch on and off at frequent intervals (i.e., African trypanosomes). Consequently, the immune system is always trying to "catch up" by generating new antibodies and memory cells.

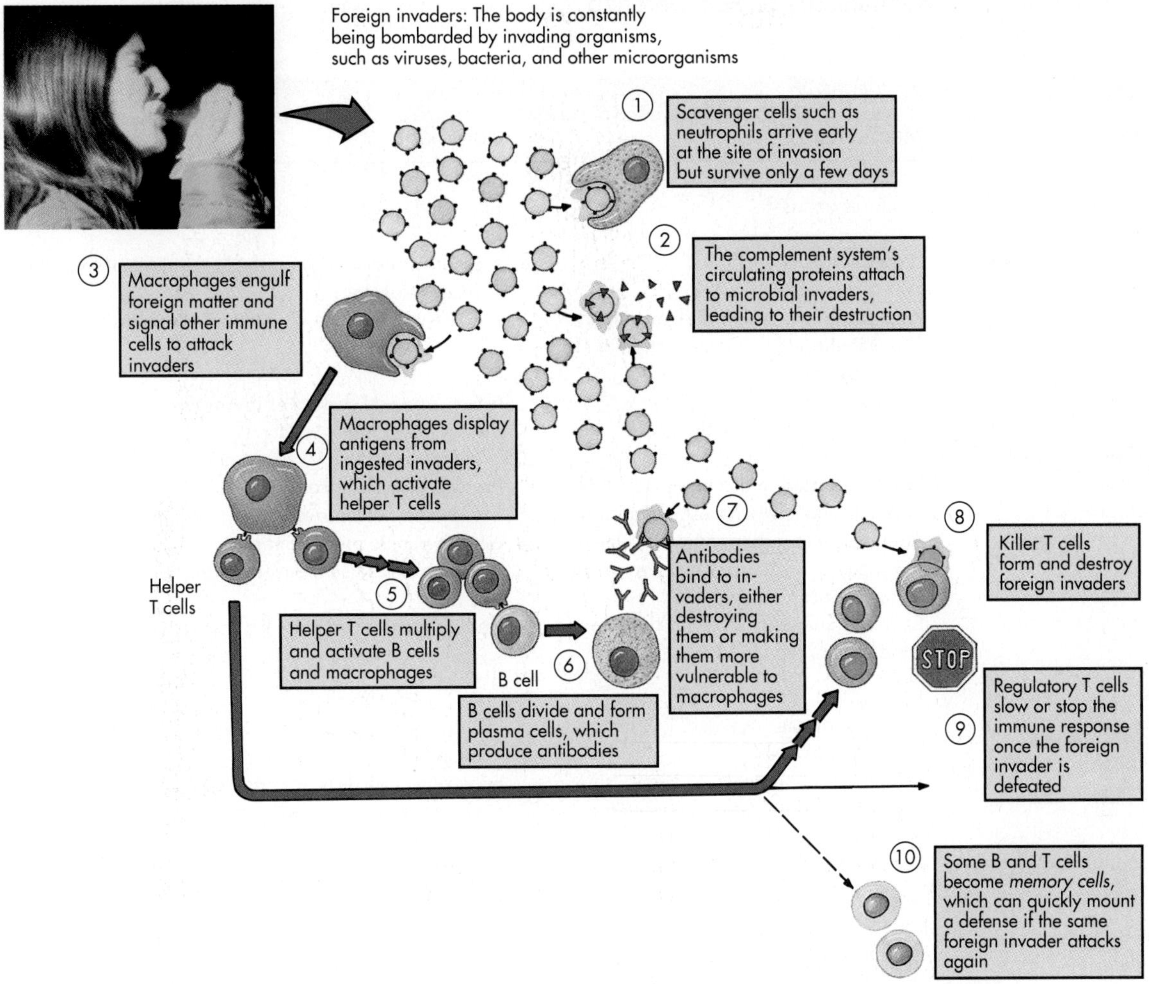

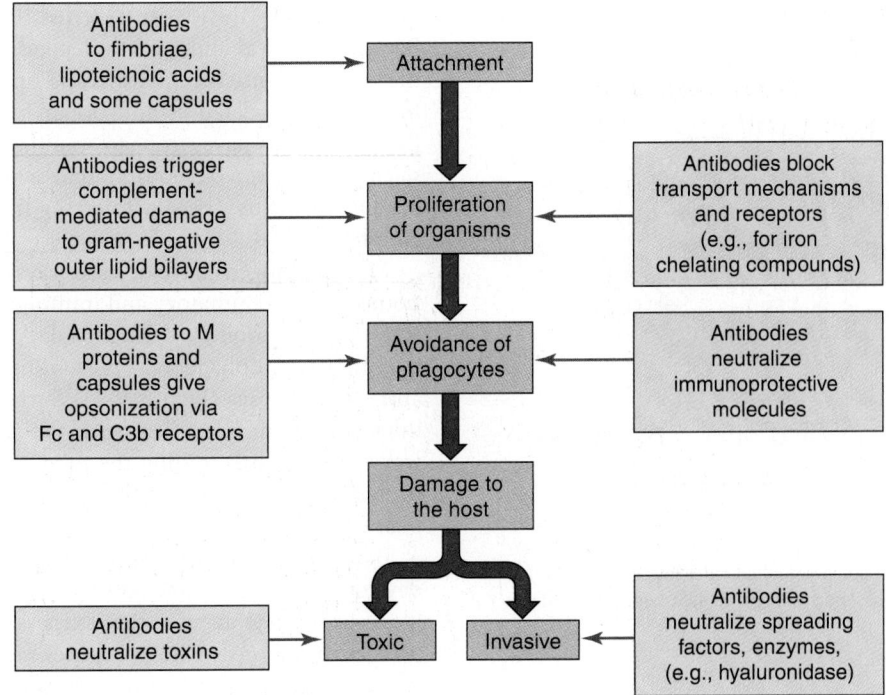

Foreign invaders: The body is constantly being bombarded by invading organisms, such as viruses, bacteria, and other microorganisms

① Scavenger cells such as neutrophils arrive early at the site of invasion but survive only a few days

② The complement system's circulating proteins attach to microbial invaders, leading to their destruction

③ Macrophages engulf foreign matter and signal other immune cells to attack invaders

④ Macrophages display antigens from ingested invaders, which activate helper T cells

Helper T cells

⑤ Helper T cells multiply and activate B cells and macrophages

B cell

⑥ B cells divide and form plasma cells, which produce antibodies

⑦ Antibodies bind to invaders, either destroying them or making them more vulnerable to macrophages

⑧ Killer T cells form and destroy foreign invaders

STOP

⑨ Regulatory T cells slow or stop the immune response once the foreign invader is defeated

⑩ Some B and T cells become *memory cells*, which can quickly mount a defense if the same foreign invader attacks again

Figure 9-2 **Biologic warfare.** A brief summary of the immune response. (Modified from Thibodeau GA, Patton KT: *Anatomy & physiology,* ed 5, St Louis, 2003, Mosby.)

Antibodies to fimbriae, lipoteichoic acids and some capsules → Attachment

Antibodies trigger complement-mediated damage to gram-negative outer lipid bilayers → Proliferation of organisms ← Antibodies block transport mechanisms and receptors (e.g., for iron chelating compounds)

Antibodies to M proteins and capsules give opsonization via Fc and C3b receptors → Avoidance of phagocytes ← Antibodies neutralize immunoprotective molecules

Damage to the host

Antibodies neutralize toxins → Toxic   Invasive ← Antibodies neutralize spreading factors, enzymes, (e.g., hyaluronidase)

Figure 9-3 **Role of antibodies in defense against bacteria.** This diagram presents the stages of bacterial invasion (red) and indicates the antibacterial effects of antibody (green) that operate at the different stages. (Redrawn from Roitt I, Brostoff J, Male D: *Immunology,* ed 6, St Louis, 2001, Mosby)

Table 9-5	Mechanisms by Which Microorganisms Fight Off the Immune System	
Organism	**Mechanism**	**Comment**
Bacteria		
Staphylococcus	Produces toxins	Either kills phagocytes or interferes with chemotaxis
Streptococcus		
Mycobacterium tuberculosis	Produces toxins	Prevents infusion of lysosomal granules and formation of phagolysosome
Toxoplasma gondii		
Mycobacteria	Produces enzymes that destroy oxygen metabolites (e.g., catalase, superoxide dismutase)	Prevents killing by O_2-dependent mechanisms
Brucella		
Salmonella typhi		
Neisseria gonorrhoeae	Produces a protease to digest IgA	Infects mucosal surface of urethra
Streptococcus pneumoniae	Produces a protease to digest IgA	Causes pneumonia
Haemophilus influenzae		
Staphylococcus	Produces surface molecules that mimic Fc receptors, which can bind antibody	Protects organism from successful activation of complement cascade and prevents antibody from functioning as an opsonin
Herpes simplex virus		
Group A streptococcus	Contains an antiphagocytic capsular antigen, M protein, that resembles human myocardial antigen	Certain people produce antibody against M protein that also reacts with cardiac tissue, resulting in rheumatic fever (carditis)
Mycoplasma pneumoniae	Expresses antigens similar to those found on human red blood cells	Antibodies also can react with human red blood cells
Viruses		
Influenza	Antigenic mutations ("drift") of antigen on a yearly basis	Immune response developed against previous year's strain is no longer protective
	Severe; virus undergoes antigenic "shift"; genetic recombination between human and avian strains of virus	Because new virus is now very distinct from those found in previous years, no protective immunity preexists, resulting in serous infection
Human immunodeficiency virus (HIV)	Can rapidly mutate its surface antigens	Antibodies produced early in disease will not react with antigens expressed later
Parasites		
Trypanosoma spp. (sleeping sickness)	Activates genes that produce different antigens on their surface	Avoids immune rejection because immune response is unable to identify parasite
Borrelia recurrentis (relapsing fever)		

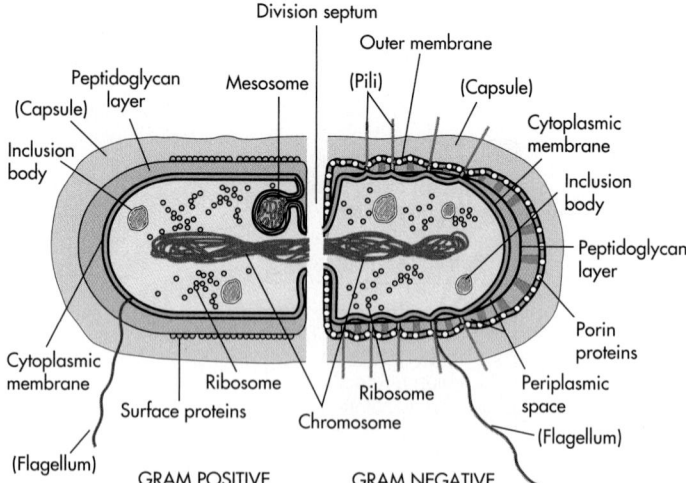

Figure 9-4 Gram-positive and gram-negative bacteria. A gram-positive bacterium has a thick layer of peptidoglycan *(left)*. A gram-negative bacterium has a thick peptidoglycan layer and an outer membrane *(right)*. (From Murray PR et al: *Medical microbiology*, ed 4, St Louis, 2002, Mosby.)

Bacterial Virulence and Infectivity

Bacterial survival and growth depend on the effectiveness of the body's defense mechanisms and on the bacterium's ability to resist those defenses and obtain nutrients and multiply. Bacteria must have iron to multiply, and some express *siderophores* (iron receptors) that acquire iron from iron-binding proteins (i.e., lactoferrin, transferrin, and hemoglobin).

Many pathogens have devised ways of preventing destruction by the inflammatory and immune systems. For example, some bacteria produce thick capsules of carbohydrate or protein that are antiphagocytic, preventing efficient opsonization and phagocytosis (Figure 9-4). Such coatings include the thick polysaccharide covering of the pneumococcus and the waxy capsule surrounding the tubercle bacillus. The long M protein on the cell wall of the streptococcus suppresses complement activation.

Because the primary immune response may take a week to develop adequately, some pathogens have developed the ability to proliferate at rates that surpass the development of a protective response. Cholera causes severe vomiting and watery diarrhea, has a 60% mortality rate, and develops within 2 to 3 days of ingestion of the bacteria. Norwalk virus and rotavirus, which cause severe diarrhea and vomiting, and *Bunyavirus* and *Hantavirus,* which cause hemorrhagic fever, have incubation periods of 24 to 48 hours. Some strains of toxin-producing group A streptococci cause destructive skin infections and pneumonia that may kill an individual within 2 days. Group B streptococci from the maternal vagina may ascend the birth canal, penetrate fetal membranes, and infect the fluid surrounding the fetus. The microorganism may have already established an active infection of the child's lungs by the time of birth, resulting in a pneumonia that is too advanced to be treated successfully by antibiotic therapy; this pneumonia has a 50% mortality rate in newborns.

Other bacteria survive and proliferate in the body by producing exotoxins and endotoxins that injure cells and tissues. **Exotoxins** are proteins released during bacterial growth. They are usually enzymes and have highly specific effects; they include cytotoxins, neurotoxins, pneumotoxins, enterotoxins, and hemolysins. Exotoxins can damage cell membranes, activate second messengers, and inhibit protein synthesis. Exotoxins are immunogenic and elicit the production of antibodies known as **antitoxins.** Consequently, vaccines are available for many of the exotoxins (i.e., tetanus, diphtheria, and pertussis). **Endotoxins** are **lipopolysaccharides (LPSs)** contained in the cell walls of gram-negative bacteria and released during lysis (or destruction) of the bacteria. Endotoxin also may be released from the membrane of the bacteria, either during bacterial growth or during treatment with antibiotics, which therefore cannot prevent the toxic effects of the endotoxin.[2,3] Bacteria that produce endotoxins are called *pyrogenic bacteria* because they activate the inflammatory process and produce fever. The innermost part of the lipo-

polysaccharide, *lipid A,* is made of polysaccharides and fatty acids and is responsible for the substance's toxic effects (Figure 9-5).

Inflammation is the body's initial response to the presence of the bacteria. Vascular permeability is increased, allowing blood-borne substances (i.e., the complement system) involved in bacterial destruction to access the site of infection. Endotoxins increase capillary permeability further by activating the anaphylotoxins (C5a and C3a) of the complement cascade. Capillary permeability may increase sufficiently to permit the escape of large volumes of plasma, contributing to hypotension and, in severe cases, cardiovascular shock (see Chapter 46). Endotoxin also can activate the coagulation cascade, leading to the syndrome of disseminated (or diffuse) intravascular coagulation (see Chapter 27).

The ability to produce immunologic hypersensitivity reactions is an important pathogenic mechanism of bacterial toxins. Tissue lesions of many chronic infections are related to the induction of hypersensitivity to the toxin or cell wall components. For example, *Mycobacterium tuberculosis* causes inflammatory chronic lesions known as *granulomas.*

Some bacteria alter antigens, initiating self-destructive (autoimmune) reactions. Other bacteria produce substances that immunologically "look like" (cross-react with) host proteins and cause the body to produce an autoimmune reaction against the cross-reactive antigen in normal tissues (see Chapter 8).

Bacteremia, or **septicemia,** is the presence of bacteria in the blood and is caused by a failure of the body's defense mechanisms. The usual cause is proliferation of gram-negative bacteria, although a few gram-positive bacteria and

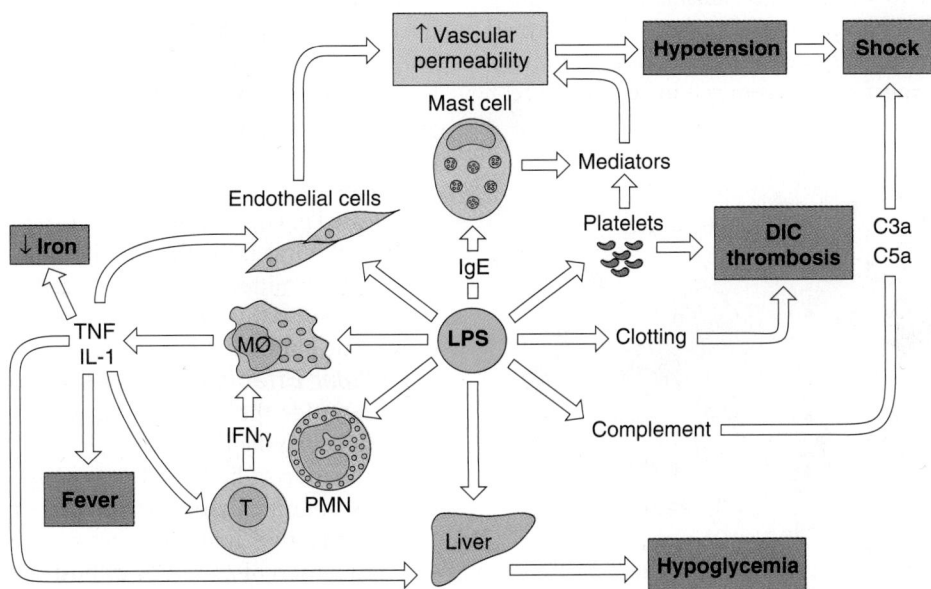

Figure 9-5 The many activities of lipopolysaccharide (LPS). Bacterial endotoxin (LPS) activates almost every immune mechanism, as well as the clotting pathway, which together make LPS one of the most powerful immune stimuli known. *IgE,* Immunoglobulin E; *DIC,* disseminated intravascular coagulation; *C3a, C5a,* complement components; *TNF,* tumor necrosis factor; *IL-1,* interleukin 1; *MØ,* macrophage; *IFNγ,* interferon-gamma; *PMN,* polymorphonuclear leukocyte; *T,* T cell. (From Mims CA et al: *Medical microbiology,* ed 3, London, 2004, Mosby.)

fungi can cause it. Symptoms of bacteremia are produced by endotoxins. Once in the blood, endotoxins cause the release of vasoactive peptides and cytokines that affect blood vessels, producing vasodilation, which reduces blood pressure, causes decreased oxygen delivery, and produces subsequent cardio-vascular shock (see Chapter 46). Bacteremia is diagnosed from evaluation of blood cultures.

Viral Infection and Injury

Viruses are obligate intracellular parasites and are entirely dependent on the host cell for replication. Viruses do not possess any of the metabolic organelles found in prokaryotes (e.g., bacteria) or eukaryotes (e.g., human cells). Unlike bacteria, viruses have no metabolism and are incapable of independent reproduction. Viral replication depends totally on their ability to infect a **permissive host cell**—a cell that cannot resist viral invasion and replication. Infection begins when a virion binds to receptors on the plasma membrane of a host cell (*attachment*) (Figure 9-6). The specificity of the virus for these receptors and the distribution of receptors throughout the host's tissues dictate the range of host cells that a particular virus can infect. Once bound, the virion penetrates the plasma membrane by receptor-mediated endocytosis, by envelope fusion with the plasma membrane, or by directly crossing the plasma membrane.

Viruses proliferate within cells by taking over the metabolic machinery of host cells and using it for their own survival and replication. Viral diseases are the most common afflictions of humans and include the common cold, the "cold sore" of herpes simplex, several forms of hepatitis, human immunodeficiency virus (HIV), and several types of cancer.

Viruses do not produce exotoxins or endotoxins. Viral pathogens bypass many defense mechanisms by developing intracellularly, thus hiding within cells and away from normal inflammatory or immune responses. In many cases, however, because viral agents must spread from cell to cell, the developing immune response eventually cures the infection so the disease is usually self-limiting. Some viruses, however, can rapidly produce irreversible and lethal injury in highly susceptible cells in an immunosuppressed host. If a symbiotic relationship is maintained between the host cell and the virus, persistent unapparent infection may result. Cell injury does not occur, and the virus persists until it is activated to replicate (e.g., the cold sores of herpesvirus infection). Immunity may protect the individual from an acute exacerbation only or may be sufficiently strong to prevent disease.

Viral Replication

Viruses contain their genetic information in either DNA or ribonucleic acid (RNA), either of which can be single stranded (ss) or double stranded (ds), and thus are known as DNA or RNA viruses. All viruses have a protein receptor binding site on their surface that adheres to specific binding sites on the host cell. For example, HIV has a glycoprotein (gp120) that attaches to CD4 antigen expressed on helper T cells, monocytes, and microglia. After penetration, the virus *uncoats* the protective nucleocapsid and releases viral genetic information into the cytoplasm. Most RNA viruses directly produce messenger RNA (mRNA), which is translated into viral proteins, and genomic RNA, which is eventually packaged into new viruses. One particular family of viruses, retroviruses (of which HIV is an example), carries an enzyme *reverse transcriptase* that creates a double-stranded DNA version of the virus. The DNA "provirus" enters the cell's nucleus, where it becomes integrated into the host cell's chromosomal DNA. DNA viruses also enter the nucleus and are transcribed into messenger RNA before protein translation. Some DNA viruses also may integrate into the host's chromosomal DNA.

The translation of viral-specific mRNA results in the production of viral proteins that self-assemble from viral genetic information. New virions then are released from the cell for transmission of the viral infection to other host cells. Enveloped viruses are released through *budding,* in which viral particles are shed enveloped in plasma membrane from the surface of the infected cell. Nonenveloped viruses commonly are released in large numbers concurrent with the destruction of the cell. Viral DNA that has become integrated with host DNA is transmitted to the host's daughter cells during host cell mitosis. By this process, viral genes can become part of the genetic information of the host cell and its progeny.

Cellular Effects of Viruses

Once inside the host cell, viruses have many harmful effects, including the following:

- Inhibition of host cell DNA, RNA, or protein synthesis
- Disruption of lysosomal membranes, resulting in release of "digestive" lysosomal enzymes that can kill the cell
- Promotion of apoptosis of host cell
- Fusion of infected, adjacent host cells, thereby producing multinucleated giant cells
- Alteration of the antigenic properties, or "identity," of the host cell, causing the host's immune system to attack the cell as if it were foreign

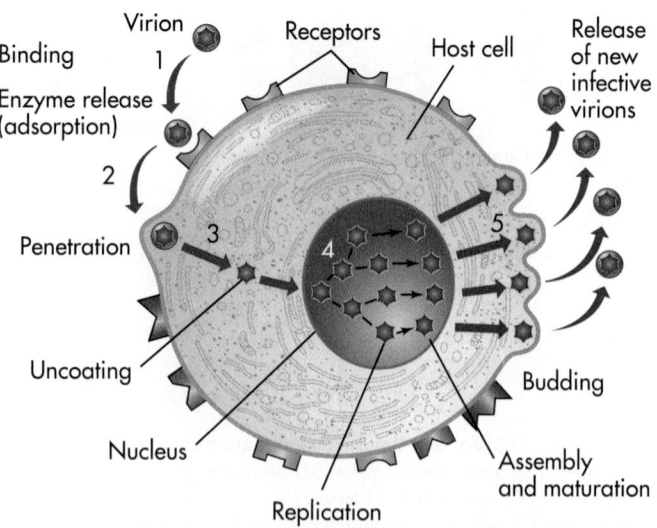

Figure 9-6 Stages of viral infection of a host cell.

- Transformation of host cells into cancerous cells, resulting in uninhibited and unregulated growth
- Promotion of secondary bacterial infection in tissues or organs damaged by viruses

Examples of human diseases caused by specific viruses are listed in Table 9-6.

Fungal Infection and Injury

Fungi (*sing.,* fungus) are relatively large microorganisms with thick walls that grow as either single-celled yeasts (spheres) or multicelled molds (filaments or hyphae) (Figure 9-7). Some fungi can exist in either form and are called **dimorphic.** The cell walls of fungi are rigid and multilayered. The wall is composed of polysaccharides different from the peptidoglycans of bacteria. The lack of peptidoglycans allows fungi to resist the action of bacterial cell wall inhibitors such as penicillin and cephalosporin. In contrast to bacteria, the cytosol of fungi contain organelles: mitochondria, ribosomes, Golgi apparatus, microtubules, microvesicles, endoplasmic reticulum, and nuclei. Molds are aerobic, and yeasts are facultative anaerobes. They usually reproduce by simple division or budding.

Pathologic fungi cause disease by adapting to the host environment. Fungi that colonize the skin can digest keratin. Other fungi can grow with wide temperature variations in lower oxygen environments. Still other fungi have the capacity to suppress host immune defenses. Phagocytes and T lymphocytes are important in controlling fungi, and low white blood cell counts promote fungal infection. Fungi have two basic structures: hyphae and yeasts. Hyphae have branching, tubular filaments. Yeasts are singular spherical cells.

Diseases caused by fungi are called **mycoses.** Mycoses (*sing.,* mycosis) can be superficial, deep, or opportunistic. Superficial mycoses occur on or near skin or mucous membranes and usually produce mild and superficial disease. Fungi that invade the skin, hair, or nails are known as **dermatophytes.** The diseases they produce are called *tineas* (ringworm), for example, tinea capitis (scalp), tinea pedis (feet), and tinea cruris (groin). Superficial dermatophytes grow in a ringlike, erythematous patch with a raised border. Itching often is intense, and cracking of tissue can occur and lead to secondary bacterial infection. Infections of the scalp are accompanied by scaling and hair loss. (Chapter 44 discusses the various skin disorders caused by fungi.)

Table 9-6	Human Diseases Caused by Specific Viruses
Virus	**Pathophysiologic Effects**
Papovaviruses (DNA) (papilloma)	Small viruses that induce tumors and cancers in animals, warts (papilloma) in humans
Adenoviruses (DNA)	Medium-sized viruses that cause various respiratory infections in humans; some cause tumors in animals
Herpesviruses (DNA) herpes simplex, herpes zoster)	Medium-sized viruses that cause various diseases in humans, such as fever blisters, chickenpox, shingles, and infectious mononucleosis; implicated in a type of human cancer called *Burkitt lymphoma*
Poxvirus (DNA) (variola, cowpox, vaccinia)	Very large, complex, brick-shaped viruses that cause diseases such as smallpox (variola), molluscum contagiosum (wartlike skin lesions), cowpox, and vaccinia; vaccinia virus gives immunity to smallpox
Hepatitis B (DNA)	Widespread throughout the world; blood and blood products are the best-documented routes for transmission; causes liver damage; may lead to liver cancer
Filoviruses (RNA)	Highly lethal human virus associated with outbreaks in Africa (e.g., Marburg and Ebola viruses)
Flavivirus (RNA)	Anthropod-borne viruses: West Nile, dengue, hemorrhagic fever, yellow fever, and hepatitis C viruses
Hantavirus (RNA)	Transmitted by infected rodent droppings; found in rural areas of the United States (i.e., *Hantavirus* pulmonary syndrome)
Picornaviruses (RNA) (poliovirus, rhinovirus)	Smallest RNA-containing viruses; at least 70 human enteroviruses are known, including the polio virus, coxsackie virus, and echovirus; more than 100 rhinoviruses exist and are the most common cause of colds
Myxoviruses (RNA) (influenza A, B, C)	Medium-sized viruses with a spiked envelope; able to agglutinate red blood cells; cause influenza
Paramyxoviruses (RNA) (measles, mumps)	Structurally similar to myxoviruses but generally larger; cause parainfluenza, measles, mumps
Coronaviruses (RNA)	Associated with upper respiratory tract infections and the common cold; causes severe acute respiratory syndrome (SARS)
Retroviruses (RNA)	Tumor-associated viruses; cause leukemia and tumors in animals; some members produce "slow" viral infections; cause of AIDS
Arenaviruses (RNA) (lassa)	Possess RNA-containing granules; some members produce "slow" viral infections in humans
Reoviruses (RNA)	Relation to human disease not clear; may be involved in mild respiratory infections and infantile gastroenteritis—diarrhea (rotavirus)
Hepatitis A (RNA)	Isolated from chimpanzees; known to be transmitted by humans by close person-to-person contact

DNA, Deoxyribonucleic acid; *RNA,* ribonucleic acid; *AIDS,* acquired immunodeficiency syndrome.

Deep infections involving internal organs can be life threatening and are most common in association with other diseases or as an opportunistic infection in immunosuppressed individuals. Fungi causing deep infection enter the body through inhalation or through open wounds. Filamentous forms can multiply extracellularly, but the spherical yeasts multiply within cells, including white blood cells. Some fungi are a part of the normal body flora and become pathologic only when immunity is compromised, allowing exaggerated growth and translocation. For example, *Candida albicans* is normally found in the mouth, gastrointestinal tract, and vagina of normal individuals. Changes in pH and use of antibiotics that kill bacteria that normally inhibit *Candida* growth permit rapid proliferation and overgrowth, which can lead to superficial or deep infection. Common pathologic fungi are summarized in Table 9-7.

Fungi are diagnosed by microscopic observation of specimens treated with potassium hydroxide and stained to enhance visualization of spheres and filaments. Specimens also can be cultured. Skin tests are available for species of *Aspergillus*. No vaccines are available to treat fungal disease. Many of the antifungal drugs (e.g., amphotericin B, ketoconazole, fluconazole) used to treat deep or systemic infection are toxic to the host because the fungal cell composition is similar to the host cell. They also can produce significant drug interactions.

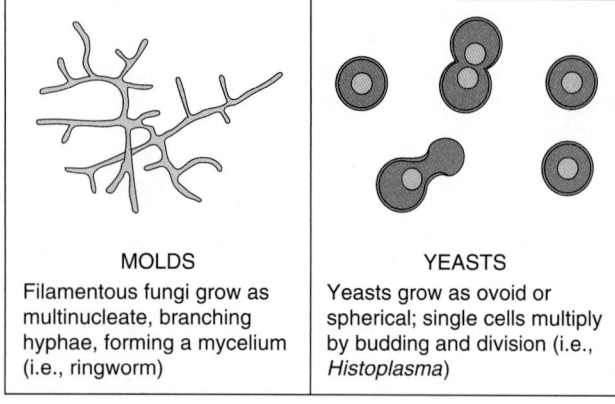

MOLDS	YEASTS
Filamentous fungi grow as multinucleate, branching hyphae, forming a mycelium (i.e., ringworm)	Yeasts grow as ovoid or spherical; single cells multiply by budding and division (i.e., *Histoplasma*)

Figure 9-7 Types of fungi. (From Mims CA et al: *Medical microbiology,* ed 3, London, 2004, Mosby.)

CLINICAL MANIFESTATIONS OF INFECTIOUS DISEASE

The progression from infection to disease follows predictable stages (Figure 9-8). Clinical manifestations of infectious disease vary, depending on the pathogen, the organ system affected, and the severity. Effects of infection may be acute, chronic, related to immune responses, or a consequence of bacterial toxins. Manifestations can arise directly from the infecting microorganism or its products; however, the majority of manifestations result from the host's inflammatory and immune responses. Infectious diseases typically begin with the nonspecific or general symptoms of fatigue, malaise, weakness, and loss of concentration. Generalized aching and loss of appetite are common complaints. However, the hallmark of most infectious diseases is fever.

Fever is not failure of the body to regulate temperature; rather, body temperature is being regulated at a higher level than normal. Body temperature is regulated by nervous system feedback to the hypothalamus, which functions as a central thermostat. A large number of agents (pyrogens) can produce fever. In current classification, those pyrogens derived from outside the host are termed **exogenous pyrogens** and those produced by the host are termed **endogenous pyrogens.** There is little evidence that exogenous pyrogens cause fever directly. Available data favor an indirect effect of such pyrogens on the hypothalamus that is mediated by endogenous pyrogen (EP) released by cells of the host.[4] A number of hormone-like mediators (cytokines) in cellular and immunologic adaptations have been identified as endogenous pyrogens. They are interleukins 1 and 6 (IL-1 and IL-6), interferon (IFN), tumor necrosis factor (TNF), and other cytokines.[4] The mechanism by which these cytokines raise the thermoregulatory set point seems to be through stimulation of prostaglandin synthesis and turnover in both thermoregulatory (brain) and nonthermoregulatory (peripheral) tissue. These mechanisms are discussed in detail in Chapter 14. Although it is generally believed that fever has a beneficial value in infection, the molecular mechanism behind the beneficial effects has not been established. Many investigators, however, consider fever as an adaptive host-defense response.

Table 9-7	Common Pathogenic Fungi		
Fungus	**Growth Form**	**Entry**	**Disease**
Superficial Dermatophytes			
Microsporum and *Epidermophyton*	Filament	Skin contact	Ringworm, jock itch, athlete's foot
Malassezia furfur	Sphere	Skin contact	Tinea versicolor
Deep			
Pneumocystis carinii	Sphere	Inhalation	Pneumonia
Histoplasma capsulatum	Sphere	Inhalation	Histoplasmosis
Aspergillus fumigatus	Filament	Inhalation	Aspergillosis and pneumonia
Coccidioides immitis	Unusual form	Inhalation	Coccidiodomycosis
Candida albicans	Sphere	Normal flora of skin, mouth, intestine	Thrush, vaginal yeast infections, systemic infections

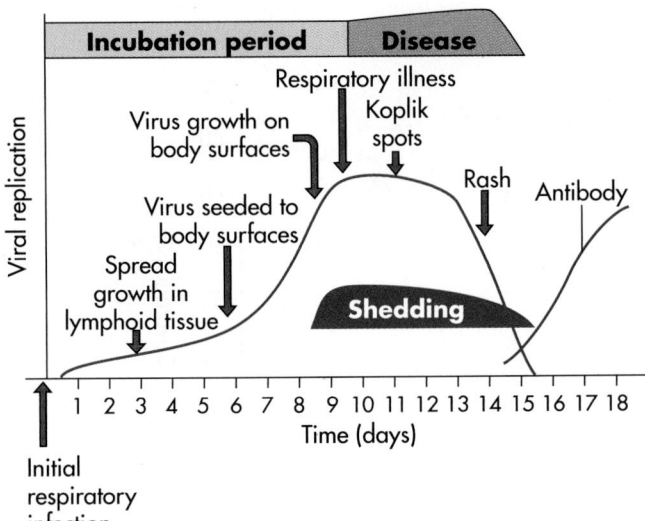

Figure 9-8 Pathogenesis of measles.

Recently recognized is the role played by TNF (cachectin) in the pathogenesis of endotoxic shock.[5] TNF is a cytokine produced by activated macrophages (e.g., large phagocytic cells) as a consequence of exposure to endotoxin (see Figure 9-5). It is sometimes called *cachectin* because of its role in promoting cachexia in individuals with cancer. (Cachexia is discussed in Chapter 11 [p. 387]; cytokines are discussed in Chapters 6 and 7.)

COUNTERMEASURES AGAINST PATHOGENS: VACCINES AND ANTIMICROBIALS

The body's innate and innovative responses against microorganisms are numerous and generally involve an interaction between the immune and inflammatory systems. Prophylactic or interventive procedures also have been developed by healthcare providers to prevent the pathogen from initiating disease (vaccines) or to destroy the pathogen once the disease process has started (antimicrobials). Most vaccine development has focused on preventing the most severe and common infections. With the initial success of antibiotic therapy, there was no perceived need for vaccination against many common and non–life-threatening infections. The more recent increasing problem of antibiotic-resistant pathogens, however, has forced a reappraisal of that strategy, and a greater emphasis now is being placed on the development of new vaccines.

Vaccines

The purpose of **vaccination** is to induce long-lasting protective immune responses under conditions that will not result in disease in a healthy recipient of the **vaccine.** The primary immune response from vaccination is generally short-lived; therefore booster injections are used to push the immune response through multiple secondary responses resulting in large numbers of memory cells and sustained protective levels of antibody or T cells, or both.

Development of a successful vaccine is costly and depends on several factors. These include identification of the protective immune response and the appropriate antigen to induce that response. For instance, patients with ongoing HIV infection produce a great deal of antibody against several HIV antigens. But, for development of a successful vaccine, we must first understand which antibody will protect against an initial infection.

Once a good candidate antigen is identified, it must be developed into an effective, cost-efficient, stable, and safe vaccine. For instance, most vaccines against viral infection (measles, mumps, rubella, varicella [chickenpox]) contain live viruses that are weakened (attenuated) so they continue to express appropriate antigens but establish only a limited and easily controlled infection. For most common vaccines against viral infections, limited replication of the virus appears to afford better long-term protection than using purified viral antigen. One current exception is the hepatitis B vaccine, which uses a recombinant viral protein. The hepatitis A vaccine is an inactivated (killed) virus and normally should not cause an infection.

Even attenuated viruses can, however, establish life-threatening infections in individuals whose immune system is congenitally deficient or suppressed (see Chapter 8). The risk of infection by the vaccine strain of virus is extremely small, but it may affect the choice of recommended vaccines. For instance, two different vaccines were developed against polio. The Sabin vaccine was an attenuated virus that was administered orally. It provided systemic protection and also induced a secretory immune response to prevent growth of the poliovirus in the intestinal tract. Being a live virus, the vaccine could cause polio in some children who had unsuspected immune deficiencies (about 1 case in 2.4 million doses). The Salk vaccine was a completely inactivated virus administered by injection. It induced protective systemic immunity, but did not provide adequate secretory immunity. Therefore, even if the individual was protected from systemic infection the "wild-type" poliovirus could transiently infect their intestinal mucosa, be shed, and spread to others. When polio was epidemic, the oral vaccine was preferred. Vaccination has been extremely effective: 2525 cases of paralytic polio were reported in the United States in 1960, 61 cases were reported in 1965, and no cases of polio due to the wild-type virus have been contracted in the United States since 1979. In 1994, the disease polio was declared officially eradicated in all the Americas. The goal of the World Health Organization (WHO) is to eradicate polio worldwide in the next few years (Figure 9-9). However, the live attenuated vaccine itself caused about 8 cases of paralytic polio per year in the United States in individuals with inadequate immune systems. As a result, the CDC currently recommends vaccination with the killed virus.

Some common bacterial vaccines are killed organisms or extracts of bacterial antigens. The vaccine against pneumococcal pneumonia consists of a mixture of capsular polysaccharides from 10 strains of *Streptococcus pneumoniae*. Of the

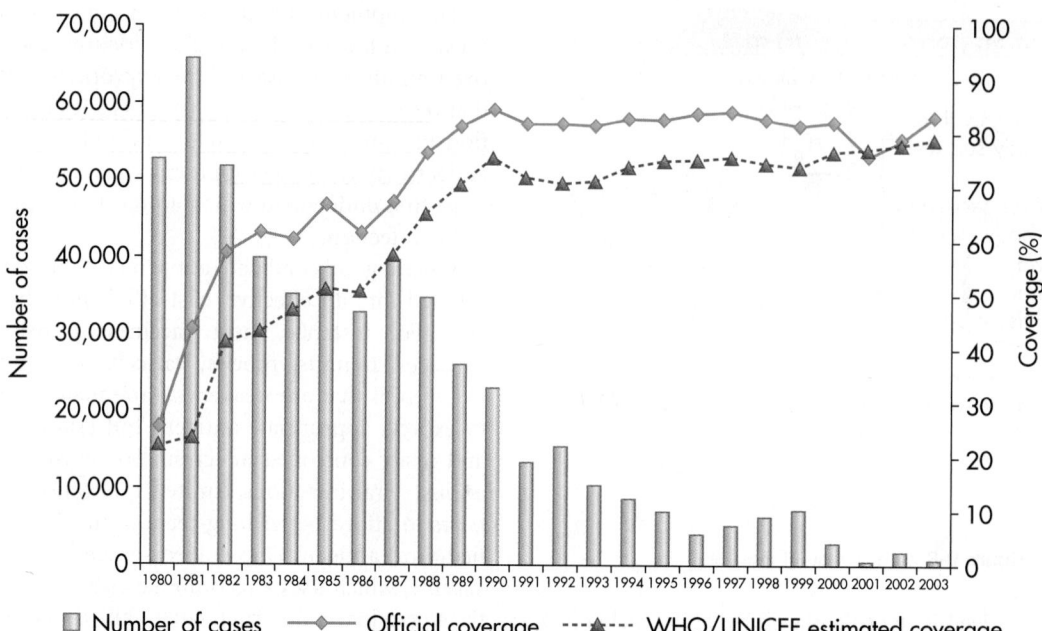

Figure 9-9 The global reported cases of polio and immunization coverage, 1980-2003. The number of global cases of polio has progressively decreased in an inverse relationship to the extent of vaccination. The "official coverage" is the percent of the world's population that has been reported to the World Health Organization (WHO) by 192 member countries as being immunized. The "WHO/UNICEF estimated coverage" indicates the best estimate of the real percentage of the population that has been immunized. (From World Health Organization: *WHO vaccine-preventable diseases: monitoring system, 2003 global summary*, Geneva, Switzerland, 2003. Additional information is available at www.who.int/vaccines-documents/.)

more than 90 known strains of this organism, only these 10 cause the most severe illnesses. However, the capsular vaccine is not very immunogenic in young children. A "conjugated" vaccine is available that contains capsular polysaccharides from 7 strains that are conjugated to carrier proteins in order to increase immunogenicity. A similar vaccine is available for *Haemophilus influenzae* type b (Hib).

Some bacterial pathogens are not invasive, but do colonize mucosal membranes or wounds and release potent toxins that act locally or systemically. These include the bacteria that cause diphtheria, cholera, and tetanus. Vaccination against systemic toxins (e.g., diphtheria, tetanus) has been achieved using **toxoids**—purified toxins that have been chemically detoxified without loss of immunogenicity. Recently, pertussis (whooping cough) vaccine has been changed from a killed whole cell vaccine to an acellular vaccine that contains the pertussis toxin and additional bacterial antigens. This change has dramatically reduced adverse side effects (fever, local inflammatory reactions, and others).

Additional difficulties associated with vaccination include allergic reactions to the vaccine antigen itself or other components of the preparation. For instance, some viral vaccines are grown in chicken eggs and many elicit a reaction in individuals who are allergic to eggs. Recently the preservative thimerosal was removed from vaccines. Thimerosal is a mercury-containing compound that has been used as a preservative since the 1930s. Although no cases of mercury toxicity have been reported secondary to vaccination, it was recommended that thimerosal be removed from vaccines (also see Chapter 2).

A more common problem is compliance of the susceptible population. Depending on the organism, a certain percentage of the population should be immunized in order to achieve protection of the total population. If this level of immunization is not achieved, outbreaks of infection can occur. For instance, an effective measles vaccine was made available in 1963 and resulted in a dramatic decrease in the number of measles cases. Many parents became complacent and did not obtain measles vaccination for their preschool children. As a result, a large increase in the number of cases and deaths in 1989 and 1990 occurred, which initiated a reemphasis on complete immunization before children could start school. Even with successful development of a vaccine, however, a certain percentage of the population will be genetically unresponsive to vaccination and therefore will not produce a protective immune response. With most vaccines, the percentage of unresponsive individuals is low, and they will benefit from successful immunization of the rest of the population.

Many vaccines are used in the United States to protect against pathogens. The vaccines and their abbreviations, as noted in Tables 9-8 and 9-9, are as follows:

Hepatitis B virus: causes cirrhosis of the liver and liver cancer; the vaccine is a recombinant viral protein.

Haemophilus influenzae type b (Hib): a bacterial infection that is commonly contracted by children younger than 5 years and infects the blood, joints, bones, and membrane covering the heart; most common cause of serious bacterial meningitis in children; the vaccine is an extracted bacterial antigen conjugated to a protein carrier.

Polio: polio is a viral infection that causes paralysis and death; the vaccine is an inactivated virus.

Diphtheria (D): a bacterial infection of the throat; produces a toxin that can lead to heart failure or paralysis; the vaccine is an inactivated form of diphtheria toxin (toxoid); part of DTaP combined vaccine.

Tetanus (T): a bacterial infection that produces a toxin that attacks the nervous system and may cause death; the vaccine is an inactivated form of the tetanus toxin (toxoid); part of DTaP combined vaccine.

Pertussis (acellular pertussis [aP]), or whooping cough: a bacterial infection that causes severe coughing in children younger than 5 years; the vaccine is an inactivated toxin and other bacterial antigens; part of DTaP combined vaccine..

Pneumococcal: *Streptococcus pneumoniae* is a bacteria that causes pneumonia, particularly in the elderly; the childhood vaccine is a protein conjugate with 7 different capsular antigens; the adult vaccine is a mixture of 10 extracted capsular polysaccharides.

Measles and mumps (MM): viruses that cause fever and rash (measles) or inflammation of the salivary glands (mumps); mumps also may cause meningitis; both vaccines are attenuated live viruses; part of MMR combined vaccine.

Rubella (R), or German measles: a viral infection that causes fever and rash; may cause severe birth defects in pregnant women infected in the first trimester; part of MMR combined vaccine.

Varicella-zoster (Varicella): a virus that causes chickenpox; vaccine is an attenuated live virus.

Influenza: a virus that causes severe upper respiratory tract infections; the most common vaccine is an injected inactivated virus.

Hepatitis A virus: a virus that causes liver disease; recommended in selected states and regions; vaccine is an inactivated virus.

Meningococcal: *Neisseria meningitides* is a major bacterial cause of meningitis, particularly in young adults; the vaccine contains four different extracted capsular polysaccharides.

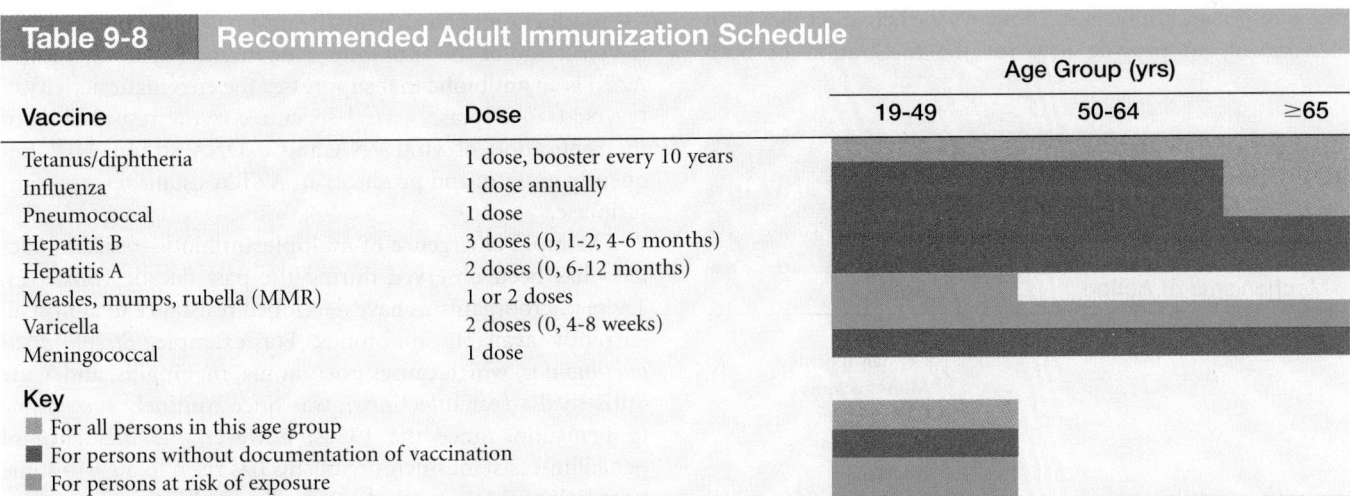

Table 9-8   Recommended Adult Immunization Schedule

Vaccine	Dose	Age Group (yrs)		
		19-49	50-64	≥65
Tetanus/diphtheria	1 dose, booster every 10 years			
Influenza	1 dose annually			
Pneumococcal	1 dose			
Hepatitis B	3 doses (0, 1-2, 4-6 months)			
Hepatitis A	2 doses (0, 6-12 months)			
Measles, mumps, rubella (MMR)	1 or 2 doses			
Varicella	2 doses (0, 4-8 weeks)			
Meningococcal	1 dose			

Key

- For all persons in this age group
- For persons without documentation of vaccination
- For persons at risk of exposure

Modified from Recommended Adult Immunization Schedule, United States, October 2004–September 2005: The Advisory Committee on Immunization Practices, Department of Health and Human Services, CDC; for additional information see www.cdc.gov/nip

Table 9-9   Recommended Childhood Immunization Schedule

Vaccine	Birth	1 mo	2 mo	4 mo	6 mo	12 mo	15 mo	18 mo	24 mo	4-6 yr
Hepatitis B	1		2			3				
Hib			1	2	3	4				
Polio			1	2		3				4
DTaP			1	2	3		4			
Pneumococcal			1	2	3	4				
MMR						1				2
Varicella						1				
Influenza								yearly		
Hepatitis A	2 doses; ≥6 m apart; children over 2 yr; selected populations									1

Modified from Recommended Childhood and Adolescent Immunization Schedule, United States, 2005: Department of Health and Human Services, CDC, for additional information see www.cdc.gov/nip

Antimicrobials

Since World War II, antibiotics have had the greatest impact on successful resistance to infection. Antibiotics are natural products of fungi, bacteria, and related microorganisms and kill or inhibit the growth of other microorganisms. Numerous chemicals or antimicrobials have been identified that either prevent the growth of microorganisms or directly destroy them (Table 9-10). Antibiotics generally act by preventing the function of enzymes or cell structures that are unique to the infecting agent. Because viruses use the enzymes of the host's cells, there has been far less success in developing antiviral antibiotics.

Recent Pathogenic Adaptations

Recently, disease-causing microbial microorganisms have emerged that have developed mechanisms for circumventing the most modern techniques for destroying or controlling infection, including microorganisms that attack the immune system (HIV) and those that are resistant to multiple antibiotics (e.g., *Mycobacterium tuberculosis*).

HIV is one of the few microorganisms that directly attacks the central processes involved in the development of an immune response. It infects and destroys the helper T cell, which is necessary to provide help for the maturation of both plasma cells and cytotoxic T cells. Therefore HIV suppresses the immune response against itself and, secondarily, creates a generalized immune deficiency by suppressing the development of immune responses against other pathogens and opportunistic microorganisms.

The development of vaccines against HIV has been frustrating because of the large number of changing antigens expressed on the viral surface. HIV also can infect by way of intercellular fusion between an infected cell in transmitted body fluids and uninfected cells near the mucosal surface. During this mechanism of infection, the virus may remain sequestered in the cell and be resistant to a vaccine-induced immune response.

Since the development of antibiotics, sensitive microorganisms have mutated and developed resistance to particular antibiotics. Resistance occurs primarily through inactivation of the drug, alteration of the bacterial membrane that prevents the antibiotic from being taken up, alteration of the target molecule, reduced uptake of the antibiotic, or active efflux of the antibiotic. These changes are generally genetic mutations and can be transmitted directly to neighboring microorganisms. Penicillin resistance, for example, results from the production of an enzyme (β-lactamase) that breaks down the structure of the antibiotic. Zidovudine (Azidothymidine, AZT) is an antibiotic that suppresses the enzymatic activity of reverse transcriptase, a viral-specific enzyme responsible for the replication of viral RNA and a DNA strand. HIV frequently mutates and produces an AZT-resistant reverse transcriptase.

The rapid emergence of multiple antibiotic–resistant bacteria has been observed during the past decade (Box 9-2). These microorganisms have developed resistance to almost all currently available antibiotics. For example, *Streptococcus pneumoniae,* which causes pneumonia, meningitis, and acute otitis media (ear infections), was once routinely susceptible to penicillin. Since the 1980s, however, the incidence of penicillin-resistant microorganisms has risen to 30% in some populations. Many of these are resistant also to multiple antibiotics. In some areas, almost 20% of tuberculosis cases are caused by multiple antibiotic–resistant *M. tuberculosis.* Also, the incidence of drug-resistant gonorrhea, malaria, pneumococcal disease, salmonellosis, shigellosis, and staphylococcal infections has increased dramatically.

Why have multiple antibiotic–resistant microorganisms appeared? Overuse of antibiotics can lead to the destruction of the normal flora, allowing the selective overgrowth of antibiotic-resistant strains or pathogens that had previously been kept under control. For example, after treatment with the antibiotic clindamycin, the normal intestinal flora can become compromised, allowing the overgrowth of *Clostridium difficile* and the development of pseudomembranous colitis. Also, individuals commonly do not comply with the instructions of healthcare providers concerning the necessity of completing the therapeutic regimen with antibiotics. This practice allows the selective resurgence of microorganisms that are more relatively resistant to the antibiotic.

Table 9-10	Examples of Chemicals or Antimicrobials that Prevent Growth of or Destroy Microorganisms	
Mechanisms of Action	**Agent**
Inhibits synthesis of cell wall	Penicillins
	Cephalosporins
	Monobactams
	Carbapenems
	Vancomycin
	Bacitracin
	Cycloserine
	Fosfomycin
Damages cytoplasmic membrane	Polymyxins
	Polyene antifungals
	Imidazoles
Alters metabolism of nucleic acid	Quinolones
	Rifampin
	Nitrofurans
	Nitroimidazoles
	Trobicin
Inhibits protein synthesis	Aminoglycosides
	Tetracyclines
	Chloramphenicol
	Macrolides
	Clindamycin
	Spectinomycin
	Mupirocin
Modifies energy metabolism	Sulfonamides
	Trimethoprim
	Dapsone
	Isoniazid

Box 9-2   Antimicrobial Resistance

Resistance to antimicrobial agents has been recognized for more than 50 years and continues to be a major cause of increased morbidity, mortality, and healthcare cost. Contributing factors include overuse of antibiotics, poor implementation of infection control measures, prolonged hospitalization, admission to intensive care units, and the use of invasive procedures.

The goal of antimicrobial therapy is to eliminate the pathogen by killing or inhibiting the bacteria. Body defenses are required for killing any remaining bacteria. Generally, antimicrobials target four cellular processes: (1) cell wall formation and maintenance, (2) protein synthesis, (3) DNA replication, and (4) folic acid metabolism. Pathogens have developed resistance for all four of these targets.

The mechanisms of resistance used by pathogens generally fall into one of three categories: (1) enzymatic inactivation of the antimicrobial (e.g., beta lactamase), (2) prevention of intracellular accumulation by active efflux of the antimicrobial (e.g., multidrug transporters are very effective in gram-negative bacteria), and (3) modification of the target site (e.g., a gene mutation) to which agents bind to exert an antimicrobial effect. Modifying the dosage regimen (e.g., using high-dose therapy) overcomes resistance to some agents or inhibits the resistance mechanism (e.g., beta-lactamase inhibitors). Other mechanisms of resistance can be overcome only by using an agent from a different class of antibiotics.

Data from Hujer AM et al: *Clin Lab Med* 24(2):343-361, 2004; Jacobs MR: *Pediatr Infect Dis J* 22(8 Suppl):S109-S119, 2003; Jacobs MR, Anon J, Appelbaum PC:, *Clin Lab Med* 24(2):419-453, 2004.

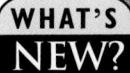

WHAT'S NEW?   Emerging Infections

In the mid-1970s many microbiologists and physicians believed that infectious disease was on the verge of being controlled as a major cause of death in the United States. That belief was based on the success of public health initiatives, vaccination programs, and the use of antibiotics. Smallpox had been eradicated from the globe (the last reported case was in 1975 in Somalia), measles was almost eradicated in the Western Hemisphere, and many diseases, such as tuberculosis and polio, were on the decline.

Since that time, however, the trend has been reversed completely. Death caused by infection in the United States rose by 58% between 1980 and 1992. Infection is the third leading cause of death in the United States after heart disease and cancer (although many individuals with cancer die of infection) and is the leading cause of death worldwide.

The reversal has occurred because of the emergence of previously unknown infections, the reemergence of old infections that were thought to be under control, and the development of infectious agents that are resistant to multiple antibiotics. The causes for this occurrence are numerous and include the following:

- Vast and rapid urbanization in many areas of the world, resulting in a breakdown in public health programs and a more rapid spread of infection
- Global travel, allowing more rapid spread of disease from isolated areas to virtually any point around the world in a few hours
- Globalization of the food supply
- Human encroachment into wilderness areas, resulting in contact with previously sequestered infectious agents
- Antibiotics that are prescribed excessively, that are not taken for a complete course of therapy, or that, even when appropriately used, result in the selection of antibiotic-resistant microorganisms
- Decreases in federal research budgets to study infectious disease
- Denial of a problem by governments, allowing infections to spread in an uncontrolled way
- Increased global warming, allowing insect vectors to spread into and breed in areas that were previously too cool for them

The emergence of previously unknown infections is not a new event. Since 1973, however, more than 40 previously unknown infections have arisen, including Lyme disease (1975), Ebola virus (1976), legionnaires disease (1978), toxic shock syndrome (1978), acquired immune deficiency syndrome (AIDS) (1981), chronic-fatigue syndrome (1985), hepatitis C virus (1989), hepatitis E virus, (1990), *Hantavirus* (1993), severe acute respiratory syndrome (SARS) (2002), and vancomycin-resistant *Staphylococcus aureus* (2002).

Concurrently, the incidence and spread of at least 20 well-known infections are increasing. A new strain of cholera that arose in Indonesia in 1961 has spread to Africa and in 1991 to South America. Malaria, dengue fever, and yellow fever are reemerging in areas where they had been eliminated or were unknown. The incidence of tuberculosis is increasing in countries that had reported declines and has risen by almost one third between the mid-1980s and early 1990s. Diphtheria has reemerged as a major health issue in Russia. In 1994 plague was reported in India after being dormant for a generation. The outbreak of SARS spread quickly through Southeast Asia to Toronto, Canada, in 2003.

Many common and reemerging infections (e.g., tuberculosis, malaria) have become antibiotic and drug resistant. *Streptococcus pneumoniae,* a common cause of otitis media, pneumonia, and bacteremia, has been treated routinely and successfully with penicillin. Now at least 25% of isolates are penicillin resistant, and some are resistant to multiple antibiotics. Multiple antibiotic–resistant forms of *Staphylococcus aureus,* a primary cause of infections of wounds, surgical incisions, and catheters, are endemic in some hospitals. Some forms of this microorganism once were sensitive only to a single antibiotic, vancomycin, and now have become vancomycin-resistant.

Bioterrorist agents, such as small pox, anthrax, and plague, are continuing threats to public health and safety. All healthcare providers should have information about the characteristics and clinical manifestations of these biologic agents.

Future of Infection Control Measures

With the development of multiple antibiotic–resistant strains, creativity in addressing this infection challenge must be rekindled. Currently available antibiotics that prove to be no longer effective must be replaced with alternative forms of therapy. New antibiotics may solve a portion of the problem or may exacerbate it further. It may be that pathogens would simply develop resistance to new antibiotics as well.

Other forms of therapy may involve the immune system. If an immune response would result in resolution of the infection, use of passive immunotherapy, in which preformed antibodies are given to the individual, may be the answer. This form of therapy has been used for decades. Horse serum–containing antibodies were given to treat diphtheria, pneumococcal pneumonia, tetanus, and other diseases in the early twentieth century. However, because of foreign proteins in the serum, many individuals developed an immune reaction against the horse proteins and an immune complex–mediated serum sickness. Passive immunotherapy has been improved by the use of purified human immunoglobulins. Individuals with an immune deficiency of B cells currently are given intravenous immunoglobulin containing various antibodies against most infectious diseases (see Chapter 8). Several diseases in persons with intact immune systems have been treated by the administration of human immunoglobulin preparations, including (1) prophylactic administration to prevent hepatitis A in travelers who will enter a region in which the virus is endemic and (2) therapeutic administration to treat hepatitis B and rabies. Recurrent administration of these preparations generally confers passive resistance to most common bacterial and viral infections. More specific therapy with monoclonal antibodies is being evaluated that would be targeted against neonatal infections with the group B streptococci and against gram-negative bacteria that cause septic shock.

Vaccines induce an active immunoprophylaxis in which the individual produces protective antibodies or T cells. In the past, vaccines were developed for only the most deadly pathogens. Now the development and widespread use of vaccines against common antibiotic-resistant microorganisms must be considered. For example, otitis media, a purulent ear infection, is caused primarily by *Streptococcus, Haemophilus,* and *Staphylococcus.* This infection routinely has been treated successfully with antibiotics; however, the now common occurrence of multiple antibiotic–resistant microorganisms makes this approach insufficient in some cases. This may force a reevaluation of the use of childhood immunization as an alternative to preventing this disease. Other vaccines used now only to a limited degree may be used more widely in the future, and others may be developed soon; these include vaccines against cholera, typhoid, malaria, West Nile virus, *Hantavirus,* severe acute respiratory syndrome (SARS), rotavirus, and several other diseases. The new infection challenge we are facing may require evaluation of even more novel therapeutic approaches such as use of bacteriophages—viruses that infect bacteria but not humans. Regardless of which solutions ultimately address the problem, expediency must be a key component.

SUMMARY REVIEW

Infectious Agents

1. Infections are the number one cause of death worldwide.
2. The stages of infection include colonization, invasion, multiplication, and spread.
3. Infection by a pathogen is influenced by a number of factors: mechanisms of action, infectivity, pathogenicity, virulence, immuncogenicity, toxigenicity, and portal of entry.
4. Classes of infectious microorganisms include viruses, bacteria, chlamydia, rickettsiae, mycoplasma, fungi, protozoa, and helminths.

Pathogen Survival Mechanisms

1. Host defenses against infection include the external barriers and the cells and biochemicals of the innate and adaptive immune systems.
2. Antigenic variation allows microorganisms to change their appearance and challenge the specificity of the immune system.
3. Bacteria injure cells by producing destructive enzymes (exotoxins) or endotoxins. Exotoxins can damage the plasma membranes of host cells or prevent phagocytosis, and endotoxins activate the inflammatory response and produce fever.
4. Bacteremia, or septicemia, is the proliferation of bacteria in the blood. Endotoxins released by blood-borne bacteria cause the release of vasoactive mediators that increase the permeability of blood vessels. Leakage from vessels causes hypotension that can result in septic shock.
5. Viruses enter host cells and use the metabolic processes of host cells to proliferate.
6. Viruses that have invaded host cells decrease protein synthesis, disrupt lysosomal membranes, form inclusion bodies where synthesis of viral nucleic acids occurs, cause intercellular fusion between host cells to produce giant cells, alter antigenic properties of the host cell, and transform host cells into cancerous cells.
7. Diseases caused by fungi are called *mycoses.* Most pathogenic fungi grow as parasites on or near skin or mucous membranes and usually produce mild and superficial disease.
8. Fungi that invade the skin, hair, or nails are known as dermatophytes.

Clinical Manifestations of Infectious Disease

1. Most clinical manifestations from infectious disease result from the host's inflammatory and immune responses. The hallmark of most infectious diseases is, however, fever.

SUMMARY REVIEW—cont'd

Countermeasures Against Pathogens: Vaccines and Antimicrobials

1. Many vaccines have been developed to protect against pathogens. Vaccines induce primary and secondary (from booster injections) immune responses under conditions that will not cause disease. Most bacterial vaccines are killed microorganisms or extracts of bacterial antigens. Most viral vaccines contain live viruses that are weakened or attenuated so that they express appropriate antigens but cause only a limited and easily controlled infection.

2. Antibiotic resistance can develop through genetic mutations that inactivate the drug, alter bacterial membranes so that the antibiotic is no longer taken up, or alter the target molecule. Overuse of antibiotics can lead to the destruction of normal flora, allowing the selective overgrowth of antibiotic-resistant strains or pathogens.

3. The development and widespread use of vaccines against common antibiotic-resistant microorganisms must now be considered.

KEY TERMS

Antigenic drift, 296
Antigenic shifts, 296
Antigenic variation, 296
Antitoxins, 299
Bacteremia (septicemia), 299
Dermatophytes, 301
Dimorphic, 301

Endogenous pyrogens, 302
Endotoxins (lipopolysaccharides [LPSs]), 299
Exogenous pyrogens (EPs), 302
Exotoxins, 299
Fungus (*pl.,* fungi), 301
Gene-switching, 296

Mutations, 296
Mycosis (*pl.,* mycoses), 301
Permissive host cell, 300
Recombination, 296
Toxoids, 304
Vaccination, 303
Vaccine, 303

MEDIA RESOURCES *evolve*

Review questions and answers for this chapter are available in the *CD Companion* included with this book. Also see the CD for an animation on the *pathogenesis of metastasis.*

WebLinks—links to Internet sites pertaining to this chapter—are available on Evolve at http://evolve.elsevier.com/McCance/.

REFERENCES

1. Mims C et al: *Medical microbiology,* London, 2004, Mosby.
2. Calandra T et al: Protection from septic shock by neutralization of macrophage migration inhibitory factor, *Nat Med* 6(2):164-170, 2000.
3. Baumgartner JD, Calandra T: Treatment of sepsis: past and future avenues, *Drugs* 57(2):127-132, 2000.
4. Conti B et al: Cytokines and fever, *Front Biosci* 9:1433-1449, 2004.
5. Beishuizen A, Thijs LG: Endotoxin and the hypothalamo-pituitary-adrenal (HPA) axis, *J Endotoxin Res* 9(1):3-24, 2003.

STRESS AND DISEASE

KATHRYN L. McCANCE • BETH A. FORSHEE • JANE SHELBY

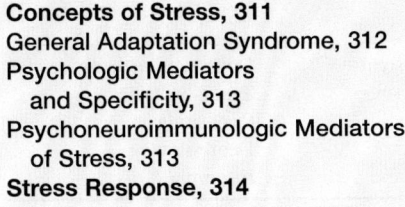
Modern society is full of stress. As a culture, Westerners are champions of the Protestant work ethic, a philosophy originating in the sixteenth century that views idleness as taboo. In Poor Richard's Almanac, Ben Franklin counseled people not to waste time. Driven by this perspective, Westerners have devoted time and energy to inventing time-saving devices. These inventions have fueled the drive of the "workaholic" American and, despite our prosperity, have not resulted in more leisure hours. Having the capacity to do something often translates into the necessity to do it. For example, replacing paper and pen with computers allows us to endlessly revise documents in pursuit of perfection. Answering machines enable us to return phone calls we would otherwise miss. We have become accustomed to an accelerated way of life that includes overstimulation, impatience, and suffering resulting from the so-called *stress-related disorders.*

It is often reported that use of the term **stress** in a biologic sense began with Hans Selye in 1946. In 1914, however, Walter B. Cannon used the term in both a physiologic and a psychologic sense in a paper reporting on his psychoendocrine studies.[1] In his report Cannon used such phrases as "great emotional stress" and "times of stress."[1] In 1935 Cannon published another paper called "Stresses and Strains of Homeostasis." In it he applied the engineering concept of stress and strain in a physiologic context.[2] Cannon thought also that stress involved psychologic factors; his paper stated that physical as well as emotional stimuli can cause stress. The *popularization* of the term, however, did begin with Hans Selye's work.

In the past decade, for the first time in history, it has been demonstrated that the interactions among social, psychologic, biologic, and behavioral factors are inherent in the causes and courses of many diseases. Molecular biologists, immunologists, neurologists, clinicians, and behavioral scientists have all begun to explore the role of the neglected half of the mind-body (dualistic) model—that is, the mind. What is

now emerging is a more holistic and complex model of health and disease states. This model involves the biochemical relationships of the central and autonomic nervous systems, the endocrine system, and the immune system and their relationships to stress-elicited coping behaviors, such as smoking and poor diet, that can also modify the integrity of the immune system. Discoveries of these complex links have, in fact, created the field of psychoneuroimmunology.

CONCEPTS OF STRESS

Psychologic stress may cause or exacerbate (worsen) several disease states, including many of the diseases (cardiovascular disease, cancer, and infectious diseases) implicated as the leading causes of death in the United States[3,4] (Table 10-1). Evidence also shows that stress is directly related to the cause of some diseases and conditions or at the least affects the severity of symptoms and outcomes in a number of diseases and conditions, including irritable bowel syndrome, ulcers, asthma, autoimmune disorders, delayed wound healing, reproductive dysfunction, diabetes (worsening of symptoms), and depression.[4,5] Chronic inflammation is suggested as being important in the functional decline that leads to frailty, disability, and untimely death. [6,7] As evidence has mounted concerning the important role that stress plays in many disease processes, research has focused on the mechanisms responsible for these mind-body interactions. Along with a greater understanding of the relationship between the human stress response and disease, new strategies for treatment of stress-related disorders are emerging. This chapter describes definitions of stress, the history of stress research, and recent findings on the role of stress in disease.

Table 10-1	Examples of Stress-Related Diseases and Conditions		
Target Organ or System	**Disease or Condition**	**Target Organ or System**	**Disease or Condition**
Cardiovascular system	Coronary artery disease Hypertension Stroke Disturbances of heart rhythm	Gastrointestinal system	Ulcer Irritable bowel syndrome Diarrhea Nausea and vomiting Ulcerative colitis
Muscle	Tension headaches Muscle contraction backache	Genitourinary system	Diuresis Impotence Frigidity
Connective tissues	Rheumatoid arthritis (autoimmune disease) Related inflammatory diseases of connective tissue	Skin	Eczema Neurodermatitis Acne
Pulmonary system	Asthma (hypersensitivity reaction) Hay fever (hypersensitivity reaction)	Endocrine system	Type 2 diabetes mellitus Amenorrhea
Immune system	Immunosuppression or deficiency Autoimmune diseases	Central nervous system	Fatigue and lethargy Type A behavior Overeating Depression Insomnia

The term *stress* has been used persistently and widely in specialties such as biology, health sciences, and social sciences despite numerous disagreements over its definition. Nevertheless, in recent years **stress** has been more usefully defined as a *transactional* or *interactional concept.* Transactionally, stress is viewed as the state of affairs arising when a person relates to (i.e., interacts or transacts with) situations in certain ways. People are not disturbed by situations per se but by the ways they appraise and react to situations. In general, a person experiences stress when a demand *exceeds* a person's coping abilities, resulting in reactions such as disturbances of cognition, emotion, and behavior that can adversely affect well-being.

General Adaptation Syndrome

Selye[8] originally sought to discover a new sex hormone when he discovered the biologic syndrome of stress. In his attempts to discover the new hormone, Selye injected crude ovarian extracts into rats. Repeatedly, he found that the following triad of structural changes occurred: (1) enlargement of the cortex of the adrenal gland, (2) atrophy of the thymus gland and other lymphoid structures, and (3) development of bleeding ulcers of the stomach and duodenal lining. Selye soon discovered that this triad of manifestations was not specific for his ovarian extracts but also occurred after he exposed the rats to other noxious stimuli, such as cold, surgical injury, and restraint. He called these stimuli **stressors.** Selye concluded that this triad or syndrome of manifestations represented a nonspecific response to noxious stimuli. Because many diverse agents caused the same syndrome, Selye suggested that it be called the **general adaptation syndrome (GAS).** In 1959 Selye wrote the following:

> Specific homeostatic mechanisms for the maintenance of body temperature, blood sugar, etc., have been under study since Claude Bernard. The principal contribution of stress research was precisely to show that if we abstract from three specific reactions, there remains a common residual response that is nonspecific in regard to its cause and can be elicited with such diverse agents as cold, heat, x-rays, adrenalin, insulin, tubercle bacilli, or muscular exercise. This is so despite the coexistence of highly specific adaptive reactions to any one of these agents.[5]

Selye later defined three successive stages in development of the GAS: (1) the **alarm stage,** in which the central nervous system (CNS) is aroused and the body's defenses are mobilized (i.e., flight or fight); (2) the **stage of resistance or adaptation,** during which mobilization contributes to flight or fight; and (3) the **stage of exhaustion,** in which continuous stress causes the progressive breakdown of compensatory mechanisms (acquired adaptations) and homeostasis. The stage of exhaustion, Selye believed, marked the onset of certain diseases he called **diseases of adaptation.**

The nonspecific physiologic response identified by Selye consists of interaction among the sympathetic branch of the autonomic nervous system (ANS) (see Chapter 14) and other neural signals that activate the endocrine system, known as the **hypothalamic-pituitary-adrenal (HPA) axis,** or interactions among the hypothalamus, pituitary gland, and the adrenal gland. The alarm phase of the GAS begins when a stressor triggers the actions of the hypothalamus and the sympathetic nervous system (SNS) (Figure 10-1). The resistance or adaptation phase begins with the actions of the adrenal hormones cortisol, norepinephrine, and epinephrine. Exhaustion occurs if stress continues and adaptation is not successful, ultimately causing impairment of the immune response, heart failure, and kidney failure, leading to death.

Selye defined **physiologic stress** as a chemical or physical disturbance in the cells or tissue fluid produced by a change, either in the external environment or within the body itself, that requires a response (i.e., begins the GAS) to counteract

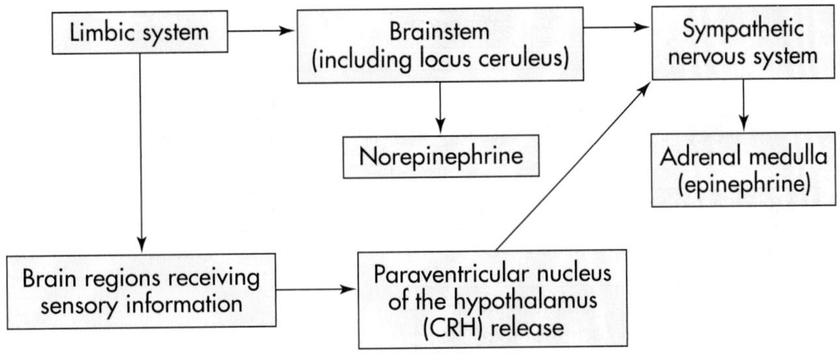

Figure 10-1 Neural recognition and response to real or predicted stressors.

the disturbance. Selye identified three components of physiologic stress: (1) the exogenous or endogenous stressor initiating the disturbance, (2) the chemical or physical disturbance produced by the stressor, and (3) the body's counteracting (adaptational) response to the disturbance.[8]

Psychologic Mediators and Specificity

Although Selye's identification of the GAS is regarded as tremendously important and the cornerstone of stress research, the idea that stress is a purely physiologic response is oversimplified. In the mid-1950s, studies showed that activation of the adrenal cortex occurred in humans in response to psychologic stressors;[9] in monkeys with conditioned emotional responses;[10] and in humans subjected to a stressful interview technique.[11] In the early 1960s, researchers found that plasma cortisol levels in groups of subjects increased while they watched war movies and decreased while they viewed Disney nature films.[12,13] Later, Mason[14] demonstrated in a series of experiments that occurrence of the GAS depended on psychologic factors surrounding the stressors. Mason demonstrated that several factors, including degrees of discomfort, unpleasantness, or suddenness of the stress, could account for the presence or absence of the physiologic stress response.

Selye believed that stressors cause a general or nonspecific response. However, research in the past 30 years has shown the remarkable sensitivity of the central nervous system and endocrine system to psychologic influences (emotional is included in psychologic and social stress and acts through psychologic mechanisms).

As with a physically mediated stress response, psychologic stressors can elicit a reactive stress response. The **reactive response** is a physiologic response derived from psychologic stressors. For example, the stress of taking an examination may produce an increased heart rate and dry mouth in the unprepared student. Although no physical stressor is involved, the psychologic stress of taking an examination elicits a reactive physiologic response in the body.

Another type of psychologic-mediated stress response is the **anticipatory response.** Rather than reacting to an obvious stressor, the body mounts a physiologic stress response in anticipation of disruption of the optimal steady-state, also known as **homeostasis.** These anticipatory responses can be generated either by species-specific innate programs, such as reacting to the presence of predators and unfamiliar situations, or by experience-dependent memory programs created by conditioning.[15] In a **conditional response,** the organism learns that specific stimuli (i.e, objects or situational context) are associated with danger, and anticipation of subsequent encounters with the stimulus produces a physiologic stress response. For example, a child that is abused by a parent may experience a physiologic stress response in anticipation of further abuse when the parent enters the room. Under some circumstances these memory programs may become so strong that psychological disorders, such as phobias, develop.

Anticipatory responses are learned responses under fine control by brain regions located in the limbic system. These regions are those most frequently associated with learning and memory and include the hippocampus, amygdala, and prefrontal cortex. In order for these regions to elicit a stress response, the paraventricular nucleus (PVN) of the hypothalamus must be stimulated (see Chapter 20). The limbic structures rarely interact directly with the PVN and are believed to influence the stress response through intermediary neurons, some of which are primarily used for the reactive response.

Psychoneuroimmunologic Mediators of Stress

Psychoneuroimmunology (PNI) is the study of the interaction of consciousness (*psycho*), brain and spinal cord (*neuro*), and the body's defense against external infection and abnormal cell division (*immunology*). Psychoneuroimmunology assumes that all immune-related disease is multifactorial, or the result of interrelationships among psychosocial, emotional, genetic, neurologic, endocrine, and immune systems and behavioral factors.[16,17] The immune system is integrated with other physiologic processes and is sensitive to changes in CNS and endocrine functioning, such as those that accompany psychologic states. Stressors can elicit the stress response or stress system through the action of the nervous and endocrine systems. Stressors include infection, noise, decreased oxygen supply, pain, malnutrition, heat, cold, trauma, prolonged exertion, radiation, responses to life events (including anxiety, depression, anger, fear, and excitement), obesity, old age, drugs, disease, surgery, and medical treatment. Specifically, **corticotropin-releasing hormone** (CRH) is released from the hypothalamus, the sympathetic nervous system, the

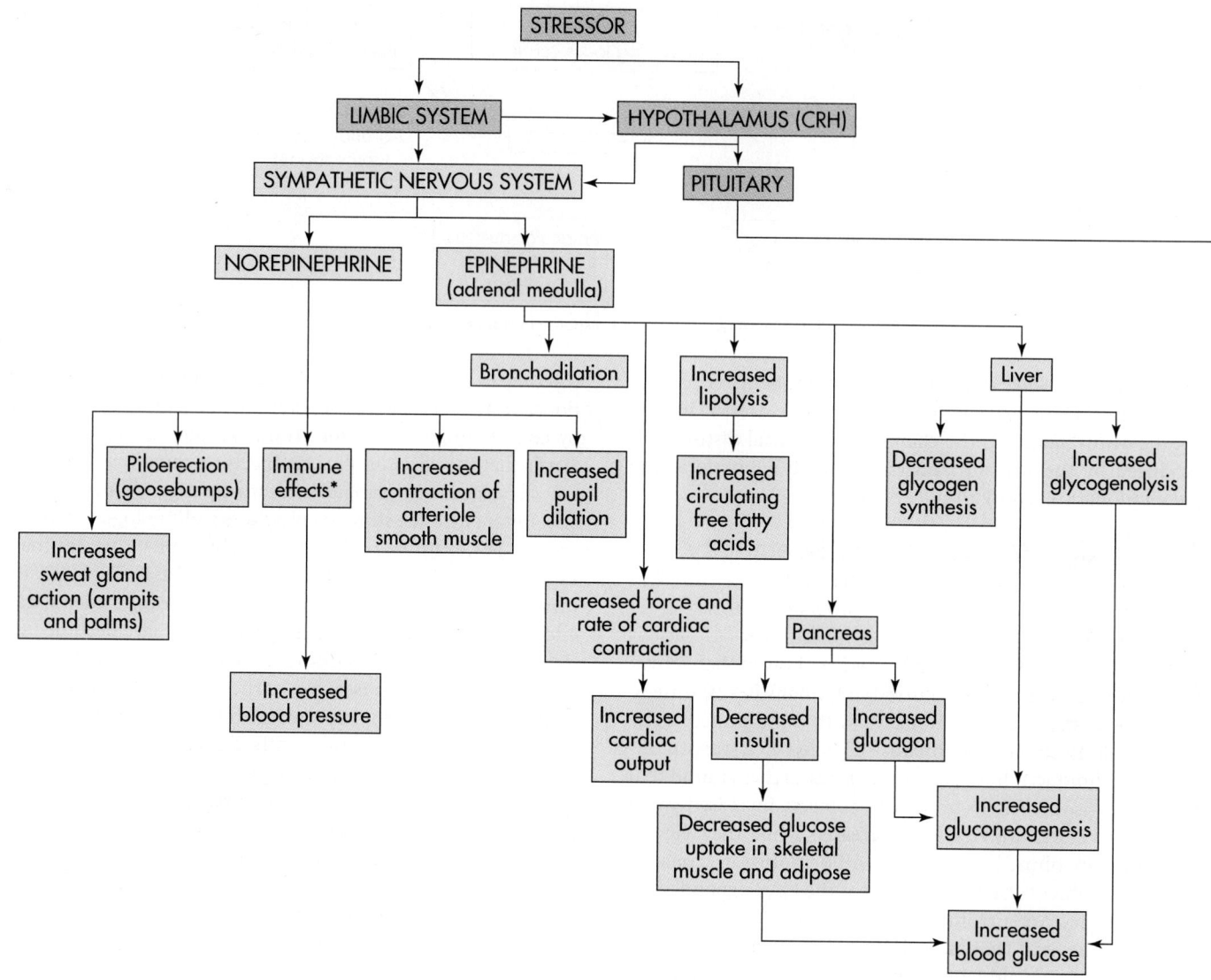

Figure 10-2 **The stress response.** *ACTH*, Adrenocorticotropic hormone; *ADH*, antidiuretic hormone; *PMNs*, polymorphonuclear leukocytes; *RNA*, ribonucleic acid; *IGF-1*, insulin-like growth factor 1. See text for explanation of hormone functions. (*See p. 317 for immune effects. †Explained in text.)

pituitary gland, and the adrenal gland (Figure 10-2). CRH is also released peripherally at inflammatory sites called **peripheral,** or **immune, CRH.** The volume of psychoneuroimmunologic research is growing rapidly and represents a substantial presence in the psychosomatic literature.[4,18-24] Sufficient data now exists to conclude that immune modulation by psychosocial stressors or interventions leads directly to health outcomes, with the strongest data found in studies of infectious disease and wound healing.[18-23]

STRESS RESPONSE

The **stress response** is initiated by the central nervous system and endocrine system (see Figure 10-1). The activation of these systems redirects adaptive energy to the CNS and stressed body sites.

Where the stress response begins depends on whether the stressor is perceived or real. Perceived stressors elicit an anticipatory response that usually begins in the limbic system of the brain, the area responsible for emotions and cognition. The limbic system indirectly elicits an endocrine stress response by stimulating neural pathways responsible for receiving sensory information and a central response by directly stimulating the locus coeruleus (LC) to release norepinephrine (see Figure 10-1). Norepinephrine release promotes arousal, increased vigilance, increased anxiety , and other protective emotional responses. Real stressors elicit a reactive response that can begin either in the limbic system or in regions of the brain receiving specific sensory information (see Figure 10-1). This information is then relayed to the PVN. The PVN stimulates the LC and both central and endocrine stress responses.

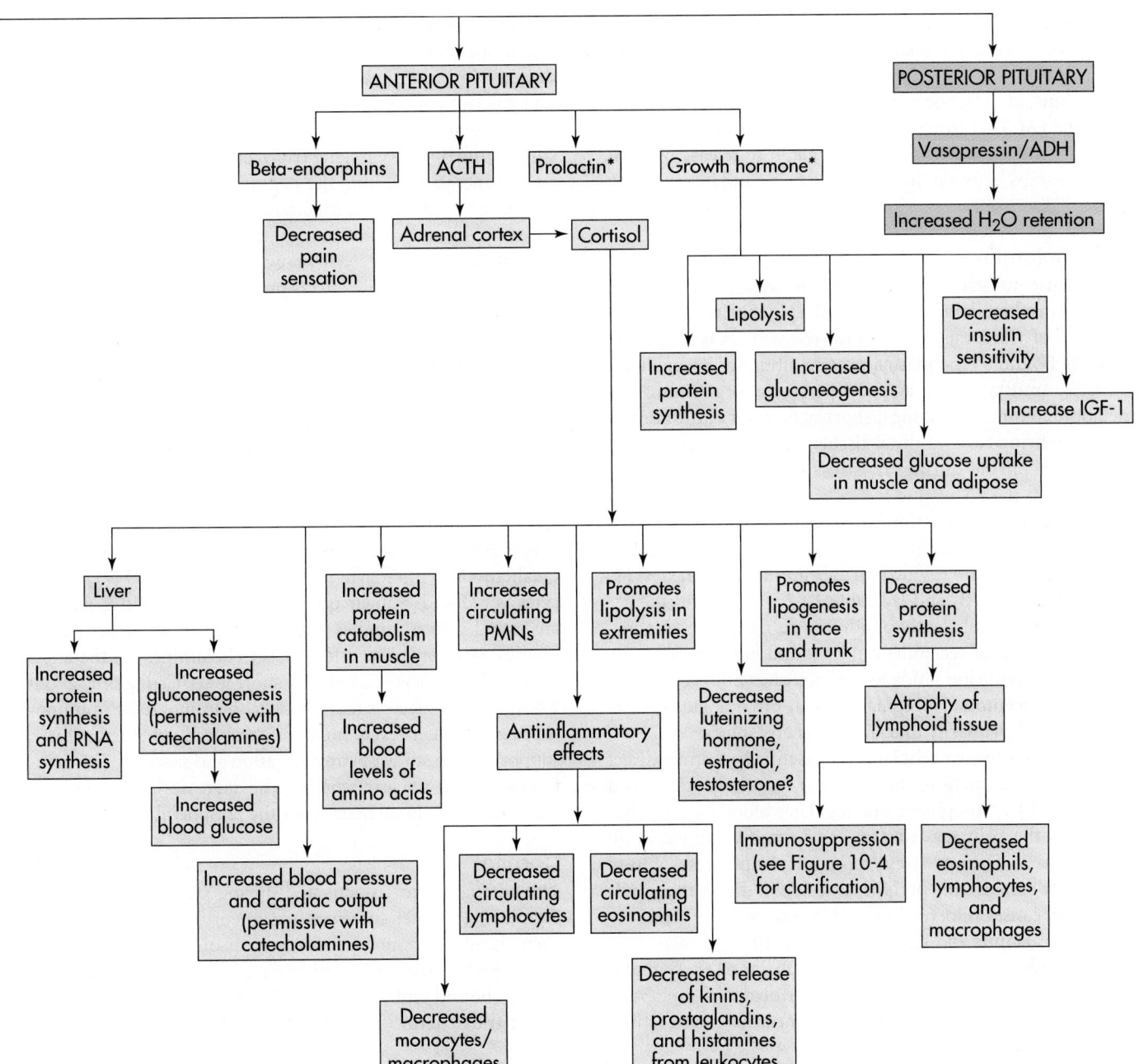

Figure 10-2, cont'd The stress response. *ACTH,* Adrenocorticotropic hormone; *ADH,* antidiuretic hormone; *PMNs,* polymorphonuclear leukocytes; *RNA,* ribonucleic acid; IGF-1, insulin-like growth factor 1. See text for explanation of hormone functions. (*See p. 317 for immune effects. †Explained in text.)

Central Stress Response

The SNS is aroused during the stress response and causes the medulla of the adrenal gland to release catecholamines (80% epinephrine and 20% norepinephrine) into the bloodstream. The adrenal medulla is actually an extension of the SNS because preganglionic fibers from the splanchnic nerve terminate in the medulla, where they innervate the chromaffin cells that produce the catecholamine hormones. Simultaneously, hypothalamic CRH stimulates the pituitary gland to release a variety of hormones, including antidiuretic hormone and oxytocin from the posterior pituitary gland, and prolactin, 3-endorphins, growth hormone (GH), and adrenocorticotropic hormone (ACTH) from the anterior pituitary gland. ACTH stimulates the cortex of the adrenal gland to release cortisol. (Relationships between the neuroendocrine and immune systems are discussed on p. 320.)

Catecholamines

In response to stress, the chromaffin cells of the adrenal medulla produce large quantities of epinephrine and small amounts of norepinephrine. Once released, catecholamines circulate bound to the plasma protein albumin. Epinephrine is rapidly transported to and acts on several organs, but it is metabolized quickly making it short-acting. Very little adrenal norepinephrine reaches distal tissue; thus the effects caused by norepinephrine during the stress response are primarily elicited from the SNS.[25,26]

The catecholamines stimulate two major classes of receptors: α-adrenergic receptors and β-adrenergic receptors. These two classes are divided further into two subclasses: (1) α_1 and α_2 and (2) β_1 and β_2. Table 10-2 summarizes the actions of the two subclasses of adrenergic receptors. (A thorough discussion of receptors can be found in Chapters 1, 20, and 29.) Epinephrine binds to and activates both α- and β-adrenergic receptors. Norepinephrine at physiologic concentrations binds primarily to α-adrenergic receptors.[27]

The circulating catecholamines essentially mimic direct sympathetic stimulation. (Sympathetic function is described in Chapter 14.) Norepinephrine regulates blood pressure because it is the primary constrictor of smooth muscle in all blood vessels. During stress, norepinephrine raises blood pressure by constricting peripheral vessels; it dilates the pupils of the eye, causes piloerection, and increases sweat gland action in the armpits and palms (see Figure 10-2).

Epinephrine has a greater influence on cardiac action and also is the principal catecholamine involved in metabolic regulation. Epinephrine enhances myocardial contractility (inotropic effect), increases the heart rate (chronotropic effect), and increases venous return to the heart, all of which increase cardiac output and blood pressure. Epinephrine dilates blood vessels of skeletal muscle allowing greater oxygenation. Metabolically, epinephrine causes transient hyperglycemia (high blood sugar) by activating enzymes whose actions promote glucose formation (gluconeogenesis) and glycogenolysis in the liver while inhibiting glycogen breakdown. Epinephrine decreases glucose uptake in the muscles and other organs and decreases insulin release from the pancreas. The decrease in insulin release prevents glucose from being taken up by peripheral tissue and thus preserves it for the CNS. Epinephrine also mobilizes free fatty acids and cholesterol by stimulating lipolysis, freeing triglycerides and fatty acids from fat stores, and inhibiting the degradation of circulating cholesterol to bile acids. The metabolic actions of epinephrine aid the metabolic actions of cortisol, which are similar. Table 10-3 summarizes other well-known effects of adrenal catecholamines. All of these effects prepare the body to take physical action: to fight or flee. Stressors commonly associated with catecholamine release by the adrenal medulla include exercise, thermal changes, and acute emotional states.

Catecholamines can modify the numbers of cells of the immune system circulating in the blood.[1] Injection of epinephrine into healthy human subjects is associated with a transient increase of the number of lymphocytes (e.g., T cells and natural killer cells) in the peripheral blood. Specifically, T cytotoxic and natural killer (NK) cells increase whereas little change occurs in B lymphocytes. The main change involves the NK cells.[1] Qualitatively, lymphocyte responsiveness of T and B lymphocytes is reduced. Similar quantitative and qualitative changes are found 5 to 6 minutes after injection of a psychologic or physical stressor.[28] The effect of catecholamines on the alteration of lymphocyte function is short lived, lasting only about 2 hours.[1] This suggests that for catecholamines to be immunosuppressive, their levels must be chronically elevated. This is supported by a study of stress duration and susceptibility to infection.[29] It is unclear whether the increase in lymphocytes comes from the bone marrow or the peripheral tissues.

Cortisol

The adrenal cortex is activated during stress by ACTH (see Figure 10-1), which increases adrenocortical secretion of glucocorticoid hormones, primarily cortisol. (Cortisol is known also as *hydrocortisone*.) Cortisol circulates in the plasma, both protein bound and free. The main plasma-binding protein is called **transcortin** or **corticosteroid-binding globulin**. The

Table 10-2	Physiologic Actions of α- and β-Adrenergic Receptors	
Receptor	**Physiologic Actions**	
α1	Increased glycogenolysis; smooth muscle contraction (blood vessels, genitourinary tract)	
α2	Smooth muscle relaxation (gastrointestinal tract); smooth muscle contraction (some vascular beds); inhibition of lipolysis, renin release, platelet aggregation, and insulin secretion	
β1	Stimulation of lipolysis; myocardial contraction (increased rate, increased force of contraction)	
β2	Increased hepatic gluconeogenesis; increased hepatic glycogenolysis; increased muscle glycogenolysis; increased release of insulin, glucagon, and renin; smooth muscle relaxation (bronchi, blood vessels, genitourinary tract, gastrointestinal tract)	

Table 10-3	Physiologic Effects of Catecholamines*
Organ/Tissue	**Process or Result**
Brain	Increased blood flow; increased glucose metabolism
Cardiovascular system	Increased rate and force of contraction
	Peripheral vasoconstriction
Pulmonary system	Bronchodilation
Skeletal muscle	Increased ventilation
	Increased glycogenolysis
	Increased contraction
	Increased dilation of muscle vasculature
	Decreased glucose uptake and utilization (decreases insulin release)
Liver	Increased glucose production
	Increased glycogenolysis
Adipose tissue	Increased lipolysis
	Decreased glucose uptake
Skin	Decreased blood flow
Gastrointestinal and genitourinary tracts	Decreased protein synthesis
	Decreased smooth muscle contraction
	Increased renin release
	Increased gastrointestinal sphincter tone
Lymphoid tissue	Acute and chronic stress inhibits several components of cellular immunity, particularly decreasing natural killer cells
Macrophages	Inhibit and stimulate macrophage activity
	Depends on availability of type 1/proinflammatory cytokines, the presence or absence of antigenic stressors, and peripheral corticotropin-releasing hormone (CRH)

Data from Elenkov IJ, Chrousos GP: *Ann N Y Acad Sci* 966:290-303, 2002; Granner DK: Hormones of the adrenal medulla. In Murray RK et al, editors: *Harper's biochemistry,* ed 25, New York, 2000.

*Some of these responses require glucocorticoids (e.g., cortisol) for maximal activity (see text for explanation).

unbound, or free, fraction is approximately 8% of the total plasma cortisol and is biologically active.[27] Cortisol mobilizes substances needed for cellular metabolism. One of the primary effects of cortisol is the stimulation of gluconeogenesis, or the formation of glucose from noncarbohydrate sources, such as amino or free fatty acids in the liver. In addition, cortisol enhances the elevation of blood glucose promoted by other hormones, such as epinephrine, glucagon, and growth hormone. This action by cortisol is said to be **permissive** for the actions of other hormones. Cortisol also inhibits the uptake and oxidation of glucose by many body cells. The overall action of cortisol increases blood glucose, thereby enabling the body energy to combat the stressor. The physiologic effects of cortisol are summarized in Table 10-4.

Cortisol also affects protein metabolism. It has an anabolic effect; that is, it increases the rate of synthesis of proteins and ribonucleic acid (RNA) in liver. The anabolic effect of cortisol, however, is countered by its catabolic effect on protein stores in other tissues. Protein catabolism acts to increase circulating amino acids, and chronic exposure to excess cortisol can severely deplete protein stores in muscle, bone, connective tissue, and skin. Further, cortisol acts to reduce protein synthesis in nonhepatic tissues, and dietary protein cannot compensate for the overall protein loss. Some evidence exists that cortisol depresses transport of amino acids into muscle cells while enhancing their uptake into the liver.

Cortisol also has a powerful effect that reverses the insulin-induced suppression of hepatic gluconeogenesis, and basal levels of cortisol stimulate the activity of hepatic enzymes responsible for glycogen and glucose production. The increased amino acid uptake into liver and glucose-producing enzymes favors the production of glucose. Although diseases of excess cortisol secretion, such as Cushing disease, produce characteristics of type 2 (noninsulin dependent) diabetes mellitus, recent studies found that chronic stress also may facilitate the development of type 2 diabetes[30,31] (see What's New? on Glucocorticoids, Insulin, Inflammation, and Obesity). The mechanism for this action is currently under investigation, but it is believed that the development of diabetes is secondary to cortisol-induced obesity. Cortisol promotes lipogenesis in certain regions of the body and to a lesser extent promotes lipolysis in other regions by increasing the actions of lipolytic hormones, such as catecholamines and growth hormone. Chronic cortisol excess induces lipogenesis in the abdomen, trunk, and face resulting in central obesity.

In the gastrointestinal tract, cortisol promotes gastric secretion. This effect is opposite that of norepinephrine, which reduces gastric secretion. Excessive cortisol may stimulate gastric secretion enough to cause ulceration of the gastric mucosa. This could account for the gastrointestinal ulceration observed by Selye.

Cortisol and the Immune System

Stress hormones, especially glucocorticoids (cortisol), have been used therapeutically as powerful antiinflammatory/immunosuppressive agents. This has lead to the conclusion that stress, in general, decreases immunity and inflammation. Data suggests, however, that glucocorticoids and catecholamines (epinephrine and norepinephrine) at concentration levels reached during stress may paradoxically result in de-

Table 10-4	Physiologic Effects of Cortisol
Functions Affected	**Physiologic Effects**
Carbohydrate and lipid metabolism	Diminishes peripheral uptake and utilization of glucose; promotes gluconeogenesis in liver cells; enhances the gluconeogenic response to other hormones; promotes lipolysis in adipose tissue
Protein metabolism	Increases protein synthesis in the liver and decreased protein synthesis (including immunoglobulin synthesis) in muscle, lymphoid tissue, adipose tissue, skin, and bone; increases plasma level of amino acids; stimulates deamination in the liver
Antiinflammatory effects (systemic effects)	High levels of cortisol used in drug therapy suppress the inflammatory response; inhibits proinflammatory activity of many growth factors and cytokines; however, over time some patients may develop tolerance to glucocorticoids causing an increased susceptibility to both inflammatory and autoimmune disease
Proinflammatory effects (possible local effects)	Cortisol levels released during the stress response may increase proinflammatory effects (this very complex physiology is reviewed on p. 317).
Lipid metabolism	Lipolysis in the extremities and lipogenesis in the face and trunk
Immune effects	Treatment levels of glucocorticoids are immunosuppressive, thus they are valuable agents used in treatment of numerous diseases; the T cell or cellular immunity system is particularly affected by these larger doses of glucocorticoids with suppression of Th1 function or cellular immunity; stress can cause a different pattern of immune response; these nontherapeutic levels can suppress cellular (Th1) and increase humoral (Th2) immunity—the so-called "Th2 shift;" several factors influence this very complex physiology and include long-term adaptations, reproductive hormones (i.e., overall, androgens suppress and estrogens stimulate immune responses), defects of the hypothalamic-pituitary-adrenal axis, histamine-generated responses, and acute versus chronic stress; thus stress seems to cause a Th2 shift *systemically* whereas *locally,* under certain conditions, it can induce proinflammatory activities and by these mechanisms may influence the onset or course of infections, autoimmune/inflammatory, allergic, and neoplastic disease
Digestive function	Promotes gastric secretion
Urinary function	Enhances excretion of calcium
Connective tissue function	Decreases proliferation of fibroblasts in connective tissue (thus delaying healing)
Muscle function	Maintains normal contractility and maximal work output for skeletal and cardiac muscle
Bone function	Decreases bone formation
Vascular system and myocardial function	Maintains normal blood pressure; permits increased responsiveness of arterioles to the constrictive action of adrenergic stimulation; optimizes myocardial performance
Central nervous system function	Somehow modulates perceptual and emotional functioning, essential for normal arousal and initiation of daytime activity
Possible synergism with estrogen in pregnancy?	Suppresses maternal immune system to prevent rejection of fetus?

creased cellular immunity and increased autoimmune (humoral) responses. These data may help explain the seemingly contradictory response to stress of immunosuppression and increased risk of infection (decreased cellular immunity) and a heightened antibody response and autoimmune disease (increased humoral immunity).

As discussed in Chapter 7, immune responses are regulated by cells of *innate immunity* called *antigen-presenting cells (APCs),* such as monocyte/macrophages, dendritic cells, and other phagocytic cells, and by cells of *adaptive immunity,* the newly described lymphocyte subclasses Th1 and Th2. These cells regulate the immune system by the secretion of chemicals called *cytokines.* Cytokines are a group of chemicals such as interferons, interleukins, and tumor necrosis factors that can stimulate or inhibit various components of the immune system. Antigen-presenting cells release cytokines that induce T cells to differentiate into Th1 cells. Th1 cells and APC cytokines work together to stimulate the immune activity of cytotoxic T cells, natural killer cells, and activated macrophages—the major components of cellular immunity. These cytokines also stimulate the synthesis of nitric oxide and other inflammatory mediators that increase chronic delayed-type inflammatory responses. Because of this effect, these cytokines are consid-

ered to be the major *proinflammatory cytokines.*[31-34] The cytokines secreted by the Th2 cells act to inhibit Th1 cells and can promote humoral immunity by stimulating growth and activation of mast cells and eosinophils, as well as the differentiation of B-cell immunoglobulins. Thus these cytokines are considered to be the major *anti-inflammatory cytokines*[32] (Figure 10-3).

Stress influences immunity by stimulating cortisol and epinephrine secretion from the adrenal glands and norepinephrine from the sympathetic nervous system. Cortisol acts to suppress the activity of Th1 cells, which leads to a decrease in cellular immunity and to the proinflammatory response. Cortisol also stimulates the activity of the Th2 cells, which leads to an increase in humoral immunity and the antiinflammatory response. Epinephrine and norepinephrine have a similar effect: the decrease in Th1 activity and the increase in Th2 activity. This decrease in Th1 activity and increase in Th2 activity is sometimes called the **Th2 shift.**

The above description of the effect of stress hormones on the Th1/Th2 balance may not be accurate for certain local responses.[32] It has been documented that catecholamines (epinephrine and norepinephrine) can cause certain epithelial cells of the lung to release cytokines that promote recruitment

Glucocorticoids, Insulin, Inflammation, and Obesity

The signs and symptoms of Cushing syndrome (e.g., excess glucocorticoids [GCs]) include truncal obesity, relatively thin extremities, a "moon face," and a "buffalo (neck) hump." In such individuals the possibility of associated hypertension is high as well as increased risk of infection and metabolic syndrome or frank type 2 diabetes. In addition, the likelihood of an elevated ratio of intraabdominal subcutaneous fat mass is high because the glucocorticoids mediate the redistribution of stored calories into abdominal fat. The specific increase in abdominal fat stores is a consequence of elevated glucocorticoids together with insulin. However, the increased glucocorticoids need not be present in the circulation, but can be generated locally in fat through conversion of inactive cortisone to active cortisol through the action of the isoenzyme 11-β-hydroxysteroid dehydrogenase (11-beta-HSD) type-1. This conversion is referred to as "pre-receptor" metabolism of cortisol. The active steroid is secreted directly to the liver through the portal vein. In vitro insulin synthesis and secretion from the pancreas are inhibited by the glucocorticoids. However, increasing glucocorticoids in vivo are associated with increasing insulin secretion possibly because of an anti-insulin effect on the liver, which appears to be vulnerable to the negative effects of glucocorticoids on insulin action. Hepatic insulin resistance is strongly associated with abdominal obesity.

Recent data reveal that the plasma concentration of inflammatory mediators, such as tumor necrosis factor-α (TNF-α) and interleukin-6 (IL-6), is increased in the insulin resistant states of obesity and type 2 diabetes. Two mechanisms might be involved in the pathogenesis of inflammation: (1) glucose and macronutrient intake (i.e., which can be mediated through chronic stress) causes oxidative stress; and (2) the increased concentrations of TNF-α and IL-6, associated with obesity and type 2 diabetes, might interfere with insulin action by suppressing insulin signal transduction. This interference might promote inflammation. Chronic overnutrition (obesity) might thus be a proinflammatory state with oxidative stress.

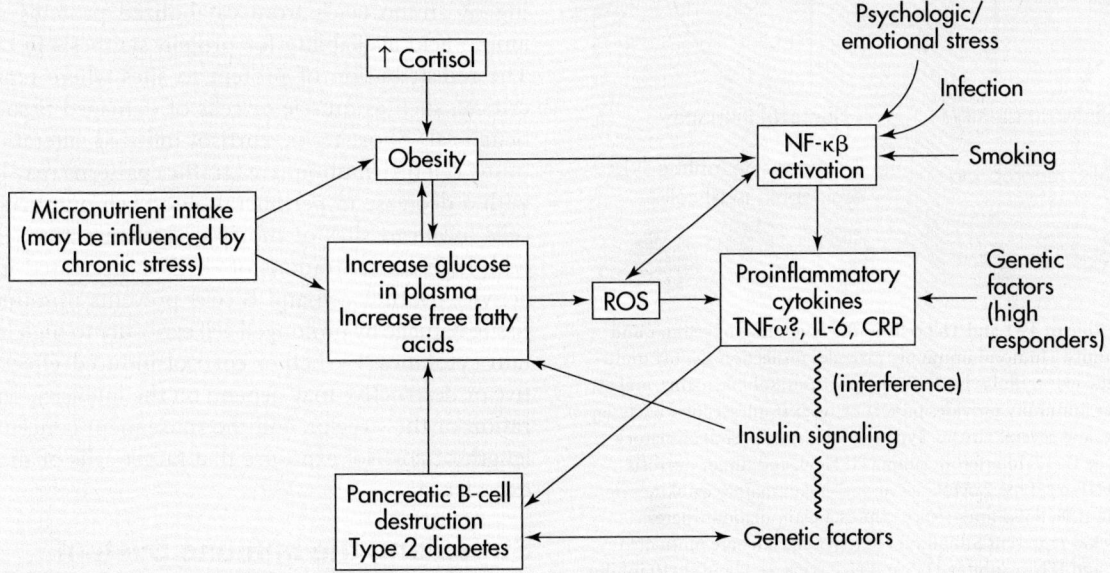

Stress, inflammation, obesity, and type 2 diabetes. The induction of reactive oxygen species (ROS) generation and inflammation through the proinflammatory transcription factor, NF-kβ, activates most proinflammatory genes. Macronutrient intake, obesity, free fatty acids, infection, smoking, psychologic stress, and genetic factors increase the production of ROS. Interference with insulin signaling (insulin resistance) leads to hyperglycemia and proinflammatory changes. Proinflammatory changes increase TNF-α, increase IL-6, and also lead to the inhibition of insulin signaling and insulin resistance. Inflammation in pancreatic B cells leads to B-cell dysfunction, which in combination with insulin resistance leads to type 2 diabetes. *CRP*, C-reactive protein; *TNF-α*, tumor necrosis factor–alpha; *IL-6*, interleukin-6. (Data from Padgett DA, Glaser R: *Trends Immunol* 24[8]:444-8, 2003.)

Data from Dallman MF et al: *Endocrinology* 145(6):2633-2638, 2004; Dandona P, Aljada A, Brandyopadhyay A: *Trends Immunol* 25(1):4-7, 2004; Kim SP et al: *Diabetes* 52:2453-2460, 2003; Masuzaki H et al: *Science* 94:2166-2170, 2001; Padgett DA, Glaser R: *Trends Immunol* 24(8):444-448, 2003; Strack AM et al: *Am J Physiol* 268:R142-149, 1995; Thakore JH et al: *Biol Psychiatry* 47:1140-1142, 1998; Wagen Knecht LE et al: *Diabetes* 52:2490-2496, 2003.

of leukocytes to the lung. This paradoxical stress-induced potentiation of inflammation in the lungs may explain why "adult respiratory distress syndrome" often develops in individuals with major infections associated with profound activity of the stress system.[35]

Corticotropic-releasing hormone (CRH) influences the immune system indirectly by the activation of cortisol (glucocorticoids) and catecholamines. CRH is secreted by the hypothalamus and also peripherally at inflammatory sites.[32,36,37] Peripheral (immune) CRH is proinflammatory, causing an increase in vasodilation and vascular permeability.[38] Therefore, it appears that mast cells are the target of peripheral CRH. Mast cells release histamine, which is a well-known mediator of acute inflammation and allergic reactions (Figure 10-4). Recent evidence has indicated that immune cells may have histamine receptors and that histamine may have an

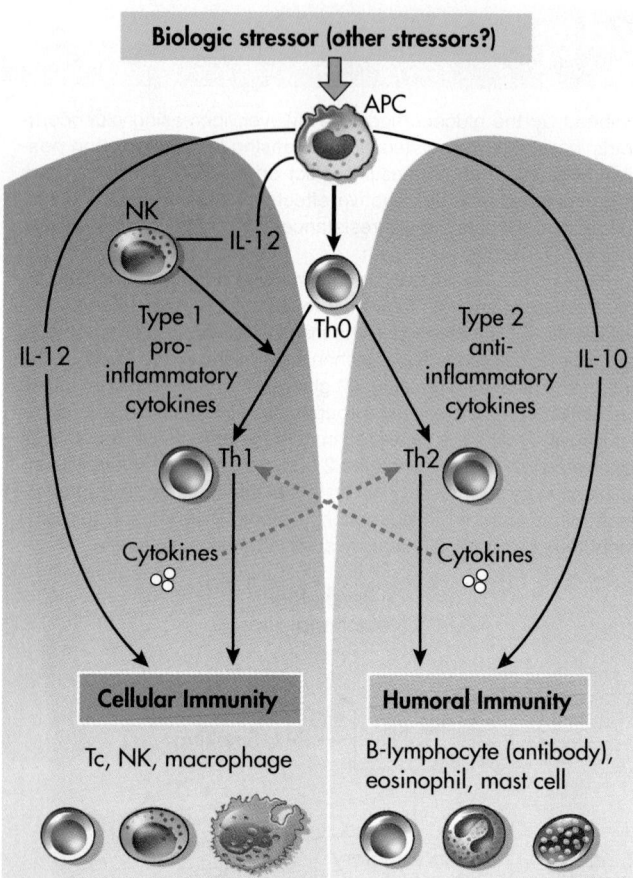

Figure 10-3 Role of Th1 and Th2 cells in the regulation of cellular and humoral immunity. Humoral immunity provides protection against multicellular parasites, extracellular bacteria, some viruses, soluble toxins, and allergens. Cellular immunity provides protection against intracellular bacteria, fungi, protozoa, and several viruses. Type 1 cytokines or proinflammatory cytokines include IL-12, interferon-gamma (IFN-γ), and tumor necrosis factor-alpha (TNF-α). Type 2 cytokines or anti-inflammatory cytokines include IL-10 and IL-4. Solid lines (black) represent stimulation whereas dashed lines (blue) represent inhibition (i.e., Th1 and Th2 are mutually inhibitory, IL-12 and IFN-γ inhibit Th2, and vice versa; IL-4 and IL-10 inhibit Th1 responses). APC, Antigen-presenting cell; IL, interleukin; NK, natural killer cell; Th, helper T cell; Tc, cytotoxic T cell; B, B cell. (Redrawn from: Elenkov IJ, Chrousos GP: *Trends Endocrinol Metab* 10[9]:359-368, 1999.)

effect similar to the catecholamines. This would indicate that histamine would induce acute inflammation and allergic reactions while at the same time it suppresses Th1 activity (decreasing cellular immunity) and promote Th2 activity (increasing humoral immunity).[38-41]

In summary, stress can activate an excessive immune response and, through cortisol and the catecholamines, suppress the Th1 response and cause a Th2 shift. Locally, stress can exert proinflammatory or antiinflammatory effects depending on what chemicals are released in the local environment and how the cells of the local environment respond to those chemicals. Finally, recent evidence indicates that stress is not a uniform, nonspecific reaction.[22] Different types of stressors might have variable effects on the immune response. Thus *systemically* stress may cause a decrease in cellular im-

munity and enhance humoral immunity, whereas *locally,* under certain conditions, it can induce proinflammatory activities that may influence the onset and cause of infection, autoimmune/inflammatory, allergic, and neoplastic disease.

Therapeutic levels of glucocorticoids inhibit the accumulation of leukocytes at the site of inflammation and inhibit the release of substances involved in the inflammatory response (i.e., kinins, plasminogen-activating factor, prostaglandins, and histamine) from the leukocytes. Glucocorticoids inhibit fibroblast proliferation and function at the site of an inflammatory response. This inhibition accounts for the poor wound healing, increased susceptibility to infection, and decreased inflammatory response that often are noted in individuals with chronic glucocorticoid excess.

It is not entirely clear why cortisol secretion during stress is beneficial. It has been suggested that gluconeogenesis promoted by cortisol ensures an adequate source of glucose (energy) for body tissues, and nerve cells in particular. The pooling of amino acids from catabolized proteins may ensure amino acid availability for protein synthesis in certain cells. The redistribution of protein to sites where replacement is critical, such as muscle or cells of damaged tissue, would be beneficial. Short-term, cortisol-induced alterations in immune cell distribution (e.g., traffic) patterns may be adaptive, with a decrease in peripheral blood cell numbers as effector cells locate to sites of injury or inflammation. In addition, with high concentrations of cortisol, decreased immune cell activity (both T cell and B cell) prevents immune-mediated tissue damage by prolonged cell exposure to high levels of certain cytokines.[24] Whether cortisol-induced effects are adaptive or destructive may depend on the intensity, type, and duration of the stressor, and the subsequent concentration and length of cortisol exposure that target cells of the individual experience.

Stress and the Immune System

Many immune-related conditions and diseases are associated with stress. Several conditions with variable pathophysiologic characteristics appear to have a common origin[42,43] relating to chronic inflammatory processes (see p. 318). These conditions include cardiovascular disease, osteoporosis, arthritis, type 2 diabetes mellitus, chronic obstructive pulmonary disease (COPD), other diseases associated with aging, and some cancers; all are characterized by the prolonged presence of proinflammatory cytokines.[42,44] (Inflammation is discussed in Chapter 6). Stress and negative emotions are associated directly with the production of increased levels of proinflammatory cytokines, providing a possible link between stress, immune function, and disease.[45-47] The specific stress-induced mechanisms causing these illnesses are not clearly defined. Recent research is focused on the regulatory interactions between the immune system and the nervous and endocrine systems, which may represent mechanistic pathways for stress-associated immune-mediated diseases (see Table 10-1).

The immune, nervous, and endocrine systems communication through similar pathways involving hormones, neuro-

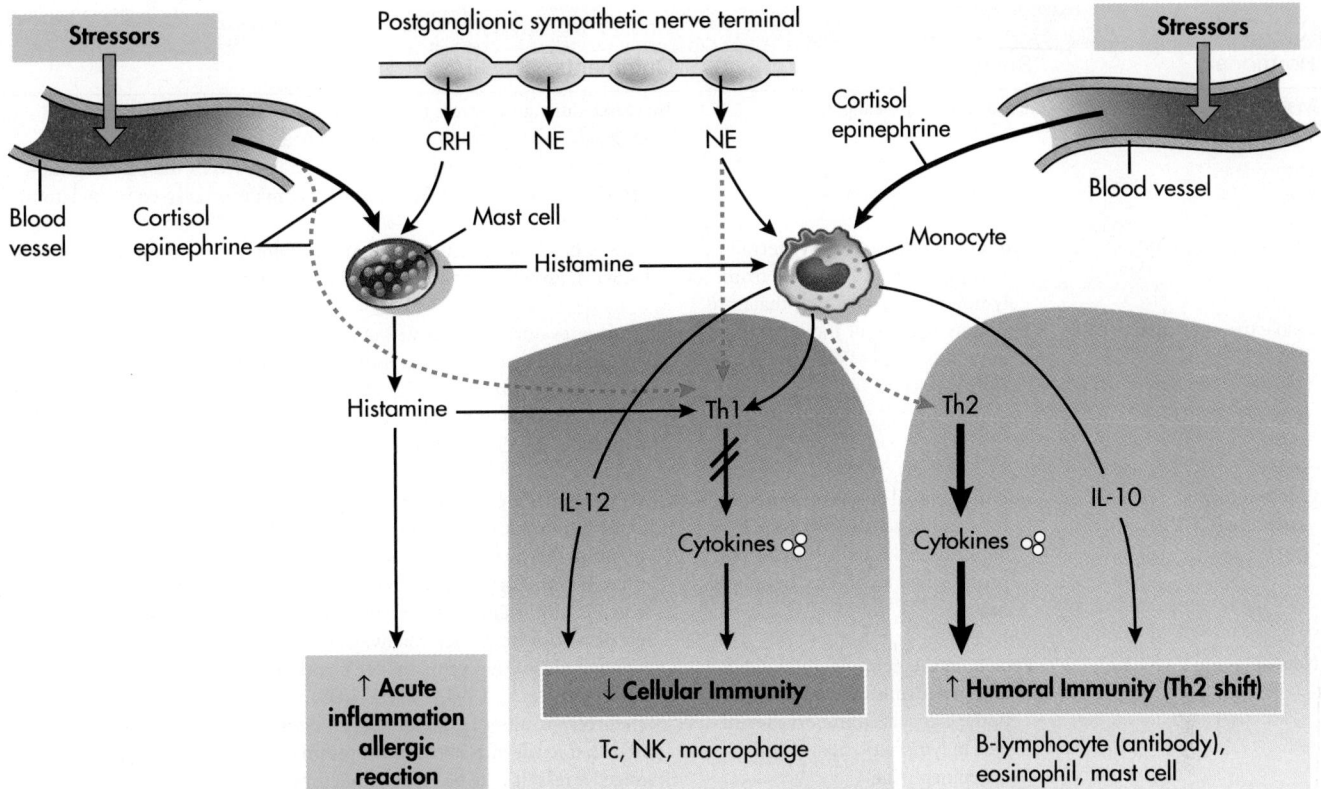

Figure 10-4 Effect of corticotropin-releasing hormone (CRH)—mast cell—histamine axis, cortisol, and catecholamines on the Th1/Th2 balance—cellular and humoral immunity. Stress and CRH modulate inflammatory/immune and allergic responses by stimulating cortisol (glucocorticoid), catecholamines, and peripheral (immune) CRH secretion and by changing the production of regulatory cytokines and histamines. Solid lines (*black*) represent stimulation and dashed lines (*blue*) represent inhibition. *CRH* (peripheral, immune), Corticotropin-releasing hormone; *NE*, norepinephrine; *Th*, helper T cell; *IL*, interleukin; *Tc*, cytotoxic T cell; *NK*, natural killer cell; *B*, B cell; ↓, decreased (inhibited); ↑, increased (stimulation). (Redrawn from Elenkov IJ, Chrousos GP: Stress hormones, Th1/Th2 patterns, pro/anti-inflammatory cytokines and susceptibility to disease, *Trends Endocrinol Metab* 10[9]:359-368, 1999.)

transmitters, neuropeptides, and immune cell products. Various components of immune system responses are potentially affected by all known neuroendocrine-produced factors involved in the stress reaction. Conversely, immune cell–derived cytokines and other products have effects on neurocrine and endocrine cells[48,49] (see Table 7-4). Several pathways regulate communication among these systems with both direct and indirect patterned effects (Figure 10-5).

The stress response directly influences the immune system through hypothalamic and pituitary peptides and through products of the sympathetic branch of the ANS. These factors include CRH, ACTH, endorphins, substance P, epinephrine, norepinephrine, dopamine, serotonin, histamine, GH, vasoactive intestinal polypeptide (VIP), β-endorphin, methionine-enkephalin, leucine-enkephalin, and somatostatin[50-53] (Table 10-5). Direct suppressive effects of CRH have been reported also on two immune cell types possessing CRH receptors—the monocyte-macrophage and CD4 (T helper) lymphocyte.[54] Release of endogenous opiates occurs during stress, and these peptides have been shown to have concentration-dependent, enhancing, and suppressive effects on various immune cells.[50] Immune cells have been shown to have surface receptors for epinephrine, serotonin, ACTH,

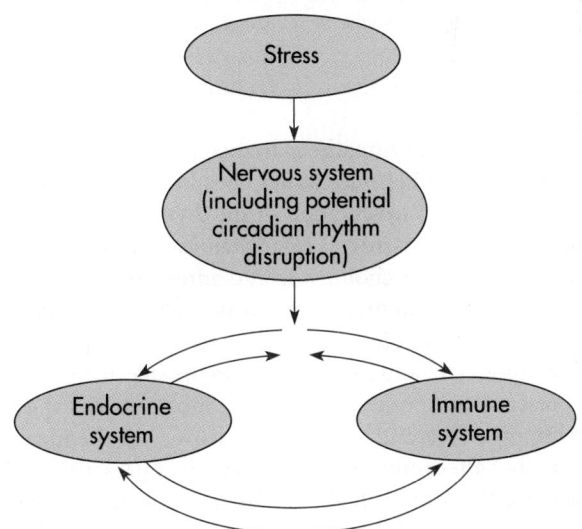

Figure 10-5 Nervous system–endocrine system–immune system interactions. Interconnections of pathways of communication among the immune, nervous, and endocrine systems.

Table 10-5	Other Hormones that Probably Influence the Stress Response	
Hormone	**Source**	**Comments**
Melatonin	Produced by pineal gland	Increases during the stress response; release is suppressed by light and increased in the dark; receptors have been identified on lymphoid cells, possibly higher density of receptors on T cells than B cells; suppression of lymphocyte function by trauma was reversed by melatonin (Maestroni, 1999)
Somatostatin (SOM)	Produced by sensory nerve terminals found in and released from lymphoid cells and hypothalamus	Natural killer (NK) function and immunoglobulin synthesis is decreased by SOM; growth hormone secretion decreased by SOM
Vasoactive intestinal peptide (VIP)	Found in neurons of the central nervous system (CNS) and in peripheral nerves	VIP increases during stress; VIP-containing nerves are located in both primary and secondary lymphoid tissues, around blood vessels, and in the gastrointestinal tract; VIP receptors are on both T and B cells; VIP may influence lymphocyte maturation; cytokine production by T cells is modified by VIP; B cells and antibody production is influenced by VIP
Calcitonin gene–related peptide (CGRP)	Found in spinal cord motor neurons and in sensory neurons near dendritic cells of the skin and in primary and secondary lymphoid tissues	CGRP receptors are present on T and B lymphocytes, thus it is likely that CGRP can modulate immune function; CGRP may enhance the acute inflammatory response because it is a vasodilator; maturation of immune B lymphocytes is inhibited by CGRP; IL-1 is inhibited by CGRP, which is important for the activation of T cells; it has been shown to interfere with lymphocyte activation
Neuropeptide Y (NPY)	Present in the neurons of the CNS and in neurons throughout the body; colocalized in nerve terminals in lymphatic tissues with norepinephrine	Lymphocytes have receptors for NPY and thus may modulate their function (Pettito et al, 1994); Several lines of evidence suggest that NPY is a neurotransmitter and neurohormone involved in the stress response; increased levels of NPY occur in plasma in response to severe or prolonged stress; it may be responsible for stress-induced regional vasoconstriction (splanchnic, coronary, and cerebral); it may also increase platelet aggregation (Rabin, 1999)
Substance P (SP)	Produced by a neuropeptide classified as tachykinin (increases heart rate subsequent to lowering blood pressure) found in the brain, as well as nerves innervating secondary lymphoid tissues	SP increases in response to stress; receptors for SP are found on the membrane of both T and B cells, mononuclear phagocytic cells, and mast cells; proinflammatory activity induces the release of histamine from mast cells during the stress response; causes smooth muscle contraction, causes macrophages and T cells to release cytokines, and increases antibody production

Data from Maestroni GJ: *Adv Exp Med Biol* 460:396, 1999; Pettito JM et al: *J Neuro Immunol* 54:81, 1994; Rabin BS: The nervous system—immune system connection. In *Stress, immune function, and health: the connection,* Wiley-Liss, 1999, New York.

CRH, endorphins, GH, and prolactin, as well as intracellular steroid receptors.

Products of the sympathetic branch of the ANS also influence immune cell behavior. It has been known for some time that there is direct innervation of the thymus, spleen, lymph nodes, and bone marrow.[53] Histochemical studies have verified the presence of cholinergic and adrenergic nerve terminals in the lymphoid organs and tissues. There is evidence for interaction of norepinephrine released from nerve endings with lymphocytes and macrophages in the spleen, implicating the presence of a route of communication between the ANS and immune system through direct delivery of chemical mediators that alter immune cell behavior in a paracrine (cell to adjacent cell) fashion in the microenvironment of the lymphoid organ.

The pineal gland regulates the immune response and mediates the apparent effects of circadian rhythm on immunity. Blockage of production of melatonin (by continuous light or by pharmacologic means) results in suppression of immune response, whereas administration of melatonin reverses these effects.[55] This immunomodulation pathway may affect immune changes found with disturbance and dysregulated circadian rhythm, which are common among elderly, acutely ill, and stressed individuals.[56] Melatonin also modulates seasonal changes in immune function and affects tumor development.[57]

The hypothalamic-pituitary-adrenal (HPA) axis may produce indirect effects on the CNS that modulate immune responses. This is the most extensively studied pathway, with original interest stemming from early studies showing profound effects of prolonged severe stress on immunologic structures.[58] It was noted that the adrenal gland enlarged with simultaneous involution of the thymus and lymph nodes. Increased levels of circulating glucocorticoids (GCSs) may be an important mechanism in stress-related immune structure alterations and in suppression of immune response.[58] The GCS level increases are attributable to pituitary ACTH production—a result of increased hypothalamic CRH. A number of stress factors initiate CRH production, including high levels of interleukin-1 (IL-1) and interleukin-6 (IL-6). Increased CRH secretion results in an increase in cortisol secretion. Cortisol feeds back to inhibit further cytokine release by macrophages and monocytes.

The observation that IL-1 can elicit changes in the nervous and endocrine systems by stimulating CRH production in the hypothalamus is part of a growing body of evidence demonstrating immune-induced regulation of the CNS. The release of immune inflammatory mediators IL-6, tumor necrosis factor–beta (TNF-β), and interferon is triggered by bacterial or viral infections, cancer, and tissue injury that in turn initiate a stress response through the HPA pathway described previously. Enhanced systemic production of these cytokines also induces other CNS and behavior changes seen frequently during the acute phase of an infectious episode, acting either directly in a distant systemic "endocrine" way or through the mediation of neuropeptides.[48,59-61] These effects include pyrogenesis (fever), induction of slow wave sleep, and anorexia, all of which are adaptive responses to infection and possibly cancer, with hyperthermia resulting in an inhospitable environment for many microorganisms and tumor cells (by slowing bacterial and tumor growth and viral replication). Slow wave sleep is associated with enhanced release of GH and a reduction in levels of cortisol, which is beneficial for tissue repair and enhanced immune response.[62] Normal and predictive changes in sleep occur in response to infections, and these changes appear to be of important recuperative value to the individual.[63]

Lymphocytes also are known to produce ACTH and endorphins in small amounts, which probably influence immune response in an autocrine or a paracrine manner in the local microenvironment of an ongoing immune response.[64] The T cell growth factor (IL-2) can up-regulate pituitary ACTH. Immune-derived cytokines have significant influence on neuroendocrine function, with evidence for direct and indirect cytokine effects on nervous and adrenal cell functions. Thus the immune system has an adaptive role as a "signal" organ to alert other systems of inner threatening stimuli (e.g., infection, tissue damage, tumor cells) that may upset the dynamic steady state.

Neuropeptides and hormones have a significant effect on the immune response. Whether this impact on immune function is suppressive or potentiating depends on the type of factor secreted, with some factors enhancing, some suppressing activities, and some doing both, depending on the concentration and length of exposure, the target cell, and the specific immune function studies.[49] Neuropeptides and neuroendocrine hormones may directly control biochemical events affecting cell proliferation, differentiation, and function or may indirectly control immune cell behavior by affecting the production or activity of cytokines.[49]

In summary, a significant body of evidence now supports a link among the nervous, endocrine, and immune systems. The bidirectional communication among these systems involves common use of signal molecules and their receptors, which in turn regulates the behavior of cells in each system. Thus the most recent findings are that (1) there are direct effects of CNS neuropeptides on immune cells; (2) stress-induced endocrine products influence immune cell and neurologic cell function; and (3) immune cell products (cytokines) affect nervous and endocrine cell function through both direct and indirect pathways.

Stress-Induced Hormonal Alterations

Elevation of glucocorticoid concentration associated with psychologic stress or physical exercise is not as high as that achieved by pharmacologic means.[1] Stress produces changes in levels of hormones other than glucocorticoids; the interaction of these various hormones in modifying the function of other physiologic systems still needs investigation.

Female Reproductive System

Cortisol exerts inhibiting effects by suppressing levels of release of luteinizing hormone, estradiol, progesterone, and possibly testosterone.[65,66] The HPA axis exerts powerful, multilevel effects on the female reproductive system. Stress generally inhibits the female reproductive system (Figure 10-6), primarily through the HPA axis by (1) suppression of hypothalamic gonadotropin-releasing hormone (GnRH) secretion by CRH and CRH stimulation of β-endorphin release; (2) inhibition of GnRH, pituitary luteinizing hormone (LH), and ovarian estradiol (E_2) secretion by cortisol; and (3) cortisol-induced target tissue resistance by estradiol.[66,67] The locus coeruleus-norepinephrine system (see Figure 10-6) provides positive input to the reproductive system, which is frequently altered by the stress-activated HPA axis. Sexual stimulation and GnRH neuron activation, however, may cause the gonadal axis to be resistant to suppression by the HPA axis. Through estradiol, the reproductive system provides positive input to both components of the stress system by stimulating CRH secretion and inhibiting reuptake and catabolism of catecholamines. Table 10-6 presents potential pathologic effects of central and peripheral corticotropin-releasing hormone in women.

Estrogen stimulates the HPA axis. Compared with controls, pregnant women and women receiving high-dose estrogen therapy had elevated levels of cortisol in both morning and evening plasma samples.[68] In addition, it appears that the HPA axis responsiveness is greater in women than men.[69] Estrogen directly stimulates the CRH gene promoter and the central noradrenergic (norepinephrine) system, which may help explain adult women's slight hypercortisolism, increases in affective anxiety and eating disorders, mood cycles, and vulnerability to autoimmune and inflammatory disease, all of which follow estradiol fluctuations. Estradiol down-regulates glucocorticoid receptor binding in the anterior pituitary, hypothalamus, and hippocampus—this tends to *increase* HPA activity by interfering with glucocorticoid negative feedback, whereas progesterone opposes these effects.[70] Thus alterations in estradiol during normal menses, perimenopause (including increases as well as decreases), and menopause alter the regulatory feedback loop, and adaptations over time develop as new equilibria are established in the relation as shown in Figure 10-6. Over time, these changes increase the incidence of mood alterations, eating disorders, anxiety, depression, weight alterations, and inflammatory and immune disorders.

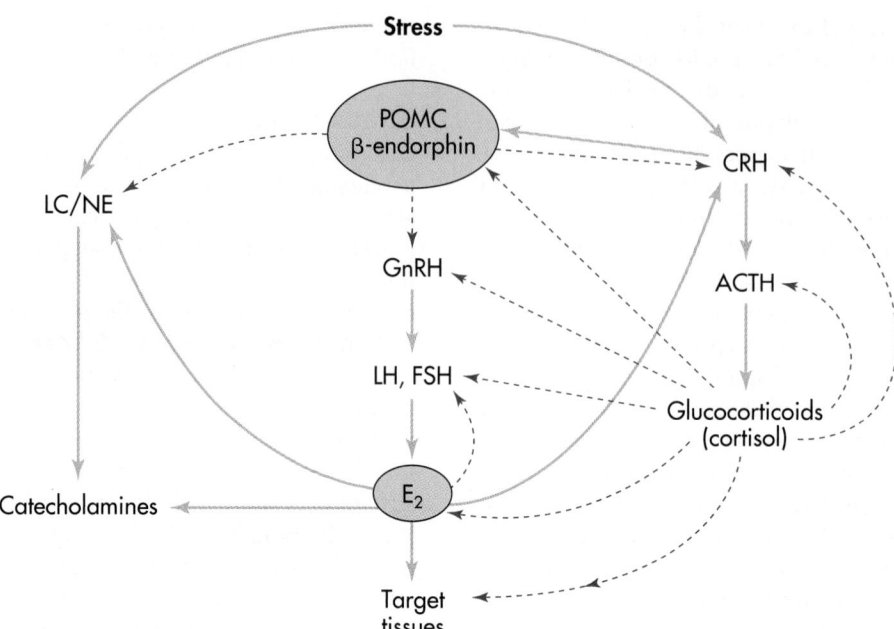

Figure 10-6 Stress and the female reproductive system. Interactions of the reproductive system with the hypothalamic–pituitary–adrenal (HPA) axis and locus ceruleus–norepinephrine system (LC/NE). Stress generally inhibits the female reproductive system primarily through the HPA by *(1)* suppressing hypothalamic gonadotropin-releasing hormone (GnRH) secretion by corticotropin-releasing hormone (CRH) and CRH-induced beta-endorphins; *(2)* inhibiting GnRH, pituitary luteinizing hormone (LH), and ovarian estradiol (E_2) secretion by cortisol; and *(3)* cortisol-induced target tissue resistance to estradiol. The LC/NE system provides positive input to the reproductive system, which can be overridden by the stress-activated HPA. Estradiol can cause the reproductive system to stimulate the stress system by stimulating CRH secretion and inhibiting reuptake and catabolism of catecholamines. Corticotroph cells of the pituitary gland express proxopiomelanocortin (POMC) peptides. (Adapted from Chrousos GP et al: Interactions between the hypothalamic-pituitary-adrenal axis and the female reproductive system, *Ann Intern Med* 129[3]:229-40, 1998.)

Table 10-6	Potential Pathologic Effects of Central and Peripheral Corticotropin-Releasing Hormone (CRH) in Women	
Changes	**Alterations**	
Central CRH		
Increased secretion	Hypercortisolism	
	Melancholic depression	
	Eating disorders	
	Chronic active alcoholism	
	Chronic active exercise	
	Consequences: osteoporosis, visceral obesity, infertility	
Decreased secretion	Atypical depression	
	Seasonal affective disorder	
	Chronic fatigue and fibromyalgia syndromes	
	Rheumatoid arthritis	
	Postpartum blues, depression, and autoimmunity	
	Premenstrual tension syndrome	
	Menopausal depression	
Peripheral CRH		
Increased secretion of immune CRH	Inflammatory disorders	
Increased secretion of placental CRH	Premature labor	
Decreased secretion of placental CRH	Delayed labor	
Decreased secretion of ovarian CRH	Ovarian dysfunction	
	Anovulation	
	Defective corpus luteum function	
Increased secretion of ovarian CRH	Early menopause	
Decreased secretion of endometrial CRH	Infertility	
	Early spontaneous abortion	

Data from Chrousos GP et al., *Ann Int Med* 129(3):229-240; Kalantaridou SN et al: *J Reprod Immunol* 62(1-2):61-68, 2004.

The adipocyte-derived peptide hormone leptin interacts directly and indirectly with both the adrenal and gonadal axes; leptin levels are higher in women than men. Leptin regulates appetite (satiety) and energy balance. It also inhibits the HPA axis at both hyopothalamic and adrenocortical levels. In addition, leptin positively influences the female reproductive axis by inhibition of the HPA axis and arcuate proopiomelanocortin (POMC) neuronal system and through activation of the locus coeruleus-norepinephrine (LC/NE) system. By promoting satiety and sympathetic system outflow, leptin is thought to provide the peripheral signal to a central mechanism regulating the size of body fat stores.[71] Thus leptin may be significant in control of the onset of puberty because of its relationship to the amount of fat mass, in the adaptive activation of the HPA axis, and inhibition of gonadal function that takes place in cases of starvation and anorexia nervosa.[72-74]

Endorphins and Enkephalins

Endorphins and enkephalins (endogenous opiates) are released into the blood as part of the response to stressful stimuli. They are proteins found in the brain that have pain-relieving capabilities. Stressful stimuli include traumatic injury and an acute, intense stress situation, such as first time parachute jumping. In inflamed tissue, immune cell–derived endorphins activate endorphin receptors on peripheral sensory nerves leading to pain relief or analgesia.[75] Hemorrhage increases β endorphin levels that appear to inhibit blood pressure increase or delay compensatory changes that would increase blood pressure.[76] Thus endogenous opiates modulate blood pressure instability and neuroendocrine and cytokine responses to blood losses.[77,78]

The secretion of ACTH and β endorphin is stimulated by corticotropin-releasing hormone; β endorphins are released from the pituitary gland.[79] Enkephalin is released from the adrenal medulla. Evidence is accumulating that β endorphins can modulate ACTH secretion and, with ACTH, inhibit hypothalamic CRH secretion, a possible down-regulation pathway of the stress response.[80]

In a number of conditions or activities in which endogenous opiate activity is increased, subjects not only experience insensitivity to pain but also report increased feelings of excitement, positive well-being, or euphoria.[81] In addition, cells of the immune system synthesize and release opioids when the lymphoid cells are activated.[82] T and B lymphocytes and mononuclear phagocytic cells have receptors for opioids.[1] Endorphins may play a role in the excitement and exhilaration produced by dancing, contact sports, and combat. There is little direct evidence, however, documenting the endorphin system in most of these activities.

Growth Hormone (Somatotropin)

Growth hormone (GH) is synthesized from the anterior pituitary gland and is also produced by lymphocytes and mononuclear phagocytic cells.[83] GH affects protein, lipid, and carbohydrate metabolism and counters the effects of insulin. It is involved in tissue repair and may participate in the growth and function of the immune system.[1] Receptors for GH are present on lymphoid cells.[84] This suggests a role for GH in regulating phagocytic function and possibly antigen presentation.[1] GH appears to have enhancing effects on immune function.[1] GH levels increase in the blood after a variety of stressful stimuli, such as cardiac catheterization, electroshock therapy, gastroscopy, surgery, fever, and physical exercise.[85,86] Psychologic stimuli associated with increased levels of GH include taking examinations, viewing of violent or sexually arousing films, anticipation of exhausting exercise, and certain psychologic performance tests. Prolonged activation of the stress response (chronic stress) leads to suppression of GH and other growth factor effects on target tissues.[87]

Prolactin

Prolactin is released from the anterior pituitary gland as well as numerous extrapituitary tissue sites.[88] It is necessary for lactation and breast development.[89] Prolactin receptors are present in many different tissues, including liver, kidney, intestine, and adrenals. Prolactin is also produced by lymphoid cells.[1,90] Prolactin levels in plasma increase as a result of a variety of stressful stimuli, including gastroscopy, proctoscopy, pelvic examination, and surgery.[91] The level of prolactin also rises during parachute jumping, during motion sickness, after taking examinations, and after receiving various sexual stimuli, for example, stimulation of the nipple or areola in women. Unlike GH, prolactin levels show little change after exercise. Like GH, however, a prolactin increase appears to require more intense stimuli than those leading to increases in catecholamine or cortisol levels. Immune cells also are influenced by prolactin. Prolactin acts as a second messenger for interleukin-2 (IL-2) and is known to have a positive influence on B cell activation and differentiation.[92] Several classes of lymphocytes have receptors for prolactin, suggesting a direct effect of prolactin on immune function.

Oxytocin

Oxytocin is well known as a hormone produced in high levels by the hypothalamus during childbirth and lactation. It is also produced during orgasm in both sexes and has been shown to promote bonding and social attachment.[93] Oxytocin also has antistress properties, as has been shown in animal experiments where elevations in endogenous oxytocin were associated with reduced hypothalamic-pituitary-adrenal (HPA) activation levels and reduced anxiety.[94] Oxytocin in some tissues works in concert with estrogen; these two hormones have a calming effect during stressful situations.[95] In contrast, another hormone closely resembling oxytocin, vasopressin, acts in concert with testosterone to increase blood pressure and heart rate, thus enhancing the "fight or flight" stress response. A recent proposal is that the oxytocin-mediated stress response may promote the "tend and befriend" response, more commonly experienced by women because estrogen is a co-mediator.[96] Studies in animals have identified a wide group of affiliative behaviors involving social encounters, pair bonding, and attachment as being increased by oxytocin.[97-99] Thus different effects of stress on males and females may be explained, in part, by gender-related hormonal profiles that dictate to some extent the characteristics, quality, and outcomes of the stress response.

Testosterone

Testosterone, a hormone secreted by Leydig cells, regulates male secondary sex characteristics and libido. Testosterone levels decrease after stressful stimuli. The decrease in testosterone occurs after stimuli such as ether or anesthesia, surgery, marathon running, and mountain climbing.[100] The mechanism causing decreased levels of testosterone is thought to be exerted by cortisol and β endorphin.

Psychologic stimuli also lead to a decrease in testosterone levels. Men engaged in rigorous combat training and those engaged in the first several weeks of officer candidate school experience significant drops in testosterone levels.[101,102] However, recent data indicate that the psychologic stress associated with some types of competition (e.g., pistol shooting) increases both testosterone and cortisol, especially in athletes older than 45 years.[103] Individuals with acute illness, such as respiratory failure, burns, and congestive heart failure, show a marked reduction in plasma testosterone.[81]

The direct immunologic effects of sex hormones contribute to the sexual dimorphism seen in the incidence of autoimmune disease[104] and the greater susceptibility to sepsis and mortality in males following injury.[105] Estrogens generally are associated with a depression of T cell–dependent immune function and enhancement of B cell functions, and androgens suppress both T and B cell responses.[104] In injury, however, males produce greater amounts of proinflammatory cytokines, a profile that is associated with poor outcome.[106] Additionally, androgens appear to induce a greater degree of immune cell apoptosis following injury, a mechanism that may elicit a greater immunosuppression in injured males versus females.[107] Table 10-5 (p. 322) lists other hormones, including melatonin, substance P, neuropeptide Y, calcitonin gene–related peptide, somatostatin, and vasoactive intestinal peptide.

STRESS, PERSONALITY, COPING, AND ILLNESS

It is not entirely clear why cortisol secretion during stress is beneficial. It has been suggested that gluconeogenesis prompted by cortisol ensures an adequate source of glucose (energy) for body tissues, and nerve cells in particular. The pooling of amino acids from catabolized proteins may ensure amino acid availability for protein synthesis in certain cells. The redistribution of protein to sites where replacement is critical, such as muscle or cells of damaged tissue, would be beneficial. Short-term, cortisol-induced alterations in immune cell distribution (e.g., traffic) patterns may be adaptive, with a decrease in peripheral blood cell numbers as effector cells locate to sites of injury or inflammation. In addition, decreased immune cell activity by cortisol may be beneficial in some situations because it prevents immune-mediated tissue damage by prolonged cell exposure to high levels of certain cytokines.

Whether cortisol-induced effects are adaptive or destructive may depend on the intensity, type, and duration of the stressor, and the subsequent concentration and length of cortisol exposure that target cells of the individual experience.

Extreme physiologic stressors, such as severe burn injury, represent a predictable stimulus for the stress responses described previously. A less severe and defined event or situation, however, can be a stressor for one person and not for another. Many stressors, such as fasting or temperature changes, do not necessarily cause a physiologic stress response if psychologic factors are minimized. Stress itself is not an independent entity but a system of interdependent processes that are moderated by the nature, intensity, and duration of the stressor and the perception, appraisal, and coping efficacy of the affected individual, all of which in turn mediate the psychologic and physiologic response to stress.

Psychosocial distress may be predictive of psychologic and physical health outcomes. In **psychologic distress** the individual feels a general state of unpleasant arousal after life events that manifests as physiologic, emotional, cognitive, and behavior changes.[108] Periods of depression and emotional upheaval often are associated with adverse life events and place the affected individual at risk for immunologic deficits, increasing the risk of ill health.[109] A meta-analysis of studies shows a relationship between depression and reduction in lymphocyte proliferation and NK cell activity.[110] Multiple moderating factors may be important in immune modulation in depressed individuals, including comorbidities such as alcoholism. Examples of triggering mechanisms include bereavement, academic pressures (including examinations), life events (positive and negative changes),[109] and aging (see p. 328). Adverse life events that have been shown to have the most negative effect on immunity have been characterized as uncontrollable, undesirable, and overtaxing the individual's ability to cope.[111,112]

Studies have strengthened the association of stress with potential for illness in humans. One study examined medical students who were immunized with hepatitis B vaccine on the third day of a stressful examination period; the time to seroconversion and level of antibody titer to the vaccine were measured later. The students with the most rapid seroconversion and the highest titers also reported being less stressed and had a good social support system (which may reduce stress).[113] Even more convincing is a study in which the psychologic stress status was determined in healthy individuals after experimentally controlled exposure to respiratory virus by nasal inoculation. Individuals reporting more stress had an increased incidence of clinical cold and respiratory symptoms compared with subjects reporting less stress, and other infections, including HIV, have been shown to be potentially influenced by psychosocial factors.[114-117]

Studies have shown adverse changes in immune function following intense exercise, with increased cortisol levels, changes in lymphocyte counts, and alterations in cytokine production.[118] Some of these immune changes could be reduced by administration of carbohydrate beverages to endurance athletes, suggesting that dehydration and decreased tissue perfusion were catalysts for the exercise stress–induced immune changes.

Other clinical situations in which the interplay between immunity and psychosocial factors may be evident include patients with cancer and heart disease.[119-121] The evidence linking cancer and psychologic distress, involving three possible mechanisms, is convincing. First, NK cell activity, an important first-line immune defense against cancer, is inhibited in stressed or depressed subjects. Stress and depression is also associated with poorer repair of damaged DNA and alterations in the rates of apoptosis of immune and cancer cells. Additional evidence showing a relationship between cancer and psychosocial factors is seen in the enhanced immune function and survival among cancer patients who undergo psychosocial interventions.[119]

New evidence is showing a relationship between immune stimulation, infections, and heart disease.[120] The relationship between stress and cardiovascular health may be mediated by stress-induced changes in immune function, which may potentiate proinflammatory processes and permit alterations that lead to heart disease.[121]

In the past decade a significant amount of evidence has accumulated linking severe psychosocial stress resulting from negative life events to a chronic syndrome with mental and physical consequences. Posttraumatic stress syndrome (PTTS) has been described in many populations.[122-124] A cascade model has been proposed to describe the pathogenesis and clinical course of the syndrome that illustrates the clinical, epidemiologic, neurobiologic, and psychosocial components of PTTS.[125] The study of PTTS has contributed to the knowledge concerning mechanisms involved in the chronic stress and disease relationship. Recently an appreciation of the association of chronic stress with high levels of cortisol production and paradoxic biounavailability (i.e., bound to plasma protein and not bioavailable) of cortisol has been gained.[126]

In addition, the interaction with health care providers in a clinical setting, the diagnosis of a major illness, and various clinical procedures (e.g., blood draws, injections, examinations, surgical procedures) may represent significant negative life events to many individuals (Figure 10-7). These additional stresses may affect the course of illness as well as interfere with the efficacy of the medical intervention. Identifying and reducing stress in the clinical setting have particular applicability in both disease prevention and illness management.

Personality characteristics are associated with individual differences in appraisal and response to stressors.[127] Specific personality characteristics, such as academic achievement, motivation, and aggression are correlated with immunologic alterations. For example, aggression was positively associated with changes in T and B cell numbers in male military personnel.[128]

The coping response of individuals may exaggerate or moderate physical consequences of the stress response. **Coping** is defined as the process of managing stressful demands

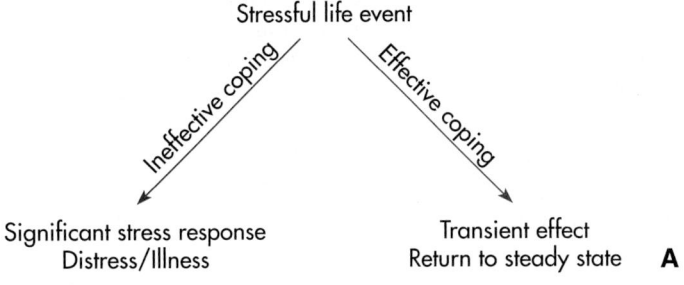

POTENTIAL EFFECTS IN HEALTHY INDIVIDUALS

Stressful life event

Ineffective coping / Effective coping

Significant stress response
Distress/Illness

Transient effect
Return to steady state   **A**

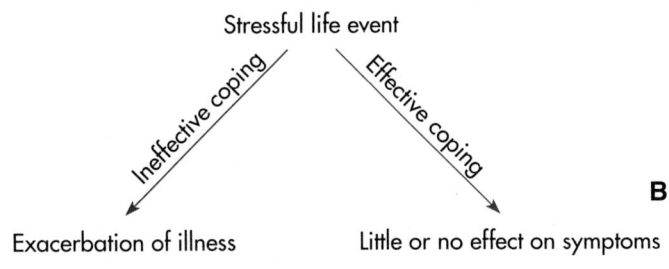

POTENTIAL EFFECTS IN SYMPTOMATIC INDIVIDUALS

Stressful life event

Ineffective coping / Effective coping

Exacerbation of illness

Little or no effect on symptoms   **B**

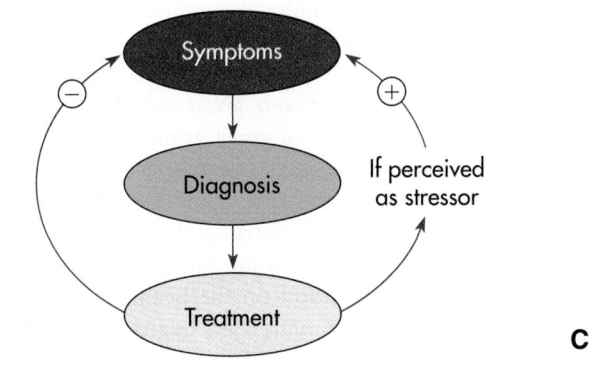

POTENTIAL EFFECTS DURING MEDICAL INTERVENTION

Symptoms

Diagnosis

If perceived as stressor

Treatment

C

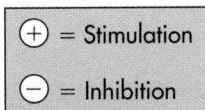

⊕ = Stimulation

⊖ = Inhibition

Figure 10-7 Health outcome determination in stressful life situations is moderated by numerous factors. Whether a life-challenged individual experiences distress or illness depends on the subject's appraisal of the event and the coping strategies used during the stressful period. Models **A** and **B** reflect possible outcomes in stressed healthy and symptomatic individuals. Model **C** illustrates the dynamic clinical setting in which the diagnosis of a serious illness and subsequent medical interventions may be perceived as stressful challenges and have potentially detrimental influences on physical outcome.

and challenges that are appraised as taxing or exceeding the resources of the person.[129] The response may be a change in behavior resulting in potentially adverse health effects (e.g., increased smoking, change in eating habits). Serious disturbances of the sleep-wake cycle are observed in many people under stress and in many clinical settings. Recent work has shown that sleep disturbance may exacerbate the pathophysiologic status of certain patient populations.[130-132] Investigators have reported that sleep deprivation and circadian disruption, even in young, otherwise healthy individuals, have detrimental influences on respiratory and immune system function. Even partial sleep deprivation was associated with reduced NK cell activity in healthy subjects, and only recently have seriously ill patients been assessed for adequacy and structure of sleep during recovery.[130]

Adaptive coping strategies, especially those that are problem focused and those that encourage seeking social support,[133,134] are beneficial during stressful experiences. The extent to which an individual responds to distress, using effective positive coping strategies, determines the degree of successful moderation of the stress challenge. Conversely, ineffective negative coping attempts may exacerbate the effects of distress on health, thus augmenting the potential for illness.[135] Mediating factors that may influence stress susceptibility or resilience include age, socioeconomic status, gender, social support status, personality and life-style, self-esteem, genetics, life events, past experiences, and current health status.[136] Evidence suggests that effective intervention may result in greater stress resilience and improved psychologic and physiologic outcomes. In a study of nursing home residents randomly assigned to control or social support intervention groups, improved psychologic measures and immune function (NK cell activity) were observed in the experimental group at 6 weeks.[137] In another study, women with recurrent metastatic breast cancer were given either routine follow-up (routine care) or weekly support group sessions. Survival in the support treatment group was an average of 19 months longer than in the routine care group, suggesting a mediating influence of additional support for these women.[31,138]

The importance of social support for seriously ill individuals has focused attention on the health and well-being of family members who function as caregivers. Significant stress manifested as depression, anxiety, and fatigue has been noted in family caregivers of those with cancer, Alzheimer disease,

and burn trauma. Individuals and caretakers exhibited suppression of various measures of immune function, with improved function associated with better perceived social support.[139-141] Gender-based coping differences may be attributed, in part, to the hormonal milieu of the individual, with females more likely to offer social support, a behavior with an oxytocin/estrogen association.[96]

Interventions to potentially prevent or manage stress-related psychologic or physical problems include both short- and long-term coping strategies. Stress management consists of educational components specific to the individual's problems and relaxation techniques, which may include meditation, imagery, massage, and biofeedback. These approaches may be used on an individual or a support group basis. Incorporation of these approaches into clinical training facilitates their use in the clinical arena. Future research should focus on the efficacy of such approaches with various populations.

AGING AND STRESS: STRESS-AGE SYNDROME
With aging, sometimes a set of neurohormonal and immune alterations, as well as tissue and cellular changes, develops. These changes, which recently have been defined as stress-age syndrome, include the following:[136,142]
- Alterations in the excitability of structures of the limbic system and hypothalamus
- Rise of the blood concentration of catecholamines, antidiuretic hormone (ADH), adrenocorticotropic hormone (ACTH), and cortisol
- Decrease of testosterone, thyroxine, and other hormones
- Alterations of opioid peptides
- Immunodepression
- Alterations in lipoproteins
- Hypercoagulation of the blood
- Free radical damage of cells

Some of the alterations are adaptational, whereas others are potentially damaging. These stress-related alterations of aging can influence the course of developing stress reactions and lower adaptive reserve and coping.

SUMMARY REVIEW

Concepts of Stress
1. Modern society is full of stress.
2. Psychologic stress may cause or exacerbate (worsen) several disease states. Stress is directly related to the cause of or effects the severity of symptoms and outcomes of diseases and conditions. Research is now focused on the mechanisms responsible for these mind-body interactions.
3. *Stress* recently has been defined as the state of affairs arising when a person relates to (i.e., interacts or transacts with) situations in a certain way. Important is how he or she appraises and reacts to situations.
4. In general, a person experiences stress when a demand *exceeds* a person's coping abilities.

5. Hans Selye identified three structural changes in rats subjected repeatedly to noxious stimuli (stressors): enlargement of the cortex of the adrenal gland, atrophy of the thymus gland and other lymphoid tissues, and gastrointestinal ulceration.
6. Selye believed that the three changes were caused by a nonspecific physiologic response to any long-term stressor. He called this response the *general adaptation syndrome (GAS)*.
7. The GAS occurs in three stages: the alarm stage, the stage of resistance or adaptation, and the stage of exhaustion. Diseases of adaptation develop if the stage of resistance or adaptation does not restore homeostasis.
8. Selye identified three components of physiologic stress: the stressor, the physiologic or chemical disturbance produced

by the stressor, and the body's adaptational response to the stressor.

9. The nonspecific physiologic response consists of interaction among the sympathetic branch of the autonomic nervous system (ANS) and other neural signals that activate the endocrine system known as the hypothalamic-pituitary-adrenal (HPA) axis.

10. The nonspecific physiologic response is a common residual response and can be elicited with diverse agents such as cold, heat, x rays, adrenalin, insulin, tubercle bacilli, and muscular exercise. Although the reactions of these stages are nonspecific, evidence supports the coexistence of highly specific, adaptive reactions to any of these agents.

11. As with a physically mediated stress response, psychologic stressors can elicit a reactive stress response, that is, a physiologic response derived from psychologic stressors.

12. Another type of psychologic-mediated stress response is the anticipatory response.

13. In a conditioned response, the organism learns that specific stimuli are associated with danger and anticipation of subsequent encounters with that particular stimulus produces a physiologic stress response.

14. Psychoneuroimmunology is the study of the interaction of consciousness (psycho), brain and spinal cord (neuro), and the body's defense against external infection and abnormal cell division (immunology).

15. Psychoneuroimmunology assumes that all immune-related disease is multifactorial. The immune system is integrated with other physiologic processes and is sensitive to changes in CNS and endocrine functioning, such as those that accompany psychologic states.

16. Important is release of corticotropin-releasing hormone (CRH) centrally from the brain and peripherally at inflammatory sites.

Stress Response

1. The stress response is initiated by the central nervous system (CNS) and endocrine system. Where the stress response begins depends on whether the stressor is perceived or real.

2. Perceived stressors elicit an anticipatory response that usually begins in the limbic system of the brain. The limbic system elicits an endocrine stress response indirectly by stimulating neural pathways responsible for receiving sensory information and elicits a central response directly by stimulating the locus coeruleus (LC) to release norepinephrine (LC/NE).

3. Real stressors elicit a reactive response that can begin either in the limbic system or in the brain in response to specific sensory information. This information is then relayed to the paraventricular nucleus (PVN). The PVN stimulates the LC and both central and endocrine stress responses.

4. The neuroendocrine response to stress consists of sympathetic stimulation of the adrenal medulla to secrete catecholamines (norepinephrine and epinephrine) and stressor-induced stimulation of the hypothalamus to secrete CRH, which in turn stimulates the pituitary to secrete ACTH, which then stimulates the adrenal cortex to secrete steroid hormones, particularly cortisol.

5. In general, the catecholamines prepare the body to act, and cortisol mobilizes energy (glucose) and other substances needed to fuel the action.

6. Epinephrine exerts its chief effects on the cardiovascular system. Epinephrine increases cardiac output and increases blood flow to the heart, brain, and skeletal muscles by dilating vessels that supply these organs. It also dilates the airways, thereby increasing delivery of oxygen to the bloodstream.

7. Norepinephrine's chief effects complement those of epinephrine. Norepinephrine constricts blood vessels of the viscera and skin; this has the effect of shifting blood flow to the vessels dilated by epinephrine. Norepinephrine also increases mental alertness.

8. CRH influences the immune system indirectly by the activation of glucocorticoids (cortisol) and catecholamines. Peripheral CRH is proinflammatory, causing vasodilation and vascular permeability. It appears that the mast cells are the target of peripheral CRH.

9. Cortisol's chief effects involve metabolic processes. By inhibiting the use of metabolic substances while promoting their formation, cortisol mobilizes glucose, amino acids, lipids, and fatty acids and delivers them to the bloodstream. Cortisol's effect on the immune system is concentration- and location-dependent and may include either stimulation or inhibition of the immune system.

10. The nervous, endocrine, and immune systems communicate through the common use of signal molecules and their receptors, which in turn regulate the behavior of cells in each system during stress challenge.

11. There are direct and indirect pathways of influence among the nervous, endocrine, and immune systems. Neuropeptides have direct effects on immune cells, as well as indirect influences through neuromediated endocrine modulation of immune function. Endocrine products (cortisol) also influence nerve cell behavior. Immune cell products affect both nerve and endocrine cell function, reflecting an adaptive role for the immune system as a "signal" organ to alert other systems of threatening stimuli.

12. Other hormones are affected by the stress response and include increased circulating levels of β endorphins, growth hormone, and prolactin and a decrease in antidiuretic hormone with extreme stress. Luteinizing hormone, estradiol, progesterone, and possibly testosterone decrease during the stress response.

Stress, Personality, Coping, and Illness

1. Stress is a system of interdependent processes that are moderated by the nature, intensity, and duration of the stressor and the coping efficacy of the affected individual, all of which in turn mediate the psychologic and physiologic response to stress.

2. Many studies have linked psychologic distress with altered immune function, and evidence now strengthens the association of stress with potential for illness in humans.

3. Adaptive coping strategies, especially those that are problem-focused and those that encourage seeking social support, are beneficial during stressful experiences.

Aging and Stress: Stress-Age Syndrome

1. With aging, sometimes a set of neurohormonal and immune alterations develop; these changes have been defined recently as stress-age syndrome.

2. These stress-related alterations of aging can influence the course of developing stress reactions and lower adaptive reserve and coping.

MEDIA RESOURCES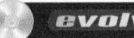

Review questions and answers for this chapter are available in the *CD Companion* included with this book.

WebLinks—links to Internet sites pertaining to this chapter—are available on Evolve at http://evolve.elsevier.com/McCance/.

REFERENCES

1. Rabin BS: The nervous system—immune system connection. In *Stress, immune function, and health: the connection,* New York, 1999, Wiley-Liss.
2. Kapcala LP et al: The protective role of the hypothalamic-pituitary-adrenal axis against lethality produced by immune, infections, and inflammatory stress, *Ann N Y Acad Sci* 771:419-437, 1995.
3. Black PH, Garbutt LD: Stress, inflammation and cardiovascular disease, *J Psychosom Res* 52(1):1-23, 2002.
4. Kiecolt-Glaser JK et al: Psychoneuroimmunology: psychological influences on immune function and health, *J Consult Clin Psychol* 70(3):537-547, 2002.
5. Liu LY et al: School examinations enhance airway inflammation to antigen challenge, *Am J Respir Crit Care Med* 165(8):1062-1067, 2002.
6. Hamerman D: Toward an understanding of frailty, *Ann Intern Med* 130(11):945-950, 1999.
7. Taaffe DR et al: Cross-sectional and prospective relationships of interleukin-6 and C-reactive protein with physical performance in elderly persons: MacArthur studies of successful aging, *J Gerontol A Biol Sci Med Sci* 55(12):M709-M715, 2000.
8. Selye H: The general adaptation syndrome and the diseases of adaptation, *J Clin Endocrinol Metab* 6:117, 1946.
9. Hill SR et al: Studies on adrenocortical and psychological responses to stress in man, *Arch Intern Med* 97:269, 1956.
10. Mason JW, Brady JV: Plasma 17-hydroxycortico-steroid changes related to reserpine effects on emotional behaviors, *Science* 124:983, 1956.
11. Hetzel BS et al: Changes in urinary 17-hydroxycorticosteroid excretion during stressful life experiences in man, *J Clin Endocrinol Metab* 15(9):1057-1068, 1955.
12. Handlon JH et al: Psychological factors lowering plasma 17-hydroxycorticosteroid concentration, *Psychosom Med* 24:535-541, 1962.
13. Wadeson RW et al: Plasma and urinary 17-OHCS responses to motion pictures, *Arch Gen Psychiatry* 14:146-156, 1963.
14. Mason JW: Organization of psychoendocrine mechanisms: a review and reconsideration of research. In Greenfield NS, Steinbach RA, editors: *Handbook of psychophysiology,* New York, 1972, Holt, Rinehart, & Winston.
15. Herman JP et al: Central mechanisms of stress integration: hierarchical circuitry controlling hypothalmo-pituitary-adrenocortical responsiveness, *Front Neuroendocrinol* 24(3):151-158, 2003.
16. Bauer-Wu SM: Psychoneuroimmunology. Part I: Physiology, *Clin J Oncol Nurs* 6(3):167-170, 2002.
17. Bauer-Wu SM: Psychoneuroimmunology. Part II: Mind-body interventions, *Clin J Oncol Nurs* 6(4):243-246, 2002.
18. Cohen S et al: Types of stressors that increase susceptibility to the common cold in healthy adults, *Health Psychol* 17(3):214-223, 1998.

19. Cohen S et al: Chronic social stress, social status, and susceptibility to upper respiratory infections in nonhuman primates, *Psychosom Med* 59(3):213-221, 1997.
20. Glaser R et al: Chronic stress modulates the immune response to a pneumococcal pneumonia vaccine, *Psychosom Med* 62(6):804-807, 2000.
21. Marucha PT, Kiecolt-Glaser JK, Favagehi M: Mucosal wound healing is impaired by examination stress, *Psychosom Med* 60(3):362-365, 1998.
22. Pacak K et al: Heterogeneous neurochemical responses to different stressors: a test of Selye's doctrine of nonspecificity, *Am J Physiol* 275(4Pt2):R1247-R1255, 1998.
23. Repka-Ramirez MS, Baraniuk JN: Histamine in health and disease, *Clin Allergy Immunol* 17:1-25, 2002.
24. Kiecolt-Glaser JK et al: Chronic stress and age-related increases in the proinflammatory cytokine IL-6, *Proc Natl Acad Sci U S A* 100(15):9090-9095, 2003
25. Dimsdale JE, Ziegler MG: What do plasma and urinary measures of catecholamines tell us about human response to stressors? *Circulation* 83(4 suppl):II36-42, 1991.
26. Herd JA: Cardiovascular response to stress, *Physiol Rev* 71(1):305-330, 1991.
27. Sapolsky RM, Romero LM, Munck AU: How do glucocorticoids influence stress responses? Integrating permissive, suppressive, stimulatory, and preparative actions, *Endocr Rev* 21(1):55-89, 2000.
28. Moyna NM et al: The effects of incremental submaximal exercise on circulating leukocytes in physically active and sedentary males and females, *Eur J Appl Physiol Occup Physiol* 74(3):211-218, 1996.
29. Cohen S et al: Types of stressors that increase susceptibility to the common cold in healthy adults, *Health Psychology* 17(3):214-223, 1998.
30. Drapeau V et al: Is visceral obesity a physiological adaptation to stress? *Panminerva Medica* 45(3):189-195, 2003.
31. Rosmond R: Stress induced disturbances of the HPA axis: a pathway to type 2 diabetes? *Med Sci Monit* 9(2):RA35-39, 2003.
32. Elenkov IJ, Chrousos GP: Stress hormones, proinflammatory and anti-inflammatory cytokines, and autoimmunity, *Ann N Y Acad Sci* 966:290-303, 2002.
33. Fearon DT, Locksley RM: The instructive role of innate immunity in the acquired immune response, *Science* 272(5258):50-53, 1996 (review).
34. Mosmann TR, Sad S: The expanding universe of T-cell subsets: Th1, Th2, and more, *Immunol Today* 17(3):138-146, 1996 (review).
35. Meduri GU, Chrousos GP: Duration of glucocorticoid treatment and outcome in sepsis: is the right drug used the wrong way? *Chest* 114(2):355-360, 1998.
36. Chrousos GP: The hypothalamic-pituitary-adrenal axis and immune-mediated inflammation, *N Engl J Med* 332(20):1351-1362, 1995.
37. Karalis K et al: Autocrine or paracrine inflammatory actions of corticotropin-releasing hormone in vivo, *Science* 254(5030):421-423, 1991.
38. Chrousos GP, Elenkov IJ: Interactions of the endocrine and immune systems. In DeGroot LG, Jameson JL, editors: *Endocrinology,* ed 4, Philadelphia, 2001, Saunders.
39. Elenkov IJ: Glucocorticoids and the Th1/Th2 balance, *Ann N Y Acad Sci* 1024:138-146 review, 2004.
40. Lagier B et al: Different modulation by histamine of IL-4 and interferon-gamma (IFN-gamma) release according to the phenotype of human Th0, Th1, and Th2 clones, *Clin Exp Immunol* 108(3):545-551, 1997.

41. Rocklin RE, editor: *Histamine and H₂ antagonists in inflammation and immunodeficiency,* New York, 1990, Mercel Dekker.
42. Rohleder N et al: Age and sex steroid-related changes in glucocorticoid sensitivity of proinflammatory cytokine production after psychosocial stress, *J Neuroimmunol* 126(1-2):69-77, 2002.
43. Bone RC: Toward an epidemiology and natural history of SIRS (systemic inflammatory response syndrome), *JAMA* 268(24):3452-3455, 1992.
44. Poynter ME, Daynes RA: Peroxisome proliferator-activated receptor alpha activation modulates cellular redox status, represses nuclear factor-kappaB signaling, and reduces inflammatory cytokine production in aging, *J Biol Chem* 273(49):32833-32841, 1998.
45. Steptoe A et al: Acute mental stress elicits delayed increases in circulating inflammatory cytokine levels, *Clin Sci (London)* 101(2):185-192, 2001.
46. Mercado AM et al: Altered kinetics of IL-1 alpha, IL-1 beta, and KGF-1 gene expression in early wounds of restrained mice, *Brain Behav Immun* 16(2):150-162, 2002.
47. Maes M et al: Platelet alpha2-adrenoceptor density in humans: relationships to stress-induced anxiety, psychasthenic constitution, gender and stress-induced changes in the inflammatory response system, *Psychol Med* 32(5):919-928, 2002.
48. Aoki N, Ohno Y, Imamura M: Physiological interactions between the immune and endocrine systems: are cytokines hormones? *Med Sci Res* 18:195-201, 1990.
49. Khansari DN, Murgo AJ: Effects of stress on the immune system, *Immunol Today* 11(5):170-175, 1990.
50. Dunn AJ: Psychoneuroimmunology for the psychoneuroendocrinologist: a review of animal studies of nervous system-immune system interactions, *Psychoneuroendocrinology* 14(4):251-274, 1989.
51. Friedman EM, Irwin MR: A role for CRH and the sympathetic nervous system in stress-induced immunosuppression, *Ann N Y Acad Sci* 771:396-418, 1995.
52. Jankovic BD: Neuroimmunomodulation: facts and dilemmas, *Immunol Lett* 21(2):101-118, 1989.
53. Rabin BS et al: Bidirectional interaction between the central nervous system and the immune system, *Clin Rev Immunol* 9(4):279-312, 1989.
54. Jain R et al: Corticotropin-releasing factor modulating the immune response to stress in the rat, *Endocrinology* 128(3):1329-1336, 1991.
55. Maestroni GJ, Conti A: Anti-stress role of the immuno-opioid network: evidence for a physiological mechanism involving T cell–derived, immunoreactive beta-endorphin and MET-enkephalin binding to thymic opioid receptors, *Int J Neurosci* 61(3-4):289-298, 1991.
56. Schwab RJ: Disturbances of sleep in the intensive care unit, *Crit Care Clin* 10(4):681-694, 1994.
57. Nelson RJ, Drazen DL: Melatonin mediates seasonal adjustment in immune function, *Reprod Nutr Dev* 39(3):383-398, 1999.
58. Ader R, Felten D, Cohen N: Interactions between the brain and the immune system, *Annu Rev Pharmacol Toxicol* 30:561-602, 1990.
59. Busbridge NJ, Grossman AB: Stress and the single cytokine: interleukin modulation of the pituitary-adrenal axis, *Mol Cell Endocrinol* 82(2-3):C209-214, 1991.
60. Hori T et al: Immune cytokines and regulation of body temperature, food intake, and cellular immunity, *Brain Res Bull* 27(3-4):309-313, 1991.
61. Navarra P et al: Interleukins-1 and -6 stimulate the release of corticotropin-releasing hormone-41 from rat hypothalamus in vitro via the eicosanoid cyclooxygenase pathway, *Endocrinology* 128(1):37-44, 1991.
62. Hall NRS, O'Grady MP: Regulation of pituitary peptides by the immune system, *BioEssays* 11(5):141-144, 1989.
63. Krueger JM et al: Sleep, microbes, and cytokines, *Neuroimmunomodulation* 1(2):100-109, 1994.
64. Weigent DA, Carr DJ, Blalock JE: Bidirectional communication between the neuroendocrine and immune systems: common hormones and hormone receptors, *Ann N Y Acad Sci* 579:17-27, 1990.
65. Chrousos GP, Gold PW: The concepts of stress and stress system disorders: overview of physical and behavioral homeostasis, *JAMA* 267(9):1244-1252, 1992.
66. Chrousos GP et al: Interactions between the hypothalamic-pituitary-adrenal axis and the female reproductive system, *Ann Intern Med* 129(3):229-240, 1998.
67. Kalantaridou SN et al: Stress and the female reproductive system. Review, *J Reprod Immunol* 62(1-2):61-68, 2004.
68. Lindholm J, Schultz-Moller N: Plasma and urinary cortisol in pregnancy and during estrogen-gestagen treatment, *Scand J Clin Lab Invest* 31(1):119-122, 1973.
69. Gallucci WT et al: Sex differences in sensitivity of the hypothalamic-pituitary-adrenal axis, *Health Psychol* 12(5):420-425, 1993.
70. Peiffer A, Lapointe B, Barden H: Hormonal regulation of type II glucocorticoid receptor messenger ribonucleic acid in rat brain, *Endocrinology* 129(4):2166-2174, 1991.
71. Caro JF et al: Leptin: the tale of an obesity gene, *Diabetes* 45(11):1455-1462, 1996.
72. Ahima RS et ak: Role of leptin in the neuroendocrine response to fasting, *Nature* 382(6588):250-252, 1996.
73. Boden G, Chen X, Mozzoli M, Ryan I: Effect of fasting on serum leptin in normal human subjects, *J Clin Endocrinol Metab* 81(9):3419-3423, 1996.
74. Grinspoon S et al: Serum leptin levels in women with anorexia nervosa, *J Clin Endocrinol Metab* 81(11):3861-3863, 1996.
75. Machelska H et al: Opioid control of inflammatory pain regulated by intercellular adhesion molecule-1, *J Neurosci* 22(13):5588-5596, 2002.
76. Molina PE: Stress-specific opioid modulation of haemodynamic counter-regulation, *Clin Exp Pharmacol Physiol* 29(3):248-253, 2002.
77. Jochem J, Josko J, Gwozdz B: Endogenous opioid peptides system in haemorrhagic shock—central cardiovascular regulation, *Med Sci Monit* 7(3):545-549, 2001.
78. Molina PE: Opiate modulation of hemodynamic, hormonal, and cytokine responses to hemorrhage, *Shock* 15(6):471-478, 2001.
79. Curtis AL et al: Previous stress alters corticotropin-releasing factor neurotransmission in the locus coeruleus, *Neuroscience* 65(2):541-550, 1995.
80. Calogero AE et al: Multiple feedback regulatory loops in hypothalamic corticotropin-releasing hormone secretion: potential clinical implications, *J Clin Invest* 82(3):767-774, 1988.
81. Rose RM: Psychoneurocrinology. In Wilson JD, Foster DW, editors: *Williams textbook of endocrinology,* ed 7, Philadelphia, 1985, Saunders.
82. Cabot PJ et al: Immune cell-derived beta-endorphin. Production, release, and control of inflammatory pain in rats, *J Clin Invest* 100(1):142-148, 1997.
83. Weigent DA et al: Characterization of the promoter-directing expression of growth hormone in a monocyte cell line, *Neuroimmunomodulation* 7(3):126-134, 2000.
84. Kelly PA et al: The prolactin/growth hormone receptor family, *Endocr Rev* 12(3):235-251, 1991.
85. Berne RM, Levy MN, editors: *Principles of physiology,* St Louis, 1990, Mosby.
86. Schalch DS: The influence of physical stress and exercise on growth hormone and insulin secretion in man, *J Lab Clin Med* 69(2):256-269, 1967.
87. Burguera B et al: Dual and selective actions of glucocorticoid upon basal and stimulated growth hormone release in man, *Neuroendocrinology* 51(1):51-58, 1990.
88. Ben-Jonathan N et al: Extrapituitary prolactin: distribution, regulation, functions, and clinical aspects, *Endocr Rev* 17(6):639-669, 1996. Review.
89. Shiu RP, Friesen HG: Mechanisms of action of prolactin in the control of mammary gland function, *Annu Rev Physiol* 42:83-96, 1980.
90. Van De Weerdt C et al: Far upstream sequences regulate the human prolactin promoter transcription, *Neuroendocrinology* 71(2):124-137, 2000.
91. Noel GL et al: Human prolactin and growth hormone release during surgery and other conditions of stress, *J Clin Endocrinol Metab* 35(6):840-851, 1972.
92. Prystowsky MB, Clevenger CV: Prolactin as a second messenger for interleukin 2, *Immunomethods* 5(1):49-55, 1994.
93. Anderson-Hunt M, Dennerstein L: Oxytocin and female sexuality, *Gynecol Obstet Invest* 40(4):217-221, 1995.
94. Neumann ID: Alterations in behavioral and neuroendocrine stress coping strategies in pregnant, parturient, and lactating rats, *Prog Brain Res* 133:143-152, 2001.
95. Liu Y et al: Differential expression of vasopressin, oxytocin, and corticotrophin-releasing hormone messenger RNA in the paraventricular nucleus of the prairie vole brain following stress, *J Neuroendocrinol* 13(12):1059-1065, 2001.
96. Taylor SE et al: Biobehavioral responses to stress in females: tend-and-befriend, not fight-or-flight, *Psychol Rev* 107(3):411-429, 2000.

97. Insel TR: A neurobiological basis of social attachment, *Am J Psychiatry* 154(6):726-736, 1997.

98. Insel TR, et al: Oxytocin, vasopressin, and the neuroendocrine basis of pair bond formation, *Adv Exp Med Biol* 449:215-224, 1998.

99. Zingg H: Oxytocin. In DeGroot LJ, Jameson JL, editors: *Endocrinology,* ed 4, Philadelphia, 2001, Saunders.

100. Matsumoto K et al: Plasma testosterone levels following surgical stress in male patients, *Acta Endocrinol* 65(1):11-17, 1970.

101. Aakvaag A et al: Testosterone and testosterone-binding globulin (TeBG) in young men during prolonged stress, *Int J Androl* 1:22, 1978.

102. Kreuz LE, Rose RM, Jennings JR: Suppression of plasma testosterone levels and psychological stress: a longitudinal study of young men in Officer Candidate School, *Arch Gen Psychiatry* 26(5):479-482, 1972.

103. Guezennec CY et al: Effect of competition stress on tests used to assess testosterone administration in athletes, *Int J Sports Med* 16(6):368-372, 1995.

104. Da Silva JA: Sex hormones and glucocorticoids: interactions with the immune system, *Ann N Y Acad Sci* 876:102-117, 1999.

105. Offner PJ, Moore EE, Biffl WL: Male gender is a risk factor for major infections after surgery, *Arch Surg* 134(9):935-938, 1999.

106. Angele MK et al: Sex steroids regulate pro- and anti-inflammatory cytokine release by macrophages after trauma-hemorrhage, *Am J Physiol* 277(1Pt1):C35-42, 1999.

107. Angele MK et al: Gender dimorphism in trauma-hemorrhage–induced thymocyte apoptosis, *Shock* 12(4):316-322, 1999.

108. Thoits PA: Dimensions of life events that influence psychological distress: an evaluation and synthesis of the literature. In Kaplan HB, editor: *Psychosocial stress: trends in theory and research,* Orlando, 1983, Academic Press.

109. Rozlog LA et al: Stress and immunity: implications for viral disease and wound healing, *J Periodontol* 70(7):786-792, 1999.

110. Irwin M: Immune correlates of depression, *Adv Exp Med Biol* 461: 1-24, 1999.

111. Irwin M et al: Impaired natural killer activity during bereavement, *Brain Behav Immun* 1:98, 1988.

112. Kiecolt-Glaser J et al: Modulation of cellular immunity in medical students, *J Behav Med* 9(1):5-21, 1986.

113. Glaser R et al: Stress-induced modulation of the immune response to recombinant hepatitis B vaccine, *Psychosom Med* 54(1):22-29, 1992.

114. Cohen S: Psychosocial stress and susceptibility to upper respiratory infections, *Am J Respir Crit Care Med* 152(4Pt2):S53-58, 1995.

115. Evans DL et al: Stress-associated reductions of cytotoxic T lymphocytes and natural killer cells in asymptomatic HIV infection, *Am J Psychiatry* 152(4):543-550, 1995.

116. Nott KH, Vedhara K, Spickett GP: Psychology, immunology and HIV, *Psychoneuroendocrinology* 20(5):451-474, 1995.

117. Sheridan JF et al: Psychoneuroimmunology: stress effects on pathogenesis and immunity during infection, *Clin Microbiol Rev* 7(2): 200-212, 1994.

118. Nieman DC: Nutrition, exercise, and immune system function, *Clin Sports Med* 18(3):537-548, 1999.

119. Kiecolt-Glaser JK, Glaser R: Psychoneuroimmunology and cancer: fact or fiction? *Eur J Cancer* 35(11):1603-1607, 1999.

120. Sharma R, Coats AJ, Anker SD: The role of inflammatory mediators in chronic heart failure: cytokines, nitric oxide, and endothelin-1, *Int J Cardiol* 72(2):175-186, 2000.

121. Sher L: Effects of psychological factors on the development of cardiovascular pathology: role of the immune system and infection, *Med Hypotheses* 53(2):112-113, 1999.

122. Bremner JD et al: Neural correlates of memories of childhood sexual abuse in women with and without posttraumatic stress disorder, *Am J Psychiatry* 156(11):1787-1795, 1999.

123. Clohessy S, Ehlers A: PTSD symptoms, response to intrusive memories and coping in ambulance service workers, *Br J Clin Psychol* 38(pt 3):251-265, 1999.

124. Donnelly CL, Amaya-Jackson L, March JS: Psychopharmacology of pediatric posttraumatic stress disorder, *J Child Adolesc Psychopharmacol* 9(3):203-220, 1999.

125. Heim C, Ehlert U, Hellhammer DH: The potential role of hypocortisolism in the pathophysiology of stress-related bodily disorders, *Psychoneuroendocrinology* 25(1):1-35, 2000.

126. Alarcon RD, Glover SG, Deering CG: The cascade model: an alternative to comorbidity in the pathogenesis of posttraumatic stress disorder, *Psychiatry* 62(2):114-124, 1999.

127. Kiecolt-Glaser JK et al: Psychoneuroimmunology and psychosomatic medicine: back to the future, *Psychosom Med* 64(1):15-28, 2002. Review.

128. Granger DA, Booth A, Johnson DR: Human aggression and enumerative measures of immunity, *Psychosom Med* 62(4):583-590, 2000.

129. Folkman S, Lazarus RS: The relationship between coping and emotion: implications for theory and research, *Soc Sci Med* 26(3):309-317, 1988.

130. Irwin M et al: Partial sleep deprivation reduces natural killer cell activity in humans, *Psychosom Med* 56(6):493-498, 1994.

131. Pollmacher T et al: Influence of host defense activation on sleep in humans, *Adv Neuroimmunol* 5(2):155-169, 1995.

132. White D et al: Sleep deprivation and the control of ventilation, *Am Rev Respir Dis* 128(6):984-986, 1983.

133. Lazarus RS, Folkman S: Coping and adaptation. In Gentry WD, editor: *The handbook of behavioral medicine,* New York, 1987, Guilford.

134. Vitaliano PP et al: Coping as an index of illness behavior in panic disorder, *J Nerv Ment Dis* 175(2):78-84, 1987.

135. Folkman S, Lazarus RS: The relationship between coping and emotion: implications for theory and research, *Soc Sci Med* 26(3):309-317, 1988.

136. Frolkis VV: Stress-age syndrome, *Mech Aging Dev* 69(1-2):93-107, 1993.

137. Kiecolt-Glaser J et al: Psychosocial enhancement of immunocompetence in a geriatric population, *Health Psychol* 4(1):25-41, 1985.

138. Spiegel D: Psychosocial intervention in cancer, *J Natl Cancer Inst* 85(15):1198-1205, 1993.

139. Baron RS et al: Social support and immune function among spouses of cancer patients, *J Pers Soc Psychol* 59(2):344-352, 1990.

140. Kiecolt-Glaser J et al: Chronic stress and immune function in family caregivers of Alzheimer's disease victims, *Psychosom Med* 45(5):523, 1987.

141. Shelby J et al: Severe burn injury: effects on psychologic and immunologic function in noninjured close relatives, *J Burn Care Rehabil* 13(1):58-63, 1992.

142. Mazzeo RS: Aging, immune function, and exercise: hormonal regulation, *Int J Sports Med* 21(suppl 1):S10-13, 2000. Review.

BIOLOGY OF CANCER

DAVID M. VIRSHUP • KATHRYN L. McCANCE

evolve

http://evolve.elsevier.com/McCance/

CHAPTER OUTLINE

Cancer is a leading disease, cause of death, and source of morbidity of adults in the Western world. The incidence of cancer increases markedly with advancing age. Over the past 30 years intensive research has lead to a significantly enhanced understanding of this complex and frightening disease. We now understand that cancer is a collection of many different diseases, caused by an accumulation of genetic alterations. Environment, heredity, and behavior interact to modify both the risk of developing cancer, and the response to treatment. Improvements in both treatment strategies and supportive care, coupled with novel therapies based on advances in our fundamental understanding of the basic pathophysiology of cancer, have contributed to an increasing number of effective options for these diverse, often lethal, disorders collectively called cancer.

CANCER CHARACTERISTICS AND TERMINOLOGY

Any discussion of cancer must start with a definition of what it is and what it is not. Although most readers may have an intuitive understanding of this disorder, composing an exact definition that encompasses this broad category is more chal-

lenging. A definition from 1922 may summarize cancer as well as any:

> The most generally accepted definition of a tumor is that it is a tissue overgrowth which is independent of the laws governing the remainder of the body. It is usual to add as a qualifying phrase to separate tumors from reparative processes, such as bone callus, that the neoplasm overgrowth serves no useful purpose to the organism.[1]

The term *cancer* derives from the Greek word for crab, *Karkinoma*, which the physician Hippocrates used to describe the appendage-like projections extending from tumors. The word **tumor** originally referred to any swelling, for example, that caused by inflammation, but is now generally reserved for describing a new growth, or **neoplasm**. Not all tumors or neoplasms, however, are cancer. The term **cancer** refers to a malignant tumor and is not used to refer to *benign* growths such as lipomas or to hypertrophy of an organ. Yet it is important to recognize that benign neoplasms also can cause life-threatening symptoms if they enlarge in critical locations. For example, a benign meningioma at the base of the skull may cause symptoms by compressing adjacent normal brain tissue. The definitions of benign versus malignant are presented below and in Table 11-1. Box 12-1 contains information on the diagnosis and clinical staging of cancer.

Table 11-1	Characteristics of Benign versus Malignant Tumors	
Benign Tumors	**Malignant Tumors**	
Grow slowly	Grow rapidly	
Have a well-defined capsule	Are not encapsulated	
Are not invasive	Invade local structures and tissues	
Well-differentiated; looks like the tissue from which it arises	Poorly differentiated; may not be able to tell what tissue it arose from	
Have a low mitotic index; dividing cells are rare	High mitotic index; many dividing cells	
Do not metastasize	Can spread distantly, often through blood vessels and lymphatics	

Tumor Classification and Nomenclature

Benign tumors, which are not referred to as cancers, are usually encapsulated and well-differentiated. They retain some normal tissue structure and do not invade the capsules surrounding them, nor do they spread to regional lymph nodes or distant locations. Benign tumors are generally named according to the tissues from which they arise, and include the suffix "oma." For example, a benign tumor of the smooth muscle of the uterus is a *leiomyoma,* and a benign tumor of fat cells is a *lipoma.*

Some tumors initially described as benign can progress to cancer and then are referred to as **malignant tumors.** These malignant tumors are distinguished from benign tumors by their more rapid growth rates and specific microscopic alterations, including loss of differentiation and absence of normal tissue organization. They lack a capsule and grow to invade nearby blood vessels, lymphatics, and surrounding structures and then spread to other distant locations *(metastasis).* The most important characteristic of malignant tumors is their ability to spread far beyond the tissue of origin. One of the hallmarks of cancer cells, as seen under the microscope, is anaplasia, the loss of cellular differentiation, irregularities of the size and shape of the nucleus, and loss of normal tissue structure (Figures 11-1 and 11-2 and see Table 11-1).

In general, cancers are named according to the cell type from which they originate. Cancers arising in epithelial tissue are called **carcinomas,** and if they arise from or form ductal or glandular structures are named **adenocarcinomas.** Hence, a malignant tumor arising from breast glandular tissue is a mammary adenocarcinoma. Cancers arising from

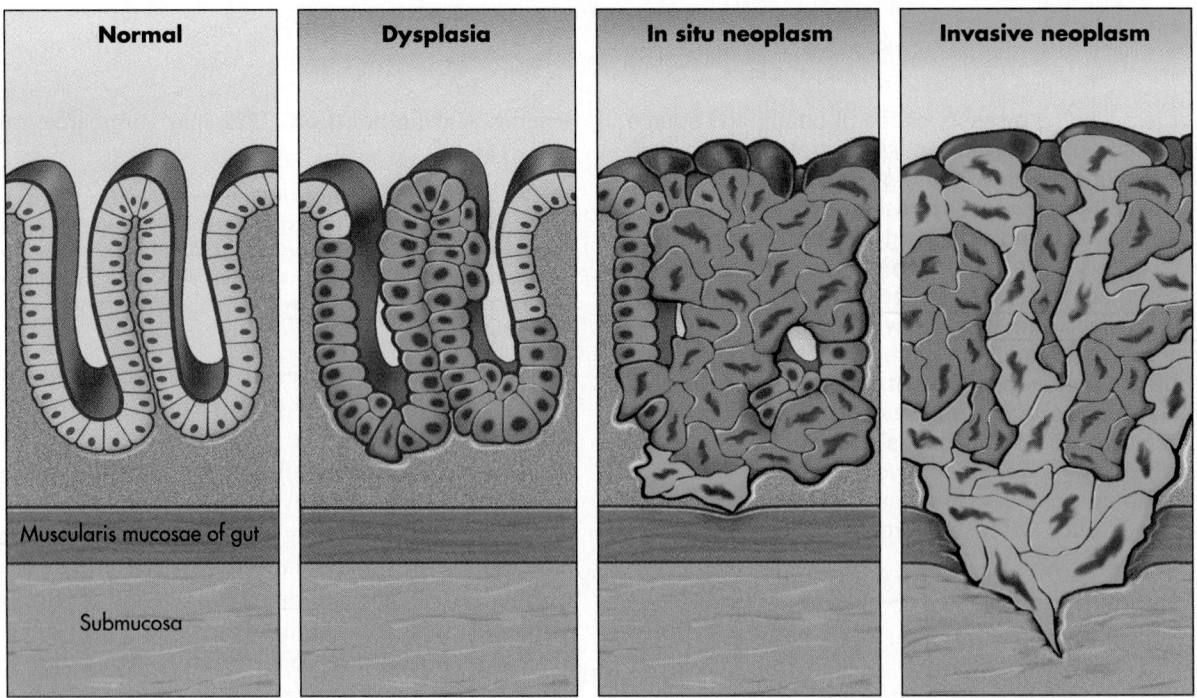

Figure 11-1 Progression of dysplasia to neoplasm. A sequence of cellular and tissue changes progressing from dysplasia to in situ neoplasia and then to invasive neoplasia is seen often in the development of cancer. In clinical specimens, distinguishing between dysplasia and in situ neoplasia is difficult. The presence of anaplastic cells and loss of normal tissue architecture signifies the development of neoplasia. This sequence of changes is most commonly seen in the squamous epithelium of the uterine cervix, the epidermis of sun-exposed skin, and colonic and gastric mucosa after long-standing inflammation. The high rate of cell turnover, local mutagens, and inflammatory mediators all contribute to the accumulation of genetic abnormalities that lead to neoplasia. (Modified from Stevens A, Lowe J: *Pathology,* ed 2, London, 2000, Mosby.)

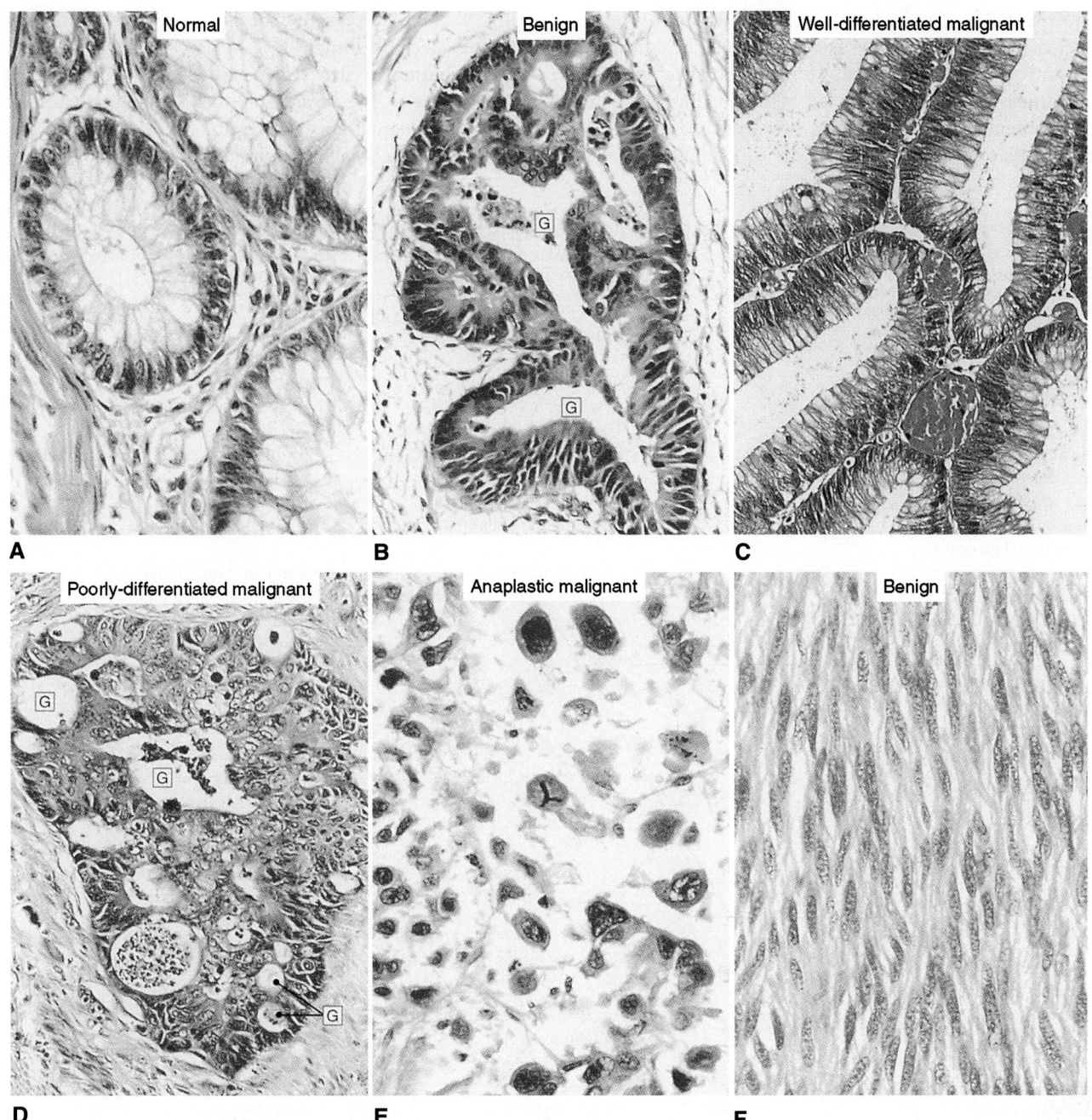

Figure 11-2 Loss of cellular and tissue differentiation during the development of cancer. The cells of a benign neoplasm (**B**) resemble those of the normal colonic epithelium (**A**), in that they are columnar and have an orderly arrangement. Loss of some degree of differentiation is evident in that the neoplasia cells do not show much mucin vacuolization. Cells of the well-differentiated malignant neoplasm (**C**) of the colon have a haphazard arrangement and although gland lumina are formed, they are architecturally abnormal and irregular. Nuclei vary in shape and size, especially when compared with panel **A.** Cells in the poorly differentiated malignant neoplasm (**D**) have an even more haphazard arrangement, with very poor formation of gland lumina. Nuclei show greater variation in shape and size compared with the well-differentiated malignant neoplasm in panel **C.** Cells in anaplastic malignant neoplasms (**E**) bear no relation to the normal epithelium, with no recognizable gland formation. Tremendous variation is found in the size of cells and their nuclei, with very intense staining (nuclear hyperchromatism) of the latter. Not knowing the site of origin would make it impossible to tell what sort of tumor this was by microscopic appearance alone. Well-differentiated tumors often resemble their cell of origin, as shown in the example of a benign tumor of smooth muscles (**F**). (From Stevens A, Lowe J: *Pathology,* ed 2, London, 2000, Mosby.)

connective tissue usually have the suffix **sarcoma.** For example, malignant cancers of skeletal muscle are known as rhabdomyosarcomas. Cancers of lymphatic tissue are called **lymphomas,** whereas cancers of blood-forming cells are called **leukemias.** Many cancers, however, are named for historical reasons that do not follow this naming convention. Table 11-2 presents the nomenclature and classification of selected tumors.

Carcinoma in situ (often abbreviated **CIS**) (see Figure 11-1) refers to pre-invasive epithelial malignant tumors of glandular or squamous cell origin. These early-stage cancers are localized to the epithelium and have not broken through

Table 11-2 Nomenclature and Classification of Benign and Malignant Tumors*		
Cell or Tissue of Origin	**Benign Tumor**	**Malignant Tumor**
Tumors of Epithelial Origin		
Squamous cells	Squamous cell papilloma	Squamous cell carcinoma
Basal cells	—	Basal cell carcinoma
Glandular or ductal epithelium	Adenoma	Adenocarcinoma
	Cystadenoma	Cystadenocarcinoma
Transitional cells	Transitional cell papilloma	Transitional cell carcinoma
Bile duct	Bile duct adenoma	Bile duct carcinoma (cholangiocarcinoma)
Liver cells	Hepatocellular adenoma	Hepatocellular carcinoma
Melanocytes	Nevus	Malignant melanoma
Renal epithelium	Renal tubular adenoma	Renal cell carcinoma
Skin adnexal glands		
Sweat glands	Sweat gland adenoma	Sweat gland carcinoma
Sebaceous glands	Sebaceous gland adenoma	Sebaceous gland carcinoma
Germ cells (testis and ovary)	—	Seminoma (dysgerminoma)
		Embryonal carcinoma, yolk sac carcinoma
Tumors of Mesenchymal Origin		
Hematopoietic/lymphoid tissue		
Leukocytes		Leukemias
Granular leukocytes and precursors		Granulocytic leukemia
		Myelocytic leukemias
		Myelogenous leukemias
Plasma cells		Multiple myeloma
Lymphoid		
Nongranular leukocytes and prelymphocytes		Lymphomas
Proliferating lymphocytes and monocytes		Lymphocytic leukemia
Proliferating immature precursor monocytes		Lymphoblastic leukemia
Solid tumors of lymph tissue (thymus, spleen, lymph nodes)		Lymphoma or lymphosarcoma
Neural and retinal tissue		
Nerve sheath	Neurilemoma, neurofibroma	Malignant peripheral nerve sheath tumor
Nerve cells	Ganglioneuroma	Neuroblastoma
Retinal cells (cones)	—	Retinoblastoma
Connective tissue		
Fibrous tissue	Fibromatosis (desmoid)	Fibrosarcoma
Fat	Lipoma	Liposarcoma
Bone	Osteoma	Osteogenic sarcoma
Cartilage	Chondroma	Chrondrosarcoma
Muscle		
Smooth muscle	Leiomyoma	Leiomyosarcoma
Striated muscle	Rhabdomyoma	Rhabdomyosarcoma
Endothelial and related tissues		
Blood vessels	Hemangioma	Angiosarcoma
		Kaposi sarcoma
Lymph vessels	Lymphangioma	Lymphangiosarcoma
Synovium	—	Synovial sarcoma
Mesathelium	—	Malignant mesothelioma
Meninges	Meningioma	Malignant meningioma
Tumors of Uncertain Origin	—	Ewing tumor

Modified from Murphy GP et al: *American Cancer Society's textbook of clinical oncology,* ed 2, New York, 1995, American Cancer Society.
*This list is intended to provide only an introduction to tumor nomenclature.

the local basement membrane nor invaded the surrounding stroma (see Figure 11-1 and Box 11-1). *Carcinoma in situ* is recognized in a number of sites, including the cervix, skin, oral cavity, esophagus, and bronchus. In glandular epithelium, *in situ* lesions occur in the stomach, endometrium, breast, and large bowel. In the breast, ductal carcinoma in situ fills the mammary ducts before progressing to local tissue invasion. These lesions are readily treatable by breast-sparing surgery. The time that such preinvasive lesions remain *in situ* before becoming invasive is unknown. Some carcinomas of the cervix are known to be preinvasive lesions *in situ* for several years before they progress to invasive carcinoma and metastatic tumors (see Figure 11-2).

Cancer Cells
Transformation and Differentiation

Cancer cells behave differently than normal cells in several important ways. **Transformation** refers to the process by which a normal cell becomes a cancer cell. **Autonomy** refers to the cancer cell's independence from normal cellular controls and is part of the transformational process. These differences are most readily seen in specialized laboratory assays, especially those examining the growth patterns of normal and cancerous cells in laboratory incubators. Transformed cells lack many of the normal "social controls" seen in nontransformed cells. Normal cells cease to divide when they fill a Petri (or tissue culture) dish, whereas transformed cells continue to crowd and eventually pile up on each other (Figure 11-3). Normal cells will not grow unless they are attached to a firm surface (like a Petri dish). However, cancer cells are often **anchorage-independent,** that is, they continue to divide even when suspended in a soft agar gel. Normal cells have a limited life span in the laboratory; they may divide in a Petri dish 10 or 50 times, but then they cease growing. Cancer cells usually are **immortal,** in that they seem to have an unlimited life span and will continue to divide for years under appropriate labo-

ratory conditions. One of the most commonly used laboratory cell lines, HeLa cells, were derived from a cervical cancer specimen in 1951 that continues to grow and divide in laboratories around the world.[2]

Cancer cells often show defects in the normal process of differentiation, that is, the process of acquiring a specialized function and organization, such as evolving into a muscle cell or a nerve cell. **Anaplasia** is the absence of differentiation (see Figure 11-2 and Figure 11-4) and means literally "without form." In clinical specimens, *anaplasia* is recognized by a loss of organization and a marked increase in nuclear size, with evidence of ongoing proliferation. In contrast to normal cells, which are uniform in size and shape, *anaplastic* cells are of variable size and shape, or **pleomorphic.** For example, a benign muscle tumor (benign myoma) will retain the ability to make muscle, whereas in a malignant muscle tumor (rhabdomyosarcoma), new muscle formation is seen only rarely, and even then appears highly disorganized. Thus the muscle cancer cells are undifferentiated as compared with the tissue they originated from (see Figure 11-5). The most malignant tumors tend to have the most *anaplasia*.

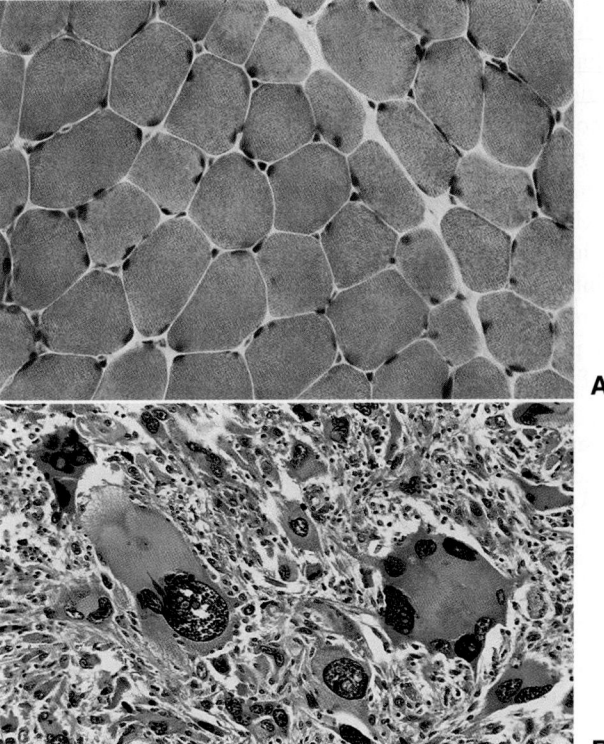

Figure 11-4 Normal and anaplastic skeletal muscle cells. **A,** Normal skeletal muscle cells. **B,** Anaplastic tumor of the skeletal muscle (rhabdomyosarcoma). Note the marked cellular and nuclear pleomorphism (cellular and nuclear variation in size and shape), hyperchromatic nuclei, and tumor giant cells. The prominent cell in the center field has an abnormal tripolar spindle. Often the tissue of origin of an anaplastic tumor can be established only by the use of molecular markers, such as immunohistochemical stains and chromosome analysis. (**A** from Damjanov I, Linder J, editors: *Anderson's pathology,* ed 10, St Louis, 1996, Mosby; **B** from Kumar V, Abbas AK, Fausto N: *Pathologic basis of disease,* ed 7, Philadelphia, 2005, Saunders; courtesy of Dr. Trace Worrell, Department of Pathology, University of Texas Southwestern Medical School.)

Density-dependent inhibition of growth in normal cells

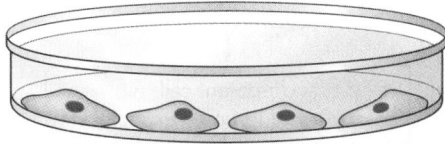

Multilayer of uninhibited cancer cells

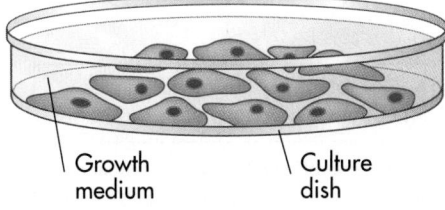

Figure 11-3 Cancerous cells show uninhibited growth. Cancer cells, unlike most normal cells, usually continue to grow and pile on top of one another after they have formed a confluent monolayer in culture.

Cancer Stem Cells

Many tissues, most notably the skin, intestines, and blood-forming cells found in the bone marrow, have a significant amount of cell division and cell death on a daily basis. This ongoing proliferation of these tissues with a high turnover rate depends on their regeneration from a small fraction of cells known as **stem cells.** Stem cells have two essential characteristics: first, they self-renew (that is, some fraction of the cell divisions create new stem cells) and second, they are **multipotent,** or have the ability to differentiate into multiple different cell types (Figure 11-5). In the bone marrow, it is estimated that only 0.05% (1 in 20,000) of the blood-forming cells are stem cells, yet this small pool of stem cells can be stimulated to divide and to repopulate the entire population of mature bone marrow–derived cells in approximately 2 weeks after bone marrow transplantation. As few as 10 stem cells are sufficient to entirely repopulate the entire bone marrow of a mouse in bone marrow transplantation experiments. Similarly, the absorptive and goblet cells lining the intestine have a life span of less than 1 week, after which they undergo cell death, or apoptosis, and slough into the intestinal lumen. They too must be replenished by ongoing proliferation of intestinal stem cells. A key feature of stem cells is that they give rise to daughter cells that ultimately terminally differentiate into diverse cell types, depending on the needs of the tissue (Figure 11-6). Multipotent bone marrow stem cells can both self-renew and differentiate into all types of bone marrow–derived cells, such as red cells, lymphocytes, and neutrophils. Controversial studies suggest that certain adult stem cells might have a broader range of potential fates. For example, a bone marrow stem cell might be able to differentiate into other types of cells, such as neurons or muscle cells. Theoretically, such a stem cell might be able to give rise to all cell types in the body, and as such, could be useful in regeneration of diseased tissues (see Figure 11-5).

The similarities between normal stem cells and cancer have led researchers to investigate whether cancer might in fact be a disease of stem cells. Like stem cells, cancer cells can proliferate indefinitely, in some cases giving rise to well differentiated cells, and in other cases giving rise to poorly differentiated cells. Experimental work in leukemia[3] and more recently in breast cancer[4] provide evidence that cancer stem cells do exist. These studies show that only a small subset of leukemia cells have the ability to divide indefinitely and give rise to full-blown leukemia. Emerging data suggests the same will be found true for breast cancer: only a small fraction of cells from a breast cancer are able to divide indefinitely and generate a full-blown breast cancer when transplanted to experimental animals. This emerging concept of the cancer stem cell as the central problem in cancer will surely generate much study in the next few years.

Tumor Markers

Tumor markers (biologic markers) are substances produced by cancer cells that are found on tumor plasma membranes or in the blood, spinal fluid, or urine (Table 11-3). Tumor mark-

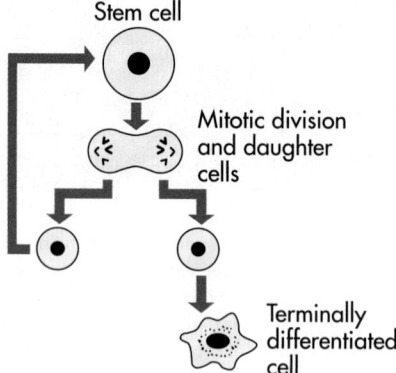

Figure 11-5 Differentiation of a stem cell. When a stem cell divides, each daughter cell has a choice: it can either continue as a stem cell or go on to become terminally differentiated, that is, completely matured (e.g., neuron, myocyte, erythrocyte).

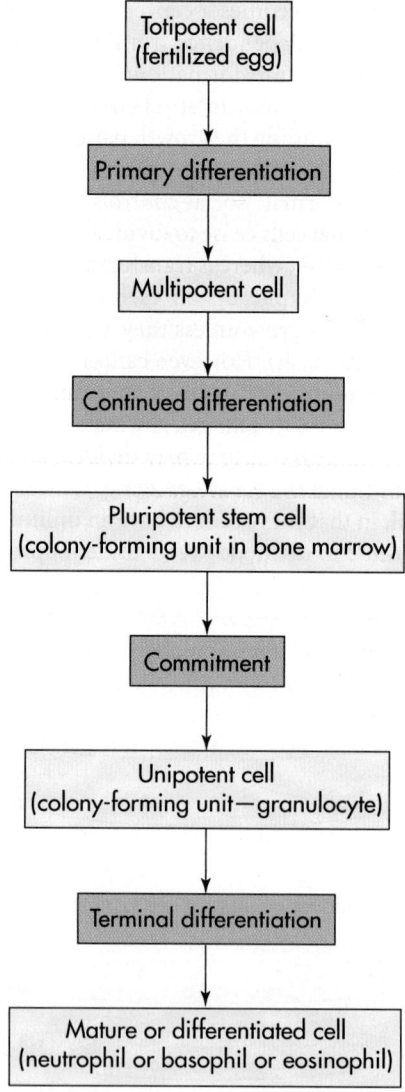

Figure 11-6 Example of differentiation. Differentiation occurs several times in the lifetime of a granulocyte, with each step further limiting the cell's potential. Eventually, the terminally differentiated cell can no longer divide, and the mature cell dies.

Table 11-3   Examples of Tumor Markers

Marker Name	Nature	Type of Cancer
α-Fetoprotein (AFP)	70 kDa protein	Hepatic, germ cell
Carcinoembryonic antigen (CEA)	200 kDa glycoprotein	GI, pancreas, lung, breast, etc.
β-Human chorionic gonadotropin (β-HCG)	Glycopeptide hormone	Germ cell
Prostate-specific antigen (PSA)	33 kDa glycoprotein	Prostate
Catecholamines	Epinephrine and precursors	Pheochromocytoma (adrenal medulla)
Homovanillic acid/vanillylmandilic acid (HVA/VMA)	Catecholamine metabolites	Neuroblastoma
Urinary Bence-Jones protein	Ig light chain	Multiple myeloma
Adrenocorticotropic hormone (ACTH)	Peptide hormone	Pituitary adenomas

GI, Gastrointestinal; *Ig*, immunoglobulin.

ers have been associated with cancer for many decades. For diseases associated with a tumor marker, there is indeed a "blood test for cancer." Tumor markers include hormones, enzymes, genes, antigens, and antibodies. For example, the adrenal medulla normally secretes the catecholamine epinephrine (adrenaline). Benign tumors of the adrenal medulla can produce catecholamines in vast excess, leading to rapid pulse, high blood pressure, sweats, and tremors. Elevated blood or urine levels of epinephrine and related compounds in someone with this set of symptoms strongly suggest the presence of an adrenal medullary tumor (pheochromocytoma). Liver and germ cell tumors secrete a protein known as *alpha fetoprotein (AFP)* into the blood, and prostate tumors secrete prostate specific antigen (PSA) into the blood. These tumor markers can be used in three ways: (1) to screen and identify individuals at high risk for cancer; (2) to help diagnose the specific type of tumor in individuals with clinical manifestations relating to cancer, as in adrenal tumors; and (3) to follow the clinical course of cancer. For example, a falling PSA after therapy for prostate cancer indicates successful treatment, and a later rise in the PSA may indicate a recurrence.

A significant problem in diagnosing cancer using tumor marker assays is that nonmalignant diseases also produce tumor markers. The presence of a tumor marker therefore may suggest a specific diagnosis, but it is not used alone as a definitive diagnostic test. Identification of ideal sensitive and specific tumor markers in common cancers remains a high priority because the early detection of cancer often improves the treatment outcome. Fortunately, new blood tests using protein fingerprinting, or **proteomic,** methods show promise in research studies as being useful for identifying individuals at high risk for specific cancers.[5]

THE GENETIC BASIS OF CANCER
Cancer-Causing Mutations in Genes
Clonal Selection

Prior to the advent of modern molecular biology, many different causes of cancer were postulated, based on epidemiologic studies, studies of carcinogens, and studies of viruses. We now understand that changes in the DNA of the cancer cell cause the cell to become cancerous. Perhaps the most telling epidemiologic data is presented in Figure 11-7.

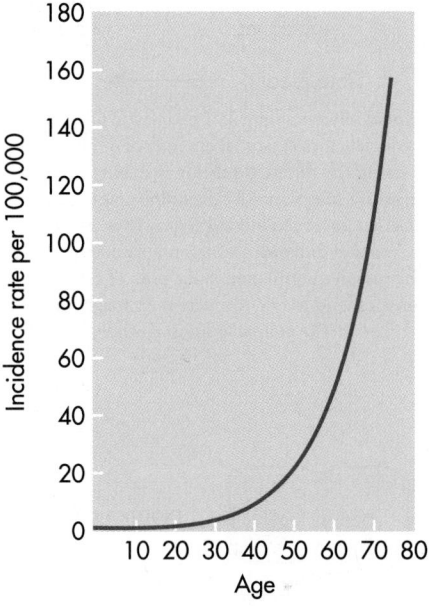

Figure 11-7 Marked increases in cancer with age. The graph depicts the number of cases of colon cancer diagnosed per 100,000 women in England and Wales in 1 year. The incidence of cancer increases dramatically with advancing age. This type of data suggests that accumulation of genetic mutations over time increases the risk of developing cancer. The slope of the curve suggests that five to seven mutations must occur before full-blown cancer develops. (Modified from Alberts B et al: *Molecular biology of the cell,* ed 4, New York, 2002, Garland.)

Cancer is predominantly a disease of aging. The incidence of cancer, that is, the fraction of individuals in each age group who develop cancer, increases dramatically with age. The best explanation for this epidemiologic data is that each individual acquires a number of genetic 'hits' or mutations over time. When sufficient mutations have occurred, cancer develops.

As an individual mutation occurs in a single cell, it may acquire some of the characteristics of a cancer cell, for example, increased growth rate, or alternatively, decreased apoptosis, or death rate. That cell may then have a selective advantage over its neighbors; its progeny can accumulate faster than its nonmutant neighbors. This is referred to as **clonal proliferation** or **clonal expansion** (Figure 11-8). As a clone with a mutation proliferates, it may become an early stage tumor, for example, a carcinoma in situ or a benign colonic polyp. Additional mutations then occur in these early lesions that permit progression

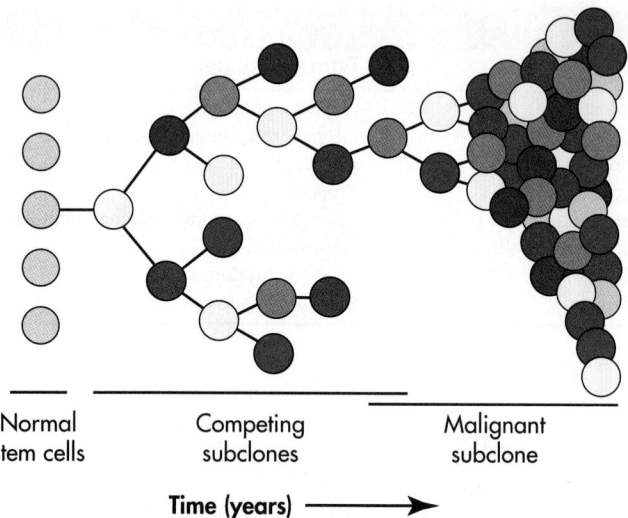

Figure 11-8 Clonal selection model of neoplastic progression. The clonal selection process depicts the sequential emergence of altered populations of cells over time. Genetically different subclones coexist for a time, and this is the basis of competitive selection. All cells of the emerging malignancy harbor the mutations that governed increased growth in earlier periods, but they can acquire new and different alterations, producing clonal heterogeneity within the invasive population. Subclones of cells with the most aggressive characteristics tend to out-compete their neighbors. (Modified from Mendelsohn J et al: *The molecular basis of cancer*, ed 2, Philadelphia, 2001, Saunders.)

to more advanced tumors. The process of tumor development is a form of Darwinian evolution; cells with a genetic change that confers a survival advantage out-compete their neighbors. The progressive accumulation of distinct advantageous (from the point of view of the cancer cell, not the individual!) mutations leads from normal cells to fully malignant cancers.

One organ in which this correlation of genetic and clinical progression has been especially well studied is the colon.[6] The colon is accessible to inspection with a colonoscope, and so neoplastic lesions of varying size can easily be detected and removed. Intestinal polyps are benign neoplasms and the first stage in development of colon cancer. Small polyps tend to have only a few detectable mutations. Large polyps have more mutations, whereas frank colon cancers have even more mutations. This type of genetic data also strongly supports the notion that it is the *accumulation* of mutations in specific genes that is required for the development of cancer (Figure 11-9).

Types of Genes that are Mutated in Cancer
Alterations in Progrowth and Antigrowth Signals

It has been established that multiple mutations are required before cancer can develop. One key question is what types of genes must be mutated to cause a cancer? The prevailing view is that a number of distinct and specific cellular control path-

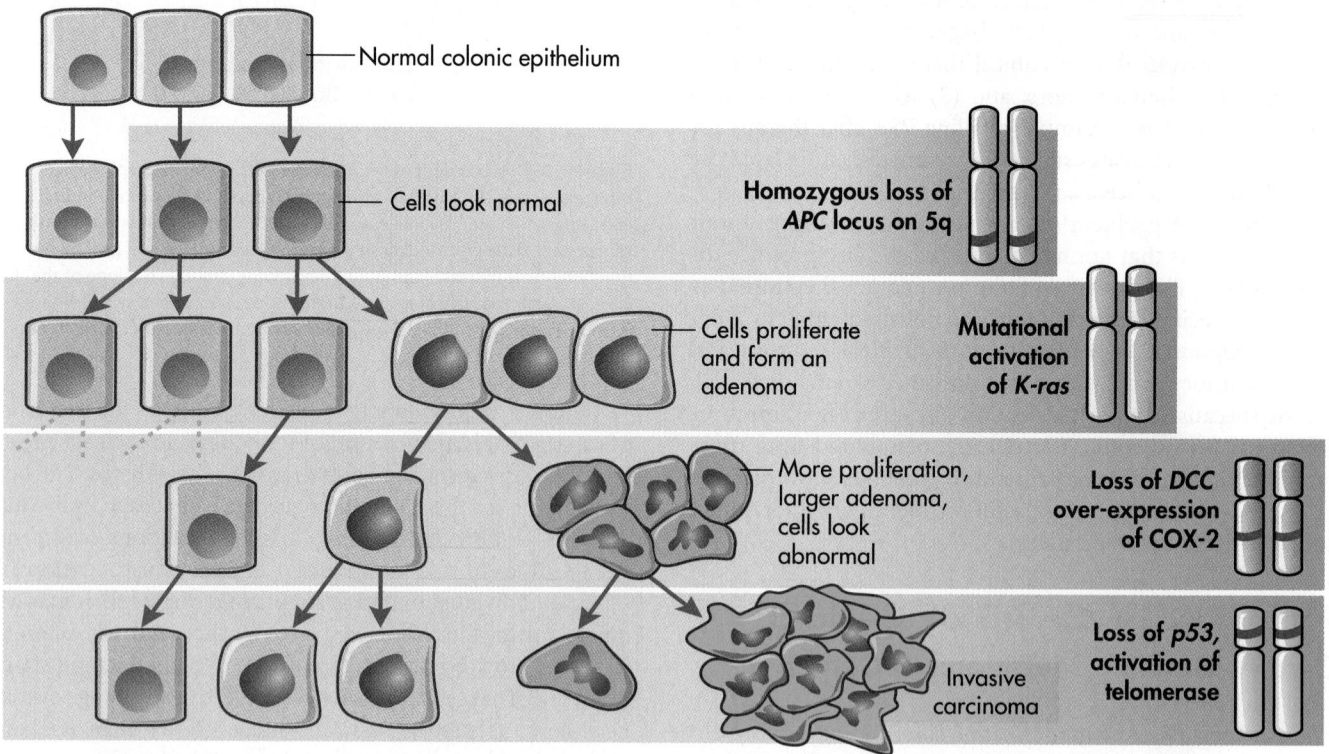

Figure 11-9 Sequential acquisition of genetic changes. Progression from a benign polyp to malignant colon cancer is accomplished by an accumulation of mutations. One of the earliest mutations in colon cancer is loss of the tumor suppressor gene *APC*. Additional mutations, often in the oncogene *ras*, activation of COX-2, and loss of the tumor suppressors *DCC* and *p53* occur as the lesion progresses from a benign polyp to an invasive carcinoma. *APC*, Adenomatous polyposis coli; *DCC*, deleted in colon cancer; *COX-2*, cyclooxygenase-2. (Modified from Kumar V, Cotran RS, Robbins SL: *Basic pathology*, ed 6, Philadelphia, 1997, Saunders.)

ways must be altered for a cell to become fully malignant[7] (see Figure 11-9 and Figure 11-10). First, cancer cells must have mutations that enable them to proliferate in the absence of external growth signals. To achieve this, some cancers acquire the ability to secrete growth factors that stimulate their own growth, a process known as **autocrine stimulation** (also see Chapter 1). Other cancers have an increase in growth factor receptors; for example, in breast cancer, the epidermal growth factor receptor HER2/neu is up-regulated, and likely sends growth signals into the cell even when growth factors are at very low levels. Alternatively, the signal cascade from the cell surface receptor to the nucleus may be mutated in the "on" position. Many cancers have an activating mutation in an intracellular signaling protein called *ras*. Mutant *ras* stimulates cell growth even when growth factors are missing (Figure 11-11).

Cells usually receive diverse "antigrowth" signals from their normal milieu. Contact with other cells, with basement membranes, and with soluble factors all normally signal cells to stop proliferating. These mechanisms can put a halt to unregulated cell growth. This normal antigrowth signal must be inactivated in cancer as well. Common mutations include inactivation of the tumor suppressor *Rb*, or conversely, activa-

tion of the protein kinases that drive the cell cycle, the cyclin-dependent kinases (see Chapter 1). Next, cells have a mechanism that causes them to self-destruct when growth is excessive and checkpoints have been ignored. This self-destruct mechanism, called **apoptosis,** is triggered by diverse stimuli, including normal development and excessive growth (see Chapter 2). The pathway to apoptosis is disabled in advanced cancers. The most common mutations conferring resistance to apoptosis occur in the *p53* gene (see Chapter 12).

Angiogenesis

As cancers grow beyond minimal size, they need their own blood supply to deliver oxygen and nutrients. However, in adults, new blood vessel growth is normally limited to areas of wound healing and to the female uterus during the proliferative phase of the menstrual cycle. Small cancers lack the ability to grow new blood vessels. More advanced cancers can secrete factors that stimulate new blood vessel growth. These **angiogenic factors,** such as *vascular endothelial growth factor* (VEGF), are required in small cancers to permit continued tumor expansion. Therapies directed against new vessel growth have proven promising in both animal and clinical

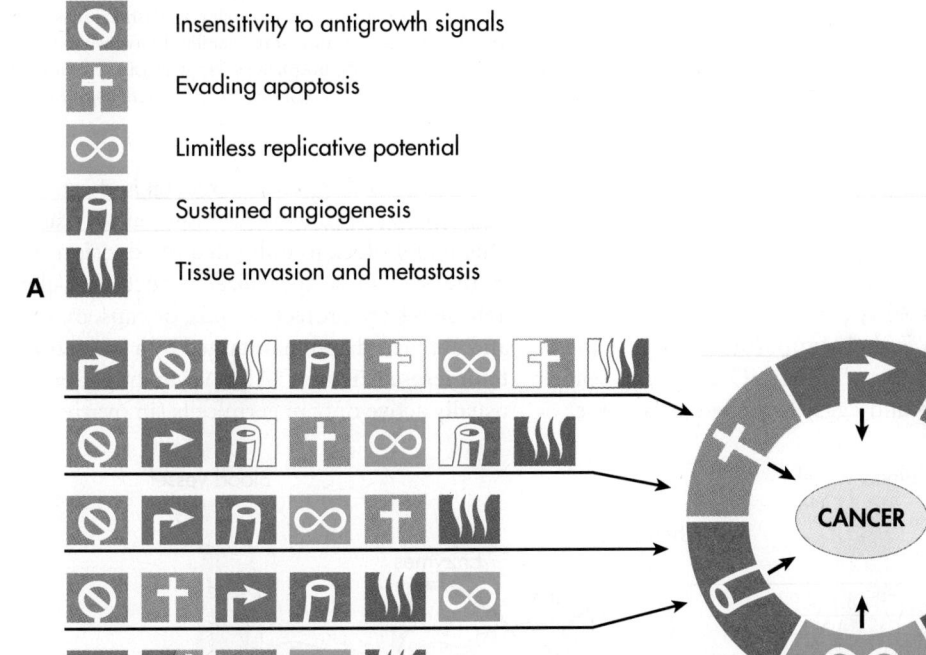

Figure 11-10 Six hallmarks of cancer. A, Most cancers acquire mutations in six distinct areas of cell control during their development. **B,** Multiple pathways of carcinogenesis. All cancers must acquire mutations in the six areas, but their means of doing so varies mechanistically and chronologically. As shown, the order in which these capabilities are acquired is variable across different cancers. In some tumors, a particular mutation may confer several capabilities simultaneously, decreasing the number of intermediate mutational steps required for full development. Loss of the *p53* tumor suppressor gene may facilitate resistance to apoptosis and angiogenesis (e.g., in the five-step pathway shown *[bottom pathway]*). In other tumors, by comparison, a collaboration of two or more distinct genetic changes may be needed to acquire a given trait. In the eight-step model *(top pathway),* invasion metastasis and resistance to apoptosis are each acquired in two steps. (Modified from Hanahan D, Weinberg, RA: *Cell* 100(1):57-70, 2000.)

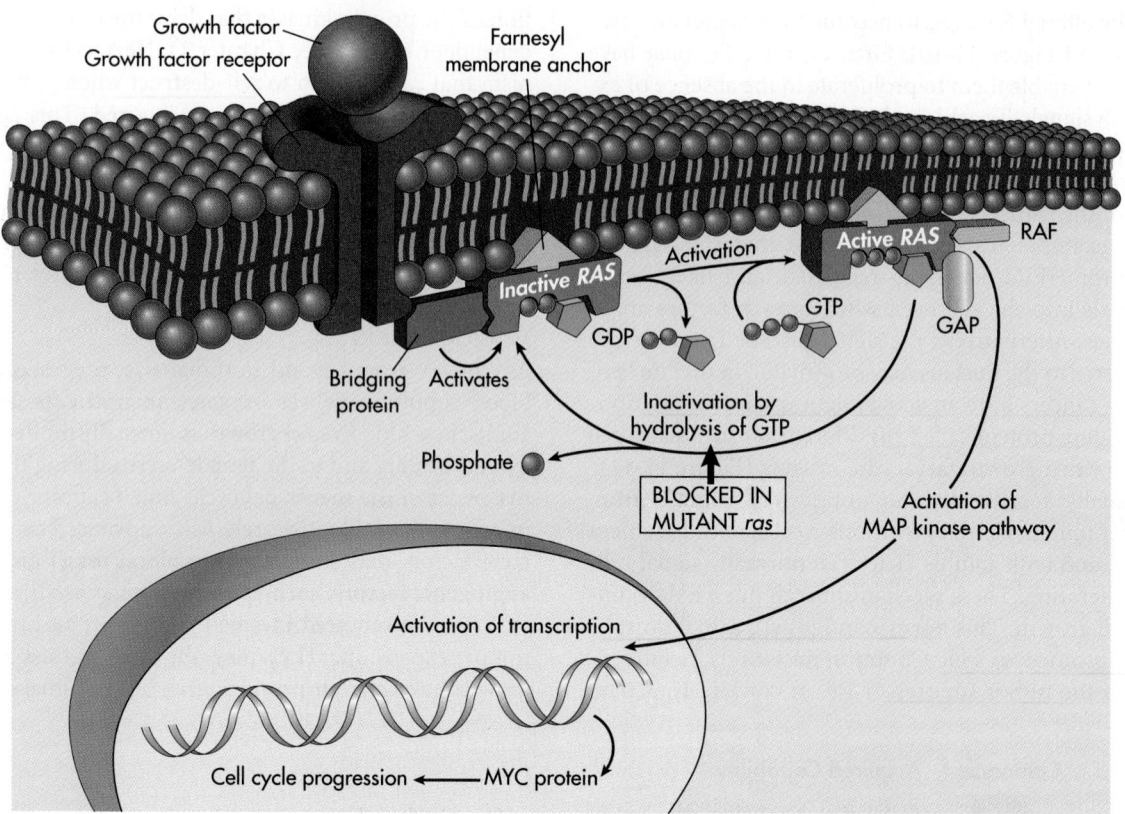

Figure 11-11 Model for action of *ras* genes. When a normal cell is stimulated through a growth factor receptor, inactive (GDP-bound) RAS is activated to a GTP-bound state. Activated RAS sends growth signals to the nucleus through cytoplasmic kinases, starting with the activation of kinase RAF. The mutant RAS protein is permanently activated because of its inability to hydrolyze GTP, leading to continual stimulation of the cell without any external trigger. *GDP,* Guanosine diphosphate; *GTP,* guanosine triphosphate; *GAP,* GTPase activating protein; *MAP,* mitogen-activated protein. (From Kumar V, Cotran RS, Robbins SL: *Basic pathology,* ed 7, Philadelphia, 2003, Saunders.)

studies and one agent, bevacizumab, a monoclonal antibody that inhibits VEGF, has been approved for use in patients with metastatic colorectal cancer[8,9] (Figure 11-12).

Telomeres and Immortality

A hallmark of cancer cells is their immortality. Usually the only cells in the body that are "immortal" are germ cells (those that generate sperm and eggs) and stem cells. Other cells in the body are not immortal and can divide only a limited number of times before they either cease dividing or die. One major block to unlimited cell division (i.e., immortality) is the size of a specialized structure called the *telomere*. **Telomeres** are protective ends, or caps, on each chromosome and are placed and maintained by a specialized enzyme called **telomerase** (Figure 11-13). As you might expect, telomerase is usually active only in germ cells (in ovaries and testes) and in

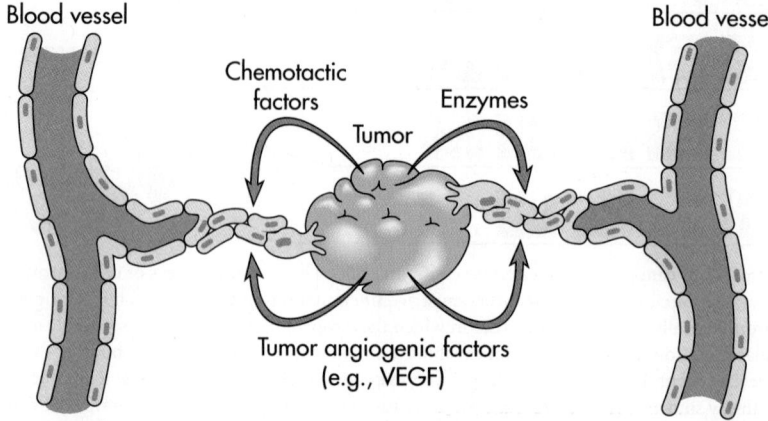

Figure 11-12 Tumor-induced angiogenesis. Malignant tumors, especially those in metastatic sites, induce formation of blood vessels, which serve as routes for the transport of nutrients into the tumor. *VEGF,* Vascular endothelial growth factor. (From Damjanov, I: *Pathology for health related professionals,* ed. 2, Philadelphia, 2000, Saunders.)

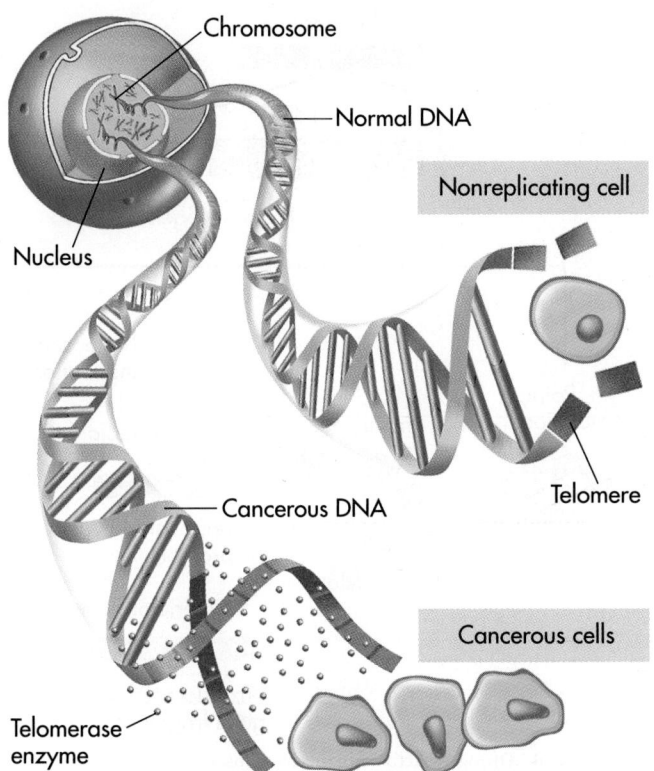

Chromosome

Normal DNA

Nonreplicating cell

Nucleus

Cancerous DNA

Telomere

Cancerous cells

Telomerase enzyme

Figure 11-13 Control of replication: telomeres. Normal cells cannot divide indefinitely. The ends of their chromosomes are capped by telomeres. In the absence of the telomerase enzyme, telomeres get shorter with each division until the cells finally stop dividing. In cancer cells the telomerase gene is "switched on," producing an enzyme that rebuilds the telomeres. Thus the cancer cell continues to divide indefinitely.

stem cells. All other cells of the body lack telomerase. Therefore, when nongerm cells begin to proliferate abnormally, their telomere caps become smaller and smaller with each cell division. When the telomeres become critically small, the chromosomes become unstable and fragment, and then the cells die. Cancer cells, when they reach a critical age, activate telomerase somehow in order to restore and maintain their telomeres and thereby make it possible to divide over and over again.[10,11]

Finally, it appears genetic differences exist between cells that successfully metastasize and those that do not.[12] It has been postulated that specific mutations activate the ability to metastasize. Decreased cell-to-cell adhesion, the secretion of various proteases that digest surrounding barriers, and the ability to grow in new locations, all contribute to successful metastasis[13] (see Chapter 12).

Oncogenes and Tumor-Suppressor Genes: Accelerators and Brakes

The previous discussion refers to the activating and inactivating of various genes as being key in the development of cancer. Just what types of mutations actually occur in cancer? First, it is useful to distinguish between oncogenes and tumor-suppressor genes. Table 11-4 compares the two types of cancer genes. **Oncogenes** are mutant genes that in their normal nonmutant state direct synthesis of proteins that positively regulate (accelerate) proliferation. Conversely, **tumor-suppressor genes** encode proteins that in their normal state negatively regulate (halt, or "put on the brakes") proliferation. Hence, they also have been referred to as anti-oncogenes.

In its normal, nonmutant state, an oncogene is referred to as a **proto-oncogene.** An example of a proto-oncogene would be a growth factor (e.g., epidermal growth factor), or a growth factor receptor (e.g., epidermal growth factor receptor). Other positive regulators of proliferation are in the signal transduction pathway that transmits the signal from the growth factor receptor to the cell nucleus. Normally, *ras* is a proto-oncogene (see Figure 11-11).

Mutation of Normal Genes into Oncogenes
Point Mutations
Several types of genetic events can activate oncogenes (Box 11-1 and Figure 11-14). Perhaps the most common events are small scale changes in DNA such as **point mutations,** the alteration of one or a few nucleotide base pairs (see Chapter 4). This type of mutation can have profound effects on the activity of proteins. A point mutation in the *ras* gene converts it from a regulated proto-oncogene to an unregulated oncogene, an accelerator of cellular proliferation. Activating point mutations in *ras* are found in many cancers, especially pancreatic and colorectal cancer.[14] Very specialized tests are usually needed to detect such point mutations.

Chromosome Translocations
Chromosome translocations, in which a piece of one chromosome is translocated to another chromosome, can activate oncogenes by way of either of two distinct mechanisms. First, a translocation can cause excess and inappropriate production of a proliferation factor. One of the best examples is the *t(8;14)* translocation found in many Burkitt lymphomas[15]; t(8;14) designates a chromosome that has a piece of chromosome 8 fused to a piece of chromosome 14 (see Chapter 27). Burkitt lymphoma is an aggressive cancer of B lymphocytes. The *myc* proto-oncogene found on chromosome 8 is normally

Table 11-4	Comparison of Cancer Gene Types	
Gene Type	Normal Function	Mutation Effect
Dominant oncogenes*	Encode proteins that promote growth (e.g., growth factors)	Overexpression, amplification, gain of function
Tumor suppressors (recessive oncogenes)	Encode proteins that inhibit proliferation and prevent or repair mutations	Loss of function of both alleles

*Nonmutant state referred to as proto-oncogene.

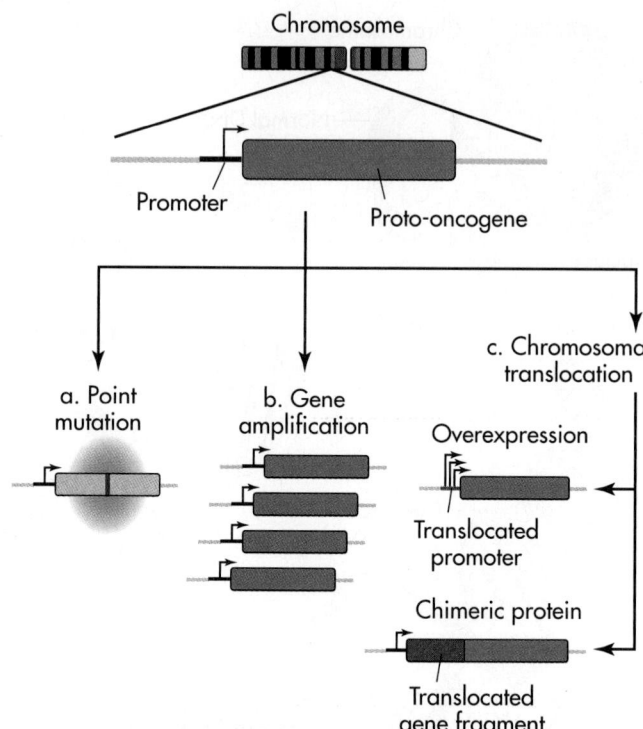

Figure 11-14 **Oncogene activation mechanisms.** Cellular genes may be activated to become cancerous oncogenes as a result of *(a) point mutations* that alter one or a few nucleotide base pairs, causing the production of a protein that is activated as a result of the reordered sequence; *(b) amplification of the cellular gene,* resulting in higher levels of protein expression; or *(c) chromosomal translocations* that either (1) lead to the juxtaposition of a strong promoter, causing increased protein expression, or (2) produce a novel fusion protein that is derived from gene fragments normally present on different chromosomes. (From Haber DA: *Molecular genetics of cancer.* In ACP Medicine, Danbury, Conn., 2004, WebMD.)

turned on at low levels in proliferating lymphocytes and is turned off in mature lymphocytes. The **MYC protein** is part of the positive signal for cell proliferation. If an accidental formation of the t(8;14) translocation occurs, the *myc* gene is aberrantly placed under the control of a B cell immunoglobulin *(Ig)* gene present on chromosome 14. The *Ig* gene is turned on high in maturing B lymphocytes. The t(8;14) alters the control of *myc;* its normal low level is switched to high levels, as directed by an *Ig* gene promoter. *MYC,* when inappropriately high, drives proliferation. Hence, the t(8;14) translocation causes cancer of maturing B cells (Figure 11-15).

Chromosome translocations also can lead to production of novel proteins with growth-promoting properties. In a different type of leukemia, chronic myeloid leukemia (CML), a specific translocation is almost invariably found. This translocation, t(9;22), was first identified in association with CML in Philadelphia in 1960 and so is often referred to as the Philadelphia chromosome.[16] This translocation fuses two chromosomes right in the middle of two genes, *bcr* on chromosome 9 and *abl* on chromosome 22. The result is production of a BCR-ABL fusion protein containing the first half of BCR and the second half of ABL. BCR-ABL is a misregulated protein tyrosine kinase that promotes growth of myeloid cells. Notably, a recently developed drug imatinib (Gleevec® [Novartis]) that specifically inhibits this tyrosine kinase has shown great efficacy in the treatment of CML, and it lacks the side effects noted with nonspecific antileukemia drugs.[17]

Gene Amplification

Another type of genetic abnormality that turns on oncogenes is **gene amplification** (Figure 11-16, and see Figure 11-14). Amplifications are the result of duplication of a small piece of a chromosome over and over again, so that instead of the normal two copies of a gene, tens or even hundreds of copies are present (see Chapter 3). Gene amplification results in increased expression of an oncogene, or in some cases, drug resistance genes. The *N-myc* oncogene is amplified in 25% of childhood neuroblastoma cases and confers a poor prognosis.[18] The epidermal growth factor receptor *erbB2* is amplified in 20% of breast cancers.[19]

Tumor-Suppressor Genes

Tumor suppressor genes are genes whose major function is to negatively regulate cell growth and prevent mutations. Tumor suppressors slow the cell cycle, inhibit proliferation resulting from growth signals, and stop cell division when cells are damaged. Examples of several tumor suppressors are given in Table 11-5. One of the first discovered tumor sup-

pressor genes, the **retinoblastoma (Rb) gene,** normally strongly inhibits the cell division cycle. When it is inactivated, the cell division cycle can proceed unchecked. *Rb* is found to be mutated in cases of childhood retinoblastoma, and in many lung, breast, and bone cancers as well.

Although oncogenes are activated by mutation, tumor suppressors first must be inactivated to allow cancer to occur (see Table 11-5 and Figure 11-17). A single genetic event can activate an oncogene. However, we have two copies, or alleles, of each gene, one from each parent. It therefore takes two 'hits' to inactivate both copies of a tumor suppressor gene. The first copy of a tumor suppressor is often inactivated by point mutations. For example, the *Rb* gene may be inactivated on one chromosome by a point mutation (e.g., the copy inherited from the father). Since the other copy of the retinoblastoma gene (in this example, the one from the mother) is intact, a functional *Rb* protein can still be made and therefore the cell division cycle can be regulated appropriately. If the remaining gene is mutated, then all Rb function is lost and another step toward cancer occurs.

Loss of Heterozygosity

For the function of a tumor suppressor to be lost, both chromosomal copies (alleles) of the gene must be inactivated.

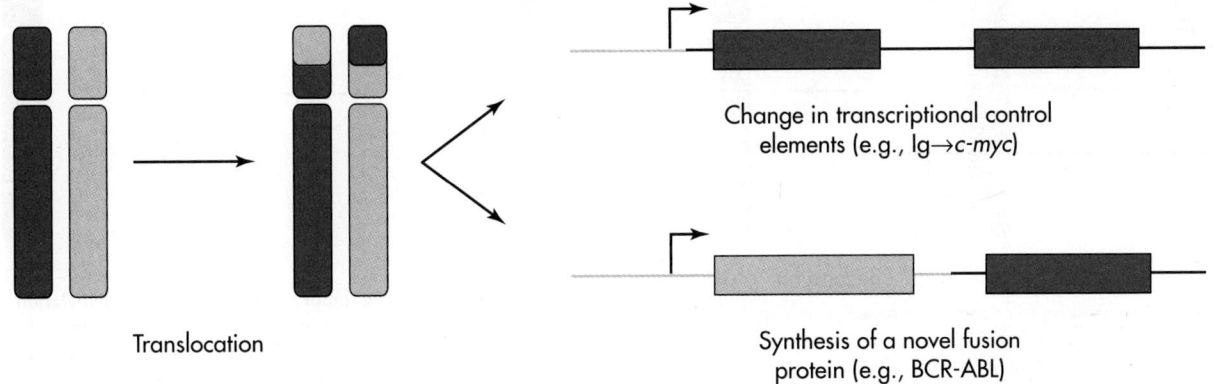

Translocation

Change in transcriptional control
elements (e.g., Ig→*c-myc*)

Synthesis of a novel fusion
protein (e.g., BCR-ABL)

Figure 11-15 **Two mechanisms of oncogenic chromosome translocations.** Chromosome translocations can lead to inappropriate activation of an oncogene by fusing the transcriptional control elements of one gene, for example, the immunoglobulin (Ig) heavy chain promoter, to the coding sequence for an oncogene, in this example, the *c-myc* oncogene. This leads to high-level expression of *c-myc* in B lymphocytes as they make immunoglobulins (antibodies). This type of translocation is found in B cell lymphomas. Chromosome translocations also can fuse two genes right in the middle, leading to synthesis of novel chimeric proteins. The fusion often creates a protein that either has new cancer-promoting properties or has lost the ability to regulate a protein kinase.

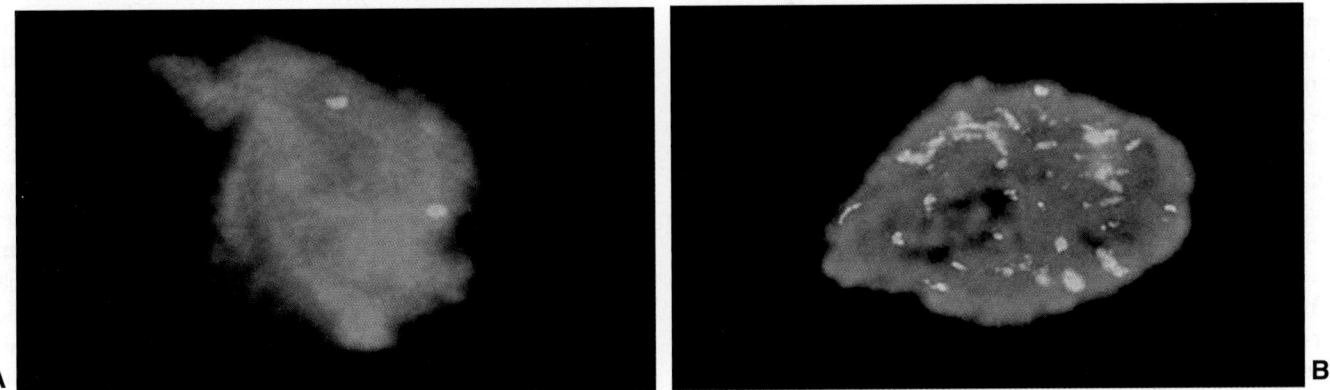

A

B

Figure 11-16 ***N-myc* gene amplification in neuroblastoma.** The *N-myc* gene is detected in human neuroblastoma cells using a technique called FISH (fluorescent in situ hybridization) **A,** A single pair of *N-myc* genes are detected in normal cells and in low-grade neuroblastoma. **B,** Multiple, amplified copies of the *N-myc* gene are detected in some cases of neuroblastoma. Amplification of the *N-myc* is strongly associated with a poor prognosis in childhood neuroblastoma. (Courtesy of Arthur R. Brothman, PhD, FACMG, University of Utah School of Medicine.)

This is because they act in a recessive manner at the level of the cell. Although it may seem intuitive that simple inactivating mutations might disrupt both alleles, in fact this is not what usually happens.[20] Instead, the first allele (in the example above, the paternal copy) is inactivated by simple mutation, but the second allele (in this example, the maternal copy) is lost because entire regions of the maternal chromosome are lost (see Figure 11-17). Because you have two chromosomes, one from each parent, you can be *heterozygous* for nearby genetic markers; loss of a chromosome region in a tumor is referred to as **loss of heterozygosity,** or **LOH.** Loss of heterozygosity unmasks inactivating mutations in recessive tumor suppressor genes. For example, the *Rb* gene resides on chromosome 13, in a region referred to as q14 (13q14). Most individuals with *Rb* mutations have a subtle mutation in one

Table 11-5	Familial Cancer Syndromes Caused by Tumor-Suppressor Gene Function Loss
Syndrome	**Gene**
Retinoblastoma	*Rb*
Li-Fraumeni syndrome	*p53*
Familial melanoma	*p16^{INK4a}*
Neurofibromatosis	Neurofibromin
Familial adenomatous polyps	*APC*
Breast cancer	*BRCA1*

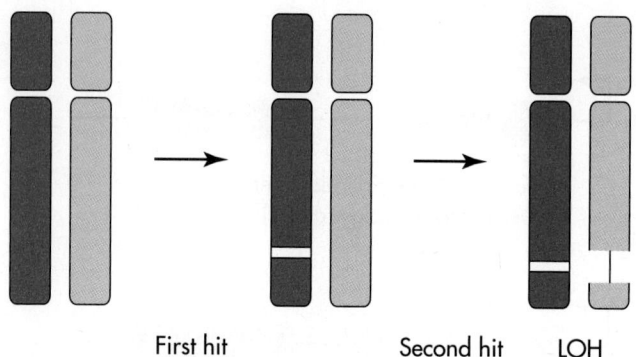

First hit   Second hit   LOH

Figure 11-17 **Inactivation of a tumor suppressor gene.** Two distinct hits are required to inactivate a tumor suppressor gene. Tumor suppressor genes are often inactivated by a mutation (1st hit) followed by complete loss of an entire region of chromosome that encompasses the remaining normal allele (2nd hit), also know as loss of heterozygosity. *LOH,* Loss of heterozygosity.

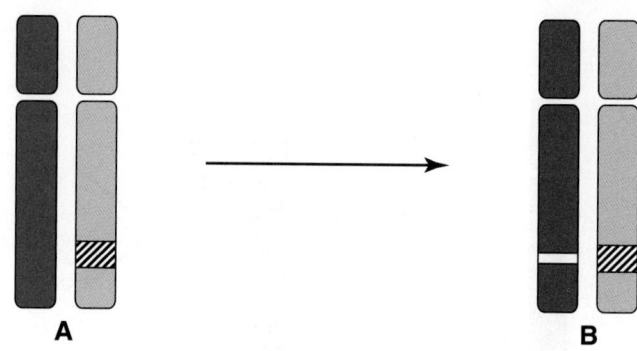

A   **B**

Figure 11-18 Silencing tumor suppressor genes by methylation. **A,** Here the gene on the paternal chromosome is methylated and therefore inactivated by gene silencing without mutation. **B,** If a mutation occurs in the other allele, no functional protein will be produced.

allele and have lost the other copy of *Rb* via loss of the 13q14 chromosome region on the other chromosome.

Gene Silencing

Gene expression can be regulated in a heritable manner (i.e., passed from a parent to a child or from a single cell to its progeny) by an **'epigenetic'** mechanism called **silencing** that does not require mutations or changes in DNA sequence. Whole regions of chromosomes are normally shut off by silencing, so that the pattern of gene expression is different than in other cells with the same genes. The boundaries of the silenced regions can spread in cancer cells, thereby shutting off previously active genes. Silencing can shut off critical tumor suppressor genes in the absence of mutations in the gene. This epigenetic silencing is associated with **methylation** (a reversible chemical modification) of both the DNA and associated chromatin. How silencing works, and how it is passed on from one generation of cells to the next, is currently an area of active research. It is clear that silencing is one important way to inactivate tumor suppressor gene expression in cancers.[21] Certain chemotherapeutic drugs such as 5-azacytidine can reverse DNA methylation and silencing and may prove useful in reactivating or turning tumor suppressor genes "back on again" in treatment of cancer[22] (Figure 11-18).

Guardians of the Genome

The previous discussion of mutations leads naturally to the question of how mutations occur in the first place. The integrity of genetic information can be compromised at several points: during each round of DNA synthesis, during each mitosis when chromosomes are segregated to daughter cells, and when external mutagens (e.g., chemicals and radiation) alter or disrupt DNA. Multiple mechanisms have evolved to protect and repair the genome.[23] These repair mechanisms are directed by **caretaker genes,** genes that are responsible for the maintenance of genomic integrity. Caretaker genes encode proteins that are involved in repairing damaged DNA, such as occurs with errors in DNA replication, mutations caused by

ultraviolet or ionizing radiation, and mutations due to chemicals and drugs. Loss of function of caretaker genes leads to increased mutation rates. If DNA damage is severe, the cell undergoes programmed cell death, or apoptosis, rather than simply divide with damaged DNA.

Inherited mutations can disrupt the caretaker genes that protect the integrity of the genome. Examples include the disorder xeroderma pigmentosum (XP); affected individuals have defects in the repair of ultraviolet light–induced DNA damage and should avoid direct sunlight exposure. They have a very high incidence of skin cancer. Hereditary nonpolyposis colorectal cancer (HNPCC) results from an inherited defect in repairing DNA base pair mismatches that occur from time to time during DNA replication. Affected individuals have an increased rate of small insertions and deletions in DNA, leading to a high rate of colon and other cancers.[24] Finally, there are inherited mutations that threaten the integrity of entire chromosomes. Bloom syndrome and Fanconi aplastic anemia are two autosomal recessive disorders in which affected individuals demonstrate marked chromosomal instability. Chromosome breaks, aberrant fusions, and loss are common. As a consequence, a high rate of cancer occurs in these individuals at an early age.

The rate of individual gene mutation is probably too low to account for the acquisition of many new mutations during the evolution of a malignant cancer clone. Instead, **chromosome instability** appears to be increased in malignant cells.[25] The underlying mechanism of this instability is not clear but may be due to malfunctions in the cellular machinery that regulates chromosome segregation at mitosis.[26] Chromosome instability results in a high rate of chromosome loss, as well as loss of heterozygosity and chromosome amplification. Each of these events can accelerate the loss of tumor suppressor genes and the overexpression of oncogenes.

Inflammation and Cancer

Chronic inflammation has been recognized for 140 years as being an important factor in the development of cancer.[27,28]

Epidemiologic studies indicate that individuals with ulcerative colitis of over 10 years duration have up to a 30-fold increase in the risk of developing colon cancer. Chronic viral hepatitis due to hepatitis B virus (HBV) or hepatitis C virus (HCV) markedly increases the risk of liver cancer. One large study found a 66% increase in risk of lung cancer among women with chronic asthma, an inflammatory disease of the airways.[29] Table 11-6 shows emerging evidence of chronic inflammatory conditions associated with neoplasms. The reasons for the association of inflammation and cancer are complex. After injury, inflammatory cells release cytokines and growth and survival factors that stimulate local cell proliferation, vascular growth, and wound healing. In chronic inflammation, these factors combine to promote continued proliferation (Figures 11-19 and 11-20). In addition, inflammatory cells release compounds such as reactive oxygen species (ROS) and other reactive molecules that can both promote mutations and block the cellular response to DNA damage. Notably, increased abundance of the enzyme cyclooxygenase 2 (COX-2) that generates prostaglandins during acute inflammation, has been associated with colon and some other cancers, and nonsteroidal anti-inflammatory drugs, such as aspirin and ibuprofen, that inhibit COX-2 protect against colon cancer development (see Chapter 5).

Genetics and Cancer Families

Genetic events are the primary basis of carcinogenesis.[30] Most of the genetic alterations that cause cancer occur during the lifetime of the individual, within their somatic tissues. The frequency of these events can be altered by exposure to **mutagens,** that is, agents causing mutations, and by defects in DNA repair that increase the rate of mutations. Because these genetic events occur in somatic cells, as opposed to germ cells, they are not transmitted to future generations. Even though they are genetic events, they are not inherited! It is possible, however, for cancer-predisposing mutations to occur in germline cells (cells that produce gametes) (Figure 11-21). Mutations present in germline cells result in the transmission of cancer-causing genes from one generation to the next, producing families with a high incidence of specific cancers. These inherited mutations that predispose to cancer are almost invariably in tumor suppressor genes (see Table 11-5).

Although rare, such "cancer families" demonstrate that inheritance of a mutated gene can cause cancer (Figure 11-22). In these families, inheritance of one mutant allele predisposes a person to a specific form of cancer: individuals who inherit the germline mutant allele will inevitably suffer loss of the normal allele by loss of heterozygosity in some cells and go on

Table 11-6	Chronic Inflammatory Conditions and Infectious Agents Associated with Neoplasms
Inflammatory Condition	**Associated Neoplasm(s)**
Asbestosis, silicosis	Mesothelioma, lung carcinoma
Bronchitis	Lung carcinoma
Cystitis, bladder inflammation	Bladder carcinoma
Gingivitis, lichens planus	Oral squamous cell carcinoma
Inflammatory bowel disease, Crohn disease, chronic ulcerative colitis	Colorectal carcinoma
Lichen sclerosus	Vulvar squamous cell carcinoma
Chronic pancreatitis, hereditary pancreatitis	Pancreatic carcinoma
Reflux esophagitis, Barrett esophagus	Esophageal carcinoma
Sialadenitis	Salivary gland carcinoma
Sjögren syndrome, Hashimoto thyroiditis	MALT lymphoma
Skin inflammation	Melanoma
Infectious Agent	**Associated Neoplasm(s)**
AIDS (HIV, herpes virus type 8)	Non-Hodgkin lymphoma, squamous cell carcinomas, Kaposi sarcoma
Chronic cholecystitis	Gallbladder cancer
Chronic cystitis (Schistosomiasis)	Bladder, liver, rectal carcinoma; follicular lymphoma of the spleen
Gastritis, gastric ulcers (*Helicobacter pylori*)	Gastric adenocarcinoma, MALT
Hepatitis	Liver carcinoma
Mononucleosis (Epstein-Barr virus)	B cell non-Hodgkin lymphoma, Burkitt lymphoma
Opis thorchis, cholangitis (liver flukes, bile acids)	Cholangiosarcoma, colon carcinoma
Osteomyelitis	Skin carcinoma in draining sinuses
Pelvic inflammatory disease, chronic cervicitis (HPV, gonorrhea, chlamydia)	Ovarian carcinoma, cervical/anal carcinoma

Modified from Coussens LM, Werb Z: *Nature* 420(6917):860-867, 2002; Dalgleish AG, O'Byrne KJ: *Adv Cancer Res* 84:231-276, 2002; Shacter E, Weitzman SA: *Oncology* 16(2):217-226, 229, 2002.
MALT, Mucosa-associated lymphoid tissue.

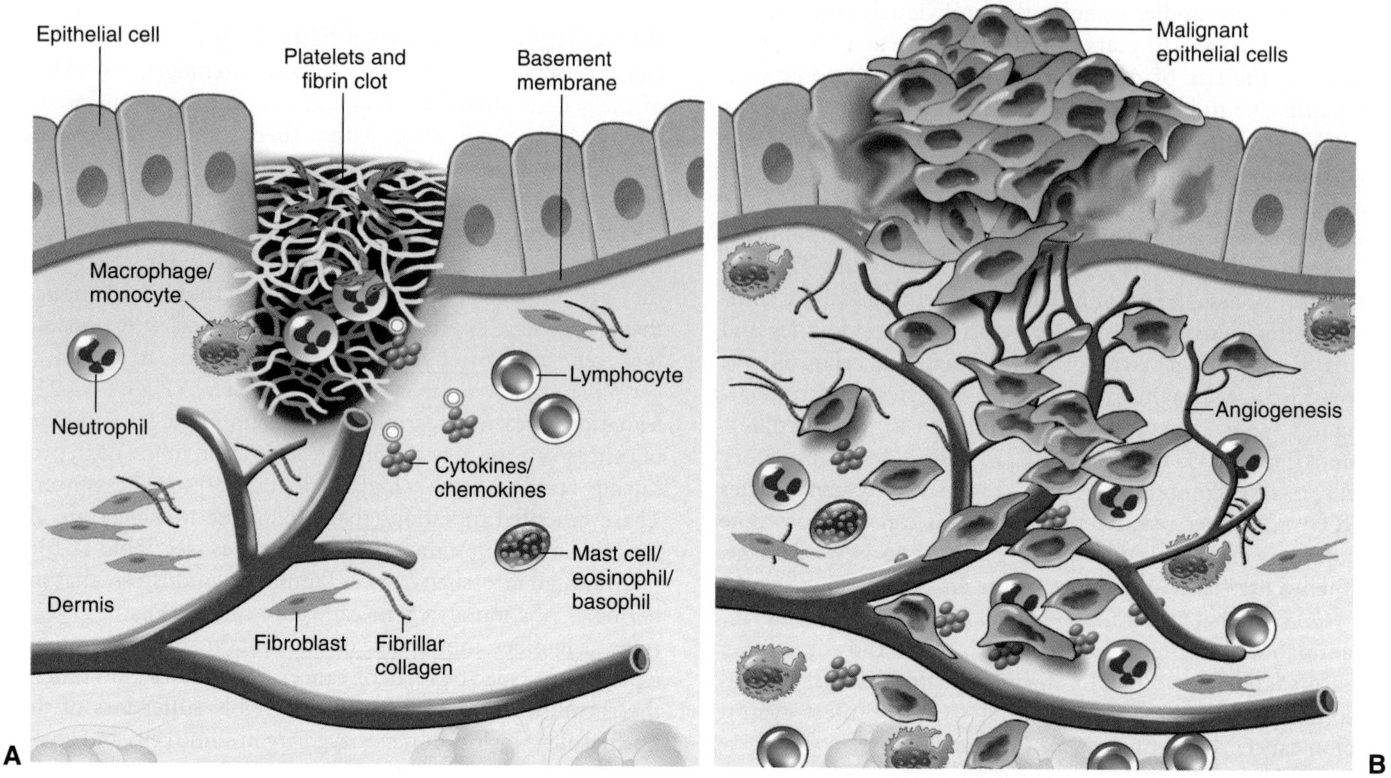

Figure 11-19 Wound healing versus invasive tumor growth. A, Normal tissues appear highly organized with recognizable architecture. Epithelial cells prominent on the basement membrane are separated from the vascularized stromal (dermis) compartment. With tissue injury, platelets are activated, wherein they release vasoactive mediators that regulate clotting. Chemotactic factors, such as transforming growth factor-β and platelet-derived growth factor, derived from activated platelets, initiate granulation tissue formation, activation of fibroblasts, and induction and activation of proteolytic enzymes necessary for remodeling of the extracellular matrix (for example, matrix metalloproteinases and urokinase-type plasminogen activator). Signaling dialogues from various cells, including stromal cells, facilitate healing. Once the wound is healed, the dialogue presumably stops. **B,** Invasive carcinomas are less organized and sometimes unrecognizable. Neoplasia-associated angiogenesis and lymphangiogenesis produce altered tissue architecture. The blood vessels and lymphatics where neoplastic cells interact with other cell types and a remodeled extracellular matrix are abnormal. Neoplastic cells produce cytokines and chemokines that are mitogenic and/or chemoattractants for numerous cells. Activated fibroblasts and infiltrating inflammatory cells also secrete proteolytic enzymes, cytokines, and chemokines, which are mitogenic for neoplastic cells, as well as endothelial cells involved in neoangiogenesis and lymphangiogenesis. These factors can enable tumor growth, stimulate angiogenesis, induce fibroblast migration and maturation, and promote metastatic spread through the venous or lymphatic networks. (Adapted from Coussens LM, Werb Z: *Nature* 420(6917):860-867, 2002.)

to develop the tumor. Examples of human cancers that can be inherited are retinoblastoma, a childhood cancer of the eye, which can be caused by germline mutations in one allele of the *Rb* gene; Wilms tumor, a childhood cancer of the kidney *(Wt1);* neurofibromatosis *(Nf1);* inherited breast cancer *(BRCA1);* and familial polyposis coli or adenomas of the colon *(APC).* A specific tumor-suppressor gene has been isolated for each of these cancers, and in many cases, these tumor-suppressor genes are then found to be inactivated in sporadic (as opposed to inherited) cancers as well. For example, inherited mutations in the *APC* gene are rare and account for only a few percent of all colon cancers. However, 85% of sporadic colon cancers also have acquired mutations of *APC,* mutations that occurred over time in the individual. Characterization of cancer-causing genes and other genetic factors helps identify individuals prone to developing cancer (see Figure 4-29) and contributes to our understanding of spo-

radic cancers. Individuals known to carry mutations in tumor suppressor genes (for example, women with a germline *BRCA1* mutation) are offered targeted cancer screening to facilitate early cancer detection and therapy.[31]

Viral Causes of Cancer

A number of viruses have been associated with human cancer[32,33] (Table 11-7). An even broader spectrum of viruses have been associated with cancer in animals. In humans, *Hepatitis B* and *C viruses (HBV, HCV), Epstein-Barr virus (EBV), Kaposi sarcoma herpesvirus (KSHV)* (also known as HHV8), and *human papillomavirus (HPV)* are associated with about 15% of all human cancers worldwide. Cancer of the cervix and hepatocellular carcinoma account for about 80% of virus-linked cancer. The initial infection with hepatitis B or C is not associated with cancer; instead, it is acquisition of a chronic viral hepatitis that markedly increases cancer risk (also see Inflam-

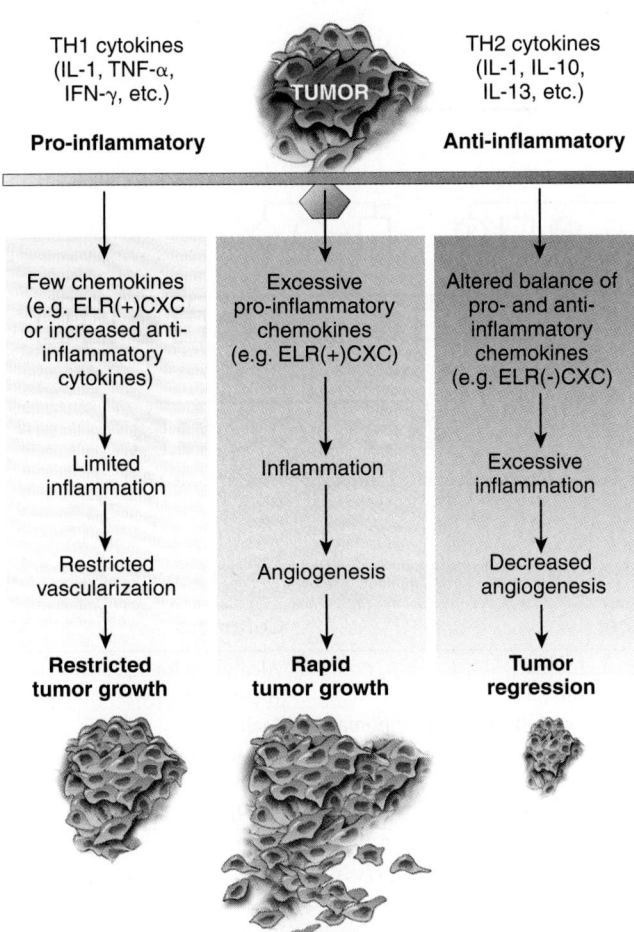

Figure 11-20 **Neoplastic outcome modulated by cytokine and chemokine balances.** The balance of cytokines in any given tumor is critical for regulating the type and extent of inflammatory infiltrate. Tumors that produce little or no cytokines or an overabundance of anti-inflammatory cytokines induce limited inflammatory and vascular responses, resulting in restricted tumor growth. In contrast, production of an excess of proinflammatory cytokines can lead to a level of inflammation that promotes angiogenesis and increasing neoplastic growth. Alternatively, high levels of monocytes and/or neutrophil infiltration, in response to an altered balance of pro- versus anti-inflammatory cytokines, can be associated with cytotoxicity, decreased angiogenesis, and tumor regression. In tumors, interleukin-10 is generally a product of tumor cells and tumor-associated macrophages. *IL,* Interleukin; *TNF,* tumor necrosis factor; *IFN,* interferon; *ELR(+)CXC,* chemokines proangiogenetic and increase endothelial cell chemotaxis vs. *ELR(−)CXC,* which are angiostatis (decrease angiogenesis). (Adapted from Coussens LM, Werb Z: *Nature* 420(6917):860-867, 2002.)

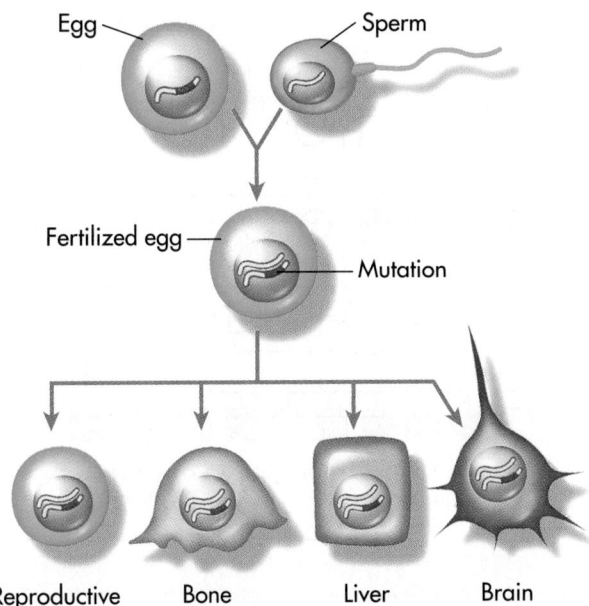

Figure 11-21 **Germline mutation.** Inherited mutations are carried in the DNA of reproductive cells. When reproductive cells containing mutations combine to produce offspring, the mutation will be present in all of the offspring's body cells. (Modified from Lea DN, Jenkins JF, Francomano CA: *Genetics in clinical practice,* Boston, 1998, Bartlett.)

mation and Cancer, p. 6). Chronic hepatitis B infections are common in parts of eastern Asia and sub-Saharan Africa and confer up to a 200-fold increased risk of developing liver cancer. Chronic hepatitis C infections have become increasingly recognized in Western countries. Up to 80% of liver cancer worldwide is associated with chronic hepatitis caused either by HBV or HCV. In both cases, it appears that a lifetime of chronic liver inflammation predisposes one to the development of hepatocellular carcinoma. Widespread use of the HBV vaccine is expected to significantly decrease the incidence of chronic hepatitis B and hence hepatocellular carcinoma. Unfortunately, a vaccine for HCV is not yet available.

Virtually all human cervical cancer is due to infection with specific subtypes of human papillomavirus (HPV). HPV infects basal skin cells and causes warts. Eighty HPV types have been sequenced and only a few (HPV16, 18, 31, 45, and a few others) are associated with cervical, anogenital, and penile cancer (see p. 358). HPV causes cancer when the viral DNA becomes accidentally integrated into the genomic DNA of the infected cervical basal cell and directs the persistent production of viral oncogenes. Early oncogenic HPV infection is readily detected by the Papanicolaou (Pap) test, an examination of cervical epithelia scrapings. Early detection of cellular atypia in a Pap test often leads to detection of cervical carcinoma in situ, which can be effectively treated. The Pap test is probably the most effective cancer screening test developed to date.

EBV and KSHV are both members of the Herpesvirus family.[32] EBV, the cause of infectious mononucleosis, infects B lymphocytes and stimulates their proliferation. In immunosuppressed individuals with HIV infection or those who have received a heart or kidney transplant, persistent EBV infection can lead to the development of B cell lymphomas. This development is known as **post-transplant lymphoproliferative disorder (PTLD)** in individuals with organ transplants. One effective therapy, where possible, for PTLD is to decrease or stop immunosuppressant drugs. EBV infection also is associated with Burkitt lymphoma in areas of endemic malaria

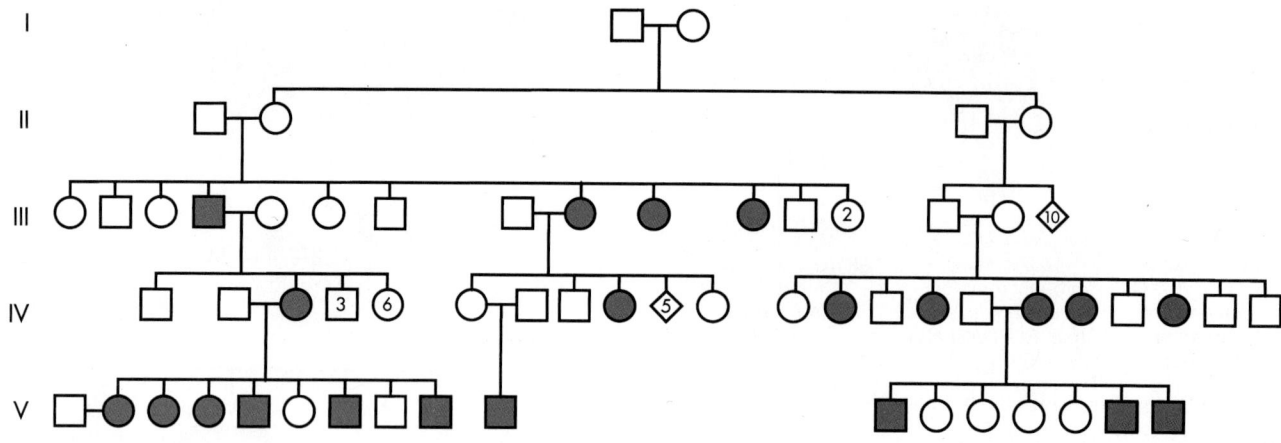

Figure 11-22 A familial colon cancer pedigree. Darkened symbols represent individuals diagnosed with cancer. (From Jorde LB et al: *Medical genetics,* ed 3, St. Louis, 2003, Mosby.)

Table 11-7	Human Viruses Associated with Cancer		
Virus Family	**Type**	**Human Cancer**	**Cofactors**
Hepatitis viruses	Hepatitis B	Hepatocellular carcinoma	Alcohol, smoking, aflatoxins
Flaviviruses	Hepatitis C	Hepatocellular carcinoma	Alcohol
Herpes viruses	Epstein-Barr	Burkitt lymphoma, nasopharyngeal carcinoma	Malaria
	KSHV/HHV-8 Immunodeficiency	Kaposi sarcoma	
Papillomaviruses	HPV-16, -18, -31, -33, other	Cervical, anogenital	Smoking, oral contraceptives
Retroviruses	HTLV-1	Adult T-cell leukemia/lymphoma	Unknown

Modified from Mendelsohn J et al, editors: *The molecular basis of cancer,* ed 2, Philadelphia, 2001, Saunders.
KSHV/HHV-8, Kaposi sarcoma–associated herpesvirus/human herpes virus-8; *HPV,* human papillomavirus; *HTLV-1,* human T-cell leukemia/lymphoma virus-1.

and is associated with nasopharyngeal carcinoma in parts of China. KSHV (also known as *HHV8*) is linked to the development of Kaposi sarcoma, a cancer that occurs in elderly men and in a markedly more virulent form in immunocompromised individuals, especially those infected with HIV. HHV8 also has been linked to several rare lymphomas.

Human T-cell leukemia-lymphoma virus (HTLV) is an oncogenic retrovirus linked to the development of adult T-cell leukemia and lymphoma (ATLL).[33] HTLV is transmitted both vertically, that is, inherited by children from infected parents, and horizontally, by breast-feeding; sexual intercourse; blood transfusions; and exposure to infected needles. Infection with HTLV may be asymptomatic, and only a small fraction of infected individuals develop ATLL, often many years after acquiring the virus. It is clear that infection by an oncogenic virus is far from sufficient to cause cancer. For example, in some industrialized regions, Epstein-Barr virus can infect 90% of the adolescent and young adult population, yet only a very small percentage of these individuals develop EBV-related cancer. For each of these infections, important co-factors increase the risk that an infection will develop into cancer.

Bacterial Cause of Cancer

Helicobacter pylori is a bacteria that infects more than half of the world's population. Chronic infection with *H. pylori* is an important cause of peptic ulcer disease and is strongly associated with stomach carcinoma, a leading cause of cancer deaths worldwide. It is also associated with a less common cancer, gastric mucosa-associated lymphoid tissue (MALT) lymphomas.[34] *H. pylori* infection is often acquired in childhood and disproportionately affects lower socioeconomic classes. Although most infections are asymptomatic, prolonged chronic inflammation can lead to atrophic gastritis that can, in a small fraction of individuals, progress to dysplastic changes and finally frank gastric adenocarcinoma. Eradication of *H. pylori* from infected individuals prior to the development of dysplasia may prevent the development of cancer.[35] However, there is no expert consensus on the value of population screening and treatment strategies.[36] The MALT lymphomas associated with chronic *H. pylori* infections may depend on chronic inflammation and antigenic stimulation associated with infections, and therefore treatment with antibiotics may be useful even in cases of early lymphoma.[37]

GENE-ENVIRONMENT INTERACTION

Environmental Risk Factors

The past two decades have led to a greater understanding of the genetic basis of neoplastic development. At the level of the cell, cancer is genetic. The frequency and consequences of these genetic mutations can be altered by a number of environmental factors. Two lines of evidence support the idea that exposure to environmental agents can increase an individual's risk of cancer. The first is based on the identification of environmental agents that have carcinogenic properties. In experimental animals, many agents have been found to cause cancer; thus these agents are called **carcinogens.** Evidence from both epidemiologic and laboratory studies show, for example, that cigarette smoke causes lung cancer. Many specific risk factors for cancer are now known, the most significant being smoking, obesity, radiation, and a few oncogenic viruses,[38,39] but whether environmental factors cause the large global variation in the incidence for such cancers as prostate, breast, and colon remains unknown.

The second line of evidence is based on comparisons of populations who have different life-styles or different rates of cancer incidence (Figure 11-23). Breast cancer, for example, is prevalent among northern Europeans and Americans, but it is relatively rare among women in developing countries. The difficulty lies in determining whether these differences between populations are attributable to life-style factors, to genetics, or to both. The influence of environmental agents was demonstrated in studies of Japanese who immigrated to Hawaii and the U.S. mainland. Researchers studied the changes in incidence of colon and stomach cancer after emigration. For example, colon cancer was, until recently, relative rare in Japan, but it is the second most common cancer in the United States. Among the first Japanese immigrants (first-generation) in Hawaii, colon cancer incidence rose several-fold but not as high as overall incidence on the U.S. mainland. Among second-generation Japanese on the U.S. mainland, colon cancer rates rose to the U.S. average. Conversely, stomach cancer is common in Japan but relatively rare in the United States. Japanese on the U.S. mainland have the same low incidence of stomach cancer as the U.S. average. Although these observations strongly implicate environment and life-style in the development of colon and stomach cancer, they do not rule out genetic factors. The difference in incidence rates could be the result of predisposing genes. One could argue that these genes are less penetrating for colon cancer in Japan because of environmental differences.[30,40]

Environmental factors play important roles in cancer development, but major gaps in current knowledge exist. Research efforts needed for shaping public policy concerning environmental exposures should focus on (1) the relationship between the timing of exposures (periods of vulnerability), multiple exposures, and chronic exposures; (2) disparities among racial groups and gender; (3) human contamination (biomonitoring); and (4) public health studies that carefully scrutinize unexplained patterns of risk. In addition, public health advocates have argued for mandating that producers of environmental hazards (chemicals, tobacco, drugs, radiologic products, etc.) assess health, safety, and environmental impacts *before* introducing them to the marketplace and make that information publicly available. Table 11-8 summarizes the estimated new cases and deaths caused by cancer, by gender, for specified sites.

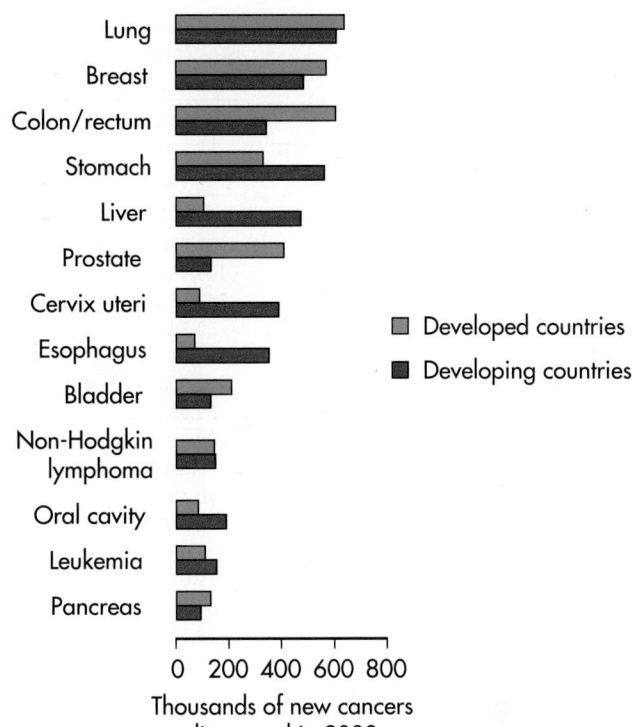

Figure 11-23 Global cancer incidence in developed and developing countries. (Modified from Parkin DM, et al: Cancer burden in the year 2000: the global picture, *Euro J Cancer* 37(suppl 8):54-66, 2001.)

Tobacco Use

Cigarette smoke is carcinogenic and remains the most important cause of cancer. The risk is greatest in those who begin to smoke when young and continue throughout life.[38] Since the 1950s, the number of deaths attributable to tobacco smoking has sharply increased, and if current smoking patterns persist, the epidemic of cancer attributable to tobacco smoking is expected to occur in developing countries.[41] Tobacco smoking is responsible for 30% of all cancer deaths in developed countries.[42] Tobacco use is associated primarily with squamous and small cell carcinomas of the lung and pulmonary adenocarcinomas. In addition, smoking causes *even more* deaths from vascular, respiratory, and other diseases than from cancer; in total, it accounts for an astonishing 4 to 5 million deaths a year worldwide.[42] The only other causes of disease with such *rapidly* increasing incidence and deaths are those related to HIV infection and, possibly, obesity in Western countries.[41]

A Centers for Disease Control report from 2004 found current smoking was most prevalent among adults aged 18 to 44 years, and declines with age.[43] Men were more likely than women to be current smokers. Men smoked more cigarettes a day ($\geq$20 cigarettes/day) than women ($\leq$16 cigarettes/day). Native-American or Alaskan-Native adults (32.6%) were more likely to be current smokers than white adults (23.7%), black adults (22.8%), or Asian adults (13.5%). Non-Hispanic black adults (22.8%) and non-Hispanic white adults (24.5%) were more likely than Hispanic adults (17.0%) to be current smokers.

Table 11-8 Estimated New Cancer Cases and Deaths by Gender, United States, 2005*

	Estimated New Cases			Estimated Deaths		
	Both Sexes	Male	Female	Both Sexes	Male	Female
All sites	1,372,910	710,040	662,870	570,280	295,280	275,000
Oral cavity and pharynx	29,370	19,100	10,270	7,320	4,910	2,410
Esophagus	14,520	11,220	3,300	13,570	10,530	3,040
Stomach	21,850	13,510	8,350	11,550	6,770	4,790
Colon	104,950	49,290	56,660	56,290†	29,540†	27,750†
Rectum	40,340	23,530	16,910			
Pancreas	32,180	1,610	16,080	31,800	15,820	15,980
Lung and bronchus	172,570	93,010	79,560	163,510	90,490	73,020
Bones and joints	2,570	1,490	1,090	1,210	670	540
Melanoma-skin	59,580	33,580	26,000	7,770	4,910	2,960
Breast	212,930	1,690	211,240	40,870	460	40,410
Uterine cervix	10,370	—	10,370	3,700	—	3,700
Uterine corpus	40,880	—	40,880	7,310	—	7,310
Ovary	22,220		22,220	1,620		1,620
Prostate	232,090	232,090		30,350	30,350	
Testis	9,010	9,010		390	390	
Urinary bladder	63,210	47,010	16,200	13,190	9,970	4,210
Brain and other nervous system	18,500	10,620	7,990	12,760	7,290	5,480
Thyroid	25,690	6,500	19,190	1,490	630	850
Hodgkin disease	7,350	3,980	3,370	1,410	780	630
Leukemia	34,810	19,640	15,170	22,570	12,540	10,030

From American Cancer Society: *Cancer facts and figures 2005*, Atlanta, 2005, The Society.

*Excludes basal and squamous cell skin cancers and in situ carcinomas except urinary bladder. Carcinoma in situ of the breast accounts for about 58,490 new cases annually, and melanoma in situ accounts for about 46,170 new cases annually.

†Estimated deaths for colon and rectum cancers are combined.

Table 11-9 Examples of Mechanistic Evidence of Carcinogenesis from Tobacco Smoke

Organ Site	Mechanisms
Lung	Polycyclic aromatic hydrocarbons (PAH) induce mutations in the *p53* gene crucial for cell cycle dysregulation and carcinogenesis[161]
	Nitroso compounds, chemicals found in tobacco smoke, are potent animal carcinogens and are found in the urine of smokers[45]
Bladder	Arylamines, particularly the potent carcinogen 4-aminobiphenyl, is present in tobacco smoke and has been shown to form DNA-adducts in bladder cells and bladder biopsy specimens
	Hemoglobin adducts formed by 4-aminobiphenyl are markedly increased in smokers, especially in smokers of black tobacco versus blonde tobacco[162, 163]
Cervix	Benzo[a]pyrene metabolites have been found in cervical mucus and as DNA adducts
	Most studies, however, were not adjusted for infection of human papillomavirus (HPV), the main etiologic agent for invasive and preinvasive cervical cancer[164]
Bone marrow: myeloid leukemia	Smokers have higher levels of benzene, an established inducer of leukemia in humans
	Six cytogenetic groups among 472 individuals with acute myeloid leukemia had increased incidence of chromosomal translocations[165]

Evidence now shows that tobacco smoke is a multipotent carcinogenic mixture that can *cause* cancer in several different organs. Tobacco smoking has been linked not only to cancers of the lung but also of the lower urinary tract (renal, penis, and bladder), upper aero-digestive tract (including the oral cavity, pharynx, larynx, nasal cavity, paranasal sinuses, esophagus, and stomach), liver, kidney, pancreas, cervix uteri, and myeloid leukemia.[42] Current evidence is not convincing for cancer of the large bowel and is inconsistent with breast cancer. Exposure to secondhand tobacco smoke (involuntary or passive smoking by persons who do not smoke) is also carcinogenic for the lungs.

Cigar and/or pipe smoking is strongly and causally related to cancers of the oral cavity, oropharynx, hypopharynx, larynx, esophagus, and lung.[42] Although the risk of dying from tobacco-associated diseases is lower for pipe smokers than cigarette smokers, pipe smoking is as harmful as and perhaps more harmful than cigar smoking.[44] Bidi smoking (a small amount of tobacco wrapped in the leaf of another plant [used in South Asia]) is mostly a habit of men. Bidi smoking delivers higher amounts of nicotine per gram of tobacco and comparable or greater amounts of tar compared to cigarettes.[42] Evidence from case controlled studies indicates bidi smoking can cause cancers of the respiratory and digestive sites including mouth, oropharynx, larynx, lung, esophagus, and stomach. Table 11-9 summarizes the mechanisms of carcinogenesis from tobacco smoke confirmed from biochemistry and molecular biology studies.

More than 50 studies have evaluated **involuntary smoking** (nonsmokers who breathe other's smoke) and the risk of lung cancer in those who have never smoked compared to risks for spouses of smokers.[42] Involuntary smoking and the risk of lung cancer is supported by evidence that the urine of nonsmokers exposed to involuntary smoking contains amounts of carcinogenic N-nitroso compounds from tobacco.[45]

Measures that prevent young adults from starting smoking would substantially avoid the future disease burden. An important public health approach is therefore needed that *prevents* young individuals from starting smoking and helps others *stop* smoking.

Ionizing Radiation

Much of the knowledge of the effects of ionizing radiation on human cancer has stemmed from observations of the Hiroshima and Nagasaki atomic bomb exposures, particularly the Life Span Study. These data provide the best estimate of human cancer risk over the dose range from 20 to 250 cGy for low linear energy transfer (LET) radiation, such as x-rays or γ-rays. Other data are derived from groups exposed for medical reasons, underground miners exposed to radon gas, and workers exposed to high doses while in the nuclear weapons program of the former USSR. The horrible atomic bomb exposures in Japan caused acute leukemias in adults and children and increased frequencies of thyroid and breast carcinomas. Lung, stomach, colon, esophageal, and urinary tract cancers and multiple myeloma have lately been added to the list. At Nagasaki and Hiroshima, leukemia incidence in individuals 15 years or younger reached its peak 6 to 7 years after the explosions and has steadily declined since 1952. Middle-aged people, 45 years and older at the time of exposure, had a latent period of 20 years before developing acute leukemia. These risks are apparently not heritable—offspring of both atomic bombs and cancer survivors do not have an increased risk of malformations, cancer, or chromosome abnormalities.[46-48]

Human exposure to ionizing radiation includes emissions from x-rays, radioisotopes, and other radioactive sources. Health risks involve not only neoplastic diseases but also somatic mutations that may contribute to other diseases (e.g., birth defects and eye maladies) and inherited mutations that may affect the incidence of diseases in future generations. The cancer risk of loss of life expectancy at doses below 20 cGy is uncertain and contentious and has been the subject of controversy for decades[49] (see p. 356). Heritable mutations are of particular concern for women because the number of oocytes are presumably fixed at birth (although this has been challenged recently) and mutations, if not repaired, are cumulative.[49]

Presently, the risks of low-dose radiation are being debated among radiobiologists, geneticists, physicists, and others because of the potential impact on the health of current and future generations.[49] Two opposing hypotheses have emerged: (1) there is no dose of radiation considered safe and the use of radiation must always be considered on the basis of risk versus benefit and (2) the health risks of diagnostic doses less than 10 cGy are not now measurable and may be nonexistent. Limiting is that general findings on the health risks of low-dose radiation are made by analyses of data on the risk of cancer alone.[49] The expression of radiation-induced damage depends not only on dose, fractionation, and protraction but also on repair mechanisms, bystander effects, radioprotective substances such as antioxidants, and how it is delivered.[49]

Radiation-Induced Cancer

Human cancers result from the accumulation of multiple hits (overexpression of genes, deletion of genes, or gene mutations), some of which occur in critical genes that regulate proliferation and differentiation (see Biology of Cancer, p. 339). Radiation-induced cancer in humans seems to have long latent periods; 10 years for leukemia and over 30 years for solid tumors.[50] This implies that radiation-induced gene mutations or chromosomal alterations that can be detected early (within 24 hours of radiation exposure) are not *solely* responsible for tumor development in normal human cells. Such mutations, however, provide a critical hit or induce genetic instability that make cells more susceptible to accumulation of genetic alterations caused by other spontaneous or induced mutations. The accumulation of mutations leads to full transformation and cancer.[49]

Two opposing dose-response models have been used to estimate cancer risk in humans.[49] The first model proposes that cancer risk from exposures 10 cGy or less (i.e., low-level radiation) is best estimated by a **linear, no-threshold, relationship** because any dose has the potential to cause mutations.[51,52] The second model proposes a threshold dose below which radiation may *not* cause cancer in humans.[53-55]

The first model estimates health threats by extrapolating from the effects of higher doses. Recent data, however, shows the linear, no-threshold, model underestimates the risk from low radiation.[56] The researchers used a precision microbeam device to fire alpha particles into nuclei of human-hamster hybrid cells in Petri dishes. When the researchers irradiated the nuclei with just *one* alpha particle each, 98 mutations of a particular gene occurred per 100,000 surviving cells. Zapping only 5% of the nuclei produced 57 such mutations per 100,000 cells, rather than the five mutations that a linear model predicts. These data suggest that the relevant target for radiation-induced mutagenesis is larger than an individual cell and, thus, supports the need to reconsider the validity of the linear extrapolation model.[56] Another study showed that pretreatment of cells with low-dose x-rays before they received alpha particle radiation reduced the alpha particle–induced mutagenesis in innocent (nonradiated) bystander cells.[57] These data further complicate and confuse interpretations of any dose-response model.[49]

The second model supports the notion of **hormesis,** or proposed stimulatory/adaptive effects of low levels of radiation (1 to 50 cGy). Thus humans are simultaneously exposed to cancer promoting and inhibiting effects of radiation. These effects are thought to be beneficial by way of producing protective feedback systems to stimulate metabolic detoxification and repair mechanisms. Interpretations, however, depend on several variables including differences in radiosensitivity, age, organs, body mass, and variations in repair-generating mechanisms.[49] Thus the validity of a dose-response model based on epidemiologic data and mathematical modeling is questionable because it cannot account for the complex biologic variability and may not provide useful data on the estimation of low-dose radiation-related cancer in humans.[49,57,58] No detectable increase in cancer was found in airline pilots or crews (expected to have higher doses of cosmic irradiation), and a very small increased cancer risk was found in nuclear energy workers.[59-61]

Carcinogenesis: Genomic Instability

Biologic consequences of exposure to ionizing radiation include cell death, gene mutations, and chromosome aberrations. Conventional dogma attributes these effects to alterations resulting from the deposition of energy to the DNA of an irradiated cell. Eventually, the cell is presumed repaired by DNA enzymatic mechanisms that also can occur during DNA replication. It was widely accepted that most of these changes took place immediately after exposure. Thus if the damage were faithfully repaired, the descendents of an irradiated cell would be normal (Figure 11-24, A). If misrepaired, however, the descendents would be expected to pass on radiation-induced genetic change and all cells derived from such a cell would have the identical genetic alteration or, more simply, the effect would be clonal (Figure 11-24, B). Yet many in vitro studies have demonstrated nonclonal chromosome aberrations and mutations in the clonal progeny of irradiated cells.[58] Furthermore, it has been known for many years that radiation-induced cellular alterations (cytotoxicity), identified as a loss of reproductive potential, might be delayed for several generations of cell replication, with death occurring randomly among the progeny cells.[58]

Now it is known that the progeny of irradiated cells can exhibit an increased death rate and loss of reproductive potential that continues for several generations and, possibly, indefinitely. This delayed cell death phenotype is known as "lethal mutation" and "delayed reproductive death." Significant is that various genetic alterations are demonstrated in cells that are *not*, themselves, irradiated but are direct descendents of cells exposed to ionizing radiation. These so-called *innocent cells* are referred to as **bystander effects** and are considered manifestations of a radiation-induced genomic instability (see below and Figure 11-24, C). This instability is similar to inherited chromosome instability syndromes with spontaneously high levels of chromosomal alterations and mutations.[62]

The genome is constantly challenged by destabilizing factors, including normal DNA replication and cell division, intracellular and extracellular environmental stresses, such as oxidative metabolism, exposure to genotoxic chemical agents and background radiation. Cells have complex mechanisms for trying to maintain genomic stability. These processes include proofreading of DNA replication, enzymatic repair of DNA damage, and checkpoints monitoring progression

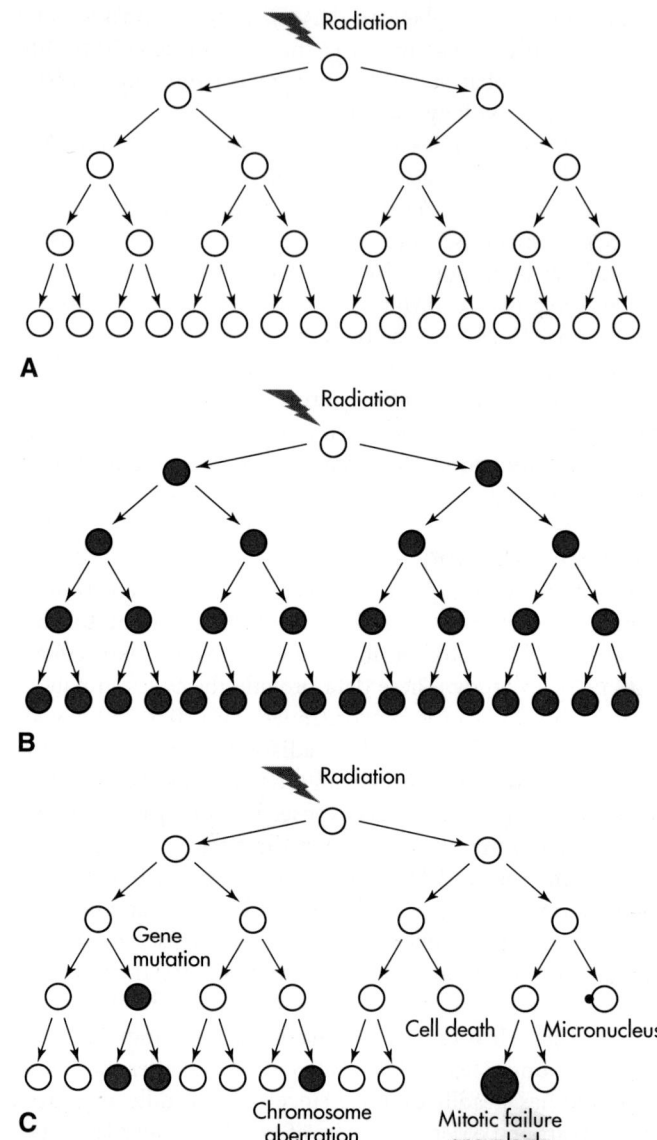

A

B

C

Figure 11-24 **Models of the responses of clonogenic cells to ionizing radiation.** Mutations and/or chromosomal aberrations are shown as filled circles and apparently normal cells as open circles. **A,** If a cell faithfully repairs DNA damage, then its clonal descendents will appear normal. **B,** If a cell is directly mutated by radiation, then all its descendents will express the same mutation. **C,** Radiation-induced genomic instability is characterized by nonclonal effects in descendant cells. (From Lorimore SA, Coates PJ, Wright EG: *Oncogene* 22(45):7058-7069, 2003.)

through the cell cycle. Failure of any of these processes can result in destabilization of the genome, deleterious mutations, and alterations in cell proliferation.

Although similar to alterations to the chromosome instability syndromes, the radiation-induced genomic instability seems to reflect epigenetic phenomena rather than mutation of genome genes.[63] Recent experiments have shown that irradiation can induce growth factors and extracellular matrix (microenvironment) remodeling. A major function of the microenvironment is to control cell differentiation and proliferation, and its disruption is required for the establishment of cancer.[64] These data suggest such epigenetic events after radiation, including alterations in pathways affecting cell adhesion, extracellular matrix interactions, and cell-to-cell communication, may override the positive or repairing influence of tissue signaling and architecture that inhibits neoplastic progression.[64] The chromosomal instability noted in mouse hematopoietic tissue[65] and mouse mammary epithelium[66] is, however, strongly influenced by genetic factors, with some genotypes being more susceptible than others.

Bystander Effects

In vivo and in vitro culture experiments performed over the past 2 decades indicate that low-dose ionizing radiation causes significantly different biologic responses than does high-dose radiation. Two important findings concerning the biologic effects of a low dose (or low fluences) of radiation occur in both the irradiated cells and in cells that are not, themselves, radiated—the so-called *bystander effect*: (1) radiation-induced genomic instability occurs in the descendant cells of the irradiated cell after several generations of cell division, and (2) radiation-induced bystander effects are caused as a consequence of damage signals transmitted from neighboring irradiated cells whereby transmission may be mediated by either direct or intercellular communication through gap junctions or by factors released into the surrounding medium.[67] In both findings, the biologic effects appear to be associated with oxidative stress and the generation of reactive oxygen species (ROS) (e.g., super oxide and hydrogen peroxide). Nitric oxide, however, may initiate intercellular signaling pathways that influence the bystander effects.[67,68]

In vivo experiments also have shown that inflammatory-type responses occur after exposure to ionizing radiation.[69] Theses studies revealed activation of macrophages and neutrophil accumulations were not *direct effects* of irradiation but were instead a consequence of the recognition and phagocytosis of radiation-induced apoptotic cells. The phagocytotic mechanism is suggested for the interactions between irradiated and nonirradiated hemopoietic cells, both in vivo and in vitro.[69] Oxidative-stress mediators also have been implicated in the cytotoxic effects observed in solid tumors located at distinct sites away from those receiving radiation.[70] Genes responsible for oxidative stress have been identified.[71] Direct evidence, however, of how these oxidative events occur is lacking. Also unclear is the source of the oxidants—are they strictly derived from cytoplasmic membranes or from the mitochondria?

Gap Junction Intercellular Communication

Confluent cell cultures respond as an integrated whole rather than separate individual cells that have been irradiated, indicating a critical role for cell-to-cell communication in mediating the bystander effect. This mediation could be controlled by gap junctions. Gap junctions consist of a cell-to-cell channel spanning two plasma membranes; they result from the bridging of two half channels, or connexons, contributed separately by each of the two participating cells.[72] Exposure of cells to low levels of radiation (≤ 0.16 cGy) significantly induces the expression of connexin 43, suggesting that oxidizing mediators increase expression of proteins involved in gap junction intercellular communication (GJIC).[71]

In conclusion, emerging data are supporting a role for both oxidative stress and GJIC in the radiation-induced bystander effects. Further, studies of the molecular mechanisms underlying bystander cells should increase our understanding of the overall risk due to ionizing radiation.

Ultraviolet Radiation

Ultraviolet sunlight *causes* basal cell carcinoma and squamous cell carcinoma (i.e., photocarcinogenesis), two common skin cancers found in white individuals. Exposure to ultraviolet radiation (UVR) can emanate from both natural and artificial sources; however, the principal source of exposure for most people is sunlight. With further depletion of the stratospheric ozone layer, people and the environment will be exposed to higher intensities of UVR. The degree of damage in skin depends on the intensity and wavelength content (i.e., ultraviolet A [UVA] or ultraviolet B [UVB]) and the depth of penetration. UV radiation is now known to cause specific gene mutations; for example, squamous cell carcinoma involves mutation in the *p53 gene*, basal cell carcinoma in the *patched* gene, and melanoma in the *p16* gene.[73] In addition, UV light induces the release of tumor necrosis factor-α (TNF-α) in the epidermis, which may reduce immune surveillance against skin cancer.[74]

Inflammation is a critical component of tumor progression. The observed inflammatory response following acute and chronic UV radiation may contribute to skin carcinogenesis by releasing free radicals.[75] Hydrogen peroxide has recently been identified in response to physiologic doses of UVB.[76] Importantly, hydrogen peroxide is required for epidermal growth factor activation and cell survival.[77,78] Reactive oxygen species, however, can injure tissue, creating oxidative stress when insufficient antioxidant defense exits. Major effects include lipid peroxidation and damage to DNA (see Chapter 2). Major antioxidants include superoxide dismutase, catalase, and glutathione peroxidase. Superoxide dismutase converts superoxide anions to hydrogen peroxide, which is metabolized by catalase or glutathione peroxidase to water (see Figure 2-10).

Thus healthy genes are needed to coordinate the levels of antioxidants and decrease the harmful ROS. Antioxidants decrease ROS and oxidative stress and other protective mechanisms including DNA repair and apoptosis (Figure 11-25). The genetic alterations in proto-oncogenes and tumor suppressor genes may make epidermal cells resistant to signals for terminal differentiation.[75] With oxidative stress, DNA damage occurs and calcium-dependent enzymes (endonucleases) are activated that produce DNA strand breaks.[75] In addition, ROS are involved in the activation of procarcinogens, such as polycyclic aromatic hydrocarbons including 7,12-dimethylbenzene(a)anthracene (DMBA). DMBA is capable of initiating a point mutation in the *ras* pro-oncogene, which is evidenced to be the triggering event in mouse carcinogenesis.[79] The essential step appears to be the activation of DMBA by NADH

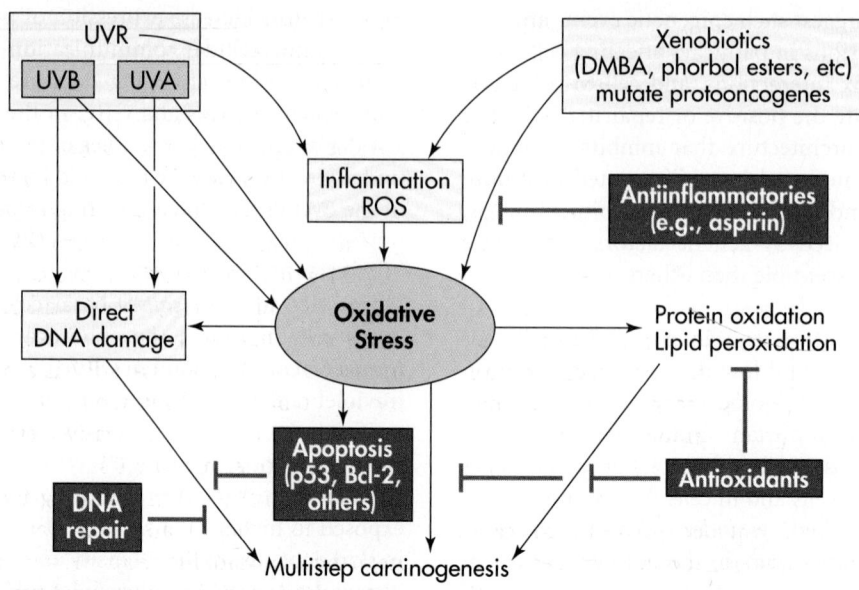

Figure 11-25 **Theoretical scheme of multistep skin carcinogenesis.** Ultraviolet radiation (UVR), inflammation, and xenobiotics (see p. 361) lead to oxidative stress, resulting in direct DNA damage, protein oxidation, lipid peroxidation, and apoptosis. The protective mechanisms shown in *red* include apoptosis, DNA repair, and antioxidants. (Adapted from Sander CD et al: *Intl J Dermatol* 43(5): 326-340, 2004.)

(nicotinamide adenine dinucleotide dehydrogenase) and cytochrome p450-dependent oxidases.[80] The pathophysiology of skin carcinogenesis is discussed further in Chapter 44.

Basal cell carcinoma commonly occurs on the head and neck. Individuals with these tumors generally have light complexions, light eyes, and fair hair. They tend to sunburn rather than tan and live in areas of high sunlight exposure. Usually these cancers arise on areas of the body that receive the greatest sun exposure, although they are not necessarily restricted to these skin sites. Squamous cell carcinoma is found more commonly in men who work outdoors. These tumors are distributed over the head, neck, and exposed areas of the upper extremities (see Chapter 44).

The incidence and mortality rates of those with melanoma have increased annually at rates of 2% to 3% for the last 3 decades.[81] Sun exposure and the risk of melanoma, a malignant pigmented mole, remain complex. Epidemiologic and case control studies suggest that UVR exposure is the most significant factor for the development of melanoma. Other evidence, however, reports rates of melanoma are uncommon in persons with outdoor occupations.[82] Although the non-melanoma skin cancers are related to cumulative exposure to UV radiation, melanoma is related to episodes of intense, intermittent exposure (measured as history of sunburn).[81] Melanomas more commonly occur in areas less continuously exposed to sunlight, like the trunks in men and back of the legs in women. Family history (i.e., genetic factors), skin type, and the density of moles are important in determining the risk of developing melanoma. For example, the incidence of melanoma in white populations is 10 times greater than in black, Asian, or Hispanic populations residing in the same area.[82] Most important, the risk of melanoma from sunlight is certainly modified by risk factors.[82] Traits associated with a high risk of melanoma are light-colored hair, eyes, and skin; an inability to tan; and a tendency to freckle, sunburn, and develop nevi.[83]

Until 1998, a direct causal relationship between UVB light and melanoma in humans had not been established. Grafted newborn human foreskin (xenograft) onto RAG-1 immune-deficient mice showed such a relationship.[84] Melanocytic hyperplasia occurred in 73% of UVB treated xenografts. One graft treated with both DMBA and UVB light developed a human malignant melanoma. This was the first experiment to show that UVB light and an exogenous carcinogen could result in a new malignant melanoma.

A similar study using UVB light and overexpression of an endogenous growth factor, basic fibroblast growth factor (bFGF), also induced human melanoma.[85] Numerous local factors may result in increased cytokine production, including trauma, infection, diet, obesity, hormones, and other causes of inflammation. Sunburn reflects an overdose of UV light, triggering inflammation with an increase in cytokine production.

A very significant finding in 2002 jolted the melanoma field. Davies and colleagues[80] detected an activating point mutation in the *B-raf* proto-oncogene in 60% to 70% of malignant melanomas. This mutation results in a marked increase in B-RAF kinase activity leading to activation of the mitogen-activated protein kinase (MAPK) pathway (see Table 1-4). Thus activation of MAPK in melanoma can occur through several mechanisms: (1) mutation in the *B-raf* gene, (2) stimulation of FGF and hepatocyte growth factor (HGF), (3) exogenous stimulation by insulin-like growth factor-1 (IGF-1), and (4) by adhesion molecule receptor signaling. The development of melanoma is associated with the loss of E-cadherin and the appearance of N-cadherin adhesion molecules. **Cad-**

herins are cell surface glycoproteins that promote calcium-dependent cell-to-cell adhesion. The major adhesion molecule between keratinocytes and normal melanocytes is E-cadherin, which disappears during melanoma progression.[86] Melanoma cells express N-cadherin, which allows them to adhere to fibroblasts and endothelial cells. Thus N-cadherin allows the melanoma cells to survive as they migrate through the dermis.[87] (For further discussion, see Chapter 44.)

Increased knowledge of the intricate cellular interactions in melanoma provides new clues for novel therapeutic approaches. These approaches may include strategies that (1) mimic keratinocytes to encourage maintenance of homeostatic control and (2) use adhesion molecules as markers for detecting melanoma behavior and determining sites for intervention.

Alcohol Consumption

Chronic alcohol consumption is a strong risk factor for cancer of the oral cavity, pharynx, hypopharynx, larynx, esophagus, and liver.[88] Although evidence is inconsistent, alcohol consumption is less strongly related to breast cancer and colorectal cancer; however, it is known to increase cell growth of human breast cancer cells in vitro.[89] In addition, although the risk is lower, breast carcinogenesis can be enhanced with relatively low daily amounts of alcohol.[88] A meta-analysis showed no consistent relationship between alcohol and cancers of the pancreas, lung, prostate, or bladder.[90] Alcohol interacts with smoke, increasing the risk of malignant tumors, possibly by acting as a solvent for the carcinogenic chemicals in smoke products. Inherited genetic factors also put some individuals at increased risk. Genetic mechanisms may include differences in DNA repair ability, carcinogen metabolism, and cell cycle control.[91] The strongest genetic associations to alcoholism are those with alcohol dehydrogenase (ADH) and mitochondrial aldehyde dehydrogenase (ALDH2). Specifically, individuals having the genes encoding 32-ADH or the dominant negative allele for ALDH2 are at reduced risk of alcoholism. However, those with ALDH2*2 are at much higher risk for oro-pharyngeal cancer.[92]

Multiple mechanisms are involved in alcohol-related carcinogenesis and include the effect of acetaldehyde, the first metabolite of ethanol oxidation; the induction of cytochrome P-4502 E1 (genetic variant CYP2EI) leading to the generation of ROS; increased procarcinogen activation (e.g., nitrosamines), as well as modulation of cellular regeneration (cell cycle); and nutritional deficiencies (retinol, retinyl esters, other vitamins). Nutritional deficiencies may give rise to altered mucosal integrity, enzyme and metabolic dysfunction, and other structural abnormalities. Women have a greater sensitivity to alcohol, progress to alcohol toxicity faster, and have increased mortality at lower levels of consumption as compared with men.[93]

Sexual and Reproductive Behavior

The last decade has demonstrated that sexually transmitted infection with carcinogenic types of human papilloma virus (HPV), referred to as high-risk types of HPV, is required for the development of most cervical cancers. HPV infections, however, are very common in sexually active women, and the majority of these infections will resolve or only cause transient, minor problems.[94] Eighty HPV types have been sequenced and 30 of these types infect both the female and male genital tract and two-thirds of these are classified as high-risk types. HPV-16, in most countries, accounts for 50% to 60% of cervical cancer cases, followed by HPV-18 (10% to 12%) and HPV-31 and HPV-45 (4% to 5% each).[95] HPV types correlated with genital warts, HPV-2 and HPV-11, are called low-risk because they are rarely associated with cancer. Persistence of infection with high-risk HPV is a prerequisite for the development of cervical intraepithelial neoplasia (CIN) 3 (see Figure 23-17) lesions and invasive cervical cancers.[94] Biologic factors that determine persistence are not understood, but risk factors include older age, long-term use of oral contraceptives (5 or more years), high parity (5 or more full-term pregnancies), smoking, and HIV infection.[94,96] Earlier reported risk factors, for example, number of sexual partners, are probably indicators of HPV exposure rather than independent risk factors. HPV can be transmitted by genital contact (oral, touching, or sexual intercourse), therefore, condoms are not necessarily protective (see Chapter 23).

About 500,000 cases of invasive cervical cancer are diagnosed each year worldwide—the majority occur in developing countries. Although HPV is the most prevalent sexually transmitted infection in the United States, fewer than one-third of women and men in the general population have heard of it and low awareness exists among women in high school and college settings.[97-99] Cervical cancer mortality has decreased over the last 5 decades in the United States by over 70%, probably due to screening with the Papanicolaou (Pap) test.[94] HIV infected individuals have demonstrated an increase in both oral and anogenital pathologic conditions because of HPV infection.[100]

The incidence of invasive cervical cancer is substantially higher in women of low socioeconomic standing and is more common in central and south America, eastern Africa, and the Caribbean.[101] Current consensus is that newborn babies can be exposed to cervical HPV infection of the mother. The possible modes of transmission in children, however, are controversial.[102]

Physical Activity

Physical activity reduces the risk of breast and colon cancers and may reduce the risk of other cancers. Several biologic mechanisms causing this effect have been proposed and include decreasing insulin and insulin-like growth factor levels; decreasing obesity; increasing free radical scavenger systems; altering inflammatory mediators; decreasing circulating estrogens and androgens; and increasing gut motility.[103,104] For colon cancer, physical activity increases gut motility, which reduces the length of time (transit time) that the bowel lining is exposed to potential mutagens.[105] For breast cancer, vigorous physical activity may decrease exposure of breast tissue to ovarian hormones, insulin, and insulin-like factor. A recent,

Table 11-10 Known Occupational Carcinogenic Agents Classified by the International Agency for Research on Cancer (IARC)

Agent, Mixture, or Circumstance	Main Industry or Use
Agents or Group of Agents	
4-Aminobiphenyl	Pigment
Arsenic and arsenic compounds	Glass, metal, pesticide
Asbestos	Insulation, filter, textile
Benzene	Chemical, solvent
Benzidine	Pigment
Beryllium and beryllium compounds	Aerospace
Bis(chloromethyl)ether and chloromethyl methyl ether*	Chemical intermediate
Cadmium and cadmium compounds	Dye/pigment
Chromium [IV] compounds	Metal plating, dye/pigment
Dioxin	Chemical
Ethylene oxide	Sterilant
Mustard gas*	War gas
2-Naphthylamine	Pigment
Nickel compounds	Metallurgy, alloy, catalyst
Plutonium-239 and its decay products*	Nuclear industry
Radium-226 and its decay products*	Luminizing industry
Radon-222 and its decay products	Mining
Silica, crystalline	Stone cutting, mining, glass
Solar radiation	Agriculture
Talc containing asbestos fibers	Paper, paints
Vinyl chloride	Plastics
X- and γ-radiation	Medical
Mixtures	
Coal-tar pitches†	Construction, electrode
Coal-tars†	Fuel, construction, chemical
Mineral oils, untreated†	Metal
Shale-oils†	Fuel
Soots†	Pigment
Wood dust	Wood
Exposure Circumstances	
Aluminum production	
Auramine, manufacture of*	Pigment
Boot and shoe manufacture and repair	
Coal gasification	
Coke production	
Furniture and cabinet making	
Hematite mining (underground) with exposure to radon	
Iron and steel founding	
Magenta, manufacture of*	
Painter (occupational exposure as a)	
Rubber industry	
Strong inorganic-acid mists containing sulfuric acid	Metallurgy

From Boffetta P: *Oncogene* 23:6392-6403, 2004.
*Agent mainly of historical interest.
†Mixture of polycyclic aromatic hydrocarbons.
IARC, International Agency for Research on Cancer.

Table 11-11 Probable Occupational Carcinogenic Agents Classified by the IARC

Agent, Mixture, or Circumstance	Main Industry or Use
Agents or Group of Agents	
Acrylamide	Chemical, construction
Benz[a]anthracene*	Combustion fumes
Benzidine-based dyes	Paper, leather, textile dyes
Benzo[a]pyrene*	Combustion fumes
1,3-Butadiene	Plastics, rubber
Captafol	Fungicide
α-Chlorinated toluenes	Chemical intermediate
4-Chloro-ortho-toluidine	Dye/pigment manufacture, textiles
Dibenz[a,h]anthracene*	Combustion fumes
Diethyl sulphate	Chemical intermediate
Dimethylcarbamoyl chloride	Chemical intermediate
Dimethyl sulphate	Chemical intermediate
Epichlorohydrin	Plastics/resins monomer
Ethylene dibromide	Chemical intermediate, fumigant
Formaldehyde	Plastics, textiles, laboratory agent
Glycidol	Chemical intermediate
4,4'-Methylene bis (2-chloroaniline) (MOCA)†	Rubber manufacture
N-Nitrosodimethylamine†	Chemical intermediate
Styrene-7,8-oxide	Plastics, chemical intermediate
Tetrachloroethylene	Solvent, dry cleaning
Ortho-Toluidine	Dyestuff, rubber
Trichoroethylene	Solvent, dry cleaning, metal
1,2,3-Trichloropropane	Solvent, chemical intermediate
Tris(2,3-dibromoprophyl) phosphate	Plastics, textiles, flame retardant
Vinyl bromide	Plastics, textiles, monomer
Vinyl flouride	Chemical intermediate
Mixtures	
Creosotes‡	Wood preservation
Diesel engine exhaust‡	Transport
Nonarsenical insecticides (spraying and application)	Agriculture
Polychlorinated biphenyls	Electrical components
Exposure Circumstances	
Art glass, glass container, and pressed ware (manufacture of)	
Hairdresser and barber	
Petroleum refining	

From Boffetta P: *Oncogene* 23(38):6392-6403, 2004.
*Component of mixtures of polycyclic aromatic hydrocarbons.
†Agent mainly of historical interest.
‡Mixture of polycyclic aromatic hydrocarbons.
IARC, International Agency for Research on Cancer.

randomized trial found after 12 months of moderate-intensity exercise, postmenopausal women had significantly decreased serum estrogens.[106] Physical activity also helps prevent type 2 diabetes that has been associated with risk of cancer of the colon and pancreas.[106,107]

Many questions are unanswered regarding frequency, intensity, and duration of exercise. Much of the literature suggests between 3.5 and 4 hours of vigorous activity per week are necessary to optimize protection for colon cancer.[104] There is likely a dose-response relationship for colon cancer and breast cancer, and 30 to 60 minutes per day of moderate to vigorous intensity is proposed to decrease breast cancer risk.[108]

Occupational Hazards as Carcinogens

Table 11-10 identifies known occupational carcinogenic agents classified by the International Agency for Research on Cancer (IARC), and Table 11-11 identifies probable occupational carcinogenic agents classified by the IARC. A substantial percentage of cancers of the upper respiratory passages, lung, bladder, and peritoneum are attributed to occupational factors, however, fewer studies of nonsmokers exist.[109] One notable occupational factor is **asbestos,** which increases the risk of mesothelioma and lung cancer. Asbestos was used in homes and buildings built before the 1970s to insulate ceiling tiles, flooring, and pipe covers. In western Europe, the epidemic of mesothelioma in building workers and other workers born after 1940 did not become apparent until the 1990s (i.e., because of long latency). Carcinoma of the bladder has been linked with the manufacture of dyes, rubber, paint, and aromatic amines, especially β-naphthylamine and benzidine. Benzol inhalation is linked to leukemia in shoemakers and in workers in the rubber cement, explosives, and dyeing industries. Other notable occupational hazards include heavy metals (e.g., high-nickel alloy, chromium VI compounds, inorganic arsenic), silica, polycyclic aromatic hydrocarbons, sulfuric acid, and chloromethyl ether. Studies of occupational exposure to diesel exhaust indicate an increased risk of lung cancer.[110] Disentangling data related to lung cancer, air pollution, and occupational risks is complex, especially in combination with active and passive smoking and the interplay of environmental factors and genetic polymorphisms at multiple loci.

Air Pollution

A person inhales about 20,000 L of air in 1 day; thus even modest contamination of the atmosphere can result in inhalation of appreciable doses of pollutants. Contaminants include outdoor and indoor air pollutants. Concerns include industrial emissions, including arsenicals, benzene, chloroform, formaldehyde, sulfuric acid, mustard gas, vinyl chloride, and acrylonitrite.[111] Living close to certain industries is a recognized cancer risk factor, although it is difficult to determine cancer risk from outdoor pollution *alone* because investigators must accurately control for smoking and radon. Studies that controlled or stratified for smoking demon-strated associations between excess lung cancer rates and heavy metal and aromatic hydrocarbon emissions in polluted air. Evidence for cancers, other than lung cancer and childhood cancer, is inconsistent.[112]

Indoor pollution generally is considered worse than outdoor pollution, partly because of cigarette smoke. Environmental tobacco smoke (ETS; passive smoking) can cause the formation of reactive oxygen free radicals and, thus, DNA damage. The IARC has classified ETS as a human carcinogen. A meta-analysis of studies found a relative risk of 1.22 (95% confidence interval) in women and 1.36 (95% confidence interval) in men resulting from workplace exposure.[112] Other meta-analyses report similar results.[113] Another significant indoor air pollutant is radon gas. **Radon** is a natural radioactive gas derived from the radioactive decay of uranium that is ubiquitous in rock and soil; it can become trapped in houses and gives rise to radioactive decay products known to be carcinogenic to humans. The most hazardous houses can be identified by testing and then modified to prevent further radon contamination. Exposure levels are greater from underground mines than from houses. Most of the lung cancers associated with radon are bronchogenic; however, small-cell carcinoma does occur with greater frequency in underground miners. Radon increases the risk of lung cancer in underground miners whether they smoke or not.

In China, some regions report very high levels of lung cancer in women who spend much of their time indoors. Exposures from heating and cooking combustion sources (e.g., oil vapors) are identified as risk factors for lung cancer.[113]

Inorganic arsenic (known as a carcinogen since the late 1960s), found principally in underground water (from 1000 to 4000 μg/L), is found in many regions of the world. According to the IARC, strong evidence indicates an increased risk of bladder, skin, and lung cancers following consumption of water with high levels of arsenic (generally above 200 μg/L).[114] Evidence for cancers of the liver, colon, and kidney are weaker. Other sources of inorganic arsenic are related to occupational exposures (see Table 11-10).

The central hypothesis, based on rat studies, for the mechanisms related to particle-induced lung carcinogenesis is that insoluble particles cause pulmonary inflammation (e.g., cytokine release, ROS), which leads to genotoxic stress, proliferative response, and tissue remodeling progressing toward fibrosis and tumor development. Much additional research is needed to understand the surface chemistry and lung tissue remodeling in relation to insoluble particles and lung carcinogenesis.[115]

Electromagnetic Fields

Health risks associated with electromagnetic fields (EMF) are controversial. Exposure to electric and magnetic fields is widespread. EMFs are a type of nonionizing radiation, low frequency radiation without enough energy to break off electrons from their orbits around atoms and ionize (charge) the atoms. Microwaves, radar, and power frequency radiation associated with electricity and radio waves, fluorescent lights, computers, and other electric equipment all create EMFs of varying strength. The major debate for over four decades has focused on the association of exposure to EMF and resultant health consequences, including cancer. Currently, no consistent body of evidence exists in support of an association between EMF and childhood cancer, albeit it warrants further investigation.[116] Evidence of an association between EMF and adult cancers, derived largely from occupational settings, is also inconsistent. In addition, little evidence indicates an association between EMF and noncancer health effects. Scientific evidence, however, is hampered by methods to accurately measure exposure, the lack of a clear dose/response relationship, and the difficulty in reproducing effects.

In 1998, however, a National Institute of Environmental Health Sciences EMF Working Group recommended that low frequency EMFs be classified as possible carcinogens.[117] A recent population-based study ($N = 5400$ women) linked residential EMF exposure from high voltage power lines to a 60% increased risk of breast cancer in Norwegian women of all ages.[118]

The controversy about potential health hazards associated with the exposure of electromagnetic fields has recently been stimulated by the increased use of mobile telecommunication devices and emissions from cell towers. Cellular telephones emit electromagnetic radiation in the range of 800 to 2000 MHz, which is in the microwave range (300 MHz to 300 GHz).

Electromagnetic radiation from a cell phone can penetrate the skull and deposit energy 4 cm to 6 cm into the brain.[119] This energy can potentially result in thermal heating of the tissue. The debate, therefore, has been whether these thermal effects could induce carcinogenesis. One thermal mechanism proposed is change in protein phosphorylation.[120,121] Exposure of human peripheral blood lymphocytes to EMFs associated with cellular phones found a linear increase in chromosome 17 aneuploidy.[122] Control experiments (without EMF) involving temperature changes from 24.5° C to 38.5° C showed that elevated temperature is not associated with genetic or epigenetic alterations. Thus these findings indicated a genotoxic effect of the EMFs is not elicited by a thermal pathway.[122] One out of three animal studies found an excess of lymphoma in genetically engineered mice exposed long term to pulsed 900-MHz electromagnetic fields.[123,124] The relevance of this study to humans is unknown. Since 2004, nine epidemiologic studies have been published concerning cell phones and cancer. Seven studies reviewed mainly brain tumors, with one examining brain tumors and salivary gland cancer, another cancer of the lymphatic tissues, and one investigating intraocular melanoma. All studies had methodological problems: (1) too short a duration (or latency period) of cell phone use to be helpful in risk assessment, (2) exposure was not rigorously determined, and (3) possibility of recall and response error. The evidence does not give clear or consistent results indicating a causal role of EMF exposures in cancer. The results, however, cannot establish the *absence* of any hazard. Particularly problematic is that the data is insufficient on individual levels or intensities of exposure.[125] Further research is desperately needed, especially for EMFs and leukemia in children and adults and cranial tumors associated with cell phone use.

Diet

Understanding dietary factors that increase the risk for cancer is complex and challenging. It is complex because of the variety of foods consumed, the many constituents of foods, the metabolic consequences of eating, and the temporal changes in the patterns of food use. Cancer risks in the elderly may also depend as much on diet in early life as on current eating practices.[38,126]

People are constantly exposed to a variety of compounds termed **xenobiotics** (Greek *xenos,* foreign; *bios,* life) that include toxic, mutagenic, and carcinogenic chemicals. Many of these chemicals are found in the human diet. Most xenobiotics are transported in the blood by lipoproteins and penetrate through lipid membranes. These chemicals can react with cellular macromolecules, such as proteins and DNA, or can react directly with cell structures to cause cell damage.[127] The body has two defense systems for counteracting these effects: (1) detoxification enzymes and (2) antioxidant systems (see Chapter 2). Enzymes that activate xenobiotics are called **phase I activation enzymes** and are represented by the multigene cytochrome P450 family, aldehyde oxidase, xanthine oxidases, and peroxidases. **Phase II detoxification enzymes** then protect further against a large array of reactive intermediates and nonactivated xenobiotics.[127] These enzymes are located predominantly in the liver and provide clearance of compounds through the portal circulation, thereby preventing the potentially carcinogenic agent(s) from entering the body through the gastrointestinal tract and portal circulation. These enzymes also occur in the skin epithelia and can be induced in other extrahepatic tissue, such as the lung.

Dietary sources of potentially toxic carcinogenic substances include compounds produced in the cooking of fat, meat, or protein, and naturally occurring carcinogens associated with plant food substances, such as alkaloids or mold byproducts.[127] The most studied and most relevant carcinogens produced by cooking are the polycyclic aromatic hydrocarbons benzo[a]pyrene and heterocyclic aromatic amines generated by meat protein. The greatest levels are found in well-done, charbroiled beef. People, likewise, ingest xenobiotics that are found in environmental or industrial contaminants (e.g., particulate matter of diesel exhaust, contaminating pesticides in food and water supplies) and in certain prescribed and over-the-counter medicines.

The strongest, most consistent and unequivocal support for diet playing a role in carcinogenesis is data related to obesity; consumption of alcohol; aflatoxin (produced by mold), which can contaminate corn, peanuts, and rice stored in hot, humid environments; and Chinese-style salted fish, which is linked to nasopharanygeal cancer.[38,128-130] A monumental amount of research from the past 2 decades has shown that rates for various cancers correlate fairly consistently with certain dietary factors, but opinions differ on the strength of the overall evidence.[38,131,132] Table 11-12 shows the relationship between dietary factors and cancer risk.

Obesity

The prevalence of overweight and obesity in most developed countries (and in urban areas of many less developed countries) has been increasing greatly over the past 20 years (Figure 11-26). The only globally accepted criteria for overweight and obesity are based on body-mass index (BMI). Widely accepted standards based on BMI criteria for overweight and obesity are recommended by the World Health Organization (WHO)[133] and supported by other panels and federal agencies (WHO classifications are shown in Table 11-13).

A recent large prospective study of 900,000 American adults showed obesity is linked to cancer. Starting with a mean age of 57 years, individuals were followed for 16 years and cancer mortality data was collected during that interval.[134] Compared with men whose body mass index was in the normal range (18.5 to 24.9), men with substantial obesity (BMI ≥40.0) had significant increases in cancer mortality. Women had a similar risk (see Figure 11-26) Although significant, people with lesser degrees of obesity had lesser increases in cancer mortality. In men with higher BMI, there were higher rates of death from esophageal, stomach, colorectal, liver, gallbladder, pancreatic, prostate, and kidney cancers and non-Hodgkin lymphoma, multiple myeloma, and leukemia.[134] Among women, high BMI was correlated with greater morbidity from colorectal, liver, gallbladder, pancreatic, breast, uterine, cervical, ovarian, and kidney cancers and

Table 11-12 Relationship of Dietary Factors with Risk of Major Cancers[a]

Diet	Colorectal	Breast	Prostate	Lung	Stomach	Esophageal	Oral	Pancreatic	Bladder	Kidney	Endometrial
Micronutrients/Energy Balance											
Obesity	↑↑	↑↑			↑[b]	↑[b]		↑		↑	↑↑
GI/GL,[c] IGF, height, or metabolic syndrome	↑↑	↑	↑					↑		↑	↑
Animal fat		↑									↑
Nutrients											
Folic acid	↓↓	↓		↓							
Alcohol	↑↑	↑↑				↑↑	↑				
Calcium	↓				↑						
Vitamin D	↓			↓							
β-carotene supplements				↑↑[e]	↓						
Lycopene-containing foods			↓		↓	↓					
Vitamin C					↓						
Vitamin E			↓								
Selenium			↓	↓							
Foods											
Red or processed meat	↑			↑							
Fruits[d]	↓		↓	↓	↓	↓	↓	↓			↓
Vegetables[d]	↓	↓	↓	↓	↓	↓	↓		↓		↓
Other											
Grilled meat	↑		↑								
Western diet pattern	↑										
High-fiber diet	↓										
Salt, preserved foods					↑						
Hot beverages						↑	↑				

From McCullough ML, Giovannucci EL: *Oncogene* 23(38):6349-6364, 2004.
[a]Two arrows indicate more consistent evidence; [b]Cancers of the gastric cardia; [c]*GI/GL,* glycemic index/glycemic load; [d]Evidence for a potential benefit from some components of fruits and vegetables (not necessarily blanket effect); [e]Increased risk limited to smokers.
IGF, Insulin-like growth factor.

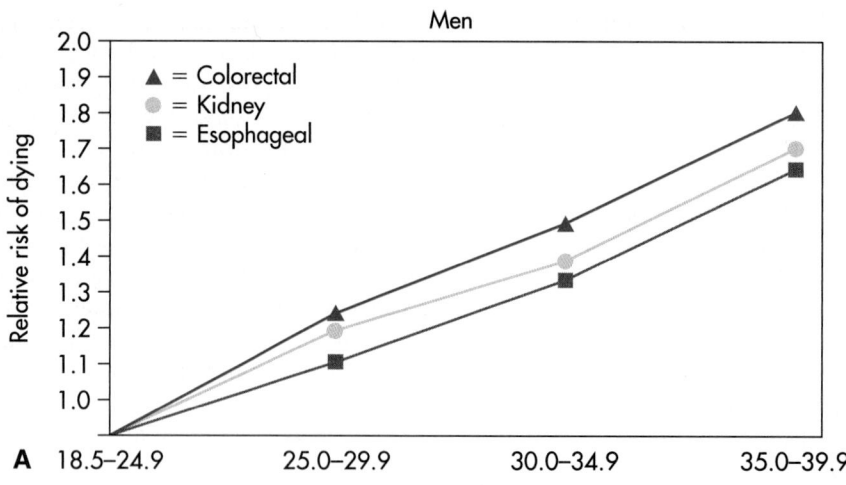

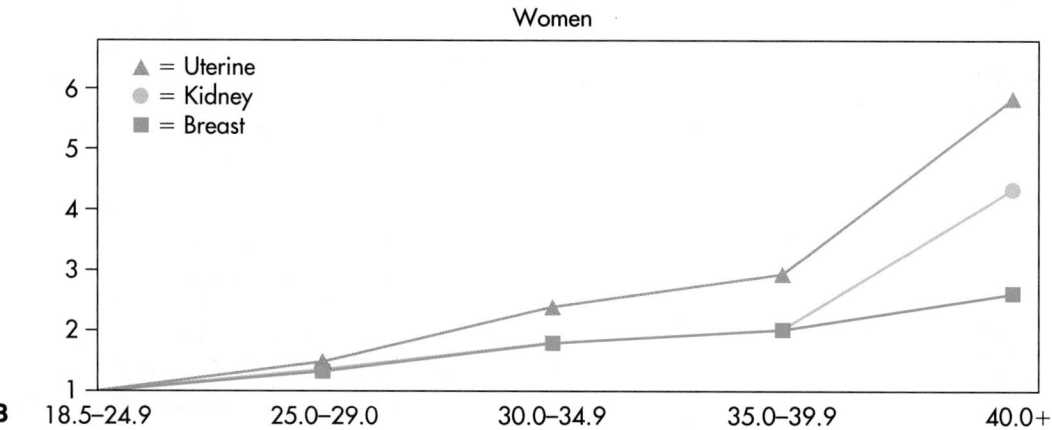

Figure 11-26 **Weight and risk of dying from cancer. A,** As a man's BMI rises above the normal range (18.5 to 24.9), his risk of dying of colorectal, esophageal, kidney, and other cancers also rises. For example, the risk of dying of colorectal cancer is 10% higher for men who are overweight (BMI 25.0 to 29.9) than for men of normal or lower BMI. For the most obese men (BMI 35 or higher) the risk is almost double (84%). **B,** As a woman's BMI rises above the normal range (18.5 to 24.9) her risk of dying of breast, kidney, uterine, and other cancers rises. For example, the risk of dying of breast cancer is 34% higher for women who are overweight. For the most obese women (BMI >40), the risk of dying of breast cancer is double. The risk of kidney disease is almost five times higher, and the risk of uterine cancer is six times higher. (Data from Calle EE et al: *N Engl J Med* 348:1625-1638, 2003.)

Table 11-13	WHO Classification of Body Mass Index (BMI)	
BMI (kg/m²)*	**WHO Classification**	**Other Descriptions**
<18.5	Underweight	Thin
18.5-24.9	Normal range	"Healthy," "normal," or "acceptable" weight
25.0-29.9	Grade 1 overweight	Overweight
30.0-39.9	Grade 2 overweight	Obesity
≥40.0	Grade 3 overweight	Morbidly overweight

*The cut-offs are somewhat arbitrary, though they are derived from epidemiologic studies of BMI and overall mortality. It is important to understand that within each category of BMI there can be substantial individual variation in total and visceral adiposity and in related metabolic factors. These variations are also true for the normal range BMI.
WHO, World Health Organization.

from non-Hodgkin lymphoma and multiple myeloma. Thus the American Cancer Society estimates that obesity accounts for 14% of cancer deaths in men and 20% in women.

Biologic Mechanisms

Adipose tissue is *active* endocrine and metabolic tissue and can have even more effects on the physiology of other tissue (see Chapter 39). In response to endocrine and metabolic signals from other organs, adipose tissue responds by increasing or decreasing the release of free fatty acids—fuel for skeletal muscle and other tissues. When triglycerides, the main storage lipid, are metabolically hydrolyzed, they release free fatty acids into the blood. Abdominal visceral adipocytes are more metabolically active than abdominal subcutaneous adipocytes and because visceral adipocytes have high lipolytic activity and release large amounts of free fatty acids, accurate measurements of adiposity needs to consider both the *amount* and the *site* of deposition of the adipose tissue. Adipose tissue is very important in the regulation of energy balance and lipid metabolism through the release of peptide hormones, including leptin, adiponectin, resistin, and tumor necrosis factor–γ (TNF-γ) (Figure 11-27). Increased release of free fatty acids, resistin, and TNF-γ by adipose tissue and *reduced* release of adiponectin give rise to *insulin resistance*— a state characterized by reduced metabolic response of tissues (muscle, liver, adipose) to insulin and to compensatory hyperinsulinemia[135] (see Figure 11-27). In addition to its role in regulating energy balance, lipid metabolism, and insulin sensitivity, adipose tissue cells produce various steroid-hormone-metabolizing enzymes and are an important source of circulating estrogens in postmenopausal women (Figure 11-28).

Excess weight, increased plasma triglyceride levels, low levels of physical activity, and certain dietary factors can all contribute to chronic hyperinsulinemia. Chronically increased insulin levels have been correlated with the pathogenesis of colon, breast, pancreatic, and endometrial cancers[136-138] (see Figure 11-28). These cancer-causing effects of insulin might be mediated by insulin receptors in the preneoplastic or neoplastic target cells or could be due to alterations in endogenous hormone metabolism secondary to hyperinsulinemia. For example, insulin promotes the synthesis and biologic activity of the growth factor **insulin-like growth factor–1 (IGF-1)**. IGF-1 is a peptide hormone with a molecular structure similar to insulin that regulates cellular proliferation in

response to available energy and nutrients from diet and body constituents (see Figure 11-28). In addition, insulin helps promote the synthesis and biologic availability of the male and female sex hormones, including estrogens, progesterone, and androgens[135] (see Figure 11-28).

In vitro studies have established that both insulin and IGF-1 act as growth factors that promote cell proliferation and inhibit apoptosis.[139-142] Epidemiologic evidence supports the hypothesis that chronic hyperinsulinemia increases cancer risk. Type 2 diabetes mellitus associated with insulin resistance and increased pancreatic insulin secretion for long periods before and after disease onset is associated with increased risks of cancer of the colon, endometrium, kidney, and pancreas.[136,138,143,144] Prospective cohort studies have shown increased risks of cancers of the colon or colorectum among individuals with increased prediagnostic blood levels of **C-peptide** (a marker for pancreatic insulin secretion), fasting glucose levels, or insulin measured 2 hours after absorption of a standard oral dose of glucose.[145] Similar data has found a direct relationship between cancer risk and prediagnostic C-peptide levels for endometrial cancer.[146] The study also found inverse relationships of cancer risk and blood levels of IGF-binding protein 1 (IGFBP1) and IGF-binding protein 2 (IGFBP2),[146] which reduce the amount of bioavailable IGF1.

The IGFBPs regulate the availability of IGF-1 because they stabilize the large pool of IGF-1 in the circulation, the efflux of IGF-1 from this circulation pool toward target tissues and binding of IGF-1 to its receptor.[135] IGBP3 increases tissue apoptosis, so decreased amounts may contribute to carcinogenesis.

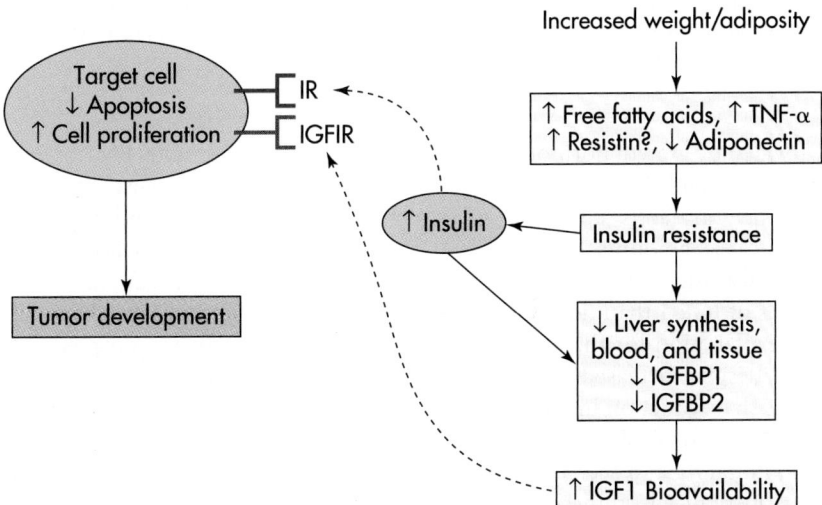

Figure 11-27 Energy balance, lipid metabolism, and insulin sensitivity and tumor development. In obesity, increased release from adipose tissue of free fatty acids (FFA), tumor necrosis factor alpha (TNF-α) and resistin, and reduced release of adiponectin lead to insulin resistance and compensatory chronic hyperinsulinemia. Increased insulin levels ultimately lead to decreased liver synthesis and blood levels of insulin-like growth factor-binding protein 1 (IGFBP1) and, theoretically, also decrease IGFBP2 synthesis locally in other tissues. Increased fasting levels of insulin in plasma are also correlated with decreased levels of IGFBP2 in the blood leading to increased levels of bioavailable IGF-1. Insulin and IGF-1 signal through the insulin receptors (IRs) and IGF-1 receptor (IGF1R) to stimulate cellular proliferation and inhibit apoptosis in many tissue types. These effects could promote tumor development. (Adapted from Calle EE, Kaaks R: *Nat Rev Cancer* 4(8):579-591, 2004.)

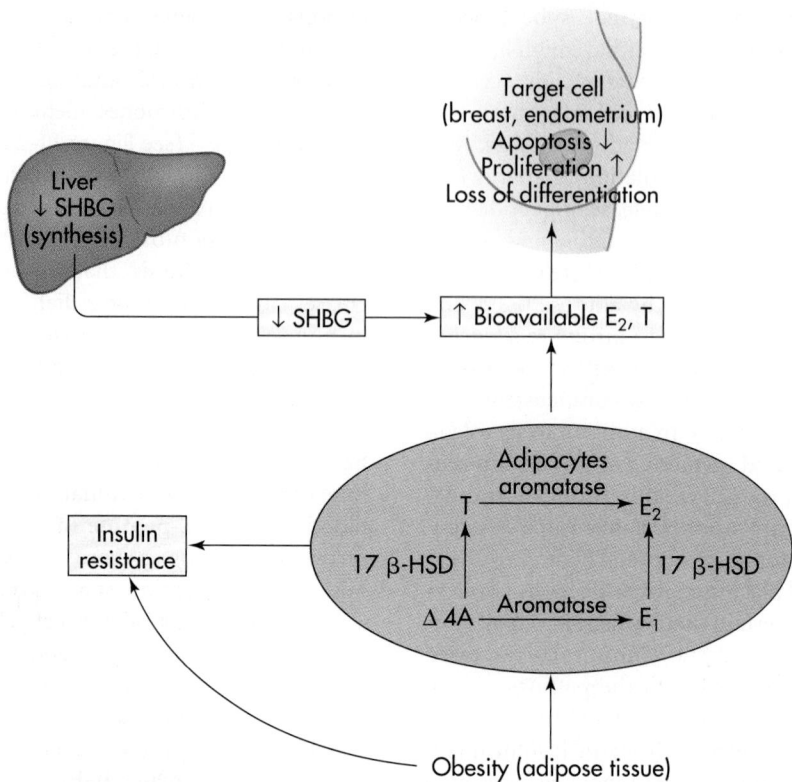

Figure 11-28 **Effects of obesity on hormone alterations.** Adipose tissue produces the enzymes aromatase and 17-beta hydroxy-steroid dehydrogenase (17-βHSD). In obese persons, therefore, there is an increased conversion of the androgens Δ4-androstenedione (Δ4A) and testosterone (T) into the estrogens estrone (E_1) and estradiol (E_2), respectively, by the enzyme aromatase. The important enzyme 17-βHSD converts the less biologically active hormones Δ4A and E_1 into the more active hormones T and E_2, respectively. In parallel, obesity leads to hyperinsulinemia, which causes a decrease in the liver synthesis and blood circulating levels of sex hormone-binding globulin (SHGB). The combined effect of increased synthesis of estrone and testosterone, along with reduced levels of SHBG (their transporter), leads to an increase in the bioavailable (or free fractions) of E_2 and T that can diffuse to target tissue where they bind to estrogen and androgen receptors. Binding to their respective receptors in some tissue (e.g., breast and endometrium) promotes cellular proliferation and inhibits apoptosis. Thus they can increase tumor development. In both men and women, adiposity-related decreases in SHGB generally increase the fraction of bioavailable or free estradiol. In contrast, decreases of SHGB in men only generally lead to reductions in testicular production of testosterone and no increase in bioavailable testosterone. (Adapted from Calle EE, Kaaks R: *Nat Rev Cancer* 4:579-591, 2004.)

Over 80% of IGF-1 is provided by growth hormone (GH). In overnourished states and in individuals with type 2 diabetes mellitus, endogenous insulin levels and liver GH-receptor levels are high and large amounts of IGF-1 are produced.[135] Contrarily and confusing, however, obese individuals have lower blood levels of IGF-1 than normal weight individuals.[147] A compelling explanation for the lower levels of IGF-1 in obese individuals, despite increased GH sensitivity of liver and other tissues, is that reduction in IGFBP1 and IGFBP2 levels lead to increased negative feedback by free IGF-1 (unbound to IGFBPs) on pituitary gland secretion of GH. Overall, this feedback results in reduced synthesis of IGF-1 and reduced plasma IGF-1 concentrations.

Epidemiologic studies have reported increased blood levels of IGF-1 as directly related to different forms of cancer. Increased levels of blood IGF-1 are related to increased risk of breast cancers, especially for premenopausal women.[148-151] Similar increased risks were reported for cancers of the prostate and colorectum.[152-155] Interestingly, however, these various types of cancer, with the exception of colon, show no clear relationship with BMI or other indices of adiposity. In addition, there is no clear linear relationship between circulating levels of IGF-1 and the degree of adiposity.[135]

Endogenous Hormones

Three mechanisms are known involving how adiposity influences the synthesis and bioavailability of endogenous sex steroids, the estrogens, progesterone, and androgens (see Figure 11-28).

1. Adipose tissue expresses various sex-steroid metabolizing enzymes that promote the formation of estrogens from androgenic precursors (secreted by the gonads and adrenal glands).
2. Adipose cells increase the circulating levels of insulin and increase IGF-1 biologic activity. This results in reduced liver synthesis and blood levels of sex hormone–binding globulin (SHBG), a binding hormone with affinity for estradiol and testosterone. The adiposity-related decrease in SHBG increases bioavailable estradiol in both men and women. In women, decreased SHBG also leads to increased levels of testos-

terone; in men, contrarily, decreases in SHBG generally lead to reduction in total testicular testosterone production and *no* increase in bioavailable testosterone.

3. High insulin levels can increase ovarian and, possibly, adrenal androgen synthesis and in some genetically susceptible, premenopausal women cause the development of polycystic ovary syndrome (PCOS).[156] PCOS is characterized by ovarian hyperandrogenism, chronic anovulation, and progesterone deficiency. PCOS is relatively common with an estimated prevalence of 4% to 6%.[135]

Epidemiologic evidence shows that adiposity-induced alterations in blood levels of sex steroids could explain the correlation noted between indices of excess weight and risks of breast cancer (postmenopausal only) and endometrium cancer (both pre- and postmenopausal).[135]

For breast and endometrial cancers, a central role of estrogens and progesterone is established from a large body of experimental and clinical evidence. These sex steroids are important regulators of cellular proliferation, differentiation, and apoptosis. Further evidence that increased endogenous estrogen levels might drive the association between BMI and breast cancer comes from studies of hormone replacement therapy (HRT). BMI is more strongly related to risk of breast cancer among postmenopausal women who have *never* received HRT compared to women who have.[157-159] Possibly, only in women whose levels of estrogen are low (after menopause with no HRT) does increased adiposity and, therefore, an increase in peripheral aromatase activity by androgenous activity and androgenous estrogen production, lead to an increase in breast cancer risk. In addition, mortality is higher among heavier women than among leaner women.[135,160]

Several case-control and prospective studies have reported increased risks among both pre- and postmenopausal women who have lower blood levels of SHBG and thus high levels of androgens and testosterone. Among postmenopausal women,

risk is also correlated to levels of estrone and total bioavailable (free) estradiol.[146]

Among men, prostate carcinogenesis is thought to be related to endogenous hormone metabolism, including androgen production and, possibly, estrogens. Yet excess weight does not appear to be a prominent risk factor except with advanced disease.[136] Other dietary factors and the outcome of studies for cancer risk are presented in Table 11-14. Hormones and cancer are discussed in Chapter 23.

NUTRITION & DISEASE

Components of a Cancer-Prevention Diet

Some foods increase the risk of cancer, whereas other foods decrease the risk. Observing the following dietary guidelines might reduce the risk of cancer:

Increase

- Fiber (limiting glycemic index)
- Fruits and vegetables (especially broccoli, cabbage, and Swiss chard)
- Foods containing vitamins A, C, D, and E; mineral selenium (not to exceed 200 mcg/day)
- Foods containing folate (fruits, vegetables, legumes, grains, supplements)
- Epigallocatechin gallate (found in green tea)

Decrease

- Fat (especially large amounts of omega-6 fatty acids)
- High glycemic index carbohydrates
- Foods with high amounts of preservatives
- Alcohol
- Grilled, blackened foods
- Fried foods
- High levels of calcium ($\geq$2000 mg)*

---

*Influences cancer risk in a complex way; lower levels $\leq$1000 mg/day may confer protection (see Table 11-14).

Table 11-14	Studies of Dietary Factors and Associated Cancer Risk
Dietary Factor	**Study Results**
Fat	Results are inconsistent
	Hypothesized to modulate sex hormone levels for breast and prostate cancers and to increase colon cancer risk by stimulating mutagenic activity secondary to bile acid secretion
	Confirming a role for fat independent of calories and other constituents of meat and dairy foods has been difficult
	Case-controlled, prospective, or intervention studies have not shown any consistent findings
	Inconsistencies may be resolved through use of biomarkers instead of questionnaires, however, markers are subject to recent intakes and inter-individual variation
	Evidence is the strongest for animal fats in prostate cancer but correlations seem to vary by the type of fat and study design
	Marine fatty acids and their sources (fish) may reduce breast and prostate cancer risk although findings are inconsistent[166]
Carbohydrates	Carbohydrates include starches, nonstarch polysaccharides, and sugars
	Because high glycemic index carbohydrates are correlated with higher postprandial blood glucose and insulin levels and higher fasting insulin levels in insulin-resistant states, they are hypothesized to increase cancer risk; epidemiologic studies have not supported this relationship to date
	Nonetheless, abnormal glucose and insulin metabolism is important in carcinogenesis, especially in obese individuals and sedentary individuals

Continued

Table 11-14	Studies of Dietary Factors and Associated Cancer Risk—cont'd
Dietary Factor	**Study Results**
Meat	Evidence for meat consumption in increasing cancer risk, especially of the colon, rectum, and prostate has fairly consistent data over time and across study designs International data with countries with higher meat consumption have higher incidence of colon cancer than those with lower meat consumption A meta-analysis with 14 prospective studies reported a significant (12% to 17%) increase in risk with each daily 100 g–increment of all meat or red meat intake (>3 oz) and a 49% increased risk for each 25 g–increment of processed meats (about 1 slice)[167] The increased risk of colon cancer associated with red and processed meats has several cancer-related hypotheses: 1. Heterocyclic amines (HCAs) 2. Polycyclic aromatic hydrocarbons (PAHs) formed at high temperatures or over an open flame 3. Mutagenic N-nitroso compounds (NOC) 4. Meat components on hormone metabolism (and possibly hormones in meat) 5. Diets high in red meat may be low in vegetables[166]
Dairy	Recent studies suggest a lower risk of cancer with higher intakes of low-fat dairy products and a higher risk of breast cancer with high-fat dairy intakes[168] Some studies have shown dairy products associated with higher risk of prostate and ovarian cancers[169] Their overall influence, however, remains inconsistent
Vitamin D	Experimental data shows a protective role for $1,25(OH)_2D$ (the active form of vitamin D) on growth regulation and cell differentiation Populations with greater exposure to ultraviolet light generally have lower risks of breast, colon, and prostate cancer Vitamin D is synthesized in the skin after exposure to UV radiation and is also obtained from fortified milk products, breakfast cereals, fatty fish, and multivitamin supplements
Calcium	Calcium has been shown to influence cancer risk in a complex way It has been inversely related to the risk of colorectal cancer and adenoma recurrence, but high amounts also have been associated with other cancers, particularly prostate[170,171] Calcium has been hypothesized to protect against colorectal cancer by binding secondary bile acids and ionized fatty acids in the colon forming insoluble soaps and reducing proliferative stimuli on the mucosa[172] Calcium also may cause terminal differentiation[173] Prospective studies of colon cancer suggest that total calcium intake above 1000 mg may not confer any additional benefit Case-control studies of calcium and prostate and breast cancer have been inconsistent One hypothesis of how high levels of calcium may increase risk of prostate cancer is by down-regulating production of $1,25(OH)_2D$, the active form of vitamin D In vitro, vitamin D reduces cell proliferation and induces cell differentiation; these functions are thought to be mediated by the vitamin D receptor (VDR)
Folate	Diet may influence carcinogenesis through its effects on DNA synthesis and methylation (see illustration below)

DNA synthesis and methylation

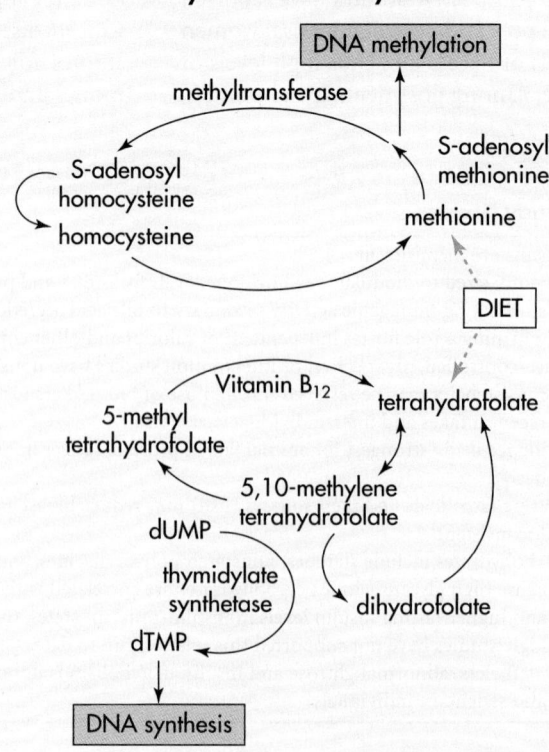

Table 11-14	Studies of Dietary Factors and Associated Cancer Risk—cont'd
Dietary Factor	**Study Results**
Folate—cont'd	Folate is essentially for the transfer of methyl groups
	Low folate (as 5-methyltetra-hydrofolate, see figure above) reduces intracellular S-adenosylmethionine (SAM), altering cytosine methylation in DNA and potentially causing inappropriate activation of proto-oncogenes[174] or inactivation of tumor-suppressor genes
	Low folate metabolites can lead to misincorporation of uracil for thymidine, which occurs during DNA synthesis,[175,176] increasing the need for DNA repair;[177] these alterations can be reversed with folic acid supplementation
	Low folate intake has been associated with several cancers, most notably colorectal,[178] breast, and cervical[179] cancers
	Folate is obtained from fruits, vegetables, and legumes and is now available in grains
	Long-term use of folate-containing supplements has been correlated with a 30% to 75% reduction in risk of colon cancer[180]
	Alcohol interferes with folate absorption and transport
	Several studies report lower risk of breast cancer with higher folate intake[179,181,182]
	Interactions of folate and folate metabolites with MTHFR (see Figure on facing page)
	Polymorphisms add additional evidence for a causal role of folate in carcinogenesis[166]
Carotenoids, including lycopene	Over 500 carotenoids are present in nature, but only 20 have been identified in human serum and only 5 are abundant (β-carotene, α-carotene, lycopene, lutein/zeaxanthin, β-cryptoxanthin;[183] they are not synthesized in animals, thus the sources are fruits and vegetables
	They act as antioxidants, pro-oxidants, nuclear transcription factors (those with provitamin activity) and can reduce tumor formation by blocking the growth factor IGF[183]
	More data is available on β-carotene and lycopene
	Prospective studies show β-carotene, and others, associated with reduced risk of lung cancer
	Studies of breast cancer are inconsistent[184]
	Intervention studies, however, have *not* isolated β-carotene as protective, and in two large chemoprevention trials found unexpected increased risk of lung cancer with larger than typical doses of β-carotene as supplements in smoker[185]
	When data reevaluated, only alcohol consumers of more than 11 g/day developed lung cancer under β-carotene supplementation[186]
	Alcohol-induced cytochrome CP-4502E1 (CYP2E1) metabolized ethanol to acetaldehyde and generates toxic and carcinogenic metabolites from retinol (i.e., β-carotene supplementation)
	β-carotene supplementation did not increase the risk of lung cancer in nonsmoking men and women
	Cigarette smoke can oxidize β-carotene in vitro, which may increase cytochrome P450 breakdown of retinoic acid, thus increasing metaplastic potential[187]
	β-carotene supplements were shown to reduce colorectal adenomas by 44% in individuals who did smoke or consume alcohol but doubled the risk among those who smoked and drank more than one drink per day[188]
	Data from the Alpha-Tocopherol Beta Carotene (ATBC) Prevention Study showed that baseline dietary intakes, as well as baseline serum β-carotene and serum retinol, were correlated with *decreased* lung cancer risk over 14 years[185]
	Lycopene from food (tomatoes, tomato products, watermelon, pink grapefruit) is related to a decreased risk of some cancers, but no long-term trials of supplementation have been done
	Lycopene is not converted to vitamin A and, therefore, may be completely available for other metabolic functions, such as antioxidation
	In some population studies, lycopene came from tomato sources, thus other protective components may be responsible or assist, including lutein and zeaxanthin[189]
Antioxidants: vitamins C and E and selenium	Oxidant metabolites (see Chapter 2) can damage DNA, protein, and lipids
	Antioxidants influence cancer risk in complicated processes
	They neutralize free radicals that can damage DNA
	Vitamin C (a major water-soluble antioxidant) is correlated with a decreased risk for cancer of the mouth, esophagus, stomach, lungs, pancreas, and cervix
	Vitamin C can interrupt the formation of nitrosamines in the stomach
	Interaction with a common bacteria, *Helicobacter pylori*, in stomach cancer is suggested as significant,[190] yet prevention trials of stomach cancer have not consistently supported vitamin C supplements; multiple antioxidant nutrients, however, were associated with regression of gastric dysplasia[191]
	Vitamin C interacts with iron to increase oxidative damage[190]
	Vitamin E (tocopherol) is known to reduce free radical damage to DNA[166]
	Fats and oils are major sources of this lipid-soluble vitamin
	Gamma-tocopherol is superior to alpha- (α-) tocopherol in altering electrophilic (free radical) oxides such as nitrogen oxides
	Recently, a very significant reduction in risk of prostate cancer was associated with higher levels of serum gamma-tocopherol[192]
	Intervention studies of vitamin E and cancers of the colon and breast have not found a significant benefit[193]

MTHFR, 5,10-Methylene tetrahydrofolate reductase; *IGF*, insulin-like growth factor.

Continued

Table 11-14	Studies of Dietary Factors and Associated Cancer Risk—cont'd
Dietary Factor	**Study Results**
Antioxidants: vitamins C and E and selenium—cont'd	Selenium is supported by epidemiologic evidence for decreasing cancer risk
	Selenoproteins, particularly selenium-dependent glutathione peroxidases, reduce production of oxidative free radicals
	Selenium content in soil can vary tremendously; therefore, investigators study biochemical markers of intake or selenium supplementation
	Selenium targets *p53*, which increases cancer cell apoptosis
	Two case-control studies of the toenail and serum biomarkers reported reduction in risk of prostate cancer[194,195]
	The SELECT trial, a continuing trial, is comparing α-tocopherol or supplemental selenium and a combination on primary prevention of prostate cancer
	A summary of dietary factors and risk of specific types of cancer is contained in Table 11-12
Fiber	Most prospective cohort studies do not support an association between dietary fiber and colon cancer risk;[166] yet a recent large European study of 10 countries found a 25% lower risk of colon cancer associated with high fiber[196]
	Intervention trials of wheat bran fiber,[197] psyllium fiber, and a high-fiber/low-fat diet failed to reduce the risk of recurrent adenomatous polyps[198,199]
	Inconsistencies may have plausible reasons because dietary fiber includes various nondigestible components with different physiologic effects; thus isolated intervention studies may not represent a true test
	Confounding by other nutrients with potential anticarcinogenic activity is problematic, for example, a high-fiber diet is correlated with other nutrients, such as folate
	Burkitt's original hypothesis that fiber may be responsible for the lower rates of colon cancer in African men, compared to men living in developed countries, also emphasized that refined grains and sugars were deleterious;[200] thus other metabolic effects such as sugar-induced insulin changes also may be operating
Fruits and vegetables	Case-control studies reveal subjects who consume diets high in certain fruits and/or vegetables have lower risk of some but not all cancers;[166] problem with case-control studies is recall bias; prospective studies of fruits and/or vegetables in stomach, breast, and colorectal cancer have weaker results[114,201,202]
	Intervention study of fruits and vegetables on recurrence of colorectal adenoma did not find a reduction in risk;[199] combining fruits and vegetables in analyses may "hide" strong protective effects of phytochemical or botanical substances; numerous substances with potential anticarcinogenic activity include folate, carotenoids, flavonoids, vitamins, isothiocyanates, dithiolthiones, glucosinolates, allium compounds, and limonene; potential protective mechanisms include modulation of DNA methylation,[174] prevention of DNA adduct formation;[203] induction of phase II carcinogen-metabolizing enzymes;[204] alteration of hormone levels;[205] and inhibition of nitrosamine formation[206]
	National Cancer Institute and the American Institute for Cancer Research recommend eating five to nine servings/day to improve health outcomes
	Improved health outcomes may be greater by maximizing fruits and vegetables by color code:
	Red-purple: red apples, grapes, berries, and wine all contain anthocyanins (antioxidants)
	Orange: carrots, mangoes, etc., contain beta-carotene
	Orange-yellow: Oranges, lemons, etc., contain citrus flavonoids, which may induce cell-cycle arrest and apoptosis, induce detoxification enzymes, and prevent oxidation
	Green: broccoli, brussels sprouts, etc., contain glucosinolates that influence detoxification enzymes
	White-green: onions, garlic, etc., contain allylic sulfides and induce glutathione transferase to increase antioxidants
	One serving of each meets the minimum recommendations
Nitrates	Strongest data in animals causing cancer of glandular stomach; dietary salts enhance metabolism to other nitrosable compounds; Chinese populations have high rates of gastric cancer and ingest large quantities of nitrates
Polyunsaturated fatty acids (PFAs)	PFAs are oxidized to yield free radicals and peroxidates that can be toxic to cells and increase tumor development
	Omega-6 fatty acids (e.g., polyunsaturated vegetable oils, etc.), promote cancer more effectively than saturated fats; however, omega-3 fatty acids (e.g., fatty fish, cod liver oil) decrease the number and size of tumors and increase the time before tumors appear
	Protective effects may be caused by enzyme and protein activity related to intracellular signaling and, ultimately, cell-to-cell proliferation or by a decrease in angiogenesis, and inflammation
	Destruction of toxic peroxides or radicals also may depend on selenium-containing enzymes
	The role of selenium appears to be inhibition of proliferation, possibly by targeting *p53* which increases apoptosis
	A safe range must be adequate (≤200 mcg/day) but not toxic (see NUTRITION & DISEASE: Essential Fatty Acids and Inflammation figure on p. 190).
Conclusions	Substantial progress has been made since the early reports from Doll and Peto[207]
	Hypotheses have been tested, clarified, refuted, and altered
	For example, a decade ago, leading hypotheses included total calories; factors in fruits and vegetables (β-carotene, fiber); fat; and vitamins A, E, and C
	The hypothesis for fat has weakened; strengthened for energy balance and obesity
	Specific phytonutrients (e.g., lycopene, folate, flavonoids, fiber) continue to be actively studied, although studies are difficult to execute (i.e., recall bias, confounding variables, extensive time requirements, expense) and identifying *the* biologic element in plant foods is daunting

Table 11-14	Studies of Dietary Factors and Associated Cancer Risk—cont'd
Dietary Factor	**Study Results**
Conclusions—cont'd	Supplemental nutrients may have different health effects than nutrients in food, and other life-style factors can interfere, such as alcohol ingestion or smoking
	In addition, varying genotypes, for example, folate metabolizing enzymes, represent complex biologic challenges
	Biologically driven hypotheses are necessary to understand diet and cancer
	For example, the importance of active vitamin D (1,25[OH]$_2$D) in tumor development lead to studies of calcium and vitamin D, and understanding DNA methylation lead to analyses of folate nutrition
	In summary, a combination of multiple exposures will be necessary to move our understanding forward, such as dietary intake, energy balance (obesity), and exercise, because they influence growth factors (e.g., IGF) in a complex and integrative fashion

SUMMARY REVIEW

Cancer Characteristics and Terminology

1. Benign tumors are usually encapsulated and well-differentiated and do not spread to distant locations.
2. Malignant tumors, compared to benign tumors, have more rapid growth rates, specific microscopic alterations (loss of differentiation), absence of normal tissue organization, and no capsule; they invade into blood vessels and lymphatics and have distant spread.
3. Carcinomas arise from lymphatic tissue, and leukemias are cancers of blood-forming cells. Carcinoma in situ (CIS) refers to preinvasive epithelial tumors of glandular or squamous cell origin.
4. Localized cancer is considered low stage, whereas cancers that have spread regionally or distantly are termed *stage 3* and *stage 4,* respectively.
5. Cancer cells are characterized by anaplasia, or loss of differentiation, and autonomy, or independence from normal cellular controls.
6. In the adult, undifferentiated cells (not totally committed to a specific function) are known as pluripotent cells, precursor cells, or stem cells. Cancer cells become more like embryonic cells and are less differentiated. Cancerous growth depends on derangements of cell differentiation.
7. Tumor markers are substances (i.e., hormones, enzymes, genes, antigens, antibodies) found on tumor plasma membranes and in blood, spinal fluid, or urine. They are used to screen and identify individuals at high risk for cancer, to help diagnose specific types of tumors, and to follow the clinical course of cancer.

The Genetic Basis of Cancer

1. Genetic events are the primary basis of carcinogenesis. Mutations in cancer-causing genes accumulate with age, causing the increasing risk of cancer with advanced age.
2. Epidemiologic and molecular data suggests it takes five or six distinct mutations in different signaling pathways to produce cancer. Mutations activate growth-promotion pathways, block antigrowth signals, prevent apoptosis, turn on telomerase and new blood vessel growth, and allow tissue invasion and distant metastasis.
3. In rare families, cancer is inherited in an autosomal dominant fashion as a result of mutations in tumor suppressor genes.
4. Proto-oncogenes encode for growth factors, growth-factor receptors, signal transducers, and nuclear growth-promoting proteins.
5. Three main genetic mechanisms have a role in human carcinogenesis: (a) mutation of proto-oncogenes resulting in hyperactivity of growth-related gene products (such genes are called *oncogenes*); (b) mutation of genes resulting in loss or inactivity of gene products that normally would inhibit growth (such genes are called *tumor suppressor genes*); and (c) mutation of genes resulting in overexpression of products that prevent normal cell death, or apoptosis, thus allowing continued growth of tumors.
6. Tumor suppressor genes encode for proteins that act as inhibitors of growth-factor stimulation. Tumor suppressor gene proteins block specific phases of the cell cycle, induce end-stage (e.g., terminal) differentiation, and stimulate cell senescence or death. Carcinogenesis, or the development of cancer, involves inactivation of tumor suppressor genes (usually by loss of heterozygosity, or by "silencing") and activation of oncogenes.
7. Caretaker genes are responsible for maintaining genomic integrity. Inherited mutations can disrupt caretaker genes and cause chromosome instability.
8. A number of viruses can cause cancer. Human cervical cancer is caused by papillomavirus infection. Kaposi sarcoma is caused by infection with a member of the herpesvirus family. Chronic hepatitis infection can cause liver cancer.
9. Chronic *H. pylori* causes stomach cancer and a rare lymphoma.

Gene-Environment Interaction

1. The frequency and consequences of genetic mutations can be altered by a number of environmental factors. The most significant factors include smoking, radiation, obesity, and a few oncogenic viruses.
2. Since the 1950s the death attributable to smoking has sharply increased. Smoking causes cancer of the lung, and is associated with cancers of the renal gland, bladder, penis, oral cavity, pharynx, larynx, nasal cavities, sinuses, esophagus, stomach, liver, kidney, uterus, and myeloid leukemia.
3. Involuntary smoking is also carcinogenic for the lungs.
4. Some mechanisms of carcinogenesis from smoking include polycyclic aromatic hydrocarbons and mutations in *p53,* nitroso compounds, arylamines form DNA adducts in bladder cells, and benzo[a]pyrene metabolites found in cervical mucus is related to DNA adducts, however, studies did not adjust for HPV, and smokers have higher levels of benzene, an inducer of leukemia.
5. Health risks from ionizing radiation involve neoplastic diseases but also birth defects and eye maladies.
6. Presently the risks of low-dose radiation are being debated.
7. Radiation-induced damage depends on dose response, LET, fractionation, protraction, repair mechanisms, bystander effects, and antioxidants.

Continued

SUMMARY REVIEW—cont'd

8. Two opposing dose-response models have been used to estimate cancer risk: (1) linear, no-threshold, relationship because any dose has the potential to cause cancer, and (2) a threshold dose below that which radiation may not cause cancer.

9. Currently, the validity of the dose-response model is questionable.

10. Progeny of irradiated cells can exhibit an increased death rate and loss of reproductive potential.

11. Low levels of radiation can induce bystander effects and genomic instability. Both findings appear to be associated with oxidative stress and cell-to-cell intercellular communication.

12. Reactive oxygen species (ROS) (oxidative stress) are involved in skin carcinogenesis from ultraviolet light (UVL).

13. UVL causes basal cell carcinoma and squamous cell carcinoma.

14. Recently an activating mutation in the B-*raf* proto-oncogene was noted in 60% to 70% of melanoma cell lines and tissues. UVB light and sunburn triggers inflammation causing cytokine release and activation of growth factors that may be related to the B-*raf* mutation.

15. Chronic alcoholism is a strong risk factor for cancer of the oral cavity, pharynx, hypopharynx, larynx, esophagus, and liver. It is less strongly related to breast cancer and colorectal cancer, however, breast carcinogenesis can be enhanced with relatively low daily amounts.

16. Multiple mechanisms are involved in alcohol-related carcinogenesis and include acetaldehyde, induction of cytochrome P-450, and ROS, increased procarcinogen activation, cell cycle effects, and nutritional deficiencies.

17. Sexually transmitted infection with high-risk types of HPV is required for the development of virtually all cervical cancers.

18. Physical activity reduces the risk of breast and colon cancers and may reduce the risk of other cancers.

19. A substantial percentage of cancers of the upper respiratory passages, lung, bladder, and peritoneum are attributed to occupational factors.

20. Air pollution is a concern in regard to cancer because of inhalation of emissions, including arsenicals, benzene, chloroform, vinyl chloride, and acrylonitrile. Indoor pollution is considered worse than outdoor pollution because of cigarette smoke and possibly radon gas.

21. Electromagnet fields (EMFs) and carcinogenesis is controversial. The evidence does not provide clear or consistent results, however, the results cannot establish the absence of any hazard.

22. Obesity is linked to cancer. High BMI is associated with higher rates of death from esophageal, stomach, colorectal, liver, breast, gallbladder, pancreatic, prostate, kidney, non-Hodgkin, ovarian, lymphoma, multiple myeloma, cervical, and leukemia.

23. Adipose tissue is active endocrine and metabolic tissue. Increased release of free fatty acids, resistin, TNF-α, and reduced release of adiponectin give rise to insulin resistance. Adipose tissue cells produce steroid-hormone-metabolizing enzymes and are an important source of estrogens in postmenopausal women. Insulin-like growth factor-1 (IGF-1) regulates cell proliferation and inhibits apoptosis and the synthesis and biologic availability of female and male sex hormones.

24. Numerous dietary factors are discussed in association with cancer risk. Table 11-14 summarizes major findings.

KEY TERMS

Adenocarcinomas, 334
Anaplasia, 337
Anchorage-independent, 337
Angiogenic factors, 341
Apoptosis, 341
Asbestos, 359
Autocrine stimulation, 341
Autonomy, 337
Benign tumors, 334
Bystander effects, 354
Cadherin, 356
Cancer, 333
Carcinogens, 351
Carcinomas, 334
Carcinoma in situ (CIS), 336
Caretaker genes, 346
Chromosome instability, 346
Chromosome translocations, 343
Clonal expansion, 339
Clonal proliferation, 339
C-peptide, 363

Epigenetic, 346
Gene amplification, 344
Hormesis, 353
Human T cell leukemia-lymphoma virus (HTLV), 350
Immortal, 337
Insulin-like growth factor–1 (IGF-1), 363
Involuntary smoking, 353
Leukemias, 336
Linear, no-threshold, relationship, 353
Loss of heterozygosity (LOH), 345
Lymphomas, 336
Malignant tumors, 334
Methylation, 346
Multipotent, 338
Mutagens, 347
MYC protein, 344
Neoplasm, 333
Oncogenes, 343
Phase I activation enzymes, 360
Phase II detoxification enzymes, 360

Pleomorphic, 337
Point mutations, 343
Post-transplant lymphoproliferative disorder, (PTLD), 349
Proteomic, 339
Proto-oncogene, 343
Radon, 359
ras, 341
Retinoblastoma *(Rb)* gene, 344
Sarcoma, 336
Silencing, 346
Stem cells, 338
Telomerase, 342
Telomeres, 342
Transformation, 337
Tumor, 333
Tumor markers, 338
Tumor-suppressor genes, 343
Xenobiotics, 360

MEDIA RESOURCES evolve

Review questions and answers for this chapter are available in the *CD Companion* included with this book. Also see the CD for an animation on the *six hallmarks of cancer.*

WebLinks—links to Internet sites pertaining to this chapter—are available on Evolve at http://evolve.elsevier.com/McCance/.

REFERENCES

1. Kern SE: Progressive genetic abnormalities in human neoplasia. In Mendelsohn J et al, editors, *The molecular basis of cancer,* Philadelphia, 2001, Saunders.

2. Skloot R: Henrietta's Dance, *Johns Hopkins Magazine,* April 2000. Available at http://www.jhu.edu/~jhumag/0400web/01.html.

3. Reya T, Morrison SJ, Clarke MF, Weissman IL: Stem cells, cancer, and cancer stem cells, *Nature* 414(6859):105-111, 2001.

4. Al-Hajj M et al: Prospective identification of tumorigenic breast cancer cells, *Proc Natl Acad Sci U S A* 100(7):3983-3988, 2003.

5. Petricoin EF et al: Use of proteomic patterns in serum to identify ovarian cancer, *Lancet* 359(9306):572-577, 2002.

6. Kinzler KW, Vogelstein B: Lessons from hereditary colorectal cancer, *Cell* 87(2):159-170, 1996.

7. Hanahan D, Weinberg RA: The hallmarks of cancer, *Cell* 100(1):57-70, 2000.

8. Folkman J: Role of angiogenesis in tumor growth and metastasis, *Semin Oncol* 29(suppl 16):15-18, 2002.

9. Fernando NH, Hurwitz HI: Inhibition of vascular endothelial growth factor in the treatment of colorectal cancer, *Semin Oncol* 30(3 suppl 6):39-50, 2003.

10. Mathon NF, Lloyd AC: Cell senescence and cancer, *Nat Rev Cancer* 1(3):203-213, 2001.

11. Shay JW, Wright WE: Telomerase: a target for cancer therapeutics, *Cancer Cell* 2(4):257-265, 2002.

12. van't Veer LJ et al: Gene expression profiling predicts clinical outcome of breast cancer, *Nature* 415(6871):530-536, 2002.

13. Kang Y et al: A multigenic program mediating breast cancer metastasis to bone, *Cancer Cell* 3(6):537-549, 2003.

14. Bos JL: *ras* oncogenes in human cancer: a review, *Cancer Res* 49(17):4682-4689, 1989.

15. Goldsby RE, Carroll WL: The molecular biology of pediatric lymphomas, *J Pediatr Hematol Oncol* 20(4):282-296, 1998.

16. Nowell P, Hungerford D: A minute chromosome in human granulocytic leukemia, *Science* 132:1497, 1960.

17. Druker BJ et al: Efficacy and safety of a specific inhibitor of the BCR-ABL tyrosine kinase in chronic myeloid leukemia, *N Engl J Med* 344(14):1031-1037, 2001.

18. Brodeur GM et al: Amplification of *N-myc* in untreated human neuroblastomas correlates with advanced disease stage, *Science* 224(4653):1121-4, 1984.

19. Berns EM et al: Prevalence of amplification of the oncogenes *c-myc*, HER2/neu, and int-2 in one thousand human breast tumours: correlation with steroid receptors, *Eur J Cancer* 28(2-3):697-700, 1992.

20. Cavenee WK et al: Expression of recessive alleles by chromosomal mechanisms in retinoblastoma, *Nature* 305(5937):779-784, 1983.

21. Esteller M et al: A gene hypermethylation profile of human cancer, *Cancer Res* 61(8):3225-3229, 2001.

22. Karpf AR, Jones DA: Reactivating the expression of methylation silenced genes in human cancer, *Oncogene* 21(35):5496-5503, 2002.

23. Rouse J, Jackson SP: Interfaces between the detection, signaling, and repair of DNA damage, *Science* 297(5581):547-551, 2002.

24. Liu B et al: Analysis of mismatch repair genes in hereditary nonpolyposis colorectal cancer patients, *Nat Med* 2(2):169-174, 1996.

25. Lengauer C, Kinzler KW, Vogelstein B: Genetic instability in colorectal cancers, *Nature* 386(6625):623-627, 1997.

26. Rajagopalan H et al: Inactivation of hCDC4 can cause chromosomal instability, *Nature* 428(6978):77-81, 2004.

27. Coussens LM, Werb Z: Inflammation and cancer, *Nature* 420(6917):860-867, 2002.

28. Fitzpatrick FA: Inflammation, carcinogenesis and cancer, *Int Immunopharmacol* 1(9-10):1651-1667, 2001.

29. Vesterinen E et al: Cancer incidence among 78,000 asthmatic patients, *Int J Epidemiol* 22(6):976-982, 1993.

30. Jorde LB et al: *Medical genetics*, ed 3, St. Louis, 2003, Mosby.

31. Schneider K: *Counseling about cancer: strategies for genetic counseling*, ed 2, Hobooken, NJ, 2001, Wiley.

32. Howley PM, Ganem D, Kieff E: Etiology of cancer: DNA viruses. In Vincent J et al, editors: *Cancer: principles and practice*, Philadelphia, 2001, Lippincott, Williams & Wilkins.

33. Poeschla EM et al: Etiology of cancer: RNA viruses. In Vincent J et al, editors: *Cancer: principles and practice of oncology*, Philadelphia, 2001, Lippincott, Williams & Wilkins.

34. Helicobacter and Cancer Collaborative Group: Gastric cancer and *Helicobacter pylori*: a combined analysis of 12 case control studies nested within prospective cohorts, *Gut* 49(3):347-353, review, 2001.

35. Wong BC et al: *Helicobacter pylori* eradication to prevent gastric cancer in a high-risk region of China: a randomized controlled trial, *JAMA* 291(2):187-194, 2004.

36. Parsonnet J, Forman D: *Helicobacter pylori* infection and gastric cancer—for want of more outcomes, *JAMA* 291(2):244-245, 2004.

37. Isaacson PG, Du MQ: MALT lymphoma: from morphology to molecules, *Nat Rev Cancer* 4(8):644-653, 2004.

38. Peto J: Cancer epidemiology in the last century and the next decade, *Nature* 411(6835):390-395, 2001.

39. zur Hausen H: Papillomaviruses and cancer: from basic studies to clinical application, *Nat Rev Cancer* 2(5):342-350, 2002.

40. Cavenee WK, White RL: The genetic basis of cancer, *Sci Am* 272(3):72-79, 1995.

41. Peto R, Lopez AD: Further worldwide health effects of current smoking patterns. In Koop CE, Pearson CE, Schwarz MR, editors: *Critical issues in global health*, San Francisco, 2001, Jossey-Bass.

42. Vineis P et al: Tobacco and cancer: recent epidemiological evidence, *J Natl Cancer Inst* 96(2):99-106, 2004.

43. Vital and Health Statistics: *Health behaviors of adults: United States, 1999-2001*, Series 10(219): 2004.

44. Henley SJ et al: Association between exclusive pipe smoking and mortality from cancer and other diseases, *J Natl Cancer Inst* 96(11):853-861, 2004.

45. Hecht SS: Human urinary carcinogen metabolites: biomarkers for investigating tobacco and cancer, *Carcinogenesis* 23(6):907-922, 2002.

46. Boice JD Jr et al: Genetic effects of radiotherapy for childhood cancer, *Health Phys* 85:6580, 2003.

47. Byrne J et al: Genetic disease in offspring of long-term survivors of childhood and adolescent cancer, *Am J Hum Genet* 62(1):45-52, 1998.

48. Winther JF et al: Chromosomal abnormalities among offspring of childhood-cancer survivors in Denmark: a population-based study, *Am J Hum Genet* 74(6):1282-1285, 2004.

49. Prasad KN, Cole WC, Hasse GM: Health risks of low dose ionizing radiation in humans: a review, *Exp Biol Med* 229(5):378-382, 2004.

50. Committee on the Biological Effects of Ionizing Radiation: Biological effects of ionizing radiation BEIR V, Washington, DC, 1990, National Academy Press.

51. Upton AC; National Council on Radiation Protection and Measurements Scientific Committee 1-6: The state of the art in the 1990s: NCRP report No 136 on the scientific basis for linearity in the dose-response relationship for ionizing radiation, *Health Phys* 85(1):15-22, 2003.

52. Sowby FD: The 1978 Stockholm meeting of the International Commission on Radiological Protection, *Phys Med Biol* 23(6):1209-1212, 1978

53. Bond VP, Benary V, Sondhaus CA: A different perception of the linear, nonthreshold hypothesis for low-dose irradiation, *Proc Natl Acad Sci U S A* 88(19):8666-8670, 1991.

54. Cohen BL: Cancer risk from low-level radiation, *AJR Am J Roentgenol* 179(5):1137-1143, review, 2002.

55. Health Physics Society: *43rd annual meeting of the Health Physics Society*, pp 12-16, Minneapolis, MN, 1998, Author.

56. Zhou H et al: Induction of a bystander mutagenic effect of alpha particles in mammalian cells, *Proc Natl Acad Sci U S A* 97(5):2099-2104, 2000.

57. Zhou H et al: Interaction between radiation-induced adaptive response and bystander mutagenesis in mammalian cells, *Radiat Res* 160(5):512-516, 2003

58. Lorimore SA, Coates PJ, Wright EG: Radiation-induced genomic instability and bystander effects: inter-related nontargeted effects of exposure to ionizing radiation, *Oncogene* 22(45):7058-7069, 2003.

59. Blettner M et al: Mortality from cancer and other causes among male airline cockpit crew in Europe, *Int J Cancer* 106(6):946-952, 2003.

60. Kendall GM et al: Mortality and occupational exposure to radiation: first analysis of the National Registry for Radiation Workers, *BMJ* 304(6821):220-225, 1992.

61. Langner I et al: Cosmic radiation and cancer mortality among airline pilots: results from a European cohort study (ESCAPE), *Radiat Environ Biophys* 42(4):247-256, 2004.

62. Futaki M, Liu JM: Chromosomal breakage syndromes and the BRCA1 genome surveillance complex, *Trends Mol Med* 7(12):560-565, 2001.

63. Nagar S, Smith LE, Morgan WF: Mechanisms of cell death associated with death-inducing factors from genomically unstable cell lines, *Mutagenesis* 18(6):549-560, 2003.

64. Park CC et al: Ionizing radiation induces heritable disruption of epithelial cell interactions, *Proc Natl Acad Sci U S A* 100(19):10728-10733, 2003.

65. Watson GE et al: In vivo chromosomal instability and transmissible aberrations in the progeny of haemopoietic stem cells induced by high- and low-LET radiations, *Int J Radiat Biol* 77(4):409-417, 2001.

66. Ponnaiya B, Cornforth MN, Ullrich RL: Radiation-induced chromosomal instability in BALB/c and C57BL/6 mice: the difference is as clear as black and white, *Radiat Res* 147(2):121-125, 1997.

67. Little JB: Genomic instability and bystander effects: a historical perspective, *Oncogene* 22(45):6978-6987, 2003.

68. Shao C et al: Targeted cytoplasmic irradiation induces bystander responses, *Proc Natl Acad Sci U S A* 101(37):13495-13500, 2004.

69. Lorimore SA et al: Inflammatory-type responses after exposure to ionizing radiation in vivo: a mechanism for radiation-induced bystander effects? *Oncogene* 20(48):7085-7095, 2001.

70. Ohba K et al: Primary biliary cirrhosis among atomic bomb survivors in Nagasaki, Japan, *J Clin Epidemiol* 54(8):845-850, 2001.

71. Azzam EI, de Toldeo SM, Little JB: Oxidative metabolism, gap junctions, and the ionizing radiation-induced bystander effect, *Oncogene* 22(45):7050-7057, 2003.

72. Spitz DR et al: Metabolic oxidation/reduction reactions and cellular responses to ionizing radiation: a unifying concept in stress response biology, *Cancer Metastasis Rev* 23(3-4):311-322, 2004.

73. Cleaver JE, Crowley E: UV damage, DNA repair, and skin carcinogenesis, *Front Biosci* 7:d1024-1043, 2002.

74. Streilein JW et al: Immune surveillance and sunlight-induced skin cancer, *Immunol Today* 15(4):174-179, 1994.

75. Sander CD et al: Role of oxidative stress and the antioxidant network in cutaneous carcinogenesis, *Intl J Dermatol* 43(5):326-335, 2004.

76. Chang H et al: The role of H_2O_2 as a mediator of UVB-induced apoptosis in keratinocytes, *Free Radic Res* 37(6):655-663, 2003.

77. Peus D et al: UBV activates ERK 1/2 and p38 signaling pathways via reactive oxygen species in cultured keratinocytes, *J Invest Dermatol* 112(5):751-756, 1999.

78. Peus D et al: UVB-induced epidermal growth factor receptor phosphorylation is critical for downstream signaling and keratinocyte survival, *Photochem Photobiol* 72(1):135-140, 2000.

79. Wei S et al: Incidence of *p53* and *ras* gene mutations in DMBA-induced rat leukemias, *J Exp Clin Cancer Res* 21(3):389-396, 2002.

80. Davies H et al: Mutations of the BRAF gene in human cancer, *Nature* 417(6892):949-954, 2002.

81. Perlis C, Herlyn M: Recent advances in melanoma biology, *Oncologist* 9(2):182-187, 2004.

82. Polsky D et al: Molecular biology of melanoma. In Mendelsohn J et al, editors: *The molecular basis of cancer*, ed 2, Philadelphia, 2001, Saunders.

83. Rees JL: The melanocortin 1 receptor (MC1R): more than just red hair, *Pigment Cell Res* 13(3):135-140, 2000.

84. Berking C et al: Basic fibroblast growth factor and ultraviolet B transform melanocytes in human skin, *Am J Pathol* 158(3):943-953, 1998.

85. Berking C et al: Basic fibroblast growth factor and ultraviolet B transform melanocytes in human skin, *Am J Pathol* 158:943-54, 2002.

86. Tang A et al: E-cadherin is the major mediator of human melanocyte adhesion to keratinocytes in vitro, *J Cell Sci* 107(pt 4):983-992, 1994

87. Li G, Satayamoorthy K, Herlyn M: N-cadherin-mediated intercellular interactions promote survival and migration of melanoma cells, *Cancer Res* 61(9):3819-3825, 2001.

88. Poschl G, Seitz HK: Alcohol and cancer, *Alcohol Alcohol* 39(3):155-165, 2004.

89. Izevbigie EB et al: Ethanol modulates the growth of human breast cancer cells in vitro, *Exp Biol Med* 227(4):260-265, 2002.

90. Bagnardi V et al: A meta-analysis of alcohol drinking and cancer risk, *Br J Cancer* 85(11):1700-1705, 2001.

91. Sturgis EM, Wei Q: Genetic susceptibility—molecular epidemiology of head and neck cancer, *Curr Opin Oncol* 14(3):310-317, 2002.

92. Crabb DW et al: Overview of the role of alcohol dehydrogenese and aldehyde dehydrogenase and their variants in the genesis of alcohol-related pathology, *Proc Nutr Soc* 63(1):49-63, 2004.

93. Brienza RS, Stein MD: Alcohol use disorders in primary care: do gender-specific differences exist? *J Gen Intern Med* 17(5):387-397, 2002.

94. Anhang R, Goodman A, Goldie SJ: HPV communication: review of existing research and recommendation for patient education, *CA Cancer J Clin* 54(5):248-259, 2004.

95. Bosch FX, de Sanjose S: Chapter 1: Human papillomavirus and cervical cancer—burden and assessment of causality, *J Natl Cancer Inst Monogr* 31:3-13, 2003.

96. Palefsky JM, Holly EA: Chapter 6: Immunosuppression and co-infection with HIV, *J Natl Cancer Inst Monogr* 31:41-46, 2003.

97. Baer H, Allen S, Braun L: Knowledge of human papillomavirus infection among young adult men and women: implications for health education and research, *J Community Health* 25(1):67-78, 2000.

98. Dell DL et al: Knowledge about human papillomavirus among adolescents, *Obstet Gynecol* 96(5 pt 1):653-656, 2000.

99. Gerhardt CA et al: Adolescent's knowledge of human papillomavirus and cervical dysplasia, *J Pediatr Adolesc Gynecol* 13(1):15-20, 2000.

100. Hagensee ME et al: Human papillomavirus infection and disease in HIV-infected individuals, *Am J Med Sci* 328(1):57-63, 2004.

101. Stuver S, Adami H-O: Cervical cancer. In Adami H, Hunter D, Trichopoulos D, editors: *Textbook of cancer epidemiology*, Oxford, 2002, Oxford University Press.

102. Syrjanen S, Puranen M: Human papillomavirus infections in children: the potential role of maternal transmission, *Crit Rev Oral Biol Med* 11(2):259-274, 2000.

103. Eyre H et al: Preventing cancer, cardiovascular disease, and diabetes: a common agenda for the American Cancer Society, the American Diabetes Association, and the American Heart Association, *Stroke* 35(8):1999-2010, 2004.

104. Slattery ML: Physical activity and colorectal cancer, *Sports Med* 34(4):239-252, 2004.

105. McTiernan A et al: Physical activity and cancer etiology: associations and mechanisms, *Cancer Causes Control* 9(5):487-509, 1998. Review.

106. McTiernan A et al: Effect of exercise on serum estrogens in postmenopausal women: a 12-month randomized clinical trial, *Cancer Res* 64(8):2923-2928, 2004.

107. Calle EE et al: Diabetes mellitus and pancreatic cancer mortality in a prospective cohort of United States Adults, *Cancer Causes Control* 9(4):403-410, 1998.

108. Lee IM: Physical activity and cancer prevention...data from epidemiologic studies, *Med Sci Sports Exerc* 35(11):1823-1827, 2003.

109. Neuberger JS, Field RW: Occupation and lung cancer in nonsmokers, *Rev Environ Health* 18(4):251-267, 2003. Review.

110. Vineis P et al: Outdoor air pollution and lung cancer: recent epidemiologic evidence, *Int J Cancer* 111(5):647-652, 2004.

111. Blair A, Kazerouni N: Reactive chemicals and cancer, *Cancer Causes Control* 8(3):473-490, 1997.

112. Boffetta P et al: Mortality among workers employed in the titanium dioxide production industry in Europe, *Cancer Causes Control* 15(7):697-706, 2004.

113. Boffetta P: Involuntary smoking and lung cancer, *Scand J Work Environ Health* 28(Suppl 2):30-40, 2002.

114. International Agency for Research on Cancer (IARC): *Cancer epidemiology*, Lyon, France, 2004, IARC Press.

115. Borm PJ, Schins RP, Albrecht C: Inhaled particles and lung cancer, part B: paradigms and risk assessment, *Int J Cancer* 110(1):3-14, 2004.

116. Habash RW et al: Health risks of electromagnetic fields. Part I: evaluation and assessment of electric and magnetic fields, *Crit Rev Biomed Eng* 31(3):141-195, 2003.

117. National Institute of Environmental Health Sciences (NIEHS) Working Group Report: *Assessment of health effects from exposure to powerline frequency electric and magnetic fields.* Washington, DC, 1998, US Government Printing Office.

118. Kliukiene J, Tynes T, Andersen A: Residential and occupational exposure to 50-Hz magnetic fields and breast cancer in women: a population-based study, *Am J Epidemiol* 159(9):852-861, 2004.

119. Christensen HC et al: Cellular telephone use and risk of acoustic neuroma, *Am J Epidemiol* 159(3):277-283, 2004.

120. Independent Expert Group on Mobile Phones: Mobile phones and health (the Stewart report). Didcot, Oxon, United Kingdom, 2000, National Radiological Protection Board. (Available at www.iegmp.org.uk/report/text.htm)

121. Repacholi MH: Radiofrequency field exposure and cancer: what do the laboratory studies suggest? *Environ Health Perspect* 105(Suppl 6):1565-1568, 1997.

122. Mashevich M et al: Exposure of human peripheral blood lymphocytes to electromagnetic fields associated with cellular phones leads to chromosomal instability, *Bioelectromagnetics* 24(2):82-90, 2003.

123. Sommer AM et al: No effects of GSM-modulated 900 MHz electromagnetic fields on survival rate and spontaneous development of lymphoma in female AKR/J mice, *BMC Cancer* 4(1):77, 2004.

124. Utteridge TD et al: Long-term exposure of E(-Pim1 transgenic mice to 898.4 MHz microwaves does not increase lymphoma incidence, *Radiat Res* 158(3):357-364, 2003.

125. Elwood JM: Epidemiological studies of radio frequency exposures and human cancer, *Bioelectromagnetics* 6:S63-73, 2003.
126. Working Group on Diet and Cancer of the Committee on Medical Aspects of Food and Nutrition Policy: *Nutritional aspects of the development of cancer,* London, 1998, Department of Health Rep Health Social Subjects 48, The Stationery Office.
127. Jones DP, Delong MJ: Detoxification and protective functions of nutrients. In Stipanuk M, editor: *Biochemical and physiological aspects of nutrition,* Philadelphia, 2000, Saunders.
128. International Agency for Research on Cancer (IARC): Some naturally occurring substances: food items and constituents, heterocyclic aromatic amines, and mycotoxins. In *IARC monographs on the evaluation of carcinogenic risks to humans,* 56, Lyon, 1993, Author.
129. Mucci L, Adami H: Oral and pharyngeal cancer. In Adami H, Hunter R, Trichopoulos D, editors: *Textbook of cancer epidemiology,* New York, 2002, Oxford University Press.
130. World Cancer Research Fund in association with the American Institute for Cancer Research: *Food, nutrition, and the prevention of cancer: a global perspective,* pp 96-106, Washington, DC, 1997, American Institute for Cancer Research.
131. Doll R, Peto R: Epidemiology of cancer. In Warrell DA et al, editors: *Oxford textbook of medicine,* ed 4, 2003, Oxford Medical Publications.
132. Parkin DM et al: Cancer burden in the year 2000: the global picture, *Eur J Cancer* 37(suppl 8):S4-66, 2001. Review.
133. World Health Organization (WHO): Global strategy on diet, physical activity, and health [online], 2004. Available at http://www.who.int/dietphysicalactivity/strategy/eb11344/en/
134. Calle EE et al: Overweight, obesity, and mortality from cancer in a prospectively studied cohort of U.S. adults, *N Engl J Med* 348(17):1625-1638, 2003.
135. Calle EE, Kaaks R: Overweight, obesity and cancer: epidemiological evidence and proposed mechanisms, *Nat Rev Cancer* 4(8):579-591, 2004.
136. Giovannucci E: Insulin and colon cancer, *Cancer Causes Control* 6(2):164-179, 1995.
137. Kaaks R, Lukanova A, Kurzer MS: Obesity, endogenous hormones, and endometrial cancer risk: a synthetic review, *Cancer Epidemiol Biomarks Prev* 11(12):1531-1542, 2002.
138. Weiderpass E et al: Occurrence, trends, and environment etiology of pancreatic cancer, *Scand J Work Environ Health* 24(3):165-174, 1998.
139. Khandwala HM et al: The effects of insulin-like growth factors on tumorigenesis and neoplastic growth, *Endocr Rev* 21(3):215-244, 2000.
140. Lawlor MA, Alessi DR: PKB/Akt: a key mediator of cell proliferation, survival, and insulin responses? *J Cell Sci* 114(pt 16):2903-2910, 2001.
141. Le Roith D: Regulation of proliferation and apoptosis by the insulin-like growth factor I receptor, *Growth Horm IGF Res* 10(Suppl A):S12-13, 2000.
142. Prisco M et al: Insulin and IGF-I receptors signaling in protection from apoptosis, *Horm Metab Res* 31(2-3):80-89, 1999.
143. Everhart J, Wright D: Diabetes mellitus as a risk factor for pancreatic cancer. A meta-analysis, *JAMA* 273(20):1605-1609, 1995.
144. Lindblad P et al: The role of diabetes mellitus in the aetiology of renal cell cancer, *Diabetologia* 42(1):107-112, 1999.
145. Schoen RE, et al: Increased blood glucose and insulin, body size, and incident colorectal cancer, *J Natl Cancer Inst* 9(13)1:1147-1154, 1999.
146. Lukanova A et al: Prediagnostic levels of C-peptide, IGF-I, IGFBP-1, -2, and -3, and risk of endometrial cancer, *Int J Cancer* 108(2):262-268, 2004.
147. Kaaks R, Lukanova A: Energy balance and cancer: the role of insulin and insulin-like growth factorI. *Proc Nutr Soc* 60(1):91-106, 2001.
148. Kaaks R et al: Prospective study of IGF-1, IGF-binding proteins, and breast cancer risk in northern and southern Sweden, *Cancer Causes Control* 13(4):307-316, 2002.
149. Keinan-Boker L et al: Circulating levels of insulin -like growth factor 1, its binding proteins-1, -2, -3, C-peptide, and risk of postmenopausal breast cancer, *Int J Cancer* 106(1):90-95, 2003.
150. Muti P et a: Fasting glucose is a risk factor for breast cancer: a prospective study, *Cancer Epidemiol Biomarkers Prev* 11(11):1361-1368, 2002.
151. Toniolo P et al: Serum insulin-like growth factor-I and breast cancer, *Int J Cancer* 88(5):828-832, 2000.
152. Chan JM et al: Plasma insulin-like growth factor-I and prostate cancer risk: a prospective study, *Science* 279(5350):563-566, 1998.
153. Kaaks R et al: Serum C-peptide, insulin-like growth factor IGF-1, IGF binding proteins, and colorectal cancer risk in women, *J Natl Cancer Inst* 92(19):1592-1600, 2000.
154. Palmqvist R et al: Plasma insulin-like growth factor 1, insulin-like growth factor binding protein 3, and risk of colorectal cancer: a prospective study in northern Sweden, *Gut* 50(5):642-646, 2002.
155. Stattin P et al: Plasma insulin-like growth factor-I, insulin-like growth factor-binding proteins, and prostate cancer risk: a prospective study, *J Natl Cancer Inst* 92(2):1910-1917, 2000.
156. Dunaif A: Insulin resistance and the polycystic ovary syndrome: mechanism and implications for pathogenesis, *Endocr Rev* 18(6):774-800, 1997.
157. Collaborative Group on Hormonal Factors in Breast Cancer: Breast cancer and hormone replacement therapy: collaborative reanalysis of data from 51 epidemiological studies of 52,705 women with breast cancer and 108,411 women without breast cancer, Lancet 350(9084):1047-1059, 1997.
158. Feigelson HS et al: Weight gain, body mass index, hormone replacement therapy, and postmenopausal breast cancer in a large prospective study, *Cancer Epidemiol Biomarkers Prev* 13(2):220-224, 2004.
159. Schairer C et al: Menopausal estrogen and estrogen-progestin replacement therapy and breast cancer risk, *JAMA* 283(4):485-491, 2000.
160. Coates RJ: Race, nutritional status, and survival from breast cancer, *J Natl Cancer Inst* 82(21):1684-1692, 1990.
161. Hainaut P, Pfeifer GP: Patterns of p53 G to T transversions in lung cancers reflect the primary mutagenic signature of DNA-damage by tobacco smoke, *Carcinogenesis* 22(3):367-374, 2001.
162. Airoldi L et al: Determinants of 4-aminobiphenyl-DNA adducts in bladder cancer biopsies, *Carcinogenesis* 23(5):861-866, 2002.
163. Talaska G et al: Detection of carcinogen-DNA adducts in exfoliated urothelial cells of cigarette smokers: association with smoking, hemoglobin adducts, and urinary mutagenicity, *Cancer Epidemiol Biomarkers Prev* 1(1):61-66, 1991.
164. Melikian AA et al: Identification of benzo[a]pyrene metabolites in cervical mucus and DNA adducts in cervical tissues in humans by gas chromatography-mass spectrometry, *Cancer Lett* 146(2(:127-134, 1999.
165. Lebailly P et al: Genetic polymorphisms in microsomal epoxide hydrolase and susceptibility to adult myeloid leukaemia with defined cytogenetic abnormalities, *Br J Haematol* 116(3):587-594, 2002.
166. McCullough ML, Giovannucci EL: Diet and cancer prevention, *Oncogene* 23(38):6349-6364, 2004.
167. Sandhu MS, White IR, McPherson K: Systematic review of the prospective cohort studies on meat consumption and colorectal cancer risk: a meta-analytical approach, *Cancer Epidemiol Biomarkers Prev* 10(5):439-446, 2001.
168. Cho E et al: Premenopausal dietary carbohydrate, glycemic index, glycemic load, and fiber in relation to risk of breast cancer, *Cancer Epidemiol Biomarkers Prev* 12(11 Pt 1):1153-1158, 2003.
169. Cramer DW et al: A case-control study of galactose consumption and metabolism in relation to ovarian cancer, *Cancer Epidemiol Biomarkers Prev* 9(1):95-101, 2000.
170. Baron JA et al: Calcium supplements for the prevention of colorectal adenomas. Calcium Polyp Prevention Study Group, *N Engl J Med* 340(2):101-107, 1999.
171. Rodriguez C et al: Calcium, dairy products, and risk of prostate cancer in a prospective cohort of United States men, *Cancer Epidemiol Biomarkers Prev* 12(7):597-603, 2003.
172. McMichael AJ, Potter JD: Dietary influences upon colon carcinogenesis, *Princess Takamatsu Symp* 16:275-290, 1985.
173. Lamprecht SA, Lipkin M: Cellular mechanisms of calcium and vitamin D in the inhibition of colorectal carcinogenesis, *Ann N Y Acad Sci* 952:73-87, 2001.
174. Duthie SJ: Folic acid deficiency and cancer: mechanisms of DNA instability, *Br Med Bull* 55(3):578-592, 1999.
175. Blount BC et al: Folate deficiency causes uracil misincorporation into human DNA and chromosome breakage: implications for cancer and neuronal damage, *Proc Natl Acad Sci U S A* 94(7):3290-3295, 1997.
176. Wickramasinghe SN, Fida S: Bone marrow cells form vitamin B_{12}- and folate-deficient patients misincorporate uracil into DNA, *Blood* 83(6):1656-1661, 1994.
177. Duthie SJ et al: Folate deficiency in vitro induces uracil misincorporation and DNA hypomethylation and inhibits DNA excision repair in immortalized normal human colon epithelial cells, *Nutr Cancer* 37(2):245-251, 2000.
178. Giovannucci E: Epidemiologic studies of folate and colorectal neoplasia: a review, *J Nutr* 132(Suppl):2350S-2355S, 2002.

179. Eichholzer M et al: Folate and the risk of colorectal, breast, and cervix cancer: the epidemiological evidence, *Swiss Med Wkly* 131(37-38): 539-549, 2001.

180. Jacobs EJ et al: Multivitamin use and colon cancer mortality in the Cancer Prevention Study II cohort (United States), *Cancer Causes Control* 12(10):927-34, 2001.

181. Feigelson HS et al: Alcohol, folate, methionine, and risk of incident breast cancer in the American Cancer Society Cancer Prevention Study II Nutrition Cohort, *Cancer Epidemiol Biomarkers Prev* 12(2):161-164, 2003.

182. Zhang SM et al: Plasma folate, vitamin B_6, vitamin B_{12}, homocysteine, and risk of breast cancer, *J Natl Cancer Inst* 95(5):373-380, 2003.

183. Arab L, Steck-Scott S, Bowen P: Participation of lycopene and beta-carotene in carcinogenesis: defenders, aggressors, or passive bystanders? *Epidemiol Rev* 23(2):211-230, 2001.

184. Toniolo P et al: Serum carotenoids and breast cancer, *Am J Epidemiol* 153(12):1142-1147, 2001.

185. Blumberg J, Block G: The Alpha-Tocopherol Beta-Carotene Cancer Prevention Study in Finland, *Nutr Rev* 52(7):242-245, 1994.

186. Albanes D et al: Alpha-tocopherol and beta-carotene supplements and lung cancer incidence in the alpha-tocopherol, beta-carotene cancer prevention study: effects of base-line characteristics and study compliance, *J Natl Cancer Inst* 88(21):1560-1570, 1996.

187. Liu C, Russel RM, Wang XD: Alpha-tocopherol and ascorbic acid decrease the production of beta-apo-carotenals and increase the formation of retinoids from beta-carotene in the lung tissues of cigarette smoke-exposed ferrets in vitro, *J Nutr* 134(2):426-430, 2004.

188. Baron JA et al: Neoplastic and antineoplastic effects of beta-carotene on colorectal adenoma recurrence: results of a randomized trial, *J Natl Cancer Inst* 95(10):717-722, 2003.

189. Mares-Perlman JA et al: The body of evidence to support a protective role for lutein and zeaxanthin in delaying chronic disease. Overview, *J Nutr* 132(3):518S-524S, 2002.

190. Jacob RA: The role of micronutrients in DNA synthesis and maintenance, *Adv Exp Med Biol* 472:101-113, 1999.

191. Correa P et al: Chemoprevention of gastric dysplasia: randomized trial of antioxidant supplements and anti-*Helicobacter pylori* therapy, *J Natl Cancer Inst* 92(23):1881-1888, 2000.

192. Helzlsouer KJ et al: Association between alpha-tocopherol, gamma-tocopherol, selenium, and subsequent prostate cancer, *J Natl Cancer Inst* 92(24):2018-2023, 2000.

193. Pryor WA: Vitamin E and heart disease: basic science to clinical intervention, *Free Radic Biol Med* 28(1):141-164, 2000.

194. Nomura AM et al: Serum selenium and subsequent risk of prostate cancer, *Cancer Epidemiol Biomarkers Prev* 9(9):883-887, 2000.

195. Yoshizawa K et al: Study of prediagnostic selenium level in toenails and the risk of advanced prostate cancer, *J Natl Cancer Inst* 90(16):1219-1224, 1998.

196. Bingham SA et al: Dietary fibre in food and protection against colorectal cancer in the European Prospective Investigation into Cancer and Nutrition (EPIC): an observational study, *Lancet* 361(9368):1496-1501, 2003.

197. Alberts DS et al: Lack of effect of a high-fiber cereal supplement on the recurrence of colorectal adenomas. Phoenix Colon Cancer Prevention Physicians' Network, *N Engl J Med* 342(16):1156-1162, 2000.

198. Bonithon-Kopp C et al: Calcium and fibre supplementation in prevention of colorectal adenoma recurrence: a randomised intervention trial. European Cancer Prevention Organisation Study Group, *Lancet* 356(9238):1300-1306, 2000.

199. Schatzkin A: Going against the grain? Current status of the dietary fiber-colorectal cancer hypothesis, *Biofactors* 12(1-4):305-311, 2000.

200. Burkitt DP: Epidemiology of cancer of the colon and rectum, *Cancer* 28(1):3-13, 1971.

201. Smith-Warner SA et al: Intake of fruits and vegetables and risk of breast cancer: a pooled analysis of cohort studies, *JAMA* 285(6): 769-776, 2001.

202. Terry P et al: 2001. Prospective study of major dietary patterns and colorectal cancer risk in women, *Am J Epidemiol* 154(12):1143-1149, 2001.

203. Ames BN, Gold LS, Willett WC: The causes and prevention of cancer, *Proc Natl Acad Sci U S A* 92(12):5258-5265, 1995.

204. Lampe JW et al: Modulation of human glutathione S-transferases by botanically defined vegetable diets, *Cancer Epidemiol Biomarkers Prev* 9(8):787-793, 2000.

205. Aldercreutz H: Phyto-oestrogens and cancer, *Lancet Oncol* 3(6): 364-373, 2002.

206. Steinmetz KA, Potter JD: Vegetables, fruit, and cancer. I. Epidemiology, *Cancer Causes Control* 2(5):325-357, 1991.

207. Doll R, Peto R: The causes of cancer: quantitative estimates of avoidable risks of cancer in the United States today, *J Natl Cancer Inst* 66(6):1191-1308, 1981.

TUMOR INVASION AND METASTASIS

KATHRYN L. McCANCE • PHILLIP BARNETTE

http://evolve.elsevier.com/McCance/

CHAPTER OUTLINE

Tumor development is a multistep process during which genetic and epigenetic events orchestrate the transition of cells from a normal to a malignant state. In the past 10 years much effort has been directed toward defining the molecular mechanisms underlying progression to the metastatic state and identifying possible molecular targets for therapy. These mechanisms include control of proliferation; the balance between cell survival and apoptosis; the communication with neighboring cells and the extracellular matrix; the induction of tumor neovascularization (angiogenesis); and finally, tumor cell migration, invasion, and metastatic dissemination.

Metastasis is the major cause of illness and death resulting from most human malignant diseases. Approximately 40% to 50% of malignant tumors are cured by current therapies.[1] Most individuals, with cancer, however, experience multiple metastases that are too small to be detected, at the time the primary tumor is treated. Consequently, an important goal is to develop new therapies or analytic approaches that can be used to accurately predict the metastatic potential of a tumor. The hope is that such therapies will be derived from the cell molecular research involving the mechanism of invasion and metastases.

HISTORICAL THEORIES OF CANCER INVASION

Critical to understanding current research approaches to invasion and metastasis is knowing, historically, where we have been. Table 12-1 reviews the evolution of research on cancer invasion and metastasis.

TUMOR SPREAD

Tumor spread throughout the body can take several forms: (1) direct invasion of contiguous organs, known as *local spread;* (2) metastases to distant organs by way of lymphatics and veins; and (3) metastases by way of implantation. Spreading of a tumor depends on its rate of growth, its degree of differentiation, the anatomic presence or absence of barriers, and other as yet unknown biologic factors. The history of progression of most malignant tumors can be divided into four phases: (1) malignant change in the initiating cell called *transformation,* (2) *growth* of the transformed cell, (3) local *invasion,* and (4) distant *metastasis.* The original transformed cell must undergo at least 30 population doublings to produce a tumor weighing about 1 g, which is the smallest clinically detectable tumor (Figure 12-1).

Table 12-1	Historical Development of the Cellular Theory of Cancer Invasion and Metastasis
Time Frame	**Theory Proposal**
Hippocrates (460-370 BC)	First theory on cancer invasion; cancer was a disease of black bile leakage into tissue; black bile diffusion theory (imbalance)
Galen (AD 131-203)	Rejected the notion of an imbalance of black bile; proposed black bile concentrated in area of invasion (humoral theory)
Paracelsus (1493-1541)	Revised humoral theory that cancer invasion was caused by diffusion of mineral salts
Morgagni (1682-1771)	Performed numerous deposits and described cancer deposits in the liver
Müller (1828)	Established cellular origin of cancer
Recamier (1829)	First to propose that invasion and metastasis were the result of translocation of cells; first to use the term *metastasis*—Recamier was not properly acknowledged for this finding
Virchow (1821-1902)	Was convinced of the cellular nature of tumors but retained the humoral diffusion theory
Thiersch (1822-1895)	Refuted the humoral concept, demonstrated that invasion was a process starting from the primary tumor; reported that cancer cells reached the lymph nodes by cellular embolism (cellular-embolic theory); by the end of the nineteenth century, the cellular theory had become firmly established
Paget (late 1800s)	First to speculate about the factors that promote cellular "seeding" of tumor cells (seed versus soil theory)
Tyzzer (early 1900s)	First scientist to develop an experimental model of metastasis
1900s-1970s	Tumor invasion and metastasis thought to be the result of passive growth pressure and low tumor cell cohesiveness
1960s-1970s	Active mechanisms of tumor growth were investigated (e.g., what mechanisms facilitated the movement of tumor cells through host barriers); possible mechanisms included tumor cell mobility, lytic enzymes, and secretions of other factors
1990s-present	Elucidation of the intracellular signaling pathways responsible for the biochemical mechanisms of invasion and metastasis, including emphasis on tumor-host signaling interaction; practical applications of therapies to interfere with these pathways.

Local Spread

Invasion, or local spread, is a prerequisite for metastasis and the first step in the metastatic process. The progression of a tumor cell from being one of benign proliferation to one that invades and develops metastatic growth is the major cause of poor clinical outcome of individuals with cancer. In its earliest stages, local invasion may occur as a function of direct tu-

mor extension. Eventually, however, cells or clumps of cells become detached or lose cell-to-cell adhesion to the primary tumor and invade the surrounding interstitial spaces. Possible mechanisms thought important in local invasion include (1) cellular multiplication, (2) mechanical pressure, (3) release of lytic enzymes, (4) decreased cell-to-cell adhesion (making cancer cells "slippery"), and (5) increased motility of

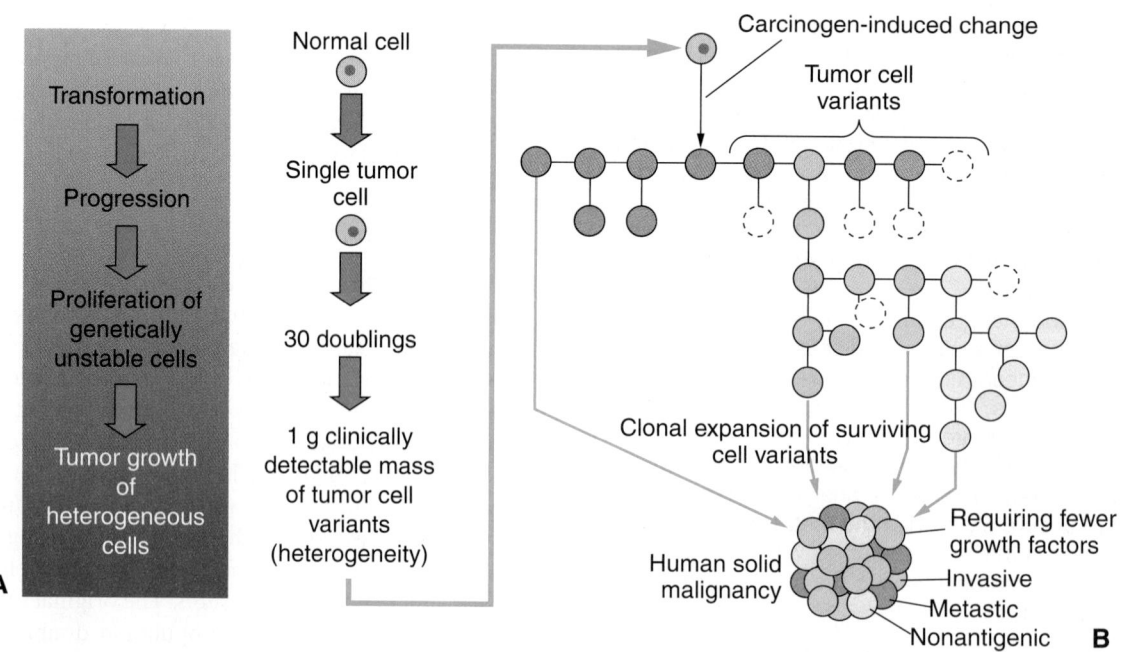

Figure 12-1 Heterogeneity of tumor growth. **A,** Tumor growth of heterogeneous cells. **B,** Multiple colors represent various cell variants becoming a solid tumor of heterogeneous cells. Heterogeneity therefore causes challenges to treatment.

individual tumor cells.[2] A recent view of invasion is that of its being a disruption of the **tumor-host microenvironment,** that is, cancer invasion is seen as an abnormal violation of tissue boundaries.

Tissue architecture, maintained by the basement membrane (BM) (a specialized form of the extracellular matrix (ECM; see Figure 1-14), delineates tissue boundaries and cell-to-cell communication. Cells usually remain close to home because they are regulated by communication with neighboring cells and the surrounding ECM. Signals from the matrix beneath normal cells tell them they are on home ground. Cross-talk between the two can elicit differentiation and development, as seen with recent examples in the study of the prostate and ovary.[3,4]

Normally, when cells detach from their home ground (matrix), they undergo apoptosis, a process called **anoikis** (Greek for *homelessness*). In contrast, neoplastic cells can survive by recruiting growth factors from the ECM and using them in a paracrine manner to suppress apoptosis, stimulate tissue invasion, and promote angiogenesis. Tumor cells also may make their own growth factors and use them in an autocrine fashion. In other words, the matrix and tumor cells *exchange* enzymes and cytokines, creating a permissive environment for the cancerous cell. For example, the autocrine mechanisms at work may include the production of TrkB protein. TrkB is a tyrosine kinase receptor best known for its role in the nervous system where, together with its main ligand, brain-derived neurotrophic factor (BDNF), it promotes proliferation, differentiation, and survival of normal neural cells[5] (Figure

12-2). Recent experiments revealed, however, that TrkB-rich epithelial cells also resist anoikis.[6] Thus TrkB generates a prosurvival signal that blocks caspases (DNA-cleaving enzymes that mediate programmed cell death [apoptosis]) allowing cells to survive and metastasize. (See Chapter 2 for a discussion of caspases.) TrkB and BDNF are often overexpressed in some human cancers, including pancreatic and prostate carcinomas, Wilms tumor, neuroblastoma, and colorectal cancers.[6-8] These observations demonstrate the oncogenic effects of TrkB and uncover a specific prosurvival mechanism that may lead to new treatment modalities. Anti-invasion treatment may target the stromal fibroblasts and endothelial cells.[9]

Cellular Multiplication

The proliferation of tumor invasion depends on the rate of cellular multiplication, which is a function of the cell generation time (evolution of the cell cycle), the number of cells that are dividing at one time (growth fraction), and the degree of cell loss from the tumor. Cells generated from malignant lesions thus can divide rapidly, but the tumor itself may not grow because a number of cells are rapidly dying. (The cell cycle is discussed in Chapters 1 and 11.)

Mechanical Invasion

Invasion, in relation to mechanical pressure, is analogous to the way in which plants force their roots through the soil (i.e., by building up pressure that forces sheets, or finger-like projections, along the lines of least mechanical resistance). Pressure from the growing mass blocks local blood vessels, lead-

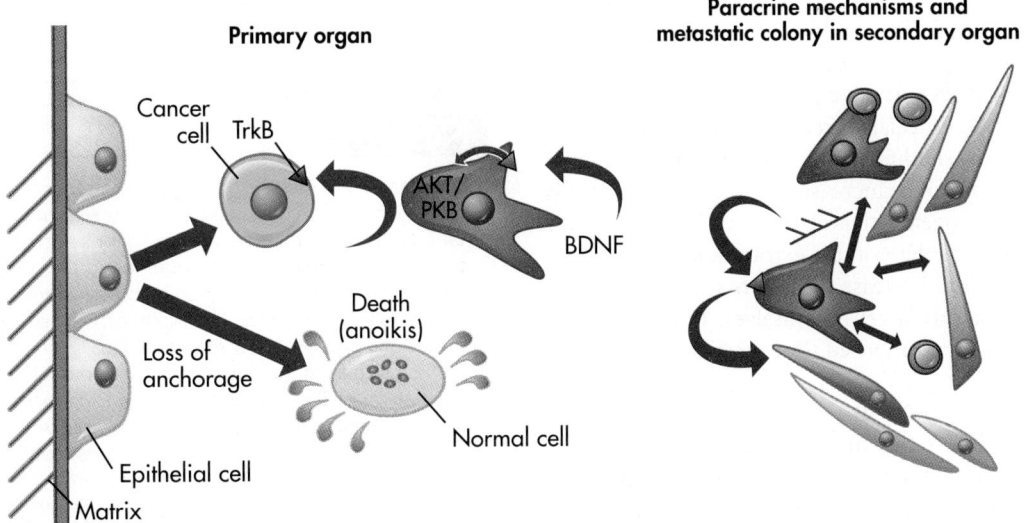

Figure 12-2 **Invasion mediated by TrkB and BDNF.** Matrix and epithelial cells intercommunicate to survive and disseminate. Epithelial cells are normally attached both to each other and to their matrix. They undergo genetically programmed cell death when detached from their home base—a process called *anoikis*. In contrast, cancer cells can survive by using autocrine or paracrine signaling mechanisms to suppress programmed cell death, stimulate tissue invasion, and promote the growth of new blood vessels to supply oxygen. Recently, investigators described an autocrine mechanism with the production of TrkB protein (a tyrosine kinase receptor), which is stimulated by brain-derived neurotrophic factor (BDNF) and in turn activates the AKT/PKB signaling pathway protein. Paracrine mechanisms involve interactions with other cells (such as immune cells, other matrices, the cells of blood vessels, and others). For simplicity, paracrine mechanisms are shown as operating only in metastatic sites, but they also may function in primary tumors.

ing to local tissue death and a reduction in mechanical resistance, which further aids the spread.

Lytic Enzymes

Malignant tumors that invade normal tissues cause significant amounts of degradation to the extracellular matrix (see Chapter 1). Because many animal and human tumors have higher levels of hydrolases (e.g., proteases and collagenases, plasminogen activators, lysosomal enzymes) than do corresponding normal tissues, the concept that malignant tumors produce and secrete lytic enzymes or induce host cells to release proteases (e.g., infiltrating macrophages) that destroy normal tissue has become firmly established.[10,11] Protease activity is regulated by antiproteases. At the invading edge of tumors, the balance between proteases and antiproteases favors proteases. Three classes of proteases have been identified: (1) serine, (2) cysteine, and (3) matrix metalloproteinases (MMPs). MMPs are increased in epithelial cancers and are involved in producing new blood vessels (angiogenesis) that aid in invasion and metastasis.[12] Collagens are the major structural elements of the extracellular matrices where invasion begins (see p. 380). One type of MMP, **type IV collagenase,** which cleaves type IV collagen of epithelial and vascular basement membranes, is increased in the cells of many highly metastatic tumors. Inhibition of collagenase activity in animal experiments has inhibited MMP, greatly reducing metastases.[12] Tumor cells can either release collagenase (e.g., digest collagen) or secrete collagenolytic substances in latent forms that are converted to activate collagenase by lysosomal proteases, such as plasmin.[13]

A number of other proteases that are attached to or released from tumor cells appear to increase tumor invasion through proteolysis, including cysteine proteinases, **cathepsin B and D,** and serine proteases such as **urokinase-type plasminogen activator (uPA).** uPA is a prognostic marker in a variety of malignancies, especially breast cancer.[14] Plasminogen activator, which converts the serum proenzyme plasminogen into the protease plasmin, is increased in tumor cells.[15,16] It is believed that plasminogen activator plays an important role in the degradation of proteins in the extracellular matrix during tumor cell invasion. Protease inhibitors can be produced by the host or by the tumor cells themselves. The use of protease inhibitors has been proposed for cancer treatment.[2]

Decreased Cell Adhesion

Cancer cells do not adhere to one another as well as normal cells do. This "slippery" trait has been related to fibronectin, which regulates cell attachment, spreading, phagocytosis, cell structure effects, and cell movement; integrin-fibronectin also stimulates and generally acts as an anchoring molecule. Cancer cells may make a defective type of integrin-fibronectin, or they may break down fibronectin as they produce it. Low levels or loss of this anchoring molecule, that is, fibronectin, may help cancer cells "slip" between normal cells in the process of invasion. Similarly, alterations in the cell-to-cell adhesion

molecule **E-cadherin** correlate with the metastatic potential of cancer cells (see "What's New? E-cadherin and Twist," and cell adhesion molecules in Chapter 1). Cadherins dominate these intercellular adhesions, but integrin-fibronectin adhesions also are important, as are cell-matrix adhesions. Recent studies suggest that these cell adhesion molecules also interact with the extracellular matrix and alter key intracellular signaling pathways, including the function of the receptor tyrosine kinases[17] (see Figure 12-2). Thus cell-matrix interactions appear to modulate this metastatic potential, thereby helping the cancer cell to become "homeless," survive, expand, and disseminate.

Increased Motility

Cell movement is a key component of tumor cell invasion. Stages of invasion include the detachment and subsequent infiltration of cells from the primary tumor into adjacent tissue, as well as the migration of cells through the vascular wall into the circulation (intravasation) and movement out of the vascular wall (extravasation) into a secondary site (Figure 12-3, A). Data suggest that tumor cells become mobile as a result of a variety of agents, including extracellular matrix components, some known (e.g., hepatocyte growth factor and epidermal growth factor) and some unknown host-derived growth and motility factors, and tumor-secreted or *autocrine motility factors.*[18] Cell migration is a complex process requiring molecular cross-talk at the invasion front, as well as the regulation of cell-to-cell attachments, cell matrix attachment, and matrix remodeling. Cell migration is often initiated in response to a chemotactic stimulus. For example, MMPs generate chemotactic signals that can act in a paracrine manner to influence the behaviors of distinct cell types (Figure 12-4).

WHAT'S NEW? E-cadherin and Twist

Metastasis is a multistep process whereby cancer cells lose attachment, disseminate, and establish secondary tumors in distant organs. Investigators searching for key regulators of metastasis using a breast tumor model found the transcription factor Twist (a major player in embryonic development) plays an essential role in metastasis. Inhibition of Twist expression in highly metastatic breast cancer cells specifically inhibits their ability to metastasize from the mammary gland to the lung. An increased expression of Twist causes a loss of E-cadherin–mediated cell-to-cell adhesion, activation of biologic markers, and initiation of cell motility. These data suggest that Twist contributes to metastasis by promoting epithelial-mesenchymal (embryonic tissue) transition (EMT). More simply, Twist induced the transmission of epithelial cells into embryonic mesodermal cells (i.e., from cobblestone-like appearance to spindle-like fibroblastic structure). High levels of Twist expression is correlated with invasive lobular carcinomas, a highly invasive tumor type associated with loss of E-cadherin expression. These results establish a mechanistic link between Twist, E-cadherin, EMT, and metastasis.

Data from Yang J et al: *Cell* 117(7):927-939, 2004.

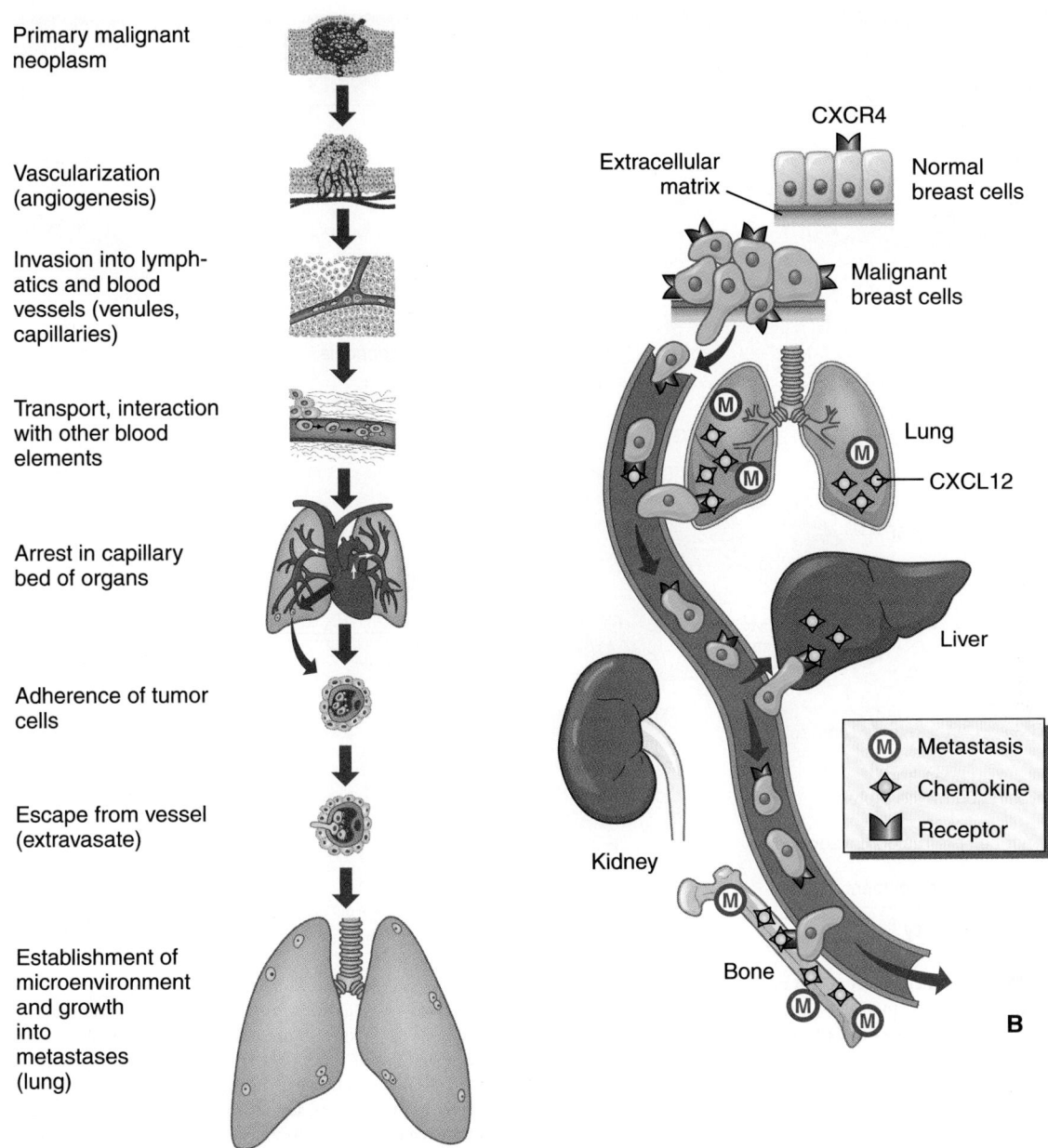

Figure 12-3 Pathogenesis of metastasis. A, Initial neoplastic transformation of susceptible cells gives rise to a small population of tumor cells. Vascularization of this initial neoplastic lesion allows further proliferation of tumor cells and enlargement of the primary tumor. Malignant cells within the primary tumor next begin to invade the surrounding host tissue or tissues. Entry of invading tumor cells into lymphatics or blood vessels serves to transport them to distant sites in the body, where they lodge and become arrested in the capillary beds of various organs. The arrested cells then exit from capillaries into the surrounding tissue where, subject to provision of a suitable environment, they proliferate to form metastases. **B,** Compared with normal breast epithelial cells (top), their malignant counterparts are enriched with chemokine receptor CXCR4. The chemokines (such as CXCL12) that are attracted to these receptors are released in high amounts only by certain organs, such as bone marrow, liver, and lung. Other organs, such as kidney (pictured), skin, and brain, contain low amounts of these chemokines. Primary breast cancer cells invade their extracellular matrix and circulate in the blood and lymphatic systems. Thus other organs, instead of the primary tumor, may *determine* metastases by allowing or attracting the tumor to invade. (**A** Redrawn from Poste G, Fidler IJ: *Nature* 20:139, 1980. **B** Redrawn from Muller A et al: *Nature* 410:50-56, 2001.)

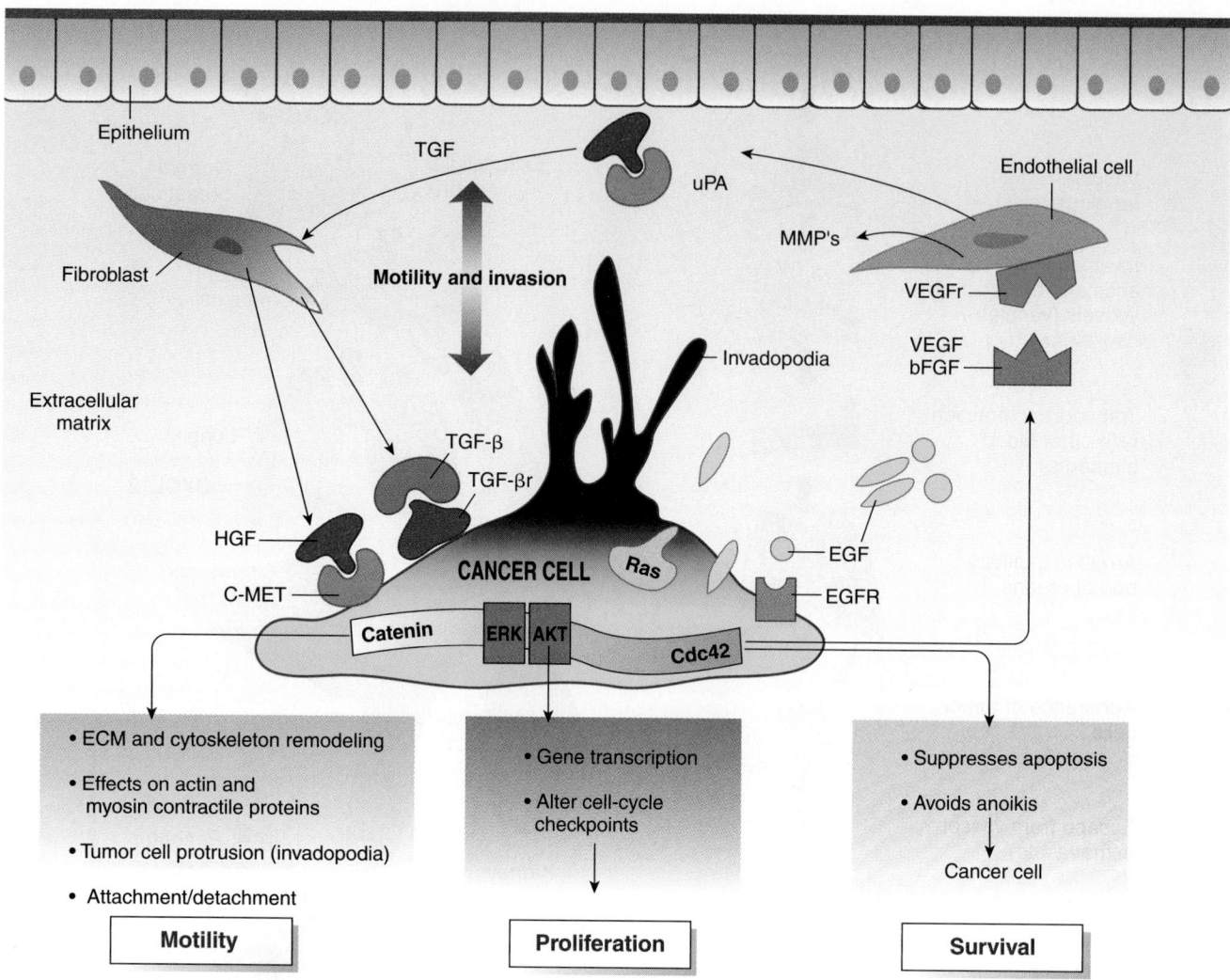

Figure 12-4 **Microenvironment of the tumor-host interface.** Molecular crosstalk at the extracellular matrix and tumor cell invasion front (only example mediators are shown). Tumor cells produce angiogenesis factors (i.e., autocrine), such as vascular endothelial growth factor (VEGF) and basic fibroblast growth factor (bFGF), which bind to receptors on stromal vascular cells (endothelial cells) and cause increased vascular permeability, endothelial proliferation, migration, and invasion. Fibroblasts produce chemoattractants, such as hepatic growth factor (HGF), which stimulate motility of tumor cells by binding to the MET receptor (c-MET). Fibroblasts and endothelial stromal cells release enzymes, including matrix metalloproteinases (MMPs) and serine proteases urokinase-type plasminogen activator (uPA), which hang out on the surface of the invading tumor cell or invadopodia and become activated. Once activated they then can degrade the ECM and clear an invading pathway. ECM degradation releases bound growth factors, such as transforming growth factor-beta (TGF-β) and epidermal growth factor (EGF), which bind to their receptors on the tumor cell. Crosstalk within the cancer cell links survival (antiapoptosis), proliferation, and motility. For example, activation of Ras, and the signaling pathway PI(3)K, B-catenin, ERK, increases cytoskeletal remodeling. ERK activation increases mitogenesis and increased tumor cell survival with phosphorylation of AKT. (Adapted from Liotta LK, Kohn EC: *Nature* 411:375-379, 2001.)

Three-Step Theory of Invasion

Although the process is actually complex, a simplified three-step theory has been proposed to describe the sequence of biochemical events during tumor cell invasion of the extracellular matrix (Figure 12-5). These steps occur after tumor cells detach from each other (see Decreased Cell Adhesion, p. 378). The three steps include tumor cell attachment to the matrix, degradation or dissolution of the matrix, and locomotion into the matrix.

The first step, attachment, is mediated by specific attachment factors such as fibronectin and laminin, a complex gly-

coprotein that is a major constituent of all basement membranes. Tissue compartments are separated from each other by two types of extracellular matrix: (1) basement membranes and (2) interstitial connective tissue. Both types, although organized differently, consist of collagens, glycoproteins, and proteoglycans. Tumor cells interact with the extracellular matrix at several stages in the metastatic process (see Figure 12-3). A tumor must first navigate the underlying basement membrane and then cross the interstitial connective tissue to eventually get access to the circulation (see Figure 12-4). Membrane vesicles on the cell surface of tumor

Attachment and dissolution

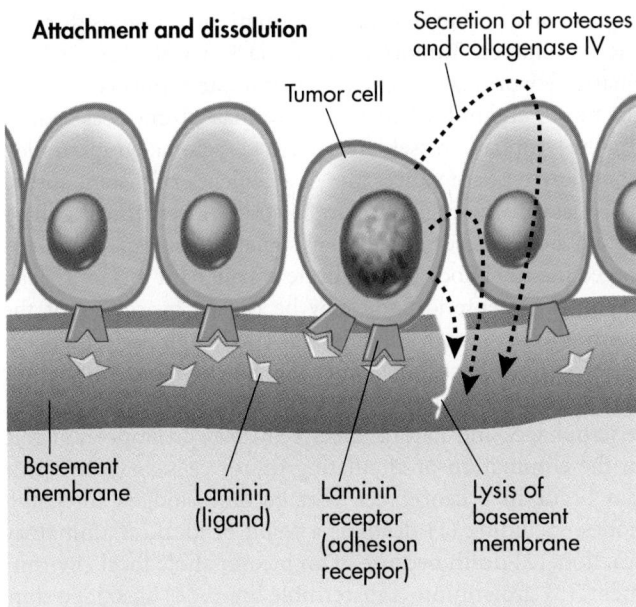

Secretion of proteases and collagenase IV

Tumor cell

Basement membrane

Laminin (ligand)

Laminin receptor (adhesion receptor)

Lysis of basement membrane

Anchoring and migration

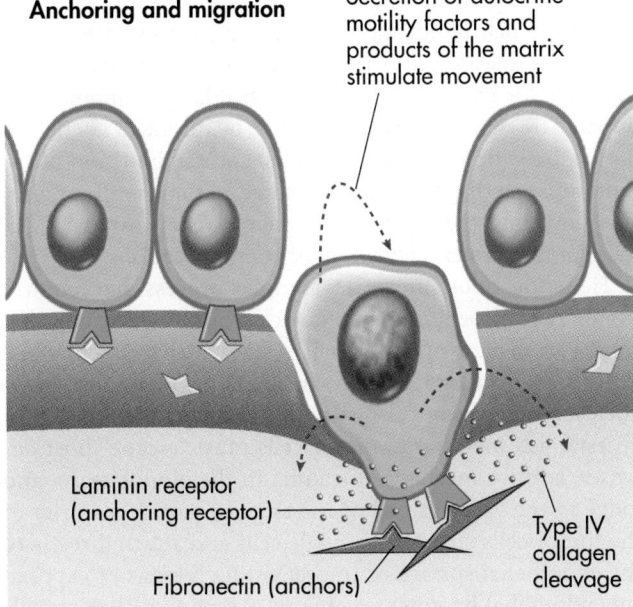

Secretion of autocrine motility factors and products of the matrix stimulate movement

Laminin receptor (anchoring receptor)

Fibronectin (anchors)

Type IV collagen cleavage

Figure 12-5 Three-step sequence of tumor invasion: attachment, dissolution, and locomotion. After tumor cells have detached from one another, the invasion process begins. Step 1, an individual tumor cell attaches to the extracellular matrix. Surface receptors on the tumor cell (laminin receptors) bind to parts of the basement membrane (laminin) in the extracellular matrix. Step 2 is degradation (dissolution) of the matrix by tumor cell proteases (collagenase IV and plasminogen activator). The anchored tumor cell either secretes proteolytic enzymes or causes the host cell to secrete the proteolytic enzymes that degrade the matrix in a region very close to the tumor cell surface. Step 3 is the migration (locomotion) of the tumor cell through the degraded basement membrane. During this phase, pseudopodia (finger-like projections) of the tumor cell cross the basement membrane, enabling the cell to extravasate from the blood vessel into the interstitial tissue.

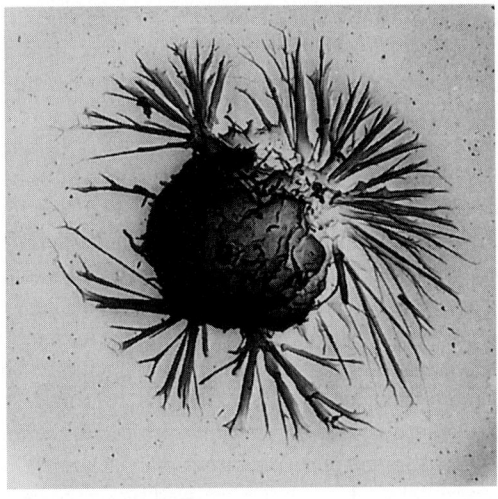

Figure 12-6 Pseudopodia. Photograph of electron microscopy of a breast cancer cell with finger-like projections called *pseudopodia*. (Courtesy National Library of Medicine.)

cells are rich in **laminin receptors** that enable their attachment to basement membrane.[2] A correlation exists between the invasiveness and the density of laminin receptors in carcinomas of the breast and colon. Laminin forms a bridge between the cell-surface laminin receptor and type IV collagen (see Figure 12-5). In addition to laminin-specific receptors, tumor cells express integrins (adhesion molecules) that can be receptors for many components of the extracellular matrix.[19]

Once anchored, the tumor cell either secretes proteolytic enzymes or induces host cells to produce them, and degradation of the matrix, or step two, begins. Such enzymes may degrade both the attachment proteins and the structural collagenous proteins of the matrix. Type IV collagenase, a powerful proteolytic enzyme, may outnumber the natural protease inhibitors present in the matrix.

The third step is tumor cell locomotion into the degraded region of the matrix. Finger-like projections called *invadopodia* (also called *pseudopodia*), which extend from the tumor cell (see Figures 12-4 and 12-6), facilitate movement by attaching to blood vessel walls that cross the basement membrane. The tumor cells then extravasate from the vasculature into the interstitial stroma. Theoretically, invasion occurs by cyclic repetition of these steps. The direction of locomotion seems to be influenced by chemotactic factors (see Figure 12-4).

Patterns of Spread: Metastasis

Metastasis, the spread of cancer cells from a primary site of origin to a distant site, is the life-threatening characteristic of malignancy. Local invasion is a condition of metastases. Methods exist for successfully eradicating **primary tumors** (original sites of tumor origin). However, the real challenge involved in reducing cancer mortality is controlling metastasis, because removal of the primary tumor does not affect the proliferating growth at other sites. Many individuals without evidence of metastatic disease on initial diagnosis will be apparently cured of their primary tumor, only to be diagnosed with distant metastases years or decades after treatment. Often the primary tumor is not even diagnosed before secondary spread occurs. Metastasis involves a series of sequential steps: (1) direct or continuous extension of local invasion of tumor cells into surrounding tissue; (2) penetration into lymphatics, blood vessels, or body cavities; (3) release into lymph or blood; (4) transport to secondary sites; and (5) entry and growth in secondary sites (see Figure 12-3, A). These mechanisms are not mutually exclusive. Tumor cell spread or dissemination through one mechanism often facilitates metastasis through other mechanisms because tumor cells move through numerous microscopic anatomic connections. Recently new findings revealed target metastasis of primary breast cancer cells. Chemokines released by certain organs attract the breast cancer cells to those organs. Breast cancer cells, compared to normal breast cells, have increased chemokine receptors that attach to those organs[20] (see Figure 12-3, B).

Direct or Continuous Extension

The earliest result of invasion could be called *continuous extension.* Cancerous tumors may extend into several areas without breaking away from the parent tumor, including (1) tissue spaces, (2) lymph vessels, (3) blood vessels, (4) body cavities (serosal seeding), and (5) cerebrospinal spaces.

Direct tumor extension, once thought to result from simple growth pressure only, now is known to be initiated by the complex sequence of events discussed earlier. They are initiated by loss of intracellular adhesion that enables cells to "slip" past one another. Movement of cells through tissue barriers is further influenced by proteases and paracrine and autocrine motility factors (see discussion of local invasion, p. 376).

Metastasis by Lymphatics and Bloodstream

Distant cancer spread involves invasion and penetration of tumor cells into blood vessels or lymphatics, or both. Lymphatics and thin-walled venules offer relatively little mechanical resistance to penetration by tumor cells. Blood vessels within tumors offer malignant cells direct access into the circulation. Clusters, single cells, and fragments of tumor cells become separated from the primary tumor site and disseminate by these routes. Clumps of cells have a better chance of successful metastasis than do single cells because clumps involve similar (homotypic) adhesions among tumor cells and heterotypic, or different, adhesions between tumor cells and blood cells, particularly platelets. Platelet tumor clumps appear to enhance tumor cell survival and implantability.[21] Those tumors that arise close to a serous surface can invade through that surface, implant, and become distant metastases, a process known as *seeding.* Cancer seeding may occur in the pleural space surrounding the lung and in the peritoneal space surrounding the abdominal cavity.

The most common route for distant metastases is through the lymphatics. Tumors generally lack a well-formed lymphatic network. Lymphatic channels occur at the periphery of the tumor and not within the tumor mass. Tumor cells entering the lymphatic vessels are carried to regional lymph nodes. For many types of cancer, the first evidence of distant spread is a mass in the regional lymph node. An enlarged axillary lymph node, for example, may signal breast cancer; an enlarged inguinal node may indicate a malignant melanoma; an enlarged mesenteric node may be caused by cancer of the gastrointestinal tract. Initially, regional lymph nodes may exert a barrier effect, preventing the further spread of tumor cells into the lymphatic system. Host defenses, such as macrophages and natural killer cells, play an important role in the elimination of circulating tumor cells. Several events can occur in a cancer cell that becomes lodged in lymph nodes, including (1) death as a result of local inflammatory reaction, (2) death because of an incompatible local environment, (3) growth into a discernible lump, (4) sustained dormancy for unknown reasons, or (5) detachment from the nodes and entrance into the efferent lymphatics.

When small lymphatic vessels are penetrated, tumor cell emboli are released into these lymphatic vessels and are responsible for lymphatic metastasis. Shedding of emboli is influenced by changes in vessel pressure, by turbulent alterations in lymphatic flow, and by movements or manipulation of the tumor during diagnostic tests or surgery. Tumor cells eventually move into the regional or systemic venous drainage because of numerous venolymphatic communications.

Hematogenous spread is a complex process that requires tumor cells to penetrate and detach from blood vessels and spread to distant organs, yet it is known that vascularized tumors shed malignant cells constantly as they grow, often releasing millions of cells without producing metastases.[21,22] To establish metastases, tumor cells must "escape" host defenses, survive mechanical trauma in the bloodstream, and lodge in the vascular bed of the target organ. A majority of the tumor cells circulate as single cells and attach directly to the endothelial surface or to preexisting regions of exposed subendothelial basement membrane. Emboli or tumor cells that contain leukocytes, fibrin, or platelets can cause direct embolization in the precapillary venules by mechanical action. The formation of a fibrin-platelet complex is thought to protect tumor cells within the emboli from host defenses and to facilitate successful attachment to the vascular epithelium. Once arrested in a blood vessel, tumor cells can actively invade the vascular wall and interstitial stroma and invade the parenchyma of the target organ. Arrest and extravasation of tumor emboli at distant sites involve adhesion to the endothelium, followed by emergence through the basement membrane. Involved in these processes are adhesion molecules (e.g., integrins) and proteolytic enzymes. Growth in the target organ parenchyma requires that a vascular network develop (angiogenesis) and that host defenses be ineffective.

Angiogenesis and Angiogenesis Factors

Growth of cancerous colonies depends on an adequate blood supply. In fact, without an adequate blood supply an in situ tumor may remain dormant indefinately.[23] Tumor implants cannot grow more than a few millimeters in diameter without developing new blood vessels to "feed" them, a process called **angiogenesis.**[24] Beyond this size, tumors fail to enlarge without vascularization because hypoxia causes apoptosis by activation of *p53* (Figure 12-7 and see p. 384). Perfusion supplies oxygen and nutrients, and newly formed endothelial cells secrete growth factors such as insulin-like growth factor and others that stimulate the growth of nearby tumor cells. It is unclear what triggers blood vessel formation. Several proangiogenic factors have been identified, including vascular endothelial growth factor (VEGF), platelet-derived growth factor (PDGF), transforming growth factor-alpha (TGF-α), basic fibroblast growth factor (bFGF), and angiopoietins.[25,26]

Specific inhibitors of angiogenesis have been identified, including platelet factor-4, angiostatin, endostatin, canstatin, tumstatin, thrombospondin, and interferon alpha/beta.[23] **Tissue factor (TF)** produced by tumor cells has been implicated in regulation of the "angiogenic switch" that, presumably, regulates the balance of positive and negative angiogenic factors.[27] It is possible that the disruption in the angiogenesis balance is determined genetically by individual cancer cells and its microen-vironment within the tumor.[23] A major factor may be a sudden drop in the cancer cell's production of **thrombospondin**—a protein that inhibits the growth of new blood vessels. Normal cells prevent the development of new blood vessels by pumping out thrombospondin.[28-30] The development of a new capillary network involves many steps and is similar to the blood coagulation cascade in that one event triggers the next through the action of specific mediators. Therapies aimed at blocking

WHAT'S NEW? VEGF Expression and Metastases

The clinical applications of vascular endothelial growth factor (VEGF) expression are being vigorously explored. Studies in ovarian carcinoma reveal a direct correlation between increasing serum VEGF levels and increasing clinical stage, tendency to metastasize, and decreased average survival times. Likewise, studies in non-small lung cancer reveal advanced clinical staging and poorer prognosis with increasing serum VEGF levels. Bevacizumab, a human monoclonal antibody against VEGF, is the most advanced of the antiangiogenic therapies and is showing promising results in clinical trials.

Data from Ferrara N: *Oncologist* 9(Suppl 1):2-10, 2004; Kaya A et al: *Respiratory Med* 98(7): 632-636, 2004; Li L et al: *Anticancer Res* 24(3b):1973-1979, 2004.

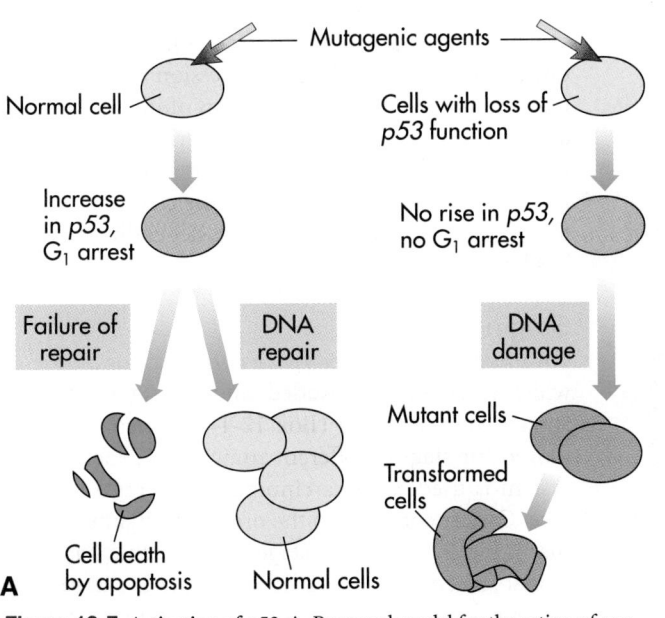

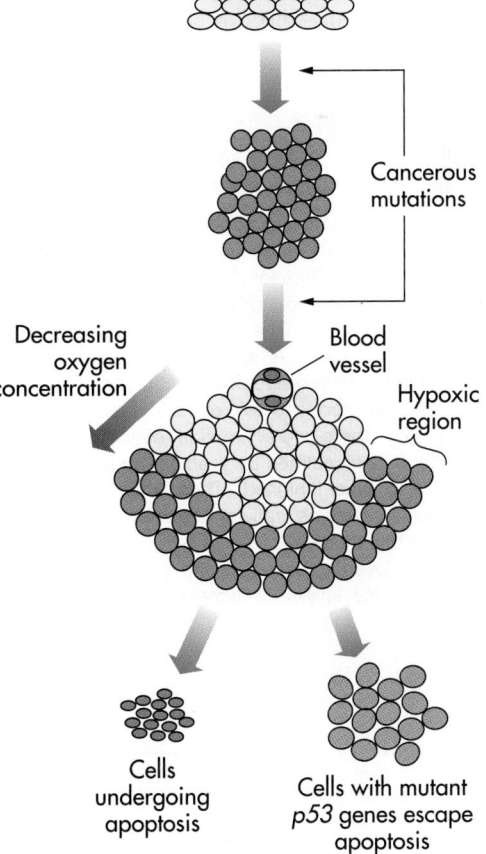

Figure 12-7 Activation of *p53*. **A,** Proposed model for the action of normal and mutant *p53*. **B,** Mutations in normal cells *(left)* result in overgrowth. In response to deoxyribonucleic acid (DNA) damage, the cells produce the protein p53. As a tumor increases in size and areas farthest from blood vessels become hypoxic, the cells undergo apoptosis. The only cells to survive and multiply are those with mutations in both copies of the *p53* gene.

angiogenesis represent a promising therapeutic target. Currently, more than 30 angiogenesis inhibitors are in clinical trials, and many promising new candidates are under investigation involving in vitro and animal models[31] (see "WHAT'S NEW? Angiogenesis and *c-Jun*").

In clinical situations, the rate of spread, as well as the growth of the tumor, is correlated with tumor vascularity. For example, small cell carcinoma of the lung arises in highly vascularized capillary beds and spreads easily and widely to other vascular organs such as the brain.

Growth of Metastases and Metastatic Potential

A metastasis grows and develops when a vascular network is developed, host defenses are evaded, and a compatible environment is available ("the soil"). The metastatic potential of many common carcinomas was formerly thought to be related to the size of the primary tumor. New data, however, suggest that the very "stresses" that cancer cells themselves endure, even in very small tumors, may promote the emergence of stronger, more aggressive tumors.[32,33] The microenvironment surrounding the tumor may play a significant role in determining how aggressive the tumor cells become. An environment such as one of low oxygen (hypoxia) can cause the production of **p53 protein.** Rather than simply arresting cell growth, the p53 protein (also called *wild-type p53*) activates a cell suicide program called *apoptosis* (see Chapter 2). In other words, p53 activates the "emergency brake" (see Figure 12-7, *A*). But if mutations occur in the *p53* gene, cells lose their "emergency brake" against uncontrolled cell growth. The af-

fected cells do not undergo apoptosis; instead they survive and may become the strongest, most aggressive cells of the tumor (see Figure 12-7, *B*). These cells may resurface as stronger renditions of their earlier selves and be able to resist drugs and radiation. More aggressive tumor cells may evolve into larger tumors, or larger tumors may overwhelm host defense mechanisms, thus favoring the survival of malignant cells.

Distribution and Common Sites of Distant Metastases

Distant metastasis in many types of cancer appears to take place in the first capillary bed encountered by the circulating cells. Table 12-2 summarizes common sites of metastases in various cancers. Patterns of metastasis for certain other tumors, however, are not related to patterns of blood flow or the location of capillary beds. Instead they show preferential growth in certain organs, a mechanism called **organ tropism.** Ocular melanoma, for example, often metastasizes to the liver, and clear cell kidney carcinomas often spread to bone and the thyroid. Organ tropism may be the result of growth factors, chemokines, or hormones present in the target organ, preferential adherence to the surface of certain target organs (sometimes called **tissue-selective homing receptors**), and the presence of chemotactic factors that diffuse from the target organ and cause circulating tumor cells to leave the vessel and gather in the target organs (see Figure 12-3, *B*). Ongoing studies are beginning to clarify the complex organ-tumor interaction involved in organ tropism. Recent work suggests differential patterns of gene expression within the cancer cell may be induced by different organs of implantation.[34] For example, the same cancer clone, experimentally grown in two different sites, will express different levels of proteolytic enzymes. In addition, the same cancer cell may experience different responses to chemotherapy, depending on which organ has been invaded.[35]

Staging

Tumor staging involves the size of the tumor, the degree to which it has locally invaded, and the extent to which it has spread (metastasized) (Box 12-1). Diverse schemes are employed for staging different tumors. In general, a four-stage system is used, with carcinoma in situ regarded as a special case. Cancer confined to the organ of origin is stage 1, cancer that is locally invasive is stage 2, cancer that has spread to regional structures such as lymph nodes is stage 3, and cancer that has spread to distant sites, such as a liver cancer spreading to lung, or a prostate cancer spreading to bone, is stage 4. One common scheme for standardizing staging is the World Health Organization's *TNM system; T* is for tumor spread, *N* is for node involvement, and *M* is the presence of distant metastasis (Figure 12-8). Prognosis for cure generally declines with increasing tumor size, lymph node involvement, and metastasis. Staging also may alter the choice of therapy, with more aggressive therapy being delivered to more invasive disease.

WHAT'S NEW?   Angiogenesis and *c-Jun*

A possible pathway for tumor angiogenesis that is under investigation involves the protein c-Jun (*Jun* oncogene) in endothelial cells. Endothelial cell proliferation, migration, invasion through collagen, and production of metalloproteinase-2 were all greatly inhibited in vitro in cells where a DNA-cleaving enzyme (DNAzyme) targeted c-Jun. A single, local injection of the DNAzyme, together with a reagent, inhibited tumor growth by 60% and significantly reduced microvessel density in the tumors. Furthermore, there were no side effects. In addition, corneal angiogenesis stimulated by vascular endothelial growth factor (VEGF) also was inhibited. Thus other angiogenesis-dependent diseases, such as macular degeneration or psoriasis, may benefit from this therapy.

When c-Jun is overexpressed, it can act as an oncogene. Several oncogenes are known to increase angiogenesis by increasing regulators of angiogenesis, such as VEFG; decreasing inhibitors of oncogenesis, such as thrombospondin-1; or initiating both mechanisms. Thus DNAzyme targeting of c-Jun could therapeutically act as both a direct and indirect inhibitor of angiogenesis.

Data from Abdollahi A et al: *Mol Cell* 13(5):649-663, 2004; Kerbel R, Folkman J: *Nat Rev Cancer* 2(10):727-739, 2002; Zhang G et al: *J Natl Cancer Inst* 96(9):683-696, 2004.

Table 12-2	Frequent Sites of Distant Metastasis in Some Types of Cancer	
Primary Tumor	**Major Anatomic Pathways**	**Frequent Site of Distant Metastasis**
Lung	Pulmonary vein, left ventricle	Multiple organs, including brain
Colorectal	Mesenteric lymphatics, portal venous system	Liver
	Inferior vena cava, right ventricle, pulmonary artery	Lungs
Testicular	Lymphatics to the periaortic area to the subclavian veins to the right ventricle	Lungs, liver
Prostate	Batson plexus of paravertebral veins; ilium, lumbar spine	Bones, lung, liver, endocrine glands, central nervous system
Breast	Batson plexus of paravertebral veins, lymph nodes, superior vena cava	Bony skeleton, lungs
Head and neck	Direct extension, Batson plexus	Lymphatics, liver, bone
Ovarian	Direct extension	Peritoneal surfaces, diaphragm
	Omentum and mesenteric veins	Omentum, liver
Sarcoma (extremity)	Inferior vena cava, right ventricle, pulmonary artery	Lungs

Box 12-1	Diagnosis and Clinical Staging of Cancer

Diagnosis

Cancer is an uncontrolled clonal proliferation of cells that can arise from virtually any cell type in the body. Because of the large variety of cell types in the body, cancer is a diverse set of different diseases that can come to medical attention by a number of routes. Some cancers can be detected at early stages by screening procedures such as skin inspection, breast self-examination, blood tests (for example, prostate-specific antigen, or PSA), and routine colonoscopy. Others come to attention because of symptoms. The symptoms a person develops depend on where the cancer occurs. Benign tumors in the brain may cause neurologic disturbances despite being quite small, whereas malignant cancers in the abdomen (for example, ovarian, pancreatic, kidney, and liver cancers) may not be detected until they are quite advanced. Symptoms can be caused by the size of the tumor, whether it presses on a nearby vital structure (e.g., pressure on nerves may cause pain, and erosion of bone can lead to pathologic fractures), or by loss of function of an organ. For example, individuals with leukemia seek medical attention when their bone marrow has been replaced by leukemia cells and no longer functions normally. This leads to pallor and fatigue due to anemia, bleeding due to low platelets, and infection due to loss of white blood cells. Sometimes cancers are detected when symptoms are caused by metastasis rather than the primary tumor, or when a small tumor secretes hormones (e.g., insulin, adrenalin) that cause symptoms.

Cancers must be diagnosed correctly to provide useful information to the individual and to the treating medical team. Accurate and in-depth diagnosis allows a better understanding of the causes of cancer, as well as optimizing the therapy. Finally, an accurate diagnosis allows predictions about how the cancer will behave over time, including how likely it is to respond to treatment (the prognosis), and where it might spread (metastasis). With very rare exceptions, the diagnosis of cancer requires the examination by a pathologist of tissue obtained from the patient. Tissue can be obtained by diverse means, including brushings (e.g., the Pap test), fine needle aspirations (for example, of a thyroid or breast mass), core needle or open biopsies that sample a small part of a mass, or complete excision of a mass. Examination of tissue by the pathologist includes, first and foremost, inspection of stained sections under the light microscope to determine whether the tissue is benign or malignant. More sophisticated testing may include immunostaining to identify the tissue of origin, various DNA tests for determination of specific genetic lesions, analysis of chromosome number and integrity, and gene expression profiling. For example, a tumor arising from muscle will react with antibodies against muscle-specific proteins, whereas a tumor arising from nerves will react with nerve-specific antibodies. In some cases, specific chromosomal or genetic alterations can be detected that help classify the tumor.

Clinical Staging

The information obtained from the pathologic diagnosis is combined with clinical information to determine the extent of the cancer. **Clinical staging** refers to the combination of physical findings, laboratory testing, and imaging studies that reveal whether the cancer has spread locally or to distant locations. The final diagnosis and clinical staging is therefore based on a broad range of information including the organ and tissue of origin (e.g., medullary thyroid versus papillary thyroid carcinoma), whether it is benign or malignant, and if it is malignant, whether it is well, moderately well, or poorly differentiated, and whether it has spread beyond the site of origin to distant sites (see Figure 12-8 on p. 386).

CLINICAL MANIFESTATIONS OF CANCER

Pain

Usually little or no pain is associated with the early stages of malignant disease, but pain occurs in 60% to 80% of individuals who are terminally ill with cancer. Pain is strongly influenced by fear, anxiety, sleep loss, fatigue, and overall physical deterioration. Pain is known to occur through an interaction among psychogenic, cultural, and physiologic components.

Recent data provide a mechanistic framework to suggest that many of the symptoms experienced by individuals with cancer may be mediated by cytokines acting on the peripheral and central nervous systems.[36] Figure 12-9 presents a biologic-physiologic framework for cytokine-induced cancer symptoms.

General mechanisms that cause pain associated with cancer include pressure, obstruction, invasion of a sensitive structure, stretching of visceral surfaces, tissue destruction, and inflammation. Although the pain may be directly related to the ma-

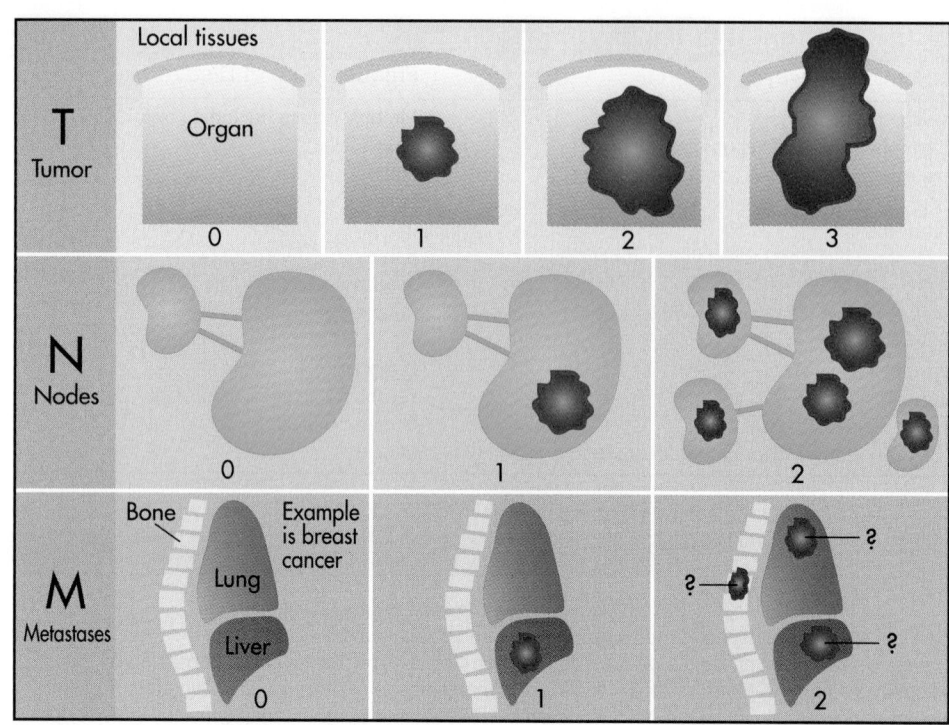

T= Primary tumor; the number equals size of tumor and its local extent. The number can vary according to site

T0= Breast free of tumor
T1= Lesion <2 cm in size
T2= Lesion 2-5 cm
T3= Skin and/or chest wall involved by invasion

N= Lymph node involvement; a higher number means more nodes are involved.

N0= No axillary nodes involved
N1= Mobile nodes involved
N2= Fixed nodes involved

M= Extent of distant metastases.

M0= No metastases
M1= Demonstrable metastases
M2= Suspected metastases

Figure 12-8 Tumor staging by the TNM system. (See figure for abbreviations.)

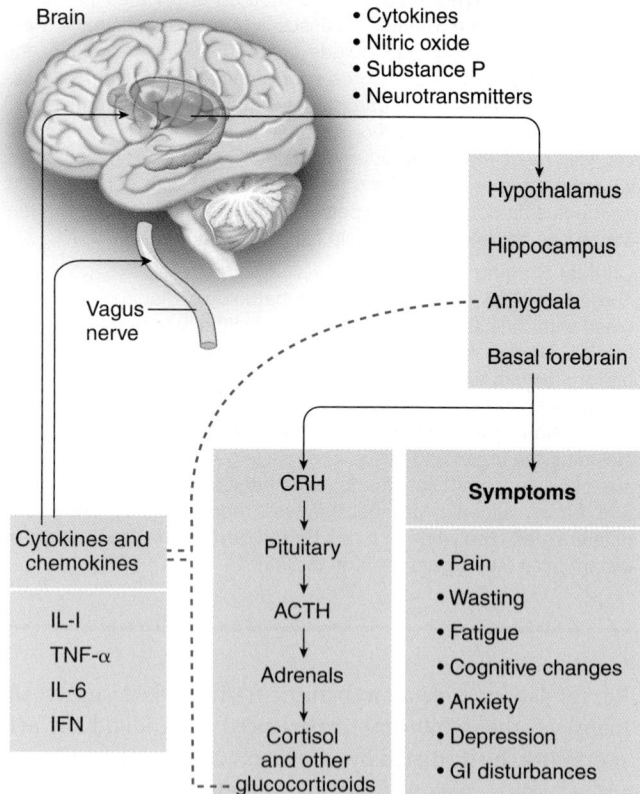

Figure 12-9 Theoretical framework for cytokine-induced cancer symptoms. Solid (red line) proinflammatory cytokines and chemokines (IL-1, TNF-α, IL-6, IFN) are released by immune cells. They exert their effect on peripheral nerves and the brain. Neurotransmitter responses by the brain are affected. The hypothalamic-pituitary-adrenal axis is activated with increased release of corticosteroids, which provide feedback (dotted lines) to decrease cytokine production. (Adapted from Cleeland CS et al: *Cancer* 97(11):2919-2925, 2003.)

lignancy, it can result from other problems, such as infection. A common cause of pain is bone metastasis, which may be referred away from the involved bone and manifest, for example, as back pain. Bone pain can be caused by periosteal irritation, medullary pressure, or pathologic fractures.

Abdominal pain often is caused by severe stretching from the tumor invasion of the hollow viscus. Tumors that obstruct and distend the bowel cause pain. Small bowel obstructions in persons with known malignant disease commonly result from recurrent cancer, surgical adhesions, or new primary tumors. Surgery is often needed to obtain relief. Hepatic malignancies stretch the liver, resulting in a dull pain or a feeling of fullness over the right upper abdominal quadrant.

Tumor compression of nerve endings against a firm surface creates pain. Brain tumors, in particular, have very little space to grow without compressing blood vessels and nerve endings between the tumor and the cranial vault. Tissue destruction from infection and necrosis can cause pain. The oral area, which often is the site of ulcerative lesions resulting from cancer and cancer treatment, can become infected and painful.

The way that pain is perceived and treated is influenced by one's ethnocultural background. The first priority of treatment is to control pain rapidly and completely as judged by the person. The second priority is to prevent recurrence of pain. Key to adequate pain control is the *continual* evaluation of pain as reported by the person. Objective measurements of pain are increasingly being included along with the reporting of more traditional vital signs. Many institutions are using specialized pain management teams that are trained to recognize different types of acute and chronic pain, as well as the individual's response to that pain. Combinations of traditional analgesics, novel agents and delivery systems, and attention to a person's psychologic responses, including depression and sleep disturbances, are sometimes addressed through a multidisciplinary approach.[37] Although cancer pain is a complex problem arising from multiple sources, individuals should be assured that suffering is not inevitable and that relief is attainable.[38]

Fatigue

Fatigue is the most frequently reported symptom of cancer and cancer treatment. The mechanisms that produce fatigue are poorly understood. Suggested causes include sleep disturbance, various biochemical changes, including cytokines and neurotransmitters, secondary to disease and treatment, numerous psychosocial factors, level of activity, nutritional status, and other environmental and physical factors.[39]

The physiologic understanding of fatigue probably includes mechanisms for decreased muscle contractility. Other areas of research include muscle function consequences from metabolic products of cancer treatment and associated muscle loss from circulating cytokines (e.g., tumor necrosis factor and interleukin-1 [IL-1]) (see Figure 12-9).

Similar to pain, fatigue is a subjective clinical manifestation. Fatigue is described by individuals with cancer as tiredness, weakness, lack of energy, exhaustion, lethargy, inability to concentrate, depression, sleepiness, boredom, lack of motivation, and decreased mental status.[40]

Individuals have reported management of fatigue by changing their expenditure of work, including planning and scheduling activities and work; decreasing nonessential activities; and increasing dependence on others for home management, transportation, and care. Much more research is needed to examine the psychophysiologic mechanisms of fatigue and develop interventions directed at these mechanisms.

Cachexia

The syndrome of **cachexia** includes anorexia; early satiety (filling); weight loss; anemia; asthenia (marked weakness); taste alterations; and altered protein, lipid, and carbohydrate metabolism (Figure 12-10). Cachexia is the most severe form of malnutrition associated with cancer and results in wasting, extensive loss of adipose tissue, emaciation, and decreased quality of life. The anorexia-cachexia syndrome is one of the most common causes of death among individuals with cancer and is present in 80% at death.[41] Recently an **acute phase response (APR)** has been linked to accelerated weight loss and a shortened survival time. The APR is possibly initiated by cytokines, including IL-6 and IL-8α.[42] Loss of adipose tissue appears to be due to an increase in catabolism of triglycerides, rather than a decrease in synthesis. A possible mechanism for triglyceride degradation is—an as yet unknown—tumor lipid mobilizing factor that stimulates lipolysis.[42] Loss of skeletal muscle occurs from both a depression in protein synthesis and an increase in protein degradation. Emerging is evidence

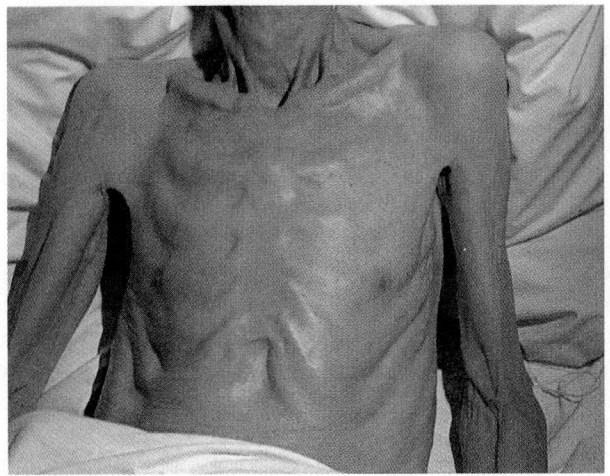

Figure 12-10 Cachexia. This severe form of malnutrition results in wasting and extensive loss of adipose tissue. (From Kamal A, Brockelhurst JC: *Color atlas of geriatric medicine*, ed 2, St. Louis, 1991, Mosby.)

that muscle wasting and weight loss is an early finding after tumor onset.[43]

One of the most significant cytokines is the activated macrophage-produced TNF-α, also called *cachectin* because of its role in the cachexia syndrome. Natural induction of TNF-α is protective; that is, it plays an important role (1) in the defense against viral, bacterial, and parasitic infections; (2) in autoimmune responses; and (3) in the selective destruction of malignant cells.[44] Unregulated TNF is now known to be involved in the development of wasting, cachexia, various inflammatory and/or autoimmune diseases, and septic shock.[44-46] (Cytokines are discussed in detail in Chapters 6 and 7.)

Alterations in taste also can account for the anorexia of cancer. Reductions in sensitivities to sweet, sour, and salty tastes make moderately seasoned foods seem bland. Persons with cancer, especially involving the liver, commonly have an aversion to red meat. Other aversions include coffee and chocolate.

Anorexia leads to a protein-energy malnutrition (PEM) of three types: (1) malnutrition similar to kwashiorkor, (2) marasmus, and (3) a combination of the two. Kwashiorkor is a form of malnutrition that evolves from a protein-deficient diet, in which calories come primarily from carbohydrates. Because the onset usually is rapid, anthropometric measurements tend to be normal but serum proteins (transferrin, albumin) are decreased. This protein serum decrease (hypoalbuminemia) causes the serum colloid osmotic pressure to decrease, so that fluid remains in the interstitium and causes edema. Marasmus is a form of malnutrition resulting from a decreased intake of calories and proteins. It is characterized by decreased anthropometric measurements caused by a prolonged and gradual wasting of muscle mass and normal serum albumin. A combination of kwashiorkor and marasmus results in hypoalbuminemia, edema, diminished immunologic competence (which depends on normal protein stores), and an overall physical deterioration. Malnutrition is a major factor contributing to death. (Malnutrition is discussed in detail in Chapter 39.)

Progressive weight loss in the person with cancer occurs despite normal or increased food intake. Starvation usually decreases the basal metabolic rate (BMR), but metabolic rates in persons with cancer are high. How increased BMR and weight loss relate to a breakdown of protein and nitrogen loss or negative nitrogen balance is unclear. Malignant cells replicate more rapidly than normal cells and require more food for their growth, but at the expense of the normal tissue. The normal tissue, over time, is sacrificed, and wasting begins to occur.

Carbohydrate metabolism is altered, causing a syndrome that resembles diabetes mellitus. Hyperinsulinemia is present, and many individuals show insulin resistance, hyperglycemia, and an abnormal glucose tolerance test result. These disturbances cause an increased gluconeogenesis, which produces glucose from amino acids. In starvation, protein usually is spared to protect vital structures, but in cancer, protein and fatty acids are used for meeting energy needs. Fatty acids are released from the breakdown of adipose tissue. An unusual and frustrating component of cancer care is the person's early satiety, or a sense of fullness after only a few mouthfuls of food.

Anemia

Anemia is a common disorder associated with malignancy. Most persons with cancer usually have a mild anemia, although 20% may have hemoglobin concentrations below 8 g/dl (normal value, 15 g/dl). Several mechanisms cause anemia in persons with cancer; these include chronic bleeding resulting in iron deficiency, severe malnutrition, medical therapies, or malignancy in blood-forming organs. Several of these mechanisms may cause suppression of the action of erythropoietin on the bone marrow, presumably by the release of cytokines.[47] Erythropoietin acts on specific erythroid progenitor cells in the bone marrow to stimulate the release of immature red blood cells (e.g., reticulocytes). Erythropoietin is effective in correcting the anemia associated with cancer. In addition, anemias that have occurred after chemotherapy or radiation therapy also have been treated successfully by erythropoietin.[48,49] Chronic bleeding and iron deficiency can accompany colorectal or genitourinary malignancy. Iron also is malabsorbed in persons with gastric, pancreatic, or upper intestinal cancer. Often there is a defect in the reuse of iron because of lack of transfer of iron from the storage pool to blood cell precursors. This defect may be caused by increased secretion of cytokines, such as IL-1, or alterations in nitric oxide regulation. Defects in erythropoietin production and shortened red cell survival also have been documented. Anorexia can cause iron deficiency, although folate deficiency is more common with anorexia.

Anemia can result from chemotherapy, but normochromic (normal hemoglobin concentration) and normocytic (average red cell size) anemias can occur after prolonged administration of alkylating agents or nitrosoureas, both classes of chemotherapeutic agents.[50] Megaloblastic (large red cell) anemias may develop after treatment with methotrexate, which causes abnormal folate metabolism.

Malignancy of the blood-forming organs is associated with a number of hemolytic anemias. An autoimmune hemolytic anemia occasionally develops in persons with chronic lymphocytic leukemia. (Anemia associated with leukemia is discussed in Chapter 27.)

Chemotherapy often worsens anemia in individuals with cancer. The administration of recombinant human erythropoietin (r-HuEPO) is safe and can significantly improve the hematocrit and quality of life of anemic individuals receiving myelosuppressive chemotherapy.[49]

Leukopenia and Thrombocytopenia

Direct tumor invasion to the bone marrow causes both leukopenia (a decreased leukocyte count) and thrombocytopenia (a decreased number of platelets). Chemotherapeutic drugs are toxic to the bone marrow, often causing both granulocytopenia and thrombocytopenia. Leukopenia can result from chemotherapy or radiation therapy of areas of the bone marrow. Thrombocytopenia is a major cause of hemorrhage in persons with cancer. It usually results from chemotherapy or bone marrow involvement by the malignancy. Thrombocytopenia is an accompanying disorder of disseminated intravascular coagulation that occurs in persons with acute promyelocytic leukemia and prostate cancer.

Infection

Infection is the most significant cause of complications and death in persons with malignant disease. When the absolute granulocyte or lymphocyte count falls, the risk of infection increases, and persons with cancer have reduced immunologic functions, debility with advanced disease, and immunosuppression from radiation therapy and chemotherapy. (Factors that predispose persons to infection are summarized in Table 12-3.) Surgery also can lower resistance to infection because removal of large quantities of tissue—together with hemorrhage, dead spaces, and poor tissue perfusion—creates favorable sites for infection. Hospital-related (nosocomial) infections increase because of indwelling medical devices, inadequate wound care, and the introduction of microorganisms from visitors and other patients.

Leukopenia resulting from bone marrow radiation dramatically increases the risk of infection. Mucous membranes and other rapidly dividing cells in the radiation field are prone to irritation and ulceration. Radiation, particularly of the cervix, bladder, and intestinal tract, also can lead to fistula formation or abnormal passages between tissue cavities. Surgery often is required to repair the fistula and eliminate continuous infectious cross-contaminations.

Paraneoplastic Syndromes

Paraneoplastic syndromes are symptom complexes that cannot be explained by the local or distant spread of the tumor or by the effects of hormones released by the tissue from which the tumor arose. About 10% of individuals with malignancy are affected. Although infrequent, paraneoplastic syn-

Table 12-3	Factors Predisposing Individuals with Cancer to Infection
Factor	**Basis**
Age	Many common malignancies occur mostly in older age.
	Immunologic functions decline with age.
	General debility reduces immunocompetence.
	Immobility predisposes to infection.
	Far-advanced cancer often results in immobility and general debility that worsens with age.
	Elderly persons are predisposed to nutritional inadequacies.
	Malnutrition impairs immunocompetence.
Tumor	Nutritional derangements can result.
	Sites and circumstances favorable to growth of microorganisms (obstruction, serous or blood effusion, ulceration) can be created.
	Far-advanced disease predisposes patients to debility and immobility.
	Humoral or cellular immune defects may result.
	Metastasis to bone marrow may cause leukopenia or other defects in immunity.
Leukemias	Inadequate granulocyte production (impaired phagocytosis) results.
	Thrombocytopenia (bleeding, breaks in skin integrity) can occur.
	Late effect: Chronic lung disease from *Pneumocystis carinii* pneumonia can develop during therapy.
Lymphomas and other mononuclear phagocyte malignancies	Humoral and cellular immune defects (anergy, altered immunoglobin production) result.
	Late effect: Splenectomy in children can cause increased susceptibility to infection.
Treatment: surgery	Invasive procedure interrupts first lines of defense.
	Radical nature of surgery (removal of large blocks of tissue in lengthy procedures) causes hemorrhage, decreased tissue perfusion, creation of dead spaces, devitalization of tissues.
	Procedure may be "dirty" surgery (bowel, infected or contaminated areas).
	Surgery patients are often older and at poor risk.
	Long preoperative hospitalization often precedes surgery.
	Patients may have had previous adrenocorticosteroid therapy.
	Patients may have infections at sites remote from operative area.
	Nutritional derangements (especially important in head and neck surgery) may result.
	Lymph node dissection may predispose patient to local infection and impair containment to area.
	Gynecologic surgery may result in fistulas.
	Lung surgery may cause bronchopleural fistulas.
	Debility and immobility may result.

Data from Donovan MI, Girton SF: *Cancer care nursing*, ed 2, New York, 1984, Appleton-Century-Crofts; Murphy GP, Lawrence W, Lenhard RE: *Clinical oncology*, ed 2, New York, 1994, American Cancer Society.

dromes are significant because (1) they may be the earliest symptom of an unknown cancer, (2) in affected individuals they may represent serious and life-threatening problems, and (3) they may mimic progression and therefore interfere with appropriate treatment. Table 12-4 presents the classifications of paraneoplastic syndromes.

CANCER TREATMENT

Cancer is treated with chemotherapy, radiation therapy, surgery, immunotherapy, and combinations of these modalities (Table 12-5). New proposed therapies are depicted in the figure in the WHAT'S NEW? box.

Chemotherapy

Although technically it includes any medicinal agent having antitumor effect, "chemotherapy" actually denotes the use of relatively nonselective cytotoxic drugs that target vital cellular machinery or metabolic pathways critical to both malignant and normal cell growth and replication. To be curative, chemotherapy must eradicate enough tumor cells so that the body's own defenses can eradicate any remaining cells. His-

torically, initial attempts to treat cancer centered on **single agent chemotherapy**. These agents were known to have significant early response rates but the duration of response was short lived.[51] Continued clinical studies have discovered several key points in chemotherapy use.

Combination chemotherapy is the synergistic use of several agents, each of which individually has an effect against a certain cancer. The primary rationale to this approach is to avoid single-agent drug resistance, which may be present even in previously untreated tumors (Figure 12-11). In addition, combination chemotherapy also may prevent acquired drug resistance. An added benefit of using lower doses of each drug in a combined manner is that the harmful effects to normal cells may be reduced. For example, much of the progress made in treating childhood acute lymphoblastic leukemia is the result of using combination chemotherapy. Whereby single-agent therapy produced remission rates of 60% with relapse within 6 to 9 months, combination therapy has led to nearly 95% remission rates with long-term remissions and cures approaching 75% to 80%.[52,53]

The **principle of dose intensity** implies there is a direct correlation between dose of a chemotherapeutic agent and killing

Table 12-4   Paraneoplastic Syndromes

Clinical Syndromes	Major Forms of Underlying Cancer	Causal Mechanism
Endocrinopathies		
Cushing syndrome	Small cell carcinoma of lung	ACTH or ACTH-like substance
	Pancreatic carcinoma	
	Neural tumors	
Syndrome of inappropriate antidiuretic hormone secretion	Small cell carcinoma of lung; intracranial neoplasms	Antidiuretic hormone or atrial natriuretic hormones
Hypercalcemia	Squamous cell carcinoma of lung	Parathyroid hormone–related peptide, TGF-α, TNF-α, IL-1
	Breast carcinoma	
	Renal carcinoma	
	Adult T-cell leukemia/lymphoma	
	Ovarian carcinoma	
Hypoglycemia	Fibrosarcoma	Insulin or insulin-like substance
	Other mesenchymal sarcomas	
	Heptaocellular carcinoma	
Carcinoid syndrome	Bronchial adenoma (carcinoid)	Serotonin, bradykinin, ?histamine
	Pancreatic carcinoma	
	Gastric carcinoma	
Polycythemia	Renal carcinoma	Erythropoietin
	Cerebellar hemangioma	
	Hepatocellular carcinoma	
Nerve and Muscle Syndromes		
Myasthenia	Bronchogenic carcinoma	Immunologic
Disorders of the central and peripheral nervous systems	Breast carcinoma	
Dermatologic Disorders		
Acanthosis nigricans	Gastric carcinoma	?Immunologic, ?secretion of epidermal growth factor
	Lung carcinoma	
	Uterine carcinoma	
Dermatomyositis	Bronchogenic, breast carcinoma	?Immunologic
Osseous, Articular, and Soft Tissue Changes		
Hypertrophic osteoarthropathy and clubbing of the fingers	Bronchogenic carcinoma	Unknown
Vascular and Hematologic Changes		
Venous thrombosis (Trousseau phenomenon)	Pancreatic carcinoma	Tumor products (mucins that activate clotting)
	Bronchogenic carcinoma	
	Other cancers	
Nonbacterial thrombotic endocarditis	Advanced cancers	Hypercoagulability
Anemia	Thymic neoplasms	Unknown
Others		
Nephrotic syndrome	Various cancers	Tumor antigens, immune complexes

From Cotran RS, Kumar V, Collins T: *Robbins pathologic basis of disease*, ed 6, Philadelphia, 1999, Saunders.
ACTH, adrenocorticotropic hormone; *TGF*, transforming growth factor, *TNF*, tumor necrosis factor; *IL*, interleukin.

of tumor cells. This relationship is often evident in a logarithmic fashion, in which small dose increases can significantly enhance the antitumor effect.[54,55] Use of maximal doses of chemotherapeutic agents is tempered by the increasing toxicities associated with their use as defined by the therapeutic index of the drug. The **therapeutic index,** that is, the relative effective dose needed to kill cancer cells as compared to the dose that would be harmful to normal cells, is generally quite low and is one of the limiting factors in the escalation of chemotherapy use.

A final key principle is the use of adjuvant chemotherapy after local treatment or removal of the primary tumor. It is in this context that chemotherapy has proven most useful, that is, in individuals who have minimal or no residual disease but who are at high risk for metastasis. Chemotherapy prevents the growth of micrometastatic deposits that are not clinically detectable at diagnosis. A variation of this approach, termed **primary,** or **neoadjuvant, chemotherapy,** is the early use of agents before definitive local control surgery or irradiation to decrease initial tumor size.[56] This approach may allow for less extensive local control measures, as well as the opportunity to begin treatment early for micrometastatic disease.

Several classes of chemotherapeutic agents are used concurrently to treat different types of cancerous tumors (Table 12-6). The mechanism by which each drug acts to eradicate

Table 12-5	Examples of Treatment of Site-Specific Cancers
Usual Treatment	**Site**
Surgery	Colon
	Breast
	Ovary
	Lung
	Thyroid
	Skin
	Uterus
Chemotherapy	Lymphoma
	Leukemia
	Choriocarcinoma
	Ovary
	Breast
Radiation	Breast (all have been combined with surgery)
	Uterus or cervix
	Lymphomas
	Lung
	Combined with surgery in many sites
Hormones	Breast
	Prostate
	Endometrium
Immunotherapy	Melanoma
	Prostate cancer
	Breast cancer?
	Leukemias
	Others?

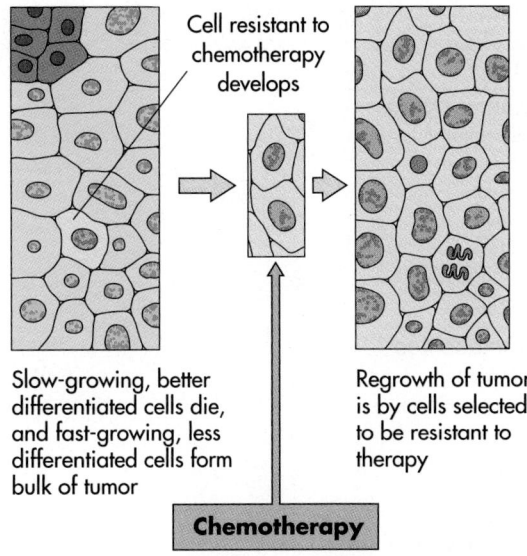

Figure 12-11 Chemotherapy and resistant cells. A cell resistant to single agent chemotherapy can develop from the pool of fast-growing tumor cells. Combination therapy helps prevent the development of resistant cells. (From Stevens A, Lowe J: *Pathology: illustrated review in color*, ed 2, London, 2000, Mosby.)

WHAT'S NEW?
Cancer Therapies in Development—Points of Attack

Cancer develops from a series of mutations. Normally a cell is inhibited from unlimited growth. With cancer the cell can lose its inhibitions to growth and multiply continuously.

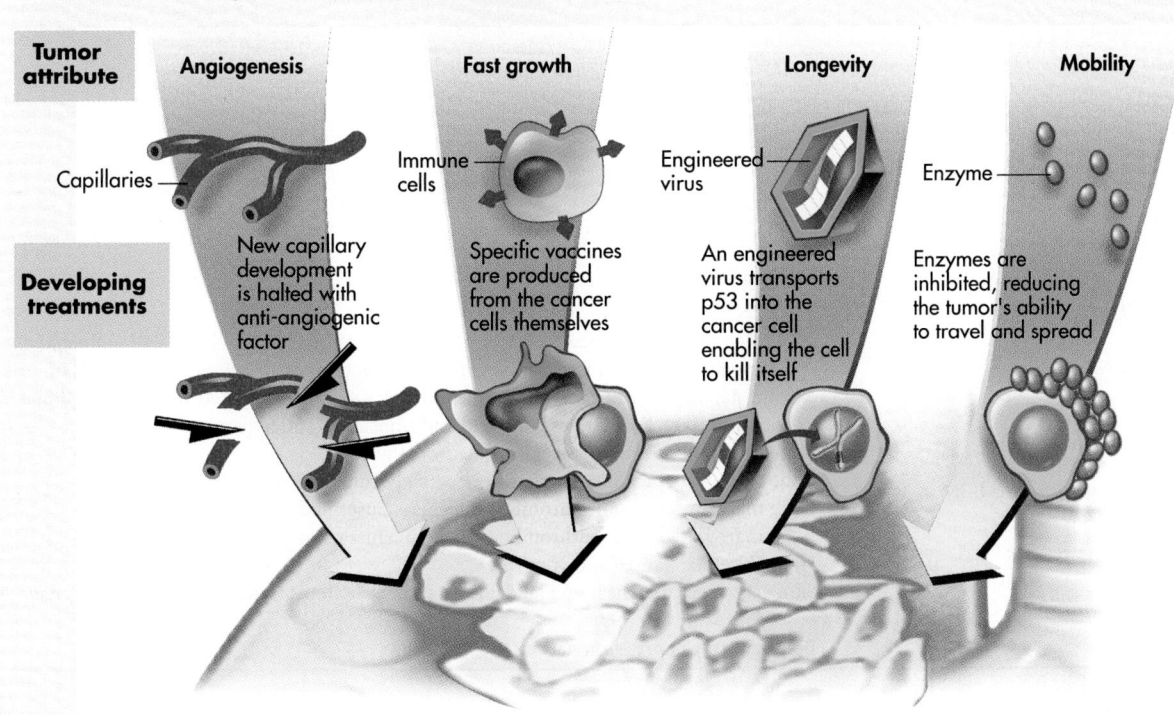

Table 12-6	Examples of Chemotherapeutic Drugs
Drug	**Major Toxicity**
Alkylating Agents	
Mechlorethamine Chlorambucil Melphalan Thiotepa Busulfan Cyclophosphamide Ifosfamide	*Therapeutic doses:* moderate depression of peripheral blood cell count; *excessive doses:* severe bone marrow depression, leukopenia, thrombocytopenia, and bleeding; maximum toxicity may occur 2-3 wk after last dose; alopecia; nausea and vomiting
Antimetabolites	
Methotrexate 6-Mercaptopurine 6-Thioguanine 5-Fluorodeoxyuridine Cytarabine Fludarabine 2-Chlorodeoxyadenosine 2'-Deoxycoformycin Gemcitabine	Oral and digestive tract ulcerations; bone marrow depression with leukopenia, thrombocytopenia, and bleeding; toxicity enhanced by impaired kidney function; alopecia
Antibiotics	
Doxorubicin Bleomycin Dactinomycin Plicamycin Mitomycin-C Mitoxantrone	Stomatitis, gastrointestinal injury; bone marrow depression; alopecia; cardiac toxicity at cumulative doses over 500 mg/m^2 (doxorubicin, daunorubicin); pneumonitis and pulmonary fibrosis at cumulative doses over 400 U (bleomycin); hypocalcemia; hepatic toxicity (plicamycin); nausea and vomiting
Steroids and Hormonally Active Agents	

Androgen
  Fluoxymesterone
Antiandrogen
  Flutamide
Estrogen
  Ethinyl estradiol
  Diethylstibestrol
Antiestrogen
  Tamoxifen
Progestin
  Megestrol acetate
Luteinizing hormone-releasing hormone agonist
  Leuprolide
Aromatase inhibitor
  Aminoglutethimide
Adrenocortical compound
  Dexamethasone
	Fluid retention; masculinization/feminization; hot flashes (sex hormones); hypertension; diabetes; adrenal insufficiency

Miscellaneous Drugs	
Asparaginase	Somnolence, lethargy, altered mental status; hypoproteinemia (including albumin and fibrinogen); hyperlipidemia, abnormal liver function tests, fatty metamorphosis of liver; pancreatitis (rare, common in children); azotemia; granulocytopenia, lymphopenia, thrombocytopenia (usually mild and transient), and hyperglycemia
Altretamine	Bone marrow depression; peripheral neuropathy
m-AMSA	Bone marrow depression; stomatitis; hepatic dysfunction; nausea and vomiting
Carmustine	Bone marrow depression; thrombocytopenia; nausea and vomiting
Lomustine	Bone marrow depression; thrombocytopenia; nausea and vomiting
Streptozocin	Hypoglycemia; nausea and vomiting
Mitotane	Skin eruptions; diarrhea; mental depression; muscle tremors; adrenal insufficiency; nausea and vomiting
Dacarbazine	Bone marrow depression; nausea and vomiting

Table 12-6	Examples of Chemotherapeutic Drugs—cont'd
Drug	**Major Toxicity**
Miscellaneous Drugs—cont'd	
Hydroxyurea	Bone marrow depression; nausea and vomiting
Etoposide	Alopecia; nausea and vomiting
Cisplatin	Bone marrow depression; renal tubular damage; deafness; nausea and vomiting
Carboplatin	Bone marrow depression; nausea and vomiting
Procarbazine	Bone marrow depression with leukopenia and thrombocytopenia; mental depression; nausea and vomiting
Vinblastine	Alopecia; areflexia; bone marrow depression
Vincristine	Areflexia; muscular weakness; peripheral neuritis; paralytic ileus; mild bone marrow depression
Levamisole	None
cis-Retinoic acid	Cheilitis; stomatitis; conjunctivitis
Paclitaxel	Leukopenia; peripheral neuropathy
Docetaxel	Leukopenia; peripheral neuropathy

tumor cells depends largely on its effect on the cell cycle (described in Chapter 1). Malignant tumors have three cellular compartments: (1) cells undergoing mitosis and cytokinesis, (2) cells capable of entering the cell cycle in the G_1 phase (see Figure 1-23), and (3) cells that do not divide and have irreversibly left the cell cycle (dying malignant cells, differentiated malignant cells, nonmalignant support cells). Cells in compartment 3 will die a natural death without chemotherapy. The specific aim of chemotherapy therefore is to kill cells from compartments 1 and 2—cells that are dividing and cells that are in interphase. Smaller tumors have a faster growth rate and generally are more sensitive to chemotherapy. Few cells in a large tumor are dividing, and as a result, these cells are largely insensitive to chemotherapy.

The development of resistance to one chemotherapeutic agent often results in the coincident development of resistance to other drugs, albeit structurally unrelated. Multidrug resistance is associated with the expression of a cell surface glycoprotein called *P-170*. Cells expressing P-170 have decreased uptake and increased efflux of the drugs to which they are resistant. Multidrug resistance–associated protein gene MRP/MRP1 and its family genes have been isolated and characterized.[57-59]

Radiation

The goals of ionizing radiation are (1) to eradicate cancer without producing excessive toxicity during treatment and (2) to avoid damage to normal structures. The application of radiation therefore requires precision and skillful application.

Ionizing radiation leads to damage of important macromolecules, especially deoxyribonucleic acid (DNA). The damage may be (1) lethal, in which the cell is killed; (2) potentially lethal, in which the cell is so severely affected by radiation that modifications in its environment will cause it to die; and (3) sublethal, in which the cell is damaged but subsequently can repair itself. Cellular compartments with rapidly renewing cells are, in general, more radiosensitive. (Cellular effects of ionizing radiation are discussed in Chapter 11.)

Surgery

Surgical therapy of cancer has several objectives. Surgical biopsy of a tumor often begins the treatment process, and intraoperative staging and sampling of adjacent lymph node regions define further therapy. **Sentinel nodes** are a limited set of lymph nodes that are first to receive drainage from any given location. Presumably, cancer metastasizes to these nodes before other nodes. Therefore, new techniques, such as sentinel node localization and biopsy, now allow less invasive tumor staging.[60]

Curative resections are performed if distant metastasis is not evident. If the tumor cannot be completely excised because of fear of causing undue morbidity, **debulking surgery** may be performed in which the majority of the tumor is removed, thereby allowing for increased success of adjuvant chemotherapy or irradiation. The goals of palliative surgery (alleviation without cure) are (1) prevention of symptoms that would have occurred if the individual were not treated and (2) relief of symptoms that are present. Surgery is indicated also for benign tumors that could progress into malignant tumors. Premalignant and in situ tumors of epithelial tissues, such as skin, mouth, and cervix, therefore are removed.

Hormonal Therapy

Hormonal therapy has been in use for a long time. Table 12-7 lists the commonly used hormonal agents and their primary indications. Their mechanism of action is presumed to include receptor activation or blockade, which interferes with intercellular growth and proliferation signaling cascades.

Immunotherapy

Chemotherapy and radiation treatments are the most common methods for managing cancer. Although these therapies are effective for certain types of cancer, they have drawbacks. In general, both therapies act by eliminating mitotically or metabolically active cells. Within a tumor mass, however, a significant portion of cells is in a part of the cell cycle that is

Table 12-7	Common Hormonal Agents and Types of Tumors
Agents	**Types of Tumors**
Corticosteroids	Leukemias
	Hodgkin disease
	Malignant lymphomas
	Breast cancer
	Multiple myeloma
Androgens	Breast cancer
Estrogens	Breast cancer
	Prostate cancer
Antiestrogens	Endometrial cancer
	Breast cancer
Aromatase inhibitors	Adrenal tumors
	Breast cancer
LH-RH analogs	Breast cancer
	Prostate cancer
Antiandrogens	Prostate cancer

LH, Luteinizing hormone; *RH,* releasing hormone.

Table 12-8	Classification of Biologic Response Modifiers
Major Classification	**Specific Examples**
Immunomodulating agents	Alkyl lysophospholipids
	BCG
	Bestatin
	Corynebacterium parvum
	Endotoxin
	Levamisole
	Muramyldipeptide
	Picibanil (OK432)
	Tuftsin
Interferons and interferon inducers	Interferons (alpha, beta, and gamma)
	Poly-ICLC
	Brucella abortus
	Viruses
Thymosins	Thymosin α_1
	Other thymosin factors
	Thymosin factor V
Antigens	Tumor-associated antigens
	Hapten-modified tumor antigens
	Vaccines
Effector cells	Macrophages
	Natural killer cells
	Cytotoxic T cells
	LAK cells
Lymphokines and cytokines	Colony-stimulating factors
	Lymphotoxin
	Interleukins (IL-1, IL-2, IL-3, etc.)
	Tumor necrosis factor
Colony-stimulating factors	G-CSF, GM-CSF, M-CSF, erythropoietin
Monoclonal antibodies	Cytotoxic antibodies
	Immunotoxins
	Phototoxins

BCG, Bacille Calmette-Guérin; *Poly-ICLC,* compound of poly-inosinic and poly-cytidylic and lysine; *LAK,* lymphokine-activated killer; *G-CSF,* granulocyte colony-stimulating factor; *GM-CSF,* granulocyte-macrophage colony-stimulating factor; *M-CSF,* macrophage colony-stimulating factor.

not affected by either metabolic inhibitors or mitotic poisons. In addition, these therapies have numerous side effects because they affect normal cell populations that, like transformed cells, have high rates of cell division. Cells of the gut epithelium, hair follicles, bone marrow, and gonads are affected by radiation and chemotherapy.

Because cancer is a dynamic disease in which the transformed cells in a tumor mass can adapt to changes in their environment, a single form of cancer therapy that is effective against all types of cancer may not be possible. More specific methods, however, eventually may eliminate transformed cells without damaging normal tissues.

In this regard, immunotherapy (immunologic treatment) holds promise. (The immune system is discussed in detail in Chapter 7.) First, the immune system has specificity for antigen recognition and is highly regulated; thus theoretically antitumor immune rejection responses can selectively eliminate cancer cells while sparing normal tissues. Second, immune memory cells are long lived and capable of providing extended protection, presumably against the emergence of recurrent primary tumor cells and foci of metastatic cancer cells. Third, numerous immunologic mechanisms are able to cause rejection of various types of cancer. Although tumor-immune surveillance can provide protection against cancer, certain evasive mechanisms allow tumor cells to escape immune rejection. Therefore current research efforts for establishing effective anticancer immunotherapies focus on characterizing the immunogenic properties of various tumor-specific antigens and developing methods to selectively enhance tumor rejection immune responses.

Immunotherapies for the treatment of cancer generally are referred to as **biologic response modifiers (BRMs)**. BRMs are mammalian gene products, agents, and clinical protocols that affect biologic responses in host/tumor interactions. BRMs have the following actions:

1. A direct cytotoxic effect on cancer cells
2. The initiation or augmentation of the host's tumor-immune rejection response

3. The modification of cancer cell susceptibility to the lytic or tumor-static effects of the immune system

The major classifications of BRMs are presented in Table 12-8. The basis of action and clinical applications of specific BRMs, selected from among the major classifications, are discussed briefly in the remainder of this section.

Immunomodulating Agents

Nonspecific stimulation of the immune system by an adjuvant (a substance that enhances the immune response) has been attempted in individuals with a variety of different cancers (Figure 12-12). This therapy consists of the administration of an adjuvant (a bacterium), such as *Corynebacterium parvum* or bacille Calmette-Guérin (BCG), an attenuated strain of *Mycobacterium bovis*. Bacterial cell wall extracts, live BCG, or nonviable *C. parvum* is injected at the tumor site. Retardation of tumor growth results through the activation of macrophages, augmentation of natural killer cells, or by some

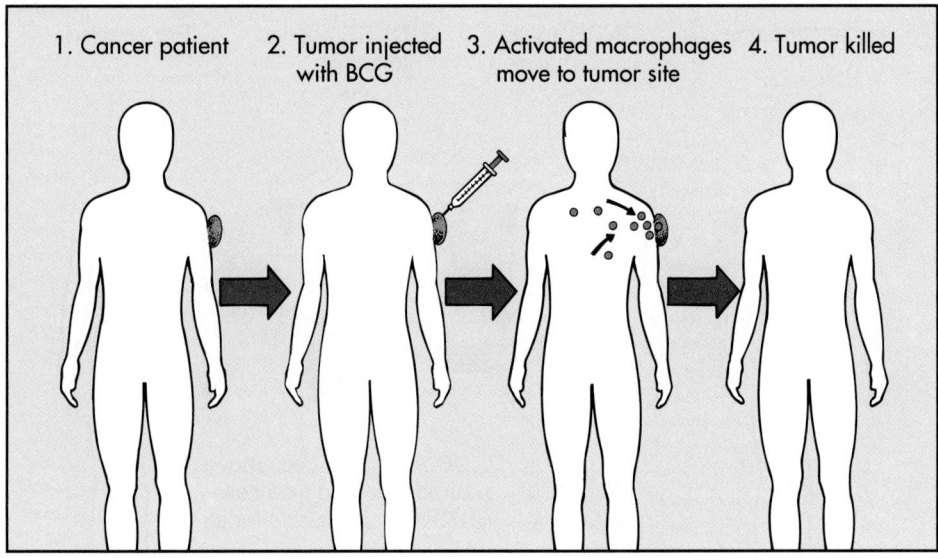

Figure 12-12 Immunostimulation in cancer therapy. *BCG*, Bacille Calmette-Guérin.

degree of antigenic cross-reactivity between the organism (BCG) and the antigen produced by certain human cancers, such as melanomas.

Some success has been observed in the treatment of genitourinary and lung cancer, usually through combined adjuvant treatments and chemotherapies. The most effective use of this type of immunotherapy, however, has been in the treatment of skin cancers.

Interferons

The interferons are a family of cell-derived proteins that have antiviral and immune modulating activities. The most successful clinical trials have come from the use of interferon-α. Interferon-α is a glycoprotein made by activated leukocytes. In addition to its antiviral activity, interferon-α inhibits tumor growth, enhances natural killer cell activity, and increases cancer cell expression of tumor antigens, thus making them more immunogenic (i.e., eliciting stronger tumor-immune rejection responses). Used either alone or in combination with other treatment modalities, interferon-α has been effective in the treatment of hairy cell leukemia, Kaposi sarcoma (a common cancer of persons with acquired immunodeficiency syndrome [AIDS]), and renal cell carcinoma. Similarly, interferon-α is effective for treating ovarian carcinoma when used after surgical removal of the tumor mass.[61] The use of interferons in cancer therapy is greatly enhanced by the ability to produce these biologic agents by recombinant gene-cloning techniques.

Antigens

Some success in treating skin tumors has been obtained by the application of contact sensitizing agents (materials that cause a hypersensitivity response in the skin), such as dinitrochlorobenzene (DNCB) (see Figure 12-13). With this approach the individual is first sensitized to DNCB through topical application to normal skin, and the tumor is subsequently painted with DNCB.

Tumor regression is thought to occur by inducing a contact hypersensitivity response to the DNCB at the tumor site. (Hypersensitivity reactions are discussed in Chapter 8.) Tumor cells probably are killed because DNCB has become associated with their cell surface and functions as an antigen. This type of therapy, however, is restricted to superficial tumors of the skin.

Research efforts are underway to identify tumor-specific antigens (the various types of antigens are described in Chapter 11) that could be used to develop anticancer vaccines. Ideally, common tumor antigens expressed by a wide range of cancers could be developed as vaccines. These vaccines could be used either as immunotherapies to augment the host's immune response against the tumor or as preventive immunization techniques for inhibiting cancer emergence in populations at risk.

Effector Cells and Lymphokines

Theoretically, an effective form of cellular immunotherapy would result from the transfer or augmentation of cytotoxic T cells (Tc cells) that are specific for the antigens expressed by the individual's tumor cells[62] (Figure 12-14). Because this represents such an attractive form of immunotherapy for cancer, a treatment protocol has been established and is undergoing extensive clinical trials. It is known as *lymphokine-activated killer (LAK) cell therapy*. The idea is to establish tumor-specific cytotoxic cell lines in tissue culture that can mediate tumor rejection when injected back into the cancer patient. The procedure takes advantage of the ability to expand LAK cells in vitro by growing them in tissue culture medium that contains interleukin-2, the T cell growth factor. LAK cells are phenotypically distinct from T lymphocytes. When injected into the patient, LAK cells are able to infiltrate the tumor and mediate lysis of cancer cells. LAK cell therapy usually is combined with interleukin-2 treatment, which is believed to both maintain LAK cell activity and enhance other antitumor im-

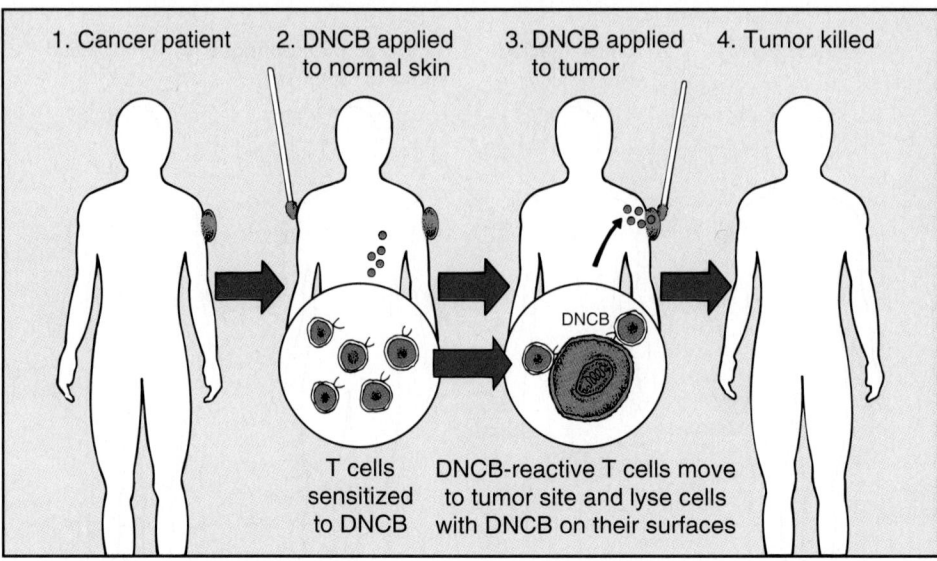

Figure 12-13 Cancer therapy through antigen modification with dinitrochlorobenzene (DNCB).

mune rejection mechanisms. Some success has been obtained by interleukin-2 treatment alone[63] or in combination with chemotherapy.[64] LAK cell therapy has been used successfully in the treatment of melanoma and renal cell carcinoma.

Monoclonal Antibodies

The development of monoclonal antibody technology has provided a method for generating highly specific antibody reagents that could not otherwise be obtained with traditional antisera. (Monoclonal antibodies are discussed in Chapter 7.) These reagents have a promising future in both the diagnosis and treatment of human cancer (Figure 12-15).

In the past, clinicians have relied on a number of methods to diagnose human cancers. For example, in the case of most skin cancers, the diagnosis can be made by visual examination of the lesion. In contrast, the diagnosis of various soft tissue cancers, such as lung tumors, may require the identification of certain clinical signs (e.g., obstruction, bleeding, pain). Cytologic methods (e.g., Papanicolaou [Pap] test) or histologic analysis of cells also can be used to diagnose various types of cancer. These diagnoses generally are confirmed by tissue biopsies and pathologic evaluations. The major problems associated with these diagnostic methods are that some tests can give false results or may detect only tumor masses that have become too large to be removed surgically, that have invaded and destroyed surrounding tissues and organs, or that have metastasized to secondary sites.

Monoclonal antibodies have been developed and used as diagnostic reagents for detecting cancer because their high specificity for antigen could reduce the number of false re-

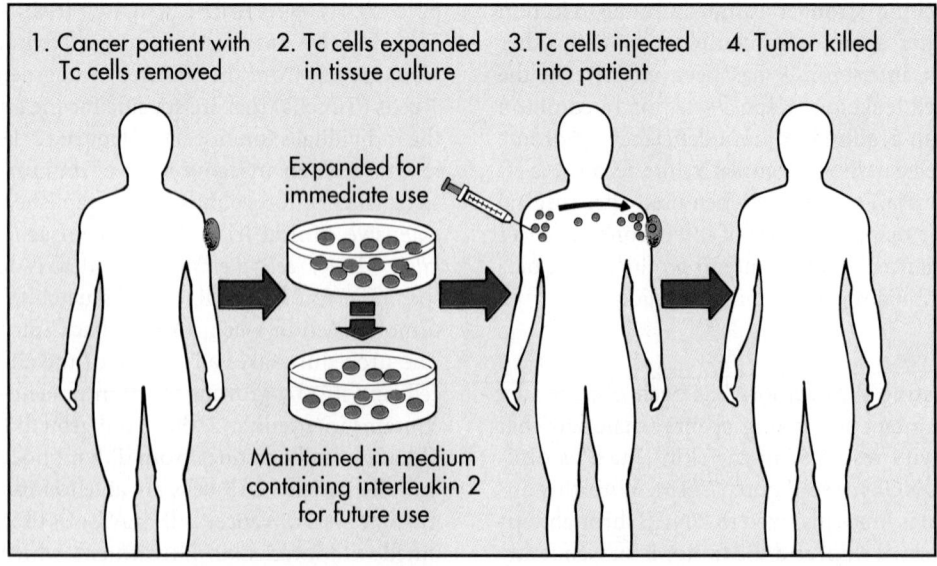

Figure 12-14 Development of cytotoxic T cell (Tc cell) lines for cancer immunotherapy.

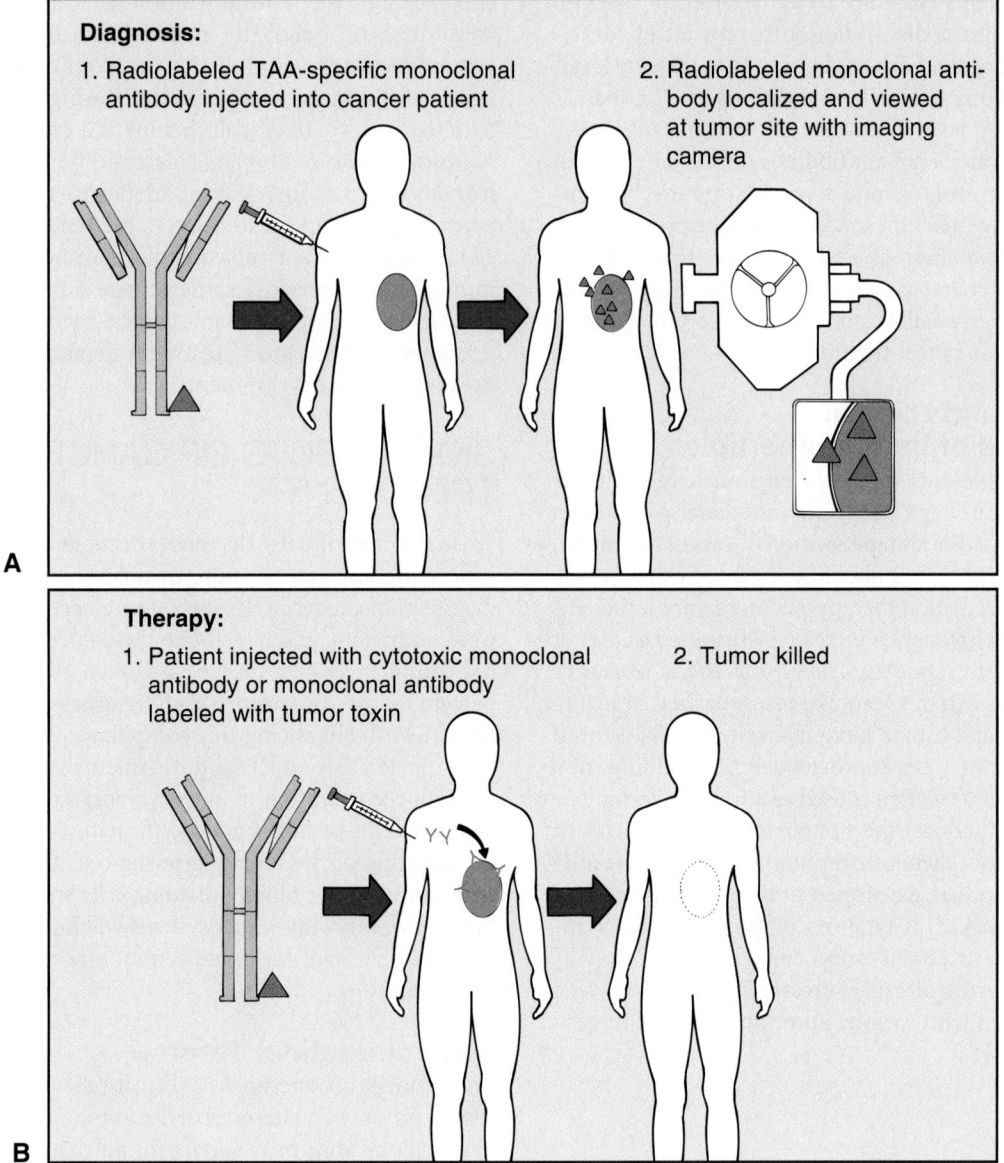

Diagnosis:

1. Radiolabeled TAA-specific monoclonal antibody injected into cancer patient

2. Radiolabeled monoclonal antibody localized and viewed at tumor site with imaging camera

A

Therapy:

1. Patient injected with cytotoxic monoclonal antibody or monoclonal antibody labeled with tumor toxin

2. Tumor killed

B

Figure 12-15 **Monoclonal antibodies. A,** Tumor immunodiagnosis. **B,** Cancer immunotherapy with monoclonal antibodies. *TAA,* Tumor-associated antigen.

sults. Coupled with the appropriate laboratory or clinical assay system, monoclonal antibodies may provide methods for earlier detection of neoplastic disease. For example, highly purified monoclonal antibodies could be used to detect circulating tumor antigens in the individual's serum and thus provide a method for periodic screening of persons at high risk for the development of a specific type of cancer. Monoclonal antibodies, when bound to a radionuclide (radioactive material), also could be used for radiologic imaging (a diagnostic process for detecting radioactive deposits in tissues). Such techniques could help in diagnosing both primary tumors and metastases in persons suspected of having disease.

Another goal is to develop monoclonal antibodies specific for tumor antigens that would mediate tumor rejection with-

out affecting normal tissues. Monoclonal antibodies have been most successful in use against hematologic and lymphatic malignancies. Certain acute myelogenous leukemia cells express the surface protein CD33, which is targeted by the antibody gemtuzumab.[65] Non-Hodgkin lymphomas expressing the CD20 surface antigen have been successfully targeted with rituximab.[66] This work is now expanding into solid-tumor immunotherapy with encouraging trials of trastuzumab for breast cancer cells expressing the Her-2 antigen.[67] The majority of these antibodies are being used in protocols incorporating standard, cytotoxic chemotherapy. A current focus of research involves **conjugated antibodies,** in which radioisotopes or toxins are attached to the antibody, thus delivering very specific doses of radiation or toxic agents to involved tissues.[68-71]

The major problems currently being faced in the attempt to use monoclonal antibodies in cancer therapy are (1) developing functional reagents with the appropriate antigen specificities; (2) overcoming clinical complications that are associated with injecting large amounts of foreign antibodies (currently, most monoclonal antibodies can be made only in rodents); and (3) controlling immunoregulatory mechanisms that would eliminate their efficacy. Certainly the potential use of monoclonal antibodies, as well as other forms of immunotherapy, has generated new interest in immune surveillance mechanisms as possible methods for development of immunotherapies for cancer treatment.

Applications and Clinical Complications of Immunotherapies

Immunotherapy represents the so-called fourth modality of cancer treatment. Although some immunotherapy protocols are designed to be used as a single method of cancer treatment, it should be appreciated that, like other types of cancer treatment (i.e., surgery, radiation therapy, chemotherapy), the efficacy of immunotherapy may be increased when used as part of a combined treatment modality. The typical effects of cancer treatment on the growth of a tumor are summarized in Figure 12-16. Typically, a solid tumor is not clinically detectable until it has reached a size of 1 cm, approximately 30 doublings of a transformed cell. Surgery often is used as a method to remove or debulk (partially reduce) the tumor mass. Other forms of therapy (i.e., radiation, chemical, immunologic) would be used to prevent clinical recurrence of the tumor mass or growth of metastatic tumor foci. This type of combined modality approach can lead to a successful cancer cure.

As with other forms of cancer treatment, numerous side effects are associated with various immunotherapies. In general, during the administration of the immunotherapy (regardless of type) the patients usually manifest flulike symptoms (i.e., fever, chills, nausea, vomiting, headache). Urticaria and skin rashes often occur during the treatment. Associated with the LAK cell therapy is a condition referred to as *vascular-leak syndrome*. This condition appears to result from the effect of interleukin-2 that causes increased vascular permeability. Thus, in addition to the symptoms listed, severe edema and cardiovascular hypotension occur. Although immunotherapies produce some adverse side effects and require extensive administration and clinical management, their potential benefit in cancer treatment demands their continued use and further development.

SIDE EFFECTS OF CANCER TREATMENT

To many individuals, the side effects and complications of cancer therapy can be quite troublesome, often rivaling the diagnosis of cancer itself. Special care needs to be directed toward addressing and alleviating these effects because individual compliance with therapy is directly linked to a person's perception of discomfort and treatment-related complications. Key to enhancing this compliance is education regarding expected side effects and treatments to alleviate them.

With the exception of surgery, most side effects can be attributed to the relatively nonspecific nature of cancer therapy—the targeting of the rapidly growing cell. Therefore organ systems consisting of rapidly dividing cells are targeted as well as the cancer. Knowing which systems will be affected allows prediction of some of the more common general therapy-related side effects.

Gastrointestinal Tract

The entire gastrointestinal (GI) tract relies on rapidly growing cells to produce an effective barrier to trauma and infection and to provide an absorptive surface for nutrients. Both chemotherapy and radiation therapy may cause a decreased cell turnover, thereby leading to oral ulcers (stomatitis), malabsorption, and diarrhea. The disruption of barrier defenses also increases the risk for infection, especially invasion by a person's own GI flora. Therapy-induced nausea, thought to be caused by an agent's direct action upon the central nervous system's vomiting centers, historically has been a major obstacle in therapy.

Aggressive antinausea (antiemetic) therapy, including the centrally acting serotonin 5-HT3 antagonists, such as ondansetron or dolasetron, have allowed better tolerance of highly emetogenic protocols. Other popular antiemetics include steroids and phenothiazines. Synthetic cannabinoids, the active ingredients in marijuana, increase appetite in addition to having antinausea properties. Analgesia often includes opiate agents, vital in treating severe cases of mucosal lesions. Supplemental nutrition through enteral or parenteral routes may be needed to combat malnutrition. Good oral care and close attention to hygiene may help prevent complications arising from mucosal membrane breakdown.

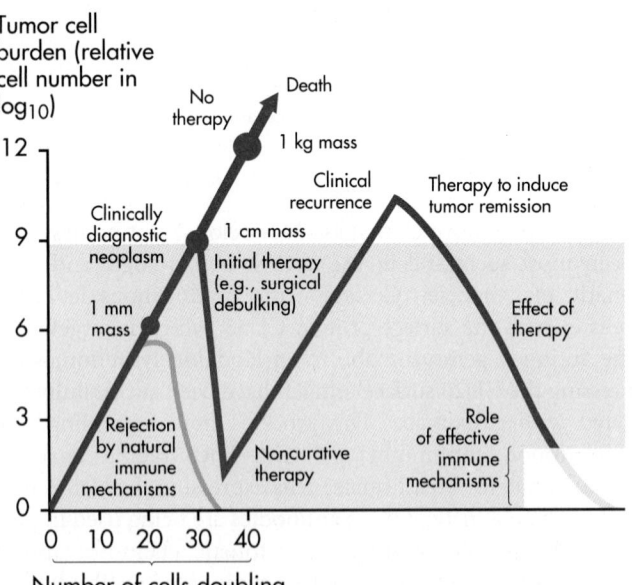

Figure 12-16 Relationship between tumor cell burden and phases of cancer treatment.

Bone Marrow

Chemotherapy is the usual offending agent causing bone marrow suppression, although radiation therapy also may contribute to suppression, especially if the two therapies are used together. The timing of suppression often can be predicted based on what agent is used. All three cell lines are usually affected (i.e., red blood cells, white blood cells, and platelets) (see anemia, p. 388). The anemia caused by red cell suppression may contribute to the generalized fatigue of the person with cancer and may require transfusion depending on the severity of the anemia or other comorbid medical conditions. Decreased platelet numbers may increase a person's tendency to spontaneously bleed and require transfusion as well. Perhaps the most potentially serious side effect is that of white blood cell suppression (neutropenia), creating for the person who already has weakened host immune defenses an even greater risk of infection. The risk of infection increases with both greater degrees of and prolonged durations of neutropenia. This infection risk mandates immediate evaluation of fever and initiation of antibiotic medication until the infection is disproved.

Red blood cell and platelet transfusions are routinely used in supportive care of marrow suppression; white blood cell transfusions are not. The development of recombinant human stimulatory cytokines are often used to stimulate the body's own regeneration of cells. These parenterally administered medications include granulocyte colony-stimulating factor (G-CSF) or granulocyte-macrophage colony-stimulating factor (GM-CSF) to aid in recovery of white blood cells, erythro-poietin to stimulate red cell production, and thrombopoietin to stimulate platelet recovery (see Chapter 25).

Hair and Skin

Alopecia (hair loss) results from chemotherapy effects on hair follicles. Alopecia is usually temporary, although hair may grow back with a different texture initially. Not all chemotherapeutic agents cause alopecia. Decreased renewal rates of the epidermal layers in the skin may lead to skin breakdown and dryness, altering the normal barrier protection against infection. Radiation therapy may cause skin erythema (redness) and contribute to breakdown.

Reproductive Tract

Radiation therapy and chemotherapy may affect the gametes, leading to varying degrees of decreased fertility and premature menopause. These effects are dose- and age-dependent, with the prepubertal gonad thought to be more resistant to damage. The potential for harm is also dependent on the agent used, with the alkylating category of chemotherapies carrying the greatest risk. Craniospinal irradiation for central nervous system tumors also may affect the hypothalamus or pituitary gland, with subsequent secondary gonadal failure because of lack of production of gonadotropin-releasing hormone, luteinizing hormone, and follicle-stimulating hormone. The potential for reproductive harm should be addressed before therapy, if possible, with provisions made for sperm or embryo banking (also see Chapter 11).

SUMMARY REVIEW

Historical Theories of Cancer Invasion

1. Historical analysis of theories of cancer invasion and metastasis began with the black bile diffusion theory of Hippocrates and later included such theories as the cellular-embolic theory and the seed-versus-soil theory.
2. Today the emphasis is on the biochemical mechanisms of metastasis, including control of proliferation, cell-cell and cell-matrix interaction, angiogenesis, migration, invasion, and dissemination.

Tumor Spread

1. Tumor spread takes several forms: (a) direct invasion, (b) metastasis of distant organs by lymphatics and veins, and (c) metastasis by implantation.
2. Invasion is the first step in the metastatic process. Mechanisms of local invasion include (a) cellular multiplication, (b) mechanical pressure, (c) release of lytic enzymes, (d) decreased adhesion (slipperiness), and (e) increased motility.
3. Recent view of invasion is disruption of the tumor-host microenvironment. Tumor cells can survive by recruiting growth factors from the extracellular matrix and using them to suppress apoptosis, stimulate tissue invasion, and promote angiogenesis. The matrix and tumor cells exchange enzymes and cytokines creating a permissive field for the cancerous cell.
4. The three-step theory of invasion includes (a) tumor cell attachment to the matrix, (b) degradation or dissolution of the matrix, and (c) tumor cell locomotion.
5. Locomotion seems to be influenced by chemotactic factors.
6. Metastasis is the life-threatening characteristic of malignancy. The sequential steps include (1) direct or continuous exten-

sion; (2) penetration into lymphatics, blood vessels, or body cavities; (3) release into lymph or blood; (4) transport to secondary sites; and (5) entry and growth into secondary sites. These mechanisms are not mutually exclusive.
7. Tumor growth is supported by the development of new blood vessels, a process called *angiogenesis*. Several angiogenic factors have been identified, including VEGF, PDGF, TGF-α, bFGF, and angiopoietins.
8. Tissue factor produced by tumor cells has been implicated in the regulation of the "angiogenic switch" regulating the balance of positive and negative angiogenic factors.
9. If mutations occur in the *p53* gene, cells have lost their "emergency brake" against uncontrolled cell growth. These cells do not undergo apoptosis; they survive and may be the strongest and most aggressive cells of the tumor.
10. Tumor staging involves the size of the tumor, the degree to which it has locally invaded, and the extent to which it has spread. A standard scheme for staging is the T (tumor spread), N (node involvement), and M (metastasis) system.

Clinical Manifestations of Cancer

1. Clinical manifestations of cancer include pain, cachexia, anemia, leukopenia, thrombocytopenia, and infection.
2. Pain generally is associated with the late stages of cancer. It can be caused by pressure, obstruction, invasion of a structure sensitive to pain, stretching, tissue destruction, and inflammation.
3. Fatigue is the most frequently reported symptom of cancer and cancer treatment.

Continued

4. Cachexia (loss of appetite, early satiety, weakness, inability to maintain weight, taste alterations; altered metabolism) leads to protein-calorie malnutrition and progressive wasting.
5. Anemia associated with cancer usually occurs because of malnutrition, chronic bleeding and resultant iron deficiency, chemotherapy, radiation, and malignancies in the blood-forming organs.
6. Leukopenia is usually a result of chemotherapy (which is toxic to bone marrow) or radiation (which kills circulating leukocytes).
7. Thrombocytopenia is usually the result of chemotherapy or malignancy in the bone marrow.
8. Infection may be caused by leukopenia, immunosuppression, or debility associated with advanced disease. It is the most significant cause of complications and death.
9. Recent data provide a mechanistic framework of symptom onset as mediated by cytokines acting on the peripheral and central nervous systems.
10. Paraneoplastic syndromes are symptom complexes that cannot be explained by the local or distant spread of the tumor or by hormones released by the tissue from which the tumor arose.

Cancer Treatment

1. Cancer is treated with surgery, radiation therapy, chemotherapy, immunotherapy, and combinations of these modalities.
2. The theoretic basis of chemotherapy is the vulnerability of tumor cells in various stages of the cell cycle. The goal of chemotherapy is to eradicate enough tumor cells so that the body's natural defenses can eradicate remaining cells.
3. Ionizing radiation causes cell damage, so that the goal of radiation therapy is to damage the tumor without causing excessive toxicity or damage to undiseased structures.
4. Surgical therapy is used for nonmetastatic disease, for which cure is possible by removing the tumor, and as a palliative measure to alleviate symptoms.
5. Immunotherapy is appropriate for cancers that cannot be effectively managed by chemotherapy or radiation, usually because enough tumor cells are inactive and invulnerable to these modalities.
6. Forms of immunotherapy known as biologic response modifiers include immunomodulating agents, interferons, antigens, effector cells, lymphokines, and monoclonal antibodies.
7. Effector cells and lymphokines provide a form of cellular immunotherapy that involves the transfer of cytotoxic T cells (Tc cells) that are specific for tumor cell antigens.

8. Immunomodulating agents provide nonspecific stimulation of the immune system by means of an adjuvant; they are most effective in treating skin cancers.
9. Antigens cause regression in skin tumors by producing a hypersensitivity response that affects the antigenic properties of the cell surface.
10. Monoclonal antibodies ultimately may be used both as diagnostic reagents for detecting cancer and as a form of cancer therapy in which antibodies specific for tumor antigens would mediate tumor rejection.

Side Effects of Cancer Treatment

1. Special care is needed to address and alleviate side effects because individual compliance with therapy is directly linked to a person's perception of discomfort and complications.
2. Key to increasing compliance is appropriate education about the side effects and treatments.
3. Most side effects are directly related to the targeting of the rapidly growing cell.
4. Both chemotherapy and radiation therapy may cause a decreased cell turnover leading to oral ulcers, malabsorption, and diarrhea.
5. Disruption of barrier defenses in the gastrointestinal tract increases risk for infection.
6. Nausea is thought to be caused by an agent's direct action on the vomiting center in the central nervous system. Thus aggressive treatment with antiemetic therapy is mandated.
7. Chemotherapy can cause bone marrow suppression of all three cell lines, red, white, and platelets. Anemia is common with red cell suppression, decreased platelet numbers can increase bleeding, and decreased white blood cells increases the risk of infection.
8. Hair loss (alopecia) results from chemotherapy effects on hair follicles. Alopecia is usually temporary and not all agents cause it.
9. Radiation and chemotherapy may affect the gametes, leading to varying degrees of decreased fertility and premature menopause. These effects are dose- and age-dependent, with the prepubertal gonad thought to be more resistant to damage.
10. Craniospinal irradiation for central nervous system tumors may affect the hypothalamus or pituitary gland resulting in gonadal failure.

KEY TERMS

Acute phase response (APR), 387
Angiogenesis, 383
Anoikis, 377
Biologic response modifiers (BRMs), 394
Cachexia, 387
Cathepsin B, 378
Cathepsin D, 378
Clinical staging, 385
Combination chemotherapy, 389
Conjugated antibodies, 397
Debulking surgery, 393

E-cadherin, 378
Fatigue, 387
Invasion, 376
Laminin receptors, 381
Metastasis, 381
Organ tropism, 384
p53 protein, 384
Paraneoplastic syndromes, 388
Primary (neoadjuvant) chemotherapy, 390
Primary tumors, 381
Principle of dose intensity, 389

Sentinel nodes, 393
Single agent chemotherapy, 389
Therapeutic index, 390
Thrombospondin, 383
Tissue factor (TF), 383
Tissue-selective homing receptors, 384
Tumor-host microenvironment, 377
Type IV collagenase, 378
Urokinase-type plasminogen activator (uPA), 378

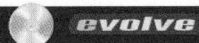
REFERENCES

1. Woodhouse EC, Chuaqui RF, Liotta LA: General mechanisms of metastasis, *Cancer* 80(8 suppl):1529-1537, 1997.
2. Liotta LA, Clair T: Cancer. Check point for invasion, *Nature* 405(6784):287-288, 2000.
3. Chung LW et al: Molecular insights into prostate cancer progression: the missing link of tumor microenvironment, *J Urol* 173(1):10-20, 2005.
4. Nilsson E, Skinner MK: Cellular interactions that control primordial follicle development and folliculogenesis, *J Soc Gynecol Investig* 8(1 Suppl Proceedings):S17-20, 2001.
5. Huang EJ, Reichardt LF: Trk receptors: roles in neuronal signal transduction, *Annu Rev Biochem* 72:609-672, review, 2003.
6. Douma S et al: Suppression of anoikis and induction of metastasis by the neutrophic receptor TrkB, *Nature* 430(70030:1034-1039, 2004.
7. Bardelli A et al: Mutational analysis of the tyrosine kinome in colorectal cancer, *Science* 200(5621):949, 2003.
8. Brodeur GM: Neuroblastoma: biological insights into a clinical enigma, *Nat Rev Cancer* 3(3):203-216, 2003.
9. Liotta LA, Kohn EC: The microenvironment of the tumour-host interface, *Nature* 411(6835):375-379, 2001.
10. Mandriota SJ et al: Vascular endothelial growth factor increases urokinase receptor expression in vascular endothelial cells, *J Biol Chem* 270(17):9709-9716, 1995.
11. Mignatti P, Rifkin DB: Biology and biochemistry of proteinases in tumor invasion, *Physiol Rev* 73(1):161-195, 1993.
12. McCawley LJ, Matrisian LM: Matrix metalloproteinases: multifunctional contributors to tumor progression, *Mol Med Today* 6(4):149-156, 2000.
13. Hubbard SM, Liotta LA: The biology of metastases. In Baird SB, McCorkle R et al, editors: *Cancer nursing: a comprehensive textbook,* ed 2, Philadelphia, 1996, Saunders.
14. Duffy MJ et al: Urokinase plasminogen activator: a prognostic marker in multiple types of cancer, *J Surg Oncol* 71(2):130-135, 1999.
15. Aguirre Ghiso JA et al: Deregulation of the signaling pathways controlling urokinase production: its relationship with the invasive phenotype, *Eur J Biochem* 263(2):295-304, 1999.
16. Woodhouse EC, Chuaqui Rf, Liotta LA: General mechanisms of metastasis, *Cancer* 80(8 suppl):1529-1537, 1997.
17. Qian X et al: E-cadherin-mediated adhesion inhibits ligand-dependent activation of diverse receptor tyrosine kinases, *EMBO J* 23(8): 1739-1784, 2004.
18. Wells A: Tumor invasion: role of growth factor-induced cell motility, *Adv Cancer Res* 78:31101, 2000.
19. Ziober BL, Lin CS, Kramer RH: Laminin-binding integrins in tumor progression and metastasis, *Semin Cancer Biol* 7(3):119-128, 1996.
20. Muller A et al: Involvement of chemokine receptors in breast cancer metastasis, *Nature* 410(6824):50-56, 2001.
21. Zhou T, Sargiannidou I, Tuszynski GP: The role of adhesive proteins in the hematogenous spread of cancer, *In Vivo* 14(1):199-208, 2000.
22. Fidler IJ, Gersten DM, Hart IR: The biology of cancer invasion and metastasis, *Adv Cancer Res* 28:149-250, 1978.
23. Folkman J, Kalluri R: Cancer without disease, *Nature* 427(6977):787, 2004.
24. Folkman J et al: Isolation of a tumor factor responsible for angiogenesis, *J Exp Med* 133(2):275-288, 1971.
25. Anan K et al: Vascular endothelial growth factor and platelet-derived growth factor are potential angiogenic and metastatic factors in human breast cancer, *Surgery* 119(3):333-339, 1996.
26. Griffioen AW, Molema G: Angiogenesis: potentials for pharmacologic intervention in the treatment of cancer, cardiovascular diseases, and chronic inflammation, *Pharmacol Revl* 52(2):237-268, 2000.
27. Abdulkadir SA et al: Tissue factor expression and angiogenesis in human prostate carcinoma, *Hum Pathol* 31(4):443-447, 2000.
28. Lahav J: The functions of thrombospondin and its involvement in physiology and pathophysiology, *Biochem Biophys Acta* 1182(1):1-14, 1993.
29. Iruela-Arispe ML, Vazquez F, Ortega MA: Antiangiogenic domains shared by thrombospondins and metallospondins, a new family of angiogenic inhibitors, *Ann N Y Acad Sci* 886:58-66, 1999.
30. Maeda K et al: Expression of vascular endothelial growth factor and thrombospondia-1 in colorectal carcinoma, *Int J Mol Med* 5(4):373-378, 2000.
31. Hagedorn M, Bikfalui A: Target molecules for anti-angiogenic therapy: from basic research to clinical trials, *Crit Rev Oncol Hematol* 34(2): 89-110, 2000.
32. Graeber TG et al: Hypoxia-mediated selection of cells with diminished apoptotic potential in solid tumors, *Nature* 379(6560):88-91, 1996.
33. Seachrist L: Only the strong survive: the evolution of a tumor favors the meanest, most aggressive cells, *Sci News* 149:216, 1996.
34. Gohji K et al: Organ-site dependence for the production of urokinase-type plasminogen activator and metastasis by human renal cell carcinoma cells, *Am J Pathol* 151(6):1655-1661, 1997.
35. Fidler IJ et al: Modulation of tumor cell response to chemotherapy by the organ environment, *Cancer Metastasis Rev* 13(2):209-222, 1994.
36. Cleeland CS et al: Are the symptoms of cancer and cancer treatment due to a shared biologic mechanism A cytokine-immunologic model of cancer symptoms, *Cancer* 97(11):2919-2925, 2003.
37. Haigh C: Contribution of a multidisciplinary team to pain management, *Br J Nurs* 10(6):370-374, 2001.
38. Cherny NI: The management of cancer pain, *CA Cancer J Clin* 50(2): 70, 2000.
39. Payne JK: A neuroendocrine-based regulatory fatigue model, *Biol Res Nurs* 6(2):141-150, 2004.
40. Winningham ML et al: Fatigue and the cancer experience: the state of the knowledge, *Oncol Nurs Forum* 21(1):23, 1994.
41. Nelson KA: The cancer anorexia-cachexia syndrome, *Semin Oncol* 27(1):64-68, 2000.
42. Tisdale MJ: Pathogenesis of cancer cachexia, *J Support Oncol* 1(3): 259-268, 2003.
43. Muscaritoli M et al: Metal therapy of muscle wasting in cancer: what is the future? *Curr Opin Clin Nutr Metab Care* 7(4):159-168, 2004.
44. Habtemariam S: Natural inhibitors of tumor necrosis factor-alpha production, secretion and function, *Planta Med* 66(4):303, 2000.
45. Kapadia SR: Cytokines and heart failure, *Cardiol Rev* 7(4):196-206, 1999.
46. Yeh SS, Schuster MW: Geriatric cachexia: the role of cytokines, *Am J Clin Nutr* 70(2):183-197, 1999.
47. Erslev AJ: Erythropoietin and anemia of cancer, *Eur J Haematol* 64(6):353-358, 2000.
48. Bragga M et al: Erythropoiesis after therapy with recombinant human erythropoietin: a dose-response study in anemic cancer surgery patients, *Vox Sang* 76(1):38, 1999.
49. Gargano G et al: The utility of a growth factor: rHuEPO as a treatment for preoperation autologous blood donation in gynecological tumor surgery, *Int J Oncol* 14(1):157-160, 1999.
50. Sabatini P: The relationship between anemia and quality of life in cancer patients, *Oncologist* 5(suppl 2):19, 2000.
51. Farber S et al: Temporary remissions in acute leukemia in children produced by folic acid antagonist 4-aminopteroylglutamic acid (aminopterin), *N Engl J Med* 28:787-789, 1948.
52. Hammond GD: Keynote address: the cure of childhood cancers, *Cancer* 58(suppl):407-411, 1986.
53. Henderson EH, Samaha RJ: Evidence that drugs in multiple combinations have materially advanced the treatment of human malignancies, *Cancer Res* 29:2272-2275, 1969.
54. Hryniuk W, Bush H: The importance of dose intensity in chemotherapy of metastatic breast cancer, *J Clin Oncol* 2:1281-1285, 1984.
55. Young RC: Mechanisms to improve chemotherapy effectiveness, *Cancer* 65(suppl):815-818, 1990.
56. Trimble EL et al: Neoadjuvant therapy in cancer treatment, *Cancer* 72:3515-3521, 1993.
57. Kumano M et al: Multidrug resistance-associated protein subfamily transporters and drug resistance, *Anticancer Drug Des* 14(2):123, 1999.
58. Roepe PD: What is the precise role of human MDR1 protein in chemotherapeutic drug resistance? *Curr Pharm Des* 6(3):241-260, 2000.
59. Sikic BI: New approaches in cancer treatment, *Ann Oncol* 10(suppl 6):149-153, 1999.

60. Krag D: Sentinel lymph node biopsy for the detection of metastases, *Cancer J Sci Am* 6(suppl 2):S121, 2000.

61. Colombo N et al: Antitumor and immunomodulatory activity of intraperitoneal IFN-gamma in ovarian carcinoma patients with minimal residual tumor after chemotherapy, *Int J Cancer* 51:42, 1992.

62. Appelbaum JW: The role of the immune system in the pathogenesis of cancer, *Semin Oncol Nurs* 8(1):51-62, 1992.

63. Melioli G et al: Perilymphatic injections of recombinant interleukin-2 (rIL-2) partially correct the immunologic defects in patients with advanced head and neck squamous cell carcinoma, *Laryngoscope* 102(5):572-578, 1992.

64. Mitchell MS: Chemotherapy in combination with biomodulation: a 5-year experience with cyclophosphamide and interleukin-2, *Semin Oncol* 19(2 Suppl 4):80-87, 1992.

65. Bernstein ID: Monoclonal antibodies to the myeloid stem cells: therapeutic implications of CMA-676, a humanized anti-CD33 antibody calicheamicin conjugate, *Leukemia* 14(3):474-475, 2000.

66. Maloney DG et al: IDEC-C2B8 (rituximab) anti-CD20 monoclonal antibody therapy in patients with relapsed low-grade non-Hodgkins lymphoma, *Blood* 90(6):2188-2195, 1997.

67. Goldenberg MM: Trastuzumab, a recombinant DNA-derived humanized monoclonal antibody, a novel agent for the treatment of metastatic breast cancer, *Clin Ther* 21(2):309-318, 1999.

68. Hursey M et al: Specifically targeting the CD22 receptor of human B-cell lymphomas with RNA damaging agents: a new generation of therapeutics, *Leuk Lymphoma* 43(5):953-959, 2002.

69. Krasner C, Joyce RM: Zevalin: 90yttrium labeled anti-CD20 (ibritumomab tiuxetan), a new treatment for non-Hodgkin's lymphoma, *Curr Pharm Biotechnol* 2(4):341-349, 2001.

70. Kreitman RJ: Toxin-labelled monoclonal antibodies, *Curr Pharm Biotechnol* 2(4):313-325, 2001.

71. Talmadge JE: Development of immunotherapeutic strategies for the treatment of malignant neoplasms, *Biotherapy* 4(3):215-236, 1992.

CANCER IN CHILDREN

ELIZABETH KASSNER • RENEE A. KLENKE

evolve

http://evolve.elsevier.com/McCance/

CHAPTER OUTLINE

Cancer in children is rare, but because so many other diseases of childhood have been conquered, cancer is now the second leading cause of death in children who have survived their first year.[1] (Trauma remains the leading killer of children and adolescents.) The unique feature of childhood cancers is the short latency time, which contrasts sharply with the long latency period common in adults. In addition, cancers among adults are categorized by the anatomic site of the primary tumor, and cancers in children are categorized by histology.[2] Table 13-1 summarizes the differences between childhood and adult cancers.

INCIDENCE AND TYPES

Both incidence rate and types of cancer that develop vary between children and adults. In 2000, approximately 10,500 children less than 20 years of age were diagnosed with cancer.[3] An estimated 9200 new cases are expected to occur among children aged less than 1 year to 14 years old in 2004, whereas approximately 1.4 million adults are expected to be diagnosed with cancer in the same year.[1,4] It is estimated that in the year 2010, 1 in every 250 persons will be a survivor of childhood cancer.[5,6]

Most childhood cancers originate from the **mesodermal germ layer** that gives rise to connective tissue, bone, cartilage, muscle, blood, blood vessels, gonads, kidney, and the lymphatic system. Thus the more common childhood cancers are leukemias, sarcomas, and embryonic tumors. Embryonic tumors originate during intrauterine life. These tumors contain abnormal cells that appear to be immature embryonic tissue unable to mature or differentiate into fully developed functional cells. Embryonic tumors are diagnosed early in life (usually by 5 years of age) and therefore are very rare in adults. **Embryonic tumors** often are named with the term **blast,** which refers to the immature nature of the cells.

Sarcomas and lymphoreticular cancers seen in childhood also occur in adults, but most adult cancers involve epithelial tissue (and are therefore carcinomas). Carcinomas almost never occur in children because these cancers most commonly result from environmental carcinogens and require a long period from exposure to the appearance of the carcinoma. However, the number of epithelial tumors begins to increase in those between 15 and 19 years of age, and epithelial tumors become the most common cancer tissue type in those beyond the age of adolescence.

By far the most common malignancy in children is leukemia, which accounts for more than one third of childhood cancers (Table 13-2). The second most common group of cancers is tumors of the nervous system, primarily brain tumors. All other pediatric malignancies occur much less often. Neuroblastoma and Wilms tumor are both embryonic tumors. Neuroblastoma is a tumor of the sympathetic nervous system. Wilms tumor is a malignancy of the kidney (named after Max Wilms, who first identified the tumor); the histologic name is *nephroblastoma*. Rhabdomyosarcoma is a soft tissue sarcoma of striated muscle. Two major bone tumors also occur in children—osteosarcoma and Ewing sarcoma (named after James Ewing, who identified this tumor type).

Childhood cancers most often are diagnosed during peak times of physical growth and maturation. In general, they are extremely fast-growing cancers, with 80% having distant spread (metastases) at diagnosis. Many childhood cancers have a peak incidence before the child is 5 years of age. Among these are the leukemias and the embryonic tumors: neuroblastomas, Wilms tumor, and retinoblastoma. Central nervous system tumors are more common in those from 5 to 10 years of age, and bone tumors, soft tissue sarcomas, and lymphomas are more likely to occur in those from 10 to 15 years of age.

Overall, cancer is 10% to 25% more common in white than in black children. This is primarily because of the lower

Table 13-1	Comparison of Usual Childhood and Adult Cancers	
Factor	Childhood Cancers	Adult Cancers
Incidence	Rare, <1% of all cancers	Common, >99% of all cancers
Sites	Involves tissue (e.g., mononuclear phagocyte system, central nervous system [CNS], muscle, bone)	Involves organs (e.g., lung, breast, colon, prostate
Histology	Most common type—nonepithelial and mesenchymal: sarcomas, embryonic tumors, leukemia, lymphoma	Most common type—epithelial: carcinomas
Latency (from initiation to diagnosis)	Relatively short period	Long period; can be well over 20 yr
Influence of environmental factors in causation	Some environmental factors known, few life-style factors; no strong influence shown overall; more likely an interaction of genetic alterations and environmental factors, called *ecogenetics*	Strong relationship to environmental exposures and life-style factors
Prevention	Minimal strategies known to date	80% estimated to be preventable
Early detection	Generally accidental; small percentage known to be genetically at high risk can be monitored more closely	Possible with adherence to early detection and screening recommendation
Stage at diagnosis	80% have metastasized	Local or regional
Response to treatment	Very responsive to chemotherapy; tolerate higher doses	Less responsive to chemotherapy
Treatment side effects	Less difficulty with acute toxicity but more significant long-term consequences	More difficulty with acute toxicity but fewer long-term consequences
Prognosis	>70% cure	<60% cure

Data from American Cancer Society: *Cancer facts and figures—2004,* http://www.cancer.org; Jemal A et al: Cancer statistics, *CA Cancer J Clin* 54(1):8-29, 2004; Pizzo PA, Poplack DG, editors: *Principles and practices of pediatric oncology,* ed 4, Philadelphia, 2002, Lippincott, Williams & Wilkins.

WHAT'S NEW? Childhood Cancer Survivors

Approximately 1 in every 250 adults will have survived childhood cancer in the year 2010. Improved cure rates are the result of multimodal therapy—radiation, chemotherapeutic agents, and surgical procedures. Survivors are at risk for physical, behavioral, or cognitive alterations related to cancer therapy. Identified health problems may include second malignancies, cardiac or endocrine abnormalities, major organ dysfunction, and neuropsychologic or physical disabilities.

It is estimated that as many as two-thirds of childhood cancer survivors will have at least one late effect. Although some late effects are obvious, many are subtle in nature. The natural aging process, existence of comorbidities, and risky health behaviors can potentiate late effects of cancer therapy. In order to decrease mortality related to late effects, childhood cancer survivors require multidisciplinary follow-up in specialty clinics by healthcare providers who are aware of potential complications survivors may experience.

Data from Aziz NM, Rowland JH: *Semin Radiat Oncol* 13(3): 248-266, 2003; Bottomley S, Kassner EA: *J Pediatr Nurs* 18(2):122-136, 2003; Hewitt M, Weiner SL, Simone JV: *Childhood cancer survivorship,* Washington, DC, 2003, National Academies Press; Hudson MM et al: *JAMA* 290(12):1583-1592, 2003.

incidence of acute lymphocytic leukemia, lymphomas, and Ewing sarcoma in black children. Blacks, however, have a higher incidence of Wilms tumor and osteosarcoma.[6] Some geographic differences also are found. Frequency of cancers by race is illustrated in Table 13-3. In the United States, childhood cancer also is slightly more common in boys than in girls. A newborn male has a 1 in 300 chance of developing cancer by age 20. A newborn female has a 1 in 333 chance of developing cancer by age 20.[6] Geographic differences exist including increases in Burkitt lymphoma in Africa, osteosarcoma in Spain, retinoblastoma in India, and Hodgkin disease in the United States and Latin America.[7]

ETIOLOGY

The causes of cancer in childhood, more so even than the causes of adult cancer, are largely unknown. Few environmental factors are known to predispose a child to cancer, but causal factors have not been established for most childhood cancers. A number of host factors, many of which are genetic risk factors or congenital conditions, have been implicated in the development of childhood cancer (Table 13-4). Because the cell types identified in childhood tumors closely resemble undifferentiated cells noted during normal development, it is hypothesized that these genetic changes alter such cells' ability to fully differentiate.[8] It has not been possible to determine whether the lack of differentiated features in tumor cells reflect arrested differentiation or dedifferentiation.[8]

Most childhood cancers, however, do not lend themselves to early cancer warning signs. Certainly the American Cancer Society's seven warning signs of cancer do not apply because they describe adult cancers. Although host factors are important in identifying populations of children at risk for cancer, most children who are diagnosed with cancer do not demonstrate any predisposing environmental or host factors.

Genetic Factors

Both oncogenes and tumor-suppressor genes have been associated with the causation of childhood cancers (Table 13-5; also see Chapter 11). Oncogenes are activated through muta-

Table 13-2 — Age-Specific Cancer Incidence Rates per Million

Type	<5 yr	5-9 yr	10-14 yr	15-19 yr
Leukemia	76.6	35	23.9	23.0
Lymphoma	7.6	13.1	24.1	51.3
CNS and miscellaneous intracranial and intraspinal neoplasms	34.5	29.8	24	19.1
Sympathetic nervous system tumors	20.0	3.0	1.1	1.0
Retinoblastoma	8.1	0.6	0.1	0.1
Renal tumors	18.9	5.9	1.3	1.2
Hepatic tumors	3.5	0.6	0.7	0.9
Malignant bone tumors	1.5	5.0	12.9	14.7
Soft tissue sarcomas	9.9	8.6	10.7	15.5
Germ-cell, trophoblastic, and other gonadal neoplasms	3.9	2.0	6.2	27.7
Carcinomas and other malignant epithelial neoplasms	1.1	3.0	11.0	42.0
Other and unspecified malignant tumors	0.6	0.3	0.7	1.6

Data from Ries LAG et al, editors: *SEER cancer review statistics review, 1975-2001*, Bethesda, Md, 2004, National Cancer Institute. Available at http://seer.cancer.gov.csr/1975_2001.
CNS, Central nervous system.

Table 13-3 — Cancers by Race/Ethnicity Incidence per Million Children Younger Than 20 Years

Cancer Type	White	Black	Hispanic	American Indian/Alaska Native	Asian/Pacific Islander
Leukemia	45.3	24.8	53.0	26.0	53.0
Lymphoma	24.4	17.5	19.2	—	19.2
CNS	28.8	21.9	21.0	13.0	21.0
Other	69.9	54.9	57.9	43.7	57.9

Data from Ries LAG et al, editors: *SEER cancer review statistics review, 1975-2001*, Bethesda, Md, 2004, National Cancer Institute. Available at http://seer.cancer.gov.csr/1975_2001.
CNS, Central nervous system.

Table 13-4 — Congenital Factors Associated with Childhood Cancer

Syndrome	Associated Childhood Cancer
Chromosome Alterations	
Down syndrome	Acute leukemia
13q syndrome	Retinoblastoma
Chromosome Instability	
Ataxia-telangiectasia	Lymphoma
Bloom syndrome	Acute leukemia, lymphoma, Wilms tumor
Fanconi anemia	Nonlymphocytic leukemia, myelodysplastic syndrome, hepatic tumors
Hereditary Syndromes	
Beckwith-Wiedemann syndrome	Wilms tumor, sarcoma, brain tumors, neuroblastoma, hepatoblastoma
Neurofibromatosis type I	Brain tumors, sarcomas, neuroblastomas, Wilms tumor, nonlymphocytic leukemia
Neurofibromatosis type II	Meningioma (malignant or benign), acoustic neuroma/schwannoma, gliomas, ependymomas
Tuberous sclerosis	Glial tumors
Li-Fraumeni syndrome	Sarcoma, adrenocortical carcinoma
Von Hippel-Lindau disease	Cerebellar hemangioblastoma, retinal angioma, renal cell carcinoma, pheochromocytomas
Ataxia-telangiectasia	Leukemia, lymphoma, brain tumors
Gorlin syndrome	Medulloblastoma, skin tumors
Immune Deficiency Disorders	
Congenital	
Agammaglobulinemia	Lymphoma, leukemia, brain tumors
Immunoglobulin A (IgA) deficiency	Lymphoma, leukemia, brain tumors
Wiskott-Aldrich syndrome	Leukemia, lymphoma
Acquired	
Aplastic anemia	Leukemia
Organ transplantation	Leukemia, lymphoma
Congenital Malformation Syndromes	
Aniridia, hemihypertrophy, hamartoma, genitourinary anomalies	Wilms tumor
Cryptorchidism	Testicular tumor
Gonadal dysgenesis	Gonadoblastoma
Family Susceptibility	
Twin or sibling with leukemia	Leukemia

TABLE 13-5	Selected Oncogenes and Tumor-Suppressor Genes Associated with Childhood Cancer
Gene	**Associated Pediatric Tumor**
Oncogenes	
bcr-abl	Acute lymphoblastic leukemia
N-myc	Neuroblastoma
c-myb	Neural tumors, leukemia lymphoma, rhabdomyosarcoma, Wilms tumor, neuroblastoma
erb B	Glioblastomas
N-ras	Neuroblastoma, leukemia
H/K-ras	Neuroblastoma, rhabdomyosarcoma, leukemia
ATM	Lymphoma, leukemia
Tumor-Suppressor Genes	
Rb1	Retinoblastoma, sarcoma
WT1, WT2	Wilms tumor, leukemia
WTC	Wilms tumor
NF-1	Sarcoma, primitive neuroectodermal tumor, juvenile chronic myelocytic leukemia
NF-2	Brain tumors, melanoma, meningiomas
p16	Brain tumors, leukemia
p53	Sarcoma, leukemia, brain tumors, lymphoma
DCC	Ewing sarcoma, rhabdomyosarcoma
$p16^{INK4a}$	Glioma, leukemia
$p15^{ARF}$	Glioblastoma, T-cell ALL
CDC2L1	Non-Hodgkin lymphoma, neuroblastoma

Data from Dome JS, Coppes MS:, *Curr Opin Pediat* 14(1):5-11, 2002; Linblom A, Nordenskjold M: *Sem Cancer Biol* 10(4):251-254, 2000; Tischkowitz M, Rosser E: *Eur J Cancer* 40:2459-2470, 2004; Look A, Kirsch IR: Molecular basis of childhood cancer. In Pizzo PA, Poplack DG, editors: *Principles and practices of pediatric oncology*, edition 4, Philadelphia, 2002, Lippincott, Williams & Wilkins.
ALL, Acute lymphocytic leukemia.

tion of a proto-oncogene that normally maintains cellular growth and control. Once activated to an oncogene, uncontrolled cell growth—the primary characteristic of cancer cells—results. Oncogenes have been identified in pediatric leukemia, lymphomas, and some solid tumors. Tumor-suppressor genes arise from genes that normally suppress cancer formation but have lost their suppressor function, thus leading to uncontrolled growth. Some childhood cancers identified with tumor-suppressor genes include osteosarcoma, rhabdomyosarcoma, leukemia, retinoblastoma, and Wilms tumor.[9]

Other genetic factors involve chromosome aberrations or single-gene defects. These chromosome abnormalities include aneuploidy, amplifications, deletions, translocations, and fragility. Examples of well-known chromosome abnormalities include the Philadelphia chromosome with chronic myelogenous leukemia and the deletion of chromosome 13q, often observed with retinoblastoma and osteosarcoma.[10]

Some congenital malformations herald the onset of pediatric malignancies. For example, certain syndromes involve easily diagnosed abnormalities, and the children can then be carefully followed and screened for tumor development. Tri-somy 21 (Down syndrome) is the most common genetic defect linked to the development of acute leukemia. Children with Down syndrome have a 10- to 20-fold increased risk of developing both acute lymphoblastic and myeloid leukemias and an even higher risk for the development of acute megakaryocytic leukemia. The risk is highest in children between 1 and 4 years of age.[11,12] Wilms tumor is associated with several congenital syndromes, such as AGR (aniridia or congenital absences of the iris of the eye, ambiguous genitalia, mental retardation), neurofibromatosis, and Beckwith-Wiedemann syndromes.[13] Retinoblastoma, a malignant embryonic tumor of the eye, occurs as an inherited defect or as an acquired mutation (see Chapter 19).

Numerous single-gene defects have been associated with the subsequent development of both childhood and adult cancers. Fanconi anemia and Bloom syndrome, two autosomal recessive conditions involving chromosomal fragility, are risk factors for the development of acute myelogenous leukemia.[14,15]

Although not determined to be genetically transmitted, a few malignancies seem to demonstrate a familial tendency, suggested by the clustering of specific cancers in a particular family. A child who has a sibling with leukemia has a risk for the development of leukemia that is two to four times greater than for children with healthy siblings. The occurrence of leukemia in monozygous twins is estimated as being as high as 25%, with an associated degree of risk relative to age.[16] The highest degree of concordance is noted in infant leukemia. Diagnosis after 7 years of age predisposes the unaffected twin to a risk similar to that of the general population. Preliminary research has suggested there may be a prenatal basis for this difference of concordance and relative age rates.[17]

In families with Li-Fraumeni syndrome (a genetic defect involving the *p53* tumor-suppressor gene), the risk of developing tumors is significantly higher when compared to the unaffected population.[18]

Environmental Factors

Although many adult cancers are associated with environmental agents, few childhood tumors share a similar strong association. Because of the lengthy latency period required between exposure and development of cancer, presumably early exposure to carcinogens does not result in a tumor until the child is an adult.

Prenatal Exposure

Prenatal exposure to some drugs and to ionizing radiation has been linked to subsequent cancers. Perhaps the most well-known such drug is diethylstilbestrol (DES), a drug once taken to avert early abortion. In 1971, DES was identified as a transplacental chemical carcinogen. Adenocarcinomas of the vagina have developed in a small percentage of the daughters of mothers who took DES while pregnant. Researchers continue to study prenatal environmental influences and their relationship with childhood cancer. Previous studies have shown a possible association linking parental factors (nonoccupational and occupational) to the risk of childhood cancer.[19] More recent research, however, has shown less evidence that exposures to environmental chemicals or toxins can lead to genetic changes of the egg or sperm or to transplacental transfer of carcinogens.[20,21] Increased parental age at the time of conception also has been linked to a higher incidence of cancer in children.[22,23]

Earlier research suggested a causal association between antenatal x-ray exposure and childhood cancer.[24-26] However, studies of children exposed to atomic fallout in uteri show no statistically significant increase in childhood cancer.[26-28] More recent studies continue to debate the possibility that development of cancer may be related to a linear dose-response relationship.[29] Consideration also must be given to the possibility that children who develop cancer may have causative factors other than the exposure to radiation in utero, or that women requiring prenatal radiographic exams may have other cancer risks that predispose the fetus to the development of cancer.

Childhood Exposure

Childhood exposure to drugs, ionizing radiation, or viruses has been implicated as a risk factor that increases susceptibility to specific cancers. Important is the risk of developing a malignancy later in life as a result of childhood radiation exposure. Retrospective research has shown a significant correlation between radiation-induced malignancies and pediatric exposure to radiotherapy for benign or malignant pediatric diseases, as well as radiation exposure from diagnostic imaging.[30-33] In addition to those drug and environmental agents that are known to cause cancer in adults and therefore also are risks for exposure during childhood, a few drugs may particularly increase cancer risk during childhood. These drugs include (1) anabolic androgenic steroids, which are used in the treatment of aplastic anemia or used for body development and have been associated with subsequent hepatocellular carcinoma; (2) cytotoxic agents used in the treatment of pediatric cancers, which may predispose the child to leukemia in later years; and (3) immunosuppressive agents, particularly those used for transplant surgeries, which have been shown to increase the risk of lymphoma.

The relationship between childhood cancer and electromagnetic field exposure from residential power lines and operation of small household appliances has been studied repeatedly, yet, no conclusive associations have been observed[34,35] (also see Chapter 11).

In children, the strongest carcinogenic relationship regarding viruses has been between the Epstein-Barr virus (EBV) and Burkitt lymphoma, nasopharyngeal carcinoma, and Hodgkin disease.[36-38] Recent research has shown that children with AIDS have an increased risk of developing certain cancers, predominantly non-Hodgkin lymphoma and Kaposi sarcoma.[39] Investigators continue to examine the role of viruses in the development of neuroblastoma, Wilms tumor, and osteosarcoma.

PROGNOSIS

Today, childhood cancer is not considered inevitably fatal. Significant progress has been made in the past 20 years; approximately 78% of children diagnosed with cancer are now cured.[6] Overall, children have a more favorable prognosis than do adults.[2] Children appear to be both more responsive to available treatments and better able to tolerate the immediate side effects. Children with cancer are more likely than adults to be enrolled and treated through clinical trials. Treatment effectiveness is more easily determined, and advances gained from clinical trials may contribute to a higher survival rate in children.[40]

Because childhood cancer should be viewed as a chronic disease rather than a fatal illness, the focus of treatment is on quality of life. Even those cancers that cannot be cured generally can be treated, thus allowing the child a significant period of quality time. These increasing survival periods have engendered more careful investigation of the long-term effects of treatment. It is imperative that more effective yet less toxic chemotherapy and radiation treatments be found.

Children who are cured still face residual and late effects of treatment. These late effects are more significant in children than in adults because childhood treatment, by definition, is administered to a physically immature, growing individual. Potential effects that need further study include physical impairments, reproductive dysfunction, soft tissue and bone atrophy, learning disabilities, secondary cancers, and psychologic sequelae. More must be learned about the genetic factors associated with childhood malignancies and about the genetic consequences of treatment. Genetic counseling is appropriate for children cured of cancers known to be transmitted genetically (e.g., retinoblastoma).

SUMMARY REVIEW

Incidence and Types
1. Although childhood cancer is rare, it is nevertheless the second leading cause of death in children.
2. The unique feature of childhood cancers is the short period of latency, which contrasts sharply with the long latency period common in adults.
3. Common childhood cancers include leukemias, central nervous system tumors, sarcomas, and embryonic tumors that contain immature fetal tissue that has not differentiated into fully developed cells.
4. Embryonic tumors are often diagnosed early and are very rare in adults.

Etiology
1. Genetic carcinomas in adults are associated with environmental exposure; these same cancers are extremely rare in children presumably because they have not lived long enough to be affected.

SUMMARY REVIEW—cont'd

2. Host factors are especially important in identifying a child at risk for cancer because environmental risk factors have had less effect on the child's short lifetime.
3. Genetic factors that place a child at risk for cancer include some congenital malformations such as chromosome aberrations, single-gene defects, or loss of tumor-suppressor genes.
4. A familial tendency is evident for a few childhood cancers, including leukemia, retinoblastoma, and Wilms tumor.
5. Environmental risk factors associated with childhood cancer include prenatal exposure to some drugs and ionizing radiation and postnatal exposure to certain drugs (particularly ana-

bolic steroids and some cytotoxic and immunosuppressive agents), to radiation, and possibly to certain viruses.

Prognosis

1. More than 78% of children diagnosed with cancer are cured.
2. Improved survival for children with cancer has led to investigations for less toxic treatments that minimize residual effects and for more research into the genetic factors associated with cancer in childhood.

KEY TERMS

Blast, 403   Embryonic tumors, 403   Mesodermal germ layer, 403

MEDIA RESOURCES *evolve*

Review questions and answers for this chapter are available in the *CD Companion* included with this book.

WebLinks—links to Internet sites pertaining to this chapter—are available on Evolve at http://evolve.elsevier.com/McCance/.

REFERENCES

1. Jemal A et al: Cancer statistics, 2004, *CA Cancer J Clin* 54:8-29, 2004.
2. American Cancer Society: *Cancer facts and figures—2002,* Atlanta, Ga, 2002, The Society.
3. US Cancer Statistics Working Group: *United States cancer statistics: 2000 incidence,* Atlanta, Ga, 2003, Department of Health and Human Services, Centers for Disease Control and Prevention and National Cancer Institute. Also available at http://www.cdc.gov/cancer/npcr/uses/2000/index.htm
4. American Cancer Society: *Cancer facts and figures—2004.* Available at http://www.cancer.org.
5. Dreyer ZE, Blatt J, Bleyer A: Late effects of childhood cancer and its treatment. In Pizzo PA, Poplack DC, editors: *Principles and practice of pediatric oncology,* ed 4, Philadelphia, 2002, Lippincott, Williams, & Wilkins.
6. Ries LAG et al, editors: *SEER cancer review statistics review, 1975-2001,* Bethesda, Md, 2004, National Cancer Institute. Available at http://seer.cancer.gov.csr/1975_2001.
7. Robinson LL: General principles of the epidemiology of cancer. In Pizzo PA, Poplack DG, editors: *Principles and practices of pediatric oncology,* ed 3, Philadelphia, 1997, Lippincott-Raven.
8. Israel M: Molecular biology of childhood neoplasms. In Mendolsohn J et al: *The molecular basis of cancer,* ed 2, Philadelphia, 2001, Saunders.
9. Look A, Kirsch IR: Molecular basis of childhood cancer. In Pizzo PA, Poplack DG, editors: *Principles and practices of pediatric oncology,* ed 4, Philadelphia, 2002, Lippincott, Williams & Wilkins.
10. Ganjavi H, Malkin D: Genetics of childhood cancer, *Clin Orthop Relat Res* 401:57-87, 2002.
11. Hasle H, Clemmensen IH, Mikkelsen M: Risks of leukemia and solid tumors in individuals with Down's syndrome, *Lancet* 355(9199):165-169, 2000.
12. Taub JW: Relationship of chromosome 21 and acute leukemia in children with Down syndrome, *J Pediat Hematol Oncol* 23(3):175-178, 2001.
13. Pritchard-Jones K: Secondary neoplasms after radiotherapy for childhood solid tumor, *Pediatr Hematol Oncolo* 87(3):241-244, 2002.
14. Poppe B et al: Chromosomal aberrations in Bloom syndrome patients with myeloid malignancies, *Cancer Genet Cytogenet* 128(1):39-42, 2001.
15. Rosenberg PS, Huang Y, Alter BP: Individualized risks of first adverse events in patients with Fanconi anemia, *Blood* 104(2):350-355, 2004.
16. Margolin J, Steuber CP, Poplack DG: Acute lymphoblastic leukemia. In Pizzo PA, Poplack DG, editors: *Principles and practice of pediatric oncology,* ed 4, Philadelphia, 2002, Lippincott, Williams, & Wilkins.
17. Greaves MF et al: Leukemia in twins: lessons in natural history, *Blood* 102(7):2321-2333, 2003.
18. Hisada M et al: Multiple primary cancers in families with Li-Fraumeni syndrome, *J Natl Cancer Inst* 90(8):606-611, 1998.
19. Feychting M et al: Paternal occupational exposures and childhood cancer, *Environ Health Perspect* 109(2):193-196, 2001.
20. Massey-Stokes M, Lanning B: Childhood cancer and environmental toxins: the debate continues, *Fam Community Health* 24(4):27-38, 2002.
21. McKinney PA, Fear NT, Stockton D: Parental occupation at periconception: findings from the United Kingdom Childhood Cancer Study, *Occup Environ Med* 60(12):901-909, 2003.
22. Jain D et al: Bloom syndrome in sibs: first reports of hepatocellular carcinoma and Wilms tumor with documented anaplasia and negphrogenic rests, *Pediatr Dev Pathol* 4(6):585-589, 2001.
23. Mueller B: Lymphoproliferative disorders and malignancies related to immunodeficiencies. In Pizzo PA, Poplack DC, editors: *Principles and practice of pediatric oncology,* ed 4, Philadelphia, 2002, Lippincott, Williams, & Wilkins.
24. Blithell JF, Stewart AM: Prenatal irradiation and childhood malignancy: a review of British data from the Oxford Survey, *Br J Cancer* 31:271-287, 1975.
25. Doll R, Wakeford R: Risk of childhood cancer from fetal irradiation, *Br J Radiol* 70:130-139, 1997.
26. Mole RH: Childhood cancer after prenatal exposure to diagnostic x-ray examinations in Britain, *Br J Cancer* 62(1):152-168, 1990.
27. Delongchamp RR et al: Cancer mortality among atomic bomb survivors exposed in utero or as young children, October 1950–May 1992, *Radiat Res* 147(3):385-395, 1997.
28. Izumi S et al: Cancer incidence in children and young adults did not increase relative to parental exposure to atomic bombs, *Br J Cancer* 89(9):1709-1713, 2003.
29. Wakeford R, Little MP: Risk coefficients for childhood cancer after intrauterine irradiation: a review, *Int J Radiat Biol* 79(5):293-309, 2003.
30. Benz MG, Benz MW: Reduction of cancer risk associated with pediatric computed tomography by the development of new technologies, *Pediatrics* 114(1):205-209, 2004.
31. Kleinerman RA et al: Risk of new cancers after radiotherapy in long-term survivors of retinoblastoma: an extended follow-up, *J Clin Oncol* 23(10):2272-2279, 2005.
32. Paulino AM, Fowler B: Secondary neoplasms after radiotherapy for childhood solid tumor, *Pediatr Hematol Oncol* 22(2):89-101, 2005.
33. Ron E: Cancer risks from medical radiation, *Health Phys* 85(1):47-59, 2003.

34. Brain JD et al: Childhood leukemia: electric and magnetic fields as possible risk factors, *Environ Health Perspect* 111(7):962-970, 2003.

35. Kheifets LI: Electric and magnetic field exposure and brain cancer: a review, *Bioelectromagnetics* (Suppl 5):S120-S131, 2001.

36. Benharroch D et al: New candidate virus in association with Hodgkin's disease, *Leuk Lymphoma* 44(4):605-610, 2003.

37. Griffin BE: Epstein-Barr virus (EBV) and human disease: facts, opinions, and problems, *Mutat Res/Rev Mutat Res* 462(2):395-405, 2000.

38. Niedobitek G, Meru N, Delecluse HJ: Epstein-Barr virus infection and human malignancies, *Int J Exp Pathol* 82(3):149-170, 2001.

39. National Cancer Institute: National Cancer Institute research on childhood cancer: cancer fact sheet 6.40, 2002 (rev 4/10/2004). Available at: http://cis.nci.nih.gov/fact/6_2.htm.

40. Ungerleider RS, Ellendber SS, Berg SL: Clinical trials: design, conduct, analysis & reporting. In Pizzo PA, Poplack DC, editors: *Principles and practice of pediatric oncology*, ed 4, Philadelphia, 2002, Lippincott, Williams, & Wilkins.

STRUCTURE AND FUNCTION OF THE NEUROLOGIC SYSTEM

RICHARD A. SUGERMAN

CHAPTER OUTLINE

The human nervous system is a remarkable structure that is responsible for the body's ability to reciprocally interact with the environment and for the regulation of activities involving internal organs. The nervous system literally *drives* the other systems of the body. It is a network composed of complex structures that transmit electrical and chemical signals between the body's many organs and tissues and the brain.

OVERVIEW AND ORGANIZATION OF THE NERVOUS SYSTEM

Although the nervous system functions as a unified whole, structures and functions of the nervous system have been divided to facilitate understanding. Structurally, the nervous system is divided into the central nervous system and the peripheral nervous system. The **central nervous system (CNS)** consists of the brain and spinal cord, enclosed within the protective cranial vault and vertebrae, respectively. The **peripheral nervous system (PNS)** is composed of the **cranial nerves,** which project from the brain and pass through foramina (openings) in the skull, and the **spinal nerves,** which project from the spinal cord and pass through intervertebral foramina of the vertebrae. Peripheral nerve pathways are differentiated into **afferent pathways (ascending pathways)** that carry sensory impulses toward the CNS and **efferent pathways (descending pathways)** that innervate **effector organs,** such as skeletal, cardiac, and smooth muscle, as well as glands, by transmitting motor impulses away from the CNS. Organs innervated by specific components of the nervous system are called *effector organs.* Cranial nerves are viewed most correctly as modified spinal nerves. Some cranial nerves function similarly to spinal nerves, whereas others have specialized sensory tasks, such as smell, taste, sight, and hearing.

Clinically, the PNS can be divided into the somatic nervous system and the autonomic nervous system. The **somatic nervous system** consists of motor and sensory pathways regulating voluntary motor control of skeletal muscle. The **autonomic nervous system (ANS)** also consists of motor and sensory components and is involved with regulation of the body's internal environment (viscera) through involuntary control of organ systems. The ANS is further divided into sympathetic and parasympathetic divisions. Today we understand that some aspects of the ANS can be controlled through mental practice with or without biofeedback techniques.

CELLS OF THE NERVOUS SYSTEM

The two basic types of cells that make up nervous tissue are neurons and supporting cells. The neuron is the primary cell of the nervous system. Working in parallel systems, neurons can scan the environment, integrate many systems at higher cognitive levels, and initiate body responses to maintain homeostasis. The supporting cells, such as the **neuroglial cells** of the CNS and the Schwann cells of the PNS, provide structural support and nutrition for neurons, increase the speed of nerve impulses, and play a significant role, along with neurons, in processing and storing information (i.e., memory).[1]

Neuron

Neuronal structure varies considerably throughout the CNS. Neurons vary in size from micrometers to several meters long and have from one cell process to many cell processes. Even the shapes and complexity of the processes can vary considerably. **Neurons** are specialized cells that share many of the same metabolic activities and constituents as other types of cells. The fuel source for the neuron is predominantly glucose; insulin, however, is not required for cellular glucose uptake in the CNS. Neurons contain many cellular constituents, namely, microtubules, neurofibrils, microfilaments, and Nissl substances. **Microfilaments** and **neurofibrils** are composed of structural proteins and are responsible for structural support within the cell and movement of neuron processes, as seen in amoebas and white blood cells. **Microtubules** also are made of protein and are believed to be involved in the transport of cellular products. **Nissl substances** consist of endoplasmic reticulum and ribosomes and are involved in protein synthesis. The CNS starts out with more neurons than it needs, and those neurons that do not become involved in functional systems die. Some neurons continue to divide after birth. Olfactory neurons in the nose continue to divide throughout life.

A neuron (Figure 14-1) has three components: a cell body (soma) and the thin processes of the cell—the dendrites and

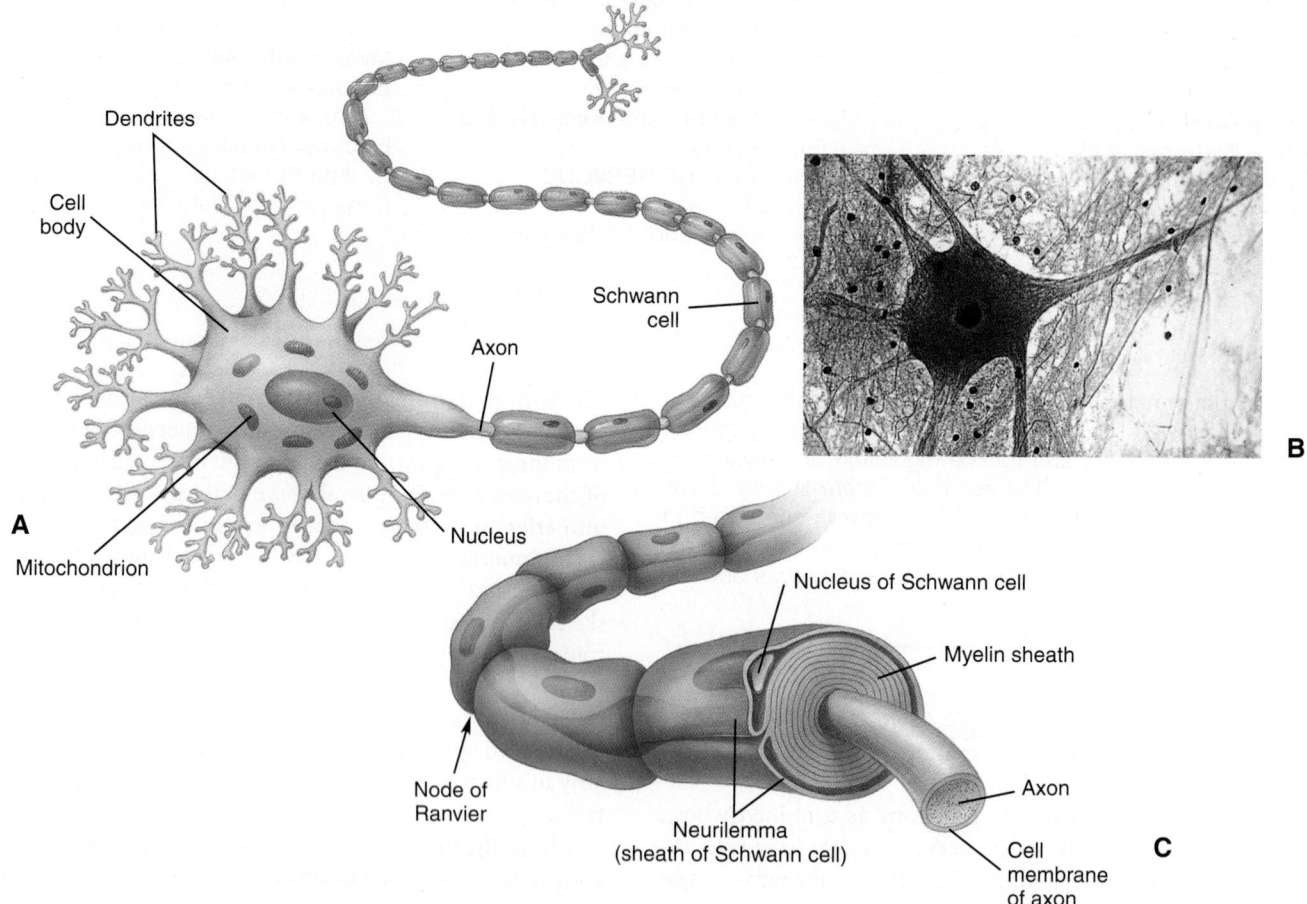

Figure 14-1 **Structure of a typical neuron. A,** Many dendrites carry nerve impulses to the cell body, which then send the nerve impulses along a single, long axon. Long axons are encased at intervals by a myelin sheath. **B,** Photomicrograph of a neuron. **C** shows a segment of myelinated fiber in cross section, showing myelin sheath composed of several layers of myelin, which insulate the axon. (**A** and **C** from Thibodeau GA, Patton KT: *Structure and function of the human body,* ed 12, St Louis, 2004, Mosby; **B,** Copyright Edward Reschke.)

axons. Most cell bodies are located within the CNS. Dense, packed cell bodies in the CNS are called **nuclei.** Cell bodies in the PNS are usually found in groups called **ganglia** or **plexuses.** The **dendrites** are extensions that carry nerve impulses *toward* the cell body. The **dendritic zone** is the receptive portion of a neuron that receives a stimulus and continues further conduction. **Axons** are long, conductive projections from the cell body that carry nerve impulses *away* from the cell body. The **axon hillock** is the cone-shaped, Nissl-free area where the axon leaves the cell body. The initial segment of the axon has the lowest threshold for stimulation, and as a result, action potentials begin there.

A typical neuron has only one axon, which may be covered with a segmented layer of lipid material called **myelin,** which acts as an insulating substance. This entire membrane is referred to as the **myelin sheath;** the thin membrane between the myelin sheath and the **endoneurium,** a delicate connective tissue around each axon in the PNS (see Figure 14-22, *B*), is the **neurilemma (Schwann sheath).** The neurilemma and the myelin sheath are interrupted at regular intervals by the **nodes of Ranvier.** The **Schwann cell** forms and maintains the myelin sheath, and the nodes of Ranvier form the spaces on either side of the Schwann cell. If the myelin layer is tightly wrapped many times around the axon forming nodes of Ranvier, it increases conduction velocity and the neuron is referred to as *myelinated* (see Figure 14-1).

Myelin acts as an insulator that allows ions to flow between segments rather than along the entire length of the membrane, resulting in increased velocity. This mechanism is referred to as **saltatory conduction.** If the Schwann cells are loosely wrapped around the axon, it is referred to as *unmyelinated* and conduction velocity is not increased. Axons are capable of extensive branching, which occurs at the nodes of Ranvier. Two major principles of information processing in the nervous system are *divergence* and *convergence.* **Divergence** refers to the ability of these branching axons to influence many different neurons. **Convergence** is the term applied to branches of numerous neurons converging on and influencing one or a few neurons. Disorders of the myelin sheath (demyelinating diseases), such as multiple sclerosis and Guillain-Barré syndrome, demonstrate the important role myelin plays in nerve function (see Chapter 17). Besides depending on the myelin coating, conduction velocities also depend on the diameter of the axon. Larger axons transmit impulses at a faster rate.

Neurons are structurally classified on the basis of the number of processes (projections) extending from the cell body. There are four basic types of cell configuration: (1) unipolar, (2) pseudounipolar, (3) bipolar, and (4) multipolar. **Unipolar neurons** have one process that branches shortly after leaving the cell body. One example is found in the retina. **Pseudounipolar neurons** (some authors call them *unipolar*) have one process that has its dendritic portion extending away from the CNS and its axon portion projecting into the CNS (Figure 14-2). The configuration is typical of sensory neurons in both cranial and spinal nerves. **Bipolar neurons** have two distinct processes arising from the cell body. This type of neuron connects to rod and cone cells of the retina. **Multipolar neurons** are the most common and have multiple processes capable of extensive branching. A motor neuron is typically multipolar (see Figure 14-2).

Functionally, there are three types of neurons (with their direction of transmission and typical configuration noted in parentheses): (1) sensory (afferent, mostly pseudounipolar), (2) associational (interneurons, multipolar), and (3) motor (efferent, multipolar). **Sensory neurons** carry impulses from peripheral sensory receptors to the CNS (Box 14-1). **Associational neurons (interneurons)** transmit impulses from neuron to neuron, that is, from sensory to motor neurons. **Motor neurons** transmit impulses away from the CNS to an effector organ. In skeletal muscle the end processes form a complex neuromuscular (myoneural) junction.

Neuroglia and Schwann Cells

Neuroglia ("nerve glue") comprise the general classification of cells that support the neurons of the CNS. They make up approximately half of the total brain and spinal cord volume and are five to ten times more numerous than neurons. Different types of neuroglia serve different functions. **Astrocytes,** for example, fill the spaces between neurons and surround blood vessels in the CNS; **oligodendroglia (oligodendrocytes)** function to deposit myelin within the CNS. Oligodendroglia are the CNS counterpart of the Schwann cells. Ependymal cells line the cerebrospinal fluid (CSF)–filled cavities of the CNS. **Microglia** remove debris (phagocytosis) in the CNS. Characteristics of neuroglia and Schwann cells are summarized in Figure 14-3 and Table 14-1.

Nerve Injury and Regeneration

When an axon is severed, a typical sequence of events, known as *wallerian degeneration,* occurs in the portion of the axon distal to the cut: (1) a characteristic swelling appears, (2) the neurofilaments hypertrophy, (3) the myelin sheath shrinks and disintegrates, and (4) this axon portion degenerates and disappears. The myelin sheaths reform into Schwann cells that line up in a column between the cut and the effector organ.

At the proximal end of the injured axon, similar changes occur, but only back as far as the next node of Ranvier. The cell body responds to trauma by swelling and then dispersing the Nissl substance (chromatolysis). During the repair process the cell increases in metabolic activity, protein synthesis, and mitochondrial activity. Approximately 7 to 14 days after the injury, new terminal sprouts project from the proximal segment and may enter the remaining Schwann cell pathway. (Figure 14-4 contains a more detailed representation of these events.) This process, however, is limited to myelinated fibers and generally occurs only in the PNS. The regeneration of axonal constituents in the CNS is limited by an increased incidence of scar formation and the different nature of myelin formation by the oligodendrocyte.

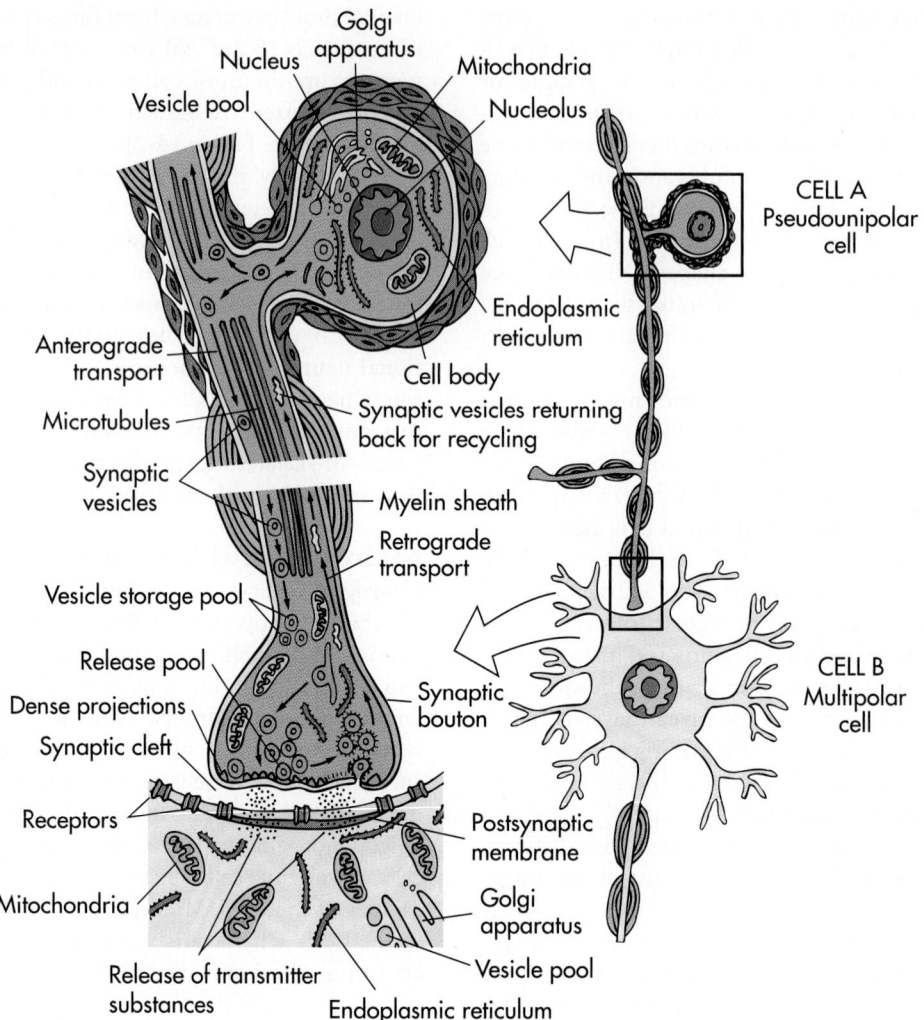

Figure 14-2 Neuronal transmission and synaptic cleft. Electrical impulse travels along axon of first neuron to synapse. Chemical transmitter is secreted into synaptic space to depolarize membrane (dendrite or cell body) of next neuron in pathway. *Cell A* represents pseudounipolar cell; *cell B* represents multipolar cell.

Box 14-1	Major Types of Sensory Receptors

Nociceptors (pain)
Mechanoreceptors (touch, pressure, and mechanical deformation or encapsulated endings)
Photochemical (light on the retina)
Chemoreceptors (flavors, odors, oxygen levels, osmolarity of body fluids, and carbon dioxide levels in the blood)
Thermoreceptors (heat and cold)
Proprioception (sensing location of body parts)
Audition and balance (sound and positional movement)

Nerve regeneration depends on many factors, such as location of the injury, type of injury, the inflammatory responses, and the process of scarring. The closer to the cell body of the nerve, the greater the chances that the nerve cell will die and not regenerate. A crushing injury allows recovery more fully than does a cut injury. Crushed nerves sometimes recover fully, whereas cut nerves often form connective tissue scars that block or slow regenerating axonal branches.

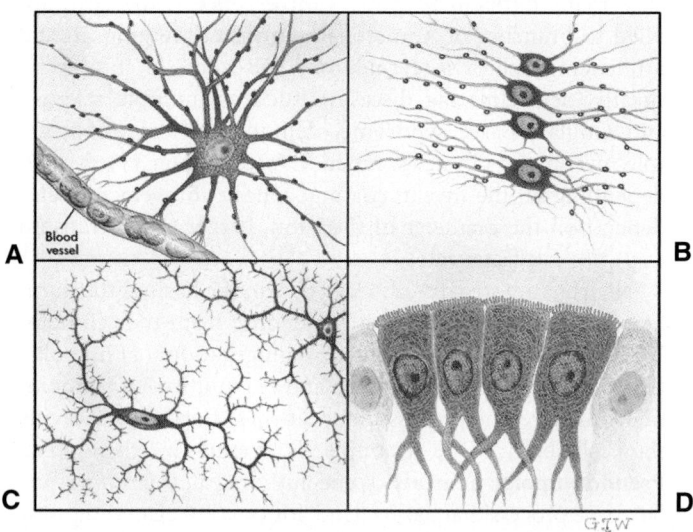

Figure 14-3 Types of neuroglia cells. A, Fibrous astrocyte; **B,** oligodendrocytes; **C,** microglia cells; **D,** ependymal cells. (Modified from Chipps E, Clanin N, Campbell V: *Neurologic disorders,* St Louis, 1992, Mosby.)

Table 14-1	Support Cells of the Nervous System
Cell Type	**Primary Functions**
Astrocytes	Form specialized contacts between neuronal surfaces and blood vessels
	Provide rapid transport for nutrients and metabolites
	Believed to form an essential component of the blood-brain barrier
	Appear to be the scar-forming cells of CNS, which may be the foci for seizures
	Appear to work with neurons in processing information and memory storage
Oligodendroglia (oligodendrocytes)	Formation of myelin sheath and neurilemma in CNS
Schwann cells (neurolemmocytes)	Formation of myelin sheath and neurilemma in PNS
Microglia	Responsible for clearing cellular debris (phagocytic properties)
Ependymal cells	Serve as a lining for ventricles and choroids plexuses involved in production of cerebrospinal fluid

CNS, Central nervous system; *PNS,* peripheral nervous system.

WHAT'S NEW?   Astrocytes

Neuroglial (glia) cells have been considered the *glue* that exists between or around neurons. Up until recently, neurons have been considered the major players in the nervous system and glia just minor support cells. Astrocytes, the most abundant glial cells in the nervous system, were considered simple nutrient support "housekeeping" cells for neurons, and it was thought they helped form the blood-brain barrier. Recent reports on astrocytes portray a "partnership" with glial cells. Astrocytes (1) can be a source for new neurons, (2) build a structural framework around neurons forming gliavascular units to provide the specific blood flow (nutrients) that a neuron requires, (3) may regulate synaptic formation and maintenance, and (4) have a two-way interaction with neurons at synapses through the release of glial neurotransmitters that could either facilitate excitation or inhibition of neuron activity at the pre- and postsynaptic membranes.

Data from Slezak M, Pfreiger FW: *Trends Neurosci* 26(10):531-535, 2003; Nedergaad M et al: *Trends Neurosci* 26(10):523-530, 2003; Newman EA: *Trends Neurosci* 26(10):536-542, 2003.

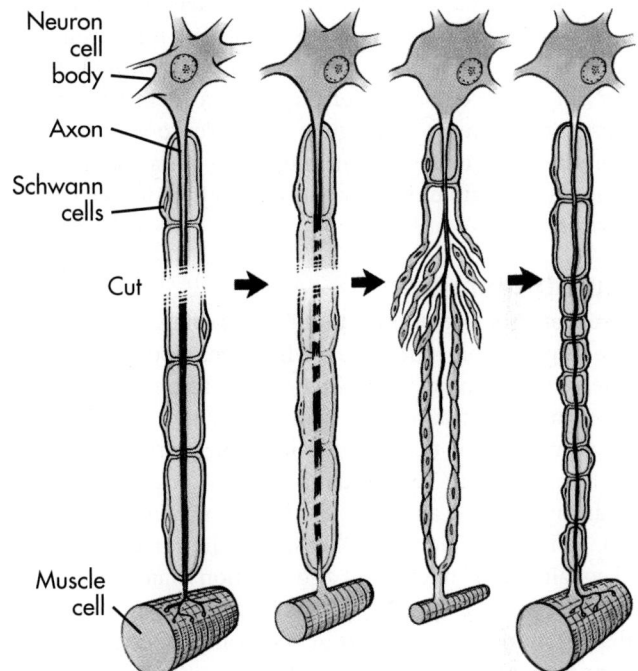

Figure 14-4 **Repair of a peripheral nerve fiber.** When cut, a damaged motor axon can regrow to its distal connection only if the neurilemma remains intact (to form a guiding tunnel) and if scar tissue does not block its way.

NERVE IMPULSE

Neurons generate and conduct electrical and chemical impulses by selectively changing the electrical portion of their plasma membranes and influencing other nearby neurons by the release of chemicals (neurotransmitters). A neuron in its unexcited state maintains a resting membrane potential (see Chapter 1). When the membrane potential is raised sufficiently, an action potential is generated (see Figure 1-32), and the nerve impulse then flows to all parts of the neuron. The action potential response occurs only when the stimulus is strong enough; if it is too weak, the membrane remains unexcited. This property is sometimes termed the *all-or-none response.*

Synapses

Neurons are not physically continuous with one another. The region between adjacent neurons is called a **synapse.** Impulses are transmitted across the synapse by chemical (see Figures 14-2 and 14-13) and electrical conduction; only chemical conduction is discussed here. The neurons that con-

WHAT'S NEW?   Brain Synthesis of Neurosteroids

Although the brain is a target site for peripheral steroids, the brain glial cells, cerebellar Purkinje, and other cells also synthesize steroids from cholesterol, such as progesterone, pregnenlone, and dehydroepiandrosterone. These steroids are called *neurosteroids* and have diverse functions, including modulation of neurotransmitters (e.g., $GABA_A$ and the glutamate and cholinergic systems). Beneficial effects have been shown for memory, learning, stress, depression, regulation of myelination, and neuroprotection and growth of axons and dendrites. Research is advancing potential pharmacologic use of neurosteroids to treat neuropathologies and support normal aging.

Data from Compagnone NA, Mellon SH: *Front Neuroendocrinol* 21(1):1-56, 2000; Tsutsui K et al: *Neurosci Res* 36(4):261-273, 2000; Dudas B et al: *Neurobiol Dis* 15(2):262-268, 2004.

duct a nerve impulse are named according to whether they relay impulses *toward* the synapse (**presynaptic neurons**) or *away* from the synapse (**postsynaptic neurons**). Four basic types of connections occur in regions of contact between the presynaptic and postsynaptic neurons. These are between axons (axoaxonic), from axon to cell body (axosomatic), from axon to dendrite (axodendritic), and from dendrite to dendrite (dendrodendritic).

Impulses are transmitted across the synapse by chemical conduction. The conducting substance is called a **neurotransmitter,** and it is often formed in the **synaptic boutons** of the presynaptic neuron's axon and stored in synaptic vesicles within the boutons. Action potentials in the presynaptic neuron cause the synaptic vesicles to release their neurotransmitter or neurotransmitters through the plasma membrane into the **synaptic cleft** (the space between the neurons), where they bind to receptor sites on the plasma membrane of the postsynaptic neuron (see Figure 14-2). Neurons can synthesize more than one neurotransmitter, and postsynaptic membranes can contain more than one type of transmitter-specific receptor.

Neurotransmitters

More than 30 substances are thought to be neurotransmitters, including norepinephrine, acetylcholine, dopamine, histamine, γ-aminobutyric acid (GABA), and serotonin.[2] Many of these transmitters have more than one function. For example, norepinephrine in the brain probably helps regulate mood, functions in dream sleep, and maintains arousal. Several neurotransmitters are amino acids, including GABA, glutamic acid, and aspartic acid. Small chains of amino acids, such as enkephalins and endorphins, also function as neurotransmitters. They (neuropeptides) are involved in the perception and integration of pain, as well as in emotional experiences. Kandel and colleagues[3] define a neurotransmitter as a chemical that "must be synthesized in the neuron, become localized in the presynaptic terminal (synaptic bouton), be released into the synaptic cleft, bind to a receptor site (binding site) on the postsynaptic membrane of another neuron or effector where it affects ion channels, and last, be removed by a specific mechanism from its site of action." Neurotransmitter and neuromodulator substances are listed in Table 14-2.

Because the neurotransmitter is stored on one side of the synaptic cleft and the receptor sites are on the other side, chemical synapses operate in only one direction. Therefore action potentials are transmitted along a multineuronal pathway in only one direction. The binding of the neurotransmitter at the receptor site changes the permeability of the postsynaptic neuron and consequently its membrane potential. Two possible scenarios can then follow: (1) the postsynaptic neuron may be excited (depolarized; **excitatory postsynaptic potentials [EPSPs]**) or (2) the postsynaptic neuron's plasma membrane may be inhibited (hyperpolarized; **inhibitory postsynaptic potentials [IPSPs]**). (Chapter 1 contains a review of electrical impulses and membrane potentials.)

Usually, a single EPSP cannot induce a neuron's action potential and the propagation of the nerve impulse. Whether an action potential occurs depends on the number and frequency of potentials the postsynaptic neuron receives—a concept known as **summation**. **Temporal summation** (time relationship) refers to the effects of successive, rapid impulses received from a single neuron on the same synapse. **Spatial summation** (spacing effect) is the combined effects of impulses from a number of neurons on a single synapse at the same time. **Facilitation** refers to the effect of EPSPs on the plasma membrane potential. The plasma membrane is facilitated when summation brings the membrane closer to the threshold potential and decreases the stimulus required to induce an action potential. The effect that a neurotransmitter has on the plasma membrane potential depends on the balance of these effects. The mechanisms of convergence, divergence, summation, and facilitation allow for the integrative processes of the nervous system.

Two points could be helpful in understanding the complexity of brain physiology. First, the aforementioned neuromodulators appear to function to raise or lower the membrane potentials of neurons. These chemicals facilitate or inhibit the effect of neurotransmitters. Second, reciprocal synapses between dendrites, that is, one dendrite being able to depolarize or hyperpolarize the membrane potential of another dendrite through the use of neurotransmitters, demonstrate that the interactions between neurons are far more complicated than postulated by simple on-off models of brain function.

CENTRAL NERVOUS SYSTEM
Brain

The human brain enables individuals to reason, function intellectually, express personality and mood, and interact with the environment. The brain is a pinkish gray organ that weighs approximately 3 pounds and has the consistency of tofu or custard. It receives approximately 15% to 20% of the total cardiac output. The three major divisions of the brain, based on embryologic origin, are (1) the forebrain, formed by the two cerebral hemispheres; (2) the midbrain, which includes the corpora quadrigemina, tegmentum, and cerebral peduncles; and (3) the hindbrain, which includes the cerebellum, pons, and medulla (Table 14-3). The midbrain, medulla oblongata, and pons make up the **brain stem,** which connects the hemispheres of the brain, cerebellum, and spinal cord. A collection of nuclei (nerve cell bodies) within the brain stem forms the **reticular formation** (Figure 14-5). The reticular formation is a large network of connected tissue nuclei that regulate vital reflexes, such as cardiovascular function and respiration. The reticular formation is essential for maintaining wakefulness and in conjunction with the cerebral cortex is referred to as the **reticular activating system.** Some nuclei within the reticular formation are involved in motor movements.[4]

In general, many major divisions of the brain are associated with specific functions, such as the occipital lobe and vi-

Table 14-2 Neurotransmitter and/or Neuromodulator Substances

Substance	Location	Effect	Clinical Example
Acetylcholine	Many parts of the brain, spinal cord, neuromuscular junction of skeletal muscle, and many ANS synapses	Excitatory or inhibitory	Alzheimer disease (a type of senile dementia) is associated with a decrease in acetylcholine-secreting neurons; myasthenia gravis (weakness of skeletal muscles) results from a reduction in acetylcholine receptors
Monoamines			
Norepinephrine	Many areas of the brain and spinal cord; also in sympathetic ANS synapses	Excitatory or inhibitory	Cocaine and amphetamines,* resulting in over-stimulation of postsynaptic neurons
Serotonin	Many areas of the brain and spinal cord	Generally inhibitory	Involved with mood, anxiety, and sleep induction; levels of serotonin elevated in schizophrenia (delusions, hallucinations, and withdrawal)
Dopamine	Some areas of the brain and ANS synapses	Generally excitatory	Parkinson disease (depression of voluntary motor control) results from destruction of dopamine-secreting neurons; drugs used to increase dopamine production induce vomiting and schizophrenia; involved in pleasure pathway
Histamine		Generally inhibitory	No clear indication of histamine-associated pathologic conditions; histamine apparently is involved with arousal, pituitary hormone secretion, control of cerebral circulation, and thermoregulation
Amino Acids			
γ-Aminobutyric acid (GABA)	Most neurons of the CNS have GABA receptors	Majority of postsynaptic inhibition in the brain	Drugs that increase GABA function have been used to treat epilepsy (excessive discharge of neurons)
Glycine	Spinal cord	Most postsynaptic inhibition in the spinal cord	Glycine receptors inhibited by strychnine
Glutamate and aspartate	Widespread in the brain and spinal cord	Excitatory	Drugs that block glutamate or aspartate are under development; might prevent seizures and neural degeneration from overexcitation
Neuropeptides			
Endorphins and enkephalins	Widely distributed in the CNS and PNS	Generally inhibitory	The opiates morphine and heroin bind to endorphin and enkephalin receptors on presynaptic neurons and reduce pain by blocking the release of neurotransmitter
Substance P	Spinal cord, brain, and sensory neurons associated with pain, GI tract	Generally excitatory	Substance P is a neurotransmitter in pain transmission pathways; blocking its release by morphine reduces pain

From Seeley R, Stephens TD, Tate P: *Anatomy and physiology,* ed 3, St Louis, 1992, Mosby.
*Increase the release and block the reuptake of norepinephrine.
ANS, Autonomic nervous system; *CNS,* central nervous system; *PNS,* peripheral nervous system; *GI,* gastrointestinal.

Table 14-3 Divisions of the Central Nervous System

Primary Vesicles	Secondary Vesicles	Associated Structures
Forebrain (prosencephalon)	Telencephalon	Cerebral hemispheres
		Cerebral cortex
		Rhinencephalon
		Basal ganglia
	Diencephalon	Epithalamus
		Thalamus
		Hypothalamus
		Subthalamus
Midbrain (mesencephalon)	Mesencephalon	Corpora quadrigemina
		Tegmentum
		Cerebral peduncles
Hindbrain (rhombencephalon)	Metencephalon	Cerebellum
		Pons
	Myelencephalon	Medulla oblongata
Spinal cord	Spinal cord	Spinal cord

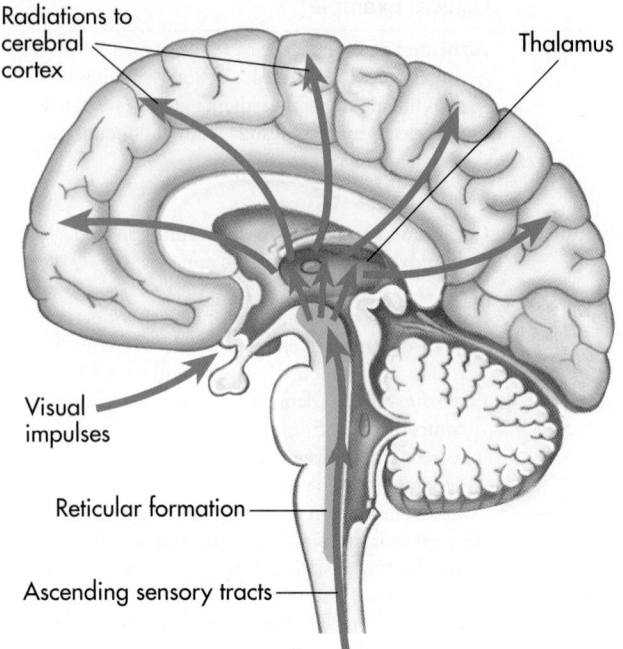

Radiations to
cerebral
cortex

Thalamus

Visual
impulses

Reticular formation

Ascending sensory tracts

Figure 14-5 Reticular activating system. System consists of nuclei in the brain stem reticular formation plus fibers (axons) that conduct to the nuclei from below and fibers that conduct from the nuclei to widespread areas of the cerebral cortex. Functioning of the reticular activating system is essential for consciousness.

sion, but attributing specific functions to definite regions of the brain is not entirely accurate. Many activities, such as motor movements and memory, may actually be performed in several regions. Understanding functional specificity is very useful to clinical personnel, especially when attempting to localize pathologic conditions in the nervous system. A neurologist often can localize the site of a tumor, stroke, or bullet wound in an individual just by performing a neurologic examination.

Many attempts have been made to ascribe function to various regions of the cerebral cortex. A German neuropsychiatrist, Brodmann (1868–1918), is credited with postulating the correlation of various activities to many regions of the cerebral cortex. (Figure 14-6, *B* and *C*, illustrates these regions and identifies some functional areas.) Another basic CNS principle, **plasticity,** holds that the CNS is capable of change. For example, children with brain damage may experience "relocation" of some functional areas to other parts of the brain. This propensity for plasticity decreases with age, which explains why older individuals tend not to recover from brain injuries as well as younger individuals. This varying balance between specificity and plasticity makes understanding brain functions difficult.

Forebrain

Telencephalon

The **telencephalon** consists of the **cerebrum** (the largest portion of the brain), which includes the cerebral cortex and **basal ganglia.** The surface of the cerebrum is characterized by

numerous convolutions called *gyri* (see Figure 14-6, *A*). The gyri greatly increase the cortical surface area. Grooves between adjacent gyri are called **sulci.** Deeper grooves are referred to as **fissures.** The **cerebral cortex** contains the cell bodies and dendrites of neurons, which often are referred to as **gray matter.** Gray matter is organized into columns perpendicular to the surface that receive, integrate, store, and transmit information. **White matter** lies beneath the cerebral cortex and is composed of myelinated nerve fibers.

The two cerebral hemispheres are separated by the longitudinal fissure. The surface of each hemisphere is divided into lobes that take their names from the region of the skull under which each of them lies. The posterior margin of the **frontal lobe** is the **central sulcus (fissure of Rolando,** central fissure); it borders inferiorly on the **lateral sulcus (sylvian fissure, lateral fissure)** (see Figure 14-6, *A*). The **prefrontal area** is responsible for goal-oriented behavior (i.e., ability to concentrate), short-term or recall memory, and the elaboration of thought and inhibition on the limbic (emotional) areas of the CNS. The **premotor area** (Brodmann area 6) (see Figure 14-6, *C*) is involved in programming motor movements. This area also contains the cell bodies that form part of the **basal ganglia system** (extrapyramidal system—efferent pathways outside the pyramids of the medulla oblongata). The frontal eye fields (the lower portion of Brodmann area 8), which are involved in controlling eye movements, are located in the middle frontal gyrus.

The **primary motor area** (Brodmann area 4) is located along the **precentral gyrus** forming the **primary voluntary motor area,** which has a somatotopic organization that often is referred to as a *homunculus* (little man) (Figure 14-7). Electrical stimulation of specific areas of this cortex causes specific muscles of the body to move. The medial part of the cortex in the **longitudinal fissure** (midline space between the two cerebral hemispheres) affects the lower limb and foot, whereas on the lateral surface, the superior third controls the torso and arm, the middle third the hand, and the lowest third the face and mouth/throat. The axons traveling from the cell bodies in and on either side of this gyrus project fibers (axons) that form the **corticospinal tracts** (pyramidal system) that descend into the spinal cord. Cerebral impulses control function in the opposite side of the body, a phenomenon called **contralateral control** (Figure 14-8, *A*). The **Broca speech area** (Brodmann areas 44, 45) is rostral to the inferior edge of the premotor area (Brodmann area 6) on the inferior frontal gyrus. It is usually on the left hemisphere and is responsible for the motor aspects of speech. Damage to this area, commonly as a result of a cerebrovascular accident (stroke), results in the inability to form, or difficulty in forming, words (expressive aphasia or dysphasia) (see Chapter 17).

The **parietal lobe** lies within the borders of the central, parietooccipital, and lateral sulci. This lobe contains the major area for somatic sensory input, located primarily along the **postcentral gyrus** (Brodmann areas 3, 1, 2), which is adjacent to the primary motor area. Communication between the motor and sensory areas (and among other regions in the cortex)

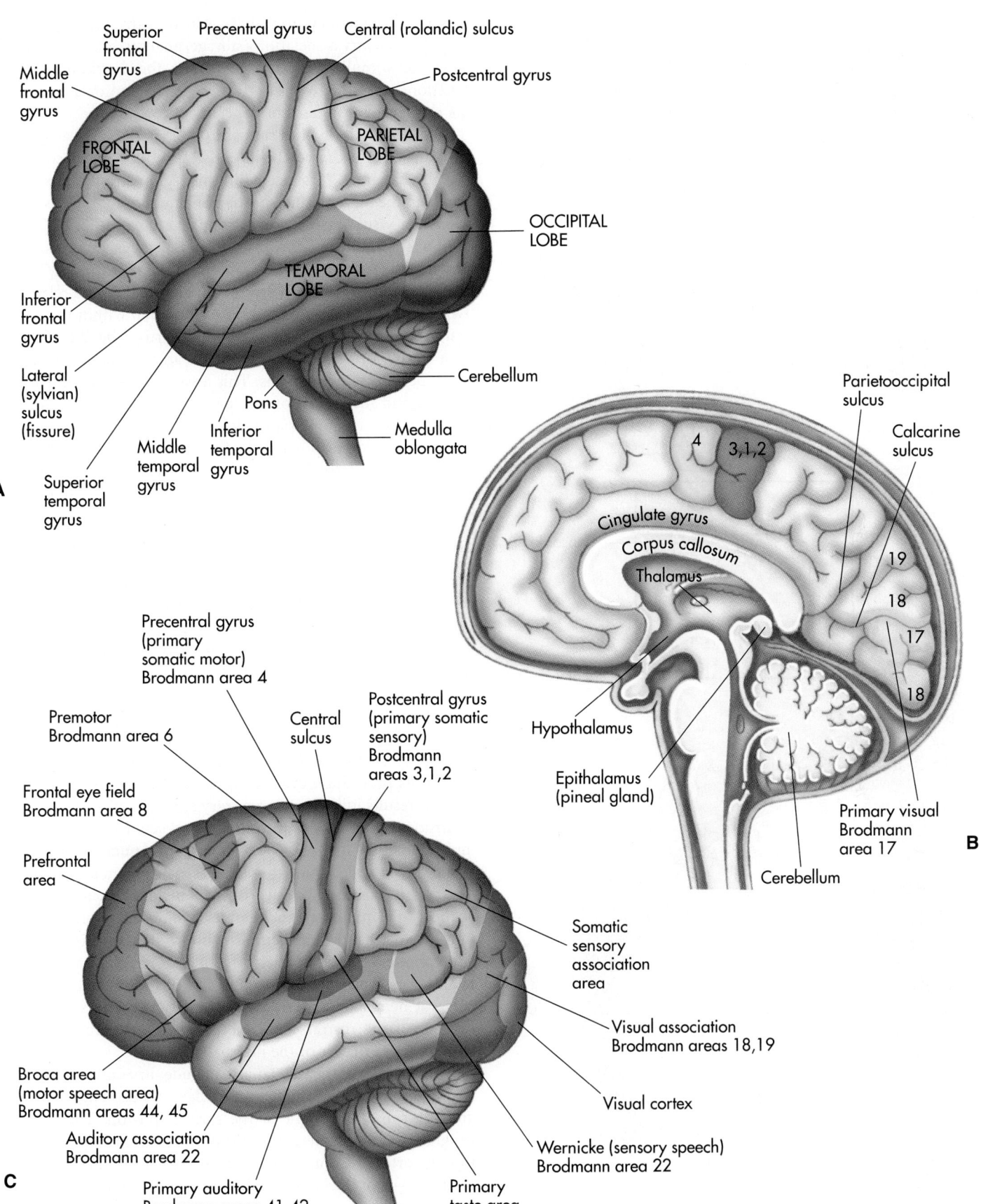

Figure 14-6 Cerebral hemispheres. A, Left hemisphere of cerebrum, lateral view. **B,** Functional areas of the cerebral cortex, midsagittal view. **C,** Functional areas of the cerebral cortex, lateral view.

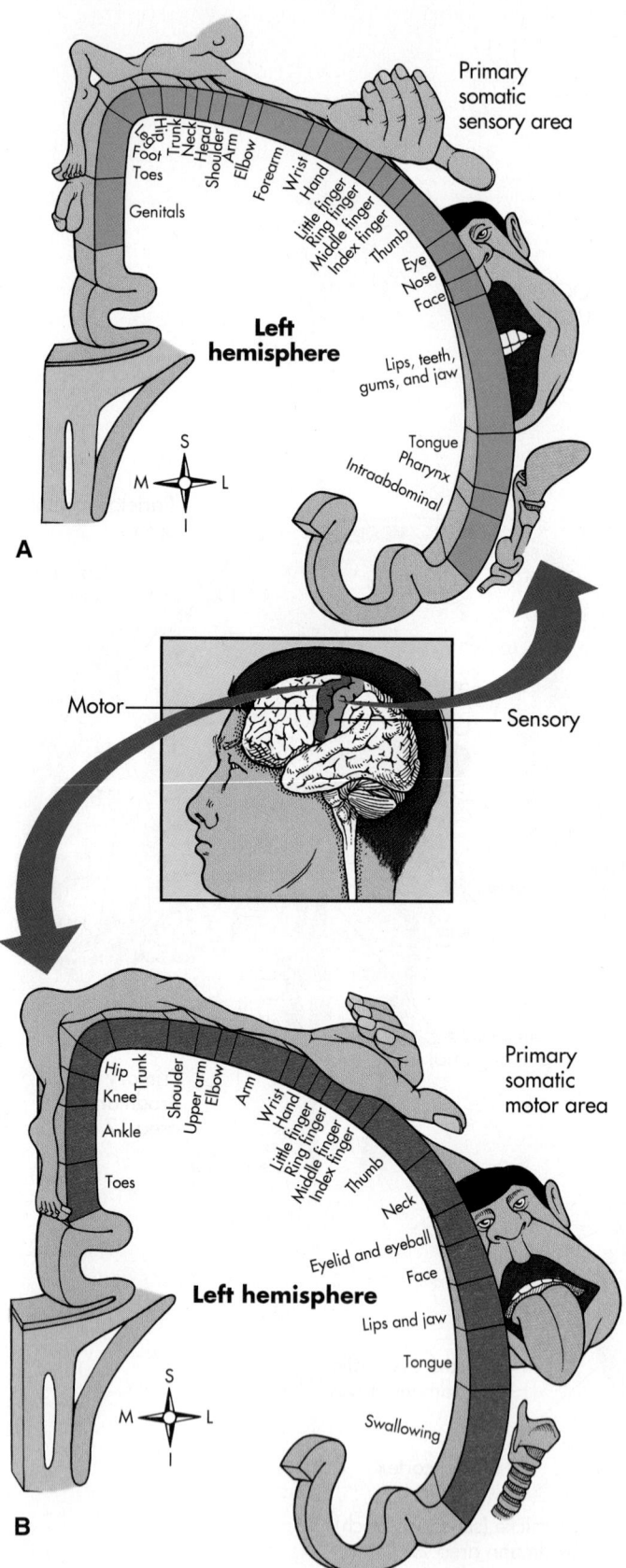

Figure 14-7 Primary somatic sensory (A) and motor (B) areas of the cortex. (From Thibodeau GA, Patton KT: *Anatomy & physiology*, ed 5, St Louis, 2003, Mosby.)

is provided by **association fibers.** Much of this region is involved in sensory association (storage, analysis, and interpretation of stimuli). (Figure 14-7 shows the distribution of functions associated with both the primary motor area and the primary sensory area of the cerebral cortex.)

The **occipital lobe** lies caudal to the parietooccipital sulci and superior to the cerebellum. The primary visual cortex (Brodmann area 17) is located in this region and receives input from the retinas. Much of the remainder of this lobe is involved in visual association (Brodmann areas 18, 19). The **temporal lobe** lies inferior to the lateral sulcus and is composed of the superior, middle, and inferior temporal gyri. The primary auditory cortex (Brodmann area 41) and its related association area (Brodmann area 42) lie deep within the lateral sulcus on the superior temporal gyrus. The **Wernicke area** (posterior portion of Brodmann area 22) is located on the superior temporal gyrus. This area is responsible for reception and interpretation of speech, and dysfunction may result in receptive aphasia or dysphasia. The Wernicke area, along with adjacent portions of the parietal lobe, constitutes a *sensory speech area.* The temporal lobe also is involved as a major area for long-term memory and secondary functions, such as balance, taste, and smell.

Another lobe, the **insula,** lies hidden from view deep in the lateral sulcus. Lying directly beneath the longitudinal fissure is a massive white matter pathway called the **corpus callosum (commissural fibers).** The corpus callosum connects the two cerebral hemispheres and is essential in the coordination of activities between hemispheres, especially specific tasks that may be present in only one hemisphere (see Figures. 14-6, *C,* and 14-14). As a last resort, part or all of the corpus callosum is cut to prevent the spread of epileptic loci (site of seizure activity) through the corpus callosum to the opposite cerebral hemisphere. Epileptic loci often are found in the temporal lobe. This procedure, evolved in the well-known split-brain studies, results initially in temporary aphasia and paralysis.

Inside the cerebrum are numerous tracts (white matter) and nuclei (gray matter). The major **cerebral nuclei** are called *basal ganglia* and include the corpus striatum and **amygdala.** The **corpus striatum** consists of the **lentiform nucleus** (lens shaped), the putamen and globus pallidus, and the ram's horn–shaped caudate nucleus. The **internal capsule** is a thick white matter region in which afferent and efferent pathways, to and from the cerebral cortex, pass through the center of the cerebral hemispheres. The corpus striatum appears striped because of the rostral connections between its gray matter and the white matter of the internal capsule.

Functionally, the basal ganglia include, in addition to the corpus striatum, the subthalamic nucleus of the diencephalon and the substantia nigra of the mesencephalon. The basal ganglia plus their interconnections with the thalamus, premotor cortex, red nucleus, reticular formation, and spinal cord are part of the basal ganglia system (extrapyramidal system). The basal ganglia system is believed to exert a fine-tuning effect on motor movements. Parkinson disease and Huntington disease are conditions associated with defects of

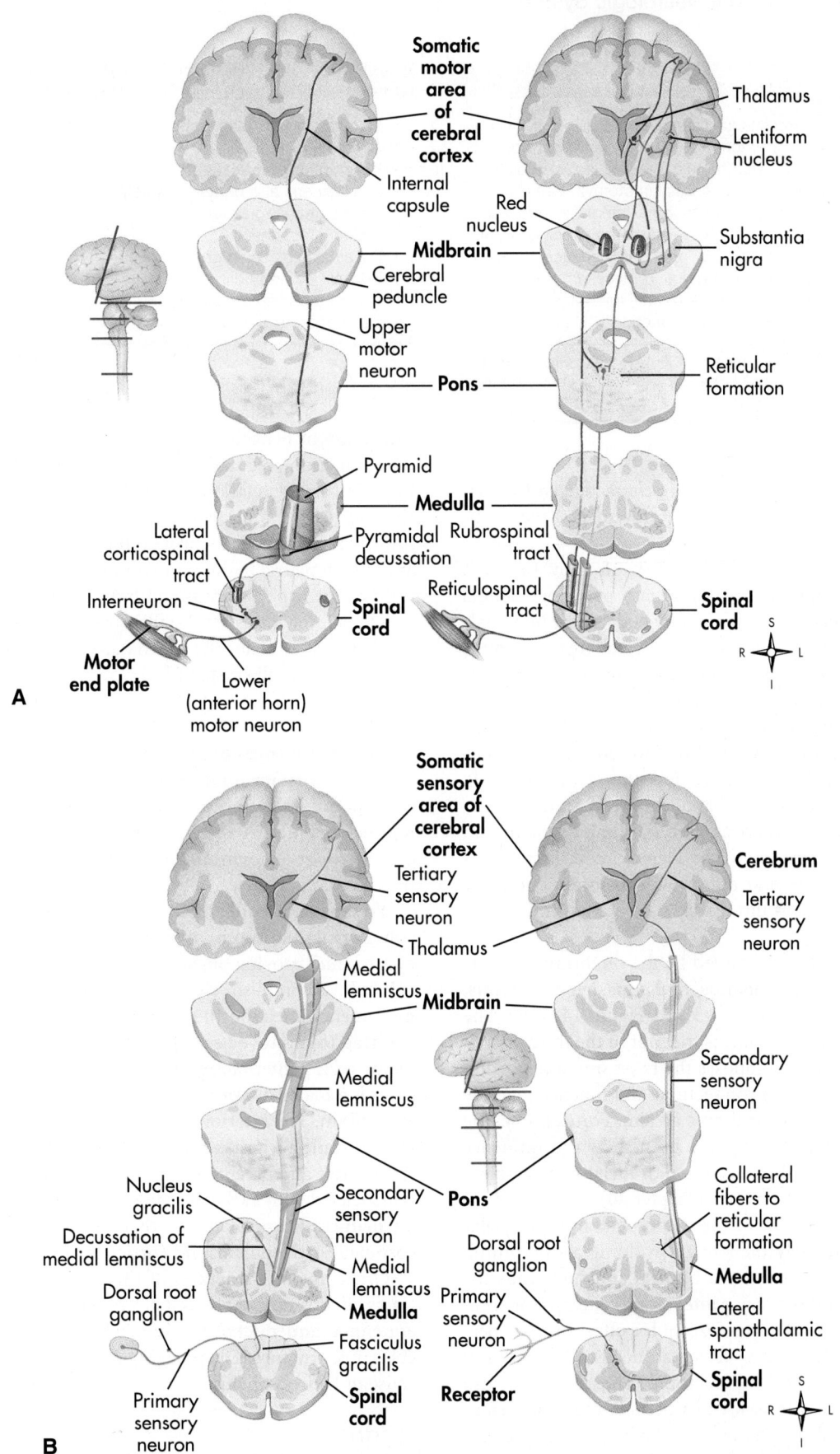

Figure 14-8 Examples of somatic motor and sensory pathways. **A,** Motor: the pyramidal pathway through the lateral corticospinal tract and the extrapyramidal pathways through the rubrospinal and reticulospinal tracts. Examples of somatic motor and sensory pathways. **B,** Sensory: pathways of the medial lemniscal system that conducts information about discriminating touch and kinesthesis and the spinothalamic pathway that conducts information about pain and temperature. (From Thibodeau GA, Patton KT: *Anatomy & physiology,* ed 5, St Louis, 2003, Mosby.)

| **Box 14-2** | Surgery for Parkinson Disease |

Surgical treatment for Parkinson disease can provide gratifying relief from the disabling symptoms of the disease when medical therapies are not effective. The forms of surgery include ablation (thalamotomy, pallidotomy, and subthalamotomy), deep brain stimulation (thalamus, globus pallidus pars internalis, and subthalamic nucleus), and cell graft and gene therapy (mainly of the striatum). Deep brain stimulation is preferred because there is symptom control without tissue destruction. Research is continuing to overcome obstacles associated with cell transplant and gene therapy that boosts dopamine production.

Data from Follett KA: *Annu Rev med* 51:135-147, 2000; Gross CE et al: *Prog Neurobiol* 59(5):509-532, 1999; Moretti R et al: *Parkinsonism Relat Disord* 10(2):73-79, 2003.

| **Box 14-3** | Functions of the Hypothalamus |

- Visceral and somatic responses
- Affectual responses
- Hormone synthesis
- Sympathetic and parasympathetic activity
- Temperature regulation
- Feeding responses
- Physical expression of emotions
- Sexual behavior
- Pleasure-punishment centers
- Level of arousal or wakefulness

the basal ganglia (Box 14-2). They are characterized by various involuntary or exaggerated motor movements (see Chapters 16 and 17).

The **limbic system,** first described in 1878 by Broca, is composed of the **Papez circuit** (amygdala, parahippocampal gyrus, **hippocampus,** fornix, mamillary body of the hypothalamus, thalamus, and cingulate gyrus), septal area, habenula, other portions of the hypothalamus, and related autonomic nuclei. It is an extension or modification of the olfactory system. Its principal effects are believed to be involved with primitive behavioral responses, visceral reaction to emotion, feeding behaviors, biologic rhythms, and the sense of smell. Expression of affect (emotional and behavioral states) is mediated by extensive connections with the limbic system and prefrontal cortex. Interestingly, the Papez circuit, first postulated in 1937, appears to have as one of its major functions the consolidation of memory through a reverberating circuit.

Diencephalon

The **diencephalon,** surrounded by the cerebrum, is made up of four divisions: **epithalamus, thalamus, hypothalamus,** and **subthalamus** (see Table 14-3 and Figure 14-6, *B*). The epithalamus (pineal gland) forms the roof of the third ventricle (a brain cavity) and composes the most superior portion of the diencephalon. It has connections and functions closely associated with those of the limbic system. For example, the hormones of the pineal body have been shown to influence reproductive ability, and the secretion of melatonin is associated with circadian rhythms (see Chapter 20).

The largest component of the diencephalon is the thalamus. It is approximately the size and volume of the thumb from the tip to the first joint. It borders and surrounds the third ventricle, and it is a major integrating center for afferent impulses to the cerebral cortex, except for olfaction. The perception of various sensations occurs at this level but requires cortical processing for interpretation. The thalamus also serves as a relay center for sensory aspects of motor information from the basal ganglia and cerebellum to appropriate cortical motor areas. Cerebral cortical information also projects to the thalamus, creating reverberating circuits.

The hypothalamus forms the base of the diencephalon. Hypothalamic function falls into two major areas: (1) main-

tenance of a constant internal environment and (2) implementation of behavioral patterns. Integrative centers control ANS function, regulation of body temperature, endocrine function, and regulation of emotional expression. (Temperature regulation is discussed in Chapter 15.) The hypothalamus exerts its influence through the endocrine system, as well as through neural pathways (Box 14-3). (For endocrine functions of the hypothalamus and pituitary, see Chapter 20.)

The subthalamus flanks the hypothalamus laterally. The subthalamus contains the **subthalamic nucleus,** which is part of the basal ganglia system.

Midbrain

The **midbrain (mesencephalon)** is composed of three structures: the **corpora quadrigemina,** or **tectum** (composed of the superior and inferior colliculi); the **tegmentum** (containing the red nucleus and substantia nigra); and the basis pedunculi. (The tegmentum and basis pedunculi are collectively the cerebral peduncles.)

The **superior colliculi** are involved with voluntary and involuntary visual motor movements (e.g., the ability of the eyes to *track* moving objects in the visual field). The **inferior colliculi** accomplish similar motor activities but involve movements affecting the auditory system (e.g., positioning the head to improve hearing). The inferior colliculus is also a major relay center along the auditory pathway. The **red nucleus** is a major motor output center that is influenced by the cerebellum. The inferior-most portion of the basal ganglia is the **substantia nigra,** which synthesizes **dopamine,** a neurotransmitter and precursor of norepinephrine. Its dysfunction is associated with Parkinson disease (see Chapter 17). The **basis pedunculi** are made up of efferent fibers of the corticospinal, corticobulbar, and corticopontocerebellar tracts.

Other notable structures of this region are the nuclei and tracts of the third and fourth cranial nerves. The **cerebral aqueduct (aqueduct of Sylvius),** which carries CSF, also traverses this structure. The plugging of this aqueduct is often the cause of hydrocephalus.

Hindbrain

Metencephalon

The major structures of the **metencephalon** are the cerebellum and the pons. The **cerebellum** (see Figure 14-6, *A* and *B*) is composed of two cerebellar hemispheres covered with small convolutions called *folia.* Each hemisphere is divided by the primary fissure into two lobes (anterior and posterior) that are connected by a midline structure called the **vermis,** meaning worm.

The cerebellum is responsible for both conscious and unconscious muscle synergy and for maintaining balance and posture. This is accomplished through extensive neural connections from the spinal cord and medulla oblongata through the inferior cerebellar peduncle and with the midbrain and higher structures through the superior cerebellar peduncle. The two cerebellar hemispheres receive massive cerebral cortical input through the middle cerebellar pedunculi. These connections allow extensive sampling of visual, vestibular, and proprioceptive data from other regions of the CNS and periphery. Damage to the cerebellum is characterized by ipsilateral (same side) loss of equilibrium, balance, and motor coordination. The cerebellum has ipsilateral control of the body, in contrast to the cerebral cortex, which has contralateral (opposite side) control of the body.

The **pons** (bridge) is easily recognized by its bulging appearance below the midbrain and above the medulla oblongata. Primarily, it transmits information from the cerebellum to the brain stem nuclei and relays motor information from the cerebral cortex to the contralateral cerebellar hemisphere. The pons is an important center for the control of respiration (i.e., rate and relationship of inspiration to expiration). The nuclei of cranial nerves V through VIII are located in this structure.

Myelencephalon

The **medulla oblongata** makes up the **myelencephalon** and is the lowest portion of the brain stem. Reflex activities, such as heart rate, respiration, blood pressure, coughing, sneezing, swallowing, and vomiting, are controlled in this area. The nuclei of cranial nerves IX through XII (see Table 14-6 for discussion) are located in this region. The lowest portion of the reticular formation is found here as well.

A major portion of the descending motor pathways (i.e., corticospinal tracts) cross to the contralateral side, or decussate, at the inferior medulla oblongata (see Figure. 14-8, *A*). These pathways, together with other areas of decussation in the CNS, are the basis for the phenomenon of contralateral control.

Spinal Cord

The **spinal cord** is the portion of the CNS that lies within the vertebral canal and is surrounded and protected by the vertebral column. The spinal cord has many functions, which include being a long nerve cable that connects the brain and body, conducting somatic and autonomic reflexes, providing motor pattern control centers, and serving as a sensory and motor modulation center. It continues from the medulla oblongata and ends at the level of the first or second lumbar vertebra in adults (Figure 14-9). The end of the spinal cord, **conus medullaris,** is cone shaped. Spinal nerves continue from the end of the spinal cord and form a nerve bundle called the **cauda equina.** The filament anchor from the conus medullaris to the coccyx is the **filum terminale** (see Figure 14-9).

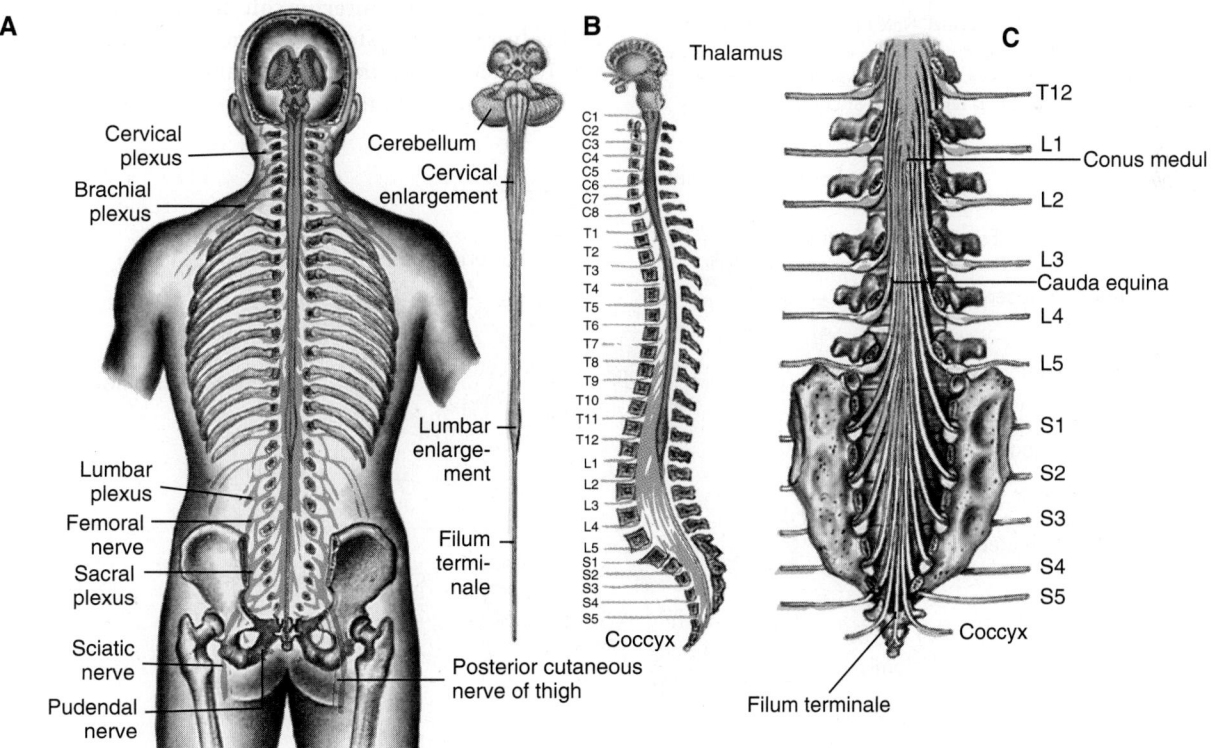

Figure 14-9 **Spinal cord within vertebral canal and exiting spinal nerves. A,** Posterior view of brain stem and spinal cord in situ with spinal nerves and plexus. **B,** Anterior view of brain stem and spinal cord. **C,** Enlargement of caudal area showing termination of spinal cord (conus medullaris) and group of nerve fibers constituting the cauda equina. (From Rudy EB, editor: *Advanced neurological and neurosurgical nursing,* St Louis, 1984, Mosby.)

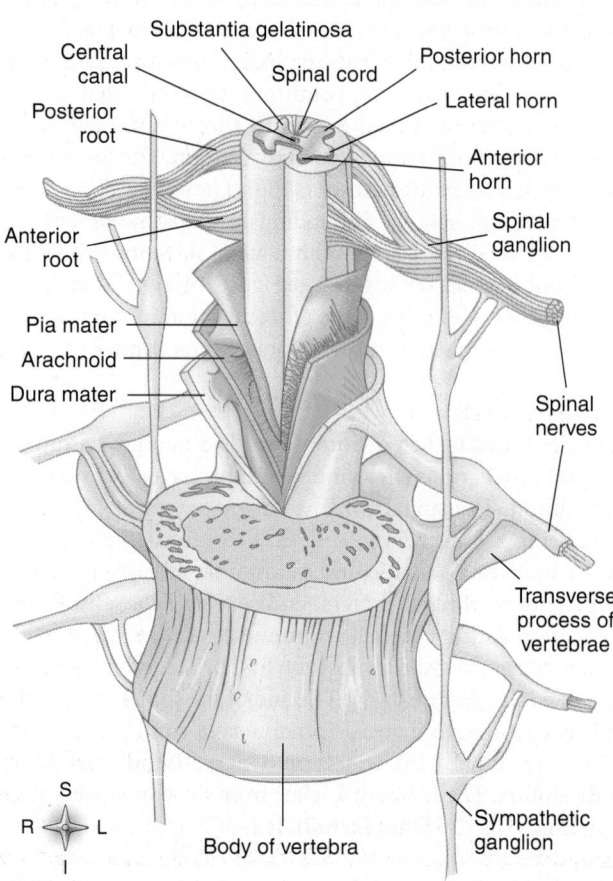

Figure 14-10 Coverings of the spinal cord. Note how the dura mater extends to cover the spinal nerve roots and nerves. The arachnoid is highlighted in *blue* and the pia mater in *pink.* (Modified from Thibodeau GA, Patton KT: *Structure and function of the body,* ed 12, St Louis, 2004, Mosby.)

Grossly, the spinal cord is divided into sections (8 cervical, 12 thoracic, 5 lumbar, 5 sacral, and 1 coccygeal) that correspond to paired nerves (see Figure 14-9). A cross section of the spinal cord (Figure 14-10) is characterized by a butterfly-shaped inner core of gray matter (containing nerve cell bodies). The **central canal** lies in the center of this region and extends through the spinal cord from its origin in the fourth ventricle. The gray matter of the spinal cord is divided into three regions with specific functional characteristics. These regions include the **posterior horn (dorsal horn),** which is composed primarily of interneurons and axons from sensory neurons whose cell bodies lie in the **sensory ganglion (dorsal root ganglion).** At the tip of the posterior horn is the **substantia gelatinosa,** a structure involved in pain transmission (see Chapter 15). The **intermediolateral gray (lateral horn)** contains cell bodies involved with the ANS. The **anterior horn (ventral horn)** contains the nerve cell bodies for efferent pathways leaving the spinal cord by way of spinal nerves. The terms *anterior* and *posterior* are preferred by many authors for describing human spinal cord anatomy, whereas *dorsal* and *ventral* are the common zoologic ("cat and dog") terms.

Surrounding the gray matter is white matter that forms ascending and descending pathways called **spinal tracts** and short ascending and descending integrative pathways. Spinal tracts are named to denote their beginning and ending points. For example, the **spinothalamic tract** carries nerve impulses from the spinal cord to the thalamus in the diencephalon. The white matter is subdivided into columns. These consist of the **anterior column (ventral column), lateral column,** and **posterior column (dorsal column).** (Figure 14-11 identifies the location and principal activities of the major spinal tracts.)

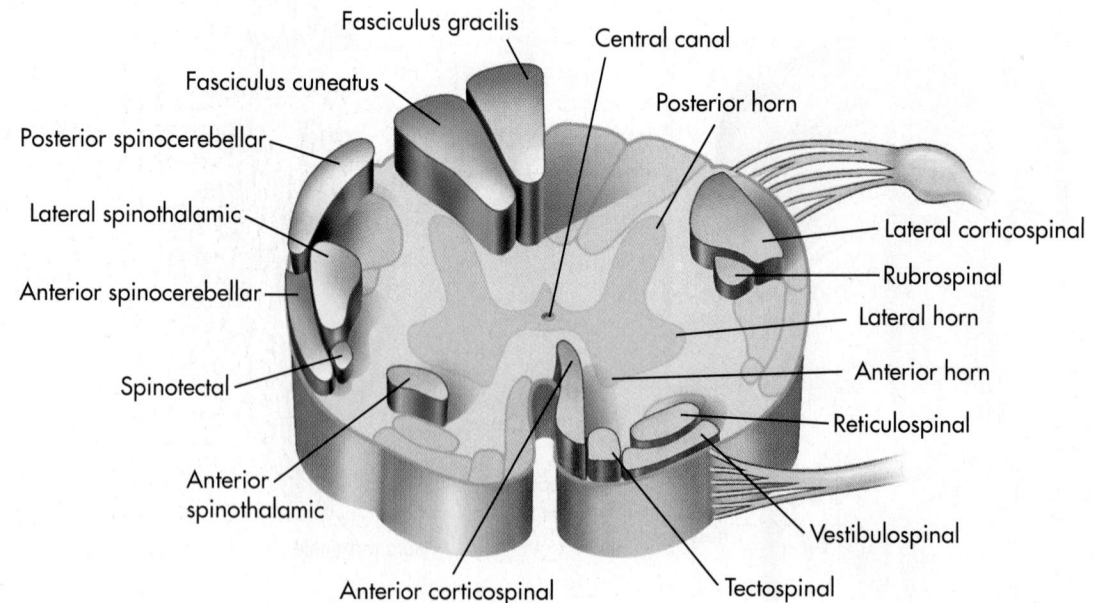

Figure 14-11 Major tracts of the spinal cord. The major ascending (sensory) tracts, shown only on the left here, are highlighted in *blue.* The major descending (motor) tracts, shown only on the right, are highlighted in *red.* (From Thibodeau GA, Patton KT: *Anatomy & physiology,* ed 5, St Louis, 2003, Mosby.)

Neural circuits in the spinal cord, when activated, display specific sets of motor responses. **Reflex arcs** form basic units that respond to stimuli and provide protective circuitry for motor output. Structures mandatory for a reflex arc are a receptor, an **afferent (sensory) neuron,** an **efferent (motor) neuron,** and an effector muscle or gland. The afferent neuron is a pseudounipolar neuron, with its cell body in the sensory ganglion. A simple reflex arc may contain only two neurons. (Figure 14-12 illustrates a simple reflex arc.) Most reflex arcs consist of three neurons that include an interneuron or association neuron between the afferent and efferent neurons. Transmission time for three-neuron reflexes is slower than in simple reflexes because there are two synaptic delays, rather than one, as well as the delay involved in crossing the interneuron. The afferent neuron of the reflex arc simultaneously sends sensory information to the effector organ and to higher CNS centers (see Figures 14-8, *B*, and 15-4). The motor effects from reflex arcs generally occur before perception of the event in the higher centers of the brain. Much of the regulation of the internal environment is mediated by ANS reflexes.

Afferent pathways transmit information from peripheral receptors and eventually terminate in the cerebral or cerebellar cortex or both. Efferent pathways primarily relay information from the cerebrum to the brain stem or spinal cord (see Figure 14-8, *A*). **Upper motor neurons** (i.e., corticospinal tract) are the classification of motor pathways completely contained within the CNS. Their primary roles include directing, influencing, and modifying reflex arcs, lower-level control centers, and motor (and some sensory) neurons. Generally, upper motor neurons form synapses with interneurons, which then form synapses with lower motor neurons

before projecting into the periphery. **Lower motor neurons** (i.e., cranial and spinal efferent neurons) are responsible for direct influence on muscles. Their cell bodies lie in the gray matter of the spinal cord, but their processes extend into the PNS (see Figure 16-20). Destruction of upper motor neurons usually results in initial paralysis followed within days or weeks by partial recovery, whereas destruction of the lower motor neurons often leads to permanent paralysis. Peripheral nerve damage may be followed by nerve regeneration and recovery. (Injury to motor neurons is discussed in Chapter 17.)

Muscle activity (i.e., stimulation and contraction) is regulated by nerve impulses. Motor neurons innervate one or more muscle cells, forming **motor units** consisting of a neuron and the skeletal muscles it stimulates. The junction between the axon of the motor neuron and the plasma membrane of the muscle cell is called the **neuromuscular (myoneural) junction** (Figure 14-13). The skeletal muscle neuromuscular junction is more elaborate than the simpler smooth muscle neuromuscular junction.

Motor Pathways

The four clinically relevant motor pathways are the **lateral corticospinal, corticobulbar,** basal ganglia, and **vestibulospinal** pathways. The corticospinal (see Figure 14-8, *A*) and corticobulbar (see Figure 16-19) are essentially the same tract and consist of a two-neuron chain. The cell bodies originate in and around the precentral gyrus; pass through the corona radiata of the cerebrum, the internal capsule, middle three fifths of the basis pedunculus, pons, and pyramid; decussate (cross contralaterally) in the medulla oblongata; and form the lateral corticospinal tract of the spinal cord (see Figure 14-11). The lateral corticospinal tract axons (upper motor

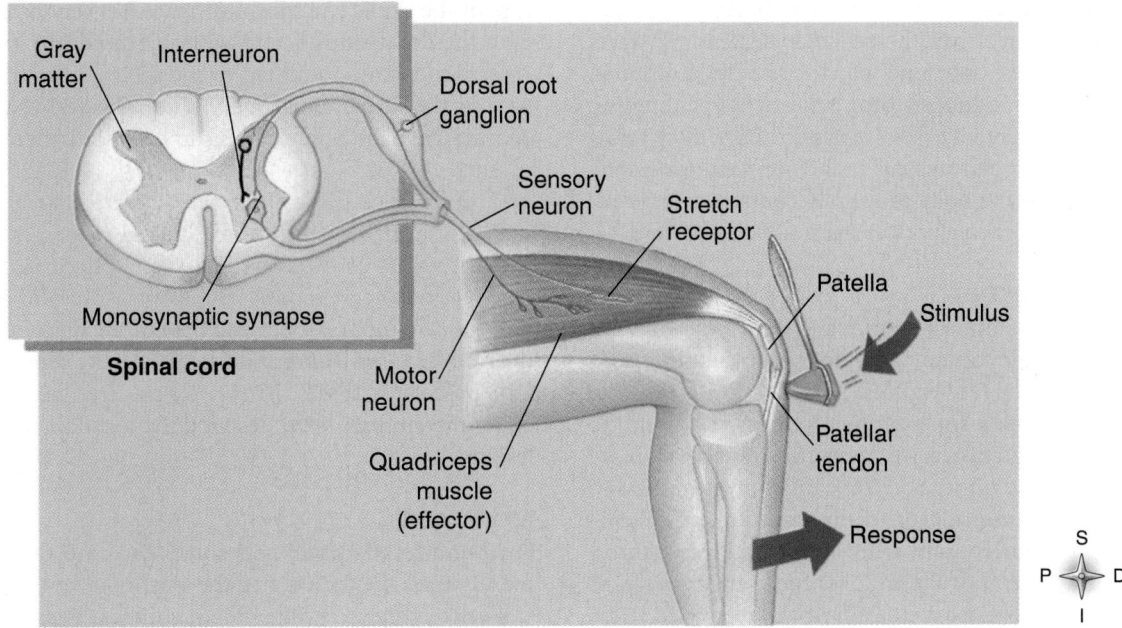

Figure 14-12 Cross section of spinal cord showing simple reflex arc. (From Thibodeau GA, Patton KT: *Anatomy & physiology,* ed 5, St Louis, 2003, Mosby.)

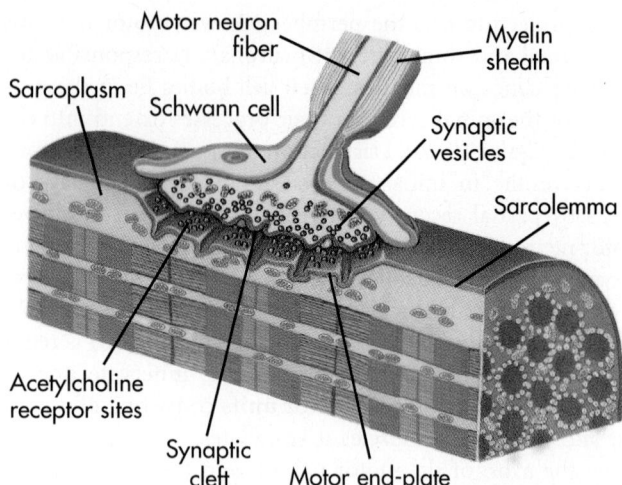

Figure 14-13 Neuromuscular junction. This figure shows how the distal end of a motor neuron fiber forms a synapse, or "chemical junction," with an adjacent muscle fiber. Neurotransmitters (specifically, acetylcholine) are released from the neuron's synaptic vesicles and diffuse across the synaptic cleft. There they stimulate receptors in the motor end-plate region of the sarcolemma. (From Thibodeau GA, Patton KT: *Anatomy & physiology*, ed 5, St Louis, 2003, Mosby.)

neurons) leave the tract to go to specific interneurons or motor neurons in the anterior horn. The lateral corticospinal tract has the same somatotopic organization as the body. These spinal motor neurons project to specific motor units and are lower motor neurons. The corticobulbar (bulbar refers to brain stem) tract can be thought of as the part of the corticospinal tract that innervates the cranial motor nuclei for eye, face, tongue, throat, and neck movement. This tract innervates all the cranial motor nuclei bilaterally except for the facial (spinal), accessory, and hypoglossal nuclei, which receive primarily contralateral innervation. These tracts are involved in precise motor movements. The basal ganglia are part of a system that drives the reticular descending tracts (Figure 14-11 shows only one of the two reticulospinal tracts.) These tracts modulate motor movement by inhibiting and exciting spinal activity. The vestibulospinal tract arises from the lateral vestibular nucleus in the pons and causes the extensor muscles of the body to rapidly contract, most dramatically witnessed when a person starts to fall backward.

Sensory Pathways

The three clinically important spinal afferent pathways are the posterior (dorsal) column, **anterior spinothalamic,** and **lateral spinothalamic** (see Figures. 14-8, *B*, and 14-11). The posterior column has a somatotopic organization with the fasciculus gracilis and fasciculus cuneatus, respectively, carrying lower body and upper body fine touch, two-point discrimination, and proprioceptive information (i.e., **epicritic**). The posterior column is formed by a three-neuron chain. The first neuron of the chain is the primary afferent neuron. It is also the sensory neuron of the reflex arc. After entering the spinal cord it sends its axon ipsilaterally up the spinal cord in a specific part of the posterior funiculus and

synapses in one of three posterior column nuclei in the hindbrain. A basketball center has primary afferent neurons that run from the great toe up to the pons, which could be over 6 feet long. The second-order neuron has its cell body in one of the posterior column nuclei and sends its axon contralaterally and ascends to a specific nucleus of the thalamus and synapses. The third-order neuron, originating in the thalamus, continues the tract into the internal capsule, corona radiata, and postcentral gyrus (Brodmann areas 3, 1, 2) (see Figure 14-6, *C*). The anterior and lateral spinothalamic tracts are responsible for vague touch and pain and temperature, respectively (see Figure 14-8, *B*). These modalities are referred to as **protopathic.**

Today, the anterior and lateral spinothalamic tracts are combined by many neuroanatomists into the anterolateral system because these modalities are difficult to localize into finite tracts in the spinal cord. These tracts also form a three-neuron chain. However, the primary afferent neurons synapse in the posterior horn of the spinal cord, not just at the level they enter the intervertebral foramen but in a number of spinal segments above and below their point of entry. This is an example of divergence. The second-order neurons in the posterior horn cross to the contralateral side in the spinal cord and ascend to the same thalamic nucleus as the posterior column pathway and continue on with the posterior column pathway to the postcentral gyrus.

Protective Structures
Cranium

The cranium is composed of eight bones. The cranial vault functions to enclose and protect the brain and its associated structures. The **galea aponeurotica,** which is a thick, fibrous band of tissue overlying the cranium between the frontal and occipital muscles, affords added protection to the bony structure of the skull. The subgaleal space has venous connections with the dural sinuses, and with increased intracranial pressure, blood can be shunted to the space, thus reducing pressure in the intracranial cavity. The subgaleal space is also a common site for wound drains to be placed after intracranial surgery.

The floor of the cranial vault is irregular and contains many foramina (openings) for cranial nerves, blood vessels, and the spinal cord to exit. The cranial floor is divided into three fossae (depressions). The frontal lobes lie in the **anterior fossa;** temporal lobes and base of the diencephalon lie in the **middle fossa (temporal fossa);** and the cerebellum lies in the **posterior fossa.** These terms are commonly used anatomic landmarks to describe the location of intracranial lesions.

Meninges

Surrounding the brain and spinal cord are three protective membranes: the dura mater, the arachnoid, and the pia mater. Collectively they are called the **meninges** (Figure 14-14). The **dura mater** (meaning literally "hard mother") is composed of two layers, with the venous sinuses formed between them.

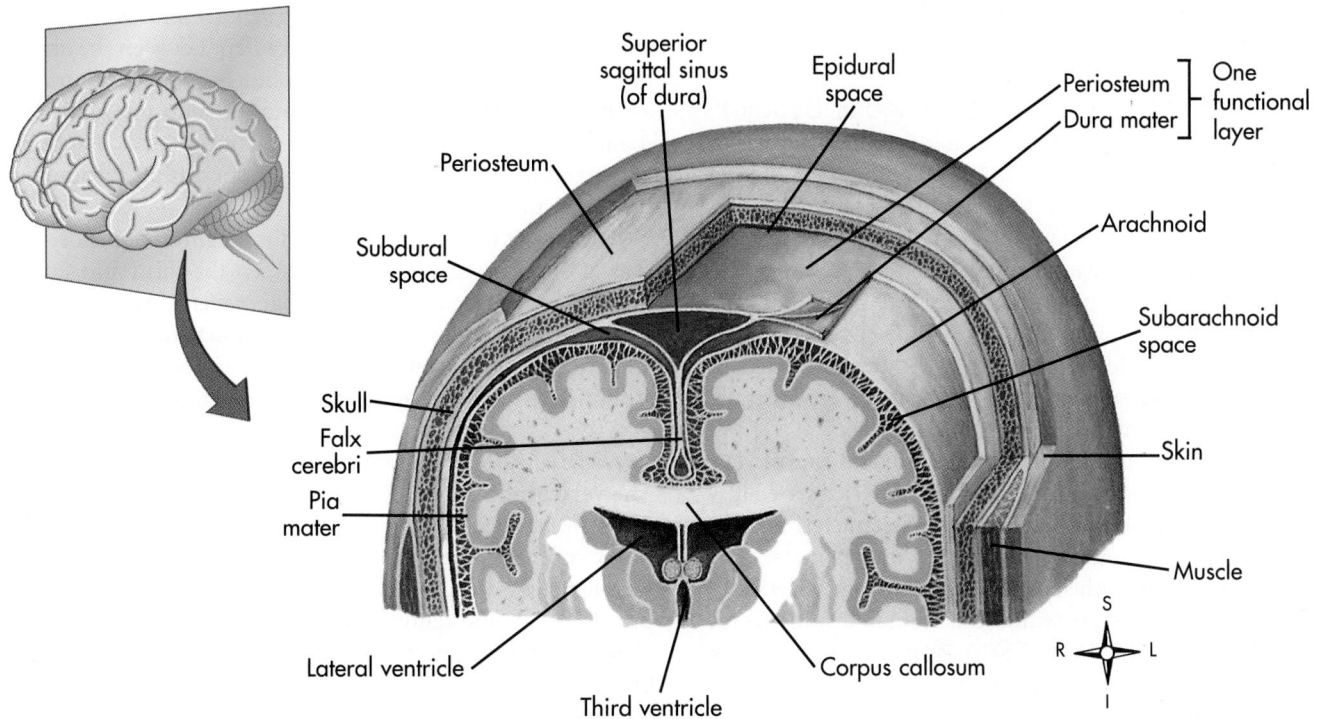

Figure 14-14 Coverings of the brain. Frontal section of the superior portion of the head, as viewed from the front. Both the bony and the membranous coverings of the brain can be seen. (From Thibodeau GA, Patton KT: *Anatomy & physiology,* ed 5, St Louis, 2003, Mosby.)

The outermost layer forms the **periosteum (endosteal layer)** of the skull, and the **inner dura,** or **meningeal layer,** is responsible for the formation of rigid, double-thickness membranous plates that serve to support and separate various brain structures.

One of these membranous plates (see Figure 14-14), the **falx cerebri,** dips between the two cerebral hemispheres along the longitudinal fissure. The falx cerebri is anchored anteriorly to the base of the brain at the crista galli of the ethmoid bone. The **tentorium cerebelli** is a membrane that separates the cerebellum below from the cerebral structures above. The tentorium may become involved during periods of increased intracranial pressure caused by an injury to the brain. An injury within the cranial cavity tends to shift intracranial contents, and as structures shift, they tend to be compressed against these rigid membranes, resulting in damage or destruction. A common example is tentorial herniation.

Below the dura mater lies the **arachnoid membrane,** characterized by its filmy, weblike structure. It loosely follows the contours of the cerebral structures but goes over the sulci.

The **subdural space** lies between the dura and arachnoid. Many small bridging veins that have little support traverse the subdural space. Their disruption results in a subdural hematoma (see Chapter 17). The **subarachnoid space,** which contains CSF, lies between the arachnoid and the pia mater (see Figure 14-14). Damage to intracranial vessels can lead to a condition called *subarachnoid hemorrhage,* which frequently results in signs of meningeal irritation, such as neck stiffness, Kernig sign, and low back pain.

Unlike the dura mater and arachnoid, the delicate **pia mater** (see Figure 14-14) closely adheres to the surface of the brain and spinal cord and even follows the sulci and fissures. It provides support for blood vessels serving brain tissue. The **choroid plexuses,** structures that produce CSF, arise from the pia mater. The spinal cord is anchored to the vertebrae by extensions of the meninges called **denticulate ligaments.** The meninges continue beyond the end of the spinal cord to the lower portion of the sacrum. CSF, contained within the subarachnoid space, also circulates down to the large **lumbar cistern,** which extends from the second lumbar vertebra to the second sacral vertebra. Cisterns are expanded areas of the subarachnoid space. The **cerebellomedullary cistern (cisterna magna)** and the pontine cisterns are two other important cisterns.

The meninges form potential and real spaces important to understanding functional and pathologic mechanisms. For example, between the dura mater and skull lies a potential space termed the **epidural space** (see Figure 14-14). In the spinal canal there is a real epidural space filled with fatty tissue and a venous plexus. The arterial supply to the meninges consists of blood vessels that lie within grooves in the skull. As a result of trauma, the skull can be fractured and the blood vessels disrupted. The ruptured vessels can lead to an accumulation of blood within the epidural space, called an *epidural hematoma* (see Chapter 17). Persons with alcoholism often fall and injure their head, resulting in an epidural hematoma. An inflammation of the meninges (meningitis) also can have life-threatening implications because of the relative proximity to the brain. (Disorders of the CNS are discussed in Chapter 17.)

Cerebrospinal Fluid and the Ventricular System

Cerebrospinal fluid (CSF) is a clear, colorless fluid similar to blood plasma and interstitial fluid. The intracranial and spinal cord structures float in CSF and are thereby protected from jolts and blows. The buoyant properties of the CSF also prevent the brain from tugging on meninges, nerve roots, and blood vessels. (Constituents of CSF are listed in Table 14-4.) Between 125 and 150 ml of CSF, approximately the quantity of a small cup of coffee, is circulating within the **ventricles** (small cavities) and subarachnoid space at any given time. Approximately 600 ml of CSF is produced daily.

The choroid plexuses in the lateral, third, and fourth ventricles produce the major portion of CSF. (Ventricles are illustrated in Figure 14-14.) These plexuses are characterized by a rich network of blood vessels, supplied by the pia mater, that lie in close contact with the ependymal cells of the ventricles.

The CSF exerts pressure within the brain and spinal cord. When a person is lying down, CSF pressure is approximately 120 to 180 mm of water pressure, or approximately 9 to 14 mm Hg pressure. CSF flow is a result of a pressure gradient between the arterial system and the CSF-filled cavities. Beginning in the lateral ventricles, the CSF flows through the **interventricular foramen (foramen of Monro)** into the third ventricle and then passes through the cerebral aqueduct (aqueduct of Sylvius) into the fourth ventricle. From the fourth ventricle, the CSF may pass through either the paired **lateral apertures (foramina of Luschka)** into the pontine cisterns, located along the basal pons, or the midline **median aperture (foramen of Magendie)** into the cerebellomedullary cistern before communicating with the subarachnoid spaces of the brain and spinal cord. The CSF does not, however, accumulate. Instead, it is reabsorbed into the venous circulation through the arachnoid villi, primarily located superior to the falx cerebri in the **superior sagittal sinus.** The **arachnoid villi** protrude from the arachnoid space, through the dura mater, and lie within the blood flow of the venous sinuses. CSF is reabsorbed by means of a pressure gradient between the arachnoid villi and the cerebral venous sinuses. The villi function as one-way valves directing CSF outflow into the blood but preventing blood flow into the subarachnoid space. Thus CSF is derived from the blood, and after circulating throughout the CNS, it returns to the blood.

Samples of CSF are withdrawn for diagnostic purposes either (1) by inserting a needle between the third and fourth lumbar vertebrae into the lumbar cistern (subarachnoid space)—a procedure called **lumbar puncture**—or (2) from an intraventricular catheter. Spinal anesthesias (blocks) are administered in a manner similar to the lumbar puncture.

Vertebral Column

The **vertebral column** (Figure 14-15) is composed of 33 vertebrae: 7 cervical, 12 thoracic, 5 lumbar, 5 fused sacral, and 4 fused coccygeal. Between each interspace (except the fused sacral and coccygeal vertebrae) is an **intervertebral disk** (Figure 14-16). At the center of the intervertebral disk is the **nucleus pulposus,** a pulpy mass of elastic fibers. The intervertebral disk functions to absorb shocks, preventing damage to the vertebrae. The intervertebral disk is also a common source of back problems. If too much stress is applied to the vertebral column, the disk contents may rupture and protrude into the spinal canal, causing compression of the spinal cord or nerve roots. The disks also can degenerate.

Table 14-4	Composition of Cerebrospinal Fluid	
Constituent	**Normal Value**	
Na⁺	148 mM	
K⁺	2.9 mM	
Cl⁻	125 mM	
HCO₃⁻	22.9 mM	
Glucose (fasting)	50-75 mg/dl (60% of serum glucose)	
pH	7.3	
Protein	15-45 mg/dl	
Albumin	80%	
Gamma globulin	6%-10%	
Cells		
White (lymphocytes)	0-6/mm³	
Red	0/mm³	

Na⁺, Sodium; *K⁺,* potassium; *Cl⁻,* chloride; *HCO₃⁻,* bicarbonate.

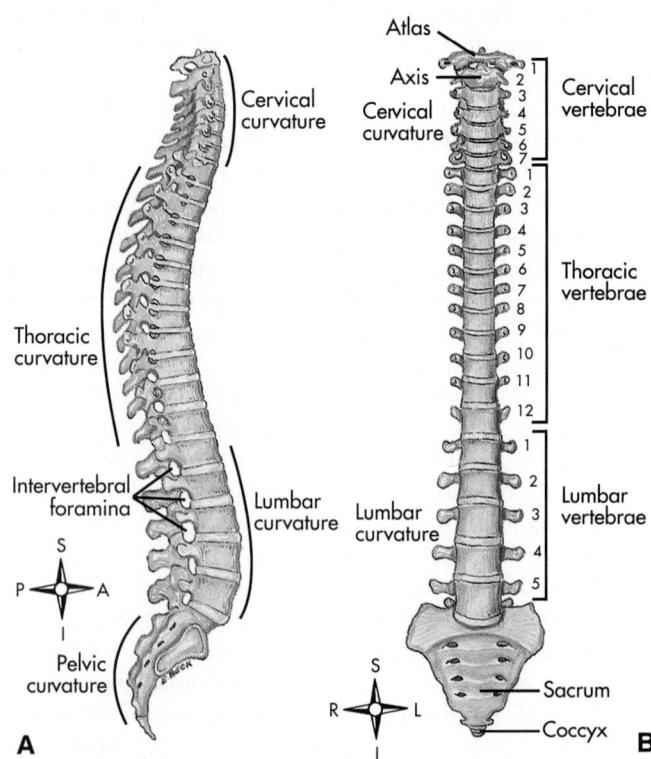

Figure 14-15 Vertebral column. **A,** Right lateral view. **B,** Anterior view. (From Thibodeau GA, Patton KT: *Anatomy & physiology,* ed 5, St Louis, 2003, Mosby.)

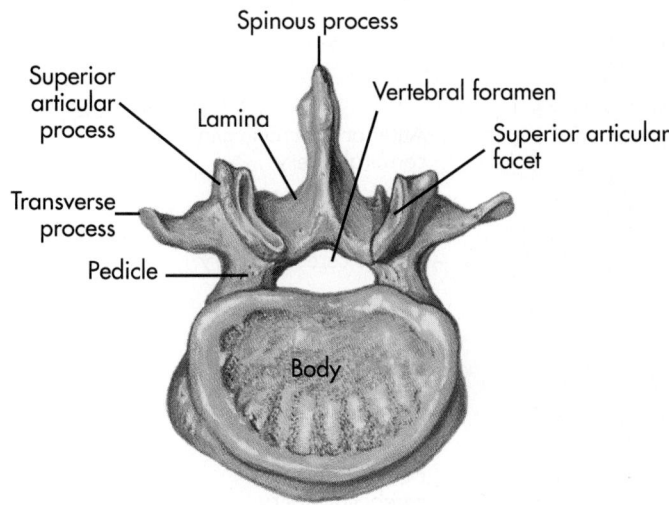

Figure 14-16 Lumbar vertebra, superior view. (From Thibodeau GA, Patton KT: *Anatomy & physiology,* ed 5, St Louis, 2003, Mosby.)

Blood Supply
Blood Supply to the Brain

The brain receives approximately 20% of the cardiac output, or 800 to 1000 ml of blood flow per minute. Carbon dioxide serves as a primary regulator for blood flow within the CNS. It is a potent vasodilator in the CNS, and its effects ensure an adequate blood supply.

The brain derives its arterial supply from two systems: the **internal carotid arteries** and the **vertebral arteries** (Figure 14-17). The internal carotid arteries, anteriorly, supply a proportionately greater amount of blood flow. They take their origin from the common carotid arteries, enter the cranium through the base of the skull, and pass through the **cavernous sinus.** After giving off some small branches, they divide into the **anterior** and **middle cerebral arteries.** The vertebral arteries, posteriorly, originate as branches off the subclavian arteries, pass through the transverse foramina of the cervical vertebrae, and enter the cranium through the foramen magnum. They join at the junction of the pons and medulla oblongata to form the **basilar artery.** The basilar artery divides at the level of the midbrain to form paired **posterior cerebral arteries.** Three major paired arteries perfuse the cerebellum and brain stem and originate from the posterior arterial supply: the posterior inferior cerebellar artery, off the vertebral artery; and the anterior inferior cerebellar and superior cerebellar arteries, off the basilar artery. The basilar artery also gives rise to small pontine arteries. The large arteries on the surface of the brain and their branches are called **superficial arteries (conducting arteries).** The small branches that project into the brain are termed **projecting arteries (nutrient arteries).** Occluding any of these vessels can cause neurologic signs and symptoms that are often diagnostically unique.

The **arterial circle (circle of Willis)** (Figure 14-18) is a structure credited with the ability to compensate for reduced blood flow from any one of the major contributors (collateral blood flow). The arterial circle is formed by the posterior

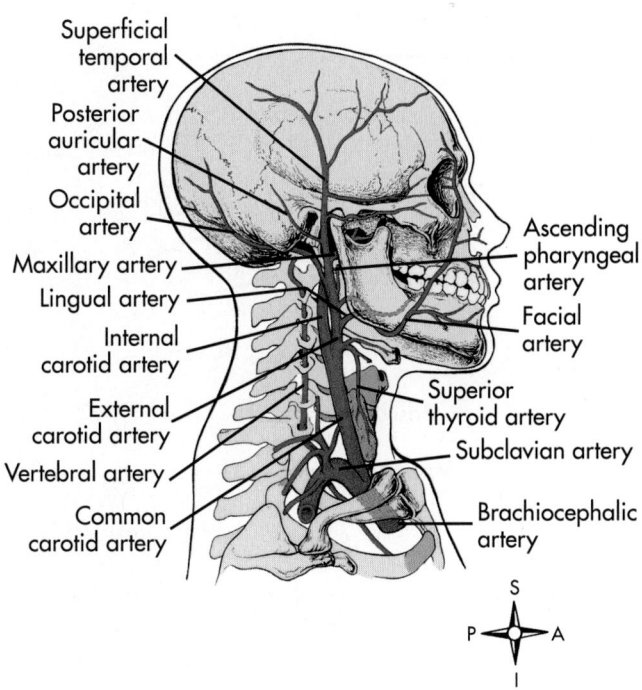

Figure 14-17 Major arteries of the head and neck. (From Thibodeau GA, Patton KT: *Anatomy & physiology,* ed 5, St Louis, 2003, Mosby.)

cerebral arteries, posterior communicating arteries, internal carotid arteries, anterior cerebral arteries, and anterior communicating artery. The anterior cerebral, middle cerebral, and posterior cerebral arteries leave the arterial circle and extend to various brain structures. (Table 14-5 and Figure 14-19 illustrate structures served, functional relationships, and pathologic considerations related to occlusion of cerebral arteries.)

Cerebral venous drainage does not parallel (lie side by side) its arterial supply, whereas the venous drainage of the brain stem and cerebellum does parallel the arterial supply of the structures. The cerebral veins are classified as superficial veins and deep cerebral veins. The veins drain into venous plexuses and dural sinuses (formed between the dural layers) and eventually join the internal jugular veins at the base of the skull (Figure 14-20). Adequacy of venous outflow can have a significant effect on intracranial pressure. For example, in individuals with head injury, turning or letting the head fall to the side partially occludes venous return and can increase intracranial pressure because of decreased flow through the jugular veins.

The blood-brain barrier is discussed in Box 14-4.

Blood Supply to the Spinal Cord

The spinal cord derives its blood supply from branches off the vertebral arteries and from branches from various regions of the aorta (Figure 14-21). The **anterior spinal arteries** and the paired **posterior spinal arteries** branch off the vertebral artery at the base of the cranium and descend alongside the spinal cord. Arterial branches from vessels exterior to the spinal cord follow the spinal nerve through the intervertebral

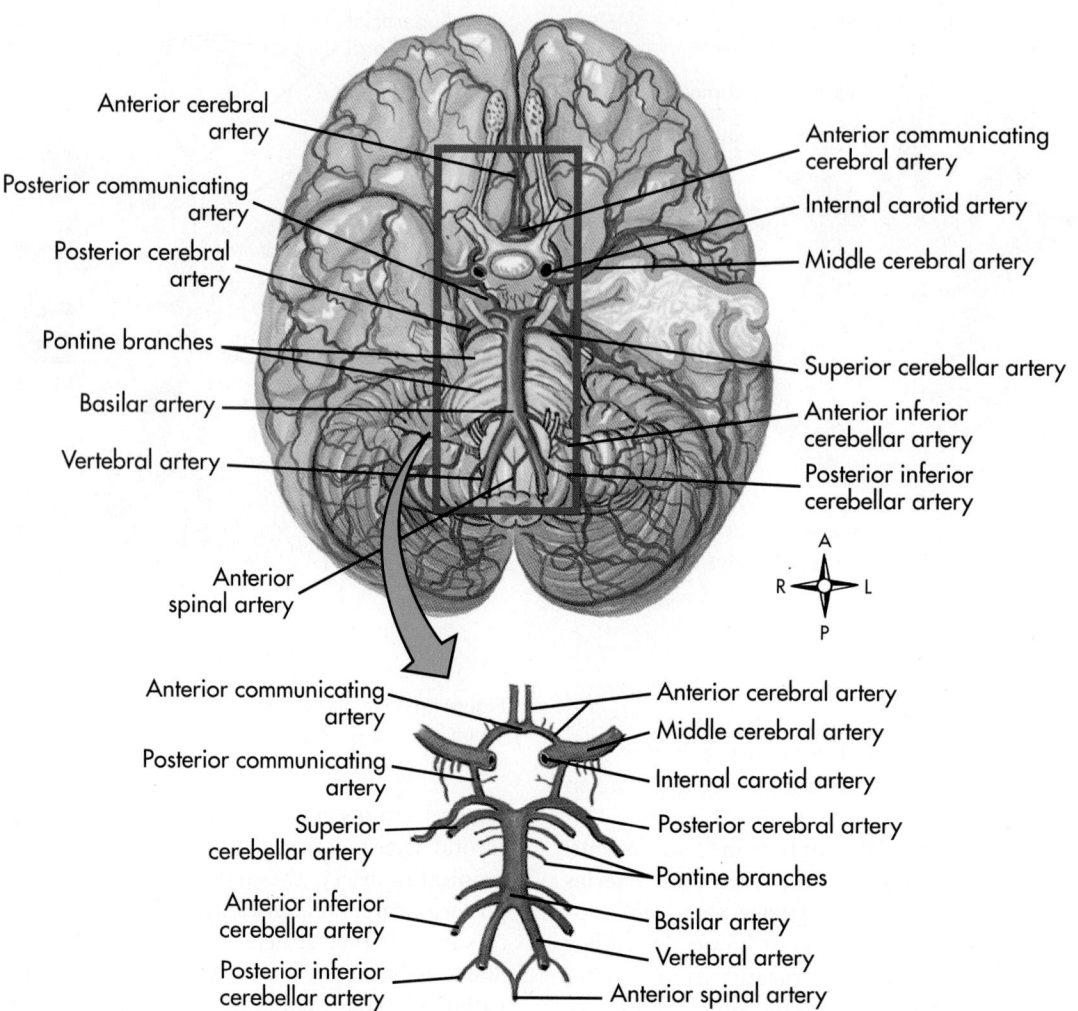

Figure 14-18 Arteries at the base of the brain. The arteries that compose the circle of Willis are the two anterior cerebral arteries, joined to each other by the anterior communicating two short segments of the internal carotids, off of which the posterior communicating arteries connect to the posterior cerebral arteries. (Modified from Thibodeau GA, Patton KT: *Anatomy & physiology,* ed 5, St Louis, 2003, Mosby.)

Table 14-5	Arterial Systems Supplying the Brain	
Arterial Origin	**Structures Served**	**Conditions Caused by Occlusion**
Anterior cerebral artery	Basal ganglia; corpus callosum; medial surface of cerebral hemispheres; superior surface of frontal and parietal lobes	Hemiplegia on contralateral side of body, greater in lower than in upper extremities
Middle cerebral artery	Frontal lobe; parietal lobe; temporal lobe (primarily cortical surfaces)	Aphasia in dominant hemisphere and contralateral hemiplegia (see Chapter 16)
Posterior cerebral artery	Part of diencephalon and temporal lobe; occipital lobe	Visual loss; sensory loss; contralateral hemiplegia if cerebral peduncle affected

foramina, pass through the dura, and divide into the anterior and posterior radicular arteries.

The radicular arteries eventually reconnect to the spinal arteries. Branches from the radicular and spinal arteries form plexuses whose branches penetrate the spinal cord, supplying the deeper tissues. Venous drainage parallels the arterial supply closely and drains into venous sinuses located between the dura and periosteum of the vertebrae.

PERIPHERAL NERVOUS SYSTEM

The cranial and spinal nerves, including their branches and ganglia, constitute the PNS. A peripheral nerve (cranial or spinal) is composed of individual axons/dendrites, with most being wrapped in a myelin sheath. These individual fibers are arranged in bundles called **fascicles** (Figure 14-22, *B*). The coverings supply structural support, a blood supply, and in-

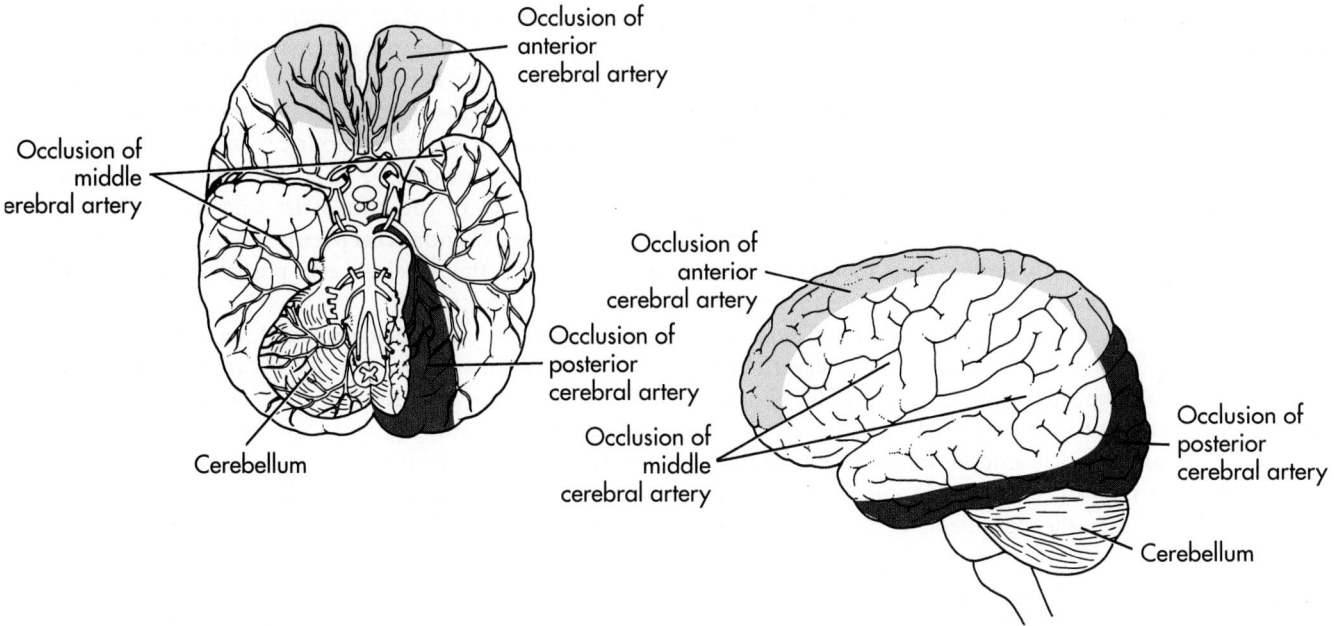

Figure 14-19 Areas of the brain affected by occlusion of the anterior, middle, and posterior cerebral artery branches. **A,** Inferior view. **B,** Lateral view. (Modified from Rudy EB, editor: *Advanced neurological and neurosurgical nursing,* St. Louis, 1984, Mosby.)

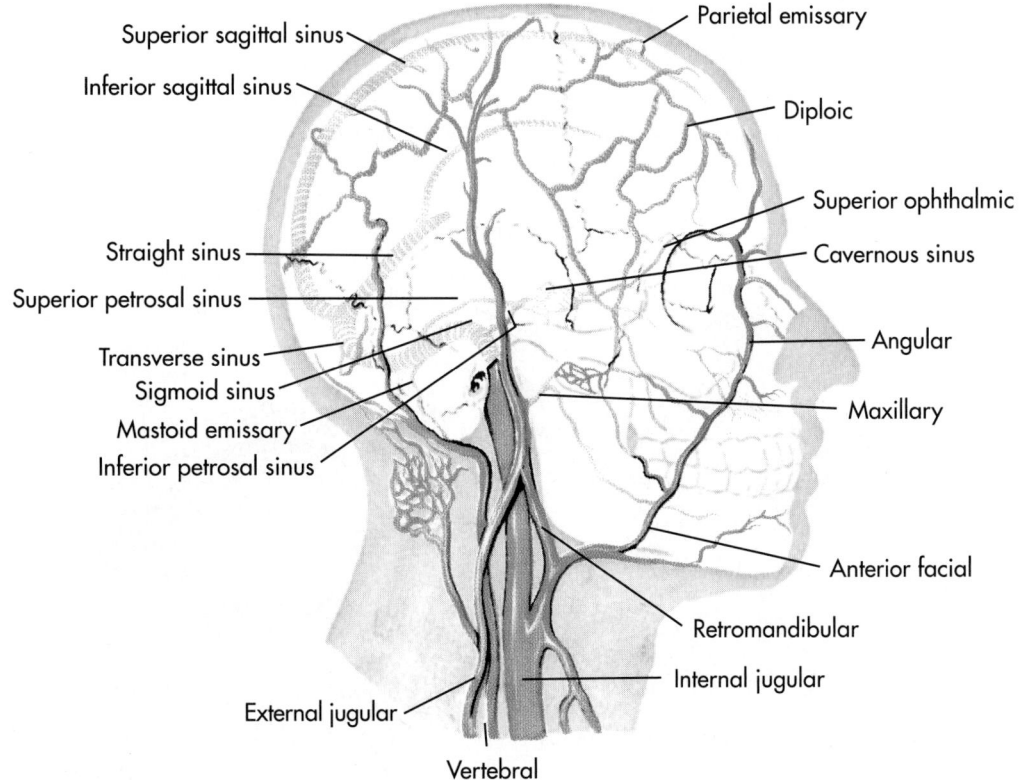

Figure 14-20 **Large veins of the head.** Deep veins and dural sinuses are projected on the skull. Note connections (emissary veins) between the superficial and deep veins. (From Rudy EB, editor: *Advanced neurological and neurosurgical nursing,* St Louis, 1984, Mosby.)

terstitial compartments necessary for the supply of essential electrolytes to support nerve impulse conduction.

The 31 pairs of spinal nerves derive their names from the vertebral level from which they exit. There are eight cervical spinal nerves. The first cervical nerve exits above the first cervical vertebra, and the rest of the spinal nerves exit below their corresponding vertebrae. From the thoracic region (and inferiorly) nerves correspond to the vertebral level above their exit.

Spinal nerves contain both sensory and motor neurons and are called **mixed nerves.** They arise as rootlets from the anterior and posterior horn cells of the spinal cord. These two spinal nerve roots converge in the region of the intervertebral foramen to form the spinal nerve (see Figure 14-10). Shortly after converging, the spinal nerve divides into anterior and posterior rami (branches). The anterior rami (except the thoracic) initially form plexuses (networks of nerve fibers), which then branch into the peripheral nerves. Instead of

---

Box 14-4   The Blood-Brain Barrier

The **blood-brain barrier** is a term used to describe cellular structures that selectively inhibit certain substances in the blood from entering the interstitial spaces of the brain or CSF. This term emphasizes the impermeability of the nervous system to large and potentially harmful molecules. It is thought that the supporting cells (neuroglia), particularly the astrocytes, and tight junctions between endothelial cells (see Chapter 1) are involved in the formation of the blood-brain barrier. It appears that certain metabolites, electrolytes, and chemicals have differing abilities to cross the blood-brain barrier. This has substantial implications for drug therapy because certain types of antibiotics and chemotherapeutic drugs show a greater propensity than others for crossing the barrier.

---

forming plexuses, the thoracic nerves pass through the intercostal spaces and innervate regions of the thorax.

The main spinal nerve plexuses innervate the skin and the underlying muscles of the limbs. The **brachial plexus,** for example, is formed by the last four cervical nerves (C5 to C8) and the first thoracic nerve (T1). The brachial plexus innervates the nerves of the arm, wrist, and hand. The **lumbar plexus** (L2 to L4) and **sacral plexus** (L5 to S5) contain nerves that innervate the anterior and posterior portions of the lower body, respectively.

The posterior rami of each spinal nerve, with their many processes, are distributed to a specific area in the body. Sensory signals thus arise from specific sites associated with a specific spinal cord segment. Specific areas of cutaneous (skin) innervation at these spinal cord segments are called **dermatomes.** The dermatomes of various spinal nerves are distributed in a fairly regular pattern, although adjacent regions between dermatomes can be innervated by more than one spinal nerve.

Like spinal nerves, cranial nerves are categorized as peripheral nerves. Most of these are mixed nerves (like the spinal nerves), although some are purely sensory or motor. Cranial nerves arise from nuclei in the brain and brain stem. (Figure 14-22, *A,* illustrates their location, and Table 14-6 describes structural and functional characteristics.)

AUTONOMIC NERVOUS SYSTEM

Components of the autonomic nervous system (ANS) are located in both the CNS and PNS; however, the ANS is considered part of the efferent division of the PNS, even though visceral afferent neurons are an important part of this system.

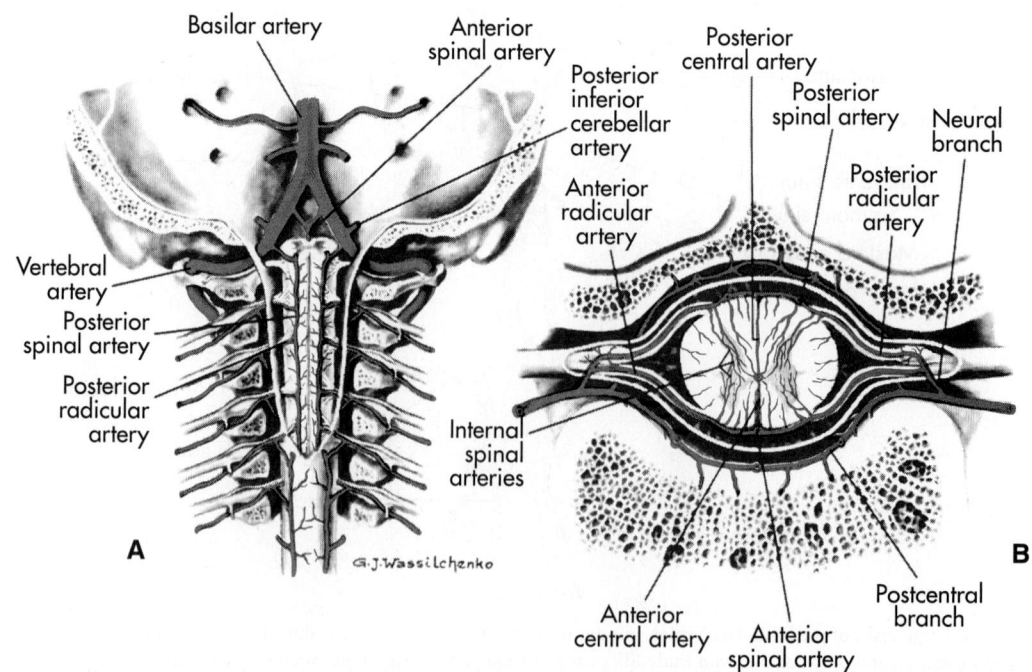

Figure 14-21 Arteries of the spinal cord. **A,** Arteries of cervical cord exposed, posterior view. **B,** Arteries of spinal cord diagrammatically shown in horizontal section. (From Rudy EB, editor: *Advanced neurological and neurosurgical nursing,* St Louis, 1984, Mosby.)

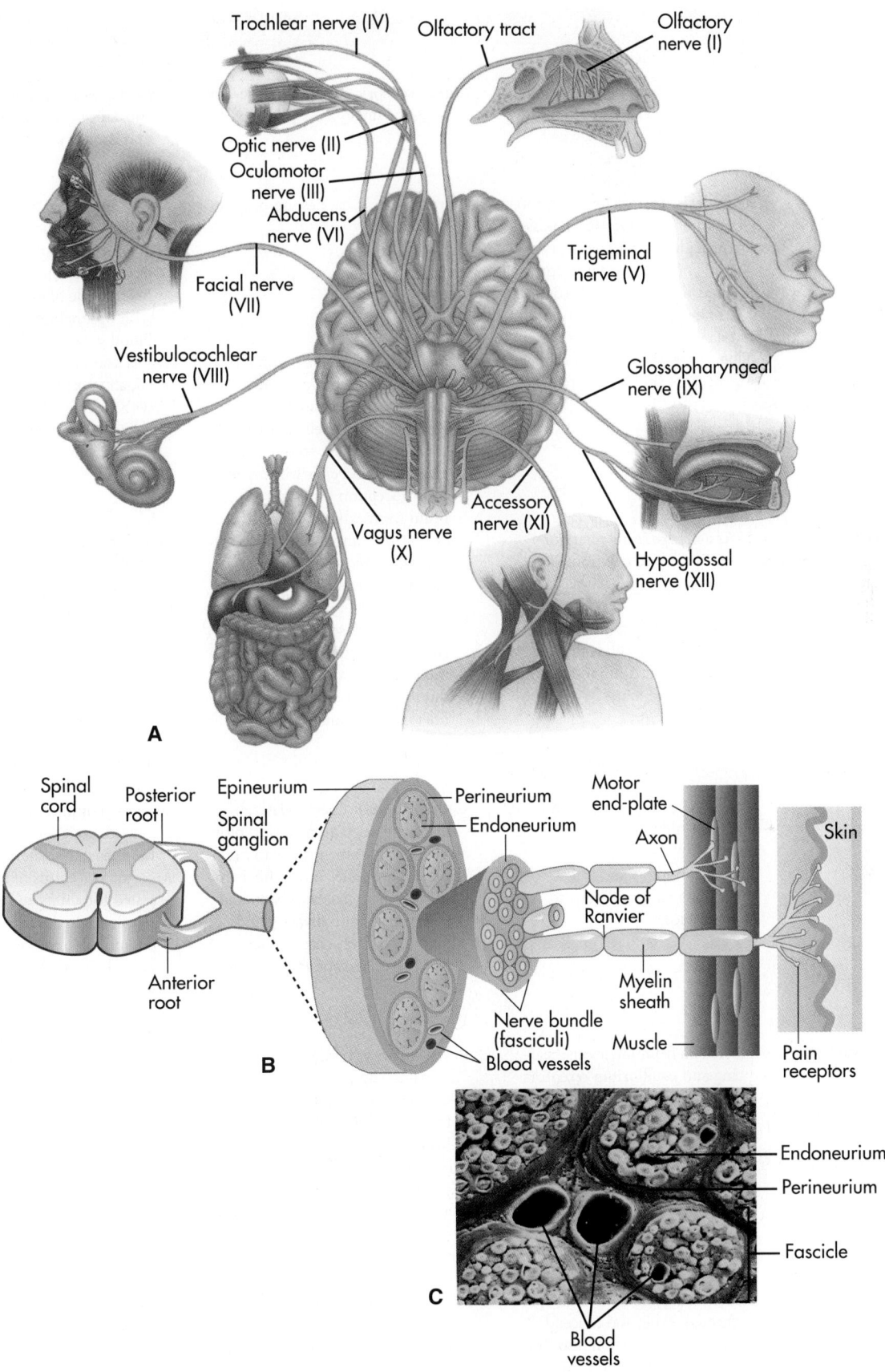

Figure 14-22 Cranial and peripheral nerves. **A,** Ventral surface of the brain showing attachment of the cranial nerves. **B,** Peripheral nerve trunk and coverings. **C,** Scanning electron micrograph of a freeze-fractured preparation of peripheral nerve. (**A** and **C** from Thibodeau GA, Patton KT: *Anatomy & physiology,* ed 5, St Louis, 2003, Mosby.)

Table 14-6	The Cranial Nerves		
Number and Name	**Origin and Course**	**Function**	**How Tested**
I. Olfactory	Fibers arise from nasal olfactory epithelium and form synapses with olfactory bulbs, which transmit impulses to temporal lobe via the olfactory tract	Purely sensory; carries impulses for sense of smell	Person is asked to sniff aromatic substances, such as oil of cloves and vanilla, and to identify them
II. Optic	Fibers arise from retina of eye to form optic nerve, which passes through sphenoid bone; two optic nerves then form optic chiasma (with partial crossover of fibers) and eventually end in occipital cortex	Purely sensory; carries impulses for vision	Vision and visual field tested with an eye chart and by testing point at which person first sees an object (finger) moving into visual field; inside of eye is viewed with ophthalmoscope to observe blood vessels of eye interior
III. Oculomotor	Fibers emerge from midbrain and exit from skull to run to eye	Contains motor fibers to inferior oblique, superior, inferior, and medial rectus extraocular muscles that direct eyeball; levator muscles of eyelid; smooth muscles of iris and ciliary body; and proprioception (sensory) to brain from extraocular muscles	Pupils examined for size, shape, and equality; papillary reflex tested with a pen light (pupils should constrict when illuminated); ability to follow moving objects
IV. Trochlear	Fibers emerge from posterior midbrain and exit from skull and run to eye	Proprioceptor and motor fibers for superior oblique muscle of eye (external eye muscle)	Tested in common with cranial nerve III relative to ability to follow moving objects
V. Trigeminal	Fibers emerge from pons and form three divisions that exit from skull and run to face and cranial dura mater	Both motor and sensory for face; conducts sensory impulses from mouth, nose, surface of eye, and dura mater; also contains motor fibers that stimulate chewing muscles	Sensations of pain, touch, and temperature tested with safety pin and hot and cold objects; corneal reflex tested with a wisp of cotton; motor branch tested by asking subject to clench teeth, open mouth against resistance, and move jaw from side to side
VI. Abducens	Fibers leave inferior pons and exit from skull to run to eye	Contains motor fibers to lateral rectus muscle and proprioceptor fibers from same muscle to brain	Tested in common with cranial nerve III relative to ability to move each eye laterally
VII. Facial	Fibers leave pons and travel through temporal bone to reach face	Mixed: (1) supplies motor fibers to muscles of facial expression and to lacrimal and salivary glands and (2) carries sensory fibers from taste buds of anterior part of tongue	Anterior two thirds of tongue tested for ability to taste sweet (sugar), salty, sour (vinegar), and bitter (quinine) substances; symmetry of face checked; subject asked to close eyes, smile, whistle, and so on; tearing tested with ammonia fumes
VIII. Vestibulocochlear (acoustic)	Fibers run from inner ear (hearing and equilibrium receptors in temporal bone) to enter brain stem just below pons	Purely sensory; vestibular branch transmits impulses for sense of equilibrium; cochlear branch transmits impulses for sense of hearing	Hearing checked by air and bone conduction by use of a tuning fork; vestibular tests: Bárány and caloric tests
IX. Glossopharyngeal	Fibers emerge from midbrain and leave skull to run to throat	Mixed: (1) motor fibers serve pharynx (throat) and salivary glands, and (2) sensory fibers carry impulses from pharynx, posterior tongue (taste buds), and pressure receptors of carotid artery	Gag and swallowing reflexes checked; subject asked to speak and cough; posterior one third of tongue may be tested for taste
X. Vagus	Fibers emerge from medulla, pass through skull, and descend through neck region into thorax and abdominal region	Fibers carry sensory and motor impulses for pharynx; a large part of this nerve is parasympathetic motor fibers, which supply smooth muscles of abdominal organs; transmits sensory impulses from viscera	Same as for cranial nerve IX (IX and X are tested in common) because they both serve muscles of throat

Table 14-6	The Cranial Nerves—cont'd		
Number and Name	**Origin and Course**	**Function**	**How Tested**
XI. Spinal accessory	Fibers arise from medulla and superior spinal cord and travel to muscles of neck and back	Provides sensory and motor fibers for sternocleidomastoid and trapezius muscles and muscles of soft palate, pharynx, and larynx	Sternocleidomastoid and trapezius muscles checked for strength by asking subject to rotate head and shrug shoulders against resistance
XII. Hypoglossal	Fibers arise from medulla and exit from skull to travel to tongue	Carries motor fibers to muscles of tongue and sensory impulses from tongue to brain	Subject asked to stick out tongue, and any position abnormalities are noted

Many neurons of the ANS travel in spinal nerves and certain cranial nerves. The widespread activity of this system indicates that its components are distributed all over the body. The peripheral autonomic nerves carry mainly efferent fibers. The motor component of the ANS is a two-neuron system consisting of **preganglionic neurons** (myelinated) and **postganglionic neurons** (unmyelinated). This arrangement contrasts with the somatic nervous system, where a single motor neuron travels from the CNS to the innervated structure. Visceral afferent neurons have their cell bodies in some sensory and cranial ganglia and their fiber processes traveling in peripheral nerves. The CNS has autonomic areas in the intermediolateral horns of the spinal cord, cardiovascular and respiratory centers in the reticular formation, and both sympathetic and parasympathetic areas in the hypothalamus. CNS pathways interconnect all these areas.

The ANS coordinates and maintains a steady state among visceral (internal) organs, such as regulation of cardiac muscle, smooth muscle, and the glands of the body. This system is considered an involuntary system because one *generally* cannot "will" these functions to happen. The ANS is separated both structurally and functionally into two divisions: (1) the **sympathetic nervous system** (Figure 14-23) and (2) the **parasympathetic nervous system** (Figure 14-24).

Anatomy of the Sympathetic Nervous System

The sympathetic nervous system functions to mobilize energy stores in times of need (e.g., in the fight-or-flight response) (see Figure 10-2; see also Chapter 10). The sympathetic division receives its innervation from cell bodies located from the first thoracic (T1) through the second lumbar (L2) regions of the spinal cord and is therefore called the **thoracolumbar division.** The preganglionic axons of the sympathetic division form synapses shortly after leaving the cord in the **sympathetic (paravertebral) ganglia.** At this point the impulse may travel several ways: (1) directly across the same ganglion level and form a synapse with the cell bodies of the postganglionic neuron, (2) up or down the sympathetic chain before forming synapses with a higher or lower postganglionic neuron (divergence), or (3) through the chain ganglion without synapsing (see Figure 14-23). Some preganglionic axons form pathways called **splanchnic nerves,** which lead to **collateral ganglia** that surround the abdominal aorta. The collateral

ganglia are named according to the branches of the aorta nearest them, namely, the **celiac, superior mesenteric,** and **inferior mesenteric.** The preganglionic neurons synapse with postganglionic neurons within the collateral ganglia. These postganglionic neurons leave the collateral ganglia and innervate the viscera below the diaphragm.

Preganglionic sympathetic neurons that innervate the adrenal medulla also travel in the splanchnic nerves and do not synapse before reaching the gland. The secretory cells in the adrenal medulla are considered modified postganglionic neurons. Because preganglionic sympathetic fibers are all myelinated, travel to the adrenal medulla is quick, and innervation causes the rapid release of epinephrine and norepinephrine. Epinephrine and norepinephrine are mediators of the fight-or-flight response (see Chapter 10).

Anatomy of the Parasympathetic Nervous System

The parasympathetic nervous system functions to conserve and restore energy. The nerve cell bodies of this division are located in the cranial nerve nuclei and in the sacral region of the spinal cord and therefore constitute the **craniosacral division.** Unlike the sympathetic division, the preganglionic fibers in the parasympathetic division travel to ganglia close to the organs they innervate before forming synapses with the relatively short postganglionic neurons (see Figure 14-24). Parasympathetic nerves arising from nuclei in the brain stem travel to the viscera of the head, thorax, and abdomen within cranial nerves—including the oculomotor (III), facial (VII), glossopharyngeal (IX), and vagus (X) nerves.

Preganglionic parasympathetic nerves that originate from the sacral region of the spinal cord run either separately or together with some spinal nerves. The preganglionic axons join together to form the **pelvic nerve,** which innervates the viscera of the pelvic cavity. These preganglionic axons synapse with postganglionic neurons in terminal ganglia located close to the organs they innervate.

Neurotransmitters and Neuroreceptors

Sympathetic preganglionic fibers and parasympathetic preganglionic and postganglionic fibers release **acetylcholine**—the same neurotransmitter released by somatic efferent neurons (Figure 14-25; also see Figure 14-22). These fibers are characterized by **cholinergic transmission.** Most postganglionic

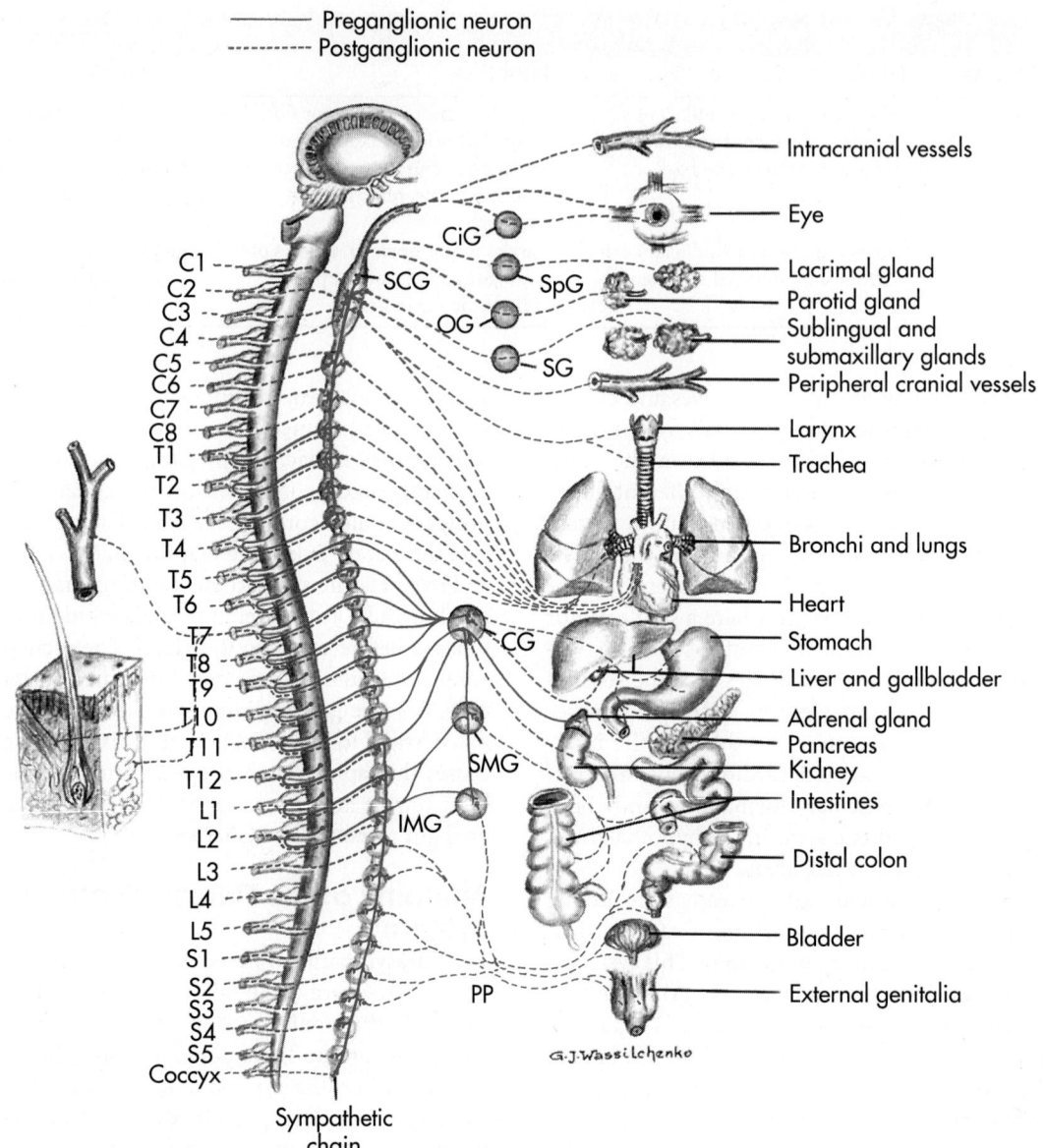

— Preganglionic neuron
----- Postganglionic neuron

Figure 14-23 Sympathetic division of the autonomic nervous system. *CiG,* Ciliary ganglion; *SpG,* sphenopalatine ganglion; *SCG,* superior cervical ganglion; *OG,* otic ganglion; *SG,* submandibular ganglion; *CG,* celiac ganglion; *SMG,* superior mesenteric ganglion; *IMG,* inferior mesenteric ganglion; *PP,* pelvic plexus. Fibers of the parasympathetic system pass through the CG and SMG, but these ganglia are not part of the parasympathetic system. (From Rudy EB, editor: *Advanced neurological and neurosurgical nursing,* St Louis, 1984, Mosby.)

sympathetic fibers release **norepinephrine** (adrenaline) and thus are considered to function by **adrenergic transmission.** A few postganglionic sympathetic fibers, such as those that innervate the sweat glands, release acetylcholine.

The action of catecholamines (epinephrine, norepinephrine, dopa) varies with the type of neuroreceptor stimulated. It should be remembered that catecholamines also are released by the adrenal medulla gland that physiologically and biochemically resembles the sympathetic nervous system. Two types of adrenergic receptors exist: α- and β-adrenergic receptors. Cells of the effector organs may have only one or both types of adrenergic receptors. The **α-adrenergic receptors** have been further subdivided according to the action

produced: α_1-adrenergic activity is associated mostly with excitation or stimulation; α_2-adrenergic activity is associated with relaxation or inhibition. Most of the α-adrenergic receptors on effector organs belong to the α_1-adrenergic class. The **β-adrenergic receptors** are classified as β_1-adrenergic receptors (which facilitate increased heart rate and contractility and cause the release of renin from the kidney) and β_2-adrenergic receptors (which facilitate all of the remaining effects attributed to β-adrenergic receptors).[5] Norepinephrine stimulates all α-adrenergic and β_1-adrenergic receptors and only certain β_2-adrenergic receptors. The primary response from norepinephrine, however, is stimulation of the α_1-adrenergic receptors that cause vasoconstriction. Epinephrine strongly

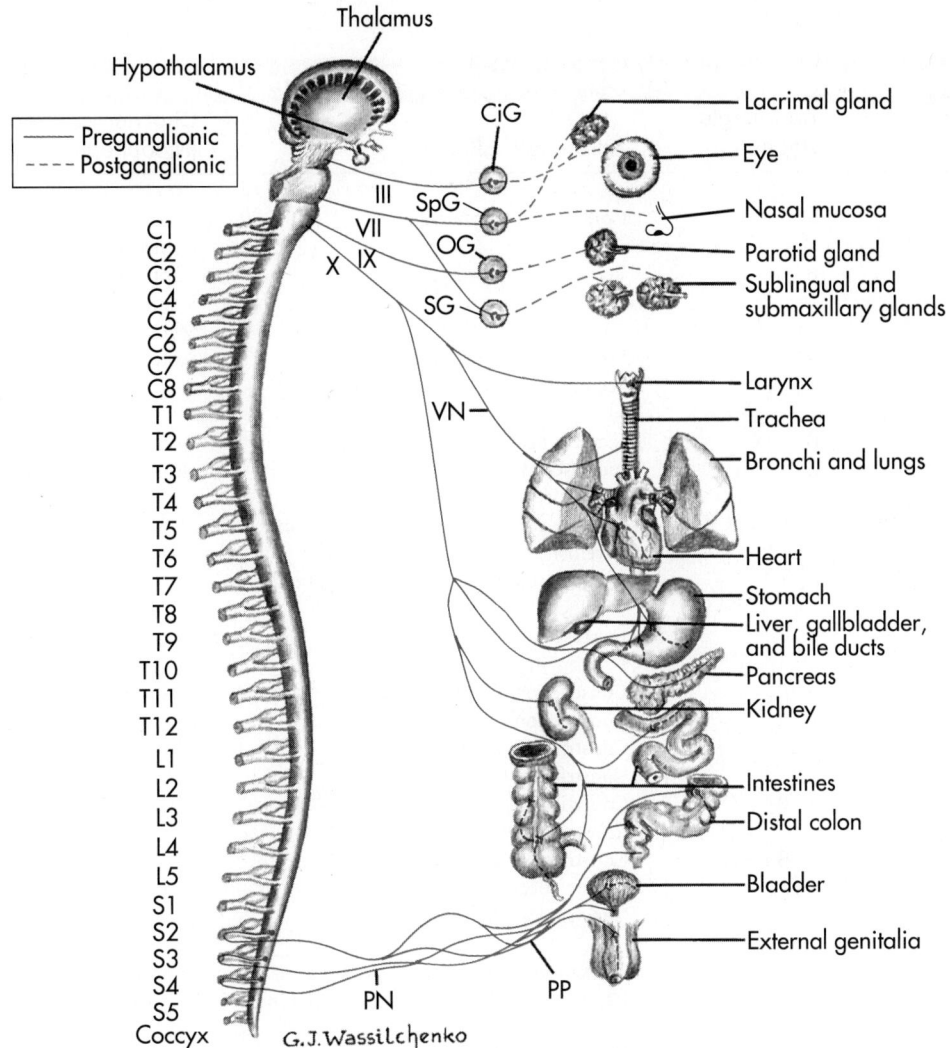

Figure 14-24 Parasympathetic division of the autonomic nervous system. *CiG*, Ciliary ganglion; *SpG*, sphenopalatine ganglion; *OG*, otic ganglion; *SG*, submandibular ganglion; *VN*, vagus nerve; *CG*, celiac ganglion; *SMG*, superior mesenteric ganglion; *PP*, pelvic plexus; *PN*, pelvic nerve. Fibers of the parasympathetic system pass through the CG and SMG, but these ganglia are not part of the parasympathetic system. (From Rudy EB, editor: *Advanced neurological and neurosurgical nursing*, St Louis, 1984, Mosby.)

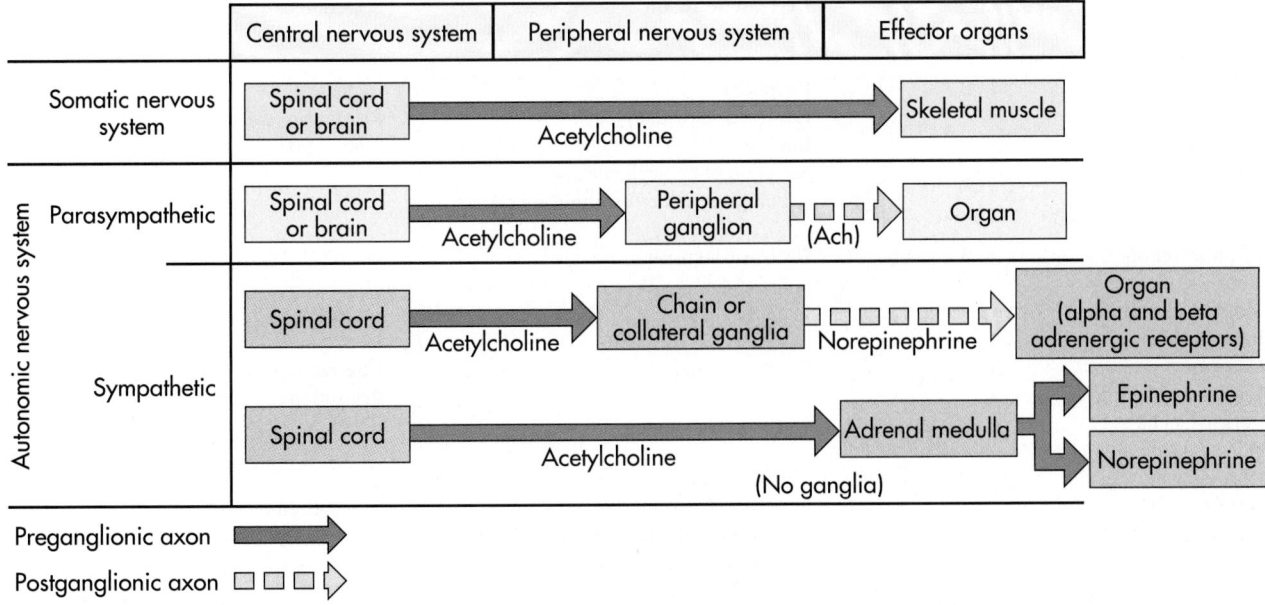

Figure 14-25 The autonomic nervous system and the type of neurotransmitters secreted by preganglionic and postganglionic fibers. Note that all preganglionic fibers are cholinergic *(Ach)*. A somatic nerve is used for comparison.

Table 14-7	Actions of Autonomic Nervous System Neuroreceptors		
Effector Organ or Tissue	**Adrenergic Receptors**	**Adrenergic Effects**	**Cholinergic Effects (Nicotine and Muscarinic Receptors)**
Eye, iris			
Radial muscle	α_1	Contraction (mydriasis)	—
Sphincter muscle		—	Contraction (miosis)
Eye, ciliary muscle	β_2	Relaxation for far vision	Contraction for near vision
Lacrimal glands	—	—	Secretion
Nasopharyngeal glands	—	—	Secretion
Salivary glands	α_1	Secretion of potassium and water	Secretion of potassium and water
	β	Secretion of amylase	—
Heart			
SA node	β_1	Increase heart rate	Decrease heart rate; vagus arrest
Atrial	β_1	Increase contractility and conduction velocity	Decrease contractility; shorten action potential duration
AV junction	β_1	Increase automaticity and propagation velocity	Decrease automaticity and propagation velocity
Purkinje system	β_1	Increase automaticity and propagation velocity	—
Ventricles	β_1	Increase contractility	—
Arterioles			
Coronary	α_1, β_2	Constriction, dilation	Dilation
Skin and mucosa	α_1, α_2	Constriction	Dilation
Skeletal muscle	α, β_2	Constriction, dilation	Dilation
Cerebral	α_1	Constriction (slight)	—
Pulmonary	α_1, β_2	Constriction, dilation	—
Mesenteric	α_1	Constriction	—
Renal	$\alpha_1, \beta_1, \beta_2, D$	Constriction, dilation	—
Salivary glands	α_1, α_2	Constriction	Dilation
Veins, systemic	α_1, β_2	Constriction, dilation	—
Lung			
Bronchial muscle	β_2	Relaxation	Contraction
Bronchial glands	α_1, β_2	Decreased secretion; increased secretion	Stimulation
Stomach			
Motility	α_1, β_2	Decrease (usually)	Increase
Sphincters	α_1	Contraction (usually)	Relaxation (usually)
Secretion	—	Inhibition (?)	Stimulation
Liver	α_1, β_2	Glycogenolysis and gluconeogenesis	Glycogen synthesis
Gallbladder and ducts	—	Relaxation	Contraction
Pancreas			
Acini	α	Decrease secretion	Secretion
Islet cells	α_2, β_2	Decreased secretion; increased secretion	—
Intestine			
Motility and tone	$\alpha_1, \beta_1, \beta_2$	Decrease	Increase
Sphincters	α_1	Contraction (usually)	Relaxation (usually)
Secretion	α_2	Inhibition (?)	Stimulation
Adrenal medulla	— —	Secretion of epinephrine and norepinephrine (nicotinic effect)	
Kidney			
Renin secretion	α_1, β_1	Decrease; increase	—
Ureter			
Motility and tone	α_1	Increase	Increase
Urinary bladder			
Detrusor	β_2	Relaxation (usually)	Contraction
Trigone and sphincter	α_1	Contraction	Relaxation
Sex organs, male	α_1	Ejaculation	Erection
Skin			
Pilomotor muscles	α_1	Contraction	—
Sweat glands	α_1	Localized secretion	Generalized secretion
Fat cells	$\alpha_2, \beta_1 (\beta_3)$	Inhibition of lipolysis; stimulation of lipolysis	—
Pineal gland	β	Melatonin synthesis	—

stimulates all four types of receptors and induces general vasodilation because of the predominance of β-adrenergic receptors in muscle vasculatures. (Table 14-7 summarizes the effects of neuroreceptors on their effector organs.)

Functions of the Autonomic Nervous System

Many body organs are innervated by both the sympathetic and parasympathetic nervous systems. The two divisions frequently cause opposite responses; for example, sympathetic stimulation of the gastrointestinal (GI) tract causes decreased peristalsis, whereas parasympathetic stimulation of the GI tract increases peristalsis. In general, sympathetic stimulation promotes responses that are concerned with the protection of the individual. For example, sympathetic activity increases blood sugar levels and temperature and raises blood pressure. In emergency situations a generalized and widespread discharge of the sympathetic system occurs. This is accomplished by an increased firing frequency of sympathetic fibers and by activation of sympathetic fibers normally silent and at rest (fibers to the sweat glands, pilomotor muscles, and the adrenal medulla, as well as vasodilator fibers to muscle). Regulation of vasomotor tone is considered the single most important function of the sympathetic nervous system. (Figure 14-26 illustrates some of the most important functions of the sympathetic nervous system; also see Figure 10-2.)

Increased parasympathetic activity promotes rest and tranquility and is characterized by reduced heart rate and enhanced visceral functions leading to digestion. Stimulation of the vagus nerve in the GI tract increases peristalsis and secretion, as well as relaxation of sphincters. Activation of parasympathetic fibers in the head, provided by cranial nerves III, VII, and IX, causes constriction of the pupil, tear secretion, and increased salivary secretion. Stimulation of the sacral division of the parasympathetic system contracts the urinary bladder and facilitates the process of genital erection.

The parasympathetic system lacks the generalized and widespread response of the sympathetic system. Specific parasympathetic fibers are activated to regulate particular functions. Although the actions of the parasympathetic and sympathetic systems usually are antagonistic, there are exceptions. Changes in the shape of the lens (for near vision) require only oculomotor parasympathetic activity. Most of the blood vessels involved in the control of blood pressure are innervated by sympathetic nerves. Peripheral vascular resistance is increased and decreased by the relative activity of the sympathetic division without a counteracting parasympathetic component. To decrease blood pressure, therefore, it is more important to block or paralyze the continuous (tonic) discharge of the sympathetic system than to promote parasympathetic activity.

AGING AND THE NERVOUS SYSTEM

The CNS mechanisms involved in the aging process are extremely complex, and many questions concerning the neurologic effects of aging have yet to be answered. Some of the identified mechanisms associated with aging are pathologic, but the distinction between these mechanisms and those that are a part of the normal aging process remains somewhat cloudy.

Structural Changes with Aging

The CNS demonstrates many structural changes during the aging process. The primary mechanism responsible for most of these structural changes is a decrease in the number of neurons. Predominant external features of the aging brain include decreased brain weight and size (primarily the frontal hemispheres), increased adherence of the dura mater to the skull, fibrosis and thickening of the meninges, narrowed gyri, and widened sulci with a corresponding increase in the size of the subarachnoid space. The basal ganglia and ventricular system are internal structures that commonly reveal changes with aging. The basal ganglia reveals aberrations in vascular structures, and the ventricles (primarily the lateral and third ventricles) are enlarged, probably because they occupy much of the space left by dead neurons.

Cellular Changes with Aging

Practically every cell type within the CNS reflects specific responses to aging. A decrease in the number of neurons characterizes aging. Although neuronal cell loss is a general feature of aging, the effects are not consistent with deteriorating mental function or age of the individual.[6] Controversy regarding the effects of neuronal cell loss is ongoing.

Principal cellular changes associated with aging include dendrite structure, lipofuscin deposition, and the presence of neurofibrillary tangles, senile plaques, and Lewy bodies. Hirano and Llena[7] described a decreased number of dendritic processes and their multiple synaptic connections. Lipofuscin, a yellow-brown fatty pigment, is found to be deposited intracellularly in increased amounts with age. Controversy still exists concerning whether increasing intracellular quantities of lipofuscin might be associated with disruption of cytoplasmic function, that is, protein synthesis.[6]

Senile plaques (areas of nerve degeneration) are found in the interstitial spaces of the cerebral cortex associated with tissue degeneration. **Neurofibrillary tangles** involve degenerative changes in neural protein fibers. These entities also are common in Alzheimer disease and some other forms of dementia. At present definitive evidence of a link between quantitative cellular changes and nervous system function in aging individuals is growing.

Closely paralleling cell function is a selective alteration in neurotransmitter function. One potentially fruitful area of research is investigation of possible correlations between the effects of acetylcholine (i.e., cholinergic transmission) and defects of memory and cognitive function associated with aging.[6]

Functional Changes with Aging

Because of integrative processes in the CNS, the consequences of aging have widespread implications for critical steady state, psychologic, and social function. Many theories have been

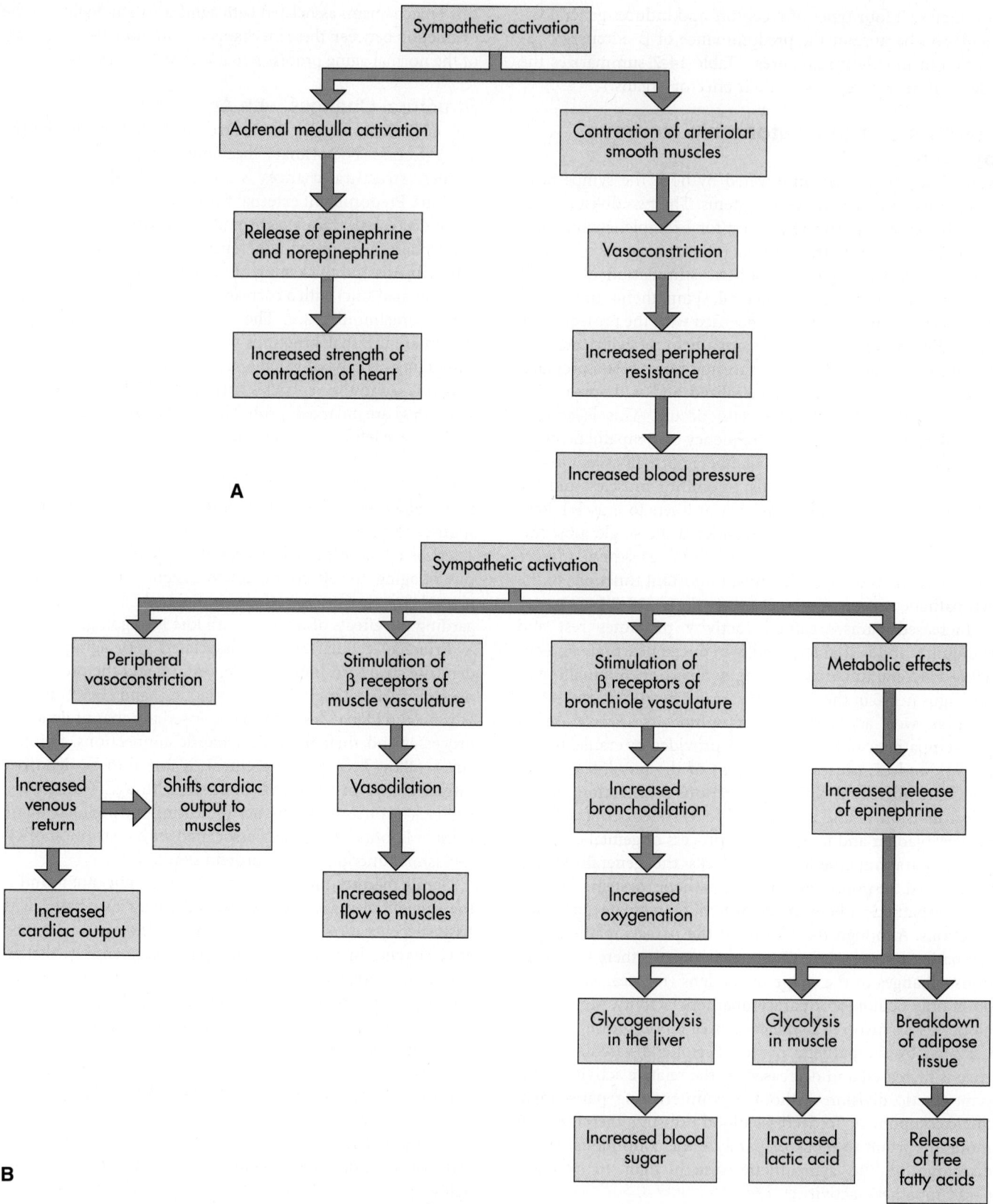

Figure 14-26 Some important functions of the sympathetic nervous system. **A,** Regulation of vasomotor tone. **B,** Regulation of strenuous muscular exercise (fight-or-flight response). (See also Chapter 10 and Figure 10-1 for more detail of the stress response.)

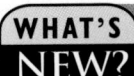

Reinforcement Center (Nucleus Accumbens)

Recently, a small nucleus (see accompanying figure) in the septal area of the frontal lobe has become a center of intense research. The nucleus accumbens is considered to be the principal site of action for addictive drugs and the anatomic basis of positive reinforcement. The nucleus accumbens has input from the mesencephalon (ventral tegmental area) and many other neural areas. Mesencephalon neurons project dopamine to the nucleus accum-

bens and can affect its activity. Other neurotransmitters involved in this positive feedback system are GABA, serotonin, and glutamate. Opiates can interfere with this system by allowing too much dopamine to go to the nucleus accumbens. The nucleus accumbens is involved in drug craving and withdrawal symptoms and therefore is clinically important.

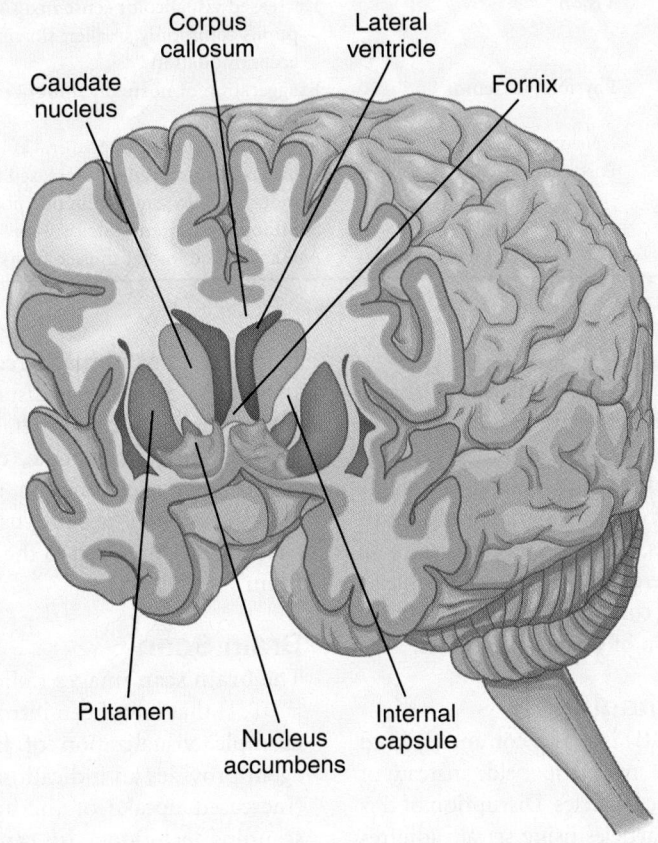

Data from Brown P. Molliver ME: *J Neurosci* 20(5):1952, 2000; Charney DS, Nestler EJ, Bunney BS, editors: *Neurobiology of mental illness,* London, 1999, Oxford University Press.

proposed to explain the observations of progressive slowing of neurologic responses seen in elderly persons (Table 14-8). Studies of changes in brain electrical activity have been helpful in determining alterations in neural function. Timiras[8] described the relationship between transmission of neural signals and slowing of responses observed in the elderly: "It is evident that the efficacy of the signals may be disturbed not only by irregularities in the action of cells carrying the signals but also by the amount of random background activity." This background activity is termed *neural noise.*

TESTS OF NERVOUS SYSTEM FUNCTION

Skull and Spine Roentgenograms

Roentgenograms (x-ray films) of the skull or spine from multiple angles (views) are used primarily to localize bony defects, bone density, erosion, or calcified structures. The pineal gland in older people becomes calcified and is useful as an internal brain landmark. X-ray films are probably the most commonly used radiologic studies.

Table 14-8	Common Neurologic Signs in Aging	
Neurologic Sign	**Examples**	**Changes in Response**
Reflexes	Ankle reflex	Usually the first tendon reflex to be lost in elderly persons
	Superficial reflex	Decreased or absent responsiveness
Primitive reflexes (reflexes seen normally in infancy but that subside with maturity)	Suck and grasp	Reappearance with aging
Sensation	Taste and smell	Progressive deficit
	Pain	Increased pain threshold, although subjective complaints increase
	Vibratory sense	Decreased
	Vision	Decreased visual color sense in a significant percentage of aged persons; pupils commonly smaller; slowing of papillary relaxation and accommodation
Motor function	Physiologic tremor	Exaggeration of normally unnoticeable resting tremor that is present at all ages
	Neuromuscular control	Decreased, resulting in postural effects
	Posture	Stance commonly shows increased flexion of hips and knees; swaying motion while standing in one position more common
	Gait	Shuffling or shortened stride; loss of arm movement with walking
	Muscular atrophy	Age-associated loss of muscle fibers

Computed Tomography

Computed tomography (CT) creates two-dimensional reconstructions from multiple radiologic images (x-rays) using computer-assisted analysis. It is capable of demonstrating fine distinctions in densities of a variety of tissues. CT imaging is a safe and noninvasive procedure used in evaluating cranial and spinal structures, as well as hemorrhages, tumors, and distortions in the brain caused by pressure differences. A variety of contrast media also are commonly used in conjunction with this procedure to aid in enhanced delineation of selected structures.

Magnetic Resonance Imaging

Magnetic resonance imaging (MRI) is now a commonly used testing modality. It uses a static magnetic field, instead of x-rays, to orient physiologic atomic particles. Disruption of this orientation by excitation of the particles using serial radiofrequency pulsations provides the image data. The specific tissue reaction is computer analyzed to give an image of exquisite detail, similar to that provided by CT. The MRI also provides reconstruction of images in three views at right angles (i.e., axial, sagittal, coronal). MRI is reported to have none of the adverse effects associated with radiation examinations.

Magnetic Resonance Angiography

A newer addition to MRI is **magnetic resonance angiography (MRA)**. Special imaging techniques allow the visualization of blood vessels in great detail. MRA is likely to become indispensable, alone or in conjunction with cerebral angiography, in detecting and localizing pathologic lesions of the circulatory system of the brain.

Positron Emission Tomography Scan

The **positron emission tomography (PET) scan** uses CT imaging to detect the emission of positive electrons from radioactive substances. These substances are injected into the bloodstream or administered as inhaled gases. As they are distributed in tissues, they display characteristic patterns that indicate physiologic and metabolic processes, for example, glucose and oxygen uptake, cerebral blood flow, neural and neurotransmitter function, and the effects of drugs. As a research tool, PET is being used to visualize the specific brain sites that are involved in the processing of information in the brain.

Brain Scan

The **brain scan** images radionuclide substances (technetium [^{99m}Tc]) that have been introduced into the bloodstream. For example, visualization of tissue uptake of the radioactive agent provides an indication of blood-brain barrier integrity (increased uptake of the agent indicates disruption). This scanning technique also can identify abnormalities in blood flow dynamics and cellular metabolic function. The brain scan is particularly helpful in detecting abnormal vascularity resulting from neoplasms, abscesses, and vascular lesions.

Isotope cisternography is another radionuclide imaging technique that uses brain scan imaging to detect CSF flow, CSF resorption, and integrity of CSF pathways. The radionuclide agent in this case is injected directly into the subarachnoid space. Under normal conditions the agent passes over the cortical surface and is resorbed through the arachnoid villi. Demonstration of the agent in the ventricular system after a specific period of time indicates CSF obstruction; that is, the CSF backflows from the subarachnoid space into the ventricles.

Cerebral Angiography

Angiography is a radiologic technique that demonstrates cerebrovascular blood flow. This technique commonly is performed by the introduction of a small catheter into the femoral artery. The catheter is then passed to the level of the cerebral circulation and through the aorta, and a contrast dye is injected. Serial x-ray films are then taken. These films demonstrate flow of the dye through the cerebral vasculature and provide information on patency, location, size, and flow pattern of the vessels. Another technique used in cerebral angiography is the retrograde (reverse flow) injection of the dye through catheterization of a brachial, axillary, subclavian, or femoral vein.

Myelography

A **myelogram** demonstrates intraspinal anatomy by the introduction of a radiographic dye into the lumbar subarachnoid space or the cerebellomedullary cistern (cisterna magna). The dye is allowed to flow in a cephalic direction, as in the case of a lumbar injection, or inferiorly in a cerebellomedullary cistern puncture. X-ray films are then obtained. The distribution of the dye delineates spinal cord and nerve root structure and integrity.

Echoencephalography (Ultrasound)

Echoencephalography, or **ultrasound**, is a safe, noninvasive procedure using sound waves that are deflected at differing rates, depending on the density of the tissue. Information is processed and displayed on an oscilloscope screen. It is useful primarily in the detection of structural characteristics of intracranial space–occupying mass lesions and the determination of ventricular dimensions, especially in newborns.

Electroencephalography

The **electroencephalograph** (EEG) is a recording of electrical impulses, arising from the cortical surface of the brain, that is detected by scalp electrodes. The recording of brain wave patterns is analyzed for alterations or localization (or both) of specific electrical activity. This test is especially useful in detecting and localizing foci that initiate seizure activity. It is also an important technique in determining, from a person's brain activity, whether the person is legally "brain dead."

Evoked Potentials

Evoked potentials (EPs) are a method of detecting electrical brain activity that results from a stimulus—primarily auditory, visual, or peripheral sensory. Electrical activity is computer formatted to display changes in trends. The primary uses of EPs include perioperative detection of sensory pathway integrity and disease- or drug-related sensory dysfunction.

Cerebrospinal Fluid Analysis

Cerebrospinal fluid (CSF) generally is obtained from the lumbar or cisternal subarachnoid space by means of a hollow needle that allows passive flow. The lumbar puncture is performed most often at the L3–4 interspace (below the level of the spinal cord at L1–2). Cisternal puncture is performed by the insertion of a needle into the cerebellomedullary cistern using an approach from the back of the neck in the region of the foramen magnum. CSF pressure is commonly measured during these procedures. The CSF can be analyzed also for gross characteristics and constituents (color, blood cells, electrolytes, and protein) and cultured for microorganisms (Table 14-9).

Table 14-9	Cerebrospinal Fluid Analysis		
Parameters	**Normal**	**Abnormal**	**Possible Cause**
Pressure (initial readings)	120-180 mm H$_2$O (9-14 mmHg)	<60 mm H$_2$O	Faulty needle placement Dehydration Spinal block along subarachnoid space Block of foramen magnum
		>200 mm H$_2$O	Muscle tension Abdominal compression Brain tumor Subdural hematoma Brain abscess Brain cyst Cerebral edema (any cause) Hydrocephalus
Color	Clear, colorless	Cloudy	Increased cell count Increased microorganisms
		Yellow	Xanthochromic (caused by red blood cell [RBC] pigments) High protein content
		Smoky	Presence of RBCs
Red blood cells	None	Blood-tinged	Traumatic tap
		Grossly bloody	Traumatic tap Subarachnoid hemorrhage

Data From Rudy EB, editor: *Advanced neurological and neurosurgical nursing*, St Louis, 1984, Mosby.

*NOTE: If CSF contains blood, this will raise the protein level.

Continued

Table 14-9	Cerebrospinal Fluid Analysis—cont'd		
Parameters	Normal	Abnormal	Possible Cause
White blood cells	0-6/mm³	>10/mm³ (Cell counts range from below 100 to many thousands depending on causative factor; all are abnormal findings.)	Occurs in many conditions: Bacterial infections of meninges Viral infections of meninges Neurosyphilis Tuberculous meningitis Metastatic neoplastic lesions Parasitic infections Acute demyelinating diseases Following introduction of air or blood into subarachnoid space
Protein*	15-45 mg/dl (1% of serum protein)	<10 mg/dl	Little clinical significance
		>60 mg/dl	Occurs in many conditions: Complete spinal block Guillain-Barré syndrome Carcinomatosis of meninges Tumors close to pial or ependymal surfaces or in cerebellopontine angle Acute and chronic meningitis Meningeal hemorrhage Demyelinating disorders Degenerative diseases
Glucose	50-75 mg/dl (approximately 60% of blood glucose level)	<40 mg/dl	Acute bacterial meningitis Tuberculous meningitis Meningeal carcinomatosis
		>100 mg/dl	Diabetes
Chloride	700-750 mg/dl; 125 mM	<625 mg/dl	Hypochloremia Tuberculous meningitis
		>800 mg/dl	Not of neurologic significance; correlates with blood levels of chloride

Data From Rudy EB, editor: *Advanced neurological and neurosurgical nursing,* St Louis, 1984, Mosby.
*NOTE: If CSF contains blood, this will raise the protein level.

SUMMARY REVIEW

Overview and Organization of the Nervous System
1. The divisions of the nervous system have been categorized as either structural (central nervous system [CNS] and peripheral nervous system [PNS]) or functional (somatic nervous system and autonomic nervous system [ANS]).
2. The CNS is contained within the brain and spinal cord.
3. The PNS is composed of cranial and spinal nerves, which carry impulses toward the CNS (afferent) and away from the CNS (efferent) to target organs or skeletal muscle.

Cells of the Nervous System
1. The neuron and neuroglial cells make up nervous tissue. The neuron is specialized to transmit and receive electrical and chemical impulses, and the neuroglial cell provides supportive functions. The neuron is further divided into unipolar, pseudounipolar, bipolar, and multipolar categories, according to structure and particular mechanics of impulse transmission.
2. The neuron is composed of a cell body, one or more dendrites, and an axon. A myelin sheath around selected axons forms an insulation that allows quicker nerve impulse conduction, referred to as *saltatory conduction.*
3. Neurons have four basic types of cell configuration: (a) unipolar; (b) pseudounipolar; (c) bipolar; and (d) multipolar. The three function types of neurons are sensory, associational, and motor.
4. Neuroglia cells ("nerve glue") support the CNS and make up approximately half of the total brain and spinal cord volume.

5. Nerve injury triggers a sequence of events known as *wallerian degeneration.* The degree of nerve regeneration that occurs depends on many factors.

Nerve Impulse
1. The region between adjacent neurons is the synapse, and the region between the neuron and muscle is the myoneural junction.
2. Neurotransmitters are responsible for chemical conduction across the synapse and myoneural junction. Nerve impulse is predominantly regulated by a balance of inhibitory postsynaptic potentials (IPSPs) and excitatory postsynaptic potentials (EPSPs), temporal and spatial summation, and convergence and divergence.

Central Nervous System
1. The brain is contained within the cranial vault and is divided into three distinct regions: (a) forebrain, (b) midbrain, and (c) hindbrain.
2. The forebrain comprises the two cerebral hemispheres and allows conscious perception of internal and external stimuli, thought and memory processes, and voluntary control of skeletal muscles. The deep portion of the forebrain is termed the *diencephalon* and processes incoming sensory data. The center for voluntary control of skeletal muscle movements is located along the precentral gyrus in the frontal lobe, whereas the center for perception is along the postcentral gyrus in the parietal lobe. The Broca area (rostral to the postcentral gyrus)

and the Wernicke area (superoposterior temporal lobe) are major speech centers.

3. The midbrain is primarily a relay center for motor and sensory tracts, as well as a center for auditory and visual reflexes.

4. The hindbrain allows sampling and comparison of sensory data from the periphery and motor impulses from the cerebral hemispheres for the purpose of coordination and refinement of skeletal muscle movement.

5. The spinal cord contains the majority of nerve fibers connecting the brain with the periphery. Reflex arcs are completed in the spinal cord and influenced by the higher centers in the brain.

6. The four clinically relevant motor pathways are the lateral corticospinal, corticobulbar, basal ganglia, and vestibulospinal.

7. The three clinically important afferent pathways are the posterior column, anterior spinothalamic, and lateral spinothalamic.

8. The CNS is protected by the scalp, bony cranium, meninges, vertebral column, and cerebrospinal fluid. Cerebrospinal fluid is formed from blood components in the choroid plexuses of the ventricles and is reabsorbed in the arachnoid villi (located in the dural venous sinuses) after circulating through the brain and spinal cord.

9. The paired carotid and vertebral arteries supply blood to the brain and connect to form the circle of Willis. The major branches projecting from the circle of Willis are the anterior, middle, and posterior cerebral arteries. Drainage of blood from the brain is accomplished through the venous sinuses and jugular veins.

10. Blood supply to the spinal cord originates from the vertebral arteries and branches arising from the aorta.

Peripheral Nervous System

1. The PNS functions to relay information from the CNS to muscle and effector organs through cranial and spinal nerve tracts arranged in fascicles (multiple fascicles bound together form the peripheral nerve).

2. The 31 pairs of spinal nerves contain both sensory and motor neurons.

Autonomic Nervous System

1. The ANS is responsible for the maintenance of a steady state in the internal environment. Two opposing systems make up the ANS: (a) the sympathetic nervous system responds to stress by mobilizing energy stores and prepares the body to defend itself, and (b) the parasympathetic nervous system conserves energy and the body's resources.

Aging and the Nervous System

1. Major structural changes with aging include a decrease in number of neurons and a decrease in brain weight and size.

2. Deposition of lipofuscin and the presence of senile plaques, multiple neurofibrillary tangles, and Lewy bodies are common cellular changes with aging.

3. A progressive slowing of neurologic function occurs with advancing age.

Tests of Nervous System Function

1. Tests of nervous system function include x-ray films, computed tomography, magnetic resonance imaging and angiography, positron emission tomography, brain scan, cerebral angiography, myelography, echoencephalography, electroencephalography, evoked potentials, and analysis of the cerebrospinal fluid.

KEY TERMS

Acetylcholine, 435
α-Adrenergic receptors, 436
β-Adrenergic receptors, 436
Adrenergic transmission, 436
Afferent pathways (ascending pathways), 411
Afferent (sensory) neuron, 425
Amygdala, 420
Angiography, 442
Anterior cerebral artery, 429
Anterior column (ventral column), 424
Anterior fossa, 426
Anterior horn (ventral horn), 424
Anterior spinal arteries, 429
Anterior spinothalamic, 426
Arachnoid membrane, 427
Arachnoid villi, 428
Arterial circle (circle of Willis), 429
Association fibers, 420
Associational neurons (interneurons), 413
Astrocytes, 413
Autonomic nervous system (ANS), 411
Axons, 413
Axon hillock, 413
Basal ganglia, 418
Basal ganglia system, 418
Basilar artery, 429
Basis pedunculi, 422
Bipolar neurons, 413
Blood-brain barrier, 432
Brachial plexus, 432

Brain scan, 442
Brain stem, 416
Broca speech area, 418
Cauda equina, 423
Cavernous sinus, 429
Celiac branch of aorta, 435
Central canal, 424
Central nervous system (CNS), 411
Central sulcus (fissure of Rolando), 418
Cerebellomedullary cistern (cisterna magna), 427
Cerebellum, 422
Cerebral aqueduct (aqueduct of Sylvius), 422
Cerebral cortex, 418
Cerebral nuclei, 420
Cerebrospinal fluid (CSF), 428
Cerebrum, 418
Cholinergic transmission, 435
Choroid plexus, 427
Collateral ganglia, 435
Computed tomography (CT), 442
Contralateral control, 418
Conus medullaris, 423
Convergence, 413
Corpora quadrigemina (tectum), 422
Corpus callosum (commissural fibers), 420
Corpus striatum, 420
Corticobulbar, 425
Corticospinal tracts, 418

Cranial nerves, 411
Craniosacral division, 435
Dendrites, 413
Dendritic zone, 413
Denticulate ligaments, 427
Dermatomes, 432
Diencephalon, 422
Divergence, 413
Dopamine, 422
Dura mater, 426
Echoencephalography (ultrasound), 443
Effector organ, 411
Efferent (motor) neuron, 425
Efferent pathways (descending pathways), 411
Electroencephalograph (EEG), 443
Endoneurium, 413
Epicritic, 426
Epidural space, 427
Epithalamus, 422
Evoked potentials (EPs), 443
Excitatory postsynaptic potentials (EPSPs), 416
Facilitation, 416
Falx cerebri, 427
Fascicles, 430
Filum terminale, 423
Fissures, 418
Frontal lobe, 418
Galea aponeurotica, 426
Ganglia, 413

KEY TERMS—cont'd

Gray matter, 418
Hippocampus, 422
Hypothalamus, 422
Inferior colliculi, 422
Inferior mesenteric branch of aorta, 435
Inhibitory postsynaptic potentials (IPSPs), 416
Inner dura (meningeal layer), 427
Insula, 420
Intermediolateral gray (lateral horn), 424
Internal capsule, 420
Internal carotid artery, 429
Interventricular foramen (foramen of Monro), 428
Intervertebral disk, 428
Lateral apertures (foramina of Luschka), 428
Lateral column, 424
Lateral corticospinal, 425
Lateral spinothalamic, 426
Lateral sulcus (sylvian fissure, lateral fissure), 418
Lentiform nucleus, 420
Limbic system, 422
Longitudinal fissure, 418
Lower motor neurons, 425
Lumbar cistern, 427
Lumbar plexus, 432
Lumbar puncture, 428
Magnetic resonance angiography (MRA), 442
Magnetic resonance imaging (MRI), 442
Median aperture (foramen of Magendie), 428
Medulla oblongata, 423
Meninges, 426
Metencephalon, 422
Microfilaments, 412
Microglia, 413
Microtubules, 412
Midbrain (mesencephalon), 422
Middle cerebral artery, 429
Middle fossa (temporal fossa), 426
Mixed nerves, 432
Motor neurons, 413
Motor units, 425
Multipolar neurons, 413
Myelencephalon, 423
Myelin, 413
Myelin sheath, 413

Myelogram, 443
Neurilemma (Schwann sheath), 413
Neurofibrils, 412
Neurofibrillary tangles, 439
Neuroglia, 413
Neuroglial cells, 412
Neuromuscular (myoneural) junction, 425
Neurons, 412
Neurotransmitter, 416
Nissl substances, 412
Nodes of Ranvier, 413
Norepinephrine, 436
Nucleus (*plural,* nuclei), 413
Nucleus pulposus, 428
Occipital lobe, 420
Oligodendroglia (oligodendrocytes), 413
Papez circuit, 422
Parasympathetic nervous system, 435
Parietal lobe, 418
Pelvic nerve, 435
Periosteum (endosteal layer), 427
Peripheral nervous system (PNS), 411
Pia mater, 427
Plasticity, 418
Plexuses, 413
Pons, 423
Positron emission tomography (PET) scan, 442
Postcentral gyrus, 418
Posterior cerebral arteries, 429
Posterior column (dorsal column), 424
Posterior fossa, 426
Posterior horn (dorsal horn), 424
Posterior spinal arteries, 429
Postganglionic neurons, 435
Postsynaptic neurons, 416
Precentral gyrus, 418
Prefrontal area, 418
Premotor area, 418
Presynaptic neurons, 416
Primary motor area, 418
Primary voluntary motor area, 418
Projecting arteries (nutrient arteries), 429
Protopathic, 426
Pseudounipolar neurons, 413
Red nucleus, 422
Reflex arcs, 425
Reticular activating system, 416

Reticular formation, 416
Roentgenograms (x-ray films), 441
Sacral plexus, 432
Saltatory conduction, 413
Schwann cell, 413
Schwann sheath (neurilemma), 413
Senile plaques, 439
Sensory ganglion (dorsal root ganglion), 424
Sensory neurons, 413
Somatic nervous system, 411
Spatial summation, 416
Spinal cord, 423
Spinal nerves, 411
Spinal tracts, 424
Spinothalamic tract, 424
Splanchnic nerves, 435
Subarachnoid space, 427
Subdural space, 427
Substantia gelatinosa, 424
Substantia nigra, 422
Subthalamic nucleus, 422
Subthalamus, 422
Sulci, 418
Summation, 416
Superficial arteries (conducting arteries), 429
Superior colliculi, 422
Superior mesenteric branch of aorta, 435
Superior sagittal sinus, 428
Sympathetic (paravertebral) ganglia, 435
Sympathetic nervous system, 435
Synapse, 415
Synaptic boutons, 416
Synaptic cleft, 416
Tegmentum, 422
Telencephalon, 418
Temporal lobe, 420
Temporal summation, 416
Tentorium cerebelli, 427
Thalamus, 422
Thoracolumbar division, 435
Unipolar neurons, 413
Upper motor neurons, 425
Ventricles, 428
Vermis, 423
Vertebral arteries, 429
Vertebral column, 428
Vestibulospinal, 425
Wernicke area, 420
White matter, 418

MEDIA RESOURCES   *evolve*

Review questions and answers for this chapter are available in the *CD Companion* included with this book.

WebLinks—links to Internet sites pertaining to this chapter—are available on Evolve at http://evolve.elsevier.com/McCance/.

REFERENCES

1. Waxman SG: *Correlative neuroanatomy,* ed 25, New York, 2002, Lange Medical Books/McGraw-Hill.
2. Nadeau SE: *Medical neuroscience,* Philadelphia, 2004, Saunders.
3. Kandel ER, Schwartz JH, Jessell TM, editors: *Principles of neural science,* ed 4, New York, 2000, McGraw-Hill.
4. Pritchard TC, Alloway KD: *Medical neuroscience,* Hershey, PA, 1999, Fence Creek Publications.
5. Benarroch EE et al: *Medical neurosciences: An Approach to Anatomy, Pathology, and Physiology by Systems and Levels,* ed 4, Philadelphia, 1999, Lippincott Williams & Wilkins.
6. Wang E, Snyder D, editors: *Handbook of the aging brain,* San Diego, 1998, Academic Press.
7. DeArmono SJ, Simko JP, Gasin DA: The molecular and genetic basis of neurodegenerative diseases. In Weidner J et al, editors: *Modern surgical pathology,* vol 2, Philadelphia, 2003, Saunders.
8. Timiras PS, editor: *Physiologic basis of aging and geriatrics,* ed 3, Boca Raton, 2003, CRC Press.

PAIN, TEMPERATURE REGULATION, SLEEP, AND SENSORY FUNCTION

CHAPTER

15

SUE E. HUETHER • CURTIS B. DEFRIEZ

http://evolve.elsevier.com/McCance/

CHAPTER OUTLINE

Alterations in sensory function may involve dysfunctions of the general or the special senses. Dysfunctions of the general senses include chronic pain, abnormal temperature regulation, tactile dysfunction, and proprioceptive dysfunction. Dysfunctions of the special senses include visual, auditory, vestibular, olfactory, and gustatory (taste) dysfunction.

The special senses of vision, hearing, touch, smell, and taste are the means by which individuals perceive stimuli that are essential in interacting with the environment. Special sensory receptors are connected to specific areas of the brain through the afferent pathways of the central nervous system (CNS). Each of the special senses thus involves a connected system of organs and tissues that receives stimuli and sends sensory messages to areas of the CNS where they are processed.

Pain is a unique sensory experience that, although universally described as unpleasant, is nonetheless essential to our survival. Pain provides protection by signaling the presence of disease or injury. Unlike pain, which need not be a part of everyday life, temperature is carefully monitored and regulated within clearly defined normal limits. Like pain, however, variations in temperature can signal disease. Fever is a common manifestation of dysfunction and is often the first symptom observed in an infectious or inflammatory condition. If the body's temperature regulatory mechanism is out of balance, the result may be death.

Sleep is a normal, cyclic process that restores the body's energy and maintains normal functioning. Sleep is so essential to both physiologic and psychologic function that sleep deprivation causes a wide range of clinical manifestations. Prolonged deprivation or disruption of sleep ultimately leads to serious dysfunction.

PAIN

Pain has various definitions. A widely accepted definition of pain is that drafted by the International Association for the Study of Pain (IASP) and accepted by the American Pain Society: "Pain is an unpleasant sensory and emotional experience associated with actual or potential tissue damage or described in terms of such damage."[1] McCaffrey maintains that "pain is whatever the experiencing person says it is, existing whenever he says it does."[2] Waddell defines pain as "a symptom, not a clinical sign, diagnosis or disease…".[3] One thing is certain: Whichever definition is used, pain is not merely a simple process or experience, and it cannot be characterized as a response to tissue damage alone. A clear understanding of the complexities of the pain experience—specifically one that encompasses an individual's emotions, cognition, motivation, prior history, and even issues of secondary gain—is needed to treat patients in pain and to further understanding in the field.

Theories of Pain

In the seventeenth century, the French philosopher and mathematician René Descartes proposed that the body works like a machine that can be studied by scientific methods and that injury activates specific pain receptors and fibers that project to the brain. He further postulated that the *intensity of pain* is directly related to the amount of associated tissue injury. For instance, pricking one's finger with a needle would cause minimal pain, whereas cutting one's hand with a knife would produce more pain. This theory—the **specificity theory**—is generally accurate when applied to certain types of injuries and the acute pain associated with them. But the specificity theory did not allow for psychologic contributions, such as attention to pain, prior experience, and the emotions involved in the "meaning" of the situation.[4] Nevertheless, it was this theory of pain, with some modification, that was still operational entering the twentieth century.

By the middle of the last century, it became evident that the specificity theory and other theories that had been advanced to that time were insufficient to explain the emotional as well as the physical dimensions of pain. Around the same time the study of chronic pain, and more specifically chronic neuropathic pain, was undergoing great upheaval. Evolving research on the nature of adaptation to pain, referred pain, and pain thresholds led to new and intriguing insights, and spawned many new questions.

The **gate control theory** proposed in 1965 by Melzack and Wall provided the first cohesive explanation for the emerging complexities of pain phenomena and has had a powerful impact on pain research and therapy.[5] Over the past 20 years exceptional progress has been made in strengthening the gate control theory of pain by elucidating the neuroanatomy and neuropharmacology of pain pathways in the peripheral and central nervous systems.

Neuroanatomy of Pain

The perception of pain is called **nociception** and depends on specifically dedicated receptors and pathways. The gate control theory describes these pathways in great detail, and explains the experience of pain by emphasizing the modulation of afferent input coming into the dorsal horn of the spinal cord and the dynamic role of the brain in pain processes.

Nociceptors

Nociceptive impulses arising from skin, muscle, joints, arteries, and the viscera are transmitted from unspecialized, bare sensory nerve endings called *nociceptors*, which respond to chemical, mechanical, and thermal stimuli (Table 15-1). The variable nature and distribution of nociceptors affects the relative sensitivity to pain in different areas of the body. For example, the tips of the fingers have more nociceptors than the skin of the back, and all skin has many more nociceptors than the internal organs. Unlike sensory neurons of the special senses of vision, gustation, and olfaction (discussed later in this chapter), which are required to detect only one type of sensory stimulus (e.g., light for the sense of vision), primary nociceptive afferents have the remarkable ability to detect a wide range of stimuli. To do this, nociceptors are equipped with an array of transduction channels that can sense different forms of noxious stimulation and at different intensities. In addition to the previously well studied voltage-gated potassium, sodium, and calcium channels, recent research has delineated the presence of up to seven other types of transmembrane receptors (called *transient receptor potential channels* or *TRP channels*), which reside on "naked nerve endings" and respond to a variety of physical, chemical, and thermal stimuli.[6]

Nociceptors are categorized not only according to the stimulus to which they respond but also by the properties of

Table 15-1	Stimuli that Activate Nociceptors (Pain Receptors)
Location of Receptor	**Provoking Stimuli**
Skin	Pricking, cutting, crushing, burning, freezing
Gastrointestinal tract	Engorged or inflamed mucosa, distention or spasm of smooth muscle, traction on mesenteric attachment
Skeletal muscle	Ischemia, injuries of connective tissue sheaths, necrosis, hemorrhage, prolonged contraction, injection of irritating solutions
Joints	Synovial membrane inflammation
Arteries	Piercing, inflammation
Head	Traction, inflammation, or displacement of arteries, meningeal structures, and sinuses; prolonged muscle contraction
Heart	Ischemia and inflammation

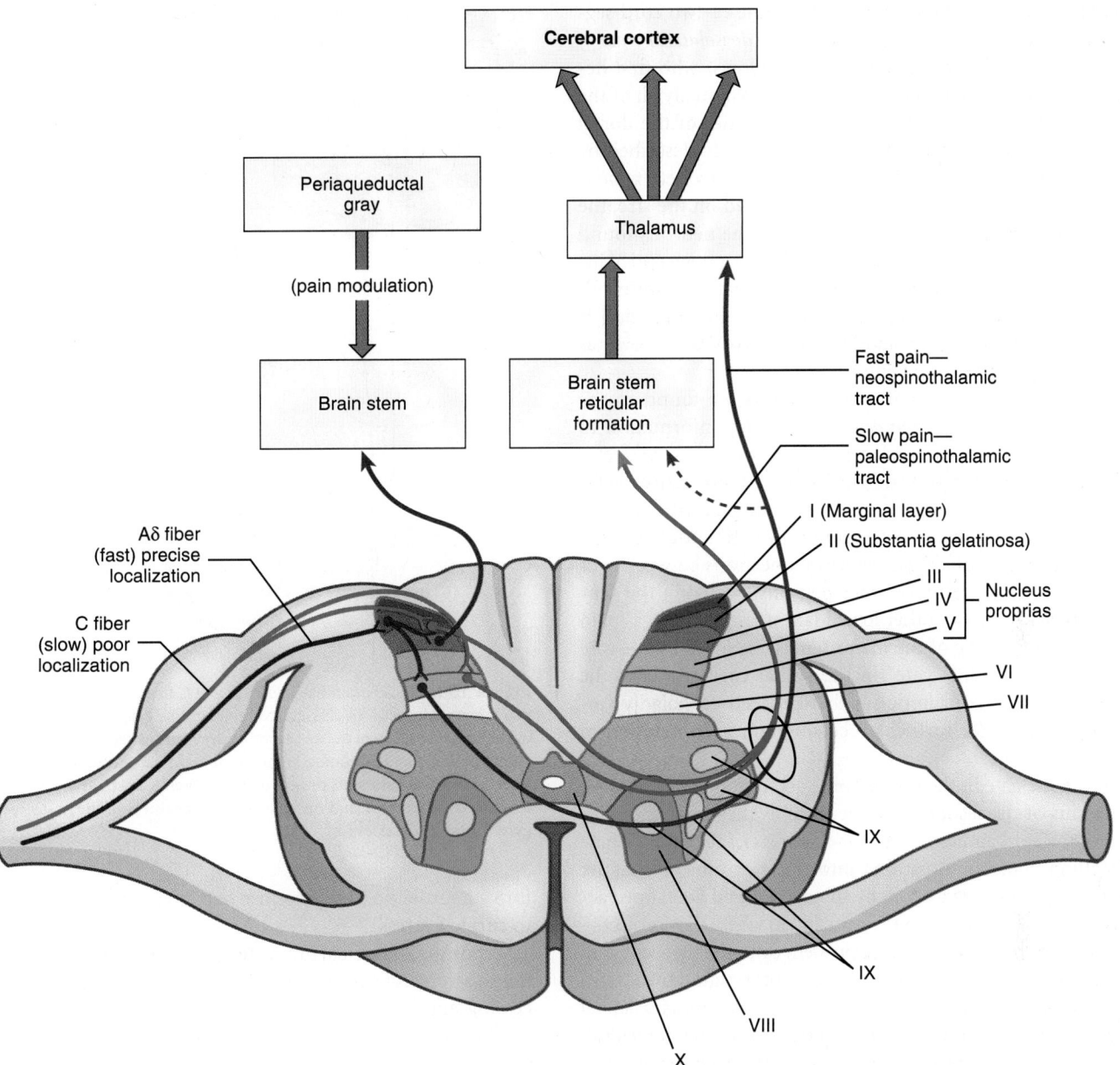

Figure 15-1 Pain fibers that terminate primarily in laminated II and V of the dorsal horn. The myelinated Aδ fibers (fast localized pain) synapse on a second set of neurons that carry the signal to the thalamus via the neospinalthalamic track. The C fibers (slow pain) synapse on laminae II and V interneurons that connect with neurons in laminae II, IV, and V and carry the pain signal to the reticular formation and midbrain via the paleospinalthalamic track. The axons of the spinothalamic tracks cross over the spinal cord to ascend in the anterior and lateral spinal cord white matter.

the axons associated with them. Severe mechanical deformation excites mechanonociceptors whereas mechanothermal nociceptors are stimulated by mechanical deformation and/or extremes of temperature. These two receptors are associated with lightly myelinated, medium-sized A-delta (Aδ) fibers. Other types of mechanical, thermal, and chemical nociception are transmitted by excitation of polymodal nociceptors and are carried on small, unmyelinated C fibers.

The nerve action potentials generated by excitation of any of these nociceptors travel along these two fiber types to reach the spinal cord. Nociceptive transmission through the Aδ fibers occurs more quickly than it does through C fibers. **Aδ**

fibers carry well-localized, sharp pain sensations and are important in initiating rapid reactions to stimuli (fast pain). The small **unmyelinated C polymodal nociceptors** are responsible for the transmission of the diffuse burning or aching sensations that follow (slow pain) (Figure 15-1).

Pathways of Nociception
The cell bodies of primary-order, pain-transmitting neurons reside in the dorsal root ganglia just lateral to the spine along the sensory pathways that penetrate into the posterior part of the cord. Once the axons of the primary afferents (Aδ and C fibers) enter the cord (see Figure 14-8), they may branch into

ascending or descending collaterals for one or two cord segments in neuronal projections called the *dorsolateral tract of Lissauer* (named after the German neurologist who first described it in the late nineteenth century). Eventually all of the primary afferents terminate in the gray matter of the dorsal horn in distinctive layers or *laminae* originally described by Rexed.[7] The gray matter of the cord has been divided by neuroanatomists into ten of these laminae based on the size, the shape, and the plane of the projection of the neurons found there. Many of the primary afferents carrying nociceptive information were originally found to terminate in lamina II, which was given the name *substantia gelatinosa*. Lamina I is called the *marginal layer*, and laminae III to V are known as the *nucleus proprius* (see Figure 15-1).

Three classes of second-order neurons are found in the dorsal horn: (1) *projection cells*, which relay information to higher brain areas (cephalad); (2) *excitatory interneurons*, which relay nociceptive transmissions to projection cells, other interneurons, or to motor cells concerned with local reflexes; and (3) *inhibitory interneurons*, which modulate nociceptive transmission. The synaptic connections between cells of primary and secondary order neurons located in the substantia gelatinosa and other Rexed lamina function as a "pain gate," providing one of the major tenets advanced by the gate control theory. This "gate" in the spinal cord regulates the transmission of pain impulses that proceed cephaladly (toward the head) for further processing and interpretation in the brain.

From the gate in the dorsal horn, nociception continues on the axons of the second-order neurons as they cross the midline of the cord and ascend to various areas of the brain. These ascending fibers are organized into tracts or funiculi that are found in the white matter of the spinal cord, and are named according to their location in the cord and to where they project—either to the higher cord and brain stem or to the diencephalon and limbic structures. Most nociceptive information travels in a cephalad direction by means of ascending columns in the lateral spinothalamic tract (also called the *anterolateral funiculus*). Other bits of nociceptive signals travel in the posterior columns of the cord to the dorsal column nuclei of the medulla, and from there ascend in the medial lemniscus to the lateral thalamus. There are several other spinal cord projection systems that convey nociceptive information directly or indirectly to the reticular formation of the brain stem and the periaquaductal gray (PAG) matter of the midbrain. These include the postsynaptic dorsal column, spinocervical, spinoreticular, spinomesencephalic, spinoparabrachial, spinohypothalamic, and other spinolimbic pathways[8] (Figure 15-3).

Although the organization of all of the ascending tracts is complex, the principal target for nociceptive afferents is the thalamus (which is the major relay station of sensory information in general). The thalamus is primarily divided into medial and lateral groups by a band of fibers called the *internal medullary lamina*. The ventral posterior lateral (VPL) and ventral posterior medial (VPM) nuclei of the thalamus facilitate the localization of pain and integrate these perceptions

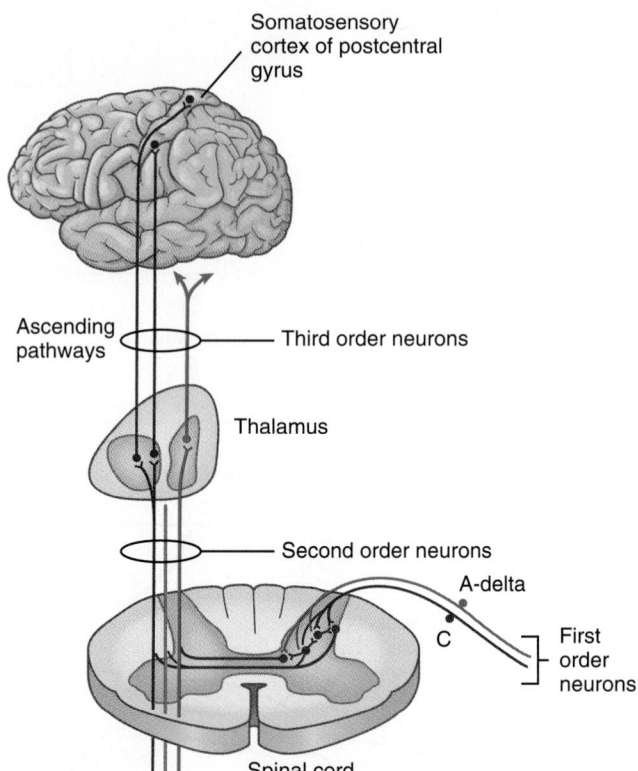

Figure 15-2 Nociception pathways. Aδ and C fibers comprise the primary, first-order sensory afferents coming into the gate at the posterior part of the spinal cord. Here we see second-order neurons crossing the cord ("decussating") and ascending to the thalamus as part of the spinothalamic tract. Third-order afferents project to higher brain centers of the limbic system, the frontal cortex, and the primary sensory cortex of the post-central gyrus of the parietal lobe.

into a neuroendocrine response (e.g., the response to fright or to surgical stress).[9,9a]

From the thalamus, brain stem, and midbrain, third-order neurons project to portions of the CNS involved in the processing and interpretation of pain, the chief areas being the cerebral cortex and the reticular and limbic systems.

Pain Processing in the Brain
Cerebral Cortex

The third-order neurons of the ventral posterior nuclear complex of the thalamus project in a highly organized manner to the primary and secondary somatosensory cortex[10] (Brodman areas 3,1,2; see Figure 14-6, *B*). On the post-central gyrus of the parietal lobe there is a topographically organized representation of the body that mirrors the concentration of peripheral sensory receptors known as the *sensory homunculus* (see Figure 14-7, p. 420). This area of the brain is thought to be involved in the discriminative and cognitive aspects of pain; that is, what we *think* about the pain.[11]

The frontal lobe of the cerebral cortex receives diffuse projections from the medial thalamic nuclei, which are thought to subserve the affective expression of pain (how your pain looks to an observer) through their frontal-limbic connections. Frontal lobectomies were once used in an effort to treat

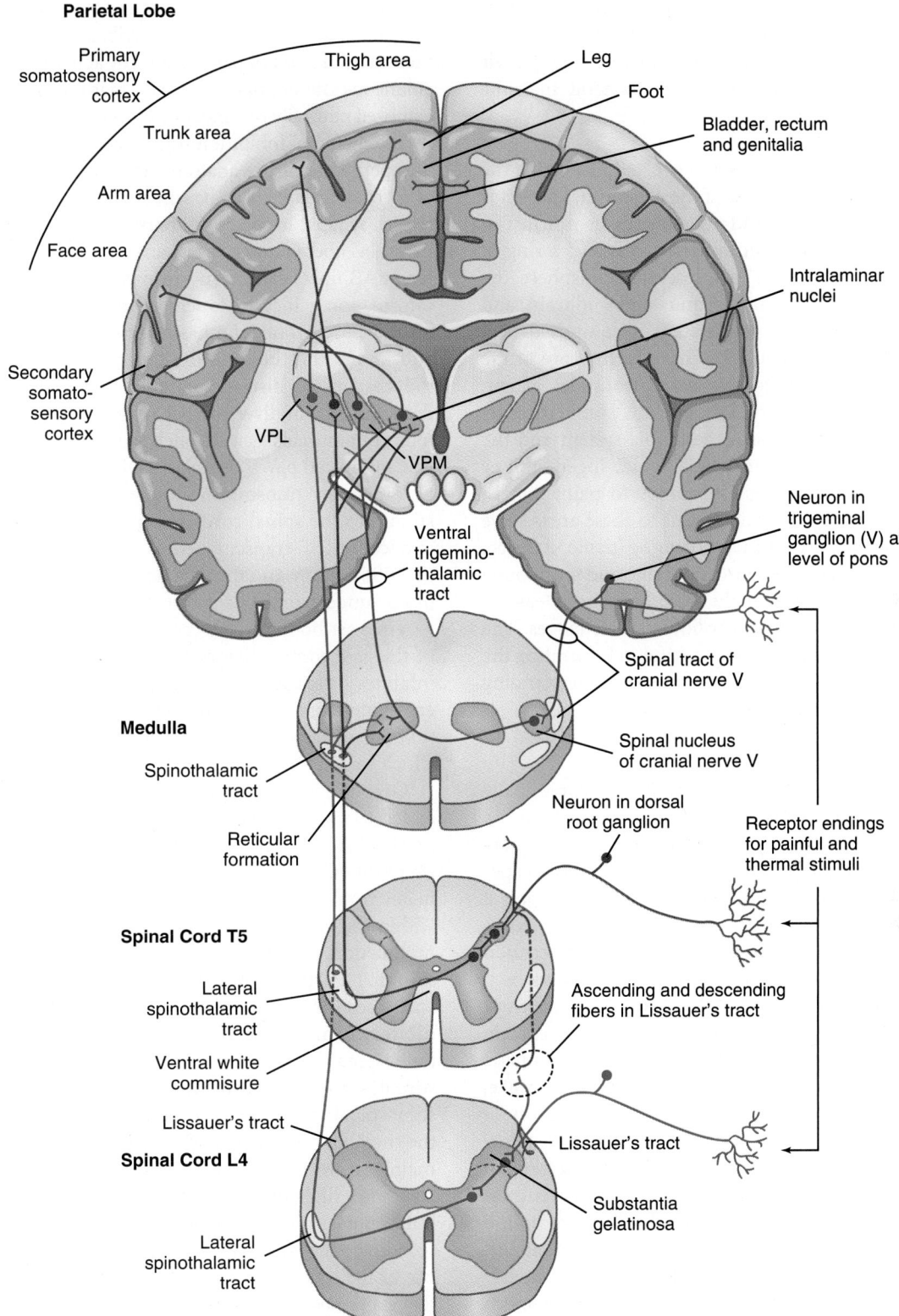

Figure 15-3 Central nervous system pathways that mediate the sensations of pain and temperature. *VPM,* Ventral posterior medial thalamic nuclei; *VPL,* ventral posterior lateral thalamic nuclei.

some cases of intractable pain. Post-surgically individuals continued to report pain if questioned, but they seldom asked for medications and no longer seemed to care about their pain. This response is also observed in bilateral thalamic lesions.[12]

Subcortical Systems

The limbic and reticular tracts are involved in alerting the body to danger, initiating arousal of the organism, and emotionally processing the perceived afferent signals not just as stimuli, but as pain. The **limbic system** consists of a ring of cortex on the medial aspect of each cerebral hemisphere, the subcortical nuclei, parts of the thalamus and midbrain, and the hypothalamus. The **reticular system** is composed of a number of vaguely defined nuclei situated in the core of the brain stem extending throughout its rostrocaudal extent. Many reticular neurons respond to noxious stimulation by initiating escape behaviors. Both the limbic system and the reticular system are phylogenetically very old. Together, they regulate the complex emotional responses to pain; that is, what we *feel* about the pain. Pain signals to these areas serve to arouse the whole organism to ongoing tissue damage, thereby activating protective neuroendocrine and autonomic reflexes such as the "fight or flight" response, the release of stress hormones, and beneficial cardiovascular changes. The gate control theory has been very successful in integrating the functions of these very "old" systems into our understanding of the emotional and motivational aspects of pain.

Neuromodulation of Pain

The extraordinary advances of gate control theory finally moved the focus of pain research away from the periphery and into the spinal cord and brain. The theory helps to better explain the psychologic component of pain—that the pain experience itself need not be proportional to the actual peripheral injury or disease. The pain pathways, no longer viewed as merely labeled lines of electric wires, were finally understood to function holistically as a single peripheral-CNS complex.

By the mid-1970s and into the 1980s, two other developments played key roles in extending the theory to explain how, under certain stressful conditions, significant traumatic injuries can be experienced as completely painless in awake, neurologically intact patients. The first was the discovery of specific descending pathways from the brain to the spinal cord that could produce significant and selective analgesia in those experiencing pain[13] (Figure 15-4). The second event was the identification of ubiquitous opioid receptors found throughout the body, and shortly thereafter, the isolation, purification, and sequencing of endogenous opioid peptides.[14] What followed was a virtual explosion of scientific research aimed at elucidating the pathways and chemicals that modify, or neuromodulate, the pain experience.

Pathways of Neuromodulation

How does central processing, including memory and interpretation of pain in the brain, lead to changes in how much algogenic (pain related) information passes through the spinal cord gate? When Melzack and Wall originally proposed the gate control theory, they described the possibility of **segmental inhibition** of pain, elicited by activity in large-diameter cutaneous afferent fibers at the dermatome level, which can be activated naturally by innocuous mechanical stimuli.[4] The reality of segmental inhibition was quickly verified when research into peripheral nerve anatomy demonstrated that stimulation of a group of large, fast, heavily myelinated A beta (Aβ) fibers (which synapse in the dorsal horn along with their nociceptive Aδ and C fiber counterparts) can close the pain gates. These afferent Aβ fibers carry non-noxious, low threshold mechanical information gained by touch, vibration, and pressure. This is intuitive to anyone who has hit their thumb with a hammer and knows that holding the thumb or putting it into their mouth conveys distraction input that lessens the pain. Indeed, this sort of diversion behavior is reflexive not just in humans but animals as well (such as the cat that will repeatedly lick an injured paw). It explains why massage therapy can relieve pain by transmitting afferent non-noxious inhibitory stimuli to the spinal cord. This principle is the basis for the application of transcutaneous electrical nerve stimulation (TENS) therapy and brought acclaim to the gate control theory by underscoring its predictive value.

The vast body of work completed since the inauguration of the gate control theory has focused on the complexity of inhibitory modulation beyond the segmental level (i.e., heterosegmental modulation). This newer work emphasizes a functional basis for pain control outside the dorsal horn, which was the focus of the original gate control hypothesis.

Over the past three decades a wealth of information has added to our understanding of heterosegmental, supraspinal mechanisms elicited by noxious and non-noxious stimuli.[15] Powerful *heterosegmental control of nociception* probably originates from the cortex because almost all nociceptive relays within the CNS are under so called corticofugal (top-down) modulation, which often occurs even in the absence of painful stimuli.[16] Further down, the caudal medulla participates in widespread inhibitory phenomena called **diffuse noxious inhibitory controls (DNIC)**.[17] Several ascending and descending bulbospinal pathways respond simultaneously to a noxious stimulus and participate in DNIC. The net effect of these supraspinal structures is to precisely encode the intensity of the noxious stimulus and transmit descending feedback, mainly to the deep dorsal horn neurons.[18] Figure 15-4 illustrates how higher brain regions participate in corticofugal and bulbospinal pain modulation as intricately incorporated descending pathways complete the circle back to the Rexed laminae of the spinal cord. Of interest is the recent demonstration that expectancy-related cortical activation also can exert control over analgesic systems of the brain stem to attenuate pain.[19,20] In other words, cognitive expectations (also known as the *placebo effect*) can cause real, measurable, often powerful physiologic effects that share some of the same descending corticofugal pathways as our pain modulation system.

The entire complex of pathways now can be visualized as an integration of peripheral sensory axon terminals, spinal

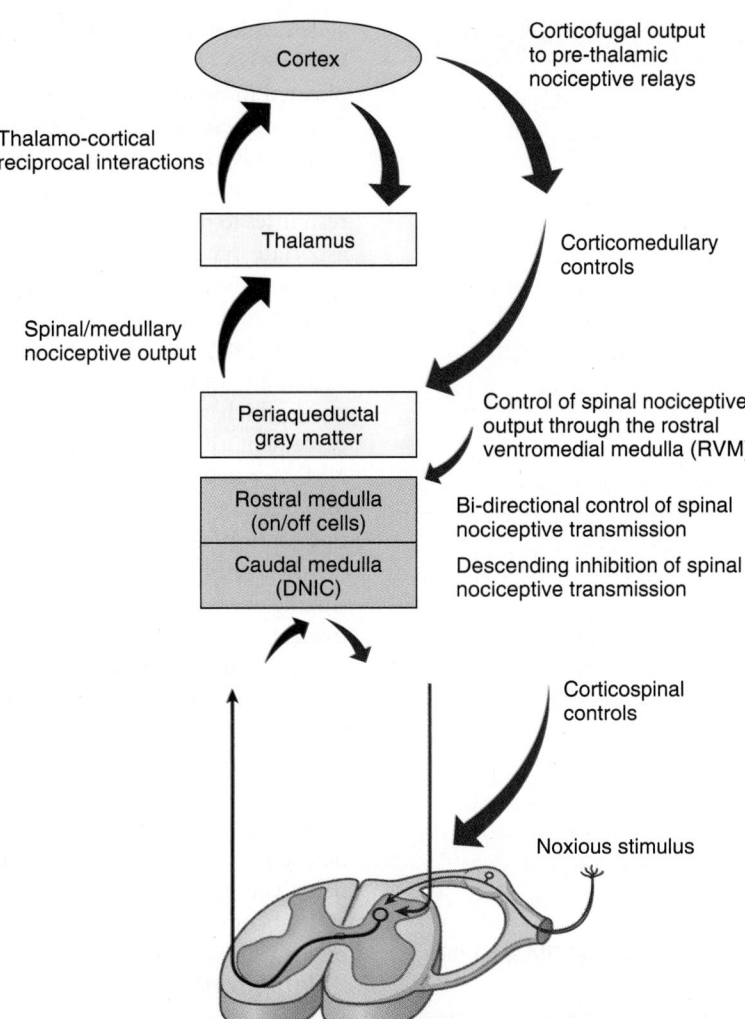

Figure 15-4 Diagram representing the central mechanisms of pain modulation. A noxious peripheral stimulus activates both segmental and bulbospinal heterosegmental modulatory mechanisms, which either accentuate or inhibit afferent pain transmission to the brain. The most important and widespread source of top-down (corticofugal) modulation arises from the cortex. Both thalamic and prethalamic nociceptive relays are under the influence of this corticofugal control. The dorsal horn of the spine is also under the influence of the caudal medulla through Descending Noxious Inhibitory Control (DNIC). (Modified from Villanueva L, Fields HL: *The pain system in normal and pathological states: a primer for clinicians,* Seattle, 2004, IASP Press.)

interneurons, and top-down control pathways that converge on the spinal dorsal horns. The result is to modify, dampen, or augment nociceptive transmission, depending on the many factors existing both within and without the organism.

Neurotransmitters and Chemicals of Neuromodulation

Many neurotransmitters mediate the transmission of pain in the periphery, the spinal cord, and the brain. In the periphery, local injury can result in direct or indirect excitation of nociceptors. Neurotransmitters can be classified as inflammatory, pain excitatory, pain inhibitory, and as modulators of pain (Box 15-1).

Direct excitation occurs when nociceptors respond with a threshold depolarization initiated by the application of heat, radiation, toxic chemicals, or tissue trauma. *Indirect excitation* occurs via the release of inflammatory mediators after the tissue is injured. The tissue injury results in the release of

prostaglandins such as PGE_2 and PGI_2, nitric oxide, bradykinins, and histamine. For example, it has been shown that lymphokines released in chronic lymphocytic inflammatory lesions contribute to some types of chronic pain. In addition, activity within the nociceptors causes them to release peptides and neurotransmitters such as substance P, neurokinin A, calcitonin-gene-related peptide (CGRP), and adenosine triphosphate (ATP), which promote the spread of pain locally and further contribute to vasodilation, increased vascular permeability, and degranulation of even more mast cell cytokines. The resultant "inflammatory soup" serves to lower the threshold for nociceptive depolarization resulting in peripheral sensitization and pain augmentation. This is readily recognized by anyone who has suffered a bad sunburn and then notices the resulting extra sensitivity of the skin to stimuli (such as mild heat or touch) that normally would be considered nonnoxious (a phenomenon referred to as *hyperalgesia*). Normally peripheral sensitization phenomena extinguish themselves as

Inflammatory Mediators
- Bradykinin
- Leukotrienes
- Prostaglandins
- Serotonin
- Substance P
- Interleukins
- Tumor necrosis factor–alpha
- Nitric oxide
- ATP
- Neurokinin
- Calcitonin–gene-related peptide

Excitatory Transmitters
- Glutamate (fast pain)
  - NMDA
  - AMDA
- Tachykinins
  - Neurokinin A
  - Neurokinin B
  - Substance P
- Other receptors
  - Calcitonin–gene-related peptide
  - Somatastatin
  - Bombesin
  - Cholecystokin

Inhibitory Transmitters
- Gamma amino butyric acid (GABA)
- Descending pain modulators
  - Norepinephrine–alpha-2 receptors
  - Serotonin (5-hydroxytryptamine)
  - Opioids (mu, delta, kappa receptors)
    - Endorphin ⎫
    - Enkephalin ⎬ Released from PAG and NRM and other areas of the brain
    - Dynorphin ⎭

ATP, Adenosine triphosphate; *NMDA,* N-methyl-D-aspartate; *AMDA,* alpha-3-hydroxy-5-methyl-4-isoxazole-propionic acid; *PAG,* peri-aqueductal gray; *NRM,* nucleus raphus mangus.

the tissue heals and inflammation subsides. However, when primary afferent function is altered in an enduring way by injury or disease of the nervous system, hyperalgesia may persist and be highly resistant to treatment.

In the spinal cord and brain, a wide variety of biogenic amines and other neurotransmitters act to modulate control over the transmission of pain impulses. Serotonin, norepinephrine, glutamate, aspartate, glycine, gamma-aminobutyric acid (GABA), and an array of endogenous opioids have been found to stimulate or inhibit interneurons in the CNS. This, in turn, may serve to stimulate or inhibit the gate and the primary nociceptive tracts.

Excitatory Neurotransmitters
Glutamate and aspartate, amino acid precursors, are the most common excitatory neurotransmitters in the brain and spinal cord. **Glutamate** activates two different kinds of receptors: AMPA/kinate (alpha-amino-3-hydroxy-5-methyl-

4-isoxazolepropionate acid) receptors, which are very fast, and NMDA (N-methyl-D-aspartate) receptors, which are implicated in memory and long-term potentiation of synapses. Both of these receptors lead to excitation of the membrane and depolarization of the cell, be it an inhibitory or excitatory neuron. Glutamate receptors mediate many spinal and central responses to painful stimulation. High levels of glutamate and aspartate have been found in the PAG as well as at the synapses of first-order nociceptors with ascending spinothalamic tract neurons. High levels of activity in the nociceptive afferents may result in an activity-dependent increase in the excitability of neurons in the dorsal horn of the cord. Glutamate, which accumulates in the dorsal horn, results in the displacement of a magnesium ion that serves to inhibit the NMDA receptor. With the loss of the blocking magnesium ion, receptor "wind up" or sensitization in the CNS to further nociception becomes evident. As a result of this *central sensitization,* activity levels that were subthreshold before the sensitizing event then become sufficient to open the more sensitive gate.

Although central sensitization is triggered in dorsal horn neurons by activity in nociceptors, the effects can generalize to other inputs into the dorsal horn as well. If this occurs, innocuous activation of fibers carrying low threshold mechanoreception (such as lightly brushing the surface of the skin with a cotton swab) will activate second-order nociceptive neurons giving rise to a sensation (often quite distressing) of pain. The induction of pain by what is normally considered an innocuous stimulus is referred to as *allodynia* and can be a major feature of neuropathic pain syndromes.

Inhibitory Neurotransmitters
GABA and glycine have major inhibitory effects in the spinal cord and brain. For example, dorsal horn laminae interneurons are rich in GABA (GABA-A, GABA-B, etc.) and function to inhibit pain by synapsing with neurons containing substance P (a major algogenic chemical found in the dorsal horn and elsewhere). Norepinephrine and 5-hydroxytryptamine (serotonin) contribute to pain modulation (inhibition) in the medulla and pons.

Endogenous opioids are a family of morphine-like neuropeptides that inhibit transmission of pain impulses in the spinal cord and brain.[21] There are four types of opioid neuropeptides: (1) *enkephalins,* (2) *endorphins,* (3) *dynorphins,* and the newest discovered (4) *endomorphins.* These substances are neurohormones that act as neurotransmitters by binding to one or more opioid receptors. Three distinct types of opioid receptors are found in the body: mu (μ) (with subtypes μ-1 and μ-2), kappa (κ), and delta (δ). Each receptor type binds differently with the various types of opioids.

Agonist activity at the opioid receptors by endogenous opioids inhibits the release of excitatory neurotransmitters such as substance P in the dorsal horn (blocking the transmission of the painful stimulus) or in other areas of the brain such as the PAG or the rostral ventromedial nuclei in the brain stem[22] (Figure 15-5). Opioids from the midbrain release adrenergic and serotonergic descending pathways from GABAergic inhibition and decrease pain.

Perhaps the best known and the most prevalent of these natural opioids are the **enkephalins.** There are two types of enkephalins, *methionine enkephalin* (met-enkephalin) and *leucine enkephalin* (leu-enkephalin), and their ratio is 4:1 respectively. They were the first endogenous opioids extracted in research. Enkephalins, which like the other endogenous opioids can be identified immunohistochemically, are found concentrated in the hypothalamus, the periaquaductal gray matter, the nucleus raphes magnus of the medulla, and the dorsal horns of the spine.

Endorphins were first discovered in the human PAG in 1979, β-endorphin being the best studied of the group. The activity of β-endorphin is concentrated in the hypothalamus and the pituitary gland; β-endorphin is purported to produce a greater sense of exhilaration, or "high," than all of the other endorphin types. It is a strong μ-receptor agonist and is generally believed to provide substantial natural pain relief.

Dynorphins (the most potent of these endogenous neurohormones) are found in the hypothalamus, the brain stem periaquaductal gray–rostral ventromedial medulla system (PAG-RVM), and the spine. Dynorphins, which bind strongly to κ receptors located in the dorsal horn of the spinal cord, generally serve to impede pain signals but can, in certain areas, incite pain.[23,24]

Endomorphin-1 (Tyr-Pro-Trp-Phe-NH$_2$, EM-1) and endomorphin-2 (Tyr-Pro-Phe-Phe-NH$_2$, EM-2) are peptides isolated from the brain and the spinal cord and show the highest affinity and selectivity for the *μ (morphine)* **opiate receptor.**[25] The **endomorphins** have potent analgesic and gastrointestinal effects. Chemical (capsaicin) and surgical (rhizotomy) disruption of nociceptive primary afferent neurons deplete levels of EM-2, implicating the peripheral nervous system as being the principal site of action. Thus EM-2 is well-positioned to serve as an anti-nociceptive modulator of pain in its earliest stages (i.e., in the peripheral transmission). In contrast to EM-2, which is more prevalent in the spinal cord and lower brain stem, EM-1 is more widely and densely distributed throughout the brain. The distribution is consistent with the role peptides play in the modulation of diverse functions, including adaptation to pain and stress and enhancement of reward perceptions.

In addition to its analgesic effects, endogenous opioids are involved in a variety of other functions throughout the body—one being maintenance of feeding behavior. This finding is supported by research indicating enhanced feeding responses being illicited after heavy exertion or injection of β-endorphin. Administration of Naloxone, a μ-receptor antagonist was found to negate this effect. Endogenous opioids also have been linked to moderation of drinking behavior and cough suppression. Stress, excessive physical exertion, acupuncture, intercourse, and other factors increase the levels of circulating endogenous opioids—serotonin, norepinephrine, and other neurotransmitters—and consequently raise the pain threshold.[23] Endogenous opioids of one type or an-

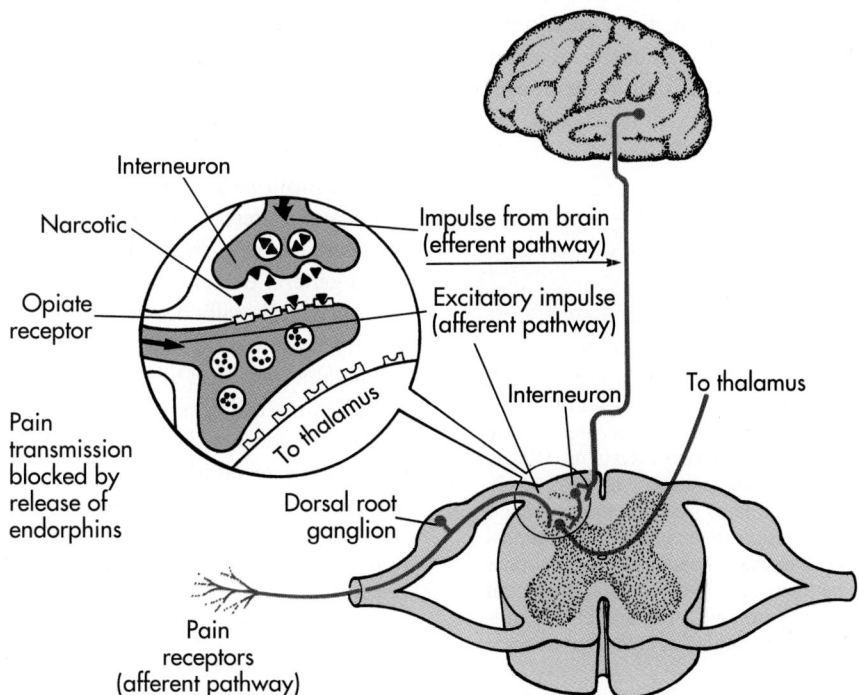

Figure 15-5 Descending pathway and endorphin response. The biologic receptors of the enkephalins and endorphins are located close to known pain receptors in the periphery and ascending and descending pain pathways.

other are found to bind to almost all tissues in the body and may be responsible for general sensations of well-being or lack thereof.[26]

Clinical Description of Pain
Pain Threshold and Pain Tolerance

The **pain threshold** is the point at which a stimulus is perceived as pain. The threshold does not vary significantly among people or in the same person over time. Intense pain at one location, however, may cause an increase in the threshold in another location. For example, a person with severe pain in one knee is less likely to experience chronic back pain that is less intense. This phenomenon is called **perceptual dominance.** Because of perceptual dominance, an individual with many painful sites may report only the most painful one. After the dominant pain is diminished, the individual may then identify other painful areas.[4]

Pain tolerance is the duration of time or the intensity of pain that an individual will endure before initiating overt pain responses. It is the amount of pain the person will tolerate before outwardly responding to it. Pain tolerance is influenced by the person's cultural perceptions, expectations, role behaviors, and physical and mental health. Pain tolerance generally is decreased with repeated exposure to pain. Tolerance is decreased also by fatigue, anger, boredom, apprehension, and sleep deprivation. Tolerance may be increased by alcohol consumption, persistant use of pain medication, hypnosis, warmth, distracting activities, and strong beliefs or faith.

Pain tolerance varies greatly among people and in the same person over time because of the body's ability to respond differently to noxious stimuli. No direct relationship exists between the objectively measured intensity of painful stimuli and an individual's perception of pain or response to pain.

WHAT'S NEW? **Dorsal Column Stimulation (DCS) and Pain Relief**

Neurostimulation of the dorsal columns of the spine have delivered pain relief to thousands of persons suffering from various types of severe, intractable chronic pain. It appears that low voltage, non-noxious electrical stimulation in the area of the posterior spine activates descending inhibitory systems. DCS is thought to close the gate in much the same way as does TENS stimulation of peripheral Aβ, which is by masking the sensation of pain with a tingling sensation (paresthesia). Implanting a dorsal column stimulator into the epidural space may be the most appropriate treatment for certain cases of failed back syndrome (FBS), complex regional pain syndrome (CRPS) and chronic adhesive arachnoiditis (from severe infections and inflammation of the cord).

Data from Taylor RS, Van Buyten JP, Buchser E. *Spine* 30(1):152-160, 2005. Palecek J: *Physiol Res* 53(Suppl 1):S125-130, 2004, Review. Carter ML. *Anaesth Intensive Care* 32(1):11-21, 2004.

Pain Classifications

The most widely used clinical classifications for pain are based on the inferred neurophysiologic mechanisms, temporal aspects, etiology, and region affected. The mechanistic approach to categorizing pain is common, but from a clinical viewpoint, this approach has shortcomings. Usually pain conditions are described clinically by mechanism as either nociceptive or non-nociceptive and by duration as either acute or chronic.

Nociceptive pain such as the pain of a crushed finger or a heart attack, is pain with a cause resulting from normal tissue injury. Nociceptive pain is either somatic (derived from the Greek word *soma* for "body" or "body wall"—meaning the whole axial portion of the body including trunk, head, and neck) or visceral (derived from the internal organs).

Non-nociceptive pain, for the purposes of this text, is defined as neuropathic pain (discussion of psychogenic pain is not covered in this chapter). Neuropathic pain is subdivided into peripheral and central categories.

Additionally, somatic, visceral, and neuropathic pains can all occur as acute or chronic presentations. These broad definitions have been summarized in Box 15-2. Some of the most common clinical pain presentations are detailed below.

Acute Pain

Acute pain is a protective mechanism that alerts the individual to a condition or experience that is immediately harmful to the body. The onset of acute pain is sudden, and usually dissipates after the stimulus is removed and the tissues have healed. A direct one-to-one relationship between physical signs of disease and accompanying symptoms is almost always present. Peripheral and central sensitization, that is, "wind-up," is not evident. Anxiety is common in acute pain states and is usually apparent in the alterations of vital signs. Tachycardia, hypertension, fever, diaphoresis, dilated pupils, and outward pain behavior such as moaning, touching, or rocking motions are discernible to an outside observer. Other physical manifestations include elevation of blood sugar levels, decreases in gastric acid secretion and intestinal motility, and a general decrease in blood flow to the viscera and skin. Nausea occasionally occurs.

The sign, symptoms, and behaviors of acute pain are a predictable response to the threat inherent in the painful experience, including issues surrounding the cause of pain, its treatment, and prognosis (Table 15-2). Individuals often psychologically respond to acute pain with fear (e.g., fear of diagnosis, fear of continued pain), anxiety, and a general sense of unpleasantness or unease. The stress of fear itself may in turn contribute to the physiologic signs of pain. Some individuals are reluctant to discuss or report their pain,[28] although hope of recovery is usually present.

Acute pain arises from cutaneous and deep somatic tissue, or from visceral organs and can be classified as (1) acute somatic, (2) acute visceral, and (3) referred.

Somatic pain arises from connective tissue, muscle or bone, and skin and is either sharp and well localized (especially fast pain carried by Aδ fibers) or dull, aching, and poorly localized pain as seen in polymodal C fiber transmissions.

Visceral pain refers to pain in internal organs and the abdomen and is transmitted by sympathetic afferents. It is poorly localized because of the lesser number of nociceptors in the visceral structures, which often can be cauterized or cut

---

Box 15-2	Categories of Pain

I. Neurophysiologic Pain
  A. Nociceptive pain
    1. Somatic
    2. Visceral
  B. Neuropathic (non-nociceptive)
    1. Central pain (lesion in brain or spinal cord)
    2. Peripheral pain (lesion in PNS)
II. Neurogenic Pain
  A. Neuralgia (pain in the distribution of a nerve)
  B. Constant
    1. Sympathetically independent
    2. Sympathetically dependent
III. Temporal Pain (time related)
  A. Acute pain
    1. Somatic
    2. Visceral
  B. Chronic
IV. Regional Pain
  A. Abdominal pain
  B. Chest pain
  C. Headache
  D. Low back pain
  E. Orofacial pain
  F. Pelvic pain
V. Etiologic pain
  A. Cancer pain
  B. Dental pain
  C. Inflammatory pain
  D. Ischemic pain
  E. Vascular pain

Adapted from Derasari MD: Taxonomy of pain syndromes: classification of chronic pain syndromes. In Raj PP, editor: *Practical management of pain,* ed 3, St Louis, 2000, Mosby.

---

without any sensation of pain being felt. However, any stretching or distension of internal organs or the abdomen will elicit a violent response.

Visceral pain is associated with nausea and vomiting, hypotension, restlessness, and, in some cases, shock. It often radiates (spreads away from the actual site of the pain) or is referred. Visceral pain that is primarily nociceptive and not referred is carried by second order neurons that travel in the dorsal column pathway to the gracilis nucleus of the medulla and then in contralateral pathways of the medial lemniscus to finally synapse in the thalamus.[29]

Referred pain is pain that is present in an area removed or distant from its point of origin. Referred pain usually, but not always, originates from the viscera and so is discussed here. The most familiar examples are pain in the shoulder from myocardial infarction, pain in the back from pancreatic or renal disease, and pain in the right shoulder from an inflamed gallbladder. Referred visceral pain is carried by second-order neurons that travel in the contralateral spinothalamic track. The area of referred pain is supplied by the same spinal segment as the actual site of pain because impulses from many cutaneous and visceral neurons converge. The presumed mechanism is one of afferent fibers from this conjoint area in the spinal cord relaying the mistaken perception that the pain arises from the referral site. Because the skin has more receptors, the painful sensation is more often experienced there instead of at the site of origin.[30] (Common areas of referred pain and their associated sites of origin appear in Figure 15-6.)

Chronic Pain

Chronic pain also can be nociceptive, but it is prolonged—usually defined as lasting at least 3 months. Perhaps even more important than the duration of the pain are the attendant physical and emotional issues that often appear to be way out of proportion to any observable tissue injury. Thus the cause of chronic pain often is unknown, and even if the cause is known or suspected, the pain does not respond to usual therapy. Chronic pain may be persistent as in chronic low back pain or occur intermittently as seen in migraine or

---

Table 15-2	Comparison of Acute and Chronic Pain	
Characteristic	**Acute Pain**	**Chronic Pain**
Experience	An event	A situation; state of existence
Source	External agent or internal disease	Unknown; if known, treatment is prolonged or ineffective
Onset	Usually sudden	May be sudden or develop insidiously
Duration	Transient (up to 6 months)	Prolonged (months to years)
Pain identification	Painful and nonpainful areas generally well identified	Painful and nonpainful areas less easily differentiated: change in sensations becomes nore difficult to evaluate
Clinical signs	Typical response pattern with more visible signs	Response patterns vary; fewer overt signs (adaptation)
Significance	Significant (informs person something is wrong)	Person looks for significance
Pattern	Self-limiting or readily corrected	Continuous or intermittent; intensity may vary or remain constant
Course	Suffering usually decreases over time	Suffering usually increases over time
Actions	Leads to actions to relieve pain	Leads to actions to modify pain experience
Prognosis	Likelihood of eventual complete relief	Complete relief usually not possible

Data from Black RG: *Surg Clin North Am* 55(4):999, 1975.

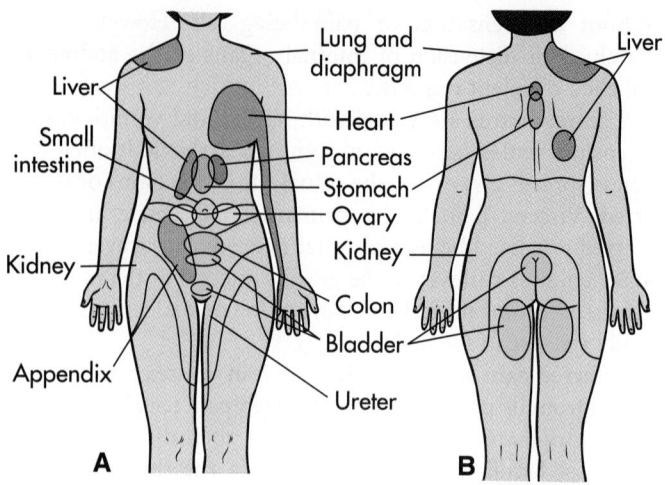

Figure 15-6 Sites of referred pain. **A,** Front. **B,** Back.

muscle tension–migraine variant headache syndromes. The onset may be sudden, but chronic pain often develops insidiously so that the individual generally experiences more suffering over time. Individual behavior is adaptive and directed toward modifying the pain. Chronic pain is often associated with a sense of hopelessness and helplessness as relief becomes more elusive and the timeframe more protracted. The pain is perceived as meaningless, and depression is often a concomitant finding, as either a result of the chronic pain state or as a contributor to its development. It is significantly more difficult to manage than acute pain, and complete relief usually is never obtained (see Table 15-2).

Physiologic responses to chronic pain depend on whether it is persistent or intermittent. Intermittent pain produces a physiologic response similar to that of acute pain (i.e., tachycardia, diaphoresis, elevated blood pressure, etc). Persistent, chronic pain, however, allows for physiologic adaptation so that a person with chronic pain may have normal heart and respiratory rates and normal blood pressure. The absence of acute physiologic responses has led many to mistakenly assume that persons in chronic pain are malingering because they do not appear to be in pain.

Chronic pain produces significant behavioral and psychologic changes.[31] Individuals with chronic pain often are depressed, have difficulty sleeping and eating, and may become preoccupied with the pain.[32] Living with chronic pain requires constant attention to the earliest signs of pain so that the pain-provoking stimuli can be identified and avoided. Persons with chronic pain generally attempt to keep pain-related behavior to a minimum so that they appear as normal as possible. A desire for the validation of the pain and the need to hide the pain are usually conflicting drives for those with chronic pain. They tend not to report pain for fear of being labeled complainers. They often deny pain and sometimes engage in activities that provoke pain in an effort to keep up with others. Even in learning to pace themselves throughout the day's activities, they may inadvertently aggravate the pain.[33]

Chronic pain states are thought to arise from a misinterpretation of nociceptive input—an imbalance of neuromodulation controls such as might occur with a decreased level of endorphins or a predominance of C-neuron stimulation[34,34a] (see Table 15-3). The following mechanisms have been implicated in the initiation and entrenchment of chronic pain states:[35]

- Changes in sensitivity of neurons—lower threshold with peripheral and central sensitization
- Spontaneous impulses from regenerating peripheral nerves
- Alterations in the dorsal root ganglion in response to peripheral nerve injury and neurotransmitters—reorganization of nociceptive neurons (deafferentation pain)
- Loss of pain inhibition in the spinal cord

The most common chronic, disabling pain condition in the United States is persistent *low back pain,* which became a medical disaster in the twentieth, and now twenty-first centuries. Over the past few decades much has been learned about back pain—where back pain fits into the pain spectrum and how people react to and are affected by it. Predictions that chronic low back pain (and the disability arising from it) would be reducing are unfounded; instead both the report of low back pain and the accompanying disability are on the rise. Recent figures estimate that 7% to 14% of adults in the United States have some disability related to back pain, and 1% to 2% of the population are totally disabled by back pain at any given time.[36,36a]

Myofascial pain syndromes (MPS) are a common cause of chronic pain. These conditions, which involve injury to the muscle and fascia, include myositis, fibrositis, myofibrositis, myalgia, and muscle strain. The pain is a result of muscle spasm, tenderness, and stiffness and leads to muscle guarding (a behavior that limits muscle motion). In turn, limited motion causes muscle weakness, stiffness, tenderness, and spasm, all of which produce more pain. The pain is described as dull and aching and may be mild to disabling. During the early stages of the disorder, the pain is localized, but as the disorder progresses it becomes more generalized.

These, like many other chronic conditions, begin as a result of poor muscle tone, inactivity, muscle strain, or sudden vigorous exercise. The acute pain of muscle agony, for reasons alluded to above, sometimes evolves into a chronic pain state.

Chronic postoperative pain occurs in a small percentage of individuals after the following:

1. Thoracotomy, with pain often caused by tumor recurrence or invasion of the chest wall (branches from the brachial plexus to the thoracic region)
2. Radical neck dissection, with pain attributable to surgical injury or interruption of the cranial nerves
3. Surgical amputation, which may be followed by phantom limb pain

Cancer pain is often chronic. Studies done at Memorial Sloan-Kettering Cancer Center indicate three major categories of pain syndromes that result in chronic pain in the individual with cancer.[37] The categories are (1) pain attributed

Table 15-3	Common Chronic Pain Conditions
Condition	**Description**
Persistent low back pain	Most common chronic pain condition
	Results from poor muscle tone, inactivity, muscle strain, or sudden, vigorous exercise
Myofascial pain syndromes	Second most common chronic pain condition
	Pain results from muscle spasm, tenderness, and stiffness
	Examples include myositis, fibrositis, myofibrositis, myalgia, and muscle strain—conditions that involve injury to the muscle and fascia
	As disorder progresses, pain becomes increasingly generalized
Chronic postoperative pain	Chronic pain that can occur with disruption or cutting of sensory nerves
Cancer pain	Can be pain attributed to advance of disease, associated with treatment, or attributed to coexisting disease entities
Deaffentiation pain	Painful condition resulting from damage to a peripheral nerve
	Common types include severe burning pain triggered by various stimuli, such as cold, light touch, or sound, and reflex sympathetic dystrophies (occur after peripheral nerve injury and are characterized by continuous, severe, burning pain associated with vasomotor changes and muscle wasting)
Hyperesthesias	Increased sensitivity and decreased pain threshold to tactile and painful stimuli
	Pain is diffuse, modified by fatigue and emotion and mixed with other sensations
	May result from chronic irritations of CNS areas
Hemiagnosia	Loss of ability to identify source of pain on one side of the body
	Painful stimuli on that side produce discomfort, anxiety, moaning, agitation, and distress but no attempt to withdraw from the stimulus
	Associated with stroke
Phantom limb pain	Pain experience in amputated limb after stump has completely healed; may be immediate or occur months later
	Influenced by emotions/sympathetic stimulation
	Trigger points—small hypersensitive regions in muscle or connective tissues that, when stimulated, produce pain in a specific area

to the advance of the disease, (2) pain associated with treatment of the disease, and (3) pain attributed to coexisting entities (e.g., osteoarthritis) that are unrelated to the disease. Cancer pain is by far the most common cause of chronic pain attributed to the advance of an identifiable disease.[37] Pain can be caused by infection and inflammation, increasing pressure of a growing tumor on nerve endings, stretching of visceral surfaces, or obstruction of ducts and intestine. Therapeutic approaches to the management of cancer pain have advanced significantly in recent years, particularly in palliative care and hospice programs.[37a] Frequent pain assessment, implementation of therapeutic strategies including pharmacotherapy, anesthetic, neuorsurgical, psychologic and rehabilitation techniques and frequent evaluations are essential to optimal cancer pain management.[37b,37c,37d]

Chemotherapy, especially treatment with vinca alkaloids, may be associated with a variety of neuropathies producing painful dysesthesias ("pins and needles" sensations) in the feet and hands. Radiation therapy may result in connective tissue fibrosis and secondary nerve injury that produces pain.[37]

Neuropathic Pain

Neuropathic pain is the result of trauma or disease of nerves and leads to abnormal processing of sensory information by the peripheral and central nervous system.[38] Most neuropathic pain seen commonly in clinical practice is chronic. Chronic neuropathic pain syndromes can be divided into two groups based on a central or peripheral location of the nervous system lesion. Although precise estimates of the prevalence of neuropathic pain are not available, it is more common than has generally been appreciated. In the United States, there may be more than 3 million people with painful diabetic neuropathy (PDN) and as many as 1 million with postherpetic neuralgia (PHN). Neuropathic pain is often paroxysmal with paresthesias (tingling sensations of pins and needles), burning, shooting, or stabbing sensations. Patients with neuropathic pain often describe a "gnawing," miserable quality to the pain. It can be evoked by movement (called *incidence pain*), and hypersensitivity and/or allodynia may be present in the involved part of the body. No single diagnostic test for neuropathic pain (or for pain in general) isavailable, and differentiating some neuropathies from certain chronic somatic pain syndromes can be difficult.

Proposed mechanisms for the development of chronic neuropathic pain focus on the development of hyperactivity of neurons in the spinal cord and thalamus. Accumulation of high numbers of sodium ion channels at sites of nerve injury and demyelination is thought to be the underlying mechanism that accounts for neuronal hyperexcitability. Neuroplastic changes (the ability of neurons to alter their structure and function) also can occur at the level of the brain and spinal cord, which results in abnormal central processing.[39-41]

When injured nerves become hyperexcitable, they generate ectopic discharges, resulting in spontaneous firing of some neurons with low thresholds for mechanical, chemical, or thermal stimuli.[42] Injury resulting in a permanent loss of sensory input from a part of the body is called *deafferentation*, and differentiates peripheral neuropathic pain syndromes from central forms of the disease.

Deafferentation pain results from tumor infiltration of nerve tissue; trauma or chemical injury to the nerve; or damage from radiation, chemotherapy, or surgical sectioning of the nerve. Deafferentation pain, which is poorly controlled by many analgesics, is usually described as a constant, dull, viselike ache, accompanied by paroxysms of burning or electric shocklike sensations.[43,44]

Sympathetically maintained pain (SMP) is another type of neuropathic pain that occurs after peripheral nerve injury and is characterized as continuous and severe with a burning quality. Sympathetically maintained pain is often associated with vasospasm and vasomotor changes in the affected limb. The diseases formerly called *causalgia* and *reflex sympathetic dystrophy*, both thought to arise from sympathetic nervous system imbalance, are now called **complex regional pain syndromes (CRPS)**, types I and II. CRPS syndromes develop 1 to 2 weeks after injury to the brachial plexus, or the median, sciatic, or other peripheral nerves. The severe, diffuse, and persistent pain occurs in the extremity supplied by the injured nerve. Discoloration and changes in the texture of the skin may appear in the affected area. Vasomotor changes usually begin with vasodilation and are followed by vasoconstriction and cool, cyanotic and edematous extremities. Excessive nail growth may be noted, and swelling and stiffness of proximate joints may occur. Hair loss is usually noted, and allodynia is often prominent and disabling.[44a,44b]

Central pain is neuropathic and is caused by a lesion or dysfunction in the CNS (brain or spinal cord). The lesions of central pain can include infarction, hemorrhage, abscess, degeneration, tumors, or traumatic injury. The pain may manifest over a large and diffuse area, or be well defined and circumscribed. It is usually irritating and constant, can be difficult to treat, and can cause considerable suffering. *Hemiagnosia pain* is one form of central pain associated with stroke that produces paralysis and a hypersensitivity/allodynia on one half of the body. In this painful condition, often a concomitant loss of ability to identify the source of pain through normal sensory pathways occurs. The result is a confusing picture in which even mild stimulation of the affected side of the body produces discomfort, anxiety, moaning, agitation, and distress, with a diminished ability to withdraw from the offending stimulus. *Thalamic pain* is another form of central pain that involves lesions in the thalamus.

Non-painful phantom limb sensations occur in almost all amputees, but the sensations usually fade with time. This is distinguished from the syndrome of phantom limb pain, a chronic pain occurring in 50% to 85% of amputees.[45,46] **Phantom limb pain** is pain that an individual feels in an amputated limb after the stump has completely healed. It is more likely to appear in individuals who experienced pain in the limb before amputation. It's been proposed that CNS integration, including reorganization of the somatosensory cortex, results in the perception of pain from receptors associated with the amputated limb even though the limb itself is no longer present.[47,48] But how do we explain the perception of pain arising from spinal gates when the gate, as in the case of complete transection of the cord, is no longer there? It appears that of all the pain phenomenon, the description of phantom limb pain by gate control theory is the least satisfactory. As Melzack points out, "It comes as a shock to conclude that you don't need a body to feel a body or that the brain itself can generate every quality of experience that is normally triggered by sensory input"[49] (see What's New? box on The Concept of a Neuromatrix).

In neuropathic pain, as well as all other chronic pain states, assessment of psychologic components (e.g., depression or anxiety), sleep disturbance, work-related issues of impairment and disability, treatment expectations, and the availability of social support from family and friends (or lack thereof) should not be overlooked. Legal entanglements need to be addressed also because very few persons involved in a court bat-

---

WHAT'S NEW?   The Concept of a Neuromatrix

Ronald Melzack proposes a neuromatrix theory of chronic pain that amends the gate control theory and provides new directions for pain research. Chronic pain is theorized to be a multidimensional experience produced by patterns of nerve impulses known as *neurosignatures*. These nerve impulses are generated in the brain by a widely distributed network known as the *body-self neuromatrix*. The *body-self* represents the unique distinction of the self with unity of feeling, experiences, and genetic predisposition. It is multidimensional, including sensory, cognitive, affective, postural, evaluative, and other components. The *neuromatrix* is composed of centers and loops of neurons in the brain whose links and synapses are initially determined genetically but can be changed and modified by sensory inputs. The neurosignature patterns may be triggered by sensory inputs from the body or may originate in the brain independently of peripheral sensory input. It is the output of the widely distributed neuromatrix, not input, that generates the neurosignature pattern of pain. This explains most types of chronic pain in which there is no discernable cause or correlation between pathology and pain (e.g., phantom limb pain and neuropathies). The neuromatrix theory also provides a rationale for various alternative approaches to pain management. In summary, neuromatrix theory suggests that the brain can detect and analyze inputs and generate perceptual experience when no external input is evoked by injury, inflammation, or other pathology. It is representative of the nervous system's plasticity. Neuromatrix theory provides a wholistic, integrated, dynamic consideration of pain.

Data from Khalsa PS: *J Electromyogr Kinesiol* 14(1):109-120, 2004; Melzack R: Toward a new concept of pain for the new millennium. In Waldman SD, editor: *Interventional pain management*, ed 2, Philadelphia, 2001, Saunders; Moseley GL: *Man Ther* 8(3):130-140, 2003; Trout KK: *J Midwifery Womens Health* 49(6):482-488, 2004; Yoo SS et al: *Neuroimage* 22(2):932-940.

tle experience any significant improvement of their chronic pain until the related legal issues are settled.[50]

PEDIATRICS AND PERCEPTION OF PAIN

Children and infants have the anatomic and functional ability to perceive pain. Pain pathways and cortical and subcortical centers for pain perception, as well as neurochemicals associated with pain transmission and modulation, are functional in preterm and newborn infants.[51] The nociceptor system is functional in fetuses by 24 weeks of gestation[52] Repetitive, painful experiences and prolonged exposure to analgesic drugs in infants during the neonatal period may permanently alter synaptic and neuronal organization,[53,54] and fetuses may "remember" pain with an enduring effect on behavior and pain perception.[55]

Change in facial expression, crying, and body movements are the most consistent expressions of pain in infants. The painful facial expression includes lowered brows drawn together; presence of a vertical bulge and furrows in the forehead between the brows; broadened nasal root; tightly closed, scourged eye fissures; and angular, squarish mouth and chin quiver[56] (Figure 15-7). Physiologic responses include an increase in heart rate, blood pressure, and respiratory rate. There may be flushing or pallor, sweating, and decreased oxygen saturation. Toddlers also express pain with crying, facial expression, and body language (body tenses, guarding, and hands holding body). Older children, between ages 5 and 18 years, tend to have a lower pain threshold than do adults. Children, like adults, have highly individual responses to pain. Any pain must be carefully and accurately assessed [57] and adequately treated for children of all ages.[58]

AGING AND PERCEPTION OF PAIN

Studies on pain perception in the elderly population have yielded conflicting evidence. Some studies show an increase in the pain threshold with aging; others show no change.[59,60] The varied results are probably a function of independent variation in the sensory/discriminative, motivational/affective, and cognitive/evaluative components of the pain experience. In general, studies confirm that an increase in the pain threshold occurs in some elderly people. This change may be caused by peripheral neuropathies and changes in the thickness of the skin.[61] (Neuropathies are discussed in Chapter 17.) A decrease in pain tolerance is also evident in some older persons, and women appear to be more sensitive to pain than are men.[62] Pain in the elderly is also influenced by liver and renal function, including alterations in metabolism of drugs and metabolites. Pain must be accurately assessed in relation to its effect on cognitive function and to reactions to treatment. Poorly managed pain can result in depression, inactivity, and failure to maintain activities of daily living.[63-65]

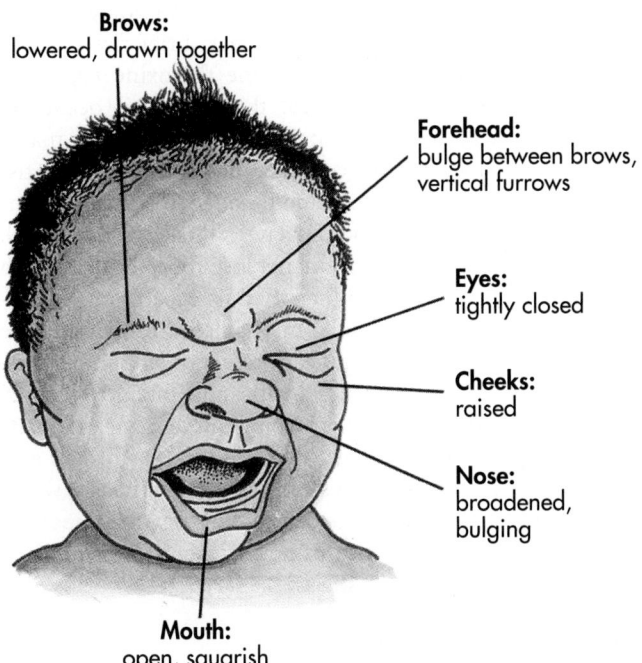

Brows:
lowered, drawn together

Forehead:
bulge between brows, vertical furrows

Eyes:
tightly closed

Cheeks:
raised

Nose:
broadened, bulging

Mouth:
open, squarish

Figure 15-7 Painful facial expression of infants. (From Hockenberry MJ: Wong's *Nursing care of infants and children*, ed 7, St. Louis, 2003, Mosby.)

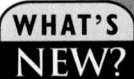

WHAT'S NEW?   Pain and Gender

Gender differences in the experience of pain have been documented in both animal and human research. Women report higher pain levels or have less tolerance for pain stimulus intensities, or both. Gender differences exist also in the prevalence of painful diseases; for example, more women are affected by intestinal cystitis, fibromyalgia, and rheumatoid arthritis, and men are more affected by cluster headache. Pain symptoms differ for men and women for diseases such as coronary artery disease, irritable bowel syndrome, appendicitis, and cancer. Sex hormones are known to have an effect on the mechanisms and outcomes of opiate analgesia, and in rodents, morphine analgesia is greater in males than in females. Pain sensitivities in women also vary across the phases of the menstrual cycle. A recent human study now suggests that kappa-opioid receptor analgesia is greater in women than in men and may reflect a difference in endogenous pain circuits activated by different opiate receptor subtypes. Gender differences with respect to pain is also influenced by role socialization, cognitive factors, and culture. Continuing research is needed to further understanding of gender differences in the operation of pain mechanisms and the development of more specific pain management strategies.

Data from Myers CD, Riley JL 3rd, Robinson ME: *Clin J Pain* 19(4):225-232, 2003; Pleym H et al: *Acta Anaesthesiol Scand* 47(3):241-259, 2003; Miaskowski C: *J Natl Cancer Inst Monogr* (32):139-143, 2004; Patel H, Rosengren A, Ekman I: *Am Heart J* 148(1):27-33, 2004; Arendt-Nielsen L, Bajai P, Drewes AM: *Eur J Pain* 8(5):465-472, 2004.

TEMPERATURE REGULATION

In all homeothermic animals, temperature regulation is achieved through precise balancing of heat production, heat conservation, and heat loss. In humans, body temperature is maintained in a range around 37° C (98.6° F) and rarely exceeds 41° C. The normal range is considered to be 36.2° to 37.7° C (97.2° to 99.9° F), but all parts of the body do not have the same temperature. The extremities, for example, are generally cooler than the trunk. The temperature at the core of the body (as measured by rectal temperature) is generally 0.5° C higher than at the surface (as measured by oral temperature). The internal temperature varies normally in response to activity, environmental temperature, and daily fluctuation of **circadian rhythm** (the pattern of each 24-hour day). Oral temperatures generally fluctuate within 0.2° to 0.5° C over a 24-hour period. Women tend to have wider fluctuations that follow the menstrual cycle, with a sharp rise in temperature just before ovulation. In both genders the daily fluctuating temperature peaks around 6 PM and is at its lowest during sleep.[66] Maintenance of body temperature within the normal range is necessary for life.

Hypothalamic Control of Temperature

Temperature regulation is mediated hormonally by the hypothalamus.[67] Peripheral thermoreceptors in the skin and central thermoreceptors in the hypothalamus, spinal cord, abdominal organs, and other central locations provide the hypothalamus with information about skin and core temperatures. If these temperatures are low, the hypothalamus responds by triggering heat production and heat conservation mechanisms.

Increased heat production is initiated by a series of hormonal mechanisms involving the hypothalamus and its connections with the endocrine system (see Chapter 20). The heat-producing mechanism begins with a hypothalamic hormone, thyrotropin-stimulating hormone-releasing hormone (TSH-RH). In turn, TSH-RH stimulates the anterior pituitary to release thyroid-stimulating hormone (TSH), which acts on the thyroid gland, stimulating release of thyroxine (T_4), one of the thyroid hormones. This hormone then acts on the adrenal medulla, causing the release of epinephrine (a catecholamine and vasopressive hormone) into the bloodstream (see Chapter 20). Epinephrine causes vasoconstriction, stimulates glycolysis, and increases metabolic rates, thus increasing heat production.

The hypothalamus also triggers heat conservation. The mechanisms of heat conservation involve stimulating the sympathetic nervous system, which is responsible for stimulating the adrenal cortex, increasing skeletal muscle tone, initiating the shivering response, and producing vasoconstriction. The hypothalamus also functions in raising body temperatures by relaying information to the cerebral cortex. Awareness of cold provokes voluntary responses such as increased body movement.

The hypothalamus responds to warmer core and peripheral temperatures by reversing the same mechanisms. The TSH-RH pathway is shut down. The sympathetic pathway is prompted to produce vasodilation, decreased muscle tone, and increased sweat production. Hypothalamic stimulation of the cerebral cortex provokes voluntary measures to reduce heat production and promote heat loss.

Mechanisms of Heat Production

Body heat is produced by the chemical reactions of metabolism, skeletal muscle tone and contraction, and chemical thermogenesis. Heat is distributed by the circulatory system.

Chemical Reactions of Metabolism

The chemical reactions that occur during the ingestion and metabolism of food and those required to maintain the body at rest (basal metabolism) require energy and give off heat. These processes occur in the body core (liver) and are in part responsible for the maintenance of core temperature.

Skeletal Muscle Contraction

Skeletal muscles produce heat through two mechanisms: (1) gradual increase in muscle tone and (2) rapid muscle oscillations (shivering—which does not occur in neonates). Both increasing muscle tone and shivering are controlled by the hypothalamus and occur in response to cold. As peripheral temperature drops, muscle tone increases and shivering begins. Shivering is a fairly effective method for increasing heat production, because no work is performed and all the energy produced is retained as heat.

Chemical Thermogenesis

Chemical thermogenesis, also called *nonshivering thermogenesis,* results from the release of epinephrine. Epinephrine produces a rapid, transient increase in heat production by raising the body's basal metabolic rate. Chemical thermogenesis seems to be different from hormone-triggered increases in the basal metabolic rate. Chemical thermogenesis—through epinephrine—produces a quick, brief rise in basal metabolic rate, whereas the hormone thyroxine triggers a slow, prolonged rise.[68] Chemical thermogenesis occurs in brown adipose tissue present mainly in small newborn mammals that have high surface/volume ratios. Brown adipose tissue is rich with mitochondria and blood vessels and is essential for nonshivering thermogenesis. Like other small newborn mammals, human infants lose more heat through **conduction** and **convection** than they are capable of generating through normal metabolic mechanisms. Brown adipose tissue therefore plays an important role in maintaining body temperature in the newborn. As with most mammals reared in a temperature-controlled environment, humans gradually lose the capacity for chemical thermogenesis as brown adipose cells dedifferentiate. This can occur as early as 4 weeks after birth.[69,69a] Because of the decrease in brown adipose tissue in the adult, the role of this mechanism of heat production in adults is under investigation.[70,71]

Mechanisms of Heat Loss

Heat loss is achieved through many mechanisms: (1) radiation, (2) conduction, (3) convection, (4) vasodilation, (5) decreased muscle tone, (6) evaporation, (7) increased respiration, (8) voluntary measures, and (9) adaptation to warmer climates.

Radiation

Radiation refers to heat loss through electromagnetic waves. These waves emanate from surfaces with temperatures higher than the surrounding air. Thus if the temperature of the skin is higher than that of the air, the skin and therefore the body lose heat to the air.

Conduction

Conduction refers to heat loss by direct molecule-to-molecule transfer from one surface to another. Through conduction, the warmer surface loses heat to the cooler surface. Thus the skin loses heat through direct contact with cooler air, water, or another surface. In the same manner, the core of the body loses heat to the cooler body surface.

Convection

Convection is the transfer of heat through currents of gases or liquids. It greatly aids heat loss through conduction by exchanging warmer air at the surface of the body with cooler air in the surrounding space. Convection occurs passively as warmer air at the surface of the body rises away from the body and is replaced by cooler air, but the process may be aided by fans or wind. (The combined effect of conduction and convection by wind is conventionally measured as the *windchill factor*.)

Vasodilation

Peripheral vasodilation increases heat loss by diverting core-warmed blood to the surface of the body. As the core-warmed blood passes through the periphery, heat is transferred by conduction to the skin surface and from the skin to the surrounding environment. Because heat loss through conduction depends on the temperature of the surrounding medium, heat loss through conduction is minimal to nonexistent if the surrounding air is warmer than the body surface.

Vasodilation occurs in response to autonomic stimulation under the control of the hypothalamus. It is useful in instances of moderate temperature elevation. As core temperature increases, vasodilation increases until maximal dilation is achieved. At that point the body must use additional heat loss mechanisms.

Decreased Muscle Tone

To decrease heat production, muscle tone may be moderately reduced and voluntary muscle activity curtailed. These mechanisms explain in part the "washed-out" feeling associated with high temperatures and warm weather. Both decreased muscle tone and reduced activity have a limited effect on decreasing heat production, however, because muscle tone and heat production cannot be reduced below basal body requirements.

Evaporation

Evaporation of body water from the surface of the skin and the linings of the mucous membranes is a major source of heat reduction. Insensible water loss (in the absence of perceptible sweating) accounts for a loss of about 600 ml of water per day. Heat is lost as surface fluid is converted to gas, so that heat loss by evaporation is increased if more fluids are

available at the body surface. To speed this process, fluids are actively secreted through the sweat glands. As much as 4 L of fluid per hour may be lost by sweating. Electrolytes are lost with the water. Therefore loss of large volumes through sweating may result in decreased plasma volume, decreased blood pressure, weakness, and fainting. (Alterations in fluid balance are discussed in Chapter 3.)

Like other heat reduction mechanisms, stimulation of sweating occurs in response to sympathetic neural activity and depends on a favorable temperature difference between the body and the environment. In addition, heat loss through evaporation is affected by the relative humidity of the air. If the humidity of the air is low, sweat evaporates quickly, but if the humidity is high, sweat does not evaporate and instead remains on the skin or drips off.

Increased Respiration

Exchanging air with the environment through the normal respiratory process provides some heat loss, although it is minimal. As air is inhaled, the air draws heat from the upper respiratory tract. The air is further warmed in the alveoli by blood in the microcirculation. This warmed air then is exhaled into the environment. This normal process occurs faster at higher body temperatures through an increase in respiratory rates. Thus hyperventilation is associated with hyperthermia. (Normal pulmonary function is discussed in Chapter 32.)

Voluntary Mechanisms

In response to high body temperatures, people typically "stretch out," thereby increasing the body surface area available for heat loss. They also "slow down" or "take it easy," thereby decreasing skeletal muscle work, and they "dress for warm weather." The most efficient dress for warm weather is a light-colored, loose-fitting garment, because light colors reflect heat from the body and loose-fitting garments allow free air movement for convection, conduction, and evaporation to occur.

Adaptation to Warmer Climates

The body of an individual who moves from a cooler to a much warmer climate undergoes a period of adjustment, a process that takes several days to weeks. At first the individual experiences feelings of lassitude, weakness, and faintness with even moderate activity. Body temperatures rise with any work. Within several days, however, the individual experiences an earlier onset of sweating; the volume of sweat is increased; and the sodium content is lowered. Heart rate is decreased and stroke volume increased so that cardiac output remains unchanged. Extracellular fluid volume increases, as does plasma volume. These physiologic adaptations result in improved warm weather functioning and decreased symptoms of heat intolerance. People's work output, endurance, and coordination increase, and their subjective feelings of discomfort decrease.[72]

Mechanisms of Heat Conservation

The body conserves heat and protects core temperature through two important mechanisms: (1) involuntary vasoconstriction and (2) voluntary mechanisms. To preserve core temperature, the skin and periphery are used as an insulating cover.[72]

Vasoconstriction

By constricting peripheral blood vessels, centrally warmed blood is shunted away from the periphery (where radiation, conduction, and convection would allow heat loss) to the core of the body, where heat can be retained. This mechanism takes advantage of the insulating layers of the skin and subcutaneous fat to protect core temperature.

Voluntary Mechanisms

In response to lower body temperatures, individuals typically "bundle up," "keep moving," or "curl up in a ball." Bundling up involves dressing with several layers of clothes that allow air to be trapped between the skin and the clothing, thus providing an additional layer of insulation. Keeping moving, stamping feet, clapping hands, jogging, and other types of physical activity increase skeletal muscle activity and thus promote heat production. Curling up in a ball decreases the amount of skin surface available for heat loss through radiation, convection, and conduction.

PEDIATRICS AND CHANGES IN TEMPERATURE REGULATION

Infants and the elderly require special attention to maintenance of body temperature. Infants produce sufficient body heat but are unable to conserve heat produced. The poor heat conservation is caused by the infant's small body size and greater ratio of body surface to body weight, which give the infant more surface area for heat loss. Infants also have a very thin layer of subcutaneous fat and thus are not as well insulated as adults.[73]

AGING AND CHANGES IN TEMPERATURE REGULATION

Elderly persons have poor responses to environmental temperature extremes as a result of slowed blood circulation, structural and functional changes in the skin, and an overall decrease in heat-producing activities. Other factors affecting thermal regulation in the elderly population include decreased shivering response (delayed onset and decreased effectiveness), slowed metabolic rate, sedentary life-style, decreased vasoconstrictor response, diminished or absent sweating, desynchronization of circadian rhythm, undernutrition, and decreased perception of heat and cold.[74,75]

Both infants and elderly people have difficulty regulating body heat through physiologic mechanisms of heat production and conservation. Health care providers need to be aware of these particular developmental differences, because infants cannot adjust to the environment to compensate for heat loss and elderly people, because of decreased peripheral sensation, may not be alerted to the need to do so.

Pathogenesis of Fever

Fever is a complex, integrated cascade of behavioral, neurologic, and endocrine responses to an immune challenge initiated by endogenous pyrogens. It is a normal adaptive response to cytokines.[76,77] The thermoregulatory mechanisms of the hypothalamus and brain stem adjust heat production, conservation, and loss to maintain body core temperature at a normal level.[78,79] During fever, this level is raised so that the thermoregulatory centers adjust heat production, conservation, and loss to maintain the core temperature at the new, higher temperature, which functions as a new "set point."[67,80]

The pathophysiology of fever begins with the introduction of **exogenous pyrogens** (i.e., endotoxins) (Figure 15-8). The most frequently encountered exogenous pyrogens are the lipopolysaccharide complex in the cell wall of gram-positive bacteria and viruses.[81] **Endogenous pyrogens,** including interleukin-1 (IL-1), interleukin 6 (IL-6), tumor necrosis factor–alpha (TNF-α), and interferon-γ, are produced by phagocytic cells as they destroy microorganisms within the host.[82] The endogenous pyrogens act on the preoptic nucleus of the hypothalamus, which release prostaglandin E$_2$ (PGE$_2$) and other cytokines.[83,84] An integrated behavioral, endocrine, and autonomic nervous system response is then initiated. Centers in the hypothalamus and brain stem signal an increase in heat production and heat conservation to raise body temperature to the new level. Peripheral vasoconstriction occurs with shunting of blood from the skin to the body core. Epinephrine release increases metabolic rate, and muscle tone increases. Decreased release of vasopressin reduces the volume of body fluid to be heated. Shivering also may occur. The individual dresses more warmly, decreases body surface area by curling up, and may go to bed in an effort to get warm. Body temperature is maintained at the new level until the fever "breaks."

During fever, arginine vasopressin (AVP), α-melanocyte-stimulating hormone (α-MSH), and corticotropin-releasing factor are released and can act as **endogenous cryogens** to help diminish the febrile response.[85,86] This antipyretic effect constitutes a negative-feedback loop[87] (see Figure 15-8). The antipyretic effect may help explain fluctuations in the febrile response. When the fever breaks, the set point is returned to normal. The hypothalamus responds by signaling a decrease in heat production and an increase in heat reduction mechanisms. The result is decreased muscle tone, peripheral vasodilation, flushing of the skin, and sweating. The individual feels very warm, replaces warm clothing with cooler clothes, throws off the covers, and stretches out. Once the body has returned to a normal temperature, the individual feels more comfortable and the hypothalamus adjusts thermoregulatory mechanisms to maintain the new temperature.

Benefits of Fever

Fever production aids responses to infectious processes through several mechanisms.[88] Simple raising of body temperature kills many microorganisms and has adverse effects on the growth and replication of others. Higher body temperatures decrease serum levels of iron, zinc, and copper, all of which are needed for bacterial replication. The body switches from burning glucose to a metabolism based on lipolysis and proteolysis, thereby depriving bacteria of a food

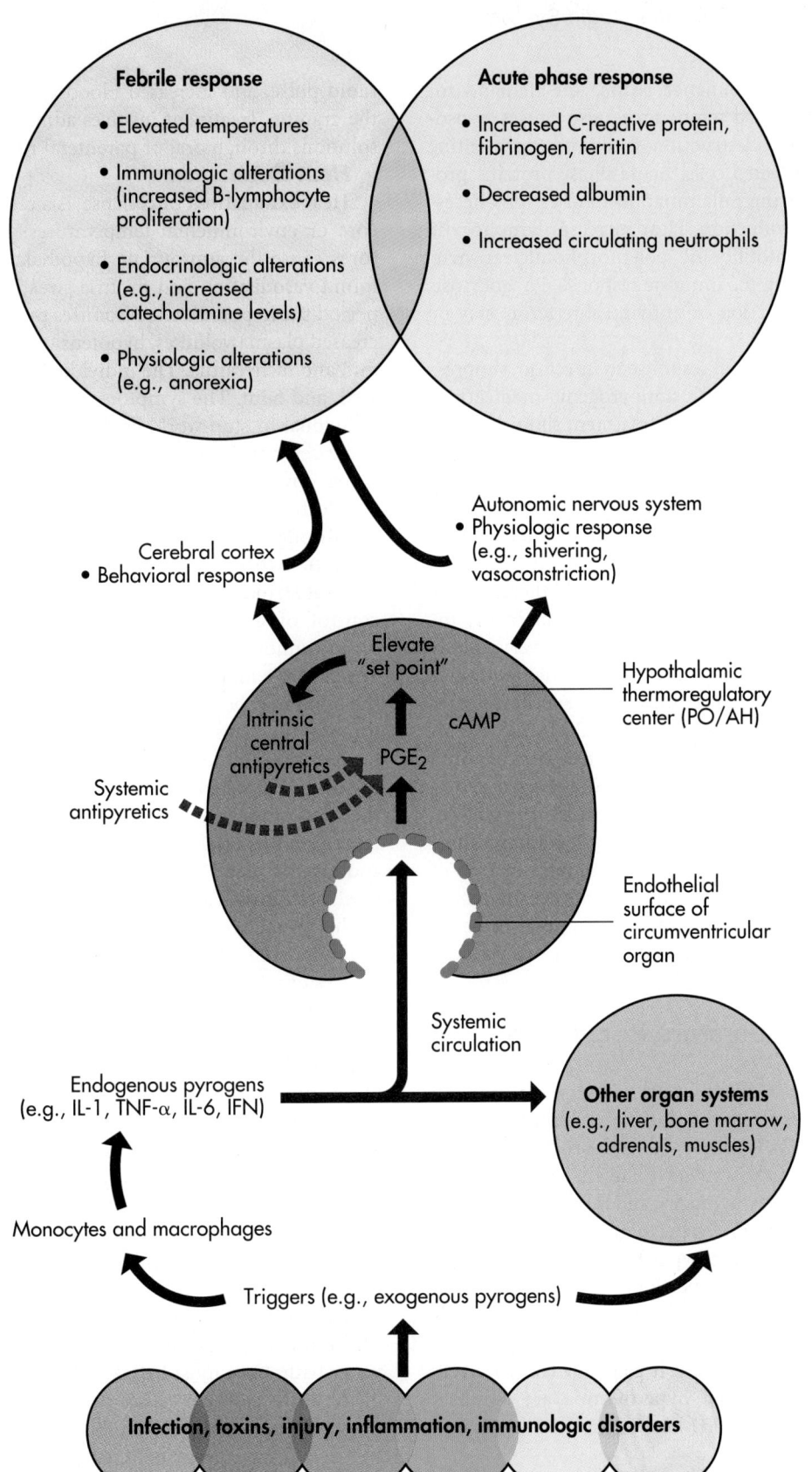

Figure 15-8 **Pathogenesis of fever and acute-phase response.** Certain disease states, through the elaboration of exogenous pyrogens, stimulate monocytes and macrophages to produce endogenous pyrogens such as IL-1, TNF-α, IL-6, and interferon-γ. These pyrogenic cytokines act at the endothelial surface of the circumventricular organ of the preoptic area of the anterior hypothalamus (PO/AH) to induce the production of PGE_2, which elevates the body's thermal set point. Intrinsic central antipyretics and systemic antipyretics exert their effects by decreasing levels of PGE_2. Physiologic and behavioral responses may be invoked to raise body temperature to a new set point. This febrile response must be considered in the context of an overlapping acute-phase response as a global nonspecific response to the original insult. *IL-1, IL-6,* Interleukin-1, interleukin-6; *TNF-α,* tumor necrosis factor–alpha; *IFN,* interferon. (Modified from Armstrong D, Cohen J: *Infectious diseases,* St Louis, 1999, Mosby.)

source. Anorexia and somnolence reduce the demand for muscle glucose.[89] Increased temperature also causes lysosomal breakdown and autodestruction of cells, thus preventing viral replication in infected cells. Acute-phase proteins produced by the liver during inflammation bind cations necessary for bacterial reproduction. Heat increases lymphocytic transformation and motility of polymorphonuclear neutrophils, thus facilitating the immune response. Phagocytosis is enhanced, and production of antiviral interferon may be augmented.[90,91]

Because fever is a beneficial response to infection, suppression of fever by treatment with antipyrogenic medications should be reviewed carefully.[92] Such treatment should be employed only if the fever produces or is high enough to produce serious side effects such as nerve damage or convulsion.

Infection and fever responses in elderly people and in children may vary from those in the normal adult. Older individuals may have decreased or no fever response to infection. The absence of fever responses to infection and therefore the beneficial aspects of fever production may explain the increase in morbidity and mortality rates seen in very elderly persons.[93] In contrast, children develop higher temperatures than adults for relatively minor infections. Febrile seizures may occur with temperatures above 39° C (102.2° F), although most children do not develop febrile seizures until temperatures are much higher. Febrile seizures are more predominant in male children before age 5 years. Febrile seizures are generally brief and self-limiting, lasting less than 5 minutes in 40% of children and less than 20 minutes in 75% of children. Authorities differ over the significance of febrile seizures. Although in most instances there appears to be no long-term effect on the child, a small percentage of children (1% to 2%) may develop epilepsy.[94]

Disorders of Temperature Regulation
Hyperthermia

Hyperthermia (marked warming of core temperature) can produce nerve damage, coagulation of cell proteins, and death. At 41° C (105.8° F), nerve damage produces convulsions in the adult. At 43° C (109.4° F), death results. Hyperthermia is not mediated by pyrogens, and there is no resetting of the hypothalamic set point. Hyperthermia may be accidental or therapeutic. Therapeutic hyperthermia is a form of local or general body-induced hyperthermia. Its purpose is to destroy pathologic microorganisms or tumor cells by facilitating the host's natural immune process through fever production. As a form of treatment, it is generally controversial. The four forms of accidental hyperthermia are (1) heat cramps, (2) heat exhaustion, (3) heat stroke, and (4) malignant hyperthermia.

Heat Cramps

Heat cramps are severe, spasmodic cramps in the abdomen and extremities that follow prolonged sweating and associated sodium loss. Heat cramps usually appear in individuals who are not accustomed to heat or in those who are performing strenuous work in very warm climates. Fever, rapid pulse, and increased blood pressure often accompany the cramps. Treatment involves administration of dilute salt solutions through oral or parenteral routes.

Heat Exhaustion

Heat exhaustion, or collapse, is a result of prolonged high core or environmental temperatures. These high temperatures cause the appropriate hypothalamic response of profound vasodilation and profuse sweating. Over a prolonged period the hypothalamic responses produce dehydration, decreased plasma volumes, hypotension, decreased cardiac output, and tachycardia. The individual feels weak, dizzy, nauseated, and faint. The symptoms of heat exhaustion cause the individual to stop work, lie down, and rest. Ceasing activity decreases muscle work, causing decreased heat production. Lying down redistributes vascular volume. The individual should be encouraged to drink warm fluids to replace fluid lost through sweating.

Heat Stroke

Heat stroke is a potentially lethal result of a breakdown in control of an overstressed thermoregulatory center. The brain cannot tolerate temperatures over 40.5° C (104.9° F). When core temperature reaches or exceeds 40.5° C (104.9° F), the brain may be preferentially cooled by maximal blood flow through the veins of the head and face, specifically the forehead. Sweat production on the face is maintained even during dehydration. Evaporation of the sweat cools the blood in the veins of the face and forehead; the blood then is returned to the endocranial venous network and sinus cavernosus, cooling the blood in the cerebral arterial vessels that lie in close proximity. Fanning the face enhances this mechanism. In this way the brain can be maintained temporarily at 40° C (104° F), even when core temperatures are higher.[72,95] In instances of very high core temperatures (40° to 43° C [104° to 109.4° F]), the cardiovascular and thermoregulatory centers may cease to function appropriately. Sweating ceases, and the skin becomes dry and flushed. The individual may be irritable, confused, stuporous, or comatose. Visual disturbances may occur.

As heat loss through the evaporation of sweat ceases, core temperatures increase rapidly. High core temperatures and vascular collapse produce cerebral edema, degeneration of the central nervous system, swollen dendrites, and renal tubular necrosis. Death results unless immediate, effective treatment is initiated.[96]

Treatment includes removing the person from the warm environment, if possible, and using a cooling blanket or cool water bath. Care must be taken to prevent too rapid cooling of the surface, which causes peripheral vasoconstriction and prevents core cooling. Individuals who recover from heat stroke may have permanent damage to the thermoregulatory center and thus may have difficulty tolerating environmental temperature changes.

Children are more susceptible to heat stroke than adults because (1) they produce more metabolic heat when exercising, (2) they have a greater surface area to mass ratio, and (3) their sweating capacity is less than that of adults.[97]

Malignant Hyperthermia

Malignant hyperthermia is a potentially lethal complication of a rare inherited muscle disorder. The condition is precipitated by the administration of volatile anesthetics and neuromuscular blocking agents. About 1 in 200 individuals may be at risk for the muscle disorder. Malignant hyperthermia is caused by either increased calcium release or decreased calcium uptake with muscle contraction. This allows intracellular calcium levels to rise, producing sustained, uncoordinated muscle contractions, which in turn increase muscle work, oxygen consumption, and lactic acid production. As a result of these contractions, acidosis develops and temperature rises (body temperature may rise 1° C [1.8° F] every 5 minutes); approximately 20% of those who develop malignant hyperthermia do not survive. Malignant hyperthermia occurs most often in children and young adults immediately after the induction of anesthesia.

Sympathetic responses and acidosis produce tachycardia and cardiac dysrhythmias, followed by hypotension, decreased cardiac output, and eventually, cardiac arrest. Increasing temperature, acidosis, hyperkalemia, and hypoxia produce coma-like symptoms in the CNS (including unconsciousness, absent reflexes, fixed pupils, apnea, and sometimes a flat electroencephalogram [EEG]). Oliguria and anuria are common, probably resulting from shock, ischemia, and low cardiac output.[98]

Treatment includes withdrawal of the provoking agents and administration of dantrolene sodium (a skeletal relaxant that inhibits calcium release during muscle contraction). Procainamide (Pronestyl) is used to treat cardiac dysrhythmias. Sodium bicarbonate also may be used. Body temperature can be decreased through use of ice bags, a cooling blanket, and iced saline lavage.[99]

Hypothermia

Hypothermia (core body temperature less than 35° C) is caused by prolonged exposure to cold and in 2002 accounted for 646 deaths in the United States.[100] Hypothermia produces vasoconstriction, alterations in microcirculation, coagulation, and ischemic tissue damage. In a controlled situation, such as a surgical procedure, most tissues can tolerate temperatures as low as 33° C. In severe hypothermia (less than 28° C), ice crystals forming on the inside of the cell cause cells to rupture and die. Tissue hypothermia slows the rate of chemical reactions (tissue metabolism), increases the viscosity of the blood, slows blood flow through the microcirculation, facilitates blood coagulation, and stimulates profound vasoconstriction. Hypothermia may be accidental or therapeutic. In accidental hypothermia, high energy phosphates (e.g., ATP) are depleted and in therapeutic hypothermia, ATP storage is preserved.[101]

Accidental Hypothermia

Accidental hypothermia (temperature below 35° C [95° F]) is generally the result of sudden immersion in cold water or prolonged exposure to cold environments.[102] At particular risk for accidental hypothermia are young persons and elderly persons, because thermoregulatory mechanisms are altered in these two groups.[103] Also at risk are individuals with conditions that diminish the ability to generate heat. Such conditions include hypothyroidism, hypopituitarism, malnutrition, Parkinson disease, and rheumatoid arthritis. Other risk factors include chronic increased vasodilation and decreased thermoregulatory control caused by cerebral injuries, ketoacidosis, uremia, and drug overdoses.[104,105]

In acute hypothermia, peripheral vasoconstriction shunts blood away from the cooler skin to the core in an effort to decrease heat loss. This peripheral vasoconstriction produces peripheral tissue ischemia. Intermittent reperfusion of the extremities (the Lewis phenomenon) helps preserve peripheral oxygenation. Intermittent peripheral perfusion continues until core temperatures drop dramatically.

The hypothalamic center stimulates shivering in an effort to increase heat production. Severe shivering occurs at core temperatures of 35° C (95° F) and continues until core temperature drops to about 30° to 32° C (86° to 89.6° F). Thinking becomes sluggish and coordination is decreased at 34° C (93.2° F). As hypothermia deepens, paradoxic undressing may occur as hypothalamic control of vasoconstriction is lost and vasodilation occurs with loss of core heat to the periphery. The hypothermic individual therefore feels suddenly warm and begins to remove clothing.[104]

At 30° C (86° F), the individual becomes stuporous; heart rate and respiratory rate decline; and cardiac output is diminished. Cerebral blood flow is decreased. Metabolic rate declines, further decreasing core temperature. Sinus node depression occurs with slowing of conduction through the atrioventricular node. In severe hypothermia (core temperature of 26° to 28° C [78.8° to 82.4° F]), pulse and respirations may be undetectable. Acidosis is moderate to severe. Ventricular fibrillation and asystole are common.[106]

If hypothermia is mild, passive rewarming may be sufficient. Passive rewarming includes provision of warm, dry clothes and warm drinks and performance of isometric exercises to increase heat production and minimize heat loss. Core temperature should be checked as soon as possible.[107,108]

If core temperature is above 30° C (86° F), active rewarming also may be required. Active rewarming employs warm water baths, warm blankets, heating pads, and warm oral fluids when the individual is fully alert. Active core rewarming is performed when core temperatures have dropped below 30° C (86° F) or when severe cardiovascular abnormalities appear. Core rewarming may be accomplished through administration of warm intravenous solutions, warm gastric lavage, warm peritoneal lavage, inhalation of warmed gases, and, in extreme cases, exchange transfusions, warming blood in a pump oxygenator circuit, and mediastinal lavage.[109,110]

Rewarming generally should proceed no faster than a few degrees per hour. (Short-term complications of rewarming are listed in Table 15-4.) Long-term complications include congestive heart failure, hepatic and renal failure, abnormal erythropoiesis, myocardial infarction, pancreatitis, and neurologic dysfunctions.

Table 15-4	Accidental Hypothermia: Complications of Rewarming
Complication	**Mechanism**
Acidosis	Rewarming stimulates peripheral vasodilation; peripheral blood, returning to the core from the ischemic peripheral tissues, causes a reduction in the pH of core blood
Rewarming shock	As rewarming and vasodilation progress, the body is unable to maintain blood pressure because of reduced fluid volume (from "cold diuresis"), catecholamine depletion (prolonged shivering), and myocardial injury
Deep-ended hypothermia	As colder surface blood is returned to the core, core temperature may drop; this is also referred to as "after fall" or "after drop"
Dysrhythmia	Rewarming places an additional stress on an already severely stressed myocardium

Therapeutic Hypothermia

Therapeutic hypothermia is used to slow metabolism and thus preserve ischemic tissue during surgery or limb reimplantation. The actual mechanism of tissue preservation has been debated.[111] It is possible that the slowed metabolism in hypothermic tissues preserves adenosine triphosphate (ATP).[112] Regardless of the mechanism, however, it is clear that hypothermic ischemic cells remain viable long after normothermic ischemic cells have died. Survival from accidental hypothermia has been reported in individuals with core temperatures at 16° C (60.8° F) and from therapeutic hypothermia with temperatures at 9° C (48.2° F).[113]

The temperature changes of hypothermia place a great deal of stress on the heart. Moderate to severe hypothermia may lead to ventricular fibrillation and cardiac arrest. (This may be the desired outcome in open heart surgery when the heart must be stopped during portions of the surgical procedure.[114]) Prolonged hypothermia may precipitate exhaustion of liver glycogen stores by prolonged shivering. Surface cooling may cause burns, frostbite, and fat necrosis.

Trauma

Major body trauma has varying effects on temperature regulation, depending on the body systems involved. Five types of traumatic injury that usually affect temperature regulation are (1) CNS trauma (discussed in Chapter 17), (2) accidental injury, (3) hemorrhagic shock, (4) major surgery, and (5) thermal burns.

Central Nervous System Trauma

CNS trauma that causes CNS damage, inflammation, increased intracranial pressures, or intracranial bleeding typically produces a fever greater than 39° C (102.2° F). This temperature, often referred to as a *central fever,* appears with or without relative bradycardia. The temperature is sustained, does not induce sweating, and is highly resistant to antipyretic therapy.

Accidental Injuries

Mild accidental injuries may produce a slight elevation in core temperature. Moderate to severe injuries result in peripheral vasoconstriction with decreased surface and core temperatures. Core temperature is thought to be inversely related to the severity of the injury and may be a result of decreased oxygen transport to the tissues. In severe injuries, shivering is absent and some alteration in thermoregulation is evident.[115]

Hemorrhagic Shock

Loss of blood volume in hemorrhage triggers peripheral vasoconstriction and a slight increase in core temperature. Subsequent decreases in core temperature have been demonstrated in individuals with hemorrhagic shock treated with unwarmed volume-expanding solutions and surgical repair. Volume expansion with warmed solutions is recommended to prevent the deleterious effects of hypothermia on cardiac output, cardiac rhythm, and the immune system.[114]

Major Surgery

Because many victims of trauma undergo major surgical repair, the effect of the surgical procedure on temperature regulation needs to be considered by health care providers. Major surgery often induces significant hypothermia through exposure of body cavities to the relatively cool operating room environment. Other mechanisms that contribute to intraoperative hypothermia include irrigation of body cavities with room temperature solutions, infusion of room temperature intravenous solutions, use of drugs that impair thermoregulatory mechanisms, and inhalation of unwarmed anesthetic agents.[114] Use of warmed irrigating and intravenous solutions may reduce intraoperative hypothermia.

Thermal Burns

Large burn injuries produce significant hypothermia because of the loss of the skin barrier to fluid evaporation and the loss of control of the microcirculation in the skin. Severe burns also compromise the normal insulation of the skin and subcutaneous tissues. (Burns are discussed in Chapter 46.)

SLEEP

Sleep is an active, multiphase process. The hypothalamus is the major sleep center and the hypocreatins (ovexins) are neuropeptides secreted by the hypothalamus that promote wakefulness and rapid eye movement (REM) sleep. Prostaglandin D_2, L-tryptophan and growth factors promote sleep.[116-118]

Normal sleep has two phases that can be documented by EEG: rapid eye movement (REM) sleep and non-REM (NREM), or slow-wave, sleep. REM and NREM sleep succeed each other in 90- to 110-minute intervals.[119] NREM sleep is divided into four stages based on changes in the EEG pattern (Figure 15-9):

Stage I—Light sleep, with alpha waves interspersed with low-frequency theta waves; slow eye movements (3% to 8% of sleep time)

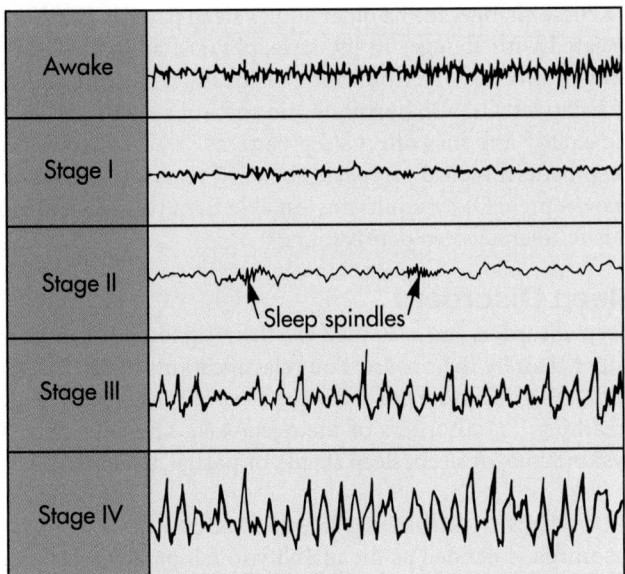

Figure 15-9 Electroencephalogram (EEG) stages of wakefulness and sleep. *Awake,* Low-voltage fast activity; *stage I,* falling asleep; *stage II,* light sleep with sleep spindles; *stage III,* moderately deep sleep; *stage IV,* deep sleep with slow delta waves. Rapid eye movement (REM) sleep looks similar to awake and stage I.

Stage II—Further slowing of the EEG with the presence of sleep spindles and slow eye movements (45% to 55% of sleep time)

Stage III—Low-frequency delta waves with occasional sleep spindles; no slow eye movements (15% to 20% of sleep time)

Stage IV—Delta waves (15% to 20% of sleep time)

Non-Rapid Eye Movement Sleep

Non-REM (slow-wave) sleep accounts for 75% to 80% of sleep time and is initiated by the withdrawal of neurotransmitters from the reticular formation and by the inhibition of arousal mechanisms in the cerebral cortex. During non-REM sleep, respiration is controlled by metabolic processes.[120] The basal metabolic rate is decreased by 10% to 15%. Temperature is decreased 0.5° to 1° C (0.9° to 1.8° F). Heart rate decreases by 10 to 30 beats per minute. Respiration, blood pressure, and muscle tone all decrease. Knee-jerk reflexes are absent. Pupils are constricted. During stages I and II, cerebral blood flow to the brain stem and cerebellum is decreased. During stages III and IV, cerebral blood flow to the cortex is decreased.[121,121a] Growth hormone is released during stage IV, and levels of corticosteroids and catecholamines are depressed.

Rapid Eye Movement Sleep

Rapid eye movement (REM) sleep accounts for 20% to 25% of sleep time and is characterized by desynchronized, low-voltage, fast activity that occurs about every 90 minutes beginning after 1 to 2 hours of non-REM sleep. This sleep is also known as *paradoxic sleep* because the EEG pattern is similar to the normal awake pattern. Alternating periods of REM and non-REM sleep occur throughout the night, with lengthening intervals of REM sleep and fewer intervals of deeper stages of non-REM sleep toward morning. REM sleep is characterized by bursts of conjugate rapid eye movement; atonia of antigravity muscles; loss of temperature regulation; alteration in heart rate, blood pressure,[122] and respiration; penile erection in men and clitoral engorgement in women; and a high rate of memorable dreams. Steroids are released in short bursts. During REM sleep, respiratory control is thought to be largely independent of metabolic requirements and oxygen variation. Loss of normal voluntary muscle control in the tongue and upper pharynx may produce some respiratory obstruction. Cerebral blood flow to both hemispheres is increased. REM sleep is controlled by the pontine reticular formation.

Many neurotransmitters are associated with excitatory and inhibitory sleep mechanisms, including gamma-aminobutyric acid, hypocretin (orexin) catecholamines, acetylcholine, serotonin, histamine L-tryptophan, prostaglandins, and adenosine.[123] Their mechanism of action is complex and not clearly understood. The reticular formation is primarily responsible for generating REM sleep, and projections from the reticular formation and other areas of the mesencephalon and brain stem produce NREM sleep.[124] Growth hormone is associated with initiation of sleep, and cortisol rises in the morning just before waking.[125]

While asleep, an individual progresses through REM and NREM sleep in a predictable cycle. Each cycle lasts approximately 90 to 110 minutes, with the individual passing through four to five cycles per night.[126] The first cycle of the night begins with stage I. The individual then progresses through stages II, III, IV, III, II, and REM sleep. A new cycle, beginning with stage II, follows each REM sleep. With each successive cycle, the amount of time spent in stage IV sleep decreases and the amount of time spent in REM sleep increases (Figure 15-10). The individual who is awakened begins the next cycle with stage I. Acetylcholine and somatostatin play a role in stages of sleep transition. Forced awakenings in the middle of the night may result in increased difficulty returning to sleep or may alter the normal progression of sleep, or both.[127,128] The purpose of sleep is unknown, although restorative processes have been proposed because growth hormone peaks are associated with slow-wave sleep. It is an important enough need that people spend about one third of their life sleeping. Loss of REM sleep impairs learning and memory.[129]

PEDIATRICS AND SLEEP PATTERNS

The sleep patterns of the newborn and young child vary from those of the adult in total sleep time, cycle length, and percentage of time spent in each sleep cycle. Newborns sleep about 16 to 17 hours per day. About 53% of that time is spent in active sleep (REM sleep), 23% in quiet sleep (non-REM sleep), and the remainder in an indeterminate phase. The infant sleep cycle is approximately 50 to 60 minutes in length, with 20 minutes of NREM sleep and 10 to 45 minutes of REM sleep, in contrast to the adult sleep cycle. Newborns enter REM sleep immediately on falling asleep.[130,131] At about 1 year

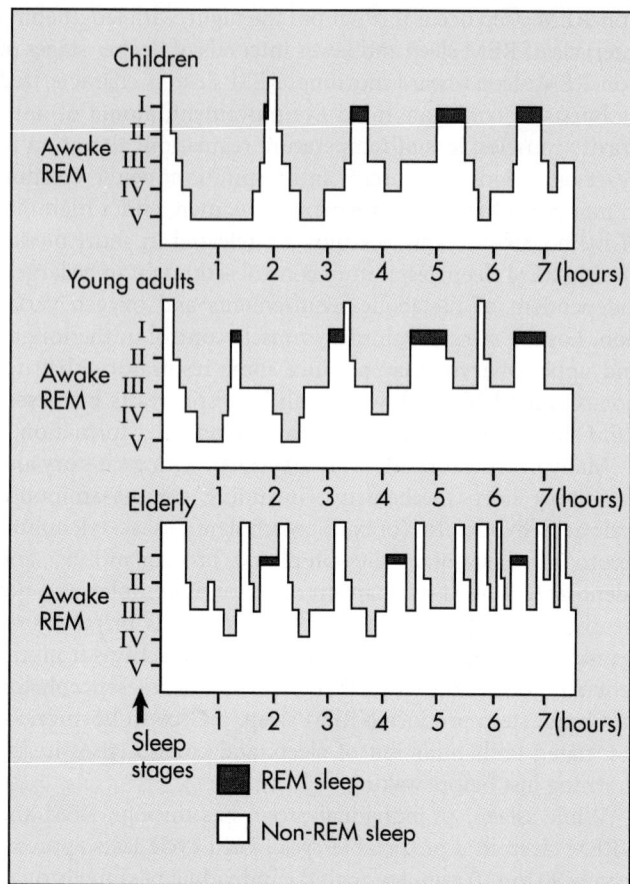

Figure 15-10 Normal sleep cycles. Rapid eye movement (REM) sleep occurs cyclically throughout the night at intervals of approximately 90 minutes in all age groups. REM sleep shows little variation in the different age groups, whereas stage IV sleep decreases with age. In addition, elderly persons awaken frequently and show a marked increase in total time awake.

of age, the infant spends approximately 45% of total sleep time in quiet sleep and 41% in REM sleep. Total sleep time decreases slightly from birth to 1 year. In the American culture, where infants are bottle fed and do not share sleeping space with the mother, infants increase maximum sleep time from 4 to 5 hours to 8 to 10 hours by 4 months of age. They begin to "sleep through the night." In other cultures, where infants are breast fed for up to 2 years and share sleeping space with the mother, they continue to sleep in short bouts and wake frequently to nurse.[132]

In the young child, the sleep cycle length is 45 to 60 minutes, in contrast to 90 to 100 minutes in the adult. The child assumes the adult sleep pattern at some point during the first 2 to 5 years of life.[133]

AGING AND SLEEP PATTERNS

The sleep pattern of the older adult differs from that of the younger adult or child. Total sleep time is decreased, and the older individual takes longer to fall asleep. Elderly people awaken earlier in the morning and more frequently during the night. Total REM and stage II time is unchanged, but stage IV sleep decreases by 15% to 30%. On EEG, the spindle indicating stage II sleep is less well formed.[134,135]

These changes in the older adult's sleep pattern may be associated with changes in life-style, physical ailments, lack of daily routine, desynchronization of circadian rhythm, and use of sedatives. Growth hormone and cortisol are diminished in the elderly and may affect sleep patterns.[136] The alteration in sleep pattern typically appears about 10 years later in women than in men. Older adults are less able than younger individuals to tolerate sleep deprivation.[133]

Sleep Disorders

Sleep disorders are classified by their signs and symptoms rather than by their cause. Four classifications of sleep disorders are (1) disorders of initiating sleep; (2) sleep disordered breathing; (3) disorders of the sleep/wake schedule; and (4) dysfunctions of sleep, sleep stages, or partial arousals.

Disorders of Initiating Sleep: Insomnia

Insomnia is defined as the inability to fall or stay asleep and is more common in women.[137] Insomnia may be transient, lasting a few days, and related to travel across time zones, or it may be caused by acute stress. Long-term insomnia is associated with drug or alcohol abuse, chronic pain disorders, or chronic depression, obesity, and aging.[138] Drugs known to produce insomnia include amphetamines, steroids, central adrenergic blockers, bronchodilating agents, and caffeine.[139]

Sleep Disordered Breathing

The disorders of breathing during sleep are related to airway resistance and exist along a continuum of severity, including upper airway resistance syndrome, obstructive sleep apnea, and obesity hypoventilation syndrome. Sleep disordered breathing affects more men than women.[140] One hypothesis to explain this is that the female hormone progesterone, a respiratory stimulant, may protect premenopausal women from sleep disordered breathing.[141,141a]

Upper airway resistance syndrome is characterized by repetitive increases in resistance to airflow within the upper airway with snoring and brief arousals from sleep and daytime somnolence. The level of negative intrathoracic pressure is the most likely stimulus for arousal, possibly mediated by mechanoreceptors in the upper airway. Hypertension is an important consequence of this disorder, probably resulting from a combination of intermittent hypoxia and hypercapnia, arousals, increased sympathetic tone, altered baroreflex control during sleep, and cardiovascular changes induced by increased negative intrathoracic pressure. Nasal continuous positive airway pressure is the most effective form of therapy,[142,143] but long-term compliance is a major problem.

Obstructive sleep apnea (OSA) syndrome affects up to 4% of middle-age adults. Symptoms of OSA include loud snoring, a decrease in oxygen saturation, fragmented sleep, chronic daytime sleepiness, and fatigue. These episodes usually last 10 to 30 seconds and result in the possible development of cardiovascular abnormalities. The obstruction is caused by the soft palate, base of the tongue, or both collapsing against the pharyngeal walls because of decreased muscle tone during sleep. Many individuals are not aware of their heavy snoring and nocturnal arousals and may remain undiagnosed. Potentially fatal systemic illnesses often associated with this disorder include hypertension, pulmonary hypertension, heart failure, nocturnal cardiac dysrhythmias, myocardial infarction, and ischemic stroke.[144]

Treatments include nasal continuous positive airway pressure and dental devices that modify the position of the tongue or jaw. Upper airway and jaw surgical procedures also may be appropriate in selected patients.[145]

Obesity hypoventilation syndrome is the most severe form of disordered breathing during sleep and is associated with severe morbidity and very high mortality. Most individuals are overweight and have a short, thick neck. Profound obesity is associated with impaired respiratory mechanics and depressed respiratory control, particularly during sleep. Systemic complications include pulmonary hypertension and ischemic heart disease. Daytime sleepiness, fatigue, car accidents, and poor work performance are common.

Continuous positive pressure and airway reconstruction are effective treatments for severe obstructive sleep apnea in the morbidly obese person. Careful selection and identification of potential coexisting obesity hypoventilation syndrome and counseling on weight reduction and avoidance of continual weight gain will improve treatment outcomes.[146]

Disorders of the Sleep/Wake Schedule

Common disorders of the sleep/wake schedule include rapid time-zone change (jet-lag syndrome), changing sleep schedule with an advance or a delay of 3 hours or more in sleep time, or a change in total sleep time from day to day. These changes in the timing of established sleep schedules have been shown to desynchronize circadian rhythm. Degree of vigilance, performance of psychomotor tasks, and subjective reports of levels of arousal are markedly depressed after alterations in the sleep/wake schedule. Individuals may experience short sleep episodes called *microsleeps* without being aware of decreased vigilance.[147]

It is well established that industrial shift workers exhibit a decrease in accuracy and increased accident proneness.[148] For similar reasons, persons suffering from jet lag require several days to adapt to the new time zone. Travel across time zones requires 2 days to adjust the sleep/wake schedule, 5 days to adjust the body temperature cycle, and 8 days to adjust cortisol secretion. Transmeridian travel requires up to 10 days to adjust the body clock when traveling from east to west. Czeisler's experiments with timed bright-light stimulation have had some success in retiming or resetting the body clock before or after time-zone shifts.[149]

Parasomnias

Parasomnias are unusual behaviors occurring during sleep, including sleepwalking, night terrors, rearranging furniture, eating food, violent behavior, and enuresis. Three dysfunctions of sleep are common in children: somnambulism (sleepwalking), night terrors (dream anxiety attacks), and enuresis (bedwetting).[150]

Somnambulism

Somnambulism is a disorder primarily of childhood and appears to resolve itself within several years of the onset of the sleepwalking episodes. Sleepwalking occurs in stages III and IV and is therefore not associated with dreaming. During the sleepwalking episode, the child functions at a very low level of arousal and has no memory of the event on awakening. The greatest concern is for the safety of the child.

Night Terrors

Night terrors are characterized by "sudden apparent arousals in which the child expresses intense fear or emotion."[133] The child, however, is not awake and is very difficult to arouse. Once awakened, the child has no memory of the night terror event. Night terrors occur during stage IV sleep and are not associated with the dreams of REM sleep. Although night terrors occur most often in children, adults may experience them as well. Unlike children, however, adults often display corresponding daytime anxiety.[149]

Enuresis

Enuresis is possibly the most disturbing of the childhood sleep dysfunctions because of the stress society places on nighttime continence and the misconception that children are bedwetting to act out against parents. Bedwetting incidents also are associated incorrectly with dreaming. Laboratory studies of sleep have demonstrated that very few incidents of bedwetting occur when the child is dreaming and that, by far, most incidents occur during non-REM sleep and during the first one third of the night, when the child is most difficult to arouse.[133] Most causes of enuresis are benign and treatable. Evaluations should be completed to detect infections, obstructions, decreased nocturnal secretion of antidiuretic hormone, and neurogenic bladder.[151] Children usually outgrow the enuretic episodes, but management is important to prevent psychologic problems.[152]

Relation Between Sleep and Disease

Sleep and disease are interrelated. Some diseases produce alterations in the quantity and quality of sleep or affect sleep stages. These are referred to as **secondary sleep disorders.** In some instances sleep stages produce alterations in certain disease states. These are referred to as **sleep-provoked disorders.** Other entities, such as sudden infant death syndrome (SIDS) and sudden unexplained nocturnal death syndrome (SUNDS), produce unexplained death almost exclusively during sleep.[149]

Secondary Sleep Disorders

The most common causes of secondary sleep disorders are depression, alterations in thyroid hormone secretion (hypothyroidism or hyperthyroidism), pain, and sleep apnea syndromes. Depressed persons have difficulty falling asleep and exhibit less slow-wave sleep, less time spent in REM sleep, early awakening, and less total sleep time. In addition, depressed individuals move through the sleep stages more quickly than do individuals who are not depressed. The same neurotransmitters that may be disturbed in depression also regulate sleep; serotonergic neuron dysfunction also is a possible mechanism.[153] Sleep deprivation paradoxically relieves depression.[149]

Changes in thyroid hormone secretion produce changes in stages III and IV sleep. An increase in thyroid secretion produces an increase in stages III and IV activity, whereas a decrease in thyroid hormone produces a decrease in both stages III and IV sleep.

Chronic pain is a cause of insomnia. Chronic pain inhibits sleep, increases arousals during sleep, and causes prolonged awake intervals during the night. Individuals with chronic pain report not only a decrease in the quantity of sleep but also a decrease in its quality.

Sleep-Provoked Disorders

Some diseases are provoked by certain aspects of sleep. Signs and symptoms of the disease appear during, or are enhanced by, sleep. Diseases that are affected by sleep include coronary artery disease, bronchial asthma, chronic obstructive pulmonary disease (COPD), diabetes, and duodenal ulcers.

Coronary artery disease is most affected during REM sleep. During REM, dreams may provoke nocturnal angina, increased heart rate, and electrocardiogram (ECG) changes. In adults, attacks of bronchial asthma may occur at any time during the night. The attacks cause the individual to spend more of the sleep period awake and thus cause a decrease in stage IV sleep. In children, bronchial asthma attacks are uncommon during the first one third of the night, when stage IV sleep predominates, and occur more frequently during the final two thirds of the night. Stage IV sleep is decreased overall in the child with bronchial asthma. In addition to these changes, asthmatics may experience bronchial spasm during REM sleep.[154]

Persons with COPD experience significantly lowered oxygen tension and increases in carbon dioxide retention during sleep. The lowered oxygen tension is most significant in the tonic phase of REM sleep when voluntary neuromuscular control, including intercostal muscle function, is depressed. Pulmonary spasm and transient pulmonary hypertension result. These changes are particularly evident in the so-called "blue bloater" individual and may contribute to early pulmonary hypertension and cor pulmonale in these persons.[155]

Because blood glucose levels vary during sleep, individuals with uncontrolled diabetes may need to pay careful attention to blood sugar levels during sleep. Studies show that people with duodenal ulcers secrete 3 to 20 times more gastric acid during REM sleep than do people without duodenal ulcers. This increased gastric acid secretion often produces nocturnal epigastric pain.[133]

SIDS affects children primarily in the first 2 years of life and may be related to central sleep apnea episodes. (For further discussion of SIDS, see Chapter 34.)

SPECIAL SENSES

Vision

The eyes are complex sense organs responsible for vision. Within a protective casing, each eye has receptors, a lens system for focusing light on the receptors, and a system of nerves for conducting impulses from the receptors to the brain. Vi-

sual dysfunction may be caused by abnormal ocular movements or alterations in visual acuity, refraction, color vision, or accommodation. Visual dysfunction also may be the secondary effect of another neurologic disorder.

External Eye Structures

The external structures protecting the eye include the eyelids (palpebrae), conjunctivae, and lacrimal apparatus (Figure 15-11). Infection and inflammatory responses are the most common conditions affecting the supporting structures of the eyes. **Blepharitis** is an inflammation of the eyelids caused by staphylococcus or seborrheic dermatitis. Redness, edema, and itching are common symptoms. A **hordeolum (stye)** is an infection of the sebaceous glands of the eyelids, and a **chalazion** is an infection of the meibomian (oil-secreting) gland. These conditions are treated symptomatically.[156]

Conjunctivitis

Conjunctivitis is an inflammation of the conjunctiva (mucous membrane covering the front part of the eyeball). Conjunctivitis may be caused by bacteria, viruses, allergies, or chemical irritations. The inflammatory response produces redness, edema, pain, and lacrimation. Treatment is related to cause.[157]

Acute bacterial conjunctivitis (pinkeye) is highly contagious and often is caused by gram-positive organisms (*Staphylococcus, Haemophilus, Proteus*), although other bacteria may be involved. The onset is acute, characterized by mucopurulent drainage from one or both eyes. Preventing spread of the organism with meticulous hand washing and use of

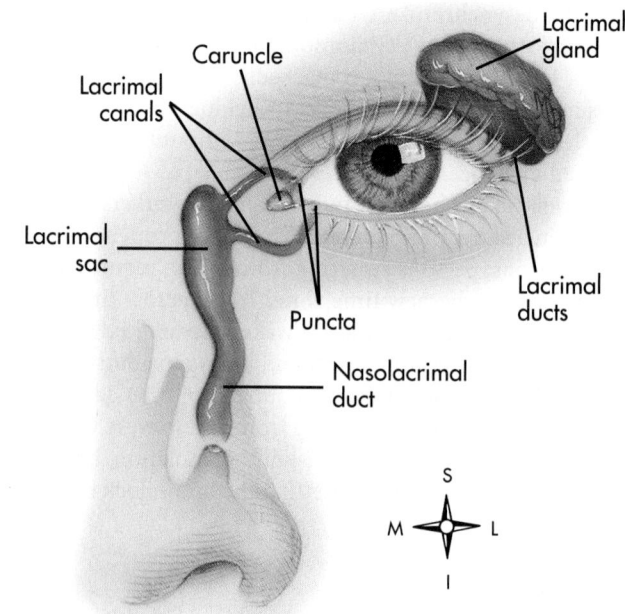

Figure 15-11 Lacrimal apparatus. Fluid produced by lacrimal glands (tears) streams across the eye surface, enters the canals, and then passes through the nasolacrimal duct to enter the nose. (From Thibodeau GA, Patton KT: *Anatomy & physiology,* ed 5, St Louis, 2003, Mosby.)

separate towels is important. The disease often is self-limiting and resolves spontaneously in 10 to 14 days. Antibiotic eye drops usually are effective.

Viral conjunctivitis is caused by an adenovirus. Symptoms vary from mild to severe. Some strains of virus cause conjunctivitis and pharyngitis (pharyngoconjunctival fever), and others cause keratoconjunctivitis. Both diseases are contagious, with watering, redness, and photophobia. Treatment is symptomatic.

Allergic conjunctivitis is associated with a variety of antigens, including pollens. There is ocular itching associated with photophobia, burning, and gritty sensations in the eye. Treatment is symptomatic and may include antihistamines, steroids, and vasoconstrictors.

Chronic conjunctivitis is the result of any persistent conjunctivitis. The cause requires identification for effective treatment.

Trachoma (chlamydial conjunctivitis) is caused by *Chlamydia trachomatis*. It often is associated with poor hygiene and is the leading cause of preventable blindness in the world. The severity of the disease varies, but it can involve inflammation and vascularization of the cornea with scarring of the conjunctiva and eyelids, leading to blindness. Chlamydial organisms are sensitive to local or systemic antibiotics. The World Health Organization aims to eliminate trachoma as a public health problem by 2020 using the SAFE Strategy: **S**urgery for inturned lashes, **A**ntibiotics, **F**acial cleanliness, and **E**nvironmental improvement.[158]

Keratitis

Keratitis is an infection of the cornea that can be caused by bacteria or viruses. Bacterial infections often cause corneal ulceration and require intensive antibiotic treatment. Type I herpes simplex virus can involve both the cornea and conjunctiva. Common symptoms include photophobia, pain, and lacrimation. Severe ulcerations with residual scarring require corneal transplantation.

The Eye

The wall of the eye is formed of three layers: sclera, choroid, and retina (Figure 15-12). The **sclera** is the thick, white, outermost layer. It becomes transparent at the **cornea,** the portion of the sclera in the central anterior region that allows light to enter the eye. The **choroid** is the deeply pigmented middle layer that prevents light from scattering inside the eye. The **iris,** part of the choroid, has a round opening, the **pupil,** through which light passes. Smooth muscle fibers control the size of the pupil so that in close vision and bright light the pupil constricts and in distant vision and dim light the pupil dilates.

The innermost layer of the eye, the **retina,** contains millions of **rods** and **cones,** special photoreceptors that convert light energy into nerve impulses. In the retina, rods mediate peripheral and dim light vision and are densest at the periphery. Cones, densest in the center of the retina, are color and detail receptors. The photoreceptive rods and cones are distributed over the entire retina, except where the optic nerve leaves the eyeball. Lack of rods and cones in this area results in the **optic disc,** or blind spot. Lateral to each optic disc is the **fovea centralis,** a tiny area that contains only cones and provides the greatest visual acuity (see Figure 15-12).

As shown in Figure 15-13, nerve impulses pass through the optic nerves after leaving the retinas. At the optic chiasm the

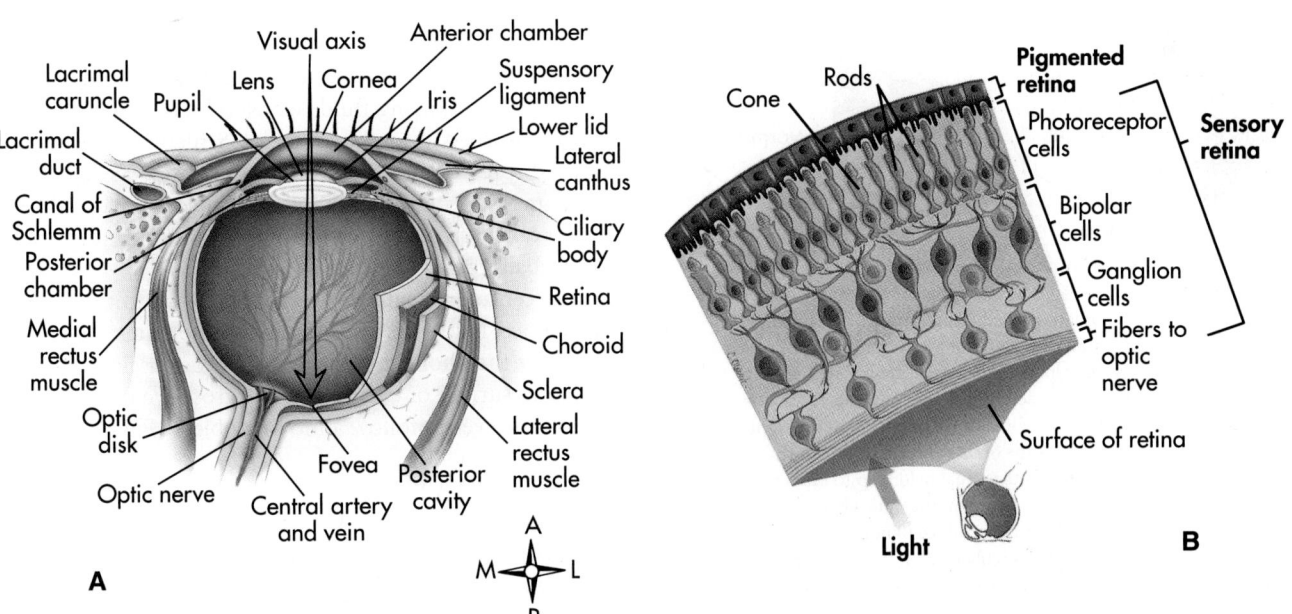

Figure 15-12 Structure of the eyeball and cell layers of the retina. **A,** Horizontal section through the left eyeball. The eye is viewed viewed from above. **B,** Pigmented and sensory layers of the retina. (From Thibodeau GA, Patton KT: *Anatomy & physiology,* ed 5, St Louis, 2003, Mosby.)

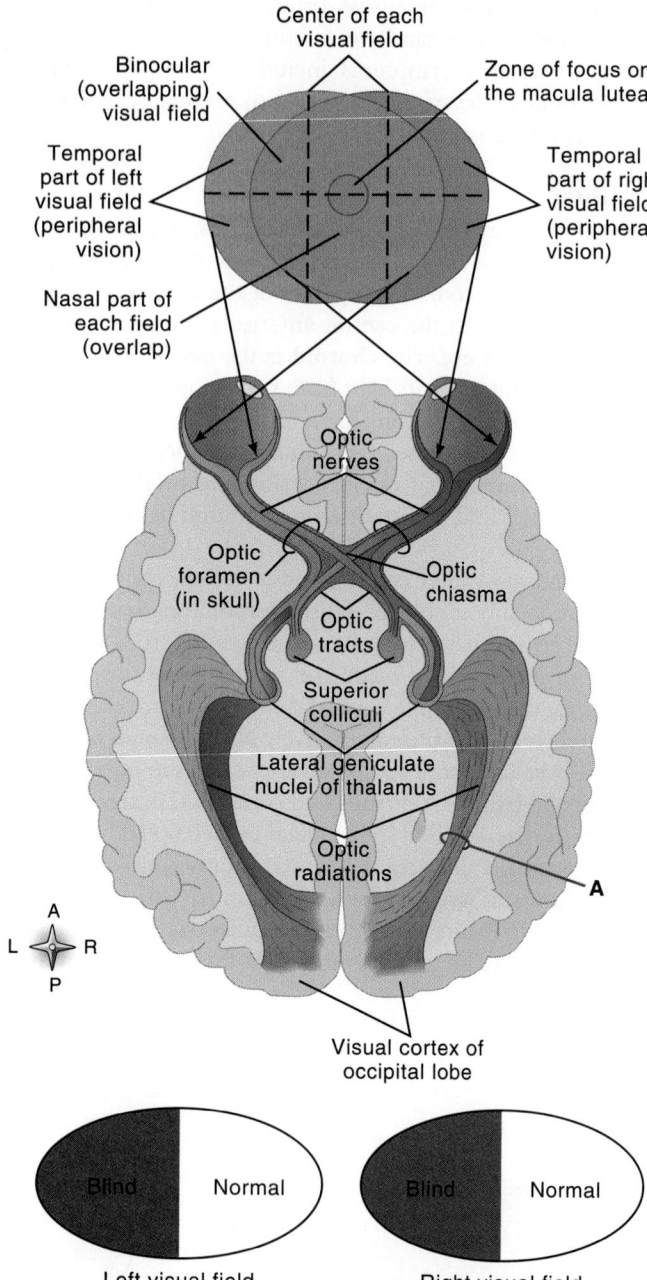

Figure 15-13 **Visual fields and neuronal pathways.** Note the structures that make up each pathway: optic nerve, optic chiasm, lateral geniculate body of thalamus, optic radiations, and visual cortex of occipital lobe. Fibers from the nasal portion of each retina cross over to the opposite side at the optic chiasma and terminate in the lateral geniculate nuclei. Location of a lesion in the visual pathway determines the resulting visual defect. Damage at *point A*, for example, would cause blindness in the right nasal and left temporal visual fields, as the ovals beneath indicate. (Trace the visual pathway from *point A* back to the visual field map to see why this is so.) What would be the effect of pressure on the optic chiasm, by a pituitary tumor, for instance? (*Answer*: It would produce blindness in both temporal visual fields. Why? Because it destroys fibers from the nasal side of both retinas.) (From Thibodeau GA, Patton KT: *Anatomy & physiology*, ed 5, St Louis, 2003, Mosby.)

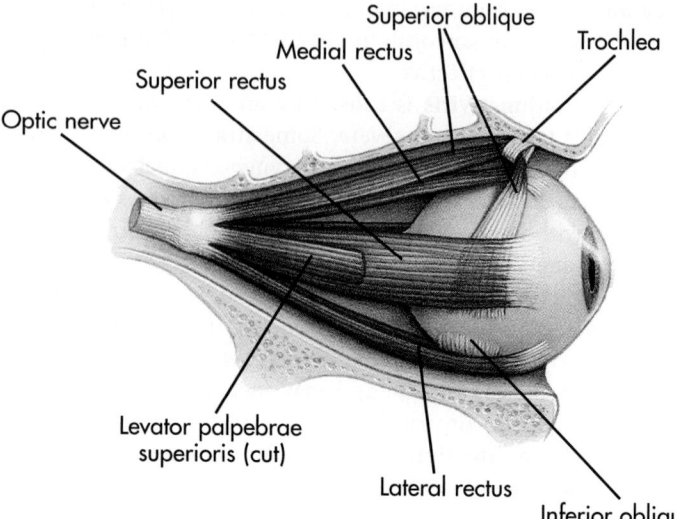

Figure 15-14 **Extrinsic muscles of the right eye. Superior view.** (From Thibodeau GA, Patton KT: *Anatomy & physiology*, ed 5, St Louis, 2003, Mosby.)

fibers from the inner (nasal) halves of the retinas cross to the opposite side, where they join fibers from the outer (temporal) halves of the retinas to form the optic tracts. The fibers of the optic tracts synapse in the dorsal lateral geniculate nucleus, and from there the geniculocalcarine fibers pass by way of the optic radiation (or geniculocalcarine tract) to the primary visual cortex in the occipital lobe of the brain.

Light entering the eye is focused on the retina by the **lens**—a flexible, biconvex, crystal-like structure. In youth the lens is transparent and has the consistency of hardened jelly. With age the lens becomes increasingly hard and opaque. The lens divides the anterior chamber into (1) the aqueous chamber and (2) the vitreous chamber. **Aqueous humor,** which fills the aqueous chamber, helps maintain the pressure inside the eye and provides nutrients to the lens and cornea. Aqueous humor is free-flowing fluid, secreted by the ciliary processes and reabsorbed into the canal of Schlemm. If drainage is blocked, pressure within the eye increases (as it does with glaucoma). The vitreous chamber is filled with a gel-like substance called **vitreous humor.** Vitreous humor helps prevent the eyeball from collapsing inward.

The central retinal artery provides blood to the inner retinal surface. Nutrients are supplied to the outer surface of the retina by the choroid. Six extrinsic eye muscles, attached to the outer surface of each eye, allow gross eye movements and permit the eyes to follow a moving object (Figure 15-14).

AGING AND VISION

Changes in the structural components of the eye caused by aging begin at an early age, particularly in the lens of the eye. Changes caused by aging are summarized in Table 15-5. The combined structural changes combined with chronic diseases including diabetes mellitus result in a decline in visual acuity.[159]

Table 15-5	Changes in the Eye Caused by Aging	
Structure	**Change**	**Consequence**
Cornea	Thicker and less curved	Increase in astigmatism
	Formation of a gray ring at the edge of cornea (arcus senilis)	Not detrimental to vision
Anterior chamber	Decrease in size and volume caused by thickening of lens	Occasionally exerts pressure on Schlemm canal and may lead to increased intraocular pressure and glaucoma
Lens	Increase in opacity	Decrease in refraction with increased light scattering and decreased color vision (green and blue); can lead to cataracts
Ciliary muscles	Reduction in pupil diameter, atrophy of radial dilation muscles	Persistent constriction (senile miosis); decrease in critical flicker frequency*
Retina	Reduction in number of rods at periphery, loss of rods and associated nerve cells	Increase in the minimum amount of light necessary to see an object

*The rate at which consecutive visual stimuli can be presented and still be perceived as separate.

Visual Dysfunction

Alterations in Ocular Movements

Abnormal ocular movements occur as a result of oculomotor, trochlear, or abducens cranial nerve dysfunction (see Table 14-6). The three types of eye movement disorders are (1) strabismus, (2) nystagmus, and (3) paralysis of individual extraocular muscles.

Strabismus is the deviation of one eye from the other when the person is looking at an object; it is caused by weak or hypertonic muscle in one of the eyes. The deviation may be upward, downward, inward, or outward. Strabismus in children requires early intervention to prevent the development of amblyopia (reduced vision in the affected eye without ocular pathology and with full optical correction). Treatment of amblyopia is patching. The primary symptom of strabismus is **diplopia** (double vision). Strabismus may be caused by a neuromuscular disorder of the eye muscle, diseases involving the cerebral hemispheres, or thyroid disease.[160,161]

Nystagmus is an involuntary unilateral or bilateral rhythmic movement of the eyes and can occur in infants (congenital) or adults (acquired). It may be present at rest, or it may occur with eye movement. The two major forms of nystagmus are pendular nystagmus and jerk nystagmus. **Pendular nystagmus** is characterized by a regular to-and-fro movement of the eyes in which both phases of the movement are equal in length. In **jerk nystagmus** one phase of the eye movement is faster than the other. Nystagmus may be caused by an imbalance in the normally coordinated reflex activity of the inner ear, vestibular nuclei (connecting the vestibular nerve with vestibulospinal tracts), cerebellum, medial longitudinal fascicle (connecting the mesencephalon with the upper portion of the spinal cord), or nuclei of the oculomotor, trochlear, and abducens cranial nerves (see Table 14-6). Drugs, retinal disease, and diseases involving the cervical cord also may produce nystagmus. Acquired untreated nystagmus can lead to loss of visual acuity.[162]

Paralysis of specific extraocular muscles may cause a variety of abnormalities, including limited abduction, abnormal closure of the eyelid, ptosis (drooping of the eyelid), and diplopia. The abnormalities occur as a result of unopposed muscle activity. Trauma or pressure in the area of the cranial nerves may cause paralysis of specific extraocular muscles. Diseases such as diabetes mellitus and myasthenia gravis also may affect specific extraocular muscles.

Alterations in Visual Acuity

Visual acuity is the ability to see objects in sharp detail. With advancing age the lens of the eye becomes less flexible and less adjustable. In addition, the sclera changes shape, causing light to fall on the **macula** (an opaque portion of the cornea). Thus visual acuity declines with age. Visual acuity also may change or diminish for many other reasons. Specific causes of visual acuity changes include (1) amblyopia, (2) scotoma, (3) cataracts, (4) papilledema, (5) dark adaptation, (6) glaucoma, (7) retinal detachment, and (8) macular degeneration.

Amblyopia is a reduction or dimness of vision for unknown reasons. It does not result from a change in refraction (i.e., deviation of light rays) or from any visible changes in the eye. Amblyopia is associated with diseases such as diabetes mellitus, renal failure, and malaria and with toxic substances such as alcohol and tobacco. Amblyopia is the most common cause of vision loss in children.[163]

A **scotoma** is a circumscribed defect of the central field of vision. It is most often a sequel to **retrobulbar neuritis**, an inflammatory lesion of the optic nerve frequently associated with multiple sclerosis (see Chapter 16). Less common causes include the compression of one optic nerve by a retroorbital tumor, neuromyelitis optica (inflammation of the optic nerve), pernicious anemia, and toxic or metabolic causes such as methyl alcohol poisoning and use of tobacco. The precise mechanisms for these conditions causing a scotoma are uncertain, but the result is always a serious impairment in visual acuity that may be related to oxidation of crystallin proteins.[164]

A **cataract** is a cloudy or opaque area in the ocular lens. The incidence of cataracts increases with age as the lens enlarges. Cataracts develop because of alterations of metabolism and transport of nutrients within the lens. Although the most common form of cataract is degenerative, cataracts also may occur congenitally as a result of infection, radiation, trauma, drugs, or diabetes mellitus. Cataracts cause decreased visual acuity, blurred vision, glare, and decreased color perception. Cataracts are treated by removal of the entire lens and replacement with an artificial lens.[165]

Papilledema is edema and inflammation of the optic nerve at its point of entrance into the eyeball. Generally, papilledema is caused by some obstruction to the venous return from the retina. An early sign is distention of the retinal vein. Obliteration of the physiologic cup (a bright area normally located in the center of the optic disc) follows. Later the optic disc becomes raised above the level of the surrounding retina, and the margins become blurred and indistinct. With severe swelling, hemorrhage and patches of white exudate develop around the disc margins. The three principal causes of papilledema are (1) increased intracranial pressure, (2) retrobulbar neuritis, and (3) changes in the retinal blood vessels. Retinal blood vessel changes are especially prevalent in individuals with diabetes mellitus or hypertension. Such changes account for a large percentage of individuals newly affected with blindness each year. Typically the blood vessels narrow, and hemorrhages and white exudate appear. Ultimately papilledema occurs.

Dark adaptation also affects visual acuity. Low illumination causes impaired visual acuity, particularly in the elderly. The average 80-year-old needs more than twice as much light as a 20-year-old to see equally well. Changes in the quantity and quality of rhodopsin, a substance found in the rods and responsible for low-light vision, are thought to be responsible for reduced dark adaptation in older adults.[166] Vitamin A deficiencies can cause the same phenomenon in individuals of any age.

Glaucoma is characterized by intraocular pressures above the normal pressures of 12 to 20 mmHg maintained by the aqueous fluid. Genetic causes of glaucoma have recently been reported and genetic testing used for diagnosis is producing promising results.[167] The mechanisms of intraocular fluid accumulation are summarized in Figure 15-15. Chronic increased intraocular pressure first causes loss of peripheral vision, followed by central vision impairment and blindness.[168] Extremely high pressures can cause blindness within days or hours. Loss of visual acuity results from pressure on the optic nerve, which is believed to block the flow of cytoplasm from neuronal bodies in the retina to peripheral optic nerve fibers entering the brain. Lack of nutrients, ischemia, cytotoxic factors and altered immune mechanisms may lead to death of the involved neurons.[169] Acute pain may result. The types of glaucoma are summarized in Table 15-6. Early detection and treatment prevents optic neuropathy and visual impairment. Glaucoma often is treated with eye drops to reduce secretion or increase absorption of aqueous humor. Surgery may be needed to open the spaces of the trabeculae[170] and reduce intraocular pressure. Neuroprotective therapies are being evaluated.[171]

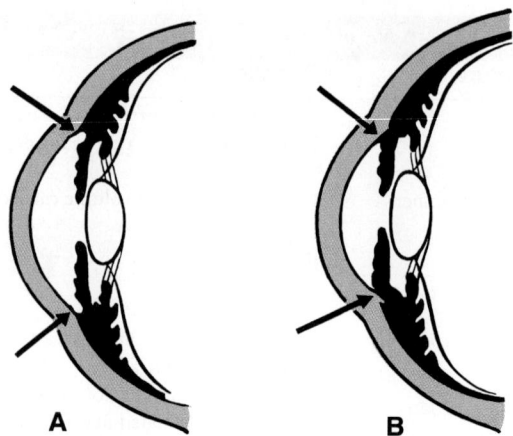

Figure 15-15 Glaucoma. **A,** Open-angle glaucoma. The obstruction to aqueous flow lies in the trabecular meshwork. **B,** Closed-angle glaucoma. The trabecular meshwork is covered by the root of the iris. (From Stein HA, Slatt BJ, Stein RM: *The ophthalmic assistant: fundamentals in clinical practice,* St Louis, 1988, Mosby.)

Retinal detachment is a common cause of visual impairment and blindness. Risk factors include retinal holes and vitreoretinal traction. Fluid (exudate, hemorrhage, or liquid vitreous) separates the photoreceptors from the retinal pigment epithelium. The separation deprives the outer retina of oxygen and nutrients because the diffusion distance is increased. Communication is also disrupted between the pigment epithelium and photoreceptors. Rhegmatogenous **retinal detachment** (retinal breaks caused by vitreoretinal traction) is the most common form of retinal detachment. Causes include intracapsular cataract extraction, severe myopia, lattice degeneration, vitreoretinal traction, and trauma. Contraction of fibrous membranes can cause tractional separation of the retinal layers as occurs in proliferative diabetic retinopathy.[172]

Age-related macular degeneration (AMD), loss of central vision, is the major cause of vision loss in individuals over age 60 years. Hypertension, cigarette smoking, and diabetes mellitus are risk factors that contribute to oxidative stress and capillary injury.[173] The atropic form of AMD involves loss of retinal pigment epithelium and photoreceptors with overall atrophy of cells. The wet exudative form involves proliferation of abnormal choroidal vessels, which leak and bleed causing retinal detachment.[174] Symptoms include blurred vision, difficulty reading, and poor night vision. Progress is being made in new treatments and in understanding genetic factors contributing to AMD.[175]

Alterations in Accommodation

Accommodation is the process whereby the thickness of the lens changes. Accommodation is needed for clear vision and is mediated through the oculomotor nerve. Pressure, inflammation, and disease of the oculomotor nerve may alter accommodation. Symptoms include diplopia, blurred vision, and headache. Accommodation is affected also by the decreased flexibility of the lens that occurs with aging. By 60 years of age the lens has become so inelastic that accommodation is not possible.

Table 15-6	Types of Glaucoma
Type	**Mechanism of Increased Pressure**
Open-angle glaucoma	Obstruction to outflow of aqueous humor at trabecular meshwork or Schlemm canal; myopia is a risk factor
Narrow-angle glaucoma (angle closure)	Forward displacement of iris toward cornea with narrowing of iridocorneal angle and obstruction to outflow of aqueous humor from anterior chamber
Acute angle closure glaucoma	Acute closure of iridocorneal angle with a sudden rise in intraocular pressure, producing nerve pain and visual disturbances

Loss of accommodation in older adults is termed **presbyopia,** a condition in which the ocular lens becomes larger, firmer, and less elastic. The major symptom is reduced near vision, causing the individual to hold reading material at arm's length. Correction is accomplished through reading glasses or bifocal lenses, accomodative intraocular lenses, or surgical treatment.[176,177]

Alterations in Refraction

Alterations in refraction are the most common visual problem. Errors in refraction are caused by irregularities of the corneal curvature, the focusing power of the lens, and the length of the eye. The major symptoms of refraction alterations are blurred vision and headache. Three types of refraction alterations are myopia, hyperopia, and astigmatism (Figure 15-16).

In **myopia** (nearsightedness), light rays are focused in front of the retina when the person is looking at a distant object resulting in burred vision. A concave lens is needed for correction. Myopia requires frequent changes of eyeglasses while the eyeball is lengthening in childhood. Myopia is a risk factor for retinal detachment.

In **hyperopia** (farsightedness), light rays are focused behind the retina when the person is looking at a near object. Hyperopia is corrected with a convex lens. **Astigmatism** is caused by an unequal curvature of the cornea. In astigmatism, light rays are bent unevenly and do not come to a single focus on the retina. Astigmatism may coexist with myopia, hyperopia, or presbyopia. Correction is accomplished with a cylinder lens.

Alterations in Color Vision

Normal sensitivity to color diminishes with age because of the progressive yellowing of the lens that occurs with aging. All colors become less intense, although color discrimination for blue and green is most greatly affected. Color vision deteriorates more rapidly for individuals with diabetes mellitus than for the general population. The deterioration is thought to be an accelerated version of senile color vision deterioration.

Abnormal color vision also may be caused by **color blindness,** an inherited trait. Color blindness is generally an X-linked, recessive characteristic affecting 8% of the male population and 0.5% of the female population. Although many forms of color blindness exist, most commonly the affected individual cannot distinguish red from green.[178,179]

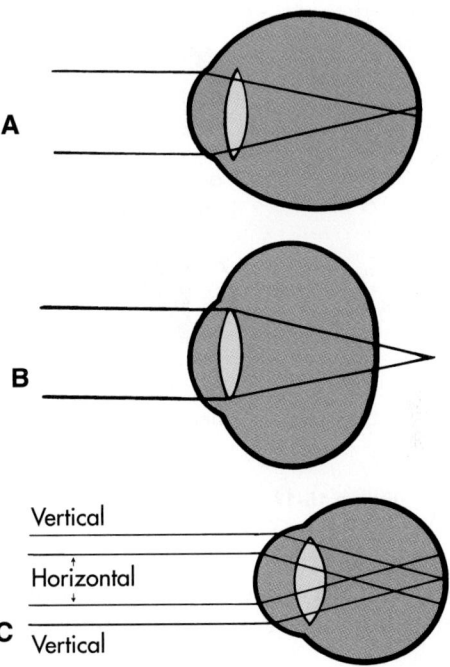

Figure 15-16 Alterations in refraction. **A,** Myopic eye. Parallel rays of light are brought to a focus in front of the retina. **B,** Hyperopic eye. Parallel rays of light come to a focus behind the retina in the unaccommodative eye. **C,** Simple myopic astigmatism. The vertical bundle of rays is focused on the retina; the horizontal rays are focused in front of the retina. (From Stein HA, Slatt BJ, Stein RM: *The ophthalmic assistant: fundamentals in clinical practice,* St Louis, 1988, Mosby.)

Neurologic Disorders Causing Visual Dysfunction

Various neurologic disorders may cause visual dysfunction. Vision may be disrupted at many points along the visual pathway, causing a variety of defects in fields of vision. Visual changes do not always cause defects or blindness in the entire visual field; **hemianopia** is the term that describes defective vision in half of a visual field. (Figure 15-17 illustrates the many areas along the visual pathway that may be damaged and the associated visual changes.)

Because of the anatomy of the optic nerves, injury to the optic nerve causes ipsilateral (same side) blindness but a normal contralateral (opposite side) visual field. Injury to the **optic chiasm** (the X-shaped crossing of the optic nerves), often caused by atherosclerotic ischemia or external compression from trauma or aneurysm, can cause a variety of defects, depending on the location of injury. These defects vary because

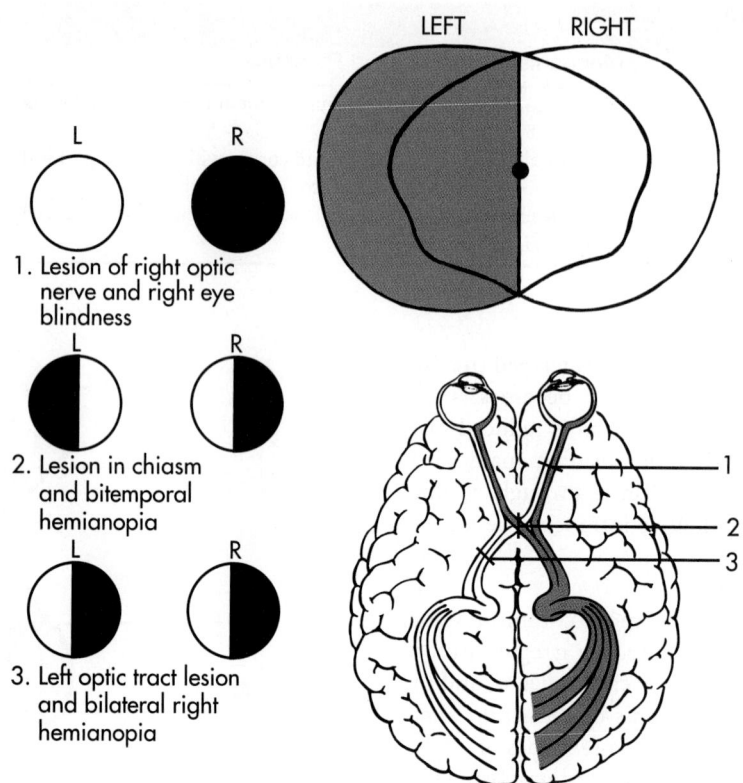

1. Lesion of right optic nerve and right eye blindness

2. Lesion in chiasm and bitemporal hemianopia

3. Left optic tract lesion and bilateral right hemianopia

Figure 15-17 **Visual pathway defects.** (From Thompson JM et al: *Mosby's clinical nursing,* ed 5, St Louis, 2002, Mosby.)

at the optic chiasm, nerve fibers from the medial half of each retina separate from the lateral half and enter the opposite optic tract.

Because of the normal structure of the visual pathways, destruction of one optic tract causes **homonymous hemianopsia** (complete loss of vision in the inner half of one eye and the outer half of the other). Thus, if an injury to the left optic tract occurs, the individual is blind in the right eye's medial (inner) field and the left eye's lateral (outer) field. If the compression of the optic tract is asymmetric, an incongruous (or uneven) homonymous defect results. Injury to one optic radiation (an ocular pathway in the internal capsule, temporal lobe, or occipital lobe) also causes a homonymous (same field) defect. A major injury in the optic radiation causes homonymous hemianopsia. A lesser injury may cause an upper quadrant homonymous defect. Generally the defects are the same size in both eyes. When the homonymous hemianopsia is caused by an occipital lobe lesion, the area of hemianopsia is split. Although visual acuity may remain unimpaired, reading is difficult because of the inability to group words.

Hearing

The **external auditory canal** is surrounded by the bones of the cranium. Its opening (meatus) is just above the **mastoid process,** which contains air-filled sinuses called **mastoid air cells.** These promote conductivity between the external and the middle ear.

The Normal Ear

The ear is divided into three areas: (1) the external ear, involved only with hearing; (2) the middle ear, involved only with hearing; and (3) the inner ear, involved with both hearing and equilibrium.

The external ear is composed of the **pinna** (auricle), which is the visible portion of the ear, and the external auditory canal, a tube that leads to the middle ear (Figure 15-18). Sound waves entering the external auditory canal hit the **tympanic membrane** (eardrum) and cause it to vibrate. The tympanic membrane separates the external ear from the middle ear.

The middle ear is composed of the **tympanic cavity,** a small chamber in the temporal bone. Three ossicles (small bones) transmit the vibration of the tympanic membrane to the inner ear. The three ossicles are termed the **malleus (hammer), incus (anvil),** and **stapes (stirrup).** When the tympanic membrane moves, the malleus moves with it and transfers the vibration to the incus, which passes it on to the stapes. The stapes presses against the **oval window,** a small membrane of the inner ear. The movement of the oval window sets the fluids of the inner ear in motion (Figure 15-19).

The **eustachian (pharyngotympanic) tube** connects the middle ear with the thorax. Normally flat and closed, the eustachian tube opens briefly when a person swallows or yawns, and it equalizes the pressure in the middle ear with atmospheric pressure. Equalized pressure permits the tympanic membrane to vibrate freely. Through the eustachian tube the

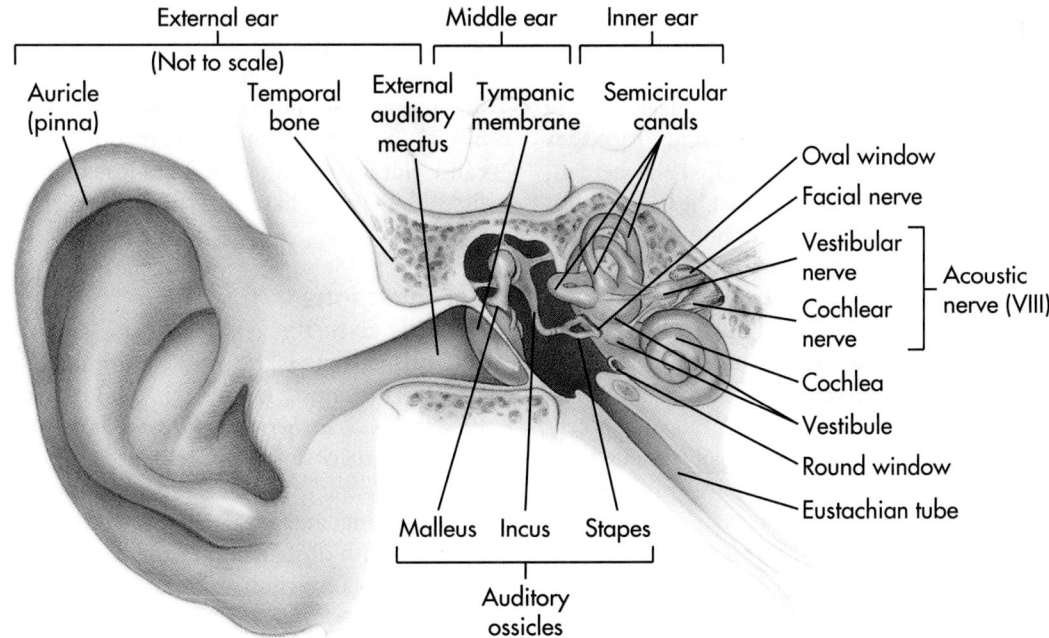

Figure 15-18 The ear. External, middle, and inner ear structures. (Anatomic structures are not drawn to scale. Middle and inner ear enlarged for better visualization here) (From Thibodeau GA, Patton KT: *Anatomy & physiology,* ed 5, St Louis, 2003, Mosby.)

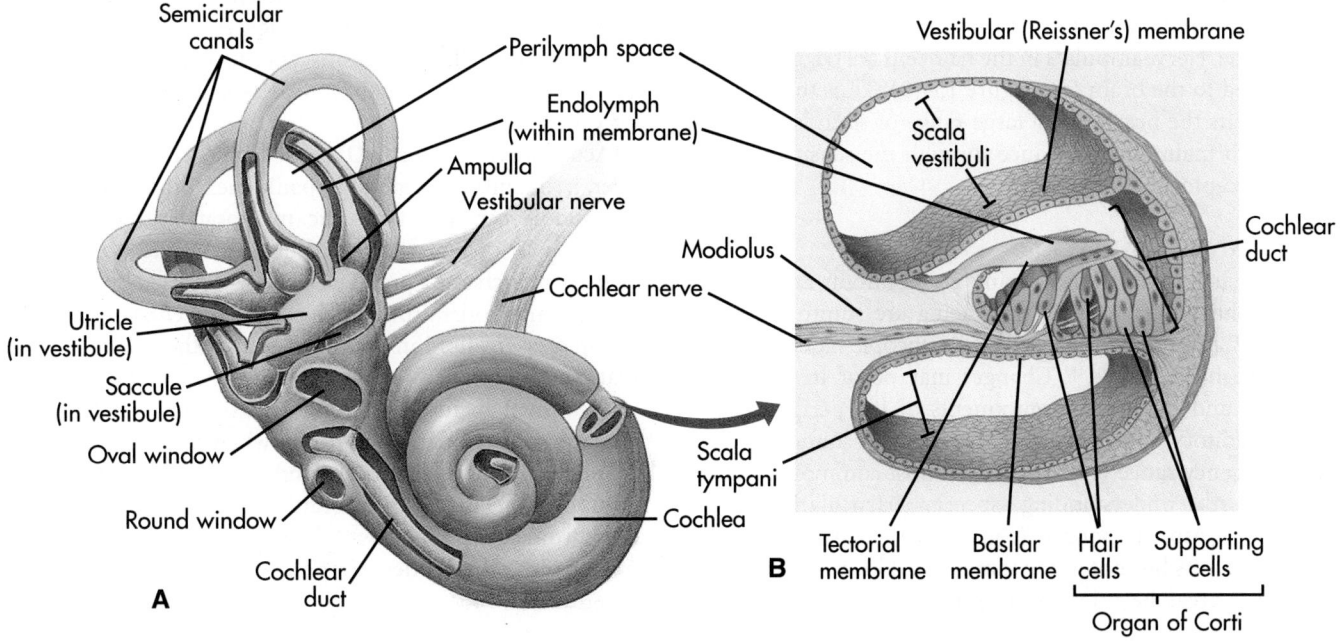

Figure 15-19 The inner ear. A, The bony labyrinth *(orange)* is the hard outer wall of the entire inner ear and includes semicircular canals, vestibule, and cochlea. Within the bony labyrinth is the membranous labyrinth *(purple),* which is surrounded by perilymph and filled with endolymph. Each ampulla in the vestibule contains a crista ampullaris that detects changes in head position and sends sensory impulses through the vestibular nerve to the brain. **B,** The inset shows a section of the membranous cochlea. Hair cells in the organ of Corti detect sound and send the information through the cochlear nerve. The vestibular and cochlear nerves join to form the eighth cranial nerve. (From Thibodeau GA, Patton KT: *Anatomy & physiology,* ed 5, St Louis, 2003, Mosby.)

mucosa of the middle ear is contiguous with the mucosal lining of the throat.

The inner ear is a system of osseous labyrinths (bony, mazelike chambers) filled with a fluid called **perilymph.** The bony labyrinth is divided into the **cochlea,** the **vestibule,** and the **semicircular canals** (see Figure 15-18). Suspended in the

perilymph is a membranous labyrinth that basically follows the shape of the bony labyrinth. The membranous labyrinth is filled with a thicker fluid called **endolymph.**

Within the cochlea is the **organ of Corti,** which contains **hair cells** (hearing receptors). Sound waves that reach the cochlea through vibrations of the tympanic membrane, ossicles, and oval window set the cochlear fluids into motion. Receptor cells on the basilar membrane are stimulated when their hairs are bent or pulled by the movement. Once stimulated, hair cells transmit impulses along the cochlear nerve (a division of the vestibulocochlear nerve) to the auditory cortex of the temporal lobe in the brain (see Figure 15-19), where interpretation of the sound occurs. Directional hearing is controlled by the angle of the sound source to both ears and axonal delay in conduction in groups of neurons.[180]

The semicircular canals and vestibule of the inner ear contain **equilibrium receptors.** In the semicircular canals the dynamic equilibrium receptors respond to changes in direction of movement. Within each semicircular canal is the **crista ampullaris,** a receptor region composed of a tuft of hair cells covered by a gelatinous cupula. When the head is rotated, the endolymph in the canal lags behind and moves in the direction opposite to the head's movement. The hair cells are stimulated, and impulses are transmitted through the vestibular nerve (a division of the vestibulocochlear nerve) to the cerebellum.

The vestibule in the inner ear contains maculae, receptors essential to the body's sense of static equilibrium. As the head moves, **otoliths** (small pieces of calcium salts) move in a gel-like material in response to changes in the pull of gravity. The otoliths pull on the gel, which in turn pulls on the hair cells in the maculae. Nerve impulses in the hair cells are triggered and transmitted to the brain (see Figure 15-19). Thus the ear not only permits the hearing of a large range of sounds but also assists with maintaining balance through the sensitive equilibrium receptors.

AGING AND HEARING

Auditory changes caused by aging are common and incremental. Changes in hearing with aging are summarized in Table 15-7. Approximately one third of people older than 65 years have hearing loss.[181] Changes may occur in both the structural and functional components of the peripheral or central auditory system. Loss of hearing for sounds in the high-frequency range (presbycusis) is most common and interferes with understanding speech, particularly high-frequency consonant sounds (e.g., *s, sh, f*). Hearing may be lost in both ears but not at the same time. Elderly individuals from rural areas have less hearing loss than those in noisy cities. The ability to discriminate localization of sound varies with high and low frequencies and diminishes with age.[182] In the low-frequency range, sound localization is a function of the timing of sound arrival between the two ears; localization of high-frequency sounds is a function of sound intensity. Because elderly individuals tend to lose high-frequency hearing first, they may have difficulty localizing high-frequency sounds.

Ear Infections

Otitis Externa

Otitis externa is the most common infection of the outer ear.[183] The most frequently found microorganisms are *Pseudomonas, Escherichia coli,* and *Staphylococcus aureus.* Infection usually follows prolonged exposure to moisture (swimmer's ear). The earliest symptoms are inflammation with swelling and clear drainage progressing to purulent drainage with obstruction of the canal. Tenderness and pain with earlobe retraction accompany inflammation.

Otitis Media

Otitis media is the most common infection of infants and children. Most children have one episode by 3 years of age. The most common pathogens are *Streptococcus pneumoniae, Haemophilus influenzae,* and *Moraxella catarrhalis.* Respiratory viruses also may have an etiologic role.[184,185] Predisposing factors include allergy, sinusitis, submucous cleft palate, adenoidal hypertrophy, and immune deficiency. Breast-feeding is a protective factor.

Acute otitis media (AOM) is associated with ear pain, fever, irritability, inflamed tympanic membrane, and fluid in the middle ear. The tympanic membrane progresses from erythema to opaqueness with bulging as fluid accumulates. There is an increasing prevalence of AOM caused by penicillin-resistant microorganisms. Otitis media with effusion (OME) is the presence of fluid in the middle ear without symptoms of acute infection.

Treatment includes antimicrobial therapy for AOM and placement of tympanotomy tubes when there is bilateral effusion persistent for 3 months and significant hearing loss.[186] Complications include mastoiditis, brain abscess, meningitis, and chronic otitis media with hearing loss. Speech, language, and cognitive disabilities may be affected by persistent middle ear effusions.[187]

Table 15-7	Changes in Hearing Caused by Aging	
Changes in Structure	**Changes in Function**
Cochlear hair cell degeneration	Inability to hear high-frequency sounds (presbycusis, sensorineural loss); interferes with understanding speech; hearing may be lost in both ears at different times
Loss of auditory neurons in spiral ganglia of organ of Corti	Inability to hear high-frequency sounds (presbycusis, sensorineural loss); interferes with understanding speech; hearing may be lost in both ears at different times
Degeneration of basilar (cochlear) conductive membrane of cochlea	Inability to hear at all frequencies, but more pronounced at higher frequencies (cochlear conductive loss)
Decreased vascularity of cochlea	Equal loss of hearing at all frequencies (strial loss); inability to disseminate localization of sound
Loss of cortical auditory neurons	Equal loss of hearing at all frequencies (strial loss); inability to disseminate localization of sound

Auditory Dysfunction

Between 5% and 10% of the general population have a hearing impairment. The major categories of auditory dysfunction are conductive hearing loss, sensorineural hearing loss, mixed hearing loss, and functional hearing loss.

Conductive Hearing Loss

A **conductive hearing loss** occurs when a change in the outer or middle ear impairs sound from being conducted from the outer to the inner ear. Conductive hearing loss occurs when there is interference in air conduction. Conditions that commonly cause a conductive hearing loss include impacted cerumen, foreign bodies lodged in the ear canal, benign tumors of the middle ear, carcinoma of the external auditory canal or middle ear, eustachian tube dysfunction, otitis media, acute viral otitis media, chronic suppurative otitis media, cholesteatoma, and otosclerosis.

Symptoms of conductive hearing loss include diminished hearing and soft speaking voice. The voice is soft because often the individual hears his or her voice, conducted by bone, as loud. In addition, although the cause is unknown, the individual often hears better in a noisy environment than in a quiet one (a condition called *paracusia willisiana*). Treatment of the underlying cause generally improves hearing.[188] A hearing aid is used if the hearing loss is greater than 40 to 50 decibels.

Sensorineural Hearing Loss

A **sensorineural hearing loss** is caused by impairment of the organ of Corti or its central connections. The hearing loss may be gradual or sudden. Conditions that commonly cause sensorineural hearing loss include congenital and hereditary factors, noise exposure, aging, Ménière disease, ototoxicity, and systemic disease (syphilis, Paget disease, collagen diseases, diabetes mellitus). Congenital and neonatal sensorineural hearing loss may be caused by maternal rubella, ototoxic drugs, prematurity, traumatic delivery, erythroblastosis fetalis, and congenital hereditary malfunction. Diagnosis often is made when delayed speech development is noted.

Presbycusis (age-related hearing loss) is the most common form of sensorineural hearing loss and is especially common in elderly people.[189,190] Presbycusis may occur because of atrophy of the basal end of the organ of Corti, a loss in the number of auditory receptors, vascular changes, or stiffening of the basilar membranes. Because of the slow progression of hearing loss, onset of symptoms is gradual. In addition, drug ototoxicities (drugs that cause destruction of auditory function) have been observed after exposure to a variety of chemicals, for example, antibiotics such as streptomycin, neomycin, gentamicin, and vancomycin; diuretics such as ethacrynic acid and furosemide; and chemicals such as salicylate, quinine, carbon monoxide, nitrogen mustard, arsenic, mercury, gold, tobacco, and alcohol. Because of increased concentrations of antibiotics in the endolymph, these drugs generally cause damage to the cells of the cristae and maculae (located in the inner ear) or the cells of the organ of Corti. The increased concentration of drugs in the endolymph is preferentially toxic to the cells.

Diuretics affect hearing primarily by altering the sodium-potassium balance, causing extracellular fluid accumulation and changes in the microstructure of secretory cells. Quinine, mercury, and lead affect the neural pathways of hearing, including the spinal ganglia, the eighth cranial nerve, and the cochlear nucleus. The site of action for the other chemicals, including alcohol and tobacco, has not yet been determined. In most instances the drugs and chemicals listed previously initially cause **tinnitus** (ringing in the ear), followed by a progressive high-tone sensorineural hearing loss. Care is aimed at prevention of further hearing loss because the loss is usually permanent.

Mixed Hearing Loss

A **mixed hearing loss** is caused by a combination of conductive and sensorineural losses.

Functional Hearing Loss

A **functional hearing loss** occurs for no organic reason. The individual does not respond to voice and appears not to hear. Functional hearing loss is thought to be caused by emotional or psychologic factors. It occurs only rarely.

Olfaction and Taste

Olfaction is a function of cranial nerve I and part of cranial nerve V. Taste is a function of multiple nerves in the tongue, soft palate, uvula, pharynx, and upper esophagus, including cranial nerves VII and IX. Olfaction (smell) dysfunction and taste (gustation) dysfunction may occur separately or jointly. The strong relationship between smell and taste creates the sensation of flavor. If either sensation is impaired, the perception of flavor is altered. (Olfactory structures are illustrated in Figure 15-20.)

Olfactory cells, which are located in the olfactory epithelium, are the receptor cells for smell. Seven primary classes of olfactory stimulants have been identified: (1) camphoraceous, (2) musky, (3) floral, (4) peppermint, (5) ethereal, (6) pungent, and (7) putrid. The primary sensations of taste are sour, salty, sweet, and bitter. Taste buds sensitive to each of the primary sensations are located in specific areas of the tongue.[191]

AGING AND OLFACTION AND TASTE

Olfaction

Sensitivity to odors declines steadily with aging.[192] A study of odor identification indicates an increasing ability from childhood to adolescence and then a decline after 60 years of age. The most significant impairments develop after 80 years.[193] Women generally have better olfactory abilities than men, but the patterns of decline are similar.[194]

The sense of smell begins to degenerate with loss of olfactory sensory neurons and loss of cells from the olfactory bulbs.[195,195a] Loss of olfactory sensitivity and odor identification may diminish appetite and food selection and thus may lead to malnutrition. Safety also may be compromised by an inability to smell toxic or hazardous gases.

Taste

The decline in taste sensation is more gradual than that of smell. Higher concentrations of flavors are required, and elderly persons have difficulty differentiating combinations of

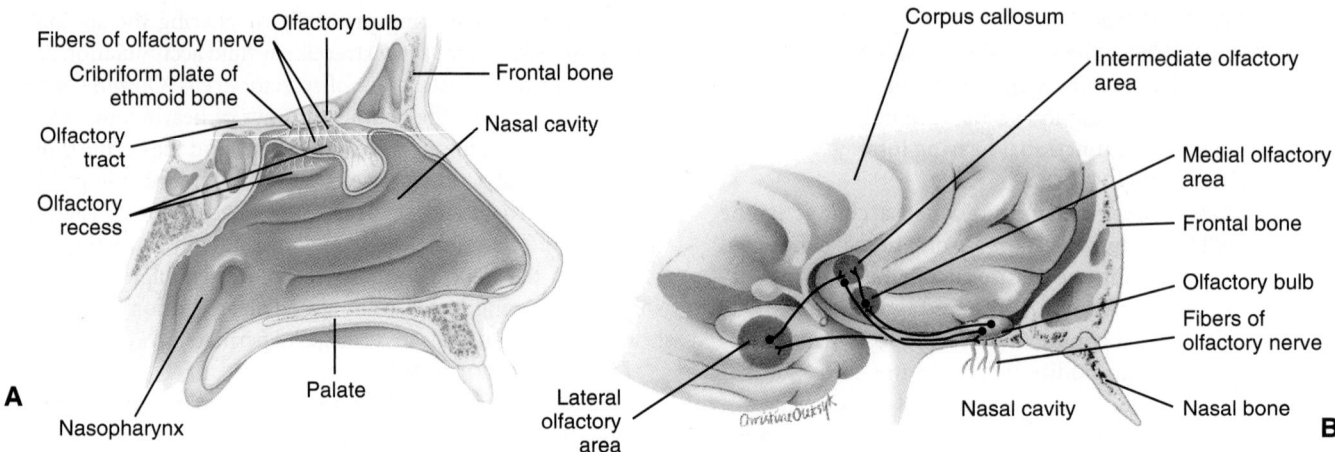

Figure 15-20 Olfaction. Location of olfactory epithelium, olfactory bulb, and neuronal pathways involved in olfaction. **A,** Midsagittal section of the nasal area shows the locations of major olfactory sensory structures. **B,** Major olfactory integration centers of the brain. (Modified from Thibodeau GA, Patton KT: *Anatomy & physiology*, ed 5, St Louis, 2003, Mosby.)

flavors.[196] The best-known change with aging is the decline in the number of fungiform papillae on the tongue, which decrease by 50% by about 50 years of age.[159] Taste also may be affected by decreased salivary gland secretion. Amylase, contained in saliva, facilitates perception of sweet sensations and also is reduced with aging.

Olfactory Dysfunction

Olfactory dysfunctions include hyposmia, anosmia, hallucinations, and parosmia. **Hyposmia** is the impaired sense of smell, and **anosmia** is the complete loss of smell. When hyposmia or anosmia occurs bilaterally, it is usually the result of rhinitis (inflammation of nasal mucosa), sinusitis, nasal polyps, or excessive smoking.[197] Unilateral hyposmia or anosmia may indicate compression of one olfactory bulb (a bulb-like portion of the olfactory nerves) or nerve tract (olfactory nerve pathway), possibly by tumor or head trauma. **Olfactory hallucinations** arise from hyperactivity in cortical neurons and involve smelling odors that are not really present. They are associated with temporal lobe seizures and rarely with schizophrenia. **Parosmia,** an abnormal or perverted sense of smell, may occur with severe depression.[198]

Taste Dysfunction

The sense of taste can be impaired by injury, medications, oral infections, or aging. An alteration in taste also may be attributable to impairment of smell associated with injury near the hippocampus.

Hypogeusia is decrease in taste sensation, and **ageusia** is the absence of taste. Ageusia affecting the entire tongue may follow head injury. Damage to the glossopharyngeal nerve (cranial nerve IX, which innervates the posterior one third of the tongue) causes the loss of the ability to detect bitterness. This loss occurs because the receptors for bitter are located on the base of the tongue. Damage to the facial nerve (cranial nerve VII, which innervates the anterior two thirds of the

tongue) causes loss of the ability to detect sour, sweet, and salt tastes. Only bitter tastes can be detected. These losses occur because sour, sweet, and salt receptors are located on the anterior portion of the tongue. **Parageusia** is a perversion of taste in which substances possess an unpleasant flavor. Parageusia occasionally develops for no apparent reason in elderly people and also is common in individuals receiving chemotherapy for cancer. In both cases, parageusia often leads to anorexia and malnutrition.

SOMATOSENSORY FUNCTION

Touch

Touch is not a uniform sensory experience. The sensation of touch involves the fusion of several qualities, including modality, intensity, location, and duration of the sensory stimulus. Receptors sensitive to touch are present in the skin. Meissner and pacinian corpuscles are rapidly adapting receptors, whereas Merkel disks and Ruffini endings are slowly adapting touch receptors. Touch receptors are most numerous in the skin of the fingers and lips and are more scarce in the skin of the trunk. Specific sensory input is carried to the higher levels of the CNS by the dorsal column of the spinal cord and the anterior spinothalamic tract.

Much of the development of the cutaneous senses takes place before birth, but structural growth of the cutaneous senses continues into early adulthood at a reduced rate. Then a gradual decline occurs. Studies have documented loss in tactile sensitivity with advancing age.[200,201] This occurs simultaneously with an increase in the size of pacinian corpuscles and a decrease in the number of corpuscles.

Abnormal tactile perception may be caused by alterations at any level of the nervous system, from the receptor to the cerebral cortex. Any factor that interrupts or impairs reception, transmission, perception, or interpretation of touch also alters tactile sensation. Trauma, tumor, infection, metabolic changes, vascular changes, and degenerative diseases thus may cause tactile dysfunction, which may involve heightened or diminished tactile perceptions.

In addition, most tactile sensations evoke affective responses that determine whether the sensation is unpleasant, pleasant, or neutral. Cerebral and hypothalamic centers influence this response. Sedative drugs and prefrontal injury, which interrupt connections between the prefrontal cortex and subcortical centers, diminish the interpretation of tactile sensations.

Proprioception

Perception and awareness of the position of the body and its parts depend on impulses from the inner ear and from receptors in joints and ligaments. The role of muscle, tendon, and cutaneous receptors is indefinite. Sensory data are transmitted to higher centers, primarily through the dorsal columns and the spinocerebellar tracts, with some data passing through the medial lemnisci and thalamic radiations to the cortex. These stimuli are necessary for the coordination of movements, the grading of muscular contraction, and the maintenance of equilibrium.

A progressive loss of proprioception has been reported in elderly persons.[202] Proprioceptive dysfunction may be caused by alterations at any level of the nervous system. As with tactile dysfunction, any factor that interrupts or impairs the reception, transmission, perception, or interpretation of proprioceptive stimuli also alters proprioception. Two common causes of proprioceptive dysfunction are vestibular dysfunction and neuropathy.

Specific vestibular dysfunctions are vestibular nystagmus and vertigo. **Vestibular nystagmus** is the constant, involuntary movement of the eyeball caused by ear disturbances. This condition occurs when the semicircular canal system is overstimulated. **Vertigo** is the sensation of spinning that occurs with inflammation of the semicircular canals in the ear. The individual may feel either that he or she is moving in space or that the world is revolving. Vertigo often causes loss of balance. Vertigo and nystagmus may occur in a variety of conditions, including labyrinthitis, vestibular neuritis, acute toxic labyrinthitis, and Ménière disease.

Ménière disease is a vestibular disorder that can cause proprioceptive dysfunction. The pathologic basis of Ménière disease is still unclear. The individual with Ménière disease may experience loss of proprioception during an acute attack, so that standing or walking is impossible.

Peripheral neuropathies also can cause proprioceptive dysfunctions. Neuropathies may be caused by a variety of conditions and commonly are associated with renal disease and diabetes mellitus. Although the exact sequence of events is unknown, neuropathies are thought to be caused by a metabolic disturbance of the neuron itself. The result is a diminished or absent sense of body position or position of body parts. Gait changes often occur. (Neuropathies are further discussed in Chapter 16.)

SUMMARY REVIEW

Pain

1. Pain is a complex phenomenon composed of sensory experiences (time, space, intensity) and emotion, cognition, and motivation.
2. The gate control theory of pain describes the modulation of pain in the dorsal horn of the spinal cord by both sensory afferent stimulation and central descending impulses that influence the "pain gate." According to the gate control theory, specialized cells within the substantia gelatinosa of the spinal cord act as a gate, opening and closing the afferent pathways to transmission of painful stimuli.
3. The portions of the nervous system responsible for the sensation and perception of pain may be divided into three areas: (a) the afferent fibers, (b) the afferent pathways and (c) the central nervous system.
4. The afferent system is composed of nociceptors, Aδ and C fibers (first order neurons), the dorsal horn of the spinal column (second order neurons), and afferent neurons in the spinothalamic tract (third order neurons).
5. Nociceptors detect a wide range of stimuli and respond to chemical, mechanical, and thermal stimulation.
6. Myelinated Aδ receptor transmission is fast and conveys mechanical and thermal sharp, localized pain. Unmyelinated polymodal C fiber transmission is slower and conveys diffuse burning and aching sensations.
7. There are three classes of second order neurons that modulate pain transmission: projection cells, excitatory interneurons, and inhibitory interneurons. The second order neurons are located in the spinal cord laminae and function as a "pain gate" to regulate pain transmission.
8. Second order neurons cross over the cord and ascend primarily in the lateral spinothalamic tract to projection centers including the reticular formation, periacquaductal gray matter and thalamus.
9. Third order neurons carry information to the sensory cortex and reticular and limbic systems for pain processing and interpretation.
10. Efferent pathways from the periaqueductal gray are responsible for modulation or inhibition of afferent pain signals. The thalamus, cortex, and postcentral gyrus perceive, describe, and localize pain. The reticular formation and limbic system control the emotional and affective response to pain.
11. Pain can be modulated by segmental inhibition, which is the peripheral stimulation of nociceptors by touch, vibration, or pressure resulting in closure of the spinal cord "pain gate." Higher brain center also can influence painful stimuli (heterosegmental control of nociception) as well as inhibition from the caudal medulla (diffuse noxious inhibitory controls). Thus pain can be modulated with stimulation from the periphery or by descending impulses from the brain.
12. Pain neurotransmitter, can be classified as inflammatory, excitatory, inhibitory and as modulators of pain. Inflammatory neurotransmitters include prostaglandins, nitric oxide, bradykinins and histamine. Glutamate, aspartate, and amino acid precursors are excitatory neurotransmitters. Endogenous opioids inhibit pain transmission and are present in varying concentrations in the neurons of the brain, spinal cord, and gastrointestinal tract. Serotonin, norepinephrine aspartate, glycine also can modulate pain processing.

Continued

13. Pain threshold is the point at which pain is perceived. Pain threshold does not vary significantly among people or within the same person over time.

14. Pain tolerance is the duration of time or the intensity of pain that an individual will endure before initiating overt pain response. Tolerance varies widely among individuals and in the same individual over time.

15. Classifications of pain include nociceptive pain (with a known physiologic cause), non-nociceptive pain (neuropathic pain), acute pain (signal to the person of a harmful stimulus), and chronic pain (persistence of pain of unknown cause or unusual response to therapy).

16. Acute pain may be (a) somatic (superficial), (b) visceral (internal), or (c) referred (present in an area distant from its origin). The area of referred pain is supplied by the same spinal segment as the actual site of pain.

17. Somatic pain arises from connective tissue, muscle, bone, and skin and is sharp and localized.

18. Visceral pain is transmitted by sympathetic afferents and is poorly localized.

19. Referred pain usually arises from the viscera and terminates in an area of the spinal cord that is conjoined with fibers originating in the skin and other areas and thereby produces the perception of pain at the referred site.

20. Physiologic responses to acute pain include increased heart rate, respiratory rate, and blood pressure; pallor or flushing; dilated pupils; and diaphoresis. Blood sugar is elevated; gastric secretion and motility are decreased; and blood flow to the viscera and skin is decreased.

21. Chronic pain is pain that generally lasts at least 3 months, and it may be persistant, for example, low back pain, or intermittent, for example, migraine headache.

22. Chronic pain conditions include myofascial pain syndromes, chronic postoperative pain, low back pain, and chronic pain associated with cancer.

23. Neuropathic pain is usually chronic and results from nerve trauma or disease and leads to abnormal peripheral and central pain processing. Types of neuropathic pain include deafferentiation pain, sympathetically maintained pain, central pain, and phantom pain.

24. Newborns and young children have the anatomic and functional ability to perceive pain. Pain experienced by infants may have prolonged effects on brain organization and responses to pain.

25. Older individuals may or may not have an increased in their pain threshold.. In all age-groups, women appear to be more sensitive to pain than men.

26. Pain in the elderly is influenced by liver and renal function, including alterations in metabolism of drugs and metabolites.

Temperature Regulation

1. Temperature regulation is achieved through precise balancing of heat production, heat conservation, and heat loss. Body temperature is maintained in a range around 37° C (98.6° F).

2. Temperature regulation is mediated by the hypothalamus. Peripheral thermoreceptors in the skin and central thermoreceptors in the hypothalamus, spinal cord, and abdominal organs provide the hypothalamus with information about skin and core temperatures.

3. Heat is produced through chemical reactions of metabolism, skeletal muscle contraction, and chemical thermogenesis.

4. Heat is lost through radiation, conduction, convection, vasodilation, decreased muscle tone, evaporation of sweat, increased respiration, and voluntary mechanisms.

5. Heat conservation is accomplished through vasoconstriction and voluntary mechanisms.

6. Infants and elderly persons require special attention to maintenance of body temperature. Because of their greater body surface/mass ratio and decreased subcutaneous fat, infants do not conserve heat well. Elderly individuals have poor responses to environmental temperature extremes as a result of slowed blood circulation, structural and functional changes in skin, and an overall decrease in heat-producing activities.

7. Fever is triggered by the release of pyrogens from leukocytes, bacteria, and other cells involved in the immune response. Fever is both a symptom of a disease and a normal immunologic mechanism.

8. Fever involves resetting the hypothalamic thermostat to a higher level. When the fever breaks, the set point is returned to normal.

9. Fever production aids responses to infectious processes. Higher temperatures kill many microorganisms and decrease serum levels of iron, zinc, and copper that are needed for bacterial replication.

10. Hyperthermia (marked warming of core temperature) can produce nerve damage, coagulation of cell proteins, and death. Forms of accidental hyperthermia include heat cramps, heat exhaustion, heat stroke, and malignant hyperthermia. Heat stroke and malignant hyperthermia are potentially lethal developments.

11. Hypothermia (marked cooling of core temperature) slows the rate of chemical reaction (tissue metabolism), increases the viscosity of the blood, slows blood flow through the microcirculation, facilitates blood coagulation, and stimulates profound vasoconstriction. Hypothermia may be accidental or therapeutic.

Sleep

1. Sleep may be divided into rapid eye movement (REM) and non-REM (NREM) stages, each of which has its own series of stages. While asleep, an individual progresses through REM and NREM (slow-wave) sleep in a predictable cycle.

2. Sleep is initiated by the withdrawal of neurotransmitters from the afferent formation and by the inhibition of arousal mechanisms in the cerebral cortex. REM sleep is controlled by mechanisms in the pontine reticular formation.

3. The sleep patterns of the newborn and young child vary from those of the adult in total sleep time, cycle length, and percentage of time spent in each sleep cycle. Elderly individuals experience a total decrease in sleep time.

4. During sleep the body is actively engaged in restoring and repairing itself. Sleep deprivation can cause profound changes in personality and functioning.

5. The restorative, reparative, and growth processes occur during slow-wave sleep.

6. Sleep disorders include (a) disorders of initiating sleep (insomnia), (b) sleep disordered breathing, (c) disorders of the sleep/wake schedule (jet lag, shift work), and (d) dysfunctions of sleep, sleep stages, or partial arousals (somnambulism, night terrors, or enuresis).

7. Ingestion of alcohol and some medications can alter or suppress sleep stages, producing sleep disorders.

8. Sleep and disease are interrelated. Some diseases may produce alterations in the quantity and quality of sleep or affect sleep stages. These are referred to as *secondary sleep disorders*. In some instances sleep stages produce alterations in certain disease states. These are referred to as *sleep-provoked disorders*.

SUMMARY REVIEW—cont'd

Special Senses

Vision

1. The eyelids, conjunctivae, and lacrimal apparatus protect the eye. Infections are the most common disorders; they include blepharitis, conjunctivitis, chalazion, and hordeolum.
2. Conjunctivitis can be acute or chronic, bacterial, viral, or allergic. Redness, edema, pain, and lacrimation are common symptoms. Chlamydial conjunctivitis is the leading cause of blindness in the world and is associated with poor sanitary conditions.
3. Keratitis is a bacterial or viral infection of the cornea that can lead to corneal ulceration. Photophobia, pain, and tearing are common symptoms.
4. The wall of the eye has three layers: sclera, choroid, and retina. The retina contains millions of photoreceptors known as rods and cones that receive light through the lens and then convey signals to the optic nerve and subsequently to the visual cortex of the brain.
5. The eye is filled with vitreous and aqueous humor, which prevent it from collapsing.
6. Structural eye changes caused by aging result in decreased visual acuity.
7. The major alterations in ocular movement include strabismus, nystagmus, and paralysis of the extraocular muscles.
8. Alterations in visual acuity can be caused by amblyopia, scotoma, cataracts, papilledema, macular degeneration, retinal detachment, and glaucoma.
9. Alterations in accommodation develop with increased intraocular pressure, inflammation, and disease of the oculomotor nerve. Presbyopia is loss of accommodation caused by loss of elasticity of the lens with aging.
10. Alterations in refraction, including myopia, hyperopia, and astigmatism, are the most common visual disorders.
11. Trauma or disease of the optic nerve pathways or optic radiations, can cause blindness in the visual fields. Homonymous hemianopsia is caused by damage of one optic tract.

Hearing

1. The ear is composed of external, middle, and inner structures. The external structures are the pinna, auditory canal, and tympanic membrane. The tympanic cavity (containing three bones: malleus, incus, and stapes), oval window, eustachian tube, and fluid compose the middle ear and transmit sound vibrations to the inner ear.
2. The inner ear includes the bony and membranous labyrinths that transmit sound waves through the cochlea to the division of the eighth cranial nerve. The semicircular canals and vestibule help maintain balance through the equilibrium receptors.
3. Approximately one third of all people older than 65 years have hearing loss.
4. Otitis extrerna is an infection of the outer ear. Otitis media, an infection of the middle ear, is common in children.
5. Hearing loss can be classified as conductive, sensorineural, mixed, or functional.
6. Conductive hearing loss occurs when sound waves cannot be conducted through the middle ear.
7. Sensorineural hearing loss develops with impairment of the organ of Corti or its central connections.
8. A combination of conductive and sensorineural loss is a mixed hearing loss.
9. Loss of hearing with no known organic cause is a functional hearing loss.

Olfaction and Taste

1. The perception of flavor is altered if olfaction or taste dysfunctions occur. Sensitivity to odor and taste decreases with aging.
2. Hyposmia is a decrease in the sense of smell, and anosmia is the complete loss of smell. Inflammation of the nasal mucosa and trauma or tumors of the olfactory nerve lead to a diminished sense of smell.
3. Hypogeusia is a decrease in taste sensation, and ageusia is the absence of taste. Loss of taste buds or trauma to the facial or glossopharyngeal nerves decreases taste sensation.

Somatosensory Function

1. The sensation of touch involves the fusion of several qualities, including modality, intensity, location, and duration of the sensory stimulus.
2. Receptors sensitive to touch are present in the skin; these include Meissner and pacinian corpuscles and Merkel disks and Ruffini endings. The sensory response is conducted to the brain through the dorsal column and anterior spinothalamic tract.
3. Abnormal tactile perception may be caused by alterations at any level of the nervous system, from the receptor to the cerebral cortex.
4. Proprioception is the position and location of the body and its parts. Proprioceptors are located in the inner ear, joints, and ligaments. Proprioceptive stimuli are necessary for balance, coordinated movement, and grading of muscular contraction.
5. Disorders of proprioception can be caused by alterations at any level of the nervous system. Two common causes of proprioceptive dysfunction are vestibular dysfunction and neuropathy.

KEY TERMS

Acute bacterial conjunctivitis (pinkeye), 472
Aδ fibers, 449
Acute otitis media (AOM), 480
Acute pain, 456
Age-related macular degeneration (AMD), 476
Ageusia, 482
Allergic conjunctivitis, 473
Amblyopia, 475
Anosmia, 482
Aqueous humor, 474

Astigmatism, 477
Blepharitis, 472
Cancer pain, 458
Cataract, 475
Central pain, 460
Chalazion, 472
Choroid, 473
Chronic conjunctivitis, 473
Chronic pain, 457
Chronic postoperative pain, 458
Circadian rhythm, 462

Cochlea, 479
Color blindness, 477
Complex regional pain syndromes (CRPS), 460
Conduction, 463
Conductive hearing loss, 481
Cones, 473
Convection, 463
Cornea, 473
Crista ampullaris, 480
Dark adaptation, 476

KEY TERMS—cont'd

Deafferentation pain, 460
Diffuse noxious inhibitory controls
   (DNIC), 452
Diplopia, 475
Dynorphins, 455
Endogenous cryogens, 464
Endogenous opioids, 454
Endogenous pyrogens, 464
Endolymph, 479
Endomorphins, 455
Endorphins, 455
Enkephalins, 455
Enuresis, 471
Equilibrium receptors, 480
Eustachian (pharyngotympanic) tube, 478
Exogenous pyrogens, 464
External auditory canal, 478
Fovea centralis, 473
Functional hearing loss, 481
Gate control theory, 448
Glaucoma, 476
Glutamate, 454
Hair cells, 479
Heat cramps, 466
Heat exhaustion, 466
Heat stroke, 466
Hemianopia, 477
Homonymous hemianopsia, 478
Hordeolum (stye), 472
Hyperopia, 477
Hyperthermia, 466
Hypogeusia, 482
Hyposmia, 482
Hypothermia, 467
Incus (anvil), 478
Insomnia, 470
Iris, 473
Jerk nystagmus, 475

Lens, 474
Limbic system, 452
Macula, 475
Malignant hyperthermia, 467
Malleus (hammer), 478
Mastoid air cells, 478
Mastoid process, 478
Ménière disease, 483
Mixed hearing loss, 481
Myofascial pain syndromes (MPS), 458
Myopia, 477
Neuropathic pain, 459
Night terrors, 471
Nociception, 448
Nociceptive pain, 456
Non-nociceptive pain, 456
Non-REM (slow-wave) sleep, 469
Nystagmus, 475
Obesity hypoventilation syndrome 471
Olfactory hallucination, 482
Opiate receptor, 455
Optic chiasm, 477
Optic disc, 473
Organ of Corti, 479
Otitis externa, 480
Otitis media, 480
Otoliths, 480
Oval window, 478
Pain threshold, 456
Pain tolerance, 456
Papilledema, 476
Parageusia, 482
Parasomnias, 471
Parosmia, 482
Pendular nystagmus, 475
Perceptual dominance, 456
Perilymph, 479
Phantom limb pain, 460

Pinna, 478
Presbycusis, 481
Presbyopia, 477
Pupil, 473
Radiation, 463
Rapid eye movement (REM) sleep, 469
Referred pain, 457
Reflex sympathetic dystrophy, 460
Reticular system, 452
Retina, 473
Retinal detachment, 476
Retrobulbar neuritis, 475
Rods, 473
Sclera, 473
Scotoma, 475
Secondary sleep disorders, 471
Segmental inhibition, 452
Semicircular canals, 479
Sensorineural hearing loss, 481
Sleep, 468
Sleep-provoked disorders, 471
Somatic pain, 456
Somnambulism, 471
Specificity theory, 448
Stapes (stirrup), 478
Strabismus, 475
Sympathetically maintained pain (SMP), 460
Tinnitus, 481
Trachoma, 473
Tympanic cavity, 478
Tympanic membrane, 478
Unmyelinated C polymodal nociceptors, 449
Vertigo, 483
Vestibular nystagmus, 483
Vestibule, 479
Viral conjunctivitis, 473
Visceral pain, 457
Vitreous humor, 474

MEDIA RESOURCES 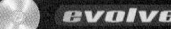 evolve

Review questions and answers for this chapter are available in the *CD Companion* included with this book.

WebLinks—links to Internet sites pertaining to this chapter—are available on Evolve at http://evolve.elsevier.com/McCance/.

REFERENCES

1. American Pain Society: www.ampainsoc.org/ce/npc/I/b_definitions.htm, accessed July 24, 2004.
2. McCaffery M: Understanding your patient's pain, *Nursing* 10(9):26-31, 1980.
3. Waddell G: *The back pain revolution*, ed 2, London, 2004, Churchill Livingstone.
4. Melzack R, Wall PD: Pain mechanisms: a new theory, *Science* 150:971, 1965.
5. Melzack R, Wall PD: Pain mechanisms: a new theory, *Science* 150: 971-979, 1965.
6. Clapham DE: TRP channels as cellular sensors, *Nature* 426(6966): 517-524, 2003.
7. Rexed B: A cytoarchitectural atlas of the spinal cord in the cat, *J Comp Neurol* 100:297, 1954.
8. Willis WD, Coggeshall RE: *Sensory mechanisms of the spinal cord*, ed 3, New York, 2004, Kluwer.
9. Romanelli P, Esposito V: The functional anatomy of neuropathic pain, *Neurosurg Clin N Am* 15(3):257-268, 2004.
9a. Herrero MT, Barcia C, Navarro JM: Functional anatomy of thalamus and basal ganglia, *Childs Nerv Syst* 18(8):386-404, 2002.
10. Partridge LD: *Nervous system actions and interactions : concepts in neurophysiology*, Boston, 2003, Kluwer.
11. Villemure C, Bushnell MC: Cognitive modulation of pain: how do attention and emotion influence pain processing? *Pain* 95(3):195-199, 2002.
12. Mayer DJ, Price DD: Central nervous system mechanisms of analgesia, *Pain* 2(4):379-404, 1976.
13. Ruda MA, Bennett GJ, Dubner R: Neurochemistry and neurocircuitry in the dorsal horn, *Prog Brain Res* 66:219-268, 1986.
14. Hughes J et al: Identification of two related pentapeptides from the brain with potent opiate agonist activity, *Nature* 258(5536):577-579, 1975.
15. Fields HL, Basbuam AI, Heinricher MM: Central nervous system mechanisms of pain modulation. In McMahon S, Koltzenburg M, editors: Wall and Melzack's *Textbook of pain*, ed 5, Edinburgh, 2005, Churchill Livingstone. In press.
16. Rainville P: Brain mechanisms of pain affect and pain modulation, *Curr Opin Neurobiol* 12(2):195-204, 2002.
17. Villenueva L, Le Bars D: The activation of bulbospinal controls by peripheral nociceptive inputs: diffuse noxious inhibitory controls (DNIC), *Biol Res* 28:113-125, 1995.

18. Fields HL, Basbuam AI, Heinricher MM: Central nervous system mechanisms of pain modulation. In McMahon S, Koltzenburg M, editors: Wall and Melzack's *Textbook of pain,* ed 5, Edinburgh, 2005, Churchill Livingstone. In press.

19. Ploghaus A et al: Neural circuitry underlying pain modulation: expectation, hypnosis, placebo, *Trends Cogn Sci* 7(5):197-200, 2003.

20. Petrovic P et al: Placebo and opioid analgesia—imaging a shared neuronal network, *Science* 295:1737-1740, 2002.

21. Sorkin LS, Wallace MS: Acute pain mechanisms, *Surg Clin North Am* 79(2):213-229, 1999.

22. von Zastrow M: Opioid receptor regulation, *Neuromolecular Med* 5(1):51-58, 2004.

23. Wollemann M, Benyhe S: Non-opioid actions of opioid peptides, *Life Sci* 75(3):257-270, 2004.

24. Laughlin TM, Larson AA, Wilcox GL: Mechanisms of induction of persistent nicoception by dynorphin, *J Pharmacol Exp Ther* 299(1):6-11, 2001.

25. Horvath G: Endomorphin-1 and endomorphin-2: pharmacology of the selective endogenous μ-opiod receptor agonists, *Pharmacol Ther* 88(3):437-463, 2000.

26. Bodnar RJ, Hadjimarkou MM: Endogenous opiates and behavior: 2002, *Peptides* 24(8):1241-1302, 2003.

27. Deleted in proofs.

28. Coward DD, Wilkie DJ: Metastatic bone pain: meanings associated with self-report and self-management decision making, *Cancer Nurs* 23(2):101-108, 2000.

29. Purves D et al: *Neuroscience,* ed 3, Sunderland, Mass, 2004, Sinauer Associates.

30. Thibodeau GA, Patton KT: *Anatomy & physiology,* ed 5, St Louis, 2003, Mosby.

31. Turk DC: The role of psychological factors in pain management, *Acta Anaesthesiol Scand* 43(9):885-888, 1999.

32. Turk DC, Okifuji A: Psychological factors in chronic pain: evolution and revolution, *J Consult Clin Psychol* 70(3):678-690, 2002.

33. Miles A et al: Managing constraint: the experience of people with chronic pain, *Soc Sci Med* 61(2):431-441, 2005.

34. Almay BG et al: Relationships between CSF levels of endorphins and monoamine metabolites in chronic pain patients, *Psychopharmacology* 67(2):139-142, 1980.

34a. Schaible HG, Richter F: Pathophysiology of pain, *Langenbecks Arch Surg* 389(4):237-243, 2004.

35. Whitehead W III, Kuhn WF: Chronic pain: an overview. In Miller TW, editor: *Chronic pain,* vol 1, Madison, Wis, 1990, International Universities.

36. Jones GT, Macfarlane GJ: Epidemiology of low back pain in children and adolescents, *Arch Dis Child* 90(3):312-316, 2005.

36a. Ehrlich GE: Back pain, *J Rheumatol* 67(Suppl):26-31, 2003.

37. Goudas LC et al.: The epidemiology of cancer pain, *Cancer Invest* 23(2):182-190, 2005.

37a. Seymour J, Clark D, Winslow M: Pain and palliative care: the emergence of new specialties, *J Pain Symptom Manage* 29(1):2-13, 2005.

37b. Cherny NI: The pharmacologic management of cancer pain, *Oncology (Huntingt)* 18(12):1499-1515, 2004.

37c. Fine PG et al: Meeting the challenges in cancer pain management, *J Support Oncol* 2(6 Suppl 4):5-22, 2004.

37d. Barrie J: The value of thorough assessment in the management of cancer pain, *Prof Nurse* 19(8):446-449, 2004.

38. Romanelli P, Esposito V: The functional anatomy of neuropathic pain, *Neurosurg Clin N Am* 15(3):257-268, 2004.

39. Ossipov MH et al: Spinal and supraspinal mechanisms of neuropathic pain, *Ann N Y Acad Sci* 909:12-24, 2000.

40. Woolf CJ, Salter MW: Neuronal plasticity: increasing the gain in pain, *Science* 288(5472):1765, 2000.

41. McMahon SB, Cafferty WB: Neutrophic influences on neuropathic pain, *Novartis Found Symp* 261:68-92, discussion 92-102, 149-154, 2004.

42. Ji RR, Strichartz G: Cell signaling and the genesis of neuropathic pain, *Sci STKE* 2004(252):reE14, 2004.

43. Backonja MM, Serra J:Pharmacologic management part 2: lesser-studied neuropathic pain diseases, *Pain Med* 5(Suppl 1):S48-S59, 2004.

44. Payne R: Anatomy, physiology, and neuropharmacology of cancer pain, *Med Clin North Am* 71(2):153-167, 1987.

44a. Ghai B, Dureja GP: Complex regional pain syndrome: a review, *J Postgrad Med* 50(4):300-307, 2004.

44b. Baron R:Mechanistic and clinical aspects of complex regional pain syndrome (CRPS), *Novartis Found Symp* 261:220-233, 2004.

45. Bittar RG, Otero S, Carter H, Aziz TZ: Deep brain stimulation for phantom limb pain, *J Clin Neurosci* 12(4):399-404, 2005.

46. Woodhouse A: Phantom limb sensation, *Clin Exp Pharmacol Physiol* 32(1-2):132-134, 2005.

47. Flor H: Cortical reorganization and chronic pain: implications for rehabilitation, *J Rehabil Med* (41 Suppl):66-72, 2003.

48. Melzack R et al: Central neuroplasticity and pathological pain, *Ann N Y Acad Sci* 933:157-174, 2001.

49. Melzack R: Phantom limbs and the concept of a neuromatrix, *Trends Neurosci* 13(3):88-92, 1990.

50. Vasedevan SV: Clinical perspectives on the relationship between pain and disability, *Neuro Clin* 7:429,1998.

51. Wolf AR: Pain, nociception and the developing infant, *Paediatr Anaesth* 9(1):7-17, 1999.

52. Modi N, Glover V: Fetal pain and stress. In Anand KJS, McGrath PJ, editors: *Pain in neonates: pain research and clinical management series,* ed 2, vol 5, New York, 2000, Elsevier.

53. Anand KJ: Effects of perinatal pain and stress, *Prog Brain Res* 122:117-129, 2000.

54. von Baeyer CL et al: Children's memory for pain: overview and implications for practice, *J Pain* 5(5):241-249, 2004.

55. Huang W et al: Management of fetal pain during invasive fetal procedures: a review, *Acta Anaesthesiol Belg* 55(2):119-123, 2004.

56. Beyer JE, Wells N: The assessment of pain in children, *Pediatr Clin North Am* 36(4):837-854, 1989.

57. Duhn JL, Medves JM: A systematic integrative review of infant pain assessment tools, *Adv Neonatal Care* 4(3):126-140, 2004.

58. Golianu B et al: Pediatric acute pain management, *Pediatr Clin North Am* 47(3):559-587, 2000.

59. Gibson SJ, Farrell M: A review of age differences in the neurophysiology of nociception and the perceptual experience of pain, *Clin J Pain* 20(4):227-239, 2004

60. Zheng Z et al: Age-related differences in the time course of capsaicin-induced hyperalgesia, *Pain* 85(1-2):51-58, 2000.

61. Gibson SJ, Farrell M.: A review of age differences in the neurophysiology of nociception and the perceptual experience of pain, *Clin J Pain* 20(4):227-239: 2004.

62. Woodrow KM et al: Pain tolerance: differences according to age, sex, and race, *Psychosom Med* 34(6):548-556, 1972.

63. Peat G et al: Social networks and pain interference with daily activities in middle and old age, *Pain* 112(3):397-405, 2004.

64. Rao A, Cohen HJ: Symptom management in the elderly cancer patient: fatigue, pain, and depression, *J Natl Cancer Inst Monogr* (32):150-157, 2004.

65. Gagliese L, Melzack R: Age-related differences in the qualities but not the intensity of chronic pain, *Pain* 104(3):597-608, 2003.

66. Dinarello CA, Wolff SM: Pathogenesis of fever in man, *N Engl J Med* 298(11):607-612, 1978.

67. Boulant JA: Role of the preoptic-anterior hypothalamus in thermoregulation and fever, *Clin Infect Dis* 31(Suppl 5):S157-S161, 2000.

68. Himms-Hagen J: Current status of nonshivering thermogenesis. In Ross Laboratories: *Assessment of energy metabolism in health and disease: a report of the first Ross conference in medical research,* Columbus, Ohio, 1980, Ross Laboratories.

69. Sell H, Deshaies Y, Richard D: The brown adipocyte: update on its metabolic role, *Int J Biochem Cell Biol* 36(11):2098-2104. 2004.

69a. Asakura H. Fetal and neonatal thermoregulation, *J Nippon Med Sch* 71(6):360-370, 2004.

70. Klaus S: Adipose tissue as a regulator of energy balance, *Curr Drug Targets* 5(3):241-250, 2004.

71. Klingenspor M: Cold-induced recruitment of brown adipose tissue thermogenesis, *Exp Physiol* 33(1):141-148, 2004.

72. Yousef MK: Effects of climatic stresses on thermoregulatory processes in man, *Experientia* 43(1):14-19, 1987.

73. Hackman PS: Recognizing and understanding the cold-stressed term infant, *Neonatal Netw* 20(8):35-41, 2001.

74. Grassi G et al: Impairment of thermoregulatory control of skin sympathetic nerve traffic in the elderly, *Circulation* 108(6):729-730, 2003.

75. Kenney WL, Munce TA: Invited review: aging and human temperature regulation, *J Appl Physiol* 95(6):2598-2603, 2003.

76. Gregson AL, Mackowiak PA: Pathogenesis of fever. In Cohen J, Powderly WG, editors: *Infectious diseases,* vol 1, St Louis, 2004, Mosby.

77. Conti B et al: Cytokines and fever, *Front Biosci* 9:1433-1449, 2004.
78. Samii A: The neurobiological basis of fever, *Surg Neurol* 45:392, 1966.
79. Saper CB, Breder CD: The neurologic basis of fever, *N Engl J Med* 330(26):1880-1886, 1994.
80. Boulant J: Thermoregulation. In Mackowiak P, editor: *Fever: basic mechanisms and management*, New York, 1991, Raven Press.
81. Steiner AA, Branco LG: Fever and anapyrexia in systemic inflammation: intracellular signaling by cyclic nucleotides, *Front Biosci* 8:s1398-s1408, 2003.
82. Dinarello CA: Cytokines as endogenous pyrogens, *J Infect Dis* 179(suppl 2):S294-S304, 1999.
83. Ivanov AI, Romanovsky AA: Prostaglandin E2 as a mediator of fever: synthesis and catabolism, *Front Biosci* 8:1977-1993, 2004.
84. Dinarello CA: Infection, fever, and exogenous and endogenous pyrogens: some concepts have changed, *J Endotoxin Res* 10(4):201-222, 2004.
85. Richmond CA: The role arginine vasopressin in thermoregulation during fever, *J Neurosci Nurs* 35(5):281-286, 2003.
86. Roth J et al: Endogenous antipyretics: neuropeptides and glucocorticoids, *Front Biosci* 9:816-826, 2004.
87. Kozak W et al: Molecular mechanisms of fever and endogenous antipyresis, *Ann N Y Acad Sci* 917:121-134, 2000.
88. Gregson AL, Mackowiak PA: Pathogenesis of fever. In Cohen J, Powderly WG, editors: *Infectious diseases*, vol 1, St Louis, 2004, Mosby.
89. Luheshi G, Rothwell N: Cytokines and fever, *Int Arch Allergy Immunol* 109(4):301-307, 1996.
90. Dinarello CA, Wolff SM: Molecular basis of fever in humans, *Am J Med* 72(5):799-819, 1982.
91. Kluger MS: The adaptive value of fever. In Mackowiak PA, editor: *Fever: basic mechanisms and management*, New York, 1991, Raven.
92. Griesman LA, Mackowiak PA: Fever: beneficial and detrimental effects of antipyretics, *Curr Opin Infect Dis* 15(3):241-245, 2002.
93. Yoshikawa TT, Norman DC: Approach to fever and infection in the nursing home, *J Am Geriatr Soc* 44(1):74-82, 1996.
94. Fruthaler GJ: Fever in children: phobia vs. facts, *Hosp Pract* 20(11A):49-53, 1985.
95. Cabanac M, Brinnel H: The pathology of human temperature regulation: thermiatrics, *Experientia* 43(1):19-27, 1987.
96. Weinmann M: Hot on the inside, *Emerg Med Serv* 32(7):34, 2003.
97. Bytomski JR, Squire DL: Heat illness in children, *Curr Sports Med Rep* 2(6):320-324, 2003.
98. Wappler F: Malignant hyperthermia, *Eur J Anaesthesiol* 18(10):632-652, 2001.
99. Ali SZ, Taguchi A, Rosenberg H: Malignant hyperthermia, *Best Pract Res Clin Anaesthesiol* 17(4):519-533, 2003.
100. Centers for Disease Control and Prevention: Hypothermia-related deaths—United States 2003-2004. *MMWR* 54(7):173-175, 2004.
101. Hildebrand F et al: Pathophysiologic changes and effects of hypothermia on outcome in elective surgery and trauma patients, *Am J Surg* 187(3):363-371, 2004.
102. Antretter H, Dapunto OE, Bonatti J: Management of profound hypothermia, *Br J Hosp Med* 54(5):215-220, 1995.
103. Reuler JB: Hypothermia: pathophysiology, clinical settings, and management, *Ann Intern Med* 89(4):519-527, 1978.
104. DeLapp TD: Accidental hypothermia, *Am J Nurs* 83(1):62-67, 1983.
105. Long WB 3rd, et al: Cold injuries, *J Long Term Eff Med Implants* 15(1):7-78, 2005
106. Tsuei BJ and Kearney PA: Hypothermia in the trauma patient, *Inury* 35(1):7-15, 2004.
107. Wittmers LE Jr: Pathophysiology of cold exposure, *Minn Med* 84(11):30-36, 2001.
108. Lee-Chiong TL Jr, Stitt JT: Accidental hypothermia: when thermoregulation is overwhelmed, *Postgrad Med* 99(1):7780, 83-84, 87-88, 1996.
109. Kempainen RR, Brunette DD: The evaluation and management of accidental hypothermia, *Respir Care* 49(2):192-205, 2004.
110. McCullough L, Arora S: Diagnosis and treatment of hypothermia, *Am Fam Pysician* 70(12); 2325-2332, 2004.
111. Osterman AL et al: Muscle ischemia and hypothermia: a bioenergetic study using 31phosphorus nuclear magnetic resonance spectroscopy, *J Trauma* 24(9):811-817, 1984.
112. Laptook AR et al: Quantitative relationship between brain temperatures and energy utilization rate measured in vivo using 31P and 1H magnetic resonance spectroscope, *Pediatr Res* 38(6):919-925, 1995.
113. Kabon B, Bacher A, Spiss CK: Therapeutic hypothermia, *Best Pract Res Clinc Anaesthesiol* 17(4): 551-568, 2003.
114. Shaver J et al: Changes in epicardial and core temperatures during resuscitation of hemorrhagic shock, *J Trauma* 24(11):957-963, 1984.
115. Little RA, Stoner HB: Body temperature after accidental injury, *Br J Surg* 68(4):221-224, 1981.
116. Dugovic C: Role of serotonin in sleep mechanisms, *Rev Neurol (Paris)*, 157(11 Pt 2):S16-S19, 2001.
117. Siegel JM: Hypocretin (orexin): role in normal behavior and neuropathology, *Annu Rev Psychol* 55:125-148, 2004.
118. Sutcliffe JG, de Lecea L: The hypocretins: setting the arousal threshold, *Nat Rev Neurosci* 3(5):339-349, 2002.
119. Voss U: Functions of sleep architecture and the concept of protective fields, *Rev Neurosci* 15(1):33-46, 2004.
120. Phillipson EA: State-of-the-art control of breathing during sleep, *Am Rev Respir Dis* 118:909, 1978.
121. Sakai F et al: Normal human sleep: regional cerebral hemodynamics, *Ann Neurol* 7(5):471, 1980.
121a. Meadows GE et al: Cerebral blood flow response to isocapnic hypoxia during slow-wave sleep and wakefulness, *J Appl Physiol* 97(4):1343-1348. 2004.
122. Sei H, Morita Y: Why does arterial blood pressure rise actively during REM sleep? *J Med Invest* 46(1-2):11-17, 1999.
123. Siegel JM: The neurotransmitters of sleep, *J Clin Psychiatry* 65(Suppl 16):4-7, 2004.
124. Siegel JM: Mechanisms of sleep control, *J Clin Neurophysiol* 7(1):49-65, 1990.
125. Friess E et al: The hypothalamic-pituitary-adrenocortical system and sleep in man, *Adv Neuroimmunol* 5(2):111-125, 1995.
126. Kryger MH, Roth T, Dement WC: *Principles and practice of sleep medicine,* ed 5, Philadelphia, 2005, Saunders.
127. Campbell SS: Evolution of sleep structure following brief intervals of wakefulness, *Electroencephalogr Clin Neurophysiol* 66(2):175-184, 1987.
128. Kedas A, Lux W, Amodeo S: A critical review of aging and sleep research, *West J Nurs Res* 11(2):196-206, 1989.
129. Dotto L: Sleep stages, memory, and learning, *CMA-1196J* 154(18):1193, 1996.
130. Anders TF, Keener M: Developmental course of nighttime sleep-wake patterns in full-term and premature infants during the first year of life, *Sleep* 8(3):173, 1985.
131. Keefe MR: Comparison of neonatal nighttime sleep-wake patterns in nursing versus rooming-in environments, *Nurs Res* 36(3):140, 1987.
132. Elias MF et al: Sleep/wake patterns of breast-fed infants in the first 2 years of life, *Pediatrics* 77(3):322, 1986.
133. Leo G: Parasomnias, *WMJ* 102(1):32-35, 2003.
134. Guazzelli M, Feinberg I, Aminoff M: Sleep spindles in the normal elderly: comparison with young adult patterns and relation to nocturnal awakening, cognitive function, and brain atrophy, *Electroencephalogr Clin Neurophysiol* 63(6):526, 1986.
135. Mourtazaev MS et al: Age and gender affect different characteristics of slow waves in sleep EEG, *Sleep* 18(7):557-564, 1995.
136. Kern W et al: Changes in cortisol and growth hormone secretion during nocturnal sleep in the course of aging, *J Gerontol A Biol Sci Med Sci* 51(1):M3-M9, 1996.
137. Voderholzer U et al: Are gender differences in objective and subjective sleep measures? A study of insomniacs and healthy controls, *Depress Anxiety* 17(3):162-172, 2003.
138. Ancoli-Israel S: Insomina in the elderly: a review for the primary care practitioner, *Sleep* 23(Suppl 1):S23-S30, discussion S36-S38, 2000.
139. Rigndahl EN, Pereira SL, Delzell JE Jr: Treatment of primary insomnia, *J Am Board Fam Pract* 17(3):212-219, 2004.
140. Jordan AS, McEvoy RD: Gender differences in sleep apnea: epidemiology, clinical presentation and pathogenic mechanisms, *Sleep Med Rev* 7(5):277-289, 2003.
141. Netzer NC, Eliasson AH, Strohl KP. Women with sleep apnea have lower levels of sex hormones, *Sleep Breath* 7(1):25-29, 2003.
141a. Saaresranta T, Aittokallio T, Polo-Kantola P, Helenius H, Polo O: Effect of medroxyprogesterone on inspiratory flow shapes during sleep in postmenopausal women, *Respir Physiol Neurobiol* 134(2):131-143, 2003.
142. Exar EN, Collop NA: The upper airway resistance syndrome, *Chest* 115(4):1127-1139, 1999.
143. Verse T et al: Recent developments in the treatment of obstructive sleep apnea, *Am J Respir Med* 2(2):157-168, 2003.

144. Friedlander AH et al: Diagnosing and comanaging patients with obstructive sleep apnea syndrome, *J Am Dent Assoc* 131(8):1178-1184, 2000.

145. Victor LD: Obstructive sleep apnea, *Am Fam Physician* 60(8): 2279-2286, 1999.

146. Gami AS, Caples SM, Somers VK: Obesity and obstructive sleep apnea, *Endorcinol Metab Clin North Am* 32(4):869-894, 2003.

147. Monk TH: Shift work. In Kryger MH, Roth T, Dement WC, editors: *Principles and practice of sleep medicine*, ed 4, Philadelphia, 2005, Saunders.

148. Taub JM, Berger RJ: The effects of changing the phase and duration of sleep, *J Exp Psychol Human Percept Perform* 2(1):30, 1976.

149. Eastman CI et al: Advancing circadian rhythms before eastward flight: a strategy to prevent or reduce jet lag, *Sleep* 28(1):33-44, 2005.

150. Sheldon SH: Parasomnias in childhood, *Pediatr Clin North Am* 51(1):69-88, vi, 2004.

151. Jalkut MW, Lerman SE, Churchill BM: Enuresis, *Pediatr Clin North Am* 48(6):1461-1488, 2001.

152. Harari MD, Moulden A: Nocturnal enuresis: what is happening? *J Paediatr Child Health* 36(1):78-81, 2000.

153. Thase ME: Treatment issues related to sleep and depression, *J Clin Psychiatry* 61(suppl 11):46-50, 2000.

154. Lewis DA: Sleep in patients with respiratory disease, *Respir Care Clin North Am* 5(3):447-460, ix, 1999.

155. McNicholas WT: Impact of sleep on COPD, *Chest* 117(2 suppl): 48S-53S, 2000.

156. Carter SR: Eyelid disorders: diagnosis and management, *Am Fam Physician* 57(11):2695-2702, 1998.

157. Coote MA: Sticky eye, tricky diagnosis, *Aust Fam Physician* 31(3):225-231, 2002.

158. Mabey DC, Solomon AW, Foster A: Trachoma, *Lancet* 362(9379):223-229, 2003.

159. Jackson GR, Owsley C: Visual dysfunction, neurodegenerative diseases, and aging, *Neurol Clin* 21(3):709-728, 2003.

160. Mittelman D: Amblyopia, *Pediatr Clin North Am* 50(1):189-196, 2003.

161. Ticho BH: Strabismus, *Pediatr Clin North Am* 50(1):173-188, 2003.

162. Tusa RJ: Nystagmus: diagnostic and therapeutic strategies, *Semin Ophthalmol* 14(2):65-73, 1999.

163. Barrett BT, Bradley A, McGraw PV: Understanding the neural basis of amblyopia, *Neuroscientist* 10(2):106-117, 2004.

164. Truscott RJ: Human cataract: the mechanisms responsible; light and butterfly eyes, *Int J Biochem Cell Biol* 35(11):1500-1504, 2003.

165. Olson RJ et al: Cataract treatment in the beginning of the 21st century, *Am J Ophthalmol* 136(1):146-154, 2003.

166. Jackson RG, Owsley C, McGwin G Jr: Aging and dark adaptation, *Vision Res* 39(23):3975-3982, 1999.

167. Cohen CS, Allingham, RR: The dawn of genetic testing for glaucoma, *Curr Opin Ophthalmol* 15(2):75-79, 2004.

168. Coleman AL: Glaucoma, *Lancet* 354(9192):1803-1810, 1999.

169. Terzel G, Yang J, Wax MB: Heat shock proteins, immunity and glaucoma, *Brain Res Bull* 62(6):473-480, 2004.

170. Shaarawy T, Flammer J, Haefliger IO: Reducing intraocular pressure: is surgery better than drugs? *Eye* 18(12):1215-1224, 2004.

171. Tezel G, Wax MB: The immune system and glaucoma, *Curr Opin Ophthalmol* 15(2):80-84, 2004.

172. Gariano RF, Kim CH: Evaluation and management of suspected retinal detachment, *Am Fam Physician* 69(7):1691-1698, 2004.

173. Zarbin MA: Current concepts in the pathogenesis of age-related macular degeneration, *Arch Ophthalmol* 122(4):598-614, 2004.

174. Hamdi HK, Kenney C: Age-related macular degeneration: a new viewpoint, *Front Biosci* 8:e305-e314, 2003.

175. Moshfeghi DM, Lewis H: Age-related macular degeneration: evaluation and treatment, *Cleve Clin J Med* 70(12):1017-1018, 1023-1025 passim, 2003.

176. Baikoff G: Surgical treatment of presbyopia: scleral, corneal, and lenticular, *Curr Opin Ophthalmol* 15(4):365-369, 2004.

177. Doane JF: Accommodating intraocular lenses, *Curr Opin Ophthalmol* 15(1):16-21, 2004.

178. Deeb SS, Kohl S: Genetics of color vision deficiencies, *Dev Ophthalmol* 37:170-187, 2003.

179. Swanson WH, Cohen JM: Color vision, *Ophthalmol Clin North Am* 16(2):179-203, 2003.

180. Javer AR, Schwartz DW: Plasticity in human directional hearing, *J Otolaryngol* 24(2):111-117, 1995.

181. Timiras PS: *Physiological basis of aging and geriatrics*, ed 3, Boca Raton, Fla, 2003, CRC Press.

182. Wiley TL et al: Aging and high-frequency hearing sensitivity, *J Speech Lang Hear Res* 41(5):1061-1072, 1998.

183. Sander R: Otitis externa: a practical guide to treatment and prevention, *Am Fam Physician* 63(5):927-936, 941-942, 2001.

184. Arrieta A, Singh J: Management of recurrent and persistent acute otitis: new options with familiar antibiotics, *Pediatr Infect Dis J* 23(2 Suppl):S115-S124, 2004.

185. Buchman CA, Brinson GM: Viral otitis media, *Curr Allergy Asthma Rep* 3(4):335-340, 2003.

186. American Academy of Pediatrics Subcommittee on Management of Acute Otitis Media: Diagnosis and management of acute otitis media, *Pediatrics* 113(5):1451-1465, 2004.

187. Kacmarynski DS et al: Complications of otitis media before placement of tympanostomy tubes in children, *Arch Otolaryngol Head Neck Surg* 130(3):289-292, 2004.

188. De la Cruz A, Angeli S, Slattery WH: Stapedectomy in children, *Otolaryngol Head Neck Surg* 120(4):487-492, 1999.

189. Borgadus ST Jr, Yueh B, Shekelle PG: Screening and management of adult hearing loss in primary care: clinical applications, *JAMA* 289(15):1986-1990, 2003.

190. Seidman MD, Ahmad N, Bai U: Molecular mechanisms of age-related hearing loss, *Ageing Res Rev* 1(3):331-343, 2002.

191. Temple EC et al: Taste development: differential growth rates of tongue regions in humans, *Brain Res Dev Brain Res* 135(1-2):65-70, 2002.

192. Finkelstein JA, Schiffman SS: Workshop on taste and smell in the elderly: an overview, *Physiol Behav* 66(2):173-176, 1999.

193. Doty RL: Influence of age and age-related diseases on olfactory function, *Ann N Y Acad Sci* 561:76-86, 1989.

194. Cain WS, Reid F, Stevens JC: Missing ingredients: aging and the discrimination of flavor, *J Nutr Elderly* 9(3):3, 1990.

195. Seiberling KA, Conley DB: Aging and olfactory and taste function, *Otolaryngol Clin North Am* 37(6):1209-1228, vii, 2004.

195a. Kovacs T: Mechanisms of olfactory dysfunction in aging and neurodegenerative disorders, *Ageing Res Rev* 3(2):215-232, 2004.

196. Winkler S et al: Depressed taste and smell in geriatric patients, *J Am Dent Assoc* 130(12):1759-1765, 1999.

197. Bromley SM: Smell and taste disorders: a primary care approach, *Am Fam Physician* 61(2): 427-438, 2000.

198. Fukunaga A, Uematsu H, Sugimoto K: Influences of aging on taste perception and oral somatic sensation, *J Gerontol A Biol Sci Med Sci* 60(1):109-113, 2005.

199. Deleted in proofs.

200. Besne I, Descombes C, Breton L: Effect of age and anatomical site on density of sensory innervation in human epidermis, *Arch Dermatol* 138(11):1445-1450, 2002.

201. Stevens JC: Age and spatial acuity of touch, *J Gerontol* 47(1):P35-P40, 1992.

202. Wolfson L: Gait and balance dysfunction: a model of the interaction of age and disease, *Neuroscientist* 7(2):178-183, 2001.

CONCEPTS OF NEUROLOGIC DYSFUNCTION

CHAPTER

16

BARBARA J. BOSS • ROBIN R. WILKERSON

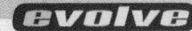
http://evolve.elsevier.com/McCance/

A person achieves functional adequacy (competence) through complex integrated processes. Three major neural systems account for this functional adequacy: cognitive systems, sensory systems, and motor systems. Alterations in any or all of these affect functional adequacy. Alterations in cognitive and motor systems are discussed in this chapter.

The neural systems basic (core) to the cognitive sphere are (1) attentional systems that provide arousal and maintenance of attention over time; (2) memory and language systems by which information is communicated; and (3) affective, or emotive, systems that mediate feeling tone. These core systems are fundamental to the processes of abstract thinking and reasoning. The products of abstraction and reasoning are organized and made operational through the executive system. The normal functioning of these systems manifests through the motor system in a behavioral array viewed by others as being appropriate to human activity and successful living.

Genetics and the genetic basis of disease are becoming increasingly important in the study of pathophysiology; selected neurologic disorders that have a genetic basis are presented in Table 16-1.

ALTERATIONS IN COGNITIVE SYSTEMS

Full consciousness, in its broadest sense, is both a state of awareness of oneself and the environment and a set of responses to that environment. Full consciousness implies that the individual responds to external stimuli with a wide array of responses. Any decrease in this state of awareness and varied responses is thus a decrease in consciousness.

Consciousness often is viewed as having two distinct components: arousal and awareness. Arousal, an attentional system, is the state of awakeness that an individual exhibits. Level of arousal is mediated by the reticular activating system, which extends from the medulla to the diencephalon. The reticular activating system provides arousal to the cerebral hemispheres (see Figure 14-5). Severe alterations in arousal can occur with brain injury, both in the acute phase of injury and on a long-term basis. Approximately 30% to 40% of survivors of severe brain injury remain in prolonged states of severely reduced consciousness. Awareness encompasses all cognitive functions that embody awareness of self, environment, and affective states (i.e., moods). **Content of thought** is mediated by attentional systems, memory systems, language systems, and executive systems.

Table 16-1	Selected Neurologic Disorders with a Genetic Basis		
Syndrome/Disorders	Currently Known Genetic Components	Pathophysiology	Major Neurologic Features
Alterations in Cognitive Systems			
Familial Alzheimer disease			
Early onset	Autosomal dominant	Three clinically indistinguishable subtypes: AD1: mutations in amyloid precursor protein (APP gene) (chromosome 12) AD3: mutations in presenilin 1 (PSEN1) gene (chromosome 14) AD4: mutations in presenilin 2 (PSEN2) gene (chromosome 1)	Adult onset progressive dementia—onset before age 60-65, often before 55
Late onset	Having 1 or 2 copies of APOE4 suggests an increased risk but is not predictive of Alzheimer	Mutations in APOE4 gene (chromosome 19); codes a cholesterol processing protein; is a susceptibility gene; several other unidentified genes and environments are thought to influence	Adult onset progressive dementia—onset after age 65
Angelman syndrome	Chromosome 15; transmission—maternal deletion, paternal UPD, imprinting center mutation, UBE3A (ubiquitin protein ligase) mutation, clinical	Genetic alteration affects the maternal expression of the UBE3A gene; UBE3A thought to have great importance in degradation of proteins in the brain	Little to no verbal language, mental retardation, seizure disorder, sleep disorder, movement/balance disorder
Batten disease	Autosomal recessive; chromosome 16	Lysosomal storage defect resulting in abnormal storage of cerebral lipofuscins	Develops normally until 6 months to 2 years of age when progressive brain disease becomes apparent; seizures, mental retardation, blindness, fatal
Branched-Chain ketoaciduria (maple syrup urine disease)	Autosomal recessive; most common type is classic caused by defect in the BCKDHA gene on chromosome 19	All types result in inability to metabolize three amino acids; these acids accumulate and are toxic at high levels	Without early diagnosis and treatment: mental retardation, seizures, and death
Cri du chat	Chromosome 5	Deletion on the short arm; deletion of multiple genes responsible for phenotype; evidence that deletion of telomerase reverse transcriptase gene contributes to phenotype	High-pitched cry; mental retardation, microcephaly, low birth weight, failure to thrive; widely spaced eyes (ocular hypertelorism), unusually small jaw (micrognathia)
Lescy-Nyhan syndrome	X-linked recessive	Metabolism disturbance of purines	Mental retardation, progressive neurologic disorder, compulsively bit lips and fingers
Neurofibromatosis NF1 (von Recklinghausen)	Autosomal dominant Chromosome 17	Variable expressivity NF1 gene produces a large, complex protein called *neurofibromin;* scientists theorize this protein acts as a switch to regulate cell growth; mutation may lessen or inhibit the normal output of this protein and allow irregular cell growth that may lead to tumor development	Multiple café au lait spots, neurofibromas, learning disability, seizure disorder
NF2 (bilateral acoustic NF)	Chromosome 22	NF2 gene produces a tumor suppressor protein (termed *merlin* or *schwannomin*)	Multiple tumors on cranial and spinal nerves, acoustic neuromas, hearing loss

Table 16-1	Selected Neurologic Disorders with a Genetic Basis—cont'd		
Syndrome/Disorders	Currently Known Genetic Components	Pathophysiology	Major Neurologic Features
Progressive myoclonus epilepsy			
Unverricht-Lundborg disease	Autosomal recessive; chromosome 21	The missing gene codes for the protein cystatin B; this protein regulates enzymes that break down other proteins	Onset at age 6-15 years, severe incapacitating stimulus-sensitive progressive myoclonus, tonic-clonic epileptic seizures and characteristic abnormalities in EEG; also develop other neurologic symptoms such as ataxia, incoordination, dysarthria
Lafora disease	Autosomal recessive; chromosome 6	Mutation in the Laforin gene; concentric amyloid (Lafora) bodies found in neurons, liver, skin, bone, and muscle	Grand mal seizures and/or myoclonus at about age 15; rapid and severe motor and coordination impairments, rapid mental deterioration, often with psychotic features; survival is short, less than 10 years after onset
Rett syndrome	X-linked dominant; appears to occur only in girls; defective gene on the x-chromosome called *MeCP2*	Caused by defects in the protein MeCP2 involved in regulation of gene expression; defects in this gene allow other genes to come on or stay on at inappropriate times in development	Progressive neurologic disorder; develops normally in first year of life, then loss of mental capacity and motor skills begins; loss of purposeful hand movements; stereotypical hand wringing and flapping
Tay-Sachs disease	Autosomal recessive; chromosome 15	Caused by a deficiency of hexosaminidase, an enzyme, which results in accumulation of a material that damages the brain	Failure to thrive, blindness, seizures, progressive paralysis; usually death by age 4
Tuberous sclerosis	Autosomal dominant; caused by mutation of either the TSC1 gene (chromosome 9) or TSC2 gene (chromosome 16)	TSC1 produces the protein hamartin, TCS2 produces the protein tuberin; these proteins act as tumor growth suppressors	Develops in early childhood; seizures, mental retardation, skin and eye lesions; multiple benign tumors in brain and other vital organs
Alterations in Motor Function			
Duchenne muscular dystrophy	X-linked recessive	Mutation of the dystrophin gene results in down-regulation or absence of dystrophin, a protein with an important structural role in muscle	Generalized weakness and muscle wasting affecting limb and trunk muscles first then progresses to respiratory system; progressive and fatal
Huntington disease	Autosomal dominant; chromosome 4	Mutation of the Huntington gene, a protein that is not well understood; results in neuron destruction in the brain	Jerky uncontrolled movements of the limbs, trunk and face (chorea); progressive loss of mental abilities; development of psychiatric disorders
Parkinson disease (early onset)	Two transmissions: Autosomal dominant—mutation in alpha-synuclein gene (chromosome 4) Autosomal recessive—mutation in the parkin gene (chromosome 6)	Too much of a normal form of the alpha-synuclein gene results in protein build-up Loss of the parkin gene, causes build-up of defective proteins	Onset before age 40; tremor, increased muscle tone, bradykinesia

Alterations in Arousal (Coma)

Possible causes of an altered level of arousal with acute onset may be separated into three major groups: **structural, metabolic,** and **psychogenic arousal alterations.** Structural causes are divided according to original location of the pathologic condition: supratentorial (above the tentorium cerebelli), infratentorial (subtentorial, below the tentorium cerebelli), subdural (below the dura mater), extracerebral (outside the brain tissue), and intracerebral (within the brain tissue).

Causes of altered level of arousal also are grouped according to a pathologic process: infectious, vascular, neoplastic, traumatic, congenital (developmental), degenerative, polygenic, and metabolic. Metabolic causes may be further divided into hypoxia, electrolyte disturbances, hypoglycemia, drugs, and toxins (both endogenous and exogenous). All the systemic diseases that eventually produce nervous system dysfunction are part of this metabolic category.

PATHOPHYSIOLOGY   Coma is produced by either (1) bilateral hemisphere damage or suppression by means of hypoxia, hypoglycemia, drugs, or toxins; or (2) a brain stem lesion or metabolic derangement that damages or suppresses the reticular activating system (RAS).[1] Supratentorial processes produce a decreased level of arousal by one of three mechanisms: (1) diffuse bilateral cortical dysfunction, (2) bilateral subcortical dysfunction, or (3) localized hemispheric dysfunction. Disease processes may produce diffuse bilateral cortical dysfunction (e.g., encephalitis) and actually may occur in either the cerebral cortex or the underlying subcortical white matter. Bilateral subcortical dysfunction involves destructive disease that compromises the RAS (e.g., brain stem trauma or cerebrovascular accident) and probably surrounding structures as well. Localized hemispheric dysfunction generally is caused by masses that directly impinge on deep diencephalic structures or that secondarily compress these structures in the process of herniation. Such localized destructive processes directly impair function of the thalamic or hypothalamic activating systems.

Extracerebral disorders also can produce diffuse bilateral cortical dysfunction. Extracerebral disorders include neoplasms, closed-head trauma with subsequent bleeding, and subdural empyema (accumulation of pus). Intracerebral disorders (those within the brain substance) function primarily as masses. These disorders include bleeding, infarcts and emboli, and tumors.

Infratentorial processes produce a reduction in arousal in one of two ways: (1) there may be direct destruction of the RAS and its pathways, or (2) the brain stem may be destroyed either by direct invasion or by indirect impairment of its blood supply. The most common cause of direct destruction is cerebrovascular disease, but demyelinating diseases, neoplasms, granulomas, abscesses, and head injury also may cause brain stem destruction. In addition, decreased level of consciousness may result from compression of the RAS by a disease process. This compression may occur because of (1) direct pressure on the pons and midbrain, producing ischemia and edema of the neurons of the RAS; (2) upward herniation of the cerebellum through the tentorial notch, thus compressing the upper midbrain and diencephalon; or (3) downward herniation of the cerebellum through the foramen magnum, compressing and displacing the medulla oblongata. Specific causes of compression of the brain stem include hematomas, hemorrhage, and aneurysm; cerebellar hemorrhage, infarcts, abscesses, and neoplasms; and demyelinating disorders.

A wide spectrum of diseases may produce a metabolically induced alteration in arousal. In encephalopathic conditions, widespread direct or indirect interference with neuronal metabolism occurs throughout much of the brain (see Chapter 17). Psychogenic unresponsiveness, although uncommon, may signal general psychiatric disorders. Despite apparent unconsciousness, the person actually is physiologically awake.

EVALUATION   Evaluating an altered level of arousal requires distinguishing between organic and functional causes. A further distinction between metabolic and structural causes then is made (Table 16-2). If the cause is structural, the pathologic condition must be localized.

CLINICAL MANIFESTATIONS   Patterns of clinical manifestations and their evolution have been identified. The patterns of clinical manifestation are important because they help in determining the extent of brain dysfunction and they serve as indexes for identifying increasing or decreasing central nervous system (CNS) function. The specific clusters of manifestations of abnormal function and their evolution suggest whether the cause of the altered arousal state is supratentorial, infratentorial, metabolic, or psychogenic (Table 16-3). Five categories of neurologic function are critical to the evaluation process: (1) level of consciousness, (2) pattern of breathing, (3) size and reactivity of pupils, (4) eye position and reflexive responses, and (5) skeletal muscle motor responses.

Level of Consciousness

Level of consciousness is the most critical clinical index of nervous system function or dysfunction. An alteration in consciousness indicates either improvement or deterioration of the individual's condition. A person who is alert and oriented to self, others, place, and time is considered to be functioning at the highest level of consciousness, which implies full use of all the person's cognitive capacities.

Because many different terms are used to indicate level of consciousness, definition becomes necessary. The term *unconscious,* for example, has no specific clinical definition and signifies different things to different people. From the normal alert state, levels of consciousness diminish in stages, each of which is clinically defined in Table 16-4.

Pattern of Breathing

Several characteristic respiratory patterns are helpful in evaluating level of brain dysfunction and level of coma. Among these characteristics are rate, rhythm, and pattern of breathing. The breathing patterns can be categorized as hemispheric or brain stem breathing patterns (Table 16-5).

Table 16-2   Clinical Manifestations of Metabolic and Structural Causes of Comas

Manifestation	Metabolically Induced Coma	Structurally Induced Coma
Blink to threat (cranial nerves II, VII)	Equal	Asymmetric
Discs (cranial nerve II)	Flat, good pulsation	Papilledema
Extraocular movement (cranial nerves III, IV, VI)	Roving eye movements; normal doll's eyes and calorics	Gaze paresis, nerve III palsy, medial longitudinal fasciculus (MLF) syndrome (internuclear ophthalmoplegia)
Pupils (cranial nerves II, III)	Equal and reactive, may be large (e.g., atropine), pinpoint (e.g., opiates), or midposition and fixed (e.g., glutethimide [Doriden])	Asymmetric and/or nonreactive; may be midposition (midbrain injury), pinpoint (pons injury), large (tectal injury)
Corneal reflex (cranial nerve V, VII)	Symmetric response	Asymmetric response
Grimace to pain (cranial nerve VII)	Symmetric response	Asymmetric response
Motor function movement	Symmetric	Asymmetric
Tone	Symmetric	Paratonic, spastic, flaccid, especially if asymmetric
Posture	Symmetric	Decorticate, especially if symmetric; decerebrate, especially if asymmetric
Deep tendon reflexes	Symmetric	Asymmetric
Babinski sign	Absent or symmetric response	Present
Sensation	Symmetric	Asymmetric

Table 16-3   Differential Characteristics of States Causing Coma

Mechanism	Manifestations
Supratentorial mass lesions compressing or displacing diencephalons or brain stem	Initiating signs usually of focal cerebral dysfunction
	Signs of dysfunction progress rostral to caudal
	Neurologic signs at any given time point to one anatomic area (e.g., diencephalon, mesencephalon, medulla)
	Motor signs often asymmetric
Infratentorial mass of destruction causing coma	History of preceding brain stem dysfunction or sudden onset of coma
	Localizing brain stem signs precede or accompany onset of coma and always include oculovestibular abnormality
	Cranial nerve palsies usually manifest "bizarre" respiratory patterns that appear at onset
Metabolic coma	Confusion and stupor commonly precede motor signs
	Motor signs usually are symmetric
	Pupillary reactions usually are preserved
	Asterixis, myoclonus, tremor, and seizures are common
	Acid-base imbalance with hyperventilation or hypoventilation is common
Psychiatric unresponsiveness	Lids close actively
	Pupils reactive or dilated (cycloplegics)
	Oculocephalic reflexes are unpredictable; oculovestibular reflexes are physiologic (nystagmus is present)
	Motor tone is inconsistent or normal
	Eupnea or hyperventilation is usual
	No pathologic reflexes are present
	Electroencephalogram (EEG) is normal

Table 16-4   Levels of Acute Coma

State	Definition
Confusion	Loss of ability to think rapidly and clearly; impaired judgment and decision making
Disorientation	Beginning loss of consciousness; disorientation to time followed by disorientation to place and impaired memory; lost last is recognition of self
Lethargy	Limited spontaneous movement or speech; easy arousal with normal speech or touch; may not be oriented to time, place, or person
Obtundation	Mild to moderate reduction in arousal (awakeness) with limited response to the environment; falls asleep unless stimulated verbally or tactilely; answers questions with minimum response
Stupor	A condition of deep sleep or unresponsiveness from which the person may be aroused or caused to open eyes only by vigorous and repeated stimulation; response is often withdrawal or grabbing at stimulus
Coma	No verbal response to the external environment or to any stimuli; noxious stimuli such as deep pain or suctioning yield motor movement
Light coma	Associated with purposeful movement on stimulation
Coma	Associated with nonpurposeful movement only on stimulation
Deep coma	Associated with unresponsiveness or no response to any stimulus

Table 16-5   Patterns of Breathing

Breathing Pattern	Description	Location of Injury
Hemispheric Breathing Patterns		
Normal	After a period of hyperventilation that lowers the arterial carbon dioxide pressure ($PaCO_2$), the individual continues to breathe regularly but with a reduced depth.	Response of the nervous system to an external stressor—not associated with injury to the CNS
Posthyperventilation apnea (PHVA)	Respirations stop after hyperventilation has lowered the PCO_2 level below normal. Rhythmic breathing returns when the PCO_2 level returns to normal (Usually an intact cerebral cortex will trigger breathing within 10 seconds regardless of PCO_2.)	Associated with diffuse bilateral metabolic or structural disease of the cerebrum
Cheyne-Stokes respirations (CSR)	The breathing pattern has a smooth increase (crescendo) in the rate and depth of breathing (hyperpnea), which peaks and is followed by a gradual smooth decrease (decrescendo) in the rate and depth of breathing to the point of apnea when the cycle repeats itself. The hyperpneic phase lasts longer than the apneic phase. (represents an amplitude change)	Bilateral dysfunction of the deep cerebral or diencephalic structures, seen with supratentorial injury and metabolically induced coma states unrelated to neurologic dysfunction, may see also in CHF
Brain Stem Breathing Patterns		
Central reflex hyperpnea (Central neurogenic hyperventilation [CNH])	A sustained deep rapid, but regular pattern (hyperpnea) occurs, with a decreased $PaCO_2$ and a corresponding increase in pH and increased PO_2.	May result from CNS damage or disease that involves the lower midbrain and upper pons; seen after increased intracranial pressure and blunt head trauma
Apneusis	A prolonged inspiratory cramp (a pause at full inspiration) occurs. A common variant of this is a brief end-inspiratory pause of 2 or 3 seconds, often alternating with an end-expiratory pause.	Indicates damage to the respiratory control mechanism located at the pontine level; most commonly associated with pontine infarction but documented with hypoglycemia, anoxia, and meningitis
Cluster breathing	A cluster of breaths has a disordered sequence with irregular pauses between breaths.	Dysfunction in the lower pontine and high medullary areas
Ataxic breathing	Completely irregular breathing occurs, with random shallow and deep breaths and irregular pauses. Often the rate is slow.	Originates from a primary dysfunction of the lower pons or upper medulla
Gasping breathing pattern (agonal gasps)	A pattern of deep "all-or-none" breaths is accompanied by a slow respiratory rate.	Indicative of a failing medullary respiratory center

CNS, Central nervous system; *CHF*, congestive heart failure.

With normal breathing, a neural center believed to be located in the forebrain (cerebrum) produces a rhythmic breathing pattern despite lowered arterial carbon dioxide pressure ($PaCO_2$). When neural control at this center is lost as consciousness decreases, the lower brain stem centers regulate the breathing pattern by responding only to changes in $PaCO_2$ levels. The result is the irregular breathing associated with posthyperventilation apnea (PHVA).

The pathophysiology of Cheyne-Stokes respirations (CSR) involves an increased ventilatory response to carbon dioxide stimulation, causing hypercapnia and a diminished ventilatory stimulus. The neural center that causes PHVA thus is related to the CSR, because changes in $PaCO_2$ produce irregular breathing that contributes to overbreathing when stimulated by carbon dioxide. As a result, the $PaCO_2$ level decreases to below normal and, because of the cerebral brain dysfunction, breathing stops until the carbon dioxide reaccumulates to

bring the $PaCO_2$ level to normal. In cases of opiate or sedative drug overdose, the respiratory center is depressed and the rate of breathing gradually decreases until respiratory failure occurs.

Certain motor activities related to breathing signify the level of brain dysfunction. Yawning, vomiting, and hiccups are complex reflex-like motor responses that are integrated by neural mechanisms in the lower brain stem. These responses may be produced by compression or diseases that involve tissues in the medulla oblongata. Such disorders include infection, neoplasm, or infarct. Similar responses are produced by dysfunction in the lower brain stem through direct stimulation.

Most CNS disorders produce both nausea and vomiting. Vomiting with no associated nausea indicates direct involvement of the central neural mechanism. Vomiting is associated particularly with CNS injuries that (1) involve the vestibular nuclei (located in the lower pons and medulla oblongata) or

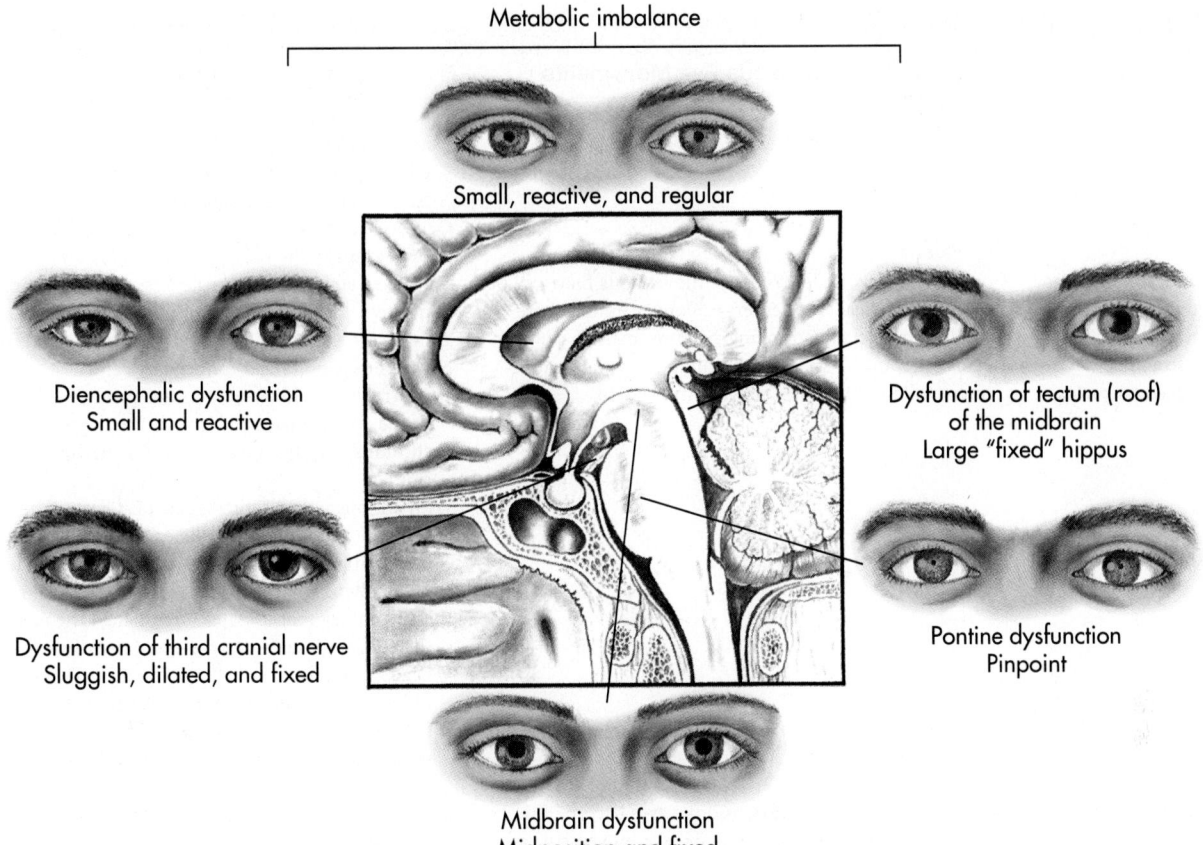

Metabolic imbalance

Small, reactive, and regular

Diencephalic dysfunction
Small and reactive

Dysfunction of tectum (roof)
of the midbrain
Large "fixed" hippus

Dysfunction of third cranial nerve
Sluggish, dilated, and fixed

Pontine dysfunction
Pinpoint

Midbrain dysfunction
Midposition and fixed

Figure 16-1 Appearance of pupils at different levels of consciousness.

their immediate projections, particularly when double vision (diplopia) also is present; (2) impinge directly on the floor of the fourth ventricle; or (3) produce brain stem compression secondary to increased intracranial pressure.

Pupillary Changes

Anatomically, brain stem areas that control arousal are adjacent to areas that control pupils. Pupillary changes thus are a valuable guide to evaluating the presence and level of brain stem dysfunction (Figure 16-1).

Certain drugs that affect pupils must be considered in the evaluation of pupillary response in comatose states. Atropine, scopolamine, amphetamines, mydriatrics, and cycloplegics in large concentrations fully dilate and fix pupils. Glutethimide in amounts sufficient to produce a coma causes the pupils to become midposition or moderately dilated (4 to 5 mm in diameter), unequal, and frequently fixed to light. Opiates (heroin and morphine) cause pinhole pupils (1.0 mm). Severe barbiturate intoxication may produce fixed pupils.

Severe ischemia and hypoxia produce bilaterally wide (5 mm) and fixed pupils in most instances. Occasionally the pupils remain small (1 to 2.5 mm) or midposition even in the presence of profound hypoxia. Hypothermia also may cause fixed pupils.

Oculomotor Responses

Resting, spontaneous, and reflexive eye movements (oculocephalic [doll's head, doll's eyes] and oculovestibular [caloric] reflexes) undergo change at various levels of brain dysfunction (Table 16-6). Persons with metabolically induced coma, except in cases of barbiturate-hypnotic and phenytoin (Dilantin) poisoning, generally do retain ocular reflexes, however, even when other signs of brain stem damage, such as central neurogenic hyperventilation, are present.

The presence of brisk oculocephalic reflexes and roving eye movements, as well as the failure to elicit nystagmus with instillation of cold or warm water into the external ear canal, indicates a decrease in consciousness (loss of cortical influence) but an intact brain stem (Figures 16-2 and 16-3).

Destructive or compressive injury to the brain stem causes specific abnormalities of the oculocephalic and oculovestibular reflexes. For example, a skewed deviation, in which one eye diverges downward and the other looks upward, indicates brain stem dysfunction. Destructive or compressive disease processes that involve an oculomotor nucleus or nerve cause the involved eye to deviate outward, producing a resting disconjugate lateral position of the eyes. Unilateral abducens paralysis (paralysis of cranial nerve VI) results in an upward deviation of the ipsilateral eye. With bilateral abducens paralysis, the eyes come together (converge). Reflexive eye movements may be suppressed by drugs, most commonly phenytoin, tricyclics, and barbiturates. Occasionally alcohol, phenothiazines, and diazepam may alter reflex eye movements.

Table 16-6	Changes in Oculomotor Responses	
State	**Resting and Spontaneous Eye Movements**	**Reflexive Eye Movements**
Full consciousness	Eyes at rest, still (cortical gaze centers inhibit spontaneous roving eye movements)	Eyes move as the head turns Oculocephalic responses not elicited or inconsistently elicited (frontal gaze centers inhibit brain stem reflexes that fix gaze straight ahead) Oculovestibular (caloric) stimulation produces nystagmus
Cortical dysfunction or disruption of efferent pathways Diffuse anoxic damage to cortex	Conjugate, horizontal, roving eye movements may well be present (cortical gaze centers no longer inhibit these brain stem–generated roving eye movements) "Ocular dipping"—slow, dysrhythmic downward movement followed by faster, upward movement	Gaze fixed straight ahead regardless of head position—positive doll's eyes reaction (normal oculocephalic reflexes are no longer inhibited by frontal gaze centers) Nystagmus is no longer induced by caloric stimulation (normally a cold water stimulus produces deviation of the eyes opposite the irrigated ear; a warm water stimulus deviates the eyes to the same [ipsilateral] side) With an injury that depresses cortical gaze center function, the eyes (and often the entire head) will deviate, or appear to look forward the side of the injured hemisphere With an injury that irritates (stimulates) the neurons of the cortical gaze center, the eyes (and often the entire head) will deviate away from the injured hemisphere (all fibers from the frontal gaze centers decussate and therefore control the function of the contralateral pontine gaze center, which moves the eyes in the ipsilateral direction)
Mesencephalon dysfunction	Roving eye movements cease, and the eyes become immobile and directed ahead (roving eye movements require an intact brain stem) Eyes may turn down and inward	Oculovestibular reflexes become inconsistent and abnormal Loss of Bell phenomenon (upward deviation of eyes on stimulation) (requires intact eye movement pathways from the mesencephalon to pons)
Pontine dysfunction	Loss of spontaneous blinking (requires an intact pons) "Ocular bobbing"—brisk, conjugate, downward movement of eyes with loss of horizontal eye movements	

Motor Responses

Motor responses contribute both to evaluating the level of brain dysfunction and to determining the side of the brain that is maximally damaged. The pattern of response is described as (1) purposeful (a defensive or withdrawal movement of limbs to noxious stimuli); (2) inappropriate, or not purposeful (generalized motor movement, posturing, grimacing, or groaning); or (3) not present (unresponsive, no motor response). Purposeful movement requires an intact corticospinal system. Nonpurposeful movement is evidence of severe dysfunction of the corticospinal system.

Motor signs indicating loss of cortical inhibition that are commonly associated with decreased consciousness include contralateral or bilateral (depending on whether the process is localized or diffuse) reflex grasping, reflex sucking, snout reflex, palmomental reflex, and rigidity (paratonia) (Figure 16-4). Abnormal flexor and extensor responses in the upper and lower extremities are defined in Table 16-7 and illustrated in Figure 16-5.

Outcomes

Categories of prognostic indicators related to outcome of coma include demographic variables, severity indices, neurologic signs, neuroimaging studies, neuromedical markers, psychologic ratings, and outcome scales.[2] Outcome domains fall into two divisions—mortality and extent of disability (morbidity). For coma, the extent of disability division has four domains—recovery of consciousness, residual cognitive dysfunction, psychosocial (functional) domain, and vocational domain. These coma outcomes differ depending on the etiology of the injury—traumatic brain injury (TBI) or nontraumatic brain injury (NTBI). The pathophysiology underlying traumatic brain injury is focal or diffuse trauma-induced injury (see Chapter 17 for further discussion). The pathophysiology of nontraumatic brain injuries is one of hypoxia and ischemia. This may be due, for example, to vascular insult, tumor, hydrocephalus, infection, or anorexia.[2]

Related to mortality, two forms of neurologic death—brain death (brain stem death) and cerebral death—may result from severe TBI and NTBI. **Brain death (brain stem death)** occurs when irreversible brain damage is so extensive that the brain has no potential for recovery and no longer can maintain the body's internal homeostasis. Destruction of the neuronal contents of the intracranial cavity includes the brain stem and cerebellum. On postmortem examination the brain is autolyzing (self-digesting) or already autolyzed.

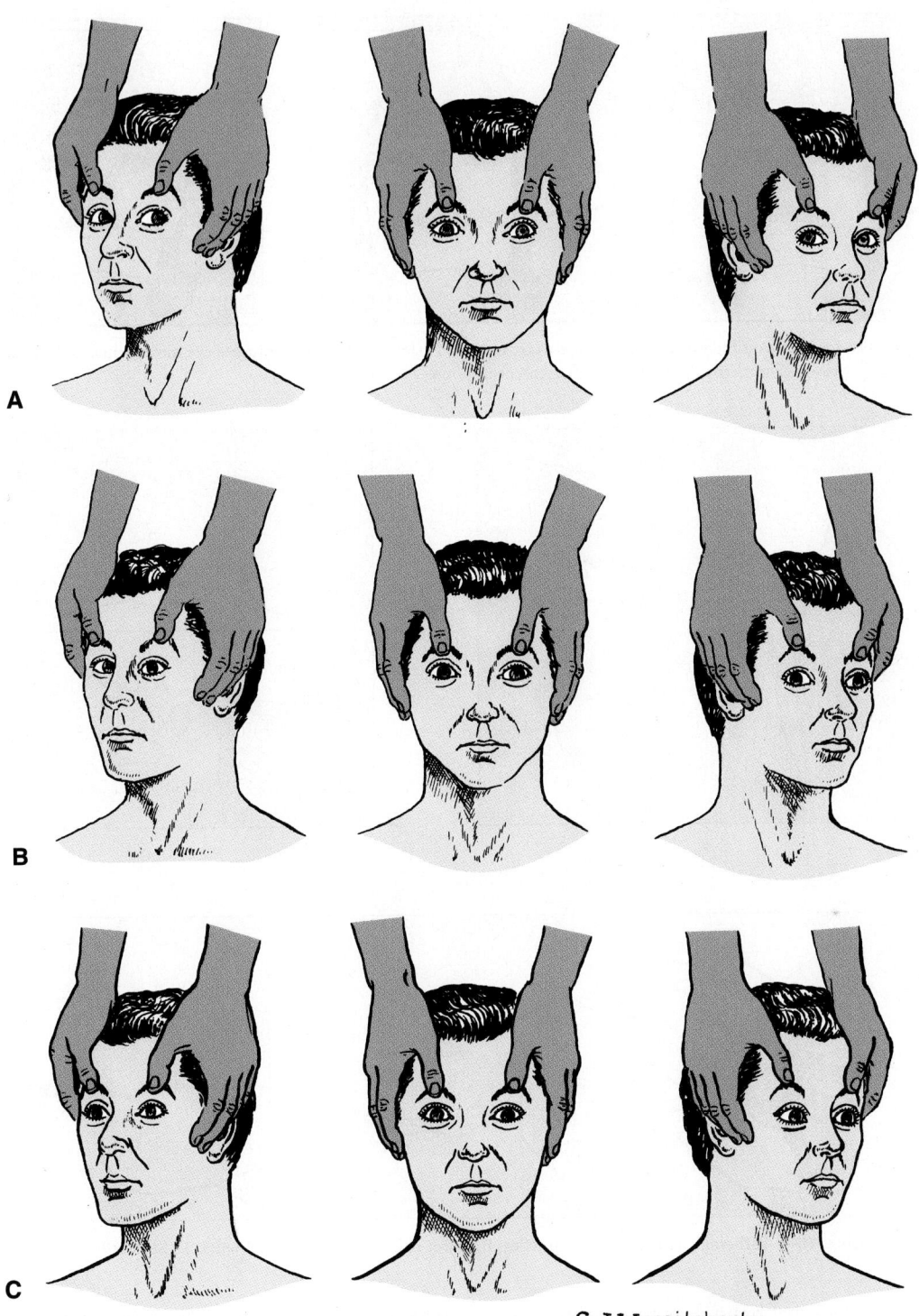

G.J.Wassilchenko

Figure 16-2 Test for oculocephalic reflex response (doll's eyes phenomenon). **A,** Normal response—eyes turn together to side opposite from turn of head. **B,** Abnormal response—eyes do not turn in conjugate manner. **C,** Absent response—eyes do not turn as head position changes. (**A** and **C** from Rudy EB: *Advanced neurological and neurosurgical nursing,* St. Louis, 1984, Mosby.)

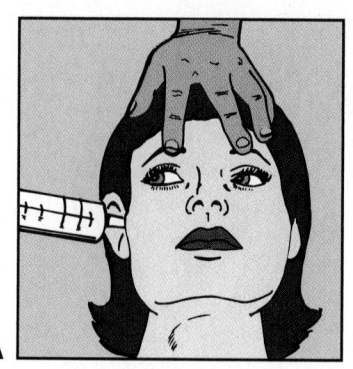
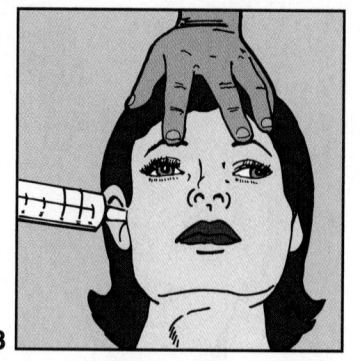
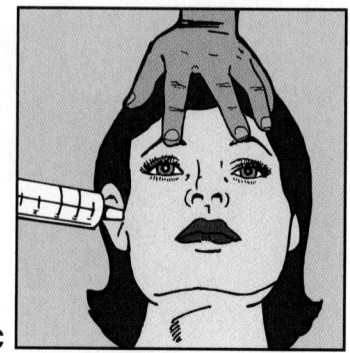

Figure 16-3 Test for oculovestibular reflex (caloric ice water test). **A,** Normal response—conjugate eye movements. **B,** Abnormal response—dysconjugate or asymmetric eye movements. **C,** Absent response—no eye movements.

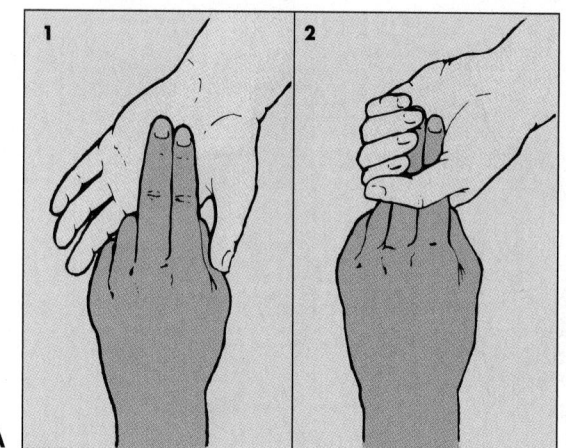
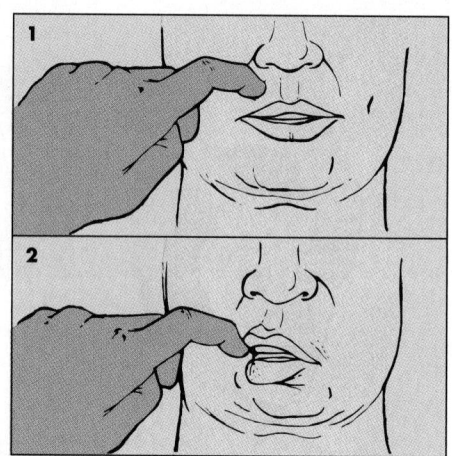
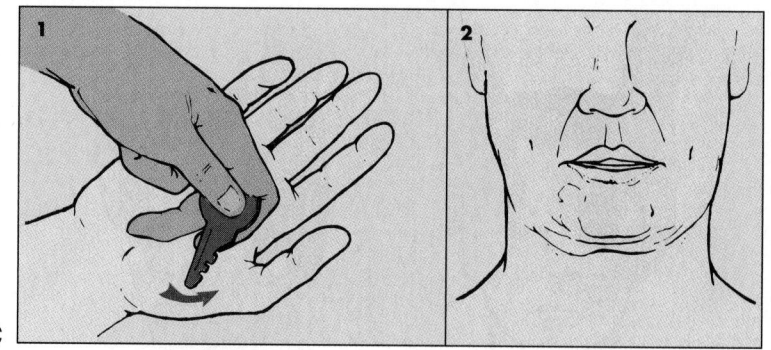
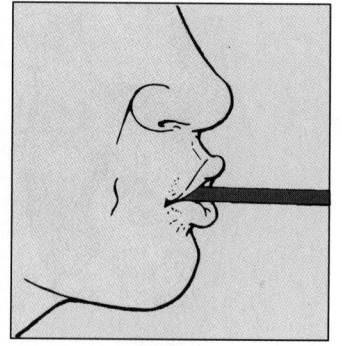

Figure 16-4 Pathologic reflexes. **A,** Grasp reflex. **B,** Snout reflex. **C,** Palmomental reflex. **D,** Suck reflex.

General agreement holds that brain death has occurred in the absence of discernible evidence of cerebral hemisphere function or function of the brain stem's vital centers for an extended period. There is no detectible function above the level of the foramen magnum.[3] In addition, the abnormality of brain function must result from structural or known metabolic disease and *not* be caused by a depressant drug, alcohol poisoning, neuromuscular blockage, or hypothermia. An isoelectric, or flat, electroencephalogram (EEG) (electrocerebral silence) for a period of 6 to 12 hours in a person who is not hypothermic and has not ingested depressant drugs indicates

that no mental recovery is possible and usually means that the brain is already dead. A task force to determine brain death in children recommended the same criteria as for adults[4] but with a longer observation period.[5]

The following clinical criteria determine brain death:[1,3,6]

1. Completion of all appropriate and therapeutic procedures
2. Unresponsive coma (absence of motor and reflex movements)
3. No spontaneous respiration (apnea)—a $PaCO_2$ that rises above 60 mmHg without breathing efforts, providing

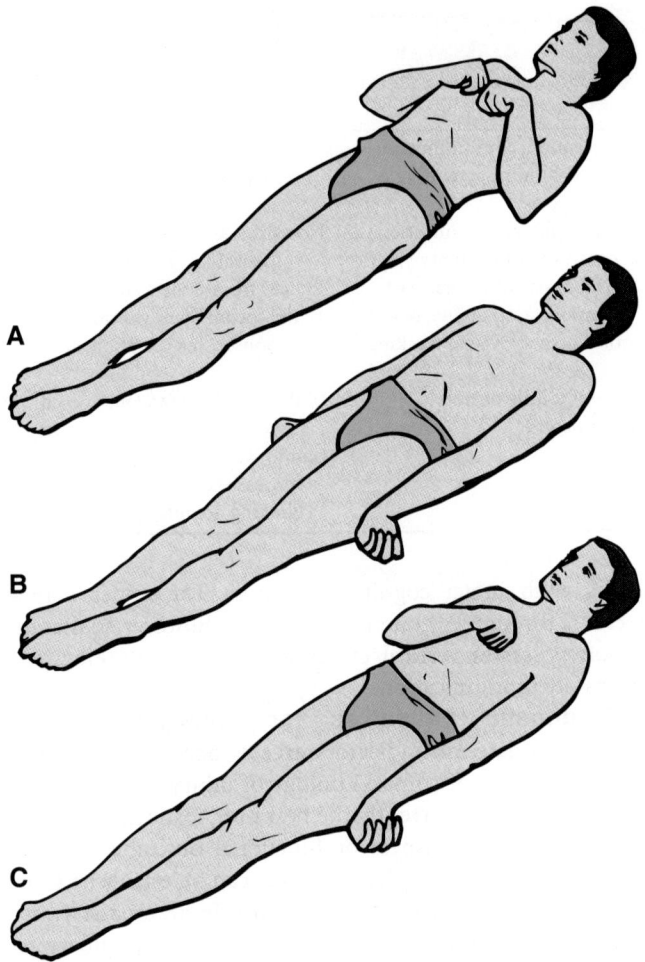

Figure 16-5 Decorticate and decerebrate responses. **A,** Decorticate response. Flexion of arms, wrists, and fingers with adduction in upper extremities. Extension, internal rotation, and plantar flexion in lower extremities. **B,** Decerebrate response. All four extremities in rigid extension, with hyperpronation of forearms and plantar extension of feet. **C,** Decorticate response on right side of body and decerebrate response on left side of body. (From Rudy EB: *Advanced neurological and neurosurgical nursing,* St Louis, 1984, Mosby.)

evidence of a nonfunctioning respiratory center (apnea challenge)

4. Absent cephalic reflexes (no ocular responses to head turning or caloric stimulation) with dilated, fixed pupils

5. Isoelectric (flat) EEG (electrocerebral silence)

6. Persistence of these signs for 30 minutes to 1 hour and for 6 hours after onset of coma and apnea

7. Confirming test indicating absence of cerebral circulation (optional)

Cerebral death (irreversible coma) is death of the cerebral hemispheres exclusive of the brain stem and cerebellum. Brain damage is permanent and sufficiently severe that the individual is unable to ever respond behaviorally in any significant way to the environment. The brain, however, may continue to maintain internal homeostasis (normal respiratory and cardiovascular functions, normal temperature control, and normal gastrointestinal function).

Related to the extent of disability, the recovery spectrum of neurobehavioral manifestations (in diagnostic terms, clinical states) after severe brain injury include (1) coma, (2) vegetative state (VS), (3) akinetic mutism, (4) minimally conscious state (MCS), and (5) locked-in syndrome[2] (Table 16-8).

The survivor of cerebral death may remain in a coma or emerge into a **vegetative state (VS).** In **coma,** a state of unarousable neurobehavioral unresponsiveness, the eyes are usually closed with no evidence of eye opening either spontaneously or in response to external stimuli.[2] The person does not follow commands, does not verbalize or mouth words, and has no goal-directed or volitional behavior. There is no sustained visual pursuit movements beyond a 45-degree arc.[2]

A VS has been called a wakeful unconscious state.[2] The Multi-Society Task Force on Persistent Vegetative States (MSTF) identified the diagnostic criteria for VS as (1) periods of eye opening (spontaneous or following stimulation); (2) the potential for subcortical responses to external stimuli, including generalized physiologic responses to pain, such as

Table 16-7	Abnormal Motor Responses with Decreased Responsiveness	
Motor Response	**Description of Motor Responses**	**Location of Injury**
Abnormal motor responses, upper extremity flexion with or without extensor responses in the leg (decorticate rigidity)	Slowly developing flexion of the arm, wrist, and fingers with abduction in the upper extremity and extension, internal rotation, and plantar flexion of the lower extremity	Suggest hemispheric damage above midbrain
Extensor responses in the upper and lower extremities (decerebrate posturing, decerebrate rigidity)	Opisthotonos (hyperextension of the vertebral column) with clenching of the teeth; extension, abduction, and hyperpronation of the arms; and extension of the lower extremities	Associated with severe damage involving caudal diencephalon or midbrain
	In acute brain injury, shivering and hyperpnea may accompany unelicited recurrent decerebrate spasms	Acute injury frequently causes limb extension regardless of location
Extensor responses in the upper extremities accompanied by flexion in the lower extremities		Indicates pontine level dysfunction
Flaccid state with little or no motor response to stimuli		Damage to lower pons and upper myelencephalon

Table 16-8	Comparison of Clinical Features of Coma, Vegetative State, and Minimally Conscious State		
Diagnosis	**Arousal**	**Awareness**	**Communication**
Coma	Eyes do not open spontaneously or in response to stimulation	No evidence of perception, communication ability, or purposeful motor activity (e.g., command following)	No evidence of yes/no responses, verbalizing, or gesture
Vegetative state	Eyes open spontaneously; sleep-wake cycle resumes; arousal often sluggish	No evidence of perception communication ability, or purposeful motor activity	No evidence of yes/no responses, verbalization, gesturing
Minimally conscious state	Eyes open spontaneously; normal to abnormal sleep-wake cycle; arousal level ranges from obtunded to normal	Reproducible but inconsistent evidence of perception, communication ability, or purposeful motor activity; visual tracking often intact	Ranges from none to unreliable and inconsistent yes/no responses, verbalization, and gesturing
Akinetic mutism	Eyes open spontaneously; normal sleep-wake cycle; arousal level is normal	Visual tracking present; little or not following of commands	Little or no spontaneous speech or gesturing
Locked-in syndrome	Eyes open spontaneously; normal sleep-wake cycle; arousal level is normal	Perceptions intact	Cannot verbalize or gesture; vertical eye movement and blinking are intact

posturing, tachycardia, and diaphoresis, and subcortical motor responses, such as grasp reflex; (3) return of so-called vegetative (autonomic) functions, including sleep-wake cycles, and normalization of respiratory and digestive system functions; and (4) occasional roving eye movements without concomitant visual tracking ability.[2] The person's eyes open spontaneously or following stimulation, or both. There may be random hand, extremity, or head movements. The individual maintains blood pressure and breathing without support. Brain stem reflexes (pupillary, oculocephalic, chewing, swallowing) are intact. No discrete localizing motor responses are present, and the individual does not speak any comprehensible words or follow commands.

Some survivors of coma progress to a minimally conscious state. The term **minimally conscious state (MCS)** was first used by the International Working Party on Vegetative States and supported by the Brain Injury Interdisciplinary Special Interest Group of the American Congress of Rehabilitation Medicine (ACRM). ACRM defined MCS as a condition of severely altered consciousness in which the person demonstrates minimal but defined behavioral evidence of self or environmental awareness.[2] The clinical features include (1) following simple commands, (2) manipulation of objects, (3) gestural or verbal "yes/no" responses, (4) intelligible verbalization, and (5) stereotypic movements (e.g., blinking, smiling) that occur in a meaningful relationship to the eliciting stimulus and are not attributable to reflexive activity.[2]

Akinetic mutism (AM) is a neurobehavioral state characterized by a severe disturbance in behavioral drive (motivation). Giacino and Zasler[2] describe this state as a subset of the MCS group. Generally, these individuals evidence eye opening with visual tracking and have little or no spontaneous speech or following of commands. Little movement is present. This is not attributable to decreased wakefulness or motor weakness or impairment.

With **locked-in syndrome,** both the content of thought and level of arousal are intact, but the efferent pathways are disrupted. Thus the individual cannot communicate either through speech or through body movement but is fully conscious, with intact cognitive function. The upper cranial nerves (I through IV) often are preserved, however, so that the person possesses vertical eye movement and blinking as a means of communication.

Prognostic Indicators for Emergence From Coma. To date, no indicators except those of brain death predict outcome of coma.[2] Etiology of injury and time since onset of coma are currently the best prognostic indicators of recovery of consciousness or functional outcome. In nontraumatic brain injury, the prognosis can be established earlier than with traumatic brain injury. In traumatic coma, there is a 95% death rate in individuals whose pupillary reflexes or reflective eye movements are absent 6 hours after onset of coma and a 91% death rate if pupils are nonreactive at 24 hours.[2] In nontraumatic coma, absence of any two of the following is an unfavorable sign in the first hours after admission: pupil reflexes, corneal reflexes, or oculovestibular responses. Absence of eye opening and muscle tone in 24 hours predicts death or severe disability.[2]

Recovery of consciousness within 2 weeks is associated with favorable outcomes. Recovery of consciousness after 6 months is correlated with severe disability on the Glasgow Outcome Scale.[2] No recovery without severe disability has ever been documented after 1 year in coma.[2] No emergence from a VS can be expected after 3 months in a VS from hypoxic-ischemic injury and after 1 year from TBI.

Emergence from MCS is confirmed when there is reliable and consistent demonstration of either (1) interactive communication, that is, the ability to answer basic yes/no questions regarding personal or environmental questions, and (2) functional use of objects, that is, the ability to appropriately discriminate among objects.[2] Failure to emerge from MCS within 12 months predicts likelihood of remaining in an MCS.[2]

Seizures

A **seizure** is a sudden, explosive, disorderly discharge of cerebral neurons and is characterized by a sudden, transient alteration in brain function, usually involving motor, sensory, autonomic, or psychic clinical manifestations and an alteration

Table 16-9	International Classification of Epileptic Seizures
Traditional Terminology	**New Nomenclature**
	I. Partial seizures (seizures beginning locally)

Focal motor; jacksonian seizures (occasionally become secondarily generalized)	A. Simple (without impairment of consciousness)
	   1. With motor signs
	   2. With special sensory or somatosensory symptoms
	   3. With autonomic symptoms or signs
	   4. With psychic symptoms

Temporal lobe or psychomotor seizures	B. Complex (with impairment of consciousness)
	   1. Simple partial onset followed by impaired consciousness
	   2. Impaired consciousness at onset—with or without automatisms
	C. Secondarily generalized (partial onset evolving to generalized tonic-clonic seizures)

	II. Generalized seizures (bilaterally symmetric and without local onset)

Petit mal	A. Absence
	   1. Typical
	   2. Atypical
	B. Myoclonic
	C. Clonic
	D. Tonic

Grand mal	E. Tonic-Clonic
Drop attack	F. Atonic (astatic, akinetic)
	III. Unclassified epileptic seizures

Table 16-10	Terminology Used to Describe a Seizure
Term	**Definition**
Aura	A partial seizure experienced as a peculiar sensation preceding the onset of a generalized seizure or complex partial seizure that may take the form of gustatory, visual, or auditory experience; a feeling of dizziness or numbness; or just "a funny feeling"
Prodroma	Early clinical manifestations, such as malaise, headache, or a sense of depression, that may occur hours to a few days before the onset of a seizure
Tonic phase	A state of muscle contraction in which there is excessive muscle tone
Clonic phase	A state of alternating contraction and relaxation of muscles
Postictal state	The time period immediately following the cessation of seizure activity

in level of arousal. The alteration in level of arousal is temporary. The term **convulsion,** sometimes applied to seizures, refers to the clonic-tonic (jerky, contract-relax) movement associated with some seizures. A seizure produces a brief disruption in brain electrical function.[7]

Types of Seizures

Seizures are classified in different ways—by clinical manifestations, site of origin, EEG correlates, or response to therapy. A simplified version of the international classification of epileptic seizures is presented in Table 16-9. **Generalized seizures,** 30% of seizures, involve neurons bilaterally, often do not have a local (focal) onset, and usually originate from a subcortical or deeper brain focus. With a generalized seizure, consciousness always is impaired or lost. **Partial seizures (focal seizures)** involve neurons only unilaterally, often have a local (focal) onset, and usually originate from cortical brain tissue, thereby having a superficial focus. Consciousness may be maintained as long as the seizure activity is limited to one hemisphere in simple partial seizures, but partial seizures may become generalized to involve neurons of the other hemisphere and the deeper brain nuclei. This process is called **secondary generalization.** Consciousness is lost at the point of generalization. In complex partial seizures, consciousness is impaired; that is, the person is unable to respond normally to exogenous stimuli. Sixty percent of seizures are either complex partial seizures or seizures with secondary generalization.

Status epilepticus is the experience of a second seizure, a third seizure, and often subsequent seizures before the person has fully regained consciousness from the preceding seizure or a single seizure lasting more than 30 minutes. The person is still in a **postictal state** (state that follows a seizure) when the next seizure begins. Status epilepticus most often results from abrupt discontinuation of antiseizure medications but also may occur in untreated or inadequately treated persons with seizure disorders. The situation is a medical emergency because of the resulting cerebral hypoxia. Mental retardation, dementia, other brain damage, and even death are serious threats. Aspiration also is a great risk. (Terminology associated with seizure activity is defined in Table 16-10.)

PATHOPHYSIOLOGY An **epileptogenic focus** appears to be a group of neurons that evidence a paroxysmal depolarization shift and sudden changes in the usual membrane potential. The plasma membranes of neuronal cells are thought to be more permeable, making them more easily activated by hyperthermia, hypoxia, hypoglycemia, hyponatremia, repeated sensory stimulation, and certain sleep phases. These neurons are hypersensitive and may even remain in a chronic partially depolarized state.

The primary abnormality may be a membrane defect leading to instability in resting potential, abnormalities of potassium conductance or calcium channels, defects of the γ-aminobutyric acid (GABA) inhibitory system, or an abnormality in excitatory transmission enhancement, particularly of the N-methyl-D-asparate type. In animal models, a defect in the GABA inhibitory system is the mechanism causing generalized seizures.

The firing of involved epileptogenic neurons becomes increasingly greater in frequency and amplitude. When the intensity of the neuronal discharge reaches a threshold point, the discharge spreads to adjacent normal neurons through corticocortical synapses. If uninhibited at this point, the cortical excitation spreads through interhemispheric tracts to the contralateral cortex and through projection pathways to the subcortical areas of the basal ganglia, thalamus, and brain stem. The excitation spread to the subcortical, thalamic, and brain stem areas corresponds to the **tonic phase** (phase of muscle contraction with increased muscle tone) and is associated with loss of consciousness. Autonomic clinical manifestations also may emerge at this point, and apnea may be present for a few seconds. The excitation is further projected downward to the spinal cord neurons through the corticospinal and reticulospinal pathways.

The **clonic phase** (phase of alternating contraction and relaxation of muscles) begins as inhibitory neurons in the cortex, anterior thalamus, and basal ganglia begin to inhibit the cortical excitation. This inhibition causes an interruption in the seizure discharge, producing an intermittent contract-relax pattern of muscle contractions. The intermittent clonic bursts gradually become more and more infrequent until they finally cease. At this point the epileptogenic neurons are exhausted and the neuronal membranes probably are hyperpolarized.

The maintenance of seizure activity demands a 250% increase in adenosine triphosphate (ATP). Cerebral oxygen consumption is increased by 60%. Although cerebral blood flow also increases approximately 250% during seizure activity, available glucose and oxygen are readily depleted. With a severe seizure the brain tissue may require more ATP than can be produced by the tissues from the available oxygen and glucose. A deficiency of ATP, phosphocreatine, and glucose then occurs, and lactate accumulates in the brain tissues. Severe seizures thus may produce secondary hypoxia, acidosis, and lactate accumulation, all of which are imbalances that may result in progressive brain tissue injury and destruction. Cellular exhaustion and destruction are consequences of these events.

If a seizure focus is active for a prolonged period, a secondary focus, called a **mirror focus,** may develop in normal tissue. This process apparently is caused by the interhemispheric communication, inasmuch as the mirror focus is located in the contralateral cortical area.

CLINICAL MANIFESTATIONS The clinical manifestations associated with seizure depend on the type of seizure (Table 16-11). Two types of symptoms often signal an impending generalized tonic-clonic seizure: an **aura,** a partial seizure that immediately precedes the onset of a generalized tonic-clonic seizure, and a **prodroma,** an early manifestation that may occur hours to days before a seizure (see Table 16-10). Both manifestations may become familiar to the person experiencing recurrent generalized seizures and so may help in preventing injuries during the seizure.

EVALUATION AND TREATMENT The health history is the most critical aspect in diagnosing a seizure disorder and establishing the cause. The health history is supplemented by the physical examination and laboratory tests of blood and urine (blood glucose, serum calcium, blood urea nitrogen, urine sodium, and creatinine clearance) to identify any systemic diseases known to have seizures as a clinical manifestation. Skull x-ray films, computed tomography (CT) scan, magnetic resonance imaging (MRI), and cerebrospinal fluid (CSF) examination are useful for identifying any neurologic diseases associated with seizures. The EEG is useful in assessing the type of seizure and may help determine its focus (Figure 16-6).

Treatment for a seizure disorder is first to correct or control its cause, if possible. If this is not possible, the major means of management is the judicious administration of antiseizure medications. The therapeutic goal is complete suppression of seizure activity without intolerable side effects of the drug. Other medical therapies may include prescription of a ketogenic diet, vagus nerve stimulation, and surgery. Folic acid supplementation is important. Some antiseizure medications decrease the effectiveness of hormonal contraceptives. In severe cases, psychologic, social, educational, and vocational counseling are often appropriate for the individual and family.

Types of Seizure Syndromes

Seizure disorders, the second most common neurologic disorder, represent a syndrome, not a specific disease entity. The term **epilepsy,** meaning "to be seized by a force from without," generally is applied to conditions in which no underlying correctable cause for the seizures is found so that the seizure activity recurs without treatment because of a primary underlying brain abnormality. Epilepsy, therefore, is a general term for the primary condition that causes the seizures. Epileptic syndromes are epileptic disorders characterized by specific clusters of signs and syndrome.[8] The three categories are based on clinical history, EEG manifestations, and etiology: (1) localization-related, (2) generalized, and (3) undetermined. Localization-related epilepsies and syndromes are typified by seizures that originate from a localized cortical region and are characterized by seizures that have a focal or partial onset. Generalized and undetermined epilepsies and epilepsy syndromes are characterized by seizures with initial activation of neurons within both cerebral hemispheres.

Table 16-11	Clinical Manifestations Related to Seizure Types	
Type	**Clinical Manifestations**	**Site**
I. Partial Seizures		
A. Simple		
1. With motor symptoms		
a. Without jacksonian march (focal motor seizure—the motor movements do not extend into adjacent areas)	Motor activity is usually clonic. Motor movement elicited by the seizure activity depends on the anatomic-physiologic portion of the irritated cortex, but motor seizures most often begin in the face and hands. Focal seizures begin with slow, repetitive jerking of the body part, which increases in strength and rate over a period of 5 to 15 sec. The seizure can cease spontaneously, with a gradual decrease in clonic movement.	Primary motor area
b. With jacksonian march (jacksonian seizure—the seizure activity spreads in an orderly fashion of adjacent areas)	Seizure activity spreads to adjacent areas after the initial clonic movement increases; motor movements, for example, would begin in the fingers of one side and spread to the hand, wrist, forearm, arm, face, and finally the lower extremity on the same side of the body. After spreading, the jerking movements in all areas would spontaneously stop.	Primary motor area
c. Adversive seizure	Turning movement of hand and eyes to the side opposite the irritative focus occurs. Often it is associated with contractions of the trunk and extremities. It may remain local or develop into a generalized seizure.	Frontal lobe anterior to the primary motor area
2. With special sensory or somatosensory symptoms (focal sensory seizure); less common than focal motor seizures; any age may be affected	Sensory experience is subjective and confined to the primary sensory modalities (somesthetic, visual, auditory-vestibular, or olfactory). If sensory seizure begins on the hand area of the sensory cortex, the patient experiences numbness, tingling, or "pins and needles" phenomena. Other sensory experiences include burning, a crawling sensation, or a feeling of movement of the body part. Areas most often affected include lips, fingers, and toes. May remain local or develop into a generalized seizure.	Sensory cortex Postcentral gyrus (parietal lobe) with involvement of the primary sensory area
B. Complex (temporal lobe or psychomotor seizure)		
1. Simple partial onset followed by impairment of consciousness—common seizures found in both children and adults but in most persons occur before 20 yr old	The person is able to interact with the environment with purposeful, although inappropriate, movements; although the body muscles stiffen, the person does not fall and may even continue the complex activity in which he or she was involved, such as driving (perseverative automatisms); the person may appear "wide eyed." A wide variety of sensory experiences precede the automatism and include illusions; formed hallucinations; primitive visceral, olfactory, and gustatory sensations; and affective and cognitive symptoms. Most characteristic event of a temporal lobe seizure is the automatism; common examples of automatisms are lip smacking, chewing, facial grimacing, swallowing movements, and patting, picking, or rubbing oneself or one's clothing. Temporal lobe seizures generally last 11 sec to 8 min (average 2 min) and are followed by several minutes of postictal confusion.	Temporal lobe and its connections Frontal lobes Other areas
2. Impaired consciousness at onset—with or without automatisms	See above.	
C. Secondarily generalized	Unconsciousness appears. General symptoms are produced.	
II. Generalized Seizures		
A. Absence (petit mal seizures) Typical	Characterized by lapses in consciousness that rarely last longer than 10 sec. Often associated additional subtle signs and symptoms such as clonic movements, changes in postural tone, automatisms, and autonomic changes. The child immediately returns to normal consciousness without a postictal period. Hyperventilation will induce a typical absence seizure.	Multifocal

Continued

Table 16-11	Clinical Manifestations Related to Seizure Types—cont'd	
Type	**Clinical Manifestations**	**Site**
II. Generalized Seizures—cont'd		
A. *Absence (petit mal seizures)— cont'd*		
Atypical	Lapses in consciousness occur almost always accompanied by motor signs, especially changes in tone and last from 10 to 25 sec. Often occurs on awakening and with drowsiness. A postictal period of confusion may follow. Hyperventilation does NOT induce an atypical absence seizure.	
B. *Myoclonus and myoclonic seizures*	Characterized by sudden, uncontrollable jerking movements of one or more extremities or the entire body. Seizures usually occur in the morning. Consciousness is thought to be preserved. Person often is flung violently to the ground so that injury is a real possibility. Myoclonic seizures can occur in clusters.	Multifocal
C. *Clonic*	Characterized by repetitive clonic jerks of constant amplitude and diminishing frequency.	
D. *Tonic (affects infants and children)*	Loss of postural tone without evidence of clonicity, with flexion of the upper limbs and extension of the lower limbs.	
E. *Tonic-clonic (grand mal seizure) (affects both children and adults)*	Child assumes an abnormal posture for seconds or minutes without losing consciousness. A prodromal period of irritability and tension may precede a tonic-clonic seizure by several hours or days; however, in most persons, seizures begin without warning. Characteristically tonic-clonic seizures begin with a sudden loss of consciousness and brief flexion; the person falls to the ground and the body stiffens in an opisthotonos position with legs and, usually, arms extended; the jaw snaps shut; a shrill cry may be heard as a result of forceful exhalation of air through the closed vocal cords as the thoracic muscles initially contract; the bladder and, less often, the bowel may evacuate; during the tonic phase, the person is apneic with subsequent cyanosis; pupils are dilated and unresponsive to light. The tonic phase lasts less than 1 min (average 10-15 sec). The clonic phase is characterized by flexion spasm of whole body interrupted by muscular relaxation, muscular contractions accompanied by strenuous hyperventilation; the face is contorted; the eyes roll, and there is excessive salivation with frothing from the mouth; profuse sweating and a rapid pulse are evident. The tongue is often bitten. The clonic jerking subsides in frequency and amplitude over a period of about 30 secs. The tonic-clonic seizure lasts 2-5 min. After the clonic phase, the person is in a stupor or coma for about 5 min; the extremities are limp; breathing is quiet; and the pupils begin to respond to light. When the person awakens, he or she may be confused and disoriented and complains of headache, muscle aching, and fatigue. There is no recollection of the attack. Tonic-clonic seizures may occur at any time of the day or night, whether the person is awake or asleep. The frequency of recurrence may vary from hours to weeks, months, or years.	Multifocal
F. *Atonic (drop attack)*	Characterized by sudden loss of postural muscle tone; the tone loss may be mild, resulting in a head nod, or more dramatic, including falls.	Multifocal

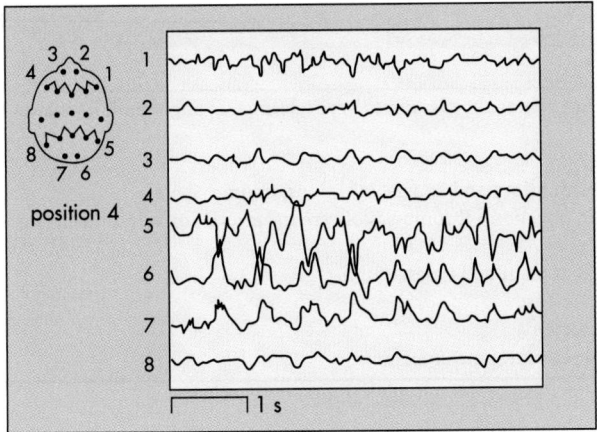

Figure 16-6 Electroencephalogram showing right posterior temporal sharp activity in individual with a microglioma. (From Perkin GD: *Mosby's color atlas and text of neurology,* London, 1998, Mosby-Wolfe.)

Epilepsy syndromes are further subdivided into idiopathic, symptomatic, or cryptogenic. **Idiopathic** refers to syndromes that arise spontaneously without a known cause, presumably having a genetic basis. The genetic basis may be through a specific inherited trait in which the seizures are the principle expression of the genetic defect (e.g., childhood absence epilepsy). In two-thirds of cases, the etiology of the epilepsy is not identified. **Symptomatic** denotes epilepsies with an identified cause. One-third of seizures can be classified as symptomatic (provoked or secondary). Some symptomatic epilepsies also have a genetic basis in which the inherited trait is expressed in a neurologic or systemic disorder that is associated with seizures (e.g., neurofibromatosis). The term **cryogenic** describes syndromes that are presumed to be symptomatic but have no known etiology, and occur in persons with or without abnormalities on neurologic examination. Box 16-1 presents the international classification of epilepsies, and Table 16-12 groups the etiology of recurrent seizures by age group.

Epilepsy is estimated to affect 6 to 7 persons per 1000 in the United States.[8] Forty to 50 new cases per 100,000 persons develop yearly. Incidence is highest in early childhood and declines to plateau in adulthood. However, incidence rises again in older people to early childhood levels. In persons with seizure disorders, seizure activity may be precipitated by hypoglycemia, fatigue or lack of sleep, emotional or physical stress, febrile illness, large amounts of water ingestion, constipation, use of stimulant drugs, withdrawal from depressant drugs (including alcohol), hyperventilation (respiratory alkalosis), and some environmental stimuli such as blinking lights, a poorly adjusted television screen, loud noises, certain music, certain odors, or merely being startled. Women may have increased seizure activity immediately before or during menses.

Alterations in Awareness

Selective attention (orienting), or a second attentional network, refers to the ability to select from available, competing environmental and internal stimuli specific information to be

---

Box 16-1   International Classification of the Epilepsies

1. Localization related (focal, partial)
   A. Idiopathic
      1. Benign childhood epilepsy with centrotemporal spikes
      2. Childhood epilepsy with occipital paroxysms
      3. Primary reading epilepsy
   B. Symptomatic
      1. Temporal lobe epilepsy
      2. Frontal lobe epilepsy
      3. Parietal lobe epilepsy
      4. Occipital lobe epilepsy
      5. Chronic progressive epilepsia partialis continua of childhood
   C. Cryptogenic defined by
      1. Seizure type
      2. Clinical features
      3. Etiology
      4. Anatomic localization
2. Generalized
   A. Idiopathic
      1. Benign neonatal familial convulsions
      2. Benign neonatal convulsions
      3. Benign myoclonic epilepsy in infancy
      4. Childhood absence epilepsy
      5. Juvenile absence epilepsy
      6. Juvenile myoclonic epilepsy
      7. Epilepsies with grand mal seizures on awakening
      8. Other generalized idiopathic epilepsies
   B. Cryptogenic or symptomatic
      1. West syndrome
      2. Lennox-Gastaut syndrome
      3. Epilepsy with myoclonic-astatic seizures
      4. Epilepsy with myoclonic absences
   C. Symptomatic
      1. Nonspecific etiology
      2. Early myoclonic encephalopathy
      3. Early infantile epileptic encephalopathy with suppression bursts
      4. Other symptomatic generalized epilepsies
3. Undetermined epilepsies
   A. Generalized and focal features
      1. Neonatal seizures
      2. Severe myoclonic epilepsy in infancy
      3. Epilepsy with continuous spike wave during slow-wave sleep
      4. Acquired epileptic aphasia
4. Special syndromes
   A. Situation-related seizures
      1. Febrile convulsions
      2. Isolated seizures or isolated status epilepticus
      3. Seizures occurring only when there is an acute or toxic event due to factors such as alcohol, drugs, eclampsia, nonketotic hyperglycemia.

Commission on classification and terminology of the International League against epilepsy: proposal for the classification of epilepsy and epileptic syndromes. *Epilepsia* 30:389-399, 1989. Used with permission of International League Against Epilepsy (ILAE).

Table 16-12	Causes of Recurrent Seizures in Different Age Groups
Age of Onset	**Probable Cause**
Neonatal	Congenital maldevelopment, birth injury, metabolic disorders (hypocalcemia, hypoglycemia), vitamin B deficiency, phenylketonuria
Infancy (1-6 mo)	As above; infantile spasms
Early childhood (3 mo-3 yr)	Infantile spasms, febrile convulsions, birth injury and anoxia, infections, trauma
Childhood (3-10 yr)	Perinatal anoxia, injury at birth or later, infections, thrombosis of cerebral arteries or veins, indeterminant cause ("idiopathic" epilepsy)
Adolescence (10-15 yr)	Idiopathic epilepsy including genetically transmitted types, trauma
Early adulthood (16-34 yr)	Trauma, neoplasm, infections, vascular disease
Middle age (35-64 yr)	Neoplasm, trauma, vascular disease, infections
Late life (>65 yr)	Vascular disease, tumor, degenerative disease, trauma, infections

From Sirven JI, Sperling MR: The epilepsies. In Corey-Bloom J, editor, *Adult neurology,* p 225, St. Louis, 1998, Mosby.

consciously processed. Certain structures have been demonstrated to contribute to selective attention. The disengagement mechanism is mediated by the right parietal lobe. The move component is mediated by the superior colliculi for visual orienting. The engage component is mediated by the pulvinar of the thalamus. A weak orienting network results in a neglect syndrome.

Sensory inattentiveness is a form of neglect and may be visual, auditory, or tactile. The person with sensory inattentiveness is able to recognize individual sensory input from the dysfunctional side when called on to do so but ignores (i.e., neglects, extinguishes) the sensory input from the dysfunctional side when stimulated from both sides. This phenomenon is called **extinction.** The entire complex of denial of dysfunction, loss of recognition of one's own body parts, and extinction is sometimes referred to as the **neglect syndrome.**

An isolated (pure) **selective attention deficit,** which manifests as a neglect syndrome, rarely, if ever, occurs clinically because typically other deficits also are present. A neglect syndrome may appear temporarily as a result of seizure activity or a postictal state. Temporary or permanent deficits may occur with contusions or subdural hematomas, encephalitis, and ischemic stroke. Progressive neglect deficits may be found with gliomas or metastatic tumor and in Alzheimer and Pick diseases.

Memory is the recording, retention, and retrieval of knowledge. Two types of memory exist, declarative and nondeclarative memory. **Declarative memory** involves the learning and remembrance of episodic memories (personal history, events, and experiences) and semantic memories (facts and information). Declarative memory is mediated by domain-specific cortical areas of the association areas of the temporal, parietal, and occipital lobes where long-term memories are thought to be stored and by domain-independent areas of the medial temporal lobe, the diencephalon, and the basal forebrain where it is thought distinct domain-specific features of an experience are related or bound.[9]

Nondeclarative memory, also called *reflexive, procedural,* or *implicit memory,* is the memory of how to carry out an action, behavior (habit), or skill. It is not a language memory but a motor memory. Nondeclarative memory involves the laying down of the motor pattern for the motor performance, so that the action, behavior, or skill becomes more and more automatic. All skills and habits are stored in this memory network. These memory stores are located in motor areas of the cerebrum, brain stem, and cerebellum.

Dysmnesia is a disorder of the domain-independent declarative memory network defined as the loss of past memories (retrograde amnesia) coupled with an inability to form new memories (anterograde amnesia) despite intact attentional networks.[9] Isolated (pure) domain-independent dysmnesia is caused by only a limited number of conditions, such as transient global dysmnesia (episodic global dysmnesia), amnestic stroke, and Korsakoff psychosis (amnestic or dysmnestic syndrome), as well as after temporal lobectomy. Many disorders may temporarily or permanently produce domain-independent dysmnesia that accompanies other deficits of the cognitive systems. A temporary domain-independent dysmnesia is found during complex partial seizures that persist for a time in the postictal state, in postconcussive states, and in mild posttraumatic brain injury states. A permanent domain-independent dysmnesia may be seen after subarachnoid hemorrhage or moderate or severe posttraumatic brain injury states; in carbon dioxide poisoning and other hypoxic or anoxic states; in Wernicke encephalopathy, viral encephalitis, and granulomatous meningitides; in tumors; and in Alzheimer and Pick diseases.

A pure auditory or visual domain-specific declarative memory deficit manifests as an isolated agnosia (see pp. 509 to 510 for etiologic factors). An isolated (pure) domain-specific declarative memory deficit of tactile sensations rarely occurs clinically because selected attention would likely be affected as well. A temporary auditory, visual, or tactile pattern recognition (remote memory) deficit may appear as a result of seizure activity or a postictal state. A temporary or permanent deficit can occur with temporal, occipital, or parietal lobe contusion; with subdural hematoma or ischemic stroke; and in encephalitis. A progressive domain-specific declarative memory deficit may occur in temporal, occipital, or parietal gliomas; in metastatic tumors; and in Alzheimer and Pick diseases.

The prefrontal areas mediate several cognitive functions, called *executive attention functions.* The vigilance system provides the person with the ability to maintain a sustained state of alertness and involves the right frontal areas and the locus ceruleus. Through the neurotransmitter norepinephrine from the locus ceruleus, the speed of the orienting (selective attention) network is increased and the detection function of the anterior cingulate lobe is decreased.

Detection is the recognition of the object's identity and the realization that the object fulfills a sought-after goal (i.e., target selection among competing, complex contingencies). There is conscious execution of an instruction, ensuring that the instructions are followed. The anterior cingulate cortex inhibits automatic responses so that a less routine response can be given. The basal ganglia and cingulate, as well as other frontal areas, function in color, motion, and form detection.

The anterior cingulate plus more lateral sites of the frontal lobes are involved in the representations of information in the absence of a stimulus, such as spatial position of visual events in memory when the event is removed from view. This is called *working memory* (short-term representation memory). Control of activation of these memories is also in these areas. This gives the person control over information processing. These temporary storage areas permit the brain to retrieve instructions and other information needed to guide behavior.

Isolated (pure) **vigilance, detection,** and **working memory deficits** have been discussed in the literature, but their individual occurrence is uncommon because these deficits generally are present simultaneously. Akinetic mutism exemplifies a detection deficit alone. The person orients to external stimuli and can follow with his or her eyes but does not initiate other voluntary activity. There are no goals generated and no plans for carrying out the goals. The combination of vigilance, detection, and working memory deficits, accompanied by other deficits of the cognitive systems, is much more common. Whether the deficits are temporary or permanent depends on the cause and severity of injury. Deficits caused by central nervous system (CNS)–depressant drugs, by seizure activity, and it is hoped, by neurosurgical procedures involving retraction of the frontal lobes are temporary. Deficits in postconcussive and mild traumatic brain injury states may prove to be temporary and resolve over time. Permanent deficits are more likely to be found with frontal lobe contusions, moderate or severe posttraumatic brain injury states, ischemic frontal lobe stroke, and neurosurgery that requires frontal lobe resection. Progressive deficits in vigilance, detection, and working memory functions are caused by frontal lobe gliomas, frontal lobe infarcts associated with hypertensive vascular disease, and late Alzheimer and Pick diseases. Persons with schizophrenia have difficulty in clearing working memory of information that is irrelevant to the current task. Additionally, recently encountered visual material that is no longer in plain view cannot be preserved in working memory.

Higher-level thought involves the same neural areas used for sensory-specific computations, but when used voluntarily in thought, these areas are activated from the detection and work memory networks (top-down processing) rather than from bottom-up processing beginning in sensory areas with a specific sensory stimulus. There is a voluntary search for a feature. By reordering component computation, a person produces novel thoughts.

PATHOPHYSIOLOGY Persons with a disease affecting the superior colliculi have a disturbance in the move operation of selective attention, which manifests as a slowness in orienting attention. Persons with parietal lobe disease may experience selective attention deficits related to disengagement from a stimulus. Persons with parietal lobe dysfunction, especially the right parietal lobe, also may experience a unilateral neglect syndrome, the prototype of a selective attention disorder. Persons with a disease affecting the pulvinar of the thalamus have a disturbance in the engage component of selective attention.

A disorder in vigilance may be produced by disease in the right frontal areas. A pathologic condition in the frontal areas also may produce detection and working memory deficits. Impaired higher-level thought may result from a pathologic process in the cortical association areas of the parietal, temporal, and occipital lobes.

The exact pathophysiology of the various disorders of cognitive systems is not fully known. Researchers currently are studying the defects in the elementary operations (components) of each cognitive system. In the past, pathophysiology related to the memory systems was the most studied. Dysmnesia, also known as *amnesia*, originates from pathologic conditions in the hippocampus and related temporal lobe structures. Orienting and the executive attentional network are currently receiving intense study.

As a highly general statement, the primary pathophysiologic mechanisms that operate in cognitive systems disorders are (1) direct destruction because of direct ischemia and hypoxia or indirect destruction as a result of compression and (2) the effects of toxins and chemicals. Disinhibition resulting in overactivity, such as seen in some drug withdrawal states, is a pathologic mechanism that can produce **detection deficits.** The pathophysiologic processes are presented in Figure 16-7.

CLINICAL MANIFESTATIONS   Clinical manifestations of selective attention deficits; domain-independent and domain-specific declarative deficits; and vigilance, detection, and working memory deficits are all presented in Table 16-13.

EVALUATION AND TREATMENT   Immediate medical management is directed at diagnosing the cause and treating reversible factors. Rehabilitative measures for cognitive system deficits generally are either compensatory in nature or restorative in nature and have of late been greatly facilitated by computer technology and other electronic-assisted devices. Approaches based on behavioral techniques tend to be compensatory, whereas process-oriented approaches, it is hoped, are restorative.

Selective attention and executive attentional deficits masquerade as other cognitive deficits. Differential diagnosis of

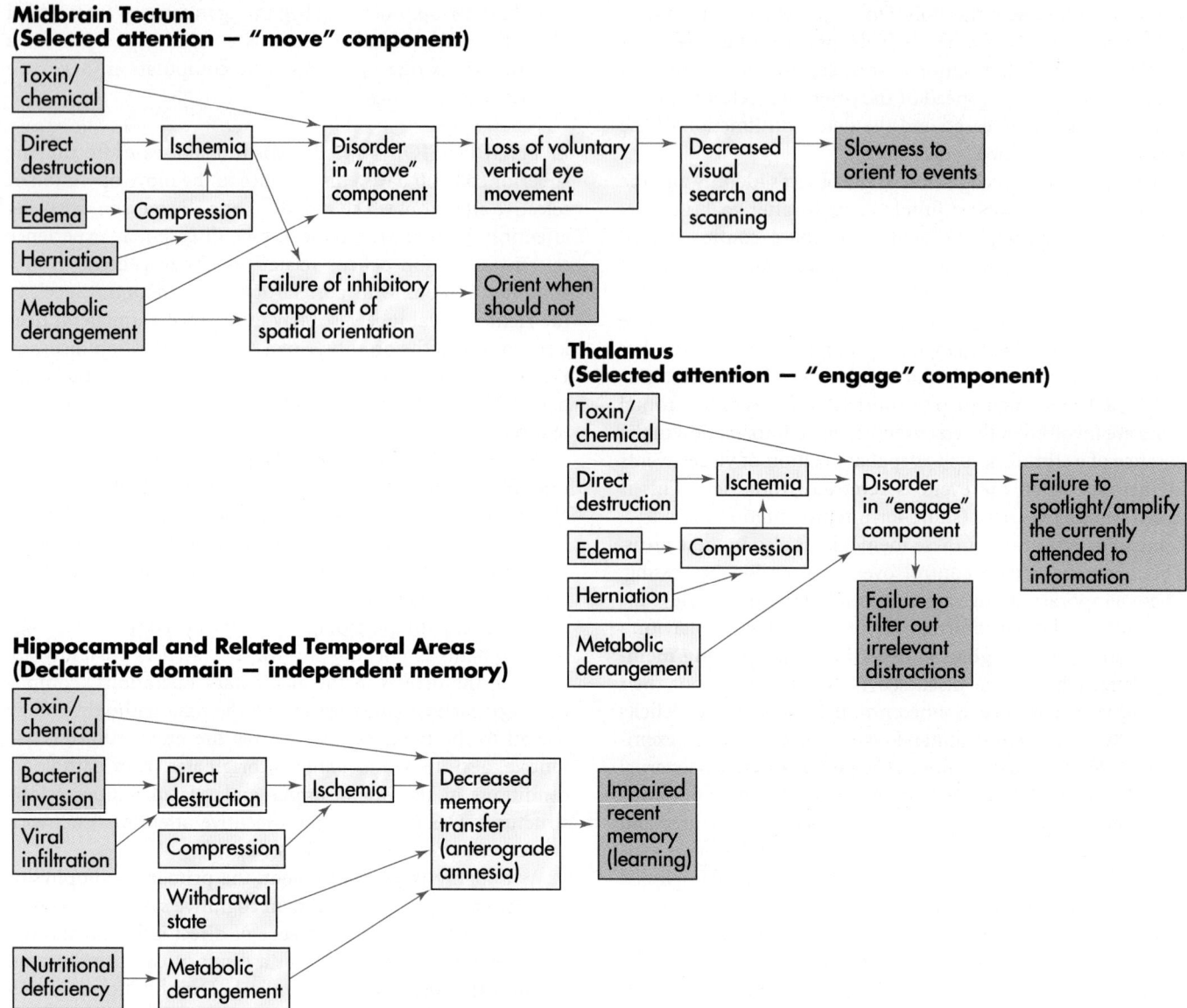

Figure 16-7 Cognitive network deficits. General pathophysiologic mechanisms underlying cognitive network deficits.

other cognitive deficits is blocked, and learning potential is largely obscured, by the presence of an attention deficit. Therefore diagnosis and treatment of attention deficits are fundamental.

Data Processing Deficits

Agnosia

Agnosia is a defect of pattern recognition—a failure to recognize the form and nature of objects. The disorder involves the loss of recognition through one sense, although the object or person may still be recognized by other senses. Agnosia can be tactile, visual, or auditory. For example, an individual may be unable to identify a safety pin by touching it with a hand but be able to name it when looking at it. Agnosia may be as minimal as a finger agnosia (failure to identify by name the fingers of one's hand) or more extensive, such as a color agnosia.

Agnosia is produced by dysfunction in the primary sensory area or in the interpretive areas of the cerebral cortex (see Figure 14-6). (The types of agnosia and the associated area that is most commonly involved with each are presented in Table 16-14.) Although agnosia most commonly is associated with cerebrovascular accidents, it may arise from any pathologic process that injures these specific areas of the brain.

Dysphasia

Dysphasia is impairment of comprehension or production of language (semantic processing). With dysphasia, comprehension or use of symbols, in either written or verbal language, is

Cortical Association Areas
(Selective attention, disengage components, declarative domain — specific memory)
(Image formation)

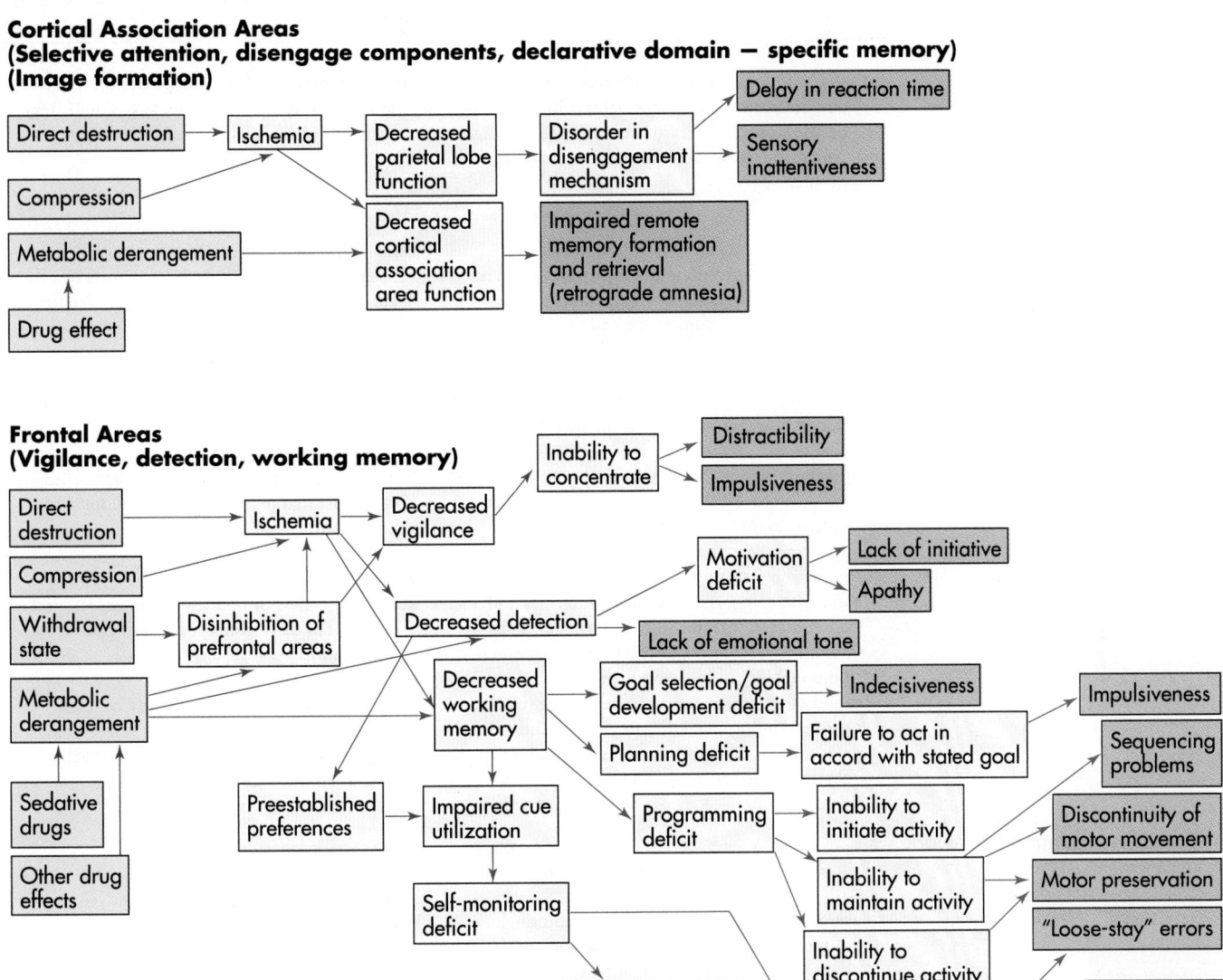

Frontal Areas
(Vigilance, detection, working memory)

Figure 16-7, cont'd Cognitive network deficits. General pathophysiologic mechanisms underlying cognitive network deficits.

disturbed or lost. **Aphasia** is loss of the comprehension or production of language.

Dysphasias usually are associated with cerebrovascular accident involving the middle cerebral artery or one of its many branches. The language disorders, however, may arise from a variety of injuries and diseases—vascular, neoplastic, traumatic, degenerative, metabolic, or infectious. Dysphasia results from dysfunction in the left cerebral hemisphere, most commonly in the frontotemporal region, particularly around the insula (Figure 16-8) (see also Figure 14-6). Most language disorders are caused by acute processes that either resolve or cause a chronic residual deficit. Some language disorders are caused by degenerative disorders that make the dysfunction progressive.

Dysphasias have been classified both anatomically and functionally. Other classifications are linguistic and describe fluency, volume, or quantity of speech. Pure forms of any language dysfunction, however, are rare. **Expressive dysphasias** are characterized primarily by expressive deficits, but a verbal comprehension (auditory-receptive element) deficit may be present. Receptive dysphasias may have expressive deficits. (Table 16-15 compares types of dysphasias; Table 16-16 illustrates some of the language disturbances.)

Dysphasias referred to as **transcortical dysphasias (transcortical sensory dysphasia, mixed transcortical dysphasia, isolated speech center)** involve the ability to repeat (called **echolalia**) and to recite. Speech is fluent but with striking paraphrases. The individual cannot read and write, and comprehension is impaired.

Transcortical dysphasias are caused by hypoxia from prolonged hypotension, carbon monoxide poisoning, or other mechanisms that destroy the border zone (watershed area) of the anterior, middle, and posterior cerebral arteries (see

Table 16-13 Clinical Manifestations of Cognitive Network Deficits

Deficit	Clinical Signs	Symptoms
Attention		
Selective attention (orienting)	Inability to focus attention; decreased eye, head, and body movements associated with focusing on the stimuli; decreased search and scanning; faulty orientation to stimuli causing safety problems	Person reports inability to focus attention, failure to perceive objects and other stimuli (history of injuries, falls, and safety problems)
Memory		
Domain-independent declarative	*Left hemisphere:* disorientation to time, situation, place, name, person (verbal identification); impaired language memory (e.g., names of objects); impaired semantic memory *Right hemisphere:* disorientation to self, person (visual), place (visual); impaired episodic memory (personal history); impaired emotional memory Either or both hemispheres: confusion; behavioral change	Person reports disorientation, confusion, "not listening," "not remembering"; reports by others of person being disoriented, not able to remember, not able to learn new information
Domain-specific declarative	*Left hemisphere:* inability to retrieve personal history, past medical history; unaware of recent current events *Right hemisphere:* inability to recognize persons, places, objects, music, etc., from past	Person reports remote memory problems; others report that person cannot recall formerly known information
Image processing (semantic processing)	Inability to categorize (identify similarities and differences), sort; inability to form concepts; inability to analyze relationships; misinterpretation; inability to interpret proverbs	Reports by others of frequent misinterpretation of data, failure to conceptualize or generalize information
	Inability to perform deductive reasoning (convergent reasoning); inability to perform inductive reasoning (divergent reasoning); inability to abstract; concrete reasoning demonstrated; delusions	Reports by others of predominantly concrete thinking; lack of understanding of everyday situations, health care regimens, and such; delusional thinking
Executive Attentional Network		
Vigilance	Failure to stay alert and oriented to stimuli	Person reports decreased alertness or ability to orient
Detection	Lack of initiative (anergy); lack of ambition; lack of motivation; flat affect; no awareness of feelings; appears depressed, apathetic, and emotionless; fails to appreciate deficit; disinterested in appearance; lacks concern about childish or crude behavior	Reports by others of laziness or apathy, flat affect or lack of emotional expression, failing to exhibit or be aware of feelings
Mild	Responds to immediate environment but no new ideas; grooming and social graces are lacking	Reports by others of lack of ambition, motivation, or initiative, failure to carry out adult tasks, lack of social graces and new ideas
Severe	Motionless, lack of responding to even internal cues, does not respond to physical needs, does not interact with surroundings	Reports by others of failure to groom or toilet self, unawareness of surroundings and own physical needs
	Inability to use feedback regarding behavior; failure to recognize omissions and errors in self-care, speech, writing, and arithmetic; impaired cue utilization; overestimation of performance	Reports by others of not changing behavior when requested; unawareness of limitations; does not recognize and correct errors in dressing, grooming, toileting, eating, and such; fails to recognize speech and arithmetic errors; careless speech
	Failure to shift response set; failure to change behavior when conditions change; cue utilization may be impaired	Reports by others of failure to use feedback; inability to incorporate feedback (does not correct when feedback is given)
Working memory	Inability to set goals or form goals; indecisiveness	Reports by others of failure to set goals, indecisiveness
	Failure to make plans; inability to produce a complete line of reasoning; inability to make up a story; appears impulsive	Reports by others of failure to plan, impulsiveness, "does not think things through"
	Failure to initiate behavior; failure to maintain behavior; failure to discontinue behavior; slowness to alternate response for the next step; motor perseveration	Reports by others of not knowing where to begin, inability to carry out sequential acts (maintain a behavior), inability to cease a behavior

Table 16-14	Types of Agnosia (Concept Disorders)	
Type of Agnosia	**Definition**	**Location of Injury**
Tactile agnosia (astereognosis)	Inability to recognize objects by touch	Parietal lobe
Spatial agnosia	Incapacity to find one's way around familiar places; disturbance of perception of space (disorders of [1] topographic [extrapersonal] orientation or [2] topographic and geographic memory [construction])	parietal lobe
Gertsmann syndrome	Loss of spatial orientation of fingers, body, sides, and numbers	Left angular gyrus (parietal lobe)
Finger agnosia (digital agnosia)	Inability to identify the names of one's fingers	
Right-left confusion	Inability to distinguish right from left	
Agraphia	Inability to write	
Acalculia	Inability to perform mathematic calculations	
Visual agnosia		
Object agnosia	Inability to recognize objects and pictures	Temporooccipital area
Prosopagnosia	Inability to recognize faces	Temporooccipital ventromesial region
Color agnosia	Inability to understand colors as qualities of objects; faulty color concepts and inability to evoke color images in the absence of color blindness; specific types: (1) "hue" problem, (2) color anomia (can not name color)	Inferior occipital cortex in left hemisphere
Body image agnosias (may be spatial)		
Anosognosia	Ignorance or denial of existence of the disease	Right parietal lobe
Autotopagnosia	Loss of ability to identify the body, in whole or in part, or to recognize relationships among various parts	Right parietal lobe
Word blindness (alexia/dyslexia)	Inability to recognize written symbols	Left parietotemporal region
Auditory agnosia (pure word deafness)	Inability to recognize speech sounds	Superior temporal area
Amusia (music deafness)	Loss of capacity to recognize tones and melodies	Right superior temporal area

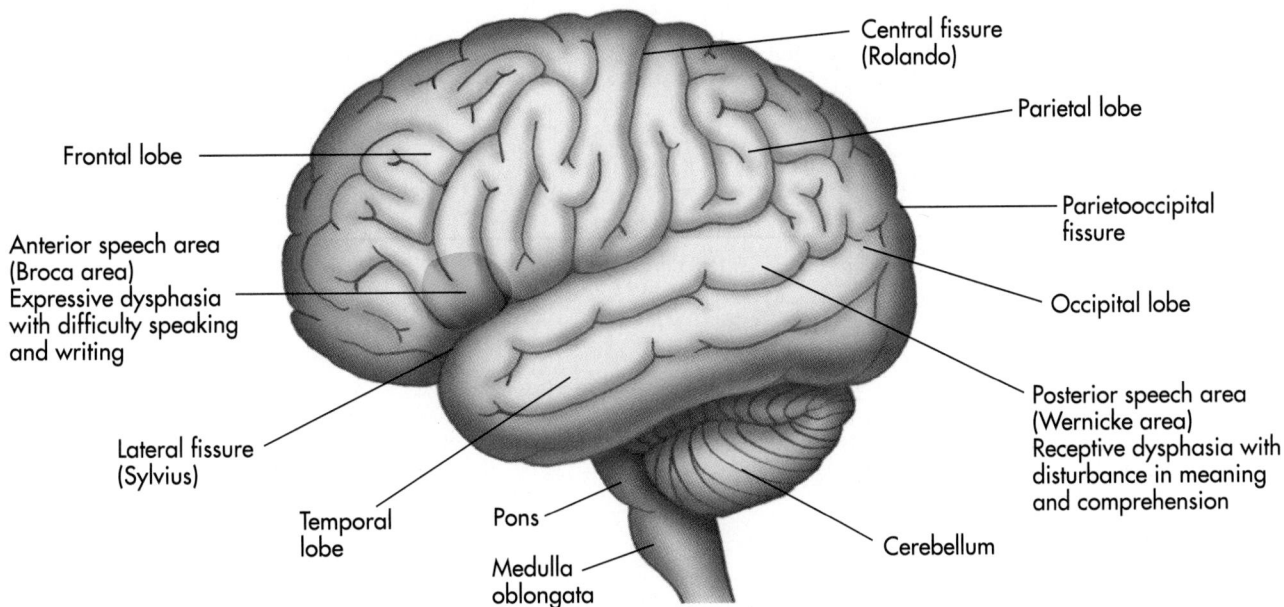

Figure 16-8 Anatomic involvement of dysphasia development. Portion of the left cerebral hemisphere considered most important in the development of dysphasia. The insula lies hidden from view, buried deep in the lateral fissure.

Table 16-15   Major Types of Dysphasia

Type	Expression	Verbal Comprehension	Repetition
Expressive (Broca Dysphasia, Motor)	Nonfluent; impairment of ability to find words, difficulty in writing	Relatively intact	Impaired
Receptive			
Wernicke dysphasia, sensory	Fluent: able to produce verbal language but language is meaningless; words are often inappropriate; words with similar sounds or words with similar meaning are substituted for the correct words; words that are not part of the language may be present; these neologisms may be so extensive as to make the speech entirely incomprehensible; because the person has no means to monitor the language for correctness, errors are not recognized; intonation, accent, cadence, rhythm, and articulation are normal	Impaired (disturbance in understanding all language)	Impaired
Global (sensory—motor receptive—expressive)	Nonfluent, produces little speech; at best speaks a few words or phrases	Impaired or completely lost; person understands only the simplest things said	Impaired; not able to repeat
Conduction	Fluent but with paraphrasia in self-initiated speech and writing or reading aloud	Relatively intact	Impaired; not able to repeat
Anomic, nominal, amnesic (anomia)	Fluent but impaired ability to name objects, persons, qualities, or characteristics; knows what he or she wants to say but cannot find words; may even use desired word in another context but still cannot isolate word when needed	Relatively intact; able to recognize word when it is given	Intact
Transcortical motor	Nonfluent	Relatively intact	Intact
Transcortical sensory	Fluent	Impaired	Intact

Name	Reading Comprehension	Writing	Location of Lesion	Cause of Lesion
Impaired	Variable	Impaired	Left posteroinferior frontal lobe (Broca area)	Occlusion of one or several branches of MCA, trauma, tumor, infection, abscess
Impaired	Impaired	Impaired	Left posterosuperior temporal lobe (Wernicke area)	Occlusion of inferior division of left middle cerebral artery, temporal abscess
Impaired	Reading out loud—impaired or completely lost. Reading silently intact	Impaired; produces little written language	Frontotemporal lobe (left sylvian region); anterior and posterior speech areas extensively impaired	Occlusion of the left middle cerebral artery of left internal carotid artery; trauma, infection, tumors, other mass lesions, and hemorrhage may cause
Impaired	Variable	Impaired	Arcuate fasciculus, deep in supramarginal gyrus, disruption of the large bundle of fibers that arise from the temporal lobe and pass posteriorly around the sylvian fissure and then project anteriorly to the premotor area	Typical cause is embolic occlusion of the ascending parietal or posterior temporal branch of the middle cerebral artery, angular branch of middle cerebral artery
Impaired	Variable	Variable	Angular gyrus—posterosuperior temporal lobe	Residual of other aphagias, degenerative disorders
Impaired	Variable	Impaired	Left dorsolateral frontal cortex (anterior presylvian fissure)	Occlusion of left anterior cerebral artery or anterior borderzone vascular infarct
Impaired	Impaired	Impaired	Left temporoparietooccipital junction (posterior presylvian fissure)	Occlusion of left internal carotid with posterior borderzone infarct, tumor, trauma, intracerebral hemorrhage, and degenerative disease

Table 16-16		Examples of Language Disturbances
Disorder		**Example**
Verbal paraphrasia	Question:	What did the car do?
	Patient:	The car would spit sweetly down the road. (The car sped swiftly down the road.)
Literal paraphrasia	Request:	Say "persistence is essential to success."
	Patient:	Mesastence is instans to success.
Neologism	Question:	What do you call this? (Pointing to a plant.)
	Patient:	It's a logper.
Circumlocution	Question:	What do you call this? (Pointing to a plant.)
	Patient:	Something that grows.
Anomia	Question:	What do you call this? (Pointing to a plant.)
	Patient:	It's . . .
		or
	Question:	What did you do this morning?
	Patient:	Reading.
	Question:	Were you reading a book or a newspaper?
	Patient:	One of those.
Telegraphic style	Question:	Where is your daughter?
	Patient:	New Orleans . . . home . . . Monday.

From Boss BJ: *J Neurosurg Nurs* 16(3):151, 1984.

Figure 14-18). Blood supply is marginal in this region. Hypoxia in this area occasionally may isolate the posterior speech areas or all the speech areas from the remainder of the cortex, although both areas remain intact. The sensory and motor speech areas therefore are functional, but connections with other sensory or motor areas are impaired. Information from the remaining areas of the cortex cannot be transmitted to the Wernicke area to be transformed into language.

Acute Confusional States

Acute confusional states (acute cerebral failure or **acute brain failure)** is an acquired mental disorder characterized by deficits in attention and coherence of thoughts and actions often associated with an altered level of arousal, global cognitive dysfunction, perceptual disturbances, sleep-wake cycle disruption, affective disturbance, and emotional liability.[10] Acute confusional states result from dysfunction secondary to such causes as drug intoxication, metabolic disorders, or nervous system disease. A common cause of an acute confusional state is withdrawal from alcohol, barbiturate, or other sedative drug ingestion. Acute confusional states of toxic origin may have either sudden or gradual onset, depending on the amount of exposure to the toxin. These states often occur with febrile illnesses, with systemic diseases such as heart failure, after head injury or anesthesia, postnatally, or with certain focal cerebral lesions.

PATHOPHYSIOLOGY Acute confusional states arise from disruption of a widely distributed neural network involving the reticular activating system of the upper brain stem and its projections to the thalamus, basal ganglion, and specific association areas of the cortex and limbic areas. Delirium (hyperkinetic confusional states) is associated with right middle temporal gyrus or left temporal-occipital junction disruption.[10] These areas receive extensive input from the limbic areas and modulate motivational and affective aspects of attention. Hypokinetic confusional states are more likely associated with right-sided frontal-basal ganglion disruption.[10] These areas modulate motor exploratory aspects of attention.

Most metabolic disturbances that produce a confusional state interfere with neuronal metabolism or synaptic transmission. Many drugs and toxins also interfere with neurotransmission function at the synapse. Cholinergic pathways critical for attention and arousal are often disrupted.

CLINICAL MANIFESTATIONS The predominant features of an acute confusional state are impaired or lost detection. Because of dysfunction of the anterior cingulate (see Figure 14-6), the ability to focus, sustain, or shift attentional focus is seriously impaired or completely lost. The person is highly distractible and unable to concentrate on incoming sensory information or on any one particular mental or motor task. Besides impaired attention, the person loses coherence of thought and actions. The person may persist in thoughts or actions that are no longer appropriate (perseveration) and be unable to monitor the environment for events of importance (impaired vigilance). The person also is unable to inhibit irrelevant or inappropriate responses.

The onset of an acute confusional state usually is abrupt rather than insidious. The first clinical manifestations are difficulty in concentration, restlessness, irritability, tremulousness, insomnia, and poor appetite. Later there are top-down processing problems, including misperception, illusion, hallucination, and delirium. Obsessions, compulsive behavior, and rituals may be evident.

In hypokinetic acute confusional states, the individual exhibits decreases in mental function. Alertness is decreased, as are attention span, accurate perception, and interpretation of the environment. Forgetfulness is prominent. Reactions to the environment are slowed and indecisive. The individual dozes frequently.

Delirium, an acute hyperkinetic confusional state, typically develops over 2 to 3 days. Early clinical manifestations include difficulty in concentrating, restlessness, irritability, insomnia, tremulousness, and poor appetite. Some persons experience seizures. Unpleasant, even terrifying, dreams may occur.

In a fully developed delirium state, the individual is completely inattentive and perceptions are grossly altered. Misperception and misinterpretation are predominant. Hallucinations may be present. The person appears distressed and often very perplexed. Conversation is incoherent. Frank tremor is evident, and a great deal of restless movement is common. Violent behavior may be present. The individual cannot sleep; is flushed; and has dilated pupils, a rapid pulse (tachycardia), temperature elevation, and perfuse sweating (diaphoresis). Delirium typically abates suddenly or gradually in 2 to 3 days, although occasional delirium states persist for several weeks.

EVALUATION AND TREATMENT   An acute confusional state is an acute medical problem. The initial goal is to establish that the individual is confused, and the cause must be distinguished as organic or functional (Table 16-17). Next, the goal is to determine whether the confusion is delirium, an acute hypokinetic confusional state, or an underlying dementia. The precise cause of an acute confusional state is established through the complete history and physical examination. Laboratory tests include an electrocardiogram and blood, urine, cerebrospinal fluid (CSF), and radiologic studies.

Once the cause is established, treatment is directed at controlling the primary disorder. In an acute confusional state, all drugs that may be contributing to or causing the condition are discontinued unless the problem is the result of drug withdrawal. Supportive measures are designed to enhance coping skills and to minimize the individual's need for altered cortical functions. Supportive and protective management also involves maintaining the person's intact cortical functions by promoting use of these functions. Agitated behavior is managed with neuroleptic medication.

Dementing Processes

Dementia is a syndrome that may be caused by a number of different illnesses. Dementia is the progressive failure of many cerebral functions that is not caused by an impaired level of consciousness.[11,12] The dementias are characterized by reduction in cognitive functions (intellectual function). Mental abilities are impaired, with a decrease in orienting, recent memory, remote memory, language, executive attentional functions, and alterations in behavior (Box 16-2).

Dementias can be classified according to etiologic factors (e.g., trauma, tumors, vascular disorders, infections) and according to associated clinical and laboratory signs. Most recently, dementing processes have been grouped as cortical, subcortical, or both (Box 16-3). The culmination of a progressive dementing process is nerve cell degeneration and brain atrophy involving the cerebral cortex, diencephalon, and basal ganglia.

PATHOPHYSIOLOGY   Mechanisms in dementing processes include (1) degeneration possibly caused by genetics, inflammation, or biochemical alterations; (2) atherosclerosis, multiple foci of infarction throughout the thalami, basal ganglia, cerebral projection pathways, and associated areas; (3) trauma, lesions in the cerebral convolutions, mainly frontal and temporal, corpus callosum, and mesencephalon; and (4) com-

Box 16-2	World Health Organization Definition of Dementia

Dementia is a syndrome due to disease of the brain, usually of a chronic or progressive nature, in which there is disturbance of multiple cortical functions, calculation, learning capacity, language, and judgment. Consciousness is not clouded. Impairments of cognitive function are commonly accompanied and occasionally preceded by deterioration in emotional control, social behavior, and motivation.

Table 16-17	Differences between Organic and Functional Confusion	
Factor	**Organic Confusion**	**Functional Confusion**
Memory impairment	Recent, more impaired than remote	No consistent difference between recent and remote
Disorientation		
Time	Within own lifetime or reasonably near future	May not be related to patient's lifetime
Place	Familiar place or one where patient might easily be	Bizarre or unfamiliar places
Person	Sense of identity usually preserved	Sense of identity diminished
	Misidentification of others as familiar	Misidentification of others based on delusion system
Hallucinations	Visual, vivid	Auditory more frequent
	Animals and insects common	Bizarre and symbolic
Illusions	Common	Not prominent
Delusions	Concern everyday occurrences and people	Bizarre and symbolic
Confusion	Spotty confusion	More consistent
	Clear intervals mixed with confused episodes	No tendency to become worse at night
	Worse at night	

From Morris M, Rhodes M: *Am J Nurs* 72(9):1632, 1972.

pression, increased intracranial pressure, and chronic hydrocephalus.

A genetic predisposition probably is a contributing factor to the dementing process. In some instances a familial history of dementia increases by four times the likelihood that dementia will develop. Environmental influences also may play a role in the pathogenesis of dementia. The exact nature of the influence of environmental factors, such as aluminum, is not clearly understood as yet. Causes of dementia are given in Table 16-18.

CLINICAL MANIFESTATIONS   A summary of the clinical manifestations of the dementias is presented in Table 16-19.

EVALUATION AND TREATMENT   Establishing the cause for a dementing process may be complicated, but all persons evidencing the clinical manifestations of dementia should be evaluated with laboratory and neuropsychologic testing to identify underlying conditions that may be treatable.

If a specific treatable cause is identified, the appropriate treatment is initiated. For example, an infectious process requires the appropriate antibiotic, and a potentially resectable mass may require neurosurgery. Nutritional deficiencies are corrected. If the cause is metabolic, the imbalance is corrected or the metabolic disorder is treated, or both.

Unfortunately, no specific treatment or cure exists for most progressive dementias. In such instances, therapy is directed at maintaining and maximizing use of the remaining capacities, restoring functions if possible, accommodating to lost abilities, and controlling behavioral changes. Delusions, paranoia, and hallucinations often respond to neuroleptic medications. If coexisting depression is suspected, a trial of antidepressants is appropriate. Assisting the family to understand the dementing process and to learn ways to assist the demented individual is an essential component of supportive management.

Alzheimer Disease

Alzheimer disease (dementia of Alzheimer type [DAT], senile disease complex) is a common neurologic disorder.[11] Formerly believed to occur mostly in persons younger than 65 years of age (familial, early-onset dementia), Alzheimer disease (AD) has now been demonstrated to be one of the most common causes of severe cognitive dysfunction in older persons. Its more prevalent forms are late-onset familial Alzheimer dementia (FAD) and nonhereditary, or sporadic, late-onset AD (70% of cases). Both FAD and sporadic, late-onset AD are known as senile dementia of the Alzheimer type (SDAT). AD is also associated with Down syndrome. It is estimated that nearly 6 million Americans had AD in 2000 with 360,000 new cases reported each year.[13] The greatest risk factor is age.[14]

PATHOPHYSIOLOGY   The exact cause of AD is unknown. Several possible theories being investigated include loss of neurotransmitter stimulation by choline acetyltransferase; mutation for encoding amyloid precursor protein; alteration in apolipoprotein E, which binds beta amyloid;[15] and pathologic activation of N-methyl-D-aspartate (NMDA) receptors resulting in an influx of excess calcium. Early-onset FAD includes at least three gene defects: amyloid precursor protein (APP) gene on chromosome 21, presenilin 1 (PSEN1) on chromosome 14, and presenilin 2 (PSEN2) on chromosome 1.[12] Late-onset FAD is linked to a defect in the apolipoprotein E (APOE4) gene on chromosome 19. Presence of the APOE4 allele is a marker of increased susceptibility rather than a genetic determinant.[14] Each of these mechanisms may be linked to aggregation and precipitation of insoluble amyloid (senile plaques, amyloid plaques, neuritic plaques) in brain tissue and blood vessels. AD also has been linked to a lysosomal pathway in the breakdown of amyloid precursor protein to yield beta amyloid, a neurotoxic substance coded by chromosome 21. A reduction in protein kinase C and the scavenging of phospholipid from the cell membrane are being studied as the cause for the lysosomal

Table 16-18	Causes of Dementia		
Illness	**Types of Damage**	**Treatment Available**	**Potential Treatment**
Dementia of Alzheimer type (DAT)	Plaques, tangles, transmitter defects, abnormal amyloid deposition	+ (?)	Anticholinesterases, nerve growth factor
Vascular dementia	Multiple infarcts, stroke, small vessel disease	+ (?)	Aspirin, lower blood pressure, lower cholesterol
Lewy body dementia	Lewy bodies, transmitter defects	+ (?)	Anticholinesterases
Parkinson disease	Lewy bodies especially in basal ganglia	—	Antiparkinsonian drugs do not help dementia
Frontal lobe dementia	Various, including Pick	—	
Normal-pressure hydrocephalus	Obstructed cerebrospinal fluid flow due to previous damage, e.g., subarachnoid hemorrhage, meningitis	+	Surgery (shunt)
Punch-drunk syndrome	Repeated head injury	+ (?)	Stop the damage
Slow-growing brain tumour	Pressure causes destruction of brain	+	Surgery
Aluminum and other metals	Direct toxic effect	+	Remove the poison
Wilson disease	Toxicity of copper	+	Penicillamine
Alcohol abuse	Toxic effect and thiamine deficiency	+	Abstinence, thiamine treatment
Huntington chorea	Genetic abnormality	—	Screening available
Syphilis (GPI)	Infective	+	Antibiotics
AIDS	Infective, secondary infection	+	Anti-AIDS drugs
CJD	Infection (?)	—	
Vitamin (e.g., B_{12}) deficiencies	Toxic (?)	+	Replacement
Hypothyroidism	Toxic (?)	+	Replacement
Parathyroid disorders	Calcium metabolism altered	+	Medical or surgical

From Jacques A, Jackson GA: *Understanding dementia*, ed 3, London, 2000, Churchill Livingstone.
AIDS, Acquired immunodeficiency syndrome; *CJD,* Creutzfeldt-Jakob disease; *GPI,* general paralysis of the insane.

pathway taking precedence. A link between the pathology of AD and aluminum has not been established. Researchers have not yet been able to isolate a virus that causes the disease, but submicroscopic proteinaceous infectious particles (prions) have been isolated. These prions already have been linked to at least one other form of degenerative brain disease. Antibrain antibodies may account for AD, and an autoimmune cause also is being investigated. One theory is that once plaques form, complement proteins attach to them, attracting microglia (the brain's immune force), which release toxins in an attempt to destroy plaques. Because plaques cannot be destroyed, the assault is endless. In addition, aging and injury also may result in changes that contribute to the development of this disease. Such changes could include decreased oxygen and glucose transport, loss of the blood-brain barrier, and mitochondrial defects that alter cell metabolism and processing of proteins, including amyloid (APOE4). APOE4 predisposes to late-onset FAD, as well as sporadic late-onset causes. The 3% of persons who are homozygous for APOE4 have an 85% risk, whereas the 25% who are heterozygous have a 45% to 50% risk.[12]

Microscopically the *Tau protein* that normally stabilizes the microtubular transport system in the neurons detaches from the microtubule and forms insoluble helical filaments[12] called a **neurofibrillary tangle** (Figure 16-9). Tangles are flame shaped. Cortical nerve cell processes become twisted and dilated because of accumulation of the same filaments that form tangles. Amyloid also is deposited in cerebral arteries, causing an amyloid angiopathy. Groups of

Table 16-19	Clinical Manifestations of Dementia
Type	**Manifestation**
Cortical dementia	Difficulty with naming
	Decreased language comprehension
	Loss of recent memory
	Agnosias
	Apraxia
	Loss of remote memory
	Decreased mathematic skill
	Altered visuospatial relationships
Subcortical dementia	Forgetfulness
	Apathy
	Depression
	Slowed thought processes
	Accident prone
	Personality changes and inappropriate affect
	Loss of motor function: wide shuffling gait with small steps, muscle rigidity, flexion posturing, tendency to fall, abnormal reflexes, bowel and bladder incontinence, immobility

nerve cells, especially terminal axons, degenerate and coalesce around an amyloid core. Microscopic examination of these areas of degeneration reveals plaquelike material known as **senile plaques.** These plaques disrupt nerve-impulse transmission. Amyloid and tau proteins also have recently been linked together. Beta amyloid binds to the seven nicotinic acetylcholine receptors on cholinergic

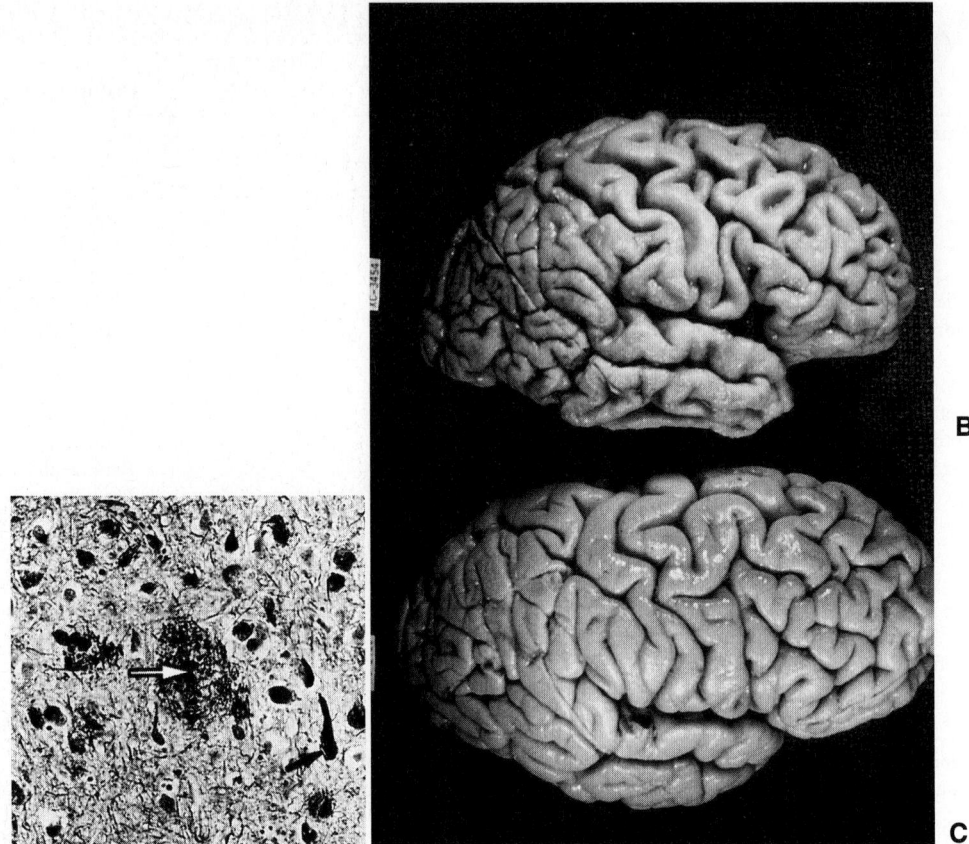

Figure 16-9 Pathologic changes in Alzheimer disease. **A,** A neuritic (mature) plaque with central amyloid core *(white arrow)* next to a neurofibrillary tangle *(black arrow)*. Alzheimer disease **(B)** compared with age-matched and sex-matched control **(C):** reduced size, narrow gyri, and wide sulci, notably in frontal and temporal lobes. (From Damjanov I, Linder J, editors: *Anderson's pathology,* ed 10, St Louis, 1996, Mosby.)

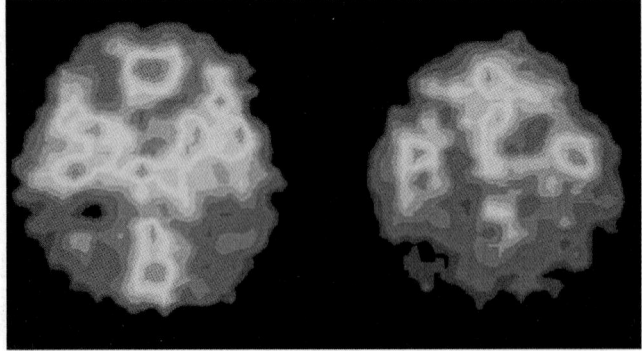

Figure 16-10 Altered cerebral blood flow in Alzheimer disease. Single photon emission computerized tomography scan showing reduction of temporoparietal blood flow *(right)* compared to normal blood flow *(left).* (From Perkin GD: *Mosby's color atlas and text of neurology,* London, 1998, Mosby-Wolfe.)

neurons. This binding induces phosphate groups to attach to tau protein. Senile plaques and neurofibrillary tangles are more concentrated in the cerebral cortex and hippocampus. The greater the number of senile plaques and neurofibrillary tangles, the more dysfunction is associated with AD. See Figure 16-10 for a visual of the disturbance in blood flow in Alzheimer disease.

CLINICAL MANIFESTATIONS Initial clinical manifestations are insidious and often attributed to forgetfulness, emotional upset, or other illness. The individual becomes progressively more forgetful over time, particularly in relation to recent events. Memory loss increases as the disorder advances, and the person becomes disoriented and confused. The ability to concentrate declines. Abstraction, problem solving, and judgment gradually deteriorate. A failure in mathematic calculation ability, language, and visuospatial orientation occurs. Dyspraxia may appear. The mental status changes induce behavioral changes, including irritability, agitation, and restlessness. Mood changes also result from the deterioration in cognition. The person may become anxious, depressed, hostile, emotionally labile, and prone to mood swings. Motor changes may occur if the posterior frontal lobes are involved. The individual exhibits rigidity (paratonia, gegenhalten), with flexion posturing, propulsion, and retropulsion. Great variability in age of onset, intensity and sequence of symptoms, and location and extent of brain abnormalities occurs among individuals with AD. Box 16-4 presents the clinical findings in each stage of AD.

EVALUATION AND TREATMENT The diagnosis of AD is made by ruling out other causes of a dementing process

Box 16-4	Clinical Findings in Each Stage of Alzheimer Disease

Stage 1 (Duration of Disease: 1 to 3 Years)
Memory—new learning defective, impaired declarative memory
Visuospatial skills—topographic disorientation, poor construction
Language—poor word list generation, anomia
Personality—apathy, irritability, depression
Motor system—normal
EEG—normal
CT—normal

Stage II (Duration of Disease: 2 to 10 Years)
Memory—more severely impaired declarative memory
Visuospatial skills—poor construction, spatial disorientation
Language—fluent aphasia
Calculation—acalculia
Praxis—ideomotor apraxia
Personality—indifference and apathy
EEG—slowing
CT—normal or ventricular dilation and sulcal enlargement

Stage III (Duration of Disease: 8 to 12 Years)
Intellectual functions—severely deteriorated
Motor—limb rigidity and flexion posture
Sphincter control—urinary and fecal incontinence
EEG—diffusely slow
CT—ventricular dilation and sulcal enlargement

From Cummings JL, Benson DF: *Dementia: a clinical approach,* Stoneham, Mass, 1992, Butterworth.
EEG, Electroencephalogram; *CT,* computed tomography.

NUTRITION & DISEASE

Alzheimer Disease

Weight loss is a major concern for elderly people with Alzheimer disease. The weight loss may be a result of (1) increased incidence of infection, (2) increased energy output because of constant pacing, (3) inadequate food intake, and (4) decreased independence and difficulty in self-feeding. Dementia may lead to memory loss, social isolation, depression, and poor food intake with resultant weight loss. Individuals may forget or refuse to eat, not communicate the need to eat, throw food or hide food, eat spoiled food or nonfood substances, eat favorite foods to the exclusion of eating other foods, take a long time to eat, have difficulty in preparing foods, and be unable to feed themselves.

Suggestions for caregivers of those with Alzheimer disease might include having a service (e.g., Home-Delivered Meals, Meals on Wheels) deliver a daily meal; taking the person to a congregate meal site; offering foods frequently; using finger foods such as Tater Tots, fish sticks, grapes, and crackers; dating refrigerated food and cleaning out the refrigerator on a regular basis; and providing a variety of foods.

Data from Riviere D, Albarede JL, Vellas B: *Am J Clin Nutr* 71(2):S67S, 2000; Wang PN et al: *J Neurol* 251(3):314-320, 2004.

by CT and blood tests. The history, including the mental status examination and the course of the illness, is used for diagnosis. The course of the disorder is highly variable, usually developing over 5 years or more.

Cholinesterase inhibitors (ChE-Is) are used in mild to moderate AD to enhance cholinergic transmission.[16] Memantine (Namenda) is a new drug with a different mechanism of action; it works as an uncompetitive NMDA receptor antagonist that blocks the activity of glutamate[17,18] and is approved for use in moderate and severe AD.

Treatment of AD also is directed at decreasing the need for the impaired cognitive function by a compensation technique, such as memory aids, maintaining those cognitive functions that are not impaired, and maintaining or improving the general state of hygiene, nutrition, and health. Environmental management, counseling, education, pharmacotherapy, and health promotion measures provide the foundation on which a comprehensive treatment program is built.

ALTERATIONS IN CEREBRAL HEMODYNAMICS

An injured brain reacts with structural, chemical, and pathophysiologic changes. Critical variables related to cerebral oxygenation include intracranial pressure, blood flow, and oxygen delivery. The pressure and oxygen delivery are critical management issues.

Cerebral Hemodynamics

Increased intracranial pressure (ICP) was the central management issue for many years. It is now recognized that cerebral oxygenation is the critical issue. Several relevant features of cerebral hemodynamics—cerebral blood volume (CBV), cerebral blood flow (CBF), and cerebral perfusion pressure (CPP)—relate to cerebral oxygenation (Box 16-5).

To guide therapeutic management, three critical categories related to cerebral hemodynamics are possible in the injured brain: (1) cerebral oligemia (also called *jugular fibrillation*), (2) CPP in the normal range (60 to 100 mmHg) but with an elevated ICP, and (3) cerebral hyperemia. In the treatment algorithms, oxygen saturation measured in the internal jugular vein (SjO_2) is categorized as less than 55%, greater than 55% but less than 70%, or greater than 75%. After SjO_2 is categorized, the ICP must be added to the equation as less than 20 mm Hg or greater than 20 mm Hg. Treatment algorithms are implemented depending on the SjO_2 and ICP that address not only ICP but also CPP.[19,20] The therapeutic goal is to balance ICP and SjO_2.[19,21] Target values for relevant clinical parameters are presented in Table 16-20.

Increased Intracranial Pressure

Intracranial pressure normally is 5 to 15 mmHg, or 60 to 180 cm H_2O. **Increased intracranial pressure** may result from an increase in intracranial content (as occurs with tumor growth), edema, excess cerebrospinal fluid (CSF), or hemorrhage. A rise in intracranial pressure necessitates an equal reduction in volume of the other contents. The most readily displaced content of the cranial vault is CSF. If intracranial pressure remains high after CSF displacement out of the

Box 16-5 Cerebral Hemodynamics

Cerebral blood volume (CBV) refers to the amount of blood in the intracranial vault at a given time (normally about 10%). Most of this CBV is in the low-pressure venous system. CBV is determined by autoregulation mechanisms that control cerebral blood flow.

Cerebral blood flow (CBF) to the brain is normally maintained at a rate that matches local metabolic needs of the brain and is normally about 750 ml/min (15% to 20% of the cardiac output). CBF is calculated as follows: CBF + CPP/CVR (cardiovascular resistance). Required CBF varies in gray and white matter and is greater in gray matter. CBF is regulated through constriction or dilation of the cerebral vessels predominantly in response to changes in arterial O_2 and CO_2 concentrations. CBF decreases 3% for every 1 mm Hg decrease in CO_2. CBF increases at a Pao_2 of less than 50 mm Hg; CBF is stable (maintained) at a Pao_2 of greater than 80 mm Hg.

Cerebral perfusion pressure (CPP) is the pressure required to perfuse the cells of the brain. The formula to calculate CPP is as follows: CPP = MAP − ICP. Normal CPP is 60 to 100 mg Hg in normal brain tissue. An injured brain requires a CPP of greater than 70 mm Hg. The CPP determines CBF. As CPP decreases to 70 to 80 mm Hg in the injured brain, vasodilation occurs, which increases CBV, also increasing ICP. An increased ICP will decrease CPP.

Oxygen saturation measured in the internal jugular vein (Sjo_2) at the jugular bulb reflects the amount of oxygen still bound as the blood leaves the cranial vault. Cerebral extraction of oxygen (CEo_2) is calculated using the formula $SAo_2 − Sjo_2/SAo_2 \times 100$.* Normal CEo_2 is 20% to 24%; normal Sjo_2 is 55% to 70%. When oxygen demand exceeds oxygen supply, extraction increases, increasing the Sjo_2. A CEo_2 less than 24% or an Sjo_2 greater than 70% to 75% indicates cerebral hyperemia. Acid-base balance and temperature influence oxyhemoglobin dissociation (see Chapter 32).

*Data from Cruz J: *Crit Care Med* 26(2):233, 1998.
CPP/CVR, Cerebral perfusion pressure/cardiovascular resistance; *MAP,* mitogen-activated protein; *ICP,* intracranial pressure; *Sjo_2,* oxygen saturation in the jugular vein; *SAo_2,* oxygen saturation in arterial blood.

Table 16-20	Therapeutic Management Goals for Patients with Altered Cerebral Hemodynamics	
Clinical Parameter	**Target Value**
Central perfusion pressure	>70 mmHg
Intracranial pressure	<20 mmHg
Arterial CO_2 pressure ($Paco_2$)	35 mmHg
Mean arterial pressure	90 mmHg
Temperature	34-36° C
Pulmonary capillary wedge pressure	10-15 mm Hg

vasoconstriction occurs in an attempt to elevate the systemic blood pressure sufficiently to overcome the increased intracranial pressure. This is stage 2 of intracranial hypertension.

As intracranial pressure begins to approach arterial pressure, the brain tissues begin to experience hypoxia and hypercapnia and the individual's condition rapidly deteriorates. Clinical manifestations include decreasing levels of arousal, Cheyne-Stokes respirations or central neurogenic hyperventilation, pupils that become sluggish and dilated, widened pulse pressure, and bradycardia.

Dramatic sustained rises in intracranial pressure are not seen until all the compensatory mechanisms have been exhausted. Once decompensation begins, dramatic rises in intracranial pressure occur over a very short period. **Autoregulation,** the compensatory alteration in the diameter of the intracranial blood vessels designed to maintain a constant blood flow during changes in cerebral perfusion pressure, is lost with progressively increased intracranial pressure. Accumulating carbon dioxide may still cause vasodilation at the local tissue level, but now, without autoregulation, this vasodilation causes the hydrostatic (blood) pressure in the vessels to drop and blood volume to increase. The brain volume is thus further enhanced, and intracranial pressure continues to rise. This is stage 3 of intracranial hypertension. Small increases in volume cause dramatic increases in intracranial pressure, and the pressure takes much longer to return to baseline. As the intracranial pressure begins to approach systemic blood pressure, cerebral perfusion pressure falls and cerebral perfusion slows dramatically. The brain tissues experience severe hypoxia and acidosis.

Increased intracranial pressure in one compartment of the cranial vault is not evenly distributed throughout the other vault compartments. In stage 4, the last stage of intracranial hypertension, brain tissue shifts (herniates) from the compartment of greater pressure to a compartment of lesser pressure (Figure 16-11). With this shift in brain tissue, the herniating brain tissue's blood supply is compromised, causing further ischemia and hypoxia in the herniating tissues. The herniated brain tissues increase the volume of content within the lower-pressure compartment, exerting pressure on the brain tissue that normally occupies that compartment, thus impairing that tissue's blood supply. Small hemorrhages frequently develop in the involved brain tissue. Obstructive hy-

cranial vault, cerebral blood volume is altered, which causes stage 1 of intracranial hypertension. Vasoconstriction and external compression of the venous system occur in an attempt to further decrease the intracranial pressure. Thus, during the first stage of intracranial hypertension, intracranial pressure may not change because of the effective compensatory mechanisms. CSF is reduced through increased reabsorption. Blood volume is reduced by compression of intracranial veins. Small increases in volume, however, cause an increase in pressure, and the pressure may take longer to return to baseline. Clinical manifestations at this stage usually are subtle and often transient and include episodes of confusion, drowsiness, and slight pupillary and breathing changes.

If intracranial pressure is still high, a state of intracranial hypertension occurs. With continued expansion of the intracranial content, the resulting increase in intracranial pressure may exceed the brain's compensatory capacity to adjust to the increasing pressure. In this state, the pressure begins to compromise neuronal oxygenation, and systemic arterial

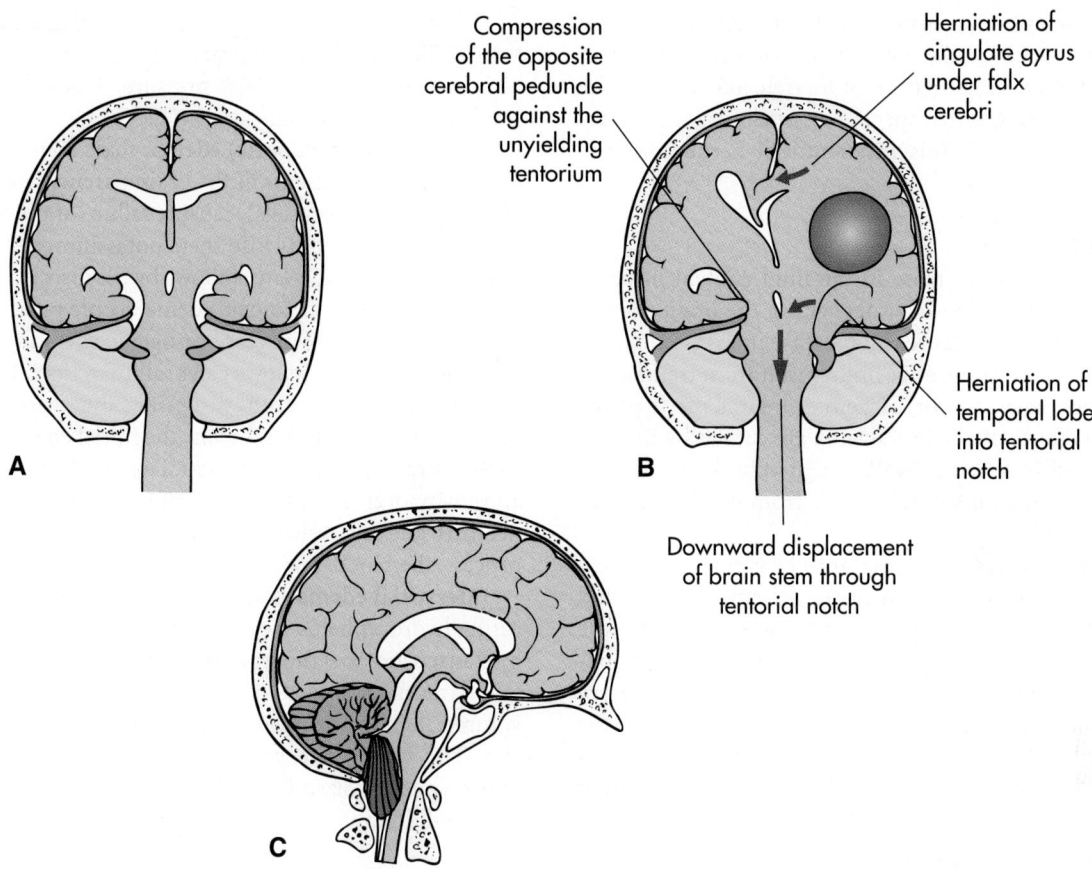

Compression
of the opposite
cerebral peduncle
against the
unyielding
tentorium

Herniation of
cingulate gyrus
under falx
cerebri

Herniation of
temporal lobe
into tentorial
notch

Downward displacement
of brain stem through
tentorial notch

Figure 16-11 Herniation resulting from increased intracranial pressure. **A,** Normal relationship of intracranial structures. **B,** Shift of intracranial structures. **C,** Downward herniation of the cerebellar tonsils into the foramen magnum.

drocephalus may develop. The herniation process markedly and rapidly increases intracranial pressure. Mean systolic arterial pressure soon equals intracranial pressure, and cerebral blood flow ceases at this point.

Herniation Syndromes

Supratentorial Herniation

The three types of supratentorial herniation syndromes are (1) uncal (temporal lobe, lateral transtentorial) herniation, (2) central (transtentorial) herniation, and (3) cingulate gyrus herniation. **Uncal herniation (hippocampal herniation, lateral mass herniation)** occurs when the uncus or hippocampal gyrus (or both) shifts from the middle fossa through the tentorial notch into the posterior fossa, compressing the ipsilateral third cranial nerve, then the contralateral third cranial nerve, and finally the mesencephalon. Uncal herniation generally is caused by an expanding mass in the lateral region of the middle fossa. The earliest signs of uncal herniation are poor concentration, drowsiness, and the bilateral corticospinal tract signs of increased tone and a positive Babinski sign.[3] The classic manifestations of uncal herniation are a decreasing level of consciousness, pupils that become sluggish before fixing and dilating (first the ipsilateral, then the contralateral pupil), Cheyne-Stokes respirations (which later shift to central neurogenic hyperventilation), the appearance of decorticate, then later decerebrate, posturing, and

ipsilateral hemiplegia because of contralateral corticospinal tract compression.[3]

Central herniation is the straight downward shift of the diencephalon through the tentorial notch. Causes of central herniation are injuries or masses located around the outer perimeter of the frontal, parietal, or occipital lobes; extracerebral injuries around the central apex (top) of the cranium; bilaterally positioned injuries or masses; and unilateral cingulate gyrus herniation. The individual experiencing transtentorial herniation rapidly passes from a conscious to an unconscious state; from Cheyne-Stokes respirations to apnea; from small, reactive pupils to dilated and fixed pupils; and from decortication to decerebration.

Cingulate gyrus herniation (subfalcine herniation) occurs when the cingulate gyrus shifts under the falx cerebri. Little is known about the clinical manifestations of this type of herniation except that there are signs of a mass causing increased intracranial pressure.[3]

Infratentorial Herniation

Two types of infratentorial herniation syndromes may occur. In the most common infratentorial herniation syndrome, a cerebellar tonsil shifts through the foramen magnum because of increased pressure within the posterior fossa. The clinical manifestations of this downward infratentorial herniation are an arched, stiff neck; paresthesias in the shoulder area;

decreased consciousness; respiratory abnormalities; and pulse rate variations. Occasionally the pressure force is such that an upward transtentorial herniation of a cerebellar tonsil or the lower brain stem results. No specific set of clinical manifestations is associated with this infratentorial herniation syndrome.

Cerebral Edema

Cerebral edema is an increase in the fluid content of brain tissue, a net accumulation of water within the brain (Figure 16-12). Cerebral edema causes an increase in extracellular or intracellular tissue volume after brain insult from trauma, infection, hemorrhage, tumor, ischemia, infarct, or hypoxia. The harmful effects of cerebral edema are caused by the distortion of blood vessels, the displacement of brain tissues, and the eventual herniation of brain tissue from one brain compartment to another.

Four types of cerebral edema are (1) vasogenic edema, (2) cytotoxic (metabolic) edema, (3) ischemic edema, and (4) interstitial edema. **Vasogenic edema** is clinically the most important type. It is caused by the increased permeability of the capillary endothelium of the brain after injury to the vascular structure. The result is a disruption in the blood-brain barrier. Plasma proteins leak into the extracellular spaces, drawing water to them, and the water content of the brain parenchyma increases. Vasogenic edema starts in the area of injury and spreads with preferential accumulation in the white matter of the ipsilateral side because the parallel myelinated fibers separate more easily. Edema then promotes more edema because of ischemia from increasing pressure.

Clinical manifestations of vasogenic edema include focal neurologic deficits, disturbances of consciousness, and a severe increase in intracranial pressure. Vasogenic edema resolves by slow diffusion.

In **cytotoxic (metabolic) edema,** toxic factors directly affect the cellular elements of the brain parenchyma (neuronal, glial, and endothelial cells), causing failure of the active transport systems. The cells lose their potassium and gain larger amounts of sodium. Water follows by osmosis into the cell, so that the cells swell. Cytotoxic edema occurs principally in the gray matter and may increase vasogenic edema.

Ischemic edema follows cerebral infarction. The ischemia has components of both vasogenic and cytotoxic edema. Soon after the onset of ischemia, the initial edema is confined to the intracellular compartment. During the following hours and then over several days, brain cells begin to undergo necrosis and die, releasing lysosomes. In this autodigestive process, the blood-brain barrier's permeability is increased.

Interstitial edema is seen most often with noncommunicating hydrocephalus (see Chapter 17). The edema is caused by transependymal movement of CSF from the ventricles into the extracellular spaces of the brain tissues. The brain fluid volume thus is increased predominantly around the ventricles. The hydrostatic pressure within the white matter increases, and the size of the white matter is reduced because of the rapid disappearance of myelin lipids.

Hydrocephalus

The term **hydrocephalus** refers to a variety of conditions characterized by an excess of fluid within the cranial vault, subarachnoid space, or both. Hydrocephalus occurs because of interference with CSF flow caused by increased fluid production, obstruction within the ventricular system, or defective reabsorption of the fluid. A papilloma (i.e., epithelial tumor) may, in rare instances, cause overproduction of CSF (Figure 16-13).

Types of Hydrocephalus

Obstruction within the ventricular system, called **noncommunicating hydrocephalus** or *internal (intraventricular) hydrocephalus,* may result from congenital abnormalities in the ventricular system or mass lesions such as a tumor that compresses one of the structures of the ventricular system (see Chapter 19 for additional discussion). Impaired absorption of CSF from the subarachnoid space occurs when an obstructive process disrupts the flow of CSF through the subarachnoid space. The fluid is prevented from reaching the convex portion of the cerebrum, where the arachnoid granulations are located.

Hydrocephalus from impaired absorption may be caused by adhesions from inflammation, as with a meningitis or subarachnoid hemorrhage; compression of the subarachnoid space by a mass, such as a tumor; congenital abnormalities of the subarachnoid space; or high venous pressure within the sagittal sinus. This type of hydrocephalus is termed **communicating (extraventricular) hydrocephalus.** The most common causes of communicating hydrocephalus are subarach-

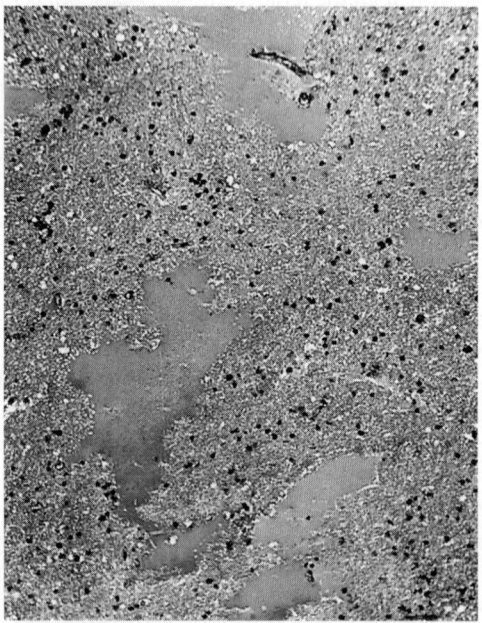

Figure 16-12 **Microscopic view of brain edema.** Note intercellular lakes of high-protein content fluid. (Hematoxylin-eosin stain; ×90.) (From Kissane JM, editor: *Anderson's pathology,* ed 9, St Louis, 1993, Mosby.)

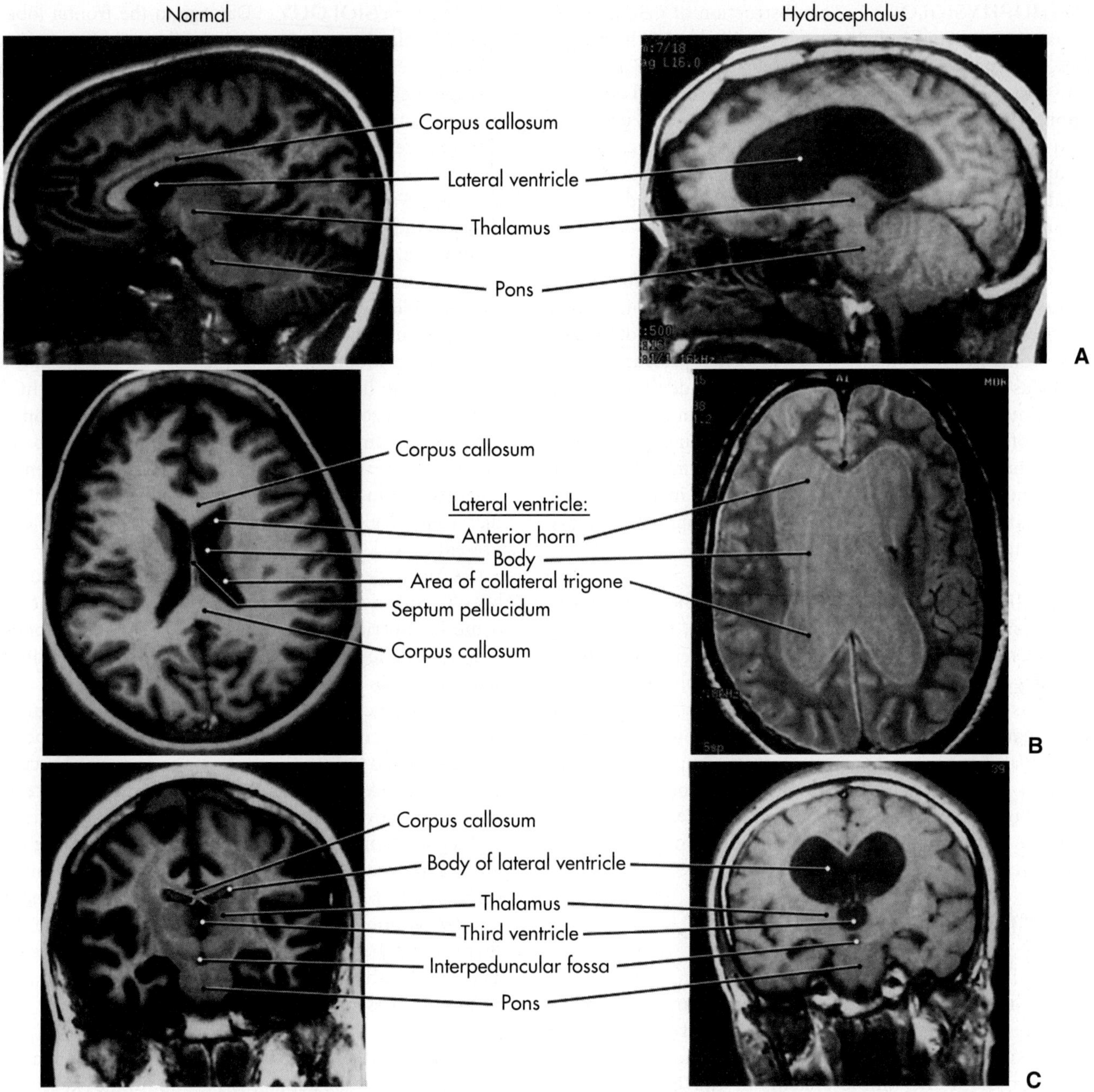

Normal   Hydrocephalus

— Corpus callosum

— Lateral ventricle —

— Thalamus —

— Pons —

A

— Corpus callosum

<u>Lateral ventricle:</u>
— Anterior horn —
— Body —
— Area of collateral trigone —
— Septum pellucidum
— Corpus callosum

B

— Corpus callosum
— Body of lateral ventricle —
— Thalamus —
— Third ventricle —
— Interpeduncular fossa —
— Pons —

C

Figure 16-13 Comparison of normal and hydrocephalic brains. **A,** Sagittal; **B,** axial; and **C,** coronal planes as seen in magnetic resonance imaging (MRI). (From Haines DE, editor: *Fundamental neuroscience,* Philadelphia, 1997, Churchill Livingstone.)

noid hemorrhage, developmental malformation, head injury, and neoplasm.

One form of communicating hydrocephalus is **hydrocephalus ex vacuo,** which arises from cerebral atrophy. CSF fills the unoccupied space. The amount of CSF is increased, but the fluid is not under pressure. Another form of communicating hydrocephalus is **normal-pressure hydrocephalus** (low-pressure, adult, or occult hydrocephalus), which occurs mostly in late middle age. The cause is thought to be arachnoid adhesions and thickening of the arachnoid that obstruct the subarachnoid space. This form of hydrocephalus is most often seen as a complication of head injury and subarachnoid hemorrhage.

Course of the Disease

Hydrocephalus may develop from infancy through adulthood. Congenital hydrocephalus (i.e., ventricular enlargement before birth) is rare. Noncommunicating hydrocephalus is more commonly seen in children. The more common type of hydrocephalus in adults is the communicating type. (Hydrocephalus in children is discussed in Chapter 19.)

Most cases of hydrocephalus develop gradually and insidiously over time. **Acute hydrocephalus,** however, may develop in several hours in persons who have sustained head injuries. Acute hydrocephalus contributes significantly to increased intracranial pressure.

PATHOPHYSIOLOGY   The obstruction of CSF flow associated with hydrocephalus produces dilation of the ventricles proximal to the obstruction. Obstructed CSF is under pressure, causing atrophy of the cerebral cortex and degeneration of the white matter tracts. There is selective preservation of gray matter. When excess CSF fills a defect caused by atrophy, a degenerative disorder, or a surgical excision, this fluid is not under pressure; therefore atrophy and degenerative changes are not induced.

CLINICAL MANIFESTATIONS   The presentation of acute hydrocephalus is one of rapidly developing increased intracranial pressure. The person deteriorates rapidly into a deep coma if not promptly treated. Normal-pressure hydrocephalus has a long-term presentation and develops slowly over time. The individual or family of the individual complains of declining memory and cognitive function. An unsteady, broad-based gait with a history of falling is common. Additional clinical manifestations are apathy; inattentiveness; and indifference to self, family, and the environment. Urinary incontinence is present.

EVALUATION AND TREATMENT   The diagnosis is made on the basis of physical examination, CT scan, and MRI. A radioisotopic cisternogram may be performed to aid in diagnosing normal-pressure hydrocephalus. Hydrocephalus can be treated by surgery to resect cysts, neoplasms, or hematomas or by ventricular bypass into the normal intracranial channel or into an extracranial compartment using a shunt. Excision or coagulation of the choroid plexus is needed occasionally when a papilloma is present. In normal-pressure hydrocephalus, reduction in CSF through a diuresis regimen often is used.

ALTERATIONS IN EMOTIONS AND MOOD

Emotions such as anger, hostility, envy, fear, and love all guide behavior and mood and are mediated largely by the limbic system. Alterations in emotions or mood arise from dysfunction in the limbic system; in the hypothalamus, which choreographs the behaviors that accompany emotional and mood states; or in the cerebral cortex, especially the temporal and frontal lobes. The neural tracts of the orbital-frontal cortex projects to the limbic system to exert inhibiting and modulating effects on social behaviors. The medial frontal-subcortical network mediates motivation.[22] The amygdala is associated with emotional memory as well as with feeding and appetite. Changes in the physical, chemical, or electrical status of the frontal lobes, limbic system, or hypothalamus may be associated with significant changes in emotions, mood, and behavior. Changes in emotions, mood, and behavior can result from abscesses, tumors, hemorrhages, metabolic disorders, degenerative disease, and intoxication states.

PATHOPHYSIOLOGY   Damage to the frontal lobes and frontolimbic tracts that project inhibitory influences to the limbic system frees the limbic system and leaves it unchecked to generate an array of emotions and mood. Behavior then becomes erratic and unpredictable. Orbitofrontal dysfunction manifests with emotional lability along with disinhibition, impaired social functioning, and obsessive-compulsive disorders. Pathologic processes within the limbic system itself may produce a deficiency in emotional response, either a lack of impulse (as in the depressive disorder) or excessive impulse, as in certain psychomotor seizures or acute anxiety states. Medial temporal dysfunction involving the limbic system, including the hippocampus and amygdala, manifest with alteration in mood, as well as memory difficulties and disinhibition. The limbic system is implicated in thought disorders.[22] In schizophrenia, the size of the cortical region, which includes the amygdala, hippocampus, and parahippocampal gyrus, is decreased while correspondingly there is ventricular enlargement in the area. Lower metabolic activity in the medial frontal region and in the dorsolateral prefrontal cortex is present as well.

Reduced dendrite branching in the frontal lobes has been found in schizophrenia.[23] A gene located on chromosome 13 contributes to at least some cases of schizophrenia, and a sequence on chromosome 8 boosts susceptibility to schizophrenia.

Likewise, increased blood flow to the anterior cingulate and lateral surface of the frontal lobes with a corresponding decrease in blood flow in the posterior brain regions occurs with depression. Overactivity in the amygdala may produce assignment of negative feelings to all thoughts and information.

Hypothalamic dysfunction may excessively arouse the limbic system by supplying too much of a neurotransmitter, resulting in an acute anxiety state or producing associated behaviors without inducing the feelings. For example, tumors that involve the tracts projecting from the hypothalamus are associated with raging behaviors, but the feeling of anger or rage is not present.

CLINICAL MANIFESTATIONS   Common among all types of frontal lobe damage is a change in the experience and expression of emotion and mood. The clinical manifestations associated with frontal lobe dysfunction range from excessive, seemingly purposeless activity to spontaneity. Irritability, impulsiveness, mood swings, mood shifts, inability to tolerate frustration, and loss of control occur frequently. Clinical manifestations can include depression, mania, hyperactivity, acute anxiety, acute confusional states, and dementia.

EVALUATION AND TREATMENT   Evaluation of alterations in emotion and mood include several strategies: physical and psychologic examinations, CT scans, MRI, EEG, and obtaining appropriate blood chemistry levels. Treatment is directed at preventing injury (including suicide), medically or surgically treating the underlying cause, instituting appropriate drug therapy and psychotherapy, and providing support and guidance to the family. Drugs used to achieve symptomatic control alter the levels of neurotransmitters within the brain tissues. For example, diazepam (Valium) and other drugs compete for the receptors ordinarily occupied by a neurotransmitter so that level of arousal is decreased. Propranolol has been used in panic and anxiety attacks.

ALTERATIONS IN MOTOR FUNCTION

Movements are complex patterns of activity controlled by the CNS. Movements are influenced by the cerebral cortex, the pyramidal system, the extrapyramidal system, and the motor units. Dysfunction in any of these areas can cause motor dysfunction. General motor dysfunctions may produce changes in muscle tone, movement, and complex motor performance.

Alterations in Muscle Tone

Normal muscle tone involves a slight resistance to passive movement. The resistance is smooth, constant, and even throughout the range of motion. Abnormalities of muscle tone are presented in Table 16-21.

Hypotonia

In **hypotonia** (decreased muscle tone), passive movement of a muscle occurs with little or no resistance. Hypotonia is thought

Table 16-21	Alterations in Muscle Tone	
Alterations	**Characteristics**	**Cause**
Hypotonia	Passive movement of a muscle mass with little or no resistance	Thought to be caused by decreased muscle spindle activity as a result of decreased excitability of neurons
	Difficult to detect; extremity is floppy and allows an excessive movement when displaced	
	Muscles may be rapidly moved without resistance	Occurs typically when nerve impulses necessary for muscle tone are lost
Flaccidity	Associated with limp, atrophied muscles and paralysis	
Hypertonia	Increased muscle resistance to passive movement	Results when the lower motor unit reflex arc continues to function but is not mediated or regulated by higher centers
	May be associated with paralysis	
	May be accompanied by muscle hypertrophy (see Figure 16-17)	
Spasticity	A gradual increase in tone causing increased resistance until tone suddenly is reduced, which results in clasp-knife phenomenon	Exact mechanism unclear; appears to arise form an increased excitability of the alpha motor neurons to any input because of absence of the descending inhibition of the pyramidal systems
	Velocity dependent (may be absent with slow speed of displacement)	
	Selective distribution (predominates in flexors of the upper extremities and extensors of lower extremities and in pronators compared with supinators)	
Gegenhalten (paratonia)	Resistance to passive movement, which varies in direct proportion to force applied	Exact mechanism unclear: associated with frontal lobe injury
Dystonia	Sustained involuntary twisting movement	Produced by slow muscular contraction
Rigidity	Muscle resistance to passive movement of a rigid limb that is uniform in both flexion and extension throughout the motion	Occurs as a result of constant, involuntary contraction of muscle
	Not velocity dependent	
	Activated by contraction of muscles in contralateral extremities	
	Uniform through range in displacement	
Plastic, or lead-pipe	Increased muscular tone relatively independent of degree of force used in passive movement; does not vary throughout the passive movement	Associated with basal ganglion damage
Cogwheel	The uniform resistance may be interrupted by a series of brief jerks resulting in movements much like a ratchet, "cogwheel" phenomenon	Associated with basal ganglion damage
Gamma	Characterized by extensor posturing (decerebrate rigidity)	Loss of excitation of extensor inhibitory areas by the cerebral cortex decreasing the inhibition of alpha and gamma motor neurons
Alpha	Impaired relaxation characterized by extensor rigidity of skeletal muscle after the contraction	Loss of cerebellum input to lateral vestibular nuclei
Myotonia	Impaired relaxation of skeletal muscle after the contraction	

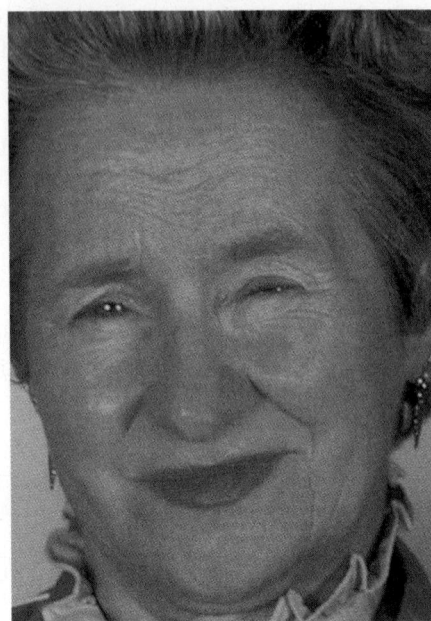

Figure 16-14 Left-sided hemifacial spasm. (From Perkin GD: *Mosby's color atlas and text of neurology*, London, 1998, Mosby-Wolfe.)

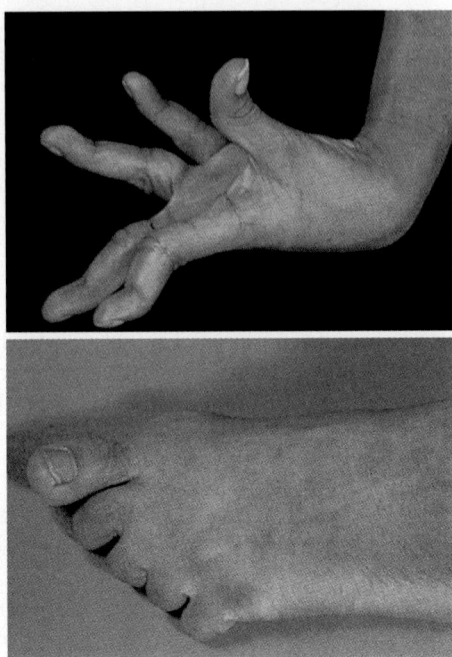

Figure 16-15 Dystonic posturing of the hand and foot. (From Perkin GD: *Mosby's color atlas and text of neurology*, London, 1998, Mosby-Wolfe.)

to be caused by decreased muscle spindle activity secondary to decreased excitability of neurons. Hypotonia is caused by pure pyramidal tract damage (a rare occurrence) and cerebellar damage. A pure pyramidal tract injury produces hypotonia and weakness. The hypotonia contributes to the ataxia and intention tremor in cerebellar damage and manifests with minimal weakness, with normal or slightly exaggerated reflexes. Hypotonia, often described as flaccidity (a state in which the muscle may be moved rapidly without resistance), occurs when nerve impulses necessary for muscle tone are lost, such as in spinal cord injury or cerebrovascular accident.

Individuals with hypotonia report that they tire easily (asthenia) or are weak, signs that can be observed during their activity attempts. They may have difficulty rising from a sitting position, sitting down without using arm support, and walking up and down stairs, as well as an inability to stand on their toes. Because of their weakness, accident proneness during locomotion and self-care activities is common. Inasmuch as the joints become hyperflexible in hypotonic states, persons with hypotonia may be able to assume positions that require extreme joint mobility. The joints may appear loose, and the knee jerks are pendulous.

The muscle mass atrophies because of decreased input entering the motor unit. Muscle cells gradually are replaced by connective tissue and fat. The muscles are flabby on palpation and are flat in appearance. Fasciculations may be present in some cases.

Hypertonia

In **hypertonia** (increased muscle tone), passive movement of a muscle occurs with resistance. Four types of hypertonia are described: spasticity, gegenhalten (paratonia), dystonia, and rigidity.

Spasticity results from hyperexcitability of the stretch reflexes (overactivation of the alpha motor neurons) and is associated with damage to the motor, premotor, and supplementary motor areas, as well as lateral corticospinal tract damage (Figure 16-14). Spasticity is accompanied by increased deep tendon reflexes (hyperreflexia) and the spread of reflexes (**clonus**).

Gegenhalten (paratonia) manifests as resistance to passive movement that varies in direct proportion to the force applied and is associated with frontal lobe injury. Paratonia is not truly an increase in tone but an increase in resistance by the person. Dystonia manifests as sustained, involuntary twisting movements caused by slow muscle contraction and may be caused by a failure in appropriate reciprocal inhibition of the muscles (Figures 16-15 and 16-16). Injury to the putamen or its outflow tracts also is associated with hemidystonia.

Rigidity produced by tonic reflex activity mediated by gamma motor neurons may be continuous or intermittent. The involved muscles are firm and tense; the increase in muscle movement is even and uniform throughout the range of passive movement. Four types of rigidity are described: plastic, or lead-pipe, rigidity; cogwheel rigidity; gamma rigidity; and alpha rigidity (see Table 16-22).

Individuals with hypertonia may tire easily (asthenia) or be weak. Passive and active movement is equally affected, except in paratonia, in which more active than passive movement is possible. As a result of hypertonia and weakness, accident proneness during locomotion and self-care activities is common.

The muscles may atrophy because of decreased use of the muscles. However, hypertrophy occasionally may occur in some diseases. Hypertrophy results from overstimulation of muscle fibers. Overstimulation occurs when the motor unit

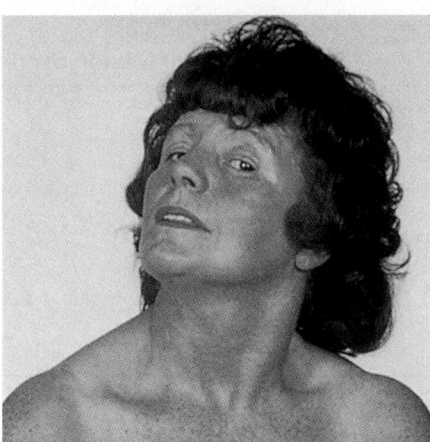

Figure 16-16 Spasmodic torticollis. A characteristic head posture. (From Perkin GD: *Mosby's color atlas and text of neurology,* London, 1998, Mosby-Wolfe.)

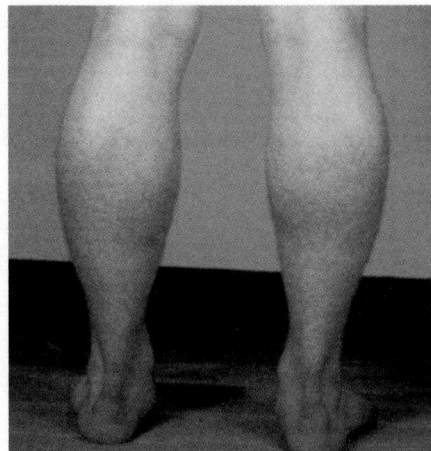

Figure 16-17 Pseudohypertrophy of the calf muscles. (From Perkin GD: *Mosby's color atlas and text of neurology,* London, 1998, Mosby-Wolfe.)

reflex arc remains intact and functioning but is not inhibited by higher centers. The loss of inhibition and the constant state of excitation cause continual muscle contraction, resulting in enlargement of the muscle mass (Figure 16-17). The muscles are firm on palpation.

Alterations in Movement

Movement requires a change in the contractile state of muscles. Abnormal movements may occur when a variety of CNS dysfunctions alter muscular innervation. Movement disorders are not well understood. Current knowledge has come predominantly from the areas of neuropharmacology and experimental therapeutics. The neurotransmitter *dopamine* has an apparent role in motor function. Some movement disorders (e.g., the akinesias) result from too little dopaminergic activity, whereas others (e.g., chorea, ballism, tardive dyskinesia) result from too much dopaminergic activity. Still others are not related primarily to dopamine function. Movement disorders are not associated necessarily with mass, strength, or tone but are neurologic dysfunctions with either a decreased amount of movement or an excess of movement. Muscle strength is quantitatively evaluated on a scale of 0 to 4+ or 0 to 5, in which 4+ or 5 is normal and 0 indicates an inability to move against gravity (Table 16-22).

Paresis and Paralysis

Paresis (weakness) is impairment of motor function, that is, partial paralysis with incomplete loss of muscle power. **Paralysis** is loss of motor function, that is, inability of a muscle group to overcome gravity. Two subtypes of paresis and paralysis are described: upper motor neuron paresis and paralysis and lower motor neuron paresis and paralysis (Table 16-23).

Upper Motor Neuron Syndromes

Upper motor neuron paresis and paralysis is known also as spastic paresis and paralysis, and many different terms are used to describe a specific paresis or paralysis. **Hemiparesis** or **hemiplegia** is paresis or paralysis, respectively, of the upper and lower extremities on one side. **Diplegia** is the paralysis of both upper or lower extremities as a result of cerebral hemi-

Table 16-22	UK Medical Research Council Classification of Muscle Power
Grade	Definition
0	Total paralysis
1	Flicker of contraction
2	Movement with gravity eliminated
3	Movement against gravity
4	Movement against resistance but incomplete
5	Normal power

UK, United Kingdom.

sphere injuries. **Paraparesis** or **paraplegia** refers to weakness or paralysis, respectively, of the lower extremities. **Quadriparesis** or **quadriplegia** refers to paresis or paralysis of all four extremities. Paraparesis or paraplegia and quadriparesis or quadriplegia may be caused by dysfunction of the spinal cord. Upper cord damage results in quadriparesis or quadriplegia, and lower cord damage preserves upper extremity function and causes paraparesis or paraplegia (spinal cord injury is discussed in Chapter 17).

Upper motor neuron paresis or paralysis is associated with a pyramidal motor syndrome. The **pyramidal motor syndrome** is a series of motor dysfunctions that result from interruption of the pyramidal system (Figures 16-18 and 16-19). The injury may be in the cerebral cortex, the subcortical white matter, the internal capsule, the brain stem, or the spinal cord. The clinical manifestations of a pure pyramidal injury without other damage are not known, but bilateral interruption of the pyramidal system in monkeys causes hypotonic paralysis, although much control of movement eventually returns. In humans, however, injury generally involves more than merely the interruption of the pyramidal system, so that an upper motor neuron paralysis occurs, which indicates involvement of several motor pathways.

The distribution of clinical manifestations varies, depending on the location of the lesion, although certain features are constant. Excessive movements such as clonus and spasms

Table 16-23	Upper and Lower Motor Neuron Syndromes	
Factor	**Upper Motor Neuron Syndromes***	**Lower Motor Neuron Syndromes†**
Distribution of affected muscles	Muscle groups are affected; when movement is possible, the proper relationship among agonists, antagonists, synergists, and fixators is preserved	Individual muscles may be affected
	Synkinesias (residual movements) are present; attempts to move paralyzed part cause a variety of associated movements; movements of normal limb may cause imitative or mirror movements in the paralyzed limb	Individual muscles may be affected
Muscle tone	Hypertonia, specifically spasticity	Hypotonia, flaccidity
Tendon reflexes	Hyperreflexia with extensor plantar reflex present	Hyporeflexia, no abnormal reflexes present
Atrophy	Slight, caused by disuse	Pronounced atrophy
Fasciculations	Absent	May be present

*Pyramidal motor syndromes.
†All are motor unit syndromes.

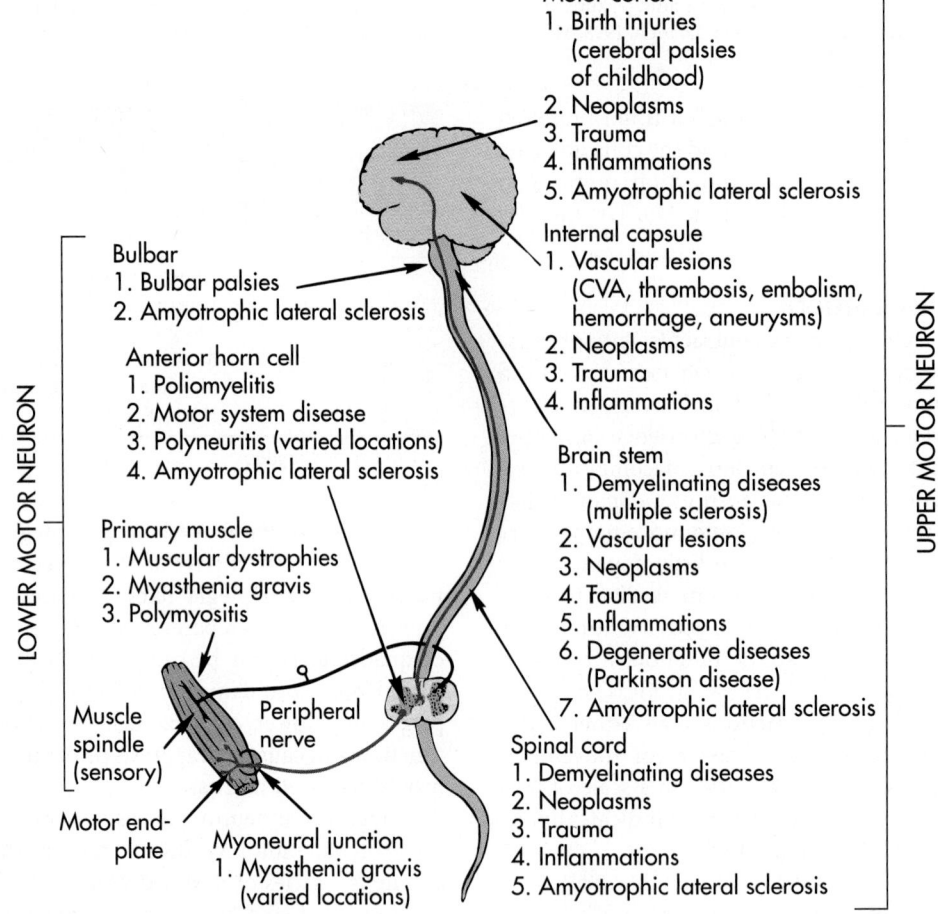

Figure 16-18 Disturbances in motor function. Disturbances in motor function are classified pathologically along upper and lower motor neuron structures. It should be noted that neoplasms occur at more than one site in an upper motor neuron, *above right*. A few pathologic conditions, such as amyotrophic lateral sclerosis, involve both upper and lower motor neuron structures. Other lesion sites include myoneural junction and primary muscle, making it possible to classify conditions as neuromuscular and muscular, respectively.

occur regularly, and much variation exists, depending on the suddenness of onset and the age of the individual.

When the pyramidal system is destroyed below the level of the pons, spinal shock occurs. **Spinal shock** is the complete cessation of spinal cord functions below the lesion. It is characterized by complete flaccid paralysis, absence of reflexes, and marked disturbances of bowel and bladder function. The

reasons for spinal shock are not fully understood, but a major factor is the sudden destruction of the efferent pathways. If destruction occurs more slowly, spinal shock may not develop (see Chapter 17).

If the pyramidal system is interrupted above the level of the pons, the hand and arm muscles are greatly affected. Paralysis rarely involves all the muscles on one side of the body, however,

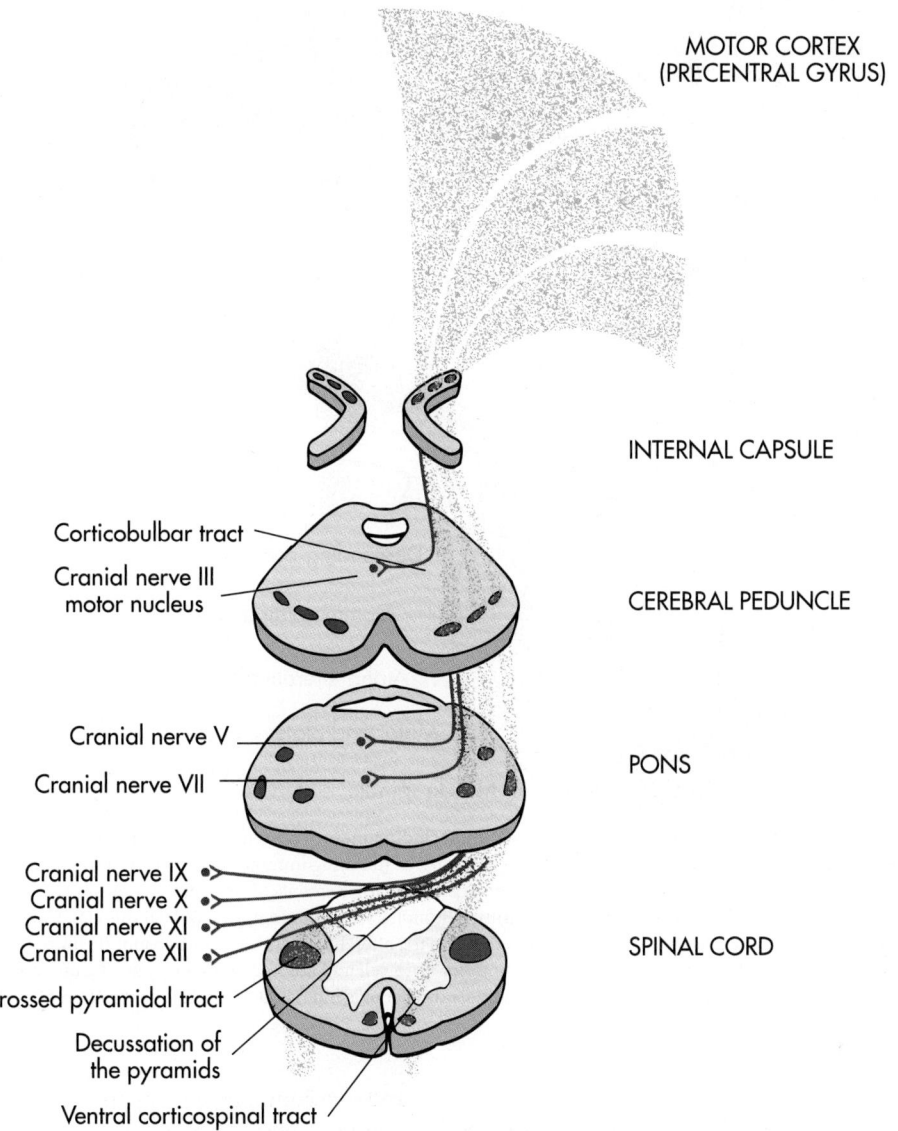

Figure 16-19 **Component structure of the upper motor neuron, or pyramidal, system.** Pyramidal system fibers are shown to originate primarily in the cells in the precentral gyrus of the motor cortex; to converge at the internal capsule; to descend to form the central third of the cerebral peduncle; to descend further through the pons, where small fibers are given off to cranial nerve motor nuclei along the way; to form pyramids at the medulla, where most of the fibers decussate; and then to continue to descend in the lateral column of the white matter of the spinal cord. A few fibers descend without crossing at the medulla level.

even when the hemiplegia results from complete damage to the internal capsule. Bilateral movements, such as those of the eye, jaw, and larynx, are affected only slightly, if at all. Predominantly the limbs are affected. Because of their bilateral control, trunk muscles are much less influenced.

Paralysis associated with a pyramidal motor syndrome rarely remains flaccid for a prolonged time. After a few days or weeks, a gradual return of spinal reflexes marks the end of spinal shock. Reflexes then become hyperactive, and muscle tone is increased significantly, particularly in antigravity muscles. Spasticity is common, although rigidity occasionally occurs. Most often, passive range of motion causes the "clasp-knife" phenomenon, probably because of the activation of the two varieties of stretch receptors: (1) the muscle spindles and (2) the Golgi tendon organ. (Muscle function is discussed in

Chapter 41.) With pyramidal motor syndrome, predominantly the flexors of the arms and extensors of the legs are affected.

Lower Motor Neuron Syndromes

Lower (primary, alpha) motor neurons are the large motor neurons in the anterior (or ventral) horn of the spinal cord, the motor nuclei of the brain stem, and the axons that originate from these nerve cell bodies (to course in the anterior spinal roots and the spine or in the cranial nerves to reach skeletal muscles) (Figure 16-20). Dysfunction in this motor system impairs movement, both voluntary and involuntary. The degree of paralysis or paresis is proportional to the number of lower motor neurons affected. If only a portion of the motor units that supply a muscle are affected, only partial paralysis or paresis results. If all the motor units are affected,

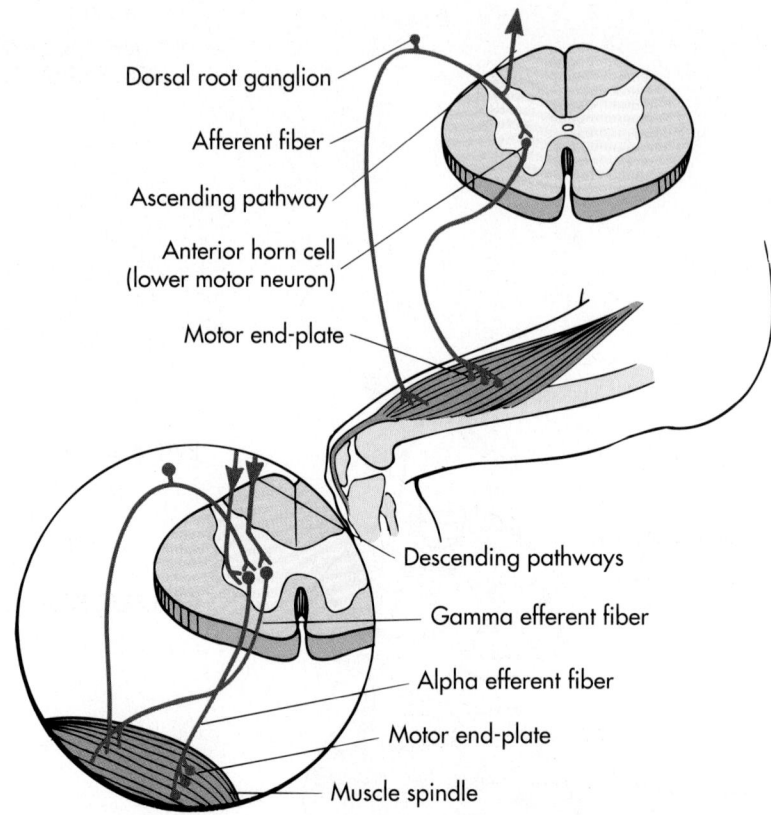

Figure 16-20 Component structure of a lower motor neuron, including motor (efferent) and sensory (afferent) elements. *Top,* Anterior horn cell (in anterior gray column of spinal cord and its axon), terminating in motor end-plate as it innervates extrafusal muscle fibers in the quadriceps muscle. *Detailed enlargement,* Sensory and motor elements of the gamma loop system. The gamma efferent fiber is shown innervating the polar, or end, region of the muscle spindle (sensory receptor of skeletal muscle). Contraction of muscle spindle fibers stretches the central portion of the spindle and causes the afferent spindle fiber to transmit the impulse centrally to the cord. Muscle spindle afferent fibers in turn synapse on the anterior horn cell and are transmitted by way of gamma-efferent fibers to skeletal (extrafusal) muscle, causing it to contract. Muscle spindle discharge is interrupted by active contraction of extrafusal muscle fibers.

a complete paralysis results. Other clinical manifestations also are proportional to the degree of dysfunction, but the precise manifestations depend on the location of the dysfunction in the motor unit and in the CNS.

Small motor (gamma) neurons, which function to maintain muscle tone and protect the muscle from injury, also are necessary for normal motor movement. These neurons depend on input from the muscle spindle (arriving through an afferent limb rising to the cord). Dysfunction in this motor system impairs tone and reduces the tendon reflexes, causing hyporeflexia. The muscle is lax and soft, with a decrease in normal tone, or hypotonia, which impairs voluntary and involuntary motor movements. The muscles become susceptible to damage from hyperextensibility because the normal protective mechanisms, which prevent muscle fiber injury, are impaired. The degree of tone loss and the loss of tendon reflexes are proportional to the dysfunction in these reflex motor units.

Generally, in a pathologic process the large and small motor neuron systems are equally affected. Therefore the paresis and paralysis caused by a disorder of the lower motor neurons is called **flaccid paresis** and **flaccid paralysis,** respectively, because the muscle has reduced or absent tone

and is accompanied by hyporeflexia or **areflexia** (loss of tendon reflexes).

A few **gamma neuropathies** (small motor neuron disorders) affect only the gamma motor system. A manifestation of these disorders is a marked reduction in the deep tendon reflexes, which are strikingly out of proportion to the degree of muscle weakness present.

Denervated muscles (i.e., muscles that have lost their nervous system input) undergo atrophy over weeks to months, mostly from disuse. Denervated muscles also demonstrate fasciculations, which are seen as muscle rippling or quivering under the skin. Occasionally, denervated muscles cramp. **Fibrillation** (isolated contraction of a single muscle fiber) also may occur, although this manifestation is not visible clinically.

Amyotrophies

Lower motor neuron syndromes originating in the anterior horn cells or the motor nuclei of the cranial nerves are called **amyotrophies.** Paralytic poliomyelitis is the prototype of these disorders. It involves a severe inflammatory reaction in motor neurons, some of which do not survive, leaving a permanent lower motor neuron syndrome.

Several pathologic processes may give rise to an amyotrophy. A virally induced or postinfectious or postvaccination inflammatory process may injure or destroy anterior horn cells or cranial nerve cell bodies. Most of these inflammatory processes are mild and are followed by rapid cellular recovery.

In the amyotrophies, muscle strength, muscle tone, and muscle bulk are affected in the muscles innervated by the involved motor neurons. The paresis and paralysis associated with anterior horn cell injury are segmental, but because each muscle is supplied by two or more roots, the segmental character of the weakness may be difficult to recognize. When cranial nerve motor nuclei are affected (these lack nerve roots and have only small rootlets near the point of exit from the brain stem), the distribution of the motor weakness follows that of the peripheral nerve. The weakness may involve distal muscles, proximal muscles, and the muscles of midline structures. Hypotonia and hyporeflexia or areflexia are present.

The atrophy associated with amyotrophy is segmental when the anterior horn cells of the spinal cord are involved and follows the distribution of the peripheral nerve when the motor nuclei of the cranial nerves are affected. The atrophy may be in distal, proximal, or midline muscles. Fasciculations are particularly associated with primary motor neuron injury, and muscle cramps are common. Mild fatigue is a common complaint. If the pathologic process is limited to the primary motor neuron, no sensory changes are evident.

Because degenerative disorders cause loss of nerve cells in the anterior horn or motor nuclei, the surviving cells are small, shrunken, and filled with lipofuscin. Lost neurons are replaced by astrocytes. The roots or rootlets are thin, and the muscles show denervation and atrophy.

Several brain stem syndromes involve damage to one or more of the cranial nerve nuclei. These are called **nuclear palsies** (Table 16-24) and may be caused by vascular occlusion, tumor, aneurysm, tuberculosis, or hemorrhage.

The anterior horn cells and the motor nuclei of the cranial nerves may be affected secondarily in many severe pathologic processes that primarily involve the peripheral nerves. The condition may extend proximally to affect the nerve roots or rootlets and the motor neurons themselves, a process commonly seen, for example, in Guillain-Barré syndrome. If sufficient numbers of motor neurons are destroyed, permanent loss of motor function results because regeneration of the damaged axons requires a living neuronal cell body.

A group of degenerative disorders principally cause progressive motor cell atrophy. One of these is **progressive spinal muscular atrophy,** in which the anterior horn cells of the spinal cord are the affected motor neurons. This disorder occurs in adults and closely resembles the familial progressive muscular atrophies that occur in infants and children and are considered inherited metabolic disorders (see Chapter 43). If the motor nuclei of the cranial nerves are affected instead of the anterior horn cells, the disorder is labeled **progressive bulbar palsy,** so named because the myelencephalon originally was called the *bulb* and a degenerative process causes a progressively more serious condition. When any lower motor neuron syndrome involves the cranial nerves that arise from the bulb (i.e., cranial nerves IX, X, and XII), the dysfunction is called a **bulbar palsy.**

The clinical manifestations of bulbar palsy include paresis or paralysis of the jaw, face, pharynx, and tongue musculature. Articulation is affected, especially articulation of the lingual *(r, n, l)*, labial *(b, m, p, f)*, dental *(d, t)*, and palatal *(k, g)* consonants. Modulation is impaired, making the voice rasping or nasal. Pharyngeal reflexes are diminished or lost. Palate and vocal cord movement during phonation is impaired, and chewing and swallowing are affected. The facial muscles are weak, and the face appears to droop. The jaw jerk is decreased. Atrophy eventually becomes apparent, as do fasciculations. All these manifestations become progressively worse, leading to aspiration, malnutrition, possible dehydration, and an inability to communicate verbally.

Hyperkinesia

Hyperkinesia (excessive movement) represents the second broad category of abnormal movements. Within this category are a number of specific hyperkinesia syndromes (Table 16-25). Also included in the general category of hyperkinesias are dyskinesias, that is, abnormal involuntary movements.

Table 16-24	Examples of Nuclear Palsy Syndromes	
Type of Nuclear Palsy	**Causes**	**Associated Clinical Manifestations**
Ocular	Upper brain stem tumor	Other cranial nerve signs
	Cerebrovascular disease in the vertebrobasilar system	Contralateral spastic hemiparesis/hemiplegia
		Contralateral hyperreflexia
	Aneurysm	Contralateral extensor plantar reflex
	Intramedullary bleeding	
Facial	Pontine tumor	Paresis/paralysis of both the upper and lower facial muscles
	Cerebrovascular disease in the vertebrobasilar system	for both voluntary movement and emotionally induced movement
Vagal	Intramedullary tumor	Ipsilateral loss of pain and temperature sensations of the face
	Cerebrovascular disease in the vertebrobasilar system	
		Contralateral spastic arm and leg paresis/hemiplegia
		Ipsilateral cerebellar signs
Hypoglossal	Intramedullary tumor	Contralateral loss of position sense and vibration in the arm and leg
	Cerebrovascular disease in the vertebrobasilar system	
		Contralateral spastic hemiparesis/hemiplegia

Table 16-25	Types of Hyperkinesia Syndromes	
Type	**Characteristics**	**Causes**
Chorea*	Nonrepetitive muscular contractions, usually of the extremities of face; random pattern of irregular, involuntary rapid contractions of groups of muscles; disappears with sleep, decreases with resting; increases with emotional stress and attempted voluntary movement	Associated with excess concentration of or a supersensitivity to dopamine within basal ganglia
Athetosis*	Disorder of distal-muscle postural fixation; slow, sinuous, irregular movements most obvious in the distal extremities, more rhythmic than choreiform movements and always much slower; movements accompany characteristic hand posture; slowly fluctuating grimaces	Occurs most commonly as a result of injury to the putamen of the basal ganglion; exact pathophysiologic mechanism is not known
Ballism	Disorder of proximal-muscle postural fixation with wild flinging movement of the limbs; movement is severe and stereotyped, usually lateral; does not lessen with sleep; ballism is most common on one side of the body, a condition termed *hemiballism*	Results from injury to subthalamus nucleus (one of the nuclei that comprise the basal ganglia); thought to be caused by reduced inhibitory influence in the nucleus, a release phenomenon; hemiballism results from injury to the contralateral subthalamic nucleus
Hyperactivity	State of prolonged, generalized, increased activity that is largely involuntary but may be subject to some voluntary control; not highly stereotyped but rather manifests as continuous changes in total body posture or in excessive performance of some simple activity, such as pacing under inappropriate circumstances	May be caused by frontal and reticular activating system injury
Wandering	Tendency to wander without regard for environment	"Release" phenomenon; associated with bilateral injury to globus pallidus or putamen
Akathisia	Special type of hyperactivity; mild compulsion to move (usually more localized to legs); severe frenzied motion possible; movements are partly voluntary and may be transiently suppressed; carrying out the movement brings a sense of relief; a frequent complication of antipsychotic drugs	Dopaminergic transmission may be involved
Tremor at Rest	Rhythmic, oscillating movement affecting one or more body parts	Caused by regular contraction of opposing groups of muscles
Parkinsonian tremor	Regular, rhythmic, slow flexion-extension contraction; involves principally the metacarpophalangeal and wrist joints; alternating movements between thumb and index finger described as "pill rolling"; disappears during voluntary movement	Loss of inhibitory influence of dopamine in the basal ganglia, causing instability of basal ganglial feedback circuit within the cerebral cortex
Postural Tremor		
Asterixis (tremor of hepatic encephalopathy)	Irregular flapping movement of the hands accentuated by outstretching arms	Due to transient inhibition of muscles that maintain posture; thought to be related to accumulation of products normally detoxified by the liver
Metabolic	Rapid, rhythmic tremor affecting fingers, lips, and tongue; accentuated by extending the body part; enhanced physiologic tremor	Occurs in conditions associated with disturbed metabolism or toxicity, as in thyrotoxicosis (hyperthyroidism), alcoholism, and chronic use of barbiturates, amphetamines, lithium, amitriptyline (Elavil); exact mechanism responsible unknown
Essential (familial)	Tremor of fingers, hands, and feet; absent at rest but accentuated by extension of body part, prolonged muscular activity, and stress	Not associated with any other neurologic abnormalities; cause unknown

*Choreoathetosis involves both chorea and athetosis; precise pathophysiology unknown.

Type	Characteristics	Causes
Table 16-25	**Types of Hyperkinesia Syndromes—cont'd**	
Intentional Tremor		
Cerebellar	Tremor initiated by movement, maximal toward end of movement	Occurs in disease of the dentate nucleus (one of the deep cerebellar nuclei responsible for efferent output) and the superior cerebellar peduncle (a stalk-like structure connected to the pons); caused by errors in feedback from the periphery and errors in preprogramming goal-directed movement
Rubral	Rhythmic tremor of limbs that originates proximally by movement	Results from lesions involving the dentatorubrothalamic tract (a spinothalamic tract connecting the red nucleus in the reticular formation and the dentate nucleus in the cerebellum)
Myoclonus	Series of shocklike, nonpatterned contractions of portion of a muscle, entire muscle, or group of muscles that cause throwing movements of a limb; usually appear at random but frequently triggered by sudden startle; do not disappear during sleep	Associated with an irritable nervous system and spontaneous discharge of neurons; structures associated with myoclonus include the cerebral cortex, cerebellum, reticular formation, and spinal cord

Paroxysmal dyskinesias are abnormal, involuntary movements that occur as spasms. The type of dyskinesia varies depending on the specific disorder.

Tardive dyskinesia is the involuntary movement of the face, trunk, and extremities. Although the condition occurs occasionally in individuals with Parkinson disease, it usually occurs as a side effect of prolonged phenothiazine drug therapy or haloperidol (Haldol). The antipsychotic drugs cause denervation hypersensitivity so that it mimics the effect of too much dopamine. The most common symptom of tardive dyskinesia is rapid, repetitive, stereotypic movements. Most characteristic is continual chewing with intermittent protrusions of the tongue, lip smacking, and facial grimacing. Stereotypic movements are believed to be a form of excessive dopaminergic activity.

Other movement disorders under this category are (1) complex repetitive movements, including automatism, stereotype, complex tics, compulsions, perseverations, and mannerisms; (2) positivism (excessive reactions to certain stimuli); and (3) paroxysmal excessive activity, including cataplexy and excessive startle reaction.

Huntington Disease

Huntington disease (HD), also known as *chorea*, is a relatively rare, hereditary-degenerative disorder diffusely involving the basal ganglia and cerebral cortex. The onset of Huntington disease is usually between 30 and 50 years of age, when the trait may already have been passed to the victim's children. The disorder has a prevalence rate of approximately 5 per 100,000 persons and occurs in all races.

PATHOPHYSIOLOGY   Huntington disease is inherited as an autosomal dominant trait with high penetrance. The genetic defect is on the short arm of chromosome 4, where there is an abnormally long, repeated trinucleotide (CAG)—40 to 70 repeats instead of 9 to 34. Age of onset of symptoms is re-

lated to the length of the repeat sequences. Increased length leads to progressively earlier presentations.

The principal pathologic feature of Huntington disease is severe degeneration of the basal ganglia, particularly the caudate and putamen nuclei, and the frontal cerebral cortex (Figures 16-21 and 16-22). Early in the disease, selective loss of the striatal γ-aminobutyric acid (GABA)/enkephalin pathway to the lateral aspect of the pallidum occurs. The basal ganglia normally contain a preponderance of GABAergic (GABA-secreting) neurons, including the pathway between the basal ganglia and substantia nigra (pallidonigral pathway). Basal ganglia and nigral depletion of GABA, an inhibitory neurotransmitter, is the principal biochemical alteration in Huntington disease. Degeneration of the GABAergic pallidonigral pathway causes GABA depletion in the substantia nigra with decreased inhibitory GABA activity on dopaminergic neurons in the substantia nigra and a relative excess of dopaminergic activity in the basal ganglial feedback circuit within the cerebral cortex. A relative excess of dopaminergic activity in this circuit, as in Huntington disease, is manifested by hypotonia and hyperkinesia (involuntary, fragmentary movements such as chorea). Loss of excitatory glutamate may liberate the pathway from the thalamus to the premotor cortex, impairing modulation of movement later in the course of the disease. Within the neurons, producing the fuel for brain activity is difficult, with a resultant buildup of lactic acid.

CLINICAL MANIFESTATIONS   The classic manifestations of Huntington disease are abnormal movement and progressive dysfunction of intellectual processes (dementia) and thought processes. Any one of these features may mark the onset of the disease. Chorea is the most common type of abnormal movement affecting individuals with Huntington disease. Choreiform movements begin in the face and arms, eventually affecting the entire body. Symptoms of frontal lobe dysfunction include executive attention deficits of short-term

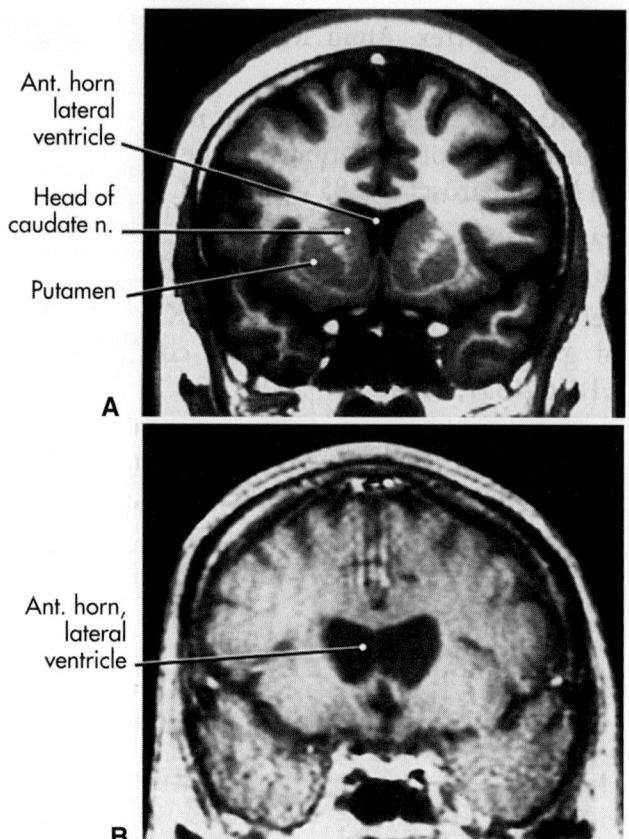

Ant. horn
lateral
ventricle

Head of
caudate n.

Putamen

A

Ant. horn,
lateral
ventricle

B

Figure 16-21 Coronal MRI through frontal lobe and head of the caudate nucleus. The head of the caudate normally forms a prominent bulge into the anterior horn of the lateral ventricle (**A,** inversion recovery image). Profound cell loss in the neostriatum of a patient with Huntington disease greatly diminishes the size of the caudate and renders the lateral wall of the ventricle flat (**B,** T1-weighted image). The slightly wavy appearance of the magnetic resonance imaging (MRI) in **B** is the result of movement (tremor) while the scan was being done. (From Haines DE, editor: *Fundamental neuroscience,* Philadelphia, 1997, Churchill Livingstone.)

memory loss (working memory); reduced capacity to plan, organize, and sequence, as well as bradyphrenia (slow thinking); and apathy. Restlessness, disinhibition, and irritability are common. Affectively, euphoria or depression or both may be present.

EVALUATION AND TREATMENT   The diagnosis of Huntington disease is based on family history and clinical presentation of the disorder. No known treatment is effective in halting the degeneration or progression of symptoms. The discovery in 1983 of the Huntington disease marker, called *G8,* on chromosome 4 paves the way for presymptomatic diagnosis of the disorder and isolation of the Huntington disease gene. Recombinant genetic techniques may someday prevent or control the disorder.

Hypokinesia

Hypokinesia (decreased movement) is loss of voluntary movement despite preserved consciousness and normal peripheral nerve and muscle function. Types of hypokinesia include akinesia, bradykinesia, and loss of associated movement.

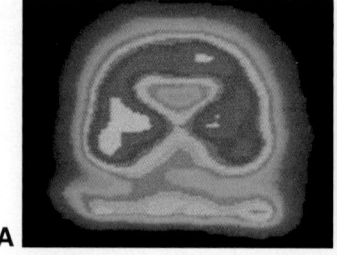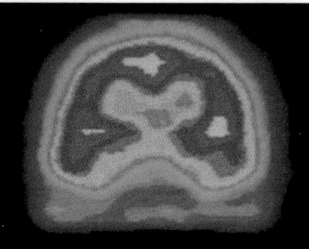

A   **B**

Figure 16-22 Caudate blood flow in Huntington disease. Single photon emission computerized tomography scan showing reduced caudate blood flow (**A**) in Huntington disease compared with normal blood flow (**B**). (From Perkin DG: *Mosby's color atlas and text of neurology,* London, 1998, Mosby-Wolfe.)

Akinesia

Akinesia is an absence, poverty, or lack of control of associated and voluntary muscle movements. There is a disturbance in the time it takes to perform a movement. Akinesia is related to dysfunction of the extrapyramidal system, as in parkinsonism. Pathogenesis is related to either a deficiency of dopamine or a defect of the postsynaptic dopamine receptors, which occurs in parkinsonism (see Chapter 17).

Bradykinesia

Bradykinesia is slowness of voluntary movements. There is a disturbance in the time it takes to perform a movement. In bradykinesia all voluntary movements become slow, labored, and deliberate. Bradykinesia consists of (1) difficulty in initiating movements, (2) difficulty in continuing movements smoothly, and (3) difficulty in performing synchronous (at the same time) and consecutive tasks. Difficulty in initiating movements ranges from slight hesitancy to severe **freezing** (transient, helpless immobility). Each intended movement requires effort. Difficulty in continuing motions smoothly causes jerky, irregular, rapid movements, which then decrease in rate and amplitude until they stop. The individual is scarcely aware of the cessation. Difficulty in performing synchronous and consecutive tasks means that each motor act is performed separately. The individual is unable to integrate two acts or to change from one motor pattern to the next with a single smooth motion.

Loss of Associated Movement

In hypokinesia the normal, habitually associated movements that provide skill, grace, and balance to voluntary movements are lost. Decreased associated movements accompanying emotional expression cause an expressionless face, a statue-like posture, absence of speech inflection, and absence of spontaneous gestures. Decreased associated movements accompanying locomotion cause reduction in arm and shoulder movements, in hip swinging, and in rotary motion of the cervical spine.

Parkinson Disease

Parkinson disease is a commonly occurring degenerative disorder of the basal ganglia (corpus striatum) involving the dopaminergic (dopamine-secreting) nigrostriatal pathway. Nigrostriatal disorders produce a syndrome of abnormal movement called **parkinsonism (Parkinson syndrome, parkinsonian syndrome)** (Figure 16-23).

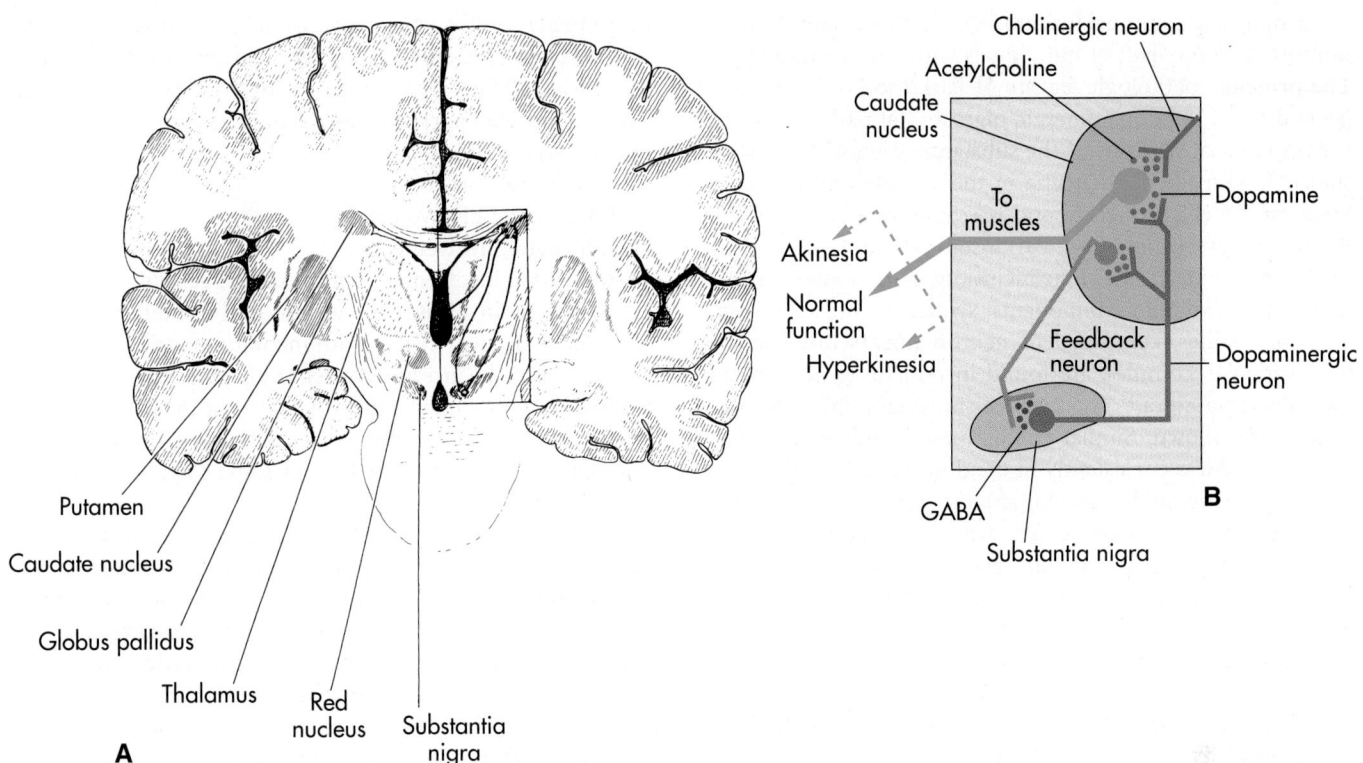

Figure 16-23 Nigrostriatal disorders produce Parkinson syndrome. Coronal section of the brain shows the basal ganglia. Pathways controlling normal and abnormal motor function are depicted in a portion of the basal ganglia *(caudate nucleus)*, **A,** and are shown enlarged in **B.** Dopaminergic synaptic activity is mediated by dopamine. Cholinergic synaptic activity is mediated by acetylcholine. A balance between the two kinds of activity produces normal motor function. A relative excess of cholinergic activity produces akinesia and rigidity. A relative excess of dopaminergic activity produces involuntary movements. Neurons in the caudate nucleus contain γ-aminobutyric acid *(GABA)* and possibly control dopaminergic neurons in the substantia nigra through a feedback pathway. (**A** from Cutler WP: *Degenerative and hereditary diseases,* ed 7, Washington, DC, 1983, Scientific American Medicine.)

Etiologic classification of parkinsonism includes primary (idiopathic) Parkinson disease and secondary parkinsonism (Box 16-6). Primary Parkinson disease involves the loss of pigmented neurons in the substantia nigra, mainly in the ventral and medial portions, associated with reactive gliosis. Secondary parkinsonism is caused by disorders other than Parkinson disease (i.e., trauma, infection, neoplasm, atherosclerosis, toxins, drug intoxication). Drug-induced parkinsonism caused by neuroleptics, antiemetics, and antihypertensives is the most common cause of the secondary form and is usually reversible. Illegal "designer drugs" containing the chemical 1-methyl-4-phenyl-1,2,3,6-tetrahydropyridine (MPTP) have produced a parkinsonian syndrome in users because of severe degeneration of the substantia nigra and locus ceruleus.

The onset of Parkinson disease occurs after 40 years of age, with mean onset between 58 and 62 years of age. Men are more affected than women. Parkinson disease is one of the most prevalent of the primary CNS disorders and a leading cause of neurologic disability in individuals older than 60 years. The prevalence rate is 107 to 187 per 100,000 persons. An estimated half-million persons in the United States are affected.

PATHOPHYSIOLOGY The pathogenesis of Parkinson disease is unknown. There is an autosomal dominant form involving a mutation in the *alpha synuclein* gene on chromo-

Box 16-6	Clinical Classification of Parkinsonian Syndromes

1. Idiopathic Parkinson disease
2. Symptomatic parkinsonism
   Postencephalitis
   Drug-induced
   Toxic
   Traumatic
   Atherosclerotic
   Normal pressure hydrocephalus
3. As part of a neuronal degenerate disorder
   Multisystem atrophy
   Progressive supranuclear palsy (PSP)
   Corticobasal degeneration
   Diffuse Lewy body disease

some 4 (4q21.23) and an autosomal recessive form (ARPD) involving a mutation in the *parkin* gene on chromosome 6 (6q25.2-27).[24] Epidemiologic data suggest possible viral and toxic causes. One hypothesis is that age predisposes the nigrostriatal pathway to damage by environmental toxins. Isolation of the neurotoxic chemical MPTP, demonstration of its ability to produce an irreversible parkinsonian syndrome, and selective destruction of substantia nigra cells have engendered a research focus on toxins as possible causative agents.

Atrophy and neuronal loss are found in the cerebral cortex in more than one half of individuals with Parkinson disease. The principle pathologic feature of Parkinson disease is degeneration of the dopaminergic nigrostriatal pathway, which is composed of neurons of the substantia nigra ("black substance"), with fibers synapsing in the caudate and putamen basal ganglia (Figures 16-24 and 16-25; see also Figure 16-23, A). In primary (idiopathic) Parkinson disease, Lewy bodies, intracytoplasmic eosinophilic inclusions composed of neurofilaments, tuberculin components, synuclein, and ubiquitin, and pale bodies, composed of neurofilaments interspersed with vacuolar granules, are found in remaining neurons of the substantia nigra.[23] The mechanism of Lewy body formation is not known. Similar changes are found in the locus ceruleus and less consistently in the dorsal vagal nucleus and in sympathetic and parasympathetic ganglia. In postencephalitis Parkinson disease, destruction of nigral neurons is widespread and associated with neurofibrillary tangles. Lewy bodies are not present. Signs of inflammation or infection are absent. The severity of Parkinson disease seems to correlate with the degree of neuronal loss in the substantia nigra. Another pathologic feature is significant reduction in certain dopamine receptors (D_1 receptors) in the basal ganglia. The mechanism of cell death is not known.

Nigral and basal ganglial depletion of dopamine, an inhibitory neurotransmitter, is the principal biochemical alteration in Parkinson disease (see Figure 16-23, B). Symptom development in basal ganglial disorders is explained as an imbalance of dopaminergic (inhibitory) and cholinergic (excitatory) activity in the caudate nucleus and putamen of the basal ganglia. Dopaminergic-cholinergic balance produces normal motor function. In Parkinson disease, degeneration of the dopaminergic nigrostriatal pathway causes dopamine depletion in the basal ganglia and a relative excess of cholinergic activity in the feedback circuit involving the cerebral cortex, basal ganglia, and thalamus. A relative excess of cholinergic activity in this circuit, as in Parkinson disease, is manifested by hypertonia (tremor and rigidity) and akinesia.

CLINICAL MANIFESTATIONS Symptoms appear after a 60% to 80% loss of pigmented nigral neurons and a loss of 60% to 90% of striatal dopamine occur. The classic manifestations of Parkinson disease are tremor at rest (resting tremor), rigidity (muscle stiffness), akinesia (poverty of movement), and postural abnormalities. These manifestations may develop alone or in combination, but as the disease progresses, all four are usually present to at least some degree. There is no true paralysis. The symptoms are staged on the Hoehn-Yale scale as follows:

0, No visible disease
1, Unilateral involvement
2, Bilateral involvement
3, Bilateral involvement with minimal gait difficulty
4, Bilateral involvement with postural instability
5, Bilateral involvement with inability to walk

Because of the insidious onset, the beginning of symptoms is difficult to document. In early stages of the disease, reflex, sensory, and mental status are usually normal. Autonomic-neuroendocrine symptoms and, in some cases, dementia are also part of the syndrome.

Parkinsonian tremor, the most conspicuous and most variable symptom, is usually the first symptom to appear. It is an asymmetric, regular, rhythmic, low-amplitude tremor, with slowly alternating flexion-extension contraction (3 to 4 cycles/sec). Later the tremor becomes symmetric at 7 to 12 cycles per second. It is a tremor at rest, disappearing briefly during the course of a voluntary movement and reappearing when the limb is held in a stationary position. Intensity and amplitude of the tremor vary. The arm is more affected than the leg. The head is involved rarely. Seventy percent of individuals with Parkinson disease have this tremor, and 20% of persons have a postural (kinesic) tremor or both tremor types. All tremors are increased by stress and anxiety.

Parkinsonian tremor appears to result from instability of feedback from the basal ganglia to the cerebral cortex caused by loss of the inhibitory influence of dopamine in the basal ganglia. Oscillation in the normal feedback cycles of the motor outflow feedback circuit when the muscles are at rest produces the tremor. When the individual performs voluntary movements, the tremor becomes temporarily blocked, presumably because other motor control signals arriving in the thalamus override the abnormal basal ganglial signals. As the disorder worsens, tremor may lessen as rigidity supervenes.

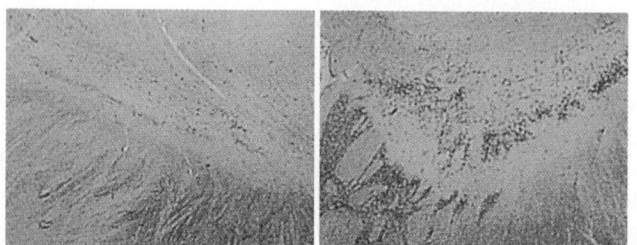

Figure 16-24 Atrophic substantia nigra (A) compared with normal control (B). (From Perkin DG: *Mosby's color atlas and text of neurology,* London, 1998, Mosby-Wolfe.)

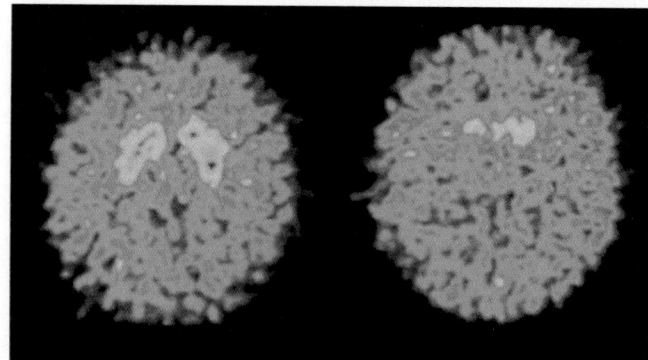

Figure 16-25 Reduced flurodopa in Parkinson disease. Positron emission tomography scan showing reduced flurodopa uptake in the basal ganglia *(right)* compared with a normal control *(left).* (From Perkin DG: *Mosby's color atlas and text of neurology,* London, 1998, Mosby-Wolfe.)

The postural tremor is associated with damage to the cerebellodentatofugal pathway to the red nucleus, a pathway that subserves communication from muscle spindles to the thalamus and motor cortex.

Parkinsonian rigidity is a state of involuntary contraction of all skeletal muscles, impedes active and passive movement. The first symptoms of rigidity may be painful muscle cramps in the toes or hands. More commonly the limb feels stiff, heavy, tired, or aching. Rigidity is felt by the examiner as lead-pipe resistance during passive movement that may be interrupted by brief jerks palpable as a cogwheel sensation. The mechanism underlying rigidity is increased resting muscle activity (enhancement of the long-latency stretch reflex).

Parkinsonian bradykinesia is poverty of associated and voluntary movements. It is the most prevalent and crippling symptom and often is overlooked in the early stages. All striated muscles—extremity, trunk, ocular, facial (Figure 16-26)—are affected eventually, including muscles of mastication (chewing), deglutition (swallowing), and articulation. The pathophysiology underlying the bradykinesia is unclear. Micrographia is present. Extreme underactivity in the patient with Parkinson disease makes the person appear stiff, even when resistance to passive movement cannot be felt. Bradykinesia is a separate phenomenon from rigidity and may be severe even in the presence of rigidity. Patients state that they feel "wooden" (as though moving against resistance) and complain of rapid, severe fatigue. Bradykinesia is attributed to

failure of the mechanism programming movement patterns manifested as a defect in the voluntary production of smooth motions at different speeds.

Hypokinesia, or decreased frequency or absence of associated movements, is one of the earliest akinetic symptoms. Individuals with Parkinson disease sit and lie motionless for long periods without the little shifts a normal person makes to prevent discomfort and stiffness. **Bradykinesia,** or slowness of voluntary movements, is characterized by difficulty initiating, continuing, or synchronizing movements. Both associated and voluntary movements are interspersed by freezing (an inability to continue movement). Freezing may be precipitated by (1) increasing the effort to move, (2) turning, and (3) initiating certain types of tactile and visual contact.

Postural Abnormalities

Postural abnormalities are caused by a loss of normal postural reflexes. Three types of postural abnormalities occur in individuals with Parkinson disease: (1) disorders of postural fixation, (2) disorders of equilibrium, and (3) disorders of righting. The disorder of postural fixation associated with Parkinson disease is involuntary flexion of the head and neck. The individual is unable to maintain an upright position of the trunk while standing or walking. The stooped (flexed, forward leaning) posture is characteristic (Figure 16-27). Postural abnormalities of the hands and feet also occur.

Disorders of equilibrium result from loss of postural stability. The person with Parkinson disease is unable to make the appropriate postural adjustment to tilting or falling and falls like a post when starting to tilt. The festinating gait (short, accelerating steps) of the patient with Parkinson disease is an attempt to maintain an upright position while walking (see Figure 16-27). Patients also are unable to right themselves when changing from a reclining or crouching position to a standing position and when rolling over from a supine to a lateral or prone position.

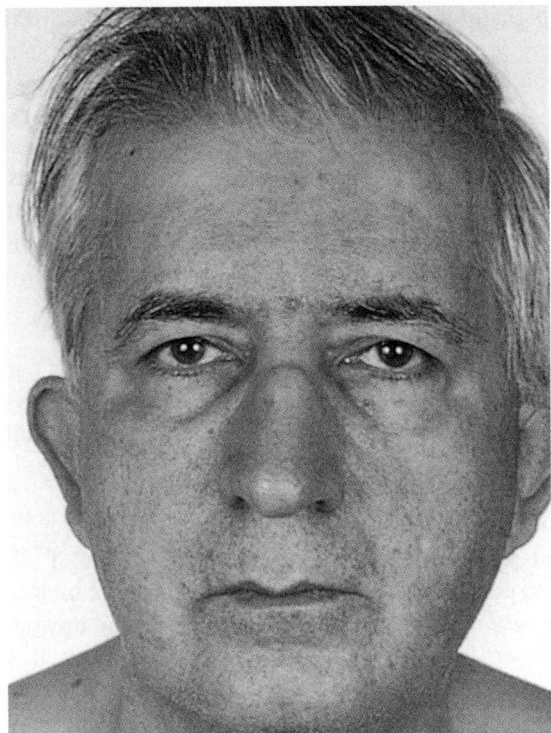

Figure 16-26 Facial appearance of Parkinson disease. Common facial characteristics include an unblinking, staring expression and smoothed-out, almost immobile, facial muscles. (From Perkin DG: *Mosby's color atlas and text of neurology,* London, 1998, Mosby-Wolfe.)

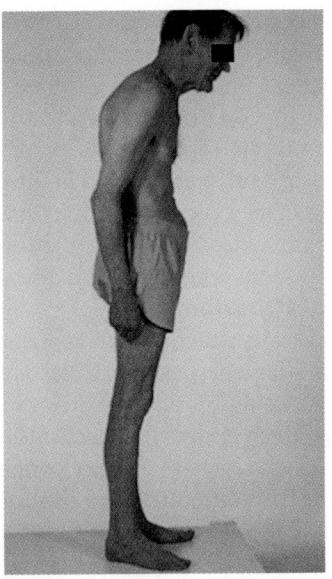

Figure 16-27 Stooped posture of Parkinson disease. (From Perkin DG: *Mosby's color atlas and text of neurology,* London, 1998, Mosby-Wolfe.)

Autonomic and Neuroendocrine Symptoms

Autonomic and neuroendocrine dysfunctions in Parkinson disease produce symptoms that are distressing but not incapacitating. The basal ganglia influence hypothalamic function (autonomic and neuroendocrine) through pathways connecting the hypothalamus with the basal ganglia and cerebral cortex. Common autonomic symptoms in Parkinson disease include inappropriate diaphoresis, orthostatic hypotension, gastric retention, constipation, and urinary retention. A symptom attributed to neuroendocrine dysfunction is seborrhea. Hypothalamic hypersecretion of hormone-releasing factors acting on the anterior pituitary causes hypersecretion of androgenotropic hormones. The androgen excess produces sebum hypersecretion by sebaceous glands. The resulting seborrhea is characterized by oily skin with seborrheic dermatitis along the hairline and in chin-nasal creases.

Cognitive-Affective Symptoms

Fifty percent of persons with Parkinson disease have a depression that is now believed to be an inherent part of the pathologic state of the disease (an endogenous depression), not a response to the situation. Thirty percent of persons treated on an outpatient basis for Parkinson disease have a dementia, and 80% of persons with Parkinson disease requiring institutional care have dementia as well. Dementia is more common in patients over 70 years of age. Pathologically, in patients with dementia, findings include loss of cholinergic cells in the basal nucleus of Meynert; neuronal loss, senile plaques, and neurofibrillary tangles in the neocortex; and amyloid changes in small blood vessels. Lewy bodies are distributed diffusely in many neocortical neurons, making this a Lewy body dementia. The patient evidences disorientation; confusion; memory loss; distractibility; and difficulty with concept formation, abstraction, calculations, thinking, and judgment. Although the symptoms fluctuate, they progressively worsen.

A cognitive disorder unassociated with either a dementia or depression, called *bradyphrenia,* is also present. This disorder may appear early in the course of the disease and may progress to dementia. Bradyphrenia is caused by disruption of the caudal basal ganglion connections and outflows. The clinical manifestations are slowness of thinking, poverty of thought (diminished imagination and insight), and difficulty formulating thoughts (decreased ability to conceptualize, plan, decide, or improvise). Sleep disturbances also have been documented in persons with Parkinson disease.

Influence of Symptoms

Early in the disease, patients often experience a sleep benefit; that is, symptoms decrease with sleep. Also, the symptoms fluctuate in an on-off pattern. Stress influences symptoms adversely, but the underlying mechanism is unclear. The patient's mental status may be further compromised by the side effects of the medication taken to control symptoms.

The combination of all the parkinsonian symptoms gives the individual a characteristic appearance: a wide-eyed, unblinking, staring expression with the facial muscles smoothed out and almost immobile. Saliva frequently drools from the corners of the slightly open mouth. The skin of the face is frequently greasy. The gait is pathognomonic: the individual walks with slow, short, shuffling steps; the arms are flexed, abducted, and held stiffly at the side; and the trunk is bent slightly forward. The person may break into a run spontaneously or when pushed forward or backward. Because of the disorder of postural fixation, the tendency is to fall to the side.

EVALUATION AND TREATMENT   The diagnosis of Parkinson disease is made on the basis of two of the four cardinal symptoms: (1) resting tremor, (2) bradykinesia, (3) cogwheel rigidity, and (4) postural instability. One of the two symptoms must be resting tremor or bradykinesia (criteria from Core Assessment Program for Intracerebral Transplantation [CAPIT]).[25] Positron emission tomography (PET) shows reduced uptake of 6-[18F]-fluoro-dopa.

The drug therapy includes administration of dopaminergic drugs, such as levodopa (L-dopa), a precursor of dopamine (dopamine does not cross the blood-brain barrier), dopamine agonists, anticholinergic drugs, antihistamines, and amantadine. These drugs are used to decrease akinesia. Because of troublesome side effects and decreased responsiveness to these drugs after 5 years, they are not initiated until symptoms become incapacitating. Apomorphine is used for the on-off phenomenon and selegiline is used for its neuroprotective properties. Implants of fetal cells are still being studied, as is some ablative surgery (e.g., destruction of a portion of the globus pallidus). Thalamotomy, pallidotomy, and thalamic stimulation are also used at times. Dysphagia and general immobility are special problems of the patient with Parkinson disease, requiring preventive, symptomatic, supportive, and rehabilitative management, such as physiotherapy and speech therapy.

Parkinson disease takes a slowly progressive course for 15 to 20 years before producing total invalidism. The course shows much variation among individuals. The prognosis has been better since the advent of levodopa, but the disorder still shortens life substantially. Pneumonia is the leading cause of death of those with Parkinson disease.

Alterations in Complex Motor Performance

The alterations in complex motor performance include disorders of posture (stance), disorders of gait, and disorders of expression.

Disorders of Posture (Stance)

An inequality of tone in muscle groups because of a loss of normal postural reflexes results in a posturing of limbs. Many reflex systems govern tone and posture, but the most important factor in posture control is the stretch reflex, in which stretching of extensor (antigravity) muscles causes increased extensor tone and inhibited flexor tone. Four types of disorders of posture are described: (1) dystonic posture, (2) decerebrate posture, (3) basal ganglion posture, and (4) senile posture. Equilibrium and balance are disrupted when postural disorders are present.

Dystonia is the maintenance of an abnormal posture through muscular contractions. When muscular contractions are sustained for several seconds, they are called **dystonic movements,** such as in choreoathetoid movements associated with high levels of L-dopa; when contractions last for longer periods, they are called **dystonic postures,** such as in torticollis. Dystonic postures may last for weeks, causing permanent fixed contractures. Dystonia has been associated with basal ganglia abnormality, but the exact pathophysiologic mechanisms are unknown. One particularly relevant dystonic posture already discussed in this chapter is decorticate (striatal posture or upper motor neuron dysfunction posture), which may be unilateral or bilateral in occurrence. **Decorticate posture** (also referred to as **antigravity posture** or **hemiplegic posture**) is characterized by upper extremities flexed at the elbows and held close to the body and by lower extremities that are externally rotated and extended. Decorticate posture is believed to occur when the brain stem, which facilitates the antigravity position, is not inhibited by the motor function of the cerebral cortex. Upper motor neuron posture is more commonly described as the arm flexed at the elbow, with a wrist-drop; the leg inadequately bent at the knee, with the hip excessively circumabducted; and the presence of a footdrop.

Decerebrate posture refers to increased tone in extensor muscles and trunk muscles, with active tonic neck reflexes. When the head is in a neutral position, all four limbs are rigidly extended. The decerebrate posture is caused by severe injury to the brain and brain stem, resulting in overstimulation of the postural righting and vestibular reflexes.

Basal ganglion posture refers to a stooped, hyperflexed posture with a narrow-based, short-stepped gait. This posture abnormality results from the loss of normal postural reflexes and not from defects in proprioceptive, labyrinthine, or visual function. Dysfunctional equilibrium results from the loss of postural stability, and thus the individual is unable to make the appropriate postural adjustment to tilting or loss of balance and falls instead. Dysfunctional righting is the inability to right oneself when changing from a lying or crouching to a standing position or when rolling from the supine to the lateral or prone position. Dysfunctional postural fixation is the involuntary flexion of the head and neck, causing the person difficulty in maintaining an upright trunk position while standing or walking. Basal ganglion dysfunction accounts for this posture.

Senile posture is characterized by an increasingly flexed posture similar to that caused by basal ganglion dysfunction. The posture is associated with frontal lobe dysfunction, but the primary pathophysiology is not well described.

Disorders of Gait
Four predominant types of gait disorder are (1) upper motor neuron dysfunction gait, (2) cerebellar (ataxic) gait, (3) basal ganglion gait, and (4) senile (frontal lobe, pseudoparkinsonian) gait. As with posture, equilibrium and balance are affected with gait disturbances.

Several upper motor neuron gaits exist. In the presence of mild upper motor neuron dysfunction, a footdrop may appear only with fatigue. The individual may complain of hip and leg pain. A **spastic gait,** which is associated with unilateral injury, is manifested by a shuffling gait with the leg extended and held stiff, causing a scraping over the floor surface. An impaired leg swing around the body rather than an appropriate lifting and placing of the leg is noted. The foot may drag on the ground, and the person tends to fall to the affected side. A **scissors gait** is associated with bilateral injury and spasticity. The legs are abducted, causing them to touch each other. As the person walks, the legs are still swung around the body but then cross in front of each other because of adduction. Injury to the pyramidal system accounts for these gaits.

A **cerebellar gait** manifests as a wide-based gait with the feet apart and often turned outward or inward for greater stability. The pelvis is held stiff, and it seems to be independent of the trunk. The individual staggers when walking. Cerebellar dysfunction accounts for this particular gait.

A **basal ganglion gait** and a **senile gait** are both broad-based gaits. The person walks with small steps and a decreased arm swing. The head and body are flexed and the arms are semiflexed and abducted, whereas the legs are flexed and rigid in more advanced states. Basal ganglion and frontal lobe dysfunction, respectively, account for these two gaits.

Disorders of Expression
Disorders of expression involve the motor aspects of communication and include (1) hypermimesis, (2) hypomimesis, and (3) dyspraxias and apraxias. Hypermimesis is a disinhibition phenomenon that most commonly manifests as pathologic laughter or crying. Pathologic laughter is associated with right hemisphere injury, and pathologic crying is associated with left hemisphere injury. The exact pathophysiology is not known. Hypomimesis manifests as aprosody, or the loss of emotional language. Receptive aprosody involves an inability to *understand* emotion in speech and facial expression, whereas expressive aprosody involves the inability to *express* emotion in speech and facial expression. Aprosody is associated with right hemisphere damage.

Dyspraxia is the partial inability and **apraxia** is the complete inability to perform purposeful or skilled motor acts in the absence of paralysis, sensory loss, abnormal posture and tone, abnormal involuntary movement, incoordination, or inattentiveness. These are disorders of learned skilled movements.[26] Dyspraxia and apraxia are associated with vascular disorders, trauma, tumor, degenerative disorders, infections, and metabolic disorders. The medial premotor cortex, including the supplementary motor area (SMA), appears to play a role in skilled movements as does the convexity premotor areas[26] (Table 16-26).

True dyspraxias occur when the connecting pathways between the left and right cortical areas are interrupted causing language-motor and motor representation disconnections between the hemispheres (Figure 16-28). Dyspraxias may result from any pathologic process that disrupts the cortical areas necessary for the conceptualization and execution of a

Table 16-26	Dyspraxias and Apraxias	
Types	**Description**	**Location**
Ideomotor apraxia	Impairment in selecting, sequencing, and spatial orientation of movements involved in gestures (spatial and temporal production errors)	Left parietal cortex (angular gyrus) or supramarginal gyrus
Posterior form	Difficulty performing in response to command and imitation; cannot discriminate well between poorly performed and well performed acts	Left parietal cortex (angular gyrus or supramarginal gyrus) lesion
Anterior form	Performs poorly to command and imitation but comprehends and discriminates pantomime	Lesions anterior to the supramarginal gyrus, which disconnects visual kinesthetic motor engrams from premotor and motor areas
Conduction apraxia	Greater impairment in performance when imitating movements than when pantomiming to command; comprehends pantomime and gesture but cannot perform the movements	Location unknown at this time
Disassociation apraxia	Inability to gesture normally to command and required verbal mediation has good performance with imitation and actual tools and objects	Callosal abnormalities but not all locations known
Ideational apraxia	Inability to carry out an ideational plan or a series of acts in the proper sequence	Location unclear at this time
Conceptual apraxia	Cannot recall type of action associated with specific tools, utensils, or objects (content and tool selection errors; may be unable to recall which tool is associated with a specific object or may have impaired mechanical knowledge)	Bilateral frontal and parietal dysfunction

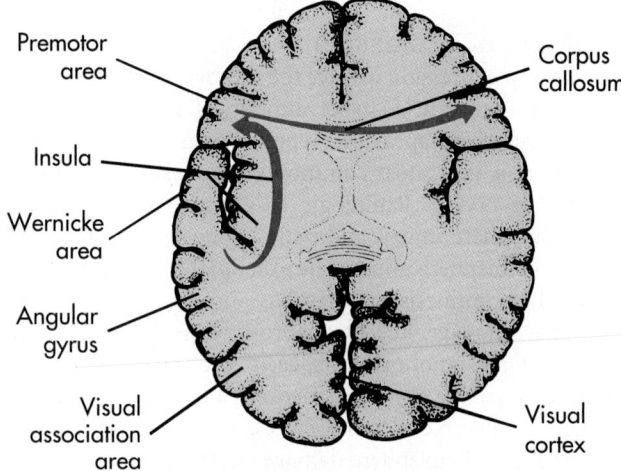

Figure 16-28 Pathways disrupted in dyspraxias. Formulation of the idea of the motor act is believed to originate in the region of the supramarginal gyrus in the inferior left parietal lobe. This area is connected via associational pathways to the left premotor cortex. The left premotor cortex is connected through the corpus callosum to the right premotor and motor areas. An injury that interrupts the pathways between the left supramarginal gyrus and the premotor region produces a dyspraxia that involves the entire body. An injury that disrupts the callosal pathways produces a dyspraxia of the left side of the body only.

complex motor act or the communication pathways within the left hemisphere or between the hemispheres.

Extrapyramidal Motor Syndromes

Because the extrapyramidal system encompasses all the motor pathways except the pyramidal system, two types of motor dysfunction make up the **extrapyramidal motor syndromes:** (1) the basal ganglia motor syndromes and (2) the cerebellar motor syndromes. Unlike pyramidal motor syndromes, both extrapyramidal motor syndromes result in movement or posture disturbance without significant paralysis, along with other distinctive symptoms (Table 16-27).

Basal Ganglia Motor Syndromes

Basal ganglia motor syndromes are movement disorders that involve either a paucity or an excess of movements. Stress and nervous tension typically worsen the symptoms, whereas relaxation improves motor performance. Akinesia may occur despite normal strength. Involuntary movements, such as tremor, chorea, ballism, athetosis, and dystonia, also may occur and probably are caused by the loss of the normal modulating effects of the corpus striatum and other parts of the basal ganglia.

Basal ganglia motor syndromes also are characterized by alterations in muscle tone and posture. Rigidity, together with the cogwheel phenomenon, is present in all muscle groups but is most prominent in those that maintain flexed position. Postural abnormalities result from the loss of normal postural reflexes. Dysfunctional equilibrium results from the loss of postural stability.

The symptoms of basal ganglia motor syndromes are explained as an imbalance of dopaminergic and cholinergic activity in the corpus striatum. A relative excess of cholinergic activity produces akinesia and hypertonia. A relative excess of dopaminergic activity produces hyperkinesia and hypotonia. The precise mechanisms by which imbalances of these striatal neurotransmitters cause specific symptoms are unknown.

Cerebellar Motor Syndromes

Cerebellar motor syndromes involve the cerebellum and may result in (1) loss of muscle tone acutely; (2) difficulty

Table 16-27   Pyramidal versus Extrapyramidal Motor Syndromes

Manifestations	Pyramidal Motor Syndrome	Extrapyramidal Motor Syndrome
Unilateral movement	Paralysis of voluntary movement	Little or no paralysis of voluntary movement
Tendon reflexes	Increased tendon reflexes	Normal or slightly increased tendon reflexes
Babinski sign	Present	Absent
Involuntary movements	Absence of involuntary movements	Presence of tremor, chorea, athetosis, or dystonia
Muscle tone	Spasticity in muscles (e.g., clasp-knife phenomenon)	Plastic (equal throughout movement) rigidity or intermittent (cogwheel) rigidity generalized but predominate in flexors of limbs and trunk
	Hypertonia present in flexors of arms and extensors of legs	Hypotonia in cerebellar disease

Table 16-28   Cerebellar Motor Syndromes

Anatomical Location of Dysfunction	Characteristics
Medial Syndromes	
Rostral vermis (so-called *anterior lobe*)	Ataxia of stance and gait with varying degrees of instability of the trunk and ataxia of legs; anteroposterior body sway; presence of a Romberg sign
Caudal vermis (including flocculonodular lobe)	Truncal, postural, and gait ataxia; omnidirectional body sway; Romberg negative; tendency to fall; saccadic slow pursuit, nystagmus; inability to suppress vestibulo-ocular reflex (Doll's eyes)
Lateral Syndrome	
Cerebellar hemisphere (neocerebellar syndrome)	Severe disturbance in ipsilateral limb movements; hypotonia in acute situation; dysmetria (extremity overshooting its target); decomposition of movement; kinetic tremor, past-pointing; deviation of gait; dysarthria

Data from Timmann D, Diener HC: Coordination and ataxia. In Goetz GC, editor, *Textbook of clinical neurology*, pp 299-315, St. Louis, 2003, Saunders.

with coordination of voluntary movements (ataxia); (3) minor degrees of muscle weakness, tendency toward fatigue, and impairment of associated movements; and (4) disorders of equilibrium, posture, and gait. Cerebellar effects are chiefly ipsilateral (primarily affecting the same side of the body), so damage to the right cerebellum generally causes symptoms on the right side of the body. Predominant symptoms depend on the area of damage within the cerebellum. The three cerebellar syndromes are the rostral vermis, caudal vermis, and lateral syndromes[27] (Table 16-28).

Diagnosis of a cerebellar motor syndrome is based on the symptoms, but these may vary because of the individual's attempts at compensation. Further, the nervous system often can operate well despite destruction of parts of the cerebellum, although the mechanisms responsible for this retained function are not fully understood.

SUMMARY REVIEW

Alterations in Cognitive Systems

1. Full consciousness is an awareness of oneself and the environment and includes an ability to respond to external stimuli with a wide variety of responses.
2. Consciousness has two components: arousal and content of thought.
3. Decreased level of arousal can occur because of diffuse bilateral cortical dysfunction, bilateral subcortical (reticular formation, brain stem) dysfunction, or localized hemispheric dysfunction.
4. An alteration in breathing pattern and level of coma reflects the level of brain dysfunction.
5. Pupillary changes reflect changes in level of brain stem function, drug action, and response to hypoxia and ischemia.
6. Abnormal eye movements, including nystagmus and divergent gaze, reflect alterations in brain stem function.
7. Level of brain function manifests by changes in generalized motor responses or no responses.
8. Loss of cortical inhibition associated with decreased consciousness includes abnormal flexor and extensor movements.
9. Cerebral death or irreversible coma represents permanent brain damage, with an ability to maintain cardiac, respiratory, and other vital functions.
10. Brain death results from irreversible brain damage that includes an inability to maintain internal homeostasis.
11. Arousal returns in vegetative states and minimally conscious states, but content of thought is absent or markedly reduced, respectively.
12. Seizures represent a sudden, chaotic discharge of cerebral neurons, with transient alterations in brain function. Seizures may be generalized or focal. There are three categories of epileptic syndrome: location-related, generalized, and undetermined.
13. With a deficit in selective attention, mediated by the brain stem, parietal lobe structures, and the pulvinar, the individual cannot focus on selective stimuli and thus neglects those stimuli.

Continued

14. In dysmnesia and amnesia, some past memories are not retrieved and new memories cannot be stored.
15. Frontal areas mediate vigilance, detection, and working memory. With a vigilance deficit, the person cannot maintain alertness. With a detection deficit, the person is unmotivated and unable to use feedback.
16. Some specific disorders of content of thought (cognition) are agnosias, dysphasias, acute confusional states, and dementias, including Alzheimer disease.
17. Agnosias are a defect of recognition and may be tactile, visual, or auditory. They are caused by dysfunction in the primary sensory area or the interpretive areas of the cerebral cortex.
18. Dysphasia is an impairment of comprehension or production of language. Dysphasia may be expressive or sensory.
19. Aphasia is loss of language comprehension or production.
20. Wernicke dysphasia is a disturbance in understanding all language—both verbal and reading comprehension.
21. Conductive dysphasias result from disruption of temporal lobe fibers, with a failure to repeat words but an ability to initiate speech, writing, and reading aloud.
22. Anomic dysphasia is an inability to name objects, persons, or qualities.
23. Transcortical dysphasias involve an ability to repeat and recite.
24. Broca aphasia is an expressive dysphasia of speech and writing but with retention of comprehension.
25. Global aphasia involves both anterior and posterior speech areas, with both expressive and receptive aphasia.
26. Acute confusional states are characterized chiefly by defects in attention and coherence of thoughts and actions and, in the case of delirium, an intense autonomic nervous system hyperactivity.
27. Alzheimer disease is a chronic, irreversible dementia.

Alterations in Cerebral Hemodynamics

1. Cerebral oxygenation is a critical management issue.
2. Cerebral perfusion pressure determines cerebral blood flow.
3. An injured brain may experience cerebral oligemia, normal cerebral blood flow but with increased intracranial pressure, or cerebral hyperemia.
4. Increased intracranial pressure may result from edema, excess CSF, hemorrhage, or tumor growth. When intracranial pressure approaches arterial pressure, hypoxia and hypercapnia produce brain damage.
5. Cerebral edema is an increase in the fluid content of the brain resulting from infection, hemorrhage, tumor, ischemia, infarct, or hypoxia.
6. The shifting or herniation of brain tissue from one compartment to another disrupts the blood flow of both compartments and damages brain tissue.
7. Supratentorial herniation involves temporal lobe and hippocampal gyrus shifting from the middle fossa to the posterior fossa; transtentorial herniation with a downward shift of the diencephalon through the tentorial notch; and shifting of the cingulate gyrus herniation under the falx.
8. The most common infratentorial herniation is a shift of the cerebellar tonsils through the foramen magnum.
9. Hydrocephalus comprises a variety of disorders characterized by an excess of fluid within the cranial vault, subarachnoid space, or both. Hydrocephalus occurs because of interference with CSF flow caused by increased fluid production or obstruction within the ventricular system or by defective reabsorption of the fluid.
10. Hydrocephalus can be treated by reducing CSF in the ventricles through the use of shunts and diuretic therapy if resection of the cause is not possible.

Alterations in Emotions and Mood

1. Disorders of the frontal lobes, limbic system, or hypothalamus may be associated with a broad range of changes in emotion and behavior.
2. Changes in emotion, mood, and behavior can result from abscesses, tumors, hemorrhages, metabolic disorders, degenerative diseases, and intoxication states.

Alterations in Motor Function

1. Motor dysfunction may be characterized as alterations of motor tone, movement, and complex motor performance.
2. Hypotonia and hypertonia are the main categories of altered tone.
3. Four types of hypertonia exist: spasticity, gegenhalten, dystonia, and rigidity.
4. Paresis, paraplegia, hyperkinesia, and hypokinesia are the main categories of altered movement.
5. Two subtypes of paresis and paralysis are described: upper motor neuron and lower motor neuron.
6. An upper motor neuron syndrome is characterized by paresis or paralysis, hypertonia, and hyperreflexia.
7. Interruption of the pyramidal tract below the pons results in spinal shock.
8. Lower motor neuron syndromes manifest with impaired voluntary and involuntary movements.
9. Partial paralysis occurs with only partial loss of alpha motor neurons, and total paralysis is complete loss of alpha motor neurons. Loss of gamma motor neurons impairs muscle tone and decreases tendon reflexes.
10. Amyotrophy (e.g., poliomyelitis) is a lower motor neuron syndrome involving the anterior horn cells, with loss of muscle tone and strength resulting in segmental paresis and hyporeflexia.
11. Nuclear palsies involve damage to the cranial nerve nuclei.
12. Bulbar palsies involve cranial nerves IX, X, and XII.
13. Included in the category of hyperkinesia are chorea, athetosis, ballism, akathisia, tremor, and myoclonus.
14. Huntington disease (chorea) is a rare hereditary disease involving the basal ganglia and cerebral cortex. It is inherited as an autosomal dominant trait and commonly manifests between 30 and 50 years of age.
15. The major pathologic feature of Huntington disease is severe degeneration of the basal ganglia and the frontal cerebral cortex. The basal ganglia and the substantia nigra exhibit a depletion of neurons that secrete γ-aminobutyric acid (an inhibitory neurotransmitter). This depletion leads to an excess of dopaminergic activity that causes involuntary, fragmentary movements.
16. No known treatment is effective in halting the degenerative process in Huntington disease.
17. Types of hypokinesia include akinesia, bradykinesia, and loss of associated movements.
18. Parkinson disease is a common degenerative disorder of the basal ganglia (corpus striatum) involving degeneration of the dopamine-secreting nigrostriatal pathway. The pathogenesis of Parkinson disease is unknown, but researchers suggest genetic, viral, and environmental toxins as possible causes.
19. Degeneration of the dopaminergic nigrostriatal pathway causes dopamine depletion in the basal ganglia and an excess of cholinergic activity in the cortex, basal ganglia, and thalamus. Tremor and rigidity are caused by the excess cholinergic activity. Progressive dementia may be associated with an advanced stage of the disease.
20. Treatment of Parkinson disease is symptomatic, involving levodopa (L-dopa), a precursor of dopamine. The disease takes a

slowly progressive course for 15 to 20 years before producing complete invalidism.

21. Alterations in complex motor performance include disorders of posture (stance), disorders of gait, and disorders of expression.
22. Disorders of posture include dystonic posture, decerebrate posture, basal ganglion posture, and senile posture.
23. Disorders of gait include upper motor neuron gaits, cerebellar gait, basal ganglion gait, and senile gait.
24. Disorders of expression include hypermimesis, hypomimesis, and dyspraxia or apraxia.
25. Dyspraxia is an impairment of the conceptualization or execution of a complex motor act.
26. Extrapyramidal motor syndromes include basal ganglia and cerebellar motor syndromes.
27. Basal ganglia disorders manifest with alterations in muscle tone and posture, including rigidity, involuntary movements, and loss of postural reflexes.
28. Cerebellar motor syndromes result in loss of muscle tone, difficulty with coordination, and disorders of equilibrium and gait.

KEY TERMS

Acute confusional states (acute cerebral failure, acute brain failure), 516
Acute hydrocephalus, 525
Agnosia, 510
Akinesia, 536
Akinetic mutism (AM), 502
Alzheimer disease (dementia of Alzheimer type [DAT], senile disease complex), 518
Amyotrophies, 532
Aphasia, 511
Apraxia, 541
Areflexia, 532
Aura, 504
Autoregulation, 522
Basal ganglia motor syndromes, 542
Basal ganglion gait, 541
Basal ganglion posture, 541
Bradykinesia, 536
Brain death (brain stem death), 498
Bulbar palsy, 533
Central herniation, 523
Cerebellar gait, 541
Cerebellar motor syndrome, 542
Cerebral death, 501
Cerebral edema, 524
Cingulate gyrus herniation (subfalcine herniation), 523
Clonic phase, 504
Clonus, 528
Coma, 501
Communicating (extraventricular) hydrocephalus, 524
Content of thought, 491
Convulsion, 503
Cryogenic, 507
Cytotoxic (metabolic) edema, 524
Decerebrate posture, 541
Declarative memory, 508
Decorticate posture (antigravity posture, hemiplegic posture), 541
Dementia, 517
Detection deficit, 509
Diplegia, 529
Dysmnesia, 508
Dysphasia, 510

Dyspraxia, 541
Dystonia, 541
Dystonic movements, 541
Dystonic postures, 541
Echolalia, 511
Epilepsy, 504
Epileptogenic focus, 503
Expressive dysphasias, 511
Extinction, 508
Extrapyramidal motor syndromes, 542
Fibrillation, 532
Flaccid paralysis, 532
Flaccid paresis, 532
Freezing, 536
Gamma neuropathies, 532
Gegenhalten (paratonia), 528
Generalized seizures, 503
Hemiparesis, 529
Hemiplegia, 529
Huntington disease (HD), 535
Hydrocephalus, 524
Hydrocephalus ex vacuo, 525
Hyperkinesia, 533
Hypertonia, 528
Hypokinesia, 536
Hypotonia, 527
Idiopathic, 507
Increased intracranial pressure, 521
Interstitial edema, 524
Intracranial pressure, 521
Ischemic edema, 524
Isolated speech center, 511
Locked-in syndrome, 502
Metabolic arousal alteration, 494
Minimally conscious state (MSC), 502
Mirror focus, 504
Mixed transcortical dysphasia, 511
Neglect syndrome, 508
Neurofibrillary tangle, 519
Noncommunicating hydrocephalus, 524
Nondeclarative memory, 508
Normal-pressure hydrocephalus, 525
Nuclear palsies, 533
Paralysis, 529
Paraparesis, 529

Paraplegia, 529
Paresis, 529
Parkinson disease, 536
Parkinsonism (Parkinson syndrome, parkinsonian syndrome), 536
Parkinsonian bradykinesia, 539
Parkinsonian rigidity, 539
Parkinsonian tremor, 538
Paroxysmal dyskinesia, 535
Partial seizures (focal seizures), 503
Postictal state, 503
Prodroma, 504
Progressive bulbar palsy, 533
Progressive spinal muscular atrophy, 533
Psychogenic arousal alteration, 494
Pyramidal motor syndrome, 529
Quadriparesis, 529
Quadriplegia, 529
Rigidity, 528
Scissors gait, 541
Secondary generalization, 503
Seizure, 502
Selective attention deficit, 508
Senile gait, 541
Senile plaques, 519
Senile posture, 541
Sensory inattentiveness, 508
Spastic gait, 541
Spasticity, 528
Spinal shock, 530
Status epilepticus, 503
Structural arousal alteration, 494
Symptomatic, 507
Tardive dyskinesia, 535
Tonic phase, 504
Transcortical dysphasias, 511
Transcortical sensory dysphasia, 511
Uncal herniation (hippocampal herniation, lateral mass herniation), 523
Vasogenic edema, 524
Vegetative state (VS), 501
Vigilance deficit, 509
Working memory deficit, 509

MEDIA RESOURCES 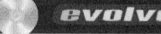 *evolve*

Review questions and answers for this chapter are available in the *CD Companion* included with this book.

WebLinks—links to Internet sites pertaining to this chapter—are available on Evolve at http://evolve.elsevier.com/McCance/.

REFERENCES

1. Plum F, Posner JB: *The diagnosis of stupor and coma,* Philadelphia, 1980, FA Davis.
2. Boss BJ, Flecher A: Severe brain injury rehabilitation: what's going to happen after critical care? *Crit Care Nurs Clin* 13(3):421-431, 2001.
3. Bleck TP: Levels of consciousness and attention. In Gottez CG, editor: *Textbook of clinical neurology,* Philadelphia, 2003, Saunders.
4. Victor M, Ropper AD: *Adam and Victor's principles of neurology,* ed 7, St. Louis, 2001, Mosby.
5. Rakel RE: *Textbook of family practice,* ed 6, Philadelphia, 2002, Mosby.
6. Walker AE: *Cerebral death,* ed 3, Baltimore, 1985, Urban & Schwarzenberg.
7. Christensen D: Endgame for epilepsy? Researchers look toward a cure, *Sci News* 160(17):259, 2001.
8. Foldvary-Schaefer N, Wyllie E: Epilepsy. In Goetz CG, editor: *Textbook of clinical neurology,* Philadelphia, 2003, Saunders.
9. Gabrieli JDE et al: Memory. In Goetz CG, editor: *Textbook of clinical neurology,* Philadelphia, 2003, Saunders.
10. Lanaska DJ: Acute confusional states. In Corey-Bloom J, editor: *Adult neurology,* St. Louis, 1998, Mosby.
11. Jacques A, Jackson GA: *Understanding dementia,* ed 3, London, 2000, Churchill Livingstone.
12. Caselli RJ, Boeve BF: The degenerative dementias. In Goetz CG, editor: *Textbook of clinical neurology,* Philadelphia, 2003, Saunders.
13. Reynolds B: Introduction: optimizing care for patients with Alzheimer's disease: emerging treatment strategies, *J Acad Nurs Pract* (suppl) 16(1):3, 2004.
14. Auerhalm C: Recognition of risk factors and screening tools: optimizing care for patients with Alzheimer's disease: emerging treatment strategies, *J Acad Nurs Pract* (suppl) 16(1):4-5, 2004.
15. Selkoe DJ: The origins of Alzheimer disease: a is for amyloid, *JAMA* 283(12):1615-1617, 2000.
16. Naslund J et al: Correlation between elevated levels of amyloid beta-peptide in the brain and cognitive decline, *JAMA* 283(12):1571-1577, 2000.
17. Mele D: Cognitive, functional and behavioral decline in Alzheimer's disease: optimizing care for patients with Alzheimer's disease: emerging treatment strategies, *J Acad Nurs Pract* (suppl) 16(1):6-7, 2004.
18. Masterman DL: The rationale behind pharmacologic management of Alzheimer's disease: optimizing care for patients with Alzheimer's disease: emerging treatment strategies, *J Acad Nurs Pract* (suppl) 16(1):8-9, 2004.
19. Molinuevo JL, Garcia-Gil V, Villar A: Memantine: an antiglutamatergic option for dementia, *Am J Alzheimers Dis Other Demen* 19(1):10-18, 2004.
20. Bullock R, Chestnut RM: *Management and prognosis of severe traumatic brain injury,* New York, 2000, Brain Trauma Foundation and American Association of Neurological Surgeons.
21. Gupta AK: Monitoring the injured brain in the intensive care unit, *J Postgrad Med* 48(3):218-225, 2002.
22. Hlatky R, Valdka AB, Robertson CS: Intracranial hypertension and cerebral ischemia after severe traumatic brain injury, *Neurol Focus* 14(4):1-4, 2003.
23. Friedman JH: Mood, emotion, and thought. In Goetz CG, editor: *Textbook of clinical neurology,* Philadelphia, 2003, Saunders.
24. Bower B: Dendrite decline in schizophrenia, *Sci News* 154:91, 2000.
25. Jankovic J: Movement disorders. In Goetz CG, editor: *Textbook of clinical neurology,* Philadelphia, 2003, Saunders.
26. Defer GL, Widner H, Marie RM et al: Core assessment program for surgical interventional therapies in Parkinson's disease (CAPSIT-PD), *Mov Disord* 14(4):572-584, 1999.
27. Heilman KM, Watson RT, Gonzalez-Rothi LJ: Praxis. In Goetz CG, editor: *Textbook of clinical neurology,* Philadelphia, 2003, Saunders.

ALTERATIONS OF NEUROLOGIC FUNCTION

BARBARA J. BOSS

CHAPTER OUTLINE

evolve
http://evolve.elsevier.com/McCance/

Alterations in central nervous system (CNS) function are caused by traumatic injury, vascular disorders, tumor growth, infectious and inflammatory processes, metabolic derangements (including those arising from nutritional deficiencies and drugs/chemicals), and degenerative processes. Alterations in peripheral nervous system function involve the nerve roots (radiculopathies), a nerve plexus, or the nerves themselves (neuropathies). Disorders of the neuromuscular junction also occur.

CENTRAL NERVOUS SYSTEM DISORDERS

Trauma

Brain Trauma

Major head injury or **traumatic brain injury (TBI)** is defined by the National Head Injury Foundation as a traumatic insult to the brain capable of producing physical, intellectual, emotional, social, and vocational changes. Of the 2 million head injuries in the United States each year, 1.6 million are mild injuries not requiring hospitalization. Of the 500,000 TBIs requiring hospitalization, 450,000 persons are admitted to the hospital alive; 80% have mild TBIs, 10% moderate TBIs, and 10% severe TBIs.[1] The Glasgow Coma Scale (GCS) is used to describe injury severity by the international and United States National Traumatic Coma Data Banks. The hallmark of a se-

vere TBI is loss of consciousness for 6 hours or more. TBI classifications using the GCS are (1) mild TBI with GCS of 13 to 15, associated with mild concussion; (2) moderate TBI with GCS of 9 to 12, associated with structural injury such as hemorrhage or contusion; and (3) severe TBI with GCS of 3 to 8, associated with cognitive and/or physical disability or death. Age and admission GCS are important diagnostic factors in traumatic brain injury.[2]

Persons at highest risk for TBI are young persons 15 to 24 years of age, infants 6 months to 2 years, young school-age children, and elderly individuals. The male/female ratio for such injury is 2:1.[3] TBI is highest among blacks and in lower-median income families. Persons living in high-crime areas are at greater risk.

Head injuries are broadly categorized into **blunt (closed, nonmissile) trauma** and **open (penetrating, missile) trauma.** Blunt trauma, the more common injury, involves the head striking a hard surface or a rapidly moving object striking the head. The dura mater remains intact, and brain tissues are not exposed to the environment. Blunt trauma may result in both focal brain injuries and diffuse axonal injuries (Table 17-1). When a break in (penetration of) the dura mater results in exposure of the cranial contents to the environment, open trauma has occurred, which results in focal brain injuries.

The most common types of brain injury are mild concussion and classic cerebral concussion (see pp. 552 to 553). Of all head injuries, 75% to 90% are not severe. Focal brain

| Table 17-1 | Severity of Trauma Related to Injury, Onset, and Persistence |

	Trauma State Induced		Onset of Clinical Manifestations	Persistence of DAI Clinical Manifestations
Severity of Trauma	Focal Injury	DAI		
Mild blunt trauma		Mild concussion	Immediate	Hours to days
Moderate blunt trauma		Classic cerebral concussion	Immediate	Up to 6 mo or longer
	Paraplegia (associated with injury to top of head)		Immediate	
	Blindness (associated with occipital injury)		Immediate	
	Delayed development of unresponsiveness (vasomotor or vasovagal syncopal episode)		Delayed	
Severe blunt trauma		Mild DAI	Immediate	Permanent residual
		Moderate DAI	Immediate	
		Severe DAI	Immediate	
	Acute epidural hemorrhage		Immediate to delayed (2-3 hr)	
	Acute contusional swelling		Delayed onset (few hours after injury)	
	Acute subdural hematoma		Delayed onset (few hours to 1 wk after injury)	
	Subacute subdural hematoma*		Delayed onset (1 to few weeks)	
	Subdural hygroma		Delayed onset	
	Traumatic cerebral hemorrhage*		Delayed onset (as late as 1 wk after injury)	

*May be seen after moderate head injury, especially in elderly persons.
DAI, Diffuse axonal injury.

injury and diffuse axonal injury (DAI) each account for one half of all injuries. Focal brain injury accounts for more than two thirds of head injury deaths; DAI, for less than one third. However, DAI accounts for the greatest number of severely disabled survivors, including persons who persist in an unresponsive state or reduced level of consciousness.

In recent years the surviving traumatic brain injury population has changed, mostly because of focus on reducing severity of injury (e.g., passive seat restraints, air bags), reduced transport time, and improved on-the-scene medical management. Improved management of secondary and tertiary injury also is influencing the situation; acute care health professionals are beginning to focus more on morbidity than mortality. As a result, persons with more severe traumatic brain injuries are being admitted to rehabilitation programs.

Causes of Brain Trauma

Most traumatic brain injuries are caused by motor vehicle accidents (MVAs) (50%) and falls (21%). Sports-related events (10%) and violence (12%) also account for a portion of craniocerebral traumatic brain injuries.[1]

Injuries related to focal brain injuries, those caused by objects (e.g., baseball bat, weapon) striking the front of the head, usually produce only coup injuries (contusions and fractures) because the inner skull in the occipital area is smooth. Objects striking the back of the head usually result in both **coup** (directly below the point of impact) and **contrecoup** (on the pole opposite the site of impact) injuries because of the irreg-

ularity of the inner surface of the frontal bones (Figure 17-1). Objects striking the side of the head may produce coup or contrecoup injuries. The same is true when the head strikes an immovable object with little velocity (e.g., a short fall).

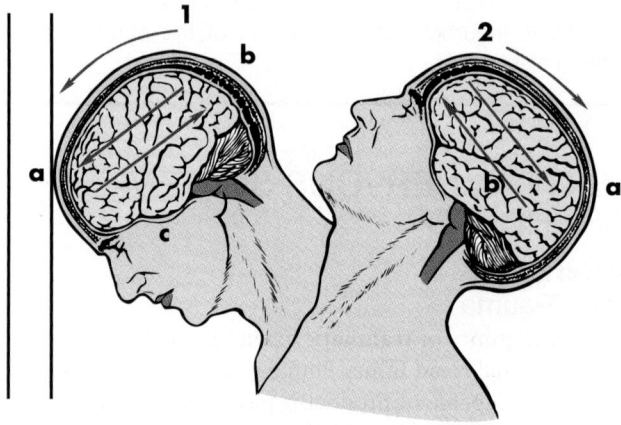

G.J. Wassilchenko

Figure 17-1 Coup and contrecoup brain injury following blunt trauma. *1,* Coup injury: impact against object; *a,* site of impact and direct trauma to brain; *b,* shearing of subdural veins; *c,* trauma to base of brain. *2,* Contrecoup injury: impact within skull, *a,* site of impact from brain hitting opposite side of skull; *b,* shearing forces through brain. These injuries occur in one continuous motion—the head strikes the wall (coup) and then rebounds (contrecoup). (Modified from Rudy EB: *Advanced neurological and neurosurgical nursing,* St Louis, 1984, Mosby.)

Extradural hematomas, a form of secondary injury, are caused most commonly by motor vehicle accidents (MVAs), occasionally by minor falls and sporting accidents. A temporal fracture causes 90% of temporal lobe extradural hematomas. Direct frontal lobe trauma is associated with frontal extradural hematomas. Posterior extradural hematomas are associated with a fracture across the transverse sinus from an occipital blow.

MVAs are the most common cause of subdural hematomas; 50% of subdural hematomas are associated with skull fractures. Falls, especially in elderly people or in persons with long-term alcohol abuse, are associated with chronic subdural hematomas.

Intracerebral hemorrhage is associated with the presence of contusions. This hemorrhage is caused by forceful impact, usually associated with MVAs and falls from some distance.

Compound fractures are caused by objects striking the head with great force or by the head striking an object forcefully. The comments regarding contusion hold true for compound fractures. Temporal blows, related to basilar skull fractures, may produce a fracture involving the middle fossa. An occipital blow may result in a basilar fracture down the occipital bone and across the petrous pyramid. The cervical vertebrae upwardly impacting the base of the skull can produce a posterior fossa **basilar skull fracture.**

Causes of penetrating injuries are missiles (most commonly bullets fired from rifles and handguns) and sharp projectiles (e.g., knives, ice picks, axes, screwdrivers). Most through-and-through injuries are from high-velocity bullets.

Related to DAI, mild concussion and classic cerebral concussion are particularly associated with a moving head striking a hard, unyielding object. A concussion may result from a moving object striking a stationary head, however. Moderate DAI is usually sustained by occupants of vehicles and pedestrians. Sagittal or horizontal (torsional) head motion produces mild or moderate DAI. Severe DAI occurs only in coronal (lateral) head motion and is caused by injuries sustained in MVAs.

PATHOPHYSIOLOGY Damage originates from three mechanisms: primary, secondary, and tertiary injury. Primary injury is caused by the impact and involves neural injury, primary glial injury, and vascular response. In primary glial injury, oligodendroglia is affected by axon injury and by direct mechanical disruption caused by debris and leakage. The vascular response is immediate at the time of injury and involves increased capillary endothelial permeability to solutes. Secondary injury includes cerebral edema, brain swelling, hemorrhage, infection, and increased intracranial pressure. Significant to secondary injury is tissue hypoxia arising from cerebral ischemia (inadequate perfusion and tissue hypoxia). Consequences of ischemia are as follows: (1) ischemic neurons release substances that produce glial permeability to sodium (cytotoxic edema); (2) with energy failure, influxes of calcium through incompetent channels produce electrophysiologic consequences and activation of phospholipases to re-

lease free fatty acids with reoxygenation, prostaglandins, and free radicals; and (3) lactic acidosis occurs. Secondary injury occurs from compromise of circulation or brain shift. Tertiary injury is caused by apnea, hypotension, change in pulmonary resistance, and change in electrocardiogram (ECG), specifically ST and T wave changes.

Primary Injury. Insight into the nature of the injury and its potential effects can be obtained from information about the causal agent and from the nature, extent, and site of damage. Knowledge of the cellular biology of head injury has progressed dramatically over the past 20 years. Previously, no explanation existed for why persons with similar computed tomography (CT) scans had different clinical pictures or for the electrophysiologic changes in concussion, and outcome was totally unexplained and unpredictable. Technologic advances set the stage for research to uncover different, more satisfactory explanations. Head injury is a process in which diffuse axonal injury is the underlying pathology on which focal injuries are superimposed.[3]

Focal Brain Injury. **Focal brain injury** is specific, grossly observable brain lesions—cortical contusions, epidural hemorrhage, subdural hematoma, and intracerebral hematoma. The force of impact (translational acceleration) typically produces **contusions** from direct contact (as well as injury to the vault, vessels, and supporting structures) that in turn produce epidural hemorrhage and subdural and intracerebral hematomas. The mechanisms of injury are depicted in Figure 17-1. Damage results from compression of the skull at the point of impact and rebound effect. Contusion and bleeding occur because of small tears in blood vessels resulting from these forces. The severity of contusion is associated with the amount of energy transmitted by the skull to underlying brain tissue. In addition, the smaller the area of impact is, the greater the severity of injury, because the force is concentrated into a smaller area. The focal injury may be coup or contrecoup. Brain edema forms around and in damaged neural tissues, contributing to the increasing intracranial pressure (ICP). Within the contused areas are infarction and necrosis, multiple hemorrhages, and edema. The tissue has a pulpy quality. The maximum effects of injury related to contusion, bleeding, and edema peak 18 to 36 hours after severe head injury.

Contusions (Figure 17-2) are found most commonly in the frontal lobes, particularly at the poles and along the inferior orbital surfaces; in the temporal lobes, especially in the anterior poles and along the inferior surface; and at the frontotemporal junction. They result in changes in attention, memory, executive attentional function (motivation, goal selection or formation, planning, self-monitoring, and use of feedback), affect, emotion, and behavior. Less commonly, contusions occur in the parietal lobes and the occipital lobes. Focal cerebral contusions are superficial, involving just the gyri. Hemorrhagic contusions may coalesce into a large, confluent intracranial hematoma.

Extradural hematomas (epidural hematomas or epidural hemorrhages) represent 1% to 2% of major head injuries and occur in all age groups, but most commonly in persons 20 to

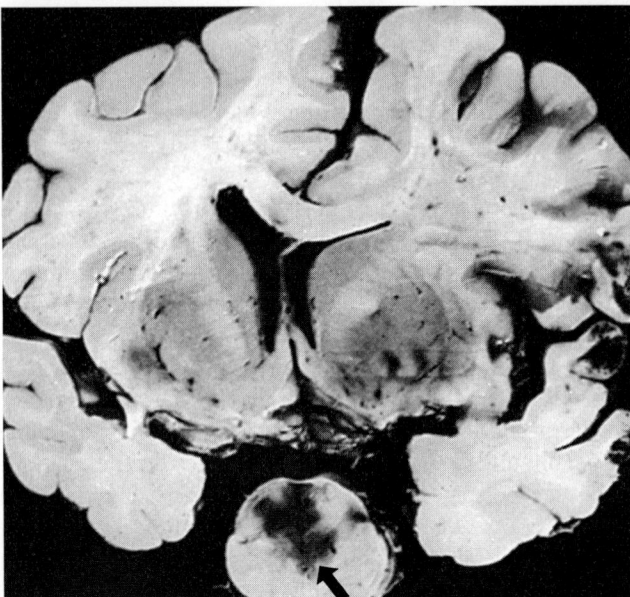

Figure 17-2 Recent contusions of frontal and temporal lobes. Displacement of cingulate gyrus and lateral ventricles are shown. Secondary hemorrhages have occurred in lower midbrain and upper pons. (From Kissane JM, editor: *Anderson's pathology,* ed 9, St Louis, 1993, Mosby.)

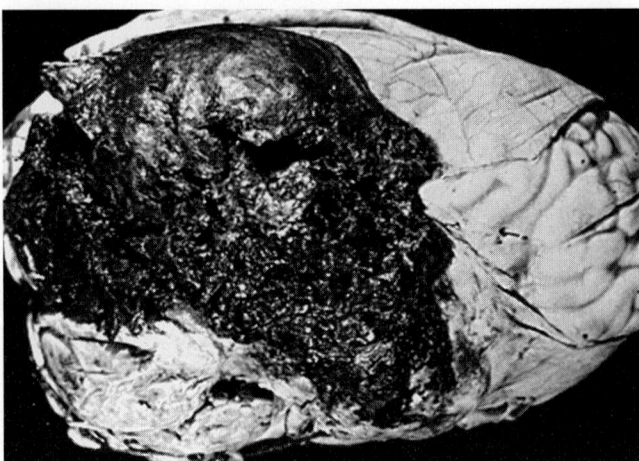

Figure 17-3 Acute epidural hematoma. Skull fracture with tear of middle meningeal artery and vein. (From Kissane JM, editor: *Anderson's pathology,* ed 9, St Louis, 1993, Mosby.)

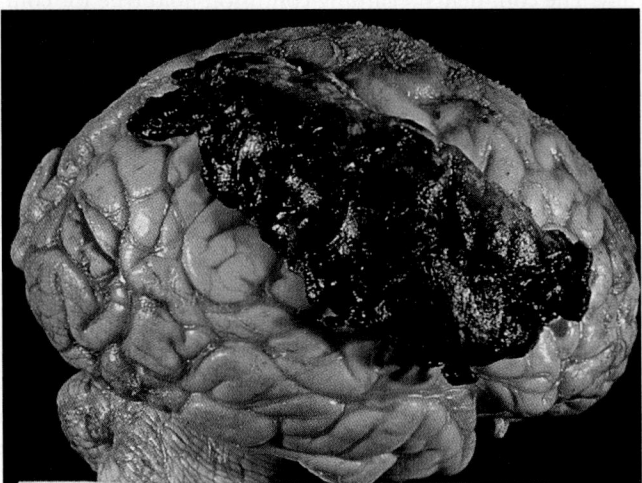

Figure 17-4 Acute subdural hematoma (dura removed). Leptomeninges are intact. (From Damjanov I, Linder J: *Anderson's pathology,* ed 10, St Louis, 1996, Mosby.)

40 years of age. An artery is the source of bleeding in 85% of extradural hematomas (Figure 17-3); 15% result from injury to the meningeal vein or dural sinus. Ninety percent of persons also have a skull fracture. The temporal fossa is the most common site of extradural hematoma caused by injury to the middle meningeal artery or vein. The resulting shift of the temporal lobe medially precipitates uncal and hippocampal gyrus herniation through the tentorial notch. Extradural hemorrhages are found occasionally in the subfrontal area (especially in the young and elderly populations), caused by injury to the anterior meningeal artery or a venous sinus, and in the occipital-suboccipital area, which results in herniation of the posterior fossa contents through the foramen magnum. Computed tomography (CT) and magnetic resonance imaging (MRI) show a lens-shaped mass over the surface of the cortex.

Subdural hematomas arise in 10% to 20% of persons with traumatic brain injury. Acute subdural hematomas rapidly develop (within 48 hours) and usually are located at the top of the skull (the cerebral convexities). On CT visualization, they appear as a high-density mass. Bilateral hematomas occur in 15% to 20% of persons. Subacute subdural hematomas develop more slowly, often over 48 hours to 2 weeks. On CT visualization, they appear as a mixed-density mass. Chronic subdural hematomas (commonly found in elderly persons and persons who abuse alcohol who have some degree of brain atrophy with a subsequent increase in the extradural space) develop over weeks to months. Tearing of the bridging veins is the major cause of rapidly developing and subacutely developing subdural hematomas, although torn cortical veins or venous sinuses and contused tissue may be the source. These subdural hematomas act as expanding masses, giving rise to increased ICP that eventually compresses the bleeding vessels (Figures 17-4 and 17-5). The displacement of brain tissue can result in a herniation syndrome.

The pathogenesis of a chronic subdural hematoma is different. The existing subdural space gradually fills with blood. A vascular membrane forms around the hematoma in approximately 2 weeks. Further enlargement takes place in some persons, but the mechanism of this enlargement is unclear.

Intracerebral hematomas (intraparenchymal hemorrhages)[3] occur in 2% to 3% of persons with head injuries, may be single or multiple hematomas, and are associated with contusions. Although most commonly located in the frontal and temporal lobes, intracerebral hematomas may occur in the hemispheric deep white matter. Small blood vessels are traumatized by penetrating injury or shearing forces. The intracerebral hematoma then acts as an expanding mass, resulting in increased ICP and compression of brain tissues with result-

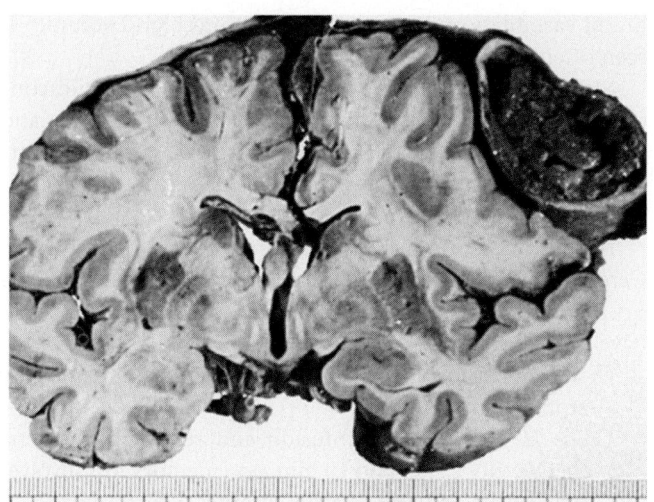

Figure 17-5 Chronic subdural hematoma. Compression of underlying brain and lateral ventricle. Note bone formation in falx and uncal herniation on side of hematoma. (From Kissane JM, editor: *Anderson's pathology,* ed 9, St Louis, 1993, Mosby.)

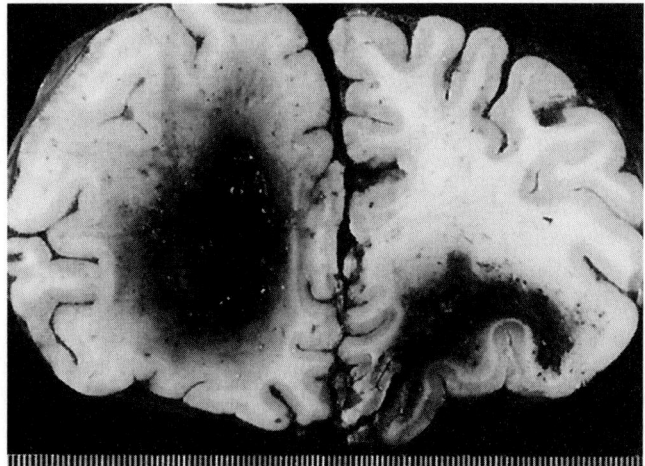

Figure 17-6 Hematomas. Recent hematomas, resulting from trauma, in frontal lobes. (From Kissane JM: *Anderson's pathology,* ed 8, St Louis, 1985, Mosby.)

ant edema (Figure 17-6). Delayed intracerebral hematomas may appear 3 to 10 days after the head injury.

Open trauma produces discrete (focal) injuries and includes compound fractures and missile injuries. A compound fracture opens a communication between the cranial contents and the environment and should be investigated whenever there are lacerations of the scalp, tympanic membrane, a sinus, an eye, or mucous membranes. Such fractures may involve the cranial vault or the base of the skull (basilar skull fracture). The injury incurred from bone fragments is mainly a tangential injury (injury caused by direct contact) and occasionally a penetrating injury. Bone fragments may lacerate or contuse brain tissues or blood vessels. In addition, cranial nerves may be damaged with a basilar skull fracture.

Missiles include bullets, rocks, shell fragments, knives, and blunt instruments. The mechanisms of injury are crush injury and stretch injury. Crush injury is the laceration and crushing of whatever tissue the missile touches, with the amount of crush related to the degree of fragmentation, deformity, size, and shape. A tangential injury is injury to the coverings of the brain (scalp lacerations), skull fractures, laceration of the meninges, and cerebral lacerations. Projectiles and debris from scalp and skull injury, when driven into the brain substance, produce a penetrating brain injury. Occasionally, projectiles are so forceful that they exit the cranial vault in addition to entering it, producing a through-and-through injury. Primary damage is localized along the path of the penetrating object, and direct tissue disruption along the projectile tract results. A high-velocity bullet produces contusions at the site of entry, caused by bone striking the brain tissue on impact. Bone fragments are driven inward.

Stretch injury involves blood vessels and nerves that are damaged without direct contact due to the amount of tissue stretched secondary to shape, deformation, and striking velocity. Air compressed in front of a bullet exerts an explosive effect on entry, producing extreme distant tissue damage and an immediate primary increase in ICP; a cavity many times greater than the size of the bullet is produced because the brain tissue is propelled away from the tract. The cavity and pressure produce contrecoup injuries. The intracranial volume is increased directly by the projectile and the debris. The temporary cavity collapses back onto itself, leaving a smaller, permanent cavity. Intracranial bleeding occurs into the permanent cavity and may cause the cavity to expand. Edema in and around the injured brain tissue rapidly develops; edema and bleeding contribute markedly to ICP. This second rise in ICP to 60 to 100 mmHg may last 2 to 5 minutes. Because of acute ischemic damage to the tract, necrosis of tissue begins. Within hours after bullet-induced injury, tissue within 1 cm adjacent to the tract disintegrates. Demyelination of white matter affected by hemorrhage and edema occurs by the second day. Unconsciousness, flaccidity, or decerebrate patients (see Chapter 16) have a 94% mortality.

Diffuse Brain Injury. Diffuse brain injury (diffuse axonal injury [DAI]) results from a shaking effect (inertial effects of mechanical input to the head associated with high levels of acceleration and deceleration, effects of head motion). Rotational acceleration (twisting movement) is the primary mechanism of injury, producing strains and distortions within the brain (see Figure 17-1). The brain tissues experience shearing stresses set up by the rotational forces that operate when a freely moving head is struck because of the skull's motion from its attachment to the neck. Shearing, tearing, or stretching of nerve fibers with subsequent axonal damage results. Forces applied axially as a result of centrifugal acceleration of the head establish a gradient of injury severity from the hemispheres to the brain stem. The most severe axonal injuries are located more peripheral to the brain stem, thus accounting for the tremendous cognitive and affective impairments seen in survivors of traumatic brain injury from MVAs. The frontal and temporal axonal tracts are particularly vulnerable. Damage reduces the speed of informational processing and responding and disrupts attention.

The common pathologic substrate in diffuse brain injury is axonal damage (disruption). Pathophysiologically, at the time of injury, the damage can be seen only with an electron microscope and involves either numerous axons alone or axonal injury in conjunction with actual tissue tears. Areas where axons and small blood vessels are torn appear as small hemorrhages, located particularly in the corpus callosum and dorsolateral quadrant of the rostral brain stem at the superior cerebellar peduncle.

Oxygen free radicals contribute to secondary injury. Free radicals damage proteins and the phospholipid components of cells and organelle membranes. Membrane depolarization caused by the trauma permits nonselective opening of voltage-sensitive calcium channels, resulting in abnormal calcium accumulation in neurons and glial cells. These calcium shifts are associated with activation of lipolytic and proteolytic enzymes, protein kinases, protein phosphatases, dissolution of microtubules, and altered gene expression. Abnormal calcium influx occurs through activation of excitatory amino acid receptors. Widespread exotoxicity occurs after trauma, resulting in cell swelling, vacuolization, and death.[3]

Progressively increasing numbers of damaged axons are visible 12 hours to several days after the injury. Chromatolysis of the neurons involving eccentric relocation of the nucleus, swelling of the axon hillock, and redistribution of the rough endoplasmic reticulum in the cell body is evident. During this time the torn axons, which resemble dilated sausage links, also regress into round balls called *retraction balls*. These retraction balls are visible with light microscopy.

The number of retraction balls increases during the first week or two but begins to diminish in 2 to 3 weeks. Clusters of microglia appear in their place. Lastly, astrocytosis (gliosis, equivalent to scarring) occurs at the sites of axonal damage. Demyelination is seen particularly in the long axon tracts of the upper brain stem.

Severity of the diffuse injury correlates with the direction and velocity of rotation, that is, how much shearing force was applied to the brain stem. Figure 17-7 illustrates the spectrum of the diffuse injury as the magnitude increases. DAI is not associated with intracranial hypertension soon after injury, but acute brain swelling (increased intravascular blood within the brain, vasodilation, and increased cerebral blood volume) is seen often.

Several categories of diffuse brain injury exist: mild concussion, classic concussion, mild DAI, moderate DAI, and severe DAI. An organic component is present within each category, in contrast to the previous conceptualization that concussion had no structural injury component.

Mild concussion involves temporary axonal disturbances. Cerebral cortical dysfunction related to attentional and memory systems results, but consciousness is not lost. Three forms have been described:

Grade I: Confusion and disorientation accompanied by amnesia (momentary)

Grade II: Momentary confusion and retrograde amnesia that develops after 5 to 10 minutes (memory loss involves only events occurring several minutes before injury)

Grade III: Confusion and retrograde amnesia present from impact (also anterograde amnesia) (persists for several minutes)

Table 17-2 contains recommended guidelines from the American Academy of Neurology for return to play after sports-related concussive injuries.

Table 17-2	American Academy of Neurology Recommended Guidelines for Return to Play After Mild Head Injury
Grade of Concussion	**Time Until Return to Play**
Multiple grade I concussion	1 week
Grade II concussion	1 week
Multiple grade II concussion	2 weeks
Grade III, brief loss of consciousness (seconds)	1 week
Grade III, prolonged loss of consciousness (minutes)	2 weeks
Multiple grade III concussion	1 month or longer based on clinical decision of evaluating health care provider

From Quality Standards Subcommittee of the American Academy of Neurology: *Neurology* 48(3):581-585, 1997. Evans RW, Wilberger JE: Traumatic disorders. In Goetz CG, editor, *Textbook of clinical neurology*, ed 2, Philadelphia, 2003, Saunders.
*Only after being asymptomatic with normal neurological assessment at rest and with exercise.

As magnitude increases, progress from:

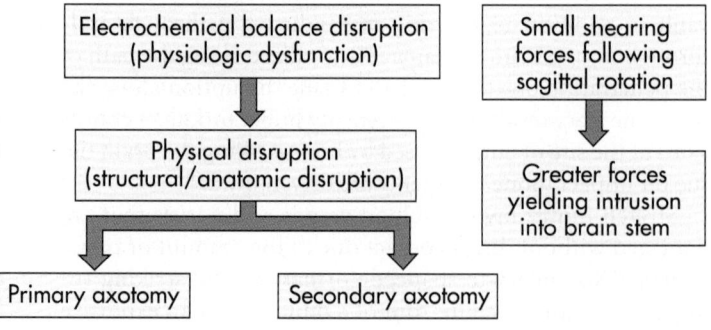

Figure 17-7 Spectrum of diffuse brain injury.

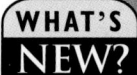

Sports-Related Concussion

Reviews of sports-related concussion suggests that athletes with three or more concussions had a slower recovery than those with only one previous concussion. In postsports-related concussion, postural stability returned to baseline levels in 3 to 5 days; cognitive function returned to baseline within 5 to 7 days; and symptoms (mostly headache) resolved within 7 days. Players with a previous history of concussions are more likely to have future concussive injuries in the same playing season and be associated with slower recovery of neurologic function.

Data from Guskiewicz KM et al *JAMA* 290(19):2549-2444, 2003; McCrea M: *JAMA* 290(19):2556-2563, 2003.

Classic cerebral concussion (*grade IV*) involves diffuse cerebral disconnection from the brain stem reticular activating system and is a phenomenon of physiologic, neurologic dysfunction without substantial anatomic disruption. Evidence of this disconnection is the immediate loss of consciousness, which lasts less than 6 hours. Retrograde and anterograde (posttraumatic) amnesia are present. This type of diffuse injury frequently is associated with focal pathologic findings, especially cerebral contusions that yield focal signs, not loss of consciousness. Two forms of classic cerebral contusion exist: uncomplicated classic cerebral concussion (without focal injury) and complicated classic cerebral concussion (accompanied by focal injury).

Diffuse axonal injury (DAI) produces prolonged traumatic coma lasting more than 6 hours because of axonal disruption. Three forms of DAI exist: mild, moderate, and severe. In **mild diffuse axonal injury (DAI),** posttraumatic coma lasts 6 to 24 hours. Death is uncommon, but residual cognitive, psychologic, and sensorimotor deficits may persist. Mild DAI is a relatively uncommon lesion, occurring in 8% of all severe head injuries and 19% of all cases of DAI.

In **moderate diffuse axonal injury (DAI),** widespread physiologic impairment exists throughout the cerebral cortex and diencephalon. Actual tearing of some axons in both hemispheres occurs. Basal skull fracture, a focal injury, commonly is associated with moderate DAI. Prolonged coma lasting more than 24 hours is present but prominent brain stem signs do not exist with moderate DAI. Recovery often is incomplete in 93% of those individuals who survive. Moderate DAI is the most common type of DAI and is found in 20% of severe head injuries and 45% of all cases of DAI.

Severe diffuse axonal injury (DAI), formerly called *primary brain stem injury* or *brain stem contusion,* involves severe mechanical disruption of many axons in both cerebral hemispheres and those extending to the diencephalon and brain stem. Severe DAI represents 16% of all severe head injuries and 36% of all cases of DAI. Sixty-four percent of persons survive. Thirty percent to 40% stay at low level or reduced states of consciousness for a prolonged period of time.

Genetics of Head Injury

Certain genes are up-regulated and others are down-regulated after head trauma. Researchers' attention has been focused predominantly on the apolipoprotein E gene and its various alleles. Certain alleles have been correlated with increased susceptibility to and severity of head injury. Other alleles have been associated with improved recovery after head injury. The clinical significance of these findings are not yet known.[3]

CLINICAL MANIFESTATIONS, EVALUATION, AND TREATMENT

Focal Brain Injury. The clinical manifestations of a contusion may include immediate loss of consciousness (generally accepted to last no longer than 5 minutes); loss of reflexes, which results in the individual falling to the ground; transient cessation of respiration; brief period of bradycardia; and decrease in blood pressure (lasting 30 seconds to a few minutes). A momentary increase in cerebrospinal fluid (CSF) pressure and ECG and electroencephalographic (EEG) changes have been demonstrated to occur on impact. Vital signs may stabilize to normal values in a few seconds. Reflexes return next, and the person begins to regain consciousness. Returning to being fully awake and alert takes variable periods, from minutes to days. Regaining a full level of consciousness may be extremely slow, and residual deficits may persist. In some persons, full level of consciousness never returns. Evaluation should include a complete history and physical examination. Skull and spinal radiographs are taken frequently, and a CT scan or MRI may be done. Large contusions and lacerations with hemorrhage may be excised surgically. Otherwise, treatment is directed at controlling ICP and managing symptoms.

Individuals with classic temporal extradural hematomas (i.e., over the temporal lobe) experience a period of loss of consciousness at the time of injury, followed by a lucid period that lasts from a few hours to a few days in one third of persons (if bleeding from a vein). As the hematoma accumulates, a headache of increasing severity, vomiting, drowsiness, confusion, seizure, and hemiparesis may develop. Level of consciousness may dwindle rapidly as the temporal lobe herniation begins. Clinical manifestations of temporal lobe herniation also include ipsilateral pupillary dilation and contralateral hemiparesis.

The diagnosis of an extradural hematoma usually is made with a CT scan or MRI. In some instances, diagnosis is made by history and clinical findings, because time for a CT scan or MRI is not available. The prognosis is usually good if intervention is initiated before bilateral dilation of the pupils. Surgical therapy is evacuation of the hematoma through burr holes, which is followed by ligation of the bleeding vessel or vessels. Extradural hematomas are almost always medical emergencies.

In acute, rapidly developing subdural hematomas, the expanding clots directly compress the brain, giving rise to the clinical manifestations. As the ICP rises, the bleeding veins are compressed and thus bleeding is self-limiting, although cerebral compression and displacement of brain tissue can cause temporal lobe herniation.

An acute subdural hematoma classically begins with headache, drowsiness, restlessness or agitation, slowed cognition, and confusion. These symptoms worsen over time and progress to loss of consciousness, respiratory pattern changes, and pupillary dilation (i.e., the symptoms of temporal lobe herniation). These manifestations are more pronounced than focal manifestations such as dysphasia, dyspraxia, or hemiparesis. Other clinical manifestations may include homonymous hemianopia (defective vision in either the right or the left field), disconjugate gaze, and gaze palsies.

Presenting manifestations of chronic subdural hematomas vary. Of persons affected, 80% have chronic headaches and tenderness over the hematoma on percussion. Most persons appear to have a progressive dementia accompanied by generalized rigidity (paratonia).

Whereas most acute and subacute subdural hematomas are treated with clot evacuation through a burr hole, chronic subdural hematomas (and some that are subacute) require a craniotomy to evacuate the gelatinous blood. The membrane around a chronic subdural hematoma is then dissected away from the dura mater and arachnoid membranes. A technique for percutaneous drainage for chronic subdural hematomas has proved successful.

A decreasing level of consciousness is associated with an intracerebral hematoma. Coma or a confusional state from other injuries, however, can make the cause of this increasing unresponsiveness difficult to detect. Contralateral hemiplegia also may occur. As the ICP rises, clinical manifestations of temporal lobe herniation may appear. In delayed intracerebral hematoma, the presentation is similar to that of a hypertensive brain hemorrhage: sudden, rapidly progressive decreased level of consciousness with pupillary dilation, breathing pattern changes, hemiplegia, and bilateral positive Babinski reflexes.

History and physical examination help to establish the diagnosis. CT scan, MRI, and cerebral angiographic visualization confirm the diagnosis. Evacuation of a singular intracerebral hematoma has only occasionally been helpful, mostly for subcortical white matter hematomas. Otherwise, treatment is directed at reducing the ICP and allowing the hematoma to reabsorb slowly.

With open-head injury, most persons lose consciousness. The depth of the coma and the length of the unresponsive state are related to the location of injury, extent of damage, and amount of bleeding. Open-head injury often requires surgery to débride the traumatized tissues to prevent infection and to remove blood clots to help reduce the ICP. ICP also is managed with steroids, dehydrating agents, osmotic diuretics, or a combination of these drugs. Broad-spectrum antibiotics are administered.

The diagnosis of a compound fracture is made through physical examination, skull radiographs, or both. The diagnosis of a basilar skull fracture is made on the basis of clinical findings. Skull radiographs often do not demonstrate the fracture, although intracranial air or air in the sinuses on radiograph, CT scan, or MRI is indirect evidence of a basilar skull fracture.

A compound linear fracture is débrided nonsurgically in cooperative adults and surgically in children and uncooperative adults. Cranioplasty with insertion of bone or an artificial graft may be necessary but often is delayed until antibiotics have been given. Antibiotics are administered after surgery.

Bed rest and close observation for meningitis and other complications are prescribed for a basilar skull fracture. Use of prophylactic antibiotics is controversial because studies have failed to demonstrate that they reduce the rate of infection.

Diffuse Brain Injury. DAI is associated with physical, cognitive, psychologic/behavioral, and social consequences. Spastic paralysis, peripheral nerve injury, swallowing disorders, dysarthria, visual and hearing impairments, and taste and smell deficits are some of the physical consequences. Common cognitive deficits include disorientation and confusion, short attention span, memory deficits, learning difficulties, dysphasia, poor judgment, and perceptual deficits. Behavioral disorders that emerge include agitation, impulsiveness, blunted affect, social withdrawal, and depression.

Mild concussion is characterized by an immediate onset of clinical manifestations at time of injury and the transitory nature of clinical manifestations. A momentary rise in CSF pressure and changes in ECG and EEG have been demonstrated to occur on impact in the laboratory. No loss of consciousness is experienced. The initial confusional state exists for a moment to several minutes. Amnesia for events preceding the trauma (retrograde amnesia) may be experienced. Anterograde amnesia may exist transiently. Persons may experience head pain and complain of nervousness and "not being oneself" for a short time up to a few days.

In classic cerebral concussion, loss of consciousness lasts as long as 6 hours and reflexes are lost, causing falls. Reflexes are regained as responsiveness returns. Transient cessation of respiration, brief periods of bradycardia, and a decrease in blood pressure lasting 30 seconds or less occur. Vital signs stabilize within a few seconds to within normal limits. Retrograde and anterograde amnesia exist. A confusional state persists for hours to days. The patient experiences head pain, nausea, and fatigue. Attentional and memory system impairments may persist for weeks to months and may include inability to concentrate and forgetfulness. Mood and affect changes may persist for weeks to months and may include nervousness, anxiety reactions, depression, irritability, fatigability, and insomnia.

Some of the effects of a concussion may persist for weeks or months, depending on the severity of the injury. Fifty percent of persons have a **postconcussive syndrome** that includes headache, cognitive impairments, psychologic and somatic complaints, and cranial nerve signs and symptoms.[3] Treatment entails reassurance and symptomatic relief. Close observation for 24 hours by a reliable individual is indicated so that immediate intervention can be obtained if delayed effects become severe.

In mild DAI, 30% of persons display decerebrate or decorticate posturing; they may experience prolonged periods of stupor or restlessness (see Figure 16-5).

In moderate DAI, the Glasgow Coma Scale (GCS) score is 4 to 8 initially and 6 to 8 by 24 hours. Thirty-five percent of victims have transitory decerebration or decortication. The person often remains unconscious for days or weeks and on awakening is confused. He or she experiences a long period of posttraumatic anterograde and retrograde amnesia and often has permanent deficits in memory, selective attention, vigilance, detection, working memory, data processing, vision or perception, and language, as well as mood and affect changes ranging from mild to severe.

Severe DAI is associated with brain stem signs that disappear in a few weeks. The person experiences immediate autonomic dysfunction that resolves in a few weeks. Increased ICP appears 4 to 6 days after injury. Pulmonary complications occur frequently, with profound sensorimotor and cognitive system deficits. Severely compromised coordinated movements and verbal and written communication, inability to learn and reason, and inability to modulate behavior also are found.

Diagnosis of focal and diffuse injury is determined by high-resolution CT scan and MRI. Medical management must include management of endocrine and metabolic derangement. Early and late seizures must be prevented and controlled. Iron from hemoglobin breakdown may increase intracellular calcium and free radical formation yielding excitotoxic damage, neuronal death, and glial scarring resulting in a seizure focus.[3] Storming (diencephalic seizures) must be diagnosed and treated. The role of fluid management has emerged as critically important in the care of individuals with severe brain injuries.

Spinal Cord Trauma

The number of persons with spinal cord injuries (SCIs) is between 30 and 40 million.[3] There are 10,000 persons injured each year. Eighty-one percent are men, mostly young adults. The average age is 33.4 years. Fifty percent of the injuries produce paraplegia and 50% produce quadriplegia.[4] MVAs account for 44% of SCIs.[5] Two-thirds of sports-related trauma are diving injuries. Violence accounts for 24% and falls 27%[3] of SCIs. Elderly persons, because of preexisting degenerative vertebral disorders, are particularly at risk for minor trauma resulting in serious spinal cord injury, especially from falls.

PATHOPHYSIOLOGY   Spinal cord injuries most commonly occur because of vertebral injuries, which are the result of acceleration, deceleration, or deformation forces most frequently applied at a distance. These forces injure the vertebral or neural tissues by compressing the tissues, pulling or exerting a traction (tension) on the tissues, or shearing tissues so that they slide into one another. These forces may be exerted on the vertebral and neural tissues by hyperextension, hyperflexion, vertical compression, or rotation of the spine (Figures 17-8 to 17-11). The bones, ligaments, and joints of the verte-

bral column may be damaged. The vertebral column may incur fracture and often compression of one or more elements, dislocation of its elements, or both fracture and dislocation. Vertebral injuries can be classified as (1) simple fracture, a single break usually affecting transverse or spinous processes; (2) compressed (wedged) vertebral fracture, in which a vertebral body is compressed anteriorly; (3) comminuted (burst) fracture, in which a vertebral body is shattered into several fragments; and (4) dislocation.

The vertebrae fracture readily with both direct and indirect trauma. When the supporting ligaments are torn, the vertebrae move out of alignment and dislocations occur. A horizontal force moves the vertebrae straight forward; if the individual is in a flexed position at the time of injury, the vertebrae are then in an angulated position. Flexion and extension injuries may result in dislocations. (Bone, ligament, and

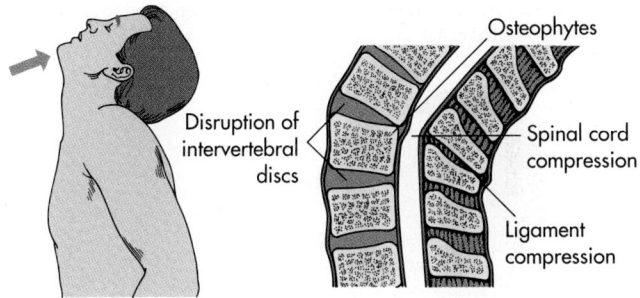

Figure 17-8 Hyperextension injuries of the spine. Hyperextension can result in fracture or nonfracture injuries with spinal cord damage.

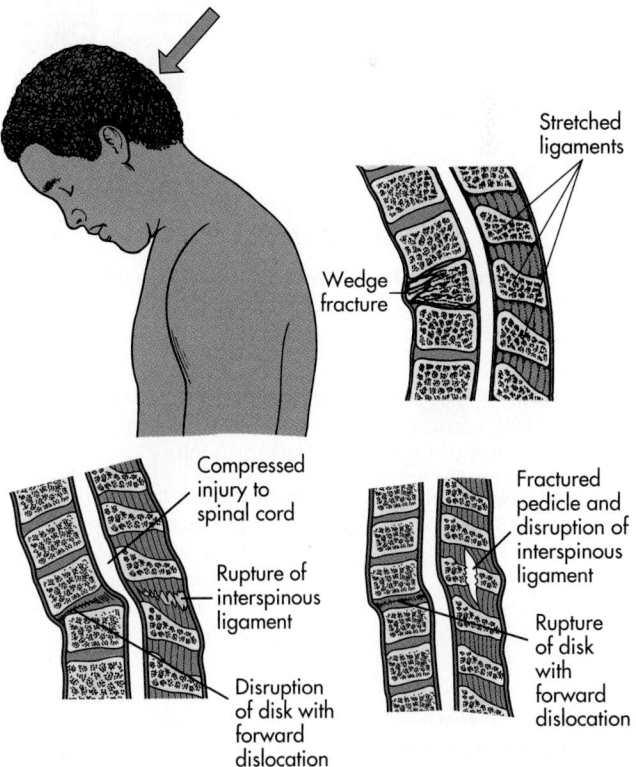

Figure 17-9 Hyperflexion injury of the spine. Hyperflexion produces translation (subluxation) of vertebrae, which compromises the central canal and compresses spinal cord parenchyma or vascular structures.

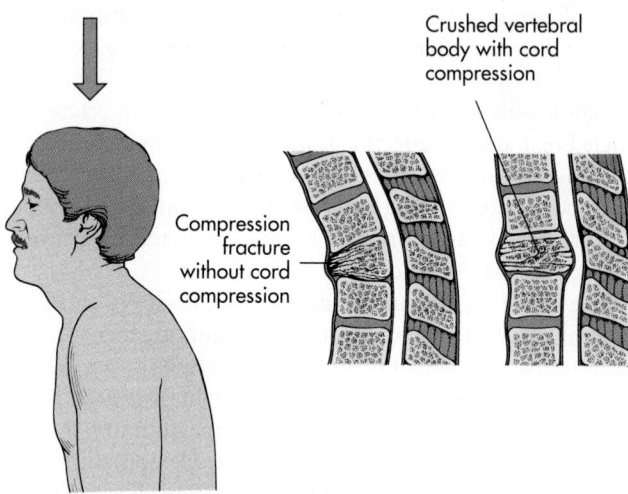

Figure 17-10 Axial compression injuries of the spine. In axial compression the spinal cord is contused directly by retropulsion of bone or disk material into the spinal canal.

Compression fracture without cord compression

Crushed vertebral body with cord compression

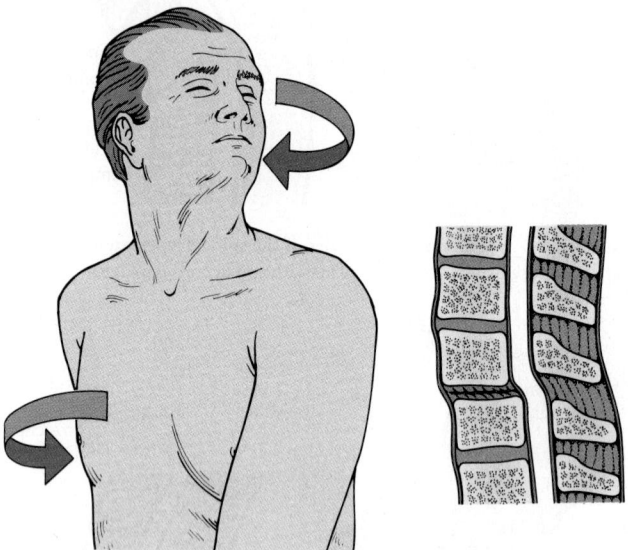

Figure 17-11 Flexion-rotation injuries of the spine.

joint injuries are presented in Table 17-3.) Vertebral injuries occur mostly at vertebrae C1 to C2 (cervical), C4 to C7, and T1 (thoracic) to L2 (lumbar) (see Figure 14-9). These are the most mobile portions of the vertebral column. The cord occupies most of the vertebral canal in the cervical and lumbar regions. The size makes the cord in these areas more easily injured. (The primary injuries to the cord are summarized in Table 17-4.) Noncontiguous vertebral injuries are not uncommon. Further, primary injury occurs if an injured spine is not adequately immobilized. A comparison of adult to child spine and spinal cord injuries are contained in Table 17-5.

The pathophysiologic cascade of secondary spinal cord injury begins within a few minutes after injury. Microscopic hemorrhages appear in the central gray matter and pia arachnoid that increase in size within 2 hours. Edema in the white matter occurs, impairing the microcirculation of the cord. Within 4 hours, numerous swollen axis cylinders develop. Localized hemorrhaging and edema therefore are followed by reduced vascular perfusion and development of ischemic areas. Oxygen tension in the tissue at the injury site is decreased. The microscopic hemorrhages and edema are maximal at the level of injury and for two cord segments above and below it.

Cellular and subcellular alterations and tissue necrosis occur. Electron microscopy has allowed cellular pathogenesis to be described. By 5 minutes after injury, venules of the gray matter are congested and distended by erythrocytes. In 15 to 30 minutes, small hemorrhages occur with extravasation of erythrocytes into perivascular spaces of postcapillary and muscular venules. Within 4 hours disruption of myelin, axonal degeneration, and ischemic endothelial injury occur.

Chemical and metabolic changes in spinal cord tissues include release of toxic excitatory amino acids, accumulation of endogenous opiates, lipid hydrolysis with production of active metabolites, and local free radical release. These changes may produce further ischemia, vascular damage, and necrosis of tissues (autodestruction). Necrosis consumes 40% of cross-sectional cord within 4 hours of trauma and 70% within 24 hours (Figure 17-12). Cord swelling increases the

Table 17-3	Mechanisms of Vertebral Injury		
Mechanisms of Injury	**Vertebral Injury**	**Forces of Injury**	**Location of Injury**
Hyperextension	Fracture and dislocation of posterior elements such as spinous processes, transverse processes, laminae, pedicles, or posterior ligaments	Results from forces of acceleration-deceleration and the sudden reduction in the anteroposterior diameter of the spinal cord	Cervical area
Hyperflexion	Fracture or dislocation of the vertebral bodies, disks, or ligaments	Results from sudden and excessive force that propels the neck forward or causes an exaggerated lateral movement of the neck to one side	Cervical area
Vertical compression (axonal loading)	Shattering fractures	Results from a force applied along an axis from the top of the cranium through the vertebral bodies	T12 to L2
Rotational forces (flexion-rotation)	Ruptures support ligaments in addition to producing fractures	Adds shearing force to acceleration—acceleration forces	Cervical area

Table 17-4	Spinal Cord Injuries
Injury	**Description**
Cord concussion	Results in a temporary disruption of cord-mediated functions
Cord contusion	Bruising of the neural tissue causing swelling and temporary loss of cord-mediated functions
Cord compression	Pressure on the cord causing ischemia to tissues; must be relieved (decompressed) to prevent permanent damage to the spinal cord
Laceration	Tearing of the neural tissues of the spinal cord; may be reversible if only slight damage sustained by the neural tissues; may result in permanent loss of cord-mediated functions if spinal tracts are disrupted
Transection	Severing of the spinal cord, causing permanent loss of function
Complete	All tracts in the spinal cord completely disrupted; all cord-mediated functions below the transection are completely and permanently lost
Incomplete	Some tracts in the spinal cord remain intact, together with functions mediated by these tracts; has the potential for recovery although function is temporarily lost
Preserved sensation only	Some demonstrable sensation below the level of injury
Preserved motor nonfunctional	Preserved motor function without useful purpose; sensory function may or may not be preserved
Preserved motor functional	Preserved voluntary motor function that is functionally useful
Hemorrhage	Bleeding into the neural tissue because of blood vessel damage; usually no major loss of function
Damage or obstruction of spinal blood supply	Causes local ischemia

Table 17-5	Comparison of Spine and Spinal Cord Injuries in Adults and Children	
Characteristics	**Adult**	**Pediatric**
Mechanism of Injury	Motor vehicle accidents	Pediatrian/falls
Level of Injury		
C1-C3	1% to 2%	60%
C3-C7	85%	30% to 40%
Thoracolumbar	10% to 15%	5%
Type of Injury		
Fracture-dislocation	>70%	25%
Subluxation	<20%	50%
SCIWORA	Rare	Up to 50%
Delayed Neurological Deficits	Rare	Up to 50%

SCIWORA, Spinal cord injury without radiological abnormalities.
From Evans RW, Wilberger JE: Traumatic disorders. In Goetz CG, editor, *Textbook of neurology,* Philadelphia, 2003, Saunders.

individual's degree of dysfunction, so that distinguishing the functions to be lost permanently from those that are impaired just temporarily becomes difficult. In the cervical region, cord swelling may be life threatening because of the possibility of resulting impairment of the diaphragm function (phrenic nerves exit C3 to C5) and vegetative functions mediated by the medulla oblongata. Within the first few days of injury, progressive axonal changes occur and necrotic zones develop. Progressive cavitation and coagulation necrosis at the site of injury are termed *posttraumatic infarction.*

Circulation in the white matter tracts of the spinal cord returns to normal in about 24 hours, but gray matter circulation remains altered. Phagocytes appear 36 to 48 hours after injury. There are proliferation of microglia and changes in astrocytes. Red cells then begin to disintegrate, and resorption of hemorrhages begins. Degenerating axons are engulfed by macrophages in the first 10 days after injury. A cyst with fluid forms. The traumatized cord is replaced by acellular collagenous tissue (a scar), usually in 3 to 4 weeks. Meninges thicken as part of the scarring process.

CLINICAL MANIFESTATIONS Normal activity of the spinal cord cells at and below the level of injury ceases because of loss of the continuous tonic discharge from the brain or brain stem and inhibition of suprasegmental impulses immediately after cord injury, thus causing spinal shock. *Spinal shock* is characterized by a complete loss of reflex function in all segments below the level of the lesion. This condition involves all skeletal muscles, bladder, bowel, sexual function, and autonomic control. Severe impairment below the level of the lesion is obvious; it includes paralysis and flaccidity in muscles, absence of sensation, loss of bladder and rectal control, transient drop in blood pressure, and poor venous circulation. The condition also results in disturbed thermal control because the sympathetic nervous system is damaged. This damage causes faulty control of sweating and radiation through capillary dilation. The hypothalamus cannot regulate body heat through vasoconstriction and increased metabolism; therefore the individual assumes the temperature of the air.

Spinal shock may last for 7 to 20 days after onset; it may persist for as short a time as a few days or as long as 3 months. Indications that spinal shock is terminating include the reappearance of reflex activity, hyperreflexia, spasticity, and reflex emptying of the bladder. In persons with cervical or upper thoracic cord injury, a form of distributive shock, called *neurogenic shock,* may be seen in addition to spinal shock, as a result of the loss of sympathetic outflow causing hypotension.

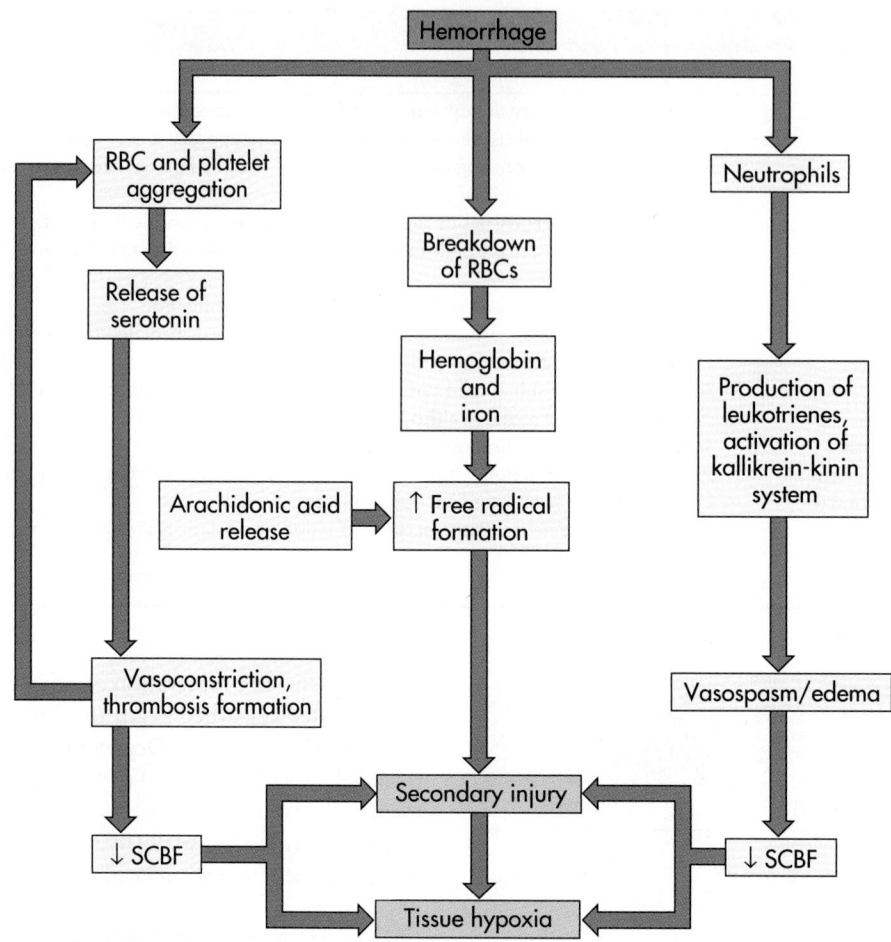

Figure 17-12 Cascade of metabolic and cellular events that leads to spinal cord ischemia and hypoxia of secondary injury. *RBC,* Red blood cells; *SCBF,* spinal cord blood flow. (Redrawn from Marciano FF et al: *BNI Quarterly* 11(2):6, 1995.)

Loss of motor and sensory function depends on the level of injury. All motor, sensory, reflex, and autonomic functions cease below any transected area and also may cease below concussive, contused, compressed, or ischemic areas (Table 17-6). Paralysis of the lower half of the body with both legs involved is termed *paraplegia.* Paralysis involving all four extremities is termed *quadriplegia* (tetraplegia). In complete quadriplegia the level of injury is above C6, and all upper extremity function is lost. In incomplete quadriplegia, function at or above C6 is preserved, leaving the shoulder, upper arm, and some forearm muscle control intact. With acceleration injuries the greatest stress point is C4-5. With a deceleration force the greatest stress point is at C5-6.

Return of spinal neuron excitability occurs slowly. Depending on the degree of damage, either of the following can occur: (1) motor, sensory, reflex, and autonomic functions return to normal; or (2) autonomic neural activity in the isolated segment develops. The sequence of hyperactivity phases, which vary in length, may include (1) minimal reflex activity, (2) flexor spasms, (3) alternation between flexor and extensor spasms, and (4) predominant extensor spasms.

The initial clinical manifestations associated with acute spinal cord injury are rapid loss of (1) voluntary movement in body parts below the level of injury, (2) sensations in the lower extremities and possibly lower trunk (depending on the level of injury), and (3) spinal and autonomic reflexes below the level of injury. The duration of this areflexic state is highly variable. In most persons, reflex activity returns in 1 to 2 weeks.

Gradually reflexes return and become increasingly easier to elicit. A pattern of flexion reflexes emerges, first involving the toes and later the feet and legs. Reflex voiding and bowel elimination appear. Flexor spasms accompanied by profuse sweating, piloerection, and automatic bladder emptying (together called a **mass reflex**) may develop. The ability to sweat when overheated may be disrupted, and extensor spasms may develop, usually after full development of flexor spasms. Sometimes after several months, episodes of autonomic hyperreflexia are elicited.

Autonomic hyperreflexia (dysreflexia) is a syndrome that may occur at any time after spinal shock resolves. The syndrome is associated with a massive, uncompensated cardiovascular response to stimulation of the sympathetic nervous system (Figure 17-13). The condition is life threatening and requires immediate treatment. Individuals most likely to be affected have lesions at the T6 level or above. Autonomic hy-

Table 17-6   Clinical Manifestations of Spinal Cord Injury

Stage	Manifestations
Spinal Shock Stage	

Complete spinal cord transection	Loss of motor function
	  1. Quadriplegia with injuries of cervical spinal cord
	  2. Paraplegia with injuries of thoracic spinal cord
	Muscle flaccidity
	Loss of all reflexes below level of injury
	Loss of pain, temperature, touch, pressure, and proprioception below level of injury
	Pain at site of injury caused by a zone of hyperesthesia above the injury
	Atonic bladder and bowel
	Paralytic ileus with distention
	Loss of vasomotor tone in lower body parts; low and unstable blood pressure
	Loss of perspiration below level of injury
	Loss or extreme depression of genital reflexes such as penile erection and bulbocavernous reflex
	Dry and pale skin, possible ulceration over bony prominences
	Respiratory impairment

Partial spinal cord transection	Asymmetric flaccid motor paralysis below level of injury
	Asymmetric reflex loss
	Preservation of some sensation below level of injury
	Vasomotor instability less severe than with complete cord transection
	Bowel and bladder impairment less severe than that seen with complete cord transection
	Preservation of ability to perspire in some portions of the body below level of injury
	Brown-Séquard syndrome (associated with penetrating injuries, hyperextension and flexion, locked facets, and compression fractures)
	  1. Ipsilateral paralysis or paresis below level of injury
	  2. Ipsilateral loss of touch, pressure, vibration, and position sense below level of injury
	  3. Contralateral loss of pain and temperature sensations below level of injury
	Central cervical cord syndrome (acute cord compression between bony bars or spurs anteriorly and thickened ligamentum flabvum posteriorly associated with hyperextension)
	  1. Motor deficits in upper extremities, especially hands, more dense than in lower extremities
	  2. Varying degrees of bladder dysfunction
	Burning hand syndrome (variant of central cord syndrome, half the time an underlying spine fracture/dislocation is present)
	  1. Severe burning parathesias and dysesthesias in the hand and/or feet
	Anterior cord syndrome (compromise of anterior spinal artery by occlusion or pressure effect of disk)
	  1. Loss of motor function below level of injury
	  2. Loss of pain and temperature sensations below level of injury
	  3. Touch, pressure, position, and vibration senses intact
	Posterior cord syndrome (associated with hyperextension injuries with fractures of vertebral arch)
	  1. Impaired light touch and proprioception
	Conus medullaris syndrome (compression injury at T12 from disk herniation or burst fracture of body of T12)
	  1. Flaccid paralysis of legs
	  2. Flaccid paralysis of anal sphincter
	  3. Variable sensory deficits
	Cauda equine syndrome (compression of nerve roots below L1 caused by fracture and dislocation of spine or large posteriocentral intervertebral disk herniation)
	  1. Lower extremity motor deficits
	  2. Variable sensorimotor dysfunction
	  3. Variable reflex dysfunction
	  4. Variable bladder, bowel, and sexual dysfunction
	Syndrome of neuropraxia (seen postathletic injury, associated with congenital spinal stenosis)
	  1. Dramatic but transiety neurologic deficits including quadriplegia
	Horner syndrome (injury to preganglionic sympathetic trunk or postganglionic sympathetic neurons of superior cervical ganglion)
	  1. Ipsilateral pupil smaller than contralateral pupil
	  2. Sunken ipsilateral eyeball
	  3. Ptosis of affected eyeball
	  4. Lack of perspiration on ipsilateral side of face

Continued

Table 17-6	Clinical Manifestations of Spinal Cord Injury—cont'd
Stage	**Manifestations**
Heightened Reflex Activity Stage	Emergence of Babinski reflexes, possibly progressing to a triple reflex; possible development of still later flexor spasms
	Reappearance of ankle and knee reflexes, which become hyperactive
	Contraction of reflex detrusor muscle, leading to urinary incontinence
	Appearance of reflex defecation
	Mass reflex with flexion spasms, profuse sweating, piloerection, and bladder and occasional bowel emptying may be evoked by an automonic stimulation of skin or from a full bladder
	Episodes of hypertension
	Defective heat-induced sweating
	Eventual development of extensor reflexes, first in muscles of hip and thigh, later in leg
	Possible paresthesias below level of transaction: dull, burning pain in lower back, abdomen, buttocks, and perineum

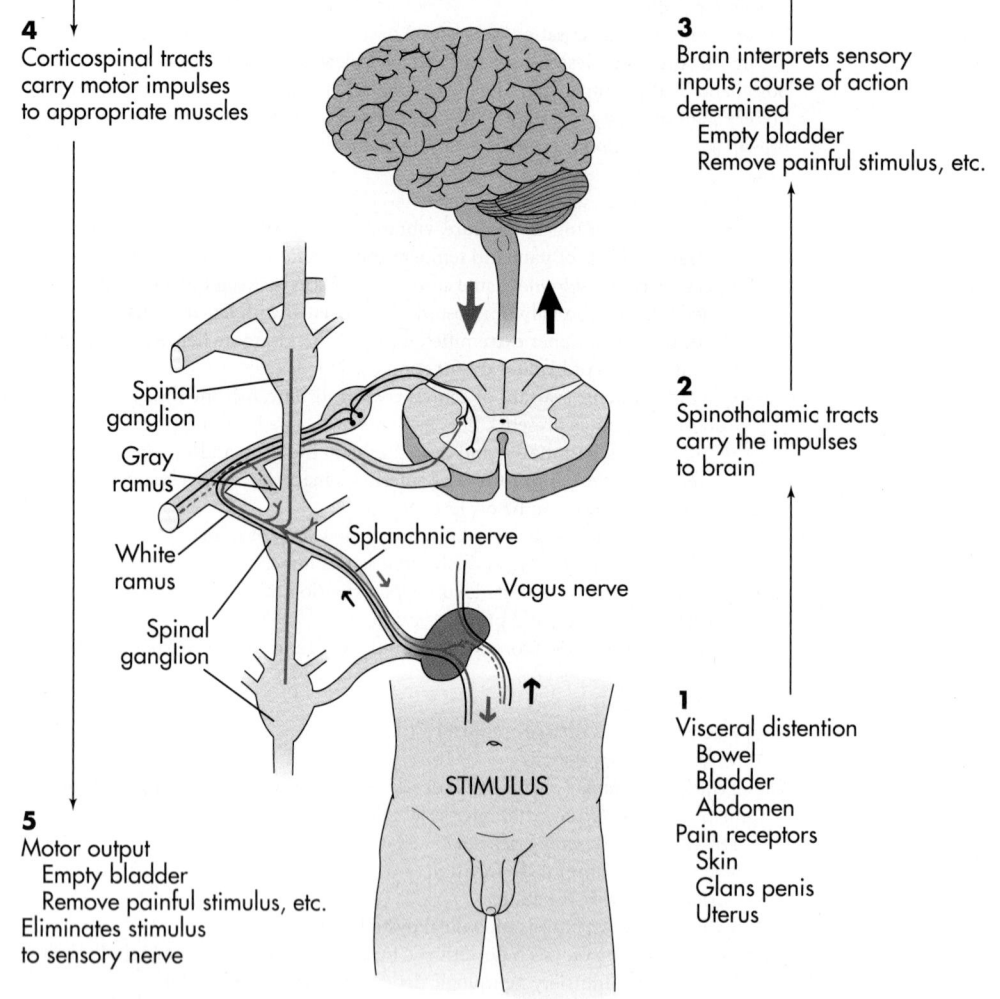

Figure 17-13 Autonomic hyperreflexia. **A,** Normal response pathway. (Modified from Rudy EB: *Advanced neurological and neurosurgical nursing,* St Louis, 1984, Mosby.)

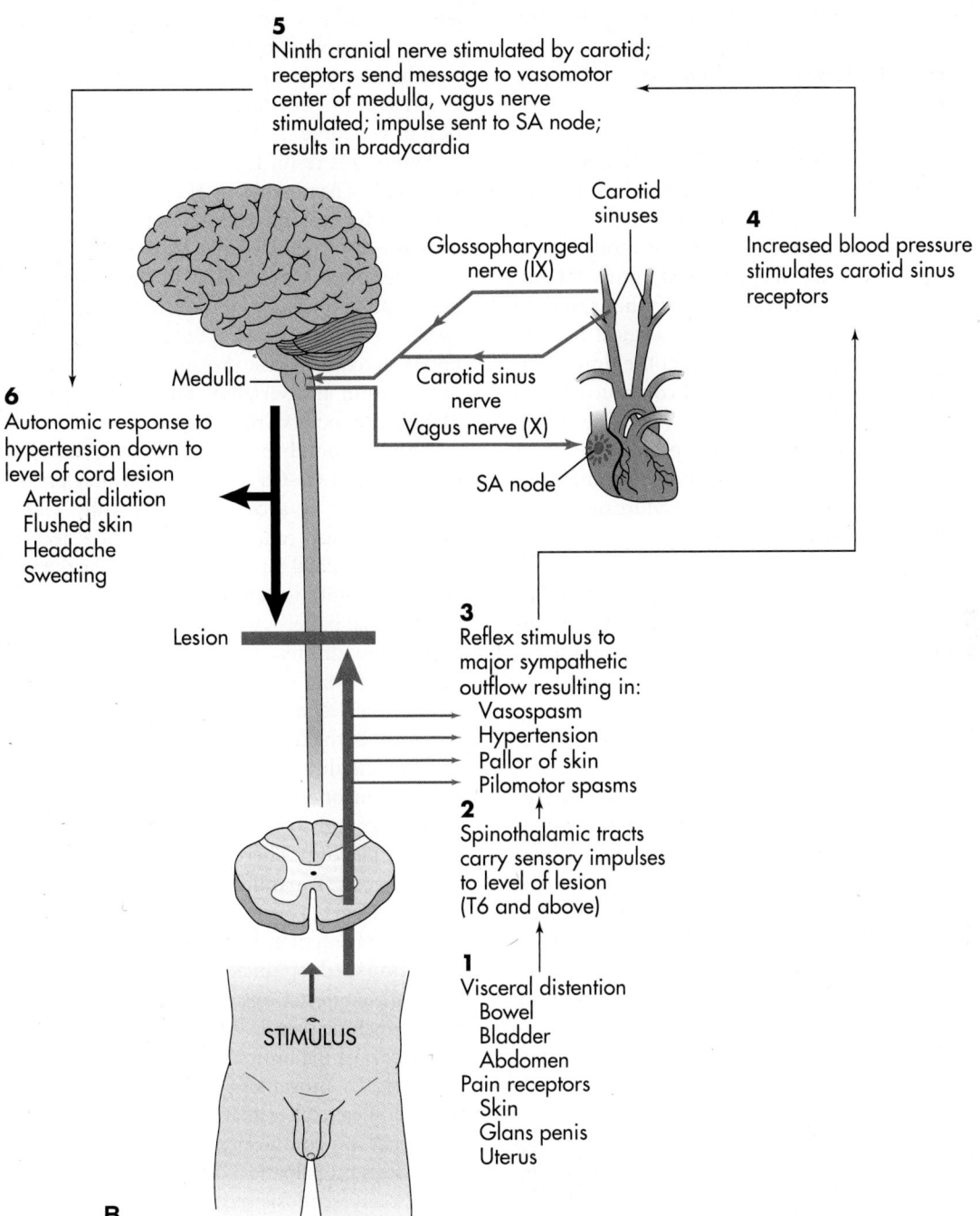

5
Ninth cranial nerve stimulated by carotid; receptors send message to vasomotor center of medulla, vagus nerve stimulated; impulse sent to SA node; results in bradycardia

Carotid sinuses

Glossopharyngeal nerve (IX)

4
Increased blood pressure stimulates carotid sinus receptors

Medulla

Carotid sinus nerve
Vagus nerve (X)

SA node

6
Autonomic response to hypertension down to level of cord lesion
  Arterial dilation
  Flushed skin
  Headache
  Sweating

Lesion

3
Reflex stimulus to major sympathetic outflow resulting in:
  Vasospasm
  Hypertension
  Pallor of skin
  Pilomotor spasms

2
Spinothalamic tracts carry sensory impulses to level of lesion (T6 and above)

STIMULUS

1
Visceral distention
  Bowel
  Bladder
  Abdomen
Pain receptors
  Skin
  Glans penis
  Uterus

B

Figure 17-13, cont'd Autonomic hyperreflexia. **B,** Autonomic dysreflexia pathway. (Modified from Rudy EB: *Advanced neurological and neurosurgical nursing,* St Louis, 1984, Mosby.)

perreflexia is characterized by paroxysmal hypertension (up to 300 mm Hg systolic), a pounding headache, blurred vision, sweating above the level of the lesion with flushing of the skin, nasal congestion, nausea, piloerection caused by pilomotor spasm, and bradycardia (30 to 40 beats/min). The symptoms may develop singly or in combination (syndrome) and often are associated with a distended bladder or rectum.

Pathophysiology of hyperreflexia involves the stimulation of sensory receptors below the level of the cord lesion. The in-

tact autonomic nervous system reflexively responds with an arteriolar spasm that increases blood pressure. Baroreceptors in the cerebral vessels, the carotid sinus, and the aorta sense the hypertension and stimulate the parasympathetic system. The heart rate decreases, but the visceral and peripheral vessels do not dilate because efferent impulses cannot pass through the cord.

The most common precipitating cause is a distended bladder or rectum, but any sensory stimulation can elicit autonomic hyperreflexia. Stimulation of the skin or stimulation of the pain receptors may cause autonomic hyperreflexia. Emptying of the bladder or bowel usually relieves the syndrome, and this may be facilitated by drugs, such as phenoxybenzamine.

EVALUATION AND TREATMENT   Diagnosis of spinal cord injury is made on the basis of physical, radiologic, and myelographic examination; CT scan; and MRI. For a suspected or confirmed vertebral fracture or dislocation, regardless of the presence or absence of spinal cord injury, the immediate intervention is immobilization of the spine to prevent further injury. Decompression and surgical fixation may be necessary. Corticosteroids are given at the time of injury to decrease secondary cord injury and continued for 24 to 48 hours, depending on time of initiation following injury. The only other agent continuing to show promise is GM-1 ganglioside (Sygen).[3] Nutrition, lung function, skin integrity, and bladder and bowel management must be addressed. Plans for rehabilitation require early consideration.

In cases of autonomic hyperreflexia, intervention must be prompt because cerebrovascular accident (CVA) is possible. The head of the bed should be elevated, and the stimulus should be found and removed. Medications may be used if these measures do not effectively reduce blood pressure.

Degenerative Disorders of the Spine
Degenerative Disk Disease

Degenerative changes occur in the vertebral disks. **Degenerative disk disease (DDD)** is a common finding in individuals 30 years of age and older. Only a small percentage of those persons have any functional incapacity because of pain. The causes of DDD include biochemical and biomechanical alterations of the tissue of the intervertebral disk. Fibrocartilage replaces the gelatinous mucoid material of the nucleus pulposus as the disk changes with age. There may be splits in the annulus fibrosis, permitting herniation of elements of nucleus pulposus. There may be shrinkage of the nucleus pulpo-

sus that produces prolapse or folding of the annulus with secondary osteophyte formation at the margins of the adjacent vertebral body. The pathologic findings in DDD include disk protrusion, spondylolysis, and/or subluxation and degeneration of vertebrae (spondylolisthesis) and spinal stenosis.

Symptoms result from either (1) disk or annulus protrusion or (2) narrowing of the spinal canal or intervertebral foramen by osteophytes. A congenital narrow canal or congenitally short pedicles may be present.

Posterior disk protrusion in the cervical and thoracic regions lead to cord compression, and cauda equine compression results in the lumbar area. Both situations are called *myelopathy*. Posterolateral disk protrusions, with or without a contribution from the vertebral body or apophyseal joint osteophytes, lead to nerve root compression (called *radiculopathy*).

Cervical spondylolysis is a DDD in the cervical spine predominately at C5-C6 and C6-C7. It may present as a cervical radiculopathy or a cervical myelopathy. Clinical manifestations of cervical radiculopathy include neck pain as well as pain in the medial aspects of the scapula, the shoulder, or arm. Sensory symptoms, such as tingling or numbness, follow a dermatomal pattern; weakness follows the pattern of innervation of the affected nerve root and occipital or suboccipital headache (some authorities refute this). Clinical manifestations of cervical myelopathy include difficulty walking, altered sensation in the feet, and sphincter disturbances (occurs late).

Thoracic disk disease is rarely symptomatic, but prolapse is found in one-seventh of scans. Lumbosacral disk disease (lumbar spondylosis) involves the lower two lumbar disks in 90% of persons. There may be (1) lateral disk protrusion (10% of cases) manifesting as pain referred to the anterior thigh and leg; (2) posterolateral disk protrusion; or (3) central disk protrusion manifesting with pain, lower extremity weakness, impaired sphincter function, and saddle anesthesia. Clinical manifestations of posterolateral protrusions (Figure 17-14) include pain in back, the sacroiliac joint, and the medial aspect of the buttock and upper thigh; radicular pain exacerbated by movement and straining (medial calf suggests L5, lateral calf suggests S1 root compression); sensory symptoms that are common and segmental in distribution; focal tenderness on palpation of the back; limited range of motion in back and scoliosis secondary to paravertebral spasms; restricted straight leg raising (root at or below L5); positive femoral stretch test (roots of L2, L3, or L4); and focal signs that are determined by root affected.

Spondylolysis

Spondylolysis is a degenerative process of the vertebral column and associated soft tissue. It is characterized by a structural defect of the spine involving the lamina or neural arch of the vertebra. The most common site affected is the lumbar spine. This defect occurs in the portion of the lamina between the superior and inferior articular facets called the *pars interarticularis*. Mechanical pressure may cause a forward displacement of the deficient vertebra called *spondylolisthesis*.

Heredity plays a significant role, and spondylolysis is associated with an increased incidence of other congenital spinal

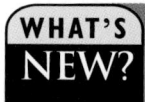

WHAT'S NEW?   Stem Cells Repair Rat Spinal Cord Damage

Advances are steadily being made in the regeneration of nerve cells in spinal cord injury. Both neuroprotective and neuro-restorative interventions for a growth permitting environment to establish reconnections between the brain and the motor and sensory neurons below the spinal lesion are being developed in animal models. Neural and embryonic stem cells, grafting of tissues, pharmacological interventions, and physiotherapy are being applied to promote nerve regeneration. The regeneration of nerve tissue is complex and involves multiple stages. Combinations of treatments will be required to achieve levels of nerve function that include modulation of pain and recovery of bowel and bladder function.

Data from Dobkin BH, Havton LA:, *Annu Rev Med* 55:255-82, 2004; McDonald JW et al: *J Neurotrauma* 21(4):383-393, 2004; Rosenzweig ES, McDonald JW: *Curr Opin Neurol* 17(2):121-131, 2004.

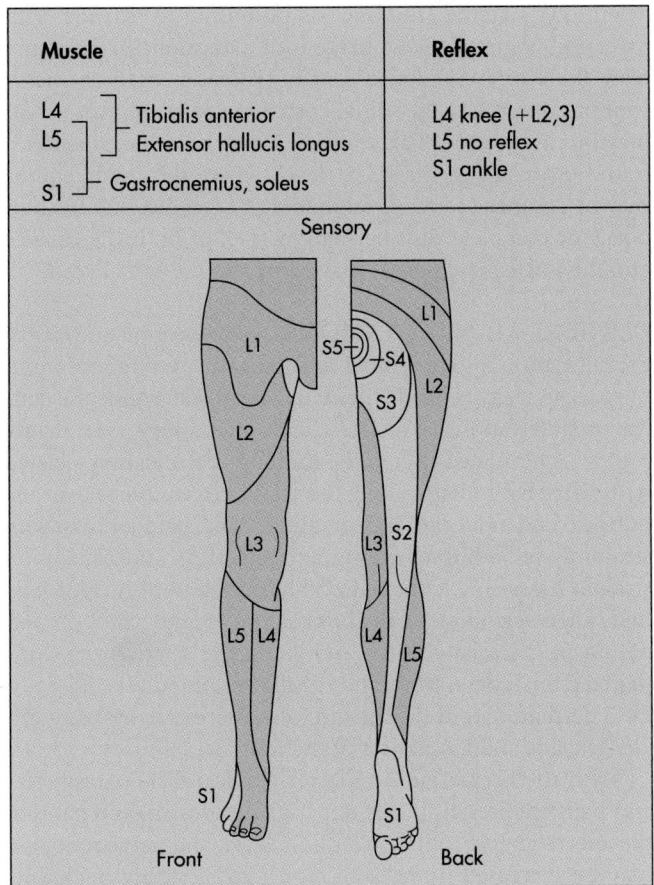

Muscle		Reflex
L4 — Tibialis anterior		L4 knee (+L2,3)
L5 — Extensor hallucis longus		L5 no reflex
S1 — Gastrocnemius, soleus		S1 ankle

Figure 17-14 Motor, sensory, and reflex changes in lumbosacral root disorders. (From Perkin dg: *Mosby's color atlas and text of neurology,* London, 1998, Mosby-Wolfe.)

defects. As a result of torsional and rotational stress, "microfractures" occur at the affected site and eventually cause dissolution of the pars interarticularis.

Spondylolisthesis

Spondylolisthesis is a stress factor allowing a vertebra to slide forward in relation to the vertebra below, commonly occurring at L5-S1. Spondylolisthesis is graded from 1 to 4 on the basis of the percentage of slip that has occurred. Individuals with grade 3 or 4 are considered for operative decompression or stabilization or both. Grades 1 and 2 usually are managed symptomatically and with nonsurgical methods.

Spinal Stenosis

In **spinal stenosis** the spinal canal may be congenitally narrowed or narrowed by a bulging annulus, a facet hypertrophy, or a thick/ossified posterior longitudinal ligament entrapping a single nerve involving many roots. It is classified as acquired (more common) or developmental (such as occurs in achondroplastic dwarfs). Surgical decompression is recommended for those with long-term symptoms and those who remain unresponsive to medical management.

Low Back Pain

Low back pain affects the area between the lower rib cage and gluteal muscles and often radiates into the thighs. About 1%

of individuals with acute low back pain have sciatica, or pain in the distribution of a lumbar nerve root. Sciatica often is accompanied by neurosensory and motor deficits, such as weakness.

The incidence of, or percentage of population affected with, low back pain at some point in life is 60% to 80%, and the annual incidence is 5%. Men and women are affected equally; however, women report low back symptoms more often after the age of 60 years.

PATHOGENESIS Most cases of low back pain are idiopathic, and clinicians are unable to provide a precise diagnosis for most individuals with this disorder. The local processes involved in low back pain range from tension caused by tumors or disk prolapse, bursitis, synovitis, rising venous and tissue pressure (found in degenerative joint disease), abnormal bone pressures, problems with spinal mobility, inflammation caused by infection (as in osteomyelitis), bony fractures, or ligamentous sprains to pain referred from viscera or the posterior peritoneum. General processes resulting in low back pain include bone diseases, such as osteoporosis or osteomalacia, and hyperparathyroidism.

Several risk factors have been identified in the pathogenesis of low back pain. They include involvement caused by occupations that require repetitious lifting in the forward bent-and-twisted position, exposure to vibrations caused by vehicles or industrial machinery, and perhaps cigarette smoking. Osteoporosis increases the risk of spinal compression fractures and may be the reason elderly women report more symptoms than men. Genetic predispositions for low back pain include isthmic spondylolisthesis (vertebra slides forward or slips in relation to a vertebra below), spinal osteochondrosis, and spinal stenosis associated with achondroplasia. Variations in posture, such as lordosis and scoliosis of less than 60 degrees, do not appear to increase the risk of low back pain or sciatica. Differences in weight, height, and leg length are controversial as risk factors.

Anatomically, low back pain must come from innervated structures, but deep pain is widely referred and varies from person to person. The nucleus pulposus has no intrinsic innervation; however, when extruded or herniated through a prolapsed disk, it irritates the dural membranes and is responsible for pain referred to the segmental area (see Figure 17-14). The interspinous bursae can be a source of low back pain between L3, L4, L5, and S1 but also may affect L1, L2, and L3 spinous processes, depending on the closeness of the adjacent pair of spines. The anterior and posterior longitudinal ligaments of the spine and the interspinous and supraspinous ligaments are abundantly supplied with pain receptors, as is the ligamentum flavum. All of these ligaments are vulnerable to traumatic tears (sprains) and fracture. The role of muscle injury in the production of low back pain remains uncertain, even though sprains and strains are the most common diagnoses. The muscle spasms that often are produced during sieges of low back pain are thought to be produced by as yet unknown sensory or motor-reflex pathways. The most commonly encountered causes of low back pain include lumbar disk herniation, degenerative disk disease, spondylolysis, spondylolisthesis, and spinal stenosis. (For a discussion of disk herniation and rupture, see below.)

EVALUATION AND TREATMENT Diagnosis of low back injury is made on the basis of physical, electromyelographic (EMG), epidurographic, diskographic, and MRI examination; CT examination with or without myelography; and nerve conduction studies. Most individuals with acute low back pain benefit from a nonspecific short-term treatment regimen including bed rest, analgesic medications, exercises, physical therapy, and education. Surgical treatments may be indicated if individuals do not respond to medical management. Surgical treatments include diskectomy and spinal fusions. Individuals with chronic low back pain can be treated with anti-inflammatory and muscle relaxant medications and exercise programs. Aerobic exercises are a popular treatment and seem to be more effective than traction or low back exercises. Spinal surgery has a limited role in curing chronic low back pain.

Herniated Intervertebral Disk

Herniation of an intervertebral disk is a protrusion of part of the nucleus pulposus (like stepping on an ice cream sandwich) through a tear in the posterior rim of the annulus fibrosus (the fibrous capsule enclosing the gelatinous center of the disk) (Figure 17-15). Rupture of an intervertebral disk usually is caused by trauma or degenerative disk disease or both. Lifting with the trunk flexed and sudden straining when the back is in an unstable position are the most common causes. Men are more affected than women, with the highest incidence among those 30 to 60 years of age. Most commonly affected are the lumbosacral disks, that is, L5-S1 and L4-5. Disk herniation occasionally occurs in the cervical area, usually at C5-6 and C6-7. Herniations at the thoracic level are extremely rare. The injury may have an immediate onset or an onset within a few hours, or the manifestations of injury may take months to years to develop.

PATHOPHYSIOLOGY   In a herniated disk the ligament and posterior capsule of the disk usually are torn, allowing the

gelatinous material (the nucleus pulposus) to extrude. This extrusion compresses the nerve root. Occasionally the injury tears the entire disk loose, and it protrudes onto the nerve root or compresses the spinal cord. One or more nerve roots may be compressed. This multiple nerve root compression is found especially at the L5-S1 level, where the cauda equina may be compressed. Large amounts of extruded nucleus pulposus or complete disk herniation (i.e., of both the capsule and the nucleus pulposus) may compress the spinal cord.

CLINICAL MANIFESTATIONS   The location and size of the herniation into the spinal canal, together with the amount of space that exists inside the spinal canal, determine the clinical manifestations associated with the injury (see Figure 17-15). A herniated disk in the lumbosacral area is associated with pain that radiates along the sciatic nerve course over the buttock and into the calf or ankle. The pain occurs with straining, including coughing and sneezing, and usually on straight leg raising. Other clinical manifestations include limited range of motion of the lumbar spine; tenderness on palpation in the sciatic notch and along the sciatic nerve; impaired pain, temperature, and touch sensation in the L5-S1 or L4-5 dermatomes of the leg and foot; decreased or absent ankle jerk; and mild weakness of the foot.

With the herniation of a lower cervical disk, paresthesias and pain are present in the upper arm, forearm, and hand in the affected nerve root distribution. Neck and nerve root pain may be increased by neck motion and straining, including coughing and sneezing. Neck range of motion is diminished. Slight weakness and atrophy of biceps or triceps may occur; the biceps or triceps reflex may decrease. Occasionally signs of corticospinal and sensory tract impairments appear. These include motor weakness of the lower extremities, sensory disturbances in the lower extremities, and presence of a Babinski reflex.

EVALUATION AND TREATMENT   Diagnosis of a herniated intervertebral disk is made on the basis of the history; physical, EMG, CT, MRI, myelographic, and diskographic examination; spinal radiographs; and nerve conduction studies. Multiple avenues of therapy are available. The conservative approach comprises traction, bed rest, heat and ice to the affected areas, and an effective analgesic anti-inflammatory regimen. The surgical approach is indicated if there is evidence of severe compression (weakness, decreased deep tendon reflexes and bladder/bowel reflexes) or if the conservative approach is unsuccessful.

Cerebrovascular Disorders

Cerebrovascular disease is the most frequently occurring neurologic disorder. More than 50% of persons admitted to general hospitals with neurologic problems have cerebrovascular disease. Any abnormality of the brain caused by a pathologic process in the blood vessels is referred to as a *cerebrovascular disease*. Included in this category are lesions of the vessel wall; occlusion of the vessel lumen by thrombus or embolus; rup-

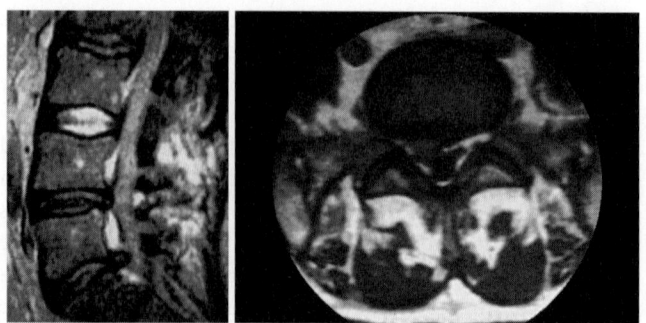

A   **B**

Figure 17-15 Posterolateral disk protrusion. Magnetic resonance imaging (MRI) scan, (**A**) sagittal and (**B**) axial sections. (From Perkin DG: *Mosby's color atlas and text of neurology*, London, 1998, Mosby-Wolfe.)

ture of the vessel; and alteration in vessel permeability, such as increased blood viscosity.

The brain abnormalities induced by cerebrovascular disease are of two types: (1) ischemia with or without infarction (death of brain tissues) accounting for 80% of CVAs and (2) hemorrhage. The common clinical manifestation of cerebrovascular disease is a **cerebrovascular accident (CVA, stroke),** which is a sudden, nonconvulsive focal neurologic deficit. Box 17-1 highlights the differences of strokes in children.

Cerebrovascular Accidents (Stroke Syndromes)

The incidence of stroke is 500,000 persons per year. Cerebrovascular accidents (CVAs) are the third leading cause of death in the United States, resulting in 150,000 deaths per year. They are the leading cause of disability in the United States. The economic cost is greater than 40 billion dollars per year.[6] Five percent to 14% of stroke survivors have a second stroke within 1 year of the first CVA. By 5 years, 24% of females and 42% of males have a second stroke.

The highest incidence of stroke is among people over 65 years of age. Strokes, however, do occur in a 3:10 ratio (28%) in individuals younger than 65 years of age. Stroke tends to run in families and is more common in men. The incidence of stroke is 2.5 times higher in blacks than whites. Blacks suffer greater physical impairments and are nearly 2 times as likely to die from their strokes. Intracranial atherosclerosis is more common in black and Asian populations, whereas extracranial disease is more common in the white population.

The mildest outcome of a CVA is so minimal as to be almost unnoticed. The most severe outcomes are hemiplegia, coma, and death. CVAs (stroke syndromes) are classified according to pathophysiology and thus are ischemic (thrombotic or embolic), global hypoprofusion (as in shock), or hemorrhagic. Risk factors for stroke include the following:

1. Arterial hypertension and both elevated systolic and diastolic blood pressures are independent risk factors.
2. Smoking increases the risk of stroke by 50%.
3. Diabetes increases the risk of ischemic stroke between 2.5 and 3.5 times.
4. Insulin resistance is an independent risk factor for ischemic stroke.[7]

5. Polycythemia and thrombocythemia increase the risk for ischemic stroke.
6. Presence of elevated lipoprotein-a is an independent risk factor for ischemic stroke.
7. Impaired cardiac function increases the risk for ischemic stroke.
8. Hyperhomocysteinemia is a strong and independent risk factor for ischemic stroke.[8]
9. Nonrheumatic atrial fibrillation is associated with a fivefold increase in the incidence of ischemic stroke.[9]
10. *Chlamydia pneumoniae* can increase the risk of stroke by infecting and injuring the endothelium.

Thrombotic Stroke

Thrombotic strokes (cerebral thrombosis) arise from arterial occlusions caused by thrombi formed in the arteries supplying the brain or in the intracranial vessels. The development of a cerebral thrombosis most frequently is attributed to atherosclerosis and inflammatory disease processes (arteritis) that damage arterial walls. Increased coagulation can lead to thrombus formation. Conditions causing inadequate cerebral perfusion (e.g., dehydration, hypotension, prolonged vasoconstriction from malignant hypertension) increase the risk of thrombosis. Over 20 to 30 years, atheromatous plaques (stenotic lesions) tend to form at branchings and curves in the cerebral circulation. The smooth stenotic area can degenerate, forming an ulcerated area of vessel wall. Platelets and fibrin adhere to the damaged wall, and clots form, gradually occluding the artery. The thrombus may enlarge both distally and proximally in the vessel. Portions of the clot break off and travel up the vessel to distant sites where occlusion occurs, producing a stroke syndrome.

Transient ischemic attacks (TIAs) are experienced by 50,000 Americans per year. They probably represent thrombotic particles causing an intermittent blockage of circulation or spasm. In a true TIA all the neurologic deficits must be completely clear within 24 hours, leaving no residual dysfunction. Recurrence of symptoms is 30% at 3 months, 60% at 6 months, and 80% at 1 year without definitive treatment.

Embolic Stroke. An **embolic stroke** involves fragments that break from a thrombus formed outside the brain or in the heart, aorta, common carotid, or thorax. Emboli infrequently arise from the ascending aorta or common carotid artery. The embolus usually involves small vessels and obstructs at a bifurcation or other point of narrowing, thus causing ischemia. An embolus may plug the lumen entirely and remain in place or break into fragments and move up the vessel. Conditions associated with the onset of an embolic stroke include atrial fibrillation; myocardial infarction; endocarditis; rheumatic heart disease; valvular prostheses; atrial-septal defects; and disorders of the aorta, carotids, or vertebral-basilar circulation. Less common contributors to embolic stroke are air, fat, and tumors. Fat emboli sometimes develop with fractures of long bones. Air emboli also can develop after certain types of surgery. In persons who experience an embolic stroke, a second stroke usually follows at some point because

---

Box 17-1	Stroke in Children

- More diverse etiologies than adults; congenital cardiac disease important cause
- Atherosclerosis is rare
- Vascular occlusion occurs more often in intracranial vessels, including internal carotid, middle cerebelar and basilar arteries; infarcts more often limited to deep regions of the cerebral hemispheres, mostly basal ganglion and internal capsule areas
- Intracerebral hemorrhage and subaracnoid hemorrhage account for a much higher percentage of strokes in children

---

Data from Chung CS, Caplan LR: Neurovascular disorders. In Goetz CG, editor, *Textbook of clinical neurology*, ed 2, Philadelphia, 2003, Saunders.

the source of emboli continues to exist. Embolization is usually in the distribution of the middle cerebral artery.

Hemorrhagic Stroke. Hemorrhagic stroke (**intracranial hemorrhage**) is the third most common cause of CVA (10% of strokes) and accounts for 10% to 15% of CVAs in whites but 30% in blacks and Asians.[9] The most common causes of hemorrhagic stroke are hypertension (56% to 81%), ruptured aneurysms, vascular malformations, bleeding into a tumor, hemorrhage associated with bleeding disorders or anticoagulation, head trauma, and illicit drug use. Risk factors for hemorrhagic stroke include hypertension, previous cerebral infarct, coronary artery disease, and diabetes mellitus.

A hypertensive hemorrhage is associated with a significant increase in systolic and diastolic pressure over several years and usually occurs within the brain tissue. A mass of blood is formed, and its volume increases. Adjacent brain tissue is displaced and compressed. Rupture or seepage into the ventricular system occurs in many cases. Hemorrhages are described as massive, small, slit, or petechial. A massive hemorrhage is several centimeters in diameter; a small hemorrhage is 1 to 2 cm in diameter; a slit hemorrhage lies in the subcortical area; and a petechial hemorrhage is the size of a pinhead bleed. The most common sites for hypertensive hemorrhages are in the putamen of the basal ganglia (a portion of the lentiform nucleus) (40%), the thalamus (15%), the cortex and subcortex (22%), the pons (8%), caudate (7%) (Figure 17-16), and cerebellar hemispheres (8%).

Lacunar Stroke. Lacunar strokes (**lacunar infarcts**) are microinfarcts smaller than 1 cm in diameter and involve the small perforating arteries, predominantly in the basal ganglia, internal capsules, and pons. Lacunar infarcts are caused by lipohyalinosis, subintimal lipid-loading foam cells, and fibrinoid materials that thicken the arterial walls and are associated with smoking,[9] hypertension and diabetes mellitus. Because of the subcortical location and small area of infarction, these strokes may have pure motor and sensory deficits.

PATHOPHYSIOLOGY

Cerebral Infarction. Cerebral infarction results when an area of the brain loses blood supply because of vascular occlusion. The pathologic manifestation is either (1) a global process that affects neurons most susceptible to ischemia (pyramidal and striatal neurons), Purkinje cells of the cerebral hemispheres, and the border zones at the very end of the arteries of circulation; or (2) a focal process with a central zone of cell loss surrounded by a zone of injured cells (a penumbra) that, if perfused in 1 hour, will survive. Proposed pathogenesis may include (1) abrupt vascular occlusion (e.g., embolus), (2) gradual vessel occlusion (e.g., atheroma), and (3) vessels that are stenosed but not completely occluded. Cerebral thrombi and cerebral emboli are the most common causes of occlusion, but atherosclerosis and hypotension are the dominant underlying processes.

Cerebral infarctions are ischemic or hemorrhagic. In ischemic infarcts (pale infarcts, "white stroke"), cytotoxic ischemic events and interaction between blood elements and blood vessels combine to produce brain injury. The affected area becomes slightly discolored and softens about 6 to 12 hours after the occlusion. Necrosis, swelling around the insult, and mushy disintegration have appeared by 48 to 72 hours after infarction. At a microscopic level, neuronal cell bodies change, myelin sheaths and axis cylinders are interrupted and disintegrate, and there is loss of oligodendrites and astrocytes.

Cellular events involve the following: (1) altered cell membranes in which cell membranes depolarize, allowing calcium influx into the cells, resulting in metabolic effects such as failure of mitochondrial oxidative phosphlylation (responsible for energy production); (2) glutamate release that alters cell membrane permeability to sodium, potassium, and calcium, and thus electrolyte influx pulls water into the cells, resulting in cytotoxic edema; and (3) fall in extra- and intracellular pH due to lactic acid production, resulting in an associated focal vasodilation. Infarcted areas may loose autoregulation.

A syndrome of luxury perfusion in areas adjacent to the infarct develops first from the loss of autoregulation. The vascular bed in this area dilates. Later, capillary sprouting (neovascularization) supports this luxury perfusion syndrome.

In hemorrhagic infarcts ("red strokes"), bleeding occurs into the infarcted area as a result of restoration of blood flow. Reperfusion occurs when the embolus fragments, or lysis or compressive forces lessen, allowing blood flow to be reestablished into the infarcted area. Most hemorrhagic infarcts are located in the cerebral cortex. Unfortunately, reperfusion has been shown to compromise recovery by accelerating the sequence of metabolically damaging events.

Cerebral Hemorrhage. The primary cause of cerebral hemorrhage is hypertension. (Aneurysms and arteriovenous malformations are discussed on pp. 567, 570, and 571.) The pathogenesis of hypertensive cerebral hemorrhage is not fully understood. Hypertension involves primarily smaller arteries and arterioles, resulting in thickening of the vessel walls, and increased cellularity of the vessels and hyalinization. Necrosis may be present. Microaneurysms in these smaller vessels or arteriolar necrosis precipitates the bleeding.

A mass of blood is formed as bleeding continues into the brain tissue. Adjacent brain tissue is displaced and compressed, producing ischemia and subsequent vasogenic edema. Increased ICP results. Rupture or seepage of blood into the ventricular system occurs in many cases.

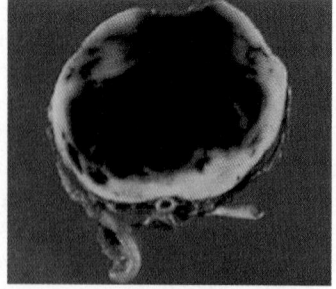

Figure 17-16 **Hypertensive hemorrhage.** Cross section of the pons showing a hypertensive hemorrhage. (From Perkin DG: *Mosby's color atlas and text of neurology,* London, 1998, Mosby-Wolfe.)

The cerebral hemorrhage resolves through reabsorption. Macrophages and astrocytes appear to clear away the blood. A cavity forms, surrounded by a dense gliosis after removal of the blood.

CLINICAL MANIFESTATIONS Because neurons surrounding the ischemic or infarcted areas undergo changes that disrupt plasma membranes, cellular edema results, causing further compression of capillaries. Cerebral edema reaches its maximum in about 72 hours and takes about 2 weeks to subside. Most persons survive an initial hemispheric ischemic stroke unless massive cerebral edema develops. However, massive brain stem infarcts, caused by basilar thrombosis or embolism, are almost always fatal.

Clinical manifestations of thrombotic stroke vary, depending on the artery obstructed. Different sites of obstruction create different occlusion syndromes (Table 17-7).

With hemorrhagic stroke, clinical manifestations vary according to the location and size of the bleed. Focal neurologic deficits are found in 80% of individuals experiencing hemorrhagic strokes, altered consciousness occurs in 50%. Once a deep unresponsive state occurs, the person rarely survives. The immediate prognosis is grave. If the person survives, however, recovery of function frequently is possible.

Individuals experiencing intracranial hemorrhage from a ruptured or leaking aneurysm have one of three sets of symptoms: (1) onset of an excruciating generalized headache with an almost immediate lapse into an unresponsive state; (2) headache, but with consciousness maintained; and (3) sudden lapse into unconsciousness. If the hemorrhage is confined to the subarachnoid space, there may be no local signs. If bleeding spreads into the brain tissue, hemiparesis/paralysis, dysphasia, or homonymous hemianopia may be present. Warning signs of an impending aneurysm rupture may include headache, transient unilateral weakness, transient numbness and tingling, and transient speech disturbance. Warning signs, however, often are not present.

EVALUATION AND TREATMENT The principle of acute stroke treatment is "time is brain." Time to treatment is often too great considering the time limits for reversibility of brain ischemia. Treatment needs to be initiated within 6 hours of symptom onset. Drug therapy is designed to prevent further thrombotic events (anticoagulation), augment blood flow (recanalization), reperfuse the tissues (vasodilators, hemodilution, thrombolytics), and protect neurons (metabolic adjustment). To provide anticoagulation and reperfusion, antiplatelets and antithrombotics such as acetylsalicylic acid (ASA), dipyridamole (Persantine), ticlopidine (Ticlid), clopidogrel (Plavix), and combination drugs; heparin; low-molecular-weight heparinoids; and warfarin sodium (Coumadin), as well as thrombolytics such as urokinase/streptokinase, tissue plasminogen (t-PA), ancrod (Arvin), and pentoxifylline may be used.[10,11] Thrombolytic therapy for acute ischemic stroke, however, has been found to be used in only 2% of persons who were eligible.[12] Metabolic protection is designed to control calcium

influx (e.g., calcium channel blockers), excitatory amine activation (e.g., glutamate inhibitors, antagonists), and free radicals (free radical scavenger agents). Cell transplants in stroke are being examined in animal models.

In thrombotic strokes, treatment is directed at supportive management to control cerebral edema and increased ICP. Ancrod (Arvin), a drug, is being tested experimentally to achieve defibrinogenation and thus increase local cerebral blood flow in the ischemic areas. Later surgical intervention to restore blood supply may be indicated. Arresting the disease process by control of risk factors is critical. In embolic strokes, treatment is directed at preventing further embolization by instituting anticoagulation therapy and correcting the primary problem. Only 11% of persons with cardioembolic strokes had been receiving anticoagulation therapy[13] as reported in one study, and women are less likely to have anticoagulation therapy for atrial fibrillation.[14] Rehabilitation is indicated in both thrombotic and embolic stroke. Treatment of an intracranial bleed, regardless of cause, is focused on stopping or reducing the bleeding, controlling the increased ICP, preventing a rebleed, and preventing vasospasm. Occasionally an attempt is made to evacuate or aspirate the blood.

Intracranial Aneurysm

Intracranial aneurysms may result from arteriosclerosis, congenital abnormality, trauma, inflammation, or infection. Cocaine use has been linked to aneurysm formation. The size of the aneurysm may vary from 2 mm to 2 or 3 cm. Most aneurysms are located at bifurcations in or near the circle of Willis, in the vertebrobasilar arteries, or within the carotid system (see Figure 14-18). Eighty-five percent are in the anterior circulation. Aneurysms may be single, but in 20% to 25% of cases, more than one aneurysm is present. In these instances the aneurysms may be unilateral or bilateral. The incidence of rupture is 11 in 100,000 persons per year. Peak incidence of rupture is among persons from 50 to 60 years of age. Women have a slightly greater incidence of aneurysms.

PATHOPHYSIOLOGY No single pathologic mechanism exists. Aneurysm development is attributed to hemodynamic stress and is believed to be exacerbated by hypertension and certain connective tissue disorders. The smooth muscle coat and elastic lamina of the intracranial artery end at the neck of the aneurysm. The aneurysm wall is composed of fibrous tissue. Aneurysms may be classified on the basis of shape and form (Figure 17-17). **Saccular aneurysms (berry aneurysms)** occur frequently (in approximately 2% of the population) and are the result of a combination of a congenital abnormality in the media of the arterial wall and degenerative changes.[9] The sac gradually grows over time. A saccular aneurysm may be (1) round with a narrow stalk connecting it to the parent artery (Figure 17-18), (2) broad based without a stalk, or (3) cylindric. Saccular aneurysms are rare in childhood; their highest incidence of rupturing or bleeding is among persons 20 to 50 years of age.

Fusiform aneurysms (giant aneurysms), by definition greater than 25 mm in diameter, make up 5% of all intracranial

Table 17-7	Stroke Syndromes Secondary to Occlusion or Stenosis	
Location/Vessel	Area of Brain Infarcted	Signs and Symptoms Noted

Anterior and Central Circulation

NOTE: The internal carotid enters the circle of Willis and supplies the lateral anterior and central portions of the cerebral hemispheres through the middle cerebral artery and the paramedical frontal lobe superior to the corpus callosum through the anterior cerebral artery; penetrating branches serve the deeper layers of the hemispheres

Location/Vessel	Area of Brain Infarcted	Signs and Symptoms Noted
Internal carotid	If collateral circulation is intact, commonly no infarction has occurred; if infarcted, location is same as in the middle cerebral artery	• Arterial pressure may be low in the retina • Bruits over the internal carotid artery • Possible retinal emboli • History of transient ischemic attacks (TIAs) • Positive noninvasive studies
Middle cerebral artery (MCA) (most common area); either stem or branches of MCA	Cortical motor area (face, arm, leg) and/or posterior limb, internal capsule, corona radiata	• **Motor:** contralateral hemiparesis or hemiplegia, greater in face and arm than leg
	Cortical sensory area (face, arm, leg) and/or posterior limb of internal capsule	• **Sensation:** contralateral loss in same distribution as motor loss
	Broca area and deep fibers in the dominant hemisphere	• **Speech:** expressive (motor) disorder with anomia (left hemisphere most commonly affected) with nonfluent aphasia and some comprehension defects
	Broca area and deep fibers in the nondominant hemisphere	• **Speech:** dysarthria
	Optic radiations deep in the temporal lobe	• **Vision:** contralateral homonymous hemianopsia or quadranopsia
	Location not known	• **Motor:** mirror movements • **Respirations:** Cheyne-Stokes respirations, contralateral hyperhidrosis, occasional mydriasis
	Posterior limb or internal capsule and adjacent corona radiata	• **Motor:** pure motor hemiplegia
	Penetrating branches of MCA (lenticulostriate branches) into the basal nuclei	• **Motor:** varying degrees of contralateral weakness of face, arm, or leg • **Sensory:** little or no loss; if present, contralateral following the motor distribution • **Speech:** transcortical sensory aphasia (communicating pathways are interrupted) • **Perception:** transient visual and sensory neglect on the left if a right lesion
Anterior cerebral artery (ACA) (least common)	Proximal segment: corona radiata (rarely)	• **Motor:** when present, a mild contralateral hemiparesis, greater in leg; with bilateral occlusion of ACA, cerebral paraplegia in both legs can occur
	Main stem (complete occlusion is uncommon, thus areas affected differ and collateral circulation may alleviate signs or symptoms); medial aspect of frontal lobes, caudate nucleus, and corpus callosum are supplied by the ACA	• **Motor:** contralateral paralysis or paresis (greater in foot and thigh); mild upper extremity weakness • **Sensory:** mild contralateral lower extremity deficiency with loss of vibratory and/or position sense, loss of two-point discrimination • **Speech:** may have transcortical motor and sensory aphasia if left hemisphere • Frontal lobe releasing signs • Apraxia

Posterior Circulation

NOTE: The posterior circulation includes the posterior cerebral artery, the vertebral arteries, and the basilar artery; the anatomic territory covered includes the posterior aspects of the hemispheres, the central areas of the thalamus and midbrain, and the brain stem; occlusion of the vessels is most commonly by emboli; effects of infarct in these vessels and their penetrating vessels can be specific or devastatingly global; many complex syndromes have been identified

Location/Vessel	Area of Brain Infarcted	Signs and Symptoms Noted
Vertebral arteries	Medulla and spinal cord tracts, anterior spinal artery and penetrating branches (medial medullary syndrome)	• **Motor:** contralateral hemiparesis (face spared) and/or impaired contralateral proprioception; flaccid weakness or paralysis of the tongue and/or dysarthria

Table 17-7	Stroke Syndromes Secondary to Occlusion or Stenosis—cont'd	
Location/Vessel	**Area of Brain Infarcted**	**Signs and Symptoms Noted**
Posterior Circulation—cont'd		
Basilar artery (three sets of branches)	Midline structures of pons (paramedian branches); three general areas of infarction are common: (1) medial inferior pontine syndrome, (2) medial midpontine syndrome, and (3) medial superior pontine syndrome	• **Motor:** contralateral hemiparesis or hemiplegia, ipsilateral lower motor neuron facial palsy, "locked-in syndrome" • **Sensory:** contralateral loss of vibratory sense, sense of position with dysmetria, loss of two-point discrimination, impaired rapid alternating movements • **Visual:** inferior pontine: diplopia; impaired abduction of ipsilateral eye: internuclear ophthalmoplegia; medial superior; diplopia, internuclear ophthalmoplegia, skewed deviation
	Corticospinal and corticobulbar tracts in pons, sensory tracts of medial and lateral lemnisci, vestibular nuclei, inferior and middle cerebellar peduncles, cranial nerve nuclei and/or fibers, cerebellar connections in tectum, descending sympathetic pathways, central brain stem, pontine tegmentum (vertebral basilar syndrome)	• **Motor:** upper motor neuron type of weakness: paralysis in combinations involving face, tongue, throat, and extremities; dysphagia, facial weakness, dysmetria, ataxia (either trunk or extremities), weak mastication muscles • **Sensation:** combinations of impaired sensation (vibratory, two-point, position sense, pain, temperature), facial hypesthesia, anesthesia of cranial nerve V
Posterior cerebral artery (PCA)	Central territory (thalamic area, dentothalamic tract, cerebral peduncle, red nucleus, subthalamic nucleus, and cranial nerve III)	• **Motor:** contralateral hemiplegia with possible dysmetria, dyskinesia, hemiballism or choreoathetosis, dystaxia, cerebellar ataxia, and tremor; contralateral upper motor neuron palsy; several syndromes are associated: (1) Weber: cranial nerve III palsy and contralateral hemiplegia; (2) thalamoperforate syndrome: superior, crossed cerebellar ataxia or inferior crossed cerebellar ataxia with cranial nerve III palsy (Claude syndrome); (3) decerebrate attacks • **Sensory:** contralateral sensory loss of all modalities without agraphia • **Function:** prosopagnosia (inability to recognize familiar faces), topographic disorientation, memory deficits, alexia, inability to read, color anomia • **Level of consciousness:** in bilateral PCA syndromes, coma with absent doll's eyes or loss of alertness may occur; if tegmentum of midbrain near hypothalamus and third ventricle is damaged, akinetic mutism may occur
Small Vessel Disease		
NOTE: Small penetrating vessels in brain parenchyma that supply areas near the basal ganglia are most vulnerable to infarction although any small vessels can occlude deep in the brain and cause injury, producing neurologic signs or symptoms; such infarcts are commonly called *lacunes* (small pit or hollow), a term that is changing in meaning; they can be caused by emboli but are most commonly associated with microatheromas; although they can be found in otherwise healthy people, those with concurrent athersclerosis, **arterial** hypertension, and/or diabetes have a higher incidence of this type of infarct		
	Internal capsule, most commonly	• **Motor:** contralateral hemiparesis on a single side, with equal deficit in face, arm, and leg; often unaccompanied by detectable signs of sensory, visual, and speech loss, depending on location; old term is "pure motor stroke" although evidence suggests that other neurologic signs are present but overlooked because of low intensity
	Thalamus, most commonly	• **Sensory:** complete or partial loss in face, arm, trunk, and leg that appears exactly midline; may be accompanied by pain, hypersthesias, and uncomfortable sensations (hemisensory stroke)
	Pons	• Dysarthria, clumsy hand
	Pons, midbrain, capsule or parietal white matter	• Hemiparesis, ataxia on same side

aneurysms. They occur as a result of diffuse arteriosclerotic changes and are found most commonly in the basilar arteries or terminal portions of the internal carotid arteries. They act as space-occupying lesions. **Mycotic aneurysms** result from arteritis caused by bacterial emboli; these aneurysms are uncommon. **Traumatic aneurysms** are caused by a weakening of the arterial wall by a fracture line, by a penetrating missile, or after neurosurgical or imaging (e.g., angiographic) procedures.

Aneurysms rupture because their walls are thin, causing hemorrhage into the subarachnoid space with rapid spread, producing localized changes in the cerebral cortex and focal irritation of nerves and arteries (see Laplace law, Chapter 29). Because of compression, bleeding ceases with the formation of a fibrin-platelet plug at the point of rupture. Blood undergoes reabsorption through arachnoid villi within 3 weeks.

CLINICAL MANIFESTATIONS Aneurysms are frequently asymptomatic. Of all persons undergoing routine autopsy, 5% are found to have one or more intracranial aneurysms. Clinical manifestations may arise from cranial nerve compression, but the signs vary, depending on the location and size of the aneurysm. Most often, cranial nerves III, IV, V, and VI are affected (see Table 14-6). Unfortunately, the most common first indication of the presence of an aneurysm is an acute subarachnoid hemorrhage, intracerebral hemorrhage, or combined subarachnoid-intracerebral hemorrhage (see p. 571).

EVALUATION AND TREATMENT Diagnosis before a bleeding episode is made using arteriographic examination. After a subarachnoid or an intracerebral hemorrhage, a tentative diagnosis of an aneurysm that has bled is based on clinical manifestations, history, CT scan, and MRI. The treatment of choice for an aneurysm is surgical management. The location and size of the aneurysm and the person's clinical status determine whether invasive therapy is feasible.[15]

Vascular Malformations

Vascular formations are one-tenth as common as aneurysms.[9] Four types of vascular malformation exist: arteriovenous malformation (AVM), cavernous angioma, capillary telangiectasis, and venous angioma. **Cavernous angiomas (malfor-**

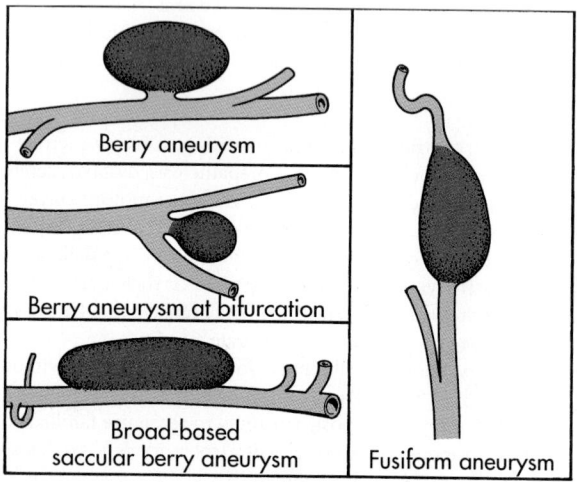

Figure 17-17 Types of aneurysms.

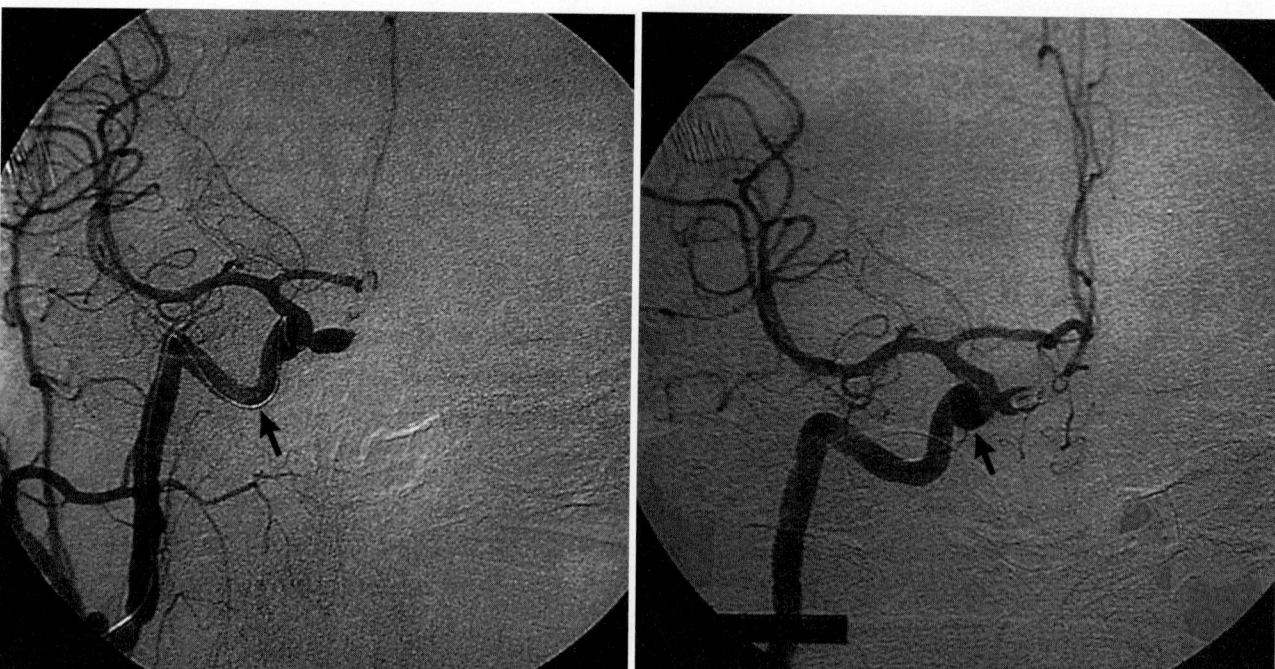

Figure 17-18 Ophthalmic artery aneyrysm. **A,** With endovascular coil; **B,** in situ. (From Perkin DG: *Mosby's color atlas and text of neurology,* London, 1998, Mosby-Wolfe.)

mations) are sinusoidal collections of blood vessels without interspersed normal brain tissue. They rarely hemorrhage and compose 8% to 15% of all vascular lesions. A **capillary telangiectasis** is dilated capillaries with interspersed normal brain tissue found deep in the brain, particularly in the brain stem. Hemorrhage is rare and these vascular malformations are associated with Rendu-Oster-Weber disease. **Venous angioma,** the most common vascular malformation found at autopsy (3% of cases), is considered a subset of developmental venous anomalies that occur secondary to arrested development.[16] The result is primitive embryologic veins in a radial pattern feeding a central vein. These rarely hemorrhage.

In an **arteriovenous malformation (AVM),** arteries feed directly into veins through a vascular tangle of malformed vessels (Figure 17-19). AVMs hemorrhage at a rate of 40% a year. AVMs occur in any part of the brain, and they are usually cone shaped. Their size is highly variable, from malformations of a few millimeters to large ones that extend from the cortex to the ventricle. The large AVMs also may involve the dura mater, including the falx cerebri and the tentorium cerebelli. AVMs occur as frequently in males as in females, and they occasionally occur in families. Although usually present at birth, AVMs exhibit a delayed age of onset and symptoms most commonly occur before 30 years of age. They most commonly rupture in the second and third decade of life.

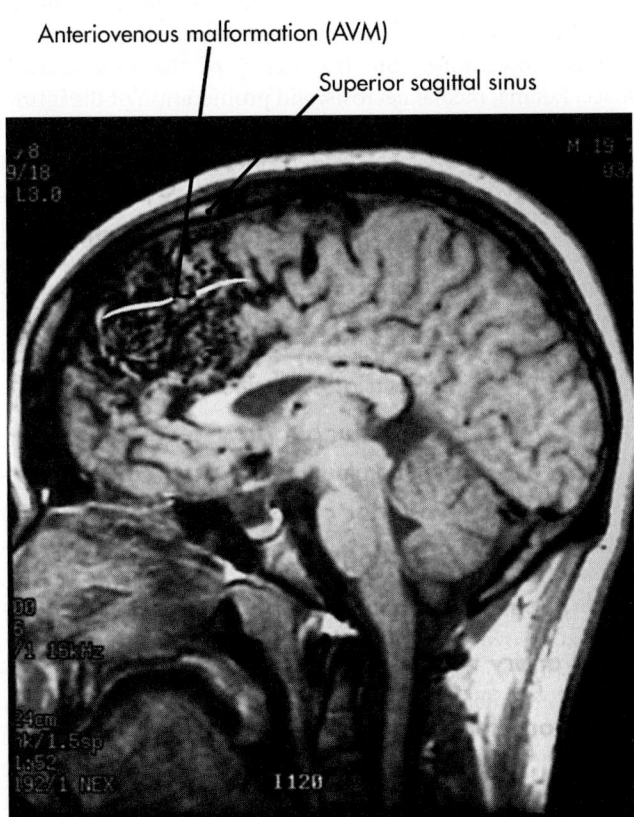

Anteriovenous malformation (AVM)

Superior sagittal sinus

Figure 17-19 Sagittal magnetic resonance imaging near the midline showing an AVM in the frontal lobe. This lesion includes branches of the anterior cerebral artery and drains into the superior sagittal sinus. *AVM,* Arteriovenous malformation. (From Haines DE, editor: *Fundamental neuroscience,* Philadelphia, 1997, Churchill Livingstone.)

PATHOPHYSIOLOGY   AVMs, which are developmental abnormalities that represent persistence of embryonic patterns of blood vessels, do not have a normal blood vessel structure and are abnormally thin. The involved vessels are thought by some to enlarge over time. The AVM may be fed by one or several arteries. These feeder vessels become tortuous over time and often are dilated. With moderate to large AVMs, sufficient blood is shunted into the malformation to deprive surrounding tissue of adequate blood perfusion.

CLINICAL MANIFESTATIONS   Clinical manifestations vary. Twenty percent of persons with an AVM have a characteristic chronic nondescript headache, although some experience migraine. Fifty percent of persons experience seizure disorders caused by compression. Initially, the seizures tend to be focal or jacksonian; generalization often occurs over time. (Seizures are discussed in Chapter 16.) The other 50% suffer an intracerebral, a subarachnoid, or a subdural hemorrhage. Bleeding from an AVM into the subarachnoid space causes clinical manifestations identical to those associated with a ruptured aneurysm. If bleeding is into the brain tissue, focal signs that develop resemble a stroke-in-evolution. Ten percent of persons experience hemiparesis or other focal signs. Hemiparesis usually is caused by compression or rupture. At times, noncommunicating hydrocephalus (see Chapter 16) develops with a large AVM that extends into the ventricle lining.

EVALUATION AND TREATMENT   A systolic bruit over the carotid in the neck, the mastoid process, or (in a young person) the eyeball is almost diagnostic of an AVM. CT, magnetic resonance angiography (MRA) and transcranial Doppler (TCD), and MRI examination are used in initial diagnosis, followed by an arteriogram to identify feeding vessels. Treatment options are direct surgical approach, embolization, or radiotherapy. The risk of bleeding is 6% in the first year and 2% to 4% each year thereafter with no intervention.

Subarachnoid Hemorrhage

With a **subarachnoid hemorrhage,** blood escapes from a defective or injured vasculature into the subarachnoid space (Figure 17-20). Individuals at risk for a subarachnoid hemorrhage are those with intracranial aneurysm (85% of cases), intracranial AVM, or hypertension and those who have sustained head injuries. There is a 50% overall mortality rate and one third of survivors are dependent. Subarachnoid hemorrhages often recur, especially from a ruptured intracranial aneurysm.

PATHOPHYSIOLOGY   When a vessel is leaking, blood oozes into the subarachnoid space. When a vessel tears, blood under pressure is pumped into the subarachnoid space. The blood is extremely irritating to the meningeal and other neural tissues and so produces an inflammatory reaction in these tissues. Additionally, the blood coats nerve roots, clogs arachnoid granulations (impairing CSF reabsorption), and clogs

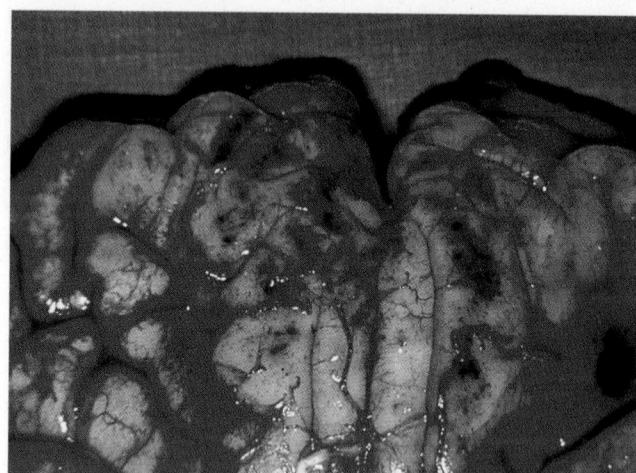

Figure 17-20 Acute subarachnoid hemorrhage. Acute subarachnoid hemorrhage with focal accentuation over superficial cortical contusions. (From Damjanov I, Linder J, editors: *Anderson's pathology,* ed 10, St Louis, 1996, Mosby.)

Table 17-8	Subarachnoid Hemorrhage Classification Scale
Category	**Description**
Grade I	Neurologic status intact; mild headache, slight nuchal rigidity
Grade II	Neurologic deficit evidenced by cranial nerve involvement; moderate to severe headache with more pronounced meningeal signs (e.g., photophobia, nuchal rigidity)
Grade III	Drowsiness and confusion with or without focal neurologic deficits; pronounced meningeal signs
Grade IV	Stuporous with pronounced neurologic deficits (e.g., hemiparesis, dysphasia); nuchal rigidity
Grade V	Deep coma state with decerebrate posturing and other brain stem dysfunction

From Cook HA: Aneurysmal subarachnoid hemorrhage: neurosurgical frontiers and nursing challenges. In Winkleman C, editor: *AACN clinical issues in critical care nursing,* Philadelphia, 1991, Lippincott.

foramina within the ventricular system (impairing CSF circulation). ICP immediately increases to almost diastolic levels. ICP returns to near baseline in about 10 minutes. Cerebral blood flow and cerebral perfusion pressure (CPP) decrease. The expanding hematoma acts like a space-occupying lesion, compressing and displacing brain tissue. Granulation tissue is formed, and scarring of the meninges with resulting impairment of CSF reabsorption and secondary hydrocephalus often results.

CLINICAL MANIFESTATIONS   Early manifestations associated with leaking vessels are episodic headache, transient changes in mental status or level of consciousness, nausea or vomiting, focal neurologic defects including visual or speech disturbances, cranial nerve palsies, or stiff neck. A ruptured vessel often is accompanied by a sudden throbbing, "explosive" headache. The headache is associated with nausea and vomiting, visual disturbances, motor deficits, and loss of consciousness. These signs all can be related to a dramatic rise in ICP. Meningeal irritation and inflammation often occur, causing neck stiffness (nuchal rigidity), photophobia, blurred vision, irritability, restlessness, and low-grade fever. A positive **Kernig sign** (in which straightening the knee with the hip and knee in a flexed position produces pain in the back and neck regions) and **Brudzinski sign** (in which passive flexion of the neck produces neck pain and increased rigidity) may appear. No localizing signs are present if the bleed is confined completely to the subarachnoid space.

The Hunt and Hess subarachnoid hemorrhage (SAH) grading system is based on description of the clinical manifestations (Table 17-8). Rebleeding is a significant risk with a high mortality (up to 70%). The period of greatest risk is the first month, with the peak incidence of rebleeding during the first 2 weeks after the initial bleed. Rebleeding is manifested by a sudden increase in blood pressure and ICP, along with a deteriorating neurologic status.

Delayed cerebral ischemia, a syndrome of progressive neurologic deterioration, is associated with cerebral artery vasospasm. In persons with a subarachnoid hemorrhage, 50% experience vasospasms in adjacent and sometimes in nonadjacent vessels. The pathophysiology of vasospasm is unclear. Vasospasm is thought to occur because of the effects of vasoactive substances (e.g., calcium, prostaglandins, serotonin, and catecholamines) on the arteries of the subarachnoid space. Edema, medial necrosis, and proliferation of the intima have been found. Vasospasm causes decreased cerebral blood flow (ischemia) and may produce infarct. The peak time of onset is 3 to 5 days, with maximal narrowing at 5 to 14 days after the initial bleed, but vasospasm may persist for 2 to 4 weeks.

Seizures occur in 25% of persons with an SAH. The incidence of hydrocephalus after a bleed is 20%. Hypothalamic dysfunction, manifested by salt wasting, hyponatremia, and ECG changes, is common.

EVALUATION AND TREATMENT   The diagnosis of a subarachnoid hemorrhage is based on the clinical presentation, a noncontrast CT scan, and a lumbar puncture, if needed. Arteriographic examination is the definitive diagnostic measure for defining and localizing an aneurysm or AVM. Treatment is directed at control of intracranial pressure, prevention of ischemia and hypoxia of neural tissues, and prevention of rebleeding episodes. Antifibrinolytic drugs may be used to stop rebleeding in selected cases. Blood pressure is allowed to remain in the high normal range or is elevated to that level. Platinum coils and balloon embolization to occlude the aneurysm are used, but microsurgical repair remains the treatment of choice. Calcium channel blockers, such as nimodipine, are used to prevent or reverse vasospasm. Volume expansion or hemodilution through continuous or bolus administration of hetastarch and plasma protein factors to maintain a hematocrit of 33% is used to expand blood volume and augment cerebral perfusion. Cerebral angioplasty can be tried for vasospasm. The primary problem must be diagnosed and corrected as well.

Headache

Headache is a common neurologic disorder and is usually a benign symptom. However, it can be associated with serious disease, such as brain tumor, meningitis, and giant cell arteritis. The headache syndromes discussed here are the chronic, recurring type not associated with structural abnormalities or systemic disease and include migraine, cluster, paroxysmal hemicrania, and tension headaches. Characteristics of the major types of headache syndromes are summarized in Table 17-9.

Migraine Headache

Migraine headache affects as many as 11 million people in the United States. The disorder occurs in 15% of women and 6% of men (a 4:1 ratio of female to male), is more common in those 25 to 55 years of age, and can occur in young children. The prevalence in women is highest at 20 to 40 years of age but remains higher than in men into older age. Onset after 50 years of age is rare. Hormonal factors account for most of the gender differences. A positive family history is a common finding, and there is a genetic predisposition to the disorder.

Migraine headache is a benign recurring headache often provoked by a trigger factor and usually is accompanied by neurologic dysfunction. Trigger factors may include stress; hunger; weather changes; spring; autumn; sunlight; noise; jet lag; foods, such as red wine, cheese, and chocolate; and menstruation, ovulation, and contraceptives. The International Headache Society[17] has classified the following different clinical subtypes of migraine:

1. Migraine without aura: common migraine
2. Migraine with aura: classic migraine
   a. Migraine with typical aura
   b. Migraine with prolonged aura
   c. Familial hemiplegic migraine
   d. Basilar migraine
   e. Migraine aura without headache
   f. Migraine with acute-onset aura
3. Ophthalmoplegic migraine
4. Retinal migraine
5. Complicated migraine
   a. Status migrainous
   b. Migraine infarction

The pathophysiologic basis for migraine is complex and includes neurologic, vascular, and hormonal and neurotransmitter components. The end point is a state of regional hypoprofusion. Several theories have been proposed to account for the pathogenesis, including cortical spreading depression and serotonergic and other neurotransmitter alterations. These theories are summarized in Table 17-10. The phases of a migraine headache are (1) a trigger phase precipitated by external factors; (2) an aura with inhibition of cortical activity and a reduction in blood flow leading to symptoms of scotoma and paresthesias; (3) release of vasoactive neuropeptides, ionic alterations, platelet release of 5-HT, and degranulation of mast cells; and (4) activation of the locus ceruleus and excitation of trigeminal nuclei resulting in vasodilation of dural arteries. The resulting perivascular inflammation leads to the typical headache. Disturbances in the blood-brain barrier in the area postrema cause nausea and vomiting.

In migraine with aura, the aura is thought to be caused by a slowly expanding area of reduced cortical activity and reduced blood flow. Reduced blood flow appears to be related to cortical arteriolar vasoconstriction and not vasospasm of larger arteries. Reductions in blood flow are not observed in migraine without aura. The pain of migraine is associated with neurotransmitters and pain fibers from the trigeminal nerve that terminate in the walls of the dural and cortical arteries. The trigeminal nucleus is controlled by the periaqueductal gray matter, which is a central modulator of pain transmission. Projections from the trigeminal nuclei also extend to the cervical spinal cord (C2) and may explain neck pain in addition to headache in migraine.

Table 17-9	Characteristics of Common Headaches			
	Migraine		**Cluster Headache/ Proximal Hemicrania**	**Tension Type of Headache**
	Without Aura	**With Aura**		
Age of onset	Childhood, adolescence, or young adulthood	Childhood, adolescence, or young adulthood	Young adulthood, middle age	Young adulthood, middle age
Gender	Female	Female	Male	Not gender specific
Family history of headaches	Yes	Yes	No	Yes
Onset and evolution	Slow to rapid	Slow to rapid	Rapid	Slow to rapid
Time course	Episodic	Episodic	Clusters in time	Episodic, may become constant
Quality	Usually throbbing	Usually throbbing	Steady	Steady
Location	Variable, often unilateral	Variable, often unilateral	Orbit, temple, cheek	Variable
Associated features	Prodrome, vomiting	Prodrome, vomiting	Lacrimation, rhinorrhea, Horner syndrome	None

Table 17-10   Pathogenic Theories of Migraine Headache

Theory	Mechanisms
Neurogenic theory of migraine (cortical spreading depression [CSD])	A primary derangement of brain function exists. A reduction in brain and electrical activity. A trigger initiates a reduction in electrical activity and decrease in blood flow that spreads across the cerebral cortex from the occipital region, moving anteriorly at a rate of 2-3 mm/min; flow abnormalities are documented in classic but not common migraine and are probably related to deranged neurologic function; reduced cortical blood flow follows the cortical surface (dural and cortical arterioles) independent of the distribution of the large arteries; reduced cortical blood flow continues after the aura and may be increased or decreased during headache; release of potassium and hydrogen ions during CSD contributes to pain by activating sensory fibers that initiate inflammation and activate trigeminal and brain stem neurons related to pain.
Serotonergic and neurotransmitter alterations	Increased release of serotonin (5-hydroxytryptamine [5-HT]), norepinephrine, substance P, nitric oxide, glutamate, and other sensory substances. Increased release of 5-HT in the dorsal raphe activates neurotransmission to cerebral arteries, altering blood flow, and also affects projections to the visual cortex and visual processing centers; brain increases in glutamate and decreases in magnesium have been documented; afferent and efferent fibers from the trigeminal nerve extend to the wall of cerebral and dural arteries, and the inflammation associated with neurotransmitter release and vascular changes may account for the pain associated with migraine. Activation of N-methyl-D-aspartate receptors by glutamine during cortical spreading depression.

Data from Lauritzen M: *Sci Med* 3(4):32, 1996; Ramadan NM et al: *Headache* 29:590, 1989.

Migraine headaches without aura, the most common type, last from 4 to 72 hours and are often located on one side. The pain is throbbing, of moderate to severe intensity, and aggravated by physical activity. In migraine with aura, the most common prodromal symptoms are visual (scotomas with luminous angles and scintillating edges, and hemianopsia). Sensory deficits and aphasia also may be present. The aura develops within 5 to 20 minutes and remits within 60 minutes, followed by headache and other symptoms, including nausea, vomiting, photophobia, scalp tenderness; 10% of persons experience diarrhea.

In susceptible women, migraine occurs most frequently before and during menstruation and is decreased during pregnancy and menopause. The cyclic withdrawal of estrogens may trigger attacks of migraine. Cyclic changes in estrogen are absent in pregnancy and after menopause, which could explain the less frequent attacks in some women. Estrogens may act directly on vascular smooth muscle, modulate activity of vasoactive substances at the neurovascular junction, and activate vasoregulatory responses in the hypothalamus. However, no direct evidence has been found to link circulating female sex hormones with the frequency and severity of migraine.

The diagnosis of migraine is made from medical history and physical examination. Clinicians must be skilled in their understanding of different types of headaches, risk factors, family history, and clinical features. Differential diagnosis is confirmed with CT and MRI scans and EEG. A significant number of individuals with migraine have depression as a comorbidity.

The management of migraine includes education that migraine is a chronic physiologic disorder and not psychosomatic. Avoidance of triggers, adequate sleep, regular eating habits, and daily relaxation and meditation can create a headache-protective environment. With the onset of acute migraine, a dark room, ice, and sleep can provide relief. The pharmacologic management of migraine varies with each individual and is related to the severity of the attack. Drug considerations should include antiemetics, nonsteroidal anti-inflammatory preparations, ergotamine and dihydroergotamine, and 5-HT antagonists (e.g., sumatriptan). Magnesium administration may help some women with menstrual migraine. Gastric absorption may be decreased during an attack, and routes of administration other than oral (e.g., nasal sprays, intravenous, and rectal) may be used.

The prophylaxis of migraine is considered when attacks cannot be treated effectively. Several drugs may be considered and should *not* be used in combination. Examples include beta-blockers, a calcium antagonist (flunarizine), serotonin antagonists (lisuride, methysergide), nonsteroidal anti-inflammatory drugs, dihydroergotamine (DHE), naproxen, valproic acid, and amitriptyline.

Cluster Headache

Cluster headaches occur primarily in men between 20 and 50 years of age. Cluster headache has been known also as *histamine cephalalgia, Horton syndrome,* and *erythromelalgia.* These headaches are known as cluster headaches because several attacks can occur during the day for a period of days followed by a long period of spontaneous remission. Cluster headache has an episodic and a chronic form.

The headache attack usually begins without warning and is characterized by severe, unilateral tearing, burning, periorbital, and retrobulbar or temporal pain lasting 30 minutes to 2 hours. One or several attacks may occur in a day, and attacks usually occur at the same time of the day or night. The same side is affected in subsequent episodes. Associated symptoms include lacrimation, reddening of the eye, nasal stuffiness, eyelid ptosis, and nausea. Pain often is referred to the midface and teeth. If the cluster of attacks occurs more frequently without sustained spontaneous remission, they are classified as *chronic cluster headaches* (20% of cases). Alcohol can stimulate an attack during a cluster headache in about 50% to 70% of cases, but it is not a triggering factor during remission.

The etiology and pathophysiology of cluster headache are unknown. There are no consistent changes in cerebral blood flow. Pathogenic mechanisms may include vascular alterations, neurogenic or neuroimmunologic dysregulation of the hypothalamus, dysregulation of the parasympathetic ganglia, sympathetic deficit, and stimulation of the trigeminal nucleus. The rhythmicity of attacks probably is related to disorders of the hypothalamus. There may be altered serotonergic nerve transmission but at different loci than in migraine headache.

Prophylactic drugs are used to treat cluster headache. The most effective are prednisone, lithium, methysergide, calcium channel antagonists, and valproate. Acute attacks are managed with oxygen inhalation, sumatriptan, and inhaled ergotamine.

Chronic Paroxysmal Hemicrania. Chronic paroxysmal hemicrania (CPH) is a cluster type of headache that occurs with more daily frequency (4 to 12 times per day) but with shorter duration (20 to 120 minutes). The remission phases are often shorter. The attacks are more common in women, usually after pregnancy. The symptoms are similar to cluster headache. As with cluster headache, there is an episodic and a chronic form. The pathophysiology involves a disorder of sympathetic hyperactivity, but the mechanism is different from cluster headache because there is effective relief of symptoms with indomethacin.

Tension-Type Headache

Tension-type headache is the most common type of headache, occurring in 69% of men and 88% of women. The average age of onset is during second decade of life. Female/male ratio is 1:1. It is a mild to moderate bilateral headache with a sensation of a tight band or pressure around the head. The onset of pain is usually gradual. The headache occurs in episodes and may last for several hours or several days. It is not aggravated by physical activity. Chronic tension headache represents headache that occurs at least 15 days per month. Many individuals have both tension-type and migraine headaches.

Both a central mechanism and a peripheral mechanism operate in causing tension headache. The central mechanism probably involves hypersensitivity of pain fibers from the trigeminal nerve. The peripheral mechanism is probably related to contraction of jaw and neck muscles, but the exact mechanisms are unknown. Headache sufferers have more localized pain and tenderness of pericranial muscles.

Mild headaches are treated with ice, and more severe forms are treated with aspirin or nonsteroidal anti-inflammatory drugs. Chronic tension headaches are best managed with a tricyclic antidepressant, such as amitriptyline. Naproxen is a second drug of choice. Long-term use of analgesics or other drugs, such as muscle relaxants, antihistamines, tranquilizers, caffeine, and ergot alkaloids, should be avoided.

Tumors of the Central Nervous System

The incidence of primary brain tumor has risen approximately 25% in the past two decades—a rise that may be attributable to better detection.[18] No proven causative agents have been established for tumors of the central nervous system. Carcinogenesis is discussed in Chapter 11.

Cranial Tumors

Tumors within the cranium can be either primary or metastatic. Primary tumors are classified as primary intracerebral tumors or primary extracerebral tumors. Primary intracerebral tumors originate from brain substance, neuroglia, neurons, cells of the blood vessels, and connective tissue. Primary extracerebral tumors originate outside the substance of the brain and include meningiomas, acoustic nerve tumors, and tumors of the pituitary and pineal glands. Metastatic tumors, or secondary tumors, can be found inside or outside the brain substance. Sites of intracranial tumors are illustrated in Figure 17-21.

CNS tumors include both brain and spinal cord tumors. The incidence is 10 per 100,000 persons. This incidence seems to increase up to 70 years of age and then decreases. These tumors represent the second most common group of tumors in children. Approximately 70% of all intracranial tumors in children are located infratentorially, and in adults 70% to 75% are located supratentorially. Peripheral nerve tumors are rare in children and common in adults.

Cranial tumors cause local and generalized clinical manifestations. The local effects are caused by the destructive action of the tumor itself on a particular site in the brain and compression causing decreased cerebral blood flow. The effects are varied and include seizures, visual disturbances, unstable gait, and cranial nerve dysfunction. The generalized effects result from increased ICP (Figure 17-22). Increased ICP may occur because of obstruction of the ventricular system, hemorrhages occurring in and around the tumor, or cerebral edema caused by tumors.

Intracranial brain tumors do not metastasize as readily as tumors in other organs because there are no lymphatic channels within the brain substance. If metastasis does occur, it is usually through seeding of cerebral blood, through CSF, during cranial surgery, or through artificial shunts.

Primary Intracerebral Tumors

Primary intracerebral tumors, also called **gliomas,** comprise 50% to 60% of all adult brain tumors and are both encapsulated and nonencapsulated or invasive tumors (Table 17-11). Typically the invasive tumors invade and destroy adjacent normal CNS tissue, whereas more distal neural and vascular tissues are displaced and compressed, causing ischemia, edema, and increased ICP. Encapsulated tumors generally do not invade adjacent tissues but displace and compress adjacent and distal CNS tissues and vasculature. As

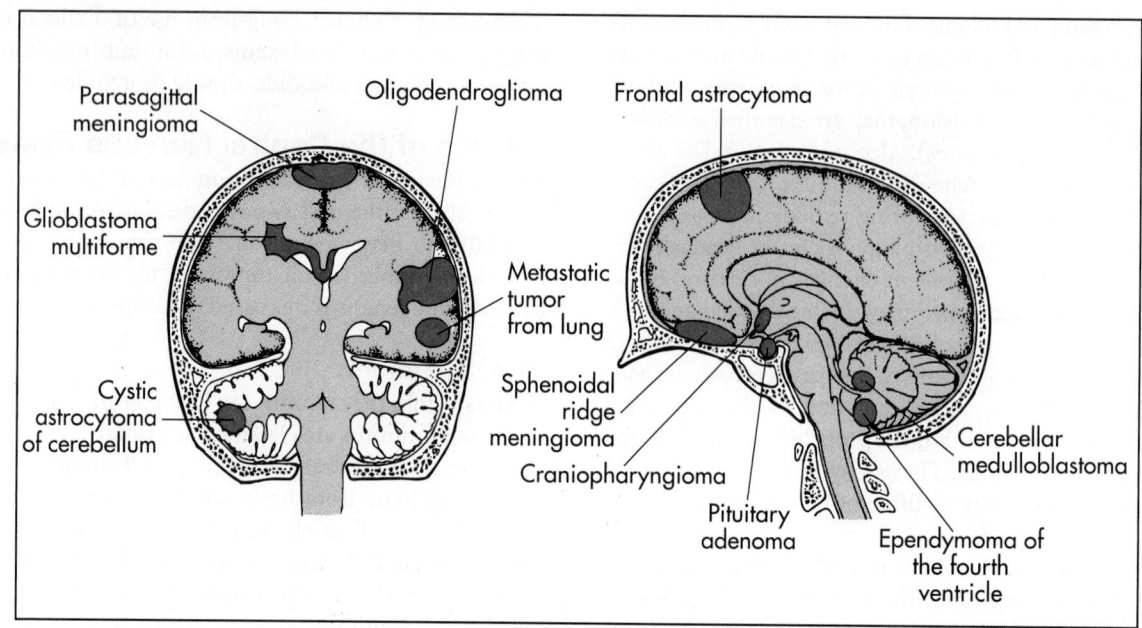

Figure 17-21 Common sites of intracranial tumors.

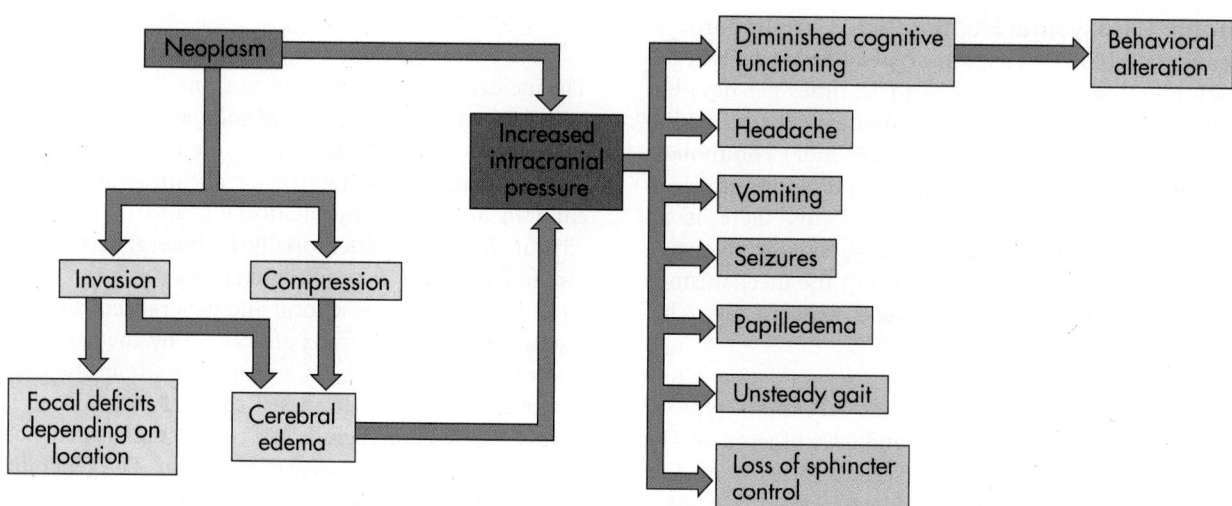

Figure 17-22 Origin of clinical manifestations associated with an intracranial neoplasm.

with invasive tumors, encapsulated tumors produce ischemia, edema, and increased pressure. Normal function of the neurons ultimately is impaired by the invasion or compression.

The principal treatment for cerebral tumors is surgical or radiosurgical excision or surgical decompression if total excision is not possible. Chemotherapy, radiation therapy, and hyperthermia also may be used. Supportive treatment is directed at reducing edema. (Cancer treatment is discussed in Chapter 11.)

Astrocytoma. Astrocytomas are the most common primary CNS tumors (50% of all brain and spinal cord tumors). Their etiology remains unknown, but environmental, occupational, and genetic factors are being studied. Multiple genetic alterations—chromosomal deletions, additions, dupli-

cations, mutations, and amplifications of specific genes—have been linked with these tumors in different stages of malignant progression. Some alterations are specific to certain types of astrocytomas. These tumors are more common in males than females. There are criteria for grading these tumors and two predominant classification systems (Table 17-12). Astrocytomas develop from astrocytes and grow by expansion and infiltration into the normal surrounding brain tissues. These tumor cells are believed to have lost normal growth restraint, and thus they proliferate uncontrollably.

One third of astrocytomas are classified at diagnosis as grade I or grade II astrocytoma. These slow-growing but infiltrative gliomas tend to form cavities (pseudocysts); however, some are firm, noncavitating, avascular, gray-white

Table 17-11   Brain and Spinal Cord Tumors

Neoplasm	Location	Characteristics	Cell of Origin
Gliomas			
Astrocytoma	Anywhere in brain or spinal cord	Slow growing, invasive	Astrocytes
Glioblastoma multiforme	Predominantly in cerebral hemispheres	Highly invasive and malignant	Thought to arise from mature astrocytes
Oligodendrocytoma	Most commonly in frontal lobes deep in white matter; may arise in brain stem, cerebellum, and spinal cord	Relatively avascular, tend to be encapsulated; more malignant form called an *oligodendroblastoma*	Oligodendrocytes
Ependymoma	Intramedullary: wall of the ventricles, may arise in caudal tail of spinal cord	More common in children, variable growth rates; more malignant, invasive form is called *ependymoblastoma;* may extend into ventricle or invade brain tissue	Ependymal cells
Neuronal Cell			
Medulloblastoma	Posterior cerebellar vermis, roof of fourth ventricle	Well demarcated, rapid growing, fills fourth ventricle	Embryonic cells
Mesodermal Tissue			
Meningioma	Intradural, extramedullary: sylvian fissure region, superior parasagittal surface of frontal and parietal lobes, olfactory groove, wing of sphenoid bone, superior surface of cerebellum, cerebellopontine angle, spinal cord	Slow growing, circumscribed, encapsulated, sharply demarcated from normal tissues, compressive in nature	Arachnoid cells, may be from fibroblast
Choroid Plexus			
Papillomas	Choroid plexus of ventricular system, lateral ventricle in children, fourth ventricle in adults	Usually benign, slow expansion inducing hemorrhage and hydrocephalus; malignant tumor is rare	Epithelial cells
Cranial Nerves and Spinal Nerve Roots			
Neurilemmoma	Cranial nerves (most commonly vestibular division of cranial nerve VIII)	Slow growing	Schwann cells
Neurofibroma	Extramedullary—spinal cord	Slow growing	Neurilemma, Schwann cells
Pituitary Tumors			
	Pituitary gland; may extend to or invade floor of the third ventricle	Age linked, several types, slow growing, macroadenomas and microadenomas	Pituitary cells, pituitary chromophobes, basophils, eosinophils
Germ Cell Tumors			
	Neurohypophysis, hypothalamus, pineal region	Rare, 0.5% of all primary brain tumors; primarily in adolescents; male>female; variable prognosis	Several types: germinoma, embryonal carcinoma, yolk sac tumor, choriocarcinoma, teratoma, mixed germ cell tumor; with different cell origins
Blood Vessel Tumors			
Angioma	Predominantly in posterior cerebral hemispheres	Slow growing	Arising from congenitally malformed arteriovenous connections
Hemangioblastomas	Predominantly in cerebellum	Slow growing	Embryonic vascular tissue

Table 17-12   Classification Systems for Astrocytomas

	Kernohan et al. System	Rigertz System	Criteria—Cellular Density, Atypia, Tumor Cell Mitosis
Astrocytoma		Well-differentiated astrocytoma	Increased number of cells
Grade I	Well-differentiated astrocytoma		Least malignant, grow slowly, near normal appearance under microscope
Grade II	More cellular and anaplastic astrocytoma		Abnormal appearance under a microscope, infiltrates, and may recur at a higher grade
Glioblastoma			
Grade III	Poorly differentiated astrocytoma	Malignant anaplastic astrocytoma	Malignant, many cells undergoing mitosis, infiltrates, and may recur at a higher grade
Grade IV	Poorly differentiated astrocytoma (glioblastoma multiforme)	Glioblastoma multiforme	Increased number of cells undergoing cell division, bizarre appearance under a microscope, widely infiltrates, neovascularization, central necrosis

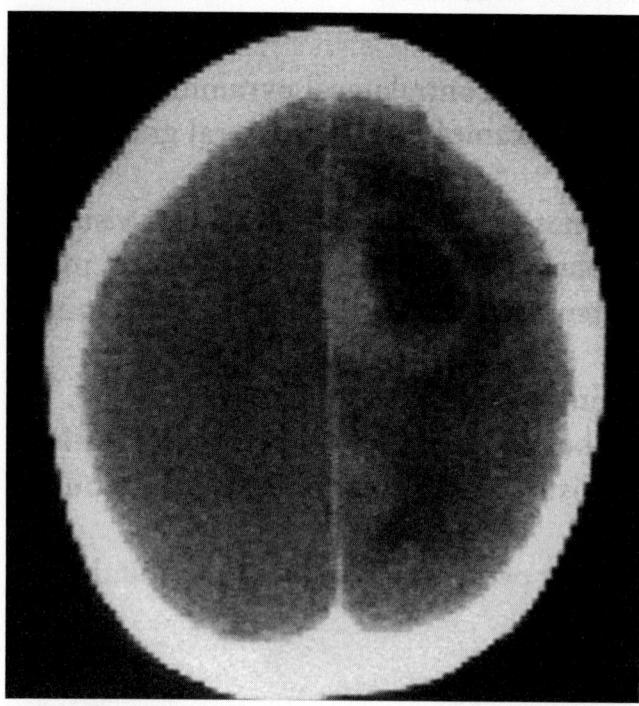

Figure 17-23 Computed tomography (CT) scan showing ring enhancement in a glioma. (From Perkin DG: *Mosby's color atlas and text of neurology,* London, 1998, Mosby-Wolfe.)

masses that are difficult to distinguish from normal white matter of the brain. Although these tumors may occur anywhere in the brain or spinal cord, they are located most commonly in the cerebrum, hypothalamus, or pons. Low-grade astrocytomas in adults tend to have a lateral or supratentorial location, and they tend to be midline or near midline in position in children, often in the posterior fossa.

Headache and subtle neurobehavioral changes may be an early symptom. Approximately half of persons with low-grade astrocytomas experience a focal or generalized seizure. Onset of a focal seizure disorder between the second and sixth

decades of life is suggestive of an astrocytoma. Other general or focal neurologic manifestations develop gradually. Increased ICP is usually a late clinical manifestation.

Grade I astrocytomas are treated with surgery and follow-up CT scans. Grade II astrocytomas are treated surgically if they are accessible or by conventional external radiation, local radiation, or stereotactic radiosurgery. Twenty-five percent of persons survive 5 years following surgery alone. Fifty percent of persons survive 5 years with surgery followed by radiotherapy.

Grades III and IV astrocytomas are found predominantly in the frontal lobes and cerebral hemispheres (Figure 17-23). These tumors also may be located in the brain stem (Figure 17-24), cerebellum, and spinal cord. They are found twice as frequently in men as in women. Grades III and IV astrocytomas are the third most common cancer in the 15 to 34 age group and the fourth most common in the 35 to 54 age group.[18] Grades III and IV astrocytomas are often large and well circumscribed with a variegated pattern. The peripheral rim is pinkish gray and solid with a soft, yellow, necrotic center and points of hemorrhage. Microscopically, there is increased cellularity, vascular proliferation, cellular pleomorphism, and necrosis. Necrosis is the principal histologic difference between an anaplastic grade III tumor and a grade IV glioblastoma multiforme.

Grade IV astrocytomas (glioblastoma multiforme) are highly vascular and extensively infiltrative. They may become large enough to extend from the meningeal surface through the ventricular wall. Fifty percent of glioblastomas are bilateral or at least occupy more than one lobe at the time of death. There are increasing reports of grade IV astrocytomas found outside the central nervous system.[18]

The typical clinical presentation for a glioblastoma multiforme is that of diffuse, nonspecific clinical manifestations, such as headache, irritability, and personality changes, that progress to more clear-cut manifestations of increased ICP, such as headache on position change; papilledema; or vomit-

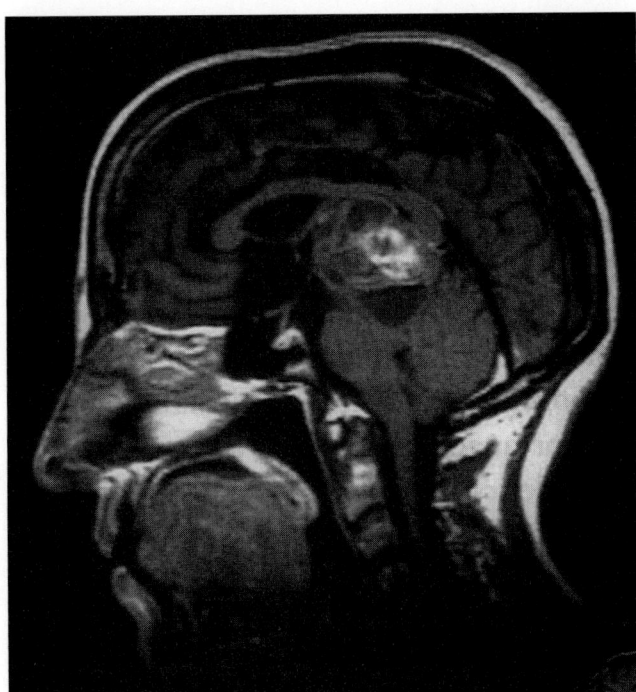

Figure 17-24 Magnetic resonance imaging (MRI) with gadolinium showing a high brain stem glioma. (From Perkin DG: *Mosby's color atlas and text of neurology,* London, 1998, Mosby-Wolfe.)

ing. Of persons affected, 30% to 40% experience seizure activity. Symptoms may progress to definite focal signs, such as hemiparesis, dysphasia, dyspraxia, cranial nerve palsies, and visual field deficits, in addition to the generalized signs from increased ICP.

Diagnosis of high-grade astrocytomas most commonly takes 3 to 6 months from onset of the first clinical manifestations because the person does not recognize the need to consult a health care provider.

Grade III astrocytomas are treated with surgery if they are accessible; radiotherapy; and chemotherapy possibly before, during, and after other therapies. Chemotherapy is given in cycles. With treatment, approximately 55% to 60% of persons with grade III astrocytomas survive 1 year, 30% to 35% survive 2 years, and 10% survive longer than 5 years. Grade IV gliomas are also treated with surgery if accessible, radiotherapy and chemotherapy, or placement of wafers. The median survival rate is 1 year.[18]

Oligodendroglioma. A far less commonly occurring glioma is **oligodendroglioma,** comprising 2% of all brain tumors and 10% to 15% of all gliomas. Oligodendrogliomas are typically slow-growing, well-differentiated tumors, often with cysts and calcification present. Most are macroscopically indistinguishable from other gliomas. They occur most commonly in persons 30 to 50 years of age and are more common in males than females. Their etiology is unknown. Most oligodendrogliomas are found in the frontal and temporal lobes, often in deep white matter. Twenty percent are in both hemispheres. They may be found also in other parts of the cerebrum, third ventricle, brain stem, cerebellum, and spinal

cord. A high incidence of this tumor is found in young adults with a history of temporal lobe epilepsy. Approximately half of these tumors generally classified as oligodendrogliomas are actually a mixed type of oligodendroglioma and astrocytoma. Malignant degeneration occurs in approximately one third of persons with oligodendrogliomas; the tumors are then referred to as **oligodendroblastomas.** The tumor rarely becomes a glioblastoma. If there is extension to the pia mater or ependymal wall (see Figure 14-14), oligodendrogliomas may metastasize to distant CNS sites through the ventriculoarachnoid spaces.

More than 50% of individuals experience a focal or generalized seizure as the first clinical manifestation. Approximately half of persons with an oligodendroglioma have experienced increased ICP at the time of diagnosis and surgery, and only one third develop any focal manifestations. The time from first clinical manifestation to surgical intervention often ranges from 2 to 6 years. Treatment options are surgery; radiotherapy (conventional external beam or stereotactic gamma knife and converged beam); and chemotherapy before, during, and after radiation. Median survival, when surgery and radiotherapy are both used, is 5 to 10 years.[18]

Ependymoma. **Ependymomas** are gliomas that arise from ependymal cells that form the walls of the ventricles and grow either into the ventricle or into adjacent brain tissue; they are not encapsulated (Figure 17-25 and see Table 17-12). They comprise 6% of all primary brain tumors in adults and 10% in children and adolescents. Among children and adolescents, 50% of those affected are under 5 years of age. Seventy percent of ependymomas occur in the fourth ventricle (i.e., in the posterior fossa) and manifest as difficulty with balance, unsteady gait, uncoordinated muscle movement, and difficulty with fine motor skills. Other common sites for ependymomas are the third ventricle, lateral ventricles, and

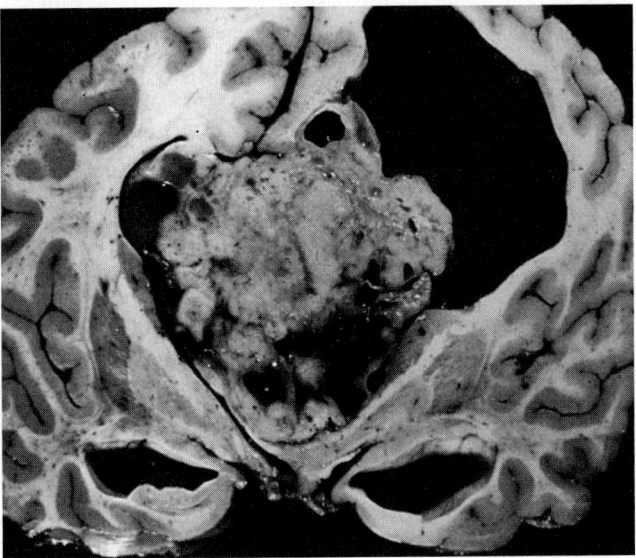

Figure 17-25 Large septal ependymoma. Note secondary hydrocephalus. (Courtesy Dr. JE Olivera-Rabiela, Mexico City, Mexico. From Rosai J: *Ackerman's surgical pathology,* ed 7, St Louis, 1989, Mosby.)

caudal portion of the spinal cord. The clinical presentation of a lateral and third ventricle ependymoma that involves the cerebral hemispheres is seizures, visual changes, and contralateral weakness of a body part or one side of the body. Approximately 40% of infratentorial ependymomas occur in children younger than 10 years. Occurrence of cerebral (supratentorial) ependymomas is distributed among all ages but more common in adults. Etiology for these tumors is unknown.

Blockage of the CSF pathway by the tumor clinically results in the presence of headache, nausea, and vomiting related to the hydrocephalus produced. Brain stem or upper spinal cord ependymomas may cause neck pain as well.

Clinical manifestations and progression of dysfunction associated with ependymomas may follow a short or long course. The interval between first manifestations and surgery may be as short as 4 weeks with some ependymoblastomas to as long as 7 to 8 years with others.

Ependymomas are treated surgically and with radiotherapy of the tumor region and operative site (possibly of the entire brain and spine); stereotactic radiosurgery focused on eradication; and chemotherapy. Between 20% and 50% of persons survive 5 years. Some persons benefit from a shunting procedure when the ependymoma has caused a noncommunicating hydrocephalus (see Chapter 16).

Primary Extracerebral Tumors

Meningioma. **Meningioma** constitutes 15% of all intracranial tumors. The peak incidence is the fifth and seventh decades, with a 2:1 female/male ratio. Meningiomas are considered benign because they are encapsulated and usually do not invade the surrounding brain (Figure 17-26). These tumors originate from the dura mater or arachnoid membranes. Rarely do meningiomas arise from arachnoid cells of the choroid plexus of the ventricles. Meningiomas most commonly are located in the olfactory grooves, on the wings of the sphenoid bone (at the base of the skull), in the tuberculum sellae (a structure next to the sella turcica), on the superior surface of the cerebellum, and in the cerebellopontine angle and spinal cord. Loss of chromosome 22 has been isolated.

Small meningiomas (less than 2 cm in diameter) often are found on postmortem examination in middle-aged and elderly individuals who had experienced no clinical manifestations and died of totally unrelated causes. The cause of meningiomas is unknown. A meningioma is a sharply circumscribed mass that derives its shape from the space it occupies. A meningioma may extend to the dural surface and erode the cranial bones or produce an osteoblastic reaction. A few meningiomas exhibit malignant, invasive qualities.

Only when meningiomas reach a certain size—at which time they begin to indent the brain parenchyma—do they begin to produce clinical manifestations. Focal seizures are frequently the first manifestation. Other clinical manifestations depend on the tumor's location. Clinical features based on site of origin are as follows:

1. *Sphenoidal wing:* ophthalmoplegia, mild proptosis, and involvement of the ophthalmic division of the trigeminal nerve

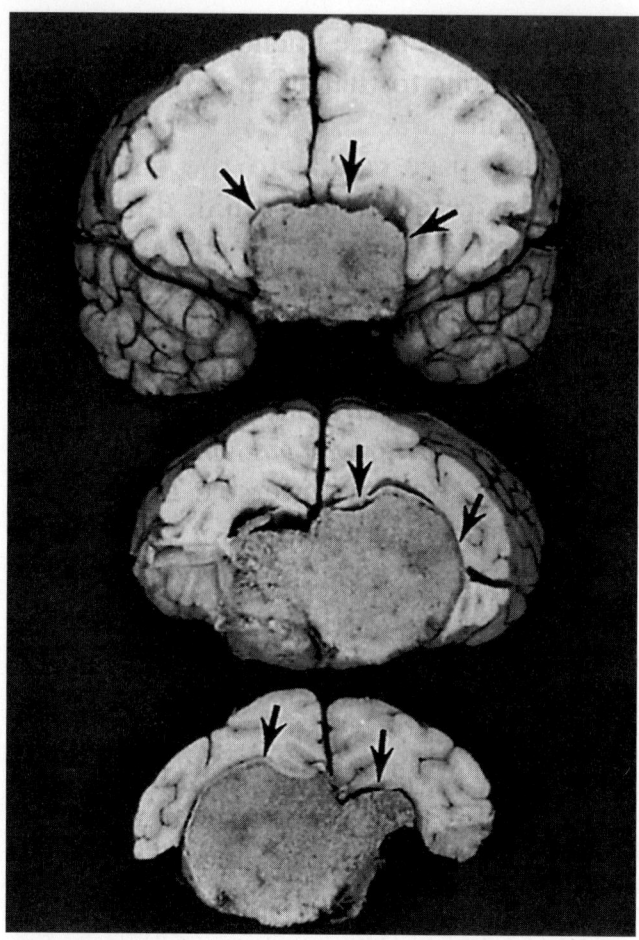

Figure 17-26 Large olfactory groove meningioma. Note that this tumor has significantly compressed (*arrows*) but not invaded the brain tissue in these sequential slices through the frontal lobe. (Courtesy Dr. Jonathan Fratkin, University of Mississippi Medical Center. From Haines DE, editor: *Fundamental neuroscience,* Philadelphia, 1997, Churchill Livingstone.)

2. *Olfactory groove:* anosmia, personality change, and visual failure
3. *Parasagittal:* focal seizures of a focal motor or sensory deficit
4. *Parasellar:* evidence of chiasmatic compression; urinary incontinence; dementia; gradual paraparesis, including hormonal failure; optic atrophy; biemporal hemianopia
5. *Lateral* convexity: variable depending on structures compressed, including slow hemiparesis, speech abnormalities[18]

Because of the extremely slow-growing nature of most meningiomas, increased ICP is less common than with gliomas.

With complete surgical excision of the tumor and its meningeal stem, the recurrence rate is still 20%. Sometimes only partial resection is possible. Radiotherapy is used to slow the tumor growth.

Nerve Sheath Tumors. Nerve sheath tumors are either neurofibroma or schwannoma (neuroma, neurolemma). Neurofibromatosis is an inherited autosomal dominant disorder. The gene for type 1 is located on chromosome 17 and the gene for type 2 is on chromosome 22. Criteria for the diagnosis of neurofibromatosis types 1 and 2 are presented in Box 17-2. Only 5% of all neuromas are attributable to neurfibromatosis; the remainder are benign tumors that arise from the sheath of Schwann cells surrounding the axons of the cranial nerves. The tumors most commonly affect persons older than 50 years of age, and women are affected more often than men. The vestibular division of cranial nerve VIII is most commonly affected, although neuroma of the acoustic division of cranial nerves VIII, V, VII, and IX are found (Figure 17-27).

The tumor originates most commonly just distal to the junction between the nerve root and the brain stem. As the tumor grows, it extends into the posterior fossa to occupy the cerebropontine angle and compress adjacent nerves. Eventually the brain stem is displaced, and the CSF flow is obstructed.

Initial clinical manifestations may include headache, tinnitus, hearing loss, impaired balance, unsteady gait, facial pain, and loss of facial sensations. Later, vertigo with nausea and vomiting, a sense of pressure in the ear, and moderate to severe unsteadiness with rapid position changes may appear. CT scan or MRI can establish the diagnosis. Posterior fossa dye studies may be required. Treatment is by surgical excision and radiotherapy of the neuroma. Pituitary tumors are discussed in Chapter 21, and cerebral tumors in children are discussed in Chapter 19.

Metastatic Carcinoma. An estimated 25% of persons with cancer develop metastasis to the brain. One half of metastatic brain tumors arise from the lung, approximately one sixth from the breast, 13% from melanomas, and 4% from the kidney. Carcinoma of the gallbladder, liver, thyroid, testes, uterus, ovary, and pancreas also may metastasize to the brain. Other tumors, besides carcinomas, that metastasize only occasionally are rhabdomyosarcomas, Ewing tumors, chorioepithelioma, and lymphoma.

Carcinomas are disseminated to the brain from the circulation. Two thirds of metastatic tumors are located within the brain and one third are located in extradural spaces. The cerebral hemispheres are the site of 75% of metastases, most predominantly in the frontal lobes followed by the parietal, occipital, and temporal lobes in order of frequency of location.

Tumors of the pelvis or retroperitoneal space have a predilection to metastasize to the cerebellum, pons, or their coverings.[19] In more than three fourths of persons with metastasis, the metastases are multiple and found in both the cerebrum and cerebellum in a scattered distribution. The metastatic tumors often are located in the meninges and near the brain surface in the gray matter and subcortical white matter. These tumors produce little glial cell reaction in the brain tissue but do cause vasogenic edema in the surrounding brain tissue.

The clinical manifestation of a metastatic brain tumor usually resembles that of a glioblastoma, although several unusual syndromes do exist. Carcinomatous encephalopathy causes headache, nervousness, depressed mood, trembling, confusion, and forgetfulness. In carcinomatosis of the cerebellum, headache, dizziness, and ataxia are found. Carcinomatosis of the craniospinal meninges (carcinomatous

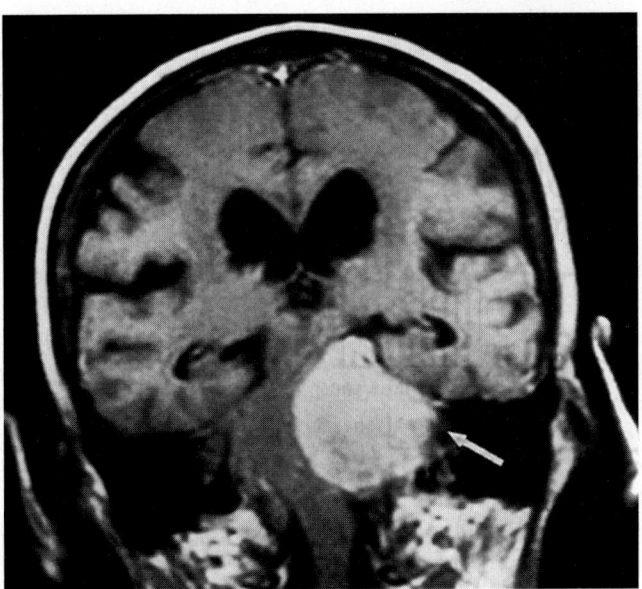

Figure 17-27 Magnetic resonance imaging (MRI) of an acoustic neuroma (neurilemmoma) of cerebellopontine angle involving the vestibular division of CN VIII. Individual complained of dizziness, nausea, and spatial disorientation. (From Haines DE, editor: *Fundamental neuroscience,* Philadelphia, 1997, Churchill Livingstone.)

Box 17-2   Criteria for Diagnosis of Neurofibromatosis Types 1 and 2

Criteria for the Diagnosis of NF-1
Two of the following eight criteria
- Six café-au-lait spots over 15 mm in diameter (adults)
- Multiple axillary or inguinal freckles
- One plexiform neurofibroma or two or more neurofibromas of other types
- Optic nerve or chiasmatic glioma
- Lisch iris nodules (two or more)
- Thinning of the cortex of long bones
- Sphenoid dysplasia
- A first-degree relative with NF-1

Criteria for the Diagnosis of NF-2
Any one of the three criteria below
- Bilateral VIIIth nerve tumors (as determined by CT or MRI)
- Unilateral VIIIth nerve tumor and first-degree relative with NF-2
- Any two of the following plus first-degree relative with NF-2
  a. Plexiform neurofibroma
  b. Neurofibroma of another type
  c. Meningioma
  d. Glioma
  e. Schwannoma
  f. Presenile posterior cataract

From Perkin GD: *Mosby's color atlas and text of neurology,* 1998, London, Mosby—Wolfe.
NF, Neurofibromatosis; *CT,* computed tomography; *MRI,* magnetic resonance imaging.

meningitis) manifests with headache, confusion, and manifestations of cranial or spinal nerve root dysfunction.

MRI with gadolinium as contrast medium is the most sensitive imaging procedure for metastatic brain tumors. Prognosis is poor. If a solitary tumor is found, surgical excision is indicated. Radiotherapy is commonly used to treat solitary as well as multiple tumors. Chemotherapy is increasingly becoming part of the treatment plan.[19]

Spinal Cord Tumors

Spinal cord tumors are relatively rare. The most common primary spine tumors are listed in Box 17-3 and shown in Figure 17-28. Spinal cord tumors are named to reflect their cell type, growth rate, and structure of origin. Spinal cord tumors are classified as **intramedullary tumors** (originating within the neural tissues) or **extramedullary tumors** (originating from tissues outside the spinal cord). Extramedullary tumors arise from the meninges or roots (forming **intradural tumors**) or from epidural tissue or vertebral structure (forming **extradural tumors**). About 5% of spinal cord tumors seen in general hospital settings are intramedullary, 40% are intradural-extramedullary, and 55% are extradural.

The axial skeleton is the third most common site for metastasis behind lung and liver metastasis. Metastatic spinal cord tumors are three to four times more common than primary spinal cord tumors. They are usually carcinomas from breast, lung, and prostate; lymphomas; or myelomas. Twenty-five percent to 70% involve the vertebral body and are asymptomatic. Metastatic spinal cord tumors are extradural in location. Of extradural tumors, 50% are metastatic and have spread to the spine through direct extension from tumors of the vertebral structures or from extraspinal sources extending through the interventricular foramen or through the bloodstream.

The most common primary extramedullary spinal cord tumors are neurofibromas and meningiomas. These tumors are intradural more often than extradural. Neurofibromas are found most commonly in the thoracic and lumbar regions. Meningiomas are more evenly distributed throughout the spine. Other extramedullary tumors in order of frequency of occurrence are sarcomas, vascular tumors, chordomas, and epidermoid and similar tumors. Of intradural-extramedullary tumors, 70% are meningiomas, neurofibromas, or sarcomas.

Box 17-3   Most Common Primary Spine Tumors

Benign Tumors
Osteoid osteoma/osteoblastoma
Giant cell tumors
Hemangiomas
Aneurysmal bone cyst

Malignant Tumors
Chondrosarcoma
Chordoma
Ewing sarcoma
Osteoarcoma

Intramedullary tumors have the same cellular origins as brain tumors. Ependymomas account for 40% of intramedullary spinal cord tumors. Astrocytomas, glioblastomas, oligodendrogliomas, ganglioneuromas, medulloblastomas, hemangiomas, and hemangioblastomas are more or less equally distributed in frequency of occurrence.

PATHOPHYSIOLOGY   Extramedullary spinal cord tumors produce dysfunction by compression of adjacent tissue, not by direct invasion. The spinal cord is compressed by the tumor from without, and destruction of the white matter tracts occurs. The spinal canal around the cord becomes filled by tumor.

Intramedullary spinal cord tumors produce dysfunction by both invasion and compression. The cord enlarges as a result of the tumor that is enlarging inside the cord. In addition, distortion of adjacent white matter tracts occurs. Metastases from spinal cord tumors occur from seeding through the CSF; medulloblastomas and ependymomas establish distant implants in this manner.

CLINICAL MANIFESTATIONS   The acute onset of clinical manifestations suggests a vascular insult caused by thrombosis of vessels supplying the spinal cord. Clinical manifestations that are gradual and progressive suggest compres-

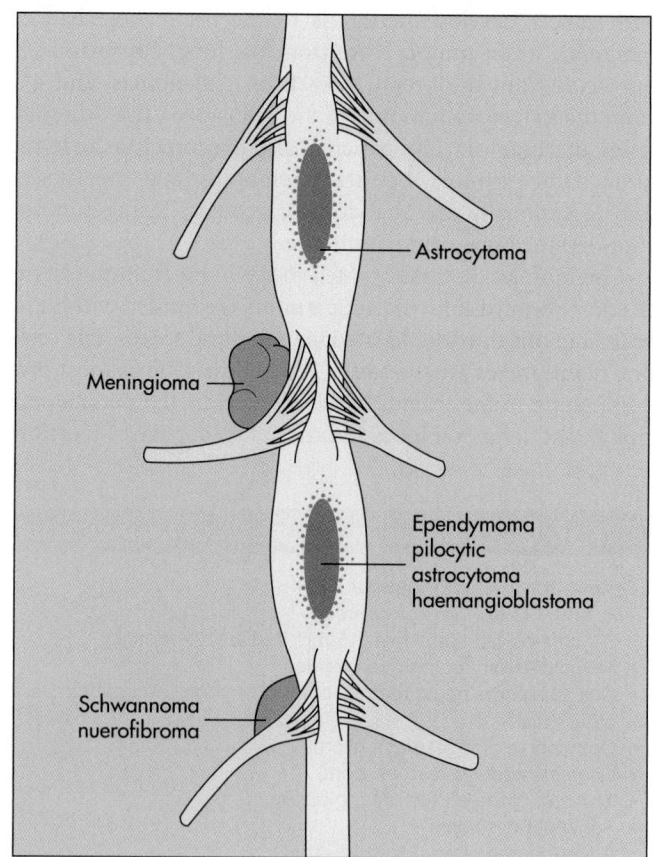

Figure 17-28 Distribution of some spinal tumors. (From Perkin DG: *Mosby's color atlas and text of neurology,* London, 1998, Mosby-Wolfe.)

sion. The clinical manifestations associated with spinal cord tumors fall into three major categories: (1) a compressive syndrome (sensorimotor syndrome), (2) an irritative syndrome (radicular syndrome), and rarely (3) a syringomyelic syndrome.

The **compressive syndrome (sensorimotor syndrome)** is associated with compression and is caused less frequently by invasion and destruction of the spinal cord tracts. Symptoms are usually gradual and progressive, and initial manifestations may be asymmetric. With tumors located in the cervical area, the motor dysfunction usually has the following pattern: ipsilateral arm involvement, followed by ipsilateral and contralateral leg involvement, and finally involvement of the opposite arm. With thoracic tumors the pattern of motor involvement is paresis and spasticity of one leg, followed by involvement of the opposite leg. The sensory clinical manifestations of tingling paresthesias have a pattern similar to that of the motor signs. Pain and temperature dysfunctions are found more commonly than touch, vibration, and proprioceptive changes, although posterior column signs also are found frequently. Pain is less well localized than with an irritative syndrome caused by root involvement. Initially the pain and temperature changes are contralateral to the motor deficit (Brown-Séquard syndrome). Bladder and bowel deficits usually appear when paresis develops in the legs.

The **irritative syndrome (radicular syndrome)** combines the clinical manifestations of a cord compression with radicular pain, which is pain in the sensory root distribution and indicates root irritation. The segmental manifestations associated with root irritation include segmental sensory changes that include paresthesias and impaired pain and touch perception; motor disturbances, including cramps, atrophy, fasciculations, and decreased or absent deep tendon reflexes; and ache in the spine. Tenderness of the spinous processes over the tumor is present in about one half of persons with extramedullary tumors. The segmental changes may appear months and sometimes years before the clinical manifestations of compression in benign tumors. The compressive clinical manifestations include an asymmetric spastic paresis of the lower extremities with tumors in the thoracic or lumbar region, paresis of the arms and legs with tumors in the cervical area, decreased or absent pain and temperature perception below the tumor site, posterior column signs, and spastic bladder.

Because they involve the central gray matter of the cord, intramedullary spinal cord tumors (notably ependymomas) may produce a **syringomyelic syndrome,** or inflammation of the spinal cord. Inflammation results in the development of tubular (syrinx) cavities in the spinal cord. Occasionally an extramedullary tumor may produce the same effect, although the mechanisms are unknown.

EVALUATION AND TREATMENT The diagnosis of a spinal cord tumor is made through bone scan, needle biopsy guided by CT and positron emission tomography (PET), or open biopsy. Benign or malignant spinal tumor staging may

be done (Box 17-4). Involvement of specific cord segments is established.

Treatment varies, depending on the nature of the tumor and the patient's clinical status. Indications for surgery include establishing a tissue diagnosis, neurologic palliation, spinal stabilization, pain relief, and cancer therapy. Surgical resection may involve curettage (piecemeal removal of the tumor) or may be performed en bloc (removal of tumor in one piece). Surgical approaches to the spine include posterior approach (decompression laminectomy), lateral approach, anterior approach (most favored), and combined approaches. Posterior and anterior reconstructive surgery may be necessary. Oncologic surgical procedures are classified as intralesional, marginal, wide excision, or radical excision. Indications for external radiation versus surgery are a radiosensitive tumor (e.g., lymphoma), soft tissue compression without instability, a patient who is a poor surgical candidate, paraplegia or advanced paraparesis of greater than 24 hours duration, and an expected survival of less than 3 to 4 months. Chemotherapy, hormonal therapy, and pain management protocols may be appropriate.

Infection and Inflammation of the Central Nervous System

The CNS may be affected directly by bacteria, viruses, fungi, protozoans, and rickettsiae. Neurologic infections produce disease by several mechanisms: direct neuronal or glial infection; mass lesions formation; inflammation with subsequent edema, interruption of cerebrospinal fluid pathways, neuronal damage, or vasculopathy; and secretion of neurotoxins. The cardinal signs of CNS infection are fever, head or spine pain, and generalized or focal neurological dysfunction.[20]

Box 17-4	Spinal Tumor Staging

Benign Spine Tumor Staging

S1	Latent, inactive, asymptomatic, are bordered by a true capsule, often confined to vertebra
S2	Active, slowly growing, mildly asymptomatic, has thin capsule and layer of reactive tissue
S3	Aggressive, rapidly growing; often symptomatic; capsule very thin, incomplete, or absent; often invades neighboring compartments

Malignant Tumor Staging

Low grade malignant: both 1A and 1B have no true capsule, but a thick pseudocapsule of reactive tissue with islands of tumor

Stage 1A	Tumor remains inside of vertebra (intracompartmental)
Stage 1B	Tumor outside of vertebra

High grade malignant: rapid growth with continuous seeding nodules

Stage IIA	Inside vertebra with skip nodules present
Stage IIB	Outside of vertebra
Stage IIIA and IIIB	Metastatic high grade intra- and extracompartmental

Meningitis

Meningitis (infection of the meninges) may be caused by bacteria, viruses, fungi, parasites, or other toxins. The infections are classified as acute, subacute, or chronic processes, and the pathophysiology, clinical manifestations, and treatment differ for each type of microorganism.

Bacterial meningitis is primarily an infection of the pia mater and arachnoid, the subarachnoid space, the ventricular system, and the CSF. A systemic or bloodstream infection or a direct extension from an infected area is the access route to the subarachnoid space. The bacterial infection originates in another part of the body. The incidence of bacterial meningitis is 2.5 to 3.5 cases per 100,000 people. The incidence is 20 per 100,000 annually for neonates, and 2 to 9 per 100,000 annually for persons over 60 years of age. The mortality is 25% in adults. Meningococcus *(Neisseria meningitidis)* and pneumococcus *(Streptococcus pneumoniae)* are the common causes of bacterial meningitis after the neonatal period. Pneumococcus and gram-negative enteric bacilli are the most common neonatal agents.

Meningococcus has been identified worldwide. Meningococcal meningitis occurs predominantly in men and boys and during the fall, winter, and spring of the year. Epidemics of meningococcal meningitis occur in approximately 10-year cycles. Children and adolescents are affected predominantly. With pneumococcal meningitis, young persons and those older than 40 years are mostly affected.

Aseptic meningitis (viral meningitis, nonpurulent meningitis, lymphocytic meningitis) is an inflammation believed to be limited to the meninges. The most at-risk populations and the time of year when occurrences are seen depends on the virus. Aseptic meningitis produces a variety of symptoms and is caused by a variety of infectious agents, most of which are viruses. They include enteroviral viruses (echovirus, coxsackievirus, and nonparalytic poliomyelitis), mumps, herpes simplex types 1 and 2, St. Louis encephalitis virus, West Nile virus, California encephalitis virus, Venezuelan equine encephalitis, Colorado tick fever, lymphocytic choriomengitis virus, Epstein-Barré virus, and influenza virus types A and B.[20] Bacterial infections not adequately treated are another cause of aseptic meningitis.

Fungal meningitis is a chronic, much less common condition than bacterial or viral meningitis. The most common fungal infections of the nervous system are histoplasmosis, cryptococcosis, coccidioidomycosis, mucormycosis, candidiasis, and aspergillosis. Fungal meningitis most frequently occurs in persons with impaired immune responses or alterations in normal body flora. Fungal meningitis develops insidiously, usually over days or weeks. Syphilis, tuberculosis, and Lyme disease also are associated with a chronic meningitis.

Tubercular (TB) meningitis, the most common and serious form of CNS tuberculosis, is again on the rise in the United States, especially in persons with acquired immunodeficiency syndrome (AIDS). Miliary tubercles form in the brain and meninges. At some point, the tuberculomas erode the pia mater, and the mycobacteria enter the CSF, producing a hypersensitivity reaction resulting in a purulent exudate involving the basal meninges, cerebrum, and spinal nerves. Cerebral ischemia and infarction occurs from vasculitis. Symptoms include headache, low-grade fever, nausea and vomiting, irritability, difficulty sleeping, and fatigue. These signs and symptoms increase to confusion, stiff neck, significant behavioral changes, and seizures. Hydrocephalus and cranial nerve palsies or cerebral infarcts may occur. Recovery rate is 90% with early diagnosis and treatment with appropriate antituberculosis therapy.

PATHOPHYSIOLOGY The bacteria that commonly cause bacterial meningitis are common inhabitants of the nasopharynx, but a predisposing factor such as a prior upper respiratory infection must be present before the bacteria become blood-borne. Bacterial meningitis also may develop as a consequence of ear, dental, or paraspinal infections; impairment in the anatomic barrier from trauma or neurosurgery; and, rarely, when a brain abscess ruptures into the ventricular system or subarachnoid space.[20] The method of CNS entry is through the choroid plexuses or areas of altered blood-brain barrier. Bacteria multiply in the subarachnoid space. The bacteria or their toxins function as irritants and induce an inflammatory reaction by the meninges (pia mater and arachnoid), the CSF, and the ventricles. The meningeal vessels undergo change, becoming hyperemic and increasingly permeable. Blood cells (neutrophils) migrate into the subarachnoid space, producing an exudate that thickens the CSF and interferes with normal CSF flow around the brain and spinal cord (Figure 17-29). The exudate has the potential to obstruct arachnoid villi and produce hydrocephalus and interstitial edema. The amount of purulent exudate increases rapidly (especially around the base of the brain), causing further inflammation. The exudate extends into the sheaths of the cranial and spinal nerves and into the perivascular spaces of the cortex. Meningeal cells become edematous. The exudate and vasogenic edema increase ICP. The small and medium-sized

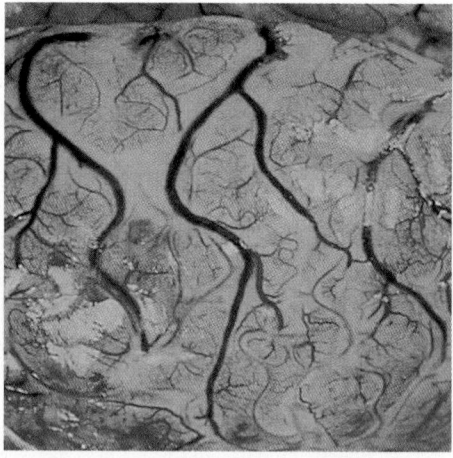

Figure 17-29 **Bacterial meningitis.** Lateral surface of the cerebral hemisphere showing a purulent exudate. (From Perkin DG: *Mosby's color atlas and text of neurology,* St Louis, 1998, Mosby-Wolfe.)

subarachnoid arteries, veins, and choroid plexuses undergo inflammatory changes and become engorged, disrupting blood flow and potentially producing thrombosis. Secondary infection of the brain may occur. The cortical neurons also show some changes, including an increase in the number of microglia and astrocytes.

Fungi in the nervous system usually produce a granulomatous reaction with formations of granulomas or gelatinous masses. These usually develop in the meninges at the base of the brain. Fungi also may extend along the perivascular sites in the subarachnoid space and into the brain tissue, producing arteritis with thrombosis, infarction, and communicating hydrocephalus. Meningeal fibrosis develops later in the inflammatory process. Cranial nerve dysfunction, caused by compression, often results from the granulomas and fibrosis.

CLINICAL MANIFESTATIONS   The clinical manifestations of a bacterial meningitis can be grouped into meningeal signs and neurologic signs. Those clinical manifestations of systemic infection include fever, tachycardia, chills, and petechial rash. The clinical manifestations that arise from the meningeal irritation are a generalized throbbing headache that becomes very severe, photophobia that becomes severe, nuchal rigidity, Kernig sign, and Brudzinski sign. The neurologic signs include a decrease in consciousness, cranial nerve palsies, focal neurologic deficits (such as hemiparesis/hemiplegia and ataxia), and seizures. The irritation and damage to the cranial nerves produced by the inflamed sheaths manifest as follows:

Cranial nerve II: papilledema, blindness
Cranial nerves III, IV, and VI: ptosis, visual field deficits, diplopia
Cranial nerve V: photophobia
Cranial nerve VII: facial paresis
Cranial nerve VIII: deafness, tinnitus, vertigo

Neck stiffness and pain, and possibly head retraction, reflect the irritability of spinal accessory and cervical spinal nerves. Often the vomiting center is irritated, causing projectile vomiting. Confusion and decreasing responsiveness are evidence of cortical involvement. In meningococcal meningitis, petechial or purpuric rash involving the skin and mucous membranes occurs. As ICP increases, papilledema may develop and delirium may progress to the point that the individual reaches an unconscious state.

The signs and symptoms of bacterial meningitis in neonates are subtle and nonspecific. Low grade fever and mild behavioral changes with few meningeal signs may be the first signs. High fever, lethargy, irritability, hypothermia, seizures, bulging fontanels, poor feeding, vomiting, and respiratory distress may be present. Children may present with either a subacute infection that worsens over several days following an ear infection or upper respiratory infection (URI), or as an acute fulminant illness that has developed rapidly over a few hours. Elders often develop low-grade fever with confusion or other mild behavioral changes. Stupor or coma may appear later.

The clinical manifestations of aseptic meningitis are mild compared with those associated with bacterial meningitis. Mild generalized throbbing headache, mild photophobia, mild neck pain, stiffness, fever, and malaise are all manifestations of aseptic meningitis.

Fungal meningitis develops slowly and insidiously. The first manifestations are often those of dementia or communicating hydrocephalus (see Chapter 16). The individual is characteristically afebrile.

EVALUATION AND TREATMENT   Diagnosis of bacterial meningitis is based on physical examination, including skin rash, nasopharyngeal smear, and antigen tests. CSF is the gold standard for diagnosis. Bacterial meningitis and fungal meningitis are treated with appropriate antibiotic therapy, but resistant strains are becoming an increasing problem. Other supportive measures may be needed. Aseptic meningitis is managed pharmacologically with antiviral drugs and steroids. Vaccinations exist for meningococcal, pneumococcal, and hemophilic meningitis. Chemoprophylaxis for persons exposed to meningococcal meningitis is rifampin.

Suppurative Cerebral Masses

Localized pus-filled masses can develop with the CNS. The mass may be an abscess within the brain or spinal cord, a subdural empyema with the infection between the dura and the subarachnoid space, or an epidural abscess with the infection between the dura and skull or vertebrae. The latter two occur less commonly but have similar predisposing conditions, infectious agents, and clinical manifestations. Treatments are also similar. Subdural empyemas and epidural abscess generally spread locally from infections in an adjoining structure.

Abscess

Abscesses are localized collections of pus within the parenchyma of the brain and spinal cord. The incidence of abscesses is about 1 per 100,000 hospital admissions. Men experience abscesses more frequently than women, with a 2:1 ratio. The median age for abscess formation is 30 to 40 years of age. Abscesses occur (1) after open trauma and during neurosurgery; (2) in association with a contiguous focus of infection, such as the middle ear, mastoid cells, nasal cavity, and nasal sinuses; (3) through metastatic or hematogenous spread from distant foci, such as the heart, lungs, pelvic organs, skin, tonsils, abscessed teeth, osteomyelitis in other than cranial bones, and dirty needles (especially in compromised hosts); and (4) cryptogenically, arising without other associated areas of infections. Streptococci, staphylococci, and bacteroids, often in combination with anaerobes, are the most common bacteria that cause abscesses; however, yeast and fungi also have been found in CNS abscesses. *Toxoplasma gondii* is producing an ever-increasing number of CNS abscesses in persons with AIDS. Eighty percent of abscesses are located in the cerebrum, and 20% are cerebellar. The frontal and temporal lobes are the most common sites. The abscesses are in more than one site in 5% to 20% of cases. Immunosuppressed persons are particularly at risk for abscesses.

Spinal cord abscesses are classified as epidural or intramedullary. Debilitated individuals with sepsis more frequently develop **intramedullary spinal cord abscesses** (those within the spinal cord).

PATHOPHYSIOLOGY Microorganisms gain entrance to the CNS from adjacent sites by direct extension from osteomyelitis or spread along the wall of a vein. Infective emboli carry the microorganisms from distant sites. Brain abscess evolves through four stages regardless of infecting microorganism except in the immunosuppressed host where the process may be incomplete. The stages are as follows:

1. *Early cerebritis* (days 1 to 3): localized inflammatory process seen where perivascular infiltration or inflammatory cells, composed of neutrophils, plasma cells, and mononuclear cells, surround a central core of coagultive necrosis; marked cerebral edema surrounds the area
2. *Late cerebritis* (days 4 to 9): necrotic center is surrounded by inflammatory infiltrate of macrophages and fibroblasts; rapid new blood vessel formation occurs around the abscess; a thin capsule of fibroblasts and reticular fibers gradually develops; the area is still surrounded by cerebral edema
3. *Early capsule formation* (days 10 to 13): necrotic center decreases in size; inflammatory infiltrate changes in character and contains an increasing number of fibroblasts and macrophages; mature collagen evolves forming a capsule
4. *Late capsule formation* (days 14 and longer): well-formed necrotic center surrounded by a dense collagenous capsule.[20]

A free (nonencapsulated) abscess is associated with a higher mortality. A mature abscess has three layers: (1) a center of polymorphonuclear leukocytes, (2) a collagenous capsule, and (3) peripheral gliosis. Existing abscesses also tend to spread and form daughter abscesses.

Abscesses arising from the ear frequently are located in the middle or inferior temporal lobe or in the anterolateral cerebellar hemispheres. Abscesses originating from the oral and nasal area most commonly are located in the frontal and temporal lobes. Abscesses from distant foci often occur in multiple numbers in the distal portion of the middle cerebral arteries. In extradural abscesses, pus and granulation tissue accumulate in the extradural space.

CLINICAL MANIFESTATIONS Clinical manifestations of brain abscesses are associated with (1) intracranial infection, such as fever and increased sedimentation rate; or (2) an expanding intracranial mass, such as headache, nausea, vomiting, decreasing cognitive abilities, paresis, and seizures. Early clinical manifestations of brain abscesses are low-grade fever, headache, neck pain and stiffness with mild nuchal rigidity, confusion, drowsiness, sensory deficits, and communication deficits. Headache is the most common early symptom. Later clinical manifestations may include inattentiveness (distractibility), memory deficits, decreased visual acuity and narrowed visual fields, papilledema, ocular palsy, ataxia, and dementia. Symptoms depend on the location of the abscess. The development of symptoms may be very insidious, often making an abscess difficult to diagnose. **Extradural brain abscesses** are associated with localized pain, purulent drainage from the nasal passages or auditory canal, fever, localized tenderness, and neck stiffness; occasionally the individual experiences a focal seizure. Clinical manifestations of spinal cord abscesses have four stages: (1) spinal aching; (2) root pain, which is usually severe, accompanied by spasms of the back muscles and limited vertebral movement because of pain and spasm; (3) weakness caused by progressive cord compression; and (4) paralysis.

EVALUATION AND TREATMENT The diagnosis is suggested on the basis of clinical features and confirmed by CT scan. MRI is helpful when the CT scan does not show an abscess even though it is suggested by clinical features. Surgery is indicated if the diagnosis is in doubt or there are space-occupying problems present. Aspiration through a burr hole or excision through craniotomy with antibiotic therapy may be used. Multiple or surgically inaccessible abscesses are treated with antibiotics, often in conjunction with steroid therapy to treat the cerebral edema. In addition, ICP may have to be managed. Because decompression is necessary, spinal cord abscesses are treated with surgical excision or aspiration. Antibiotic and support therapy also is instituted.

Encephalitis

Encephalitis is an acute febrile illness, usually of viral origin, with nervous system involvement. The most common encephalitides are caused by arthropod-borne (mosquito-borne) viruses and herpes simplex, almost exclusively herpes simplex type I in adults (Figure 17-30). Etiological agents for viral encephalitis are presented in Box 17-5. Referred to as *infectious viral encephalitides,* encephalitis also may occur as a complication of systemic viral diseases such as poliomyelitis, rabies, or mononucleosis, or it may arise after recovery from some viral infection such as rubella or rubeola. Encephalitis also may follow vaccination with a live attenuated virus vaccine if the vaccine has an encephalitis component. Such vaccines include measles, mumps, and rubella. Typhus, trichinosis, malaria, and schistosomiasis also are associated with encephalitis. Toxoplasmosis may acutely reactivate in immunosuppressed persons when the once-dormant parasite in cyst form disseminates in brain tissues (see pp. 590 to 591).

With the exception of the California viral encephalitis, which is endemic, the arthropod-borne encephalitides occur in epidemics, varying in geographic and seasonal incidence (Table 17-13). Eastern equine encephalitis is the most serious but least common of the encephalitides.[20] West Nile virus is presented in Box 17-6.

PATHOPHYSIOLOGY Viruses gain access to the CNS through the bloodstream or through an intraneuronal route from peripheral nerves.[21] Evidence of meningeal involvement appears in all encephalitides. The arthropod-

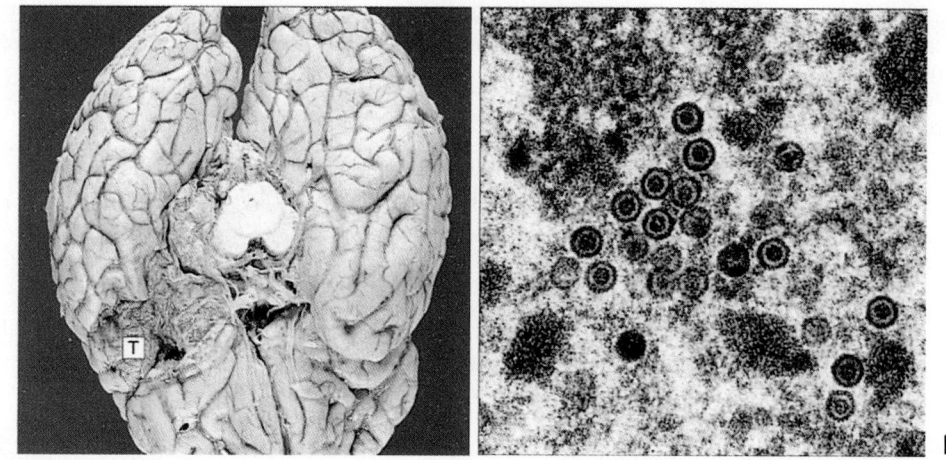

Figure 17-30 Herpes encephalitis. In herpes simplex encephalitis (**A**) necrosis of the temporal lobes *(T)* is a typical development. Brain biopsy is useful in diagnosis when the virus can be seen by electron microscopy (**B**) as rounded particles with a dense core. Virus also can be identified by immunostaining or culture. In early cases, polymerase chain reaction (PCR) can be used to identify viral deoxyribonucleic acid (DNA) in cerebrospinal fluid samples. (From Stevens A, Lowe J: *Pathology,* ed. 2, London, 2000, Mosby.)

Box 17-5	Etiological Agents of Viral Encephalitis

Herpes Simplex Viruses
Herpes simplex virus type 1
Herpes simplex virus type 2 (neonates)

Arthropod-Borne
Mosquito-borne
  California encephalitis virus
  St. Louis encephalitis virus
  West Nile virus
  Japanese B encephalitis virus
  Eastern equine encephalitis virus
  Western equine encephalitis virus
  Dengue viruses
Tick-borne
  Powassan virus
  Colorado tick fever

Enteroviruses (Neonates, Young Adults, Agammaglobulinemic Patients)
Coxsackieviruses
Echoviruses
Enteroviruses 70 and 71

Immunocompromised
Varicella-zoster virus
Epstein-Barr virus
Cytomegalovirus
Human herpesvirus type 6
Measles virus (postmeasles encephalomyelitis, subacute sclerosing panencephalitis)
Rubella virus
Lymphocytic choriomeningitis virus

Focal Encephalitis
Herpes simplex virus
Enterovirus
California encephalitis virus
Powassan virus
Measles (subacute measles encephalitis)
Human herpesvirus type 6
Varicella-zoster virus

From Roos KL: Viral infections. In CG Goetz: *Textbook of clinical neurology,* ed 2, Philadelphia, 2003, Saunders.

---

borne viral encephalitides cause widespread nerve cell degeneration. Edema and areas of necrosis with or without hemorrhage develop. Increased ICP develops and may progress to herniation. Large degenerative injuries are found in Eastern equine encephalitis, whereas the other arthropod-borne viral encephalitides have microscopic areas of injury and degeneration.

Infectious encephalitis may result from a postinfectious autoimmune response to the virus or from direct invasion of the CNS by the virus. Herpes simplex type I has a tendency to infect the inferomedial surfaces of the temporal and frontal lobes and causes hemorrhagic necrosis.

CLINICAL MANIFESTATIONS   Encephalitis may range from a mild infectious disease to a life-threatening disorder.

The dramatic clinical manifestations of encephalitis are fever, delirium or confusion progressing to unconsciousness, seizure activity, cranial nerve palsies, paresis and paralysis, involuntary movement, and abnormal reflexes. Signs of marked ICP may be present.

EVALUATION AND TREATMENT   Diagnosis is based on medical history and clinical presentation aided by CSF examination and culture, serologic examination, WBC count, CT scan, or MRI. Until very recently, no definitive treatment was available for the viral encephalitides, but herpes encephalitis now is being treated with antiviral agents such as acyclovir and steroids. Ribavirin treats LaCrosse encephalitis.[21] Supportive therapy is initiated, and measures to control ICP are paramount.

Table 17-13   Classification and Characteristics of Arthropod Viruses Causing Encephalitis

Viruses	Incubation Period (days)	Virus	Location	Vector	Season	Affected Population
Eastern equine encephalitis	5-15	*Togaviridae* Alphavirus (formerly group A arbovirus)	Atlantic, Gulf Coast, and Great Lake regions	Mosquito	Midsummer to early fall	Infants, children, and adults >50 yr
Western equine encephalitis	5-10	Same as above	All parts of United States, especially western two thirds of country	Mosquito	Summer to early fall	Infants and young children
Venezuelan equine encephalitis	2-5	Same as above	Texas, Florida, Mexico; Central and South America	Mosquito	Year round	Infants and young children
St. Louis encephalitis	4-21	*Flaviviridae* Flavivirus group B (formerly group B arbovirus)	United States and Canada, especially Mississippi River, Pacific Coast, Texas, and Florida	Mosquito	Summer and fall	Adults >40 yr; elderly more often affected than younger ages
California encephalitis including LaCross	5-15	*Bunyaviridae* Bunyavirus (California virus serogroup)	Midwestern United States, eastern seaboard, and Canada	Woodland mosquito	Late summer and early fall	Children <15 yr
West Nile encephalitis	3-14	Same as above	Lower 48 states of the United States	Mosquito	Summer and fall	Elderly most seriously

---

Box 17-6   Emergence of West Nile Virus

West Nile virus, a flavivirus transmitted predominantly by the *Culex* mosquito, emerged in New York State in 1999. By July 2004, human cases had been found in 45 states. Humans and horses, as well as other mammals, are incidental hosts. Birds and mosquitoes are life cycle hosts. Summer and fall are peak times of infection incidence.

Stages of Infection

Stage 1: febrile illness of acute onset that is clinically unrecognizable as West Nile virus infection

Stage 2: mild infection (20% of cases) after a 3- to 4-day incubation period; symptoms last 4 to 6 days

Stage 3: severe infection (1 in 150 cases); identified risk factor for developing this stage is advanced age

Most West Nile virus infections are mild with symptoms including fever (90% of cases), weakness (56%), nausea (51%), vomiting (51%), headache (47%), mental status changes (46%), diarrhea (27%), rash (19%), and lymphadenopathy (2%). Severe infections are marked by meningeal signs of severe headache, high fever, and nuchal rigidity; and encephalitis signs of disorientation, stupor, coma, seizures, and movement disorders including tremor, ataxia, extrapyramidal signs, and paralysis. Myelitis and polyradiculitis also may be present. Myocarditis, pancreatitis, and fulminant hepatitis are rare. Abnormalities in the thalamus, basal ganglia, and cerebellum are often seen on MRI in persons with severe infection.

A preliminary diagnosis is made if IgM for the virus is found in serum or CSF. Plaque reduction neutralization assay (PRA) is the confirmatory test. Interferon-alpha is used during treatment along with supportive care for those with severe infection. A new vaccine is currently being tested.

MRI, Magnetic resonance imaging; *CSF,* cerebrospinal fluid.
Data from Hall RA, Khromykh AA: *Expert Opin Biol Ther* 4(8):1295-1305, 2004; National Institute on Allergy and Infectious Disease, Department of Health Human Services, National Institutes of Health: *NIAID research on West Nile Virus,* April 2004, available at http://www.niaid.nih.gov; West Nile virus activity United States, July 7-13, 2004, *MMWR* 53(27):615, 2004.

Neurologic Complications of Acquired Immunodeficiency Syndrome

Approximately 40% to 60% of all persons with AIDS have neurologic complications. On postmortem examination, 75% of AIDS victims have nervous system pathologic findings. The CNS pathologic findings in persons with AIDS result from (1) the primary human immunodeficiency virus (HIV) infection; (2) the immune dysregulation of early HIV infection and progressive immunosuppression in late HIV infections resulting in opportunistic infections, neoplasms, and systemic illness; and (3) complications of therapy.[22]

A variety of CNS complications of AIDS exist (Box 17-7). Multiple CNS pathologic conditions may be experienced by one person. The most common neurologic disorder is HIV-associated cognitive dysfunction. Other common neurologic disorders are peripheral neuropathies, vacuolar (spongy softening) myelopathy, opportunistic infections of the CNS, and neoplasms.

HIV-infected macrophages/monocytes in blood are attracted to the brain by up-regulation of proinflammatory mediators such as monocyte chemoattractant protein-1 (MCP-1), tumor necrosis factor-alpha (TNF-α), and adhesion molecules on endothelial cells. Up-regulation enables transendothelial migration of activated macrophages/monocytes. CNS neuropathologic findings in HIV are listed in Box 17-8.

Human Immunodeficiency-Associated Cognitive Dysfunction

HIV-associated cognitive dysfunction (HIV encephalopathy, subacute encephalitis, HIV-associated dementia complex, HIV cognitive motor complex, AIDS encephalopathy, AIDS dementia complex, or AIDS-related dementia) may affect both adults and children and is charac-

Box 17-7	Nervous System Complications of HIV-1 Infections

CNS Complications of HIV-1 Infection
Diffuse cerebral disorders
   HIV-1–associated cognitive dysfunction
Meningitis
   Atypical aseptic meningitis
      Acute: typical meningitis signs
      Chronic: headache syndrome
   Nonviral infection
      Cryptococcus neoformans
   Other fungal infections
      Mycobacterial infections
Myelopathy
   Spinal vacuolar myelopathy
Focal brain disorders
   Opportunistic viral infections
      Progressive multifocal leukoencephalopathy
      Herpesviruses
   Nonviral infections
      Toxoplasma gondii
   Bacterial infections
   Neoplasms
      Primary CNS neoplasms
      Metastatic neoplasms
   Cerebrovascular complications
   Complications resulting from systemic AIDS therapy

Peripheral Nervous System Complications of HIV-1 Infections
Distal symmetric peripheral neuropathy
Inflammatory demyelinating polyradiculoneuropathy
Mononeuropathy multiplex
Progressive polyradiculopathy
Other causes of peripheral nervous system dysfunction
   Herpes zoster radiculitis
Cranial neuropathies

CNS, Central nervous system.

Box 17-8	CNS Neuropathological Findings in HIV

Gross Examination
Cerebral atrophy of variable degrees
   Ventricular enlargement
   Widening of sulci
   Attenuation of deep cerebral white matter

Microscopic Examination
HIV-1 encephalitis
   Perivascular foci of inflammatory cells, microglia, macrophages, MGC involving the basal ganglia and subcortical white matter predominantly
HIV-1 leukoencephalopathy
   Diffuse myelin pallor and white matter damage, reactive astrogliosis, macrophages
Calcific vasculopathy
   Small vessel mineralization of basal ganglia, frontal white matter (children > adults)
   Leukoencephalopathy and gliosis
   Basal ganglia calcific vasculopathy (infants and children)
   Diffuse poliodystrophy
   Multinucleated giant cells (MGC)

Modified from Budka, H et al: *Brain Pathol* 1(3):143-152, 1991.

terized by progressive cognitive dysfunction in conjunction with motor and behavioral alterations[22] (Table 17-14). The syndrome typically develops later in the disease but may be an early or a singular manifestation in some persons.

The viral route of entry into the CNS is unclear, but it is believed that HIV-associated cognitive dysfunction is the result of direct brain tissue infection by the virus. HIV is found mostly in white matter subcortical areas affecting macrophages, macrophage-derived multinucleated cells, and microglia, causing an immune-mediated demyelination process in white matter. Some viral replication occurs in some of the glial cells and, occasionally, within neurons. Multiple small nodules containing inflammatory cells are found scattered throughout the white matter and in subcortical gray matter, such as the basal ganglia and thalami. Multinucleated giant cells are present, as is perivascular inflammation. Focal and diffuse demyelination of white matter and spongy changes of the spinal cord are present. Factors other than direct cell damage are involved, such as released toxins, lymphokines, or other substances. Elevation in CSF levels of quinolinic acid, a neurotoxic metabolite of tryptophan, is cor-

related with the degree of dementia present. A decreased concentration of adenosine triphosphate (ATP) and inorganic phosphates in the CNS produces a decrease in metabolism.

HIV-associated cognitive dysfunction is insidious in onset and unpredictable in its course. Most persons experience a steady progression characterized by abrupt accelerations of signs over several months to more than 1 year, although some individuals experience an abrupt onset or an accelerated course.

Early clinical manifestations of HIV-associated cognitive dysfunction may be vague. Impaired concentration and short-term memory and retrieval deficits commonly occur. Apathy and lack of motivation may appear; social withdrawal, irritability, and emotional lability appear. Later, difficulties with language, spatial or temporal disorientation, and visual construction appear. Some persons manifest an organic psychosis with agitation, inappropriate behavior, and hallucinosis.

Generalized cognitive system deficits occur later in the course of HIV-associated cognitive dysfunction, often accompanied by psychomotor slowing and decreased speech spontaneity and fluency. Progressive loss of balance, ataxia, spastic paraparesis or paralysis, and generalized hyperreflexia are common motor signs. Decreased writing ability, tremor, myoclonus, and seizure are less commonly seen.

Diagnosis is difficult, especially in early stages. The patient's medical history along with physical examination findings and supporting CSF, CT, and MRI data help to establish the diagnosis. Antiretrovirae, protease inhibitors, reverse transcriptase inhibitors, and adjunctive agents may be effective along with supportive treatment.

HIV Myelopathy

HIV myelopathy involving diffuse degeneration of the spinal cord may occur in persons with AIDS. **Vacuolar**

Table 17-14	Classification of HIV-Associated Cognitive Dysfunction
Category	Dysfunction
1 (HIV-associated, minor)	0.5 SD below normal on standardized neuropsychologic tests
	Decline in work or other activities of daily living (ADLs)
	Symptoms for 1 month
	Criteria for HIV-1–associated dementia or delirium is absent
	No other etiology
2 (HIV-associated dementia)	Marked impairment in at least two ability domains
	Significant impairment in work and other ADLs
	Symptoms for 1 month
	No other etiology
	Free of delirium for a period sufficient to establish the presence of dementia
3 (HIV-associated delirium)	Clouding of consciousness
	Marked, rapid worsening of cognitive function in ≥2 domains

From Belman AL, Mirjana-Savatic M. Human immunodeficiency virus and acquired immunodeficiency syndrome. In CG Goetz, *Textbook of clinical neurology*, ed 2, Philadelphia, 2003, Saunders.
SD, Standard deviation.

myelopathy is believed to be a direct consequence of HIV. The lateral and posterior columns of the lumbar spinal cord are affected. A progressive spastic paraparesis with ataxia is the predominant clinical manifestation. Leg weakness, upper motor neuron signs, incontinence, and posterior column sensory loss may be present. Diagnosis is made on the basis of history, physical findings, and supporting data from diagnostic procedures. Vacuolar myelopathy is treated supportively and does not respond to antiretrovirals.

HIV Neuropathy

HIV neuropathy may have one or a combination of several presentations: a predominantly sensory neuropathy, an autonomic neuropathy, a mononeuritis multiplex, a Guillian-Barré-like syndrome, and a myopathy. The peripheral nervous system may sustain injury in AIDS, manifesting as a peripheral neuropathy or radiculopathy. A progressive radiculopathy of predominantly the dorsal roots of the lumbar and sacral nerves may occur, involving severe myelin and axonal loss. The most common neuropathy is a sensory neuropathy that most commonly occurs later in the disease and is unresponsive to treatment.

HIV has been isolated from peripheral nerves, so it is believed that the virus may directly infect nerves. Patients experience painful, burning dysesthesias and paresthesias, typically in the extremities. Weakness and decreased or absent distal reflexes may be present. Diagnosis is established through history, physical findings, laboratory data, nerve conduction studies, EMG, and possibly biopsy. The most common myopathy is polymyositis; it may be present initially, or it may be a later development. The muscle fiber is infiltrated, initiating inflammation that leads to cellular degeneration and necrosis. The patient experiences muscle weakness of extremities with myalgia and fatigue. Steroids are used therapeutically in polymyositis.

Aseptic Viral Meningitis

Some persons develop an acute aseptic meningitis at approximately the time of seroconversion. This may well represent the initial infection of the nervous system by the HIV. Symptoms include headache, fever, and meningismus. Cranial nerve involvement, especially of nerves V and VII, may appear, but the disease is self-limiting and requires only symptomatic treatment. Aseptic meningitis may occur at any point in the disease.

Opportunistic Infections

Opportunistic infections may be bacterial, fungal, protozoan, or viral in origin and produce nervous system disease. Typically, bacterial infections are caused by unusual microorganisms. Cryptococcal infection is the most common fungal disorder and the third leading cause of neurologic disease in persons with AIDS. In *Cryptococcus neoformans*, small granulomas and cysts are found in the cerebral cortex and later may be present in deep cerebral tissues. The symptoms are vague, such as fever, headache, malaise, and meningismus. Herpes encephalitis and herpes varicella zoster radiculitis may develop. Papovavirus (especially JC virus) in the immunocompromised person with AIDS may produce a demyelinating disorder called *progressive multifocal leukoencephalopathy (PML)*. This virus is found in 90% of healthy persons but is dormant. The virus reactivates to cause PML in 15% of persons with AIDS. Sensory and motor deficits, aphasia, and apraxia are common clinical manifestations. The condition is progressive.

Cytomegalovirus Infection. Cytomegalovirus encephalitis is common in persons with AIDS but often not diagnosed while the person is alive. The encephalitis may be present as an acute illness with encephalitis features accompanied by nystagmus and cranial nerve signs. Retinitis is found in 50% of those affected.

Parasitic Infection. Toxoplasmosis is the most common opportunistic infection and occurs in one third of persons with AIDS. CNS toxoplasmosis typically manifests as focal encephalitis. *Toxoplasma gondii*, a protozoan, is thought to reactivate from latent lesions to produce a well-demarcated necrotizing process. Inflammatory infiltrates, thrombotic lesions, and fibrinoid vascular walls are present at the necrotic edge. Marked edema is present adjacent to necrotic areas. Lesions may be multiple and exist throughout the cerebral hemispheres.

Clinical manifestations of CNS toxoplasmosis are focal but highly variable and include clumsiness to hemiplegia, aphasia, seizures, ataxia, cognitive changes, and constitutional symptoms. Fever and headache are common. Toxoplasmosis is difficult to diagnose but is treated effectively with pyrimethamine and sulfadiazine. Allergic response to sulfadiazine can be a problem, and other drugs can be substituted. Persons with AIDS may develop meningitis; encephalitis; or brain abscesses of fungal, mycobacterial, and bacterial origin.

Central Nervous System Neoplasms

CNS neoplasms associated with AIDS include primary CNS lymphoma, systemic non-Hodgkin lymphoma, and metastatic Kaposi sarcoma. The precise mechanism of lymphoproliferation is not known. Primary CNS lymphoma is a large-cell lymphoma that presents as rapidly developing and expanding multicentric intracranial mass lesions. The meninges are invaded and, possibly, the cranial nerves and spinal cord are invaded as well in systemic non-Hodgkin lymphoma. Metastasis of a Kaposi sarcoma to the CNS is uncommon.

Other Central Nervous System Complications

Persons with AIDS may develop multifocal ischemic infarctions, hemorrhagic infarctions, hemorrhage into tumors, subdural hematomas, and epidural hemorrhage. The precise mechanism of these cardiovascular complications is not yet known. Reported neurologic symptoms produced by AIDS therapeutics include extrapyramidal movements, myoclonus, dysphasia, delirium, and acute myelopathy.

Lyme Disease

Lyme disease, a tick-borne spirochete bacterial infection, is a common arthropod-borne infection in the United States. It affects all age groups and involves the peripheral and central nervous systems. Lyme disease is caused by *Borrelia burgdorferi* introduced into the person by tick bite. Infected ticks are endemic in the Midwest, western wooded and coastal areas, and the northeast coast. The microorganism incubates for 3 to 32 days and then migrates to the skin, lymph nodes, and other body systems. The pathologic process progresses through three stages:

Stage I (acute localized). Three weeks after the bite, the disease is characterized by a bull's-eye-like (5 cm in diameter) burning rash, general malaise, flulike symptoms (fever, muscle pain), stiff neck, and headache

Stage II. With acute widespread dissemination of antibodies and immune complexes, cardiac and neurologic involvement predominates. About 10% of persons have cardiac signs and symptoms (palpitations, dizziness, shortness of breath, dysrhythmias, and first-degree heart block). Neurologic signs occur in 10% to 15% of persons and include headache, chronic aseptic (lymphocytic) meningitis, Bell's palsy, encephalitis, and radiculitis. Pathologically, there is a meningeal inflammation, perivascular inflammatory cell formation, and focal demyelination.

Stage III (chronic stage). The third stage may occur up to 2 years after the bite and involves arthritis and involvement of brain parenchyma with encephalitis, chronic neuropathy, and encephalopathy.

Treatment of choice is antibiotic therapy. Minor recurring symptoms are common in 50% of patients.

Demyelinating Disorders
Multiple Sclerosis

Multiple sclerosis (MS) is a relatively common dysimmune disorder diffusely involving CNS myelin. The peripheral nervous system is not involved. MS is one of many chronic heterogenous demyelinating disorders of the CNS.[23] They are acquired conditions and are characterized by degeneration of previously normal myelin with relative preservation of axons. CNS demyelinating disorders are subclassified as primary and secondary. MS and its variants are primary demyelinating disorders. In secondary disorders, CNS demyelination is caused by disorders other than multiple sclerosis.

The onset of MS is usually between 20 and 40 years of age with a peak of age 30. Male/female ratio is about 1:2. MS is the most prevalent CNS demyelinating disorder and a leading cause of neurologic disability in early adulthood. The disease is most prevalent in areas far from the equator. In the United States the prevalence rate ranges from 250,000 to 350,000 persons.[23] MS occurs in all races, but it is chiefly a disorder of whites. Although the disorder does not exhibit a defined inheritance pattern, 15% of persons with MS have an affected relative. A single gene, DR2, is implicated in this genetic susceptibility.[23] All epidemiologic data point to a relationship between MS and some environmental factor encountered in childhood.

PATHOPHYSIOLOGY   MS is currently described as occurring when a previous viral insult to the nervous system has occurred in a genetically susceptible individual with a subsequent abnormal immune response in the central nervous system. T cells become autoreactive to a single myelin protein. Thus the disease is associated with a genetic predisposition and interaction with an environmental risk factor (see Chapter 5). Genetically determined susceptibility is determined by a pattern (haplotype) of histocompatibility antigens (HLA, DR15, DQ6). Histocompatibility antigen is discussed in Chapter 6. Pathogenesis of demyelination may be heterogenous within different plaques and among different MS patterns.[24] Infiltrates of CD4 T cells and, possibly, CD8 cells across the blood-brain barrier is followed by chemotaxis and infiltration of monocytes and macrophages.[25] In the rat model, immune cells, arriving at the site of myelin sheath damage, discharge glutamate routinely. The glutamate binds to the oligodendrocyte's receptor site and the cell takes it in, accumulating too much glutamate.[26] This in turn causes excessive cell excitation.

Demyelinating lesions (plaques and diffuse lesions) are the second pathologic feature and produce slowing of conduction and finally a conduction block. Plaques characteristically involve the CNS white matter, especially around periventricular regions, optic nerves, brainstem, cerebellum, and spinal cord, but occasionally they may extend into the adjacent gray matter. They often coalesce into much larger plaques. In established disease the multifocal, multistaged feature of plaques gives rise to the aphorism that the lesions are "scattered in space and time." Symptoms therefore are multiple and variable. Whether plaques are multiple from the onset of the disease is not known. In many individuals the initial symptoms suggest a single lesion.

The acute (early) stage of plaque formation is characterized by the process of perivenous demyelination. Most of the neurologic deficits in the acute stage are attributed to inflammatory edema in and around the plaque and to partial demyelination. Symptoms usually remit, partially or completely, weeks after the onset of an early episode. The chronic stage of demyelination and plaque formation is characterized by the process of **gliosis** (glial scarring with late degeneration of axons). Progressive loss of function leads to permanent disability, usually over 20 years.

Although plaques are considered diagnostic of MS, diffuse lesions are common pathologic findings in actively progressive cases. Diffuse lesions are small, widespread areas of perivenular demyelination that do not progress through gliosis. These lesions are sometimes accompanied by edema of surrounding normal brain tissue. The relationship of plaques to diffuse lesions is unknown.

CLINICAL MANIFESTATIONS   A variety of events (e.g., infection, trauma, or pregnancy) occurring immediately before the onset or exacerbation of symptoms are regarded as precipitating factors related to MS. Most of the pregnancy-related exacerbations occur 3 months postpartum, suggesting a relation to the stresses of labor and the increased fatigue during the postpartum period rather than to the pregnancy itself.

The major classifications of MS are relapsing-remitting, primary progressive, secondary progressive, and progressive-relapsing (Box 17-9). Initially, 90% of persons present with a relapsing, remitting course. The major manifestations of MS are initial syndromes followed by remissions and established syndromes with no remissions (Box 17-10). Usually persons with late MS have predominantly one of the established syndromes—mixed, spinal, or cerebellar. The initial syndrome depends on the portion of the CNS that is most involved. After years, 50% of individuals appear to have established syndromes of mixed involvement.

Mixed (General) Type

Twenty-five percent of persons initially experience retrobulbar or optic neuritis, the manifestations of optic nerve demyelination. The condition usually evolves rapidly over hours to days and is highly suggestive of MS. Involvement may be unilateral or bilateral. Subjective symptoms are impaired central vision (blurring, fogginess, haziness) and impaired color perception. Signs are decreased central visual acuity; central or paracentral scotoma (area of diminished vision); acquired color vision deficit, especially to red and green; and defective pupillary reaction to light. A variety of field defects may occur. In the acute phase these symptoms may reflect optic papillitis (inflammation and swelling of the optic disc) or retrobulbar neuritis with a normal disc. One third of persons recover completely, and most others improve significantly. Later, pallor of the temporal half of the disc occurs from demyelination of a portion of the optic nerve. (Normal visual function is discussed in Chapter 15.)

The brain stem lesions involve cranial nerves III through XII at the root, nuclear, or corticobulbar (upper motor neuron) level. Internuclear ophthalmoplegia, nystagmus, and dysarthria are the most common brain stem symptoms, followed by deafness, vertigo and vomiting, tinnitus, facial weakness, and facial sensory deficit. Internuclear ophthalmoplegia is lateral gaze paralysis caused by involvement of the medial longitudinal fasciculus, the brain stem pathway that coordinates eye movement. Diplopia and eyeball pain are common complaints. Bilateral internuclear ophthalmoplegia in a young adult is virtually diagnostic of MS.

Cognitive dysfunction recently has been demonstrated to occur early in the disease course. The person experiences decreased short-term memory, recent memory impairment, decreased concentration, word-finding problems, and planning difficulties. Mood alterations are common in MS. Depression is far more common than euphoria.

Box 17-9	**Clinical Course of Multiple Sclerosis (MS)**

Relapsing-Remitting (RR) MS
Clear relapses (called *acute attacks* or *excerbations*) with either full recovery, or with partial recovery and lasting disability. Between attacks, there is no progression (or worsening) of disease. The most common course of MS (85% of cases).

Primary Progressive (PP) MS
Steady progression (or worsening) from onset, with only occasional plateaus or minor recovery. This is a fairly uncommon disease course, and one that may involve different brain and spinal cord damage than do other forms of MS.

Secondary Progressive (SP) MS
Begins with a pattern of clear-cut relapses and recovery but becomes steadily progressive over time with continued worsening between acute attacks (develops in two thirds of patients eventually).

Progressive-Relapsing (PR) MS
A rare type that is steadily progressive from onset but also has clear acute attacks.

Box 17-10	**Established Syndromes of Multiple Sclerosis**

Mixed or Generalized Type (50% of Persons)
Optic signs—optic neuritis
Brain stem signs—internuclear ophthalmoplegia, diplopia, vertigo (vomiting), nystagmus, dysarthria
Cerebellar signs—see text

Spinal Type (30% to 40% of persons)
Spastic ataxia
Deep sensory changes in the extremities
Bladder and bowel symptoms

Cerebellar or Pontobulbar-Cerebral Type (5% of persons)
Motor ataxia
Hypotonia
Asthenia

Amaurotic Form (5% of persons)
Blindness

Spinal Type

The spinal type of MS is the second most common type, chiefly involving the spinal tracts and dorsal column. Weakness, numbness, or both in one or more limbs are initial symptoms in 50% of persons with MS. Subjective corticospinal (upper motor neuron) symptoms (stiffness, slowness, weakness) are often unilateral and are a component of fatigability. Spinal signs are usually bilateral (symmetric), with lower limbs more often and more severely affected than upper limbs; spastic paraparesis is probably the most common single neurologic finding in MS.

Bladder and bowel symptoms occur with major spinal cord involvement. Urgency and hesitancy generally precede incontinence. Bladder dysfunction most often involves a small, spastic bladder, although occasionally a large, flaccid bladder may result with retention problems. Neurogenic impotence is often present when sphincter symptoms are present. Bowel incontinence is rare, but constipation is common with severe disease. Subjective dorsal column symptoms are symmetric paresthesias (tingling and numbness) in an unpredictable pattern but with a predilection for lower extremities over upper extremities. Dorsal column signs are vibration, position, and two-point discrimination deficits. Sensory complaints often are not substantiated by objective physical findings but by further diagnostic tests.

Cerebellar Type

A nystagmus and ataxia presentation initially is not uncommon and reflects cerebellar and corticospinal involvement. Cerebellar deficits are usually symmetric, with all four limbs involved. With combined corticospinal and cerebellar involvement, the individual has a spastic ataxic gait and ataxia of the arms. Pure cerebellar symptoms are those of motor ataxia, hypotonia, and asthenia (weakness). Manifestations of motor ataxia are decomposition of movement, inability to perform rapid alternating movements (dysdiadochokinesia), and dysmetria. Charcot triad describes a combination of dysarthria, intention tremor, and nystagmus. Hypotonia is manifested by decreased resistance to passive movement, hypoactive deep tendon reflexes, and pendular knee jerk.

Short-lived attacks of neurologic deficits are the temporary appearance or worsening of symptoms. The mechanism of these attacks is complete, reversible conduction block in partially demyelinated axons. Conditions that cause short-lived attacks include (1) minor increases in body temperature or serum Ca^{++} concentration and (2) functional demands exceeding conduction capacity. An increase in body temperature or serum Ca^{++} level increases current leakage through demyelinated neurons. Persons with MS may become dramatically worse when body temperature is raised. Hypercalcemia induced by decreased serum pH may aggravate symptoms of MS. Physical and emotional stress impose functional demands that may exceed conduction capacity of affected neurons.

Paroxysmal attacks are sensory or motor symptoms of abrupt onset and short duration (few seconds or minutes). These symptoms include paresthesias, dysarthria and ataxia, and tonic head turning. The mechanism of paroxysmal attacks is nonsynaptic transmission in which nerve impulses are directly transmitted between adjacent demyelinated axons. These impulses arise focally and spuriously in the cervical portion of the spinal cord or in the brain stem. A common paroxysmal symptom, called *Lhermitte sign*, is the momentary paresthesia (shocklike or tingling sensation) that shoots down the trunk or limbs during active or passive flexion of the neck. Bending the neck evokes nonsynaptic impulses in demyelinated axons of the dorsal column in the spinal cord. A person with MS may have many paroxysmal attacks each day. Inciting events include sensory stimulation, voluntary movement, hyperventilation, and emotional stress. Paroxysmal attacks tend to persist for weeks or months and may be followed by progressive symptoms of MS.

EVALUATION AND TREATMENT The diagnosis of MS (MS, possible MS, not MS) is based on the history and physical examination supported by findings from CSF examination (Table 17-15), evoked response (ER) studies (Figure 17-31), CT scans of the head, and MRI. Persistently elevated CSF immunoglobulin G (IgG) is found in about two thirds of individuals with MS, and oligoclonal (IgG) bands on electrophoresis are found in more than 90% (Figure 17-32). ER studies aid diagnosis by detecting decreased conduction

Table 17-15	Typical Cerebrospinal Fluid Findings in a Multiple Sclerosis Patient	
CSF Component	**Typical Value in MS**
Protein	0.80 g/L
Cell count (all lymphocytes)	15/mm³
Immunoglobulin G/albumin	0.30
Immunoglobulin G index	1.05
Oligoclonal bands	positive

From Perkin GD: *Mosby's color atlas and text of neurology,* 1998. London, Mosby-Wolfe.
CSF, Cerebrospinal fluid; *MS,* multiple sclerosis.

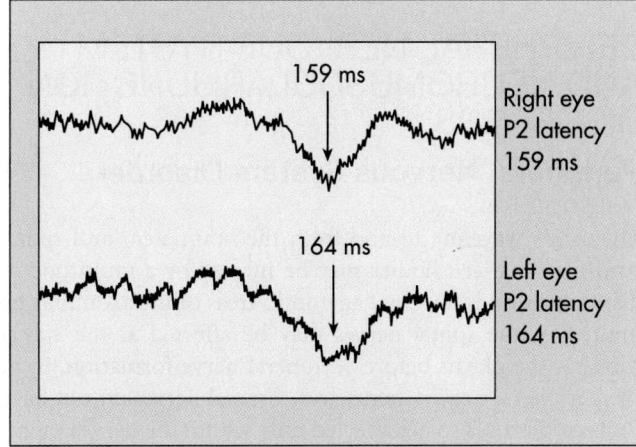

Figure 17-31 Visual evoked responses showing bilateral delay. (From Perkin DG: *Mosby's color atlas and text of neurology,* London, 1998, Mosby-Wolfe.)

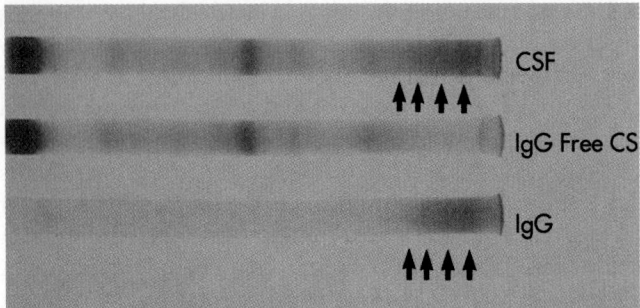

Figure 17-32 Oligoclonal bands in the cerebrospinal fluid. (From Perkin DG: *Mosby's color atlas and text of neurology,* London, 1998, Mosby-Wolfe.)

velocity in visual, auditory, and somatosensory pathways. MRI is the most sensitive available method of detecting the disease. MRI shows brain stem, optic nerve, and spinal cord lesions not detected by CT. MRI is a good tool with which to monitor progression of the disease.

Treatment has three purposes: (1) acute management of relapses to prevent disability, (2) reducing the frequency of relapses and/or minimizing disease progression ("disease burden"), and (3) management of symptoms. Methylprednisolone (Solu-Medrol) and plasma exchange are used in acute episodes to shorten the duration of the acute relapses. Disease modifying drugs (DMD) are used early to reduce the relapse rate. Interferon beta-1b (Betaseron), interferon beta-1a (Avonex), glatiramer acetate (Copaxone), interferon beta-1a (Rebif), and intravenous immunoglobulins are used in relapse-remitting MS.[27,28] Interferon beta-1b and mitoxantrone (Novantrone) are used in secondary progressive MS.[27]

Symptom management for fatigue, weakness, vertigo, ataxia, tremor, heat intolerance, spasticity, bladder dysfunction, bowel dysfunction, sexual dysfunction, sensory sensations, pain, cognitive difficulties, depression, and psychosocial issues is essential. Supportive and rehabilitative management are directed toward preventing the complications of immobility, especially pressure sores and infections of the pulmonary and genitourinary systems. The average duration of the disease is 30 years.

PERIPHERAL NERVOUS SYSTEM AND NEUROMUSCULAR JUNCTION DISORDERS

Peripheral Nervous System Disorders
Neuropathies
The axons traveling to and from the brain stem and spinal cord neuronal cell bodies may be injured by a multitude of disease processes. Distinct anatomic areas of the axon may be injured or the spinal nerves may be affected at the spinal roots, at the plexus before peripheral nerve formation, or at the peripheral nerves themselves. Cranial nerves do not have roots or plexuses so are affected only within the nerves themselves. Autonomic nerve fibers may be injured as they travel within certain cranial nerves or emerge through the ventral root and plexuses to travel in the peripheral nerves of the body.

Neuropathies can be classified as (1) generalized symmetric polyneuropathies, (2) generalized neuropathies, and (3) focal or multifocal neuropathies.[28,29] **Generalized symmetric polyneuropathies** are characterized by symmetric involvement of sensory, motor, or autonomic fibers although, with clinical signs, one type of fiber may predominate. Generalized symmetric polyneuropathies further subdivide into **distal axonal polyneuropathy** and **demyelinating polyneuropathy.**[29] Distal axonal polyneuropathy affects peripheral axons and is the generalized peripheral neuropathy commonly seen. The clinical feature of distal axonal polyneuropathy is involvement of the longest nerve of the body, those going to the feet, first. Sensory impairment is greater than motor impairment. Symptoms are burning pain, tingling, and numbness of the feet. Small nerve fiber damage produces decreased pain and temperature, as well as burning, numbness, and tingling. Large nerve fiber injury causes decreased light touch, vibration, and position sense. The two most common causes are diabetes mellitus and alcohol abuse; occasionally, neurotoxic therapeutic agents also are the cause. Within the classification of distal axonal neuropathies is another group of neuropathies called *autonomic neuropathy.*[30] This neuropathy can involve virtually any sympathetic or parasympthetic nerve fiber. Autonomic neuropathies have a progressive course and are usually reversible. The myelin or Schwann cells are affected in demyelinating polyneuropathy, which occurs far less frequently. Weakness is the predominant sign with far less sensory impairment. Acute and chronic inflammatory demyelinating neuropathies comprise this group, of which Guillain-Barré syndrome is the most widely recognized disorder.

Generalized neuropathies affect the cell body of only one type of peripheral neuron. The dorsal root ganglion cell is affected in sensory neuropathies producing numbness that may begin in a focal or asymmetric distribution or in a distal symmetric pattern. **Sensory neuropathies** are seen in leprosy, some industrial solvent poisonings, some hereditary disorders, and chloramphenicol toxicity. The anterior horn in motor neuropathy is affected causing weakness that may be symmetric or asymmetric. Motor neuropathies are caused by anterior horn cell disease, such as amyotrophic lateral sclerosis (ALS) or paralytic poliomyelitis.

Focal or **multifocal neuropathies** affect sensory and motor fibers in one or more nerves as is seen in common compression neuropathies such as carpal tunnel syndrome (median nerve compression), ulnar nerve compression (at the elbow), peroneal nerve compression, or sciatic nerve compression. Focal neuropathies can involve one or more cranial nerves. Plexus injuries and radiculopathies also fall into this category.

PATHOPHYSIOLOGY   Although distinct pathophysiologic processes are recognized in a neuropathy, these are not disease specific and may exist simultaneously in any one neuropathy. Wallerian degeneration, in which the axon and myelin distal to the site of axonal interruption degenerate, may be present (see Chapter 14). This type of degeneration is characteristic of a traumatic nerve injury in which the nerve is severed. In demyelinating neuropathies the axon may be spared and only the myelin degenerates. In **axonal degeneration,** distal degeneration of the axon occurs first and is followed by degeneration of the myelin and the axis cylinder. Many pathologic processes may give rise to neuropathy, and one or more nerves may be involved.

CLINICAL MANIFESTATIONS   When the axons are affected, muscle strength, muscle tone, and muscle bulk also are affected. Whole muscles or groups of muscles are paretic or paralyzed, and the muscles of the feet and legs often are affected first and more severely. These long, large axons are thought to (1) be more vulnerable to injury because of their size and length, (2) have more Schwann cells available to be injured, and (3) exhibit a "dying back" phenomenon caused by difficulty of the nerve cell body in maintaining the terminal portion of the axon. If unchecked, the pathologic process tends to involve the hands and arms because these have the next longest and largest axons.

Tone and the deep tendon reflexes in the affected muscles generally are decreased in a neuropathy. Atrophy is distributed according to the peripheral nerves involved. The degree and distribution of the atrophy probably depend on the extent of the injury. Fasciculation may be present, especially with associated ventral root or motor neuron changes or both, as in Guillain-Barré syndrome, diabetic neuropathy, and porphyric neuropathy. Mild fatigue may be experienced. A few disorders, notably Guillain-Barré syndrome, produce a pattern of paresis and paralysis that involves all limbs, the trunk, and the neck. Peripheral bifacial and other cranial nerve palsies may be seen with a variety of disorders. Tenderness of the nerve trunks and associated sensory alterations help to distinguish neuropathy from amyotrophy. These include paresthesias and dysesthesias as well as decreased or absent primary sensations (e.g., of temperature, touch, light pain, position, or vibration). Ataxia of gait or limb may arise from the loss of position and vibratory sensations (i.e., proprioceptive sensory loss) and may be enhanced by motor weakness.

Reflexes may be altered. Reflex-mediated autonomic nervous system functions, such as sweating and pupillary size, may be affected. Neuropathies associated with autonomic disturbances include diabetes mellitus, alcoholism and related nutritional neuropathies, amyloidosis, porphyria, Guillain-Barré syndrome, Riley-Day syndrome, and familial sensory neuropathy. In many chronic polyneuropathies the feet, hands, and spine become deformed. Metabolic changes may arise secondary to nerve dysfunction.

EVALUATION AND TREATMENT   The diagnostic workup to determine the cause of a neuropathy is often extensive. Early diagnosis and treatment before irreversible neuronal cell damage ensues are of paramount importance. Although axonal regrowth and recovery of function may take months, many neuropathies can be reversed. The therapeutic management is directed first at elimination of the cause, if possible. At least the primary disorder, such as diabetes melli-

tus, should be controlled. Further damage to the axon must be prevented by avoiding (1) trauma from too-early demand for reuse of the nerve, (2) accidents that cause tissue damage, and (3) hypoxia and ischemia or other deprivation of essential substrates.

Guillain-Barré Syndrome

Guillain-Barré syndrome (Landry-Guillain-Barré syndrome, idiopathic polyneuritis, acute inflammatory demyelinating polyradiculopathy, acute autoimmune neuropathy) is an acquired inflammatory disease that results in demyelination of the peripheral nerves with relative sparing of axons. The disease is characterized by the acute onset of a motor paralysis, usually of an ascending nature. This neurologic disorder occurs throughout the world, affects children and adults of both genders and all age groups equally, and occurs in all seasons of the year.

The annual incidence rate is 1 to 2 per 100,000 persons with a 4% to 6% mortality rate, and a 5% to 10% morbidity rate (permanent disabling weakness, imbalance, or sensory loss). Precipitating, or at least preceding, events include a mild respiratory or gastrointestinal viral or bacterial infection or other viral illness 1 to 3 weeks or longer before onset of neurologic manifestations, surgical procedures, viral immunizations, and lymphoma or other viral illness. In 60% of patients, *Campylobacter jejuni* is identified as the cause of the preceding infection. Guillain-Barré syndrome is now classified as the acute subtype of acquired demyelinating disorders of the peripheral nervous system, under which falls the following classification:

Acute inflammatory demyelinating polyradiculoneuropathy (AIDP)

Acute axon loss ("axonal") polyradiculopathy

Acute motor axonal neuropathy

Acute motor-sensory axonal neuropathy[31]

PATHOPHYSIOLOGY   The neurologic dysfunctions in Guillain-Barré syndrome (GBS) are probably caused by both a humoral- and cell-mediated immunologic reaction directed at peripheral nerve myelin. Lymphocytes infiltrate precedes the influx of macrophages, the cell believed to be responsible for destruction. Macrophages migrate into the areas adjacent to the nerve and attack the myelin surrounding the nerve fibers, causing variable degrees of demyelination of nerve segments. The humoral-mediated component blocks the conduction of nerve impulses to muscles and results in paralysis. Later, there are focal and segmental areas of cellular infiltration by T cell lymphocytes and macrophages in the motor, sensory, autonomic, and cranial nerve pathways. Evidence of reduced suppressor T cell response and abnormal lymphocyte reaction directed against peripheral nervous system myelin has been found. Immunoglobulin M (IgM) antibodies against myelin glycolipid have been found in the serum of GBS patients. Anti-GM1 is more prominent in individuals without sensory symptoms and with prodromal diarrheal illness. Anti-GD1b is more prominent in individuals with prominent sensory symptoms and ataxia. Anti-GQ1b is found in almost all individuals with cranial nerve signs and the Miller-Fisher variant. Antibodies that are cell-mediated responses are thought to be responsible for peripheral nerve demyelination and inflammation. If the process continues, the axons themselves are destroyed by wallerian degeneration. The muscle innervated by the damaged peripheral nerves undergoes denervation and atrophy. If the cell body survives, regeneration of the peripheral nerve takes place and recovery of motor function is likely. If the cell body dies from intense ventral root involvement in the inflammatory-degenerative process, no regeneration is possible. Collateral reinnervation from surviving axons and regenerating axons may take place. In this case, motor recovery is less complete and residual deficits persist.

CLINICAL MANIFESTATIONS   Clinical manifestations may vary from paresis of the legs to complete quadriplegia, respiratory insufficiency, and autonomic nervous system instability. Motor signs manifest as an acute or subacute progressive paralysis. Proximal muscles may be involved earlier and more significantly than distal muscles. The paresis/paralysis may be present in an ascending pattern involving limbs, respiratory muscles, and bulbar muscles. Only bulbar muscles may be involved, resulting in dysphagia and dysarthria. Weakness usually plateaus or improves by the fourth week in 90% of persons. After weakness plateaus, strength improves over a period of days to months, with the majority of individuals reaching activity levels similar to their predisease state. Sensory symptoms are common and include paresthesias/dysthesias (tingling, burning, shocklike sensations, particularly in the limbs), pain (throbbing, aching, particularly in the lower back, buttocks and legs), and numbness. Position and vibratory sensations are more affected than superficial sensation. Deep tendon reflexes are absent or greatly diminished. Respiratory muscle weakness leads to the need for ventilatory support in 10% to 30% of patients. Cranial nerve weakness manifests as facial weakness and bulbar weakness involving chewing, swallowing, and cough. Autonomic dysfunction may manifest as tachycardia or, less frequently, bradycardia; hypotension or hypertension; and loss of or significant increase in sweating in those more severely affected. Patients may undergo a respiratory arrest or cardiovascular collapse. Hyponatremia caused by the syndrome of inappropriate antidiuretic hormone (SAIDH) is common, especially in ventilated individuals.

EVALUATION AND TREATMENT   The individual's clinical history helps to diagnose the disorder. Significant signs include paresthesias, paralysis, and CSF findings. The major diagnostic tests are the examination of the CSF, nerve conduction studies, and EMG. The CSF findings include an unusually high protein level (500 mg/dl) without cellular abnormality. Ventilatory support and management of the autonomic nervous system dysfunction are two dominant aspects of the therapeutic management. Plasmapheresis or plasma exchanges within the first 2 weeks of onset of clinical manifestations are indicated. Intravenous immune globulin is used as well as combination therapy. After the disorder begins to remit, aggressive rehabilitation should be instituted.

Amyotrophic Lateral Sclerosis

Amyotrophic lateral sclerosis (ALS, sporadic motor system disease, sporadic motor neuron disease, motor neuron disease) is a worldwide degenerative disorder diffusely involving lower and upper motor neurons resulting in progressive muscle weakness leading to respiratory failure and death, usually 2 to 5 years from symptom onset.[32] There are no racial, ethnic, or socioeconomic boundaries. The prevalence rate is 6 to 8 cases per 100,000, with 2 deaths per 100,000. There are 5000 newly diagnosed cases per year in the United States. The term *amyotrophic* (without muscle nutrition or progressive muscle wasting) refers to the predominant lower motor neuron component of the syndrome. Lateral sclerosis, or scarring of the corticospinal tract in the lateral column of the spinal cord, refers to the upper motor neuron component of the syndrome. ALS differs from other motor neuron disorders in that both upper and lower motor neurons are involved.

Classic ALS (Lou Gehrig disease) may begin at any time from the fourth decade of life; its peak occurrence is in the early 50s. Male/female ratio is 3:2, equalizing after menopause. Of persons with ALS, 10% have a familial ALS involving an autosomal dominant pattern with an age-dependent penetrance. ALS is linked to chromosome 21. A defective superoxide dismutase (SOD) gene is responsible for 25% of cases of familial ALS.[33]

ALS presentations include crural ALS, proximal or shoulder girdle ALS, and hemiplegic (Mills) ALS. Of persons with ALS, 20% have a benign form of the disease. Subtypes of ALS include primary lateral sclerosis, progressive bulbar palsy, and progressive muscular atrophy.

PATHOPHYSIOLOGY   The pathogenesis of ALS is not fully clear. Current data suggest a genetic factor. Persons with familial ALS have a genetic defect on chromosome 21 in the gene that codes for superoxide dismutase, an enzyme that helps destroy free radicals. Abnormal glutamate metabolism and hydrogen peroxide production are also under study as part of the pathogenesis of ALS. RNA strands of echovirus have been isolated in the spinal cord tissue of 15 of 17 persons with ALS who did not have familial ALS.[34]

The principal pathologic feature of ALS is lower and upper motor neuron degeneration, although without inflammation. The number of large motor neurons in the spinal cord, brain stem, and cerebral cortex (premotor and motor areas) is reduced, with ongoing degeneration in the remaining motor neurons. The nuclei of cranial nerves III, IV, and VI are not involved. Death of the motor neuron results in axonal degeneration and secondary demyelination with glial proliferation and sclerosis (scarring) along the corticospinal tract. Inclusion bodies containing the protein *uliquitin* are found in surviving neurons.

Lower motor neuron degeneration denervates motor units. Adjacent, still-viable lower motor neurons attempt to compensate by a process of distal intramuscular sprouting, reinnervation, and enlargement of motor units. The initial symptoms of the disease may be related to lower or upper motor neuron dysfunction or both. Fifty percent of persons with ALS present with hand weakness or incoordination, dysarthria, or leg weakness or incoordination.[35]

CLINICAL MANIFESTATIONS   Weakness may begin in any or all muscles of the body. Muscle weakness in ALS exhibits the following characteristics:

1. Paresis usually begins in a single muscle group.
2. Corresponding muscle groups are asymmetrically affected in a mottled distribution.
3. Gradual involvement occurs in all striated muscles except extraocular muscles and heart and progresses to paralysis with no remissions.
4. Flaccid and spastic paresis may coexist in a single muscle group; flaccid paresis may mask spasticity, which is usually mild.
5. Urethral and anal sphincter weakness is uncommon.
6. No associated mental, sensory, or autonomic symptoms are present. Normal intellectual and sensory functions are sustained until death.

The lower motor neuron syndrome of flaccid paresis consists of weakness of individual muscles, progressing to paralysis, associated with hypotonia and primary muscle atrophy (i.e., atrophy caused by denervation). Hypotonia is manifested by (1) decreased resistance to passive movement, (2) hypoactive or absent deep tendon reflexes, (3) absent abdominal and cremasteric reflexes, and (4) absent Babinski sign. Primary atrophy is manifested by (1) severe, irreversible muscular wasting; (2) fasciculations; (3) metabolically related changes in the skin and appendages; and (4) specific EMG findings. Fasciculations, along with fibrillations, are prominent features of ALS. Metabolic changes include (1) thinning of the skin, (2) thickening of the nails, (3) loss of body hair, and (4) decreased perspiration.

The upper motor neuron syndrome of spastic paresis consists of weakness of movement patterns, progressing to paralysis, associated with spasticity and, in some cases, atrophy secondary to disuse. Spasticity is manifested by (1) clasp-knife phenomenon, evident with passive movement; (2) hyperactive deep tendon reflexes and clonus with severe spasticity; (3) absent abdominal and cremasteric reflexes; and (4) presence of Babinski sign.

EVALUATION AND TREATMENT   The diagnosis of the syndrome is based predominantly on medical history and physical examination. EMG and muscle biopsy verify lower motor neuron degeneration and denervation. Muscle biopsy usually is not needed to confirm the diagnosis. Rilutek (Riluzole), an antiglutamate, is the first treatment for ALS.[36] It prolongs life. Treatment is also directed at symptom relief, prevention of complications, maintenance of maximal function, and maintenance of optimal quality of life.[37] Special problems requiring preventive and symptomatic management are communication difficulty caused by dysmasesis and dysphonia, salivation problems with either thick saliva or excessively thin saliva (sialorrhea), and dyspnea caused by diaphragmatic and intercostal weakness. Ventilatory issues become prominent. Supportive and rehabilitation management is directed toward preventing complications of immobility. Psychologic support of the affected individual and the family is extremely important in this disorder. A booklet, *Facts about ALS* (1999), is available from the ALS Association in Calabasas Hills, California. An ALS severity scale is also available.

The average duration of life is approximately 2 to 3 years from the appearance of symptoms, but the course of the disease may run from a few months to 15 years. Twenty percent of persons survive 5 years (benign form) and 10% survive 10 years.

Radiculopathies

As the spinal roots emerge from or enter the vertebral canal, they may be injured or damaged by compression, inflammation, or direct trauma whereby the roots are stretched or torn. **Radiculopathies** are disorders of roots of spinal nerves. **Radiculitis (radiculoneuritis)** refers to an inflammatory disorder of the spinal nerve roots. One or more roots may be affected.

PATHOPHYSIOLOGY   Many different pathologic conditions may cause compression, inflammation, or tearing of nerve roots. Roots may be traumatized by a forceful tearing of a nerve, termed *avulsion,* often associated with injuries to the head and shoulders. An acute intervertebral disk prolapse (herniated disk) or a benign tumor may compress nerve roots. Metastatic tumors of the lung, breast, and gastrointestinal tract may produce a carcinomatous meningitis, causing compression and inflammatory changes in nerve roots. Other causes of inflammatory changes in nerve roots are chronic meningitis, neurosyphilis, sarcoidosis, and **inflammatory arachnoiditis** produced by myelography and lumbar punctures.

CLINICAL MANIFESTATIONS   The strength, tone, and bulk of the muscles innervated by the involved roots are affected. The pattern and distribution of weakness and atrophy are similar to those of the amyotrophies. Tone and deep tendon reflexes are decreased, but rarely absent, because the involved muscles are usually innervated by two or more spinal roots. Fasciculations often are present, and mild fatigue may be experienced. Because pathologic processes usually affect both the ventral and dorsal roots, sensory alterations are common.

Diseases that involve spinal roots typically produce local pain; pain on local percussion; pain and paresthesias in the sensory root distribution (called **radicular pain** and **radicular paresthesia**); increased pain with movement, stretching of the root, and maneuvers that transiently increase CSF pressure; sensory loss in a radicular pattern; and spasms of the muscles surrounding the vertebral column (i.e., paravertebral muscle spasms).

EVALUATION AND TREATMENT   Diagnostic measures may include spinal films, EMG, lumbar puncture with CSF examination, myelography, and biopsy of tumor masses.

Treatment is directed at the cause of the injury and may take the form of surgery, antibiotics, removal of the injurious agent, steroids, and radiation therapy and chemotherapy. Supportive management may include control of the discomfort, protection from further injury, prevention of complications, and rehabilitation where appropriate.

Plexus Injuries

Plexus injuries involve the nerve plexus distal to the spinal roots but proximal to the formation of the peripheral nerves. Such injuries may be caused by trauma, compression, or infiltration, or they may be iatrogenic, caused by positioning during surgery or by an intramuscular injection. Clinical manifestations include motor weakness, muscle atrophy, and sensory loss in affected areas. Paralysis can occur with complete plexus lesions.

The diagnosis is made on the basis of history and clinical manifestations. Therapeutic treatment is directed at removal of the cause, repair and approximation of nervous tissue, prevention of further injury, control of discomfort, prevention of complications, and rehabilitation where appropriate.

Neuromuscular Junction Disorders

Transmission of the nerve impulse at the neuromuscular junction requires the release of adequate amounts of neurotransmitter from the presynaptic terminals of the axon and effective binding of the released transmitter to the receptors on the membranes of muscle cells (see Figure 14-13). Nutritional deficits, certain drugs (e.g., reserpine or methyldopa [Aldomet]), and certain disorders that interfere with the synthesis or packaging of the neurotransmitter or its release into the synaptic cleft may result in weakness. Likewise, any pathologic process or drug that interferes with the binding of the neurotransmitter to the receptor may cause weakness.

Marked weakness results from interference with neuromuscular transmission. The distribution of affected muscles is mainly in the bulbar, respiratory, and proximal muscle groups. Botulism toxin has a predilection for the cranial nerves. Eaton-Lambert syndrome affects limb musculature, whereas myasthenia gravis predominantly involves ocular, bulbar, and proximal upper extremity muscles. There is marked fatigability. Muscle tone may be slightly reduced, as may deep tendon reflexes, but the muscle cells are not denervated. Atrophy, if present, is only mild, probably because the small motor system is intact so that tone is maintained to a large degree. Fasciculations or sensory alterations are not present.

The weakness associated with presynaptic dysfunction (as in botulism or Eaton-Lambert syndrome) and that associated with postsynaptic dysfunction (as in myasthenia gravis) are difficult to distinguish clinically, although theoretically some difference should be evident.

Myasthenia Gravis

Myasthenia gravis is a chronic autoimmune disease mediated by antiacetylcholine receptor antibodies that act at the neuromuscular junction; it affects 20,000 to 70,000 persons in the United States. The disease is characterized by exertional fatigue and weakness that worsens with activity, improves with rest, and recurs with resumption of activity. The female/male ratio is 3:2 in younger-aged persons. More males in the older age-group (over 50 years of age) have myasthenia gravis. In 10% to 25% of persons with myasthenia gravis, thymic tumors are found. Of persons with myasthenia gravis, 70% to 80% have pathologic changes in the thymus. Such tumors are more common in males than in females. Myasthenia gravis is an autoimmune disease associated with an increased incidence of other autoimmune diseases, including systemic lupus erythematosus, rheumatoid arthritis, polymyositis, and thyrotoxicosis. (Autoimmune mechanisms are discussed in Chapter 8.) Transitory signs of myasthenia gravis are present in 10% to 15% of infants born to mothers with myasthenia gravis.

Classification of presentations for myasthenia gravis are neonatal myasthenia, congenital myasthenia (neonatal persistent myasthenia), juvenile myasthenia, ocular myasthenia, and generalized autoimmune myasthenia. In **neonatal myasthenia,** onset of signs is 1 to 3 days after birth and the signs persist for a few days to a few weeks. Myasthenia immune globulin is transferred from the mother to the neonate through the placenta. **Congenital myasthenia** presents in infancy and continues into adulthood. The maternal side of the family usually has a positive history for myasthenia gravis. **Juvenile myasthenia** is an autoimmune disorder with a childhood onset usually about 10 years of age. **Ocular myasthenia,** which is more common in males, involves muscle weakness of the eye muscles and eyelids and may include swallowing difficulties and slurred speech as well. **Generalized autoimmune myasthenia** involves the proximal musculature throughout the body and has several courses: (1) a course with periodic remissions, (2) a slowly progressive course, (3) a rapidly progressive course, or (4) a fulminating course. Classification by disease severity is:

> *Grade I:* ocular disease
> *Grade II:* generalized mild weakness
> *Grade IIa:* mild weakness
> *Grade IIb:* moderate weakness
> *Grade III:* severe generalized weakness
> *Grade IV:* myasthenic "crisis" with respiratory failure[38]

PATHOPHYSIOLOGY Myasthenia gravis results from a defect in nerve impulse transmission at the neuromuscular junction. The postsynaptic acetylcholine receptors (ACh-R) on the muscle cell's plasma membrane for an unknown reason are no longer recognized as "self" and therefore elicit the generation of antibodies. Acetylcholine receptor antibodies (an IgG antibody) is produced against the acetylcholine receptors. These fix onto the receptor sites and block the binding of acetylcholine. Eventually the antibody action causes the destruction of receptor sites, and the number of receptors on the plasma membrane is reduced. The destruction of receptor sites causes diminished transmission of the nerve impulse across the neuromuscular junction. Muscle depolarization is incomplete or not achieved. The cause of this autosensitization is not known. Evidence supports the autoimmune theory. Clinical and laboratory data show the following:

1. Receptor-binding antibodies are present in 85% to 90% of persons with myasthenia gravis.
2. Passive transfer of myasthenia gravis to animals is possible by injecting serum and IgG from humans with myasthenia gravis.
3. Myasthenia gravis frequently is associated with other autoimmune disorders, such as rheumatoid arthritis, systemic lupus erythematosus, and thyroid disease.
4. Transitory neonatal myasthenia gravis occurs.
5. A strong association between myasthenia gravis and thymus gland hyperplasia exists (0.80).
6. Steroid therapy, antimetabolite drugs, plasma exchange, and thoracic duct drainage all improve the clinical status of the patient with myasthenia gravis.
7. Correlation exists with specific HLA types (HLA-B8).

CLINICAL MANIFESTATIONS   Myasthenia gravis typically has an insidious onset. Clinical manifestations may first appear during pregnancy, during the postpartum period, or in conjunction with the administration of certain anesthetic agents. The foremost complaint is muscular fatigue and progressive weakness. The patient often complains of fatigue after exercise and has a recent history of recurring upper respiratory tract infections. The muscles of the eyes, face, mouth, throat, and neck usually are affected first. The extraocular (eye) muscles and the levator muscles are most affected. Manifestations include diplopia, ptosis, and ocular palsies.

The muscles of facial expression, mastication, swallowing, and speech are the next most involved. The results are facial droop and an expressionless face; difficulty chewing and swallowing associated with dietary changes and weight loss; drooling; episodes of choking and aspiration; and a nasal, low-volume but high-pitched monotonous speech pattern.

The muscles of the neck, shoulder girdle, and hip flexors are affected less frequently. When these muscles do become involved, however, the person experiences fatigue requiring periods of rest, weakness of the arms and legs that improves with rest, and difficulty in maintaining head position. The respiratory muscles of the diaphragm and chest wall become weak, and ventilation is impaired. Impairment in deep breathing and coughing predisposes the individual to atelectasis and congestion. In the advanced stage of the disease, all the muscles are weak.

Myasthenic crisis occurs when severe muscle weakness causes extreme quadriparesis or quadriplegia, respiratory insufficiency with shortness of breath and a markedly decreased tidal volume and vital capacity, and extreme difficulty in swallowing. The individual in myasthenic crisis is in danger of respiratory arrest. Myasthenic crisis usually occurs 3 to 4 hours after the patient takes medication.

Cholinergic crisis may arise secondary to drug overdose (anticholinerase drug toxicity). The clinical picture resembles that of myasthenic crisis but the weakness occurs 30 to 60 minutes after taking anticholinergic medication. Other symptoms are also present. Intestinal motility increases and is associated with episodes of diarrhea and complaints of cramping; fasciculation, bradycardia, pupillary constriction, increased salivation, and increased sweating are present. These clinical manifestations are caused by the smooth muscle hyperactivity secondary to excessive accumulation of acetylcholine at the neuromuscular junctions and excessive parasympathetic-like activity. As in myasthenic crisis, the individual is in danger of respiratory arrest.

EVALUATION AND TREATMENT   The diagnosis of myasthenia gravis is made on the basis of a response to edrophonium chloride (Tensilon), repetitive single-fiber EMG, and antistriated muscle antibodies. The antibodies are found in 80% of persons with generalized autoimmune myasthenia and 70% of persons with occular myasthenia. With intravenous administration of Tensilon, immediate improvement in muscle strength usually persists for 5 to 10 minutes (Figure 17-33). The EMG is diagnostic in that the muscle fiber weakens readily. Mediastinal CT and MRI are used to determine whether a thymoma is present. Thymus gland abnormalities are seen in 75% of all persons with myasthenia. The progression of myasthenia gravis is highly variable. In some individuals it is mild and spontaneously remits. There is usually a series of relapses, with symptom-free intervals ranging from weeks to months. Over time the disease can progress, leading to death. Ocular myasthenia has a very good prognosis.

Anticholinesterase drugs, steroids, immunosuppressant drugs, azathioprine, and cyclosporine are used to treat myasthenia gravis and myasthenic crisis.[38] Plasmapheresis may be

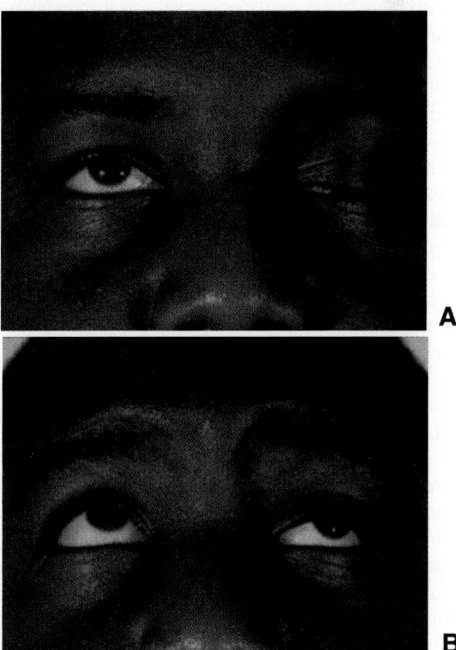

Figure 17-33 Appearance of the eyes (A) before and (B) after injection of intravenous Tensilon. (From Perkin DG: *Mosby's color atlas and text of neurology,* London, 1998, Mosby-Wolfe.)

lifesaving during myasthenic crisis, before and after thymectomy, and at the start of immunosuppressant therapy. For individuals with cholinergic crisis, treatment is to withhold anticholinergic drugs until blood levels fall out of the toxic range, while providing ventilatory support and preventing respiratory complications. Thymectomy is the treatment of choice in individuals with a thymoma.

Myopathies

Myopathy is the term applied to a primary muscle disorder. Many pathologic processes affect muscles and cause loss of functional muscle cells. Within myopathies, muscle strength, tone, and bulk are affected. Primary muscle disease is invariably associated with weakness—usually marked weakness. The distribution of the weakness in myopathy is usually symmetric and proximal, although occasionally the weakness is predominantly distal, such as in myotonic dystrophy. The weakness is associated with mild fatigue. Tone is decreased, as are the tendon reflexes. Atrophy may be present. Some myopathies are associated with muscle hypertrophy as in cretinism and the familial progressive muscular dystrophies of childhood, in which hypertrophied muscles are rubbery and weak. Fasciculations are not present with myopathy because no denervation is present. No sensory changes are found. (Specific myopathies are discussed in Chapter 16.)

SUMMARY REVIEW

Central Nervous System Disorders

1. Motor vehicle accidents (MVAs) are the major cause of traumatic CNS injury. Traumatic injuries are classified as closed-head trauma (blunt) or open-head trauma (penetrating). Closed-head trauma is the more common type of trauma.
2. Different types of focal brain injury include contusion (bruising of the brain), laceration (tearing of brain tissue), extradural hematoma (accumulation of blood above the dura mater), subdural hematoma (blood between the dura mater and arachnoid membrane), intracerebral hematoma (bleeding into the brain), and open-head trauma.
3. Open-head trauma involves a skull fracture with exposure of the cranial vault to the environment. The types of open-head trauma (compound fracture, perforated fracture) are linear, comminuted, compound, and basilar skull fracture (in the cranial vault or at the base of the skull).
4. Diffuse axonal injury (DAI) results from the effects of head rotation. The brain experiences shearing stresses resulting in axonal damage ranging from concussion to a severe DAI state.
5. Spinal cord injuries occur most often in young men who sustain various kinds of injuries (recreational or travel related) and elderly persons because of preexisting degenerative vertebral disorders.
6. Spinal cord injury involves damage to vertebral or neural tissues by compressing tissue, pulling or exerting tension on tissue, or shearing tissues so that they slide into one another.
7. Spinal cord injury often causes spinal shock with cessation of all motor, sensory, reflex, and autonomic functions below any transected area. Loss of motor and sensory function depends on the level of injury.
8. Paralysis of the lower half of the body with both legs involved is called *paraplegia*. Paralysis involving all four extremities is called *quadriplegia*.
9. Return of spinal neuron excitability occurs slowly. Reflex activity can return in 1 to 2 weeks in most persons with acute spinal cord injury. A pattern of flexion reflexes emerges, involving first the toes and then the feet and the legs. Eventually, reflex voiding and bowel elimination appear and mass reflex (flexor spasms accompanied by profuse sweating, piloerection, and automatic bladder emptying) may develop.
10. Immobilization of the spine is the immediate intervention for a suggested or confirmed vertebral fracture.
11. The pathologic findings in degenerative disk disease (DDD) include disk protrusion, spondylosis, and/or subluxation and degeneration of the vertebrae (spondylolisthesis) and spinal stenosis.
12. Low back pain is pain between the lower rib cage and gluteal muscles and often radiates into the thigh.
13. Low back pain has a high prevalence, affecting 75% to 90% of the population at some time. Sciatica affects about 1% of those with low back pain.
14. Most causes of low back pain are unknown; however, some secondary causes are disk prolapse, tumor, bursitis, synovitis, DDD, osteoporosis, fracture, inflammation, and sprain.
15. Diagnosis of injury to the lower back is made on the basis of physical examination, electromyography (EMG), myelography, computed tomography (CT), and magnetic resonance imaging (MRI).
16. Treatment for low back pain includes bed rest, use of analgesics and anti-inflammatory agents, exercise, physical therapy, education, and surgery.
17. Herniation of an intervertebral disk is a protrusion of part of the nucleus pulposus. Herniation most commonly affects the lumbosacral disks (L5-S1 and L4-5). The extruded pulposus compresses the nerve root, causing pain that radiates along the sciatic nerve course.
18. The conservative approach to treatment of an intervertebral rupture is traction and bed rest. Surgery is indicated if there is evidence of severe compression (weakness, chronic pain, decreased deep tendon reflexes, and bladder/bowel reflexes).
19. Cerebrovascular disease is the most frequently occurring neurologic disorder. Any abnormality of the blood vessels of the brain is referred to as a cerebrovascular disease.
20. Cerebrovascular disease is associated with two types of brain abnormalities: (a) ischemia with or without infarction and (b) hemorrhage.
21. The most common clinical manifestation of cerebrovascular disease is a cerebrovascular accident (CVA, stroke syndrome).
22. Cerebrovascular accidents are classified according to pathophysiology and include global hypoperfusion and thrombotic (arterial occlusions caused by thrombi), embolic (fragments that break from a thrombus outside the brain), hemorrhagic (intracranial hemorrhage), and lacunar strokes.
23. Treatment for an ischemic CVA includes preventing further thrombotic events, augmenting blood flow, reperfusing tissues, and protecting neurons, as well as supportive management for cerebral edema and increased intracranial pressure. Surgical intervention may be required to restore blood supply.
24. Intracranial aneurysms result from defects in the vascular wall and are classified on the basis of form and shape. They are commonly asymptomatic, but the signs vary according to the location and size of the aneurysm.

25. In cerebral aneurysms, surgical intervention is the treatment of choice before rupture.
26. An arteriovenous malformation (AVM) is a tangled mass of dilated blood vessels. Although sometimes present at birth, AVM exhibits a delayed age of onset.
27. Clinical manifestations of AVM range from headache and dementia to seizures and intracerebral or subarachnoid hemorrhage.
28. A subarachnoid hemorrhage occurs when blood escapes from defective or injured vasculature into the subarachnoid space. When a vessel tears, blood under pressure is pumped into the subarachnoid space. The blood produces an inflammatory reaction in these tissues.
29. Clinical manifestations of a subarachnoid hemorrhage include headache, changes in mental status, transient motor weakness, and numbness and tingling. Vasospasm is a serious complication and may cause ischemia and infarct. Treatment of vasospasm includes use of calcium channel blockers to prevent or reverse vasospasm and augmenting cerebral perfusion by volume expansion and hemodilution.
30. Migraine headache occurs with and without aura and is precipitated by a triggering event. The aura is associated with a spreading wave of cortical depression and decreased blood flow accompanied by scotomas and jagged flashes of light and sensory changes.
31. Etiologic theories of migraine include a central alteration in neurotransmitters, ions, and hormones with altered neural function and blood flow. In women, migraine is associated with the cyclic withdrawal of estrogen.
32. The headache of migraine is throbbing and intense; it may be accompanied by photophobia, nausea, and vomiting.
33. Cluster headaches occur in episodes several times during a day for a period of days at different times of the year. The pain is unilateral, intense, tearing, and burning. Associated symptoms include ptosis, lacrimation, reddening of the eye, and nausea. The etiology is unknown but involves hyperactivity of the sympathetic nervous system; the two forms are acute and chronic.
34. Chronic paroxysmal hemicrania is a cluster headache with more frequent daily attacks; it occurs primarily in women. It responds to treatment with indomethacin.
35. Tension-type headache is the most common type of headache. Both a central mechanism and a peripheral mechanism are associated with the etiology. The headache is bilateral, with the sensation of a tight band around the head. The pain may last for hours or days. There are acute and chronic forms.
36. Two main types of tumors occur within the cranium: primary and metastatic. Primary tumors are classified as intracerebral or extracerebral. Metastatic tumors can be found inside or outside the brain substance.
37. Central nervous system (CNS) tumors cause local and generalized manifestations. The effects are varied; local manifestations include seizures, visual disturbances, loss of equilibrium, and cranial nerve dysfunction.
38. The principal treatment for brain tumors is surgical or radiosurgical excision or decompression if total excision is not possible. Chemotherapy and radiation therapy also are used.
39. Spinal cord tumors are classified as intramedullary (within the neural tissues) or extramedullary (outside the spinal cord). Metastatic spinal cord tumors are usually carcinomas, lymphomas, or myelomas.
40. Extramedullary spinal cord tumors produce dysfunction by compression of adjacent tissue, not by direct invasion. Intramedullary spinal cord tumors produce dysfunction by both invasion and compression.

41. The onset of clinical manifestations of spinal cord tumors is gradual and progressive, suggesting compression. Specific manifestations depend on the location of the tumor; for example, there may be paresis and spasticity of one leg with thoracic tumors, followed by involvement of the opposite leg.
42. Spinal cord tumors are treated by surgery, radiation therapy, chemotherapy, and hormonal therapy.
43. Infection and inflammation of the CNS can occur by bacteria, viruses, fungi, protozoans, and rickettsiae. The resulting infection of bacterial infections is pus producing, or pyogenic.
44. Meningitis (infection of the meninges) is classified as bacterial, aseptic (nonpurulent), or fungal. Bacterial meningitis is primarily an infection of the pia mater and arachnoid and of the fluid of the subarachnoid space. Aseptic meningitis is believed to be limited to the meninges. Fungal meningitis is a chronic, less common type of meningitis.
45. The meningeal vessels become hyperemic, and neutrophils migrate into the subarachnoid space with bacterial meningitis. An inflammatory reaction occurs, and exudation ensues and increases rapidly.
46. The variety of clinical manifestations depends on the type of meningitis and ranges from throbbing headache to neck stiffness and rigidity and decreasing responsiveness. Specific cranial nerve dysfunction is a common occurrence.
47. Bacterial meningitis and fungal meningitis are treated with appropriate antibiotic therapy; aseptic meningitis is treated with antibiotics, antiviral drugs, and steroids.
48. Brain abscesses often originate from infections outside the CNS. Microorganisms gain access to the CNS from adjacent sites or spread along the wall of a vein. A localized inflammatory process develops with exudate formation, thrombosis of vessels, and degenerating leukocytes. After a few days the infection becomes delimited, with a center of pus and a wall of granular tissue.
49. Clinical manifestations of brain abscesses include headache, nuchal rigidity, confusion, drowsiness, and sensory and communication deficits. Treatment includes antibiotic therapy and surgical excision or aspiration.
50. Encephalitis is an acute, febrile illness of viral origin with nervous system involvement. The most common encephalitides are caused by arthropod-borne viruses and herpes simplex virus. Meningeal involvement appears in all encephalitides.
51. Clinical manifestations of encephalitis include fever, delirium, confusion, seizures, abnormal and involuntary movement, and increased intracranial pressure.
52. Herpes encephalitis is treated with antiviral agents. Ribavirin is used for LaCrosse encephalitis. No definitive treatment exists for the other encephalitides.
53. The common neurologic complications of acquired immunodeficiency syndrome (AIDS) are human immunodeficiency virus (HIV) neuropathy, HIV myelopathy, opportunistic infections, cytomegalovirus infection, parasitic infection, and neoplasms. Pathologically, there may be diffuse CNS involvement, focal pathologic findings, and obstructive hydrocephalus.
54. Multiple sclerosis (MS) is a relatively common degenerative disorder involving CNS myelin. Although the pathogenesis is unknown, the demyelination is thought to result from an immunogenetic-viral cause. A previous viral insult to the nervous system in a genetically susceptible individual yields a subsequent abnormal immune response in the CNS.
55. The clinical manifestations of MS involve different types: mixed or generalized, spinal, and cerebellar.
56. No treatment is available to cure MS. Steroid and immune therapy is used to acutely manage relapses or reduce frequency of relapses.

Continued

Peripheral Nervous System and Neuromuscular Junction Disorders

1. Neuropathies are the syndromes that result when the peripheral nerves are affected. Axon and myelin degeneration may be present. Neuropathies are classified as generalized symmetric polyneuropathies, generalized neuropathy, and focal or multifocal neuropathies.
2. Therapy for the neuropathies is directed at the primary cause, such as diabetes mellitus. Axonal regrowth and recovery of function may take months, but many neuropathies can be reversed.
3. Guillain-Barré syndrome is a demyelinating disorder caused by a humoral and cell-mediated immunologic reaction directed at the peripheral nerves. The clinical manifestations may vary from paresis of the legs to complete quadriplegia, respiratory insufficiency, and autonomic nervous system instability. Plasmapheresis or plasma exchange is used in severe disease, followed by aggressive rehabilitation.
4. Amyotrophic lateral sclerosis (ALS) is a degenerative disorder diffusely involving lower and upper motor neurons. The pathogenesis of ALS is not fully known; however, both lower and upper motor neuron degeneration occur.
5. Clinical manifestations of ALS may include weakness in all muscles. Flaccid paresis progressing to paralysis is characteristic of the lower motor neuron syndrome. One treatment is currently available to alter the time course of the ALS syndrome.
6. Radiculopathies are disorders of the roots of spinal cord nerves. The roots may be compressed, inflamed, or torn. Clinical manifestations include local pain or paresthesias in the sensory root distribution. Treatment may involve surgery, antibiotics, steroids, radiation therapy, and chemotherapy.
7. Plexus injuries involve the plexus distal to the spinal roots. Paralysis can occur with complete plexus involvement.
8. Myasthenia gravis is a disorder of voluntary muscles characterized by muscle weakness and fatigability. It is considered an autoimmune disease and is associated with an increased incidence of other autoimmune diseases.
9. Myasthenia gravis results from a defect in nerve impulse transmission at the neuromuscular junction. Acetycholine receptor antibody is secreted against the "self" and blocks the binding of acetylcholine. The antibody action destroys the receptor sites, causing decreased transmission of the nerve impulse across the neuromuscular junction.
10. Clinical manifestations of myasthenia gravis include weakness of the muscles of the face and throat and may involve muscles of the diaphragm and chest wall.
11. Treatment of myasthenia gravis involves symptom relief and immunotherapy. The progression of the disease is highly variable; in some individuals it is mild and spontaneously remits.
12. Primary disorders with weakness and atrophy are known as myopathies.

MEDIA RESOURCES  evolve

Review questions and answers for this chapter are available in the *CD Companion* included with this book. Also see the CD for an animation on *pathogenesis of metastasis.*

WebLinks—links to Internet sites pertaining to this chapter—are available on Evolve at http://evolve.elsevier.com/McCance/.

REFERENCES

1. Marion DW: *Traumatic brain injury,* New York, 1999, Thieme.
2. van der Naalt J et al: One year outcome in mild to moderate head injury: the predictive value of acute injury characteristics related to complaints and return to work, *J Neurol Neuros Psychiatry* 66(2):207-213, 1999.
3. Evans RW, Wilberger JE: Traumatic disorders. In Goetz CG, editor, *Textbook of clinical neurology,* ed 2, pp 1129-1153, Philadelphia, 2003, Saunders.
4. Sullivan J: Spinal cord injury research: review and synthesis, *Crit Care Nurs Q* 22(2):80-99, 1999.
5. Mitcho K, Yanko JR: Acute care management of spinal cord injury, *Crit Care Nurs Q* 22(2):60-79, 1999.
6. Sarasin FP, Gaspoz JM, Bornameaux H: Cost effectiveness of antiplatelet regimens used as secondary prevention of stroke or transient ischemic attack, *Arch Intern Med* 160(18):2773-2778, 2000.
7. Pyorala M et al: Insulin resistance syndrome predicts the risk of coronary heart disease and stroke in healthy middle-aged men: the 22-year follow-up results of the Helsinki Policeman Study, *Arterioscler Thromb Vasc Biol* 20(2):538-544, 2000.
8. Eikelboom JW: Association between high homocyst(e)ine and ischemic stroke due to large- and small-artery disease but not other etiologic subtypes of ischemic stroke, *Stroke* 31(5):1069-1075, 2000.
9. Chung CS, Caplan LR: Neurovascular disorders. In Goetz CG, editor, *Textbook of clinical neurology,* ed 2, Philadelphia, 2003, Saunders.
10. Osborn TM, LaMonte MR, Gaasch WR: Intravenous thrombolytic therapy for stroke: a review of recent studies and controversies, *Ann Emerg Med* 34(2):244-255, 1999.
11. Mohr JP et al: A comparison of warfarin and aspirin for the prevention of recurrent ischemic stroke, *New Engl J Med* 345(20):1444-1451, 2001.
12. Kothari R et al: Acute stroke: delays to presentation and emergency department evaluation, *Ann Emerg Med* 33(1):3-8, 1999.
13. Roquer J, Campello AR, Gomis M: Sex differences in first-ever acute stroke, *Stroke* 34(7):1581-1585, 2003.
14. Glader EL et al: Sex differences in management and outcome after stroke: a Swedish national perspective, *Stroke* 34(8):1970-1975, 2003.
15. Gupta J: To clip or to coil, *Time* 159(9), 2002.
16. Kealy KA, Dilger K: Unsuspected venous angioma infarct:. a case study. In *AANN 32nd annual meeting program book,* New Orleans, 2000, AANN.
17. Headache Classification Committee of the International Headache Society: Classification and diagnostic criteria for headache disorders, cranial neuralgias, and facial pain, *Cephalagia* 8(suppl 7):1, 1988.
18. Janus TJ, Yung KA: Primary neurological tumors. In Goetz CG, editor, *Textbook of clinical neurology,* ed 2, Philadelphia, 2003, Saunders.
19. Benjamin RK, Das A, Hochberg FH: Metastatic neoplasms and paraneoplastic syndrome. In Goetz CG, editor, *Textbook of clinical neurology,* ed 2, Philadelphia, 2003, Saunders.
20. Roos KL: Nonviral infections. In Goetz CG, editor, *Textbook of clinical neurology,* ed 2, Philadelphia, 2003, Saunders.
21. Roos KL: Viral infections. In Goetz CG, editor, *Textbook of clinical neurology,* ed 2, Philadelphia, 2003, Saunders.
22. Belman AL, Maleti-Savatic M: Human immunodeficiency virus and acquired immunodeficiency syndrome. In Goetz CG, editor, *Textbook of clinical neurology,* ed 2, Philadelphia, 2003, Saunders.
23. Calabresi PA: Diagosis and management of multiple sclerosis, *Am Fam Physician,* 70(10):1934-1944, 2004.
24. Lucchinetti C et al: Heterogeneity of the multiple sclerosis lesions: implications for the pathogenesis of demyelination, *Ann Neurol* 47(6):707-717, 2000.
25. Huseby ES et al: A pathogenic role for myelin specific CD8(+) T cells in a model for multiple sclerosis, *J Exp Med* 194(5):669-776, 2001.
26. Seppa N: The give and take of Parkinson's disease, *Sci News* 156:342, 1999.
27. Pirko I, Noseworthy JH: Demyelinating disorders of the central nervous system. In Goetz CG, editor, *Textbook of clinical neurology,* ed 2, Philadelphia, 2003, Saunders.
28. Chabus D et al: The influence of the proinflammatory cytokine, osteopontin, on autoimmune demyelinating disease, *Sci* 294:1731-1735, 2001.
29. McCarthy RJ, Olney RK: Neuromuscular diseases. In Corey-Bloom J, editor, *Adult neurology,* St. Louis, 1998, Mosby.
30. Reges T: Gastroparesis, an autonomic neuropathy: recognition, diagnosis and treatment, *AACN News* 21(2):14, 2004.
31. Shields Jr RW, Wilbourn AJ: Demyelinating disorders of the peripheral nervous system. In Goetz CG, editor, *Textbook of clinical neurology,* ed 2, Philadelphia, 2003, Saunders.
32. Walling AD: Amyotrophic lateral sclerosis: Lou Gehrig's disease, *Am Fam Physician* 59(6):1489-1496, 1999.
33. Morrison BM, Morrison JH: Amyotrophic lateral sclerosis associated with mutations in superoxide dismutase: a punative mechanism of degeneration, *Brain Res Brain Res Rev* 29(1):121-135, 1999.
34. Seppa N: Nerve cells of ALS patients harbor virus, *Sci News* 157:37, 2000.
35. Siddique N, Sufit R, Siddique T: Degenerative motor, sensory and autonomic disorders. In Goetz CG, editor, *Textbook of clinical neurology,* ed 2, Philadelphia, 2003, Saunders.
36. Bromberg MG: Ongoing trials in motor neuron disease, *Expert Opin Invest Drugs* 8(6):885-902, 1999.
37. Miller RG et al: Practice parameters: the care of the patient with amyotrophic lateral sclerosis (an evidence-based review): report of the Quality Standards Subcommittee of the American Academy of Neurology: ALS Practice Parameters Task Force, *Neurol* 52(7):1311-1323, 1999.
38. Bartt R, Shannon KM: Autoimmune and inflammatory disorders. In Goetz CG, editor, *Textbook of clinical neurology,* ed 2, Philadelphia, 2003, Saunders.

NEUROBIOLOGY OF SCHIZOPHRENIA, MOOD DISORDERS, AND ANXIETY DISORDERS

LOREY K. TAKAHASHI

evolve

CHAPTER OUTLINE

Mental illnesses are common and have a long history of afflicting humanity. They appear in different cultures and across the socioeconomic spectrum. When mental disorders are left untreated, the consequences can be devastating. This chapter provides an introduction to the neurobiology of schizophrenia, mood disorders, and anxiety disorders. The etiology and pathophysiology of these major mental illnesses are diverse and complex. Diagnostic criteria are constantly being updated to more precisely diagnose and effectively treat the disorders. Every mental disorder manifests a range of symptoms that vary in intensity for each individual. Symptom variations likely reflect individual differences in neural pathologic brain structures and functions, which impact the options for treatment. To further complicate diagnosis and treatment, comorbidity of disorders such as depression and anxiety are often present.

Insight into the pathophysiologic basis of mental disorders has been greatly aided by the development of structural and functional neuroimaging techniques that provide a visual and quantitative evaluation of diseased brain regions. In schizophrenia, neuroanatomic, functional, and neurochemical alterations associated with this debilitating disorder have been uncovered along with a host of candidate genes that confer risk. Similarly, in mood and anxiety disorders, brain scans are providing new information on structural and functional abnormalities. Many of the altered brain regions found in those with schizophrenia, mood, and anxiety disorders involve structures implicated in normal cognitive and emotional processes, suggesting that their exaggerated or diminished functions underlie the illness.

Knowledge of the pathophysiology associated with a specific mental illness has guided the development of pharmacologic medications. Although more effective second- and third-generation drugs with fewer side effects are currently available, many individuals continue to suffer. Future identification and characterization of diseased genes and how they contribute to psychopathology may eventually lead to medications that produce effective relief of symptoms and stop or reverse the neural alterations that produce the disorder.

SCHIZOPHRENIA

Schizophrenia is a serious psychiatric illness that strikes 1% of the world's population. **Schizophrenia** is the term coined originally by Eugene Bleuler in 1911 to describe a collection of illnesses characterized by thought disorders. According to Bleuler, **thought disorders** reflected a break in reality or splitting of the cognitive from the emotional side of one's personality. A schizophrenic individual may exhibit a feeling of happiness when recollecting a terrible event or emotional indifference when describing a joyful occasion. Thought disorders are manifested also by incoherent speech, delusions (abnormal beliefs), and hallucinations (imaginary perceptions). These so-called *positive symptoms* (Box 18-1) commonly

Box 18-1 Major Symptoms of Schizophrenia

Positive Symptoms

Hallucinations
Auditory
Somatic-tactile
Visual

Delusions
Delusions of being controlled
Delusions of mind reading
Delusions of reference
Guilt
Grandiose
Persecutory
Religious
Somatic
Thought broadcasting
Thought insertion
Thought withdrawal

Positive formal thought disorder
Circumstantiality
Derailment
Distractible speech
Illogicality
Incoherence
Pressure of speech
Tangentiality

Bizarre behavior
Aggressive, agitated
Clothing, appearance
Repetitive, stereotyped
Social, sexual behavior

Negative Symptoms

Affective flattening
Affective nonresponsivity
Decreased spontaneous movements
Inappropriate affect
Lack of vocal inflections
Paucity of expressive gestures
Poor eye contact
Unchanging facial expression

Alogia
Blocking
Increase in response latency
Poverty of speech
Poverty of speech content

Anhedonia-asociality
Few recreational interests
Few social relationships
Impaired intimacy
Little sexual interest

Attention
Social inattentiveness
Inattentiveness during testing

Avolition-apathy
Impaired personal hygiene
Lack of persistence
Physical anergia

---

occur during a **psychotic episode,** when the individual loses touch with reality.

In addition to psychotic episodes, individuals may exhibit blunted affect, apathy, poverty of speech, and lack of social interactions. There characteristics are termed *negative symptoms* (see Box 18-1). Thus schizophrenia is an illness of multiple symptoms (see Clinical Manifestations). The illness emerges in young adults during the late teens and early twenties, with a slightly earlier onset in males than in females.

Etiology and Pathophysiology
Genetic Predisposition

Genetic epidemiologic studies demonstrate that schizophrenia is a heritable disorder. In monozygotic twins, the concordance rate varies from 30% to 50%. This variability may stem from different diagnostic criteria and methodological or sampling differences across studies. In dizygotic twins and siblings, the concordance rate decreases to 15%, which is still considerably higher than the 1% figure found in the general population.

Nonetheless, schizophrenia is not a simple genetic disorder in which inherited disease alleles generally lead to illness. Schizophrenia likely involves several genes located on different chromosomes and differs from Mendelian disorders, in which genes are fully penetrant. That is, in Mendelian disorders, individuals with genes for a disease (e.g., Huntington disease) will usually develop the disorder. In contrast, as indi-

cated by the 50% concordance rate in monozygotic twins, the genes for schizophrenia show reduced penetrance resulting in individuals who may carry the disease genes without manifesting the illness. Further complicating the search for the genes that confer risk of schizophrenia is the variability in biologic and phenotypic traits among individuals who manifest the illness.

Prenatal and Perinatal Factors

A leading hypothesis for the etiology of schizophrenia suggests that the illness results from neurodevelopmental defects that occur in fetal life. According to this hypothesis, environmental factors interfere with genetically programmed neural development leading to alterations in brain structure and function.[1] An early brain defect may remain silent and not affect the individual until subsequent development requires extensive use of that brain structure.[2] Several early environmental factors have been suggested to increase the risk of developing schizophrenia including viral infection during pregnancy, prenatal nutritional deficiencies, and perinatal complications, such as birth defects and neonatal hypoxia.

Neuroanatomic and Functional Abnormalities
Neuroanatomic Alterations

The use of advanced neuroimaging techniques has provided strong evidence for structural brain abnormalities of individuals with schzophrenia.[3,4] A consistent finding is the enlargement of the lateral and third ventricles and widening of frontal cortical fissures and sulci (Figure 18-1). In addition, some imaging studies reveal reductions in the thalamus and temporal lobe, which includes the amygdala, hippocampus, and parahippocampal gyrus, brain areas important in emotional regulation and memory functions. Postmortem brain examinations support the brain imaging studies and provide further evidence for an early neurodevelopmental defect in schizophrenia.[5] For example, in the hippocampal formation, there is a marked reduction in dentate granule cell density and a disarray of pyramidal cells in the horn of Ammon. In addition, a significant reduction is found in cell density and volume of the entorhinal cortex, a major subfield of the hippocampal formation receiving diverse cortical information. These temporal lobe alterations may be linked to the positive schizophrenic symptoms, such as hallucinations, delusions, thought disorder, and bizarre behavior. Indirect support for this view comes from studies showing that in nonpsychotic individuals, electrical stimulation of the temporal lobe induces hallucinations and delusions.

The abnormalities documented in schizophrenic brains are believed to originate during the prenatal period of cell proliferation and migration. Reelin, an extracellular matrix protein involved in neuronal migration during development and synaptic function in the adult, is reduced in the prefrontal cortex and hippocampus of schizophrenic individuals.[6,7] Reelin is concentrated in interneurons that contain **γ-aminobutyric acid (GABA),** the most widespread inhibitory neurotransmitter in the brain. Furthermore, in the dorsal prefrontal cortex of schizophrenic brains, glutamic acid decarboxylase, the major enzyme in GABA biosynthesis, is diminished, which likely impairs synaptic performance and cognitive and behavioral functions associated with this brain region.

Data suggest that the pathophysiologic processes in the dorsal prefrontal cortex are responsible for the negative symptoms of schizophrenia (Figure 18-2). In particular, the **dorsal lateral prefrontal cortex (DLPFC)** is intricately involved in the initiation and maintenance of goal-directed activities and is actively involved in solving cognitive problems related to working memory. **Working memory** involves the brief storage and use of information that may be important in simple number calculations as well as complex tasks such as winning a chess match. Working memory is also essential in verbal comprehension and reasoning. During cognitive problem solving, blood flow and metabolism normally increase in the DLPFC. However, individuals with schizophrenia often perform poorly on these tests and fail to show an increase in cortical blood flow and metabolism. These studies suggest that the dorsal prefrontal cortex is hypoactive in schizophrenia.

Recent brain imaging work indicates that brain abnormalities, which are evident by the time the patient seeks treatment, progressively worsen throughout the course of the illness despite the use of antipsychotic medication.[8] In particular, the frontal lobe undergoes a progressive loss in volume that is accompanied by increased severity of negative symptoms and reduced cognitive functioning. These results

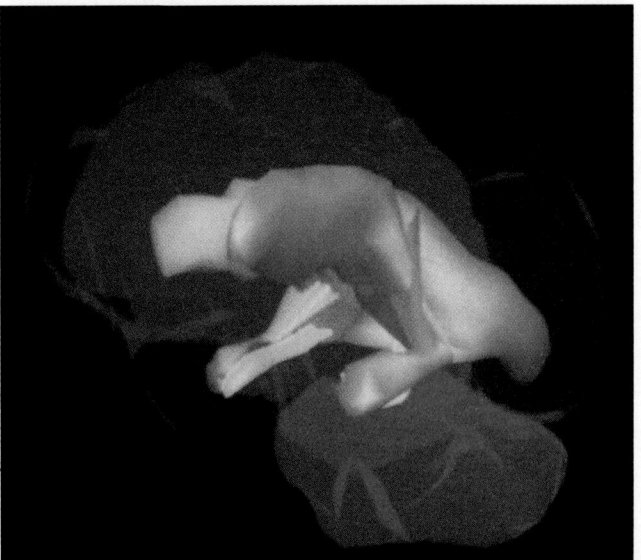

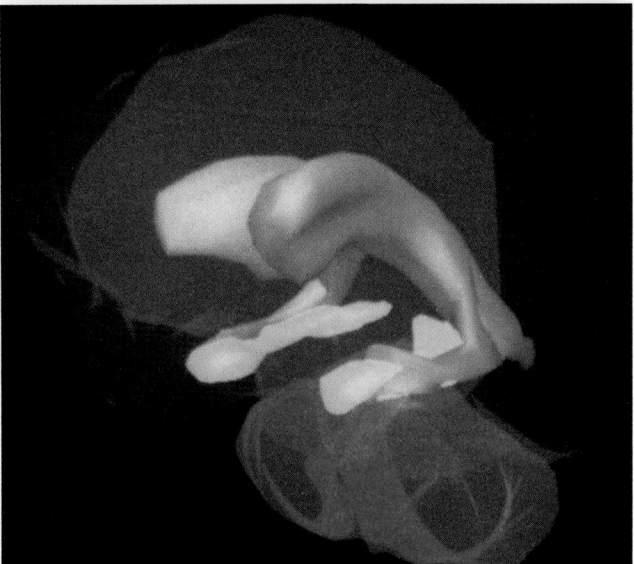

Figure 18-1 MRI comparison of normal brain and brain with schizophrenia. Three-dimensional magnetic resonance imaging (MRI) reconstructions showing, **A,** the cerebroventricles (*gray regions*) and hippocampus (*yellow regions*) of a schizophrenic, and **B,** a normal individual. Note enlarged cerebroventricles and reduced hippocampal volume of the brain of the schizophrenic individual. (From Gershon ES, Rieder RO: *Sci Am* 267:128, 1992. Original illustrations by Nancy C. Andreason, University of Iowa.)

highlight the progressive nature of the structural brain abnormalities and the ineffectiveness of current treatments in attenuating or reversing the frontal brain alterations present in schizophrenia.

Neurotransmitter Alterations

Alterations in different neuroanatomic regions may act in concert to compromise neurotransmitter functions leading to the onset of schizophrenia. A long-standing neurotransmitter hypothesis of schizophrenia involves dopamine. The **dopamine hypothesis** initially suggested that abnormal elevation in dopaminergic transmission contributes to the onset of schizophrenia. This hypothesis was based on pharmacologic studies

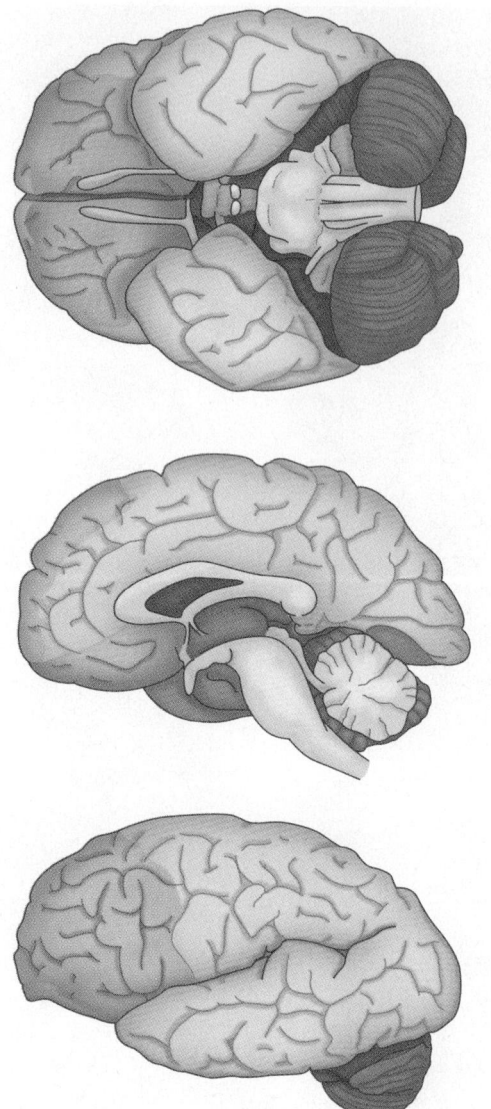

Figure 18-2 **The prefrontal cortex.** The prefrontal cortex consists of a dorsolateral *(blue)* and an orbitofrontal *(green)* region.

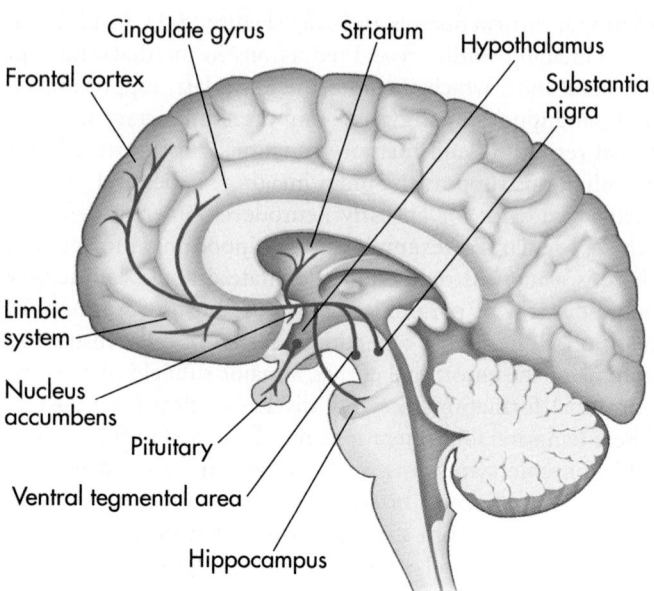

Figure 18-3 **The dopamine system.** Dopamine cell bodies are located in the substantia nigra where they project to the stratum (nigrostriatal pathway); and in the ventral tegmental area where they project to the frontal and cingulate cortex (mesocortical pathway), the striatum, the hippocampus and other limbic structures (mesolimbic pathway). Dopamine nuclei are also located in the hypothalamus and project to the pituitary.

showing that antipsychotic drugs are potent blockers of brain dopamine receptors. A strong positive correlation is found between the clinical potencies of traditional antipsychotic drugs (e.g., chlorpromazine, fluphenazine, and haloperidol) and their affinity for the dopamine D_2 receptor. In addition, drugs that increase dopaminergic transmission—such as levodopa (L-dopa), cocaine, and amphetamine—produce schizophrenic-like psychosis at high doses. Dopamine blockers reverse these drug-induced psychotic states.

A more current view of the dopamine hypothesis of schizophrenia is that brain dopamine pathways are altered in different ways (Figure 18-3). For example, the mesocortical dopamine pathway plays an essential role in dorsal prefrontal cortical functions. Depletion of prefrontal cortical dopamine in monkeys produces deficits in cognition and affect. Some investigators suggest that negative symptoms of schizophrenia result from decreased dopaminergic neurotransmission in frontal cortical regions.[9] This hypodopaminergic transmis-

sion in the dorsal prefrontal cortex contrasts with the hypothesized hyperdopaminergic secretion in mesolimbic pathways. The mesolimbic dopamine pathway innervates temporal lobe structures including the hippocampal formation and amygdala, as well as the nucleus accumbens and anterior cingulate cortex. Hypersecretion of mesolimbic dopamine may contribute to the manifestation of positive symptoms.

Of additional relevance to brain dopamine systems and schizophrenia is the potential involvement of a genetic loci at chromosome 22q11.[10] Microdeletion of 22q11 causes velocardiofacial syndrome characterized by cardiac defects, learning impairments, and deformities of the palate and face. In addition, 25% to 30% of individuals with velocardiofacial syndrome exhibit psychotic symptoms. Deletion of 2q11 is also found in 2% of schizophrenic patients, a rate much higher than the .025% estimate occurring in the general population. Interestingly, 22q11 contains a gene encoding catechol-O-methyl transferase (COMT), an enzyme that catabolizes dopamine. COMT is normally active in dorsal prefrontal brain regions linked to schizophrenia. Thus deletion of a gene encoding an enzyme involved in dopamine regulation increases the risk of schizophrenia.

Another neurotransmitter system that may be involved in schizophrenia is the excitatory neurotransmitter glutamate and its actions on the N-methyl-D-aspartate (NMDA) receptor subtype.[9] This receptor is implicated in learning and memory, and NMDA antagonists, such as the cyclohexylamine anesthetics phencyclidine and ketamine, cause psychosis in healthy subjects and exacerbate symptoms in schizophrenic individuals. In schizophrenia, glutamate concentrations in the cerebrospinal fluid (CSF) are reduced along with a reduction in cortical glutamate synthesis. These data suggest that a reduction in NMDA receptor function occurs in schizophrenia. Notably, glutamateric neurotransmission is tightly coupled with GABAergic neurotransmission. As indicated earlier, there is a loss of GABA synthesis in schizophrenic brains that may have pathophysiologic consequences for NMDA receptor actions underlying cognitive functions.

Clinical Manifestations

Although traditionally a distinction has been made between positive and negative symptoms (see Box 18-1) of schizophrenia, the current focus is on three symptom dimensions. The three core groupings include (1) psychotic symptoms, such as hallucinations and delusions; (2) disorganized symptoms that include thought disorder and bizarre or inappropriate behavior; and (3) negative symptoms.

Hallucinations

A **hallucination** is a perception experienced without external stimulation of the sense organs. Sensory hallucinations involve auditory, tactile, visual, gustatory, and olfactory features. For example the schizophrenic individual may hear voices, experience touch or electrical sensations, report images of animate and inanimate objects, or complain of unpleasant tastes and odors. These hallucinations may occur alone or together.

Delusions

A **delusion** is a persistent belief contrary to the educational and cultural background of the individual. Delusions may involve grandiose, nihilistic, persecutory, somatic, sexual, and religious themes. A common delusion revolves around paranoid beliefs that may involve spying, conspiracy, persecution, and ridicule. Delusions also may be referential in that certain stimuli or events become highly personalized. For example, schizophrenic individuals may believe that a television talk show host is directing information specifically at them.

Disorganized Behavior

Disorganized Speech

A common form of disorganized speech is **formal thought disorder,** which involves fluent speech that is difficult to comprehend. The speech is often incoherent as the individual moves from one topic to another unexpectedly (loose associations). Answers to questions are illogical or unrelated, and the person becomes easily distracted when talking.

Another form of disorganized speech is called **poverty of content.** In this case, the use of vocabularies to convey information is severely retarded despite a fair amount of spoken words. For instance, the same phrases are used repeatedly throughout a conversation.

Disorganized Behavior

Disorganized behavior is the conceptual equivalent of disorganized speech. The individual has difficulty engaging in goal-directed activities. Behavior may be repetitive (e.g., stereotyped rocking) or aimless, and personal hygiene is poorly maintained. Another aspect is the manifestation of inappropriate situational affect as exemplified by hostility without provocation or childlike silliness in sober situations.

Negative Symptoms

Negative symptoms reflect a deficit in normal functioning. These symptoms are disabling and include affective flattening, anhedonia, alogia (poverty of speech) and avolition. **Affective flattening** is the near absence of emotional or facial expression. A fixed expression is maintained throughout a conversation or in different situations. In **anhedonia,** individuals are unable to experience emotions such as pleasure or pain and report a sense of detachment from the environment. **Alogia** is the absence of spontaneous speech production for the purpose of answering questions or expressing one's self. **Avolition** is a deficit in spontaneous or goal-directed behavior in which an individual may sit for prolonged periods of time and must be prodded into completing simple daily tasks.

Treatment

Prior to the early 1950s, there was a steady increase in the number of schizophrenic patients requiring extensive hospitalization in mental institutions. The use of chlorpromazine dramatically changed the treatment of schizophrenia. The drug was especially effective in reducing positive symptoms such as hallucinations and delusions, as well as thought disorders and hyperactivity. The widespread use of chlorpromazine and similar drugs such as haloperidol lead to a marked reduction in the number of patients requiring hospitalization. These antipsychotic drugs are also known as **neuroleptics** from the Greek term *"to clasp the neuron."* The beneficial effects of these first-generation neuroleptics on positive symptoms were due to their ability to block the dopamine D_2 receptor subtype, especially in limbic and prefrontal brain regions associated with emotionality. As indicated earlier, the mesolimbic dopamine pathways are hypothesized to be overly active in schizophrenia, which contributes to the expression of positive symptoms. However, blockade of the D_2 receptor in brain regions such as the striatum also produced a notable neurologic side effect resembling Parkinson disease, a disorder associated with degeneration of dopamine cell bodies in the substantia nigra that projects to striatum. Other side effects may include sedation, hypotension, akathisia (motor restlessness), constipation, weight gain, amenorrhea, and less frequently, hepatotoxicity and electrocardiographic changes. Although the pharmacologic blockade of D_2 receptors occurs rapidly, clinical efficacy does not appear until after 1 or 2 weeks of treatment. Thus the antipsychotic effects are not related directly to D_2 receptor blockade or acute suppression of dopamine hypersecretion.

Although the majority of schizophrenic individuals obtained some positive symptom relief from the first-generation or conventional antipsychotic drugs, approximately 20% failed to respond to D_2-blocking drugs. Some of these treatment-resistant individuals responded to a new class of drugs that became known as atypical antipsychotic drugs.[11] Clozapine was the first of this class of atypical medications that was found to be superior to chlorpromazine. Other atypical drugs that followed include risperidone, olanzapine, quetiapine, and ziprasidone. Some studies suggest that atypical antipsychotic drugs have superior efficacy in reducing not only the positive symptoms but also the negative symptoms in comparison to conventional neuroleptics. In addition, the notable neurologic side effects that accompany the use of the conventional neuroleptics were diminished.

Although the mechanism of action of these drugs is not known, atypical medications clearly differ from conventional antipsychotic drugs in blocking a range of neurotransmitter receptors. For example, clozapine blocks a variety of receptors that include D_2 receptors, as well as D_1, D_3, D_4, and D_5 receptors and serotonin ($5-HT_2$, $5-HT_6$, $5-HT_7$); norepinephrine; cholinergic, and histamine receptors. Risperidone and ziprasidone have higher affinity for blocking $5-HT_2$ than D_2 receptors. The higher $5-HT_2$:D_2 receptor binding ratio of atypical antipsychotics in comparison to conventional neuroleptics may reflect a normalization of serotonin-dopamine interactions leading to clinical efficacy not observed with D_2 receptor blockade alone.

In conjunction with antipsychotic medication, psychosocial therapy can facilitate the management of schizophrenia. Psychosocial relationships may assist the individual in developing coping strategies and in identifying stressors and relapse symptoms. The addition of cognitive behavioral therapy (CBT) may alleviate some of the schizophrenic symptoms resistant to medication.[12] An important benefit of psychosocial and family support is the encouragement of compliance with antipsychotic medication that requires a period of time before the emergence of clinical efficacy.

MOOD DISORDERS: DEPRESSION AND MANIA

Mood refers to a sustained emotional state as opposed to brief emotional feelings, which are termed *affective states.* Healthy individuals are normally capable of experiencing a variety of affective states including euphoria, joy, surprise, fear, sadness, anxiety, and depression. When emotional states, such as sadness became predominant and uncontrollable, individuals may be diagnosed with a mood disorder called *depression.* The two major categories of mood disorder are (1) unipolar or major depressive disorder, also known as *major depression* or *clinical depression,* which consists of episodes of depression; and (2) bipolar disorder, also known as *manic-depressive illness,* characterized by recurrent episodes of depression and mania.

Box 18-2 presents the major symptoms of depression and mania. **Major (unipolar) depression** is the most common mood disorder and the leading cause of disability in the United States and throughout the world. Unipolar depression appears in all age groups including young children. In the United States, the lifetime prevalence rate for depression ranges from 8% to 20% of the population, with a twofold

greater risk in women than men after adolescence. In children and adolescents, 2% to 6% suffered from depression. Individuals with major depression experience an intense, unpleasant mood that lasts for several months and gradually terminates. During the depressive episode, they are unable to experience pleasure and show a loss of motivation and outside interest. Appetite and sleep patterns are disrupted, and if depression becomes too intense and unremitting, individuals may commit suicide.

Approximately 25% of individuals with major depression develop **bipolar disorder.** The incidence is 1% in the general population and occurs equally in males and females. During mania, the individual talks excessively and experiences intense euphoria, elevated self-esteem, restlessness, hyperactivity, and impulsivity and may become easily distracted and engage in reckless behavior. Psychotic symptoms are common. A manic episode usually begins and ends abruptly and will last for a period of days to months. In some bipolar individuals, moods alternate rapidly from one to another.

Etiology and Pathophysiology
Genetic Predisposition and Environmental Influences

A strong genetic basis exists for the development of mood disorder. For unipolar depression, twin studies reveal concordance rates of approximately 40% and 11% for monozygotic and dizygotic twins, respectively. For bipolar disorder, concordance rates as high as 72% and 40% have been reported in monozygotic and dizygotic twins, respectively. Even among adoptees with a biologic family history of mood disorders, the incidence of developing major depression or manic-depressive illness is higher than among control adoptees. The strong tendency for mood disorders to run in families has encouraged a search for the abnormal gene or genes. Some promising molecular genetic studies suggest that regions on chromosome 4, 12, 18, 21, and/or 22 may be involved in bipolar disorder. Interestingly, loci on chromosomes 18 and 22 have been linked to both bipolar disorder and schizophrenia. Bipolar individuals, who exhibit psychotic behavior, have deficits in Reelin expression linked to genetic loci, located on chromosome 22, which confers susceptibility to schizophrenia (see section on Schizophrenia).

Although genetic influences are important in the etiology of mood disorders, environmental factors, such as psychosocial stressors, play a significant role in elevating risk.[13] For example, the first episode of major depression is often precipitated by exposure to psychosocial stress. The trend toward an earlier age onset of depression also is attributed to an increased incidence of stress occurring in the past several decades. A current view of mood disorders is that the illness stems from a complex interplay between susceptible genes and environmental influences. The development of a mood disorder appears to depend on how individuals with a genetic risk respond and interact with their environment (see What's New?: A Gene Increases Vulnerability to Stress-Induced Depression).

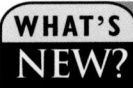

A Gene Increases Vulnerability to Stress-Induced Depression

Stressful life events involving loss, humiliation, or threat may lead to major depression. Not all people who experience stress, however, develop depression. Researchers have identified a gene linked to the serotonin transporter that exists either as a short (s) allele or long (l) allele. The serotonin transporter serves in the reuptake of serotonin at the synapse and may moderate the serotonergic response to stress. Individuals with one or two copies of the s allele were more likely to develop major depression and have suicidal thoughts in response to stressful events than individuals homozygous for the l allele. In addition, among individuals who carry two s alleles, the risk of major depressive episodes increased twofold after experiencing four or more stressful events. This work clearly illustrates the gene-by-environment interaction conferring risk of major depression.

Data from Caspi A et al:, *Sci* 301:386, 2003.

Neurochemical Dysregulation

Modern theories of the pathophysiology of mood disorders began with the important observation that imipramine reduced the reuptake of norepinephrine into presynaptic neurons, and the resultant increase in norepinephrine within the synapse was then responsible for antidepressant effects. This key finding, along with other work showing that drugs (e.g., reserpine) that deplete monoamines produce depression, lead to the dominant **monoamine hypothesis** of depression. Accordingly, depression occurs following a deficit in brain norepinephrine, dopamine, and/or serotonin, whereas mania results from elevated concentrations of monoamines. The three major classes of antidepressant medications include the monoamine oxidase inhibitors (MAOIs), the tricyclic antidepressants (TCAs), and the selective serotonin reuptake inhibitors (SSRIs). These different types of medications share the common property, albeit through different mechanisms, that of increasing neurotransmitter level within the synapse, which is the basis for their antidepressant effects (Figure 18-4).

Further support for the monoamine hypothesis of depression came from examination of the major metabolites of norepinephrine (3-methoxy-4-hyudroxyphenylethyleneglycol [MHPG]), dopamine (homovanillic acid [HVA]), and serotonin (5-hydroxyindole acetic acid [5-HIAA]), in depressed individuals. The major metabolites of these monoamines were reduced in the CSF of depressed individuals. Other work demonstrated that dietary depletion of tryptophan, the precursor of serotonin synthesis, or alpha-methylparatyrosine (AMPT), a drug that inhibits dopamine and norepinephrine synthesis, produced a rapid return to depression in individuals who had been treated successfully with antidepressants.[14]

As is the case with antipsychotic medications, the time course of the pharmacologic effects of antidepressants differs from the therapeutic effects. Whereas TCAs and SSRIs rapidly block synaptic reuptake of monoamines, thereby resulting in elevations in synaptic monoamine concentrations, the onset of clinical efficacy may require several weeks or months of treatment. Thus the pathophysiology of depression cannot be attributed to mere reductions in neurotransmitter levels as proposed by the monoamine hypothesis.

Analysis at the cellular and molecular levels that accompany long-term antidepressant treatment may someday provide a clearer understanding of the mechanism of action of antidepressants. For example, the cyclic adenosine monophosphate (cAMP) signal transduction pathway is regulated by direct coupling of receptors to adenylyl cyclase or indirectly through other second messenger pathways. Chronic administration of antidepressants increases adenylyl cyclase leading to increased cAMP signal transduction. Chronic lithium administration, which is used in the treatment of bipolar disorders, produces similar effects. Because elevated cAMP activates protein kinases that lead to phosphorylation of intracellular proteins and transcription factors, which produce genomic effects, antidepressant-induced gene effects on cell function can then be linked to therapeutic actions.

Neuroendocrine Dysregulation
Hypothalamic-Pituitary-Adrenal System Dysregulation

Hypothalamic-pituitary-adrenal (HPA) hormones are elevated in a large percentage of individuals (30% to 70%) with major depression suggesting that mechanisms responsible for the hormone alterations contribute to the pathophysiology of depression. Altered HPA function can be demonstrated in the dexamethasone suppression test. Administration of dexamethasone, a potent synthetic glucocorticoid, normally suppresses adrenal cortisol secretion because of its negative-feedback effects on the HPA system. Individuals with depression, however, fail to suppress cortisol secretion after dexamethasone administration. In addition, whereas healthy individuals typically exhibit a diurnal rise in cortisol secretion at the onset of wakefulness followed by a trough 12 hours later, depressed people continue to exhibit elevated plasma cortisol levels throughout the evening and early morning hours. Notably, antidepressant drugs effective in normalizing the HPA system are associated with a good clinical response, whereas persistent HPA system dysregulation, as evidenced in the dexamethasone suppression test, is related to continued depression or relapse.

The basis of the hypercortisolemia in major depression has sparked interest in corticotropin-releasing hormone (CRH), the major neuropeptide secretotogue released from hypothalamic nerve endings in the median eminence to control pituitary adrenocorticotropic hormone (ACTH) secretion (see Chapter 10). CRH and CRH-related peptides and their receptors are also present in a wide variety of peripheral tissues, including immune, cardiovascular, and reproductive tissues (see Chapter 10). In comparison to healthy controls, depressed individuals have elevated levels of CRH in CSF and plasma suggesting increased hypothalamic CRH production and release. Indeed, cells expressing CRH are increased in the hypothalamic paraventricular nucleus of depressed and

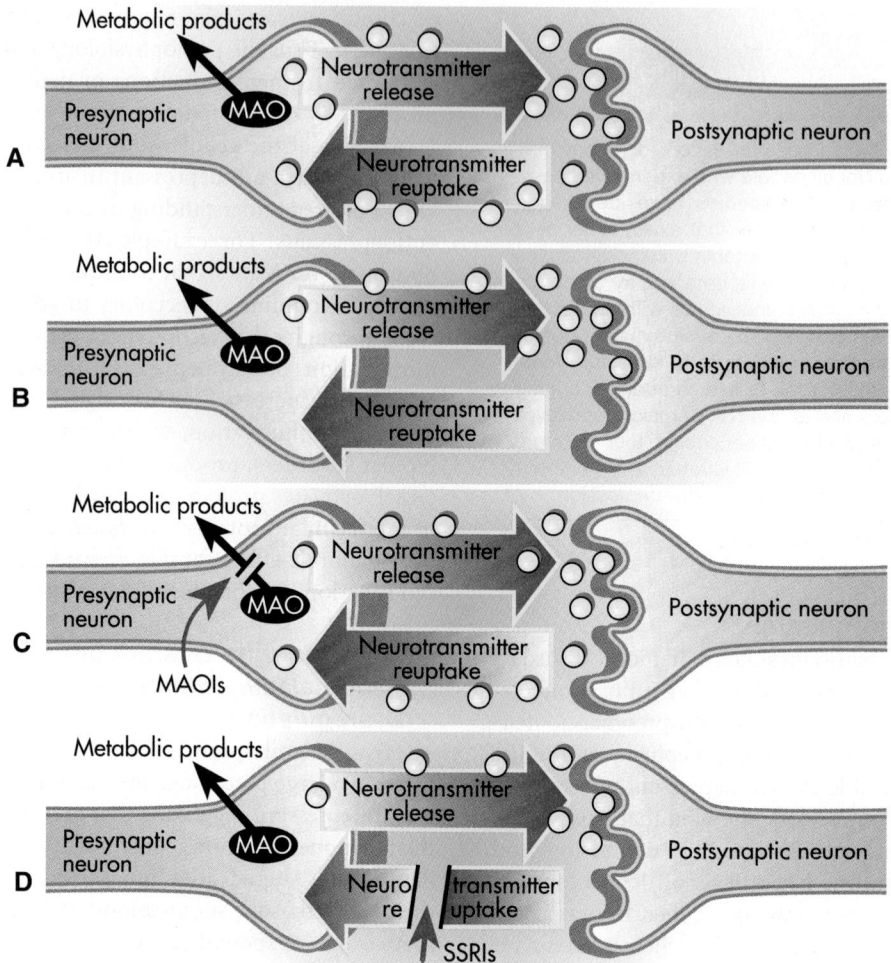

Figure 18-4 Schematic diagrams showing the sites of actions of antidepressants and their effects on neurotransmitter levels. **A,** In normal individuals an action potential generated in the presynaptic neuron results in neurotransmitter release into the synapse. Some neurotransmitters bind to receptors on the postsynaptic neuron that leads to activation of second messenger systems (not shown). Neurotransmitters are also removed from the synapse by reuptake into the presynaptic neuron and deaminated by monoamine oxidase (MAO). **B,** In depressed individuals, neurotransmitter levels are hypothesized to be reduced. The mechanisms responsible for this reduction are not understood. **C,** Monoamine oxidase inhibitors (MAOIs) act by preventing the degradation of neurotransmitters, such as norepinephrine and serotonin. As a result, neurotransmitter levels are elevated. **D,** The tricyclic antidepressants (TCAs) and selective serotonin reuptake inhibitors (SSRIs) act by reducing the uptake of neurotransmitters from the synapse, leading to increased neurotransmitter levels. TCAs, such as nortriptyline and desipramine, tend to block norepinephrine reuptake, whereas amitriptyline and imipramine also have effects on serotonin reuptake. SSRIs are highly effective in blocking serotonin reuptake.

bipolar individuals. Prolonged elevations in CRH secretion may down-regulate CRH receptors in both the pituitary and brain as shown in depressed suicide victims. Whether dysregulation of CRH secretion is a primary contributing factor to depression has yet to be determined. CRH secretion is regulated by monoamines that may have a more fundamental role in the pathophysiology of depression (see previous section). Nevertheless, small molecule CRH receptor antagonists are currently under development as a new class of antidepressants that have been shown to be effective in animal models.

Hypothalamic-Pituitary-Thyroid System Dysregulation

Approximately 20% to 30% of persons with unipolar depression have an altered hypothalamic-pituitary-thyroid (HPT) system. These individuals exhibit increased CSF levels of thyrotropin-releasing hormone (TRH), blunted thyrotropin-stimulating hormone (TSH) response to TRH challenge, and decreased nocturnal rise in TSH that normally occurs between midnight and the early morning hours.[15] Persistent blunting of the TSH response to TRH is associated with an increased probability of relapse. Although the pathophysiologic significance of an altered HPT system to depression is not clear, studies have demonstrated the clinical efficacy of 1-triiodothyronine (T_3), a thyroid hormone, in facilitating the effects of antidepressant drugs in depressed nonresponders.

Neuroanatomic and Functional Abnormalities

The dorsal and median raphe nuclei, located in the central gray of the caudal mesencephalon and rostral pons, contain a large group of serotonin-synthesizing neurons that project extensively to all regions of the cortex, basal ganglia, limbic system, hypothalamus, cerebellum, and brain stem (Figure

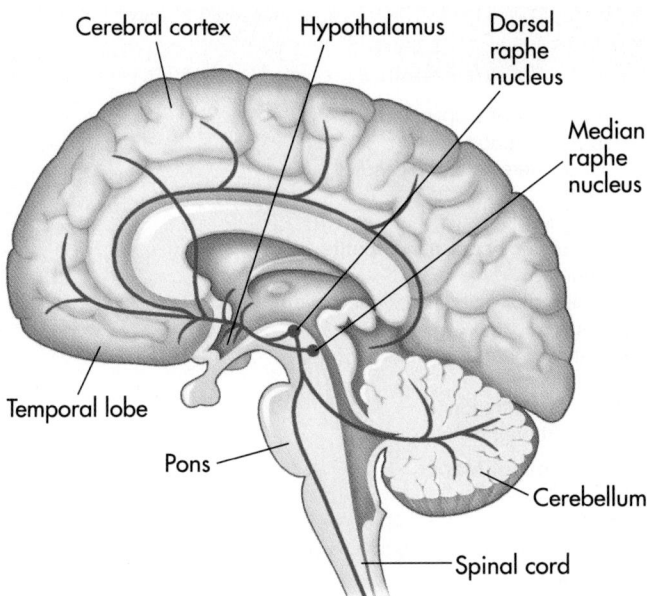

Figure 18-5 The serotonin system. Serotonin neurons are located in the brain stem raphe nuclei. They project diffusely to all regions of the cortex, temporolimbic regions, hypothalamus, basal ganglia, cerebellum, the brain stem, and spinal cord.

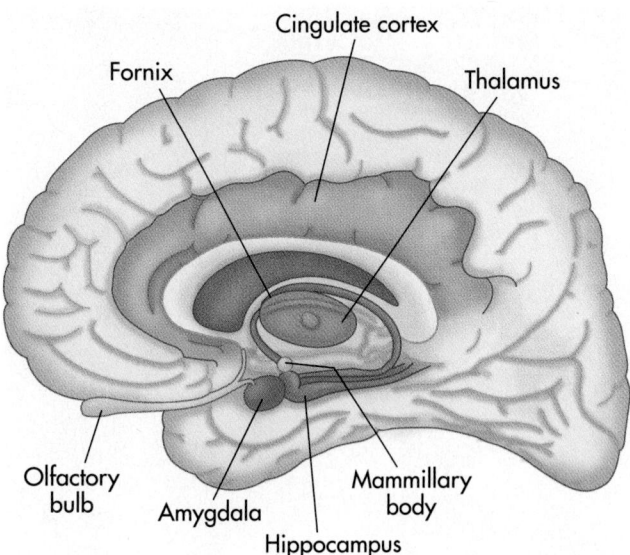

Figure 18-6 The limbic system. Structures of the limbic system play important roles in emotion, learning, and memory. Pathophysiology in limbic structures is frequently found in mental disorders.

18-5). Postmortem and/or brain imaging studies of depressed individuals revealed a widespread decrease in serotonin 5-HT$_{1A}$ receptor binding in frontal, temporal, and limbic cortex as well as serotonin transporter binding in cerebral cortex and hippocampus. Mood disorders may reflect a dysfunctional raphe-serotonin system, which normally modulates homeostasis, emotionality, and tolerance to aversive experiences activated by the amygdala, a limbic structure involved in evaluating and coupling sensory information with emotions or affect (Figure 18-6).

A group of norepinephrine-containing cells located in the locus coeruleus of the rostral pons project to vast areas of the forebrain, brain stem, and spinal cord. The locus coeruleus-norepinephrine system is implicated in global psychologic processes including attention, vigilance, and orientation to novel, aversive, or threatening stimuli. Activation of the locus coeruleus-norepinephrine system is also capable of inhibiting the raphe-serotonin system suggesting an indirect role in modulating serotonin functions. Norepinephrine receptor alterations (e.g., α- and β-adrenergic receptor subtypes) are found in the frontal cortex of some suicide victims with major depression. Alterations in norepinephrine systems may be linked to attention or concentration difficulties as well as sleep and arousal disturbances in depression.

Postmortem and brain imaging studies further reveal structural and functional abnormalities associated with mood disorders, especially in frontal and limbic regions such as the amygdala.[16,17] Postmortem studies reported a reduction in glial cell numbers in persons with unipolar and bipolar disorders. There are also reports of reduced frontal lobe volume in depressed individuals and decreased or asymmetric temporal lobe volume in bipolar illness and depression. One

study reported an increased volume of the amygdala in bipolar illness. In some cases, specific brain abnormalities are associated with a subtype of depression. For instance, enlarged lateral ventricles are found more often in late onset or elderly depressed persons than in mid-life depressives, elderly depressives with an early age of illness, or bipolar individuals.

Functional neuroimaging studies indicate decreased cerebral blood flow and glucose metabolism in the dorsal lateral and dorsal medial prefrontal cortex of major and bipolar depressives. Dorsal lateral abnormalities in depression may be responsible for the retardation in cognitive processing and speech deficits similar to those found in schizophrenia. Dorsal medial frontal dysfunction may be associated with mnemonic and attentional impairments that accompany mood disorders. Other frontal cortical regions, including the ventrolateral, ventromedial, and orbital areas, exhibit increased blood flow and metabolism in unipolar depression (Figure 18-7). These frontal brain areas have extensive interconnections with the amygdala, and increased blood flow and metabolism, especially in the right amygdala, is positively related to negative affect in depressed individuals. These functional changes in brain activity begin to normalize with successful antidepressant treatments suggesting they are state rather than trait related.

Clinical Manifestations
Depression

Major **depression** is characterized by unremitting feelings of sadness and despair.[18] The **dysphoric** or intensely painful mood is accompanied frequently by insomnia, loss of appetite and body weight, and reduced interest in pleasurable activities and interpersonal relationships. Sleep disturbances may include difficulty in initially falling asleep, awakening in the middle of the night and lying awake for several hours, and

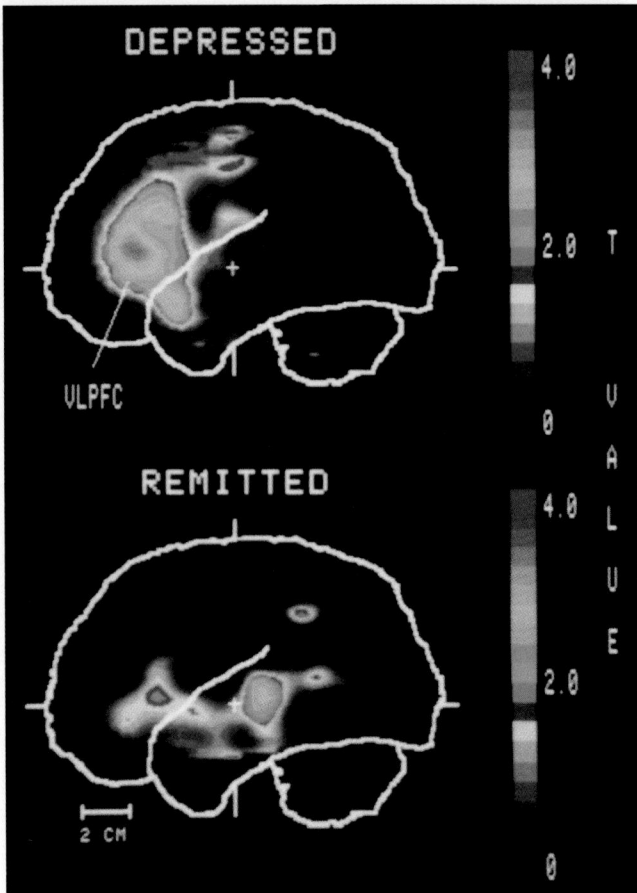

Figure 18-7 PET comparison of brain activity in depression and in remittance. Positron emission tomography (PET) scan showing increased activity in the left prefrontal cortex in a depressed person but not in the remitted person. *VLPFC,* Ventrolateral prefrontal cortex. (From Drevets WC et al: *J Neurosci* 12:3628, 1992. Copyright ©1992 by the Society for Neuroscience.)

early morning wakefulness with an inability to subsequently fall asleep. Individuals may have reduced motor activity and suffer marked fatigue. Others complain of restlessness and agitation. Feelings of worthlessness and guilt are common, and pessimistic or negative outcomes are often perceived even in routine situations. The ability to function (e.g., work) and concentrate is greatly diminished. Severe depression may increase suicide thoughts and the risk of suicide. The symptoms of major depression are summarized in Box 18-2. Major depression is defined as the occurrence of five or more of these symptoms during a 2-week period in which at least one of the symptoms includes depressed mood or loss of interest or pleasure.[18]

Mania

Manic individuals experience elevated levels of euphoria. Self-esteem and feelings of grandiosity are abnormally elevated and may result in psychoses such as delusions and hallucinations. Energy levels are greatly enhanced even after only a few hours of sleep each night. The increased energy, however, does not lead to organized plans and thoughts. The in-

---

Box 18-2   Major Symptoms of Depression and Mania

Symptoms of Depression
Depressed mood
Loss of interests and pleasure
Irritability
Sadness
Decrease or increase in appetite
Insomnia
Psychomotor agitation or retardation
Fatigue
Feelings of worthlessness
Excessive guilt
Poor concentration
Suicide thoughts

Symptoms of Mania
Elevated mood
Irritability
Inflated self-esteem or grandiosity
Decreased need for sleep
Flight of ideas
Excessive talking
Pressured speech
Distractibility
Increased physical activities
Increased pleasurable activities
Psychomotor agitation

Data from American Psychiatric Association: *Diagnostic and statistical manual of mental disorders,* ed 4, Washington, DC, 1994, The Association.

---

dividual shows poor judgment in spending money, may become hypersexual, and makes poor business commitments. Other hallmarks of mania are excessive, rapid, loud, and pressured speech. The manic person frequently skips from one topic of conversation to another and is easily distracted both when speaking and when performing tasks. The DSM-IV diagnostic criteria for manic episodes is a period lasting at least 1 week in which the individual experiences an abnormal and persistently elevated, expansive, or irritable mood.[18] During this period, at least three (four if the mood is only irritable) of the manic symptoms listed in Box 18-2 must be exhibited.

Treatment
Depression

Unipolar depression is one of the more treatable psychiatric disorders. Approximately 80% of depressed persons will respond to antidepressant drugs, psychotherapy, or a combination of both. MAOIs, TCAs, and SSRIs are used in the treatment of depression (Box 18-3). In addition, there are atypical antidepressants, such as nefazodone, trazodone, and mirtazapine, which presumably produce their clinical effects by blocking specific receptors (e.g., 5HT$_{2A}$). A new generation of antidepressants that selectively block serotonin and norepinephrine reuptake has become available in the United States (i.e., venlafaxine) or Europe (i.e., milnacipran, reboxetine) or awaits further development (i.e., duloxetine). Although SSRIs have become the standard first-line treatment for major de-

Box 18-3	Medications Used in the Treatment of Depression and Anxiety Disorders

Monoamine Oxidase Inhibitors
Isocarboxazid
Phenelzine
Tranylcypromine

Tricyclics
Amitriptyline
Clomipramine
Desipramine
Imipramine
Nortriptyline

Selective Serotonin Reuptake Inhibitors
Citalopram
Fluoxetine
Fluvoxamine
Paroxetine
Sertraline

Norepinephrine Reuptake Inhibitors
Reboxetine

Serotonin and Norepinephrine Reuptake Inhibitors
Venlafaxine

Atypical Antidepressants
Buproprion
Mirtazapine
Nefazodone
Trazodone

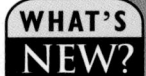

WHAT'S NEW?   SSRIs and Suicide Risk

Selective serotonin reuptake inhibitors (SSRIs) are among the most commonly used medications in the treatment of depression. The widespread use of SSRIs is attributed to its safety profile and reduced side effects in comparison to other antidepressants. The popularity of SSRIs, however, also has led to claims of increased risk of attempted and committed suicides. This suicidal risk issue was first raised in the early 1990s and continues to attract the attention of the medical community and general public. The issue is difficult to tease apart because major depression is highly associated with increased suicidal ideation, attempts, or impulses, and the illness is strongly associated with the use of SSRIs.

Two recent reports suggest that SSRIs or other classes of antidepressants do not significantly increase the risk of suicide rate. In one study, data from Food and Drug Administration (FDA)–controlled clinical trials were evaluated for several FDA-approved antidepressants and the rate of committed suicide. Of 48,177 depressed individuals who were not suicidal or did not have other psychiatric illnesses or substance abuse problems at the start of the study, 77 committed suicide (38 suicides [0.15%] in the SSRI group, 34 suicides [0.20%] in the non-SSRI group, and 5 suicides [0.10%] in the placebo group). However, the rates of committed suicides across the three groups were not statistically significant. In the other study, based on the United Kingdom General Practice Research Database, suicide risk was examined in 158,810 first-time users of SSRIs and tricyclic antidepressants. Results indicated that nonfatal suicides were four times more likely to occur during the first 10 days after start of antidepressant medication and nearly three times more likely to occur within 10 to 29 days after start of medication, regardless of antidepressant type, than after more than 90 days after start of medication. Rather than suggesting that SSRIs or antidepressants rapidly increase the risk of suicidal behavior, these results may, instead, reflect the individual's vulnerability to the distress of depression during the first few weeks of antidepressant treatment when clinical drug efficacy has not yet been resolved. Specifically, energy and cognition may improve before mood improves making it possible for individuals to follow through on suicidal thoughts. Clinicians should carefully monitor all clients on antidepressant therapy for an increase in suicidal risk, particularly when initiating drug treatment because the reduced risk of suicide associated with several weeks of antidepressant use is likely linked to an improved clinical situation after several weeks.

Data from Jick H, Kaye JA, Jick SS: *JAMA* 292(3):338-343, 2004; Khan A et al:, *Am J Psychiatry* 160(4):790-792, 2003.

pression, initial selection of an antidepressant often includes an assessment of the person's symptoms, age, side effects, safety, cost, and convenience. For example, medications that produce sedation may be helpful for the treatment of sleep disturbances. Approximately 50% of depressed individuals may not show a favorable response during initial treatment to an antidepressant drug, and 10% to 20% may continue to exhibit symptoms after 2 years. Individuals who are nonresponsive to a specific antidepressant during a 2-month period may be given another antidepressant medication. At present, there are no criteria that indicate whether selection of the next antidepressant drug will be efficacious. Among children and adolescents, only fluoxetine, which is approved for use in children by the US Food and Drug Administration, appears to have a favorable risk-benefit profile.[19]

In bipolar depression, antidepressant medications may lead to cycle acceleration or induction of mania. However, SSRIs and bupropion, which have effects on norepinephrine (NE) and dopaminergic function, may be less like to induce these effects than MAOIs or TCAs.

A number of side effects are reported with MAOIs, TCAs, and SSRIs. Commonly reported side effects of MAOIs include sedation or agitation, insomnia, dry mouth, impotence, and weight gain. MAOIs also may induce acute and heightened elevations in blood pressure (e.g., hypertensive crisis) after intake of tyramine-rich foods, such as aged cheeses, sour cream, pods of broad beans, pickled herring, liver, canned figs, raisins, and avocados. In addition, MAOI interactions with

TCAs, SSRIs, stimulants, and over-the-counter flu medications are dangerous and should be avoided. Due to these adverse side effect issues, MAOIs are used less often than other antidepressant medications.

TCAs may produce sedation, insomnia, orthostatic hypotension, seizures, and weight gain. Some TCAs have moderate anticholinergic side effects, including constipation, urinary hesitancy or retention, dry mouth, blurred vision, and memory impairment. These side effects may be an issue when considering TCA treatment of the elderly. In that case, the TCAs desipramine and nortriptyline may be preferred due to their reduced anticholinergic, cardiovascular, and sedating effects.

Common side effects of SSRIs include sleep disturbances (e.g., insomnia) and nausea. However, agitation, allergic skin reactions, dry mouth, anxiety, altered appetite, and sexual dysfunction have been reported. Unlike MAOIs and TCAs, SSRIs do not have pronounced effects on the cardiovascular or cholinergic systems. SSRIs are potent inhibitors of cytochrome P-450 isoenzymes, which are involved in drug metabolism. Therefore, SSRIs may lead to dangerous elevations in blood concentrations of other psychiatric medications when taken together. SSRIs should not be taken with MAOIs or immediately after discontinuing MAOI treatment. A serotonin syndrome characterized by excitement or autonomic hyperactivity, abdominal pain, rigidity, and hyperthermia may develop leading to coma or death.

Side effects of atypical antidepressants may include sedation, dry mouth, weight gain, and constipation. Nefazodone and trazodone have been associated with hepatic toxicity. Venlafaxine and reboxetine lack many of the serious side effects associated with TCAs. However, sweating, dry mouth, and some sedation may occur.

Electroconvulsive therapy (ECT) is used when individuals fail to respond to antidepressants or when they are severely depressed, pregnant, suicidal, or psychotic. ECT is effective in alleviating depressive symptoms in about 50% to 80% of people who may then begin to respond to antidepressant medications. Although the mechanism of action of ECT is not clear, the procedure is known to produce alterations in monoamine systems.

Mania

Individuals with bipolar disorder are treated with lithium or other mood stabilizers (e.g., carbamazepine or valproic acid) when they do not respond to lithium treatment. The full clinical effects of lithium usually require about 1 week of treatment.

In some cases, lithium in combination with SSRIs are used in the treatment of bipolar disorder. As in depression, ECT is administered when manic individuals fail to respond to medication, are pregnant, or have cardiovascular disease.

Frequently reported side effects of lithium treatment include increased thirst, tremors, diarrhea, and weight gain, which diminishes over time. A potentially serious side effect is lithium toxicity. Lithium is normally removed from the kidneys. However, when the body is sodium depleted, the kidneys will reabsorb sodium along with lithium. Individuals receiving lithium treatment are advised to avoid physically demanding activities that may dehydrate the body and to seek medical attention during fever or other conditions that may increase sweating.

Newer treatments for bipolar disorder include the use of lamotrigine and gabapentin.[20] Lamotrigine decreases the presynaptic release of excitatory neurotransmitters and may have effects on bipolar depression and reduce rapid cycling in bipolar individuals. The gabapentin effects of promoting sleep and reducing anxiety may be useful in some individuals. Lamotrigine is metabolized by the liver and must be titrated over a period of 2 to 4 weeks because of adverse effects, including dizziness, headaches, somnolence, double vision, and rash. Gabapentin is relatively safe, well tolerated, and excreted by the kidneys.

In addition to pharmacotherapy, psychotherapy can be beneficial for those who have difficulty with psychosocial stressors, such as self-esteem, legal problems, fear of recurrence, and interpersonal conflicts. Treatment involves a combination of making the individual aware of the bipolar disorder, coping with psychosocial stressors, facilitating drug compliance, and monitoring symptom recurrences.

ANXIETY DISORDERS

Fear and anxiety are normal feelings expressed in threatening or harmful situations. The symptoms may include arousal, tenseness, and increased autonomic activity such as heart rate, blood pressure, and respiration. In addition, individuals often engage in protective behavioral responses such as flight or avoidance. These physiologic and behavioral responses reflect the individuals' evolutionary heritage. Their expression allowed humans to adapt and cope under a variety of situational challenges. However, when fear and anxiety become too intense and undermine the ability to function on a daily basis, the individual may develop an anxiety disorder. Anxiety disorders are the most prevalent psychiatric disorder, occurring in approximately 10% to 30% of the general population. Notably, many individuals with anxiety disorders develop major depression and individuals with major depression often suffer from anxiety disorders. Comorbidity of anxiety disorders and depression suggest a common neural pathophysiologic basis linking these two mental illnesses. This section presents an overview of panic disorder, generalized anxiety disorder, posttraumatic stress disorder, and obsessive-compulsive disorder.

Panic Disorder

Panic disorder is a well-studied psychiatric condition that consists of multiple disabling panic attacks. Approximately 2% to 3% of women and 0.5% to 1.5% of men have panic disorder. Between panic attacks the individual spends an excessive amount of time worrying about future panic attacks. Panic attacks are characterized by intense autonomic arousal involving a wide variety of symptoms, including lightheadedness, a racing heart, difficult breathing, chest discomfort, generalized sweating, general weakness, trembling, abdominal distress, and chills or hot flashes. In addition, the individual experiences the fear of losing control and dying. Symptoms originally occur spontaneously and vary in length from several minutes to an hour. If the symptoms are prolonged, they can be disabling.

A notable complication of panic disorder is the development of **agoraphobia** or phobic avoidance of places or situations where escape or help are not readily available. The agoraphobic individual will avoid being away from home; standing in line or in a crowd; or riding a train, plane, or automobile. Severe agoraphobia leads to individuals being housebound.

Etiology and Pathophysiology

Genetic factors appear to play a major role in panic disorder. The risk is nearly 20% among relatives of panic disorder individuals. In contrast, the risk of panic disorder with or without agoraphobia is about 4% among individuals with no family history of the illness. Some studies suggest that the cholecystokinin receptor gene on chromosome 11p may be linked to panic disorder.[21]

Although the etiology of panic attacks is not known, some factors may be acting on vulnerable brain stem regions to provoke symptoms. For example, physiologic information from the peripheral cardiovascular and respiratory systems is regulated closely by cells in the brain stem, which may activate central autonomic pathways. Fearful perceptions and thoughts emanating from the cerebral cortex may further contribute by activating neural circuits in the temporal lobe and brain stem, which may then facilitate the production of panic symptoms.

Brain regions likely to be involved in panic attacks include the locus coeruleus–norepinephrine (NE) system and temporal lobe structures, including the amygdala and hippocampus[22] (see Figure 18-6). Both the hippocampus and locus coeruleus monitor internal and external signals and increase their activity when aroused. The locus coeruleus is sensitive to respiratory and cardiovascular changes in the periphery, such as hyperventilation. Abnormal firing of locus coeruleus neurons in response to peripheral autonomic signals may contribute to the onset of panic attacks.

Panic disorder also may involve the GABA-benzodiazepine (BZ) receptor system. BZ receptors and $GABA_A$ receptors are functionally coupled. BZ increases the $GABA_A$ ion channel response to GABA, thereby elevating chloride ion influx and producing a neuronal inhibitory effect. Brain imaging work reveals a reduction in BZ receptor binding in brain regions including the hippocampus, insular, and prefrontal cortex.[23] Thus an alteration in inhibitory neuromodulation may contribute to panic disorder.

Individuals with panic disorder respond to some pharmacologic challenges differently than healthy controls. Physical symptoms of panic attacks are reproduced to a certain degree in panic-prone persons by inhalation of carbon dioxide, caffeine ingestion, sodium lactate, and NE receptor compounds. Many of these agents appear to directly or indirectly modulate the locus coeruleus-NE system, thereby contributing to the production of panic. For example, panic-prone individuals are sensitive to the anxiety provoking effects of yohimbine, an α_2–adrenergic receptor antagonist, and exhibit elevated levels of plasma MHPG (a norepinephrine metabolite), cortisol, and cardiovascular responses. Clonidine, the α_2–adrenergic receptor agonist, produces less sedation and less plasma MHPG, but greater hypotension, when given to individuals with panic disorder. Other drugs that block the benzodiazepine receptor or stimulate the cholecystokinin receptor are reported to increase panic attacks and feelings of anxiety in persons with panic disorder. As indicated previously, these receptor systems may be involved in the pathophysiology of panic disorder.

Treatment

Panic disorder is highly treatable. Up to 80% of panic disorder individuals respond to cognitive behavioral therapy (CBT) and antidepressant medication, either separately or in combination. In CBT, the individual learns that the physical symptoms are not fatal and attempts to exert control over the anxiety and panic. For example, breathing exercises to control the hyperventilation serve to lessen the intense physiologic symptoms of panic, such as elevated heart and respiration rates. Another benefit of CBT is awareness of the benefits associated with drug medications and compliance. For those individuals who have mild agoraphobia, CBT alone may be effective.

Antidepressants such as TCAs and SSRIs are considered first-line medications for panic disorder with SSRIs having a somewhat superior antipanic efficacy over TCAs. Among the SSRIs, paroxetine and sertraline have received FDA approval specifically for panic disorder. Similar safety and side effect issues of SSRIs and TCAs that apply to major depression are relevant for those with panic disorder. MAOIs are not often prescribed because of their potentially adverse effects.

BZs such as alprazolam and clonazepam are another class of medications used in the treatment of panic disorder; their efficacy may be related in part to their inhibitory effects on locus coeruleus neuronal activity. These drugs also are used as an adjunct or augmentation therapy for individuals who do not fully respond to SSRIs or TCAs. Short-term effects of BZ treatment include sedation, ataxia, and cognitive impairments. A potential complication of long-term BZ treatment is physiologic and psychologic dependence. Abrupt BZ withdrawal may produce a withdrawal syndrome that includes a heightened reemergence or rebound of anxiety, insomnia, photophobia, and diarrhea. These symptoms may be lessened with gradual tapering off of BZ medication. Individuals taking BZs may benefit from CBT, which could reduce their reliance on these drugs.

Generalized Anxiety Disorder

Excessive and persistent worries are the hallmarks of **generalized anxiety disorder (GAD)**. The individual worries about life events such as marital relationships, job performance, health, money, or social status. The lifetime prevalence rates of GAD range from 4.1% to 6.6%, with somewhat higher rates in women than in men. GAD usually emerges in the early 20s, but can occur in childhood. Symptoms include restlessness, motor tension, irritability, fatigue, difficulty concentrating, and sleep disturbance. The individual startles easily and frequently suffers from depression and panic attacks. The severity of symptoms fluctuates over time and may be linked to the changing nature of environmental stress. Although GAD tends to be a chronic disorder, the symptoms may become less severe with age.

Etiology and Pathophysiology

The etiology and pathophysiology of GAD are poorly understood. Female twin studies suggest a concordance rate of 30%, but disease genes linked to specific chromosomes have yet to be identified. Abnormalities in the norepinephrine and serotonin systems were reported in GAD.[24] For example, there is a reduction in α_2 adrenergic receptor binding, a decrease in serotonin levels in CSF, and reduced platelet binding of paroxetine, an SSRI.

A prominent alteration of GAD involves the GABA-BZ receptors. In GAD, there is a reduction in peripheral BZ receptors, which increase after treatment with BZ drugs. Brain imaging work indicates GAD subjects have greater homogeneity of the cerebrum, BZ receptor distribution, and a significant reduction in the left temporal hemisphere.[25] The therapeutic effects of BZs may lie, in part, in their ability to normalize these BZ receptor alterations.

Treatment

GAD is diagnosed when the individual spends at least 6 months worrying excessively. 5-HT/NE reuptake inhibitors, such as venlafaxine or paroxetine, have become first-line therapeutics for managing GAD. These medications may produce relief of GAD symptoms within a period of 1 week and are also effective in treating comorbid symptoms of depression. Buspirone, which has affinity for serotonin receptors ($5\text{-}HT_{1A}$) is another treatment option, although the onset of clinical efficacy may take 2 weeks. The primary side effects of buspirone, which lessen over time, include dizziness, headaches, nausea, and mild nervousness. GAD nonresponders to 5-HT/NE reuptake inhibitors or buspirone may be placed on benzodiazepines. However, because GAD tends to be chronic, and comorbid with depression or other anxiety disorders,[26] benzodiazepines are usually limited to uncomplicated cases of GAD. SSRIs also have been used in the treatment of the young with GAD. In addition to drug therapy, treatment of GAD may involve behavioral therapy. During behavioral therapy, the individual learns relaxation techniques to control his or her anxiety.

Posttraumatic Stress Disorder

Exposure to a terrifying or life-threatening trauma may produce **posttraumatic stress disorder (PTSD)**.[27,28] Although the disorder was initially described in combat situations and called "shell shock," "war neurosis," or "traumatic neurosis," PTSD does not arise solely from exposure to the battlefield. Exposure to any serious trauma, including serious accidents, natural disasters (such as earthquakes), child abuse, kidnapping, and violent attacks (such as rape or muggings), that involves intense fear, threat of death, or helplessness may induce PTSD. The disorder may develop within hours of the traumatic experience or after several months or years. In PTSD, the individual reexperiences the traumatic event as intrusive recollections or flashbacks during the day and during persistent nightmares. During a flashback, images, odors, sounds, and negative emotions are recalled and lead to marked distress. The duration of the flashback varies from seconds to hours or, in rare cases, several days. Nightmares replicate the traumatic experiences and often prevent further sleep. Exposure to cues associated with the life-threatening event also may trigger psychologic distress, intense autonomic arousal, and avoidance behavior. For instance, the individual avoids activities that may lead to a recollection of thoughts, feelings, places, or people involved in the trauma. Persistent symptoms of PTSD include sleeping difficulties, irritability, lack of concentration, hypervigilance, and exaggerated startle response.

The lifetime prevalence rate of PTSD is 7% to 8%. In men, PTSD is usually found among combat veterans, whereas PTSD in women is often related to rape or assault. Abused children also may develop PTSD. Certain individuals appear to be vulnerable to PTSD. Persons with a history of psychiatric illness (major depression, panic disorder) or those lacking strong social support are at increased risk and may be more sensitive to the effects of traumatic stress.

Etiology and Pathophysiology

The primary etiology of PTSD is exposure to a terrifying life-threatening event and may involve several neural structures and neurotransmitter systems. Structural brain imaging studies reported that combat-related PTSD victims have a smaller hippocampus, a brain structure susceptible to the damaging effects of the stress hormone cortisol and excitatory amino acids. Pediatric PTSD studies reveal a more generalized effect of trauma on reducing total brain volume. In functional imaging studies, PTSD individuals exposed to trauma-related stimuli generally exhibit increased activation in the amygdala and diminished activity in some prefrontal cortical areas. Reduced activation of the anterior cingulate cortex also has been reported in some but not all studies.[29]

As in panic disorder, benzodiazepine binding is altered in those with PTSD. Individuals with PTSD have reduced distribution of benzodiazepine receptor binding in the prefrontal cortex in comparison to healthy controls.[30] This reduction in benzodiazepine receptor distribution was not found in other brain regions.

These structural and functional data involving the hippocampus, amygdala, and prefrontal cortex are highly relevant to the pathophysiology of PTSD because these brain regions normally play important roles in how fearful memories are stored, retrieved, and forgotten (see Figures 18-2 and 18-6). The pathogenesis of PTSD is hypothesized to stem from an altered fear learning process that may involve, for example, amygdala hyperresponsiveness, lack of prefrontal cortical inhibition, hippocampal dysfunction, and/or susceptibility to the adverse effects of stress. Continued dysfunction and deterioration of this fear-based memory system may underlie chronic PTSD.

Treatment

PTSD is diagnosed when symptoms persist for over a month.[18] Although the disorder may be short lived and ultimately disappear, in 30% of individuals, PTSD may become chronic and last for years. As in GAD, the severity of symptoms fluctuates over time. Current treatment methods involve drug medications and psychotherapy. During psychotherapy, the individual learns to control the anxiety symptoms. Among war veterans, group or family therapy is supported by the Veterans Administration.

Paroxetine, and sertraline are considered first-line SSRI medications for chronic PTSD because of their tendency to lessen the recurrent nightmares and flashbacks. For chronic PTSD, long-term SSRI therapy is required for steady improvement of symptoms and quality of life. Other antidepressants such as the TCAs (amitriptyline and imipramine) have moderate effects and are second-line drugs. Some data suggest that nefazodone and bupropion may provide benefits. The tendency to use antidepressants is due to the high prevalence of comorbid depression and substance abuse. Benzodiazepines may be used during the aftermath of a traumatic event to control hyperarousal symptoms such as irritability, insomnia, and muscle tension. However, there is no clear evidence that benzodiazepines have clinical efficacy or provide prophylaxis against the development of chronic PTSD. Benzodiazepines should be carefully monitored among individuals with a history of drug abuse.

Obsessive-Compulsive Disorders

Repetitive, intrusive thoughts and/or compulsions are the hallmarks of **obsessive-compulsive disorder (OCD).** These thoughts and acts are irrational, impair normal functioning, and may cause marked distress. Obsessions may involve a preoccupation with contamination, doubting, religious or sexual themes, or the belief that a negative outcome will occur if a specific act is not performed. Compulsions are physical and mental ritualized acts such as washing, cleaning, checking, counting, organizing, hoarding, and repeating specific thoughts or prayers.

The lifetime prevalence rates of OCD range from 1.2% to 3.3%. Although the age of onset is between 20 to 25 years, many begin to experience symptoms during childhood or adolescence.

OCD individuals are often diagnosed with at least one other psychiatric illness.[31] In adulthood, comorbidity with major depression, other anxiety disorders (especially panic disorders and GAD), and Tourette syndrome are common. Among children, tic disorders, attention deficit hyperactivity disorder, and depression coexist with OCD.

Etiology and Pathophysiology

Family studies indicate a risk of about 10% to 12% among first-degree relatives. These first-degree relatives are also at increased risk (4.6%) of Tourette disorder and tics in comparison to control relatives (1%). Thus OCD and Tourette syndrome may share a common pathophysiology.

Abnormalities of the basal ganglia–frontal cortical circuitry are found in OCD.[32] Some studies have shown increased orbitofrontal and thalamic volumes in OCD but not in the caudate nucleus of the basal ganglia (Figure 18-8).

More consistent data are obtained from functional imaging studies, which report an increase in orbitofrontal and anterior cingulate cortical activity. Orbitofrontal and anterior cortical hyperactivity may be responsible for intrusive thoughts, obsessions, and anxiety, which drives the basal ganglia to engage in compulsive ritualized acts as a means to alleviate the anxious obsessions. Studies further suggest that when provoked, OCD individuals consistently show increased activity in the orbitofrontal, anterior cingulate, and caudate nucleus areas of the brain. Of particular relevance to prognosis, OCD individuals with very high frontal cortical activity are likely to respond more poorly to treatment than persons with lower pretreatment activity in the orbitofrontal cortex.

Abnormalities in serotonin and dopamine functions may contribute to the pathophysiology of OCD. Serotonin agonists exacerbate the symptoms of OCD, and serotonin synthesis is decreased in the prefrontal cortex and caudate nucleus. Stimulation of the dopamine system increases repetitive acts, which may be blocked by dopamine antagonists. However, the dopamine stimulant-induced compulsions were not accompanied by anxiety, which led some investigators to suggest that lack of serotonin control over the dopamine system may be a primary defect in OCD.

Treatment

Because of the chronic nature of OCD, long-term treatment consisting of a combination of pharmacotherapy and cognitive-behavioral therapy (CBT) is often required. SSRIs are the first drug of choice for OCD.[33] Approximately 70% to 80% of OCD individuals will show a partial response that may be further improved by other medications. For example, clonazepam, a benzodiazepine, is found to improve the effects of fluoxetine and clomipramine therapy. Antipsychotic drugs, haloperidol and risperidone, in combination

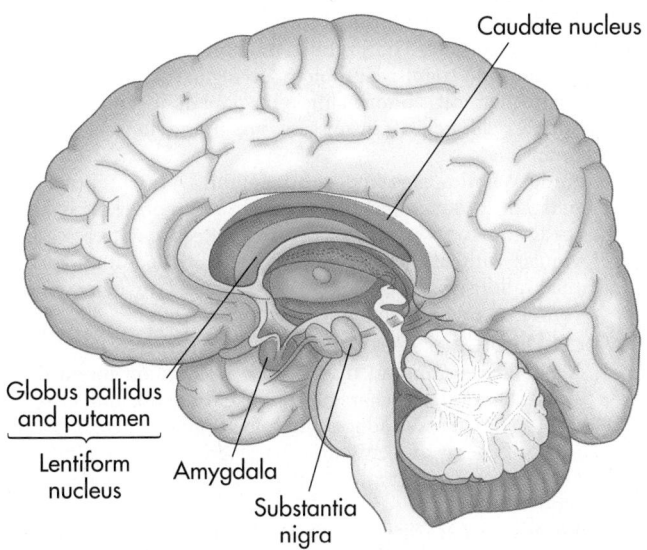

Figure 18-8 Basal ganglion. Structures of the basal ganglion, which include the caudate nucleus, putamen, globus pallidus, and substantia nigra, are important in movement.

with SSRIs are also found to be effective especially in co-morbid OCD and tic disorders. Normalization of dysfunctional serotonin and dopamine systems in OCD may be the basis for the therapeutic effects of SSRIs and dopamine receptor related drugs.

CBT involves daily exposure to cues that elicit distress followed by preventing the individual from engaging in compulsive rituals for a least an hour or until the anxiety subsides. This exposure and response prevention therapy can produce long-term symptom remission and is effective in adults and children who are able to tolerate the exposure-induced anxiety component.

For individuals with severe OCD, neurosurgery is performed to disconnect the basal ganglia from the frontal cortex.[34] This lesioning procedure results in significant relief of obsessions and compulsions and provides further evidence of a pathophysiology in the basal ganglia–frontal cortical circuitry in OCD.

SUMMARY REVIEW

Schizophrenia

1. Schizophrenia is a collection of symptoms characterized by thought disorders. Thought disorders reflect a break between the cognitive and the emotional sides of one's personality.
2. Schizophrenic symptoms are generally classified into positive and negative symptoms. Positive symptoms include hallucinations, delusions, formal thought disorder, and bizarre behavior. Negative symptoms include flattened affect, alogia, anhedonia, attention deficits, and apathy.
3. There is a genetic predisposition to acquire schizophrenia.
4. Schizophrenia may result from neurodevelopmental defects occurring in the fetus. During early development, environmental factors (viral infection, nutritional deficiencies, or prenatal birth complications) may interfere with genetically programmed neural development leading to alterations in brain structure and function.
5. Structural brain abnormalities are present in schizophrenia. Brain imaging studies reveal an enlargement of the cerebroventricles and widening of the fissures and sulci in the frontal cortex. In addition, there is a reduction in the volume of the thalamus and temporal lobe. Within the temporal lobe, the hippocampus, a structure linked to memory and cognitive functions, shows a reduced number of granule cells and disarray of pyramidal neurons. Temporal lobe alterations may be responsible for the manifestation of positive symptoms.
6. In schizophrenia, the frontal lobe shows a progressive loss in volume and a worsening of negative symptoms despite the used of antidepressant medications. Functional alterations in the dorsal lateral prefrontal cortex, such as reduced blood flow and metabolism, compromise the ability to engage in goal-directed and cognitive problem solving behavior.
7. Neurochemical abnormalities in dopamine and excitatory amino acid neurotransmission are found in schizophrenic brains.
8. Antipsychotic drugs block the dopamine D_2 receptor or a combination of dopamine and serotonin receptors. Antipsychotic medications, however, are not always effective in treating individuals with severe negative symptoms. In addition to drug medications, psychosocial therapy is used to increase drug compliance and to encourage coping strategies.

Mood Disorders: Depression and Mania

1. Major depression and mania are two common mood disorders. The former is characterized by an intense and sustained unpleasant state of sadness and hopelessness, whereas extreme levels of energy and euphoria characterize the latter. Individuals with recurrent patterns of depression and mania have a bipolar illness.
2. Environmental triggers such as psychosocial stress appear to facilitate the onset of depression in individuals with a genetic vulnerability.
3. A reduction in brain monoamine neurotransmission is linked to depression, whereas an elevated monoamine level is associated with mania.
4. Individuals with major depression commonly have elevated levels of the stress hormone cortisol, which appears to be due to increased secretion of corticotropin-releasing hormone. Neuroendocrine abnormalities involving thyroid hormones also are found in depression.
5. Structural brain alterations that include reduced frontal lobe and limbic system volumes are found in depression and bipolar illness. Functional brain imaging studies show that depressed individuals have alterations in blood flow to prefrontal and limbic brain regions that include the amygdala, a structure implicated in emotional behavior.
6. Pharmacotherapy involving the use of MAOIs, TCAs, SSRIs, and atypical antidepressants is effective in the treatment of mood disorders. Manic and bipolar individuals are treatable with lithium or mood stabilizers. The clinical effects of drugs used in the treatment of mood disorders often take several weeks to develop. Severely depressed and manic people who do not respond to medication are administered ECT.

Anxiety Disorders

1. Fear and anxiety are normal emotional states that reflect individuals' evolutionary heritage. However, an anxiety disorder may develop when these states become intrusive and uncontrollable. Panic disorder, generalized anxiety disorder, post-traumatic stress disorder (PTSD), and obsessive-compulsive disorder (OCD) are examples of uncontrollable fear and anxiety states that require medical attention.
2. Panic disorder consists of panic attacks characterized by intense autonomic arousal that occurs spontaneously and may last for up to 1 hour. During a panic attack the individual experiences multiple symptoms including light-headedness, a pounding heart, and difficulty breathing. In addition, the intense occurrence of autonomic responses is accompanied by heightened fear and anxiety that often continue between panic attacks.
3. Brain regions involved in the production of panic attacks are the locus coeruleus, hippocampus, and amygdala. A reduction in $GABA_A$-benzodiazepine receptor binding also may contribute to the pathophysiology of panic disorder.
4. Panic disorder can generally be treated with cognitive behavioral therapy and antidepressant medications such as TCAs and SSRIs. Benzodiazepines are used as an adjunct or augmentation therapy for individuals who are nonresponsive to SSRIs or TCAs.
5. Generalized anxiety disorder is characterized by excessive and persistent worries about life events. Individuals exhibit varying levels of motor disturbances, irritability, and fatigue that may be linked to fluctuations in psychosocial stress. Many GAD individuals manifest symptoms of depression.

SUMMARY REVIEW—cont'd

6. Pathophysiology in norepinephrine, serotonin, and GABA$_A$-benzodiazepine systems are found in those with generalized anxiety disorder.
7. Treatment of generalized anxiety disorder usually involves a combination of behavioral therapy and drug medications, especially serotonin/norepinephrine reuptake blockers.
8. PTSD develops after exposure to a life-threatening or traumatic experience. Individuals experience recurring thoughts and flashbacks and nightmares of the terrifying event.
9. In PTSD structural and/or functional alterations exist in the hippocampus, amygdala, and prefrontal cortex, which are neural components of a fear-based memory system.
10. Treatment of chronic PTSD is difficult. Current methods involve psychotherapy and SSRI pharmacotherapy.
11. OCD is characterized by irrational thoughts and ritualized acts that impair normal functioning and cause distress.
12. Pathophysiology in the basal ganglia–frontal cortical circuitry and serotonin and dopamine functions is linked to OCD.
13. OCD is a chronic illness that requires long-term treatment consisting of cognitive-behavioral therapy and drug medication, such as SSRIs. Severe OCD may require neurosurgery to disconnect the basal ganglia from the frontal cortex.

KEY TERMS

γ-Aminobutyric acid (GABA), 607
Affective flattening, 609
Agoraphobia, 616
Alogia, 609
Anhedonia, 609
Avolition, 609
Bipolar disorder, 610
Delusion, 609
Depression, 613
Dopamine hypothesis, 607

Dorsal lateral prefrontal cortex (DLPFC), 607
Dysphoric mood, 613
Formal thought disorder, 609
Generalized anxiety disorder (GAD), 617
Hallucination, 609
Major (unipolar) depression, 610
Manic, 614
Monoamine hypothesis, 611
Mood, 610

Neuroleptic drug, 609
Obsessive-compulsive disorder, 619
Panic disorder, 616
Posttraumatic stress disorder (PTSD), 618
Poverty of content, 609
Psychotic episode, 606
Schizophrenia, 605
Thought disorder, 605
Working memory, 607

REFERENCES

1. Lewis DA, Levitt P: Schizophrenia as a disorder of neurodevelopment, *Annu Rev Neurosci* 25:409-432, 2002.
2. Marenco S, Weinberger DR: The neurodevelopmental hypothesis of schizophrenia: following a trail of evidence from cradle to grave, *Dev Psychopathol* 12(3):501-527, 2000.
3. Berman KF, Meyer-Lindenberg A: Functional brain imaging studies in schizophrenia. In Charney DS, Nestler EJ, editors: *Neurobiology of mental illness*, ed 2, New York, 2004, Oxford.
4. Shenton ME, Dickey CC, Frumin M et al: A review of MRI findings in schizophrenia, *Schizophr Res* 49(1-2):1-52, 2001.
5. Falkai P, Bogerts B: The neuropathology of schizophrenia. In Hirsch SR, Weinberger DR, editors: *Schizophrenia*, Cambridge, 1995, Blackwell.
6. Costa E, Davis J, Grayson DR et al: Dendritic spine hypoplasticity and downregulation of reelin and GABAergic tone in schizophrenia vulnerability, *Neurobiol Dis* 8(5):723-742, 2001.
7. Fatemi SH, Earle JA, McMenomy T: Reduction in reelin immunoreactivity in hippocampus of subjects with schizophrenia, bipolar disorder, and major depression, *Mol Psychiatry* 5(6):654-663, 2000.
8. Ho BC, Andreasen NC, Nopoulos P et al: Progressive structural brain abnormalities and their relationship to clinical outcome: a longitudinal magnetic resonance imaging study early in schizophrenia, *Arch Gen Psychiatry* 60(6):585-594, 2003.
9. Duncan GE, Sheitman BB, Lieberman JA: An integrated view of pathophysiological models of schizophrenia, *Brain Res Brain Res Rev* 29(2-3):250-264, 1999.
10. Kennedy JL, Farrer LA, Andreasen NC et al: The genetics of adult-onset neuropsychiatric disease: complexities and conundra? *Sci* 302:822, 2003.
11. Tamminga CA: Principles of the pharmacotherapy of schizophrenia. In Charney DS, Nestler EJ, editors: *Neurobiology of mental illness*, ed 2, New York, 2004, Oxford.
12. Sensky T, Turkington D, Kingdon D et al: A randomized controlled trial of cognitive-behavioral therapy for persistent symptoms in schizophrenia resistant to medication, *Arch Gen Psychiatry* 57(2):165-172, 2000.
13. Sullivan PF, Neale MC, Kendler KS: Genetic epidemiology of major depression: review and meta-analysis, *Am J Psychiatry* 157(10):1552-1562, 2000.
14. Heninger GR, Delgado PL, Charney DS: The revised monoamine theory of depression: a modulatory role for monoamines, based on new findings from monoamine depletion experiments in humans, *Pharmacopsych* 29(1):2-11, 1996.
15. Bartalena L, Placidi GF, Martino E et al: Nocturnal serum thyrotropin (TSH) surge and the TSH response to TSH-releasing hormone: disassociative behavior in untreated depressives, *J Clin Endocrinol Metab* 71(3):650-655, 1990.
16. Drevets WC: Prefrontal cortical-amygdalar metabolism in major depression, *Ann N Y Acad Sci* 877:614-637, 1999.
17. Rajkowska G: Depression: what we can learn from postmortem studies, *Neuroscientist,* 9(4):273-284, 2003.
18. American Psychiatric Association: *Diagnostic and statistical manual of mental disorders*, ed 4, Washington, DC, 1994, American Psychiatric Association.
19. Whittington CJ et al: Selective serotonin reuptake inhibitors in childhood depression: systematic review of published versus unpublished data, *Lancet* 363(9418):1341-1345, 2004.
20. Hilty DM, Brady KT, Hales RE: A review of bipolar disorder among adults, *Psychiatr Serv* 50(2):201-213, 1999.
21. Kennedy JL, Bradwejn J, Koszycki D et al: Investigation of cholecystokinin system genes in panic disorder, *Mol Psychiatry* 4(3):284-285, 1999.
22. Goddard AW, Charney DS: Toward an integrated neurobiology of panic disorder, *J Clin Psychiatry* 58(suppl 2):4-11, 1997.
23. Malizia AL, Cunningham VJ, Bell CJ et al: Decreased brain GABA$_A$-benzodiazepine receptor binding in panic disorder: preliminary results from a quantitative PET study, *Arch Gen Psychiatry* 55(8):715-720, 1998.
24. Jetty PV, Charney DS, Goddard AW: Neurobiology of generalized anxiety disorder, *Psychiatr Clin North Am* 24(1):75-97, 2001.
25. Tiihonen J et al: Cerebral benzodiazepine receptor binding and distribution in generalized anxiety disorder: a fractal analysis, *Mol Psychiatry* 2(6):463-471, 1997.
26. Bruce SE: Infrequency of "pure" GAD: impact of psychiatric comorbidity on clinical course, *Depress Anxiety* 14(4):219-225, 2001.
27. Charney DS, Deutch AY, Krystal JH et al: Psychobiologic mechanisms of posttraumatic stress disorder, *Arch Gen Psychiatry* 50(4):295-305, 1993.

28. Southwick SM, Paige S, Morgan CA III et al: Neurotransmitter alterations in PTSD: catecholamines and serotonin, *Semin Clin Neuropsychiatry* 4(4):242-248, 1999.

29. Pissiota A, Frans O, Fernandez M et al: Neurofunctional correlates of posttraumatic stress disorder: a PET symptom provocation study, *Eur Arch Psychiatry Clin Neurosci* 252(2):68-75, 2002.

30. Bremner JD, Innis RB, Southwick SM et al: Decreased benzodiazepine receptor binding in prefrontal cortex in combat-related posttraumatic stress disorder, *Am J Psychiatry* 157(7):1120-1126, 2000.

31. Fireman B, Koran LM, Leventhal JL et al: The prevalence of clinically recognized obsessive-compulsive disorder in a large health maintenance organization, *Am J Psychiatry* 158(11):1904-1910, 2001.

32. Saxena S, Rauch SL: Functional neuroimaging and the neuroanatomy of obsessive-compulsive disorder, *Psychiatr Clin North Am* 23(3):563-586, 2000.

33. Swedo SE, Snider LA: The neurobiology and treatment of obsessive-compulsive disorder. In Charney DS, Nestler EJ, editors: *Neurobiology of mental illness*, ed 2, New York, 2004, Oxford.

34. Greenberg BD, Murphy DL, Rasmussen SA: Neuroanatomically based approaches to obsessive-compulsive disorder: neurosurgery and transcranial magnetic stimulation, *Psychiatr Clin North Am* 23(3):671-686, 2000.

ALTERATIONS OF NEUROLOGIC FUNCTION IN CHILDREN

KATHERINE PADGETT

evolve

http://evolve.elsevier.com/McCance/

CHAPTER OUTLINE

Central nervous system (CNS) malformations are responsible for 75% of fetal deaths and 40% of deaths during the first year of life. During the perinatal period, CNS malformations account for 33% of all apparent congenital malformations, and 90% of CNS malformations are defects of neural tube closure. Although embryology is a highly complex and often difficult science to understand fully, having a basic knowledge of this science is essential because it is the process of embryonic development that explains many of the malformations that occur in children.

Environmental influences also play a significant role in nervous system development. Nutrition, hormones, oxygen levels, and external stimulation all affect normal growth. The proper proportions of essential nutrients are necessary for proliferation of the nervous system tissue. Maternal life-style, nutrition, and state of health also have a crucial impact on nervous system development at certain critical periods of maturation.

STRUCTURE AND FUNCTION OF THE NERVOUS SYSTEM IN CHILDREN

The CNS develops from a dorsal thickening of the ectoderm known as the **neural plate.** This plate appears around the middle of the third gestational week and unfolds to form a neural groove and neural folds. During the fourth gestational week the neural groove deepens; its folds develop laterally; and it closes dorsally to form the **neural tube,** epithelial tissue that ultimately becomes the CNS. The neural tube closes first in the cervical region and then "zippers" in two directions—cranially and caudally (Figure 19-1).

In the developmental process, some neuroectodermal cells separate from the neural tube but remain between the tube and the surface ectoderm, creating the **neural crest.** This cellular band develops into the cranial and spinal ganglia, more commonly referred to as the *peripheral nervous system.* Other structures associated with the nervous system arise from mesoderm (**somite**) and include blood vessels, microglial cells, dural and arachnoid layers of the meninges, the capsule of some peripheral sensory nerve endings, and peripheral nerve coverings.

The cranial end of the neural tube forms the brain, and the remainder develops into the spinal cord. The lumen of the neural tube becomes the ventricles of the brain and the central canal of the spinal cord (Figure 19-2). On either side of the neural tube's inner surface is a longitudinal groove (**sulcus limitans**). Anterior to this region (**basal plate**) the gray matter differentiates into the nuclei of the lower motor neurons. The region posterior to the sulcus (**alar plate**) differentiates into the sensory nuclei of the spinal cord.

Embryonic development of the nervous system occurs in six stages: (1) dorsal (posterior) induction, (2) ventral (ante-

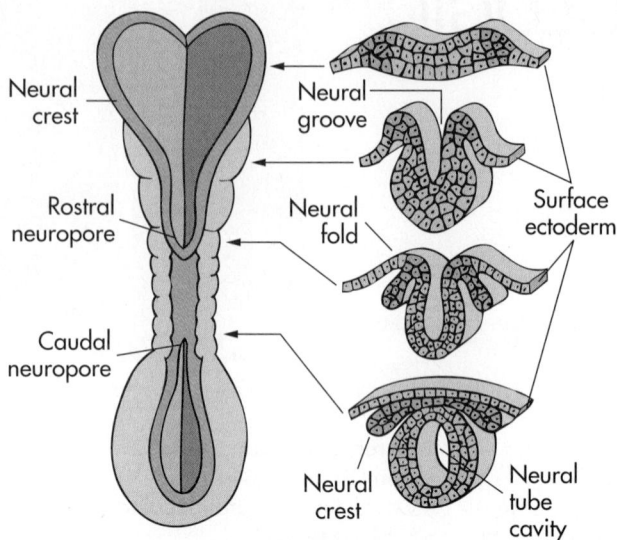

Figure 19-1 **Neural tube at three weeks of gestation.** Neural folds have begun to fuse at the cervical level of the future spinal cord. *Right,* Cross sections of the neural tube at four different levels; at any given level the embryonic central nervous system (CNS) goes through a series of stages resembling these four cross sections. Total length of neural tube at this time is about 2.5 mm.

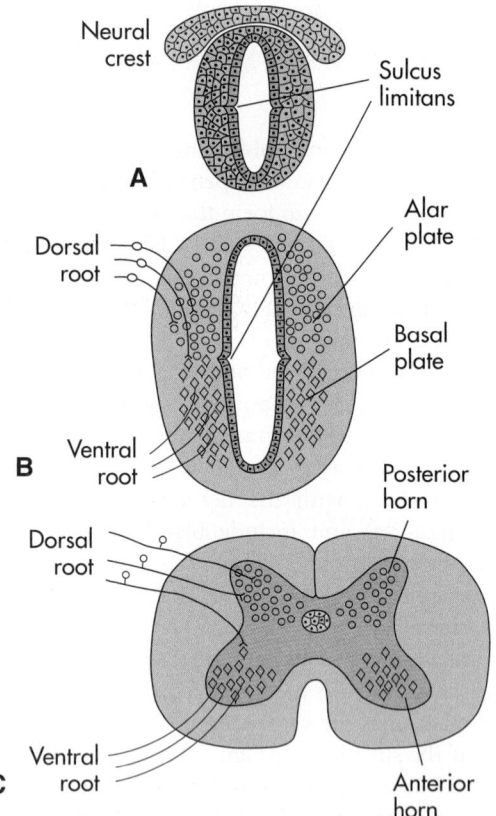

Figure 19-2 **Sulcus limitans and alar and basal plates. A,** Neural tube during the fourth week of gestation. **B,** Embryonic spinal cord during the sixth week of gestation; dorsal root ganglion cells, derived from the neural crest, send their central processes into the spinal cord to terminate mainly in alar plate cells; basal plate cells become motor neurons, whose axons exit in the ventral roots. **C,** Adult spinal cord.

rior) induction, (3) proliferation, (4) migration, (5) organization, and (6) myelination. (Figure 19-3 summarizes the embryonic development of the nervous system and identifies disorders associated with interference in any of these stages.) Many different events happen simultaneously, and critical periods must pass uninterrupted if the vulnerable fetus is to develop normally.

In the newborn the bones of the skull are separated, but definite **sutures** (bands of connective tissue) form shortly thereafter. The edges are several millimeters wide to allow for normal growth. At the junctions of the sutures are wider spaces of unossified membranous tissue called **fontanelles.** Sutures and fontanelles close as the skull and brain grow and develop.

On average the posterior fontanelle closes within the first 3 months of life. By 6 months of age, a fibrous union of suture lines occurs and serrated edges interlock. By approximately 20 to 24 months, the anterior fontanelle is closed (Figure 19-4). At approximately 8 years of age, ossification of the cranial bones is complete; the sutures usually are completely fused and cannot be separated by 12 years of age, even in the presence of increased intracranial pressure (IICP).

Myelin Sheath

Axons are wrapped in concentric layers of myelin, a lipid-protein sheath (see Chapter 14). Specialized connective tissue cells, which in the peripheral nervous system are called **Schwann cells,** form membranes that wrap around the axon during embryonic development, laying down the lipoprotein lamellae of the myelin sheath. These axons are myelinated, whereas the axons that lack a sheath are thinner, unmyelinated fibers and conduct nerve impulses more slowly. During the first year of life, the presence or absence of various reflexes is indicative of the myelination that has occurred with growth of the infant.

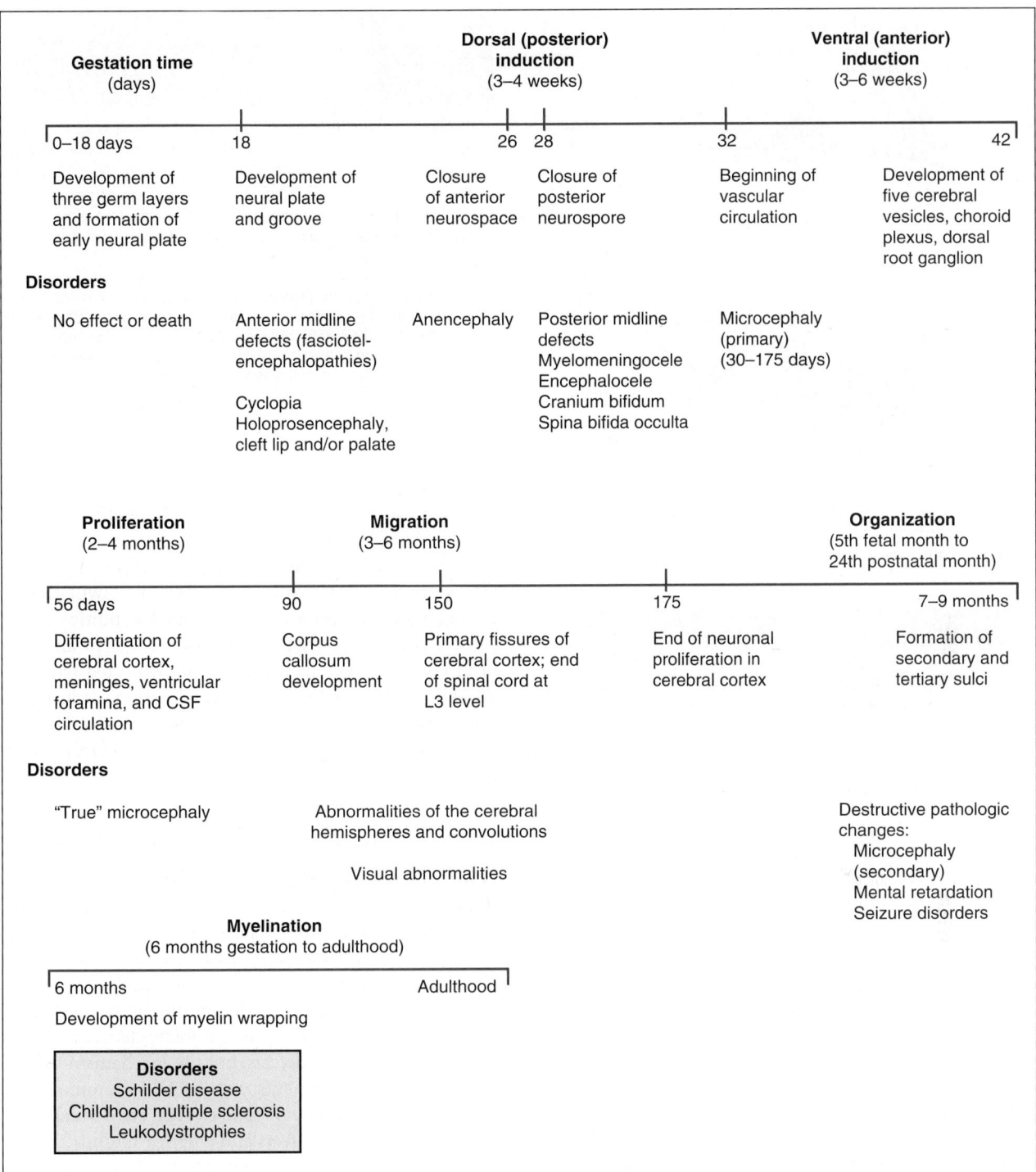

Figure 19-3 Disorders associated with specific stages of embryonic development. *CSF,* Cerebral spinal fluid.

Normal Growth and Development

Human neurologic functioning is primarily at a subcortical level at birth (impulses are handled by the brain stem and spinal cord). Many reflex patterns mediated by brain stem and spinal cord mechanisms are present at birth and disappear at predictable times during infancy. Table 19-1 summarizes the ages at which reflexes appear and disappear.

Absence of expected reflex responses at the appropriate age indicates general depression of central or peripheral motor functions. Asymmetric responses may indicate lesions in the motor cortex or may occur with fractures of bones after traumatic delivery or postnatal injury. As the infant matures, the neonatal reflexes disappear in a predictable order as voluntary motor functions supersede them. Abnormal persistence of

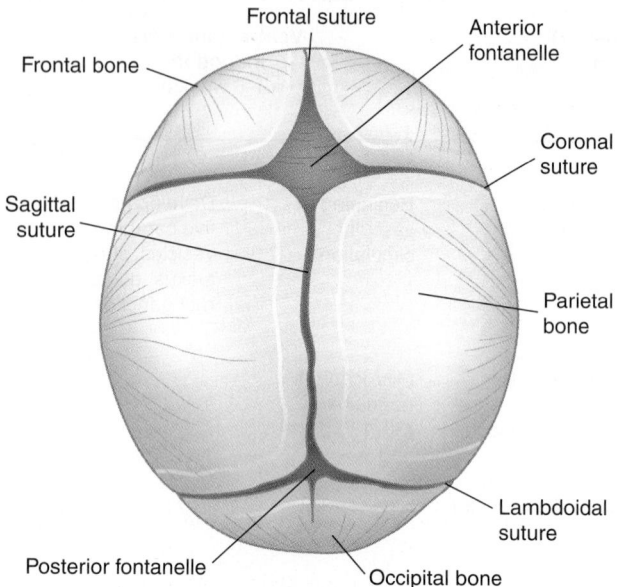

Figure 19-4 **Cranial sutures and fontanelles in infancy.** Fibrous union of suture lines and interlocking of serrated edges (occurs by 6 months; solid union requires approximately 12 years).

Table 19-1	Reflexes of Infancy	
Reflex	Age at Appearance of Reflex	Age at Which Reflex Should No Longer Be Obtainable
Moro	Birth	3 months
Stepping	Birth	6 weeks
Sucking	Birth	4 months awake 7 months asleep
Rooting	Birth	4 months awake 7 months asleep
Palmar grasp	Birth	6 months
Plantar grasp	Birth	10 months
Tonic neck	2 months	5 months
Neck righting	4-6 months	24 months
Landau	3 months	24 months
Parachute reaction	9 months	Persists for life

these reflexes is seen in infants with developmental delays or with central motor lesions.

Several differences between adults and children illustrate the pathophysiology of the nervous system in children. First, the head of a normal infant accounts for approximately one fourth of the total height, whereas an adult's head is one eighth of the total body height. Second, the bones of the infant's skull are separated at the suture lines, thus forming two fontanelles or "soft spots:" one diamond-shaped anterior fontanelle and one triangular-shaped posterior fontanelle. The posterior fontanelle may be open until 2 to 3 months of age, whereas the anterior fontanelle normally closes by 18 months. Whereas the adult cranium is a closed cavity with sutures firmly holding the cranial bones together, the infant cranium has room for expansion through the fontanelles. An

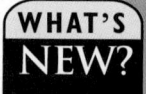

WHAT'S NEW? Reduction of Risks for Neural Tube Defects

Studies indicate that ingestion of multivitamins with folic acid before conception or early in pregnancy may offer protection against the occurrence of neural tube defects. Recent repeated studies demonstrate a 60% to 86% reduction of risks for neural tube defects with periconceptional ingestion of vitamins containing the U.S. recommended daily allowance of 400 mg folic acid.

Data from Centers for Disease Control: Use of vitamins containing folic acid among women of childbearing age—United States, 2004, *MMWR* 53(36):847-850, 2004; Lumley J et al: Periconceptional supplementation with folate and/or multivitamins for preventing neural tube defects, *Cochrane Database Syst Rev* (3):CD001056, 2001.

adult's head size will not expand, regardless of intracranial events such as trauma or increased production of cerebrospinal fluid (CSF). The infant's head circumference, on the other hand, increases in size as a result of normal growth up to 5 years of age. The head is the fastest growing body part during infancy. Abnormal intracranial conditions, such as those characterized by IICP, also may result in an increased head circumference in excess of that expected with normal growth. Healthcare providers carefully monitor head growth during the first 5 years of life by measuring head circumference and comparing the results with a standardized growth chart.

STRUCTURAL MALFORMATIONS

Defects of Neural Tube Closure

Neural tube defects, which are caused by an arrest of the normal developmental process, have an incidence rate of approximately 0.7 to 1.0 for every 1000 live births in the United States each year. There is a strong association of fetal death with neural tube defects, reducing the actual prevalence of neural defects at birth.[1] Maternal folate deficiency is associated with neural tube defects, but the mechanism that relates to how folate supplements prevent these anomalies is unknown.[2] Defects of neural tube closure are divided into two categories: posterior defects and anterior midline defects.

Posterior defects are more common. These include anencephaly (*an* = without; *enkephalos* = brain) and a group of disorders collectively referred to as the *myelodysplasias* (*dys* = bad; *plassein* = to form). Although **myelodysplasia** is defined as a defective formation of the spinal cord, the term is used to refer to anomalies of both the vertebral column and the spine.

Anterior midline defects are less common because the inductive processes occur in a relatively short period (2 to 3 days). These developmental defects may cause brain and skull abnormalities. The most extreme form is **cyclopia**, in which the child has a single midline orbit and eye with a protruding noselike appendage above the orbit.

Anencephaly

Anencephaly is an anomaly in which the soft, bony component of the skull and part of the brain are missing. This is a relatively common disorder, with an incidence rate of approximately 0.36 per 1000 total live births in the United States each year.[3] When development is arrested early in anterior closure of the neural tube, the cerebral hemispheres, diencephalon, mesencephalon, cerebellum, brain stem, or spinal cord may be affected. At birth the infant's head, viewed face-on, has a froglike appearance. These infants are stillborn or die within a few days after birth.

Encephalocele

Encephalocele refers to a herniation or protrusion of brain and meninges through a defect in the skull, resulting in a saclike structure. The incidence rate is approximately 1 in 5000 live births in the United States each year.[4] When the defect contains only meninges, it is referred to as a **cranial meningocele**. Most encephaloceles occur in the occipital area, with the remainder found in the frontal, parietal, or nasopharyngeal regions.

CLINICAL MANIFESTATIONS   Encephalocele usually is seen at birth as a midline skull defect through which a large mass protrudes (Figure 19-5). If the defect is located in the nasopharynx, no external anomaly is visible, but the child may experience nasal airway obstruction. On examination with a nasal speculum, a smooth, round mass will be visible in the nasal passages. A frontal encephalocele may extend into the orbit of the eye and produce proptosis on the affected side.

EVALUATION AND TREATMENT   Diagnosis is based on clinical manifestations and examination of the meningeal sac. With cranial meningocele, surgical repair of the cranial

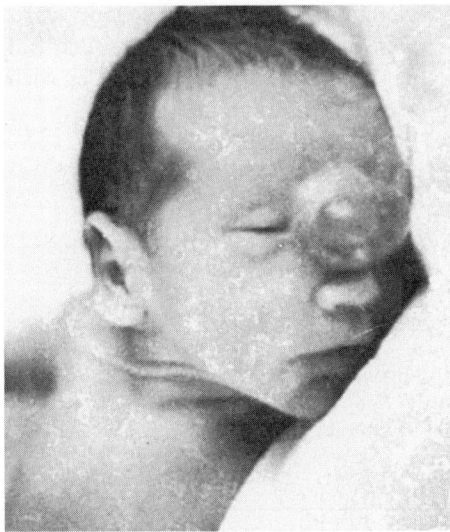

Figure 19-5 Newborn with frontal, nasal, interocular encephalocele. (Courtesy Dr. Charles Linder, Medical College of Georgia.)

defect affords a good prognosis for most affected infants whose intellectual and motor functioning is normal. An occipital encephalocele may be associated with other findings, such as blindness and cognitive impairment. The size, location, and involvement of the encephalocele help to determine the child's development and intellectual outcome.

Meningocele

A **meningocele,** which is a saclike cyst of meninges filled with spinal fluid, occurs when the neural tube fails to close completely (Figure 19-6). This cystic dilation of meninges protrudes through the vertebral defect and around the malformed tube. This defect does not involve the spinal cord. Meningoceles occur with equal frequency in the cervical, thoracic, and lumbar spine areas.

CLINICAL MANIFESTATIONS   At birth the infant has a protruding sac on the back at the level of the defect. The sac may be covered by a thin layer of muscle and skin and usually

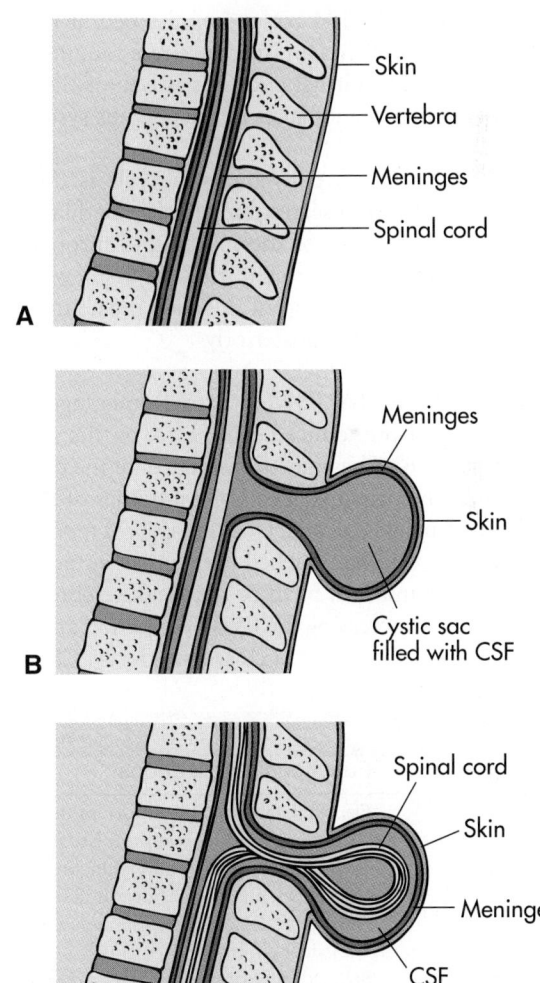

Figure 19-6 Comparison of normal spine and meningocele and myelomeningocele neural tube defects. Diagram depicts section through normal spine (**A**), spine with meningocele (**B**), and spine with myelomeningocele (**C**).

appears as raw, fluid-filled tissue. Abnormal neurologic function sometimes is present. Talipes equinovarus (clubfoot), gait disturbance, bladder dysfunction, and upper extremity weakness also have been associated with meningocele. Hydrocephalus commonly is associated with this diagnosis.

EVALUATION AND TREATMENT The diagnosis is made on the basis of clinical manifestations and examination of the meningeal sac. In an effort to preserve neuronal function and minimize potential damage that may occur from infection and manipulation of the fragile sac, surgical closure is optimal during the first 72 hours of life. Functional implications depend on the level and severity of the defect (Table 19-2).

Myelomeningocele

Myelomeningocele (meningomyelocele; spina bifida cystica) is a hernial protrusion of a saclike cyst (containing meninges, spinal fluid, and a portion of the spinal cord with its nerves) through a defect in the posterior arch of a vertebra. Eighty percent of myelomeningoceles are located in the lumbar and lumbosacral regions, the last regions of the neural tube to close. Myelomeningocele has an incidence rate ranging from 0.2 to 0.4 per 1000 live births[5] and thus is one of the most common developmental anomalies of the nervous system.

PATHOPHYSIOLOGY A myelomeningocele is the failure of the neural tube to close, resulting in a cystic dilation of meninges and protuberance of the spinal cord through the vertebral defect. This defect occurs during the first 4 weeks of the gestational period; at the end of this time the neural tube is closed both anteriorly and posteriorly.

CLINICAL MANIFESTATIONS A myelomeningocele is evident at birth as a pronounced skin defect on the infant's back (see Figure 19-6). The bony prominences of the unfused neural arches can be palpated at the lateral border of the defect. The defect usually is covered by a transparent membrane that may have neural tissue attached to its inner surface. This membrane may be intact at birth or may leak cerebrospinal fluid (CSF), thereby increasing the risks of infection and neuronal damage. Until the defect is closed surgically, CSF may

accumulate, resulting in further dilation and enlargement of the sac, which may risk further damage to neuronal function.

The actual involvement of the spinal cord has greater implications for the overall function of the infant throughout childhood (see Table 19-2). An absence of neurologic function may occur in some infants with myelomeningocele. Function may be attained if underlying fluid or pus accumulation is prevented from stretching and applying pressure to the neural tissue or if the biochemical alterations do not cause neural tissue to die. Residual neural tissue also may be lost temporarily or permanently at birth because of trauma to the tissue during delivery.

One serious, potentially life-threatening problem associated with myelomeningocele is the **Arnold-Chiari type II malformation.**[6] This deformity involves the downward displacement of the cerebellum, cerebral tonsils, brain stem, and fourth ventricle (Figure 19-7). (Chiari type I malformations also involve downward displacement but are not as great as those in type II; type I is seen more commonly in adults.) Arnold-Chiari II malformation compresses and essentially stretches the posterior region of the cerebellum and brain stem downward through the foramen magnum and into the cervical space. The brain stem houses the 12 cranial nerves. Pressure on this region may result in altered function of these nerves or actual palsies. Dysfunction of the lower cranial nerves is common, and the displacement of this area of the brain results in the compression and elongation of nerves and tissue, which in turn restrict neuronal performance in varying degrees.[7]

Hydrocephalus occurs in 85% of these infants.[8] Seizures also occur in 30% of those with myelodysplasia.[9] Visual and perceptual problems, including ocular palsies, astigmatism, and visuoperceptual deficits, are common.[10] Motor and sensory functions below the level of the lesions are altered. This dysfunction may include degrees of weakness, paralysis, spasticity, and bowel and bladder dysfunction. Often these problems worsen as the child grows and the cord ascends within the vertebral canal, pulling primary scar tissue and tethering the cord.[11] Several musculoskeletal deformities are related to this diagnosis, including clubfoot, dislocation of hip or hips, and poor spinal alignment. Spinal deformities, such as scoliosis and kyphosis, are common.[12]

Table 19-2	Functional Alterations in Myelodysplasia Related to Level of Lesion
Level of Lesion	**Functional Implications**
Thoracic	Flaccid paralysis of lower extremities; variable weakness in abdominal trunk musculature; high thoracic level may mean respiratory compromise; absence of bowel and bladder control
High lumbar	Voluntary hip flexion and adduction; flaccid paralysis of knees, ankles, and feet; may walk with extensive braces and crutches; absence of bowel and bladder control
Midlumbar	Strong hip flexion and adduction; fair knee extension; flaccid paralysis of ankles and feet; absence of bowel and bladder control
Low lumbar	Strong hip flexion, extension, and adduction and knee extension; weak ankle and toe mobility; may have limited bowel and bladder function
Sacral	Normal function of lower extremities; normal bowel and bladder function

Data from Farley JA, Dunleavy MJ. Myelodysplasia. In Allen PJ, Vessey JA, editors: *Primary care of the child with a chronic condition,* ed 4, St Louis, 2004, Mosby.

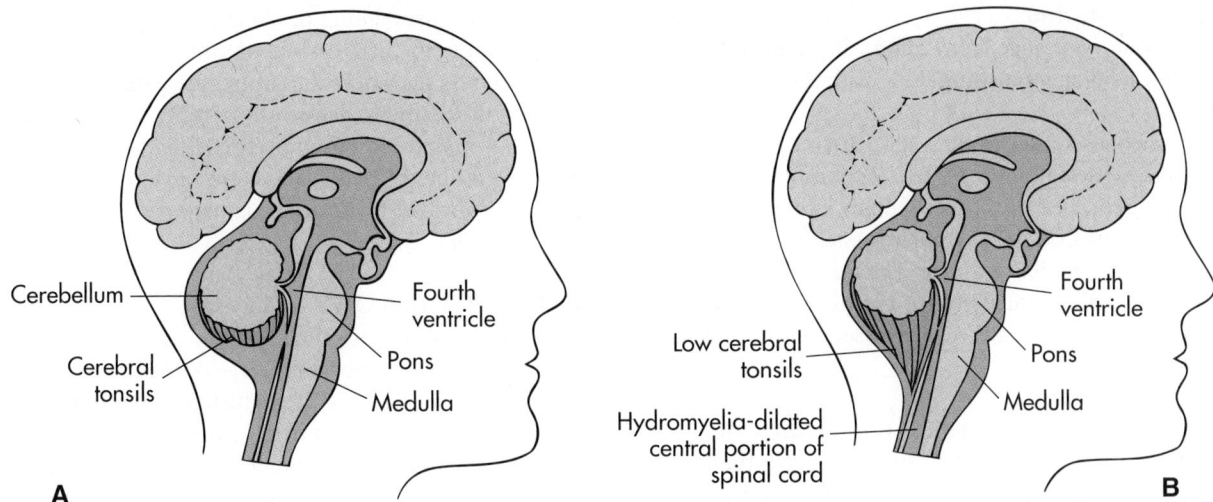

Figure 19-7 Comparison of normal brain and Arnold-Chiari type II malformation. Diagram depicts normal brain (**A**) and brain with Arnold-Chiari malformation (**B**).

Tethered cord syndrome may develop in children with myelomeningocele, particularly after surgical correction.[13] The cord becomes caught or tethered as a result of scar tissue as it transcends the vertebral canal with growth. Symptoms are related to excessive tension on the lumbosacral cord and can include scoliosis, altered gait pattern, changes in muscle strength at or below the lesion, disturbance in urinary and bowel patterns, and back pain.[14]

EVALUATION AND TREATMENT   Diagnosis is based on clinical manifestations and examination of the meningeal sac. However, because the pathophysiology of myelodysplasia is determined early in gestation, prenatal diagnosis is possible through ultrasonography. In addition, the presence of a neural tube defect may result in an elevated amniotic fluid α-fetoprotein (AFP) level and subsequent maternal serum AFP levels. Prenatal diagnosis offers the parents the option to terminate the pregnancy or become a candidate for fetal intrauterine repair.[15,16] If they choose to continue the pregnancy, prenatal diagnosis provides the family and the healthcare team the opportunity to prepare both physically and emotionally for the birth of the child. Cesarean delivery may be recommended to minimize trauma to the open myelomeningocele.[17]

Treatment for the infant with myelomeningocele is early surgical closure of the defect. Intrauterine endoscopic surgery is under investigation.[18] Because myelodysplasia affects several other body systems (e.g., renal, gastrointestinal, musculoskeletal), these infants require a lifetime, comprehensive, multidisciplinary approach to treatment. The prognosis depends on the extent of the involvement at birth and the success of prophylactic and acute treatment for potential and actual complications that affect the many body systems. Symptomatic Arnold Chiari II malformations require surgical decompression and/or placement of cerebrospinal fluid shunts.[19]

Malformations of the Axial Skeleton
Spina Bifida Occulta

When defects of neural tube closure occur, such as meningocele and myelomeningocele, an accompanying vertebral defect allows the protrusion of the neural tube contents. Such a defect is called **spina bifida.** The cause of spinal bifida is unknown. Periconceptual maternal folate deficiency and genetic alterations are commonly associated with the defect.[20] It also is possible for a defect to occur without any visible exposure of meninges or neural tissue. Because the defect is not apparent to the naked eye (i.e., it is "occult" or hidden), the term **spina bifida occulta** is used. In spina bifida occulta the posterior vertebral laminae have failed to fuse. This extremely common defect occurs to some degree in 10% to 25% of infants. Approximately 80% of these vertebral defects are located in the lumbosacral regions, most commonly in the fifth lumbar vertebra and the first sacral vertebra, and may be detected prenatally with ultrasonic scanning and AFP testing. About 3% of normal adults have spina bifida occulta of the atlas (cervical vertebra 1). The following cutaneous or subcutaneous abnormalities suggest underlying spina bifida:

- Abnormal growth of hair along the spine, which often is either very coarse or very silky
- A midline dimple with or without a sinus tract
- A cutaneous angioma, usually of the "port wine" variety
- A subcutaneous mass, usually representing a lipoma or dermoid cyst

Spina bifida occulta usually causes no serious neurologic dysfunctions.[5] The spinal cord and spinal nerves generally are anatomically and functionally normal. When dysfunctions occur, the common lumbosacral defects cause gait abnormalities, positional deformities of the feet as a result of muscle weakness, or sphincter disturbances of the bladder and bowel. These dysfunctions become evident during periods of rapid growth. Surgical closure is usually completed in the neonatal period and techniques are being developed for intrauterine closure.[21]

Cranial Deformities

Skull malformations range from minor, insignificant defects to major defects that are incompatible with life.

Acrania

In **acrania** the cranial vault is almost completely absent and an extensive defect of the vertebral column often is present. Acrania associated with anencephaly (absence of brain and spinal column) occurs in approximately 1 per 1000 live births and is incompatible with life. The malformation results from a failure of the cranial end of the neural tube to close during the fourth gestational week. Subsequently, the cranial vault fails to form.

Craniosynostosis

Craniosynostosis (craniostenosis) is the premature closure of one or more of the cranial sutures during the first 18 to 20 months of the infant's life. The incidence of craniosynostosis is 1 in 2100 live births.[22] Males are affected twice as often as females. Craniosynostosis prevents normal skull expansion and causes asymmetric skull growth. Premature closure of a suture causes failure of the growth of the bone located at a right angle to the involved suture. Compensatory growth occurs in regions where the sutures are patent, and this causes the various cosmetic deformities. In the absence of adequate sutures, cerebral growth may exceed the space present. Brain growth may be restricted, and compression may cause neurologic dysfunction from brain damage after 6 months of age (Figure 19-8).

PATHOPHYSIOLOGY The exact causes of craniosynostosis are unknown, but the condition represents more than a single disorder of embryonic development. One possible explanation is a germ layer disturbance involving the mesenchyma (embryonic connective tissue that gives rise to the connective tissues, blood vessels, and lymphatics). This mesenchymal defect may be caused by a deficiency in enzyme inhibition of ossification. A number of metabolic disorders are accompanied by premature or delayed ossification of cranial bones, suggesting a metabolic mechanism. A genetic defect of

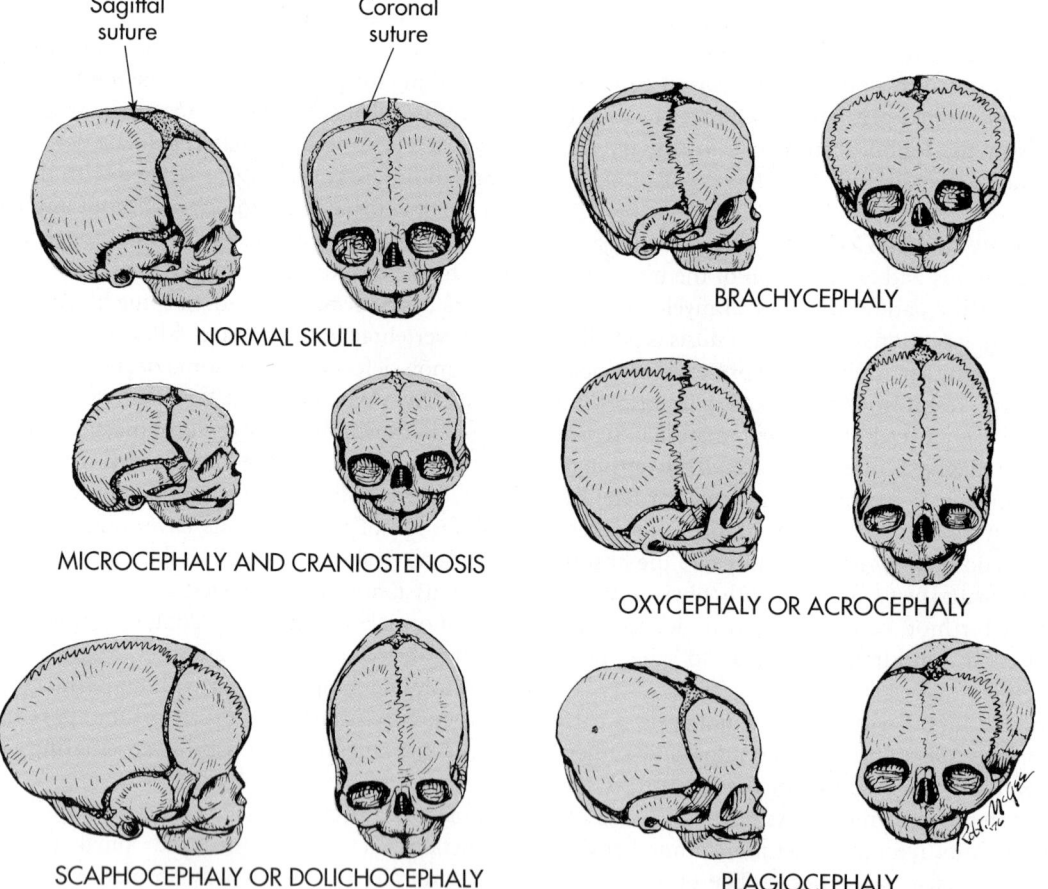

Figure 19-8 Craniosynostosis. Abnormal head configuration resulting from premature closing of cranial sutures. *Normal skull,* Bones separated by membranous seams until sutures gradually close. *Microcephaly and craniostenosis,* Microcephaly is head circumference more than 2 standard deviations below the mean for age, gender, race, and gestation and reflects a small brain; craniosynostosis is premature closure of sutures. *Scaphocephaly or dolichocephaly* (frequency 56%), Premature closure of sagittal suture, resulting in restricted lateral growth. *Brachycephaly,* Premature closure of coronal suture, resulting in excessive lateral growth. *Oxycephaly or acrocephaly* (frequency 5.8%-12%), Premature closure of all coronal and sagittal sutures, resulting in accelerated upward growth and small head circumference. *Plagiocephaly* (frequency 13%), Unilateral premature closure of coronal suture, resulting in asymmetric growth. (From Hockenberry JH et al: *Wong's nursing care of infants and children,* ed 7, St Louis, 2003, Mosby.)

hormonal or mineral metabolism may create ossification centers at abnormal sites. Mechanical factors also appear to play a role in craniosynostosis because secondary premature fusion of sutures occurs in microcephaly and after shunting in hydrocephalus.

CLINICAL MANIFESTATIONS   Craniosynostosis is classified according to head contour or suture involvement.[23] Final skull contour is determined by the sutures that close, the duration and order of closure, and the ability of other sutures to compensate by expansion. (The frequency and types of craniosynostosis are depicted in Figures 19-8 and 19-9.)

Premature closure of the sagittal suture, the most common form of craniosynostosis, causes elongation of the skull in the anteroposterior direction. Other anomalies are seen in 25% of these children. When the coronal suture fuses prematurely, the brain expands in a lateral direction. This type of craniosynostosis is associated with a 33% to 66% incidence of associated anomalies. Approximately half of these children are mentally retarded.

EVALUATION AND TREATMENT   Diagnosis is made on the basis of physical examination, head circumference measurements, and radiologic examination. Surgical treatment is indicated when closure of multiple sutures causes chronic IICP. Surgery then limits the extent of brain damage. In children with craniosynostosis of one suture, surgery often is performed for cosmetic purposes to limit the appearance of deformity.

Microcephaly

Microcephaly is a defect in brain growth as a whole (see Figure 19-8). The word *microcephaly* is derived from the Greek (*mikro* = small; *kephale* = head). Cranial size is significantly below average for the infant's age, gender, race, and gestation. The small size of the skull reflects a small brain, except in infants with premature closure of the sutures. The condition is not treatable.

True (primary) microcephaly can be caused by an autosomal recessive disorder, by a chromosomal abnormality, or by toxin exposure during the period of induction and major cell migration (Box 19-1). Radiation, maternal infection, or chemical exposure may be the initiating factor. Secondary microcephaly is associated with a variety of causes. Infection, trauma, metabolic disorders, and anorexia experienced during the third trimester of pregnancy, the perinatal period, or early infancy may be responsible.

Brain weight may be as low as 25% of normal in the microcephalic brain. Both the number and the size of the cortical gyri may be diminished. Growth of the frontal lobes is severely stunted, and the cerebellum often is disproportionately large. In microcephaly caused by perinatal or postnatal disorders, neuronal loss and gliosis may be present in the cerebral cortex. The neurologic manifestations of microcephaly range from decerebrate posture, complete unresponsiveness, and autistic behavior to mild motor impairment, **mental retardation,** and hyperkinesis.

Congenital Hydrocephalus

Congenital hydrocephalus is characterized by an increased volume of CSF. This increase in volume may be caused by a blockage within the ventricular system in which the CSF flows, an imbalance in production of the CSF, or a reduced reabsorption of the CSF that results in ventricular enlargement and IICP. The pressure within the ventricular system pushes and compresses the brain tissue against the skull cavity. When hydrocephalus develops before fusion of the cranial sutures, the skull has the capacity to increase its effort to accommodate this additional space-occupying volume and to preserve neuronal function. The overall incidence of hydrocephalus is approximately 3 per 1000 live births.[24] The incidence of hydrocephalus, excluding the hydrocephalus associated with myelomeningocele, is approximately 0.5 to 1 per 1000 live births, with aqueductal stenosis as the cause for ap-

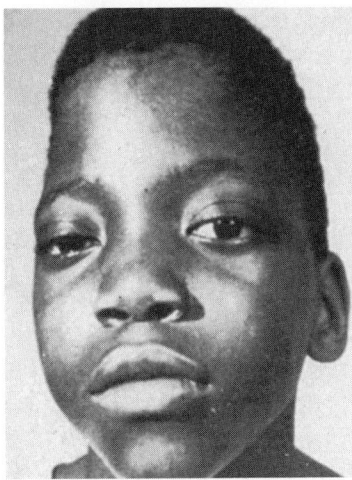

Figure 19-9 Dolichoscaphocephaly in 14-year-old boy. One of the less threatening of the craniosynostoses. (From Dyken PR, Miller MD: *Facial features of neurologic syndromes,* St Louis, 1980, Mosby.)

Box 19-1	Causes of Microencephaly

Defects in Brain Development
Hereditary (recessive) microcephaly
Down syndrome and other trisomy syndromes
Fetal ionizing radiation exposure
Maternal phenylketonuria
Seckel syndrome
Cornelia de Lange syndrome
Rubinstein-Taybi syndrome
Smith-Lemli-Opitz syndrome
Fetal alcohol syndrome

Intrauterine Infections
Congenital rubella
Cytomegalovirus infection
Congenital toxoplasmosis
Congenital syphilis

Perinatal and Postnatal Disorders
Intrauterine or neonatal anoxia
Severe malnutrition in early infancy
Neonatal herpesvirus infection

proximately one third of these cases.[25] (Types of hydrocephalus are discussed in Chapter 16.)

PATHOPHYSIOLOGY Obstructive hydrocephalus is caused most commonly by congenital aqueduct stenosis. The cerebral aqueduct is narrowed or replaced by multiple channels, or "forks," that end blindly. In a small number of children the stenosis is transmitted as an X-linked recessive trait. The **Dandy-Walker deformity** is a congenital defect of midline cerebellar structures in which hydrocephalus is caused by atresia of the foramina of Luschka or Magendie, leading the ventricular flow of CSF into a "blind pouch." Other causes of obstructions within the ventricular system that can result in hydrocephalus include brain tumors, cysts, trauma, arteriovenous malformations, blood clots, and infections.

CSF travels throughout the ventricular system, surrounds the brain, and is reabsorbed into the venous system by the arachnoid villi. Blockage of the arachnoid villi may occur in conditions such as bacterial or viral meningitis, intraventricular hemorrhage, and subarachnoid hemorrhage, or blockage may result from congenital malformations within this area. In that instance CSF flows or communicates effectively but is unable to be reabsorbed, resulting in hydrocephalus.

CLINICAL MANIFESTATIONS Congenital hydrocephalus may cause fetal death in utero, or the increased head circumference may require cesarean delivery of the infant. Symptoms of this condition depend directly on the cause and rate of hydrocephalus development. Infants may have no symptoms at birth. During the early weeks of life, the head begins to grow at an abnormal rate. Significant dilation of the ventricles may occur before an abnormal increase in head growth develops. The fontanelles enlarge and become full and bulging (Figures 19-10

and 19-11). The separation of the cranial sutures leads to a resonant note when the skull is tapped, a manifestation termed **Macewen sign ("cracked-pot" sign).** The eyes may assume a staring expression, with sclera visible above the cornea, called *sunsetting.*

The infant may have difficulty holding the head upright. The scalp skin is thin and shiny, and scalp veins may become prominent. The large cranial vault and the face are disproportionate, and frontal bossing may be present. The infant's cry becomes high pitched as intracranial pressure (ICP) rises;

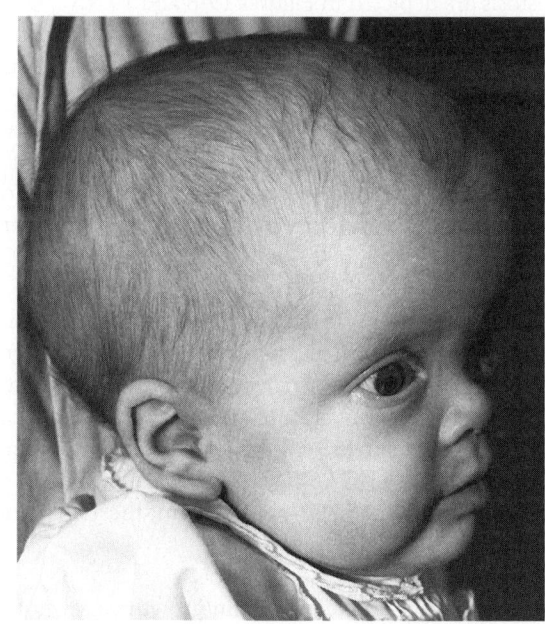

Figure 19-11 Child with enlarged head caused by hydrocephalus. (From McLaurin DC: *Pediatric neurosurgery,* ed 2, Philadelphia, 1989, Saunders.)

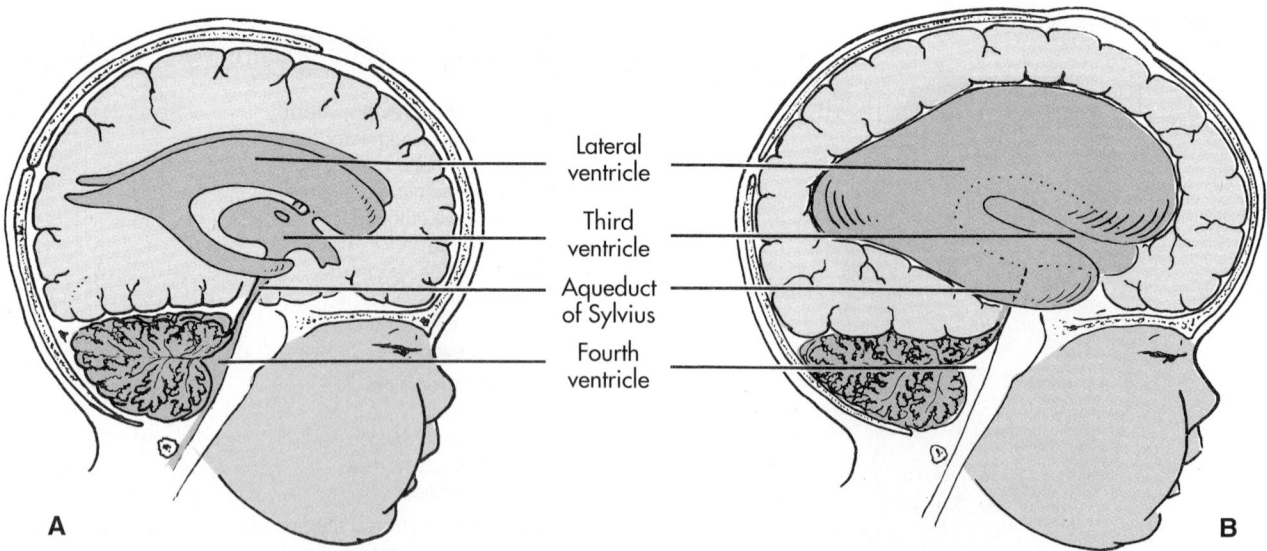

Lateral ventricle

Third ventricle

Aqueduct of Sylvius

Fourth ventricle

Figure 19-10 Hydrocephalus. A block in the flow of cerebrospinal fluid (CSF). **A,** Patent cerebrospinal fluid circulation. **B,** Enlarged lateral and third ventricles caused by obstruction of circulation—stenosis of aqueduct of Sylvius. (From Hockenberry MJ et al: *Wong's nursing care of infants and children,* ed 7, St Louis, 2003, Mosby.)

irritability, lethargy, vomiting, and other signs of IICP may develop. Dramatic head growth and enlargement, compression of the optic nerves, and optic chiasm occur in chronic, untreated hydrocephalus. However, because of early surgical intervention, these signs of hydrocephalus rarely are seen. When hydrocephalus develops late in childhood, the head may not have the capacity to enlarge and evidence of IICP is present (see Chapter 16).

The relationship between hydrocephalus and mental retardation has been heavily debated. Correlation between the degree of hydrocephalus and impaired cognitive function often is a result of additional complications, such as severe congenital malformations, acute or chronic infections, or progressive brain tumors. Approximately two thirds of children with uncomplicated congenital hydrocephalus treated successfully with shunting may have normal to borderline intelligence.[26]

EVALUATION AND TREATMENT   The definitive diagnostic tool for hydrocephalus is computed tomography (CT), and magnetic resonance imaging (MRI) may add information about the specific cause of the hydrocephalus. In infancy, head circumference measurements also are obtained and monitored. The treatment is surgical placement of a shunt to divert the excess CSF from the ventricular cavity to other areas of the body. Several types of shunts are available. The main objective of any shunt system is to decrease ICP and preserve neuronal function. With neurosurgical intervention and follow-up, the 5-year survival usually is greater than 80%. Most deaths that occur within this category result from severe congenital malformations and/or progressive disorders such as brain tumors. Children with hydrocephalus depend on the internal shunt system to maintain safe ICPs and therefore are forever at risk for sudden failure of this system, which leads to acute IICP and death.

ENCEPHALOPATHIES

Encephalopathy, a disorder involving the brain, is a general category that includes a number of syndromes and diseases (see Chapter 16). Encephalopathies in children are associated with a great variety of known and suspected causes. These disorders may be acute or chronic and static or progressive.

Static Encephalopathies

Brain injury may occur during gestation or birth or at any time during childhood growth and development, causing a static, nonprogressive disorder. The clinical manifestations depend on the site and extent of the injury, as well as the age of the child and stage of development at the time of injury. Varying degrees of impairment may result from diffuse or localized injury to the cortex. For example, cerebral palsy results when the motor areas of the brain are injured. Injury to the occipital lobe of the cerebral cortex early in gestation can interfere with normal cerebral maturation and result in future blindness. Cognitive impairment may follow diffuse cerebral

injury. Seizures also may develop from cortical injury, particularly if scar tissue remains.

Prenatal factors that affect the developing nervous system may be endogenous or exogenous. The fetus may be affected by impaired embryo implantation, chromosomal abnormalities, infection, trauma, radiation, and toxic substances. Maternal toxemia, diabetes mellitus, and maternal nutritional deficiencies can produce neurologic damage in the fetus. The developing nervous system is most susceptible to injury occurring during the first trimester of pregnancy. Anoxia, trauma, and infections are the most common factors that cause injury to the nervous system in the perinatal period. Infections, metabolic disturbances (acute or a result of inborn errors), trauma, toxins, and vascular disease may injure the nervous system in the postnatal period.

Cerebral Palsy

Cerebral palsy is the term given to a diverse group of nonprogressive syndromes that affect the brain and cause motor dysfunction beginning in early infancy. Cerebral palsy can be classified on the basis of neurologic signs and symptoms. The major types are spasticity, ataxia, dyskinesia, and a mix of one or more of the three. Although cerebral palsy is, by definition, nonprogressive, its clinical manifestations change with growth and maturation of the child.

Cerebral palsy is one of the most common crippling disorders of childhood, affecting nearly 500,000 children in the United States alone. Although the exact incidence is unknown, studies suggest that the incidence is 1 to 2.3 cases of cerebral palsy per 1000 live births.[27,28] Causes of cerebral palsy are numerous, and both genetic and environmental factors may be responsible. These factors can occur during the prenatal, perinatal, or postnatal period (Table 19-3).

PATHOPHYSIOLOGY   Several factors, alone or in combination, can produce brain damage that leads to cerebral palsy. Prenatal cerebral hypoxia can be responsible for systemic degeneration of immature areas of the brain and can interfere with cell maturation. The severity of the damage depends on the gestational age at the time of the injury and the degree of injury sustained.

Low birth weight and birth asphyxia are commonly identified risk factors for cerebral palsy.[29,30] Hypoxia and asphyxia are known to cause edema in the brain. Lack of oxygen and the incorporation of amino acids during protein synthesis lead to acidosis. Carbon dioxide and lactic acid accumulate with acidosis, causing osmotic pressure changes. This condition contributes to generalized cerebral swelling and CNS damage.

Vascular abnormalities, arterial or venous stasis, and thrombosis can occur as a result of tissue hypoxia or as unrelated structural alterations. These anomalies may result in direct brain trauma that leads to infarction, intraventricular hemorrhage, and subarachnoid hemorrhage. Intraventricular hemorrhage is a common cause of death in newborn infants. Such injuries contribute to CNS damage.

Table 19-3	Cerebral Palsy: Predisposing Factors and Known Causes	
Risk Factors	**Associated Causes**	
Prenatal		
Maternal	Metabolic diseases	
	Nutritional deficiencies (e.g., anemia)	
	Twin or multiple births	
	Bleeding	
	Toxemia	
	Blood incompatibilities	
	Exposure to radiation	
	Infection (e.g., rubella, toxoplasmosis, cytomegalic inclusion disease)	
	Premature labor	
Prematurity	Asphyxia leading to cerebral hemorrhage	
Genetic factors	Absence of corpus callosum, aqueductal stenosis, cerebellar hypoplasia	
Congenital anomalies of the brain	Unknown causes not evident on clinical examination	
Perinatal	Anesthesia or analgesia during labor and delivery	
	Mechanical trauma during delivery	
	Immaturity at birth	
	Metabolic disorders (e.g., hyperbilirubinemia, hypoglycemia, amino acid disorders, hyperosmolality)	
	Electrolyte disturbances (e.g., hypernatremia, hypoglycemia)	
Postnatal	Head trauma	
	Infections (e.g., meningitis, encephalitis)	
	Cerebrovascular accidents	
	Toxicosis	
	Environmental toxins (e.g., lead ingestion, methyl mercury ingestion from contaminated fish)	

Physical trauma to the central or peripheral nervous system can occur during the birthing process. Linear and depressed fractures are seen in newborn infants when head molding is extreme, with resultant hemorrhages and tears of the tentorium or falx cerebri. Tearing of the superficial cerebral veins is a relatively common occurrence and causes a thin layer of blood over the cerebral convexity. This blood may irritate the brain and result in CNS dysfunction. The infant's position during delivery may cause stretching and damage to nerves. Breech deliveries can cause traumatic injury to the brain stem or spinal cord, resulting in a more localized area of impairment. Malformations of the CNS play an important role in brain injury from perinatal trauma, and they predispose the infant to a greater probability of sustained injury to the CNS. Both faulty maturation of the nervous system and a greater vulnerability to perinatal trauma and hypoxia are responsible for a high incidence of neurologic dysfunction in the preterm infant. Genetic, teratogenic, and early pregnancy influences on the development of cerebral palsy are not yet fully understood.[31]

CLINICAL MANIFESTATIONS   The syndromes associated with cerebral palsy are classified according to the predominant clinical manifestations. **Spastic cerebral palsy** is associated with increased muscle tone, prolonged primitive reflexes, exaggerated deep tendon reflexes, clonus, rigidity of the extremities, scoliosis, and contractures. This results from motor neuron involvement and injury to the cerebral cortex in either one or both hemispheres and accounts for approximately 65% to 75% of cerebral palsy cases.

Dyskinetic cerebral palsy is associated with extreme difficulty in fine motor coordination and purposeful movements. Movements are jerky, uncontrolled, and abrupt, resulting from injury to the basal ganglia or extrapyramidal tracts. This form of cerebral palsy accounts for approximately 20% to 25% of cases. **Ataxic cerebral palsy** manifests with gait disturbances and instability. The infant with this form of cerebral palsy may have hypotonia at birth, but stiffness of the trunk muscles develops by late infancy. This lack of flexibility exaggerates the infant's inability to balance body position without support. Persistence of this increased tone in truncal muscles affects the child's gait and ability to maintain equilibrium. This form of cerebral palsy accounts for approximately 5% of cases. A child may have symptoms of each of these cerebral palsy types, which leads to a mixed-variety disorder that accounts for approximately 13% of cases.

Children with cerebral palsy often have associated neurologic disorders, such as seizures (35% to 50%), intellectual impairment ranging from mild to severe (50% to 75%), and visual impairment (50%). Because standardized intelligence tests do not allow for the physical handicaps of cerebral palsy, the incidence of associated cognitive impairment is uncertain. Other associated complications include but are not limited to hearing impairment, communication disorders, respiratory problems, bowel and bladder problems, and orthopedic disabilities.[32]

EVALUATION AND TREATMENT   Diagnosis of cerebral palsy is made on the basis of neurologic examination and history. The management of children with cerebral palsy varies with age, type and severity of involvement, and associated disorders. Thus the scope of care required by the child and family includes social and educational intervention and a multidisciplinary team approach.

Although the brain injury is static, the clinical picture of cerebral palsy may change with growth and development. Therefore a fundamental component of an effective treatment regimen includes ongoing assessment, evaluation, and revision of the child's overall management plan. The use of intrathecal baclofen pumps and botulinum toxin has shown some improvement in selected children with cerebral palsy.[33,34] Family-focused interdisciplinary team management provides the best treatment outcomes.[35,36]

Inherited Metabolic Disorders of the Central Nervous System

A large number of inherited metabolic disorders have been identified. Because these disorders are inherited, their manifestations usually occur in infancy and childhood. Typically these metabolic disorders damage the entire CNS so extensively that these children do not survive to adulthood. The clinical syndromes of the inherited metabolic disorders depend on the nature of the biochemical defect and the stage of nervous system maturation. (Table 19-4 lists some of these inherited metabolic disorders.) Defects in amino acid and lipid metabolism are more common than rarely occurring defects in carbohydrate metabolism.

Defects in Amino Acid Metabolism

Biochemical defects in amino acid metabolism may be classified as (1) those in which the transport of amino acid is impaired, (2) those involving an enzyme or cofactor deficiency, and (3) those grouped around certain chemical components, such as sulfur-containing amino acids.[37] Most of the disorders in the literature described to date suggest that the absence of enzymatic activity most often is caused by the genetically determined absence of the enzyme protein.

Diseases caused by an enzymatic deficiency are associated with increased blood concentrations of the amino acid whose degradation pathway is impaired and with the presence of the amino acid in the urine. Because the normal pathway is blocked, small amounts of certain metabolites are found in the blood. Thus in certain diseases, an increase of compromised amino acids and unusual metabolites may appear in blood and urine concentrates.[38]

Phenylketonuria. Phenylketonuria (PKU) is an inborn error of metabolism characterized by the inability of the body to convert the essential amino acid phenylalanine to tyrosine (Figure 19-12). PKU is caused by phenylalanine hydroxylase deficiency and has a prevalence rate of 1 per 14,000 worldwide.[39] Because of its genetic component and distribution, this statistical prevalence varies widely on the basis of geographic and ethnic differences.[40] Most natural food proteins contain about 15% phenylalanine, an essential amino acid. Phenylalanine hydroxylase controls the conversion of this essential amino acid to tyrosine in the liver. The body uses tyrosine in the biosynthesis of protein, melanin, thyroxine, and the catecholamines in the brain and adrenal medulla. Phenylalanine hydroxylase deficiency causes an accumulation of phenylalanine in the serum and, subsequently, in the urinary excretion of abnormal metabolites called *phenyl acids*. One of these phenyl acids, phenylpyruvic acid, gives the urine a characteristic musty odor and is responsible for the name given to the disorder. Such high blood levels of phenylalanine prevent sufficient neutral amino acid entry into the brain, which contributes to the neuropathologic process of PKU.[41] Abnormalities occur, such as anomalous development of the CNS, defective myelination, cystic degeneration of the gray and white matter, and disturbances in cortical layers. Unfortunately, brain damage occurs before the metabolites can be detected in the urine, and damage continues as long as phenylalanine levels remain high.

Clinical manifestations related to CNS damage range from mild to severe behavioral disturbances, self-abusive tendencies, and seizures. Because of the lack of tyrosine and its relationship to the biosynthesis of melanin, children with PKU have a characteristic phenotype that includes blond hair, blue

Table 19-4	Inherited Metabolic Disorders of the Central Nervous System
Age of Onset	**Disorder**
Neonatal period	Pyridoxine dependency, galactosemia, maple syrup urine disease and its variant, phenylketonuria (PKU)
Early infancy	Tay-Sachs disease and its variants, infantile Gaucher disease, infantile Niemann-Pick disease, Krabbe disease (leukodystrophy), Farber lipogranulomatosis, Pelizaeus-Merzbacher disease and other sudanophilic leukodystrophies, spongy degeneration, Alexander disease, Alpers disease, Leigh disease (subacute necrotizing encephalomyelopathy), congenital lactic acidosis, Zellweger encephalopathy, Lowe disease (oculocerebrorenal disease)
Late infancy and early childhood	Disorders of amino acid metabolism, metachromatic leukodystrophy, late infantile GM1 gangliosidosis, late infantile Gaucher and Niemann-Pick diseases, neuroaxonal dystrophy, mucopolysaccharidosis, mucolipidosis, fucosidosis, mannosidosis, aspartylglycosaminuria, amaurotic idiocy (Jansky-Bielschowsky disease, Batten disease, Vogt-Spielmeyer disease, neuronal ceroid lipofuscinosis), Cockayne syndrome
Later childhood and adolescence	Progressive cerebellar ataxias of childhood and adolescence, hepatolenticular degeneration (Wilson disease), Hallervorden-Spatz disease, Lesch-Nyhan syndrome and other uremic states, familial calcification of vessels in basal ganglia and cerebellum, familial polymyoclonus, chronic familial leukodystrophy, homocystinuria, Fabry disease

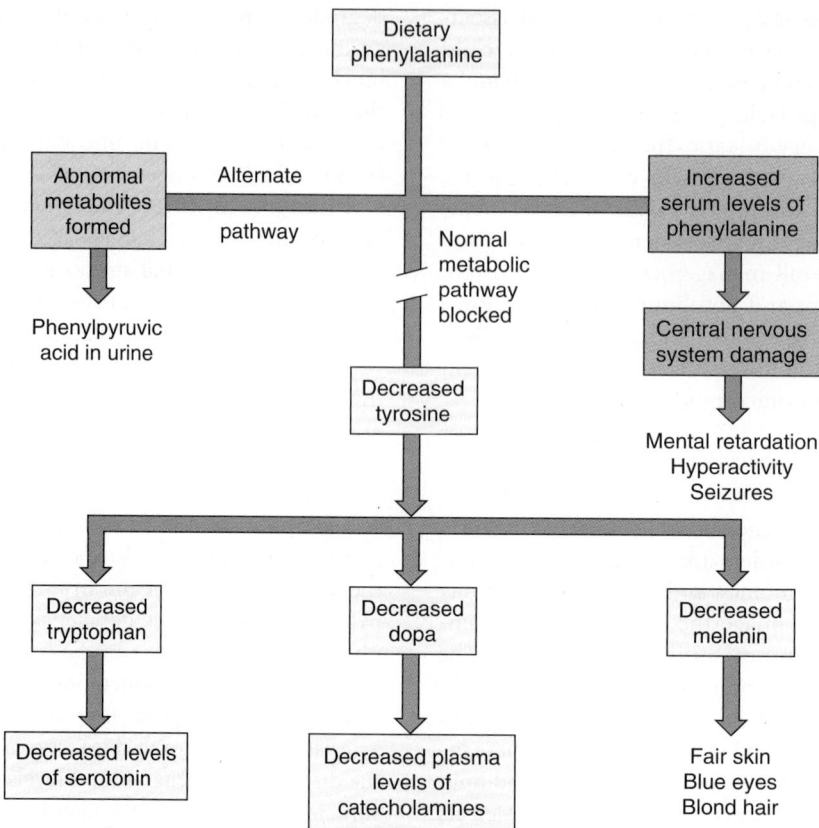

Figure 19-12 Metabolic errors and consequences in phenylketonuria. (Redrawn from Hockenberry MJ et al: *Wong's nursing care of infants and children*, ed 7, St Louis, 2003, Mosby.)

eyes, and fair skin. Children with genetically darker complexions may be red haired or brunette.

Less severe variants of this disorder are caused by defects in the phenylalanine hydroxylase system rather than the phenylalanine hydroxylase itself. This related disorder, known as **hyperphenylalaninemia (HPA),** occurs when plasma phenylalanine levels rise above normal but do not rise as high as in PKU.

Nonselective newborn screening is used to detect PKU and HPA in the United States and in more than 30 countries. Such programs are the greatest source of referrals and allow for accurate interpretation and follow-up of test results, including appropriate genetic and nutrition counseling.[40]

Treatment for PKU involves restriction of phenylalanine in the diet to maintain a nontoxic level. The diet must be supplemented with adequate sources of energy, protein, and nutrients to allow for optimum growth and brain development. Supplementation of tyrosine also may be required if plasma levels are low. The child benefits from ideal management that begins at birth and continues throughout the life span, especially before conception and throughout the mother's pregnancy.[42] Enzyme replacement and PKU gene therapy are both under investigation.[43,44]

Defects in Lipid Metabolism

Disorders of lipid metabolism are termed **lysosomal storage diseases** because each disorder in this group can be traced to a missing lysosomal enzyme. (Lysosomes, the vesicles within the cell whose primary function is to degrade the breakdown products of cellular metabolism, are discussed in Chapter 1.) An estimated 25 to 30 enzymes within the lysosomes participate in the breakdown of lipids, carbohydrates, proteins, and proteolipids (see Chapter 2). A genetic defect results in missing or defective enzyme and causes an excessive accumulation of a particular cell function. The enzyme defect may occur in the brain, liver, spleen, bone, or lung, thus involving several organ systems. Prenatal diagnosis is available. Therapy has been unsuccessful to date.

Tay-Sachs Disease. Perhaps the best known of the lysosomal storage disorders is **Tay-Sachs disease,** an autosomal recessive disorder.[45] Approximately 80% of individuals diagnosed are of Jewish ancestry, although sporadic cases appear in the non-Jewish population.[38]

In Tay-Sachs disease the pathologic changes predominate in the CNS, but neurons throughout the body contain characteristic changes in the cytoplasm. With time, neurons become distorted and balloon, and microglial cells, which also are swollen and filled with large granules, proliferate. Cystic degeneration of the cerebral white matter and atrophy of the cerebellar hemispheres often occur. The number of neurons is diminished. Changes in the spinal cord, particularly in the motor cells of the anterior horn of the cord, also are characteristic. Involvement of this region of the spinal cord results in hypotonia, hyporeflexia, and overall weakness.

Onset of this disease usually occurs when the infant is 3 to 6 months old. A loss of milestones is associated with an excessive startle response. Seizures, muscular rigidity, and blindness become prominent after the first year of life, and head size may increase. Death usually occurs by 2 to 5 years of age. No beneficial therapy has been developed. Genetic counseling programs are available, and some states require screening techniques for couples and those at risk who may be carriers. One in 25 Ashkenazi Jews carry this recessive gene.

Seizure Disorders in Children

Epilepsy

The incidence of epilepsy varies greatly with age. The incidence of epilepsy is estimated to be 0.5% to 1% of children with onset during infancy or childhood.[40] Infants are particularly susceptible during the first 12 months of life. The incidence decreases with age; 75% to 80% of epilepsy cases initially occur before 20 years of age, with 30% of the cases initially occurring within the first 4 years of life. Approximately 181,000 persons in the United States are newly affected each year.[46]

PATHOPHYSIOLOGY Seizures are the abnormal discharge of electrical activity within the brain. When a sufficient number of neurons become overexcited, they discharge abnormally, which sometimes results in clinical manifestations. If clinical manifestations do occur, the specific physical activity that occurs may depend on the origin of the electrical activity and its extent within the brain. Repeated recurrence of seizure activity is known as **epilepsy.** Seizures may result from an underlying disorder of the CNS or a disorder that directly or indirectly affects normal CNS function. Certain types of seizures may have a genetic component or familial predisposition, or they can result from maternal diseases or congenital structural anomalies of the CNS. During the newborn period, asphyxia, intracranial hemorrhage, CNS infections, injury, electrolyte imbalances, and inborn errors of metabolism may cause seizures. Etiologic factors of seizures in older infants and children generally are the same as during the first month of life. Often the cause of seizures is unknown.

Seizures and seizure patterns may change as a child grows and develops. The differences between the immature and mature nervous systems may help to explain the changing patterns of clinical seizures with age. The immature nervous system has a reduced capacity for sustaining well-organized seizures. Intracortical connections are poorly developed, and the sending of impulses throughout the cortex is limited. At the cellular level, neurons are less capable of firing in repetitive high-frequency bursts. The excitatory output of a seizure focus is further diminished because the affected neurons do not act synchronously. In addition, changing neurotransmitters, immaturity of cells, and ongoing postnatal factors affect seizure expression in children.

CLINICAL MANIFESTATIONS The clinical manifestations at the time of diagnosis vary depending on the primary cause and the extent and involvement of abnormal electrical discharges within the neuronal tissue. Because of the diversities and complexities that seizure activity invariably displays, an international classification system (see Table 16-9, p. 503) was adopted. This classification system groups seizures with similar clinical manifestations (see Table 16-11, p. 505). Its general purpose is to assist the clinician with the assessment of the clinical course, the identification of the most appropriate treatment, and the evaluation of the individual's response to treatment.

The international classification system of epilepsy contains three major groupings: (1) partial seizures, (2) generalized seizures, and (3) unclassified epileptic seizures. Each major grouping is then divided into subsets on the basis of clinical manifestations and electroencephalogram (EEG) findings.

Partial seizures are characterized by seizure activity that begins in and usually is limited to one part of either the left or right hemisphere. A *simple partial seizure* refers to seizure activity that occurs without loss of consciousness. A *complex partial seizure* refers to seizure activity that occurs with impairment of consciousness. The clinical activity displayed by the individual is contingent on the particular part of the cortex from which the seizure is generated. For example, partial seizures may result in abnormal motor activity, such as twitching or loss of tone, or sensory changes, such as tingling or numbness.

Simple partial seizures generally are confined to one hemisphere, whereas a complex partial seizure involves both cerebral hemispheres. A simple or complex partial seizure may evolve into a generalized tonic-clonic, tonic, or clonic convulsion.

Generalized seizures are those in which the first clinical manifestations indicate that the seizure activity starts in or involves both cerebral hemispheres. Consciousness may be impaired in this grouping of seizures. The clinical manifestations may include convulsive activity (tonic-tonic, tonic, or clonic activity) or nonconvulsive activity (absence seizures). Absence seizures do not follow a Mendelian pattern of inheritance that results from a single gene defect but, rather, have an autosomal dominant inheritance pattern.[47] Because both hemispheres are involved, the clinical manifestations almost always are bilateral.

Not all seizure disorders fit neatly into a classified grouping. These seizures are referred to as **unclassified epileptic seizures** and characteristically have a wide variety of abnormal clinical activity. Examples of this activity include rhythmic eye movements, chewing, and swimming movements. These activities are commonly seen in neonatal seizures.[48]

In addition to the seizures classified by the international system, there are several types of epileptic syndromes. These are seizure disorders that display a group of signs and symptoms that occur collectively and that characterize or indicate a particular condition. Several syndromes associated with epilepsy occur in infants and children. The three syndromes that occur most often are infantile spasms, Lennox-Gastaut syndrome, and juvenile myoclonic epilepsy.

Infantile spasms are a severe form of epilepsy characterized by a variety of clinical manifestations.[49] The infant may have episodes of sudden flexion or extension movements involving the neck, trunk, and extremities. Clinical manifestations of the resulting spasms may range from subtle head nods to violent body contractions, commonly referred to as *jackknife seizures*. Onset of infantile spasms usually is between 4 and 8 months of age and may be idiopathic or may occur in response to a CNS insult.[50] An EEG will display the classic hypsarrhythmic pattern of epileptic spike and wave discharges on a slow, disorganized background. Infantile spasm manifests a typical clinical course. The "spasms" usually happen in clusters and occur 5 to 150 times per day. They usually are worse when the infant is waking up or falling asleep. Once begun, the seizure activity increases in intensity and severity over time. Invariably a loss of developmental milestones and disability is associated with this syndrome. Infantile spasms are also common (30%) in those with **tuberous sclerosis complex (TSC)**.[51] TSC develops from mutations in hamartin and tuberin genes. *Tubers* are cortical developmental malformations in the brain; they also form in other organs.[51] Epilepsy associated with TSC is often difficult to treat and requires surgical intervention.[52]

Lennox-Gastaut syndrome is an epileptic syndrome characterized by an onset of seizures early in childhood, usually in males and around 1 to 5 years of age. This syndrome includes a variety of generalized seizures—predominantly tonic-clonic, atonic (drop attacks), akinetic, absence, and myoclonic activity. Mental retardation, delayed psychomotor development, and personality disorders often are associated with this syndrome.[53]

Juvenile myoclonic epilepsy is a primary generalized epilepsy that usually affects adolescents and young adults. Studies have indicated a possible locus on chromosome 6p and 15q14 as a cause for this type of epilepsy.[54] It is a relatively benign form of epilepsy involving myoclonic jerks of the neck, shoulders, and arms. The seizures may occur singularly or repetitively. This form of epilepsy commonly is associated with a normal neurologic examination, normal intelligence, and a positive family history of seizures and is often underdiagnosed.[55]

EVALUATION AND TREATMENT Diagnosis of epilepsy and seizure classification are based on history, clinical presentation, physical and developmental examination, and the record of milestone achievements. Evaluation and testing include an EEG to isolate the focus or origin and involvement of seizure activity, CT scan, and/or MRI of the brain to investigate the presence of a lesion or abnormal tissue. A complete metabolic workup must be reviewed to explore the possibility of deficiency or malabsorption.

Specific treatment for epilepsy is directed at the particular clinical manifestations or syndrome of seizure activity and its underlying causes. Treatment usually begins with the use of anticonvulsant medications. Often the epileptic pattern and clinical course require more than one drug to control the ab-

NUTRITION & DISEASE

Ketogenic Diet in Children With Epilepsy

The goal of the ketogenic diet in some children with epilepsy is to create and maintain a state of ketosis, which appears to facilitate reduced seizure activity, particularly for epilepsy that is refractory to medical treatment. The diet may be helpful to children who do not respond to conventional therapy or have intolerable side effects. The two basic approaches to the ketogenic diet are (1) a traditional approach with four parts fat to one part carbohydrate/protein in the diet and (2) the medium-chain triglyceride (MCT) approach, in which MCTs make up about 50% to 70% of the diet. Either diet may be unpalatable and difficult to follow, particularly if the child has free access to food. Carbohydrates can be added by 5-g increments after 3 to 6 months if there has been no seizure activity, provided ketosis is maintained. Both dietary approaches include adequate protein for growth. The mechanism is not clearly understood, but it may be caused by a change in neuronal metabolism in which a ketone body behaves as an inhibitory neurotransmitter, producing an anticonvulsant effect on the body. The benefits of the diet usually last less than 2 to 3 years and appear to be less effective with older children.

Data from Katyal NG et al: T Clin Pediatr (Phil) 39(3):153-159, 2000; Lefevre F, Aronson N: Pediatrics 105(4):E46, 2000; Vaisleib II, Buchhalter JR, Zupanc, ML: Pediatr Neurol 31(3):198-202, 2004.

normal discharges.[48] A ketonic diet may be effective as a supplement treatment for epilepsy that is difficult to control with drugs[56,57] (see Nutrition & Disease box).

Surgery provides treatment for some forms of epilepsy that cannot be controlled with drugs. As with medical interventions, surgical therapy focuses on the particular clinical manifestations of seizure activity. Surgical interventions include resection of the epileptogenic zone of brain tissue (i.e., the temporal lobe for partial seizures or partial or complete severing of the corpus callosum for intractable generalized epilepsy).[58-60] Children with intractable epilepsy have benefited somewhat from using the vagal nerve stimulator.[61]

Prognosis for epilepsy depends greatly on the type and severity of the disorder, the age of onset, coexisting factors, and the type and success of medical, surgical, and nutritional therapy. Several studies have estimated that approximately 40% to 50% of children diagnosed with epilepsy eventually will be seizure free.

Benign Febrile Seizures

Benign febrile seizures occur in 3% to 4% of children younger than 5 years. These seizures usually are brief and self-limited and occur most often between the ages of 6 months and 5 years, with peak age at 14 to 18 months.[5,62]

PATHOPHYSIOLOGY The pathogenesis of benign febrile seizures is unknown. A familial incidence of benign febrile seizures indicates a genetic predisposition to the problem. Factors that contribute to susceptibility include age, degree and rate of temperature elevation, and nature of the particular fever-inducing illness. Any disorder producing a high fever may provoke benign febrile seizures in susceptible children.[63]

CLINICAL MANIFESTATIONS   Characteristic features distinguish benign febrile seizures from seizures precipitated by fever:

1. Benign febrile seizures are rare before 9 months or after 5 years of age.
2. The convulsion occurs with a rise in temperature greater than 39° C.
3. An acute respiratory or ear infection usually is present, with no evidence of CNS infection or inflammation.
4. Most seizures occur during the first 24 hours of the illness.
5. The convulsion is short (15 minutes or less), generalized, and predominantly tonic.
6. Interictal electroencephalogram (EEG) is normal.
7. The seizure usually does not recur during the same infection.
8. No acute systemic metabolic disorder is present.

Complex febrile seizures have characteristic features similar to these, except that (1) they have a longer duration than do benign febrile seizures, usually longer than 15 minutes; (2) they have focal characteristics; and (3) they usually occur more than once in a 24-hour period. Complex febrile seizures are considered a risk factor for the development of epilepsy.[64]

EVALUATION AND TREATMENT   Reduction of elevated body temperature usually controls benign febrile seizures without anticonvulsant medication. In selected individuals, phenobarbital is the most effective medication for preventing recurrence of benign febrile seizures.

Status Epilepticus

Status epilepticus is defined as the state of continuing or recurring seizure activity in which the recovery from seizure activity is incomplete. Seizure activity is unrelenting and usually lasts for 30 minutes or more. Any one of the seizure activities discussed can evolve into status epilepticus. Status epilepticus is a medical emergency that requires immediate intervention.

Acute Encephalopathies
Reye Syndrome

Reye syndrome is characterized by encephalopathy and fatty changes in a variety of organs, especially the liver. The incidence of Reye syndrome has declined sharply over the past 20 years, coinciding with increased public awareness of the association between ingestion of aspirin during illness and subsequent development of Reye syndrome.[65] Although Reye syndrome is becoming increasingly rare in the population, a brief overview of it is important for the following reasons:

1. It may be considered a prototype for acute hepatic encephalopathies.
2. The potential for recurrence is a factor.
3. The use of acetaminophen over aspirin should be considered important and discussed with the parents when obtaining a history.

PATHOPHYSIOLOGY   Reye syndrome usually is associated with influenza B or varicella virus infections in children who have taken aspirin or aspirin-containing products. A distinct clinical syndrome is apparent. The profound hypoglycemia, hyperammonemia, and an increase in short-chain fatty acids in the serum after liver involvement are responsible for the cerebral manifestations. The liver shows diffuse deposits of lipids and absence of any inflammatory reaction or necrosis. Fatty degeneration of the kidneys leads to azotemia (excess urea in the blood). The brain is extremely edematous.[66,67]

The cause and pathogenesis of Reye syndrome remain unclear. The development of Reye syndrome has been linked to the administration of salicylates (aspirin). The American Association of Pediatrics has recommended not administering aspirin to children who have varicella or flulike symptoms. A direct relationship clearly exists between this recommendation and the overall decrease in incidence of Reye syndrome. A further reduction has occurred with administration of the varicella vaccine to children between 12 to 18 months of age.[68]

CLINICAL MANIFESTATIONS   Typically Reye syndrome develops in a previously healthy child who is recovering from varicella, influenza B, or upper respiratory infection, or gastroenteritis. The various clinical states are as follows:

Stage I—Vomiting, lethargy, drowsiness

Stage II—Disorientation, delirium, aggressiveness and combativeness, central neurologic hyperventilation, shallow breathing, hyperactive reflexes, stupor

Stage III—Obtundation, coma, hyperventilation, decorticate rigidity

Stage IV?—Deepening coma, decerebrate rigidity, loss of ocular reflexes, large fixed pupils, divergent eye movements

Stage V?—Seizures, loss of deep tendon reflexes, flaccidity, respiratory arrest

EVALUATION AND TREATMENT   According to the Centers for Disease Control and Prevention (CDC), the following conditions must be present for diagnosis of Reye syndrome:

1. Acute, noninflammatory encephalopathy documented by (a) alteration in level of consciousness and, if available, (b) a record of CSF containing leukocytes ($8/mm^3$) and (c) a histologic specimen demonstrating cerebral edema without perivascular or meningeal irritation
2. Hepatomegaly documented by either a liver biopsy or autopsy
3. No more reasonable explanation for cerebral and hepatic abnormalities

The severity of the condition is inversely related to the age of the child at the onset of the illness.

The management of children with Reye syndrome ranges from simple monitoring to extremely complex neurointensive care. Treatment and outcome vary depending on the stage of involvement and the individual child's symptoms.

Box 19-2	Common Poisons	
Pharmacologic Agents	**Heavy Metals**	**Miscellaneous Agents**
Acetaminophen	Lead	Botulinum toxin
Amphetamines	Acute	Alcohols
Anticonvulsants	Chronic	Ethyl, isopropyl,
Antidepressants	Mercury	methyl
Antihistamines	Thallium	Pesticides
Atropine	Arsenic	Organophosphates
Barbiturates		Chlorinated
Methadone		hydrocarbons
Phencyclidine		Mushrooms
Salicylates		Venoms
Tranquilizers		Snake bite
		Tick paralysis
		Ethylene glycol

Data from Swaiman KF, Ashwal S: *Pediatric neurology: principles and practice,* vol 2, ed 3, St Louis, 1999, Mosby.

Intoxications of the Central Nervous System

Drug-induced encephalopathies always must be considered a possibility in the child with unexplained neurologic changes. Such encephalopathies may result from accidental ingestion, therapeutic overdose, intentional overdose, or ingestion of environmental toxins (the most commonly ingested poisons are listed in Box 19-2). About 2 million childhood poisonings that require medical attention occur each year. Approximately 1000 children die each year of poisonings.

High blood levels of lead occur in lead poisoning. If lead poisoning is not treated, lead encephalopathy will result and cause serious and irreversible neurologic damage[69,70] (Figure 19-13). Those at greatest risk are children 2 to 3 years of age and those prone to picas and living in lead-contaminated environments. **Pica** is the habitual, purposeful, and compulsive ingestion of nonfood substances such as clay, dirt, and paint chips. Lead intoxication also may occur from long-term exposure to smelters, sniffing of gasoline, and ingestion of airborne lead.[71]

An estimated 225,000 children in the United States and 4% of children 6 months to 5 years of age have excessive amounts of lead in their blood. Black children have a six times greater incidence of symptoms than white children. Most lead exposure is preventable.[72]

Meningitis

Meningitis refers to inflammation of the meningeal coverings of the brain. The origin of such inflammation and acute encephalopathy can be bacterial or viral.

Bacterial Meningitis

Bacterial meningitis is one of the most serious infections to which infants and children are susceptible.[73] In the United States there are approximately 6000 cases per year of bacterial meningitis, of which half occur in children younger than 18 years of age. The microorganisms accountable for this illness are *Streptococcus pneumoniae* (1.1 per 100,000) and

Haemophilus influenza type B (0.2 per 100,000), especially in children beyond the neonatal period.

Haemophilus influenza type B was once the most common pathogen of bacterial meningitis in children younger than 5 years old. The occurrence has dropped 95% with the advent of the Hib vaccine. Otitis media or sinusitis may be a precursor because the infections are almost always associated with a bacterium in the blood.

The most common microorganism causing bacterial meningitis is *Neisseria meningitidis* (meningococcus).[74] Approximately 2% to 5% of healthy children are carriers of *N. meningitidis*. The risk of meningitis in day-care center contacts of children with meningococcal disease is 1 per 1000.[75] During epidemics among military personnel, nasal and oral secretions from as many as 90% of those examined reveal *N. meningitidis*, suggesting a high rate of infectious transmission.

The third microorganism is *Streptococcus pneumoniae*, which is likely to be found in children older than 4 years. Staphylococcal or streptococcal meningitis can occur in children of any age but shows a predilection for children who have had neurosurgery, skull fracture, or a complication of systemic bacterial infection. Infections that originate in the middle ear, sinuses, or mastoid cells also may lead to *S. pneumoniae* infection in children. In addition, this microorganism tends to occur in children with sickle cell disease or splenectomy. One in every 24 children with sickle cell disease develops pneumococcal meningitis by the age of 4 years. This incidence is 36 times greater than that found in the black population without sickle cell disease and 314 times greater than in white children. *Escherichia coli* and group B β-hemolytic streptococci are the most common causes of meningitis in the newborn period.

PATHOPHYSIOLOGY The cause of bacterial meningitis is related to the age of the child and to a number of factors that predispose the child to bacterial infection or that alter the child's response to an invading microorganism. Any microorganism may be pathogenic under the appropriate circumstances in a given individual.

During the first 2 months of life, the causative microorganisms are those that reflect the maternal flora or the environment in which the infant has been placed (e.g., gram-negative intestinal bacilli and group B streptococci). Most bacterial meningitis in children 2 months to 12 years of age is caused by *H. influenzae* type B, *S. pneumoniae*, or *N. meningitidis*. In children older than 12 years, meningitis usually is caused by *S. pneumoniae* or *N. meningitidis*. When the child's response has been compromised or when anatomic defects are present, other microorganisms may be responsible, including *Pseudomonas*, staphylococci, salmonellae, and *Serratia*.

Meningitis may follow bacterial infections of the paranasal sinuses or mastoid cells. Bacterial meningitis in children with otitis media generally follows bacteremia. Direct invasion of the meninges is rare. Infection may spread through the blood to the meninges in children with infective endocarditis, pneumonia, or thrombophlebitis.

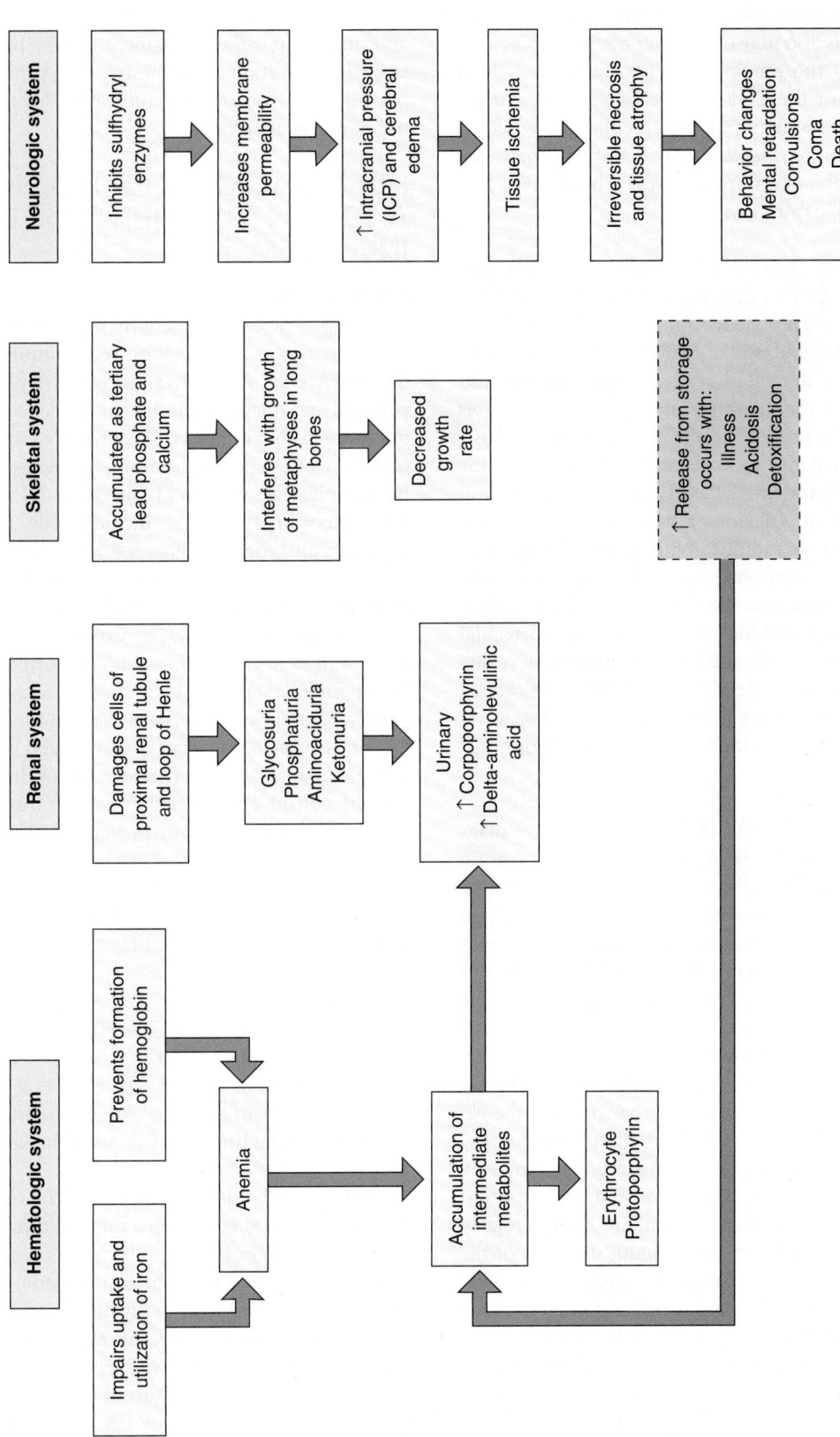

Figure 19-13 Systemic effects of increased lead absorption in children.

Direct invasion of the CNS occurs with fracture of the paranasal sinus, dermoid sinus tracts, or myelomeningoceles if direct communication occurs between the skin and meninges. Meningitis also may occur after neurosurgical procedures, particularly those involving CSF diversion such as shunting. Infection of the CNS may be caused by environmental contamination or manipulation. Meningitis caused by *Staphylococcus aureus* or *Pseudomonas aeruginosa* may develop in the child with cystic fibrosis or severe burns. (For further discussion, see Chapter 17.)

CLINICAL MANIFESTATIONS   Acute bacterial meningitis often is preceded by an upper respiratory or a gastrointestinal infection. Fever, headache, vomiting, irritability, photophobia, and nuchal and spinal rigidity develop and can progress rapidly to a decreased level of consciousness and seizures. Irritation of the meninges and spinal roots causes pain and resistance to neck flexion (nuchal rigidity), a positive Kernig sign (resistance to knee extension in the supine position with the hips and knees flexed against the body), and a positive Brudzinski sign (flexion of the knees and hips when the neck is flexed forward rapidly). With severe meningeal irritation the child may demonstrate opisthotonic posturing (rigid arching of the back with the head extended). Meningococcal meningitis can produce a characteristic petechial rash.[76] IICP is caused by cerebral edema and may be increased further by obstruction to the CSF circulation. Thickened meninges and fibrous exudate in the subarachnoid space at the base of the brain obstruct the CSF, resulting in communicating hydrocephalus.

EVALUATION AND TREATMENT   A definitive diagnosis is made only by examination of CSF obtained from a lumbar puncture. The principles of treatment are similar to those followed for adults (see Chapter 17) and are based on the culture results in which the causative microorganisms is identified. The conjugate vaccines against *H. influenzae* and *N. meningitidis* (serogroups A, C Y, and W-135) decrease the rate and spread of this disease.[76] Vaccines for serogroup B *N. meningitidis* are not yet available.[77]

The factors that influence outcomes are the age of the child (mortality is highest in infants younger than 1 year), the infective microorganisms (the lowest mortality is in meningococcal meningitis and the highest in meningitis caused by gram-negative enteric microorganisms), and the duration and extent of inflammation before treatment. Approximately 8% of children with *H. influenzae* meningitis die; 35% of the survivors have serious and permanent sensory or motor dysfunction caused by pressure on the peripheral nerves during the early phases of the illness. Approximately 5% of the children who survive meningitis have hearing deficits; 10% to 15% have cerebral damage, hydrocephalus, motor deficits, or sensory impairments.[78]

Viral Meningitis

The hallmark of viral meningitis, or aseptic meningitis, is a mononuclear response in the CSF and the presence of normal blood glucose level. In some cases the findings with aseptic meningitis are consistent with bacterial meningitis. The clinical manifestations are similar to those in bacterial meningitis, although usually milder. Isolation of the virus is difficult and often impossible. Treatment usually begins with aggressive administration of antibiotics (potential bacterial meningitis) until the diagnosis is confirmed. Treatment may include use of antiviral agents.

HUMAN IMMUNODEFICIENCY VIRUS AND CENTRAL NERVOUS SYSTEM INVOLVEMENT

The human immunodeficiency virus (HIV) subjects the body to multiple, repeated infections. The end stage of this infectious process is called **acquired immunodeficiency syndrome (AIDS)**. Through a process of replication, HIV perpetuates and integrates itself into the genetic materials of the microorganisms it infects. The primary pathologic condition of HIV causes specific immunodeficiency that destroys the host's ability to withstand infection. HIV directly invades most major organ systems, including the CNS.[79,80] (HIV and AIDS are discussed in Chapter 8.)

Infants and children have become infected with HIV through a variety of sources. Transmission may occur perinatally through the placenta, by exposure to infected maternal blood and vaginal secretions, and by postpartum ingestion of breast milk.[81] Perinatal transmission accounts for approximately 90% of pediatric AIDS cases in the United States. Infection also can occur from contaminated blood products, although new safeguards with blood products have lessened this risk considerably over the past few years.

The actual incidence of pediatric HIV is not known because no national statistics have been compiled. The CDC estimates that through 2003, 9348 children under the age of 13 years in the United States had HIV with 5406 resulting deaths. Worldwide in 2003, an estimated 2.2 million children acquired HIV.[82,83,93a]

PATHOPHYSIOLOGY   The HIV infects T lymphocytes, in particular the CD4 T cells. The virus replicates itself, rendering the CD4 cell nonfunctional. The child is at great risk because the immune system is still developing and therefore has little or no ability to fight this virus (discussed in Chapter 8).

CLINICAL MANIFESTATIONS   The clinical diagnosis of HIV in children is very often a difficult task. The CDC revised the classification in 1994 for HIV infection in children younger than 13 years (Box 19-3). The HIV infection may be identified by viral culture of blood or tissue, and the diagnosis is confirmed by the presence of specific antibodies to the virus. However, the presence of passive maternal antibody limits the use of HIV antibody testing in infants in the high-risk category up to 15 months of age. Therefore two definitions of infection in children are necessary: one for prenatally exposed infants up to 15 months of age and one for older children.[84]

HIV affects all body systems. Therefore the clinical manifestations vary greatly from child to child. The initial signs and symp-

Box 19-3	Pediatric Human Immunodeficiency Virus (HIV) Classification			
Immunologic Categories	N: No Signs/Symptoms	A: Mild Signs/Symptoms	B: Moderate Signs/Symptoms	C: Severe Signs/Symptoms
1. No evidence	N1	A1	B1	C1
2. Evidence of moderate suppression	N2	A2	B2	C2
3. Severe suppression	N3	A3	B3	C3

Clinical Categories for Children With HIV Infection

Category N: Not symptomatic
   Children who have no signs or symptoms considered to be the result of HIV infection or who have only one of the conditions listed in Category A

Category A: Mildly symptomatic
   Children with two or more of the conditions listed below but none of the conditions listed in Categories B or C:
      Lymphadenopathy
      Hepatomegaly
      Splenomegaly
      Dermatitis
      Parotitis
      Recurrent or persistent upper respiratory infection, sinusitis, or otitis media

Category B: Moderately symptomatic
   Children who have symptomatic conditions other than those listed for Category A or C that are attributed to HIV infection; examples of conditions in clinical Category B include but are not limited to:
      Anemia ($\leq$8 g/dl), neutropenia ($\leq$1000mm^3), or thrombocytopenia ($\leq$100,000mm^3) persisting $\geq$30 days
      Bacterial meningitis, pneumonia, or sepsis (single episode)
      Candidiasis or oropharyngeal (thrush) persisting ($\geq$2 months) in children $\geq$6 months of age
      Cardiomyopathy
      Cytomegalovirus infection with onset before 1 month of age
      Diarrhea, recurrent or chronic
      Hepatitis
      Herpes simplex virus (HSV), somatitis, recurrent (more than 2 episodes within 1 year)
      HSV bronchitis, pneumonitis, or esophagitis with onset before 1 month of age
      Herpes zoster (shingles) involving at least two distinct episodes or more than 1 dermatone
      Lieomyosarcoma
      Lymphoid interstitial pneumonia (LIP) or pulmonary lymphoid hyperplasia complex
      Neuropathy
      Nocardiosis
      Persistent fever (lasting $\geq$1 month)
      Toxoplasmosis, onset before 1 month of age
      Varicella, disseminated (complicated chickenpox)

Category C: Severely symptomatic
   Children who have any condition listed in the 1987 surveillance case definition of acquired immunodeficiency with the exception of LIP.

Data from Centers for Disease Control and Prevention: 1994 revised classification system for human immunodeficiency virus infection in children less than 13 years of age, *MMWR* 43(12):1, 1994.

toms may be nonspecific and subtle, and they may progress slowly or rapidly to an acute, life-threatening condition.

A particularly vulnerable site of HIV infection in infants and children is the CNS. HIV encephalopathy is more common in the advanced stages.[85,86] Since survival of children with HIV has been prolonged with effective treatment, the incidence of progressive encephalopathy has increased.[87] The 1994 classification from the CDC requires one of the following progressing findings to be present for at least 2 months,[88] in the absence of a concurrent illness other than HIV that could explain the findings:

1. Failure to attain or loss of developmental milestones, or loss of intellectual ability, verified by standard developmental scale or neuropsychologic tests
2. Impaired brain growth or acquired microcephaly demonstrated by head circumference measurements or brain atrophy demonstrated by CT or MRI with serial imaging required in children less than 2 years of age
3. Acquired symmetric motor deficits manifested by affecting a child 1 month of age or older

The onset of progressive encephalopathy may be a prognostic indicator of a poor outcome.

It may be difficult to completely differentiate the impact of HIV infection on the CNS from the impact of prenatal and perinatal exposure. In addition, other insults may accompany HIV in a young child and affect growth and development, such as drug exposure, prematurity, chronic illness, and a chaotic social atmosphere.[79,84] The pathogenesis of HIV encephalopathy in children is poorly understood, but the presence of inflammatory mediators may be a contributing factor.[89]

EVALUATION AND TREATMENT A definite diagnosis of HIV is made by patient history, viral culture, and clinical manifestations. Monitoring CD8(+) T lymphocytes and monocytes, in addition to CD4(+) T lymphocytes, has been suggested for predicting risk for progressive encephalopathy. Decreases in CD8(+) T lymphocytes diminish defenses against viral infection and facilitate infected monocytes to cross the blood-brain barrier.[87] A growing number of investigational protocols are available for treatment of children with HIV. In general, treatment is focused on the preservation and maintenance of the immune system, aggressive response to opportunistic infections, and support and relief of symptomatic occurrences and administration of highly active antiretroviral therapy (HAART).[90,91] (HIV treatment is discussed in Chapter 8.)

Acquired immunodeficiency syndrome (AIDS) was the seventh most common cause of death in children 1 to 4 years of age in 2002.[92] In 1994 the United States Public Health Service (PHS) encouraged the use of Zidovudine to reduce perinatal HIV transmission. The following year (1995), the PHS published guidelines for universal, routine HIV counseling and voluntary HIV testing of pregnant women. This has resulted in a decrease in perinatal HIV transmission.[93] Outcome may depend on the child's age at diagnosis and subsequent onset of symptoms and complications of AIDS.

CEREBROVASCULAR DISEASE IN CHILDREN

Cerebrovascular disease in children differs from that in adults in three ways:

1. An absence of predisposing factors, such as high blood pressure and arteriosclerosis
2. Significant differences in the clinical response related to the developing nervous system and thus a greater capacity for the pediatric brain to recover from vascular insult
3. The anatomic site of the pathologic condition

Cerebrovascular disease can be divided into two categories: occlusive and hemorrhagic.

Occlusive Cerebrovascular Disease

Occlusive cerebrovascular disease may result from embolism, sinovenous thrombosis, or congenital or iatrogenic narrowing of vessels, which leads to a decreased flow of blood and oxygen to areas of the brain. Sickle cell disease and cardiac anomalies are the most common disorders that lead to complications of cerebral occlusion.[94]

Moyamoya disease is a rare, chronic, progressive vascular disease that results in the progressive stenosis of arterial flow to the brain. Moyamoya, a Japanese term, means "puff of smoke," which describes its appearance on CT examination. The vascularity may be a congenital anomaly, or it can develop as a result of cranial radiation therapy. Complications are developmental delay and mental retardation.[95] Treatment is surgical bypass of the occluded region. Regardless of the

cause, failure of blood flow to the brain results in an ischemic stroke. Strokes are relatively rare in the pediatric population, with an incidence of approximately 0.63 per 100,000 annually in the United States.

Hemorrhagic Cerebrovascular Disease

PATHOPHYSIOLOGY Congenital arteriovenous malformations are the most common cause of intracranial bleeding and hemorrhagic stroke in children.[96] Hemorrhagic disease may result from vascular anomalies that lead to rupture, such as aneurysm, or from congenital arteriovenous malformation. The rupture and symptomatic development of a cerebral aneurysm are rare in children younger than 19 years. Treatment is surgical repair of the weakened vessel and does not differ from that for the adult population (see Chapter 17).

CLINICAL MANIFESTATIONS The extent of the pathologic condition usually is less extensive in children than in adults. Symptoms may include degrees of hemiplegia (flaccid, spastic), weakness, seizures, high fever, nuchal rigidity, hemianopia, sensory changes, facial palsy, and temporary aphasia.

EVALUATION AND TREATMENT Diagnosis of cerebrovascular disease is made through a series of tests, including CT, MRI, magnetic resonance angiogram (MRA), angiogram, and echocardiogram.[97] History of evolving symptoms and past medical history are of vital importance in attaining an accurate diagnosis. Causative factors in the change in vascular flow often are not determined. Malformations vary in size, location, and symptoms, and these factors determine treatment. Options include surgery, radiation therapy, and occlusion of the malformation (see Chapter 17).

Excellent collateral circulation in the child's brain allows for more rapid recovery of motor function. The developing brain, however, may suffer more global, long-term effects, leading to mental retardation, behavior disorders, and seizures.

CHILDHOOD TUMORS

Brain Tumors

Brain tumors are the most common solid tumor and the second most common primary neoplasm in children, second only to leukemia. Approximately 50% of solid tumors in children are nonmalignant.[98] Overall, brain tumors account for nearly 20% of all childhood cancers, with an annual incidence of 2.4 to 4 per 100,000 in the United States; approximately 2000 cases are diagnosed each year.[99] Brain tumors remain the leading cause of death from disease in children ages 1 to 15 years.[100]

The cause of brain tumors is largely unknown, although genetic, environmental, and immune factors have been implicated in some tumor development. Other considerations and factors that have been investigated in the cause of brain tumors include familial tendencies, radiation, oncologic viruses, and chemical carcinogens.[101] An important area of study has been the relationship of parental occupation to subsequent brain tumors in offspring. Associations have been found with tumors and parental employment, for example, parental exposure to hydrocarbons and employment in the aircraft and paper/pulp industries. Alterations in embryologic development also may play a part in the development of childhood brain tumors. This theory suggests that tumors arise from cells that are "misplaced" during embryonic development, never maturing but later proliferating in this immature form. Chromosomal work has implicated the deletion of chromosomes 22 and 17 in some pediatric brain tumors. Further studies are being conducted that may affect the course of treatment for these children.[102] None of these factors, however, has proved significant.

PATHOPHYSIOLOGY Most childhood brain tumors arise from glial tissue, the supportive tissue of the brain. Tumors also may originate in other tissue such as nerve cells, cranial nerves, the pineal and pituitary glands, blood vessels, or neuroepithelium. Brain tumors are classified by the tissue and location from which they arise. Because a uniform pathologic nomenclature has yet to be established, inconsistencies occur when statistical data are compared.

Two thirds of all pediatric brain tumors are found in the posterior fossa region of the brain. This area also may be referred to as *infratentorial* because it is located below the ten-

torium. The tentorium is the layer of dura mater that separates the cerebellum from the cortex or cerebrum. Thus the area above the tentorium is referred to as the *supratentorial region*. Approximately one third of childhood brain tumors are located in the supratentorial space. On the other hand, in the adult population two thirds of brain tumors are located in the supratentorial region and only one third in the infratentorial region. The types and characteristics of childhood brain tumors are summarized in Table 19-5.

Brain tumors, by virtue of their location, have unique characteristics that distinguish them from tumors found elsewhere in the body. A number of brain tumors in children may be considered histologically benign yet clinically malignant and life threatening because of their location. For example, a tumor located in the brain stem region may appear benign under the microscope, but the clinical presentation threatens and all too often overrides the vital functions of the brain stem.

Types

Medulloblastoma, ependymoma, astrocytoma, brain stem glioma, craniopharyngioma, and optic nerve glioma make up approximately 75% to 80% of all pediatric brain tumors.[103] The location of brain tumors in children is illustrated in Figure 19-14; specific characteristics, treatment strategies, and prognoses are listed in Tables 19-5 and 19-6.

Table 19-5	Treatment Strategies for Childhood Brain Tumors
Tumor Type	**Treatment and Prognosis**
Cerebellar astrocytoma	Surgery; possibly curative
	Radiation and chemotherapy not proved successful but may delay recurrence
	Survival rate of more than 5 years in 50%-75%; if tumor recurs, it does so very slowly
Medulloblastoma	Surgery, primarily as a partial resection to relieve increased intracranial pressure and "debulk" the tumor
	Type of treatment is age dependent
	Radiation as the primary treatment; may include spinal radiation
	Chemotherapy showing some promise in conjunction with craniospinal radiation
	35% 5-year survival rate
Brain stem glioma	Surgery, resection occasionally possible
	Radiation, primarily palliative treatment
	Chemotherapy not yet proved beneficial, but new protocols being studied
	20% to 40% 5-year survival rate dependent upon total resection
Ependymoma	Tumor possibly indolent for many years
	Surgery rarely curative; risk of resecting an infratentorial tumor too great
	Radiation for palliation (current controversy regarding whether local or craniospinal radiation is best)
	Chemotherapy used for recurrent disease but with disappointing results
	20%-80% 5-year survival rate dependent upon total resection
Craniopharyngioma	Surgery possibly successful when a complete resection is performed (partial resection usually requires further treatment)
	Radiation after partial surgical resection
	Chemotherapy not commonly used
	75% to 85% 5-year survival rate
Optic nerve glioma	Initial treatment controversial
	Surgery used for diagnosis or relief of hydrocephalus
	Radiation useful, particularly if the tumor is not treated by surgery
Cerebral astrocytoma	Surgery used if resection is possible
	Radiation useful for all grades of astrocytoma
	Chemotherapy beneficial in higher-grade tumors, but further study required

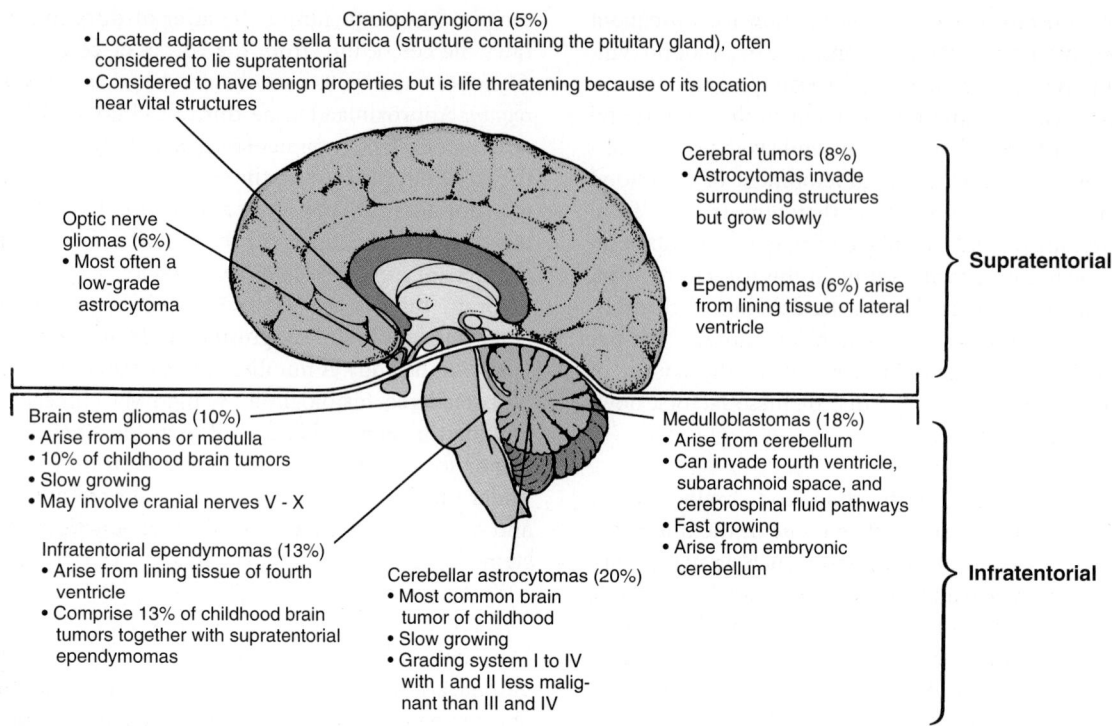

Figure 19-14 Location of brain tumors in children.

Table 19-6	Brain Tumors in Children
Type	Characteristics
Astrocytoma	Arises from astrocytes, often in the cerebellum or lateral hemisphere
	Slow growing, solid or cystic
	Often very large before diagnosed
	Varies in degree of malignancy
Optic nerve glioma	Arises from optic chiasm or optic nerve
	Slow-growing, low-grade astrocytoma
Medulloblastoma (infiltrating glioma)	Often located in cerebellum, extending into fourth ventricle and spinal fluid pathway
	Rapidly growing malignant tumor
	Can extend outside of central nervous system
Brain stem glioma	Arises from pons or myeloencephalon
	Numerous cell types
	Compresses cranial nerves V through X
Ependymoma	Arises from ependymal cells lining ventricles
	Circumscribed, solid, nodular tumors
Craniopharyngioma	Arises near pituitary gland, optic, chiasm, and hypothalamus
	Cystic and solid tumors that affect vision, pituitary, and hypothalamic functions

CLINICAL MANIFESTATIONS The actual location of the brain tumor dictates the presenting signs and symptoms (discussed in greater detail with each particular brain tumor type). In addition to tumor location and cell type, the rate of growth of the tumor also determines the presenting signs and symptoms. The ability of the brain and intracranial cavity to compensate for tumor growth is directly related to the rate of its growth. This compensatory mechanism allows the components of the intracranial space (blood, brain, and CSF) to adapt temporarily to slow changes in ICP. Therefore slow-growing tumors can grow to enormous size before signs and symptoms are apparent. Conversely, fast-growing tumors al-

low little time for compensation of the space-occupying lesion, and clinical symptoms occur quickly.

Signs and symptoms of brain tumors in children vary from generalized and vague to those that are localized and related specifically to the anatomic area. If the tumor is located in the posterior fossa region, the fourth ventricle may become blocked, which leads to hydrocephalus and signs of IICP. IICP also may occur because of the additional mass volume within the fixed container of the skull vault. The symptoms of IICP include headache, vomiting, lethargy, and irritability. If a young child complains of a headache, a thorough investigation should take place because headache is an uncommon complaint in young children. Headache caused by IICP usually is worse in the morning and gradually improves during the day when the child is upright and venous drainage is enhanced. Frequency of headache and other symptoms worsens as the tumor grows. A headache related to IICP generally occurs because of expansion of the lateral ventricle and cerebral hemisphere, which causes a stretching of the pain-sensitive dura mater. Irritability or possible apathy and increased somnolence also may result from IICP. Like headache, vomiting occurs more commonly in the morning. It frequently is not preceded by nausea and may become projectile, differing from a gastrointestinal disturbance in that the child may be ready to eat immediately after vomiting. Other signs and symptoms that can accompany IICP include increased head circumference with bulging fontanelle in children younger than 2 years of age, cranial nerve palsies, and papilledema.

Localized findings relate to the degree of disturbance in physiologic functioning in the area where the tumor is located (see Table 17-10). Infratentorial tumors exhibit localized signs of impaired coordination and balance, including ataxia, gait difficulties, truncal ataxia, and loss of balance. The **medulloblastoma** is the most common childhood malignant tumor and occurs as an invasive tumor that develops in the vermis of the cerebellum and may extend into the fourth ventricle.[104] The **ependymoma** develops in the fourth ventricle and arises from the ependymal cells that line the ventricular system. The histology of the ependymoma varies, which makes the treatment course and prognosis difficult to establish. Because both tumors are located in the posterior fossa region along the midline, presenting signs and symptoms are similar. In addition to those already described, they may obstruct the fourth ventricle, resulting in hydrocephalus and generalized IICP, headache, nausea and vomiting, and nystagmus (involuntary eye movement).

In contrast, **cerebellar astrocytomas** are located on the surface of the right or left cerebellar hemisphere and cause unilateral symptoms (occurring on the same side of the tumor), such as head tilt, limb ataxia, and nystagmus when the eyes are turned toward the tumor.

Brain stem gliomas often cause a combination of cranial nerve involvement, cerebellar signs of ataxia, and corticospinal tract dysfunction. A common clinical pattern includes unilateral paralysis of cranial nerves with contralateral paralysis of the arm and leg, hyperreflexia, and extensor plantar responses. IICP generally does not occur.

The area of the sella turcica, the structure containing the pituitary gland, is the site of several childhood brain tumors; most common of this group is the **craniopharyngioma.** These tumors may originate from the pituitary gland or the hypothalamus. They are usually slow-growing tumors and may be quite large by the time of diagnosis. Symptoms include headache, seizures, diabetes insipidus, early onset of puberty, and growth delay. Other tumors located in this region of the brain include **optic gliomas.** Tumors that involve the optic tract may cause complete unilateral blindness and hemianopia of the other eye. Optic atrophy is another common finding.

Supratentorial tumors of the cerebral hemispheres in children are not very common. Tumors located in the cortex may cause focal cerebral dysfunction, weakness, hemiparesis, seizures, and visual changes. Involvement of particular lobes may result in more specific localized symptoms. For example, a tumor located in the frontal lobe may cause changes in affect and behavior, and a tumor in the occipital lobe may cause cortical blindness or blindness in one half of the visual field.

EVALUATION AND TREATMENT   A child with signs and symptoms of a brain tumor requires a complete workup, including a neurologic, developmental, and ophthalmic examination. CT with contrast enhancement allows direct visualization of the tumor mass. MRI now provides advanced, dramatic examination of the brain and neoplasms. Small, low-grade tumors not seen on CT may be detected by MRI. Although less commonly used, MRA is very helpful in assessing vascularity of the tumor and its relationship to major blood vessels. Myelographic examination may be used to evaluate tumor dissemination along the spinal column. Lumbar puncture to examine CSF for tumor cells also is an option. Tumors more likely to spread throughout the neuraxis include medulloblastomas and ependymomas.

The most useful treatment for brain tumors is surgical resection. Surgery to establish the diagnosis by biopsy or to excise the tumor is part of the initial treatment for most brain tumors. Some brain tumors may be cured with complete resection alone, such as low-grade cerebellar astrocytomas. Contraindications to such interventions are tumors in which surgical resection and biopsy carry a high risk of mortality or serious morbidity (brain stem gliomas). In these instances, diagnosis is made on radiologic evidence and clinical manifestations.

Most brain tumors require additional radiation and chemotherapy. Although these treatments are essential for potential eradication of the brain tumor, radiation to the child's brain is associated with significant morbidity, including both acute and long-term sequelae. Much research and persistence and many investigations are directed at uncovering the secrets to successful treatment of this disease. Prognosis varies according to the type and location of the brain tumor. Historically, survival rates have been low; however, advances have been made with the combination of surgery, radiation therapy, and chemotherapy. Comprehensive care and management of these children and their families are vital. Multidisciplinary teams composed of neurosurgeons, neurologists, neuropathologists, radiation therapists, oncologists, nurses, social workers, physical therapists, and other providers are necessary to provide the continuity and consistency needed to care for these children.

Embryonal Tumors
Neuroblastoma

Neuroblastoma is an embryonal tumor that originates in neural crest cells that normally give rise to the sympathetic ganglia and the adrenal medulla. The primitive neural crest cells (also called *sympathogonia*) are pluripotential (i.e., they give rise to several cell types). They mature into ganglion cells, pheochromocytes (which are found in the sympathetic nervous system), or neurofibrous tissue. Thus tumors that develop from neural crest cells reflect the varying degrees of differentiation of the cells. **Ganglioneuroblastomas** are tumors of an intermediate level of cellular differentiation. The most differentiated tumor is a **ganglioneuroma,** which is considered benign and does not metastasize.

Because neuroblastoma involves a defect of embryonal tissue, it is diagnosed most commonly in young children and infants. Most tumors are diagnosed during the first 2 years of life, and 75% are found before the child is 5 years of age. Occasionally these tumors have been diagnosed at birth with metastasis apparent in the placenta. Neuroblastomas also are known to regress or mature into benign lesions.[105] Neuroblastoma is seen more commonly in white children (9.6 per million) than in black children (7 per million). Although it accounts for 8% to 10% of pediatric malignancies, neuroblastoma causes 15% of cancer deaths in children.[106]

PATHOPHYSIOLOGY   Neuroblastoma is the most primitive, or immature, form of the sympathetic nervous system tumors. Areas of necrosis and calcification often are present in the tumor.

Neuroblastoma, more than any other cancer, has been associated with spontaneous remission, commonly in infants who have liver, bone marrow, or skin involvement in addition to the primary site. Remission has been estimated to occur in approximately 7% of cases, but it may occur much more often. Neuroblastoma in situ (i.e., noninvasive tumor) has been found during autopsies of infants who died of other causes.

The cause of neuroblastoma is elusive. The tumor has been associated with a number of conditions, including neurofibromatosis and Hirschsprung disease, but most children with neuroblastoma have neither of these conditions. Although familial tendency has been noted in individual cases, a nonfamilial or sporadic pattern occurs in most children with neuroblastoma. Familial cases of neuroblastoma are considered to have an autosomal dominant pattern of inheritance (mechanisms of inheritance are discussed in Chapter 4).

Intense genetic study of neuroblastoma cells has led to some interesting findings. Often these cells show a deletion of the short arm of chromosome 1, which is believed to represent the loss of a tumor response gene. In addition, an oncogene, the *Myc-N* oncogene, is present and amplified in neuroblastoma. There is an association between the number of *Myc-N* copies present in the neuroblastoma cells and the child's prognosis. The greater the number of copies of the *Myc-N* oncogene, the more rapidly progressive and lethal the disease is.[107] Further, a gene, the human multidrug-resistant gene (*MDR1* at chromosomes 3p and 11q1), has been identified and is associated with chemotherapy failure. The *MDR1* gene has been found to be amplified in some neuroblastoma cells after initial treatment with chemotherapy, and the increased presence of *MDR1* is associated with chemotherapy resistance. Chromosome 17q may be overexpressed.[108] Other

molecular markers (i.e., neurotrophins) for neuroblastoma are being considered to support risk stratification and guidance of treatment.[109,110]

CLINICAL MANIFESTATIONS   The clinical manifestations of neuroblastoma depend on the location of the tumor. Because neuroblastoma originates where there are elements of sympathetic nervous tissue, the tumor can arise in the sympathetic chain (column of sympathetic ganglia that parallels the spinal column), ganglia of effector organs, peripheral ganglia, adrenal medulla, bladder, and inner genitalia. The most common location is in the retroperitoneal region (65% of cases) and most often the adrenal medulla. The tumor is evident as an abdominal mass and may cause anorexia, bowel and bladder alteration, and sometimes spinal cord compression.[111]

The second most common location of neuroblastoma is the mediastinum (area separating the lungs) (15% of cases). There the tumor may cause dyspnea or infection related to airway obstruction. If the tumor is large, compression of the trachea, bronchi, lymphatic vessels, and mediastinal veins often results. Neck and facial edema may then be caused by superior vena cava syndrome. Less commonly, neuroblastoma may arise from the cervical sympathetic ganglion (3% to 4% of cases). Cervical neuroblastoma often causes Horner syndrome, which consists of miosis (pupil contraction), ptosis (drooping eyelid), enophthalmos (backward displacement of the eyeball), and anhidrosis (sweat deficiency).

The initial signs and symptoms of neuroblastoma often are related to metastatic disease. Two thirds of children have metastatic disease at the time of diagnosis. Common sites of metastasis include the skin, with characteristic blue or purple nodules; the liver, causing enlargement; bone, causing pain and pathologic fracture; and bone marrow infiltration, occurring in more than 50% of children. A unique but uncommon site of metastasis is the orbit of the eye, causing an ecchymotic discoloration of the upper and lower eyelids and a "raccoon" eye appearance.

A number of systemic signs and symptoms are characteristic of neuroblastoma, including weight loss, irritability, fatigue, and fever. Intractable diarrhea occurs in 7% to 9% of children and is caused by tumor secretion of a hormone called *vasoactive intestinal polypeptide (VIP)*.

More than 90% of children with neuroblastoma have increased amounts of catecholamines and associated metabolites in their urine. High levels of urinary catecholamines and serum ferritin are associated with a poorer prognosis.

EVALUATION AND TREATMENT   Initial diagnostic studies are dictated by the location of the primary tumor. Diagnosis begins with a complete physical and neurologic examination. Visualizing examinations, including intravenous pyelogram, CT scan, and MRI of the primary site, provide further information. Investigation of metastatic disease includes skeletal survey, bone scan, liver scan, and bone marrow aspiration and examination. Newer nuclear medicine imaging studies for neuroblastoma, such as ^{131}I-metaiodobenzyl-guanidine (^{131}I-MIBG) and tumor-specific monoclonal antibody scan, may be helpful. Urinary catecholamine levels are measured by two metabolites, vanillylmandelic acid (VMA) and homovanillic acid (HVA). Measurement of these levels requires a 24-hour urine collection. Other laboratory analyses are likely to include ferritin; serum neuron-specific enolase (NSE), an enzyme produced by neuronal tissues; and gangliosides, lipid molecules that may be shed from the surface of tumor cells.

The diagnosis of neuroblastoma is confirmed by surgical biopsy. Occasionally the biopsy may be avoided if bone marrow aspiration shows tumor infiltration and significant elevation of urinary catecholamines. For many years there was no agreement on a staging system for neuroblastoma. Finally in 1986, an international group proposed a single staging system that was adopted in 1987. A special stage (IV-S) is designated for infants who otherwise would be classified as having early-stage disease but who also have metastatic disease involving the liver, skin, or bone.

Treatment is based on the extent of the disease and prognostic markers, such as age, *Myc-N* copy numbers, and high serum ferritin or NSE levels. Early-stage disease is treated by primary excision of the tumor. Because neuroblastoma is a radiosensitive tumor, postoperative radiation therapy may be used for residual disease; however, multiagent chemotherapy is now the predominant treatment modality.[112] The success of radiation therapy in early-stage disease, however, is controversial.

High-risk neuroblastomas are being treated with high-dose chemotherapy and radiotherapy followed by transplantation of purged autologous bone marrow. Additional treatment may include 13-*cis* retinoic acid. These combined treatments have increased survival rate in some to 3 years.

Stage IV-S disease requires very little treatment, primarily because of the high rate of spontaneous regression. Low-dose radiation treatment or single-course chemotherapy may be used to reduce large tumors. Approximately 60% of children with high stage disease will die despite intensive therapy.[112]

Retinoblastoma

Retinoblastoma is a rare congenital eye tumor of young children that originates in the retina of one or both eyes (Figure 19-15). It has been intensively studied and is of much interest to geneticists. Retinoblastoma demonstrates both an inher-

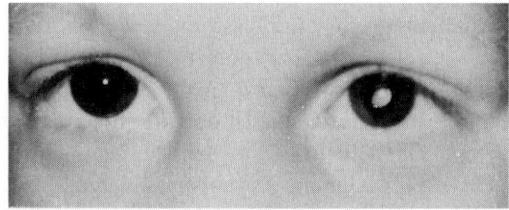

Figure 19-15 Retinoblastoma. Prominent white reflex (caused by retinoblastoma) in dilated pupil of left eye. (From Kissane JM, editor: *Anderson's pathology,* ed 9, St Louis, 1990, Mosby.)

ited and an acquired form. Retinoblastoma rarely is diagnosed after the child is 5 years of age. The inherited form of the disease generally is diagnosed during the first year of life and often involves multiple tumors and sometimes both eyes. The acquired disease most commonly is diagnosed in children 2 to 3 years of age and involves unilateral disease. Although retinoblastoma is the most common pediatric intraocular tumor, the prevalence rate is estimated between 1 in 17,000 and 1 in 34,000 live births.[113]

PATHOPHYSIOLOGY   Approximately 40% of retinoblastomas are inherited as an autosomal dominant disorder caused by mutations in the *RB1* gene.[114] The remaining 60% are acquired. In the early 1970s Knudson[115] proposed the "two-hit" hypothesis to explain the occurrence of both hereditary and acquired forms of the disease. This hypothesis predicts that two separate transforming events or "hits" must occur in a normal retinoblast cell to cause the cancer. Further, it proposes that in the inherited form the first "hit" or mutation occurs in the germ cell (inherited from either parent), and the mutation is contained in every cell of the child's body. Only a second, random mutation in a retinoblast cell is necessary to transform that cell into cancer. Multiple tumors are observed in the inherited form because these second mutations are likely to occur in several of the approximately 1 to 2 million retinoblast cells. In contrast, the acquired form of retinoblastoma requires that two independent "hits" or mutations occur in the same somatic cell (after the egg is fertilized) for transformation to cancer. This is much less likely to happen. Figure 19-16 illustrates the two-mutation model for these two patterns of mutation.

The gene location in which the initial retinoblastoma mutation occurs is on the long arm of chromosome 13, band q14.[116] The gene responsible for retinoblastoma, a tumor suppressor gene, is called the *Rb gene.* The first "hit" inactivates one allele of the *Rb* gene, and the second "hit" inactivates the other allele of the gene. Without the normal functioning of the *Rb* gene, production of protein growth regulators that control retinal cell growth is lacking. Because the gene is inactivated, lack of cell growth control results in unregulated proliferation and tumor development.[117]

The *Rb* gene also has been implicated in other cancers, and survivors of hereditary retinoblastoma may be at increased risk for second cancers, particularly osteosarcoma but also cancer of the lung, breast, prostate, and bladder. Although retinoblastoma occurs in the very young child, second tumors can develop when survivors are in their 20s and 30s; such tumors generally are resistant to therapy.

CLINICAL MANIFESTATIONS   Retinoblastoma grows as one or more tumors in the retina and extends into the vitreous humor. Free-floating, small tumors in the vitreous humor may attach to the surface of the retina in multiple areas and proliferate (Figure 19-17). The tumor also can invade the optic nerve by infiltrating through the cribriform plate of the ethmoid bone or can spread through the sheath around the nerve. In either case the tumor can gain access to the

Inherited

Sporadic

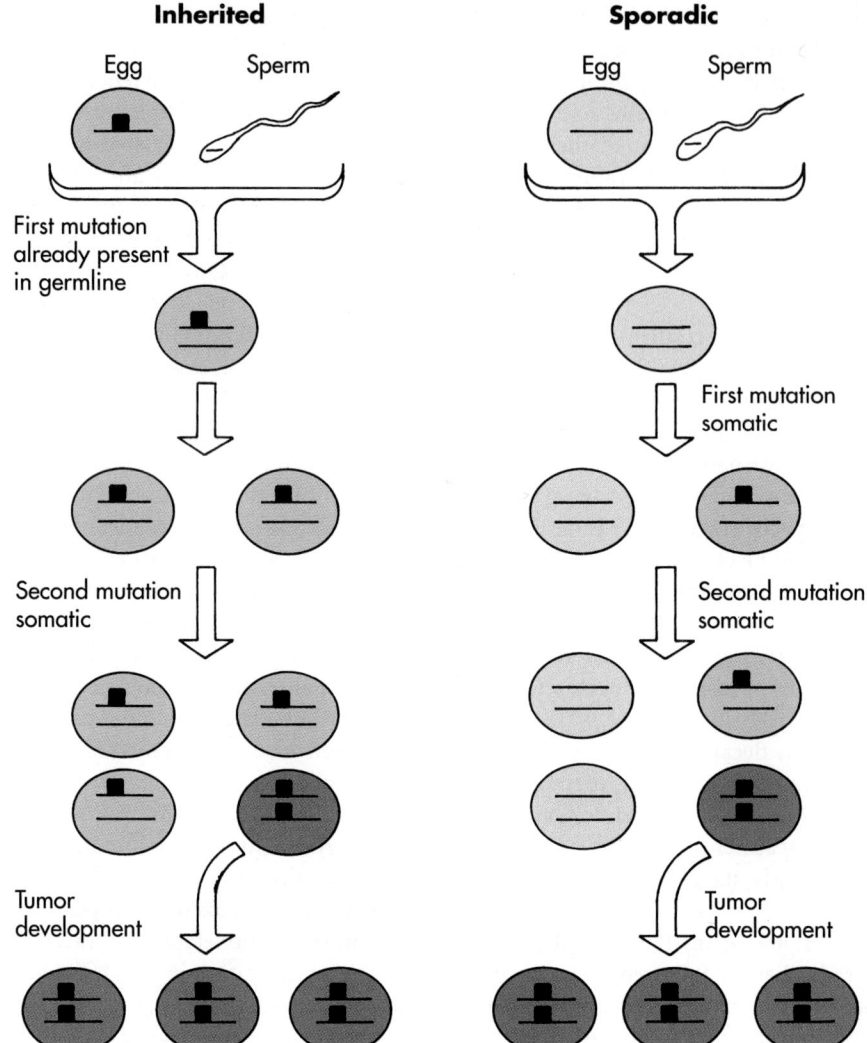

Figure 19-16 The two-mutation model of retinoblastoma development. In inherited retinoblastoma, the first mutation is transmitted through the germline of an affected parent. The second mutation occurs somatically in a retinal cell, leading to development of the tumor. In sporadic retinoblastoma, development of a tumor requires two somatic mutations.

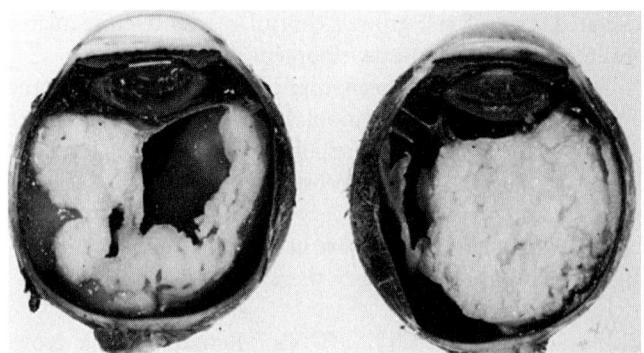

Figure 19-17 Bilateral retinoblastoma. Presence of white mass consisting of detached retina and neoplastic tissue immediately behind lens in each eye. (From Kissane JM, editor: *Anderson's pathology,* ed 8, St Louis, 1985, Mosby.)

subarachnoid space and the CNS. The tumor spreads into the choroid in 25% of children with retinoblastoma. Because the choroid is highly vascular, metastasis by means of hematogenous spread is possible. When hematogenous spread occurs, metastatic sites include the bone marrow, long bones, lymph nodes, and liver. If the tumor invades the orbit, lymphatic spread is possible. Spontaneous regression occurs, although infrequently, and may be caused by the tumor outgrowing its blood supply.

The primary sign of retinoblastoma is leukokoria, a white pupillary reflex also called *cat's eye reflex,* that is caused by the mass behind the lens (see Figure 19-15). At that point the tumor is large enough that a light shone into the eye is reflected back by the tumor, making the pupil appear white. Other signs and symptoms include strabismus; a red, painful eye; and limited vision. Any of these signs and symptoms in a child younger than 4 years of age warrants careful ophthalmologic examination of both eyes. Similarly, any newborn with a known genetic risk for retinoblastoma should have routine ophthalmologic examinations.

EVALUATION AND TREATMENT   Diagnostic evaluation for retinoblastoma includes documentation of family history; complete ophthalmologic examination; and metastatic studies that include bone marrow aspiration, lumbar puncture for spinal fluid examination, bone scan, and additional radiologic and CT studies of the orbit and brain. Because of the potential hereditary risk to a child's siblings, all siblings younger than 4 years also should receive ophthalmologic evaluations.

Because retinoblastoma is a treatable tumor, dual priorities are saving the child's life and restoring useful vision. Early diagnosis and new chemotherapeutic agents have led to a more conservative approach to treatment. Chemoreduction of the tumor occurs with intravenous chemotherapy to reduce tumor volume. Focal treatments using hyperthermia, laser photocoagulation, or cryotherapy then destroy residual tumor. Large or multiple tumors, indicating more advanced disease, require external beam or plaque radiotherapy and, in some cases, enucleation (removal) of the eye. Every attempt is made to preserve vision in at least one eye without jeopardizing the child's survival.[118,119]

The prognosis for most children with retinoblastoma is excellent, with a greater than 90% long-term survival, although children with metastatic disease at diagnosis have a poor prognosis. Approximately 75% of children have useful vision in the treated eye.

SUMMARY REVIEW

Structure and Function of the Nervous System in Children

1. The central nervous system develops from the neural tube, which is ectodermal in origin. The cranial end of the tube forms the brain, and the spinal cord is formed from the remainder of the tube.
2. The cranial and spinal ganglia form the neural crest.
3. The nervous system develops in six stages, and disruption of any of the stages can lead to malfunction of the nervous system.
4. The bones of the skull are joined by sutures; the wide, membranous junctions of the sutures, known as *fontanelles*, close by 20 months of age.
5. Myelin is a sheath that develops around axons to facilitate speed of nerve impulse conduction. Progressive development of reflexes corresponds to normal maturation of nerve tissue.
6. At birth neurologic functioning is at the subcortical level, with reflex patterns mediated by the brain stem and spinal cord. With maturation, neonatal reflexes disappear and voluntary motor functions develop.
7. Head circumference is one fourth of the total height in infants compared to one eighth in adults. The fontanelles allow for cranial expansion because the head is the fastest growing body part during infancy.

Structural Malformations

1. Defects of neural tube closure include anencephaly, encephalocele, meningocele, and myelomeningocele.
2. Failure of the vertebra to close with protrusion of neural tube contents is known as *spina bifida*.
3. Acrania is nearly complete absence of the cranial vault.
4. Premature closure of the cranial sutures causes craniosynostosis and prevents normal skull expansion and compression of growing brain tissue.
5. Microcephaly is lack of brain growth and retarded mental and motor development.
6. Congenital hydrocephalus results from an imbalance between the production and reabsorption of cerebrospinal fluid.

Encephalopathies

1. Static encephalopathies are nonprogressive disorders of the brain that can occur during gestation, birth, or childhood and can be caused by endogenous or exogenous factors.
2. Cerebral palsy can be caused by prenatal cerebral hypoxia or perinatal trauma with symptoms of mental retardation, seizure disorders, or developmental disabilities.
3. Inherited metabolic disorders that damage the nervous system include defects in amino acid metabolism (phenylketonuria) and lipid metabolism (Tay-Sachs disease) and result in abnormal behavior, seizures, and deficient psychomotor development.
4. Seizure disorders are associated with numerous nervous system disorders and more often are a generalized rather than a partial type of seizure.
5. Generalized forms of seizures include tonic-clonic, myoclonic, atonic, akinetic, and infantile spasms.
6. Partial seizures suggest more localized brain dysfunction.
7. Febrile seizures usually are limited to the ages of 9 months to 3 years with a pattern of one seizure per febrile illness.
8. Reye syndrome is associated with influenza B and varicella viruses and symptoms of hypoglycemia, hyperammonemia, and increased serum short-chain fatty acids. Progressive manifestations include lethargy, stupor, rigidity, seizures, and respiratory arrest.
9. Accidental poisonings from a variety of toxins can cause serious neurologic damage.
10. Bacterial meningitis is commonly caused by *Haemophilus influenzae, Neisseria meningitidis,* or *Streptococcus pneumoniae* and may result from respiratory or gastrointestinal infections, with symptoms of fever, headaches, photophobia, seizures, rigidity, and stupor.

Human Immunodeficiency Virus and Central Nervous System Involvement

1. Human immunodeficiency virus (HIV) may be transmitted to infants and children through the placenta, by exposure to infected blood or vaginal secretions, or by ingestion of infected breast milk.
2. The incidence of HIV among children is increasing. The classic symptoms are related to progressive encephalopathy.
3. Acquired immunodeficiency syndrome (AIDS) was the seventh most common cause of death among children 1 to 4 years of age in developing countries in 2002.

Cerebrovascular Disease in Children

1. Occlusive cerebrovascular disease may result from embolism, sinovenous thrombosis, or congenital or iatrogenic vessel narrowing.
2. Congenital arteriovenous malformations are the most common cause of intracranial bleeding and hemorrhagic stroke in children.

Continued

SUMMARY REVIEW—cont'd

Childhood Tumors

1. Brain tumors are the most common tumors of the nervous system and the second most common type of childhood cancer.
2. Tumors in children most often are located below the tentorial membrane.
3. Fast-growing tumors produce symptoms early in the disease, whereas slow-growing tumors may become very large before symptoms appear.
4. Symptoms of brain tumors may be generalized or localized. The most common general symptom is increased intracranial pressure (headache, irritability, vomiting, somnolence, and bulging of fontanelles).

5. Localized signs of infratentorial tumors in the cerebellum include impaired coordination and balance. Cranial nerve signs occur with tumors near the brain stem.
6. Supratentorial tumors may be located near the cortex or deep in the brain. Symptoms depend on the specific location of the tumor.
7. Neuroblastoma is an embryonal tumor of the sympathetic nervous system and can be located anywhere there is sympathetic nervous tissue. Symptoms are related to tumor location and size of metastasis.
8. Retinoblastoma is a congenital eye tumor that has both a hereditary and a nonhereditary form.

KEY TERMS

Acquired immunodeficiency syndrome (AIDS), 642
Acrania, 630
Alar plate, 623
Anencephaly, 627
Arnold-Chiari type II malformation, 628
Ataxic cerebral palsy, 634
Basal plate, 623
Benign febrile seizures, 638
Brain stem gliomas, 647
Cerebellar astrocytomas, 647
Cerebral palsy, 633
Congenital hydrocephalus, 631
Cranial meningocele, 627
Craniopharyngioma, 647
Craniosynostosis, 630
Cyclopia, 626
Dandy-Walker deformity, 632
Dyskinetic cerebral palsy, 634
Encephalocele, 627
Encephalopathy, 633

Ependymoma, 647
Epilepsy, 637
Fontanelles, 624
Ganglioneuroblastomas, 648
Ganglioneuroma, 648
Generalized seizures, 637
Hyperphenylalaninemia (HPA), 636
Infantile spasms, 638
Juvenile myoclonic epilepsy, 638
Lennox-Gastaut syndrome, 638
Lysosomal storage disease, 636
Macewen sign (cracked-pot sign), 632
Medulloblastoma, 647
Meningocele, 627
Mental retardation, 631
Microcephaly, 631
Moyamoya disease, 644
Myelodysplasia, 626
Neural crest, 623
Neural folds, 623
Neural groove, 623

Neural plate, 623
Neural tube, 623
Neuroblastoma, 647
Optic gliomas, 647
Partial seizures, 637
Phenylketonuria (PKU), 635
Pica, 640
Retinoblastoma, 649
Reye syndrome, 639
Schwann cells, 624
Somite, 623
Spastic cerebral palsy, 634
Spina bifida, 629
Spina bifida occulta, 629
Sulcus limitans, 623
Sutures, 624
Tay-Sachs disease, 636
Tethered cord syndrome, 629
Tuberous sclerosis complex (TSC), 638
Unclassified epileptic seizures, 637

MEDIA RESOURCES evolve

Review questions and answers for this chapter are available in the *CD Companion* included with this book.

WebLinks—links to Internet sites pertaining to this chapter—are available on Evolve at http://evolve.elsevier.com/McCance/.

REFERENCES

1. Kaufman BA: Neural tube defects, *Pediatr Clin North Am* 51(2):389-419, 2004.
2. Stover PJ: Physiology of folate and vitamin B₁₂ in health and disease, *Nutr Rev* 62(6 Pt 2):S3-S12, discussion S13, 2004.
3. Merserau P et al: Spina bifida and ancephaly before and after folic acid mandate—United States 1995-1996 and 1999-2000, *MMWR* 53(17):362-365, 2004.
4. Pollack IF: Management of encephaloceles and craniofacial problems in the neonatal period, *Neurosurg Clin N Am* 9(1):121-139, 1998.
5. Behrman RE, Kleigman RM, Jenson HB: *Nelson's textbook of pediatrics,* ed 17, Philadelphia, 2004, Saunders.
6. Stevenson KL: Chiari Type II malformation: past, present and future, *Neurosurg Focus* 16(2):E5, 2004.
7. Adzick NS, Walsh DS: Myelomeningocele: prenatal diagnosis, pathophysiology and management. *Sem Pediatr Surg* 12(3):168-174, 2003.
8. Wakhlu A, Ansari NA: The predicting of postoperative hydrocephalus in patients with spina bifida, *Childs Nerv Syst* 20(2):104-106, 2004.
9. Reigel, DH: Infancy through the school years. In Rowley-Kelly F, Reigel DH, editors: *Teaching the student with spina bifida,* Baltimore, 1993, Brookes.
10. Loller DJ: *Learning among children with spina bifida. Spina Bifida Spotlight: 1-6,* Washington, DC, 1993, Spina Bifida Association of America.
11. Yamada S et al: Pathophysiology of tethered cord syndrome and other complex factors, *Neurol Res* 26(7):722-726, 2004.
12. Jobe AH: Fetal surgery for myelomeningocele, *N Engl J Med* 347(4):230-231, 2002.
13. Yamada S, Won DJ, Yamada SM: Pathophysiology of tethered cord syndrome: correlation with symptomatology, *Neurosurg Focus* 16(2):E6, 2004.
14. Hudgins RJ, Gilreath CL: Tethered spinal cord following repair of myelomeningocele, *Neurosurg Focus* 16(2):E7, 2004.
15. Bliton MJ: Ethics "life before birth" and moral complexity in maternal-fetal surgery for spina bifida, *Clin Perinatol* 30(3):449-464, 2003.
16. Simpson JL: Fetal surgery for myelomeingocele: promise, progress and problems, *JAMA* 282(19):1873-1874, 1999.
17. Rintoul NE et al: A new look at myelomeningocele: functional level, vertebral level, and the implication for fetal intervention, *Pediatrics* 109(3):409-413, 2002.
18. Tulipan N: Intrauterine closure of myelomeningocele: an update, *Neurosurg Focus* 16(2)E2, 2004.

19. Tubbs RS, Oakes WJ: Treatment and management of the Chiari II malformation: an evidence-based review of the literature, *Childs Nerv Syst* 20(6):375-381, 2004.
20. Mitchell LE et al: Spina bifida, *Lancet* 364(9448):1885-1895, 2004.
21. Bruner JP et al: Intrauterine repair of spina bifida: preoperative predictors of shunt-dependent hydrocephalus, *Am J Obstet Gynecol* 190(5):1305-1312, 2004.
22. Cartwright C: Assessing asymmetrical infant head shapes, *Nurse Pract* 27(8):33, 35-36, 39, 2002.
23. Ehet FW et al: Differential diagnosis of trapezoid head, *Cleft Palate Craniofac J* 41(1):13-19, 2004.
24. Garton HJ, Platt JH Jr: Hydrocephalus, *Pediatr Clin North Am* 51(2):305-325, 2004.
25. Jackson PL: Hydrocephalus. In Jackson PL, Vessey JA, editors: *Primary care of the child with a chronic condition,* ed 4, St Louis, 2003, Mosby.
26. Kestle JR: Pediatric hydrocephalus—current management, *Neurol Clin* 21(4):883-895, 2003.
27. Jacobsson B, Hagberg G: Antenatal risk factors for cerebral palsy, *Best Pract Res Clin Obstet Gynaecol* 18(3):425-436, 2004.
28. Murphy N, Such-Neibar T: Cerebral palsy diagnosis and management: the state of the art, *Curr Probl Pediatr Adolesc Health Care* 33(5):146-169, 2003.
29. Lawson RD, Badawi N: Etiology of cerebral palsy, *Hand Clin* 19(4):547-556, 2003.
30. Palmer FB: Strategies for early diagnosis of cerebral palsy, *J Peds* 145(2 Suppl):8-11, 2004.
32. Russman BS, Ashwal S: Evaluation of the child with cerebral palsy, *Sem Pediatr Neurol* 11(1):47-57, 2004.
32. Steele S: Cerebral palsy. In Jackson PL, Vessey JA, editors: *Primary care of the child with a chronic condition,* ed 3, St Louis, 2000, Mosby.
33. Wong AM et al: Clinical effect of botulinum toxin A and phenol block on gait in children with cerebral palsy, *Am J Phys Med Rehabil* 83(4):284-291, 2004.
34. Tilton AH: Management of spasticity in children with cerebral palsy, *Semin Pediatr Neurol* 11(1):58-65, 2004.
35. Koman LA, Smith BP, Shilt JS: Cerebral palsy, *Lancet* 363(9421):1619-1631, 2004.
36. Singhi PD: Cerebral palsy-management, *Indian J Pediatr* 71(7):635-639, 2004.
37. Menkes JH, Sarnat HB: *Child neurology,* ed 6, Philadelphia, 2000, Lippincott William & Wilkins.
38. Swainman KF, Ashwal S: *Pediatric neurology: principles and practice,* ed 3, St Louis, 1999, Mosby.
39. Fusetti F et al: Structure of tetrameric human phenylalanine hydroxylase and its implications for phenylketonuria, *J Biol Chem* 273(27):16962-16927, 1998.
40. Schmidt K: Phenylketonuria. In Jackson PL, Vessey, JA, editors: *Primary care of the child with a chronic condition,* ed 4, St Louis, 2003, Mosby.
41. Kaufman S: An evaluation of the possible neurotoxicity of metabolites of phenylalanine, *J Pediatr* 114(5):895-900, 1989.
42. Macdonald A et al: Protein substitutes for PKU: what's new? *J Inherit Metab Dis* 27(3):363-371, 2004.
43. Ding Z, Harding CO, Thony B: State-of-the-art 2003 on PKU gene therapy, *Mol Genet Metab* 81(1):3-8, 2004.
44. Kim W et al: Trends in enzyme therapy for phenylketonuria, *Mol Ther* 10(2):220-224, 2004.
45. Wille MC et al: Advances in preconception genetic counseling, *J Perinat Neonatal Nurs* 18(1):28-40, 2004.
46. Jarrar RG, Buchhalter JR: Therapeutics in pediatric epilepsy. Part 1: the new antiepileptic drugs and the ketogenic diet, *Mayo Clin Proc* 78(3):359-370, 2003.
47. Leppik E: The expanding role of genetics in epilepsy, *Am J Electroneurodiagnostic Tech* 43(2):70-73, 105-107, 2003.
48. Pellock JM: Managing pediatric epilepsy syndromes with new antiepileptic drugs, *Pediatrics* 104(5 Pt1):1106-1116, 1999.
49. Frost JD Jr, Hrachovy, RA: Pathogenesis of infantile spasms: a model based on developmental desynchronization, *J Clin Neurophysiol* 22(1):25-36, 2005.
50. Rantala H et al: Risk factors of infantile spasms compared with other seizures in children under 2 years of age, *Epilepsia* 37(4):362, 1996.
51. Thiele EA: Managing epilepsy in tuberous sclerosis complex, *J Child Neurol* 19(9):680-686, 2004.
52. Weiner HL et al: Epilepsy surgery for children with tuberous sclerosis complex, *J Child Neurol* 19(9):687-689, 2004.

53. Hancock E, Cross H: Treatment of Lennox-Gastaut syndrome, *Cochrane Database Syst Rev* (3):CD003277, 2003.
54. Ghingo J, Neidermeyer E: Juvenile myoclonic epilepsy, *Am J Electroneurodiagnostic Tech* 40(4):225-267, 292-294, 2000.
55. Renganathan R, Delanty N: Juvenile myoclonic epilepsy: underappreciated and under-diagnosed, *Postgrad Med J* 79(298):78-80, 2003.
56. Levy R, Cooper P: Ketogenic diet for epilepsy, *Cochrane Database Syst Rev* (3):CD00192, 2003.
57. Stafstrom CE, Bough KJ: The ketogenic diet for the treatment of epilepsy: a challenge for nutritional neuroscientists, *Nutr Neurosci* 6(2):67-79, 2003.
58. Cascino GD: Surgical treatment for epilepsy, *Epilepsy Res* 60(2-3):179-186, 2004.
59. Devinsky O, Laff R: Callosal lesions and behavior: history and modern concepts, *Epilepsy Behav* 4(6):607-617, 2003.
60. McKhann GM 2nd: Novel surgical treatments for epilepsy, *Curr Neurol Neurosci Rep* 4(4):335-339, 2004.
61. Buchhalter JR, Jarrar RG: Symposium on seizures. Therapeutics in pediatric epilepsy part 2: epilepsy surgery and vagus nerve stimulation, *Mayo Clin Proc* 78(3):371-378, 2003.
62. Champi G, Gaffney-Yocum PA: Managing febrile seizures in children, *Dimens Crit Care Nurs* 20(5):2-10, 2001.
63. Waruiru C, Appleton R: Febrile seizures: an update, *Arch Dis Child* 89(8):751-756, 2004.
64. Baulac S et al: Fever, genes, and epilepsy, *Lancet Neurol* 3(7):421-430, 2004.
65. Monto AS: The disappearance of Reye's syndrome—a public health triumph, *N Engl J Med* 340(18):1423-1424, 1999.
66. Belay ED et al: Reye's syndrome in the United States from 1981 though 1997, *New Eng J Med* 340(18):1377, 1999.
67. Ward MJ: Reye's syndrome: an update, *Nurs Pract* 22(12):45, 1997.
68. Bhutta AT et al: Reye's syndrome: down but not out, *South Med J* 96(1):43-45, 2003.
69. Bernard SM: Should the Center for Disease Control and Prevention's childhood lead poisoning intervention level be lowered? *Am J Public Health* 94(1):8-9, 2004.
70. Meyer PA et al: Surveillance for elevated blood lead levels among children—United States, 1997-2001, *MMWR* 52(10):1-21, 2003.
71. Needleman H: Lead poisoning, *Annu Rev Med* 55:209-222, 2004.
72. Bellinger DC: Lead, *Pediatrics* 113(4 Suppl):1016-1022, 2004.
73. Chang CJ et al: Bacterial meningitis in infants: the epidemiology, clinical features and prognostic factors, *Brain Dev* 26(3):168-175, 2004.
74. Zimmer SM, Stephens DS: Meningococcal conjugate vaccines, *Expert Opin Pharmacother* 5(4):855-863, 2004.
75. Nigrovic LE, Kuppermann N, Malley R: Development and validation of a multivariable predictive model to distinguish bacterial from aseptic meningitis in children in post-*Haemophilus influenzae* era, *Pediatrics* 110(4):712-719, 2002.
76. Feigin RD et al: Bacterial meningitis beyond the neonatal period. In Feigin RD et al editors: *Textbook of pediatric infectious diseases,* ed 5, Philadelphia, 2003, Saunders.
77. Duke T, Curtis N, Fuller DG: The management of bacterial meningitis in children, *Expert Opin Pharmacother* 4(8):1227-1240, 2004.
78. Ahmed MN, Steele RW: Meningitis in a young infant, *Clin Pediatr* (Phila) 43(5):495-497, 2004.
79. Fahrner R: Pediatric HIV infections and AIDS. In Jackson PL, Vessey JA, editors: *Primary care of the child with a chronic condition,* ed 4, St Louis, 2003, Mosby.
80. Tamula MA et al: Cognitive decline with immunologic and virologic stability in four children with human immunodeficiency virus disease, *Pediatrics* 112(3Pt1):679-684, 2003.
81. Newell ML, Brahmbhatt H, Ghys PD: Child mortality and HIV infection in Africa: a review, *AIDS* 18(Suppl 2):S27-S34, 2004.
82. National Institute of Allergy and Infectious Diseases (NIAID), Institutes of Health: *HIV infection in infants and children,* 2003. Available at www.thebody.com/niaid/pediatri.html
83. Takebe Y, Kusagawa S, Motomura K: Molecular epidemiology of HIV: tracking AIDS pandemic, *Pediatr Int* 46(2):236-244, 2004.
84. Tardieu M: HIV-1 and the developing central nervous system, *Dev Med Child Neurol* 40(12):843-846, 1998.
85. Hanson IC, Shearer WT: Lentiviruses human immunodeficiency virus type I and acquired immunodeficiency syndrome). In Feigin RD et al, editors: *Textbook of pediatric infectious diseases,* ed 5, Philadelphia, 2003, Saunders.

86. Civitello L: Neurologic aspects of HIV infection in infants and children: therapeutic approaches and outcome, *Curr Neurol Neurosci Rep* 3(2):120-128, 2003.

87. Sanchez-Ramon S et al: Low blood CD8+ T-lymphocytes and high circulating monocytes are predictors of HIV-1 associated progressive encephalopathy in children, *Pediatrics* 111(2):E168-175, 2003.

88. Centers for Disease Control and Prevention: 1994 revised classification system for human immunodeficiency virus infection in children less than 13 years of age, *MMWR* 43(12):1, 1994.

89. McCoig C et al: Cerebrospinal fluid and plasma concentrations of proinflammatory mediators in human immunodeficiency virus-infected children, *Pediatr Infect Dis J* 23(2):114-118, 2004.

90. McKinney RE Jr, Cunningham CK: New treatments for HIV in children, *Curr Opin Pediatr* 16(1):76-79, 2004.

91. Resino S et al: Impact of highly active antiretroviral therapy on CD4+ T cells and viral load of children with AIDS: a population-based study, *AIDS Res Hum Retroviruses* 20(9):927-931, 2004.

92. UNAIDS/WHO AIDS Update, December 2004: www.unaids.org/wad2004/report.html.

93. Mofenson LM et al: Treating opportunistic infections among HIV exposed and infected children: recommendations fro CDC, the National Institutes of Health, and the Infectious Disease Socity of America, *MMWR* 53(14):1-92, 2004.

93a. Centers for Disease Control and Prevention: National Center for HIV, STD and TB Prevention Divisions of HIV/AIDS Prevention AIDS Surveillance—General Epidemiology L178 slide series; accessed March 3, 2005.

94. Hutchinson JS et al: Cerebrovascular disorders, *Semin Pediatr Neurol* 11(2):139-146, 2004.

95. Horn P et al: Arterio-embolic ischemic stroke in children with moyamoya disease, *Childs Nerv Syst* 21(2):104-107, 2004.

96. Meyer-Heim AD, Boltshauser E: Spontaneous intracranial haemorrhage in children: aetiology, presentation and outcome, *Brain Dev* 25(6):416-421, 2003.

97. Golomb MR et al: Neonatal arterial ischemic stroke and cerebral sinovenous thrombosis are more commonly diagnosed in boys, *J Child Neurol* 19(7):493-497, 2004.

98. Rashidi M et al: Nonmalignant pediatric brain tumors, *Curr Neurol Neurosci Rep* 3(3):200-205, 2003.

99. Walter AW: Brain tumors in children, *Curr Oncol Rep* 6(6):438-444, 2004.

100. Kline ME: Solid tumors in children, *J Pediatr Nurs* 18(2):96-102, 2003.

101. Baldwin RT, Preston-Martin S: Epidemiology of brain tumors in childhood—a review, *Toxicol Appl Pharmacol* 199(2)118-131, 2003.

102. Biegel JA: Genetics of pediatric central nervous system tumors, *J Pediatr Hematol Oncol* 19(6):492-501, 1997.

103. Sklar CA: Childhood brain tumors, *J Pediatr Endocrinol Metab* 15(Suppl 2):669-673, 2002.

104. Gilbertson RJ: Medulloblastoma: signalling a change in treatment, *Lancet Oncol* 5(4):209-218, 2004.

105. Kushner BH: Neuroblastoma: a disease requiring a multitude of imaging studies, *J Nucl Med* 45(7):1172-1188, 2004.

106. Schwab M et al: Neuroblastoma: biology and molecular and chromosomal pathology, *Lancet Oncol* 4(8):472-480, 2003.

107. Weinstein JL, Katzenstein HM, Cohn SL: Advances in the diagnosis and treatment of neuroblastoma, *Oncologist* 8(3):278-292, 2003.

108. Goldstein LJ et al: Expression of the multidrug resistance, MDR1, gene in neuroblastomas, *J Clin Oncol* 8(1):128, 1990.

109. Henry MC, Tashjian DB, Breuer C: Neuroblastoma update, *Curr Opin Oncol* 17(1):19-23, 2005.

110. Vasudevan SA, Nuchtern JG: Gene profiling of high risk neuroblastoma, *World J Surg* [Epub ahead of print], 2005.

111. Golden CG, Feusner JH: Malignant abdominal masses in children: quick guide to evaluation and diagnosis, *Pediatr Clin North Am* 49(6):1369-1392, 2002.

112. Goldsby RE, Matthay KK: Neuroblastoma: evolving therapies for a disease with many faces, *Paediatr Drugs* 6(2):107-122, 2004.

113. Butros LJ, Abramson DH, Dunkel IJ: Delayed diagnosis of retinoblastoma: analysis of degree, cause, and potential consequences, *Pediatrics* 109(3):5, 2002.

114. Lohmann DR, Gallie BL: Retinoblastoma: revising the model prototype of inherited cancer, *Am J Med Genet C Semin Med Genet* 129(1):23-28, 2004.

115. Knudson AG: Mutation and cancer: a statistical study of retinoblastoma, *Proc Natl Acad Sci USA*, 68:620, 1971.

116. Kivela T et al: Retinoblastoma associated with chromosome 13q14 deletion mosaicism, *Ophthalmology* 110(10):1983-1988, 2003.

117. Rubnitz JE, Crist WM: Molecular genetics of childhood cancer: implications for pathogenesis, diagnosis, and treatment, *Pediatrics* 100(1):101, 1997.

118. Shields CL et al: Continuing challenges in the management of retinoblastoma with chemotherapy, *Retina* 24(6):849-862, 2004.

119. Yanagisawa T: Systemic chemotherapy as a new conservative treatment for intraocular retinoblastoma, *Int J Clin Oncol* 9(1):13-24, 2004.

MECHANISMS OF HORMONAL REGULATION

SUE E. HUETHER

CHAPTER OUTLINE

The endocrine system is composed of various glands located throughout the body (Figure 20-1). These glands are capable of synthesizing and releasing special chemical messengers called **hormones.** The endocrine system has five general functions:

1. Differentiation of the reproductive and central nervous systems in the developing fetus
2. Stimulation of sequential growth and development during childhood and adolescence
3. Coordination of the male and female reproductive systems, which makes sexual reproduction possible
4. Maintenance of an optimal internal environment throughout the life span.
5. Initiation of corrective and adaptive responses when emergency demands occur

Hormones convey specific regulatory information among cells and organs and are integrated with the nervous system to maintain communication and control. The mechanisms of communication include autocrine (within cell), paracrine (between local cells), and endocrine (between remote cells).

MECHANISMS OF HORMONAL REGULATION

The endocrine glands respond to specific signals by synthesizing and releasing hormones into the circulation. Although a wide variety of hormones function within the body, they share certain general characteristics:

1. Hormones have specific rates and rhythms of secretion. Three basic secretion patterns are (a) diurnal patterns, (b) pulsatile and cyclic patterns, and (c) patterns that depend on levels of circulating substrates (e.g., calcium, sodium, potassium, or the hormones themselves).
2. Hormones operate within feedback systems, either positive or negative, to maintain an optimal internal environment.
3. Hormones affect only cells with appropriate receptors and then act on those cells to initiate specific cell functions or activities.
4. The kidneys excrete hormones, whereas the liver metabolizes hormones—inactivating them and rendering the hormone more water soluble for renal excretion.

Hormones may be classified according to their structure, gland of origin, effects, or chemical composition. (Table 20-1 categorizes hormones based on structure.) The secretion and mechanisms of action of hormones represent an extremely complex system of integrated responses. Although much has been learned about these complex systems, many of the specific mechanisms of action are not yet understood. The endocrine and nervous systems work together to regulate responses to the internal and external environments.

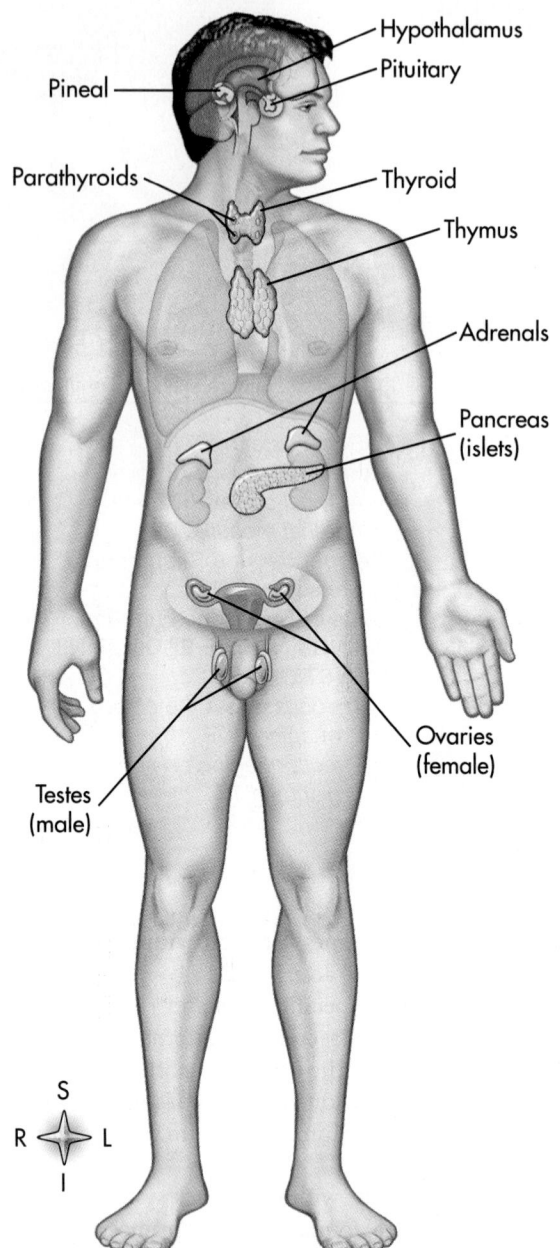

Figure 20-1 Principal endocrine glands. (From Thibodeau GA, Patton KT: *Anatomy & physiology,* ed 5, St Louis, 2003, Mosby.)

Labels on figure:
- Pineal
- Hypothalamus
- Pituitary
- Parathyroids
- Thyroid
- Thymus
- Adrenals
- Pancreas (islets)
- Ovaries (female)
- Testes (male)

Table 20-1	Structural Categories of Hormones	
Structural Category	**Examples**	
Water Soluble		
Peptides	Growth hormone	
	Insulin	
	Leptin	
	Parathyroid hormone	
	Prolactin	
Glycoproteins	Follicle-stimulating hormone	
	Luteinizing hormone	
	Thyroid-stimulating hormone	
Polypeptides	Adrenocorticotropic hormone	
	Antidiuretic hormone	
	Calcitonin	
	Endorphins	
	Glucagon	
	Hypothalamic hormones	
	Lipotropins	
	Melanocyte-stimulating hormone	
	Oxytocin	
	Somatostatin	
	Thymosin	
	Thyrotropin-releasing hormone	
Amines	Epinephrine	
	Norepinephrine	
	Thyroxine (both thyroxine [T_4] and triiodothyronine [T_3])	
Lipid Soluble		
Steroids (cholesterol is a precursor for all steroids)	Estrogens	
	Glucocorticoids (cortisol)	
	Mineralocorticoids (aldosterone)	
	Progestins (progesterone)	
	Testosterone	
Derivatives of arachidonic acid (autocrine or paracrine action)	Leukotrienes	
	Prostacyclins	
	Prostaglandins	
	Thromboxanes	

Regulation of Hormone Release

The release of hormones occurs either in response to an alteration in the cellular environment or in the process of maintaining a regulated level of certain hormones or certain substances. Hormone release is regulated by chemical factors, endocrine or hormonal factors (a hormone from one endocrine gland controlling another endocrine gland), and neural control. Of these regulatory mechanisms, endocrine regulation by way of feedback circuits (systems) is one of the most important ways in which hormonal secretion is maintained within a physiologic range.

  Negative feedback is the most common type of feedback system. In a negative-feedback system, plasma levels of one type of hormone influence the level of other types of hor-

mones. An example of hormone negative feedback is shown in Figure 20-2, *A.* Increased anterior pituitary release of thyroid-stimulating hormone (TSH) stimulates the synthesis and secretion of thyroid hormones. TSH is inhibited by thyroxine (T_4) and to a lesser extent by triiodothyronine (T_3). TSH secretion is regulated by thyrotropin-releasing hormone primarily in the hypothalamus and by negative feedback inhibition from thyroid hormones.

Negative-feedback systems are important in maintaining hormones within physiologic ranges. The lack of negative-feedback inhibition on hormonal release often results in pathologic conditions. As discussed in Chapter 21, various hormonal imbalances and related conditions are caused by excessive hormone production, which is the result of failure to "turn off" the system. These negative-feedback regulatory systems are diagrammed in Figure 20-2, *B.*

An example of neural regulation is the release of epinephrine from the adrenal medulla as a result of activation of the sympathetic division of the autonomic nervous system in re-

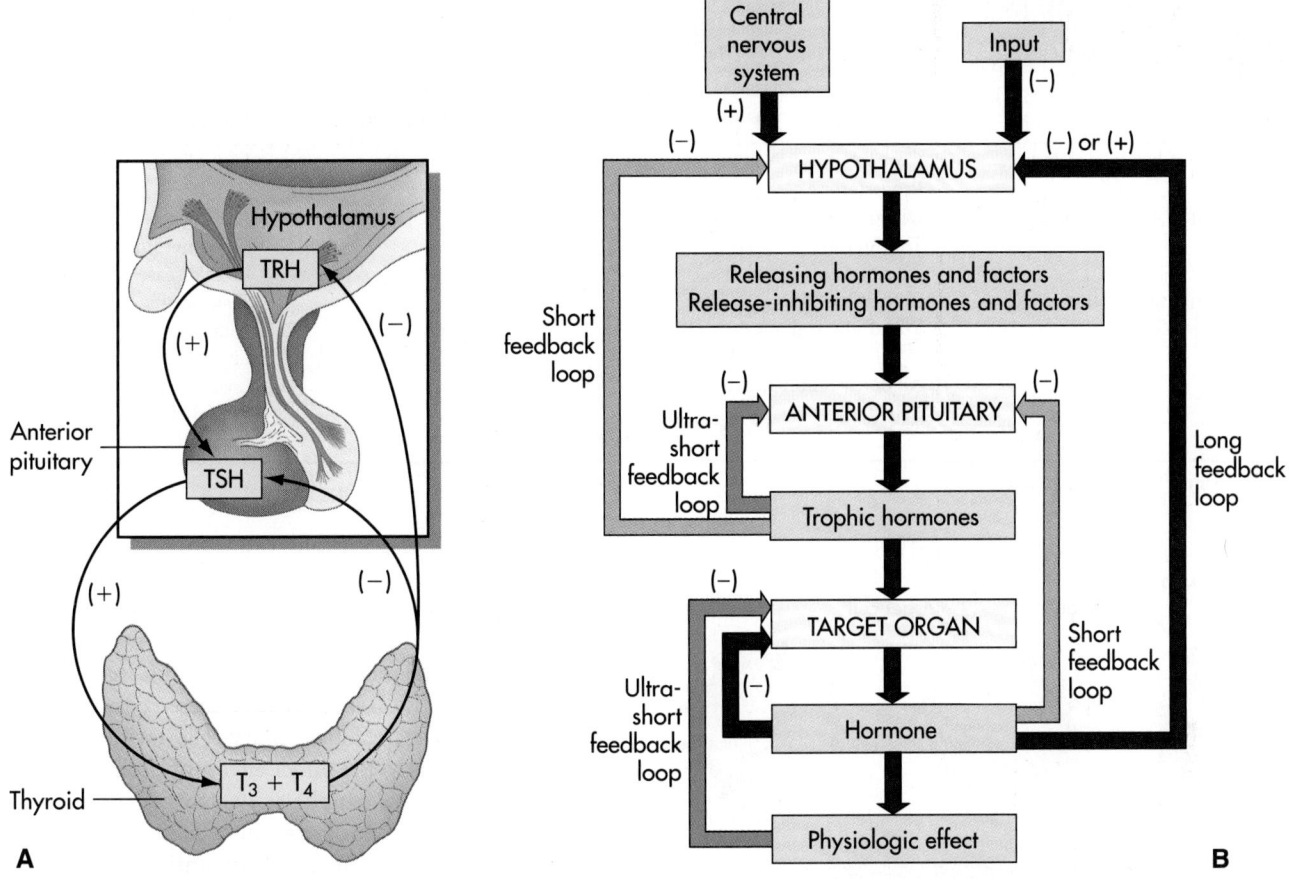

Figure 20-2 Feedback loops. A, Endocrine feedback loops involving the hypothalamus-pituitary gland and end organs, in this example, the thyroid gland (endocrine regulation). **B,** General model for control and negative feedback to hypothalamic–pituitary target organ systems. Negative-feedback regulation is possible at three levels: target organ (ultrashort feedback), anterior pituitary (short feedback), and hypothalamus (long feedback). *TRH,* Thyroid releasing hormone; *TSH,* thyroid stimulating hormone; T_3, triiodothyronine; T_4, tetraiodothyronine.

sponse to stress. When the stress is removed, the nervous stimulation decreases and less epinephrine is released.

Hormone Transport

Once hormones are released into the circulatory system by the endocrine glands, they are circulated throughout the body. Peptide or protein hormones (insulin, pituitary, hypothalamic, parathyroid) are water soluble and circulate in free (unbound) forms. Water-soluble hormones generally have a short half-life because they are catabolized by circulating enzymes. For example, insulin has a half-life of 3 to 5 minutes and is catabolized by insulinases. Lipid-soluble hormones, such as cortisol and adrenal androgens, are primarily circulated bound to a carrier or binding protein (Table 20-2). A small percentage of the lipid-soluble hormone circulates in a free or active form. For example, approximately 10% of the circulating cortisol is free, whereas 75% is bound to corticosteroid-binding globulin. A large change in the concentration of binding protein can affect the concentration of free hormone and, therefore, hormone effects (see Table 20-2). As discussed later, water-soluble hormones bind to one of four classes of cell surface receptors, whereas lipid-soluble hormones bind to plasma membrane receptors or diffuse

through the plasma membrane and bind to cytosolic or nuclear receptors.

Cellular Mechanisms of Hormone Action

When a hormone is released into the circulatory system, it is distributed throughout the body, but only those cells with appropriate receptors for that hormone are affected. The **target cell** hormone receptors have two main functions: (1) to recognize and bind with high affinity to their particular hormones and (2) to initiate a signal to appropriate intracellular effectors. See Chapter 1 for cell signaling pathways, particularly Figures 1-16 and 1-17 on page 18. The binding of hormones with their receptors generally stimulates three general types of responses by:

1. Acting on pre-existing channel forming proteins to alter membrane channel permeability
2. Activating pre-existing proteins through a second messenger system
3. Activating genes to cause protein synthesis

The sensitivity of the target cell to a particular hormone is related to the total number of receptors per cell. Low concentrations of hormone increase the number of receptors per cell; this is called **up-regulation** (Figure 20-3, *A*). High concentrations of

Table 20-2	Binding Proteins, Their Hormones, and Variables that Affect Their Circulating Levels		
Binding Protein	**Hormone**	**Factors that Increase Binding Protein Levels**	**Factors that Decrease Binding Protein Levels**
Corticosteroid-binding globulin	Cortisol Progesterone	Estrogen	Liver disease
Sex hormone–binding globulin	Dihydrotestosterone Testosterone Estradiol	—	Androgens Hypothyroidism Liver disease
Thyroid-binding globulin	Thyroxine (T_4) Triiodothyronine (T_3)	Estrogen Hyperthyroidism	Testosterone Glucocorticoids Liver disease
Albumin	All lipid-soluble hormones	Estrogen	Liver disease Malnutrition Renal disease

T_4, Thyroxine; T_3, triiodothyronine.

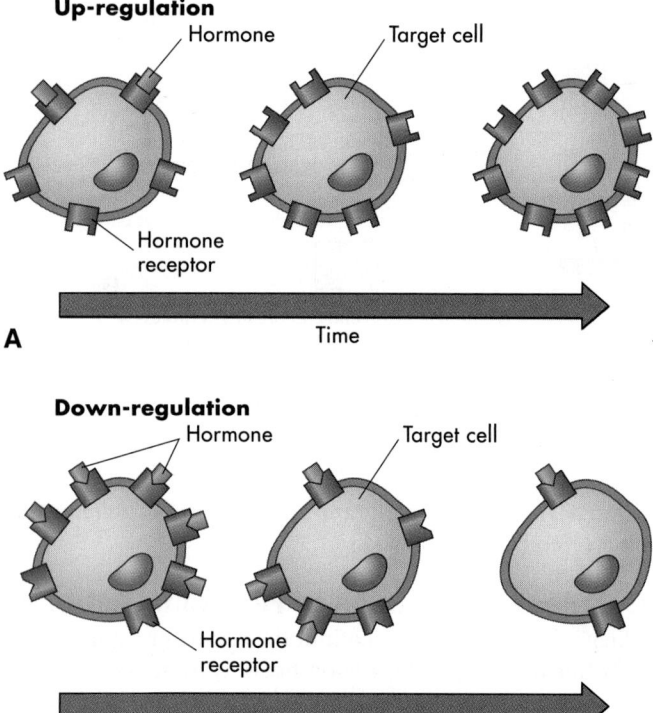

Figure 20-3 Regulation of target cell sensitivity. If synthesis of new receptors occurs faster than degradation of old receptors, the target cell will have more receptors and thus be more sensitive to the hormone. This phenomenon, **A**, often is called *up-regulation* because the number of receptors goes up. If the rate of receptor degradation exceeds the rate of receptor synthesis, the target cell's number of receptors will decrease, **B**. Because the number of receptors and thus the sensitivity of the target cell go down, this phenomenon often is called *down-regulation*. Shading in box represents hormone concentration. (Modified from Thibodeau GA, Patton KT: *Anatomy & physiology,* ed 5, St Louis, 2003, Mosby.)

hormone decrease the number of receptors; this is called **down-regulation** (Figure 20-3, *B*). Thus the cell can adjust its sensitivity to the concentration of the signaling hormone.

Hormones have two general types of effects on target cells: direct and permissive. **Direct effects** are the obvious changes in cell function that specifically result from stimulation by a particular hormone. **Permissive effects** are less obvious hormone-induced changes that facilitate the maximal response or functioning of a cell. For example, insulin has a direct effect on skeletal muscle cells with insulin receptors, causing increased glucose transport into these cells. Insulin also has a permissive effect on mammary cells, facilitating the response of these cells to the direct effects of prolactin.

Some hormones have biphasic pharmacologic effects that are dependent on the concentration of the hormone. For example, low or physiologic levels of antidiuretic hormone (ADH or arginine vasopressin; i.e., levels that are secreted in response to dehydration) stimulate renal tubular reabsorption of sodium and water. However, at supraphysiologic levels (i.e., those that can be achieved by exogenous administration), ADH acts as a vasoconstrictor.

Hormone Receptors

Hormone receptors may be located in or on the plasma membrane or in the intracellular compartment of the target cell. Water-soluble hormones (see Table 20-1) have a high molecular weight and cannot diffuse across the cell membrane. They interact or bind with receptors in or on the cell membrane. Steroid hormones are lipid soluble. These hormones easily diffuse across the plasma membrane and bind to either cytosolic or nuclear receptors. The hormone–receptor complex binds to a specific region in the deoxyribonucleic acid (DNA) and alters the expression of a specific gene (Figure 20-4). The recent discovery of nongenomic rapid actions of steroid hormones indicates plasma membrane receptors that activate second messenger systems are also present.[1-3] (Types of hormones, their corresponding receptors, and the mechanisms by which they affect the cell are summarized in Table 20-3.)

Plasma Membrane Receptors and Signal Transduction

First Messenger

Receptors for most water-soluble hormones are located on the plasma membrane of a target cell. Sometimes a hormone or ligand that binds to a receptor is referred to as a **first mes-**

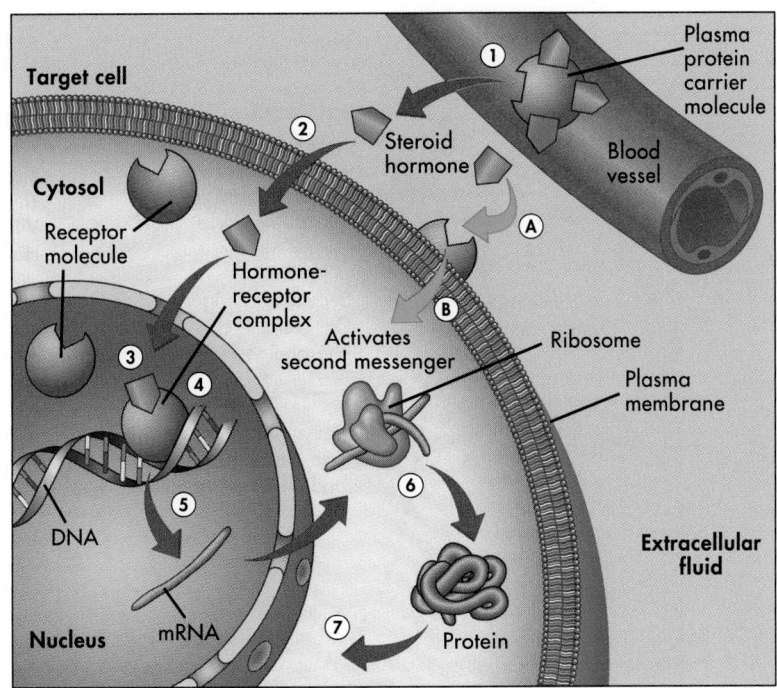

Figure 20-4 Steroid hormone mechanism. Lipid-soluble steroid hormone molecules detach from the carrier protein *(1)* and pass through the plasma membrane *(2)*. Hormone molecules then diffuse into the nucleus where they bind to a receptor to form a hormone–receptor complex *(3)*. This complex then binds to a specific site on a deoxyribonucleic acid (DNA) molecule *(4)*, triggering transcription of the genetic information encoded there *(5)*. The resulting messenger ribonucleic acid (mRNA) molecule moves to the cytosol, where it associates with a ribosome, initiating synthesis of a new protein *(6)*. This new protein—usually an enzyme or channel protein—produces specific effects on the target cell *(7)*. The classical genomic action is typically slow *(red arrows)*. Steroids also may exact rapid effects by binding to receptors on the plasma membrane *(A)* and activating an intercellular second messenger *(B)*. (Modified from Thibodeau GA, Patton KT: *Anatomy & physiology*, ed 5, St Louis, 2003, Mosby.)

Table 20-3	Types of Hormones, Their Receptors, and Their Mechanisms of Action	
Hormone	**Type of Receptor**	**Mechanism of Action**
Water-Soluble Hormones		
Glycoproteins, amines, small peptides and proteins (except insulin)	Plasma membrane receptors	Second messengers; cAMP, cGMP, Ca^{++}, IP_3, DAG
Insulin	Plasma membrane receptors	Involves receptor autophosphorylation and activation of the receptor protein tyrosine kinase
Growth hormone, prolactin, ceptin	Plasma membrane receptors	Involves intracellular JAK and activation of STAT pathway
Lipid-Soluble Hormones		
Steroid hormones	Plasma membrane receptors	Rapid nongenomic action
	Nuclear receptors	Nuclear translocation and altered genome transcription
Thyroid hormones (iodothyronines)	Nuclear receptor	Altered genome transcription
	Cytosolic receptors	

cAMP, Cyclic adenosine monophosphate; *cGMP,* cyclic guanosine monophosphate; *IP_3,* inositol triphosphate; *DAG,* diacylglycerol; *JAK,* Janus family of tyrosine kinases; *STAT,* signal transducers and activators of transcription.

senger. This is because a hormone binding to its specific receptor represents the first signal within an elaborate signal transduction cascade. **Signal transduction** is the process by which extracellular signals (e.g., hormones) are communicated into a cell. In general, signal transduction involves a series of steps that includes receptor activation or binding of a hormone to its receptor, activation of a G protein (transducer) and membrane-associated enzyme (effector enzyme), and production of a second messenger (Figure 20-5). The final event is activation of an intracellular enzyme, such as pro-

tein kinase A or C, usually leading to alterations in gene transcription.

The signal transduction process begins at the receptor, which is a protein. Receptors on the plasma membrane are continuously synthesized and degraded, so the receptor number can vary from one cell type to another. Various physiochemical conditions can affect both the receptor number and the affinity at which the hormone binds to its receptor. Some of these physiochemical conditions are the fluidity and structure of the plasma membrane, pH,

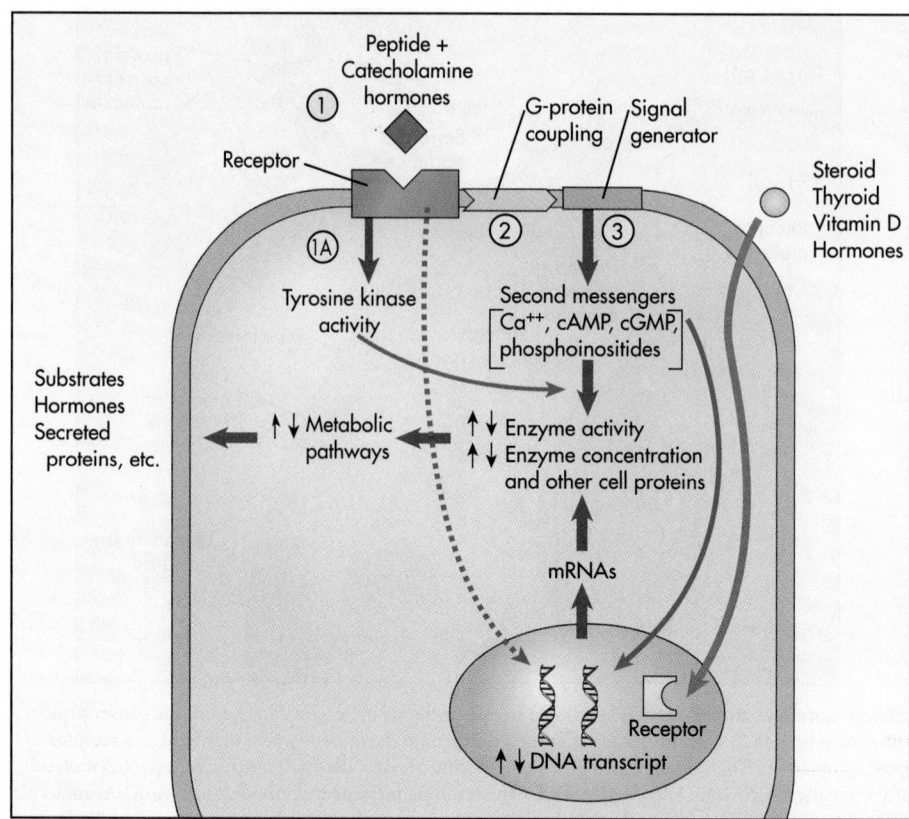

Figure 20-5 **Example of a second-messenger mechanism.** Hormones interact with either the plasma membrane or intracellular receptors. Hormones may generate second messengers within the receptor (e.g., tyrosine kinase activity), cytoplasm (e.g., cyclic AMP [cAMP]), or nucleus (i.e., gene expression). Metabolic pathways can be regulated by altering the activities or concentrations of enzymes. Cell growth and architecture also may be modulated. *cGMP*, Cyclic guanosine monophosphate; *mRNA*, messenger ribonucleic acid; *DNA*, deoxyribonucleic acid. (From Berne RM, Levy ML: *Principles of physiology*, ed 3, St Louis, 2000, Mosby.

temperature, ion concentration, diet, and the presence of other chemicals (e.g., drugs).

Cell surface receptors usually are classified according to their function: (1) G protein–linked receptors, (2) ion-channel receptors, and (3) enzyme-linked receptors (including tyrosine-kinase and the cytokine-receptor superfamily with intrinsic enzyme activity—such as the Janus family of tyrosine kinases [JAK] and signal tranducers and activators of transcription [STAT] molecules). With the exception of insulin, growth hormone, and prolactin, most water-soluble hormones—such as adrenocorticotropic hormone (ACTH), glucagon, norepinephrine, and epinephrine—activate G protein–linked receptors. Other hormones, such as angiotensin II, activate both G protein–linked and ion-channel receptors. Insulin activates a tyrosine-kinase receptor. Growth hormones, prolactin, and cytokines—such as interleukins—activate the JAK/STAT receptors.

Second-Messenger Molecules: cAMP, Ca++, and cGMP

Cyclic Adenosine Monophosphate (cAMP). Second-messenger molecules are the initial link between the first signal (hormone) and the inside of the cell (Table 20-4). For example, binding of epinephrine to a β-adrenergic receptor subtype activates (through a stimulatory G protein [G_s]) the

enzyme adenylyl cyclase. Adenylyl cyclase catalyzes the conversion of adenosine triphosphate (ATP) to the second messenger, 3′,5′-cAMP. Elevation of cAMP activates the enzyme cAMP-dependent *protein kinase A (PKA)*. Kinase enzymes, by adding a phosphate moiety to cellular proteins, either activate or deactivate intracellular proteins or enzymes. In cardiac muscle, cAMP-dependent protein kinase phosphorylation of cellular membrane proteins associated with the L-type channel increase the influx of Ca^{++} into the cell. Increased intracellular Ca^{++} levels increase myocardial contractility. The actions of cAMP are terminated by the enzyme phosphodiesterase (PDE) III, which hydrolyzes cAMP into inactive adenosine monophosphate (AMP).

Calcium (Ca++). In addition to being an important ion that participates in a multitude of cellular actions, calcium (Ca^{++}) is also considered an important second messenger. The binding of a hormone (such as norepinephrine or angiotensin II) to a surface receptor activates the enzyme *phospholipase C* through a G protein inside the plasma membrane. This enzyme breaks down membrane phospholipid phosphatidylinositol biphosphate (PIP_2) into second messengers **inositol triphosphate (IP_3)** and **diacylglycerol (DAG)** (Figure 20-6). IP_3 mobilizes Ca^{++} from intracellular stores (endoplasmic reticulum). In several cell types an increase in intra-

Table 20-4	Second Messengers Identified for Specific Hormones
Second Messenger	**Associated Hormones**
Cyclic AMP	Adrenocorticotropic hormone (ACTH)
	Luteinizing hormone (LH)
	Human chorionic gonadotropin (hCG)
	Follicle-stimulating hormone (FSH)
	Thyroid-stimulating hormone (TSH)
	Antidiuretic hormone (ADH)
	Thyrotropin-releasing hormone (TRH)
	Parathyroid hormone (PTH)
	Glucagon
Cyclic GMP	Atrial natriuretic peptide
Calcium	Angiotensin II
	Gonadotropin-releasing hormone (GnRN)
	Antidiuretic hormone (ADH)
IP₃ and DAG	Angiotensin II
	Antidiuretic hormone (ADH)
	Luteinizing hormone-releasing hormone (LHRH)
Tyrosine phosphorylation	
Tyrosine kinase	Insulin
JAK-STAT	Growth hormone
	Leptin
	Prolactin

AMP, Adenosine monophosphate; *GMP,* guanosine monophosphate; *IP₃,* inositol triphosphate; *DAG,* diacylglycerol; *JAK,* Janus family of tyrosine kinases; *STAT,* signal transducers and activators of transcription.

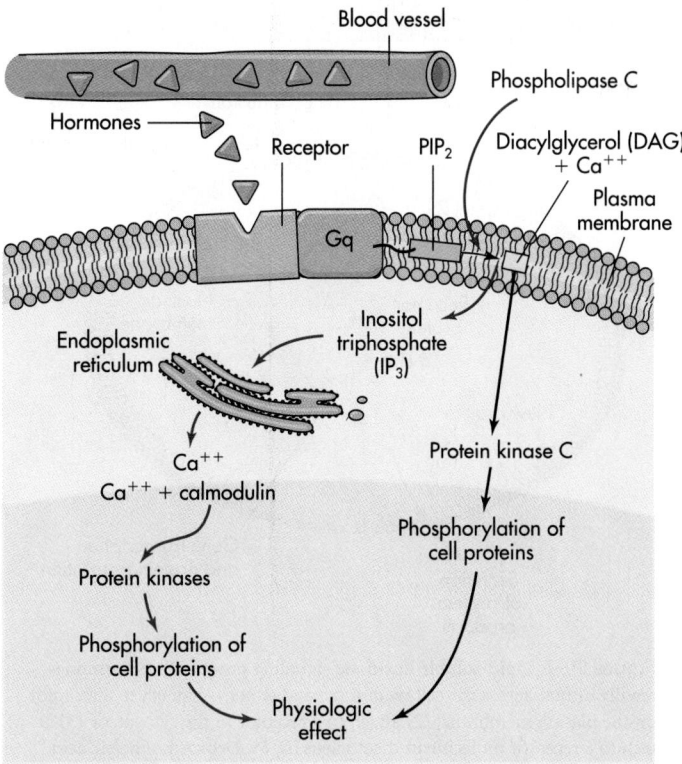

Figure 20-6 Calcium (Ca⁺⁺), inositol triphosphate (IP3), and diacylglycerol (DAG) as second messengers. See text for details. *Gq,* G protein; *PIP₂,* phosphatidylinositol biphosphate.

cellular Ca^{++} activates specific physiologic effects. For example, when Ca^{++} binds with intracellular calmodulin, the Ca^{++}-calmodulin complex activates specific proteins.

DAG, together with Ca^{++}, activates *protein kinase C (PKC)*. Similar to other kinase enzymes, PKC either activates (by phosphorylation) or deactivates (dephosphorylates) other proteins or enzymes. PKC initiates a variety of cellular responses that are linked to cell metabolism and growth. For example, PKC activates glycogen synthase in liver cells to convert glucose to glycogen.

Cyclic Guanosine Monophosphate (cGMP). The production of the second messenger 3′,5′-cGMP is associated with the activation of the intracellular enzyme guanylyl cyclase. cGMP activates cGMP-dependent kinase, which in turn activates a number of physiologic processes. The effects of various ligands, such as atrial natriuretic factor and nitric oxide (endothelium-derived relaxing factor), are mediated by the second messenger cGMP. A summary of second messenger systems is presented in Figure 20-5.

Steroid (Lipid-Soluble) Hormones
The lipid-soluble hormones are classified as steroid hormones and include androgens, estrogens, progestins, glucocorticoids, mineralocorticoids, and thyroid hormones. Steroid hormones are relatively small hydrophobic molecules (synthesized from

cholesterol) and therefore cross the plasma membrane by simple diffusion (see Chapter 1). Some steroid hormones bind to receptor molecules in the cytoplasm and then diffuse into the nucleus, whereas others bind to receptors in the nucleus. The resulting hormone–receptor complex binds to a specific site on the promoter region of deoxyribonucleic acid (DNA). This binding activates ribonucleic acid (RNA) polymerase, which stimulates DNA transcription and increased synthesis of specific proteins (increased gene expression) (Figure 20-7). Modulation of gene expression can take hours to days.

Recent studies indicate there are steroid hormone receptors in the plasma membrane associated with rapid response (seconds or minutes) that have nongenomic and genomic effects. The receptors are still being identified; the nongenomic actions involve many second messengers. Cross talk between gene transcription and nongenomic responses modulate each other allowing cells to adapt rapidly to environmental changes.[2,4-6]

STRUCTURE AND FUNCTION OF THE ENDOCRINE GLANDS

Hypothalamic–Pituitary Axis
The hypothalamic–pituitary axis forms one of the most important and prominent portions of the endocrine system. The hypothalamic–pituitary axis produces a number of

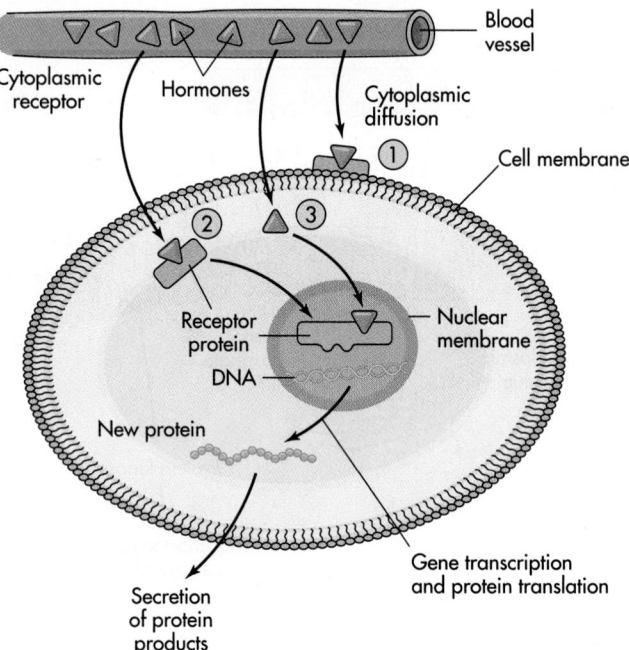

Figure 20-7 **Lipid-soluble hormone signaling process.** Free hormones readily diffuse across the cell membrane and either *(1)* attach to a receptor on the plasma membrane, *(2)* attach to a receptor in the cytosol, or *(3)* attach to a receptor molecule in the nucleus. *DNA,* Deoxyribonucleic acid.

releasing/inhibitory hormones and tropic hormones, respectively, that affect a number of diverse body functions (Figure 20-8). For example, the functions of the thyroid gland, adrenal gland, and male and female reproductive glands, as well as somatic growth and lactation, are regulated by hormones originating from the hypothalamic–pituitary axis.

Hypothalamus

The hypothalamus is divided into several nuclei and nuclear areas and is located at the base of the brain (Figures 20-9 and 20-11). The pituitary gland is located at the sella turcica (a saddle-shaped depression on the superior surface of the sphenoid bone). The communication or anatomic connection (blood vessels and neural tract) between the hypothalamus and anterior and posterior pituitary is quite elaborate and well described. However, simply described, the hypothalamus is connected to the anterior pituitary by way of portal hypophysial blood vessels (Figure 20-10), whereas the hypothalamus is connected to the posterior pituitary by way of a nerve tract referred to as the *hypothalamohypophysial tract* (Figure 20-11). These connections are vital to the functioning of the hypothalamus–pituitary system. For example, first, ADH and oxytocin are synthesized in hypothalamic neurons but are stored and secreted by the posterior pituitary. ADH and oxy-

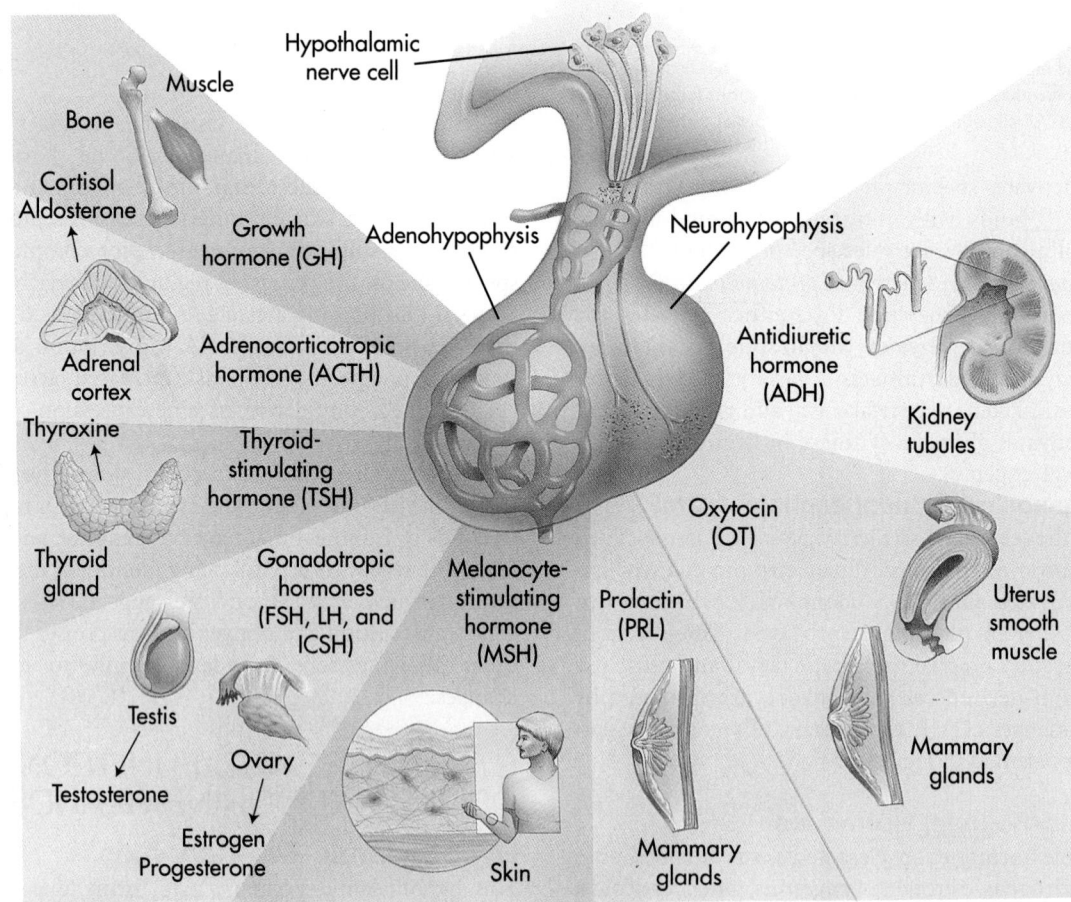

Figure 20-8 **Pituitary hormones and their target organs.** *FSH,* Follicle-stimulating hormone; *LH,* luteinizing hormone; *ICSH,* male analog of LH (interstitial cell–stimulating hormone). (Modified from Thibodeau GA, Patton K: *Anatomy & physiology,* ed 5, St Louis, 2003, Mosby.)

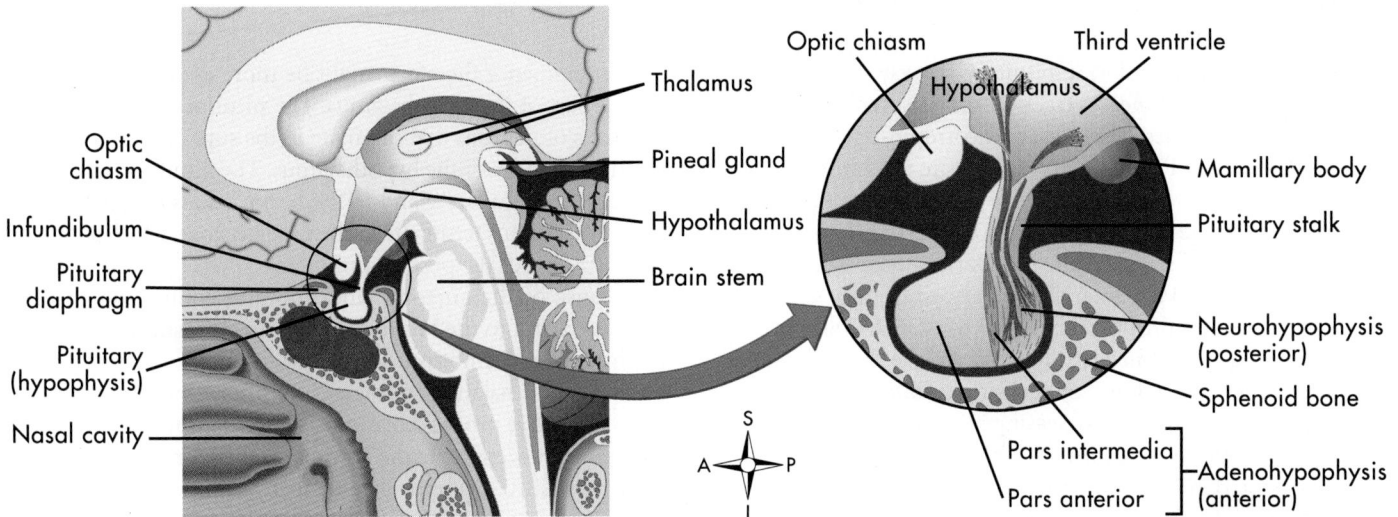

Figure 20-9 Location and structure of the pituitary gland (hypophysis). The pituitary gland is located within the sella turcica of the skull's sphenoid bone and is connected to the hypothalamus by a stalklike infundibulum. The infundibulum passes through a gap in the portion of the dura mater that covers the pituitary (the pituitary diaphragm). The inset shows that the pituitary is divided into an anterior portion, the adenohypophysis, and a posterior portion, the neurohypophysis. The adenohypophysis is further subdivided into the pars anterior and pars intermedia. The pars intermedia is almost absent in the adult pituitary. (Modified from Thibodeau GA, Patton KT: *Anatomy & physiology,* ed 5, St Louis, 2003, Mosby.)

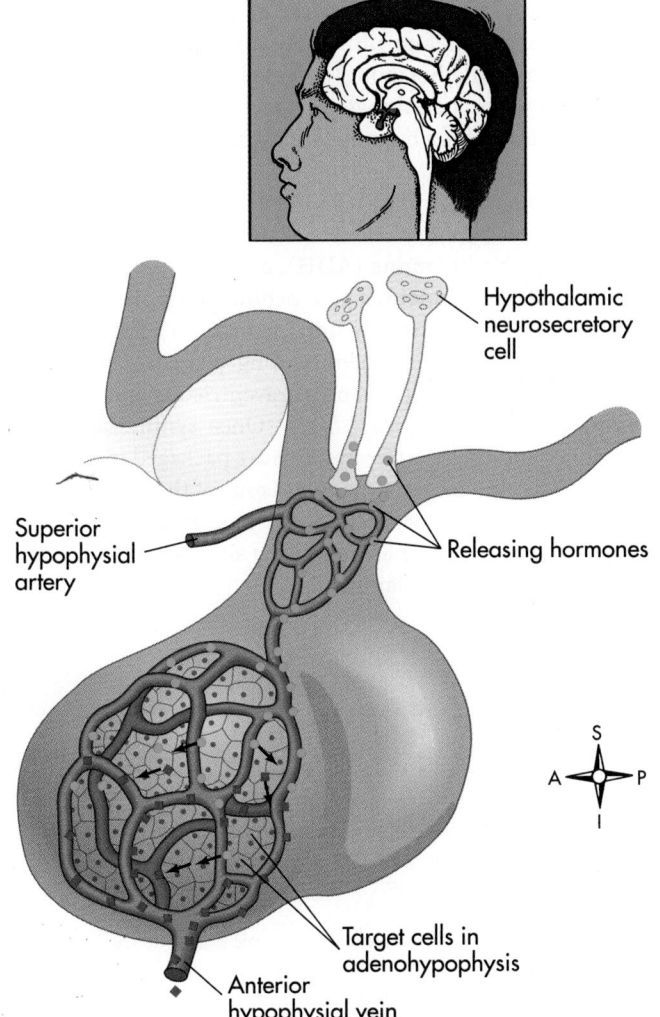

Figure 20-10 Hypophysial portal system. Neurons in the hypothalamus secrete releasing hormones into veins that carry the releasing hormones directly to the vessels of the adenohypophysis, thus bypassing the normal circulatory route. (From Thibodeau GA, Patton KT: *Anatomy & physiology,* ed 5, St Louis, 2003, Mosby.)

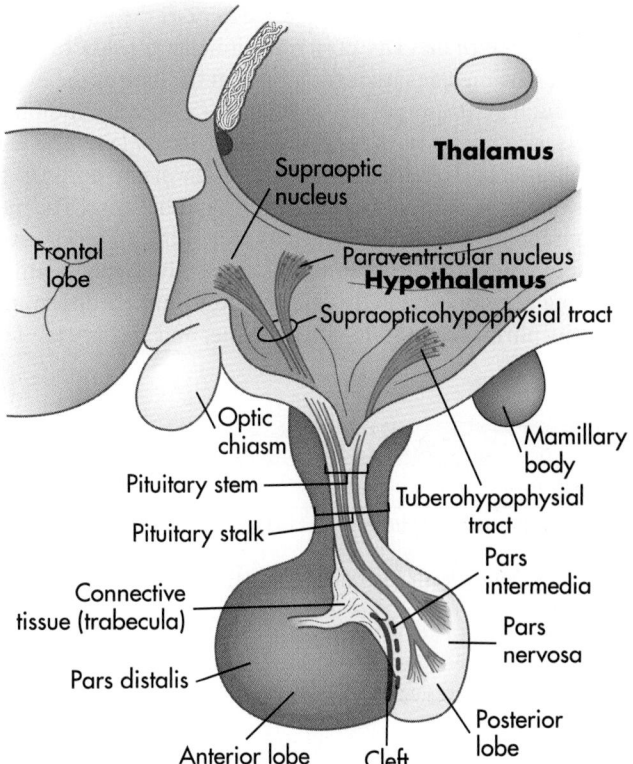

Figure 20-11 Nerve tracts from hypothalamus to posterior lobe of pituitary gland.

tocin travel to the posterior pituitary by way of the hypothalamohypophysial nerve tract. Second, several releasing/inhibitory hormones, such as corticotropin-releasing hormone (CRH) (see Figure 20-18, p. 672), are synthesized in the hypothalamus and control the release of tropic hormones, such as ACTH, from the anterior pituitary (Table 20-5). These releasing hormones are secreted into the portal hypophysial blood vessels and travel to the anterior pituitary, where they stimulate the secretion of tropic hormones such as ACTH. Other releasing/inhibiting hormones synthesized in the hypothalamus that influence the release of anterior pituitary tropic hormones include thyrotropin-releasing hormone (TRH), growth hormone–releasing hormone (GHRH), gonadotropin-releasing hormone (GnRH), somatostatin, dopamine, and substance P. These are also referred to as the **hypophysiotropic hormones.**

Pituitary Gland

The **anterior pituitary** (adenohypophysis) accounts for 75% of the total weight of the pituitary gland. It is composed of three regions: (1) the pars distalis, (2) the pars tuberalis, and (3) the pars intermedia. The **pars distalis** is the major component of the anterior pituitary and the source of the anterior pituitary hormones. The **pars tuberalis** is a thin layer of cells on the anterior and lateral portions of the pituitary stalk. The **pars intermedia** lies between the two lobes of the pituitary gland. In the adult the distinct intermediate lobe disappears, and the individual cells are distributed diffusely throughout the pars distalis and pars nervosa (neural lobe).[7]

The **posterior pituitary** (neurohypophysis) arises embryologically from an outpouching of the floor of the third ventricle within the brain. The posterior pituitary consists of three parts: (1) the median eminence located at the base of the hypothalamus, (2) the pituitary stalk, and (3) the infundibular process, also known as the *pars nervosa* or *neural lobe*. The **median eminence** is composed largely of the nerve endings of axons that arise primarily in the ventral hypothalamus. The median eminence often is designated as part of the posterior pituitary but contains at least 10 biologically active hypothalamic-releasing hormones, as well as the neurotransmitters dopamine, norepinephrine, serotonin, acetylcholine, and histamine. The

median eminence therefore might be more appropriately considered part of the hypothalamus. The **pituitary stalk** contains the axons of neurons that originate in the supraoptic and paraventricular nuclei of the hypothalamus. The pituitary stalk thus connects the pituitary gland to the brain. Axons originating in the hypothalamus terminate in the **pars nervosa,** which secretes the hormones of the posterior pituitary.

Because of the anatomic location and connection of the pituitary gland to the brain, several neurotransmitters as well as physical and emotional stressors influence the release of specific hypothalamic releasing/inhibitory hormones and their respective tropic hormones. For example, the neurotransmitter norepinephrine stimulates the secretion of CRH, TRH, and GnRH, whereas the neurotransmitter γ-aminobutyric acid (GABA) inhibits CRH, TRH, and GnRH secretion. In terms of tropic hormone release from the anterior pituitary, norepinephrine stimulates the secretion of thyroid-stimulating hormone (TSH), growth hormone (GH), luteinizing hormone (LH), and follicle-stimulating hormone (FSH), whereas the secretion of ACTH is inhibited. Physical (trauma) and emotional (pain) stress, as well as hypoglycemia, can influence the release of stimulating hormones such as CRH, therefore ultimately affecting the amount of ACTH (the tropic hormone) released by the anterior pituitary. This example emphasizes the integrated and coordinated function of the hypothalamic–pituitary axis.

Hormones of the Posterior Pituitary

The posterior pituitary secretes two polypeptide hormones: (1) **antidiuretic hormone (ADH),** also called *arginine vasopressin,* and (2) **oxytocin.** These peptide hormones are similar in structure, differing by only two amino acids. They are synthesized, along with their binding proteins, the neurophysins, in the supraoptic and paraventricular nuclei of the hypothalamus (see Figure 20-11). Once synthesized, these hormones and their carrier proteins are packaged in secretory vesicles. They are moved down the axons of the pituitary stalk to the pars nervosa for storage. The posterior pituitary thus can be seen as a storage and releasing site for hormones synthesized in the hypothalamus.

Table 20-5	Hypothalamic Hormones (Hypophysiotropic Hormones)	
Hormone	**Target Tissue**	**Action**
Thyrotropin-releasing hormone (TRH)	Anterior pituitary	Stimulates release of thyroid-stimulating hormone (TSH) Modulates prolactin secretion
Gonadotropin-releasing hormone (GnRH)	Anterior pituitary	Stimulates release of follicle-stimulating hormone (FSH) and luteinizing hormone (LH)
Somatostatin	Anterior pituitary	Inhibits release of growth hormone (GH) and TSH
Growth hormone–releasing hormone (GHRH)	Anterior pituitary	Stimulates release of GH
Corticotropin-releasing hormone (CRH)	Anterior pituitary	Stimulates release of adrenocorticotropic hormone (ACTH) and β-endorphin
Substance P	Anterior pituitary	Inhibits synthesis and release of ACTH Stimulates secretion of GH, FSH, LH, and prolactin
Dopamine	Anterior pituitary	Inhibits synthesis and secretion of prolactin
Prolactin-releasing factors (PRF)	Anterior pituitary	Stimulates secretion of prolactin

Similar to the anterior pituitary hormones, the release of ADH and oxytocin is influenced by neurotransmitter release. In well-defined areas within the hypothalamus and other brain stem areas, norepinephrine–containing fibers innervate vasopressin and oxytocin neurons. Stimulation of these areas results in an increase in ADH and oxytocin release.

Antidiuretic Hormone

The major homeostatic function of the posterior pituitary is the control of plasma osmolality, as regulated by ADH, or arginine vasopressin (see Chapter 3). At physiologic levels, ADH acts to increase the permeability of renal collecting ducts (see Chapter 35). This increased permeability leads to an increase in water reabsorption and the production of more concentrated urine. These effects may be inhibited by hypercalcemia, prostaglandin E, and hypokalemia. ADH has no direct effect on electrolyte levels.

ADH originally was named *vasopressin* because in extremely high doses it does cause vasoconstriction and a resulting increase in arterial blood pressure. These levels are not reached physiologically, but this effect may be achieved pharmacologically. For example, high doses of ADH (as the drug vasopressin) may be administered to achieve hemostasis during hemorrhage.

The secretion of ADH is regulated primarily by the osmoreceptors of the hypothalamus, located near or in the supraoptic nuclei (osmoreceptors are stimulated by increased osmolality). The plasma osmolality is maintained at the mean set point of approximately 280 mOsm/kg. As plasma osmolality increases, the rate of ADH secretion increases.

Other mechanisms also affect ADH secretion. ADH secretion is increased by changes in intravascular volume. Intravascular volume changes are monitored by mechanoreceptors in the left atrium and in the carotid and aortic arches. A volume loss of 7% to 25% acts through these receptors to stimulate ADH secretion. This mechanism for regulating ADH secretion is much less sensitive than that of the osmoreceptors. Stress, trauma, pain, exercise, nausea, nicotine, exposure to heat, and drugs such as chloroform and morphine also increase ADH secretion, apparently by activating cholinergic neurotransmitters in the hypothalamus. ADH secretion decreases with a decrease in plasma osmolality, an increase in intravascular volume, hypertension, estrogen, progesterone, angiotensin II, and alcohol ingestion.

Oxytocin

Oxytocin is primarily responsible for contraction of the uterus and milk ejection in lactating women and may have a role in sperm motility in men, although this effect has not yet been clearly elucidated. In both genders, oxytocin has an antidiuretic effect similar to that of ADH. The mechanisms by which this effect is achieved appear to be similar to those of ADH, but the physiologic significance is not clear. (The function of this hormone is discussed in Chapter 22.)

The release of oxytocin has been studied more extensively in women than in men. In the woman, oxytocin is secreted in response to suckling and mechanical distention of the female reproductive tract. Oxytocin is required for the milk "let-down" reflex. Stimulated by sucking, oxytocin binds to its receptors on myoepithelial cells in the mammary tissues and causes contraction of those cells. This results in increased intramammary pressure and milk expression.

Oxytocin also acts on the uterus to stimulate contractions. Its role in initiating labor has been debated because levels of oxytocin do not increase until near the end of labor. However, it is used clinically to induce uterine contraction. It is hypothesized that near the end of labor oxytocin functions to enhance effectiveness of contractions, to promote delivery of the placenta, and to stimulate postpartum contractions to prevent excessive bleeding.[8]

Hormones of the Anterior Pituitary

The anterior pituitary is composed of two main cell types: (1) the **chromophobes,** which appear to be nonsecretory; and (2) the **chromophils,** which are considered the secretory cells of the adenohypophysis. The chromophils are subdivided into six secretory cell types, and each cell type secretes one or more specific hormones (Table 20-6).

The tropic hormones secreted by the anterior pituitary include ACTH, melanocyte-stimulating hormone (MSH), LH, GH, prolactin, FSH, and TSH. The actions of these anterior pituitary tropic hormones are summarized in Table 20-6. Even though six major stimulatory hormones are released by the anterior pituitary, they can be grouped into three categories: corticotropin-related hormones (ACTH, β-lipoprotein, MSH, and related endorphins), somatomammotropins (GH and prolactin), and glycoproteins (LH, FSH, and TSH). The corticotropin-related hormones are all derived from the precursor pro-opiomelanocortin (POMC). POMC is the precursor for ACTH and β-lipotropin; MSH exists within the ACTH amino acid sequence. β endorphin and metenkephalin are derived from β-lipotropin. In general, the regulation of the anterior pituitary hormones is achieved by (1) feedback of hypothalamic releasing/inhibitory hormones and factors, (2) feedback from target gland hormones (i.e., cortisol, estrogen), and (3) direct effects of neurotransmitters.

Thyroid and Parathyroid Glands

The thyroid gland, located in the neck just below the larynx, produces hormones that control the rates of metabolic processes throughout the body. The parathyroid glands are located near the posterior side of the thyroid. The four parathyroid glands function to control serum calcium levels.

Thyroid Gland

The **thyroid gland** is composed of two lobes that lie on either side of the trachea, inferior to the thyroid cartilage (Figure 20-12). The lobes are joined by a small band of tissue, the **isthmus,** which crosses the anterior surface of the trachea and larynx at the cricoid cartilage. The normal thyroid gland is not visible on inspection, but it may be palpated on swallowing, which causes upward displacement of the gland.

The thyroid gland is composed of **follicles** (Figure 20-13). The follicles are composed of follicular cells that surround a

Table 20-6	Tropic Hormones of the Anterior Pituitary and Their Functions		
Hormone	**Secretory Cell Type**	**Target Organs**	**Functions**
Adrenocorticotropic hormone (ACTH)	Corticotropic	Adrenal gland	Increased steroidogenesis Synthesis of adrenal proteins contributing to maintenance of the adrenal gland
Melanocyte-stimulating hormone (MSH)	Melanotropic	Anterior pituitary	Promotes secretion of melanin and lipotropin by anterior pituitary; makes skin darker
Somatotropic hormones			
Growth hormone (GH)	Somatotropic	Muscle, bone, liver	Regulates metabolic processes related to growth and adaptation to physical and emotional stressors, muscle growth, increased protein synthesis, increased liver glycogenolysis, increased fat mobilization
		Liver	Induces formation of somatomedins, or insulin-like growth factors (IGF) that have actions similar to insulin
Prolactin	Lactotropic	Breast	Milk production
Glycoprotein hormones			
Thyroid-stimulating hormone (TSH)	Thyrotropic	Thyroid gland	Increased production and secretion of thyroid hormone Increased iodide uptake
Luteinizing hormone (LH)	Gonadotropic	In women: granulosa cells In men: Leydig cells	Ovulation, progesterone production Testicular growth, testosterone production
Follicle-stimulating hormone (FSH)	Gonadotropic	In women: granulosa cells In men: Sertoli cells	Follicle maturation, estrogen production Spermatogenesis
β-Lipotropin	Corticotropic	Adipose cells	Fat breakdown and release of fatty acids
β-Endorphins	Corticotropic	Adipose cells Brain opioid receptors	Analgesia; may regulate body temperature, food and water intake

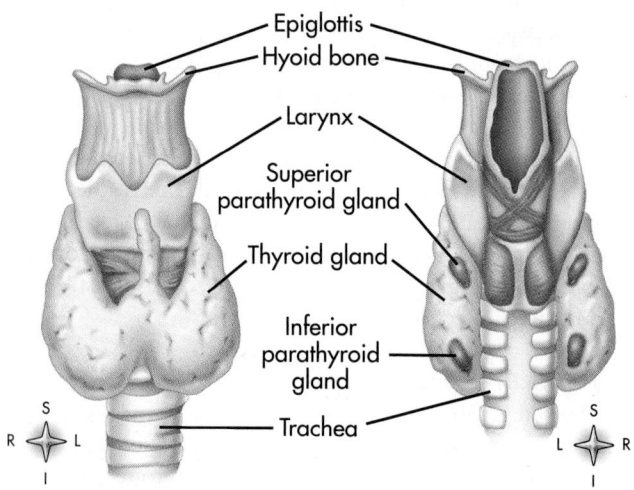

Figure 20-12 Thyroid and parathyroid glands. Note the relationship of the thyroid and parathyroid glands to each other, to the larynx (voice box), and to the trachea. (From Thibodeau GA, Patton KT: *Anatomy & physiology,* ed 5, St Louis, 2003, Mosby.)

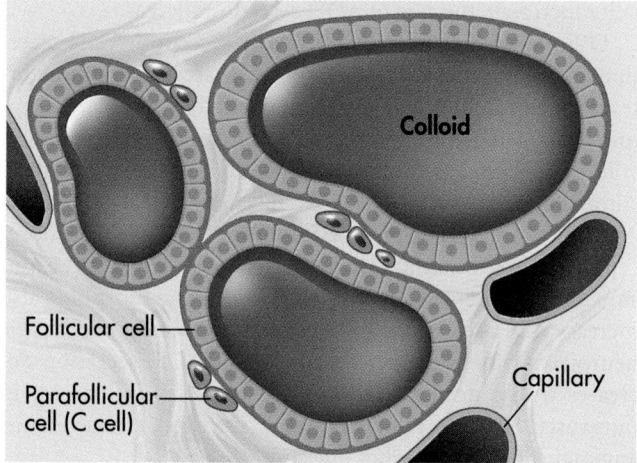

Figure 20-13 Thyroid follicle cells.

viscous substance called *colloid.* The follicular cells synthesize and secrete some of the thyroid hormones. Neurons terminate on blood vessels within the thyroid gland and on the follicular cells themselves. Acetylcholine, catecholamines, and other peptides directly affect secretory activity of the follicular cells and thyroid blood flow.[9]

Also found in the tissue of the thyroid are parafollicular cells, or **C cells** (see Figure 20-13). The C cells secrete various polypeptides, including calcitonin and somatostatin.[9] **Calcitonin,** also called *thyrocalcitonin,* acts to lower serum calcium levels by inhibition of bone-resorbing osteoclasts. High levels of calcitonin are required for these effects, and deficiencies of calcitonin do not lead to hypocalcemia. (Bone resorption is explained in Chapter 42.) Consequently, the metabolic consequences of calcitonin deficiency or excess does not appear to be significant in humans (Table 20-7). However, calcitonin is used for treatment of osteoporosis, Paget bone disease, hypercalcemia, osteogenesis imperfecta, and bone pain.[10,11]

Table 20-7	Thyroxine (T$_4$) and Triiodothyronine (T$_3$): Their Regulation and Function	
Regulation	**Functions**
T$_4$ and T$_3$ levels are controlled by TSH	Regulates protein, fat, and carbohydrate catabolism in all cells
Hormones show diurnal variation with a peak during late evening	Regulates metabolic rate of all cells
Influences on amount secreted	Regulates body heat production
Gender	Acts as insulin antagonist
Pregnancy	Maintains growth hormone secretion, skeletal maturation
Gonadal- and adrenal cortical–increased steroids = ↑ levels	Affects CNS development
Exposure to extreme cold = ↑ levels	Necessary for muscle tone and vigor
Nutritional state	Maintains cardiac rate, force, and output
Chemicals	Maintains secretion, motility, and absorption of GI tract
Somatostatin = ↓ levels	Affects respiratory rate and oxygen utilization
Dopamine = ↓ levels	Maintains calcium mobilization
Catecholamines = ↑ levels	Affects RBC production
	Stimulates lipid turnover, free fatty acid release, and cholesterol synthesis

TSH, Thyroid-stimulating hormone; *CNS,* central nervous system; *GI,* gastrointestinal; *RBC,* red blood cell.

Regulation of Thyroid Hormone Secretion

Thyroid hormone (TH) is regulated through a negative-feedback loop involving the hypothalamus, the anterior pituitary, and the thyroid gland (see Figure 20-2). (Figure 20-12 illustrates the thyroid and parathyroid glands.) The initiating hormone is termed **thyrotropin-releasing hormone (TRH),** and it is synthesized and stored within the hypothalamus. TRH is released into the hypothalamic–pituitary portal system and circulates to the anterior pituitary, where it stimulates the release of thyroid-stimulating hormone (TSH). TRH is increased with exposure to cold, stress, and decreased levels of thyroxine (T$_4$).

Thyroid-stimulating hormone (TSH) is a glycoprotein hormone synthesized and stored within the anterior pituitary. Once TSH is secreted by the anterior pituitary, it circulates to bind with TSH receptor sites located on the outer side of the thyroid cell's plasma membrane. The effects of TSH on the thyroid include (1) an immediate increase in the release of stored thyroid hormones, (2) an increase in iodide uptake and oxidation, (3) an increase in thyroid hormone synthesis, and (4) an increase in the synthesis and secretion of prostaglandins by the thyroid. Thyroid gland hormones and their regulation and function are summarized in Table 20-7.

When TH is secreted by the thyroid gland, it acts on the thyroid gland, the anterior pituitary, and the median eminence to regulate further TH production. Thyroid hormones have a negative-feedback effect and inhibit TRH and TSH, which decreases TH synthesis and secretion.

Synthesis of Thyroid Hormone

The thyroid gland is stimulated to produce thyroid hormone by pituitary TSH, by low serum iodide levels, or by drugs interfering with the thyroid gland's uptake of iodide from the blood. (Iodide is the inorganic or ionic form of iodine and is the form in which iodine enters the thyroid gland.) Iodide is oxidized to iodine in the presence of thyroidal peroxidase. The major naturally occurring source of iodine is seafood; in the United States iodine is added to salt and flour. Approximately 25% of ingested iodine is trapped by the thyroid gland.

Thyroid hormone synthesis is summarized in the following steps:

1. Uniodinated thyroglobulin (a large glycoprotein) is produced by the endoplasmic reticulum of the follicular cells.
2. Tyrosine is incorporated into the thyroglobulin as it is synthesized.
3. Iodide is actively transferred (pumped) from the blood into the colloid by carrier proteins located in the outer membrane of the follicular cells. This active transport system is called the *iodide trap* and is very efficient at accumulating the trace amounts of iodide from the blood.
4. Iodide quickly attaches to tyrosine within the thyroglobulin molecule.
5. Coupling of iodinated tyrosine forms thyroid hormones. Triiodothyronine (T$_3$) is formed from coupling of monoiodotyrosine (one iodine atom and tyrosine) and diiodotyrosine (two iodine atoms and tyrosine). Tetraiodothyronine (T$_4$) is formed from coupling of two diiodotyrosines.
6. Thyroid hormones are stored attached to thyroglobulin within the colloid until it is released into the circulation.

The thyroid gland normally produces 90% T$_4$ and 10% T$_3$. In the body tissues, however, T$_4$ is converted to T$_3$, and T$_3$ has the greatest metabolic effects. Once released into the circulation, T$_3$ and T$_4$ are transported bound to one of three carrier proteins: thyroxine-binding globulin, thyroxine-binding prealbumin (transthyretin), or albumin.

Thyroid hormones affect many body tissues, primarily by affecting growth and maturation of tissues. Similar to some steroid hormones, thyroid hormones bind to intracellular receptor complexes and then influence the genetic expression of specific proteins. Thyroid hormones also affect cell metabolism by altering protein, fat, and glucose metabolism and, as a result, heat production and oxygen consumption are increased.[12]

It is important to note that thyroid hormones exert a number of permissive effects on many organs, which are rather modest at physiologic thyroid hormone levels. However, these effects can become very pronounced when there is either high or low levels of circulating thyroid hormones. For example, in the heart, T_3 stimulates the synthesis of specific contractile proteins (e.g., α-myosin heavy chain), sarcolemmal ion pumps (Na^1-K^1–ATPase pump, Ca^{++}–ATPase pump) and membrane receptors (β-adrenergic receptors). Therefore in hyperthyroidism, which is associated with elevated levels of thyroid hormones, cardiac effects include increased heart rate and cardiac output, as well as the development of a cardiomyopathy. Thyroid hormones also affect the respiratory center, contributing to the normal hypoxic and hypercapnic drive. In severe hypothyroidism, ventilation can become very depressed. Thyroid hormone also stimulates bone resorption, and hyperthyroidism is associated with osteopenia, hypercalcemia, and hypercalciuria. Other manifestations of thyroid hormone alteration are explained in Chapter 21.

Parathyroid Glands

Two pairs of parathyroid glands normally are present. They are small and located behind the upper pole of the thyroid gland and behind the lower pole (see Figure 20-12). The number of parathyroid glands, however, may range from two to six.

The parathyroid glands produce **parathyroid hormone (PTH)**, a regulator of serum calcium. PTH is regulated primarily by the level of ionized plasma calcium, although how these regulatory mechanisms work is not precisely clear. Calcium also increases intraparathyroid destruction of PTH but apparently does not affect the rate of PTH synthesis.

Magnesium and phosphate levels also affect PTH secretion. Hypomagnesemia in persons with normal calcium levels acts as a mild stimulant to PTH secretion. In hypocalcemic persons, hypomagnesemia decreases PTH secretion. Hyperphosphatemia leads to hypocalcemia, probably because of calcium-phosphate precipitation in soft tissue and bone. Alterations in serum phosphate levels therefore may indirectly influence PTH secretion by affecting serum calcium levels (Figure 20-14). The overall effect of PTH is to decrease serum phosphate concentration.

Once the parathyroid gland is stimulated, PTH is secreted. On release, PTH enters the circulation in unbound form. The hormone attaches to plasma membrane receptors in target tissues, where the biologic effects of PTH are mediated primarily by activation of the adenylyl cyclase system (see Chapter 1).

PTH is the single most important factor in the regulation of serum calcium levels (Figure 20-15). To achieve regulation of serum calcium, PTH acts directly on bone and on the kidneys. In bone, PTH has at least two effects. The effect of intense acute stimulation involves the breakdown and resorption of bone (see Chapter 42). Chronic stimulation by PTH results in bone remodeling, a process in which bone is broken down and re-formed.

In the kidneys, PTH acts on its plasma membrane receptor in the distal and proximal tubules of the nephron to increase reabsorption of calcium and to decrease reabsorption of phosphorus, respectively. PTH also decreases proximal tubule reabsorption of bicarbonate. In the kidney, PTH stimulates the synthesis of a biologically active form of vitamin D (1,25 dihydroxy vitamin D), a potent stimulator of calcium and phosphate absorption in the intestine. In this way PTH apparently increases gastrointestinal absorption of calcium.

Endocrine Pancreas

The **pancreas** is both an endocrine gland that produces hormones and an exocrine gland that produces digestive enzymes. (The exocrine pancreas is discussed in Chapter 38.) The pancreas therefore is responsible for much metabolism within the body. A major disorder of the endocrine pancreas is diabetes mellitus.

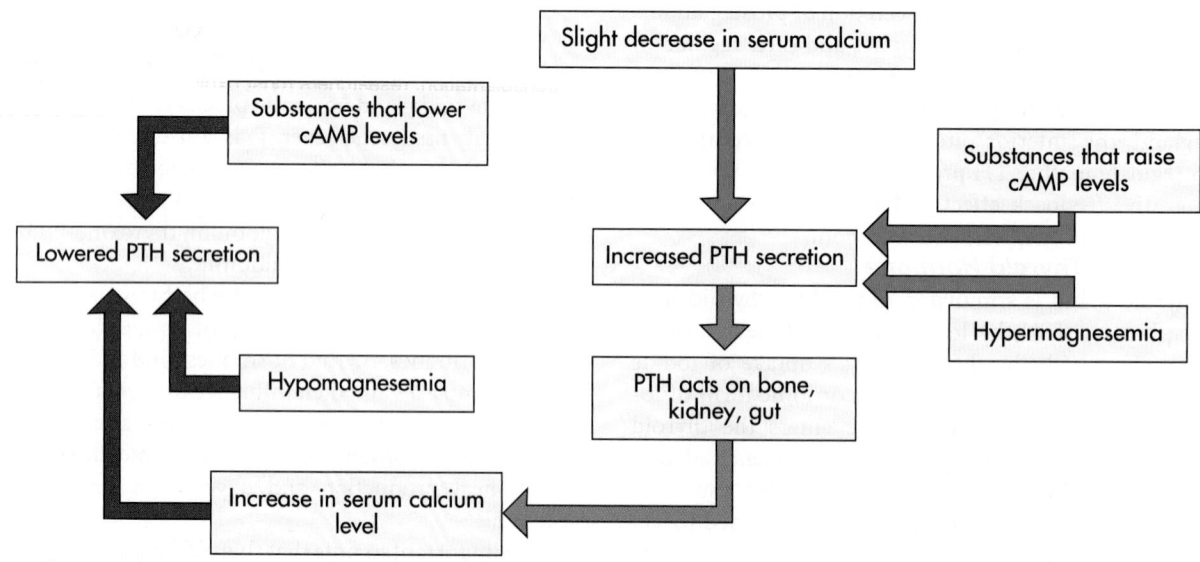

Figure 20-14 Variables affecting parathyroid hormone (PTH) secretion. *cAMP,* Cyclic adenosine monophosphate.

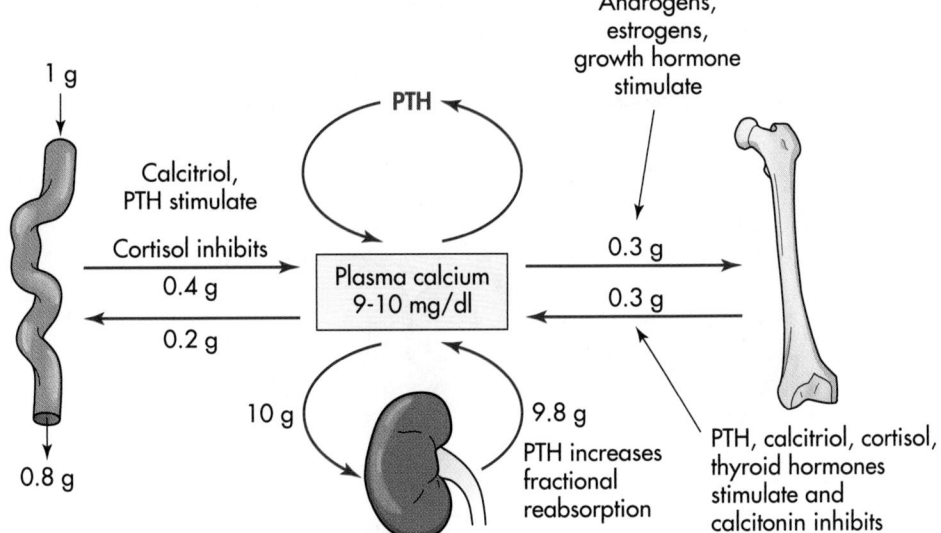

Figure 20-15 Normal calcium metabolism regulated by parathyroid hormone (PTH). (Redrawn from Porterfield SP: *Endocrine physiology*, ed 2, 2001, Mosby.)

The pancreas is located behind the stomach, between the spleen and the duodenum. It houses the **islets of Langerhans,** which secrete **glucagon** and **insulin,** hormones that help to regulate much of the carbohydrate metabolism within the body. The islets of Langerhans have three types of hormone-secreting cells: alpha cells, which secrete glucagon; beta cells, which secrete insulin; and delta cells, which secrete somatostatin and gastrin. The alpha cells and delta cells are located at the periphery of the islet, and beta cells are located in the middle. F cells, a fourth type of pancreatic cell, secrete pancreatic polypeptide. (The pancreas is illustrated in Figure 20-16.) Nerves from both divisions of the autonomic nervous system innervate the pancreatic islets.

The parasympathetic nervous system stimulates hormonal secretion and the sympathetic nervous system inhibits secretion. The perfusion of the anterior lobe of the pancreas where alpha, beta, and delta cells are most numerous comes from branches of the superior mesenteric artery. The posterior lobe is perfused by branches of the celiac artery. The pancreatic islets receive 10% of the pancreatic blood flow but represent only 1% of pancreatic mass. This is necessary for oxygenation and delivery of islet hormones to target cells.

Insulin

The **beta cells** of the pancreas synthesize insulin from the precursor, proinsulin. Proinsulin is formed from a larger and earlier precursor molecule, preproinsulin. Proinsulin is composed of an A peptide and a B peptide connected by a C peptide and two disulfide bonds. C peptide is cleaved by proteolytic enzymes, leaving the A and B peptide chains connected by the disulfide bonds. The bonded A and B chains become insulin. Insulin circulates freely in the plasma and is not bound to a carrier.

Secretion of insulin is regulated by chemical, hormonal, and neural control. Insulin secretion is promoted by increased blood levels of glucose, amino acids (arginine and ly-

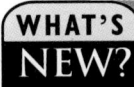

WHAT'S NEW? **Diabetes and Pancreatic Islet Cell Transplant**

Whole pancreas transplantation can effectively restore endogenous insulin secretion and achieve long-term normoglycemia in people with type 1 diabetes mellitus. The development of new procedures and new immunosuppressive therapies for pancreatic transplant during the past two decades has contributed to the prevention, delay, or reversal of diabetic complications. However, the secondary complications of long-standing diabetes are often irreversible at the time of whole organ transplant.

Pancreatic islet transplantation provides a safer and less invasive alternative for beta cell replacement and can be implemented earlier in the course of diabetes to prevent the development of secondary complications. Research is in progress to promote longevity of transplanted pancreatic islets and the further development of immunosuppressive regimens that are not toxic to the islets, which would prevent recurrent autoimmune destruction of the transplanted pancreatic beta cells.

Because of the lack of available cadaveric islet cells for transplantation, researchers must explore alternative sources of graft material. Cell engineering of non-beta cells and selective expansion of stem cells are key potential sources. For pancreatic islet cell transplant to be successful as a standard therapy for type 1 diabetes mellitus, the shortage of suitable donor tissues must be resolved and the requirement of lifelong immunosuppression must be minimized.

Data from Burke GW, Ciancio G, Sollinger HW: *Transplantation* 77(9 Suppl):S62-67, 2004; Kobayashi N et al: *J Artif Organs* 7(1):1-8, 2004; Shamblott MJ, Clark GO: *Expert Opin Biol Ther* 4(3):269-277, 2004; Stock PG, Bluestone JA: *Annu Rev Med* 55:133-156, 2004.

sine), serum free fatty acids, and gastrointestinal hormones, and by parasympathetic stimulation of the beta cells. Insulin secretion diminishes in response to low blood levels of glucose (hypoglycemia), high levels of insulin (through negative feedback to the beta cells), and sympathetic stimulation of the

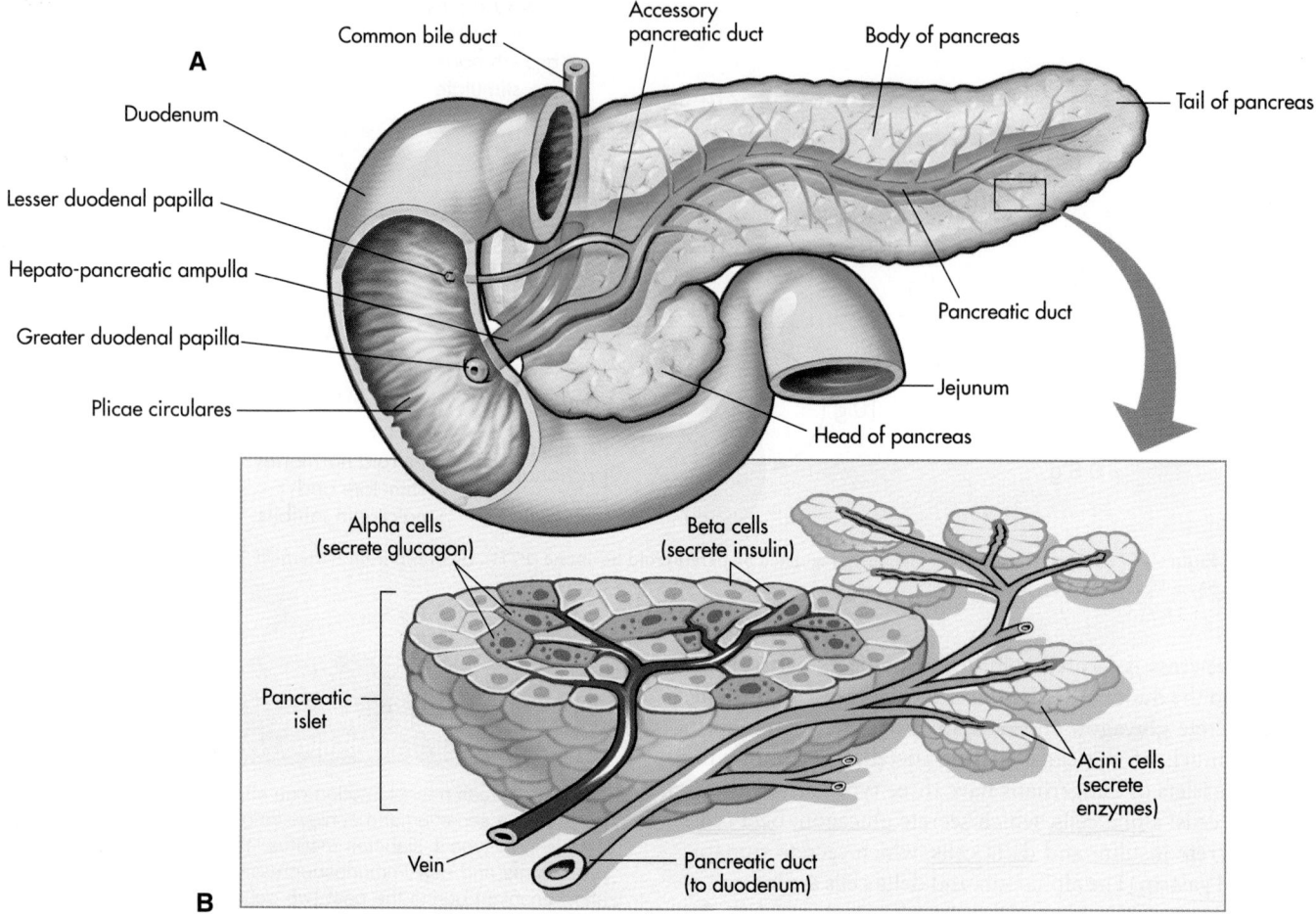

A

Common bile duct

Accessory pancreatic duct

Body of pancreas

Tail of pancreas

Duodenum

Lesser duodenal papilla

Hepato-pancreatic ampulla

Greater duodenal papilla

Plicae circulares

Pancreatic duct

Jejunum

Head of pancreas

Alpha cells (secrete glucagon)

Beta cells (secrete insulin)

Pancreatic islet

Acini cells (secrete enzymes)

Vein

Pancreatic duct (to duodenum)

B

Figure 20-16 **The pancreas. A,** Pancreas dissected to show main and accessory ducts. The main duct may join the common bile duct, as shown here, to enter the duodenum by a single opening at the major duodenal papilla, or the two ducts may have separate openings. The accessory pancreatic duct is usually present and has a separate opening into the duodenum. **B,** Exocrine glandular cells (around small pancreatic ducts) and endocrine glandular cells of the pancreatic islets (adjacent to blood capillaries). Exocrine pancreatic cells secrete pancreatic juice, alpha endocrine cells secrete glucagon, and beta cells secrete insulin. (From Thibodeau GA, Patton K: *Anatomy & physiology,* ed 5, St Louis, 2003, Mosby.)

alpha cells in the islets. Prostaglandin (PGE$_2$) also inhibits insulin secretion.[13]

Insulin facilitates the rate of glucose uptake into many cells within the body. Binding of insulin to its tyrosine-kinase receptor subtype initiates a series of events that involves autophosphorylation of the insulin receptor substrate 1 (IRS-1) and the activation (phosphorylation) of other proteins, including GRB2, a PI-3 kinase, and a tyrosine phosphatase. The net effect is that glucose transporters (GLUT) migrate from the cytosol to the cell surface. Translocation of the GLUT4 transporter is associated with a tenfold to twentyfold increase in glucose diffusion into the cell, particularly in skeletal and cardiac muscle, liver, and adipose cells (Figure 20-17).

Insulin is an anabolic hormone that promotes the synthesis of proteins, lipids, and nucleic acids. The major sites of insulin-promoted synthesis are the liver, muscle, and adipose tissue (Table 20-8). The net effect of insulin in these tissues is to stimulate cellular metabolism. Overall, however, the major consequence of insulin release is to decrease blood glucose. Insulin also facilitates the intracellular transport of potas-

sium. The brain and red blood cells do not require insulin for glucose transport.

Insulin is metabolized in the liver and kidney by enzymes that split disulfide bonds. Very little insulin is excreted unchanged in the urine.

Glucagon

Glucagon is produced by the alpha cells of the pancreas and by a number of cells lining the gastrointestinal tract. High glucose levels cause glucagon release to be inhibited; low glucose levels and sympathetic stimulation promote glucagon release, particularly in the liver. Amino acids, such as alanine, glycine, and asparagine, also stimulate glucagon secretion. A protein-rich meal has the same effect.

Glucagon acts primarily in the liver and increases blood glucose by stimulating glycogenolysis and gluconeogenesis. Glucagon acts as an antagonist to insulin. Much controversy exists regarding the role of glucagon in carbohydrate regulation, both normally and in diabetes mellitus. Glucagon also stimulates lipolysis, which has a ketogenic effect caused by the metabolism of free fatty acids in the liver.

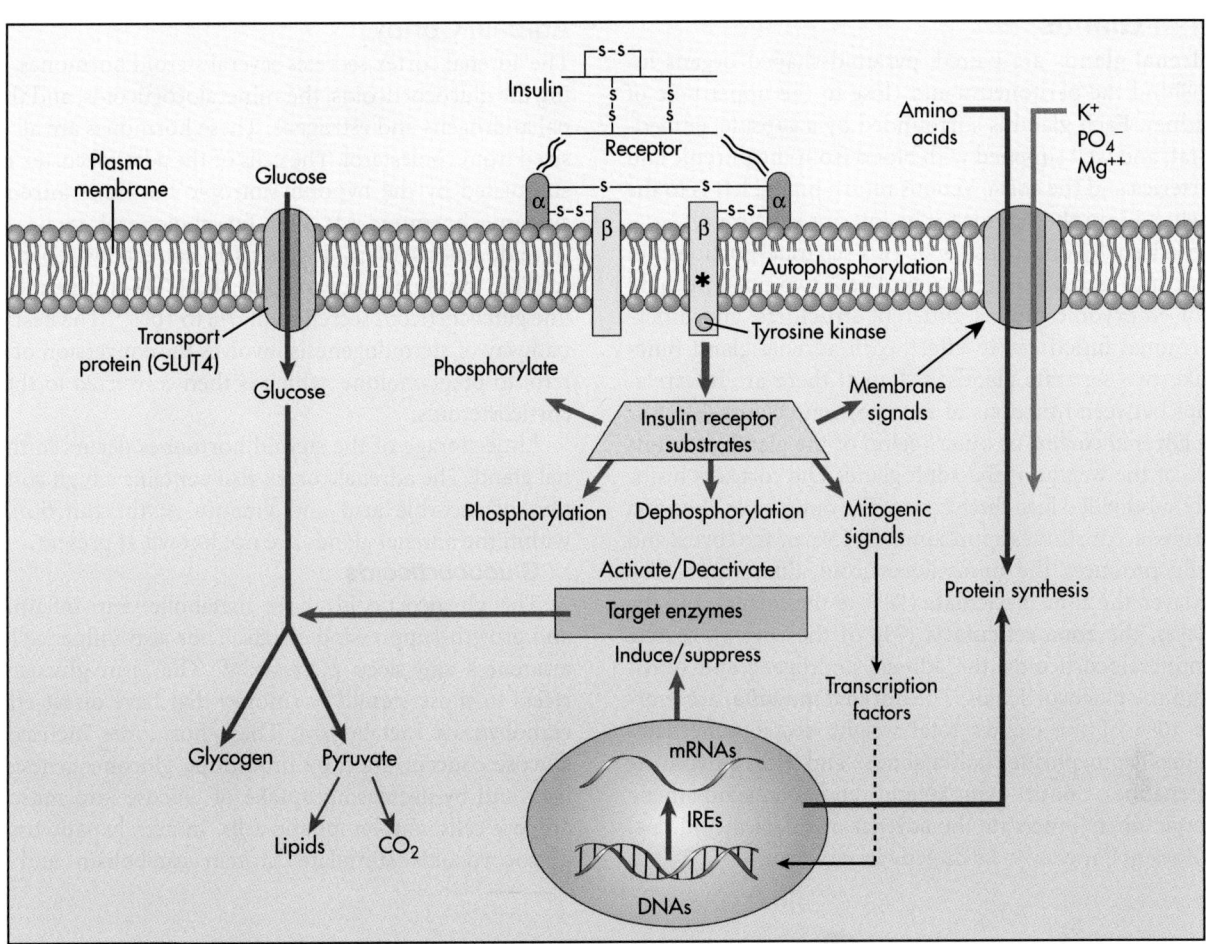

Figure 20-17 Insulin action on cells. Binding of insulin to its receptor causes autophosphorylation of the receptor, which then itself acts as a tyrosine kinase that phosphorylates insulin receptor substrate 1 (IRS-1). Numerous target enzymes, such as protein kinase B and MAP kinase are activated and these enzymes have a multitude of effects on cell function. The glucose transporter, GLUT4, is recruited to the plasma membrane, where it facilitates glucose entry into the cell. The transport of amino acids, potassium, magnesium, and phosphate into the cell is also facilitated. The synthesis of various enzymes is induced or suppressed, and cell growth is regulated by signal molecules that modulate gene expression. *mRNA,* Messenger ribonucleic acid; *IREs,* insulin responsive elements. (From Berne RM, Levy MN: *Principles of physiology,* ed 3, St Louis, 2000, Mosby.)

Table 20-8	Insulin Actions		
	Sites of Insulin-Promoted Synthesis		
Actions	**Liver Cells**	**Muscle Cells**	**Adipose Cells**
Glucose uptake	Increased	Increased	Increased
Glucose use	—	—	Increased glycerol phosphate
Glycogenesis	Increased	Increased	—
Glycogenolysis	Decreased	Decreased	—
Glycolysis	Increased	Increased	Increased
Gluconeogenesis	Increased	—	—
Other	Increased fatty acid synthesis	Increased amino acid uptake	Increased fat esterification
	Decreased ketogenesis	Increased protein synthesis	Decreased lipolysis
	Decreased urea cycle activity	Decreased proteolysis	Increased fat storage

Somatostatin

The somatostatin produced by delta cells is a hormone essential in carbohydrate, fat, and protein metabolism (i.e., homeostasis of ingested nutrients). It differs from hypothalamic somatostatin, which inhibits release of growth hormone and TSH. Little is known about pancreatic somatostatin, but it probably is involved in the regulation of alpha cell and beta cell function within the islets. Presumably, somatostatin inhibits both glucagon and insulin secretion, and it may prevent excess secretion of insulin.

Adrenal Glands

The **adrenal glands** are paired, pyramid-shaped organs located behind the peritoneum and close to the upper pole of each kidney. Each gland is surrounded by a capsule, embedded in fat, and well supplied with blood from the phrenic and renal arteries and the aorta. Venous return on the left is to the renal vein and on the right is to the inferior vena cava.

Each adrenal gland consists of two separate portions: an inner medulla and an outer cortex. These two portions have different embryonic origins, different structures, and different hormonal functions. In effect, each adrenal gland functions like two separate glands, although there are interrelationships between functions of each portion (Figure 20-18).

The **adrenal cortex,** or outer region of the gland, accounts for 80% of the weight of the adult gland. The cortex is histologically subdivided into three zones. The outer layer, the **zona glomerulosa,** constitutes approximately 15% of the cortex and primarily produces the mineralocorticoid aldosterone. The middle layer, the **zona fasciculata** (78% of the cortex), and the inner layer, the **zona reticularis** (7% of the cortex), secrete other mineralocorticoids, the adrenal androgens and estrogens, and the glucocorticoids. The **adrenal medulla,** accounting for 20% of the gland's total weight, secretes the catecholamines epinephrine (adrenaline), and norepinephrine (noradrenaline). Both sympathetic and parasympathetic cholinergic fibers innervate the adrenal medulla; the adrenal cortex does not appear to be directly innervated.

Adrenal Cortex

The adrenal cortex secretes several steroid hormones, including the glucocorticoids, the mineralocorticoids, and the adrenal androgens and estrogens. These hormones are all synthesized from cholesterol. The cells of the adrenal cortex must be stimulated by the hypophysiotropic hormone **adrenocorticotropic hormone (ACTH)** for cholesterol to be used in steroidogenesis. Steroidogenesis is not totally dependent on ACTH,[14] but there appears to be an ACTH-independent baseline glucocorticoid secretion of 3% to 10%.[15] The best-known pathway of steroidogenesis involves the conversion of cholesterol to pregnenolone, which is then converted to the major corticosteroids.

Little storage of the steroid hormones occurs in the adrenal gland. The adrenal cortex also contains a high concentration of ascorbic acid and vitamin A; the functional roles within the adrenal glands are not known at present.

Glucocorticoids

The glucocorticoids have metabolic, anti-inflammatory, and growth-suppressing effects. They also influence levels of awareness and sleep patterns.[16,17] The term **glucocorticoid** refers to those steroid hormones that have direct effects on carbohydrate metabolism. These hormones increase blood glucose concentration by promoting gluconeogenesis in the liver and by decreasing uptake of glucose into muscle cells, adipose cells, and lymphatic cells. In extrahepatic tissues the glucocorticoids stimulate protein catabolism and inhibit

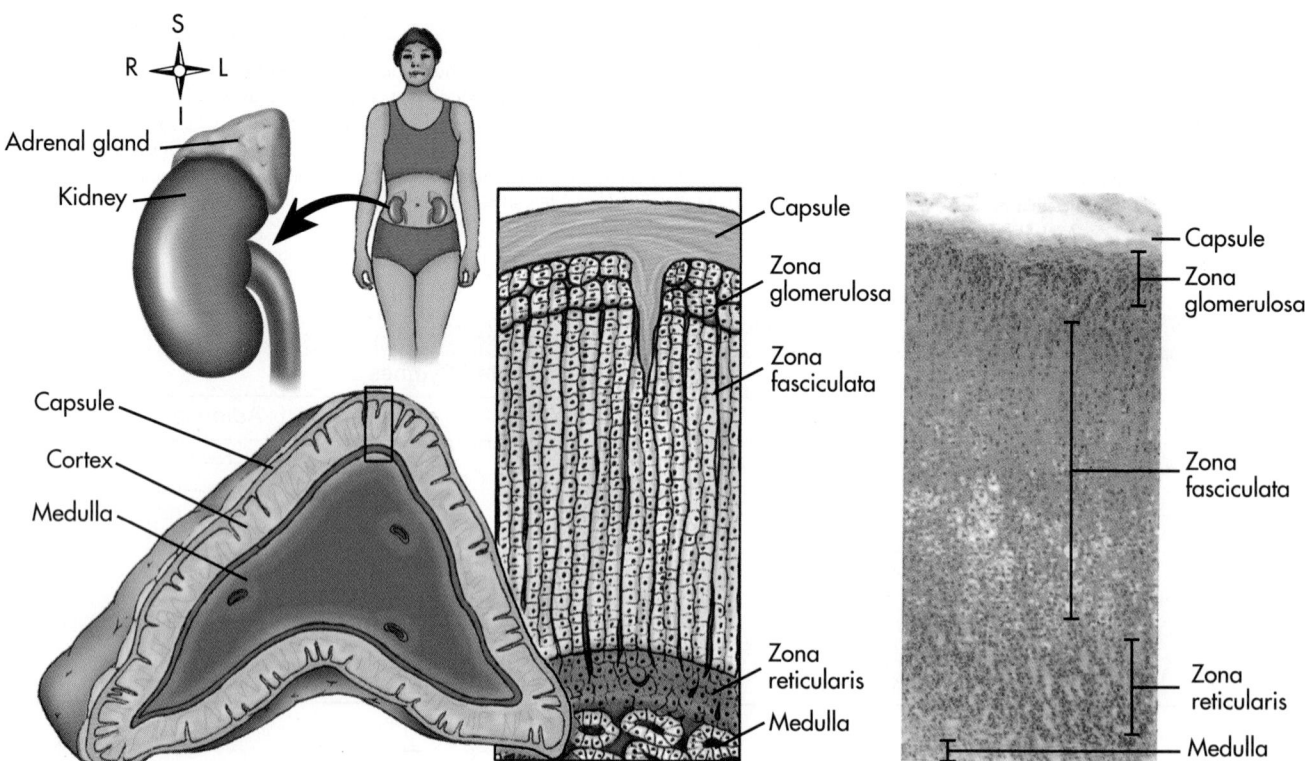

Figure 20-18 Structure of the adrenal gland showing cell layers (zonae) of the cortex. Zona glomerulosa secretes aldosterone. Zona fasciculata secretes abundant amounts of glucocorticoids, chiefly cortisol. Zona reticularis secretes minute amounts of sex hormones and glucocorticoids. A portion of the medulla is visible at lower right in the photomicrograph (×35) and at the bottom of the drawing. (From Thibodeau GA, Patton KT: *Anatomy & physiology,* ed 5, St Louis, 2003, Mosby.)

amino acid uptake and protein synthesis. In hepatic tissue, however, glucocorticoids act primarily to stimulate glucose formation and synthesis of enzymes that mediate glucocorticoid effects. The ultimate effect on the body is protein breakdown (catabolism).

The glucocorticoids act at several sites to influence immune and inflammatory reactions (described in Chapters 6 and 10). These include depressing proliferation of T lymphocytes, including those that produce the antiviral protein interferon; decreasing natural killer cell activity; promoting microphage phagocytosis of apoptotic granulocytes; and suppressing the synthesis, secretion, and actions of chemical mediators involved in inflammatory and immune responses. These chemical mediators include leukotrienes, bradykinin, serotonin, and histamine.[18-21]

Glucocorticoids stimulate anti-inflammatory cytokines (i.e., IL4, IL10, and transforming growth factor beta). Glucocorticoids suppress the inflammatory response by blocking phospholipase A_2, synthesis of prostaglandins, thromboxanes, and leukotrienes, and inhibiting inflammatory gene expression.[22] Lysosomal membranes are also stabilized, decreasing the release of proteolytic enzymes. Conversely, glucocorticoids potentiate humoral immunity and the production of antibodies.[23]

Other actions of the glucocorticoids include increasing circulating erythrocytes, leading to polycythemia; increasing the appetite; promoting fat deposits in the face and cervical areas; increasing uric acid excretion; decreasing serum calcium levels, possibly by inhibiting gastrointestinal absorption of calcium; suppressing the secretion and synthesis of ACTH; and suppressing growth hormone (GH) secretion so that somatic growth is inhibited. The glucocorticoids also have important "permissive" effects, sensitizing arterioles to the vasoconstrictive effects of norepinephrine.

Glucocorticoids appear to potentiate the effects of catecholamines, thyroid hormone, and GH on adipose tissue. It also has been speculated that a metabolite of cortisol may act like a barbiturate and depress nerve cell function in the brain. This may account for the noted effects on mood associated with steroid fluctuation in disease or stress.[24]

The most potent of the naturally occurring glucocorticoids is **cortisol.** It is the main secretory product of the adrenal cortex and is necessary for the maintenance of life and for protection from stress (see Chapter 10, particularly Figure 10-6). Cortisol has a biologic half-life of approximately 90 minutes, with the liver primarily responsible for its deactivation.

The secretion of cortisol is regulated primarily by the hypothalamus and the anterior pituitary gland (Figure 20-19). In the hypothalamus, corticotropin-releasing hormone (CRH) is produced in several nuclei and stored in the median eminence. Once released, CRH travels through the portal vessels to stimulate the production of ACTH from POMC, β-lipotropin, γ-lipotropin, endorphins, and enkephalins by the anterior pituitary. ACTH is the main regulator of cortisol secretion and adrenocortical growth.

Three factors appear to be primarily involved in regulating the secretion of ACTH: (1) high circulating levels of cortisol and synthetic glucocorticoids suppress both CRH and ACTH, whereas low cortisol levels stimulate their secretion; (2) diurnal rhythms affect ACTH and cortisol levels (in persons with regular sleep/wake patterns, ACTH peaks 3 to 5 hours after sleep begins and declines throughout the day; and cortisol levels follow a similar pattern, peaking right before awakening); and (3) stress has been shown to increase ACTH secretion, leading to increased cortisol levels. (Neuroendocrine mechanisms regulating sleep are discussed in Chapter 15.) A form of ACTH (i.e., ir ACTH) also is produced by the cells of

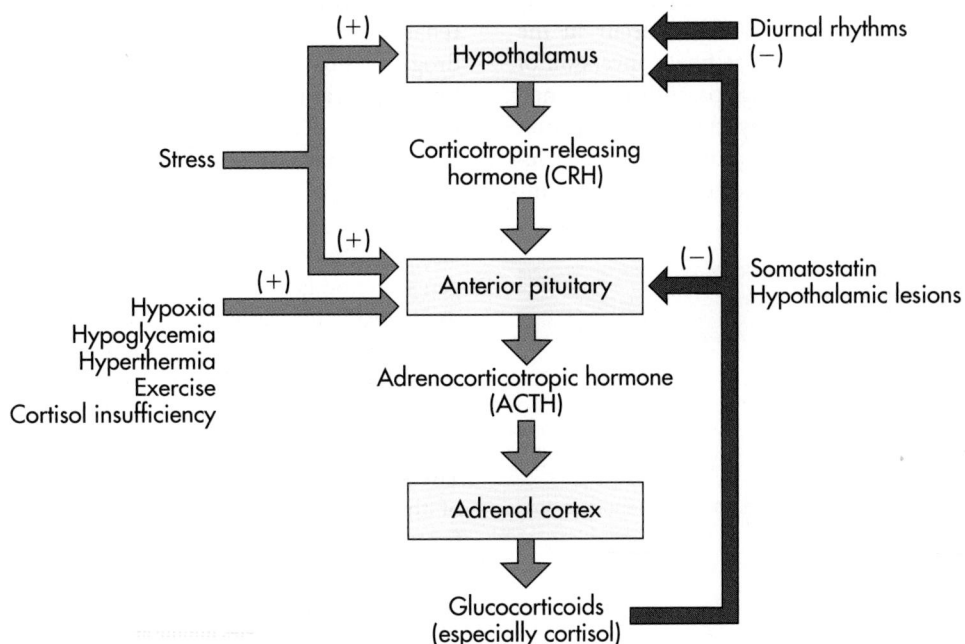

Figure 20-19 Feedback control of glucocorticoid synthesis and secretion.

the immune system. It is detectable through laboratory techniques, and physiologically it appears to exert the usual feedback effects (see Chapter 10). This mechanism may account in part for integration of the immune and endocrine systems.

Once ACTH is secreted, it binds to specific plasma membrane receptors on the cells of the adrenal cortex and on other extraadrenal tissues. Because both adrenal and extraadrenal tissues have ACTH receptors, a number of effects result from stimulation by ACTH. (These are summarized in Box 20-1.) Both adrenal and extraadrenal effects appear to be mediated through the activation of the adenylyl cyclase system. Melanocyte-stimulating hormone is also synthesized from the precursor POMC and increases skin pigmentation.[25]

Once ACTH stimulates the cells of the adrenal cortex, cortisol synthesis and secretion immediately occur. In the normal person the secretory patterns of ACTH and cortisol are nearly identical. After secretion, most cortisol circulates in bound form. Fifteen to thirty percent is bound to albumin, and 55% to 75% is tightly but reversibly bound to a plasma glycoprotein called *transcortin,* or corticosteroid-binding globulin. Transcortin levels are significantly elevated by increased estrogen levels that occur with pregnancy and hormone therapy. Ten to fifteen percent of the cortisol secreted circulates unbound. The unbound portion is free to diffuse into cells, but only those cells with specific intracellular glucocorticoid receptors respond to cortisol stimulation. ACTH is rapidly inactivated in the circulation, and the liver and kidneys remove the deactivated hormone.

Mineralocorticoids: Aldosterone

Mineralocorticoid steroids directly affect ion transport by epithelial cells, causing sodium retention and potassium and hydrogen loss. **Aldosterone** is the most potent of the naturally occurring mineralocorticoids and acts to conserve sodium by increasing the activity of the sodium pump of the epithelial cells. (The sodium pump is described in Chapter 1.)

The initial stages of aldosterone synthesis occur in the zona fasciculata and zona reticularis. The final conversion of corticosterone to aldosterone, however, apparently is confined to the zona glomerulosa. Aldosterone synthesis and secretion are regulated primarily by the renin–angiotensin system (described in Chapter 35), although other factors also may be in-

volved. Sodium and potassium levels may directly affect aldosterone secretion; however, the mechanisms involved are not understood. ACTH may transiently stimulate aldosterone synthesis but does not appear to be a major regulator of aldosterone secretion.

Aldosterone synthesis and secretion is stimulated by angiotensin II. The conversion of angiotensin I to angiotensin II is stimulated by the enzyme angiotensin I–converting enzyme (Figure 20-20). The conversion of angiotensinogen to angiotensin I is stimulated by renin (see Figure 20-20). Renin secretion is stimulated primarily by sodium and water depletion, or a diminished effective blood volume or increased potassium.

When sodium and potassium levels are within normal limits, approximately 50 to 250 mg of aldosterone are secreted daily. Fifty to seventy-five percent of the secreted aldosterone binds to plasma proteins, including albumin, transcortin, and an α_1-acid glycoprotein (AAG). The relatively large proportion of unbound aldosterone contributes to its rapid metabolic turnover in the liver, its low plasma concentration, and its short half-life of approximately 15 minutes. The main site of aldosterone degradation is the liver, with the metabolic end products being excreted by the kidney.

In the kidney, aldosterone primarily acts on the epithelial cells of the nephron collecting duct to increase sodium ion reabsorption (thus promoting water reabsorption) and increase potassium and hydrogen ion excretion. High levels of aldosterone may result in alkalosis and hypokalemia (see Chapter 3). (Kidney function is discussed in Chapter 35.) This renal effect takes $1\frac{1}{2}$ to 6 hours to occur after stimulation by aldosterone. Aldosterone also reduces sodium in sweat, saliva, and gastric juice.

Adrenal Estrogens and Androgens

Estrogen secretion by the normal adrenal cortex is so minimal as to be considered physiologically unimportant. The adrenal cortex also secretes androgens. Some of the weakly androgenic substances secreted by the cortex are then converted by peripheral tissues to stronger androgens, such as testosterone, thus accounting for some androgenic effect initiated by the adrenal cortex. An increased capacity for peripheral conversion of adrenal androgens to estrogens occurs in particular cases, however, including aging, obesity, liver disease, and hyperthyroidism.[26,27] The modulation of adrenal androgen secretion is not well understood. ACTH appears to be the major regulator rather than the gonadotropins. The biologic effects and metabolism of the adrenal sex steroids do not vary from those produced by the gonads (see Chapter 22).

Adrenal Medulla

The adrenal medulla, together with the sympathetic divisions of the autonomic nervous system, is embryonically derived from neural crest cells. **Chromaffin cells (pheochromocytes)** are the cells of the adrenal medulla. The major products secreted by the chromaffin cells are the catecholamines epinephrine (adrenaline) and norepinephrine, although the medulla is only a minor source of norepinephrine. The adrenal medulla

Box 20-1	Effects of Adrenocorticotropic Hormone

Adrenal
Maintenance of gland size
Depletion of ascorbic acid
Activation of adenylyl cyclase
Conversion of cholesterol to pregnenolone
Maintenance of enzymes active in converting pregnenolone to other steroids
Accumulation of cholesterol
Secretion of cortisol and adrenal androgens

Extraadrenal
Activation of tissue lipase

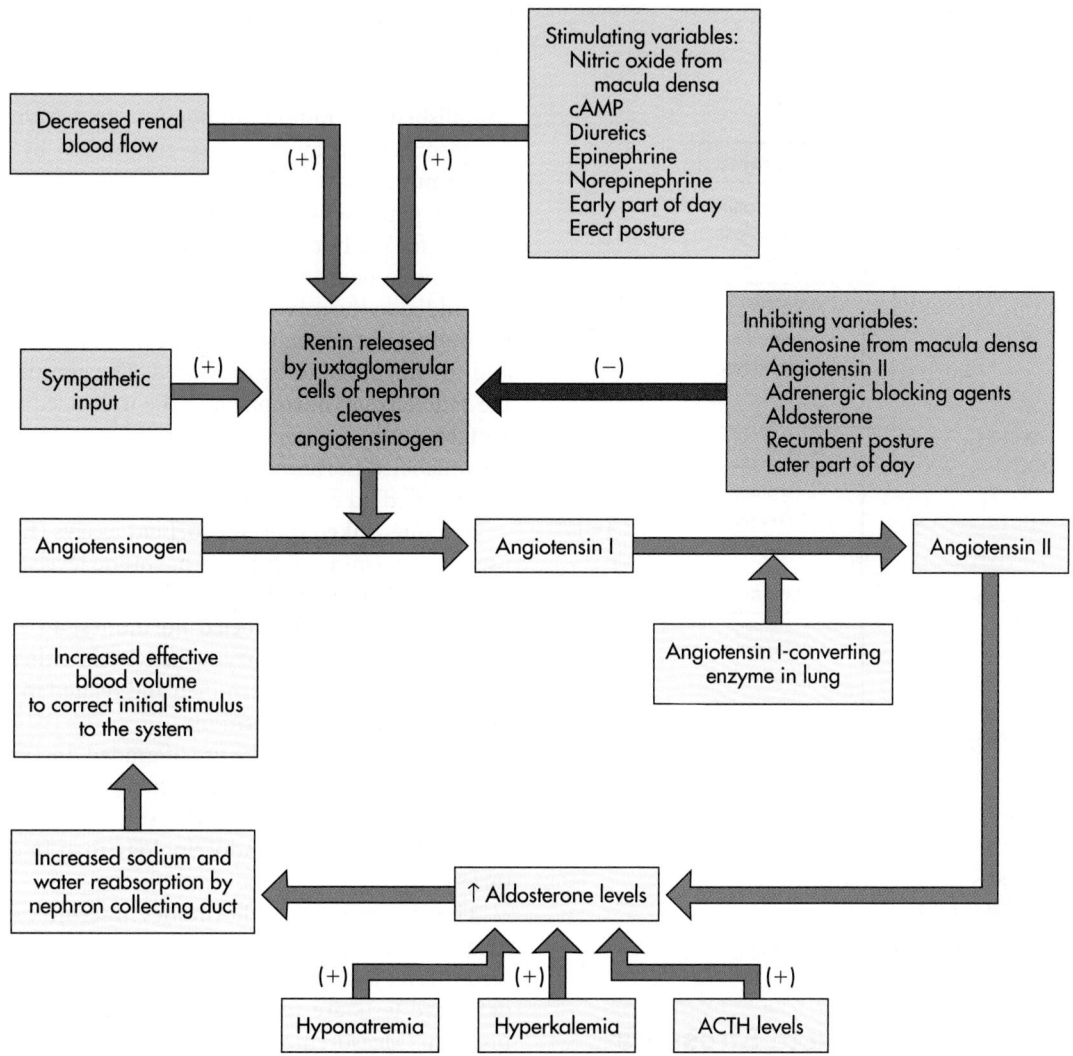

Figure 20-20 The feedback mechanisms regulating aldosterone secretion. *cAMP,* Cyclic adenosine monophosphate; *ACTH,* adrenocorticotropic hormone.

functions as a sympathetic ganglion without postganglionic processes. Sympathetic cholinergic preganglion fibers terminate on the chromaffin cells and secrete catecholamines directly into the bloodstream. The catecholamines are therefore hormones and not neurotransmitters.

Catecholamine production in the adrenal medulla consists of approximately 75% to 85% epinephrine and approximately 15% to 25% norepinephrine. Epinephrine is about 10 times more potent than norepinephrine in producing direct metabolic effects. The adrenal medulla synthesizes the catecholamines from the amino acid phenylalanine (Figure 20-21). Only 30% of circulating epinephrine comes from the adrenal medulla. The other 70% is released from nerve terminals.

The regulation of adrenal catecholamine release is complex. Secretion is increased by ACTH and the glucocorticoids. The catecholamines apparently exert a direct inhibiting influence on their own secretion by decreasing the formation of the rate-limiting enzyme tyrosine hydroxylase. Other stimuli to adrenal medullary secretion include sympathetic nerve stimulation, hypoglycemia, hypoxia, hypercapnia, acidosis, hemorrhage, glucagon, nicotine, pilocarpine, histamine, and angiotensin II. On stimulation of the adrenal medullary cell, cytoplasmic storage granules that contain the catecholamines migrate to the cell surface and undergo exocytosis. The control of exocytosis probably involves calcium, although this mechanism is not fully understood.

Once released, the catecholamines may bind to various target cells, may be taken up by neurons for storage in new cytoplasmic granules, or may be metabolically inactivated and excreted in the urine. The catecholamines exert their biologic effects after binding to a plasma membrane receptor in target cells. This binding activates the adenylyl cyclase system.

Catecholamines have diverse effects on the entire body. Their release and the body's response have been characterized as the "fight or flight" response (see Chapter 10). In general, the metabolic effects of catecholamines promote hyperglycemia through a variety of mechanisms and through interfering with usual glucose regulatory feedback mechanisms.

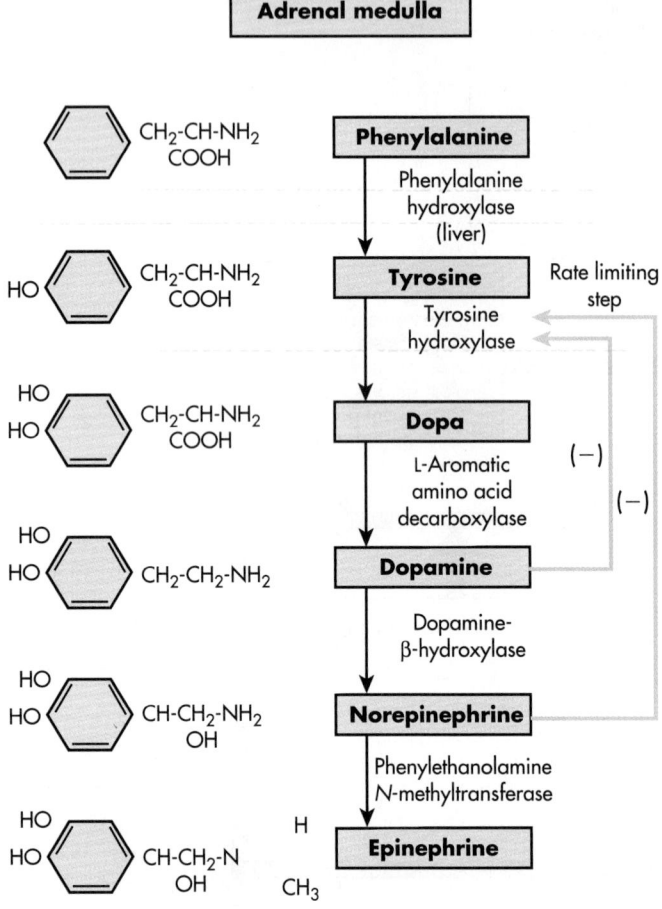

Figure 20-21 Synthesis of catecholamines.

Neuroendocrine Response to Stressors

The endocrine system acts together with the nervous system to respond to stressors. The integrated response to stressors also includes the immune system. Hormones of the neuroendocrine system affect components of the immune system, and mediators produced by immune components regulate the neuroendocrine response.

Perception that an event is stressful may be essential to the emotional arousal and initiation of the stress response (discussed in Chapter 10). Some events, such as bacterial invasion, can activate the stress response without emotional arousal. The hypothalamus receives input from a variety of areas within the brain and ultimately directs the neuroendocrine response to stress through the actions of corticotropin-releasing hormone (CRH), the locus ceruleus–norepinephrine autonomic (sympathetic) nervous system, and the pituitary–adrenal axis. In addition to the neuroendocrine components of the stress response, the gamma motor neuron system is activated to increase skeletal motor tone. Enhanced availability of vital substrates occurs, and growth and reproduction are inhibited to preserve energy for protective responses.[28] Details of the stress response are presented in Chapter 10.

Tests of Endocrine Function

Tests of the endocrine system involve several general types of clinical evaluation.[29] Measurement of hormone level is accomplished by radioimmunoassay, by enzyme-linked immunosorbent assay, and less commonly by bioassay. **Radioimmunoassay (RIA)** is a technique for measuring the minute quantities of hormones in the blood. Antibody that is specific for the hormone is mixed with plasma containing the hormone to be measured. Standard radiolabeled hormone is also added to the mixture. The amount of antibody present in the body is not enough to bind with both the tagged hormone and the hormone to be measured. The competition between the radiolabeled hormone and the unlabeled hormone in an antigen-antibody reaction determines the concentration of the unlabeled hormone. A quantitative value is established by use of standard reference curves.

Enzyme-linked immunosorbent assays (ELISAs) also are used to determine circulating hormone levels. The method is similar to that of RIA but is less expensive and easier to conduct. Instead of radiolabeled hormones, an enzyme-labeled hormone is used. The enzyme activity in either the bound or unbound fraction is determined and related to the concentration of the unlabeled hormone.

A **bioassay** involves the use of graded doses of hormone in a reference preparation and then comparison of the results with an unknown sample. Bioassays are used more commonly in investigative endocrinology than in clinical laboratories.

The concentration of hormones in serum can be measured to assess endocrine function in health and disease. If the serum level is greater or less than the reference values, more definitive tests are required to determine the source of the problem. Measurement of individual hormones does not always permit differentiation between normal and abnormal when hormone levels are changing over time. For an accurate interpretation, the broad normal range of some hormones requires a knowledge of previous hormonal levels and timed sampling.[30]

The major problems in evaluating the endocrine system include (1) the complexity of the clinical presentation because of multiple organ system involvement, (2) the nonspecific nature of complaints frequently associated with endocrine dysfunction, and (3) the inappropriate use of laboratory test interpretations.

AGING AND THE ENDOCRINE SYSTEM

The precise relationship between aging and the endocrine system is not clear. Perhaps most important, the question of whether changes in endocrine function are a consequence or a cause of aging has yet to be resolved.[31] These relationships have been difficult to identify, in part because of a number of age-related variables that may coexist, such as acute and chronic nonendocrine disease; use of medications; alterations in diet, body composition, and weight; and changes in sleep/wake cycles.[16,17]

Theories About the Effects of Aging

Investigation into the role of the endocrine glands and their interactions in the aging process has generated much data, although the evidence is contradictory. Altered biologic activity of hormones, altered circulating levels of hormones, altered secretory response of the endocrine glands, altered metabolism of hormones, and loss of circadian control of hormone secretion are among the findings.[32]

Theories of cellular damage deal with adverse cellular conditions that produce the biologic effects associated with aging. (These theories are discussed in Chapter 2.) The endocrine system has not been specifically implicated in any of these theories, particularly as a causative variable. The cellular changes or consequences described by these theories, however, do affect specific endocrine glands and might contribute to endocrine gland dysfunction or alterations in responsiveness of target organs.

Theories of stress and adaptation suggest that body structures wear out from overuse or are no longer able to adapt to the cumulative effects of physiologic stress. One such endocrine function that may be affected is the sympathoadrenal axis. Exhaustion of this axis may be associated with an inability of the body to respond effectively to stressors.

Theories of programmed change are concerned with genetic control of cell function. Certain secretory cells may be programmed genetically to secrete hormones for a prescribed length of time. Changes seen with female reproductive function may represent the phenomenon of programmed change. Reduced signaling of insulin and insulin-like peptides is associated with increased lifespans.[33,34]

All changes in cellular activity—as a result of damage, programmed change, or wear and tear—may affect neuroendocrine regulation. Changes in secretion of hypothalamic regulatory factors and hormones or changes in hypothalamic feedback sensitivity may contribute to alterations in control of an optimal internal environment. The dynamic equilibrium of the endocrine system also may be affected by altered secretion of neurotransmitters within certain areas of the brain, affecting hypothalamic and pituitary function. Such alterations may include an excess or deficit in secretion of pituitary hormones and loss of appropriate secretory pattern of those hormones. Loss of endocrine steady states may be associated with or contribute to aging.

Effects of Aging on Specific Glands

Thyroid Gland

Changes in thyroid structure and function occur with aging. Structurally, some glandular atrophy and fibrosis occur with nodularity and increasing inflammatory infiltrates. These infiltrative changes may reflect age-related autoimmune damage.[35] The presence of thyroid nodules increases over the age of 70 years.[36]

Changes relative to thyroid hormone and its function are more difficult to assess. One difficulty is finding older adults who are free of all systemic and thyroid-related illness, so that the resulting changes can be attributed to aging. Much of the available data is contradictory. Most evidence, however, supports the following age-related changes:[37,38]

1. Overall TSH secretion is diminished.
2. Responsiveness of plasma TSH concentration to TRH administration is reduced, especially in men.
   a. T_4 secretion and turnover are decreased.
   b. Plasma levels of T_3 decline, especially in men, but are generally in the normal range.
   c. Hypothyroidism is seen with increasing frequency as age advances.

In addition, the average dose for TH replacement appears to be lower in elderly persons because the peripheral metabolism of TH decreases with age.[35] TH must be replaced slowly in elderly individuals with coronary artery disease to prevent angina and myocardial infarction.[39] Clinical signs of thyroid disease are more difficult to detect in elderly persons.[40]

Parathyroid Glands

An age-related alteration in PTH secretion has been proposed to explain alterations in calcium homeostasis that have been noted in older adults. Such an alteration, however, has not been documented consistently. Calcium intake, especially in women, tends to decrease with aging and may contribute to osteoporosis (see Chapter 42). The average daily intake of 450 to 500 mg/day causes a negative calcium balance greater than 40 mg/day and may be related to the absolute bone loss of approximately 1.5% per year. Older adults show decreased intestinal adaptation to variations in calcium intake. Hyperparathyroidism may occur secondary to calcium malabsorption and hypocalcemia with increased bone remodeling that results in cortical bone thinning and porosity. Many older adults also have a mild, persistent hypercalciuria, which indicates a defective renal mechanism for responding to decreased calcium intake. Decreased circulating levels of vitamin D also have been documented.[41]

The decrease in calcium intake, an age-related decrease in circulating vitamin D, and a blunted response of older persons to PTH may explain these changes seen in aging.[42] Additional investigation into mechanisms of altered calcium metabolism is required before the age-associated alterations can be explained.

Adrenal Glands

The adrenal cortex loses some weight and has more fibrous tissue after the age of 50 years. Age does not appear to affect the feedback mechanisms involved in maintaining glucocorticoid levels, but the decrease in the metabolic clearance rate of the glucocorticoids is age related.

The metabolic clearance of cortisol decreases with an age-related decline in liver and kidney function. Further, less cortisol appears to be used by the body when aging is accompanied by a loss of lean body mass. Both decreased clearance and reduced use of cortisol contribute to higher circulating cortisol levels, but diurnal variation is maintained.[43] Because feedback mechanisms are intact, the higher cortisol levels cause a decrease in cortisol secretion. Plasma levels of the adrenal androgens, as well as urinary excretion of the metabolic end products, decrease gradually but dramatically with age, to as much as 50% to 70% of the young adult level. This change appears to reflect a decline in the function of the zona reticularis. The effects of decreased secretion are obscured, however, by the effects of aging on gonadal androgen secretion (see Chapter 22). Because cortisol secretion does not vary significantly with aging, the decrease in secretion of adrenal androgens probably is independent of ACTH. Change in both the testis and hypothalamic–pituitary axis may be responsible for decreased testosterone levels.[44] Circadian patterns of ACTH and cortisol secretion may change with aging.[45]

Posterior Pituitary

Although hyponatremia is a common finding in older persons,[46] it appears related to changes in renal function rather than to ADH-related mechanisms. Morphologic studies have not shown significant age-related degenerative changes in the neuroendocrine pathways that regulate the synthesis and secretion of ADH. It appears that ADH secretion is augmented when stimulated by changes in osmotic concentration, whereas baroreceptor-mediated ADH secretion is reduced.[16,17]

Anterior Pituitary

The anterior pituitary in older persons is characterized by a number of morphologic changes, including increases in fibrosis, focal necrosis, iron deposits, and microadenoma formation and a moderate decrease in size.[47] Growth hormone may be reduced in the elderly and accounts, in part, for increased visceral fat, decreased lean body mass, and decreased bone density.[48]

SUMMARY REVIEW

Mechanisms of Hormonal Regulation

1. The endocrine system has diverse functions, including sexual differentiation, growth and development, and continuous maintenance of the body's internal environment.
2. Hormones are chemical messengers synthesized by endocrine glands and released into the circulation.
3. Hormones have specific negative- and positive-feedback mechanisms. Most hormone levels are regulated by negative feedback, in which tropic hormone secretion raises the level of a specific hormone, which feeds back causing secretion of the tropic hormone to subside.
4. Endocrine feedback is described in terms of short, long, and ultrashort feedback loops.
5. Water-soluble hormones circulate throughout the body in unbound form, whereas lipid-soluble hormones (i.e., steroid and thyroid hormones) circulate throughout the body bound to carrier proteins.
6. Hormones serve as first messengers and affect only target cells with appropriate receptors and then act on those cells to initiate specific cell functions or activities.
7. Hormones have two general types of effects on cells: direct effects, or obvious changes in cell function, and permissive effects, or less obvious changes that facilitate cell function.
8. Receptors for hormones are proteins and may be located on or in the plasma membrane or in the cytosol or nucleus of the target cell. Receptors may be G protein–linked, ion channels, or enzyme-linked.
9. Water-soluble hormones act as first messengers, binding to receptors on the cell's plasma membrane. The signals initiated by hormone–receptor binding are then transmitted into the cell by the action of second messengers.
10. Second messengers that have been identified include cyclic adenosine monophosphate (cAMP), cyclic guanosine monophosphate (cGMP), and calcium which associates with inositol triphosphatase (IP$_3$), and diacylglycerol (DAG) to produce physiologic effects.
11. For cells that have cAMP as their second messenger, a series of interactions within the plasma membrane must activate adenylyl cyclase.
12. For cells that have calcium as their second messenger, a rise in intracellular calcium causes calcium to bind with calmodulin, a regulatory protein. This step then initiates other intracellular processes.
13. Cells that have cGMP as their second messenger are activated by the enzyme guanylyl cyclase.
14. Lipid-soluble hormones (including steroid and thyroid hormones) may have rapid effects by binding to a plasma membrane or receptor or crossing the plasma membrane through diffusion. These hormones then either bind to cytoplasmic proteins or diffuse directly into the cell nucleus and bind to nuclear receptors.

Structure and Function of the Endocrine Glands

1. The pituitary gland, consisting of anterior and posterior portions, is connected to the central nervous system through the hypothalamus.
2. The hypothalamus regulates anterior pituitary function by secreting releasing hormones into the portal circulation.
3. Hypothalamic hormones include dopamine, which inhibits prolactin secretion; thyrotropin-releasing hormone, which affects release of thyroid hormones; gonadotropin-releasing hormone (GnRH), which facilitates release of adrenocorticotropic hormone (ACTH) and endorphins; and substance P, which inhibits ACTH release and stimulates release of a variety of other hormones.
4. The posterior pituitary secretes antidiuretic hormone (ADH), also called *arginine vasopressin,* and oxytocin.
5. ADH controls serum osmolality, increases permeability of the renal tubules to water, and causes vasoconstriction when administered pharmacologically in high doses. ADH also may regulate some central nervous system functions.
6. Oxytocin causes uterine contraction and lactation in women and may have a role in sperm motility in men. In both men and women, oxytocin has an antidiuretic effect similar to that of ADH.
7. Hormones of the anterior pituitary are regulated by (a) secretion of hypothalamic-releasing hormones or factors, (b) negative feedback from hormones secreted by target organs, and (c) mediating effects of neurotransmitters.
8. Hormones of the anterior pituitary include ACTH, melanocyte-stimulating hormone (MSH), somatotropic hormones (growth hormone [GH] and prolactin), and glycoprotein hormones (follicle-stimulating hormone [FSH], luteinizing hormone [LH], and thyroid-stimulating hormone [TSH]).
9. The two-lobed thyroid gland contains follicles, which secrete some of the thyroid hormones, and C cells, which secrete calcitonin and somatostatin.

10. Regulation of thyroid hormone (TH) levels is complex and involves the hypothalamus, anterior pituitary, thyroid gland, and numerous biochemical variables.

11. Thyroid hormone (TH) secretion is regulated by thyroid-releasing hormone through a negative-feedback loop that involves the anterior pituitary and hypothalamus.

12. TSH, which is synthesized and stored in the anterior pituitary, stimulates secretion of TH by activating intracellular processes, including uptake of iodine necessary for the synthesis of TH.

13. Once secreted, TH acts on the thyroid gland, the anterior pituitary, and the median eminence to regulate further TH production.

14. Synthesis of TH depends on the glycoprotein thyroglobulin, which contains a precursor of TH, tyrosine. Tyrosine then combines with iodide to form precursor molecules of the thyroid hormones thyroxine (T_4) and triiodothyronine (T_3).

15. When released into the circulation, T_3 and T_4 are bound by carrier proteins in the plasma, which store these hormones and provide a buffer for rapid changes in hormone levels.

16. Thyroid hormones alter protein synthesis and have a wide range of metabolic effects on proteins, carbohydrates, lipids, and vitamins. TH also affects heat production and cardiac function.

17. The paired parathyroid glands normally are located behind the upper and lower poles of the thyroid. These glands secrete parathyroid hormone (PTH), an important regulator of serum calcium levels.

18. PTH secretion is regulated by levels of ionized calcium in the plasma and by cAMP within the cell. Some other substances—hormones, neurotransmitters, and ions—affect PTH secretion by inhibiting cAMP or by changing calcium levels.

19. In bone, PTH causes bone breakdown and resorption. In the kidney, PTH increases reabsorption of calcium, decreases reabsorption of phosphorus and bicarbonate, and stimulates synthesis of vitamin D.

20. The endocrine pancreas contains the islets of Langerhans, which secrete hormones responsible for much of the carbohydrate metabolism in the body.

21. The islets of Langerhans consist of alpha cells, beta cells, and delta cells. Delta cells secrete somatostatin, which inhibits glucagon and insulin secretion. Beta cells secrete preproinsulin, which is ultimately converted to insulin.

22. Insulin is a hormone that regulates blood glucose concentrations and overall body metabolism of fat, protein, and carbohydrates.

23. Alpha cells produce glucagon, which is secreted inversely to blood glucose concentrations.

24. The paired adrenal glands are situated on the kidneys. Each gland consists of an adrenal medulla, which secretes catecholamines, and an adrenal cortex, which secretes steroid hormones.

25. The steroid hormones secreted by the adrenal cortex are all synthesized from cholesterol. These hormones include glucocorticoids, mineralocorticoids, and adrenal androgens and estrogens.

26. Glucocorticoids directly affect carbohydrate metabolism by increasing blood glucose concentration through gluconeogenesis in the liver and by decreasing use of glucose. Glucocorticoids also inhibit immune and inflammatory responses.

27. The most potent naturally occurring glucocorticoid is cortisol, which is necessary for the maintenance of life and for protection from stress. Secretion of cortisol is regulated by the hypothalamus and anterior pituitary.

28. Cortisol secretion is related to secretion of adrenocorticotropic hormone (ACTH), which is stimulated by corticotropin-releasing hormone (CRH). ACTH binds with receptors of the adrenal cortex, which activates intracellular mechanisms (specifically cAMP) and leads to cortisol release.

29. Mineralocorticoids are steroid hormones that directly affect ion transport by epithelial cells, causing sodium retention and potassium and hydrogen loss.

30. Aldosterone is the most potent of the naturally occurring mineralocorticoids. Its primary role is to conserve sodium. Aldosterone secretion is regulated by the renin–angiotensin system.

31. Aldosterone acts by binding to a site on the cell nucleus and altering protein production within the cell. Its principal site of action is the kidney, where it causes sodium reabsorption and potassium and hydrogen excretion.

32. Androgens and estrogens secreted by the adrenal cortex act in the same way as those secreted by the gonads.

33. The adrenal medulla secretes the catecholamines epinephrine and norepinephrine. Catecholamines are synthesized from the amino acid phenylalanine. Their release is stimulated by sympathetic nervous system stimulation, ACTH, and glucocorticoids.

34. Catecholamines bind with various target cells and are taken up by neurons or excreted in the urine. They cause a range of metabolic effects that generally are characterized as the "flight or fight" response.

35. The endocrine system acts together with the nervous and immune systems to respond to stressors providing an integrated and protective response.

36. Several assay methods are used to measure levels of hormones in the plasma. Radioimmunoassay (RIA) compares the proportion of radiolabeled vs. non-radiolabeled hormone against standard reference curves.

37. Enzyme-linked immunosorbent assay uses a method similar to RIA, but uses a radiolabeled enzyme rather than a radiolabeled hormone.

38. Bioassays use graded doses of hormone in a reference preparation and then compare the results with an unknown sample to determine hormone level.

Aging and the Endocrine System

1. Endocrine changes that may be associated with aging include altered biologic activity of hormones, altered circulating levels of hormones, altered secretory responses of endocrine glands, altered metabolism of hormones, and loss of circadian control of hormone release.

2. Cellular damage associated with aging, genetically programmed cell change, and chronic wear and tear may contribute to endocrine gland dysfunction or alterations in responsiveness of target organs.

3. Aging apparently causes atrophy of the thyroid gland and is associated with infiltrative glandular changes. Secretion of thyroid hormones may diminish with age.

4. Aging is associated with alterations in calcium steady states, which may be related to alterations in PTH secretion from the parathyroid glands.

5. Age-related changes in adrenal function include decreased clearance of glucocorticoids and a decrease in levels of adrenal androgens. The effects of these changes, however, are offset by feedback mechanisms that maintain glucocorticoid levels and by gonadal secretion of androgens.

KEY TERMS

MEDIA RESOURCES evolve

REFERENCES

1. Losel RM et al: Nongenomic steroid action: controversies, questions, and answers, *Physiol Rev* 83(3):965-1016, 2003.
2. Losel R, Wehling M: Nongenomic actions of steroid hormones, *Nat Rev Mol Cell Biol* 4(1):46-56, 2003.
3. Sak K, Everaus H: Nongenomic effects of 17beta-estradiol—diversity of membrane binding sites, *J Steroid Biochem Mol Biol* 88(4-5):323-35, 2004.
4. Limbourg FP, Liao JK: Nontranscriptional actions of the glucocorticoid receptor, *J Mol Med* 81(3):168-74, 2003.
5. Schiff R et al: Cross-talk between estrogen receptor and growth factor pathways as a molecular target for overcoming endocrine resistance, *Clin Cancer Res* 10(1 Pt 2):331S-336S, 2004.
6. Watson CS, Gametchu B: Proteins of multiple classes may participate in nongenomic steroid actions, *Exp Biol Med (Maywood)* 228(11):1272-1281, 2003.
7. Reichlin S: Neuroendocrinology. In Wilson JD et al, editors: *Williams textbook of endocrinology*, ed 9, Philadelphia, 1998, Saunders.
8. Kacson B: *Endocrine physiology*, New York, 2000, McGraw-Hill.
9. Braverman LE, Utiger RD: *Werner and Ingbar's The thyroid: a fundamental and clinical text*, ed 8, Philadelphia, 2000, Lippincott Williams and Wilkins.
10. Inzerillo AM, Zaidi M, Huang CL: Calcitonin: physiological actions and clinical applications, *J Pediatr Endocrinol Metab* 17(7):931-940, 2004.
11. Mehta NM, Malootian A, Gilligan JP: Calcitonin for osteoporosis and bone pain, *Curr Pharm Des* 9(32):2659-2676, 2003.
12. Yen PM: Physiological and molecular basis of thyroid hormone action, *Physiol Rev* 81(3):1097-1142, 2001.
13. Robertson RP: Dominance of cyclooxygenase-2 in the regulation of pancreatic islet prostaglandin synthesis, *Diabetes* 47(9):1379-1383, 1998.
14. Weber MM et al: Interleukin-3 and interleukin-6 stimulate cortisol secretion from adult human adrenocortical cells, *Endocrinology* 138(5):2207-2210, 1997.
15. Neville AM, O'Hare MJ: *The human adrenal cortex*, New York, 1982, Springer Verlag.
16. Rupprecht R, Holsboer F: Neuroactive steriods: mechanisms of action and neuropsychopharmacological perspectives, *Trends Neurosci* 22(9):410-416, 1999.
17. Steiger A et al: Effects of hormones on sleep, *Horm Res* 49(3-4):125-130, 1998.
18. Heasman SJ et al: Glucocorticoid-mediated regulation of granulocyte apoptosis and macrophage phagocytosis of apoptotic cells: implications for the resolution of inflammation, *J Endocrinol* 178(1):29-36, 2003.
19. Heasman SJ, Giles KM, Rossi AG et al: Interferon gamma suppresses glucocorticoid augmentation of macrophage clearance of apoptotic cells, *Eur J Immunol* 34(6):1752-1761, 2004.
20. Morand EF, Leech M: Glucocorticoid regulation of inflammation: the plot thickens, *Inflamm Res* 48(11):557-560, 1999.
21. Rook GA: Glucocorticoids and immune function, *Baillieres Best Pract Res Clin Endocrinol Metab* 13(4):567-581, 1999.
22. Saklatvala J, Dean J, Clark A: Control of the expression of inflammatory response genes, *Biochem Soc Symp* 70:95-106, 2003.
23. Elenkov IJ, Chrousos GP: Stress hormones, proinflammatory and anti-inflammatory cytokines, and autoimmunity, *Ann N Y Acad Sci* 966:290-303, 2002.
24. Gard PR, Pelagatti S: *Human endocrinology*, Old Tappan, NJ, 1998, Pearson Education.
25. Abel-Malek Z et al: The melanocortin-1 receptor and human pigmentation, *Ann N Y Acad Sci* 885:117-133, 1999.
26. Meikle AW, Daynes RA, Araneo BA: Adrenal androgen secretion and biologic effects, *Endocrinol Metab Clin North Am* 20(2):381-400, 1991.
27. Bulun SE et al: Aromatase in aging women, *Semin Reprod Endocrinol* 17(4):349-358, 1999.
28. Sapolsky RM, Romero LM, Munck AU: How do glucocorticoids influence stress responses? Integrating permissive, suppressive, stimulatory, and preparative actions, *Endocr Rev* 21(1):55-89, 2000.
29. Hall JE, Nieman J: *Handbook of diagnostic endocrinology*, Totowa, NJ, 2000, Humana Press.
30. Kronenberg H. et al: Principles of endocrinology. In Larsen PR et al, editors: *Williams textbook of endocrinology*, ed 10, Philadelphia, 2003, Saunders.
31. Morley JE: Hormones and the aging process, *J Am Geriatr Soc* 51(7 Suppl):S333-S3337, 2003.
32. Quau WB, Timiras PA: *Hormones and aging*, 3rd ed., Boca Raton, Fla, 2003, CRC Press.
33. Chang AM, Halter JB: Aging and insulin secretion, *Am J Physiol Endocrinol Metab* 284(1):E7-12, 2003.
34. Tatar M, Bartke A, Antebi A: The endocrine regulation of aging by insulin-like signals, *Sci* 299(5611):1346-1351, 2003.
35. Mariotti S et al: Thyroid autoimmunity and aging, *Exp Gerontol* 33(6):535-541, 1998.
36. Mariotti S et al: The aging thyroid, *Endocr Rev* 16(6):686-715, 1995.
37. Chiovato L, Mariotti S, Pinchera A: Thyroid diseases in the elderly, *Baillieres Clin Endocrinol Metab* 11(2):251-270, 1997.
38. Samuels MH: Subclinical thyroid disease in the elderly, *Thyroid* 8(9):803-813, 1998.

39. Urban JR: Neuroendocrinology of aging in the male and female, *Endocrinol Metab Clin North Am* 21(4):921-931, 1992.

40. Trivalle C et al: Differences in the signs and symptoms of hyperthyroidism in older and younger patients, *J Am Geriatr Soc* 44(1):50-53, 1996.

41. Seeman E: Pathogenesis of bone fragility in women and men, *Lancet* 359(9320):1841-1850, 2002.

42. Haden ST et al: The effects of age and gender on parathyroid hormone dynamics, *Clin Endocrinol* 52(3):329-338, 2000.

43. Van Cauter E, Leproult R, Kupfer DJ: Effects of gender and age on the levels and circadian rhythmicity of plasma cortisol, *J Clin Endocrinol Metab* 81(7):2468-2473, 1996.

44. Veldhuis JD: Nature of altered pulsatile hormone release and neuroendocrine network signalling in human ageing: clinical studies of the stomatotropic, gonadotropic, corticotropic, and insulin axes, *Novartis Found Symp* 227:163-185, 2000.

45. Deuschle M et al: With aging in humans the activity of the hypothalamus-pituitary-adrenal system increases and its diurnal amplitude flattens, *Life Sci* 61(22):2239-2246, 1997.

46. Miller M et al: Apparent idiopathic hyponatremia in an ambulatory geriatric population, *J Am Geriatr Soc* 44(4):404-408, 1996.

47. Lurie SN et al: In vivo assessment of pituitary gland volume with magnetic resonance imaging: the effect of age, *J Clin Endocrinol Metab* 71(2):505-508 1990.

48. Nass R, Thorner MO: Impact of the GH-cortisol ratio on the age-dependent changes in body composition, *Growth Horm IGF Res* 12(3):147-161, 2002.

ALTERATIONS OF HORMONAL REGULATION

ROBERT E. JONES • SUE E. HUETHER

CHAPTER OUTLINE

Function of the endocrine system involves complex interrelationships and interactions that maintain dynamic steady states and provide growth and reproductive capabilities. Dysfunction of the endocrine system initially was described in terms of excessive or insufficient function of the endocrine gland with alterations in hormone levels. Alterations in function were thought to be caused by either hypersecretion or hyposecretion of the various hormones, leading to abnormal hormone concentrations in the blood. Techniques for studying the various components of the endocrine system have improved, and evidence has shown that dysfunction may result from abnormal receptor function or from altered intracellular response to the hormone-receptor complex.

MECHANISMS OF HORMONAL ALTERATIONS

Significantly elevated or depressed hormone levels may result from a variety of causes (Figure 21-1). Feedback systems that recognize the need for a particular hormone may fail to function properly or may respond to inappropriate signals (see Chapter 20). Dysfunction of an endocrine gland may involve the gland's failure to produce adequate amounts of biologically free or active hormone forms. This failure may occur when the secretory cells are unable to produce or obtain an adequate quantity of required hormone precursors or when they are unable to convert the precursors to the active hormone. A gland also may synthesize or release excessive amounts of hormone. Once hormones are released into the circulation, they may be degraded at an altered rate or they may be inactivated by antibodies before reaching the target cell. Ectopic sources of hormones (hormones produced by nonendocrine tissues) may result also in abnormally elevated

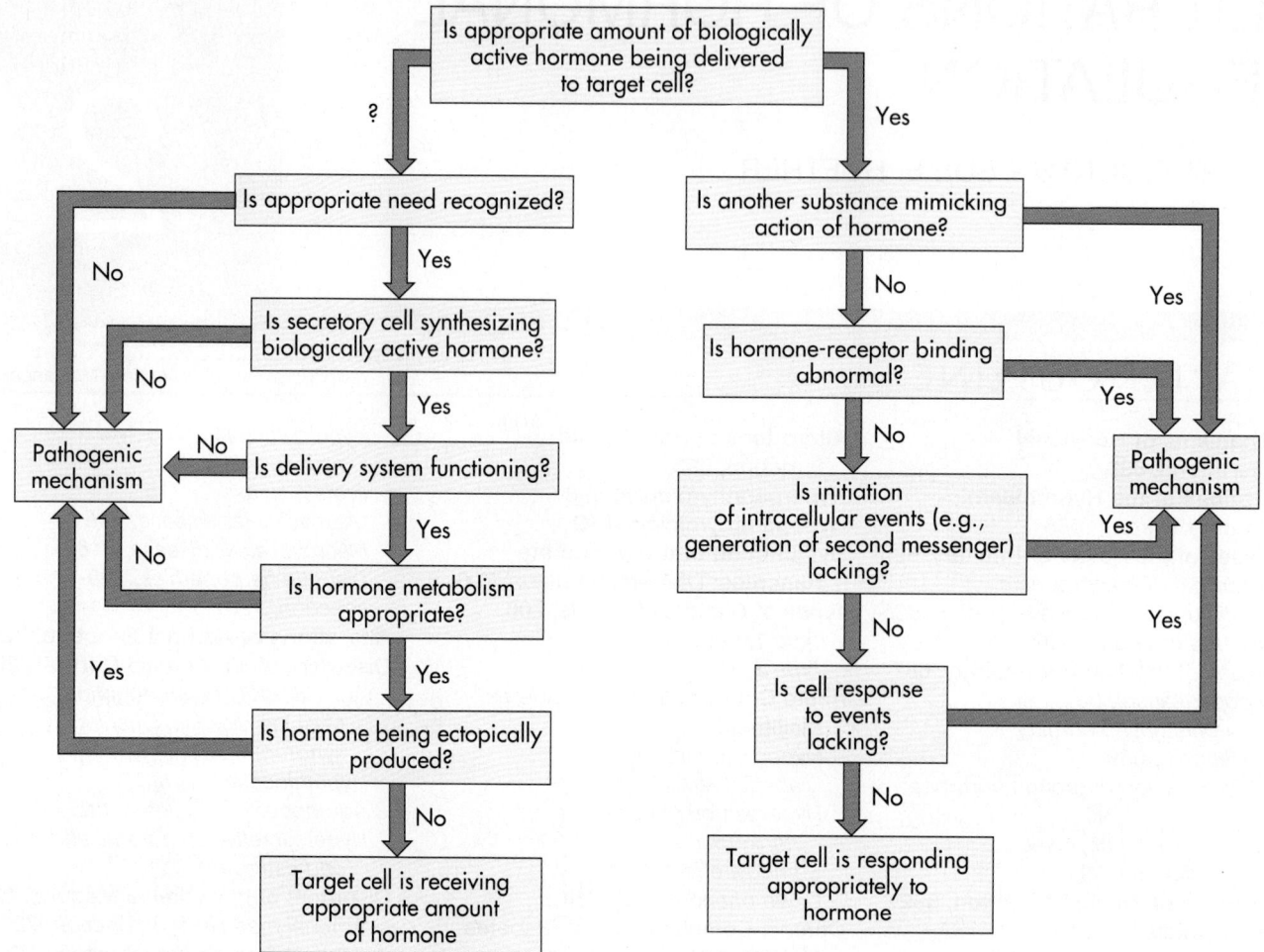

Figure 21-1 Hormone delivery to cells. Phases at which pathogenic mechanisms may develop in delivering appropriate amounts of hormone to the cells.

hormone levels. This mechanism operates without benefit of the normal feedback system for hormone control. In these cases the ectopic hormone production is said to be *autonomous.*

Recently, research has been directed toward understanding causes for the failure of the target cell to respond to its hormone. The general types of abnormal target cell responses currently recognized are receptor-associated disorders and intracellular disorders. Receptor-associated disorders have been identified primarily in water-soluble hormones, such as insulin.[1] These types of disorders usually involve one of the following: (1) a decrease in the number of receptors, leading to decreased or defective hormone-receptor binding; (2) impaired receptor function, resulting in insensitivity to the hormone; (3) presence of antibodies against specific receptors that either reduce available binding sites or mimic hormone action, exaggerating target cell response; or (4) unusual expression of receptor function, as occurs in some tumor cells with abnormal receptor activity.

Intracellular disorders may involve inadequate synthesis of the second messenger, such as cyclic adenosine monophosphate (cAMP), needed to transduce the hormonal signal into intracellular events. The target cell for water-soluble hormones may have a faulty response to hormone-receptor binding and thus fail to generate the required second messenger. The cell also may have an abnormal response to the second messenger if levels of intracellular enzymes or proteins are altered. (Second messengers for various hormones are listed in Table 20-4.) Both of these pathogenic mechanisms result in failure of the target cell to express the usual hormonal effect.

Pathogenic mechanisms affecting target cell response for lipid-soluble hormones, such as thyroid hormone or glucocorticoids, either occur less often or are recognized less often than those affecting the water-soluble hormones. These hormone-resistant states have been generally linked to mutations in the nuclear receptor for the hormone or, in some instances, to alterations in nuclear coregulators.[2,3] The number of receptors may be decreased, or those receptors may have an altered affinity for hormones. Both mechanisms would affect hormone-receptor binding. Alterations in generation of new messenger ribonucleic acid (mRNA) or absence of substrates for new protein synthesis also may occur, resulting in altered target cell response.

ALTERATIONS OF THE HYPOTHALAMIC–PITUITARY SYSTEM

Documenting abnormal release of hypothalamic-releasing hormones has been difficult because of the relative inaccessibility of the hypothalamic–pituitary unit in the brain and the short half-life and small concentrations of the hypothalamic hormones. The most common hypothalamic diseases probably result from interruption in the pituitary stalk caused by destructive lesions of the stem, rupture of the stem after head injury, surgical transection of the stem, or stem tumor. In these cases, interruption of the physical connections between the hypothalamus and the pituitary gland causes apparent pituitary disease. For example, diabetes insipidus (antidiuretic hormone [ADH] insufficiency) may result, depending on the location at which the infundibular stem is interrupted. If the lesion is close to the hypothalamus, diabetes insipidus is likely; the farther away the lesion is from the hypothalamus, the less likely is the occurrence of diabetes insipidus.

The absence of hypothalamic releasing or inhibiting hormones (Figure 21-2) causes a variety of manifestations. In women the menses cease, and in men spermatogenesis is impaired because of the absence of gonadotropin-releasing hormone (GnRH) stimulation of gonadotropin follicle-stimulating hormone (FSH) and luteinizing hormone (LH). Spontaneous mutations of the prophet of pituitary transcription factor (PROP-1) gene involved in early embryonic pituitary development leads to combined hormonal deficiencies. The hormones include thyroid-stimulating hormone (TSH), growth hormone (GH), adrenocorticotropic hormone (ACTH), and prolactin (PRL), and cause failure-to-thrive and short stature in children.[4,5]

Diseases of the Posterior Pituitary
Syndrome of Inappropriate Antidiuretic Hormone Secretion

Diseases of the posterior pituitary that cause clinically observable symptoms are rare. If they do occur, they usually are related to abnormal secretion of antidiuretic hormone (ADH, arginine vasopressin) **Syndrome of inappropriate ADH (SIADH) secretion** is characterized by high levels of ADH in the absence of normal physiologic stimuli for its release.[6] In order to make the diagnosis of SIADH, the individual should have both normal adrenal and thyroid function because thyroid hormone and glucocorticoids are essential for free water clearance by the kidneys.[7]

The most common cause of elevated levels of ADH is ectopically produced ADH. SIADH is associated with some forms of cancer, apparently because of the ectopic secretion of ADH by tumor cells. Tumors that have been reported in association with SIADH include small cell adenocarcinoma of the lung, carcinoma of the duodenum and pancreas, leukemia, lymphoma, Hodgkin disease, sarcoma, and squamous cell carcinoma of the tongue.

Transient SIADH may follow pituitary surgery, because stored ADH is released in an unregulated fashion. When postoperative fluid volume shifts occur after any type of surgery, ADH secretion is increased for 5 to 7 days. The precise mechanism is uncertain, but it is likely related to fluid and volume changes following surgery, the amount and type of intravenous fluids given, and the use of narcotic analgesics. SIADH secretion may be seen in individuals with a variety of infectious pulmonary diseases. It may be caused by the ectopic production of ADH by infected lung tissue[8] or by increased posterior pituitary secretion of ADH in response to a hypoxia-induced decrease in pulmonary perfusion.[9]

SIADH secretion may be associated with psychiatric disease and also may occur after treatment with a variety of drugs.[10] These include hypoglycemic medications (chlorpropamide), barbiturates, general anesthetics, vincristine, nicotine, morphine, diuretics, and synthetic ADH analogs. These drugs serve either to simulate ADH release or to enhance the physiologic effects of ADH or have a biologic action similar to ADH.

PATHOPHYSIOLOGY The cardinal features of SIADH are symptoms of water intoxication caused by enhanced renal

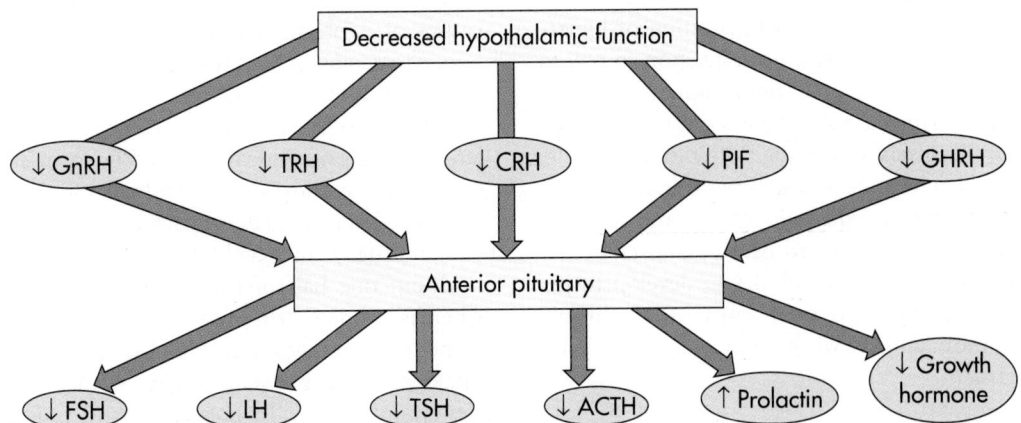

Figure 21-2 Loss of hypothalamic hormones. *GnRh,* Gonadotropin-releasing hormone; *TRH,* thyrotropin-releasing hormone; *CRH,* corticotropin-releasing hormone; *PIF,* prolactin-release inhibiting factor; *GHRH,* growth hormone releasing hormone *FSH,* follicle-stimulating hormone; *LH,* luteinizing hormone; *TSH,* thyroid-stimulating hormone; *ACTH,* adrenocorticotropic hormone.

water retention or increases in total body water that lead to hyponatremia (low serum sodium), hypoosmolarity, and urine that is inappropriately concentrated with respect to serum osmolarity. These features lead to hyponatremia and hypoosmolality.[11] In SIADH, ADH is released continually. Water retention results from the normal action of ADH on collecting ducts, increasing their permeability to water and increasing water reabsorption by the kidneys. (Renal function is discussed in Chapter 36.) An expansion of extracellular fluid volume results, and a dilutional hyponatremia develops.

CLINICAL MANIFESTATIONS   A diagnosis of SIADH requires the following signs: (1) serum hypoosmolality and hyponatremia; (2) urine hyperosmolarity (i.e., the osmolality of the urine is greater than expected for the concomitant serum osmolality); (3) urine sodium excretion that matches sodium intake; (4) normal renal, adrenal, and thyroid function; and (5) absence of conditions that can alter volume status (e.g., congestive heart failure, hypovolemia from any cause, or renal insufficiency).

The symptoms of SIADH are primarily the result of hyponatremia. The severity and the sudden onset of the hyponatremia determine the extent of the symptoms. Even if hyponatremia develops slowly, serum sodium levels below 110 to 115 mEq/L are likely to cause severe and sometimes irreversible neurologic damage. Thirst, impaired taste, anorexia, dyspnea on exertion, fatigue, and dulled sensorium occur when the serum sodium decreases rapidly from 140 to 130 mEq/L. Severe gastrointestinal symptoms, including vomiting and abdominal cramps, occur with a drop in sodium from 130 to 120 mEq/L. With a serum sodium level below 115 mEq/L, confusion, lethargy, muscle twitching, and convulsions may occur. Symptoms usually resolve with correction of hyponatremia.

EVALUATION AND TREATMENT   Serum electrolyte levels, serum osmolality and urine volume, urine electrolyte levels, and urine osmolality are adequate measures of the presence of SIADH. The treatment of SIADH involves the correction of the underlying causal problems; emergency correction of severe hyponatremia by administration of hypertonic saline; and, most important, fluid restriction to 600 to 800 ml/day. Careful monitoring is important. If hyponatremia is too rapidly corrected, a severe neurologic syndrome, central pontine myelinolysis, can ensue.[12] Resolution usually occurs within 3 days, with a 2- to 3-kg weight loss resulting from enhanced free water clearance. No drug therapy is available to suppress ectopically produced ADH; however, demeclocycline, which causes the renal tubules to develop resistance to ADH, may be used to treat resistant or chronic SIADH. ADH receptor agonists, when approved, will be a significant new treatment.[13]

Diabetes Insipidus

Diabetes insipidus is an insufficiency of ADH, leading to polyuria (frequent urination) and polydipsia (frequent drinking). There are two forms, neurogenic, or central, and nephrogenic, or renal.[14] Neurogenic diabetes insipidus is the category encountered most often in clinical practice and is caused by insufficient amounts of ADH. The nephrogenic form is caused by an inadequate response to ADH. Psychogenic polydipsia, commonly referred to as compulsive water drinking, may be difficult to differentiate from true diabetes insipidus.

The neurogenic form of diabetes insipidus occurs when any organic lesion of the hypothalamus, pituitary stalk, or posterior pituitary interferes with ADH synthesis, transport, or release. These lesions include primary brain tumors, hypophysectomy, aneurysms, thrombosis, infections, and immunologic disorders. Diabetes insipidus is a well-recognized complication of closed-head trauma associated with a high mortality rate.[15]

The nephrogenic form of diabetes insipidus is usually an acquired disorder. An idiopathic form also has been documented and usually occurs in genetically predisposed individuals. Nephrogenic diabetes insipidus is usually associated with end-organ failure, with an insensitivity of the renal tubule to ADH, particularly the collecting tubules. Nephrogenic diabetes insipidus is generally related to disorders and drugs that damage the renal tubules or inhibit the generation of cAMP in the tubules. These disorders include pyelonephritis, amyloidosis, destructive uropathies, polycystic disease, and intrinsic renal disease, all of which lead to irreversible diabetes insipidus. Drugs that may induce a generally reversible form of nephrogenic diabetes insipidus include lithium carbonate, general anesthetics such as methoxyflurane, and demeclocycline.

PATHOPHYSIOLOGY   Individuals with diabetes insipidus have partial or total inability to concentrate urine. In individuals with psychogenic polydipsia, polyuria results from both the volume of fluids ingested plus an effective washout of the renal medullary concentration gradient (see Chapter 36). In nephrogenic diabetes insipidus, ADH levels are normal or high, but the collecting ducts do not increase their permeability to water in response to ADH. Genetic causes of nephrotic diabetes insipidus are related to alterations in acquaporin-2, the signaling protein for ADH in the collecting duct.[16]

Insufficient ADH secretion causes immediate excretion of large volumes of dilute urine, leading to an increase in plasma osmolality. In conscious individuals the thirst mechanism is stimulated and induces polydipsia. For unknown reasons the person usually craves cold drinks. The urine output is varied. In about one half of cases, urine volume is 4 to 8 L/day, whereas in one fourth of the cases, it is 8 to 12 L/day. Normal urine output ranges from 1 to 2 L/day depending on volume intake and sensible water losses. With profound ADH deficiency, output may be greater than 12 L/day. The urine specific gravity is low, from 1.00 to 1.005, which is consistent with the failure to reabsorb water. If the individual with diabetes insipidus cannot keep up with the urinary loss of water, hypernatremia occurs. Other serum electrolytes generally are not affected. Dehydration develops rapidly without ongoing fluid replacement.

CLINICAL MANIFESTATIONS   The clinical manifestations of diabetes insipidus are caused by the absence of ADH. These signs and symptoms include polyuria, nocturia, continuous thirst, polydipsia, low urine specific gravity, low urine osmolality,[17] and high-normal plasma osmolality (300 mOsm or more).[9] Plasma osmolality is always higher than urine osmolality in diabetes insipidus after 8 hours of water deprivation. Untreated individuals with long-standing diabetes insipidus may develop a large bladder capacity and hydronephrosis (see Chapter 36).

Idiopathic neurogenic diabetes insipidus usually has an abrupt onset, and many individuals can specifically recall the date of onset of their symptoms. Those with posttraumatic or postneurosurgical diabetes insipidus may develop a classic three-phase syndrome. Initially, significant diuresis occurs, apparently as a result of acute damage to the hypothalamic centers involving ADH secretion. The second phase is one of antidiuresis, which may represent necrosis of denervated tissue of the posterior pituitary with release of ADH into the circulation. The final phase is one of polyuria and polydipsia, reflecting a permanent loss of the ability to secrete adequate amounts of ADH. Antidiuretic hormone does not have to be completely absent for polyuria and polydipsia to occur.

EVALUATION AND TREATMENT   Diabetes insipidus must be distinguished from other polyuric states, including diabetes mellitus, osmotically induced diuresis, and psychogenic polydipsia. Water restriction is a useful test because people without diabetes insipidus respond with a rapid decrease in urine volume and urine osmolarity (800 mOsm/kg). Persons with diabetes insipidus have no decrease in urine volume and maintain a urine osmolarity of approximately 100 mOsm/kg. The diagnosis of diabetes insipidus is generally established through water deprivation testing or by correlating the clinical presentation with serum osmolarity and plasma ADH levels. In individuals with true diabetes insipidus, water deprivation testing can be hazardous. If the individual loses more than 3% of their pretest body weight, circulatory collapse and shock can ensue. The diagnosis of psychogenic polydipsia can be extremely difficult, and differentiation from nephrogenic diabetes insipidus (caused by the washout of renal concentrating gradient) is based upon plasma ADH levels.[17]

Treatment of neurogenic diabetes insipidus is based on the extent of the ADH deficiency and on individual variables such as age, endocrine and cardiovascular status, and life-style.[18] Individuals who have a urine output in excess of 9 L/day and a urine osmolality of less than 100 mOsm/kg after a dehydration or water restriction test generally require ADH replacement.

Replacement therapy for symptomatic central or neurogenic diabetes insipidus includes administration of the synthetic vasopressin analog DDAVP (desmopressin) given intranasally or orally. Drugs that potentiate the action of otherwise insufficient amounts of endogenous ADH, such as chlorpropamide, may be used in individuals with incomplete ADH deficiency.

Diseases of the Anterior Pituitary

Disorders of the anterior pituitary may involve either hypofunction or hyperfunction of the gland. **Hypopituitarism** is defined as a range of dysfunction, from the absence of selective pituitary trophic hormones to complete failure of hormonal functions of the anterior pituitary. Pituitary hypofunction may result from intrinsic pituitary process or from a hypothalamic disorder. The most common causes of hypopituitarism lie within the pituitary. Functional hypopituitarism may be seen in systemic illnesses such as anorexia nervosa; starvation; or severe, systemic illness. **Hyperpituitarism** generally is caused by a pituitary adenoma.

Anterior pituitary hypofunction may result from infarction of the gland, removal or destruction of the gland, or space-occupying lesions such as pituitary adenomas or aneurysms that compress otherwise normal secreting pituitary cells and lead to compromised hormonal output. Growth hormone–secreting cells are most sensitive to pressure. Hyperfunction of the anterior pituitary generally implies an adenoma composed of secretory pituitary cells.

Hypopituitarism

In terms of endocrine replacement therapy, it is not important to differentiate the level of functional loss (hypothalamic vs. pituitary), but it is critical to address the underlying lesion if either neurosurgical intervention or special medical therapy is warranted to treat a neoplastic process.

One cause of hypopituitarism is pituitary infarction (death of tissue). Infarction may be seen in conjunction with Sheehan syndrome (ischemic pituitary necrosis) caused by severe postpartum hemorrhage. Pituitary infarction is also seen with shock; pituitary apoplexy; sickle cell disease; and rarely, during pregnancy in women with diabetes mellitus. Other causes of hypopituitarism are head trauma; infections (e.g., meningitis, syphilis, tuberculosis); vascular malformations; surgical ablation related to tumor removal; and rarely, granulomatous lesions. The pathogenesis and consequences of Sheehan syndrome illustrate the anatomic relationships and physiologic consequences of panhypopituitarism.

PATHOPHYSIOLOGY   The pituitary gland is highly vascular and is therefore extremely vulnerable to ischemia and infarction. In addition, the pituitary relies heavily on portal blood flow from the hypothalamus. The likelihood of infarction is increased with the increased size and vasculature of the gland, which occurs during pregnancy, and a rare condition known as **Sheehan syndrome** may develop. In 1961 Sheehan and Stanfield proposed that the primary pathologic mechanism in postpartum pituitary infarction is vasospasm of the artery supplying the anterior pituitary. A commonly identified cause is some event that leads to circulatory collapse (such as postpartum hemorrhage) and compensatory vasospasm. If vasospasm is sustained for more than several hours, tissue necrosis occurs. The pituitary gland may be particularly susceptible to necrosis because its blood supply, through the hypophyseal system, is already partially deoxygenated and, especially in the hyperplastic pituitary of pregnancy, oxygen demands are increased.

After tissue necrosis, edema occurs. Expansion of the pituitary within the fixed compartment of the sella turcica further impedes blood supply to the pituitary. A second mechanism, which may be involved in pituitary infarction in the postpartum woman (Sheehan syndrome), is an increased risk for intravascular coagulation. In such individuals, excessive fibrin is deposited in the pituitary vessels, predisposing the woman to decreased blood supply and infarction of the pituitary.[19]

CLINICAL MANIFESTATIONS The signs and symptoms of hypofunction of the anterior pituitary are highly variable and depend on the affected hormones. If all hormones are absent (a condition termed **panhypopituitarism**), the individual experiences cortisol deficiency from lack of ACTH; thyroid deficiency from lack of TSH; and gonadal failure and loss of secondary sex characteristics from absence of FSH and LH. GH and, consequently, insulin-like growth factor I levels are low, resulting in delayed growth in children (Figure 21-3) and a vague, multisymptom syndrome in

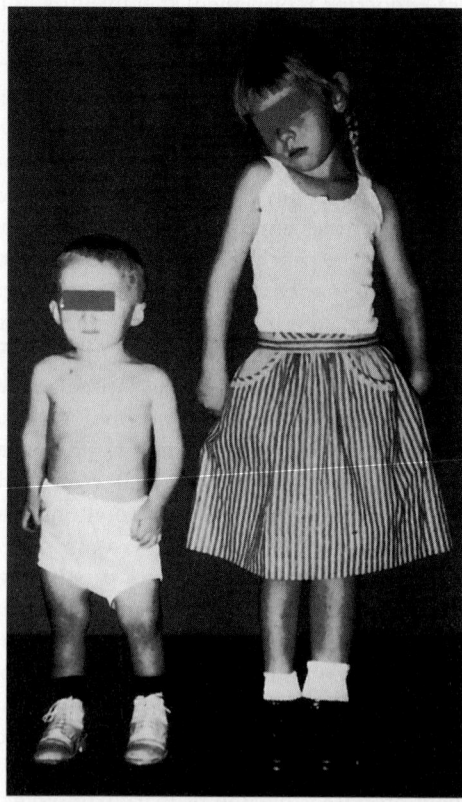

Figure 21-3 Hypopituitary dwarfism. A 4-year-old boy whose height is 25 inches. Girl is also 4 years old and has a normal height of 39 inches. Dwarf has a normal face, as well as head, trunk, and limbs of approximately normal proportions. (From Brashear HR, Raney RB: *Shand's handbook of orthopaedic surgery,* ed 10, St Louis, 1986, Mosby.)

adults.[20] Children also have **dwarfism** with GH insensitivity or resistance (Laron syndrome), in which the GH receptor is altered.[21,22] In addition, postpartum women are unable to lactate because of the absence of prolactin. Menses may cease from absence of FSH and LH.

ACTH deficiency is a potentially life-threatening disorder because cortisol is required for functional maintenance. ACTH deficiency is usually encountered with generalized pituitary hypofunction; it rarely occurs as an isolated event. Within 2 weeks of the complete absence of ACTH, symptoms of cortisol insufficiency develop, including nausea, vomiting, anorexia, fatigue, and weakness. The resulting hypoglycemia is caused by increased insulin sensitivity, decreased glycogen reserves, and decreased gluconeogenesis associated with hypocortisolism. In women, loss of body hair and decreased libido may be caused by decreased adrenal androgen production. ACTH deficiency has a limited effect on aldosterone secretion.

TSH deficiency is rarely seen in isolation but often occurs in conjunction with other pituitary hormone deficiencies. The effects of decreased TSH levels may become apparent 4 to 8 weeks after the onset of hypothyrotropinemia. Cold intolerance, dryness of skin, mild myxedema, lethargy, and decreased metabolic rate occur as a result of hypothyroidism induced by decreased TSH levels. The symptoms are usually less severe than those associated with primary hypothyroidism, in which lack of thyroxine is related to disease in the thyroid gland (see p. 692).

The onset of **FSH** and **LH deficiencies** in women of reproductive age is associated with amenorrhea and atrophic vagina, uterus, and breasts. In postpubertal males, atrophy of the testes and decreased beard growth occur. Both men and women experience a decrease in body hair and diminished libido. FSH and LH deficiencies often occur as a result of pressure on the gonadotropes from other sources, such as tumors. If there is enlargement caused by tumor, symptoms may include headache and visual disturbances with blurring and field defects from pressure on the optic chiasm.

GH deficiency occurs in both children and adults. In children it may be genetic or it may be the result of tumors such as craniopharyngiomas. In adults it is caused by structural or functional abnormalities of the pituitary, but a decline in growth hormone production is an inevitable consequence of aging and the significance of this phenomenon is poorly understood.[23]

GH deficiency in children is manifested by growth failure, but not all children with short stature have growth hormone deficiency. Other causes of growth failure not related to GH deficiency include systemic illness, hypothyroidism, malnutrition, and emotional deprivation. Another feature of GH deficiency in children is fasting hypoglycemia, likely due to impaired substrate mobilization for gluconeogenesis and enhanced insulin sensitivity. Several genetic defects have been identified in the growth hormone axis that account for impaired GH action. The more common type is a recessive mutation in the GHRH gene resulting in a failure of growth hormone secretion. A rare mutation, loss of the growth hormone gene itself, also has been observed. Mutations that cause GH insensitivity also have been reported. These mutations may involve the GH receptor, insulin-like growth factor 1 (IGF-1) biosynthesis, IGF-1 receptors, or defects in GH signal transduction. Individuals with GH sensitivity do not respond normally to exogenously administered growth hormone. Lastly, structural lesions of the pituitary or hypothalamus also may cause GH deficiency and may be associated with other anterior pituitary hormone deficiencies.[24]

An adult GH deficiency syndrome has been described in those who have complete or even partial failure of the anterior pituitary. Symptoms of adult GH deficiency syndrome are extremely vague and include social withdrawal, fatigue, loss of motivation, and a diminished feeling of well-being.[25] Several studies also have documented increased mortality in adults who are GH deficient.[26] Osteoporosis and alterations in body composition (i.e., reduced lean body mass) are common concomitants of adult GH deficiency.[26]

GH replacement therapy has become relatively simple with the introduction of recombinant human growth hormone. In children, GH replacement therapy is monitored by measuring linear growth and IGF-1 levels. GH replacement in adults is much more controversial and is generally reserved for those with symptomatic hypopituitarism.[20]

EVALUATION AND TREATMENT The diagnostic tests evaluating hypopituitarism are well defined and must be interpreted together with the individual's signs and symptoms. Radioimmunoassay is used to measure hormone levels, and both the trophic pituitary and target hormones must be assessed. Radiographic assessment of the pituitary (magnetic resonance imaging [MRI] or computed tomography [CT] scans) may demonstrate enlargement of the pituitary, abnormal areas of enhancement suggestive of an adenoma, deviation of the pituitary stalk, or evidence of a locally aggressive tumor. However, some radiographic findings may be nonspecific and require clinical correlation to establish a diagnosis.

In general, treatment of hypopituitarism involves replacing target gland hormone(s) that are deficient because of lack of tropic anterior pituitary hormones, and thyroid and cortisol replacement therapy must be maintained. Gender-specific sex steroid replacement therapy is also initiated to improve general well-being and to prevent osteoporosis. In cases of circulatory collapse, immediate therapy with glucocorticoids and intravenous fluids is critical.

Hyperpituitarism: Primary Adenoma

Pituitary adenomas are usually benign, slow-growing tumors that arise from cells of the anterior pituitary. The incidence of pituitary adenomas may be as high as 22%, but most of these adenomas are microscopic and asymptomatic.[27] Before the widespread use of higher resolution MRI scanning, most of these incidentally discovered lesions (incidentalomas) were found on postmortem examination. The vast majority of pituitary incidentalomas are hormonally silent and do not pose

significant hazards to the individual.[28] The molecular pathogenesis of pituitary adenomas is not clearly understood. The mortality associated with pituitary tumors usually is attributable to alterations in hormone secretion or to invasion or impingement of surrounding structures caused by expanding adenomas.[29] Primary pituitary carcinomas are rare, representing about 0.2% of all pituitary tumors.[29a]

PATHOPHYSIOLOGY Local expansion of pituitary adenomas may cause both neurologic and secretory defects. Neurologically, the tumor may impinge on the optic chiasm if it extends upward from the sella turcica. This causes a variety of visual disturbances, depending on the area of the optic chiasm that is compressed. If the tumor is locally aggressive, it may invade the cavernous sinus and cause cavernous sinus thrombosis with impairment of the function of the oculomotor, trigeminal, trochler, and abducens cranial nerves, evoking symptoms relative to their function. Extension also may involve the hypothalamus, disturbing hypothalamic control of wakefulness, thirst, appetite, and temperature.

The adenomatous tissue secretes the hormone of the cell type from which it arose, without regard to physiologic needs and without benefit of regulatory feedback mechanisms. GH-, LH-, and FSH-secreting cells in the pituitary are most sensitive to pressure from expanding tumors within the rigid sella turcica, and as a consequence, hyposecretion of these hormones is most often seen in people with a large pituitary gland.

CLINICAL MANIFESTATIONS The clinical manifestations of pituitary adenomas are related to tumor growth and hormone hypersecretion or hyposecretion. Effects from an increase in tumor size include such nonspecific complaints as headache and fatigue. Visual changes produced by pressure on the optic chiasm include visual field impairments (occasionally beginning in one eye and progressing to the other) and temporary blindness. If the tumor infiltrates other cranial nerves, neurologic function is affected.

The pressure produced by a pituitary adenoma is also associated with a paradoxical effect on neighboring anterior pituitary cells, which results in hyposecretion of other anterior pituitary hormones. For example, hyposecretion of GH almost always occurs, and in adults the symptoms of growth hormone deficiency are subtle and include fatigue. Gonadotropic hyposecretion often results in menstrual irregularity in women, decreased libido, and receding secondary sex characteristics in both men and women. If the tumor exerts sufficient pressure, thyroid and adrenal hypofunction may occur because of lack of TSH and ACTH. These result in the symptoms of hypothyroidism and hypocortisolism.

EVALUATION AND TREATMENT Diagnosis of pituitary adenoma involves physical and laboratory evaluations, including pertinent hormone assays and radiographic examination of the skull. This may be accomplished by CT scanning or dynamic MRI used in conjunction with contrast material. Dynamic MRIs provide superior imaging and greater sensitivity for small lesions in comparison to CT scans.[30]

The goal of treatment is to protect the individual from the effects of tumor growth and to control hormone hypersecretion or hyposecretion while minimizing damage to appropriately secreting portions of the pituitary. Individuals can be treated with specific medications to suppress tumor growth, transsphenoidal tumor resection, or radiation therapy, depending on the tumor type, extent of tumor growth, and the suitability of the individual for specific types or combinations of treatment.[31]

Hypersecretion of Growth Hormone: Acromegaly

Acromegaly occurs in adults who are exposed to continuously excessive levels of GH and concomitant elevation of IGF-1. In children and adolescents whose epiphyseal plates have not yet closed, the effect of increased GH levels on long bone growth is termed **giantism** (Figure 21-4).

Acromegaly is a relatively uncommon disease, estimated to occur in about 40 persons per million.[32,33] Approximately 15% of all pituitary tumors release excessive GH. The most common cause of acromegaly is a primary autonomous GH-secreting pituitary adenoma. Acromegaly occurs more often in women than men and is diagnosed most often in adults in

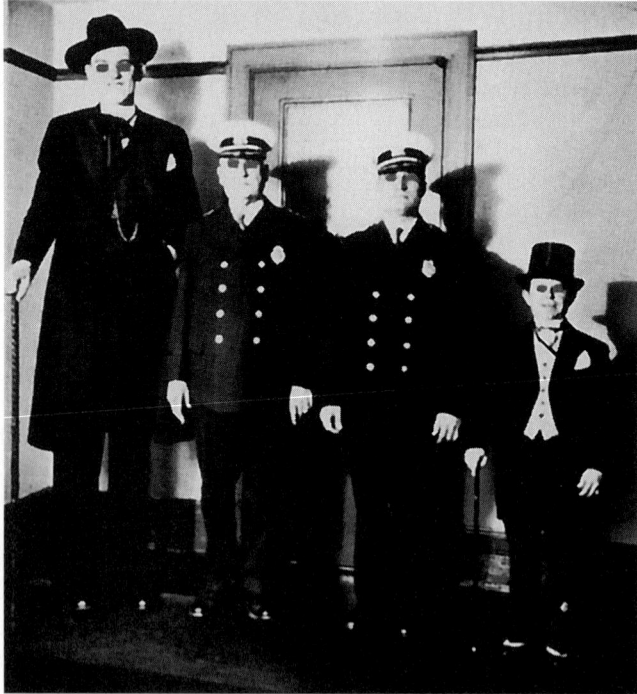

Figure 21-4 **Giantism.** A pituitary giant and dwarf contrasted with normal-size men. Excessive secretion of growth hormone by the anterior lobe of the pituitary gland during the early years of life produces giants of this type, whereas deficient secretion of this substance produces well-formed dwarfs. (From Thibodeau GA, Patton K: *Anatomy & physiology*, ed 5, St Louis, 2003, Mosby.)

their 40s and 50s, although the disease is usually present for years preceding the diagnosis.

Acromegaly is a slowly progressive disease that, if untreated, is associated with a decreased life expectancy. An increased number of deaths associated with acromegaly are caused by cardiac hypertrophy, hypertension, atherosclerosis, and insulin-resistant type 2 diabetes mellitus that lead to coronary artery disease. Malignancies, in particular colon cancer evolving from colonic polyps, are also more common in individuals with acromegaly.[34]

PATHOPHYSIOLOGY   With a GH-secreting adenoma, the usual GH baseline secretion pattern is lost, as are sleep-related GH peaks. A totally unpredictable secretory pattern ensues. With only slight elevations of GH, IGF-1 levels increase, stimulating growth. In the adult, epiphyseal closure has occurred and increased amounts of GH and IGF-1 cannot stimulate further long bone growth. Instead, these elevations cause connective tissue proliferation, an increase in the extra-cytoplasmic matrix, and bony proliferation.

GH acts on the renal tubules to increase phosphate reabsorption, leading to mild hyperphosphatemia. The metabolic effects of GH hypersecretion include impaired carbohydrate tolerance and increased metabolic rate. Hyperglycemia may be seen as a result of GH's inhibition of peripheral glucose uptake and increased hepatic glucose production, followed by insulin resistance and, finally, compensatory hyperinsulinism. **Type 2 diabetes mellitus** occurs when the pancreas is unable to secrete enough insulin to offset the effects of GH. Not surprisingly, because of the aforementioned changes in glucose use, approximately one third of people with GH abnormalities have glucose intolerance and half of those individuals develop type 2 diabetes mellitus.[35,36]

CLINICAL MANIFESTATIONS   As a result of connective tissue proliferation, individuals with acromegaly have enlarged tongues, interstitial edema, increase in the size and function of sebaceous and sweat glands (leading to increased body odor), and coarse skin and body hair. The coarse skin condition becomes very apparent when procedures such as inserting an intravenous needle are performed; the skin is very thick and difficult to penetrate (Figure 21-5). Bony proliferation involves periosteal vertebral growth and enlargement of the facial bones and the bones of the hands and feet (Figure 21-6). The associated growth results in protrusion of the lower jaw and forehead and a need for increasingly larger sizes of shoes, hats, rings, and gloves.

Because IFG-1 stimulates cartilaginous growth, the increased IGF-1 levels cause elongation of ribs at the bone-cartilage junction, leading to a barrel-chest appearance and increased proliferation of cartilage in joints. This in turn causes backache, arthralgia, and arthritis. These are early manifestations of acromegaly. When shaking hands with an individual with acromegaly, one can palpate the large soft tissues. With bony and soft tissue overgrowth, entrapment of nerves may occur, leading to peripheral nerve damage as

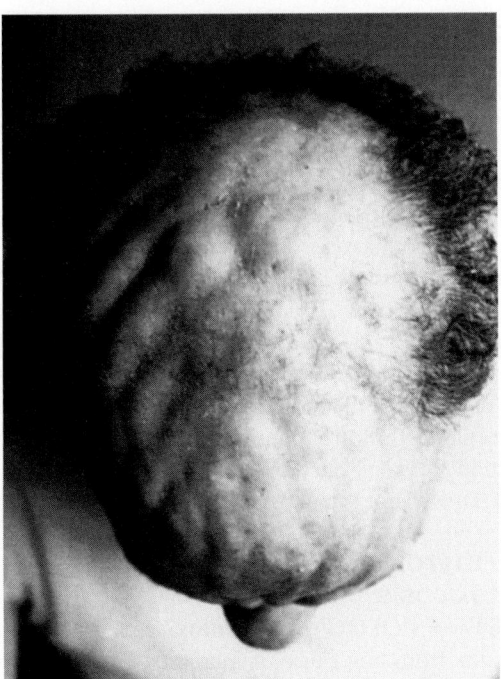

Figure 21-5 Acromegaly. Note thickening of skin on scalp. (From Thibodeau GA: *Anatomy & physiology,* St Louis, 1987, Mosby.)

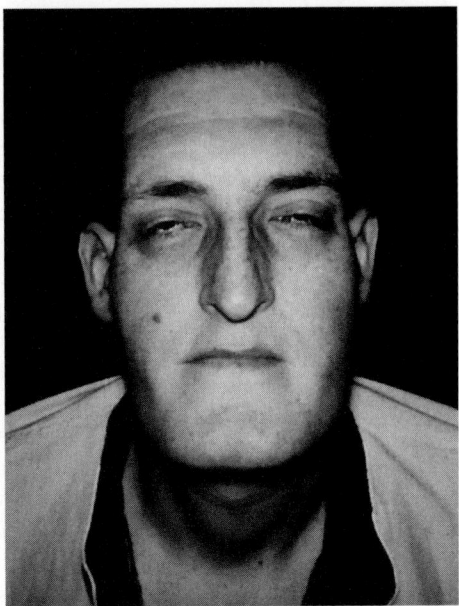

Figure 21-6 Acromegaly. Note large head, forward projection of jaw, and protrusion of frontal bone. (From Thibodeau GA: *Anatomy & physiology,* St Louis, 1987, Mosby.)

manifested by weakness, muscular atrophy, footdrop, and sensory changes in the hands.

Although the associated pathophysiology is not clearly understood at present, hypertension and left heart failure are seen in one third to one half of individuals with acromegaly. Cardiomyopathy associated with progressive and unrestrained myocardial growth is a significant factor.[37] Headache occurs in 50% to 87% of cases and does not appear related to GH levels, size, or extension of the tumor or presence of hypertension. Because of a space-occupying lesion, central nervous system symptoms of headache, seizure activity, visual disturbances (e.g., bitemporal hemianopia from compression of the optic chiasm), papilledema, and compression hypopituitarism may occur.[38]

If compression hypopituitarism does occur because of a large GH-secreting adenoma, the secretion of the gonadotropins may be affected. This causes amenorrhea in women and loss of libido and erectile dysfunction in men because of pituitary stalk compression. Dopamine delivery to the anterior pituitary is impaired in 30% to 40% of individuals with acromegaly resulting in hyperprolactinemia. In addition, cosecretion of GH and prolactin by the same neoplastic cell line has been documented.[39,40]

EVALUATION AND TREATMENT   Diagnosis of acromegaly requires growth hormone suppression during oral glucose tolerance testing and elevated IGF-1 levels.[41] The goals of treatment are to normalize GH and IGF-1 serum levels, if possible, allowing normal pituitary function and relieving or preventing complications related to tumor expansion. The treatment of choice in acromegaly is transsphenoidal surgical removal of the GH-secreting adenoma. Treatment by radiation therapy may be effective when rapid control of GH levels is not essential, when the individual is not a good surgical candidate, or when hyperfunction persists after subtotal resection. Octreotide, a long-acting somatostatin analog, has been shown to be extremely effective in lowering elevated growth hormone levels, reversing many of the clinical manifestations of the disease, and causing tumor shrinkage in nearly one half of individuals.[42] Pegvisomant is a new and effective drug that inhibits dimerization (the joining of two identical molecules) of GH receptors.[43]

Hypersecretion of Prolactin: Prolactinoma

Pituitary tumors that secrete prolactin, **prolactinomas,** are the most common of the hormonally active pituitary tumors encountered in clinical medicine.[44] Prolactin is under tonic inhibitory hypothalamic control through the secretion of dopamine. The physiologic actions of prolactin include breast development during pregnancy, postpartum milk production, and suppression of ovarian function in nursing women. Pathologic elevation of prolactin in women results in amenorrhea, nonpuerperal milk production (galactorrhea), hirsutism (excessive body hair in a masculine distribution pattern), and osteopenia caused by estrogen deficiency. Hyperprolactinemia in men causes hypogonadism, erectile dysfunction, impaired libido, oligospermia, and diminished ejaculate volume.[45]

Approximately 30% of pituitary tumors secrete prolactin; however, many conditions or medications can elevate prolactin in the absence of pituitary pathologic condition. For example, renal failure, polycystic ovarian disease, primary hypothyroidism, breast stimulation, or even venipuncture can increase prolactin levels. Medications that can increase prolactin block the effects of dopamine at the pituitary or stimulate proliferation of prolactin-secreting cells (lactotrophes). These include antipsychotics (risperidone, chlorpromazine), metoclopramide, tricyclic antidepressants, methyldopa, and estrogens. Any process that interferes with the delivery of dopamine from the hypothalamus to the lactotrophes (pituitary stalk tumor, pituitary stalk transection, or compressive pituitary tumor) also results in hyperprolactinemia. Because thyrotropin-releasing hormone (TRH) stimulates prolactin secretion in addition to enhancing TSH release, prolactin may be elevated in individuals with primary hypothyroidism.

PATHOPHYSIOLOGY   The hallmark of a prolactinoma is sustained increases in serum prolactin. Indeed, tumor size roughly correlates with the degree of prolactin elevation. Hyperprolactinemia has several reproductive consequences. Prolactin suppresses GnRH pulses at the hypothalamus, impairs pulsatile pituitary gonadotropin release, and blunts the gonadal responsiveness to gonadotropins. In estrogen- and progesterone-primed breasts, milk production is stimulated.

CLINICAL MANIFESTATIONS   Women with hyperprolactinemia generally present with galactorrhea (nonpuerperal milk production) and menstrual disturbances including amenorrhea. In susceptible women, hirsutism develops as a result of estrogen deficiency. If detected after many years, estrogen deficiency also may result in osteoporosis. Menstrual abnormalities and galactorrhea are alarming symptoms in women, and, as a result, women generally present earlier in the course of the illness and are found to have microadenomas (<1 cm in size) that are less likely to have associated compressive or impingement symptoms. Men, on the other hand, often present with headache or visual impairment. Symptoms of hypogonadism, erectile dysfunction, loss of libido, oligospermia, and decreased ejaculate volume are commonly associated with hyperprolactinemia in men.[45,46]

EVALUATION AND TREATMENT   The diagnostic evaluation of hyperprolactinemia starts with a careful history to exclude medications that may cause elevations in prolactin. Symptoms of hypothyroidism should be elicited, and screening with a serum TSH is mandatory. A careful search for a nonpituitary cause should be pursued if prolactin is less than 50 ng/ml. Prolactin levels over 200 ng/ml are usually associated with a prolactinoma. MRI scanning of the pituitary is often helpful in detecting prolactinoma, but the chance of finding an unrelated incidentaloma must always be considered.

Dopaminergic agonists (bromocriptine, cabergoline, and pergolide) are the treatment of choice for prolactinomas,[47] and their use is often associated with both a rapid reduction in the size of the tumor and a reversal of the gonadal effects of hyperprolactinemia. Restoration of fertility in previously anovulatory women is common. In individuals resistant or intolerant to these medications, transsphenoidal surgery and radiotherapy are options.

ALTERATIONS OF THYROID FUNCTION

Disorders of thyroid function develop as a result of primary dysfunction or disease of the thyroid gland or, secondarily, as a result of pituitary or hypothalamic alterations. Primary thyroid disorders result in alterations of thyroid hormone (TH) levels with secondary feedback effects on pituitary thyroid-stimulating hormone (TSH). For example, when there are primary elevations in TH, TSH will secondarily decrease because of negative feedback. When TH is decreased because of a condition affecting the thyroid gland, TSH will be elevated. Secondary disorders of the thyroid gland are related to disorders of pituitary gland TSH production. When there is excessive TSH production, TH is elevated secondary to the primary elevation of TSH. The reverse is true with inadequate TSH production.

Hyperthyroidism
Thyrotoxicosis
PATHOPHYSIOLOGY   **Thyrotoxicosis** is a condition that results from any cause of increased levels of circulating thyroid hormone (TH).[48] The terms *thyrotoxicosis* and *hyperthyroidism* are often used interchangeably. Primary hyperthyroidism is a form of thyrotoxicosis in which excess thyroid hormones are secreted by the thyroid gland. Thyrotoxicosis has a variety of causes. Identifying the cause is important because the treatment and expected outcome vary accordingly. Specific diseases that can cause hyperthyroidism include Graves disease; toxic multinodular goiter; solitary hyperfunctioning nodules; and very rarely, follicular thyroid carcinoma. Secondary hyperthyroidism is very rare and is caused by TSH-secreting pituitary adenomas. Thyrotoxicosis not associated with hyperthyroidism (because thyroid hormone is not being actively synthesized) includes thyroiditis (either subacute or painless) or ingestion of excess TH. Each of these conditions is associated with specific pathophysiology and manifestations. All forms of thyrotoxicosis share some common characteristics.

CLINICAL MANIFESTATIONS   The clinical features of thyrotoxicosis are attributable to the metabolic effects of increased circulating levels of thyroid hormones. This usually results in an increased metabolic rate with heat intolerance and an increased tissue sensitivity to stimulation by the sympathetic division of the autonomic nervous system. The major manifestations are summarized in Table 21-1. Goiter is almost always present in thyrotoxicosis.

EVALUATION AND TREATMENT   The diagnosis of thyrotoxicosis is based upon symptoms of thyroid hormone excess and documentation of increased circulating thyroid hormone levels. Elevated serum free thyroxine (T_4), triiodothyronine (T_3), and radioactive iodine uptake (RAIU) are common in hyperthyroid states.

Treatment is directed at controlling excessive TH production, secretion, or action. The major types of therapy cur-

Table 21-1	Systemic Effects of Hyperthyroidism	
System	Clinical Manifestations	Mechanisms Underlying Clinical Manifestations
Endocrine	Enlarged thyroid gland (goiter) (97%-99% of cases); systolic or continuous bruit over thyroid; increased cortisol degradation; hypercalcemia and decreased PTH secretion; diminished sensitivity to exogenous insulin	Hyperactivity of the thyroid gland; excess bone resorption leading to hypercalcemia and a disruption of PTH-regulating mechanisms; increased insulin degradation
Reproductive	Oligomenorrhea or amenorrhea in women, erectile dysfunction and decreased libido in men; increased serum estradiol and estrone but lower than normal levels of free estradiol and estrone	Menstrual cycle alterations that may be related to hypothalamic or pituitary disturbances; increase in sex hormone–binding globulin
Gastrointestinal	Weight loss; increased peristalsis leading to less formed and more frequent stools; nausea, vomiting, anorexia, abdominal pain; increased use of hepatic glycogen stores and of adipose and protein stores; decrease in serum lipid levels (including triglycerides, phospholipids, and cholesterol); changes in vitamin metabolism leading to decrease in tissue stores of vitamins	Increased catabolism leading to the body's inability to meet its metabolic needs; increased glucose absorption; increase in cholesterol excretion in feces and cholesterol conversion to bile salts; impaired conversion of B vitamins to their coenzymes, causing increased need for water-soluble and fat-soluble vitamins
Integumentary	Excessive sweating, flushing, and warm skin; heat intolerance; hair fine, soft, and straight; temporary hair loss; nails that grow away from nail beds, palmar erythema	Hyperdynamic circulatory state
Sensory (eyes)	Ocular manifestations including elevated upper eyelid leading to decreased blinking and a staring quality; fine tremor of lid; infiltrative ocular changes associated with Graves disease	Overactivity of Müller muscle; inflammation of retro-orbital contents
Cardiovascular	Increased cardiac output and decreased peripheral resistance; tachycardia at rest; loud heart sounds; supraventricular dysrhythmias, left ventricular dilation and hypertrophy	Hypermetabolism and need to dissipate heat
Nervous	Restlessness; short attention span; compulsive movement; fatigue; tremor; insomnia; increased appetite; emotional lability	Not clearly defined; alterations in cerebral metabolism resulting from excess thyroid hormone
Pulmonary	Dyspnea; reduced vital capacity	Weakness of respiratory muscles

PTH, Parathyroid hormone.

rently used to achieve these goals include antithyroid drug therapy (methimazole or propylthiouracil), radioactive iodine therapy, and surgery.

Graves Disease

Graves disease is an autoimmune disease and is the most common cause of hyperthyroidism. Genetic factors play an important role in the pathogenesis of autoimmune thyroid disease.[49] This disease is characterized as a multisystem syndrome consisting of one or more of the following: (1) hyperthyroidism, (2) diffuse thyroid enlargement (goiter), (3) ophthalmopathy, and (4) dermopathy. The prevalence is less than 1% in the U.S. population.[50] It occurs more commonly in women.

The pathology of Graves disease indicates that normal regulatory mechanisms are overridden by abnormal immunologic mechanisms. Substances termed *thyroid autoantibodies* (or *thyroid-stimulating immunoglobulins*) of the immunoglobulin G (IgG) class are found in more than 95% of subjects with Graves disease.[51] The disease is slowly progressive. T lymphocytes are sensitized to thyroid antigens and stimulate B cells to produce the stimulatory antibodies that cause hyperthyroidism.[52] The stimulating antibodies function like TSH by binding to the TSH receptor, thus stimulating TH synthesis and secretion. The hyperfunction of the thyroid

gland leads to suppression of TSH and TRH, because of the normal negative feedback from elevated levels of thyroid hormone. The hyperfunction of the thyroid gland is reflected in a dramatically increased iodide uptake and increased rate of thyroid gland metabolism, which may in turn contribute to the hypervascularity and enlargement of the gland (goiter). The disproportionate increase in T_3 production reflects long-term hyperstimulation of the thyroid gland. A decrease in the concentration of thyroid-binding globulin, combined with the increased production of thyroid hormone, causes increased circulating levels of thyroid hormone responsible for many of the thyrotoxic symptoms previously described.

A small number of individuals with Graves disease experience **pretibial myxedema (Graves dermopathy)**, characterized by subcutaneous swelling on the anterior portions of the legs and by indurated and erythematous skin. These manifestations occasionally appear on the hands as well.

Many individuals with Graves disease experience ocular manifestations (Figure 21-7). Two categories of ocular manifestations are associated with Graves disease: (1) functional abnormalities resulting from hyperactivity of the sympathetic division of the autonomic nervous system and (2) infiltrative changes involving the orbital contents with enlargement of the ocular muscles. Functional abnormalities occur in most individuals with Graves disease. These abnormalities include

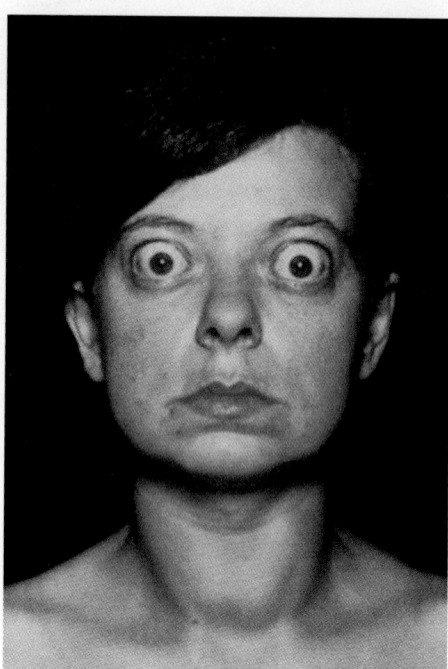

Figure 21-7 Thyrotoxicosis (Graves disease). Note large and protruding eyeballs in association with a large goiter. (Seidel et al: *Mosby's guide to physical examination,* ed 4, St Louis, 1999)

a lag of the globe on upward gaze or a lag of the upper lid on downward gaze and are caused by overactivity of Mueller's (eyelid) muscles. This manifestation does not affect ocular function and resolves with treatment for hyperthyroidism. Thyroid-associated dermopathy and ophthalmopathy are associated with thyrotropin receptor antigen on fibroblasts and recruited T lymphocytes.[53]

Infiltrative ophthalmopathy may occur with Graves disease.[54] It appears in 50% to 70% of individuals with Graves disease[55] and is characterized by edema of the orbital contents; protrusion of the globe (exophthalmos); paralysis of the extraocular muscles; and damage to the retina and optic nerve, which may lead to blindness. These changes result in exophthalmos, periorbital edema, and extraocular muscle weakness leading to diplopia (double vision). The individual may experience irritation, pain, lacrimation, photophobia, and blurred vision. Occasionally, decreased visual acuity, papilledema (edema of the optic nerve), visual field impairment, exposure keratopathy, and corneal ulceration may occur.

Unfortunately, current treatment for Graves disease does not reverse the infiltrative ophthalmopathy or the pretibial myxedema. Therapy for Graves disease includes antithyroid drugs (propylthiouracil and methimazole), radioactive iodine, and surgery. Skin lesions rarely require treatment.

Hyperthyroidism Resulting From Nodular Thyroid Disease

Enlargement of the thyroid gland is referred to as a **goiter.** The thyroid gland normally enlarges in response to an increased secretion of TSH that may occur in puberty, pregnancy, or iodine deficiency. The increased number of follicles is a compensatory mechanism in response to increased TSH

levels. When the condition requiring increased TH resolves, TSH secretion normally subsides and the thyroid gland returns to its original size.

Irreversible changes may have occurred in some follicular cells, however, so that such cells then function autonomously. Hyperthyroidism may result from these irreversible changes. On the other hand, some of these clusters of cells may cease to function, and the remainder of the gland then functions to supply the remainder of the body's need, and a euthyroid state is achieved and maintained. If the autonomously functioning cells produce sufficient or excessive TH for usual body requirements, the remainder of the gland undergoes involution, becoming normal but inactive tissue. This condition may result in euthyroidism or hyperthyroidism, depending on the amount of TH produced.

Once thyrotoxicosis results, the condition generally is termed **toxic multinodular goiter;** however, only one nodule may become hyperfunctioning. This is termed a **toxic adenoma.** Mutations of the TSH receptor have been found in most of the solitary, hyperfunctioning thyroid adenomas.[56] Manifestations of hyperthyroidism resulting from toxic multinodular goiter or a toxic adenoma are similar to those of Graves disease, although infiltrative ophthalmopathy and myxedema do not occur. The symptoms usually develop slowly and appear over time.[57]

Thyrotoxic Crisis

Thyrotoxic crisis (thyroid storm) is a rare but dangerous worsening of the thyrotoxic state, in which death occurs within 48 hours without treatment.[58] The condition may develop spontaneously, but it occurs most often in individuals who have undiagnosed or partially treated severe hyperthyroidism and who are subjected to excessive stress from other causes. These causes may include infection, pulmonary or cardiovascular disorders, emotional distress, dialysis, plasmapheresis (mechanical removal of antibodies from the bloodstream), or inadequate preparation for thyroid surgery.

The systemic symptoms of thyrotoxic crisis include hyperthermia; tachycardia, especially atrial tachydysrhythmias; high-output heart failure; agitation or delirium; and nausea, vomiting, or diarrhea contributing to fluid volume depletion. The symptoms may be attributed to increased β-adrenergic receptors and catecholamines. The treatment is designed (1) to reduce both circulating TH levels by inducing a block of thyroid hormone synthesis (i.e., propylthiouracil) and thereby reducing their effects to eliminate the precipitating disorder, (2) use of beta blockers for control of cardiovascular symptoms, and (3) supportive care.[59]

Hypothyroidism

Hypothyroidism is the most common disorder of thyroid function. **Hypothyroidism** is caused by a deficient production of TH by the thyroid gland. Hypothyroidism may be primary or secondary. Primary causes include (1) defective hormone synthesis resulting from autoimmune (circulating antithyroid antibodies) thyroiditis, endemic iodine deficiency, or antithyroid drugs (goitrous hypothyroidism); and

(2) congenital defects or loss of thyroid tissue after treatment for hyperthyroidism. Secondary hypothyroidism, which is less common, includes conditions that cause either pituitary or hypothalamic failure.

PATHOPHYSIOLOGY   In primary hypothyroidism the loss of functional thyroid tissue leads to a decreased production of TH. The response is an increased secretion of TSH that may lead to goiter. On the other hand, the cellular infiltration that occurs in autoimmune thyroiditis also may cause thyroid enlargement independently of the trophic actions of TSH. Secondary hypothyroidism is caused most commonly by failure of the pituitary to synthesize adequate amounts of TSH. Pituitary tumors or the results of their treatment are the most common causes of secondary hypothyroidism.

Hypothyroid Conditions
Primary Hypothyroidism

There are several causes of primary hypothyroidism. Some are associated with spontaneous recovery and resultant euthyroidism, whereas others are linked to permanent hypothyroidism. Spontaneous recovery of thyroid function is seen in three conditions—subacute thyroiditis, painless thyroiditis, and postpartum thyroiditis.[60] **Subacute thyroiditis** is a nonbacterial inflammation of the thyroid, often preceded by a viral infection. It is accompanied by fever, tenderness, and enlargement of the thyroid. The inflammatory process results initially in elevated levels of thyroid hormone caused by release of stored thyroglobulin and later in hypothyroidism before the gland recovers normal activity. Symptoms may last for 2 to 4 months, and nonsteroidal antiinflammatory agents, beta-blockers, and possibly thyroid hormone supplementation may be required during the course of the illness. **Autoimmune thyroiditis (Hashimoto disease, chronic lymphocytic thyroiditis)** results in gradual destruction of thyroid tissue by infiltration of lymphocytes and circulating thyroid autoantibodies (antithyroid peroxidase and antithyroglobulin antibodies). Hashimoto disease also has a genetic disposition.[61] Autoreactive T lymphocytes, natural killer cells, and cytokines also may be involved in tissue destruction.[62] Other causes of primary hypothyroidism include radioiodine ablation, thyroidectomy, and medications (lithium and amiodarone). Goiter formation is commonly observed. **Painless thyroiditis** has a course similar to subacute thyroiditis, but it is pathologically identical to Hashimoto disease. **Postpartum thyroiditis** generally occurs within 6 months of delivery, occurs in up to 7% of all women, and has a course similar to painless thyroiditis. Pathologic specimens suggest it is related to Hashimoto disease as well. Spontaneous recovery is seen in over 95% of individuals affected with these forms of thyroiditis.

CLINICAL MANIFESTATIONS   Hypothyroidism generally affects all body systems, with the extent of the symptoms closely related to the degree of TH deficiency. The onset is usually insidious over months or years. The lowered levels of TH result in decreased energy metabolism and heat production. The individual develops a low basal metabolic rate, cold intolerance, lethargy, tiredness, and slightly lowered basal body temperature. Many organ systems are affected (Table 21-2). The decrease in TH leads to increases in TSH production and may cause goiter.

The characteristic sign of severe or long-standing hypothyroidism is **myxedema,** which is histologically similar to the pretibial myxedema deposits that often occur with Graves disease. Myxedema is a result of an alteration in the composition of the dermis and other tissues. The connective fibers are separated by an increased amount of protein and mucopolysaccharides.

This protein-mucopolysaccharide complex binds water, producing nonpitting, boggy edema, especially around the eyes, hands, and feet and in the supraclavicular fossae (Figure 21-8). Myxedema is also responsible for thickening of the tongue and the laryngeal and pharyngeal mucous membranes. This results in thick, slurred speech and hoarseness, both common in hypothyroidism.

Myxedema coma, a medical emergency, is a diminished level of consciousness associated with severe hypothyroidism.[63] Signs and symptoms include hypothermia without shivering, hypoventilation, hypotension, hypoglycemia, and lactic acidosis. Older individuals with severe vascular disease and with moderate or untreated hypothyroidism are particularly at risk for developing myxedema coma. It also may occur after overuse of narcotics or sedatives or after an acute illness in hypothyroid individuals.

EVALUATION AND TREATMENT   In addition to the clinical symptoms of hypothyroidism, a decrease in both total and free T_4 is present in myxedema; however, **subclinical hypothyroidism,** defined as an elevation in TSH with normal levels of circulating TH, is more common and also responds to levothyroxine supplementation.[64] TSH concentration increases from loss of negative feedback from thyroid hormone. When hypothyroidism is caused by pituitary deficiencies, serum TSH levels are decreased or are inappropriately normal in the face of low levels of TH. Hormone replacement therapy is the treatment of choice for hypothyroidism. Thyroid hormone is available as a synthetic hormone (levothyroxine), which is preferred over the crude extract from animal thyroid glands (desiccated thyroid).

The restoration of normal TH levels should be timed appropriately; a regimen of hormonal therapy depends on the individual's age; the duration and severity of the hypothyroidism; and the presence of other disorders, particularly cardiovascular disorders. The goal is maximal metabolic restoration consistent with the individual's overall well-being and normalization of TSH levels in individuals with primary hypothyroidism.

Congenital Hypothyroidism

Congenital hypothyroidism, classified as a rare form of primary hypothyroidism, occurs in infants as a result of absent thyroid tissue (thyroid agenesis) and hereditary defects in thyroid hormone synthesis. Thyroid agenesis occurs more

Table 21-2	Systemic Manifestations of Hypothyroidism	
System	Clinical Manifestations	Mechanisms Underlying Clinical Manifestations
Neurologic	Confusion, syncope, slowed speech and thinking, memory loss; lethargy, headaches, hearing loss, night blindness; slow, clumsy movements; cerebellar atazia; slow alpha-wave activity and loss of amplitude in EEG; reduced cAMP response to epinephrine, glucagons, and PTH stimulation; decreased appetite	Decreased cerebral blood flow leading to cerebral hypoxia; reduced intracellular processes caused by decreased β-adrenergic activity that may be related to a decrease in the number of β-adrenergic receptor sites
Endocrine	Increased TSH production in primary hypothyroidism; enlarged pituitary thyrotropes, increase in serum prolactin levels with galactorrhea; decreased rate of cortisol turnover but with normal serum cortisol levels	Impaired TH synthesis or defects in iodide trapping leading to compensatory TSH production; chronic overstimulation of thyrotropes of TRH and by TSH synthesis; stimulation of lactotropes by TRH related to increased prolactin levels; decreased deactivation of cortisol
Reproductive	Decreased androgen secretion in men, increased estriol formation in women; low total hormone values but with increased amounts of unbound hormone; anovulation, decreased libido, and a high incidence of spontaneous abortion in women; erectile dysfunction, decreased libido, and oligospermia in men	Altered metabolism of estrogens and androgens; decreased levels of sex hormone–binding globulin
Hematologic	Decrease in red cell mass leading to normocytic, normochromic anemia; macrocytic anemia associated with vitamin B_{12} deficiency and inadequate folate or iron absorption in the gastrointestinal tract	Decreased basal metabolic rate and reduced oxygen requirements, decreased production of erythropoietin, possible relationship between TH and optimal hematologic response to vitamin B_{12}
Cardiovascular	Reduction in stroke volume and heart rate causing lowered cardiac output; increased peripheral vascular resistance to maintain systolic blood pressure; normal response to exercise but with alterations in circulatory system at rest (prolonged circulation time and decreased blood flow to tissues); cool skin and cold tolerance; enlarged heart; decreased intensity of heart sounds and variety of ECG changes (sinus bradycardia, prolonged PR interval, depressed P waves, flattened or inverted T waves, and low-amplitude QRS complexes); cardiac tamponade (although rare) (See Chapter 30)	Decreased metabolic demands and loss of regulatory and rate-setting effects of TH; protein-mucopolysaccharide-rich fluid in the pericardial sac associated with enlarged heart; pericardial effusions associated with heart sounds and ECG changes
Pulmonary	Dyspnea; myxedematous changes in respiratory muscles leading to hypoventilation and carbon dioxide retention, which contribute to myxedema coma	Pleural effusions associated with dyspnea, although effusions may be asymptomatic
Renal	Reduced renal blood flow and glomerular filtration rate leading to decreased renal excretion of water; increase in total body water and dilutional hyponatremia; reduced production of erythropoietin	Hemodynamic alterations associated with reduced blood flow and filtration; increased total body water related to decreased excretion and mucinous deposits in tissue
Gastrointestinal	Constipation, weight gain, and fluid retention; decreased absorption of most nutrients; decreased protein metabolism leading to retarded skeletal and soft-tissue growth and slightly positive nitrogen balance; edema; decreased glucose absorption and delayed glucose uptake; elevated serum lipid values	Reduced intake and reduced peristaltic activity that may progress to fecal impaction; water absorption related to prolonged transit time; fluid retention associated with myxedematous changes; edema associated with high concentrations of exchangeable albumin in the extravascular space caused by increased capillary permeability to proteins; depressed insulin degradation; depressed lipid synthesis and degradation
Musculoskeletal	Muscle aching and stiffness; slow movement and slow tendon jerk reflexes; decreased bone formation and resorption, increased bone density; aching and stiffness in joints	Decreased rate of muscle contraction and relaxation contributing to slow movement and reflexes
Integumentary	Dry, flaky skin; dry, brittle head and body hair; reduced growth of nails and hair, slow wound healing	Reduced sweat and sebaceous gland secretion
	Myxedema	Accumulation of hyaluronic acid, which binds water and causes a puffy appearance
	Cool skin	Decreased circulation to skin

EEG, Echoencephalogram; *cAMP,* cyclic adenosine monophosphate; *PTH,* parathyroid hormone; *TH,* thyroid hormone; *TSH,* thyroid-stimulating hormone; *TRH,* thyrotropin-releasing hormone; *ECG,* electroencephalogram.

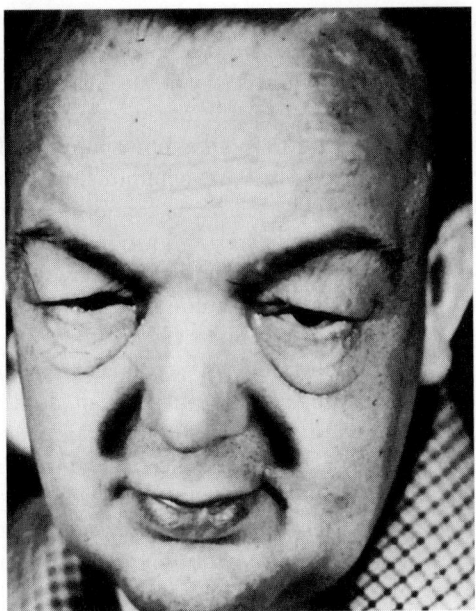

Figure 21-8 Myxedema. Note edema around eyes and facial puffiness. (From Thibodeau GA: *Anatomy & physiology,* St Louis, 1987, Mosby.)

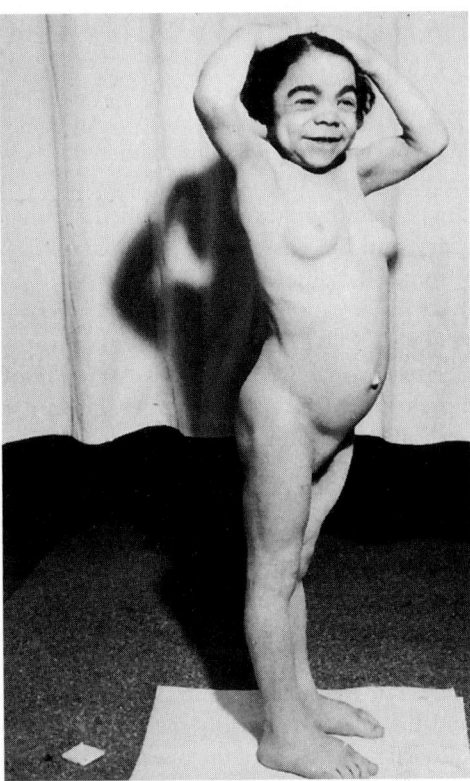

Figure 21-9 Adult cretin. Note characteristic facial features, dwarfism (44 inches), absent axillary and scant pubic hair, poorly developed breasts, potbelly, and small umbilical hernia. (From Schneeberg NG: *Essentials of clinical endocrinology,* St Louis, 1970, Mosby.)

often in female infants, with permanent abnormalities in 1 of every 3000 to 4000 live births.[65,66]

Thyroid hormone is essential for embryonic growth, particularly of brain tissue. The infant will be mentally retarded if there is no thyroxine (T_4) during fetal life, but this can be significantly reversed with administration of T_4 immediately after birth.

Clinical manifestations of hypothyroidism may not be evident until after 4 months of age. Signs and symptoms include difficulty eating, hoarse cry, and protruding tongue caused by myxedema of oral tissues and vocal cords; hypotonic muscles of the abdomen with constipation, abdominal protrusion, and umbilical hernia; subnormal temperature; lethargy; excessive sleeping; slow pulse; and cold, mottled skin. Skeletal growth is stunted because of impaired protein synthesis, poor absorption of nutrients, and lack of bone mineralization. The child will be dwarfed, with short limbs, if not treated (cretinism) (Figure 21-9). Dentition is often delayed. Mental retardation is a function of the severity of hypothyroidism and the delay before initiation of treatment.

Hypothyroidism is difficult to identify at birth, but high birth weight, hypothermia, delay in passing meconium, and neonatal jaundice are suggestive signs. Cord blood can be examined in the first days of life for T_4 and TSH levels. Treatment is administration of T_4. The probability of normal growth and intellectual function is high if treatment is started before the child is 3 or 4 months old.

Thyroid Carcinoma

Thyroid carcinoma is the most common endocrine malignancy but is relatively rare, accounting for 25,690 estimated new cases annually in 2005 and 1490 estimated cancer deaths in the United States.[67] The most consistent causal risk factor in the development of thyroid cancer appears to be exposure to ionizing radiation,[68] especially exposure during childhood or puberty.[69] Papillary and follicular thyroid carcinomas are the most frequent and medullary and anaplastic thyroid carcinomas are less common. Most tumors are well differentiated.

Most individuals with thyroid carcinoma have normal T_3 and T_4 levels and are therefore euthyroid. Thyroid cancer typically is discovered as a small thyroid nodule or as a metastatic tumor most commonly occurring in the regional lymph nodes, lungs, brain, or bone. Changes in voice and swallowing and difficulty in breathing are related to tumor growth impinging on the trachea or esophagus. The diagnosis of thyroid carcinoma is generally made by fine-needle aspiration of a thyroid nodule. Ultrasonography and radioisotope scanning are rarely helpful in assessing the malignant potential of a thyroid nodule; however, ultrasound-guided aspiration biopsy of small (<1 cm) thyroid nodules is very helpful in providing an earlier diagnosis and earlier institution of therapy.

Treatment for thyroid carcinoma remains controversial, primarily because of the rarity of the disease, its protracted nature, and the relatively low mortality regardless of the method of treatment. Treatment of well-differentiated tumors includes a near-total or total thyroidectomy, postoperative radioactive iodine, and suppression of TSH with levothyroxine. Anaplastic thyroid carcinoma carries a grave prognosis, and palliation with surgical debulking, external beam radiotherapy, or chemotherapy may be offered.[70]

ALTERATIONS OF PARATHYROID FUNCTION

Hyperparathyroidism

In general, **hyperparathyroidism** is characterized by a greater than normal secretion of parathyroid hormone (PTH). The causes of hyperparathyroidism are classified as either primary or secondary, and their associated pathophysiologic mechanisms are somewhat different.

PATHOPHYSIOLOGY   **Primary hyperparathyroidism** is characterized by inappropriate excess secretion of PTH by one or more of the parathyroid glands.[71] In primary hyperparathyroidism, normal feedback mechanisms, such as elevated serum levels of ionized calcium, fail to normally inhibit PTH secretion by the parathyroid gland.

The cause of primary hyperparathyroidism is unknown; however, recent data suggest that there are two mechanisms for the development of this condition. The first is a clonal proliferation of parathyroid cells with a higher threshold for calcium feedback, and the second is generalized growth of parathyroid tissue. The former is most likely the cause of adenomas, and the latter is probably the cause for hyperplasia. There is also a familial form of the disease that has an autosomal dominant pattern of inheritance.[72] Hypercalcemia and hyperphosphatemia are the hallmarks of primary hyperparathyroidism. The effects of excessive PTH secretion and primary hyperparathyroidism on various organ systems are summarized in Table 21-3.

Secondary hyperparathyroidism is caused by an increase in PTH secondary to a chronic disease state, such as chronic renal failure or intestinal malabsorption, which causes a decrease in serum ionized calcium levels (hypocalcemia). The chronic renal failure–induced hypocalcemia serves as the stimulus for increased PTH secretion and renal and gastrointestinal calcium absorption in an attempt to reestablish normal ionized calcium levels. Since vitamin D metabolism is impaired in renal failure, eucalcemia cannot be restored unless vitamin D supplements are administered. Hypercalcemia does not occur in secondary hyperparathyroidism because the parathyroid tissue is not autonomous and is only responding to a physiologic stimulus (hypocalcemia).

The most common cause of secondary hyperparathyroidism is chronic renal failure (with failure of glomerular filtration), which results in hyperphosphatemia, reduced levels of activated vitamin D, and hypocalcemia, which stimulates parathyroid hormone secretion. Other causes include dietary deficiency in vitamin D or calcium; decreased intestinal absorption of vitamin D or calcium; and ingestion of drugs, such as phenytoin, phenobarbital, and laxatives, which decrease intestinal absorption of calcium.[73]

CLINICAL MANIFESTATIONS   Hypersecretion of PTH causes excessive osteoclastic activity, resulting in bone resorption. (Bone resorption is discussed in Chapter 41.) Pathologic bone changes include pathologic fractures, kyphosis (curvature) of the dorsal spine, and compression fractures of the vertebral bodies. Parathyroid hormone hypersecretion and its resulting hypercalcemia increase the renal filtration load of calcium, leading to hypercalciuria.

Hypercalcemia also affects proximal renal tubular function, causing metabolic acidosis and production of an abnor-

---

Table 21-3   Manifestations of Primary Hyperparathyroidism

Symptoms	Responsible Derangements	Mechanisms
Renal colic, nephrolithiasis, recurrent urinary tract infections, renal failure	Hypercalcemia, hyperphosphaturia, proximal renal tubular bicarbonate leak, urine pH >6	Calcium phosphate salts precipitate in alkaline urine, renal pelvis, and collecting ducts; calcium oxalate stones also formed
Abdominal pain, peptic ulcer disease	Hypercalcemia-stimulated hypergastrinemia	Elevated hydrochloric acid secretion
Pancreatitis	Hypercalcemia	Etiology of relationship unknown
Bone disease, osteitis fibrosa and cystica, osteoporosis	PTH-stimulated bone resorption, metabolic acidosis	Osteoporosis now more commonly encountered, but other disorders more specific for hyperparathyroidism
Muscle weakness, myalgia	PTH excess, possible direct effect on striated muscle and on nerves	Characteristic myopathic changes in muscle histology (neuropathy of type I and type II muscle fibers)
Neurologic and psychiatric problems (impaired memory, confusion, stupor, coma)	Hypercalcemia	Neuropathy; electroencephalographic changes present
Polyuria, polydipsia	Hypercalcemia	Direct effect on renal tubule to decrease responsiveness to antidiuretic hormone
Constipation	Hypercalcemia	Decreased peristalsis of gastrointestinal tract
Anorexia, nausea, and vomiting	Hypercalcemia	Central stimulation of vomiting center
Hypertension	Renal disease, direct effect of calcium on arterial smooth muscle, pheochromocytoma	Plasma rennin activity elevated or normal
Arthralgia and arthritis	Gout, pseudogout, periarticular classification	Hyperuricemia, chronic renal failure with high calcium × phosphate product

From Harden RH et al, editors: *William's textbook of endocrinology,* ed 10, Philadelphia, 2002, Saunders.

mally alkaline urine. PTH also enhances the renal excretion of phosphate, which results in hypophosphatemia (low serum phosphate) and hyperphosphaturia (increased urine phosphate). The combination of these three variables—hypercalciuria, alkaline urine, and hyperphosphaturia—predisposes the individual to the formation of calcium stones. Kidney stones are often formed in the renal pelvis or in the renal collecting ducts and may be associated with infections. Both kidney stones and renal infection may lead to impaired renal function. Hypercalcemia also impairs the concentrating ability of the renal tubule by decreasing its response to ADH.

Chronic hypercalcemia of hyperparathyroidism is associated with mild insulin resistance, necessitating increased insulin secretion to maintain normal glucose levels. Hypercalcemia also affects the muscular, nervous, and gastrointestinal systems. (The clinical symptoms of primary hyperparathyroidism are summarized in Table 21-3.)

EVALUATION AND TREATMENT   The diagnosis of hyperparathyroidism is relatively straightforward. The concurrent findings of increased ionized calcium in the face of elevated or inappropriately normal intact PTH (which documents an abnormal feedback mechanism) are suggestive. The definitive treatment of hyperparathyroidsm is surgery.[74] Surgery is generally reserved for individuals with documented complications of hyperparathyroidism (osteoporosis, nephrolithiasis, or gastrointestinal or neuropsychiatric complications) or severely elevated serum calcium levels (>1 mg/dl above the upper limit or normal for the laboratory). Hypercalciuria (>4 mg/kg/24 hours) caused by a benign inherited condition, familial hypocalciuric hypercalcemia (FHH), is not treated surgically. FHH is caused by a mutation in the transmembrane calcium receptor and is not associated with the classic complications of hyperparathyroidism but must be differentiated from primary hyperparathyroidism to avoid unnecessary surgery.

If intact PTH levels are low, the differential diagnosis shifts to hypercalcemia of malignancy, granulomatous diseases (sarcoidosis), excessive calcium ingestion, or to hypervitaminosis A or D. Treatment of these conditions depends on the underlying cause.

Hypoparathyroidism

Hypoparathyroidism (abnormally low PTH levels) most commonly is caused by damage to the parathyroid glands during thyroid surgery.[75] Postoperative hypoparathyroidism occurs in approximately 1% of all individuals undergoing thyroid surgery, with the incidence increasing to 10% after repeated neck explorations. This is caused by the anatomic proximity of the parathyroid gland to the thyroid gland.

PATHOPHYSIOLOGY   In hypoparathyroidism a lack of circulating PTH causes a depressed serum calcium level and an increased serum phosphate level. In the absence of PTH the abilities to resorb calcium from bone and to regulate calcium reabsorption from the renal tubules are impaired. The phosphaturic effects of PTH are lost, resulting in hyperphosphatemia.

Hypoparathyroidism can occur also as a result of hypomagnesemia, although the effects of hypomagnesemia on the peripheral metabolism and clearance of PTH are not clearly understood. Once serum magnesium levels return to normal, however, PTH secretion returns to normal, as does peripheral tissues' responsiveness to PTH. Hypomagnesemia may be related to chronic alcoholism, malnutrition, malabsorption, increased renal clearance of magnesium caused by the use of aminoglycoside antibiotics or certain chemotherapeutic agents, or prolonged magnesium-deficient parenteral nutritional therapy.

CLINICAL MANIFESTATIONS   Symptoms associated with hypoparathyroidism are related to hypocalcemia. Hypocalcemia causes a lowering of the threshold for nerve and muscle excitation so that a nerve impulse may be initiated by a slight stimulus anywhere along the length of a nerve or muscle fiber. This is manifested as muscle spasms; hyperreflexia; clonic-tonic convulsions; laryngeal spasms; and in severe cases, death from asphyxiation.

Other symptoms of hypocalcemia are caused by mechanisms that are not yet understood. These symptoms include dry skin; loss of body and scalp hair; hypoplasia of developing teeth; horizontal ridges on the nails; cataracts; basal ganglia calcifications (which may be associated with a parkinsonian syndrome); and bone deformities, including brachydactyly and bowing of the long bones.

Phosphate retention caused by increased renal reabsorption of phosphate is associated also with hypoparathyroidism. Hyperphosphatemia is associated with inhibition of the renal enzyme necessary for the conversion of vitamin D to its most active form. This tends to depress serum calcium levels further by reducing gastrointestinal absorption of calcium.

EVALUATION AND TREATMENT   A low serum calcium level and high phosphorus level in the absence of renal failure, intestinal disorders, or nutritional deficiencies are diagnostic of hypoparathyroidism. Intact PTH levels are low in hypoparathyroidism, but they are elevated in an inherited condition associated with hypocalcemia, pseudohypoparathyroidism. There is a defect in the tissue responsiveness to PTH in pseudohypoparathyroidism.[76]

The treatment of hypoparathyroidism is directed toward the alleviation of hypocalcemia. In acute states this involves parenteral administration of calcium, which allows correction of serum calcium within minutes. Maintenance of serum calcium is achieved with pharmacologic doses of an active form of vitamin D and oral calcium. The recommended daily dose of calcium is 1 to 3 g.

Hypoplastic dentition, cataracts, bone deformities, and basal ganglia calcifications do not respond to the correction of hypocalcemia, but the other symptoms of hypocalcemia are reversible. As serum calcium levels return to normal, phosphaturia usually is stimulated. This leads to a return to normal serum phosphate levels. In some individuals, however, the absence of the phosphaturic effect of PTH causes a persistent hyperphosphatemia.

Significant elevations of phosphorus should be treated with drugs that inhibit gastrointestinal absorption of phosphate (phosphate binders) and thus prevent ectopic calcifications.

DYSFUNCTION OF THE ENDOCRINE PANCREAS: DIABETES MELLITUS

Diabetes mellitus is not a single disease but a group of clinically heterogeneous disorders with glucose intolerance in common. It encompasses many causally unrelated diseases and includes many different etiologies of disturbed glucose tolerance.[77,77a,77b] The term *diabetes mellitus* is used to describe a syndrome characterized by chronic hyperglycemia and other disturbances of carbohydrate, fat, and protein metabolism. Types 1 and 2 diabetes are the most common and are discussed in greatest detail in this text. Table 21-4 describes the terminology and characteristics of the conditions associated with abnormal glucose metabolism including gestational diabetes (GDM), impaired glucose tolerance (IGT), and impaired fasting glucose (IFG).

Normal blood glucose levels are maintained within a narrow range of 70 to 120 mg/dl. The diagnosis of diabetes is based on one of the following:[78]

1. More than one fasting plasma glucose level greater than or equal to 126 mg/dl
2. Plasma glucose value in the 2-hour sample (2hPG) of the standard oral glucose tolerance test (OGTT) greater than or equal to 200 mg/dl, confirmed on subsequent day
3. Random (any time of day without regard to time since last meal) plasma glucose level greater than 200 mg/dl, combined with classic symptoms of polydipsia, polyphagia, and polyuria

IFG is defined as a fasting glucose greater than or equal to 110 mg/dl but less than 126 mg/dl. Glucose tolerance is normal if the 2-hour postload glucose level is less than 140 mg/dl. IGT is defined as a 2-hour postload glucose level greater than or equal to 140 but less than 200 mg/dl. Any abnormality of glucose tolerance has potentially serious consequences. Numerous epidemiologic studies have shown an increased risk of cardiovascular disease and premature death in individuals with glucose intolerance.[79] In addition, individuals with abnormal glucose tolerance have a 3% to 7% yearly risk of developing overt diabetes. In comparison, the individual's *lifetime* risk of acquiring diabetes is around 7% to 10%. This has led several organizations to adopt the term *prediabetes* to describe both IGT and IFG.[80]

In nonpregnant women, an OGTT consists of the administration of a 75-g oral glucose load after a 10-hour fast followed by measurement of plasma glucose 2 hours later. It is unnecessary and potentially harmful to perform an OGTT in individuals who already meet criteria for diabetes based upon their fasting plasma glucose level. IGT results from reduced suppression of hepatic glucose output and reduced pancreatic islet cell function.[81] Intravenous glucose tolerance tests are rarely used because they are generally less sensitive than OGTTs and may cause painful venous thrombosis.

Another mechanism used primarily to identify the plasma glucose concentration over time is the measurement of **glycosylated hemoglobin** or, more precisely, hemoglobin A_{1c}, but because of the lack of standardization of this measurement, it is not considered a diagnostic test for diabetes. In the normal 120-day life span of the red blood cell, glucose molecules join hemoglobin, forming glycosylated hemoglobin. In individuals with persistent hyperglycemia, increases in the quantities of three glycosylated hemoglobins (A_{1a}, A_{1b}, and A_{1c}) are noted. A buildup of glycosylated hemoglobin within the red cell reflects the average level of glucose to which the cell has been exposed during its life cycle (approximately 120 days). Measuring glycosylated hemoglobin (HgbA1c) assesses the effectiveness of therapy by monitoring long-term serum glucose regulation.[82,83]

Types of Diabetes Mellitus
Type 1

Type 1 diabetes mellitus accounts for approximately 10% of all diabetes mellitus in the Western world. There is pancreatic atrophy and specific loss of beta cells with small islets in type 1 diabetes. Macrophages, T and B lymphocytes, and natural killer cells are often present. The incidence of the condition is increasing in some areas, with other areas showing no change in incidence.[84] Several studies suggest that the incidence and prevalence are higher for whites than for nonwhites, with the highest rate found in Finland and the lowest rate in Japan. Variations occur, however, even within individual countries. (Table 21-5 summarizes the epidemiology of diabetes mellitus.)

Type 1 diabetes mellitus is thought to be the result of a genetic-environmental interaction. Between 10% and 13% of individuals with newly diagnosed type 1 diabetes have a first-degree relative (parent or sibling) with type 1 diabetes. Diagnosis has a seasonal distribution, with more cases reported during autumn and winter in the northern hemisphere. Diagnosis is rare during the first 9 months of life and peaks at 12 years of age.

PATHOPHYSIOLOGY   Two distinct types of type 1 diabetes have been identified: immune and nonimmune. In immune-mediated diabetes mellitus, environmental-genetic factors are thought to result in cell-mediated destruction of pancreatic beta cells. In the common form, markers of immune destruction, including autoantibodies to islet cells and/or to insulin, glutamic acid decarboxylase (GAD_{65}), and protein tyrosine phosphatase IA-2,[85,86] are found in 85% to 90% of individuals when fasting hyperglycemia is initially detected. Nonimmune type 1 diabetes occurs secondary to other diseases such as pancreatitis or to a more fulminant disorder termed *idiopathic (type 1B) type 1 diabetes*. Autoimmune type 1 diabetes is called *type 1A*.[87]

Table 21-4	Classification and Characteristics of Diabetes Mellitus	
Name	Previous Synonyms	Characteristics
Type 1: Primary B Cell Defect or Failure Immune-mediated diabetes common form (~90%)	Juvenile diabetes Juvenile-onset diabetes Ketosis-prone diabetes Brittle diabetes Idiopathic diabetes Insulin-dependent diabetes mellitus (IDDM)	Cellular mediated autoimmune destruction of pancreatic B cells Individual prone to ketoacidosis Little or no insulin secretion Insulin dependent 75% of individuals develop before 30 yr of age, can occur up to the tenth decade Usually not obese
Idiopathic (~10%)	Other types	No defined etiologies; absolute requirement for insulin replacement therapy in affected individuals may come and go
Type 2 Diabetes: Insulin Resistance with Inadequate Insulin Secretion	Adult-onset diabetes Maturity-onset diabetes Stable diabetes Ketosis-resistant diabetes Non-insulin-dependent diabetes mellitus (NIDDM)	Usually not insulin-dependent but may be insulin requiring Individual not ketosis prone (but may form ketones under stress) Obesity common in the abdominal region Generally occurs in those older than 40 yr, but the frequency is rapidly increasing in children Strong genetic predisposition Often associated with hypertension and dyslipidemia
Other Forms Genetic defects of the B cell	Secondary diabetes Maturity-onset diabetes of the young (MODY)	Genetic abnormalities such as inability to convert proinsulin to insulin, mutation of insulin molecules or mitochrondrial deoxyribonucleic acid (DNA), glucokinase abnormalities
Genetic defects in insulin action		Mutations in the insulin receptor with hyperinsulinism or hyperglycemia or severe diabetes
Pancreatic diseases Drug- or chemical-induced B cell dysfunction Endocrinopathies Infections	Secondary diabetes	Any process that diffusely injures the pancreas Impaired insulin secretion or antagonism of insulin by counter-excess regulatory hormones Inhibition of insulin secretion B cell destruction by viruses: *cytomegalovirus, congenital rubella*
Uncommon forms of immune-mediated diabetes mellitus		Few known conditions Anti-insulin receptor antibodies Reported with "stiff man syndrome" and individuals receiving interferon-α
Other genetic syndromes sometimes associated with diabetes mellitus		Down, Klinefelter, Turner and Wolfram syndromes
Gestational Diabetes Mellitus	Asymptomatic diabetes Subclinical diabetes Latent diabetes	Glucose intolerance first recognized during pregnancy, most likely in the third trimester Following pregnancy, glucose may normalize, remain impaired, or progress to diabetes mellitus Occurs in 1%-14% of all pregnancies; 40%-60% will develop diabetes mellitus within 15 yr after gestation
Impaired fasting glucose (IFG) Impaired glucose tolerance (IGT)		Fasting plasma glucose ≥100 and <126 mg/dl Abnormal response to oral glucose tolerance test: 2hPG ≥140 and <200 mg/dl 10%-25% will convert to type II diabetes within 10 yr Many with IGT are obese

Data from American Diabetes Association (Committee Report): Report of the expert committee on the diagnosis and classification of diabetes mellitus, *Diabetic Care* 26(Suppl. 1):S5-S20, 2003.

Table 21-5	Epidemiology and Etiology of Diabetes Mellitus	
	Type 1 Diabetes: Primary B Cell Defect or Failure	**Type 2 Diabetes: Insulin Resistance with Inadequate Insulin Secretion**
Incidence		
Frequency	One of the most common childhood diseases (5%-10% of all cases of diabetes mellitus) Range from 29.5/100,000 (Finland) to 1.6/100,000 (Japan)	Accounts for most cases ($\approx$90%-95%) Prevalence rate in United States (for age 18 yr and older): 6.6% Prevalence for American Indian/Alaska Native; non-Hispanic black; Hispanic/Latino American; Asian American): 39.9%
Change in incidences	Increased incidences in British Isles, Finland, Norway, Denmark, Israel, Germany, and Poland; stable elsewhere	Incidence has risen in United States since 1940
Characteristics		
Age at onset	Peak onset at age 11 to 13 yr (slightly earlier for girls than for boys) Rare in children younger than 1 yr and adults older than 30 yr	Risk of developing diabetes increases after age 40 yr; in general, incidence increases with age into the 70s; among Pima Indians, incidence peaks between ages 40 and 50 yr, then falls
Gender	Similar in males and females	In the United States, more females than males
Racial distribution	Rates for whites 1.5-2 times higher than for nonwhites Higher rates for those of Scandinavian descent than for those of central or southern European descent	Certain racial groups may be more likely to develop type 2 diabetes when exposed to a particular environment Common in migrant groups encountering a different environment (e.g., Polynesians moving from traditional to western life-style) In the United States, risk is highest for American Indians; rates are higher for Pacific Islanders, Japanese, Puerto Ricans, Hispanics, and blacks than for whites
Socioeconomic status	Conflicting data	A disease of the affluent in developing nations but more common among those of lower incomes and less education in the United States
Seasonal distribution	More new cases documented during fall and winter in the northern hemisphere	No known association
Childbirth association	No association documented	Effect of parity on subsequent development of type 2 diabetes varies among different populations
Obesity	Generally normal or underweight	Frequent contributing factor to precipitate type 2 diabetes among those susceptible; a major factor in populations recently exposed to westernized environment Increased risk related to duration, degree, and distribution of obesity
Etiology		
Common theory	*Autoimmune:* genetic and environmental factors, resulting in gradual process of autoimmune destruction in genetically susceptible individuals *Nonautoimmune:* Unknown Strong association with HLA-DQA and HLA-DQB genes Monogenic β-cell defect	Disease results from genetic susceptibility (although the precise gene or genes have not yet been determined) combined with environmental determinants and other risk factors Associated with long-duration obesity
Heredity	Risk to sibling: 5%-10%; risk to offspring: 2%-5%	Risk to first-degree relative (child or sibling): 10%-15%
Presence of antibody	Islet cell autoantibodies (ICA) and/or autoantibodies to insulin, and autoantibodies to glutamic acid decarboxylase (GAD_{65}) and tyrosine phosphatases IA-2 and IA-2β are present in 85%-90% of individuals when fasting hyperglycemia is initially detected	Islet cell antibodies not present
Insulin resistance	Insulin resistance rare	Insulin resistance is generally caused by altered cellular metabolism and an intracellular postreceptor defect
Insulin secretion	Severe insulin deficiency or no insulin secretion at all	Typically increased at time of diagnosis, but progressively declines over the course of the illness

Data from American Diabetes Association: Diagnosis and classification of diabetes mellitus, *Diabetic Care* 28(Suppl 1): S37-S42, 2005.

Historically, type 1 diabetes mellitus has been thought to have an abrupt onset. More recently, however, prospective studies show a distinctive natural history involving genetic susceptibility; a long preclinical period; immunologically mediated destruction of beta cells, eventually leading to insulin deficiency; and hyperglycemia. Generally, this latent period is longer in older individuals and often results in misclassification of an older type 1 individual as having type 2 diabetes.

Genetic Susceptibility

The exact nature of genetic susceptibility is not clearly understood. The strongest association with type 1 diabetes is with major histocompatibility complex (MHC) (histocompatibility leukocyte antigen [HLA]) class II alleles HLA-DQ and HLA-DR. The HLA-DR marker is associated with other autoimmune disorders, such as Graves, Hashimoto, and Addison diseases.[88] The risk of developing type 1 diabetes increases five to eight times when one of those specific loci is present. When the individual is heterogenous for HLA-DR3 and HLA-DR4, the risk is 20 to 40 times higher than that of the general population. Specific human antigens also are thought to decrease the risk of developing type 1 diabetes, with HLA-DR2 associated with an unusually low risk. Current theories of causation hold that islet cell destruction occurs predominantly in genetically susceptible people.

Environmental Factors

Environmental factors are thought to have a significant contribution to the development of type 1 diabetes mellitus. Some types of viral infections have been implicated with autoimmune damage to beta cells, including cytomegaloviruses, mumps, and Epstein-Bar virus. Bovine serum albumin, a major constituent of cow's milk, may be involved in triggering beta cell autoantibodies. Stress may advance development of type 1 diabetes mellitus by stimulating secretion of counterregulatory hormones and affecting immune responses (see Chapter 10). Specific environmental factors linked to type 1 diabetes mellitus are presented in Box 21-1.

Immunologically Mediated Destruction of Beta Cells

Research has demonstrated the presence of islet cell autoantibodies (ICAs) for years before the occurrence of symptoms. These immune markers precede evidence of beta cell deficiency and have been found in 85% to 90% of type 1 diabetes cases at the time of clinical onset.[89] Autoantibodies against insulin (insulin autoantibodies [IAAs]) also have been noted. Researchers speculate that IAAs may form during the process of active islet cell and beta cell destruction. ICAs and IAAs are probably the result of the autoimmune process rather than the cause.[82,83] They tend to disappear with time. Antiglutamic acid decarboxylase (antiGAD$_{65}$) antibodies are more persistent, which makes them clinically useful in differentiating the etiology of diabetes in a given individual.[85] (Glutamic acid decarboxylase promotes the synthesis of gamma aminobutyric acid from islet cells, which inhibits both glucagon and somatostatin secretion.)

Type 1 diabetes mellitus is a slowly progressive T cell–mediated disease accompanied by autoantibodies against

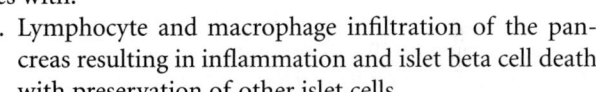

Box 21-1	Specific Environmental Factors Linked to Type 1 Diabetes

Drugs and Chemicals
Alloxan
Streptozotocin
Pentamidine
Vacor (a rodenticide)

Nutritional Intake
Bovine milk
High levels of nitrosamines

Viruses
Mumps and coxsackievirus—type 1 diabetes does occur rarely as a complication of viral infections, but no evidence of substantial relationship exists
Rubella—40% of individuals with congenital rubella infection develop type 1 diabetes later
Cytomegalovirus (CMV)—persistent CMV infections appear to be relevant to pathogenesis of some cases of type 1 diabetes

Data from Lees Murdock DJ, Barnett YA, Barnett CR: *Biochem Pharmacol* 68(3):523-530, 2004; Drescher KM et al: *Virology* 329(2):381-394, 2004; Marshall AL et al: *U K Diabet Med* 21(9):1035-1040, 2004.

pancreatic beta cells in genetically susceptible individuals[90] (Figure 21-10). Islet cells express MHC class II molecules that are recognized by specific T-cell receptors. Both CD4+ and CD8+ T cells are involved in beta cell death, as well as activation of macrophages and inflammatory cytokines, including interleukin-1 (IL-1), tumor necrosis factor (TNF), and interferon[91-93] (see Figure 21-10). The precise sequence of events that trigger migration or attachment of immune cells to the pancreatic islets has not yet been determined. The result is ketoacidosis. The destruction of beta cells progresses through stages with:

1. Lymphocyte and macrophage infiltration of the pancreas resulting in inflammation and islet beta cell death with preservation of other islet cells
2. Production of autoantibodies against insulin, glutamic acid decarboxylase (GAD), and other cytoplasmic proteins

Environmental mechanisms are thought to play a role in the destruction by direct toxicity, increasing the susceptibility of beta cells to another mechanism or triggering an autoimmune response to beta cells.

Hyperglycemia and Other Symptoms

Before hyperglycemia occurs, 80% to 90% of the function of the insulin-secreting beta cells in the islet of Langerhans must be lost. Beta cell abnormalities are present long before the acute clinical onset of type 1 diabetes. The initiating events of beta cell destruction may differ from the final event that precipitates clinical symptoms.

Regardless of the cause, a disequilibrium of hormones produced by the islets of Langerhans occurs in diabetes mellitus. Considerable evidence suggests that both alpha cell and beta cell functions are abnormal and that both a lack of insulin and a relative excess of glucagon (produced by alpha

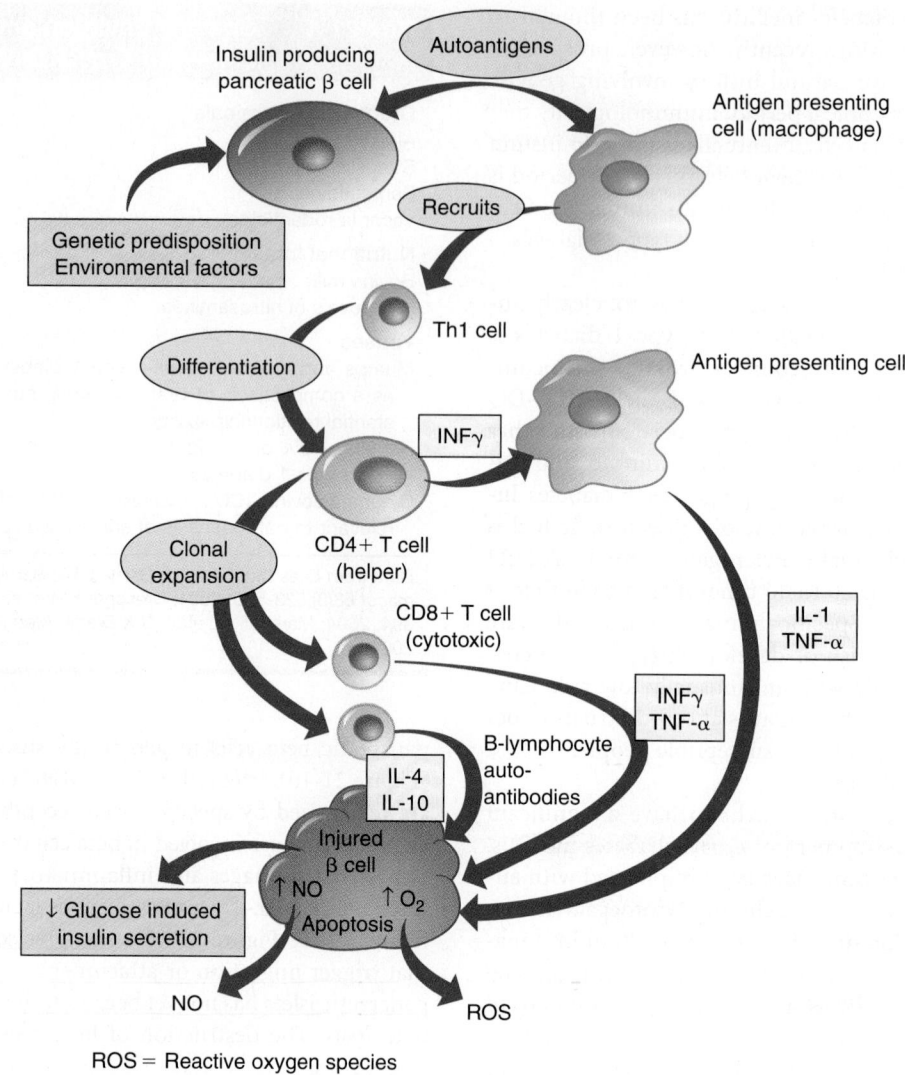

ROS = Reactive oxygen species
NO = Nitric oxide

Figure 21-10 Cell-mediated autoimmune injury of pancreatic beta cells in type 1 diabetes. *IL-1,* Interleukin-1; *TNF-α,* tumor necrosis factor alpha; *IFNγ,* interferon gamma; *NO,* nitric oxide; *O₂,* superoxide; *IL-4,* interleukin 4; *IL-10,* interleukin 10. (Modified from Belchetz P, Hammond P: *Mosby's color atlas of diabetes and endocrinology,* Edinburgh, 2003, Mosby.)

cells) exist in type 1 diabetes. Normally, the paracrine action of insulin suppresses secretion of glucagon.

Considerable data has documented that, in the absence of glucagon, the generation of both hyperglycemia and hyperketonemia is considerably delayed compared to conditions in which glucagon is present. Thus the full metabolic syndrome is caused by both hormones, a finding that ultimately may provide an entirely new therapeutic approach to the management of diabetes mellitus. Relative hyperglucagonemia occurs in every form of diabetes mellitus. The concentration of glucagon therefore is relatively high in comparison with the relative or absolute deficiency of insulin, and elevated blood glucose levels fail to suppress the production of glucagon. Overproduction of glucose and ketones, as occurs in uncontrolled diabetes mellitus, results from excessive glucagon relative to the amount of effective insulin. The ratio of insulin to

glucagon in the portal vein—and not the concentration of each hormone—controls hepatic glucose and fat metabolism.

Insulin normally stimulates lipogenesis and inhibits lipolysis, thus preventing fat catabolism. With insulin deficiency, lypolysis is enhanced and there is an increase in the amount of nonesterified fatty acids delivered to the liver. The consequence is increased glyconeogenesis contributing to hyperglycemia and production of ketone bodies (acetoacetate, hydroxybutyrate, and acetone) by the mitochondria of the liver at a rate that exceeds peripheral use.

CLINICAL MANIFESTATIONS   Type 1 diabetes mellitus affects the metabolism of fat, protein, and carbohydrates (Figure 21-11). Glucose accumulates in the blood and appears in the urine as the renal threshold for glucose is exceeded, producing an osmotic diuresis and symptoms of polyuria and

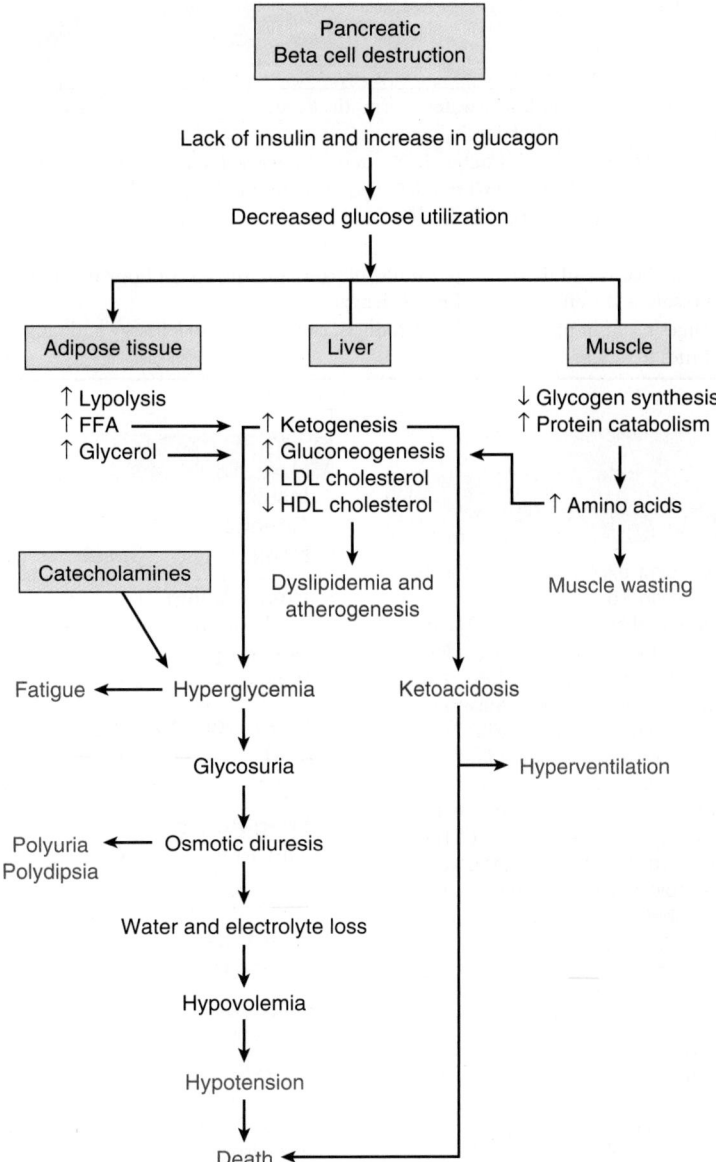

Figure 21-11 Pathophysiology of type 1 diabetes mellitus.

thirst. In addition, protein and fat breakdown occur because of the lack of insulin, resulting in weight loss.

Initial clinical manifestations of type 1 diabetes are generally acute. The individual often has the classic symptoms of polyuria, polydipsia, and polyphagia (Table 21-6). Weight loss and wide fluctuations in blood glucose levels occur.

Ketoacidosis, caused by increased levels of circulating ketones in the absence of the antilipolytic effect of insulin, is also common. Accumulation of ketone bodies causes a drop in pH and triggers the buffering system associated with metabolic acidosis (see Chapter 3). Acetone then is blown off, giving the breath a sweet or fruity odor. Occasionally, diabetic coma caused by ketoacidosis is the initial presenting manifestation of the disease.

EVALUATION AND TREATMENT   The diagnosis of diabetes is not difficult when the symptoms of polydipsia, polyuria, polyphagia, weight loss, and hyperglycemia are present in fasting and postprandial states. Under the above circumstances, an OGTT is not needed and its use is contraindicated. In fact, an OGTT is rarely needed to diagnose type 1 diabetes.[94]

Currently, treatment regimens are designed to avoid high and low levels of glucose. The Diabetes Control and Complications Trial (DCCT) was designed to evaluate the effects of tighter glucose control on the appearance or progression of the early vascular and neurologic complications of type 1 diabetes.[95] In June 1993 the National Institutes of Health announced research results showing a link between glycemic con-

Table 21-6	Clinical Manifestations and Rationale for Type 1 Diabetes Mellitus
Manifestations	**Rationale**
Polydipsia	Because of elevated blood sugar levels, water is osmotically attracted from body cells, resulting in intracellular dehydration and stimulation of thirst in the hypothalamus
Polyuria	Hyperglycemia acts as an osmotic diuretic; the amount of glucose filtered by the glomeruli of the kidneys exceeds that which can be reabsorbed by the renal tubules; glycosuria results, accompanied by large amounts of water lost in the urine
Polyphagia	Depletion of cellular stores of carbohydrates, fats, and protein results in cellular starvation and a corresponding increase in hunger
Weight loss	Weight loss occurs because of fluid loss in osmotic diuresis and the loss of body tissue as fat and proteins are used for energy as a result of the effects of insulin deficiency
Fatigue	Metabolic changes result in poor use of food products, contributing to lethargy and fatigue; sleep loss from severe nocturia also contributes to fatigue

WHAT'S NEW?

Incretin Hormones for Diabetes Mellitus Therapy

The incretin hormone system is being explored as a possible therapeutic target in diabetes. Incretin hormones are secreted by enteroendocrine cells of the large and small intestine. The major component of this system, glucagon-like peptide-1 (GLP-1), has many positive effects on glucose metabolism. GLP-1 augments glucose-dependent insulin secretion without causing hypoglycemia, stimulates insulin gene expression, inhibits glucagon secretion, delays gastric emptying, and induces a feeling of satiety through an effect on the central nervous system. GLP-1 also has been shown to induce new beta cell differentiation (neogenesis) from pancreatic ductal cells and to protect beta cells from apoptosis (programmed cell death). Considering the actions of GLP-1, it should be able to dramatically improve metabolic control in people with diabetes, assist individuals with weight loss, and augment endogenous insulin secretion. Because GLP-1 has an extremely short half-life (1 to 3 minutes), analogs with similar properties have been developed, and compounds, such as dipeptidylpeptidase-IV (DPP-IV) inhibitors, that inhibit the degradation of GLP-1 are being explored. Exenatide, a DPP-IV resistant GLP-1 receptor agonist, has shown considerable promise in clinical trials in individuals with type 2 diabetes. FDA-approval of Exenatide is pending.

Data from Bulotta A et al: *Cell Biochem Biophys* 40(3 suppl):65-78, 2004; D'Alessio DA, Vahl TP: *Am J Physiol Endocrinol Metab* 286(6):E882-890, 2004.

Table 21-7	Human Insulin Preparations			
Insulin Generic Name	**Onset**	**Peak (Hours)**	**Form**	**Duration of Action (Hours)**
Rapid Acting				
Insulin lispro	<15 min	1-2	Analog*	3-4
Insulin aspart			Analog	
Regular	0.5-1 hr	2-3	Human	3-6
Intermediate-Acting				
NPH	2-4 hr	4-10	Human	10-16
Lente	3-4 hr	4-12	Human	12-18
Long-Acting				
Ultra lente	6-10	Varies with dose	Human	18-20
Insulin glargine	2-4 hr	Peakless	Analog	20-24
Mixtures				
70% NPH/30% regular			Human	Action based on insulin mixes
75% lispro protamine/ 25% lispro			Analog	
70% aspart protamine/ 30% aspart			Analog	

*Analog insulins have an amino acid in a different position in the molecule than the natural hormone and are more readily absorbed.

trol and development of diabetic complications. The research compared individuals whose blood sugars were tightly controlled (with blood glucose checks four times per day, three or more insulin injections daily or insulin pump, and meal planning) with those who received standard treatment. Intensively treated individuals who achieve similar metabolic control of near-normal glucoses can expect a 50% to 75% reduction in the risk of developing or progression of retinopathy, neuropathy, and nephropathy after 8 to 9 years. These changes start to appear at 3 to 4 years in nonintensively treated individuals.[94] Although long-term complications were decreased in the tightly controlled group,[95] achieving near-normal glucose levels was accompanied by risks, such as severe hypoglycemia and weight gain.[95] The detailed management of diabetes mellitus is beyond the scope of this text. Successful management requires individual planning according to type of disease, age, and ac-

tivity level and all type 1 individuals require some combination of insulin, meal planning, exercise, and self-monitoring of blood glucose. Table 21-7 summarizes the human insulin preparations. Individuals should be screened at least yearly for complications of diabetes.

Type 2

Type 2 diabetes mellitus is much more common than type 1. The incidence of the disease has risen in the United States since 1940. Current U.S. disease prevalence in those older than 20 years is 8.7%. Diabetes is the most common chronic disease in children. About one in every 400 to 500 children and adolescents have type 1 diabetes and there is an increasing frequency of type 2 diabetes. Type 2 diabetes is difficult to diagnose in children because they often have no symptoms. Among children and adults one case is undiagnosed for each known case in the United States. Additionally prevalence varies by ethnic group, with the condition being more common in native Americans, Hispanic/Latino Americans, Pacific Islanders, and African Americans.[84] A genetic-environmental interaction appears to be responsible for the condition Risk factors include obesity, increased body mass index, family history of type 2 diabetes, member of an ethnic minority, puberty, female, and metabolic syndrome.[96-98]

Individuals with **maturity-onset diabetes of youth (MODY)**, a subset of type 2 diabetes, are normal weight to underweight. There are several specific subtypes of MODY, and each has been traced to a mutation in a gene responsible for insulin secretion or action.[99] For example, MODY2 is associated with mutations in the B cell glucose sensor, glucokinase.

Gestational diabetes mellitus (GDM) develops when diabetes appears during pregnancy, and pregnant women at risk should be screened. Risk factors include a family history of diabetes, membership in a high-risk ethnic group, obesity, high maternal age, and a previous complicated pregnancy or poor obstetric outcome. Aggressive treatment is required to prevent morbidity and fetal mortality.[100]

PATHOPHYSIOLOGY   The cause of the common form of type 2 diabetes mellitus is unknown; the genetics of this form of diabetes are complex and not clearly defined. It affects people primarily after the age of 40 years, many of whom are obese.[101]

Insulin resistance in glucose and lipid metabolism and decreased insulin secretion by beta cells are the main abnormalities of type 2 diabetes mellitus (Figure 21-12). **Insulin resistance** is defined as a suboptimal response of insulin-sensitive tissues (especially liver, muscle, and adipose tissue) to insulin. Several mechanisms are involved in abnormalities of the insulin signaling pathway and contribute to insulin resistance.[101a] They include an abnormality of the insulin molecule, high amounts of insulin antagonists, down regulation of the insulin receptor, decreased tyrosine kinase and insulin receptor, phosphorylation, and alteration of glucose transporter (GLUT) proteins. Several adipokines also have been proposed to be associated with insulin resistance, including leptin, adiponectin, and restin. Many years of compensatory hyperinsulinemia are thought to exist before the clinical appearance of diabetes (see Figure 21-12). The insulin resistance is

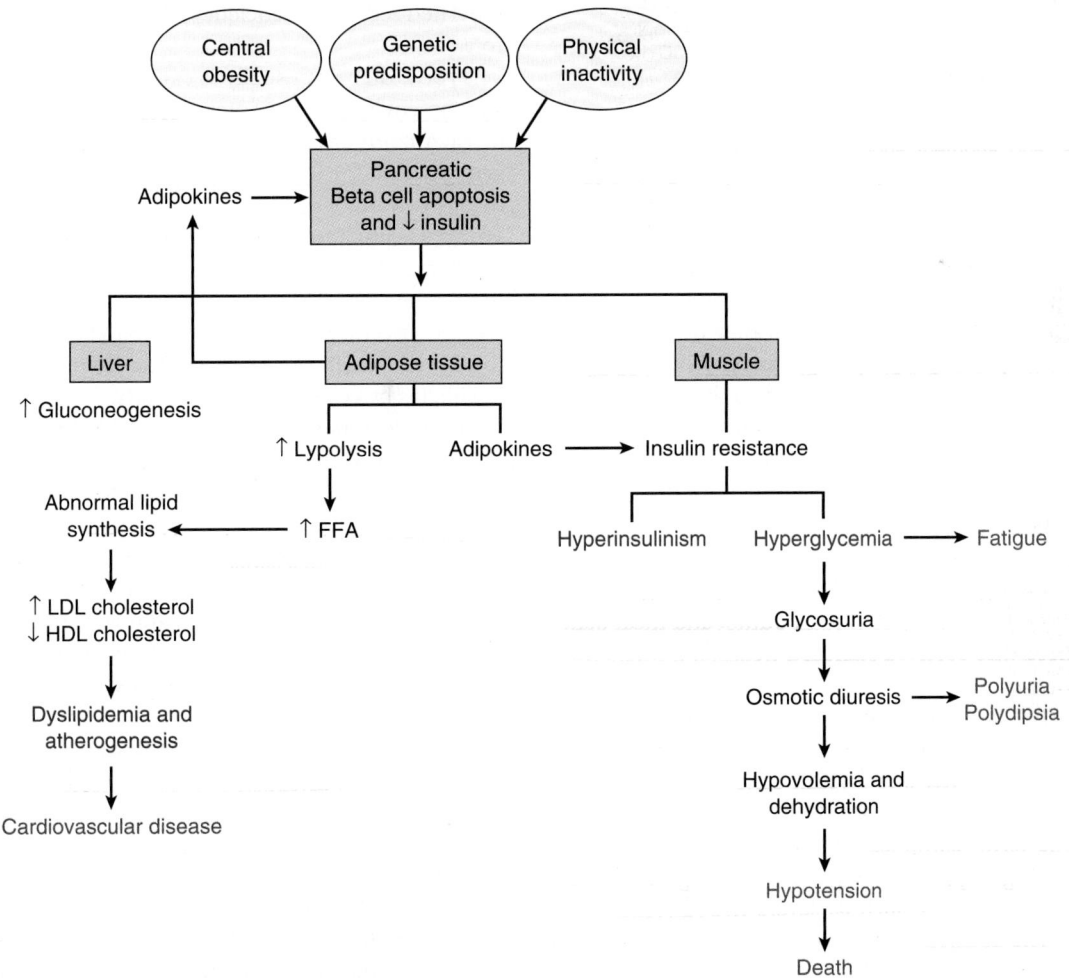

Figure 21-12 Pathophysiology of type 2 diabetes mellitus.

WHAT'S NEW?   Metabolic Syndrome and Diagnosis

The metabolic syndrome also has been called the *insulin resistance syndrome* or *syndrome "X."* It is a clustering of clinical traits occurring together that increase the risk for accelerated cardiovascular disease and type 2 diabetes mellitus. Metabolic syndrome was recently defined by the National Cholesterol Education Program's Adult Treatment Panel III as the identification of three of the following five traits:

- Increased waist circumference (>40 inches in men; >35 inches in women)
- Plasma triglycerides ≥15 mg/dl
- Plasma high-density lipoprotein (HDL) cholesterol <40 mg/dl (men) or <50 mg/dl (women)
- Blood pressure ≥130/85 mmHg
- Fasting plasma glucose ≥100 mg/dl

The syndrome is associated with insulin resistance and behaviorally modifiable risk factors, such as smoking, exercise, and diet. Approximately 55 million Americans meet the criteria for metabolic syndrome. These individuals should be screened on a regular basis for diabetes mellitus. Recent studies indicate that the syndrome develops during childhood and is highly prevalent among overweight children and adolescents. Early recognition and treatment, including vigorous life-style changes, are critical to reducing cardiovascular events and improving clinical outcomes. Treatment includes decreasing dietary calories, exercise, weight loss, treating dyslipidemias, and enhancing insulin sensitivity.

Data from Bonrow RO, Gheorghiade M: *Am J Med* 116(Suppl 5A):2S-10S, 2004; Davidson, MH: *Am J Cardiol* 93(11A):3C-11C, 2004; Devaraj S, Rosenson RS, Jialal I: *Endocrinol Metab Clin North Am* 33(2):431-453, 2004.

heightened by obesity (present in 60% to 80% of type 2 individuals), inactivity, illnesses, medications, and age. Abnormal glucagon secretion also has been demonstrated with increased hepatic production of glucose.[102] A significant body of evidence has accumulated that indicates that defects in insulin secretion can lead to insulin resistance and vice versa. Once type 2 diabetes has become established, it is impossible to determine in any given individual whether the primary defect originated in the beta cell or in peripheral or hepatic tissues.[103] Eventually the beta cell responsiveness to the glucose stimulus diminishes and hyperglycemia supervenes; yet most type 2 individuals, obese or lean, are still hyperinsulinemic at the time of diagnosis but have a relative deficiency of insulin activity. The islet dysfunction may be caused by a decrease in beta cell mass, abnormal function of the beta cells, or some combination.

Pancreatic changes in individuals with type 2 diabetes mellitus are nonspecific and have been observed to a lesser degree in nondiabetic persons. Amyloid infiltration of the islets occurs in 10% to 40% of the pancreata from individuals with type 2 diabetes. The extent of amyloid deposits is positively correlated with the age of the individual and the duration and severity of the disease.[104] Amyloid formation is associated with islet cell destruction.[105] However, the role of amyloid accumulation in the pathogenesis of type 2 diabetes is unclear.

Amylin is a hormone cosecreted with insulin by the beta cells. There is a deficiency of amylin in type 1 and type 2 diabetes that parallels the reduction in insulin secretion. Amylin inhibits glucagon secretion, and problems with glycemic control may be related to altered glucagon control or assimilation of nutrients in relation to the deficit of amylin. Amyloid deposition also may be related to amylin loss.[106]

The initial hepatic lesion is fatty infiltration (also called *nonalcoholic steatohepatitis* or *NASH*) and has been linked in several epidemiologic studies to risk factors associated with insulin resistance including obesity and elevated serum triglycerides.[107] NASH may progress to varying degrees of cirrhosis resulting in alterations of portal blood flow and diminished intrahepatic concentrations of insulin, which may negatively affect hepatic glucose output.

A decrease in the weight and number of beta cells generally occurs in type 2 diabetes, but the cause is unclear. The decrease in beta cells is progressive over time. To confuse the issue further, the ratio of alpha cells to beta cells may be completely normal in the individual with type 2 diabetes, and most individuals with type 2 diabetes have plasma and pancreatic insulin levels that are not decreased. This latter finding supports the hypothesis that diabetes is a disorder caused by both insulin and glucagon, so that a deficiency of insulin and an excess of glucagon may be either relative or absolute. An inherited secretory deficiency of the beta cells also may play a role.[101]

Type 2 diabetes usually is caused by some combination of genetic-environmental interaction, although the contribution of each component varies under different circumstances. A gene specific for insulin resistance has not been isolated. The most powerful risk factor for type 2 diabetes, identified by a World Health Organization study group,[108] is obesity. (Risk factor analysis is discussed in Chapter 5.) Abdominal adiposity, defined as a waist-to-hip ratio greater than 1, and increased visceral adiposity[108] appears to be the greatest risk factor. Excessive caloric intake predisposes an individual to type 2 diabetes by contributing to obesity.

In obese persons, insulin is less able to facilitate the entry of glucose into the liver, skeletal muscles, and adipose tissue. Multiple theories have been presented to explain this phenomenon[109,110] as follows:

1. A decreased number of insulin receptors in the plasma membrane causes decreased insulin binding.
2. Postreceptor events in insulin-sensitive cells are responsible for insulin resistance in obese people.[111]
3. Hyperinsulinemia, which occurs often in the early stages of type 2 diabetes, is a compensatory adaptation to insulin resistance in tissues, so elevated levels of circulating insulin are induced by obesity until the pancreas cannot continue to overproduce insulin.
4. Release of free fatty acids from adipocytes reduces tissue responses to insulin.
5. Overeating leads to hyperinsulinemia, which necessitates the development of peripheral insulin resistance to protect against hypoglycemia.[101]

6. Intracellular satiety factors (e.g., hexosamines) reduces tissue responsiveness to insulin.

In any event the mechanism responsible for insulin receptor binding or postreceptor activity may be improved through weight loss. Other forms of type 2 diabetes mellitus range from genetic defects in insulin action to association with other genetic syndromes (see Table 21-4). The overwhelming problem associated with all type 2 diabetes is insulin resistance with inadequate insulin secretion.

CLINICAL MANIFESTATIONS   Clinical manifestations of type 2 diabetes are often nonspecific. Although younger people may develop the condition, it generally affects those older than 30 years. The individual often is overweight, dyslipidemic, hyperinsulinemic, and hypertensive. A unique manifestation of insulin resistance in women of reproductive age is the polycystic ovary syndrome (POS).[112] Women with POS have a risk seven times the average for developing diabetes later in life. The onset is commonly slow and insidious. Some studies show that the onset of type 2 diabetes occurs at least 7 years before its diagnosis.[113] The individual with type 2 diabetes may show some classic symptoms of diabetes but more often will have nonspecific symptoms such as fatigue, pruritus, recurrent infections, visual changes, or paresthesias (Table 21-8).

EVALUATION AND TREATMENT   The diagnosis of type 2 diabetes is similar to that of type 1 (see pp. 700, 703 to 704). As with type 1 diabetes, the goal of treatment for individuals with type 2 diabetes is the restoration of near-euglycemia (a normal blood glucose level) and correction of related metabolic disorders. Dietary measures, including restriction of the total caloric intake, are of primary importance in the overweight individual. As the obese individual loses weight, the body's resistance to insulin often diminishes so that weight loss results in improved glucose tolerance. Nonobese individuals with type 2 diabetes should consume calories consistent with their ideal weight and pattern of activity. The emphasis of medical nutrition therapy (MNT) in type 2 diabetes mellitus should be focused on achieving glucose, lipid, and blood pressure goals.

Although the first approach to treatment of the individual with type 2 diabetes is appropriate meal planning, exercise and medication are usually needed for optimal management. Sulfonylurea, biguanide, thiazolidinediones, and α-glucosidase inhibitors are useful in treating some individuals with type 2 diabetes (Table 21-9). Use of oral hypoglycemic agents requires a pancreas capable of secreting insulin. Sulfonylureas acutely augment beta cell insulin secretion. Biguanides (metformin) inhibit hepatic glucose production and increase the sensitivity of peripheral tissue to insulin.[114] α-Glucosidase inhibitors decrease postprandial hyperglycemia through delaying carbohydrate digestion and absorption. The thiazolidinedione class of insulin-sensitizing compounds activate a nuclear receptor termed the *peroxisome proliferator activator receptors (PPARγ)*, which in turn regulates cellular carbohy-

---

NUTRITION & DISEASE

Diet and Metabolic Syndrome

The primary goal of dietary change in regard to metabolic syndrome is to reduce or prevent risk of diabetes and cardiovascular disease. No single diet has been proven effective, and individual metabolic alterations must be considered in dietary recommendations. Low sodium diets help to maintain lower blood pressure after antihypertensive medication withdrawal. The Dietary Approaches to Stop Hypertension (DASH) study indicated that a diet low in saturated fat and high in carbohydrates significantly reduced blood pressure. The DASH diet emphasizes fruits, vegetables, low-fat dairy products, whole grains, poultry, fish, nuts and reduced saturated fats, red meats, and sugar-containing drinks, candies and refined-grain breads and pastries. Increased intake of dietary fiber and foods with monosaturated fats reduces hypertriglyceridemia and increases HDL cholesterol. Low glycemic index foods produce lower levels of postprandial glucose and insulin. The Coronary Artery Risk Development in Young Adults study indicated consumption of dairy products was associated with reduced risk of metabolic syndrome. Overall consuming fewer calories than calories expended promotes weight loss and improves metabolic syndrome.

Data from Hooper L et al: *Cochrane Database Syst Rev* (2):CD003656, 2004; Jenkins DJ et al: *Am J Med* 113(Suppl 9B):30S-37S, 2002; Pereira MA et al: *JAMA* 287(16):2081-2089, 2002; Szapary PO, Hark LA, Burke FM: *Patient Care* 36:75-88, 2002; Vollmer WM et al: *Ann Intern Med* 135(12):1019-1028, 2001.

Table 21-8   Clinical Manifestations and Rationale for Type 2 Diabetes Mellitus

Manifestation	Rationale
Recurrent infections (e.g., boils and carbuncles; skin infections) and prolonged wound healing	Growth of microorganisms is stimulated by increased glucose levels; impaired blood supply hinders healing
Genital pruritus	Hyperglycemia and glycosuria favor fungal growth; candidal infections, resulting in pruritus, are a common presenting symptom in women
Visual changes	Blurred vision occurs as water balance in the eye fluctuates because of elevated blood glucose levels; diabetic retinopathy is another cause of visual loss
Paresthesias	Paresthesias are common manifestations of diabetic neuropathies
Fatigue	Metabolic changes result in poor use of food products, contributing to lethargy and fatigue

drate and lipid metabolism.[115] Because the pathogenesis of type 2 diabetes involves a combination of insulin resistance and a relative insulin deficiency, it is common to combine therapeutic agents from different classes of oral agents in order to achieve acceptable glycemic control.[116]

Table 21-9	Types of Oral Hypoglycemic Drugs	
Drug Type	**Mechanism of Action**	
α-glycosidase inhibitor	Delays carbohydrate absorption in gut by inhibiting disaccharidases	
Biguanide (metformin)	Decreases hepatic glucose production Increases insulin sensitivity and peripheral glucose uptake	
Meglitinides Amino acid derivatives	Stimulates insulin release from pancreatic beta cells	
Sulfonylureas	Stimulates insulin release from pancreatic beta cells	
Thiazolidinediones	Increases insulin sensitivity, particularly in adipose tissue	

Exercise is an important aspect of treatment for the individual with type 2 diabetes. Physical training improves glucose control.[117] Exercise reduces postprandial blood glucose levels, diminishes insulin requirements, lowers triglyceride and cholesterol levels, and increases the level of high-density lipoprotein (HDL) cholesterol. In addition, exercise is a valuable adjunct to weight loss for the overweight individual. Hypoglycemia may result, however, when the exercising individual receives sulfonylurea or insulin therapy. Research suggests that regular, vigorous exercise is associated with a decreased incidence of type 2 diabetes, thus helping prevent the condition.[118,119]

Acute Complications of Diabetes Mellitus
Hypoglycemia

Hypoglycemia is a lowered plasma glucose level. Its causes may be exogenous, endogenous, or functional (Tables 21-10, 21-11, and 21-12 for a summary of causes). In general, hypoglycemia occurs when blood glucose levels are below 35 mg/dl in newborns for the first 48 hours of life and below 45 to 60 mg/dl in children and adults. Evidence also indicates that some individuals may become symptomatic before glucose

Table 21-10	Exogenous Causes of Hypoglycemia	
Exogenous Cause	**Predisposing Factor**	**Occurrence**
Insulin	Intentional or accidental overdose; may be combined with inadequate food intake, unusually increased exercise, decrease in insulin requirement, or potentiating medications	Most common cause of hypoglycemia
Sulfonylurea agents	Intentional or accidental overdose; may be combined with inadequate food intake, increased exercise, or potentiating medications	Frequent cause of hypoglycemia
Alcohol	Particularly likely in chronically malnourished or acutely food-deprived individuals	Occurs within 6-36 hr of ingesting moderate to large amounts of alcohol
Other agents	Salicylates, hypoglycines, pentamidine	Common in children younger than 2 yr
Exercise	Increased duration and intensity of exercise increase glucose uptake and normally decrease insulin secretion	Occurs with both insulin and sulfonylurea administration, and intense exercise but may be unpredictable in onset

Table 21-11	Endogenous Causes of Hypoglycemia	
Endogenous Cause	**Predisposing Factor**	**Occurrence**
Organic hypoglycemia	Insulinoma	Uncommon neoplasm of B cells of islets of Langerhans
	Nesidioblastosis and B cell hyperplasia	Rare disease causing persistent hypoglycemia of infancy
Extrapancreatic neoplasms	May be mesenchymal tumors, hepatomas, adrenocortical carcinomas, gastrointestinal tumors, lymphomas, or leukemias	Rare; most common in adults 40-70 yr of age
Inborn errors of metabolism	Hereditary fructose intolerance	Rare autosomal recessively inherited inborn error of metabolism
	Fructose-1,6-disphosphatase deficiency	Rare autosomal recessive disease
	Galactosemia	Autosomal recessive disease; hypoglycemia less common than in fructose intolerance
	Phosphoenolpyruvate carboxykinase deficiency	Reported in a few infant cases
	Inborn errors in glycogen metabolism, leucine sensitivity	Reported in von Gierke disease, Hers disease, and type IXb glycogen storage disease

Table 21-12	Functional Causes of Hypoglycemia	
Dysfunction	Precipitating Factor	Occurrence
Alimentary hypoglycemia	Rapid dumping of carbohydrates into the upper small intestine	Postgastrectomy
Spontaneous reactive hypoglycemia	Syndrome of unknown cause with symptoms such as diaphoresis, tachycardia, tremulousness, headache, fatigue, drowsiness, and irritability	Rarely diagnosed throughout the world; widely diagnosed in United States, prompting American Diabetes Association and Endocrine Society to issue statement that entity is probably overdiagnosed; it is a benign condition
Alcohol-promoted reactive hypoglycemia	Drinking on an empty stomach	More common with drinks containing both alcohol and glucose or saccharin (e.g., beer, gin and tonic, rum and cola, whisky and ginger ale)
Posthyperalimentation hypoglycemia	Rapid discontinuation of total parenteral alimentation	Easily prevented by gradually reducing parenteral administration (alimentation)
Endocrine-deficiency states	Glucocorticoid deficiency Growth hormone deficiency	A danger for any person with adrenal insufficiency Particularly during a prolonged fast
Severe liver deficiency	Insufficient glucose output by the liver	Fasting hypoglycemia
Lack of body stores for protein, fat, and carbohydrates	Profound malnutrition	Frequent; also found with relative frequency in kwashiorkor
Prolonged muscular exercise	Metabolism of energy-producing substances	Occurs if exercise is too prolonged or severe or if nutritional intake and carbohydrate stores are insufficient
Functional or transient hypoglycemia in infancy	Transient neonatal hypoglycemia	Occurs in 10% of live births, during first 3 days of life
	Maternal diabetes	Caused by beta-cell hyperplasia and possibly relative hypoglucagonemia
	Erythroblastosis fetalis	Frequently associated with erythroblastosis fetalis
	Leucine-induced hypoglycemia	Generally in infants younger than 6 months of age; severe hypoglycemia attacks may occur postprandially or after short periods of fasting
	Ketotic or ketogenic hypoglycemia	One of the most common forms of hypoglycemia in childhood, occurs after food deprivation in children 1-8 yr old; generally, spontaneous recovery before 10 yr old

levels decrease to 60 mg/dl if the decrease is relatively rapid.[120] Hypoglycemia occurs most often in individuals with diabetes mellitus treated with insulin (Table 21-13 lists predisposing factors). It occurs in more than 90% of those with type 1 diabetes and limits the management of the disease.[120] Hypoglycemia in diabetes is sometimes called *insulin shock* or *insulin reaction.* Individuals with type 2 diabetes are at risk when treatment involves two oral hypoglycemic drugs or increasing drug doses.

Symptoms result from either activation of the sympathetic nervous system (adrenergic symptoms) or from an abrupt cessation of glucose delivery to the brain (neuroglycopenic symptoms) or both. Symptoms commonly vary among individuals but tend to be consistent for each person. Adrenergic reactions occur when the decrease in blood glucose is rapid with tachycardia, palpitations, diaphoresis, tremors, pallor, and arousal anxiety. The response is probably generated when the hypothalamus senses decreased glucose levels. Reduced substrate delivery to the brain (neuroglycopenia) produces further symptoms, including headache, dizziness, irritability, fatigue, poor judgment, confusion, visual changes, hunger, seizures, and coma. Hypoglycemia unawareness is a phenomenon that occurs in individuals without appropriate autonomic warning symptoms before development of neuroglycopenia. These individuals have reduced counterregulatory hormone responses.[121] If an individual is receiving a beta-blocking medication, the autonomic symptoms may be blunted, and recovery from hypoglycemia may be delayed because of impaired glycogenolysis and hampered delivery of gluconeogenic substrates to the liver.

When hypoglycemic symptoms are nonspecific, the safest treatment is to provide some form of glucose, because failure to provide glucose may precipitate convulsions, coma, and death. Prevention of hypoglycemia episodes through alternate therapeutic regimens, individualizing target blood glucose levels, frequent self-monitoring of blood glucose, and proper education should be the goal.

Diabetic Ketoacidosis

Ketoacidosis, a serious complication of diabetes mellitus, is a common cause for hospital admissions, and average mortality rates throughout the United States are less than 5%. **Diabetic ketoacidosis (DKA)** develops when there is an absolute or relative deficiency of insulin and an increase in insulin counterregulatory hormones: catecholamines, cortisol, glucagon, and growth hormone. Under these conditions, hepatic

Table 21-13   Common Acute Complications of Diabetes Mellitus (DM)

	Hypoglycemia in Persons with DM	Diabetic Ketoacidosis	Hyperglycemic Nonketotic Syndromes
Synonyms	Insulin shock, insulin reaction	Diabetic coma syndrome	Hyperosmolar hyperglycemia nonketotic coma
Persons at Risk	Individuals taking insulin Individuals with rapidly fluctuating blood sugar Individuals with type 2 diabetes taking sulfonylurea agents	Individuals with type 1 diabetes Individuals with nondiagnosed diabetes	Elderly or very young individuals with type 2 diabetes, nondiabetics with predisposing factors, persons with renal insufficiency, individuals with undiagnosed diabetes
Predisposing Factors	Excessive insulin or sulfonylurea agent intake, lack of sufficient food intake, excessive physical exercise, abrupt decline in insulin needs (e.g., renal failure, immediately postpartum), simultaneous use of insulin-potentiating agents or beta-blocking agents that mask symptoms	Stressful situation such as infection, accident, trauma, emotional stress; omission of insulin; medications that antagonize insulin	High-carbohydrate diets (e.g., tube feedings, total parenteral nutrition), prolonged mannitol diuresis, peritoneal dialysis or hemodialysis with hyperosmolar dialysate, medications antagonizing insulin
Typical onset	Rapid	Slow	Slowest
Presenting Symptoms	Adrenergic reaction: pallor, sweating, tachycardia, palpitations, hunger, restlessness, anxiety, tremors Neurogenic reaction: fatigue, irritability, headache, loss of concentration, visual disturbances, dizziness, hunger, confusion, transient sensory or motor defects, convulsions, coma, death	Malaise, dry mouth, headache, polyuria, polydipsia, weight loss, nausea, vomiting, pruritus, abdominal pain, lethargy, shortness of breath, Kussmaul respirations, fruity or acetone odor to breath	Polyuria, polydipsia, hypovolemia, dehydration (parched lips, poor skin turgor), hypotension, tachycardia, hypoperfusion, weight loss, weakness, nausea, vomiting, abdominal pain, hypothermia, stupor, coma, seizures
Laboratory Analysis	Serum glucose below 30 mg/dl in newborn (first 2-3 days) and below 55-60 mg/dl in adults	Glucose levels 300-750 mg/dl, reduction in bicarbonate concentration, increased anion gap, increased plasma levels of β-hydroxybutyrate, acetoacetate, and acetone	Glucose levels 600-4800 mg/dl, lack of ketosis, serum osmolarity above 350 mOsm/L, elevated blood urea nitrogen and creatinine

glucose production increases, peripheral glucose usage decreases, fat mobilization increases, and ketogenesis is stimulated (Figure 21-13). The most common precipitating factor is intercurrent illness, such as infection, trauma, surgery, or myocardial infarction. Interruption of insulin administration also may result in DKA. In 20% to 30% of the cases, no precipitating factors are noted. Emotional factors and stress, particularly in children, are thought to contribute to the development of DKA.[122] The frequency of DKA peaks in adolescence.[123]

PATHOPHYSIOLOGY   Catecholamines, cortisol, glucagon, and growth hormone antagonize insulin by increasing glucose production. In addition, catecholamines, cortisol, and growth hormones decrease use of glucose. Insulin deficiency results in decreased glucose uptake, an increased release of fatty acids, and accelerated gluconeogenesis and ketogenesis. Relatively increased glucagon levels are simultaneously responsible for activation of the gluconeogenic (glucose-forming) and ketogenic

(ketone-forming) pathways in the liver. Because of the insulin deficiency, hepatic overproduction of α-hydroxybutyrate and acetoacetic acids causes increased ketone concentrations. Ordinarily, ketones are used by tissues as an energy source regenerate bicarbonate. This balances the loss of bicarbonate, which occurs when the ketone is formed. Hyperketonemia (increased blood ketone levels) may be a result of impairment in the use of ketones by peripheral tissue, which permits strong organic acids to circulate freely.[122] Bicarbonate buffering then does not occur, and the individual develops a metabolic acidosis.

CLINICAL MANIFESTATIONS   The signs and symptoms of DKA are fairly nonspecific, and an individual rarely progresses to complete coma without intervention. Polyuria and dehydration result from the osmotic diuresis associated with hyperglycemia. Here the plasma glucose level is higher than the individual's renal threshold, allowing much glucose to be lost in the urine. Although water deficits may reach 100 ml/kg of body weight, they generally are not as severe as those

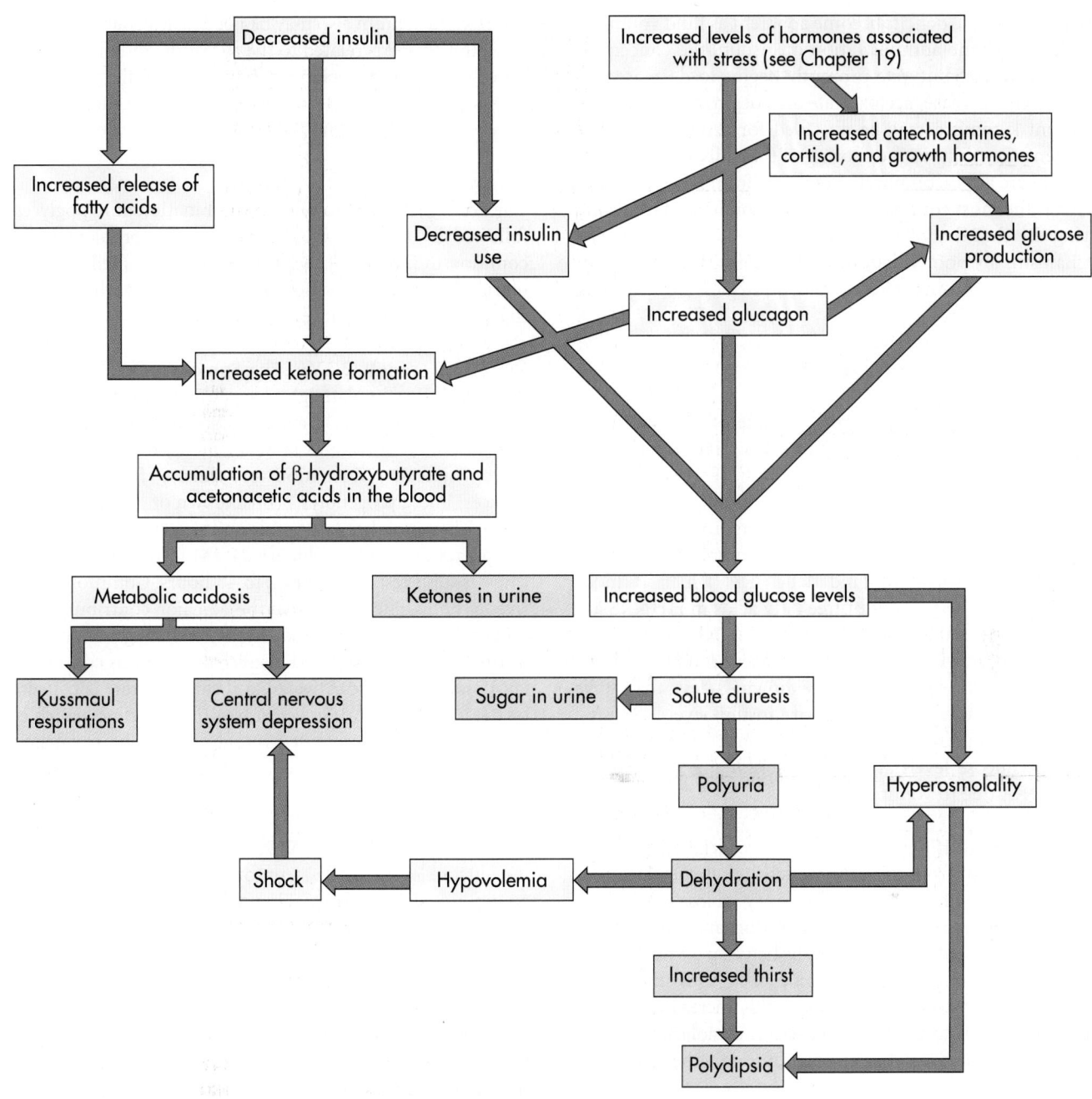

Figure 21-13 Diabetic ketoacidosis.

experienced by the individual with hyperosmolar nonacidotic diabetes. Sodium, phosphorus, and magnesium deficits are common. The most important electrolyte disturbance, however, is a marked deficiency in total body potassium. Although the serum potassium may appear normal or elevated because of volume contraction and a shift of potassium from the cell caused by metabolic acidosis, the total body deficiency of potassium may reach 3 to 5 mEq/kg. Symptoms of diabetic ketoacidosis include Kussmaul respirations (hyperventilation in an attempt to compensate for the acidosis), postural dizziness, central nervous system depression, ketonuria, anorexia, nausea, abdominal pain, thirst, and polyuria.

EVALUATION AND TREATMENT   The diagnosis of ketoacidosis is suggested when individuals have symptoms of vomiting, abdominal pain, dehydration, and an acetone odor on the breath. Laboratory findings include serum glucose more than 300 mg/dl, reduced serum bicarbonate, increased anion gap, arterial pH less than 7.30, and presence of urine and serum ketones.

Treatment of DKA involves continual administration of low-dose insulin to decrease glucose levels. Fluids are administered to replace lost fluid volume, and electrolytes—particularly sodium, potassium, and phosphorus—are administered as needed. Fluids and electrolytes should be monitored closely. Electrolyte deficits become apparent as fluid volume is replaced. After the administration of insulin, the concentration of β-hydroxybutyrate promptly begins to decrease and after a slight increase, acetoacetate also begins to decrease. A persistent ketonuria may be observed for several days after treatment. Continuous monitoring of the individual is essential to ensure an uncomplicated recovery from DKA. Cerebral edema is the most common cause of morbidity and mortality during the first day of treatment for DKA in children. The mechanisms are poorly understood.[124,125] Health teaching emphasizes predisposing factors and strategies for avoiding DKA.

Hyperosmolar Hyperglycemic Nonketotic Syndrome

Hyperosmolar hyperglycemic nonketotic syndrome (HHNKS)[103] was first described in 1886. HHNKS is more commonly seen with type 2 diabetes.[126]

PATHOPHYSIOLOGY   HHNKS differs from DKA in the degree of insulin deficiency (which is more profound in DKA) and the degree of fluid deficiency (which is more marked in HHNKS). Levels of free fatty acids in HHNKS are consistently lower than those found in DKA. HHNKS is characterized also by a lack of ketosis. Because the amount of insulin required to inhibit fat breakdown is less than that needed for effective glucose transport, insulin levels are sufficient to prevent excessive lipolysis but not to use glucose properly. Glucose levels are considerably higher in HHNKS than in DKA due to volume depletion.

CLINICAL MANIFESTATIONS   Glycosuria and polyuria in HHNKS result from the extreme serum glucose elevation. As much as 19 g of glucose per hour may be lost in diuresis, which also causes severe volume depletion and intracellular dehydration. Water losses are generally between 4.8 and 12.6 L, and although some electrolytes are lost with the fluid, the urine is hypotonic. This, along with increased glucose levels, contributes to the increased serum osmolarity. Neurologic changes, such as stupor, correlate with the degree of hyperosmolarity.

EVALUATION AND TREATMENT   The serum ketone concentration is normal or only mildly elevated in HHNKS. In addition to the depressed mental state, laboratory findings include serum glucose levels higher than 600 mg/dl, serum osmolarity higher than 310 mOsm/L (normal = 285 mOsm/L), and blood urea nitrogen (BUN) of 70 to 90 mg/dl. DKA and HHNKS show considerable overlap in symptoms and treatment. An important distinction, however, is that the dehydration in HHNKS is far more severe than that in DKA. Thus fluid replacement, with both crystalloids and colloids, is more rapid. As much as 2000 ml may be given the first hour, together with monitoring of the response to therapy. Potassium deficits may be so extreme in HHNKS that more than 1 week may be needed to correct the total body deficits. Phos-phorus and sodium also may be needed. Mortality is also high in HHNKS, and is related to the age of the individual and co-morbid conditions including the severity of the precipitating illness.[127] (Table 21-13 compares the three acute complications described thus far.)

Somogyi Effect

The **Somogyi effect** is a unique combination of hypoglycemia followed by rebound hyperglycemia. The problem is more common in individuals with type 1 diabetes mellitus, particularly in children, and should be investigated whenever fluctuations in blood sugar levels are serious.

PATHOPHYSIOLOGY   The Somogyi effect occurs when hypoglycemia stimulates glucose counterregulation, including epinephrine, growth hormone, cortisol, and glucagon release.[120] These hormones serve to increase blood glucose by gluconeogenesis (formation of glucose from nonglucose sources) and glycogenolysis (breakdown of glycogen into glucose). They mobilize fatty acids and proteins while inhibiting peripheral glucose use (Figure 21-14). These hormones may cause insulin resistance for 12 to 48 hours. Commonly, excessive carbohydrate intake may be a major contributor to rebound hyperglycemia. Also, hypoglycemia generally occurs during the peak of injected insulin; therefore, as counterregulatory hormones are activated and carbohydrate is consumed by the individual, insulin levels are on the decline, which contributes to the subsequent hyperglycemia. The frequency of this phenomenon is debated, and recent studies suggest that it is much less common than previously reported.[94]

CLINICAL MANIFESTATIONS   In addition to fluctuating glucose levels, subtle symptoms of hypoglycemia occur. If an individual has nocturnal hypoglycemia, there may be complaints of nightmares and early morning headaches. Both symptoms probably reflect a hypoglycemic state. Ketonuria may occur if the mobilization of energy sources overshoots the body's need for glucose and exogenous insulin is depleted.

EVALUATION AND TREATMENT   If the individual has nocturnal hypoglycemia, diagnosis involves the documentation of nighttime hypoglycemia by several plasma glucose analyses at 2 AM, 4 AM, and 7 AM or by using monitors capable of continuous glucose sensing. Treatment consists of decreasing insulin dosage or changing the time of administration.

Dawn Phenomenon

The **dawn phenomenon** is an early morning rise in blood glucose concentration with no hypoglycemia during the night. It appears to be related to nocturnal elevations of growth hormone. Growth hormone is a counterregulatory hormone that causes hyperglycemia by decreasing peripheral (other than liver) glucose uptake. Increased clearance of plasma insulin also may be involved. Altering the time and dose of insulin manages the problem. Treating dawn phenomenon may result in the Somogyi effect and vice versa.

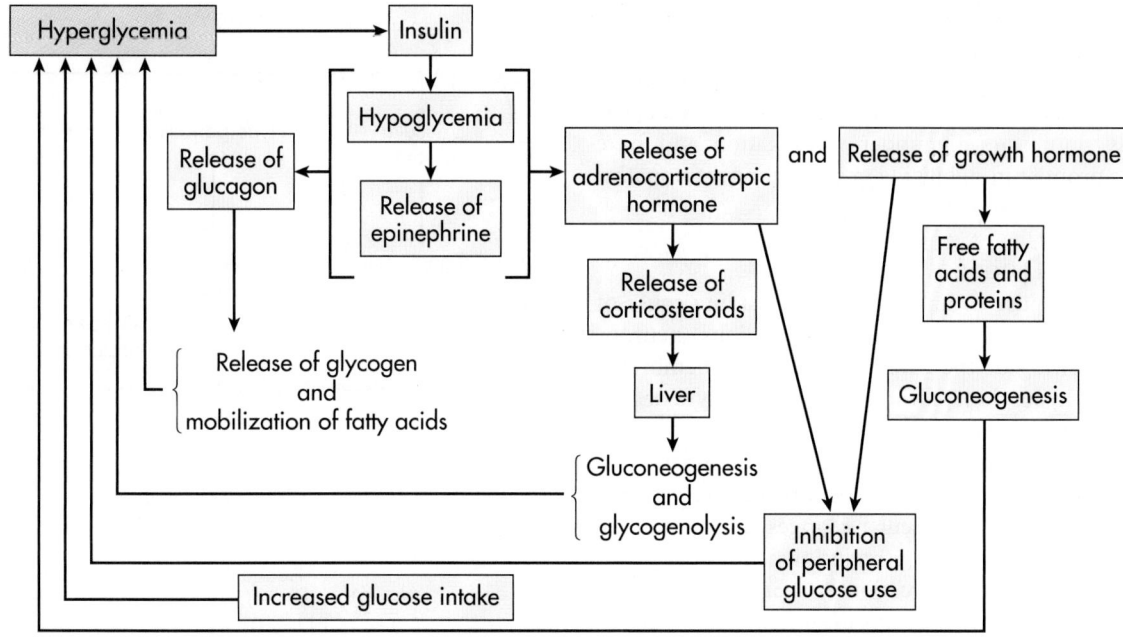

Figure 21-14 The Somogyi effect.

Chronic Complications of Diabetes Mellitus

A number of serious complications are associated with any type of diabetes mellitus and include microvascular (retinopathy and nephropathy) and macrovascular disease (e.g., coronary artery disease, stroke, and peripheral vascular disease), neuropathies, and infection. Most complications are associated with metabolic alterations, primarily hyperglycemia. Strict control of blood glucose significantly reduces complications. Three metabolic events associated with chronic hyperglycemia are involved in the pathogenesis of diabetic complications: nonenzymatic glycosylation, shunting of glucose to the polyol pathway, and activation of protein kinase C.

Hyperglycemia and Nonenzymatic Glycosylation

Nonenzymatic glycosylation is the reversible attachment of glucose to proteins, lipids, and nucleic acids without the action of enzymes. With recurrent or persistent hyperglycemia, glucose becomes irreversibly bound to collagen and other proteins in red blood cells, blood vessel walls, and interstitial tissue. The products of this binding are known as **advanced glycosylation end-products (AGE).** AGEs have a number of properties that may cause tissue injury or pathologic conditions associated with diabetes:[128-130]

1. Cross-linking and trapping of proteins, including albumin, low-density lipoprotein (LDL), immunoglobulin, and complement, with thickening of the basement membrane or increased permeability in blood vessels and nerves
2. Binding to cell receptors, such as macrophages and glomerular mesangial cells, and inducing release of cytokines and growth factors that stimulate cellular proliferation in the glomeruli, smooth muscle of blood vessels, and collagen synthesis with fibrosis
3. Induction of lipid oxidation and oxidative stress
4. Inactivation of nitric oxide with loss of vasodilation and diminished endothelial function
5. Procoagulant changes on endothelial cells with promotion of platelet adhesion and reduced fibrinolysis

Pharmacologic agents, such as aminoguanidine, inhibited AGE formation in experimental trials.

Hyperglycemia and the Polyol Pathway

Tissues that do not require insulin for glucose transport, such as kidney, red blood cells (RBCs), blood vessels, eye lens, and nerves, use an alternate metabolic pathway for glucose metabolism known as the **polyol pathway.** With hyperglycemia, glucose is shunted to this pathway and is converted to sorbitol (a polyol) by the enzyme aldose reductase. Sorbitol is then slowly converted to fructose by sorbitol dehydrogenase. The accumulation of sorbitol and fructose increases intracellular osmotic pressure and attracts water, leading to cell injury. This is particularly evident in the lens of the eye and leads to swelling with visual changes and cataracts. In nerves, sorbitol interferes with ion pumps, damages Schwann cells, and disrupts nerve conduction. RBCs become swollen and stiff and interfere with perfusion.

Aldose reductase inhibitors can slow or prevent some diabetic complications,[131,132] although their toxicity has limited their therapeutic usefulness.

Protein Kinase C

Protein kinase C (PKC) is an enzyme that is inappropriately activated in different tissues by hyperglycemia. Various consequences have been observed, including insulin resistance, production of extracellular matrix and cytokines, vascular cell proliferation, enhanced contractility, and increased permeability.[133] These effects may contribute to the macrovascular, microvascular, and neurologic complications of diabetes. Specific PKC inhibitors are under investigation and have shown some promise in stabilizing or preventing retinopathy, nephropathy, and neuropathy.[134,135]

Microvascular Disease

Diabetic microvascular complications are a leading cause of blindness, end-stage renal failure, and various neuropathies.[136] Thickening of the capillary basement membrane, endothelial cell hyperplasia, thrombosis, and pericyte degeneration are characteristic of diabetic microangiopathy and emerges over a period of 1 to 2 years. The thickening eventually results in decreased tissue perfusion. Hyperglycemia is a prerequisite for these microvascular changes and may be related to glycation of structural proteins, which results in the accumulation of advanced glycation end-products (AGEs). The frequency of the lesions appears to be proportional to the duration of the disease and blood glucose levels. In the DCCT study, individuals with tightly controlled blood glucose were half as likely to have renal and eye complications as those who received standard treatment.[95] Hypoxia and ischemia of various organs may result from microangiopathy. Two areas often affected are the retina and the kidney.

Retinopathy

The retina is the most metabolically active structure per weight of tissue in the body. Thus the retina is a vulnerable target for microvascular disease in diabetes mellitus. **Diabetic retinopathy** appears to be a response to retinal ischemia resulting from blood vessel changes and red blood cell aggregation (Figure 21-15). In addition, poorly controlled hypertension is a risk factor for worsening of retinopathy. Growth hormone appears to play a permissive role in developing retinopathy, and therapeutic strategies have been developed to exploit this phenomenon. The prevalence and severity of the retinopathy are strongly related to the age of the individual and duration of the diabetes and glycemic control. Retinopathy may be present in individuals at the time of diagnosis of type 2 diabetes as a result of the long preclinical latency of this form of diabetes. The vast majority of individuals with diabetes mellitus have some degree of retinopathy,[137] and retinopathy is closely associated with **diabetic nephropathy,** the so-called *renal retinal syndrome.*

The three stages of retinopathy are described in Table 21-14. Nonproliferative retinopathy (stage I) is characterized by an increase in retinal capillary permeability, vein dilation, microaneurysm formation, and superficial (flame-shaped) and deep (blot) hemorrhages. Preproliferative retinopathy (stage II) is a progression of retinal ischemia with areas of poor perfusion that culminate in infarcts. Proliferative diabetic retinopathy (stage III) is the result of neovascularization and fibrous tissue formation within the retina or optic disc.[138] Traction of the new vessels on the vitreous humor may cause retinal detachment or hemorrhage into the vitreous humor.

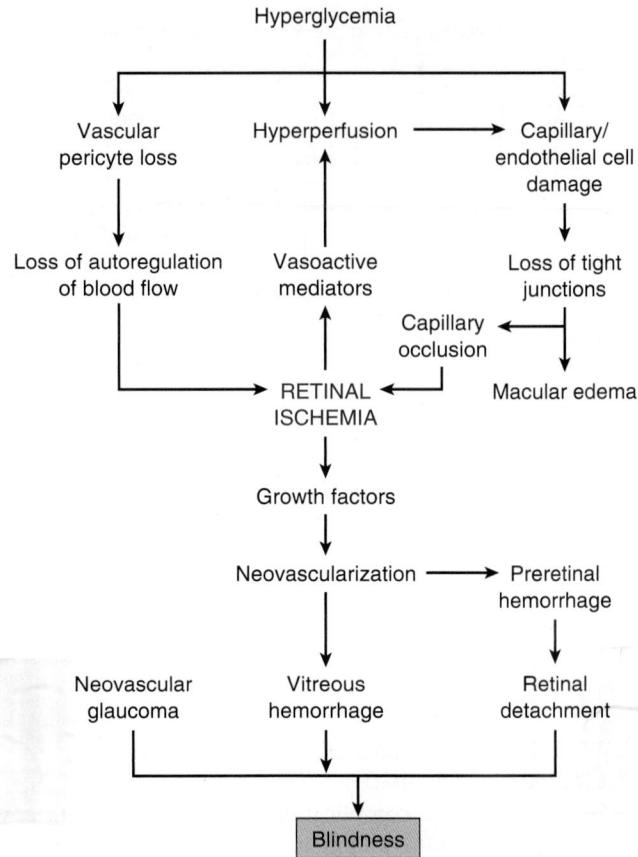

Figure 21-15 Diabetic retinopathy.

Maculopathy is a progressive process that may accompany the increased retinal capillary permeability, vessel occlusion, and ischemia. If formation of exudates, edema, or ischemia occurs near the fovea, serious loss of vision may result. Laser treatments are used to reduce the rate of vision loss from diabetic macular edema and neovascularization. Vitrectomy is a surgical procedure used to treat an intravitreal hemorrhage secondary to rupture of a neovascular capillary tuft.

Diabetic Nephropathy

Diabetes is the most common cause of end-stage renal disease in the Western world. Approximately 30% of individuals with type 1 and 40% of those with type 2 diabetes develop nephropathy.[139] The early phases of nephropathy are asymptomatic and begin to develop after 10 years in type 1 diabetes or 5 to 8 years in type 2 diabetes.

The exact process responsible for destruction of kidneys in diabetes is unknown. Mechanisms such as hyperglycemia, hyperfiltration, increased blood viscosity, increased glomerular pressure, albumin, protein kinase C, growth factors, advanced glycation end products, oxidative stress, and hypercholesterolemia are being investigated.[140-143] The glomeruli are injured by at least two mechanisms: protein denaturation by high glucose levels and adverse effects of intraglomerular hypertension. Renal glomerular changes can occur early in diabetes mellitus and occasionally may precede the overt manifestations of the disease (Figure 21-16). Glomerular

Table 21-14	Findings in Diabetic Retinopathy
Stages of Retinopathy	**Pathologic Findings**
Nonproliferative Retinopathy (Stage I)	
Venous abnormalities	Increased tortuosity, dilation with irregular constriction; frequency increases with increased severity of retinopathy
Microaneurysms	Mostly thin walled, 15-50 mcg in diameter, pathogenesis controversial
Interretinal hemorrhage	Circular and small; may take several months to resorb
Macular edema	Caused by serum leakage through incompetent vessel walls, may resorb in several weeks
Hard exudates	Characteristically "hard" exudates with pattern of exudation irregular in shape and sharply defined may appear and disappear over months to years; common with hypertension; "soft" exudates may appear and disappear more often; related to increased retinal capillary permeability
Preproliferative Diabetic Retinopathy (Stage II)	
Cotton-wool patches	Infarcts of the nerve fiber layer caused by retinal ischemia
Intraretinal microvascular shunts	Tortuous shunts between patent and occluded retinal vessels
Proliferative Diabetic Retinopathy (Stage III)	
Neovascularization	New vessels surrounded by connective tissue; five distinct groups representing different hazards to the eye
Glial proliferation	Often produced to reinforce neovascularization; may occur on optic disc and along vascular arcades
Vitreoretinal traction hemorrhage; retinal detachment	Traction occurring from the vitreous jelly; eventually causes small blood vessels to hemorrhage and retinal detachment to occur

enlargement and glomerular basement membrane thickening, resulting in diffuse intercapillary glomerulosclerosis, develop during the first few years of diabetes. The Kimmelstiel-Wilson nodule, with thickening at the center of the glomerular lobules and thickening of the peripheral basement membrane, is distinctive in individuals with diabetes.[144]

Microalbuminuria is the first manifestation of renal dysfunction. Continuous untreated proteinuria generally heralds a life expectancy less than 10 years. Microalbuminuria is also an independent risk factor for cardiovascular disease.[145] Scanty information is available to explain the determinants of proteinuria in diabetic nephropathy. Leakage of albumin into glomerular filtrate results from factors other than increased membrane pore size, although these other factors are not yet defined. As renal failure progresses, extensive vascular and extravascular changes occur.

Before the development of proteinuria, no clinical signs or symptoms of progressive glomerulosclerosis are likely to be evident. Later, hypoproteinemia, reduction in plasma oncotic pressure, fluid overload, anasarca (generalized body edema), and hypertension may occur.[146] As renal function continues to deteriorate, individuals with type 1 diabetes may experience hypoglycemia, which necessitates a decrease in insulin therapy. The hypoglycemia occurs because the kidney's ability to metabolize insulin is lost along with other renal functions. As the glomerular filtration rate drops below 10 ml/min, uremic signs such as nausea, lethargy, acidosis, anemia, and uncontrolled hypertension occur (see Chapter 36 for a discussion of renal failure). Impaired kidney function also accelerates retinopathy. Death from renal failure is much more common in individuals with type 1 diabetes mellitus than in those with type 2, because of the association between microalbuminuria and coronary artery disease in individuals with type 2 diabetes.

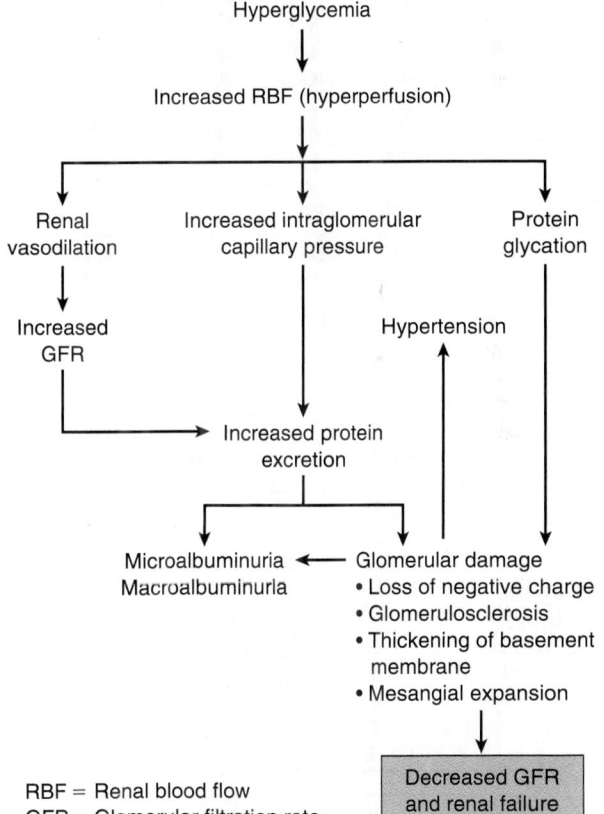

RBF = Renal blood flow
GFR = Glomerular filtration rate

Figure 21-16 Diabetic nephropathy.

The development of more sensitive tests has permitted the detection of small amounts of urinary albumin, microalbuminuria. Earlier intervention with tight glucose control and angiotensin-converting enzyme (ACE) inhibitors or angiotensin II receptor blockers has reduced proteinuria and slowed the progression of nephropathy. Aggressive treatment of hypertension is another therapeutic intervention definitively shown to slow the progression of established renal disease.[147]

Macrovascular Disease

Macrovascular disease is a major cause of morbidity and mortality among individuals with type 2 diabetes mellitus. Children with poorly controlled type 2 diabetes have high risk for macrovascular disease within one or two decades.[148] The premature atherosclerosis of diabetes has many contributing factors, such as hyperinsulinemia, hypertriglyceridemia, low HDL, lipoprotein oxidation, vascular consequences of advanced glycation end products, and altered endothelial function. The fibrous plaques of atherosclerosis result from the

proliferation of subendothelial smooth muscle in the arterial wall. Other factors in the serum of individuals with diabetes also stimulate this proliferation (Figure 21-17).

In addition, deposition of lipids in the lesions may be facilitated in individuals with diabetes. Triglyceride elevations with low levels of the protective high-density lipoprotein (HDL) cholesterol are common in individuals with type 2 diabetes mellitus in association with increased quantities of small, dense (very atherogenic) low-density lipoprotein (LDL) cholesterol and endothelial cell and platelet abnormalities.[149] Increased levels of the atherogenic oxidized LDL also are seen in hyperglycemic individuals. Hypertension can increase capillary wall pressure, damage endothelium, increase capillary permeability, decrease nitric oxide synthesis, and decrease autoregulation of blood flow.[150-151] Further work is needed to clarify the complexities of macrovascular complications.

Coronary Artery Disease

The risk of coronary artery disease (CAD) for those individuals with type 2 diabetes is higher than for the general population even when hypertension and hyperlipidemia are taken into account. CAD is the most common cause of death in individuals with type 2 diabetes and also is common in those with type 1.[152] Whereas the cardiovascular mortality is increased in all age groups, mortality is most marked at or before middle age and is higher for both men and women.[153] In general, the prevalence of CAD increases with the duration but not the severity of diabetes.

Myocardial infarction (death of heart muscle as a result of coronary artery occlusion) is the cause of death in 20% of those with diabetes, and individuals with diabetes mellitus have a higher mortality during the acute phase of myocardial infarctions than do nondiabetic individuals. In addition, the

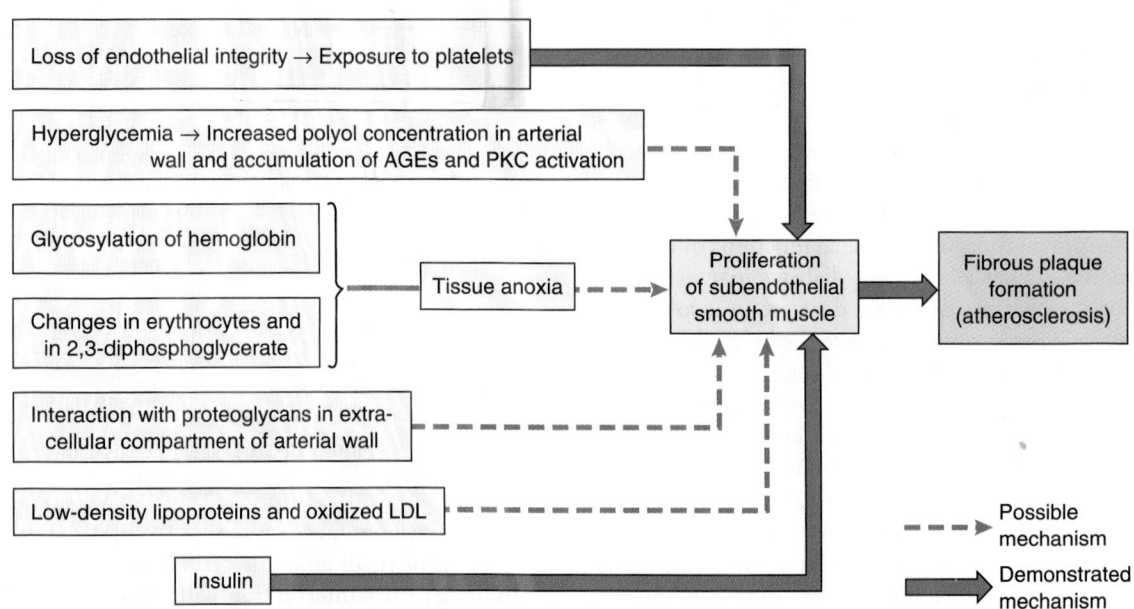

Figure 21-17 Diabetes mellitus and atherosclerosis. Contributing causes of proliferation of subendothelial smooth muscle in arterial wall, resulting in atherosclerosis. *AGEs,* Advanced glycosylation end-products; *PKC,* protein kinase C.

incidence of congestive heart failure is higher in individuals with diabetes, even without myocardial infarction. The reason is unclear but may be related to the presence of increased amounts of collagen in the ventricular wall, which reduces the mechanical compliance of the heart during filling. Increased platelet adhesion and decreased fibrinolysis promote thrombus formation and vascular occlusion.[154]

Stroke

Stroke is twice as common in those with diabetes as in the nondiabetic population.[155] Ischemic stroke is more common than hemorrhagic stroke. The survival rate for an individual with diabetes after a massive stroke is typically shorter than for a person without diabetes. Hypertension and dyslipidemia are definite risk factors (see Chapter 30), and aggressive management of blood pressure and lipidemia in individuals with diabetes has been shown to reduce the incidence of stroke.[156,157]

Peripheral Arterial Disease

The increased incidence of peripheral arterial disease (PAD), gangrene, and amputation in diabetic persons has been documented in many studies, particularly in individuals with type 2 diabetes.[158,159] Figure 21-18 illustrates how foot lesions of diabetes can lead to amputation. Many individuals with type 2 diabetes have evidence of peripheral vascular disease at the time of their initial diagnosis. The atherosclerotic process in diabetic persons is more common, appears at a younger age, and advances more rapidly than vascular changes in nondiabetic persons. The prevalence of PAD is nearly equal in males and females with diabetes. Age, duration of diabetes, genetics, and additional risk factors influence the development of PAD.

Because of occlusions of the small arteries and arterioles, most of the gangrenous changes of the lower extremities occur in patchy areas of the feet and toes.[160] Smaller vessels often have more advanced disease than larger vessels in the same individuals. Fifty percent of nontraumatic amputations in the United States are performed on individuals with diabetes. Hospital mortality for individuals with diabetes who undergo major amputation is between 10% and 23%. The survival rate after surgery is only about 40% at the end of 5 years.[158]

Diabetic Neuropathies

Diabetic neuropathy is the most common cause of neuropathy in the Western world and is probably the most common complication of diabetes. The prevalence is similar for type 1 and type 2,[161] yet the disease remains poorly understood. Neuropathy and other long-term complications are thought

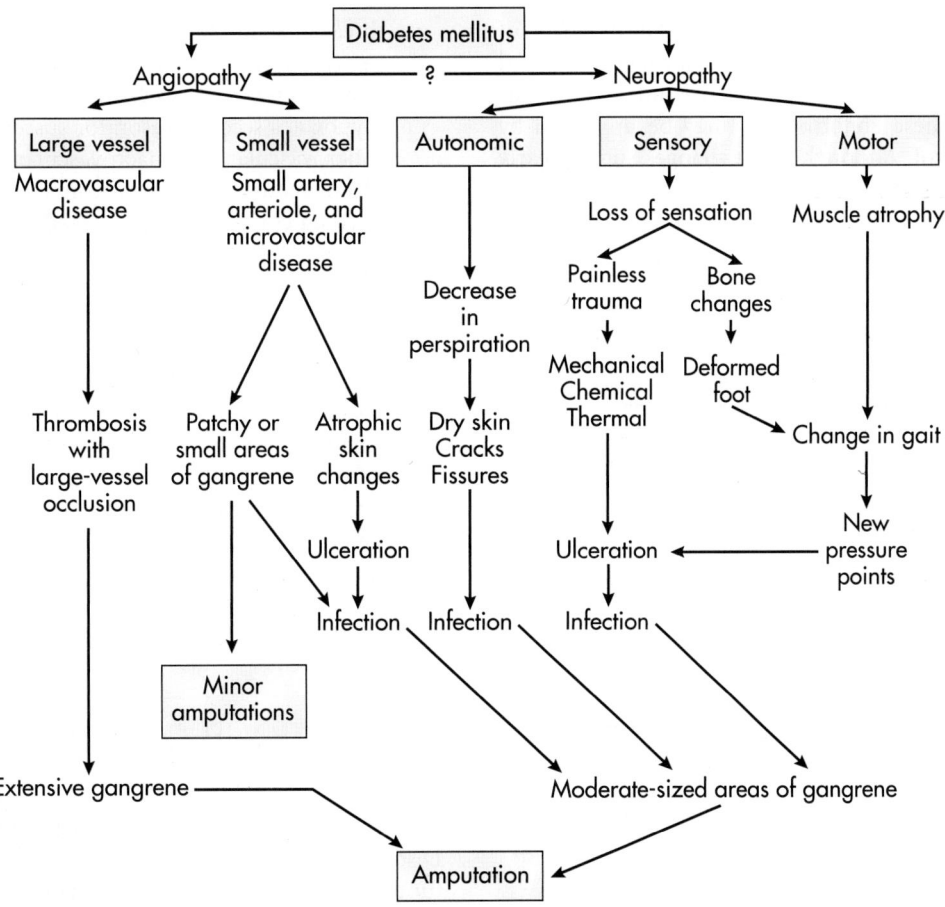

Figure 21-18 How foot lesions of diabetes can lead to amputation. (From Levin ME, O'Neal LW, Bowker JH: *The diabetic foot,* ed 5, St Louis, 1993, Mosby.)

to result from the interaction of multiple metabolic, genetic, and environmental factors. The underlying pathologic mechanism may be vascular, metabolic, or a combination of both mechanisms and is related to hyperglycemia.[162] Neuropathy is classified into two stages: subclinical and clinical. In the subclinical stage, there is evidence that peripheral nerve dysfunctions such as slowed motor and sensory nerve conduction exist without clinical signs. In the clinical stage, symptoms or clinically detectable neurologic deficits are present. Generally, sensory deficits and symptoms are more common than motor involvement.

Diabetic neuropathy is considered to be a form of a "dying back" neuropathy, in which the distal portions of the neurons are initially and eventually more severely affected. The earliest morphologic change in both peripheral nerves and the central nervous system is axonal degeneration that preferentially involves unmyelinated nerve fibers. Schwann cell abnormalities then occur because of changes in the axons they support. Metabolic activity of the Schwann cell is disturbed, causing segmental loss of myelin and the characteristic pattern of demyelination and remyelination observed in long-term diabetic neuropathy (Figure 21-19). The location of the pathologic condition may include the spinal cord, the posterior root ganglia, or the peripheral nerves. These changes may occur alone or in combination.

Motor nerve conduction velocity, electromyography, and sensory perception have shown abnormalities at the onset of diabetes. Sensory nerve conduction also may be impaired at this stage and is probably the most sensitive index of peripheral neuropathy. These abnormalities may be improved by good glucose control. Although these changes suggest early involvement of the nervous system in individuals with diabetes, they generally are not accompanied by clinical symptomatology.

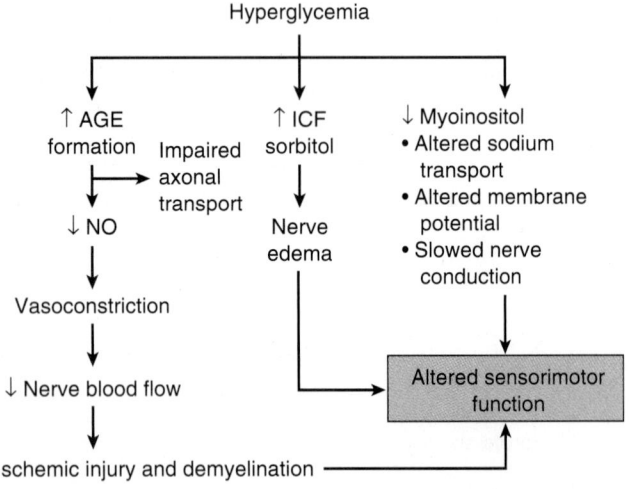

AGE = advanced glycation end products
ICF = intracellular fluid
NO = nitric oxide (vasodilator)

Figure 21-19 Diabetic neuropathy

Various diabetic neuropathies occur, with varying causes, pathogenesis, and clinical backgrounds (Table 21-15). Some of the diabetic neuropathic syndromes are progressive, but many—such as painful peripheral neuropathy, mononeuropathy (wristdrop, footdrop), diabetic amyotrophy, diabetic neuropathic cachexia, and visceral manifestations associated with autonomic neuropathy (e.g., diabetic diarrhea and orthostatic hypotension)—may spontaneously improve. This suggests that metabolic changes are not completely responsible for the neuropathies. In fact, acute neuropathic syndromes caused by nerve infarction may occur during periods of good glucose control. Obviously, much investigation regarding diabetic neuropathies remains to be done. The Diabetes Control and Complications Trial (DCCT) demonstrated a 60% reduction in results related to the appearance of clinical neuropathy and parameters of subclinical nerve dysfunction in the intensive insulin therapy cohort.[95] Similar results are seen in the Kumamoto trial.[163]

Infection

Increased morbidity and mortality from infectious agents have been documented in those with diabetes.[164] The individual with diabetes is at increased risk for infection throughout the body for at least five reasons:

1. Impaired vision caused by retinal changes and impaired touch caused by neuropathy diminish the prevention of breaks in the skin by decreasing the early warning systems. Once breaks in skin integrity occur, tissues may have increased susceptibility to infection because of hypoxia, a second reason for susceptibility to infection.
2. Microvascular and macrovascular complications cause decreased oxygen supply to tissues. In addition, the increased content of glycosylated hemoglobin in the red blood cell impedes the release of oxygen to tissues.
3. Pathogens are able to multiply rapidly once they have gained access to the tissues. Some pathogens proliferate rapidly because the increased glucose in body fluids provides an excellent source of energy.
4. Decreased blood supply resulting from vascular changes decreases the supply of white blood cells to the affected area.
5. Function of the white cells is impaired by ischemia and hyperglycemia. Chemotaxis is abnormal, and phagocytosis is defective.

The risk of infection is especially high for individuals undergoing surgery and for those taking immunosuppressant medications.[165,165a]

ALTERATIONS OF ADRENAL FUNCTION

Disorders of the Adrenal Cortex

Disorders of the adrenal cortex are related to either hyperfunction or hypofunction. Hyperfunction that causes increased levels of circulating cortisol leads to Cushing disease, or Cushing syndrome; hyperfunction that causes increased

Table 21-15   Classification of Diabetic Neuropathies

Location	Characteristics
Somatic (Peripheral) Neuropathies	
Lower extremities	Most commonly bilateral, symmetric, and sensory
Asymptomatic	Paresthesias, progressive and irreversible, underlie the development of neuropathic ulcers and Charcot joints
Painful	Pain and paresthesias, particularly nocturnally; anorexia, depression, and irritability; absence of knee and ankle jerk reflexes
Upper extremities	Involves muscle atrophy, asthenia, sensory impairment, and radiculitis
Asymmetric neuropathies	Predominantly motor involvement, absent sensory involvement, sudden onset, severe pain, good prognosis
Diabetic neuropathic cachexia	Profound weight loss with severe pain, spontaneous recovery
Visceral Neuropathies (Generally Occur with Peripheral Neuropathies)	
Cranial nerves	Involves cranial nerve III, leading to pain, diplopia, and ptosis; involvement of cranial nerve VII leads to Bell palsy
Gastrointestinal tract	Involves decreased esophageal motility, delayed gastric emptying, and diabetic constipation and diarrhea
Genitourinary tract	Insidious and progressive bladder paralysis with urinary retention; sexual dysfunction in males, including retrograde ejaculation and erectile dysfunction
Autonomic nervous system	Includes cardiovascular reflexes, anhidrosis, gustatory sweating, and orthostatic hypotension
Radiculopathy	Spinal cord or root compression, transverse myelitis

secretion of adrenal androgens and estrogens leads to virilization or feminization; and hyperfunction that causes increased levels of aldosterone leads to hyperaldosteronism, which may be primary or secondary. Hypofunction of the adrenal cortex leads to Addison disease.

Adrenocortical Hyperfunction: Cushing Disease, Cushing Syndrome

Cushing disease is caused by excessive anterior pituitary secretion of ACTH. **Cushing syndrome** is an uncommon disorder and occurs whenever there is an excessive level of cortisol regardless of the cause. Cushing syndrome is the most common complication of Cushing disease. Cushing syndrome resulting from ectopic ACTH secretion is more common in older adults, particularly men. Adrenal tumors, rather than pituitary tumors, are more common in children, especially girls. Cushing syndrome can occur at any age but usually occurs between 30 and 50 years of age. In addition, a Cushing-like syndrome may develop as a result of the exogenous administration of glucocorticoids.[166] ACTH-induced Cushing disease is more common in adults and is two to three times more common in women than in men.

PATHOPHYSIOLOGY Hypercortisolism usually is caused by Cushing disease, ectopic ACTH-secreting tumors, or cortisol-secreting adrenal tumors. Approximately 75% to 80% of individuals with hypercortisolism have Cushing disease, whereas both ectopic ACTH-secreting tumors and cortisol-secreting adrenal tumors are less often the cause of hypercortisolism.[167]

Although the origin of Cushing disease remains incompletely understood, the vast majority of individuals with Cushing disease have a pituitary microadenoma, which secretes ACTH.[168] In Cushing disease there is a loss of normal feedback inhibition by cortisol because there appears to be a higher set-point for cortisol feedback on corticotropin-releasing hormone (CRH) and ACTH secretion.

Ectopic ACTH-secreting tumors are nonpituitary tumors that synthesize and hypersecrete ACTH, leading to hypercortisolism. Some tumors may hypersecrete CRH, which results in oversecretion of ACTH from the pituitary. Tumors associated with episodic secretion of ACTH and hypercortisolism include small cell carcinomas of the lung, thymoma, pancreatic cell tumors, carcinoid tumors, medullary carcinoma of the thyroid, and pheochromocytoma tumors. Even though the secretion of ectopic ACTH from the neoplasm is not under hypothalamic–pituitary control, the normal pituitary release of ACTH is inhibited by the elevated levels of cortisol. However, cortisol fails to inhibit the release of ACTH from the ectopic source.

Autonomous secretion of cortisol can be the result of either an adrenal adenoma or, less commonly, adrenal cortical carcinoma.[169] Elevated cortisol levels suppress CRH and ACTH release secretion from the hypothalamus and anterior pituitary, respectively, which leads to low levels of ACTH. Low levels of ACTH cause atrophy of the remaining normal portions of the adrenal cortex, which over time will alter the cortisol-secreting activity of normal cells. The normal diurnal variation in cortisol secretion is lost in individuals with hypercortisolism regardless of the underlying cause.

CLINICAL MANIFESTATIONS Most of the clinical signs and symptoms of Cushing syndrome are caused by hypercortisolism.[170] Weight gain is the most common feature and results from the accumulation of adipose tissue in the trunk, facial, and cervical areas. These characteristic patterns of fat deposition have been described as "truncal obesity," "moon face," and "buffalo hump" (Figures 21-20 and 21-21). Transient weight gain from sodium and water retention may be present because of the mineralocorticoid effects of cortisol, exhibited when cortisol is present in high levels.

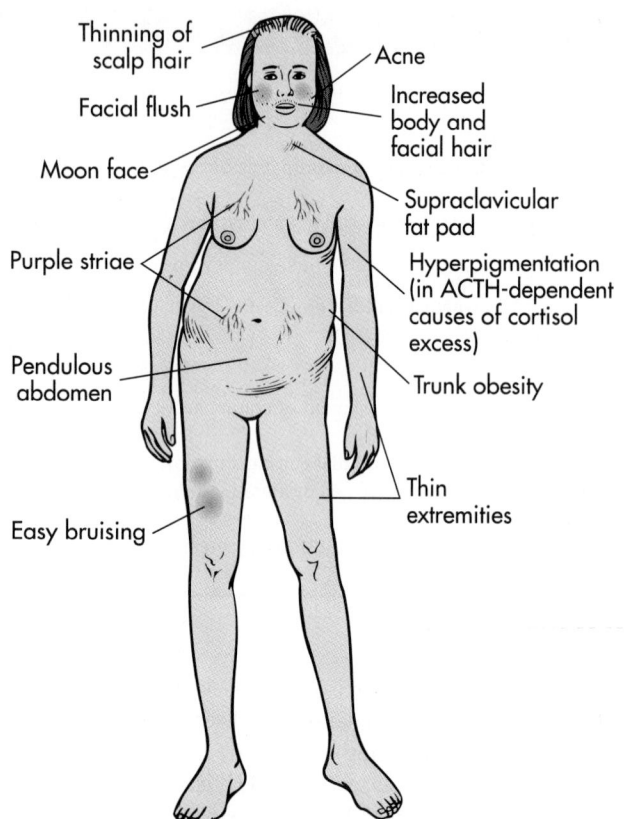

Figure 21-20 Symptoms of Cushing disease. *ACTH*, Adrenocorticotropic hormone.

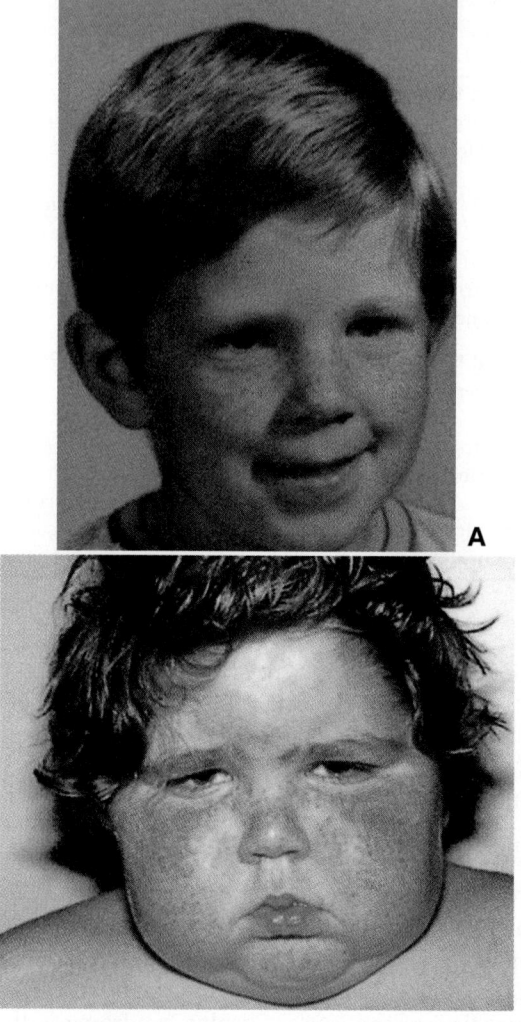

Figure 21-21 Cushing syndrome. **A,** Patient before onset of Cushing syndrome. **B,** Patient 4 months later. Moon facies is clearly demonstrated. (From Zitelli BJ, Davis HW: *Atlas of pediatric physical diagnosis,* ed 4, London, 2002, Gower.)

Glucose intolerance occurs because of cortisol-induced insulin resistance and increased gluconeogenesis and glycogen storage by the liver. Overt diabetes mellitus develops in approximately 20% of individuals with hypercortisolism. Polyuria, which is sometimes seen in hypercortisolism, is a manifestation of hyperglycemia and resultant glycosuria.

Protein wasting is commonly observed in hypercortisolism and is caused by the catabolic effects of cortisol on peripheral tissues. Muscle wasting, especially obvious in the muscles of the extremities, leads to muscle weakness. Hypercortisolism increases bone resorption, inhibits bone formation, decreases intestinal calcium absorption, and increases renal calcium excretion. This leads to osteoporosis, with pathologic fractures, vertebral compression fractures, bone and back pain, kyphosis, and reduced height. Hypercalciuria may result in renal stones, which are experienced by approximately 20% of individuals with this disease. Loss of collagen also leads to thin, weakened integumentary tissues through which capillaries are more visible; the tissues are easily stretched by adipose deposits. Together these changes account for the characteristic purple striae most often observed in the trunkal area. Loss of collagenous support around small vessels makes them susceptible to rupture, leading to easy bruising, even with minor trauma. Thin, atrophied skin is also easily damaged, leading to skin breaks and ulcerations.

Hyperpigmentation in Cushing syndrome is associated with very high serum levels of ACTH, believed to be caused by increased melanocyte-stimulating hormones resulting from excess conversion of pro-opiomelanocortin when ACTH is elevated.[171] The pigmentation involves the mucous membranes, hair, and skin, all of which acquire a characteristic brownish or bronze color.

Cortisol has a permissive effect on the actions of the catecholamines. With elevated cortisol levels, vascular sensitivity to catecholamines is increased significantly, leading to vasoconstriction and hypertension. Elevated blood pressure occurs in most individuals with Cushing syndrome. Chronically elevated cortisol levels also cause suppression of the immune system and increased susceptibility to infections. Consequently, individuals with hypercortisolism experience poor wound healing and are particularly susceptible to superficial fungal infections.

Approximately 50% of individuals with Cushing syndrome experience alterations in their mental status and include effects of cortisol on hippocampal neurons and the implications for learning and memory and other neurologic functions when cortisol is elevated. These may range from irritability and depression to severe psychiatric disturbances such as schizophrenia.[172,173] The effects of glucocorticoids on mood are complex.

Females may experience symptoms of increased adrenal androgen levels, increased hair growth (especially facial hair), acne, and oligomenorrhea. Androgen levels rarely become high enough to cause changes of the voice, recession of the hairline, and clitoral hypertrophy unless an adrenal carcinoma is involved. Routine laboratory examinations may reveal hyperglycemia, glycosuria, hypokalemia, and metabolic alkalosis.

EVALUATION AND TREATMENT   A variety of laboratory tests must be used to diagnose hypercortosolism and to determine the underlying disorder. These include urinary free cortisol higher than 100 mcg per 24 hours, abnormal dexamethasone suppressibility of either urinary or serum cortisol, and simultaneous measurement of ACTH and cortisol. Visualizing procedures, including pituitary MRI or abdominal scanning, are essential in the evaluation. Selective catheterization of the veins draining the pituitary (inferior pertrosal sinus sampling) is very helpful in determining the cause of hypercortisolism and in localizing pituitary tumors.[170] The diagnosis and evaluation of hypercortisolism is one of the most challenging problems in endocrinology.[174]

Without treatment, approximately 50% of individuals with Cushing syndrome die within 5 years of onset. Major causes of death are overwhelming infection, suicide, complications from generalized arteriosclerosis, and hypertensive disease. Treatment is specific for the cause of hypercorticoadrenalism and includes medication, radiation therapy, and surgery. Therefore it is essential to differentiate between pituitary, adrenal, and ectopic causes of the hypercortisolism.

Hyperaldosteronism

Hyperaldosteronism is characterized by excessive aldosterone secretion by the adrenal cortex. The excessive secretion can result from a primary adrenal disorder, such as an aldosterone-secreting adenoma, or from excessive stimulation of the normal adrenal cortex by substances such as angiotensin II, ACTH, or elevated potassium. Both primary and secondary forms of hyperaldosteronism can occur in individuals. **Primary hyperaldosteronism** refers to an excessive secretion of aldosterone caused by an abnormality of the adrenal cortex. **Secondary hyperaldosteronism** involves excessive aldosterone secretion from an extraadrenal stimulus, most often angiotensin II through a renin-dependent mechanism.

Primary hyperaldosteronism (Conn disease, primary aldosteronism) presents a clinical picture of hypertension, hypokalemia, renal potassium wasting, and neuromuscular manifestations. The most common cause of primary aldosteronism is the benign, single adrenal adenoma (80% to 90% of cases), followed by multiple tumors or idiopathic hyperplasia of the adrenals (10% to 15% of cases). Adrenal carcinomas and unknown causes account for the remainder of cases. The incidence of primary hyperaldosteronism is not known, but 5% to 13% of individuals with hypertension have primary aldosteronism.[175]

Because aldosterone secretion normally is stimulated by the renin-angiotensin system, secondary hyperaldosteronism can be expected to result from sustained elevated renin release and activation of angiotensin II. (Factors that affect renin and aldosterone secretion are summarized in Table 21-16.) Increased renin-angiotensin secretion occurs in a variety of situations. In general, these include decreased circulating blood volume (e.g., in dehydration, shock, or hypoalbuminemia) and decreased delivery of blood to the kidneys (e.g., renal artery stenosis, heart failure, or hepatic cirrhosis). In many of these instances the activation of the renin-angiotensin system and subsequent aldosterone secretion may be seen as compensatory, although in some instances (e.g., congestive heart failure) the increased circulating volume may further worsen the condition.

Increased estrogen levels associated with pregnancy and use of oral contraceptives also increase renin-angiotensin levels, apparently by stimulating renin substrate production by the liver. These pregnancy-induced changes, however, may represent adaptation to pregnancy and are therefore not representative pathophysiologic alterations.

Other causes of secondary hyperaldosteronism include Bartter syndrome, which is a heterogenous autosomal recessive disorder associated with reduced or absent salt transport by the thick ascending limb of Henle. Symptoms include salt wasting and low blood pressure, hypokalemia, metabolic acidosis, and hypercalciuria.[176] Renin-secreting tumors of the kidney also cause secondary hyperaldosteronism. Diuretic use is perhaps the most common cause of secondary hyperaldosteronism. (Renal disorders are discussed in Chapter 36.)

PATHOPHYSIOLOGY   In primary hyperaldosteronism, pathophysiologic alterations are caused by excessive aldosterone secretion and the fluid and electrolyte imbalances that ensue. Hyperaldosteronism promotes increased sodium reabsorption with corresponding hypervolemia (see Chapter 3). The extracellular fluid volume overload and suppression of

Table 21-16	Physiologic Factors Affecting Renin and Aldosterone Secretion	
Factors	**Renin Secretion**
Age	Highest in infants; lowest in the elderly
Menstrual cycle	Highest in luteal phase (see Chapter 22)
Sodium intake	Increased by salt restriction
	Decreased by salt loading
Potassium status	Increased by K⁺ excess
Posture	Increased with erect posture
Sympathetic nervous stimulation	Renin increased by catecholamines
Time of sampling	Highest before noon; lowest in evening

ACTH, Adrenocorticotropic hormone.

normal feedback mechanisms of renin secretion are characteristic of primary disorders.

Edema usually does not occur with primary aldosteronism, possibly because of the renal tubular "escape" phenomenon that is activated in chronic hyperaldosteronism. The escape phenomenon changes or resets the rate of sodium excretion and prevents more severe sodium retention. The escape phenomenon operates in the proximal tubules and causes additional sodium to pass to the distal tubules, where the sodium is, to some extent, reabsorbed in exchange for potassium. This mechanism, while protecting from excessive sodium reabsorption and edema, increases urinary losses of potassium (Figure 21-22).

In secondary hyperaldosteronism the effect of increased extracellular volume on renin secretion may vary. If renin secretion is being stimulated by variables other than pressure-initiated cellular changes at the juxtaglomerular apparatus (see Chapter 35), increased circulating blood volume may not decrease renin secretion through feedback mechanisms. This physiologic process is normal in pregnancy and related to increased plasma estrogen.

In Bartter syndrome a state of hypokalemia develops because of defective renal tubular reabsorptive mechanisms. The hypokalemic state may induce the formation of prostaglandins (especially PGE_2) by the renal cells, which stimulates renin and hence aldosterone secretion. The stimulatory effect on aldosterone secretion is offset somewhat by the aldosterone-suppressing effects of hypokalemia.

Potassium secretion also is promoted by aldosterone, so that with excessive circulating levels of aldosterone, hypokalemia occurs (see Chapter 3). In hyperaldosteronism, hypokalemic alkalosis, changes in myocardial conduction, and skeletal muscle alterations may be seen, particularly with severe potassium depletion (i.e., the renal tubules may become insensitive to ADH, thus promoting excessive loss of free water). Rarely, this may result in mild hypernatremia because water is not able to follow the sodium that is reabsorbed.

CLINICAL MANIFESTATIONS Hypertension, hypokalemia, and less commonly, metabolic alkalosis are the hallmarks of hyperaldosteronism.[177] Hypertension may result from increased intravascular volume or from a state of aldosterone-mediated vasoconstriction, although the latter mechanism requires very high levels of aldosterone. If hypertension is sustained, the long-term effects of elevated arterial pressure become evident, which include the development of left ventricular dilation and hypertrophy. Because of the increased arterial pressure, renin secretion is typically suppressed, although it is elevated in secondary hyperaldosteronism, which provides a means to clearly differentiate between these conditions.

Aldosterone-stimulated potassium loss can be substantial. Serum potassium levels below 3.0 mEq/L result in the typical manifestations of hypokalemia: hypokalemic alkalosis caused by the movement of potassium from the intercellular to extracellular space in exchange for hydrogen ions as well as renal loss of hydrogen ions to facilitate sodium reabsorption (see Chapter 3). Individuals with hypokalemic alkalosis may experience the following:

1. Tetany and paresthesia caused by an alkalosis-induced lowering of ionized calcium levels
2. Skeletal muscle weakness that can be so severe as to mimic flaccid paralysis
3. Cardiovascular alterations consistent with hypokalemia (see Chapter 4), including depressed T waves and ST

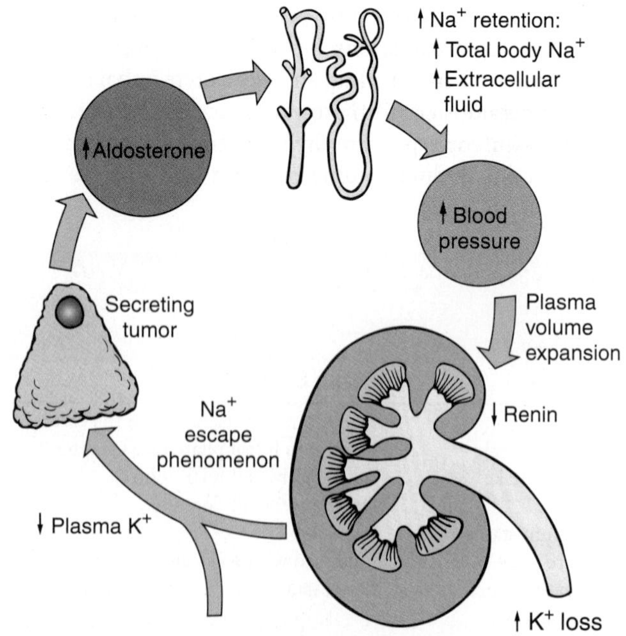

Figure 21-22 **Primary hyperaldosteronism.** Pathophysiology of mineralocorticoid excess syndromes in primary hyperaldosteronism.

WHAT'S NEW? Aldosteronism and Cardiovascular and Renal Toxicity

Chronic inappropriate elevations of aldosterone are associated with cardiac fibrosis, vascular remodeling, endothelial cell dysfunction, and renal vascular injury with proteinuria independent of hypertensive effects. In animal models, sustained elevated aldosterone induces vascular smooth muscle cell hypertrophy in the right and left heart, including invasion of monocytes, macrophages, and lymphocytes, with evidence of oxidative and nitrosative stress, myofibroblasts and perivascular fibrosis. There may be a link between cardiovascular toxicity and an aldosterone-stimulated immunoregulatory state. The development of vasculitis requires salt that is inappropriate for aldosterone levels and may involve nonepithelial mineralocorticoid receptors and rapid nongenomic effects of aldosterone. Mineralocorticoid receptor agonists (i.e., eplerenone) provide end-organ protection in addition to their diuretic and secondary blood pressure lowering effects.

Data from Fritsch Neves M, Schiffrin EL: *Curr Hypertens Rep* 5(1):59-65, 2003; Losel R et al: *Steroids* 69(8-9):575-578, 2004; Sato A, Saruta T: *Hypertens Res* 27(5):303-310, 2004; Schmidt BM, Schmieder RE: *Am J Hypertens* 16(1):80-86, 2003.

segment, appearance of U waves on the electrocardio-gram, and ventricular ectopy, which may or may not be associated with syncopy

4. Loss of urine-concentrating mechanisms, leading to polyuria or nocturia

EVALUATION AND TREATMENT   A variety of clinical and laboratory measurements are useful in the assessment of hyperaldosteronism.[178,179] These include blood pressure, serum and urinary electrolyte levels, serum and urinary levels of aldosterone and renin, plasma aldosterone concentration to plasma renin activity ratio, and aldosterone suppression testing. Blood pressure is elevated; serum sodium may be normal or elevated; and serum potassium is depressed, whereas urinary potassium is elevated (i.e., >30 mmol/day). Serum aldosterone, as measured by radioimmunoassay, usually is greater than 20 ng/dl. Plasma renin activity is generally less than 1 ng/ml/hr for individuals with primary aldosteronism. Serum aldosterone and plasma renin activity both must be measured under controlled situations and after careful dietary regulation of sodium and potassium intake (see Table 21-16). Aldosterone suppression testing commonly is accomplished with fludrocortisone acetate (Florinef) or salt loading. Imaging techniques, such as CT and nuclear magnetic resonance (NMR), may be used to localize an aldosterone-secreting adenoma. Selective venous catheterization of both adrenal veins is also useful.

Treatment includes management of hypertension and hypokalemia, as well as correction of any underlying causal abnormalities. If an aldosterone-secreting adenoma is present, it is generally approached surgically; however, medical management with spironolactone or eplerenone, a new drug without the side effects of spironolactone, is a viable option in complicated cases.[180-181]

Adrenocortical Hypofunction

Hypocortisolism (low levels of cortisol secretion) develops because of either inadequate stimulation of the adrenal glands by ACTH or a primary inability of the adrenals to produce and secrete the adrenocortical hormones. In some syndromes, however, there is partial dysfunction of the adrenal cortex so that only synthesis of aldosterone or the adrenal androgens is affected. Hypofunction of the adrenal cortex may affect glucocorticoid or mineralocorticoid secretion or a combination of both.

Primary adrenal insufficiency is termed **Addison disease.** Addison disease is a relatively rare disease, occurring most often in adults 30 to 60 years of age, although it may appear at any time throughout the life span. Addison disease, caused by autoimmune mechanisms, is more common in women.

The most common cause of Addison disease in the United States is autoimmune destruction of the adrenal cortex. Other causes include infections (tuberculosis, fungal, HIV), infiltrative diseases (amyloidosis, metastatic carcinoma), or bilateral adrenal hemorrhage. Adrenoleukodystrophy and adrenomyeloneuropathy are two rare types of X-linked adrenal deficiency that lead to symptoms of hypocortisolism and progressive neurologic symptoms.

PATHOPHYSIOLOGY   Addison disease is characterized by elevated serum ACTH levels with inadequate corticosteroid synthesis and output. Before clinical manifestations of hypocortisolism are evident, more than 90% of total adrenocortical tissue must be destroyed.

Idiopathic Addison Disease

Idiopathic Addison disease (organ-specific autoimmune adrenalitis), which causes adrenal atrophy and hypofunction, generally is recognized as an organ-specific autoimmune disease. (Autoimmunity is discussed in Chapter 8.) Autoantibodies are present in 50% to 70% of individuals with idiopathic Addison disease, and this percentage increases in younger persons and in those with other autoimmune diseases. The autoantibodies are specific for the cells of the adrenal cortex and 21-hydroxylase (the enzyme that produces cortisol and aldosterone).[182] A combination of cell membrane and cytoplasmic antibodies and cell-mediated immune mechanisms contributes to the pathologic findings of the disease. Apparently a genetic defect in immune surveillance mechanisms causes a deficiency of immune-suppressor cells. This deficiency allows the proliferation of immunocytes directed against specific antigens within the adrenocortical cells.

Idiopathic Addison disease often is associated with other autoimmune diseases and in such cases is known as *autoimmune polyendocrine syndrome (APS)*. ASPI (APS type I) is inherited as autosomal recessive and includes Addison disease, hypoparathyroidism, candidias, and other less common symptoms. ASPII (APS type II) is more common and involves Addision disease, immune thyroid disease, diabetes mellitus, and hypogonadism.[183] (Mechanisms of inheritance are described in Chapter 4.)

The adrenal glands in idiopathic Addison disease are smaller than normal and may be misshapen. Microscopically, gland atrophy is evident throughout the cortex, although the medulla appears intact. Extensive diffuse cortical lymphocytic infiltrate supports the immune component of the disease process.

Secondary Hypocortisolism

Secondary hypocortisolism is characterized by low to absent ACTH levels, which cause inadequate adrenal stimulation, adrenal atrophy, and ultimately decreased corticosteroidogenesis. The exogenous administration of glucocorticoids for nonendocrine disease results in this form of hypocortisolism. Successful surgical removal of cortisol-secreting tumors also results in postoperative hypocortisolism. In these cases, increased glucocorticoid levels suppress ACTH production through normal feedback mechanisms. With decreased ACTH levels, corticosteroid synthesis by remaining adrenal tissue is suppressed. Pituitary hypofunction (as occurs in postpartum pituitary infarction [Sheehan syndrome] and panhypopituitarism, hypophysectomy, or isolated ACTH deficiency) causes inadequate ACTH production and secretion and absence of pituitary responsiveness to normal stimulatory mechanisms. In all instances of low ACTH levels, adrenal atrophy occurs, and endogenous adrenal steroidogenesis is depressed.

Clinical manifestations of secondary hypocortisolism are similar to those of Addison disease. One difference is that with the typically low levels of ACTH seen in secondary hypocortisolism, hyperpigmentation does not occur. Second, the renin-angiotensin system is usually normal in these individuals; therefore aldosterone and potassium levels also tend to be normal.

CLINICAL MANIFESTATIONS   The symptoms of Addison disease are primarily a result of hypocortisolism and hypoaldosteronism and include weakness and fatigue, anorexia, weight loss, nausea, diarrhea, and orthostatic hypotension. Hyperpigmentation is associated with elevated ACTH levels. Decreased adrenal androgen secretion is usually not clinically obvious in males because the adrenals are not a major source of male androgens. Females may experience a loss of some secondary sex characteristics, such as pubic and axillary hair, normally maintained by the adrenal androgens. The symptoms of Addison disease are summarized in Table 21-17.

EVALUATION AND TREATMENT   Serum and urine levels of cortisol are depressed with hypocortisolism. In primary adrenal insufficiency (Addison disease), ACTH levels are clearly elevated, and ACTH levels are low in secondary adrenal insufficiency. ACTH levels can be interpreted only in the face of a simultaneous measurement of cortisol. Individuals may develop azotemia caused by dehydration, and hyponatremia is common. Hyperkalemia is seen only in Addison disease, but hypoglycemia may be seen in hypocortisolism from any cause. Anemia, eosinophilia, and lymphocytosis are also common with symptoms of fatigue. The ACTH stimulation test may be used to evaluate adrenocortical function. This is achieved by administering ACTH and monitoring the serum cortisol levels.

The treatment of Addison disease involves glucocorticoid and possibly mineralocorticoid replacement therapy, together with dietary modifications.[184] All individuals with hypocortisolism require lifetime daily glucocorticoid replacement therapy. In the event of acute stressors, additional cortisol must be administered to approximate the amount of cortisol that might be expected to be secreted if normal diurnal adrenal function were present (approximately 100 to 300 mg/day).

The individual's diet should include at least 150 mEq of sodium per day, with sodium intake increased in the event of excessive sweating or diarrhea. Treatment also must include correction of any underlying disorders.

Hypersecretion of Adrenal Androgens and Estrogens

Hypersecretion of adrenal androgens and estrogens may be caused by adrenal tumors, either adenomas or carcinomas, Cushing syndrome, or defects in steroid synthesis. The clinical syndrome that results depends on the hormone secreted, the gender of the individual, and the ages at which the hypersecretion was initiated. Hypersecretion of estrogens causes **feminization,** the development of female sex characteristics. Hypersecretion of androgens causes **virilization,** the development of male sex characteristics (Figure 21-23).

The effects of an estrogen-secreting tumor are most evident in males and result in gynecomastia (breast enlargement) (98% of cases), testicular atrophy, and decreased libido. In female children such tumors may lead to early development of secondary sex characteristics. An androgen-secreting tumor indicates changes more easily observed in females, including hirsutism, clitoral enlargement, deepening of the voice, amenorrhea, acne, and breast atrophy. In children, virilizing tumors promote precocious sexual development and bone aging. Treatment of androgen-secreting tumors usually involves surgical excision.

Disorders of the Adrenal Medulla
Adrenal Medulla Hypofunction

No known physiologic alterations are associated with hypofunction of the adrenal medulla. Bilateral adrenalectomy, for example, is followed by a rapid decrease in urinary excretion

Table 21-17 Clinical Manifestations and Pathophysiologic Mechanisms of Addison Disease	
Clinical Manifestations	**Pathophysiologic Mechanism**
Weakness and easy fatigability that worsens as the day progresses, seen especially after exposure to stressors	Not known, may be related to hypoglycemia, hypotension, decreased metabolism of proteins
Gastrointestinal disturbances: anorexia, nausea, vomiting, diarrhea, abdominal pain, weight loss	May be associated with celiac disease
Hypoglycemia, manifested by fatigue, mental confusion, apathy, psychosis	Absence of cortisol leads to decreased gluconeogenesis, decreased glycogen storage by liver, decreased metabolism of proteins, increased insulin sensitivity
Hyperpigmentation	Elevations of ACTH, which lead to stimulation of melanocytes
Vitiligo (white patchy areas of depigmented skin)	Autoimmune destruction of melanocytes
Addisonian crisis: severe hypotension and vascular collapse	Combined effects of hypocortisolism, hypoaldosteronism, extracellular volume depletion, and some precipitating stressor (e.g., infection, vomiting, diarrhea); decreased vasomotor tone caused by cortisol deficiency

ACTH, Adrenocorticotropic hormone.

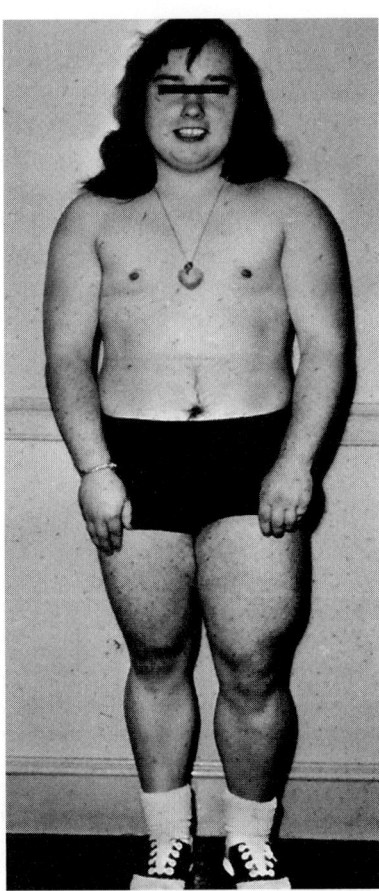

Figure 21-23 Virilization. Virilization of a young girl by an androgen-secreting tumor of the adrenal cortex. Masculine features include lack of breast development, increased muscle bulk, and hirsutism. (From Thibodeau GA: *Anatomy & physiology*, St Louis, 1987, Mosby.)

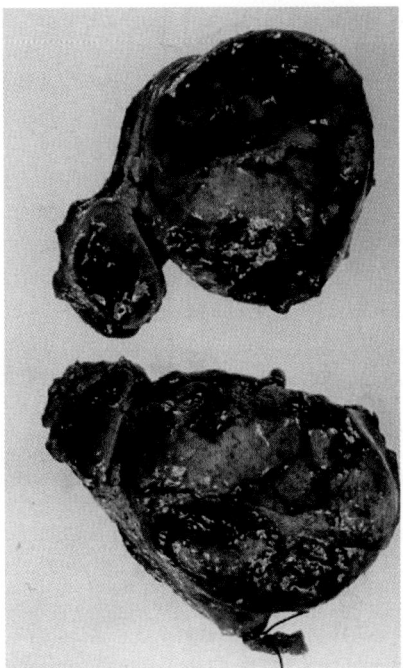

Figure 21-24 Pheochromocytoma. Gross appearance of adrenal pheochromocytoma. (From Rosai J: *Akerman's surgical pathology*, ed 8, St Louis, 1996, Mosby.)

of epinephrine, but excretion of norepinephrine remains relatively stable. Pathophysiologic alterations are instead associated with hyperfunctioning of the adrenal medulla.

Adrenal Medulla Hyperfunction

Adrenomedullary hyperfunction is caused by tumors derived from the chromaffin cells of the adrenal medulla. These tumors, **pheochromocytomas,** secrete catecholamines on a continual or episodic basis (Figure 21-24). Less than 10% of these tumors are malignant; those that are malignant may metastasize to the lungs, liver, bones, or paraaortic lymph nodes. Most pheochromocytomas produce norepinephrine, although large tumors secrete both epinephrine and norepinephrine.

The true incidence of pheochromocytoma in the general population is not known. One tenth of one percent of the hypertensive population have a pheochromocytoma.[185] The tumors are most common in people 40 to 60 years of age, with men and women equally affected.

PATHOPHYSIOLOGY Pheochromocytomas cause excessive production of catecholamines attributable to autono-

mous functioning of the tumor. Approximately 5% of people with pheochromocytomas have no symptoms because the tumor appears to be nonfunctioning; however, these tumors can release catecholamines in response to stressors, such as abdominal surgery.

CLINICAL MANIFESTATIONS The clinical manifestations of a pheochromocytoma are related to the chronic effects of catecholamine secretion and include persistent hypertension associated with diaphoresis, tachycardia, palpitations, and severe headache.[186] Hypertension is a result of increased peripheral vascular resistance and may be sustained or paroxysmal. Headaches appear because of sudden changes in catecholamine levels in the blood, affecting cerebral blood flow. Hypermetabolism is related to chronic activation of sympathetic receptors in adipocytes, hepatocytes, and other tissues. Glucose intolerance may occur because of catecholamine-induced inhibition of insulin release by the pancreas. Complaints of warmth, heat intolerance, weight loss, and constipation are common despite a normal or an increased appetite.

An acute episode of hypertension related to hypersecretion of catecholamines may follow specific events. Exercise, excessive ingestion of tyrosine-containing foods (aged cheese, red wine, beer, yogurt), ingestion of caffeine-containing foods, external pressure on the tumor, and induction of anesthesia all can increase secretion of catecholamines by the tumor.

These tumors tend to be extremely vascular and can rupture. Such an event can cause massive and potentially fatal hemorrhage. Rupture of a pheochromocytoma is characterized by a sudden, unexplained decrease in blood pressure; sudden, severe abdominal pain; and a rigid abdomen.

EVALUATION AND TREATMENT A diagnosis of pheochromocytoma is made when increased catecholamine production is demonstrated in the blood or urine. Individuals with this disorder can have total urine catecholamine levels above 250 mg/day. After elevation of urinary or plasma

catecholamines is documented, the site of the tumor is determined using MRI; because of the possibility of metastasis, whole-body scanning may be done.

The usual treatment of pheochromocytoma is laparoscopic surgical excision of the tumor. Medical therapy is used to stabilize blood pressure before surgery. Drugs used include α-adrenergic blocking agents and, possibly later, β-adrenergic blocking agents. Open resection is completed for large tumors or when metastasis is suspected.[187]

SUMMARY REVIEW

Mechanisms of Hormonal Alterations
1. Abnormalities in endocrine function may be caused by hypersecretion or hyposecretion of hormones, causing alterations in normal hormone levels.
2. Endocrine abnormalities also may be caused by alterations in receptor function through a variety of mechanisms: (a) a decrease in number of receptors, (b) receptor insensitivity to the hormone, (c) antibodies against specific receptors, and (d) defects in second messenger generation or postreceptor defects.
3. Abnormally high levels of circulating hormones sometimes are caused by hormone release from tissues outside the endocrine system (ectopic foci), which may not respond to normal feedback mechanisms, in which case they are said to function autonomously.

Alterations of the Hypothalamic–Pituitary System
1. Dysfunction in the release of hypothalamic hormones probably is related to interruption of the connection between the hypothalamus and pituitary—namely, the pituitary stalk.
2. Disorders of the posterior pituitary include syndrome of inappropriate antidiuretic hormone (SIADH) secretion and diabetes insipidus. SIADH secretion is characterized by abnormally high ADH secretion; diabetes insipidus is characterized by abnormally low ADH secretion.
3. In SIADH, high ADH levels interfere with renal free water clearance, leading to hyponatremia and hypoosmolality. SIADH secretion is associated with certain forms of cancer, apparently because of ectopic secretion of ADH by tumor cells.
4. Diabetes insipidus may be neurogenic, caused by insufficient amounts of ADH, or nephrogenic, caused by an inadequate response to ADH. Its principal clinical features are polyuria and polydipsia.
5. Hypopituitarism is dysfunction of the anterior pituitary that causes failure of hormonal functions. Symptoms may be mild to severe.
6. The most common cause of hypopituitarism is a tumor of the pituitary or subsequent treatment of the tumor (surgical or radiation therapy). Symptoms are variable depending on which hormones are deficient (i.e., TSH, ACTH, GH, etc.).
7. Hyperpituitarism is caused by pituitary adenomas. These are usually benign, slow-growing tumors that arise from cells of the anterior pituitary.
8. Expansion of a pituitary adenoma causes both neurologic and secretory effects. Pressure from the expanding tumor causes hyposecretion of cells, dysfunction of the optic chiasm (leading to visual disturbances), and dysfunction of the hypothalamus and some cranial nerves.
9. Hypersecretion of growth hormone (GH) causes acromegaly, in which GH secretion becomes high and unpredictable. Pituitary adenoma is the most common cause of acromegaly.
10. Prolonged, abnormally high levels of GH lead to proliferation of body and connective tissues. Renal, thyroid, and reproductive dysfunction develop slowly, together with a change in bony proportions.
11. Growth hormone (GH) deficiency in children results in growth failure and fasting hypoglycemia. Adult GH deficiency results in fatigue, osteoporosis, and increased mortality.
12. Pituitary prolactinomas result in increased prolactin and affects reproductive organs and function in both men and women.

Alterations of Thyroid Function
1. Thyrotoxicosis is a general condition in which thyroid hormone (TH) levels are elevated and produce an exaggerated physiologic response in tissues. The condition can be caused by a variety of specific diseases, each of which has its own pathophysiology and course of treatment.
2. In general, hyperthyroidism has a range of endocrine, reproductive, gastrointestinal, integumentary, and ocular manifestations. These are caused by increased circulating levels of TH and by stimulation of the sympathetic division of the autonomic nervous system.
3. Graves disease, the most common form of hyperthyroidism, is caused by an autoimmune mechanism that overrides normal mechanisms for control of TH secretion.
4. Manifestations of Graves disease can include symptoms of hyperthyroidism, diffuse thyroid enlargement, disorders of the skin, and enlargement of extraoccular muscles.
5. The cutaneous manifestation of Graves disease is pretibial myxedema, a condition characterized by subcutaneous swelling of the legs and, occasionally, the hands.
6. Ocular manifestations of Graves disease are caused by hyperactivity of the sympathetic division of the autonomic nervous system and by immune-induced infiltration of extraoccular muscles.
7. Toxic nodular goiter and toxic multinodular goiter occur when hyperplastic regions of the thyroid become autonomous.
8. Toxic nodular goiters are follicular-cell adenomas that produce symptoms similar to those of Graves disease.
9. Toxic multinodular goiters result from multiple functioning adenomas.
10. Thyrotoxic crisis is a severe form of hyperthyroidism that often is associated with physiologic stress. Without treatment, death occurs quickly.
11. Hypothyroidism is caused by deficient production of TH by the thyroid gland. The condition may be primary or secondary.
12. Primary hypothyroidism transiently occurs in either subacute or painless thyroiditis and spontaneous resolution of hypothyroidism is nearly universal. Chronic lymphocytic thyroiditis, an autoimmune disease, is associated with permanent hypothyroidism.
13. Subacute thyroiditis, a form of hypothyroidism, is a self-limited nonbacterial inflammation of the thyroid gland. The inflammatory process damages follicular cells, causing leakage

of triiodothyronine (T3) and thyroxine (T4). Hyperthyroidism then is followed by transient hypothyroidism, which is corrected by cellular repair and a return to normal levels in the thyroid.

14. Autoimmune thyroiditis is associated with infiltration or fibrosis of the thyroid, circulating thyroid antibodies, and gradual loss of thyroid function. Autoimmune thyroiditis occurs in those individuals with a genetic susceptibility to an autoimmune mechanism that causes thyroid damage and eventual hypothyroidism.

15. Hypothyroidism also can be caused by hypothalamic–pituitary dysfunction in which TRH and TSH are not produced in sufficient amounts.

16. Thyroid carcinoma is a relatively rare cancer. The most consistent causal risk factor associated with thyroid carcinoma is exposure to ionizing radiation, especially in childhood.

17. Hypothyroidism affects all body systems. Symptoms depend on the degree of TH deficiency. Common manifestations include decreased energy metabolism and heat production.

18. Myxedema is the characteristic sign of hypothyroidism. Myxedema is caused by alterations in connective tissue with water-binding proteins. The excess water leads to edema and thickened mucous membranes.

19. Myxedema coma is a severe form of hypothyroidism, which may be life threatening without emergency medical treatment.

20. Congenital hypothyroidism occurs with thyroid agenesis and results in hypothyroidism, growth failure, and mental retardation from absence of thyroxine.

21. Thyroid carcinoma is probably caused by exposure to ionizing radiation with the development of nodules and normal thyroxine levels.

Alterations of Parathyroid Function

1. Hyperparathyroidism may be primary or secondary and is characterized by greater than normal secretion of parathyroid hormone (PTH).

2. Primary hyperparathyroidism is caused by an interruption of the normal mechanisms that regulate calcium and PTH levels. Manifestations include chronic hypercalcemia, increased bone resorption, and hypercalciuria.

3. Secondary hyperparathyroidism is a compensatory response to hypocalcemia and often occurs with chronic renal failure.

4. Hypoparathyroidism, defined by abnormally low PTH levels, is caused by thyroid surgery, autoimmunity, or genetic mechanisms.

5. The lack of circulating PTH in hypoparathyroidism causes depressed serum calcium levels, increased serum phosphate levels, decreased bone resorption, and eventual hypocalciuria.

Dysfunction of the Endocrine Pancreas: Diabetes Mellitus

1. Diabetes mellitus is a complex syndrome that causes a number of physiologic changes, some of which are metabolic processes and others of which are vascular.

2. A diagnosis of diabetes mellitus is based on elevated plasma glucose concentrations. Classic signs and symptoms may be present as well.

3. The two most common types of diabetes mellitus are type 1 and type 2.

4. Type 1 diabetes mellitus is characterized by a lack of insulin and a relative excess of glucagon, which causes improper metabolism of fat, protein, and carbohydrates. There is an immune type and a nonimmune type. The immune type is associated with autoantibodies.

5. Type 1 diabetes mellitus is diagnosed most commonly among whites younger than 30 years of age.

6. In type 1 diabetes mellitus, beta cells are destroyed, and islet cell autoantibodies (ICAs and GAD65) appear. The function of these antibodies is unknown, and they tend to disappear with time.

7. Type 1 diabetes mellitus seems to be caused by a gradual process of autoimmune destruction in genetically susceptible individuals.

8. In type 1 diabetes mellitus, lack of insulin and excess glucagon cause hyperglycemia and subsequent loss of glucose in the urine. Polyuria and polydipsia result from osmotic diuresis. Weight loss is a classic symptom of type 1 diabetes.

9. Ketoacidosis is caused by abnormally low levels of insulin and increased levels of glucagon and lipids and is associated with increased levels of glucose and ketones.

10. Type 2 diabetes mellitus is caused by genetic susceptibility that is triggered by environmental factors. The most compelling environmental risk factor is obesity.

11. In the obese, insulin has a diminished ability to influence glucose uptake and metabolism.

12. In type 2 diabetes, amyloid deposits in the islets, fatty atrophy of the pancreas and liver, and vascular sclerosis (causing ischemia) generally are present.

13. Some insulin production continues in type 2 diabetes mellitus, but the weight and number of beta cells decrease.

14. Because the ratio of alpha cells to beta cells may be normal in the individual with type 2 diabetes, hypotheses suggest that the disease is caused by dysfunctional levels of both insulin and glucagon.

15. Acute complications of diabetes mellitus include hypoglycemia, diabetic ketoacidosis, hyperosmolar hyperglycemic nonketotic syndrome, the Somogyi effect, and the dawn phenomenon.

16. Hypoglycemia is a lowered blood glucose level, which may be related to exogenous, endogenous, or functional causes.

17. Symptoms of hypoglycemia are divided into adrenergic, caused by activation of the sympathetic nervous system, and neuroglycopenic, reflecting defective CNS metabolism resulting from impaired energy generation.

18. Diabetic ketoacidosis develops when there is an absolute or relative deficiency of insulin and an increase in the insulin counterregulatory hormones of catecholamines, cortisol, glucagon, growth hormone, and free fatty acids.

19. Hyperosmolar hyperglycemic nonketotic syndrome (HHNKS) is pathophysiologically similar to diabetic ketoacidosis, although levels of free fatty acids are lower in HHNKS and lack of ketosis indicates that some level of insulin is present.

20. The Somogyi effect is a combination of hypoglycemia with rebound hyperglycemia. It is most common in persons with type 1 diabetes mellitus and in children.

21. The dawn phenomenon is an early morning rise in glucose levels caused by nocturnal elevations of growth hormone.

22. Chronic sequelae of diabetes mellitus include diabetic neuropathies, microvascular disease (e.g., retinopathy, nephropathy), macrovascular disease (e.g., coronary artery disease, stroke, peripheral vascular disease), and infection. Metabolic changes contributing to complications include formation of advanced glycosylation end-products, shunting of glucose to the polyol pathway, and activation of protein kinase C.

23. Diabetic neuropathies may be caused by vascular or metabolic mechanisms or a combination of both.

24. In diabetic neuropathy, axonal and Schwann cell degeneration and metabolic aberrations are related to abnormalities in motor nerve conduction velocity, electromyography, and sensory perception.

Continued

SUMMARY REVIEW—cont'd

25. Microangiopathy is caused by thickening of the capillary basement membrane and eventual decreased tissue perfusion, affecting the microcirculation.
26. Diabetic retinopathy is caused in part by retinal ischemia related to microvascular occlusion associated with diabetes mellitus.
27. Diabetic nephropathy is related to glomerular enlargement and glomerular basement membrane thickening, which in turn cause diffuse intercapillary glomerulosclerosis.
28. Macrovascular disease associated with diabetes mellitus probably is related to the proliferation of fibrous plaques in the arterial wall and to elevated lipid levels.
29. Incidence of coronary heart disease, peripheral vascular disease, and stroke is greater in persons with diabetes than in non-diabetic individuals.
30. Individuals with diabetes are at risk for a variety of infections.
31. Infection may be related to sensory impairment and resulting injury, hypoxia, increased proliferation of pathogens in elevated concentrations of glucose, decreased blood supply associated with vascular damage, and impaired white cell function.

Alterations of Adrenal Function

1. Disorders of the adrenal cortex are related to hyperfunction or hypofunction. No known disorders are associated with hypofunction of the adrenal medulla, but medullary hyperfunction causes clinically defined syndromes.
2. Hypercortisolism is divided into ACTH-dependent (Cushing disease or ectopic ACTH syndrome) and ACTH-independent (adrenal adenoma or adenocarcinoma) mechanisms.
3. Cushing disease is most commonly caused by an ACTH-secreting pituitary microadenoma and either ectopic CRH or ACTH production results in a similar clinical syndrome. Cushing syndrome is the result of autonomous cortisol production by adrenal tissue.
4. Individuals with Cushing disease lose diurnal and circadian patterns of ACTH and cortisol secretion, and they lack the ability to increase secretion of these hormones in response to a stressor. Individuals experience weight gain, glucose intolerance, protein wasting, bone disease, hyperpigmentation, and immune suppression.
5. Excessive aldosterone secretion causes hyperaldosteronism, which may be primary or secondary. Primary hyperaldosteronism is caused by an abnormality of the adrenal cortex. Secondary hyperaldosteronism involves an extraadrenal stimulus, driven by the renin-angiotensin system.
6. Primary hyperaldosteronism usually is caused by an adrenal adenoma or bilateral nodular hyperplasia. The condition is characterized by hypertension, hypokalemia, renal potassium wasting, and neuromuscular manifestations.
7. Secondary hyperaldosterone secretion is related to a variety of conditions associated with elevated renin release and activation of angiotensin. These include decreased circulating blood volume and decreased renal blood supply, elevated estrogen levels, Bartter syndrome, and renin-secreting tumors.
8. Hyperaldosteronism promotes increased sodium reabsorption, corresponding hypervolemia, increased extracellular volume (which is variable), and hypokalemia related to renal reabsorption of sodium.
9. Adrenal tumors, either adenomas or carcinomas, can autonomously secrete androgens or estrogens.
10. Hypofunction of the adrenal cortex can affect glucocorticoid or mineralocorticoid secretion or both. Hypofunction can be caused by a deficiency of ACTH or by a primary deficiency in the gland itself.
11. Hypocortisolism (low levels of cortisol) is caused by inadequate adrenal stimulation by ACTH or by primary cortisol hyposecretion. Primary adrenal insufficiency is termed Addison disease.
12. Addison disease is characterized by elevated ACTH levels with inadequate corticosteroid synthesis and output.
13. Causes of Addison disease include idiopathic autoimmune disease, tuberculosis of the adrenal gland, familial adrenal insufficiency, amyloidosis, metastatic destruction of the adrenal glands, and adrenal hemorrhage.
14. Secondary hypercortisolism is characterized by low to absent ACTH levels, leading to inadequate adrenal stimulation, adrenal atrophy, and decreased corticosteroidogenesis. The most common cause is withdrawal of exogenous administration of glucocorticoids.
15. Manifestations of Addison disease are related to hypocortisolism and hypoaldosteronism. Symptoms include weakness, fatigability, hypoglycemia and related metabolic problems, lowered response to stressors, vitiligo, hyperpigmentation, and manifestations of hypovolemia and hyperkalemia.
16. Hyperfunction of the adrenal medulla is caused by a pheochromocytoma, which is a catecholamine-producing tumor. Symptoms of catecholamine excess are related to their sympathetic nervous system effects and include hypertension, palpitations, tachycardia, glucose intolerance, excessive sweating, and constipation.

KEY TERMS

Acromegaly, 690
ACTH deficiency, 688
Addison disease (primary adrenal insufficiency), 725
Advanced glycosylation end-products (AGE), 715
Amylin, 708
Autoimmune thyroiditis (Hashimoto disease, chronic lymphocyte thyroiditis), 695
Cushing disease, 721
Cushing syndrome, 721
Dawn phenomenon, 714
Diabetes insipidus, 686
Diabetes mellitus, 700

Diabetic ketoacidosis (DKA), 711
Diabetic nephropathy, 716
Diabetic neuropathy, 720
Diabetic retinopathy, 716
Dwarfism, 688
Feminization, 726
FSH deficiency, 688
Gestational diabetes mellitus (GDM), 707
GH deficiency, 688
Giantism, 690
Glycosylated hemoglobin, 700
Goiter, 694
Graves disease, 693
Hyperaldosteronism, 723

Hyperosmolar hyperglycemic nonketotic syndrome (HHNKS), 714
Hyperparathyroidism, 698
Hyperpituitarism, 687
Hypocortisolism, 725
Hypoglycemia, 710
Hypoparathyroidism, 699
Hypopituitarism, 687
Hypothyroidism, 694
Idiopathic Addison disease (organ-specific autoimmune adrenalitis), 725
Insulin resistance, 707
LH deficiency, 688

KEY TERMS—cont'd

MEDIA RESOURCES evolve

Review questions and answers for this chapter are available in the *CD Companion* included with this book. Also see the CD for an animation of *type 2 diabetes mellitus.*

WebLinks—links to Internet sites pertaining to this chapter—are available on Evolve at http://evolve.elsevier.com/McCance/.

REFERENCES

1. Fujimoto WY: The importance of insulin resistance in the pathogenesis of type 2 diabetes, *Am J Med* 108(Suppl 16a):9S, 2000.
2. Chrousos GP: A new 'new' syndrome in the world: is multiple postreceptor steroid hormone resistance due to a coregulator defect? *J Clin Endocrinol Metab* 84(12):4450-4453, 1999.
3. Nagaya T, Seo H: Molecular basis of resistance to thyroid hormone (RTH), *Endocr J* 45(6):709-718, 1998.
4. Paracchini R et al: Two new PROP1 gene mutations responsible for compound pituitary hormone deficiency, *Clin Genet* 64(2):142-147, 2003.
5. Salemi S et al: New N-terminal located mutation (Q4ter) within the POU1F1-gene (PIT-1) causes recessive combined pituitary hormone deficiency and variable phenotype, *Growth Horm IGF Res* 13(5):264-268, 2003.
6. Haycock GB: The syndrome of inappropriate secretion of antidiuretic hormone, *Pediatr Nephrol* 9(3):375-381, 1995.
7. Keenan AM: Syndrome of inappropriate secretion of antidiuretic hormone in malignancy, *Semin Oncol Nurs* 15(3):160-167, 1999.
8. Kovacs L, Lichardus B: *Vasopressin: disturbed secretion and its effects,* Boston, 1989, Dordrecht.
9. Labhart A: *Clinical endocrinology: theory and practice,* Berlin, 1986, Springer-Verlag.
10. Riggs AT et al: A review of disorders of water homeostasis in psychiatric patients, *Psychosomatics* 32(2):133-148, 1991.
11. Miller M: Syndromes of excess antidiuretic hormone release, *Crit Care Clin* 17(1):11-23, 2001.
12. Kozniewska E, Podlecka A, Rafalowska J: Hyponatremic encephalopathy—some experimental and clinical findings, *Folia Neuropathol* 41(1):41-45, 2003.
13. Janicic Nm, Verbalis JG: Evaluation and management of hypo-osmolality in hospitalized patients, *Endocrinol Metab Clin North Am* 32(2):459-481, vii, 2003.
14. Blevins LS Jr, Want GS: Diabetes insipidus, *Crit Care Med* 20(1):69-79, 1992.
15. Boughey JC, Yost MJ, Bynoe RP: Diabetes insipidus in the head-injured patient, *Am Surg* 70(6):500-503, 2004.
16. Nguyen MK, Nielsen S, Kurtz I: Molecular pathogenesis of nephrotic diabetes insipidus, *Clin Exp Nephrol* 7(1):9-17, 2003.
17. Goldman L, Bennett JC, editors: *Cecil textbook of medicine,* ed 21, Philadelphia, 2000, Saunders.
18. Verbalis JG: Disorders of body water homeostasis, *Best Pract Res Clin Endocrinol Metab* 17(4):471-503, 2003.
19. Kelestimur F: Sheehan's syndrome, *Pituitary* 6(4):181-188, 2003.

20. Cook DM: Shouldn't adults with growth hormone deficiency be offered growth hormone replacement therapy? *Ann Intern Med* 137(3):197-201, 2002.
21. Laron Z: Laron syndrome (primary growth hormone resistance or insensitivity): the personal experience 1958-2003, *J Clin Endocrinol Metab* 89(3):1031-1044, 2004.
22. Randian R, Nakamoto JM: Rational use of the laboratory for childhood and adult growth hormone deficiency, *Clin Lab Med* 24(1):141-74, 2004.
23. Harman SM, Blackman MR.: Use of growth hormone for prevention or treatment of effects of aging, *J Gerontol A Biol Sci Med Sci* 59(7):652-658, 2004.
24. Rosenfeld RG: Growth hormone deficiency in children. In Melmed S, editor: *Endocrinology,* ed 4, Philadelphia, 2001, Saunders.
25. Sheppard MC: Growth hormone—from molecule to mortality, *Clin Med* 4(5):437-440, 2004.
26. Rosen T, Bengtsson BA: Premature mortality due to cardiovascular disease in hypopituitarism, *Lancet* 336(8710):285-288, 1990.
27. Ezzat S et al: The prevalence of pituitary adenomas: a systemic review, *Cancer* 101(3):613-619, 2004.
28. Aron DC, Howlett TA: Pituitary incidentalomas, *Endocrinol Metab Clin North Am* 29(1):205-221, 2000.
29. Aron DC, Tyrrell JB, Wilson CB: Pituitary tumors: current concepts in diagnosis and management, *West J Med* 162(4):340-352, 1995.
29a. Kaltsas GA et al: Diagnosis and management of pituitary carcinomas, *Clin Endocrinol Metab* Mar 1, 2005. [Epub ahead of print]
30. Di Sarno A et al: An evaluation of patients with hyperprolactinemia: have dynamic tests had their day? *J Endocrinol Invest* 26(7 Suppl):39-47, 2003
31. Hurley DM, Ho KK: MJA practice essentials—endocrinology. 9: Pituitary disease in adults, *Med J Aust* 180(8):419-25, 2004.
32. Melmed S: Acromegaly, *N Engl J Med* 322(14):966-977, 1990.
33. Ben-Shlomo A, Melmed S: Acromegaly, *Endocrinol Metab Clin North Am* 30(3):565-583, vi, 2001.
34. Terzolo M et al: Colonoscopic screening and follow-up in patients with acromegaly: a multicenter study in Italy, *J Clin Endocrinol Metab* 90(1):84-90, 2005; Epub Oct 26, 2004.
35. Colao A et al: Systemic complications of acromegaly: epidemiology, pathogenesis, and management, *Endocr Rev* 25(1):102-152, 2004.
36. Holdaway IM, Rajasoorya RC, Gamble GD: Factors influencing mortality in acromegaly, *J Clin Endocrinol Metab* 89(2):667-674, 2004
37. Sacca L, Napoli R, Cittadini A: Growth hormone, acromegaly, and heart failure: an intricate triangulation, *Clin Endocrinol* 59(6):660-671, 2003.
38. Hennessey JV, Jackson IM: Clinical features and differential diagnosis of pituitary tumors with emphasis on acromegaly, *Baillieres Clin Endocrinol Metab* 9(2):271-314, 1995.
39. Hofland LJ et al: The novel somatostatin analog SOM230 is a potent inhibitor of hormone release by growth hormone- and prolactin-secreting pituitary adenomas in vitro, *J Clin Endocrinol Metab* 89(4):1577-1585, 2004.
40. Teramoto A et al: Pathological study of thyrotropin-secreting pituitary adenoma: plurihormonality and medical treatment, *Acta Neuropathol (Berl)* 108(2):147-153, 2004.

41. Wass JA: Dynamic testing in the diagnosis and follow-up of patients with acromegaly, *J Endocrinol Invest* 26(7 Suppl):48-53, 2003.

42. Freda PU: How effective are current therapies for acromegaly? *Growth Horm IGF Res* 132(Suppl A):S144-S151, 2003.

43. Stewart PM: Pegvisomant: an advance in clinical efficacy in acromegaly, *Eur J Endocrinol* 148(Suppl 2):S27-S32, 2003.

44. Xu RK et al: Pituitary prolactin-secreting tumor formation: recent developments, *Biol Signals Recept* 9(1):1-20, 2000.

45. De Rosa et al: Hyperprolactinemia in men: clinical and biochemical features and response to treatment, *Endocrine* 20(1-2):75-82, 2003.

46. Luciano AA: Clinical presentation of hyperprolactinemia, *J Reprod Med* 44(12 suppl):1085-1090, 1999.

47. Davis JR: Prolactin and reproductive medicine, *Curr Opin Obstet Gynecol* 16(4):331-337, 2004.

48. Roberts CG, Ladenson PW: Hypothyroidism, *Lancet* 363(9422): 793-803, 2004.

49. Prummel MF, Strieder T, Wiersinga WM: The environment and autoimmune thyroid diseases, *Eur J Endocrinol* 150(5):605-618, 2004.

50. McDougall IR: Graves disease: current concepts, *Med Clin North Am* 75(1):79-95, 1991.

51. Tonacchera M et al: Patient with monoclonal gammopathy, thyrotoxicosis, pretibial myxedema, and thyroid-associated ophthalmopathy; demonstration of direct binding of autoantibodies in the thyrotropin receptor, *Eur J Endocrinol* 134(1):97-103, 1996.

52. Prabhakar BS, Bahn RS, Smith TJ: Current perspective on the pathogenesis of Graves' disease and ophthalmopathy, *Endocr Rev* 24(6):802-835, 2003.

53. Weetman AP: Grave's disease 1935-2002, *Horm Res* 59(Suppl 1): 114-118, 2003.

54. Bahn RS: Understanding the immunology of Graves ophthalmopathy: is it an autoimmune disease? *Endocrinol Metab Clin North Am* 29(2):287-296, 2000.

55. Braverman LE, Utiger RD: *Werner and Ingbar's The thyroid: a fundamental and clinical text,* ed 8, Philadelphia, 2000, Lippincott Williams & Wilkins.

56. Corvilain B: The natural history of thyroid autonomy and hot nodules, *Ann Endocrinol (Paris)* 64(1):17-22, 2003.

57. Gavin LA: Thyroid crises, *Med Clin North Am* 75(1):179-193, 1991.

58. Smallridge RC: Metabolic and anatomic thyroid emergencies: a review, *Crit Care Med* 20(2):276-291, 1992.

59. Langely RW, Burch HB: Perioperative management of the thyrotoxic patient, *Endocrinol Metab Clin North Am* 32(2):519-354, 2003.

60. Schubert MF, Kountz DS: Thyroiditis: a disease of many faces, *Postgrad Med* 98(2):101-103, 107-108, 1995.

61. Barbesino G, Chiovato L: The genetics of Hashimoto's disease, *Endocrinol Metab Clin North Am* 29(2):357-374, 2000.

62. Ciampolillo A et al: Modifications of the immune responsiveness in patients with autoimmune thyroiditis: evidence for a systemic immune alterations, *Curr Pharm Des* 9(24):1946-1950, 2003.

63. Wall CR: Myxedema coma: diagnosis and treatment, *Am Fam Physician* 62(11):2485-2490, 2000.

64. Ayala AR, Danese MD, Ladenson PW: When to treat mild hypothyroidism, *Endocrinol Metab Clin North Am* 29(12):399-415, 2000.

65. DeGroot LJ: *Endocrinology,* ed 4, Philadelphia, 2001, Saunders.

66. Gruters A, Biebermann H, Krude H: Neonatal thyroid disorders, *Horm Res* 59(Suppl 1):24-29, 2003.

67. American Cancer Society: Estimated new cancer cases and deaths by sex for all sites, US, 2005. Available at www.cancer.org/docroot/MED/content/downloads/MED_1_1x_CFF2005_Estimated_New_Cases_Deaths_by_Sex_US.asp.

68. Mizuno T et al: Preferential induction of RET/PTC1 rearrangement by x-ray irradiation, *Oncogene* 19(3):438-443, 2000.

69. Farahati T et al: Inverse association between the age at the time of radiation exposure and extent of disease in cases of radiation-induced childhood thyroid carcinoma in Belarus, *Cancer* 88(6):1470-1476, 2000.

70. Pasieka JL: Anaplastic thyroid cancer, *Curr Opin Oncol* 15(1):78-83, 2003.

71. Bringhurst ER, Demay MB, Kronenberg HM: Hormones and disorders of mineral metabolism. In Larsen RP et al, editors: *William's textbook of endocrinology,* ed 10, Philadelphia, 2003, Saunders.

72. Dwarakanathan AA et al: Isolated familial hyperparathyroidism with a novel mutation of the MEN1 gene, *Endocr Pract* 6(3):268-270, 2000.

73. Carling T: Molecular pathology of parathyroid tumors, *Trends Endocrinol Metab* 12(2):53-58, 2001.

74. Walgenbach S, Hommel G, Junginger T: Outcome after surgery for primary hyperparathyroidism: ten year prospective follow-up study, *World J Surg* 24(5):564-569, 2000.

75. Pallotti F et al: Diagnostic and therapeutic aspects of iatrogenic hypoparathyroidism, *Tumori* 89(5):547-549, 2003.

76. Rosenbloom AL et al: Autosomal dominant pseudohypoparathyroidism type Ib is associated with a heterozygous microdeletion that likely disrupts a putative imprinting control element of GNAS, *J Clin Invest* 112(8):1255-1263, 2003.

77. DeFronzo RA: Pathogenesis of type 2 diabetes mellitus, *Med Clin North Am* 88(4):787-835, ix, 2004.

77a. Rewers M, Norris J, Dabelea D: Epidemiology of type 1 diabetes mellitus, *Adv Exp Med Biol* 552:219-246, 2004.

77b. Korc M.: Update on diabetes mellitus, *Dis Markers* 20(3):161-165, 2004.

78. American Diabetes Association: Diagnosis and classification of diabetes mellitus, *Diabetes Care* 27:S5-S10, 2004.

79. The DECODE Study Group, European Diabetes Epidemiology Group, Diabetes Epidemiology Collaborative Analysis of Diagnostic Criteria in Europe: Glucose tolerance and mortality: comparison of WHO and American Diabetes Association diagnostic criteria, *Lancet* 354(9179):617-621, 1999.

80. The Expert Committee on the Diagnosis and Classification of Diabetes Mellitus: Follow-up report on the diagnosis of diabetes mellitus, *Diabetic Care* 26(11):3160-3167, 2003.

81. Mitrakou A et al: Role of reduced suppression of glucose production and diminished early insulin release in impaired glucose tolerance, *N Engl J Med* 326(1):22-29, 1992.

82. Anand SS et al: Diagnostic strategies to detect glucose involerance in a multiethnic population, *Diabetes Care* 26(2):290-296, 2003.

83. Woerle HJ et al: Diagnostic and therapeutic implications of relationships between fasting, 2-hour postchallenge plasma glucose and hemoglobin a1c values, *Arch Intern Med* 164(15):1627-1632, 2004.

84. National Center for Chronic Disease Prevention and Health Promotion: *National diabetes fact sheet: national estimates on diabetes, 2002.* Available at www.cdc.gov/diabetes/pubs/estimates.htm.

85. Falorni A, Brozzetti A.: Diabetes-related antibodies in adult diabetic patients, *Best Pract Res Clin Endocrinol Metab* 19(1):119-133, 2005.

86. Achenbach P, Ziegler AG: Diabetes-related antibodies in euglycemic subjects, *Best Pract Res Clin Endocrinol Metab* 19(1):101-117, 2005.

87. Imagawa A et al: A novel subtype of type 1 diabetes mellitus characterized by a rapid onset and an absence of diabetes-related antibodies, *N Engl J Med* 342(5):301-307, 2000.

88. Huang W et al: Although DR3-DQB1*0201 may be associated with multiple component diseases of the autoimmune polyglandular syndromes, the human leukocyte antigen DR4-DQB1*0302 haplotype is implicated only in beta-cell autoimmunity, *J Clin Endocrinol Metab* 81(7):2559-2563, 1996.

89. Roep BO et al: HLA-associated inverse correlation between T cell and antibody responsiveness to islet autoantigen in recent-onset insulin-dependent diabetes mellitus, *Eur J Immunol* 26(6):1285-1289, 1996.

90. Panagiotopoulos C, Trudeau JD, Tan R: T-cell epitopes in type 1 diabetes, *Curr Diab Rep* 4(2):87-94, 2004.

91. Fridlyand LE, Philipson LH: Does the glucose-dependent insulin secretion mechanism itself cause oxidative stress in pancreatic beta-cells? *Diabetes* 53(8):1942-1948, 2004.

92. Roep BO: The role of T-cells in the pathogenesis of type 1 diabetes: from cause to cure, *Diabetologia* 46(3):305-321, 2003.

93. Sakai K et al: Mitochondrial reactive oxygen species reduce insulin secretion by pancreatic beta-cells, *Biochem Biophys Res Commun* 300(1):216-222, 2003.

94. Santiago J et al, editors: *Medical management of insulin-dependent (type I) diabetes,* ed 2, Alexandria, Va, 1994, American Diabetes Association.

95. Diabetes Control and Complications Trial Research Group: The effect of intensive treatment of diabetes on the development and progression of long-term complications in insulin-dependent diabetes mellitus, *N Engl J Med* 329(14):977-986, 1993.

96. National Center for Chronic Disease Prevention and Health Promotion: *Epidemiology of type 1 and type 2 diabetes mellitus among North American children and adolescents;* retrieved January 18, 2005. Available at www.cdc.gov/diabetes/projects/cda2.htm.

97. Aye T, Levitsky LL: Type 2 diabetes: an epidemic disease in childhood, *Curr Opin Pediatr* 15(4):411-415, 2003.

98. Reusch JE: Current concepts in insulin resistance, type 2 diabetes mellitus, and the metabolic syndrome, *Am J Cardiol* 90(5A):19G-26G, 2002.

99. Bellanne-Chantelot C et al: Clinical spectrum associated with hepatocyte nuclear factor 1-beta mutations. *Ann Intern Med* 140(7):510-517, 2004.

100. American Diabetes Association: Gestational diabetes mellitus, *Diabetes Care* 412(Suppl 1):288-290, 2004.

101. Patti ME: Gene expression in the pathophysiology of type 2 diabetes mellitus, *Curr Diab Rep* 4(3):176-181, 2004.

101a. Porter JR, Barrett TG: Monogenic syndromes of abnormal glucose homeostasis: clinical review and relevance to the understanding of the pathology of insulin resistance and (beta) cell failure, *J Med Genet*, Mar 16, 2005. (Epub ahead of print).

102. Larsson H, Ahren B: Islet cell dysfunction in insulin resistance involves impaired insulin secretion and increased glucagon secretion in postmenopausal women with impaired glucose tolerance, *Diabetes Care* 23(5):650-657, 2000.

103. Raskin P et al, editors: *Medical management of noninsulin-dependent (type II) diabetes,* ed 3, Alexandria, Va, 1994, American Diabetes Association.

104. Hull RL et al: Islet amyloid: a critical entity in the pathogenesis of type 2 diabetes, *J Clin Endocrinol Metab* 89(8):3629-3643, 2004.

105. Clark A et al: Autoantibodies to islet amyloid polypeptide in diabetes, *Diabetic Med* 8(7):668-673, 1991.

106. Weyer C et al: Amylin replacement with pramlintide as an adjunct to insulin therapy in type 1 and type 2 diabetes mellitus: a physiological approach toward improved metabolic control, *Curr Pharm Des* 7(14):1353-1373, 2001.

107. Bellentani S et al: Prevalence of and risk factors for hepatic steatosis in Northern Italy, *Ann Int Med* 132(2):112-117, 2000.

108. World Health Organization (WHO) Study Group: Diabetes mellitus report of a WHO study group, *Tech Rep Series* 727:1, 1985.

109. Cefalu WT: Insulin resistance. In Leahy JL, Clark NG, Cefalu WT, editors: *Medical management of diabetes mellitus,* New York, 2000, Marcel Dekker.

110. Goldstein BJ: Insulin resistance as the core defect in type 2 diabetes mellitus, *Am J Cardiol* 90(5):3G-10G, 2002.

111. Hsueh WA, Law RE: Insulin signaling in the arterial wall, *Am J Cardiol* 84(1A):21J-24J, 1999.

112. Dunaif A: Insulin action in the polycystic ovary syndrome, *Endocrinol Metab Clin North Am* 28(2):341-359, 1999.

113. Harris MI: Epidemiologic studies on the pathogenesis of noninsulin-dependent diabetes mellitus (NIDDM), *Clin Invest Med* 18(4):231-239, 1995.

114. DeFronzo RA, Goodman AM, The Multicenter Metformin Study Group: Efficacy of metformin in patients with non-insulin-dependent diabetes mellitus, *N Engl J Med* 333(9):541-549, 1995.

115. Komers R, Vrana A: Thiazolidinediones—tools for the research of metabolic syndrome X, *Physiol Res* 47(4):215-225, 1998.

116. DeFronzo RA: Pharmacologic therapy for type 2 diabetes mellitus, *Ann Intern Med* 131(4):281-303, 1999.

117. Sheaves R et al: *Clinical endocrine oncology,* Oxford, 1997, Blackwell.

118. Manson JE et al: A prospective study of exercise and incidence of diabetes among US male physicians, *JAMA* 268(1):63-67, 1992.

119. Diabetes Prevention Research Group: Reduction in the incidence of type 2 diabetes with lifestyle intervention or metformin, *N Engl J Med* 346(6):393-403, 2002.

120. Murata GH et al: Hypoglycemia in type 2 diabetes: a critical review, *Biomed Pharmacother* 58(10):551-559, 2004.

121. Dagogo-Jack S: Hypoglycemia in type 1 diabetes mellitus: pathophysiology and prevention, *Treat Endocrinol* 3(2):91-103, 2004.

122. Newton CA, Raskin P: Diabetic ketoacidosis in type 1 and type 2 diabetes mellitus: clinical and biochemical differences, *Arch Intern Med* 164(17):1925-1931, 2004.

123. Skinner TC: Recurrent diabetic ketoacidosis: causes, prevention and management, *Horm Res* 57(Suppl 1):78-80, 2002.

124. Carlotti AP, Bohn D, Halperin ML: Importance of timing of risk factors for cerebral edema during therapy for diabetic ketoacidosis, *Arch Dis Child* 88(2):170-173, 2003.

125. Levitsky LL et al: ESPEL/WPES consensus statement on diabetic ketoacidosis in children and adolescents, *Arch Dis Child* 89(2):188-194, 2004.

126. Magee MF, Bhatt BA: Management of decompensated diabetes. Diabetic ketoacidosis and hyperglycemic hyperosmolar syndrome, *Crit Care Clin* 17(1):75-106, 2001

127. Gaglia JL, Wyckoff J, Abrahamson MJ: Acute hyperglycemic crisis in the elderly, *Med Clin* 88(4):1063-1084, xii, 2004.

128. Jerums G et al: Evolving concepts in advanced glycation, diabetic nephropathy, and diabetic vascular disease, *Arch Biochem Biophys* 419(1):55-62, 2003.

129. Li JH et al: Advanced glycation end products activate Smad signaling via TGF-beta-dependent and independent mechanisms: implications for diabetic renal and vascular disease, *FASEB J* 18(1):176-178, 2003.

130. Vlassara H, Palace MR: Diabetes and advanced glycation endproducts, *J Intern Med* 251(2):87-101, 2002.

131. Okamoto H et al: Effects of epalrestat, an aldose reductase inhibitor, on diabetic neuropathy and gastroparesis, *Intern Med* 42(8):655-664, 2003.

132. Petrash JM: All in the family: aldose reductase and closely related aldo-keto reductase, *Cell Mol Life Sci* 61(7-8):737-749, 2004.

133. Schmitz-Peiffer C: Protein kinase C and lipid-induced insulin resistance in skeletal muscle, *Ann N Y Acad Sci* 967:146-157, 2002.

134. Dang L, Seale JP, Qu X: Reduction of high glucose and phorbol-myristate-acetate-induced endothelial cell permeability by protein kinase C inhibitors LY379196 and hypocrellin A, *Biochem Pharmacol* 67(5):855-864, 2004.

135. Tuttle KR, Anderson PW: A novel potential therapy for diabetic neuropathy and vascular complications: protein kinase C beta inhibition, *Am J Kidney Dis* 42(3):456-465, 2003.

136. Colucciello M: Diabetic retinopathy: control of systemic factors preserves vision, *Postgrad Med* 116(1):57-64, 2004.

137. Grassi G: Diabetic retinopathy, *Minerva Med* 94(6):419-435, 2003.

138. Khan ZA, Chakrabarti S: Growth factors in proliferative diabetic retinopathy, *Exp Diabesity Res* 4(4):287-301, 2003.

139. Lewis EJ, Lewis JB: Treatment of diabetic nephropathy with angiotensin II receptor antagonist, *Clin Exp Nephrol* 7(1):1-8, 2003.

140. Hsu CY et al: Diabetes, hemoglobin A(1c), cholesterol, and the risk of moderate chronic renal insufficiency in an ambulatory population, *Am J Kidney Dis* 36(2):272-281, 2000.

141. Odoni G, Ritz E: Diabetic nephropathy—what have we learned in the last three decades? *J Nephrol* 12(suppl 2):S120-S124, 1999.

142. Prabhakar SS: Role of nitric oxide in diabetic nephropathy, *Semin Nephrol* 24(4):333-344, 2004.

143. Rossert J, Terraz-Durasnel C, Brideau G: Growth factors, cytokines, and renal fibrosis during the course of diabetic nephropathy, *Diabetes Metab* 26(suppl 4):16-24, 2000.

144. Harris RD et al: Global glomerular sclerosis and glomerular arteriolar hyalinosis in insulin dependent diabetes, *Kidney Int* 40(1):107-114, 1991.

145. Battisti WP, Palmisano J, Keane WE: Dyslipidemia in patients with type 2 diabetes. Relationships between lipids, kidney disease and cardiovascular disease, *Clin Chem Lab Med* 41(9):1174-1181, 2003.

146. Steffes MW, Mauer SM: Diabetic nephropathy: a disease causing and complicated by hypertension, *Clin Chem* 37(10 Pt 2):1838-1842, 1991.

147. Sonkodi S, Mogyorosi A: Treatment of diabetic nephropathy with angiotensin II blockers, *Nephrol Dial Transplant* 18(Suppl 5):v21-23, 2003.

148. Chiarelli F, Mohn A: Angiopathy in children with diabetes, *Minerva Pediatr* 54(3):187-201, 2002.

149. Ghosh J et al: Diabetes mellitus and coronary artery disease: therapeutic considerations, *Heart Dis* 5(2):119-128, 2003.

150. Sowers JR: Insulin resistance and hypertension, *Am J Physiol Heart Circ Physiol* 286(5):H1597-H1602, 2004.

151. Winer N, Sowers JR: Vascular compliance in diabetes, *Curr Diab Rep* 3(3):230-234, 2003.

152. Schoenhagen P, Nissen SE: Coronary atherosclerosis in diabetic subjects: clinical significance, anatomic characteristics, and identification with in vivo imaging, *Cardiol Clin* 22(4):527-540, vi, 2004.

153. Kanaya AM, Grady D, Barrett-Connor E: Explaining the sex difference in cornary heart disease mortality among patients with type 2 diabetes mellitus: a meta-analysis, *Arch Intern Med* 162(15):1737-1745, 2002.

154. Vinik A, Flemmer M: Diabetes and macrovascular disease, *J Diabetes Complications* 16(3):235-245, 2002.

155. Bell DS: Stroke in the diabetic patient, *Diabetes Care* 17(3):213-219, 1994.

156. Levetan CS: Effect of hyperglycemia on stroke outcomes, *Endocr Pract* 10(Suppl 2):34-39, 2004.

157. Mankovsky BN, Ziegler D: Stroke in patients with diabetes mellitus, *Diabetes Metab Res Rev* 20(4):268-287, 2004.

158. Gazis A et al: Mortality in patients with diabetic neuropathic osteoarthropathy (Charcot foot), *Diabetes Med* 21(11):1243-1246, 2004.

159. Al-Delaimy WK et al: Effect of type 2 diabetes and its duration on the risk of peripheral arterial disease among men, *Am J Med* 116(4):236-240, 2004.

160. Bowering CK: Diabetic foot ulcers: pathophysiology, assessment, and therapy, *Can Fam Physician* 47:1107-1116, 2001.

161. Vinik AI, Mehrabyan A: Diabetic neuropathies, *Med Clin North Am* 88(4):947-999, xi, 2004.

162. Cameron NE et al: Vascular factors and metabolic interactions in the pathogenesis of diabetic neuropathy, *Diabetologia* 44(11):1973-1988, 2001.

163. Ohkabo Y et al: Intensive insulin therapy prevents the progression of diabetes microvascular complications in Japanese patients with non-insulin–dependent diabetes mellitus: a randomized, prospective 6-year study, *Diabetes Res Clin Pract* 28(2):103-117, 1995.

164. Jude EB, Unsworth PF: Optimal treatment of infected diabetic foot ulcers: *Drugs Aging* 21(13):833-850, 2004.

165. Piazza O et al: Candidemia in intensive care patients: risk factors and mortality, *Minerva Anestesiol* 70(1-2):63-69, 2004.

165a. Furnary AP et al: Continuous intravenous insulin infusion reduces the incidence of deep sternal wound infection in diabetic patients after cardiac surgical procedures, *Ann Thorac Surg* 67(2):352-362, 1999.

166. Bolland MJ et al: Cushing's syndrome due to interaction between inhaled corticosteroids and itraconazole, *Ann Pharmacother* 38(1):46-49, 2004.

167. Sippel RS, Chen H: Subclinical Cushing's syndrome in adrenal incidentalomas, *Surg Clin North Am* 84(3):875-885, 2004.

168. Hentschel SJ, McCutcheon IE: Stereotactic radiosurgery for Cushing disease, *Neurosurg Focus* 16(4):E5, 2004.

169. Barzon L et al: Prevalence and natural history of adrenal incidentalomas, *Eur J Endocrinol* 149(4):273-285, 2003.

170. Schuff KG: Issues in the diagnosis of Cushing's syndrome for the primary care physician, *Prim Care* 30(4):791-799, 2003.

171. Newell-Price J: Proopiomelanocortin gene expression and DNA methylation: implications for Cushing's syndrome and beyond, *Endocrinol* 177(3):365-372, 2003

172. Findling JW, Raff H: Diagnosis and differential diagnosis of Cushing's syndrome, *Endocrinol Metab Clin North Am* 30(3):729-747, 2001.

173. Sonimo N, Fava GA: Psychiatric disorders associated with Cushing's syndrome. Epidemiology, pathophysiology, and treatment, *CNS Drugs* 15(5):361-373, 2001.

174. Davies JS et al: Diagnostic dilemmas in Cushing's syndrome, *Ann Clin Biochem* 37(Pt1):85-89, 2000.

175. Young WF Jr: Minireview: primary aldosteronism—changing concepts in diagnosis and treatment, *Endocrinology* 144(6):2208-2213, 2003.

176. Herbert SC: Bartter syndrome, *Curr Opin Nephrol Hypertens* 12(4):527-532, 2003.

177. Moneva MH, Gomez-Sanchez CE: Pathophysiology of adrenal hypertension, *Semin Nephrol* 22(1):44-53, 2002.

178. Mulatero P et al: Increased diagnosis of primary aldosteronism, including surgically correctable forms, in centers fro five continents, *J Clin Endocrinol Metab* 89(3):1045-1050, 2004.

179. Seiler L et al: Diagnosis of primary aldosteronism: value of different screening parameters and influence of antihypertensive medication, *Eur J Endocrinol* 150(3):329-337, 2004.

180. Magni P, Motta M: Aldosterone receptor antagonists: biology and novel therapeutical applications, *J Endocrinol Invest* 26(8):788-798, 2003.

181. Stowasser M, Gordon RD: Primary aldosteronism, *Best Pract Res Clin Endocrinol Metab* 17(4):591-605, 2003.

182. Falorni A et al: Italian Addison network study: update of diagnostic criteria for the etiological classification of primary adrenal insufficiency, *J Clin Endocrinol Metab* 89(4):1598-604, 2004.

183. Larsen RP et al: *Williams textbook of endocrinology,* ed 10, Philadelphia, 2003, Saunders.

184. Lovas K, Husebye ES: Replacement therapy in Addison's disease, *Expert Opin Pharmacother* 4(12):2145-2149, 2003.

185. Opocher G et al: Clinical and genetic aspects of phaeochromocytoma, *Horm Res* 59(Suppl 1):59-61, 2003.

186. Bravo EKL: Pheochromocytoma, *Cardiol Rev* 10(1):44-50, 2002.

187. Veglio F et al: Recent advances in diagnosis and treatment of pheochromocytoma, *Minerva Med* 94(4):267-271, 2003.

STRUCTURE AND FUNCTION OF THE REPRODUCTIVE SYSTEMS

ANGELA DENERIS • SUE E. HUETHER

evolve

http://evolve.elsevier.com/McCance/

CHAPTER OUTLINE

The male and female reproductive systems have several anatomic and physiologic features in common. Most obvious is their major function, reproduction, through which a 23-chromosome female gamete, the **ovum,** and a 23-chromosome male gamete, the **spermatozoon (sperm cell),** unite to form a 46-chromosome zygote that is capable of developing into a new individual. The male reproductive system produces sperm and delivers them to the female reproductive tract. The female reproductive system produces the ovum and, if it is fertilized, can nurture and protect it (at that point called the *embryo* and *developing fetus*) and expel it at birth. These functions are determined not only by anatomic structures but also by complex hormonal, neurologic, and psychogenic factors.[1]

DEVELOPMENT OF THE REPRODUCTIVE SYSTEMS

The structure and function of both male and female reproductive systems depend on steroid hormones called **sex hormones.** Hormonal effects on the reproductive systems begin well before birth and continue for life.

Sexual Differentiation in Utero

During embryonic development, the initial reproductive structures of male and female embryos are homologous (the same) and consist of one pair of primary sex organs, or **gonads,** and two pairs of ducts, the mesonephric ducts (wolffian ducts) and the paramesonephric ducts (müllerian ducts) (Figure 22-1). Both pairs of ducts empty into an opening called the *urogenital sinus.*

At about 7 to 8 weeks of gestation, the gonads of genetically male embryos produce testosterone. Under the influence of testosterone, the male gonads develop into two testes, which produce sperm after puberty. The paramesonephric ducts degenerate and the mesonephric ducts develop into the vas deferens—the two tubes that carry sperm from the testes to the urethra.

In female embryos the gonads produce the primary female sex hormone, estrogen. In the absence of testosterone the two gonads develop into ovaries, which produce ova. In females the mesonephric ducts deteriorate and the lower ends of the paramesonephric ducts join to become the uterus. The upper portions of the paramesonephric ducts develop into the fallopian (uterine) tubes. These two ducts carry ova from the ovaries to the uterus.

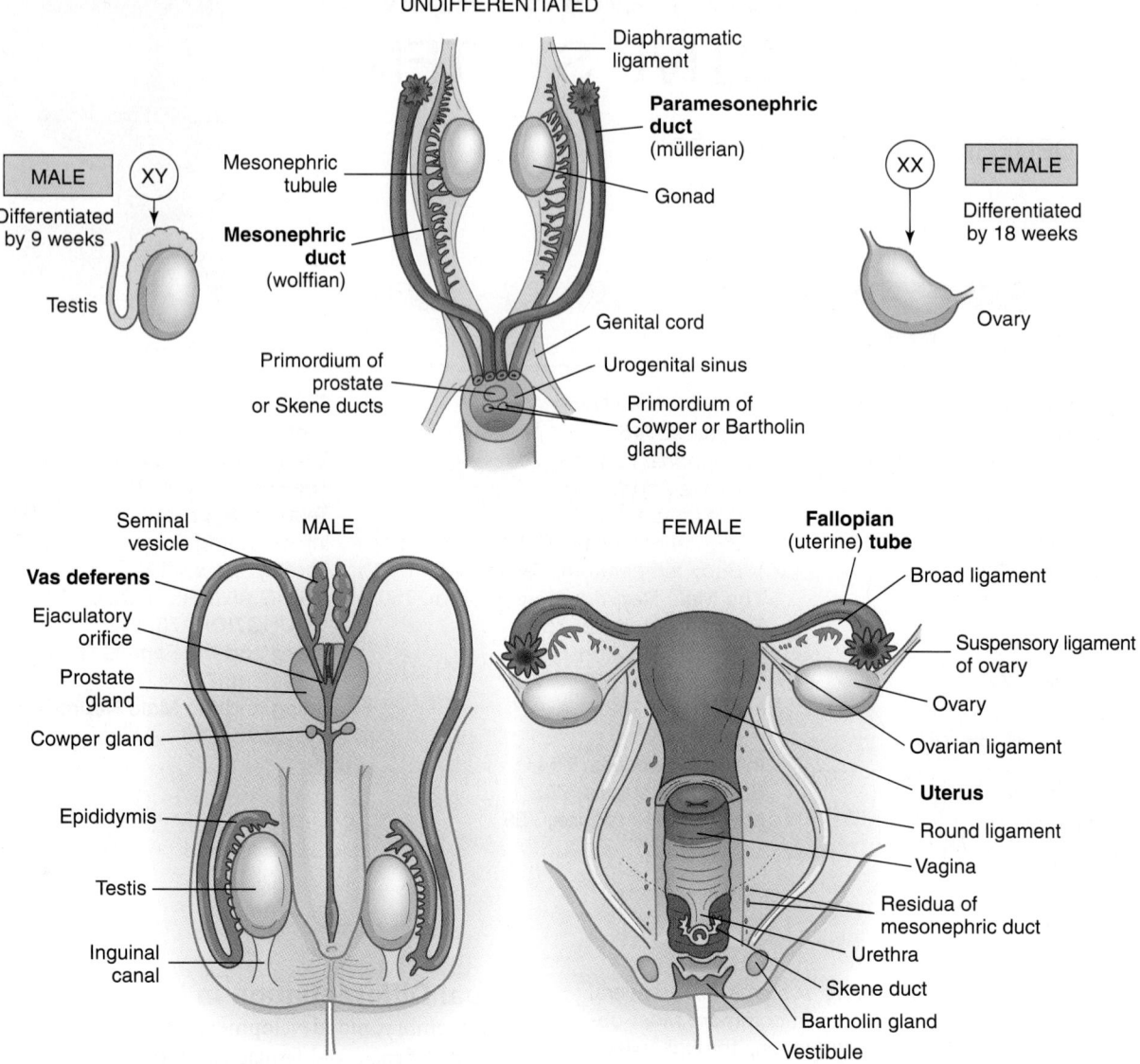

UNDIFFERENTIATED

Diaphragmatic
ligament

**Paramesonephric
duct**
(müllerian)

MALE · XY
Differentiated
by 9 weeks

Mesonephric
tubule

Gonad

**Mesonephric
duct**
(wolffian)

Testis

XX · FEMALE
Differentiated
by 18 weeks

Ovary

Primordium of
prostate
or Skene ducts

Genital cord

Urogenital sinus

Primordium of
Cowper or Bartholin
glands

Seminal
vesicle

MALE

Vas deferens

Ejaculatory
orifice

Prostate
gland

Cowper gland

Epididymis

Testis

Inguinal
canal

FEMALE

Fallopian
(uterine) **tube**

Broad ligament

Suspensory ligament
of ovary

Ovary

Ovarian ligament

Uterus

Round ligament

Vagina

Residua of
mesonephric duct

Urethra

Skene duct

Bartholin gland

Vestibule

Figure 22-1 **Internal genitalia development.** Embryonic and fetal development of the internal genitalia.

Like the internal reproductive structures, the external structures develop from homologous embryonic tissues. During the first 7 to 8 weeks of gestation, both male and female embryos develop an elevated structure called the *genital tubercle*. Figure 22-2 shows how the undifferentiated genital tubercle develops into the external reproductive organs.

Anterior pituitary development starts between the 4th and 5th weeks of fetal life and the vascular connection between the hypothalamus and the pituitary is established by the 12th week. In the female fetus, high levels of two gonadotropins, **follicle-stimulating hormone (FSH)** and **luteinizing hormone (LH)** are excreted by the anterior pituitary. **Gonadotropin-releasing hormone (GnRH)** is produced in the hypothalamus by 10 weeks gestation; this controls the production of the gonadotropins LS and FSH.[1] This cycle is referred to as the *hypothalamic-pituitary axis (HPA)* and stimulates the production of estrogen and progesterone

by the ovary. The production of FSH and LH rise until midgestation, until the production of estrogen and progesterone by the ovaries and placenta is high enough to result in the decline of gonadotropin production.

Testosterone, which is converted to estrogen in the brain,[2] is necessary for the genital tubercle to differentiate into external male genitalia. By 9 months of gestation the internal and external genital structures are all present and the male gonads (the testes) have descended into the scrotum. Although male differentiation is dependent on testicular hormones and their metabolites, female differentiation occurs in the absence of testosterone; it may even occur in the absence of ovaries,[3] possibly as a result of the presence of placental estrogens.

At term, a sensitive negative-feedback system, which includes the **gonadostat** (also known as the *gonadotropin-releasing hormone pulse generator*), is operative in the human fetus. The gonadostat responds to high placental estrogens by

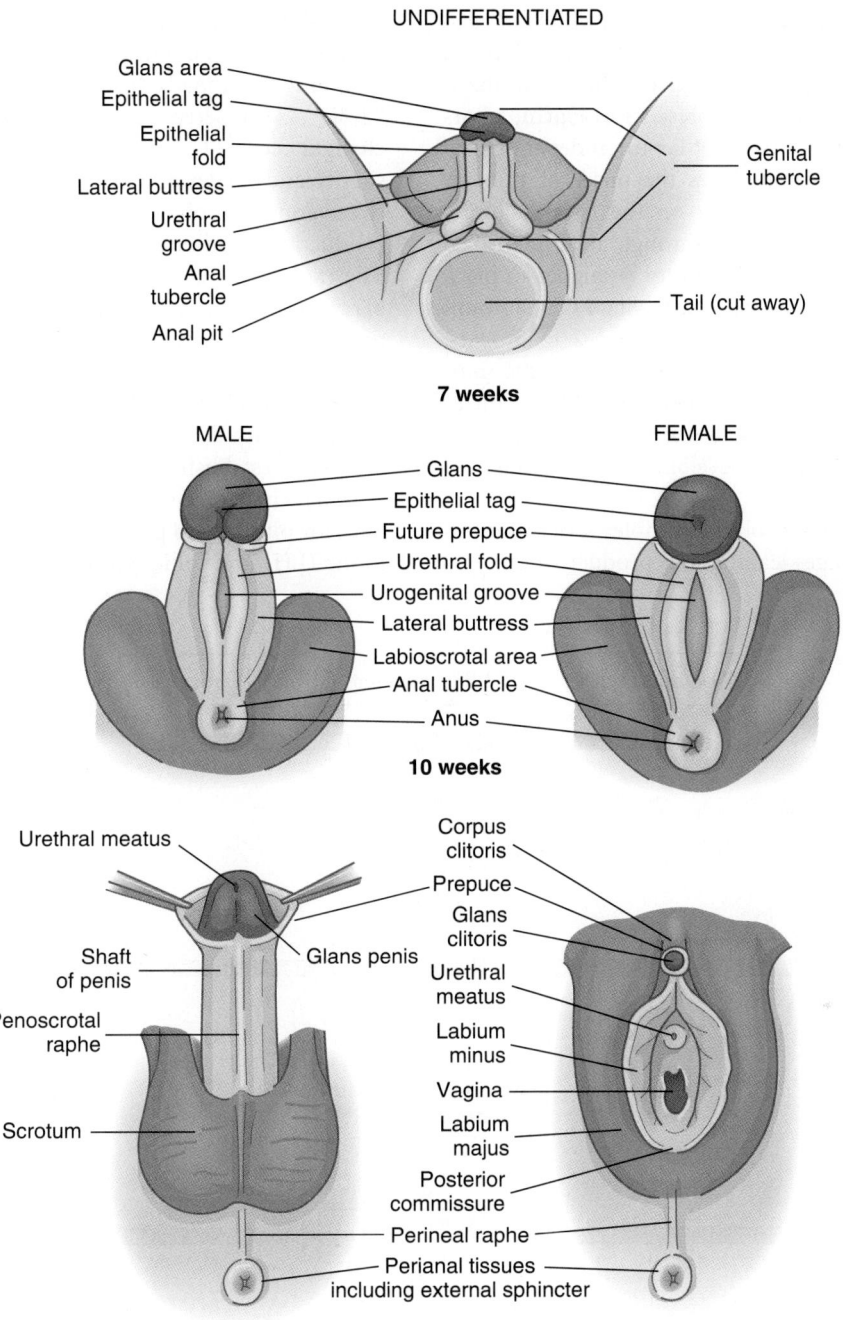

UNDIFFERENTIATED

Glans area
Epithelial tag
Epithelial fold
Lateral buttress
Urethral groove
Anal tubercle
Anal pit

Genital tubercle

Tail (cut away)

7 weeks

MALE

FEMALE

Glans
Epithelial tag
Future prepuce
Urethral fold
Urogenital groove
Lateral buttress
Labioscrotal area
Anal tubercle
Anus

10 weeks

Urethral meatus

Shaft of penis

Glans penis

Penoscrotal raphe

Scrotum

Corpus clitoris
Prepuce
Glans clitoris
Urethral meatus
Labium minus
Vagina
Labium majus
Posterior commissure
Perineal raphe
Perianal tissues including external sphincter

Near 40 weeks

Figure 22-2 External genitalia development. Embryonic and fetal development of the external genitalia.

releasing low levels of gonadotropin-releasing hormone. Soon after birth, sex hormones drop precipitously; negative feedback action of the sex steroids on the hypothalamus and pituitary is removed; and gonadotropins are released. During infancy and early childhood, the gonadostat is remarkably sensitive (6 to 15 times more sensitive than in the adult) to negative feedback,[1] and GnRH secretion is restrained by extraordinarily low levels of estrogen or testosterone. This feedback mechanism is probably an intrinsic neuronal inhibitory system, which suppresses endogenous GnRH secretion and

gonadotropin synthesis.[1,3] By age 4, low levels of gonadotropins parallel low levels of sex steroids.

Puberty

Although the exact trigger for puberty is unknown, the first steroids in girls to rise in the blood are dehydroepiandrosterone (DHA) and its sulfate (DHAS), beginning at 6 to 8 years of age. Between ages 8 and 12, the gonads begin to produce more sex hormones, initiating sexual maturation, or puberty. In the United States, puberty begins with thelarche (breast development) at about 9 years of age in white girls and 8 years of age in black girls. In boys thelarche begins later, at approximately 11 years of age. Early puberty has been linked to obesity and more recently to the presence of **leptin,** a hormone secreted from adipose tissue.[3,4] Leptin, independent of sex hormone production, influences the onset of puberty purportedly through a direct effect on the hypothalamic-pituitary-gonadal axis or indirectly through an unidentified intermediary factor.[4] Leptin levels tend to be higher in black girls than in white girls of the same age, which may account for timing of puberty.[5] Puberty usually lasts 2 to 3 years, longer for early developers, and is complete when the individual is capable of reproduction. Puberty is not the same as adolescence. *Puberty* refers solely to sexual maturation; adolescence refers to all aspects of development that occur between ages 11 and 19 years.

Puberty is a process that involves a complex series of interrelated physiologic changes leading to reproductive matura-tion.[3] Reproductive maturation involves the hypothalamic-pituitary axis—the central nervous system, the endocrine system, and the gonads (ovaries or testes) themselves (Figure 22-3). As puberty approaches, three critical endocrine changes occur: (1) adrenarche, (2) decreased gonadostat sensitivity, and (3) development of a positive feedback system between gonadotropins and GnRH. **Adrenarche** is the increased production of adrenal androgens and occurs in both sexes.[1,3] The exact role that adrenarche plays in the initiation of puberty is unclear. Of interest is that adrenarche and **gonadarche** are overlapping but independent developmental processes; that is, adrenarche may occur without gonadarche, and vice versa.[1,3] Next, through unclear mechanisms, gonadostat sensitivity declines and a pulsatile pattern of GnRH secretion is established. This leads to the third essential endocrine change. GnRH levels increase and stimulate the anterior pituitary to produce gonadotropins: luteinizing hormone (LH) and follicle-stimulating hormone (FSH). An in-

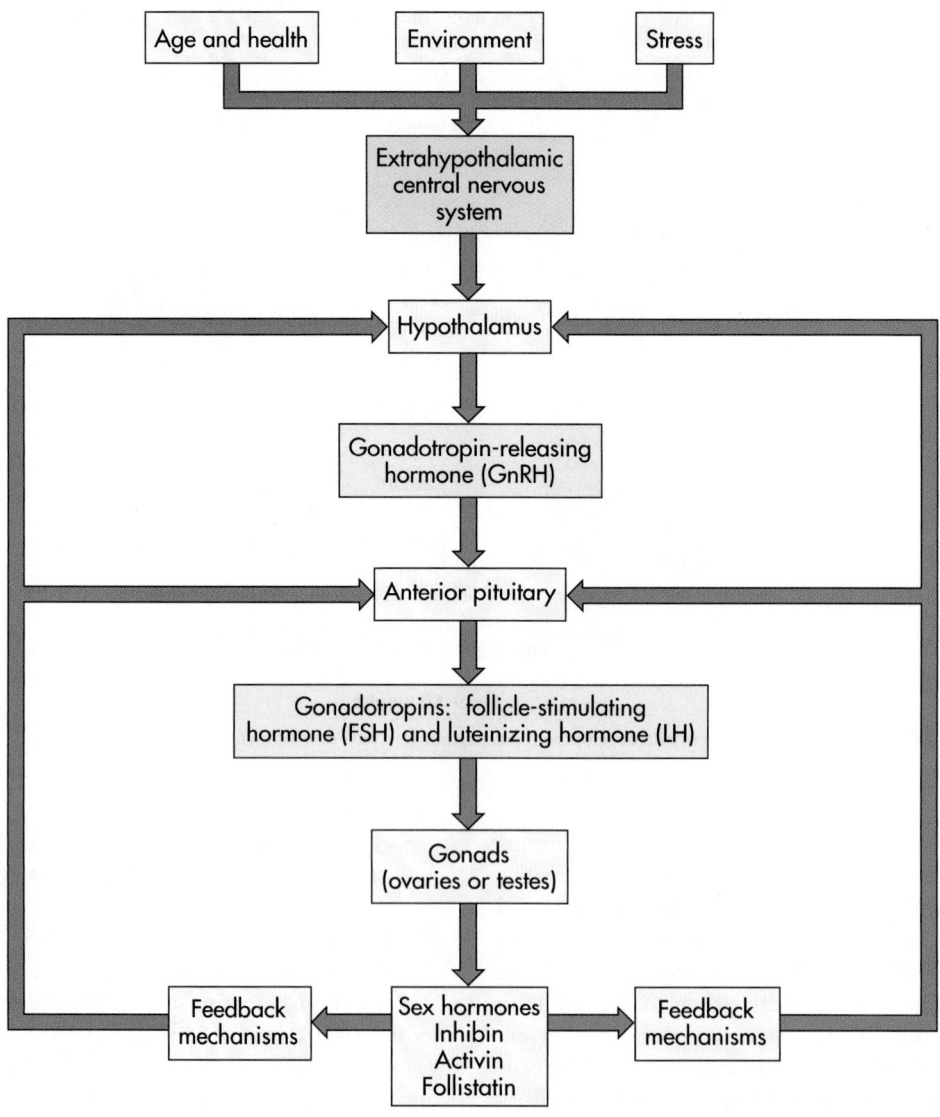

Figure 22-3 Hormonal stimulation of the gonads. The hypothalamic-pituitary-gonadal axis.

crease in nocturnal LH secretion is characteristic of puberty in both boys and girls. A positive feedback loop is created with gonadotropins stimulating the gonads to produce more sex hormones. (The sex hormones are discussed in the sections on the female and male systems.)

Increased sex hormone production causes the genitalia to grow to adult proportions. It also stimulates the develop-

ment of male and female secondary sex characteristics (increased body hair, voice changes, and breast development). The most important hormonal effects occur in the gonads, however. In males, the testes begin to produce mature sperm that are capable of fertilizing an ovum. Male puberty is complete with the first ejaculation that contains mature sperm. In females, the ovaries begin to release mature ova. Female puberty is complete at the time of the first ovulatory menstrual period.

THE FEMALE REPRODUCTIVE SYSTEM

The function of the reproductive system is to produce mature ova and, when they are fertilized, to protect and nourish them through embryonic and fetal life and expel them at birth. In females the most important reproductive organs, or genitalia, are internal. They are the ovaries, fallopian tubes, uterus, and vagina. These organs are essential to reproduction. The external genitalia have accessory functions. They protect body openings and play an important role in sexual functioning.[1,6,7]

External Genitalia

Figure 22-4 shows the external female genitalia, which are known collectively as the **vulva**, or pudendum. The major structures are as follows.

The **mons pubis** (also known as *mons veneris*) is a fatty layer of tissue over the pubic symphysis (joint of the pubic bones). During puberty the mons pubis becomes covered with pubic hair, and its sebaceous and sweat glands become

WHAT'S NEW? Race and Puberty

Girls in the United States begin puberty at a younger age than previously documented. White girls enter stage 2 of breast and pubic hair development about 1 year and black girls about 2 years earlier than documented standards suggest. Breast development is considered the most reliable sign of pituitary-gonadal axis activation. Pubertal changes do not seem to be related to body weight or adipose tissue, but may be activated by leptin levels. Higher leptin levels are found in black girls and may account for earlier onset of puberty in this population. Although breast and pubic hair development may occur at a younger age, average age of menarche remains at 13 years (12.54 years) for white girls and 12 years (12.30 years) for black girls. An inverse relationship between the length of the maturation process and onset of puberty seems to exist. Recent studies of young boys between ages 10 and 15 years do not show a significant difference in the timing of puberty based on race.

Data from Anderson SE, Dallal GE, Must A: *Pediatrics* 111(4 Pt 1):844-850, 2003; Chumlea WC et al: *Pediatrics* 111(1):110-113, 2003; Mayett K, Moore WV, Jacobson JD: *Pediatrics* 111(1):47-51, 2003.

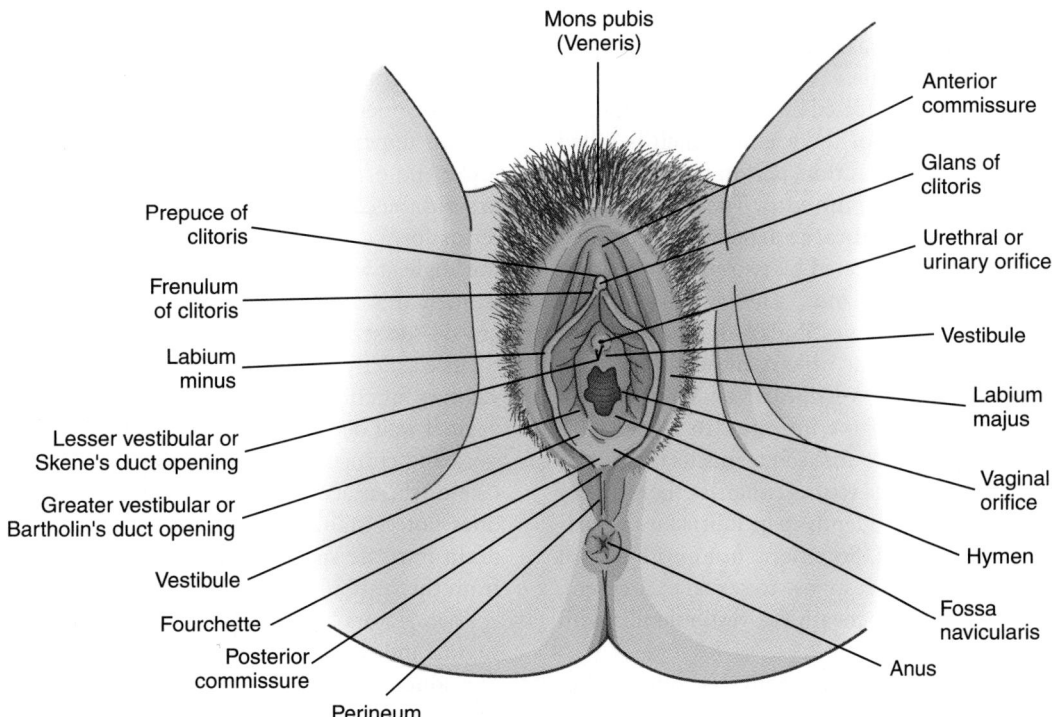

Figure 22-4 External female genitalia.

more active. Estrogen causes fat to be deposited under the skin, giving the mons pubis a moundlike shape. This cushion of tissue protects the pubic symphysis during sexual intercourse.

The **labia majora** (*singular,* **labium majus**) are two folds of skin that arise at the mons pubis and extend back to the fourchette, forming a cleft. Like the mons pubis, the labia majora undergo changes at puberty: the amount of fatty tissue increases, pubic hair grows on the lateral surfaces, and sebaceous glands on the hairless medial surfaces begin to secrete lubricants. Because of an extensive network of nerve endings, the labia majora are highly sensitive to temperature, touch, pressure, and pain and are homologous to the male scrotum (see Figure 22-2). The principal function of the labia majora is to protect the inner structures of the vulva.

The **labia minora** (*singular,* **labium minus**), two smaller, thinner folds of skin, lie within the labia majora. Anteriorly, they form the clitoral hood, or prepuce, and frenulum, then split to enclose the vestibule, and converge near the anus, forming the fourchette. The labia minora are hairless, pink, and moist and are well supplied with nerves, blood vessels, and sebaceous glands. These glands secrete a bactericidal fluid that has a distinctive odor and that lubricates and waterproofs the vulvar skin. During sexual arousal the labia minora become swollen with blood.

The **clitoris** is a richly innervated, erectile organ that lies anterior, between the labia minora. It is a small, cylindric structure having a glans that is visible and a shaft that lies beneath the skin (see Figure 22-4). The clitoris is homologous to the male penis. Like the penis, the clitoris is a major site of sexual stimulation and orgasm. With sexual arousal, erectile tissues in the clitoris fill with blood, causing it to enlarge somewhat. Similar to other vulvar glands, the clitoris secretes a fluid, called *smegma,* which has a unique odor and may be erotically stimulating to the male.

The **vestibule** is the area protected by the labia minora and contains the external opening of the vagina, which is called the **introitus,** or vaginal orifice. A thin, perforated membrane called the **hymen** may cover the introitus. The vestibule also contains the opening of the urethra, or **urinary meatus** (orifice). These structures are lubricated by two pairs of glands: Skene glands and Bartholin glands. The ducts of **Skene glands** (also called the **lesser vestibular** or **paraurethral glands**) open on both sides of the urinary meatus. The ducts of **Bartholin glands (greater vestibular** or **vulvovaginal glands)** open on either side of the introitus. In response to sexual stimulation, Bartholin glands secrete mucus that lubricates the inner labial surfaces, as well as enhances the viability and motility of sperm. Skene glands help lubricate the urinary meatus and the vestibule. Secretions from both sets of glands facilitate coitus. Also, in response to sexual excitement, the highly vascular tissue just beneath the vestibule fills with blood and becomes engorged.

The less hairy skin and the subcutaneous tissue that lie between the vaginal orifice and the anus are referred to as the **perineum.** Unlike the rest of the vulva, this area has little sub-cutaneous fat so that the skin is close to the underlying muscles. The perineum covers the muscular **perineal body,** a fibrous structure that comprises elastic fiber, connective tissue, and the common attachment of the bulbocavernosus, the external anal sphincter, and the levator ani muscles (see Figure 22-4). The perineum varies in length from 2 to 5 cm or more and stretches remarkably. The length of the perineum and the elasticity of the perineal body influence tissue resistance and injury during childbirth.

Internal Genitalia
Vagina

The **vagina** is an elastic, fibromuscular canal, 9 to 10 cm long, which extends up and back from the introitus to the lower portion of the uterus. As Figure 22-5 shows, it lies between the urethra (and part of the bladder) and the rectum. Mucosal secretions from the upper genital organs, menstrual fluids, and products of conception leave the body through the vagina, which also receives the penis during coitus. During sexual excitement the vagina lengthens and widens and the anterior third becomes congested with blood.

The vaginal wall is composed of four layers:

1. Its lining is a mucous membrane of squamous epithelial cells. (Types of epithelium are described and illustrated in Chapter 1, Table 1-7.) This layer thickens and thins in response to hormones, particularly estrogen. The squamous epithelial membrane is continuous with the membrane that covers the lower part of the uterus. In women of reproductive age, the mucosal layer is arranged in transverse wrinkles, or folds, called **rugae** (*singular,* **ruga**) that permit stretching during coitus and childbirth.
2. Fibrous connective tissue containing numerous blood and lymphatic vessels.
3. Smooth muscle.
4. Connective tissue and a rich network of blood vessels.

The upper part of the vagina surrounds the cervix, the lower end of the uterus (see Figure 22-5). The recessed space around the cervix is called the **fornix** of the vagina. The posterior fornix is "deeper" than the anterior fornix because of the angle at which the cervix meets the vaginal canal. In most women this angle is about 90 degrees. A pouch called the **cul-de-sac** separates the posterior fornix and the rectum.

Its elasticity and relatively sparse nerve supply enhance the vagina's function as the birth canal. During sexual arousal the vaginal wall becomes engorged with blood, like the labia minora and clitoris. Engorgement pushes some fluid to the surface of the mucosa, enhancing lubrication. The vaginal wall does not contain mucus-secreting glands; rather, secretions drain into the vagina from the endocervical glands or enter from the vestibule, from the Bartholin and Skene glands.

Two factors help maintain the self-cleansing action of the vagina and defend it from infection, particularly during the reproductive years: (1) an acid-base balance that discourages the proliferation of most pathogenic bacteria and (2) the thickness of the vaginal epithelium. Before puberty, vaginal

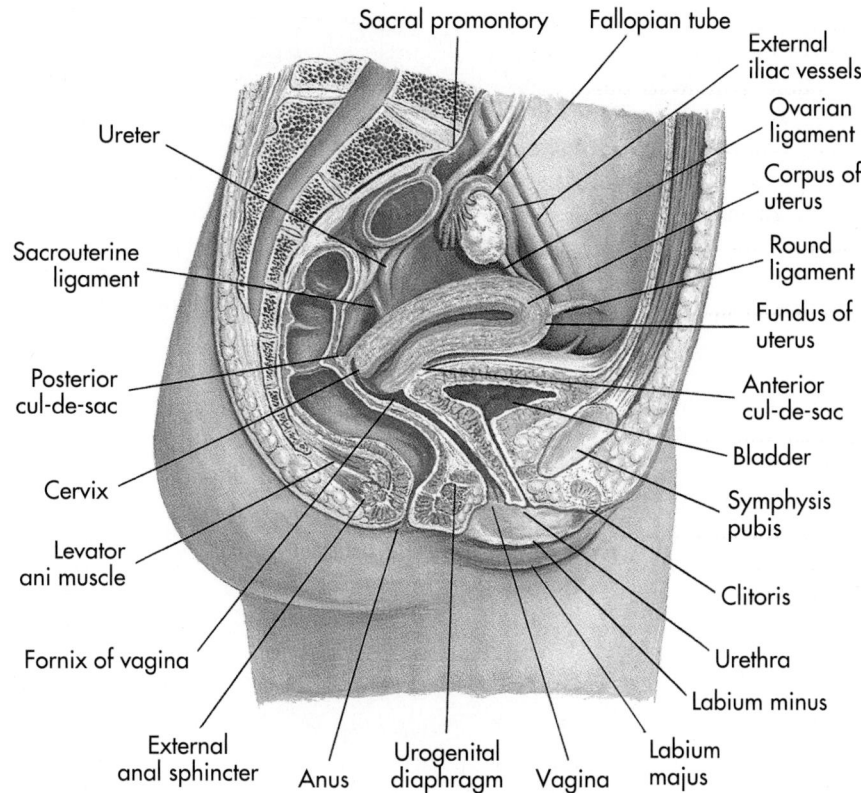

Figure 22-5 Internal female genitalia and other pelvic organs. Midsagittal view. (Modified from Seidel HM et al: *Mosby's guide to physical examination,* ed 5, St Louis, 2003, Mosby.)

pH is about 7.0 (neutral) and the vaginal epithelium is thin. At puberty, the pH becomes more acidic (4.0 to 5.0) and the squamous epithelial lining thickens. These changes are maintained until menopause (cessation of menstruation), at which time the pH rises again to more alkaline levels and the epithelium thins out. Therefore protection from infection is greatest during the years when a woman is most likely to be sexually active. Between puberty and menopause, vulnerability to infection varies somewhat with cyclic changes in pH and epithelial thickness. Both defenses are greatest when estrogen levels are high and the vagina contains a normal population of *Lactobacillus acidophilus,* a harmless resident bacterium that helps maintain pH at acidic levels. Any condition that causes vaginal pH to rise, such as douching or use of vaginal sprays or deodorants, low estrogen levels, or destruction of *L. acidophilus* by antibiotics, lowers vaginal defenses against infection.

Uterus

The **uterus** is a hollow, pear-shaped organ whose lower end opens into the vagina. The functions of the uterus are to anchor and protect a fertilized ovum, provide an optimal environment while it develops, and push the fetus out at birth. In addition, the uterus plays an important role in sexual response and conception. During sexual excitement the opening of the uterus (the cervix) dilates slightly. At the same time, the uterus increases in size and moves upward and backward, creating a tenting effect in the midvagina that results in the

cervix "sitting" in a pool of semen. During orgasm, rhythmic contractions facilitate movement of sperm through the cervical os while also enhancing physical pleasure.

At puberty the uterus attains its adult size and proportions and descends from the abdomen to the lower pelvis, between the bladder and the rectum (see Figure 22-5). The uterus of a mature, nonpregnant female is approximately 7 to 9 cm long and 6.5 cm wide, with muscular walls 3.5 cm thick. It is held loosely in position by ligaments, peritoneal tissue folds, and pressure of adjacent organs, especially the urinary bladder, sigmoid colon, and rectum. In most women the uterus is anteverted; that is, it is tipped forward so that it rests on the urinary bladder. However, it may be retroverted, or tipped backward. Various degrees of flexion are normal (Figure 22-6).

Figure 22-7 shows a cross section of the uterus. The uterus has two major parts: the body, or **corpus,** and the cervix. The top of the corpus, above the insertion of the fallopian tubes, is called the **fundus.** The diameter of the uterine cavity is widest at the fundus and narrowest at the **isthmus,** which is the narrowed part of the corpus just above the cervix. The **cervix,** or "neck of the uterus," extends from the isthmus to the vagina. The passageway between the cervix's upper opening (the internal os) and its lower opening (the external os) is called the **endocervical canal.** The entire uterus, like the upper vagina, is innervated exclusively by motor and sensory fibers of the autonomic nervous system.

The uterine wall is composed of three layers: the perimetrium, the myometrium, and the endometrium (see

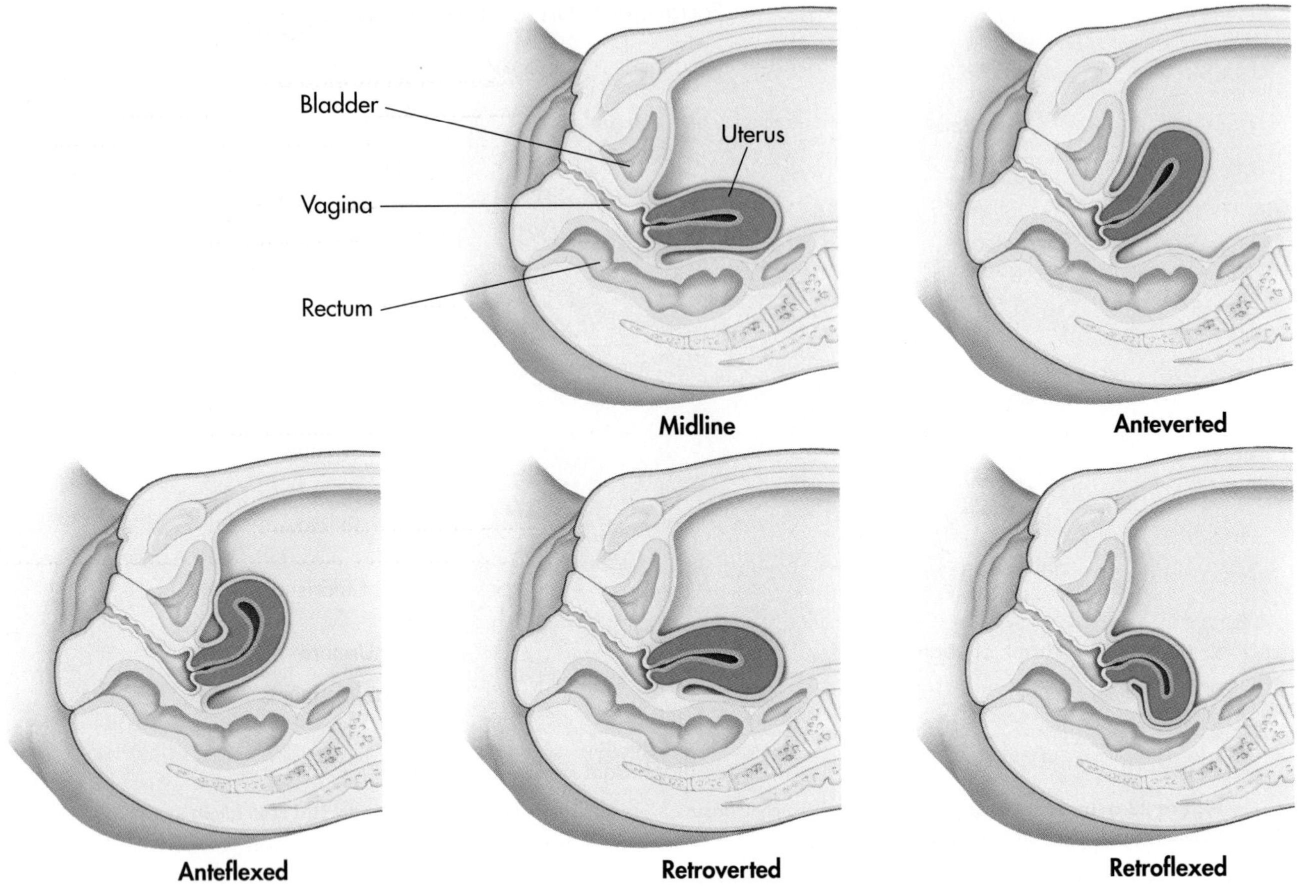

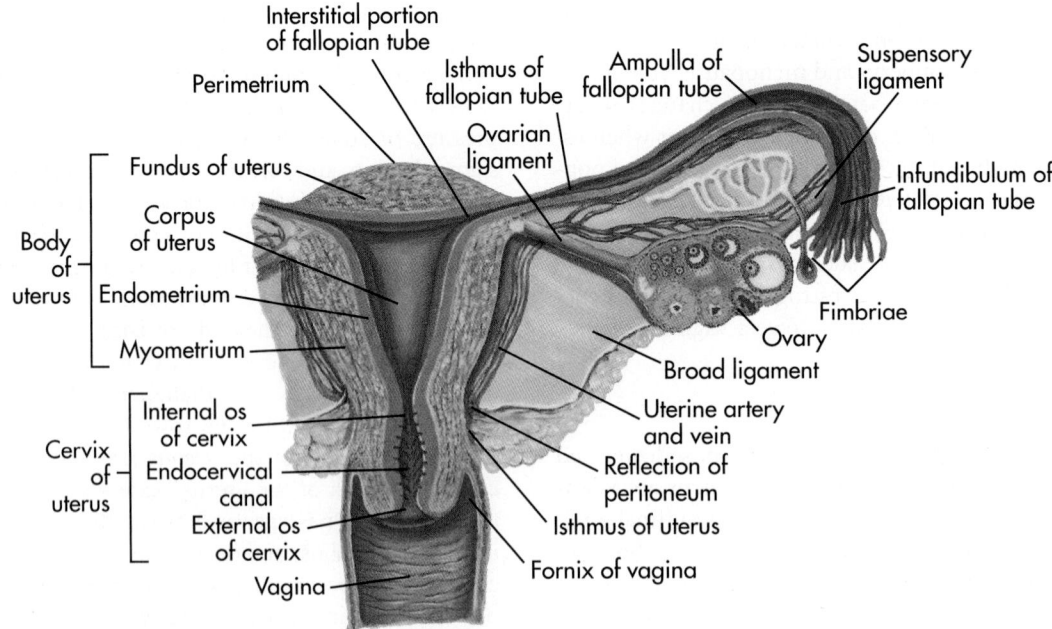

Figure 22-6 Variations in uterine position.

Figure 22-7 Cross section of uterus, fallopian tube, and ovary. (From Seidel HM et al: *Mosby's guide to physical examination*, ed 5, St Louis, 2003, Mosby.)

Figure 22-7). The **perimetrium (parietal peritoneum)** is the outer serous membrane that covers the uterus. The **myometrium** is the thick, muscular middle layer. The myometrium is thickest at the fundus, apparently to facilitate birth. The **endometrium,** or uterine lining, is composed of a functional layer (superficial compact layer and spongy middle layer) and a basal layer. The functional layer of the endometrium is responsive to sex hormones. Between puberty and menopause this layer proliferates and sloughs off monthly. The basal layer, which is attached to the myometrium, regenerates the functional layer after it sloughs (menstruation).

The endocervical canal does not have an endometrial layer. Rather, it is lined with columnar epithelial cells (see Table 1-7). The endocervical lining is continuous with that of the outer cervix and vagina, but it is not made up of the same type of epithelial cells. The point at which the columnar epithelium of the cervix meets the squamous epithelium of the vagina is called the *transformation zone,* or the **squamous-columnar junction.** The transformation zone is the usual site of cervical dysplasia or carcinoma in situ; these are the cells sampled during a Papanicolaou test (Pap test).[1]

The cervix acts as a mechanical barrier to infectious microorganisms that may be present in the vagina. The external cervical os is a very small opening that contains thick, sticky mucus (the *mucous plug*) during most of the menstrual cycle and all of pregnancy. During ovulation, the mucus changes under the influence of estrogen and forms watery strands, or spinnbarkeit mucus, to facilitate the transport of sperm into the uterus. In addition, the downward flow of cervical secretions moves microorganisms away from the cervix and uterus. In women of reproductive age, the pH of these secretions is inhospitable to most bacteria. Further, mucosal secretions contain enzymes and antibodies (mostly immunoglobulin A) of the secretory immune system. (The secretory immune system is discussed in Chapter 7.) These defenses do not always prevent infection, even if they are intact. Besides infection, uterine pathophysiology includes displacement of the uterus within the pelvis, benign growths (fibroids) of the uterine wall, hyperplasia of the endometrium, endometriosis, and cancer.

Fallopian Tubes

The two **fallopian tubes (oviducts, uterine tubes)** enter the uterus bilaterally just beneath the fundus (see Figure 22-7). Their function is to conduct the ova from the spaces around the ovaries to the uterus. From the uterus the fallopian tubes curve up and over the two ovaries. Each tube is 8 to 12 cm long and about 1 cm in diameter, except at its ovarian end, which flares out like the bell of a trumpet. This widened end, called the **infundibulum,** is fringed or fimbriated. The **fimbriae** (fringes) move, creating a current that draws the ovum into the infundibulum. Once the ovum has entered the fallopian tube, cilia and peristalsis (muscle contractions) keep it moving toward the uterus.

The ampulla, or distal third, of the fallopian tube is the usual site of fertilization (see Figure 22-7). Sperm released into the vagina travel upward through the endocervical canal and uterine cavity and enter the fallopian tubes. If an ovum is present in either tube, fertilization can occur. Whether or not the ovum encounters sperm, it continues to travel through the fallopian tube to the uterus. If fertilized, the ovum (then called a *blastocyst*) implants itself in the endometrial layer of the uterine wall. If not fertilized, the ovum breaks down within 12 to 24 hours.

Disorders that affect the fallopian tubes can block the path of both sperm and ovum and cause infertility or ectopic (tubal) pregnancy. Such disorders include congenital malformations, infection, and inflammation.

Ovaries

The **ovaries,** or the female gonads, are the primary female reproductive organs. They have two main functions: secretion of female sex hormones and development and release of female gametes, or ova.

The almond-shaped ovaries are located on both sides of the uterus and are suspended and supported by the mesovarian portions of the broad ligament, ovarian ligaments, and suspensory ligaments (see Figure 22-7). The ovaries are smaller than their male homologs, the testes. In women of reproductive age, each ovary is 3 to 5 cm long, 2.5 cm wide, and 2 cm thick and weighs 4 to 8 g. Size and weight vary somewhat from phase to phase of the menstrual cycle (see p. 746).

Figure 22-8 shows a cross section of an ovary. The central part, or medulla, is composed of connective tissue and contains many small arteries, veins, and lymphatics, which enter at the hilum. Surrounding the medulla is the cortex. At birth the cortex of each ovary contains approximately 1 million ova within immature **ovarian follicles.** Follicles grow and undergo atresia continuously and irrevocably during a woman's life. By puberty the number ranges between 200,000 and 400,000 ova. During puberty some of the follicles and the ova within them begin to mature. Between puberty and menopause the ovarian cortex always contains follicles and ova in various stages of development. Once every menstrual cycle (about every 28 days), usually only one of the follicles reaches maturation and discharges its ovum through the ovary's outer covering, the germinal epithelium. During the reproductive years, 300 to 500 ovarian follicles mature completely and release an ovum, an event termed **ovulation.** The rest either fail to develop at all or degenerate without maturing completely.[1]

Having ejected a mature ovum, the follicle develops into another structure, the **corpus luteum** (see Figure 22-8). The immediate fate of the corpus luteum depends on whether the ejected ovum is fertilized. If fertilization occurs, the corpus luteum enlarges and begins to secrete hormones that maintain and support pregnancy. If fertilization does not occur, the corpus luteum secretes these hormones for approximately 14 days and then degenerates, which triggers the maturation

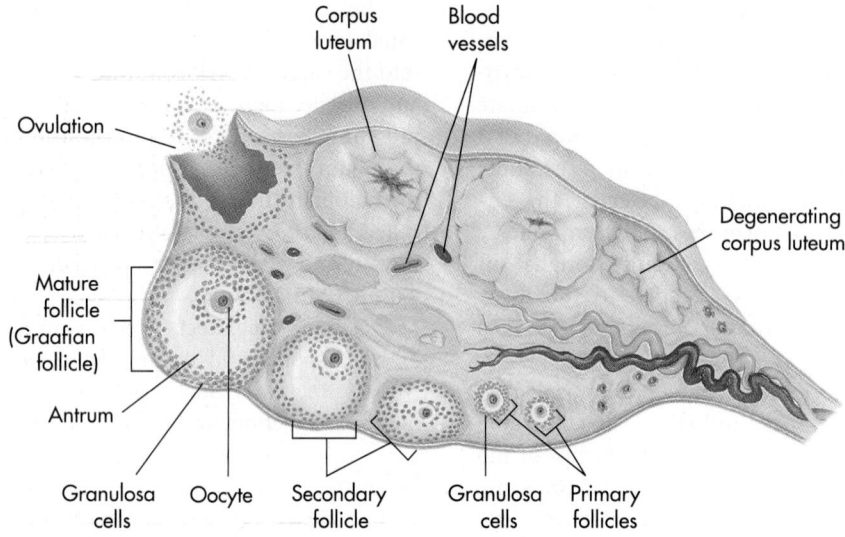

Figure 22-8 Cross section of ovary during reproductive years. (From Thibodeau GA, Patton KT: *Anatomy & physiology,* ed 5, St Louis, 2003, Mosby.)

of another follicle. The **ovarian cycle**—the process of follicular maturation, ovulation, corpus luteum development, and corpus luteum degeneration—is continuous from puberty to menopause, except during pregnancy or hormonal contraceptive use. At menopause, this process ceases and the ovaries atrophy to the point that they cannot be felt during pelvic examination.

Four types of cells within the ovarian cortex secrete sex hormones: cells of the stroma, or tissue matrix; two types of cells in the ovarian follicle, **granulosa cells** and **theca cells,** and cells of the corpus luteum (Figure 22-9). These cells all contain receptors for the gonadotropins (LH and FSH) or for the sex hormones, which are discussed in the next section.

Because gonadotropins and hormones regulate ovarian function, any disorder that disrupts this process, such as abnormal pituitary or thyroid function, or reception by target cells can cause ovarian dysfunction and infertility. Benign or malignant growths, cysts, infection, or inflammation also can cause ovarian pathologic conditions.[1]

Female Sex Hormones

The sex hormones are all steroid hormones, that is, they are synthesized from cholesterol (see Chapter 20). Both male and female sex hormones are present in all adults. However, the female body contains low levels of testosterone and other androgens, and the male body contains low levels of estrogen. Individual effects of sex hormones depend on their amount and concentration in the blood.

The dominant female sex hormones, estrogen and progesterone, are produced by the ovaries. During fetal development, infancy, and childhood, sex hormone production is low. At puberty, hormone production surges, triggering sexual maturation and development of secondary sex characteristics. From puberty to menopause, the sex hormones control the menstrual cycle and are produced cyclically, that is, production surges and diminishes monthly, creating the ovarian

and uterine changes associated with the menstrual cycle. These hormones are also produced in higher levels during pregnancy by the placenta and inhibit ovulation. Androgens are produced in small amounts by the ovaries and the adrenals and also have important functions in women.

Estrogens

Estrogen is a generic term for three similar hormones: estradiol, estrone, and estriol. **Estradiol (E2)** is the most potent and plentiful of the three and is principally produced by the ovaries (ovarian follicle and corpus luteum). The ovary secretes about 95% of circulating estradiol, with limited amounts secreted by the adrenal cortex. Androgens are converted to estrone in ovarian and peripheral adipose tissue, and estriol is the peripheral metabolite of estrone and estradiol.

Estrogen has numerous biologic effects, many of which involve interactions with other hormones. Estrogen is needed for maturation of reproductive organs, development of secondary sex characteristics, closure of long bones after the pubertal growth spurt, regulation of the menstrual cycle, and endometrial regeneration after menstruation. Estrogen also has metabolic effects on the bones, liver, blood vessels, brain and central nervous system, kidneys, and skin. After menopause, ovarian production of estradiol and estrone is markedly diminished. For this reason, postmenopausal women are susceptible to osteoporosis, a condition in which bone density is reduced. At this time, the majority of estrogen is derived from extraovarian and extraglandular production of estrones.[1] (Hormone levels during the perimenopause are discussed in the section on menopause, p. 761.)

Like other steroid hormones, estrogens are derived from cholesterol in a complex, enzyme-mediated series of reactions. (Mechanisms of hormone synthesis and action are described in Chapter 20.) The hypothalamus secretes GnRH in a pulsating manner that stimulates gonadotropin (LH and

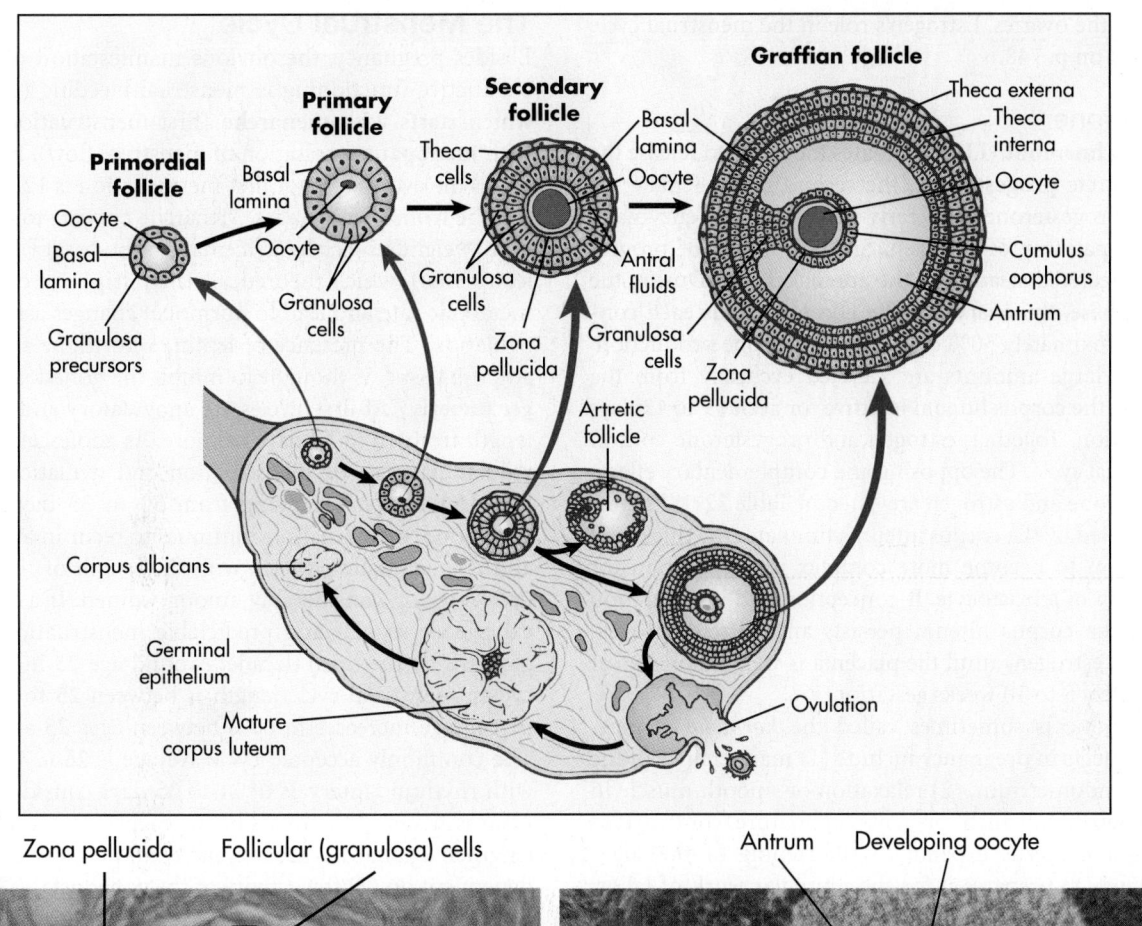

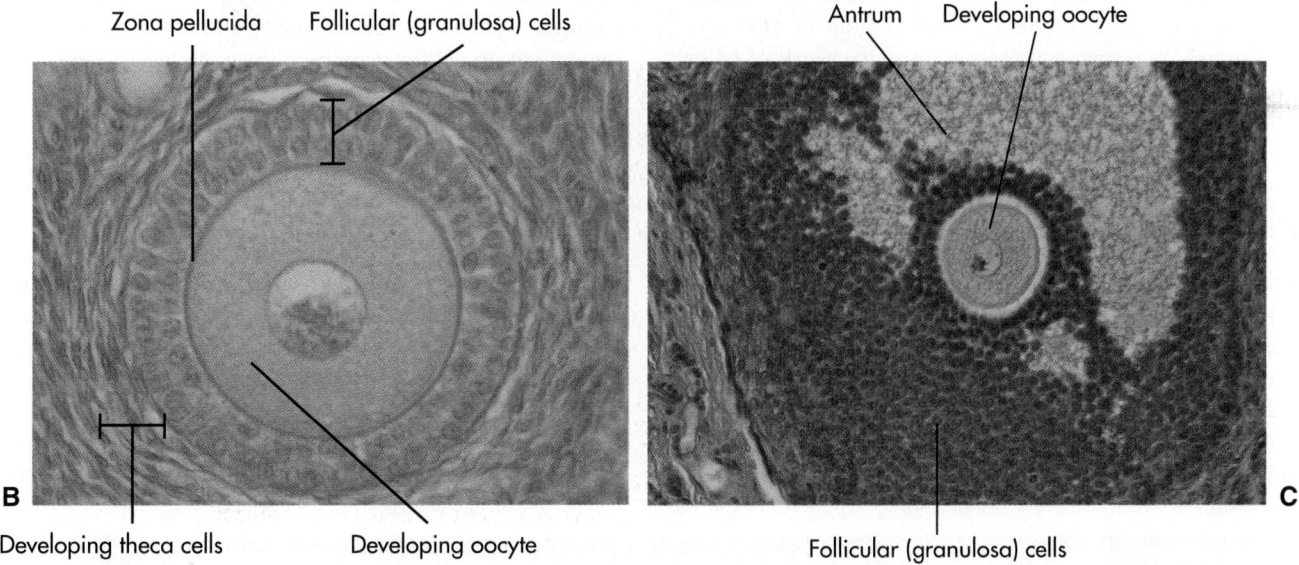

Figure 22-9 Development of an ovarian follicle. **A,** Schematic representation (not to scale) of the structure of the ovary, showing the various stages in the development of the follicle and its successor structure, the corpus luteum. **B,** A developing oocyte surrounded by hormone-secreting follicular (granulosa) cells. **C,** More mature ovarian follicle has a fluid-filled cavity called the *antrum*. (**A,** From Berne RM, Levy MN, editors: *Physiology,* ed 5, St Louis, 2003, Mosby. **B** and **C,** From Thibodeau GA, Patton KT: *Anatomy & physiology,* ed 5, St Louis, 2003, Mosby.)

FSH) release from the anterior pituitary. Gonadotropins trigger ovarian production of estrogen. The primary function of LH is to stimulate theca cells of the ovarian follicle to produce androgens, mainly androstenedione. (Androgens are discussed further on p. 755 and in the section on male reproductive function.) Some of these androgens are converted to estrogen by the theca cells themselves, and others diffuse into the granulosa cells. Within the granulosa layer, FSH induces conversion (aromatization) of androgens to estrogens. Estrogens are then released into the bloodstream.

Disturbances of estrogen production can be caused by abnormalities that affect (1) secretion of GnRH by the hypothalamus, (2) secretion of LH or FSH by the anterior pituitary, (3) hormonal feedback mechanisms, or (4) structural integrity of the ovaries. Estrogen's role in the menstrual cycle is described on p. 748.

Progesterone

Luteinizing hormone (LH) stimulates the ovary to release the ova and secrete **progesterone,** the second major female sex hormone. Progesterone is an early product in the enzymatic conversion pathway of estrogen. Small amounts of progesterone are secreted steadily by the adrenal cortex. During the follicular phase, the ovary and the adrenal glands each contribute approximately 50% of total progesterone production. Conversely, large amounts are secreted cyclically from the ovary while the corpus luteum is active for about 9 to 13 days after ovulation. Together, estrogen and progesterone control the menstrual cycle. The opposing and complementary effects of progesterone and estrogen are listed in Table 22-1. Progesterone secreted by the corpus luteum stimulates the thickened endometrium to become more complex in preparation for implantation of a blastocyte. If conception and implantation do occur, the corpus luteum persists and secretes progesterone (and estrogen) until the placenta is well established at approximately 8 to 10 weeks gestation.

Progesterone is sometimes called the *hormone of pregnancy*. Its effects in pregnancy include (1) maintenance of the thickened endometrium; (2) relaxation of smooth muscle in the myometrium, which prevents premature contractions and helps the uterus expand; (3) thickening of the myometrium, which prepares it for the muscular work of labor; (4) prevention of lactation until the fetus is born; and (5) prevention of additional maturation of ova by way of suppressing FSH and LH, thereby stopping the menstrual cycle.

Androgens

Although **androgens** are primarily male sex hormones, small amounts are produced in the ovary and adrenal cortex in women. Some androgens are precursors of female sex hormones, notably androstenedione. At puberty, androgens contribute to the skeletal growth spurt and cause growth of pubic and axillary hair. The androgens also activate sebaceous glands, accounting for some cases of acne during puberty, and play a role in libido.

The Menstrual Cycle

Besides pregnancy, the obvious manifestation of female reproductive functioning is menstrual bleeding (the menses), which starts with **menarche** (first menstruation) and ends with **menopause** (cessation of menstrual flow). In the United States the average age of first menstruation is 12.5 years, with a range from 9 to 17 years. Menarche appears to be related to body weight, especially percentage of body fat (ratio of fat to lean tissue), which theoretically may trigger a change in the metabolic rate and lead to hormonal changes associated with ovulation. The presence of leptin, a hormone secreted from adipose tissue, is thought to inhibit the gonadostat and trigger puberty.[3] At first, cycles are anovulatory and may vary in length from 10 to 60 days or more. As adolescence proceeds, regular patterns of menstruation and ovulation are established at intervals ranging from 30 to 35 days.[8-10] During adulthood, menstruation continues to recur in a recognizable and characteristic pattern, with the length of the menstrual cycle varying considerably among women. If a woman is to experience regular and predictable menstruation, it usually happens by the third decade. Around age 25 in over 40% of cycles, menstrual cycle length is between 25 to 28 days; the percentage increases to 60% between ages 25 and 35 years.[1] The commonly accepted cycle average is 28 (27 to 30) days, with rhythmic intervals of 21 to 35 days considered normal. Approximately 2 to 4 years before menopause, cycles begin to lengthen again. Menstrual cyclicity and regular ovulation are dependent on (1) the activity of the gonadostat (GnRH pulse generator); (2) the pituitary secretion of gonadotropins; and (3) estrogen (estradiol) positive feedback for the preovulatory LH surge, oocyte maturation, and corpus luteum formation.[3]

Phases

The menstrual cycle consists of three phases of one event, ovulation. During ovulation, an ovum from a mature ovarian follicle is released. The three phases are the follicular/proliferative phase, the luteal/secretory phase, and the ischemic/menstrual phase, known as *menstruation* (Figure 22-10).

During **menstruation (menses),** the functional layer of the endometrium disintegrates and is discharged through the vagina. Menstruation is followed by the **follicular/**

Table 22-1	Complementary and Opposing Effects of Estrogen and Progesterone	
Structure	**Effect of Estrogen**	**Effect of Progesterone**
Vaginal mucosa	Proliferation of squamous epithelium; increase in glycogen content of cells; layering (cornification) of cells	Thinning of squamous epithelium; decornification
Cervical mucosa	Production of abundant fluid secretions that favor survival and enhance motility of sperm	Production of thick, sticky secretions that tend to "plug" the cervical os
Fallopian tube	Increase of motility and ciliary action	Decrease of motility and ciliary action
Uterine muscle	Increase of blood flow; increase of contractile proteins and uterine muscle and myometrial excitability and action potential; increase of sensitization to oxytocin	Relaxation of myometrium; decrease of sensitization to oxytocin
Endometrium	Stimulation of growth; increase in number of progesterone receptors	Activation of glands and blood vessels; accumulation of glycogen and enzymes; decrease in number of estrogen receptors
Breasts	Growth of ducts; promotion of prolactin effects	Growth of lobules and alveoli; inhibition of prolactin effects

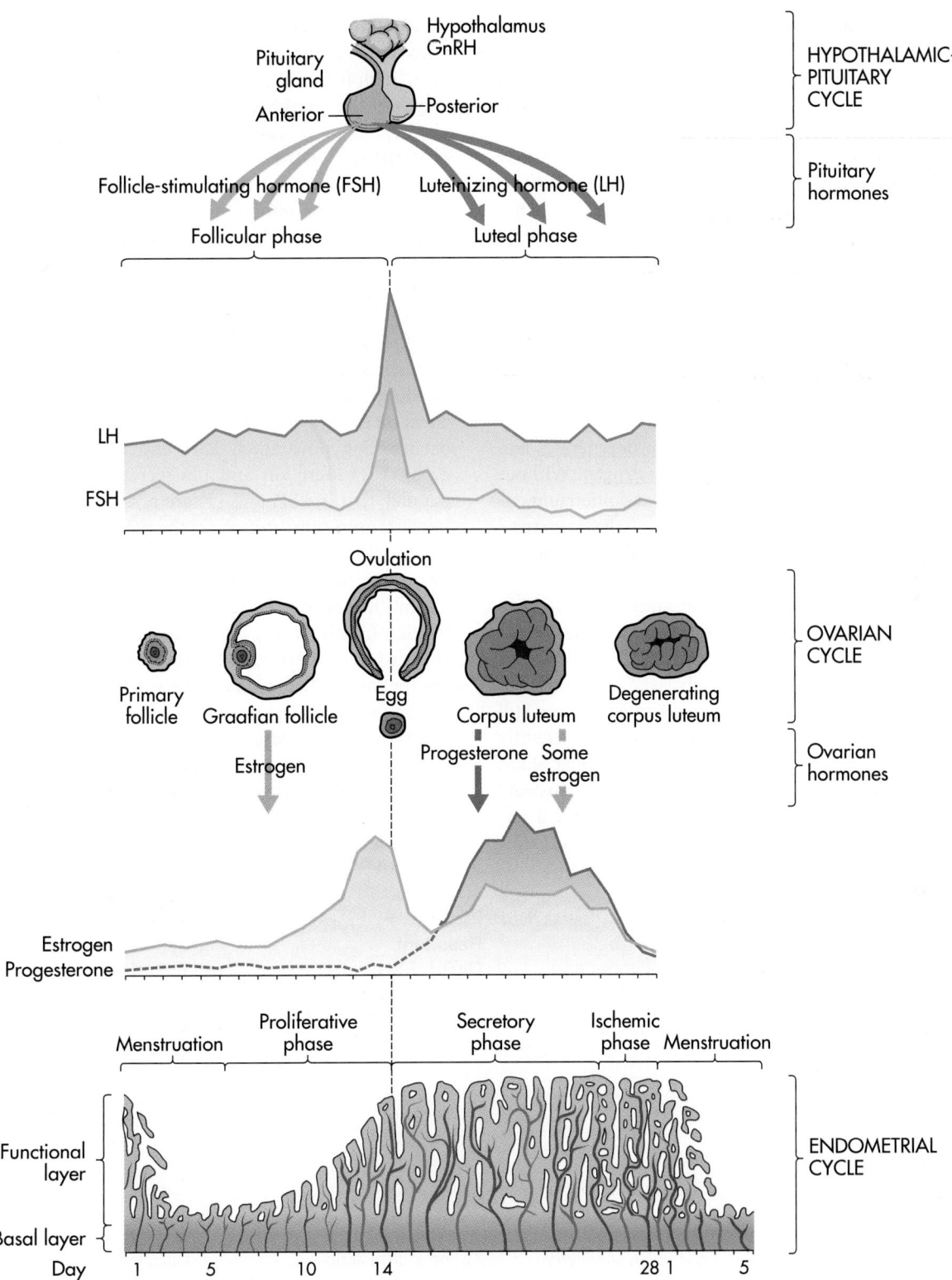

Figure 22-10 **The menstrual cycle.** (From Lowdermilk DL, Perry SE, Bobak IM: *Maternity and women's health care*, ed 8, St Louis, 2004, Mosby.)

proliferative phase. This phase is named for two simultaneous processes: maturation of an ovarian follicle and proliferation of the endometrium (see Figure 22-10). During the follicular/proliferative phase, the anterior pituitary gland secretes FSH, which causes a dominant ovarian follicle to develop. While the follicle is developing, its granulosa cells se-

crete estrogen and estrogen causes cells of the endometrium to proliferate and induces an LH surge causing progesterone production in the granulosa layer of the ovary. By the time the ovarian follicle is mature, the endometrial lining is restored. At this point ovulation occurs.[3] When the lesser follicles fail to achieve full maturity, they retain their ability to respond to

LH and steroid production, even though they return to stromal tissue. Increase in stromal tissue in the late follicular phase is associated with a rise in androgen levels. Androgen production enhances the process of follicle atresia and may stimulate libido at the point of ovulation.[1]

Ovulation marks the beginning of the **luteal/secretory phase** of the menstrual cycle. The ovarian follicle begins its transformation into a corpus luteum (see Figure 22-8), hence the name *luteal phase.* LH from the anterior pituitary stimulates the corpus luteum to secrete progesterone, which in turn initiates the secretory phase of endometrial development. Glands and blood vessels in the endometrium branch and curl throughout the functional layer, and the glands begin to secrete a thin, glycogen-containing fluid, hence the name *secretory phase.* If conception occurs, the nutrient-laden endometrium is ready for implantation. If conception and implantation do not occur, the corpus luteum degenerates and ceases its production of progesterone and estrogen. Without progesterone or estrogen to maintain it, the endometrium enters the ischemic (blood-starved) portion of the menstrual phase and disintegrates. Menstruation occurs, marking the beginning of another cycle.

Ovarian cycles appear to have a minimum length of 24 to 26.5 days: the ovarian follicle requires 10 to 12.5 days to develop, and the luteal phase appears relatively fixed at 14 days (±3 days). Menstrual blood flow usually lasts 3 to 7 days, but it may last as long as 8 days or stop after 1 to 2 days and still be considered within normal limits. Bleeding is consistently scant to heavy and varies from 30 to 80 ml, with most blood loss occurring during the first 3 days of menses. Menstrual discharge consists of blood, mucus, and desquamated endometrial tissue and does not clot under normal circumstances. It is usually dark and produces a characteristic musty odor on oxidation. Factors such as severe emotional stress, illness, malnutrition, and seasonal variation may affect the length of the menstrual cycle.[9-11]

Hormonal Controls

Hormonal control of the menstrual cycle depends on complex interactions among the hypothalamus, the anterior pituitary, and the ovaries (or hypothalamic-pituitary-ovarian [H-P-O] axis).[11] GnRH is secreted by the hypothalamus into the hypophyseal portal system and travels to the anterior pituitary, where it stimulates the secretion of LH and FSH. FSH and LH are released from the anterior pituitary in pulses that correspond to the pulsatile secretion of GnRH.

Blood levels of estrogen and progesterone exert a feedback effect on the hypothalamus and the anterior pituitary, thereby determining how much FSH and LH are secreted (Table 22-2). FSH secretion and LH secretion are not completely parallel; that is, FSH and LH are not secreted simultaneously in equal amounts throughout the menstrual cycle. Nonparallel secretion is caused by cyclic changes in feedback mechanisms. During the early follicular phase, low levels of estrogen inhibit the FSH-secreting cells of the anterior pituitary. As the ovarian follicle grows, it produces more and more estrogen. Higher levels of estrogen further suppress FSH release. During the late follicular phase, the preovulatory rise in progesterone facilitates the positive feedback of estrogen; estrogen levels begin to increase, stimulating a surge of FSH and LH secretion from the anterior pituitary. (Progesterone may be necessary also to induce the midcycle FSH peak.) The midcycle surge of LH causes ovulation. Rising estrogen and progesterone levels during the luteal phase may have some in-

Table 22-2	Hormonal Feedback Mechanisms of the Menstrual Cycle		
Phase of Cycle and Ovarian Hormone Levels	Feedback to Hypothalamus and Anterior Pituitary	Resultant GnRH, FSH, and LH Levels	Ovarian and Menstrual Events
Early follicular phase: estrogen levels low; minute amount of progesterone secreted	Negative and inhibitory	All low	Ovarian follicle develops; endometrium proliferates
Late follicular (preovulatory) phase: estrogen levels high; progesterone increases with small surge before ovulation	Positive and stimulatory	All surge; LH dominates	Process of ovulation begins; endometrial proliferation complete
Ovulatory phase: estrogen levels dip; progesterone levels begin to rise	Negative and inhibitory	All fall sharply	Corpus luteum begins to develop; endometrium enters secretory phase
Early luteal phase: estrogen and progesterone levels high; progesterone dominates	Negative and inhibitory	All continue to decline, but gradually	Corpus luteum fully developed; endometrium ready for implantation
Late luteal phase: estrogen and progesterone levels fall sharply	Negative and inhibitory; feedback lessens slightly	All rise slightly	Corpus luteum regresses; endometrium breaks down; menstruation begins
Menstrual phase: estrogen levels low; minute amount of progesterone secreted	Negative and inhibitory	All low	More ovarian follicles begin to develop; functional layer of endometrium is shed

GnRH, Gonadotropin-releasing hormone; *FSH,* follicle-stimulating hormone; *LH,* luteinizing hormone.

hibitory effect on the anterior pituitary, thereby reducing LH and FSH secretion. Just before the onset of menstruation, FSH and LH levels begin to increase slightly, probably because of declining estrogen and progesterone levels (Figure 22-11).

A variety of growth factors and autocrine/paracrine peptides influence hormonal control and follicular response.[1,12] During the early follicular stage, FSH stimulates FSH and LH receptors, insulin-like growth factor–I, and production of inhibin and activin; after ovulation, inhibin release comes under the control of LH. **Activin** stimulates FSH release in the pituitary and augments its action in the ovary, possibly by increasing FSH receptors. **Inhibin** inhibits FSH synthesis and secretion, restrains prolactin and growth hormone release, interferes with GnRH receptors, and promotes breakdown of intracellular gonadotropins.[13,14] To a lesser degree, **follistatin,** a polypeptide produced by the pituitary but found primarily in the follicles, suppresses FSH activity, probably by binding to activin. In summary, the balance between activin and inhibin regulates FSH secretion, and follistatin inhibits activin and boosts inhibin activity. Inhibin and activin also regulate LH stimulation of androgen synthesis in theca cells. Figure 22-11 depicts fluctuating estrogen, progesterone, gonadotropin, and inhibin levels.[1]

Interestingly, inhibins, activins, and follistatins are structurally similar, belonging to the same family of nonsteroidal polypeptides, and are synthesized by granulosa cells in response to FSH. Inhibin is synthesized and secreted from both granulosa and luteal ovarian cells, activin from granulosa cells only, and follistatin from pituitary cells. These peptides are secreted into the follicular fluid and ovarian venous effluent. The expression of these peptides is not limited to the ovary; they are present in many tissues throughout the body and serve as regulators. Inhibin messenger RNA and activin are also found within the pituitary. Dimers of the β subunits of inhibin (activin) stimulate FSH secretion, whereas a,β-inhibin inhibits FSH.[3] Understanding of the function and structural complexity of these polypeptides and their interaction with GnRH, gonadotropins, and sex hormones has increased monumentally over the past decade. New information is gained through research and published on a regular basis.

Ovarian Cycle

By stimulating follicles, gonadotropins initiate their growth and maturation. The most important hormonal event is a rise in FSH. The decline in the late luteal phase of estrogen, progesterone, and inhibin secretion allows FSH to rise; concurrently there is a slight increase in LH levels (see Figure 22-11). More specifically, FSH stimulates granulosa cell growth and initiates estrogen production in these cells in the next cycle. At this time a group of ovarian follicles is recruited and begins to mature; the exact number depends on the remaining pool of inactive follicles. As the follicles mature, granulosa cells mul-

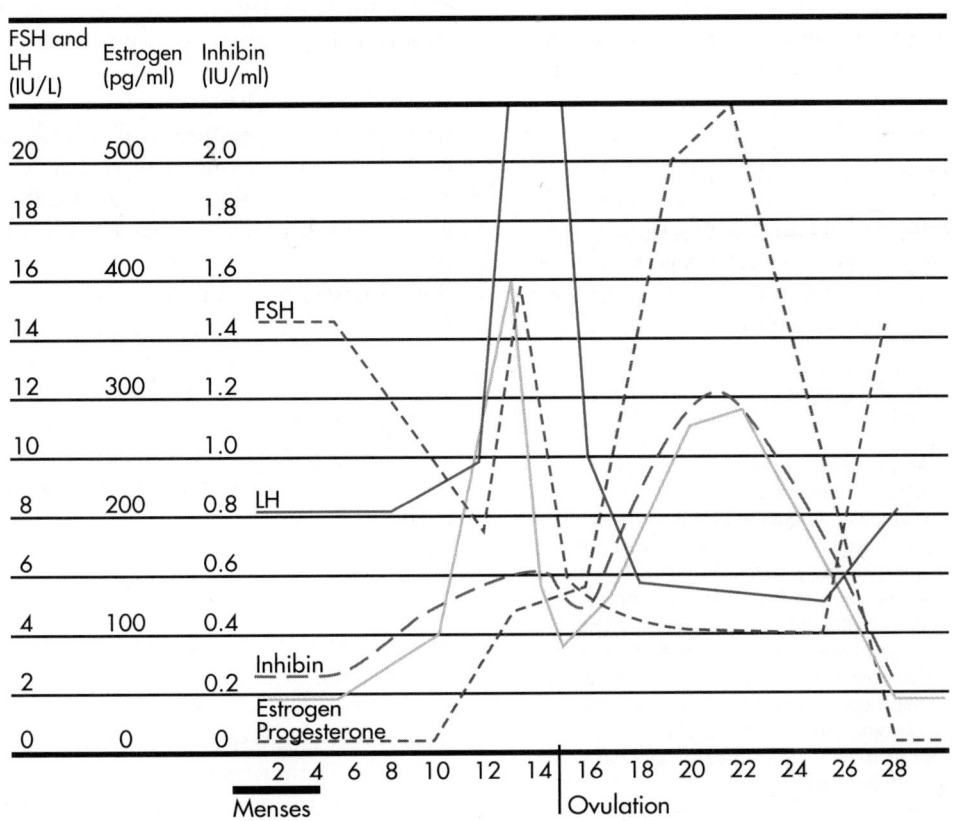

Figure 22-11 Estrogen, progesterone, gonadotropin, and inhibin fluctuations over the menstrual cycle. Inhibin rises slowly but steadily throughout the follicular phase, peaking at midcycle and again during the midluteal phase. The midcycle peak coincides with surges of luteinizing hormone (LH) and follicle-stimulating hormone (FSH).

tiply, increasing estradiol secretion. Within a few days of the cycle, one follicle becomes dominant and the others atrophy. The mechanism for follicular recruitment or dominance is unknown. Once dominance is acquired, it is not transferable but may be related to FSH receptors, blood supply, or the ability to convert androgens to estradiol. The dominant follicle begins to secrete progressively larger amounts of estradiol, which exerts a positive-feedback effect causing the LH surge. (The dynamic process of follicular growth is outlined in Box 22-1.) Ovulation generally occurs 1 to 2 hours before the final progesterone surge, or about 12 to 36 hours after the onset of the LH surge; specific timing may reflect seasonal variations. Progesterone, proteolytic enzymes, and prostaglandins (E and F series) trigger mechanisms controlling follicular rupture and release of the ovum.[1] Possible mechanisms include thinning, stretching, degradation, and digestion of the follicular wall and contraction of smooth muscle cells of the follicle. The role of prostaglandins is essential to ovulation, and infertility patients should be advised to avoid the use of drugs that inhibit prostaglandin synthesis.[15]

The LH surge also transforms the granulosa cells of the ovulatory follicle into the corpus luteum. The corpus luteum secretes both estrogen and progesterone in amounts that depend, in part, on adequate development of the follicle before ovulation. Progesterone acts both centrally and locally within the ovary to suppress new follicular growth during the early and midluteal phases. If pregnancy does not occur, the corpus luteum persists for 11 to 14 days and then regresses and eventually disappears. An increase in pulse frequency of GnRH from a low level reactivates hormonal control of the menstrual cycle.

Uterine Phases

Uterine phases of the menstrual cycle—proliferative, secretory, and ischemic/menstrual phases—involve cyclic endometrial changes controlled by estrogen and progesterone. Hormonal effects are influenced by the presence of receptors and numerous growth factors, peptides, and enzymes that act as intermediaries between the sex steroids and the endometrium.[3] During the midfollicular phase, increasing levels of estrogen contribute to endometrial repair and proliferation, thus increasing endometrial thickness. Once ovulation occurs and serum progesterone levels increase, the endometrial tissue develops secretory characteristics. If implantation of a fertilized ovum does not take place, endometrial tissue begins to break down approximately 11 days after ovulation. The period of breakdown is sometimes called the *ischemic phase* (see Figure 22-10). Sloughing of tissue (menstrual bleeding) begins about 14 days after ovulation.

Cervical mucus also undergoes cyclic changes. During the proliferative phase the cervical mucus is thin and watery. Peak estrogen levels occur just before ovulation and maximally stimulate the cervical glands to produce mucus. Cervical mucus becomes thicker and more elastic (spinnbarkeit). In the presence of estrogen, tiny channels develop in the mucus, which allows sperm access to the interior of the uterus. Changes in the consistency of cervical mucus can be used to identify fertile intervals.

Vaginal Response

Vaginal endothelium also responds to cyclic hormonal changes. Under the influence of estrogen, epithelial cells of the vagina grow maximally during the follicular/proliferative phase. After ovulation, layers of keratinized cells overgrow the basal epithelium, a process known as **cornification**. Near the end of the luteal phase, leukocytes invade vaginal epithelium, removing the outer layers in a process termed **decornification**.

Body Temperature

Basal body temperature (BBT) undergoes characteristic biphasic changes during menstrual cycles in which ovulation occurs. During the follicular phase the BBT fluctuates around 98° F (37° C). During the luteal phase, the average temperature increases by 0.4° to 1.0° F (0.2° to 0.5° C). At the end of the luteal phase, 1 to 3 days before the onset of menstruation, BBT declines to follicular-phase levels. The shift in temperature is related to ovulation, corpus luteum formation, and increased serum progesterone levels. Progesterone probably acts on the thermoregulatory center of the hypothalamus to increase body temperature. Changes in BBT are used to document ovulatory cycles but are not useful to predict the exact timing of ovulation.

THE MALE REPRODUCTIVE SYSTEM

In men the external genitalia perform the major functions of reproduction, which are to produce sperm and deliver them to the female reproductive tract.[16] Sperm are produced in the male gonads, the testes, and delivered to the female vagina by the penis. The internal male genitalia have a more accessory function. They consist of conducting tubes and fluid-producing glands, all of which aid in the transport of sperm from the testes to the urethral opening of the penis. The male reproductive and urinary structures are shown in Figure 22-12.

Box 22-1	Dynamic Process of Follicular Growth

Follicles grow and undergo atresia under all physiologic circumstances. Growth and atresia continue during pregnancy, ovulation, or periods of anovulation and occur at all ages from fetal development to menopause. Maximum number of oocytes (follicles) is found in the fetus at approximately 16 to 20 weeks of gestation. By birth, the number has diminished from 6 to 7 million to 2 million. By puberty, only about 300,000 oocytes remain. During a woman's reproductive years, fewer than 500 oocytes will mature and be released during ovulation. The number of follicles that begin developing during each cycle depends on the residual pool. As a woman ages, fewer numbers of follicles are recruited. Follicular loss accelerates about 10 to 15 years before menopause and seems to coincide with a follicular pool of 25,000.

Data from Kirtley Jones (reproductive endocrinologist): Personal communication, December 2000; Speroff L et al: *Clinical gynecologic endocrinology and fertility,* ed 6, Baltimore, 1999, Lippincott.

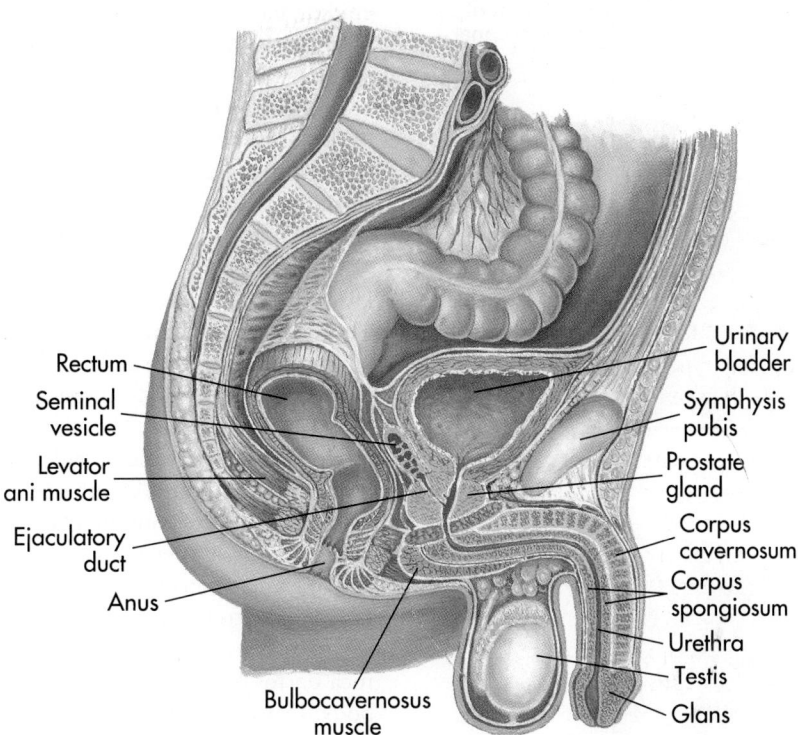

Figure 22-12 Structure of the male reproductive organs. (From Seidel HM et al: *Mosby's guide to physical examination,* ed 5, St Louis, 2003, Mosby.)

External Genitalia

Testes

In men the testes are the essential organs of reproduction. Like the ovaries, the testes have two functions: (1) production of gametes (in this case, sperm) and (2) production of sex hormones (in this case, androgens and testosterone). The testes are suspended outside the pelvic cavity because sperm production requires an environment that is 1° or 2° C cooler than body temperature.

During embryonic and fetal life, the testes develop within the abdomen (see Figure 22-1). Then, about 3 months before birth, the testes start to descend toward the developing scrotum. About 1 month before birth, they enter twin passageways called **inguinal canals.** The inguinal canals are vaginal processes created by outpouchings of the peritoneum (lining of the abdominal cavity). The descent of a **testis** is shown in Figure 22-13. Each testis moves down outside the peritoneum until it is suspended in the scrotal sac by its supply lines: the ducts, blood vessels, lymphatic vessels, and nerves of the **spermatic cord.** When descent is complete, the abdominal end of each vaginal process closes up and the inguinal canal disappears. If peritoneal closure at the site of the inguinal canal is incomplete or weak, an inguinal hernia may occur later in life. The scrotal end of each vaginal process becomes the outer covering of the testis, the **tunica vaginalis.**

Figure 22-14 shows a sagittal section of a mature testis. The adult testis is ovoid and varies considerably in length (3 to 6 cm), width (2 to 3.5 cm), depth (3 to 4 cm), and weight (10 to 40 g). The testis is almost entirely surrounded by an outer covering, the tunica vaginalis, which separates the testis from the scrotal wall, and an inner covering, the **tunica albuginea.** Inward extensions of the tunica albuginea form septa that separate the testis into about 250 compartments, or lobules, each of which contains several tortuously coiled ducts called **seminiferous tubules.** The seminiferous tubules constitute the bulk (80%) of testicular volume and are the site of sperm production. (Sperm production, termed **spermatogenesis,** is described on p. 755.) Tissue surrounding these ducts contains blood and lymphatic vessels, fibroblastic support cells, macrophages, mast cells, and Leydig cells. **Leydig cells,** which occur in clusters and account for about 1% to 5% of testicular volume, produce androgens, chiefly testosterone.

The two ends of each seminiferous tubule join and leave the lobule through a short, straight section called the **tubulus rectus.** Sperm travel from the seminiferous tubules into these straight sections, which lead to the central portion of the testis, the **rete testis.** From the rete testis, sperm move through the **efferent tubules,** or vasa efferentia, to the epididymis, where they mature.

The testes are innervated by adrenergic fibers, whose sole function apparently is to regulate blood flow to the Leydig cells. The testes receive arterial blood from the internal spermatic and differential arteries. Arterial blood flows over the surface of the testes before entering the parenchyma (functional tissues). Surface flow cools the blood to temperatures that promote spermatogenesis, approximately 1.8° to 3.6° F (1° to 2° C) below body core temperature.

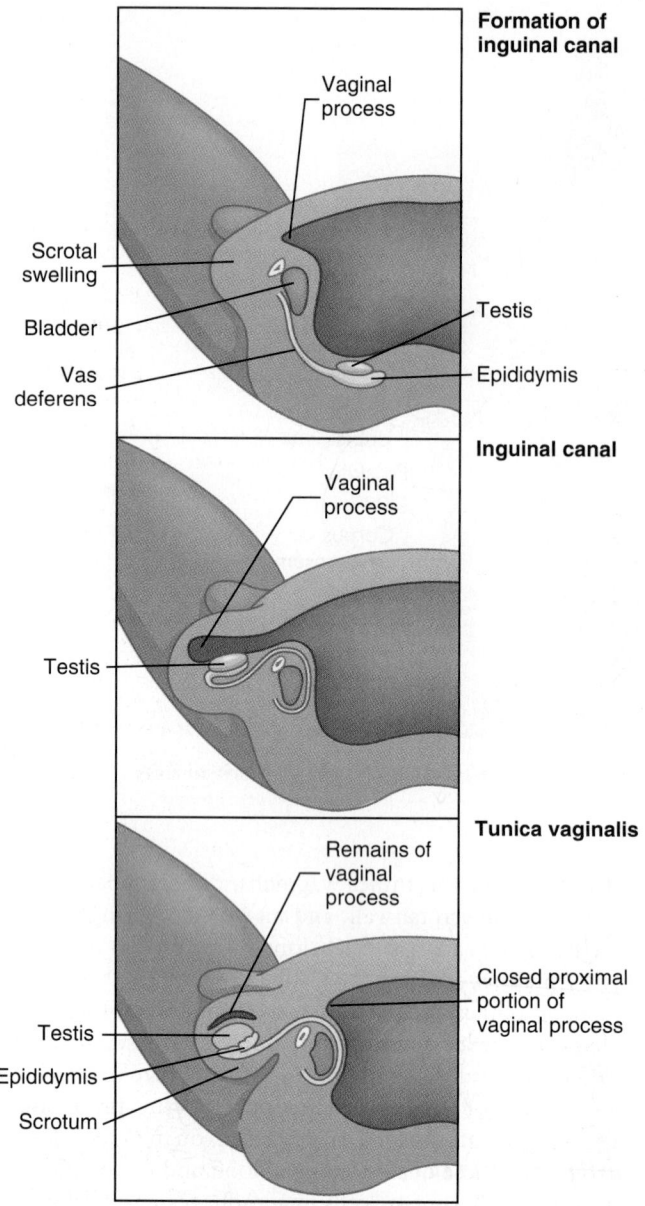

Figure 22-13 Descent of a testis. The testes descend from the abdominal cavity to the scrotum during the last 3 months of fetal development.

Epididymis

The **epididymis** (*plural,* epididymides) is a comma-shaped structure that curves over the posterior portion of each testis (see Figure 22-14). It consists of a single, highly packed, and markedly coiled (60 to 70 cm when uncoiled) duct measuring 5 cm long, whose structural function is to conduct sperm from the efferent tubules to the vas deferens. The duct can become inflamed from infection by microorganisms that ascend the urethra or from the prostate, causing epididymitis. The epididymis has physiologic functions as well. When sperm enter the head of the epididymis, they are not fully mature or motile, nor are they capable of fertilizing an ovum. During the 12 days (or more) sperm take to travel the length of the epididymis, they receive nutrients and testosterone from the

epididymal epithelium, and some biochemical or physiologic mechanism enhances their capacity for fertilization.

The tail of the epididymis is continuous with the **vas deferens (ductus deferens),** a duct with muscular layers capable of powerful peristalsis that transports sperm toward the urethra. After traveling the length of the epididymis, sperm are stored in the epididymal tail and vas deferens. The vas deferens enters the pelvic cavity through the spermatic cord.

Scrotum

The testes, epididymides, and spermatic cord are enclosed and protected by the scrotum. The **scrotum** is a skin-covered, fibromuscular sac that is homologous to the female labia majora (see Figure 22-2). The skin of the scrotum is thin and has rugae (wrinkles or folds), which enable it to enlarge or relax away from the body. At puberty the scrotal skin darkens, develops active sebaceous glands, and becomes sparsely covered with hair. Just under the skin lies a layer of connective tissue (fascia) and smooth muscle, the tunica dartos (see Figure 22-14). The **tunica dartos** also forms a septum that separates the two testes. Exposure to cold temperatures causes the tunica dartos to contract, pulling the testes close to the warm body. In warm temperatures the tunica dartos relaxes, suspending the testes away from body heat. These mechanisms promote optimal temperatures for spermatogenesis. In addition, scrotal sensitivity to touch, pressure, temperature, and pain protects the testes against potential harm. During sexual excitement, the scrotal skin and tunica thicken, the scrotum tightens and lifts, and the spermatic cords shorten, partially elevating the testes toward the body. As excitement plateaus, the engorged testes increase 50% in size, rotate anteriorly, and flatten against the body, signaling impending ejaculation.

Penis

The **penis** has two main functions: delivery of sperm to the female vagina and elimination of urine. (Urine formation and excretion are the subjects of Chapter 35.) Embryonically, the penis is homologous to the female clitoris (see Figure 22-2).

Figure 22-12 shows a sagittal section of the adult penis and its anatomic relation to other urogenital structures. Externally the penis consists of a shaft with a tip, the **glans,** which contains the opening of the urethra. For protection, the skin of the glans folds over the tip of the penis, forming the prepuce, or **foreskin.** At birth, the foreskin is adhered to the glans. Penile erections, which commonly occur, cause the adhesions to break so that by age 3 years the foreskin becomes completely retractable. The skin of the penis is continuous with that of the groin, scrotum, and inner thighs. It is hairless, movable, and darker than surrounding skin.

Internally, the penis consists of the urethra and three compartments: two **corpora cavernosa** and the **corpus spongiosum** (Figure 22-15). The three compartments are separated by Buck fascia and, like the testes, are enclosed by a tunica albuginea. The **urethra** passes through the corpus spongiosum and ends at a sagittal slit in the glans. If the urethra is not completely surrounded by the corpus spongiosum, the mea-

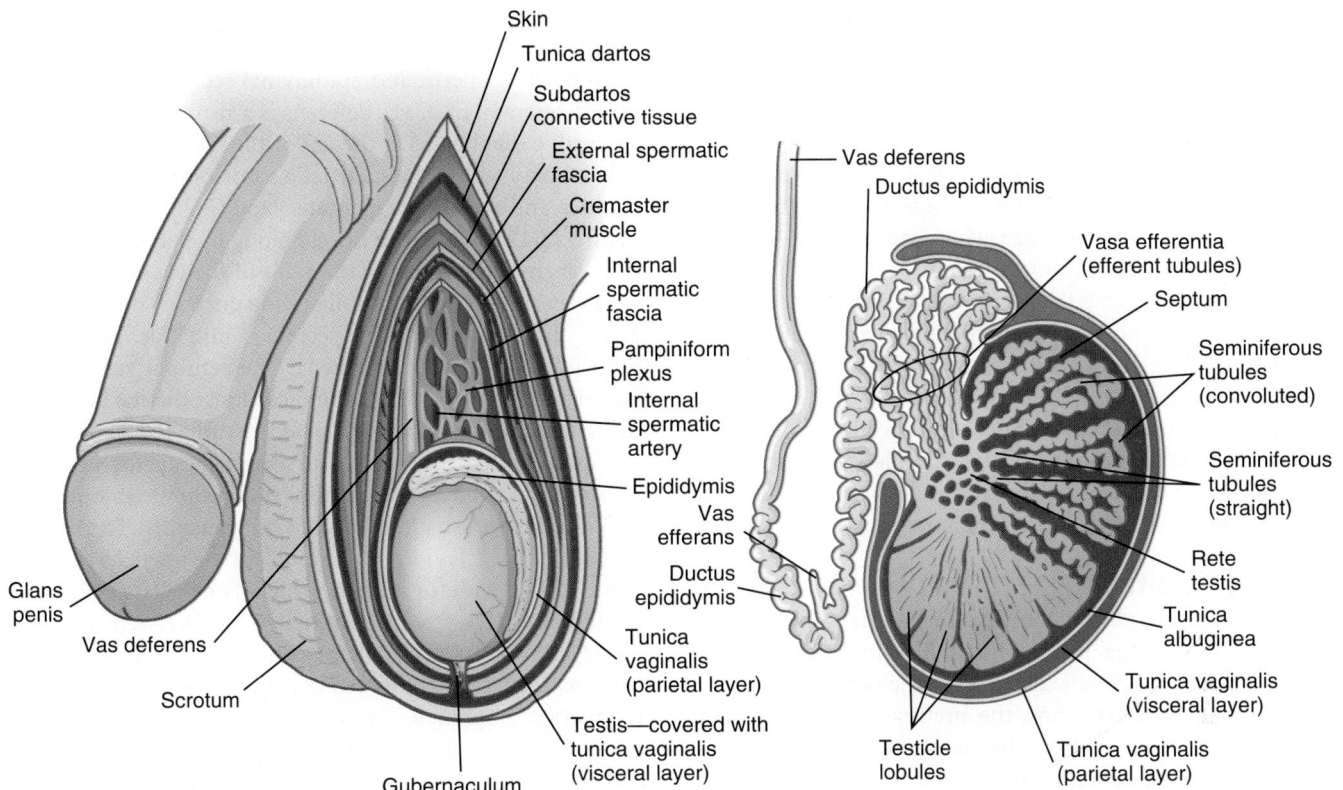

Figure 22-14 **The testes.** External and sagittal views showing interior anatomy. (Redrawn from Seidel HM et al: *Mosby's guide to physical examination,* ed 5, St Louis, 2003, Mosby.)

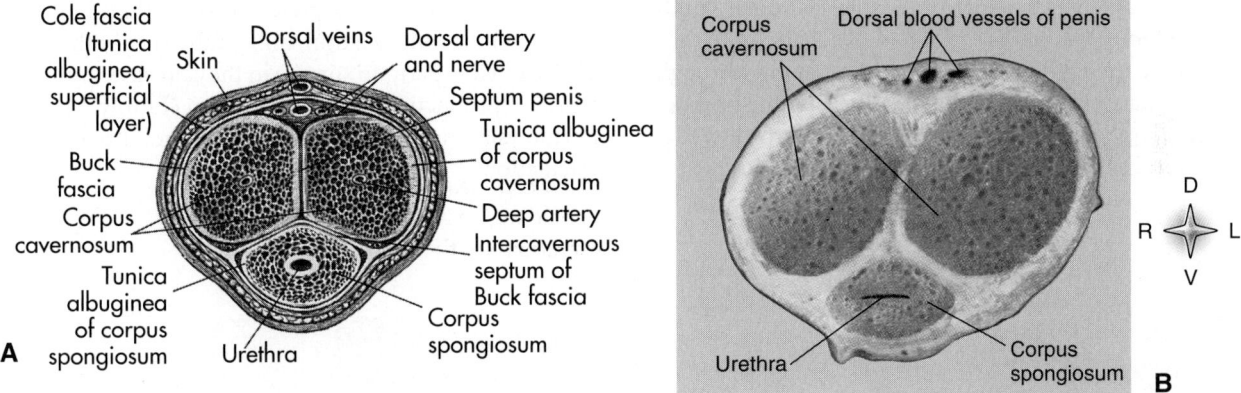

Figure 22-15 **The penis. A,** Cross section of the penis. **B,** Cross section of the shaft of the penis showing three columns of erectile, or cavernous, tissue. (**A,** From Thompson JM et al: *Mosby's clinical nursing,* ed 5, St Louis, 2002, Mosby. **B,** From Thibodeau GA, Patton KT: *Anatomy & physiology,* ed 5, St Louis, 2003, Mosby.)

tus may open on the ventral surface of the penile shaft (hypospadias) or on the dorsal surface (epispadias).

Penetration of the female vagina is made possible by the **erectile reflex,** a process in which erectile tissues within the corpora cavernosa and corpus spongiosum become engorged with blood, generally 20 to 50 ml. The erectile tissues consist of vascular spaces, or chambers, which are supplied with blood by arterioles (small arteries). Most of the time the arterioles are constricted, so that not much blood flows through the erectile tissues. Sexual stimulation, however, causes the arterioles to dilate and fill with blood. Their rapid expansion

fills the erectile tissues, causing an erection. Erection apparently is maintained by compression or constriction of veins that drain the corpora cavernosa and corpus spongiosum. When sexual stimulation ceases or orgasm and ejaculation occur, these veins open up, blood flows out of the arterioles, and the penis becomes flaccid (soft and pendulous).

Erection is under the control of the autonomic nervous system but can be stimulated or inhibited by central nervous system input. Stimulation of mechanoreceptors of the penis, particularly of the glans, causes parasympathetic nerves of the autonomic nervous system to relax smooth muscle in the walls of penile arterioles. At the same time the effects of sympathetic nerves, which normally cause arteriolar smooth muscle to constrict, are inhibited.

Erections begin in utero and continue throughout life, but ejaculation does not occur until sperm production begins at puberty. Growth of the penis and scrotal contents continues well past puberty, however, and may not be complete until the late teens or early 20s. Penis size, when flaccid, varies considerably; with an erection, differences in penis size diminish. Sexual excitement causes the corpora cavernosa to increase in length and width and become rigid; the penis becomes erect. Stimulation of the glans, which is endowed with copious sensitive nerve endings, provides maximum erotic sensation. With sexual arousal, skin color deepens, the glans doubles in size, and the urethral meatus dilates. Ejaculation occurs with frequent, strong contractions of the vas deferens, epididymis, seminal vesicles, prostate, urethra, and penis.[17]

Internal Genitalia

Figure 22-14 shows the anatomy of the internal genitalia and their relation to other pelvic organs. The internal genitalia consist of ducts and glands. The ducts—the two vasa deferentia, the ejaculatory duct, and the urethra—conduct sperm and glandular secretions from the testes to the urethral opening of the penis. The glands—the prostate gland, two seminal vesicles, and two Cowper (or bulbourethral) glands—secrete fluids that serve as a vehicle for sperm transport and create an alkaline, nutritious medium that promotes sperm motility and survival. Together, the sperm and the glandular fluids compose **semen.**

Sperm leave the epididymides and travel rapidly through the internal ducts in a process called **emission.** Emission occurs just seconds before ejaculation, at the moment when sexual arousal peaks. Emission always leads to ejaculation.

Emission occurs as smooth muscle in the walls of the epididymides and vasa deferentia begins to contract rhythmically, pushing sperm and epididymal secretions through the vasa deferentia. Each vas deferens is a firm, elastic, fibromuscular tube that begins at the tail of the epididymis, enters the pelvic cavity within the spermatic cord, loops up and over the bladder, and ends in the prostate gland (Figure 22-16; see also Figure 22-12). Sperm are moved along by peristaltic contractions of smooth muscle in the walls of the vas deferens.

As sperm leave the ampulla (wide portion) of the vas deferens, the seminal vesicles secrete a nutritive, glucose-rich fluid into the ejaculate (semen). The **seminal vesicles** are a pair of glands, each about 4 to 6 cm long, that lie behind the urinary bladder and in front of the rectum. The seminal vesicles provide fructose as a source of energy for ejaculated sperm, and secrete prostaglandins that promote smooth muscle contraction assisting with sperm transport. The ducts of the seminal vesicles join the ampulla of the vas deferens to become the **ejaculatory duct,** which contracts rhythmically during emission and ejaculation. As can be seen in Figures 22-12 and 22-16, the ejaculatory duct joins the urethra, where both pass through the prostate gland. During emission and ejaculation a sphincter (muscle surrounding a duct) closes, preventing urine from entering the prostatic urethra.

The **prostate gland** is composed of alveoli and ducts embedded in fibromuscular tissue. It measures 4 cm in diameter and weighs approximately 20 g. While semen moves through the prostatic portion of the urethra, the prostate gland contracts rhythmically and secretes prostatic fluid into the mixture. Prostatic fluid is a thin, milky substance with an alkaline pH that helps sperm to survive in the acid environment of the female reproductive tract. In addition, clotting enzymes and fibrinolysin in prostatic fluids help mobilize sperm after ejaculation.

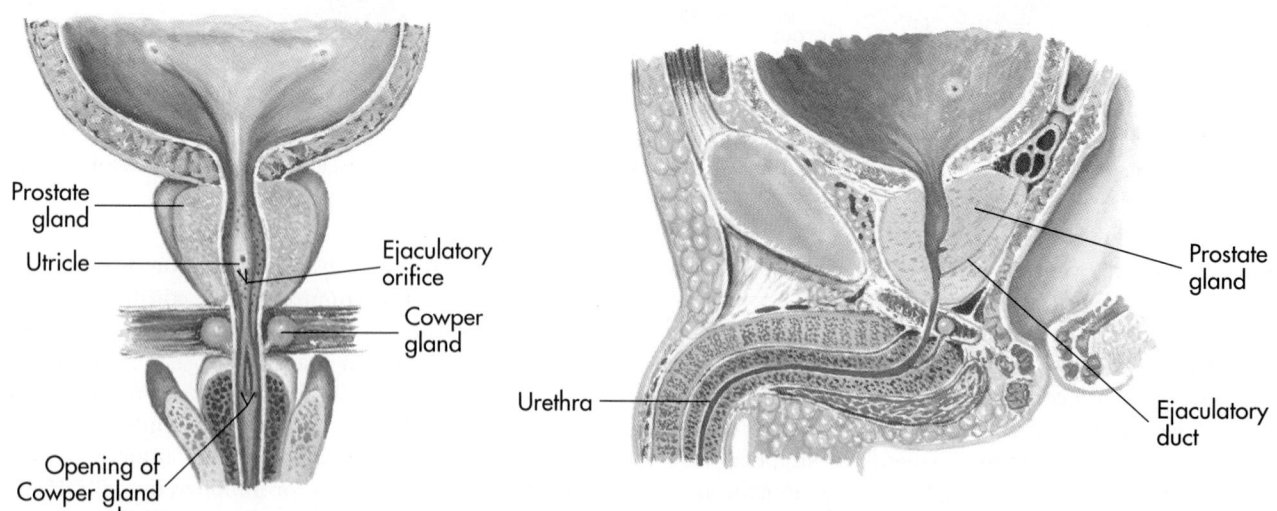

Figure 22-16 Anatomy of the prostate gland and seminal vesicles. (From Seidel HM et al: *Mosby's guide to physical examination,* ed 5, St Louis, 2003, Mosby.)

Cowper glands (bulbourethral glands), whose ducts secrete mucus into the urethra near the base of the penis, are the last pair of glands to add fluid to the ejaculate. Ejaculation occurs as semen reaches the base of the penis and muscles there begin the rhythmic contractions that push semen out. Normally a man ejaculates between 2 and 6 ml of semen, containing 75 million to 400 million sperm. About 98% of the ejaculate consists of glandular fluids; 60% to 70% of volume comes from the seminal vesicles and 20% from the prostate. Therefore the ejaculate of a man who has undergone vasectomy (a surgical procedure that prevents sperm from entering the vas deferens) is not reduced by much: about 2%.

Spermatogenesis

Spermatogenesis begins at puberty and continues for life. In this respect, spermatogenesis differs markedly from oogenesis (production of primordial ova), which occurs during fetal life only.

Spermatogenesis takes place within the seminiferous tubules of the testes (see Figure 22-14). The basement membrane of each seminiferous tubule is lined with diploid (46-chromosome) germ cells called **spermatogonia** (*singular,* spermatogonium). These cells undergo continuous mitotic division. (Mitotic division, in which a cell divides into two identical cells, is described in Chapter 1.) Some of the spermatogonia move away from the basement membrane and mature, becoming **primary spermatocytes** (Figure 22-17). The primary spermatocytes undergo meiosis, a type of cell division that results in two haploid (23-chromosome) cells called **secondary spermatocytes.** (Meiosis is described and illustrated in Chapter 4.) The two secondary spermatocytes then undergo meiosis, resulting in four **spermatids.** It is the spermatids that differentiate into spermatozoa, or sperm, each of which contains 23 chromosomes (Figure 22-18).

The development of spermatids into sperm depends on the presence of **Sertoli cells (nondividing support cells)** within the seminiferous tubules. The spermatids attach themselves to Sertoli cells, from which they receive the nutrients and the hormonal signals they need to develop into sperm.

The process of spermatogenesis, from mitotic division of a spermatogonium to maturation of the spermatids, takes about 70 to 80 days. Mature sperm migrate from the seminiferous tubules to the epididymis, where their capacity for fertilization continues to develop. Although they are completely mature by the time they are ejaculated, the sperm do not become motile (capable of movement) until they are activated by biochemicals in semen and in the female reproductive tract.

Male Sex Hormones

The male sex hormones are androgens. **Testosterone,** the primary male sex hormone, is an androgen. Mainly Leydig cells of the testes and, to a lesser degree, the adrenal glands produce testosterone and other androgens. In men, sex hormone production is relatively constant with some diurnal variation.

The androgens have a number of physiologic actions related to growth and development of male tissues and organs.

They are responsible for fetal differentiation and development of the male urogenital system and have some effects on the fetal brain. After birth, the Leydig cells become quiescent until activated by the gonadotropins during puberty. At puberty, androgens cause the sex organs to grow and secondary sex characteristics to develop.

Testosterone affects nervous and skeletal tissues, bone marrow, skin and hair, and sex organs. It has an anabolic effect on skeletal muscle tissue, thereby contributing to the difference in body weight and composition between men and women. Testosterone also stimulates growth of the musculature and cartilage of the larynx, causing a permanent deepening of the voice. Testosterone directly stimulates the bone marrow and indirectly stimulates renal erythropoietin production to achieve increased hemoglobin and hematocrit levels. Because sebaceous gland activity is stimulated by testosterone, acne may develop. In the presence of testosterone, hair becomes coarser in texture and facial hair, axillary hair, and pubic hair grow in male patterns. Later in life, testosterone causes baldness in genetically susceptible individuals. Testosterone is required for spermatogenesis and for secretion of fluid by the prostate gland, seminal vesicles, and Cowper glands. Testosterone is also associated with an increase in **libido** (sex drive). Other, less-understood, effects of testosterone include alterations in fatty acid and cholesterol metabolism.

The regulation of androgen production and spermatogenesis is achieved by a complex feedback system involving the extrahypothalamic central nervous system, the hypothalamus, the anterior pituitary, the testes, and the androgen-sensitive end organs. These relationships, which are essentially the same in women, are summarized in Figure 22-3. Extrahypothalamic influences include such variables as physiologic and psychologic stress, which may inhibit or augment hypothalamic activity. In the hypothalamus, neurotransmitters regulate GnRH synthesis and pulsatile release (about every 3 hours) into the hypophyseal portal veins. Norepinephrine stimulates GnRH secretion, and serotonin and dopamine inhibit GnRH secretion. GnRH is transported by portal flow to the median eminence of the pituitary gland, where it binds to receptors and stimulates the synthesis and secretion of gonadotropins, LH, and FSH. LH and FSH, which are named for their effects in the female reproductive system, have important effects on the male system as well. LH acts on the Leydig cells to regulate testosterone secretion. FSH acts on the seminiferous tubule Sertoli cells to promote spermatogenesis. FSH secretion is inhibited by inhibin secreted by the Sertoli cells. Similar to their action in the female gonad, inhibin functions as an autocrine/paracrine regulator in the male gonad. Inhibin inhibits proliferation of spermatogonia by regulating pituitary FSH levels. In addition, inhibin facilitates LH stimulation of androgen biosynthesis in Leydig cells.

Ninety-eight percent of testosterone, the major steroid hormone produced by the testis, binds to either **sex hormone–binding globulin (SHBG)** (40%) or albumin (48%). The remaining 2% remains unbound in the plasma and is free

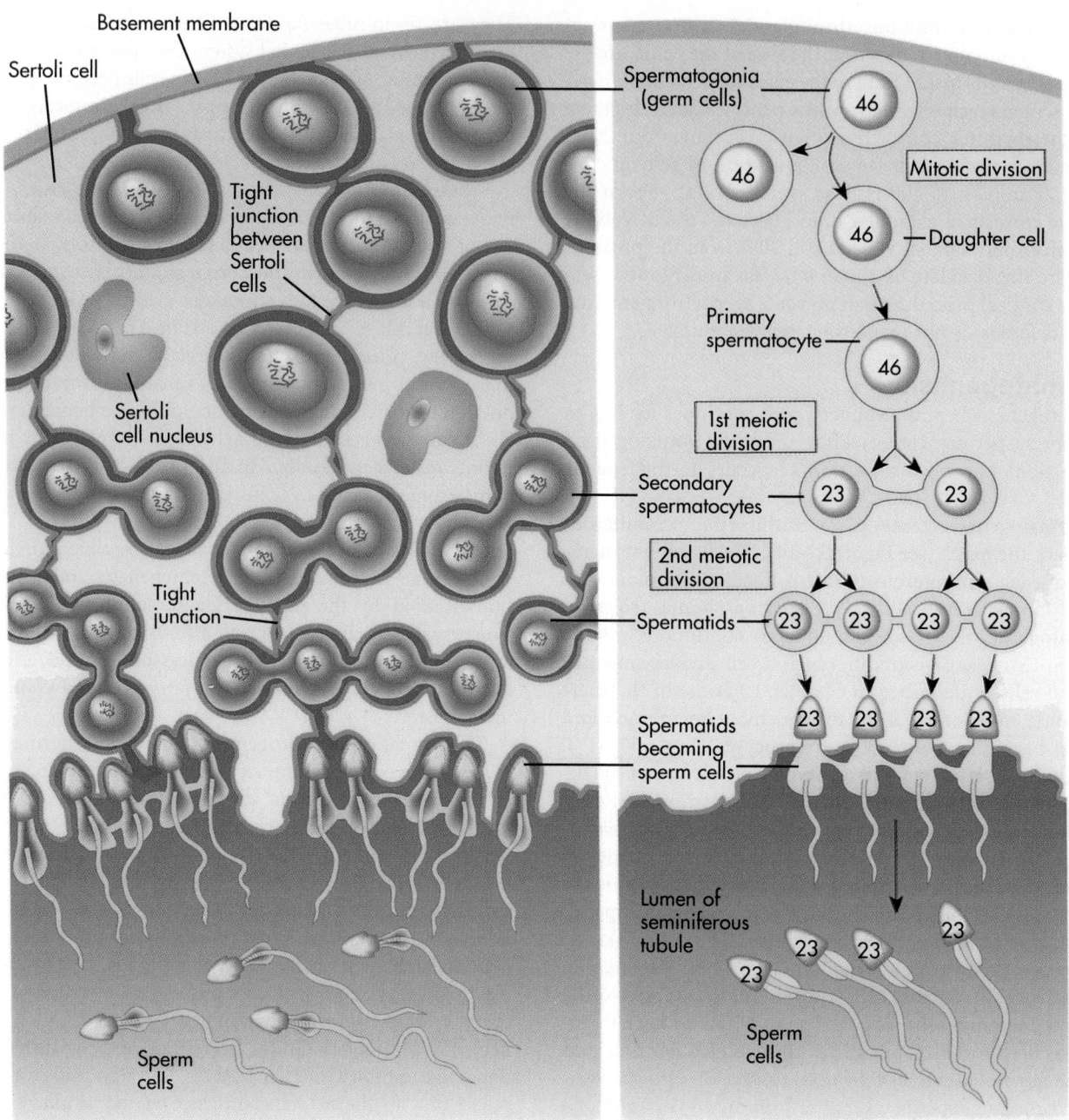

Figure 22-17 **Seminiferous tubule.** Section shows process of meiosis and sperm cell formation. (From Thibodeau GA, Patton KT: *Anatomy & physiology,* ed 5, St Louis, 2003, Mosby.)

to enter cells and wield its metabolic effects. Changes in the amount of available SHBG affect the amount of testosterone within tissues. The testis secretes only 25% of circulating estrogen (estradiol). The majority is produced by peripheral conversion of testosterone and androstenedione. Estrogens help regulate GnRH and LH secretion. Peripheral conversion of testosterone by 5-alpha-reductase also produces **dihydrotestosterone (DHT),** another potent androgen. DHT is necessary for external virilization during embryogenesis and androgen activity beginning at puberty and continuing throughout adulthood. **Prolactin,** a polypeptide synthesized and secreted from the pi-

tuitary, helps maintain biosynthesis of testosterone. However, elevated prolactin levels may suppress biosynthesis.[18]

In summary, hormones secreted at each level of the hypothalamic-pituitary-testicular (H-P-T) axis control and coordinate testicular function (Figure 22-19) This control is exerted through positive and negative feedback signals by (1) sex steroids that inhibit hypothalamic GnRH secretion and pituitary LH responsiveness to GnRH; and (2) testicular inhibin that inhibits pituitary FSH and, possibly, circulating estrogens (E2). Any disruption along the H-P-T axis may lead to hypogonadism or infertility.

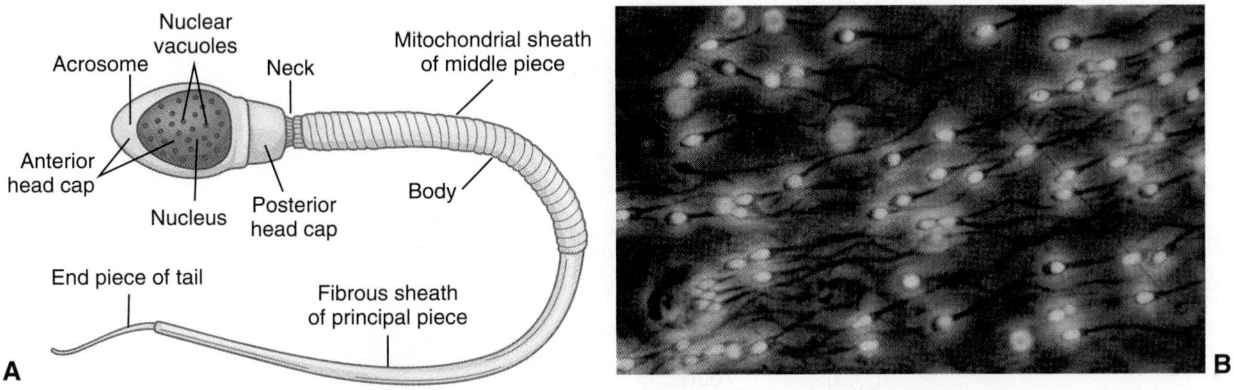

Figure 22-18 Mature sperm cell (**spermatozoon**). **A,** Anatomy of mature sperm cell. **B,** Human sperm with nuclear material glowing with a fluorescent dye. (**B,** From Thibodeau GA, Patton KT: *Anatomy & physiology,* ed 5, St Louis, 2003, Mosby.)

STRUCTURE AND FUNCTION OF THE BREAST

The **breasts** are modified sebaceous glands that lie on the ventral surface of the thorax, within the superficial fascia of the chest wall. They extend vertically from the second rib to the sixth or seventh intercostal space and laterally from the side of the sternum to the midaxillary line. Breast tissue also may extend into the axilla; this tissue is known as the *tail of Spence.*

The Female Breast

The female breast is composed of 15 to 20 pyramid-shaped lobes that are separated and supported by Cooper ligaments (Figure 22-20). Each lobe contains 20 to 40 lobules (alveoli), which subdivide further into many functional units called **acini** (*singular,* acinus). Each acinus is lined with a layer of epithelial cells capable of secreting milk and a layer of subepithelial cells capable of contracting to squeeze milk from the acinus. The acini empty into a network of lobular collecting ducts, which empty into interlobular collecting and ejecting ducts. These ducts reach the skin through openings (pores) in the nipple. The lobes and lobules are surrounded and separated by muscle strands and fatty connective tissue. The amount of fatty connective tissue varies from individual to individual, depending on weight and genetic and endocrine factors, and contributes to the diversity of breast size and shape.

An extensive capillary network surrounds the acini and is supplied by the internal and lateral thoracic arteries and the intercostal arteries. Venous return follows arterial supply, with relatively rapid emptying into the superior vena cava. The breasts receive sensory innervation from branches of the second through sixth intercostal nerves and the cervical plexus. This accounts for the fact that breast pain may be referred to the chest, back, scapula, medial arm, and neck. Lymphatic drainage of the breast occurs largely through axillary nodes, but approximately 25% occurs through transpectoral and internal mammary routes (Figure 22-21).

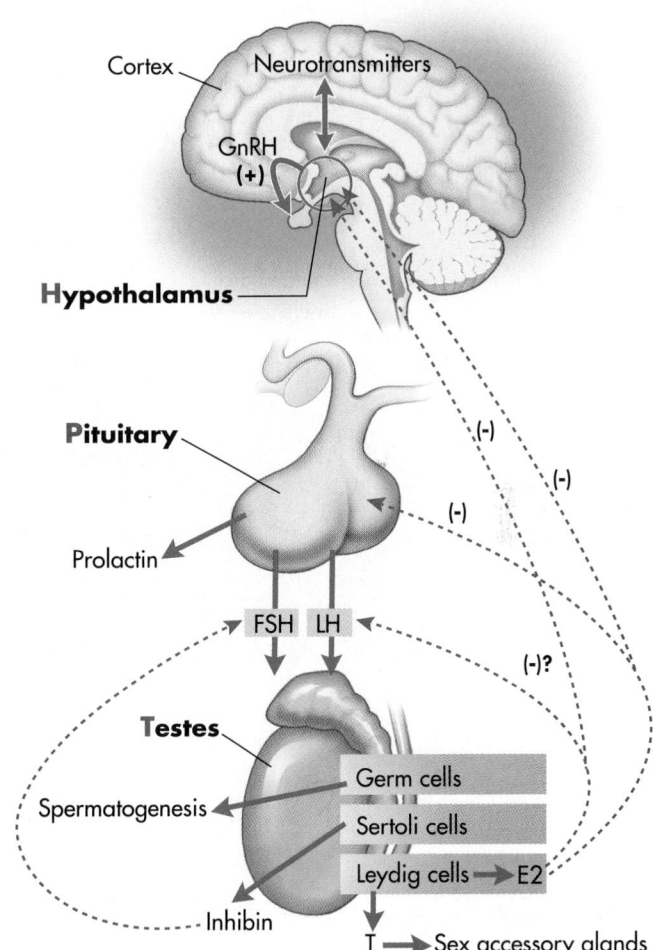

Figure 22-19 Schematic representation of activity along the H-P-T axis. *E2,* Estrogen; *T,* testosterone.

The **nipple** is a pigmented, cylindrical structure that is usually located at the fourth or fifth intercostal space. It measures 0.5 to 1.3 cm in diameter and is approximately 10 to 12 mm in height when erect. On its surface lie multiple openings, one from each lobe. The **areola** is the pigmented, circular area around the nipple. It may be 15 to 60 mm in diame-

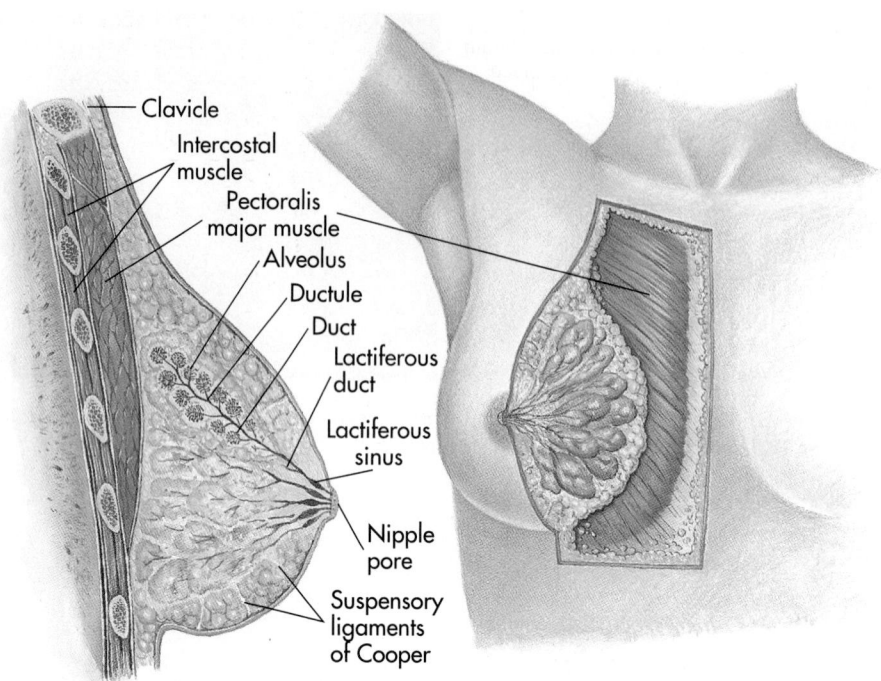

Figure 22-20 The female breast. (From Seidel HM et al: *Mosby's guide to physical examination,* ed 5, St Louis, 2003, Mosby.)

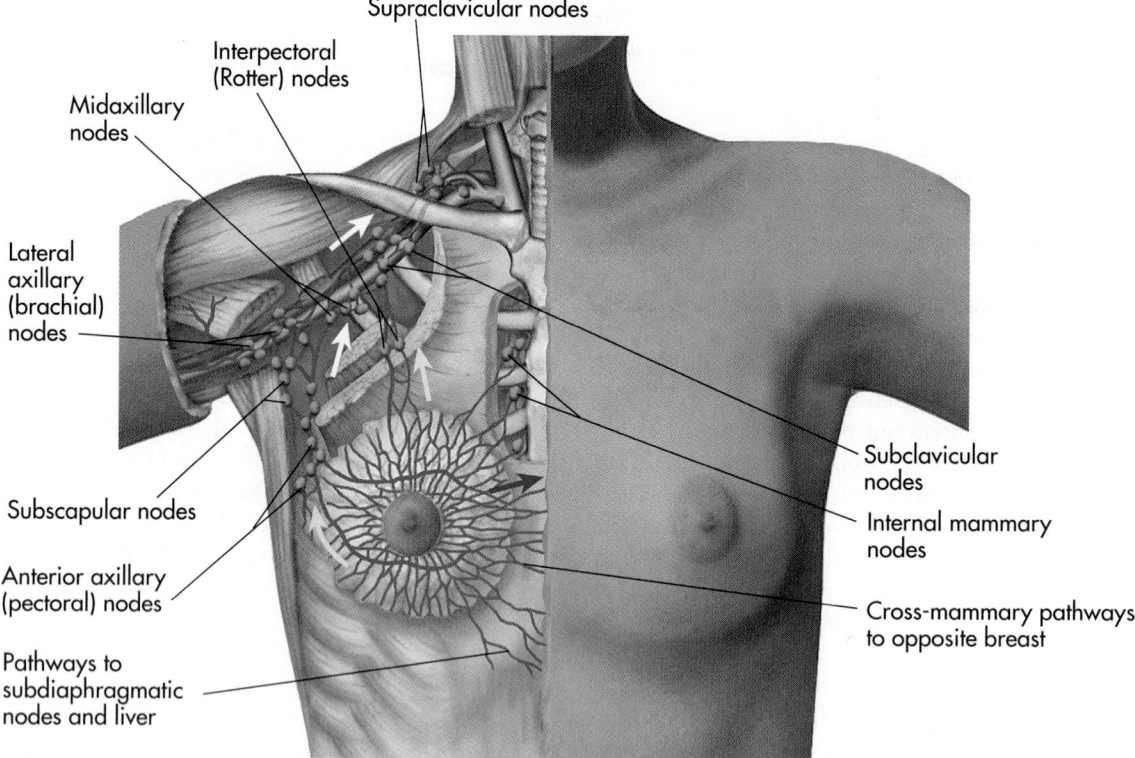

Figure 22-21 Lymphatic drainage of the female breast. (From Seidel HM et al: *Mosby's guide to physical examination,* ed 5, St Louis, 2003, Mosby.)

ter. A number of sebaceous glands, the **glands of Montgomery,** are located within the areola and aid in lubrication of the nipple during lactation. The nipple and areola contain smooth muscles, which receive motor innervation from the sympathetic nervous system. Sexual stimulation and exposure to cold cause the nipple to become erect.

The fetal and early postnatal development of breast tissue does not depend on hormones, although fetal breast tissue does become progressively responsive to hormonal stimulation. During childhood, breast growth is latent and growth of the nipple and areola keeps pace with body surface growth. (Male breast development normally does not progress any further.) At the onset of puberty in the female, estrogen secretion stimulates mammary growth. Breast development, or **thelarche,** is usually the first sign of puberty in the female. Full differentiation and maturation of breast tissue occur over approximately 4 years and are mediated by a variety of hormones, including estrogen, progesterone, prolactin, growth hormone, thyroid and parathyroid hormones, insulin, and cortisol. Estrogen promotes development of the lobular ducts; progesterone stimulates development of cells lining the acini. Lactation (milk production) occurs after childbirth in response to increased levels of prolactin. Prolactin secretion, in turn, increases by continued breast-feeding. Oxytocin, another hormone released during and after delivery, controls milk ejection from acini cells. Variations in breast development are listed in Box 22-2.

During the reproductive years, the breast undergoes cyclic changes in response to changes in the levels of estrogen and progesterone associated with the menstrual cycle. During the follicular/proliferative phase of the menstrual cycle, high estradiol levels increase the vascularity of breast tissue and stimulate proliferation of ductal and acinar tissue. This effect is sustained into the luteal/secretory phase of the cycle. During this phase, progesterone levels increase and contribute to the breast changes induced by estradiol. Specific effects of progesterone include dilation of the ducts and conversion of the acinar cells into secretory cells. Most women experience some degree of premenstrual breast fullness, tenderness, and increased nodularity. Breast volume may increase as much as 10 to 30 ml. Because the length of the menstrual cycle does not allow for complete regression of new cell growth, breast growth continues at a slow rate until approximately 35 years of age. Because of the cyclic changes that occur in breast tissue, breast examination should be conducted at the conclusion of or a few days after menses, when hormonal effects are minimal and breasts are at their smallest and least tender.

Box 22-2	Variations in Breast Development

- Ectopic breast development may occur in the axilla, abdomen, labia, or back and buttocks (less common) due to development of breast tissue from the milk line, an embryonic mammary ridge of ectoderm.
- Accessory nipples (polythelia) or mammary glands (polymastia) are due to cellular migration along the milk line; polythelia occurs in approximately 1% of the population.
- Failed development of the nipple (athelia) or entire mammary gland (amastia) is rare and may include a complete lack of development, unilateral failure, or extreme asymmetry.
- Symmetric or asymmetric hyperplasia occurs in approximately 1% to 4% of all females.
- In testicular feminization syndrome, the biologic action of testosterone is blocked and full mammary development occurs in a genetic male at puberty.
- In pubescent males, androgens fail to block the development of the mammary bud, which leads to transient unilateral or bilateral gynecomastia.

Data from Runowicz CD: Benign breast disease and screening for malignant tumors. In Copeland JL, Farrell JF, editors: *Textbook of gynecology,* ed 2, Philadelphia, 2000, Saunders.

The function of the female breast is primarily to provide a source of nourishment for the newborn. Physiologically, breast milk is the most appropriate nourishment for newborns. Not only does its composition change over time to meet the changing digestive capabilities and nutritional requirements of the infant but also breast milk contains specific immunoglobulins, especially IgA, and nonspecific antimicrobial factors, such as lysosomes and lactoferrin, which protect the infant against infection and allergies/asthma. Ongoing research suggests breast-feeding decreases future incidence in the infant of adult obesity, lowers cardiac disease, and lowers the incidence of types 1 and 2 diabetes. During lactation, high prolactin levels interfere with hypothalamic-pituitary hormones that stimulate ovulation. This mechanism suppresses the menstrual cycle and prevents ovulation. In many parts of the world (so-called underdeveloped or Third World countries), continuous and constant breast-feeding is the major means of contraception. Breasts are also a source of pleasurable sexual sensation and in Western cultures have become a sexual symbol.

The Male Breast

Until puberty, development of the male breast is similar to that of the female breast. In the absence of sufficiently high levels of estrogen and progesterone, the male breast does not develop any further. The normal male breast consists of a small, underdeveloped nipple; some fatty and fibrous tissue; and a few ductlike structures in the subareolar area. The male breast may appear enlarged in obese men because of accumulation of fatty tissue. During puberty some males experience gynecomastia, a condition in which the breasts enlarge temporarily as a result of hormonal fluctuations.

TESTS OF REPRODUCTIVE FUNCTION

Diagnostic tests of the male and female reproductive systems are performed to determine the cause of infertility, to detect the presence of cancerous lesions, or to identify the presence of sexually transmitted infections. (Alterations of the reproductive systems are discussed in Chapter 23; sexually transmitted infections are discussed in Chapter 24.) Procedures include laboratory tests, such as cultures, tests, stains, biopsies, serologic testing, and hormonal assays. Radiographic procedures are performed to identify abnormal growths or structures. Direct observation of reproductive organs is completed by laparoscopy or colposcopy.

Infection and Cancer Tests

Tests, stains, cultures, and serologic testing commonly are used to detect infectious diseases. Tests are prepared by spreading a layer of specimen material on a glass slide. The specimen may be evaluated microscopically as a wet mount or dried and stained with different dyes. Gram staining is a technique that allows the differential identification of two categories of bacteria according to the tendency of the microorganism to selectively absorb different components of the stain. Fluorescent antibody testing and deoxyribonucleic acid (DNA) probe testing (nucleic acid hybridization detection method) are fairly quick, inexpensive, and accurate methods that can be used to detect some bacterial and viral infections.

A **culture** is the growth of microorganisms in a nutrient medium selectively prepared to support the growth of particular microorganisms that are obtained from body secretions or tissues. Both bacteria and viruses, such as cytomegalovirus, can be cultured.

Serologic testing identifies whether an antigen-antibody reaction has occurred in response to an infectious microorganism. Several different techniques can be used to identify the formation of antigen-antibody complexes. With immunofluorescent testing, fluorescein-labeled antibodies react with specific antigen, such as the spirochetes of syphilis. The fluorescent pattern of the reaction can be microscopically observed under ultraviolet light. The flocculation (agglutination) test is the precipitation of clumped cells caused by the reaction of antigen with homologous antiserum. The Venereal Disease Research Laboratory (VDRL) test for syphilis is a type of flocculation test. Certain viral diseases can be diagnosed using specific serologic antibody markers, for example, the diagnosis of hepatitis A and hepatitis B viruses. Radioimmunoassay (RIA) and enzyme-linked immunosorbent assay (ELISA) are more specific tests used to document viral infections. Tests used for the diagnosis of sexually transmitted infections are presented in Table 22-3.

Table 22-3	Diagnosis of Sexually Transmitted Infections	
Test	**Description**	**Normal Value**
Serologic Test for Syphilis	Detection of antibodies to *Treponema pallidum*	Negative or nonreactive
VDRL	Venereal Disease Research Laboratory (nonspecific)	
RPR	Rapid plasma reagin (more specific)	
FTA	Fluorescent treponemal antibody absorption test (more specific; confirmatory test)	
Other Test for Syphilis		
Darkfield examination	Direct smear of serous exudate from moist lesions to detect *Treponema pallidum* with corkscrew appearance	Negative
Tests for Gonorrhea		
Culture	Isolation and detection of *Neisseria gonorrhoeae* in urethral, anal, or pharyngeal secretions	No growth
Gram stain	Direct smear and staining of cervical or urethral discharge to identify gram-negative intracellular diplococci with polymorphonuclear (PMN) leukocytes	Negative
DNA probe	Direct detection of DNA (inexpensive and quick)	Negative
Tests for *Chlamydia*		
Tissue culture	Isolation and detection of *Chlamydia trachomatis* from epithelial cells of endocervix and urethra (expensive, time extensive)	No growth
Cervical wet mount	A wet mount preparation of endocervical secretions (EC) can accurately rule out the presence of gonococci and *Chlamydia trachomatis*	EC WBC <5
Antigen detection of DNA probe	Direct immunofluorescent staining of cervical or urethral specimens to detect monoclonal antibodies or genetic probe to detect DNA sequence (both are inexpensive, quick)	Negative
Urine DNA amplification	Universal screening is more effective; future studies are recommended	Negative
Tests for HIV Infection		
ELISA (enzyme-linked immunosorbent assay)	Detects the presence of antibodies to human immunodeficiency virus (HIV)	Nonreactive
IFA (indirect fluorescent antibody)	A more specific test for HIV	Nonreactive
WB (Western blot)	A more specific test for HIV	Nonreactive
Tests for Viral Infections		
TORCH test	Detects elevations of IgA or IgM caused by *Toxoplasma*, rubella, cytomegalovirus, syphilis, and herpes simplex in mother and newborn infant; herpes requires more specific testing when result is positive	No elevation in antibodies
Cytomegalovirus (herpes virus 5)	Can be grown in cell culture with samples from urine, cervix, semen, saliva, blood	No growth
HPV testing	Detects human papillomavirus, a primary cause of cervical cancer	Negative

DNA, Deoxyribonucleic acid; *TORCH*, toxoplasmosis, other, cytomegalovirus, herpes simplex; *IgA*, immunoglobulin A; *IgM*, immunoglobulin M.

Tissue biopsy is the surgical resection of a tissue specimen from a suspected site. The biopsy provides cells and tissues to be used to identify infectious processes and to differentiate benign from malignant conditions and primary from metastatic lesions. In the reproductive tract, tissue may be obtained from the vagina, cervix (by cone or brush biopsy), endometrium of the uterus (by curettage), ovary, testis, prostate, or penis.

Needle biopsy is a technique of aspirating small amounts of tissue by positioning a needle in the tissue and applying negative pressure by pulling back on the plunger of the attached syringe as the needle is moved back and forth at the biopsy site. There is relatively less discomfort with this procedure than with a tissue biopsy that requires opening the surface of the skin to localize the tissue site. Normal findings indicate no abnormal cells or tissues on histologic examination.

The **Papanicolaou (Pap) test** is a procedure commonly used for the **cytologic examination** of the female reproductive tract. Cells from body tissues and fluids (from the vagina or cervix) are stained and examined for the number and types of cells and abnormalities in their morphology. Specimens also may be obtained from the mouth; nipple discharge; or amniotic, pleural, or spinal fluid aspirations. The Pap test is particularly useful for diagnosis of premalignant (dysplastic), malignant, atypical, and inflammatory cells. Because of the increased prevalence of Pap test screening, the rate of invasive cervical cancer has declined steadily over the past 30 years from 55% to 16%. Pap test screening is no longer necessary annually if the woman is over 30, has had 3 negative Pap tests, and is in a mutually monogamous relationship. She may consider Pap tests every 2 to 3 years.[19]

Evaluations of the breast are commonly performed to detect tumors or to differentiate solid masses from cysts and benign from malignant tumors. Screening or diagnostic **mammography,** surgical or **fine needle biopsy,** and **ultrasonography** are specific examination techniques. Less common tests include thermography, which is used for screening; chest x-rays, which are used to detect pulmonary metastases; and computed tomography (CT) scanning, which is used when liver or brain metastases are suspected. Mammography is a low-dose radiographic examination used to identify nonpalpable (less than 1 cm) or unrecognized lesions. Breast cancer can be detected by radiography 2 to 3 years before its clinical presentation, providing an excellent prognosis for cure. The American Cancer Society recommends a baseline mammogram of all women at 40 years of age, annual or biannual mammograms between 40 and 49 years of age, and yearly mammograms after 50 years of age.[20]

Ultrasonography is performed chiefly to differentiate cystic from solid lesions; it is not diagnostic of malignancy. Fine needle aspiration, an inexpensive and relatively simple procedure, is used to aspirate cysts or to obtain a specimen for cytologic examination. The main problem with any needle biopsy, or aspiration, is sampling error caused by improper positioning of the needle, which creates false-negative test results. The rate of false-positive results with fine needle aspiration is 1% to 2%; the rate of false-negative results is 10%.[7]

Fertility Tests

Tests of reproductive function are performed most commonly when infertility exists. Both the male and female partners are examined, and several diagnostic evaluations may be completed. The types of tests and their normal values are summarized in Tables 22-4 and 22-5. The man is evaluated for number, amount, structure, and motility of sperm and obstruction along the reproductive tract. Tests for women determine whether (1) the reproductive tract (cervix, uterus, fallopian tubes) is adequately patent to allow for passage of ovum and sperm, (2) ovulation occurs normally, (3) the endometrium is responding normally to hormones, and (4) reproductive tissues are free of tumors or infections. Hormonal assays evaluate the adequacy of pituitary function and target organ response. The position and size of organs or the presence of tumors can be detected by direct observation procedures using a laparoscope or by radiographic studies, such as plain films, computerized scans, or tomography.

AGING AND REPRODUCTIVE FUNCTION
Aging and the Female Reproductive System

Menopause is a normal developmental event that is experienced universally by midlife women. In the United States, women reach menopause between ages 48 and 55 years, at a median age of 51.4 years.[12] The mean age for smokers is 2 years sooner than nonsmokers (50 versus 52 years).[12,21] Age of menopause tends to be genetically predetermined and does not appear to be affected by age at menarche, childbearing or lactation, use of oral contraceptives, socioeconomic class, or race. Besides smoking, younger age at menopause has been associated with abnormal chromosome karyotype (Turner syndrome, gonadal dysgenesis) and undernourishment. Thinner women experience menopause at a slightly younger age, probably related to body fat. Irregular menses in women in their early forties also may be a predictor of an earlier menopause. Alcohol consumption has been associated with later menopause, perhaps because of higher blood and urinary levels of estrogen.[12]

Perimenopause is the transitional period between reproductive and nonreproductive years, a transition lasting 2 to 8 years.[12] Five to 10 years before menopause, approximately 90% of women note mild to extreme variability in frequency and quality of menstrual flow. Perimenopause symptoms depend on the sensitivity of the target tissue receptors. Symptoms usually begin with a shortening of the menstrual cycle, which correlates with shorter follicular phase (FP) lengths, followed by unpredictable or irregular ovulation and a lengthening of the menstrual cycle. Whether early or late, lengthening of cycles uniformly precedes menopause.[1] The perimenopause experience varies between women and from cycle to cycle in the same woman, just as the menstrual experience does in younger, fertile women. It is not uncommon

Table 22-4	Tests and Normal Values of Reproductive Function/Fertility	
Test	**Description**	**Normal Value**
Basic Assessment		
Semen analysis (2 samples at least 2 weeks apart)	Determines number, motility, and structure of sperm cells	Volume = 2-6 ml Number = >20 million/ml Motility = >50% with forward progression Morphology = >30% normal shape Immunobead test = <20% with adherent particles Sperm Mar test = <10% with adherent particles
	Determines presence of bacteria/leukocytes	<10^6 WBC/ml
Antisperm antibody	Detects antibody to sperm	No sperm agglutinins present
Intermediate Assessment		
Basal body temperature	Determines whether ovulation has occurred	Decrease in basal body temperature before ovulation followed by a rise in temperature at the time of ovulation
FSH level	Day 3 of cycle	Lab specific results
Cervical mucus	Evaluates presence of ovulation from estrogenic effects at ovulation; mucus also may be examined for pH, glucose, or proteins or cultured for presence of infection	Fern pattern appears when cervical mucus dries on a clean slide; mucus is clear, watery, and elastic (spinnbarkeit ≥8-10 cm) with no inflammatory cells
Postcoital cervical mucus (Sims-Huhner test)	Tests ability of sperm to penetrate and maintain motility in cervical mucus 2-4 hours after coitus approximately 1 day before ovulation	≥10 motile sperm in each high-power field; motility in one direction; previous sperm analysis normal
Zona binding test or Hamster penetration test	Nonliving oocytes are surgically removed and bisected; sperm added to the hemioocyte to test fertilizing capability	Bonding <30% predicted failed fertilization 70% of the time Bonding >30% predicted successful fertilization 85% of the time Results may vary with lab
Ultrasound vaginal scanning	Provides superior quality resolution of the uterine, fallopian, and ovarian structures; also can be used to study folliculogenesis, ovulation, and luteogenesis to detect abnormalities	Normal structures visualized
More Specialized Tests		
Endometrial biopsy	Determines whether ovulation has occurred by obtaining endometrial tissue on day 26 of 28-day menstrual cycle (or postovulatory day 12)	Finding is "secretory-type" endometrium if ovulation has occurred; read in conjunction with day of cycle and serum progesterone levels
Hysterosalpingogram	Assessment of uterus and fallopian tubes for obstructions using transuterine injection of contrast material and radiography; performed 1-2 days after cessation of menses	No obstruction evident
Laparoscopy (pelvic endoscopy)	Visualization of reproductive organs using a laparoscope inserted within the pelvic cavity through the abdomen to assess structure or determine presence of adhesions, endometriosis, tumors, or infection	Normal structure and position of organs
Hysteroscopy	Visualization of uterine cavity using modified cystoscope inserted through cervical os; best done during first 14 days of cycle	Absence of intrauterine lesions

WBC, White blood cells.

for a woman to experience a short cycle with shortened FP, ovulation, and insufficient luteal phase (LP); followed by a long cycle with extended FP, anovulation, and high E2 levels in the premenstrual phase; followed by a short FP, anovulatory cycle. Variability in cycle length is the norm, and response to the ever-changing hormonal milieu is individual.

Around 37 to 38 years of age, 10 to 15 years before menstruation ceases, women experience accelerated follicular loss that begins when the total number of follicles reaches about 25,000 and ends when the supply of follicles is depleted (see discussion under Hormonal Controls, earlier in this chapter). This loss correlates with a subtle but definite increase in FSH and a decrease in inhibin. Increased FSH stimulation seems to accelerate follicular loss, and declining inhibin production disturbs the negative feedback influence over pituitary secretion of FSH. Perimenopausal cycles are marked by elevated FSH, decreased inhibin, normal LH, and slightly elevated estradiol levels[1] (Figure 22-22). A hallmark characteristic of

Table 22-5   Serum Hormone Values

Hormone	Value
Serum progesterone	Normal = >10 ng/dl, presumptive evidence of ovulation; draw level between days 20-25 of 28-day cycle or 6-10 days post ovulation <10 ng/ml = inadequate luteal function <3 ng/ml suggests anovulation
Serum testosterone	Normal = 300-1200 ng/dl; must be interpreted with serum LH and FSH levels
Resulting from diurnal and pulsatile pattern, need serial blood draws	Low values in male hypogonadism
Serum FSH and LH	FSH = <22 international units/L
Resulting from diurnal and pulsatile pattern, need serial blood draws	LH = 4-24 international units/L High levels in males indicate primary testicular disease; low levels in males indicate hypogonadism caused by hypothalamic-pituitary dysfunction

LH, Luteinizing hormone; *FSH,* follicle-stimulation hormone.

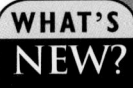

WHAT'S NEW? Women's Health Initiative (WHI) Study and Hormone Replacement Therapy (HRT)

The WHI was a randomized primary-prevention trial of 0.625 mg/day conjugated equine estrogen plus 2.5 mg/day of medroxyprogesterone acetate (*n* = 8506) or placebo (*n* = 8102). After 5.2 years of study (planned duration 8.5 years), the data and safety monitoring board recommended terminating the estrogen-plus-progestin trial because the overall risks exceeded the benefits. Coronary heart disease (in women with previous coronary heart disease) and venous thromboembolism both increased after 1 year of HRT use. Breast cancer and stroke increased beyond the threshold of acceptable risk after 5 years of use. Colorectal cancer and osteoporosis both declined. Current recommendations include using the smallest dose of hormones and only when there is quality of life issues associated with the onset of menopause (hot flashes, night sweats, etc.) and discontinuing use within 1 to 4 years. Long-term effects of even low-dose hormone levels have not been studied. Bioidentical hormones, herbs, foods and supplements containing isoflavones, omega-3, exercise, and SSRIs are currently under investigator for safety and effectiveness for treatment of perimenopausal/postmenopausal symptoms.

Data from Krebs EE et al: *Obstet Gynecol* 104(4):824-836, 2004; Manson JE et al: *N Engl J Med* 349(6):523-534, 2003; Nelson HD: *JAMA* 291(13):1621-1625, 2004; Warren MP: *Am J Obstet Gynecol* 190(4):1141-1167, 2004; Wassertheil-Smoller S et al: *JAMA* 289(20):2673-2684, 2003.

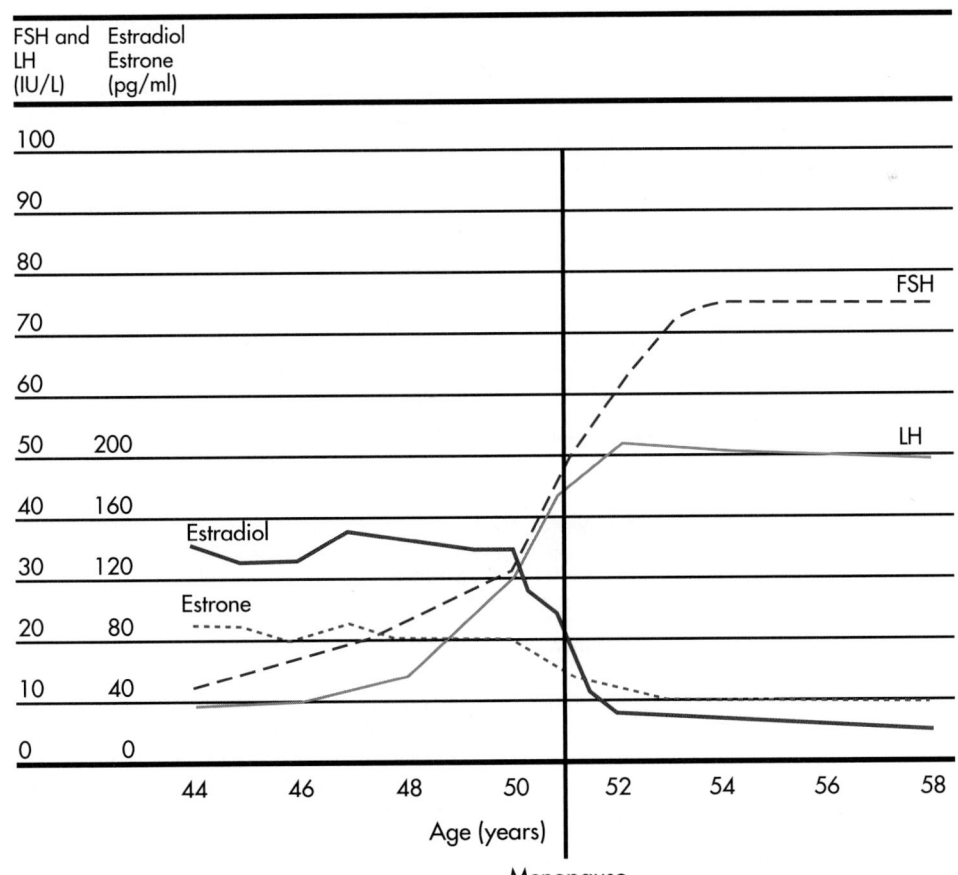

Figure 22-22 The perimenopausal transition. Mean circulating hormone levels. (From Speroff L et al: *Clinical gynecologic endocrinology and fertility,* ed 6, Baltimore, 1999, Lippincott.)

impending menopause is the initial "monotropic" FP increase in FSH without corresponding changes in LH levels. Lower inhibin B and increased activin A (a potent stimulator of FSH) levels contribute to this phenomenon.[1]

Increased FSH levels and reduced ovarian secretion of inhibin reflect quality and capability of aging follicles. In a study of pregnancy rates during in vitro fertilization (IVF), women over 40 years of age had as many oocytes recovered during laparoscopy, equal estrogen and progesterone levels, and similar pregnancy rates when compared with younger women. Yet, despite similar estradiol (E2) levels, inhibin response to exogenous hyperstimulation was significantly lower in the older women. Further, inhibin levels were significantly related to progesterone levels. In this study, 60% of women over 40 years of age who became pregnant through IVF spontaneously aborted, compared with 30% of younger women.[22]

In summary, hormonal findings during the years surrounding menopause indicate that the process of folliculogenesis changes (Box 22-3). Initially, FSH levels are significantly elevated whereas pulsatile secretion by the pituitary is maintained. Later, LH levels rise. In younger women, FSH stimulates inhibin, which in turn suppresses FSH. However, through an undetermined mechanism, perimenopausal women produce high levels of FSH in early FP and lower FP inhibin levels. The ovary, in response to high FSH, recruits increasing numbers of follicles; these follicles only partially develop, with a net effect of irregular ovulation, lower progesterone levels, and depleted follicle reserve. The increase in developing follicles leads to increased E2 levels. It is believed that lower levels of inhibin and higher levels of activin counteract the usual impact of the negative feedback loop found in younger women.[22] Table 22-6 summarizes endocrine events occurring during the perimenopause.

The majority of health concerns and public health issues focus on menstrual cycle changes, **vasomotor symptoms,** or hot flashes/flushes, potential for bone loss (osteoporosis is discussed in Chapter 42), and the emotional symptoms that may accompany the perimenopausal transition.[22,23] Heavy menstrual bleeding, menorrhagia (flooding), is one of the most distressing complaints and affects approximately 50% of women. It is also the complaint that in the past put women at high risk for hysterectomy. Increased endometrial bleeding is correlated with a change from ovulatory to anovulatory cycles and is associated with unopposed high E2 levels the week before menses. Estrogen causes endometrial tissue to thicken. Because women with anovulatory cycles have longer exposure to periods of unopposed estrogen, the mean thickness of their endometrium, as measured by ultrasound, can be greater than that of ovulatory women.[22,23] Thicker endometrium without corresponding stromal support from progesterone production leads to heavier periods, menorrhagia, or midcycle bleeding, metrorrhagia[7] (Table 22-7).

In the United States, most women and clinicians link hot flashes/flushes, or **vasomotor flush,** with menopause and low estrogen levels. However, a rapid change in estrogen levels (withdrawal or increase), rather than low estrogen levels, induces hot flushes. Vasomotor symptoms are characterized by a rise in skin temperature, dilation of peripheral blood vessels, increased blood flow to the hands, increased skin conductance, and transient increase in heart rate (average of 9 beats per minute and up to 20), followed by a temperature drop and profuse perspiration over the area of flush distribution. Vasomotor flush usually occurs in the face and neck and may radiate into the chest and other parts of the body. Dizziness, nausea, headaches, or palpitations may accompany the flush. Vasomotor symptoms vary in frequency, intensity, and duration, lasting 1 to 5 minutes (mean 2.7 minutes). Any-

---

Box 22-3	Changes in Ovarian Folliculogenesis During the Perimenopause Leading to Endogenous Overstimulation

- ↑ FSH → ovarian hyperstimulation → ↑ number of follicles recruited (net effect of follicular depletion) → ↑ estrogen (E2)
- ↓ Follicular reserve → ↓ inhibin and ↑ activin in FP and LP → ↑ FSH → ↑ number of follicles recruited, partial development, infrequent ovulation → ↑ estrogen (E2) and ↓ progesterone

FP, Follicular phase; *LP,* luteal phase; *FSH,* follicle-stimulating hormone.

Table 22-6	Endocrine Events Associated With Perimenopause
Hormone Changes	**Effects**
Estradiol (E2) levels	Erratic and intermittent increase
Mean FP level 1 greater than mean FP level in younger women	First in FP (inverse relationship between length of FP and estradiol level)
FP level may be greater than midcycle peak level in fertile women	Later during premenstrual phase
Ovulatory cycles	Short or insufficient LP (decreased fertility)
Progesterone levels	Decreased in ovulatory cycle; minimal during anovulatory cycles
Anovulatory cycles	Increased to about 50%; perhaps more in later perimenopause
FSH levels	Variable, then increased
LH levels	Normal initially, then increased
Inhibin levels	Correlate with progesterone levels

FP, Follicular phase; *FSH,* follicle-stimulating hormone; *LH,* luteinizing hormone; *LP,* luteal phase.

Table 22-7   Impact of High Estrogen Levels on Menstrual Cycle and Symptomatology

Associated Physiologic Change	Signs/Symptoms
Short follicular phase (FP)	Short cycles
Long FP	Long cycles
Thickened endometrium*	Heavy, long, or unpredictable flow (including clotting and flooding)*
Increase in glandular cells without stromal support produced by progesterone → unstable endometrium	Midcycle spotting
Possible increased production of prostaglandins within endometrial tissue	Menorrhagia
	Metrorrhagia
	Dysmenorrhea
	Breast tenderness, modularity, enlargement
	Water retention
	Emotional stress; new or unpredictable mood swings
	Weight gain
	Vasomotor symptoms
	New onset of migraine headaches; exacerbation of headaches
	Increased premenstrual symptoms

*Symptoms aggravated by anovulatory cycles; leads to dysfunctional uterine bleeding (see Chapter 23.)

where from 11% to 85% of menopausal women experience vasomotor flushes.[22,23] Most (about 60% to 65%) have symptoms for 1 to 5 years, 25% for 6 to 10 years, and 10% to 15% for 10 to 15 years or longer.

Women with higher cyclic E2 levels, that is, premenopausal women with premenstrual vasomotor symptoms and women who report breast, fluid, and premenstrual mood symptoms during the early stages of the perimenopause, are predisposed to withdrawal vasomotor symptoms later in the perimenopausal transition. Anecdotal reports from participants in various research studies suggest that vasomotor symptoms occur just before flow and may be used to predict menstruation.[23] Cyclic vasomotor symptoms, which typically begin early in the perimenopausal transition, differs from noncyclic vasomotor symptoms, which are experienced in late perimenopause. Early vasomotor symptoms typically occur during sleep, often in the early hours of the morning, with few or no daytime vasomotor symptoms; are occasionally preceded by an aura (feelings of anxiety, anger, or panic); and may be associated with nausea, palpitations, dizziness, or faint feelings. Cyclic symptoms tend to occur over several days before and during menses, whereas midcycle vasomotor symptoms are less common and more likely to occur in anovulatory cycles when progesterone does not follow high estrogen midcycle peak. In summary, vasomotor symptoms commonly start when estrogen levels are erratic in the early perimenopause, and are highly correlated with a decreased quality of life, especially when sleep is disturbed. Understanding the physiology of vasomotor symptoms and developing a range of nonhormonal and hormonal strategies for control are important priorities in perimenopause research.

Based on the integration of collected data, a temporal chart outlining phases of the perimenopausal transition and associated endocrine changes and symptoms has been developed.[22] Although the transition is divided into five phases, the vast variability in timing and degree of symptoms experienced by individual women may make clear predictions impossible. The information outlined in Table 22-8 provides a template to visualize the complex physiology of the perimenopause and the dynamic changes that occur during this time.

Several other physiologic changes are associated with the postmenopausal period. These changes affect breast tissue, urogenital structures, bone density or risk for osteoporosis, risk for heart disease, possible memory loss or Alzheimer disease, and others. Only changes in the breast and urogenital structures will be addressed here (other topics are addressed in appropriate chapters).

As ovarian function changes, breast tissue involutes. Two phases of involution have been described: the premenopausal phase and the postmenopausal phase. The premenopausal phase occurs between 35 and 45 years of age. During this phase, there is a moderate decrease in mammary tissue. During the postmenopausal phase, glandular breast tissue is significantly reduced and there is some increase of fat deposits and connective tissue. These changes contribute to the reduction in size and firmness of breast tissue.

The urogenital tract undergoes a number of changes. The ovaries begin to decrease in size around age 30 years, and shrinkage accelerates after age 60 years. Gradually, over the years, the uterus atrophies and decreases in size. The vagina shortens, narrows, and loses some of its elasticity. Vaginal walls lose their ability to lubricate quickly. Intercourse before adequate lubrication may be painful. The vaginal pH, usually maintained at 4.0 to 6.0 before menopause, increases to between 6.5 and 8.0 and contributes to a higher incidence of vaginitis. The cervix atrophies and the cervical os decreases in size. The vaginal epithelium also atrophies; this atrophy can cause vaginal irritation, burning, itching (pruritus), white discharge (leukorrhea), painful intercourse (dyspareunia), and vaginal bleeding. The labia majora and minora become less prominent, and some pubic hair is lost. Urethral tone

Table 22-8	Postulated Perimenopausal Transition Timeline		
Phase	**Menstrual Physiology**	**Hormonal Changes**	**Symptomatology**
A	Regular, ovulatory cycles Short cycles, short FP	Intermittent ↑ E2 FSH usually normal Intermittent ↑ FP FSH Low inhibin	Increased breast tenderness, mood swings, fluid retention, premenstrual symptoms Early morning night sweats (vasomotor symptoms) Weight gain, migraine headaches, heavy flow
B	Regular cycles with disturbances in ovulation Short LP Insufficient LP Anovulatory cycles	Intermittent ↑ FP FSH E2 often ↑ Inhibin inappropriately low	Heavy flow ↑ premenstrual symptoms ↑ dysmenorrhea Predictable or ↑ vasomotor symptoms before flow
C	Onset of perimenopause Alternating short, long, or skipped cycles	E2 often quite ↑ E2 normal or low ↑ FSH (slight) ↑ LH Low inhibin	Vasomotor symptoms during waking hours Vasomotor symptoms more persistent, remain cyclic before flow
D	Onset of oligomenorrhea 50% of cycles anovulatory Heavy flow may predict onset of oligomenorrhea	↑ progesterone with ovulation Persistent ↓ FSH ↑ LH ↑ E2 Low inhibin	↑ vasomotor symptoms ↑ signs/symptoms of high estrogen after long periods without flow Flow light but unpredictable
E	Final menstrual period plus 1 year	↑ FSH and LH ↓ or normal E2 Consistent low inhibin ↓ progesterone	↑ intensity and frequency of vasomotor symptoms (although vasomotor symptoms may disappear) ↓ cramps and premenstrual-type symptoms without subsequent flow ↓ breast, mood, and fluid symptoms

E2, Estradiol; *FP,* follicular phase; *FSH,* follicle-stimulating hormone; *LP,* luteal phase.

declines, as does muscle tone throughout the pelvic area. Urinary frequency, urgency, and incontinence are associated with estrogen deficiency.

Sexually active women have less vaginal atrophy; presumably, sexual activity and stimulation maintains vaginal vasculature and circulation.[1] Regular intercourse (once or twice per week) and masturbation are associated with vaginal pliability, vaginal function, and continued lubrication with arousal.

Aging and the Male Reproductive System

Men maintain reproductive capacity longer than women. There is no known discrete event, comparable to menopause, that characterizes aging of the male reproductive system. Gradual changes do occur, however, in male sexual behavior and in testicular structure and function, including hormonal secretion and spermatogenesis. Aging changes are also influenced by chronic diseases and use of medications.

Components of male sexual behavior include both sexual drive and erectile and ejaculatory capacity. Libido, or sexual drive, is a complex phenomenon that requires a baseline hormonal milieu but is influenced significantly by health status and environmental, social, and psychologic factors. Aging causes specific physical changes that influence erectile and ejaculatory capabilities. Alterations in sexual response include the need for longer stimulation to achieve full erection; slower and less forceful ejaculation, with less pelvic muscle involvement; decreased vasocongestive response; and longer refractory period (time during which erection and ejaculation are not possible), up to 24 hours in some men.

The testes undergo several age-related structural changes, including decreased weight, atrophy, and softening. Degenerative changes in the seminiferous tubules may include thickening of the basement membrane; increase in lumen size; germ cell (spermatogonium) arrest and a decrease in spermatogenic activity; and collapse of tubules, followed by complete obstruction caused by sclerosis and fibrosis. Areas of mild to severe degenerative change may be interspersed with areas having intact tubules. These morphologic changes may result from atherosclerosis (arterial clogging) in the testicular vascular bed.[17] Alterations of the seminiferous tubules do not appear to diminish sperm counts, but they do reduce fertility because a greater percentage of the sperm lack motility or have structural abnormalities.

Aging probably causes changes in the production of male sex hormones, levels of SHBG, and responsiveness of target tissues. Hormone synthesis by the testes, testicular responsiveness to the gonadotropins (FSH and LH), and pituitary secretion of these gonadotropins are altered.[24] Most studies of testosterone levels in aging men show that their serum testosterone levels are lower than levels in younger men,[25-27] and has been defined as androgen deficiency in the aging male (ADAM).[28]

The reduced levels of testosterone may be related to alterations in the Leydig cells, the testosterone producers of the testes. The number of Leydig cells decreases as age increases, perhaps because of atherosclerotic changes in arteries that supply blood to the testes.[29] Even if testosterone levels are not decreased, older men may have less unbound testosterone in their blood, decreasing the amount of unbound hormone available to stimulate target tissues. Decreased testosterone levels have several effects, including functional deterioration of the accessory sex organs (the prostate gland, seminal vesicles, epididymis, and ductus deferens); loss of muscle mass, strength, and endurance; increased visceral fat, osteopenia, and cognitive decline; and, in many men, decrease in libido. This last effect also may be caused by alterations in other variables that affect libido.

Serum levels of the gonadotropins, particularly FSH, increase with age. The change in gonadotropin secretion may be similar to that in women and may result from some hypothalamic-pituitary dysregulation of the gonadotropins related to inhibin levels.

SUMMARY REVIEW

Development of the Reproductive Systems

1. Differentiation of female and male genitalia begins around weeks 7 to 8 of embryonic development, when the gonads of genetically male embryos begin to secrete male sex hormones, primarily testosterone. Until that time, the primitive reproductive organs of males and females are homologous (the same).
2. The structure and function of both male and female reproductive systems are controlled by the hypothalamic-pituitary-gonadal [H-P-G] axis, a set of complex neurologic and hormonal interactions that accelerate at puberty and lead to sexual maturation and reproductive capability.
3. Extrahypothalamic factors cause the hypothalamus to secrete gonadotropin-releasing hormone (GnRH), which stimulates the anterior pituitary to secrete gonadotropins—follicle-stimulating hormone (FSH) and luteinizing hormone (LH)—that stimulate the gonads (ovaries or testes) to secrete female or male sex hormones. Paracrine hormones (inhibin, activin, and follistatin) influence the positive and negative feedback loops that occur along the H-P-G axis.
4. Production of primitive female gametes (ova) occurs solely during fetal life. From puberty to menopause, one female gamete matures per menstrual cycle. Production of the male gametes (sperm) begins at puberty; after that, millions are produced daily, usually for life.

The Female Reproductive System

1. The function of the reproductive system is to produce mature ova and, when fertilized, to protect and nourish them through embryonic and fetal life, and expel them at birth.
2. The external female genitalia are the mons pubis, labia majora, labia minora, clitoris, vestibule (urinary and vaginal openings), Bartholin glands, and Skene glands.
3. The internal female genitalia are the vagina, uterus, fallopian tubes, and ovaries.
4. The vagina is a fibromuscular canal that receives the penis during sexual intercourse and is the exit route for menstrual fluids and products of conception. The vagina leads from the introitus (its external opening) to the cervical portion of the uterus.
5. The uterus is the hollow, muscular organ in which a fertilized ovum develops. The uterine walls have three layers: the endometrium (lining), myometrium (muscular layer), and perimetrium (outer covering, which is continuous with the pelvic peritoneum). The endometrium proliferates (thickens) and sloughs off in response to cyclic hormonal changes. The cervix is the narrow, lower portion of the uterus that opens into the vagina.
6. The two fallopian tubes extend from the uterus to the ovaries. Their function is to conduct ova from the spaces around the ovaries to the uterus. Fertilization normally occurs in the distal third of the fallopian tubes.
7. From puberty to menopause, the ovaries are the site of (1) ovum maturation and release and (2) production of female sex (estrogen and progesterone) and male (androgens) hormones. Female sex hormones predominate and are involved in sexual differentiation and development, the menstrual cycle, pregnancy, and lactation. Androgens in women contribute to prepubertal growth spurt, pubic and axillary hair growth, and activation of sebaceous glands.
8. Developing ovarian follicles (structure that encloses the ovum) produce estrogen (primarily estradiol). The corpus luteum, the structure that develops from the ruptured ovarian follicle after ovulation or ovum release, produces progesterone. Androgens are produced within the ovarian follicle, adrenal glands, and adipose tissue.
9. The average menstrual cycle lasts 27 to 30 days and consists of three phases, which are named for ovarian and endometrial changes: the follicular/proliferative phase, the luteal/secretory phase, and menstruation.
10. Ovarian events of the menstrual cycle are controlled by gonadotropins. High FSH levels stimulate follicle and ovum maturation (follicular phase); then a surge of LH causes ovulation, which is followed by development of the corpus luteum (luteal phase).
11. Ovarian hormones control the uterine (endometrial) events of the menstrual cycle. During the follicular phase of the ovarian cycle, estrogen produced by the follicle causes the endometrium to proliferate (proliferative phase) and induces the LH surge and progesterone production in the granulosa layer. During the luteal phase, estrogen maintains the thickened endometrium while progesterone causes it to develop blood vessels and secretory glands (secretory phase). As the corpus luteum degenerates, production of both hormones drops sharply, and the "starved" endometrium degenerates and sloughs off, causing menstruation.
12. Cyclic changes in hormone levels also cause thinning and thickening of the vaginal epithelium, thinning and thickening of cervical secretions, and changes in basal body temperature.

The Male Reproductive System

1. The function of the male reproductive system is to produce male gametes (sperm) and deliver them to the female reproductive tract.
2. The external male genitalia are the testes, epididymides, scrotum, and penis. The internal genitalia are the vas deferens, ejaculatory duct, prostatic and membranous sections of the urethra, seminal vesicles, prostate gland, and Cowper glands.
3. The testes (male gonads) are paired glands suspended within the scrotum. The testes have two functions: spermatogenesis (sperm production) and production of male sex hormones (androgens, chiefly testosterone).

Continued

4. The epididymis is a long, coiled tube arranged in a comma-shaped compartment that curves over the top and rear of the testis. The epididymis receives sperm from the testis and stores them while they develop further. Sperm travel the length of the epididymis and then are ejaculated into the vas deferens.

5. The scrotum is a skin-covered, fibromuscular sac that encloses the testes and epididymides, which are suspended within the scrotum by the spermatic cord. The scrotum keeps these organs at optimal temperatures for sperm survival (about 1° to 2° C lower than body temperature) by contracting in cold environments and relaxing in warm environments.

6. The penis is a cylindrical organ consisting of three longitudinal compartments (two corpora cavernosa and one corpus spongiosum) and the urethra. The urethra runs through the corpus spongiosum. The corpora cavernosa and corpus spongiosum consist of erectile tissue. Externally the penis consists of a shaft and a tip, which is called the *glans*. The glans contains sebaceous glands and the opening of the urethra and is covered by a flap of skin (the foreskin).

7. The penis has two functions: delivery of sperm to the female vagina and elimination of urine. Although semen (sperm and glandular secretions) and urine both exit the penis through the urethra, these two fluids are never in the urethra at the same time.

8. Sexual intercourse is made possible by the erectile reflex, in which tactile or psychogenic stimulation of the parasympathetic nerves causes arterioles in the corpora cavernosa and corpus spongiosum to dilate and fill with blood, causing the penis to enlarge and become firm.

9. Emission, which occurs at the peak of sexual arousal, is the movement of semen from the epididymides to the penis. Ejaculation, which is a continuation of emission, is the pulsatile ejection of semen from the penis. Both emission and ejaculation involve rhythmic contractions of smooth muscle within the internal glands and ducts.

10. Spermatogenesis is a continuous process because spermatogonia, the primitive male gametes, undergo continuous mitosis within the seminiferous tubules of the testes. Some of the spermatogonia develop into primary spermatocytes, which divide meiotically into secondary spermatocytes and then spermatids. The spermatids develop into sperm with the help of nutrients and hormonal signals from Sertoli cells.

11. Production of the male sex hormones is controlled (like production of the female sex hormones) by the hypothalamic-pituitary-gonadal axis and by complex feedback mechanisms. The male hormones are produced steadily, with diurnal variations.

Structure and Function of the Breast

1. Until puberty the female and male breasts are similar, consisting of a small, underdeveloped nipple, some fatty and fibrous tissue, and a few ductlike structures under the areola. At puberty, however, a variety of hormones (estrogen, progesterone, prolactin, growth hormone, insulin, cortisol) cause the female breast to develop into a system of glands and ducts that is capable of producing and ejecting milk.

2. The basic functional unit of the female breast is the lobe, a system of ducts that branches from the nipple to milk-producing units called *lobules*. The lobules contain acini, which are convoluted spaces lined with epithelial cells that secrete milk and subepithelial cells that contract, moving the milk into the system of ducts that leads to the nipple.

3. Each breast contains 15 to 20 lobes, which are separated and supported by Cooper ligaments.

4. Milk production occurs in response to prolactin, a hormone that is secreted in larger amounts after childbirth. Milk ejection is under the control of oxytocin, another hormone of pregnancy and parturition.

5. During the reproductive years, breast tissue undergoes cyclic changes in response to hormonal changes of the menstrual cycle.

Tests of Reproductive Function

1. Diagnostic tests are performed to evaluate fertility or presence of tumors, infection, or sexually transmitted infections.

2. Tests, stains, cultures, and serologic tests are used to diagnose infections. These tests specifically identify microorganisms or types of infections.

3. Tissue biopsy can be performed by resection or needle aspiration. Specimen analysis permits identification of abnormal cells.

4. The Papanicolaou test (Pap test) is a cytologic examination of cells taken from body fluids and tissues. Although cells can be obtained from many sites, the test is most commonly used (with endocervical cells) for diagnosis of cervical carcinoma.

5. Mammography is a low-dose radiographic examination of the breast for cancer detection.

6. Evaluation of fertility includes reproductive hormone assays and assessment of structural alteration or infections and the determination of normal ovulation or adequate sperm motility and count.

Aging and Reproductive Function

1. In women, the transition from fertility to menopause (perimenopause) starts about 5 years before the last menstrual period and ends the following year. During this transition period, the ovaries produce erratic and high levels of estrogen that contribute to such symptoms as hot flush, breast tenderness and nodularity, and migraine headaches. Menstrual cycles shorten and then become irregular as anovulation occurs. Menstruation ceases, and women move into menopause.

2. Menopause begins 1 year after the cessation of menstruation and occurs at the average age of 51.4 years. Levels of sex hormones decrease with the last menstrual cycle.

3. In response to reduced levels of female sex hormones, the reproductive organs atrophy, the vaginal epithelium thins, and glandular secretions diminish and become more alkaline. Continued sexual activity and orgasm reduce vaginal changes.

4. Nonreproductive effects of reduced estrogen levels may include increased risk of osteoporosis and coronary artery disease.

5. Male reproductive function diminishes with age, but it does not cease in healthy men.

6. The testes atrophy and produce less testosterone, and some seminiferous tubules may degenerate and become fibrotic. These changes affect sex drive (libido) and sperm morphology. Although sperm count remains normal, the semen tends to contain more defective and nonmotile sperm.

7. The erectile reflex is somewhat diminished and occurs more slowly as age advances.

8. Reduced testosterone levels cause some loss of function in the internal genitalia and enlargement (hypertrophy) of the prostate gland.

KEY TERMS

MEDIA RESOURCES evolve

Review questions and answers for this chapter are available in the *CD Companion* included with this book.

WebLinks—links to Internet sites pertaining to this chapter—are available on Evolve at http://evolve.elsevier.com/McCance/.

REFERENCES

1. Speroff L, Glass RH, Kase NG: *Clinical gynecology, endocrinology, and infertility,* ed 6, Baltimore, 1999, Williams & Wilkins.
2. Persaud TVN: Embryology of the female genital tract and gonads. In Copeland LJ, Farrell JF, editors: *Textbook of gynecology,* ed 2, Philadelphia, 2000, Saunders.
3. Gordon K, Oehninger S: Reproductive physiology. In Copeland LJ, Farrell JF, editors: *Textbook of gynecology,* ed 2, Philadelphia, 2000, Saunders.
4. Klein KO et al: Effect of obesity on estradiol level, and its relationship to leptin, bone maturation, and bone mineral density in children, *J Clin Endocrinol Metab* 83(10):3469, 1998.

5. Wong WW et al: Serum leptin concentrations in Caucasian and African-American girls, *J Clin Endocrinol Metab* 83(10):3574-3577, 1998.
6. Berne RM, Levy MN, editors: *Physiology,* ed 5, St Louis, 2003, Mosby.
7. Lowdermilk DL, Perry SE: *Maternity and women's health care,* ed 8, St Louis, 2004, Mosby.
8. Rics FJ et al: A cross-cultural study of menstrual cycle characteristics of women practicing the sympto-thermal method of natural family planning. In Komenich P et al, editors: *The menstrual cycle,* vol 2, New York, 1981, Springer.
9. Trealor AE et al: Variation of the human menstrual cycle through reproductive life, *Int J Fertil* 12:77-126, 1970.
10. Adams Hillard PJ: Menstruation in young girls: a clinical perspective, *Obstet Gynecol* 99(4):655-662, 2002.
11. Golub S: *Periods: from menarche to menopause,* Newbury Park, NJ, 1992, Sage.
12. Speroff L et al: *Clinical gynecologic endocrinology and fertility,* ed 6, Baltimore, 1999, Lippincott.
13. deKretser DM et al: Inhibins, activans and follistatin in reproduction, *Hum Reprod Update* 8(6):529-541, 2002.
14. Stenchevor MA et al: *Comprehensive gynecology,* ed 4, St Louis, 2001, Mosby.

15. Sirois J et al: Cyclooxygenase-2 and its role in ovulation: a 2004 account, *Hum Reprod Update* 19(5):373-385, 2004.
16. Tanango EA, McAninch JW: *Smith's general urology,* ed 16, Norwalk, Conn, 2003, McGraw-Hill.
17. Hafez ESE, Hafez B, Hafez SD: *An atlas of reproductive physiology in men,* London, 2003, Taylor & Francis Group.
18. Buvat J: Hyperprolactinemia and sexual function in men: a short review, *In J Impot Res* 15(5):373-377, 2003.
19. American College of Obstetrics and Gynecologists: ACOG practice bulletin. Cervical cytology screening, Number 45, August 2003, *Int J Gynaecol Obstet* 83(2):237-247, 2003.
20. American Cancer Society: *Cancer facts & figures,* New York, 2003, Author. Available online: www.cancer.org
21. Runowicz CD: Benign breast disease and screening for malignant tumors. In Copeland LJ, Farrell JF, editors, *Textbook of gynecology,* ed 2, Philadelphia, 2000, Saunders.
22. Prior JC: Perimenopause: the complex endocrinology of the menopause transition, *Endvoc Rev* 19(4):397, 1998.
23. Dagwood MY: Menopause. In Copeland LJ, Farrell JE, editors, *Textbook of gynecology,* ed 2, Philadelphia, 2000, Saunders.
24. Shulman C, Lunenfeld B: The ageing male. *World J Urol* 20(1):4-10, 2002.
25. Juul A, Skakkebaek NE: Androgens and the ageing male. *Hum Reprod Update* 8(5):423-433, 2002.
26. Harman SM, Blackman MR: Use of growth hormone for prevention or treatment of effects of aging, *J Gerontol A Biol Sci Med Sci* 59(7): 652-658, 2004.
27. Tenover JS: Declining testicular function in aging men, *Int J Impot Res* 15(Suppl 4):S3-S8, 2003.
28. Morales A, Tenover JL: Androgen deficiency in the aging male: when, who, and how to investigate and treat, *Urol Clin North Am* 29(4): 975-982, x, 2002.
29. Haider SG: Cell biology of Leydig cells in the testis, *Int Rev Cytol* 233:181-241, 2004.

ALTERATIONS OF THE REPRODUCTIVE SYSTEMS

KATHERINE MORGAN • KATHRYN L. McCANCE

CHAPTER OUTLINE

Alterations of the reproductive system span a wide range of concerns, from delayed sexual development and suboptimal sexual performance to structural and functional abnormalities. Many common reproductive disorders carry potentially serious physiologic or psychologic consequences. Sexual or reproductive dysfunction, such as impotence or infertility, can dramatically affect self-concept, relationships, and overall quality of life. Conversely, organic and psychosocial problems, such as alcoholism, depression, situational stressors, chronic illness, and medications, can affect ovulation and menstruation, sexual performance, and fertility and may be risk factors for the development of some types of reproductive tract cancers.[1] Prostate cancer is the second leading cause of cancer death in men, breast cancer is the second leading cause of cancer death in women. Diagnosis and treatment of reproductive system disorders are complicated because of the stigma and symbolism associated with the reproductive organs and the emotion-laden beliefs and behaviors related to reproductive health. Treatment and diagnosis for any problem may be delayed because of embarrassment, guilt, fear, or denial.

ALTERATIONS OF SEXUAL MATURATION

The process of sexual maturation, or puberty, is marked by the development of secondary sexual characteristics, rapid growth, and, ultimately, the ability to reproduce. The average age of puberty has been occurring earlier than previously defined. A variety of congenital and endocrine disorders can disrupt the timing of puberty, or sexual maturation. These disorders may cause puberty to occur too late (delayed puberty) or too early (precocious puberty). Both types of disorders involve the inappropriate onset of sex hormone production by the gonads.

Delayed Puberty

About 3% of children in North America experience delayed development of secondary sex characteristics.[2] The first sign of puberty in girls is thelarche, or breast development. Thelarche should begin by the time a girl is 13 years old. Normally boys tend to mature later than girls, around 14 to 14.5 years of age. In boys the first sign is enlargement of the testes and thinning of the scrotal skin. In **delayed puberty** these secondary sex characteristics have not appeared by age 13 in girls or age 14 in boys (2 SD [standard deviation] above the mean age of pubertal onset). Clinical diagnosis also can be made in the absence of menarche within 5 years of thelarche or by 16 years of age. Boys especially tend to be embarrassed by sexual immaturity;[3] therefore early diagnosis and treatment is recommended, as well as reassurance for both boys and girls.

In 95% of cases, delayed puberty is a constitutional delay; that is, hormonal levels are normal and the hypothalamic-pituitary-ovarian axis is intact, but maturation is happening slowly. Physiologic or constitutional delay tends to be familial and is much more common in boys than in girls (Box 23-1). Constitutional delay is difficult to distinguish from isolated gonadotropin deficiency and can be diagnosed only retrospectively once pubertal progression is complete. Delayed puberty may be related to consequences of chronic disease, such as lung disease, renal failure, or cystic fibrosis, or as a consequence of treatment such as corticosteroid use in asthma.[4] For constitutional delay, many clinicians recommend a trial of exogenous sex hormones to reduce embarrassment and enhance self-image and as a diagnostic measure for irreversible hypogonadotropism.[2,3]

The other 5% of cases are caused by some disruption of the hypothalamic-pituitary-gonadal axis (either congenital or acquired) or by a systemic disease. Human gonadal function is partially controlled by luteinizing hormone (LH) and follicle-stimulating hormone (FSH), and the release of which is regulated by the pulsatile secretion of hypothalamic gonadotropin-releasing hormone (GnRH).[5,6] Most recently, the G-protein–coupled receptor (GPR) 54 has been identified as the gatekeeper gene for activation of the GnRH axis based on loss of function studies in mice and humans. GPR54 is required for the normal function of this axis, and data suggests that the ligand kisspeptin-1 may act as a neurohormonal regulator of the GnRH axis.[5] The mechanisms of childhood inhibition of GnRH release and activation are poorly understood but appear to involve feedback inhibition by sex steroids and presumably other CNS pathways.[7] A thorough physical examination, including precise body measurements and accurate assessment of sexual maturation, should be done. Careful questioning is imperative to elicit a history of chronic illness, eating disorder, strenuous exercise, drug abuse, anosmia (decreased or absent smell that accompanies Kallmann syndrome), signs and symptoms of hypopituitarism, hypothyroidism, Turner syndrome, Klinefelter syndrome, and Tanner staging.[8] Laboratory workup generally consists of x-ray studies for bone age, measurement of thyroid function, serum levels of prolactin and adrenal and gonadal steroids, radioimmunoassay of plasma gonadotropins, and

---

Box 23-1	Causes of Delayed Puberty

Hypergonadotropic Hypogonadism (Increased Follicle-Stimulating Hormone [FSH] and Luteinizing Hormone [LH])
1. Gonadal dysgenesis, most commonly Turner syndrome (45,X/46,XX; structural X or Y abnormalities; or mosaicism)
2. Klinefelter syndrome (47,XXY)
3. Bilateral gonadal failure
   a. Traumatic or infectious
   b. Postsurgical, postirradiation, or postchemotherapy
   c. Autoimmune
   d. Idiopathic empty-scrotum or vanishing-testes syndrome (congenital anorchia) or resistant-ovary syndrome

Hypogonadotropic Hypogonadism (Decreased LH, Depressed FSH)
1. Reversible
   a. Physiologic delay
   b. Weight loss/anorexia
   c. Strenuous exercise
   d. Severe obesity
   e. Illegal drug use, especially marijuana
   f. Primary hypothyroidism
   g. Congenital adrenal hyperplasia
   h. Cushing syndrome
   i. Prolactinomas
2. Irreversible
   a. Gonadotropin-releasing hormone (GnRH) deficiency (Kallmann syndrome) or idiopathic hypogonadotropic hypogonadism (IHH)
   b. Hypopituitarism
   c. Congenital central nervous system (CNS) defects
   d. Other pituitary adenomas
   e. Craniopharyngioma
   f. Malignant pituitary tumors

Eugonadism
1. Congenital anomalies
   a. Müllerian agenesis
   b. Vaginal septum or imperforate hymen
2. Androgen insensitivity syndrome
3. Inappropriate positive feedback

Data from Rudolph AM, Hoffman JIE, Rudolph CD: *Rudolph's pediatrics,* ed 20, Stamford, Conn, 1996, Appleton & Lange; Speroff L, Glass RH, Kase NG: *Clinical gynecologic endocrinology and infertility,* ed 5, Baltimore, 1994, Williams & Wilkins; Rosen DS, Foster C: *Pediatr Rev* 22(9): 309-315, 2001; Pozo J, Argente J: *Horm Res* 60(Suppl 3): 35-48, 2003.

---

screening for systemic disorders. Adolescents with high gonadotropin levels require a karyotype, and those with low levels need skull imaging (lateral skull film, computed tomography, or magnetic resonance imaging) to rule out pituitary or other central nervous system infiltrate or tumor.[2] Treatment of pathophysiologic delayed puberty depends on the cause; the goal of treatment is the development of secondary sex characteristics and fertility, when possible.[9,10] Insufficient sex hormone secretion can be corrected by hormone replacement therapy; idiopathic hypogonadotropic hypogonadism and Kallmann syndrome,[11] which may be different expressions of the same X-linked chromosomal disorder, are treated with synthetic GnRH. Treatment of Turner syndrome consists of long-term growth hormone therapy with late estrogen therapy.

Precocious Puberty

Precocious puberty is a rare event, affecting about 1 in 10,000 girls and less than 1 in 50,000 boys. Recently, precocious puberty has been redefined as sexual maturation before 6 in black girls or age 7 in white girls, and before age 9 in boys.[12] This reflects the overall trend toward earlier puberty. All cases of precocious puberty require thorough evaluation.

Precocious puberty occurs in many forms, including isosexual, heterosexual, and incomplete. **Isosexual precocious puberty** is premature development of appropriate characteristics for the child's sex and may be GnRH dependent or GnRH independent. True isosexual precocious puberty is GnRH dependent and occurs when the hypothalamic-pituitary-gonadal axis is working normally but prematurely. Besides the premature development of secondary sex characteristics, precocity causes premature closure of the epiphysis of long bones, which results in short stature. Idiopathic precocity, or central precocious puberty, results from failure of central inhibition of the GnRH pulse generator (the gonadostat). The diagnosis of central precocious puberty is one of exclusion. Because a central nervous system (CNS) lesion may be missed, children with presumed idiopathic precocious puberty require long-term surveillance. More serious causes of central or GnRH dependent sexual precocity are listed in Box 23-2. Pseudoprecocious puberty, also known as *peripheral* or *GnRH independent precocious puberty,* develops when sex hormones are produced by some mechanism other than stimulation by the gonadotropins. One cause is glandular insufficiency syndromes such as severe hypothyroidism or adrenal insufficiency; others are listed in Box 23-2.

Heterosexual precocious puberty (virilization of a girl or feminization of a boy) causes the child to develop some secondary sex characteristics of the opposite sex. This condition is usually evident at birth and is rare in older children.

Incomplete precocious puberty is the partial development of appropriate secondary sex characteristics. A girl with incomplete precocious puberty might undergo thelarche or adrenarche and, rarely, premature menarche. Premature thelarche is seen in girls between 6 months and 2 years of age. Premature adrenarche tends to occur between ages 5 and 8 years. Premature adrenarche is the consequence of an early increase in the adrenal androgens that leads to early growth of pubic hair and possibly a transient acceleration in growth and bone maturation that has no significant effect on timing of puberty or final height. Sparse hair growth on the genitalia does not represent precocious puberty.

The diagnosis and cause of premature development are often obvious. A thorough history and physical examination are done to determine the velocity of the process and to rule out life-threatening CNS, ovarian, or adrenal neoplasms. Family occurrence helps exclude tumors. The majority of children with precocious puberty are obese.

Treatment for all forms of precocious puberty includes identifying and removing the underlying cause or administering appropriate hormones (Boxes 23-3 and 23-4; see also Box 23-2). In many cases, precocious puberty can be reversed. Management goals include diagnosing and treating intracranial disease; arresting maturation until early teen years; maximizing eventual adult height; reducing emotional problems; and providing contraception, if necessary. The most common form, central precocious puberty, is usually treated with potent GnRH agonist analogues, which induce reversible, selective suppression of the pituitary-gonadal axis.[13] Treatment does not seem to affect body composition or increase obesity in children with central precocious puberty.[14] Because the

---

Box 23-2	Causes of Isosexual Precocious Puberty

Central (Gonadotropin-Releasing Hormone [GnRH] Dependent)
1. Idiopathic, including familial
2. Central nervous system (CNS) abnormalities
   a. Congenital anomalies (hydrocephalus)
   b. Tumors (hypothalamic, pineal, other)
   c. Hypothalamic hamartoma
   d. Postinflammatory/infectious condition
   e. Trauma
   f. Syndromes
      (1) Neurofibromatosis
      (2) Tuberous sclerosis
3. Hypothyroidism (severe)

Pseudoprecocious Puberty (GnRH Independent)
1. Exogenous sex steroids
2. Gonadal tumors or cysts
3. Adrenal hyperplasia or tumor
4. Ectopic gonadotropin-secreting tumors (chorioepithelioma, hepatoblastoma, teratoma)
5. Familial Leydig cell hyperplasia
6. McCune-Albright syndrome

From Hoekelman RA et al: *Primary pediatric care,* ed 4, St Louis, 2001, Mosby.

Box 23-3	Causes of Heterosexual Precocious Puberty

Female
1. Congenital adrenal hyperplasia
2. Androgen-secreting tumors
   a. Adrenal
   b. Ovarian
   c. Teratoma
3. Exogenous androgens

Male
1. Estrogen-producing tumors
   a. Adrenal
   b. Teratoma
   c. Hepatoma
   d. Testicular
2. Exogenous estrogens
3. Increased peripheral conversion of androgens to estrogens

From Hoekelman RA et al: *Primary pediatric care,* ed 4, St Louis, 2001, Mosby.

Box 23-4	The Three Forms of Precocious Puberty

Isosexual Precocious Puberty
Premature development of appropriate characteristics for the child's sex
Hypothalamic-pituitary-ovarian axis working normally but prematurely
In about 10% of cases, lethal central nervous system tumor may be the cause*

Heterosexual Precocious Puberty
Causes the child to develop some secondary sex characteristics of the opposite sex
Common causes: adrenal hyperplasia or androgen-secreting tumors

Incomplete Precocious Puberty
Partial development of appropriate secondary sex characteristics
Premature thelarche (breast budding) seen in girls between 6 months and 2 years of age
Does not progress to complete puberty (ovulation and menstruation)
Premature adrenarche (growth of axillary and pubic hair) tends to occur between 5 and 8 years of age
Can progress to complete precocious puberty; may be caused by estrogen-secreting neoplasms or may be a variant of normal pubertal development

*Kaplowitz PB et al: *Pediatrics* 104(4):936, 1999. Kaplowitz, PB: *Early puberty in girls,* New York, 2004, Random House.

majority of these children are obese and childhood obesity is predictive of morbidity in adolescence and adulthood, it is important for clinicians to include assessment and management of obesity as part of the treatment for central precocious puberty.

DISORDERS OF THE FEMALE REPRODUCTIVE SYSTEM

Hormonal and Menstrual Alterations

Primary Dysmenorrhea

Primary dysmenorrhea is painful menstruation associated with the release of prostaglandins in ovulatory cycles, but not with pelvic disease. The severity of dysmenorrhea is directly related to the duration and amount of menstrual flow. Between 50% and 75% of women ages 15 to 25 years are affected, some (up to 15%) severely enough to miss work or school. Primary dysmenorrhea usually begins with the onset of ovulatory cycles, around age 15 or 16 years. The incidence steadily rises, peaks in women in their mid twenties, and decreases slowly thereafter. **Secondary dysmenorrhea** is related to pelvic pathology, manifests in later reproductive years, and may occur any time in the menstrual cycle.[15]

PATHOPHYSIOLOGY   Dysmenorrhea is the result of excessive endometrial prostaglandin production and effect. Women with painful periods produce 10 times as much prostaglandin F ($PGF_{2\alpha}$), a potent myometrial stimulant and vasoconstrictor, as asymptomatic women. Elevated levels of prostaglandins (especially $PGF_{2\alpha}$ and $PGE_{2\alpha}$) are found in endometrial fluid of dysmenorrheic women and correlate positively with pain. Compared with proliferative endometrium, secretory endometrium produces three times the amount of prostaglandins, and the discharged endometrium produces even more.[16] In addition, leukotrienes heighten sensitivity of pain fibers in the uterus and vasopressin contributes to myometrial hypersensitivity, constriction of endometrial blood vessels, and resultant ischemia, endometrial bleeding, and pain caused by prostaglandins.[17] Prostaglandins are primarily released during the first 48 hours of menstruation, when symptoms are the most intense. Women who are anovulatory because they use oral contraceptives do not have primary dysmenorrhea. Secondary dysmenorrhea results from disorders such as endometriosis, pelvic adhesions, inflammatory disease, cervical stenosis, uterine fibrosis, or adenomyoma.

CLINICAL MANIFESTATIONS   The chief symptom of dysmenorrhea is pelvic pain associated with the onset of menses. The pain often radiates into the groin and may be accompanied by backache, anorexia, vomiting, diarrhea, syncope, and headache. The latter symptoms are caused by entry of prostaglandins and prostaglandin metabolites into the systemic circulation. Usually, the discomfort associated with primary dysmenorrhea begins shortly before the onset of menstruation and rarely persists beyond the second day.

EVALUATION AND TREATMENT   Primary dysmenorrhea can be differentiated from secondary dysmenorrhea by a thorough history and pelvic examination. In women who desire contraception, dysmenorrhea may be relieved with hormonal contraceptives. Hormonal contraception stops ovulation and creates an atrophic endometrium, thereby decreasing prostaglandin synthesis and myometrial contractility. Prostaglandin inhibitors work in the majority of women with primary dysmenorrhea and are most effective if started at the first sign of bleeding or cramping. Regular exercise is thought to prevent or reduce symptoms. Other comfort measures include local application of heat, massage, and relaxation techniques. Orgasm may relieve or worsen symptoms.

Primary Amenorrhea

Amenorrhea means lack of menstruation. **Primary amenorrhea** is the failure of menarche and the absence of menstruation by age 14 years without the development of secondary sex characteristics or by age 16 years regardless of the presence of secondary sex characteristics (see p. 772 for discussion of delayed puberty). Primary amenorrhea differs from delayed puberty in that most cases of delayed puberty require only reassurance, but when the diagnosis of primary amenorrhea is reached, a thorough evaluation must be undertaken.

PATHOPHYSIOLOGY   There are numerous classifications of the etiologies of primary amenorrhea. One approach to understanding the pathophysiology is through compartmentalization. *Compartment IV disorders* include CNS disorders, in particular hypothalamic disorders. In some of the congenital syndromes that cause primary amenorrhea, the hypothalamic-pituitary-ovarian (H-P-O) axis is dysfunctional. The hypothalamus is unable to synthesize GnRH, so the pituitary fails to secrete luteinizing hormone (LH) and follicle-stimulating hormone (FSH). Therefore the ovary does not receive the hormonal signals that normally initiate the ovarian and endometrial changes of the menstrual cycle, and ovulation and menstruation do not occur. Because the ovarian hormones are absent, secondary sex characteristics do not develop.

Compartment III disorders are disorders of the anterior pituitary, including tumors. Some anatomic defects of the CNS, whether congenital or acquired, impinge on the hypothalamic-pituitary unit so as to interfere with or interrupt the secretion of GnRH or FSH and LH. Examples of such defects include hydrocephalus, craniopharyngiomas, and other space-occupying lesions of the CNS (see Box 23-1). Again the target organ, the ovary, does not receive the necessary signals, and ovulation and menstruation do not occur. In some cases these lesions develop between the onset and conclusion of puberty. Therefore skeletal growth may occur and secondary sex characteristics may develop, but sexual maturation is interrupted before menarche, which normally concludes puberty.

Compartment II disorders involve the ovary. Several genetic disorders are associated with primary amenorrhea. These include gonadal dysgenesis (Turner syndrome), androgen insensitivity syndrome (AIS), formerly known as testicular feminizing syndrome or male pseudohermaphroditism. Among all the chromosomal abnormalities of Turner syndrome (45,X/46,XX; structural X or Y abnormalities; mosaicism),[10] the ovaries lack gametes and ovarian failure is complete. Without primitive gametes and follicles, follicular development and estrogen secretion cannot occur. Lack of estrogen accounts for failure of secondary sex characteristic development, and amenorrhea, although there are high levels of circulating FSH and LH. In AIS, the individual is male genetically but female morphologically. The individual does not develop male genitalia because androgen receptors are absent in undifferentiated target organs. The gonads are found either in the abdomen or in the inguinal canal, and they produce both androgens and estrogens. Because target tissues lack androgen receptors but have estrogen receptors, most individuals with AIS have female external genitalia and female secondary sex characteristics. With the exception of a small vagina, internal female genitalia are absent, accounting for amenorrhea and infertility.

Compartment I disorders are anatomic defects of the outflow tract associated with primary amenorrhea. They include congenital absence of the vagina and uterus and congenital uterine hypoplasia (infantile uterus). Females without a uterus or vagina usually have normal ovarian function. Therefore skeletal growth occurs and secondary sex characteristics develop in the proper sequence, but menstruation does not occur. In cases of uterine hypoplasia the uterus does not respond to hormonal stimulation during puberty.

CLINICAL MANIFESTATIONS   The major clinical manifestation of primary amenorrhea is the absence of the menses. The cause of the amenorrhea determines whether secondary sex characteristics and height are affected.

EVALUATION AND TREATMENT   Diagnosis of primary amenorrhea is based on history and physical examination. If ovarian steroid hormone levels are low, the individual has the appearance of an immature female. Physical examination may show structural or physiologic alterations. Laboratory studies may be required to document karyotype, abnormal levels of gonadotropins, and ovarian hormones. Diagnostic imaging is used to document structural abnormalities (Figure 23-1).

Treatment involves correction of any underlying disorders and hormone replacement therapy to induce the development of secondary sex characteristics (see p. 772 for a discussion of delayed puberty). Although surgical alteration of the genitalia may be undertaken to correct structural abnormalities, surgery should be delayed until the affected individual can make a truly informed decision. Hormonal manipulation or embryo transplantation may make pregnancy possible for women with primary amenorrhea who have a uterus.

Secondary Amenorrhea

Secondary amenorrhea is the absence of menstruation for a time equivalent to three or more cycles or 6 months in women who have previously menstruated. A wide variety of disorders and physiologic conditions are associated with secondary amenorrhea. Besides disease, secondary amenorrhea can be triggered by dramatic weight loss, whether the loss results from malnutrition or excessive exercise. Secondary amenorrhea is normal during early adolescence and the perimenopausal period, pregnancy, and lactation.

PATHOPHYSIOLOGY   The causes of secondary amenorrhea are summarized in Figure 23-2. In women with normal ovarian steroid hormone levels, secondary amenorrhea may be caused by structural abnormalities (müllerian anomalies), Asherman syndrome (removal of the endometrial decidua basalis), or removal of the uterus. In women with elevated ovarian steroid hormone levels, inhibited ovulation leads to amenorrhea. An excess of ovarian hormones disrupts feedback relationships within the H-P-O axis, preventing ovulation. Depressed ovarian hormone levels, which are associated with a variety of clinical disorders, also cause amenorrhea by preventing ovulation. Lack of ovulation, termed **anovulation,** may result from increased levels of prolactin, decreased levels of gonadotropins, irregular secretion of gonadotropins, or abnormally low levels of CNS neurotransmitters. Any of these variables alters the feedback effects that the ovarian hormones have on the hypothalamus and pituitary.

Hyperprolactinemia (overproduction of prolactin by the pituitary) may have short-loop feedback effects that lead to decreased secretion of GnRH by the hypothalamus. The result is a loss of pulsatile LH secretion and an overall reduction in

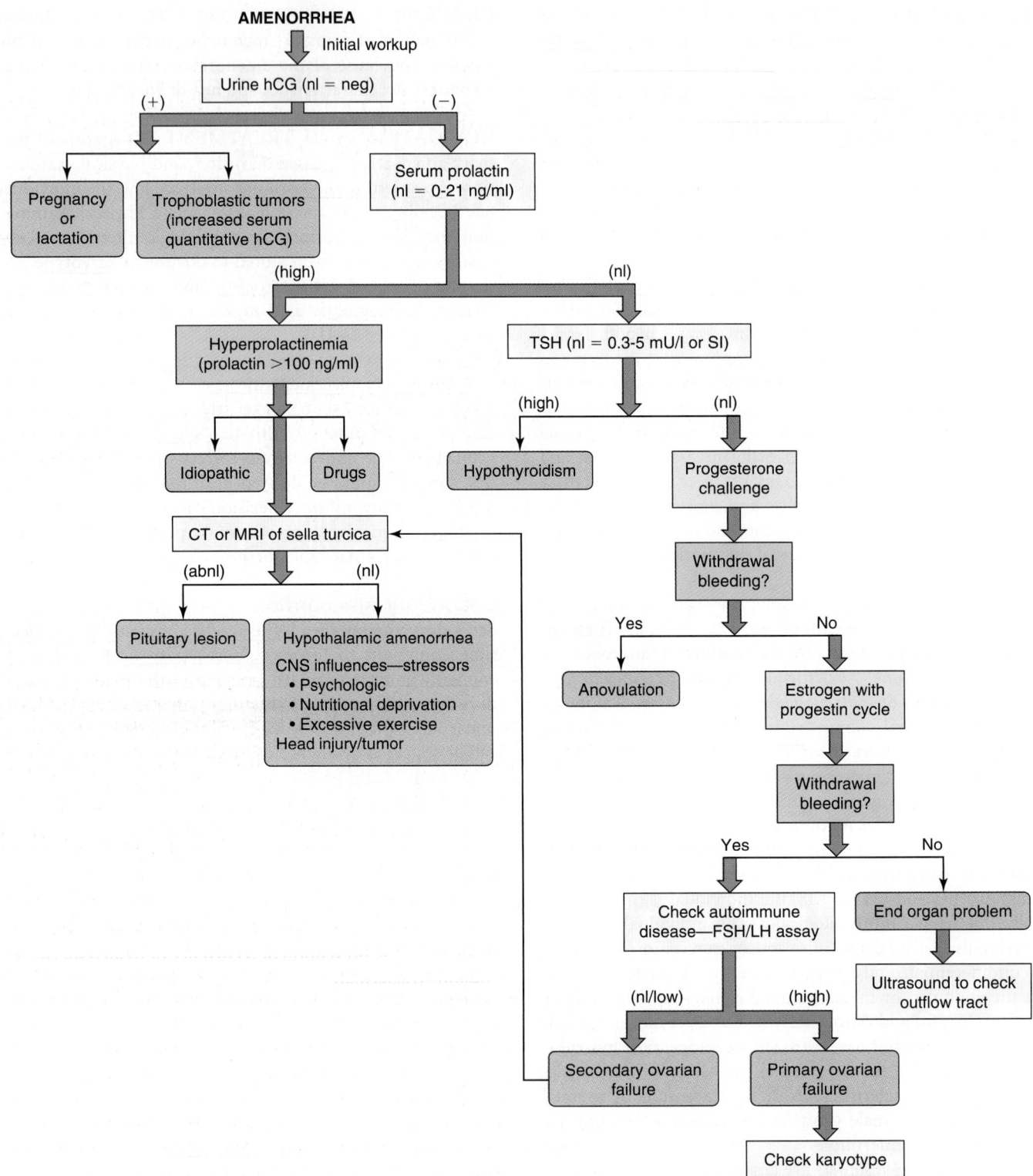

Figure 23-1 **Diagnosis of amenorrhea.** Pregnancy is the most common cause of amenorrhea. *abnl,* Abnormal; *nl,* normal.

LH levels. Anovulation and secondary amenorrhea may result. In the ovary, elevated prolactin levels appear to inhibit the secretion of progesterone by the granulosa cells of the follicle. This leads to anovulation caused by follicular atresia. These abnormalities may act singly or in combination to cause other alterations in the menstrual cycle.

CLINICAL MANIFESTATIONS The major manifestation of secondary amenorrhea is the absence of menses. Infertility, vasomotor flushes, vaginal atrophy, acne, osteopenia, and **hirsutism** (abnormal hairiness) also may be present, depending on the underlying cause of the amenorrhea.

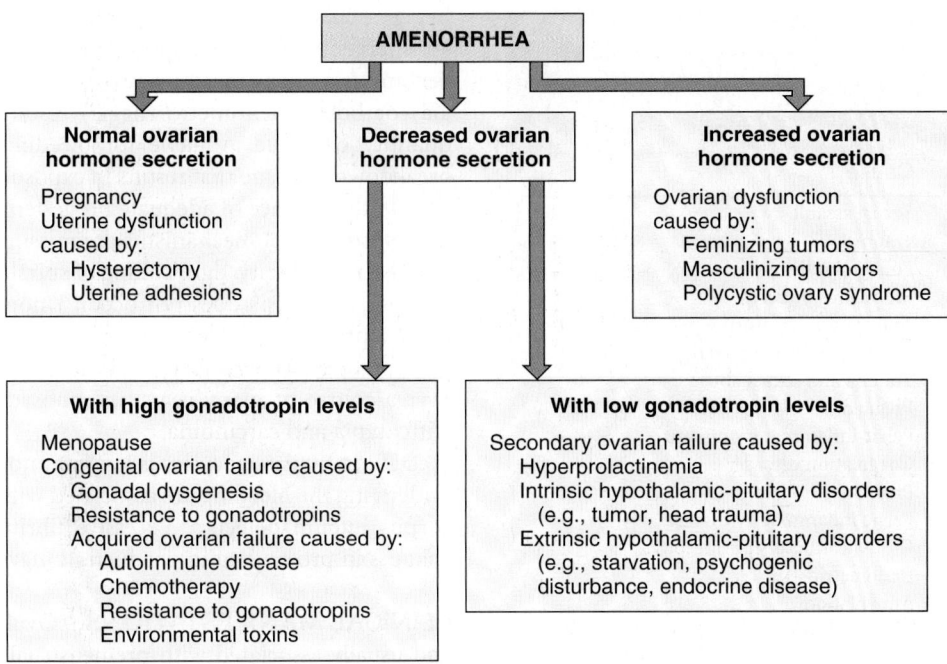

Figure 23-2 Causes of amenorrhea.

Table 23-1	Abnormal Menstrual Bleeding
Term	Definition
Polymenorrhea	Cycles shorter than 3 wk; may indicate disturbance in endocrine control of ovulation
Oligomenorrhea	Cycles longer than 6-7 wk; may indicate disturbance in endocrine control of ovulation
Metrorrhagia	Intermenstrual bleeding or bleeding of light character occurring irregularly between cycles; may be a sign of organic disease
Hypermenorrhea	Excessive flow; may be a sign of organic disease
Menorrhea	Prolonged duration of flow
Menorrhagia	Increased amount and duration of flow
Menometrorrhagia	Prolonged flow associated with irregular and intermittent spotting between bleeding episodes

EVALUATION AND TREATMENT   Pregnancy is the most common cause of amenorrhea and must be ruled out prior to other evaluations. Diagnosis of secondary amenorrhea involves the identification of underlying hormonal or anatomic alterations. A woman with secondary amenorrhea and normal secondary sex characteristics should have a complete history and physical examination. Pregnancy is ruled out before any further workup is undertaken. Initial evaluation begins with a measurement of thyroid-stimulating hormone, a prolactin level, and a progesterone challenge to induce withdrawal bleeding. Radioimmunoassay levels of gonadotropins, computed tomography (CT) or magnetic resonance imaging (MRI) imaging of the sella turcica, and ultrasound of the outflow tract may be necessary to determine the cause of amenorrhea[18,19] (see Figure 23-1). Depending on the cause of the amenorrhea, treatment may involve oral, vaginal, or injectable hormone replacement therapy[16,18,20,21] (e.g., estrogens, thyroid hormone, glucocorticoids, gonadotropins, bromocriptine) or a corrective procedure, such as surgical removal of pituitary tumors. New evidence suggests that insertion of a copper intrauterine device (IUD) may be effective in the prevention of recurrence of treated uterine adhesions (Asherman syndrome).[22]

Abnormal Uterine Bleeding

Menstrual irregularity or abnormal bleeding patterns (Table 23-1) account for approximately 33% of all gynecologic visits. This proportion increases to 69% in the perimenopausal and postmenopausal age-groups.[23] Failure to ovulate as an expression of age, stress, or endocrinopathy is the most common cause of cycle irregularity. Other causes include intrinsic uterine pathologic conditions, including malignancy, pregnancy and its complications, and hematologic disorders. Common causes of abnormal uterine bleeding based on age-group and frequency are listed in Table 23-2.

Dysfunctional uterine bleeding (DUB) is heavy or irregular bleeding and a diagnosis of exclusion. It is not associated with other causes of abnormal uterine bleeding, such as submucous fibroids, endometrial polyps, blood dyscrasias, pregnancy, infection, or systemic disease, such as hepatic disease

Table 23-2	Common Causes of Abnormal (Vaginal/Genital) Bleeding in Descending Order of Frequency
Age Group	Cause
Prepubescence	Sexual assault
	Trauma
	Foreign bodies
	Precocious puberty
Adolescence	Anovulation (maturing hypothalamic-pituitary-ovarian axis)
	Trauma and sexual abuse
Reproductive years	Pregnancy
	Pelvic inflammatory disease
	Coagulation disorder
	Pregnancy
	Pelvic inflammatory disease
	Complication of contraceptives
	Endometriosis
	Anovulation
Perimenopause	Anovulation
	Malignancy
	Pregnancy
	Endometriosis
	Benign neoplasms (myomas, adenomyosis)
Postmenopause	Malignancy

or endocrinopathies. The diagnosis of DUB is made once these other causes have been excluded. DUB affects 15% to 20% of all women at some time during their menstrual life and accounts for 25% of gynecologic surgeries.[24]

PATHOPHYSIOLOGY   Greater than 80% of DUB is associated with anovulatory cycles, and the remaining 20% is due to corpus luteum defects or atrophic endometrium.[25] Although DUB may occur at any time during the reproductive years, 20% of cases occur in adolescents, and more than 50% of cases occur in perimenopausal women ages 40 to 50 years. Symptoms of hypomenorrhea, followed by missed periods or prolonged intervals between menses, could mark the onset of physiologic perimenopause or may be an early sign of pathologically premature ovulatory failure and secondary amenorrhea. Other conditions associated with chronic anovulation include polycystic ovary syndrome, immaturity of the H-P-O axis, obesity, hyperthyroidism and hypothyroidism, and estrogen-secreting ovarian neoplasms.

DUB secondary to ovarian dysfunction is a result of either progesterone deficiency or relative estrogen excess. In perimenopausal women in their forties and fifties, progesterone secretion is absent or low, yet estrogen (estradiol [E2]) continues to be secreted by the granulosa–theca cell complex, and levels are often erratic and high.[26] (See Chapter 22 for a description of the many hormonal changes associated with the time before and just after menopause.) In the absence of growth-limiting progesterone and periodic desquamation, the endometrium attains an abnormal height with increasing

hypervascularity and back-to-back glandularity, but without an intervening stromal support matrix. Menstrual flow may become irregular (metrorrhagia) and excessive (menorrhagia) or both (menometrorrhagia) resulting from the large quantity of tissue available for bleeding and the random breakdown of tissue that results in exposure of vascular channels. In the absence of adequate progesterone levels, usual endometrial control mechanisms are missing, such as vasoconstrictive rhythmicity, tight coiling of spiral vessels, and orderly collapse, and stasis does not occur. Unopposed estrogen induces a progression of endometrial responses beginning with proliferation, hyperplasia, and adenomatous hyperplasia; over a course of many years, unopposed estrogen may end with atypia and carcinoma.

DUB in ovulatory cycles is less common, and mechanisms underlying the bleeding are associated with organic lesions or corpus luteum defects.[25] Excessive fibrinolytic activity and changes in prostaglandin production may be implicated.

CLINICAL MANIFESTATIONS   Ovulatory DUB is cyclic and usually associated with premenstrual symptoms such as breast tenderness, water retention, and cramping. Anovulatory DUB is characterized by unpredictable and variable bleeding in terms of amount and duration. Especially during perimenopause, dysfunctional bleeding also may involve flooding and the passage of large clots, which often indicate excessive blood loss. It is difficult to estimate the severity of blood loss in otherwise healthy women because such women do not become anemic until blood loss exceeds 1.6 L over a short interval.

EVALUATION AND TREATMENT   Treatment goals include preventing or controlling abnormal bleeding, identifying underlying disease, and inducing regular menstrual cycles.[27] Usual therapy is hormonal and may consist of progestin-estrogen combination therapy, estrogen-only therapy (for acute episodes only), or progesterone-only therapy.[17,20,21,25,26,28] For the woman with idiopathic menorrhagia not associated with anovulatory cycles, prostaglandin synthetase inhibitors may be effective in decreasing blood loss. Desmopressin, a synthetic analog of arginine vasopressin, is used to treat abnormal uterine bleeding in women with coagulation disorders (von Willebrand disease, which affects about 1% of the population).[25,28] Recalcitrant bleeding may be controlled by suppression of the endometrium followed by ablation. Total or partial ablation of the endometrium has replaced dilation and curettage (D & C) or hysterectomy as the surgical technique of choice for treatment of menorrhagia. Various techniques have been developed, including laser, a resectoscope with a loop or rolling ball electrode, partial roller-ball or radiofrequency-induced balloon, and microwave thermal destruction.[25,29-32] The best results are obtained if the endometrium is suppressed for 4 to 6 weeks with either high-dose progestin, GnRH agonist, or danazol. Endometrial ablation is successful in approximately 90% of women; only 50% become amenorrheic. Routine treatment of DUB with D & C or hysterectomy is not recommended. The major indication for a D & C is diagnostic or as a curative procedure in the removal of products of conception, polyps, or focal endometrial hyperplasia.

Polycystic Ovary Syndrome

Polycystic ovary syndrome (PCOS) is a syndrome with at least two of the following conditions present: oligoovulation or anovulation, elevated levels of androgens or clinical signs of hyperandrogenism and polycystic ovaries.[33] Polycystic ovaries do not have to be present to diagnose PCOS; and conversely their presence alone does not establish the diagnosis.[33] PCOS remains one of the most common endocrine disturbances affecting women, especially young women, and is a leading cause of infertility in the United States. Prevalence rates are estimated at between 5% and 10% in the United States, afflicting between 3.2 and 5.4 million young women.[33] PCOS appears to be familial, and various features of the syndrome may be differentially inherited.[34,36] Confusing the issue is the frequency, expression, and timing of PCOS (polycystic ovaries can be detected in prepubescent children). From 22% to 30% of women have polycystic ovaries on ultrasound, with 80% having one or more symptoms of the syndrome; 80% of women with normal ovaries also experience one or more PCOS symptoms. Signs and symptoms of women with PCOS may change over time. In addition, polycystic ovaries may be associated with Cushing syndrome, acromegaly, premature ovarian failure, simple obesity, congenital adrenal hyperplasia, thyroid disease, androgen-producing adrenal tumors or ovarian tumors (Figure 23-3), and syndromes with hyperprolactinemia. Thus several factors contribute to difficulties in the diagnosis.

PATHOPHYSIOLOGY   No single factor fully accounts for the abnormalities of PCOS.[33] Hyperinsulinemia plays a key role in androgen excess, anovulation, and pathogenesis of PCOS.[34,35,37,39-42] Insulin stimulates androgen secretion by the ovarian stroma and reduces serum sex hormone–binding globulin (SHBG) directly and independently.[35] The net effect is an increase in free testosterone levels. Excessive androgens affect follicular growth, and insulin affects follicular decline by suppressing apoptosis and enabling follicles, which would normally disintegrate, to survive[34] (Figure 23-4). Further, there seems to be a genetic ovarian defect in PCOS, which makes the ovary either more susceptible to or sensitive to insulin's stimulation of androgen production. Recent research suggests that decreased intraovarian receptors for estrogen receptor-α[38] or insulin-like growth factor–I,[43] increased leptin levels,[44] or direct insulin resistance within selective ovarian cells (fibroblasts)[42] may contribute to this phenomenon.

Several interlinking factors affect the expression of PCOS. Weight gain tends to aggravate symptoms, whereas weight loss may ameliorate some of the endocrine and metabolic events and thus decrease symptoms. Women with PCOS tend to have increased leptin levels (leptin levels are increased in both thin and overweight women with PCOS).[45] Leptin influences the hypothalamic pulsatility of GnRH and consequent interaction along the entire H-P-O axis. Feedback from the polycystic ovary is disturbed because of changes in ovarian steroid and nonsteroidal (inhibins and related proteins) hormones.

In PCOS, there is dysfunction in follicle development. Inappropriate gonadotropin secretion triggers the beginning of a vicious cycle that perpetuates anovulation. Typically, levels of FSH are low or below normal and LH levels and LH bioactivity are elevated. An increased frequency of GnRH pulses appears to cause increased frequency of LH pulses.[33] Persistent LH elevation causes an increase in androgens (dehydroepiandrosterone sulfate [DHEAS] from the adrenal glands and testosterone, androstenedione, and dehydroepiandrosterone [DHEA] from the ovary). Androgens are converted to estrogen in peripheral tissues, and increased testosterone levels cause a significant reduction (approximately 50%) in SHBG, which, in turn, causes increased levels of free estradiol. Elevated estrogen levels trigger a positive-feedback response

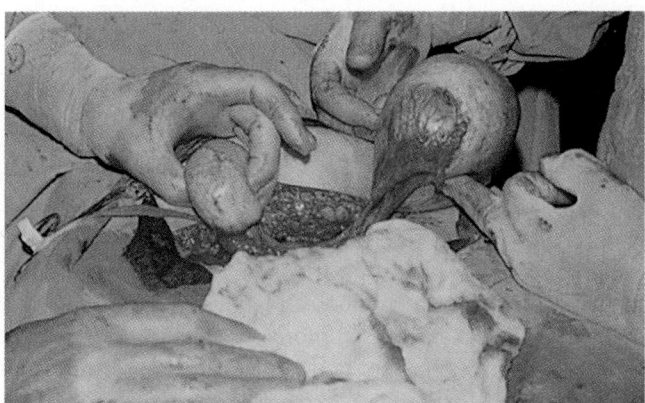

Figure 23-3 Polycystic ovary. (From Symonds EM, Macpherson MBA: *Diagnosis in color: obstetrics and gynecology,* London, 1997, Mosby-Wolfe.)

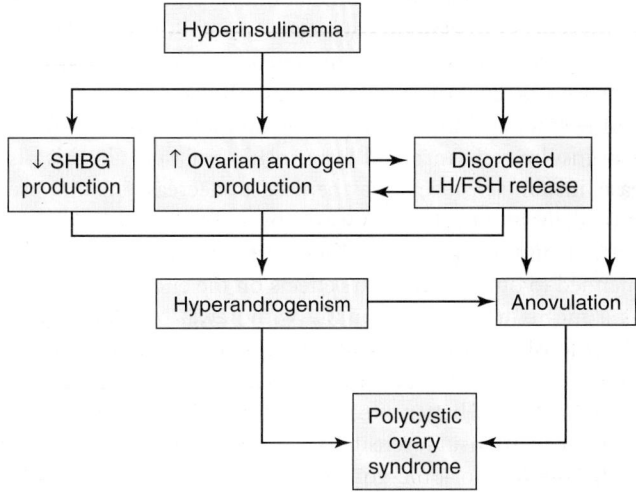

Figure 23-4 Insulin resistance and hyperinsulinemia in PCOS. See text. *SHBG,* Sex hormone-binding globulin; *LH,* luteinizing hormone; *FSH,* follicle-stimulating hormone.

in LH and a negative-feedback response in FSH. Because FSH levels are not totally depressed, new follicular growth is continuously stimulated, but not to full maturation and ovulation. The accumulation of follicular tissue in various stages of development allows an increased and relatively constant production of steroids in response to gonadotropin stimulation. Thus PCOS is characterized by excessive production of both androgen and estrogen.

Increased androgen secretion by the ovaries contributes to premature follicular failure (atresia) and persistent anovulation. In turn, persistent anovulation causes enlarged polycystic ovaries characterized by a smooth, pearly white capsule. This characteristic appearance is caused by an increase of surface area and increased volume of up to 2.8 times, doubling of growing and atretic follicles, thickening of the tunica (outermost area) by 50%, increasing cortical stromal thickening by one third and a fivefold increase in subcortical stroma, and escalating hyperplasia.

CLINICAL MANIFESTATIONS Clinical manifestations of PCOS usually appear at puberty but may appear after a variable period of normal menstrual function and, possibly, pregnancy. The symptoms are related to anovulation and include dysfunctional bleeding or amenorrhea, hirsutism, and infertility. Approximately 38% of women with PCOS are obese.[34,37] Box 23-5 contains a list of signs and symptoms, summary of hormonal disturbances, and complications of PCOS.

EVALUATION AND TREATMENT Diagnosis of PCOS is based on evidence of androgen excess, chronic anovulation, and inappropriate gonadotropin secretion. Tests for impaired glucose tolerance are recommended. As stated earlier, polycystic ovaries do not have to be present and, conversely, their presence alone does not establish the diagnosis. Goals of treatment include reversing signs and symptoms of androgen excess, instituting cyclic menstruation, restoring fertility, and ameliorating any associated metabolic or endocrine, or both, disturbances.[36] Traditionally, treatment of PCOS focused on correcting anovulation and the effects of hyperandrogenism with combined oral contraceptives (COCs), antiandrogens, and fertility agents. With a greater understanding of the role that insulin resistance and hyperinsulinemia play in this disease, insulin sensitizers may be used to decrease insulin, prevent diabetes and heart disease (by reducing microvascular events), and restore fertility.[46] Progesterone therapy is recommended to oppose estrogen's effects on the endometrium and as a means to initiate monthly withdrawal bleeding (at the expense of continued hirsutism). For infertile women, clomiphene citrate, an antiestrogen, can be used to facilitate ovulation, although better effects are achieved if therapy is combined with an insulin sensitizer.[35,36,39] Women who are primed with human chorionic gonadotropin (hCG) before in vitro fertilization have greater success in achieving and maintaining pregnancy.[47] For women who do not desire pregnancy, low-dose oral contraceptives may be used to suppress androgen

production and hirsutism. Approximately 40% of women with PCOS can become pregnant with the proper medical management; this number may increase with current changes in the therapeutic management of PCOS.

Premenstrual Syndrome

Premenstrual syndrome (PMS) is the cyclic recurrence (in the luteal phase of the menstrual cycle) of distressing physical, psychologic, or behavioral changes that impair interpersonal relationships or interfere with usual activities.[48] The prevalence of PMS is difficult to determine. It has been estimated that 5% to 10% of menstruating women have severe to disabling premenstrual symptoms, 3% to 8% have cyclic dysphoria warranting treatment,[49] and 50% or more have mild to moderately distressing symptoms. To confuse matters, it seems that (1) symptoms are experienced to some degree by most adolescent and adult women and can occur throughout all menstrual phases, (2) the presence and severity of symptoms in any one woman may be inconsistent from month to month, and (3) menstrual phase for peak symptom severity may differ depending on the population studied.[50-52]

Past theories of PMS causes have focused on ovarian, pituitary, and adrenal hormones, as well as insulin, endogenous opioids, prostaglandins, yeast, and bacteria. Support for these varying theories is nonexistent or inconclusive. It is thought that PMS is the result of abnormal tissue response to the normal changes of the menstrual cycle. This biologic response may be triggered by fluctuating estrogen and progesterone levels, which are important but not sufficient to produce PMS. Other mediating factors must exist. The effectiveness of selective serotonin reuptake inhibitors (SSRIs) in relieving premenstrual mood, behavior, or somatic symptoms strongly suggests that PMS is a disorder of decreased synaptic serotonin levels as a mechanism of action. Endorphins and neurosteroids have also been implicated.[49,53,54] A predisposition to PMS runs in families, perhaps because of genetics or shared environment. A woman's menstrual experience tends to be similar to her mother's or her sister's experience. Although research is limited, further evidence supports a relationship between the severity and frequency of premenstrual symptoms and reports of low general well-being, history of major affective disorder, and personality characteristics, such as perfectionism, increased stress, poor nutrition, lack of exercise, low self-esteem, history of sexual abuse, and family conflict. In turn, when premenstrual symptoms are perceived as distressing, the quality of interpersonal relationships and self-image are negatively affected.

CLINICAL MANIFESTATIONS   The pattern of symptom frequency and severity is more important than specific complaints. More than 200 physical, emotional, and behavioral symptoms have been attributed to PMS. Emotional symptoms, particularly depression, anger, irritability, and fatigue, have been reported as the most prominent and the most distressing, whereas physical symptoms seem to be the least prevalent and problematic. Approximately 6% of women have classic PMS, as defined earlier, and 7% report premenstrual magnification of symptoms that occur during the entire cycle. A typical premenstrual symptom pattern may appear after the treatment of a systemic disease. Likewise, underlying physical or psychologic disease may be aggravated premenstrually.

EVALUATION AND TREATMENT   Diagnosis of PMS is based on prospective health history and symptoms. Research and diagnostic criteria for premenstrual dysphoric disorder (PMDD) are presented in Boxes 23-6 and 23-7. Because

---

Box 23-6   General Criteria for Premenstrual Dysphoric Disorder

Premenstrual dysphoria is the predominant feature of Premenstrual Dysphoric Disorder (PMDD) and is triggered (not caused) by the endocrine changes that occur in the late luteal phase of the menstrual cycle. Although PMDD is not an accepted diagnostic entity in the *Diagnostic and Statistical Manual of Mental Disorders* (DSM-IV-TR[2000]) text, recognition is given to the severe and incapacitating dysphoria that characterizes the disorder by listing PMDD as an example under "Mood Disorders, Depression, Not Otherwise Specified" in the main text. To encourage further research, PMDD remains in the appendix of DSM-IV. Criteria for PMDD include a rigorous prospective assessment confirming a regular premenstrual pattern of severe depressive symptoms.

Data from American Psychiatric Association: *DSM-IV-TR diagnostic and statistical manual of mental disorders,* ed 4, Washington, DC, 2000, American Psychiatric Association.

Box 23-7   Research Criteria for Premenstrual Dysphoric Disorder

A. In most menstrual cycles during the past year, five (or more) of the following symptoms were present for most of the time during the last week of the luteal phase, began to remit within a few days after the onset of the follicular phase, and were absent in the week postmenses, with at least one of the symptoms being either (1), (2), (3), or (4):
   (1) Markedly depressed mood, feelings of hopelessness, or self-deprecating thoughts
   (2) Marked anxiety, tension, feelings of being "keyed up," or "on edge"
   (3) Marked affective lability (e.g., feeling suddenly sad or tearful or increased sensitivity to rejection)
   (4) Persistent and marked anger or irritability or increased interpersonal conflicts
   (5) Decreased interest in usual activities (e.g., work, school, friends, hobbies)
   (6) Subjective sense of difficulty in concentrating
   (7) Lethargy, easy fatigability, or marked lack of energy
   (8) Marked change in appetite, overeating, or specific food cravings
   (9) Hypersomnia or insomnia
   (10) A subjective sense of being overwhelmed or out of control
   (11) Other physical symptoms, such as breast tenderness or swelling, headaches, joint or muscle pain, a sensation of "bloating," weight gain
   NOTE: In menstruating females, the luteal phase corresponds to the period between ovulation and the onset of menses, and the follicular phase begins with menses. In nonmenstruating females (e.g., those who have had a hysterectomy), the timing of luteal and follicular phases may require measurement of circulating reproductive hormones.
B. The disturbance markedly interferes with work or school or with usual social activities and relationships with others (e.g., avoidance of social activities, decreased productivity and efficiency at work or school).
C. The disturbance is not merely an exacerbation of the symptoms of another disorder, such as Major Depressive Disorder, Panic Disorder, Dysthymic Disorder, or a Personality Disorder (although it may be superimposed on any of these disorders).
D. Criteria A, B, and C must be confirmed by prospective daily ratings during at least two consecutive symptomatic cycles. (The diagnosis may be made provisionally prior to this confirmation.)

Data from American Psychiatric Association: *DSM-IV-TR diagnostic and statistical manual of mental disorders,* ed 4, Washington, DC, 2000, American Psychiatric Association.

the cause of PMS is complex and cannot be reduced to a single biologic explanation and because the occurrence and severity of PMS are mediated by lifestyle, social, and psychologic factors, current treatment for PMS is symptomatic. Nonpharmacologic therapies, with or without medication, tend to be more effective in controlling symptoms than medication alone.

Initial treatment focuses on validation of the premenstrual experience, education on PMS and self-help techniques, and elimination of contributing factors or treatment of coexisting disorders. Individual, marriage, or family counseling; anger management and conflict resolution; and stress-reduction techniques, including biofeedback, relaxation and imagery, regular exercise, adequate rest, and time management, are all recommended. Dietary changes, such as eating six small meals each day; increasing intake of complex carbohydrates, fiber, and water; and decreasing caffeine, alcohol, sugar, and animal fat consumption are beneficial.

After a trial of nonpharmacologic therapies or if criteria for PMDD is met, medications may be added to the treatment regimen. Drugs often prescribed include vitamin and mineral supplements, SSRIs, antiprostaglandins, and alprazolam. SSRIs relieve symptoms in about 60% of women and may be given continuously or only during the premenstrual period. Long-acting SSRIs, such as fluoxetine, should be tapered to prevent withdrawal symptoms. Progesterone has been used for its muscle relaxant and sedative properties but has failed to show efficacy for severe PMS/PMDD in large, randomized placebo controlled trials.[55] Because the edema associated with PMS is a result of local fluid shifts rather than fluid retention, diuretics are not recommended. Women tend to respond immediately to SSRIs whether prescribed intermittently or consistently, suggesting that premenstrual depression is mediated differently than major mood disorders.[53]

In severe cases, menses is abolished, which eliminates cyclic ovarian hormones and thus the biologic trigger for PMS. Elimination of menses can be accomplished with the use of oral contraceptives, medroxyprogesterone acetate, or GnRH agonists; emotional symptoms may not be relieved with the latter. In addition, if GnRH analogues are used, then continuous estrogen replacement therapy is needed. Of interest is that women with PMS may experience similar symptoms with synthetic hormones.[53]

Infection and Inflammation

Infections of the genital tract may result from exogenous or endogenous microorganisms. Exogenous pathogens are most often sexually transmitted (see Chapter 24). Endogenous causes of infection include microorganisms that are normally present in the vagina, bowel, or vulva. Infection occurs if these microorganisms migrate to a new location or overproliferate or if the immune system and other defense mechanisms are impaired.

A number of skin disorders can affect the vulva. They include reactive dermatitis, contact dermatitis, psoriasis, and impetigo. (For a discussion of skin disorders, see Chapter 44.) Most infectious disorders that affect the vulva and vagina are sexually transmitted, however. These disorders are described in Chapter 24.

Pelvic Inflammatory Disease

Pelvic inflammatory disease (PID) is an acute inflammatory process caused by infection (Figure 23-5). PID may involve any organ, or combination of organs, of the upper genital tract—the uterus, fallopian tubes, or ovaries—and, in its most severe form, the entire peritoneal cavity. (Inflammation of the fallopian tubes is termed **salpingitis** [Figure 23-6]; inflammation of the ovaries is called **oophoritis**.) Sexually transmitted microorganisms that migrate from the vagina to the uterus, fallopian tubes, and ovaries cause most cases of PID.

PATHOPHYSIOLOGY   The development of upper genital tract infections is mediated by the failure of a number of defense mechanisms that usually are effective in preventing PID (see Chapter 22). Virulence of the organism, size of the inoculum, and defense status of the individual all determine whether an infectious process results.

PID usually is considered a polymicrobial infection.[56-58] Although initiated by gonorrhea or chlamydia, the majority of cases (up to 84%) are caused by mixed nongonococcal/nonchlamydial bacteria, including anaerobes (*Bacteroides* species and peptostreptococci), facultative organisms (*Gardnerella vaginalis, Haemophilus influenzae,* and streptococci),

---

NUTRITION & DISEASE

Premenstrual Syndrome

Women who are affected by premenstrual syndrome (PMS) often are looking for ways to decrease their symptoms. Dietary interventions that can help are multiple. Dietary changes, such as eating six small meals each day; increasing intake of complex carbohydrates, fiber, and water; and decreasing caffeine, alcohol, refined sugar, and animal fat consumption are beneficial. Recently, a low-fat vegetarian diet was associated with decreased symptoms, possibly because of an increase in serum sex hormone–binding globulin concentration that lowers serum estrogen levels. It also may be helpful to limit sodium intake, and some limited evidence suggests that moderate doses (50 mg/day) of vitamin B_6 may reduce emotional symptoms of depression, irritability, and tiredness. This finding needs to be confirmed.

Some researchers have suggested links between serotonin, endorphins, and high sugar intake and PMS risk. One interesting craving is chocolate. Some researchers suggest that a craving for chocolate is an unconscious desire for a compound called phenyl-ethylamine (PEA) in chocolate that stimulates the release of the neurotransmitter dopamine, which regulates mood.

Data from Mahan LK, Escott-Strump S: *Krause's food, nutrition, and diet therapy,* ed 10, Philadelphia, 2000, Saunders; Barnard ND et al: *Obstet Gynecol* 95(2):245, 2000.

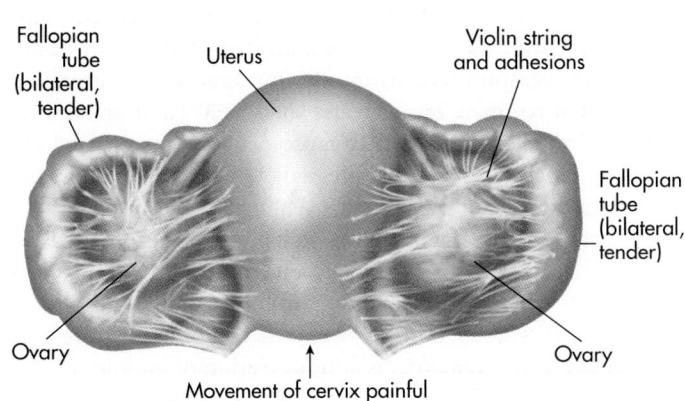

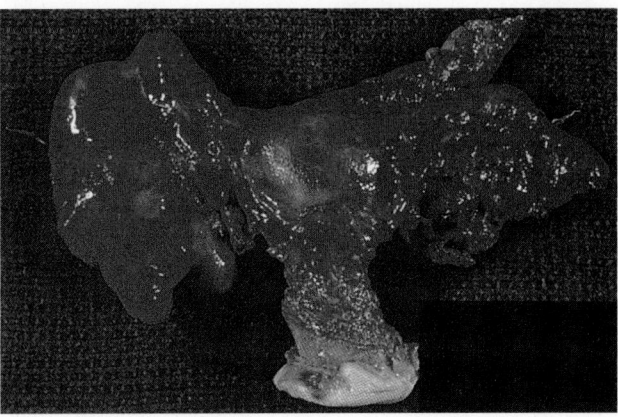

Figure 23-5 Pelvic inflammatory disease. **A,** Involvement of both ovaries and fallopian tubes. **B,** Total abdominal hysterectomy and bilateral salpingo-oophorectomy specimen showing unilateral pyosalpinx. (**A,** From Seidel H et al: *Mosby's guide to physical examination,* ed 4, St Louis, 1999, Mosby. **B,** From Morse SA, et al: *Atlas of sexually transmitted diseases and AIDS,* ed 3, London, 2003, Mosby.)

and genital tract mycoplasmas *(Mycoplasma hominis, Mycoplasma genitalis,* and *Ureaplasma urealyticum). Mycoplasma hominis* and *Ureaplasma urealyticum* have been isolated from the endocervix but not the fallopian tubes. *Escherichia coli* has been overemphasized as a causal agent but may contribute to pelvic infections in older women. Recovery of *Neisseria gonorrhoeae* (37% to 44%), *Chlamydia trachomatis* (10% to 45%), or both (9% to 12%) is variable; however, facultative or anaerobic bacteria have been isolated in about 50% of women with acute PID. About 25% to 50% of the time, only facultative or anaerobic organisms are recovered.

PID develops when pathogenic microbes ascend from an infected cervix along the endometrial tissue to infect the uterus and adnexae. Gonorrhea or chlamydia may induce changes in the columnar epithelium that lines the upper reproductive tract, causing damage and facilitating invasion by other microorganisms. This observation is supported from the recovery of cytokines, such as interleukin 6, from the cervix and endometrium of women with acute PID,[59] and the presence of antibodies to a chlamydial protein (CHSP60) in animal studies of chronic PID.[60] The resultant inflammatory response leads to tubonecrosis with repeated infections and may predispose a woman to PID.[56,57] Other mechanisms that may contribute to PID include lymphatic drainage with parametrial spread of the infection or the adherence of sexually transmitted bacteria to sperm that travel through the genital tract. Several investigators report that bacterial vaginosis (BV), a bacterial overgrowth of the vagina, has been linked to clinical findings of PID and histologic endometritis. Women with BV are nine times more likely to develop PID.[56,61] (See Chapter 24 for further discussion of BV.) After one episode of pelvic infection, 15% to 25% of women develop long-term sequelae, such as infertility, ectopic pregnancy, chronic pelvic pain, dyspareunia, pelvic adhesions, perihepatitis, and tuboovarian abscess. The incidence of complications increases markedly with repeated infections. Tubal infertility occurs in 8% to 11% of women after one episode, 20% to 30% after two episodes, and 40% to 50% after three episodes.[56] The mortal-

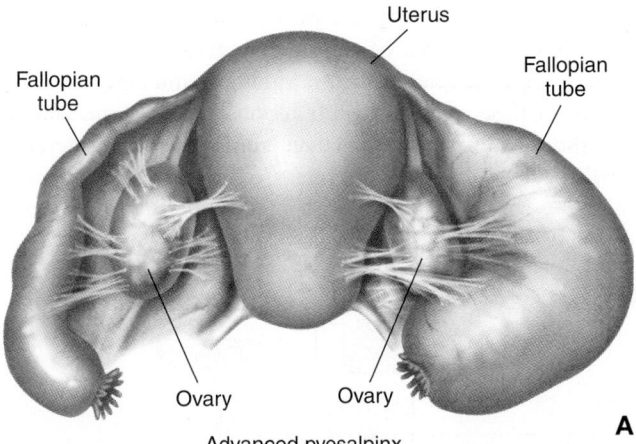

Advanced pyosalpinx

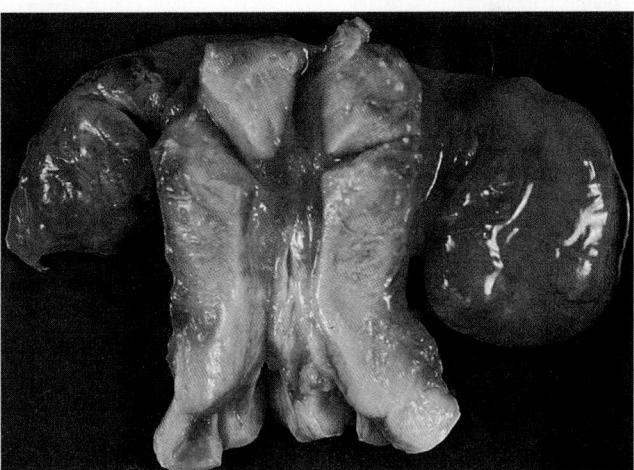

Figure 23-6 Salpingitis. **A,** Note the swollen fallopian tubes. **B,** Bilateral, retort-shaped, swollen, sealed tubes and adhesions of ovaries are typical of salpingitis. (**A,** From Seidel H et al: *Mosby's guide to physical examination,* ed 4, St Louis, 1999, Mosby. **B,** From Damjanov I, Linder J, editors: *Anderson's pathology,* ed 10, St Louis, 1996, Mosby.)

ity rate associated with PID is 0.29 deaths per 100,000 women aged 14 to 44.[62] Most deaths resulting from PID are caused by septic shock (see Chapter 46).

CLINICAL MANIFESTATIONS   The clinical manifestations of PID vary from sudden, severe abdominal pain with fever to no symptoms at all. An asymptomatic cervicitis may be present for some time before PID develops. Of women with salpingitis, 67% to 75% may have a subclinical infection. The first sign of the ascending infection may be the onset of low bilateral abdominal pain, most often characterized as dull and steady with a gradual onset. Symptoms are more likely to develop during or immediately after menstruation. The pain of PID may worsen with walking, jumping, or intercourse. Other manifestations of PID include dysuria (difficult or painful urination) and irregular bleeding.

EVALUATION AND TREATMENT   The diagnosis of PID is based on history, abdominal tenderness with or without rebound, presence of uterine and cervical movement tenderness on bimanual pelvic examination, mucopurulent discharge at the cervical os, white blood cells on Gram stain or wet mount of cervical discharge, leukocytosis, and increased erythrocyte sedimentation rate. To support the diagnosis,

chlamydia and gonorrhea testing is done; sonography, laparoscopy, and culdocentesis are indicated when a woman has recurrent symptoms or symptoms unresponsive to outpatient treatment regimen, fever greater than 38.3° C, or an adnexal mass. Other conditions that cause pelvic pain must be excluded, including ectopic pregnancy, threatened abortion, ovarian torsion, or appendicitis (Figure 23-7).

Because of the significance of the complications of PID, aggressive treatment is recommended. Treatment involves bed rest, avoidance of intercourse, and combined antibiotic therapy (Box 23-8). From 25% to 40% of women require hospitalization for intravenous administration of antibiotics and treatment of peritonitis or a tuboovarian abscess. To prevent recurrence, sexual partners also are treated with antibiotic combinations.[58]

Vaginitis

Vaginitis is infection of the vagina. The major causes of vaginitis are sexually transmitted pathogens (see Chapter 24) and *Candida albicans (C. albicans)*. The incidence of sexually transmitted vaginitis remains highest in young women 10 to 24 years of age.[63,64]

The development of vaginitis is related to loss of local defense mechanisms, such as skin integrity, immune reaction,

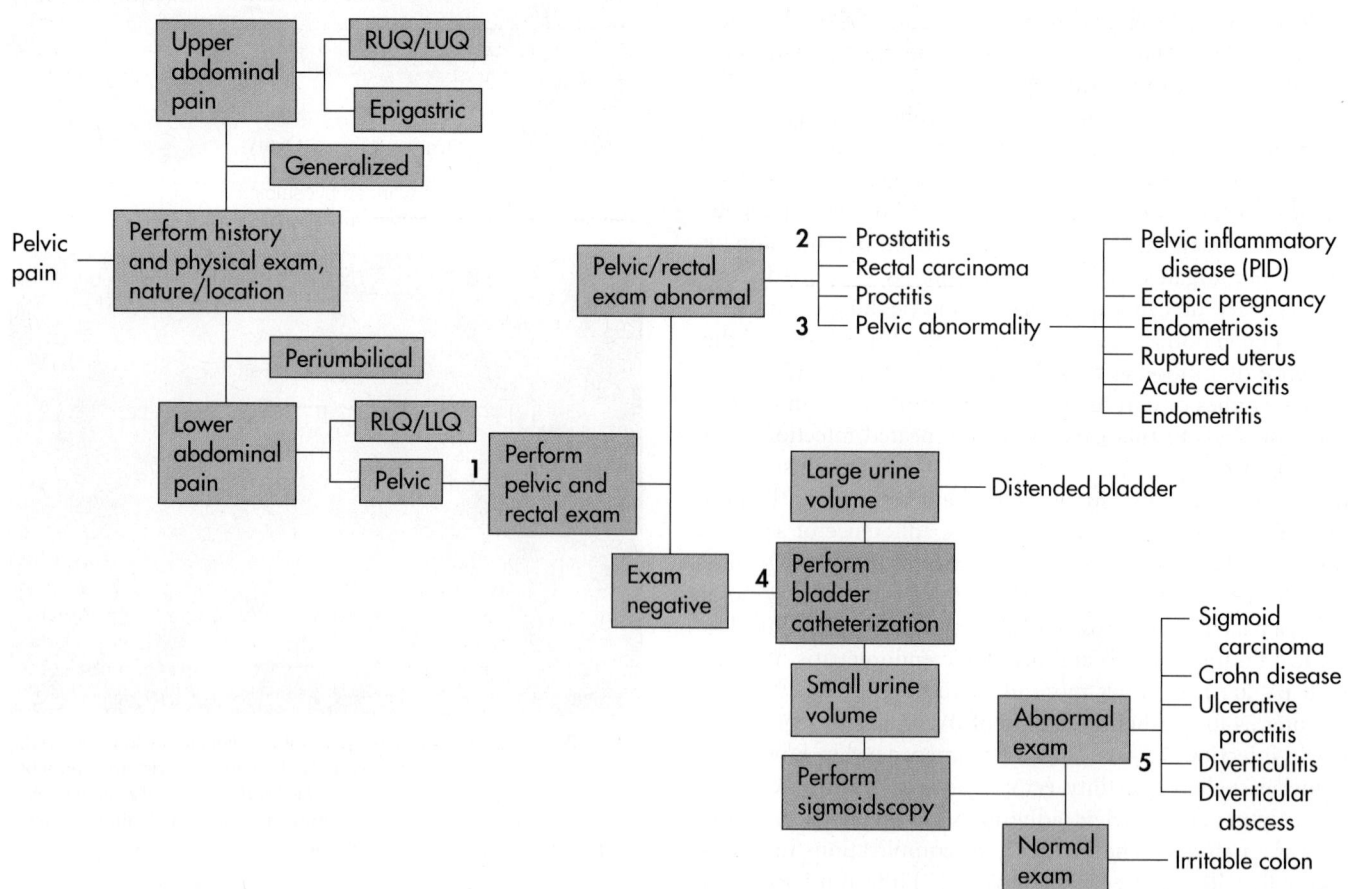

Figure 23-7 Diagnostic algorithm for pelvic pain. *RUQ,* Right upper quadrant; *LUQ,* left upper quadrant; *RLQ,* right lower quadrant; *LLQ,* left lower quadrant.

| **Box 23-8** | Centers for Disease Control and Prevention Recommended Treatment for Acute Pelvic Inflammatory Disease (2002) |

Parenteral

Regimen A

Cefotetan, 2 g IV every 12 hours

or

Cefoxitin, 2 g IV every 6 hours

plus

Doxycycline, 100 mg orally or IV every 12 hours

NOTE: Because of pain associated with infusion, doxycycline should be administered orally when possible, even when the patient is hospitalized. Both oral and IV administration of doxycycline provide similar bioavailability.

Parenteral therapy may be discontinued 24 hours after a patient improves clinically, and oral therapy with doxycycline (100 mg twice a day) should continue to complete 14 days of therapy. When tubo-ovarian abscess is present, many health-care providers use clindamycin or metronidazole with doxycycline for continued therapy rather than doxycycline alone, because it provides more effective anaerobic coverage.

Clinical data are limited regarding the use of other second- or third-generation cephalosporins (e.g., ceftizoxime, cefotaxime, and ceftriaxone), which also may be effective therapy for PID and may replace cefotetan or cefoxitin. However, these cephalosporins are less active than cefotetan or cefoxitin against anaerobic bacteria.

Regimen B

Clindamycin, 900 mg IV every 8 hours

plus

Gentamicin, loading dose IV or IM (2 mg/kg of body weight) followed by a maintenance dose (1.5 mg/kg) every 8 hours; single daily dosing may be substituted

Although use of a single daily dose of gentamicin has not been evaluated for the treatment of PID, it is efficacious in other analogous situations. Parenteral therapy can be discontinued 24 hours after a patient improves clinically; continuing oral therapy should consist of doxycycline 100 mg orally twice a day or clindamycin 450 mg orally four times a day to complete a total of 14 days of therapy. When tubo-ovarian abscess is present, many health-care providers use clindamycin for continued therapy rather than doxycycline, because clindamycin provides more effective anaerobic coverage.

Alternative Parenteral Regimens

Limited data support the use of other parenteral regimens, but the following three regimens have been investigated in at least one clinical trial, and they have broad spectrum coverage.

Ofloxacin, 400 mg IV every 12 hours

or

Levofloxacin, 500 mg IV once daily

with or without

Metronidazole, 500 mg IV every 8 hours

or

Ampicillin/sulbactam, 3 g IV every 6 hours

plus

Doxycycline, 100 mg orally or IV every 12 hours

Intravenous ofloxacin has been investigated as a single agent; however because of concerns regarding its spectrum, metronidazole may be included in the regimen. Preliminary data suggest that levofloxacin is as effective as ofloxacin and may be substituted; its single daily dosing makes it advantageous from a compliance perspective.[a] Ampicillin/sulbactam plus doxycycline has good coverage against *C. trachomatis, N. gonorrhoeae*, and anaerobes and is effective for patients who have tubo-ovarian abscess.

Oral Treatment

As with parenteral regimens, clinical trials of outpatient regimens have provided minimal information regarding intermediate and long-term outcomes. The following regimens provide coverage against the frequent etiologic agents of PID, but evidence from clinical trials supporting their use is limited. Patients who do not respond to oral therapy within 72 hours should be reevaluated to confirm the diagnosis and should be administered parenteral therapy on either an outpatient or inpatient basis.

Regimen A

Ofloxacin, 400 mg orally twice a day for 14 days

or

Levofloxacin, 500 mg orally once daily for 14 days

with or without

Metronidazole, 500 mg orally twice a day for 14 days

Oral ofloxacin has been investigated as a single agent in two well-designed clinical trials, and it is effective against both *N. gonorrhoeae* and *C. trachomatis*.[b,c] Despite the results of these trials, lack of anaerobic coverage with ofloxacin is a concern; the addition of metronidazole to the treatment regimen provides this coverage. Preliminary data suggest that levofloxacin is as effective as ofloxacin and may be substituted[a]; its single daily dosing makes it advantageous from a compliance perspective.

Regimen B

Ceftriaxone, 250 mg IM in a single dose

or

Cefoxitin, 2 g IM in a single dose and **Probenecid**, 1 g orally administered concurrently in a single dose

or

Other parenteral third-generation **cephalosporin** (e.g., **ceftizoxime** or **cefotaxime**)

plus

Doxycycline, 100 mg orally twice a day for 14 days

with or without

Metronidazole, 500 mg orally twice a day for 14 days

The optimal choice of a cephalosporin for Regimen B is unclear; although cefoxitin has better anaerobic coverage, ceftriaxone has better coverage against *N. gonorrhoeae*. Clinical trials have demonstrated that a single dose of cefoxitin is effective in obtaining short-term clinical response in women who have PID; however, the theoretical limitations in its coverage of anaerobes may require the addition of metronidazole to the treatment regimen.[d] The metronidazole also will effectively treat BV, which is frequently associated with PID. No data have been published regarding the use of oral cephalosporins for the treatment of PID.

Modified from Centers for Disease Control and Prevention: *2002 Sexually transmitted diseases: treatment guidelines, 2002,* US Department of Health and Human Services.

[a]Matsuda: *Chemotherapy* 40:311-323, 1992.

[b]Martens MG, et al: *South Med J* 86:604-610, 1993.

[c]Peipert JF, et al: *Infect Dis Obstet Gynecol* 7:138-144, 1999.

[d]Walker CK, et al: *Clin Infect Dis* 28(Suppl 1):S29-S36, 1999.

Continued

Box 23-8 Centers for Disease Control and Prevention Recommended Treatment for Acute Pelvic Inflammatory Disease (2002)—cont'd

Limited data suggest that the combination of oral metronidazole plus doxycycline after primary parenteral therapy is safe and effective.[e,f]

Alternative Oral Regimens

Although information regarding other outpatient regimens is limited, one other regimen has undergone at least one clinical trial and has broad spectrum coverage. Amoxicillin/clavulanic acid plus doxycycline was effective in obtaining short-term clinical response in a single clinical trial; however, gastrointestinal symptoms might limit compliance with this regimen. Several recent investigations have evaluated the use of azithromycin in the treatment of upper reproductive tract infections; however, the data are insufficient to recommend this agent as a component of any of the oral treatment regimens for PID.

Follow-Up

Patients should demonstrate substantial clinical improvement (e.g., defervescence; reduction in direct or rebound abdominal tenderness; and reduction in uterine, adnexal, and cervical motion tenderness) within 3 days after initiation of therapy. Patients who do not improve within this period usually require hospitalization, additional diagnostic tests, and surgical intervention.

If the health-care provider prescribes outpatient oral or parenteral therapy, a follow-up examination should be performed within 72 hours using the criteria for clinical improvement described previously. If the patient has not improved, hospitalization for parenteral therapy and further evaluation are recommended. Some specialists also recommend rescreening for *C. trachomatis* and *N. gonorrhoeae* 4 to 6 weeks after therapy is completed in women with documented infection with these pathogens.

Modified from Centers for Disease Control and Prevention: *2002 Sexually transmitted diseases: treatment guidelines, 2002,* US Department of Health and Human Services.

[e]Witte EH, et al: *Eur J Obstet Gynecol Reprod Biol* 50:153-158, 1993.

[f]Ridgway GL, et al: Azithromycin with or without metronidazole compared with cefoxitin, doxycycline and metronidazole in the treatment of laparoscopy confirmed acute pelvic inflammatory disease [Abstract]. In: *Proceedings of the 11th International Meeting of the International Society for STD Research* (New Orleans), Fort Lee, New Jersey, 1995, International Society for STD Research.

---

and particularly vaginal pH. The pH of the vagina depends on cervical secretions and the presence of normal flora that help maintain an acidic environment. A neutral or alkaline pH normally occurs before puberty, after menopause, and during pregnancy. The acidic nature of vaginal secretions during the reproductive years provides protection against a variety of sexually transmitted pathogens. Therefore variables that alter the vaginal pH or the bactericidal nature of secretions (see Chapter 22) may predispose a woman to infection. These variables include douching; use of soaps, spermacides, feminine hygiene sprays, or deodorant menstrual pads or tampons; and conditions associated with increased glycogen content of vaginal secretions, such as pregnancy or diabetes. Antibiotics may destroy normal vaginal flora, facilitating *C. albicans,* causing a yeast vaginitis.

Normally, vaginal discharge is a clear, milky, or cloudy secretion with a slippery or clumpy texture. It is nonirritating, has a mild inoffensive odor, and turns yellow after drying. Throughout the menstrual cycle, the amount and texture of a woman's discharge will change in response to hormonal fluctuation. Vaginal secretions increase at the time of ovulation, during pregnancy, and with sexual arousal; just before menstruation, vaginal discharge becomes thick and sticky. Although the amount of vaginal discharge alone is not an indication of infection, any other change in discharge may indicate a problem. Infection is suggested with a marked change in color or if the discharge becomes copious, malodorous, or irritating.

Diagnosis is based on history, physical examination, and examination of the discharge by wet mount. Treatment involves developing and maintaining an acidic environment, relieving symptoms (usually pruritus), and administering an-

timicrobial or antifungal medications to eradicate the infectious organism. If the infection can be sexually transmitted, a woman's partner also will be treated.

Cervicitis

Cervicitis is a nonspecific term used to describe inflammation of the cervix prior to the identification of pathogens. **Mucopurulent cervicitis (MPC)** usually is caused by one or more sexually transmitted pathogens, such as *Trichomonas,* gonorrhea, *Chlamydia, Mycoplasma,* or *Ureaplasma.* Infection causes the cervix to become red and edematous. A mucopurulent (mucus- and pus-containing) exudate drains from the external cervical os, and the individual may report vague pelvic pain, bleeding, or dysuria. The infectious organisms are cultured or identified by immunoassay. Definitive diagnosis is followed by oral antibiotic therapy to prevent reinfection; sexual partners are treated as well.[58]

Vulvitis

Inflammation of the vulva is termed **vulvitis.** Acute vulvitis is an inflammation of the skin (dermatitis) of the vulva and often of the perianal area. Vulvitis can be caused by contact with soaps, detergents, lotions, hygienic sprays, shaving, menstrual pads, perfumed toilet paper, or nonabsorbent or tight-fitting clothes. Vulvitis may increase susceptibility to vaginal infection, likewise, vulvitis also may be caused by vaginal infections (e.g., candidiasis, trichomoniasis) that spread to the labia, where they cause inflammation and edema. Other skin diseases, such as tinea cruris, psoriasis, lichen sclerosis, and inflammation of the apocrine (sweat) glands, can involve the vulva (see Chapter 44).

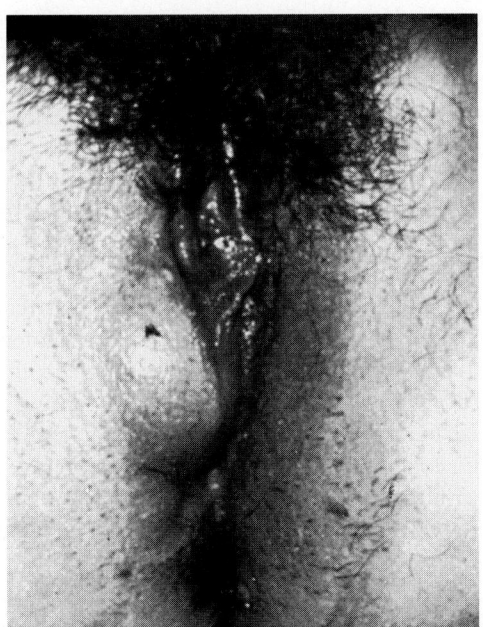

Figure 23-8 **Inflammation of Bartholin glands.** (From Gardner HL, Kaufman RH: *Benign diseases of the vulva and vagina,* St Louis, 1969, Mosby.)

Avoidance of irritants; wearing loose, cotton clothing; and appropriate antimicrobial or antifungal treatment for recurrent vaginitis are usually effective cures for acute vulvitis. Chronic vulvitis usually is treated with fluorinated hydrocortisone. Biopsy specimens of persistent lesions are examined for the presence of malignancy.

Bartholinitis

Bartholinitis, or **Bartholin cyst,** is an inflammation of one or both of the ducts that lead from the introitus (vaginal opening) to the Bartholin glands (Figure 23-8). The usual causes of bartholinitis are microorganisms that infect the lower female reproductive tract, such as streptococci, staphylococci, and sexually transmitted pathogens. Acute bartholinitis may be preceded by an infection, such as cervicitis, vaginitis, or urethritis.

Infection or trauma causes inflammatory changes that narrow the distal portion of the duct, leading to obstruction and stasis of glandular secretions. The obstruction, or cyst, varies from 1 to 8 cm in diameter and is located in the posterolateral portion of the vulva. The cyst is usually reddened and painful, and pus may be visible at the opening of the duct; this exudate should be cultured. The individual may have symptoms of the initiating infection, fever, and malaise.

Most Bartholin cysts are asymptomatic and require no treatment. Chronic bartholinitis is characterized by the presence of a small cyst that is slightly tender but otherwise is asymptomatic. Symptoms occur if an exacerbation of infection causes an abscess to form in the gland itself.

Diagnosis of bartholinitis is based on the clinical manifestations and the identification of infectious microorganisms.

Antibiotics are given to treat infection, and pain is relieved with analgesics and warm sitz baths. If an abscess forms, it is surgically drained.

Pelvic Relaxation Disorders

The bladder, urethra, and rectum are supported by the endopelvic fascia and the perineal muscles. This muscular and fascial tissue loses tone and strength with aging and may fail to maintain the pelvic organs in the proper position. Progressive relaxation of the pelvic support structures may cause uterine displacement. Uterine displacement also can result if trauma, such as childbirth or pelvic surgery, damages or weakens the supporting structures. Pelvic relaxation is progressive and is related to the inherent strength or weakness of the woman's musculofascial tissue. Malpositioning of the bladder, urethra, or rectum (and hence the uterus) may occur many years after an initial injury to the supporting structure. A strong familial tendency and possibly a multifactorial genetic component place some women at risk for the development of prolapse. Genital prolapse is 80 times more prevalent in whites than in blacks, and, despite grand multiparity, pelvic relaxation is rare in Canadian Indians. Risk factors in nulliparous women, which mimic the impact of childbirth, tend to be occupational activities that require heavy lifting or chronic medical conditions, such as chronic lung disease or refractory constipation. Some women at risk for pelvic organ prolapse have neural abnormalities that interfere with the innervation of the levator ani (see Chapter 22 for a discussion of pelvic support structures).

Approximately one in nine women in the United States will undergo at least one surgery to treat pelvic organ prolapse or urinary incontinence.[65] At least 30% will have repeat surgical procedures. Because physical examination is an unreliable measure of visceral abnormalities, the trend is to replace urethrocele, cystocele, rectocele, and enterocele with precise terminology that reflects examination findings (Box 23-9). Having a woman stand and strain maximally provides the best information about the degree of pelvic organ relaxation. Physical examination is augmented with imaging by ultrasound, fluoroscope, or magnetic resonance. The urinary, sexual, anorectal (USA) review of systems for pelvic floor disorders provides comprehensive historical data (Box 23-10).

Box 23-9   Physical Examination Terms for Description of Support Abnormalities

- Anterior wall support abnormality (further specified as lateral, midline, upper/transverse)
- Apical support abnormalities (with or without uterus present)
- Posterior wall support abnormality (specify as distal or proximal)

Data from Brubaker L: Abnormalities of pelvic support. In Copeland LJ, Farrell JF, editors: *Textbook of gynecology,* ed 2, Philadelphia, 2000, Saunders.

Uterine prolapse is decent of the cervix or entire uterus into the vaginal canal (Figure 23-9). In severe cases the uterus falls completely through the vagina and protrudes from the introitus. First-degree uterine prolapse is not treated unless it causes discomfort. Second- and third-degree prolapse cause feelings of fullness, heaviness, and collapse through the vagina. Symptoms of other pelvic relaxation disorders also may be present. Treatment in these cases is the insertion of a **pessary,** which is a removable mechanical device that holds the uterus in position. The pelvic fascia may be strengthened through Kegel exercises (repetitive, isometric tightening and relaxing of the pubococcygeal muscles) or by a course of estrogen therapy in menopausal women. Maintaining a healthy body mass index, prevention of constipation, and treatment of chronic cough may help prevent prolapse. Surgical repair with or without hysterectomy is the treatment of last resort.

Figure 23-10 shows vaginal prolapse caused by cystocele and rectocele. **Cystocele** is decent of a portion of the posterior bladder wall and trigone into the vaginal canal and usually is caused by the trauma of childbirth. In severe cases the bladder and anterior vaginal wall bulge outside the introitus. Usually symptoms are insignificant; increased bulging and descent of the anterior vaginal wall and urethra can be aggravated by vigorous activity, prolonged standing, sneezing,

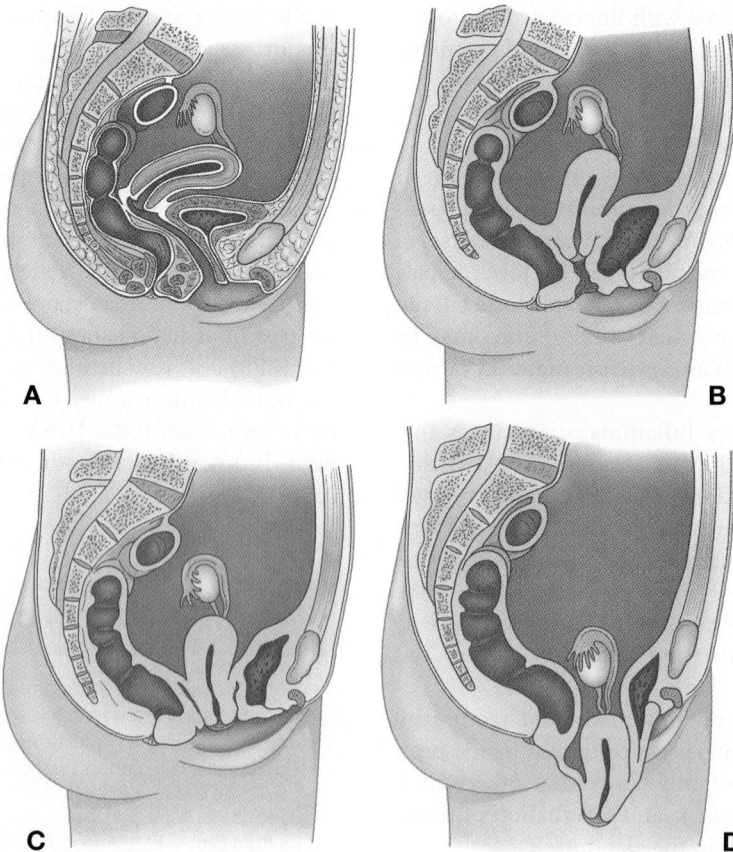

Figure 23-9 Degrees of uterine prolapse. **A,** Normal uterus. **B,** First-degree prolapse: descent within the vagina. **C,** Second-degree prolapse: the cervix protrudes through the introitus. **D,** Third-degree prolapse: the vagina is completely everted.

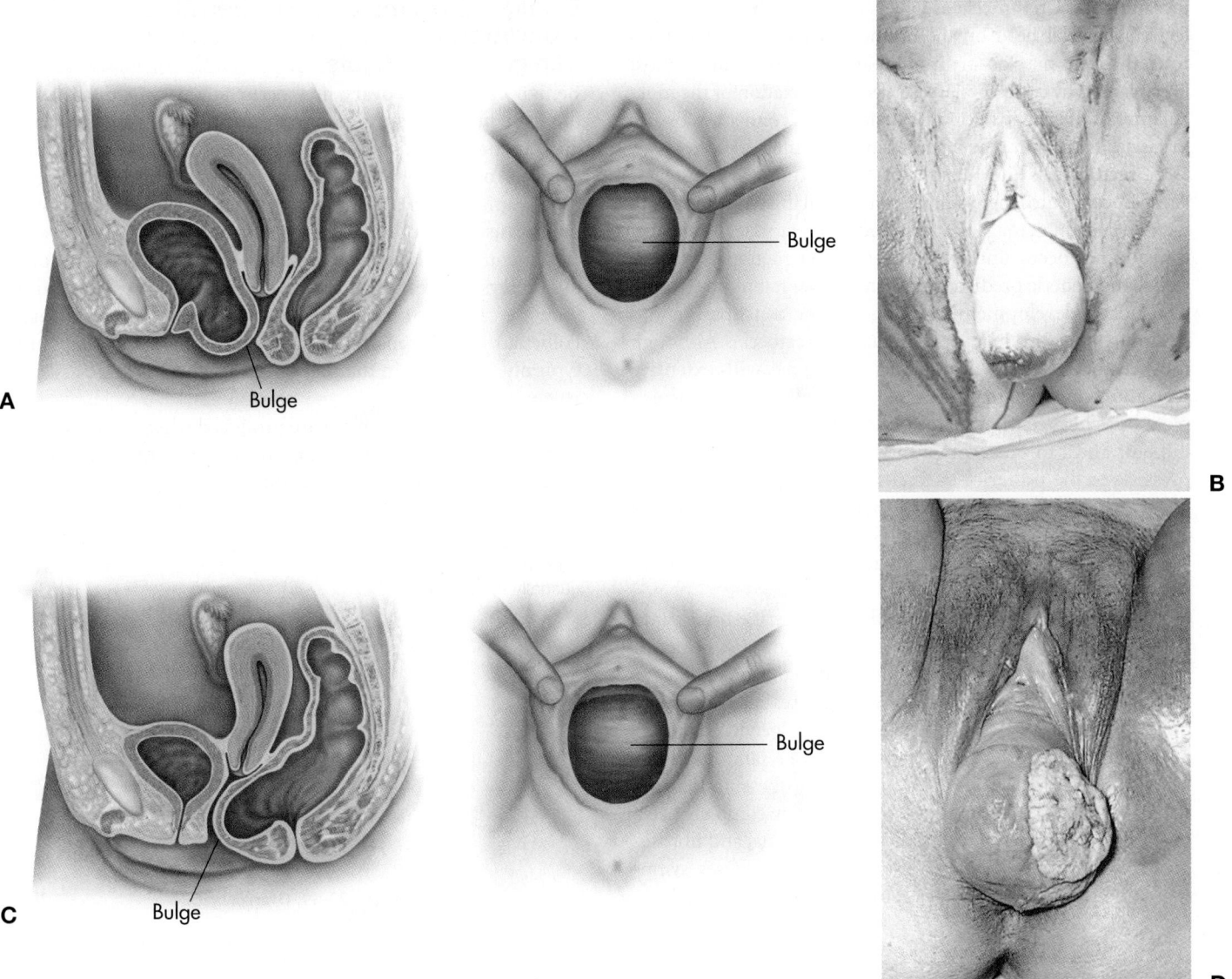

Figure 23-10 Cystocele and rectocele. **A,** Cystocele. **B,** Large cystocele. **C,** Rectocele. **D,** Rectocele associated with ulceration of vaginal wall. (**A** and **C,** From Seidel H et al: *Mosby's guide to physical examination,* ed 4, St Louis, 1999, Mosby. **B** and **D,** From Symonds EM, Macpherson MBA: *Color atlas of obstetrics and gynecology,* London, 1994, Mosby-Wolfe.)

coughing, or straining and can be relieved by rest or assumption of a recumbent or prone position. If the cystocele is large, women may complain of vaginal pressure or the feeling of "sitting on a ball." Vaginal pressure may be interpreted as incomplete bladder emptying, which can be controlled by a second voiding a few minutes after the first void or by manually reducing the cystocele before voiding. Occasionally a cystocele causes significant residual urine and bladder infection.

Although commonly associated with urinary stress incontinence, cystocele does not cause it. Dorr[66] states that "stress incontinence is the result of relaxation of the musculofascial supporting tissues of the urethra. Unless special attention is directed to the urethral supports, operative correction of a large cystocele may cause rather than correct stress incontinence."

Medical management includes vaginal pessary; Kegel exercises (prophylactic use produces best outcome); estrogen therapy for postmenopausal women; and, most important, reassurance that pressure symptoms are not the result of a serious condition. Surgical correction is used for severe anatomic injury unresponsive to medical treatment, and its success depends on treatment of generalized urogenital musculofascial supporting tissue relaxation, correction of underlying paravaginal defects, and elimination or prevention of contributing factors that increase intraabdominal pressure, such as pregnancy, constipation, obesity, large pelvic tumors, bronchitis, and heavy manual labor.[66]

Urethrocele, or sagging of the urethra, is commonly associated with cystocele, especially in women with urinary stress incontinence. Like cystocele, urethrocele does not cause urinary incontinence. Urethrocele usually is caused by the shearing effect of the fetal head on the urethra during childbirth. **Cystourethrocele** may occur in nulliparous women and is most likely caused by congenital weakness and relaxation of the musculature of the pelvic floor or the endopelvic connective tissues or fascia. Treatment may be necessary after menopause.

A **rectocele** is the bulging of the rectum and posterior vaginal wall into the vaginal canal. During childbirth, all women sustain damage that can lead to a rectocele, but symptoms do not occur until several years after menopause.[66] Familial and genetic predisposition and bowel habits contribute to rectocele development. Lifelong chronic constipation and straining may produce or aggravate a rectocele. Although most rectoceles are asymptomatic, larger ones with extensive relaxation cause vaginal pressure, rectal fullness, and incomplete bowel evacuation. If rectoceles are severe, defecation is difficult and can be accomplished only by applying manual pressure to the posterior vaginal wall. Medical treatment focuses on the management and prevention of constipation and, if needed, the use of a pessary. Rectocele alone (without associated enterocele, uterine prolapse, and cystocele) seldom requires surgery.

An **enterocele** is herniation of the rectouterine pouch into the rectovaginal septum (between the rectum and posterior vaginal wall). It can be congenital or acquired. Congenital enterocele rarely causes symptoms or progresses in size; the acquired form usually is associated with other pelvic relaxation disorders such as uterine prolapse, cystocele, and rectocele. Most large enteroceles are found in grossly obese and elderly persons and can be complicated by rupture or complete eversion of the vagina with trophic ulceration, edema, and fibrosis. Treatment is surgical. Table 23-3 summarizes the causes, symptoms, and treatment of cystocele, urethrocele, and rectocele.

Benign Growths and Proliferative Conditions

Benign Ovarian Cysts

Benign cysts of the ovary may occur at any time during the life span, but are most common during the reproductive years and, in particular, at the extremes of those years (Figure 23-11). An increase in benign ovarian cysts occurs when hormonal imbalances are more common, around puberty and menopause.[62] Two common causes of benign ovarian enlargement in ovulating women are follicular cysts and corpus luteum cysts. These cysts are called **functional cysts** because they are caused by variations of normal physiologic events. Follicular and corpus luteum cysts are unilateral. They are typically 5 to 6 cm in diameter but can grow as large as 8 to 10 cm.

Benign cysts of the ovary are produced when a follicle or a number of follicles are stimulated but no dominant follicle develops and completes the maturity process. Every month

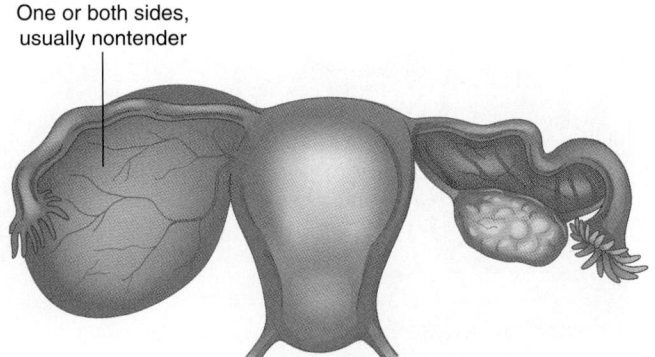

One or both sides, usually nontender

Figure 23-11 Ovarian cyst.

Table 23-3	Cystocele, Urethrocele, and Rectocele		
Condition	Etiology	Symptoms	Treatment
Cystocele	Laceration, stretching, or weakening of supporting fascial tissue; usually caused by prolonged labor, multiple births, or birth of a large baby Paravaginal defects	Usually insignificant Sensation of incomplete emptying of bladder Vaginal pressure or feeling of "sitting on a ball"	Reassurance Depending on age of woman and severity of the condition, includes: Isometric exercise to strengthen the pubococcygeal muscle Estrogen to improve tone and vascularity of fascial support Pessary (a removable device) to hold bladder in position Surgical correction (rarely indicated)
Urethrocele	Pressure of fetal head on urethra and attachments beneath symphysis pubis Familial or genetic predispositions Commonly associated with cystocele in women with stress incontinence	Usually asymptomatic	Isometric exercises (see Cystocele)
Rectocele	Trauma to fascia and levator muscles; usually caused by childbirth Familial or genetic predisposition Lifelong chronic constipation	Constipation or feeling of rectal fullness Difficult defecation Pressure and sensation of fullness in vagina	Isometric exercises and prevention of constipation Surgery (rarely indicated)

about 120 follicles are stimulated, but normally only one succeeds in ovulation of a mature ova.

Normally, during the early follicular phase of the menstrual cycle, follicles of the ovary respond to hormonal signals from the brain. The pituitary produces FSH to mature follicles in the ovary. As the follicles enlarge, granulosa cells in the follicle multiply and secrete estradiol. As a dominant follicle develops, it secretes higher levels of estradiol, which stimulates the LH surge that comes from the pituitary. The LH surge stimulates the follicle to rupture, releasing the ova and transforming the granulosa cells of the dominant follicle into the corpus luteum. If the dominant follicle develops properly before ovulation, the corpus luteum becomes vascularized and secretes progesterone. Progesterone arrests development of other follicles in both ovaries in that cycle. Progesterone, proteolytic enzymes, and prostaglandins trigger follicular rupture and release of the ovum.

Follicular cysts can be caused by a transient condition in which the dominant follicle fails to rupture or one or more of the nondominant follicles fail to regress. This disturbance is not well understood. It may be that the hypothalamus does not receive or send a message strong enough to increase FSH levels to the degree necessary to develop or mature a dominant follicle. The hypothalamus monitors blood levels of estradiol and progesterone; when FSH is low, estradiol does not increase enough to stimulate LH. Recent evidence indicates that when progesterone is not being produced, the hypothalamus releases gonadotropin-releasing hormone (GnRH) to increase the FSH level.[67] FSH continues to stimulate follicles to mature, and the granulosa cells grow and, presumably, estradiol increases. This abnormal cycle continues to stimulate follicular size and causes follicular cysts to develop. Clinical symptoms of follicular cysts or even a single cyst is bloatedness, swollen and tender breasts, and heavy or irregular menses. After several subsequent cycles in which hormone levels once again follow a regular cycle and progesterone levels are restored, cysts usually will be absorbed or will regress.

Follicular cysts can vary in size and symptoms from one episode to the next. Often, follicular cysts will recur. Most follicular cysts are fluid filled; the more solid an ovarian cyst, the greater the chance of malignancy.

A **corpus luteum cyst** may develop because of a hormonal imbalance in low LH and progesterone levels causing an inadequate development of the corpus luteum. There is an intracystic hemorrhage that occurs in the vascularization stage, and the affected cyst then consists of blood. In normal cysts the blood is replaced by a clear fluid that accumulates in the cavity of the corpus luteum.

Corpus luteum cysts are less common than follicular cysts, but luteal cysts typically cause more symptoms, particularly if they rupture. Manifestations include dull pelvic pain and amenorrhea or delayed menstruation, followed by irregular or heavier-than-usual bleeding. Rupture can cause massive bleeding with excruciating pain and can require immediate surgery. Corpus luteum cysts usually regress spontaneously in

nonpregnant women. Oral contraceptives may be used to prevent cysts from forming in the future.

Dermoid cysts are ovarian teratomas that contain elements of all three germ layers; they are common ovarian neoplasms. These growths may contain mature tissue including skin, hair, sebaceous and sweat glands, muscle fibers, cartilage, and bone. Dermoid cysts are usually asymptomatic and are found incidentally on pelvic examination. Dermoid cysts have malignant potential and should be removed.

Torsion of the ovary may occur as a complication of ovarian cysts or tumors or enlargement of the ovary associated with infertility treatments. Ovarian torsion is rare but is a gynecologic emergency when present. Individuals present with acute, severe unilateral abdominal or pelvic pain related to a change of position.

Endometrial Polyps

An **endometrial polyp** is a benign mass of endometrial tissue and contains a variable amount of glands, stoma, and blood vessels. Endometrial polyps are usually solitary and originate at the fundus but also may be multiple (20% of the time) or originate from the lower uterine segment or upper endocervix and contain mixed epithelium. Polyps are morphologically diverse and are usually classified as hyperplastic, atrophic (or inactive), or functional. In the latter case, the surface epithelium may be "out of phase" with other endometrial tissue. Hyperplastic polyps are often pedunculated and may be mistaken for endometrial hyperplasia or, if large, adenosarcoma (Figure 23-12). Although polyps most often develop in women between ages 40 and 60 years, they can occur at all ages.[68]

Endometrial polyps are a common cause of intermenstrual or excessive menstrual bleeding. Diagnosis is made by hysteroscopy or direct examination of tissue obtained by curettage. The lesions are removed with small, curved forceps. Malignancy is extremely rare, and coexistence of a separate

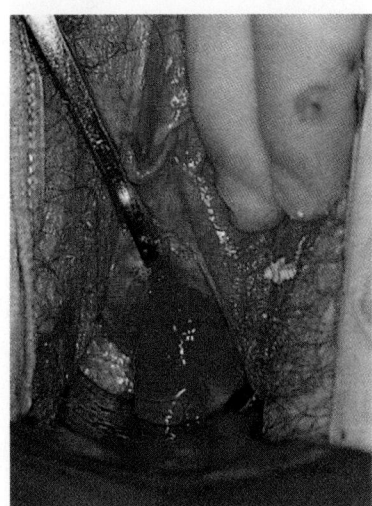

Figure 23-12 Endometrial polyp. It is protruding through the cervical os. (From Symonds EM, Macpherson MBA: *Color atlas of obstetrics and gynecology,* London, 1994, Mosby-Wolfe.)

endometrial atypical hyperplasia or adenocarcinoma is common.

Leiomyomas

Leiomyomas, commonly called **uterine fibroids,** are benign tumors that develop from smooth muscle cells in the myometrium (Figure 23-13). Leiomyomas are the most common benign tumors of the uterus, and most remain small and asymptomatic. Prevalence increases in women ages 30 to 50 years but decreases with menopause. In the United States it is estimated that myomas develop in 30% of white and 50% of black women by age 50 years. The incidence of leiomyomas in black and Asian women is two to five times higher than that in white women.[68]

The cause of uterine leiomyomas is unknown, although their size appears to be related to hormonal fluctuations (particularly estrogen). Uterine leiomyomas are not seen before menarche, and those that develop during the reproductive years generally decrease in size after menopause. Tumors in pregnant women enlarge rapidly but often decrease in size after termination of the pregnancy.

PATHOPHYSIOLOGY   Most leiomyomas occur in multiples in the fundus of the uterus, although they may occur singly and throughout the uterus. Leiomyomas are classified as subserous, submucous, or intramural according to their location within the various layers of the uterine wall (Figure 23-14). Uterine leiomyomas are usually firm and surrounded by a pseudocapsule composed of compressed but otherwise normal uterine myometrium. Degenerative changes, such as ulceration and necrosis, may occur when the leiomyoma outgrows its blood supply and therefore are more common in larger tumors.

CLINICAL MANIFESTATIONS   The major clinical manifestations of leiomyomas are abnormal uterine bleeding, pain, and symptoms related to pressure on nearby structures. The leiomyoma tends to make the uterine cavity larger, thereby increasing the endometrial surface area. This increase may account for the increased menstrual bleeding that is associated with leiomyomas. Pain is not an early symptom but tends to occur with the devascularization of larger leiomyomas. It is also associated with blood vessel compression that limits blood supply to adjacent structures. Symptoms of abdominal pressure are slow to develop, apparently because the tumor is relatively slow growing, enabling adjacent structures to adapt to pressure. Pressure on the bladder may contribute to urinary frequency, urgency, and dysuria. Pressure on the

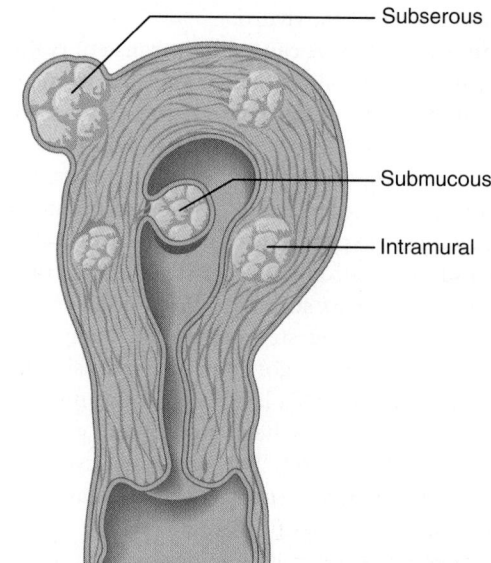

A

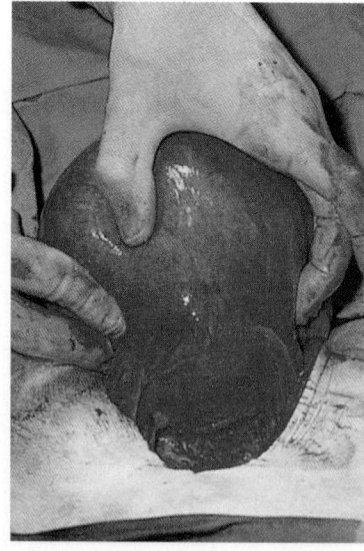

Figure 23-13 **Uterine fibroid.** The uterus is irregular because it contains multiple fibroids. (From Symonds EM, Macpherson MBA: *Color atlas of obstetrics and gynecology,* London, 1994, Mosby-Wolfe.)

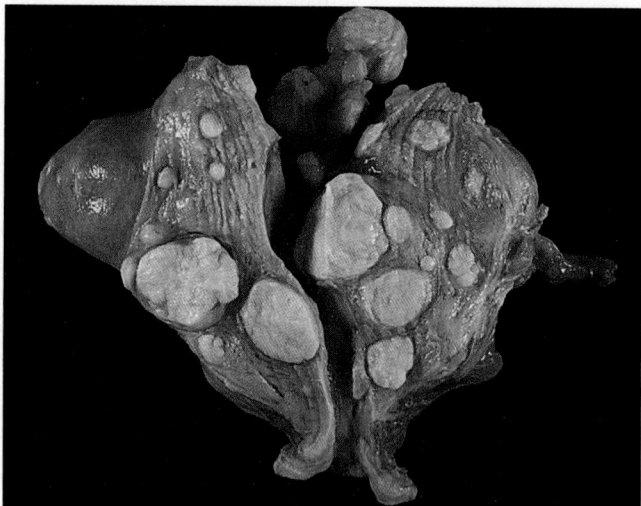

B

Figure 23-14 **Leiomyomas. A,** Uterine section showing whorl-like appearance and locations of leiomyomas, which are also called *uterine fibroids.* **B,** Multiple leiomyomas in sagittal section. Typical, well-circumscribed, solid, light gray nodules distort uterus. (**B** from Damjanov I, Linder J: *Pathology: a color atlas,* St Louis, 2000, Mosby.)

ureter may cause it to become distended "upstream" from the pressure point; rectosigmoid pressure may lead to constipation. A sensation of abdominal or genital heaviness may be felt with larger tumors.

EVALUATION AND TREATMENT   Uterine leiomyomas are suspected when the bimanual examination discloses irregular, nontender nodularity of the uterus. Pelvic sonography or MRI confirms diagnosis.[69] Treatment depends on the symptoms, tumor size, age, reproductive status, and overall health of the individual. Most myomas can be treated conservatively. Conservative treatment is aimed at shrinking the myoma. Some leiomyomas shrink in response to oral contraceptives because progestin is the dominant hormone, however, the estrogen in OCPs may enhance growth so should be monitored carefully. GnRH agonists may be used but have several side effects related to decreased estrogen, including hot flashes and osteoporosis. Various selective estrogen receptor modulators have been studied in conjunction with GnRH agonists and appear safe and effective.[70] Myomectomy may be undertaken and remains the standard of cure for women wishing to preserve their fertility. Newer experimental treatments that show promise include uterine artery embolization, laser ablation treatment with mifepristone, and the levonorgestrel intrauterine system. With each of these new therapies, benefits and risks should be carefully explored.[71]

Adenomyosis

Adenomyosis is the presence of islands of endometrial glands surrounded by benign endometrial stroma within the uterine myometrium. Unlike endometriosis, this tissue does not respond to cyclic hormone changes. It commonly develops during the late reproductive years, with the highest incidence among women in their forties and women on tamoxifen. Adenomyosis has been found in 18% of hysterectomy specimens and 53% of specimens from women taking tamoxifen. Adenomyosis may be asymptomatic or may be associated with abnormal menstrual bleeding, dysmenorrhea, uterine enlargement, and uterine tenderness during menstruation. Secondary dysmenorrhea becomes increasingly severe as disease progresses. On bimanual examination, the uterus is diffusely enlarged, globular, and most tender just before or after menstruation. Diagnosis is confirmed with ultrasonography or MRI.[72] Treatment is symptomatic and, when necessary, is surgical and includes resection of localized areas of adenomyosis or, if severe, hysterectomy. Adenomyosis is unresponsive to hormone treatment, yet three cases of severe adenomyosis treated successfully with GnRH have been reported.[68]

Endometriosis

Endometriosis is the presence of functioning endometrial tissue or implants outside the uterus. Like normal endometrial tissue, the ectopic (out of place) endometrium responds to the hormonal fluctuations of the menstrual cycle.

The incidence of endometriosis is difficult to determine, particularly in asymptomatic adolescent and fertile women. It is estimated that 10% to 15% of reproductive-age women and 2% to 4% of menopausal women have endometriosis. In addition, as many as 50% of women evaluated for pelvic pain, infertility, or a pelvic mass are diagnosed as having endometriosis. Conversely, endometriosis is found in as many as 31% of fertile asymptomatic women undergoing laparoscopy and 11.3% having hysterectomies.[73] Moreover, the frequency and severity of symptoms do not correlate with the extent or site of lesions.[74] A large study has found that endometriosis outside the ovary, pelvis, or uterus causes an increased risk for endocrine cancers (breast, ovarian, and non-Hodgkin lymphoma).[75]

The cause of endometriosis is not known, but several theories have been proposed. In 1927 Sampson[76] proposed that endometriosis is caused by the implantation of endometrial cells during **retrograde menstruation,** in which menstrual fluids move through the fallopian tubes and empty into the pelvic cavity (Figure 23-15). It is now known that retrograde menstruation occurs in almost all women; however, not all women develop endometriosis.

Another theory is that women with endometriosis have a slightly depressed cytotoxic T cell response to endometrial cells or some other defect of the immune response. These alterations may cause the body to tolerate ectopic implantation of endometrial cells. Researchers also have proposed that endometrial cells spread through the lymphatic system or that multipotential cells in the epithelial coverings of reproductive organs are somehow stimulated to develop into endometrial cells. A genetic predisposition to endometriosis has been documented. Studies show that incidence and severity of disease are greatest among women with female relatives who also have endometriosis.[73]

PATHOPHYSIOLOGY   Endometrial implants can occur throughout the body but generally occur in the pelvic and abdominal cavities. The most common sites of implantation are the ovaries, uterine ligaments, rectovaginal septum, and

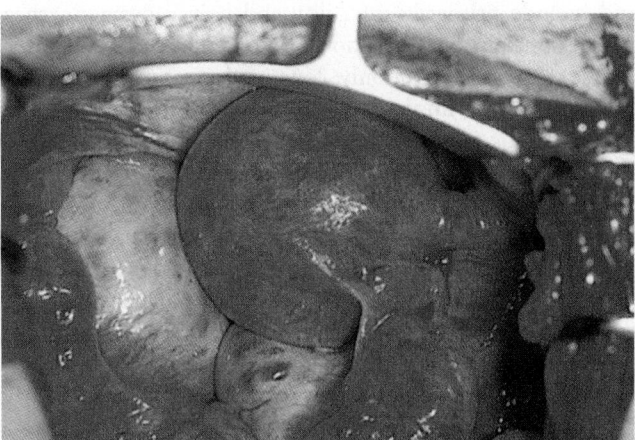

Figure 23-15 Endometriosis. The uterus is distended, and retrograde spill of menstrual loss has led to the development of endometriosis (*dark purple patches*). (From Symonds EM, Macpherson MBA: *Color atlas of obstetrics and gynecology,* London, 1994, Mosby-Wolfe.)

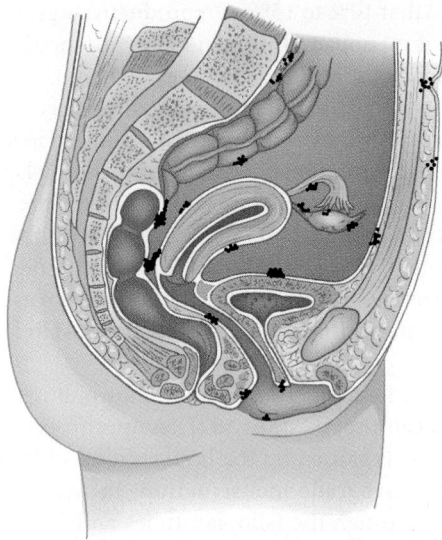

Figure 23-16 Pelvic sites of endometrial implantation. Endometrial cells may enter the pelvic cavity during retrograde menstruation.

pelvic peritoneum (Figure 23-16). Other sites of implantation are the sigmoid colon, small intestine, rectum, appendix, bladder, uterus, vulva, vagina, cervix, lymph nodes, extremities, pleural cavity, lungs, laparotomy scars, and hernial sacs.

Cyclic changes depend on the blood supply of the implants and the presence of both glandular and stromal cells. Given that blood supply is sufficient, the ectopic endometrium proliferates, breaks down, and bleeds in conjunction with the normal menstrual cycle. The bleeding causes inflammation, triggering a cascade of cellular inflammatory mediators, including cytokines, chemokines, growth factors, and protective factors such as secretory leukocyte protease inhibitor[77] and superoxide dismutase.[78] Pain occurs in surrounding tissues. The inflammation may lead to fibrosis, scarring, and adhesions.

CLINICAL MANIFESTATIONS   The clinical manifestations of endometriosis are variable in frequency and severity and include primarily infertility and pain,[73] dysmenorrhea, dyschezia (pain on defecation), dyspareunia (pain on intercourse), and less commonly, constipation, abnormal vaginal bleeding, and if implants are located within the pelvis, an asymptomatic pelvic mass having irregular, movable nodules and a fixed, retroverted uterus. Most symptoms of endometriosis can be explained by the proliferation, breakdown, and bleeding of the ectopic endometrial tissue with subsequent formation of adhesions. In many instances, however, the degree of endometriosis is not related to the frequency or severity of symptoms. Dysmenorrhea, for example, does not appear to be related to the degree of endometriosis. With involvement of the rectovaginal septum or the uterosacral ligaments, dyspareunia develops. Dyschezia, a hallmark symptom of endometriosis, occurs with bleeding of ectopic endometrium in the rectosigmoid musculature and subsequent fibrosis.

Up to one third of women with infertility have endometriosis.[16,73] The link between endometriosis and infertility is strong, yet the degree of disease and infertility are not as closely associated. That is, women with untreated minimal to mild disease may have high pregnancy rates or may experience infertility. The exact mechanism for infertility in women with endometriosis is unknown. Infertility may result from mechanical interference with ovulation or ovum transport through the fallopian tube, yet mechanical interference is an unlikely cause of infertility in women with mild endometriosis. Another possible cause is phagocytosis of sperm by macrophages in the reproductive tract. It is known that endometriosis causes macrophages in the peritoneal fluid to become more aggressive phagocytes (see Chapter 6). However, similar numbers of motile sperm have been recovered from the peritoneal cavity of fertile and infertile women. Elevated cytokines in the peritoneal fluid and interleukin-1 secreted from macrophages of infertile women may play a role by affecting sperm motility and survival, sperm-oocyte interactions, ovum pickup by the fimbriae, or early embryonic development.[73] Other explanations include changes in prostaglandin secretion, luteal phase defect, unruptured luteinizing follicle syndrome, hyperprolactinemia, and autoimmune and genetic factors.

EVALUATION AND TREATMENT   A presumptive diagnosis can be made based on clinical manifestations but laparoscopy is required for definitive diagnosis of endometriosis. Because treatment and prognosis are based on the extent and severity of the disease, a uniform classification system that includes both extent and severity is desirable. However, currently there is no satisfactory classification system for endometriosis.[73,79] Treatment is aimed at preventing or decreasing progression and spread, alleviating pain, and restoring fertility. Current therapies include suppression of ovulation with noncyclic estrogen-progestin COCs, depot medroxyprogesterone acetate (DMPA), danazol (which diminishes midcycle LH and FSH surge), GnRH agonists/analogues (to create a medical oophorectomy), gestrinone (a 19-nortestosterone derivative and antiprogestational steroid), mifepristone (RU 486) (an antiprogestational and antiglucocorticoid agent that can inhibit ovulation and disrupt endometrial integrity), and atrophy of endometrium with progestogens. A newer therapy is injectable GnRH antagonist, which produces immediate inhibition of gonadotropin release. GnRH antagonists are shorter acting than GnRH but release histamine at the site of injection. Conservative surgical treatment includes laparoscopic removal of endometrial implants with conventional or laser techniques and presacral neurectomy for severe dysmenorrhea. Effectiveness of therapy can be monitored by CA-125 (carcinoembryonic antigens shed into blood; see p. 801) and may be increased when medical regimens are combined with surgical techniques. All treatments have risks or side effects, and recurrent symptoms develop in as many as 45% of women within 5 years.[73,74]

Cancer

Malignant tumors of the female reproductive system are common. Endometrial carcinoma accounts for approximately 6% of all cancers in women, ovarian tumors account for 3% of all cancers, and cervical cancers account for 1.8%.[80] Malignant neoplasms of the female reproductive tract account for about 1 of 8 (12.5%) diagnosed cancers and 1 of 13 (7.7%) cancer deaths in women in the United States.[80]

Cervical Cancer

Cancer of the cervix is the most common cancer in women worldwide; however, in the United States, it is the 14th most common type of cancer in women.[80] Mortality rates caused by cervical cancer have declined more than 45% since the early 1970s. The incidence rate in black women (11.2 per 100,000) exceeds the rate in white women (7.3 per 100,000). In 2005 the American Cancer Society estimated 10,370 new cases of cervical invasive cancer and 3710 cervical cancer deaths.[80]

Because of increased prevalence of Papanicolaou (cytologic) screening, rates of invasive cancer have declined steadily over the past 30 years (greater than 55% since the early 1970s). Although mortality for blacks declined more rapidly than for whites, mortality risks for black women continue to be more than two times those of white women.[80]

Precancerous dysplasia, also called *cervical intraepithelial carcinoma [CIN]* or *cervical carcinoma in situ,* is more common than invasive cancer and occurs more often in younger women. An estimated one in eight young women will have cervical dysplasia by age 20, most likely caused by human papillomavirus (HPV) infection.[81] Infection with high risk types of human papilloma virus (HPV) is a necessary precursor to developing CIN and cervical cancer (also see Chapter 11). Smoking, immunosuppression, and poor nutrition are considered cofactors. Infection with *Chlamydia trachomatis* may be a cofactor in the development of one type of cervical cancer; squamous cell invasive cervical cancer.[82] Human immunodeficiency virus (HIV)–positive women are at greater risk for developing cervical cancer.[83,84] Specific CDC guidelines for screening and follow-up of abnormal Papanicolaou testing for HIV-positive women are available and incorporate the use of HPV DNA testing.[85]

PATHOGENESIS   Cervical cancer is a progressive disease that is staged according to histology (Table 23-4). Premalignant lesions usually occur 10 to 12 years before the development of invasive carcinoma. Other than HPV infection, the genetics of cervical cancer remains poorly understood. Several chromosome regions with recurrent loss of heterozygosity (LOH) have been identified (also see Chapter 11). However, the problematic tumor suppressor genes located on these chromosomal locations are yet to be identified. Recurrent amplifications have been mapped to the short arm of chromosome 3 in invasive cancer. Like other cancers, cervical cancer requires the accumulation of genetic alterations for carcinogenesis to occur.

Table 23-4	Clinical Staging for Cancer of the Cervix	
Stage	**Characteristics**	
0	Cancer in situ, intraepithelial carcinoma; earliest stage of cancer; cancer confined to its original site	
I	Carcinoma confined to cervix (extension to corpus disregarded)	
IA	Earliest form of stage I; there is very small amount of cancer, which is visible only under a microscope	
IA1	Area of invasion is <3 mm (about 1/8 inch) deep and <7 mm (about 1/3 inch) wide	
IA2	Area of invasion is between 3 mm and 5 mm (about 1/5 inch) deep, and <7 mm (about 1/3 inch) wide	
IB	Includes cancers that can be seen without a microscope; also includes cancers seen only with a microscope that have spread deeper than 5 mm (about 1/5 inch) into connective tissue of the cervix or are wider than 7 mm	
IB1	A IB cancer that is no larger than 4 cm (about 1 3/5 inches)	
IB2	A IB cancer that is >4 cm	
II	Cancer has spread beyond the cervix to the upper part of the vagina; cancer does not involve the lower third of the vagina	
IIA	Cancer has spread beyond the cervix to the upper part of the vagina; cancer does not involve the lower third of the vagina	
IIB	Cancer has spread to the tissue next to the cervix, called the *parametrial tissue*	
III	Cancer has spread to the lower part of the vagina or the pelvic wall; cancer may be blocking the ureters (tubes that carry urine from the kidneys to the bladder)	
IIIA	Cancer has spread to the lower third of the vagina but not to the pelvic wall	
IIIB	Cancer extends to the pelvic wall, blocks urine flow to the bladder, or both	
IV	Most advanced stage of cervical cancer; cancer has spread to other parts of the body	
IVA	Cancer has spread to the bladder or rectum, which are organs close to the cervix	
IVB	Cancer has spread to distant organs beyond the pelvic area, such as the lungs	

Reprinted from the American Cancer Society's Cancer Information Database with permission.

The progressive changes of cervical cells are classified on a continuum from cervical intraepithelial neoplasia, to cervical carcinoma in situ, to invasive carcinoma. **Cervical intraepithelial neoplasia (CIN),** commonly called **cervical dysplasia,** is replacement of some epithelial cells by atypical, neoplastic cells. CIN is graded as mild dysplasia (CIN 1), moderate dysplasia (CIN 2), or severe dysplasia and carcinoma in situ (CIN 3), depending on the depth of epithelial involvement (Figure 23-17).

In **cervical carcinoma in situ,** all or most of the cervical epithelium shows cellular features of carcinoma, but underlying tissue is not affected. Risk of progression to invasive car-

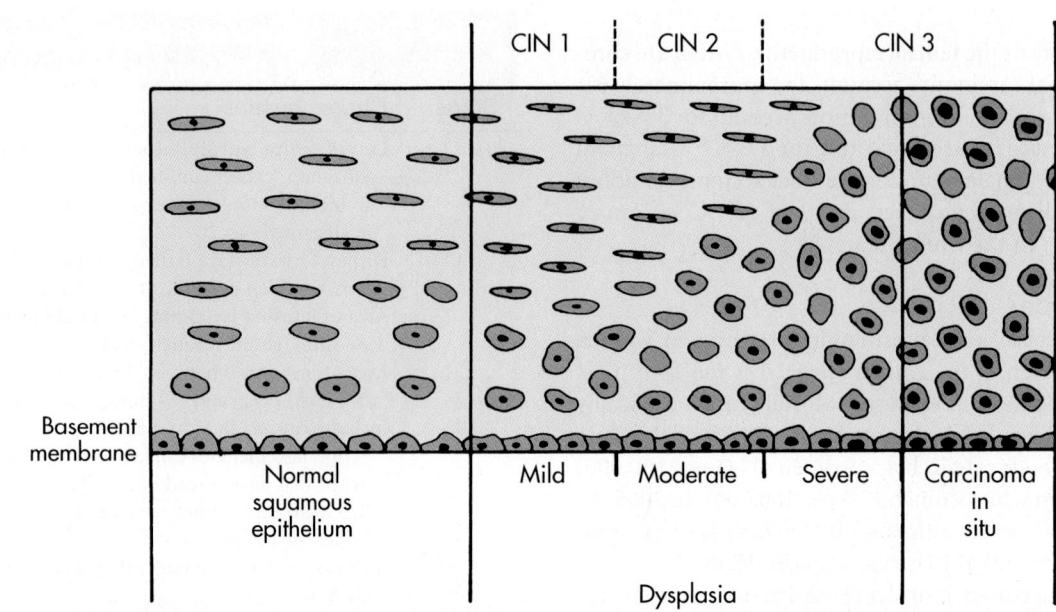

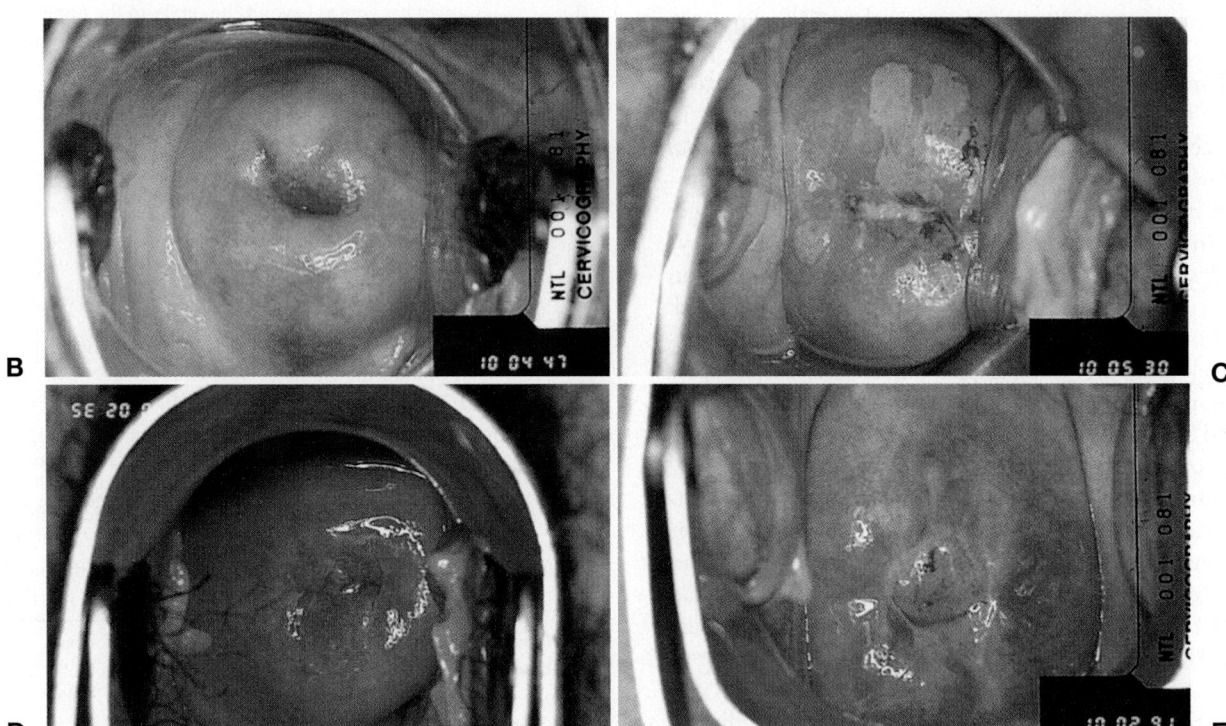

Figure 23-17 Cervical intraepithelial neoplasia (CIN). **A,** Diagram of cervical endothelium showing progressive degrees of CIN. **B,** Normal multiparous cervix. **C,** CIN stage 1. Note the white appearance of part of the anterior lip of the cervix associated with neoplastic changes. **D,** CIN stage 2. Lesions reflected in distant capillaries. **E,** CIN stage 3. Lesion predominantly around the external os. (**A,** From Herbst AL et al: *Comprehensive gynecology,* ed 2, St Louis, 1992, Mosby. **B–E,** From Symonds EM, Macpherson MBA: *Color atlas of obstetrics and gynecology,* London, 1994, Mosby-Wolfe.)

cinoma rises steadily with the severity of dysplasia. Women with CIN 1 have a 15% chance of developing malignant lesions. This rate increases to 75% in women with CIN 3.

Carcinoma in situ is most likely to develop in the squamous-columnar junction—the so-called transformation zone—where the columnar epithelium of the cervical lining meets the squamous epithelium of the outer cervix and vagina (Figure 23-18). In this zone, columnar epithelium is constantly being replaced by squamous epithelium in a process known as *metaplasia*. Metaplasia is thought to be affected by hormonal levels; change in cervical epithelium is not understood as well as endometrial tissue change in response to fluctuating hormones. Because metaplastic cells are at increased risk of incorporating foreign or abnormal genetic

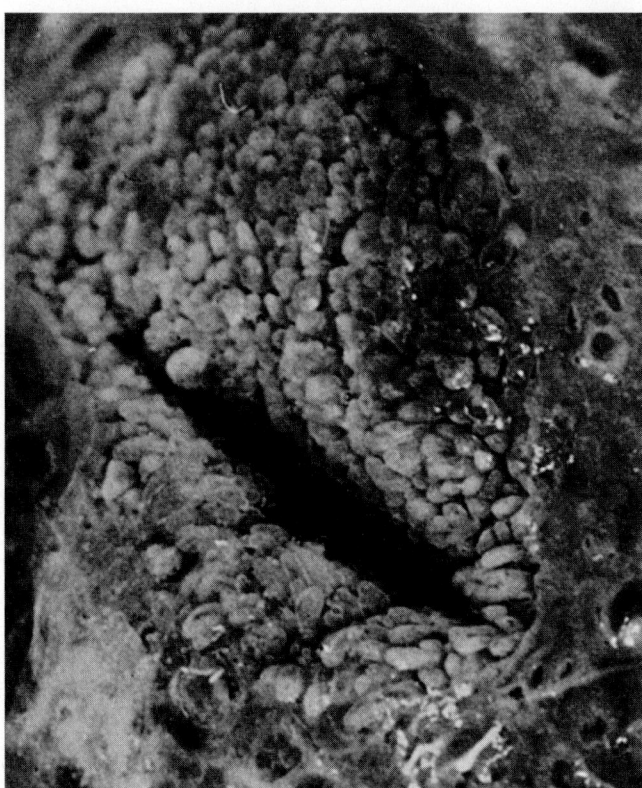

Figure 23-18 Cervical carcinoma in situ. Typical transformation zone, where the columnar (grapelike) epithelium is replaced by metaplastic epithelium. At its outer edge, the metaplastic epithelium adjoins the squamous epithelium, which extends into the vagina. (From Coppleson M, Pixley E, Reid B: *Colposcopy: a scientific approach to the cervix in health and disease,* Springfield, Ill, 1971, Charles C Thomas.)

material, neoplastic changes are most common in the transformation zone.

The spontaneous regression of carcinoma in situ is extremely rare. Carcinoma in situ is generally a precursor of invasive carcinoma of the cervix. A number of factors, including tumor type, contribute to the rate at which carcinoma in situ becomes invasive. **Invasive carcinoma of the cervix** consists of direct invasion into adjacent tissues and metastasis through the lymphatics. Adjacent tissues most often involved are the ureters and structures of the lateral pelvic wall, the vaginal stroma and epithelium, and the lower uterine segment and myometrium. The internal, external, and common iliac lymph nodes and the obturator nodes are common sites of lymphatic involvement. A staging system for carcinoma of the cervix is shown in Table 23-4.

CLINICAL MANIFESTATIONS   Because cervical neoplasms are asymptomatic, regular cytologic screening (Papanicolaou [Pap] test) is necessary. About 90% of cervical cancer cases can be detected early through the use of Pap tests.[86] If symptoms exist they may include vaginal bleeding or abnormal discharge. Bleeding is variable and may occur after intercourse or between menstrual periods. At times, women will complain of abnormal menses or postmenopausal bleeding.

Vaginal discharge is a less common presenting symptom and may be serosanguineous or yellowish in color. A new or foul odor also may be present. Bleeding and discharge are subtle and are likely to be disregarded by premenopausal women, who mistake these signs for variations of normal processes. Postmenopausal women are more likely to seek medical attention if these signs appear. With severe bleeding, symptoms of anemia may occur. Pelvic or epigastric pain is experienced only with large lesions. Advanced disease may cause urinary or rectal symptoms and pelvic or back pain.

EVALUATION AND TREATMENT   Cervical cytology is most accurate if cells are obtained from both the endo- and ectocervix. When dysplasia is detected, cervical biopsy and curettage are required. Colposcopy is used to identify suggestive sites for biopsy. The transformation zone moves higher into the cervix as age increases, making biopsy more difficult. If invasive carcinoma is found, lymphangiography, CT scan, ultrasonography, or radioimmunodetection methods are used to assess lymphatic involvement. Cystoscopy and proctoscopy also may be performed.

The treatment depends on the degree of neoplastic change, the size and location of the lesion, and the extent of metastatic spread. For premalignant change or early cancer (stage 0), cryosurgery or carbon dioxide laser therapy is commonly used; laser treatment may produce better results in the multiparous cervix. Loop diathermy conization and the loop electrosurgical excision procedure (LEEP) are alternative treatments. In LEEP, a small, looped wire with electric current generates heat and burns off cancer cells. Conization is removal of a cone-shaped section of tissue that includes the cancer; high-frequency current is used with cold-knife conization. The amount of tissue removed depends on the location of the lesion. None of these measures affects fertility or childbearing.

For invasive cervical carcinoma, treatment depends on the stage of the tumor (Table 23-5). Surgical intervention may include a hysterectomy, pelvic lymphadenectomy, and pelvic exenteration (radical removal of contents of body cavity). Radiation therapy is used most often in cases of small cell cancer with lymphatic involvement. External radiation usually is combined with one or two intracavity implants. Multidrug chemotherapy regimens also have been used. Recent phase 3 trials suggest significant improvement in survival with combined chemotherapy and radiation therapy.[87] Smokers tend to have a higher stage of disease at diagnosis, and their cancer is more resistant to radiation treatment.

With early detection and treatment, prognosis is excellent. Overall, the 5-year survival rate is 70% and increases to 92% with early diagnosis. A cure rate of 100% is possible for women with dysplasia or carcinoma in situ.[88]

Vaginal Cancer

Cancer of the vagina is the rarest of the female genital cancers and accounts for 0.2% of gynecologic cancers.[80] About 75% to 85% are squamous cell–type cancers; the remaining tumors,

Table 23-5	Cervical Cancer Treatment Options
Stage	**Treatment**
0	Cryosurgery, laser surgery, loop diathermy conization, or loop electrosurgical excision procedure (LEEP)
IA	Surgery (total abdominal hysterectomy, may include oophorectomy), radiation therapy
IB	Surgery (radical hysterectomy with lymph node dissection), internal and external radiation therapy combined
IIA	Surgery (radical hysterectomy with lymph node dissection), internal and external radiation therapy combined
IIB	Internal and external radiation therapy combined
III	Internal and external radiation therapy combined
IVA	Internal and external radiation therapy combined; surgery (exenteration) for removal of uterus, vagina, cervix; could include bladder, colon, or rectum depending on the area of malignant spread
IVB	Radiation therapy for pain symptoms

in descending order of frequency, are adenocarcinomas (15% to 20%), sarcomas (rare), and melanomas (rare). Women with either an in situ or an invasive cervical or vulvar squamous cell cancer are at increased risk for squamous cell abnormality of the vagina.[86] The mean age of women with invasive cancer of the vagina is 55 years; carcinoma in situ occurs about 10 years earlier. Invasive squamous cell cancer affects postmenopausal women, usually in the sixth or seventh decade. Vaginal sarcomas develop in children younger than 5 years and in women in the fifth to sixth decades. Clear-cell carcinomas, the most common form of adenocarcinomas, occur in conjunction with vaginal adenosis in young women with a history of in utero diethylstilbestrol (DES) exposure. Metastatic adenocarcinomas arise from the urethra, Bartholin gland, rectum, bladder, endometrium endocervix, ovary, or a distant organ.[86]

Vaginal and cervical cancers are thought to have similar epidemiology. Both start as intraepithelial lesions, occur in sexually active women, and are associated with HPV infection.[83] As mentioned previously, prior carcinoma of the cervix places a woman at higher risk for developing vaginal cancer. In utero exposure to nonsteroidal estrogens also has been considered a risk factor. It has been estimated that 100,000 to 160,000 women were exposed in utero to such nonsteroidal estrogens as DES, dienestrol, or hexestrol from 1960 to 1970. Apparently, exposure to such hormones during the first 3 months of gestation inhibits the normal replacement of columnar epithelium by squamous epithelium in the vagina of the fetus. The columnar epithelium, which is not normally found in the vagina, then may undergo malignant transformation. Not all women exposed to DES in utero develop neoplastic changes in the vagina, however. Between 0.14 and 1.4 cases of vaginal cancer develop per 1000 women at risk. Nineteen years is the average age at which clear-cell carcinoma develops as a result of DES exposure.

Like cervical neoplasms, vaginal cancers are classified as intraepithelial neoplasia (dysplasia), carcinoma in situ, or invasive carcinoma and are staged based on extension into local tissues and metastasis to distant organs. Vaginal cancer is generally asymptomatic, discovered by vaginal cytologic examination, and confirmed by colposcopy and biopsy. The major symptom of invasive cancer, independent of type, is vaginal bleeding (bloody discharge). Advanced disease causes vaginal discharge, vulvar pruritus, rectal or bladder symptoms, and pain or leg edema.

Biopsy techniques confirm the tumor type and determine its size, location, and extent. Treatment depends on these findings and the age of the individual. Vaginal dysplasia or carcinoma in situ is excised with upper vaginectomy, laser ablation or loop electrosurgical excision, cryotherapy, or laser surgery.[86] Topical 5-fluorouracil (5-FU) also may be used. If the lesion is invasive, surgery may include hysterectomy and pelvic bilateral inguinal lymphadenectomy. Radiation and chemotherapy may follow surgery. Approximately 40% of individuals with invasive vaginal cancer develop recurrent cancer, which usually is confined to the pelvic area. The 5-year survival rate is 70% to 75% for early disease, 30% to 40% for stage III, and rare for stage IV.

Vulvar Cancer

Cancer of the vulva is responsible for approximately 0.4% of gynecologic cancers; an incidence of 3970 new cases were estimated for 2004.[88] The majority (90%) are squamous cell carcinomas, although melanoma (5%), Bartholin gland carcinoma (2%), sarcoma (2%), and adenosquamous carcinoma (1%) may occur.[89] A history of HPV infection or squamous dysplasia of the vagina or cervix is a major risk factor;[83] smoking and coffee use also are considered risk factors.[89] Although it usually affects postmenopausal women (median age of presentation is women in their sixties), vulvar cancer has been diagnosed in women between ages 30 and 90 years. Although leukoplakia and lichen scleroses were believed to be precursors, no prospective studies have been able to confirm such a relationship. Usually, women have a long history of vulvar irritation and pruritus (70%); urinary symptoms and discharge are less common. In addition, women may have a hard ulcerated area of the vulva, large cauliflower lesions, or lesions similar to those of chronic dermatitis. Biopsy confirms the diagnosis. Treatment options include surgery primarily and sometimes radiation with or without chemotherapy.[89] Prognosis depends on lesion size and location, histology, and lymph involvement; risk of metastasis increases with tumor size. The 5-year survival rate is 85% to 90% for stage I and decreases to 20% for stage IV cancer.[89]

Endometrial Cancer and Uterine Sarcoma

Endometrial carcinomas arise within the glandular epithelium of the uterine lining. Cancer of the endometrium is the most common cancer of the pelvic region in women and accounts for 6% of all cancers in women.[80] Estimates include 40,880 new cases in 2005, with approximately 7310 deaths.[80] Although incidence rates are higher in white than in black women, mortality rates in black women are nearly twice as high. Most cases occur in postmenopausal women (Figure 23-19), with peak incidence occurring in the late fifties to early sixties.[90] The primary risk factor is unopposed estrogen exposure with resultant hyperplasia.[90] The World Health Organization has divided endometrial hyperplasia into two major categories according to whether cytologic atypia is present; only atypical hyperplasia has a significant risk of progressing to well-differentiated endometrial carcinoma.[91] Estrogen-related exposures include estrogen replacement therapy, tamoxifen, early menarche, late menopause, never having children, and a failure to ovulate. Other risk factors include infertility, diabetes, gallbladder disease, hypertension, and obesity. Hereditary nonpolyposis colon cancer, a genetic syndrome, also has been associated with endometrial and ovarian cancer.

Pregnancy and the use of COCs containing synthetic estrogen and progestin have a protective effect.[90] After 12 months of COC use, the risk of endometrial cancer is half that among women who have never used COCs; this effect seems to persist for at least 10 years after birth control pills are discontinued.[57] In addition, controlling obesity, hypertension, and diabetes may reduce an individual's risk of endometrial cancer.

About 75% of endometrial cancers are adenocarcinomas. Abnormal vaginal bleeding is the most common clinical manifestation of endometrial cancer. The bleeding is caused by disruption of the endometrial surface by neoplastic processes. Pain and weight loss are symptoms of late disease.

Screening methods for early detection of endometrial cancer are as effective as those for cervical cancer. Pap tests, which are highly effective in detecting cervical dysplasia, are ineffective in detecting early endometrial cancer.[80] Endometrial biopsies, which allow for direct cytologic sampling of the endometrium, are required for diagnosis and are recommended to screen high-risk women at menopause and periodically. Transvaginal ultrasound (TVUS) is used to measure endometrial thickness and also may be used to screen postmenopausal and high-risk premenopausal women. An endometrial depth of less than 5 mm is suggestive of atrophic endometrium.[26,91] Although serum CA-125 is not a useful screen for endometrial cancer, it may predict the presence of

extrauterine disease in women with endometrial cancer.[91] Once cancer is confirmed by biopsy, a laparoscopy may be performed to determine stage of disease. Evaluation for metastasis includes routine blood work, metabolic studies, chest x-ray films, intravenous pyelography (IVP), barium enema, ultrasonography, lymphangiography, CT, MRI, and bone scans.

Treatment is based on the extent of the disease and includes surgical removal of the obvious tumor and radiation for control of residual microscopic disease. Surgical interventions include curettage for carcinoma in situ, total abdominal hysterectomy with bilateral salpingo-oophorectomy, and lymphadenectomy. Chemotherapy or hormone therapy with progesterone may be used. Treatment options for recurrent cancer include radiation and hormone therapy with progestins. Progesterone may benefit individuals with advanced or recurrent disease. The 1-year relative survival rate for endometrial cancer is 93%; the 5-year relative survival rate is 95% with early diagnosis and 64% if diagnosis occurred in the late stage. Relative survival rates for white women exceed those for black women by at least 18% at every stage.

Uterine sarcomas are rare neoplasms that arise from myometrial smooth muscle, endometrial stroma, or more rarely ubiquitous connective tissue elements. Uterine sarcomas constitute 2% to 6% of all uterine malignancies. The average age at diagnosis is the early fifties. There is no epidemiologic association with parity, systemic disease, or prior radiation exposure. However, there is a difference in race-specific incidence; the relative risk for black women compared with white women is 1.6. Symptoms include abnormal uterine bleeding, awareness of a mass, and pelvic pressure or pain. Vaginal discharge is rare. Most commonly, serendipitous diagnosis occurs at the time of surgery for leiomyomas. Treatment consists of total hysterectomy with bilateral salpingo-oophorectomy and selective lymphadenectomy followed by radiation therapy. Five-year survival rates range from 50% in early disease to 5% in advanced disease. Like most cancers, stage is the most important determinant of prognosis. The survival rate at 5 years for stage I disease is 50%. Few women survive advanced-stage disease.[92]

Ovarian Cancer

The incidence of ovarian cancer is estimated as 22,220 women in the United States in 2005[80] (Figure 23-20). In 2005 ovarian cancer accounted for 3% of all cancers among women and caused more deaths than any other female reproductive cancer.[80] During 1985 to 2001, the incidence declined at a rate of 0.8% per year. The decline was greater in women 65 and older.[80] Ovarian cancer in women older than 40 years is associated with early menarche, late menopause, nulliparity, and the use of fertility drugs. Factors that suppress ovulation decrease the risk of ovarian cancer and include multiple pregnancies, prolonged lactation, and the use of oral contraceptives. Oral contraceptives increase apoptosis of ovarian surface epithelium in primates, and progestin appears to be the crucial component.[93]

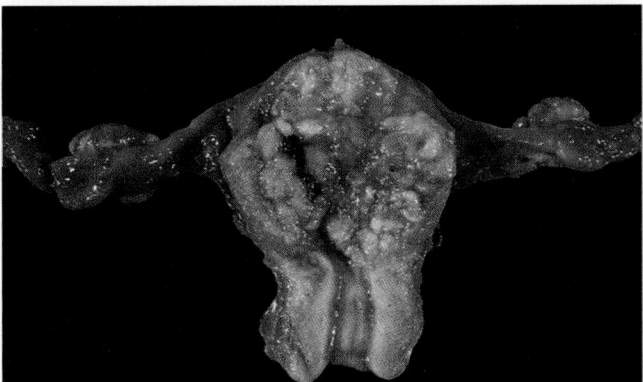

Figure 23-19 **Endometrial cancer.** Tumor fills the endometrial cavity. Obvious myometrial invasion is seen. (From Damjanov I, Linder J, editors: *Anderson's pathology,* ed 10, St Louis, 2000, Mosby.)

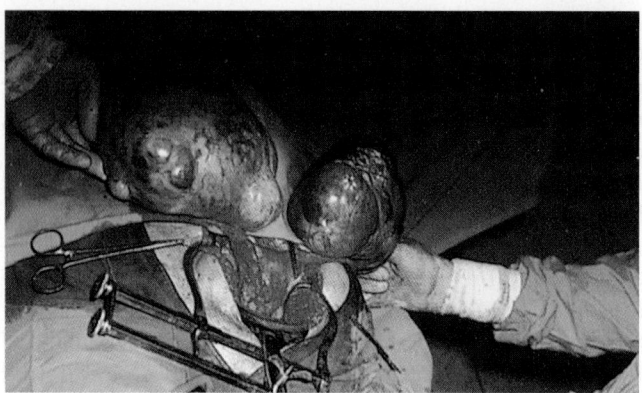

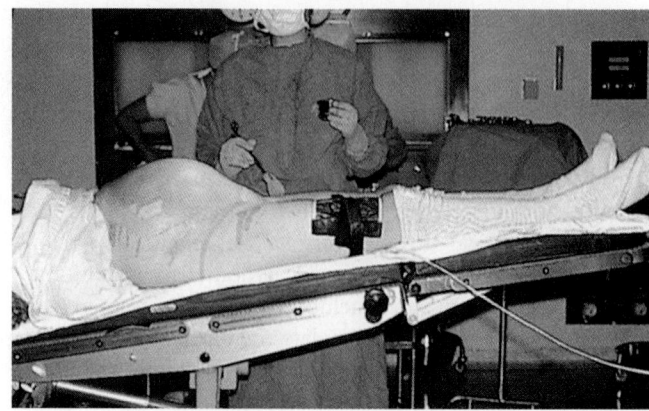

A

Figure 23-20 **Ovarian tumors.** Bilateral multicystic ovarian tumors. (From Symonds EM, Macpherson MBA: *Color atlas of obstetrics and gynecology*, London, 1994, Mosby-Wolfe.)

PATHOGENESIS   The cause of ovarian cancer is unknown at present. The great majority (approximately 90%) of ovarian cancers are sporadic and not associated with a known pattern of inheritance.[94] Of the 5% to 10% that are familial, the majority are associated with the breast cancer susceptibility gene 1 *(BRCA1)* and a smaller number with mutations of *BRCA2* or mismatch repair genes (hereditary nonpolyposis colorectal cancer syndrome). Germline mutations of *p53* are rarely associated with ovarian cancer (i.e., Li-Fraumeni syndrome). However, frequent abnormalities in *p53* occur in sporadic ovarian cancers. In sporadic ovarian cancer, *BRCA1* and *BRCA2* are rarely mutated.[95]

The two major types of ovarian cancer are epithelial ovarian neoplasms and germ-cell neoplasms. Most ovarian malignancies are epithelial ovarian neoplasms that usually develop from the surface epithelium of the ovary or that which lines cysts immediately beneath the ovarian surface. Most epithelial cancers arise from a single cell (i.e., clonal), involve loss of tumor suppressor genes, and activation of oncogenes (see Chapter 11). Therefore a number of abnormalities, including LOH, and amplification of several chromosomes are observed. Epithelial ovarian tumors may be serous, mucinous, endometrioid, or undifferentiated. These tumors are classified as (1) benign, (2) borderline malignant, or (3) frankly malignant. The malignant forms are collectively classed as ovarian adenocarcinomas and account for 90% of all ovarian malignancies. Of the ovarian adenocarcinomas, 40% to 50% are serous epithelial malignancies, which usually involve both ovaries and tend to be bulky. Serous tumors generally affect women from 50 to 55 years of age and are extremely rare in prepubertal girls. The 5-year survival rate is 90% if treated in stage I; however, only 25% of ovarian cancers are diagnosed this early. Five-year survival rates decline with stage of disease: 40% to 60% of women with stage II disease survive 5 years, 15% to 20% with stage III disease survive 5 years, and less than 5% with stage IV disease survive 5 years.[96]

Germ-cell tumors are derived from the primitive germ cells (gametes) of the embryonic gonad and may be either malignant or benign. The benign cystic teratoma accounts for

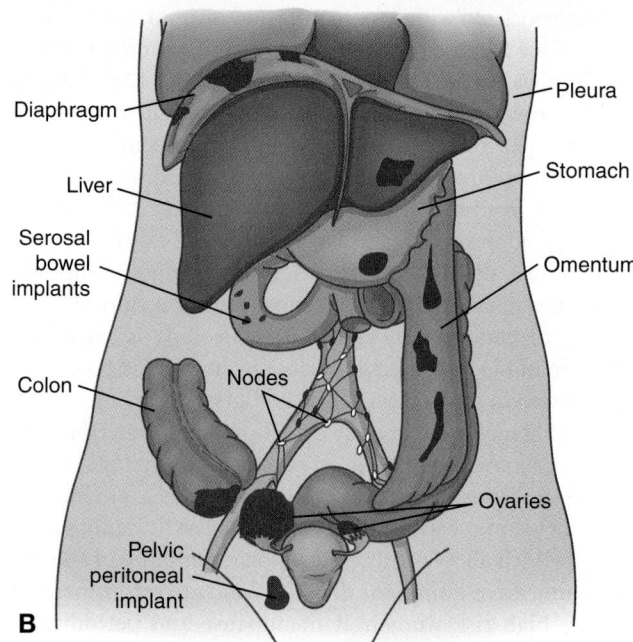

B

Figure 23-21 Large malignant ovarian tumor and metastasis of ovarian cancer. **A,** Tumor has caused massive abdominal distention. **B,** Pattern of spread for epithelial cancer of the ovary. (**A** from Symonds EM, Macpherson MBA: *Color atlas of obstetrics and gynecology*, London, 1994, Mosby-Wolfe.)

approximately 10% of all ovarian tumors. If the germ-cell tumor is malignant, it tends to be a highly aggressive and rapidly growing tumor with a poor prognosis. Germ-cell tumors almost always occur in children or adolescents.

CLINICAL MANIFESTATIONS   Given the location of the ovaries, assessing abnormalities on routine gynecologic examination poses difficulty, and thus, the disease is mostly diagnosed after metastases have occurred. The intrapelvic location of the ovaries and the range of tumor activity (from slow to rapid and relentless growth) cause diverse signs and symptoms. The most obvious symptoms are pain and abdominal swelling that arise from the primary ovarian mass or ascites and abdominal distention (Figure 23-21). Gastrointestinal manifestations may include dyspepsia, vomiting, and

Table 23-6	FIGO Staging of Carcinoma of the Ovary
Stage	Characteristics
I	Growth limited to the ovaries
IA	Growth limited to one ovary; no ascites
i	No tumor on the external surface; capsule intact (90% 5-year survival with treatment)
ii	Tumor present on the external surface, or capsule(s) ruptured, or both
IB	Growth limited to both ovaries; no ascites
i	No tumor on the external surface; capsule intact
ii	Tumor present on the external surface, or capsule(s) ruptured, or both
IC	Tumor either stage IA or stage IB, with ascites present or with positive peritoneal washings
II	Growth involving one or both ovaries with pelvic extension
IIA	Extension and/or metastases to the uterus and/or tubes
IIB	Extension to other pelvic tissues
IIC	Tumor either stage IIA or stage IIB but with ascites present or with positive peritoneal washings
III	Growth involving one or both ovaries with intraperitoneal metastases outside the pelvis, or positive retroperitoneal nodes, or both; tumor limited to the true pelvis with histologically proven malignant extension to small bowel or omentum
IV	Growth involving one or both ovaries with distant metastases; if pleural effusion is present, there must be positive cytology to allot a case to stage IV; parenchymal liver metastases indicate stage IV
Special category	Unexplored cases that are thought to be ovarian carcinoma

FIGO, International Federation of Gynecologists and Obstetricians.

alterations in bowel habits caused by mechanical obstruction. Abnormal vaginal bleeding may occur if the postmenopausal endometrium is stimulated by a hormone-secreting tumor. The tumor also may cause ulcerations through the vaginal wall that result in bleeding. There also can be a feeling of pressure in the pelvis and leg pain.

Systemic manifestations of nonmetastatic malignant disease include connective tissue inflammation (dermatomyositis), abnormal pigmentation (acanthosis nigricans), and subacute cerebellar degeneration. Tumor obstruction of vascular channels can cause venous and, occasionally, arterial thrombosis. Alterations in coagulability also occur, contributing to clot formation. Metastasis often causes pleural effusion.

EVALUATION AND TREATMENT Because ovarian cancer has no early symptoms and no effective screening techniques can detect it, disease usually is advanced by the time treatment is sought. Diagnosis is confirmed by biopsy, and extent of the disease is determined by ultrasound, CT, MRI, or other imaging techniques. Women undergoing surgery for early-stage ovarian cancer need thorough checking for spread to the abdomen and lymph nodes. Staging of disease requires exploratory surgery. The International Federation of Gynecologists and Obstetricians (FIGO) staging system is described in Table 23-6. Other preoperative studies may be used to determine the extent of metastasis. These include an upper gastrointestinal series, barium enema, intravenous pyelogram (IVP), mammography, and lymphography.

The search for a tumor marker that could be used as a screening tool for ovarian cancer is ongoing. Some types of germ cells and, rarely, adenocarcinoma may be associated with increased levels of α-fetoprotein (AFP), human chorionic gonadotropin (hCG), or carcinoembryonic antigen (CA-125). Increased CA-125 levels are found in about 78% to 80% of nonmucinous ovarian cancers; however, elevated levels are produced in 29% of nongynecologic tumors and in a variety of noncancerous conditions, for example, endometriosis, PID, benign ovarian cysts, myomas, and pregnancy. Carcinoembryonic antigen is a nonspecific, nonsensitive test for ovarian cancer; when combined with transvaginal ultrasound, it is more sensitive and accurate than pelvic examination alone. Using a panel of markers may be more sensitive and specific. Further research is needed.[96]

The initial approach to treatment is surgery, which is performed to determine the stage of disease and remove as much of the tumor as possible. Radiation therapy may follow if the tumor is smaller than 2 cm in size and is confined to the abdominopelvic area without involvement of the kidneys or liver. Radiation therapy may be administered externally, intraperitoneally, or in both ways. The success of chemotherapy depends on whether the tumor is a discrete mass, the extent of disease, and whether there has been prior exposure to chemotherapeutic agents. The gold standard for previously untreated individuals is taxane and platinum.[97] Most people, however, suffer relapses and less than 20% survive long term with stage III or IV disease. New therapies have extended clinical trials, including small molecular-weight inhibitors, monoclonal antibodies, antisense therapy, and gene therapy.[97]

Sexual Dysfunction

Increased awareness of female sexual dysfunction is relatively new, and most of what is known comes from clinical observations and anecdotal reports from women. Adequate research is still needed. Both organic and psychosocial disorders can be implicated in sexual dysfunction. Organic problems may be the underlying cause in 10% to 20% of cases and can contribute to another 15%. The exact cause may not always be identified.

As in men, chronic illness can affect sexual functioning and response in women. For example, neuropathy in the

Table 23-7	Possible Effects of Chronic Disease on Sexual Functioning in Women
Disease	**Sexual Function**
Cerebral palsy	Intact genital sensations, decreased lubrication; difficulty with sexual activity/positioning because of muscle spasticity, rigidity, and/or weakness; pain with positioning caused by contracture of knees and hips or because of increased spasms with arousal
Cerebrovascular accident (CVA)	Difficulties in sexual positioning and sensitivity because of impaired motor strength, coordination or paralysis; decreased sex drive with stroke on the dominant side of the brain
Diabetes	Diminished intensity of orgasm and gradual decline in ability to achieve orgasm; decreased lubrication and/or recurrent vaginal infections with resultant dyspareunia
Chronic renal failure	Decreased arousal; increasingly rare and less intense orgasms; decreased lubrication
Rheumatoid arthritis (RA)	Painful sexual activity/positions because of swollen, painful joints, muscular atrophy and joint contracture; decreased sex drive because of pain, fatigue, and/or medication; genital sensations remain intact
Systemic lupus erythematosus (SLE)	Similar to RA; decreased lubrication and vaginal lesions result in painful penetration
Myocardial infarction (MI)	Most literature male oriented; problems related to medications
Multiple sclerosis (MS)	Diminished genital sensitivity; decreased lubrication; declining orgasmic ability; difficulty with sexual activity because of muscle weakness, pain, or incontinence
Spinal cord injury	Reflex sexual response with injury above sacral area; disrupted response with lesion at or below sacrum; loss of sensation, decreased lubrication; spasticity, incontinence, or pain with arousal; continued orgasmic sensations or sensations diffused in general or to specific body parts, such as breast or lips

pelvic region may increase the threshold for orgasm in diabetic women. Diminished intensity and gradual decline in orgasm may be analogous to the development of impotence in diabetic men. For women with heart disease, problems in sexual functioning more often are related to drug therapy than the disease itself. Table 23-7 outlines possible effects of specified chronic diseases on female sexual functioning.

Disorders of desire (inhibited sexual desire, decreased libido) may be a biologic manifestation of depression, alcohol or other substance abuse, prolactin-secreting pituitary tumors, or testosterone deficiency. β-adrenergic blockers used for heart disease also may inhibit sexual desire.

Vaginismus is an involuntary muscle spasm in response to attempted penetration. Common causes include prior sexual trauma or fear of sex; organic causes are less common and are similar to those that cause dyspareunia. Even after the underlying organic problem is detected and successfully treated, vaginismus may persist.

Anorgasmia or **orgasmic dysfunction** is the inability of the woman to reach or achieve orgasm. Dysfunction follows a continuum from difficulty in arousal to lack of orgasm. Any chronic illness may affect arousal. Orgasmic dysfunction is linked to organic causes in less than 5% of cases. Diabetes, alcoholism, neurologic disturbances, hormonal deficiencies, and pelvic disorders, such as infections, trauma, and surgical scarring, are specific disorders that may block orgasm. Drugs, such as narcotics, tranquilizers, antidepressants, and antihypertensive medications, also can inhibit orgasm.

Rapid orgasm is a relatively new diagnosis and seems to be rare. In this instance, once orgasm occurs there is little interest in further sexual activity. Rapid orgasm has no known organic cause.

Dyspareunia (painful intercourse) is common. Women may experience pain during arousal, at the time of orgasm, at the initiation of intercourse, midway during intercourse, or after intercourse. The pain may have a burning, sharp, searing, or cramping quality and may be described as external, vaginal, deep abdominal, or pelvic. A variety of psychosocial and organic causes have been identified. Inadequate lubrication may make penetration or intercourse difficult or painful. Drugs with a drying effect, such as antihistamines, certain tranquilizers, and marijuana, and disorders such as diabetes, vaginal infections, and estrogen deficiency can decrease lubrication. Other causes of dyspareunia include skin problems around the introitus or affecting the vulva; irritation or infection of the clitoris; disorders of the vaginal opening, such as scarring from episiotomy, intact hymen, or chronically infected hymenal remnants; bartholinitis; disorders of the urethra or anus; disorders of the vagina, such as infections, thinning of the walls caused by aging or decreased estrogen, or irritation caused by spermacides or douches; and pelvic disorders, such as infection, tumors, cervical or uterine abnormalities, and torn uterine ligaments.

Sexual dysfunction may develop as a coping mechanism. Women with a history of sexual trauma—rape, incest, or molestation—often have problems of desire, arousal, or orgasm or experience pain with sexual activity. In extreme cases, total sexual aversion may develop. At other times, sexual dysfunction may be a symptom of marital or relationship problems. Unresolved anger may manifest as inhibited desire or diminished arousal.

Impaired Fertility

Infertility affects approximately 15% of all couples and is defined as the inability to conceive after 1 year of unprotected intercourse with the same partner. Fertility can be impaired by factors in the man or the woman or both partners. Male factors include diminished quality and production of sperm and female factors are associated with malfunctions of the fallopian tubes, ovaries, or reproductive hormones. Adhesions from pelvic infection may cause blockage of one or both fallopian tubes, preventing access of the sperm to the ovum. Hormonal or local factors may disrupt ovulation or prevent a fertilized egg from implantation. Hyperthyroidism in males may affect production of sperm and motility.[98] Hypothyroidism in females is also related to infertility. For unclear reasons, endometriosis also may contribute to infertility. These factors have been discussed previously. A number of diagnostic procedures are required in the routine investigation of the infertile couple (see Table 22-4). In many instances no cause may be identified.

Treatment of infertility is aimed toward correcting problems identified during the diagnostic workup. The best treatment for infertility is prevention, specifically prevention of sexually transmitted infection that can result in scarring and adhesion formation in the reproductive tract of either the man or the woman.

Fertility Tests

Tests of reproductive function are performed most commonly when infertility exists. Both the male and female partners are examined, and several diagnostic evaluations may be completed. The types of tests and their normal values are summarized in Tables 21-4 and 21-5. The man is evaluated for number, amount, structure, and motility of sperm and obstruction along the reproductive tract. Tests for women determine whether (1) the reproductive tract (cervix, uterus, fallopian tubes) is adequately patent to allow for passage of ovum and sperm, (2) ovulation occurs normally, (3) the endometrium is responding normally to hormones, and (4) reproductive tissues are free of tumors or infections. Hormonal assays evaluate the adequacy of pituitary function and target organ response. The position and size of organs or the presence of tumors can be detected by direct observation procedures using a laparoscope or by radiographic studies, such as plain films, computerized scans, or tomography. Before testing and treatment, assessing knowledge of fertility with timing of sexual intercourse is essential. A mature ovum remains viable for 12 to 24 hours, and sperm retain their fertility for up to 5 days. A prospective study showed that almost all pregnancies resulted from sexual intercourse during a 6-day period ending on the day of ovulation.[99]

DISORDERS OF THE MALE REPRODUCTIVE SYSTEM

Disorders of the Urethra

Urethritis and urethral strictures are common disorders of the male urethra. Urethral carcinoma occurs in men older than 60 years, but it is an extremely rare form of cancer.

Urethritis

Urethritis is an inflammatory process of the urethra without concurrent bladder infection that is usually, but not always, caused by a sexually transmitted microorganism. Biologic agents associated with infectious urethritis in males include

Neisseria gonorrhoeae and *Chlamydia trachomatis, Ureaplasma urealyticum,* and other, less common, mycobacteria; parasites (e.g., *Trichomonas vaginalis*); and viruses (herpes simplex virus [HSV]).[100] Infectious urethritis caused by *N. gonorrhoeae* often is called *gonococcal urethritis (GU);* infection caused by other microorganisms is called *nongonococcal urethritis (NGU).*[58] (Sexually transmitted urethritis is described in Chapter 24.) Nonsexual origins of urethritis include inflammation or infection as a result of urologic procedures, insertion of foreign bodies into the urethra, anatomic abnormalities, or trauma.

Noninfectious urethritis is rare and is associated with the ingestion of wood alcohol, ethyl alcohol, or turpentine. It is seen also with Reiter syndrome, which involves a number of mucocutaneous lesions.

Symptoms of urethritis include urethral tingling, itching, or burning sensation on urination (dysuria), frequency, and urgency. The individual may note a purulent or clear mucuslike discharge from the urethra. Nucleic acid detection amplification tests allow easy detection of *N. gonorrhoeae* and *C. trachomatis* in first-void urine.[58] Treatment consists of appropriate antibiotic therapy for infectious urethritis and avoidance of future chemical or mechanical irritation.

Urethral Strictures

A **urethral stricture** is a fibrotic narrowing of the urethra caused by scarring. The scars may be congenital but are more likely to result from trauma or untreated or severe urethral infections, most often from long-term use of indwelling urinary catheters. Large catheters and instruments cause internal trauma and ischemia, whereas external trauma, such as pelvic fracture, can partially or completely sever the urethra and cause severe and complex strictures.[101] Urethral carcinoma is a less common cause of urethral stricture. Prostatitis and infection secondary to urinary stasis are common complications. Severe and prolonged obstruction can result in hydronephrosis and renal failure. In addition, chronic, severe strictures may lead to urethral fistulas and periurethral abscesses.[101]

The clinical manifestations of urethral stricture are caused by bladder outlet obstruction. The primary symptom is diminished force and caliber of the urinary stream; other symptoms include urinary frequency and hesitancy, mild dysuria, double urine stream or spraying, and postvoiding dribbling. Symptoms of acute urinary retention may occur in the presence of infection or urinary obstruction. Induration at the stricture site may be palpable. Tender, enlarged masses along the urethra usually indicate periurethral abscesses.

Urethral stricture is diagnosed on the basis of history, physical examination, urinary flow rates, voiding cystourethrogram, and urethroscopy; biopsy confirms carcinoma. Treatment is usually surgical and may involve urethral dilation, urethrotomy, or a variety of open surgical techniques. The choice of surgical intervention depends on the age of the individual and the severity of the problem. Strictures may recur up to 1 year after treatment. Follow-up is necessary during this time; urinary flow measurements and urethrogram help determine extent of residual obstruction.

Disorders of the Penis
Phimosis and Paraphimosis

Phimosis and paraphimosis are both disorders in which the foreskin (prepuce) is "too tight" to be moved easily over the glans penis. **Phimosis** is a condition in which the foreskin cannot be retracted back over the glans, whereas **paraphimosis** is the opposite: the foreskin is retracted and cannot be moved forward (reduced) to cover the glans (Figure 23-22). Both conditions can cause penile pathologic conditions.

The inability to retract the foreskin is normal in infancy and is caused by congenital adhesions. During the first 3 years of life, these adhesions separate naturally with penile erections and are not an indication for circumcision. Although most cases occur in uncircumcised males, stenosis and resultant phimosis can occur in males with excessive skin remaining after circumcision.[101] Phimosis can occur at any age and is caused most commonly by poor hygiene and chronic infection. Chronic balanoposthitis (inflammation of the glans and prepuce) predisposes older diabetic men to phimosis. It rarely occurs with normal foreskin.

Edema, erythema, and tenderness of the prepuce and purulent discharge are usually the reasons for seeking treatment; inability to retract the foreskin is a less common complaint. Circumcision, if needed, is performed after infection has been eradicated. Complications of phimosis include inflammation of the glans (balanitis) or prepuce (posthitis) and paraphimosis. There is a higher incidence of penile carcinoma in uncircumcised males, but chronic infection, most likely with HPV, is usually the underlying factor in such cases.[102]

Paraphimosis, in which the foreskin is retracted, can constrict the penis, causing edema of the glans. If edema is such that the foreskin cannot be reduced manually, surgery must be performed to prevent necrosis of the glans caused by constricted blood vessels. Severe paraphimosis is a surgical emergency.

Peyronie Disease

Peyronie disease (bent nail syndrome) is a fibrotic condition that causes lateral curvature of the penis during erection (Figure 23-23). Peyronie disease develops slowly and is character-

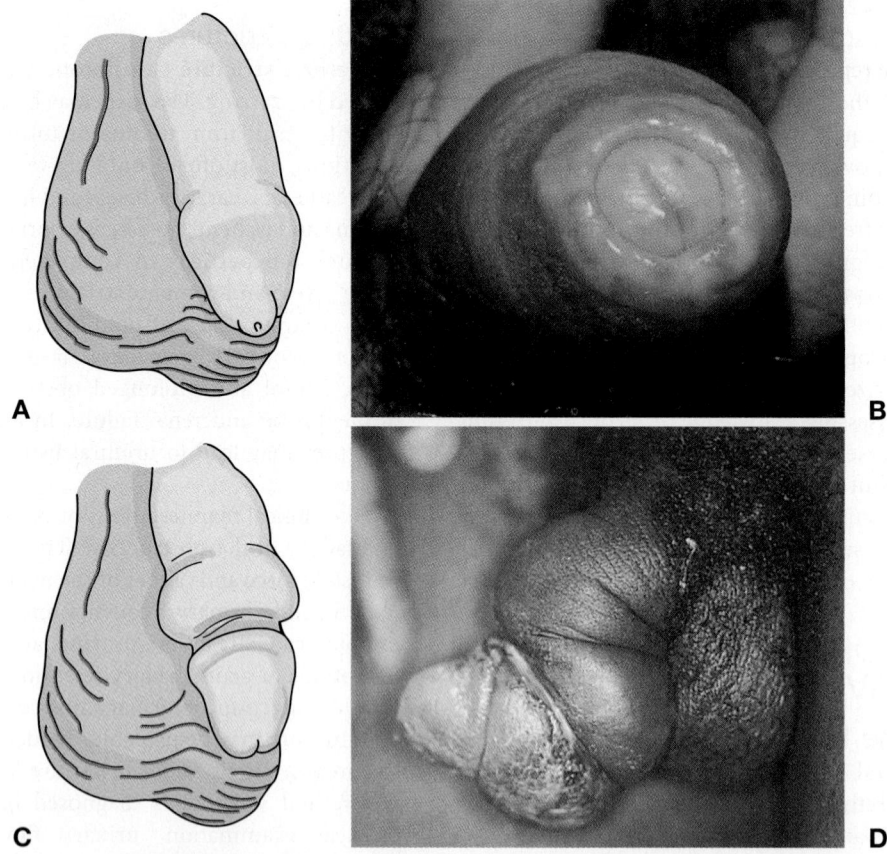

Figure 23-22 Phimosis and paraphimosis. A, Phimosis: the foreskin has a narrow opening that is not large enough to permit retraction over the glans. **B,** Lesions on the prepuce secondary to infection cause swelling, and retraction of foreskin may be impossible. **C,** Paraphimosis: the foreskin is retracted over the glans but cannot be reduced to its normal position. Here it has formed a constricting band around the penis. **D,** Ulcer on the retracted prepuce with edema. (**A, C,** From Phipps WP, Sand JK, Marek JF: *Medical-surgical nursing: concepts and clinical practice*, ed 6, St Louis, 1999, Mosby. **B,** From Taylor PK: *Diagnostic picture tests in sexually transmitted diseases*, London, 1995, Mosby. **D,** From Morse SA, Moreland AA, Holmes KK: *Atlas of sexually transmitted diseases and AIDS*, ed 2, London, 1996, Mosby-Wolfe.)

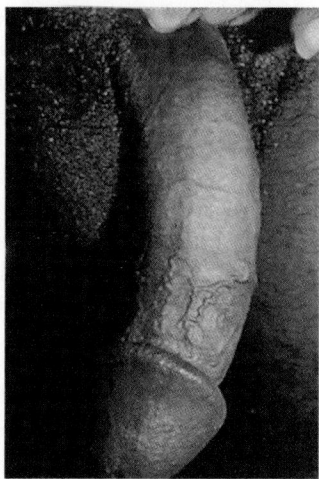

Figure 23-23 Peyronie disease. (From Taylor PK: *Diagnostic picture tests in sexually transmitted diseases,* London, 1995, Mosby-Wolfe.)

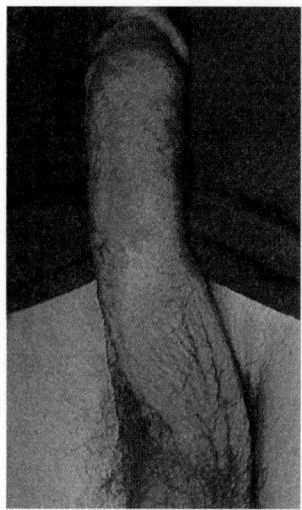

Figure 23-24 Priapism. (From Lloyd-Davies RW et al: *Color atlas of urology,* ed 2, London, 1994, Mosby-Wolfe.)

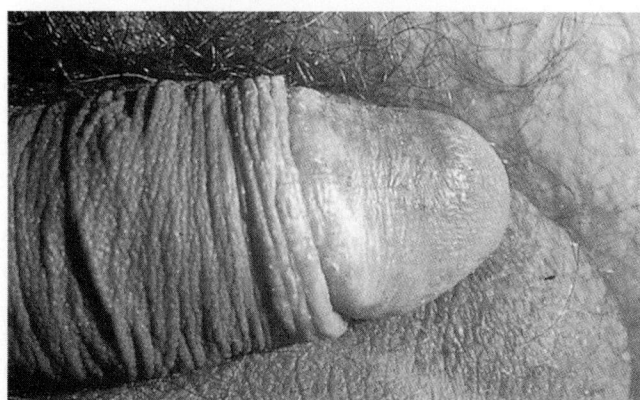

Figure 23-25 Balanitis. Itchy, red rash on glans of penis secondary to *Candida albicans.* (From Taylor PK: *Diagnostic picture tests in sexually transmitted diseases,* London, 1995, Mosby-Wolfe.)

ized by tough, fibrous thickening of the fascia in the erectile tissue of the corpora cavernosa. A dense, fibrous plaque is usually palpable on the dorsum of the penile shaft. The problem usually affects middle-age men and is associated with painful erection, painful intercourse (for both partners), and poor erection distal to the involved area. In some cases, impotence or unsatisfactory penetration occurs. There is no pain when the penis is flaccid.

Although the exact cause is unknown, a local vasculitis-like inflammatory reaction occurs and decreased tissue oxygenation results in fibrosis and calcification. Peyronie disease is associated with Dupuytren contracture (a flexion deformity of the fingers or toes caused by shortening or fibrosis of the palmar or plantar fascia), diabetes, tendency to develop keloids, and in rare cases, use of β-blocker medications.

There is no definitive treatment for Peyronie disease. Spontaneous remissions occur in as many as 50% of the cases. Pharmacologic therapies that increase oxygenation, such as vitamin E and aminobenzoate potassium (Potaba), may hasten self-resolution if used several times daily for prolonged periods. Placation, as well as surgical resection of the fibrous plaque followed by grafting, has been successful.[101]

Priapism

Priapism is an uncommon condition of prolonged penile erection. It is usually painful and is not associated with sexual arousal (Figure 23-24). Priapism is idiopathic in 60% of cases; the remaining 40% of cases are associated with spinal cord trauma, sickle cell disease, leukemia, pelvic tumors or infections, or penile trauma. Priapism also has been associated with cocaine use.[103] Currently, intracavernous injection therapy for impotence seems to be the most common cause. Prolonged sexual stimulation often is associated with initial development of the idiopathic type.[101] The two corpora cavernosa within the erect penis are filled with blood and are tender to palpation; neither the corpus spongiosum nor the glans is engorged. The vascular congestion is thought to be as-

sociated with venous obstruction. If the erection remains over a period of days, edema and fibrosis develop, leading to erectile dysfunction (impotence).

Priapism is a urologic emergency. Treatment within hours is effective and prevents impotence. Conservative approaches include iced saline enemas, ketamine administration, and spinal anesthesia. Needle aspiration of blood from the corpus through the dorsal glans is often effective and is followed by catheterization and pressure dressings to maintain decompression. More aggressive surgical treatments include the creation of vascular shunts to maintain blood flow.[88] Erectile dysfunction results in up to 50% of prolonged cases.

Balanitis

Balanitis is an inflammation of the glans penis (Figure 23-25) and usually occurs in conjunction with posthitis, an inflammation of the prepuce. (Inflammation of the glans and the prepuce is called *balanoposthitis.*) It is associated with poor hygiene and phimosis. The accumulation under the foreskin of glandular secretions (smegma), sloughed epithelial cells, and *Mycobacterium smegmatis* can irritate the glans directly or lead to infection. Skin disorders (e.g., psoriasis, lichen planus, eczema) and candidiasis must be differentiated from inflammation resulting from poor hygienic practices. Balanitis is seen most commonly in men with poorly controlled diabetes mellitus and candidiasis. Antimicrobials are used to treat infection. Circumcision can prevent recurrences and can be considered after the inflammation has subsided.

Penile Cancer

In the United States, carcinoma of the penis is rare and affects about 1 in 100,000 men (Figure 23-26). Estimates by the American Cancer Society indicated that approximately 270 men would die of penile cancer and 1470 new cases would be diagnosed in the year 2005.[80] Although rare in North America and Europe, where it accounts for about 0.2% of cancers and 0.1% of cancer deaths in men, penile cancer may account for up to 10% of cancers in African and South American men.

In the United States, it is twice as common in black men compared with white men[102] and men over age 50.[104] Major risk factors include infection with HPV (mainly serotypes 16, 18, 33, 35, and 45), smoking, and psoriasis treated with a combination involving the drug psoralen and ultraviolet light. About 3/4 of men with penile cancer are diagnosed at over 55 years.[80]

Before the development of penile cancer, signs of premalignant cancer or epidermal cancer in situ are present.[105] These include thick, white plaque (leukoplakia) that typically involves the meatus; red, inflamed areas of Paget disease; red, velvety, ulcerative lesions of erythroplasia of Queyrat that usually involve the glans; large, invasive, scaly growths of Buschke-Löwenstein tumor; red plaque with encrustations of Bowen disease; and in situ carcinoma that generally affects the penile shaft. Men with leukoplakia or erythroplasia of Queyrat may have concurrent invasive penile carcinoma.[102,106] Pain and bleeding are late signs of penile cancer. Condylomata (genital warts) caused by the HPV may be involved in the development of precancerous lesions (see Chapter 24 for a discussion of HPV). At times the penis might be the site of metastatic spread of solid tumors from the bladder, prostate, rectum, or kidney. Early squamous cell carcinoma and premalignant epidermal lesions are easily treated but are often ignored. Delays in seeking treatment are attributed to denial, embarrassment, failure to detect lesions under a phimotic foreskin, fear, guilt, and ignorance.

Penile cancer is mostly squamous cell carcinoma. Squamous cell carcinoma usually begins as a small, fat, ulcerative or papillary lesion on the glans or foreskin that grows to involve the entire penile shaft. Extensive lesions are associated with metastases and a poor prognosis. These lesions are not as painful as the amount of tissue involvement would seem to indicate. The regional femoral and iliac nodes are common metastatic sites. Rarely, the urethra and bladder are involved. Weight loss, fatigue, and malaise accompany chronic suppurative lesions. Untreated, progressive disease causes death within 2 years.

The specific diagnosis is made by biopsy after examination to document the location, size, and fixation of the lesion. After a positive biopsy, the extent of cancer spread is determined by imaging tests such as ultrasound, CT, or MRI. Fine-needle aspiration of lymph tissue confirms absence or presence of regional adenopathy.[102] About 30% of penile cancers spread to lymph nodes before diagnosis.[104] Distant metastases occur in fewer than 10% of cases and may involve lung, liver, bone, or brain.[106] Staging of penile cancer uses a system created by the American Joint Committee on Cancer (AJCC) and the International Union Against Cancer (UICC). The AJCC/UICC staging system is also known as the tumor, node, metastasis (TNM) system[80] (see Chapter 12). Although this system initially seems cumbersome, it is a simple and an easy method of communicating degree of cancer (Box 23-11).

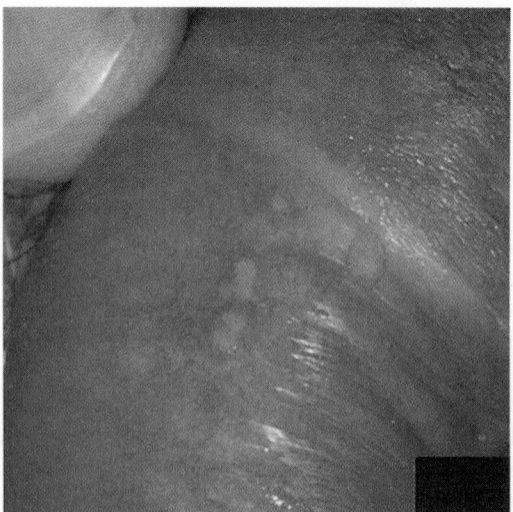

Figure 23-26 **Carcinoma in situ of penis.** Flat papules turn white after diagnostic treatment with acetic acid. (From Morse SA, et al: *Atlas of sexually transmitted diseases and AIDS,* ed 3, London, 2003, Mosby.)

Box 23-11	Tumor, Node, Metastasis (TNM)* Staging for Penile Cancer

Stage 0	**Stage III**
T_{is}, N_0, M_0	T_1, N_2, M_0
T_a, N_0, M_0	T_2, N_2, M_0
Stage I	T_3, N_0, M_0
T_1, N_0, M_0	T_3, N_1, M_0
	T_3, N_2, M_0
Stage II	T_2, N_1, M_0
T_1, N_1, M_0	
T_2, N_0, M_0	**Stage IV**
T_2, N_1, M_0	$T_4,$ any N, M_0
	Any T, N_3, M_0
	Any T, any N, M_1
Recurrent	

Any local or distant penile cancer that returns after treatment

*See Figure 12-8, p. 386 for T, N, and M definitions.

For invasive penile carcinoma, complete excision leaving adequate tumor-free margins is the goal. A simple circumcision may be sufficient for localized lesions of the prepuce. If the primary site is glans and distal shaft, the penis is amputated, leaving a 2-cm margin proximal to the tumor. Inguinal lymph nodes also are removed if metastasis to these structures is known or suspected. Palliative treatment with radiation or chemotherapy may be used when the disease is inoperable and bulky inguinal metastases have occurred. Options for individuals with carcinoma in situ include local excision, radiation, laser surgery, cryosurgery, chemosurgery, or chemotherapy with topical (5%) 5-FU. Differentiation, tumor stage, and age influence prognosis.[107] The 5-year survival rate for stage I disease is greater than 80%;[80,104] average 5-year survival rate for all stages is 50%.[80,102]

Disorders of the Scrotum, Testis, and Epididymis

Disorders of the Scrotum

Men may seek treatment for painful or painless scrotal masses. Masses may be serious (cancer or torsion) or benign (hydrocele or cyst); they may require immediate surgical intervention or allow for careful observation. A flow diagram for diagnosing scrotal masses[108] is provided in Figure 23-27.

Varicocele, hydrocele, and spermatocele are common intrascrotal disorders.[109-111] A **varicocele** is an abnormal dilation of a vein within the spermatic cord and is classically described as a "bag of worms" (Figure 23-28). Most (95%) occur on the left side and may be painful or tender. Varicocele occurs in 10% of males and is seen most often after puberty. Sudden development of a varicocele in an older man is a late sign of renal tumor.[110] Unilateral right-sided varicoceles are rare and result from compression or obstruction of the inferior vena cava by a tumor or thrombus. Color Doppler ultrasonography is used to confirm the diagnosis.[108]

The cause of varicocele is incompetent or congenitally absent valves in the spermatic veins. The valves that normally prevent backflow are absent or do not close adequately, permitting blood to pool in the veins rather than flow into the venous system. Varicocele decreases blood flow through the testis. This interferes with spermatogenesis and is a cause of infertility.[109,110] If infertility is a problem, treatment consists of ligation of the spermatic vein or occlusion of the vein by percutaneous methods, such as balloon catheter and sclerosing

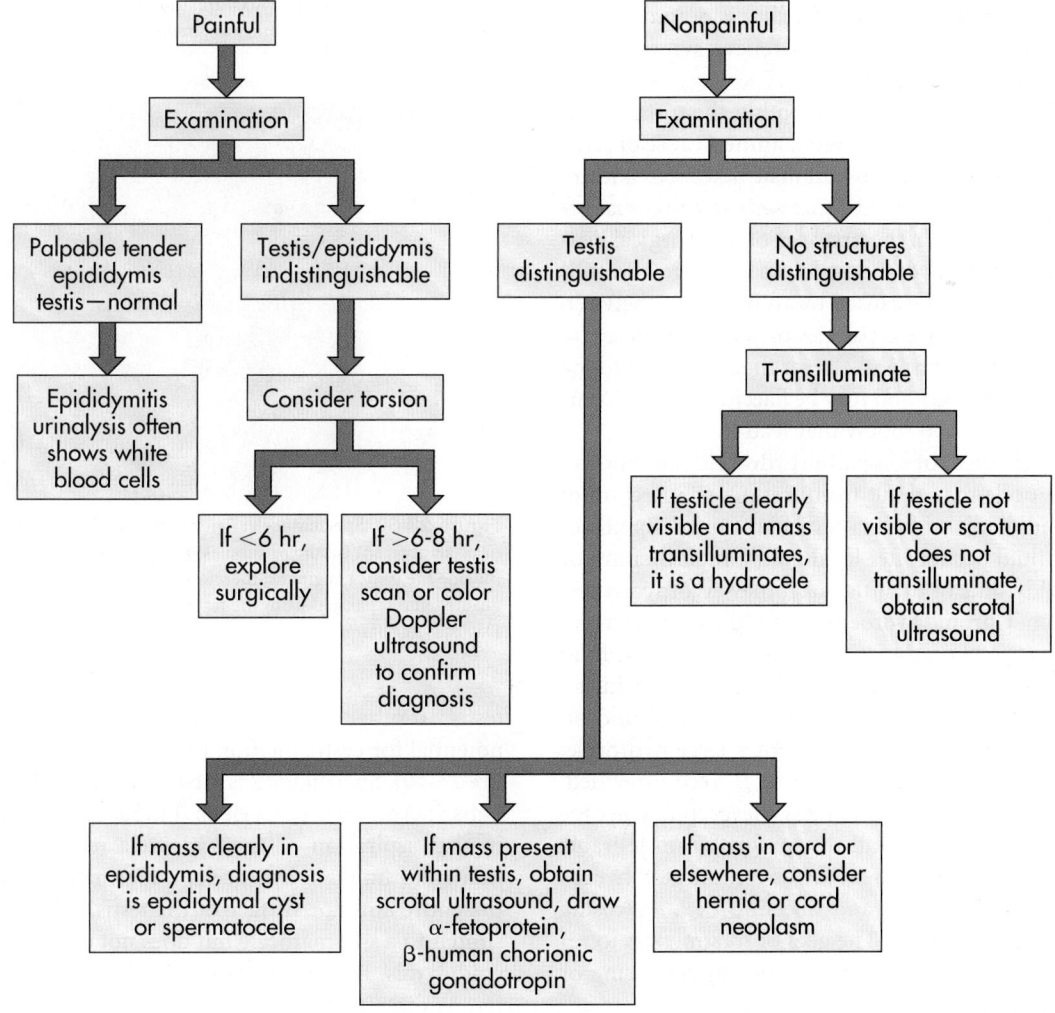

Figure 23-27 Diagnostic algorithm of a scrotal mass.

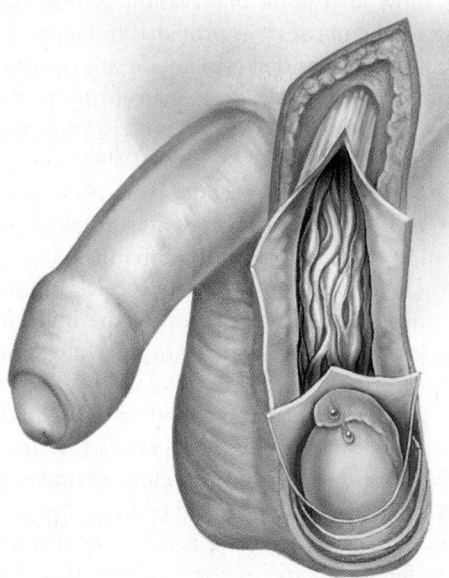

Figure 23-28 Varicocele. Dilation of veins within the spermatic cord. (From Seidel H et al: *Mosby's guide to physical examination*, ed 4, St Louis, 1999, Mosby.)

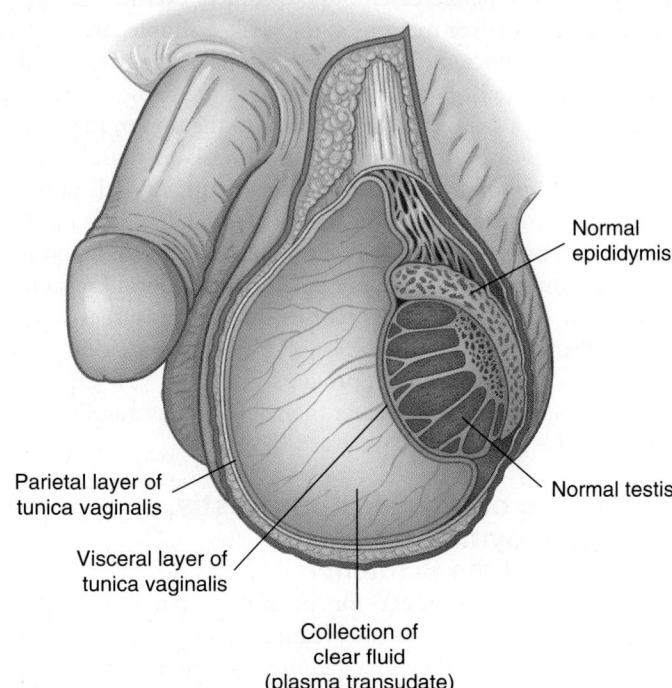

Normal epididymis

Normal testis

Parietal layer of tunica vaginalis

Visceral layer of tunica vaginalis

Collection of clear fluid (plasma transudate)

Figure 23-29 Hydrocele. Accumulation of clear fluid between the visceral and parietal layers of the tunica vaginalis.

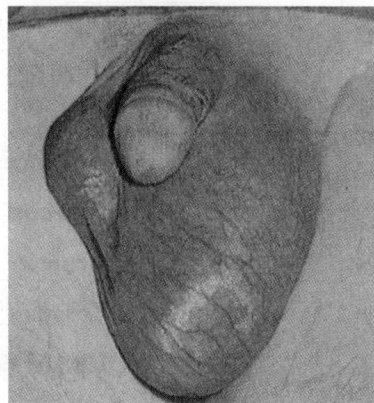

Figure 23-30 Spermatocele. Retention cyst of the head of the epididymis or of an aberrant tubule or tubules of the rete testis. The spermatocele lies outside the tunica vaginalis; therefore on palpation it can be readily distinguished and separated from the testis. (From Lloyd-Davies RW, Gow JG, Davies DR: *Color atlas of urology*, ed 2, London, 1994, Mosby-Wolfe.)

fluids.[110,112] If varicocele is mild and fertility is not an issue, a scrotal support usually is sufficient to relieve symptoms of scrotal heaviness or "dragging."

A **hydrocele** is a collection of fluid within the tunica vaginalis[108-110] (Figure 23-29). It is the most common cause of scrotal swelling. Hydroceles occur in 6% of male newborns and are congenital malformations (patent processes vaginalis) that often resolve spontaneously in the first year of life. Surgical ligation is recommended if hydrocele persists after age 1 year.[111] Hydroceles in adults may be caused by an imbalance between the secreting and absorptive capacities of scrotal tissues. Hydroceles range in size from slightly larger than the testes to the size of a grapefruit or larger and may be flaccid or tense. Compression of testicular blood supply may lead to atrophy.

The exact mechanism of idiopathic hydrocele is unknown. Secondary hydrocele may result from trauma or infection of the testis or epididymis or from a testicular tumor. Rapid accumulation of fluid occurs after local injury, radiotherapy, or infection (epididymitis or orchitis), or it may accompany testicular neoplasm. Chronic hydroceles are more common and occur in men over 40 because of an imbalance between fluid secretion and reabsorption in the tunica vaginalis. A painless, extratesticular mass that easily transilluminates is found on physical examination. Ultrasonography of a large hydrocele, which may conceal a testicular tumor, is recommended. Treatment is usually not required unless a large, bulky hydrocele causes considerable physical discomfort or undesirable cosmetic appearance.[109] Treatment for uncomplicated hydrocele is aspiration of the fluid and injection of a sclerosing agent into the scrotal sac.[108,113] The goal of treatment is to remove the hydrocele and prevent recurrence by sclerosing or excising the tunica vaginalis.

A **spermatocele** is a painless diverticulum of the epididymis located between the head of the epididymis and the testis. In other words, efferent ducts of the epididymis have potential for cystic dilation to form a spermatocele[108,110] (Figure 23-30). Spermatoceles are filled with milky fluid that contains sperm. Spermatocele is differentiated from a hydrocele in that aspiration of the hydrocele recovers a clear, yellow fluid, and unlike a hydrocele, a spermatocele does not cover the entire anterior surface of the testis. An epididymal cyst is similar to a spermatocele but does not communicate with the epididymis. Both spermatoceles and epididymal cysts manifest as discrete, firm, freely mobile masses distinct from the testis that may be transilluminated. Epididymal cysts do not require treatment.[108] A spermatic cord tumor may feel like a tense spermatocele but does not contain fluid and will not transilluminate.[110] Spermatoceles that cause pain or discomfort are excised. Usually, however, spermatoceles are asymptomatic or produce mild discomfort that is relieved by scrotal support. Neither hydroceles nor spermatoceles are associated with infertility.

Cryptorchidism and Ectopy

Cryptorchidism is a condition of testicular maldescent, whereas an **ectopic testis** has strayed from the normal pathway of descent. Ectopy may be caused by an abnormal connection at the distal end of the gubernaculum testis that leads the gonad to an abnormal position, usually at the superficial inguinal site. In cryptorchidism the descent of one or both testes is arrested, with unilateral arrest occurring more often than bilateral arrest.[110] The testes may remain in the abdomen, or testicular descent may be arrested in the inguinal canal or the puboscrotal junction. About 3% to 6% of full-term and 20% to 30% of premature male infants have undescended testes at birth;[111] half of such testes descend in the first month of life and a few more at puberty. The incidence of cryptorchidism in adults is 0.7% to 0.8%.[110] Cryptorchidism is commonly associated with vasal or epididymal abnormalities. These congenital anomalies affect about one third to two thirds of newborns with cryptorchidism. Other structural anomalies include posterior urethral valves (less than 5%), upper tract abnormalities (less than 5%), and hypospadias. The presence of both hypospadias and cryptorchidism raises the suspicion of mixed gonadal dysgenesis (intersex infant). It has been hypothesized that cryptorchidism may result from an absence or abnormality of the gubernaculum, a cordlike structure that extends from the lower pole of the testis to the scrotum; a congenital gonadal or dysgenetic defect that makes the testis insensitive to gonadotropins (a likely explanation for unilateral cryptorchidism); or lack of maternal gonadotropins (a likely explanation for bilateral cryptorchidism of prematurity).[110] Mechanical possibilities include a short spermatic cord, fibrous bands or adhesions in the normal path of the testes, or a narrowed inguinal canal. Chromosomal studies do not support a genetic component. Physiologic cryptorchidism, also called *retractile* or *migratory testis,* is an involuntary retraction of the testes out of the scrotum that occurs with excitement, physical activity, or exposure to cold and is caused by the small mass of prepubertal testis and the strength of the cremaster muscle. This is a common phenomenon that is self-limiting (descent occurs at puberty).

Physical examination discloses the absence of one or both testes in the scrotum and an atrophic scrotum on the affected side. If the undescended testis is in a vulnerable position, for example, over the pubic bone, an individual may complain of severe pain secondary to trauma. The adult male with bilateral cryptorchidism may be infertile. Ultrasonography, CT, or MRI can be used to locate an intraabdominal or nonpalpable testis.

Undescended testes are susceptible to neoplastic processes: the risk of testicular cancer is 35 to 50 times greater for men

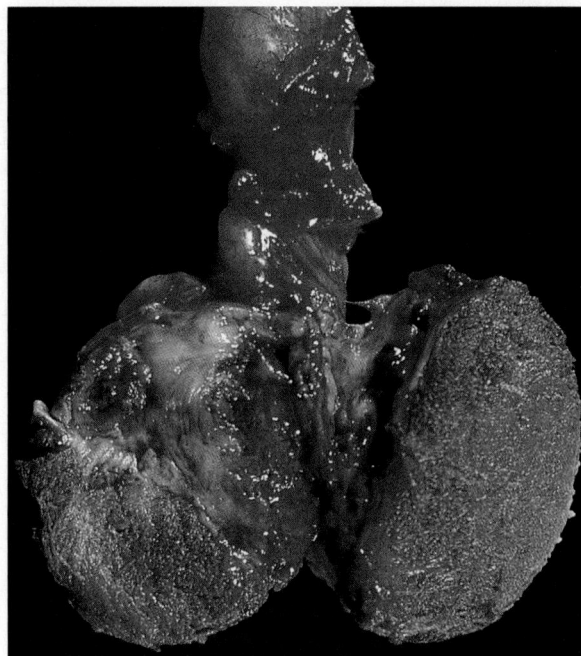

Figure 23-31 Torsion of the testes. The testes appear dark red and partially necrotic owing to hemorrhagic infarction. (From Damjanov I, Linder J, editors: *Anderson's pathology,* ed 10, St Louis, 1996, Mosby.)

with cryptorchidism or a history of cryptorchidism than for the general male population. Because definite histologic change (decreased Leydig cells, loss of germ cells, and peritubular fibrosis) occurs in the cryptorchid testis by 1 year of age, surgical correction is recommended around that age.[110,114] Treatment often begins with administration of GnRH or hCG, hormones that may initiate descent, making surgery unnecessary. GnRH is given as a nasal spray in Europe and may enhance germ-cell counts even when the testis does not descend.[114] If hormonal therapy is not successful, the testis is located and moved surgically (orchiopexy) in young children or removed (orchiectomy) in adults and children over 10 years of age.[110,114] The testis that is properly placed in the scrotum provides adequate hormonal function and gives the scrotum a normal appearance. A successful operation does not ensure fertility if the testis is congenitally defective. Approximately 20% of males with unilateral undescended testis remain infertile even though orchiopexy is performed by age 1 year; most individuals with treated or untreated bilateral testicular maldescent have poor fertility. In addition, placement of the cryptorchid testis into the scrotal sac does not decrease the potential for malignancy; it does facilitate examination and tumor detection.

Torsion of the Testis

Torsion of the testis is rotation of a testis, which twists blood vessels in the spermatic cord. It causes an acute scrotum, which is testicular pain and swelling (Figure 23-31). Differentiation between testicular torsion and two other common causes of an acute scrotum is based on physical examination and history[108,111] (Table 23-8). This event is most common among neonates and pubertal adolescents, but it can occur in

Table 23-8	Diagnosis of Selected Conditions Responsible for the Acute Scrotum					
Condition	Onset of Symptoms	Age	Tenderness	Urinalysis	Cremasteric Reflex	Treatment
Testicular torsion	Acute	Early puberty	Diffuse	Negative	Negative	Surgical exploration
Appendiceal torsion	Subacute	Prepubertal	Localized to upper pole	Negative	Positive	Bed rest and scrotal elevation
Epididymitis	Insidious	Adolescence	Epididymal	Positive or negative	Positive	Antibiotics

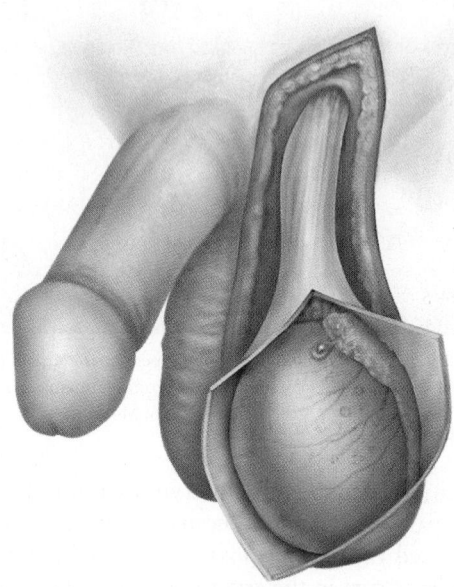

Figure 23-32 Orchitis. (From Seidel H et al: *Mosby's guide to physical examination,* ed 4, St Louis, 1999, Mosby.)

males at any age.[108,111] Onset may be spontaneous or follow physical exertion or trauma. Torsion twists the arteries and veins in the spermatic cord, reducing or stopping circulation to the testis. Vascular engorgement and ischemia develop, causing scrotal swelling and pain. These manifestations are not relieved by scrotal elevation (Prehn sign), rest, or scrotal support. On physical examination, men have a tender, high-riding testis, a thickened spermatic cord, and an absent cremasteric reflect. Unlike epididymitis, the epididymis cannot be differentiated from the testis.[111] Diagnostic testing includes urinalysis (to rule out infection) and color Doppler ultrasonography.[99,110,111] Torsion of the testis is a surgical emergency. If the torsion cannot be reduced manually, surgery must be performed within 6 hours after the onset of symptoms to preserve normal testicular function. Surgery includes untwisting the spermatic cord and anchoring both testes in correct position within the scrotum to prevent recurrences. With successful manual detorsion, surgical fixation should be done within a few days.

Orchitis

Orchitis is an acute inflammation of the testes (Figure 23-32) and is uncommon except as a complication of systemic infection or as an extension of an associated epididymitis[100] (see

p. 813). Infectious microorganisms may reach the testes through the blood or the lymphatics or, most commonly, by ascent through the urethra, vas deferens, and epididymis. Most cases of orchitis are actually cases of epididymo-orchitis. Occasionally, in middle-age men, a nonspecific, apparently noninfectious, inflammatory process (called *granulomatis orchitis*) can occur. It seems to be an autoimmune disease that triggers a granulomatous response to spermatozoa.

Mumps is the most common infectious cause of orchitis and usually affects postpubertal males. The onset is sudden, occurring 3 to 4 days after the onset of parotitis. Signs and symptoms include high fever, reaching 40° C (104° F), marked prostration, bilateral or unilateral erythema, edema and tenderness of the scrotum, and leukocytosis. An acute hydrocele may develop. Urinary signs and symptoms, which accompany epididymitis, are absent. Atrophy with irreversible damage to spermatogenesis may result in 30% of affected testes. Bilateral orchitis does not affect androgenic function but may cause permanent sterility.

Treatment is supportive and includes bed rest, scrotal support, elevation of the scrotum, hot or cold compresses, and analgesic agents for relief of pain. If an acute hydrocele develops, it is aspirated. Testicular abscess usually requires orchiectomy (removal of the testis). Appropriate antimicrobial drugs should be used for bacterial orchitis, and corticosteroids are indicated in proved cases of nonspecific granulomatous orchitis.

Cancer of the Testis

Testicular cancer is among the most curable of cancers; for nearly all common types, cure rates are more than 95%. Overall, testicular cancers are rare, accounting for only 1% of cancers and 0.24% of cancer deaths[80] in men, yet they are the most common form of cancer in young men between ages 15 and 35. Approximately 8980 cases and 360 deaths were estimated for 2004.[80] In the United States, the lifetime probability of developing testicular cancer is 0.2% for white men, an incidence that is four times higher than for blacks. Testicular tumors are slightly more common on the right side than on the left, a pattern that parallels the occurrence of cryptorchidism; about 1% to 2% of primary testicular cancers are bilateral (Figure 23-33), and 50% of these tumors arise from treated or untreated cryptorchid testes.

PATHOGENESIS Ninety percent of testicular cancers are germ-cell tumors arising from the male gametes. Germ-cell tumors constitute 90% of testicular cancers and can be

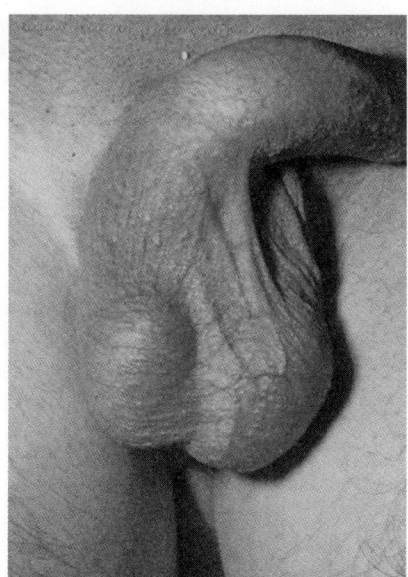

Figure 23-33 Testicular tumor. (From *400 self-assessment picture tests in clinical medicine,* London, 1984, Wolfe Medical Publications.)

broadly classified into two types: seminomas and nonseminomas. Seminomas are the most common, are the least aggressive, and make up about 30% to 35% of testicular cancers. Nonseminomas include embryonal carcinomas, teratomas, and choriocarcinomas, the most aggressive but rare (less than 1%) form of testicular cancer. Testicular cancers can include a mix of types.[115] In addition, testicular tumors can arise from specialized cells of the gonadal stroma. These tumors, which are named for their cellular origins, are Leydig cell, Sertoli cell, granulosa cell, and theca cell tumors and constitute less than 10% of all testicular cancers.[116]

The cause of testicular neoplasms is unknown. A genetic predisposition is suggested by the fact that the incidence is higher among brothers, identical twins, and other close male relatives. Genetic predisposition is supported further by statistics showing that the disease is relatively rare among black Africans, black Americans, Asians, and native New Zealanders. Risk factors include history of cryptorchidism, abnormal testicular development, Klinefelter syndrome, and history of testicular cancer.[115]

CLINICAL MANIFESTATIONS   Painless testicular enlargement commonly is the first sign of testicular cancer. Enlargement is usually gradual and may be accompanied by a sensation of testicular heaviness or dull ache in the lower abdomen.[115,116] Occasionally, acute pain occurs because of rapid growth, resulting in hemorrhage and necrosis. Ten percent of affected men have epididymitis, 10% have hydroceles,[116] and 5% have gynecomastia or hydrocele. Incidence of gynecomastia increases considerably (30% to 45%) in men with Sertoli or Leydig tumors. Approximately 10% of individuals already have symptoms related to metastases at the time of initial diagnosis, which correlates with the typical delay of 3 to 6 months from initial recognition to definitive treatment. Lum-

bar pain may be present and usually is caused by retroperitoneal node metastasis. Signs of metastasis to the lungs include cough, dyspnea, and bloody sputum (hemoptysis). Supraclavicular node involvement may cause difficulty swallowing (dysphagia) and neck swelling. Alterations in vision or mental status, papilledema, and seizures may be experienced with metastasis to the CNS. Approximately 10% of affected individuals are asymptomatic; the tumor may be detected by the man's sexual partner or incidentally following trauma.

EVALUATION AND TREATMENT   An incorrect diagnosis at the initial examination occurs in as many as 25% of men with testicular cancer. Epididymitis and epididymoorchitis are the most common misdiagnoses; others include hydrocele and spermatocele. Evaluation begins with careful physical examination, including palpation of the scrotal contents with the individual in the erect and supine positions. The abdomen and lymph nodes are palpated to rule out metastases. Signs of testicular cancer include abnormal consistency, induration, nodularity, or irregularity of the testis. A firm, nontender testicular mass or diffuse enlargement is found in the majority of cases. Primary testicular cancer can be assessed rapidly and accurately by scrotal ultrasonography. Tumor markers are higher than normal in the presence of a tumor and may help detect a tumor that is too small to be palpated during physical examination or seen on imaging.[115] Tumor type is identified after inguinal biopsy or orchiectomy. Scrotal incisions may cause dissemination of the tumor and increase the risk of local recurrence and therefore are avoided. Chest x-ray, lymphangiogram, IVP, abdominal ultrasound, and CT are used in clinical staging of disease. Treatment is based on type of tumor, stage of disease, general health, and age. Besides surgery, treatment involves radiation and chemotherapy singly or in combination. A number of factors influence the prognosis (Table 23-9). They include histology of the tumor, stage of the disease, and selection of appropriate treatment. Serum markers, such as AFP, β-hCG, and lactate dehydrogenase, are useful for detecting metastases and assessing responses to therapy. Most individuals treated for cancer of the testis can expect a normal life span, although some have persistent paresthesias, Raynaud phenomenon, or infertility. Almost 90% of disease-related deaths occur in the first 2 years after cessation of therapy; disease-free survival of 3 years is considered a cure. Approximately 10% of men treated for testicular cancer will experience a relapse; if the relapse is discovered early and treated, 99% can be cured. Orchiectomy does not affect sexual function, but infertility can result from chemotherapy or surgical removal of affected abdominal lymph nodes if nerves necessary for ejaculation are severed. After orchiectomy, testicular silicone implants may be used to restore "normal" scrotal appearance.

Epididymitis

Epididymitis, or inflammation of the epididymis, generally occurs in sexually active young males (younger than 35 years) and is rare before puberty (Figure 23-34). In young men the

Table 23-9   Testicular Tumors of Germ-cell Origin

Cell Types	Occurrence	Metastatic Pattern	Prognosis/Remission Rate
A. Seminoma (germinoma)	30%-35% of all testicular tumors	Rarely to retroperitoneal lymph nodes	Excellent; tumor usually remains localized and is responsive to radiation; cure rate stages I and II >95%; stages III and IV >80%
B. Nonseminomatous tumors	60% of all testicular tumors		
1. Single cell			
a. Embryonal carcinoma	20%-25% of all testicular tumors; most common testicular tumor in infants and children	Earlier to regional lymphatics, also lung, liver, bone	Good; complete remission rate stages I and II >95%; stages III and IV >70%-80%
b. Teratoma	5%-10% of all testicular tumors (occurs in children and adults)	Through lymphatics and bloodstream; affects same organ systems as embryonal type	Fair
c. Choriocarcinoma	<1% of all testicular tumors	Earliest and widest, initially through bloodstream	Poor; early metastasis
2. Mixed tumors	30%-40% of all testicular tumors		
a. Teratocarcinoma	20%-25% of all testicular tumors	Mixed pattern; depends on cell types	Variable; prognosis becomes that of the most malignant element
b. Other	10%-15% of all testicular tumors	Mixed pattern; depends on cell types	Variable; prognosis becomes that of the most malignant element
i. Teratocarcinoma with seminoma			
ii. Embryonal cancer with seminoma			
iii. Teratoma with seminoma			
iv. Any combination with choriocarcinoma			
3. Non–germ-cell tumors (Leydig cell, Sertoli cell, granulose cell, and theca cell tumors)	<10%		

Data from American Cancer Society. In *Cancer response system document #10029,* New York, 1995, The Society; Fresti et al with Lanum DL: Carcinoma of the genitourinary system. In Nseys UO, Weinman E, Lamm DL, editors: *Urology for primary care physicians,* Philadelphia, 1999, Saunders; Cancer Net: *Cancer facts: questions and answers about testicular cancer,* National Cancer Institute, 2000. Available at www.cancernet.nci.nih.gov/.

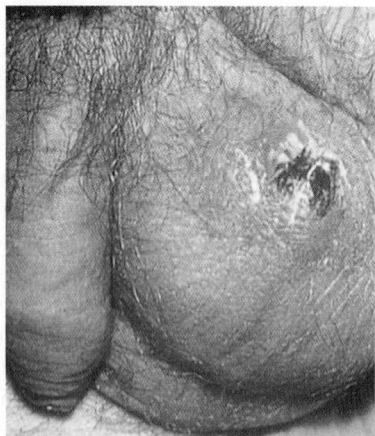

Figure 23-34 Epididymitis secondary to gonorrhea or nongonococcal urethritis. Secondary to gonorrhea or nongonococcal urethritis, this infection spread to the testes, and rupture through the scrotal wall is threatened. (From Taylor PK: *Diagnostic picture tests in sexually transmitted diseases,* London, 1995, Mosby-Wolfe.)

usual cause is a sexually transmitted microorganism, such as *N. gonorrhoeae* or *C. trachomatis.* Men who practice unprotected anal intercourse may acquire sexually transmitted epididymitis because of *E. coli, H. influenzae,* tuberculosis (especially in regions where incidence of pulmonary tuberculosis is high), *Cryptococcus,* or *Brucella.*[117] In men older than 35 years, Enterobacteriaceae (intestinal bacteria) and *Pseudomonas aeruginosa* associated with urinary tract infections and prostatitis also may cause epididymitis. Besides an infectious etiology, epididymitis may result from a chemical inflammation caused by the reflux of sterile urine into the ejaculatory ducts.[117,118] It is associated with urethral strictures, congenital posterior valves, and excessive physical straining in which increased abdominal pressure is transmitted to the bladder. Chemical epididymitis is usually self-limiting and does not require evaluation or intervention unless it persists.

PATHOPHYSIOLOGY   The pathogenic microorganism usually reaches the epididymis by ascending the vasa deferentia from an already infected urethra or bladder. The presence of bacteria initiates the inflammatory response, causing symptoms of bacterial epididymitis. Epididymitis caused by heavy lifting or straining results from reflux of urine from the bladder into the vas deferens and epididymis. Urine is extremely irritating to the epididymis and initiates an inflammatory response called *chemical epididymitis.*

CLINICAL MANIFESTATIONS   Pain is the main symptom of epididymitis. Scrotal or inguinal pain is caused by inflammation of the epididymis and surrounding tissues. The pain is usually acute and severe. Flank pain may occur if, as the urethra passes over the spermatic cord, edematous swelling of the cord obstructs the urethra. The individual may have pyuria and bacteriuria and a history of urinary symptoms, including urethral discharge. The scrotum on the involved side is red and edematous as a result of inflammatory changes. The tail of the epididymis near the lower pole of the testis usually swells first; then swelling ascends to the head of the epididymis. The spermatic cord also may be swollen and tender.

Complications of epididymitis include abscess formation, infarction of the testis, recurrent infection, and infertility. Infarction probably is caused by thrombosis (obstruction by blood clots) of the prostatic vessels secondary to severe inflammation. Recurrent epididymitis may result from inadequate initial treatment or failure to identify or treat predisposing factors. Chronic epididymitis can cause scarring of the epididymal endothelium. Once scarring has occurred, treatment with antibiotics is ineffective because adequate antibiotic levels cannot be achieved within the epididymis.[117,118]

EVALUATION AND TREATMENT   A history of recent urinary tract infection or urethral discharge suggests the diagnosis of epididymitis. The relief of pain when the inflamed testis and epididymis are elevated (Prehn sign) is also diagnostic. Definitive diagnosis is based on culture or Gram stain of a urethral swab. Epididymal aspiration may be necessary to obtain a specimen, especially if the individual has been taking antibiotics and has sterile urine.

Treatment includes antibiotic therapy for the infection itself (see Chapter 24) and various measures to provide symptomatic relief. Bed rest and scrotal elevation are recommended until the scrotum is no longer tender. Scrotal elevation facilitates maximal lymphatic and venous drainage. Abscess formation is rare with antibiotic therapy. If an abscess occurs and persists, it is drained surgically and an orchiectomy may be indicated. Complete resolution of swelling and pain may take several weeks to months. The individual's sexual partner should be treated with antibiotics if the causative microorganism is a sexually transmitted pathogen.

Disorders of the Prostate Gland
Benign Prostatic Hyperplasia
Benign prostatic hyperplasia (BPH), also called **benign prostatic hypertrophy,** is the enlargement of the prostate gland (Figure 23-35). (Because the major prostatic changes are

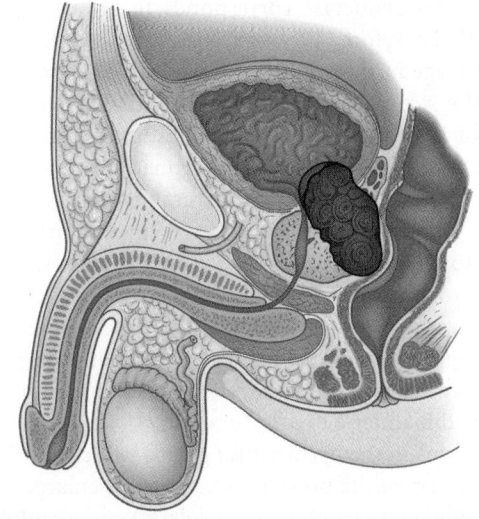

A

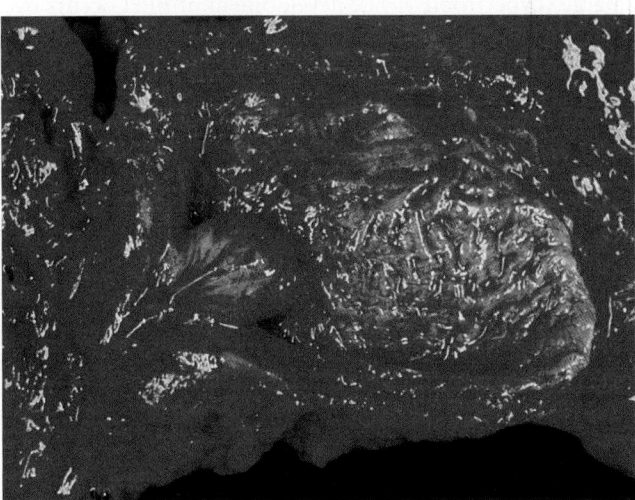

B

Figure 23-35 Benign prostatic hyperplasia. **A,** Condition becomes a problem as prostatic tissue compresses the urethra. **B,** Gross appearance of BPH showing transition zone resulting from bulging nodules of varying size. (**B** from Damjanov I, Linder J, editors: *Anderson's pathology,* ed 10, St Louis, 1996, Mosby.)

caused by hyperplasia, not hypertrophy, benign prostatic hyperplasia is the preferred term.) This condition becomes problematic as prostatic tissue compresses the urethra, where it passes through the prostate. Approximately 80% of men will have prostatic enlargement before age 80 years, and there is a 25% to 30% lifetime chance of needing prostatectomy for BPH once a man reaches 50 years of age.[119] Although BPH is common, its cause remains obscure. Its relationship to aging is well documented, however. At birth the prostate is pea sized, and growth of the gland is gradual until puberty. A period of rapid development continues until the third decade of life, when the prostate reaches adult size (see Chapter 22). Around 40 to 45 years of age, benign hyperplasia begins and continues slowly until death. Although dihydrotestosterone (DHT) is necessary for normal prostatic development, its role in BPH remains unclear. Among all androgen-metabolizing enzymes within the human prostate, 5α-reductase is the most powerful. This reductase corresponds to an age-dependent DHT level. Therefore, although 5α-reductase and DHT decrease with age in the epithelium, they remain relatively constant in the stroma of the prostate gland. Current causative theories of BPH focus on levels and ratios of endocrine factors such as androgens, estrogens, gonadotropins, and prolactin and changes in the balance between autocrine/paracrine growth-stimulatory and growth-inhibitory factors. These factors include insulin-like growth factors (IGFs), epidermal growth factor, nerve growth factor, IGF binding proteins, and transforming growth factor–beta.[120] Other relationships being explored include the interrelationship of the prostatic capsule with α-adrenergic innervation of the prostate and bladder detrusor function.[119]

BPH begins in the periurethral glands, which are the inner glands or layers of the prostate. The prostate enlarges as nodules form and grow (nodular hyperplasia) and glandular cells enlarge (hypertrophy). The development of BPH occurs over a prolonged period, and changes within the urinary tract are slow and insidious. Pathophysiologic effects are a result of complex interactions involving prostatic urethral resistance to the mechanical and spastic effects of BPH, intravesical pressure during voiding, detrusor muscle strength, neurologic functioning, and general physical health.

During the early stages of urethral obstruction, the detrusor muscle hypertrophies to help the bladder force urine out against increasing resistance. Symptoms are considered obstructive (weak urinary stream, prolonged voiding, abdominal straining, hesitancy, intermittency, incomplete bladder emptying, postmicturitional dribble) or irritative (frequency and repeated urination, nocturia, urgency, incontinence, and bladder pain and dysuria)[121] and may wax and wane.[122] As obstruction progresses, often over a period of several years, the detrusor muscle decompensates and the bladder is unable to empty all of the urine. Increasing volumes of urine are retained until urine retention is chronic. The volume of urine retained may be great enough to produce uncontrolled "overflow incontinence" with any increase in intraabdominal pressure. At this stage the force of the urinary stream is reduced significantly and much more time is required to initiate and complete voiding.

Progressive bladder distention causes sacculations or diverticular outpouchings of the bladder wall, and some neural degeneration of smooth muscle cells occurs. The ureters may be obstructed where they pass through the hypertrophied detrusor muscle. Hematuria, bladder or kidney infection, bladder calculi, acute urinary retention hydroureter, hydronephrosis, and renal insufficiency are common complications.[121] Some men initially have signs of uremia and renal failure. On digital rectal examination (DRE) the hyperplastic prostate is a soft or firm enlargement with smooth mucosal surface and no discernible distinction between lobes; asymmetry is common. The palpated prostate does not always reflect the degree of BPH because a substantial portion of the enlargement is intravesicular.[123] Thirty percent of men with mild to moderate symptoms improve with watchful waiting.

There is no way to reverse progressive BPH, but the hyperplasia is not always progressive. For these reasons, timing of intervention is variable and depends on severity of symptoms and the presence of complications. Annual DREs are used to screen men over 40 years of age for BPH. If marked enlargement, moderate to severe symptoms, or complications are present, transrectal ultrasonography (TRUS) is used to determine bladder and prostate volume and residual urine. Urinalysis, serum creatinine and blood urea nitrogen, uroflowmetry, postvoid residual (PVR) urine, pressure-flow study, cystometry, and cystourethroscopy are used to determine kidney and bladder function.[121] Physical examination with DRE and **prostate-specific antigen** (PSA) is conducted to determine hyperplasia.[124] PSA density (PSAD) is helpful in differentiating BPH from prostatic cancer. PSAD is calculated by dividing PSA serum levels by the volume of prostate tissue, which is determined by TRUS. When necessary, the hyperplastic tissue may be removed surgically to prevent the serious consequences of urethral obstruction. Glands less than 60 g are treated by transurethral resection, laser therapy, or microwave thermotherapy,[125] whereas larger glands are removed surgically (prostatectomy). A permanent indwelling catheter is inserted if the individual cannot tolerate surgery. Recently, BPH has been treated successfully with drugs. α₁-Adrenergic blockers (Prazosin and Tamsulosin) are used to relax the smooth muscle of the bladder and prostate. Antiandrogen agents, such as finasteride (Proscar), selectively block androgens at the prostate cellular level and cause the prostate gland to shrink.[126] These drugs offer an alternative to surgery for as many as 75% of men with mild prostate enlargement.[126] Neither α₁-adrenergic blockers nor finasteride seems to affect sexual desire or potency; finasteride may cause bone loss and lower levels of PSA. Because of the effect of finasteride on PSA levels, new recommendations for men on finasteride for 6 months or longer state that the serum PSA level should be multiplied by 2 and compared with either age-independent or age-specific upper limits of normal for serum PSA in untreated men with BPH. PSA is used as a screen for prostate cancer. (See Chapter 11 for a discussion of antigens as tumor markers.)

The standard nonsurgical approach to the management of prostatic neoplasm is to decrease androgen levels and trigger involution of the gland. Although men with BPH respond favorably to this approach, androgen ablation in men with prostatic cancer is less effective than surgery. One explanation is that local and independent growth factors fully or partially replace the androgen-driven growth signal. Prostatic fibromuscular stroma is a rich source of IGF-II and possesses an abundance of IGF receptors. Recent research supports inhibition of normal IGF-I functions as an alternative or supplement to standard steroid-based therapies for BPH.

Prostatitis

Prostatitis is an inflammation of the prostate. Some degree of prostatic inflammation is present in 4% to 36% of the male population. This percentage increases to 50% in older men.

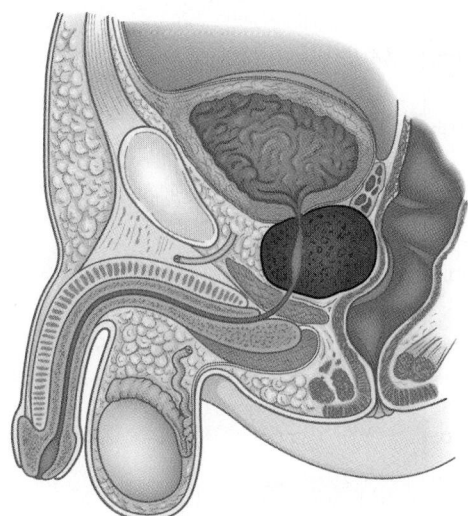

Figure 23-36 Prostatitis.

Inflammation is usually limited to a few of the gland's excretory ducts (Figure 23-36).

Prostatitis is characterized as (1) acute bacterial prostatitis, (2) chronic bacterial prostatitis, or (3) nonbacterial prostatitis. **Prostatodynia** (pain in the prostate) is sometimes considered a form of nonbacterial prostatitis. Men with prostatodynia have the same clinical manifestations as those with nonbacterial prostatitis, but physical and laboratory examinations do not show prostatic pathology. Prostatodynia may not be caused by a pathologic condition of the prostate but rather by spasms in the genitourinary tract or tension in the muscles of the pelvic floor.

A number of defense mechanisms normally protect the lower urogenital tract from infection. Mechanical defenses include urethral length, micturition (urination), and ejaculation. Structural malformations and instrumentation of the genitourinary tract may weaken these defense mechanisms. Chemical defenses include antimicrobial substances in the prostatic fluid. The most important of these is a zinc-containing polypeptide known as *prostatic antibacterial factor.* Coliform bacteria, particularly *Enterobacter, E. coli, Enterococcus, Klebsiella,* and *Pseudomonas,* are common pathogens of bacterial prostatitis. *Ureaplasma* and *C. trachomatis* also may be causative agents of infectious prostatitis.[118]

Bacterial Prostatitis

Acute bacterial prostatitis is an ascending infection of the urinary tract that tends to occur in men between ages 30 and 50 years but is also associated with BPH in older men. Infection stimulates an inflammatory response in which the prostate becomes enlarged, tender, and firm or boggy. The onset of prostatitis may be acute and unrelated to previous illnesses, or it may follow catheterization or cystoscopy.

Clinical manifestations of acute bacterial prostatitis are those of acute cystitis or pyelonephritis. Sudden onset of malaise, low back and perineal pain, high fever (up to 40° C [104° F]), and chills is common, as are dysuria, inability to empty the bladder, nocturia, and urinary retention. Myalgia and arthralgia also may occur. The individual also may have symptoms of lower urinary tract obstruction, such as a slow, small, "narrowed" urinary stream, which may be a medical emergency. Men are acutely ill and may look toxic. Prostatic pain may occur, especially when the individual is in an upright position, because the pelvic floor muscles tighten with standing and compression of the prostate gland occurs. Some individuals experience low back pain, painful ejaculation, and rectal or perineal pain. Palpation discloses an extremely tender, swollen prostate with normal to "boggy" consistency that may be warm to the touch.

Because acute bacterial prostatitis usually is associated with a bladder infection caused by the same microorganism, urine cultures disclose its identity. Prostatic massage may express enough secretions from the urethra for direct bacterial examination, but massage may be painful and increases the risk that the infection will ascend to adjacent structures or enter the bloodstream and cause septicemia. For these reasons, prostatic massage generally is contraindicated; transurethral instrumentation also is contraindicated.

Long-term, broad-spectrum antibiotic therapy with fluoroquinolone agents or trimethoprim-sulfamethoxazole for at least 30 to 42 days is recommended to resolve the infection and control its spread. In severe cases the individual is hospitalized and treated with combination intravenous antibiotics, usually an aminoglycoside (gentamicin sulfate, kanamycin sulfate, or tobramycin) and ampicillin for 1 week followed by 4 to 6 weeks of oral antibiotics. Pain relievers, antipyretics, bed rest, and adequate hydration are also therapeutic. Complications include urinary retention that resolves with antibiotic therapy; prostatic abscess that may rupture into the urethra, rectum, or perineum; epididymitis; bacteremia; and septic shock. Urinary retention requiring drainage is best managed with a suprapubic catheter; Foley catheterization is contraindicated during acute infection.

Chronic bacterial prostatitis is characterized by recurrent urinary symptoms and persistence of pathogenic bacteria (usually gram negative) in urine or prostatic fluid.[118] This form of prostatitis is the most common recurrent urinary tract infection in men. Symptoms are variable and may be similar to those of an acute bladder infection: frequency, urgency, dysuria, perineal discomfort, low back pain, and sexual dysfunction. The prostate may be only slightly enlarged or boggy, but fibrosis caused by repeated infections can cause it to be firm and irregular in shape.

When the initial urine sample is bacteria free, prostatic massage is used to express secretions. Subsequently, the first 10 ml of voided urine is collected and examined microscopically. Prostatic secretions showing more than 10 white blood cells per high-power field and macrophages containing fat indicate bacterial infection; diagnosis is confirmed by culture. Prostatic calculi may be seen on pelvic x-ray or TRUS.

Treatment of chronic bacterial prostatitis is difficult because it is often caused by prostatic calculi. Calculi are silent and are found in up to 50% of men with prostatitis, and infected calculi can serve as a source of bacterial persistence and relapsing urinary tract infections.[118] Calculi harbor pathogens within the stone, and consequently pathogens cannot be eradicated from the urinary tract. Permanent cure is achieved by surgical removal of the stones through transurethral prostatectomy, which may not be a viable option for young men. More common symptoms are tempered with chronic suppressive therapy. Quinolones, because of their bioavailability and penetration into prostatic tissue, are the treatment of choice; drug therapy lasts for a minimum of 3 to 4 weeks. If symptoms do not subside, other infectious microorganisms are considered and treated accordingly.[118] Comfort measures include nonsteroidal antiinflammatory drug therapy and liberal use of sitz baths.

Nonbacterial Prostatitis

Nonbacterial prostatitis is the most common prostatitis syndrome and consists of prostatic inflammation without evidence of bacterial infection. Symptoms tend to be milder but are persistent and annoying. Presumably, noninfectious prostatitis or prostatodynia is caused by reflux of sterile urine into the ejaculatory ducts as a result of high-pressure voiding.[118] Reflux may be triggered by spasms of the external or internal sphincters. Some men may actually have interstitial cystitis and should be treated accordingly.

Men with nonbacterial prostatitis may complain of pain or a dull ache that is continuous or spasmodic in the suprapubic, intrapubic, scrotal, penile, or inguinal area. Other symptoms are pain on ejaculation and urinary symptoms, such as frequency of urination. The prostate gland generally feels normal on palpation.

Digital examination of the prostate, bacterial cultures of the urogenital tract, microscopic examination of expressed prostatic fluid, urethroscopy, and urodynamic studies are used to verify the diagnosis of nonbacterial prostatitis. Nonbacterial prostatitis is a diagnosis by exclusion.

Therapy is individualized and aimed at decreasing symptoms. α_1-Adrenergic blockers (e.g., terazosin, doxazosin, and tamsulosin) may be helpful in decreasing spasms of the prostate muscle. Other treatments include skeletal muscle relaxants, pelvic floor relaxation using biofeedback, and prostatic thermotherapy.[118] Additional treatments may include hot sitz baths, bed rest, anticholinergics, and anti-inflammatory drugs.

Cancer of the Prostate

Prostate cancer is among the most common male cancers but the incidence varies greatly worldwide (Figure 23-37). It is the most common cancer in American males but the third most common cancer worldwide. In the United States, it accounts for more than 14% of all cancer deaths; only lung cancer accounts for more deaths. Among countries with reliable cancer statistics, prostate cancer rates are highest in Westernized countries, such as the United States and Western Europe and lowest in Asian countries. It also is rare in Africa, Central America, and South America. Screening with PSA can amplify the incidence of prostate cancer by allowing detection of prostate lesions that, while meeting the pathologic criteria for

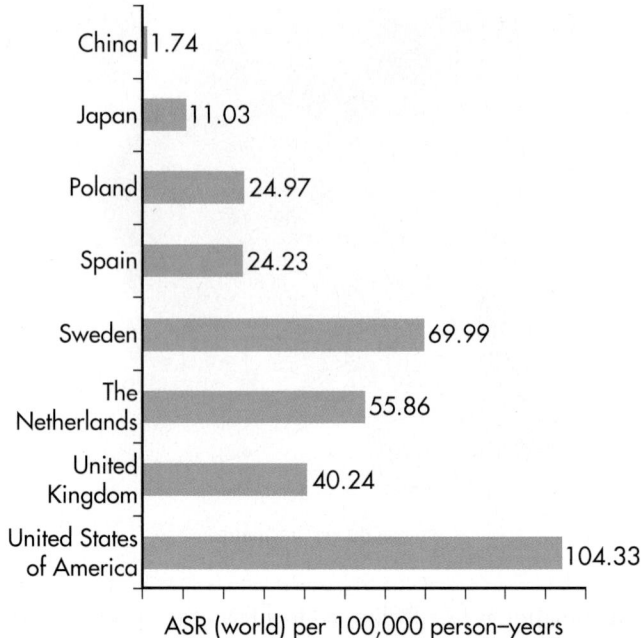

Figure 23-37 Selected world population age-standardized (to the world population) incidence rates of prostate cancer. *ASR*, Age-standardized rate. (Data from Ferlay J et al: *GLOBOCAN 2000: cancer incidence, mortality, and prevalence worldwide,* Lyon, 2001, International Agency for Research on Cancer.)

malignancy, many believe to have low potential for growth and metastasis; however, this is controversial. Thus screening can amplify the incidence of prostate cancer by including the detection of these localized lesions. Therefore the incidence rates in some countries, such as the United States, reflect both clinical and latent (preclinical) disease compared to other countries that report only clinical disease. Comparing data in the pre-PSA era does reflect less extreme incidence rates, but the United States still has the highest rates. Data from the Surveillance, Epidemiology, and End Results (SEER) program show that incidence rates in the United States for white men increased 80% from 1983 to 1987 and 1988 to 1992 (possibly because of increased screening in asymptomatic men).[127]

A small decline in the death rate has been noted during the past few years in the United States and other developing countries. The overall mortality rates are mostly in men over the age of 65; within younger groups, mortality has been stable across decades. Incidence increases with advancing age; more than 75% of all prostate cancer is diagnosed in men older than 65.[88] By age 85, about one in six American men will develop prostate cancer in their lifetime and about 3% will die from it. With aging, most of the androgen-metabolizing enzymes undergo significant alteration. The incidence is low in black African men worldwide; however, black African-American men have the highest rate of prostate cancer in the world and in the United States.

Dietary Factors

The worldwide distribution of prostate cancer suggests that diet may play a role in the development of prostate cancer, especially if the diet affects hormone levels. Consistency across studies indicates that a high intake of fat (total and especially saturated fat) is a risk factor for prostate cancer, but the strength of the associations is modest and may be greater for African-Americans than for European-Americans.[119-128] Several hypotheses exist concerning the enhancing effect of fat on prostate carcinogenesis, including hormonal mediation and the generation of free radicals. Fat intake from dairy products increases calcium, itself a proposed risk factor. Calcium can suppress circulating levels of dihydroxyvitamin D, a possible protective factor for prostate cancer.[129] In addition, a low intake of dietary fiber and complex carbohydrates and a high intake of protein are associated with an increased risk of prostate cancer.[128] Some data suggest a slight increase in risk of advanced prostate cancer or death among individuals with a high body mass index.[130,131] High-energy intake (consumption of excess calories) indicates that this may indeed increase insulin levels and insulin-like growth factors (IGF-1). IGF-1 is known to be a powerful carcinogenic agent[132] (see Pathogenesis).

Individual nutrients or foods and their associations with prostate cancer risk are not strong, yet migration of individuals from low-risk geographic areas of the world, such as Japan, to high-risk countries, such as the United States, increases risk considerably.[133] These changes in risk probably reflect differences in lifestyle and dietary habits. Geographically, individuals who reside in regions with less sunlight have a higher risk of prostate cancer. The highest rates of mortality from prostate cancer in the world are in Scandinavian countries, where exposure to ultraviolet light is low; the possible link is less vitamin D induced by less sun exposure. The Cure of Cancer of the Prostate (CaP CURE) Report[134] states that of all the risk factors for prostate cancer, only nutrition seems to explain the differences in global distribution of prostate cancer.

Animal studies suggest a protective effect of retinoids (vitamin A) and prostate carcinogenesis; however, consistency is lacking among epidemiologic studies. Vegetarian men have a lower incidence of prostate cancer than omnivorous males.[135] Low levels of dietary selenium are associated with increased prostate cancer risk.[136] Vitamin D (1,25-[OH]2D3) inhibited the growth of certain human prostate cancer cell lines by an androgen-dependent mechanism.[137] Lycopene, a carotenoid found in large amounts in tomatoes that gives them their red color, has been associated with a lower risk of prostate cancer.[138,139]

Hormones

Prostate cancer develops in an androgen-dependent epithelium and is usually androgen sensitive. In addition, a few case reports exist of prostate cancer in men who used androgenic steroids as anabolic agents or for medical purposes, suggestive of a causal relationship.[133,140-142] Population studies have not, however, provided clear and convincing patterns about associations between circulating hormone concentrations and prostate cancer risk.[133] Only a few associations with prostate cancer risk have been observed consistently (in at least three studies), and their associations are weak: (1) slightly higher circulating testosterone and estrogen levels and lower DHEA (sulfate) levels in high-risk African-American men as compared with lower-risk European-American men; and (2) a cytosine-adenine-guanine (CAG) repeat-length polymorphism in the androgen-receptor gene associated with increased risk and increased receptor activity (androgen receptor). Evidence for involvement of activity of the enzyme 5α-reductase, which is critical in androgen activity in the prostate, is contradictory and inconsistent.[133] In men younger than 50 years, circulating levels of androgens and estrogens appear to be higher in men of African descent than in European-American men.

Androgens promote prostatic epithelial growth during fetal and prepubertal periods. In adults androgens act through reciprocal homeostatic stromal (microenvironment; see Chapter 11) epithelial interactions to maintain normal differentiation and halt growth[143] (see Pathogenesis).

Investigations directed at understanding the hormonal basis of prostate (as well as breast) carcinogenesis have numerous problems. The complexities of interacting hormones and separating out the effects of a single hormone are profound. In addition, only single *blood* samples are generally available, *tissue* hormone samples important for paracrine signaling are not consistently measured, and within-subject variations over time and differences in circadian rhythms cannot be adequately measured. The results of several animal studies do support elevation of bioavailable and bioactive androgens in the circulation and in target tissue as an important risk factor. Animal studies also indicate that increased biologic activity of

---

NUTRITION & DISEASE

Nutrition and Risk Reduction for Prostate Cancer

- Avoid saturated fat
- Avoid specific polyunsaturated fats, including omega-6 fat, linoleic acid (found in safflower and soybean oil), and omega-3 fat α-linolenic acid (found in red meat, mayonnaise, soybean oil, rapeseed oil, and margarine)
- Avoid foods with hydrogenated or partially hydrogenated oil
- Substitute oils with olive oils (use sparingly)
- Decrease total energy intake from calories; avoid refined sugars*
- Increase antioxidants, vitamin E (400 IU/day), selenium (from grains, garlic, supplements), green tea, cruciferous vegetables, and fruits
- Increase lycopene (reddest tomatoes available, tomato juice, soup, salads)
- Increase soy (genistein)
- Increase sunshine exposure for daily requirement of vitamin D (200 to 400 IU/day)
- Maintain calcium intake at 1000 mg (19 to 50 years old), 1200 mg (51 and older); switch from cow's milk to soy milk
- Increase fiber (whole grains, beans, cereals)

For documented studies see Arnot R: *The prostate cancer protection plan: the foods, supplements and drugs that could save your life,* Boston, 2000, Little, Brown.
*Emerging as very important for decreasing IGF-1.

the androgen receptor may be associated with prostate cancer. See the "Pathogenesis" section for a more thorough discussion of the role of hormones in the pathogenesis of prostate cancer.

Vasectomy

Vasectomy has been identified as a possible risk factor for prostate cancer in both case-controlled studies and cohort studies.[144,145] Three mechanisms by which vasectomy could increase risk are (1) elevation of circulating androgens; (2) immunologic mechanisms involving antisperm antibodies; and (3) reduction of seminal fluid levels of 5α-dihydrotestosterone, the active metabolite of testosterone in the prostate, in vasectomized men. Other investigators reported a decrease in sex hormone–binding globulin (SHBG) and an increase in the ratio of testosterone to SHBG.[146] These results suggest an elevation of circulating free testosterone following vasectomy.[133] However, with these combined mechanisms it is unlikely that vasectomy plays a causal role.[129]

Familial Factors

Other possible causes are genetic predisposition (familial and hereditary forms). Recent genetic studies suggest that strong familial predisposition may be responsible for 5% to 10% of prostate cancers.[80] Hereditary cancer is an autosomal dominant disease caused by a rare but highly penetrant gene; that is, 88% of gene carriers develop prostate cancer by age 85 years. Hereditary cancer differs from the familial form, which occurs in individuals with a positive family history but who do not exhibit early age of onset.[147] The hereditary form constitutes about 9% of all prostate cancers and approximately 43% of cancers in men less than 55 years of age.[123] There is no clear evidence of a causal link between BPH and prostate cancer even though they may often occur together. Recent data substantiate that tobacco use has a significant impact on the occurrence of fatal prostate cancer.[148]

PATHOGENESIS More than 95% of prostatic neoplasms are adenocarcinomas,[149] and most occur in the periphery of the prostate. Several histologic grading systems have been developed on the basis of the glandular pattern, the degree of differentiation (anaplasia) of the cancer cells, or both. The biologic aggressiveness of the neoplasm appears to be related to the degree of differentiation rather than the size of the tumor (see Box 23-12 on p. 821).

Just as the testicles are the male equivalent of the female ovaries, the prostate is the male equivalent of the female uterus; in both situations they originate from the same embryonic cells. This may be important in understanding the role of the associated hormones testosterone, dihydrotestosterone, and estradiol in prostate carcinogenesis. Testosterone and dihydrotestosterone (DHT) are the most important androgens in the adult male. Testosterone is the major *circulating* androgen, whereas DHT predominates in prostate tissue and binds to the androgen receptor (AR) with greater affinity than does testosterone.[150]

Testosterone is the major androgen from the interstitial cells of the testis (Leydig cells). Its production in men is almost 5 mg/day. The adrenal cortex contributes the far less potent androstenedione as its major androgen, at about 3 mg/day. In the target tissues and, to a lesser extent, in the testes themselves, testosterone is converted to DHT by the enzyme 5α-reductase (Figure 23-38). Thus DHT is the most potent intraprostatic androgen. About half of circulating testosterone is bound to sex hormone-binding globulin (SHBG), about half binds to albumin, and about 1% to 2% exists in a free state. Free testosterone, including testosterone disassociated from albumin and possibly SHBG, enters the prostate cell where it is converted to DHT.[150] DHT is a paracrine hormone because it affects the local environment or stroma. Several intraprostatic enzymes encoded by genes, *HSD3A* and *HDS3B*, are activated by DHT and are important components of intraprostatic androgen regulation. The conjugated byproduct, 3α-androstenediol glucuronide (AAG), a terminal metabolite of DHT, can be measured in the circulation and used as an indicator of DHT levels. The drug finasteride, an inhibitor of intraprostatic 5α-reductase type II enzyme, decreases AAG levels. Thus AAG is a marker of intraprostatic 5α-reductase activity and androgen levels.

Normally, a small amount of estrogen is produced per day—65 mcg of estrone and 45 mcg of estradiol—by the aromatization of androstenedione and testosterone, respectively. This reaction is catalyzed by the enzyme system aromatase. A very small quantity of estradiol is released by the testes (see Figure 23-40); the rest of the estrogens in males are produced by adipose tissue, liver, skin, brain, and other nonendocrine tissue. Thus testosterone is a precursor of the two hormones, DHT and estradiol.

Most of the androgen-metabolizing enzymes undergo a significant age-dependent alteration. In epithelium, both the 5α-reductase activity and the DHT level decrease with age; whereas in stroma not only is 5α-reductase activity rather constant over the whole age range but also the DHT level is constant as well. In contrast to the relatively unaltered DHT level, the estrogen content follows an age-dependent increase. Thus the age-dependent decrease of the DHT accumulation in epithelium and the concomitant increase of the estrogen accumulation in stroma lead to a tremendous increase with age of the estrogen/androgen ratio in the human prostate. In animal studies, chronic exposure to testosterone plus estradiol is strongly carcinogenic, whereas testosterone alone is weakly carcinogenic.[133] The mechanism is not clearly understood but appears to involve estrogen-generated oxidative stress and DNA toxicity, and it requires androgen and estro-

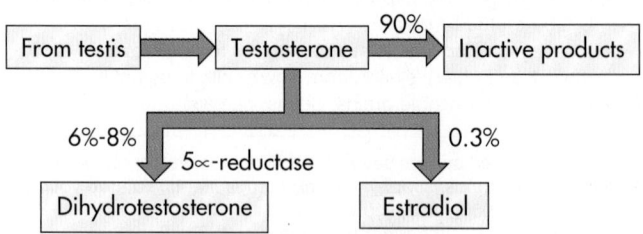

Figure 23-38 Testosterone and conversion to DHT.

gen receptor–mediated processes, such as changes in sex steroid metabolism and receptor status.[133] In addition, there are changes in the balance between autocrine/paracrine growth-stimulatory and growth-inhibitory factors, such as IGFs, epidermal growth factor (EGF), nerve growth factor (NGF), IGF-binding proteins, and transforming growth factor–beta (TGF-β).

The microenvironment (stroma) surrounding the prostatic tumor actively fuels the progression of prostate cancer from localized growth, to invasion, to development of distant metastases.[151] Androgens drive prostatic epithelial growth during fetal and prepubertal periods and in adulthood androgens participate through reciprocal homeostatic stromal-epithelial interactions to maintain differentiation but *arrest* growth.[143] Recent data support the idea that *newly acquired* and *not* preexisting tumor cells are the dominant mechanisms of prostate cancer progression.[151] Intercellular communication between prostate tumor cells and organ-specific stroma involve diffusible molecules that interact as mediators leading to the development of metastasis[151] (also see Chapter 12). Thus a new opportunity arises for therapeutic targeting of the microenvironment, especially of testosterone and estradiol (T+E$_2$) through paracrine mechanisms. In addition, the periepithelial stroma undergoes progressive loss in smooth muscle with the appearance of carcinoma-associated fibroblasts (CAFs). Abnormal stroma was shown to promote carcinogenesis in genetically abnormal epithelial cells in vitro. Thus the stromal microenvironment is a necessary determinant of benign versus malignant growth.[143]

From all of these observations, the following multifactorial general hypothesis of prostate carcinogenesis emerges: (1) androgens act as tumor promoters through androgen receptor–mediated mechanisms to (2) enhance the carcinogenic activity of strong endogenous DNA toxic carcinogens, including reactive estrogen metabolites and estrogen—and prostatic-generated reactive oxygen species—(3) alterations in autocrine/paracrine growth-stimulating and growth-inhibiting factors and (4) possibly unknown environmental-lifestyle carcinogens. All of these factors are modulated by diet and genetic determinants, such as hereditary susceptibility genes and polymorphic genes (especially steroid 5α-reductase type II [SRD5A2]), that encode receptors and enzymes involved in the metabolism and action of steroid hormones.[133,150]

The most common sites of distant metastasis are the lymph nodes, bones, lungs, liver, and adrenals. The pelvis, lumbar spine, femur, thoracic spine, and ribs are the most common sites of bone metastasis. Local extension is usually posterior, although late in the disease the tumor may invade the rectum or encroach on the prostatic urethra and cause bladder outlet obstruction (Figure 23-39; see Clinical Manifestations). The spread through blood vessels is illustrated in Figure 23-40.

CLINICAL MANIFESTATIONS
Prostatic cancer often causes no symptoms until it is far advanced. The first manifestations of disease are those of bladder outlet obstruction:

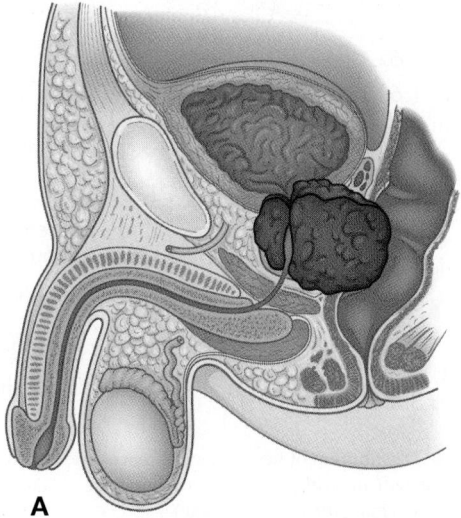

A

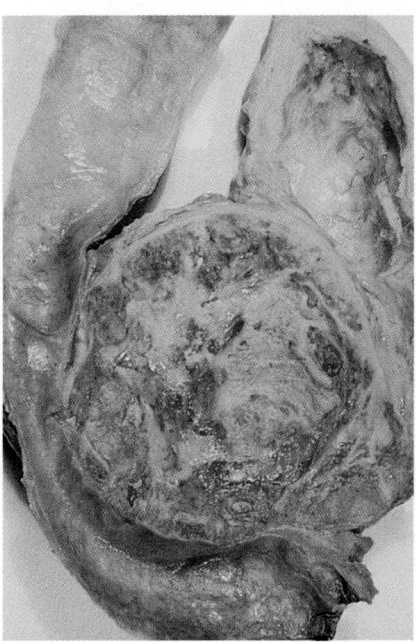

B

Figure 23-39 **Carcinoma of prostate. A,** Common sites of distant metastasis are the lymph nodes, bones, lungs, liver, and adrenals. **B,** Carcinoma of the prostate extending into the rectum and urinary bladder. (**B** from Damjanov I, Linder J, editors: *Pathology: a color atlas,* St Louis, 2000, Mosby.)

slow urinary stream, hesitancy, incomplete emptying, frequency, nocturia, and dysuria. Unlike the symptoms of obstruction caused by BPH, the symptoms of obstruction caused by prostatic cancer are progressive and do not remit. Local extension of prostatic cancer can obstruct the upper urinary tract ureters as well. If rectal obstruction occurs, the individual may experience a large bowel obstruction or difficulty in defecation. Symptoms of late disease include bone pain at sites of bone metastasis, edema of the lower extremities, enlargement of lymph nodes, liver enlargement, pathologic bone fractures, and mental confusion associated with brain metastases.

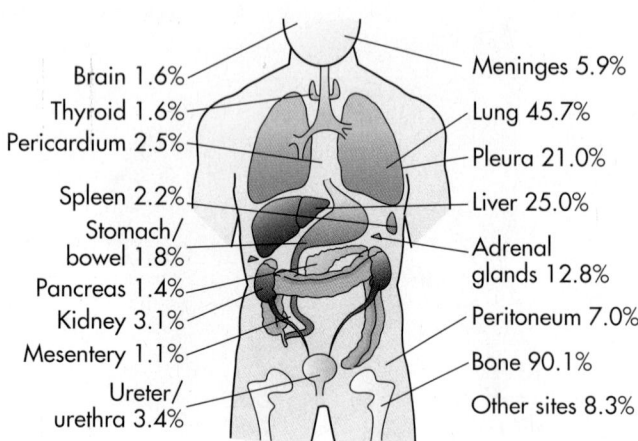

Brain 1.6%
Thyroid 1.6%
Pericardium 2.5%
Spleen 2.2%
Stomach/bowel 1.8%
Pancreas 1.4%
Kidney 3.1%
Mesentery 1.1%
Ureter/urethra 3.4%

Meninges 5.9%
Lung 45.7%
Pleura 21.0%
Liver 25.0%
Adrenal glands 12.8%
Peritoneum 7.0%
Bone 90.1%
Other sites 8.3%

Figure 23-40 Distribution of hematogenous metastases in prostate cancer. Study of 556 patients with metastatic prostate cancer. (Adapted from Budendorf L et al: *Hum Pathol* 31:578, 2000.)

EVALUATION AND TREATMENT Screening for prostatic cancer includes DRE, PSA blood tests, and TRUS. The American Cancer Society recommends annual DREs for men older than 40 years and an annual DRE and PSA blood test for men older than 50 years (with at least a 10-year life expectancy).[152] Earlier screening with the PSA test is recommended for men at high risk for prostate cancer, such as blacks or relatives of men who have had prostate cancer.[123,147,152,153] It is important to note that PSA levels tend to be higher in blacks at baseline and all stages of cancer.[154] When TRUS is added to the annual DRE and PSA testing, the ability to predict cancer rises significantly, from 41% to greater than 78%. Cancer diagnosis is confirmed through tissue biopsy and microscopic examination of tissue. Lymph node biopsy, bone scans, MRI, and CT may be used to determine metastasis to lymph, bone, or other adjacent tissue.

The 5-year survival rate of men with localized cancer is 100% with or without treatment.[152] However, before screening most men with prostate cancer had advanced disease and died within a few years of diagnosis. Therefore it is unclear which men will benefit from early screening and which will not. Currently, there are no prospective studies to demonstrate benefit or disadvantage of screening. Because of the decreased mortality rate and incidence of advanced disease, some authorities continue to recommend regular screening[152,153] (see What's New? box on PSA screening). If a mass is found on DRE or if PSA is greater than 10, TRUS is recommended to confirm presence of mass and to assist with biopsy.[149] New screening alterations may appear, such as PCA3 (prostate cancer-specific gene 3, formerly called DD3).[155] The most important observation for pathologists to make to facilitate cure of any individual of prostate cancer is that of accurately measuring the size of the index (longest) tumor and its percentage of Gleason grade 4/5 (degree of differentiation).[156] The annual rate by which PSA rises (i.e., PSA velocity) is one way to improve the prognostic accuracy of PSA screening[157] (Box 23-12).

Treatment of prostatic cancer depends on the stage of the neoplasm (see Box 23-12); the anticipated effects of treatment; and the age, general health, and life expectancy of the individual. The tumor, node, metastasis (TNM) method of staging has been used to determine extent of disease (see Chapter 12, p. 386). Options include no treatment; surgical treatments such as total prostatectomy, transurethral resection of the prostate (TURP), or cryotherapy; nonsurgical treatments such as radiation therapy, hormone therapy, or chemotherapy; watchful waiting; and any combination of these.[152] In addition, new approaches are using immunotherapy.[158] Palliative treatment is aimed at relieving urinary, bladder outlet, or colon obstruction; spinal cord compression; and pain. Treatments at an early stage can cure the disease in most, if not all, men, and treatment for advanced stage cancer can extend life and reduce tumor size, thus preventing or relieving pain. Prognosis and survival rates have improved steadily over the past 50 years. Currently, 85% of all prostate cancers are discovered in the local and regional stages; in these stages the 5-year survival rate is 100%; survival rates decline at 10 years (84%) and 15 years (56%).[159]

Treatment for prostate cancer may lead to loss of urinary control, which often returns to normal after several weeks or months. Stress incontinence can occur after surgery and mild urge incontinence can occur after radiation therapy. Prostate cancer and its treatment can affect sexual functioning. Most men will need assistance (medication) with obtaining an erection for 3 to 12 months after surgery. Sensation of orgasm is not usually affected, but smaller amounts of ejaculate will be produced or men may experience a "dry" ejaculate because of retrograde ejaculation.

Sexual Dysfunction

In males the normal sexual response involves three processes: erection, emission, and ejaculation. **Sexual dysfunction** is the impairment of any or all of these processes. Impairment can be caused by a number of physiologic, psychologic, and emotional factors.

Until the late 1970s, most cases of male sexual dysfunction were thought to be psychogenic. Studies of this problem indicate that, in men older than 40 years, organic factors are involved in more than 50% of cases. The causes of organic sexual dysfunction include (1) vascular, endocrine, and neurologic disorders; (2) chronic disease, including renal failure and diabetes mellitus; (3) penile diseases and penile trauma; and (4) iatrogenic factors, such as surgery and pharmacologic therapies. Most of these disorders cause erectile dysfunction.

PATHOPHYSIOLOGY   Vascular disorders can prevent erection. Some arterial diseases diminish or interrupt circulation to the penis. This prevents engorgement of erectile tissues in the corpora cavernosa and corpus spongiosum. Rarely, excessive venous drainage of the corpora cavernosa prevents erection.

Endocrine disorders that reduce testosterone production affect sexual function and libido. The reduction may be caused by inadequate secretion of the gonadotropins caused by pituitary dysfunction or hyperprolactinemia. Feminizing tumors and estrogen therapy reduce relative levels of testosterone. Testicular atrophy from any cause also decreases testosterone levels and contributes to sexual dysfunction.

Neurologic disorders can interfere with the important sympathetic, parasympathetic, and CNS mechanisms required for erection, emission, and ejaculation. They include spinal cord injury or tumor, multiple sclerosis, and disorders that cause peripheral neuropathies, such as diabetes mellitus and chronic renal failure. Spinal cord injuries or tumors can alter one or more components of the sexual response, depending on the location of the lesion. For example, in most men with upper motor neuron lesions, reflexogenic erection is possible but emission and ejaculation (i.e., orgasm) are not possible. Lesions affecting the lower motor neurons usually prevent erection. In approximately 40% of such cases, emission and ejaculation are prevented.

Many chronic diseases are associated with sexual dysfunction. In some conditions the sexual dysfunction has a specific physiologic cause. Diabetes mellitus, for example, causes both peripheral vascular and neurologic pathology that can lead to erectile dysfunction. Impotence occurs in about 50% of men undergoing dialysis. Multiple factors are involved, including decreased testosterone levels, autonomic neuropathy, accelerated vascular disease, multiple medications, worsening of primary disease, and psychologic stress. Potency may be restored by successful renal transplantation, except in bilateral transplantation if arterial flow is diminished or interrupted. Cirrhosis of the liver, scleroderma, chronic debilitation, and cachexia also are known to cause impotence. Emotional and psychologic response to chronic illness, such as anxiety, depression, and loss of self-esteem, can affect sexual functioning. In other chronic conditions, sexual dysfunction is associated with low energy levels and loss of libido. The pathophysiologic mechanisms responsible for such changes are not known.

Priapism causes fibrosis of trabeculae (erectile tissues) within the corpora cavernosa, making erection difficult. The penile curvature caused by Peyronie disease does not make erection impossible but may make it extremely painful and intercourse impossible. Penile trauma can damage the erectile tissue, disrupt the posterior urethra, and disrupt the pudendal arteries or nerves.

Iatrogenic factors, including drugs and surgery, have a significant impact on erectile function. The following surgical procedures all carry the risk of erectile dysfunction: radical pelvic surgery; radical prostatectomy; transurethral, suprapubic, or simple retropubic prostatectomy; and aortoiliac surgery. Erectile dysfunction is caused by the severing of small nerve branches that are essential for erection. Aortoiliac surgery, retroperitoneal lymphadenectomy, and sympathectomy cause the loss of ejaculation capacity in some individuals.

A few pharmacologic agents enhance the sexual response, but most have the opposite effect. Men who are taking antihypertensives, antidepressants, antihistamines, antispasmodics, sedatives or tranquilizers, barbiturates, diuretics, sex hormone preparations, narcotics, or psychoactive drugs may experience some degree of sexual dysfunction. Drug-induced sexual dysfunction consists of decreased desire, decreased erectile ability, or decreased ejaculatory ability. Ethyl alcohol may induce alcoholic neuropathy or increased estrogens because of hepatic dysfunction; marijuana depresses testosterone levels; and cigarette smoking contributes to vasoconstriction and venous leakage. A number of pharmacologic agents also diminish the quality or quantity of sperm. A few may cause priapism. Drugs can assist in maintaining an erection.

EVALUATION AND TREATMENT   Evaluation of sexual dysfunction includes a physical examination, with particular attention to the genitalia, prostate, and nervous system, and basic laboratory tests to identify the presence of endocrinopathies or other underlying disorders that can cause the dysfunction. If no physiologic cause is found and the condition does not improve with psychotherapy, the man is referred for further investigation of organic causes. Psychologic evaluation is indicated for younger men with a sudden onset of sexual dysfunction or men of any age who are able to achieve but not maintain an erection.

Sophisticated diagnostic techniques can be used to assess penile blood flow, erectile tissue anatomy, nervous system function, and occurrence of erection or emission during sleep (nocturnal emission). Penile blood flow is measured by Doppler techniques and penile arteriography. Corpus cavernosography, in which contrast material is injected into the corpora cavernosa, provides anatomic information about the erectile tissue of the penis. Neuropathic causes of sexual dysfunction are evaluated by measuring the speed of the bulbocavernous reflex. Nocturnal penile tumescence monitoring measures the frequency of nocturnal erections. Depending on the equipment used, this information may be correlated to rapid eye movement (REM) or non-REM sleep.

Treatments for organic sexual dysfunction include both medical and surgical interventions. Nonsurgical interventions include correction of underlying disorders, particularly drug-induced dysfunction and endocrinopathy-related (e.g., reduced testosterone associated with chronic renal failure) dysfunction. Vasodilators and cessation of smoking can benefit individuals with vasculogenic erectile dysfunction. Surgical interventions include penile implants, penile revascularization, and correction of other anatomic defects contributing to sexual dysfunction.

Impairment of Sperm Production and Quality

Spermatogenesis requires adequate secretion of FSH and LH by the pituitary; sufficient secretion of testosterone by the Leydig cells; sufficient function of the Sertoli cells, including secretion of androgen-binding protein, growth factors, inhibin B, and a number of other important (but poorly understood) peptides; and adequate spermatogonia.[160,161] The Leydig cells are located in the testicular interstitium *between* the tubules, and the Sertoli cells and spermatogonia are located

within the seminiferous tubules. The Sertoli cells extend from the basement membrane to the lumen, display tight junctions between adjacent cells, and form the blood-testis barrier. Inadequate secretion of gonadotropins may be caused by hypothyroidism, hyperadrenocortisolism, hyperprolactinemia, or hypogonadotropic hypogonadism. In these situations, gonadotropin levels are low because of feedback inhibition or idiopathic hyposecretion. In the absence of adequate gonadotropin levels, the Leydig cells are not stimulated to secrete testosterone and sperm maturation is not promoted in the Sertoli cells. Spermatogenesis depends not only on appropriate stimulation by the gonadotropins but also on an appropriate response by the testes. Defects in testicular response to the gonadotropins result in decreased secretion of testosterone and inhibin B and, as a result of normal feedback mechanisms, high levels of circulating gonadotropins. In the absence of adequate testosterone levels, spermatogenesis is impaired. Newer research demonstrates the significance of inhibin B as an important marker of the competence of Sertoli cells and spermatogenesis. Inhibin B is strongly correlated with severity of spermatogenic effects. A positive correlation exists between serum inhibin B levels and sperm concentration and testicular volume, and lower levels have been associated with azoospermia, testicular disorders, and infertility.[161]

Impaired spermatogenesis also can be caused by genetic disorders (such as Klinefelter syndrome), myotonic dystrophy, or testicular trauma. Other conditions associated with impaired spermatogenesis include systemic illness, such as renal failure, hepatic disease, or sickle cell disease; exposure to gonadotoxins, such as chemotherapy or radiation; varicocele; and cryptorchidism.

Fertility is adversely affected if spermatogenesis is normal but the sperm are chromosomally or morphologically abnormal or are produced in insufficient quantities. Chromosomal abnormalities are caused by genetic factors and by external variables, such as exposure to radiation or toxic substances. A sperm count of 20 million sperm per milliliter of semen has been suggested as the minimum concentration required for fertility. Average fertile men have 50 to 100 million sperm per milliliter.[112,160]

Sperm motility is another important variable affecting fertility. Motility appears to be affected by the sperm's chemical environment, that is, the characteristics of semen. Prostatic dysfunction, excessive semen viscosity, presence of drugs or toxins in the semen, and presence of antisperm antibodies are associated with impaired sperm motility. Approximately 3% to 7% of infertile males have antisperm antibodies in their semen. Antisperm antibodies may develop as a result of epididymitis or other inflammation of the genitourinary tract, testicular injury or torsion, a previous vasectomy or biopsy, and cryptorchidism. Antisperm antibodies may be (1) cytotoxic antibodies, which attack sperm and reduce their number in the semen; or (2) sperm-immobilizing antibodies, which impair sperm motility and reduce their ability to traverse the endocervical canal. Intrinsic, biologic factors leading to the production of antisperm antibodies seem to play a greater role than extrinsic factors. The exact mechanism remains unclear.[160]

Thorough history and physical, including imaging for varicocele
Two semen analyses and quantification of serum FSH, LH, testosterone levels, and prolactin if indicated
Semen and urethral cultures
Serum assays or monoclonal antibody testing for white blood cells
Immunobead monoclonal antibody test
Postcoital testing of semen activity and function
Sperm penetration assay
Inhibin B assays or testicular biopsy
Vasogram, TRUS, or other imaging studies

For an in-depth discussion see Kim ED, Lipshultz ED: Male infertility. In Copeland LJ, Farrell JF, editors: *Textbook of gynecology,* ed 2, Philadelphia, 2000, Saunders.
FSH, Follicle-stimulating hormone.

A male factor contributes to the cause of up to 50% of cases of infertility. As understanding of the male factor in infertility increases, evaluation becomes more complex and essential to appropriate treatment (Box 23-13). Treatment for impaired spermatogenesis involves correction of any underlying disorders and avoidance of radiation or toxins. Androgens, human gonadotropins, and antiestrogens (e.g., clomiphene citrate, tamoxifen citrate) may enhance spermatogenesis. Semen can be modified to improve sperm motility. If conception is desired, the semen is obtained by masturbation (or mechanical device),[160] after which it can be diluted, concentrated, or washed to remove antisperm antibodies. These alterations are followed by artificial insemination.

DISORDERS OF THE BREAST
Disorders of the Female Breast
Galactorrhea

Galactorrhea (inappropriate lactation) is the persistent and sometimes excessive secretion of a milky fluid from the breasts of a woman who is not pregnant or nursing an infant. Galactorrhea, which also can occur in men, may involve one or both breasts and is not associated with breast cancer.

The incidence of galactorrhea is difficult to estimate because of differences among definitions of the condition, examination techniques, and populations of women who have been studied. Prevalence has been documented as 0.1% to 32% of all women.

PATHOPHYSIOLOGY   Galactorrhea is not a breast disorder per se. Rather, it is a manifestation of pathophysiologic processes elsewhere in the body. These processes are chiefly hormone imbalances caused by hypothalamic-pituitary disturbances, pituitary tumors, or neurologic damage. Exogenous causes include drugs, estrogen, and manipulation of the nipples. Inappropriate lactation caused by hyperprolactinemia is manifested by the spontaneous appearance of a milky secretion from multiple duct openings, usually from both breasts. Galactorrhea caused by oral contraceptives (OCs) is more likely to occur with high-dose OC use; is characterized by clear, serous, or milky discharge from multiple ducts; and is noticeable during the drug-free interval between OC packets. In premenopausal women, unilateral or bilateral spontaneous multiple duct discharge that increases before menstruation often is caused by fibrocystic change. Unilateral, spontaneous, serous or serosanguineous discharge from a single duct usually is caused by an intraductal papilloma; bloody discharge suggests cancer; bilateral, sticky, multicolored discharge from multiple ducts is often caused by duct ectasia; and purulent discharge indicates a subareolar abscess.[162]

The most common cause of galactorrhea is **nonpuerperal hyperprolactinemia,** or excessive amounts of prolactin in the blood not related to pregnancy or childbirth. Prolactin is a pituitary hormone that stimulates milk production. Nonpuerperal hyperprolactinemia can be caused by any factor that (1) stimulates or overstimulates the prolactin-secreting units of the pituitary gland; (2) interferes with production of **prolactin-inhibiting factor (PIF),** a neurotransmitter (probably dopamine) that inhibits prolactin secretion; or (3) interferes with pituitary receptors for PIF. A variety of exogenous agents and disorders can trigger one of these three mechanisms, thereby causing hyperprolactinemia (Box 23-14).

Several drugs can cause nonpuerperal hyperprolactinemia. They include phenothiazines, reserpine, methyldopa, exogenous estrogens (particularly in high-dose OCs), narcotics, and tricyclic antidepressants.

Hypothyroidism causes increased secretion of hypothalamic thyroid-releasing hormone (TRH), which stimulates prolactin release from the pituitary. Hypothyroidism also is associated with reduced metabolic clearance of prolactin, which prolongs its effects.

Many types of pituitary tumors cause hyperprolactinemia. Prolactinomas cause hyperprolactinemia by secreting prolactin, decreasing production of PIF, or putting pressure on the pituitary stalk such that delivery of PIF to the anterior pituitary is prevented. Growth hormone–secreting pituitary tumors may cause galactorrhea through the intrinsic lactogenic effect that growth hormone appears to have on mammary tissue. Prolactin-secreting lung and kidney tumors also cause hyperprolactinemia.

Chronic stress may cause hyperprolactinemia by inhibiting PIF release. Cervical spinal injuries, head trauma, encephalitis, meningitis, herpes zoster, or thoracotomy scars may stimulate the afferent portion of the suckling reflex arc, which is carried in the second to sixth thoracic nerves. The suckling reflex increases prolactin secretion.

Galactorrhea can be induced by persistent and repeated sucking or squeezing of the nipples and has been documented in women who manipulate their breasts and nipples daily.[163] Monthly examination of the breasts for nipple discharge usually is not associated with the development of galactorrhea.

CLINICAL MANIFESTATIONS   A small amount of breast milk expressed from the nipple of parous women usually is not a concern, and normal breast milk can be colors other than white. Inappropriate lactation is manifested by the

Box 23-14 | Common Causes of Hyperprolactinemia

Physiologic Causes
Exercise
Idiopathic
Pregnancy and postpartum period
Sleep (rapid eye movement [REM] phase)
Stress (trauma, surgery)
Suckling

Drug Causes
Amoxapine
Amphetamines
Anesthetic agents
Butyrophenones
Cimetidine
Estrogens
Hydroxyzine
Methyldopa
Metoclopramide
Narcotics
Phenothiazines
Progestins
Reserpine
Tricyclic antidepressants
Verapamil

Pathophysiologic Causes
Acromegaly
Chronic chest wall stimulation (e.g., postthoracotomy, postmastectomy, herpes zoster)
Cirrhosis
Hypothalamic disease
Hypothyroidism
Pressure on pituitary stalk
Prolactin-secreting tumors
Pseudocyesis (false pregnancy)
Renal failure (especially with zinc deficiency)
Spinal cord lesions

appearance of a milky breast secretion in nonpregnant, nonlactating women from one or both breasts. Most women with galactorrhea experience menstrual abnormality. If a pituitary process is involved, the woman usually experiences hirsutism and infertility; if a hypothalamic lesion is present, she may report such CNS symptoms as intractable headache, visual field disturbances, sleep disturbances, and abnormal temperature, thirst, or appetite.[164]

EVALUATION AND TREATMENT Galactorrhea requires evaluation (1) when it occurs in nulliparous women or in parous women who have not been pregnant or have not breast-fed for 12 months or (2) when it is associated with amenorrhea, headache, visual field abnormalities, or other symptoms implying systemic illness. The evaluation of galactorrhea includes a variety of diagnostic tests. When amenorrhea accompanies galactorrhea, the assessment is the same as for amenorrhea. Breast secretions are examined for fat globules and neoplastic cells to verify their source. Serum prolactin levels are measured. Because such variables as eating, sleeping, stress, and breast examinations all increase prolactin levels, at least two positive results are needed for a diagnosis

of hyperprolactinemia. Prolactin levels greater than 25 to 30 ng/ml (by radioimmunoassay) are considered elevated. Those in the range of 75 to 100 ng/ml are considered to be caused by a pituitary tumor until proved otherwise. Serum thyroxine and thyroid-stimulating hormone levels are measured to rule out hypothyroidism, and LH and FSH levels are obtained if the individual is amenorrheic. CT, MRI, and carotid angiography may assist in the localization of adenomas.

Treatment for galactorrhea consists of identification and treatment of the cause. Medical and surgical therapies may be involved. If a pituitary microadenoma is found, it may be surgically removed, particularly if there has been progressive tumor growth, loss of visual field or acuity, cranial nerve dysfunction, increased intracranial pressure, cerebrospinal fluid leak or obstruction, or infertility. A microadenoma may be treated medically with bromocriptine (Parlodel). This drug controls the tumor but does not cure it, and it must be taken indefinitely. A pituitary macroadenoma usually is treated medically because surgical and radiologic therapies seldom succeed.

Benign Breast Conditions

Numerous benign alterations in ducts and lobules occur in the breast. The most common symptoms reported by women are pain, palpable mass, or nipple discharge; the majority of these prove to have a benign cause. Benign epithelial lesions can be broadly classified according to their future risk of developing breast cancer as (1) nonproliferative breast lesions, (2) proliferative breast disease, and (3) atypical (atypia) hyperplasia.

Nonproliferative Breast Lesions

The term "nonproliferative" is used to discriminate from the "proliferative" changes associated with increased risk for development of breast cancer. This group includes **fibrocystic changes (FCC)**—the most widely accepted term—for physiologic nodularity and breast tenderness that waxes and wanes with the menstrual cycle. On palpation, breasts are lumpy or bumpy and, from radiology studies, breast tissue appears dense with cysts. These lesions mimic carcinoma and women seek medical attention because they produce palpable lumps or nipple discharge. **Cysts,** fluid-filled sacs, are a specific type of lump that commonly occurs in women in their 30s, 40s, and early 50s. Cysts feel squishy-like when they occur close to the surface of the breast but when deeply embedded they can feel hard (Figure 23-41). It has become increasingly clear that FCC is a heterogeneous group of lesions that should be diagnosed separately. An estimated 50% to 80% of women normally experience some of these changes. The prevalence of fibrocystic lesions is probably related to hormonal changes, which in turn are affected by genetic background, age, parity, history of lactation, caffeine, and use of exogenous hormones.[165] Cystic change can be induced in experimental animals by altering ratios of estrogens and progesterone. It is assumed, therefore, that breast cysts are the result of ovarian alterations but the exact mechanism is unknown. Calcifications, found in cysts and adenosis or an increase in the number of acini per lobule, can form mammographically suspicious alterations.[166] Cysts also can be associated with unilateral nipple discharge. A variety of substances are secreted into cyst fluid, including polypeptide

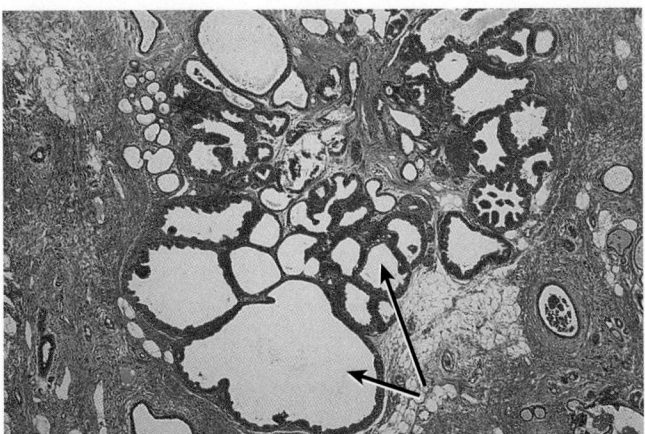

Figure 23-41 Fibrocystic change. Dilated terminal duct and lobules *(arrows)* are lined by epithelium that is either flattened or shows metaplasia. (From Damjanov I, Linder J: *Pathology,* St Louis, 2000, Mosby.)

<table>
<tr><td colspan="2">**Box 23-15** Classification of Breast Biopsy Tissue According to Risk for Breast Cancer</td></tr>
</table>

No Increased Risk
Adenosis (sclerosing or florid)
   Apocrine metaplasia
   Macrocysts or microcysts
   Fibroadenoma
   Fibrosis
Mild hyperplasia
   Mastitis or periductal mastitis
   Squamous metaplasia

Slightly Increased Risk (1.5 to 2.0 times)
Moderate or florid hyperplasia
   Papilloma

Moderately Increased Risk (4 to 5 times)
Atypical hyperplasia (ductal or lobular)

hormones and both male and female sex steroid hormones. Cystic changes by themselves do not appear to be premalignant alterations. Cysts often rupture with release of secretory material into the adjacent tissue. The resulting chronic inflammation and scarring fibrosis contribute to the palpable firmness of the breast.[166] Fibrous tissue increases progressively until menopause and regresses thereafter.

The College of American Pathologists has classified biopsy tissue according to breast cancer risk. These classifications are listed in Box 23-15. In addition to FCC, many women experience benign breast tumors; these are outlined in Table 23-10 and illustrated in Figure 23-42. In general, the frequency of chromosome abnormalities is lower in benign lesions than in breast cancer. Genetic aberrations are more common in proliferative than in nonproliferative lesions.[166]

Proliferative Breast Lesions without Atypia

These disorders are characterized by proliferation of ductal epithelium and/or stroma without cellular signs of malignancy. The following structurally diverse lesions are included: (1) moderate or florid epithelial hyperplasia, (2) sclerosing adenosis, (3) complex sclerosing lesions (radial scar), (4) papillomas, and (5) fibroadenoma with complex features.[166] **Epithelial hyperplasia** is defined by the presence of *more* than two cell layers above the basement membrane. In the normal breast, only myoepithelial cells and a single layer of luminal cells are present above the basement membrane.[166] Moderate to **florid hyperplasia** is more than four cell layers above the basement membrane. The proliferating epithelium fills and distends the ducts and lobules by both luminal and myoepithelial cells.

Sclerosing adenosis is present when the number of acini per terminal duct is greater than twice the number found in uninvolved lobules.[166] Commonly present within the lumens is calcification, however, the normal lobular arrangement is maintained. The acini are structurally altered and myoepithelial cells are prominent. Occasionally, stromal fibrosis may mimic the appearance of invasive carcinoma.[166]

Complex sclerosing lesion (radial scar) refers to an irregular, radial proliferation of ductlike small tubules entrapped in a dense central fibrosis. The term *scar* refers to the structural ap-

pearance only because these lesions are not associated with prior injury or surgery. Radial scar also has been called *radial sclerosing lesions* and *sclerosing papillary proliferation*. Among women with atypical hyperplasia, as compared to women with nonproliferative disease, the relative risk of breast cancer was 5.8 for those with radial scars and 3.8 for those without radial scars. Radial scars are now considered an independent histologic risk factor for breast cancer.[167] The appearance in mammograms, as well as the gross and microscopic appearance, can cause it to be confused with infiltrating ductal carcinoma.[168]

Papillomas consist of multiple, finger-like projections or branching axis lined by myoepithelial cells and luminal cells. Hyperplasia and metaplasia are often present within the ducts. Small duct papillomas increase the risk of subsequent carcinoma; it is unknown whether large duct papillomas do as well.

Proliferative Breast Lesions with Atypia

Proliferative breast lesions with some abnormal structure or *atypia* include atypical ductal hyperplasia (ADH) and atypical lobular hyperplasia (ALH).[166] **Atypical hyperplasia** is an increase in the number of cells and the cells have some variation in structure. **Ductal hyperplasia** is an increased number of cells mostly within the lumen of the terminal ducts (Figure 23-43, *A*). It includes a continuum of changes— cell structure and placement—ranging from an increase in cellularity to features of ductal carcinoma in situ (DCIS; see p. 845). In ADH, the cells fail to completely fill ductal spaces as compared to DCIS.

Lobular hyperplasia refers to proliferation of small, uniform cells in the lumen of lobular units. The abnormal cells of ALH and lobular carcinoma in situ (LCIS) are identical, but the cells in ALH do not distend more than 50% of the acini within a lobule[166] (see Figure 23-43, *B*). ALH can extend into ducts and this is associated with an increased risk of invasive carcinomas.[166]

Clinical Importance of Benign Epithelial Changes

Nonproliferative changes do not increase the risk of breast cancer. Proliferative disease is correlated with a mild increase in risk. Table 23-11 classifies benign histologic changes with

Table 23-10	Benign Breast Tumors			
Benign Breast Tumor	**Risk Factors**	**Pathophysiology**	**Clinical Manifestations**	**Treatment**
Fibroadenoma	Puberty, early adulthood; occurs earlier and more frequently in young black women	Slow-growing lesion composed of variable proportions of epithelial and connective tissue; thought to be under influence of estrogen	Painless, firm, elastic, solitary, well-circumscribed mass ~1-5 cm in diameter	Excision with person under local anesthesia; or careful observation
Phyllodes tumor	Middle age	Fibroepithelial tumor characterized by marked proliferation of connective tissue stroma and great size; initially slow growing; 10%-25% may be malignant	Spheric, firm, usually well-circumscribed, multinodular tumor with a diameter of 2-20 cm; trophic cutaneous ulceration is a late manifestation	Local excision of benign or small tumor; simple mastectomy if voluminous or malignant tumor
Intraductal papilloma	Ages 30-50 yr; relatively uncommon	Subareolar tumor consists of epithelial vegetation with central connective tissue axis; found in lactiferous duct	Spontaneous or induced watery, serous, or bloody nipple discharge; small soft, friable, yellow or red, ~5 mm, papillomatous growth attached to duct wall by short, thin stalk; rare nipple retraction	Excision of involved duct
Mammary duct ectasia	After menopause or during pregnancy and lactation	Principal lactiferous ducts become dilated and filled with cellular debris; secondary inflammatory reaction; possible rupture of ducts	Subareolar induration or nipple retraction; spontaneous, bloody, sticky, thick, multiple duct discharge; burning pain and swelling of areolar area; palpable mass after rupture	Antibiotic and anti-inflammatory therapy
Fat necrosis	Ages 14-80 yr; average age 50 yr; increased in women with fatty, voluminous breasts; trauma	50% are posttraumatic; necrosis secondary to inflammation is more rare	Poorly circumscribed indurated area with yellow or gray necrotic foci	Leave alone or local excision

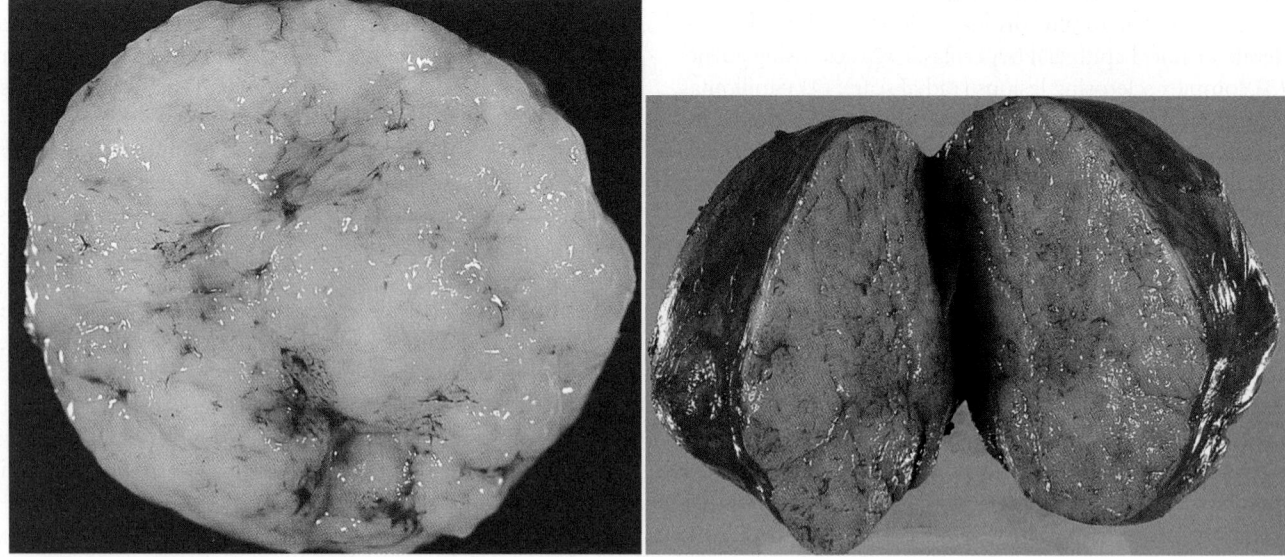

Figure 23-42 Fibroadenoma. **A,** Myxoid type of fibroadenoma, showing pale, lobulated, translucent tissue. **B,** Juvenile fibroadenoma showing well-circumscribed mass of tan, fleshy, lobulated tissue. (From Damjanov I, Linder J, editors: *Anderson's pathology,* ed 10, St Louis, 1996, Mosby.)

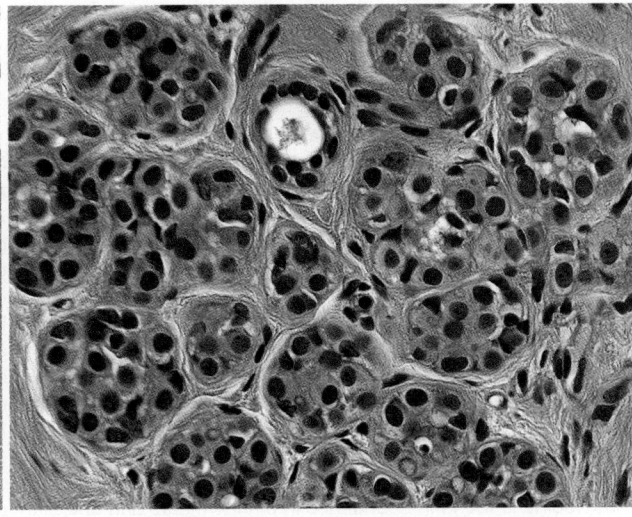

A   B

Figure 23-43 **Atypical ductal and lobular hyperplasias. A,** Atypical ductal hyperplasia. A duct is filled with a mixed population of cells. Although some of the spaces are round and regular, the peripheral spaces are irregular and slitlike. These features are highly atypical but fall short of a diagnosis of DCIS. **B,** Atypical lobular hyperplasia. A population of monomorphic small, rounded, loosely cohesive cells partially fill a lobule. (From Kumar V, Abbas AK, Fausto N: *Robbins and Cotran pathologic basis of disease,* ed 7, Philadelphia, 2005, Saunders.)

Table 23-11	Other Benign Breast Conditions
Type	**Comment**

Developmental	
Milk-line remnants	Increase in number of nipples or breasts results from persistent epidermal thickening along the milk line
Accessory axillary breast tissue	Ductal system may extend into subcutaneous tissue of the chest wall and axillary region; this tissue can undergo lactational changes and give rise to tumors
Congenital nipple inversion	Is common and may be unilateral; can spontaneously correct during pregnancy; can be confused with retraction of nipple which is sometimes part of invasive cancer or inflammation
Macromastia	Juvenile hypertrophy may be caused by unusual tissue response to hormonal stimulus
Iatrogenic	
Reconstruction or augmentation	Breast tissue can be replaced or augmented by skin and muscle flaps for synthetic prostheses; silicone implants, the most common, are rubbery silicone filled with either silicone gel or saline; a common complication of implants is formation of a thick fibrous capsule (i.e., chronic inflammatory responses) that can cause cosmetic deformity; the capsule can limit the spread of a ruptured implant but if the capsule ruptures silicone gel can escape; long-term consequences of rupture are unknown
Inflammation	
Acute mastitis	Inflammatory diseases of the breast are rare; acute mastitis is confined to the lactating period of nursing; the nipples can become dry, cracked, and fissure increasing risk of bacterial infection; infection may lead to abscess formation
Periductal mastitis	Women or men present with a painful subareolar mass thought to be infectious; not associated with lactation, 90% of individuals are smokers; vitamin A deficiency associated with smoking may alter the differentiation of the ductal epithelium; keratin is trapped within the ductal system causing dilation and rupture; antibiotic therapy and surgery is usually indicated
Mammary duct ectasia	Affects 50- and 60-year-olds, usually multiparous women, not associated with smoking; dilation of ducts with chronic granulomatous inflammatory reaction; fibrosis may eventually lead to skin and nipple retraction, thus mistaken for cancer; may have white nipple secretions
Fat necrosis	Painless, palpable mass, skin thickening or retraction; mammographic density or calcification; may have hemorrhage; most women will give a history of prior surgery or trauma; can be confused with breast carcinoma
Lymphocytic mastopathy	Single or multiple hard, palpable masses; can be so hard that interferes with biopsy; lesion includes collagenized stroma surrounding atrophic ducts and lobules; the breast membrane is frequently thickened; a prominent lymphocytic infiltrate surrounds epithelium and blood vessels; most common in women with type 1 diabetes or autoimmune thyroid disease

Data from Lester SC: The breast. In Kumar V, Abbas AK, Fausto N, editors: *Robbins & Cotran pathologic basis of disease,* ed 7, Philadelphia, 2005, Saunders.

NUTRITION & DISEASE

Revisiting Iodine and Breast Alterations

The last national nutritional survey revealed that 15% of the U.S. adult female population are iodine deficient by the World Health Organization (WHO) standard, that is, less than 0.05 mg/L urine.[382] Recommendations by the WHO, United Nations International Children's Emergency Fund, and the International Council for the Control of Iodine Deficiency Disorders set 10 mcg/dl as the minimum urinary iodine concentration for iodine sufficiency.[383] This amount corresponds to a daily intake of 150 mcg iodine. Large segments of Europe continue to have iodine deficiency. Significant deficiency is present in 45 countries in Africa, 15 in the Americas, 24 in Europe and Central Asia, 11 in Southeast Asia, 10 in the Middle East, and 9 in the Far East. Iodine deficiency is a common endocrine problem, presumably easy to correct, and the most preventable cause of mental retardation in many underdeveloped countries. Iodine is found in abundance in marine plants and animals in deposits of organic origin, in certain natural mineral waters, in phosphate rock, and in association with mineral deposits. A small fraction is from drinking water. Important factors in the depletion of iodine has been glaciation, which removes old soil and scrapes virgin rocks, the substitution of bromine for iodine in bread manufacturing, and decreases in iodinated salt intake.

Although several extrathyroidal organs and tissues can concentrate and organify iodine, compelling evidence for iodine is its effects on the mammary gland. Intriguing is the concept that iodine deficiency causes fibrocystic changes in rodents and that iodine, and to a lesser extent iodide, induced relief of breast pain in two large uncontrolled trials and in one placebo-controlled trial.[384,385]

Most studies on iodine function in humans and animals have focused on thyroid function. Little attention has been devoted to extrathyroidal tissues where an important function of iodine is as an antioxidant in humans, including the eye, thyroid, and breast. The antioxidant properties of dietary iodide depend on redox reactions from iodination of tyrosine to the formation of thyroid hormones.[386]

Although thyroid-stimulating hormone has no role in promoting iodide intake into mammary cells, these cells have been shown to possess the sodium iodide symporter (transporter).[387,388] Uptake of iodide into mammary cells can be promoted by prolactin and other hormones (oxytocin, estrogens). Iodoproteins have been detected in breast tissue but it is not known how their facilitation occurs. Free radicals have been associated with carcinogenesis, including breast cancer. Although no direct evidence exists that iodide acts as an antioxidant in the breast, increased rates of breast cancer have been reported in iodine deficient populations.[389] Iodine deficiency also has been linked to increased fibrosis and adenosis of the mammary gland and administration of iodine has been used in the treatment of breast pain.[390,384] It has been suggested that a combination of deficiency of iodine and selenium may facilitate the development of breast cancer.[391,386] Funahashi and colleagues[392,393] found that administration of Lugal's iodine or iodine-rich Wakame seaweed to rats treated with dimethylbenz(a)-anthracene (DMBA, a carcinogen) suppressed the development of mammary tumors. In addition, the same researchers documented that seaweed-induced apoptosis in human breast cancer cells had a stronger effect than fluorouracil (a strong chemotherapeutic agent) used to treat breast cancer. This finding led these authors and others to hypothesize that "seaweed may be applicable for prevention of breast cancer."[394] This hypothesis is intriguing because of the relatively low incidence of breast cancer in Japan in both females and males where the diet is rich in seaweed and with increasing breast cancer rates in Japanese women who emigrate to the West or consume a Western diet.[395-397] The antioxidant potential of iodide may require its oxidation to iodine. Eskin and colleagues[398] have postulated that normal physiologic function of mammary tissue requires iodine. Careful consideration of iodine deficiency is warranted because iodine replacement can promote problems with thyroid and extrathyroidal tissue function.

---

later development of invasive cancer. Proliferative disease with atypia (ADH and ALH) confers a moderate increase in risk. Carcinoma in situ (DCIS and LCIS) is associated with a substantial risk if untreated.[166] Other benign breast conditions also are summarized in Table 23-12.

EVALUATION AND TREATMENT Breast problems should be diagnosed from a multimodal approach that combines physical examination, mammogram where applicable, sonogram, aspiration of lumps, and surgical or needle biopsy if warranted. Breast biopsy is used to make a definitive diagnosis and assess an individual's risk for the development of breast cancer. The principle mammographic signs of breast carcinoma are densities and calcifications. Mammography can detect masses before they become palpable, however, the dense breast tissue often seen in young women can make interpretation extremely difficult (also see Radiation and Breast Cancer Risk, p. 836). Ultrasonography (ultrasound) is used to differentiate a solid mass from a cystic (fluid-filled) mass.

Treatment consists largely of relieving symptoms. The individual can minimize breast pain by wearing a brassiere that provides good support. Cystic pain is reduced by draining the

cysts with the person under local anesthesia; however, given time the cysts may disappear without treatment. Caffeinated beverages, methylxanthines in cola, root beer, and chocolate can cause overstimulation of breast tissue for some women. Reduction of these substances in the diet may reduce both the pain and nodularity. Iodine deficiency may increase fibrocystic breast change and iodine may be important for normal breast physiology (see Nutrition & Disease). Decreasing intake of dairy products also may help. Although unknown, increasing omega-3 fatty acids may decrease associated pain caused by inflammation as well as the application of castor oil packs to the breasts. The use of aspirin for decreasing breast alterations is currently a hot topic (see What's New?). Drugs used to treat severe breast pain are listed in Table 23-12.

Cancer

Breast cancer, the most common cancer in American women, is the leading cause of death in women ages 40 to 44 years and the second most common killer after lung cancer of women of all ages. The incidence of breast cancer has risen steadily since 1950 and is leveling off at about 110 cases per 100,000 women (30% of new cancers) (Figure 23-44). The highest ab-

The role of inflammation in breast disorders and cancer is a hot topic. Specifically the role of the inflammatory enzymes COX-1 and COX-2 and drugs that inhibit COX-2 (see Chapters 6 and 11). COX-2 has been found to be associated with some cancers, including breast cancer. Recently, investigators reported that aspirin use in women is associated with a significant reduction in the risk of breast cancer, especially for hormone receptor–positive tumors.[374] This was the first report to examine whether the protective effects of aspirin varied with estrogen receptor (ER) or progesterone receptor (PR) status. Aspirin has been associated with a reduction in mortality from cardiovascular disease and colorectal cancer.[375,376] Observational studies showing a protective effect of aspirin on breast cancer have been inconsistent. In mice, Chang and colleagues[377] defined the molecular mechanisms by which COX-2 derived prostaglandin E_2 (PGE$_2$; proinflammatory) induced tumor-associated angiogenesis and initiation or progression of mammary cancer. These investigations reported that PGE$_2$ induced angiogenesis at the earliest stage of tumor development, even before PGE$_2$-induced *mammary gland hyperplasia!* The current study by Terry and colleagues[374] found the inverse association between aspirin use and breast cancer was evident for every patient subgroup except those with negative hormone receptor status (ER−, PR−). The association was strongest among frequent aspirin users, unfortunately the dose was not identified. Acetaminophen was not associated with protection in any group. Aspirin showed more effects than ibuprofen (nonsteroidal anti-inflammatory drug [NSAID]). These findings suggest possible mechanistic connections between aspirin and estrogen. In 1996, investigators suggested genetic activation of COX-11 in transformed mammary epithelial cells.[378] The COX-2 gene is normally inactive (quiescent) but becomes active in response to infection, inflammation (e.g., from arthritis), and growth factors. COX-2 has been found in precancerous breast disease (hyperplasia, hyperplasia with atypia) and both noninvasive and invasive breast cancer. In the same year, Zhao and colleagues[379] demonstrated that PGE$_2$ can induce the enzyme aromatase leading to increased estrogen production in mammary adipose stromal cells. In 1999, investigators found that COX-2 is up-regulated in the *normal adjacent* epithelium to ductal carcinoma in situ and that COX-2 overexpression correlates with local areas of p16(INKa) hypermethylation (see Chapter 11) in vivo that might represent *early* neoplastic changes leading to breast cancer.[380,381] Altogether and significant, these studies provide a notable rationale for a role of COX and prostaglandins in breast cancer, particularly among postmenopausal women. Blocking COX activity with aspirin and NSAIDs would inhibit the production of aromatase and result in lower estrogen levels (see illustration below). Emerging is evidence supporting a protective effect of aspirin in ER+ and PR+ breast cancers. Questions about the dosage; timing and duration of treatments; and management of side effects, such as gastric irritation and bleeding, and aspirin allergies and how to manage this risk need to be evaluated. Studies are ongoing to determine whether COX-2 selective inhibitors, either alone or in combination with other drugs, help prevent breast cancer.

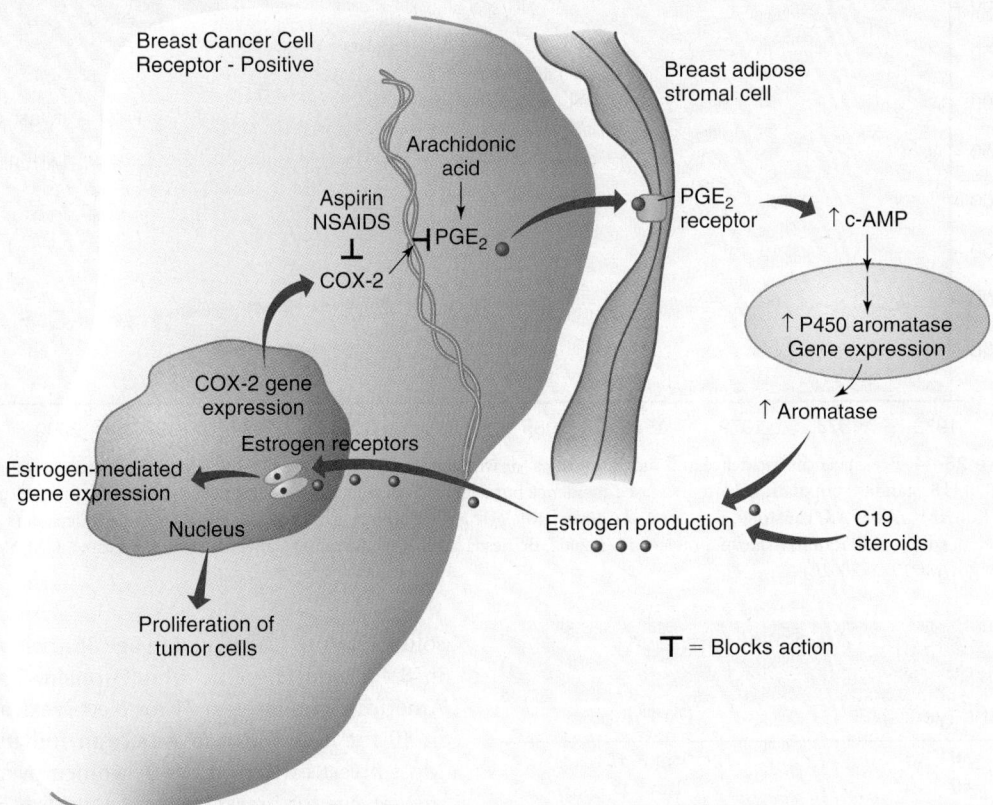

Proinflammatory prostaglandin E$_2$ (PGE$_2$) produced by breast cancer cells stimulates aromatase in breast stromal cells. Increased cyclooxygenase 2 (COX-2) can occur in precancerous breast disease (hyperplasia, hyperplasia with atypia) and noninvasive and invasive cancer. Here COX-2 in breast cancer cells leads to changes in tumor biology from increased PGE$_2$ levels (i.e., can affect apoptosis, cell invasion, immune function, and angiogenesis. PGE$_2$ can induce expression of local tissue levels of aromatase through increased cyclic adenosine monophosphate (c-AMP) production in breast stromal cells. Thus estrogen synthesis is enhanced, which can increase proliferation of tumor cells. This paracrine loop (which is not associated with blood levels of estrogen) could explain why inhibition of COX-2 activity could decrease estrogen and decrease proliferation of hormone receptor-positive breast cancers. (Adapted from DuBois RN: *JAMA* 291:2488-2489, 2004.)

Table 23-12	Drugs Used to Treat Severe Breast Pain (Mastalgia)
Agents	**Comments**

Definitely Effective

Danazol	Causes a decrease in cyclic pain and nodularity believed to reduce estrogen; also used for endometriosis; some side effects include changes in menstrual cycle regularity, weight gain, acne, and flushing
Bromocriptine	Decreases cyclic pain, nodularity, and tenderness; decreases prolactin levels and may alter dopamine receptors; is also used to suppress lactation after childbirth; can cause nausea, vomiting, hypotension, and dizziness
Tamoxifen	As an antiestrogen it can decrease cyclic pain; increase clot formation (phlebitis, emboli, strokes); cause hot flashes, amenorrhea, weight gain, and increased risk of uterine cancers
Evening Primrose Oil (linoleic acid)	Can decrease cyclic pain, nodularity, and tenderness; women with mastalgia believed to have low levels of breast linoleic acid; reduces PGE_2 prostaglandins and inflammation; too much oil, however, has been associated with increasing inflammation (>1000 mg/day)

Possibly Effective

Iodine	Can decrease cyclic pain and nodularity (see Nutrition & Disease box, p. 828)
Vaginal progesterone	Decrease in cyclic pain and tenderness; not as effective for decreasing tenderness; antagonist to estrogen; can cause weight gain

Insufficiently Studied

Progestins	May decrease estrogenic effects, however, related to endothelial vasospasms, weight gain, and increased risk of breast cancer

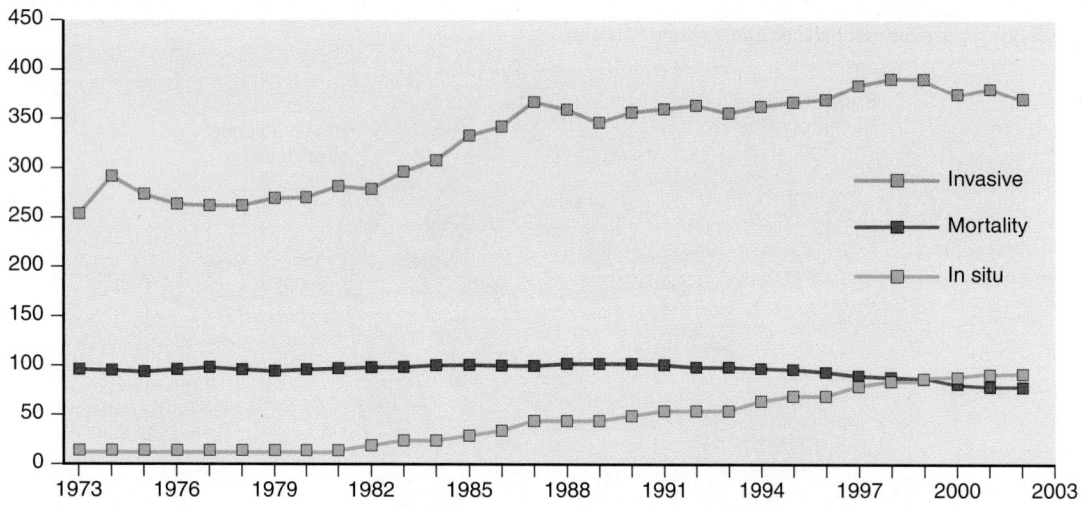

Figure 23-44 **Breast cancer incidence and mortality rates for women over 50.** Rates are per 100,000 women and are age-adjusted to the 2000 U.S. standard population. Note increased incidence but slightly declining mortality rate over the past 30 years. (Updated from Kumar V, Abbas AK, Fausto N: *Robbins and Cotran pathologic basis of disease,* ed 7, Philadelphia, 2005, Saunders; data from Ries LAG et al, editors: *SEER cancer statistics review, 1975-2002,* Bethesda, Md, 2005, National Cancer Institute. Accessed at http://seer.cancer.gov/csr/1975_2002/.)

Table 23-13	Risk of Developing Breast Cancer
By Age (years)	**By Ratio**
30	1 in 2212
40	1 in 235
50	1 in 54
60	1 in 23
70	1 in 14
80	1 in 10
Ever*	1 in 8

Data from National Institute of Health, 2004.
*Absolute lifetime risk.

solute lifetime (calculated to age 85) risk of breast cancer is 1 in 8 for non-Hispanic white women, 1 in 14 for African-American women, 1 in 21 for New Mexican Hispanics, and 1 in 40 for New Mexican American Indians[169] (Table 23-13). Most breast cancer occurs in women over 50 years old. The median age for breast cancer diagnosis is 64 years of age. Because ductal carcinoma in situ (DCIS) is almost exclusively detected by mammography, DCIS accounts for the large increase in incidence by screening.

Risk factors and possible causes of breast cancer can be classified as reproductive, hormonal, environmental and lifestyle, and familial (Table 23-14). Although high-risk pop-

Table 23-14   Factors Associated with Increased Risk of Breast Cancer*

Category	Risk Factor	Relative Risk†
Race	Blacks have higher incidence up to age 40 yr; whites have higher incidence over age 40 yr	1.1-1.9
Family history	Breast cancer in first-degree relative before age 60 yr	2.0-3.0
	Premenopausal or bilateral breast cancer	>4.0
	Postmenopausal in first-degree relative	≤2.0
	Breast cancer in two first-degree relatives	4.0-6.0
	BRCA1 or *BRCA2*	≥4.0
	p53 (Li Fraumeni syndrome)	≥4.0
Previous medical history	Moderate or florid mammary hyperplasia	1.5-2.0
	Mammary papilloma	1.5-2.0
	Atypical mammary hyperplasia	4.0-5.0
	DCIS, LCIS‡	8.0-10.0
Estrogen exposure	Early menarche (before age 12 yr)	1.1-1.9
	Late menopause (after age 55 yr)	1.1-1.9
	Postmenopausal estrogen therapy	1.4
	Oral contraceptive use	1.5
Pregnancy	Nulliparous or late first pregnancy (after age 35 yr)	1.1-1.9
Radiation	Atomic bomb	3.0
	Repeated fluoroscopy	1.5-2.0§
Obesity and stature	Postmenopausal	1.2
	Tallness	≤2.0
Dietary/alcohol	High alcohol consumption	1.4-2.0
	High energy intake	≤2.0
	Advanced age	2.0-4.0
	Xenobiotics	≤2.0
Social	Smoking	2.0-4.0
	Higher socioeconomic status	≤2.0
	Low physical activity	≤2.0
Environmental	Excess radiation to breasts	??‡
	Chemical carcinogens	≤2.0-??
	Infectious agents	≤2.0-??

*Normal lifetime risk in white non-Hispanic women: 1 in 8.

†Relative risk is defined and discussed in Chapter 5.

‡Data from Lester SC: The breast. In Kumar V, Abbas AK, Fausto N, editors: *Robbins and Cotran pathologic basis of disease*, ed 7, Philadelphia, 2005, Saunders.

‡Currently being debated.

DCIS, ductal carcinoma in situ; *LCIS*, lobular carcinoma in situ.

ulations can be identified, the majority (75%) of breast cancers occur in women whose only risk factors are gender and age.[21,170]

Reproductive Factors

A woman's age when her first child is born affects her risk for developing breast cancer—the younger she is, the lower the risk. The main mechanisms for the protective effect of pregnancy are controversial including (1) induction of breast differentiation with lasting protective genetic changes, (2) removal or modification of vulnerable cells that are prone to breast cancer, (3) enhancement of the ability for DNA repair, (4) reduction in hormones *within* breast tissue and consequently a reduction in growth regulation receptors, and (5) decreased tumor growth.[171] The most widely accepted explanation proposes that the development and differentiation of the breast are completed *only* by the end of the first term pregnancy. The important factor concerning pregnancy at a younger age being protective seems to be the *interval* of time between menarche and the first pregnancy because the increased risk of breast cancer is greater with an interval of

more than 14 years. The protection conveyed early persists in subsequent years, even in women over 75 years old. The protective effect is possibly the induction of lasting genetic changes through differentiation.[171]

Lobule formation, which is the hallmark of differentiation, usually starts 1 to 2 years after the first menstrual period. The lobular composition is determined by numerous factors, including menstrual cycles, endogenous hormone levels and imbalances, use of exogenous hormones, environmental endocrine disruptions, and pregnancy. In nulliparous women, the breast contains a moderate number of undifferentiated structures, such as terminal ducts and Lob 1, although occasionally Lob 2 and Lob 3 are present. The percentage of Lob 1 remains mostly constant throughout the lifespan of nulliparous women.[171] Having a full-term pregnancy between the ages of 14 to 20 years correlates with a significant increase in the number of Lob 3. Lob 3 remains the predominant structure until a woman reaches 40 years of age. However, the percentage decreases after age 40, and with increasing age breast tissue involutes to predominantly Lob 1. Pregnancy further increases differentiation and the formation of Lob 4, which are important for secretory activity (lactation) of the breast. Thus nulliparous women seldom reach the Lob 3 stage and never the Lob 4 stages. Even though during menopause the major structure of the breast in both nulliparous and parous women is Lob 1, the nulliparous women are at a higher risk of breast cancer whereas the parous women have reduced risk. Ductal carcinoma in situ (DCIS) may originate in Lob 1, indicating that Lob 1 is biologically different in these two groups of women[171] (see p. 845). In addition, the presence of Lob 1 in the breast of parous women has been postulated as a failure of the breast tissue to respond to biologic changes induced by pregnancy and lactation.[171]

Other explanations may be that pregnancy may cause the removal or modification of a population of cells that are all prone to breast carcinogenesis or after pregnancy mammary cells have an enhanced ability for DNA repair.[172] (Other biologic factors of pregnancy are discussed in the Pathogenesis section.)

Pregnancy also has been found to cause a subsequent reduction of hormones *within* breast tissue in women and rats and a decrease in receptors for epidermal growth factor and estrogen in mammary tissue of parous rats.[173] These findings challenge the notion that protection by an early pregnancy causes lasting genetic changes through differentiation. Most recent are the findings of Thordarson and colleagues[174] that show gene expression is altered in parous mice and nulliparous rats compared to virgin rats. Treatment with pregnancy levels of bioidentical estrogen and progesterone significantly decreased their risk of chemically induced breast tumor development. These treatments also were associated with alterations in gene expression in breast tissue. Their conclusion is that pregnancy-associated protection against breast cancer can be abolished by changing the hormonal environment of the animal.[174] Further studies demonstrated that treatment with IGF-1 increased breast carcinogenesis in parous rats compared to nulliparous rats that had no treatment. IGF-1 elevated the signaling cascade through the Raf/Ras/mitogen-activated protein kinase, which resulted in activation of the estrogen receptor alpha (ERα). Finally, they hypothesized that cancerous breast tissue sustains a defect in ERα causing uncontrolled growth. Of fundamental importance to breast cancer progression could be the IGF-1–stimulated increase in ERα. Regulation of ERα in normal tissues is under tight control; that is, increased ERα activity induced by estrogen administration (17β-estradiol in rat studies) causes a sharp down-regulation in ERα.[60,73] Administration of *low* doses of 17β-estradiol to parous rats, however, caused a significant stimulation of mammary development and a large increase in breast tumor development, but caused a significant reduction in ERα in *normal* breast tissue as compared to those in untreated parous rats that cannot develop breast tumors and age-matched virgin animals.[174] More simply, the tight regulation of ERα appears to be diminished in breast tumors compared with normal breast tissue in that its ligand-mediated down-regulation (feedback from IGF-1 and estradiol) is lost or significantly decreased.

Furthermore, growth hormone (GH) deficient rats exhibit the same protection to breast tumor development that is seen in parous rats.[174,175] and when treated with GH the rats acquire the same high susceptibility seen in virgin rats. Thus it appears unequivocal that the activity of the GH/IGF-1 axis is fundamental in determining the level of breast carcinogenesis.

In conclusion, these new data support the notion that there might not be any difference in susceptibility to tumor initiation between parous and virgin *animals*. Tumor formation does occur in parous rats; however, these tumors stay latent at a microscopic size and grow to a palpable size only upon hormonal stimulation. So the tumor formation does occur in parous rats, but tumor progression is slowed or nonexistent. The difference between parous and virgin animals thus may be the promotion of growth. Transformation and protection of tissue conferred either by pregnancy or by hormonal treatment is equally effective regardless of whether it takes place before or after exposure to a carcinogen.[174]

Hormonal Factors

The link between breast cancer and hormones is based on five factors that affect risk: (1) the protective effect of an early (i.e., in the twenties) first pregnancy; (2) the protective effect of removal of the ovaries and pituitary gland; (3) the increased risk associated with early menarche, late menopause, and nulliparity; (4) the relationship between types of fat, free estrogen levels, and oxidative changes in estrogen metabolism; and (5) the hormone-dependent development and differentiation of mammary gland structures (see Pathogenesis). A vast majority of breast cancers are *initially* hormone-dependent (estrogen positive [ER+] and/or progesterone positive [PR+]), with estrogens playing a crucial role in their development.[171]

Most of our current understandings of carcinogenicity of estrogens is based on animal systems, epidemiologic data, and observational studies. These data reveal a greater risk of endometrial hyperplasia and neoplasia associated with exogenous estrogen usage or polycystic ovarian syndrome.[176,177] Two main mechanisms of carcinogenicity of estrogens involve (1) a receptor-mediated hormonal activity shown to stimulate cellular proliferation resulting in increased opportunities for accumulation of genetic damage, and (2) oxidative catabolism of estrogens mediated by various cytochrome p450 (CYP) complexes that eventually activate and generate reactive oxygen species (ROS). ROS can cause oxidative stress and genomic damage directly (Figure 23-45). A third mechanism is that of estrogens functioning as inducers of aneuploidy (gain or loss of chromosomes). DNA alterations, that is, loss of heterozygosity (LOH), and aneuploidy is a crucial event during carcinogenesis. Still not clear, however, is whether aneuploidy is a result of neoplastic development or a cause.

Estrogens affect microtubules that are essential for establishing cell shape and cell polarity, processes necessary for epithelial gland organization.[171] In addition, the centrosomes, which are necessary for segregating chromosomes into daughter cells, are affected by estrogen. Centrosomes facilitate the coordination of intracellular activities, including cell cycle

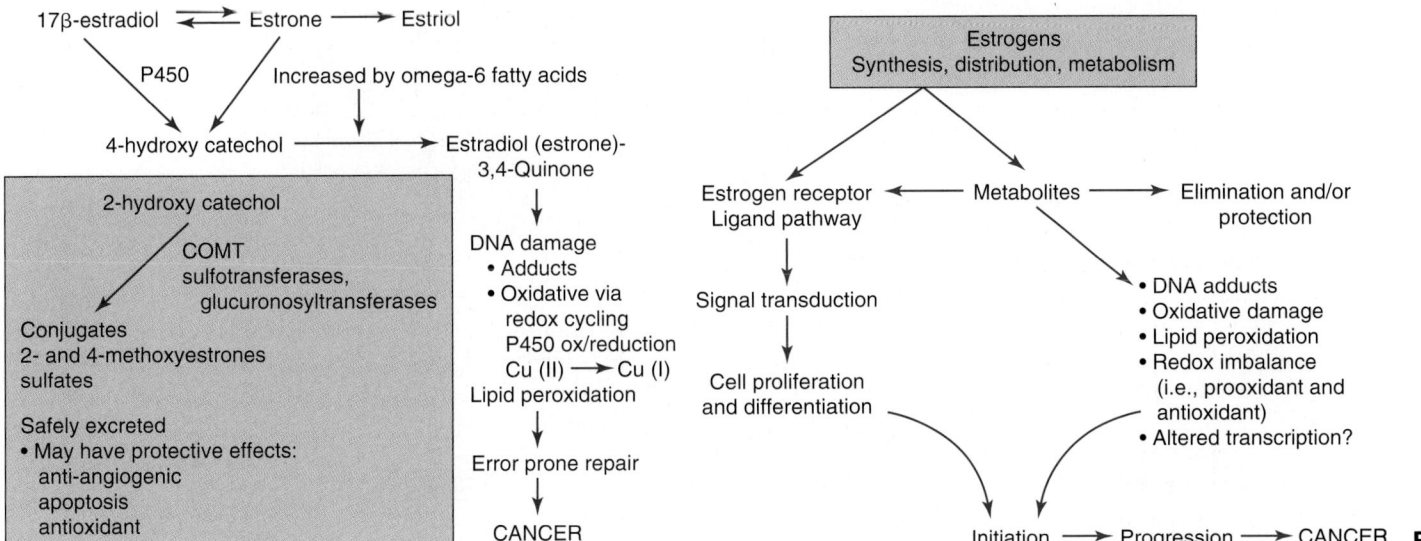

Figure 23-45 Metabolites of estrogen and their associated carcinogenic effects. **A,** Metabolites of estrogen and carcinogenic pathway. Genotoxicity can be produced by the 4-hydroxy catechol metabolite. A redox cycle catalyzed by microsomal P450 and cytochrome P450-reductase can locally generate superoxide (O_2^-) and hydroxyl radicals to produce additional DNA damage. Catechol estrogens also have been shown to interact with breast tissue nitric oxide, a potent oxidant that induces DNA strand breakage. Unstable polyunsaturated fats (omega-6) can increase the production of quinones. Unstable omega-6 fatty acids can be transformed by the effects of oxygen and heat into carriers of free radicals. 2-Hydroxy catechol, when methylated, may have protective effects against tumor development. Several enzymes are involved with the metabolism of estrogen, including specific cytochrome P450 isoforms, sulfotransferases, and catecholamine O-methyltransferase (COMT). These enzymes may be influenced by environmental factors, including fats, alcohol, and xenobiotic exposures. These enzymes also are polymorphic and their distributions may differ among different ethnic populations. **B,** Estrogen receptor and estrogen metabolites on cancer initiation and progression. (**B** adapted from Yager JD: *J Natl Cancer Institute Monogr* 27:67, 2000; additional data from Russo J, Russo I: *Molecular basis of breast cancer: prevention and treatment,* Germany, 2004, Springer; and Cavalieri EL, Rogan EG: *Ann N Y Acad Sci* 1028:247-257, 2004.)

progression and cell cycle checkpoints (see Chapter 1). Although the mechanisms that promote the formation of abnormal centrosomes are unclear, several possibilities have been proposed in regard to the development of cancer.[171] A recent report indicates that progestin also may facilitate aneuploidy.[178] Also, women on hormone replacement therapy (HRT) (i.e., including progestin) have increased mammographic breast density and increased breast cancer risk compared with women taking only estrogen.[179-181] Thus the role of progestin is currently being debated (see p. 835 for summary discussion).

Hormones were originally believed to function as promoters of carcinogenesis. Emerging now in research are their roles (estrogen and other hormones) as initiators. By stimulating cell proliferation, hormonal agents increase the amount of DNA. Evidence pointing to a direct genotoxic effect of estrogen involves its ability to induce DNA adducts.[182]

Recent studies suggest that *local* (in situ; paracrine) formation of estrogens in breast tumors is more important than circulating estrogens in *plasma* for the growth and survival of estrogen-dependent breast cancer in postmenopausal women.[171,183-185] The rationale for the importance of local tissue formation of estrogens is based on the following evidence: (1) estradiol (E_2) levels in breast tumors are equivalent to those of premenopausal women, despite plasma E_2 levels being lower after menopause; (2) E_2 concentrations in breast tumors of postmenopausal women are 10 to 40 times higher

than serum levels; and (3) biosynthesis of estrogens in breast tumors occurs through two different routes, one is the aromatase pathway and the other the steroid sulfate (STS) pathway[171,184] (see Figure 23-46).

An explanation for the estradiol levels (17β-estradiol) in breast cancer tissues being equivalent in premenopausal and postmenopausal women despite plasma levels decreasing significantly after menopause is that enzymatic transformation of circulating precursors in peripheral tissues contribute 75% of estrogen in premenopausal women and almost 100% in postmenopausal women.[186,187] The specific enzyme complexes involved in the most biologically active estrogen, 17β-estradiol, in breast tissue include (1) aromatase, which converts androstenedione to estrone; (2) estrone sulfatase, which hydrolyses estrogen sulfate to estrone; and (3) 17β-estradiol hydroxysteroid dehydrogenase (HSD), which reduces estrone to 17β-estradiol in tumor tissues[171] (Figure 23-46).

Breast tissue (endogenous) metabolism of estrogens through the aromatase-mediated pathway is correlated with the risk of breast carcinogenesis.[188,189] Although the main pathway of estrone synthesis is through aromatization of the androgens present in the ovary and peripheral tissue, much of the estrone synthesized is converted to estrone by estrone sulfatase–mediated hydrolysis. Sulfation is important to estrogens, as well as other steroids, because the addition of the charged sulfonate group protects the hormones from binding to their receptors, thereby increasing reserve substances for

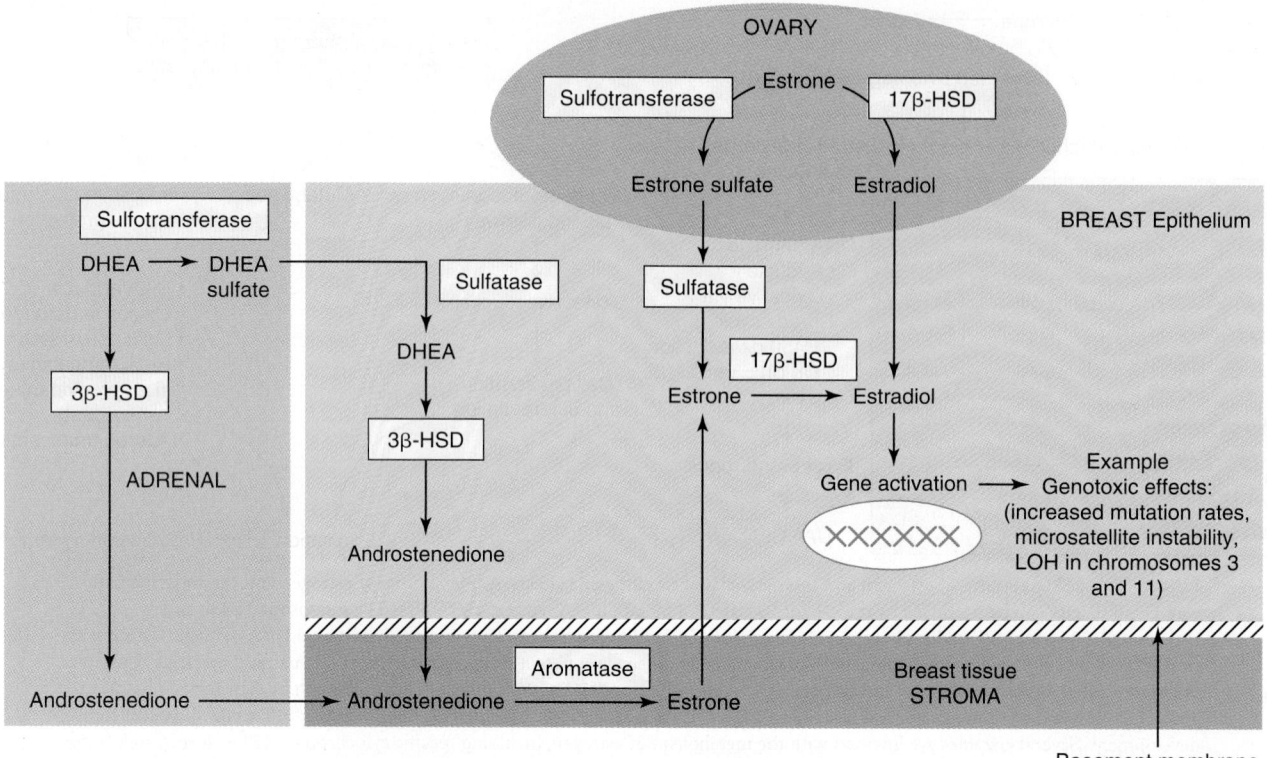

Figure 23-46 Local biosynthesis of estrogens. Three main enzyme complexes (yellow) involved in estrogen formation in breast tissue, including aromatase, sulfatase, and 17β-estradiol hydroxysteroid dehydrogenase (HSD). Thus despite low levels of circulating estrogens in postmenopausal women with breast cancer, the tissue levels are several-fold higher than these in plasma suggesting tumor accumulation of these estrogens. Data suggest that most abundant is sulfatase in both premenopausal and postmenopausal women with breast cancer. Numerous agents can block the aromatase action, exploration of progesterone, and various progestins to inhibit sulfatase and 17β-HSD or stimulate sulfotransferase (i.e., breast cancer cells cannot inactivate estrogens because they lack sulfotransferase) to provide new possibilities for treatment. (Adapted from Russo J, Russo I: *Molecular basis of breast cancer: prevention and treatment,* Germany, 2004, Springer.)

the biosynthesis of active hormones through the action of endogenous sulfatases.

Breast cancer tissues may contain higher sulfatase activity than aromatase activity and produce estrone through the hydrolysis of estrone sulfate[171,190-192] (see Figure 23-46). In addition, estrone sulfate has a longer half-life than estrone.[192] Thus quantitatively estrone sulfate may be the most important circulating estrogen in women; it increases the reservoir for the production of estrone and, ultimately, estradiol. Furthermore, sulfatase levels have independently predicted breast cancer relapse-free survival.[192,193] The association between sulfatase and poor prognosis was significant only in individuals with estrogen receptor (ER+) tumors.[193] Miyoshi and colleagues[193] found high sulfatase expression was associated with a poorer prognosis in *both* premenopausal and postmenopausal women with ER+ tumors. These results suggest a possibility that, even in premenopausal women, the intratumoral estrogen biosynthesis plays an important role in the growth stimulation of breast tumors.[193] Unknown are the relative contributions of estradiol to the intratumoral synthesized estradiol from the ovary versus the total intratumoral quantities. Aromatase inhibitors (anastrozole, letrozole, and exemestane) are extremely effective in inhibiting aromatase

and being very selective (targeted) for this enzyme. In fact the anastrozole, tamoxifen, alone or in combination (ATAC) trial showed that disease-free survival was significantly greater with anastrozole alone than with tamoxifen alone.[194] Estrogen formation from estrone sulfatase cannot be blocked by aromatase inhibitors. Thus new molecular targets of the sulfatase pathway needs development and testing.

Insulin-like growth factors (IGFs) regulate cellular functions involving cell proliferation, differentiation, and apoptosis. Emerging evidence indicates that members of the IGF family, including IGF-I, IGF-II, the IGF-I receptor (IGF-IR), and IGF-binding proteins, play important roles in the development and progression of cancer. IGF-IR, overexpressed in cancer cells, mediates the effects of IGFs and plays a role in cell transformation.[195] IGFs are potent mitogens for estrogen receptor–positive (ER+) breast cell lines. Interruption of IGF action can inhibit estrogenic stimulation of breast cancer cells. Thus there is cellular crosstalk between the insulin growth factors and estrogen receptors.[196] Insulin-like growth factor binding protein 3 (IGFBP-3) regulates the mitogenic and metabolic effects of IGFs; *p53* may regulate apoptosis in tumors cells through IGFBP-3.[171] The protective effects of IGFBP-3 may be modulated by human chorionic gonadotropin (hCG) that facilitates differentiation of the mammary gland. Increased levels of IGFBP-3 in the more differentiated Lob 3 compared to Lob 1 is a new finding that requires further study.[171]

Human chorionic gonadotropin (hCG) increases during the first trimester of pregnancy and then rapidly declines to a slow steady state maintained throughout the rest of pregnancy. The action of hCG is mediated by a G-protein–coupled receptor, which also binds luteinizing hormone (LH). Low levels of these receptors are present in breast tissue. This coupled with the epidemiologic findings of a decreased breast cancer risk in women who complete full-term pregnancy at a young age and a protective effect of hCG against carcinogen-induced mammary tumor development in rats, suggests that hCG may be protective against breast cancer.[171,197] Recently, treatment of human breast cancer cells (MCF-7) with hCG resulted in a modest dose-dependent decrease in cell proliferation but a dramatic decrease of cell invasion.[197] The antiproliferative and anti-invasive effects prevented NF-κB (i.e., transcription factor) activation through a cyclic adenosine monophosphate [c-AMP]–dependent signaling pathway. In addition, experiments showed not only inhibition of genes involved in cell proliferation and invasion but also activation of genes involved in cell differentiation, apoptosis, and DNA repair.[197] Treatment with hCG, however, can stimulate breast cancer growth in animals with overexpressed *Her-2/neu* oncogene.[198] Nonetheless, the antiproliferative and anti-invasive effect may be useful in developing new therapies.

Exogenous estrogen use has decreased since 2002 when the first randomized, controlled trial released findings that women using conjugated equine estrogen (CEE) and medroxyprogesterone had small but significant increases in their risk of coronary heart disease events, strokes, and breast cancer.[199] There also were small decreases in the risks of hip fracture and colon cancer. After 5 years of treatment, the risk was one serious adverse event per 100 women treated.[200] In terms of invasive breast cancer with combined hormone therapy, the relative risk was 1.26 (follow-up of 5.2 years; 199 cases in the treated group versus 150 in the placebo group) and a trend toward increasing risk with increasing duration was noted. DCIS was slightly increased in the treated group (47 cases) versus the placebo group (37 cases). Another study found that the combined estrogen/progestin formulation doubled the risk of breast cancer in women who took it for 20 years.[201] Also, taking progestin plus estrogen increased the risk of breast cancer more than if women took estrogen alone.[202]

The Women's Health Initiative (WHI) estrogen-only study (conjugated equine estrogen alone) found no increase in breast cancer incidence; in fact, this study found a slight decrease (94 cases in the treated group versus 124 cases in the control group) but the observational Million Women Study found an increase with estrogen only.[203] These conclusions may not apply to women taking other estrogen and progesterone/progestin formulations.[204]

In summary, the WHI agrees with some case-control and cohort studies indicating that long-term current use (≥5 years) of combined estrogen and progestin have a slightly increased risk of breast cancer. Whether exogenous estrogen only increases the risk of breast cancer is still controversial. However, the combination of continuous estrogen with interrupted or cyclic progestin (synthetic) does increase sensitivity to both estrogen and progestin receptors in breast tissue.[205] And progestin added to estrogen appears to increase breast density on mammogram. This is a problem for two reasons: first, it is more difficult to see lumps on the mammogram and, second, it demonstrates that stroma tissue is being stimulated (see Chapter 12).

Depending on the tissue, progesterone is classified as either a proliferative or differentiative hormone. Its effects also vary depending on whether it is used in combination with estrogen or alone. Investigators report that in cell cultures progesterone alone (no estrogen) rushes the cell through the cell cycle and stops it at the G_1 phase but leaves it ready to proceed. It stays in the G_1 phase unless estrogen or another growth factor, like epithelial grow factor, prompts the cell to divide and proliferate.[206,207] The conclusion from these studies is that progesterone is neither inherently proliferative nor antiproliferative but it is capable of stimulating or inhibiting cell growth depending on whether treatment is transient or continuous. Continuous treatment may decrease sensitivity of the cells to the proliferative effects of epidermal growth factor. The activity of the cell cycle–dependent protein kinase cdK2 is regulated biphasically by progesterone; it increases initially, then decreases.[206] Recently investigators reported that different signal transduction pathways are used by natural versus synthetic progestins for the induction of vascular endothelial growth factor (VEGF), which promotes angiogenesis. This distinction may represent the different pathologies reported in progesterone versus synthetic progestin medroxyprogesterone acetate (MPA)–induced breast tumors in mice or the different potencies exhibited by natural and synthetic progestins for inducing proliferation of breast cancer cells in vitro.[208] The safe use of progesterone/progestins, in terms of breast cancer, however, is not now established.

Some studies have shown that oral contraceptive (OC) use increases a young woman's risk of breast cancer, especially current use.[209,210] Other studies have found that the most important variable is the total months of use, with an increase of 38% (relative risk) for 10 years of use.[211] A recent study of women between 35 and 64 years of age that included both current and former OC users showed no significant association with increased breast cancer risk.[212] A small study ($N = 25$) showed that baby boomers who took OCs for 10 years and then took hormone therapy for 3 or more years (the first group to do this) had a relative risk of 3.2—more than triple the risk of women who never used either.[213] Controversy remains about the relationship between OC use and breast cancer risk; however, the efficacy of OCs in protecting against ovarian cancer and endometrial cancer is well established.

Environmental Factors and Lifestyle

The environmental causes of breast cancer possibly affect the glandular epithelial cells of the breast during the early differential stages—that is, undifferentiated cells to alveolar buds and then lobules (see Pathogenesis). During these early phases, mitotic activity and cell division are greater than later in life.

Radiation. Radiation from nature is everywhere—cosmic rays; elements from the soil and rocks, such as radon; and terrestrial radiations. To date only accidentally or medically induced radiation has been demonstrated to exert a carcinogenic effect on the breast. There are many sources of ionizing radiation, including x-rays, CT scans, fluoroscopy, and other medical radiologic procedures. According to the National Cancer Institute (NCI), CT scans "comprise about 10% of diagnostic radiologic procedures in large U.S. hospitals;" however, they contribute an estimated 65% of the effective radiation dose to the public from all medical x-ray examinations.[214]

Although such an assumption is controversial, some suggest increased radiation exposure from multiple sources *may* have contributed to a rising incidence of breast cancer between 1950 and 1991. During this period, the incidence of breast cancer in the United States increased dramatically but so did screening.[215] Since the 1980s, screening has resulted in increased detection of small invasive carcinomas and in situ carcinomas. Ionizing radiation is a known risk factor for breast cancer. Decades of research has confirmed a link between breast cancer and radiation, beginning with the work of Ian MacKenzie, a physician, who studied 800 women who had received repeated fluoroscopy examinations for tuberculosis. Published in 1965, his study found that irradiated women had 24 times the risk of breast cancer compared to those individuals with tuberculosis who had not been radiated.[216] The link between radiation and cancer found in the breast has been documented in other conditions, including benign breast disease,[217] acute postpartum mastitis,[218] enlarged thymus,[219] skin hemangiomas,[220] scoliosis,[221] and Hodgkin disease.[222-224] The duration of increased risk from radiation is unknown, but increased risk appears to have lasted at least 35 years in women treated for mastitis, those treated with fluoroscopy, and A-bomb survivors.

The type of cancer that can result from radiation exposure depends on the area directly exposed and the age of the individual at time of exposure. The younger the age, the higher the risk. Radiologic exposure of the upper spine, heart, ribs, lungs, shoulders, and esophagus also exposes breast tissue to radiation. X-rays and fluoroscopy of infants may constitute whole body irradiation. Evidence indicates that childhood exposure to radiation creates the greatest cancer risk whereas exposure after age 40 confers the lowest.[214] Breast cancer rates in atomic bomb survivors in Japan were highest among women under 20 years of age at time of exposure. The relative risk was 14.6 per unit of radiation if exposure occurred before 20 years of age and was 3.0 if exposure occurred when people were older.[225] An important finding among the A-bomb survivors is that those who had early full-term pregnancies were at significantly lower risk than those who had not.[226]

Currently, a hot topic of discussion is the effects of low-dose ionizing radiation. Radiobiologists have long been strug-

gling to estimate the health risks for low doses of radiation as evidenced by six BEIR (Biological Effects of Ionizing Radiation) reports, animal and human studies on somatic and heritable mutations, and the incidence of neoplasms and birth defects found after radiation exposures. New biologic understanding related to low doses of radiation are presented in Chapter 11. Relevant here, however, is a discussion about mammography. Renewed debate is emerging concerning the benefits of routine screening mammography.[227,228] The debate has centered on whether screening mammography actually saves lives; that is, does early detection matter? Less discussion has concerned the risk of radiation-induced breast cancer. Glandular doses from screening mammography are low, typically around 3 mGy of 26 to 30 kVp low energy x-rays.[229] The debate, however, is that very low-energy x-rays may be more hazardous, per unit dose, than high-energy x-ray or γ-rays.

Much of the data on the effects of low-dose radiation that were extrapolated from epidemiologic data concerning A-bomb survivors are now being questioned. Low-dose radiation–induced cancer depends on several variables not possible to account for in epidemiologic studies, including (1) interaction of radiation with other physical (UV light), chemical and biologic mutagens, and carcinogens in a synergistic involvement; (2) variation in bystander cells (see Chapter 11); (3) variation in repair mechanisms; and (4) variation in adaptive responses that depend on dose and protective substances (antioxidants).[230] An important assumption in question and implied by the International Commission of Radiation Protection (ICRP) is that all low-linear energy transfer (LET) radiations (specifically x-rays and electrons) have the *same* radiobiologic effectiveness (RBE). The ICRP (publication 60) has emphasized that setting the radiation weighing factor equal to unity of photons is merely practical, an estimate used to simplify the quantity effective dose, E, which is important for regulatory purposes, such as the setting of dose limits.[231] Straume[232] has suggested that the risk coefficient derived for the high-energy gamma rays from the A-bombs may underestimate the risk coefficient for conventional x-rays by a factor of up to 4. In this regard, Frankenberg and colleagues[233] reported data on in vitro oncogenic transformation frequencies induced by low levels of radiation comparable to mammography suggesting that low-energy x-rays are considerably more biologically effective. Thus some argue that the low levels used in screening mammography (26-30 kVp) can be expected to be more hazardous per unit dose than high-energy x- or γ-rays, such as those to which A-bomb survivors were exposed.[234]

Other in vitro studies have shown oncogenic transformation and chromosome aberration end-points using low doses of low-energy x-rays. Because human cancers arise from the accumulation of multiple genetic abnormalities, the earlier the initial mammogram and the total number of mammograms received may be important factors. Even with the low doses involved in screening mammography, the risk-benefit ratio for older women ($\geq$50 years) would still be expected to be large (i.e., greater benefits for screening), though for younger women the benefits are decreased. In addition, in younger women, because their breasts are denser, finding abnormalities by use of mammogram is more difficult. Over 25% of invasive breast cancers are not detected by mammography in the 40 to 49 year olds, compared to 10% to 12% not detected in women over age 50.[235] The pro–early-mammography professionals argue that cancers that occur between the ages 40 and 49 seem to be faster growing ones. They report that the reasons many studies are not showing the value of mammography in this age group is that mammograms are not done often enough. Eight randomized control trials have, however, consistently shown a reduction in mortality in women between the ages of 50 and 69 of about 30%. That is, for every 100 women over the age of 50 with undetected breast cancer, 30 would have died had they not be screened. Still unknown are the risk-benefits in women older than 70 years.

In summary, the magnitude of risk per unit dose depends strongly on when radiation exposure occurs: exposure before the age of 20 years carries the greatest risk (presumably because of immature tissue). Other factors that also may influence risk include age at first term pregnancy, parity, possibly a history of benign breast disease and injury, exposure while pregnant, endogenous hormone levels and ratios, and genetic factors.[236] Young women carriers of breast susceptibility genes are being screened in some medical centers with MRIs.

In conclusion, risk of cancer caused by radiation, based on statistical models from epidemiologic studies of high-dose exposures that are currently being questioned (i.e., using the process of extrapolation), is low. The actual risk at lower doses, based on new biologic studies, could, however, be higher. The hypothesis that early detection by mammography significantly saves lives is questionable, especially in women below the age of 50 years. Mammography for mass screening may be useful *only* because it is *all* we have. Thus less controversial methods with higher specificity and no risk need to be developed.

Diet. Prospective studies do not support the concept that fat intake in middle life has a major relation to breast cancer risk.[237] Moreover, there is limited evidence that modest reductions in fat intake (less than 20% of caloric intake) reduces breast cancer risk.[238] Even so, because breast cancer incidence varies widely around the world (Figure 23-47), and offspring that migrate from countries with low incidence to countries with high incidence have the same rates as those in the new country, nutrition remains an important area of study. The dominant hypothesis has been that high fat intake increases risk.[237] Studies in animal models, and recent observations in humans, however, have provided evidence that a high intake of omega-6–polyunsaturated fatty acids (omega-6 PUFAs) stimulates several stages in the development of mammary and colon cancer and possibly prostate cancer—from an increase in oxidative DNA damage that effects cell proliferation and increased free estrogen levels that effect hormonal catabolic products.[239-242] Conversely, fish oil–derived omega-3 fatty acids may *prevent* cancer by influencing the activity of

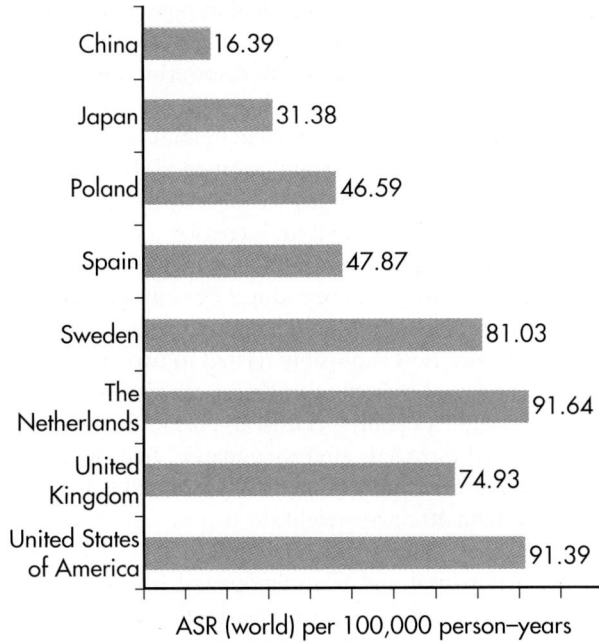

Figure 23-47 Selected world population age-standardized (to the world population) incidence rates of breast cancer among women. *ASR,* Age-standardized rates. (Data from Ferlay J et al: *GLOBOCAN 2000: cancer incidence, mortality, and prevalence worldwide,* Lyon, 2001, International Agency for Research on Cancer.)

enzymes and proteins related to intracellular signaling and, eventually, cell proliferation.[232,243] Studies that show protective effects of fish oil and decreased cancer risk have been confined to countries with high fish intake.

Investigators have identified potential carcinogens in breast fluid in normal women, especially cholesterol derivatives.[244] Breast fluid is the result of secretions from the cells lining the breast ducts. Breast ductal cells are where the majority of breast cancers develop.[245] These breast secretions have been related to the fat content of the diet. The levels of estrogens are also substantially higher in breast secretions than in blood.[245] Thus fat tissue in the breast may be a source of high concentrations of fat-soluble chemicals (including estrogens), some of which may be carcinogens.[245]

Further studies are needed to evaluate the benefits of substantially lowering fat intake (20% or less of total calories) and the roles of micronutrient imbalances and childhood nutrition in the development of breast cancer. The role of obesity in breast cancer is complex and seems to be related to fat distribution, type of fatty acids consumed, and sex hormone levels.[246]

Obesity has been associated with a *reduced* risk of *premenopausal* breast cancer. One mechanism suggested is the direct relationship between irregular menstrual cycling, especially anovulatory cycling and obesity. The anovulatory cycling would result in a decrease in both estrogens and progesterone and thus a decreased risk of breast cancer. Some obese women have polycystic ovaries. With this condition they may have anovulatory cycling, abnormal menstrual periods, elevated androgens, hyperinsulinemia, and alterations in gonadotropic secretions. It is possible that higher insulin levels increase the enzymatic conversion of testosterone to dihydrotestosterone, rather than estradiol, lowering their estrogen levels.[245]

Obesity, however, is weakly related to increasing the risk of breast cancer in *postmenopausal* women.[237] Despite strong links with endogenous estrogen levels, body fat has been consistently but *weakly* related to increased postmenopausal risk.[237] This observation has been surprising because obese postmenopausal women have endogenous estrogen levels (estrone and estradiol) nearly double those of lean women.[237,247] This weak association is possibly related to two factors. First, the premenopausal reduction in breast cancer risk related to being overweight possibly persists, opposing the adverse effect of elevated estrogens after menopause. Thus *weight gain* should be more strongly related to postmenopausal breast cancer risk than attained weight. In two case-control studies and prospective studies, this was indeed true.[248-251] Weight gain premenopausal and postmenopausal is also associated with higher estradiol and estrone levels and lower sex-hormone–binding globulin (SHBG) as a transporter protein; low levels cause higher bioavailable estrogen.[252] The increase in estrogens, particularly estradiol, is from aromatization in the adipose tissue. Second, use of exogenous hormones postmenopausally obscures the variation in endogenous estrogens caused by adiposity and elevates breast cancer risk regardless of body weight.[237] Among newer users of postmenopausal hormones, those gaining at least 55 pounds after age 18 years had double the breast cancer risk of women who maintained their weight.

Obesity is associated with poor survival among women with breast cancer and the association of obesity with mortality from breast cancer appears to be stronger than its association with incidence.[237,250] Thus the increase in breast cancer risk with increasing BMI among postmenopausal women is largely the result of increases in estrogen, especially with estradiol.[237]

Energy restriction significantly reduces mammary tumors in rodents.[237] Data from the World War II Norwegian famine found that those females who lived through the famine had a slightly lower breast cancer risk at all ages—13% reduction in risk.[253] Energy-deprived children do not attain full height and observation studies of height and breast cancer risk suggest a modest positive correlation.[254-256] Age at menarche also indicates childhood energy balance. Prospective studies document weight, height, and body fat as predictors of age at menarche.[257,258] Age at menarche is 12 to 13 years in Western countries; in rural China (where the risk of breast cancer is low) the typical age of menarche has been 17 to 18.[259]

Most prospective studies have not supported a link between fiber intake and breast cancer.[260,261] Carbohydrate quality, however, rather than absolute amount may be important for breast cancer risk, especially for premenopausal women. One case-control study of premenopausal bilateral breast cancer subjects reported an increased risk for intake of sweetened beverages.[262] An Italian population-based case-control study demonstrated women with either pre- or postmenopausal breast cancer had a higher mean dietary glycemic index.[263] Other studies, however, have not shown a significant association.[237]

Substantial evidence exists that alcohol consumption increases breast cancer risk. In a pooled analysis of the six largest cohort studies, the risk of breast cancer increased incrementally with increasing intake of alcohol.[264] Beer, wine, and liquor all contribute to the positive association. Differences in alcohol intake, however, explain only a small fraction of breast cancer rates.[265,266] In large prospective studies, high intake of folic acid appeared to decrease completely the excess risk for breast cancer caused by alcohol.[267-269]

The mechanisms by which alcohol intake increases the risk of breast cancer are unknown. Alcohol may hinder the liver's ability to rid the body of cancer-causing agents, impair the body's immune system, or make breast tissue more susceptible to cancer cells. Alcohol stimulates liver enzyme activity, and greater sulfation of estrone thus increases the availability of estrone and possibly breast exposure to greater levels of estrone/estradiol.[265] In intervention studies, intake of one or two alcoholic drinks per day increased estrogen levels in premenopausal and postmenopausal women.[270,271] Alcohol combined with estrogen replacement therapy may synergistically enhance the risk. Alcohol can down-regulate the expression of *BRCA1* (i.e., the unmutated tumor-suppressor gene), a potent inhibitor of estrogen receptor-α activity, thus increasing estrogen responsiveness.[272] Growth factor systems (ligands and receptors) may be targets of ethanol toxicity.[273] Another mechanism is the possibility that increasing levels of alcohol decrease melatonin levels at night, which might increase circulating estrogen (as well as decrease sleep).[274] It is not known whether decreasing or stopping alcohol consumption in midlife decreases the risk of breast cancer.

Data from observational studies suggest a possible protection effect of vitamin A intake, particularly carotenoids, on breast cancer risk. This effect is only noted for premenopausal women.[237] Vitamin E has inhibited breast tumors in some animal studies.[275] None of the prospective studies, however, have reported a significant association.[237] Yet, epidemiologic evidence indicates a higher risk of breast cancer development with a combination of low vitamin E and low selenium levels.[171,276,277] No significant overall association between vitamin C and breast cancer was observed in prospective studies.[278,279] Selenium, an important antioxidant component of glutathione peroxidase, inhibits cell proliferation in animal studies. Selenium intake cannot be measured accurately because it depends on the measurement of selenium in soil in geographic areas in which foods are grown. In tissues, measurements of selenium in blood and toenails (prospective studies) has not shown any association. Chemoprevention of mammary tumors in laboratory animals, however, indicates that naturally occurring organoseleniums (e.g., selenomethionine and selenocysteine) are effective.[171,280,281]

Soy products are a hot topic because of their consumption in Asian countries that have low rates of cancer. These isoflavone compounds, including diadzen and genistein, can bind estrogen receptors but are far less potent than estradiol. Researchers have found that soy binds to both ERα and ERβ. Compared to estradiol, the affinity for soy binding is stronger to ERβ (87% compared to 4% for ERα).[282] Soy may act like other antiestrogens, tamoxifen for example, by blocking the action of endogenous estrogens to reduce breast cancer risk. Thus depending on the estradiol concentration, soy exhibits weak estrogenic or antiestrogenic activity. Isoflavones can influence transcription and cell proliferation. They modulate enzyme activities, as well as signal transduction, and have antioxidant properties.[282] Results of clinical studies on the effects of soy products or isolated isoflavones on vasomotor symptoms are contradictory. Epidemiologic studies, however, have shown a decrease in the prevalence of hot flashes in women from countries with high isoflavone intake, such as Japan, more so than in Western countries. Evidence from epidemiologic, animal, in vitro data, and human clinical trials show isoflavones are promising agents for breast cancer prevention.[283-288] Concerns, however, are that soy or isoflavones may increase proliferating cells. From a study of nipple aspirate fluid from women who had ingested high soy diets and were either premenopausal or took estrogen replacement therapy showed an increase in proliferating cells.[289] Controversy has ensued on whether breast stimulation can equal breast cancer growth. Soy may cause breast cells to grow; however, in vitro properties of soy for blocking invasion and antiangiogenesis may be more important in preventing breast cancer. In vitro and animal studies show soy to inhibit breast cancer growth, and additional work showed this effect on cancer cells that are both ER+ and ER−.[288] In addition, soy may optimize extrarenal 1,25(OH)2 cholecalciferol or vitamin D_3 (a prodifferentiating vitamin D metabolite), which could result in growth control and, conceivably, inhibition of tumor progression.[283]

Environmental Chemicals. Evidence for linking chemicals to the cause of breast cancer is difficult. It is challenging because it is a life history of exposure that is important—not just a single chemical but complex mixtures of chemicals and their interaction with endogenous hormones. The highest rates of breast cancer are found in superindustrialized countries—North America and Europe—and the lowest rates in Central Africa and Asia. With development, breast cancer rates increase. An estimated 85,000 synthetic chemicals are registered for use today in the United States, and toxicologic screening for these chemicals is minimal. Chemicals persist in the environment, accumulate in adipose tissue, interact with local adipose tissue physiology in an endocrine/paracrine manner, and remain in breast tissue for decades. Some of these chemicals have been linked to breast tumors in animals. Women who emigrate to the United States from Asian countries experience an enormous percent increase in risk within one generation. A generation later, the rate of their daughter's risk approaches that of women born in the United States. This change in risk suggests that utero exposures affect subsequent disease risk. It is difficult to know whether these changes in risk come from nutritional content, pollutants, food additives, or other factors.

Xenoestrogens are synthetic chemicals that mimic the actions of estrogens and are found in many pesticides, fuels, plastics, detergents, and drugs.[168] Because many factors correlated with breast cancer (early menarche, delayed pregnancy and breastfeeding, late menopause, etc.) are associated with lifetime exposure to estrogens, investigators reasoned that environmental chemicals affect estrogen metabolism and contribute to breast cancer. The most significant chemicals may be polychlorinated biphenyls (PCBs), such as dichloro-diphenyltrichloroethane (DDT). Such chemicals are fat soluble, and the estrogenic effect would require that they bind to either the nuclear estrogen receptor and then cause cell division or gene transcription or that they activate ROS through exudative catabolism of estrogens (see p. 833). Because the amount of these environmental estrogens is presumably minute, their effect must be secondary to an abnormal (e.g., mutagenic) response of the estrogen receptor and DNA or catabolize products of estrogen. Thus far, however, human studies have not found an increased risk of breast cancer with exposure to chemicals.[290,291] Because fat-soluble chemicals are transported with lipoproteins (e.g., high-density lipoproteins [HDLs]) in blood and will be higher in women with high lipoprotein levels, as well as in obese women, investigators must include these measures in studies. Further, a long-term follow-up (30 years) of women who were exposed to diethylstilbestrol (DES) shows a minute increased risk of breast cancer (relative risk 1.35) and no increasing risk over time.[245] Table 23-15 contains information on selected studies, chemicals, and risk of breast cancer.

Physical Activity. Regular physical activity may reduce overall risk of breast cancer, especially in premenopausal or young postmenopausal women.[292-294] Mechanisms for this protective effect are not known but include alterations in endogenous free radical formation and oxidative damage, effects on DNA repair capacity, alteration in carcinogen-metabolizing enzymes, increased intestinal transit times (i.e.,

---

NUTRITION & DISEASE

Indol 3-Carbinol (I3C) Decreases Estrogen

Epidemiologic, laboratory, and animal and translational studies all support the efficacy of indol 3-carbinol (I3C). I3C decreases the development of estrogen-enhanced cancers including breast, endometrial, and cervical cancers. I3C is a derivative of indol glucosinate, a secondary plant metabolite in cruciferous vegetables. Administration of I3C at 400 mg/day for 3 months to women volunteers altered estrogen metabolism in vivo, indicating a chemopreventive effect against breast cancer without side effects. I3C induced apoptosis with a concomitant increase of p53.

Data from Grubbs C et al: *Anticancer Res* 15:709-716, 1995; Katdare M, Osborne MP, Telang NT: *Oncol Report* 5:311-315, 1998; Telang NT et al: *Adv Exp Med Biol* 400A:409-418, 1997.

Table 23-15	Selected Chemicals and Risk of Breast Cancer
Chemical	**Comments**
Bisphenol-A (BPA)	Studies have shown altered reproductive systems and breast tissue when exposed to BPA in utero
	BPA is commonly found in plastics[362]
Polyvinyl chloride (PVC)	Used in food packaging, medical products, appliances, cars, toys, credit cards, rain wear
	Has been found in the air near waste sites, landfills, and tobacco smoke
	Has been linked to increased mortality from breast and liver cancer among manufacturing workers[349,358]
Pesticides: aldrin and dieldrin (organochlorines)	Used in crops like corn and cotton from 1950s to 1970s
	Banned by the EPA in 1975 except for termite control; completely banned in 1987
	In vitro assays showed estrogenic activity and dieldrin found in 78% of women diagnosed with breast cancer[357]
	High incidence of breast cancer in Massachusetts study found associations with higher income and regular use of lawn services, termite treatments, and home pesticides[363]
Household products: methylene chloride	Spray paints and paint removers may contain methylene chloride, documented breast cancer in lab animals[365]
Diethylstilbestrol (DES)	Prescribed for women to avert miscarriages between 1941 and 1971
	Exposed daughters known to have higher rates of vaginal cancer and in the mothers slight increased risk of breast cancer[350,356]
	Daughters now known to have slight increased risk of breast cancer[367]
Solvents (e.g., benzene, toluene, trichloroethylene, chlorinated organic solvents)	Used in manufacture of computers, also some in cosmetics
	In 2003 a Taiwanese study documented increased risk of breast cancer among electronic workers exposed to chlorinated organic solvents[348]
	Danish study of women 22 to 55 years of age employed in industries (fabricated metal, lumber, furniture, printing, textiles) using solvents double the risk of breast cancer[354]
Styrene, carbon tetrachloride, formaldehyde	1995 study suggested increased risk with occupational exposure—validation in Finland, Sweden, and Italy[344,369,371,372]
Ethylene glycol methyl ether (EGME)	Duke University study found they act as hormone sensitizers both in vivo and in vitro[342,359]
	Compounds are found in semiconductor industry, varnishes, paints, dyes, and fuel additives
Valproic acid (anticonvulsant medication)	Found to be hormone sensitizing and prescribed for migraines and bipolar disorder[342,359]
1,3-butadiene	Air pollutant and synthetic rubber product and some fungicides and tobacco smoke
	Causes mammary and ovarian tumors in female mice and rats[364,366]
Aromatic amines (heterocyclic, polycyclic, moncyclic)	Plastics, tobacco smoke, grilled meats and fish, combustion of wood chips and rubber
	Exposure in adolescence before full-term pregnancy may increase risk[351]
DDT (dichlorodiphenyl-trichloroethane) and PCB (polychlorinated biphenyls)	PCB used in manufacture of electrical equipment[352]
	PCB and DDT both banned in the United States since 1970s but are still found in body fat, as well as breast milk[373]
	DDT used as pesticide for insects on farms and swamps
	PCB deteriorates slowly in soil
	PCB difficult to study because diverse class of compounds
	1999 in vitro study showed PCBs proliferate breast cancer cells[355]
	Conflicting results; several large studies failed to show relationship with PCBs
Polycystic aromatic hydrocarbons (PAH, including tobacco)	Found in soot and fumes from fuels
	Increased DNA damage (DNA adducts) implicated from the Long Island Breast Cancer Study Project[353]
	Tobacco smoke also contains PAHs
	Smokers smoking as adolescents have an increased risk of breast cancer[343,347,360]
	In 2004 the California EPA concluded that environmental tobacco smoke (ETS) increases the risk of breast cancer and the association appears stronger for premenopausal women[346]
	Tobacco smoke also contains the carcinogens polonium-210, vinylchloride, benzene, and 1-3 butadiene[361]
Dioxin	Products containing polyvinyl chloride (PVC), PCBs, or other chlorinated compounds release dioxin from incineration
	Declared a known carcinogen by EPA in 2000
	It may be the most prevalent of all toxic chemicals
	Occurs in meat, poultry, dairy products, and human breast milk
	United Kingdom study linked dioxin to the development of mammary tumors in mice[345]
	Seveso, Italy, study connected dioxin with breast cancer[370]
Ethylene oxide	Used to sterilize surgical instruments and in some cosmetics
	Linked to breast cancer in women exposed to ethylene oxide in commercial sterilization facilities[368]

reduced exposures to carcinogens), weight loss, and changes in endogenous sex hormone levels.[293,294]

Familial Factors and Tumor-Related Genes

Genetically, breast cancer can be divided into three main groups: (1) sporadic, the majority or 40% of women with breast cancer have no known family history; (2) inherited dominant cancer gene syndromes, where the gene is passed to future generations by an autosomal dominant mechanism; and (3) probable polygenic, where there is family history but it is not passed on to future generations as a dominant gene. Yet to be determined are the number of genes in the polygenic model that could be involved, the nature of the interactions among these genes, and their interaction with environmental factors. The major risk factors for sporadic cancer are related to hormone exposure including gender, age at menarche and menopause, reproductive history, breastfeeding history, and endogenous and exogenous estrogens (see p. 832). Radiation exposure is known to increase risk. The majority of these cancers occur in postmenopausal women with increased ER expression.

A history of breast cancer in first-degree relatives (mother or sister) increases a woman's risk two to three times. Risk increases even more if two first-degree relatives are involved, especially if the disease occurred before menopause and was bilateral. In some families, breast cancer occurs at an earlier age and the frequency of bilateral tumors is greater. Women with inherited breast/ovarian cancer have tumors characterized by alterations in particular genes, mainly *BRCA1* and *BRCA2* breast cancer susceptibility genes, but also *CHEK2* (Li-Fraumeni syndrome), *ATM* (ataxia telangiectasia) *STK11* (Puetz-Jeghers syndrome), and others. An obvious hereditary predisposition and strongly penetrant mutations in genes such as *BRCA1* and *BRCA2* is responsible for 5% to 10% of all breast cancer, or 18,000 individuals per year.[295] The probability that a mutation will be present in family kindred increases if the family history includes disease at early ages, clustering of both breast and ovarian cancers *(BRCA1)*, male breast cancer *(BRCA2)*, and other rare cancers, such as sarcomas.[295] Even in families with more than four individuals with breast cancer, a germline mutation in *BRCA1* or *BRCA2* was found in only 65% of people.[296] Unexplained familial breast cancer possibly includes other more common lower-penetrant genes.

Investigators estimate that 45% of families with apparent autosomal dominant transmission of breast cancer susceptibility and about 90% of families with dominant inheritance of both breast and ovarian cancer have *BRCA1* germline mutations[297] (Figure 23-48). The *BRCA1* and *BRCA2* genes include several "founder" mutations identified in various populations. Most common in the United States are three mutations of the Eastern European population: two in *BRCA1* (185delAg and 5382insC) and the 6174delT mutation in *BRCA2*.[295] Founder mutations in other populations have been noted. The penetrance, or lifetime risk, of developing breast cancer and ovarian cancer from *BRCA* mutations is still the subject of intense research. Breast cancer risk associated with mutations in *BRCA1* have been estimated in the range of

50% to 80% and in 40% to 70% for *BRCA2*.[296,298] The ovarian cancer risk among *BRCA1* carriers is about 40% lifetime, exceeding the risk of 20% for *BRCA2* carriers. The risk for ovarian cancer is not the same for all *BRCA2* mutations, which depend on the location of the gene mutation.[299] In premenopausal women, a modifier of risk for breast cancer has been prophylactic oophorectomy, reducing lifetime risk by 50%.[300,301] Thus the risk associated with an inherited predisposition can be reduced significantly by modifying endogenous, and possibly exogenous, hormonal exposures. The risk for other cancers, such as pancreatic, prostate, melanoma, and others, are increased in *BRCA2* carriers.[295]

Recently, *BRCA1* action has been linked to the Fanconi anemia (FA) pathway.[302] A second surprising link between *BRCA2* and FA is a rare recessive pediatric disorder associated with childhood leukemia, called the D1 form of FA.[303] Pediatric medulloblastoma and Wilms tumor also is found in children carrying different mutations in *BRCA2* genes.[304]

Genes important to the development of cancer regulate diverse cellular pathways, including the progression of cells through the cell cycle, resistance to apoptosis, and the response to signals that direct cellular differentiation.[305] The inactivation of genes (e.g., tumor-suppressor genes) that contribute to the stability of the genome itself can favor errors in other genes that regulate proliferation. The importance of this latter pathway is exemplified by two studies linking the function of the *BRCA1* gene with that of the gene for ataxia-telangiectasia mutation (ATM) (Figure 23-49).

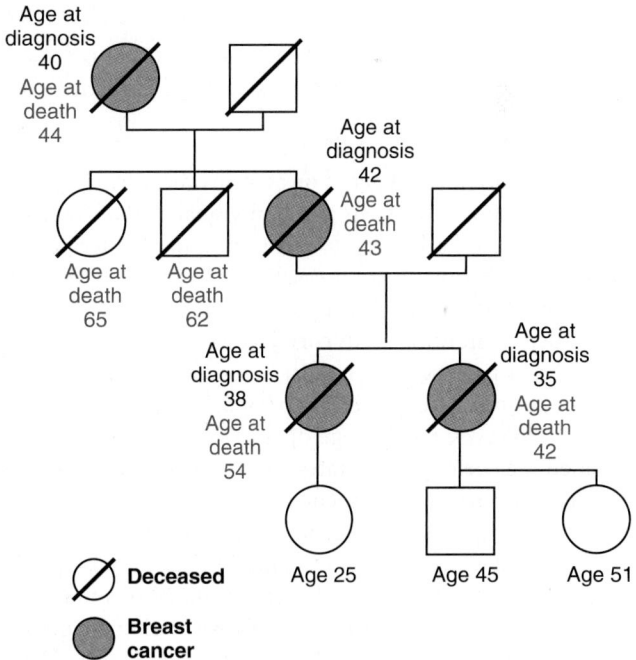

Figure 23-48 Example of family pedigree for breast cancer. Family pedigree showing cases of breast cancer associated with typical dominant transmission of breast cancer. Other possible genetic alterations related to risk of breast cancer include changes in *p53* and alterations in the estrogen receptor. Numerous somatic mutations in the expression of oncogenes in breast cancer cells have been reported.

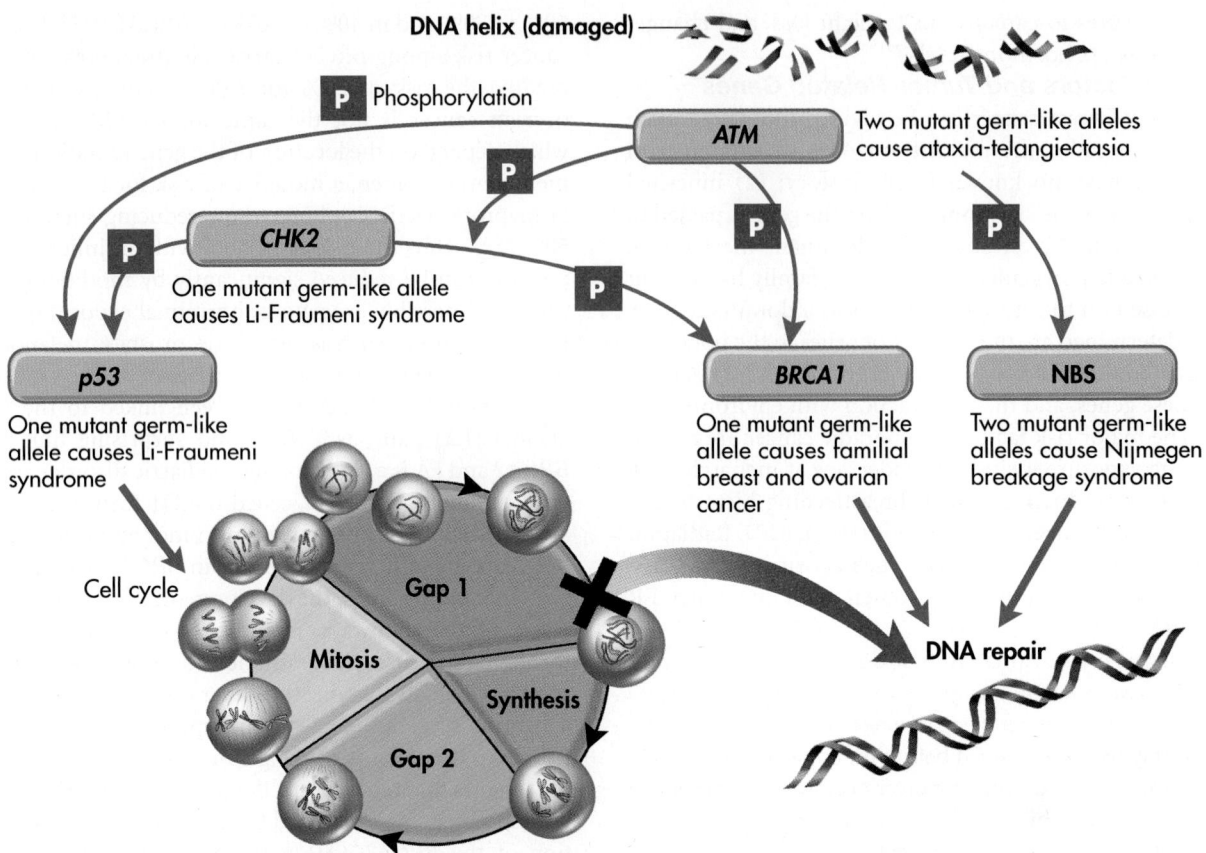

Figure 23-49 Mutations in genes that regulate cellular proliferation and repair of DNA and lead to breast carcinogenesis. The ataxia-telangiectasia mutated (ATM) gene encodes a protein kinase that activates (through phosphorylation) the tumor-suppressor *p53* protein either directly or indirectly by activating *CHK2* (a gene that encodes a protein kinase that activates *p53* by adding a phosphate group to it) in response to damage to DNA. The *p53* protein then triggers the arrest of the cell cycle, increasing time for DNA to be repaired. More simply, the *ATM* gene is necessary to accomplish DNA repair. The *BRCA1* and Nijmegen breakage syndrome (NBS) proteins are also activated by the *ATM* gene and are thought to be directly involved in the repair of damaged DNA. The inactivating mutations in the genes that encode these proteins increase the risk of breast cancer. (Redrawn from Haber D: *N Engl J Med* 343(21):1566, 2000.)

Other tumor-related genes or proteins include *p53, Bcl-2, HER-2/neu,* and *c-myc*. Cells with functional *p53* die by apoptosis, whereas cells lacking *p53* continue to proliferate (see Figure 12-7). About 40% of breast carcinomas reveal high levels of stabilized, often mutant *p53* protein in their cells; *p53*-related defects in tumor cells correlate with a poor prognosis.

Bcl-2 is a proto-oncogene. *Bcl-2* production decreases or inhibits apoptosis and thereby promotes breast and other cancers. However, the College of American Pathologists has classified it as belonging to category III, meaning insufficient evidence supports it as a prognostic factor.[306]

Her-2/neu, another oncogene, is overexpressed in 25% to 30% of breast cancer cells. It transmits a growth signal to the nucleus. The drug trastuzumab (Herceptin) blocks the signal in about 35% of those affected, thereby decreasing the growth of the tumor.

C-myc is a proto-oncogene expressed in cells and is one of the immediate, early growth response genes that are rapidly induced when quiet cells receive a signal to divide. Mutation of *c-myc* is amplified in breast, colon, lung, and many other cancers.

PATHOGENESIS   Breast cancer is as diverse as the breast itself. Table 23-16 lists the different types of breast carcinomas and summarizes their major characteristics. Most breast cancers arise from the ductal epithelium. Tumors of the infiltrating ductal type do not grow to a large size, but they metastasize early. This type accounts for 70% of breast cancers.

Breast cancer is a disease of the glandular epithelium, and pathogenesis probably involves several steps. First, modifications of the DNA of the breast epithelial ductal cells are caused by either genetic alterations, environmental agents, or their interactions. The initiated changes in DNA may occur early in a woman's life—before full differentiation of the breast tissue.[265] Second, growth factors increase the rate of growth of premalignant to malignant cells—the most important of which are estrogen and possibly progesterone. Breast cells produce other growth factors, including IGF, TGF-α, EGF, platelet-derived growth factor, and TGF-β (Figure 23-50). The production of these factors is to some degree regulated by estrogen.[265] Third, specific oncogenes are progressively modified or specific suppressor genes are lost, leading to advanced metastatic disease.

Table 23-16	Types of Breast Carcinomas and Major Distinguishing Features
Histologic Type	**Distinguishing Features**

Carcinoma of Mammary Ducts

Papillary	Well delineated cystic masses in multiple areas; hemorrhage often present; majority appear in 40- to 60-year age group; often involves skin
Intraductal (comedo)	Often accompanied with evidence of inflammation; well circumscribed tumors within the duct; well-differentiated tumor cells; rarely ulcerates the skin

Infiltrating Carcinoma

Ductal (no specific type [NST])	Fibrous, firm, glistening, gray-tan mass with chalky streaks, mixture of patterns; may cause discharge from the nipple; represents about 79% of all breast cancer
Mucinous	Usually large (>3 cm in diameter), circumscribed, and encapsulated, glistening appearance, varies in color; two types: pure and mixed; pure tumor is surrounded by mucin; infrequent; found in the lateral half of the breast; tends to occur in women after age 70 years
Medullary	Encapsulated and grows to be very large (7-8 cm in diameter); commonly surrounded by lymphocytic inflammatory infiltrate; occurs after age 50 years
Tubular	Well differentiated with orderly tubules in center (stroma) of mass; can be associated with noninfiltrating ductal carcinoma; occurs in women about 50 years of age; nodal metastasis infrequent; occurrence rare
Adenoid cystic	Very rare; well-circumscribed, painless mass arising from the nipple and areola
Metaplastic	Involves cartilage or bone; mixed tumors or osteogenic sarcomas
Squamous cell	Frequent in blacks; originates in ductal epithelium

Carcinoma of Mammary Lobules

Lobular carcinoma in situ	Found in individuals with fibrocystic disease; localized to upper breast quadrants; risk of 15%-35% becoming invasive; occurs frequently in mid-40s; infiltrating variety occurs in early 50s
Infiltrating lobular	Infiltrates from duct; firm mass with chalky streaks
Paget disease	Eczema of the nipple that extends to the areola; cancer usually found underneath the nipple; poorly circumscribed; large Paget cells arise from the duct and directly invade nipple; history of scaly, red rash spreading from the nipple; lesion palpable beneath the nipple, often bilateral; occurs in middle age
Inflammatory carcinoma	Not a histologic type; fairly diffuse within the breast tissue, diffuse edema of the overlying skin; extremely undifferentiated, very rare, most metastasize to axilla

Sarcoma of the Breast

Cytosarcoma phyllodes	Usually large (>17 cm in diameter); mostly localized but can rupture through the skin; rarely metastasizes to lymph nodes; history of painless nodule present for years before it forms a large mass; ulceration and bleeding of skin often present; occurs in wide age range (ages 13-77 years)
Fibrosarcoma	Well circumscribed, firm, and usually does not involve the skin or nipple; well differentiated to extremely undifferentiated; arises from connective tissue; extremely rare (e.g., liposarcoma, angiosarcoma)

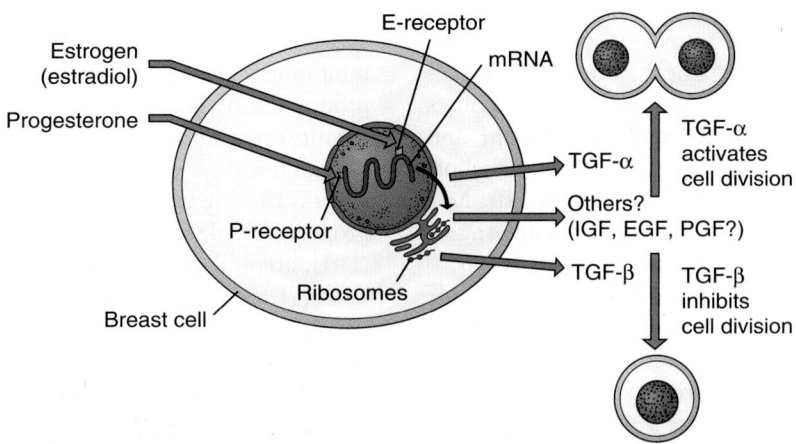

Figure 23-50 Control of breast cell growth. Two levels of control of breast cell growth: *(1)* paracrine signaling by estrogen *(E-receptor)* and progesterone *(P-receptor)* steroids and *(2)* autocrine signaling by locally secreted growth factors, such as transforming growth factor *(TGF-α and TGF-β)* and others, including insulin-like growth factor *(IGF)*, epidermal growth factor *(EGF)*, and platelet-derived growth factor *(PGF)*. *mRNA*, Messenger ribonucleic acid.

Unlike most human organs, which are differentiated by the end of fetal life, development and differentiation of the mammary gland occur after puberty. Factors that affect full differentiation of the breast may be essential for countering development of breast cancer (see p. 831 for a discussion of differentiation and pregnancy).

Mammary epithelial cells achieve rapid renewal by a small number of mitotic divisions of immortal stem cells. (Cell renewal is discussed in Chapters 1 and 11.) Because the number of mutations is proportional to the rate and number of stem cell divisions, factors that accelerate cell division can have a carcinogenic effect. Hormones may act as accelerators and influence the susceptibility of the breast epithelium either endogenously or to environmental carcinogens, because hormones control the differentiation of the mammary gland epithelium and thereby regulate the rate of stem cell division. Current knowledge of the mechanisms of differentiation of the mammary gland suggests that especially estrogens and possibly progesterone may be involved in breast carcinogenesis. This hypothesis is supported by two facts: (1) the increased incidence of breast cancer in women (e.g., 100 times more frequent in women than in men) and (2) the association of breast cancer with the events of reproductive life.

The period of highest proliferative activity of mammary epithelium stem cells is during each ovulatory cycle between puberty and either the first full-term pregnancy or menopause among nulliparous women (also see p. 831). The greatest increase in mitotic activity in the breast is during the luteal phase. During the estrogen follicular phase, terminal ductules are few and there is no mitotic activity. During the luteal phase, because of the increased progesterone levels, perhaps resulting from the estrogen priming (i.e., cyclic progesterone increases sensitivity of estrogen receptors), or as a result of cooperation between the two hormones, there is increased mitotic activity.[265,307,308] A large body of evidence is accumulating that indicates estrogens induce various types of DNA damage in vitro and in vivo. Although estrogen-induced cell proliferation undoubtedly has an important role in estrogen carcinogenesis, other pathways involving indirect or direct DNA toxicity (i.e., genotoxicity) originate from estrogen metabolites (Box 23-16). Among the metabolites formed during the process of estrogen metabolism and elimination, some are estrogenic (i.e., 4-hydroxycatechol) and some may be protective (i.e., 2-methoxyestrones) through their antioxidant properties or growth and angiogenesis inhibitory activities and promotion of apoptosis.[309] Conversely, the more reactive quinone metabolites are able to form direct adducts (i.e., when carcinogen binds to the DNA) with DNA and may cause oxidative damage to lipids and DNA through redox cycling processes producing reactive oxygen species[309-311] (see Figure 23-49). Estrogen-dependent breast cancer growth may be regulated by positive growth stimulators, such as TGF-α, and negative (inhibiting) growth stimulators, such as TGF-β.[306,312] (The role of other growth factors and hormones on breast mitotic activity also may be important.)

Box 23-16   Estrogen Carcinogenesis

Standard Theory
Estrogen and perhaps progesterone affect the rate of cell division and thus affect the risk of breast cancer by causing proliferation of breast epithelial cells. Proliferating cells are susceptible to genetic errors during DNA replication; if uncorrected, these errors can ultimately lead to a malignant phenotype.

Updated Theory
Although estrogen-induced proliferation undoubtedly has an important role in the carcinogenic process, mounting evidence supports a complementary pathway involving direct and indirect genotoxicity originating from estrogen metabolites (for example, 4-hydroxy catechol):
- *Indirect:* Oxidative DNA damage through redox cycling leads to reactive oxygen species
- *Direct:* Estrogen-quinone DNA adducts (see Figure 23-45)
Protective effects: perhaps through 2-methoxy catechol estrogen-mediated growth inhibition, apoptosis, and antiangiogenesis

Data from Feigelson HS, Henderson BE: Estrogens and breast cancer, *Carcinogenesis* 17:2279, 1996; Russo J, Russo I: *Molecular basis of breast cancer: prevention and treatment,* Germany, 2004, Springer.

Thus it can be suggested that the risk of carcinogenic mutations is proportional to the *time* required for all stem cells to undergo differentiation. The risk then would be proportional to the duration of the interval separating menarche from the first full-term birth and to the number of ovulatory cycles during this period of time.[313] In human studies, an increased risk of breast cancer is associated with young age at menarche, later age at menopause, or longer duration of ovulatory activity. Likewise, a protective effect or decreased risk of breast cancer is associated with young age at first live birth; full-term birth presumably shifts the mammary gland from a proliferative state with high susceptibility to carcinogens to a low-proliferative, low-risk state.[171] Lesions with an increased number of epithelial cells (proliferative changes) are associated structurally with a small increased risk of cancer.[166] These early changes may be related to evasion of growth-inhibiting signals, resistance to apoptosis, and autonomous production of growth signals. Invasive ductal carcinoma is the most commonly diagnosed malignancy in women and, although this theory is controversial, is considered to be the result of a histopathologically defined multistep process that progressively develops through stages of ductal hyperplasia (DH), atypical ductal hyperplasia (ADH), ductal carcinoma in situ (DCIS), invasive ductal carcinoma (IDC) and metastatic disease.[314,315] Data are strongest for atypical hyperplasia and in situ carcinoma as precursor lesions.[316] Unknown are the genetic alterations that correlate with these defined histopathologic stages of cancer progression.

Genetic instability, in the form of loss of heterozygosity (LOH) may be a later change and is rarely detected in proliferative changes. LOH, however, becomes more frequent in atypical hyperplasias and is almost always present in carcinoma in situ.[166] Another controversial supposition is that early genomic alterations observed in ductal hyperplasia are the result of the activation of the ferritin H chain gene, which may provide iron necessary for abnormal cell growth that is associated with oxidative damage and the S100P protein that may be involved in the transport of calcium and, therefore, a regulator of cell proliferation.[171]

Aneuploidy observed as nuclear enlargement and irregularity with increased chromatin is seen only in high-grade DCIS and some invasive carcinomas. Clonal populations of the cells of DCIS can fill the ductal system, suggesting limitless replicative potential.[166] Surrounding the basement membrane of some ducts is increased angiogenesis.

Emerging is the understanding that the biologic and structural features of carcinomas usually begin at the in situ stage, which is evident in the majority of cases.[166] The in situ lesion closely resembles the developing invasive carcinoma.[166] For example, low-grade DCIS with well differentiated carcinomas, high-grade DCIS with high-grade carcinomas, and lobular carcinomas are associated with lobular carcinoma in situ (LCIS).[166] Several lines of evidence, however, support the concept that different types of DCIS show different genetic alterations suggesting that there may be multiple pathways for the evolution of DCIS.[317-319]

Also emerging are the complex interactions between the luminal cells, myoepithelial cells, and stromal cells. These interactions are necessary for normal development of new ductal branches and lobes during puberty and pregnancy—interrupting or nullifying the basement membrane, increased proliferation, escape from growth inhibition, angiogenesis, and invasion of stroma—can all be preempted by abnormal epithelial cells, stromal cells, or both during tumor development. While all of these changes are occurring, parallel changes also occur because of mutation, epigenetic alterations (e.g., DNA methylation, see Chapter 11), or abnormal signaling pathways resulting in altered cellular interactions and tissue structure. Important is that loss of these normal functions also occurs with aging, which may contribute to breast cancer in older women.

The last step in carcinogenesis, the transition of carcinoma in situ to invasive carcinoma, is the least understood. The genetic alterations permitting invasion are unknown. The transition may be caused by loss of the basement membrane and tissue integrity because of abnormal function of myoepithelial and stromal cells rather than the "classic view" of the malignant cell gaining the ability to invade through the basement membrane and into stroma (Figure 23-51).

New techniques, such as microarray technologies (gene chips) that survey many changes in DNA, RNA, and proteins of carcinomas, have provided molecular patterns of the overall biologic diversity of invasive breast carcinomas. These technologies reveal ER+ and ER− tumors as separate categories. The majority (70% to 80%) of breast carcinomas are ER+ and thought to arise from ER+ luminal cells. Many genes (possibly hundreds) may be under transcriptional control by ER, for example, those genes governing IGF-1. Important for treatment is that the expression of downstream genes in ER+ tumors might be more predictive of tumor behavior and respond to estrogen-blocking agents than the presence of the estrogen receptor itself. Additional genetic or epigenetic factors modulate estrogen response or cell survival or both including oncoproteins, growth factors, and signaling molecules, such as Ha-Ras, Raf1, FGF-1 and 4, TGF-β, HER-2/neu, and cyclin D1.[171] For a discussion of different mechanisms considered responsible for the carcinogenicity of estrogens see p. 831.

Estrogen receptor (ER) tumors comprise two major groups—basal-like carcinomas and HER-2 (proteins from oncogene *Her-2/neu*) positive carcinomas. Basal-like carcinomas, so termed because the myoepithelial cell is located in the basal area of the lobules, have characteristics suggestive of myoepithelial cell differentiation. *BRCA1* carcinomas tend to fall into this category.[166] A second ER group is diagnosed by amplification of HER-2/protein. Other subgroups also have been identified.

Stromal cells interacting with cancer cells are possibly responsible for important components of these gene expressions, thus supporting the significance of cell-to-cell communication in the overall behavior of cancer. Carcinomas are divided into in situ and invasive carcinomas. Carcinoma in situ, however, does not involve lymphatics and blood vessels. Invasive carcinoma infiltrates beyond the basement membrane into the stroma.

Ductal carcinoma in situ (DCIS) refers to a malignant heterogenous group of lesions limited to ducts and lobules. The cells sometimes can extend to the overlying skin without crossing the basement membrane and mistakenly appear as Paget disease[166] (see Table 23-16). Before 1980, DCIS was a rare disease and usually presented as a palpable lesion, nipple discharge, or Paget disease (eczema-like lesions of the nipple). Since 1980, with the increased use of mammography, the incidence and presentation has changed dramatically.[320] Today, DCIS represents at least 15% to 30% of all newly diagnosed cases of breast cancer and about half of all cases diagnosed by mammography. It is still not clear whether the increase in incidence reflects an increase in cancer or increased detections by mammography. DCIS presents as calcifications on a mammogram (Figure 23-52).

DCIS is a clonal proliferation usually confined to a single ductal system. The natural history of DCIS is unknown because in the past women with DCIS were treated with mastectomy. The main issue revolves around which lesions of the category DCIS become invasive and how soon does that happen.[320] In a study of 110 autopsies of young and middle-aged women (20 to 54 years), 14% were found to have DCIS,[321] suggesting that the preclinical prevalence (subtle histologic distortion and/or nonpalpable mass) is significantly higher than the clinical expression. Other autopsy series show that not all DCIS lesions progress to invasion or become clinically significant.[128,134,321,322] The consensus today seems to be that DCIS progresses eventually to invasive carcinoma, emphasizing appropriate diagnosis and therapy.[166] DCIS is detected more often in younger women than in older women.

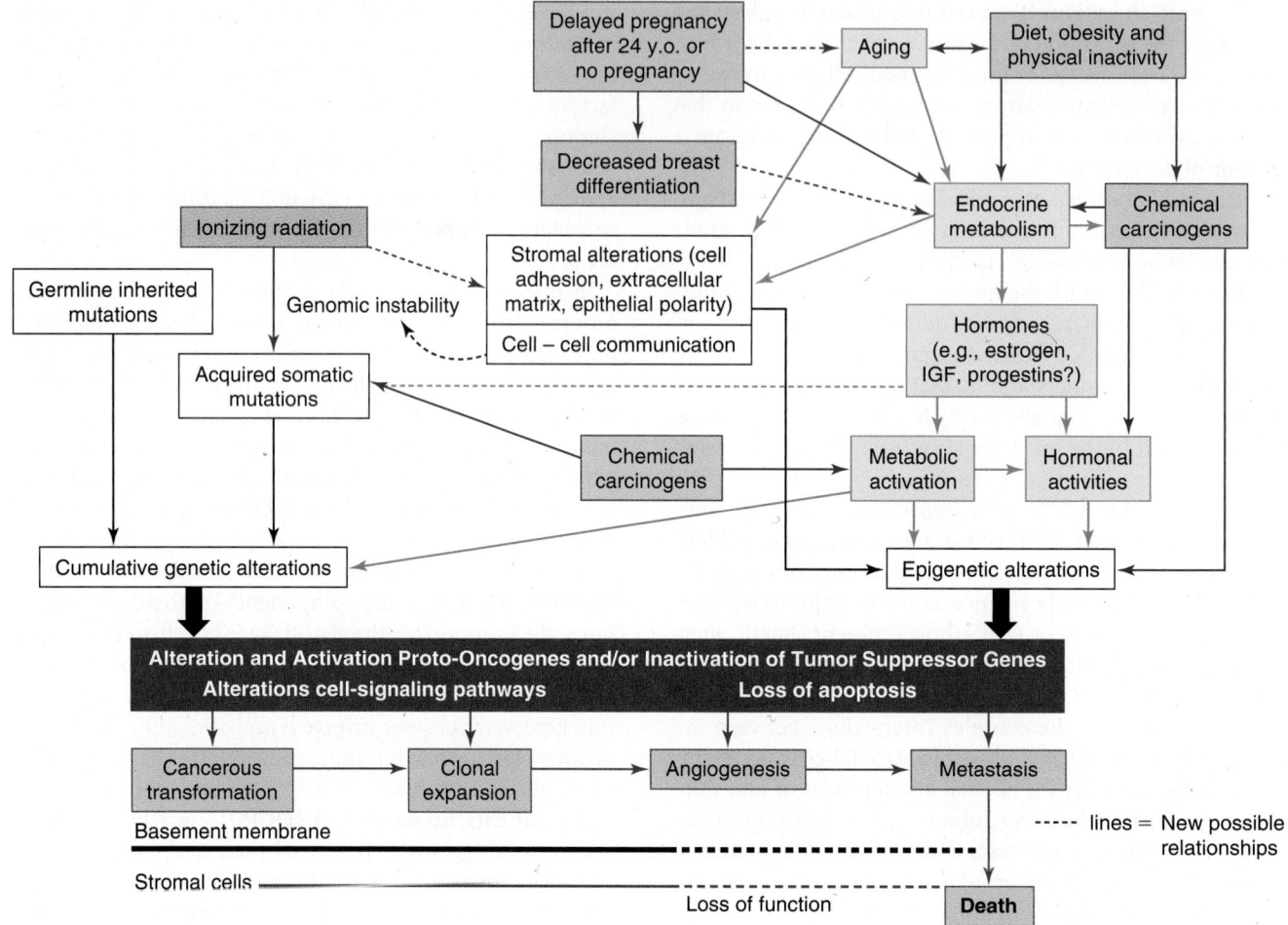

Figure 23-51 **Model of breast carcinogenesis.** Molecular mechanisms underlying each of the risk factors for breast cancer are not completely defined. Breast carcinogenesis involves uncontrolled cellular proliferation, alterations in cell signaling pathways, aberrance or loss of apoptosis as a consequence of accumulated genetic damage that lead to activation, and alteration of germline mutation *(black)* or acquired *(black)* as somatic mutations as a result of environmental physical *(red)* (e.g., ionizing radiation), chemical *(blue)* (e.g., carcinogenesis), lifestyle *(purple)* (e.g., pregnancy, diet, obesity, physical inactivity, and biologic factors *(green)* (e.g., aging, endocrine/hormonal mileu). The expression of the transformed phenotype requires cumulative genetic alterations and epigenetic alterations. The normal breast is maintained by a complex set of interactions among luminal cells, myoepithelial cells, the basement membrane, and stromal cells. Changes in malignant cells are accompanied or preceded by alterations in the supporting myoepithelial and stromal cells because of genetic and epigenetic events and disruption of normal signaling pathways. The final alteration, invasion of the stroma, is the least understood. Emerging is the possibility that invasion is a result of the loss of myoepithelial and stromal cells to maintain the basement membrane.

Although there is no universally accepted histopathologic classification, most pathologists divide DCIS into five subtypes (papillary, micropapillary, cribriform, solid, and comedo) and often compare the first four types, noncomedo, with comedo. **Comedo** is generally considered more aggressive and is associated with a high nuclear grade, aneuploidy, a higher proliferation rate, diagnostic gene amplification, and protein over expression (HER-2/neu).[320] In a single biopsy, however, several types may be mixed and some noncomedo types may express characteristics of the comedo type.

Recently, the characteristic of higher nuclear grade has assumed more importance. Nuclear grade (degree of differentiation) is emerging as a key factor for determining aggressiveness, that is, the higher the grade the less differentiated and

the more aggressive. Grade 3 is being used to define the most aggressive group.

Comedo DCIS tends to have "casting calcifications" on mammography, which are linear, branching, or bizarre (see Figure 23-52, *A*). When noncomedo lesions are calcified they tend to have mostly fine but also some course granular calcifications (see Figure 23-52, *B*).

Lobular carcinoma in situ (LCIS), unlike DCIS, has a uniform appearance in which the cells occur in noncohesive clusters in ducts and lobules. LCIS is not associated with calcifications or a stromal involvement that would form a density. Thus it is usually an incidental finding from biopsy for something else. LCIS is less common (1% to 2% of all carcinomas).[166] LCIS is bilateral in 20% to 40% of women and the

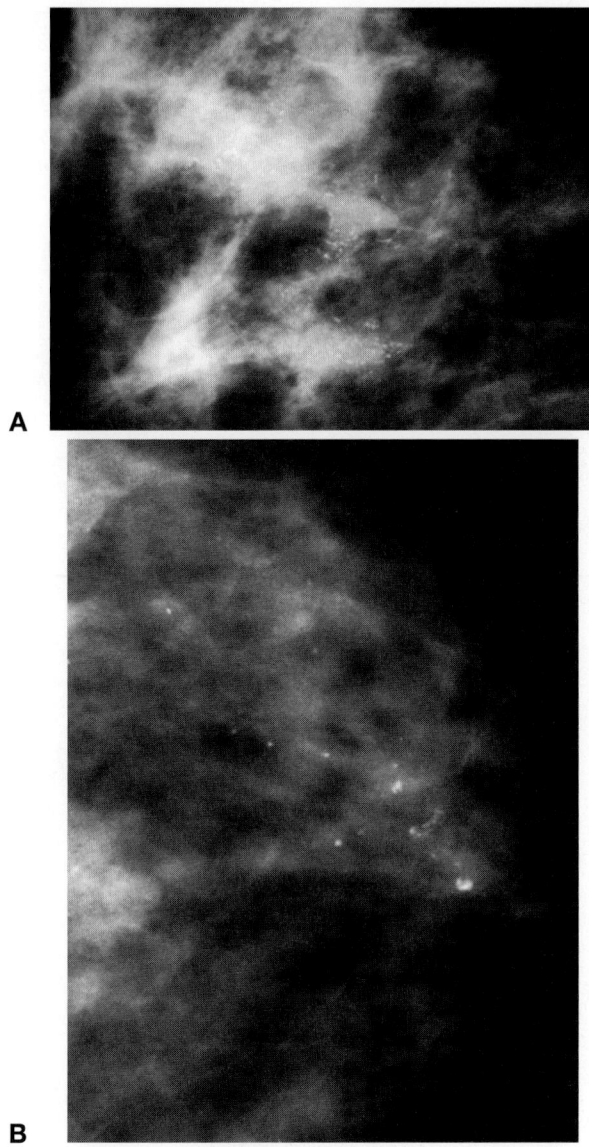

A

B

Figure 23-52 Ductal carcinoma in situ. **A,** Magnification mammography reveals pleomorphic, linear, and casting calcifications. Histopathology revealed high-grade comedo ductal carcinoma in situ (DCIS). **B,** Craniocaudal mammography reveals fine and course granular calcifications. Histopathology revealed low-grade DCIS. (From Donegan WL, Spratt JS: *Cancer of the breast,* ed 5, Philadelphia, 2002, Saunders.)

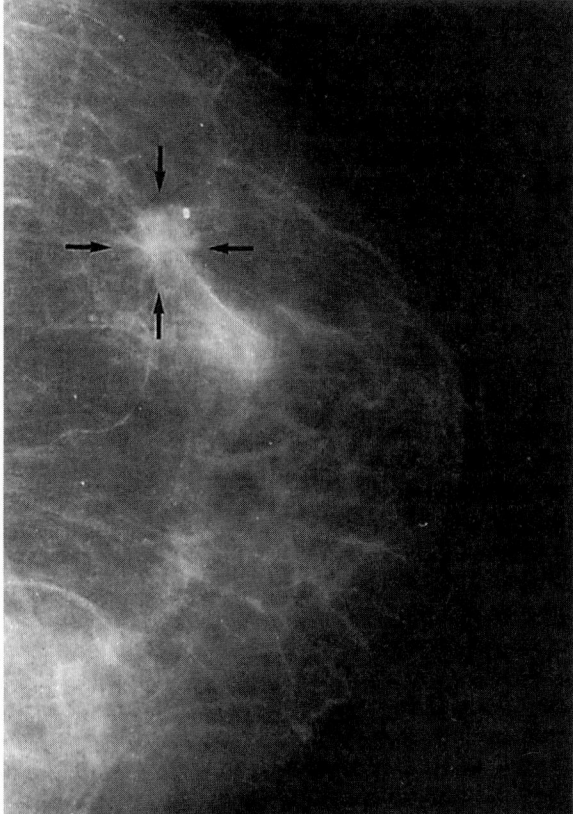

Figure 23-53 Invasive ductal carcinoma. This mammogram shows a density with an irregular border. There is a small, superimposed, accidental calcification. Over 90% of such masses will prove to be invasive carcinomas. Rarely, complex sclerosing lesions, prior surgical scars, and fibromatosis may present in this fashion. (From Kumar V, Abbas AK, Fausto N: *Robbins and Cotran pathologic basis of disease,* ed 7, Philadelphia, 2005, Saunders.)

majority (80% to 90%) occurs before menopause. Although the cells of LCIS and invasive lobular carcinoma are identical,[166] controversial is whether LCIS is a true neoplasm or a marker of breast cancer risk. Evidence to support LCIS as a precursor lesion of invasive carcinoma is that LOH on chromosome 16q is present in both LCIS and invasive carcinoma.[323] Invasive carcinoma develops in 25% to 35% of women with LCIS and the uninvolved breast may be at greater risk.[324] Treatment choices include bilateral mastectomy, estrogen antagonists, or more commonly, close follow-up and screening.

CLINICAL MANIFESTATIONS   In women of all ages not undergoing mammography, invasive carcinoma presents as a palpable mass.[166] Most carcinomas cause a marked increase in dense, fibrous stroma resulting in a hard consistency on palpation that replaces fat and is identified on mammography as density. By the time a cancer becomes palpable, it is estimated that 50% of individuals will have axillary node metastasis.[166] In postmenopausal women undergoing mammography, invasive carcinomas present as density (Figure 23-53). Dimpling of the skin or fixation to the chest wall occurs with larger carcinomas. If the local lymphatics are blocked, the subsequent lymphedema and thickening of the skin causes a change called *peau d'orange* (orange peel skin). Tethering of the skin by Cooper ligaments to the breast mimics the look of an orange peel. If the central portion of the breast is involved, retraction of the nipple can occur.

The most common histologic types of breast carcinomas are listed in Table 23-16 (p. 843). Invasive carcinomas of no special type (NST) constitute the majority (70% to 80%) of tumors, however, they cannot be specifically classified. Carcinomas of NST have varying amounts of DCIS. In the future, gene expression profiling may specifically identify subtypes

Table 23-17	Clinical Manifestations of Breast Cancer
Clinical Manifestation	**Pathophysiology**
Chest pain	Metastasis to the lung
Dilated blood vessels	Obstruction of venous return by a fast-growing tumor; obstruction dilates superficial veins
Dimpling of the skin	Can occur with invasion of the dermal lymphatics because of retraction of Cooper ligament or involvement of the pectoralis fascia
Edema	Local inflammation or lymphatic obstruction
Edema of the arm	Obstruction of lymphatic drainage in the axilla
Hemorrhage	Erosion of blood vessels
Local pain	Local obstruction caused by the tumor
Nipple/areolar eczema	Paget disease
Nipple discharge in a nonlactating woman	Spontaneous and intermittent discharge caused by tumor obstruction
Nipple retraction	Shortening of the mammary ducts
Pitting of the skin (similar to the surface of an orange [*peau d'orange*])	Obstruction of the subcutaneous lymphatics, resulting in the accumulation of fluid
Reddened skin, local tenderness, and warmth	Inflammation
Skin retraction	Involvement of the suspensory ligaments
Ulceration	Tumor necrosis

Data from Griffiths MJ, Murray KH, Russo PC: *Oncology nursing: pathophysiology, assessment, and intervention*, New York, 1984, Macmillan.

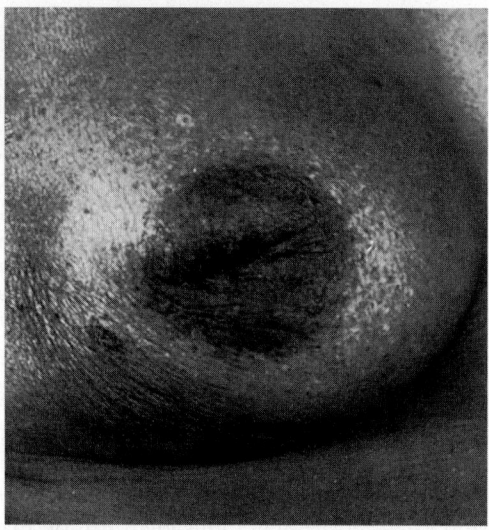

Figure 23-54 Retraction of nipple caused by carcinoma. (From del Regato JA, Spjut HJ, Cox JD: *Ackerman and del Regato's cancer: diagnosis, treatment, and prognosis,* ed 6, St Louis, 1985, Mosby.)

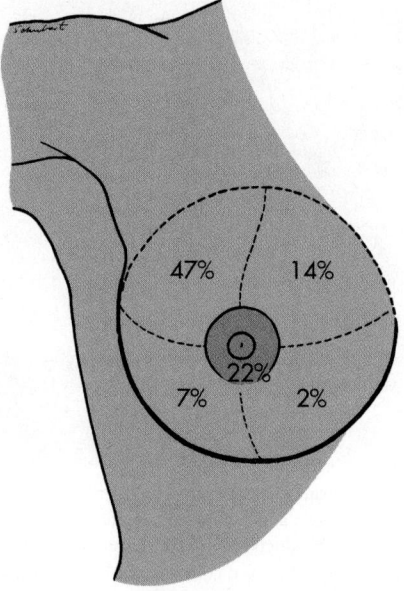

Figure 23-55 Distribution of carcinomas in different areas of the breast. (From del Regato JA, Spjut HJ, Cox JD: *Ackerman and del Regato's cancer: diagnosis, treatment, and prognosis,* ed 6, St Louis, 1985, Mosby.)

and enable understanding of the clinical relevance (e.g., etiology, presentation, prognosis, or treatment).

The first sign of breast cancer is usually a painless lump. Lumps caused by breast tumors do not have any classic characteristics. Other signs include palpable nodes in the axilla, retraction of tissue (dimpling) (Figure 23-54), thickening of the skin, or bone pain caused by metastasis to the vertebrae. Table 23-17 summarizes the clinical manifestations of breast cancers. Manifestations vary according to the type of tumor and stage of disease.

EVALUATION AND TREATMENT Approximately 50% of carcinomas of the breast occur in the upper outer quadrant because most of the glandular tissue of the breast is

there (Figure 23-55). The lymphatic spread of cancer to the opposite breast, to lymph nodes in the base of the neck, and to the abdominal cavity is caused by obstruction of the normal lymphatic pathways or destruction of lymphatic vessels by surgery or radiation. The less common inner-quadrant tumors may spread to mediastinal nodes or Rotter nodes, which are located between the pectoral muscles. Internal mammary chain nodes are common sites of metastasis. Metastases from the vertebral veins can involve the vertebrae, pelvic bones, ribs, and skull. The lungs, kidneys, liver, adrenal glands, ovaries, and pituitary gland are also sites of metastasis.

Mammography, digital mammography, percutaneous needle aspiration, biopsy or minimally invasive biopsy called *mammotome*, palpation, ultrasonography, and hormone receptor assays are generally used in evaluating breast cancer. Mammography has low specificity in distinguishing between malignant and benign lesions.[325] Responding to the need for earlier, more accurate, and cost-effective methods for cancer detection, investigators are studying alternative methods, including digital mammography, MRI, and ultrasound.[326] The benefits of mammography are unknown in women over 70 years of age and are still debated in those between 40 and 49 years of age. Biopsy is the definitive diagnostic test.

Treatment is based on the extent or stage of the cancer (Box 23-17). The extent of the tumor at the primary site, the presence and extent of lymph node metastasis, and the presence of distant metastases are all evaluated to determine the stage of disease.

Little is known regarding how dietary factors affect the survival of women with breast cancer. As previously discussed, an increased ratio of omega-3 to omega-6 fatty acids can possibly decrease growth of breast cancer. It is postulated that to minimize oxidative radicals, further dietary supplementation with vitamin E and a retinoid may increase the effectiveness of such a diet.[327] In addition, a recent study found that women eating more protein (but not red meat) increased their survival.[328] Avoidance of hyperinsulinemia, insulin resistance, and the production of insulin-like growth factors (e.g., via physical activity) also may provide new approaches to cancer prevention.[195]

Surgery, radiation, chemotherapy, hormone therapy, and biologic therapy may be used to treat breast cancer. The extent of the surgery depends on the tumor's histology, predictability, and stage and the individual's age and medical and psychologic history. Beginning with the most conservative, the surgical procedures commonly used are as follows:

1. Tylectomy or lumpectomy, in which the tumor and a small amount of surrounding tissue are removed
2. Quadrant excision, in which a quadrant of the breast is removed
3. Partial mastectomy or segmental mastectomy, in which a larger amount of tissue is removed
4. Total or simple mastectomy, in which the tumor and all breast tissue are removed (the nipple may or may not be removed)
5. Modified radical mastectomy, in which the breast, pectoralis minor, and axillary contents are removed
6. Radical mastectomy, in which the breast, axillary contents, and pectoralis major and minor are removed

Radiation therapy is used to prevent metastasis of a small tumor (0.2 cm) or if the cancer is near bone or the edge of the breast that has been surgically excised. Not all women with breast cancer need radiation. It is especially important to protect the heart and lungs from unnecessary radiation exposure. Chemotherapy and hormone therapy are most successful as an adjunct to surgery in premenopausal women with hormone-dependent tumors. They are also used in individuals with advanced disease. Herceptin, the antibody to the *Her-2* oncogene, is available and blocks the growth-promoting signal produced by *Her-2/neu.* Endocrine therapy (androgens, estrogens, progesterones, and steroids) may be used to prolong survival time and is thought to be most effective in women with estrogen receptor– and progesterone receptor–positive tumors. Estrogen receptor– and progesterone receptor–negative tumors are unlikely to respond to hormonal therapy. Long-term antiestrogen therapy, such as tamoxifen, has proven efficacy in individuals with ER+ tumors. Use of tamoxifen for many years, however, can increase its resistance.

Box 23-17   Staging of Breast Cancer

T—Primary Tumor Size

T_x Primary tumor cannot be assessed

T_0 No evidence of primary tumor

T_{is} Carcinoma in situ: intraductal carcinoma, lobular carcinoma in situ, or Paget disease of the nipple with node

T_1 Tumor 2 cm or less in greatest dimension

T_2 Tumor more than 2 cm but not more than 5 cm in greatest dimension

T_3 Tumor more than 5 cm in greatest dimension

T_4 Tumor of any size with direct extension to chest wall or skin

NOTE: Paget disease associated with a tumor is classified according to the size of the tumor

N—Regional Lymph Nodes

N_x Regional lymph nodes cannot be assessed (e.g., previously removed)

N_0 No regional lymph node metastasis

N_1 Metastasis to movable ipsilateral axillary lymph node or nodes

N_2 Metastasis to ipsilateral axillary lymph node(s) fixed to one another or to other structures

N_3 Metastasis to ipsilateral internal mammary lymph node or nodes

M—Distant Metastasis

M_x Presence of distant metastasis cannot be assessed

M_0 No distant metastasis

M_1 Distant metastasis (includes metastasis to ipsilateral supraclavicular lymph node or nodes)

Stage Grouping

Stage	T	N	M
Stage 0	T_{is}	N_0	M_0
Stage 1	T_1	N_0	M_0
Stage IIa	T_0	N_0	M_0
	T_1	N_1	M_0
	T_2	N_0	M_0
Stage IIB	T_2	N_1	M_0
	T_3	N_0	M_0
Stage IIIA	T_0	N_2	M_0
	T_1	N_2	M_0
	T_2	N_2	M_0
	T_3	N_1	M_0
	T_3	N_2	M_0
Stage IIIB	T_4	Any N	M_0
	Any T	N_3	M_0
Stage IV	Any T	Any N	M_1

Data from Beahrs OH, Hutter RV, Kennedy BJ, editors: *Breast manual for staging of cancer,* ed 45, Philadelphia, 1992, Lippincott.

Thus it is recommended for only 5 years. Tamoxifen can have estrogenic effects in the uterus and cause endometrial cancer. It is not recommended for women intending to become pregnant. In addition, in postmenopausal women, tamoxifen increases the risk of cataracts and blood clots in leg veins. Currently, tamoxifen is not recommended as an agent for prevention of breast cancer in those without breast cancer. Aromatase inhibitors, such as anastrozole, have increased disease-free survival rates more than has tamoxifen[329] (see p. 834). Of need are data on the long-term safety of aromatase inhibitors. New strategies are being studied that have high affinity for breast estrogen receptors but weak affinity for receptors in the uterus. Such a drug, raloxifene, is currently under investigation. Results from the Multiple Outcomes of Raloxifene Evaluation (MORE), a randomized study, found that among postmenopausal women with osteoporosis the risk of invasive breast cancer was decreased by 76% (13 cases in 5129 women vs. 27 in the 2579 placebo group). Results are anticipated for the STAR (study of tamoxifen and Raloxifene) trial in 2006. Newer treatments that include biologic response modifiers (see Chapter 12) are being used in clinical research trials. The effectiveness of sulfatase inhibitors needs to be studied.

Disorders of the Male Breast

Gynecomastia

Gynecomastia is the overdevelopment of breast tissue in a male. Gynecomastia accounts for approximately 85% of all masses that develop in the male breast and affects 32% to 40% of the male population. If only one breast is involved, it is typically the left. Incidence is greatest among adolescents and men older than 50 years.

Gynecomastia results from hormonal alterations, which may be idiopathic or caused by systemic disorders, drugs, or neoplasms. Gynecomastia usually involves an imbalance of the estrogen/testosterone ratio. The normal estrogen/ testosterone ratio can be altered in one of two ways. First, estrogen levels may be excessively high, although testosterone levels are normal. This is the case in drug-induced and tumor-induced cases of hyperestrogenism. Second, testosterone levels may be extremely low although estrogen levels are normal, as is the case in hypergonadism. Gynecomastia also can be caused by alterations in breast-tissue responsiveness to hormonal stimulation. Breast tissue may have increased responsiveness to estrogen or decreased responsiveness to androgen. Alterations of responsiveness may cause many cases of idiopathic gynecomastia.

Besides puberty and aging, estrogen/testosterone imbalances are associated with hypogonadism, Klinefelter syndrome, and testicular neoplasms. Hormone-induced gynecomastia is usually bilateral. Pubertal gynecomastia is a self-limiting phenomenon that usually disappears within 4 to 6 months. Senescent gynecomastia usually regresses spontaneously within 6 to 12 months.

Systemic disorders associated with gynecomastia include cirrhosis of the liver, infectious hepatitis, chronic renal failure, chronic obstructive lung disease, hyperthyroidism, tuberculo-

sis, and chronic malnutrition. It may be that these disorders ultimately alter the estrogen/testosterone ratio, initiating the gynecomastia.

Gynecomastia is often seen in males receiving estrogen therapy, either in preparation for a sex-change operation or for prostatic carcinoma. Other drugs that can cause gynecomastia include digitalis, cimetidine, spironolactone, reserpine, thiazide, isoniazid, ergotamine, tricyclic antidepressants, amphetamines, vincristine, and busulfan. Gynecomastia is usually unilateral in these instances.

Malignancies of the testes, adrenals, or liver can cause gynecomastia if they alter the estrogen/testosterone ratio. Pituitary adenomas and lung cancer also are associated with gynecomastia.

PATHOPHYSIOLOGY The breast enlargement consists of hyperplastic stroma and ductal tissue. Hyperplasia results in a firm, palpable mass, at least 2 cm in diameter and located beneath the areola.

EVALUATION AND TREATMENT The diagnosis of gynecomastia is based on physical examination. Identification and treatment of the cause are likely to be followed by resolution of the gynecomastia. The man should be taught to perform breast self-examination and is examined at 6- and 12-month intervals if the gynecomastia persists. All unilateral breast enlargement in men warrants an evaluation for malignancy; workup includes fine-needle aspiration, cytology, mammography, ultrasound, and biopsy.

Cancer

Male breast cancer (MBC) accounts for 1% of all male cancers and less than 1% of all breast cancers. Breast cancer in men is seen most commonly after age 60 years, with the peak incidence between 60 and 69 years. It has, however, been reported in males as young as 6 years and in adolescents. Possible risk factors include gynecomastia, radiation of the chest wall, family history of breast cancer, Klinefelter syndrome, and especially in those with germline mutation in *BRCA1* or *BRCA2*. Other genetic factors include CYP17 polymorphism, Cowden syndrome, *CHEK2,* and *AR* gene mutations.[330] Obesity increases the risk of MBC. Testicular disorders, including cryptorchidism, mumps, orchitis, and orchiectomy are related to risk.[330] The relationship between these factors and risk of disease is not clearly defined.

Male breast tumors often resemble carcinoma of the breast in women (see p. 828). The majority of MBCs express estrogen and progesterone receptors.[331] The malignant male breast lesion is usually a unilateral solid mass located near the nipple. Because the nipple is commonly involved, crusting and nipple discharge are typical clinical manifestations. Other findings include skin retraction, ulceration of the skin over the tumor, and axillary node involvement. Patterns of metastasis are similar to those in females.

The diagnosis of cancer is confirmed by biopsy. Because of delays in seeking treatment, male breast cancer tends to be advanced at the time of diagnosis and therefore tends to have a poor prognosis. Treatment protocols are similar to those for female breast cancer, but endocrine therapy is used more often for males because a higher percentage of male tumors are hormone dependent. The mainstay of treatment is modified mastectomy with axillary node dissection to assess stage and prognosis.[332] Orchiectomy is performed to treat metastatic disease.

SUMMARY REVIEW

Alterations of Sexual Maturation

1. Sexual maturation, or puberty, should begin in girls between ages 8 and 13 years and in boys between ages 9 and 14 years. Delayed puberty is the onset of sexual maturation after these ages; precocious puberty is onset before these ages. The average age of puberty has been occurring earlier than previously defined.

2. Alterations of sexual maturation can be idiopathic or caused by a disease or congenital anomaly. In most cases of delayed puberty, the hypothalamic-pituitary-gonadal axis is intact but the surge of activity that stimulates puberty is delayed. This situation is common in boys. Precocious puberty, more common in girls, also can be caused by mistiming of the stimulatory surge in a child whose hypothalamic-pituitary-ovarian system is otherwise normal.

3. Precocious puberty can be isosexual (sex appropriate), heterosexual (not sex appropriate), or incomplete (development of one secondary sex characteristic only). Causes of delayed or incomplete puberty can be divided into categories based on gonadotropic secretion: hypergonadotropism (increased levels of follicle-stimulating hormone [FSH] and luteinizing hormone [LH]), hypogonadotropism (decreased LH and FSH levels), and eugonadism.

Disorders of the Female Reproductive System

1. The female reproductive system can be altered by hormonal imbalances, infectious microorganisms, inflammation, structural abnormalities, and benign or malignant proliferative conditions.

2. Menstrual disorders usually involve some disruption of the hypothalamic-pituitary-ovarian axis and subsequent alteration of hormone production, reception by target organs, or feedback mechanisms.

3. Primary dysmenorrhea is painful menstruation not associated with pelvic disease. It results from excessive synthesis of prostaglandins, which cause the myometrium to contract and constrict blood vessels, resulting in ischemic pain.

4. Primary amenorrhea is the continued absence of menarche and menstrual function by 14 years of age without the development of secondary sex characteristics or by age 16 years if these changes have occurred.

5. Secondary amenorrhea is the absence of menstruation for a time equivalent to more than three cycles or 6 months in women who have previously menstruated. Secondary amenorrhea is associated with anovulation.

6. Categorization of amenorrhea as primary or secondary has no clinical significance. Instead, amenorrhea is divided into compartments that reflect the underlying disorder: compartment I, disorders of the outflow tract or uterine target organ; compartment II, disorders of the ovary; compartment III, disorders of the anterior pituitary; and compartment IV, disorders of the central nervous system (CNS) or hypothalamic factors.

7. Dysfunctional uterine bleeding (DUB) is heavy or irregular bleeding caused by a disturbance of the menstrual cycle.

8. Polycystic ovary syndrome (PCOS) is a difficult syndrome to diagnose because several factors are involved. PCOS is a syndrome when at least two of the following are present: oligoovulation or anovulation, elevated levels of androgens, or clinical signs of hyperandrogenism and polycystic ovaries. Prolonged anovulation leads to infertility, menstrual bleeding disorders, hirsutism, acne, endometrial hyperplasia, cardiovascular disease, and diabetes mellitus in women with hyperinsulinemia. PCOS affects females between 15 and 30 years of age.

9. Premenstrual syndrome (PMS) is the cyclic recurrence of physical, psychologic, or behavioral changes distressing enough to disrupt normal activities or interpersonal relationships. More than 200 emotional, physical, and behavioral symptoms have been attributed to PMS. Emotional symptoms, particularly depression, anger, irritability, and fatigue, are reported as the most distressing symptoms; physical symptoms tend to be less problematic. Treatment is symptomatic and includes self-help techniques, lifestyle changes, counseling, and selective serotonin reuptake inhibitors (SSRIs).

10. Infection and inflammation of the female genitalia can result from microorganisms from the environment or overproliferation of microorganisms that normally populate the genital tract.

11. Pelvic inflammatory disease (PID) is an acute ascending polymicrobial infection of the upper genital tract and is sexually transmitted.

12. Vaginitis, or vaginal infection, is usually caused by sexually transmitted pathogens or *Candida albicans*, which causes candidiasis. Development is related to the overall health of a woman and local defense mechanisms, particularly vaginal pH. Variables, such as antibiotics, douching, soaps, feminine hygiene sprays, and pregnancy, alter vaginal pH or the bactericidal nature of secretions and predispose a woman to infection.

13. Cervicitis, which is inflammation of the cervix, can be acute (mucopurulent cervicitis) or chronic. Its most common cause is a sexually transmitted pathogen.

14. Vulvitis is an inflammation of the skin of the vulva. It can be caused by chemical and mechanical irritants, allergens, skin disorders, or spread of vaginal infections, such as candidiasis.

15. Bartholinitis, also called Bartholin cyst, is an inflammation of the ducts that lead from the *Bartholin glands* to the surface of the vulva. Inflammation blocks the glands, preventing the outflow of glandular secretions, and is caused by trauma or infection.

16. The pelvic relaxation disorders—uterine prolapse, cystocele, rectocele, and urethrocele—are caused by the relaxation of muscles and fascial supports, usually with age or after childbirth or other trauma, and are more likely to occur in women with a familial or genetic predisposition.

17. Benign growths and proliferative conditions of the female reproductive tract tend to affect the ovaries (benign ovarian cysts) or uterine tissues (endometrial polyps, leiomyomas, and endometriosis).

18. Benign ovarian cysts develop from mature ovarian follicles that do not release their ova (follicular cysts) or from a corpus luteum that persists abnormally instead of degenerating (corpus luteum cyst). Cysts usually regress spontaneously.

19. Endometrial polyps consist of overgrowths of endometrial tissue and often cause abnormal bleeding in the premenopausal woman.

Continued

20. Leiomyomas, also called *uterine fibroids,* are tumors arising from the muscle layer of the uterus, the myometrium. Incidence increases in women between ages 30 and 50 years; most myomas remain small and asymptomatic. Adenomyosis is the presence of endometrial glands and stroma within the uterine myometrium.

21. Endometriosis is the presence of functional endometrial tissue (i.e., tissue that responds to hormonal stimulation) at sites outside the uterus. Endometriosis causes an inflammatory reaction at the site of implantation and is a cause of infertility.

22. Most cancers of the female genitalia involve the uterus (particularly the cervix) and the ovaries. Cancer of the vagina is rare.

23. Infection with high-risk human papillomavirus (HPV) is a necessary precursor to developing CIN and cervical cancer. Smoking, immunosuppression, and poor nutrition are considered cofactors.

24. Cervical cancer arises from the cervical epithelium and is considered a sexually transmitted disease. The progressively serious neoplastic alterations are (a) cervical intraepithelial neoplasia (cervical dysplasia), (b) cervical carcinoma in situ, and (c) invasive cervical carcinoma.

25. Risk factors for cancer of the vagina are in utero diethylstilbestrol (DES) exposure and prior or concurrent cervical cancer. Like cervical cancers, vaginal cancers arise from the epithelium and are identified as intraepithelial neoplasia (dysplasia), carcinoma in situ, or invasive carcinoma. Most vaginal cancers are secondary in nature. Mean age is 55 years for invasive cancer and 45 years for precursor lesions.

26. The major risk for vulvar cancer is a history of HPV infection or squamous dysplasia of the vagina or cervix. Symptoms include chronic vulvar irritation, pruritus, bloody discharge, and a hard, ulcerated area of the vulva or large cauliflower lesions. Peak incidence is in postmenopausal women, but women age 40 years or younger can be affected.

27. Endometrial cancer is the most common cancer of the pelvic region. Risk factors for endometrial cancer include unopposed estrogen exposure, obesity, infertility, failure to ovulate, early menarche or late menopause, and tamoxifen. Oral contraceptive use protects against endometrial and ovarian cancers. Peak incidence occurs at 58 to 60 years of age, approximately 10 years later than peak incidence of precursor lesions.

28. Risk factors for ovarian cancer include early menarche, late menopause, nulliparity, use of fertility drugs, and associations with breast cancer susceptibility genes. Ovarian cancer causes more deaths than any other genital cancer in women.

29. Awareness of sexual dysfunction is relatively new. Chronic illness, medications, infection, sexual trauma, and a variety of psychosocial concerns have been implicated as causes.

30. Infertility, or the inability to conceive after 1 year of unprotected intercourse, affects approximately 15% of all couples. Fertility can be impaired by factors in the male, female, or both partners.

Disorders of the Male Reproductive System

1. Disorders of the urethra include urethritis (inflammation of the urethra) and urethral strictures (narrowing or obstruction of the urethral lumen caused by scarring).

2. Although noninfectious urethritis can occur, most cases of urethritis result from sexually transmitted pathogens. Symptoms of urethritis include dysuria, frequency, urgency, urethral tingling or itching, and clear or purulent discharge. Treatment consists of appropriate antibiotic therapy and avoidance of future chemical or mechanical irritation.

3. Acquired or congenital scarring that causes urethral stricture can be caused by trauma or by severe or untreated urethral infection. The primary symptom is diminished force and caliber of the urinary stream; other symptoms include urinary frequency and hesitancy, mild dysuria, double urine stream or spraying, and postvoiding dribbling. Treatment is usually surgical.

4. Phimosis and paraphimosis are penile disorders involving the foreskin (prepuce). In phimosis the foreskin cannot be retracted over the glans. In paraphimosis the foreskin is retracted and cannot be returned to its normal anatomic position over the glans. Phimosis is caused by poor hygiene and chronic infection and can lead to paraphimosis. Paraphimosis can constrict the penile blood vessels, preventing circulation to the glans.

5. Peyronie disease consists of fibrosis, affecting the corpora cavernosa, which causes penile curvature during erection. Fibrosis prevents engorgement on the affected side, causing a lateral curvature that can prevent intercourse.

6. Priapism, a prolonged painful erection not stimulated by sexual arousal, is a urologic emergency. The corpora cavernosa (but not the corpus spongiosum) fill with blood that does not drain out, probably because of venous obstruction. Priapism is associated with spinal cord trauma, sickle cell disease, leukemia, and pelvic tumors. It can also be idiopathic.

7. Balanitis is an inflammation of the glans penis and usually occurs in conjunction with posthitis. It is associated with phimosis, inadequate cleansing under the foreskin, skin disorders, and infections.

8. Cancer of the penis is rare; major risk factors include HPV, smoking, and consequences of treatment for psoriasis. Penile carcinoma in situ tends to involve the glans; invasive carcinoma of the penis involves the shaft as well.

9. A varicocele is an abnormal dilation of the veins within the spermatic cord caused by either congenital absence of valves in the internal spermatic vein or acquired valvular incompetence.

10. A hydrocele is a collection of fluid between the testicular and scrotal layers of the tunica vaginalis. Hydroceles can be idiopathic or caused by trauma or infection of the testes.

11. A spermatocele is a cyst located between the testis and epididymis that is filled with fluid and sperm.

12. Cryptorchidism is a congenital condition in which one or both testes fail to descend into the scrotum. Treated or untreated cryptorchidism is associated with infertility and a significantly increased risk of testicular cancer.

13. Testicular torsion is the rotation of a testis, which twists blood vessels in the spermatic cord. This interrupts blood supply to the testis, resulting in edema and, if not corrected within 4 to 6 hours, necrosis and atrophy of testicular tissues.

14. Orchitis is an acute inflammation of the testes. Pathogenic organisms may reach the testes through the blood or the lymphatics; most commonly, they reach the testes by ascending through the vas deferens and epididymis. Complications of orchitis include hydrocele and atrophy. Granulomatis orchitis, an autoimmune disease, is a nonspecific, noninfectious, inflammatory process that occurs in middle-age men.

15. Testicular cancer is the most common malignancy in males ages 15 to 35 years. Although its cause is unknown, high androgen levels, genetic predisposition, and a history of cryptorchidism, trauma, or infection may contribute to tumorigenesis. Most testicular neoplasms are germ-cell tumors.

16. Epididymitis, an inflammation of the epididymis, is usually caused by a sexually transmitted pathogen that ascends through the vasa deferentia from an already infected urethra or bladder.

17. Benign prostatic hyperplasia (BPH) is an enlargement of the prostate gland. Symptoms are obstructive or irritative in nature and include urge to urinate often, delay in starting urination, and decreased force of stream. BPH can be treated surgically, with laser therapy, microwave thermotherapy, or medications.

18. Prostatitis can be bacterial or nonbacterial and chronic or acute. Bacterial prostatitis is an infection of the prostate. Acute bacterial prostatitis causes an inflammatory response in which the prostate becomes enlarged, tender, and firm. Chronic bacterial prostatitis is recurrent prostatic infection that eventually causes fibrosis. Nonbacterial prostatitis is prostatic inflammation without evidence of bacterial infection.

19. Prostate cancer is the most common cancer in American males and the incidence varies greatly worldwide. Possible causes involve dietary and hormonal factors, obesity, and age. Only nutrition seems to explain the differences in global incidence. Incidence is greatest among northwestern European and North American men (particularly blacks) older than 65 years.

20. Most cancers of the prostate are adenocarcinomas that develop at the periphery of the gland. Because there are no early symptoms, disease is often advanced at the time of diagnosis.

21. A multifactorial model of prostate carcinogenesis includes (1) androgens act as tumor promoters through receptor mechanisms; (2) to enhance endogenous DNA toxic carcinogens, including ROS and reactive estrogen metabolites and estrogen; and (3) unknown environmental carcinogens. In addition, there are changes in the balance between autocrine/paracrine growth promoting and inhibiting factors, such as IGFs.

22. The microenvironment fuels the metastatic growth of prostate cancer.

23. Sexual dysfunction in males can be caused by any physical or psychologic factor that impairs erection, emission, or ejaculation. Impairment can be caused by a number of physiologic, psychologic, and emotional factors.

24. Spermatogenesis (sperm production by the testes) can be impaired by disruptions of the hypothalamic-pituitary-testicular axis that reduce testosterone secretion and by testicular trauma or atrophy from any cause. Sperm production is also impaired by neoplastic disease, cryptorchidism, or any factor that causes testicular temperature to rise.

25. Sperm quality is impaired by chromosomal abnormalities resulting from genetic factors, irradiation, or toxins. Sperm motility can be impaired by unfavorable constituents or characteristics of semen.

Disorders of the Breast

1. Most disorders of the breast are disorders of the mammary gland, that is, the female breast.

2. Galactorrhea, or inappropriate lactation, is the persistent secretion of a milky substance by one or both breasts in nonpregnant, nonlactating women. Its most common cause is nonpuerperal hyperprolactinemia, a rise in serum prolactin levels that is not associated with pregnancy and childbirth. Hyperprolactinemia can be caused by medications, pituitary tumors, hypothyroidism, chronic stress, or persistent and repeated suckling.

3. Numerous benign conditions occur in ducts and lobules in the breast. Benign lesions are broadly classified as (1) nonproliferating breast lesions, (2) proliferative breast disease, and (3) atypical (atypia) hyperplasia.

4. The term *nonproliferative lesions* is used to discriminate such lesions from the "proliferative" changes associated with increased risk of breast cancer.

5. *Fibrocystic changes (FCC)* is the most widely accepted term for physiologic nodularity and breast tenderness that waxes and wanes with the menstrual cycle. These changes are nonproliferative. Symptoms of FCC affect women ages 30 to 50 years and include cyclic bilateral breast tenderness and transient breast lumps.

6. Proliferative breast lesions without atypia are characterized by proliferation of ductal epithelium and/or stroma without cellular signs suggestive of malignancy. These diverse lesions include (1) moderate or florid hyperplasia, (2) sclerosing adenosis, (3) complex sclerosing (radial scar), (4) papillomas, and (5) fibroadenoma.

7. Proliferative breast lesions with atypia include atypical ductal hyperplasia (ADH) and atypical lobular hyperplasia (ALH). ADH is an increased number of cells mostly within the lumen of the terminal ducts. It includes a continuum of changes—cell structure and placement—ranging from an increase in cellularity to features of ductal carcinoma in situ (DCIS). The cells in ALH do not distend more than 50% of the acinii within a lobule.

8. Breast cancer is the most common form of cancer in American women and second only to lung cancer as the most frequent cause of cancer death. Most breast cancer occurs in women over 50 years of age. The major risk factors for breast cancer are reproductive factors, such as nulliparity; familial factors, such as inherited gene syndromes; and environmental and lifestyle factors, such as radiation exposure. New data on estrogen, estrogen metabolites, and estrogen-dependent growth factors are also implicated.

9. Most breast cancers arise from the ductal epithelium and then may metastasize to the lymphatics, opposite breast, abdominal cavity, lungs, bones, kidneys, liver, adrenal glands, ovaries, and pituitary glands.

10. Pathogenesis of breast cancer probably involves several steps: (1) modification of DNA, (2) growth factors increase the rate of growth, and (3) specific oncogenes that are progressively modified or specific suppressor genes that are lost, leading to metastatic disease. In addition, metastatic growth may be related to resistance to apoptosis and stromal cell interactions with cancer cells.

11. Ductal carcinoma in situ (DCIS) refers to a malignant heterogenous group of lesions limited to ducts and lobules. Because not all DCIS lesions progress to invasion or become clinically significant, the main concern is which DCIS lesions become invasive.

12. The first clinical manifestation of breast cancer is usually a small, painless lump in the breast. Other manifestations include palpable lymph nodes in the axilla, dimpling of the skin, nipple and skin retraction, nipple discharge, ulcerations, reddened skin, and bone pain associated with bony metastases.

13. Treatment is based on the extent or stage of the cancer and includes surgery, radiation, chemotherapy, hormone therapy, and biologic therapy.

14. Gynecomastia is the overdevelopment (hyperplasia) of breast tissue in a male. It is first seen as a firm, palpable mass at least 2 cm in diameter located in the subareolar area. Gynecomastia affects 32% to 40% of the male population. Incidence is greatest among adolescents and men older than 50 years.

15. Gynecomastia is caused by hormonal or breast tissue alterations that cause estrogen to dominate. These alterations can result from systemic disorders, drugs, neoplasms, or idiopathic causes.

16. Although breast cancer is relatively uncommon in males, it has a poor prognosis because men tend to delay seeking treatment. Most breast cancers in men are estrogen receptor positive. Incidence is greatest in men in their sixties.

KEY TERMS

Acute bacterial prostatitis, 815
Adenomyosis, 793
Amenorrhea, 774
Anorgasmia (orgasmic dysfunction), 802
Anovulation, 775
Atypical hyperplasia, 825
Balanitis, 805
Bartholinitis (Bartholin cyst), 787
Benign prostatic hyperplasia (BPH)
     (benign prostatic hypertrophy), 813
Cervical carcinoma in situ, 795
Cervical intraepithelial neoplasm (CIN)
     (cervical dysplasia), 795
Cervicitis, 786
Chronic bacterial prostatitis, 815
Comedo, 846
Complex sclerosing lesion (radial scar), 825
Corpus luteum cyst, 791
Cryptorchidism, 809
Cysts, 824
Cystocele, 788
Cystourethrocele, 790
Delayed puberty, 772
Dermoid cysts, 791
Disorders of desire (inhibited sexual
     pleasure, decreased libido), 802
Ductal carcinoma in situ (DCIS), 845
Ductal hyperplasia, 825
Dysfunctional uterine bleeding (DUB), 777
Dyspareunia (painful intercourse), 802
Ectopic testis, 809
Endometrial polyp, 791

Endometriosis, 793
Enterocele, 790
Epididymitis, 811
Epithelial hyperplasia, 825
Fibrocystic changes (FCC), 824
Florid hyperplasia, 825
Follicular cysts, 791
Functional cysts, 790
Galactorrhea (inappropriate lactation), 823
Gynecomastia, 850
Heterosexual precocious puberty, 773
Hirsutism, 776
Hydrocele, 808
Hyperprolactinemia, 775
Incomplete precocious puberty, 773
Infertility, 802
Invasive carcinoma of the cervix, 797
Isosexual precocious puberty, 773
Leiomyomas (uterine fibroids), 792
Lobular carcinoma in situ (LCIS), 846
Lobular hyperplasia, 825
Mucopurulent cervicitis (MPC), 786
Nonbacterial prostatitis, 816
Nonpuerperal hyperprolactinemia, 823
Oophoritis, 782
Orchitis, 810
Papillomas, 825
Paraphimosis, 804
Pelvic inflammatory disease (PID), 782
Pessary, 788
Peyronie disease (bent nail syndrome), 804
Phimosis, 804

Polycystic ovary syndrome (PCOS), 779
Precocious puberty, 773
Premenstrual syndrome (PMS), 780
Priapism, 805
Primary amenorrhea, 774
Primary dysmenorrhea, 774
Prolactin-inhibiting factor (PIF), 823
Prostate-specific antigen (PSA), 814
Prostatitis, 814
Prostatodynia, 815
Rapid orgasm, 802
Rectocele, 790
Retrograde menstruation, 793
Salpingitis, 782
Sclerosing adenosis, 825
Secondary amenorrhea, 775
Secondary dysmenorrheal, 774
Sexual dysfunction, 821
Spermatocele, 808
Torsion of the testis, 809
Urethral stricture, 803
Urethritis, 803
Urethrocele, 789
Uterine prolapse, 788
Uterine sarcomas, 799
Vaginismus, 802
Vaginitis, 784
Varicocele, 807
Vulvitis, 786
Xenoestrogens, 839

MEDIA RESOURCES

Review questions and answers for this chapter are available in the *CD Companion* included with this book. Also see the CD for animations on *prostate cancer* and *breast cancer*.

WebLinks—links to Internet sites pertaining to this chapter—are available on Evolve at http://evolve.elsevier.com/McCance/.

REFERENCES

1. American Cancer Society: Estimated new cancer cases and deaths by sex, US, 2005. In *Cancer facts & figures—2005*, Atlanta, 2005, American Cancer Society.
2. Reid RL: Amenorrhea. In LJ Copeland, JF Farrell, editors: *Textbook of gynecology*, ed 2, Philadelphia, 2000, Saunders.
3. Healtheon/WebMD: Hypothalamic disorders. In *Scientific American Medicine*, 1999. Available at www.samed.com/sam/forms/index.htm.
4. Simon D: Puberty in chronically diseased patients, *Horm Res* 57(Suppl 2):53-56, 2002.
5. Bo-Abbas Y et al: Autosomal recessive idiopathic hypogonadotropic hypogonadism: genetic analysis excludes mutations in the gonodotrapin-releasing hormone (GnRH) and GnRh receptor genes, *J Clin Endocrinol Metab* 88(6):2730-2737, 2003.
6. Bernanova M et al: Prevalence, phenotypic spectrum, and modes of inheritance of gonadotripin-releasing hormore receptor mutations in idiopathic hypogonadotropic hypogonadism. *J Clin Endocrinol Metab* 86(4):1580-1588, 2001.
7. Parent AS et al: The timing of normal puberty and the age limits of sexual precocity: variations around the world, secular trends, and changes after migration, *Endocr Rev* 24(5):668-693, 2003.

8. Rudolph AM, Hoffman JIE, Rudolph CD: *Rudolph's pediatrics*, ed 20, Stamford, Conn, 1996, Appleton & Lange.
9. Cacciari E, Mazanti L, Italian Study Group for Turner Syndrome: Final height of patients with Turner's syndrome treated with growth hormone (GH): indications for GH therapy alone at high doses and late estrogen therapy, *J Clin Endocrinol Metab* 84(12):4510, 1999.
10. Saenger P: Growth-promoting strategies in Turner's syndrome, *J Clin Endocrinol Metab* 84(12):4345, 1999.
11. Seminara SB, Hayes FJ, Crowley WF: Gonadotropin-releasing hormone deficiency in the human (idiopathic hypogonadotropic hypogonadism and Kallman's syndrome): pathophysiological and genetic considerations, *Endocr Rev* 19(5):521, 1998.
12. Kaplowitz PB et al: Reexamination of the age limit for defining when puberty is precocious in girls in the United States: implications for evaluation and treatment, *Pediatrics* 104(4):936, 1999.
13. Massachusetts General Hospital Pediatric Endocrine Research Unit. Available at http://mghra-partners.org/narratives/BoepplePA2.html.
14. Palmert MR et al: Is obesity an outcome of gonadotropin-releasing hormone agonist administration? *J Clin Endocrinol Metab* 84(12):4480, 1999.
15. Marjoribanks J, Proctor ML, Farquhar C: Nonsteroidal anti-inflammatory drugs for primary dysmenorrhoea, *Cochrane Database Syst Rev* (4):CD001751, 2003.
16. Speroff L, Fritz MA: *Clinical gynecologic endocrinology and infertility*, ed 7, Philadelphia, 2005, Lippincott Williams & Wilkins.
17. Wolf LL, Schumann L: Dysmenorrhea, *J Am Acad Nurse Pract* 11(3):125, 1999.
18. Reid RL: Amenorrhea. In Copeland LJ, Farrell JF, editors: *Textbook of gynecology*, ed 2, Philadelphia, 2000, Saunders.
19. Healey PM, Jacobson EJ: *Common medical diagnoses: an algorithmic approach*, ed 3, Philadelphia, 2000, Saunders.
20. Wetzel W: Micronized progesterone: a new option for women's health care, *Nurse Pract* 24(5):62, 1999.

21. Warren MP, Biller MK, Shangold MD: A new clinical option for hormone replacement therapy in women with secondary amenorrhea: effects of cyclic administration of progesterone from the sustained-release vaginal gel Crinone (45 and 8%) on endometrial morphologic features and withdrawal bleeding, *Am J Obstet Gynecol* 180(1):42, 1999.

22. Al-Inany H: Intrauterine adhesions: an update, *Acta Obstet Gynecol Scand* 80(11):986-993, 2001.

23. Mencaglia L, Perino A, Hamou J: Hysteroscopy in perimenopausal and postmenopausal women with abnormal uterine bleeding, *J Reprod Med* 32(8):577, 1987.

24. Weingold AB: Abnormal bleeding. In Kase N, Weingold AB, Gershenson DM, editors: *Principles and practice of clinical gynecology*, New York, 1990, Churchill Livingstone.

25. Kim MH: Dysfunctional uterine bleeding. In Copeland LJ, Farrell JF, editors: *Textbook of gynecology*, ed 2, Philadelphia, 2000, Saunders.

26. Prior JC: Perimenopause: the complex endocrinology of the menopausal transition, *Endocr Rev* 19(4):397, 1998.

27. Dealy MF: Dysfunctional uterine bleeding in adolescents, *Nurse Pract* 23(5):12, 1998.

28. Oriel KA, Schager S: Abnormal uterine bleeding, *Am Fam Physician* 60(5):1371, 1999.

29. Hodgson DA et al: Microwave endometrial ablation: development, clinical trials, and outcomes at three years, *Br J Obstet Gynaecol* 106(7):684, 1999.

30. Aberdeen Endometrial Ablation Trials Group: A randomised trial of endometrial ablation versus hysterectomy for the treatment of dysfunctional uterine bleeding: outcome at four years, *Br J Obstet Gynaecol* 106(4):360-366, 1999.

31. Hawe JA et al: Cavaterm thermal balloon ablation for the treatment of menorrhagia, *Br J Obstet Gynaecol* 106(11):1143-1148, 1999.

32. McCausland AM, McCausland VM: Partial rollerball endometrial ablation: a modification of total ablation to treat menorrhagia without causing complications from intrauterine adhesions, *Am J Obstet Gynecol* 180(6):1512, 1999.

33. Ehrmann DA: Polycystic ovary syndrome, *N Engl J Med* 352(12):1223-1236, 2005.

34. Balen A: Pathogenesis of polycystic ovary syndrome—the enigma unravels? *Lancet* 354(9183):966-967, 1999.

35. Nestler J: *Insulin resistance and women's health: new insights into polycystic ovary syndrome*. Paper presented at the 14th Annual National Conference of the American Academy of Nurse Practitioners, Atlanta, June 17, 1999.

36. Patel SR, Korykowski MT: Treating polycystic ovary syndrome: today's approach, *Womens Health Prim Care* 3(2):109, 2000.

37. Diamanti-Kandarakis E et al: A survey of the polycystic ovary syndrome in the Greek island of Lesbos: hormonal and metabolic profile, *J Clin Endocrinol Metab* 84(11):4006, 1999.

38. Couse JF et al: Prevention of the polycystic phenotype and characterization of ovulatory capacity in the estrogen receptor—a knockout mouse, *Endocrinology* 140(12):5855, 1999.

39. Pugeat M, Ducluzeau PH: Insulin resistance, polycystic ovary syndrome and metformin, *Drugs* 58(suppl 1):41, 1999.

40. Gordon CM: Menstrual disorders in adolescents: excess androgens and the polycystic ovary syndrome, *Pediatr Clin North Am* 46(3):519, 1999.

41. Radon PA, McMahon MJ, Meyer WR: Impaired glucose tolerance in pregnant women with polycystic ovary syndrome, *Obstet Gynecol* 94(2):194, 1999.

42. Book CB, Dunaif A: Selective insulin resistance in the polycystic ovary syndrome, *J Clin Endocrinol Metab* 84(9):3110, 1999.

43. Amato G et al: Lack of insulin-like growth factor binding protein-3 variation after follicle-stimulating hormone stimulation in women with polycystic ovary syndrome undergoing in vitro fertilization, *Fertil Steril* 72(3):454, 1999.

44. Orabi HE et al: Serum leptin as an additional possible pathogenic factor in polycystic ovary syndrome, *Clin Biochem* 32(1):71, 1999.

45. Mendonca HC et al: Positive correlation of serum leptin with estradiol levels in patients with polycystic ovary syndrome, *Braz J Med Biol Res* 37(5):729-735, 2004.

46. Iuorno MJ, Nestler JE: Insulin-lowering drugs in polycystic ovary syndrome, *Obstet Gynecol Clin North Am* 28(1):153-164, 2001.

47. Chian RC et al: Pregnancies from in vitro matured oocytes retrieved from patients with polycystic ovary syndrome after priming with human chorionic gonadotropin, *Fertil Steril* 72(4):639, 1999.

48. Reid R: *Premenstrual syndrome: current problems in obstetrics, gynecology, and fertility*, St Louis, 1985, Mosby.

49. Zerbe KJ: *Women's mental health in primary care*, Philadelphia, 1999, Saunders.

50. Woods NF et al: *Prevalence of perimenstrual symptoms: final report*, Seattle, 1989, University of Washington.

51. York R et al: Characteristics of premenstrual syndrome, *Obstet Gynecol* 73(4):601, 1989.

52. Roca C, Schmidt PJ, Rubinow DR: A follow-up study of premenstrual syndrome, *J Clin Psychiatry* 60(11):763, 1999.

53. Rapkin AJ: *Update on the treatments for PMS/PMDD*. Paper presented at the 8th International Nurse Practitioner Conference, San Diego, September 30, 2000.

54. Freeman EW et al: Differential response to antidepressants in women with premenstrual syndrome/premenstrual dysphoric disorder: a randomized controlled trial, *Arch Gen Psychiatry* 56(10):932-939, 1999.

55. Freeman EW: Luteal phase administration for agents for the treatment of premenstrual dysphoric disorder, *CNS Drugs*, 18(7):435-468, 2004.

56. Lawson MA, Blythe MJ: Pelvic inflammatory disease in adolescents, *Pediatr Clin North Am* 46(4):767, 1999.

57. Hatcher RA et al: *Contraceptive technology*, New York, 1998, Ardent Media.

58. Centers for Disease Control and Prevention: *Sexually transmitted diseases: treatment guidelines*, 1998, Washington, DC, 1998, DHHS.

59. Richter HE et al: The association of interleukin-6 with clinical and laboratory parameters of acute pelvic inflammatory disease, *Am J Obstet Gynecol* 181(4):940, 1999.

60. Peeling RW et al: Antibody response to the chlamydial heat-shock protein 60 in an experimental model of chronic pelvic inflammatory disease in monkeys, *J Infect Dis* 180(3):774-779, 1999.

61. Hillier SL et al: Role of bacterial vaginosis-associated microorganisms in endometritis, *Am J Obstet Gynecol* 175(2):435-441, 1996.

62. Stenchever MA et al: *Comprehensive gynecology*, ed 4, St. Louis, 2001, Mosby

63. Division of STD Prevention, US Department of Health and Human Services: *Sexually transmitted disease surveillance*, 1998, Atlanta, 1998, Centers for Disease Control and Prevention.

64. Division of STD Prevention, US Department of Health and Human Services: *Sexually transmitted disease surveillance*, 1995, Atlanta, 1996, Centers for Disease Control and Prevention.

65. Brubaker L: Abnormalities of pelvic support. In Copeland LJ, Farrell JF, editors: *Textbook of gynecology*, ed 2, Philadelphia, 2000, Saunders.

66. Dorr CH: Relaxation of pelvic supports. In DeCherney AH, Pernoll ML, editors: *Current obstetric and gynecologic diagnosis and treatment*, ed 8, Norwalk, Conn, 1994, Appleton & Lange.

67. McCartney CR et al: Hypothalamic regulation of cyclic ovulation: evidence that the increase in gonadotropin-releasing hormone pulse frequency during the follicular phase reflects the gradual loss of the restraining effects of progesterone, *J Clin Endocrin Metab* 87(5):2194-2200, 2002.

68. Adelson MD, Adelson KL: Miscellaneous benign disorders of the upper genital tract. In Copeland LJ, Farrell JF, editors: *Textbook of gynecology*, ed 2, Philadelphia, 2000, Saunders.

69. Ueda H et al: Unusual appearances of uterine leiomyomas: MR imaging findings and their histopathologic backgrounds, *Radiographics* 19:S131-145, 1999.

70. Palomba S et al: Long-term effectiveness and safety of GnRH agonist plus raloxifene administration in women with uterine leiomyomas, *Hum Reprod* 19(6):1308-1314, 2004.

71. Olive DL, Lindeheim SR, Pritts EA: Non-surgical management of leiomyoma: impact on fertility, *Curr Opin Obstet Gynecol* 16(3):239-243, 2004.

72. Reinhold C et al: Uterine adenomyosis: endovaginal US and MR imaging features with histopathologic correlation, *Radiographics* 19:S147, 1999.

73. Guarnaccia MM, Silverberg K, Olive DL: Endometriosis and adenomyosis. In Copeland LJ, Farrell JF, editors: *Textbook of gynecology*, ed 2, Philadelphia, 2000, Saunders.

74. Wardle PG, Hull MG: Is endometriosis a disease? *Baillieres Clin Obstet Gynaecol* 7(4):673, 1993.

75. Brinton LA et al: Cancer risks after a hospital discharge diagnosis of endometriosis, *Am J Obstet Gynecol* 176(3):572-579, 1997.

76. Sampson JA: Peritoneal endometriosis due to the menstrual dissemination of endometrial tissue into the peritoneal cavity, *Am J Obstet Gynecol* 14:422, 1927.

77. Suzumori N et al: Expression of secretory leukocyte protease inhibitor in women with endometriosis, *Fertil Steril* 72(5):889, 1999.

78. Ota H et al: Immunohistochemical assessment of superoxide dismutase expression in the endometrium in endometriosis and adenomyosis, *Fertil Steril* 72(1):129, 1999.

79. Canis M et al: Classification of endometriosis, Baillieres Clin Obstet Gynaecol 7(4):759, 1994.

80. American Cancer Society: *Cancer facts and figures—2005,* Atlanta, 2005, American Cancer Society.

81. Kjaer SK et al: Human papillomavirus—the most significant risk determinant of cervical intraepithelial neoplasia, *Int J Cancer* 65(5):601-606, 1996.

82. Smith JS et al: Chlamydia trachomatis and invasive cervical cancer: a pooled analysis of the IARC multicentric case-control study, *Int J Cancer* 111(3):431-439, 2004.

83. Center for Disease Prevention and Epidemiology: Anogenital papillomavirus infections, *CD Summary* 47(2), 1998.

84. Klaus BD, Grodesky MJ: Cervical dysplasia in women with HIV, *Nurse Pract* 24(8):79, 1999.

85. Wright TC Jr et al: 2001 consensus guidelines for the management of women with cervical cytological abnormalities, *Am J Obstet Gynecol* 189(6):295-304, 2003.

86. Hopkins MP: Vaginal neoplasms. In Copeland LH, Farrell JF, editors: *Textbook of gynecology,* ed 2, Philadelphia, 2000, Saunders.

87. Research report: combination therapy for cervical cancer, *Womens Health Prim Care* 2(60):479, 1999.

88. American Cancer Society: *Cancer facts and figures—2004,* Atlanta, 2004, American Cancer Society.

89. Gordon AN: Vulvar neoplasms. In Copeland LJ, Farrell JF, editors: *Textbook of gynecology,* ed 2, Philadelphia, 2000, Saunders.

90. Burke TW, Morris M: Adenocarcinoma of the endometrium. In Copeland LJ, Farrell JF, editors: *Textbook of gynecology,* ed 2, Philadelphia, 2000, Saunders.

91. Steren AJ: Improved ways of screening for gynecologic cancers, *Contemp Ob Gyn* 75:42, 1995.

92. Nickline JL, Copeland LJ: Uterine sarcomas. In Copeland LJ, Farrell JF, editors: *Textbook of gynecology,* ed 2, Philadelphia, 2000, Saunders.

93. Rodriquez GC et al: Effect of progestin on the ovarian epithelium of macaques: cancer prevention through apoptosis? *J Soc Gynecol Invest* 5(5):271-276, 1998.

94. Blast RC, Mills GB: Molecular pathogenesis of ovarian cancer. In Mendelsohn J et al, editors: *The molecular basis of cancer,* ed 2, Philadelphia, 2001, Saunders.

95. Lancaster JM et al: *BRCA2* mutations in primary breast and ovarian cancer, *Nat Genet* 13(2):238-240, 1996.

96. Gershenon D: Epithelial ovarian cancer. In Copeland LJ, Farrell JF, editors: *Textbook of gynecology,* ed 2, Philadelphia, 2000, Saunders.

97. See HT, Kavanagh JJ: Novel agents in epithelial ovarian cancer, *Cancer Invest* 22(Suppl 2):29-44, 2004.

98. Krassas GE, Pontikides N: Male reproductive function in relation with thyroid alterations, *Best Pract Res Clin Endocrinol Metab* 18(2):183-195, 2004.

99. Wilcox AJ, Weinberg CR, Baird DD: Timing of sexual intercourse in relation to ovulation, *N Engl J Med* 33(23):1517, 1995.

100. LaRock DR, Sant GR: Lower urinary tract infections in men. In Nseyo UO, Weinman E, Lamm DL, editors: *Urology for primary care physicians,* Philadelphia, 1999, Saunders.

101. McAninch JW: Disorders of the penis and male urethra. In Tanagho EA, McAninch JW, editors: *Smith's general urology,* ed 14, Norwalk, Conn, 1995, Appleton & Lange.

102. American Cancer Society: *Penile cancer resource center,* 1999. Available at www3.cancer.org/cancerinfo.

103. Altman AL et al: Cocaine associated priapism, *J Urol* 161(6):1817-1818, 1999.

104. American Cancer Society: Penile cancer. In *Cancer response system document #10005,* New York, 1995, The Society.

105. Nasca MR, Innocenzi D, Micali G: Penile cancer among patients with genital lichen sclerous, *J Am Acad Dermatol* 41(6):911-914, 1999.

106. Presti JC, Herr HW: Genital tumors. In Tanagho EA, McAninch JW, editors: *Smith's general urology,* ed 14, Norwalk, Conn, 1995, Appleton & Lange.

107. Lindegarrds JC et al: A retrospective analysis of 82 cases of cancer of the penis, *Br J Urol* 77(6):883, 1996.

108. Kolon TF, Albertsen PC: Diagnosis and treatment of scrotal abnormalities, *Clin Advisor* 47:47-48, 53-56, 2000.

109. Franklin G, Nseyo UO: Anatomic basis of common urologic diseases. In Nseyo UO, Weinman E, Lamm DL, editors: *Urology for primary care physicians,* Philadelphia, 1999, Saunders.

110. McAninch JW: Disorders of the testis, scrotum, and spermatic cord. In Tanagho EA, McAninch JW, editors: *Smith's general urology,* ed 14, Norwalk, Conn, 1995, Appleton & Lange.

111. Galejs LE, Usaf M: Diagnosis and treatment of the acute scrotum, *Am Fam Physician* 59(4):817, 1999.

112. Del Pizzo JJ, Jarow JP: Management of male infertility. In Nseyo UO, Weinman E, Lamm DL, editors: *Urology for primary care physicians,* Philadelphia, 1999, Saunders.

113. Rosenthal MS: *The fertility sourcebook,* Los Angeles, 1998, Lowell House.

114. Schenkman EM, Tarry WT: Congenital anomalies. In Nseyo UO, Weinman E, Lamm DL, editors: *Urology for primary care physicians,* Philadelphia, 1999, Saunders.

115. CancerNet: *Cancer facts: questions and answers about testicular cancer,* National Cancer Institute, 2000. Available at www.cancernet.nci.nih.gov/.

116. Lanum DL: Carcinoma of the genitourinary system. In Nseyo UO, Weinman E, Lamm DL, editors: *Urology for primary care physicians,* Philadelphia, 1999, Saunders.

117. Gebrosky NP, Nseyo UO: Sexually transmitted diseases. In Nseyo UO, Weinman E, Lamm DL, editors: *Urology for primary care physicians,* Philadelphia, 1999, Saunders.

118. LaRock DR, Sant GR: Lower urinary tract infections. In Nseyo UO, Weinman E, Lamm DL, editors: *Urology for primary care physicians,* Philadelphia, 1999, Saunders.

119. Partin AW: Benign prostratic hyperplasia. In Lepor H, editor: *Prostatic diseases,* Philadelphia, 2000, Saunders.

120. Untergasser G et al: Proliferative disorders of the aging human prostate: involvement of protein hormones and their receptors, *Exp Gerontol* 34(2):275, 1999.

121. Jepson JV, Bruskewitz RC: Clinical manifestations and indications for treatment. In Lepor H, editor: *Prostatic diseases,* Philadelphia, 2000, Saunders.

122. Barry MJ, Meigs JB: Benign prostatic hyperplasia. In Lepor H, editor: *Prostatic diseases,* Philadelphia, 2000, Saunders.

123. Narayan P: Neoplasms of the prostate gland. In Tanagho EA, McAninch JW, editors: *Smith's general urology,* ed 14, Norwalk, Conn, 1995, Appleton & Lange.

124. Roehrborn CG: In Lepor H, editor: *Prostatic diseases,* Philadelphia, 2000, Saunders.

125. Foratos DL, de La Rosette JJ: Heat treatment for the prostate: where do we stand in 2000? *Curr Opin Urol* 11(1):35, 2000.

126. Chiu KY, Yong CR: Effects of finasteride on prostate volume and prostate specific antigen, *J Chin Med Assoc* 67(11):571-574, 2004.

127. Shibata A, Ma J, Whittemore AS: Prostate cancer incidence and mortality in the United States and the United Kingdom, *J Natl Can Inst* 90(16):1230-1231, 1998.

128. Kolonel LN, Nomura AM, Cooney RV: Dietary fat and prostate cancer: current status, *J Natl Cancer Inst* 91(5):414, 1999.

129. Signorello LB, Adami H: Prostate cancer. In Adami H, Hunter D, Trichopoulos D, editors: *Textbook of cancer epidemiology,* New York, 2002, Oxford Press.

130. Calle EE et al: Overweight, obesity, and mortality from cancer in a prospectively studied cohort of U.S. adults, *N Engl J Med* 348(17):1625-1638, 2003.

131. Rodriquez C et al: Body mass index, height, and prostate cancer mortality in two large cohorts of adult men in the United States, *Cancer Epidemiol Biomarkers Prev* 10(4):345-353, 2001.

132. Platz EA: Energy imbalance and prostate cancer, *J Nutr* 132(11 suppl):3471S-3481S, 2002.

133. Bosland MC: The role of steroid hormones in prostate carcinogenesis, *J Natl Cancer Inst Monogr* 27:39-66, 2000.

134. Heber D, Fair WR, Ornish D: *Nutrition and prostate cancer: a monograph from the CaP CURE Nutrition Project,* ed 2, Santa Monica, Calif, 1998, CaP CURE.

135. Denis L et al: Diet and its preventive role in prostatic disease, *Eur Urol* 35(5-6):377, 1999.

136. Yang M, Sytkowski AJ: Differential expression and androgen regulation of the human selenium-binding protein gene hSP56 in prostate cancer cells, *Cancer Res* 58(14):3150, 1998.

137. Zhao XY et al: 1-Alpha,25-dihydroxyvitamin D3 inhibits prostate cancer cell growth by androgen-dependent and androgen-independent mechanisms, *Endocrinology* 141(7):2548, 2000.
138. Arnot R: *The prostate cancer protection plan: the powerful foods, supplements, and drugs that could save your life,* Boston, 2000, Little, Brown.
139. Giovannucci E et al: Intake of carotenoids and retinol in relation to risk of prostate cancer, *J Natl Cancer Inst* 87(23):1767, 1995.
140. Ebling DW et al: Development of prostate cancer after pituitary dysfunction: a report of 8 patients, *Urology* 49(4):564, 1998.
141. Oosthuzien JM et al: Melatonin and steroid-dependent carcinomas, *Andrologia* 21(5):429, 1989.
142. Roberts JT, Essehigh DM: Adenocarcinoma of prostate in 40-year-old body builders, *Lancet* 2(8509):742, 1986.
143. Cunha GR et al: Role of the stromal microenvironment in carcinogenesis of the prostate, *Int J Cancer* 107(1):1-10, 2003.
144. Giovannucci E et al: A prospective cohort study of vasectomy and prostate cancer in US men, *JAMA* 269(7):873, 1993.
145. Peterson RE et al: Vasectomy and the risk of prostate cancer, *Am J Epidemiol* 135(3):324, 1992.
146. Honda GD et al: Vasectomy, cigarette smoking, and age at first sexual intercourse as risk factors for prostate cancer in middle-aged men, *Br J Cancer* 57(3):326, 1988.
147. Klein EA: An update on prostate cancer, *Cleve Clin J Med* 62(5):325, 1995.
148. Giovannucci E et al: Smoking and risk of total fatal prostate cancer in United States health professionals, *Cancer Epidemiol Biomarkers Prev* 8(4 pt 1):277, 1999.
149. Brown SL, Resnick MI: Transrectal ultrasound and the prostate biopsy: clinical and pathologic issues. In Lepor H, editor: *Prostatic diseases,* Philadelphia, 2000, Saunders.
150. Parnes HL, Thompson IM, Ford LG: Review article: prevention of hormone -related cancers: prostate cancer, *J Clin Oncol* 23(2):368-377, 2005.
151. Chung LW et al: Molecular insights into prostate cancer progression: the missing link of tumor microenvironment, *J Urol* 173(1):10-20, 2005.
153. Tanejo SS: The rationale for early detection of prostate cancer. In Lepor H, editor: *Prostatic diseases,* Philadelphia, 2000, Saunders.
154. Moule JW et al: Prostate-specific antigen values at the time of prostate cancer diagnosis in African-American men, *JAMA* 274(16):1277, 1995.
155. Kirby R, Fitzpatrick J: Prostate-specific antigen testing for the early detection of prostate cancer, *BJU Int* 94(7):966-967.
156. Stamey TA: The era of serum prostate specific antigens as a marker for biopsy of the prostate and detecting prostate cancer is now over in the USA, *BJU Int* 94(7):963-964, 2004.
157. Schwenk TL: PSA screening lacks value, *J Watch N Engl J Med* 25(10):7-8, 2005.
158. Salgaller ML: Prostate cancer immunotherapy at the dawn of the new millennium, *Expert Opin Investig Drugs* 9(6):1217, 2000.
159. American Cancer Society: *Cancer facts and figures—2005,* Atlanta, 2005, American Cancer Society. Available at www.cancer.org/docroot/stt/stt_0.asp.
160. Kim ED, Lipshultz ED: Male infertility. In Copeland LJ, Farrell JF, editors: *Textbook of gynecology,* ed 2, Philadelphia, 2000, Saunders.
161. Pierik FH et al: Serum inhibin B as a marker of spermatogenesis, *J Clin Endocrinol Metab* 83(9):3110, 1998.
162. Harney KA, Smith LF: The breast. In DeCherney AH, Pernoll ML, editors: *Current obstetric and gynecologic diagnosis and treatment,* ed 8, Norwalk, Conn, 1994, Appleton & Lange.
163. Haagensen CD: *Diseases of the breast,* Philadelphia, 1986, Saunders.
164. Kase N, Weingold AB, Gershenon DM, editors: *Principles and practice of clinical gynecology,* ed 2, New York, 1990, Churchill Livingstone.
165. Friedenreich C et al: Risk factors for benign proliferative breast disease, *Int J Epidemiol* 29(4):634, 2000.
166. Lester SC: The breast. In Kumar V, Abbas AK, Fausto N, editors: *Robbins & Cotran pathologic basis of disease,* ed 7, Philadelphia, 2005, Elsevier-Saunders.
167. Jacobs TW: Radial scars in benign breast-biopsy specimens and the risk of breast cancer, *N Engl J Med* 340(6):430, 1999.
168. Sharkey FE, Allred DC, Valente PT: Breast. In Damjanov I, Linder J, editors: *Anderson's pathology,* ed 10, St Louis, 1996, Mosby.
169. Berg JW: Clinical implications of risk factors for breast cancer, *Cancer* 53(3 Suppl):589-591, 1984.

170. Guiliano AE: Breast. In Tierney LM, McPhee SH, Papadakis MA, editors: *Current medical diagnosis and treatment,* ed 35, Norwalk, Conn, 1996, Appleton & Lange.
171. Russo J, Russo I: *Molecular basis of breast cancer: prevention and treatment,* Germany, 2004, Springer.
172. Russo I, Russo J: Mammary gland neoplasia in long-term rodent studies, *Environ Health Perspect* 104(19):938-967, 1996.
173. Thordarson G et al: Refractoriness to mammary tumorigenesis in parous rats: is it caused by persistent changes in the hormonal environment or permanent biochemical alterations in the mammary epithelia, *Carcinogenesis* 16(11):2847-2853, 1995.
174. Thordarson G et al: Mammary tumorigenesis in growth hormone deficient dwarf rats: effects of hormonal treatments, *Breast Cancer Res Treat* 87(3):277-290, 2004.
175. Swanson SM, Unterman TG: The growth hormone deficient spontaneous dwarf rat is resistant to chemically induced mammary carcinogenesis, *Carcinogenesis* 23(6):977-982, 2002.
176. Beral V, Hannaford P, Kay C: Oral contraceptive use and malignancies of the genital tract, *Lancet* ii:1331-1334, 1988.
177. Shaw RW: Adverse long term effects of oral contraceptives—a review, *Br J Obst Gynecol* 94(8):724-730, 1987.
178. Goepfert TM et al: Progesterone facilitates chromosome instability (aneupoloidy) in *p53* null normal mammary epithelial cells, *FASEB J* 14(13):2221-2229, 2000.
179. Greendale GA et al: Effects of estrogen and estrogen-progestin on mammographic parenchymal density, *Ann Int Med* 130(4 Pt1):262-269, 1999.
180. Ross RK et al: Effect of hormone replacement therapy on breast cancer risk: estrogen versus estrogen plus progestin, *J Natl Cancer Inst* 92(4):328-332, 2000.
181. Schairer C et al: Menopausal estrogen and estrogen-progestin replacement therapy and breast cancer risk, *JAMA* 283(4):485-491, 2000.
182. Saeed M et al: Slow loss of deoxyribose from the N7 deoxyguanosine adducts of estradiol-3,4-quinone and hex Estrol-3,(4(-quinone. Implications for mutagenic activity, *Steroids* 70(1):29-35, 2005.
183. Chetrite GS et al: Comparison of estrogen concentrations, estrone sulfatase and aromatase activities in normal and in cancerous, human breast tissues, *J Steroid Biochem Mol Biol* 72(1-2):23-27, 2000.
184. Nakata T et al: Role of steroid sulfatase in local formation of estrogen in postmenopausal breast cancer patients, *J Steroid Biochem Mol Biol* 86(3-5):455-460, 2003.
185. Pasqualine JR et al: Concentrations of estrone, estradiol, and estrone sulfate and evaluation of sulfatase and aromatase activities in pre- and postmenopausal breast cancer patients, *J Clin Endocrinol Metab* 81(4):1460-1464, 1996.
186. Labrie F: Intracrinology, *Mol Cell Endocrinol* 78:C113-C118, 1991.
187. Labrie F et al: Structure, regulation and role of 3 beta-hydroxysteroid dehydrogenase, 17 beta-hydroxysteroid dehydrogenase and aromatase enzymes in the formation of sex steroids in classical and peripheral intracrine tissues, *Bailliere's Clin Endocrinol Metab* 8(2):451-474, 1994.
188. Dowsett M: Future uses for aromatase inhibitors in breast cancer, *J Steroid Biochem Mol Biol* 61(3-6):261-266, 1997.
189. Miller WR, O'Neill J: The importance of local synthesis of estrogen within the breast, *Steroids* 50(4-6):537-548, 1987.
190. Falany JL, Falany CN: Regulation of estrogen activity by sulfation in human MCF-7 breast cancer cells, *Oncol Res* 9(11-12):589-596, 1997.
191. Martel C et al: Distribution of 17 beta-hydroxysteroid dehydrogenase gene expression and activity in rat and human tissues, *J Steroid Biochem Mol Biol* 41(3-8):597-603, 1992.
192. Utsumi T et al: Steroid sulfatase expression is an independent predictor of recurrence in human breast cancer, *Cancer Res* 59(2):377-381, 1999.
193. Miyoshi Y et al: High expression of steroid sulfatase in mRNA predicts poor prognosis in patients with estrogen receptor-positive breast cancer, *Clin Cancer Res* 9(6):2288-2293, 2003.
194. Baum M: Anastrozole alone or in combination with tamoxifen versus tamoxifen alone for adjuvant treatment of postmenopausal women with early breast cancer: first results of the ATAC randomized trial, *Lancet* 359(9324):2131-2139, 2002.
195. Yu H, Berkel H: Insulin-like growth factors and cancer, *J La State Med Assoc* 151(4):218, 1999.
196. Yee D, Lee AV: Crosstalk between the insulin-like growth factors and estrogens in breast cancer, *J Mammary Gland Biol Neoplasia* 5(1):107, 2000.

197. Rao ChV et al: Human chorionic gonadotropin decreases proliferation and invasion of breast cancer MCF-7 cells by inhibiting NF-κB and AP-1 activation, *J Biol Chem* 279(24):25503-25510, 2004.

198. Tanaka Y et al: Gonadotropins stimulate growth of MCF-7 human breast cancer cells by promoting intercellular conversion of adrenal androgens to estrogens, *Oncol* 59(Suppl 11):19-23, 2000.

199. Rossouw JE et al: Risks and benefits of estrogen plus progestin in healthy postmenopausal women: principle results from the Women's Health Initiative randomized controlled trial, *JAMA* 288(3):321-333, 2002.

200. Grady D: Postmenopausal hormones—therapy for symptoms only, *N Engl J Med* 348(19):1835-1937, 2003.

201. Ettinger B et al: Reduced mortality associated with long-term postmenopausal estrogen therapy, *Obstet Gynecol* 87(1):6-12, 1996.

202. Schairer C et al: Menopausal estrogen and estrogen-progestin replacement therapy and brteast cancer risk, *JAMA* 283(4):485-491, 2000.

203. Beral V, Million Women Study Collaborators: Breast cancer and hormone-replacement therapy in the Million Women Study, *Lancet* 362(9382):419-427, 2003.

204. de Lignieres B et al: Combined hormone replacement therapy and risk of breast cancer in a French cohort study of 3175 women, *Climacteric* 5(4):332-340, 2002.

205. Casper RF: Estrogen with interrupted progestin HRG: a review of experimental and clinical studies, *Maturitas* 34(2):97, 2000.

206. Groshong SD et al: Biphasic regulation of breast cancer cell growth by progesterone: role of the cyclin-dependent kinase inhibitors, p21 and p27 (Kip1), *Molecular Endocrinol* 11(11):1593-1607, 1997.

207. Lange CA, Richer JK, Horwitz, KB: Hypothesis: progesterone primes breast cancer cells for cross-talk with proliferative or antiproliferative signals, *Molecular Endocrinol* 13(6):829-836, 1999.

208. Wu J, Brandt S, Hyder SM: Ligand- and cell-specific effects of signal transduction pathway inhibitors on progestin-induced vascular endothelial growth factor levels in human breast cancer cells, *Molecular Endocrinol* 19(2):312-326, 2005.

209. Collaborative Group on Hormonal Factors in Breast Cancer (CGHFBC): Breast cancer and hormonal contraceptives: collaborative reanalysis of individual data on 53,297 women with breast cancer and 100,239 women without breast cancer from 54 epidemiological studies, *Lancet* 347(9017):1713-1727, 1996.

210. Ursin G et al: Use of oral contraceptives and risk of breast cancer in young women, *Breast Cancer Res Treat* 50(2):175-184, 1998.

211. Bernstein L, Ross R, Henderson B: Relationship of hormone use to cancer risk, *Monogr Natl Cancer Inst* 12:137, 1992.

212. Marchbanks PA et al: The NICHD Women's Contraceptive and Reproductive Experiences Study: methods and operational results, *Ann Epidemiol* 12(4):213-221, 2002.

213. Brinton LA et al: Breast cancer risk among women under 55 years of age by joint effects of usage of oral contraceptives and hormone replacement therapy, *Menopause* 5(3):145-151, 1998.

214. National Cancer Institute: *Radiation risks and pediatric computed tomography (CT): a guide for health care providers,* 2002. Available at www.cancer.gov.

215. National Cancer Institute: *SEER cancer statistics review 1975-2001,* 2001. Available at http://seer.cancer.gov/csr1975_2001/results_merged/topic_inc_mor_trends.pdf.

216. MacKenzie I: Breast cancer following multiple fluoroscopies, *Br J Cancer* 19:1-8, 1965.

217. Mattsson A et al: Dose- and time-response for breast cancer risk after radiation therapy for benign breast disease, *Br J Cancer* 72(4):1054-1061, 1995.

218. Shore RE et al: Breast cancer among women given x-ray therapy for acute postpartum mastitis, *J Natl Cancer Inst* 77(3):689-696, 1986.

219. Hildreth NG, Shore RE, Dvoretsky PM: The risk of breast cancer after irradiation of the thymus in infancy, *N Engl J Med* 321(19):1281-1284, 1989.

220. Lundell M et al: Breast cancer risk after radiotherapy in infancy: a pooled analysis of two Swedish cohorts of 17,202 infants, *Radiation Res* 151(5):626-632, 1999.

221. Merin-Doody M et al: Breast cancer mortality after diagnostic radiography: findings from the U.S. Scoliosis Cohort Study, *Spine* 25(16):2052-2063, 2000.

222. Bhatia S et al: High risk of subsequent neoplasms continues with extended follow-up of childhood Hodgkin's disease: report from the Late Effects Study Group, *J Clin Oncol* 21(23):4386-4394, 2003.

223. Bhatia S et al: Breast cancer and other second neoplasms after childhood Hodgkin's disease, *N Engl J Med* 334(12):745-751, 1996.

224. Travis LB et al: Breast cancer following radiotherapy and chemotherapy among young women with Hodgkin's disease, *JAMA* 290(4):465-475, 2003.

225. Tokunaga M et al: Incidence of female breast cancer among atomic bomb survivors, 1950-1985, *Radiation Res* 138(2):209-223, 1994.

226. Land CD: Radiation and breast cancer risk, *Prog Clin Biol Res* 396:115-124, 1997.

227. Miettinen OS et al: Mammographic screening: no reliable supporting evidence? *Lancet* 359(9304):404-405, 2002.

228. Olsen O, Gøtzsche PC: Cochrane review of screening for breast cancer with mammography, *Lancet* 358(9290):1340-1342, 2001.

229. Young KC, Burch A: Radiation doses received in the UK Breast Screening Programme in 1997 and 1978, *Br J Radiol* 73(867):278-287, 2000.

230. Prasad KN, Cole WC, Hasse GM: Health risks of low dose ionizing radiation in humans: a review, *Exp Biol Med* (Maywood) 229(5):378-382, 2004.

231. Kellerer AM, Roos H: Are all photon radiations similar in large absorbers? A comparison of electron spectra, *Radiat Prot Dosimetry,* 2005. Advanced access at doi:10.1093/rpd/nch458

232. Straume T: High-energy gamma rays in Hiroshima and Nagasaki: implications for risk and war, *Health Phys* 69(6):954-956, 1995.

233. Frankenberg D et al: Enhanced neoplastic transformation my mammography x-ray relative to 200 kVp x-rays: indication for a strong dependence on photon energy of the RBE(M) for various end points, *Radiat Res* 157(1):99-105, 2002.

234. Brenner DJ et al: Routine screening mammography: how important is the radiation-risk side of the benefit-risk equation? *Int J Radiat Biol* 78(12):1065-1067, 2002.

235. Kerlikowske K et al: Effect of age, breast density, and family history on the sensitivity of first screening mammography, *JAMA* 276(1):33-38, 1996.

236. Ronckers CM, Erdmann CA, Land CE: Radiation and breast cancer: a review of current evidence, *Breast Cancer Res* 7(1):21-32, 2005.

237. Holmes MD, Willett WC: Does diet affect breast cancer risk? *Breast Cancer Res* 6(4):170-178, 2004.

238. Byers T: Nutritional risk factors for breast cancer, *CA Cancer J Clin* 74(suppl 1):288, 1994.

239. Bartsch H et al: Dietary polyunsaturated fatty acids and cancer of the breast and colorectum: emerging evidence for their role as risk modifiers, *Carcinogenesis* 20(12):2209, 1999.

240. Cognault S et al: Effect of an alpha-linolenic acid–rich diet on rat mammary tumor growth depends on the dietary oxidative status, *Nutr Cancer* 36(1):33, 2000.

241. Nakagawa H et al: Effects of genstein and synergistic action in combination with eicosapentaenoic acid on the growth of breast cancer cell lines, *J Cancer Res Clin Oncol* 126(8):448, 2000.

242. Thoennes SR et al: Differential transcriptional activation of peroxisome proliferator-activated receptor gamma by omega-3 and omega-6 fatty acids in MCF-7 cells, *Mol Cell Endocrinol* 160(1-2):67, 2000.

243. Simopoulos AP: The importance of the ratio of omega-6/omega-3 essential fatty acids, *Biomed Pharmacother* 56(8):365-379, 2002.

244. Petrakis NL: Nipple aspirate fluid in epidemiologic studies of breast disease, *Epidemiol Rev* 15(1):188-195, 1993.

245. Kuller LH: The etiology of breast cancer—from epidemiology to prevention, *Public Health Rev* 23(2):157-213, 1995.

246. Deslypere JP: Obesity and cancer, *Metabolism* 44(suppl 9):14, 1995.

247. Hankinson SE et al: Alcohol, height, and adiposity in relation to estrogen and prolactin levels in post-menopausal women, *J Natl Cancer Inst* 87(17):1297-1302, 1995.

248. Wenten M et al: Associations of weight, weight change, and body mass with breast cancer risk in Hispanic and non-Hispanic white women *Ann Epidemiol* 12(6):435-444, 2002.

249. Trentham-Diaz A et al: Weight change and risk of postmenopausal breast cancer (United States), *Cancer Causes Control* 11(6):533-542, 2000.

250. Le Marchand L et al: Body size at different periods of life and breast cancer risk, *Am J Epidemiol* 128(1):137-152, 1988.

251. Morimoto LM et al: Obesity, body size, and risk of postmenopausal breast cancer: the Women's Health Initiative (United States), *Cancer Causes Control* 13(8):741-751, 2002.

252. Endogenous Hormones Breast Cancer Collaborative Group: Body mass index, serum sex hormones, and breast cancer risk in postmenopausal women, *J Natl Cancer Inst* 95(6):1218-1226, 2003.

253. Tretli S, Gaard M: Lifestyle changes during adolescence and risk of breast cancer: an ecologic study of the effect of World War II in Norway, *Cancer Causes Control* 7(5):507-512, 1996.

254. Hunter DJ, Willett WC: Diet, body size, and breast cancer, *Epidemiol Rev* 15(1):110-132, 1993.

255. Swanson CA et al: Breast cancer risk assessed by anthropometry in the NHANES I epidemiological follow-up study, *Cancer Res* 48(18):5363-5367, 1988.

256. Vatten LJ, Kvinnsland S: Body height and risk of breast cancer: a prospective study of 23,831 Norwegian women, *Br J Cancer* 61(6):881-885, 1990.

257. Meyer F et al: Dietary and physical determinants of menarche, *Epidemiology* 1(5):377-381, 1990.

258. Merzenich H, Boeing H, Wahrendorf J: Dietary fat and sports activity as determinants of age at menarche, *Am J Epidemiol* 138(4):217-224, 1993.

259. Chen J, Campbell TC, Junyao L: *Diet, lifestyle, and mortality in China: a study of the characteristics of 65 Chinese counties,* Oxford, England, 1990, Oxford University Press.

260. Cho E et al: *Premenopausal dietary carbohydrate, glycemic index, glycemic load, and fiber in relation to risk of breast cancer,* Toronto, Canada, 2003, American Association for Cancer Research.

261. Terry P et al: No association among total dietary fiber, fiberfractions, and risk of breast cancer, *Cancer Epidemiol Biomarkers Prev* 11(11):1507-1508, 2002.

262. Witte JS et al: Diet and premenopausal bilateral breast cancer: a case-control study, *Breast Cancer Res Treat* 42(3):243-251, 1997.

263. Augustin LS et al: Dietary glycemic index and glycemic load, and breast cancer risk: a case-control study, *Ann Oncol* 12(11):1533-1538, 2001.

264. Smith-Warner SA et al: Alcohol and breast cancer in women: a pooled analysis of cohort studies, *JAMA* 279(7):535-540, 1998.

265. Kuller LH: The etiology of breast cancer—from epidemiology to prevention, *Public Health Rev* 23(2):157-213, 1995.

266. Stampfer MJ, Bechtel SD, Hunter D: Fat, alcohol, selenium, and breast cancer risk, *Contemp Oncol* 3(7):28, 33-35, 1993.

267. Rohan TE et al: Dietary intake folate consumption and breast cancer risk, *J Natl Cancer Inst* 92(3):266-622, 2000.

268. Sellers TA et al: Dietary folate intake, alcohol, and risk of breast cancer in a prospective study of postmenopausal women, *Epidemiology* 12(4):420-428, 2001.

269. Zhang S et al: A prospective study of folate intake and the risk of breast cancer, *JAMA* 281(17):1632-1637, 1999.

270. Ginsburg ES et al: The effect of acute ethanol ingestion on estrogen levels in postmenopausal women using transdermal estradiol, *J Soc Gynecol Investig* 2(1):26-29, 1995.

271. Reichman ME et al: Effects of alcohol consumption on plasma and urinary hormone concentration in pre-menopausal women, *J Natl Cancer Inst* 85(9):722-727, 1993.

272. Fan S et al: Alcohol stimulates estrogen receptor signaling in human breast cancer cell lines, *Cancer Res* 60(20):5635-5639, 2000.

273. Lou J, Miller MW: Ethanol enhances erb B–mediated migration of human breast cancer cells in culture, *Breast Cancer Res Treat* 63(1): 61, 2000.

274. Stevens RG et al: Alcohol consumption and urinary concentration of 6-sulfatoxymelatonin in healthy women, *Epidemiology* 11(6):660, 2000.

275. Thompson HJ: Effects of combined deficiencies of selenium (Se) and vitamin E (VitE) on the initiation and promotion phases of 7,12-dimethylbenz(a)anthracene (DMBA)–induced mammary tumorigenesis, *Proc Am Assoc Cancer Res* 32:146, 1993.

276. Takada H et al: Inhibition of 7,12-dimethyl-benz(a)anthracene–induced lipid peroxidation and mammary tumor development in rats by vitamin E in conjunction with selenium, *Nutr Cancer* 17(2): 115-122, 1992.

277. Willett WC et al: Relation of serum vitamins A and E and carotenoids to the risk of cancer, *N Engl J Med* 310(7):430-434, 1983.

278. Verhoeven DT et al: Vitamins C and E, retinol, beta-carotene, and dietary fibre in relation to breast cancer risk: a prospective cohort study, *Br J Cancer* 75(1):149-155, 1997.

279. Wu K et al: A prospective study of plasma ascorbic acid concentrations and breast cancer (United States), *Cancer Causes Control* 11(3): 279-283, 2000.

280. Ip C, Hayes C: Tissue selenium levels in selenium-supplemented rats and their relevence in mammary cancer protection, *Carcinogenesis* 10(5):921-925, 1989.

281. Thompson HJ, Meeker LD, Kokoska S: Effect of an inorganic and organic form of dietary selenium on the promotional stage of mammary carcinogenesis in the rat, *Cancer Res* 44(7):2803-2806, 1984.

282. Wolters M, Hahn A: Soy isoflavones—a therapy for menopausal symptoms, *Wein Med Wochenschr,* 2004.

283. Cross HS et al: Phytoestrogens and vitamin D metabolism: a new concept for the prevention and therapy of colorectal, prostate, and mammary carcinomas, *J Nutr* 134(5):1207S-1212S, 2004.

284. Ito T, Warnken SP, May WS: Protein synthesis inhibition of flavinoids: roles of eukaryotic initiation factor 2 alpha kinase, *Biochem Biophys Res Com* 265(2):3890-594, 1999.

285. Kumar N et al: Isofavones in breast cancer chemoprevention: where do we go from here? *Front Biosci* 9:2927-2934, 2004.

286. Lu LJ et al: Effects of soy consumption for one month on steroid hormones in premenopausal women: implications for breast cancer risk reduction, *Cancer Epidemiol Biomarkers Prev* 5:63-70, 1996.

287. McMichael-Phillips DF et al: Effects of soy-protein supplementation on epithelial proliferation in the histologically normal human breast, *Am J Clin Nutr* 68(Suppl):1431S-1435S, 1998.

288. Shao Z-M et al: Genistein experts multiple suppressive effects on human breast carcinoma cells, *Cancer Res* 58(21):4851-4857, 1998.

289. Petrakis NL et al: Stimulatory influence of soy protein isolate on breast secretion in pre- and postmenopausal women, *Cancer Epidemiol Biomarkers Prev* 5(10):785-794, 1996.

290. Krieger N et al: Breast cancer and serum organochlorines: a prospective study among white, black, and Asian women, *J Natl Cancer Inst* 86(8):589-599, 1994.

291. Wolff MS et al: Blood levels of organochlorine residues and risk of breast cancer, *J Natl Cancer Inst* 85(8):648-652, 1993.

292. Dorn J et al: Lifetime physical activity and breast cancer risk in pre- and postmenopausal women, *Med Sci Sports Exercise* 35(2):278-285, 2003.

293. Friedenreich CM, Orenstein MR: Physical activity and cancer prevention: etiologic evidence and biological mechanisms, *J Nutr* 132(11 Suppl):3464S-3465S, 2002.

294. Kaaks R, Lukanova A: Effects of weight control and physical activity in cancer prevention: role of endogenous hormone metabolism, *Ann N Y Acad Sci* 963:268-81, 2002.

295. Garber JE, Offit K: Hereditary cancer predisposition syndromes, *J Clin Oncology* 23(2):276-292, 2005.

296. Ford D et al: Genetic heterogeneity and penetrance analysis of the *BRCA1* and *BRCA2* genes in breast cancer families. The Breast Cancer Linkage Consortium, *Am J Hum Genet* 62(3):676-689, 1998.

297. Weber B: Genetic testing for breast cancer, *Sci Am Sci Med* 3(1):12, 1996.

298. Antoniou A et al: Average risks of breast and ovarian cancer associated with *BRCA1* and *BRCA2* mutations detected in case series unselected for family history: a combined analysis of 22 studies, *Am J Hum Genet* 72(2):1117-1130, 2003.

299. Thompson D, Easton D, Breast Cancer Linkage Consortium: Variation in cancer risks by mutation position in *BRCA2* mutation carriers, *Am J Hum Genet* 68(2):410-419, 2001.

300. Kauff ND et al: Risk reducing salpingo-oophorectomy in women with *BRCA1* or *BRCA2* mutation, *N Engl J Med* 346(21):1609-1615, 2002.

301. Rebbeck TR et al: Prophylactic oophorectomy in carriers of *BRCA1* or *BRCA2* mutations, *N Engl J Med* 346(21):1616-1622, 2002.

302. Garcia-Higuera I et al: Interaction of the Fanconi anemia proteins and *BRCA1* in a common pathway, *Mol Cell* 7(2):249-262, 2001.

303. Howlett NG et al: Bialleic inactivation of *BRCA2* in Fanconi anemia, *Science* 297:609, 2002.

304. Offit K et al: Shared genetic susceptibility to breast cancer, brain tumors, and Fanconi anemia, *J Natl Cancer Inst* 95(20):1548-1551, 2003.

305. Haber D: Roads leading to breast cancer, *N Engl J Med* 343(21):1566, 2000.

306. Waxman J: A new understanding of the hormonal regulation of endocrine dependent cancer, *Br Med Bull* 47(1):197, 1991.

307. Kainu T et al: Somatic deletions in hereditary breast cancers implicate 13q21 as a putative novel breast cancer susceptibility locus, *Proc Natl Acad Sci U S A* 97(17):9603-9608, 2000.

308. Russo IH, Calaf G, Russo J: Hormones and proliferative activity in breast tissue. In Stoll BA, editor: *Approaches to breast cancer prevention,* Dordrecht, Netherlands, 1991, Kluwer Academic Publishers.

309. Zhu BT, Conney AH: Is 2-methoxyestradiol an endogenous estrogen metabolite that inhibits mammary carcinogenesis? *Cancer Res* 58(11):2269-2277, 1998.

310. Cavalieri E et al: Chapter 4: estrogens as endogenous genotoxic agents—DNA adducts and mutations, *J Natl Cancer Inst Monogr* 27:75-93, 2000.

311. Yager JD: Chapter 3: endogenous estrogens as carcinogens through metabolic activation, *J Natl Cancer Inst Monogr* 27:67-73, 2000.

312. Knabbe C et al: Evidence that transforming growth factor-β is a hormonally regulated negative growth factor in human breast cancer cells, *Cell* 48(3):417-428, 1987.

313. Morabia A, Wynder EL: Epidemiology and natural history of breast cancer, *Surg Clin North Am* 70(4):739, 1990.

314. Lakhani SR: The transition from hyperplasia to invasive carcinoma of the breast, *J Pathol* 187(3):272-278, 1999.

315. Russo J et al: Breast cancer multistage progression, *Front Biosci* 3:944-960, 1998.

316. Reiss-Filho JS, Lakhani SR: The diagnosis and management of pre-invasive breast disease: genetic alterations in pre-invasive lesions, *Breast Cancer Res* 5:313-319, 2003.

317. Boecker W et al: Ductal epithelial proliferation of the breast: a biological continuum? Comparative genomic hybridization and high molecular-weight cytokeratin expression patterns, *J Pathol* 195:415-421, 2001.

318. Buerger H et al: Different genetic pathways in the evolution of invasive breast cancer are associated with distinct morphological subtypes, *J Pathol* 189(4):521-526, 1999.

319. Buerger H et al: Genetic characterisation of invasive breast cancer: a comparison of CGH and PCR based multiplex microsatellite analysis, *J Clin Pathol* 54(11):836-840, 2001.

320. Silverstein MJ, Baril NB: In situ carcinoma of the breast. In Donegan WL, Spratt JS, editors: *Cancer of the breast,* Philadelphia, 2002, Saunders.

321. Nielsen M et al: Breast cancer and atypia among young and middle-aged women: a study of 110 medicolegal autopsies, *Br J Cancer* 56(6):814-819, 1987.

322. Alpers CE, Wellings SR: The prevalence of carcinoma in situ in normal and cancer-associated breasts, *Hum Pathol* 16(8):796-807, 1985.

323. Lakhani SR: Molecular genetics of solid tumors: translating research into clinical practice. What we could do now: breast cancer, *Mol Pathol* 54(5):281-284, 2001.

324. Page DL et al: Atypical lobular hyperplasia as a unilateral predictor of breast cancer risk: a retrospective cohort study, *Lancet* 361(9352):125-129, 2003.

325. Antman K, Shea S: Screening mammography under age 50, *JAMA* 281(16):1470, 1999.

326. Conant EF, Maidment ADA: Breast cancer imaging, *Sci Am Sci Med* 3(1):22, 1996.

327. Stoll BA: Breast cancer and the western diet: role of fatty acids and antioxidant vitamins, *Eur J Cancer* 34(12):1852, 1998.

328. Holmes MD et al: Dietary factors and the survival of women with breast carcinoma, *Cancer* 86(5):826, 1999.

329. Baum M: Anastrozole alone or in combination with tamoxifen versus tamoxifen alone for adjuvant treatment of postmenopausal women with early breast cancer: first results of the ATAC randomized trial, *Lancet* 359(9324):2131-2129, 2002.

330. Weiss JR, Moysich KB, Swede H: Epidemiology of male breast cancer, *Cancer Epidemiol Biomarkers Prev* 14(1):20-26, 2005.

331. Clark JL et al: Prognostic variables in male breast cancer, *Am Surg* 66(5):501, 2000.

332. Jepson AS, Fentiman IS: Male breast cancer, *Int J Clin Pract* 52(8):571, 1998.

333. Diamanti-Kandarakis E et al: A survey of the polycystic ovary syndrome in the Greek island of Lesbos: hormonal and metabolic profile, *J Clin Endocrinol Metab* 84(11):4006, 1999.

334. Gordon CM: Menstrual disorders in adolescents: excess androgens and the polycystic ovary syndrome, *Pediatr Clin North Am* 46(3):519, 1999.

335. Orabi HE et al: Serum leptin as an additional possible pathogenic factor in polycystic ovary syndrome, *Clin Biochem* 32(1):71, 1999.

336. Kurioka H et al: Diagnostic difficulty in polycystic ovary syndrome due to an LH-β-subunit variant, *Eur J Endocrinol* 140(3):235-238, 1999.

337. Couse JF et al: Prevention of the polycystic phenotype and characterization of ovulatory capacity in the estrogen receptor-α knockout mouse, *Endocrinology* 140(12):5855, 1999.

338. Amato G et al: Lack of insulin-like growth factor binding protein-3 variation after follicle-stimulating hormone stimulation in women with polycystic ovary syndrome undergoing in vitro fertilization, *Fertil Steril* 72(3):454, 1999.

339. Speroff, L, Fritz MA: *Clinical gynecologic endocrinology and infertility,* ed 7, Philadelphia, 2005, Lippincott Williams & Wilkins.

340. Patel, SR, Korykowski MT: Treating polycystic ovary syndrome: today's approach, *Womens Health Prim Care* 3(2):109, 2000.

341. Radon, PA, McMahon MJ, Meyer WR: Impaired glucose tolerance in pregnant women with polycystic ovary syndrome, *Obstet Gynecol* 94(2):194, 1999.

342. Almekinder JL et al: Toxicity of methoxyacetic acid in cultured human luteal cells, *Fund Appl Toxicol* 38(2):191-194, 1997;

343. Band PR et al: Carcinogenic and endocrine disrupting effects of cigarette smoke and risk of breast cancer, *Lancet* 360(9339):1044-1049, 2002.

344. Belli S et al: Mortality study of workers employed by the Italian National Institute of Health, 1960-1989, *Scand J Work Environ Health* 18(1):64-67, 1992;

345. Brown NM et al: Prenatal TCDD and predisposition to mammary cancer in rats, *Carcinogenesis* 19(9):1623-1629, 1998.

346. California Environmental Protection Agency, Air Resources Board: Proposed identification of environmental tobacco smoke as a toxic air contaminant, *Draft Report Part B,* chap 7, p 147, 2004.

347. Calle EE et al: Cigarette smoking and risk of fatal breast cancer, *Am J Epidemiol* 139(10):1001-1007, 1994.

348. Chang YM et al: A proportionate cancer morbidity ratio study of workers exposed to chlorinated organic solvents in Taiwan, *Indust Health* 41(2):77-87, 2003.

349. Chiazze L Jr, Ference LD: Mortality among PVC fabricating employees, *Env Health Perspect* 41:137-143, 1981.

350. Colton T et al: Breast cancer in mothers prescribed diethylstilbestrol in pregnancy. Further follow-up, *JAMA* 269(16):2096-2100, 1993.

351. DeBruin LS, Josephy PD: Perspectives on the chemical etiology of breast cancer, *Environ Hlth Perspect* 110:(S1):119-128, 2002.

352. Evans N: *State of the evidence: what is the connection between the environment and breast cancer?* ed 3, San Francisco, Calif, 2004, Breast Cancer Fund.

353. Gammon MD et al: Environmental toxins and breast cancer on Long Island. I. Polycyclic aromatic hydrocarbon DNA adducts, *Cancer Epidemiol Biomark Prev* 11(8):677-685, 2002.

354. Hansen J: Breast cancer risk among relatively young women employed in solvent-using industries, *Am J Ind Med* 36(1):43-47, 1999.

355. Hatakeyama M, Matsumura F: Correlation between the activation of Neu tyrosine kinase and promotion of foci formation induced by selected organochlorine compounds in the MCF-7 model system, *J Biochem Molec Toxicol* 13(6):296-302, 1999.

356. Herbst AL, Scully RE: Adenocarcinoma of the vagina in adolescence: a report of 7 cases including 6 clear cell carcinomas (so-called mesonephromas), *Cancer* 25(4):745-757, 1970.

357. Hoyer AP et al: Organochlorine exposure and risk of breast cancer, *Lancet* 352(9143):1816-1820, 1998.

358. Infante PF, Pesak J: A historical perspective of some occupationally related diseases of women, *J Occup Med* 36(8):826-831, 1994.

359. Jansen MS et al: Short-chain fatty acids enhance nuclear receptor activity through mitogen-activated protein kinase activation and histone deacetylase inhibition, *Proc Natl Acad Sci* 101(18):7199-7204, 2004.

360. Johnson KC, Hu J, Mao Y: Passive and active smoking and breast cancer risk in Canada, 1994-1997, The Canadian Cancer Registries Epidemiology Research Group, *Cancer Causes Control* 11(3):211-221, 2000.

361. Kilthau GF: Cancer risk in relation to radioactivity in tobacco, *Radiol Tech* 67(3):217-222, 1996;

362. Markey CM et al: In utero exposure to bisphenol A alters the development and tissue of organization of the mouse mammary gland, *Biol Reproduct* 65(4):1215-1223, 2001.

363. Maxwell NI et al: *Newton Breast Cancer Study,* Newton, Mass, 1999, Silent Spring Institute.

364. Melnick RL et al: Multiple organ carcinogenicity of inhaled chloroprene (2-chloro-1,3-butadiene) in F334/N rats and B6C3F1 mice and comparison of dose-response in 1,3-butadiene in mice, *Carcinogenesis* 20(5):867-878, 1999.

365. National Toxicology Program (NTP): *Chemicals associated with site-specific tumor induction in mammary gland,* 2003. Available at http://ntp-server.niehs.nih.gov/htdocs/sites/MAMM.html.

366. National Toxicology Program (NTP), US Department of Health and Human Services: *Toxicology and carcinogenesis studies of 1,3-butadiene (CAS No 106-99-0) in B6C3F1 mice (inhalation studies),* NTP TR 434, NIH Pub No 93-3165, Research Triangle Park, NC, 1993, National Institute of Health.

367. Palmer JR et al: Risk of breast cancer in women exposed to diethyl-stilbestrol in utero: preliminary studies (United States), *Cancer Causes Control* 13(8):753-758, 2002.

368. Steenland K et al: Ethylene oxide and breast cancer incidence in a cohort study of 7576 women, *Cancer Causes Control* 14(6):531-539, 2003.

369. Walrath J et al: Causes of death among female chemists, *Am J Public Health* 75(8):883-885, 1985,

370. Warner MB et al: Serum dioxin concentrations and breast cancer risk in the Seveso Women's Health Study, *Environ Health Perspect* 110(7):625-628, 2002,

371. Weiderpass E et al: Breast cancer and occupational exposures in women in Finland, *Am J Ind Med* 36(1):48-53, 1999,

372. Wennborg H et al: Mortality and cancer incidence in biomedical laboratory personnel in Sweden, *Am J Ind Med* 35(4):382-389, 1999,

373. Zheng T et al: DDE and DDT in breast adipose tissue and risk of female breast cancer, *Am J Epidemiol* 150(5):453-458, 1999.

374. Terry MB et al: Association of frequency and duration of aspirin use and hormone receptor status with breast cancer risk, *JAMA* 291(20):2433-2440, 2004.

375. Mueller RL, Scheidt S: History of drugs for thrombotic disease: discovery, development, and directions for the future, *Circulation* 89(1):432-449, 1994.

376. Smalley WE, DuBois RN: Colorectal cancer and nonsteroidal anti-inflammatory drugs, *Adv Pharmacol* 39:1-20, 1997.

377. Chang SH et al: Role of prostaglandin E2-dependent angiogenic switch in cyclooxygenase-2-induced breast cancer progression, *Proc Natl Acad Sci U S A* 101(2):591-596, 2004.

378. Subbaramaiah K et al: Transcription of cyclooxygenase-2 is enhanced in transformed mammary epithelial cells, *Cancer Res* 56(19):4424-4429, 1996.

379. Zhao Y et al: Estrogen biosynthesis proximal to a breast tumor is stimulated by PGE$_2$ via cyclic AMP, leading to activation of promoter II of the CYP19 (aromatase) gene, *Endocrinology* 137(12):5739-5742, 1996.

380. Crawford YG et al: Histologically normal human mammary epithelia with silenced p16(INK4a) overexpress COX-2, promoting a premalignant program, *Cancer Cell* 5(3):263-273, 2004.

381. Shim V et al: Cyclooxygenase-2 expression is related to nuclear grade in ductal carcinoma in situ and is increased in its normal adjacent epithelium, *Cancer Res* 63(10):2347-2350, 2003.

382. Hollowell JG et al: Iodine nutrition in the United States. Trends and public health implications: iodine excretion data from National Health and Nutrition Examination Surveys I and II (1971-1974 and 1988-1994), *J Clin Endocrinol Metab* 83(10):3401-3408, 1998.

383. World Health Organzation, United Nations International Children's Emergency Fund, International Council for the Control of Iodine Deficiency Disorders: *Indicators for assessing iodine deficiency disorders and their control thorugh salt iodination*, Geneva, 1994, World Health Organization.

384. Ghent WR et al: Iodine replacement in fibrocystic disease, *Can J Surg* 36(5):453-460, 1993.

385. Medeiros-Neto G: Iodine deficiency disorders. In GeGroot LJ, Jameson JL, editors: *Endocrinology*, ed, 4, Philadelphia, 2001, Saunders.

386. Smyth PP: Role of iodine in antioxidant defense in thyroid and breast disease, *Biofactors* 19(3-4):121-130, 2003.

387. Tazebay UH et al: The mammary gland iodide transporter is expressed during lactation and in breast cancer, *Nat Med* 6(8):871-878, 2000.

388. Wapnir IL et al: Immunohistochemical profile of the sodium/iodide symporter in thyroid, breast, and other carcinomas using high density tissue microarrays and conventional sections, *J Clin Endocrinol Metab* 88(4):1880-1888, 2003.

389. Bogardus GM, Finley JW: Breast cancer and thyroid disease, *Surgery* 49:461-468, 1961.

390. Eskin BA et al: Iodine metabolism and breast cancer, *Trans NY Acad Sci* 11:911-947, 1970.

391. Cann SA, van Netten JP, van Netten C: Hypothesis: iodine, selenium, and the development of breast cancer, *Cancer Causes Control* 11(2):121-127, 2000.

392. Funahashi H et al: Suppressive effect of iodine on DMBA-induced breast tumor growth in the rat, *J Surg Oncol* 61(3):209-213, 1996.

393. Funahashi H et al: Wakame seaweed suppresses the proliferation of 7,12-dimethylbenz(a)-anthracene-induced mammary tumors in rats, *Jpn J Cancer Res* 90(9):922-927, 1999.

394. Funahashi H et al: Seaweed prevents breast cancer? *Jpn J Cancer Res* 92(5):483-487, 2001.

395. LeMarchand K, Kolonel LN, Nomura AM: Breast cancer survival among Hawaii Japanese and Caucasian women: ten-year rates and survival by place of birth, *Am J Epidemiol* 122(4):571-578, 1985.

396. Minami Y et al: Trends in the incidence of female breast and cervical cancer in Miyagi Prefecture, Japan 1959-1987, *Jpn J Cancer Res* 87(1):10-17, 1996.

397. Tajima N, Tsukuma H, Oskima A: Descriptive epidemiology of male breast cancer in Osaka, Japan, *J Epidemiol* 11(1):1-7, 2001.

398. Eskin BA et al: Different tissue repsonses for iodine and iodide in rat thyroid and mammary glands, *Biol Trace Elem Res* 49(1):9-19, 1995.

SEXUALLY TRANSMITTED INFECTIONS

KATHERINE MORGAN

Throughout recorded history, infectious diseases have threatened humans. Even into the twentieth century, epidemics of diphtheria, typhoid, tuberculosis, cholera, and other catastrophic infections have decimated entire communities almost overnight. Despite medical advances, improved living standards, and better nutrition, new epidemics still arise as major public health problems, and some pose lethal threats to individuals and communities. Some of these epidemics are caused by sexually transmitted infections (STIs). At this time, many people consider the number of individuals with acquired immunodeficiency syndrome (AIDS) and human immunodeficiency virus (HIV) and human papillomavirus (HPV) infections to be at epidemic levels.

Sexually contracted infections affect over 15 million Americans per year, 3 million of whom are teenagers,[1] and account for about one third of the reproductive mortality in the United States. Complications of STIs include pelvic inflammatory disease, infertility, ectopic pregnancy, chronic pelvic pain, neonatal morbidity and mortality, and genital cancers. Long-term sequelae of untreated or undertreated STIs may be disastrous and can affect a person's physical, emotional, and financial well-being.

In the past an infection transmitted through sexual intercourse was called a *venereal disease.* Because of its limited scope, the term venereal disease has been replaced with *sexually transmitted infection (STI).* STIs are infections contracted by intimate, as well as sexual, contact and include systemic infections, such as tuberculosis and hepatitis, that can be spread to a sexual partner. Etiology of an STI may be bacterial, viral, protozoan, parasitic, or fungal (Table 24-1). Al-

though the majority of STIs can be treated, virally induced STIs are considered incurable. The current increase in severity and incidence of STIs can be attributed to earlier onset of sexual activity and a greater number of lifetime sexual partners. Many infected individuals do not seek treatment because symptoms are absent, minor, or transient or because health services are inaccessible. Increased numbers of single individuals, bisexuality, and premarital or extramarital sexual affairs contribute to rising numbers of lifetime sexual partners and exposure to STIs. Indulgence in high-risk sexual behaviors and poor health habits, such as failure to use a condom in nonmonogamous or new relationships, and drug use, increases an individual's risk of exposure or the severity of infection if exposed. Perhaps partly because of risk-taking behavior (unprotected intercourse or selection of high-risk partners), adolescents have the greatest risk for STI exposure and infection. In addition, adolescent women may have a physiologically increased susceptibility to infection because of increased cervical immaturity and lack of immunity. Rates of gonorrhea, chlamydia, vaginitis, cervical condyloma, genital warts, and pelvic inflammatory disease (PID) are all highest in adolescents and young women and decline exponentially with increasing age. Women and infants bear the greatest burden from STIs.

STIs are stereotyped as occurring only among urban poor and minority populations. Because the Centers for Disease Control and Prevention (CDCP) does not require that all STIs be reported, private physicians may not report them. Thus reported STIs often come from public health clinics, giving the impression that a greater number of the urban poor and mi-

Table 24-1	Currently Recognized Sexually Transmitted Infections
Causal Microorganism	Infection
Bacteria	
Campylobacter	Campylobacter enteritis
Calymmatobacterium granulomatis	Granuloma inguinale
Chlamydia trachomatis	Urogenital infections; lymphogranuloma venereum
Polymicrobial	
Gardnerella vaginalis interaction with anaerobes (*Bacteroides* and *Mobiluncus* species) and genital mycoplasmas	Bacterial vaginosis
Haemophilus ducreyi	Chancroid
Mycoplasma	Mycoplasmosis
Neisseria gonorrhoeae	Gonorrhea
Shigella	Shigellosis
Treponema pallidum	Syphilis
Viruses	
Cytomegalovirus	Cytomegalic inclusion disease
Hepatitis B virus (HBV)	Hepatitis
Hepatitis C (HCV)	Hepatitis
Herpes simplex virus (HSV)	Genital herpes
Human immunodeficiency virus (HIV)	Acquired immunodeficiency syndrome (AIDS)
Human papillomavirus	Condylomata acuminata, cervical dysplasia, and cervical cancer
Molluscum contagiosum virus	Molluscum contagiosum
Protozoa	
Entaboeba histolytica	Amebiasis; amebic dysentery
Giardia lambia	Giardiasis
Trichomonas vaginalis	Trichomoniasis
Ectoparasites	
Phthirus pubis	Pediculosis pubis
Sarcoptes scabiei	Scabies
Fungus	
Candida albicans	Candidiasis

nority populations are infected with STIs. In fact, STIs are prevalent among individuals in all socioeconomic groups.

SEXUALLY TRANSMITTED UROGENITAL INFECTIONS

Bacterial Infections

Gonorrhea

Gonorrhea is caused by **gonococci** (singular, *gonococcus*), which are microorganisms of the species *Neisseria gonorrhoeae*. Neisser first identified gonococci in stained smears of vaginal, urethral, and conjunctival exudate in 1879. Until 1994 gonorrhea was the most commonly reported communicable infection in the United States. Numbers of reported cases have declined to 335,104 cases in 2003,[2] but, when unreported infections are included, the annual number of cases is estimated to be about twice as high.

The incidence of gonorrhea has dropped remarkably since the peak of the gonorrhea epidemic in the mid-1970s. Infection rates remain highest in the southern region of the coun-

try, however, rates in the South have since declined by 2.3%.[3] Although the number of reported cases declined in all racial and ethnic groups, the gonorrhea rate remains about 20 times greater for blacks than for non-Hispanic whites, down from 30 times higher in 1999. Other demographic and life-style risk factors may include transient or urban residence, early onset of sexual activity, multiple serial or consecutive sex partners, drug use, prostitution, and previous gonorrheal or concurrent STI.[2] The overall rate of gonorrhea has declined 74.3% since 1975. The risk of developing gonorrhea from intercourse with an infected male partner is 50% to 80% for females, and with an infected female partner, it is 20% to 30% for males. The risk increases threefold to fourfold for males after four exposures to an infected partner.

Transmission of gonococcal infection generally requires contact of epithelial (mucosal) surfaces, such as occurs during sexual, oral, or anal intercourse. A pregnant woman also can transmit gonorrhea to her fetus. The infection passes from mother to child across the amniotic membranes, by direct inoculation with a fetal scalp electrode during labor monitoring, or during passage through the birth canal. **Fomites** (contaminated objects) are rarely involved in the transmission of

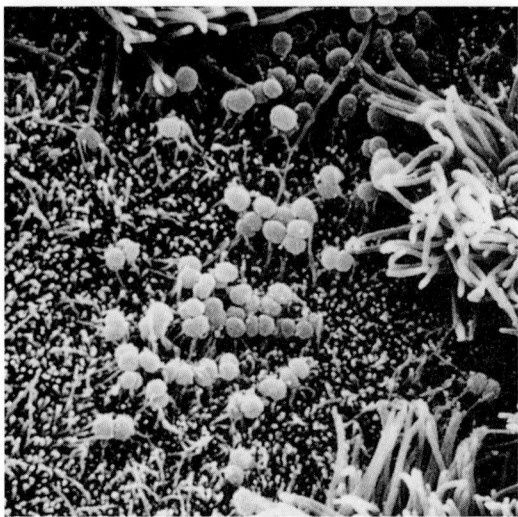

Figure 24-1 Gonococci. Scanning electron microscopy showing gonococci attaching to the nonciliated cells of human fallopian tube mucosa. (From Morse SA, Ballard RC, Holmes KK, Moreland AA, editors: *Atlas of sexually transmitted diseases and AIDS,* ed 3, London, 2003, Mosby.)

N. gonorrhoeae, primarily because the gonococcus requires a rich medium (e.g., body fluids) and an environment high in carbon dioxide (5% to 10%) for growth.

PATHOPHYSIOLOGY Humans are the only natural hosts for *N. gonorrhoeae,* which is an aerobic, non-spore-forming, oxidase-positive, gram-negative coccal (round) microorganism that usually appears in pairs (diplococci), with the adjacent sides slightly flattened. Hairlike filaments, called *pili,* appear to help the microorganisms attach themselves to host cells: the epithelial cells of mucous membranes (Figure 24-1). Columnar, transitional, and stratified squamous epithelial cells are infected most often. First the microorganisms become attached to the plasma membranes (cell walls) of these cells, and then they invade the cells and begin to damage the mucosa. Generally a quick leukocytic (inflammatory) response and exudation at the site of infection occur.

In females the endocervical canal (inner portion of the cervix) is the usual site of original gonococcal infection, although urethral colonization and infection of Skene or Bartholin glands also are common. Several factors can facilitate ascent of gonococci into the uterus and the fallopian tubes, where they cause pelvic inflammatory disease (PID). Among these factors are (1) disintegration of the cervical mucus plug and a rise in vaginal pH above 4.5 during menstruation, (2) uterine contraction that may cause retrograde menstruation into the fallopian tubes, and (3) various microbes that possess virulent potentiating factors for chlamydia or gonococcal PID. Bacteria (*N. gonorrhoeae, Chlamydia tra-*

chomatis) also may adhere to sperm and be transported to the fallopian tubes. In the fallopian tubes, progressive mucosal and submucosal invasion and sloughing of normal, ciliated tubal epithelium are accompanied by marked inflammatory response, causing the fallopian tubes to fill with exudate. In males the gonococci typically infect the urethra. Untreated urethral infection causes epididymitis in 1% to 2% of men and, rarely, urethral stricture and sterility. Commonly, concurrent oropharyngeal and anorectal infection can be found in infected men and women.[4-6] Virulence is determined by variations in the bacterial properties and host response.

CLINICAL MANIFESTATIONS The clinical manifestations of gonorrhea can be categorized as local or systemic and uncomplicated or complicated. Uncomplicated local infections are seen as urethral infections in males and urogenital infections in females. In males the incubation period for urethritis is 3 to 10 days with a range of 12 hours to 3 months.[7] Without treatment, urethritis persists for 3 to 7 weeks, with 95% of men becoming asymptomatic after 3 months. Approximately 60% of men infected suddenly experience marked dysuria (painful or difficult urination) and spontaneous, profuse, mucopurulent discharge from the urethra. However, some individuals have little discharge or urethral itching only, and 5% to 10% never have signs or symptoms. Most cases of untreated gonococcal urethritis resolve spontaneously after several weeks, and more than 95% of individuals are asymptomatic by 6 months after infection. Some men develop urethritis even after being appropriately treated.

In females the incubation period varies, but those who typically develop symptoms do so within 10 days of exposure or within 1 to 2 days after the next menstrual period. The clinical manifestations of uncomplicated gonorrhea in women may be absent (50% of women have asymptomatic

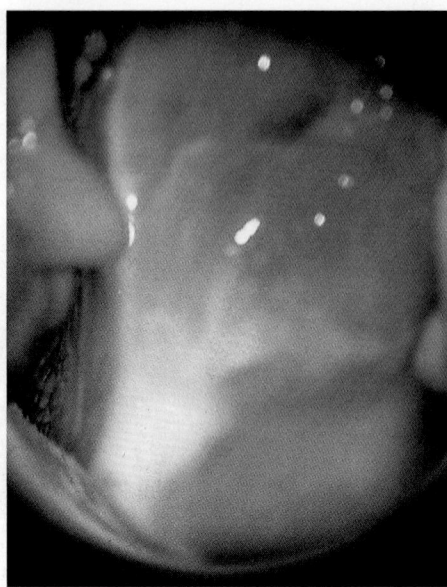

Figure 24-2 Gonococcal cervicitis. The cervix is involved in 85% to 90% of cases in females, but the resultant discharge is profuse enough to be recognized in only 10%. (From McMillan A, Scott GR: *Sexually transmitted infections,* ed 2, London, 2000, Churchill Livingstone.)

infection) or severe; they can include dysuria, increased vaginal discharge, abnormal menses (increased flow or dysmenorrhea), or dyspareunia. Physical examination may disclose cervical friability and erythema (redness) and purulent or mucopurulent discharge from the cervical os (Figure 24-2). There may be a discharge from the Skene or Bartholin glands if these sites are involved.

Anal and rectal gonococcal infection is found in 30% to 50% of women diagnosed with urogenital gonorrhea. In women, anorectal infection is usually asymptomatic and not necessarily related to anal intercourse. Anorectal gonorrhea most commonly occurs in homosexual men with a history of receptive anorectal intercourse. About 50% of these infected men have symptoms.[7]

Symptoms of anorectal gonorrhea range from mild anal pruritus (itching), mucopurulent rectal discharge, and slight rectal bleeding to severe rectal pain, tenesmus (painful and ineffectual straining at stool), and constipation. Physical examination may disclose anal erythema and discharge and evidence of mucosal damage to the anus and rectum, such as friability, edema, and purulent exudate.

Gonococcal pharyngitis occurs primarily in homosexual or bisexual men or heterosexual women after fellatio (oral sexual contact) with an infected partner. Symptomatic pharyngitis is indistinguishable from any other bacterial pharyngitis and can include fever, lymphadenopathy, and tonsillitis. Approximately 60% of these infections are asymptomatic.

Other sites of uncomplicated local infections include the eye, leading to conjunctivitis; however, this is rare in adults. Primary cutaneous infection also has been reported and is usually manifested as a localized ulcer of the genitalia, per-

ineum, proximal lower extremities, or fingers. It is important to determine whether such infections are the result of *N. gonorrhoeae* or secondary colonization by a preexisting lesion.

Localized gonococcal infections can be complicated by prostatitis, epididymitis, lymphangitis, and urethral stricture in men and salpingitis, PID, and bartholinitis in women. Chronic salpingitis or perididymitis can cause scarring and tubal adhesions that lead to sterility. Anyone who is infected and remains untreated is at risk for disseminated gonococcal infection.[4-6]

Before the advent of antimicrobial therapy, approximately 20% of infected males developed acute epididymitis. Men with this condition report unilateral testicular pain and swelling and commonly have overt urethritis at the same time. Penile lymphangitis is a rare complication with an unclear pathogenesis.[4] Before modern antibiotics, individuals with this condition were at risk for developing urethral strictures; however, this complication is now uncommon if treatment is sought and therapy instituted properly.

Acute salpingitis, or PID, is the most common local complication in females. Approximately 10%[2] of women with untreated cervical gonorrhea develop this condition. Salpingitis is significant in its development because of the potential long-term sequelae associated with it, namely, infertility and ectopic pregnancy.

The onset of symptoms may be rapid and usually occurs during menses. Women may experience chills, fever, nausea, vomiting, and lower abdominal pain that worsen with coughing, sneezing, or intercourse. Abdominal palpation often discloses bilateral lower quadrant tenderness and rebound tenderness resulting from peritoneal irritation caused by tubal exudate. Marked tenderness of the internal genitalia is often noted during pelvic examination. Enlargement or masses also may be palpable in the upper genital tract. Abscess of Skenes and Bartholins glands is also a local complication associated with gonococcal infection in females. Tubal infertility is found in 8% of women after one episode of PID. If a woman has three or more episodes of PID, she has a 40% risk of tubal infertility.[8] Apart from PID, abscess formation of Bartholin gland is the most common complication of gonorrhea in females.

Disseminated gonococcal infection (DGI) is a rare systemic complication brought about by the spread of infection through the bloodstream. Less than 1% of individuals with untreated gonococcal infection develop this complication.[9] Males are affected more than females. Symptoms include fever, rash, and joint swelling or pain.

Spread of *N. gonorrhoeae* to the liver causes a condition known as **perihepatitis** or Fitz-Hugh-Curtis syndrome. *C. trachomatis* also has been identified as a causative agent. Inflammation of the capsule of the liver is the primary pathologic manifestation and produces sudden and intense right upper quadrant pain.[10] This complication usually develops after acute salpingitis and is very rare in men.

Newborns are at risk most commonly for gonococcal eye infection (**ophthalmia neonatorum**) (Figure 24-3) but also

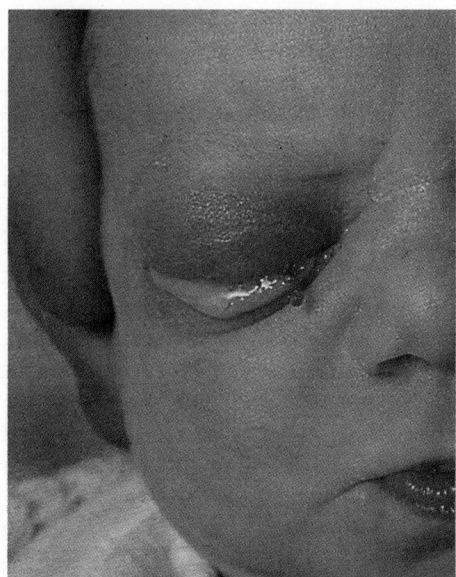

Figure 24-3 Gonococcal ophthalmia neonatorum. (Examiner would be gloved.) (From McMillan A, Scott GR: *Sexually transmitted infections,* ed 2, London, 2000, Churchill Livingstone.)

may acquire rhinitis, anorectal infection, or an abscess at the site of electrode placement for fetal monitoring. Onset of symptoms generally occurs 1 to 12 days after birth, with a mean of 4 to 6 days. Affected newborns usually are born to mothers who have had prolonged ruptured membranes. In these cases, immediate treatment with a topical antibiotic is not effective, because the infection is already established. Established infection causes bilateral corneal ulceration, with a profuse yellow or gray purulent exudate and is followed by necrosis, scarring, and compromised vision. Signs of systemic disease are seldom apparent.

EVALUATION AND TREATMENT   Clinical signs and symptoms are not sufficient for the differential diagnosis of gonococcal infections. Microscopic evaluation of gram-stained slides of clinical specimens is deemed positive for *N. gonorrhoeae* if gram-negative diplococci with typical "kidney bean" morphology are seen inside polymorphonuclear leukocytes. Such a finding is considered adequate for the diagnosis of gonococcal urethritis in a symptomatic male. For females the Gram stain technique is less accurate and reliable and is replaced with a single culture of endocervical secretions. Most clinic settings now use ligase chain reaction (LCR), polymerase chain reaction (PCR) testing, or deoxyribonucleic (DNA) testing because these samples do not require an anaerobic incubation, are highly sensitive, and can be easily transported to a laboratory for testing. Because of the large percentage of infected women without symptoms, routine screening for at-risk women is recommended. Tests should be obtained from any site that may be exposed.[11]

The many different strains of *N. gonorrhoeae* vary with respect to pathogenicity, virulence, and susceptibility to antibiotics. Several types of drug-resistant strains have been identi-

fied; they are penicillinase-producing *N. gonorrhoeae* (PPNG), which is resistant to penicillin; chromosomal control of mechanisms of resistance of *N. gonorrhoeae* (CMRNG), which is resistant to penicillin and tetracycline; and the emerging drug-resistant strain quinolone-resistant *N. gonorrhoeae* (QRNG).[12,13] Of all the isolates collected in 2002 by the Gonococcal Isolate Surveillance Project (GISP), 18%[14] were resistant to penicillin, tetracycline, or both.[15] In the United States the overall percentage of PPNG isolates has declined every year since 1998.[4] However, QRNG is increasing in Asia, the Pacific Islands, and Hawaii. The CDC no longer recommends fluoroquinolone treatment for those individuals for whom infection may have been acquired in any of those areas.[16]

Another major concern is the coexistence of chlamydial infection with gonorrhea.[17] (Chlamydial infections are discussed on p. 875.) Approximately 20% to 30% of males and a higher proportion of females have coexistent chlamydia infections. In the absence of gonorrhea, chlamydia may go undetected until complications such as PID or urethritis manifest themselves.

Treatment for gonorrhea is influenced by three factors: (1) the spread of infection caused by drug-resistant strains, (2) the high frequency of chlamydia infection accompanying gonorrhea, and (3) recognition of the serious complications of chlamydia and gonorrheal infections. CDC treatment guidelines are updated regularly and the most recent edition should be used. Current CDC treatment guidelines for uncomplicated gonorrheal infections are listed in Box 24-1; complicated infections require intravenous antibiotic therapy and possibly hospitalization.

Sexual partners also are assessed and treated according to these protocols, and sexual contact is avoided until treatment is completed. Condoms are strongly recommended to prevent future infection.

Box 24-1   Outpatient Treatment for Uncomplicated Gonorrhea Infection

One of the following:
  Ceftriaxone, 124 mg IM
  or
  Ciprofloxacin, 500 mg PO in a single dose
  or
  Spectinomycin, 2 g IM (if allergic to penicillin)
  or
  Cefiximine, 400 mg PO
  or
  Ofloxacin, 400 mg PO in a single dose
Followed by one of these regimens for presumptive coexistent chlamydia:
  Azithromycin, 1 g PO in a single dose
  or
  Doxycycline, 100 mg PO bid × 7 days
  or
  Erythromycin, 500 mg PO qid × 7 days

Syphilis

Syphilis, a disease with local and systemic manifestations, has been well known throughout history. Many famous figures from the ancient world and from the royal families of Europe were thought or known to have had syphilis.[16] In the early half of the 1900s, an estimated 1 in 4 to 1 in 20 Americans were infected.[18] With the advent of antibiotics and intensive public health efforts during and after World War II, the prevalence of syphilis declined sharply to 3 in 100,000 Americans in 2002. Rates of syphilis declined in the 1990s and reached an all-time low in 2000. However, there has been an increase in cases identified in men who have sex with men (MSM) between 2000 and 2002.[3] Although the incidence in the United States has diminished significantly in the past 3 decades, syphilis remains a problem in certain geographic regions, particularly in the South. Syphilis facilitates the transmission of HIV infection and seems to contribute to HIV transmission in those parts of the United States where rates of both infections are high. Rates of syphilis have declined dramatically in African-Americans because of efforts begun in 1999.[19] Rates in non-Hispanic whites have increased 0.5 per 100,000 to 1.5 per 100,000 persons. Rates in women have declined 27.3%.[19] During pregnancy, untreated early syphilis results in perinatal death in as many as 40% of cases and, if acquired in the previous 4 years, may lead to fetal infection in more than 70% of cases.[20]

Race and ethnicity alone do not alter STI risk but rather act as risk markers that correlate with other more fundamental determinants of health status, such as poverty, access to quality care, and health-seeking behavior. Higher infection rates have been associated with urban areas and with the exchange of sex for drugs, especially crack cocaine.[21] A growing concern is the incidence of coinfection with HIV among MSM.[19]

The current rate of **congenital syphilis (CS)** has paralleled the decline of primary and secondary syphilis diagnosed in women over the past 10 years. CS has declined 17% annually since 1991.[2] The *Healthy People 2010* objective is to reduce CS to 1 new case per 100,000 live births.

PATHOPHYSIOLOGY *Treponema pallidum,* the cause of syphilis, is an anaerobic bacterium that cannot be cultured in vitro. The treponema (individual microorganism) looks like a corkscrew, with regular, tight spirals and a rotary motion; it can infect any body organ or tissue. Because the bacterium is present in exudate from moist mucosal or cutaneous lesions, the spirochete is transmitted during the first few years of infection. Transmission generally occurs through minor abrasions during sexual intercourse but can occur extragenitally as well. Approximately 30% to 50% of partners who have sexual intercourse with an individual in early-stage syphilis develop the disease.[22]

Syphilis becomes a systemic disease shortly after infection and can be transmitted from a pregnant woman to her fetus as early as the ninth week of gestation. The risk of transmission to the fetus gradually declines with each subsequent pregnancy; therefore a mother who has had several children with severe congenital syphilis may go on to bear a healthy child. After about 8 years, even without treatment, the mother's infection is not transmitted to her fetus.[18]

The course of untreated syphilis consists of four stages: primary, secondary, latent, and tertiary (Box 24-2). **Primary syphilis** begins at the site of bacterial invasion (Figure 24-4). There *T. pallidum* multiplies in the epithelium, producing a granulomatous tissue reaction called a **chancre.** Some microorganisms drain with lymph into adjacent lymph nodes. Within the nodes and at the site of the chancre, the cell-mediated and humoral immune responses are stimulated.

Secondary syphilis is systemic. During this stage, blood-borne bacteria spread to all major organ systems. The secondary stage is followed by a period during which the immune system is able to suppress the infection. Even without treatment, spontaneous resolution of the skin lesions occurs and the individual enters the latent stage of infection. **Latent syphilis** may be subdivided into early and late stages; however, no specific criteria delineate one from the other.[21] Medical history and serologic studies show that syphilis is present, but the individual has no clinical manifestations. Transmission is possible during the late and early latent stages.

Tertiary syphilis is the most severe stage, involving significant morbidity and mortality. The pathogenesis of syphilitic manifestations at this stage remains unclear. The destructive skin, bone, and soft tissue lesions (called **gummas**) of tertiary syphilis probably are caused by a severe hypersensitivity reaction to the microorganism. Within the cardiovascular system, infection with *T. pallidum* may cause aneurysms, heart valve insufficiencies, and heart failure. Within the central nervous system (CNS), the presence of *T. pallidum* in cerebrospinal fluid may cause the manifestations of **neurosyphilis.**[18]

The risk of acquiring CS is estimated at 50% in primary and secondary syphilis, 40% in early latent syphilis, and 10% in late latent syphilis.[23] Intrauterine infection causes fetal or perinatal death in 40% of affected infants.[20,24]

CLINICAL MANIFESTATIONS

Primary Stage. In adults the incubation period of syphilis ranges from 12 days to 12 weeks after exposure and

---

Box 24-2 **Progression of Untreated Syphilis**

Stage I, primary syphilis—local invasion: *T. pallidum* multiplies in epithelium, producing granulomatous tissue reaction (chancre); lymph-containing microorganisms drain into adjacent lymph nodes and stimulate immune responses

Stage II, secondary syphilis—systemic disease: blood-borne bacteria spread to all major organ systems; immune system suppresses infection and symptoms regress spontaneously

Stage III, latent syphilis—silent infection: transmission of infection possible even though there are no clinical signs of infection

Stage IV, tertiary syphilis—noninfectious disease: significant morbidity and mortality occur; destructive skin, bone, and soft tissue lesions, or gummas, result from severe hypersensitivity; cardiovascular complications (aneurysms, heart valve insufficiency, heart failure) and neurosyphilis develop

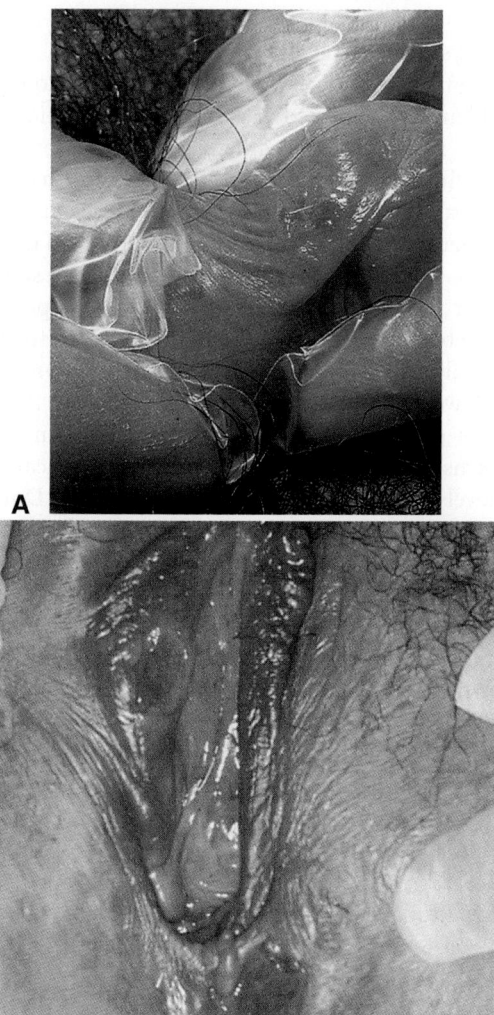

A

B

Figure 24-4 Primary syphilis. **A,** Penile chancre. **B,** Vulval chancres; labia and the perineum show induration and edema of chancres. (**A,** from McMillan A, Scott GR: *Sexually transmitted infections,* ed 2, London, 2000, Churchill Livingstone; **B,** from Morse SA, Ballard RC, Holmes KK, Moreland AA, editors: *Atlas of sexually transmitted diseases and AIDS,* ed 3, London, 2003, Mosby.)

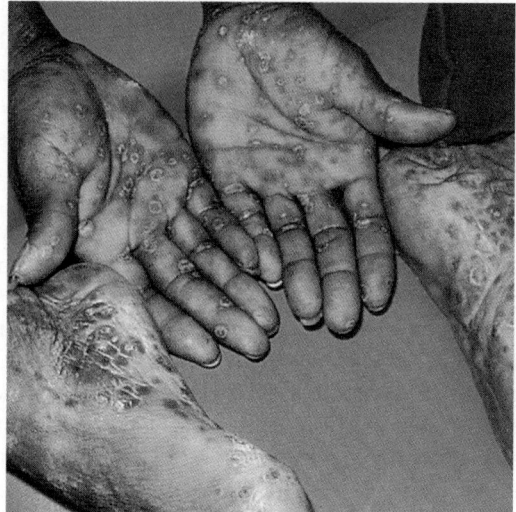

Figure 24-5 Secondary syphilis. Secondary syphilis to the palms and plantar surfaces. (From Morse SA, Ballard RC, Holmes KK, Moreland AA, editors: *Atlas of sexually transmitted diseases and AIDS,* ed 3, London, 2003, Mosby.)

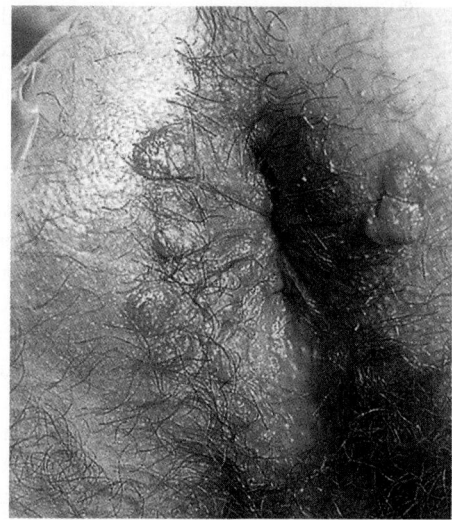

Figure 24-6 Condylomata lata. Broad-based, moist, darkfield-positive condylomata lata of the perineum. (From McMillan A, Scott GR: *Sexually transmitted infections,* ed 2, London, 2000, Churchill Livingstone.)

averages 3 weeks. At the site of treponemal entry a sore, or *hard chancre,* develops. Typically the chancre is an eroded, painless, firm, and indurated (hard) ulcer that may be a few millimeters to 2 cm in diameter. Firm, enlarged, and nontender regional lymph nodes accompany chancres. Figure 24-4 shows typical chancres of the penis and vulva. Syphilitic chancres are not always typical, however, and syphilis should be considered in the presence of any open lesion. Secondary infection can cause chancres to become necrotic and painful, and lesions on the fingers may be dry, scaly, and papular or moist and vegetative. If left untreated, the chancre of primary syphilis heals in 2 to 8 weeks and then spontaneously disappears, usually without leaving a scar.

Secondary Stage. Clinical manifestations of secondary syphilis usually develop 6 weeks after the first appearance of the chancre but may overlap with those of the primary stage. Typically this stage presents with variable systemic symptoms, including low-grade fever, malaise, sore throat, hoarseness, anorexia, generalized adenopathy, headache, joint pain, and skin or mucous membrane lesions or rashes. Cutaneous (skin) rashes are generally papulosquamous (raised and scaly), but any variation or combination of macular (flat), papular (raised), and pustular (pus-filled) lesions may be seen. Often lesions are widespread and bilateral and appear on the palms and soles (Figure 24-5). Some lesions become hypertrophied, flat, moist, and wartlike or vegetative (e.g., cauliflower-like). These lesions, called **condylomata lata,** are highly contagious and develop on the perineum, vulva, and groin of women (Figure 24-6) and around the inner thigh and the anal area in both men and women. Besides skin sores, oral mucous membrane lesions (known as mucous patches), lymphadenopathy, pruritus, and alopecia are common. Some individuals develop anemia, leukocytosis, increased sedimentation rate, hepatitis, transitory proteinuria, arthritis, electrocardiographic abnormalities, and CNS symptoms. Regardless of whether treatment is given, the cutaneous lesions generally heal in 2 to 10 weeks, but relapses may occur for several years.[23]

Latent and Tertiary Stages. The asymptomatic, latent stage of syphilis may be as short as 1 year or as long as a lifetime. After the latent stage, tertiary syphilis may present with gummas, cardiovascular lesions, and neurosyphilis. These manifestations of tertiary syphilis are quite rare because antibiotics can cure syphilis.

Congenital Syphilis. CS is characterized by vasculitis, necrosis, fibrosis, and distribution of *T. pallidum* throughout the tissues; it is divided into early and late stages. Signs and symptoms of early CS manifest in the first 2 years of life, and clinical manifestations of the late stage often occur near puberty. Affected newborns often are premature and show evidence of intrauterine growth retardation, hepatosplenomegaly, bone marrow depression, destructive bone and skin lesions (see Figure 24-5), retinal inflammation, glaucoma, blood dyscrasia, nephrotic syndrome, and varying degrees of CNS involvement.[18] Late manifestations of classic congenital syphilis correspond to those of tertiary syphilis in the adult and are rare.

EVALUATION AND TREATMENT   Because *T. pallidum* cannot be cultured in vitro, early definitive diagnosis of primary or secondary syphilis depends on dark-field microscopy of a specimen taken from a chancre, regional lymph node, or other lesion. If the initial result is negative, the dark-field examination is repeated on two successive days. When suspicion of syphilis—based on history and physical examination—persists, serologic testing is required. An algorithmic approach to the diagnosis of genital ulcers is presented in Figure 24-7.

Two categories of serologic testing exist: nontreponemal antigen tests and treponemal antibody tests.[25] Nontreponemal antigen tests, which demonstrate the presence of *reagin* (a group of antibodies present in syphilis) in serum, provide indirect evidence of infection. Examples of nontreponemal analysis are the Venereal Disease Research Laboratory (VDRL) antigen and the rapid plasma reagin (RPR) tests (Box 24-3). These tests yield a positive result (presence of reagin) in more than 50% of individuals with primary syphilis and 100% of individuals with secondary disease. When the serologic test is negative and another stage of syphilis is suspected, the test is repeated. If latent or tertiary syphilis is suspected, a treponemal serologic test is done. Treponemal tests are serologic-specific tests that are used to assess antibody response to *T. pallidum* and include the fluorescent treponemal antibody absorption (FTA-ABS) test and the microhemagglutination (MHA-TP) test.

Numerous dermatologic disorders can mimic the skin lesions of secondary syphilis, making differential diagnosis difficult. Again, laboratory confirmation is important; dark-field microscopy of scrapings from the condylomata lata or other skin lesions discloses the treponemata. Serologic tests are almost always strongly positive in this stage.

During the latent stage, individuals continue to have serologic evidence of untreated disease, but confirmation through dark-field microscopy is difficult. Examination of cerebrospinal fluid may confirm that the treponemata are present and the insidious onset of neurosyphilis has begun.

Treatment for all stages of syphilis is parenteral injection of benzathine penicillin G. If the individual has had signs of the disease for less than 1 year, a single dose is appropriate. If signs have been present for more than 1 year, the treatment is three weekly injections. This therapy is also appropriate for pregnant women. There is no evidence to date that *T. pallidum* has developed resistance to penicillin. In fact, it is highly sensitive but because of the slow replication time serum levels must be maintained for 7 to 14 days. Duration of therapy depends on estimated length of infection. Treatment for 14 days is recommended if the individual has been infected less than 1 year; treatment is for 28 days if the individual has been infected for longer than 1 year. Individuals who are allergic to penicillin receive oral doxycycline, 100 mg twice daily; or if the individual is pregnant, she receives oral erythromycin, 500 mg four times daily. Because treatment failures do occur, all individuals should have follow-up evaluation. Sexual partners also are examined and treated, and the use of condoms is recommended.

Definitive diagnosis of CS is made by microscopic identification of *T. pallidum* in material from skin lesions or nasal discharge. Probable diagnosis is assumed on the basis of a rising or persistently reactive FTA-ABS value and clinical manifestations. In all cases of maternal syphilis, the goal is to treat the mother to prevent CS. Maternal treatment with penicillin before delivery usually prevents CS. If the infant requires treatment, penicillin is the drug of choice, because allergy does not pose a problem in the neonatal period. Such infants are then given serologic tests for syphilis at 3, 6, and 12 months. Nearly all tests become nonreactive (negative) by the time the infant is 6 months of age.[20]

Chancroid

Chancroid, or soft chancre, is an acute infectious disease that was first differentiated from syphilis in 1852. It is caused by *Haemophilus ducreyi,* a gram-negative bacillus. Chancroid occurs most often in underdeveloped or developing tropical countries. Although incidence in the United States is low, 54 cases were reported to the CDC in 2003[2]; sporadic outbreaks can occur and tend to be associated with conditions such as poverty, urban prostitution, and illicit drug use, in which individuals continue to engage in intercourse in spite of the presence of a lesion.[26]

PATHOPHYSIOLOGY   *H. ducreyi* is a gram-negative bacillus with rounded ends. Under a microscope it is commonly observed in small chains or clusters along mucous strands. Transmission can occur through sexual contact and autoinoculation. There is no evidence of maternal-fetal trans-

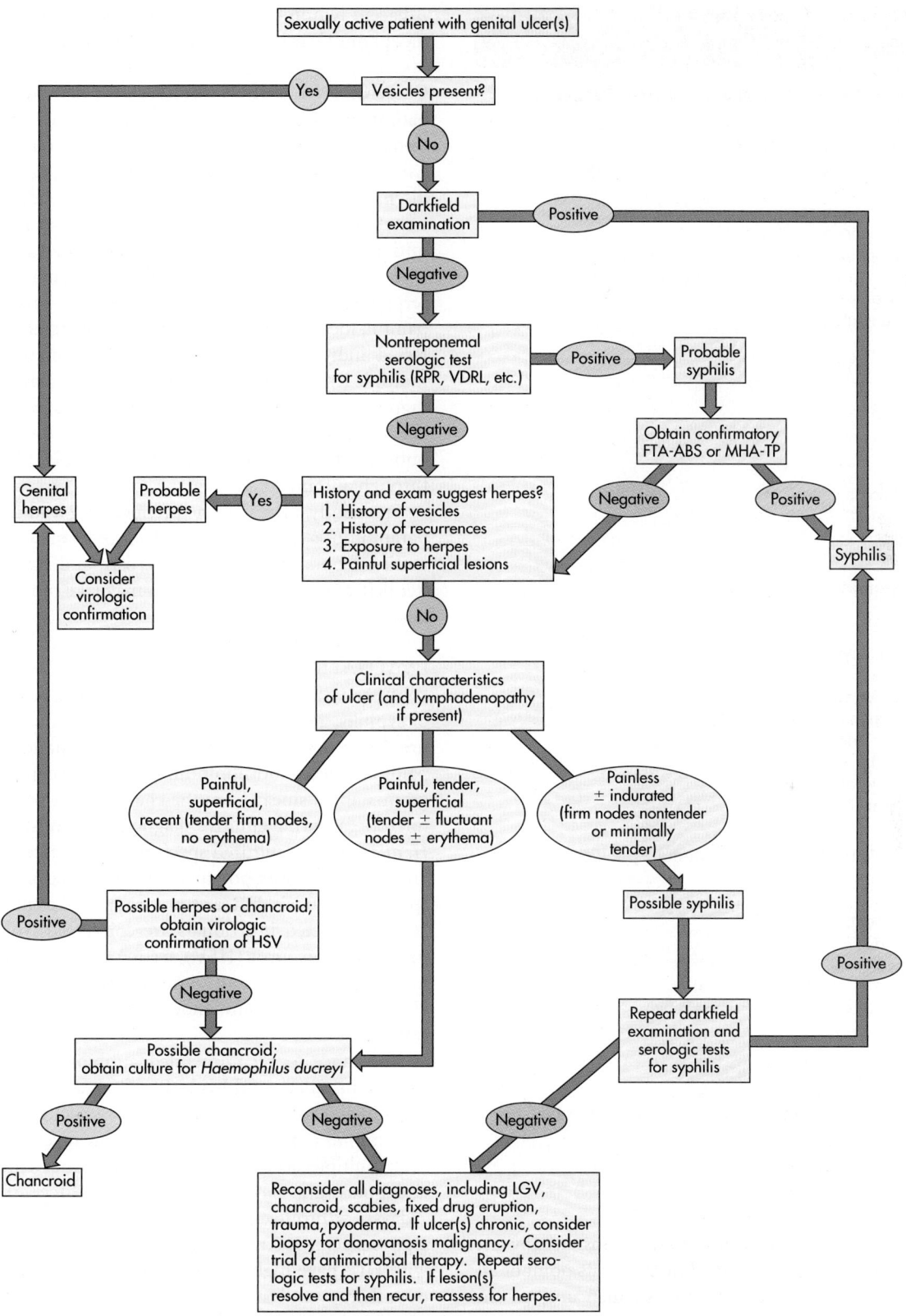

Figure 24-7 Genital ulceration. Algorithm outlining an approach to the diagnosis of an individual who presents with a genital ulceration. *RPR,* Rapid plasma reagin test; *VDRL,* Venereal Disease Research Laboratory test; *FTA-ABS,* fluorescent treponemal antibody absorption test; *MHA-TP,* microhemagglutination test; *HSV,* herpes simplex virus; *LGV,* lymphogranuloma venereum. (Redrawn from Pitot P, Plummer FA. In Holmes KK et al, editors: *Sexually transmitted diseases,* ed 2, New York, 1990, McGraw-Hill.)

fer before or after delivery. Chancroid lesions usually are found on the internal surface of the foreskin or its point of attachment to the penis (the frenulum) in men and on the labia, clitoris, or fourchette in women. Initially the papule enlarges; it then erodes into a soft, circumscribed ulcer containing a superficial exudate. Beneath the ulcer is a lesion characterized by edema, endothelial proliferation, and a base of granulation tissue that is full of lymphocytes and plasma cells.

Adjacent lymph nodes are acutely inflamed and full of polymorphonuclear leukocytes and necrotic cells.[27]

CLINICAL MANIFESTATIONS   Chancroid has an incubation period of 3 to 10 days.[28] Generally, women are asymptomatic, but depending on the site of infection, can present with less obvious symptoms (dysuria, dyspareunia, vaginal discharge, pain on defecation, or rectal bleeding). Constitutional symptoms are unusual. At the site of inoculation, an initial vesicopustule lesion forms and erodes into a soft ulcer with a necrotic base, surrounding erythema, and a ragged, serpiginous (spreading) border (Figure 24-8). Unilateral, painful, local lymphadenopathy presents in about half of infected individuals—primarily men. (Women tend to have multiple lesions.) Inguinal **buboes** (unilocular abscess of the inguinal lymph nodes) develop 7 to 10 days after the initial chancre and fill with exudate. In 25% to 60% of cases, the buboes spontaneously rupture. Multiple lesions spread through autoinoculation.

Frequently, ulcers on the prepuce may lead to phimosis or paraphimosis. Other complications of chancroid include balanitis, secondary infections, necrosis, and fistula formation. Recalcitrant, serpiginous lesions may take months or years to heal.

EVALUATION AND TREATMENT   Chancroid is easily confused with other types of genital ulcers, particularly those of syphilis, genital herpes, and granuloma inguinale (see Figure 24-8). Unlike the syphilitic ulcer, chancroidal ulcer is painful, tender, and nonindurated. Microscopic analysis of a gram-stained smear from the chancroid helps to identify the microorganism. Definitive diagnosis depends on recovery of *H. ducreyi* from cultured specimens. Fluorescent monoclonal antibody stains and polymerase chain reaction provide more specific diagnosis but are not routinely available. Because 10% of infected individuals are coinfected with syphilis or herpes simplex virus (HSV), testing includes serologic examination for syphilis and viral culture for HSV. In addition, HIV testing is recommended: chancroid is a cofactor for transmission of HIV.

Resistance to recommended antibiotics has emerged in isolated instances worldwide. Recent treatment recommendations include a single intramuscular injection of ceftriaxone (250 mg) or a single dose of oral azithromycin (1 g). Effective oral multiple-dose regimens include amoxicillin (500 mg) and potassium clavulanate (125 mg) three times daily for 7 days; erythromycin, 500 mg four times daily for 7 days; or ciprofloxacin, 500 mg twice daily for 3 days. Persons infected with HIV have higher rates of treatment failure with single-dose therapy and may require a longer treatment regimen. As a palliative measure, buboes can be aspirated through adjacent, healthy skin. In approximately 5% of cases, relapses at the site of original ulcer have occurred.[28,29] Simultaneous treatment of sexual partners and condom use are recommended to prevent reinfection.

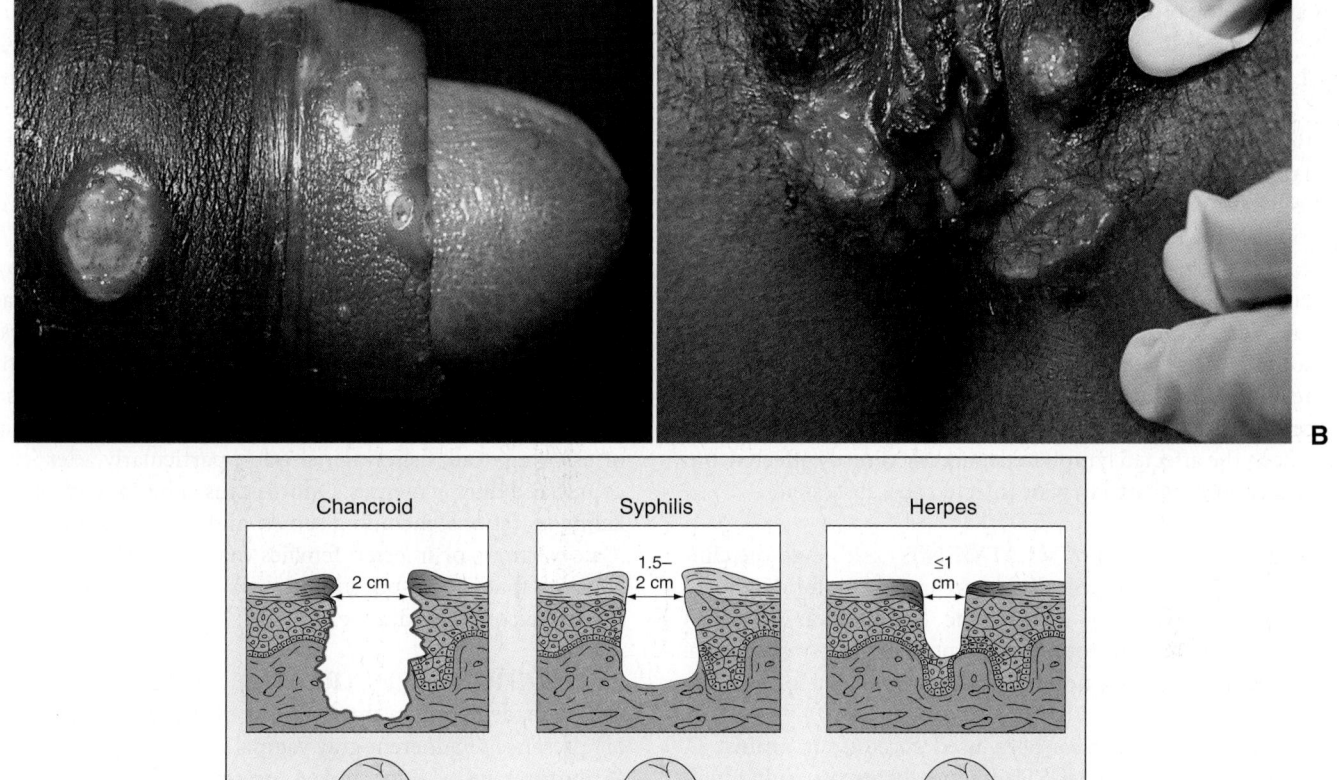

Figure 24-8 Chancroid. **A,** Ulcers on the penile shaft. **B,** Multiple vulvar lesions. **C,** Differences in clinical appearance among chancroid, syphilis, and genital herpes. (From Morse SA, Ballard RC, Holmes KK, Moreland AA, editors: *Atlas of sexually transmitted diseases and AIDS,* ed 3, London, 2003, Mosby.)

Granuloma Inguinale

Granuloma inguinale (donovanosis) is a chronic, progressively destructive bacterial infection caused by *Calymmatobacterium granulomatis,* recently reclassified as *Klebsiella granulomatis.*[26] Although sexually transmissible, granuloma inguinale is only mildly contagious and repeated exposure is necessary to cause disease. Often, individuals are coinfected with syphilis.[30]

Indigenous granuloma inguinale no longer occurs in the United States (cases that occur are imported).[28] Yet, in some parts of the world (India, New Guinea, Africa, and to a lesser extent the Caribbean and Brazil), granuloma inguinale is among the most prevalent of the present STIs. Incidence of infection is found in tropical and subtropical environments with sustained high temperature and high relative humidity. Infection is usually acquired through sexual intercourse with an individual who has active disease or asymptomatic rectal infection. As with all genital ulcerative diseases, granuloma inguinale plays a role in HIV transmission.[26]

PATHOPHYSIOLOGY *C. granulomatis* is a gram-negative, nonsporing, nonmotile, encapsulated rod that is not easily isolated in the laboratory. After exposure the bacteria survive and multiply within vacuoles of large histiocytic cells or polymorphonuclear leukocytes. The bacteria reproduce within these cells until a vacuole may contain 20 to 30 microorganisms. These bacteria-filled vacuoles were identified by Donovan in 1905 and are termed **Donovan bodies.** The presence of Donovan bodies in tissue smears of material from the lesions is considered the "gold standard" for diagnosis of lymphogranuloma inguinale.[30,31]

The initial lesion is an indurated subcutaneous nodule that is often preceded and accompanied by itching. The primary sites for development of the lesions are the distal penis in males and the introitus in females. Single lesions often coalesce with nearby lesions or form new lesions by autoinoculation of nearby skin surfaces. Progression from the initial nodule to a large, granuloma-heaped ulcer occurs slowly. Secondary infection may occur, increasing tissue damage and residual scarring. The disease may spread to the bones, joints, and liver.

CLINICAL MANIFESTATIONS   The incubation period of granuloma inguinale is 8 to 80 days. The initial lesion is an indurated, sharply defined, painless, subcutaneous nodule that is often preceded and accompanied by itching. Nodules bleed easily and contain abundant red, beefy-looking granulation tissue. Progression to a large, granuloma-heaped ulcer occurs slowly; single lesions coalesce or form new lesions by autoinoculation of nearby skin surfaces. Secondary infection may occur, increasing tissue damage and residual scarring. Although systemic symptoms are rare, the disease may spread to the bones, joints, and liver. In some cases, infection spreads to the inguinale area and produces **pseudobuboes.** In these instances, the affected lymph nodes are not directly affected, but the surrounding area may be infected and abscessed.

EVALUATION AND TREATMENT   Although the clinical manifestations of this disease are important for diagnosis, confirmation involves microscopic examination in which Donovan bodies are found in a smear or biopsy specimen. Polymerase chain reaction tests are now available for research only.[26]

Many antibiotics have been used successfully against *C. granulomatis.* Since other STIs frequently coexist, individuals should be tested for chlamydia, gonorrhea, syphilis, Hepatitis B, and HIV. Because of the indolent nature of the disease, duration of therapy tends to be relatively long. With effective antibiotic treatment, lesions begin to heal in 7 days, but treatment is continued for 21 days or until all lesions are healed. Therapy includes oral erythromycin (500 mg) four times daily, or doxycycline (100 mg) or trimethoprim-sulfamethoxazole twice daily for 21 days. Gentamicin and ciprofloxacin are reserved for resistant infections. Relapses can occur 6 to 18 months later despite effective initial therapy, so prolonged follow-up is necessary, as is treatment of sexual partners.

Bacterial Vaginosis

Bacterial vaginosis (BV)—previously called nonspecific vaginitis; nonspecific vaginosis; or *Haemophilus, Corynebacterium,* or *Gardnerella* vaginitis—is a sexually associated condition, but is not necessarily considered an STI. Bacterial vaginosis occurs almost exclusively in sexually active women of reproductive age and is uncommon in sexually inexperienced women. Prevalence rates vary from 17% among women in family planning clinics to 37% among some groups of pregnant women.[1] Fifty percent of women with signs of BV are asymptomatic.

PATHOPHYSIOLOGY   The exact etiology of BV is unknown. *Gardnerella vaginalis* and various anaerobes, including *Mycoplasma hominis, Bacteroides,* and *Mobiluncus,* interact and proliferate when lactobacilli (the normal predominant vaginal flora) are decreased or absent. Bacteria adhere to vaginal epithelium, and massive overgrowth occurs

and causes a noninflammatory response. Catabolic enzymes degrade proteins into amines. In turn, amines elevate vaginal pH and produce the characteristic fishy odor associated with BV. BV has been implicated in PID, chorioamnionitis, preterm labor, and postpartum endometritis. Sexual intercourse is believed to be the primary method of initiating BV, but definitive proof is lacking and the syndrome has been identified in virgins.[28,32]

CLINICAL MANIFESTATIONS   BV is characterized by a thin, gray, homogenous, and malodorous discharge that adheres to the vaginal walls but is often copious enough to drain into the vulva. Occasionally the discharge is bubbly or frothy. Usually the vaginal pH is 5.0 to 5.5 and there are no signs of vaginal or cervical inflammation. Individuals often complain of a strong, foul, fishy vaginal odor, particularly after intercourse and during menses. Odor is caused by contact with alkaline secretions, including semen and menstrual discharge. Male partners of infected females may harbor the microorganisms that are responsible for BV but have no signs or symptoms of active disease.

EVALUATION AND TREATMENT   Diagnosis of BV can be made based on three of four of the following criteria: (1) presence of adherent gray vaginal discharge, (2) pH >4.5, (3) positive amine odor, and (4) presence of clue cells on wet mount.[33] Clue cells are considered pathognomonic for BV. The saline wet mount also may show absence of lactobacilli and few or no leukocytes. Clue cells are vaginal epithelial cells that are covered with bacteria and look as if pepper has been sprinkled on them. When a drop of potassium hydroxide (KOH) solution is added to the slide, a characteristic amine odor is released immediately. Cultures are neither useful nor recommended; however, individuals should be screened for gonorrhea and chlamydia.

The most commonly used treatment for *Gardnerella*-associated BV is a course of oral metronidazole (Flagyl),

---

WHAT'S NEW?   **Is Bacterial Vaginosis a Risk Factor for Preterm Delivery?**

Eighteen studies with 20,232 subjects were reviewed as a meta-analysis to evaluate bacterial vaginosis as a risk factor for preterm delivery. It was found that bacterial vaginosis increased the risk of preterm delivery twofold. Higher risks were calculated for subgroups of studies that screened for bacterial vaginosis at <16 weeks of gestation or at <20 weeks of gestation. Bacterial vaginosis also significantly increased the risk of spontaneous abortion and maternal infection. No significant results however, were calculated for the outcome of neonatal infection or perinatal death. In conclusion, it was determined that bacterial vaginosis, early in pregnancy, is a strong risk factor for preterm delivery and spontaneous abortion.

Data from Leitich H et al: *Am J Obstet Gynecol* 289(1):139-247, 2003.

500 mg twice daily for 7 days, or 0.75% vaginal gel twice daily for 5 days. Alternative regimens include oral clindamycin, 300 mg twice daily for 7 days, or 2% vaginal cream once daily for 7 days. Clindamycin vaginal suppositories have been newly approved for use as a 3-day treatment regimen in nonpregnant women. Clindamycin cream is oil based, and for up to 72 hours after completing therapy, it may weaken latex condoms. For high-risk pregnant women, metronidazole, 750 mg divided into 3 doses daily for 7 days, is the preferred treatment. BV treatment in women infected with HIV is the same for HIV-negative patients. It is especially important in women who are pregnant, because BV and chorioamnionitis may increase the risk of perinatal transmission of HIV.[28] No evidence indicates that treatment of sexual partners reduces recurrence and is not recommended.[33]

Chlamydial Infections
Urogenital Infections

Chlamydia is the common name for infections caused by *Chlamydia trachomatis* (CT). *C. trachomatis* is responsible for a variety of syndromes, including acute urethral syndrome, nongonococcal urethritis (NGU), mucopurulent cervicitis, and pelvic inflammatory disease (PID). Chlamydia, the most common bacterial STI in the United States, affects about 3 million individuals annually[2] and is the leading cause of preventable infertility and ectopic pregnancy. In 2003, 877,478 cases of chlamydial infections were reported. This is more than twice the number of gonorrhea infections.[2] The rate of chlamydia has risen from 78.5 cases/100,000 women to 46.65/100,000 women—probably reflecting improved sensitivity in testing as well as a frank increase in incidence.[34] Approximately 75% of women with CT infection are asymptomatic. In addition, *C. trachomatis* can be recovered from the urethra in 25% to 60% of men with nongonoccal urethritis (NGU), in 4% to 35% of men with gonorrhea, in 28% of asymptomatic men whose partners have chlamydial cervicitis, and in 0% to 7% of men without urethritis who are seen in STI clinics.

Chlamydia is most common among young (less than 20 years old) heterosexuals who have new or multiple partners or who have been diagnosed with gonorrhea. The incidence of CT infection in pregnancy has been estimated at between 2% and 30%. Age younger than 25 years (with highest rates in women younger than 20 years), a new sexual partner, and first pregnancy were strongly and independently associated with infection in a study of over 7000 pregnant women who were screened for CT at their first prenatal visit. Like gonorrhea, *Chlamydia* infection is transmitted from mother to infant through the infected birth canal. Estimated rate of transmission ranges from 60% to 70%.[35]

PATHOPHYSIOLOGY   *C. trachomatis* is an obligate, gram-negative, intracellular bacterium that lacks the ability to reproduce independently. Like viruses, *Chlamydia* can reproduce only within host cells. It is differentiated from other bacteria by its unique two-part growth cycle. The first part consists of an elementary body that is small, resilient, metabolically inert, and able to survive extracellularly. Once this elementary body attaches itself to a receptor host cell, it is able to enter by endocytosis. Once inside the cell, the second part of the cycle begins and the organism becomes a metabolically active parasite, reproducing within the cell until the cell is destroyed and ruptures, disseminating up to 1000 new elementary bodies. Rarely does this cause a secondary infection. Infection with *C. trachomatis* produces a mononuclear inflammatory reaction rather than a polymorphonuclear inflammatory reaction. The former reaction produces permanent scarring of tissues.[36]

Chlamydia microorganisms are always pathogens; they are not part of the normal flora of the urogenital tract, despite the fact that infection is often asymptomatic. Numerous serotypes, or strains, of *C. trachomatis* have been identified. Some cause urogenital infection; some, ocular trachoma; and others, lymphogranuloma venereum, which is discussed in the next section.

The strains of *C. trachomatis* that cause urogenital infection apparently require squamous-columnar and columnar epithelial cells as hosts. *C. trachomatis* infects and disrupts epithelial tissues but does not seem to invade or destroy deeper tissues or organs. Urogenital chlamydial infections may have a fairly self-limited acute course followed by a chronic, low-grade, persistent infection that lasts for years.[36]

In newborns, several sites may be inoculated with *Chlamydia* during passage through the infected maternal cervix. These include the eye, nasopharynx, rectum, and vagina. The infant also may aspirate infected secretions with its first breaths, resulting in chlamydial pneumonitis and substantial newborn morbidity.

CLINICAL MANIFESTATIONS   Asymptomatic chlamydial infection is common. Urogenital infections caused by *Chlamydia* closely parallel those caused by gonorrhea. Both microorganisms infect superficial genital tract tissues, such as mucosa of the urethra and cervix, and both can invade the epididymides, fallopian tubes, and hepatic capsule. Table 24-2 lists the pathophysiologic similarities of chlamydial and gonococcal infections.

Chlamydial infection accounts for 50% to 60% of cases of NGU in men. Clinically, urethritis caused by gonorrhea and chlamydia cannot be differentiated: both have a 7- to 21-day incubation period and cause dysuria. Although urethral discharge in men may be similar in the two infections, chlamydial discharge tends to be more clear and gonococcal discharge more purulent. Men might note a clear, mucous discharge on rising in the morning; dry, clear discharge on their underwear; or mild burning with urination. Chlamydial urethritis is generally milder than gonorrheal urethritis and more likely to be asymptomatic. Symptoms may be intermittent or unnoticeable. Gram-stained smears of the urethral discharge show numerous polymorphonuclear leukocytes, which indicates ongoing inflammation. Screening men without symptoms is not cost effective at this time.

Table 24-2	Similarity of Clinical Syndromes Caused by *Chlamydia trachomatis* and *Neisseria gonorrhoeae*	
	Clinical Syndrome	
Site of Infection	N. gonorrhoeae	C. trachomatis
Men		
Urethra	Urethritis	Nongonococcal urethritis; postgonococcal urethritis
Epididymis	Epididymitis	Epididymitis
Rectum	Proctitis	Proctitis
Conjunctiva	Conjunctivitis	Conjunctivitis
Systemic	Disseminated gonococcal infection	Reiter syndrome
Women		
Urethra	Acute urethral syndrome	Acute urethral syndrome
Bartholin gland	Bartholinitis	Bartholinitis
Cervix	Cervicitis	Cervicitis; cervical atypia
Fallopian tube	Salpingitis	Salpingitis
Conjunctiva	Conjunctivitis	Conjunctivitis
Liver capsule	Perihepatitis	Perihepatitis
Systemic	Disseminated gonococcal infection	Arthritis-dermatitis syndrome

Data from Stamm WE, Holmes KK. In Holmes KK et al, editors: *Sexually transmitted diseases,* ed 2, New York, 1990, McGraw-Hill.

Chlamydial epididymitis can accompany chlamydial urethritis and is characterized by fever and a unilaterally painful, swollen scrotum. Chlamydial infection also causes proctitis (rectal inflammation) in homosexual men and occasionally in heterosexual women and is linked to the practice of receptive anal intercourse. Chlamydial proctitis is generally mild, although it may, like gonorrheal proctitis, cause rectal bleeding, mucous discharge, and diarrhea. Reiter syndrome (urethritis, conjunctivitis, arthritis, and characteristic mucocutaneous lesions) is also associated with untreated chlamydial infections of the urogenital tract.

Chlamydia infection is the leading cause of tubal infertility in women. Risk factors for infertility include numbers of chlamydial infections and duration and severity of infection. Even women with asymptomatic salpingitis have a risk of subsequent infertility. This may reflect an antigen-antibody response rather than inflammatory damage.[37]

In young, sexually active women, *C. trachomatis* is a cause of **acute urethral syndrome** (dysuria, urinary frequency, and presence of sterile pus in the urine). *C. trachomatis* also causes asymptomatic urethral infection in women. Chlamydial infection of Bartholin glands can cause purulent discharge and formation of a Bartholin cyst. Women with chlamydial cervicitis may be asymptomatic or may have a yellow mucopurulent discharge from the cervical os and a hypertrophic, edematous, and friable area of cervical ectopy. The woman also may report intermenstrual or postcoital spotting. Although ectopy alone does not indicate a pathologic condition, a raised, erythematous, raw, and friable ectopy is abnormal and strongly suggestive of chlamydial cervicitis (Figure 24-9).

The most common clinical manifestations of chlamydial infections in the newborn are conjunctivitis and pneumonia. Like gonococcal infection, prophylactic treatment with antibiotic eye ointment at birth does not provide complete pro-

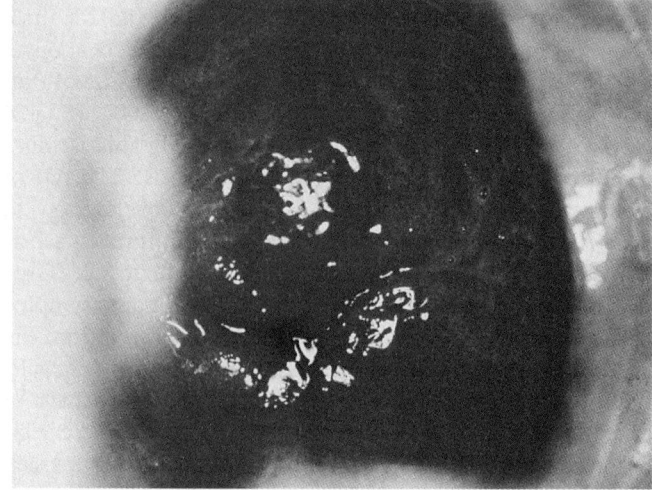

Figure 24-9 Chlamydial cervicitis. Beefy red mucosa of columnar epithelium of cervix. (From Morse SA, Ballard RC, Holmes KK, Moreland AA, editors: *Atlas of sexually transmitted diseases and AIDS,* ed 3, London, 2003, Mosby.)

tection against neonatal conjunctivitis and does not protect against neonatal pneumonia. Chlamydial conjunctivitis begins between 5 and 14 days after delivery, when the infant's eyes begin to water. This discharge may become purulent, and both eyes may become red and swollen (Figure 24-10). Scarring of the conjunctivae may result, but this infection does not cause blindness, as does the ophthalmia neonatorum caused by *N. gonorrhoeae*. The pneumonia is mild or severe and may accompany the conjunctivitis. Infants with chlamydial pneumonia are seen at 3 to 11 weeks of age with staccato coughing spells, nasal congestion, dyspnea, and minimal fever. Other signs include otitis media, tachypnea, wheezing, bronchospasm, crepitant inspiratory rales, and apneic spells.

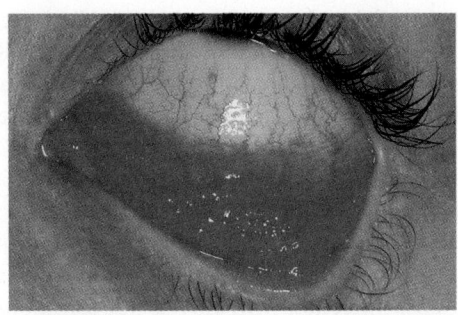

Figure 24-10 Chlamydial ophthalmia. (From McMillan A, Scott GR: *Sexually transmitted infections*, ed 2, London, 2000, Churchill Livingstone.)

EVALUATION AND TREATMENT   Methods for diagnosing chlamydial infections include tissue culture techniques, direct chlamydia enzyme immunoassay, fluorescein-labeled monoclonal antibody tests, and DNA probe testing. Currently, tests using chlamydia-specific nucleic acid sequences (LCR, PCR, and DNA) are the most sensitive and cost-effective tests available.[34] Concurrent DNA testing for gonorrhea can be done using the same swab.

C. trachomatis is susceptible to inexpensive, readily accessible antibiotics. Treatment includes antibiotic therapy for infected individuals and all sexual contacts; abstinence or use of condoms during treatment is recommended. Azithromycin, 1 g orally, as a single dose or a 7-day course of oral doxycycline, 100 mg twice daily; or oral erythromycin or tetracycline, 500 mg four times daily, is effective.[2] Azithromycin is the drug of choice in pregnancy. Because of the asymptomatic nature of *Chlamydia* and the potential sequelae of untreated infection, extensive widespread screening is warranted.

Lymphogranuloma Venereum

C. trachomatis (invasive serovars of strains L1, L2, or L3) can cause a chronic STI known as **lymphogranuloma venereum (LGV),** which may be confused with syphilis, herpes, or chancroid. Although LGV is rare in the United States, it has been endemic in Asia and Africa. The infection is acquired during sexual intercourse or through contact with contaminated exudate from active lesions. Inapparent infections and latent disease are rare.[38]

PATHOPHYSIOLOGY   The strain of *C. trachomatis* that causes LGV probably penetrates skin and mucous membranes through tiny abrasions. LGV begins as a skin lesion and spreads to genital and rectal lymphatic tissue, where it causes marked inflammation, necrosis, buboes, abscesses of inguinal lymph nodes, and infection of surrounding tissues. Healing occurs by fibrosis after several weeks or months and results in scarring, which damages the lymph nodes and disrupts nodal function. Affected nodes become chronically swollen, hardened, and enlarged. *C. trachomatis* also spreads systematically through the bloodstream and can enter the CNS.[39]

CLINICAL MANIFESTATIONS   The primary lesion of LGV appears after an incubation period of 5 to 21 days. The lesion is most commonly a herpetiform (multivesicular) ulcer, but it can take various forms. The ulcer generally is asymptomatic and inconspicuous and heals rapidly, leaving no scar. In men the lesion is found most commonly on the penis or scrotum; in women it is found on the vaginal wall, cervix, or labia. Other signs of primary LGV include a large, tender lymphatic nodule or bubo, urethritis, and cervicitis.

The secondary stage of untreated LGV in men is characterized by inflammation and swelling of the lymph nodes. At first the inguinal bubo is a firm, somewhat painful mass. As the bubo gradually enlarges, it becomes very painful, thereby restricting mobility, and takes on a deep blue color. This color change signals impending rupture of the bubo through the skin. Thick yellow pus may drain from the site for weeks or months. Healing is slow and results in scar formation. Systemic manifestations of secondary LGV include meningitis, pneumonitis, and other major infections. In some cases the bubo does not rupture but rather involutes and becomes firm. Bubo formation is most common in men. In women the inguinal lymph nodes are involved in fewer than one third of cases.

Anorectal LGV may be caused by direct inoculation during anal intercourse, or it may be a chronic or late manifestation of lymphatic spread from the inguinal area. Most individuals with anorectal LGV are women and homosexual men. Clinical symptoms include multiple ulcerations of the rectal mucosa, chronic inflammation, mucopurulent rectal discharge, and rectovaginal fistulas in women. Individuals may have fever, rectal pain, and tenesmus. Rectal strictures, perirectal abscesses, and anal fissures may develop and are the cause of most of the severe morbidity associated with LGV.

EVALUATION AND TREATMENT   Clinical manifestations and laboratory tests are used to diagnose LGV. Tests include the LGV complement-fixation tests, isolation of the microorganism in tissue culture, and monoclonal antibody tests. The diagnosis usually is made serologically and by excluding other causes of genital ulcers or inguinal lymphadenopathy. LGV is treated with oral doxycycline, 100 mg twice daily for 21 days. A 21-day course of erythromycin is also effective. Sex partners also should be treated.

Nongonococcal or Nonspecific Urethritis

Nongonococcal urethritis (NGU), also known as *nonspecific urethritis,* is a nonreportable STI. In student health centers and STI clinics, more than 50% of individuals with urethritis have NGU. The morbidity is equal to or greater than that associated with gonorrhea. Approximately 2 million men are affected each year. Most commonly, it affects heterosexual men and men of higher socioeconomic status. NGU may be complicated by epididymitis in heterosexual men under age 35 years, proctitis in homosexual men, and Reiter syndrome.

PATHOPHYSIOLOGY   Nongonococcal urethritis is a syndrome caused by a variety of microbes, including *C. trachomatis* and *Ureaplasma urealyticum.* Postgonococcal urethritis occurs in 15% to 35% of men diagnosed with gonorrhea. These men usually have coexistent gonorrheal and chlamydial infection and develop biphasic illness because of the longer incubation period of CT. Chlamydial infections are discussed earlier in this chapter (see p. 875).

C. trachomatis is the most common cause of NGU (23% to 55%). *Trichomonas vaginalis* and HSV sometimes cause NGU. However, *Ureaplasma, U. urealyticum,* and possibly *Mycoplasma* are implicated in as many as one third of the cases of NGU.[2] Genital colonization with *U. urealyticum* occurs with an increasing number of sexual partners. That is, urethral cultures of men with a history of three to five lifetime sexual partners yield *U. urealyticum* whether those men have urethritis or not. The difference in symptomatology may be the result of infection by different serotypes. Some of the 14 different serotypes of *U. urealyticum* may be more pathogenic than others. Twenty to thirty percent of men with acute urethritis are negative for *N. gonorrhoeae, C. trachomatis,* and *U. urealyticum.* Some of these men respond to antibiotic treatment; others experience persistent and recurrent infection. No clear association has been found between NGU and infection caused by herpes simplex virus, trichomonads, cytomegalovirus, and other microorganisms.

CLINICAL MANIFESTATIONS   Clinically, NGU infection caused by CT cannot be differentiated from NGU caused by another microbe. In both cases, men present after a 7- to 21-day incubation period with complaints of dysuria and mild to moderate white or clear urethral discharge. Discharge may be absent, and urethral itching may be the only symptom. Asymptomatic infection is common.

EVALUATION AND TREATMENT   NGU is a diagnosis of exclusion. Urethral exudate is gram stained, and an endourethral swab is taken for testing or culture. Urine sediment also may be examined. All individuals who have urethritis should be evaluated for the presence of gonococcal and chlamydial infection. A treatment of a single 1 g oral dose of azithromycin should be initiated as soon as possible after diagnosis. Doxycycline, 100 mg orally twice a day for 7 days, is also effective. Single-dose regimens have the advantage of improved compliance and of directly observed therapy.[2]

Viral Infections
Genital Herpes
Genital herpes, which causes blisters (cold sores), is the most common infectious genital ulceration in the United States. In fact, genital infection with the herpes simplex virus (HSV) is an epidemic in the United States. Genital herpes can be caused by either of the two serotypes of HSV-type 1 (HSV-1) or type 2 (HSV-2). Although infections caused by the serotypes are clinically indistinguishable, serologic studies show that more than 80% of initial and 98% of recurrent genital HSV infections are caused by HSV-2.

Herpes simplex virus is not a reportable disease, and any reporting that is done is nonstandardized, so national statistics are not available. However, primary HSV infections are estimated to affect 1 million individuals each year. Recurrent infections are mostly asymptomatic (50% to 70%) and affect an estimated 45 million Americans annually.[1] The seroprevalence of HSV-2 is estimated to range from 16% to 20% of the total adult population to 35% to 60% for subgroups, for example, STI clinic patients and black women. The incidence of HSV infection tends to be highest in the teen to young adult age group (12 to 29 years) and in nonwhite lower socioeconomic groups.[2] Infection with HSV is not commonly associated with other STIs, for example, gonorrhea.[20]

Herpes simplex virus infection is transmitted through intimate contact with a person who is shedding the virus in a secretion or from a peripheral lesion or mucosal surface. Persons without symptoms probably transmit most infections. Transmission rates are not well identified; however, it is estimated that a woman has an 80% to 90% risk of developing genital herpes after being exposed to an infected male. In 1992 Mertz and colleagues[40] studied monogamous heterosexual couples in which one partner had HSV-2 infection. The noninfected partner seroconverted in 10% of couples over a 1-year period. As many as 70% of such infections seem to be acquired during periods of asymptomatic shedding. Uninfected female partners were at greater risk than males, especially if they were seronegative for HSV-1 antibodies as well. The likelihood of nonsexual transmission of genital herpes, through aerosolized secretions of other fomites, is quite rare and unlikely.[5,36]

Neonatal infections can occur in utero or, more commonly, during the intrapartum or postpartum period. The incidence of neonatal infections has been estimated to be 1 in 2500 to 1 in 20,000 births.[41] Perinatal transmission can cause extensive morbidity and mortality.

Intrauterine transmission can occur through transplacental or ascending infection and can cause spontaneous abortion or premature delivery.[20] Most infections are transmitted intrapartally. Infants are at greatest risk if the mother has a primary infection acquired near the time of delivery (30% to 50%) rather than a recurrent infection or an infection acquired during the first half of pregnancy (3%). Ruptured membranes have a role in the development of HSV. Membranes that have been ruptured for more than 4 hours increase the risk for contracting HSV. Internal fetal monitoring devices also increase the risk of the infant contracting HSV.[42]

PATHOPHYSIOLOGY   After initial exposure and entry of the virus at mucocutaneous sites or abraded skin, the virus undergoes replication locally in the dermis and epidermis. This leads to cell destruction, transudation, and vesicle formation. The virus spreads to contiguous cells and eventually into sensory nerves. Eventually the virus is transported intraaxonally to the dorsal root, where it remains in a latent stage until it becomes reactivated. During the latent period the genome for the virus is maintained in the host cell nucleus without causing the death of the cell. After oral infection the latent virus resides in the trigeminal ganglion; after genital infection it resides in the dorsal sacral nerve roots.

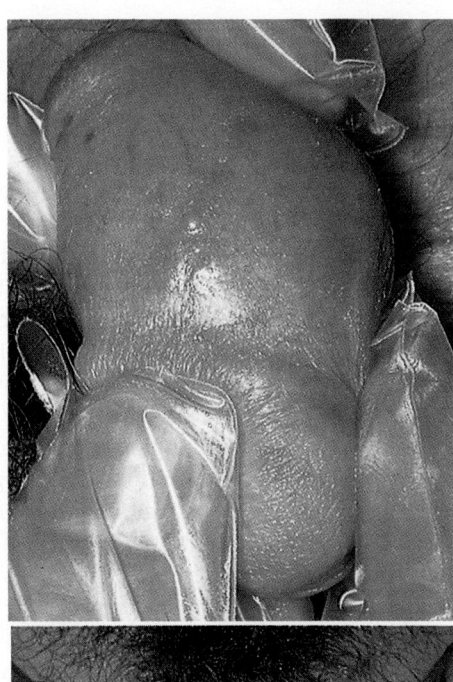

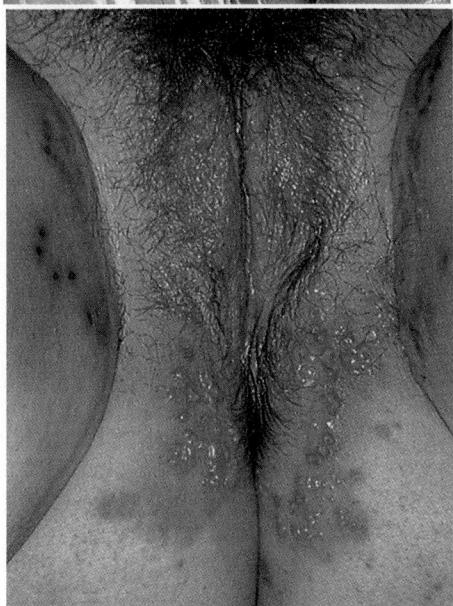

Figure 24-11 Herpes lesions. **A,** Herpetic vesicles on the penis. **B,** Herpetic ulceration of the vulva. (From McMillan A, Scott GR: *Sexually transmitted infections,* ed 2, London, 2000, Churchill Livingstone.)

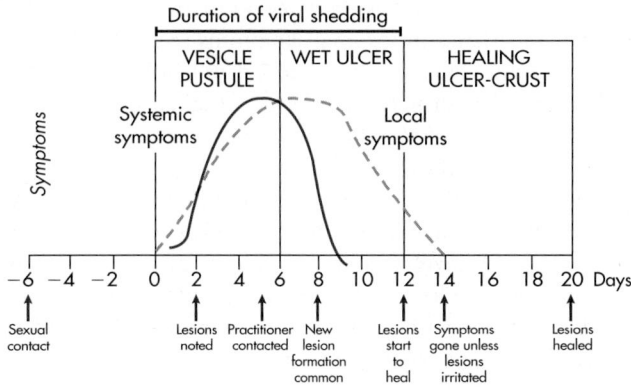

Figure 24-12 Clinical course of primary genital herpes. (From Corey L: Genital herpes. In Holmes KK et al, editors: *Sexually transmitted diseases,* ed 2, New York, 1990, McGraw-Hill.)

Latent infections can become reactivated and cause a recurrent infection with similar manifestations. Reactivation of the HSV-2 infection is twice as common as HSV-1 infections, and the likelihood of HSV-2 recurrent infections is 8 to 10 times. Reactivation of HSV is not well understood but may be attributable to physical, hormonal, and immunologic stimuli. Other triggering events may be menstruation, stress, and sun exposure.[35] During reactivation the viral genomes are transported through the peripheral sensory nerves back to the dermal surface.

CLINICAL MANIFESTATIONS   Three distinct syndromes associated with HSV infection are first-episode primary genital

infection, first-episode nonprimary HSV, and recurrent infections. The manifestations of each one depend on the individual's previous immune state. First-episode primary genital infection occurs when an individual has no antibodies to HSV-1 or HSV-2. Up to 60% of primary infections with HSV-2 and one-third of primary infections with HSV-1 are asymptomatic.[43] If symptoms occur, the individual may have small (1 to 2 mm), multiple, vesicular lesions, which are generally located on the labia minora, fourchette, or penis (Figure 24-11). They also may appear on the cervix, buttocks, and thighs and are often painful and pruritic. These lesions usually last about 10 to 20 days. The lesions of HSV-1 and HSV-2 are indistinguishable to the naked eye. These wet lesions actively shed virus for about 10 to 14 days, after which they heal by reepithelialization. Small lesions may coalesce into larger ulcers and become secondarily infected.

Systemic manifestations often accompany primary HSV infection, and an individual may experience fever, malaise, myalgias, lymphadenopathy, and urinary retention. Pharyngitis, aseptic meningitis, and hepatitis also may accompany primary HSV infection. Figure 24-12 illustrates the clinical course of primary genital HSV.

First-episode nonprimary HSV occurs in individuals who have preexisting antibodies. In some individuals the primary infection may not have had any clinical manifestations. The HSV becomes latent within the nerve root and is reactivated at a later date. Compared with primary infection, the first episode of nonprimary HSV is often milder with fewer lesions that are less painful and heal faster. Fewer systemic manifestations occur and viral shedding is of shorter duration.

Recurrent infections produce mild local symptoms. The number of lesions is greatly reduced, and the lesions are less painful. Lesions are often unilateral, with crusting within 4 to 5 days. Recovery and healing are usually complete within 10 days.[44] Asymptomatic viral shedding can occur with both HSV-1 and HSV-2.

Individuals affected with HSV-2 are more likely to experience recurrent infections. Recurrent infections occur an average of five to eight times per year but may be as frequent as every month or as rare as every few to many years. Individuals may experience prodromal symptoms (e.g., pruritus, tingling, dysesthesias) a few hours to 2 days before the eruption of lesions. Women may experience a vaginal discharge and dysuria, and 44% of men have dysuria. Symptomatic HSV infection of the newborn may occur any time in the first month of life. Manifestations range from a local infection of the eyes, skin, or mucous membranes to a severe, disseminated infection with CNS involvement. About 70% of affected infants present with skin lesions. CNS involvement includes seizures and is associated with a mortality of more than 50% and extensive neurologic sequelae in survivors.

EVALUATION AND TREATMENT Genital HSV infection is suggested if typical genital lesions are present. A presumptive diagnosis of HSV-associated infection is supported by the identification in a Papanicolaou (Pap) test of multinucleated giant cells with intranuclear inclusions. Definitive diagnosis is made after viral tissue culture. HSV-1 and HSV-2 are distinguished by fluorescent antibody, neutralization, or serologic tests. Serologic testing may be useful in identifying symptomatic carriers of HSV, for use in discordant couples and to screen pregnant women.

Currently no curative treatment for HSV infection is known. A vaccine is in development but is only effective in women who have not been infected with HSV-1; however, it is not currently available.[45] Oral acyclovir, valacyclovir, penciclovir, and famciclovir are used for primary and periodic outbreaks and to prevent recurrences. Neither valacyclovir or famciclovir is approved by the U.S. Food and Drug Administration for use in children under age 12.[4] Intravenous acyclovir is reserved for severely immunocompromised individuals.[46] Acyclovir-resistant strains of HSV have been identified periodically; no specific definitive resistant strains are known to exist. Suppressive treatment is recommended for individuals with more than six recurrences per year. Suppressive treatment also may reduce asymptomatic viral shedding. Although condoms offer some protection, individuals with HSV should refrain from all genital contact when symptomatic and understand that an undetermined risk of transmission exists even during asymptomatic periods.

Human Papillomavirus Infection

Human papillomavirus (HPV) infection is the most common symptomatic viral STI in the United States. Although over 5.5 million cases are diagnosed yearly, prevalence is considered underestimated because HPV infection is often subclinical. More sensitive measures of HPV indicate that 57% to 60% of all sexually active young women are infected with the virus. Currently the incidence of HPV is at epidemic proportions; an estimated 75% of the reproductive-age population has been infected with HPV.[1]

Over 120 different types of HPV have been identified. Over 30 serotypes are unique to the stratified squamous epitheliums of the genital area. These are divided into serotypes that have a high risk of causing cervical cancer and low-risk

serotypes, which are associated with benign lesions; *condyloma acuminata* of the vulva, vagina, penis, and perianal areas. High-risk types 16 and 18 are the most common found in more than half of cases of cervical dysplasia.[47] High-risk type 18 is associated with adenocarcinoma of the cervix.[47] Serotypes associated with genital warts include types 6 and 11, among others. These lesions can coexist with the high-risk types but do not cause cancer. Although rare, these types also may cause oral lesions. It is now known that infection with persistent, high-risk serotypes of HPV are necessary for the development of cervical cancer (also see Chapter 11). Fortunately, most cases of HPV are transient and resolve by two years.[47] Persistence of the virus, immune response, and the presence of cofactors, including smoking and hormonal contraceptive exposure, may play a role in the development of cervical dysplasia and cancer following HPV exposure.[48] HPV infection is closely associated with multiple sexual partners and early onset of sexual activity and is most common in teens and young adults, 16 to 25 years of age.

Genital warts are quite contagious, with transmission rates between individuals estimated to be between 38% and 95%. Such a wide range is attributable to the subclinical nature of some infections and various influencing factors that include number of exposures, HPV type, location of lesions, and cellular immunity response. Infants and children also have been identified as being infected with HPV. Infants can be infected in utero and by passage through an infected birth canal. HPV infection in children has been traced to child sexual abuse; however, reports vary in making this connection.[4,49]

PATHOPHYSIOLOGY HPV is a nonenveloped, circular, double-stranded DNA virus, one of the papovaviruses, that belongs to the Papovaviridae family.[50] Information about HPV was not readily available until the late 1970s, when it became possible to clone the viral genomes directly from infected tissues by recombinant DNA technology.[51]

Transmission of the virus is believed to occur through sexual contact; however, the exact transmissibility of the virus into the cell is unknown. The initial infection follows trauma to the epithelium that allows the virus to reach and infect the basal cells of the epithelium, which appear to be supportive of viral propagation. Such minor trauma may occur during sexual intercourse. Epithelial cells that are infected with HPV undergo transformation, proliferate, and form a warty growth. HPV manifestations appear in about 2 to 3 months.

CLINICAL MANIFESTATIONS **Condylomata acuminata** are soft, skin-colored, whitish pink to reddish brown, discrete growths. They may occur singly or in clusters and may be broad based or pedunculated and feathery or smooth (Figure 24-13). Sometimes the warts enlarge to form cauliflower-like masses on the male frenulum, glans, foreskin, urinary meatus, shaft, scrotum, or anus and on the female labia, clitoris, perineum, vagina, or anus (Figure 24-14). Although the lesions are usually not painful, they may cause dyspareunia (painful intercourse) and may be friable and bleed easily.

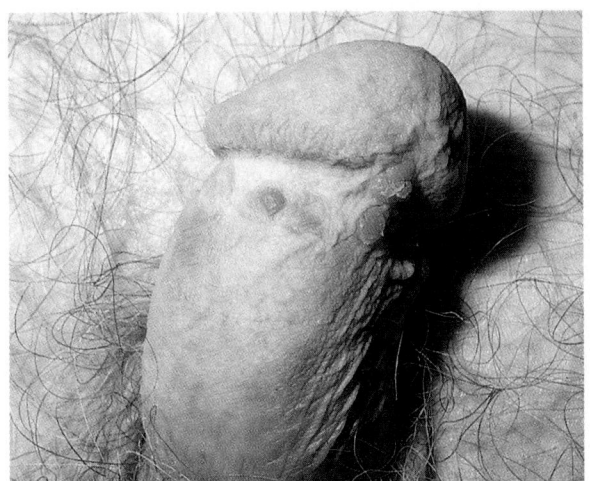

Figure 24-13 Condylomata acuminata—penile. Asymptomatic, flesh-colored papules are present on the shaft of the penis. (From Morse SA, Ballard RC, Holmes KK, Moreland AA, editors: *Atlas of sexually transmitted diseases and AIDS*, ed 3, London, 2003, Mosby.)

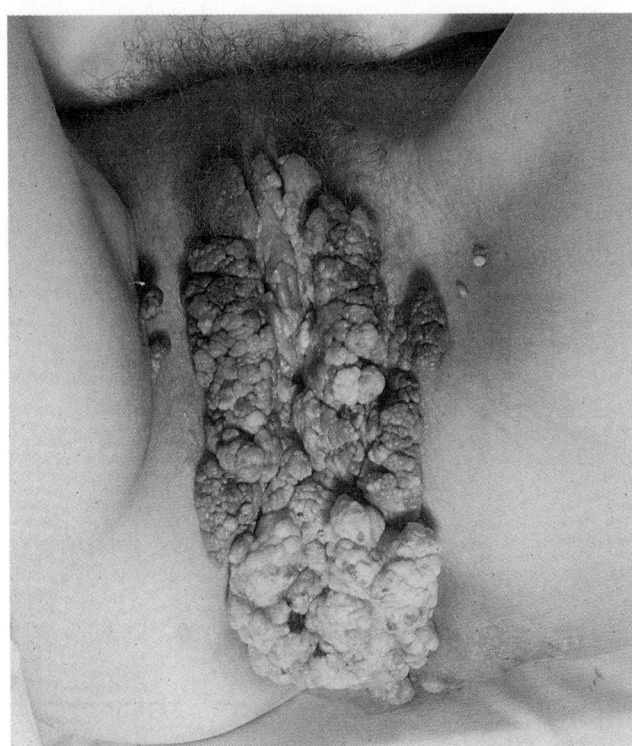

Figure 24-14 Condylomata acuminata—vulva and perineum. The clinical diagnosis was giant condylomata of Buschke and Löwenstein. Such large and confluent lesions should be carefully examined and multiple biopsies obtained to rule out underlying malignancy. (From Morse SA, Ballard RC, Holmes KK, Moreland AA, editors: *Atlas of sexually transmitted diseases and AIDS*, ed 3, London, 2003, Mosby.)

Some individuals complain of pruritus. Cervical lesions are generally flattened and may not be seen easily without colposcopy.[16] Urethral condylomata may occur in men, are always preceded by skin lesions, and can become cancerous.[52] Ninety percent of lesions are found in the distal urethra.

Laryngeal papillomas can occur in infants whose mothers had genital warts at the time of delivery. Clinical manifestations of laryngeal warts include stridor, hoarseness, abnormal cry, cough, and respiratory distress.[41] Many women with HPV may develop cytologic changes detected by Pap testing. These cell changes may be transient or may progress to dysplasia and, ultimately, cancer.

EVALUATION AND TREATMENT   Generally, diagnosis of condylomata acuminata is made on the basis of clinical manifestations. Verrucose, fleshy pink lesions caused by HPV must be differentiated from condylomata lata (the whitish gray, flat lesions) of secondary syphilis. Because HPV infection often accompanies other STIs, gonorrhea culture, chlamydia culture, serologic test for syphilis, and wet mount for other vaginal microorganisms also should be performed.

HPV infection is associated with the development of squamous cell carcinoma; therefore all atypical or persistent lesions should have a biopsy examination. HPV testing can be useful in the triage of abnormal Pap tests or can be used in conjunction with Pap testing to identify women at risk for the development of cervical dysplasia.

Treatments for external genital warts are considered cosmetic—not curative—and include patient-applied therapies (podofilox and imiquimod) and provider-administered therapies (cryotherapy, podophyllin resin, trichloroacetic acid [TCA], bichloroacetic acid [BCA], interferon, and surgery). Cervical and extensive vaginal lesions may be treated with 5-fluorouracil cream or surgical excision with CO_2 laser surgery, cryosurgery, or electrosurgery. Interferons that have gen-eral antiviral, antiproliferative, and immunomodulating effects have been used successfully in treating stubborn genital warts. Success of treatment depends on response of the immune system. Approximately one third of individuals experience a cure, and another one third experience a decrease in wart size.[20] Surgical excision is the treatment for laryngeal warts in infants. A vaccine against HPV serotypes 16 and 18 is in development and has shown to be effective in prevention of primary cervical infection with those strains, which are associated with cervical cancer[53] (Table 24-3).

Molluscum Contagiosum

Molluscum contagiosum is a benign viral infection of the skin in children and adults. Primarily the face, hands, lower abdomen, and genitalia are affected; papules found on other parts of the skin or widely distributed are not uncommon. Individuals with AIDS may develop extensive lesions over the face, neck, and genital region.

Molluscum contagiosum occurs throughout the world and has been a common childhood disease in Papua New Guinea and Fiji. It is much less common in the United States, where incidence is highest among young adults. The childhood disease is transmitted by skin-to-skin contact and fomites (swimming pools, towels, gymnasium equipment) and affects the face, trunk, and limbs. Adult disease is more commonly sexually transmitted and affects the lower abdomen, genitalia,

Table 24-3   Recent Recommendations for Cervical Cancer Screening

Parameter	American Cancer Society (ACS) Guidelines	American College of Obstetricians and Gynecologists (ACOG) Practice Bulletin
Age to start screening	3 years after onset of sexual activity but no later than 21 years of age	3 years after onset of sexual activity but no later than 21 years of age
Age to stop screening	At 70 years—if three consecutive normal Paps and no history of CIN in last 10 years and no history of DES exposure or immunosuppression	It is difficult to set an upper age limit—determine on an individual basis as regards medical history and risk factors for CIN
Screening post-hysterectomy for benign disease	Not indicated if documented that hysterectomy was for benign disease	Not indicated if documented that hysterectomy was for benign disease
Cytologic screening—interval up until age 30 years	Annually with conventional Paps or every 2 years with liquid-based cytology	Annual screening
Cytologic screening—interval after age 30 years	After three consecutive negative Paps on screen every 2-3 years unless history of CIN, DES exposure, or immunosuppression	After three consecutive negative Paps on screen every 2-3 years; women with HIV, immuno-suppression, or DES exposure may require more frequent screening
Use of HPV DNA testing and Pap after age 30 years	HPV DNA testing and cervical cytology is an acceptable screening approach	Acknowledges the FDA approval for using a combination of HPV DNA testing and cervical cytology
HPV DNA testing and Pap after age 30—screening interval	No more frequently than every 3 years	If negative on both tests—repeat no more frequently than every 3 years

Data from American Cancer Society Guidelines, *CA—Cancer J Clinicians* 52:320, 2002; Cervical cytology screening, *ACOG Pract Bull* 45, 2003.

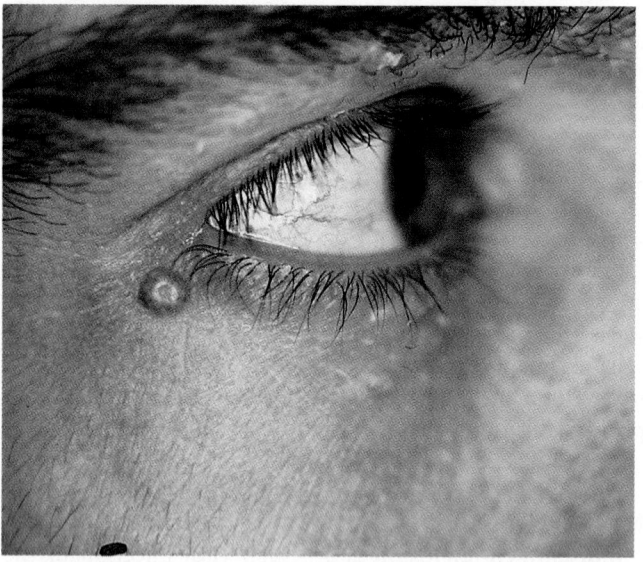

Figure 24-15 **Molluscum contagiosum.** Flesh-colored papules of molluscum may be distinguished by their umbilicated centers. The papules contain a white, cheesy substance, which may be stained for the presence of viral inclusion bodies. (From Morse SA, Ballard RC, Holmes KK, Moreland AA, editors: *Atlas of sexually transmitted diseases and AIDS*, ed 3, London, 2003, Mosby.)

and perianal area.[54] Molluscum contagiosum is most common in males 20 to 29 years of age and in those with multiple sexual partners. The molluscum contagiosum virus is taken into epithelial cells by phagocytosis and replicates within the cytoplasm, where it produces cytoplasmic inclusions (**molluscous bodies**) and cellular hyperplasia. The underlying skin usually is not affected.[55]

After an incubation period of 2 to 7 weeks, white or flesh-colored, round or oval, dome-shaped papules appear. The lesions are relatively small (3 to 5 mm) but occasionally may coalesce to form larger lesions up to 15 mm. The surface has a characteristic central umbilication, from which a thick, creamy core material can be expressed (Figure 24-15). Generally the lesions are not painful or pruritic unless secondarily infected. The papules may last several months or several years and spread by autoinoculation.

The appearance of the lesions is generally all that is needed to make the diagnosis, although direct microscopic examination of stained material from the core of the papule discloses molluscous bodies within the swollen and rounded epithelial cells. The lesions often heal spontaneously after several months. Other effective means of removing the lesions include curettage and application of liquid nitrogen (cryotherapy) or silver nitrate. Topical acids have been used also but cause scarring. Individuals tend to have lifetime immunity once lesions are healed completely.

Parasitic Infections
Trichomoniasis

Originally discovered in 1836, *Trichomonas vaginalis* was at first thought to be a harmless commensal microorganism. *T. vaginalis* is now known to be a common cause of sexually transmitted lower genital tract infection and urethritis.

Because **trichomoniasis** (infection by *T. vaginalis*) is not a reportable disease, its prevalence can only be estimated. The latest estimates suggest that as many as 5 million cases of trichomoniasis occur each year in the United States,[1] and that *T. vaginalis* accounts for one of four cases of infectious vaginitis.

Trichomoniasis is usually found in both sexual partners and often coexists with gonorrhea. Although sexual transmission is clearly the most common means of disease spread, transmission through fomites is theoretically possible. To cause infection, the fomite would have to introduce an inoculum of about 10,000 microorganisms directly into the vagina.[56]

PATHOPHYSIOLOGY   *T. vaginalis* is an anaerobic, unicellular, flagellated, parasitic protozoan that adheres to and damages squamous epithelial cells. Because this protozoan selectively affects squamous epithelia, vaginal and urethral tissue is often infected, as are Skene and Bartholin glands. The endocervical canal is not affected because it is lined with columnar epithelium. In men the urethra is the most common site of infection, although the protozoa, called **trichomonads,** also can infect the epididymis and (rarely) the prostate. Zinc, which has potent antibacterial properties, is found in high concentrations in the prostate. Hence many trichomonads are cleared from the male urethra during ejaculation. This action makes urethral trichomoniasis a fairly self-limiting infection in men. Most infections of the male urethra clear up within 2 weeks.

Trichomoniasis is most common in men and women of reproductive age, and it is primarily an infection of the vagina. *T. vaginalis* can induce a marked inflammatory response in the vagina, causing a copious discharge that contains large numbers of polymorphonuclear neutrophils. Trichomonads adhere to but do not invade the squamous epithelial cells.

CLINICAL MANIFESTATIONS   Manifestations of vaginal trichomoniasis range from none to severe, with some women reporting an increase in distressing symptoms immediately after menses. Vaginal discharge and internal pruritus are the most common complaints. Dyspareunia and dysuria are also fairly common. Secretions are usually copious, frothy, malodorous, and yellow-green to a gray-green. The vaginal walls may appear erythematous and sore. Rarely, small, punctate red marks, sometimes called *strawberry spots,* are visible. Vaginal pH is usually more than 4.2.

Most men with trichomoniasis remain asymptomatic. Possible clinical manifestations include scant intermittent discharge, slight pruritus, and mild dysuria.

EVALUATION AND TREATMENT   History and symptoms are inadequate for diagnosis of trichomoniasis. Fresh secretions have a pH higher than 4.7 and a positive amine odor when mixed with 10% KOH (positive "whiff test").

Microscopic confirmation of the presence of the trichomonads in vaginal secretions or urine provides a definitive diagnosis. In a fresh wet mount preparation that has been warmed slightly, the epithelial cells have relatively clean and sharp edges, the ratio of polymorphonuclear leukocytes to epithelial cells exceeds 1:1, and the trichomonads are visible. The ovoid microorganism is slightly larger than a polymorphonuclear leukocyte and has one rounded, flagellated end and one slightly pointed, flagellated end. The flagella give the trichomonads their characteristic twisting motility. In an acidic environment, such as urine, the trichomonads assume a "balled-up" or spherical shape and become less motile.

The treatment of choice for trichomoniasis is a single dose of metronidazole (Flagyl). The single-dose therapy is effective, has few side effects, and obviates the need for individual compliance with longer regimens. Sexual partners, even if asymptomatic, also are treated and examined for coexisting STIs. The 2-g single dose of metronidazole can be used to treat pregnant women. However, lactating women should suspend breastfeeding for 24 hours after single-dose therapy.[57]

Scabies

Scabies is a rather benign, common parasitic infection that can be spread by skin-to-skin and sexual contact. Discovered by Bonomo in 1687, it is considered to be the first human disease with a known cause.[58]

Scabies has a worldwide distribution, but actual prevalence is unknown.[25] Traditionally the disease was attributed to conditions of poverty, overcrowding, uncleanliness, and sexual promiscuity. Today it is recognized that scabies occurs in individuals with good personal hygiene and is not limited to any social class. Outbreaks of scabies occur every 30 years or so and last about 15 years. The most recent outbreak in the United States began in 1971 and subsided in the 1980s.

Transmission of scabies requires prolonged close skin-to-skin contact, which typically occurs within families or between sexual partners. Nonsexual transmission from patient to nurse has been reported in hospitals during sponge baths and lotion application, and mites have been transferred through infested bedding, clothes, and other fomites.[5]

PATHOPHYSIOLOGY   The adult female itch mite, *Sarcoptes scabiei,* is 0.3 to 0.4 mm long and has a life span of about 30 days. Once deposited on human skin, it burrows through the horny layer of the stratum granulosum. Within hours of burrowing, the female begins laying two or three large eggs per day, each of which progresses through larval and nymphal stages to become an adult itch mite in about 10 days. The most common places for scabies to burrow are on the hands (between the fingers) and on the flexor surfaces of the wrists and the extensor surfaces of the elbows. Characteristic lesions may occur on the nipples of women and as pruritic papules on the penile shaft and glans and on the scrotum.[54,59] Pruritic papules may be seen on the buttocks also.[59] Figure 24-16 shows the typical sites of scabies burrows.

CLINICAL MANIFESTATIONS   The classic symptom of scabies is intense pruritus, which may be pronounced at night. The typical burrow of the *S. scabiei* is a short, linear, curved, or S-shaped line (Figure 24-17). There may be small, erythematous, excoriated larval papules near the burrows. Secondary infections are common and are caused by scratching. In some individuals a hypersensitivity reaction occurs a month or more after the infestation and causes multiple, reddish brown, pruritic nodules to develop on the covered portions of the body—most commonly, the upper thighs, buttocks, male gen-

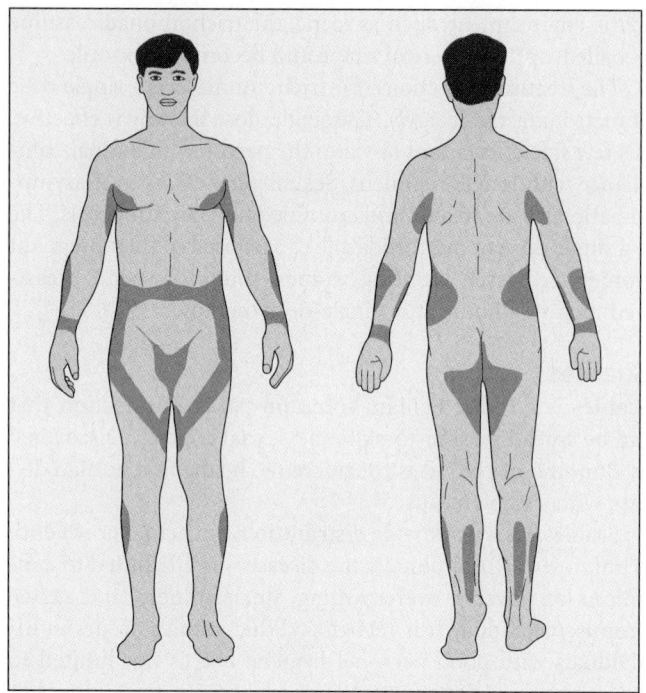

Figure 24-16 Distribution of skin lesions of *Sarcoptes scabiei* infestation. Unshaded areas are rarely affected in healthy adults. (From Morse SA, Ballard RC, Holmes KK, Moreland AA, editors: *Atlas of sexually transmitted diseases and AIDS,* ed 3, London, 2003, Mosby.)

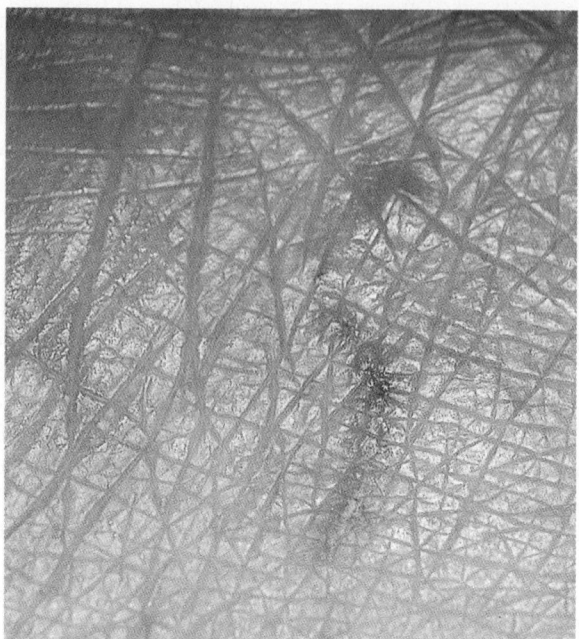

Figure 24-17 Scabies burrow. An S-shaped burrow with a tiny vesicle at one end. (From Habif TP et al: *Skin disease: diagnosis and treatment,* St Louis, 2001, Mosby.)

italia, and axillary regions. These nodules may persist for more than 1 year despite treatment with a scabicide.

EVALUATION AND TREATMENT Although the diagnosis is often made on clinical grounds, microscopic identification of the mite or its eggs, larvae, or feces is recommended because the symptoms of scabies can imitate those of many other dermatologic conditions. Superficial scrapings from a recently developed, unexcoriated papule or burrow can be observed easily under the microscope; the addition of potassium hydroxide allows easier visualization of the mite.

Preferred treatment is topical application of 5% permethrin massaged and left for 8 to 14 hours. Lindane (1%) lotion or cream applied thinly to all areas of the body below the neck and washed thoroughly at 8 hours and 10% crotamiton applied to the body below the neck nightly for 2 nights and washed thoroughly 24 hours after the second application are effective also.[57,59] Close household and sexual contacts should be treated also. Permethrin has been used safely in infants as young as 2 months and is the treatment of choice for children. Pregnant women should be treated with permethrin only if infestation with scabies can be documented.[57,59] To prevent reinfestation, clothing and bed linens should be machine washed and dried at high temperatures, or dry-cleaned.

Pediculosis Pubis

Phthirus pubis, the crab louse, is one of three species of lice that infest humans. *P. pubis* is commonly transmitted sexually and causes **pediculosis pubis,** or "crabs." Adolescents and young children are most commonly infected.

P. pubis is transmitted primarily by intimate sexual contact or contact with infected bed linens or clothing. It is highly contagious; there is a 95% chance of contracting the disease during a single sexual encounter. The transfer of lice from pubic hair is probably mechanical, assisted by animated scratching; fingernails; towels; and other similar means rather than by self-propulsion. Pubic lice usually infect the perineal and axillary hair and occasionally the hair of the trunk, beard, scalp, and eyelashes.

PATHOPHYSIOLOGY The crab louse has a 25- to 30-day life cycle from egg to egg that consists of five stages: an egg (or nit) stage, three nymphal stages, and an adult stage, all of which occur in the host. The nits of crab lice are found "glued" to hairs; they are oval, 0.8 by 0.3 mm, and whitish, and they hatch in 5 to 10 days (Figure 24-18). In the adult stage, pubic lice are grayish, are approximately 1 mm in length, and have a segmented body and claws particularly designed for clinging to pubic hairs. Because lice depend on blood for nutrition, they bite into the skin to obtain food.

CLINICAL MANIFESTATIONS Symptoms range from mild pruritus to severe, intolerable itching, depending on the individual's sensitivity to louse bites. Allergic sensitization occurs in about 5 days, when itching, erythema, and inflammation may worsen. Excessive scratching may lead to secondary infection.

EVALUATION AND TREATMENT The individual's history usually discloses a recent exposure and the typical symptoms of infestation. Because both the lice and nits are visible to the naked eye, a thorough clinical examination per-

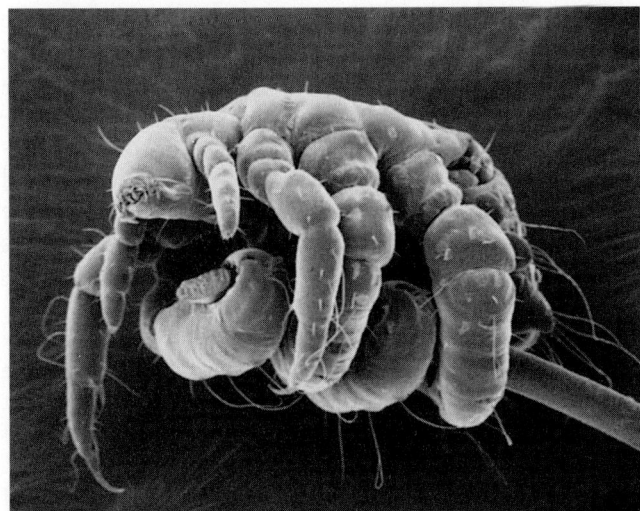

A

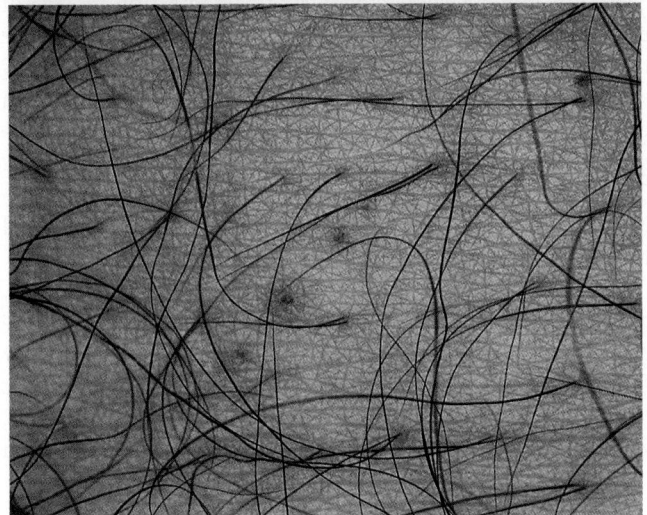

B

Figure 24-18 **Pubic louse and crab louse. A,** Pubic louse *(Phthirus pubis)* encircling a pubic hair; the clawlike legs produce a firm grip. **B,** Crab louse bites *(Phthirus pubis)*. (From Morse SA, Ballard RC, Holmes KK, Moreland AA, editors: *Atlas of sexually transmitted diseases and AIDS,* ed 3, London, 2003, Mosby.)

mits definitive diagnosis. Pediculosis pubis is treated with 1% permethrin cream rinse or 1% lindane lotion, cream, or shampoo or with over-the-counter pyrethrin or piperonyl butoxide. The pediculicide is applied to infested and adjacent hairy areas and removed after a specified length of time by thorough washing. Remaining nits can be removed with a fine-tooth comb. Permethrin is recommended for young children and pregnant women and has less potential toxicity with inappropriate use. On the other hand, lindane is the least expensive and nontoxic if used correctly. Lindane should not be used after a bath, or by persons with extensive dermatitis, by pregnant or lactating women, or by children less than 2 years of age.[57] Sexual contacts and any other intimate household contacts also should be examined and treated, and clothing and bed linens should be dry-cleaned or machine washed and dried at high temperatures. Treatment can be repeated in 7 days to eradicate any newly hatched lice.

SEXUALLY TRANSMITTED INFECTIONS OF OTHER BODY SYSTEMS

Gastrointestinal Infections

Shigellosis and *Campylobacter* Enteritis

A variety of enteric bacterial pathogens are now recognized as being sexually transmitted, particularly among homosexual men. The bacteria most commonly involved include species of *Shigella* and *Campylobacter*. *Shigella* infection, termed **shigellosis,** is transmitted by contact with infected feces. Few microorganisms are needed to cause infection. Anal-oral spread occurs easily through household contact and anal-oral sexual practices. *Campylobacter jejuni,* which causes ***Campylobacter* enteritis,** is primarily an animal pathogen but also may be transmitted among humans through anal-oral sexual practices. Again, few microorganisms are necessary for inoculation and infection.

PATHOPHYSIOLOGY　　*Shigella* microorganisms are nonmotile, gram-negative rods that are related to *Escherichia coli*. They invade and kill intestinal epithelial cells, thereby inducing a marked inflammatory response and diarrhea. *Campylobacter* microorganisms are highly motile, curved, gram-negative rods that also invade and kill intestinal cells and cause bloody, inflammatory exudate and diarrhea.

CLINICAL MANIFESTATIONS　　Either microorganism may cause a mild, self-limited gastroenteritis or severe dysentery. After a 24- to 48-hour incubation period, shigellosis begins with fever, abdominal distress, and diarrhea. It may resolve completely or progress to dysentery with severe cramping, abdominal pain, tenesmus, and bloody mucoid discharge from the rectum. *Campylobacter* enteritis typically begins, after a 1- to 7-day incubation period, with sudden fever and abdominal pain followed by diarrhea. Malaise, anorexia, headache, arthralgia, and myalgia are common.

EVALUATION AND TREATMENT　　Clinical manifestations and cultures of fresh stool samples are used to diagnose shigellosis. Culturing *Campylobacter* is expensive; therefore microscopic analysis of a gram-stained smear of rectal exudate may be used as a diagnostic aid.

　　Treatment for mild illness includes correction of fluid and electrolyte imbalance. Antidiarrheals are avoided because they may delay clearance of the microorganism. Because both *Shigella* and *Campylobacter* are highly contagious, antibiotic treatment may be advisable even for mild cases. The preferred treatment for shigellosis is oral ciprofloxacin, 500 mg, or norfloxacin, 400 mg, twice daily for 3 days. Oral ciprofloxacin, 500 mg twice daily for 3 to 5 days, or erythromycin, 500 mg four times daily for 5 days, is effective against *Campylobacter* enteritis.[57] Sexual partners are examined and treated, and individuals are instructed to avoid oral-anal contact until the infection is cured.

Giardiasis and Amebiasis

Two enteric protozoa that are sexually transmitted, primarily among homosexual men, are *Giardia lamblia,* the cause of **giardiasis,** and *Entamoeba histolytica,* the cause of **amebiasis.** The incidence of these infections in the male homosexual population has decreased over the past years, presumably because of safer sex practices.[60] Although the principal route of transmission is contaminated drinking water, giardiasis and amebiasis are transmitted also by anal-oral or genital-anal contact.

PATHOPHYSIOLOGY *G. lamblia* and *E. histolytica* are both parasites having two forms, cysts and **trophozoites** (uncysted protozoa). The cysts are the infective form because they can survive in moist environments outside the host. Giardiasis commonly begins with ingestion of a small number of *G. lamblia* cysts. Once in the upper small bowel, each cyst becomes a trophozoite, which multiplies and attaches to the bowel mucosa. Enzyme deficiencies, inflammation, and immunologic damage then apparently occur, resulting in intestinal malabsorption. Amebiasis begins similarly: the ingested cysts pass to the small or large bowel, where each returns to the trophozoite state, multiplies quickly, and begins to invade the mucosa through cytotoxic activity. Mucosal invasion results in the development of ulcers and an inflammatory response. Individuals infected with *E. histolytica* may excrete up to 45 million cysts per day.

CLINICAL MANIFESTATIONS Giardiasis begins with sudden, explosive diarrhea, distention, and flatulence. Upper gastrointestinal symptoms are also prominent and may include epigastric pain; vomiting; foul, sulfuric burping; and nausea. After the acute illness, which usually lasts several days, milder symptoms may persist for months, with evidence of malabsorption and weight loss. Amebiasis is often asymptomatic. Symptoms that do occur range from mild diarrhea to severe dysentery. Amebiasis may spread from the intestine to other organs, such as the liver.

EVALUATION AND TREATMENT Diagnosis of both entities usually is made by history and microscopic examination of fresh stool specimens for either trophozoites or cysts. Small bowel biopsy may aid in the diagnosis of giardiasis; rectal biopsy may aid in the diagnosis of amebiasis. Serologic testing is useful in the differential diagnosis of symptomatic individuals with amebiasis. Metronidazole is the treatment of choice in the United States, usually 250 mg three times daily for 5 to 7 days.[65] Other nitroimidazoles as well as other agents including Quinacrine are also effective. The dosage of metronidazole for amebiasis depends on the severity of the infection.[57]

Hepatitis B

Hepatitis is a liver infection that can be caused by six types of viruses: hepatitis A, hepatitis B, hepatitis C, hepatitis D, hepatitis E, and hepatitis G. Each virus causes a syndrome of acute, icteric (jaundice-producing) liver inflammation. Of the three types, the **hepatitis B virus (HBV)** is known to be sexually transmitted. (Hepatitis A, like most other predominantly enteric infections, may be considered an STI because of oral-anal transmission.) Although hepatitis C (HCV) is not currently recognized as an STI, the CDC has listed sexual exposure as an HCV risk factor (Figure 24-19). Data indicate sexual transmission of HCV appears to occur, but the virus is inefficiently spread through this manner.[61] Additional information about hepatitis is found in Chapter 39.

The prevalence of HBV infection varies dramatically worldwide. In Southeast Asia and Africa, 60% to 80% of the population may harbor serologic evidence of past or current infection. In the United States, approximately 5% to 20% of the general population have evidence of HBV infection. Seropositivity generally increases with age. Serologic tests of STI clinic patients show evidence of past infection in 28% of individuals ages 25 years and older and 7% in those younger than 25 years.[57] At risk for HBV infection are those with low socioeconomic status, blacks, Indochinese refugees, health care workers, and male homosexuals. In groups of male homosexuals, the seropositivity rates may be as high as 80%. Other groups at risk are intravenous drug users, institutionalized mentally retarded persons, hemodialysis patients, and heterosexual partners of HBV carriers.[62]

Transmission of HBV can occur through needle puncture, blood transfusion, cuts or abrasions in the skin, and absorption by mucosal surfaces. Direct contact with infected body fluids, such as tears, cerebrospinal fluid, synovial fluid, gastric juices, pleural fluid, semen, and urine, may pass the infection. Fomites also can transmit hepatitis: HBV can survive on inanimate objects for up to 1 week.[63]

Perinatal transmission of HBV is relatively common. Neonates whose mothers are infectious have a 70% to 90% chance of becoming infected with HBV during labor or delivery and a 90% chance of becoming chronic carriers.[63] Hepatitis B virus can be found in maternal vaginal secretions, blood, amniotic fluid, saliva, and breast milk.[63]

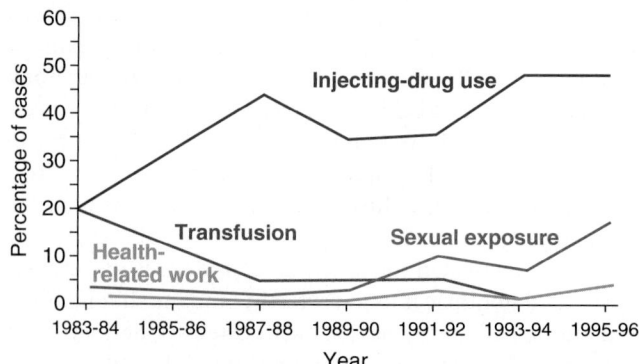

Figure 24-19 **Risk for hepatitis C exposure.** Comparison of injecting drug use *(green),* transfusions *(red),* health-related work *(blue),* and sexual exposure *(gold).* Note the rise in sexually transmitted incidences. (From Centers for Disease Control and Prevention: *Hepatitis C: what clinicians and other health professionals need to know,* 2000. Available at www.cdc.gov/ncidod/diseases/hepatitis/c_training/edu/intro.)

Hepatitis delta agent is a defective virus that is similar to HBV antigen but cannot cause hepatitis B by itself, requiring the presence of HBV to cause hepatitis. Hepatitis delta infection is rare in the United States, but cases have been documented in intravenous drug users and their sexual contacts and also in recipients of contaminated blood. It commonly is found in homosexuals, persons requiring kidney dialysis, and health care workers.

PATHOPHYSIOLOGY   After exposure, HBV passes through the bloodstream to the liver, where it infects liver cells and multiplies. The infection is usually self-limiting, with most patients mounting an effective immune response. Approximately 6% to 10% of infected individuals cannot eradicate the virus and become chronic carriers of HBV.

CLINICAL MANIFESTATIONS   Most HBV infections are clinically inapparent and result in solid and permanent immunity. Symptoms of hepatitis usually develop only after a certain HBV antigen has been circulating in the blood for 3 to 6 weeks. Approximately 15% to 20% of individuals develop a prodromal syndrome that is similar to serum sickness. This syndrome is characterized by an erythematous rash, urticaria, polyarthralgias, and arthritis. Symptoms of infection also may include lassitude, anorexia, nausea, vomiting, headache, fever, dark urine, jaundice, and moderate liver enlargement with tenderness. Long-term sequelae include chronic persistent and chronic active hepatitis, cirrhosis, hepatocellular carcinoma, hepatic failure, and death. In neonates who contract HBV, the disease may be manifested in many ways, from mild illness to a severe, fulminant infection with a mortality of 75%.

EVALUATION AND TREATMENT   Hepatitis B virus infection is clinically indistinguishable from other types of hepatitis. Diagnosis can be made only through serologic testing.

No specific therapy exists for HBV infection in adults. Treatment consists of supportive care and relief of symptoms. Vaccinations of only high-risk groups has proven to be ineffective. Thus a comprehensive strategy to eliminate HBV and its sequelae has been implemented by the Centers for Disease Control and Prevention. This involves testing of all pregnant women and vaccinations of susceptible infants, children, and high-risk adults.[64]

The infant who is born to a mother with infectious HBV is given HBV immune globulin and HBV vaccine within 12 hours of birth. The HBV vaccine is administered again at 1 and 6 months if serologic tests show that a chronic carrier state has not developed.

Systemic Diseases
Epstein-Barr Virus
Recent investigations have indicated that the **Epstein-Barr virus (EBV),** which is transmitted orally, is also capable of being harbored within the male and female genital tracts and transmitted sexually. Further research is needed to specifically identify the role that EBV plays in STIs; however, the significance of EBV infection of the genital tract relates to its ability to transform cells and potentially contribute to the development of cancers in the genital tract.[66]

Acquired Immunodeficiency Syndrome
Epidemiology, modes of transmission, pathophysiology, clinical manifestations, and evaluation and treatment of AIDS are discussed in detail in Chapter 8.

Cytomegalovirus Infection
Cytomegalovirus (CMV) is a sexually transmissible herpesvirus. It is associated with a number of clinical syndromes in newborns, otherwise healthy adults, and immunosuppressed individuals.

CMV infection causes no specific genital disease, but its incidence is high in individuals being treated for other STIs. CMV infection is prevalent worldwide, especially in developing countries and lower socioeconomic groups. The virus is found in semen, cervical secretions, urine, blood, saliva, breast milk, and stool, and transmission is associated with close (although not always genital) interpersonal contact or direct transfer of cells or body fluids. It is more common in homosexual men and in young women with multiple sexual partners. Intrauterine CMV infection is the most common congenital infection and occurs in 0.5% to 3% of all live births. Like HSV, primary maternal infection carries the greatest risk of transmission and severe consequences. Infected infants can be asymptomatic or may experience varying degrees of sensorineural hearing loss or severe cognitive and psychomotor developmental deficits.[2,67] Perinatal transmission of CMV may occur across the placenta, by contamination with infected secretions during passage through the birth canal, or during breast-feeding.

PATHOPHYSIOLOGY   After CMV infects a human cell, it may replicate and destroy the infected cell or become incorporated into the host cell's DNA. Local CMV infections can persist despite the presence of large quantities of systemic antibody to CMV. Cell-mediated immunity seems to have a particular role in protecting against CMV infections. Depression of CMV-specific cell-mediated immunity has been noted in otherwise normal hosts with CMV infection. This may be caused by injury of T cells or macrophages by the cytomegalovirus.[68]

CLINICAL MANIFESTATIONS   In healthy individuals, CMV infection can cause a number of mild subclinical or nonspecific illnesses, including mononucleosis, pneumonitis, hemolytic anemia, and thrombocytopenia purpura. In contrast, a CMV infection in an immunocompromised individual, such as a transplant recipient or an individual with AIDS, can cause a devastating, life-threatening illness.

Congenital CMV infection is the most common serious viral infection among infants. Approximately 1% of all infants (40,000) are born with congenital CMV. Of these, 10%

(4000) demonstrate typical manifestations of the infection, such as hepatosplenomegaly, intracranial calcifications, microcephaly, smallness for gestational age, and hearing impairments. An additional 10% to 15% of these are asymptomatic at birth; however, they begin to develop manifestations of the infection within the first few months of life. Recent evidence suggests that symptomatic infection of infants is caused by a primary infection of the mother during her pregnancy and not necessarily by reinfection or reactivation of a prior infection.

EVALUATION AND TREATMENT   The most definitive diagnostic test for CMV is isolation of the virus, usually through growth in human fibroblast cell culture. Several methods for measuring antibodies to CMV are available, including complement-fixation (CF) tests and indirect im-munofluorescent antibody (IFA) tests. These methods commonly are used in clinical situations.

With the increased incidence of CMV infection among immunocompromised individuals (persons with AIDS or transplants), various treatment modalities have been investigated. Ganciclovir is similar to acyclovir and inhibits viral DNA polymerase (see Chapter 4). Relapses of CMV infection are frequent after therapy ceases; thus lifelong therapy is particularly indicated in individuals with AIDS.[51] Acyclovir has been used, but optimum therapeutic benefits have not been established. Future therapies still under investigation include ganciclovir plus CMV immune globulin and vaccine.

Experimental antiviral drugs may prove helpful in the treatment of severe CMV infection, and preliminary studies to develop a vaccine appear promising. No treatment is indicated, however, in most cases of CMV infection.

SUMMARY REVIEW

Sexually Transmitted Urogenital Infections

1. Gonorrhea is a sexually transmitted communicable disease that can be local or systemic. Complications include pelvic inflammatory disease (PID); sterility; and disseminated infection, which is spread through the bloodstream to the skin, joints, and heart.
2. Gonorrhea passed to the fetus from the mother typically manifests as an eye infection and develops 1 to 12 days after birth. Usually ophthalmic antibiotic prophylaxis is not sufficient to prevent infection.
3. Antibiotic coverage for penicillin-resistant strains and chlamydial coinfection is recommended for all individuals diagnosed with gonorrhea and their partners.
4. Syphilis is a sexually transmitted infection (STI) that becomes systemic shortly after infection. The four stages of the disease are (a) primary syphilis with a chancre at the site of infection; (b) secondary syphilis with systemic spread to all body systems; (c) latent syphilis with minimal symptoms or the development of skin lesions; and (d) tertiary syphilis, the most severe stage, with destruction of bone, skin, and soft and neurologic tissues.
5. Congenital syphilis contributes to prematurity of the newborn with bone marrow depression, central nervous system (CNS) involvement, renal failure, and intrauterine growth retardation. Late clinical manifestations are those of tertiary syphilis and are rare.
6. Syphilis is diagnosed by serologic testing and treated with injectable penicillin. Sexual partners are treated also.
7. With chancroid infection, women are generally asymptomatic and men may develop inflamed, painful genital ulcers and inguinal buboes. Incubation period is 1 to 14 days. Single-dose therapy with injectable ceftriaxone or oral azithromycin for both partners is recommended. Persons with human immunodeficiency virus (HIV) may require a longer treatment regimen.
8. Granuloma inguinale (donovanosis) is rare in the United States. The bacteria are gram-negative and survive within macrophages. Localized nodules coalesce to form granulomas and ulcers on the penis in men and labia in women. Antibiotics provide effective treatment. Although rare and mildly infectious, granuloma inguinale is a chronic, progressively destructive bacterial infection. Often individuals diagnosed with granuloma inguinale are coinfected with syphilis.
9. Bacterial vaginosis (BV) is a sexually associated condition caused by an overgrowth of anaerobic bacteria that produce aromatic amines and raise the pH of the vagina, promoting further bacterial growth (without an inflammatory response) and a fishy-smelling odor. "Clue cells" are found on the wet mount. Metronidazole (Flagyl) provides effective treatment. BV has been associated with PID, chorioamnionitis, preterm labor, and postpartum endometritis. Treatment of male sexual partners is not recommended.
10. Chlamydia is the most common bacterial STI in the United States and the leading preventable cause of infertility and ectopic pregnancy. The causative organism, *C. trachomatis*, localizes to epithelial tissue and can spread throughout the urogenital tract or pass from infected mother to the eyes and respiratory tract of newborn infants during birth. As with gonorrhea, prophylactic eye antibiotic treatment is insufficient to prevent infection. *C. trachomatis* is susceptible to inexpensive, readily accessible antibiotics. Single-dose azithromycin is the drug of choice. Antibiotic therapy for infected individuals and all sexual contacts is recommended. Because of the asymptomatic nature of chlamydia and the potential sequelae of untreated infection, extensive and widespread screening is warranted.
11. Lymphogranuloma venereum is a chronic STI that is uncommon in the United States. The lesion begins as a skin infection and spreads to the lymph tissue, causing inflammation, necrosis, buboes, and abscesses of the inguinal lymph nodes. Primary lesions appear on the penis and scrotum in men and on the cervix, vaginal wall, and labia in women. Secondary lesions involve inflammation and swelling of the lymph nodes with formation of large blue buboes that rupture and form draining ulcerative lesions. A 21-day course of oral doxycycline or erythromycin is effective. Treatment of sexual partners is recommended.
12. Genital herpes is the most common genital ulceration in the United States and is caused by either type 1 (HSV-1) or type 2 (HSV-2) herpesvirus. Lesions initially appear as groups of vesicles that progress to ulceration with pain, lymphadenopathy, and fever. Herpes simplex virus passes from mother to fetus and can cause spontaneous abortion or prematurity. Acyclovir reduces symptoms but does not cure the disease.
13. Three distinct syndromes are associated with HSV infection: (a) first-episode primary infections, (b) first-episode nonpri-

SUMMARY REVIEW—cont'd

mary infections, and (c) recurrent infections. Recurrent infections are most often attributable to HSV-2 and are generally milder and of shorter duration.

14. Human papillomavirus (HPV) is associated with both the development of cervical dysplasia and cancer and condylomata acuminata. The high-risk strains of HPV (HR-HPV) that are precursors to the development of cervical cancer do not cause genital warts. Testing is available to detect HR-HPV.

15. Condylomata acuminata (genital warts) are associated with multiple sexual partners and are highly contagious. The velvety, cauliflower-like lesions occur in the genital and anal areas, vagina, and cervix and are painless. They can be transmitted to the infant at birth.

16. Molluscum contagiosum is a benign viral infection of the skin. It is transmitted by skin-to-skin contact in children and adults. In adults it tends to occur on the genitalia and to be transmitted by sexual contact.

17. Trichomoniasis *(T. vaginalis)* causes vaginitis in women, and urethritis in men. Both partners usually are infected. Women usually have a copious, malodorous, gray-green discharge with pruritus. Men usually are asymptomatic. Metronidazole is the treatment for both partners.

18. Scabies is a common parasitic infection that can be spread by skin-to-skin contact and sexual contact. The scabies mite burrows through the skin, depositing two or three large eggs per day. Intense pruritus, especially at night, is the most pronounced clinical manifestation. Treatment consists of topical application of a pediculicide.

19. Pediculosis pubis (crabs) is commonly transmitted sexually and is caused by the crab louse, *Phthirus pubis.* The lice bite into the skin for nutrition. Symptoms include mild and severe pruritus. Topical application of prescription or over-the-counter pediculicides is effective treatment.

20. Hepatitis B infection poses significant health risks including chronic ulcer disease and hepatocellular cancer. Immunization against hepatitis B is the most effective means of preventing transmission. Universal vaccination of infants and children is recommended, as well as vaccination of high-risk adults.

21. Hepatitis C is generally transmitted percutaneously but sexual transmission appears possible.

Sexually Transmitted Infections of Other Body Systems

1. Various enteric bacterial pathogens are now recognized as being sexually transmitted, particularly among homosexual men. The infections include shigellosis, *Campylobacter* enteritis, giardiasis, amebiasis, and hepatitis A.

2. Shigellosis is transmitted by contact with infected feces. *Campylobacter* enteritis can be transmitted through anal-oral sexual practices.

3. Giardiasis and amebiasis are transmitted primarily through contaminated drinking water, but they can be transmitted by anal-oral and genital-anal contact.

4. Transmission of hepatitis B virus (HBV) can occur through needle puncture, blood transfusion, cuts in the skin, and contact with infected body fluids.

5. Perinatal transmission of HBV is relatively common.

6. Systemic diseases known to be sexually transmitted include acquired immunodeficiency syndrome (AIDS) (see Chapter 8), cytomegalovirus infection, and Epstein-Barr virus.

7. Epstein-Barr virus may be harbored in the genital tract and passed on through sexual encounters.

8. Cytomegalovirus (CMV) is a sexually transmissible herpesvirus. The infection causes no specific genital disease, but its incidence is high in individuals being treated for other sexually transmitted infections (STIs). The virus is found in semen, cervical secretions, urine, blood, saliva, breast milk, and stool.

9. CMV infection is more common in homosexual men and in young women with multiple sexual partners. It is the most common congenital infection.

10. CMV infection can cause mononucleosis, pneumonitis, hemolytic anemia, and thrombocytopenia purpura. A CMV infection in an immunosuppressed individual can cause a life-threatening illness. No treatment is indicated in most cases of CMV infection.

KEY TERMS

Acute urethral syndrome, 876
Amebiasis, 886
Bacterial vaginosis (BV), 874
Buboes, 872
Campylobacter enteritis, 885
Chancre, 868
Chancroid, 870
Chlamydia, 875
Condylomata acuminata, 880
Condylomata lata, 869
Congenital syphilis (CS), 868
Cytomegalovirus (CMV), 887
Disseminated gonococcal infection (DGI), 866
Donovan bodies, 873

Epstein-Barr virus (EBV), 887
Fomites, 864
Genital herpes, 878
Giardiasis, 886
Gonococcus, 864
Gonorrhea, 864
Granuloma inguinale, 873
Gummas, 868
Hepatitis B virus (HBV), 886
Hepatitis delta agent, 887
Human papillomavirus (HPV), 880
Latent syphilis, 868
Lymphogranuloma venereum (LGV), 877
Molluscous bodies, 882
Molluscum contagiosum, 881

Neurosyphilis, 868
Nongonococcal urethritis (NGU), 877
Ophthalmia neonatorum, 866
Pediculosis pubis, 884
Perihepatitis, 866
Primary syphilis, 868
Pseudobuboes, 874
Scabies, 883
Secondary syphilis, 868
Shigellosis, 885
Syphilis, 868
Tertiary syphilis, 868
Trichomonads, 883
Trichomoniasis, 882
Trophozoites, 886

REFERENCES

1. National Center for HIV, STD, and TB Prevention: *Tracking the hidden epidemics: trends in the STD epidemics in the United States,* Atlanta, 2000, Centers for Disease Control and Prevention. Available at www.cdc.gov/nchstp/dstd/STD_Index.htm.
2. Centers for Disease Control and Prevention: *Sexually transmitted disease surveillance 2003,* Atlanta, 2003, US Department of Heath and Human Services. Available at www.cdc.gov/std/stats/.
3. Centers for Disease Control and Prevention: Trends in reportable sexually transmitted diseases in the United States, 2003: National data on chlamydia, gonorrhea and syphilis. In *STD surveillance 2003.* Available at www.cdc.gov/std/stats/trends2003.htm.
4. Hook EW III, Handsfield HH: Gonococcal infections in the adult. In Holmes KK et al, editors: *Sexually transmitted diseases,* ed 2, New York, 1990, McGraw-Hill.
5. Pelouze PS: *Gonorrhea in the male and female,* Philadelphia, 1941, Saunders.
6. Whittington W et al: Gonorrhea. In Morse SA, Moreland AA, Holmes KK, editors: *Atlas of sexually transmitted diseases and AIDS,* ed 2, London, 1996, Mosby-Wolfe.
7. Berger TG, Rothman I: Sexually transmitted diseases in men. In Tanagho EA, McAninch JW, editors: *Smith's general urology,* Norwalk, Conn, 1995, Appleton & Lange.
8. Westrom L et al: Pelvic inflammatory disease and fertility: a cohort study of 1,844 women with laparoscopically verified disease and 657 control women with normal laparoscopic results, *Sex Trans Dis* 19(4):184-1982, 1992.
9. Zenilman JM: Gonorrhea: clinical and public health issues, *Hosp Pract* 28(2a):29, 1993.
10. Sperling RS: Infection protocols: perihepatitis, *Contemp OB/GYN* 37(6):51, 1992.
11. Emmert DH, Kirchner JT: Sexually transmitted diseases in women: gonorrhea and syphilis, *Postgrad Med* 107(2):181-184, 189-190, 193-197, 2000.
12. Centers for Disease Control and Prevention: *Sexually transmitted disease surveillance 2003 supplement, gonococcal isolate surveillance project (GISP) annual report,* Atlanta, Ga, 2004, US Department of Health and Human Services.
13. Centers for Disease Control and Prevention: *Sexually transmitted disease surveillance 2003 supplement, syphilis surveillance report,* Atlanta, Ga, 2004, US Department of Health and Human Services.
14. Division of STD Prevention, Department of Health and Human Services: *Sexually transmitted disease surveillance 1998 supplement,* Atlanta, 2000, Centers for Disease Control and Prevention. Available at www.cdc.gov/nchstp/dstd/Stats_Trends.
15. Centers for Disease Control and Prevention: Sexually transmitted diseases treatment guidelines 2002, *MMWR* 51(RR-6):1-73, 2002.
16. Brandt AM: *No magic bullet: a social history of venereal disease in the United States since 1880,* expanded edition, New York, 1987, Oxford University Press.
17. Leu RH: Complications of coexisting chlamydial and gonococcal infections, *Postgrad Med* 89(7):56-60, 1991.
18. Sparling PF: Natural history of syphilis. In Holmes KK et al, editors: *Sexually transmitted diseases,* ed 2, New York, 1990, McGraw-Hill.
19. Centers for Disease Control and Prevention: *Sexually transmitted disease surveillance 2003 supplement: syphilis surveillance project,* Atlanta, Ga, 2004, US Department of Health and Human Services.
20. Schultz KF et al: Congenital syphilis. In Holmes KK et al, editors: *Sexually transmitted diseases,* ed 2, New York, 1990, McGraw-Hill.
21. Hook EW, Marra CM: Medical progress: acquired syphilis in adults, *N Engl J Med* 326(16):1060, 1992.
22. Thin RN: Early syphilis in the adult. In Holmes KK et al, editors: *Sexually transmitted diseases,* ed 2, New York, 1990, McGraw-Hill.
23. Wooldridge WE: Syphilis: a new visit from an old enemy, *Postgrad Med* 89(1):193-196, 199-202, 1991.
24. Tillman J: Syphilis an old disease, a contemporary problem, *J Obstet Gynecol Neonat Nurs* 21(3):209, 1992.
25. Jacobs RA: Infectious diseases: spirochetal. In McTierney LM, McPhee SJ, Papadakis MS, editors: *Current medical diagnosis & treatment,* ed 35, Norwalk, Conn, 1996, Appleton & Lange.
26. O'Farrell N: Tropical medicine series: donovanosis, *Sex Transm Infect* 78(6):452-457, 2002.
27. Para MF, Baird IM: Genital ulcer syndromes. In Spagna VA, Prior RB, editors: *Sexually transmitted diseases: a clinical syndrome approach,* New York, 1985, Marcel Dekker.
28. Committee on Infectious Disease: *Red Book 2000,* Elk Grove Village, Ill, 2000, American Academy of Pediatrics.
29. Ronald AR, Albritton W: Chancroid and *Haemophilus ducreyi.* In Holmes KK et al, editors: *Sexually transmitted diseases,* ed 2, New York, 1990, McGraw-Hill.
30. Richens J: The diagnosis of treatment of donovanosis (granuloma inguinale), *Genitourin Med* 67(6):441-452, 1991.
31. Hart G: Donovanosis. In Holmes KK et al, editors: *Sexually transmitted diseases,* ed 2, New York, 1990, McGraw-Hill.
32. Hillier SL et al: Association between bacterial vaginosis and preterm delivery of a low-birth-weight infant, *N Engl J Med* 333(26):1737-1742, 1995.
33. Amsel R et al: Nonspecific vaginitis. Diagnostic criteria ad microbial and epidemiologic associations, *Am J Med* 74(1):14-22, 1983.
34. Kellogg ND et al: Comparison of nucleic acid amplification tests and culture techniques in the detection of *Neisseria gonorrhoeae* and *Chlamydia trachomatis* in victims of suspected child sexual abuse, *J Pediatr Adolesc Gynecol* 17(5):331-339, 2004.
35. Sargent SJ: The "other" sexually transmitted diseases: chlamydial, herpes simplex virus, and human papillomavirus infections, *Postgrad Med* 91(4):359-362, 371-374, 377, 1992.
36. Schachter J, Barnes R: Infections caused by *Chlamydia trachomatis.* In Morse SA, Moreland AA, Holmes KK, editors: *Atlas of sexually transmitted diseases and AIDS,* ed 2, London, 1996, Mosby-Wolfe.
37. Westrom LV: Chlamydia and its effect on reproduction, *J Br Fer Soc* 1(1):23-30, 1996.
38. Chambers HF: Infectious diseases: bacterial and chlamydial. In McTierney LM, McPhee SJ, Papadakis MA, editors: *Current medical diagnosis and treatment,* ed 35, Norwalk, Conn, 1996, Appleton & Lange.
39. Perine PI, Osoba AO: Lymphogranuloma venereum. In Holmes KK et al, editors: *Sexually transmitted diseases,* ed 2, New York, 1990, McGraw-Hill.
40. Mertz GJ et al: Risk factors for the sexual transmission of genital herpes, *Ann Intern Med* 116(3):197, 1992.
41. Camisa C: Condyloma acuminatum and other human papillomavirus-induced diseases. In Spagna VA, Prior RB, editors: *Sexually transmitted disease: a clinical syndrome approach,* New York, 1985, Marcel Dekker.
42. Stagno S, Whitley RJ: Herpesvirus infection in the neonate and children. In Holmes KK et al, editors: *Sexually transmitted diseases,* ed 2, New York, 1990, McGraw-Hill.
43. Landenberg AG et al: A prospective study of new infections with herpes simplex virus type 1 and type 2. Chiron HSV Vaccine Study Group, *N Engl J Med* 341(19):1432-1438, 1999.
44. Koelle DM, Wald A: Herpes simplex virus: the importance of asymptomatic shedding, *J Antimicrob Chemother* 45(Suppl T3):1-8, 2000.
45. Stephenson J: Genital herpes vaccine shows limited promise, *JAMA* 284(15):1913-1914.
46. Rose FB, Camp CJ: Genital herpes: how to relieve patients' physical and psychological symptoms, *Postgrad Med* 84(3):81-86, 1988.
47. Wright TC, et al: Interim guidance for the use of human papillomavirus DNA testing as an adjunct to cervical cytology for screening, *Obstet Gynecol* 103(2):304-309, 2004.
48. Woodman CB et al: Natural history of cervical human papillomavirus infection in young women: a longitudinal cohort study, *Lancet* 357(9271):1831-1836, 2001.
49. Derksen DJ: Children with condylomata acuminata, *J Fam Pract* 34(4):419-423, 1992.
50. Alary M et al: Strategy for screening pregnant women for chlamydial infection in a low-prevalence area, *Obstet Gynecol* 82(3):399, 1993.
51. Shah KV: Biology of genital tract human papillomaviruses, *Urol Clin North Am* 19(1):63-69, 1992.
52. McAninch JW: Disorders of the penis and male urethra. In Tanagho EA, McAninch JW, editors: *Smith's general urology,* Norwalk, Conn, 1995, Appleton & Lange.

53. Harper DM et al: Efficacy of a bivalent L1 virus-like particle vaccine in prevention of infection with human papillomavirus types 16 and 18 in young women: a randomised controlled trial, *Lancet* 364(9447):1757-1765, 2004.

54. Berger TG: Skin diseases of the external genitalia. In Tanagho EA, McAninch JW, editors: *Smith's general urology,* Norwalk, Conn, 1995, Appleton & Lange.

55. Lambert DR, Yoder FW: Ectoparasites and molluscum contagiosum. In Spagna VA, Prior RB, editors: *Sexually transmitted diseases: a clinical syndrome approach,* New York, 1985, Marcel Dekker.

56. Rein MR, Holmes KK: Nonspecific vaginitis, vulvovaginal candidiasis, and trichomoniasis: clinical features, diagnosis, and management. In Remington J, Schwartz MN, editors: *Current clinical topics in infectious diseases,* New York, 1983, McGraw-Hill.

57. Bartlett JG: *Pocket book of infectious disease therapy,* Baltimore, 1995, Williams & Wilkins.

58. Orkin M, Maibach HI: Scabies. In Holmes KK et al, editors: *Sexually transmitted diseases,* ed 2, New York, 1990, McGraw-Hill.

59. Hammerschlag MR, Laraque D: Inappropriate use of nonculture tests for the detection of chlamydia trachomatis in suspected victims of child sexual abuse: a continuing problem, *Pediatrics* 104(5):1137, 1999.

60. Quinn TC, Stamm WE: Proctocolitis, enteritis, and esophagitis in homosexual men. In Holmes KK et al, editors: *Sexually transmitted diseases,* ed 2, New York, 1990, McGraw-Hill.

61. Centers for Disease Control and Prevention: *Hepatitis C: what clinicians and other health professionals need to know,* 2000. Available at www.cdc.gov/ncidod/diseases/hepatitis/c_training/edu/intro

62. Lemon SM, Newbold JE: Viral hepatitis. In Holmes KK et al, editors: *Sexually transmitted diseases,* ed 2, New York, 1990, McGraw-Hill.

63. Klein MB: Hepatitis B virus: perinatal management, *J Perinat Neonat Nurs* 1(4):12, 1988.

64. Immunization Practices Advisory Committee: Hepatitis B virus: a comprehensive strategy for eliminating transmission in the United States throughuniversal childhood vaccination: recommendations of the Immunization Practice Advisory Committee (ACIP), *MMWR* 40(RR-13):1-19, 1991.

65. Gardner TB, Hill DR: Treatment of giardiasis, *Clin Microbiol Rev* 14(1):114-128, 2001. Available at http://cmr.asm.org/cgi/content/full/14/1/114?view=long&pmid=11148005

66. Naher H et al: Subclinical Epstein-Barr virus infection of both the male and female genital tract: indication for sexual transmission, *J Invest Dermatol* 98(5):791-793, 1992.

67. Baker ER, Shephard B: Neonatal resuscitation and care of the newborn at risk. In DeCherney AH, Pernoll ML, editors: *Current obstetric and gynecologic diagnosis and treatment,* ed 8, Norwalk, Conn, 1994, Appleton & Lange.

68. Wilson CB: The cellular immune system and its role in host defense. In Mandell G, Douglas RG, Bennett JE, editors: *Principles and practice of infectious diseases,* ed 3, New York, 1990, Churchill Livingstone.

STRUCTURE AND FUNCTION OF THE HEMATOLOGIC SYSTEM

KATHRYN L. McCANCE

CHAPTER OUTLINE

Blood cells travel long distances through sometimes rough terrain and thus must be flexible (i.e., adapt to the road conditions) or blood would hardly be able to flow at all. Blood cells act as vehicles—cells and chemicals—that travel along the tens of thousands of miles of blood vessels packed into the human body. Most of these cells are red blood cells that, like tanker trucks, function as carriers; yet although red blood cells are carriers, they maneuver more like sports cars, flexing and deforming as they travel along to squeeze through capillaries smaller than their own diameters. White blood cells are larger than red blood cells and less flexible. Spherical and stiffer in nature, white blood cells therefore create more resistance in the blood vessels and are much more likely to create "traffic jams." Consequently, white blood cells tend to travel the "main highways," avoiding the small capillaries that red blood cells are so expertly able to squeeze through. However, disease can make the white cells "sticky," thereby hampering their movements even in the larger blood vessels, which creates blockades that cause the red blood cells to inadvertently "lose their cargo." These alterations in blood cell function can lead to difficulties in oxygenation, acid-base balance, and immune function and, like a major thoroughfare at rush hour, may alter the usual streamlined flow of blood.

COMPONENTS OF THE HEMATOLOGIC SYSTEM

Composition of the Blood

Blood consists of a variety of formed elements (cells and proteins) that circulate in the cardiovascular system suspended in plasma, which is approximately 90% water and 10% dissolved substances (solutes). All of these elements constitute blood volume, which in adults amounts to about 6 quarts (5.5 L). Approximately 45% to 50% of blood volume consists of formed elements, and the remainder is plasma. The continuous movement of blood keeps the formed elements dispersed throughout the plasma, where they are available to carry out their chief functions: (1) delivery of substances needed for cellular metabolism in the tissues, (2) defense against invading microorganisms and injury, and (3) acid-base balance.

Plasma and Plasma Proteins

In adults, plasma accounts for 55% to 60% of blood volume. Plasma is a complex aqueous liquid containing a number of organic and inorganic elements (Table 25-1). The concentration of these elements varies depending on diet, metabolic demand, hormones, and vitamins. Plasma differs from serum in that serum is plasma that has been altered in the laboratory to remove fibrinogen (a clotting factor) or some other element that is unwanted or unneeded in the sample.

Table 25-1	Organic and Inorganic Components of Arterial Plasma	
Constituent	Amount/Concentration	Major Functions
Water	93% of plasma weight	Medium for carrying all other constituents
Electrolytes	Total <1% of plasma weight	Maintain H_2O in extracellular compartment; act as buffers; function in membrane excitability
Na^+	142 mEq/L (142 mM)	
K^+	4 mEq/L (4 mM)	
Ca^{++}	5 mEq/L (2.5 mM)	
Mg^{++}	3 mEq/L (1.5 mM)	
Cl^-	103 mEq/L (103 mM)	
HCO_3^-	27 mEq/L (27 mM)	
Phosphate (mostly HPO_4^{--})	2 mEq/L (1 mM)	
SO_4^-	1 mEq/L (0.5 mM)	
Proteins	7.3 g/dl (2.5 mM)	Provide colloid osmotic pressure of plasma; act as buffers; bind other plasma constituents (lipids, hormones, vitamins, minerals, etc.); clotting factors; enzymes; enzyme precursors; antibodies (immune globulins); hormones; transporters
Albumins	4.5 g/dl	
Globulins	2.5 g/dl	
Fibrinogen	0.3 g/dl	
Transferrin	250 mg/dl	
Ferritin	15-300 mcg/L	
Gases		
CO_2 content	22-20 mmol/L plasma	By-product of oxygenation, most CO_2 content is from HCO_3 and acts as a buffer
O_2	Pao_2 80 torr or greater (arterial); Pvo_2 30-40 torr (venous)	Oxygenation
N_2	0.9 ml/dl	By-product of protein catabolism
Nutrients		Provide nutrition and substances for tissue repair
Glucose and other carbohydrates	100 mg/dl (5.6 mM)	
Total amino acids	40 mg/dl (2 mM)	
Total lipids	500 mg/dl (7.5 mM)	
Cholesterol	150-250 mg/dl (4-7 mM)	
Individual vitamins	0.0001-2.5 mg/dl	
Individual trace elements	0.001-0.3 mg/dl	
Iron	50-150 mcg/dl	
Waste products		
Urea (blood urea nitrogen [BUN])	7-18 mg/dl (5.7 mM)	End product of protein catabolism
Creatinine (from creatine)	1 mg/dl (0.09 mM)	End product from energy metabolism
Uric acid (from nucleic acids)	5 mg/dl (0.3 mM)	End product from protein metabolism
Bilirubin (from heme)	0.2-1.2 mg/dl (0.003-0.018 mM)	End product of red blood cell destruction
Individual hormones	0.000001-0.05 mg/dl	Functions specific to target tissue

Data from Vander AJ, Sherman JH, Luciano DS: *Human physiology: the mechanisms of body function*, ed 8, New York, 2001, McGraw-Hill.

In circulating plasma the dominant elements by weight are the plasma proteins, which constitute about 7% of the total plasma weight. The plasma proteins vary in structure and function but can be classified into three major groups: the albumins, globulins, and clotting factors. The albumins are the most numerous, followed by the various globulins (immune globulins or g-globulins) and the clotting factors, chiefly fibrinogen. The plasma proteins are synthesized in the liver, with the exception of the immune globulins, which are synthesized by lymphocytes in the lymph nodes and other lymphoid tissues (see Chapter 7).

Albumin is present at a concentration of about 4 g/dl and is essential for regulating the passage of water and solutes through the capillaries. Because albumin molecules are large and do not diffuse freely through the vascular endothelium, they provide the critical colloid osmotic or oncotic pressure that regulates the passage of water and solutes through the microcirculation (arterioles, capillaries, and venules) (see Chapters 1 and 3). Water and solute particles diffuse out of the arterial portions of the capillaries because blood pressure is greater in arterial than in venous blood vessels (see Chapter 3). Water and solutes move from tissue cells into the venous portions of the capillaries, where the pressures are reversed, with oncotic pressure being greater than intravascular pressure. Albumin also serves as a carrier molecule for both normal components of blood and exogenous agents, such as drugs.

The immune globulins, or antibodies, are synthesized by mature lymphocytes called *plasma cells* in the lymphoid organs, chiefly lymph nodes. The immune globulins include IgA, IgG, IgM, IgD, and IgE. Most of them are critical for defense against infectious microorganisms. (Lymphocyte and antibody function is described in Chapter 7.)

The third important class of plasma proteins is the **clotting factors,** which promote coagulation and stop bleeding from damaged blood vessels. Fibrinogen is the most plentiful of the clotting factors and is the precursor of the fibrin clot (see p. 914). Other plasma proteins include complement proteins, a group of proteins involved in the immune response, a variety of enzymes and their inhibitors, and specific carriers of such elements as iron and copper. The plasma lipids, triglycerides, phospholipids, cholesterol, and fatty acids are carried through the blood as complexes with plasma proteins; they are known as *lipoproteins* (see Chapters 1 and 30).

The electrolytes (electrically charged solutes) of the plasma maintain the osmolarity and pH of blood within a physiologic range (see Table 25-1). (Electrolytes are described in Chapters 1 and 3.)

Cellular Components of the Blood

The cellular elements of the blood are broadly classified as erythrocytes (red blood cells [RBCs]), leukocytes (white blood cells [WBCs]), and platelets (thrombocytes). The components of blood are listed in Table 25-2.

Erythrocytes

In 1628 Robert Burton described blood as a "hot, temperate red humor whose office is to nourish the whole body, to give it strength and color being dispersed by the veins through every part of it."[1] A few years later, with the invention of the microscope, researchers learned that erythrocytes give blood its red color.

Erythrocytes (red blood cells [RBCs]) are the most abundant cells of the blood, occupying approximately 48% of the blood volume in men and about 42% in women. Erythrocytes are responsible primarily for tissue oxygenation. Their shape, size, and structure reflect their unique function as deliverers of gases throughout the body. The erythrocyte's cytoplasm consists of a solution containing protein (mostly hemoglobin [Hb], which carries the gases) and electrolytes, which regulate diffusion through the cell's plasma membrane. The mature erythrocyte lacks the cytoplasmic organelles—a nucleus, mitochondria, and ribosomes—that would enable it to divide or carry out metabolic functions. Therefore it cannot synthesize protein or carry out oxidative reactions. Because it cannot undergo mitotic division, it lives out its life span (approximately 120 days) in the circulation, dies, and is replaced by a new erythrocyte.

The erythrocyte's size and shape are ideally suited to its function as a gas carrier. It is a small disk with two unique properties: (1) biconcavity and (2) reversible deformability (Figure 25-1). The flattened, biconcave shape provides a surface area–to–volume ratio that is optimal for gas diffusion into and out of the cell. Reversible deformity enables the erythrocyte to alter its shape to squeeze through the microcirculation and then return to normal. During its 120-day life

Table 25-2	Cellular Components of the Blood			
Cell	Structural Characteristics*	Normal Amounts of Circulating Blood	Function	Life Span
Erythrocyte (red blood cell)	Nonnucleated cytoplasmic disk containing hemoglobin	4.2-6.2 million/mm³	Gas transport to and from tissue cells and lungs	80-120 days
Leukocyte (white blood cell)	Nucleated cell	5000-10,000/mm³	Body defense mechanisms	See below
Lymphocyte	Mononuclear immunocyte	25%-33% of leukocyte count (leukocyte differential)	Humoral and cell-mediated immunity (see Chapter 6)	Days or years depending on type
Monocyte and macrophage	Large mononuclear phagocyte	3%-7% of leukocyte differential	Phagocytosis; mononuclear phagocyte system	Months or years
Eosinophil	Segmented polymorphonuclear granulocyte	1%-4% of leukocyte differential	Phagocytosis, antibody-mediated defense against parasites, allergic reactions, associated with Hodgkin disease, recovery phase of infection	Unknown
Neutrophil	Segmented polymorphonuclear granulocyte	57%-67% of leukocyte differential	Phagocytosis, particularly during early phase of inflammation	4 days
Basophil	Segmented polymorphonuclear granulocyte	0%-0.75% of leukocyte differential	Secretes chemicals chemotactic for neutrophils†, but associated with allergic reactions and mechanical irritation	Unknown
Platelet	Irregularly shaped cytoplasmic fragment (not a cell)	140,000-340,000/mm³	Hemostasis following vascular injury; normal coagulation and clot formation/retraction	8-11 days

*See bottom row of Figure 25-7 for illustrations of cells.
†Recent data.

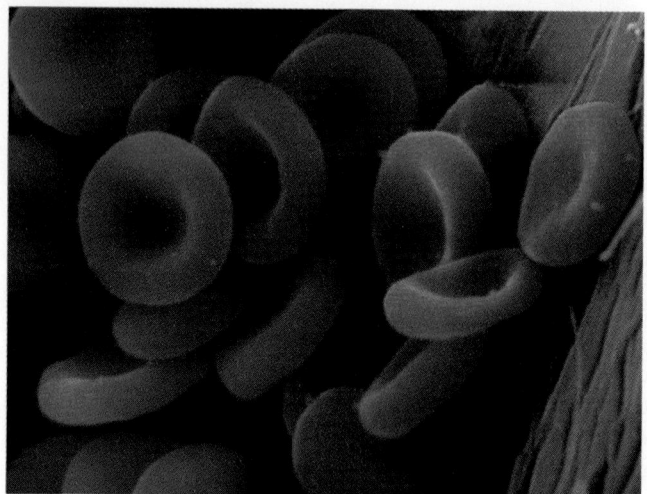

Figure 25-1 Mature erythrocytes. Scanning electron micrograph of mature erythrocytes on cell wall. (Copyright Dennis Kunkel Microscopy, Inc.)

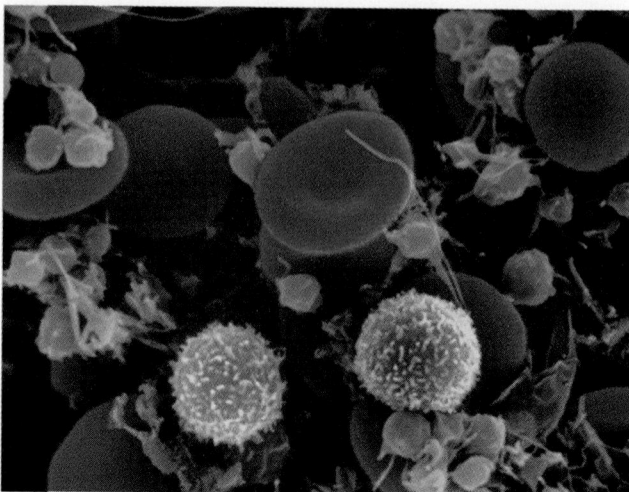

Figure 25-2 Blood cells. Leukocytes are spherical and have irregular surfaces with numerous extending pili (appears as yellow). Erythrocytes are flattened spheres with a depressed center. Activated platelets are green. (Copyright Dennis Kunkel Microscopy, Inc.)

span, where most of its time is spent within the capillary channels, the erythrocyte, which is 8 mm in diameter, must repeatedly circulate through splenic sinusoids and capillaries that are only 2 mm in diameter. To do this, the erythrocyte assumes a torpedo-like conformation. The physical arrangement of membrane proteins is responsible for the biconcave shape of the resting cell.

Leukocytes

Leukocytes (white blood cells [WBCs]) defend the body against organisms that cause infection and remove debris, including dead or injured host cells of all kinds (Figure 25-2). The leukocytes act primarily in the tissues but are transported in the circulation. They are fewer in number than erythrocytes; the average adult has approximately 5000 to 10,000 leukocytes per mm^3 of blood.

Leukocytes are classified according to structure as either granulocytes or agranulocytes and according to function as either phagocytes or immunocytes. The granulocytes, which include neutrophils, basophils, and eosinophils, are all phagocytes. Of the agranulocytes, the monocytes and macrophages are phagocytes, whereas the lymphocytes are immunocytes (cells that create immunity; see Chapter 7).

Granulocytes. The **granulocytes** are so called because of the many membrane-bound granules in their cytoplasm. The granules contain enzymes capable of killing microorganisms and catabolizing debris ingested by the process of phagocytosis. The granules also contain powerful biochemical mediators with a variety of inflammatory and immune functions. These mediators, along with the digestive enzymes, are released from some granulocytes in response to specific stimuli and from all granulocytes as they reach the end of their natural life span and die. The biochemical mediators have various vascular and intercellular effects, and the enzymes participate in the breakdown of free-floating debris from sites of infection or injury.

Granulocytes are capable of ameboid movement, by which they migrate through vessel walls and then to sites where their

action is needed. Migration through vessel walls, called *diapedesis*, and movement through the tissues, which occurs in response to chemotactic factors, are described and illustrated in Chapter 6.

The **neutrophil (polymorphonuclear neutrophil [PMN])** is the most numerous and best understood of the granulocytes (Figure 25-3, *A*). Neutrophils constitute about 55% of the total leukocyte count in adults. The cytoplasm of neutrophils contains small lysosomal granules and a central nucleus with two to five distinct lobes. Immature neutrophils are called *bands* or *stabs*. Mature neutrophils are called *segmented neutrophils* because of the characteristic appearance of their nucleus. Neutrophils reach a fully mature state in the bone marrow, and these mature neutrophils are called the *marrow neutrophil reserve*. Normally it takes about 14 days for neutrophils to develop from early precursors, but this process is accelerated by infection and treatment with colony stimulating factors.

Neutrophils are the chief phagocytes of early inflammation. Soon after bacterial invasion or tissue injury, neutrophils migrate out of the capillaries and into the inflamed site, where they ingest and destroy microorganisms and debris and then die in 1 or 2 days. The dissolution of dead neutrophils releases digestive enzymes from their cytoplasmic granules. These enzymes dissolve cellular debris and prepare the site for healing. (This final function, called *débridement*, is described in Chapter 6).

Eosinophils, which have large, coarse granules, constitute only 1% to 4% of the normal leukocyte count in adults (see Figure 25-3, *B*). Like neutrophils, eosinophils are capable of ameboid movement and phagocytosis. Unlike neutrophils, which ingest cellular debris, eosinophils ingest antigen-antibody complexes and are induced by IgE-mediated hypersensitivity reactions to attack parasites. Eosinophils also help to control inflammatory processes. (Their function in inflam-

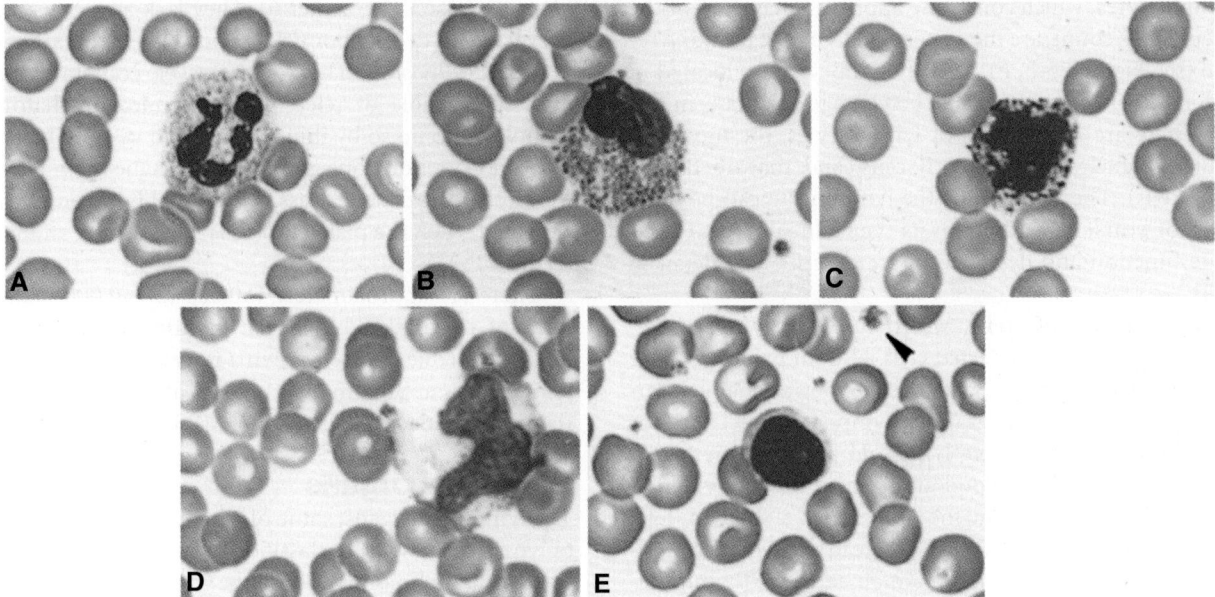

Figure 25-3 Leukocytes. An example of leukocytes in a human blood smear. **A,** Neutrophil. **B,** Eosinophil. **C,** Basophil. **D,** Monocyte. **E,** Lymphocyte. (From Erlandsen S, Magney J: *Color atlas of histology,* St Louis, 1992, Mosby.)

mation and defense against parasites is described in Chapter 6.) High eosinophil counts in atopic (allergy-prone) individuals experiencing type I allergic reactions, such as asthma or allergic rhinitis, demonstrate that eosinophils participate in hypersensitivity reactions to allergens as well as parasites (see Chapter 8).

Mast cells are large cells with cytoplasmic granules that contain an abundant mixture of biochemical mediators, including histamine, chemotactic factors, and cytokines. Mast cells act rapidly to make blood vessels more permeable. Mast cells are a central cell in inflammation (see Chapter 6 and Figure 6-8). They are found in high concentrations in vascularized connective tissues just beneath body epithelial surfaces, including the submucosal tissues of the gastrointestinal and respiratory tracts and the dermal layer that lies just below the surface of the skin. Being in close proximity to blood vessels, mast cells make their mediators available to a large variety of cell types, including fibroblasts, glandular cells, nerves, vascular endothelial cells, smooth muscle cells, and other cells of the immune system. It used to be believed that mast cell activation was all-or-nothing, with IgE cross-linking inducing the miseries of allergy and anaphylaxis. The activity of mast cells, however, is now known to be present in different pathologies, such as chronic inflammatory processes, fibrotic disorders, wound healing, and neoplastic tissue transformation.[2-5] A number of stimuli cause mast cells to become activated resulting in initiation of the inflammatory response. **Mastocytosis** is an increased accumulation of mast cells.

Basophils, which make up less than 1% of the leukocytes, are structurally similar to the mast cells found throughout extravascular tissue (see Figure 25-3, *C*). Like the mast cells, whose role in stimulating the inflammatory response is described in Chapter 6, the basophils have cytoplasmic granules

that contain vasoactive amines (histamine, bradykinin, serotonin) and an anticoagulant (heparin). The precise function of basophils is poorly understood.

Agranulocytes. The **agranulocytes**—monocytes, macrophages, and lymphocytes—differ from the granulocytes in that they do not contain lysosomal granules in their cytoplasm. The lymphocytes do not contain any enzyme-filled digestive vacuoles, and the digestive vacuoles of the monocytes and macrophages are larger and fewer than those of the granulocytes.

The monocytes and macrophages make up the **mononuclear phagocyte system (MPS),** formerly called the *reticuloendothelial system (RES)*. (The MPS is described on p. 900.) Both monocytes and macrophages participate in the immune and inflammatory response because they are powerful phagocytes. They also ingest dead or defective host cells, particularly blood cells.

Monocytes are the largest normal blood cell and have a horseshoe-shaped nucleus. Monocytes appear to be precursors of macrophages that are fixed in tissues. Monocytes migrate to the inflammatory site, where they develop into macrophages. Macrophages are generally larger and are more active as phagocytes than monocytes. **Macrophages,** particularly those residing in tissues, are significant initiators of the inflammatory response (see Chapter 6) (see Figure 24-3, *D*). After monocytes are formed and released by the bone marrow, they enter the bloodstream. They participate in immune responses. Monocytes ingest and "process" antigens so that the antigens can be recognized by T and B lymphocytes (described in Chapter 7). Monocytes have many other biologic properties, including the ability to release tissue thromboplastin and to activate plasminogen, proteolytic enzymes, and other active agents.

Lymphocytes, which constitute approximately 36% of the total leukocyte count, are the primary cells of the immune response (see Figure 25-3, *E*). Most lymphocytes are located in lymphoid tissues; only a small percentage circulate in the blood. There are many types of lymphocytes, the most important of which are T cells, B cells, and mature B cells (plasma cells). The life span of the lymphocyte can be days, months, or years, depending on its type and subtype. (Lymphocyte function and dysfunction are described in detail in Unit III.)

Natural killer (NK) cells, which resemble lymphocytes, kill some types of virus-infected cells without prior exposure to them and tumor cells in vitro. Hence they are named *natural killer cells*. These large granular lymphocytes account for 5% to 10% of the circulating lymphoid pool and are found mainly in the peripheral blood and spleen. Recent evidence, however, has shown that in the absence of a thymus, fetal thymocytes develop into NK cells instead of T-helper or T-regulatory cells. The same cells maintained in the thymus develop into mature T cells, also called *NKT cells*. Therefore, it is believed that immature thymocytes give rise to T cells or NK cells, depending on the microenvironment. Recently identified and cloned are three distinct NK-specific molecules termed *natural cytotoxicity receptors (NCR)*. They mediate NK cell activation in the interaction and lysis of infected cells or tumor cells. These cells are discussed in Chapters 6 and 7.

Platelets

Platelets are not cells; they are disk-shaped cytoplasmic fragments. They are formed by fragmentation of very large (40 to 100 (m) cells known as **megakaryocytes** (Figure 25-4). Platelets are essential for blood coagulation and control of bleeding (also see Chapter 6). They lack a nucleus; therefore they have no deoxyribonucleic acid (DNA) and are incapable of mitotic division. They do, however, contain cytoplasmic granules capable of releasing biochemical mediators when stimulated to do so by injury to a blood vessel. Thrombopoietin (TPO), a hormone growth factor, is the main regulator of the circulating platelet mass.[6,7] Presumably, thrombopoietin is activated when the platelet mass is low, causing an increase in serum TPO.[6]

There are approximately 140,000 to 340,000 platelets per mm³ of circulating blood. An additional one third of the body's available platelets are in a reserve pool in the spleen. A platelet lives approximately 10 days, after which it dies and is removed by macrophages of the MPS, mostly in the spleen.

Lymphoid Organs

The lymphoid organs, some of which are merely aggregations of lymphoid tissue, are classified as primary or secondary. The primary lymphoid organs are the thymus and the bone marrow. The secondary lymphoid organs consist of the spleen, lymph nodes, tonsils, and Peyer patches of the small intestine (see Figure 7-3). All of the lymphoid organs link the hematologic and immune systems in that they are sites of residence, proliferation, differentiation, or function of lymphocytes and mononuclear phagocytes (monocytes and macrophages). (The liver, which also has hematologic functions, is primarily a digestive organ and is described in Chapter 38.)

Spleen

The spleen is the largest of the secondary lymphoid organs. It is a site of fetal hematopoiesis; its mononuclear phagocytes filter and cleanse the blood; its lymphocytes mount an immune response to blood-borne microorganisms; and it serves as a blood reservoir (see Chapter 27).

The spleen is a concave, encapsulated organ that weighs about 150 g and is about the size of a fist (see Figure 7-3). It is located in the left upper abdominal cavity, curved around a portion of the stomach. Strands of connective tissue (trabeculae) extend throughout the spleen from the splenic capsule, dividing the spleen into compartments. The compartments contain masses of lymphoid tissue called *splenic pulp*. The spleen is interlaced with many blood vessels, some of which are capable of distending to store blood.

Blood that circulates through the spleen comes from the splenic artery, which branches from the descending aorta and reenters the circulatory system through the splenic vein, which feeds into the portal vein. The portion of arterial blood that enters the spleen first encounters the white splenic pulp, which consists of masses of lymphoid tissue containing lymphocytes and macrophages. The white pulp forms clumps around the splenic arterioles and is the chief site of immune and phagocytic function within the spleen. Here blood-borne antigens encounter lymphocytes, initiating the immune response (see Chapter 7).

Some of the blood that enters the terminal capillaries of the spleen continues through the microcirculation and enters

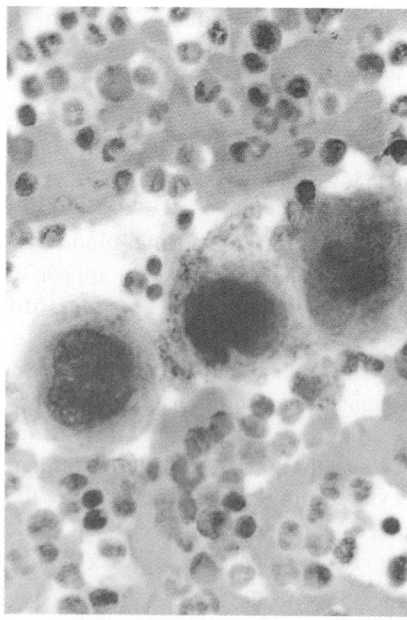

Figure 25-4 Megakaryocyte and platelets. Note the large number of platelets (purple) surrounding the large megakaryocytes in the center. (From Miale JB, *Laboratory medicine: hematology,* ed 6, St Louis, 1982, Mosby.)

highly distensible storage areas called *venous sinuses.* Most of the blood, however, oozes through the extremely permeable capillary walls into the principal site of splenic filtration, the red pulp (Figure 25-5). Here the resident macrophages of the MPS phagocytose old, damaged, or dead blood cells of all kinds (but chiefly erythrocytes); microorganisms; and particles of debris. Hemoglobin from phagocytosed erythrocytes is catabolized, and heme (iron) is stored in the cytoplasm of the macrophages or released back into the blood plasma (see p. 908 and Figure 25-13). The macrophages also can remove certain particulate inclusions from erythrocytes without harming the cells themselves. Blood that filters through the red pulp also finds its way into the venous sinuses and hence into the portal circulation.

The venous sinuses (and the red pulp) are capable of storing more than 300 ml of blood. Passive dilation of the venous sinuses enables the spleen to increase its storage capacity as needed by the body. Sudden reductions in blood pressure cause the sympathetic nervous system to stimulate constriction of the sinuses. Constriction, which can expel as much as 200 ml of blood into the venous circulation, helps restore blood volume and increases the hematocrit.

The spleen is not necessary for life or for adequate hematologic function. However, splenic absence from any cause (atrophy, traumatic injury, or removal because of disease) has several effects on the body that indicate what its function once was. For example, leukocytosis (high levels of circulating leukocytes) often occurs after splenectomy. This suggests that the spleen exerts some control over the rate of proliferation of leukocyte stem cells in the bone marrow or their release into the bloodstream. Splenic absence is associated also with decreased levels of iron in the circulation, reflecting the spleen's role in the iron cycle (see p. 908). Immune function decreases in the absence of the spleen. Antibody production in response to small doses of soluble (i.e., blood-borne) antigen diminishes. Finally, the splenic function of removing old and defec-

tive blood cells seems to be confirmed by the fact that the blood of individuals lacking spleens contains more morphologically defective blood cells than normal.

Lymph Nodes

Structurally, lymph nodes are part of the lymphatic system. Thousands of them are clustered around the lymphatic veins, the vessels that collect interstitial fluid from the tissues and transport it, as lymph, back into the circulatory system near the heart. Functionally, however, lymph nodes are part of the hematologic and immune systems because they are the site of development or activity of large numbers of lymphocytes, monocytes, and macrophages. As the lymph filters through the bean-shaped lymph nodes clustered in the inguinal, axillary, and cervical regions of the body, it is cleansed of foreign particles and microorganisms by the monocytes and macrophages. The microorganisms in lymph stimulate the resident lymphocytes to develop into antibody-producing plasma cells (see Chapter 7). Lymphocytes, monocytes, and macrophages proliferate in the lymph nodes and are released into the lymphatic stream. During an infection the rate of proliferation of macrophages within the nodes is so great that the nodes enlarge and become tender.

Each lymph node is enclosed in a fibrous capsule (Figure 25-6). Strands of connective tissue (trabeculae) extend inward from the capsule, dividing the node into several compartments. Reticular fibers that extend between the trabeculae divide the compartments into smaller sections. The reticular fibers trap and store large numbers of lymphocytes, monocytes, and macrophages. The node is composed of an outer cortex area and an inner medullary area. Within the cortex of each node are germinal centers, or separate masses of lymphoid tissue. Lymph enters the node through several

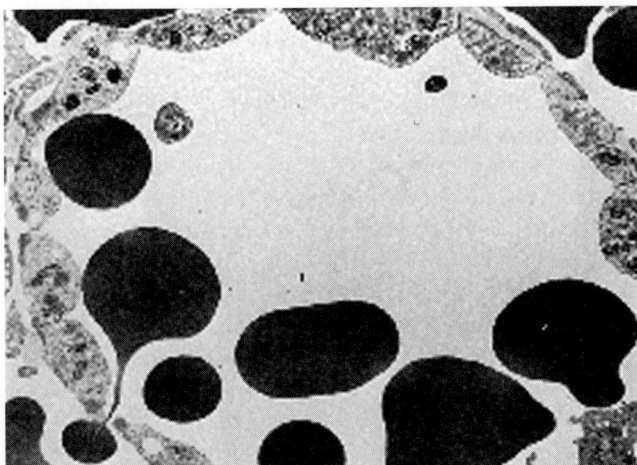

Figure 25-5 Red cells in the spleen. Transmission electron micrograph of a normal red blood cell traversing the sinus wall in a human spleen. Note how it must deform to reenter the sinus. (From Damjanov I, Linder J, editors: *Anderson's pathology,* ed 10, St Louis, 1996, Mosby.)

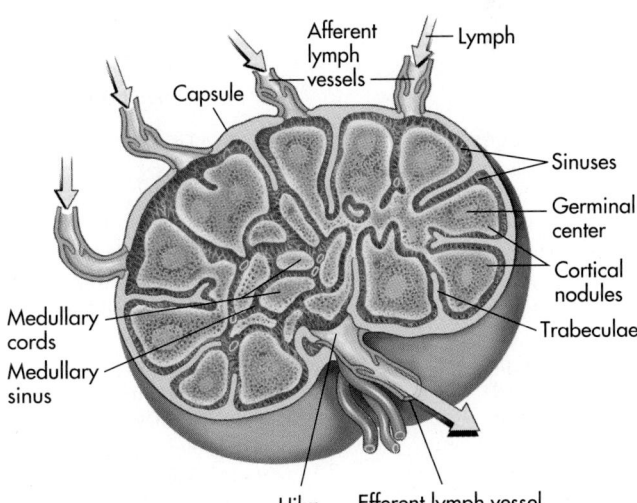

Figure 25-6 Structure of a lymph node. Several afferent valved lymphatics bring lymph to the node. A single efferent lymphatic leaves the node at the hilus. Note that the artery and vein also enter and leave at the hilus. Arrows show direction of lymph. (From Thibodeau GA, Patton K: *Anatomy & physiology,* ed 5, St Louis, 2003, Mosby.)

afferent lymphatic vessels, filters through the sinuses in the node, and leaves by way of efferent lymphatic vessels. Lymph flows slowly through the nodes, which facilitates the phagocytosis of foreign substances within the node and prevents them from reentering the bloodstream.

Mononuclear Phagocyte System

The **mononuclear phagocyte system (MPS)** consists of a line of cells that originate in the bone marrow; are transported by the bloodstream; and after differentiation into blood monocytes, finally settle in the tissues as mature macrophages. It is composed of monoblasts, promonocytes, and monocytes in bone marrow, monocytes in peripheral blood, and macrophages in tissue. The journey from bone marrow stem cell to chemotactic macrophages in tissue is regulated by growth and differentiation factors, adhesion molecules, and cellular interactions. Table 25-3 lists the various names given to macrophages localized in specific tissues.

The cells of the MPS ingest and destroy (by phagocytosis) unwanted materials in the blood and in organs. During inflammation they engulf and digest foreign protein particles, microorganisms, debris from dead or injured cells, defective or injured erythrocytes, and dead neutrophils (see Figure 6-13). The MPS (mostly in the liver and spleen) also is the main line of defense against bacteria in the bloodstream. In addition, the MPS cleanses the blood by removing old, injured, or dead erythrocytes, leukocytes, platelets, coagulation products, antigen-antibody complexes, and macromolecules

Table 25-3	Mononuclear Phagocyte System*	
Name of Cell	**Location**	
Committed Stem Cells†	Bone marrow	
Monoblasts	Bone marrow	
Promonoblasts	Bone marrow	
Monocytes	Bone marrow and peripheral blood	
Macrophages	Tissue	
Kupffer cells (inflammatory macrophages)	Liver	
Alveolar macrophages	Lung	
Histiocytes	Connective tissue	
Macrophages	Bone marrow	
Fixed and free macrophages	Spleen and lymph nodes	
Pleural and peritoneal macrophages	Serous cavities	
Microglial cells	Nervous system	
Mesangial cells	Kidney	
Osteoclasts	Bone	
Langerhan cells	Skin	
Dendritic cells	Lymphoid tissue	

Data from Kumar V et al: *Robbins and Cotran's pathologic basis of disease,* ed 7, Philadelphia, 2005, Saunders.
*Formerly called the reticuloendothelial system.
†Development of blood cells from stem cells in the marrow is described on this page and illustrated in Figure 25-7.

(such as lipids and carbohydrates synthesized by the body as the result of faulty metabolism, as in storage diseases). Macrophages are the key cellular player in inflammation. Activated macrophages secrete a large array of biologically active chemicals that if uncontrolled, result in chronic inflammation and tissue injury (see Chapter 6). Macrophages also play a role in blood coagulation, wound healing, tissue remodeling, and the control of blood production.

Multiple cell types, including endothelial cells, fibroblasts, and lymphocytes, produce substances called **colony-stimulating factors (CSFs),** or **hematopoietic growth factors,** that are soluble mediators secreted by cells for the purpose of cell-to-cell communication. These factors control the production, maturation, and function of granulocytes and monocyte-macrophages (Figure 25-7) and the development of blood cells.

The origin and turnover of all the tissue macrophages named in Table 25-3 are not precisely known. It seems clear that once monocytes leave the circulation, they do not return. In the tissues, monocytes differentiate into macrophages without dividing. They can survive many months or even years. Monocytes migrating into inflamed tissues give rise to most of the reactive macrophage population. Under normal circumstances, macrophages show little evidence of mitotic division, probably because the levels of CSF production normally are low, but production can be rapidly elevated in response to need, such as an infection.

DEVELOPMENT OF BLOOD CELLS

Hematopoiesis

Blood cell production, termed *hematopoiesis,* occurs in the liver and spleen of the fetus, but after birth it normally occurs only in bone marrow and is then known as *medullary hematopoiesis* (see Chapter 28). It is still a mystery as to why hematopoiesis is restricted to bone marrow after birth.

Hematopoiesis is a two-stage process that involves mitotic division (or proliferation) and maturation (or differentiation). In the maturation stage, cell division stops, but maturation changes continue before cells enter the blood. Each type of blood cell has parent cells, called *stem cells,* that undergo mitosis when they receive specific biochemical signals indicating that populations of circulating blood cells have diminished to a certain point. The stem cells continue to proliferate until the requisite number of mature daughter cells has entered the circulation. The stem cells of lymphocytes and possibly monocytes are stimulated to proliferate and differentiate by other mechanisms, particularly activation of the immune response, but they too originate in bone marrow.

Hematopoiesis can be divided by activity in the bone marrow by two separate pools: the stem cell pool and the bone marrow pool, with eventual release of mature cells into the peripheral circulation (Figure 25-8). In the bone marrow microenvironment a stem cell pool exists where structurally unidentifiable multipotential stem cells and unipotential committed colony-forming units (CFUs) reside. In addition,

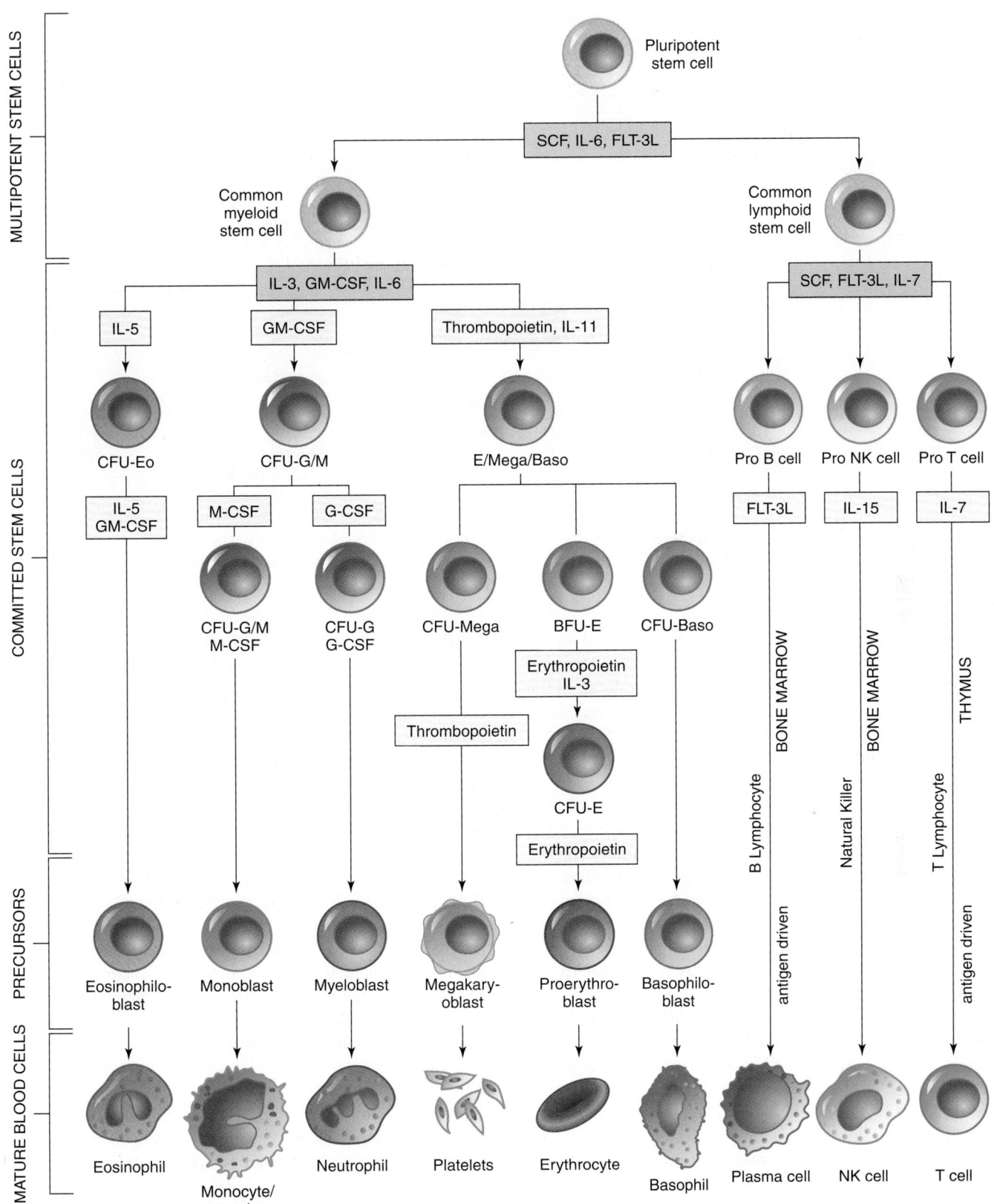

Figure 25-7 Differentiation of hematopoietic cells. *SCF,* Stem cell factor; *FTL-3L,* fms-like tyrosine kinase 3 ligand; *GM-CSF,* granulocyte-macrophage colony-stimulating factor; *M-CSF,* macrophage colony-stimulating factor; *G-CSF,* granulocyte colony-stimulating factor; *CFU,* colony-forming unit; *Eo,* eosinophil; *G,* granulocyte; *M,* macrophage; *BFU,* burst-forming unit; *IL,* interleukin; *E,* erythrocyte; *Mega,* megakaryocyte; *Baso,* basophil.

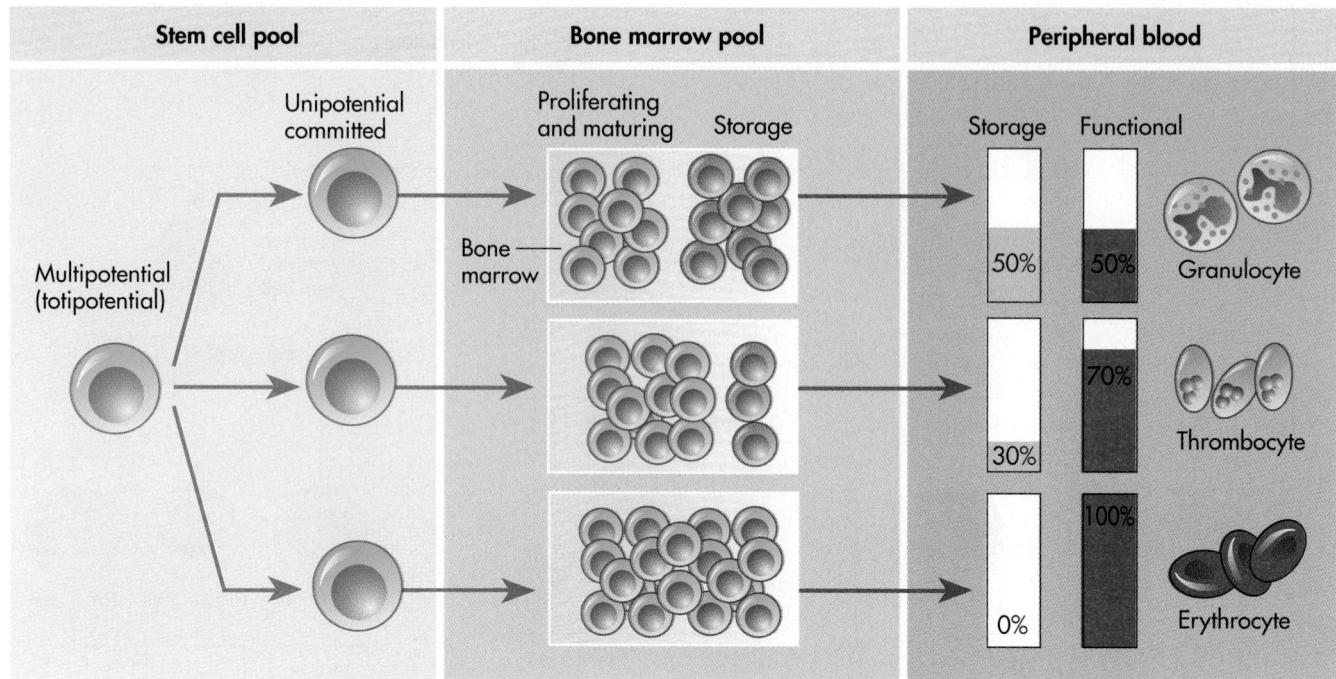

Figure 25-8 **Hematopoiesis.** Hematopoiesis from the stem cell pool; activity mainly in the bone marrow and in the peripheral blood. (Modified from Harmening DM, editor: *Clinical hematology and fundamentals of hemostasis,* ed 3, Philadelphia, 1997, FA Davis.)

there is a bone marrow pool that can be divided into two cell pools: cells that are proliferating and maturing and cells that are stored and later released into the peripheral blood. In the peripheral blood, two pools of cells are also categorized: those circulating and those in storage. Those cells stored around the walls of the blood vessels are often called the *marginating storage pool* (see Figure 25-8).

Certain blood cells proliferate and differentiate simultaneously for a period. Proliferation usually ceases after a number of doubling divisions, but differentiation continues. Evidence indicates that separate signaling pathways for proliferation and differentiation exist in erythroid cells.[8,9] Erythrocytes and neutrophils usually are mature before entering the blood. Monocytes and other leukocytes are not. They enter the bloodstream and continue to mature as they travel to the spleen, peritoneal cavity, and lung.

Hematopoiesis continues throughout life to replace blood cells that grow old and die, are killed by disease, or are lost through bleeding. Medullary hematopoiesis increases in response to proliferative disease, hemorrhage, hemolytic anemia (in which erythrocytes are destroyed), chronic infection, idiopathic thrombocytopenic purpura (bleeding caused by platelet insufficiency; see Chapter 27), and other disorders that deplete blood cells. In general, long-term stimuli, such as chronic diseases, cause a greater increase in hematopoiesis than acute conditions, such as hemorrhage. Abnormal proliferation of erythrocytes occurs in polycythemia vera, a myeloproliferative disease.

Medullary hematopoiesis can be accelerated by any or all of three mechanisms: (1) conversion of yellow bone marrow,

which does not produce blood cells, to red marrow, which does; (2) faster differentiation of daughter cells; and presumably (3) faster proliferation of stem cells. Marrow conversion is stimulated by erythropoietin, the hormone that stimulates erythrocyte production. An increase in blood cell production occurs in response to emergencies, such as infection (see the next section).

In adults, extramedullary hematopoiesis—blood cell production in tissues other than bone marrow—is usually a sign of disease. Extramedullary production of one or more types occurs in disease states that affect erythrocytes (e.g., pernicious anemia, sickle cell anemia, thalassemia, hemolytic disease of the newborn [erythroblastosis fetalis], hereditary spherocytosis) and leukocytes (certain leukemias). Extramedullary hematopoiesis of apparently normal blood cells has been reported also to occur in the spleen and liver and, less frequently, in lymph nodes, adrenal glands, cartilage, adipose tissue, intrathoracic areas, and kidneys.

Stem Cell System

The processes by which blood cells develop from a common ancestor, or stem cell, are known collectively as the *stem cell system*. This system is a hierarchy in which the earliest, most primitive ancestor is a stem cell (see Figure 25-7). Because these cells have the potential to develop into many types of blood cells—and other cells, for example, osteoclasts, as well as a new stem cell like itself—they also are called **pluripotent stem cells.** One pathway of development leads to various lymphoid tissues, in which T and B lymphocytes mature. The other pathway leads to myeloid tissue—the bone marrow.

The common myeloid stem cell triggers differentiation of eosinophils, monocyte/macrophages, neutrophils, platelets, erythrocytes, and basophils (see Figure 25-7). The common lymphoid stem cell triggers differentiation of B cells, NK cells and T cells.

Blood cell production in any one pathway requires numerous amplifying cell divisions coupled with complex maturation changes to produce the mature cells that are released into the blood. Regulation of hematopoiesis possibly occurs in two ways: (1) by **stromal** (covering or supportive tissue) **cells** in the marrow that control some of the cellular events by "cell contact processes" and (2) by the interaction of cytokines or regulatory molecules. Stromal cells apparently express **steel factor,** a stem cell factor, which activates stem cells to develop. Recently, stromal cells were shown to differentiate into myocytes, muscle cells, hepatocytes, and glial cells.[10] In vitro, stromal cells can differentiate into neural cells.[11] Stem cells possess two properties that other cells lack: (1) they are uncommitted to being any one cell type, such as skin, liver, or muscle and (2) they can multiply, possibly indefinitely, making descendent cells that retain this uncommitted state or adapt their commitment in appropriate circumstances. **Embryonic stem cells,** from the fertilized egg, are the most flexible stem cells—they can create any cell in the body. The challenge of getting stem cells to differentiate reliably involves coaxing them with identical chemical signals that the body uses naturally for differentiation. This is a daunting task with potentially astonishing clinical implications. For example, bone marrow might become the reservoir from which stem cells are harvested and then stimulated to produce nerve cells to help with the treatments of spinal cord injuries.

In vitro, hematopoietic cells will survive, proliferate, and differentiate only if they are provided with specific growth factors. These factors are glycoproteins usually called *hematopoietic growth factors* or *colony-stimulating factors (CSFs)*. These factors (cytokines) act as hormones and stimulate the proliferation of progenitor cells and their progeny and initiate the maturation events necessary to produce fully mature cells (i.e., activating specialized functions). Specific CSFs are necessary for the adequate growth of myeloid, erythroid, lymphoid, and megakaryocytic pathways and also are required to keep cells alive. CSFs are thought to play a role in preventing programmed cell death (apoptosis)[12,13] (Table 25-4 and Figure 25-9).

Clinical Uses of Colony-Stimulating Factors

Blood granulocyte numbers (e.g., eosinophils, neutrophils, basophils/mast cells) are normally present in the blood in the range of 4000 to 6000 cells per microliter, and susceptibility to

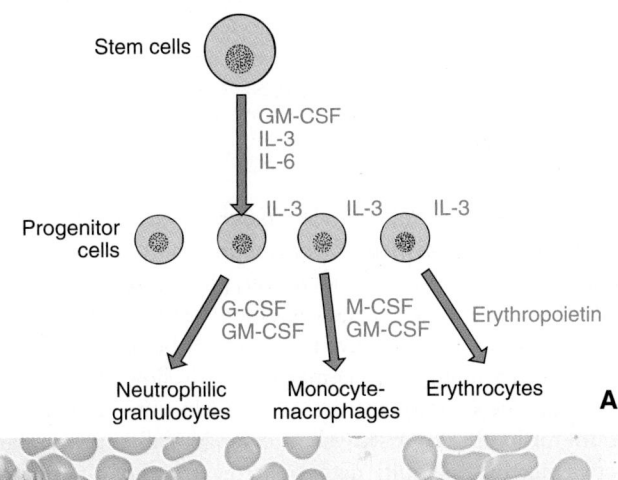

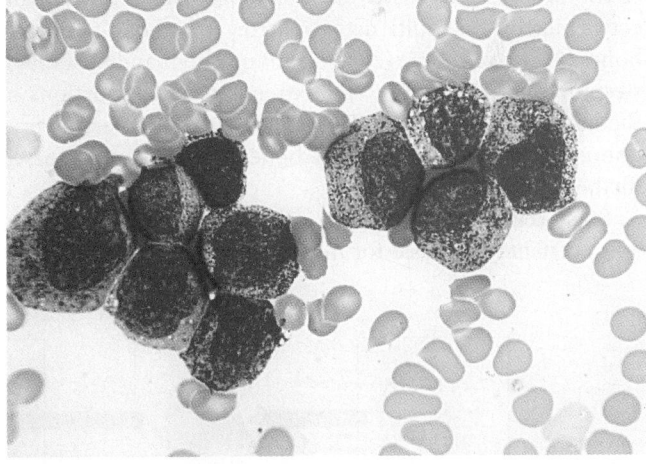

Table 25-4	Human Colony-Stimulating Factors (CSFs)	
CSF	**Cell Origin**	**Cell Stimulated**
M-CSF	Macrophage, fibroblast, endothelial cells	Macrophage, GM progenitor cells
GM-CSF	T cell, endothelial cells, fibroblast	Neutrophil, macrophage, eosinophil, GM progenitor cells
G-CSF	Macrophage, fibroblast	Neutrophils and GM progenitor cells
IL-3	T cell, epidermal cells	Pluripotent stem cell, progenitor cells, many differentiated cells
Erythropoietin	Kupffer and peritubular kidney cells	Erythrocyte
Steel factor (stem cell factor)	Stromal cells in bone marrow and many other cells	Stem cells

M-CSF, Macrophage; *GM-CSF,* granulocyte-macrophage; *G-CSF,* granulocyte; *IL-3,* interleukin-3.

Figure 25-9 Colony-stimulating factor (CSF) effects. **A,** Physiologic effects of some CSFs. **B,** Morphologic effects of growth factor. Marrow aspirate from a patient receiving G-CSF showing an early neutrophil response. There is a marked shift toward immaturity in the neutrophils with the majority at the promyelocyte and early myelocyte stages of maturation (Wright-Giemsa stain). *IL,* Interleukin; *G-CSF,* granulocyte colony-stimulating factor; *M-CSF,* macrophage colony-stimulating factor; *GM-CSF,* granulocyte-macrophage colony-stimulating factor. (**B** from Damjanov I, Linder J, editors: *Anderson's pathology,* ed 10, St Louis, 1996, Mosby.)

infection develops when they number below 1000 cells per microliter. During a natural response to a bacterial infection, granulocytes usually increase in number to 10,000 to 20,000 cells per microliter. The CSFs can raise white cell numbers even higher. No advantage, however, is gained from extreme numbers because of the resulting formation of toxic products and tissue damage.[12,14] CSFs have been studied in individuals with subnormal hematopoiesis either as a result of diseases such as acquired immunodeficiency syndrome (AIDS), aplastic anemia, or congenital neutropenia or as a consequence of cytotoxic therapy for cancer, including lymphoma and leukemia. The CSFs can stimulate increases in granulocyte-macrocyte populations in such individuals, but responses are quantitatively restricted if the available numbers of stem and progenitor cells have been drastically depleted by chemotherapy or disease. Responses to CSF treatment are evident in the correction of a preexisting disorder, such as in congenital neutropenia, or in a hematopoietic response after cytotoxic therapy (e.g., after bone marrow transplantation). CSF treatment can result in shorter periods of intensive nursing and hospitalization.[14] Currently, some CSFs are being mass-produced in recombinant form and are used to stimulate hematopoiesis; these include G-CSF, GM-CSF, and erythropoietin.

Bone Marrow

Bone marrow, also called *myeloid tissue* (myelos = marrow), is confined to the cavities of bone. Bone marrow consists of blood vessels, nerves, mononuclear phagocytes, stem cells, blood cells in various stages of differentiation, and stromal and fatty tissue. Adults have two kinds of bone marrow: red (or active [hematopoietic]) marrow and yellow (or inactive) marrow. The large quantities of fat in inactive marrow account for its characteristic yellow color. Not all bones contain active marrow. In adults, active marrow is found in the pelvic bones (34%), vertebrae (28%), cranium and mandible (13%), sternum and ribs (10%), and extreme proximal portions of the humerus and femur (4% to 8%).[15] Inactive marrow predominates in cavities of other bones. (Bones are discussed further in Chapter 41.)

Stem cells in hematopoietic marrow receive the oxygen and nutrients they need for mitosis and maturation from the primary or nutrient arteries of the bones. Branches of these arteries terminate in a capillary network that coalesces into large venous sinuses, which eventually drain into a central vein. Hematopoietic marrow and fat fill the spaces surrounding the network of venous sinuses. Some mechanism of transport enables the newly produced blood cells to traverse narrow openings in venous sinus walls and thus enter the circulation. It is not known whether the movement of the new blood cells forces an opening or whether certain sites open in response to the presence of the newly formed cells. Normally, cells do not enter the circulation until they have differentiated to a certain extent, but premature release is known to occur in certain diseases.

Development of Erythrocytes

For almost 100 years it was believed that erythrocytes developed from lymphocytes that were transformed in the spleen. It was not until the 1850s that the bone marrow was accepted as the site of erythropoiesis. It is now known that erythrocytes are derived from precursor cells called *erythroblasts* (Figure 25-10). Normal erythroblasts are also called *normoblasts*, whereas abnormal ones are called *megaloblasts*.

Erythrocyte development is shown in detail in Figure 25-10. The proerythroblast (pronormoblast) possesses a huge nucleus, is rich in ribosomes, and can synthesize protein. The signal that causes an increase in circulating erythrocytes is the glycoprotein erythropoietin. Erythropoietin stimulates uncommitted stem cells to differentiate into proerythroblasts. Whether hemoglobin has been synthesized at this stage is controversial. Hemoglobin is, however, readily apparent and increases in quantity as nuclear size shrinks throughout the basophilic and polychromatophilic stages. The orthochromatic erythroblast (normoblast) is the smallest of the nucleated erythrocyte precursors. Once the nucleus is lost, the cell that remains is called a **reticulocyte.** Although it lacks a nucleus, the reticulocyte contains polyribosomes (for globin synthesis) and mitochondria (for oxidative metabolism and heme synthesis). The reticulocyte matures into an erythrocyte within 24 to 48 hours. During this period, mitochondria and ribosomes disappear and the cell becomes smaller and more disklike. With these final changes, the erythrocyte loses its capacity for hemoglobin synthesis and oxidative metabolism.

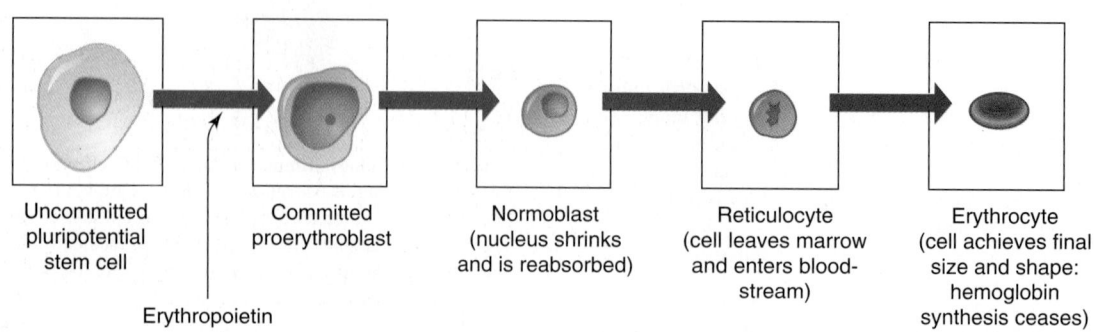

| Uncommitted pluripotential stem cell | Committed proerythroblast | Normoblast (nucleus shrinks and is reabsorbed) | Reticulocyte (cell leaves marrow and enters bloodstream) | Erythrocyte (cell achieves final size and shape: hemoglobin synthesis ceases) |

Erythropoietin

Figure 25-10 **Erythrocyte differentiation.** Erythrocyte differentiation from large, nucleated stem cell to small, nonnucleated erythrocyte.

Reticulocytes remain in the marrow approximately 1 day and then are released into the venous sinuses before maturation is complete. Reticulocytes continue to mature in the bloodstream and may travel to the spleen for several days of additional maturation. The normal reticulocyte count is 1% of the total red blood cell count. Approximately 1% of the body's circulating erythrocyte mass normally is generated every 24 hours. Therefore the reticulocyte count is a useful clinical index of erythropoietic activity and indicates whether new red blood cells are being produced. The concept of "erythron" has been used to describe all the tissues that produce erythrocytes and their precursors. Thus included in this term are stem cells, all stages of developing erythrocytes, and mature red blood cells.

One of the most significant advances in the study of hematopoietic growth factors has been the development of erythropoietin for use in individuals with chronic renal failure. In 1986 large amounts of recombinant human erythropoietin (r-HuEPO) became widely available for clinical research. Erythropoietin is administered intravenously or subcutaneously for the treatment of anemia caused by decreased production of erythropoietin. The most significant side effect associated with r-HuEPO is increased blood pressure.[16] Other features that can affect the response to r-HuEPO include blood loss (occult); infection; inflammation; hyperparathyroidism with marrow fibrosis; aluminum toxicity; vitamin B_{12}/folate deficiency; hemolysis; bone marrow disorders; underdialysis; and possibly, angiotensin-converting enzyme inhibitors.[17] An immediate effect of increased endogenous or exogenous erythropoietin is an increase in the blood reticulocyte count.

Hemoglobin Synthesis

Hemoglobin, the oxygen-carrying protein of the erythrocyte, constitutes approximately 90% of the cell's dry weight. The cytoplasm of a single erythrocyte can contain as many as 300 hemoglobin molecules. Hemoglobin enables the blood to transport 100 times more oxygen than could be transported dissolved in plasma alone. Hemoglobin is not one molecule but a family of molecules whose members differ slightly in primary structure. Nonetheless, each member is composed of two pairs of polypeptide chains (the globins) and four colorful complexes of iron plus protoporphyrin (the hemes) (Figure 25-11).

Hemoglobin synthesis is precisely coordinated by mechanisms not completely understood. Three requisites for hemoglobin synthesis are (1) formation of protoporphyrin, (2) availability of iron (heme), and (3) generation of the proteinaceous globin. Several genes dictate the synthesis of globin in maturing human erythroblasts, each gene resulting in the formation of a structurally different polypeptide chain (alpha, beta, gamma, delta, epsilon, or zeta). Each polypeptide chain contains approximately 150 amino acids and is arranged in the knotted-sausage configuration shown in Figure 25-11. The chains assemble to form a tetrahedron containing two pairs of identical chains. Hemoglobin A, the most common type of hemoglobin in adults, is composed of two α-polypeptide and two β-polypeptide chains. Seven different types of hemoglobin have been identified in healthy human blood at all stages, from fetal life to adulthood—testimony to the heterogeneity of the molecule (Table 25-5). The timing of synthesis and the relative amount of each type of hemoglobin are determined by complex developmental processes.

Heme is a large, flat, iron-protoporphyrin disk that is capable of carrying one molecule of oxygen (O_2). Recall that hemoglobin contains four heme groups; thus it is capable of

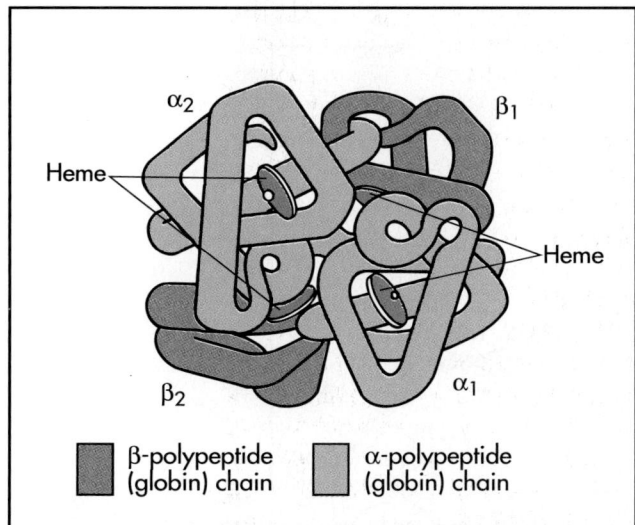

Figure 25-11 **Molecular structure of hemoglobin.** Molecule is a spherical tetramer weighing approximately 64,500 daltons. It contains a pair of α-polypeptide and a pair of β-polypeptide chains and several heme groups.

Table 25-5	Structure of Normal Hemoglobin Molecules	
Type of Hemoglobin (Hb)	**Identity of Polypeptide Chain**	**Significance**
Hb A	$\alpha_2\beta_2$	92% of adult Hb
Hb A_{1c}	$\alpha_2(\beta\text{-NH-glucose})$	5% of adult Hb; increased in diabetes (see Chapter 21)
Hb A_2	$\alpha_2\delta_2$	2% of adult Hb; increased in β-thalassemia (see Chapter 26)
Hb F	$\alpha_2\gamma_2$	Major fetal Hb from the third through ninth month of gestation; promotes oxygen transfer across platelets; increase in β-thalassemia
Hb Gower I	ϵ_4 or $\zeta_2\epsilon_2$	Present in early embryo; function unknown
Hb Gower II	$\alpha_2\epsilon_2$	Present in early embryo; function unknown
Hb Portland	$\zeta_2\gamma_2$	Present in early embryo; function unknown

Recent data indicate that nitrite (NO_2) reacts with deoxyhemoglobin to form nitric oxide (NO) and methemoglobin (met-Hb) and other NO compounds. NO can then either diffuse out of the erythrocyte directly or via an intermediate NO metabolite.[37] Nitric oxide was identified as a mediator of vascular tone in 1987. NO produced by endothelial cells promotes vasodilation and inhibits platelet aggregation and leukocyte adhesion. Thus it executes multiple functions that maintain vascular homeostasis (see Figure 25-12).

carrying four oxygen molecules. Through a series of complex biochemical reactions, protoporphyrin, a complex four-ringed molecule, is produced and abounds with ferrous iron. The biochemical reactions of heme synthesis include condensation, oxidation, and reduction, all of which are powered by catalytic enzymes. It is crucial that the iron be correctly charged. Presence of the reduced ferrous iron (Fe^{II}) allows the formation of normal hemoglobin, which is capable of binding oxygen where it is plentiful (in the lungs) and releasing it where it is less plentiful (in the tissues).

Oxidized ferric iron (Fe^{III}) carries an extra positive charge and results in the formation of methemoglobin, an unstable

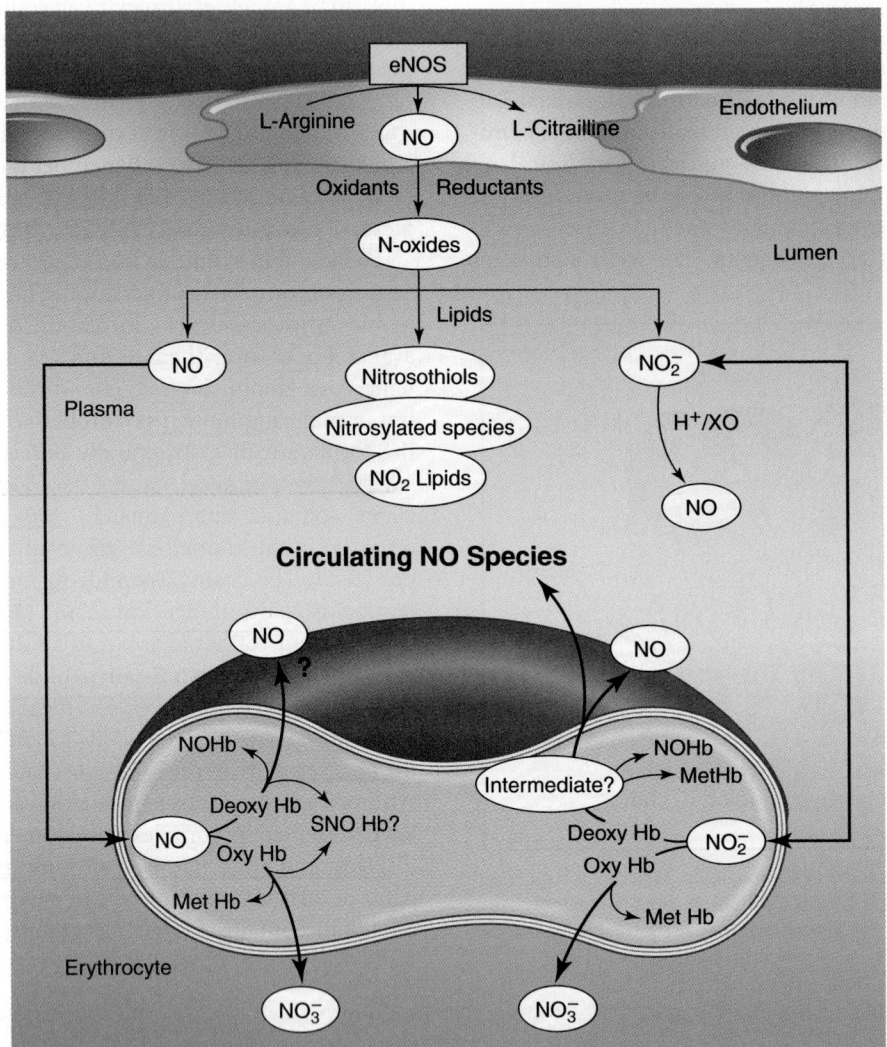

Figure 25-12 Erythrocytes and nitric oxide: a recent model. Nitric oxide (NO) produced by endothelial NO-synthase (eNOS) may diffuse into the vascular lumen as well as the underlying smooth muscle where it promotes vasodilation. Most of this NO enters the erythrocyte and reacts with oxyhemoglobin (oxy Hb) to form nitrate (NO_3^-); a small amount may escape the hemoglobin and react with plasma constituents to form nitros(yl)ated species (RXNO, nitrosothiols: RSNO) nitrated lipids (NO_2 lipids), and nitrate (NO_2). Each of these species is capable of promoting NO bioactivity far from its location of formation. Nitrate *may* diffuse into the erythrocytes where it appears in a higher concentration than in plasma. In the erythrocyte nitrite reacts with deoxyhemoglobin (deoxy Hb) to form nitric oxide and methemoglobin (met-Hb) and other NO compounds. NO can then either diffuse out of the erythrocyte directly or via an intermediate NO metabolite. The question mark after "Intermediate" in the oval refers to the possibility of an intermediate during nitrite bioactivation. *H+/XO,* hypoxanthine/xanthine oxidase; *NOHb,* iron nitrosylhemoglobin; *SNO Hb,* nitrosohemoglobin. (Modified from Dejam A et al: Erythrocytes are the major intravascular storage sites of nitrite in human blood, *Blood (First Edition Paper),* March 17, 2005 [E-pub ahead of print].)

type of hemoglobin that is not capable of binding oxygen. An excess of ferric iron occurs in the presence of certain drugs and chemicals, such as nitrates and sulfonamides.

Hemoglobin that is carrying oxygen is called **oxyhemoglobin.** If all four oxygen-binding sites on the oxyhemoglobin's hemes are occupied by oxygen, the molecule is said to be saturated. Oxyhemoglobin that has released its oxygen or is not bound to oxygen for some other reason is called reduced hemoglobin, or **deoxyhemoglobin.**

Nutritional Requirements for Erythropoiesis

Normal development of erythrocytes and synthesis of hemoglobin depend on an optimal biochemical milieu and adequate supplies of the necessary building blocks, including protein, vitamins, and minerals (Table 25-6). If these components are lacking, it is usually the result of a nutritional deficiency or a metabolic imbalance in which other organs or tissues use up a disproportionate share of these nutrients or are unable to absorb the needed nutrients. If abnormal distribution of nutrients is prolonged, erythrocyte production slows and anemia (insufficient numbers of functional erythrocytes) may result (see Chapter 26).

Protein is an important structural component of the erythrocyte's plasma membrane, contributing to its strength, flexibility, and elasticity. Amino acid chains form hemoglobin. Without proteins and amino acids, erythrocyte production decreases and the life span of cells that are produced may be shortened because of structural defects. One of the most important proteins is intrinsic factor (IF), a glycoprotein nec-

essary for gastrointestinal absorption of vitamin B_{12}. Lack of vitamin B_{12} causes pernicious anemia. IF is secreted by the parietal cells in the gastric mucosa and facilitates vitamin B_{12} uptake at its absorptive site, the ileum.

Erythropoiesis cannot proceed in the absence of vitamins, especially B_{12}, folate (folic acid), B_6, riboflavin, pantothenic acid, niacin, ascorbic acid, and vitamin E. Vitamin B_{12} is a large molecule; therefore it requires assistance from IF to penetrate the gastrointestinal mucosa. Once absorbed, vitamin B_{12} is stored in the liver and used as needed in erythropoiesis.

Folate is the second most important vitamin for erythrocyte production and maturation. Folate is necessary for DNA synthesis, being a component of three of the four DNA bases (thymine, adenine, and guanine). Folate also is needed for ribonucleic acid (RNA) synthesis. IF is not required for folate absorption, which occurs principally in the upper small intestine. Folate is stored in and circulates through the liver. Folate deficiency is more common than vitamin B_{12} deficiency and occurs more rapidly. Folate stores can be depleted within a few months, whereas vitamin B_{12} depletion can take years. Folate supplements are prescribed for pregnant women because pregnancy increases the demand for folate and deficiency can cause anemia.

Iron Cycle

Approximately 67% of total body iron is bound to heme in erythrocytes and muscle cells, and approximately 30% is stored bound to ferritin or hemosiderin mononuclear phagocytes (i.e., macrophages) and hepatic parenchymal cells. The

Table 25-6	Nutritional Requirements for Erythropoiesis	
Nutrient	**Role in Erythropoiesis**	**Consequence of Deficiency**
Protein (amino acids)	Structural component of plasma membrane	Decreased strength, elasticity, and flexibility of membrane; hemolytic anemia
	Synthesis of hemoglobin	Decreased erythropoiesis and life span of erythrocytes
Cobalamin (vitamin B_{12})	Synthesis of DNA, maturation of erythrocytes, facilitator of folate metabolism	Macrocytic (megaloblastic) anemia
Folate (folic acid)	Synthesis of DNA and RNA, maturation of erythrocytes	Macrocytic (megaloblastic) anemia
Vitamin B_6 (pyridoxine)	Heme synthesis	Hypochromic-microcytic anemia
Vitamin B_2 (riboflavin)	Oxidative reactions	Normochromic-normocytic anemia
Vitamin C (ascorbic acid)	Iron metabolism, acts as a reducing agent to maintain iron in its ferrous (Fe^{++}) form	Normochromic-normocytic anemia
Pantothenic acid	Heme synthesis	Unknown in humans*
Niacin	None, but needed for respiration in mature erythrocytes	Unknown in humans
Vitamin E	Heme synthesis (?); protection against oxidative damage in mature erythrocytes	Hemolytic anemia with increased cell membrane fragility; shortens life span of erythrocytes in individuals with cystic fibrosis
Iron	Hemoglobin synthesis	Iron deficiency anemia
Copper	Required for optimal mobilization of iron from tissues to plasma	Hypochromic-microcytic anemia

Data from Strine-Martin EA, Lotspeich-Steininger CA, Koepke JA: *Clinical hematology: principles, procedures, correlations,* ed 2, Philadelphia, 1998, Lippincott.
DNA, Deoxyribonucleic acid; *RNA,* ribonucleic acid.
*Although pantothenic acid is important for optimal synthesis of heme, experimentally induced deficiency *failed* to produce anemia or other hematopoietic disturbances.

remaining 3% (less than 1 mg) is lost daily in urine, sweat, bile, and epithelial cells shed from the gut. Iron not lost is continuously recycled (Figure 25-13). Recycling is made possible by **transferrin,** a glycoprotein synthesized primarily by the liver but also by tissue macrophages, submaxillary and mammary glands, and ovaries or testes. **Apotransferrin** is transferrin without attached iron. Apotransferrin from the hepatocyte is the source of almost all the circulating apotransferrin. Transferrin receptors are on the plasma membrane of all nucleated cells and thought to be the only route of cellular entry for transferrin-attached iron.

Dietary iron is absorbed primarily in the duodenum and proximal jejunum. Some of it passes into the bloodstream, and the rest is sequestered in intestinal epithelial cells as ferritin. This iron is lost when epithelial cells are sloughed off in the intestinal lumen. Iron that is released to the bloodstream is picked up by transferrin, which is the body's major iron-transport molecule. Iron for hemoglobin production is delivered to erythroblasts in erythropoietic bone marrow. Under normal conditions, only one third of the iron-binding sites on transferrin molecules are occupied. It is postulated that iron is transferred from transferrin to erythroblasts in the marrow as follows:

1. The transferrin-iron complex binds to a transferrin receptor on the erythroblast's plasma membrane.
2. The complex moves into the cell, possibly by active transport.

3. Iron is released (dissociated) from transferrin.
4. The dissociated transferrin is returned to the bloodstream (see Figure 25-13).

Another source of iron for erythropoiesis is the iron stored by the protein **ferritin** and possibly hemosiderin in the cytoplasm of mononuclear phagocytes (macrophages) resident in the marrow.

Apoferritin, which is ferritin without attached iron, can store thousands of atoms of iron. Several (24) apoferritin complexes combine to form the micelle ferritin. Large aggregates of micelles (if a large amount of iron is present) produce numerous ferritin micelles, which are known as **hemosiderin.** Hemosiderin is visible as an iron-based pigment under a light microscope as cell inclusions. The iron within deposits of hemosiderin is poorly available to supply iron when needed. Conditions leading to large amounts of iron include hemolysis, severe congestion, unusual increases in dietary iron consumption, increased absorption, or decreased loss. The most common cause of hemosiderin deposition is simple bruising (see Figure 2-15). Hemosiderin in small amounts within iron-rich tissues (i.e., spleen, liver, bone marrow) is considered normal. Large aggregates or its presence in tissue such as the lungs or subcutaneous tissue suggest a pathologic condition. Once the iron is released into the marrow and incorporated into the erythroblast's mitochondria, the enzyme heme synthetase inserts ferrous iron into protoporphyrin to form heme. Heme then is bound to globin to form hemoglobin.

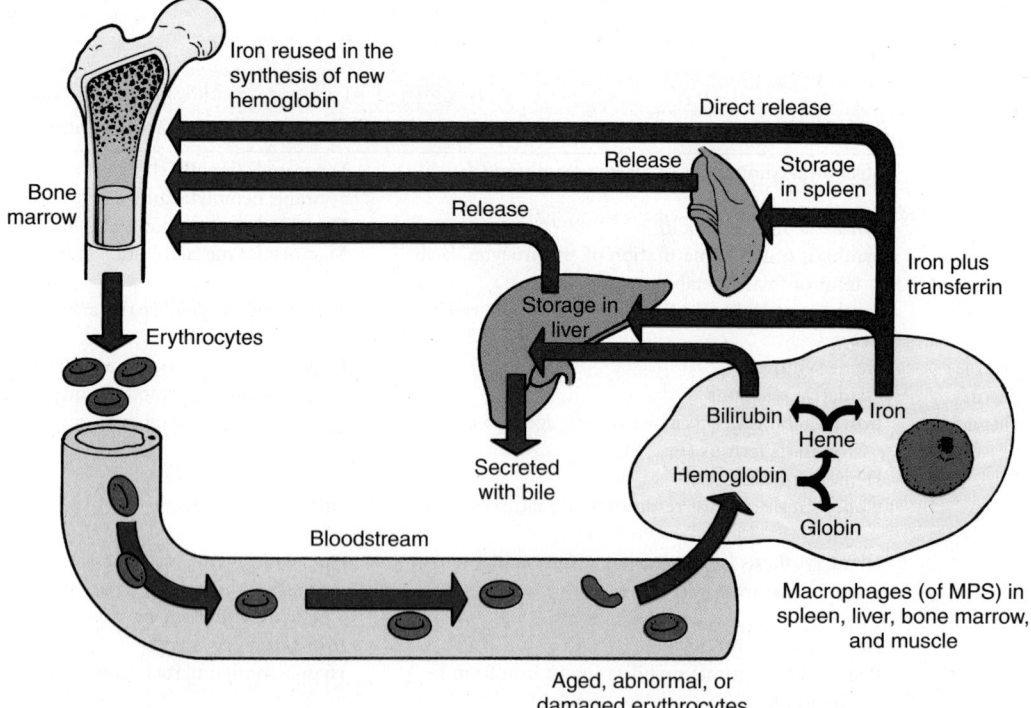

Figure 25-13 Iron cycle. Iron (Fe) released from gastrointestinal epithelial cells circulates in bloodstream associated with its plasma carrier, transferring. It is delivered to erythroblasts in bone marrow, where most of it is incorporated into hemoglobin. Mature erythrocytes circulate for approximately 100-120 days, after which they become senescent and are removed by the mononuclear phagocyte system (MPS). Macrophages of MPS (mostly in spleen) break down ingested erythrocytes and return iron to bloodstream directly or after storing it as a ferritin or hemosiderin.

Iron not used in erythropoiesis is stored temporarily as ferritin or hemosiderin and later excreted.

After mature erythrocytes have circulated for 100 to 120 days, they are removed from the bloodstream by macrophages of the MPS—chiefly in the spleen. Within the phagolysosomes (digestive vacuole) of the macrophage, the erythrocyte is catabolized and the iron in hemoglobin is oxidized, forming Fe^{111} (methemoglobin). The heme and globin of methemoglobin dissociate easily, and globin may be reduced to its component amino acids. The iron released by methemoglobin dissociation is stored in the macrophage's cytoplasm as ferritin or hemosiderin or released into the bloodstream, where it is free to bind again to transferrin (see Figure 25-13). A minute amount of iron is stored in muscle cells by the heme-containing protein myoglobin. Unavailable stores of iron are present in cytochromes, catalases, and peroxidase enzymes.

Iron balance is achieved through mechanisms controlling its absorption rather than its excretion. Regulation of iron transport across the plasma membrane of gastrointestinal epithelial cells is related to the cell's iron content and the overall rate of erythropoiesis. If the body's iron stores are low or the demand for erythropoiesis is increased, iron passes rapidly through the epithelial cell and into the plasma, probably by mechanisms of active transport. (Transport mechanisms are described in Chapter 1.) If the body stores are high and erythropoiesis is not increased, iron crosses the epithelial cell's plasma membrane passively and is stored there bound to ferritin. Excretion of iron occurs when the epithelial cells of the intestinal mucosa slough off.

Regulation of Erythropoiesis

In healthy humans the total volume of circulating erythrocytes remains surprisingly constant. The feedback mechanism that maintains an optimal population of erythrocytes is mediated by erythropoietin. The peritubular cells of the kidney are the primary site for erythropoietin production. In response to hypoxia, transcription of the erythropoietin gene in these cells results in increased secretion of erythropoietin (Figure 25-14). After transportation through the blood to the marrow, erythropoietin induces the selective proliferation and differentiation of proerythroblasts (see Figure 25-10). Its earliest effects are to stimulate RNA synthesis, after either binding to receptors on the erythroblast's plasma membrane or entrance into the cell. Hemoglobin synthesis begins hours after initial stimulation by erythropoietin.

Erythropoietin causes a compensatory increase in erythrocyte production if the oxygen content of blood decreases because of anemia, high altitude, or pulmonary disease. The normal steady-state rate of production of approximately 2.5 million erythrocytes per second in humans can increase up to about 17 million per second under anemic or low-oxygen states.[18] Unlike the peripheral chemoreceptors of the carotid body and aortic arch that send messengers to the brain to increase respiration in individuals with hypoxia, receptors in the kidney are on cells that synthesize and secrete erythropoi-

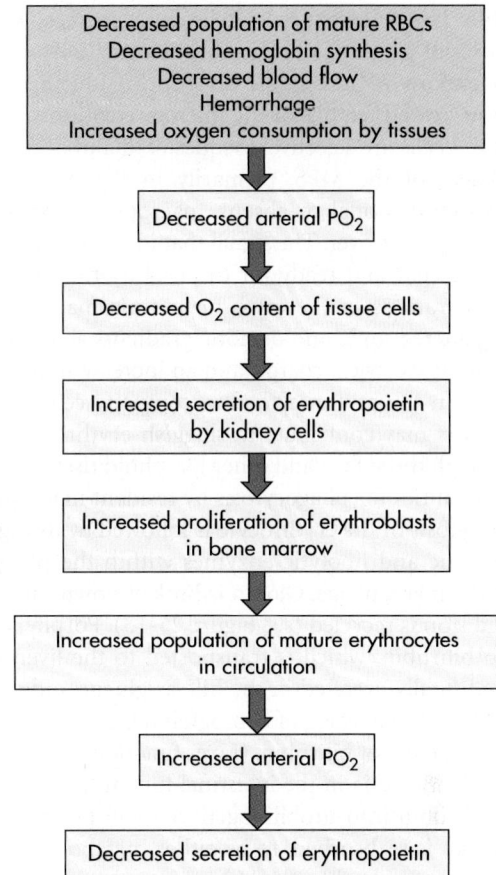

Figure 25-14 Role of erythropoietin in regulation of erythropoiesis. Decreased arterial oxygen levels stimulate production of erythropoietin, which in turn stimulates red cell production and expansion of the erythron. The increase in red cells frequently corrects the problem of low oxygen levels (hypoxia). This restoration to normal oxygen levels alerts the kidney to stop producing erythropoietin (negative feedback). Further erythrocyte production is not needed. *RBCs*, Red blood cells; *PO₂*, partial pressure of oxygen in the blood (see Chapter 32).

etin. Thus the body responds to reduced oxygenation of blood in two ways: by increasing intake of oxygen through increased respiration and by increasing the oxygen-carrying capacity of the blood through increased erythropoiesis. Erythropoietin not only stimulates proliferation of committed stem cells in the marrow but also accelerates maturation of existing erythroblasts. (Erythropoiesis also is discussed in the hematopoiesis section.)

Normal Destruction of Senescent Erythrocytes

Although mature erythrocytes lack nuclei, mitochondria, and endoplasmic reticulum, they do have cytoplasmic enzymes capable of glycolysis (anaerobic glucose metabolism) and production of small quantities of adenosine triphosphate (ATP). The ATP provides the energy necessary to keep the cell alive and its plasma membrane pliable (see Figure 25-1). Metabolic processes diminish as the erythrocyte ages. Consequently, less ATP is available to maintain the functions essential for life. The senescent red cell becomes increasingly fragile and loses its property of reversible deformability. Its membrane therefore is susceptible to rupture during passage through narrowed regions of the microcirculation.

Aged red cells are selectively sequestered and destroyed by macrophages of the MPS, primarily in the spleen. If the spleen is dysfunctional or absent, macrophages in the liver (Kupffer cells) take over. The signal that identifies an erythrocyte as senescent and ready for disposal by the MPS is not known. Alterations in the erythrocyte's plasma membrane, including altered ionic and osmotic gradients across it and a decrease in its electrical charge, and an increase in methemoglobin within the erythrocyte all accompany cellular aging. These factors may contribute to sluggish erythrocyte movement through the spleen and other lymphoid tissues, increasing opportunities for phagocytosis by resident macrophages.

Phagocytosis of the erythrocyte is followed by its digestion by proteolytic and lipolytic enzymes within the phagolysosome of the macrophage. Globin is broken down into amino acids, and iron is recycled (see Figure 25-13). Porphyrin is reduced to bilirubin, which is transported to the liver, conjugated, and finally excreted in the bile as glucuronide (Figure 25-15). Approximately 6 g of hemoglobin is catabolized daily, producing 200 mg of bilirubin. (Liver function is described in Chapter 38.) Bacteria in the intestinal lumen transform conjugated bilirubin into urobilinogen. A small portion of this urobilinogen is reabsorbed, to be either metabolized further by the liver or excreted by the kidney into the urine. Most of the urobilinogen is excreted in feces.

Conditions causing accelerated erythrocyte destruction increase the load of bilirubin for hepatic clearance, leading to increased serum levels of unconjugated bilirubin and increased urinary excretion of urobilinogen. Gallstones (cholelithiasis) can result from a chronically elevated rate of bilirubin excretion.

Development of Leukocytes

All of the leukocytes arise from stem cells in the bone marrow (their pathways of differentiation are shown in Figure 25-7). The granulocytes (neutrophils, eosinophils, and basophils/mast cells) normally mature fully in the marrow and then are released into the bloodstream. The agranulocytes (monocytes and lymphocytes), however, are released into the bloodstream before they undergo their final phase of maturation. The monocytes mature into macrophages within 1 or 2 days of release, and the lymphocytes travel to lymphoid tissues, where they are stimulated to differentiate into T cells or B cells (see Chapter 7).

The bone marrow exhibits selective retention of immature granulocytes. Hematopoietic growth factors, granulocyte-macrophage colony-stimulating factor (GM-CSF), and granulocyte colony-stimulating factor (G-CSF) are required for granulocyte growth and differentiation. G-CSF increases neutrophil production (see Figure 25-7). (Recall that neutrophils are always increased with infection.)

Maintenance of optimal levels of granulocytes and monocytes in the blood depends on the availability of pluripotential stem cells in the marrow, induction of these into commit-

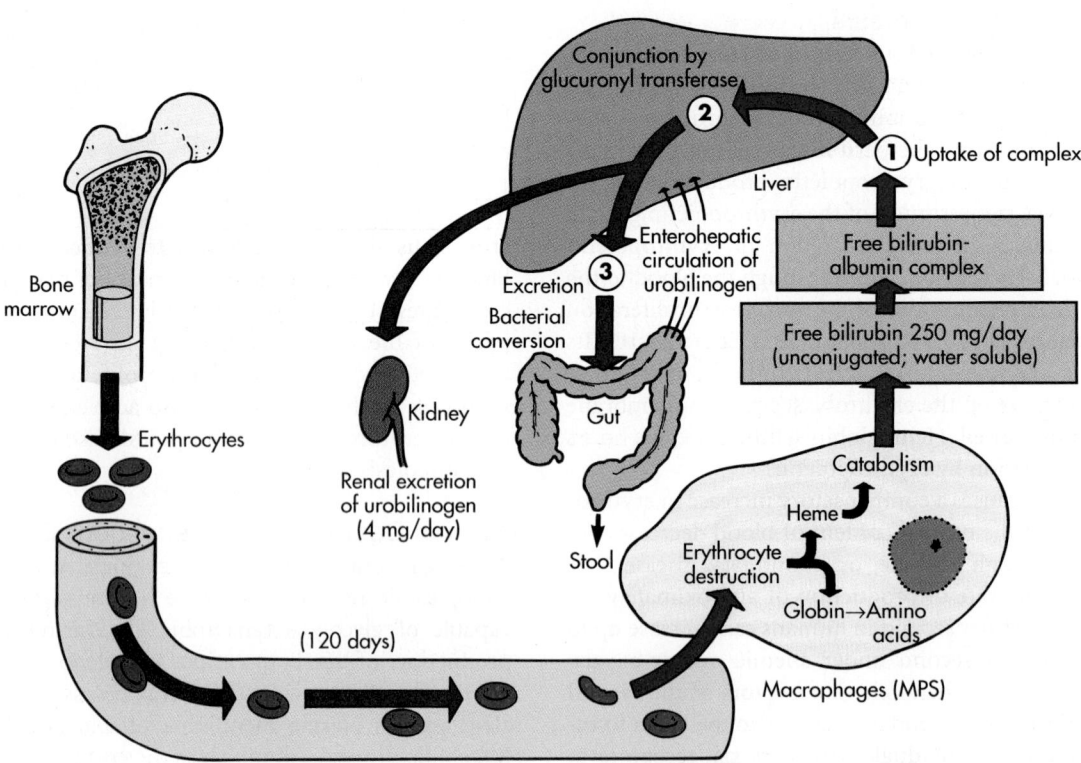

Figure 25-15 Metabolism of bilirubin released by heme breakdown.

ted stem cells, and timely release of new cells from the marrow. The marrow contains a reserve pool that can be rapidly mobilized in response to the body's needs. Once cells are released from the marrow, they join the marginating pool or the circulating pool. The cells in the marginating pool lie along the capillary walls and can move into tissues and mucous membranes. Cells from the circulating pool join the marginating pool to replace the cells that have migrated out of the capillaries. Leukocyte production increases in response to infection, to the presence of steroids, and to reduction or depletion of reserves in the marrow. It is also associated with strenuous exercise, convulsive seizures, heat, intense radiation, paroxysmal tachycardias, pain, nausea and vomiting, and anxiety.

Normally, some leukocytes are lost in saliva, urine, lungs, liver, spleen, and gastrointestinal tract. Most exist in the body from days to years, depending on type (see Table 25-2).

Development of Platelets

Platelets (thrombocytes) develop from megakaryocytes by a unique process of proliferation termed **endomitosis.** In endomitosis the megakaryocyte undergoes the nuclear phase of cellular division (mitosis) but fails to undergo the cytoplasmic phase (cytokinesis) (see Chapter 1). Without cytokinesis the cell does not divide into two daughter cells. Rather, the megakaryocyte expands to accommodate the doubling of its DNA (nuclear) content and breaks up into fragments known as platelets.

An optimal number of platelets and committed platelet precursors (megakaryoblasts) in the bone marrow is maintained in part by the actions of thrombopoietin and IL-II (see Figure 25-7). Thrombopoietin stimulates committed cells at further stages of differentiation to differentiate faster. Rates of the processes of megakaryocyte development, endomitosis, and platelet release are increased.

Platelets, once released, circulate for 10 days before they begin to lose their capacity to carry out biochemical reactions. The initial alteration of function is possibly attributable to proteolytic enzymes present at sites of chronic vascular inflammation. The inflammatory mediator, IL-6 increases platelet production and newly formed platelets are more thrombogenic.[19] Platelet activation increases the inflammatory response by releasing CD 40 ligand, which increases inflammatory cytokines.[19] Senescent platelets are phagocytosed by neutrophils and monocytes if they are circulating freely or by neutrophils and macrophages if they are part of a clot, or thrombus. Senescent platelets may be removed also by tissue macrophages of the MPS in the liver or spleen.

MECHANISMS OF HEMOSTASIS

Hemostasis means arrest of bleeding. Mechanisms of hemostasis maintain a relatively steady state of blood volume, pressure, and flow through injured blood vessels after vascular damage and bleeding. Hemostasis requires platelets, the clotting cascade, blood flow and shear forces, endothelial cells, and

fibrinolysis. After vascular damage and bleeding, hemostasis involves a complex sequence of events: (1) vasoconstriction (vasospasm); (2) formation of a platelet plug; (3) activation of the coagulation (or clotting) cascade; (4) formation of a blood clot; and (5) clot retraction and clot dissolution (fibrinolysis). All of these events involve platelets, clotting, and the blood vessels (vasculature). Platelets must be adequate in number and function to stop bleeding. The normal platelet count ranges from 140,000 to 340,000/mm³ depending on the laboratory.

At the site of vascular injury platelets are activated and form a plug (**platelet plug**) to arrest bleeding. This step occurs temporally with the activation of the coagulation system (thrombin activation), which occurs in response to the rupture of endothelium and exposure of blood to the extravascular tissue.[20] Platelet stimuli include adenosine diphosphate (ADP), epinephrine, thrombin, and collagen. Thrombin and

---

NUTRITION & DISEASE

Chocolate, Red Wine, Platelet, and Antioxidant Functions

An increasing number of foods have been reported to have platelet-inhibitory actions including flavanol-rich foods like cocoa and chocolate. Flavonoids are polyphenolic compounds—water soluble plant pigments—found in fruits, vegetables, and certain beverages (tea, coffee, beer, wine, and fruit drinks) with diverse beneficial biochemical and antioxidant effects. Antioxidant effects depend on their molecular structure. Recent studies showed flavanol-rich cocoa *inhibited* several measures of platelet activity—epinephrine- and ADP-induced glycoprotein (GP) IIb/IIIa and P-selection expression, platelet micro-particle formation, and epinephrine-collagen– and ADP-collagen–induced primary hemostasis.[38,39] Although less dramatic than low dose (81 mg) aspirin, the epinephrine-induced inhibitory effects on GPIIb/IIIa and primary hemostasis were similar. Flavonoids found in chocolate include the flavanols which include epicatechin and catechin. Not all chocolate is created equal. Dark chocolate contains much more cocoa than does light chocolate. A recent study at the University of California at San Francisco is the largest clinical trial to date to show improvement in blood vessel function from rich dark chocolate.[40] Dark chocolate intake was associated with increased epicatechin levels. Additional cardio-protective effects may include antioxidant properties and activation of nitric oxide (NO).[40] Flavanols are one subclass of polyphenols and include many major groups.

Low to moderate consumption of red wine reportedly has a greater benefit than other alcoholic beverages on cardioprotective mechanisms.[41] Decreases in mortality from alcohol have been attributed (by epidemiologic and metaanalytic studies) to change in lipid profiles, decreased coagulation, increased fibrinolysis, inhibition of platelets, increased NO, and antioxidant properties. Emerging are the effects of the polyphenol resveratol (3,5,4-trihydroxy-*trans*-stilbene) known to be abundant in red wine. Investigators documented that the polyphenolic antioxidants, resveratrol and proanthocyanidins, provide cardioprotection by their function in vivo as antioxidants.[42] Secondarily to antioxidant properties are decreases in platelet aggregation, vasodilation, changes in prostacyclin thromboxane ratios, and increased fibrinolytic effects.[42,43]

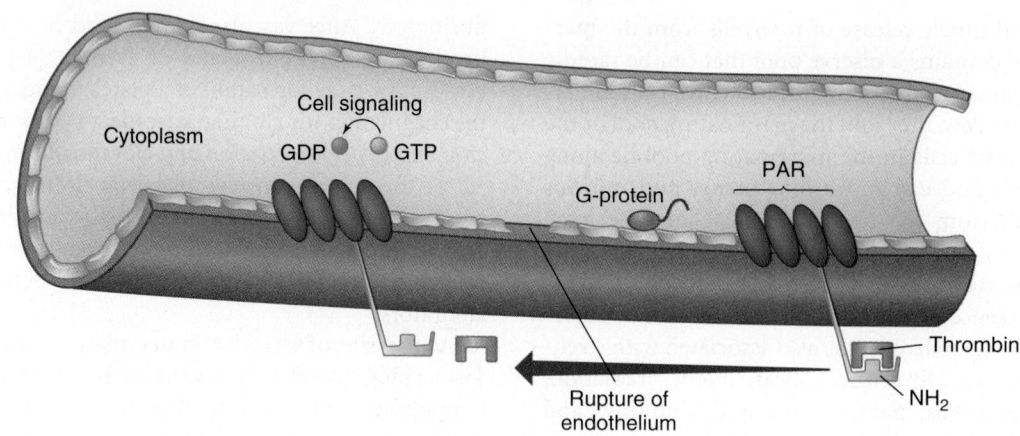

Figure 25-16 **Thrombin activation.** Thrombin activation is mediated by G-protein, which is coupled to protease-activated receptor (PAR). Thrombin cleaves the NH$_2$-end region of the PAR, which uncovers a new NH$_2$ end. The new NH$_2$ end then serves as an attached ligand and binds intracellularly to the PAR initiating transmembrane signaling. Thrombin activation occurs in response to the rupture of endothelium and exposure of blood to the extravascular tissue.

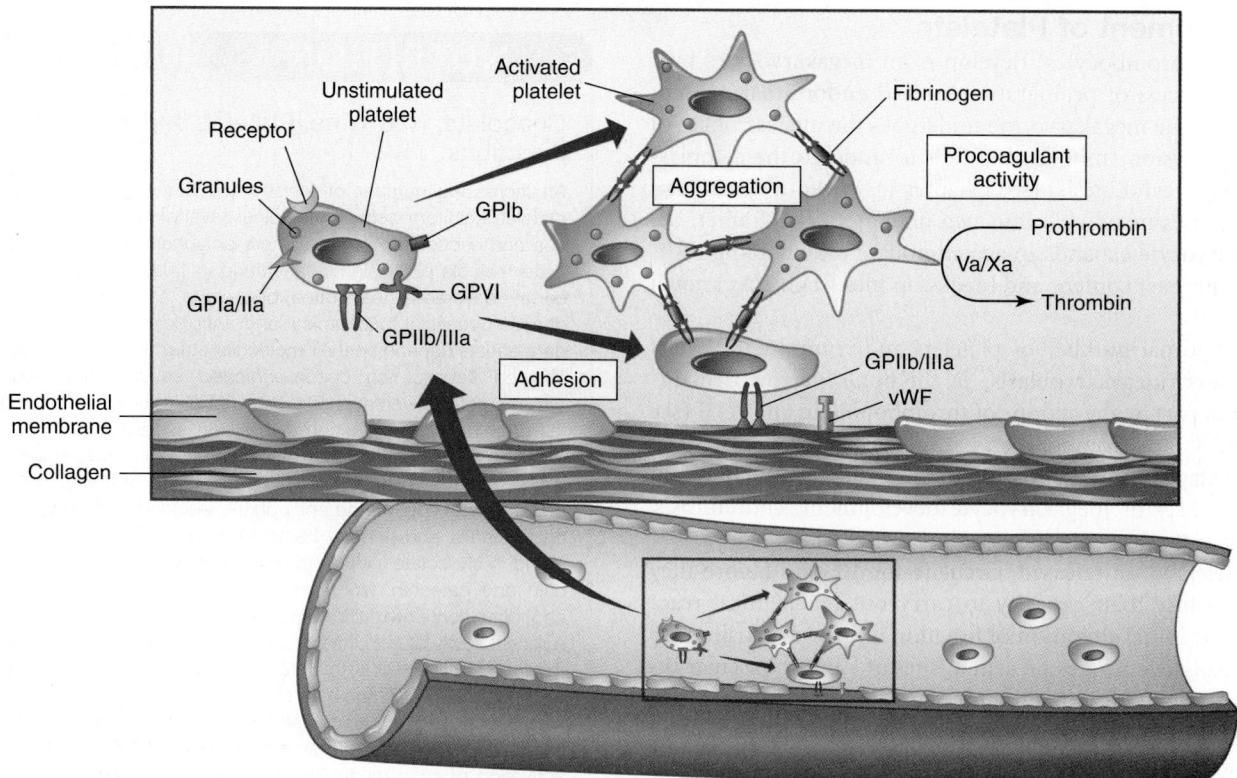

Figure 25-17 Platelet activation. *vWF,* von Willebrand factor; *ADP,* adenosine diphosphate; *PDGF,* platelet-derived growth factor; *GP,* glycoproteins; *GPIb,* GPIb-IX-V complex.

collagen are particularly strong stimuli. Thrombin activation is mediated by G-protein–coupled protease-activated receptors (PAR). Thrombin cleaves the external domain, the NH$_2$-terminal domain of PAR, thereby initiating transmembranous signaling[21] (Figure 25-16). Also important are receptors for ADP, epinephrine, and collagen.

If blood vessel injury is minor, hemostasis is achieved temporarily by the platelet plug, which usually forms within 3 to 5 minutes of injury. Platelet plugs seal the many minute ruptures that occur daily in the microcirculation, particularly in capillaries. With too few platelets small hemorrhagic areas

called *purpuras* develop under the skin and throughout tissue (see Chapter 27).

Platelet activation involves four separate processes: (1) *adhesion* (attachment of platelets on subendothelial matrix); (2) *aggregation* (complexing [cohesion] of platelets; (3) *secretion* (release of granule proteins from platelet); and (4) *procoagulant activity* (promotion of thrombin generation) (Figures 25-17 and 25-18).

Platelet adhesion is mostly mediated by the binding of platelet surface receptor glycoprotein GPIb-IX-V complex to **von Willebrand factor (vWF),** an adhesion protein in the

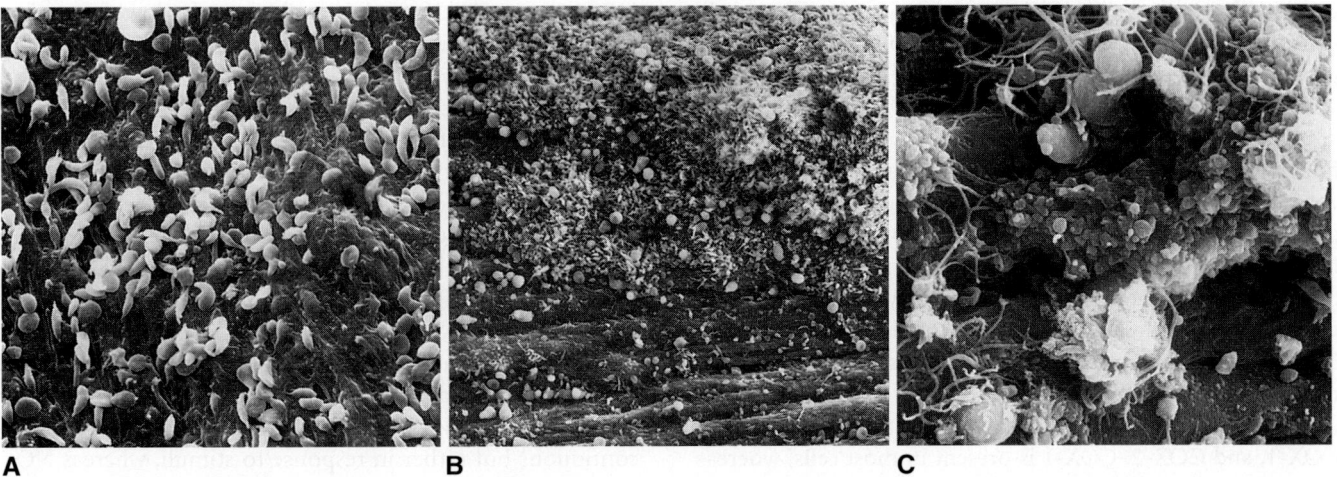

Figure 25-18 Platelet degranulation. **A,** After simple endothelial denudation, platelets adhere to the subendothelium in a monolayer fashion. **B,** Platelet-fibrin thrombus formation. **C,** Higher magnification of the thrombus shows a mixture of red cells and platelets incorporated into the fibrin meshwork. (From Damjanov I, Linder J, editors: *Anderson's pathology*, ed 10, St. Louis, 1996, Mosby.)

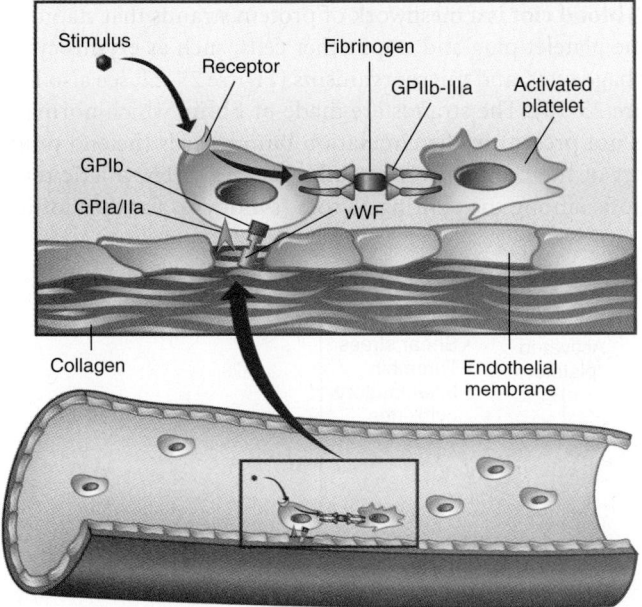

Figure 25-19 Fibrinogen and GPIIb-IIIa. Binding of fibrinogen to the platelet fibrinogen receptor (the GPIIb-IIIa complex) facilitates platelet aggregation. After platelet stimulation, GPIIb-IIIa becomes a high-affinity fibrinogen receptor. The intracellular portion of the activated GPIIb-IIa complex can mediate platelet spreading and clot retraction. *vWF,* von Willebrand factor.

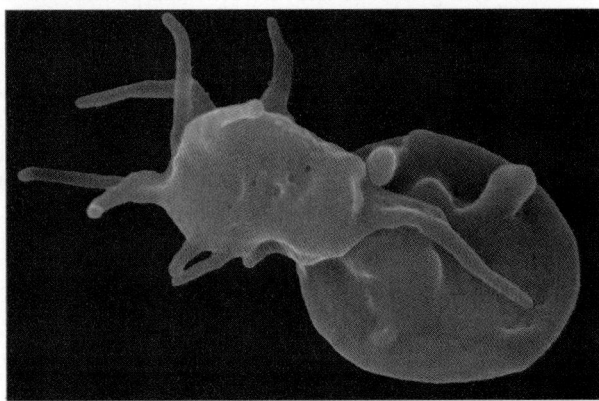

Figure 25-20 Micrograph of an active and moderately active platelet. (Copyright Dennis Kunkel Microscopy, Inc.)

subendothelial matrix (Figure 25-19). Deficiency of the proteins (GPIb-IX-V complex, vWF) leads to congenital bleeding disorders, Bernard-Soulier disease and von Willebrand disease, respectively.[21] Platelet adhesion is also facilitated by binding of platelet collagen receptor GPVI to collagen in the matrix.[22]

Platelet aggregation involves binding of fibrinogen to the platelet fibrinogen receptor **GPIIb-IIIa complex** (also called αIIbβ) a member of the integrin receptor family. GPIIb-IIIa complex is the most abundant receptor on the platelet surface

and it does *not* bind fibrinogen on nonstimulated platelets.[21] Fibrinogen bridges the activated platelets (see Figure 25-19). GPIIb-IIIa complex binding to the platelet cytoskeleton mediates the dynamic changes in shape from smooth to spiny spheres that develop protrusions (pseudopods) exposing receptors on their surface that mediate clot retraction (Figure 25-20). The GPIIb-IIIa–fibrinogen pathway is the final common pathway for platelet aggregation, so blockage by antiplatelet drugs is an important therapeutic strategy.

Secretion involves platelet granule release (also called *platelet-release reaction*) of ADP and serotonin, which recruits and stimulates more platelets, adhesive proteins that stabilize platelet aggregates, factor V (from clotting cascade) and growth factors (i.e., platelet-derived growth factor [PDGF]) which stimulate smooth muscle cells and promote tissue repair. ADP promotes the adherence and subsequent degranulation of nearby platelets by causing their plasma membranes to become ruffly and sticky (see Figure 25-20). The newly activated platelets cause a platelet plug to seal the injured endothelium. If the effects of ADP were not counteracted and laminar flow were not sufficient, platelet aggregation could continue indefinitely. This is determined by two antagonistic prostaglandin derivatives, **thromboxane (TXA₂)** in platelets and **prostacyclin I₂ (PGI₂)**, produced by endothelial cells. TXA₂, a potent stimulator of platelet aggregation increases fibrinogen receptors on platelet membranes and causes vasoconstriction and promotes the degranulation of other platelets, which then release more ADP. PGI₂ inhibits the effects of TXA₂ by promoting vasodilation and inhibiting platelet degranulation. PGI₂ activates adenylate cyclase, which increases intracellular adenylate monophosphate (cAMP). PDGF may increase atherogenesis and reocclusion after coronary angioplasty.[21]

Cyclooxygenase is an enzyme that exists in two isoforms, COX-1, and COX-2. COX-1 is present in most cells, whereas COX-2 is normally absent from cells but is rapidly induced in response to inflammatory stimuli in endothelial cells and monocytes.

Procoagulation involves the extremely close interaction between the clotting cascade and the activated platelet surface. Specifically it involves the assembly of the enzyme complexes of the clotting cascade on the platelet surface (see p. 916).

Aspirin decreases platelet aggregation by inhibiting COX-1 in platelets, preventing arachidonic acid from reaching the COX-1's binding and catalytic sites. Prevention of the binding results in reduced prostaglandin synthesis, especially TXA₂, for the life span of the platelet (8 to 10 days). Because COX-1

inhibition in platelets is *irreversible,* regular low doses of aspirin lead to more than 95% inhibition of TXA₂ generation after several day's dosing.[23] After a single dose of aspirin, platelet COX-1 activity recovers minimally (10% per day), similarly with platelet turnover (i.e., platelets are without a nucleus and cannot resynthesize COX-1).[24] Other additional mechanisms are proposed for some of aspirin's effects in cardiovascular disease, including decreased platelet aggregation by neutrophils, other unknown effects on the endothelium, and antioxidant effects.[12-14]

Nitric oxide (NO) is formed from L-arginine in endothelial cells. NO, via cGMP, causes vasodilation and inhibits platelet adhesion and aggregation (Figure 25-21). Synergism between PGI₂ and NO is significant. PGI₂ production is not continuous but rather in response to stimuli, whereas NO is released continually to regulate vascular tone. NO has other biologic functions including cell signaling, free radical production, and possibly others.

Function of Clotting Factors

A **blood clot** is a meshwork of protein strands that stabilizes the platelet plug and traps other cells, such as erythrocytes, phagocytes, and microorganisms (Figure 25-22; see also Figure 25-18). The strands are made of fibrin, which normally is not present in the circulation but rather is the end product of the **coagulation cascade,** a series of enzymatic reactions among the clotting factors (synonyms for the clotting

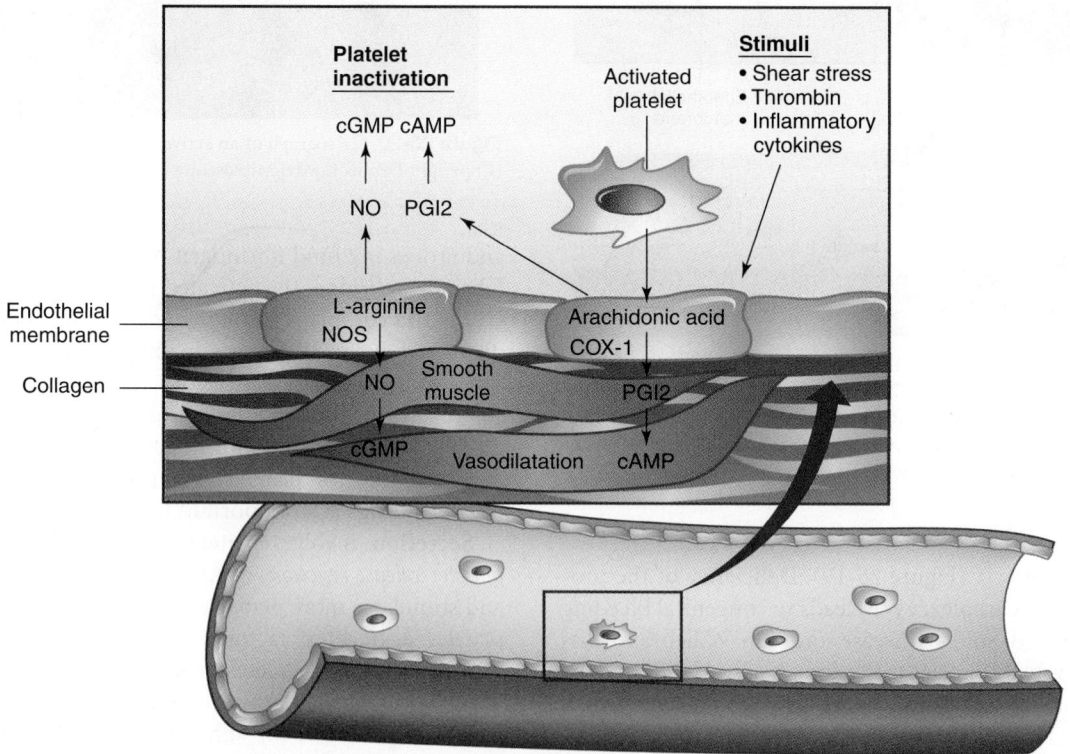

Figure 25-21 **Prostacyclins and inhibition of platelet aggregation.** Injury activates inflammation (COX-1 arachidonic acid). Enzymes convert arachidonic acid into prostacyclin I₂ (PGI₂) in endothelial cells. PGI₂ eventually increases intracellular cyclic adenosine monophosphate (cAMP), cAMP inhibits platelet aggregation and induces vasodilation. Nitric oxide (NO) formation is induced by NO synthases (NOS) and NO causes increased cyclic guanosine monophosphate (cGMP).

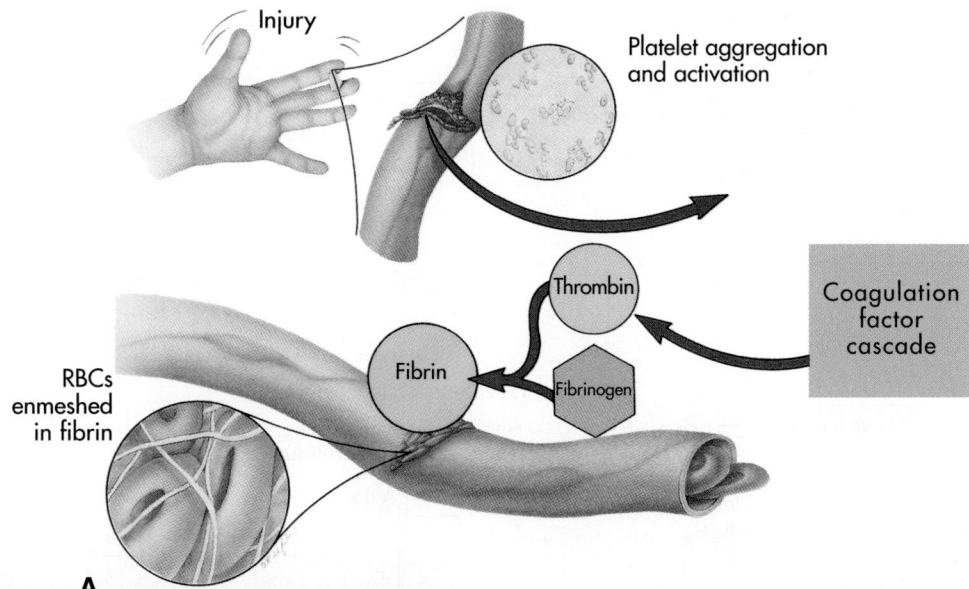

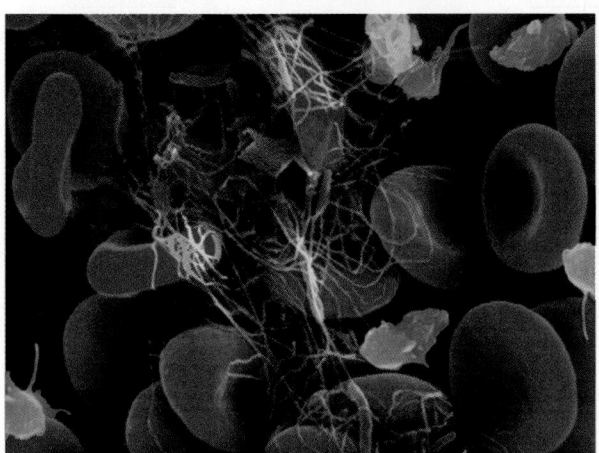

Figure 25-22 Blood clotting mechanism. **A,** The clotting mechanism involves release of platelet factors at the injury site, formation of thrombin and trapping of red blood cells (RBCs) in fibrin to form a clot. **B,** An electron micrograph showing entrapped RBCs in a fibrin clot. (**A** from Thibodeau GA, Patton KT: *Anatomy & physiology,* ed 5, St Louis, 2003, Mosby; **B,** copyright Dennis Kunkel Microscopy, Inc.)

factors are listed in Table 25-7). All procoagulants are synthesized in the liver except von Willebrand factor, which is synthesized in megakaryocytes and endothelial cells. According to the cascade theory of coagulation, each coagulation factor is converted to its active form by the preceding factor until fibrin is produced, which reinforces the platelet plug. Key is the concept of amplification, which enables rapid hemostasis but requires tight regulation to prevent problematic thrombosis. In effect, soluble clotting factors become insoluble fibrin.

The classical view of coagulation is the coagulation cascade comprised of both intrinsic and extrinsic pathways (Figure 25-23). The intrinsic pathway is activated when Hageman factor (factor XII) in plasma contacts with subendothelial substances exposed by vascular injury; whereas the extrinsic pathway is activated when **tissue factor (TF),** also called *tissue thromboplastin,* a substance released by damaged endothelial cells, contacts with one of the clotting factors, serum prothrombin conversion factor (factor VII); together they are known as the **TF:F VIIa complex.** Both pathways lead to a final common pathway when each has activated factor X

Table 25-7	Coagulation Factors and Synonyms
Factor	**Synonym**
I	Fibrinogen
II	Prothrombin
V	AC-Globulin
VII	Prothrombin conversion accelerator
VIII:C	Antihemophilic factor
IX	Christmas factor (PTC)
X	Stuart-Prower factor
XI	Thromboplastin antecedent (PTA)
XII	Hageman (contact) factor
XIII	Profibrinoligase
Fletcher factor	Prekallikrein
Fitzgerald factor	High-molecular-weight kininogen
Protein C	Xa inhibitor
Protein S	None

From Bick RL et al, editors: *Hematology: clinical and laboratory practice,* vol II, St Louis, 1993, Mosby.

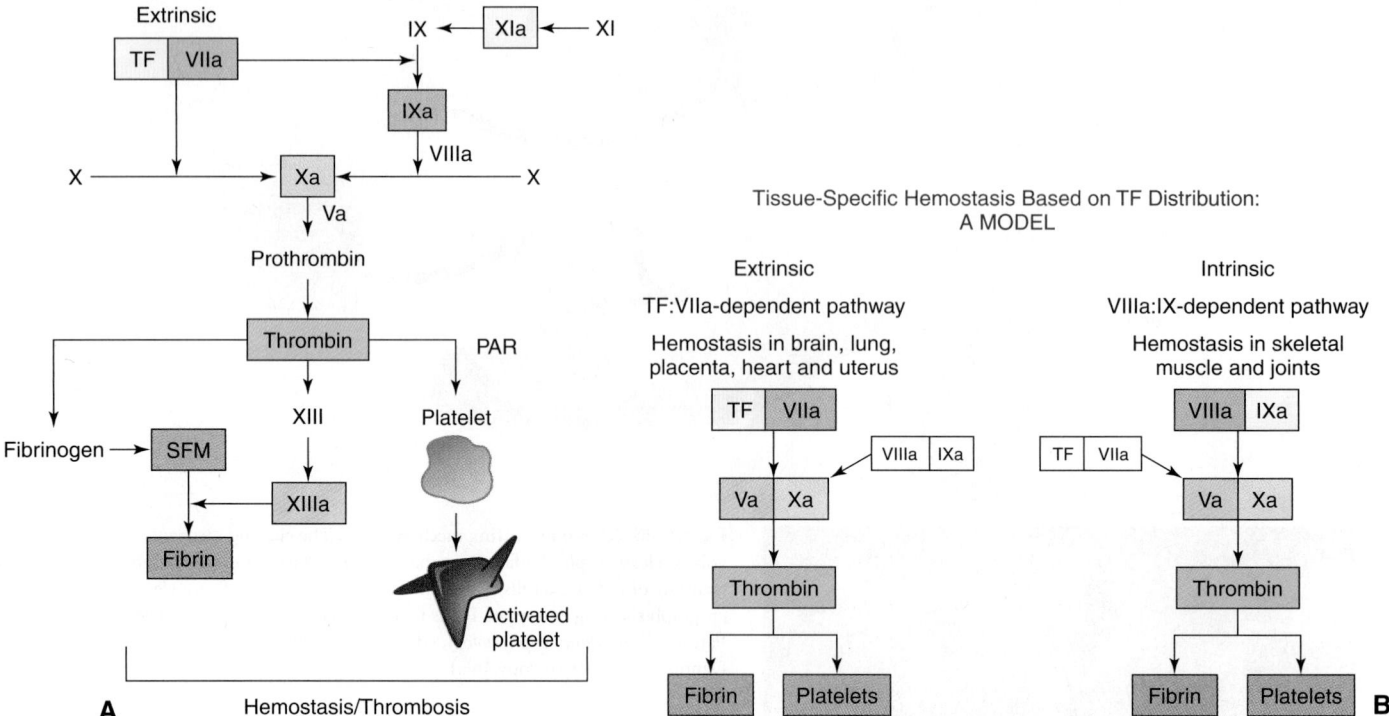

Figure 25-23 **The coagulation cascade. A,** TF: FVIIa complex initiates clotting by activating factors X and IX. Alternatively, factor XI can activate IXa. Factors Va:Xa, known as the *prothrombinase complex* activates prothrombin. Thrombin activates several other proteases and cofactors. Clot formation finally occurs when thrombin cleaves fibrinogen to soluble fibrinogen monomers (SFM), which are cross-linked by factor XIIIa, and with activation of protease-activated receptors (PARs) on platelets. Abnormal tissue factor (TF) expression within the vasculature initiates life-threatening thrombosis in various conditions, such as sepsis and diseases, for example, atherosclerosis and cancer. **B,** TF distribution is different depending on tissue type. High levels exist in the brain, lung, placenta, intermediate levels in the heart, kidney, intestine, uterus, and testes, and low levels in the spleen, thymus, skeletal muscle, and liver. Perhaps the differing amounts of TF provide a "safety" factor in vital organs to limit bleeding after injury in, for example, the brain, lung, and placenta. Tissues that express low levels of TF rely on the VIIIa:IXa complex of the intrinsic pathway to prevent bleeding. This model helps explain why hemophilia patients deficient in either factor VIII or IX often bleed into joints and soft tissues (Modified from Mackman N: *Arterioscler Thromb Vasc Biol* 24(6):1015-1022, 2004.)

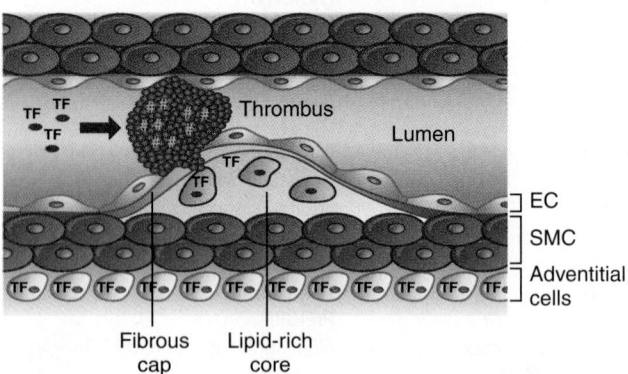

Figure 25-24 **Tissue factor (TF) in thrombus formation after rupture of an atherosclerotic plaque.** In atherosclerosis, TF is expressed by macrophage-derived foam cells and within atherosclerotic plaque. High levels of TF exposed upon rupture trigger thrombosis and myocardial infarction. In addition, blood-borne TF may contribute to thrombus propagation. TF is also expressed by adventitial cells (blue). *EC,* Endothelial cells; *SMC,* smooth muscle cells. (Modified from Mackman N: *Arterioscler Thromb Vasc Biol* 24(6):1015-1022, 2004.)

(Stuart-Prower factor), which then activates prothrombin (factor II) to thrombin, the final enzyme. Although this view of the clotting cascade has been useful clinically for interpreting clotting times, it lacks accuracy. Individuals severely deficient in factor XII—as well as patients deficient in fact XI—do not bleed clinically; this indicates that the contact phase or initiation point of the intrinsic pathway is not important invivo.[21] It is now known that the primary physiologic event that initiates clotting is the generation or exposure of tissue factor at the wound site. Tissue factor (TF) is the primary cellular initiator of blood coagulation. After vessel injury the TF:FVIIa complex activates the coagulation cascade leading to fibrin deposition and activation of platelets. In vitro studies have showed that TF:FVIIa complex activates protease-activated receptors (PARs); thus TF may contribute to other biologic processes by facilitating signaling in vascular cells (Figure 25-24). Abnormal TF expression in the vessel wall and/or low circulating cells initiates life-threatening thrombosis in various diseases (Figure 25-25). Data is emerging on

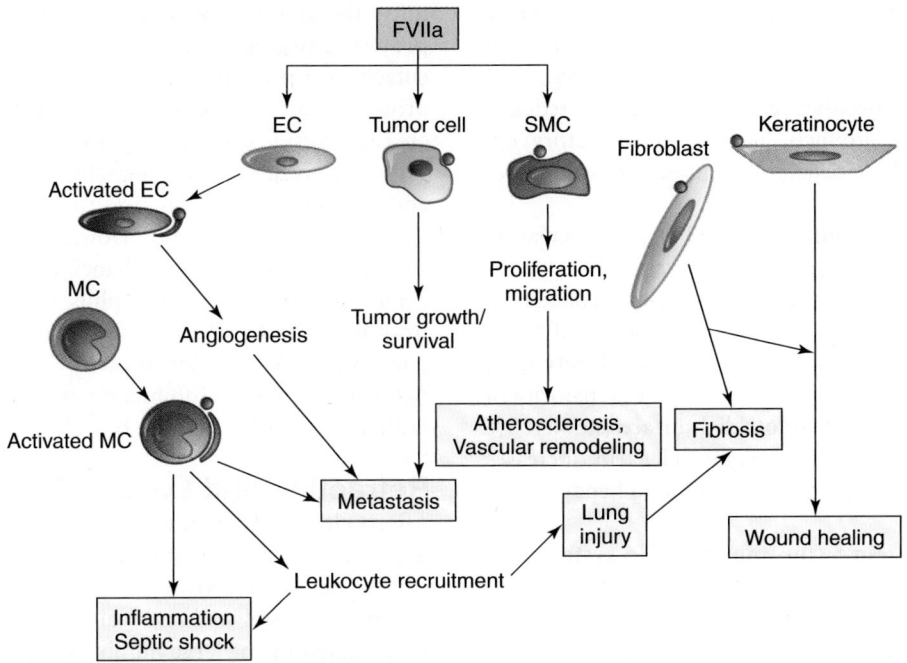

Figure 25-25 TF-VIIa signaling mediated cellular effects and various pathogenic alterations. *EC,* Endothelial cell; *SMC,* smooth muscle cell; *MC,* monocyte/macrophage. (Modified from Rao LV, Pendurthi UR: *Arterioscler Thromb Vasc Biol* 25(1):47-56, 2005.)

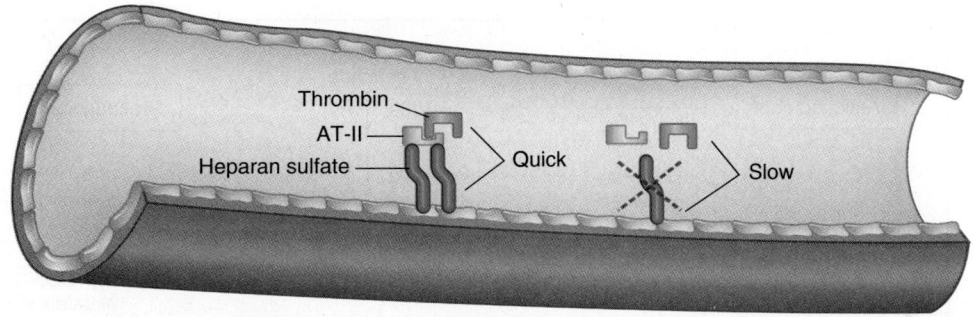

Figure 25-26 Antithrombin III-heparan sulfate system. Antithrombin III (AT-III) inhibits thrombin slowly when heparan sulfate (HS) is absent. When HS is present, it quickly activates thrombin because it binds to a specific site on AT-III that causes an instant conformational change in AT-III, allowing it to quickly activate thrombin.

how TF contributes to inflammation, tumor angiogenesis and metastasis, and cell migration.[25]

Control of Hemostatic Mechanisms

The major regulatory events in the clotting processes, including the activation of the clotting factors, the inhibition of these active clotting factors, and the production of circulating anticoagulant proteins, take place on membrane surfaces. The endothelium is a major site of hemostasis. Despite the continual presence of clotting factors and platelets in the circulation, blood normally remains fluid. To prevent unwanted clot formation, several natural anticoagulant mechanisms are in place including the antithrombin-heparin mechanism, the tissue factor pathway inhibitor mechanism, and the protein C anticoagulant pathway.[19] Additional antithrombotic mechanisms are listed in Table 25-8.

Antithrombin III (AT-III) is a circulating plasma protease inhibitor. Specifically, it inhibits thrombin and factor Xa. In

Table 25-8	Antithrombotic Mechanisms of Endothelial Cells	
Function Regulated	**Substances Involved**
Clotting cascade	Tissue factor pathway inhibitor
	Antithrombin III
	Protein C/protein S
Vessel and platelet activity	Prostacyclin (PGI$_2$)
	Nitric oxide (NO)
Eliminate fibrin clot	Fibrinolysis

addition, it inhibits factor XII and factor XI. If heparin is present, heparin binds to AT-III, causes a conformational change in AT-III, which then instantly inhibits thrombin[21] (Figure 25-26). Heparin inhibition of thrombin and factor Xa is the basis of its use clinically. Endothelial cells are normally coated with a layer of AT-III that is already activated by the heparan sulfate proteoglycans that are *also* on the surface of endothelial cells. Thus the AT-III heparin sulfate system is readied to instantly inactivate any thrombin in the circulating blood.[21] AT-III heparan sulfate system can be down-regulated by inflammation.[19] The heparan sulfate system can be reduced by neutrophil release products and by inflammatory cytokines. In addition, these heparin-like molecules can be degraded by sepsis.[19]

Tissue factor pathway inhibitor (TFPI) is a circulating plasma protease inhibitor synthesized by endothelial cells. TFPI inhibits factor Xa, but has a very low plasma concentration. TFPI/factor Xa complex becomes an inhibitor of tissue factor/factor VIIa, which mediates feedback inhibition of both tissue factor and factor VIIa.[21] Although the majority of TFPI remains associated with endothelial surfaces, about 20% circulates in plasma with lipoproteins. Heparin increases plasma levels of TFPI, which may contribute to heparin's antithrombotic effects.[21]

Protein C and Protein S (thrombomodulin system) is a membrane protein found on the surface of the endothelium in the microcirculation[21] (Figure 25-27). When thrombin binds to thrombomodulin, thrombin undergoes a conformational change resulting in a significant change—it no longer clots fibrinogen or activates platelets. It does, however, ac-quire the ability to activate protein C in plasma. Activated **protein C** degrades factor Va and factor VIIIa. **Protein S** is a cofactor for protein C. Deficiencies of AT-III, protein C, and protein S are important causes of hypercoagulation (increased clotting). Thrombomodulin and the endothelial cell protein C receptor are especially sensitive to inflammation and are inhibited by IL-1α, tumor necrosis factor–alpha (TNF-α), and endotoxin.[26] Down-regulation decreases protein C activation, thereby enhancing clot formation.[19] The enzyme elastase from neutrophils cleaves thrombomodulin from the endothelial cell surface, causing a less active thrombomodulin. With sepsis, protein C decreases significantly.[19] Activated protein C inhibits neutrophil adhesion to the endothelium possibly because of inflammatory cytokines.[19]

Retraction and Lysis of Blood Clots

After a clot is formed it retracts or "solidifies." Clot retraction is the final stage of hemostasis. Fibrin strands shorten, becoming denser and stronger, which approximates the edges of the injured vessel wall and seals the site of injury. Retraction is facilitated by the large numbers of platelets trapped within the fibrin meshwork. The platelets, which contain actin-like contractile protein, contract and "pull" the fibrin threads

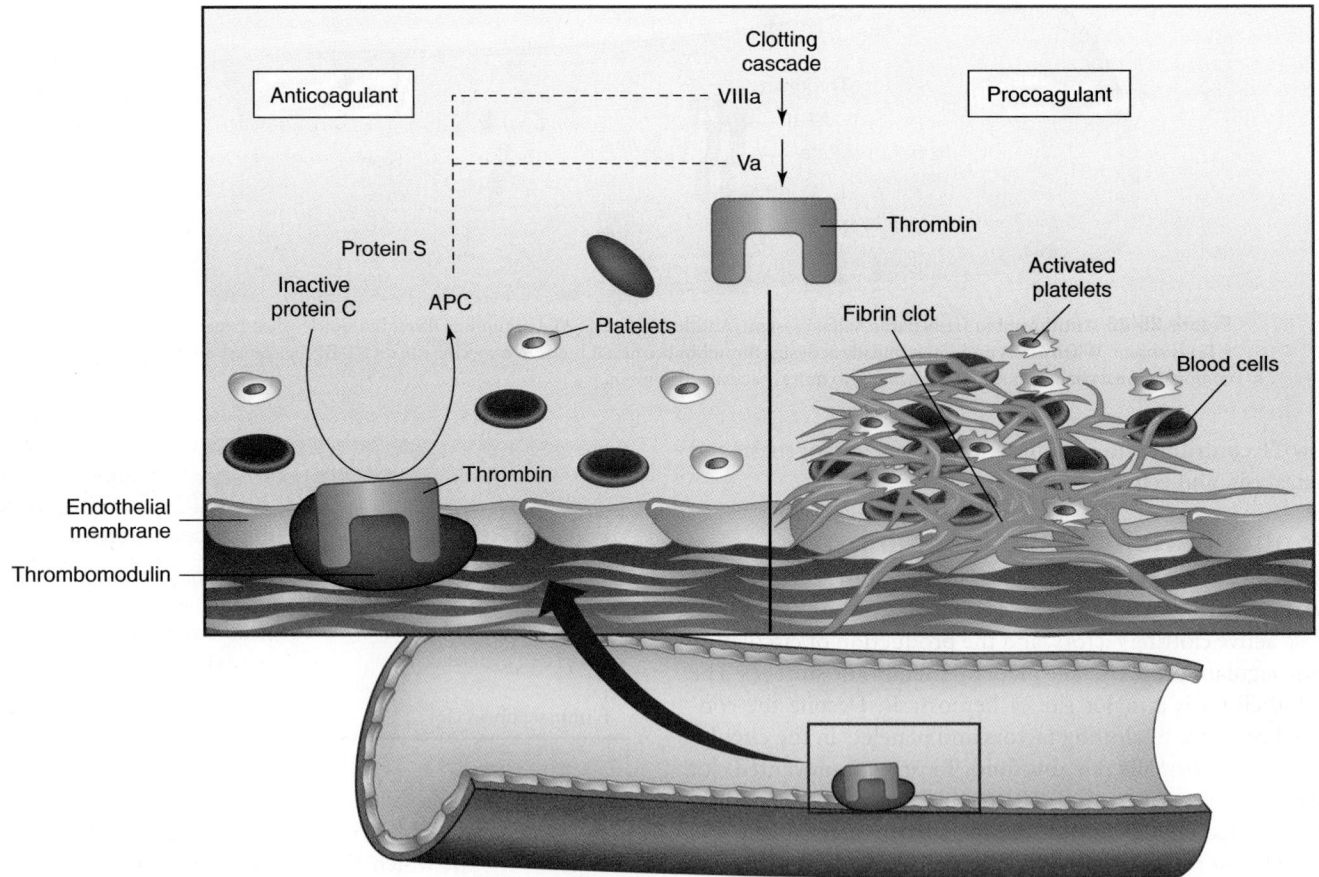

Figure 25-27 Protein C/protein S pathway (**thrombomodulin**). With thrombin binding to thrombomodulin (protein C/protein S pathway) thrombin undergoes a conformational change and eventually no longer clots fibrinogen or activates platelets. However, it does acquire the ability to activate protein C in plasma. Protein S is a cofactor for activated protein C (APC). APC inhibits activated factors V and VIII, cofactors in the clotting cascade.

closer together while releasing a factor that stabilizes the fibrin. Contraction expels protein-free serum from the fibrin meshwork. This process usually begins within a few minutes after a clot has formed, and most of the serum is expressed within 1 hour.

Lysis (breakdown) of blood clots is carried out by the **fibrinolytic system (plasminogen/plasmin system)** (Figure 25-28). **Tissue plasminogen activator (t-PA)** is released from perturbed endothelial cells near the site of vascular injury and converts plasminogen to plasmin. Similar to the AT-III interaction with thrombin, which is quickened in the presence of heparan sulfate on the endothelial cell surface, generation of plasmin optimally takes place on a surface, such as the fibrin clot.[21] Both t-PA and plasminogen bind to fibrin causing plasmin generation and localized fibrinolysis. **Plasmin** also called *fibrinase* or *fibrinolysin* is a degrading enzyme (serine protease) of many proteins of blood plasma, but specifically of fibrin clots. It is released as **plasminogen** into the circulation and activated by t-PA, thrombin, fibrin, and factor XII (Hageman factor). It is inactivated by a serine protease inhibitor, alpha 2-antiplasmin. Plasmin proteolyses proteins in other systems, it activates collagenases, some mediators of the complement system, cleaves fibronectin, fibrin, thrombospondin, laminin , and von Willebrand factor. Urokinase is another plasminogen activator, thus called **urokinase type plasminogen activator (u-PA);** u-PA binds to a specific cellular receptor (u-PAR) causing enhanced activation of cell-bound plasminogen resulting in plasmin generation. This urokinase is the major activator of fibrinolysis in the *extravascular* or tissue compartment, whereas t-PA is largely involved in *intravascular* fibrinolysis.[21,27] The main role of u-PA appears to be the induction of proteolysis via the degradation of matrix components or via latent proteases or growth factors.[27] Although the plasminogen activator-plasmin system provides cells with a powerful fibrinolytic system, the occurrence of plasminogen deficiency without evidence of massive clot formation (i.e., deposition of fibrin) indicates the presence of alternate routes of fibrin degradation. Emerging is evidence of direct fibrinolytic activity of various other enzymes including leukocyte elastase and cathepsin G, and metalloproteinases (MMPs).[28,29] Cross-linked fibrin is deposited in tissues around wounds, inflammatory sites, and tumors. Fibrin removal is an important biological process, for both intravascular and extravascular spaces, with various controlling mechanisms that can lead to abnormalities of fibrin accumulation, thrombotic events and also as a structural barrier to tumor invasion (see Chapter 12). Inhibition of the fibrinolytic system may occur either at the level of plasminogen activator by specific plasminogen activator inhibitors (PAI), or at the level of plasmin, mainly by α_2-antiplasmin.[27] Plasmin splits fibrin and fibrinogen into **fibrin degradation products (FDPs),** which dissolve the clot. The fibrinolytic system removes clotted blood from tissues and dissolves small clots (thrombi) in blood vessels. A major FDP is D-dimer. **D-dimer** is two D domains from adjacent fibrin monomers that are cross-linked by activated factor, XIII. Analysis of D-dimer has been used to diagnose deep

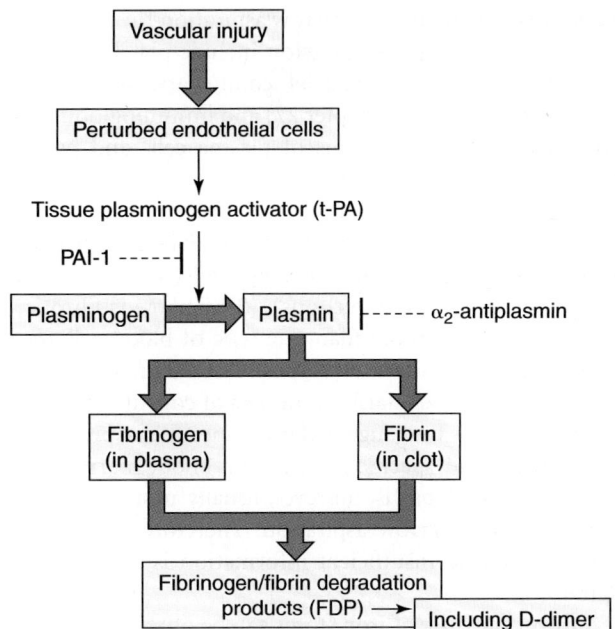

Figure 25-28 The fibrinolytic system. Although tissue plasminogen activator (t-PA) initiates intravascular fibrinolysis, urokinase plasminogen activator (u-PA) is the major activator of fibrinolysis in tissue (extravascular). Inhibitors of fibrinolysis include α_2-antiplasmin that inhibits plasmin and plasminogen activator inhibitor-1 (PAI-1) that inhibits t-PA. - - - - (dotted line) = inhibition.

venous thrombosis (DVT) or pulmonary embolism (PE). Despite extensive literature, the diagnostic role of D-dimer is unclear because of multiple D-dimer assays and varying sensitivities and variability.[30] A balance between amounts of thrombin and plasmin in the circulation maintains normal coagulation and lysis.

CLINICAL EVALUATION OF THE HEMATOLOGIC SYSTEM

Tests of Bone Marrow Function

In tests of marrow function, or hematopoiesis, small amounts of myeloid tissue are removed from the bone cavity and examined under a microscope. Cells contained in the marrow specimen are assessed with respect to (1) relative numbers of stem cells and their developing daughter cells and (2) morphologic structure.

Bone marrow aspiration, in which marrow is withdrawn using a hollow needle, provides information on gross cellular structure; estimation of iron stores in reticulocytes; determination of the ratio of erythrocyte precursor cells to myeloid cells (the normal ratio is 1:3); and the presence or absence of abnormal cells, such as tumor cells. A marrow aspirate that is richly cellular implies normal or increased hematopoiesis but does not indicate whether marrow activity is effective.

Bone aspiration is an important diagnostic test for several anemias (see Chapter 26) and the presence of infiltrative cells (i.e., leukemias) (see Chapters 27 and 28). (Chronic leukemias can be diagnosed from blood samples alone.)

Other disorders requiring marrow aspiration for diagnosis or monitoring of disease progression include platelet disorders (to determine whether platelet counts are increased, decreased, or normal; see Chapter 27) and immunoglobulin disorders (to gauge populations of plasma cells and lymphocytes; see Chapter 8).

Bone marrow biopsy, a surgical procedure in which a "slice" of marrow is removed, is performed if (1) aspiration is not diagnostic, (2) tumors are suggested (tumors are more easily detected in biopsy sections), (3) marrow is fibrotic, or (4) populations of more than one type of blood cell are reduced. Because marrow aspiration disturbs marrow structure, only general cellularity (numbers of constituent cells) of the marrow can be gauged. Biopsy specimens provide the most reliable and specific information about marrow cellularity. Marrow biopsy is, however, usually more painful and expensive than marrow aspiration. Therefore biopsy is not performed unless insufficient information is obtained from aspiration.

A direct measure of iron stores can be obtained only from liver or marrow biopsy specimens. The bone marrow technique is preferred, not only because it is safer than liver biopsy but also because the red blood cell is the immediate source of plasma iron destined for erythrocyte production. Examination of biopsy specimens and aspirate routinely includes a differential cell count (Table 25-9).

The differential cell count involves examining approximately 400 nucleated cells under oil-immersion magnification and counting populations of different stem cells. The relative number of each type of stem cell is expressed as a fraction of 400.

Blood Tests

Blood tests provide information about the absolute and relative numbers of blood cells in a specimen of blood, as well as various structural and functional characteristics of the cells. Deviations from normal can reflect disease, phys-

iologic states (e.g., pregnancy, infancy, old age), injury, or dysfunction in almost any part of the body. Blood tests that reflect chiefly hematologic disorders are listed in Table 25-10.

PEDIATRICS AND THE HEMATOLOGIC SYSTEM

Blood cell counts tend to rise above adult levels at birth and then decline gradually throughout childhood. Table 25-11 lists normal ranges during infancy and childhood. The immediate rise in values is the result of accelerated hematopoiesis during fetal life, increased numbers of cells that result from the trauma of birth, and cutting of the umbilical cord.

Average blood volume in the full-term neonate is 85 ml per kilogram of body weight. The premature infant has a slightly larger blood volume of 90 ml per kilogram of body weight, with the mean increasing to 150 mg/kg during the first few days after birth. In both full-term and premature infants, blood volume decreases during the first few months. Thereafter the average blood volume is 75 to 77 ml/kg, which is similar to that of older children and adults.

The hypoxic intrauterine environment stimulates erythropoietin production in the fetus and accelerates fetal erythropoiesis, producing polycythemia (excessive proliferation of erythrocyte precursors) of the newborn. After birth the oxygen from the lungs saturates arterial blood, and more oxygen is delivered to the tissues. In response to the change from a placental to a pulmonary oxygen supply during the first few days of life, levels of erythropoietin and the rate of blood cell formation decrease. The very active rate of fetal erythropoiesis is reflected by the large numbers of immature erythrocytes (reticulocytes) in the peripheral blood of full-term neonates. After birth the number of reticulocytes decreases about 50% every 12 hours so that it is rare to find an elevated reticulocyte count after the first week of life. During this period of rapid growth, the rate of erythrocyte destruction is greater than that in later childhood and adulthood. In full-term infants, normal erythrocyte life span is 60 to 80 days; in premature infants it may be as short as 20 to 30 days; and in children and adolescents it is the same as that in adults—120 days.

In premature infants the postnatal fall in hemoglobin and hematocrit values is more marked than in the full-term infant. In the preschool and school-age child, hemoglobin, hematocrit, and red blood cell counts gradually rise. Metabolic processes within the erythrocytes of neonates differ significantly from those of erythrocytes in the normal adult. The relatively young population of erythrocytes in the newborn consumes greater quantities of glucose than do erythrocytes in adults.

The lymphocytes of children tend to have more cytoplasm and less compact nuclear chromatin than do the lymphocytes of adults. A possible explanation is that children tend to have more frequent viral infections, which are associated with atypical lymphocytes. Even minor infections, in which the child fails to exhibit clinical manifestations of illness, and ad-

Table 25-9	Differential Cell Counts in Bone Marrow with Age				
Developing Cells in Marrow	Birth	1 mo- 1 yr	1-4 yr	4-12 yr	Adult
Erythrocytic series	14	8	19	21	20
Lymphocytic series	14	47	22	18	17
Eosinophilic series	3	3	6	3	3
Neutrophilic series	60	33	50	52	57
Myeloid/erythroid ratio	4:3	4:0	1:3	2:5	1:3

NOTE: Values are percentages of cell types counted during examination of a marrow specimen containing approximately 400 nucleated cells.

Table 25-10 Blood Tests for Hematologic Disorders

Cell Type and Test	Properly Evaluated by Test	Possible Hematologic Cause of Abnormal Findings
Erythrocyte		
Red cell count	Number (in millions) of erythrocytes/μL of blood	Altered erythropoiesis, anemias, hemorrhage, Hodgkin disease, leukemia
Mean corpuscular volume	Size of erythrocytes	Anemias, thalassemias
Mean corpuscular hemoglobin (MCH)	Amount of hemoglobin in each erythrocyte (by weight)	Anemias, hemoglobinopathy
Mean corpuscular hemoglobin concentration (MCHC)	Concentration of hemoglobin in each erythrocyte (percentage of erythrocyte occupied by hemoglobin)	Anemias, hereditary spherocytosis
Hemoglobin determination	Amount of hemoglobin (by weight)/dl of blood	Anemias
Hematocrit determination	Percentage of a given volume of blood that is occupied by erythrocytes	Hemorrhage, polycythemia, erythrocytosis, anemias, leukemia
Reticulocyte count	Number of reticulocytes/μL of blood (also expressed as percentage of reticulocytes in total red cell count)	Hyperactive or hypoactive bone marrow function
Erythrocyte osmotic fragility test	Cellular shape (biconcavity), structure of plasma membrane	Anemias, hemolytic disease caused by ABO or Rh incompatibility, Hodgkin disease, polycythemia vera, thalassemia major
Hemoglobin electrophoresis	Relative percentage of different types of hemoglobin in erythrocytes	Sickle cell disease, sickle cell trait, hemoglobin C disease, hemoglobin C trait, thalassemias
Sickle cell test	Presence of hemoglobin S in erythrocytes	Sickle cell trait, sickle cell anemia
Glucose-6-phospahte dehydrogenase (G6PD) deficiency test	Deficiency of G6PD in erythrocytes	Hemolytic anemia
Hemoglobin Metabolism		
Serum ferritin determination	Depletion of body iron (potential deficiency of heme synthesis)	Iron deficiency anemias
Total iron-binding capacity (TIBC)	Amount of iron in serum plus amount of transferring available in serum (mcg/dl)	Hemorrhage, iron deficiency anemia, hemochromatosis, hemosiderosis, iron overload, anemias, thalassemia
Transferrin saturation	Percentage of transferring that is saturated with iron	Acute hemorrhage, hemochromatosis, hemosiderosis, sideroblastic anemia, iron deficiency anemia, iron overload, thalassemia
Porphyrin analysis (protoporphyrin analysis)	Concentration of protoporphyrin in erythrocytes (mcg/dl); an indicator of iron-deficient erythropoiesis	Megaloblastic anemia, congenital erythropoietic porphyria
Direct antiglobulin test (DAT)	Antibody binding to erythrocytes	Hemolytic disease of the newborn, autoimmune hemolytic anemia, drug-induced hemolytic anemia, transfusion reaction
Antibody screen (indirect Coombs test)	Detection of antibodies to erythrocyte antigens (other than the ABO antigens)	Same as for DAT
Leukocytes: Differential White Cell Count (Absolute Number of a Type of Leukocyte/μL of Blood)	See below	See below
Neutrophil count	Neutrophils/μL	Myeloproliferative disorders, hematopoietic disorders, hemolysis, infection
Lymphocyte count	Lymphocytes/μL	Infectious lymphocytosis, infectious mononucleosis, hematopoietic disorders, anemias, leukemia, lymphosarcoma, Hodgkin disease
Plasma cell count	Plasma cells/μL	Infectious mononucleosis, lymphocytosis, plasma cell leukemia
Monocyte count	Monocytes/μL	Hodgkin disease, infectious mononucleosis, monocytic leukemia, non-Hodgkin lymphoma, polycythemia vera
Eosinophil count	Eosinophils/μL	Hematopoietic disorders
Basophil count	Basophils/μL	Chronic myelogenous leukemia, hemolytic anemias, Hodgkin disease, polycythemia vera

Data from Byrne CJ et al: *Laboratory tests: implications for nursing care,* Menlo Park, Calif, 1986, Addison-Wesley; Bick RL et al: *Hematology: clinical and laboratory practice,* St Louis, 1993, Mosby.

NOTE: See Figure 25-23 and Table 25-7 for information about clotting factors and their sequence of activation in the coagulation cascade.   *Continued*

Table 25-10   Blood Tests for Hematologic Disorders—cont'd

Cell Type and Test	Properly Evaluated by Test	Possible Hematologic Cause of Abnormal Findings
Platelets and Clotting Factors		
Platelet count	Number of circulating platelets (in thousands)/ μL of blood	Anemias, multiple myeloma, myelofibrosis, polycythemia vera, leukemia, disseminated intravascular coagulation (DIC), hemolytic disease of the newborn, idiopathic thrombocytopenic purpura, transfusion reaction, lymphoproliferative disorders
Bleeding time	Duration of bleeding following a standardized superficial puncture wound of the skin, integrity of the platelet plug, measured in minutes following puncture	Leukemia, anemias, DIC, fibrinolytic activity, purpuras, hemorrhagic disease of the newborn, infectious mononucleosis, multiple myeloma, clotting factor deficiencies, thrombasthenia, thrombocytopenia, von Willebrand disease
Clot retraction test	Platelet number and function, fibrinogen quantity and use, measured in hours required for expression of serum from a clot incubated in a test tube	Acute leukemia, aplastic anemia, factor XIII deficiency, increased fibrinolytic activity, Hodgkin disease, hyperfibrinogenemia or hypofibrinogenemia, idiopathic thrombocytopenic purpura, multiple myeloma, polycythemia vera, secondary thrombocytopenia, thrombasthenia
Platelet adhesion studies	Ability of platelets to adhere to foreign surfaces	Anemia, macroglobulinemia, Bernard-Soulier syndrome, multiple myeloma, myeloid metaplasia, plasma cell dyscrasias, thrombasthenia, thrombocytopathy, von Willebrand disease
Platelet aggregation tests	Ability of platelets to adhere to one another	Afibrinogenemia, Bernard-Soulier syndrome, thrombasthenia, hemorrhagic thrombocythemia, myeloid metaplasia, plasma cell dyscrasias, platelet release defects, polycythemia vera, preleukemia, sideroblastic anemia, von Willebrand disease, Waldenström macroglobulinemia, hypercoagulability
Whole blood clotting time (Lee-White coagulation time)	Overall ability of blood to clot, as measured in minutes in a test tube	Afibrinogenemia, clotting factor deficiencies, excessive fibrinolysis, hemorrhagic disease of the newborn, hypofibrinogenemia, hypoprothrombinemia, leukemia
Circulating anticoagulants (immune globulin G [IgG] antibodies that inhibit coagulation)	Presence of antibodies that neutralize clotting factors and inhibit coagulation, as indicated by prolonged clotting time, prothrombin time, or partial thromboplastin time	Afibrinogenemia, presence of fibrin-fibrinogen degradation products, macroglobulinemia, multiple myeloma, DIC, plasma cell dyscrasias
Partial thromboplastin time (PTT)	Effectiveness of clotting factors (except factors VII and VIII), effectiveness of intrinsic pathway of coagulation cascade, as measured by a test tube (in seconds)	Presence of circulating anticoagulants, DIC, clotting factor deficiencies, excessive fibrinolysis, hemorrhagic disease of the newborn, hypofibrinogenemia and afibrinogenemia, prothrombin deficiency, von Willebrand disease, acute hemorrhage
Prothrombin time	Effectiveness of activity of prothrombin, fibrinogen, and factors V, VII, and X; effectiveness of vitamin K–dependent coagulation factors of the extrinsic and common pathways of the coagulation cascade as measured in a test tube (in seconds)	Hypofibrinogenemia, dysfibrinogenemia, and afibrinogenemia; presence of circulating anticoagulants; DIC; deficiency of factors V, VII, or X; presence of fibrin degradation products, increased fibrinolytic activity, hemolytic jaundice, hemorrhagic disease of the newborn; acute leukemia, polycythemia vera, prothrombin deficiency, multiple myeloma

Data from Byrne CJ et al: *Laboratory tests: implications for nursing care,* Menlo Park, Calif, 1986, Addison-Wesley; Bick RL et al: *Hematology: clinical and laboratory practice,* St Louis, 1993, Mosby.

NOTE: See Figure 25-23 and Table 25-7 for information about clotting factors and their sequence of activation in the coagulation cascade.

Table 25-10   Blood Tests for Hematologic Disorders—cont'd

Cell Type and Test	Properly Evaluated by Test	Possible Hematologic Cause of Abnormal Findings
Platelets and Clotting Factors—cont'd		
Thrombin time	Quantity and activity of fibrinogen as measured in a test tube (in seconds)	Hypofibrinogenemia, dysfibrinogenemia, and afibrinogenemia; presence of circulating anticoagulants; hemorrhagic disease of the newborn, polycythemia vera; increase in fibrinogenfibrin degradation products; increased fibrinolytic activity
Fibrinogen assay	Amount of fibrinogen available for fibrin formation	Acute leukemia, congenital hypofibrinogenemia or afibrinogenemia, DIC, increased fibrinolytic activity, severe hemorrhage
Fibrin-fibrinogen degradation products (fibrin-fibrinogen split products)	Fibrinogenic activity as measured by levels of fibrin-fibrinogen degradation products (in mcg/ml of blood)	Transfusion reactions, DIC, internal hemorrhage in the newborn, deep vein thrombosis, pulmonary embolism

Table 25-11   Hematologic Values During Infancy and Childhood

Age	Hemoglobin (g/dl):Mean	Hematocrit (%):Mean	Reticulocytes (%):Mean	Leukocytes (WBC/mm³): Mean	Neutrophils (%):Mean	Lymphocytes (%):Mean	Eosinophils (%):Mean	Monocytes (%):Mean	Platelets (10³/mm³)
Cord blood	16.8	55	5.0	18,000	61	31	2	6	290
2 wk	16.5	50	1.0	12,000	40	48	3	9	252
3 mo	12.0	36	1.0	12,000	30	63	2	5	140-340
6 mo-6 yr	12.0	37	1.0	10,000	45	48	2	5	140-340
7-12 yr	13.0	38	1.0	8,000	55	38	2	5	140-340
Adult	13.0	40	1.0	8,000	55	35	2	5	140-340
Female	14	41	0.8-4.1	7,400	54-62	25-33	1-4	3-7	140-340
Male	16	47	0.8-2.5	7,400	54-62	25-33	1-4	3-7	140-340

Differential Counts

ministration of immunizations may result in lymphocyte changes.[31]

The lymphocyte count is high at birth, continues to rise during the first year of life, and then steadily declines until lower adult values are reached. It is unknown whether these developmental variations are physiologic or a pathologic response to frequent viral infections and immunizations in children.

At birth the neutrophil count is very high and rises further during the early days of life.[32] After 2 weeks, neutrophil counts fall to within or below normal adult ranges. By approximately 4 years of age, the neutrophil count is the same as that of an adult.

Eosinophil count is high in the first year of life and is higher in children than in teenagers or adults.[33] Monocyte counts are high in the first year of life and then decrease to adult levels. Platelet counts in full-term neonates are comparable to platelet counts in adults and remain so throughout infancy and childhood.[34]

AGING AND THE HEMATOLOGIC SYSTEM

Blood composition changes little with age. Erythrocyte life span is normal, although erythrocytes are replenished more slowly after bleeding, probably because of iron depletion. Total serum iron, total iron-binding capacity, and intestinal iron absorption are all decreased in the elderly.[35] Iron deficiency is often responsible for the low hemoglobin levels noted in elderly people. The plasma membranes of erythrocytes become increasingly fragile, with portions being lost, presumably because of physical trauma inflicted during circulation.

Lymphocyte function decreases with age (see Chapters 7 and 8), causing changes in cellular immunity with some decline in T cell function. The humoral immune system is less able to respond to antigenic challenge.

No changes in platelet numbers or structure have been observed in elderly persons, yet evidence shows that platelet adhesiveness probably increases.[36] Although fibrinogen levels and factors V, VII, and IX tend to be increased in the elderly population, evidence concerning hypercoagulability is inconclusive.

Components of the Hematologic System

1. Blood consists of a variety of formed elements: about 90% water and 10% solutes. In adults the total blood volume is approximately 5.5 L.
2. Plasma, a complex aqueous liquid, contains three major groups of plasma proteins: albumins, globulins, and clotting factors.
3. The cellular elements of blood are the erythrocytes, leukocytes, lymphocytes, and platelets.
4. Erythrocytes are the most abundant cells of the blood, occupying approximately 48% of the blood volume in men and approximately 42% in women. Erythrocytes are responsible for tissue oxygenation.
5. Leukocytes are fewer in number than erythrocytes and constitute approximately 5000 to 10,000 cells per mm^3 of blood. Leukocytes defend the body against infection and remove dead or injured host cells.
6. Leukocytes are classified as either granulocytes (neutrophils, basophils, eosinophils) or agranulocytes (monocytes, macrophages and lymphocytes).
7. Natural killer cells, which resemble lymphocytes, kill some types of virus-infected cells, without being exposed to them beforehand, and tumor cells in vitro.
8. Platelets are not cells; rather they are disk-shaped cytoplasmic fragments. Platelets are essential for blood coagulation and control of bleeding.
9. The lymphoid organs are classified as primary (thymus and bone marrow) or secondary (spleen, lymph nodes, tonsils, and Peyer patches of the small intestine).
10. The lymphoid organs are sites of residence, proliferation, differentiation, or function of lymphocytes and mononuclear phagocytes.
11. The spleen is the largest of the secondary lymphoid organs and functions as the site of fetal hematopoiesis, filters and cleanses the blood, and is a reservoir for lymphocytes and other blood cells.
12. The lymph nodes are the site of development or activity of large numbers of lymphocytes, monocytes, and macrophages.
13. The mononuclear phagocyte system (MPS), previously called the *reticuloendothelial system (RES)*, is composed of monoblasts, promonocytes, and monocytes in bone marrow, monocytes in peripheral blood, and macrophages in tissue.
14. The MPS is the main line of defense against bacteria in the bloodstream and cleanses the blood by removing old, injured, or dead blood cells; antigen-antibody complexes; and macromolecules.

Development of Blood Cells

1. Hematopoiesis, or blood cell production, occurs in the liver and spleen of the fetus and in the bone marrow after birth.
2. Hematopoiesis involves two stages: (a) proliferation and (b) differentiation, or maturation. Each type of blood cell has parent cells called *stem cells.*
3. Hematopoiesis continues throughout life to replace blood cells that grow old and die, are killed by disease, or are lost through bleeding.
4. Regulation of hematopoiesis possibly occurs two ways: (1) by stromal cells involved in cell contact processes, and (2) by cytokines or regulatory molecules.
5. Specific humoral colony-stimulating factors (CSFs) are necessary for the adequate growth of myeloid, erythroid, lymphoid, and megakaryocytic lineages.
6. Bone marrow consists of blood vessels, nerves, mononuclear phagocytes, stem cells, blood cells in various stages of differentiation, stromal cells and fatty tissue.

7. Hemoglobin, the oxygen-carrying protein of the erythrocyte, enables the blood to transport 100 times more oxygen than could be transported dissolved in plasma alone.
8. Erythropoiesis depends on the presence of vitamins (especially vitamin B_{12}, folate, B_6, riboflavin, pantothenic acid, niacin, ascorbic acid, and vitamin E).
9. Regulation of erythropoiesis is mediated by erythropoietin. Erythropoietin is secreted by the kidneys in response to tissue hypoxia and causes a compensatory increase in erythrocyte production if the oxygen content of the blood decreases because of anemia, high altitude, or pulmonary disease.
10. Maintenance of optimal levels of granulocytes and monocytes in the blood depends on the availability of pluripotential stem cells in the marrow, induction of these into committed stem cells, and timely release of new cells from the marrow.
11. Platelets develop from megakaryocytes by a process called *endomitosis.* In endomitosis the megakaryocytes undergo mitosis but not cytokinesis; thus the cell does not divide into two daughter cells.
12. Platelet activation increases the inflammatory response.

Mechanisms of Hemostasis

1. Hemostasis, or arrest of bleeding, involves (a) vasoconstriction (vasospasm), (b) formation of a platelet plug, (c) activation of the clotting cascade, (d) formation of a blood clot, and (e) clot retraction and clot dissolution.
2. Platelet activation involves four separate processes: (1) adhesion; (2) aggregation; (3) secretion; and (4) procoagulant activity.
3. A blood clot is a meshwork of protein strands that stabilizes the platelet plug. The strands are made of fibrin. Fibrin is the end product of the coagulation cascade.
4. The classical view of coagulation is that the coagulation cascade is comprised of both intrinsic and extrinsic pathways. It is now known that tissue factor (TF) is the primary cellular initiator of blood coagulation after vessel injury. The TF:FVIIa complex activates the coagulation cascade.
5. To prevent unwanted clots, several anticoagulant mechanisms exist including antithrombin-heparan mechanism, the tissue factor pathway inhibitor mechanism, and the protein C anticoagulant pathway.
6. Lysis of blood clots is the function of the fibrinolytic system. Plasmin is a degrading enzyme of fibrin clots. It is released as plasminogen and activated by tissue plasminogen activator (t-PA), thrombin, fibrin, and factor XII.

Clinical Evaluation of the Hematologic System

1. Tests of bone marrow function include bone marrow aspiration and bone marrow biopsy.
2. Cells contained in the marrow specimen are assessed with respect to (1) relative numbers of stem cells and their developing daughter cells and (2) morphologic structure.

Pediatrics and the Hematologic System

1. Blood cell counts rise above adult levels at birth and then gradually decline throughout childhood.
2. The average blood volume of an infant is 75 to 77 ml/kg, which is similar to that of older children and adults.
3. In response to the change from a placental to a pulmonary oxygen supply during the first few days of life, levels of erythropoietin and the rate of blood cell formation decrease.
4. During the first week of life with rapid growth, the rate of erythrocyte destruction is greater than later in childhood and adulthood.
5. The normal erythrocyte life span is 60 to 80 days in full-term infants, 20 to 30 days in premature infants, and 120 days in children, adolescents, and adults.

SUMMARY REVIEW—cont'd

6. The lymphocyte count is high at birth, rises further during the first year of life, and steadily declines until lower adult volumes are reached.
7. The neutrophil count is very high at birth, falls to adult ranges after 2 weeks, and is the same as for adults by 4 years of age.
8. The eosinophil count is high in the first year of life and is higher in children than in adolescents and adults. Monocyte counts are high in the first year of life and decrease to adult levels.
9. Platelet counts in full-term infants are comparable with those in adults and remain so throughout childhood.

Aging and the Hematologic System
1. Blood composition changes little with age. A delay in erythrocyte replenishment may occur after bleeding, presumably because of iron deficiency.
2. Lymphocyte function appears to decrease with age. Particularly affected is a decrease in cellular immunity.
3. Platelet adhesiveness probably increases with age.

KEY TERMS

Agranulocytes, 897
Antithrombin III (AT-III), 917
Apoferritin, 908
Apotransferrin, 908
Basophils, 897
Blood clot, 914
Clotting factors, 895
Coagulation cascade, 914
Colony-stimulating factors (CSFs), 900
Cyclooxygenase, 914
D-dimer, 919
Deoxyhemoglobin, 907
Embryonic stem cells, 903
Endomitosis, 911
Eosinophils, 896
Erythrocytes (red blood cells [RBCs]), 895
Ferritin, 908
Fibrin degradation products (FDPs), 919
Fibrinolytic system (plasminogen/plasmin system), 919
GPIIb-IIIa complex, 913
Granulocytes, 896

Hematopoietic growth factors, 900
Hemosiderin, 908
Hemostasis, 911
Leukocytes (white blood cells [WBCs]), 896
Lymphocytes, 898
Macrophages, 897
Mast cells, 897
Mastocytosis, 897
Megakaryocytes, 898
Monocytes, 897
Mononuclear phagocyte system (MPS), 897, 900
Natural killer (NK) cells, 898
Neutrophil (polymorphonuclear neutrophil [PMN]), 896
Nitric oxide (NO), 914
Oxyhemoglobin, 907
Plasmin, 919
Plasminogen, 919
Platelets, 898
Platelet activation, 912
Platelet adhesion, 912

Platelet aggregation, 913
Platelet plug, 911
Pluripotent stem cells, 902
Procoagulation, 914
Prostacyclin I_2 (PGI$_2$), 914
Protein C, 918
Protein S, 918
Protein C and Protein S (thrombomodulin system), 918
Reticulocyte, 904
Secretion, 913
Steel factor, 903
Stromal cells, 903
TF:F VIIa complex, 915
Thromboxane (TXA$_2$), 914
Tissue factor (TF), 915
Tissue factor pathway inhibitor (TFPI), 918
Tissue plasminogen activator (t-PA), 919
Transferrin, 908
Urokinase type plasminogen activator (u-PA), 919
von Willibrand factor (vWF), 912

MEDIA RESOURCES

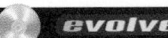

Review questions and answers for this chapter are available in the *CD Companion* included with this book.

WebLinks—links to Internet sites pertaining to this chapter—are available on Evolve at http://evolve.elsevier.com/McCance/.

REFERENCES

1. Babior BM, Stossel TP: *Hematology: a pathophysiological approach,* New York, 1984, Churchill Livingstone.
2. Bischoff SC, Sellge G: Mast cell hyperplasia: role of cytokines, *Int Arch Allery Immunol* 127(2):118-122, 2002.
3. Metcalfe DD, Akin C: Mastocytosis: molecular mechanisms and clinical disease heterogeneity, *Leuk Res* 25(7):577-582, 2001.
4. Li CY, Baek JY: Mastocytosis and fibrosis: role of cytokines, *Int Arch Allergy Immunol* 127(2):123-126, 2002.
5. Wimazal F et al: Increased angiogenesis in the bone marrow of patients with systemic mastocytosis, *Am J Pathol* 160(5):1639-1645, 2002.
6. Hobisch-Hagen P et al: Low platelet count and elevated serum thrombopoietin after severe trauma, *Eur J Haematol* 64(3):157, 2000.
7. Wang Q et al: Interferon-alpha directly represses megakaryopoiesis by inhibiting thrombopoietin-induced signaling through induction of SOCS-1, *Blood* 96(6):2093, 2000.
8. Burke LJ, Baniahmad A: Co-repressors 2000, *FASEB J* 14(13): 1876-1888, 2000.

9. Grandori C et al: The Myc/Max/Mad network and the transcriptional control of cell behavior, *Annu Rev Cell Dev Biol* 16:653-699, 2000.
10. Kraus, DS: Plasticity of marrow-derived stem cells, *Gene Therapy* 9(11):754-758, 2002.
11. Sanchez-Ramos, JR: Neural cells derived from adult bone marrow and umbilical cord blood, *J Neuroscience Res* 69(6): 880-893, 2002.
12. Alberts B et al: *Molecular biology of the cell,* ed 4, New York, 1999, Garland.
13. Ogilvy S et al: Constitutive Bcl-2 expression throughout the hematopoietic compartment affects multiple lineages and enhances progenitor cell survival, *Proc Natl Acad Sci* 96(26):14943, 1999.
14. Metcalf D: Cellular hemoatopoiesis in the twentieth century, *Semin Hematol* 36(4 suppl 7):5, 1999.
15. Russell WJ et al: Active bone marrow distribution in the adult, *Br J Radiol* 39(466):735-739, 1966.
16. Winearls GC: Recombinant human erythropoietin: 10 years of clinical experience, *Nephrol Dial Transplant* 13(suppl 2):3, 1998.
17. Macdougall IC: Meeting the challenges of a new millennium: optimizing the use of recombinant human erythropoietin, *Nephrol Dial Transplant* 13(suppl 23):23, 1998.
18. Jai L, Bonaventura J, Stamler JS: S-nitrosohaemoglobin: a dynamic activity of blood involved in vascular control, *Nature* 380(6571):221, 1996.
19. Esmon CT: Coagulation inhibitors in inflammation, *Biochem Soc Trans* 33(2):401-405, 2005.
20. Dahlback B: Blood coagulation and its regulation by anticoagulant pathways: genetic pathogenesis of bleeding and thrombonic diseases, *J Intern Med* 257(3):209-223, 2005.

21 Leung LLK: Hemostasis and its regulation, *ACP Medicine,* New York, 2003, WebMD.

22. Andrews RK, Berndt MC: Platelet physiology and thrombosis, *Thrombosis Res* 114(5-6):447-453, 2004.

23. Sanderson S et al: Narrative review: aspirin resistance and its clinical implications *Ann Intern Med* 142(5):370-380, 2005.

24. Harmening DM, editor: *Clinical hematology and fundamentals of hemostasis,* ed 3, Philadelphia: 1997, F.A. Davis.

25. Mackman N: Rose of tissue factor in hemostasis, thrombosis, and vascular development, *Arterioscler Thromb Vac Biol* 24(6):1015-1022, 2004.

26. Fishbach D, Fogdall R: *Coagulation: the essentials,* Baltimore, 1981, Williams & Wilkins.

27. Lijnen, HR: Elements of the fibrinolytic system, *Ann N Y Acad Sci* 936:226-236, 2001.

28. Hotary KB et al: matrix metalloproteinases (MMPs) regulate fibrin-invasive activity via MTI-MMP-dependent and independent processes, *J Exp Med* 195(3):295-308, 2002.

29. Kluft C: The fibrinolytic system and thrombotic tendency, *Pathophysiol Haemost Thromb* 33(5-6):425-429, 2003.

30. Stein PD et al: D-dimer for the exclusion of acute venous thrombosis and pulmonary embolism: a systematic review, *Ann Intern Med* 140(8):589-602, 2004.

31. Mauer AM: *Pediatric hematology,* New York, 1969, McGraw-Hill.

32. Manroe BL et al: The neonatal blood count in health and disease. I. Reference values for neutrophilic cells, *J Pediatr* 95(1):89-98, 1979.

33. de Sauvage FJ et al: Stimulation of megakaryocytopoiesis and thrombopoiesis by the c-mpl ligand, *Nature* 369(6481):533, 1994.

34. Ablin AR et al: Platelet enumeration in the neonatal period, *Pediatrics* 28:822-824, 1961.

35. Garry PJ, Hunt WC, Baumgartner RN: Effects of iron intake on iron stores in elderly men and women: longitudinal and cross-sectional results, *J Am Coll Nutr* 19(2):262-269, 2000.

36. McBane RD et al: Fibrinogen, fibrin, and crosslinking in aging arterial thrombi, *Thromb Haemost* 84(1):83, 2000.

37. Dejam A et al: Erythrocytes are the major intravascular storage sites of nitrite in human blood, *Blood (First Edition Paper),* March 17, 2005 [Epub ahead of print].

38. Pearson DA et al: Flavanols and platelet reactivity, *Clin Dev Immunol* 12(1):1-9, 2005.

39. Holt RR et al: Chocolate consumption and platelet function, *JAMA* 287(17):2212-2213, 2002.

40. Engler MB: Flavonoid-rich dark chocolate improves endothelial function and increases plasma epicatechin concentrations in health adults, *J Am Coll Nutr* 23(3):197-204, 2004.

41. de lange DW, van de Wiel A: Drink to prevent: review on the cardioprotective mechanisms of alcohol and red wine polyphenols, *Semin Vasc Med* 4(2):173-186, 2004.

42. Sato M, Maulik N, Das DK: Cardioprotection with alcohol: role of both alcohol and polyphenolic antioxidants, *Annals N Y Acad Sci* 957: 122-135, 2002.

43. Wang Z et al: Effects of red wine and wine polyphenol resveratol on platelet aggregation in vivo and in vitro, *Int J Mol Med* 9(1):77-79, 2002.

ALTERATIONS OF ERYTHROCYTE FUNCTION

CHAPTER

26

THOM J. MANSEN • KATHRYN L. McCANCE

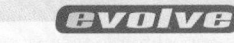

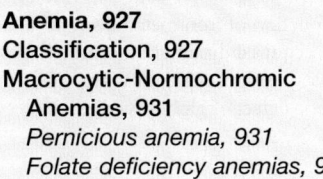lterations of erythrocyte function involve either insufficient or excessive numbers of erythrocytes in the circulation or normal numbers of cells with abnormal components. Anemias are conditions in which there are too few erythrocytes or an insufficient volume of erythrocytes in the blood. Polycythemias are conditions in which erythrocyte numbers or volume is excessive. Each of these two conditions has many causes, and in turn each is known by many names. Anemia and polycythemia are not diseases per se but rather are pathophysiologic manifestations of a variety of disease states.

ANEMIA

Strictly speaking, **anemia** is a reduction in the total number of erythrocytes in the circulating blood or a decrease in the quality or quantity of hemoglobin. Anemias commonly result from (1) impaired erythrocyte production, (2) blood loss (acute or chronic), (3) increased erythrocyte destruction, or (4) a combination of these three.

Classification

Anemias are classified in two ways, according to their etiology or to their morphology (Box 26-1). Morphologic classification is based on two cellular characteristics: size and hemoglobin content. Therefore, morphologic classification is most commonly used (Table 26-1). Cellular size is identified by terms that end in "cytic," whereas hemoglobin content is identified by terms that end in "chromic" (Table 26-2). Additional descriptions of erythrocytes associated with some ane-

Box 26-1	Etiologic (Pathophysiologic) Classification of Anemias

Decreased or Defective Production of Erythrocytes
Altered hemoglobin synthesis
  Iron deficiency
  Thalassemia
  Anemia of chronic inflammation
Altered deoxyribonucleic acid (DNA) synthesis resulting from deficient nutrients
  Pernicious anemia (decreased B_{12}, folate)
Stem cell dysfunction
  Aplastic anemia
  Myeloproliferative leukemia
Bone marrow infiltration
  Carcinoma
  Lymphoma
Pure red cell aplasia

Increased Erythrocyte Destruction
Blood loss
  Acute—hemorrhage, trauma
  Chronic—gastrointestinal bleeding, menorrhagia
Hemolysis (intracorpuscular defect)
  Membrane—hereditary spherocytosis
  Hemoglobin—sickle cell trait or disease
  Glycolysis—pyruvate kinase
  Oxidation—glucose-6-phosphate dehydrogenase (G6PD) deficiency
Hemolysis (extracorpuscular defect)
  Immune mechanisms—warm antibody/cold antibody
  Infection—clostridial, malarial
  Trauma to erythrocyte—hemolytic uremic syndrome
  Splenic sequestration—hypersplenism

Table 26-1	Morphologic Classification of Anemias	
Morphology and Cause of Reduced Oxygen-Carrying Capacity of the Blood	**Name and Mechanism of Anemic Condition**	**Primary Cause of Associated Disorder**
Macrocytic-normochromic anemia: large, abnormally shaped erythrocytes but normal hemoglobin concentrations	Pernicious anemia: lack of vitamin B_{12} (cobalamin) for erythropoiesis; abnormal deoxyribonucleic acid (DNA) and ribonucleic acid (RNA) synthesis in the erythroblast; premature cell death	Congenital or acquired deficiency of intrinsic factor (IF); genetic disorder of DNA synthesis
	Folate deficiency anemia: lack of folate for erythropoiesis; premature cell death	Dietary folate deficiency
Microcytic-hypochromic anemia: small, abnormally shaped erythrocytes and reduced hemoglobin concentration	Iron deficiency anemia: lack of iron for hemoglobin production; insufficient hemoglobin	Chronic blood loss; dietary iron deficiency, disruption of iron metabolism or iron cycle (see Chapter 25)
	Sideroblastic anemia: dysfunctional iron uptake by erythroblasts and defective porphyrin and heme synthesis	Congenital dysfunction of iron metabolism in erythroblasts, acquired dysfunction of iron metabolism as a result of drugs or toxins
	Thalassemia: impaired synthesis of alpha or beta chain of hemoglobin A; phagocytosis of abnormal erythroblasts in the marrow	Congenital genetic defect of globin synthesis
Normocytic-normochromic anemia: destruction or depletion of normal erythroblasts or mature erythrocytes	Aplastic anemia: insufficient erythropoiesis	Depressed stem cell proliferation resulting in bone marrow aplasia
	Posthemorrhagic anemia: blood loss	Acute or chronic hemorrhage that stimulates increased erythropoiesis, which eventually depletes body iron
	Hemolytic anemia: premature destruction (lysis) of mature erythrocytes in the circulation	Any condition that increases fragility of erythrocytes
	Sickle cell anemia: abnormal hemoglobin synthesis, abnormal cell shape with susceptibility to damage, lysis, and phagocytosis	Congenital dysfunction of hemoglobin synthesis
	Anemia of chronic disease: abnormally increased demand for new erythrocytes	Chronic infection or inflammation; malignancy

Table 26-2	Terms Used in Assessment of Erythrocytes	
	Erythrocyte Volume	**Hemoglobin Content**
Normal	Normocytic	Normochromic
Increased	Macrocytic (higher mean corpuscular volume [MCV])	Hyperchromic (higher mean corpuscular hemoglobin concentration [MCHC])
Decreased	Microcytic (lower MCV)	Hypochromic (lower MCHC)

mias include **anisocytosis** (assuming various sizes) or **poikilocytosis** (assuming various shapes) (Figure 26-1).

CLINICAL MANIFESTATIONS The major physiologic manifestation of anemia is a reduced oxygen-carrying capacity of the blood, which produces tissue hypoxia. Symptoms of anemia vary in severity and number depending on the body's ability to compensate for hypoxia (Figure 26-2). Previous reasoning suggested that individuals would adapt to low hemoglobin levels if anemia developed gradually, so-called *asymptomatic anemia*. However, asymptomatic still represents impairments in physical condition, quality of life, and cogni-

tive functions not recognized by individuals and health care providers.[1] As the reduction in red blood cells (RBCs) continues, symptoms become more evident and alterations of specific organs and compensatory manifestations become more apparent. Compensation for anemias is primarily executed by the cardiovascular, respiratory, and hematologic systems. Hematologic findings associated with various anemias are listed in Table 26-3 on p. 938 and progression and manifestations of anemias are shown in Figure 26-2.

The initial manifestations of anemia are apparent in the cardiovascular system. With hemorrhage, a reduction in the number of RBCs results in reduced blood volume. Compensation for a reduced blood volume causes fluids to move from the interstitium into the intravascular space (osmotic gradient), expanding plasma volume. This compensatory mechanism maintains adequate blood volume, increasing venous return, preload, and stroke volume, but the viscosity (thickness) decreases causing the blood to become diluted. The diluted blood flows faster and more turbulently than normal blood.

Hypoxia further contributes to cardiovascular alterations by causing systemic arterial dilation leading to decreased vascular resistance, which effectively reduces afterload. Additionally, anemia activates the sympathetic nervous system causing the heart rate to increase.

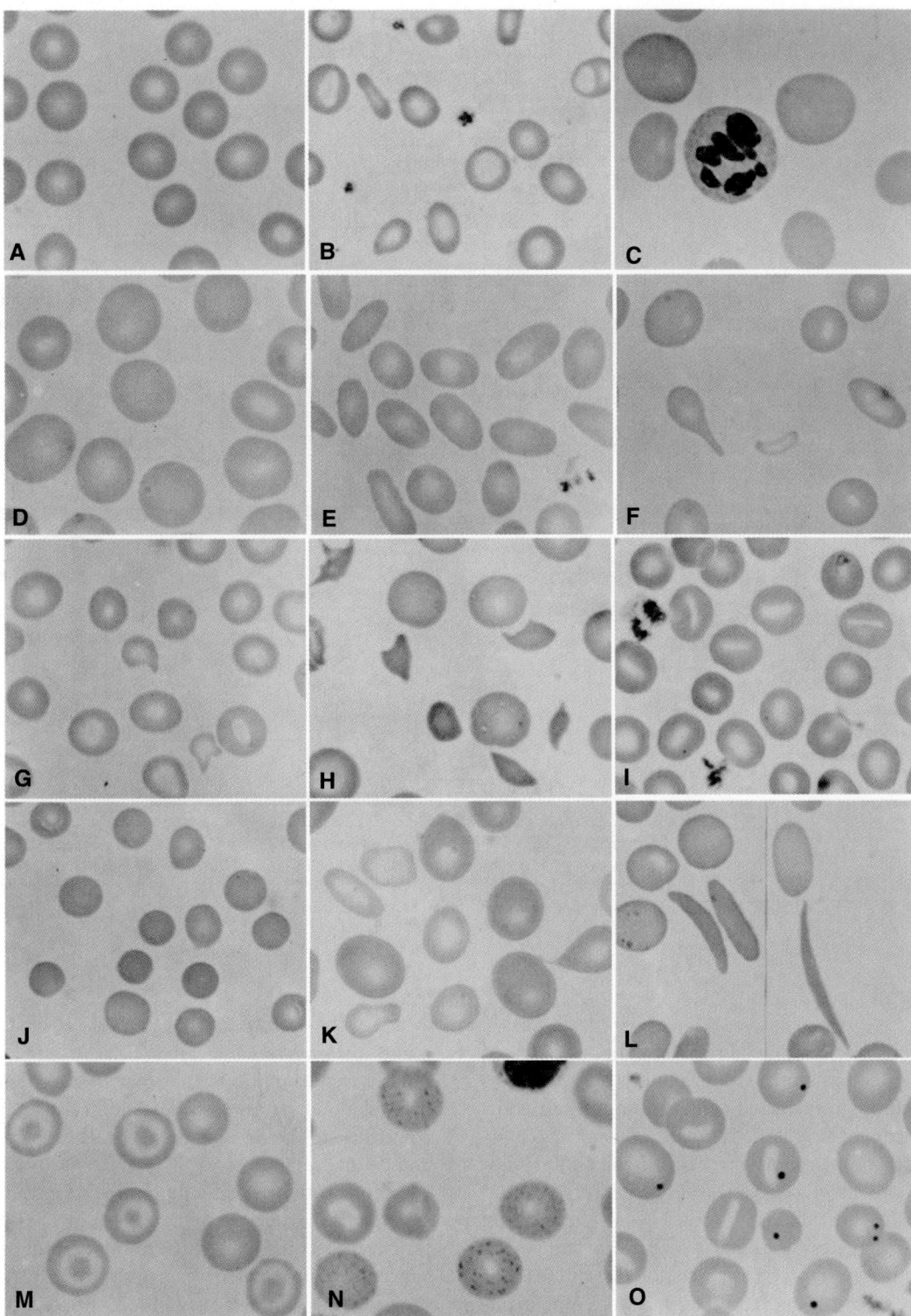

Figure 26-1 **Appearance of red blood cells in various disorders. A,** Normal blood smear. **B,** Hypochromic-microcytic anemia (iron deficiency). **C,** Macrocytic anemia (pernicious anemia). **D,** Macrocytic anemia in pregnancy. **E,** Hereditary elliptocytosis. **F,** Myelofibrosis (teardrop). **G,** Hemolytic anemia associated with prosthetic heart valve. **H,** Microangiopathic anemia. **I,** Stomatocytes. **J,** Spherocytes (hereditary spherocytosis). **K,** Sideroblastic anemia; note the double population of red blood cells. **L,** Sickle cell anemia. **M,** Target cells (after splenectomy). **N,** Basophil stippling in case of unexplained anemia. **O,** Howell-Jolly bodies (after splenectomy). (From Wintrobe MM et al: *Clinical hematology,* ed 8, Philadelphia, 1981, Lea & Febiger.)

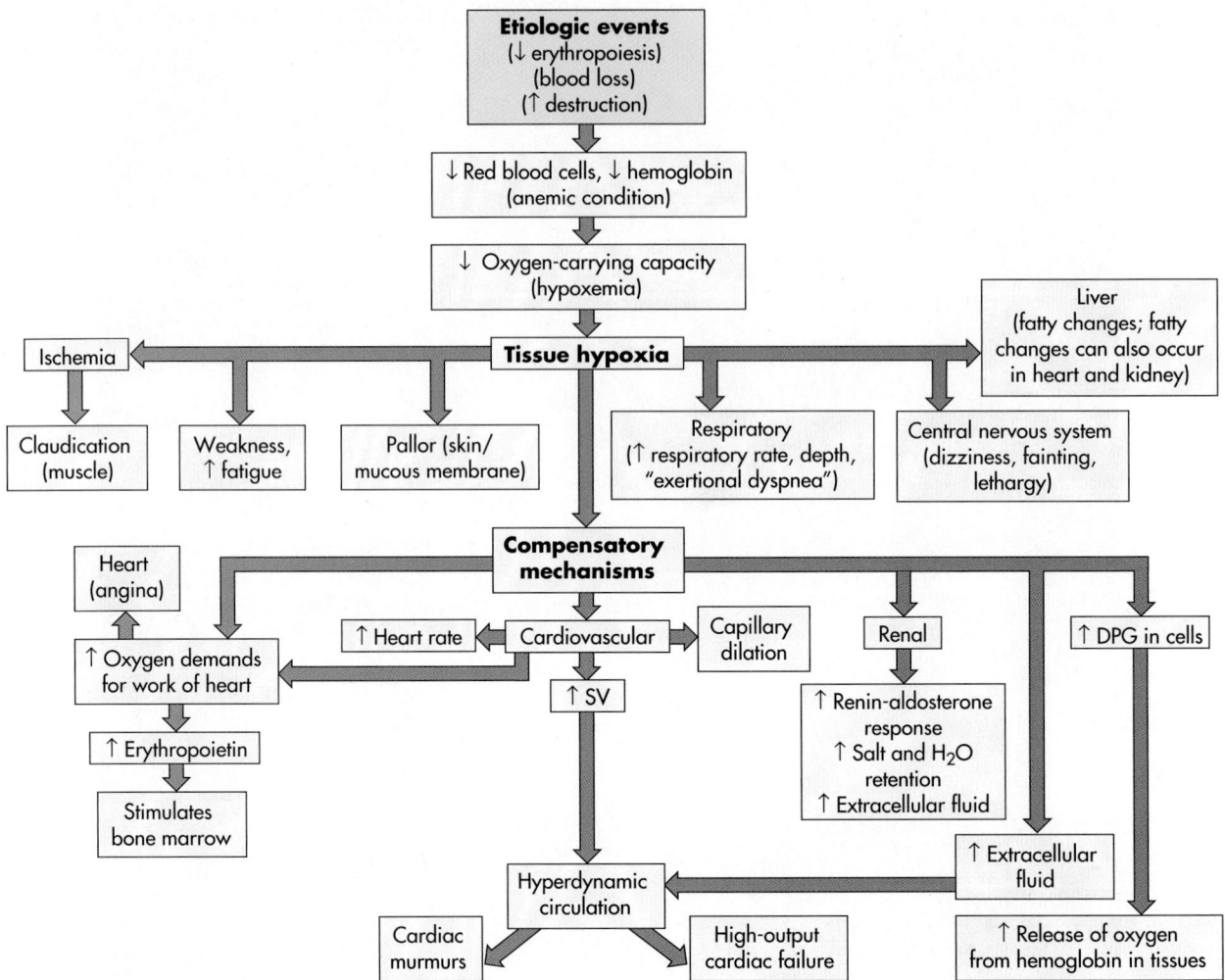

Figure 26-2 Progression and manifestations of anemia. *SV,* Stroke volume; *DPG,* diphosphatidylglycerol.

The result of these hemodynamic alterations—increased preload, heart rate, and stroke volume, and a reduced afterload—all contribute to increased cardiac output in an effort to maintain adequate oxygen delivery. Without timely interventions, cardiac compensatory mechanisms fail and precipitate the development of congestive heart failure.[2] (Mechanisms of congestive heart failure are described in Chapter 30.)

Tissue hypoxia creates additional demands and compensatory actions on the pulmonary and hematologic systems. The rate and depth of breathing increases in an attempt to increase the availability of oxygen. These demands are accompanied by an increase in the release of oxygen from hemoglobin because of an increase in diphosphatidylglycerol (DPG) in the erythrocytes.[2] (Mechanisms of oxygen transport and release by hemoglobin are described in Chapter 32.) When compensatory mechanisms fail, shortness of breath (dyspnea), a rapid, pounding heartbeat (palpitations), dizziness, and fatigue even at rest are evident. In mild, chronic conditions, these symptoms might be experienced only when de-

mand for oxygen is increased (i.e., during physical exertion) but in severe conditions, they may be experienced at rest. Decreased blood supply to skeletal and cardiac muscle also may contribute to the development of muscle pain (claudication) and cardiac angina.

Manifestations of anemia may be observed in other organ systems. Skin, mucous membranes, lips, nail beds, and conjunctivae become pale as a result of reduced hemoglobin concentration. If anemia is caused by RBC destruction (hemolysis), the skin also may become yellowish because of accumulation of the products of hemolysis. Tissue hypoxia also affects the skin causing impaired healing and loss of elasticity, as well as thinning and early graying of the hair.

Anemia caused by a vitamin B_{12} deficiency can affect the nervous system. Myelin degeneration may occur with the resultant loss of fibers in the spinal cord producing paresthesias (numbness), gait disturbances, extreme weakness, spasticity, and reflex abnormalities. Decreased oxygen supply to the gastrointestinal (GI) tract often produces abdominal pain, nausea, vomiting, and anorexia. A low-grade fever (less than 101° F) occurs in some anemic individuals and may be the result of leukocyte pyrogens released from ischemic tissues.

When the anemia is severe or rapid in onset (i.e., hemorrhage), peripheral blood vessels constrict diverting blood flow to vital organs. Decreased blood flow detected by the kidneys activates the renal renin-angiotensin response. This life-saving maneuver causes vasoconstriction and increases salt and water retention to increase blood volume and improve kidney perfusion. Situations such as this are emergencies and require immediate intervention to correct the underlying problem causing the acute blood loss; consequently, long-term compensatory mechanisms do not develop.

Treatment for an anemic condition requires identification and resolution of the underlying disorder and palliation of symptoms. Therapeutic interventions include control of bleeding, transfusions, dietary correction, and administration of supplemental vitamins or iron.

Macrocytic-Normochromic Anemias

The **macrocytic anemias,** also termed **megaloblastic anemias,** are characterized by defective DNA synthesis that results in ineffective erythropoiesis manifested by unusually large stem cells (megaloblasts) in the marrow that mature into unusually large stem cells (macrocytes) in the circulation. In addition to an increase in size (diameter), the thickness and volume of the cell also increase.[3,4] Defective DNA synthesis is caused by deficiencies of vitamin B_{12} (cobalamin) or folate, coenzymes that are required for nuclear maturation and the DNA synthesis pathway. Vitamin B_{12} deficiency is present in less than 20% of elderly persons but often goes unrecognized because of the subtle nature of manifestations that are potentially serious, particularly hematologically and neurologically.

In spite of defective DNA synthesis in megaloblasts, ribonucleic acid (RNA)–controlled processes (RNA replication and hemoglobin synthesis) occur at a normal rate, resulting in the unequal growth and development of the cytoplasm and nucleus. Asynchronous cytoplasmic and nuclear development produces megaloblastic stem cells that are larger than normal stem cells (normoblasts) and contain a nucleus that is immature and disproportionately small when compared to the size of the normal RBC. Each cell division causes the disproportion between RNA and DNA to become more obvious.

As the megaloblastic cell matures and begins to synthesize hemoglobin, chromatin in the nucleus fails to clump normally, resulting in finely distributed chromatin throughout the nucleus. This altered pattern of chromatin deposition allows for differentiation of normoblasts from megaloblasts. Hemoglobin increases in proportion to the size of the cell; thus the mean corpuscular hemoglobin concentration (MCHC) remains normal and the megaloblastic anemias, in the absence of complications, are normochromic.[4]

Ineffective erythropoiesis also contributes to premature cell death of all cell lines within the bone marrow. Immature precursors of the megaloblastic RBCs, white blood cells

(WBCs), and probably platelets have a greater chance of dying during maturation than do normoblastic precursors. Phagocytosis of these cells occurs within the bone marrow; thus a reduction of reticulocytes and erythrocytes occurs, further contributing to the anemia. Additionally there is an increase in lactic dehydrogenase, reflecting cellular destruction, and indirect bilirubin, from the breakdown of heme. Both of these substances may be measured in the blood, providing biochemical evidence of ineffective erythropoiesis.[3]

Defective DNA synthesis also may affect the white cells (neutrophils) causing them to demonstrate significant enlargement (giant metamyelocytes) with a tendency to have more nuclear lobes than normal.[3] Other cells throughout the body also may demonstrate enlargement and nuclear abnormalities. Cells lining epithelium and those with high turnover rates are most affected.

Pernicious Anemia

Pernicious anemia (PA), the most common type of megaloblastic anemia, is caused by vitamin B_{12} deficiency, which is often associated with the end stage of type A chronic atrophic (autoimmune) gastritis[5] (Figures 26-1, *C,* and 26-3). *Pernicious* means highly injurious or destructive and reflects the fact that this condition was once fatal. PA is generally considered a condition of the elderly, predominantly occurring in those over 60 years of age. It also is more common in females than males and those of Northern European descent. Blacks and Hispanics also demonstrate a tendency toward PA, with an earlier onset occurring in black females.[3]

PATHOPHYSIOLOGY   The principle disorder in PA is an absence of **intrinsic factor (IF),** an enzyme required for absorption of dietary vitamin B_{12}. Vitamin B_{12} catalyzes the ac-

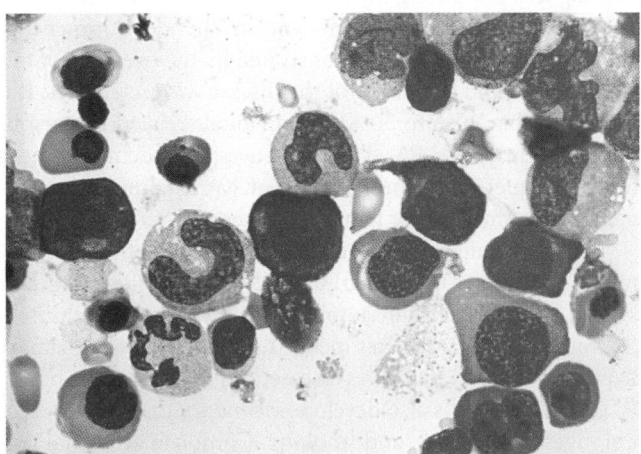

Figure 26-3 Bone marrow aspirate from individual with pernicious anemia. Bone marrow aspirate smear from an individual with megaloblastic red blood cell precursors and giant metamyelocytes. The chromatin in the red blood cell nuclei is more dispersed than in normal red blood cell precursors at comparable stages of maturation; the giant metamyelocytes have dispersed nuclear chromatin in contrast to a normal metamyelocyte, which has condensed chromatin (Wright-Giemsa stain). (From Damjanov I, Linder J, editors: *Anderson's pathology,* ed 10, St Louis, 1996, Mosby.)

tion of methionine synthase and R-methylmalonyl-CoA mutase,[6] which acts to promote nuclear maturation and DNA synthesis in erythrocytes. IF, along with hydrochloric acid, is secreted by gastric parietal cells. Deficiency in IF secretion may be congenital or result from adult onset gastric mucosal atrophy, which causes destruction of parietal cells. Congenital IF deficiency is a genetic disorder that demonstrates an autosomal recessive inheritance pattern.[7] Gastric atrophy commonly occurs in the presence of type A chronic gastritis. Autoimmunity plays a significant role in the development of this condition because of autoantibodies to gastric parietal cells that are present in the serum and gastric juice. The antigen recognized by chronic gastric autoantibodies has been identified as H^+/K^+ ATPase, an enzyme responsible for secretion of hydrogen ions by parietal cells in exchange for potassium ions.[8] Other characteristics associated with chronic gastric atrophy include achlorhydria, low serum levels of pepsinogen I, hypergastrinemia, and gastric carcinoids.

Early manifestations of atrophic gastritis lesions begin with chronic infiltration of the gastric submucosa with inflammatory cells; eventually extending into the lamina propria causing degeneration of the parietal and zymogenic cells. Late in the course of the disease, the parietal and zymogenic cells are destroyed and replaced by mucus-containing cells (intestinal metaplasia). The mechanism of cellular destruction in autoimmune gastritis is unknown, but it is thought to involve signaling through death-inducing pathways (e.g., Fas/FasL[Fas ligand] and TNF/TFNR [tumor necrosis factor/tumor necrosis factor receptor] pathways).[9] Loss of parietal cells results in IF deficiency, the major factor in the development of vitamin B_{12} deficiency and PA. A direct correlation exists between the severity of the gastric lesion and the degree of malabsorption of vitamin B_{12}. Contributing further to malabsorption, autoantibodies present in gastric juice bind with vitamin B_{12} at its IF binding site, preventing the formation of the B_{12}/IF complex.

Genetic factors are significant in the development of chronic gastritis and PA demonstrated by the presence of autoantibodies and clustering of the disease within families. It is estimated that 20% to 30% of individuals related to persons with PA also have PA. These relatives also demonstrate a higher frequency of the presence of gastric autoantibodies, particularly first-degree female relatives.

Pernicious anemia also is associated with other autoimmune conditions, particularly those affecting the endocrine system, including chronic autoimmune thyroiditis (Hashimoto thyroiditis), type 1 diabetes mellitus, Addison disease, primary hypoparathyroidism, Graves disease, and myasthenia gravis.[5]

Chronic gastritis also develops secondary to excessive alcohol ingestion, hot tea, and smoking. Complete or partial gastrectomy also causes IF deficiency. Helicobacter pylori (H. pylori) has recently been identified as a causative agent in the development of vitamin B_{12} deficiency.[10] Drugs known as proton pump inhibitors (PPIs), used to decrease gastric acidity, also have been identified as a factor in decreasing cobalamin absorption; however, it is not thought that they actually cause PA.[11] Individuals with type A chronic gastritis PA are at risk for developing gastric adenocarcinoma of the non-cardia stomach from intestinal metaplasia and esophageal squamous cell carcinoma.[12] The incidence of carcinoma in these individuals is 2% to 3%. Type B gastritis is caused by H. pylori with a decreased risk for development of cancer.[13]

CLINICAL MANIFESTATIONS Pernicious anemia develops slowly—possibly from 20 to 30 years; 60 years of age is the median age at time of diagnosis. Because symptoms develop slowly, PA is usually severe by the time treatment is sought. Early symptoms are vague and often ignored and consist of infections, mood swings, and gastrointestinal, cardiac, or kidney ailments. When the hemoglobin has decreased significantly (7 to 8 g/dl), the classic symptoms of anemia—weakness, fatigue, paresthesias of the feet and fingers, and difficulty in walking—are experienced.

Neurologic manifestations result from nerve demyelination that may produce neuronal death. The posterior and lateral columns of the spinal cord also may be affected, causing a loss of position and vibration sense, ataxia, and spasticity. These complications pose a serious threat because they are not reversible, even with appropriate treatment. The cerebrum also may be involved with manifestations of affective disorders, most commonly of the depressive types.[14] An increased prevalence of serum vitamin B_{12} deficiency has been reported among individuals with Alzheimer disease.[15]

Additionally, the individual may experience a loss of appetite, abdominal pain, and a beefy red tongue caused by atrophic glossitis. The skin may become "lemon yellow" (sallow) as a result of a combination of pallor and icterus. The liver may be enlarged, especially in the elderly, indicating right-sided heart failure. The spleen also may enlarge but remains nonpalpable.

EVALUATION AND TREATMENT Diagnosis of PA is based on a variety of tests (see Table 26-3, p. 938), which include blood tests, bone marrow aspiration, serologic studies, gastric biopsy, clinical manifestations, and the Schilling test. The Schilling test indirectly evaluates vitamin B_{12} absorption by measuring the urinary excretion of vitamin B_{12}. Low urinary excretion is significant for PA. A second test often is done to confirm the diagnosis. In the second test, IF may be administered to see whether urinary excretion increases. If urinary excretion does not increase, other causes must be considered.[16]

Serologic studies, however, have replaced the Schilling test for diagnosing PA. Measuring methylmalonic acid and homocysteine levels, which are elevated early in PA, is a more sensitive test. Serologic testing also identifies the presence of parietal cells and intrinsic factor antibodies.[17] These antibodies also may be present in gastric juices. Gastric biopsy reveals total achlorhydria (absence of hydrochloric acid), which is diagnostic for PA because it occurs only in the presence of this gastric lesion.

Treatment is replacement of vitamin B_{12} (cobalamin). Cyanocobalamin or hydroxocobalamin (1000 mcg) is administered parenterally on a monthly schedule. Initial injections are administered weekly until the deficiency is corrected. Conventional wisdom and practice assumed that oral preparations were ineffective because there was no IF to facilitate absorption. Recent practice, however, has determined that oral administration is beneficial in dosages higher than parenteral dosages.[17] Vitamin B_{12} will pass across and be absorbed in the small bowel.[18]

The effectiveness of cobalamin replacement therapy is measured by a rising reticulocyte count. Within 5 to 6 weeks, blood counts return to normal. PA cannot be cured, so maintenance therapy is lifelong. Blood transfusions are given if the individual shows signs of circulatory collapse, heart failure, or severe angina pectoris.

Untreated PA is fatal, usually because of heart failure. Death occurs after a course of remissions and exacerbations lasting from 1 to 3 years. Since 1926, when replacement therapy began, mortality has been reduced significantly. Today, death from PA is rare and any relapses that occur are usually the result of noncompliance with therapy.

Folate Deficiency Anemia

Folate (folic acid) is an essential vitamin that is required for erythrocyte production and maturation. Humans totally depend on dietary intake of folate, requiring 50 to 200 mcg/day, with pregnant and lactating females requiring increased amounts. Folate synthesis takes place in the human intestine, however, not in quantities sufficient to make any significant contribution.[19]

Absorption of folate occurs primarily in the upper small intestine and does not depend on the presence of any other facilitating factor. From the small intestine it is circulated to and through the liver where it is stored. Folate deficiency is more common than cobalamin deficiency and commonly is associated with alcoholism and other conditions that cause chronic malnourishment in individuals. Alcohol interferes with folate metabolism in the liver causing a profound depletion of folate stores.[20] Fad diets and diets low in vegetables are also causes of folate deficiency caused by the absence of plant sources of folate.[21] Folate deficiency, however, has been on the decrease in the United States since the fortification of food with folate and the increased use of folate supplements.[22]

The primary biochemical function of folate coenzymes involves the synthesis of purines and pyrimidines (thiamine, adenine, and guanine), which form the structural elements of DNA and RNA. DNA synthesis requires preformed thymidine monophosphate. In the absence of thymidine monophosphate, DNA is synthesized from deoxyuridine monophosphate, which is catalyzed by thymidylate synthetase and uses methylenetetrahydrofolate as the methyl donor. A folate deficiency results in impaired synthesis of thymidylate.[21] The clinical manifestations of folate deficiency become apparent when the synthesis of thymidylate is critically impaired and progresses to the development of megaloblastic anemia.[19]

PATHOPHYSIOLOGY   The mechanisms causing impaired DNA synthesis and destruction of hematopoietic cells in folate deficiency are not well understood. Apoptosis of erythroblasts in the late stages of differentiation is thought to occur.[23,24] In addition to anemia, folate deficiency is associated with neural tube defects of the fetus and heart disease, and also is implicated in the development of cancers, specifically colorectal cancers.[25]

CLINICAL MANIFESTATIONS   Clinical manifestations of folate deficiency anemia are similar to the cachectic, malnourished appearance characteristic of those with PA. Accompanying the wasted appearance is severe cheilosis (fissures of the lips and corners of the mouth), stomatitis, and painful ulcerations of the buccal mucosa and tongue. Gastrointestinal symptoms may be present and include dysphagia (difficulty swallowing), flatulence, and watery diarrhea. In addition, there may be histologic changes and roentgenographic presentations of the GI tract suggestive of the malabsorption syndrome, sprue.

Neurologic manifestations, such as those that occur in PA, are generally not seen in folate deficiency anemia. If they are present, another vitamin deficiency (e.g., thiamine deficiency, which often accompanies folate deficiency) is possibly the cause.

EVALUATION AND TREATMENT   Treatment for folate deficiency anemia requires daily oral administration of folate preparations. One milligram per day is sufficient for most individuals, although persons with alcoholism may require 5 mg. Prophylactic dosages of 0.1 to 0.4 mg/day are sometimes given during pregnancy. Parenteral administration of folic acid (citrovorum factor or leucovorin) generally is not used except in situations where an individual has been using drugs that inhibit dihydrofolate reductase.[22] After administration of folate, the manifestations of anemia disappear within 1 to 2 weeks.

After the folate deficiency has been corrected, long-term treatment with folate is not necessary if the appropriate dietary adjustments needed to maintain adequate intake are made. Increasing the intake of folate (400 mcg/day) is recommended as a measure to prevent heart disease because of its ability to reduce homocysteine, a risk factor for the development of atherosclerosis (see Chapter 30).

Microcytic-Hypochromic Anemias

The **microcytic-hypochromic anemias** are characterized by erythrocytes that are abnormally small and contain abnormally reduced amounts of hemoglobin (see Figure 26-1, *B*). Hypochromia occurs even in cells of normal size.

Microcytic-hypochromic anemia results from a wide variety of conditions that are related to (1) disorders of iron metabolism, (2) disorders of porphyrin and heme synthesis, or (3) disorders of globin synthesis. Specific disorders include iron deficiency anemia, sideroblastic anemia, and thalassemia.

Iron Deficiency Anemia

Iron deficiency anemia (IDA) is the most common type of anemia worldwide, occurring in developing and developed countries. It is estimated that one-fifth of the world population has iron deficiency.[26] Populations at risk for developing hypoferremia and IDA include those living in chronic poverty, women of childbearing age, and children. Iron deficiency in children is associated with numerous adverse health-related manifestations, specifically cognitive impairment, which may be irreversible. Recent research has identified that teens who had iron deficiency as infants are likely to score lower on cognitive and motor tests. These scores are found even if the iron deficiency was identified and treated in infancy.[27]

Children in developing countries often are affected by chronic parasite infestations that result in intestinal blood and iron loss that outpaces dietary intake.[28] Treatment of helminth infections results in an improvement in the anemia as well as in appetite and growth.[26] Iron deficiency also occurs in individuals with lead poisoning. Treatment of the iron deficiency is associated with a decrease in lead levels.[29] In the United States, 720,000 children (9%) aged 1 to 2 years are estimated to be iron deficient, of whom 240,000 (3%) are anemic.[30]

In the United States, females demonstrate a higher incidence of hypoferremia (13.9%) than do males (8.3%). The incidence of IDA is also higher in females (4% to 6%) than in males (4%). The incidence peaks in females during their reproductive years and decreases after menopause. Those at highest risk are African-American females living in urban poverty.[31] Males demonstrate a higher incidence during childhood and adolescence, with a decrease occurring during young adulthood and an upswing during late adulthood.[20] An increased prevalence of iron deficiency has been demonstrated in overweight children.[32] Children under 2 years are often affected because of their increasing requirement for iron associated with growth.

The most common cause of IDA in well-developed countries is pregnancy and chronic blood loss. Blood loss of 2 to 4 ml/day (1 to 2 mg of iron) is sufficient to cause iron deficiency and may result from erosive esophagitis, gastric and duodenal ulcers, colon adenomas, and cancers.[33] *H. pylori* infections also have been found to cause IDA and are associated with anemia of unknown origin.[34] *H. pylori* has been found to impair iron uptake.[35]

In females, menorrhagia (excessive bleeding during menstruation) is a common cause of primary IDA. Related causes of IDA are (1) medications that cause gastrointestinal bleeding (aspirin, nonsteroidal antiinflammatory drugs [NSAIDs]); (2) surgical procedures that decrease stomach acidity, intestinal transit time, and absorption; (3) insufficient dietary intake of iron; and (4) eating disorders, such as pica, which is the craving and eating of nonnutritional substances.

Iron is the essential component of hemoglobin and is in constant demand for use in normal erythropoiesis. Iron is recyclable, therefore the body maintains a balance between iron that is contained in hemoglobin and iron that is in storage and available for future hemoglobin synthesis.

Iron also is recognized as contributing to immune function by regulating immune effector mechanisms (i.e., cytokine activities [IFN-γ], nitric oxide formation, and T-cell proliferation).[36] Pathogen survival also is iron-dependent; thus hypoferremia has been hypothesized to be an adaptive response initiated to protect against infectious diseases; however, knowledge related to the precise interaction between iron deficiency and immunity is still controversial.[37] The pathogenesis of anemia is recognized as being part of the nonspecific acute phase response to any type of inflammation of sufficient degree.[38]

Iron metabolism is complex and not well understood. Sources of iron include a small portion absorbed from the duodenum and, to a lesser extent, from the stomach, ileum, and colon. A second source, and a much larger portion, becomes available through recycling of iron from senescent RBCs. Iron recycling is carried out by specialized reticuloendothelial macrophages that ingest aged erythrocytes, lyse them, and catabolize the hemoglobin.[39] Iron that is ingested or removed from destroyed blood cells is bound to the protein transferrin and transported in the plasma to storage sites in the liver, spleen, bone marrow, and skeletal muscle. Iron is stored as ferritin or hemosiderin.

PATHOPHYSIOLOGY Iron deficiency anemia can be classified as arising from one or two different etiologies or a combination of both. Nutritional iron deficiency is the first category and results from inadequate dietary intake or excessive blood loss. In both instances, there is no intrinsic dysfunction in iron metabolism; however, they both deplete iron stores and result in IDA caused by reduced hemoglobin synthesis. The second category is best described as a metabolic or functional iron deficiency in which various metabolic disorders lead to either insufficient iron delivery to bone marrow or impaired iron use within the marrow. Paradoxically, iron stores are sufficient, but iron delivery is inadequate to maintain heme synthesis, thus producing a functional or relative iron deficiency.[40]

Iron deficiency anemia is present when the demand for iron exceeds the supply, developing slowly through three overlapping stages. In stage I, the body's iron stores are depleted. Erythropoiesis proceeds normally with the hemoglobin content of RBCs remaining normal. In stage II, iron transportation to bone marrow is diminished resulting in iron deficiency erythropoiesis. Stage III begins when the small hemoglobin-deficient cells enter the circulation in sufficient numbers to replace the normal mature erythrocytes that have been removed from the circulation. Manifestations of IDA appears in stage III when iron stores are depleted and there is diminished hemoglobin production.[41]

CLINICAL MANIFESTATIONS Symptoms of IDA begin gradually, and individuals often do not seek medical attention until hemoglobin has decreased to a certain level (about 7 to 8 g/dl). Early symptoms include fatigue, weakness, and shortness of breath. Pale earlobes, palms, and conjunctivae (Figure 26-4) are also common signs.

Progression of IDA causes more severe alterations, with structural and functional changes apparent in epithelial tissue (see Figure 26-4). The nails become brittle, thin, coarsely ridged, and spoon-shaped or concave (koilonychia) as a result

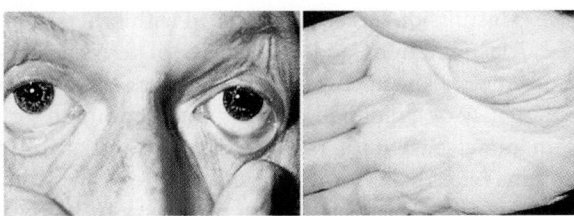

Figure 26-4 Pallor and iron deficiency. Pallor of the skin, mucous membranes, and palmar creases in an individual with hemoglobin of 9 g/dl. Palmar creases become as pale as the surrounding skin when the hemoglobin level approaches 7 g/dl. (Courtesy Hoffbrand AV, Pettit JE, editors: *Sandoz atlas of clinical hematology,* London, 1988, Gower Medical.)

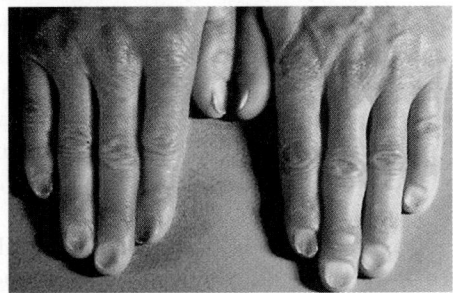

Figure 26-5 Koilonychia. The nails are concave, ridged, and brittle. (Courtesy Hoffbrand AV, Pettit JE, editors: *Sandoz atlas of clinical hematology,* London, 1988, Gower Medical.)

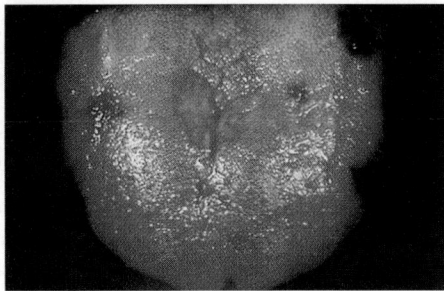

Figure 26-6 Glossitis. Tongue of individual with iron deficiency anemia has bald, fissured appearance caused by loss of papillae and flattening. (Courtesy Hoffbrand AV, Pettit JE, editors: *Sandoz atlas of clinical hematology,* London, 1988, Gower Medical.)

of impaired capillary circulation (Figure 26-5). The tongue becomes red, sore, and painful, which is caused by atrophy of the papillae (glossitis) (Figure 26-6). The degree of pain experienced is directly associated with the amount of iron deficiency.[42] Individuals also experience dryness and soreness in the epithelium at the corners of the mouth, known as *angular stomatitis.* Difficulty in swallowing is associated with an esophageal "web," a thin, concentric, smooth extension of normal esophageal tissue consisting of mucosa and submucosa at the juncture between the hypopharynx and esophagus. The association between IDA and web formation is questionable, fueled by the uncertainty in duration of iron deficiency required for web formation.[43] Dysphagia also is exacerbated by hyposalivation. The pathophysiology associated with these epithelial lesions is not well understood, but they are recognized as having the potential to become malignant. Recent studies also have documented that IDA is associated with malignancies, particularly of the GI tract.[44]

Iron also is a component of compounds other than hemoglobin (e.g., cytochromes, myoglobin, catalases, peroxidases). Nonheme iron is found in many important enzymes, particularly those involved in the metabolism of amine neurotransmitters, reduction of nucleotides, and biosynthesis of methionine. Abnormalities and deficiencies of iron-dependent enzymes may account for many of the clinical manifestations of IDA.[41] Individuals with IDA also exhibit gastritis, neuromuscular alterations, irritability, headache, numbness, tingling, and vasomotor disturbances. The pathogenesis of neurologic symptoms is unknown but may be caused by hypoxia in already compromised cerebral vessels. Gait disturbances are rare. Mental confusion, memory loss, and disorientation often are associated with anemia in the elderly population and may be wrongly perceived as "normal" events related to aging.

EVALUATION AND TREATMENT Initial evaluation is based on the presence of a decreased hemoglobin and hematocrit. Additional measurements, however, are needed to make the diagnosis (see Table 26-3, p. 938). Iron stores may be measured directly by bone marrow biopsy and iron staining. Indirect tests measure serum ferritin, transferrin saturation, or total iron-binding capacity. Serum ferritin is a widely accepted and available measurement of iron status that has been used for the past 25 years; 1 mcg/L serum ferritin corresponds to 8 to 10 mg or 120 mcg of storage iron/kg body weight.[45] The serum ferritin level has demonstrated its superiority over other measures (i.e., mean corpuscular volume [MCV], transferrin saturation). One limit to the serum ferritin is the elevation of values independent of iron status that accompanies acute or chronic inflammation, malignancy, liver disease, or alcoholism.

A more recent indicator of iron levels is the serum transferrin receptor (sTfR). Transferrin receptors are membrane glycoproteins that function as the entrance point to cells for circulating transferrin. Using the ratio of serum transferrin receptor to serum ferritin (R/F), estimation of body iron stores is becoming more reliable and accurate. A major drawback to the use of sTfR is the lack of proper standardization for the sTfR assay. A major advantage to using sTfR is that it allows for the differentiation of IDA as a primary condition or a condition occurring in the presence of anemia or chronic disease. Additionally, it is capable of identifying IDA when it occurs in the presence of anemia related to chronic disease.[45,46]

The first step in treatment of IDA is to identify and eliminate, or rule out, sources of blood loss. Without this strategy, any pharmacologic therapy is likely to be ineffective. Iron replacement therapy is very effective in the treatment of nutritional deficient anemia. In fact, the most conclusive evidence for the diagnosis of IDA is an increase in hemoglobin of 1 to 2 g/dl after iron therapy is initiated. Iron is available in ferrous or ferric forms; however, ferrous is preferable because it is more readily absorbed. The ferrous form is available as sulfate, gluconate, or fumarate. The sulfate form is the cheapest and most commonly used.[47]

Initial iron replacement therapy is 150 to 200 mg/day; however, recent studies have found that dosages as low as 60 mg/day are effective in certain individuals.[48] Once therapy has begun, individuals demonstrate a rapid decrease in fatigue, lethargy, and other associated symptoms. Hematocrit levels should improve within 1 to 2 months of therapy; however, the serum ferritin level is a more precise measurement of improvement and total body stores of iron. Once the serum ferritin level reaches 50 mcg/L, adequate replacement of iron has occurred.[48] Replacement therapy is usually continued for 3 to 6 months after bleeding has been contained; however, therapy may continue for as long as 24 months. Daily therapy (325 mg/day) for menstruating females may be required until menopause.

Parenteral iron therapy is used in instances of uncontrolled blood loss, intolerance to oral iron, intestinal malabsorption, and poor adherence to oral therapy.[49] Iron dextran has been the only parenteral agent available in the United States. Intramuscular injection is the recommended method; however, intravenous administration is generally preferred because of the ability to administer larger doses. A significant concern in the use of IV dextran is the potential for severe anaphylactic reaction. Delayed reaction is also a major concern.[45]

Newer medications that have recently been approved for parenteral therapy in treating IDA are sodium ferric gluconate complex in sucrose (Ferriecit) and iron sucrose injection (Venofer). Iron dextran is recommended as the first choice in spite of its higher rate of adverse reactions. For individuals who are intolerant of iron dextran, the two newer agents are safe and effective alternatives. Drawbacks to their use include higher cost and the need for multiple infusions.[49]

Sideroblastic Anemia

Sideroblastic anemias (SAs) are a heterogenous group of disorders characterized by anemia of varying severity caused by a deviation in mitochondrial metabolism.[50] Altered mitochondrial metabolism causes ineffective iron uptake resulting in dysfunctional hemoglobin synthesis. Ringed sideroblasts within the bone marrow are diagnostic of SA. **Ringed sideroblasts** are erythroblasts that contain iron granules that have not been synthesized into hemoglobin, but instead are distributed in a perinuclear collar arrangement around one third or more of the nucleus (see Figure 26-1, *K*). Individuals with SA also have increased tissue levels of iron.

PATHOPHYSIOLOGY SAs have multiple etiologies; however, they share the commonality of altered heme synthesis in the erythroid cells in bone marrow. SAs are either hereditary or acquired.

Hereditary SAs occur almost exclusively in males, supporting a recessive X-linked transmission; however, autosomal re-

cessive transmission has been associated with genetic and mitochondrial mutations and deficiencies of ferrochelatase in both genders.[51] The anemia in all conditions is usually present in infancy or childhood, but it is not uncommon for it to remain undetected until midlife. In some instances, other symptoms (e.g., diabetes or cardiac failure resulting from tissue iron overload) may be the first manifestation of SA. Differentiation of SA from idiopathic hemachromatosis needs to be confirmed because both are characterized by tissue iron deposition.

The severity of the anemia is quite variable; even when there is little to no anemia present, qualitative alterations of the erythrocytes (e.g., decreased MCV and increased RBC volume distribution width) may be evident.[51] **Dimorphism,** in which both normocytic and normochromic cells are seen concomitantly with microcytic-hypochromic cells, may be present and is seen more commonly in individuals with mild anemia, female carriers, or those receiving treatment with pyridoxine. Anisocytosis and poikilocytosis also are seen on examination of the blood smear.

Hereditary SA (X-linked sideroblastic anemia [XLSA]) has been linked to missense mutations in the erythroid-specific aminolevulinic acid (ALA) synthase (ALAS-E) gene *Xp11.21*. Currently more than 25 missense mutations are recognized to cause decreased ALAS activity.[52] ALAS is the first and rate-limiting enzyme used in the heme biosynthesis pathway. ALAS uses pyridoxal phosphates as cofactors for the synthesis of protoporphyrin IX. Protoporphyrin IX is normally combined with iron to produce heme. Reduction in the synthesis of protoporphyrin IX results in the characteristic accumulation of iron in the erythrocyte.

Acquired idiopathic sideroblastic anemias (AISAs) represent the greatest incidence of SAs, with drugs and toxins being the leading cause.[50] The next largest subgroup of AISAs are conditions that can be categorized as myelodysplastic syndrome. **Myelodysplastic syndrome (MDS)** is a group of disorders that demonstrate hematopoietic stem cell dysfunction. All three stem cell lines demonstrate dysplastic characteristics. Initially, AISA associated with MDS was considered to be one in the same and was identified as refractory anemia with ringed sideroblasts (RARS). This classification proved unsatisfactory because different outcomes were observed in individuals. Further investigations discovered morphologic and chromosomal characteristics that predicted different clinical courses. Two different subsets of myelodysplastic ringed sideroblasts were identified based on which cell line was affected. One subset demonstrates dysplastic features of the erythroid line classified as pure sideroblastic anemia (PSA) making anemia the dominant manifestation in PSA. Individuals with PSA require transfusions, which may produce iron overload, but with adequate chelation therapy, they are able to survive and thrive for many years. A significant outcome of this condition is the rare occurrence of conversion to leukemia.

The second group demonstrates abnormalities of all three cell lines in addition to ringed sideroblasts. In addition to anemia, neutrophil and platelet alterations are the dominant problems. Infections are common and often are the cause of death due to neutropenia and neutrophil dysfunction. Bleeding from thrombocytopenia and platelet dysfunction also are prevalent. Of those who survive, 40% develop acute (myeloblastic) leukemia.

The ineffective erythropoiesis characteristic of AISAs results in a paradox—anemia in the presence of increased blood cells. Bone marrow hyperplasia results from increased proliferation of erythroid progenitors and precursors to compensate for reduced peripheral blood cell counts and anemia. The anemic condition is hypothesized as being caused by increased intramedullary stem cell apoptosis.[53] Apoptosis may occur because of disruption of the mitochondrial membrane potential or an increase in caspase activation (enzymes that play an active role in apoptosis, see Chapter 2).

Disruptions to the mitochondria that contribute to development of AISA appear to be related to alterations in mitochondrial iron metabolism. The actual mechanisms of mitochondrial iron metabolism are still poorly understood;[54] however, mitochondrial damage is known to be caused by iron not converted (reduced) from the ferric form (Fe^{+3}) to the ferrous form (Fe^{++}). Iron is stored as ferric but requires conversion to ferrous by ferrochelatase for use in heme synthesis. The electrons required for conversion are provided by the mitochondrial electron chain present on the mitochondrial DNA (mDNA) located near the inner mitochondrial membrane, making it vulnerable to damage by oxygen-free radicals generated by the respiratory chain. This disrupted electron chain transport is caused by the decline of mitochondrial membrane potential ($\Delta\psi_m$). Total collapse of $\Delta\psi_m$ is apparently an explicit marker for apoptosis.[55]

The most prevalent causes of AISA are caused by toxins that are often associated with alcoholism, drugs, nutritional deficiencies, and hypothermia. Anemia resulting from these causes is also considered reversible. Alcohol-induced AISA is uncommon, however, the use and abuse of alcohol is pervasive. Alcohol impairs the synthesis of heme by direct antagonism of pyridoxal 5'-phosphate (PLP), which is required for ALA synthase synthesis. Alcohol also produces inhibitory effects at several steps throughout the heme biosynthetic pathway. Alcohol or acetylaldehyde, or both, also inhibits protein synthesis within hepatic mitochondria. Folate deficiency often accompanies alcoholism, which also reduces the availability of PLP, further contributing to impaired heme synthesis.[51]

Specific drugs causing AISA include antituberculosis agents (isoniazid [INH], pyrazinamide, and cycloserine) and chloramphenicol. Antituberculous agents interfere with vitamin B_6 metabolism, which reduces ALA synthesis, thus decreasing heme generation. Chloramphenicol causes direct mitochondrial injury by inhibiting mitochondrial membrane proteins and thus mitochondrial respiration. Additionally, therapeutic drug levels are known to inhibit erythroid colony growth but not granulocyte colony growth.[51]

Nutritional deficiencies causing AISA are related to folate and copper (discussed previously). Copper deficiency in humans as a cause of AISA is extremely rare and is associated with gastrectomy, prolonged parenteral nutrition without additional copper supplements, and excessive chelation therapy. Copper deficiency is thought to interfere with conversion of ferric iron to ferrous iron. Hypothermia may be a contributing factor because it causes diminished heme synthesis and incorporation of iron into hemoglobin.

CLINICAL MANIFESTATIONS The anemias of SA are generally moderate to severe with hemoglobin levels varying from 4 to 10 g/dl. In addition to the cardiovascular and respiratory manifestations common to all anemias, individuals with SA demonstrate signs of iron overload known as **erythropoietic hemochromatosis.**[51] Mild to moderate enlargement of the spleen (splenomegaly) and liver (hepatomegaly) occur; however, liver function remains normal or only slightly impaired. Occasionally abnormal skin pigmentation (bronze colored) is seen. Neurologic and epithelial alterations commonly associated with anemias are nonexistent. Heart rhythm disturbances, along with congestive heart failure, are major life-threatening complications related to cardiac iron overload. These manifestations are fortunately rare and occur late in the progression of the disease. Young children and infants who are severely affected may demonstrate growth and developmental impairment.

EVALUATION AND TREATMENT Initially, SA may be mistaken for deficiency of stem cells in the marrow (**hypoplastic anemia**) or iron deficiency anemia. (Laboratory findings are listed in Table 26-3). Bone marrow examination establishes the diagnosis. The marrow is packed with erythrocyte stem cells, and mononuclear phagocytes in the marrow are loaded with iron in the form of hemosiderin. Platelet and leukocyte values are generally normal; however, they may be reduced if splenomegaly is evident. The presence of sideroblasts confirms the diagnosis of SA.

Initial treatment of SA is directed toward identification of a causative agent (i.e., drugs or toxins). Treatment is supportive, with transfusions being the primary intervention. Following removal of the agent, oral pyridoxine (100 mg/day) may be administered on a trial basis. Acquired SAs related to alcohol abuse and pyridoxine antagonists often demonstrate a complete response to pyridoxine. SAs caused by other etiologies do not demonstrate the same improvement.

Individuals with hereditary X-linked SA also are initially treated with pyridoxine therapy in doses of 50 to 200 mg/day. Approximately one third of individuals with hereditary SA respond to this therapy. An optimal response is related to reticulocytosis with blood hemoglobin levels returning to normal within 1 to 2 months and low free erythrocyte protoporphyrin (FEP) levels also returning to normal. Morphologic abnormalities of cells (microcytosis), however, do not disappear, even in the presence of normal ALA synthetase activity and hemoglobin. A less than optimal response also may be seen in which hemoglobin levels are elevated but stabilize at less than normal levels. When a response to pyridoxine ther-

| Table 26-3 | Laboratory Findings for Various Anemias | | | | | | | |

Test	Pernicious Anemia	Folate Deficiency Anemia	Iron Deficiency Anemia	Sideroblastic Anemia	Aplastic Anemia	Posthemorrhagic Anemia	Hemolytic Anemia	Anemia of Chronic Disease
Hemoglobin	Low	Low	Low	Low	Low or normal	Normal or low	Low	Low
Hematocrit	Low	Low	Low	Low	Low or normal	Normal or low	Low	Low
Reticulocyte count	Low	Low	Normal or slightly high or low	Normal or slightly high	Low	Increased	High	Normal
Mean corpuscular volume	High	High	Low	Low	Normal or slightly high	Slightly low	Normal or high	Normal or low
Plasma iron	High	High	Low	High	High	Normal	Normal or high	Low
Total iron-binding capacity	Normal	Normal	High	Normal	Normal	Normal	Normal	Low
Ferritin	High	High	Low	High	Normal	Normal	Normal	Normal
Serum B_{12}	Low	Normal	Normal	Normal	Normal	Normal	Normal	Normal
Folate	Normal	Low	Normal	Normal	Normal	Normal	Normal	Normal
Bilirubin	Slightly high	Slightly high	Normal	High	Normal	Normal	Slightly high	Normal
Free erythrocyte protoporphyrin	Normal	Normal	High	Increased or normal	High	Normal	Normal	Normal or slightly high
Transferrin	Slightly high	Slightly high	Low	High	Normal	Normal	Normal	Slightly low

apy is observed, lifelong maintenance therapy at a lowered dosage is instituted. Discontinuing therapy initiates a relapse. Individuals not responding to pyridoxine require blood transfusions to relieve symptoms and permit growth and development.

Individuals who demonstrate evidence of iron overload require iron depletion therapy to prevent or minimize organ damage. Phlebotomies are generally well tolerated and preferable for individuals who have a mild to moderate anemia without other complications, such as heart disease. Once all the stored iron is removed, maintenance phlebotomies are performed on a continuing basis. Individuals who have severe anemia and/or depend on transfusions become extremely overloaded with iron. When this occurs, iron chelation therapy with desferrioxamine is necessary to eliminate excess iron.

As previously stated, individuals with acquired SA infrequently respond to pyridoxine. Fortunately, these individuals are rarely incapacitated by SA. In the absence of abnormalities of other blood cells and without iron overload, progression takes place over many years. Transfusion and chelation therapy are the same as for hereditary SA when indicated.

Recent advances in treatment for SAs include prolonged administration of erythropoietin and stem cell transplant. Treatment with recombinant human erythropoietin has been found to improve anemia in 20% of those with myelodysplastic syndrome. Those with the subset of MDS identified as

refractory anemia (RA) had the overall best response rate. Stem cell transplant has been found to successfully treat congenital SA; however, this treatment is in the early stages of use and long-term efficacy has not yet been established. Death from SA is relatively rare and is often secondary to complications, such as infection; bone marrow failure; liver failure; or cardiac failure or arrhythmias, or both.

Normocytic-Normochromic Anemias

Normocytic-normochromic anemias (NNAs) are characterized by erythrocytes that are relatively normal in size and hemoglobin content but insufficient in number. These anemias have no common etiology, pathologic mechanisms, or morphologic characteristics. They are less common than macrocyticnormochromic and microcytic-hypochromic anemias. The diversity of this group of anemias is exemplified by five distinct groups: aplastic, posthemorrhagic (acute blood loss), hemolytic, sickle cell, and anemia of chronic inflammation. (Sickle cell anemia is discussed in Chapter 28.)

Aplastic Anemia

Aplastic anemia (AA) is a critical condition characterized by pancytopenia, a reduction or absence of all three blood cell types. Pancytopenia results from failure or suppression of bone marrow to produce adequate amounts of blood cells (Figure 26-7). The rate or decline in the quantity of blood cells is related to their respective life span; thus RBCs are last to demonstrate a reduction in numbers. The rate of decline is often moderated sufficiently to allow the individual to adapt to the reduction and maintain a new level of hematologic function. This condition is referred to as *hypoplastic anemia* rather than aplastic. Approximately 50% of AA cases progress rapidly, leading to death from overwhelming infection or bleeding.

The incidence of AA is relatively rare, with an annual incidence rate of 2 to 5 new cases per million per year.[56] The incidence in developing countries is somewhat higher and is thought to be caused by unregulated use of and exposure to certain chemicals known to cause AA. The incidence is biomodal, with one peak occurring between 15 and 25 years of age and a second peak occurring in individuals over the age of 60. AA is equally distributed between genders.[57]

Acquired aplastic anemias are the most common type, with idiopathic AA (primary acquired) accounting for approximately 75% of all confirmed cases. Secondary AA, which accounts for approximately 15% of cases, is caused by a variety of known chemical agents and ionizing radiation. Chemical agents include benzene, arsenic, and multiple drugs, including chloramphenicol and alkylating and antimetabolite

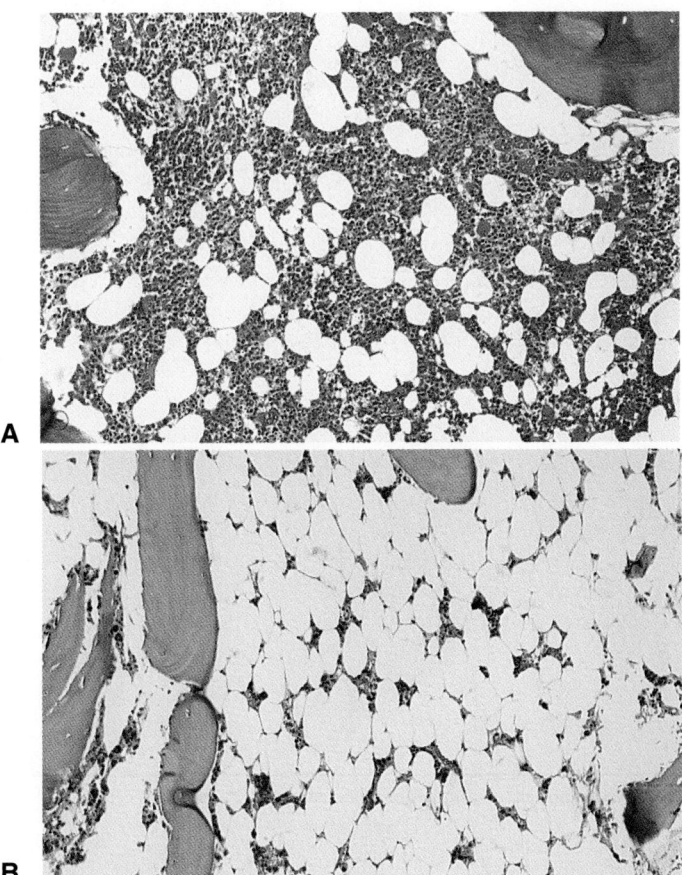

Figure 26-7 Aplastic anemia. **A,** Normal bone marrow of an adult. Hematopoietic cells account for approximately 40% of marrow's cellularity. **B,** There is a marked reduction in hematopoietic cells with expansion of fat cells. (From Damjanov I, Linder J: *Pathology: a color atlas,* St Louis, 2000, Mosby.)

chemotherapeutic drugs (6-mercaptopurine, vincristine, and busulfan). Other drugs known to cause AA are identified in Table 26-4. The development of AA with use of these agents is generally dose-related, and the effect can be controlled with appropriate dosages. In other instances, AA might develop after the use of small amounts of these drugs (idiosyncratic), with the anemia following a severe, rapid, irreversible progression. Liver disease is also recognized as a cause of AA.

AA is constitutional or familial in origin or is associated with one or more somatic abnormalities in approximately 5% to 10% of affected individuals. A subset of these are found to have defective telomerase RNA resulting in shortened telomeres. This abnormality also is found in some individuals with idiopathic AA.[56]

Total body irradiation also causes AA and, in certain instances, may be used therapeutically for this effect. Infections are also known to cause AA, with viruses being the most common agent. Viral infections identified as causing AA include the human immunodeficiency virus (HIV) infections, Epstein-Barr virus, and hepatitis (non-A, non-B, non-C, and non-G virus). Persistent parvovirus B19 infection also has been identified as producing bone marrow failure resulting in AA.[58] Parvovirus B19 has been identified as the cause of aplastic crisis in children who have sickle cell hemaglobinopathies and hereditary spherocytosis.[59]

Another condition associated with AA is **pure red cell aplasia (PRCA),** in which only the RBCs are affected. PRCA is a rare disorder and has been associated with autoimmune, viral, and neoplastic (leukemias) disorders; infiltrative disorders of the bone marrow (myelofibrosis); renal failure; hepatitis; mononucleosis; and systemic lupus erythematosus. It also is a well recognized but infrequent complication of allogenic bone marrow transplantation, particularly when there is donor-recipient ABO mismatch.[60] A thymoma often is found in association with PRCA and is also present in Diamond-Blackfan syndrome, a congenital disorder.

A very small percentage of AA cases is linked to genetic alterations or predisposition. **Fanconi anemia** is a rare genetic anemia characterized by pancytopenia resulting from defects in DNA repair. This anemia develops early in life and is accompanied by multiple congenital anomalies.

PATHOPHYSIOLOGY The characteristic lesion of AA is a hypocellular bone marrow that has been replaced with fat. Currently, AA is hypothesized to be an autoimmune disease directed against hematopoietic stem cells; however, the causative antigen has yet to be identified.[61] Recent evidence relates to suppression of hematopoiesis by activated cytotoxic T cells that produce a soluble inhibitory factor identified as interferon-gamma (IFN-γ).[62] Tumor necrosis factor (TNF) also is produced by T cells and exerts an inhibitory effect on hematopoiesis.[63]

Hematopoietic suppression by lymphokines IFN-γ and TNF is thought to occur during early and late hematopoiesis of progenitor CD34 and stem cells.[64] The crucial feature of suppression is proposed as being apoptosis. Both lym-

Table 26-4	Anemias Secondary to Drug Effects			
Drug	**Hemolytic**	**Megaloblastic**	**Sideroblastic**	**Aplastic**
Antibiotics				
Amphotericin B				X
Trimethoprim-sulfamethoxazole (Bactrim)		X		
Chloramphenicol (Chloromycetin)			XX	XXXX
Erythromycin	X			X
Sulfisoxazole (Gantrisin)				X
Penicillin	XXX			X
Sulfanilamide/sulfonamides	XX			X,X*
Streptomycin	X			X
Anticonvulsants				
Phenytoin (Dilantin)		XXX		XXX,X*
Mephenytoin		XXX		XXX
Primidone (Mysoline)		XX		
Phenobarbital		XX		
Trimethadione (Tridione)				XXX
Antiinflammatories				
ASA (aspirin)				X*
Colchicine		X?		
Gold compounds				XX
Ibuprofen (Motrin)	X			X
Indomethacin (Indocin)				X
Phenacetin	XXX			X
Phenylbutazone				XX,X*
Antihypertensive/Diuretics				
Methyldopa (Aldomet)	XXX			
Acetazolamide (Diamox)				X
Thiazides	X			
Tranquilizers				
Chloridazepoxide (Librium)				X
Chlorpromazine (Thorazine)	XX			X
Meprobamate				X
Oral Hypoglycemics				
Chlorpropamide (Diabinese)	X			
Tolbutamide (Orinase)				X,X*
Immunosuppressants				
Azathioprine (Imuran)			X	X*
Cyclosporine	X			
Miscellaneous Agents				
Benzene	XX			XX
Cimetidine (Tagamet)				X
Heparin				X*
INH (isoniazid) } Anti-TB agents	XX			
PASA (paraaminosalicylic acid) } Anti-TB agents	XX	X		
Pyridium (phenazopyridine HCl)				XX
Potassium perchlorate				XX
Quinine/quinidine	XX			
Acetaminophen (Tylenol)	X			X

X, Rare number of reported cases; *XXXX*, substantial number of reported cases; *XX, XXX*, intermediate number of reported cases; *X**, "pure red cell" aplasia.

phokines have demonstrated triggering of the Fas receptor on CD34 progenitor cells, which initiates apoptosis.[62,65] Additionally, inactivation of intracellular pathways leads to cell cycle arrest.[66] IFN-γ and TNF also induce the production of nitric oxide synthase and nitric oxide by marrow cells, which also contributes to immune-mediated cytotoxicity and removal of hematopoietic cells.[64] The process by which antigens control the pathologic immune response is unknown.

CLINICAL MANIFESTATIONS   The onset of symptoms is insidious and related to the rapidity with which the bone marrow is destroyed and replaced. Initial symptoms depend on which cell line is affected. When the onset is rapid, symptoms associated with hypoxemia, pallor, and weakness along with fever and dyspnea may be the first manifestations of a decreased RBC population. A slower onset is characterized by progressive weakness and fatigue advancing toward infection and hemorrhaging when white blood cell and platelet populations are affected. Common sites for hemorrhaging include the nose, mouth, or GI tract. Major hemorrhage may occur from any organ; however, it is generally observed in the late stages and is often secondary to other events.[57] Menorrhagia and purpura also may be evident; however, purpura is not necessarily a classic indication of AA and may not be representative of the degree of thrombocytopenia.

A waxy pallor of the skin is generally demonstrated by the time the condition has been diagnosed. The skin also may demonstrate a brownish pigmentation. Late manifestations of the condition include ulcerations of the mouth and pharynx or a low-grade cellulitis in the neck. Splenomegaly is extremely rare, and if present, other conditions that may imitate AA should be ruled out. Neurologic changes are only evident when hemorrhages have occurred within the system; however, some individuals have complained of paresthesias.

Commonly, the RBCs appear normal in spite of the severity of the anemia. Occasionally, the RBCs are macrocytic, with anisocytosis and poikilocytosis, and also may appear immature. Diagnosis of AA requires that two of the following be present: a granulocyte count <500/μL, a platelet count <20,000/μL, an absolute reticulocyte count ≤40 × 10^9/L, and a bone marrow with <25% normal cellularity. Both a bone marrow biopsy and aspirate are necessary for a diagnosis. The biopsy evaluates cellularity and architecture, and the aspirate is used to evaluate cell morphology.[57] Pancytopenia occurs when stem cell and progenitor cell populations have decreased to approximately 1% or less of normal.[66]

EVALUATION AND TREATMENT   Bone marrow biopsy is necessary to determine whether the specimen is true bone marrow and not blood so that fat content and stromal elements may be examined and determined. Marrow biopsied from individuals with typical AA contains yellowish white material consisting mainly of fat, fibrous tissue, and lymphocytes.[67] Bone marrow characteristics may vary widely and range from aplastic, hypoplastic, normal, or hyperplastic. Individuals with these various types of bone marrow are diffi-cult to document because descriptive and diagnostic criteria vary.[67]

Up until the last 20 years, treatment involved determining the cause, removal of exposure to the potential causative agent, transfusion, and prevention and treatment of infection and hemorrhage. Stimulation of blood cell production also was used and in some instances splenectomy was recommended. The prognosis with these forms of treatment was extremely poor. In acute cases, 25% of individuals succumbed within 4 months, demonstrating a rapid and fatal progression. Approximately 70% died within 5 years and only about 10% experienced complete recovery. Newer forms of treatment, such as bone marrow transplant (BMT), immunotherapy, and identification of high-risk individuals, has decreased mortality significantly.[68]

Bone marrow and, most recently, peripheral blood stem cell transplantation from a histocompatible sibling often cures the underlying bone marrow failure.[66] Survival rates of 75% to 80% have been reported, and mortality rates within the first 100 days have decreased. Graft-versus-host disease (GVHD), however, remains the primary limiter of success and is a major contributor to premature death. Children demonstrate higher survival than adults.

Allogenic BMT remains the preferred and most successful method for treatment of AA.[69,70] For those individuals unable to undergo such treatment or who lack a suitable sibling donor, immunosuppression remains the treatment of choice. Current therapies with immunosuppression include antithymocyte globulin (ATG). Response rates, that is, increased blood cell counts, of 40% to 50% have been reported in individuals who receive ATG. The addition of cyclosporine has increased the response and survival rates to as much as 70% to 80%, with a 5-year survival rate between 80% and 90%. Cyclosporine as a single therapeutic agent is not as effective. Cyclophosamide also has been used as an immunosuppressive agent and produced the same effects as ATG; however, its use has been discontinued because of its toxicity. The addition of recombinant hematopoietic growth factors, such as granulocyte-macrophage colony-stimulating factor, IL-6, and epoetin, to immunosuppressive therapy has produced significant results in both children and adults.[71] Survival rates of 80% have been reported for both types of treatment.[69]

A more recent form of treatment is that of inducing immunologic tolerance. Mycophenolate mofetil is used to inhibit T-cell proliferation and generation of cytotoxic T cells. Thus activated lymphocytes are subject to elimination because of their cell antigens that are recognized by ATG and their mitotic activity.[66]

Immunosuppressive therapy is not without risk. Individuals receiving immunosuppressive therapy are at risk of experiencing treatment failure or late clonal/malignant conditions or both. Late clonal/malignant conditions include paroxysmal nocturnal hemoglobinuria (PNH), myelodysplastic syndrome (MDS), acute leukemia, or solid tumor.[72] Although quite rare (<3%), administration of ATG may cause an anaphylactic reaction in some individuals.[73]

Posthemorrhagic Anemia (Acute Blood Loss)

Posthemorrhagic anemia is a normocytic-normochromic anemia caused by acute blood loss from the vascular space. Initial manifestations of this event depend on the severity of blood loss. If blood loss is severe, the manifestations are related to loss of blood volume rather than loss of hemoglobin. The immediate effects of volume depletion are more significant than loss of circulating blood cells. Volume loss reduces mean systemic filling pressure, resulting in decreased venous return.

A normal, healthy young adult can tolerate a blood loss of 500 to 1000 ml (10% to 20%) without experiencing any symptoms. Additional losses up to 1500 ml do not cause obvious symptoms if the individual is recumbent—symptoms only appear when assuming an upright position. When blood loss exceeds 1500 ml, symptoms are apparent even in a recumbent position (Table 26-5).

The initial manifestations (increased sympathetic nerve activation and a reduction in blood pressure, cardiac output, and central venous pressure) are caused by cardiovascular adaptations to blood volume depletion (e.g., thirst, shortness of breath and clouding or loss of consciousness, and sweating). If blood loss exceeds 2000 ml, severe shock, lactic acidosis, and death occur.[4] (Shock is discussed in Chapter 46).

If the acute blood loss is not severe (does not cause the preceding manifestations), recovery from the initial insult is possible. Within 24 hours of blood loss, lost plasma is replaced by mobilizing water and electrolytes from tissues and interstitial spaces into the vascular system. The hemodilution that results lowers the hematocrit; concurrently, there is often a rapid elevation of circulating neutrophils and platelets. Neutrophils can rise to levels between 10,000 to 30,000/μL within a few hours as a result of a shift of marginated leukocytes into the circulation and a release of leukocytes from the bone marrow.[74] The platelet count can rise to levels of about 1,000,000/μL. In severe hemorrhage, more immature cells—metamyelocytes, myelocytes, and nucleated red blood cells—may enter the circulation. Tissue oxygenation reduction stimulates production of erythropoietin, and the bone marrow responds by increasing production of RBCs (reticulocytes).

Iron recovery from destroyed RBCs may occur if the acute blood loss is internal; however, if blood is lost externally, iron stores may be depleted and erythropoiesis may be impeded. Hemorrhage that is chronic (occult [i.e., bleeding ulcer or neoplasm]) produces adaptations that are less prominent and the individual experiences an iron deficiency anemia when iron reserves become depleted.

Initial treatment for acute blood loss is restoration of blood volume by intravenous administration of saline, dextran, albumin, or plasma. Large volume losses may require transfusion of fresh whole blood; however, allergenic substances within the plasma or cells can interfere with volume expansion and even produce volume contraction.[74] The actual anemia may not require treatment unless it is associated with iron, folate, or cobalamin deficiency.

Evidence that normality has resumed is noted by erythrocytes returning to their normal size and shape. However, as the bone marrow begins to produce more erythrocytes, an increase in reticulocytes (10% to 15% after 7 days) is seen. Changes in the appearance of RBCs (polychromatophilia and macrocytosis) associated with reticulocytosis may give the impression that an underlying hemolytic process is occurring. A normal erythrocyte count is usually noted in 4 to 6 weeks, but hemoglobin restoration may take 6 to 8 weeks.

Hemolytic Anemia

Premature, accelerated destruction of erythrocytes, either episodically or continuous, is a clinical manifestation of many disease states and is the predominant event in **hemolytic anemias.** Adaptation to red cell destruction is facilitated by increased red cell production. Bone marrow is capable of increasing red cell production up to eight times its normal rate. Accommodation by increasing red cell production results in identifying the condition as a hemolytic disorder. Accelerated RBC production that is incapable of keeping up with destruction develops into a true hemolytic anemia.[75]

PATHOPHYSIOLOGY   Classification of hemolytic anemias is somewhat problematic because there is not one system that is entirely satisfactory. Dividing these anemias into

Table 26-5	Clinical Manifestations of Acute Blood Loss of Increasing Severity	

Volume Lost		
% TBV	ml	Clinical Manifestations
10	500	None; rarely notice vasovagal syncope in blood donors
20	1000	When person at rest, difficult, if not impossible, to detect volume loss; tachycardia is common with exercise and a slight drop in blood pressure with postural change
30	1500	Neck veins are flat in supine position; exercise tachycardia and postural hypotension are usually present; resting supine blood pressure and pulse can still be normal
40	2000	Central venous pressure, cardiac output, and arterial blood pressure are below normal even at rest and supine position; individual commonly has air hunger; a rapid, thready pulse; and cold, clammy skin
50	2500	Severe shock, lactic acidosis, death

Adapted from Hillman RS: Acute blood loss anemia. In Beutler E et al, editors: *William's hematology,* ed 5, New York, 1995, McGraw-Hill.
Data based on a 70-kg person with a total blood volume of 5000 ml.
TBV, Total blood volume.

inherited or acquired is the preferred and most useful method.[75] Hereditary hemolytic anemias are caused by intrinsic (cellular) abnormalities, typically of the erythrocyte's plasma membrane or cytoplasmic contents (enzymes) and hemoglobin structure and synthesis. Acquired hemolytic anemias are caused by extrinsic (extracellular) defects such as infection, chemical agents (drugs, toxins, and venom), trauma, physical agents, and abnormal immune responses. Causes of acquired and hereditary hemolytic anemias are listed in Table 26-6.

Hemolysis occurs within blood vessels (intravascular) or lymphoid tissues (extravascular) that filter blood—that is, spleen and liver. Intravascular hemolysis is the least common and typically is caused by physical destruction of RBCs or complement-mediated lysis facilitated by antibodies acting as a lysin, opsonin, or agglutinin.

Extravascular hemolysis, occurring within lymphoid tissue, is most common and is caused by macrophage destruction and/or digestion by the mononuclear phagocyte system (MPS). Erythrocytes continuously circulate through the spleen, passing through the thin-walled splenic cords into the splenic sinusoids, a sponge-like labyrinth of macrophages with long dendritic processes. Normally, RBCs are able to alter their shape to allow passage through openings in the splenic cords. RBCs with structure alterations of the membrane surface or that have become more rigid are incapable of maneuvering through this network, making them more vulnerable to phagocytosis and destruction by macrophages. Erythrocytes coated with immunoglobulin G (IgG) are particularly vulnerable.[76]

Autoimmune hemolytic anemias (AIHAs) are acquired disorders caused by extravascular hemolysis and are most often associated with autoimmune mechanisms, although in some instances they are mediated by drugs; thus the term **immunohemolytic anemia.** Recent studies propose various mechanisms of these anemias including loss of recognition of RBC antigens, molecular mimicry, polyclonal T- and B-cell activation, errors in central or peripheral tolerance, and disturbances in cytokines.[77] Th1 and Th2 cytokine imbalances are related to decreased Th1 cytokines (IL-12) and increased Th2 cytokines (IL-4 and IL-10).[77] The incidence of immunohemolytic anemia is approximately 1 in 100,000 persons per year with peak incidence in those between 60 and 70 years of age.[78] Immunohemolytic anemias are classified in various ways, most significantly are classifications based on the responsible antibody: (1) warm antibody type, (2) cold agglutinin type, and (3) cold hemolysins.

Warm antibody immunohemolytic anemia, the most common form, primarily affects females over the age of 40. Immunoglobulin G (IgG) is the mediating antibody specific

Table 26-6	Causes of Hemolytic Anemias	
Type of Hemolytic Disorder	**Primary Cause or Associated Disorder**	**Mechanisms of Erythrocyte Destruction**
Acquired Forms		
Immune system–mediated hemolysis	Transfusion reaction Hemolytic disease of the newborn (see Chapter 28) Autoimmune hemolytic anemia (see text)	Antibody-mediated erythrocytes by enzymes of the complement system (see Chapter 8)
Traumatic hemolysis	Presence of prosthetic heart valves Structural abnormalities of the heart Hemolytic uremic syndrome Disseminated intravascular coagulation Hemodialysis	Physical destruction of erythrocytes by "mechanical" means (trauma)
Infectious hemolysis	Bacterial infection (clostridia, cholera, typhoid fever) Protozoal infection (malaria, toxoplasmosis)	Infection of erythrocytes
Drug or toxic (chemical) hemolysis	Exposure to toxic chemical agents Hemodialysis or uremia Venoms	Chemical injury of erythrocytes (see Chapter 2)
Physical hemolysis	Burns Radiation	Heat or radiation injury (see Chapter 2)
Hypophosphatemic hemolysis	Hypophosphatemia (phosphate deficiency in plasma; see Chapter 3)	Diminished cellular production of substances required for erythrocyte life and function
Hereditary Forms		
Structural defects	Plasma membrane defects	Fragility of the erythrocyte
Enzyme deficiencies	Deficiency of glycolytic enzymes Deficiency of metabolic enzymes (i.e., glucose-6-phosphate dehydrogenase deficiency)	Diminished cellular function
Defects of globin synthesis or structure	Sickle cell anemia	Increased membrane fragility and deformation during sickle crises
	Thalassemia	Defective hemoglobin structure and function
	Miscellaneous hemoglobin defects	Defective hemoglobin structure and function

From Lee GR et al: *Wintrobe's clinical hematology,* ed 9, Philadelphia, 1993, Lea & Febiger.

for erythrocyte antigens and has a maximum binding capacity to the surface of the erythrocyte at body temperature (37° C). This condition is idiopathic and primary in approximately half of affected individuals; in the remaining half, some underlying predisposing condition is present, such as lymphoma, leukemia (chronic lymphocytic leukemia [CLL]), other neoplastic disorders, systemic lupus erythematosus, or exposure to a drug or drugs, producing a secondary form of the anemia. RBC destruction is usually not caused by intravascular hemolysis but rather by extravascular processes. IgG-coated RBCs bind to the Fc receptors on monocytes and splenic macrophages. Attempted phagocytosis of the IgG-coated cells results in partial loss of the cell membrane causing erythrocytes to undergo spheroidal transformation. These RBCs are sequestered in the spleen, removing them from the circulation.

Drug-induced hemolytic anemia is classified as warm antibody type according to three mechanisms of action: the hapten model, immune complex, and autoantibody model (Figure 26-8). The *hapten model,* based on penicillin and cephalosporins, proposes that these drugs act as hapten and combine with the RBC membrane to induce antibody formation (IgG) that is directed against the cell-bound drug. RBC destruction is mostly extravascular as noted in warm antibody immunohemolytic anemia. This form of drug-induced anemia usually follows a large intravenous infusion of an antibiotic and occurs 1 to 2 weeks after the initiation of therapy.

Drug-induced anemias may precipitate intravascular hemolysis because of complement fixation or extravascular hemolysis in the MPS. The *immune complex model* is based on the drug quinidine. Hemolysis occurs when the drug induces IgM antibody production. This drug-antibody complex binds to the RBC membrane, which then activates complement causing intravascular hemolysis. The *autoantibody model* is based on the prototype drug α-methyldopa, which somehow initiates production of antibodies that become directed against intrinsic RBC antigens, particularly Rh blood group antigens. It is estimated that 10% of individuals taking α-methyldopa develop detectable antibodies, but only 1% actually develop clinically significant hemolysis.[79]

Cold agglutinin immunohemolytic anemia is mediated by IgM and occurs less often than warm antibody hemolysis, affecting mostly older females. Cold antibodies have a RBC binding capacity that occurs at colder temperatures (lower than 31° C) with maximal binding capacity at 0° to −4° C. Autoantibodies appear acutely during recovery of certain infectious disorders, including infectious mononucleosis and mycoplasma pneumonia. With these conditions, the anemia is self-limiting and rarely produces hemolysis. Other infections include HIV, cytomegalovirus, and influenza virus. Chronic cold agglutinin immunohemolytic anemias can occur in association with lymphoid neoplasms and other unknown or idiopathic conditions.

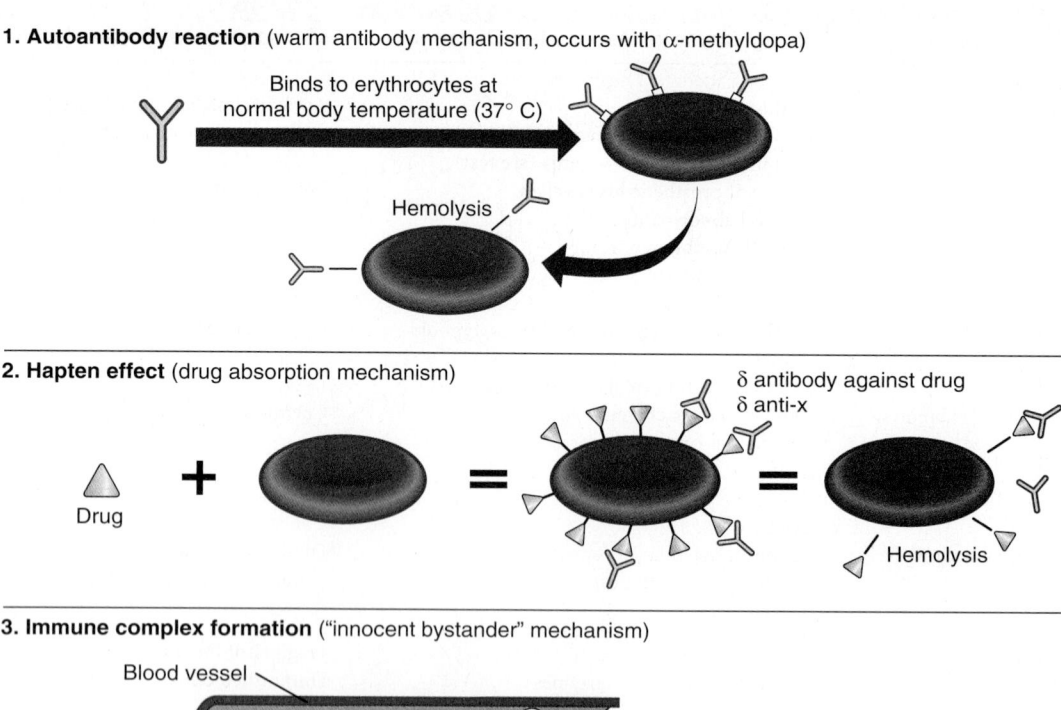

Figure 26-8 Drug-induced hemolytic anemia. *Xp,* Drug–plasma protein complex, *RBC,* red blood cell. (See discussion in text.)

IgM binding agglutinates RBCs and rapidly fixes (attaches) complement on their surface. IgM is rapidly released when the blood recirculates and warms, usually before complement-mediated hemolysis can occur. However, the temporary interaction with IgM allows the deposition of C3b on the RBC surface, which results in rapid phagocytosis by mononuclear phagocytes in the liver and spleen (also see Chapter 8). The severity of hemolysis is variable. Clinical manifestations result from binding of IgM to RBCs at exposed sites, such as fingers, toes, and ears, when temperatures are below 30° C. Obstruction of blood flow caused by RBC agglutination results in pallor, Raynaud phenomenon, and cyanosis of body parts.

Cold hemolysin hemolytic anemia is a rare disorder involving IgG autoantibodies and is associated with *paroxysmal cold hemoglobinuria*. This anemia involves acute, intermittent but massive intravascular hemolysis and often hemoglobinuria after exposure to cold temperatures. Destruction or lysis is clearly complement-dependent. Ironically, complement-mediated intravascular lysis occurs when cells begin to warm because the enzymes of the complement cascade are more efficient at warmer temperatures. The involved antibody, also called *Donath-Landsteiner antibody*, was first recognized with chronic syphilis infection. Today other infections involving paroxysmal cold hemoglobinuria are known, including measles, mumps, mycoplasma pneumonia, and other viral and flu syndromes.

Hemolysis related to alloimmunity is best characterized by an acute blood transfusion reaction because of ABO incompatibility of RBCs (also see Chapter 8). The IgM antibodies activate complement resulting in a rapid intravascular hemolysis. The individual may immediately experience fever, chills, dyspnea, and hypotension and may progress to shock. A delayed hemolytic transfusion may develop 3 to 10 days after transfusion. The delayed reaction is caused by a low titer of antibodies to minor RBC antigens.

CLINICAL MANIFESTATIONS

The presence and severity of signs and symptoms of hemolytic anemia depend on the degree of anemia and hemolysis and the success of compensatory erythropoiesis. The severity of anemia varies widely from individual to individual, even in individuals who have the same illness. Severe disease is commonly diagnosed shortly after birth or within the first year of life. Mild to moderate anemia is more common because the shortened erythrocyte survival time is offset by increased erythropoiesis. Some individuals have no symptoms of anemia, and it remains undetected unless some other complication develops during the course of the disease.

Jaundice (icterus) is present when heme destruction exceeds the liver's ability to conjugate and excrete bilirubin. Jaundice is first noticed in the neonatal period. Children and adults with congenital hemolytic anemia may not have icterus, or it may be mild enough that it goes unnoticed. In some individuals, faint scleral icterus may be the only indication of hemolytic disease.

Acute conditions that disrupt the delicate equilibrium of accelerated erythropoiesis and RBC destruction may precipitate a crisis. The most common type of crisis is aplastic and results from failure of bone marrow RBC production. The most common cause of aplastic crisis is human parvovirus B19 infection.

Commonly individuals with congenital hemolytic disorders demonstrate splenomegaly, which is often only mild in nature. In some cases the spleen may become quite enlarged and may cause discovery of the underlying hemolytic disorder. Another underlying condition which may be the cause of inadvertently determining the presence of the anemic disorder is the development of gallstones.

Children who have hemolytic anemia often demonstrate skeletal abnormalities caused by expansion of erythroid bone marrow during the active phase of growth and development. These alterations are more pronounced in the bony structures of the face and skull (see Chapter 28). In some instances, pathologic fractures also may result. Cardiovascular and respiratory manifestations vary with the degree of anemia. In spite of the disorder being characterized as hemolytic in nature, the presence of thromboembolism also is demonstrated. Autopsies of individuals with immunohemolytic anemia have revealed that pulmonary embolism is a common finding.[78]

EVALUATION AND TREATMENT   Evaluation is based on clinical manifestations, bone marrow studies, and blood tests (see Table 26-3, p. 938). Abnormally increased numbers of erythrocyte stem cells are found in the marrow, a finding termed *erythroid hyperplasia*. Accelerated erythropoiesis causes large numbers of fragile and immature erythrocytes (stem cells and reticulocytes) to be released prematurely into the circulation. These cells are observed in blood smears. If the bone marrow is able to consistently maintain adequate compensation, the hemoglobin may remain stable. The mean corpuscular volume, however, may be decreased in the presence of reticulocytes. A blood smear is helpful in determining the presence of spherocytes or schistocytes, as well as examining white blood cells and platelets for coexisting hematologic or malignant conditions.

Acquired hemolytic anemias are treated by removing the cause or treating the underlying disorder. Acute fulminating hemolytic anemia (hemolytic crisis) is treated with fluid and electrolyte replacement to prevent shock and renal damage, which may be caused by RBC debris clogging the kidney tubules. Transfusions of blood products sometimes are given. Splenectomy is performed if the spleen is the major site of hemolysis and splenomegaly is significant.

Folate also is used in treating chronic hemolytic disease to prevent megaloblastic crisis because long-term erythrocyte turnover increases folate requirements. Recent studies with selected monoclonal antibodies (MoAbs) have yielded positive preliminary data. Rituximab, an MoAb directed against CD20 antigen, may be effective and safe for certain immunohemolytic anemias.[80] In addition, manipulation of IL-10/IL-12 balance may be warranted for therapeutic control.

Anemia of Chronic Disease

Anemia of chronic disease (ACD) is a mild to moderate anemia in individuals with chronic conditions that include acquired immunodeficiency disease (AIDS); chronic inflammatory disorders, including RA, systemic lupus erythematosus (SLE), and acute and chronic hepatitis; chronic renal failure; and malignancies. ACD also is commonly noted in the presence of congestive heart failure (CHF).[81] The anemia develops after 1 to 2 months of active disease. The severity of anemia is related to that of the underlying disorder. Individuals with ACD may be asymptomatic, or ACD may be a coincidental clinical finding. Morphologically, ACD is initially normocytic-normochromic, but as the condition progresses, it becomes hypochromic and microcytic. ACD, by definition, is characterized by normal iron stores with low circulating iron (<60 mcg/dl).[82]

Anemia of chronic disease is one of the most common conditions encountered in medicine and is probably only secondary to iron deficiency anemia in overall incidence.[83] Estimates of anemia in the elderly is 11% in males and 10.2% in females over the age of 65. Of the elderly with anemia, two thirds were identified as having ACD or unexplained anemia. The elderly may be predisposed to ACD related to age-associate hematopoietic restriction. Additionally, the elderly demonstrate increased concentrations of inflammatory cytokines, which play a significant role in the development of ACD.[84] Elderly females who present with characteristics of ACD without an underlying malignancy or inflammatory condition are described as having primary defective iron-utilization syndrome.[85]

PATHOPHYSIOLOGY   Three pathologic mechanisms associated with ACD include (1) decreased erythrocyte life span, (2) ineffective bone marrow response to erythropoietin, and (3) altered iron metabolism. Overall, the manifestations of ACD appear to be mediated by activation of the cellular immune response (Th1) which causes release of specific cytokines (also see Chapter 7). The Th1 response appears to be the common factor among the various inflammatory and infectious conditions associated with ACD. Activation of macrophages is the initial step, after which proinflammatory cytokines are released. These cytokines then act on other cells, such as lymphocytes, endothelial cells, and fibroblasts, to cause erythropoietic suppression or act directly on effector cells.[86] Specific cytokines implicated in ACD include tumor necrosis factor–α (TNF-α), interferon-γ (IFN-γ), interleukin-1β (IL-1β), and interleukin-6 (IL-6).[87]

The precise mechanism by which RBC destruction is mediated remains unclear, but it is thought to be activated by macrophages.[86] Various causes have been suggested. Decreased erythrocyte life span may be attributed to RBC destruction mediated by some extrinsic factor that renders the erythrocyte more vulnerable to phagocytosis. Hemolysis caused by bacterial toxins or tumor secretions also have been suggested as factors that contribute to RBC destruc-

tion.[88] Individuals with RA who have ACD demonstrate increased levels of IL-1, suggesting that RBC destruction is facilitated by this factor. An increase in erythroid apoptosis induced by TNF-α also has been identified, as well as an inappropriate low production of erythropoietin. Decreased erythropoietin responsiveness also contributes to erythroid apoptosis in chronic diseases.[87] Increased levels of TNF-α, which inhibits erythropoiesis, have been found in CHF.[89] The severity of the anemia is directly related to the severity of the disease.

The erythropoietic defect in ACD is failure to increase erythropoiesis in response to decreased numbers of RBCs. Instead of accelerating production of erythrocytes, RBC production proceeds at a normal rate. Erythropoietic failure results from suppression of erythroid progenitor cells in bone marrow by the release of proinflammatory cytokines. Tryptophan degradation also results from IFN-γ. Tryptophan is required for protein synthesis and cell growth, thus with a reduced amount of tryptophan available, suppression of erythroid progenitor cells occurs.[90] Concomitant with suppression of bone marrow function, the amount of iron in the blood is reduced, thereby impairing the ability of bone marrow to synthesize hemoglobin.

Impaired iron metabolism is the third factor contributing to the pathogenesis of ACD (Figure 26-9). Lactoferrin is hypothesized to be the cause of this dysfunction. **Lactoferrin**, is a member of the transferring family of nonheme iron-binding glycoproteins, and resides in the polymorphonuclear cells that play a significant role in maintaining host defense at the mucosal surface.[91] Under normal conditions lactoferrin is present in the blood in only small amounts. During periods of inflammation and infection neutrophils release lactoferrin to bind iron and reduce its availability for bacteria. However, it also is more available to compete with transferrin and transports iron away from RBCs that have lactoferrin receptors.[92] The affinity of iron for lactoferrin is 260 times greater than for transferrin. Lactoferrin-bound iron is removed by the MPS and converted into ferritin, the storage form of iron.

Another protein, **apoferritin,** is implicated in altered iron metabolism. Apoferritin is produced in greater amounts in inflammatory and malignant conditions and also has a greater affinity for iron than transferrin. Apoferritin-bound iron also is converted to ferritin and stored, further contributing to a reduction of iron available for hemoglobin synthesis.

CLINICAL MANIFESTATIONS   Anemia of chronic disease has fewer and milder manifestations than most other anemias. Manifestations depend on the degree of anemia. As a rule, disability caused by chronic disease limits physical activity; consequently, hemoglobin levels remain adequate to accommodate activities of an affected individual. If hemoglobin levels drop significantly, clinical manifestations of iron deficiency anemia appear.

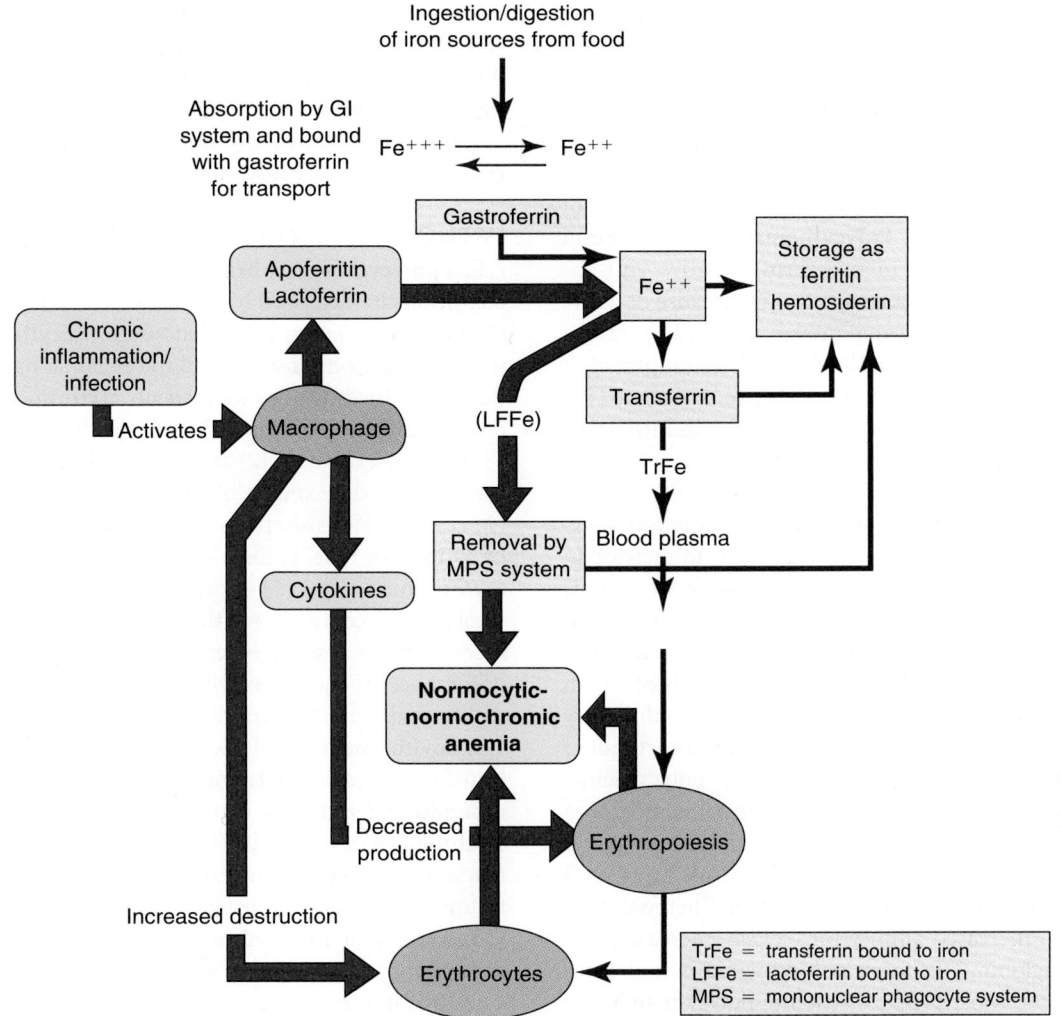

Ingestion/digestion
of iron sources from food

Absorption by GI
system and bound
with gastroferrin
for transport

$Fe^{+++} \longrightarrow Fe^{++}$

Gastroferrin

Apoferritin
Lactoferrin

Fe^{++}

Storage as
ferritin
hemosiderin

Chronic
inflammation/
infection

Activates

Macrophage

(LFFe)

Transferrin

TrFe

Cytokines

Removal by
MPS system

Blood plasma

**Normocytic-
normochromic
anemia**

Decreased
production

Erythropoiesis

Increased destruction

Erythrocytes

TrFe = transferrin bound to iron
LFFe = lactoferrin bound to iron
MPS = mononuclear phagocyte system

Figure 26-9 Pathophysiology of anemia of chronic disease. Normal iron metabolism is indicated by the narrow arrows. Abnormal mechanisms that are instrumental in the development of anemia of chronic inflammation are indicated by thick arrows. (See discussion in text.)

EVALUATION AND TREATMENT The significant findings of ACD are low serum iron, low or normal total iron binding capacity (TIBC), normal or high serum ferritin levels, and low concentrations of soluble transferrin receptor. Additionally, an iron deficiency is present in the bone marrow despite normal or increased iron stores elsewhere in the body. (Blood test findings are listed in Table 26-3, p. 938). Occasionally it may be difficult to differentiate ACD from IDA; however, the ability to measure sTfR has provided a means for differentiating between the two. Soluble transferrin receptor (sTfR) is nonresponsive to ACD but is responsive to IDA. Individuals who have ACD but demonstrate no evidence of inflammatory or infectious conditions are screened for the presence of malignancies.

Anemia of chronic disease does not respond to conventional iron replacement therapy because of dysfunctional transportation of iron to the bone marrow. Use of erythropoietin in treatment of ACD associated with arthritis, malignancies, and AIDS has met with limited success.[93]

WHAT'S NEW?   Hepcidin and Iron Regulation

The recent discovery of hepcidin, a liver-derived antimicrobial protein, has provided new insights into iron regulation, maternal-fetal iron transport across the placenta, and its role in anemia of chronic disease (ACD) (see Box 26-1). Hepciden inhibits iron uptake in the duodenum, modifies intestinal iron absorption, and inhibits iron release from macrophages. Thus an increase in hepcidin would explain iron deficiency and inadequate erythropoiesis resulting in anemia. Inflammation and IL-6 are strong stimuli for hepcidin production, adding further insight into its relationship to ACD. Hypoxia also has been identified as a stimulus to hepcidin activity. Hepcidin levels are reduced in individuals with hemochromatosis because of mutation in genes involved with iron metabolism, for example, the *HFE* gene, which encodes an HLA-like (human leukocyte antigen–like) transmembrane protein involved in iron absorption.

Data from Ganz T: *Curr Opin Hematol* 11(4):251-254, 2004; Robson KJ et al: *J Med Genet* 41(10):721-730, 2004.

The principal treatment is alleviation of the underlying disorder.

MYELOPROLIFERATIVE RBC DISORDERS (POLYCYTHEMIA)

Hematologic dysfunction results from an overproduction of RBCs as well as a deficiency. **Polycythemia** is an increase in RBC production and exists in two forms: relative and absolute. **Relative polycythemia** results from any cause of dehydration such as decreased water intake, diarrhea, excessive vomiting, or increased use of diuretics. Its development is temporary; usually affects obese, hypertensive, or stressed individuals; and resolves with appropriate fluid administration or treatment of the underlying condition.

Absolute polycythemia is *primary* when it results from an abnormality of the bone marrow stem cells. *Secondary polycythemia,* the most common type, is caused by an increase in erythropoietin as a normal physiologic response to chronic hypoxia or inappropriately (pathologically) to erythropoietin-secreting tumors. Individuals who live at higher altitudes (i.e., above 10,000 ft), smokers (who have increased levels of CO in their blood), individuals with chronic obstructive pulmonary disease (COPD), and those who have congestive heart failure develop secondary polycythemia. Secondary polycythemia also develops in individuals who have abnormal hemoglobin (e.g., $Hb_{San Diego}$ or $Hb_{Chesapeake}$). Over 100 possible hemoglobin mutations can result from genetic mutations in the α or β chains of hemoglobin.[94] These abnormal hemoglobins demonstrate an increased affinity for oxygen, increasing the need for hemoglobin.[95] Primary polycythemia is known as *polycythemia vera.* Most primary absolute polycythemias are acquired and occur at various ages; however, some are hereditary, present at birth, and identified as familial and congenital polycythemias.[96]

Polycythemia vera (PV) belongs to a group of disorders known as *chronic myeloproliferative disorders (CMPD).* These disorders are marrow expansive disorders with a dysregulated hypersensitivity to endogenous hormones, growth factors, or failure of the feedback loop, which causes a single cell proliferative advantage.[97] In addition to PV, CMPDs include idiopathic myelofibrosis (IM), essential thrombocytosis (ET), and chronic myeloid leukemia (CML). The major characteristics shared by these disorders are (1) involvement of a multipotent hematopoietic progenitor cell; (2) dominance of the transformed progenitor cell over the nontransformed progenitor cells; (3) overproduction of one or more of the formed elements of the blood in the absence of a defined stimulus; (4) marrow hypercellularity; (5) megakaryocyte hyperplasia and dysplasia; (6) chromosome 1, 8, 9, 13, and 20 abnormalities; (7) predisposition to thrombus formation and hemorrhage; and (8) spontaneous transformation to acute leukemia or development of marrow fibrosis.[98]

Determining a precise distinction between the CMPDs is difficult if not impossible because of similarities in their manifestations and a lack of specific molecular markers. As a result, diagnosis is quite challenging. One characteristic that does differentiate PV, IF, and ET from CML is the absence of the Philadelphia chromosome.

The CMPDs affect all three cell lines causing increases in erythrocytes, leukocytes, and megakaryocytes.

PATHOPHYSIOLOGY   Polycythemia vera **(PV),** also called **polycythemia rubra vera,** is a neoplastic, nonmalignant condition characterized by an increase in red blood cells, white blood cells, platelets, and splenomegaly. Erythrocytosis is the most serious complication and the essential manifestation for diagnosis. Investigators focused on erythropoiesis have produced conflicting findings. Findings include (1) the life of the RBC is not extended; (2) the erythroid progenitor cell is not expanded at the expense of the myeloid progenitor cell pool; (3) erythropoiesis suppression does not occur in the presence of hypoxia or renal failure; (4) phlebotomy does not stimulate erythropoiesis; and (5) erythropoietin levels are lower. Laboratory evidence has shown that erythroid progenitor cells proliferate in the absence of erythropoietin, suggesting that the dominance of the PV erythroid clone may be caused by its ability to differentiate more efficiently in a lower erythropoietin environment.[98] This dominance also may be affected by transforming growth factors that are produced by the PV mononuclear cells and increased sensitivity of polycythemia erythroid progenitor cells to interleukin 3 (IL-3), granulocyte macrophage-colony-stimulating factor (GM-CSF), stem cell factor (SCF), and insulin-like growth factor (IGF-1). Recently found was that PV erythroid progenitor cells overexpressed the antiapoptotic protein Bc1-x1, rendering them resistant to apoptosis in the absence of erythropoietin.[98]

CLINICAL MANIFESTATIONS   PV is relatively rare, with an estimated incidence of 2.3 per 100,000 individuals,[94] peak incidence is between the ages of 60 and 80 years of age, with a median incidence of 55 to 60. However, PV has been observed in individuals under the age of 40.[99,100] Males appear to have an increased incidence, although it is not overwhelmingly significant, and PV is more common in whites, particularly those of Northern European Jewish ancestry, than in African Americans. PV is rarely found in children or in multiple members of a single family; however, an autosomal dominant form exists that is characterized by increased production of erythropoietin. A rare form of congenital PV results from a deficiency of 2,3-bisphosphoglycerate (BPG), which increases oxygen affinity to hemoglobin that leads to decreased tissue oxygenation and compensatory polycythemia.[94]

The clinical course of PV occurs in four stages:

1. *Stage 1:* Prediagnostic (developmental) but symptomatic; generally 1 to 2 years.
2. *Stage 2:* Polycythemic or proliferative phase; begins at the time of diagnosis and initial treatment with remissions characterized by amelioration of symptoms; return of peripheral blood counts and bone marrow; re-

duction of spleen size, often to the point of being non-palpable; this stage is more descriptive of remissions with myelosuppressive and interferon regimens than phlebotomy alone.

3. *Stage 3:* Myeloid-metaplasia (spent phase): characterized by anemia, leukocytosis, splenomegaly, and myeloid metaplasia (myelofibrosis).

4. *Stage 4:* Acute leukemia.[101]

Clinical manifestations of absolute PV result from marrow erythropoiesis causing increased cellularity of the blood, which increases blood volume and viscosity. The major complication of PV is development of thrombi with occlusion of major and minor blood vessels leading to tissue and/or organ ischemia or infarction (tissue injury and/or death). Thrombosis and occlusion of vessels occur in approximately 40% of individuals, which is directly correlated with hematocrit levels. Increases in thrombocytes as well as dysfunctional platelets also contribute to this hypercoagulable state.

Circulatory alterations prevalent in PV, caused by thick, sticky blood, give rise to specific manifestations, such as plethora (ruddy, red color of the face, hands, feet, ears, and mucous membranes) and engorgement of the retinal and cerebral vessels. Individuals also experience headache, drowsiness, delirium, mania, psychotic depression, chorea, and visual disturbances. Death from cerebral thrombosis is approximately five times greater in individuals with PV.

Cardiac workload and output remain essentially unchanged; however, increased blood volume may lead to elevated blood pressure. Coronary blood flow may be affected and lead to the onset of angina; however, myocardial infarctions caused by PV are relatively rare. Other evidence of cardiovascular involvement is the development of Raynaud phenomenon and thromboangiitis obliterans.

Additionally, gastrointestinal involvement may occur, indicated by the development of gastric and duodenal thrombosis with resultant hemorrhaging. The development of mesenteric thrombosis requires immediate medical intervention. Splenomegaly and hepatomegaly are common as a result of pooling of blood in these organs; consequently individuals may develop portal hypertension. The respiratory system, generally not affected by PV, becomes involved if thrombosis and embolization occur.

A unique feature of PV, one that is potentially instrumental in diagnosis, is extreme, painful itching upon exposure to water (aquagenic pruritis) The involvement of mast cells in the cause and development of pruritis is speculative because the evidence of its role is contradictory.[98] Treatment is challenging because no specific effective modality is known. Various treatments include phlebotomy for minor itching, antihistamines, and ataractics; these may be effective but no single treatment has been found to produce consistent results. Interferon has been used when other forms of treatment have failed but is not consistently effective. Ultraviolet A light therapy may be useful but does have some toxic effects. Other drugs, such as hydroxyurea and Danazol, which reduce leuko-

cyte count, have been used but have potential lethal side effects (i.e., leukemia, hyperviscosity).[98]

EVALUATION AND TREATMENT Diagnosis of PV is made from blood and laboratory findings (Box 26-2). Blood manifestations include an absolute increase in RBCs, with hematocrits ranging from 18 to 24 g/dl and RBC counts of 7 to 10×10^{12}. Absolute total blood volume also is increased as well as possibly moderate increases of white blood cells and platelets. Erythrocytes appear normal, but anisocytosis may occur occasionally. Bone marrow examination may be done, but its use is controversial and no definitive criteria are known that can be used to establish the diagnosis. Typically the marrow is hypercellular but not in such a manner as to differentiate it from other myeloproliferative disorders.

Treatment of PV is guided by two objectives: minimize the risk of thrombosis and prevent progression to myelofibrosis and acute leukemia.[98] Treatment modalities are not universally agreed upon and consistent outcomes have not been obtained. Erythrocytosis and increased blood volume are reduced by phlebotomy. Three hundred to 500 ml are removed to maintain hematocrit at a safe level (<45). Phlebotomy remains the primary treatment modality and its safety and efficacy have been validated. Prior concerns related to its potential to cause thrombosis and iron deficiency have been eliminated.[98] Generally, individuals may not require further intervention unless there is evidence of increasing splenomegaly and increasing leukocyte or platelet counts. Cytoreductive drugs then may be used.

Box 26-2	Diagnostic Criteria for Polycythemia Vera

Major Criteria (A)
Increased total red blood cell (RBC) volume (RBC mass):
>25% above normal predicted value
  M ≥36 ml/kg (Hgb >18.5 g/dl)
  F ≥32 ml/kg (Hgb >16.5 g/dl)
O_2 saturation ≥92%
Splenectomy
Clonal genetic abnormality other than Philadelphia chromosome or BRC/ABL fusion gene in marrow*
Endogenous erythroid formation in vitro*

Major Criteria (B)
Platelets ≥400,000 µL
WBC count ≥12,000 µL
LAP score >100
Serum B_{12} >900 pg/ml
$UB_{12}BC$ >2200 pg/ml
Panmyelosis (myeloid metaplasia with abnormal immature blood cells in spleen and/or liver) with prominent erythroid/megakaryocytic hyperplasia on marrow biopsy*
Decreased serum erythropoietin levels*

---

*WHO Criteria for Diagnosis: elevated red cell mass (RCM) and any other major criteria or elevated RCM and any two minor criteria.
WBC, White blood cell; *LAP,* leukocyte alkaline phosphatase; $UB_{12}BC$, unbound B_{12} binding capacity.

Radioactive phosphorus (^{32}P) also is used to suppress erythropoiesis. It is generally effective for an extended time, and as many as 18 months may elapse between treatments. Side effects of ^{32}P treatment include suppression of hematopoiesis resulting in anemia, leukopenia, or thrombocytopenia. Development of acute leukemia is also a major side effect of ^{32}P, occurring after 7 or more years of treatment, making this therapy more useful in elderly individuals. Chlorambucil and busulfan have been discontinued as myelosuppressive agents because of leukemogenic effects and toxicity.[101] Hydroxyurea, a nonalkylating myelosuppressive drug, replaced chlorambucil and busulfan as the drug of choice because its safety was questioned and is no longer prescribed. Interferon alpha (IFN-α) also is gaining in popularity. Interferon inhibits the growth of the abnormal clone, which leads to the reduction of the clinical and laboratory signs of myeloproliferation.[102] IFN-α is the drug of choice and is most effective in relieving pruritus. Response to interferon includes a reduction in hematocrit with a decrease in splenomegaly and, if the individual has been on a phlebotomy-only regimen, the need for phlebotomy has been decreased.[101] Anagrelide, developed and used to reduce platelet counts, was effective in obtaining complete remissions but is now considered a risk for developing leukemia.

Causes of the conversion of PV to myelofibrosis or acute leukemia have not been completely identified. It is unclear whether it is part of the natural progression of the disease or whether it is related to the use of cytotoxic drugs.[103]

More recent therapeutic interventions have included the use of aspirin and stem cell transplantation. Aspirin is used for its antithrombotic (decrease thromboxane) properties. Recent findings have identified an increase in thromboxane biosynthesis in PV, and it is considered a major risk factor in the development of thrombosis.

Without proper treatment, 50% of individuals with PV die within 18 months of the onset of initial symptoms. The primary cause of death is thrombosis, which is more prevalent in older individuals and those with prior vascular complications.[98] Hemorrhage is rare and more common in individuals with high platelet counts and those taking antiplatelet drugs. Conversion to acute myeloid leukemia (AML) occurs in 10% of individuals within 15 years, increasing to 50% within 20 years. This leukemia is generally refractory to conventional treatment and remains a significant potential adverse outcome of PV.[104] Conversion to AML has been shown to increase when individuals are treated with alkylating agents, whereas those treated only with IFN or hydroxyurea had the same incidence of conversion as those who received no treatment.[98]

Although PV is a chronic disorder, remissions occur with appropriate therapy, and prevention of significant morbidity and mortality is possible. Survival for 10 to 15 years is common.

SUMMARY REVIEW

Anemia

1. Anemia is defined as a reduction in the number or volume of circulating red blood cells (RBCs) or an alteration in hemoglobin. Polycythemias are excessive RBCs or volume.
2. Anemias can be classified according to (a) erythrocyte size or concentration of hemoglobin, (b) cause of low blood count, or (c) the kinetics of why constant and adequate numbers of mature erythrocytes are not maintained in the circulation.
3. Clinical manifestations of anemia may be demonstrated in all organs and tissues throughout the body. Decreased oxygen delivery to tissues causes fatigue, dyspnea, syncope, angina, compensatory tachycardia, and organ dysfunction.
4. Macrocytic- (or megaloblastic-) normochromic anemias, characterized by larger than normal RBCs with smaller than normal nuclei, most commonly are caused by deficiency of vitamin B$_{12}$ (caused by a lack of intrinsic factor [IF]) or folate. Pernicious anemia can be fatal unless vitamin B$_{12}$ is replaced; replacement is generally done by injection but larger than normal doses given orally may be just as effective. Folate deficiency anemia is due to inadequate dietary intake of folate. After treatment with replacement therapy, no further treatment, other than adequate dietary intake, is required.
5. Microcytic-hypochromic anemias are characterized by abnormally small RBCs with insufficient hemoglobin content. The most common cause is iron deficiency.
6. Iron deficiency anemia is the most common type of anemia worldwide. It usually develops slowly, with gradual insidious onset of symptoms. Fatigue, weakness, dyspnea, alteration of various epithelial tissues, and vague neuromuscular complaints result.
7. Iron deficiency anemia (IDA) is usually a result of blood loss or poor nutritional intake. Individuals at highest risk for developing IDA are the elderly, females, infants, and those living in poverty. Anemia is also recognized as part of the nonspecific acute phase response to any type of inflammation. Once the source of blood loss is identified and corrected, oral iron replacement therapy can be initiated.
8. Elevated reticulocyte count is a good index of response to iron therapy. A recently discovered indicator of iron levels is serum transferrin receptor (sTfR).
9. Sideroblastic anemia (SA) results from impaired iron metabolism resulting in dysfunctional hemoglobin synthesis that produces abnormal cellular sequestration of iron. SAs may be hereditary or acquired, and treatment varies depending on the cause.
10. Normocytic-normochromic anemias are characterized by insufficient numbers of normal erythrocytes. Included in this category are aplastic, posthemorrhagic, and hemolytic anemias and anemia of chronic disease.
11. Aplastic anemia is a critical condition characterized by pancytopenia or a reduction or absence of all three blood cell types. Unless the cause is determined, bone marrow aplasia results in death.
12. Acute blood loss from hemorrhage results in a normocytic-normochromic anemia (posthemorrhagic anemia). Restoration of blood volume by plasma expanders or transfusions may diminish subjective symptoms of anemia. Hemoglobin restoration may take 6 to 8 weeks.
13. Premature destruction of erythrocytes (hemolytic anemia) may be acquired or hereditary. Of the acquired forms, autoim-

SUMMARY REVIEW

mune reaction (immunohemolytic) and drug-induced hemolysis are the most common.

14. Immunohemolytic anemias include (1) warm antibody type, (2) cold agglutinin type, and (3) cold hemolysins.

15. Failure of erythropoiesis in anemia of chronic disease may result in release of cytokines and lactoferrin by phagocytic cells. Lactoferrin has been shown to cause abrupt decreases in plasma iron levels by interfering with the normal iron cycle.

16. Anemia of chronic disease (ACD) is a mild to moderate anemia in individuals with chronic conditions that include AIDS, inflammatory disorders, acute and chronic hepatitis, chronic renal failure, and malignancies. ACD is one of the most common conditions encountered in medicine.

17. The Th1 response appears to be the common factor among the various inflammatory and infectious conditions associated with ACD.

18. Mechanisms associated with ACD include (1) decreased erythrocyte lifespan, (2) ineffective bone marrow response to erythropoietin, and (3) altered iron metabolism.

Myeloproliferative RBC Disorders (Polycythemia)

1. Polycythemia vera is characterized by excessive proliferation of erythrocyte precursors in the bone marrow. Signs and symptoms result directly from increased blood volume and viscosity.

2. Therapeutic phlebotomy to remove excessive blood volume and use of radioactive phosphorus have been helpful in decreasing the excessive RBC population.

KEY TERMS

Absolute polycythemia, 948
Anemia, 927
Anemia of chronic disease (ACD), 946
Anisocytosis, 928
Aplastic anemia (AA), 938
Apoferritin, 946
Autoimmune hemolytic anemia (AIHA), 943
Cold agglutinin immunohemolytic anemia, 944
Cold hemolysin hemolytic anemia, 945
Dimorphism, 936
Drug-induced hemolytic anemia, 944
Erythropoietic hemochromatosis, 937

Fanconi anemia, 939
Hemolytic anemias, 942
Hypoplastic anemia, 937
Immunohemolytic anemia, 943
Intrinsic factor (IF), 931
Iron deficiency anemia (IDA), 933
Lactoferrin, 946
Macrocytic anemia (megaloblastic anemia), 931
Microcytic-hypochromic anemias, 933
Myelodysplastic syndrome (MDS), 936
Normocytic-normochromic anemias (NNAs), 938

Pancytopenia, 938
Pernicious anemia (PA), 931
Poikilocytosis, 928
Polycythemia, 948
Polycythemia vera (PV) (polycythemia rubra vera), 948
Posthemorrhagic anemia, 942
Pure red cell aplasia (PRCA), 939
Relative polycythemia, 948
Ringed sideroblasts, 936
Sideroblastic anemias (SAs), 936
Warm antibody immunohemolytic anemia, 943

MEDIA RESOURCES  *evolve*

Review questions and answers for this chapter are available in the *CD Companion* included with this book. Also see the CD for an animation on *anemia*.

WebLinks—links to Internet sites pertaining to this chapter—are available on Evolve at http://evolve.elsevier.com/McCance/.

REFERENCES

1. Gasche C et al: Iron, anaemia, and inflammatory diseases, *Gut* 53(8):1190-1197, 2004.
2. Pereira AA, Sarnak MJ: Anemia as a risk factor for cardiovascular disease, *Kidney Int* 64(Suppl 87):S32-S39, 2003.
3. Carmel R, Rosenblatt DS: Disorders of cobalamin and folate metabolism. In Handen RI, Lux SE, Stossel TP, editors: *Blood: principles and practice of hematology*, Philadelphia, 2003, Lippincott, Williams & Wilkins.
4. Glader B: Anemia: general considerations. In Greer JP et al, editors: *Winbrobe's clinical hematology*, Baltimore, 2004, Williams & Wilkins.
5. Toh B, van Driel IR, Gleeson PA: Pernicious anemia, *N Engl J Med* 337(20):1441-1448, 1997.
6. Martens JH et al: Microbial production of vitamin B_{12}, *Appl Microbiol Biotechnol* 58(3):275-285, 2002.
7. Gordon MM et al: A genetic polymorphism in the coding of the gastric intrinsic factor gene (GIF) is associated with congenital intrinsic factor deficiency, *Hum Mutat* 23(1):85-91, 2004.
8. Bergman MP et al: Characterization of H^+, K^+-ATPase T cell epitopes in human autoimmune gastritis, *Eur J Immunol* 33(2):539-545, 2003.

9. Alderuccio F, Toh BH: Immunopathology of autoimmune gastritis: lessons from mouse models, *Histol Histopathol* 15(3):869-879, 2000.
10. Kaptan K et al: *Helicobacter pylori*—is it a novel causative agent in vitamin B_{12} deficiency? *Arch Intern Med* 160(9):1349-1353, 2000.
11. Howden CW: Vitamin B_{12} levels during prolonged treatment with proton pump inhibitors, *J Clin Gastroenterol* 30(1):29-33, 2000.
12. Ye W, Nyren O: Risk of cancers of the oesophagus and stomach by histology or subsite in patients hospitalised for pernicious anaemia, *Gut* 52(7):938-941, 2003.
13. Carmel R et al: Cobalamin deficiency with and without neurologic abnormalities: differences in homocysteine and methionine metabolism, *Blood* 101(8):3302-3308, 2003.
14. Fafouti M et al: Mood disorder with mixed features due to vitamin B_{12} and folate deficiency, *Gen Hosp Psychiatry* 24(2):106-109, 2002.
15. Malouf R, Areosa Sastre A: Vitamin B_{12} for cognition, *Cochrane Database Syst Rev* (3):CD004326, review, 2003.
16. Brigden ML: Shilling test still useful in pernicious anemia? *Postgrad Med J*106(5):37-38, 1999.
17. Oh R, Brown DL: Vitamin B_{12} deficiency, *Am Fam Physician* 67(5): 993-994, 2003.
18. Nyholm EP et al: Oral vitamin B_{12} can change our practice, *Postgrad Med J* 79:218-220, 2003.
19. McNulty H: Folate requirements for health in different population groups, *Br J Biomed Sci* 52(2):110-119, 1995.
20. Lee GR: Iron deficiency and iron deficiency anemia. In Lee GR et al, editors: *Wintrobe's clinical hematology*, Baltimore, 1999, Williams & Wilkins.
21. Bender DA: Megaloblastic anaemia in vitamin B_{12} deficiency, *Br J Nutr* 89(4):439-441, 2003.
22. Carmel R: Megaloblastic anemias: disorders of impaired DNA synthesis, In Greer JP et al, editors: *Winbrobe's clinical hematology*, Baltimore, 2004, Williams & Wilkins.

23. Huang RF et al: Folate deficiency induces a cell cycle-specific apoptosis in HepG2 cells, *J Nutr* 129(1):25-31, 1999.
24. Koury MJ, Horne DW: Apoptosis mediates and thymidine prevents erythroblast destruction in folate deficiency anemia, *Proc Natl Acad Sci U S A* 91(9):4067-4071, 1994.
25. Duthie SJ: Folic acid deficiency and cancer: mechanisms of DNA instability, *Br Med Bull* 55(3):578-592, 1999.
26. Stoltzfus RJ et al: Low dose daily iron supplementation improves iron status and appetite but no anemia, whereas quarterly anthelminthic treatment involves growth, appetite, and anemia in Zanaibari preschool children, *J Nut* 134:348-356, 2004.
27. Iron-deficient infants score worse on cognitive, motor tests as teens, *Blood Weekly*, May 27, 2004. Available online by subscription at www.NewsRx.com (accessed April 2005).
28. Andrews NC: Iron metabolism: iron deficiency and iron overload, *Annu Rev Genomics Hum Genet* 1:75-98, 2000.
29. Wolf AW, Jimenez E, Lozoff B: Effects of iron therapy on infant blood levels, *J Pediatr* 143(6):789-795, 2003.
30. Geltman PL et al: Daily multivitamins with iron to prevent anemia in high-risk infants: a randomized clinical trial, *Pediatrics* 114(1):86-93, 2004.
31. Hord J: Anemia and coagulation disorders in adolescents, *Adolesc Med* 10(3):359-367, 1999.
32. Nead KG et al: Overweight children and adolescents: a risk group for iron deficiency, *Pediatrics* 114(1):104-108, 2004.
33. Coppola A et al: A 69-year-old woman with persistent iron deficiency anemia, *Ann Hematol* 83(7):474-476, 2004.
34. Russo-Mancuso GF et al: Iron deficiency anemia as the only sign of infection with *Helicobacter pylori*: a report of 9 pediatric cases, *Int J Hematol* 78(5):429-431, 2003.
35. Ciacci C et al: Helicobacter pylori impairs iron absorption in infected individuals, *Dig Liver Dis* 36(7):455-460, 2004.
36. Weiss G et al: Possible role of cytokine-induced tryptophan degradation in anaemia of inflammation, *Eur J Haematol* 72(2): 130-134, 2004.
37. Berger J et al: Effect of daily iron supplementation on iron status, cell-mediated immunity, and incidence of infections in 6-36 month old Togolese children, *Eur J Clin Nutr* 54(1):29-35, 2000.
38. Eskeland B et al: Influence of mild infections on iron status parameters in women of reproductive age, *Scand J Prim Health Care* 20(1):50-56, 2002.
39. Weinstein DA et al: Inappropriate expression of hepcidin is associated with iron refractory anemia: implications for the anemia of chronic disease, *Blood* 100(10):3776-3781, 2002.
40. Labbe RF, Dewanji A: Iron assessment tests; transferrin receptor vis-a-vis zinc protoporphyrin, *Clin Biochem* 37(3):165-174, 2004.
41. Andrews NC: Disorders of iron metabolism. In Handin, RI, Lux SE, Stossel TP, editors: *Blood: principles and practice of hematology*, Philadelphia, 2003, Lippincott, Williams & Wilkins.
42. Osaki T et al: The pathophysiology of glossal pain in patients with iron deficiency anemia, *Am J Med Sci* 318(5):324-329, 1999.
43. Wong P: Esophageal webs and rings, retrieved November 17, 2004 from www.emedicine.com/med/topic3413.htm.
44. Lindsay JO et al: The investigation of iron deficiency anemia—a hospital based audit, *Hepatogastronenterology* 46(29):2887-2890, 1999.
45. Beutler E, Hoffbrand AV, Cook JD: Iron deficiency and overload, *Hematology* 40-61, 2003.
46. Joosten E: Strategies for the laboratory diagnosis of some common causes of anaemia in elderly patients, *Gerontology* 50(2):49-56, 2004.
47. Conrad ME: Iron deficiency anemia, retrieved November 17, 2004 from www.emedicine.com/med/topic1188.htm.
48. Little DR: Ambulatory management of common forms of anemia, *Am Fam Physician* 59(6):1598-1604, 1999.
49. Silverstein SB, Rodgers GM: Parenteral iron therapy options, *Am J Hematol* 76(1):74-78, 2004.
50. Alcindor T, Bridges KR: Sideroblastic anemias, *Br J Haematol* 116(4):733-743, 2002.
51. Bottomley SS: Sideroblastic anemias. In Greer JP et al, editors: *Wintrobe's clinical hematology*, Philadelphia, 2004, Lippincott, Williams & Wilkins.
52. Yamamoto M, Nakajima O: Animal studies for x-linked sideroblastic anemia, *Int J Hematol* 72(2):157-164, 2000.

53. McKenna R: Abnormal coagulation in the postoperative period contributing to excessive bleeding, *Med Clin North Am* 85(5):1277-1310, 2001.
54. Cazzola M et al: Mitochondrial ferritin expression in erythroid cells from patients with sideroblastic anemia, *Blood* 101(5):1996-2000, 2003.
55. Matthes TW et al: Increased apoptosis in acquired sideroblastic anemia, *Br J Haematol* 111(3):843-852, 2000.
56. Vulliamy T et al: Association between aplastic anaemia and mutations in telomerase RNA, *Lancet* 359(9324): 2168-2470, 2002.
57. Guinan EC, Shimamura A: Acquired and inherited aplastic anemia. In Greer JP et al, editors: *Wintrobe's clinical hematology*, Philadelphia, 2004, Lippincott, Williams & Wilkins.
58. Goto H et al: Successful bone marrow transplantation for severe aplastic anemia in a patient with persistent human parovirus B19 infection, *Intl J Hematol* 79(4):384-386, 2004.
59. Kellermayer R et al: Clinical presentation of parovirus B19 infection in children with aplastic crisis, *Ped Infect Dis J* 22(12):1100-1101, 2003.
60. Maschan AA et al: Successful treatment of pure red cell aplasia in a single dose of rituximab in a child after major ABO incompatible peripheral blood allogenic stem cell transplantation for acquired aplastic anemia, *Bone Marrow Transplant* 30(6):405-407, 2002.
61. Nissen C, Schubert J: Seeing the good and bad in aplastic anemia: is autoimmunity in AA disregulated or antineoplastic? *Hematol J* 3(4):169-175, 2002.
62. Marsh JCW, Gordon-Smith EC: Insights into the autoimmune nature of aplastic anemia, *Lancet* 364(9431):308-309, 2004.
63. Hara T et al: Excessive production of tumor necrosis factor-alpha by bone marrow T lymphocytes is essential in causing bone marrow failure in patients with aplastic anemia, *Eur J Haematol* 73(1):10-16, 2004.
64. Young NS: Hematopoietic cell destruction by immune mechanisms in acquired aplastic anemia, *Semin Hematol* 37(1):3-14, 2000.
65. Testa U: Apoptotic mechanisms in the control of erythropoiesis, *Leukemia* 18(7):1176-1199, 2004.
66. Young NA: Acquired aplastic anemia, *Ann Intern Med* 36(7):534-546, 2002.
67. Williams DM: Pancytopenia, aplastic anemia, and pure red cell aplasia, In Lee GR et al, editors: *Wintrobe's clinical hematology*, Baltimore, 1999, Williams & Wilkins.
68. Frickhofen N, Rosenfeld SJ: Immunosuppressive treatment of aplastic anemia with antithymocyte globulin and cyclosporine, *Semin Hematol* 37(1):56-68, 2000.
69. Bacigalupo A et al: Treatment of acquired severe aplastic anemia: bone marrow transplantation compared with immunosuppressive therapy—the European group for blood and marrow transplantation experience, *Semin Hematol* 37(1):69-80, 2000.
70. Tisdale JF, Dunn DE, Maciejewski J: Cyclophosphamide and other new agents for the treatment of severe aplastic anemia, *Semin Hematol* 37(1):102-109, 2000.
71. Locasciulli A: Acquired aplastic anemia in children: incidence, prognosis and treatment options, *Paediatr Drugs* 4(11): 761-766, 2002.
72. Socie G et al: Late clonal diseases of treated aplastic anemia. *Semin Hematol* 37(1):91-101, 2000.
73. Bevans MF, Shlabi RA: Management of patients receiving antithymocyte globulin for aplastic anemia and myeloplastic syndrome, *Clin J Oncol Nurs* 8(4):377-382, 2004.
74. Hillman RS: Acute blood loss. In Beutler E et al, editors: *William's hematology*, ed 5, New York, 1995, McGraw-Hill.
75. Lee GR: Hemolytic disorders: general considerations. Megaloblastic and nonmegaloblastic macrobytic anemias. In Lee GR et al, editors: *Wintrobe's clinical hematology*, Baltimore, 1999, Williams & Wilkins.
76. Delamaire M et al: Is there a mechanical factor of haemolysis in patients with positive IgG type direct antiglobulin test? *Br J Haematol* 80(1):91-96, 1992.
77. Fagiolo E: Immunological tolerance loss vs. erythrocyte self antigens and cytokine network disregulation in autoimmune hemoytic anaemia, *Autoimmun Rev* 3(2):53-59, 2004.
78. Hendrick AM: Auto-immune haemolytic anaemia—a high risk disorder for thromboembolism, *Hematology* 8(1):53-56, 2003.
79. Aster JC: Red blood cell and bleeding disorders. In Kumar VK, Abbas AK, Fausto N: *Robbins Cotran pathologic basis of disease*, ed 7, Philadelphia, 2005, Elsevier.

80. Robak T: Monoclonal antibodies in the treatment of autoimmune cytopenias, *Eur J Haematol* 71(2):79-88, 2004.

81. Komajda M: Prevalence of anemia in patients with chronic heart failure and their clinical characteristics, *J Card Fail* 10(1 Suppl):S1-S4, 2004.

82. Guralink JM et al: Prevalence of anemia in persons 65 years and older in the United States: evidence for a high rate of unexplained anemia, *Blood* 104(9):2263-2268, 2004.

83. Dallalio G, Fleury T, Means RT: Serum hepcidin in clinical specimens, *Br J Haematol* 122(6):996-1000, 2003.

84. Balducci L: Epidemiology of anemia in the elderly: information on diagnostic evaluation, *J Am Geriatr Soc* 51(3 Suppl):S2-S9, 2003.

85. Besa EC, Kim PW, Hauvani FI: Treatment of primary defective iron-reutilization syndrome: revisited, *Ann Hematol* 79(8):465-468, 2000.

86. Means RT: Anemias secondary to chronic disease and systemic disorders. In Greer JP et al, editors: *Wintrobe's clinical hematology*, Philadelphia, 2004, Lippincott, Williams & Wilkins.

87. Brugnara C: Iron deficiency and erythropoiesis: new diagnostic approaches, *Clin Chem* 49(10):1573-1578, 2003.

88. Richer S: A practical guide for differentiating between iron deficiency anemia and anemia of chronic disease in children and adults, *Nurs Pract* 22(4):82, 85-86, 91-96, 1997.

89. van der Meer P et al: Erythropoietin in cardiovascular diseases, *Eur Heart J* 25:285-291, 2004.

90. Weiss G et al: Possible role of cytokine-induced tryptophan degradation in anaemia of inflammation, *Eur J Haematol* 72(2):130-134, 2004.

91. Ward PC: Modern approaches to the investigation of B_{12} deficiency, *Clin Lab Med* 22(2):435-445, 2002.

92. Lux SE: Hematologic aspects of systemic disease. In RI Handin, Lux SE, Stossel TP, editors: *Blood: principles and practice of hematology*, Philadelphia, 2003, Lippincott, Williams & Wilkins.

93. Drueke TB: Modulating factors in the hematopoietic response to erythropoietin, *Am J Kidney Dis* 18(4 Suppl 1):87-92, 1991.

94. Prchal JT: Classification and molecular biology of polycythemias (erythrocytes) and thrombocytosis, *Hematol Oncol Clin North Am* 17(5):1151-1158, 2003.

95. Nagel RL: Disorders of hemoglobin function and stability. In Handin, RI, Lux SE, Stossel TP, editors: *Blood: principles and practice of hematology*, Philadelphia, 2003, Lippincott, Williams & Wilkins.

96. VanMaerkan T et al: Familial and congenital polycythemias: a diagnostic approach, *J Pediatr Hematol Oncol* 26(7):407-416, 2004.

97. Bennett JM: The myelodysplastic/myeloproliferative disorders: the interface, *Hematol Oncol Clin North Am* 17(5):1095-1100, 2003.

98. Spivak JL et al: Chronic myeloproliferative disorders, *Hematology* 20:200-224, 2003.

99. Means JRT: Polycythemia vera. In Lee GR et al, editors: *Wintrobe's clinical hematology*, p 2374 Baltimore, 1999, Williams & Wilkins.

100. Provan D, Weatherall D: Red cells II: acquired anaemias and polycythemia, *Lancet* 355(9211):1260-1268, 2000.

101. Berlin NI: Polycythemia vera, *Hematol Oncol Clin North Am* 17(5):1191-1210, 2003.

102. Lengfelder E, Berger U, Hehlmann R: Interferon alpha in the treatment of polycythemia vera, *Ann Hematol* 79(3):103-109, 2000.

103. Barbui T, Finazzi G: Clinical parameters for determining when and when not to treat essential thrombocythemia, *Semin Hematol* 36(1 Suppl 2):14-18, 1999.

104. George TI, Arber DA: Pathology of the myeloproliferative diseases, *Hematol Oncol Clin North Am* 17(5):1101-1127, 2003.

ALTERATIONS OF LEUKOCYTE, LYMPHOID, AND HEMOSTATIC FUNCTION

THOM J. MANSEN • KATHRYN L. McCANCE

evolve

http://evolve.elsevier.com/McCance/

CHAPTER OUTLINE

The many disorders involving leukocytes range from purely reactive alterations, such as leukocytosis, to proliferative disorders, such as leukemia. An event of importance to hematology has been its increasing relationship with oncology. Many hematologic disorders are malignancies, and many nonhematologic malignancies metastasize to bone marrow. Thus a large portion of this chapter is devoted to malignant disease.

Because the only role of clotting (hemostasis) is to stop bleeding, this interesting self-regulatory system is obviously essential to survival. It is remarkable that blood clots when shed and normally does not clot within blood vessels. Platelets—through a renaissance of research interest—are now known to have roles in clotting, wound healing, inflammation, and phagocytosis of foreign matter. They also play deleterious roles, however, in the pathogenesis of many diseases. This chapter also discusses various clotting factors and their control systems.

ALTERATIONS OF LEUKOCYTE FUNCTION

Leukocyte function is affected if too many or too few cells are present in the blood or if the cells that are present are structurally or functionally defective. Increases or decreases in cell numbers, the **quantitative disorders,** result from bone marrow dysfunction or premature destruction of cells in the circulation. Many quantitative alterations, however, originate in the circulation or lymphoid organs in response to invasion by infectious microorganisms.

The **qualitative disorders** consist of disruptions of leukocyte function in mechanisms of self-defense. Phagocytic cells (granulocytes, monocytes, macrophages) may lose their capacity to function as effective phagocytes. Lymphocytes may lose their capacity to respond to antigens. (Qualitative disruptions of inflammatory and immune processes caused by leukocyte disorders are described in Chapter 8.) Other leukocyte alterations, not considered to be primarily immune or inflammatory defects, are described as hematologic defects. These disorders include infectious mononucleosis and cancers of the blood—leukemia and multiple myeloma.

Quantitative Alterations of Leukocytes

Leukocytosis is present when the leukocyte count is higher that normal; conversely, **leukopenia** develops when the count is lower than normal. Leukocytosis or leukopenia may affect all cell types or only a specific type of leukocyte.

Leukocytosis and leukopenia result from a variety of physiologic conditions and alterations. Leukocytosis is a normal protective response to physiologic stressors, such as invading microorganisms, strenuous exercise, emotional changes, temperature changes, anesthesia, surgery, pregnancy, and some drugs, hormones, and toxins. It is also caused by pathologic conditions, such as malignancies and hematologic disorders. Unlike leukocytosis, leukopenia is never normal or beneficial. When the leukocyte count decreases to below 1000/mm³, the individual is at risk for infection. With counts below 500/mm³, very serious life-threatening infections occur. Leukopenia can be caused by radiation, anaphylactic shock, systemic lupus erythematosus, and certain chemotherapeutic agents.

Granulocytes and Monocytes

Increased numbers of circulating granulocytes (neutrophils, eosinophils, basophils) and monocytes are primarily a response to microbial invasion. Increased numbers also occur as a result of myeloproliferative disorders (polycythemia vera, chronic myelocytic leukemia) that increase stem cell proliferation in bone marrow.

Decreased numbers occur when infectious processes exhaust the supply of circulating granulocytes and monocytes by drawing them out of the circulation and into infected tissues faster than they can be replaced. Decreases also can be caused by disorders that suppress marrow function.

Granulocytosis begins with the release of white cells that have been stored in the venous sinuses of the marrow. Because the neutrophil is the most numerous of the granulocytes, the term *granulocytosis* often is used to describe **neutrophilia** (Table 27-1). Neutrophilia occurs in the early stages of infection or inflammation and is confirmed when the absolute neutrophil count exceeds 7500/µL.[1] Stored neutrophils are approximately 20 to 40 times greater in number than circulating neutrophils. When the neutrophil count increases greatly—more than 100,000/µL (usually seen only in those with myelocytic leukemia)—the blood viscosity may increase greatly so that thrombosis or occlusion of blood vessels occurs. Emptying of the venous sinuses stimulates granulopoiesis to replenish neutrophil stores in the marrow. Specific conditions associated with neutrophilia are identified in Table 27-1.

When the demand for circulating neutrophils exceeds the supply, the marrow begins to release immature neutrophils (and other leukocytes) into the blood. Premature release of the immature white cells is responsible for the phenomenon identified as a **shift-to-the-left.** The shift-to-the-left refers to the microscopic detection of disproportionate numbers of immature leukocytes in peripheral blood smears. The phenomenon is best understood by visualizing cellular differentiation and maturation progressing from left to right, as shown in Figure 25-7. (This phenomenon is sometimes called a **leukemoid reaction** because it resembles morphologic findings in blood smears of individuals with leukemia.) As infection or inflammation diminishes and granulopoiesis replenishes circulating granulocytes, a **shift-to-the-right,** or return to normal, occurs.

Neutropenia is the condition associated with a reduction in circulating neutrophils. Clinically, neutropenia exists when the neutrophil count is less than 2000/µL (2.0). A reduction in neutrophils occurs in severe prolonged infections when production of granulocytes cannot keep up with demand. Neutropenia is considered mild with a neutrophil count between 1.0/µL and 1.5/µL. Moderate neutropenia is a neutrophil count between 0.5/µL and 1.0/µL, and severe neutropenia is a count <0.5/µL.[2] Neutrophil reduction results from severe or prolonged infections when granulocyte production does not keep up with demand.

Other causes of neutropenia not related to infection may be (1) decreased neutrophil production or ineffective granulopoiesis, (2) reduced neutrophil survival caused by increased turnover or use, and (3) abnormal neutrophil distribution and sequestration.[2,3] Neutropenia also is categorized as primary or secondary; primary disorders are further identified as congenital or acquired.

Ineffective or defective neutrophil production is caused by primary hematologic disorders. Congenital causes are cyclic neutropenia and neutropenia with congenital immunodeficiency diseases, as well as multiple syndromes (Kostmann, Schwachman-Diamond, Diamond-Blackfan, Griscelli, Chédiak-Higashi, and Barth). Primary acquired neutropenia is associated with multiple conditions, for example, hypoplastic anemia or aplastic anemia, leukemia (acute myelogenous leukemia [AML]/chronic lymphocytic leukemia [CLL]), lymphomas (Hodgkin, non-Hodgkin), myelodysplastic syndrome. The megaloblastic anemias (vitamin B_{12} and folate deficiency) are also known to cause neutropenia.[4] Starvation and anorexia nervosa also cause neutropenia because of an inadequate supply of protein building blocks.[5]

Reduced neutrophil survival and abnormal distribution and sequestration are associated with secondary disorders. Neutropenia occurs in immune and autoimmune disorders, particularly systemic lupus erythematosus, rheumatoid arthritis, Felty and Sjögren syndrome, splenomegaly, and drug-related causes.

If neutrophils are drastically reduced to less than 100/µL, a serious condition called **granulocytopenia** or **agranulocytosis** results. Agents that may cause agranulocytosis include drugs, chemicals, infective agents, ionizing radiation, immune mechanisms, and genetic alterations. Clinical manifestations of agranulocytosis include infection (particularly of the respiratory system), general malaise, septicemia, fever, tachycardia, and ulcers in the mouth and colon. If untreated, sepsis caused by agranulocytosis results in death within 3 to 6 days.

Eosinophilia, an absolute increase (greater than 450/µL) in the total numbers of circulating eosinophils, has a variety of causes. Allergic disorders (type I) associated with asthma, hay fever, and drug reactions are often cited as causes. Hypersensitivity reactions trigger the release of eosinophilic chemotaxic factor of anaphylaxis (CTF-A) and histamine from mast cells, attracting eosinophils to the area. Areas abundant in mast cells, such as the respiratory and gastrointestinal tracts, are particularly common sites for eosinophil invasion. Other causes of eosinophilia are associated with dermatologic disorders, such as atopic dermatitis, eczema, and pemphigus. Various types of eosinophilic scleroderma-like diseases also have been reported to occur in association with hemato-oncogenic disorders (i.e., eosinophilic cellulitis [Well syndrome] and eosinophilic fasciitis [Schulman syndrome]).[6,7] Most recently, increased numbers of eosinophils have been identified with eosinophilia-myalgia syndrome (EMS), which is associated with ingestion of tryptophan, and

Table 27-1	Other Conditions Associated with Neutrophils, Eosinophils, Basophils, Monocytes, and Lymphocytes	
Condition	**Cause**	**Example**
Neutrophil		
Neutrophilia	Inflammation or tissue necrosis	Surgery, burns, MI, pneumonitis, rheumatic fever, RA
	Infection	Gram-positive (staphylococci, streptococci, pneumococci), gram-negative (*Escherichia coli, Pseudomonas* species)
	Physiologic	Exercise, extreme heat or cold, third-trimester pregnancy, emotional distress
	Hematologic	Acute hemorrhage, hemolysis, myeloproliferative disorder, CGL
	Drugs or chemicals	Epinephrine, steroids, heparin, histamine, endotoxin
	Metabolic	Diabetes (acidosis), eclampsia, gout, thyroid storm
	Neoplasms	Liver, GI tract, bone marrow
Neutropenia	Decreased marrow production	Radiation, chemotherapy, leukemia, aplastic anemia, abnormal granulopoiesis (megaloblastic anemia)
	Increased destruction	Splenomegaly, hemodialysis, immune reaction
	Infection	Gram-negative (typhoid), viral (influenza, hepatitis B, measles, mumps, rubella), severe infection, protozoal infections (malaria)
Eosinophil		
Eosinophilia	Allergy (type I)	Asthma, hay fever, drug sensitivity
	Infection	Parasites (trichinosis, hookworm), chronic (fungal, leprosy, TB)
	Malignancies	CML, lung, stomach, ovary, Hodgkin lymphoma
	Dermatoses	Pemphigus, exfoliative dermatitis (drug induced)
	Drugs	Digitalis, heparin, streptomycin, tryptophan (eosinophilia−myalgia syndrome), penicillins, propranolol
Eosinopenia	Stress response	Trauma, shock, burns, surgery, mental distress
	Drugs	Steroids (Cushing syndrome)
Basophil		
Basophilia	Inflammation	Infection (measles, chickenpox), hypersensitivity reaction (immediate)
	Hematologic	Myeloproliferative disorders (CGL, polycythemia vera, Hodgkin lymphoma, hemolytic anemia)
	Endocrine	Myxedema, antithyroid therapy
Basopenia	Physiologic	Pregnancy, ovulation, stress
	Endocrine	Graves disease
Monocyte		
Monocytosis	Infection	Bacterial: SBE, TB, recovery phase of infection
		Rickettsiae: Rocky Mountain spotted fever, typhoid fever
		Protozoa: malaria
	Hematologic	Monocytic leukemia, myeloproliferative disorders, Hodgkin lymphoma agranulocytosis
	Physiologic	Normal newborn
Monocytopenia	Rare	Chronic diseases: ulcerative colitis, Crohn disease, RA, SLE
Lymphocyte		
Lymphocytosis	Physiologic	4 months to 4 years
	Acute infections	Infectious mononucleosis, CMV infection, pertussis, hepatitis, mycoplasma pneumonia, typhoid
	Chronic infections	Congenital syphilis, tertiary syphilis
	Endocrine	Thyrotoxicosis, adrenal insufficiency
	Malignancies	ALL, CLL, lymphosarcoma cell leukemia
Lymphocytopenia	Immune deficiency syndromes	AIDS, agammaglobulinemia
	Lymphocyte destruction	Steroids (Cushing syndrome), radiation, chemotherapy
	Malignancies	Hodgkin lymphoma
	Debilitating illness	CHF, renal failure, TB, SLE, aplastic anemia

MI, Myocardial infarction; *RA,* rheumatoid arthritis; *CGL,* chronic granulocytic leukemia; *GI,* gastrointestinal; *TB,* tuberculosis; *CML,* chronic myelocytic leukemia; *SBE,* subacute bacterial endocarditis; *SLE,* systemic lupus erythematosus; *CMV,* cytomegalovirus; *ALL,* acute lymphocytic leukemia; *CLL,* chronic lymphocytic leukemia; *AIDS,* acquired immunodeficiency syndrome; *CHF,* congestive heart failure.

a relationship between EMS and fibromyalgia syndrome (FMS) has been suggested.[8]

Parasitic invasion also is associated with eosinophilia, particularly metazoan parasites. Eosinophils are attracted out of the circulation to the site of infestation, where they degranulate powerful enzymes onto the parasites. (This process is described and illustrated in Chapter 7.) Other conditions that cause eosinophilia are detailed in Table 27-1.

Eosinopenia, a decrease in circulating numbers of eosinophils, generally is caused by migration of eosinophils into inflammatory sites. It also may be seen in Cushing syndrome and as a result of stress caused by surgery, shock, trauma, burns, or mental distress. Other conditions causing eosinopenia are detailed in Table 27-1.

Basophilia, an increase in circulating numbers of basophils, is rare and when present generally is seen as a response to inflammation and hypersensitivity reactions of the immediate type. Basophils contain histamine that is released during an allergic reaction. An increase in basophils is seen also in myeloproliferative disorders, such as chronic myeloid leukemia and myeloid metaplasia. Other conditions associated with basophilia are listed in Table 27-1.

Basopenia (also known as *basophilic leukopenia*), a decrease in circulating numbers of basophils, is seen in hyperthyroidism, acute infection, and long-term therapy with steroids. A decrease in basophils is seen also during ovulation and pregnancy. Other conditions associated with basopenia are listed in Table 27-1.

Monocytosis, an increase in numbers of circulating monocytes, is often transient and correlates poorly with disease states. When present, it most commonly occurs with neutropenia associated with bacterial infections, particularly in the late stages or recovery stage, when monocytes are needed to phagocytize surviving microorganisms and debris. Increased numbers of monocytes also may indicate marrow recovery from agranulocytosis. Monocytosis often is seen in chronic infections such as tuberculosis (TB) and subacute bacterial endocarditis (SBE). Recently, peripheral monocytosis has been found to correlate with the extent of myocardial damage following myocardial infarction.[9] Other conditions associated with monocytosis are identified in Table 27-1.

Monocytopenia, a decrease in numbers of circulating monocytes, is rare, and not much is known about this condition because of the small numbers of monocytes generally present in the blood. Monocytopenia, however, has been identified with hairy cell leukemia and prednisone therapy.

Lymphocytes

Quantitative alteration of lymphocytes occurs when lymphocytes are activated by antigenic stimuli, usually microorganisms (see Chapter 7). A **lymphocytosis** is rare in acute bacterial infections and occurs most commonly in acute viral infections, particularly those caused by the Epstein-Barr virus (EBV, a causative agent in infectious mononucleosis). Other specific disorders associated with lymphocytosis are listed in Table 27-1.

Lymphocytopenia may be attributable to abnormalities of lymphocyte production associated with neoplasias and immune deficiencies, as well as destruction by drugs, viruses, or radiation. It also is known to occur in individuals for no apparent reason. Other conditions associated with lymphocytopenia are identified in Table 27-1. It has been hypothesized that the lymphocytopenia associated with heart failure and other acute illnesses may be caused by elevated levels of cortisol. The mechanisms in other disease states are not well understood.[10]

The most recent condition in which lymphocytopenia is a major problem is acquired immunodeficiency syndrome (AIDS). The lymphocytopenia associated with this condition is caused by the human immunodeficiency virus (HIV), which is cytopathic for T-helper lymphocytes. (For a more detailed discussion of AIDS, see Chapter 8.)

Infectious Mononucleosis

Infectious mononucleosis (IM) is an acute, self-limiting, neoplastic lymphoproliferative clinical syndrome characterized by acute infection of B lymphocytes (B cells). The most common etiologic agent is the Epstein-Barr virus (EBV), a ubiquitous, lymphotrophic, gamma-group herpesvirus,[11] which was first recognized as the causative agent in IM in the late 1960s.[12] EBV accounts for approximately 85% of all IM cases.[13] Other etiologic agents that may cause symptoms resembling IM are viruses (cytomegalovirus [CMV], adenovirus, HIV, hepatitis A, influenza A and B, and rubella), as well as the bacteria *Toxoplasma gondii, Corynebacterium diphtheriae,* and *Coxiella burnetti.*[14,15] IM caused by CMV is generally noted in older individuals, with fever and malaise being the major complaints; the major manifestations of EBV-induced IM are the classic triad of symptoms of pharyngitis, lymphadenopathy, and fever.[16]

IM usually affects young adults between ages 15 and 35 years, with the peak incidences occurring between 15 and 19 years; males have a later peak (18 to 23 years) than females. The overall incidence rate for this age group is 6 to 8 cases per 1000 persons per year.[17] Children from low socioeconomic environments are particularly susceptible to infections with EBV. Infection with EBV at this early state is usually asymptomatic and provides the individual with immunity to later infections.[18] IM is uncommon in individuals over age 40 years, but if it does occur, it is more commonly caused by CMV.

Saliva is the primary route of transmission for EBV through close personal contact (e.g., kissing, hence the term "kissing disease"). However, the virus may be present in other mucosal secretions of the genital, rectal, and respiratory tract, as well as blood. No evidence of aerosol transmission has been documented.[19] The infection begins with widespread invasion of B lymphocytes, all of which possess an EBV receptor site. Sites of invasion are initially the oropharynx, nasopharynx, and salivary epithelial cells with simultaneous spread to the lymphoid tissue and B cells.[14] Infection of B cells permits the virus to enter the bloodstream, which systematically spreads the infection.[20]

In the immunocompetent individual, EBV invasion triggers an *immunopathologic* response. Unaffected B cells are transformed into immortal plasmacytoid cells that produce antibodies (immunoglobulins A, M, and G [IgA, IgM, and IgG]) against the virus. Concomitantly, there is a massive activation and proliferation of cytotoxic T cells (CD8) that can account for greater than 50% of the total circulating lymphocytes. CD8 cells also release cytokines, primarily of a Th1 type (interferon-γ, interleukin), which are thought to cause the clinical features.[21] Lymphocyte activation is regulated by surface lymphocyte activation marker (SLAM)–associated protein (surface antigen [SA]) by signals sent from the cell surface CD244 and SLAM. Recent evidence suggests a relationship between the proliferation of CD4 and CD8 cells and the up-regulation of SLAM and CD244 that ultimately influences the manifestations of IM.[21]

The proliferation of clones of B and T cells and removal of dead and damaged leukocytes are largely responsible for the swelling of lymphoid tissues (lymph nodes, spleen, tonsils, and, occasionally, liver) characteristic of IM. Sore throat and fever, two of the earliest manifestations, are caused by inflammation at the site of viral entry and initial infection (the mouth and throat).

CLINICAL MANIFESTATIONS   The incubation period of IM is approximately 30 to 50 days (4 to 8 weeks). Initial symptoms, including headache, malaise, fatigue, arthralgia, fever, chills, dysphagia, and anorexia, may appear within the first 3 to 5 days after introduction of EBV. These symptoms may vary in severity for the next 7 to 20 days. At the time of diagnosis the individual usually has the classic triad of symptoms: fever, pharyngitis, and lymphadenopathy of the cervical lymph nodes.[16] The pharyngitis is usually diffuse and often accompanied by a whitish or grayish green, thick exudate. It also is quite painful and is the symptom that most often causes the individual to seek treatment.[22] Enlargement of the spleen and liver also may occur. Splenomegaly is clinically evident 50% of the time and is demonstrated radiologically 100% of the time.[16] Difficulty in detecting splenomegaly with physical examination contributes to the underestimation of actual enlargement.[23]

On rare occasions, individuals with IM may have other organ systems affected by EBV. These include neurologic alterations, such as meningitis, encephalitis, Guillain-Barré syndrome, Bell palsy, optic neuritis, mental impairment, transverse myelitis, cerebellar ataxia, and demyelinating diseases. Ocular manifestations also may develop, including eyelid and periorbital edema, dry eyes, keratitis, uveitis, conjunctivitis, retinitis, occuloglandular syndrome, choroiditis, papillitis, and ophthalmoplegia.[24] In children, Reye syndrome also has been associated with EBV infection.

Pulmonary manifestations may develop; however, these are rare. When present, they may include hilar and mediastinal lymphadenopathy, interstitial pneumonitis, and pleural effusion. Incidences of pneumonia and respiratory failure have been documented; however, they are more likely to develop in immunocompromised individuals. Approximately 3% to 10% of adults over 40 years of age have never been infected with EBV and are susceptible to IM later in life.[23] In these individuals, the classic symptoms are not generally present making diagnosis more difficult. If an older individual has an elevated temperature that cannot be explained and persists for greater than 2 weeks, EBV infection should be suspected, particularly in the presence of abnormal liver function tests with hepatomegaly and jaundice. Other neurologic manifestations that may be present include peripheral neuropathy and Guillain-Barré syndrome.[25]

EVALUATION AND TREATMENT   Diagnosis of IM is commonly based on Hoagland's criteria of at least 50% lymphocytes and at least 10% atypical lymphocytes in the presence of fever, pharyngitis, and adenopathy confirmed by a positive serologic test. Serologic tests are used to determine a heterophile antibody response. **Heterophilic antibodies** are a heterogeneous group of IgM antibodies that are agglutinins against nonhuman red blood cells (e.g., sheep, horse). These antibodies may be detected by either qualitative methods (Monospot) or qualitative methods (heterophile antibody test).

The Monospot test is limited because other infections (e.g., CMV, adenovirus) and toxoplasmosis also produce heterophilic antibodies. The percentage of individuals with IM who have heterophilic antibodies in their blood increases relative to the time of onset of symptoms. Some individuals do not produce heterophilic antibodies, and children under age 4 years also do not produce heterophilic antibodies.[15] For these reasons, 5% to 15% of Monospot tests yield a false-positive result.[26] Specificity for EBV infection may be increased with newer viral-specific serology tests that identify EBV-specific antibodies (e.g., viral capsid antigen [VCA], IgG and IgM, and EBV nuclear antigen [EBNA], and IgG). These tests are more expensive and labor intensive and thus should be used in instances where the Monospot test is not appropriate.

IM is usually self-limiting, and recovery occurs in a few weeks. Severe clinical courses with complications are rare, occurring in only 5% of cases. Fatalities associated with IM involve fulminant hepatitis, hemophagocytic syndrome, and splenic rupture.[27] Splenic rupture is the most common cause of death and appears to be the only gender-related factor associated with IM, with 90% of cases occurring in males.[20] Rupture of the spleen may occur spontaneously without evidence of trauma and most often occurs between 4 and 21 days after onset of symptoms.[14] Fortunately, splenic rupture is rare, occurring in only 0.1% to 0.15% of all cases. Conventional treatment for splenic rupture has been removal of the spleen and continues to be the choice in hemodynamically unstable individuals. More recent practice has been to repair the spleen to avoid overwhelming postoperative infection (OPSI). Children are at greater risk of OPSI than adults. Postsplenectomy vaccinations for *S. pneumoniae*, *H. influenza*, and *Meningococcus* are essential because these microorganisms are responsible for 92% of fatal infections.[16] Airway obstruction from massive edema of the Waldeyer ring is another complication associated with IM,[20] as is autoimmune hemolytic anemia, which occurs in approximately 3% to 5% of cases.[28]

Fatal IM also is expressed with the inherited X-linked lymphoproliferative syndrome (XLP). The underlying cause leading to death is the absence of a functional SAP protein that allows for the unregulated proliferation of cytotoxic T cells and the concomitant production and release of cytokines.[21]

Treatment of IM is supportive and includes rest and alleviation of symptoms with analgesics and antipyretics. Ibuprofen and acetaminophen, *not aspirin,* are used with children and adolescents because of the reported incidence of Reye syndrome associated with EBV infection. Pharyngitis of streptococcal origin, which occurs in 20% to 30% of cases, is treated with penicillin or erythromycin. Ampicillin is contraindicated because it causes a rash in most individuals with IM.[29]

Bed rest and avoidance of strenuous activity should be included in the therapy. Steroids may be used, but only in the presence of severe complications (e.g., impending airway obstruction)[17] or other organ system involvement (e.g., nervous system manifestations, thrombocytopenic purpura, myocarditis, pericarditis).[25] Acyclovir has been used with immunosuppressed individuals; however, clinical improvement has been minimal and therefore it is not recommended for standard treatment. The relationship between EBV and IM has been controversial and somewhat inconsistent, however, recent evidence supports a causal relationship between EBV and IM and also between EBV and the development of Hodgkin lymphoma.[30]

Leukemias

Leukemia is a clonal malignant disorder of the blood and blood-forming organs causing an accumulation of dysfunctional cells and a loss of cell division regulation. The excessive accumulation of leukemic cells results in an overcrowding of bone marrow, which causes a decreased production and function of normal hematopoietic cells. The first description of a "leukemic" individual was written by Velpeauin 1827.[31] Virchow, a pathologist, coined the term *white blood (Weissus blut)* and later he originated the term *leukemia.* Since Virchow's initial discovery, the overall classification of leukemia has become increasingly complex and includes the dominant cell affected, lymphoid or myeloid (myelogenous), and the point at which cell maturation is arrested, acute or chronic (Figure 27-1). Thus, there are four types of leukemia: acute lymphoid (lymphocytic), acute myelogenous, chronic lymphoid (lymphocytic), and chronic myelogenous.

Both types, either acute or chronic leukemia, have a variety of subtypes. **Acute leukemia** is characterized by undifferentiated or immature cells, usually a blast cell. The onset of disease is abrupt and rapid with a progression resulting in a short survival time. In **chronic leukemia** the predominant cell is mature but does not function normally. The onset of disease is gradual and the prolonged clinical course results in a relatively longer survival time. In 1976 the French-American-British Cooperative Group developed more extensive criteria for the classification of acute leukemias. This system is based on structure, number of cells, genetics, identification of surface markers, and histochemical staining that provide significant therapeutic and prognostic information.

Leukemia occurs with varying frequencies at different ages and is more common in adults than children. Acute lymphocytic leukemia is the most common type in children and accounts for approximately 50% of cases occurring after the age of 67.[33] Acute myelogenous leukemia and chronic lymphocytic leukemia are the most common types in adults (Table 27-2). In all types of leukemia males have a higher incidence rate (56%) as do Americans of European descent. White children have the highest rates of leukemia.[34]

Acute Leukemias

Acute lymphocytic leukemia (ALL) is a progressive neoplasm defined by the presence of >30% lymphoblasts in the bone marrow or blood.[35] ALL is the most common leukemia in children (80%) and most often occurs in the first decade. Although adults with ALL account for only 20%, their mortality rate is significantly higher (see Table 27-2). The significant difference between the incidence of ALL in adults and children is thought to be determined by differences in the biology of the disease. Philadelphia (Ph) chromosome–positive ALL carries the worst prognosis of all types of ALL and is found in 25% to 30% of adult ALL cases but less than 5% of childhood ALL cases. Conversely, there is a molecular abnormality of the *TEL* and *AML1* genes (*TEL-AML1*) in childhood ALL. This abnormality is present in 25% to 30% of childhood ALL cases but in only 2% of adult ALL cases. This molecular alteration of genes significantly impacts the prognosis of childhood ALL. Children with ALL and *TEL-AML1* arrangement have a cure rate of 90%, whereas those without the rearrangement have only a 60% cure rate. These unique alterations associated with adult and childhood ALL and their contrasting outcomes help explain the significant differences between children and adults with ALL.[36]

PATHOPHYSIOLOGY Leukemias are considered clonal disorders in that a single progenitor cell undergoes malignant transformation.[37] An interesting paradox is that leukemic cells apparently divide more *slowly* and take longer to synthesize deoxyribonucleic acid (DNA) than other blood precursors. Acute leukemia therefore is not caused by rapid cellular proliferation but is instead caused by the blocking of cellular differentiation. Leukemic cells accumulate relentlessly in the bone marrow causing overcrowding of the marrow, and they compete with cellular proliferation and function of normal hematopoietic cells. Thus acute leukemia has been termed an *accumulation* disorder, as well as a *proliferation* disorder. In the majority of cases, leukemic cells are ejected into the blood where they accumulate. These cells also may infiltrate and accumulate in the liver, spleen, lymph nodes, and other organs throughout the body. The presentation of large numbers of leukemic cells in the blood may be one of the most dramatic indicators of leukemia; however, leukemia is still a primary disruption of the bone marrow.

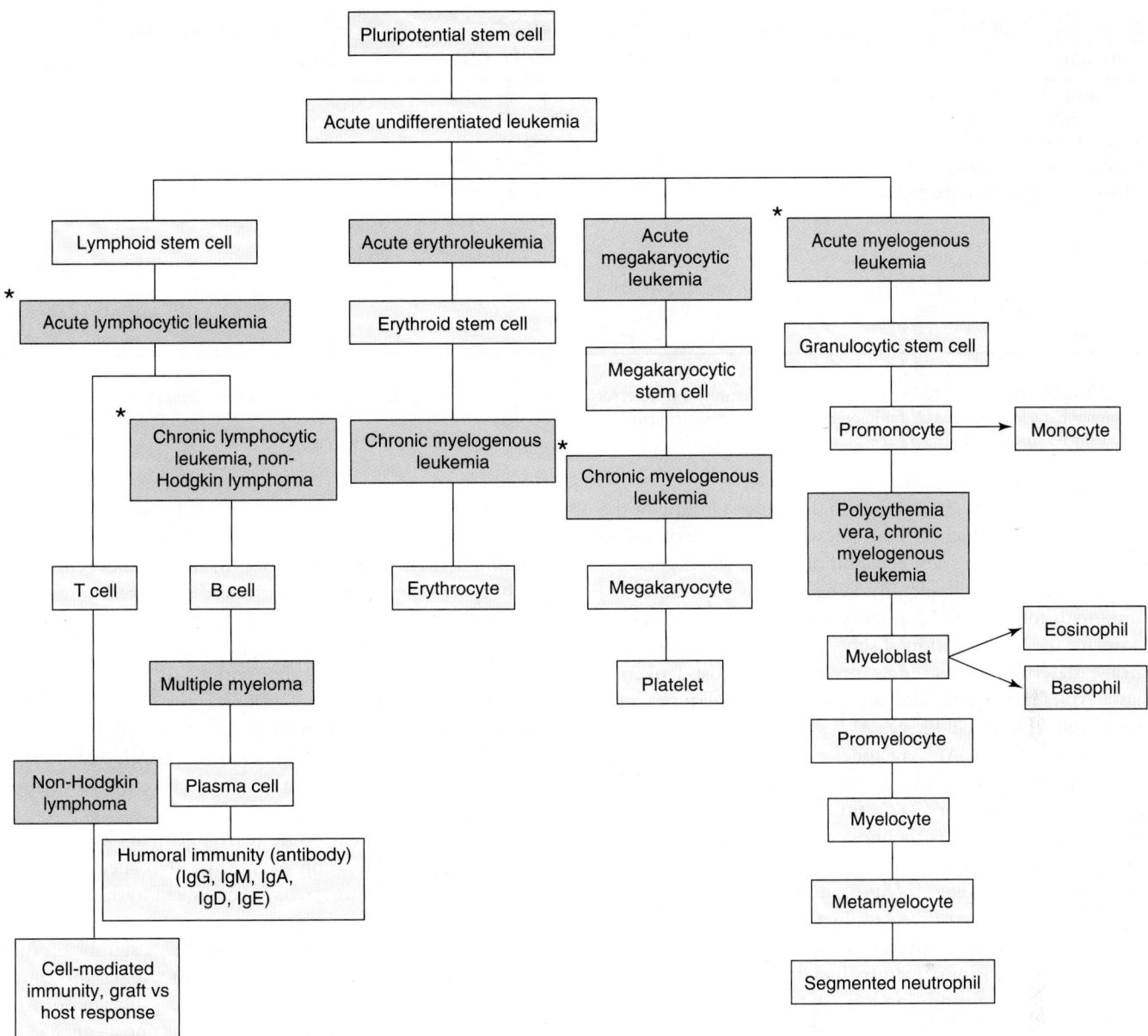

Figure 27-1 Cell-specific leukemias. Differentiation pathways of blood-forming cells and reported sites of block resulting in cell-specific leukemias. *Ig,* Immunoglobulin. *Major types

Table 27-2	Epidemiology of Major Types of Leukemia in the United States							
	Estimated New Cases of Leukemia in the U.S.			Estimated Number of Deaths Attributed to Leukemia in the U.S. (2002)			Survival Rate in the U.S. (1995-2000)	
Type	Number and Proportion (%) of New Cases in 2002	Male (2005)	Female (2005)	Total	Male	Female	Overall	<5 years of age
Acute lymphocytic leukemia	3970 (11.4%)	2180	1790	1490	850	640	64.8%	89.1%
Chronic lymphocytic leukemia	9730 (28%)	5780	3950	4600	2520	2080	72.7%	
Acute myelogenous leukemia	11,960 (34.3%)	6530	5430	9000	5040	3960	19.5%	53.0%
Chronic myelogenous leukemia	4600 (13.2%)	2640	1960	850	430	420	36.7%	
Other	4550 (13%)	2510	2040	6630	3700	2930		
Totals	34,810 (99.9%)	19,640	15,170	22,570	12,540	20,880		

Data from *Cancer Facts and Figures 2005,* American Cancer Society.

Table 27-3	Immunophenotype of Adult Acute Lymphocytic Leukemia						
Lineage	TdT	HLA–DR	CD34	CD19	CD22	CD79a
Precursor–B cell ALL						
Pro-B ALL	+	+	+	+	+	+
cALL	+	+	−	+	+	−
Pre-B ALL	+	+	−	+	+	−
Transitional precursor–B cell ALL	±	+	−	+	+	−
Mature–B cell ALL	−	+	−	+	±	−
T-lineage ALL						
Pro-T ALL	+	±	±			
Pre-T ALL	+	±	±			
Cortical-T ALL	+	−	−			
Mature-T ALL	+	−	−			

From Faderl S et al: *Cancer* 98:1337-1354, 2003.

TdT, Terminal deoxynucleotidyl transferase; *cy*, cytoplasmic; *s*, surface; *IgH*: immunoglobulin heavy chain; *Igl*, immunoglobulin light chain; *ALL*, acute lymphoblastic leukemia; *cALL*, common acute lymphoblastic leukemia.

*Usually no surface light chain (L) expression.

Much progress has been made in the understanding of the biology of ALL, which is now known to be an expanding group of different entities. Recognition of particular gene expression patterns will identify subgroups with unique requirements for therapy. Immunotyping of leukemic blast cells allows for the identification of subtypes of ALL. A distinct cell lineage determination is now possible for most leukemic blasts. ALL blasts are divided into precursor B cell types, mature–B cell ALL, and T-lineage ALL (Table 27-3).

Precursor B-cell ALL includes pre–pre-B ALL (pro-B ALL), common ALL (cALL), and pre B ALL. Pro-B ALL blasts express *CD19, CD79,* or *CD22,* but no other B-cell differentiation antigens.[38] cALL is the most common immunophenotype in adults and children and is positive for *CD10.* The presence of *CD10 (common ALL antigen)* accounts for the worse prognosis of CD10-positive ALL in adults compared to children. Pre-B ALL blasts express cytoplasmic immunoglobulins (Igs). The blasts are more mature than in early pre-B ALL, and more cases have translocation *t*(1;19).[38]

Mature B-cell ALL is classified by the expression of surface cell immunoglobulin (Ig), usually IgM and by the absence of staining for the enzyme—terminal deoxynucleotidyl transferase (TdT). Genetic translocations between the *c-myc* locus on chromosome 8 and one of the loci for the Ig heavy (IgH) or light chain genes (14q32, 2p12, and 22q11) are characteristic (also see Chapters 7 and 11). About 80% to 85% of ALL arise from the B-cell line.

The T cell lineage subtypes (T-ALL) are distinguished according to the stage of normal thymocyte development. Cytoplasmic CD3 (cCD3) is the most common T cell lineage specific marker.[38]

In addition to lymphoid markers, ALL blast cells also can express myeloid markers in 15% to 50% of adults and 5% to 35% of children.[38]

Over the last two decades more than 15 distinct cytogenetic abnormalities, which occur in up to 50% of individuals with ALL, have been identified. These defects include mostly disrupted genes that encode transcription factors that regulate cellular growth and involve principally two major types of alterations. The first type of alteration is the result of recombination between intron sequences of two distinct genetic loci resulting in novel gene fusion. These novel rearrangements include the *BCR-ABL E2A-PBX1, E2A-HLF, MLL,* and *TEL-AMI* fusion genes. The second type of recombination results in alteration of a structural gene with regulatory sequences of either immunoglobulin or T cell receptor (TCR) loci. These rearrangements result in neoplastic transformation and include *SCL, MYC, LMO2, HOX11, IL-3, TAN1, LYL 1, LCK,* and *TAL2* genes. The altered regulatory genes then determine the subtype of ALL.

T cell receptor (TCR) gene rearrangements are the most common genetic alteration in T-ALL.[38] No specific cytogenetic abnormality, however, has been linked to the subtype of T-ALL.

In addition to the above genetic lesions a significant incidence of mutational changes in proto-oncogenes and tumor suppressor genes are characteristic of many subtypes of ALL. These alterations include defects in the *ras* oncogene, *p53* tumor-suppressor gene, and *INK4A,* the gene encoding a cell cycle regulatory protein. Finally, variability in chromosomal number is often observed.

The most common genetic abnormality in adult ALL is the reciprocal translocation between chromosomes 9 and 22 t (9;22)(q34;q11), the **Philadelphia chromosome.** This translocation results in the novel fusion of the *BCR* gene and a portion of the proto-oncogene *abl;* thus two different oncoproteins BCR-ABL are observed in ALL (see Figure 11-15 on p. 345). The abnormal oncoproteins have deregulated and abnormally increased receptor tyrosine kinase activity with eventual involvement of downstream signaling pathways.[38] **Receptor tyrosine kinases** (RTKs) are transmembranous proteins that span the entire plasma membrane. Certain ligands that bind with RTKs cause gene transcription by entering the nucleus, transferring their phosphate to continual transcription factors, thus activating them. Activation can lead to uncontrolled mitosis and proliferation consistent with leukemia.

CD10	cyμ	cgκ/λ	sIgH/L	cyCD3	CD7	CD1a	CD2	CD5	sCD3	Frequency (%)
										5-10
−	−	−	−							40-50
+	−	−	−							10
±	+	−	−							1
−	−	−	+*							1
−	−	+	+							5
				+	+	−	−	−	−	5
				+	+	−	+	+	−	
				+	+	+	+	+	−	10-15
				+	+	−	+	+	+	5-10

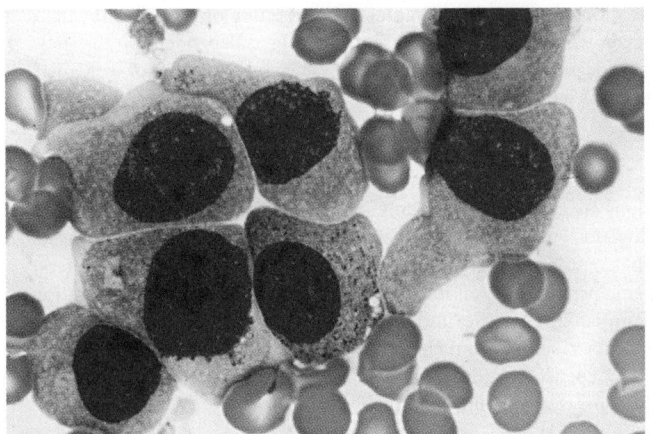

Figure 27-2 Acute monoblastic leukemia (M5A). The bone marrow contains monoblasts, which are larger than normal myeloblasts and usually have abundant cytoplasm, often with scattered granules. (From Damjanov I, Linder J: *Pathology: a color atlas,* St Louis, 2000, Mosby.)

Box 27-1	Classification of Acute Myeloid Leukemias

Acute myeloblastic leukemia, minimally differentiated (AML-M0)
Acute myeloblastic leukemia without maturation (AML-M1)
Acute myeloblastic leukemia with maturation (AML-M2)
Acute promyelocytic leukemia (AML-M3)
   Hypergranular type
   Microgranular variant
Acute myelomonocytic leukemia (AML-M4)
   Increased marrow eosinophils (AML-M4-EO)
Acute monocytic leukemia (AML)
   Acute monoblastic leukemia (AML-M5A)
   Acute monocytic leukemia, differentiated (AML-M5B)
Erythroleukemia (AML-M6)
Acute megakaryoblastic leukemia (AML-M7)

From Damjanov I, Linder J: *Pathology: a color atlas,* St Louis, 2000, Mosby.

Specific causes of ALL are unknown, but it is thought that multiple factors contribute to its development. Life-style and environmental factors remain the target of interest, however, no direct relationships between these factors have been discovered. A unique characteristic of ALL, unlike other forms, is that ALL develops at different rates in different locations. Individuals in developed countries and in higher socioeconomic categories have an increased incidence of ALL. Prevention is almost impossible because there are no known causes.

Acute myelogenous leukemia (AML) involves an abnormal proliferation of myeloid precursor cells, decreased rate of apoptosis, and an arrest in cellular differentiation (Figure 27-2). Therefore the bone marrow and peripheral blood are characterized by leukocytosis and a predominance of blast cells. As the immature blasts increase, they replace normal myelocytic cells, megakaryocytes, and erythrocytes. This displacement eventually leads to complications of bleeding, anemia, and infection. AML increases with age, peaking in the sixth decade of life. Certain risk factors have been identified

as possible causes, including exposure to radiation, benzene, and chemotherapy. Hereditary conditions, such as Down syndrome, Fanconi aplastic anemia, Bloom syndrome, ataxia-telangiectasis, trisomy 13 (Patau syndrome), Wiskott-Aldrich syndrome, and congenital X-linked agammaglobulinemia, are known to be associated with a higher risk for AML (see Table 27-2).

Current molecular studies of AML reveal a heterogenous disorder of the myeloid cell lineage. The AML subtypes are classified based on the stage of development myeloblasts have reached at the time of diagnosis. These subtypes are included in Box 27-1.

Several kinds of mutations have been found in AML; however, a mutation in the receptor tyrosine kinase **FLT3** occurs in about one third of AML patients. FLT3 conveys a proliferation signal normally expressed early in the development of bone marrow stem cells, but mutated FLT3 remains active and promotes blast cell proliferation.[39] Several FLT3 inhibitors are in various stages of clinical development. Another

Table 27-4   Clinical Manifestations and Related Pathophysiology in Leukemia

Clinical Manifestations	Laboratory Abnormalities	Cause	Comments
Anemia	Either a decrease or normal number of erythroblasts; key is the relative *proportion* of erythroblasts to total count; decreased iron in mature RBC	Decreased RBC production may be caused by decreased stem cell input or ineffective erythropoiesis or both; proposed reasons are: 1. Replacement of ESCs by leukemic clone 2. Inhibition of ESCs by leukemic cells 3. Inhibition of pluripotent stem cell 4. Decreased erythropoietin responsiveness from impaired interaction of ESCs with T lymphocytes (in leukemia there is an increase in T lymphocytes) 5. Hemorrhage 6. Splenic pooling of RBC 7. Drug therapy	In acute leukemia, anemia is usually present from beginning, often the first symptom noticed, and severe; mild form without symptoms is common in CML and CLL; hemorrhage is common in acute forms, occasionally in CML, but rare in CLL
Bleeding, purpura, petechiae, ecchymosis, thrombosis, or hemorrhage	Decreased and possibly abnormal platelets; abnormal clotting	Reduction in megakaryocytes leading to thrombocytopenia	Bleeding occurs more commonly in acute than in chronic leukemia
DIC	Abnormal promyelocytes; hypofibrinogenemia; prolonged prothrombin, thrombin, and reptilase times; elevated fibrin degranulation products; and decreased levels of factor V, fibrinogen, and platelets	Proliferation of promyelocytic granulocytes with an excessive release of procoagulants from granules within the leukemic promyelocyte	Correction of coagulopathy in DIC is dependent on the successful treatment of leukemia
Infection	Infection is likely with an AGC below 500/mm³ (AGC is the proportion of neutrophils and bands to the total white blood cell count)	Infections are caused by organisms endogenous to the host or present in the environment; granulocytopenic persons have an impaired inflammatory response; immune deficiency resulting from chemotherapy, corticosteroids, and the disease process contributes to the infection	Major sites of infection are the alimentary tract sinuses, lungs, and skin; prevention of infection focuses on the restoration of host defenses, decreasing invasive procedures, and reducing colonization of organisms
Weight loss	Decreased 24-hr urinary creatinine excretion; hypoalbuminemia	Condition can be attributed to pain, depression, chemotherapy, radiation therapy, some unknown circulating inhibitor, and alterations in taste	Causes of weight loss are poorly understood; severe alterations in taste; highly seasoned foods seem bland, aggravate condition; patients with liver involvement often detest red meat; some patients have good appetites in the morning but become satiated later; increased metabolism also aggravates the condition
Bone pain	Frequently no radiographic evidence of bone problems	Result of bone infiltration by leukemic cells or intramedullary infarction	If combination drug regimens are ineffective, radiation therapy is used
Elevated uric acid	Normal excretion of uric acid is 300-500 mg/day; the leukemic patient can excrete 50 times more; uric acid precipitates (urates) are commonly found in the proximal collecting tubules and pelvises of the kidney; oliguria and concentrated urine are sometimes found	Uric acid is a normal by-product of protein catabolism; nucleic acid catabolism is accelerated in the leukemic patient; uric acid precipitation occurs at an acidic, or low, pH; urate precipitation in the leukemic patient is increased from dehydration caused by anorexia or fever and drug therapy	Hyperuricemia is present in both acute leukemia and CML; kidney pathologic manifestations can be prevented by ensuring increased urine flow, increasing urine pH by administering sodium bicarbonate, or decreasing acid production through allopurinol, which inhibits the enzyme xanthine oxidase
Liver, spleen, and lymph node enlargement	Biopsy is abnormal for liver and spleen	Leukemic cell infiltration causes splenic, hepatic, and lymph node enlargement; lymph nodes also undergo leukemic proliferation as in CLL	

RBC, Red blood cell; *ESC*, erythropoietic stem cell; *CML*, chronic myelocytic leukemia; *CLL*, chronic lymphocytic leukemia; *DIC*, disseminated intravascular coagulation; *AGC*, absolute granulocyte count.

mutation in receptor tyrosine kinases is **c-KIT,** which also provides a proliferative and/or survival signal to progenitor cells. Together these mutations result in proliferation but not differentiation.[40]

CLINICAL MANIFESTATIONS   The clinical manifestations of all the varieties of acute leukemia are generally similar. (Mechanisms associated with common manifestations are summarized in Table 27-4.) Signs and symptoms related to bone marrow depression include fatigue caused by anemia, bleeding resulting from thrombocytopenia (reduced numbers of circulating platelets), and fever caused by infection. Bleeding can occur in skin, gums, mucous membranes, and gastrointestinal and genitourinary tracts. Signs of bleeding include petechiae and ecchymosis visible in dependent areas, discoloration visible through the skin, gingival bleeding, hematuria, and midcycle menstrual bleeding or heavy bleeding associated with menstruation.

Sites of infection include the oral cavity, throat, respiratory tract, lower colon, urinary tract, and skin. Common organisms include the gram-negative bacilli *Escherichia coli,* *Pseudomonas aeruginosa,* and *Klebsiella pneumoniae.* Fever is an early sign. Chills and tissue infiltration are common.

Anorexia can occur in all varieties of acute leukemia and is associated with weight loss, diminished sensitivity to sour and sweet tastes, wasting away of muscle, and difficulty in swallowing. Liver, spleen, and lymph node enlargement are more common in ALL than in acute myelogenous leukemia (AML). Splenomegaly and hepatomegaly usually occur together. The leukemic individual often experiences abdominal pain and tenderness and breast tenderness. Pain in the bones and joints are thought to result from leukemia infiltration with secondary stretching of the periostium.[41]

Central nervous system (CNS) involvement and manifestations are common and may be caused by either leukemic infiltration or cerebral bleeding. Headache, vomiting, papilledema, facial palsy, blurred vision, auditory disturbances, and meningeal irritation can occur if leukemic cells infiltrate the cerebral or spinal meninges. CNS involvement at the time of diagnosis is rare, and less than 5% of children and less than 10% of adults are affected. Without CNS prophylaxis, approximately one third of individuals will develop CNS complications. Interventions associated with CNS prophylaxis include cranial irradiation, chemotherapy, and high doses of systemic chemotherapy. Specific treatment modalities or combinations of treatment vary and are determined by age and risk status.[42]

EVALUATION AND TREATMENT   Leukemia is often confused with other conditions, making early detection difficult. Persistent symptoms indicate the need for intensive medical investigation. The diagnosis is made through examination of blood cells and bone marrow (Figure 27-3). A stained peripheral blood smear will exhibit low red blood cell and platelet counts along with the presence of leukemic blast cells. Examination of bone marrow demonstrates hypercellu-

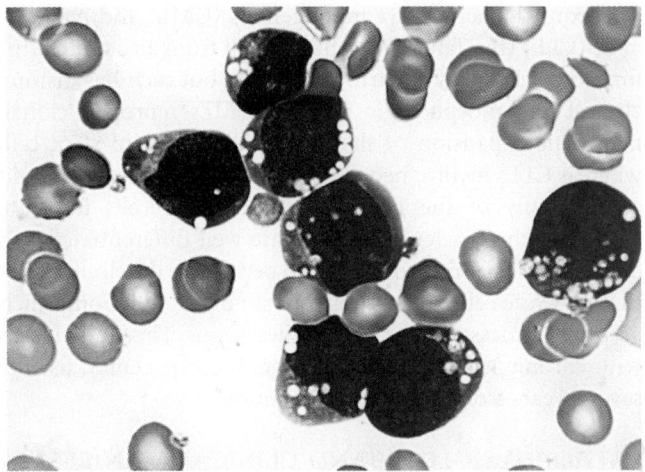

Figure 27-3 Acute lymphocytic leukemia. L3 lymphoblasts in a marrow aspirate. The cytoplasm contains sharply outlined cytoplasmic vacuoles (Wright-Giemsa stain). (From Damjanov I, Linder J, editors: *Anderson's pathology,* ed 10, St Louis, 1996, Mosby.)

larity with 60% to 100% blast cells, an occasional normal myeloid, and erythroid precursors and rare to no megakaryocytes.

Chemotherapy in varying combinations is the treatment of choice for leukemia. Two controversial treatments are immunotherapy agents that induce differentiation of immature granulocytes (i.e., *cis*-retinoic acid) and marrow transplants. Stem cell transplantation, instituted about 35 years ago, is now considered standard therapy for selected individuals with leukemia. Supportive measures include blood transfusions, antibiotics, antifungals, and antivirals. Allopurinol is used for preventing production of uric acid (which is elevated from cellular death because of treatment). Bone marrow transplantation as a treatment has been increasing during the past two decades. Although there has not been a marked improvement in response or survival of AML, dramatic improvements in survival and response of people with ALL have occurred.

Improved survival rates in individuals with ALL have occurred in the past three decades.[36] Factors influencing increased survival rates include the use of combined and multimodality treatment regimens, improved supportive services such as blood banking and nutritional support, improvements in histocompatibility testing, and microbial treatment.[43,44] Hematopoietic growth factors also have increased neutrophil recovery in myeloablative therapy and bone marrow transplant.[45] Newer approaches to treatment include the development of new drugs that target abnormal tyrosine kinases. Antibody treatment, immune cell administration, and vaccine development are three types of immunotherapy currently under investigation.[32]

Chronic Leukemias

Chronic leukemias have a presentation and progression different from acute leukemias. Chronic leukemia advances slowly and insidiously without warning. The two main types of chronic leukemias are myelogenous (CML) and lymphocytic (CLL) (see Table 27-2). Both result from an acquired injury to the DNA of a marrow stem cell, but each has distinct clinical and morphologic features. CMLs represent clonal, neoplastic expansion of the multipotent myeloid stem cell, whereas CLLs involve neoplastic transformation of lymphoid cells, mainly of the B cell lineage. Unlike cells in acute leukemia, chronic leukemic cells are well differentiated and can be readily identified. They also permit the development of mature white cells that are capable of normal function, which accounts for less severe early manifestations. Thus individuals with chronic leukemia have a longer life expectancy, usually several years from the time of diagnosis.

PATHOPHYSIOLOGY AND CLINICAL MANIFESTATIONS

Chronic lymphocytic leukemia (CLL) involves malignant transformation and progressive accumulation of monoclonal B lymphocytes that express CD5 and CD23 molecules and low amounts of surface membrane Ig and CD79b molecules.[46] The major pathophysiologic deficit in CLL is therefore failure of B cells to mature into plasma cells that synthesize immunoglobulins. B cells are the predominant cell involved although T cell CLL occasionally occurs. Unlike the other three major types of leukemia, CLL is not associated with exposure to radiation or benzene. However, there is a familial tendency with first-degree relatives having a 3 times greater risk of developing the disease. It is rare in individuals less than 45 years of age, and when diagnosed, 95% of individuals are over the age of 50.

Leukemic cells that accumulate in the marrow do not interfere with normal blood cell production to the extent found in acute leukemias. This is a significant feature explaining the reduced severity in the beginning stage of disease. Accumulation of malignant B cells is the result of cell cycle arrest in the G_0/G_1 phase creating B cells that are resistant to apoptosis.[46,47] Because the major pathophysiologic deficit in CLL is the failure of B cells to mature into plasma cells that synthesize immunoglobulin, this often results in hypogammaglobulinemia.[48] It is thought that aberrant T cell regulation is a contributing factor to hypogammaglobulinemia, however, studies on helper and regulatory T cells are inconclusive and fail to establish a relationship.

Suppression of humoral immunity caused by reduction in normally functioning B cells is the most significant effect of CLL. Individuals are at risk both for infections commonly combated by B cell-produced immunoglobulins and development of autoimmune diseases resulting in secondary cancers. Anemia, thrombocytopenia, and neutropenia are typically present with overt CLL. Invasion of most organ cells is uncommon but infiltration does occur in lymph nodes, liver, spleen, and salivary glands. CNS involvement is rare. Elevated levels of the enzyme lactic dehydrogenase and hyperuricemia are common, whereas hypercalcemia is rare. Symptoms, when they do appear, include splenomegaly, extreme fatigue, weight loss, night sweats, and low grade fever.

Chronic myelogenous leukemia (CML) is a myeloproliferative disorder, as are polycythemia vera, primary thrombocytosis, and idiopathic myelofibrosis (invasion of bone marrow by fibrous tissue) (see Chapter 26). A unique distinguishing and diagnostic marker for CML is the presence of the Philadelphia chromosome (Figure 27-4, *A*). It is not clear why myeloid cells predominate (i.e., in the chronic phase) with such strong evidence that CML begins in a stem cell. The translocation of genetic material from genes 9 and 22 creates an abnormal, fused gene identified as *BCR-ABL*.[39] In spite of the genetic alterations, the *BCR-ABL* gene functions, but the tyrosine kinase protein produced is abnormal. The abnormal protein is elongated resulting in dysfunctional regulation of cell growth and survival, and it is this abnormal protein that is thought to cause leukemic conversion (see Chapter 11).

Identifying the Philadelphia chromosome allows the clinician to follow the transformation process. Transformation occurs and is identified in erythroid, megakaryocytic, and macrophage cell lines; however, erythrocyte and megakaryocyte production and function is relatively normal. Other structural cellular abnormalities are not readily identified in transformed CML cells. Absent or low levels of the enzyme neutrophil alkaline phosphatase, with subsequent decreased phagocytic capabilities, do, however, indicate that cells fail to differentiate normally.[49]

The acute effects of CML resemble those of acute leukemia but with more prominent and painful splenomegaly. Liver function rarely is altered despite enlargement, and lymphadenopathy generally is found only in the acute phase of the disease. Hyperuricemia invariably is present and produces gouty arthritis. Infections, fever, and weight loss are common findings in patients with CML.

EVALUATION AND TREATMENT

Diagnosis of chronic leukemia depends on laboratory analyses of peripheral blood and bone marrow.

Once CLL has been diagnosed, decisions of how and when to treat need to be made. Staging of CLL facilitates the decision, but treatment outcomes are not necessarily consistent with predictions related to disease stage.[46] Chlorambucil, administered with or without corticosteroids, on a daily or intermittent schedule is the most common treatment.[32] Symptom relief is often achieved, but there is no substantial data that survival is improved. Combination therapy that includes cyclophosphamide, hydroxydaunomycin (Adriamycin), vincristine (Oncovin), and prednisone (CHOP) has an improved response rate but still does not demonstrate improved survival.[46] Fludarabine, a purine analog, has demonstrated promising results with higher response rates and incidence of complete remission as well as improved quality of life.[32] Promising results also have been obtained with the use of monoclonal antibodies (rituximab and alemtuzumab). Stem cell (autogenic and allogenic) transplant also is being investigated as treatment; however, the advanced age at which individuals contract CLL make its use less desirable.

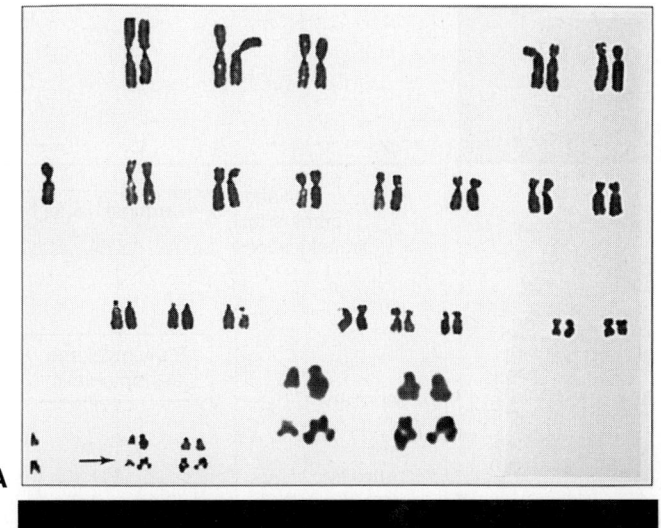

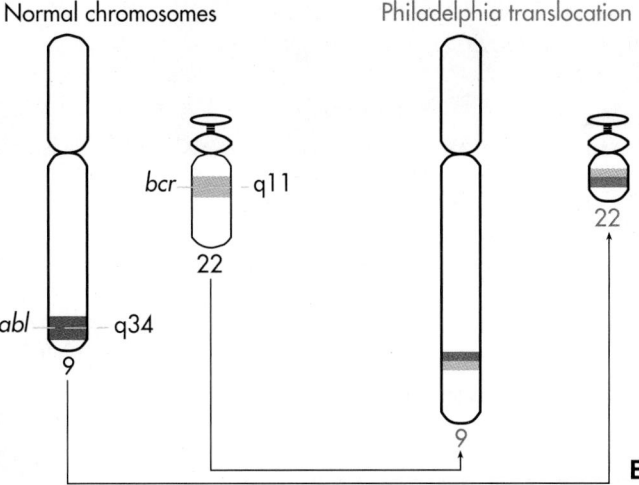

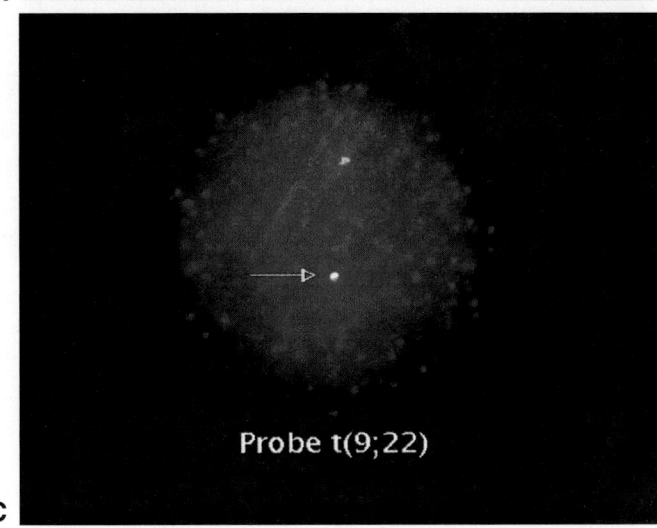

Probe t(9;22)

Figure 27-4 **Philadelphia chromosome. A,** Metaphase spread of marrow cell in chronic myelocytic leukemia. Ph1 chromosome *(arrow and enlarged inset)* is recognized by partial deletion of long arm. **B,** Schema of the Philadelphia (Ph) translocation (1) seen in chronic myelocytic leukemia. The Ph1 chromosome results from an exchange of materials between chromosomes 9 and 22, that is, t(9;22)(q34;q11). Because chromosome 22 gives up much more of its long arm than that translocated to it from chromosome 9, chromosome 22 becomes much abbreviated and known as Ph1. **C,** Chronic myelogenous leukemia (CML) is characterized by a reciprocal exchange of chromosomal material (translocation) between chromosomes 9 and 22. Probes specific for the involved regions, that is, *abl* gene (chromosome 9) and *bcr* (breakpoint cluster region on chromosome 22), are labeled with a green- and red-emitting signal, respectively (made by ONCOR, Gaithersburg, Md). If a translocation is present (bringing abl and bcr into proximity), a yellow-white signal is seen, as in this cell from an individual with CML. (**A,** Courtesy Dr. A.K. Sinha, Houston, Texas. From del Regato JA, Spjut HJ, Cox JD: *Ackerman and del Regato's cancer,* ed 2, St Louis, 1985, Mosby. **B** and **C,** From Damjanov I, Linder J, editors: *Anderson's pathology,* ed 10, St Louis, 1996, Mosby.)

Present treatment modalities for CML do not cure the disease, prevent blastic transformation, or prolong the average survival time. Standard treatment consists of chemotherapy and allogenic stem cell transplant. Although transplantation is potentially curative, its use is limited by donor availability and high toxicity in older adults thus limiting use to those over 65 years of age. Interferons in combination with other chemotherapy agents prolongs life. Traditional chemotherapy agents used are hydroxyurea (HU) and busulfan. The development and introduction of imatinib mesylate (Gleevec) as a treatment modality has changed current management of CML.[50] Response rates achieved with its use have made it the standard of care for CML, particularly in individuals who have failed to respond to interferon (IFN). Several new agents are under investigation as treatments for CML.

Myeloma

Myeloma is a neoplastic proliferation of immunocytes called *plasma cells.* Myeloma is the most common of primary malignant tumors of the skeleton and accounts for 27% of bone tumors and 1% of all malignancies. The tumor may be solitary or multifocal, known as **multiple myeloma (MM).** Approximately 15% of detected myelomas are multiple myelomas. The incidence in the United States is estimated at 16,000 persons in 2005.[51] Myeloma is more common in persons older than 40 years. Males are affected twice as often as females, and blacks have a higher incidence than whites.

PATHOGENESIS   Multiple myeloma is a disease of either (1) transformed precursor plasma cells (plasmablasts) that have completed functional rearrangement of immunoglobulin heavy chain (IgH) (see Chapter 7) in the germinal center of the lymph node before migrating to the bone marrow or (2) transformed, terminally differentiated, long-lived plasma cells in the bone marrow[51] (Figure 27-5). The genetics of MM are complex and include numerous chromosomal changes. Emerging is the understanding that continued genomic instability and the progression of genetic alterations progress to frank MM (Figure 27-5, *B*). The low mitotic index of malignant plasma cells may, however, contribute to the lack of finding or to the underestimating of genetic alterations in laboratory studies of individuals with MM.[51] Chromosome 13

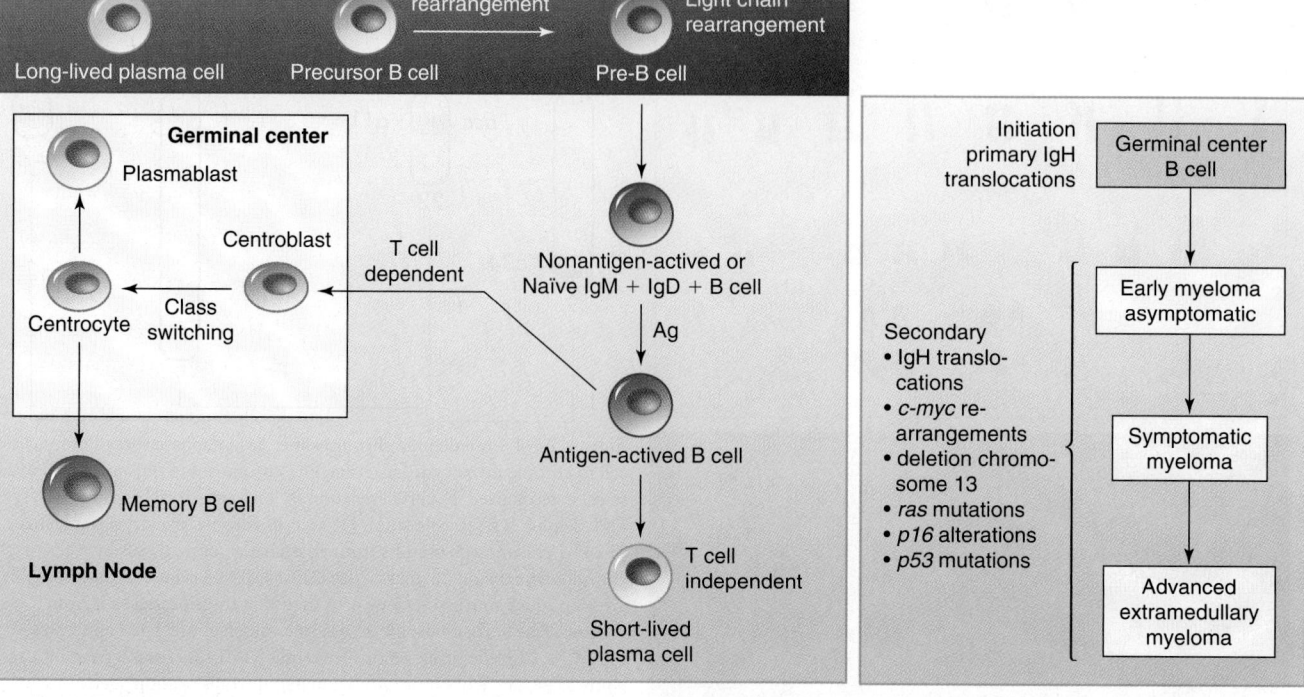

Figure 27-5 Normal plasma cell development and alterations in multiple myeloma. **A,** Precursor B cells undergo genetic rearrangement of *VDJ* chain of the IgH (heavy chains) and IgL (light chains) genes in the bone marrow *(dark shading)* before exiting to the lymph node as naïve B cells *(light shading)*. With antigen interaction, these B cells differentiate into short-lived plasma cells during the early immune response and mainly secrete IgM. Later in the immune response, some antigen-activated B cells enter a germinal center (dependent on T cell) and undergo genetic alterations with Ig heavy chain (IgH) switching (also see Chapter 7). These cells are now plasma cells, able to secrete all the different classes of immunoglobulins. Eventually, the B cells develop into either long-lived plasma cells or memory B cells. **B,** The progression of multiple myeloma is initiated by a genetic event, often an IgH translocation causing the formatting of a malignant plasma cell clone. Stepwise progression and genetic instability progresses to other altered genetic and epigenetic changes developing to frank multiple myeloma. (Adapted from Chng WJ et al: *Cancer Control* 12(2):91-104, 2005.)

abnormality is the most common alteration found in 86% of those affected.[52]

The molecular pathogenesis of multiple myeloma involves chromosomal translocations, proto-oncogene mutations, and rarely inactivation of tumor-suppressor genes. Recently proposed are two types of genetic translocations in MM, primary, or initiation, and secondary, or progression.[53,54] The primary translocation involves chromosome 14 (IgH or class switch; see Chapter 7). Secondary translocations and insertions involve other chromosomes (e.g., *c-myc*) associated with increased proliferation and disease progression.[55] In addition to *c-myc*, other genetic and epigenetic alterations are correlated with MM progression and include loss of chromosome 13, hypermethylation of *p16^{INK4A}* (cell cycle regulator), *ras* oncogenes, inactivation or deletion of *p53*, and inactivation of PTEN (pentaerythritol tetranitrate, a tumor-suppressor gene, phosphatase, and tensin homolog).[53]

Malignant plasma cells arise from one clone of B cells that then produce abnormally large amounts of one class of immunoglobulin (usually IgG, occasionally IgA, and rarely IgM, IgD, or IgE). Recent studies identify primitive B lymphocytes as the origin of MM, which implies that B cell transformation occurs in the bone marrow. Subsequent migration of these transformed B cells through the circulation to and from extramedullary sites, most likely lymph nodes, is required for their maturation and development. Eventually, the matured myeloma cells return to the bone marrow or other soft tissues. Their return is aided by cell adhesion receptors that promote "homing" to a nurturing environment site for further expansion and maturation.

The microenvironment of MM consists of myeloma cells, extracellular matrix proteins, bone marrow stromal cells, osteoclasts, and osteoblasts. Crucial in the progression of MM is the interaction of the MM cells with the microenvironment through adhesion molecules and cytokines. Interleukin 6 (IL-6) is the most significant cytokine produced in a paracrine way by MM cells and bone marrow stromal cells. Normally, IL-6 causes B-cell differentiation, but in MM it inhibits apoptosis and enhances myeloma cell proliferation. The role of IL-6 is shown in Figure 27-6.

The lysis of bone found in MM is the consequence of abnormal bone remodeling leading to increased osteoclastic bone destruction (Figure 27-7). The binding of *RANKL* (receptor activator of nuclear factor–κB ligand) to its receptor *RANK* plays a central role in promoting osteoclast differentiation and maturation (see Chapters 41 and 42). It activates

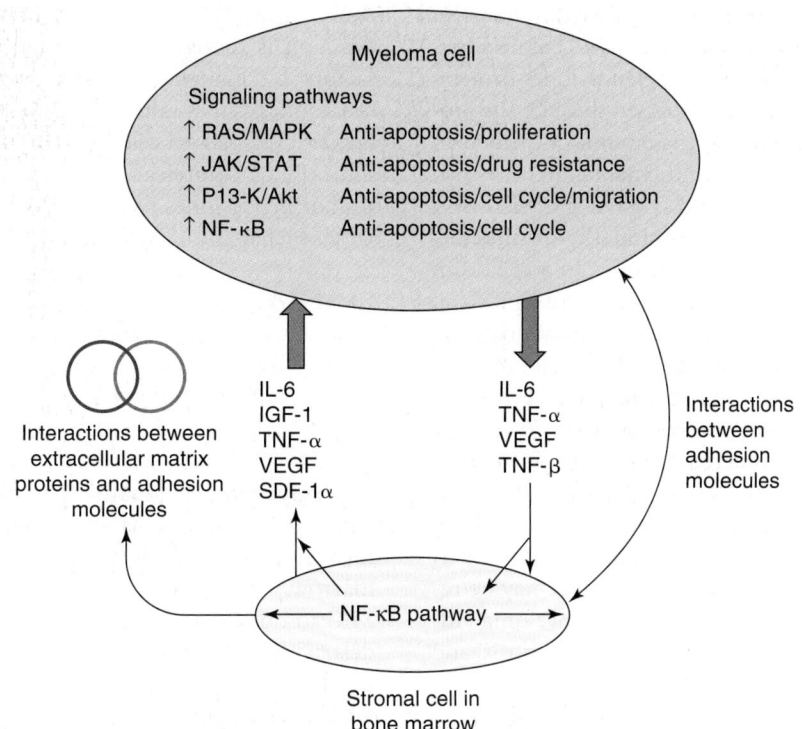

Figure 27-6 **Myeloma cell proliferation and disease progression.** This illustrates the bone marrow microenvironment (extracellular matrix) and the interaction with myeloma cells. Binding of myeloma cells to bone marrow stromal cells occurs through adhesion molecule–induced secretion of cytokines. Cytokines modulate myeloma cell proliferation, survival (antiapoptosis), drug resistance, and migration by activating various signaling pathways. Interactions between extracellular matrix proteins and adhesion factors up-regulates the NF-κB pathway (a transcription factor of the Rel family proteins) further increasing adhesion molecule expression, anti-apoptotic pathways, and cytokine secretion. *IL-6,* Interleukin; *IGF-1,* insulin-like growth factor-1; *TNF-α,* tumor necrosis factor-α; *VEGF,* vascular endothelial growth factor; *SDF-1α,* stromal-derived factor-1 α. (Adapted from Chng WJ et al: *Cancer Control* 12(2):91-104, 2005.)

mature osteoclasts and increases bone resorption (see pp. 1509-1511). The decoy receptor osteoprotegerin (OPG) binds RANKL, thus inhibiting its binding to RANK and preventing osteoclast formation and activation. Thus normally a delicate balance between RANKL and OPG regulates osteoclast activity. Adhesion of MM cells to bone marrow stromal cells induces the stromal cells to secrete osteoclast-activating factors such as IL-6, IL-1, TNF-α, and others. These factors increase RANKL resulting in greater bone breakdown, or osteolysis. The destruction of the bone matrix further increases release of cytokines that stimulate MM cell growth. The drug thalidomide disrupts the stromal marrow–MM cell interaction by modulating cell surface adhesion molecules and inhibiting angiogenesis. In addition, it increases apoptosis and G_1 growth arrest (i.e., the cell cycle gap 1, see Chapter 1) of MM cells.

In addition to the bone lesions, the malignant transformed plasma cells produce an abnormal protein—monoclonal immunoglobulin—that is responsible for many of the clinical manifestations of MM. Monoclonal immunoglobulin is present in the blood and may be used as a measure of the extent of the disease. The intact immunoglobulin resembles normal immunoglobulins with two heavy and two light chains. In certain instances, the combining and attachment of the light

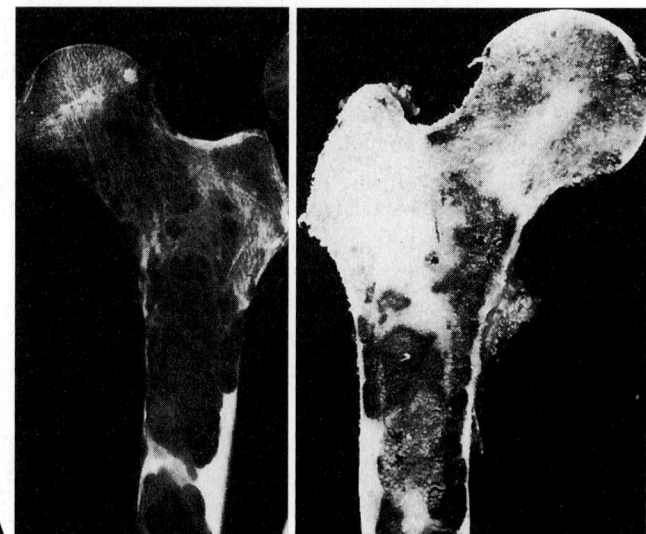

A   **B**

Figure 27-7 **Multiple (plasma cell) myeloma. A,** Roentgenogram of femur showing extensive bone destruction caused by tumor. Note absence of reactive bone formation. **B,** Gross specimen from same individual; myelomatous sections appear as dark granular sections. (From Kissane JM, editor: *Anderson's pathology,* ed 9, St Louis, 1990, Mosby.)

and heavy chains is disrupted, allowing the light chains to leave the cell unattached. This unattached light chain is identified as the **Bence-Jones protein.** The Bence-Jones protein, unlike the intact immunoglobulin, is passed through the kidneys and excreted into the urine. Large amounts of the Bence-Jones protein causes renal damage and renal failure.

MM is a progressive disorder and is often preceded by a condition known as **monoclonal gammopathy of undetermined significance (MGUS).** MGUS belongs to a spectrum of diseases known as plasma cell dyscrasias. The diagnosis of MGUS denotes the presence of a monoclonal immunoglobulin in the blood or urine without additional evidence of MM. MGUS is estimated to be present in approximately 1% of the general population and in 3% of individuals over 70 years of age. Although MGUS is considered nonpathologic and requires no treatment, about 16% of individuals with MGUS progress to malignant plasma cell disorders.[56] Progression of MM following MGUS advances to asymptomatic MM and finally symptomatic MM. Asymptomatic MM also may be referred to as **smoldering myeloma** and indolent myeloma. Additionally, MM is staged to help determine prognosis and appropriate treatment (Table 27-5).

CLINICAL MANIFESTATIONS   Myelomas characteristically cause cortical and medullary bone lysis and infiltrate the bone marrow (Figure 27-8). The most common initial symptom of myeloma is pain, which may be felt in a single bone of the entire skeleton. The usual sites of pain are the lower back, upper spine, pelvis, ribs, and sternum. Renal failure or recurrent bacterial infections also are common. The pain is initially aching, intermittent, and aggravated by weight-bearing. As the disease progresses, pain becomes severe and prolonged. It is common for the individual with myeloma to be treated for a slipped disk or arthritis before the correct diagnosis of myeloma is established. The individual also may complain of weakness, fatigue, weight loss, and anorexia in addition to pain.

In addition to bone pain, bone destruction contributes to the development of hypercalcemia. This may be characterized by neurologic disturbances such as confusion, lethargy, and weakness, as well as contributing to renal complications.

Recurring infections is another major clinical manifestation. These result from suppression of the humoral immune response. Cell-mediated immune function, that is, T cell function, is relatively normal. Suppressed humoral immune function is thought to be caused by secretion of unknown factors by malignant plasma cells. These factors activate macrophages that inhibit maturation of B cells into normally functioning plasma cells capable of producing immunoglobulins. Renal complications are thought to result from excretion of Bence-Jones protein, which may be toxic to the tubular epithelial kidney cells.

EVALUATION AND TREATMENT   Diagnosis of myeloma is made by radiographic studies, laboratory studies, and biopsy. Laboratory studies are done on blood and urine to determine the presence of abnormal immunoglobulins, as well as the Bence-Jones protein. The presence of another protein found on the surface of white blood cells, **β_2-microglobulin,** also may be present in myeloma but is present in other diseases as well. A bone marrow biopsy is performed to confirm the presence of myeloma cells in the marrow. Radiographic studies include x-ray, CT scans, and MRI to document the presence of bone lesions and areas of destruction. Diagnosis is based on findings and the degree of involvement. The individual must have at least one major criteria or three minor criteria (Box 27-2).

Table 27-5	New International Staging System	
Stage	**Criteria**	
I	Serum β_2-microglobulin <3.5 mg/L Serum albumin ≥3.5 g/dL	
II	Not stage I or III*	
III	Serum β_2-microglobulin ≥5.5 mg/L	

From Greipp PR et al: *J Clin Oncology* 23(15):3412-3420, 2005.
*There are two categories for stage II: serum β_2-microglobulin <3.5 mg/L but serum albumin <3.5 g/dL; or serum β_2-microglobulin 3.5 to <5.5 mg/L irrespective of the serum albumin level.

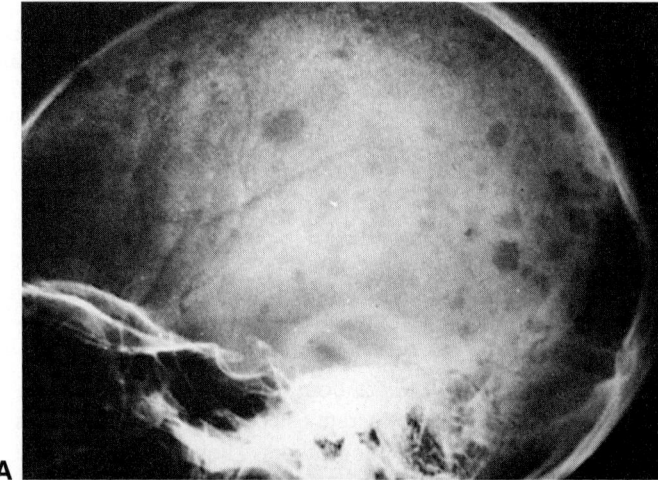

A

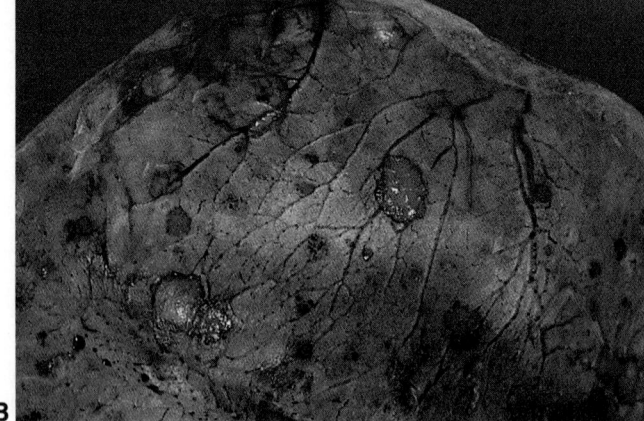

B

Figure 27-8 Lytic lesions in multiple myeloma. **A,** The radiograph shows lytic lesions. **B,** The skull contains lytic (punched-out) lesions. (From Damjanov I, Linder J: *Pathology: a color atlas,* St Louis, 2000, Mosby.)

Box 27-2	Diagnostic Criteria for Multiple Myeloma

Major Criteria
Positive biopsy result
Over 30% plasma cells in bone marrow sample
Monoclonal antibody in blood/urine

Minor Criteria
10% to 30% plasma cells in bone marrow sample
Monoclonal antibody present but not enough to be a major criteria
Holes in bone from tumor seen on imaging studies
Normal antibody in blood abnormally low

Chemotherapy, radiation therapy, and plasmapheresis (exchange), and marrow transplantation have been the standards of treatment. Conventional chemotherapeutic agents have been melphalan and prednisone with the addition of vincristine, carmustine, cyclophosphamide, doxorubicin, and dexamethasone in various combinations. Dose intensification improves the outcomes in younger patients; however, long-term remissions are obtained in a minority of patients. Thus intensive research measuring the impact of novel new therapies is the objective of ongoing trials. Gene expression profiling (GEP) will help improve the treatment of MM because it will identify prognostic subgroups and define the molecular pathways associated with these subgroups. New agents (thalidomide, Revimid, Velcade) have broadened the therapeutic regimens for end-stage myeloma.

High-dose chemotherapy and blood-forming stem cell transplantation [SCT] has become standard treatment for individuals up to age 70. Survival is increased with SCT compared to chemotherapy alone. SCT uses the patient's own blood-forming stem cells (autologous) or a donor's cells (allogenic). Survival may be prolonged by performing a second autologous transplant within 6 to 12 months from the first transplant

Radiation is used more for a localized effect rather than systemic. It is most often used to treat areas of the bone that have been damaged and are not responding to chemotherapy. In addition, it may be used to treat spinal cord compression.

Additional interventions are used to prevent and/or treat complications arising from progression of the disease. Drugs that inhibit bone resorption—bisphosphonates—reduce the incidence of skeletal damage, which also reduces hypercalcemia and decreases bone pain. Hydration and diuretics may be used to maintain a high urine output, and antibiotics may be used to treat recurring infections.

ALTERATIONS OF LYMPHOID FUNCTION

Lymphadenopathy

Lymph nodes that are characteristically small and not palpable or only barely palpable are classified as tender or nontender. **Lymphadenopathy** is characterized by enlarged lymph nodes that become palpable and tender (Figure

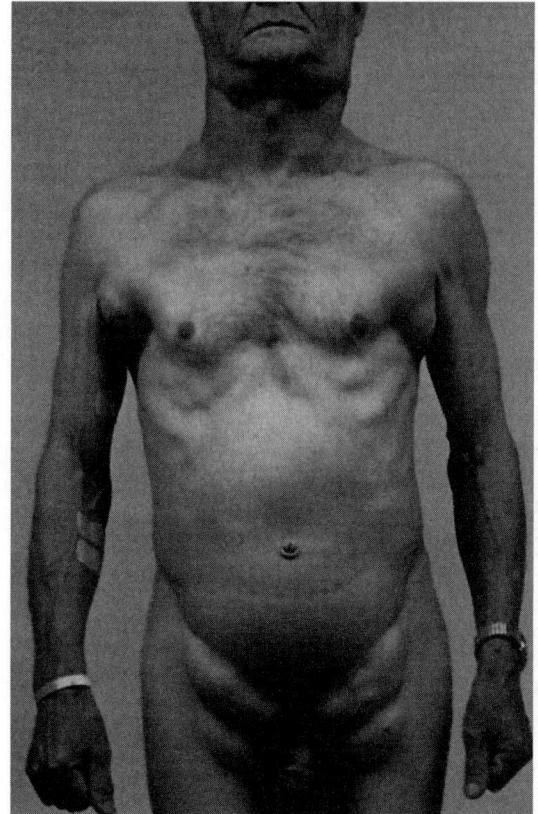

Figure 27-9 Lymphadenopathy. Individual with lymphocyte leukemia with extreme but symmetric lymphadenopathy. (Courtesy Dr. A.R. Kagan, Los Angeles. From del Regato JA, Spjut HJ, Cox JD: *Ackerman and del Regato's cancer*, ed 2, St Louis, 1985, Mosby.)

27-9). Localized lymphadenopathy usually indicates drainage of an inflammatory lesion located near the enlarged node. Generalized lymphadenopathy associated with infection occurs less often and is generally seen in the presence of malignant or nonmalignant disease. Lymphadenopathy reflects significant diseases more often in adults than in children.

Enlargement of the lymph node often is caused by an increase in size and number of the germinal centers within the node caused by proliferation of lymphocytes or monocytes (immature macrophages). Enlargement also may be caused by invasion of the node by malignant cells or cells not normally present within the node. Palpable nodes, however, do not always indicate serious disease and may indicate only a reaction to minor trauma or infection of a specific structure. The location and size of the enlarged node are important factors in diagnosing the cause of the lymphadenopathy, as are the individual's age, gender, and geographic location. Generalized lymphadenopathy occurs with non-Hodgkin lymphomas, CLL, histiocytosis, and disorders that produce lymphocytosis. In general, lymphadenopathy results from four types of conditions: (1) neoplastic diseases, (2) immunologic or inflammatory conditions, (3) endocrine disorders, or (4) lipid storage diseases. Diseases of unknown cause, including autoimmune diseases and reactions to drugs, also may lead to generalized lymphadenopathy.

Malignant Lymphomas

Lymphomas are cancers that begin with the malignant transformation of a lymphocyte and involve the proliferation of lymphocytes, histiocytes and their precursors, and derivatives in lymphoid tissues. Lymphomas display a wide spectrum of clinical and histologic patterns. There are two major categories of lymphoid malignancies, Hodgkin lymphoma and other (non-Hodgkin) lymphoma. Subtypes within each disease category may be further categorized into prognostic groups indicating the range of clinical aggressiveness or behavior of the tumor (Table 27-6). Histopathologic parameters in Hodgkin lymphoma do not predict or have prognostic value. Lymphomas and lymphocytic leukemia share some pathobiologic similarities but differ in the site of origin. When the lymphatic malignance occurs within the lymphatic tissue in the bone marrow it is designated as *lymphocytic leukemia*. When the malignancy transformation occurs within the lymph node or other lymphatic structure in the skin, gastrointestinal (GI) system, or other sites, it is designated as a *lymphoma*.

Lymphomas, including Hodgkin lymphoma, are the result of injury to the DNA of a lymphocyte. This malignant transformation produces an uncontrolled and excessive growth of the cell. These cells also possess a survival advantage allowing

Table 27-6 Classification of Lymphoid Neoplasms	
Lymphoid Neoplasms	**Prognostic Group**
B Cell Neoplasms	
1. Precursor B cell neoplasm	
a. Precursor B lymphoblastic leukemia	Highly aggressive
b. Precursor B lymphoblastic lymphoma	Highly aggressive
2. Peripheral B cell neoplasms	
a. B cell chronic lymphocytic leukemia (CLL),	Indolent
prolymphocytic leukemia (PLL),	Moderately aggressive
small lymphocytic lymphoma (SLL)	Indolent
b. Lymphoplasmacytoid lymphoma/immunocytoma	Indolent
c. Mantle cell lymphoma	Moderately aggressive
d. Follicle center lymphoma, follicular	
(1) Grade I or II	Indolent
(2) Grade III	Moderately aggressive
e. Marginal zone B cell lymphoma	Indolent
Extranodal (MALT type +/− monocytoid B cells)	
f. Hairy cell leukemia	Indolent
g. Plasmacytoma/plasma cell lymphoma	Indolent
h. Diffuse large cell lymphoma*	Aggressive
i. Burkitt lymphoma	Highly aggressive
T Cell and Putative Natural Killer (NK) Cell Neoplasms	
1. Precursor T cell neoplasms	
a. Precursor T lymphoblastic lymphoma	Highly aggressive
b. Precursor T lymphoblastic leukemia	Highly aggressive
2. Peripheral T cell and NK cell neoplasms	
a. T cell chronic lymphocytic leukemia/promyelocytic leukemia	Moderately aggressive
b. Large granular lymphocytic leukemia (LGL)	
(1) T cell type	Indolent
(2) NK cell type	Aggressive
c. Mycosis fungoides/Sezary syndrome	Indolent
d. Peripheral T cell lymphomas, unspecified*	Aggressive
e. Angioimmunoblastic T cell lymphoma (AILD)	Moderately aggressive
f. Angiocentric lymphoma	Moderately aggressive or aggressive
g. Intestinal T cell lymphoma (+/− enteropathy associated)	Aggressive
h. Adult T cell lymphoma/leukemia (ATL/L)	
(1) Smoldering	Indolent
(2) Chronic	Moderately aggressive
i. Anaplastic large cell lymphoma (ALCL), CD30+, T cell and null cell types	Aggressive
Hodgkin Lymphoma (HL)	
1. Lymphocyte predominance	
2. Nodular sclerosis	
3. Mixed cellularity	
4. Lymphocyte depletion	

*This subtype is more likely to include more than one disease entity.

them to accumulate in the lymph nodes and other sites, producing tumor masses. Lymphomas usually start in the lymph nodes or lymphatic tissues of the stomach or intestines.

Malignant lymphomas are the fifth most common cause of death from cancer in the United States. Incidence rates differ with respect to age, gender, geographic location, and socioeconomic class. New estimates for 2005 are 63,740 new cases, including 7350 cases of Hodgkin lymphoma and 56,390 cases of non-Hodgkin lymphoma. Since 1976, age-adjusted incidence rates for non-Hodgkin lymphoma have increased more than 71%. A large portion of this increase has been attributed to lymphomas developing in association with immunodeficiencies, including those with AIDS and organ transplants.[57]

Hodgkin Lymphoma

Hodgkin lymphoma (HL) is a malignant lymphoma first characterized by Thomas Hodgkin in 1832. Classification of Hodgkin as a disease or lymphoma remains inconsistent. The Lymphoma and Leukemia Society identifies Hodgkin as a lymphoma, whereas the American Cancer Society identifies it as a disease. HL is used for this chapter to be consistent with the Leukemia and Lymphoma Society. The incidence of HL is approximately 2.6 per 100,000 men and 2.2 per 100,000 women. Incidence rates for HL have declined, especially among the elderly population. The decrease in incidence in the older population is attributed to improved diagnostic accuracy. The incidence is greater in whites than blacks. Denmark, the Netherlands, and the United States have the highest incidence of HL, and Japan and Australia have the lowest incidence. The overall incidence is lower in economically disadvantaged countries with proportionately more cases occurring at older ages. HL peaks at two different ages: early in life in the second and third decades and later in life during the sixth and seventh decades.

PATHOPHYSIOLOGY HL can be distinguished from other lymphomas by the presence of Reed-Sternberg (RS) cells surrounded by a background of benign-appearing host inflammatory cells (Figure 27-10). It is widely accepted that the RS cells or their variant represents the malignant transformation of cells. The molecular events causing malignant transformation remain controversial; however, there is evidence of proto-oncogene involvement in the transformation of RS cells of HL. The origin of the RS cell may differ for various subtypes of the disease, such as activated lymphoid cells with features of B cell, T cell, or monocytic cell lines. RS cells represent a clonal proliferation of B cells as determined by their immunoglobulin gene rearrangements.[58] Characteristically, B cells are microscopically larger than normal B lymphocytes and do not resemble the cells of other non-Hodgkin lymphoma or other cancers. B cells have lost their ability to express their antibodies because of their multiple somatic mutations. Additionally, B cells constantly express CD15 (Leu-M1) and CD30 (Ki1) antigens.[59]

Although the RS cell is necessary for diagnosis, it is not specific to HL, and in rare instances cells resembling Reed-

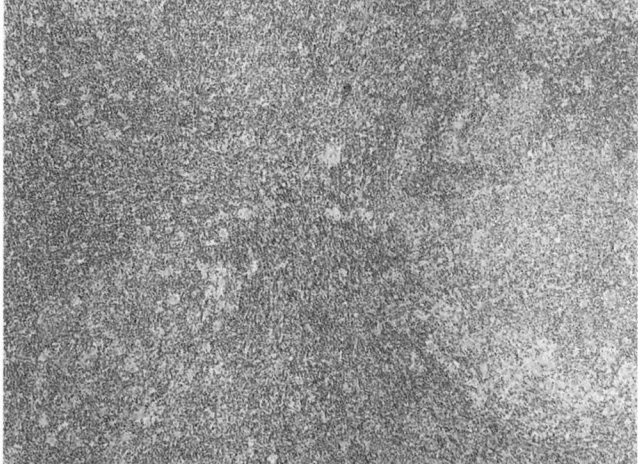

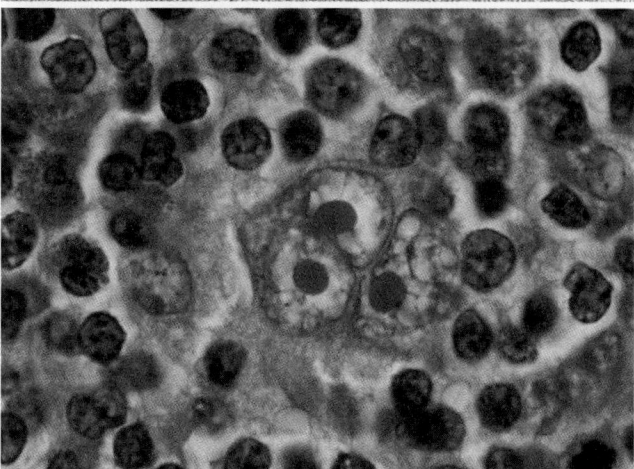

Figure 27-10 Lymph nodes. **A,** Lymphocytes (L) and histiocytes (H) Hodgkin lymphoma, nodular type. Large nodules with small, round lymphocytes, histiocytes, and scattered L&H cells. **B,** Diagnostic Reed-Sternberg cell. A large multinucleated or multilobed cell with inclusion body–like nucleoli surrounded by a halo of clear nucleoplasm. (From Damjanov I, Linder J, editors: *Anderson's pathology,* ed 10, St Louis, 1996, Mosby.)

Sternberg cells can be found in benign illness as well as other forms of neoplasia, including non-Hodgkin lymphoma and carcinoma. HL is subcategorized into two main types: classical Hodgkin and nodular lymphocyte predominant Hodgkin. Classical Hodgkin is further categorized into four distinct types based on their histologic characteristics. The four subtypes of Hodgkin lymphoma (Table 27-7) are based on the nonmalignant background of the involved node rather than the appearance of the malignant cell.

CLINICAL MANIFESTATIONS Many of the characteristic clinical features (Box 27-3) of HL can be explained by the expression of cytokines and hematopoietic growth factors by the malignant cells. The transformed cells secrete and release cytokines (IL-1, IL-2, IL-5, IL-6, tumor necrosis factor-β, interferon gamma, granulocyte colony-stimulating factor [G-CSF], and tumor growth factor-beta) that result in local and systemic reactions. The production and secretion of these cytokines has been linked to T cell transcription factors (TF).[58]

Table 27-7   Subtypes of Hodgkin Lymphoma

Subtype	Incidence	Clinical Presentation
Lymphocyte predominance	Found in all ages, but more common in adults than in children Incidence in males exceeds that in females	Peripheral node involvement Spares the mediastinum Usually localized at diagnosis Survival is long with or without treatment Late relapses common
Nodular sclerosing	Found in all ages, but most common in adolescents and young adults Incidence in females equals or exceeds that in males	Mediastinal involvement Stage and bulk of disease have prognostic significance
Mixed cellularity	Common in adults Incidence in males exceeds that in females	Stage more advanced than in nodular sclerosis and lymphocyte predominance subtypes Involves lymph nodes, spleen, liver or marrow
Lymphocyte depletion	Least common variant Most common type in elderly persons, human immunodeficiency virus (HIV)–positive individuals, and persons in nonindustrialized countries	Abdominal lymphadenopathy; spleen, liver, and bone marrow involvement, without peripheral lymphadenopathy Stage is more advanced at diagnosis

Box 27-3   Clinical Manifestations of Hodgkin Lymphoma

Physical Findings
Adenopathy
Mediastinal mass
Splenomegaly
Abdominal mass

Symptoms
Fever, weight loss, night sweats
Pruritus

Laboratory Findings
Thrombocytosis
Leukocytosis
Eosinophilia
Elevated erythrocyte sedimentation rate (ESR)
Elevated alkaline phosphatase

Paraneoplastic Syndromes

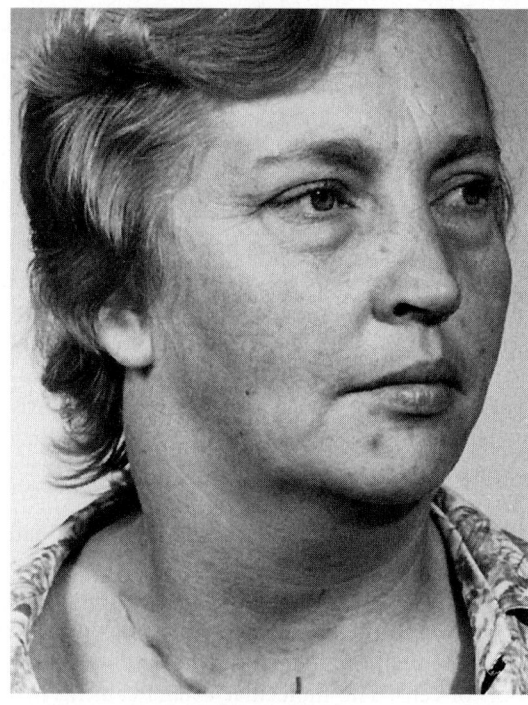

Figure 27-11 Hodgkin lymphoma and enlarged cervical lymph node. Typical enlarged cervical lymph node in the neck of a 35-year-old woman with Hodgkin lymphoma. (From del Regato JA, Spjut HJ, Cox JD: *Ackerman and del Regato's cancer,* ed 2, St Louis, 1985, Mosby.)

These cytokines are hypothesized to act in a complex autocrine and paracrine loop, stimulating both the malignant and nonmalignant stromal cells.

An enlarged painless mass, found most commonly in the neck, is often an initial sign of HL (Figure 27-11). Pain may accompany the enlarged node associated with HL. Rarely, pain may be brought on or exacerbated with the ingestion of alcohol. The discovery of an asymptomatic mediastinal mass on routine chest x-ray is not unusual. The cervical, axillary, inguinal, and retroperitoneal lymph nodes are most commonly affected in HL (Figure 27-12). Local symptoms caused by pressure and obstruction are produced by lymphadenopathy. Intermittent fever, without other symptoms of infection, and drenching night sweats are relatively common clinical presentations of HL. These constitutional symptoms and weight loss have been associated with poor diagnosis.

Once a diagnosis of HL has been made, the next step is to identify what stage it is in. Staging is done to help determine treatment and prognosis. The Cotswold Staging Classification

System is used for Hodgkin lymphoma (Table 27-8). HL and non-Hodgkin lymphomas can be divided into four stages based upon location and distribution of lymph node involvement, other organs involved, and the location of any large masses. Additionally, each stage is subclassified as to A or B, based on the symptoms of fever, exaggerated sweating, and weight loss. *A* indicates the absence of these symptoms and *B* indicates their presence and requires more aggressive treatment. Staging system is based on medical examination and radiographic results (CT scans, MRI, and PET scans). The staging system has been able to establish a correlation between

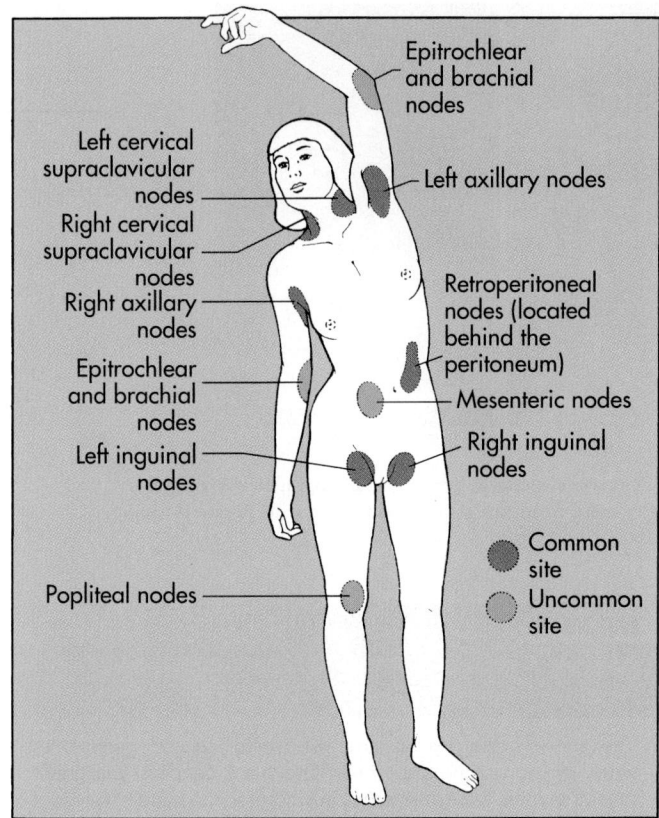

Figure 27-12 Common and uncommon involved lymph node sites for Hodgkin lymphoma.

Table 27-8	Cotswold Staging Classification System
Stage	**Criteria**
I	Involvement of a single lymph node region or lymphoid structure (i.e., spleen, thymus, Waldeyer ring)
II	Involvement of two or more lymph node regions on the same side of the diaphragm (the mediastinum is a single site, hilar lymph nodes are lateralized); the number of anatomic sites should be indicated by a suffix (i.e., II_3)
III	Involvement of lymph node regions or structures on both sides of the diaphragm Stage III_1: with or without splenic hilar, celiac, or portal nodes Stage III_2: with paraaortic, iliac, mesenteric nodes
IV	Involvement of extranodal site(s) beyond that designated "E" Modifying characteristics A: no symptoms B: fever, drenching sweats, weight loss X: bulky disease >1/3 widening of mediastinum >10-cm maximum dimension of nodal mass E: involvement of a single extranodal site contiguous or proximal to known nodal site CS: clinical stage PS: pathologic stage

Data from Lister TA, Crowther D: Staging for Hodgkin's disease, *Semin Oncol* 17:696, 1990.

anatomic extent of the disease and prognosis. Prognostic factors include clinical stage, histologic type, tumor cell concentration and tumor burden, constitutional symptoms, and age.

Although HL rarely arises in the lung, mediastinal and hilar node adenopathy can cause secondary involvement of the trachea, bronchi, pleura, or lungs. Retroperitoneal nodes can involve vertebral bodies and nerves, causing displacement of ureters. Spinal cord involvement is more common in the dorsal and lumbar regions than in the cervical region. Although uncommon, skin manifestations include psoriasis and eczematoid lesions, causing itching and scratching.

As a result of direct invasion from mediastinal lymph nodes, pericardial involvement can cause pericardial friction rub, pericardial effusion, and engorgement of the neck veins. The gastrointestinal tract and urinary tract rarely are involved. Anemia often is found in individuals with low serum iron and iron-binding capacity. Other laboratory findings include elevated sedimentation rate, leukocytosis, and eosinophilia. With advanced stages of HL, leukopenia occurs.

Splenic involvement of HL depends on histopathologic type (see Table 27-6, p. 972). The spleen is involved in 60% of cases of mixed cellularity and lymphocytic depletion types. With lymphocyte predominance and nodular sclerosis types, only 34% of cases reveal splenic involvement.

EVALUATION AND TREATMENT Because of the variability in symptoms, early definitive detection may be dif-

ficult. Asymptomatic lymphadenopathy can progress undetected for several years. Careful evaluation, including chest x-ray films, lymphangiography, and biopsy, should be done for individuals with fever of unknown origin and peripheral lymphadenopathy. About three of every four individuals diagnosed with HL are cured. Irradiation and chemotherapy have been responsible for the successful treatment of HL (Figure 27-13). More recent treatments include high-dose chemotherapy with bone marrow or stem cell transplant. Monoclonal antibodies also are being developed and nonmyeloablative allogenic stem cell transplant has been found to help certain individuals even though this treatment is still under development

The 5-year survival rate varies depending on which stage is identified at diagnosis. The 5-year survival rate for stage I and II is 90% to 95%, 80% to 85% for stage III, and 75% for stage IV. Other factors, if present, have an influence on survival. Poorer survival is related to a high white blood cell count (>15,000) or low hemoglobin (Hgb) (<10.5); low lymphocyte count (<600); and being male.[60] Cure for HL can be achieved in 70% of cases with current therapies.[61,62]

Non-Hodgkin Lymphoma

Non-Hodgkin lymphoma (NHL) is the generic term for a diverse group of clinicopathologic disorders that may be differentiated based on etiology, unique features, and response to therapy. NHL is characterized by the malignant transforma-

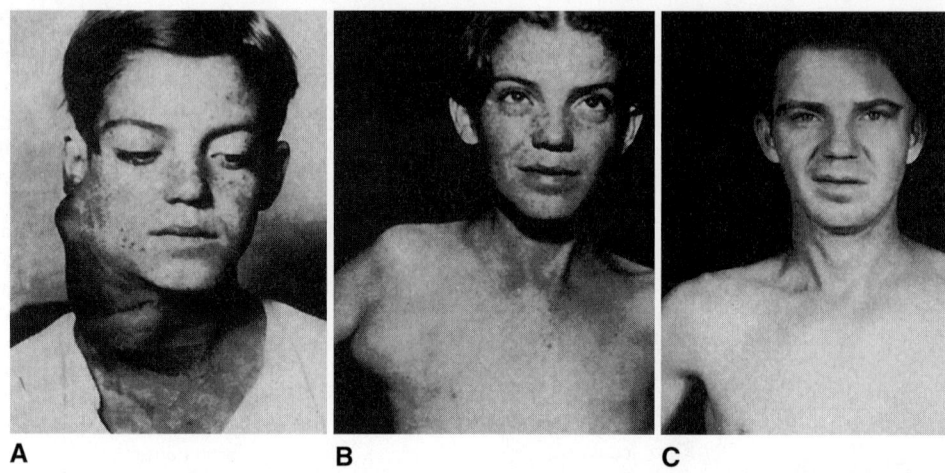

Figure 27-13 Cervical Hodgkin lymphoma. **A,** Young boy with extensive cervical Hodgkin lymphoma. **B,** Appearance several years later, when axillary manifestations developed. **C,** Appearance 23 years after initial treatment with radiation. (From del Regato JA, Spjut HJ, Cox JD: Ackerman and del *Regato's cancer,* ed 2, St Louis, 1985, Mosby.)

tion of the lymphoid tissues, primarily lymph nodes. Presently there is no primary classification system that captures the complex diversity of NHLs. The molecular rearrangements and chromosomal translocations of specific oncogenes and immunoglobulin genes are important to understanding the development of NHL.

Currently, five recognized chromosomal translocations exist that potentially set in motion the transformation or loss of critical oncogenes and tumor-suppressor genes. In addition, multiple viruses are associated with development of NHL, primarily because of their ability to provoke chronic antigenic stimulation and cytokine dysregulation resulting in unrestrained B- and T-cell stimulation, proliferation, and lymphomagenesis.[63] Viruses associated with NHLs are Epstein-Barr (EBV), human T cell leukemia virus type 1 (HTLV-1), hepatitis C virus (HCV), and Kaposi sarcoma-associated herpesvirus (KSHV) and possibly polyomavirus simian virus 40 (SV40) (see What's New? Emergent Human Simian Virus 40 and Cancer). In addition, environmental agents (chemicals, chemotherapy, and radiation exposure) and congenital or acquired immunodeficiency states are associated with increased risk for NHLs. Autoimmune disorders with chronic inflammation (Sjögren syndrome, Hashimoto thyroiditis) and *H. pylori* infection also are related to NHLs. High grade NHL is seen with increasing frequency in persons with AIDS and has an extremely poor prognosis. NHL appears to be multicentric in origin with an early tendency to spread widely.

The incidence of NHL has doubled from 8 persons per 100,000 in 1973 to 16 per 100,000 in 1995. Lymphomas from HIV and EBV have accounted for some of the increase but an actual cause has yet to be determined. Conversely, the mortality rate has risen by only half of the incidence rate. It is thought that newer treatment modalities are improving survival rates.[64]

PATHOPHYSIOLOGY   NHL is best described as a progressive clonal expansion of B cells, T cells, and/or natural killer (NK) cells. The genetic lesions affecting proto-oncogenes

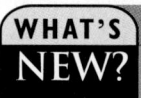
WHAT'S NEW?   **Emergent Human Simian Virus 40 and Cancer**

The polyomavirus simian virus 40 (SV40), an oncogenic DNA virus, is known to induce brain and bone cancers, malignant mesothelioma, and lymphomas in laboratory animals.[145] A recent meta-analysis of clinical data, molecular and pathologic data of 1793 cancer patients indicates a significant excess risk of SV40 and cancer. The Institute of Medicine recently concluded that the biologic evidence is of "moderate strength" that SV40 exposure could lead to human cancers. The discovery of the SV40 as well as its introduction as a pathogen to humans was related to its contamination in the polio vaccine. Inactivated (Salk) and early live attenuated (Sabin) forms of polio vaccine were inadvertently contaminated with SV40 from 1955 through 1963. Millions of people worldwide were potentially exposed because the polio vaccine was distributed worldwide. In vitro studies established that the oncogenic potential of SV40 possibly reflects disruption of cell cycle control pathways. During the last decade, independent and numerous laboratories have shown SV40 large tumor antigen (T-ag) or DNA in primary human brain and bone cancers and malignant mesothelioma.[146-149]

Recently, studies have demonstrated SV40 T-ag significantly associated with non-Hodgkin lymphoma (NHL).[150-152] Although the prevalence of SV40 infections in humans is unknown, three decades of studies reveal SV40 infections are occurring in child and adult populations today. Now, prospective studies are greatly needed to determine the prevalence of SV40 infections as well as the exact biologic mechanisms sufficient for the virus to induce human cancers.[145]

or tumor-suppressor genes result in cell immortalization and the resultant increase in malignant cells. Oncogenes may be activated by chromosomal translocations or the tumor-suppressor loci may be inactivated by deletion or mutation of chromosomes. Oncogenic viruses also may alter the genome of certain subtypes. The various subtypes of NHL may be identified by specific diagnostic markers related to various cytogenic lesions.

B cells account for approximately 85% of NHLs, with T cells and NK cells accounting for the remaining 15%. A very small percent originates from macrophages. NHL tumors are categorized by the level of differentiation, cell of origin, and rate of cellular proliferation. Tumor aggressiveness of many B cell NHLs may be predicted by the pattern of cell growth and size. Tumors with a characteristic nodular pattern, vaguely resembling lymphoid follicular structures, are generally less aggressive than lymphomas with a diffuse pattern of proliferation. Small lymphocyte lymphomas are less aggressive than large cell lymphomas, which are generally intermediate to high grade in aggressiveness. However, small cells are characteristic of some subtypes of high grade lymphomas.

CLINICAL MANIFESTATIONS   Clinical manifestations of individuals with NHL are primarily determined by the type of NHL as classified by the *Working Formulation Classification* (Table 27-9). Lymphomas are classified as low, intermediate, or high grade. A low-grade lymphoma, which also may be termed *indolent,* has a slow progression. Individuals with low-grade lymphoma commonly present with a painless, peripheral adenopathy. Spontaneous regression of these nodes may occur, mimicking the presence of an infection. Night sweats with an elevated temperature ($>38°$ C) and weight loss, as well as extranodular involvement, are not commonly present in the early stages but are common in advanced or end stage. Cytopenia, reflective of bone marrow involvement, is often observed. Hepatomegaly is common; however, splenomegaly is present in approximately 40% of individuals. Fatigue and weakness are more prevalent with advanced stages.

Immediate and high-grade lymphomas, which are more progressive, have a more varied clinical presentation. A

Table 27-9   A Comparison of the Working Formulation Classification and the Proposed Revised European-American Classification

Working Formulation	Revised European-American Classification	
	B Cell Neoplasms	**T Cell Neoplasms**
1. Small lymphocyte consistent with CLL	**B cell CLL/PLL/SLL**	**T cell CLL/PLL**
	Marginal zone/MALT	LGL
	Mantle cell	ATL/L (chronic and smoldering types)
Plasmacytoid	**Lymphoplasmacytoid marginal zone/MALT**	
	B cell CLL/PLL, SLL	
2. Follicular, predominantly small cleaved cell	**Folliclular center, follicular grade II**	
	Marginal zone/MALT	
3. Follicular, mixed small cleaved and large cell	**Follicle center, follicular grade II**	
	Marginal zone/MALT	
4. Follicular, large cell	Follicle center, follicular grade III	
5. Diffuse, small cleaved cell	**Mantle zone**	**T cell CLL/PLL**
	Follicle center, diffuse small cell	LGL
	Marginal zone/MALT	ATL/L
		Angioimmunoblastic
		Angiocentric
6. Diffuse, mixed small and large cell	**Large B cell lymphoma (rich in T cells)**	**Peripheral T cell, unspecified**
	Follicle center, diffuse small cell	ATL/L
	Lymphoplasmacytoid	Angioimmunocentric
	Marginal zone/MALT	Angiocentric
	Mantle cell	Intestinal T cell lymphoma
7. Diffuse, large cell	Diffuse large B cell lymphoma	**Peripheral T cell, unspecified**
		ATL/L
		Angioimmunoblastic
		Angiocentric
		Intestinal T cell lymphoma
8. Large cell immunoblastic	Diffuse large B cell lymphoma	**Peripheral T cell, unspecified**
		ATL/L
		Angioimmunoblastic
		Angiocentric
		Intestinal T cell
		Anaplastic large cell
9. Lymphoblastic	Precursor B lymphoblastic	Precursor T lymphoblastic
10. Small noncleaved cell	Burkitt	Peripheral T cell, unspecified
Burkitt	High-grade B cell, Burkitt-like	
Non-Burkitt	Diffuse large B cell	

From Harris NL: A practical approach to the pathology of lymphoid neoplasms: a revised European-American Classification from the International Lymphoma Study Group. In DeVita VT, Hellman S, Rosenberg SA, editors: *Important advances in oncology 1995,* Philadelphia, 1995, Lippincott.

Table 27-10 Clinical Differences Between Non-Hodgkin Lymphoma and Hodgkin Lymphoma

Characteristic	Non-Hodgkin Lymphoma	Hodgkin Lymphoma
Nodal involvement	Multiple peripheral nodes	Localized to single axial group of nodes (i.e., cervical, mediastinal, para-aortic)
	Mesenteric nodes and Waldeyer ring commonly involved	Mesenteric nodes and Waldeyer ring rarely involved
Spread	Noncontiguous	Orderly spread by contiguity
B symptoms*	Uncommon	Common
Extranodal involvement	Common	Rare
Extent of disease	Rarely localized	Often localized

*Fever, weight loss, night sweats.

Table 27-11 Ann Arbor Staging for Hodgkin Lymphoma

Stage	Criteria
I	Involvement of single lymph node
II	Involvement of 2 or more lymph node regions
III	Involvement of lymph nodes on both sides of diaphragm
IV	Diffuse involvement of one or more extra lymphatic organs with or without associated lymph node involvement

Subclassifications

E	Involvement of adjacent extra lymphatic site
S	Involvement of spleen
A	Asymptomatic
B	Fever, night sweats, weight loss

high-grade lymphoma also may be termed *aggressive*. Adenopathy is common with more than one-third of individuals having extra nodal involvement. Common sites are the GI tract, skin, bone marrow, sinuses, genitourinary (GU) tract, thyroid, and central nervous system (CNS). Night sweats, with an increased temperature ($>38°$ C), as well as weight loss ($>10\%$ from baseline within 6 months) are present in approximately 30% to 40% of individuals. Some individuals have retroperitoneal and abdominal masses with symptoms of abdominal fullness, back pain, ascites (fluid in the peritoneal cavity), and leg swelling. Hepatomegaly and splenomegaly are often present. Differences in clinical features are noted in Table 27-10.

EVALUATION AND TREATMENT Biopsy is considered the primary means for diagnosis of NHL. Staging of NHL is necessary to identify treatment and make a prognosis. In addition to biopsy, CT scans of the neck, chest, abdomen, and pelvis, as well as bilateral bone marrow aspirate, are per-

formed. Data from all three procedures is necessary for appropriate staging. A common finding in NHL is noncontiguous lymph node involvement, which is not common in HL. The Ann Arbor Staging System is most commonly used to stage NHL (Table 27-11). Treatment for NHL is quite diverse and depends on type (B cell or T cell) of tumor stage, histologic status (low, intermediate, or high grade), symptoms, age, and any comorbidities.

The goal of therapy is to cause a complete remission by eliminating all or as many malignant cells as possible. In general, treatment is initiated at the time of diagnosis; however, some low-grade lymphomas are widely disseminated at diagnosis, and because current therapy is not curative, observation without treatment may be the most appropriate choice. A partial remission may be achieved in some cases in which evidence of the disease remains but it does not progress.

Chemotherapy, radiation therapy, and immunotherapy remain the keystone forms of treatment. Single drugs or combinations of chemotherapeutic agents are used depending on the aggressiveness of tumor growth. Radiation is used commonly in conjunction with chemotherapy but may be used alone in rare instances. Immunotherapy that stimulates the individual's immune system to treat the disease is a recent addition to the arsenal of treatment modalities. Stem cell transplantation (allogenic) also is a newer treatment and is used most commonly when the lymphoma is resistant to other forms of treatment and is used more often in individuals with high-grade lymphoma.

Individuals with NHL can survive for long periods. Survival with nodular lymphoma ranges up to 15 years. Individuals with diffuse disease generally do not survive as long. The relative 1-year survival rate is 77%, 59% at 5 years, and 42% at 10 years. Many investigators believe that more aggressive treatment increases the cure rate.

Burkitt Lymphoma

Burkitt lymphoma, the most common type of NHL in children, is a tumor with unique clinical and epidemiologic features. It comprises about 2% of all lymphomas and occurs in children from east-central Africa and New Guinea. It is a very fast growing tumor and involves primarily the jaw and facial bones (Figure 27-14). Epstein-Barr virus (EBV), found in nasopharyngeal secretions, is associated with Burkitt lymphoma in African children.

The American type of Burkitt lymphoma usually involves the abdomen and is characterized by extensive marrow replacement. The cancerous cell is a B cell that undergoes cancerous transformation and progression. The African variety has been treated successfully with radiation therapy and cyclophosphamide. The American type is more resistant to treatment.

Conditions that Mimic Lymphomas

Certain other clinical conditions mimic the malignant lymphomas. These conditions include tuberculosis (TB), syphilis, systemic lupus erythematosus, lung cancer, and bone cancer.

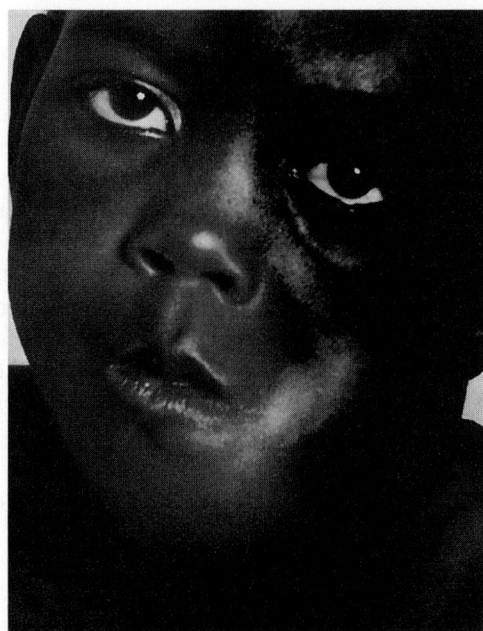

Figure 27-14 Burkitt lymphoma. Burkitt lymphoma involving the jaw in young African boy. (Courtesy Dr. J.N.P. Davies, Albany, NY. From del Regato JA, Spjut HJ, Cox JD: *Ackerman and del Regato's cancer,* ed 2, St Louis, 1985, Mosby.)

An important distinction between lymphomas and other conditions is that lymphomas usually involve localized lymphadenopathy. Infectious precursors of malignant lymphomas are characterized by more generalized lymphadenopathy with systemic signs and symptoms.

ALTERATIONS OF SPLENIC FUNCTION

The spleen has been an organ of mystery and perplexity in the study of medicine. Its relationship to other organs and disease processes, particularly the immune and hematologic systems, was not identified until the eighteenth century. The complexities of splenic function are still not totally understood, and its mysteries are still being explored. The spleen is a useful organ, but its functions overlap those of other organs so that one is capable of living a normal, healthy life without the spleen.[65] The relationship between asplenia and a higher risk for infection was not recognized until the early 1950s.[66]

In the past, enlargement of the spleen (**splenomegaly**) was considered a pathologic manifestation of various disease states. It is now recognized that splenomegaly is not necessarily pathologic because some individuals may have an enlarged spleen without any evidence of disease. It is still considered abnormal and may be one of the first physical signs of underlying conditions; therefore, when present, identification of an underlying cause is a priority.[67] In conditions where splenomegaly is present, the normal functions of the spleen may become overactive and produce a condition known as **hypersplenism.**

The concept of an overactive spleen dates to 1866; however, the term *overactive spleen* was not uniformly applied to specific conditions and confusion existed over the clinical use and

Box 27-4	Diseases Related to Classification of Splenomegaly

Inflammation or Infections
1. Acute
   a. Viral (hepatitis, infectious mononucleosis, cytomegalovirus)
   b. Bacterial (salmonella, gram negative)
   c. Parasite (typhoid)
2. Subacute or chronic
   a. Bacterial (subacute bacterial endocarditis, tuberculosis)
   b. Parasite (malaria)
   c. Fungal (histoplasmosis)
   d. Felty syndrome
   e. Systemic lupus erythematosus
   f. Rheumatoid arthritis

Congestive
1. Cirrhosis
2. Heart failure
3. Portal vein obstruction (portal hypertension)
4. Splenic vein obstruction

Infiltrative
1. Gaucher disease
2. Amyloidosis
3. Diabetic lipemia

Tumors or Cysts
1. Malignant
   a. Polycythemia rubra vera
   b. Thrombocytopenia
   c Chronic leukemia (chronic myelocytic leukemia, chronic lymphocytic leukemia)
   d. Hodgkin disease
   e. Acute leukemia
   f. Metastatic solid tumors
2. Nonmalignant: hamartoma
3. Cysts
   a. True: lymphangiomas, hemangiomas, epithelial, endothelial
   b. False: hemorrhagic, serous, inflammatory

meaning of the term. Current criteria for overactive spleen include (1) anemia, leukopenia, thrombocytopenia, or combinations of these; (2) cellular bone marrow; (3) splenomegaly; and (4) improvement after splenectomy.[67,68] It is recognized that individuals may seek treatment for problems without having met all these clinical criteria; therefore there is still uncertainty as to the relevance and clarity of this condition. Hypersplenism is further categorized as either primary, when no etiologic factor is identified, or secondary, when splenomegaly results from some other identified condition.[67]

PATHOPHYSIOLOGY   Splenomegaly without a specific etiology is seen in 7% to 15% of individuals who are being evaluated for primary splenomegaly and is generally a diagnosis of exclusion.[69] Specific conditions causing secondary splenomegaly and resulting hypersplenism are many and are related to all other categories of disease that affect individuals. Secondary splenomegaly may be classified according to the underlying cause. Specific conditions related to these various classifications of splenomegaly are detailed in Box 27-4. Different pathologic processes that produce splenomegaly are described briefly.

Acute inflammatory or infectious processes cause splenomegaly because of an increased demand for defensive activities. Acutely enlarged spleens secondary to infection may become so filled with erythrocytes that their natural rubbery resilience is lost and they become fragile and vulnerable to blunt trauma.[70] Traumatic rupture of the spleen is a complication in individuals with infectious mononucleosis; rupture occurs mostly in males between the fourth and twenty-first day of acute illness.[19]

Congestive splenomegaly is accompanied by ascites, portal hypertension, and esophageal varices and is most commonly seen in those with hepatic cirrhosis. Splenic hyperplasia (neoplasia) develops in disorders that increase splenic workload and is associated most commonly with various types of anemia (hemolytic) and chronic myeloproliferative disorders (i.e., polycythemia vera).

Infiltrative splenomegaly is caused by engorgement of the macrophages with indigestible materials associated with various "storage diseases." Tumors and cysts cause actual growth of the spleen. Metastatic tumors of the spleen are rare and may result from skin, lung, breast, and cervical primary sites.[10]

CLINICAL MANIFESTATIONS Overactivity of the spleen results in hematologic alterations that affect all blood components. Sequestering of red blood cells, granulocytes, and platelets results in a reduction of all circulating blood cells. The spleen may sequester up to 50% of the red blood cell population, thereby upsetting the normal physiologic concentration of red blood cells in the circulating blood.[70] The rate of splenic pooling is directly related to spleen size and the degree of increased blood flow through it. In addition to this pooling, the sequestered red blood cells also are exposed to splenic conditions that accelerate destruction, further contributing to the decreased red blood cell concentration. These combined activities result in anemia.

Anemia may be further potentiated by an increase in blood volume, which produces a dilutional effect on the already reduced concentration of red blood cells. Anemia has been identified as the result of sequestering. The dilutional effect, as well as the removal and destruction of red blood cells, depends primarily on the degree of splenomegaly.

White blood cells and platelets also are affected by sequestering, although not to the same degree as the red blood cell. Again, the size of the spleen is the determining factor in the number of cells sequestered.

EVALUATION AND TREATMENT Treatment for hypersplenism is splenectomy; however, it is not always the treatment of choice. It is generally beneficial to perform a splenectomy when the spleen is exerting destructive effects on the red blood cells and is not performed when the spleen is exerting favorable effects, such as antibody production and hematopoiesis.[10] The initial goal of treatment should be to treat the underlying disorder causing the splenomegaly.

Splenectomy should be performed for clinical indicators and not necessarily for specific conditions.[65] Splenectomy for splenic rupture no longer is considered mandatory in light of the possibility of overwhelming sepsis after removal. Repair and preservation of the ruptured spleen is now considered before the decision to remove the spleen is made. Splenectomy also may be performed to establish a diagnosis, particularly in cases of lymphoma. Recent studies have determined that a substantial number of persons with idiopathic splenomegaly will progress to develop a lymphoma.[69] In addition to establishing a diagnosis, splenectomy for lymphoma also is a part of treatment. Splenectomy also may be performed as treatment for hairy cell leukemia, Felty syndrome, agnogenic myeloid metaplasia, thalassemia major, Gaucher disease, hemodialysis splenomegaly, splenic venous thrombosis, and thrombotic thrombocytopenia purpura (TTP).[71]

Individuals are able to lead normal lives after splenectomy, but hematologic abnormalities often exist after removal of the spleen. The red blood cells become thinner, broader, and wrinkled as a result of increases in surface area and membrane lipids.[70] The white blood cell count increases dramatically 1 week after removal and then levels off to approximately 40% above normal. Platelets also rise immediately after surgery and then level off to above-normal levels for the duration of the individual's life. Increased platelet levels have been implicated in ischemic heart disease in males because of increased thrombocytosis and hypercoagulability.[70]

A major postoperative complication following splenectomy is overwhelming postsplenectomy infection (OPSI). Unless treated in time, OPSI rapidly progresses to septic shock and possibly disseminated intravascular coagulation (DIC). Initial statistics indicate a mortality rate of 50% to 70%, with most deaths occurring within the first 48 hours after hospitalization. Prompt medical attention can reduce the mortality rate to 10%.[71]

ALTERATIONS OF PLATELETS AND COAGULATION

Hemostasis is affected by alterations of platelets and coagulation, either by preventing hemostasis or by causing it to occur when it is not needed. (Hemostasis is described in Chapter 25.) Prevention of hemostasis results in either internal or external hemorrhage. Diffuse hemorrhage into skin tissues that is visible through the skin causes a red-purplish discoloration identified as a **purpura.** Purpuric disorders occur when there are not enough normal platelets to plug damaged vessels or prevent leakage from the many minute tears that occur daily in normal capillaries. Coagulation disorders tend to result in more serious internal bleeding and usually are caused by a deficiency of one or several clotting factors.

Disorders in which hemostasis proceeds needlessly tend to result from vascular abnormalities that stimulate clotting.

These disorders are known collectively as **thromboembolic disease.**

Disorders of Platelets

Quantitative or qualitative abnormalities of platelets can interrupt normal blood coagulation and prevent hemostasis. The quantitative abnormalities are thrombocytopenia, a decrease in the number of circulating platelets, and **thrombocythemia,** an increase in the number of platelets. Qualitative disorders affect the structure or function of individual platelets and can coexist with the quantitative disorders. Qualitative disorders usually prevent platelet adherence and aggregation, preventing formation of a platelet plug.

Thrombocytopenia

Thrombocytopenia is defined as a platelet count below 100,000 platelets/mm³ of blood. A count of 50,000/mm³ or less increases the potential for hemorrhage associated with minor trauma. Spontaneous bleeding can occur with counts between 10,000/mm³ and 15,000/mm³, resulting in petechiae, ecchymoses, larger purpuric spots, or frank bleeding from mucous membranes.[72] Severe bleeding results if the count is below 10,000/mm³ and can be fatal if it occurs in the gastrointestinal tract, respiratory system, or central nervous system.

Before the diagnosis of thrombocytopenia is made, it is important to determine whether a **pseudothrombocytopenia** is present. This phenomenon occurs in approximately 1 in 1000 to 1 in 10,000 situations and is an in vitro artifact that occurs when platelets counted in a blood smear by automatic cell counting are agglutinated by IgG, IgM, or IgA in the presence of ethylenediamine tetraacetic acid (EDTA), a preservative in banked blood.[73] The agglutinated platelets are not counted, and it appears that the individual may have thrombocytopenia when in fact it is a false representation of the total platelet count.

Another situation that mimics thrombocytopenia is a dilutional effect observed after massive transfusion of packed cells, which are generally platelet poor. This occurs when an individual has received more than 10 units of blood within a 24-hour period. The hemorrhage that necessitated the transfusion accelerates a loss of platelets, which further contributes to the thrombocytopenic state.

Thrombocytopenia is also the result of increased sequestering of platelets by the spleen secondary to hypersplenism (congestive) (hypersplenism is discussed on p. 979). Hypothermia also has been identified as a cause of thrombocytopenia. Temperatures below 25° C appear to be necessary for this condition to be present. After rewarming, levels of platelets return to normal, suggesting that the platelets are sequestered and later released.[73]

Thrombocytopenia is often secondary to other acquired or congenital conditions that may cause decreased production of platelets or decreased platelet survival. Congenital conditions are rare and include thrombocytopenia with absent radii (TAR) syndrome, Wiskott-Aldrich syndrome, May-Hegglin syndrome, and autosomal recessive thrombocytopenia. The acquired states are more common and include such conditions as viral infections (e.g., EBV, rubella, CMV, and HIV). Thrombocytopenia also may accompany nutritional deficiency states associated with vitamin B₁₂, folic acid, and iron. Bone marrow replacement and bone marrow hypoplasia (aplastic anemia) also may precipitate thrombocytopenia. Drugs (e.g., thiazides, estrogens, quinine-containing medications) and chemotherapy and toxins (e.g., ethanol, cocaine-specific toxins) are also implicated as causing thrombocytopenia.

Heparin is a common cause of drug-induced thrombocytopenia. Approximately 8% of individuals treated with unfractionated heparin develop the antibody associated with heparin-induced thrombocytopenia (HIT) but do not become thrombocytopenic. Of these, 1% to 5% will develop HIT and 33% will develop thrombosis.[74] HIT is an immune-mediated, adverse drug reaction resulting in a hypercoaguable state. It is caused by IgG antibodies that recognize complexes of heparin and platelet factor 4, leading to platelet activation through platelet Fc γIIa receptors.[75] The hallmark of HIT is a decrease in platelets beginning 5 to 10 days after administration of heparin.[75] A decrease of approximately 50% in the platelet count is seen in more than 95% of individuals. Other clinical features that indicate HIT are the development of thrombosis and the instance of other causes of thrombocytopenia being ruled out or in. Bleeding is uncommon in HIT, even with low platelet counts.[76] Diagnosis of HIT is primarily based on clinical presentation because no definitive criteria have been established for diagnosis. HIT antibody titers may be measured, but the titers must be evaluated in the context of the clinical presentation.[77] If HIT is not recognized and treated, intravascular aggregation of platelets causes rapid development of arterial and venous thrombosis. Although rare, heparin antibodies have caused anaphylactic shock.[78]

Venous thrombosis is most common and results in deep venous thrombosis and pulmonary emboli. A majority of arterial thromboses affect the large arteries of the lower extremities, causing acute limb ischemia. In addition, arterial thrombosis leads to cerebrovascular accidents and myocardial infarctions. Other major arteries (renal, mesenteric, upper limb) also may be affected.[75]

Treatment for HIT has been discontinuation of heparin and use of other anticoagulants. Two newer thrombin inhibitors—lepirudin and argatroban—have been used with relative success. Both agents can be monitored by an activated partial thromboplastin time (a PTT).[79]

Thrombocytopenia also is caused by increased platelet destruction most commonly associated with **immune thrombocytopenic purpura (ITP).** The incidence of ITP is estimated to be 5.8 to 6.6 per 100,000 in the general population. ITP was formerly known as *idiopathic thrombocytopenic purpura;* however, it is widely recognized now as an autoimmune process, hence the change from idiopathic to immune. IgG is identified as the antibody in the majority of cases, however, IgA and IgM antibodies also have been identified.[80] The autoantibodies target either platelet glycoprotein (GP)IIb/IIIa or GPIb/IX[81] (see Chapter 25). T cell activation also is recognized as a critical event in ITP. B cell activation through T cell depends on the interaction of T cell CD154 with B cell CD40. CD154 also is expressed intracellularly in platelets; however, on activation it is expressed on the surface membrane of the platelet. Expression of CD154 on the surface provides a target for antigens and a stimulus for B cell antibody production.[82]

The antibody-coated platelets are removed from the circulation by mononuclear phagocytes in the spleen through the Fc receptor. The specific mechanisms for platelet destruction are not completely clear. Autoantibodies also are thought to affect platelet development within bone marrow. The characteristic manifestation of bone marrow is a normal or increased number of megakaryocytes. Immature platelets, thought to be more hemostatically active, are released into the circulation. Their "stickiness" may account for the lower incidence of bleeding.[80]

ITP is a common disease in adults and children; however, the characteristics of each group differ considerably. It is commonly a chronic condition in adults and is more prevalent in females. The incidence is highest in the young adult group (20 to 40 years old), but ITP is found in all age categories. The onset is variable and vague, often with no preceding illness.

The acute form of ITP is more prevalent in children, often developing after a viral illness, and is one of the most common childhood bleeding disorders.[83] In children, the disease is self-limiting and approximately 80% to 90% recover completely within 6 months. The remaining 10% to 20%, who are thrombocytopenic beyond 6 months, are considered to have chronic ITP.[84] Females over age 10 with initial elevated platelet count (>200,000/μL) are more likely to develop chronic ITP.[85] However, even those with chronic ITP have a recovery rate of 58% to 79% over the subsequent years.

Initial manifestations include minor problems, such as development of petechiae and purpura over the course of several days, that progress to major hemorrhage from mucosal sites, epistaxis, hematuria, menorrhagia, and bleeding gums. Initial platelet counts are generally <150,000/μL. Rarely will an individual present with intracranial bleeding or other sites of internal bleeding.

No specific guidelines existed for the diagnosis and treatment of ITP until recently. Since 1994, guidelines established by a panel of the American Hematological Society have been used for diagnosis and treatment of ITP in children and adults.[86] Diagnosis of ITP is based on a history of bleeding and associated symptoms, such as weight loss, fever, and headache. Risk factors are also identified, such as HIV infection, and medications are screened as a potential cause of ITP, as well as any family history of bleeding. Physical examination signs are also evaluated for types of bleeding, location, and severity. Evidence of other infections (bacterial, HIV) and

thrombosis are also assessed. Other diagnostic tests include complete blood count (CBC) and peripheral blood smear.

Treatment of ITP is controversial because of the fact that it is palliative and not curative. There are two schools of thought in the treatment of ITP—interventionist and observational. There is no body of evidence that supports one over the other, therefore treatment is often dictated by the specific individual's course of disease. The overall course of the disease is variable, particularly in children, and even in the chronic form the platelet count may be decreased. However, the individual experiences no major consequences. The presence of bleeding is a manifestation that requires immediate attention. Treatment is initiated when platelet counts are less than 20,000 to 30,000 or less than 50,000 with evidence of bleeding from mucous membranes or when the individual is at high risk to develop bleeding.[87]

The overall goal of therapy is to reduce or eliminate platelet destruction. The majority of drugs used in treatment of ITP impair clearance of IgG autoantibody-coated platelets by Fcγ receptors expressed by tissue macrophages.[88] Initial therapy for ITP is infusion of glucocorticoids (prednisone), which prevents sequestering and further destruction of platelets. If platelet counts do not increase appropriately, splenectomy is considered. Splenectomy generally produces response rates of 60% to 70%; however, it is not without risk, and approximately 10% to 20% of individuals who undergo splenectomy suffer a relapse and require further treatment.[89] In these relapsed individuals, it is thought that other reticuloendothelial organs, particularly the liver, have emerged as a reservoir for platelets.[90]

Further treatment for ITP includes intravenous immunoglobulin (IVIg), anti–(Rh) D, danazol, and vinca alkaloids (chemotherapeutic agents). Anti–(Rh) D is used as an alternative to splenectomy or to delay the need for one. It is also hoped that its use may induce a remission of ITP.[91] Immunosuppressives (azathioprine and cyclophosphamide) also are used, but only for individuals who are intolerant of other therapies.[89] Monoclonal antibodies have recently been identified as successfully treating relapsing or refractory ITP.[92]

Thrombocytopenia is also a manifestation of **thrombotic thrombocytopenic purpura (TTP)**, a thrombotic microangiopathy in which platelets aggregate and cause occlusion of arterioles and capillaries within the microcirculation. This is a relatively uncommon syndrome occurring in about 1;1,000,000 individuals with a preference for females in their thirties.[93] TTP is rarely observed in infants and the elderly. TTP is increasing in incidence, and this appears to be a true increase rather than a result of improved recognition.[94]

Platelet aggregation and microthrombi formation are the key pathologic features resulting in microthrombi causing occlusion of arterioles and capillaries within the microcirculation. The thrombi are found throughout the entire vascular system causing damage to multiple organs. Organs most susceptible to damage are the kidney, brain, and heart. Other organs often affected are the pancreas, spleen, and adrenal glands.[95]

The thrombi are primarily composed of platelets with minimal fibrin and red cells, differentiating them from thrombi secondary to intravascular coagulation.[96] The etiology of TTP remains a mystery; however, recent evidence points to the presence of von Willebrand factor (vWf) and its effect on platelets causing them to clump and aggregate. Failure to cleave vWf, leaving it in larger than normal size, allow it to become entangled in the subendothelial fibrous components potentiating vWf-mediated platelet adhesion to the subendothelium.[95] A deficiency of vWf cleaving protease (metalloprotease) has been identified as the major cause of failure to cleave vWf. Antibodies (IgG) have been identified against metalloprotease, linking the condition to an autoimmune process.[73,95]

TTP is clinically related to other thrombotic microangiopathic conditions, including hemolytic uremic syndrome; malignant hypertension; and preeclampsia, or the pregnancy-induced HELLP (hemolysis, elevated liver enzymes, low platelet count) syndrome. Hemolytic uremic syndrome (HUS) shares many of the clinical characteristics of TTP; however, HUS often follows a hemorrhagic, diarrheal illness. Certain drugs also have been identified that may precipitate TTP or HUS. The specific mechanism of action is unknown. Pregnancy also has been identified with the development of TTP.

Typical presentation of the individual with TTP is identified as the "pathognomonic pentad." These clinical features include hemolytic anemia, thrombocytopenia, neurologic abnormalities, fever, and renal alterations. It is not mandatory that all five be present to make an official diagnosis because the earlier the diagnosis is made the earlier treatment can be initiated—earlier treatment results in more positive outcomes.

There are two types of TTP: chronic relapsing and acute idiopathic. **Chronic relapsing TTP** is the more rare type and is usually seen in children. When recognized early enough and successfully treated, the child will experience recurring episodes at approximately 3-week intervals that are usually predictable and responsive to treatment.

Acute idiopathic TTP is much more common and more severe. Early diagnosis and treatment is important because if left untreated it may prove to be fatal within 90 days of onset. Individuals with acute idiopathic TTP have extreme thrombocytopenia, intravascular hemolytic anemia from red cell fragmentation (schistocytosis, an elevated LDL level from tissue injury), and ischemic signs and symptoms most often involving the central nervous system.[94] Central nervous system symptoms may include memory disturbances, behavioral irregularities, headaches, or coma.

Untreated TTP has a mortality rate of 90%; however, mortality is reduced to 12% to 20% with treatment. Plasma exchange (PE) with fresh frozen plasma is the treatment of choice for acute idiopathic TTP, achieving a response rate of 70% to 85%. In the absence of major organ damage, individuals may make a complete recovery with no long-term complications. Relapses do occur at a rate of 13% to 36%, and recurrences have been reported, some as far out as 9 years.[96] In addition to PE, steroids (glucocorticoids) are administered.

Individuals who do not respond to conventional treatment may be candidates for splenectomy; however, postoperative hemorrhage remains a dangerous complication. Some individuals have responded to immunosuppressive (azathioprine) therapy.[94]

Thrombocythemia

Essential (primary) thrombocythemia (ET) is a proliferative clonal myeloproliferative disorder that belongs to the chronic myeloproliferative disorders that also include polycythemia vera, chronic myelogenous leukemia, and chronic idiopathic myelofibrosis. As with all other myeloproliferative disorders, ET is caused by an alteration of a multipotent stem cell causing platelets to be produced in greater numbers than normal, resulting in platelet counts in excess of 600,000/mm[3]. The bone marrow of affected individuals with ET is characterized by hyperplasia of megakaryocytes. Additional manifestations include splenomegaly and periodic episodes of hemorrhage or thrombosis or both.[97]

The exact incidence of essential thrombocythemia is unknown because extensive epidemiologic studies are not available; however, recent statistics demonstrate the overall incidence to be 0.8 per 100,000 in the United Kingdom, 2.53 in the United States, and 0.59 in Denmark.[98] It is more common in middle-age individuals, with the majority of cases occurring between ages 50 and 60 years. There is no known gender preference, although the above reports indicate a greater female prevalence. There also is a rare hereditary type of EG called *familial essential thrombocythemia (FET)* that is inherited in an autosomal dominant pattern.[99]

Precise mechanisms causing essential thrombocythemia are unknown. There is no specific diagnostic test for ET, therefore, it is important to differentiate between reactive (physiologic) thrombocythemia, noted after exercise, postpartum, and as a result of epinephrine. There also are conditions in which platelets increase as a result of some other conditions, such as postsplenectomy and infectious/inflammation conditions. The platelets of affected individuals appear to have a normal survival time, and evidence suggests that the disorder is caused by increased megakaryocyte production originating at the pluripotential hematopoietic stem cell. Essential thrombocythemia has not been associated with erythrocytosis, which is the hallmark of polycythemia vera; however, recent evidence suggests that, along with an increase in platelets, there may be a concomitant increase in red blood cells reflecting a close association with myeloproliferative disorders.[100] The presence and degree of erythrocytosis appears to correlate with altered stem cell commitment and development.

Clinical manifestations of essential thrombocythemia vary significantly among individuals. As many as two thirds of affected individuals are diagnosed from a routine CBC. After diagnosis, these individuals may recall events related to thrombosis or hemorrhage. Manifestations of ET may be mistaken for CML, therefore, differentiation of the two is important because treatment varies significantly. Identification of the Philadelphia chromosome is recommended in all cases of ET.[101]

The primary presenting symptoms of **microvasculature thrombosis** are erythromyalgia, headache, and paresthesias. **Erythromyalgia** is characterized by unilateral or bilateral warm, congested, red hands and feet with painful burning sensations, particularly in the forefoot sole and one or more toes. The pain is initiated by standing, exercise, or warmth and relieved by elevation and cooling. In extreme situations, erythromyalgia may lead to acrocyanosis and gangrene.[102]

Arterial thrombosis is more common than venous thrombosis and may involve other arteries, such as the coronary and renal arteries. Also reported is involvement of the carotid, mesenteric, and subclavian arteries. Myocardial ischemia and myocardial infarction, without clear evidence of coronary artery disease, also have been observed in individuals with essential thrombocythemia. Deep venous thrombosis of the lower extremities and pulmonary embolism are the major sites for venous involvement. Intra-abdominal venous thrombosis (portal and hepatic) also account for a significant proportion of venous thrombotic events.[102]

Other manifestations of ET related to microvascular thrombosis include neurologic symptoms, of which headache and dizziness are the most common. Other reported symptoms include paresthesias, transient ischemic attacks, strokes, visual disturbances, and seizures.[103] Major thrombotic events that are not directly related to the platelet count are estimated to occur in 20% to 30% of individuals with ET. Other risk factors (e.g., prior history of thrombotic events, advanced age, and duration of thrombocytosis) are identified as better predictors of future thrombotic complications.[104] Individuals over the age of 60 are at greatest risk.

In contrast to thrombosis, hemorrhagic manifestations also are part of the clinical course but occur less frequently than thrombosis. Primary sites of hemorrhage are the skin and mucus membranes, observed as ecchymosis, epistaxis, menorrhagia, and gingival bleeding.[102] Other sites of bleeding include skin, eyes, urinary tract, gums, tooth sockets (after extraction), joints, and the brain. Hemorrhage is most often not severe, occurring more often in individuals with very high platelet counts,[103] and occasionally requires transfusion. Important is recognition that bleeding and clotting may exist simultaneously and individuals will not necessarily be "bleeders" or "clotters."[105]

A major concern for individuals with ET is conversion to acute myelogenous leukemia or myelofibrosis. Conversion to myelofibrosis occurs approximately 8% of the time and conversion to AML occurs approximately 3.5% of the time when treated with hydroxyurea as a single cytotoxic but increases to 14% when more than one cytotoxic agent is used.[106]

Treatment of ET does not cure the underlying disease or prevent clonal evolution, therefore treatment is directed toward preventing thrombosis or hemorrhage. Whether to reduce platelet count or not remains the significant treatment issue. Historically treatment of ET relied on the use of alkylating agents (busulfan) or radiophosphorus (^{32}P) to suppress platelet production. Since 1980, hydroxyurea (HU), a nonalkylating myelosuppressive agent, has been the drug of choice. HU is relatively effective in causing platelet produc-

tion suppression; however, safety for long-term use is questioned as to its association with conversion to other myelodysplastic disorders.

Interferon (IFN) also may be used and has a response rate of 80%. IFN may not work for everyone because it has many side effects and 20% of individuals may be intolerant. Anagrelide is now considered to be the drug of choice. Anagrelide appears to be platelet specific, interfering with platelet maturation rather than production, and as such does not affect red blood cell and white blood cell growth and development.[107]

Aspirin also is used in the treatment of ET; however, its action is not to reduce the platelet count but to prevent adherence of platelets to each other and prevent thrombus formation. Early studies with aspirin found hemorrhage to be a major contraindication for its use; however, in lower doses it has been found to be effective in alleviating erythromyalgia and transient neurologic manifestations.[108]

Prognosis and survival of individuals with ET has been somewhat difficult to establish.[108] The diagnosis of ET is not necessarily considered life-threatening, but complications are more common and have a higher risk of morbidity and mortality, particularly in those over 60 years of age and who have had previous incidences of thrombosis.

Alterations of Platelet Function

Qualitative alterations in platelet function occur with an increased bleeding time in the presence of a normal platelet count. Qualitative alterations may be acquired or congenital. Congenital alterations (thrombocytopathies) are rare and may be categorized into four types: disorders of platelet adhesion, platelet aggregation, platelet secretion, and procoagulant activity.[109] Clinical manifestations of platelet alterations include petechiae and purpura, mild to moderate mucosal bleeding (bilateral epistaxis, gastrointestinal, genitourinary, and pulmonary), gingival bleeding, and spontaneous bruising.

Disorders of platelet adhesion result from deficiency of a platelet membrane glycoprotein complex Ib/IX (Bernard-Soulier syndrome) or von Willebrand factor (vWf). Lack of these proteins prevents platelets from adhering to collagen, resulting in impaired hemostasis and clinical hemorrhage.[110]

Disorders of platelet aggregation are manifested by failure of platelets to aggregate with adenosine diphosphate (ADP), collagen, epinephrine, or thrombin because of a deficiency in the glycoprotein (IIb/IIIa) that acts as a fibrinogen receptor (Glanzmann thrombasthenia). Lack of this protein results in a failure to build "fibrinogen bridges" between platelets (see Figure 25-19 on p. 913).

Disorders of platelet secretion are characterized by initial normal platelet aggregation with collagen or ADP; however, there is failure of subsequent processes, specifically secretion of prostaglandins and release of granule-bound–alpha or –delta ADP (Gray platelet syndrome, Storage pool disease). Disorders of platelet procoagulant activity are extremely rare and are characterized by lack of procoagulant factors normally present on activated platelets and promote the activation of factor X of the coagulation pathway and prothrombin.

| Box 27-5 | Common Drugs or Agents* that Inhibit Platelet Function† |

Box 27-5	Common Drugs or Agents* that Inhibit Platelet Function†

Nonsteroidal antiinflammatories
  Acetylsalicylic acid (ASA)
  Ibuprofen
  Naproxen
  Indomethacin
β-Lactam antibiotics
  Penicillin G (all penicillin derivatives ending in "cillin")
  Cephalosporins
Cardiovascular drugs
  Nitroglycerin
  Propranolol
  Nifedipine
  Verapamil
  Quinidine
  Diltiazem
Psychotropic drugs
  Tricyclic antidepressants: imipramine
  Phenothiazines: chlorpromazine, promethazine
Anesthetics
  Local: lidocaine, procaine
  General: halothane
Antihistamines
  Diphenhydramine
Food additives or foods
  Ethanol
  Cumin
  Turmeric
  Clove

*Of these drugs and agents, only ASA causes significantly increased bleeding time. Other drugs affect platelet aggregation or bleeding time.
†Generic drug names used in this box.

Acquired disorders of platelet function are more common than the congenital disorders and may be categorized into three principal causes: drugs, systemic conditions, and hematologic alterations.

Multiple drugs are known to affect platelet function and are listed in Box 27-5. Of this vast array of drugs, aspirin is the only known drug specifically used for its antithrombotic activity.[86] Drugs interfere with platelet function in three ways: inhibition of platelet membrane receptors, inhibition of prostaglandin pathways, and inhibition of phosphodiesterase activity.[111]

Systemic disorders that affect platelet function are chronic renal disease, cardiopulmonary bypass surgery, and antiplatelet antibodies associated with autoimmunity disorders. Hematologic disorders that cause platelet dysfunction are chronic myeloproliferative disorders, leukemias, myelodysplastic syndromes, and dysproteinemias.

Disorders of Coagulation

Disorders of coagulation usually are caused by defects or deficiencies of one or more of the clotting factors. (Normal function of the clotting factors is described in Chapter 25.) Qualitative or quantitative abnormalities of clotting factors prevent the enzymatic reactions by which these factors are normally transformed from circulating plasma proteins to a stable fibrin clot (see Figure 25-23 on p. 916).

Some clotting factor defects are inherited and usually involve a single factor. Two of the most common inherited disorders, the hemophilias and von Willebrand disease, are caused by deficiencies of specific clotting factors (see Chapter 28). Other coagulation defects are acquired and tend to result from deficient synthesis of clotting factors by the liver. Liver disease is one cause of acquired coagulation deficiency. Another is a dietary deficiency of vitamin K, which is necessary for normal synthesis of the clotting factors.

Other coagulation disorders not caused by quantitative or qualitative clotting factor defects are attributed to pathologic conditions that trigger coagulation inappropriately, engaging the clotting factors and causing detrimental clotting within blood vessels. For example, any cardiovascular abnormality that alters normal blood flow by speeding it up, slowing it down, or obstructing it can create conditions in which coagulation proceeds within the vessels. This is a cause of thromboembolic disease, in which blood clots obstruct blood vessels. Coagulation is also stimulated by the presence of tissue factor, which is released by damaged or dead tissues. Therefore any condition in which tissue decay or damage releases a great deal of tissue thromboplastin, such as occurs in complications of pregnancy, including death of the fetus and placental decay within the mother, can cause widespread and possibly fatal intravascular coagulation. Another cause of detrimental coagulation processes is vasculitis, or inflammation of the blood vessels. Damage to inflamed vessels causes platelet activation, which in turn activates the coagulation cascade. In extensive or prolonged vasculitis, blood clot formation can overcome mechanisms that normally control clot formation and breakdown, leading to clogging of the vessels. In each of these acquired conditions, normal hemostatic function proves detrimental to the body by consuming coagulation factors excessively or by overwhelming normal control of clot formation and breakdown (fibrinolysis).

Impaired Hemostasis

Impaired hemostasis, or the inability to promote coagulation and the development of a stable fibrin clot, is commonly associated with either the lack of vitamin K or specific liver disorders.

Vitamin K Deficiency

Vitamin K, a fat-soluble vitamin, is necessary for synthesis and regulation of normal prothrombin, the prothrombin factors (II, VII, IX, X), and the anticoagulant regulators (proteins C and S) within the liver. Vitamin K is found in green leafy vegetables and is the primary dietary source. Vitamin K also is synthesized by intestinal flora, but contributions to the overall supply of vitamin K is uncertain. The most common cause of vitamin K deficiency is parenteral nutrition in combination with broad-spectrum antibiotics that destroy normal gut flora. Rarely is a deficiency caused by lack of dietary intake;[112] however, bulimia can suppress vitamin K dependent activity. Clinical manifestations of vitamin K deficiency are caused by a reduction of vitamin K-dependent proteins. The severity of manifestations are related to the degree of deficiency and range from laboratory abnormalities to significant hemorrhage.[113]

Parenteral administration of vitamin K is the treatment of choice and usually results in correction. Improvement of clotting tests is usually noted within 8 to 12 hours. Fresh frozen plasma (FFP) also may be administered and usually is reserved for individuals with life-threatening hemorrhages or who require emergency surgery. Infusion of prothrombin complex concentrations is not recommended because of their thrombogenic activity.[114]

Liver Disease

Individuals with liver disease have a broad range of hemostasis derangements that may be characterized by defects in the clotting or fibrinolytic systems and by platelet function.[114] The usual sequence of events is an initial reduction in clotting factors, which parallels the degree of hepatic parenchymal cell damage or destruction. Factor VII is the first to decline because of its rapid turnover, followed by declines in prothrombin and factor X. Factor IX levels are less affected and do not decline until liver destruction is well advanced. Protein C levels also decline early, similar to levels of factor VII; protein S levels decline in the later stages of liver disease. Factor V reduction is of special importance because its plasma level appears to be a direct reflection of liver cell damage.[114] Factor VIII levels are not affected because of extrahepatic synthesis.[115]

Other hemostatic alterations in liver disease include increased fibrinolytic activity, which may be primary in origin or a result of disseminated intravascular coagulation (DIC). Increased fibrinolysis results from increased levels and impaired clearance of fibrinolytic activators and decreased levels of inhibitors, such as α_2-antiplasmin.

Thrombocytopenia and thrombocytopathies also occur with liver disease. Thrombocytopenia is related to splenomegaly, which often accompanies liver disease and is associated with portal hypertension. Splenic pooling of platelets is the major cause of thrombocytopenia. Thrombocytopathies are associated with elevated levels of fibrin split products, ethanol, and drugs.

Treatment of hemostatic alterations in liver disease must be comprehensive to cover all aspects related to platelet, clotting, and fibrinolytic dysfunctions. FFP administration is the treatment of choice, but not all individuals tolerate the volume needed to adequately replace all deficient factors. Alternative modalities include the addition of exchange transfusions and platelet concentration to FFP administration.

Consumptive Thrombohemorrhagic Disorders

Consumptive thrombohemorrhagic disorders are a heterogeneous group of conditions that demonstrate the entire range of hemorrhagic and thrombotic pathologic conditions.[116] Symptoms range from subtle to devastating, and these disorders generally are considered to be intermediary disease processes that complicate many primary disease states. Confusion and controversy also exist regarding diagnosis, treatment, and management of consumptive thrombohemorrhagic disorders. No one definition can cover all possible varieties of these disorders; however, disseminated intravascular coagulation is the most common term used in the clinical setting to describe a pathologic condition associated with hemorrhage and thrombosis.

Disseminated Intravascular Coagulation

Disseminated intravascular coagulation (DIC) is a complex and highly variable, acquired clinical syndrome with manifestations that are the result of increased protease activity in the blood caused by unregulated release of thrombin with subsequent fibrin formation and accelerated fibrinolysis. The Subcommittee on DIC of the International Society on Thrombosis and Hemostasis defined DIC as, "An acquired syndrome characterized by the intravascular activation of coagulation with loss of localization arising from different causes. It can originate from and cause damage to the microvasculature, which if sufficiently severe, can produce organ dysfunction."[117,118]

The clinical course of DIC ranges from an acute, severe, life-threatening process that is characterized by massive hemorrhage and thrombosis to a chronic, low-grade condition. The chronic condition is characterized by minor laboratory abnormalities with subacute hemorrhage and diffuse microcirculatory thrombosis. The clinical course and outcomes of DIC are determined largely by the intensity of the stimulus, host response, and comorbid conditions.[119]

Because of the complexity and wide variations in manifestations of DIC, diagnosis has been confusing and difficult. Diagnosing DIC has been aided by the development of minimally acceptable criteria that is characteristic of DIC. Based on these criteria, DIC can be further defined as "a systemic thrombohemorrhagic disorder seen in association with well-defined clinical situations and laboratory evidence of (1) procoagulant activation, (2) fibrinolytic activation, (3) inhibitor consumption, and (4) biochemical evidence of end-organ damage or failure."[119]

DIC is an intermediary mechanism of disease that is associated with a wide variety of well-defined clinical conditions, specifically those capable of activating the clotting cascade. The potential for procoagulant activity exists in clinical situations that present with (1) arterial hypotension, frequently accompanying shock; (2) hypoxemia; (3) acidemia; and (4) stasis of capillary blood flow.[120] Whatever the precipitating cause, DIC is initiated by release of tissue factor.

Tissue factor (TF) is a 47-kD membrane glycoprotein present in numerous sites throughout the body, primarily in tissues not in contact with blood, such as the endothelial layer of blood vessels and subcutaneous tissue.[121,122] Release of TF from either endothelial damage or direct tissue damage (ischemia and necrosis, surgical manipulation, and crushing injury) activates the coagulation cascade (see Chapter 25).

Endothelial damage is the primary instigator of DIC in the presence of sepsis. Sepsis is the most common condition associated with DIC. Symptoms of DIC are estimated to be evident in 7.5% to 49% of individuals diagnosed with sepsis. Gram-negative microorganisms, as well as gram-positive microorganisms, fungi, protozoan (malaria) and viruses (flu, herpes), have all been identified as infectious agents capable of precipitating DIC. Potent endotoxins are the primary cause of endothelial damage. Once endothelial damage occurs the negatively charged basement membrane is exposed, which then acts as a hemostatically active vascular surface, precipitating activation of factor XII.

Endotoxin also triggers the release of multiple cytokines that play a significant role in the development and maintenance of DIC. These proinflammatory cytokines (tumor necrosis factor–alpha [TNF-α], interleukins [IL-1, IL-6, IL-8], and platelet activating factor [PAF]) are largely, possibly completely, responsible for the clinical signs and symptoms associated with sepsis. Their major role is activating epithelial cells, causing release of TF and von Willebrand factor, and they have been shown in vitro to increase plasminogen activator inhibitor–1 (PAI-1) synthesis, increase tissue factor activity, and decrease thrombomodulin expression, thereby promoting development of thrombi. TF also may be released directly into the bloodstream from circulating white blood cells (monocyte/endotoxin interaction) or immune complexes. Cancer is the cause of DIC in approximately 10% to 20% of individuals with cancer. Solid tumor and leukemic cells, particularly acute promyelocytic leukemia, express TF on their membranes.[123,124] Tumor infiltrating and circulating monocytes may express TF.[125]

Direct tissue damage in which normal structures are broken down (ischemia and necrosis, surgical manipulation, and crushing injury) also result in release of TF. Tissue damage causes damage to the endothelium complicating the situation and predisposing the processes leading to the development of DIC.

In addition to endothelial or tissue damage, DIC may be precipitated by direct proteolytic activation of factor X that has been identified as thrombin mimicry[126] and results in proteases directly converting fibrinogen to fibrin. Proteases may come from snake venom, as well as tumor cells. Enzymes from the pancreas and liver also have a direct proteolytic effect and are released during pancreatitis and various stages of liver disease. It appears that direct proteolytic activity does not depend on any type of damage to either the endothelium or tissue.

Miscellaneous causes of DIC also have been identified, most notably blood transfusion. Transfused blood dilutes the clotting factors, as well as circulating naturally occurring antithrombins. In hemolytic transfusion reactions, the endothelium is damaged as a result of the assembly of the complement membrane attack complex rather than the intravascular destruction of red blood cells.[127] Antibody-antigen reactions are also responsible for the development of DIC after anaphylaxis.

PATHOPHYSIOLOGY   The pathophysiology of DIC is shown in Figure 27-15. DIC is initiated by one of the previ-

ously identified etiologies (Box 27-6), activating either the intrinsic or extrinsic clotting cascade. The extrinsic system appears to be the predominant system that is activated. The significant substances produced during DIC—thrombin and plasmin—are the primary factors in the pathophysiology of DIC. Once TF is released it complexes with factor VIIa and directly generates the enzymatic components of the tenase and prothrombinase complexes that are capable of causing an explosive generation of thrombin.[128,127]

The amount of thrombin produced during DIC exceeds the ability of the body's naturally occurring anticoagulants (proteins C and S; antithrombin [AT]) to regulate it. Antithrombin is unable to adequately regulate thrombin activity in DIC because of three impaired functions. First, continuous consumption of antithrombin occurs because of persistent thrombin formation and other activated proteases susceptible to antithrombin complex formation. Second, antithrombin is degraded by elastase released by activated neutrophils. Third, hepatic dysfunction in sepsis results in decreased antithrombin synthesis and extravascular leakage of this protease inhibitor because of capillary leakage, which contributes further to reduced levels of antithrombin.[115] When the clotting factors are expended, hemorrhage ensues resulting in the primary pathophysiologic paradox of DIC—thrombosis in the presence of hemorrhage (see What's New? Antithrombin Levels in Disseminated Intravascular Coagulation).

Thrombin, initially released at the beginning of the clotting cascade, causes platelet aggregation and consumption of clotting factors. It also cleaves fibrinogen into fibrin monomers that polymerize into fibrin clots that become deposited in the microcirculation. This results in microvascular and macrovascular thrombosis, obstructing blood flow and causing peripheral ischemia and end-organ damage.[119]

Once clotting is initiated, the fibrinolytic pathway is activated and begins degrading the formed clots. After the coagulation and fibrinolytic systems are activated, large amounts of circulating prothrombin and plasminogen are converted to thrombin and plasmin. Once thrombin and plasmin are circulating systemically, DIC results.[119] Circulating thrombin and plasmin is tantamount to DIC.

Plasmin is a potent proteolytic enzyme that digests fibrin and fibrinogen and is produced when plasminogen is activated by tissue plasminogen activators (t-PA), which is present in endothelial cells and released during tissue damage. Overstimulation of the clotting cascade is also responsible for an abundance of plasmin.

As fibrin is degraded by plasmin, fibrin degradation products (FDPs) are released into the circulation. FDPs interfere with fibrin monomer polymerization, which further impairs hemostasis and may cause clinically significant hemorrhage. They also have a high affinity for platelets causing extensive platelet dysfunction that also contribute to hemorrhaging. FDPs, along with thrombin, induce further cytokine release from monocytes, further contributing to endothelial damage and TF release. FDPs normally are cleared from the blood by the macrophage system; however, they are not cleared as read-

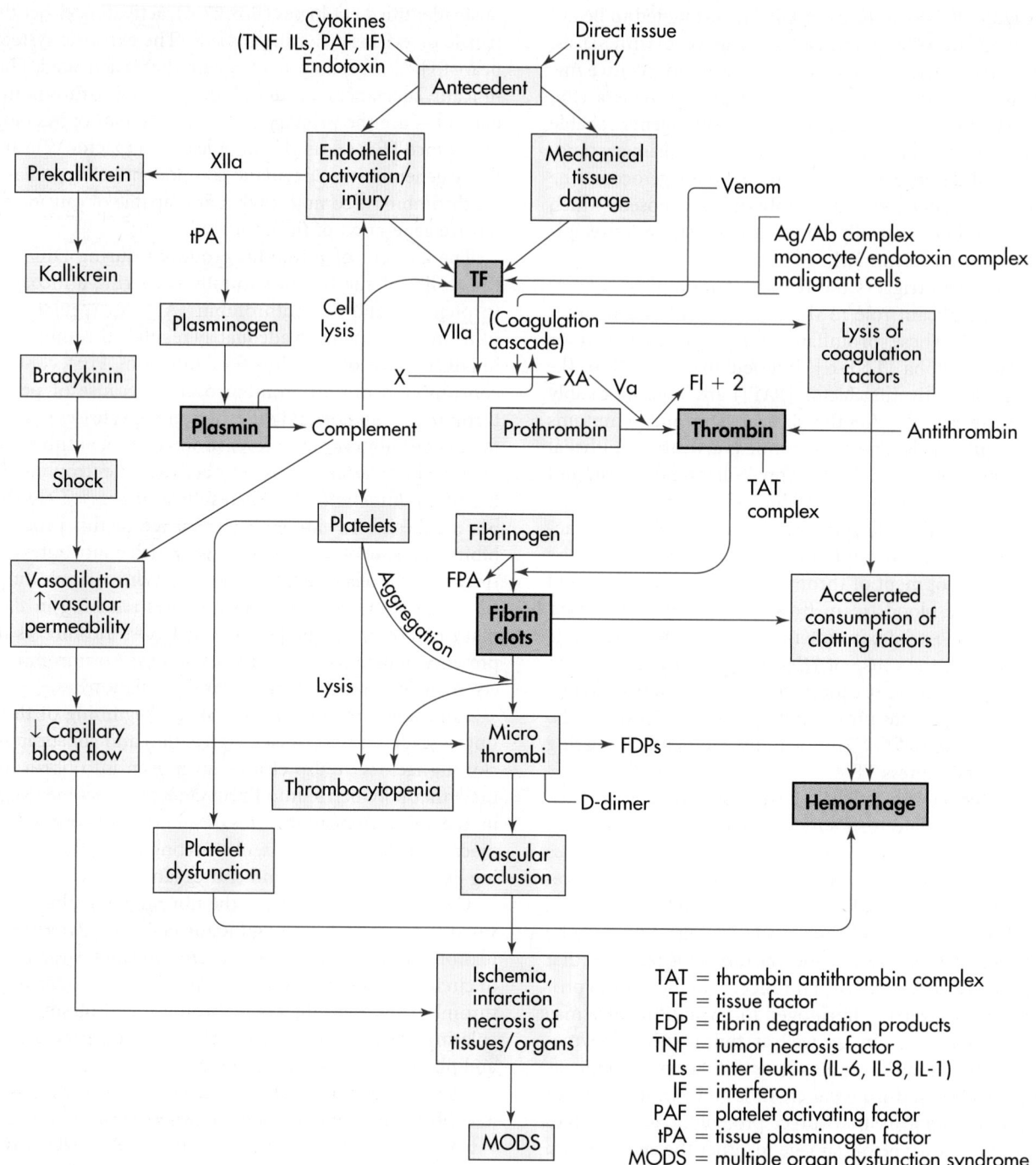

Figure 27-15 Pathophysiology of disseminated intravascular coagulation (DIC). DIC is initiated by endothelial damage, either directly (tissue damage) or indirectly (activation) causing release of tissue factor (TF). TF initiates the coagulation cascade, which ultimately activates plasmin and thrombin, leading to accelerated use of clotting factors causing clotting and hemorrhage at the same time. TF also may be released by dead tissue. Conversion of X to Xa may also be initiated by venom.

ily in DIC, which is thought to be caused by a lack of fibronectin. Fibronectin is a glycoprotein with adhesive properties that mediate removal of particulate matter (e.g., fibrin clumps). Low levels of fibronectin in individuals with DIC carry a poor prognosis.[120]

In addition, plasmin activates the kallikrein-kinin and complement systems. Factor XIIa, generated in DIC, acts to convert prekallikrein to kallikrein with later conversion to high-molecular-weight kininogen into circulating kinins.[119] All of these activated systems further contribute to the thrombosis and hemorrhage of DIC. Complement and kinin system activation increases vascular permeability, leading to hypotension and shock. Additional affects of complement activation are formation of the membrane attack complex

Box 27-6	Major Etiologies Identified as Antecedents to the Initiation and Development of Disseminated Intravascular Coagulation (DIC)

Acute Fulminant DIC
Obstetric complications
   Abruptio placentae
   Retained fetus syndrome
   Eclampsia
   Septic abortion
Intravascular hemolysis
   Hemolytic transfusion reactions
   Massive transfusions
Infections
   Sepsis (gram negative or positive)
   Viremias (HIV, varicella, CMV, hepatitis)
Malignancies
   Leukemia (acute promyelocytic)
Crush injuries/tissue necrosis
   Burns
   Trauma
Acute liver disease
   Obstructive jaundice
   Acute hepatic failure
Prothesis
   LeVeen/Denver shunts
   Aortic balloon pump
Vascular disorders
Chronic Low-Grade DIC
Cardiovascular disease
Autoimmune disease
Renal vascular disorders
Hematologic disorders
Inflammatory disorders
Malignancies

HIV, Human immunodeficiency virus; *CMV*, cytomegalovirus.

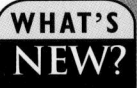

WHAT'S NEW? Antithrombin Levels in Disseminated Intravascular Coagulation (DIC)

Acquired antithrombin (AT) deficiency, most notably with DIC, is being used as a predictor of morbidity and mortality in the presence of sepsis. Normal levels of AT are between 75% and 120%. Levels of AT below 70% in plasma were associated with 90% mortality in trauma patients with sepsis; plasma levels below 60% were associated with 100% mortality. The lowest AT levels were found in individuals with sepsis, and AT levels below 65% predicted mortality.

Data from Mammen EF: *Semin Thromb Hemost* 24(1):19-25, 1998.

(MAC) that attaches to cell membranes and punches holes in it, and activation of C3a and C5a (anaphylatoxins) that exert proinflammatory effects, including leukocyte recruitment.[129]

Platelet interaction with thrombin also plays a significant role in the clotting-bleeding scenario. Thrombin-induced platelet aggregation that occurs early in the clotting cascade initially plays a role in microcirculatory coagulation and obstruction. Eventually the platelets are consumed, causing a thrombocytopenia that increases the hemorrhaging.

The obstruction that results from circulatory deposition of thrombin and clot formation impedes with blood flow, causing widespread organ hypoperfusion that can lead to tissue ischemia, infarction, and necrosis. The tissue damage that results from circulatory obstruction further potentiates and complicates the existing DIC process. Because organ perfusion is drastically impaired, manifestations of multisystem organ dysfunction and failure ultimately result.[130] Multisystem organ dysfunction and failure are discussed in Chapter 46.

The positive feedback loop that perpetuates the cycle of thrombosis and hemorrhage persists until the underlying mechanism that precipitated DIC is removed or appropriate therapeutic interventions terminate the process.

CLINICAL MANIFESTATIONS Clinical signs and symptoms of DIC present a wide spectrum of possibilities. The initial manifestation depends on whether it manifests as an acute or a chronic condition and what the etiology was that precipitated its onset. Initial signs of acute DIC are rapid development of hemorrhaging, such as oozing from venipuncture sites, arterial lines, and surgical wounds or development of ecchymotic lesions (purpura, petechiae) and hematomas. Other sites of bleeding include the eyes (sclera and conjunctiva), the nose (epistaxis), and the gums. An average individual with DIC demonstrates bleeding at three unrelated sites, and any combination may be observed.[119] Individuals with DIC also manifest a variable level of shock that is out of proportion to the amount of apparent blood loss.[131]

DIC has been conceptualized as a systemic hemorrhagic disorder because this is initially evident and often impressive.[119] Manifestations of thrombosis are not always as evident, even though thrombosis is often the first pathologic alteration to occur ultimately determines morbidity and mortality. A large amount of microvascular and macrovascular occlusion may occur that is not clinically obvious. Organ systems that are susceptible to microvascular thrombosis associated with dysfunction include the cardiovascular, pulmonary, central nervous, renal, and hepatic systems. Quick and accurate clinical interpretation are critical to prevent further disruption and destruction. Manifestations of these system dysfunctions include changes in level of consciousness, behavior, and mentation; confusion; seizure activity; oliguria; hematuria; hypoxia; hypotension; hemoptysis; chest pain; and tachycardia. Hemorrhaging into closed compartments of the body, such as the gastrointestinal system, also can occur and may preclude the development of shock.

Symmetrical cyanosis of the fingers and toes ("blue finger/ toe syndrome") and, in some instances, of the nose and breasts may be present. Symmetric parts are often affected and are indicative of microvascular thrombosis. This may progress to infarction and gangrene, requiring amputation.[128]

Jaundice also may be present and is believed to result from red blood cell destruction rather than hepatic dysfunction.

Individuals with chronic or low-grade DIC who do not have the overt manifestations of hemorrhaging and thrombosis but instead have subacute bleeding and diffuse thrombosis are described as having a **compensated DIC,** or non-overt DIC.[132,133] Individuals with this type of DIC demonstrate an increased turnover and decreased survival time of the components of hemostasis. On occasion, an individual may have diffuse or localized thrombosis, but this is not often noted.

EVALUATION AND TREATMENT   Diagnosis of DIC is based primarily on clinical manifestations with confirmation provided by laboratory evidence. Because of the complex nature of DIC, laboratory results are highly variable and difficult to interpret without understanding the pathophysiology of DIC.

In general, coagulation tests (prothrombin time [PT], activated partial thromboplastin time [aPTT], reptilase time) provide unreliable data and do not confirm the diagnosis. It would be expected that these tests would be abnormal; however, the results range from shortened times to prolonged times and in many cases are normal. Coagulation factor assay does not contribute further meaningful data to confirm the diagnosis. Coagulation assays done by the standard aPTT- or PT-derived laboratory techniques give uninterpretable results.

FDPs are elevated in 85% to 100% of individuals with DIC; however, presence of FDPs is not necessarily diagnostic for DIC because they may be elevated in other clinical conditions. Presence of FDPs in the blood is diagnostic only for the presence of plasmin and the result of its action on fibrinogen.

The D-dimer test has been used more recently to diagnose DIC. **D-dimer** is a neoantigen produced by plasmin lysis of cross-linked fibrin clots.[117] Monoclonal antibodies are formed against this D-dimer antigen and identified, documenting the activity of thrombin (cross-linking) and plasmin (fibrinolysis). The D-dimer test is the most reliable and specific test for the diagnosis of DIC. The D-dimer antigen is recognized as an indicator of fibrin formation rather than fibrin degradation.[132] The presence of fibrin complexes in plasma is an early indicator of DIC and also indicates ongoing intravascular coagulation. Identifying specific molecular markers associated with thrombin activity facilitates the diagnosis of DIC. Normal conversion of prothrombin to thrombin produces an inactive prothrombin fragment 1.2 (PF1+2). This fragment is released from the prothrombin molecule generating an intermediate factor, prethrombin 2. Once generated, prethrombin 2 can be split to produce thrombin that can then proteolyze fibrinogen, liberating fibrinopeptide A (FPA) or combine with its major antagonist, antithrombin, and form a stable inactive enzyme inhibitor complex, the thrombin-antithrombin (TAT) complex. Assays of these factors (PF1+2, FPA, TAT) are now generally available to quantify their blood levels, providing evidence of excessive factor Xa (F1+2) and thrombin (FPA) generation.[119]

A new assay that is highly sensitive to early procoagulant activity is thrombin precursor protein. This assay detects circulating soluble-fibrin polymer. Initial results are promising; however, additional assessment in individuals with DIC needs to be performed.[119]

Antithrombin III (AT III) levels are also assessed for diagnosing and monitoring therapy for DIC. Low levels of antithrombin have been found to be associated with increased mortality in septic individuals.[134] Assays of blood detect this decrease and provide reliable data for diagnosing DIC.

Laboratory diagnosis of DIC is complex and requires evidence of (1) procoagulant activity, (2) fibrinolytic system activation, (3) inhibitor consumption, and (4) end-organ damage. The relationships among these four criteria are summarized in Box 27-7. Despite development of molecular marker tests for DIC, their use is still not seen as completely diagnostic because of issues related to specificity and standardization.[135]

Treatment of DIC, like diagnosis, is complex and individualized; it is based on the person's condition, the underlying etiology and the progression of the condition, and changes in the laboratory tests caused by therapy. Clinical trials of DIC treatment do not exist, which complicates treatment modalities, so evidence of effectiveness is not available to assist with treatment. Treatment goals are directed toward (1) eliminat-

---

Box 27-7	**Laboratory Diagnostic Criteria for Disseminated Intravascular Coagulation (DIC)**

Group I Tests (Indicators of Procoagulant Activation)
1. Elevated prothrombin fragment 1 + 2
2. Elevated fibrinopeptide A
3. Elevated fibrinopeptide B
4. Elevated thrombin-antithrombin (TAT) complex
5. Elevated D-dimer

Group II Tests (Indicators of Fibrinolytic Activity)
1. Elevated D-dimer
2. Elevated fibrin degradation products (FDPs)
3. Elevated plasmin
4. Elevated plasmin-antiplasmin (PAP) complex

Group III Tests (Indicators of Inhibitor Consumption)
1. Decreased antithrombin III
2. Decreased alpha-2 antiplasmin
3. Decreased heparin cofactor II
4. Decreased protein C or S
5. Elevated TAT complex
6. Elevated PAP complex

Group IV Tests (Indicators of End-Organ Damage/Failure)
1. Elevated lactic dehydrogenase (LDH)
2. Elevated creatinine
3. Decreased pH
4. Decreased Pao_2

Satisfactory criteria for laboratory diagnosis of DIC requires one abnormality in each of groups I through III and at least two abnormalities in group IV.

Data from Bick RL: *Semin-Thromb Hemost* 24(1):3, 1998.

ing the underlying pathology, (2) restoring hemostasis, and (3) maintaining organ viability.[120,136] Specific and vigorous treatment of the underlying pathology is the essential intervention.[137] In some instances treatment is all that is needed, however, further treatment is needed in most cases.[138]

Restoration of hemostasis is more difficult to attain. Heparin has been used frequently; however, its use is controversial and indicated only in certain situations related to DIC. In clinical trials using heparin, results vary widely, therefore no standards for its use have been developed. Heparin's anticoagulant effect depends on the concentration of functionally active AT III, which is reduced in DIC, and on heparin-neutralizing substances, such as platelet factor 4, that are released from activated platelets in DIC.[136]

Heparin use seems to be effective in DIC caused by a retained dead fetus and acute promyelocytic leukemia. It also is indicated when there is a predisposition to thromboembolism and organ function is compromised, or there is a risk of losing an extremity because of vascular occlusion. Heparin's effectiveness in reducing mortality and morbidity in DIC that is precipitated by septic shock has not been established, and its use is contraindicated where there is evidence of postoperative bleeding, peptic ulcer, or central nervous system bleeding. Heparin use in chronic DIC has been established.

AT III has been available for a number of years and appears to be most useful in DIC related to sepsis. Low levels of AT III correlate with sepsis-initiated DIC; therefore its use in this situation is strongly recommended.[128] AT III is an α_2-globulin that inactivates thrombin, plasmin, and other serine proteases of coagulation, including factors IXa, Xa, XIa, XIIa, and VIIa, thus inhibiting coagulation.[117] AT III augments the activity of heparin; therefore use of AT III with heparin has not been established. Use of AT III is still relatively new, and clinical guidelines for its efficacy in DIC have not been fully established.

Replacement therapy (interventions based on restoring the balance of coagulation factors, deficient coagulation factors, platelets, and other coagulation elements) is gaining importance as a treatment modality. Components used in replacement therapy include platelets, FFP, and cryoprecipitate. Platelets are given for thrombocytopenia, FFP provides volume and replaces clotting factors, and cryoprecipitate replaces fibrinogen.[139] A major concern with using replacement therapy was "adding fuel to the fire." This fear has not been validated; therefore replacement therapy has become accepted treatment in individuals who demonstrate bleeding and coagulation parameters consistent with DIC.[137]

Antifibrinolytics are another group of drugs that may be used in the treatment of DIC but should be used only if other treatment modalities have been unsuccessful. No clear evidence exists to justify their use except in instances of life-threatening hemorrhaging that is not controlled by blood component replacement therapy.[128]

Maintenance of organ viability is accomplished primarily by adequate fluid replacement to sustain adequate circulating blood volume and to maintain optimal tissue and organ perfusion. Fluid resuscitation also may be required to restore blood pressure, cardiac output, and urine output to normal parameters.

Thromboembolic Disease

Abnormal blood clots may form occasionally within the vascular system. A stationary clot that adheres to the vessel wall is called a **thrombus** (Figure 27-16). Thrombi are composed of fibrin and blood cells. The proportion of each depends on the location of their formation and the hemodynamics of the blood flow in that particular area. **Arterial thrombi** formation occurs under conditions of high blood flow and are composed mostly of platelet aggregates held together by fibrin strands. **Venous thrombi** formation occurs in conditions of low flow and are composed mostly of red blood cells with larger amounts of fibrin and very few platelets.[140]

Thrombi may eventually grow large enough to interfere with or obstruct blood flow to tissues or organs critical to survival, such as the heart, brain, or lungs. A thrombus has the potential to separate from the vessel wall and travel within the bloodstream to a different location. When this occurs, the thrombus becomes an **embolus.**

The mobile embolus travels within the bloodstream until it comes to a point in a blood vessel that is smaller than itself, causing it to lodge at that location in the vessel. Once it is lodged, blood flow beyond the embolus is blocked; thus tissues and organs that depend on delivery of blood from that particular section of the circulatory system are deprived of oxygen and nutrients. Deprivation of an adequate blood supply has the potential to cause injury (ischemia) and/or death (infarction).

Prethrombotic conditions predispose an individual to the development of thrombi. The prethrombotic state in general is caused by **hypercoagulability** or thrombophillic disor-

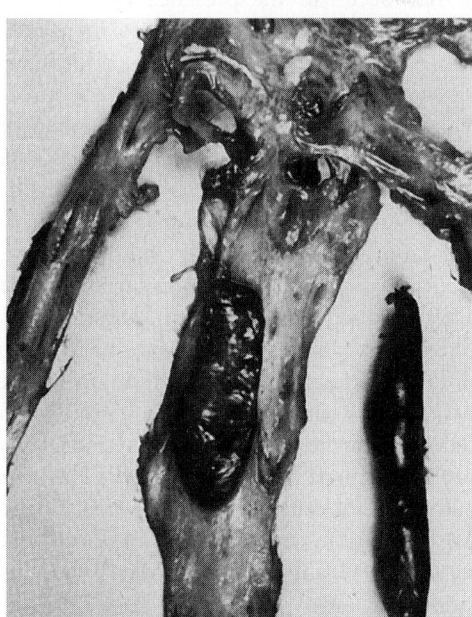

Figure 27-16 Thrombus. Thrombus arising in valve pocket at upper end of superficial femoral vein. Postmortem clot on the right is shown for comparison. (From McLachlin J, Paterson JC: *Surg Gynecol Obstet* 93:1, 1951.)

ders,[119] a tendency to coagulate more rapidly than is normal, within the vasculature. Hypercoagulability may be attributable to hereditary or acquired causes. (Congenital hypercoagulability and thrombosis are discussed in Chapter 28.)

Acquired Hypercoagulability and Thrombosis. The acquired hypercoagulable states are caused mostly by conditions that promote venous stasis. The most common clinical states that predispose to thromboembolic phenomena are major surgery (orthopedic), acute myocardial infarction, congestive heart failure, limb paralysis, spinal injury, malignancy, advanced age, the postpartum period, and bed rest longer than 1 week. These clinical states present the greatest risk because of the presence of predisposing factors that promote thrombus formation. Risk of developing thromboemboli is increased by age, previous thrombi development, and hereditary risk factors related to hypercoagulable states.[141] During these clinical states, development of thrombi is greatest because of predisposing factors that promote thrombus formation. Factors that predispose thrombus formation are referred to as the **triad of Virchow** and are (1) injury to the blood vessel endothelium, (2) abnormalities of blood flow, and (3) hypercoagulability of the blood.[129]

Endothelial injury to blood vessels from a variety of sources is the most significant cause of thrombus formation and may, by itself, precipitate the development of thrombi.[140] Initial endothelial injury exposes subendothelial collagen (and other platelet activators) and causes release of tissue factor. These activities initiate platelet adhesions and aggregation, promoting the individual development of atherosclerotic plaques that progress to further vessel damage and occlusion. Specific causes of vessel endothelial injury are hemodynamic alterations associated with hypertension and turbulent blood flow that occurs in other arterial disorders. Injury also may occur in the presence of radiation injury, exogenous chemical agents (cigarette toxins), endogenous agents (cholesterol), bacterial toxins or endotoxins, or immunologic complex deposits. Whatever the precipitating cause of endothelial injury, it is a potent thrombogenic agent.

Abnormalities of blood flow, specifically turbulence and stasis, contribute to thrombus formation by interfering with laminar flow. Laminar flow is such that the cellular components of blood are located centrally within the vessel, separated from the vascular endothelium by a slower-moving, clear zone of plasma.[18] Interruption of laminar flow by turbulence and stasis promotes thrombus formation by bringing platelets into contact with the endothelium. In addition, clotting factors that may become activated are inhibited from being diluted by fresh-flowing blood, and clotting factor inhibitors are not brought into the area to prevent formation of thrombi. Endothelial cells are also activated by turbulence and stasis, creating an environment for local thrombosis, leukocyte adhesion, and multiple other endothelial cell manifestations.

Clinical conditions in which stasis and turbulence occur include ulcerated atherosclerotic plaques (myocardial infarction), aneurysms, cardiac valve disorders, hyperviscosity conditions (polycythemia vera), and deformed red blood cells (sickle cell anemia).

Hypercoagulability is the condition in which an individual is at risk for but does not necessarily develop thrombosis.[142] By itself it is a rare cause of thrombosis and is due to primary or secondary causes. Primary causes include congenital conditions related to protein C, protein S, and AT III deficiencies, abnormal clotting factor V, and fibrinogen variants (see Chapter 28). Secondary causes include a variety of clinical disorders or conditions (Box 27-8). A recent discovery is the positive relationship between hyperhomocysteinemia and thrombus development. Individuals with homocysteine levels above the 95th percentile were 2.5 times more likely to experience an episode of deep venous thrombosis.[143] It is not well understood why there is not a greater incidence of thrombosis formation in hypercoagulable states associated with various disease states and conditions (Box 27-9).

Whether episodes of thromboembolism are life threatening depends on the site of vessel occlusion. Therapy consists of removal or breakdown of the clot and supportive measures. Anticoagulant therapy is effective in preventing arterial thrombosis; it is not useful in treating arterial thrombosis. Parenteral heparin is the major anticoagulant used to treat thromboembolism; however, it may contribute to thrombus formation. Oral coumarin drugs also are widely used, particularly for outpatients.

Box 27-8	Hereditary and Acquired Thrombophilic Disorders

Inherited Disorders (Primary)
Activated protein C resistance
   Factor V Leiden mutation
   Factor V Cambridge mutation
   Factor V Hong Kong
   Factor V HR2 mutation
   Prothrombin 20210A mutation
Factor XII deficiency (Hageman trait)
Dysfibrinogenemia
Hyperhomocyst(e)inemia
Platelet defects
   Wein-Penzing defect
   Sticky platelet syndrome

Inherited and Acquired Disorders
Antithrombin deficiency
Heparin cofactor II deficiency
Protein C deficiency
Protein S deficiency
Plasminogen deficiency
Other fibrinolytic system defects

Acquired Disorders (Secondary)
Antiphospholipid antibodies
   Anticardiolipin antibodies
   Lupus anticoagulant
   Subgroup phospholipids antibodies
Myeloproliferative syndromes
Trousseau syndrome

From Bick RL: *Hematol Oncol Clin North Am* 17(1):115-147, 2003.

Box 27-9	Clinical Conditions Associated with High-Risk for Thrombosis/ Thromboembolism

Arterial	**Venous**
Atherosclerosis	General surgery
Cigarette smoking	Orthopedic surgery
Hypertension	Arthroscopy
Diabetes mellitus	Trauma
LDL cholesterol	Malignancy
Hypertriglyceridemia	Immobility
Positive family history	Sepsis
Left ventricular failure	Congestive heart failure
Oral contraceptives	Nephrotic syndrome
Estrogens	Obesity
Lipoprotein A	Varicose veins
Polycythemia	Postphlebotic syndrome
Hyperviscosity syndrome	Oral contraceptives
Leukostasis syndrome	Estrogens
Thrombocythemia	Thrombocythemia

More aggressive therapy may be indicated for such conditions as pulmonary embolism, coronary thrombosis, or deep venous thrombosis (DVT). Streptokinase and urokinase activate the fibrinolytic system and are administered to accelerate the lysis of known thrombi. Thrombolytic therapy has limited uses and is prescribed cautiously because it can cause hemorrhagic complications.

In addition, protein S and C conditions and AT III deficiency also may be acquired and contribute to a hypercoagulable state (see Chapter 28). Conditions associated with an acquired protein deficiency include DIC, liver disease, infection, deep venous thrombosis, adult respiratory distress syndrome, L-asparaginase therapy, hemolytic uremic syndrome, and thrombocytic thrombocytopenic purpura. The postoperative state also predisposes an individual to protein C or S deficiency; however, its role in contributing to deep venous thrombosis remains unclear.[144]

SUMMARY REVIEW

Alterations of Leukocyte Function

1. Quantitative alterations of leukocytes (too many or too few) can be caused by bone marrow dysfunction or premature destruction of cells in the circulation. Many quantitative changes in leukocytes occur in response to invasion of microorganisms.
2. Leukocytosis (a leukocyte count higher than normal) is usually a response to stress or physiologic response, or both, to invasion of microorganisms.
3. Leukopenia (a leukocyte count lower than normal) is caused by pathologic conditions, such as malignancies and hematologic disorders.
4. Granulocytopenia, a condition resulting in a severe decrease in neutrophils, can be a life-threatening condition if sepsis occurs; often it is caused by chemotherapeutic agents, severe infection, and radiation.
5. Eosinophilia results most commonly from parasitic invasion and ingestion or inhalation of toxic foreign particles.
6. Monocytosis occurs during the late or recuperative phase of infection when macrophages (mature monocytes) phagocytose surviving microorganisms and debris.
7. Infectious mononucleosis (IM) is a self-limiting, nonneoplastic, lymphoproliferative syndrome caused by infection of B cells, most commonly the Epstein-Barr virus (EBV), a herpestype virus.
8. IM most commonly affects young adults between 15 and 35 years of age who have not had previous EBV infection during childhood.
9. Most cases of EBV infectious mononucleosis start with fever and sore throat, a temperature elevation lasting 7 to 10 days, and enlargement and tenderness of the cervical lymph nodes from inflammation at the site of viral entry.
10. The common pathologic feature of all forms of leukemia is an uncontrolled proliferation of leukocytes.
11. All leukemias can be designated as (a) lymphocytic, (b) myelocytic or myelogenous, or (c) monocytic. The acute leukemias are divided into two major types: (a) acute myelogenous leukemia (AML) and (b) acute lymphocytic leukemia (ALL).
12. The two principal types of chronic leukemia are (a) chronic myelocytic leukemia (CML) and (b) chronic lymphocytic leukemia (CLL).
13. Although the exact cause of leukemia is unknown, it is considered a clonal disorder. A high incidence of acute leukemias and CLL is reported in certain families, suggesting a genetic predisposition. The most common genetic abnormality in adult ALL is the Philadelphia chromosome. In about a third of patients with AML there is a mutation in the receptor tyrosine kinase FLT3.
14. In leukemia, blasts (precursor cells) "crowd out" the marrow and cause cellular proliferation of the other cell lines to cease.
15. Acute leukemias involve abnormal proliferation of precursor cells, decreased rate of apoptosis and an arrest in differentiation.
16. CLL involves transformation and accumulation of monoclonal B lymphocytes. Accumulation is the result of cell cycle arrest in the G_0/G_1 phase creating B cells resistant to apoptosis.
17. Cellular abnormalities in CML often include the Philadelphia chromosome.
18. The major clinical manifestations of leukemia include fatigue caused by anemia, bleeding caused by thrombocytopenia, fever secondary to infection, anorexia, and weight loss.
19. Chemotherapy is the treatment of choice for leukemia. Acute leukemias are associated with a 20% to 50% long-term survival rate. Chronic leukemias are associated with a longer life expectancy.
20. Chronic leukemias progress differently from acute leukemias, advancing slowly and without warning.
21. Myeloma is a neoplasm of immunocytes called *plasma cells*. The tumor may be solitary or multifocal, known as *multiple myeloma (MM)*.
22. Multiple myeloma is a disease of transformed precursor plasma cells that have completed rearrangement of immunoglobulin heavy chain in the lymph node or transformed fully matured (differentiated) plasma cells in the bone marrow.
23. The exact cause of multiple myeloma is unknown, but genetic factors and chronic stimulation of the mononuclear phagocyte system by bacteria, viral agents, and chemicals have been suggested.
24. Chromosome 13 abnormality is the most common alteration found in 86% of those with MM.

Continued

SUMMARY REVIEW—cont'd

25. The major clinical manifestations for multiple myeloma include recurrent infections caused by suppression of the humoral immune response and renal disease, presumably, as a result of Bence-Jones proteinuria.
26. Chemotherapy, stem cell transplant, thalidomide, and dexamethasone are treatments for multiple myeloma. Astonishing has been the positive effects of these treatments.

Alterations of Lymphoid Function

1. The number of lymphocytes is decreased (lymphocytopenia) in most acute infections and in some immune deficiency syndromes.
2. Lymphocytosis occurs in viral infections, infectious mononucleosis, infectious hepatitis, leukemia, lymphomas, and some chronic infections.
3. Lymphomas are tumors of primary lymphoid tissue (thymus and bone marrow) or secondary tissue (lymph nodes, spleen, tonsils, and intestinal lymphoid tissue). The two major types of malignant lymphomas are Hodgkin and non-Hodgkin.
4. Distinctive abnormal chromosomes are present in multiple cells of the lymph nodes of an individual with Hodgkin lymphoma. The abnormal cell is called a *Reed-Sternberg cell.*
5. Viruses are suspected to be involved in the pathogenesis of Hodgkin lymphoma. Some familial clustering suggests an unknown genetic mechanism.
6. An enlarged, unilateral painless mass or swelling, most commonly in the neck, is an initial sign of Hodgkin lymphoma. Local symptoms are produced by lymphadenopathy, usually caused by pressure or obstruction.
7. Treatment of Hodgkin lymphoma includes radiation therapy and chemotherapy. A cure is possible regardless of the stage of Hodgkin lymphoma; however, individuals treated with chemotherapy who relapse in less than 2 years have a poor prognosis.
8. The cause of lymph node enlargement and cancerous transformation in non-Hodgkin lymphoma is unknown. Immunosuppressed persons have a greater incidence of non-Hodgkin lymphoma, suggesting an immune mechanism.
9. Generally, with non-Hodgkin lymphoma, the swelling of lymph nodes is painless and the nodes have enlarged and transformed over a period of months or years.
10. Individuals with non-Hodgkin lymphoma can survive for long periods. Treatment consists of chemotherapy.
11. Burkitt lymphoma involves the jaw and facial bones and occurs in children from east-central Africa and New Guinea.

Alterations of Splenic Function

1. Splenomegaly (enlargement of the spleen) is not necessarily considered pathologic but may indicate underlying pathology.
2. Splenomegaly results from a wide variety of conditions, most notably those caused by acute inflammatory or infectious processes or those that produce splenic congestion or infiltration.
3. Hypersplenism (overactivity) is associated with splenomegaly and pancytopenia.

Alterations of Platelets and Coagulation

1. Thrombocytopenia is characterized by a platelet count below 100,000 platelets/mm³ of blood; a count below 50,000/mm³ increases the potential for hemorrhage associated with minor trauma. Thrombocytopenia exists in primary and secondary forms.
2. Secondary thrombocytopenia commonly is associated with autoimmune diseases and viral infections; bacterial sepsis, which may cause disseminated intravascular coagulation (DIC), also results in thrombocytopenia.
3. Heparin-induced thrombocytopenia develops in approximately 2% to 15% of individuals receiving heparin.
4. Immune thrombocytopenic purpura (ITP) is a major cause of platelet destruction, often affecting females, and results in hemorrhaging that ranges from minor development of petechiae to major bleeding from mucosal sites.
5. Thrombotic thrombycytopenic purpura (TTP) causes platelet aggregation leading to microcirculatory occlusion.
6. Thrombocythemia is characterized by a platelet count greater than 600,000/mm³ of blood and is symptomatic when the count exceeds 1,000,000/mm³ and when the risk for intravascular clotting (thrombosis) is high.
7. Primary thrombocythemia is caused by accelerated platelet production in the bone marrow characterized by hyperplasia of megakaryocytes.
8. Alterations in normal platelet adherence or aggregation prevent platelet plug formation and may result in prolonged bleeding times.
9. Qualitative platelet dysfunction results from disorders of platelet adhesion, platelet aggregation platelet secretion and procoagulant activity.
10. Disorders of coagulation usually are caused by defects or deficiencies of one or more of the clotting factors.
11. Coagulation is impaired when there is a deficiency of vitamin K because of insufficient hepatic production of prothrombin and clotting factors II, VII, IX, and X.
12. Liver disease accounts for a pattern of hemostatic derangement caused by a disruption of the synthesis of clotting factors.
13. DIC is a complex syndrome resulting from a variety of clinical conditions that cause release of tissue factor and results in activation and circulation of plasmin and thrombin.
14. DIC is characterized by a cycle of intravascular clotting followed by active bleeding because of accelerated consumption of coagulation factors, platelets, and diffuse fibrinolysis.
15. Thromboembolic disease results from a fixed (thrombus) or moving (embolism) clot that obstructs blood flow within a vessel, denying nutrients to tissues distal to the occlusion; death can result when clots are lodged in the heart, brain, or lungs.
16. Hypercoagulability is the result of deficient anticoagulation proteins. Secondary causes are conditions that promote venous stasis.
17. The term *triad of Virchow* refers to three factors that can cause thrombus formation: (1) loss of integrity of the vessel wall, (2) abnormalities of blood flow, and (3) alterations in the blood constituents.

KEY TERMS

KEY TERMS—cont'd

MEDIA RESOURCES evolve

Review questions and answers for this chapter are available in the *CD Companion* included with this book.

WebLinks—links to Internet sites pertaining to this chapter—are available on Evolve at http://evolve.elsevier.com/McCance/.

REFERENCES

1. Chandrasoma P, Taylor CR: *Concise pathology,* Norwalk, Conn, 1995, Lange.
2. Dale DC, Liles WC: Neutrophils and monocytes: normal physiology and disorders of neutrophil and monocyte production. In Handin RI et al, editors: *Blood: principles and practice of hematology,* Philadelphia, 2003, Lippincott, Williams & Wilkins.
3. Russin SJ, Fillipo BH, Alder AG: Neutropenia in adults: what is its clinical significance? *Postgrad Med* 88:209, 1990.
4. Munshi HG, Montgomery RB: Severe neutropenia: a diagnostic approach, *Western J Med* 172(4):248-252, 2000.
5. Watts RG: Neutropenia. In Lee GR et al, editors: *Wintrobe's clinical hematology,* Baltimore, 1999, Williams & Wilkins.
6. Bohme A, Wolter M, Hoelzer D: L-tryptophan–related eosinophilia-myalgia syndrome possibly associated with a chronic B-lymphocyte leukemia, *Ann Hematol* 77(5):235-238, 1998.
7. Weller PF, Tsai M, Galli SJ: Eosinophils, basophils, and mast cells. In Handin RI, Lux SE, Stossel TP, editors: *Blood: principles and practice of hematology,* ed 2, 2003, Lippincott, Williams, & Wilkins.
8. Barth H, Berg PA, Klein R: Is there any relationship between eosinphilia myalgia syndrome (EMS) and fibromyalgia syndrome (FMS)? An analysis of clinical and immunological data, *Adv Exper Med Biol* 467:487-496, 1999.
9. Meisel SR et al: Peripheral monocytosis following acute myocardial infarction: incidence and its possible role as a bedside marker of the extent of cardiac injury, *Cardiology* 90(1):52-57, 1998.
10. Athens JW: Variations of leukocytes in disease. In Lee GR et al, editors: *Wintrobe's clinical hematology,* ed 9, Philadelphia, 1993, Lea & Febiger.
11. Sitki-Green DL et al: Biology of Epstein-Barr virus during infectious mononucleosis, *J Infect Dis* 189(3):483-492, 2004.
12. Grotto I et al: Clinical and laboratory presentation of EBV-positive infectious mononucleosis in young adults, *Epidemiol Infect* 131(1):683-689, 2003.
13. Willis JL: Mono: tough for teens and twenty-somethings, *FDA Consumer* 32(3):32, 1998.
14. Godshall SE, Kirchner JT: Infectious mononucleosis: complexities of a common syndrome, *Postgrad Med* 107(7):175-179, 183-184, 186, 2000.
15. Ventura KC, Hudnall SD: Hematologic differences in heterophile-positive and heterophile-negative infectious mononucleosiws, *Am J Hematol* 76(4):315-318, 2004.
16. Stockinger ZT: Infectious mononucleosis as spontaneous splenic rupture without other symptoms, *Military Med* 168(9):722-723, 2003.
17. Ebell M: Epstein-Barr virus infectious mononucleosis, *Am Fam Phys* 70(7):1279-1286, 2004.
18. Cotran RS et al: *Robbins' pathologic basis of disease,* ed 6, Philadelphia, 1999, Saunders.
19. Hickey SM, Strasburger VC: What every pediatrician should know about infectious mononucleosis in adolescents, *Pediatr Clin North Am* 44(6):1541, 1997.
20. Omori M: *Mononucleosis,* 2000. Available at www.emedicine.com.
21. Williams H et al: Analysis of immune activation and clinical events in infectious mononucleosis, *J Infect Dis* 190(1):63-71, 2004.
22. Roy M et al: Dexamethasone for the treatment of sore throat in children with suspected infectious mononucleosis: a randomized, double-blind, placebo-controlled clinical trial, *Arch Pediatr Adol Med* 158(3):250-254, 2004.
23. Auwaerter PG: Infectious mononucleosis in middle age, *JAMA* 281(5):454, 1999.
24. Gross TG: Infectious mononucleosis and other Epstein Barr virus related disorders. In Greer JP et al, editors: *Wintrobe's clinical hematology,* Philadelphia, 2004, Lippincott, Williams, & Wilkins.
25. Zidovec Lepej S et al: Increased numbers of CD38 molecules on bright DC8 T lymphocytes in infectious mononucleosis caused by Epstein-Barr virus infection, *Clin Experiment Immunol* 133(3):384-390, 2003.
26. Bailey RE: Diagnosis and treatment of infectious mononucleosis, *Am Fam Physician* 49(4):879, 1994.
27. Haller A et al: Severe respiratory insufficiency complicating Epstein-Barr virus infection: case report and review, *Clin Infect Dis* 21(1):206, 1995.
28. Bates S, Friedman J: Index of suspicion, *Pediatr Rev* 19(4):137, 1998.
29. Vincent MT, Celestin N, Hussain AN: Pharyngitis, *Am Fam Physician* 69(6):1465-1470, 2004.
30. Hjalguim H et al: Characteristics of Hodgkin's lymphoma after infectious mononucleosis, *New Engl J Med* 349(14):1324-1332, 2003.
31. Gunz FW: The dread leukemias and the lymphomas: their nature and their prospects. In Wintrobe MM, editor: *Blood, pure and eloquent: a story of discovery, of people, and of ideas,* New York, 1980, McGraw-Hill.

32. Ferrajoli A, Keating MJ: Current guidelines in defining therapeutic strategies, *Hematol Oncol Clin North Am* 18(4):881-893, 2004.

33. Pui CH: Acute lymphoblastic leukemia, *Ped Clin North Am* 44(4):831-846, 1997.

34. The Leukemia and Lymphoma Society: *Facts 2004.* Available at www.leukemia-lymphoma.org.

35. Lai R et al: Pathologic diagnosis of acute lymphocytic leukemia, *Hematol Oncol Clin North Am* 14(6):1209-1235, 2000.

36. Kantarjian HM: Adult acute lymphocytic leukemia, *Hematol Oncol Clin North Am* 14(6):1205-1207, 2000.

37. Fialkow PJ et al: Clonal remission in adult nonlymphocytic leukemia: evidence for a multistep pathogenesis of the malignancy, *Blood* 77(7):1415-1417, 1991.

38. Faderl S, Jeha S, Kantarjian HM: The biology and therapy of adult acute lymphoblastic leukemia, *Cancer* 98(17):1337-1354, 2003

39. Gilliland DG, Jordan CT, Felix CA: The molecular basis of leukemia, *Hematology (Am Soc Hematol Educ Program)*:80-97, 2004.

40. Advani AS: C-kit as a target in the treatment of acute myelogenous leukemia, *Curr Hematol Rep* 4(1):51-58, 2005.

41. Silverman LB, Sallan SE: Acute lymphoblastic leukemia. In Handin RI et al, editors: *Blood: principles and practice of hematology,* Philadelphia, 2003, Lippincott, Williams & Wilkins.

42. Cortes J: Central nervous system involvement in adult acute lympho-cytic leukemia, *Hematol Oncol Clin North Am* 15(1):145-161, 2001.

43. Gorin NC et al: Feasibility and recent improvement of autologous stem cell transplantation for acute myelocytic leukemia in patients over 60 years of age: importance of the source of stem cells, *Br J Haematol* 110(4):887, 2000.

44. Williams M: Gastrointestinal manifestations of graft-versus-host dis-ease: diagnosis and management, *AACN Clin Issues* 10(4):500-506, 1999.

45. Laport GF, Larson RA: Treatment of acute lymphoblastic leukemia, *Sem Oncol* 24(1):70-82, 1997.

46. Dighiero G: Perspectives in chronic lymphocytic leukemia biology and management, *Hematol Oncol Clin North Am* 18(4):927-943, 2004.

47. Caligaris-Cappio F, Ghia P: The nature and origin of the B-chronic lymphocytic leukemia cell: a tentative model, *Hematol Oncol Clin N Am* 18(4):849-862, 2004.

48. Saffa MM, Foon KA: Chronic lymphoid leukemia. In Handin RI et al, editors: *Blood: Principles and practice of hematology,* Philadelphia, 2003, Lippincott, Williams & Wilkins.

49. Kantarjian HM et al: Clinical course and therapy of chronic myeloge-nous leukemias with interferon alpha and chemotherapy, *Hematol On-col Clin North Am* 12(1):34-80, 1998.

50. Cortes J, Kantarjian HM: Beyond chronic myelogenous leukemia, *Cancer* 100(10):2064-2078, 2004.

51. Chng WJ et al: Targeted therapy in multiple myeloma, *Cancer Control* 12(2):91-104, 2005.

52. Shaughnessy J et al: Continuous absence of metaphase-defined cytoge-netic abnormalities, especially of chromosome 13 and hypodiploidy, ensures long-term survival in multiple myeloma treated with Tital Therapy I: interpretation in the context of global gene expression, *Blood* 101(10):3849-3856, 2003.

53. Kuehl WM, Bergsagel PL: Multiple myeloma: evolving genetic events and host interactions, *Nat Rev Cancer* 2(3):175-187, 2002.

54. Hideshima T et al: Advances in biology of multiple myeloma: clinical applications, *Blood* 104(3):607-618, 2004.

55. Avet-Loiseau H et al: Rearrangements of the *c-myc* oncogene are pres-ent in 15% of primary human multiple myeloma tumors, *Blood* 98(10):3082-3086, 2001.

56. Ablashi DV et al: Lack of serologic association of human herpesvirus-8 (KSHV) in patients with monoclonal gammopathy of undertermined significance with and without progression to multiple myeloma, *Blood* 96(6):2304-2306, 2000.

57. The Leukemia and Lymphoma Society: Lymphoma. Available at http:www.leukemia-lymphoma.org/all_page?item_id=7030.

58. Atayar CS et al: Expression of the T-cell transcription factors, GATA-2 and T-bet, in the neoplastic cells of Hodgkin lymphomas, *Am J Pathol* 166(1):127-134, 2005.

59. Argiris A, Kaklamani V: Hodgkin disease. Available at http://www.emedicine.com/med/topic1022.htm. Accessed 3/16/2005.

60. American Cancer Society: *Cancer facts and figures 2005,* Atlanta, 2005, Author.

61. Ambinder R: Infection and lymphoma, *New Engl J Med* 349(14):1309-1311, 2003.

62. Gobbi PG et al: The clinical value of tumor burden at diagnosis in Hodgkin lymphoma, *Cancer* 101(8):1824-1834, 2004.

63. Estrada DA et al: Lymphoma, non-Hodgkin. Available at http://www.emedicine.com/MED/topic1363.htm. Accessed 3/16/2005.

64. Bociek RG, Armitage JO: Non-Hodgkin's lymphomas. In Handin RI et al, editors: *Blood: principles and practice of hematology,* Philadelphia, 2003, Lippincott, Williams & Wilkins.

65. Shurin SB: The spleen and its disorders. In Hoffman R et al, editors: *Hematology: basic principles and practice,* New York, 2000, Churchill Livingstone.

66. Jacobsen CT, Shurin SB: Disorders of Spleen. In Handin RI, Lux SE, Stossel TP, editors: *Blood: principles and practice of hematology,* ed 2, 2003, Lippincott, Williams, & Wilkins.

67. Goodman TG et al: Disorders of the spleen. In Greer JP et al, editors: *Wintrobe's clinical hematology,* Philadelphia, 2004, Lippincott, Williams & Wilkins.

68. Erslev AJ: Hypersplenism and hyposplenism. In Beutler MA et al, edi-tors: *Williams hematology,* New York, 2003, McGraw-Hill.

69. Carr JA, Shurafa M, Velanovich V: Surgical indications in idiopathic splenomegaly, *Arch Surg* 137(1):64-68, 2002.

70. Jandl JH: *Blood: textbook of hematology,* ed 2, Boston, 1996, Little, Brown.

71. Kaplan LJ, Coffman D: Splenomegaly. Available at http://www.emedi-cine.com/med/topic2156.htm. Accessed March 30, 2005.

72. Cines D, Bussel JB: How I treat: ITP, *Blood* June 7, 2005: (Epub ahead of print, 2005.)

73. Warkentin TE, Kelton JG: Platelet life cycle: quantitative disorders. In Handin RI et al, editors: *Blood: principles and practice of hematology,* Philadelphia, 2003, Lippincott, Williams & Wilkins.

74. Lathan LO, Staggers SL: Ancrod: the use of snake venom in the treat-ment of patients with heparin-induced thrombocytopenia and throm-bosis undergoing coronary artery bypass grafting: nursing manage-ment, *Heart Lung* 25(6):451-460, 1996.

75. Warkentin TE: Heparin-induced thrombocytopenia: a ten-year retro-spective, *Annu Rev Med* 50:129-147, 1999.

76. Horner BM, Myers SR: Don't miss HIT (heparin-induced thrombocy-topenia), *Burns* 30(1):88-90, 2004.

77. Warkentin TE: New approaches to the diagnosis of heparin-induced thrombocytopenia, *Chest* 127(Suppl 2):35S-45S, 2005.

78. Mims M, Manian P, Rice L: Acute cardiorespiratory collapse from hep-arin: a consequence of heparin-induced thrombocytopenia, *Eur J Haematol* 72(5):366-369, 2004.

79. Ayala E et al: Heparin-induced thrombocytopenia presenting with thrombosis of multiple saphenous vein grafts and myocardial infarc-tion, *Am J Hematol* 76(4):383-385, 2004.

80. Di Paola JA, Buchanan GR: Immune thrombocytopenic purpura, *Pe-diat Clin North Am* 49(5):911-928, 2002.

81. McMillan R: The pathogenesis of chronic immune (idiopathic) thrombocytopenic purpura, *Semin Hematol* 37(1 suppl 1):5, 2000.

82. Solanilla A et al: Platelet-associated CD154 in immune thrombo-topenic purpura, *Blood* 105(1):215-218, 2005.

83. Bolton-Maggs P et al: The child with immune thrombocytopenic pur-pura: is pharmacotherapy or watchful waiting the best initial manage-ment? *J Pediat Hematol Oncol* 26(2):146-151, 2004.

84. Jayabose S et al: Long-term outcome of chronic idiopathic thrombocy-topenic purpura in children, *J Pediat Hematol Oncol* 26(11):724-726, 2004.

85. Ahmed S et al: Prognostic variables in newly diagnosed childhood im-mune thrombocytopenia, *Am J Hematol* 77(4):358-362, 2004.

86. George JN, Shatti SJ: Acquired disorders of platelet function. In Hoffman R et al, editors: *Hematology: basic principles and practice,* ed 2, New York, 1995, Churchill Livingstone.

87. George JN et al: Idiopathic thrombocytopenia purpura: a practice guideline developed by explicit methods for the American Society of Hematology, *Blood* 88(1):30, 1996.

88. Cines DB et al: Mechanisms of action of therapeutics in idiopathic thrombocytopenic purpura, *J Ped Hematol Oncol* 20(Suppl 1):S52-S56, 2003.

89. Bussel J, Cines D: Immune thrombocytopenia purpura, neonatal al-loimmune thrombocytopenia, and post-transfusion purpura. In Hoff-man R et al, editors: *Hematology: basic principles and practice,* ed 2, New York, 1995, Churchill Livingstone.

90. Karpatkin S: Autoimmune (idiopathic) thrombocytopenic purpura, *Lancet* 349(9064):1531-1536, 1997.

91. George JN: Treatment options for chronic idiopathic (immune) thrombocytopenic purpura, *Semin Hematol* 37(Suppl 1):31, 2000.

92. Robak T: Monoclonal antibodies in the treatment of autoimmune cytopenias, *Eur J Haematol* 72(2):79-88, 2004.

93. Rock G et al: Thrombotic thrombocytopenic purpura treatment in the year 2000, *Haematologica* 85(4):410, 2000.

94. Moake JL: Thrombotic thrombocytopenic purpura today, *Hosp Pract* 34(7):53, 1999.

95. Nabhan C, Kwaan HC: Current concepts in the diagnosis and management of thrombotic thrombocytopenic purpura, *Hematol Oncol Clin North Am* 17(1):177-199, 2003.

96. Wun T, Bahou WF: Thrombotic thrombocytopenic purpura. Available at http://www.emedicine.com/med/topic2265.htm. Accessed March 29, 2005.

97. Jantunen RE et al: Essential thrombocythemia at diagnosis: causes of diagnostic evaluation and presence of positive diagnostic findings, *Ann Hematol* 77(3):101-106, 1998.

98. Spivak JL: Myeloproliferative disorders. In Handin RI et al, editors: *Blood: principles and practice of hematology*, Philadelphia, 2003, Lippincott, Williams & Wilkins.

99. Ding J et al: Familial essential thrombocythemia associated with a dominant-positive activating mutation of the c-MPL gene, which encodes for the receptor for thrombopoietin, *Blood* 103(11):4198-4200, 2004.

100. Jantunen RE: Development of erythrocytosis in the course of essential thrombocythemia, *Ann Hematol* 78(5):219-222, 1999.

101. Rice L: Heparin-induced thrombocytopenia: myths and misconceptions (that will cause trouble for you and your patient), *Arch Intern Med* 164(18):1961-1964, 2004.

102. Elliott MA, Tefferi A: Thrombosis and haemorrhage in polycythemia vera and the essential thrombocythaemia, *Br J Haematol* 128(3):275-290, 2005.

103. Barbui T, Finazzo G: Clinical parameters for determining when and when not to treat essential thrombocythemia, *Semin Hematol* 36(1 suppl 2):14, 1999.

104. Murphy S: Diagnostic criteria and prognosis in polycythemia vera and essential thrombocythemia, *Semin Hematol* 36(1 suppl 2):9, 1999.

105. Hoffman R, Silverstein MN, Hromas R: Primary thrombocythemia. In Hoffman R et al, editors: *Hematology: basic principles and practice*, ed 2, New York, 1995, Churchill Livingstone.

106. Spivak JL: The chronic myeloproliferative disorders: clonality and clinical heterogeneity, *Semin Hematol* 41(2 Suppl 3):1-5, 2004.

107. Silverstein MN, Tefferi A: Treatment of essential thrombocythemia with Anagrelide, *Semin Hematol* 36(1 suppl 2):23, 1999.

108. Harrison CN, Green AR: Essential thrombocythemia, *Hematol Oncol Clin North Am* 17(5):1175-1190, 2003.

109. Simmons ED: Bleeding and hemostasis. In Michelson EA et al, editors: *Current critical care: diagnosis and treatment*, pp 443-465, New York, 2004, Lange Medical Books/McGraw-Hill.

110. Wyrick-Glatzel J: Quantitative and qualitative vascular and platelet disorders, both congenital and acquired. In Harming DM, editor: *Clinical hematology and fundamentals of hemostasis*, Philadelphia, 1997, Davis.

111. Bick RL: Platelet function defects associated with hemorrhage or thrombosis, *Med Clin North Am* 78(3)577, 1994.

112. Staudinger T et al: Management of acquired coagulation disorders in emergency and intensive care medicine, *Semin Thromb Hemost* 22(1):93, 1996.

113. Furie B et al: Vitamin K dependent blood coagulation proteins: normal function and clinical disorders. In Handin RI et al, editors: *Blood: principles and practice of hematology*, Philadelphia, 2003, Lippincott, Williams & Wilkins.

114. Mammen EF: Coagulation defects in liver disease, *Med Clin North Am* 78(3):545, 1994.

115. Hambleton J, Leung LL, Levi M: Coagulation: consultative hemostasis, *Hematology (Am Soc Hematol Educ Program)*, 335-342, 2002.

116. Marder VJ et al: Consumptive thrombohemorrhagic disorders. In Colman RW et al, editors: *Hemostasis and thrombosis: basic principles and clinical practice*, ed 3, Philadelphia, 1994, Lippincott.

117. Furlong MA, Furlong BR: Disseminated intravascular coagulation. Available at www.emedicine.com/emerg/topic150.htm. Accessed March 16, 2005.

118. Taylor FB Jr et al: Towards definition, clinical and laboratory criteria, and a scoring system for disseminated intravascular coagulation, *Thromb Hemost* 86(5):1327-1330, 2001.

119. Bick RL et al: Disseminated intravascular coagulation: current concepts of etiology, pathophysiology, diagnosis, and treatment, *Hematol Oncol Clin North Am* 17(1):149-176, 2003.

120. Labelle CA, Kitchens CS: Disseminated intravascular coagulation: treat the cause, not the lab values, *Cleve Clin J Med* 72(5):377-378, 383-385, 390 passim, 2005.

121. Gando S et al: Imbalances between the levels of tissue factor and tissue factor pathway inhibitor in ARDS patients, *Thromb Res* 109(2-3):119-124, 2003.

122. Levi M et al: Sepsis and disseminated intravascular coagulation, *J Thrombosis Thrombolysis* 16(1-2):43-47, 2003.

123. Ruf W: Tissue factor-dependent signaling in tumor biology, *Pathophysiol Haemost Thromb* 33(Suppl 1):28-30, 2003.

124. Seligsohn U: Disseminated intravascular coagulation. In Beutler E et al, editors: *Williams Hematology*, New York, 2003, McGraw-Hill.

125. Donati MB: Coagulation factors and tumor cell biology: the role of tissue factor, *Pathophys Haemost Thromb* 33(Suppl 1):22-25, 2003.

126. Johnson PC: Disseminated intravascular coagulation. In Fry DE, editor: *Multiple system organ failure*, St Louis, 1996, Mosby.

127. Baglin T: Disseminated intravascular coagulation: diagnosis and treatment, *BMJ* 312(7032):683-687, 1996.

128. Joist JH: Disseminated intravascular coagulation. In Baue AD, Faist E, Fry DE, editors: *Multiple organ failure*, New York, 2000, Springer.

129. Norman KE: Alternative treatments for disseminated intravascular coagulation, *Drug News Perspect* 17(4):243-250, 2004.

130. Mammen EF: Natural coagulation inhibitors and inflammation, *Turkish J Haematol* 19(2):97-102, 2002.

131. Grosset ABM, Rodgers GM: Acquired coagulation disorders. In Lee GR et al, editors: *Wintrobe's clinical hematology*, Baltimore, 1999, Williams & Wilkins.

132. Dempfle CE: Coagulopathy of sepsis, *Thromb Haemost* 91(2):213-224, 2004.

133. Hoots WK: Non-overt disseminated intravascular coagulation: definition and pathophysiological implications, *Blood Rev* 16(Suppl 1):S3-S9, 2002.

134. Levi M: Platelets at a crossroad of pathogenic pathways in sepsis, *J Thromb Haemost* 2(12):2094-2095, 2004.

135. Toh CH: Performance and prognostic importance of a new clinical and laboratory scoring system for identifying non-overt disseminated intravascular coagulation, *Blood Coagul Fibrinolysis* 16(1):69-74, 2005.

136. Riewald M, Reiss H: Treatment options for clinically recognized disseminated intravascular coagulation, *Semin Thromb Hemost* 24(1):53, 1998.

137. Francini M, Manzato F: Update on the treatment of disseminated intravascular coagulation, *Hematol Oncol Clin North Am* 9(2):81-85, 2004.

138. Levi M, DeJonge E: Current management of disseminated intravascular coagulation. Available at www.hospprract.com/issues/2000/08/celevi.htm. Accessed May 13, 2005.

139. Maxson JH: Management of disseminated intravascular coagulation, *Crit Care Nurs Clin North Am* 12(3):341-352, 2000.

140. Mitchell RN: Hemodynamic disorders, thromboembolic diseases, and shock, In Kumar VK, Abbas AK, Fausto N: *Robbins and Cotran Pathophysiologic Basis of Disease*, ed 7, Philadelphia, 2005, Saunders.

141. Toulon P, Perez P: Screening for risk factors for thrombosis using a new generation of assays developed to evaluate the functionality of the protein C anticoagulant pathway, *Hematol Oncol Clin North Am* 14(2):379, 2000.

142. Whiteman T, Hassouna HI: Hypercoagulable states, *Hematol Oncol Clin North Am* 14(2):355, 2000.

143. Bauer KA, Zwiker JI: Natural anticoagulants and the prethrombotic state, In Handin RI, Lux IV SE, Stossel TP, *Blood: Principles and Practice of Hematology*, Philadelphia, 2003, Lippincott.

144. Bick RL, Kaplan H: Syndromes of thrombosis and hypercoagulability: congenital and acquired causes of thrombosis, *Med Clin North Am* 82(3):409, 1998.

145. Vilchez RA, Butel JS: Emergent human pathogen simian virus 40 and its role in cancer, *Clin Microbiol Rev* 17(3):495-508, 2004.

146. Butel JS, Lednicky JA: Cell and molecular biology of simian virus 40: implications for human infections and disease, *J Natl Cancer Inst* 91(2):119-134, 1999.

147. Jasani B et al: Association of SV40 with human tumours, *Semin Cancer Biol* 11(1):49-61, 2001.

148. Vilchez RA, Kozinetz CA, Butel JS: conventional epidemiology and the link between SV40 and human cancers, *Lancet Oncol* 4(3):188-191, 2003.

149. Lednicky JA, Garcea RL: Detection of SV40 DNA sequences in human tissue, *Methods Mol Biol* 165:257-267, 2001.

150. Shivapurka N et al: Presence of simian virus 40 DNA sequences in human lymphomas, *Lancet* 359(9309):851-852, 2002.

151. Vilchez RA et al: Detection of polyomavirus simian virus 40 tumor antigen DNA in AIDS-related systemic non-Hodgkin lymphoma, *J Acquir Immune Defic Syndr* 29(2):109-116, 2002.

152. Vilchez RA et al: Association between simian virus 40 and non-Hodgkin lymphoma, *Lancet* 359(9309):817-823, 2002.

ALTERATIONS OF HEMATOLOGIC FUNCTION IN CHILDREN

NANCY E. KLINE

CHAPTER OUTLINE

This chapter briefly explains fetal and neonatal hematopoiesis and postnatal changes in blood as a foundation for understanding the pathophysiology of specific blood disorders in childhood. Among the diseases that affect erythrocytes are acquired disorders, such as iron deficiency anemia, hemolytic disease of the newborn, and anemia of infectious disease, and inherited disorders, such as glucose-6-phosphate dehydrogenase (G6PD) deficiency, hereditary spherocytosis, sickle cell disease, and the thalassemias. Disorders of coagulation and platelets include inherited hemorrhagic diseases, such as the hemophilias, and antibody-mediated hemorrhagic diseases, which include idiopathic thrombocytopenic purpura, autoimmune neonatal thrombocytopenias, and autoimmune vascular purpuras. Finally, leukocyte disorders, such as leukemia and the lymphomas (both non-Hodgkin lymphoma and Hodgkin disease), are discussed.

FETAL AND NEONATAL HEMATOPOIESIS

As the developing embryo becomes too large for oxygenation of tissues by simple diffusion, the production of erythrocytes begins within the vessels of the yolk sac. Shortly after 2 weeks of gestation, circulating erythrocytes play a major role in delivering oxygen to the tissues. At approximately the eighth week of gestation, the site of erythrocyte production shifts from the vessels to the liver sinusoids and the production of leukocytes and platelets begins in the liver and spleen. Erythropoiesis in the liver and, to a lesser extent, in the spleen and lymph nodes reaches a peak at approximately 4 months. Hepatic blood formation declines steadily thereafter but does not disappear entirely during the remainder of gestation. By the fifth month of gestation, hematopoiesis begins to occur in the bone marrow and increases rapidly until hematopoietic (red) marrow fills the entire bone marrow space. By the time of delivery, the marrow is the only significant site of hematopoiesis.

In neonates and young infants, hematopoietic marrow progressively fills the bony cavities of the entire axial skeleton (skull, vertebrae, ribs, sternum), the long bones of the limbs, and many intramembranous bones. (These structures are described in Chapter 43.) Fatty (yellow) marrow gradually replaces hematopoietic marrow in some bones. During childhood, hematopoietic tissue retreats centrally to the vertebrae, ribs, sternum, pelvis, scapulae, skull, and proximal ends of the femur and humerus.

In diseases characterized by hemolysis, erythrocyte production can increase as much as eight times the normal because erythropoietin causes hematopoietic marrow to increase in volume. Initially, hematopoietic marrow expands from the ends of the long bones toward the middle of the shafts, replacing fatty marrow. Next, blood cell production begins to occur outside the marrow cavities, especially in the liver and spleen. Extramedullary hematopoiesis is more likely to occur in children than in adults because the bony cavities of children already are filled with red marrow (Figure 28-1). This is why hemolytic disease causes especially pronounced enlargement of the spleen and liver in children.

The erythrocytes undergo striking changes during gestation, particularly during the first two trimesters, at which time they nearly double in numbers and in hemoglobin content. A proportionate increase in hematocrit also occurs. By the end of gestation the erythrocyte count has more than tripled but the size of each erythrocyte has decreased.

A biochemically distinct type of hemoglobin is synthesized during fetal life. The three **embryonic hemoglobins (Gower 1, Gower 2, and Portland)** and the **fetal hemoglobin (Hb F)** are composed of two alpha and two gamma chains of polypeptides, whereas the adult hemoglobins (Hb A and Hb A_2) are composed of two alpha and two beta chains. (The structure of an adult hemoglobin molecule is illustrated in Figure 25-11, and types of hemoglobin are defined in Table

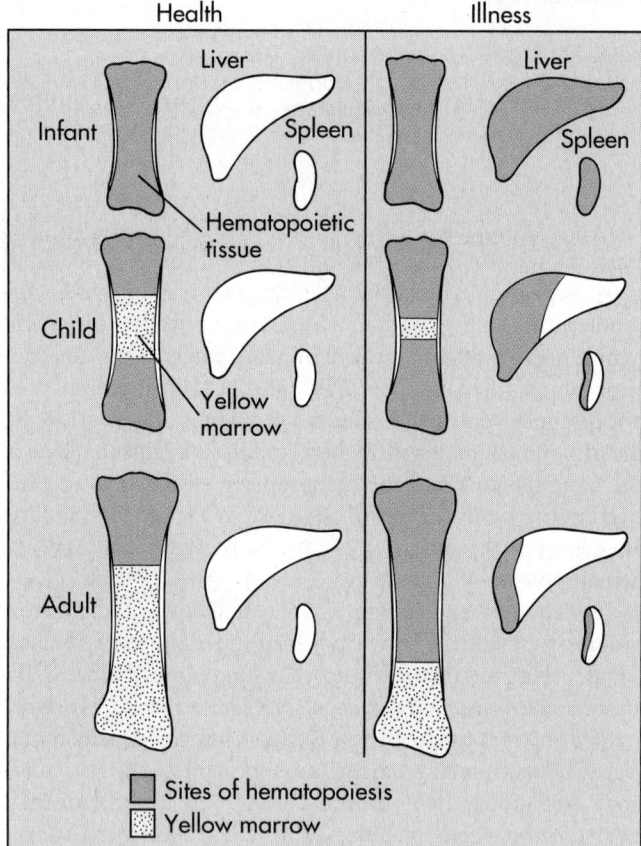

Figure 28-1 Sites of hematopoiesis in health and illness. With normal maturation, red marrow is partly replaced by yellow marrow in the shafts of the long bones. In adults, red marrow is largely restricted to the proximal ends of the femur and humerus. In response to hemolysis, red marrow replaces yellow marrow in the long bones. In infants, whose long bones already are filled with red marrow, additional hematopoiesis takes place in the liver and spleen. In children and adults, red marrow can replace yellow marrow in response to hemolysis, necessitating less hematopoiesis in the liver and spleen.

25-5.) Some unknown regulatory mechanism promotes gamma chain synthesis and inhibits beta and delta chain synthesis in utero. This results in production of embryonic or fetal hemoglobin. After birth, gamma chain synthesis is inhibited, whereas beta and delta chain synthesis is facilitated, resulting in production of adult hemoglobins.

Fetal hemoglobin has greater affinity for oxygen than does adult hemoglobin because it interacts less readily with an enzyme (2,3-diphosphoglycerate [2,3-DPG]) that inhibits hemoglobin-oxygen binding. The decreased inhibitory effects of 2,3-DPG enable fetal blood to transport oxygen despite the relative lack of oxygen in the uterine environment. The increased affinity for oxygen enables Hb F to bind with maternal oxygen in the placental circulation.

During the first trimester, nearly all of the hemoglobin in the fetus is embryonic, but some Hb A can be detected. Therefore it is possible to identify as early as 16 to 20 weeks of gestation some disorders of adult hemoglobin, such as sickle cell anemia and thalassemia major. In the 6-month fetus, Hb F constitutes 90% of the total. This percentage then begins to decline. At birth, neonatal hemoglobin consists of 70% Hb F, 29% Hb A, and 1% Hb A_2. Between 6 and 12 months of age, normal adult hemoglobin percentages are established (see Chapter 25).

POSTNATAL CHANGES IN THE BLOOD

Blood cell counts tend to rise above adult levels at birth and then decline gradually throughout childhood. Table 28-1 lists normal ranges during infancy and childhood. The immediate rise in values is the result of accelerated hematopoiesis during fetal life, increased numbers of cells that result from the trauma of birth, and cutting of the umbilical cord. These events surrounding the birth also are accompanied by a "shift to the left," that is, the presence of large numbers of immature erythrocytes and leukocytes (particularly granulocytes) in peripheral blood (see Chapter 27). The shift to the left disappears as the infant develops, usually within the first 2 to 3 months of life. Other unique postnatal characteristics, particularly of lymphocytes, may be caused by exogenous factors, such as viral infections.

Average blood volume in the full-term neonate is 85 ml/kg of body weight. The premature infant has a slightly larger blood volume of 90 ml/kg of body weight, with the mean increasing to 150 mg/kg during the first few days after birth. In both full-term and premature infants, blood volume decreases during the first few months. Thereafter the average blood volume is 75 to 77 ml/kg, which is similar to that of older children and adults.

Erythrocytes

The hypoxic intrauterine environment stimulates erythropoietin production in the fetus. This accelerates fetal erythropoiesis, producing polycythemia (excessive proliferation of erythrocyte precursors) of the newborn. After birth the oxy-

Table 28-1	Hematologic Values During Infancy and Childhood

Age	Hemoglobin (g/dl)		Hematocrit (%)		Reticulocytes (%)	MCV (fl)	Leukocytes (WBC/mm³)		Neutrophils (%)		Lymphocytes (%)	Eosinophils (%)	Monocytes (%)
	Mean	Range	Mean	Range	Mean	Lowest	Mean	Range	Mean	Range	Mean*	Mean	Mean
Cord blood	16.8	13.7–20.1	55	45-65	5.0	110	18,000	(9,000–30,000)	61	(40-80)	31	2	6
2 wk	16.5	13.0–20.0	50	42-66	1.0		12,000	(5,000–21,000)	40		63	3	9
3 mo	12.0	9.5–14.5	36	31–41	1.0		12,000	(6,000–18,000)	30		48	2	5
6 mo to 6 yr	12.0	10.5–14.0	37	33–42	1.0	70–74	10,000	(6,000–15,000)	45		48	2	5
7–12 yr	13.0	11.0–16.0	38	34–40	1.0	76–80	8,000	(4,500–13,500)	55		38	2	5
Adult													
Female	14	12.0–16.0	42	37–47	1.6	80	7,500	(5,000–10,000)	55	(35–70)	35	3	7
Male	16	14.0–18.0	47	42–52		80							

From Behrman R et al, editors: *Nelson textbook of pediatrics,* 17th ed. Philadelphia, 2004, Saunders.
*Relatively wide range.
MCV, Mean corpuscular volume; *fl,* femtoliters; *WBC,* white blood cells.

gen from the lungs saturates arterial blood and the amount of oxygen delivered to the tissues increases. In response to the change from a placental to a pulmonary oxygen supply during the first few days of life, levels of erythropoietin and the rate of blood cell formation decrease. The very active rate of fetal erythropoiesis is reflected by the large numbers of immature erythrocytes (reticulocytes) in the peripheral blood of full-term neonates. After birth the number of reticulocytes decreases about 50% every 12 hours so that it is rare to find an elevated reticulocyte count after the first week of life. A decrease in extramedullary hematopoiesis also occurs at this time. In the peripheral blood the erythrocyte count drops for 6 to 8 weeks after birth. During this period of rapid growth the rate of erythrocyte destruction is greater than that in later childhood and adulthood. In full-term infants, normal erythrocyte life span is 60 to 80 days; in premature infants it may be as short as 20 to 30 days; and in children and adolescents, it is the same as that in adults—120 days. (Mechanisms of hemolysis are described in Chapter 25.)

In the premature infant the postnatal fall in hemoglobin and hematocrit values is more marked than in the full-term infant. In the preschool and school-age child, there is a gradual rise in hemoglobin, hematocrit, and red blood cell count. Values in males and females first begin to diverge in adolescence. In the female the gradual hemoglobin increase continues into early puberty, at which time it stabilizes. In the male the hemoglobin increase keeps pace with growth and maturation and eventually surpasses that of the female. This higher value in the mature male is related to androgen secretion.

Metabolic processes within the erythrocytes of neonates differ significantly from those of erythrocytes in the normal adult. The relatively young population of erythrocytes in the newborn consumes greater quantities of glucose than do erythrocytes in adults. Several enzymes that regulate glucose consumption are increased in the erythrocytes of neonates, with a subsequent increase in the rate of glycolysis.

Leukocytes and Platelets

The lymphocytes of children tend to have more cytoplasm and less compact nuclear chromatin than do the lymphocytes of adults. The significance of these differences is unknown. One possible explanation is that children tend to have more frequent viral infections, which are associated with atypical lymphocytes. Even minor infections, in which the child fails to exhibit clinical manifestations of illness, and administration of immunizations may result in lymphocyte changes.[1]

The lymphocyte count is high at birth and continues to rise in some healthy infants during the first year of life. Then a steady decline occurs throughout childhood and adolescence until lower adult values are reached. It is unknown whether these developmental variations are physiologic or are a pathologic response to frequent viral infections and immunizations in children.

At birth the neutrophil count is very high and rises further during the early days of life.[2] After 2 weeks, neutrophil counts fall to within or below normal adult ranges. By approximately 4 years of age, the neutrophil count is the same as that of an adult. White children have slightly higher counts than black children.[3]

Eosinophil count is high in the first year of life and is higher in children than in teenagers or adults.[4] Monocyte counts are high in the first year of life and then decrease to adult levels. No relationship between age and basophil count has been found.

Platelet counts in full-term neonates are comparable to platelet counts in adults and remain so throughout infancy and childhood.[5] Controversy exists as to whether premature infants tend to have thrombocytopenia.

DISORDERS OF ERYTHROCYTES

Anemia is the most common blood disorder in children. Like the anemias of adulthood, the anemias of childhood are caused by ineffective erythropoiesis or premature destruction of erythrocytes. The most common cause of insufficient erythropoiesis is iron deficiency, which may result from insufficient dietary intake or chronic loss of iron caused by bleeding. The hemolytic anemias of childhood may be divided into two large categories. The first category consists of disorders that result from premature destruction caused by intrinsic abnormalities of the erythrocytes, and the second category consists of disorders that result from damaging extraerythrocytic factors. The hemolytic anemias are inherited, congenital, or both.

The most dramatic form of acquired congenital hemolytic anemia is **hemolytic disease of the newborn (HDN),** also termed **erythroblastosis fetalis.** HDN is an alloimmune disease in which maternal blood and fetal blood are antigenically incompatible, causing the mother's immune system to produce antibodies against fetal erythrocytes. Fetal erythrocytes that have been attacked by (i.e., bound to) maternal antibodies are recognized as foreign or defective by the fetal mononuclear phagocyte system and are removed from the circulation by phagocytosis, usually in the fetal spleen. (For a complete discussion of HDN, see p. 1003. Other acquired hemolytic anemias—some of which begin in utero—include those caused by infections or the presence of toxic chemicals.

The inherited forms of hemolytic anemia result from intrinsic defects of the child's erythrocytes, any of which can lead to erythrocyte removal by the mononuclear phagocyte system. Structural defects include abnormal cellular size and abnormalities of plasma membrane structure (spherocyto-sis). Intracellular defects include enzyme deficiencies, the most common of which is G6PD deficiency, and defects of hemoglobin synthesis, which manifest as sickle cell disease or thalassemia, depending on which component of hemoglobin is defective. These and other causes of childhood anemia, some more common than others, are listed in Table 28-2.

Acquired Disorders
Iron Deficiency Anemia

Iron deficiency anemia is the most common blood disorder of infancy and childhood, with the highest incidence occurring between 6 months and 2 years of age. Incidence is not related to gender or race, but socioeconomic factors are important because they affect nutrition. Recent studies document the risk of iron deficiency anemia in children of single, homeless women.[6] Iron deficiency anemia is a common disorder in children because of their extremely high need for iron for normal growth to occur.

Between 4 years of age and the onset of puberty, dietary iron deficiency is uncommon. During adolescence, however, it is relatively common, especially in menstruating females. Rapid growth, together with the average teenager's dietary habits, causes iron depletion. (Mechanisms of iron depletion are described in Chapter 25.)

PATHOPHYSIOLOGY   Although inadequate intake of iron is the most common cause of iron deficiency anemia during the first few years of life and during adolescence, blood

Table 28-2	Anemias of Childhood	
Cause	**Anemic Condition**
Deficient Erythropoiesis or Hemoglobin Synthesis	
Decreased stem cell population in marrow (congenital or acquired pure red cell aplasia)	Normocytic-normochromic anemia
Decreased erythropoiesis despite normal stem cell population in marrow (infection, inflammation, cancer, chronic renal disease, congenital dyserythropoiesis)	Normocytic-normochromic anemia
Deficiency of a factor or nutrient needed for erythropoiesis	
Cobalamin (vitamin B_{12}), folate	Megaloblastic anemia
Iron	Microcytic-hypochromic anemia
Increased or Premature Hemolysis	
Alloimmune disease (maternal-fetal Rh, ABO, or minor blood group incompatibility)	Hemolytic disease of the newborn (HDN)
Autoimmune disease (idiopathic autoimmune hemolytic anemia, symptomatic systemic lupus erythematosus, lymphoma, drug-induced autoimmune processes)	Autoimmune hemolytic anemia
Inherited defects of plasma membrane structure (spherocytosis, elliptocytosis, stomatocytosis) or cellular size or both (pyknocytosis)	Hemolytic anemia
Infection (bacterial sepsis, congenital syphilis, malaria, cytomegalovirus infection, rubella, toxoplasmosis, disseminated herpes)	Hemolytic anemia
Intrinsic and inherited enzymatic defects (deficiencies of glucose-6-phosphate dehydrogenase [G6PD], pyruvate kinase, 5'-nucleotidase, glucose phosphate isomerase)	Hemolytic anemia
Inherited defects of hemoglobin synthesis	Sickle cell anemia
	Thalassemia
Disseminated intravascular coagulation (see Chapter 27)	Hemolytic anemia
Galactosemia	Hemolytic anemia
Prolonged or recurrent respiratory or metabolic acidosis	Hemolytic anemia
Blood vessel disorders (cavernous hemangioma, large vessel thrombus, renal artery stenosis, severe coarctation of the aorta) (see Chapter 31)	Hemolytic anemia

loss is the most common cause in childhood. Chronic iron deficiency anemia from occult (hidden) blood loss may be caused by a gastrointestinal lesion, parasitic infestation, or hemorrhagic disease. As many as one third of infants with severe iron deficiency anemia have chronic intestinal blood loss induced by exposure to a heat-labile protein in cow's milk. Such exposure causes an inflammatory gastrointestinal reaction that damages the mucosa and results in diffuse hemorrhage.

The amount of iron available for hemoglobin synthesis in the infant depends on iron stores present at birth, rate of growth, the amount of dietary iron absorbed, and physiologic or pathologic loss of iron. During the period of inactive erythropoiesis immediately after birth, iron from erythrocytes that die at the end of their normal life span is stored, as hemosiderin, in bone marrow and liver tissue. This creates an iron reserve that can be used in lieu of dietary intake. The greatest stores are present 4 to 8 weeks after birth. Until erythropoiesis resumes, these iron stores are mobilized. In the premature infant, resumption of erythropoiesis depletes iron stores within 6 to 12 weeks; in the full-term infant, depletion takes longer—about 16 to 20 weeks. Once iron stores have been used, the infant depends on dietary iron.

The amount of dietary iron available for erythropoiesis depends on which foods are consumed. Iron-fortified cereals, green and yellow vegetables, fruits, and milk are common in the average 6-month-old infant's diet and provide iron in the amount of 0.9 to 1.5 mg/kg/day, amounts that satisfy the normal average daily requirement. Iron-fortified formulas are available commercially.

CLINICAL MANIFESTATIONS   The symptoms of mild anemia—lethargy and lassitude—usually are not present or detectable in infants and young children, who are unable to describe these symptoms. Therefore parents usually do not notice any change in the child's behavior or appearance until moderate anemia has developed. General irritability, decreased activity tolerance, weakness, and lack of interest in play are nonspecific indications of anemia. In mild to moderate iron deficiency anemia (hemoglobin of 6 to 10 g/dl), compensatory mechanisms of tissue oxygenation, such as increased amounts of 2,3-DPG within erythrocytes and a shift of the oxyhemoglobin dissociation curve, may be so effective that few clinical manifestations are apparent. When the hemoglobin falls below 5 g/dl, however, pallor, anorexia, tachycardia, and systolic murmurs may occur.

Splenomegaly is evident in 10% to 15% of children with iron deficiency anemia, and if the condition is long-standing, the sutures of the skull may be widened. Chronic anemia also may result in decreased physical growth and developmental delays. Some children exhibit pica, a behavior in which nonfood substances are eaten. Because children with iron deficiency anemia may be obese, underweight, or of normal weight, other manifestations of undernutrition must be identified.

Iron deficiency anemia may affect neurologic and intellectual function. Some research findings indicate that low iron in the blood affects attention span, alertness, and learning ability, even when anemia is not severe.[7]

EVALUATION AND TREATMENT   The most definitive test for differentiating iron deficiency from other microcytic states is the absence of iron stores in the bone marrow. However, measurement of serum ferritin iron concentration, transferrin saturation, iron-binding capacity, and, more recently, serum transferrin receptors may prevent proceeding to actual bone marrow evaluation.[8] Evaluation and treatment of iron deficiency anemia in children are similar to evaluation and treatment in adults (see Chapter 26). Oral administration of simple ferrous salts usually is satisfactory, but additional vitamin C may be needed to promote absorption.[9] Administration of supplementary trace metals or other vitamins is not necessary. If malabsorption is the cause of the anemia (or if oral administration has not been successful), iron dextran (Imferon) is given intravenously. Iron therapy is continued for at least 2 months after erythrocyte indexes have returned to normal in order to replenish iron stores.[10,11]

Dietary modification is required to prevent recurrences of iron deficiency anemia. The child's intake of iron-rich foods is increased, and the intake of cow's milk may be restricted, with the exact amount depending on the child's age (from 16 to 32 ounces). Limiting milk intake makes the child hungrier for other iron-rich foods and prevents gastrointestinal blood loss in children whose anemia is aggravated or caused by inflammatory reactions to proteins in cow's milk.

Hemolytic Disease of the Newborn

HDN can occur only if antigens on fetal erythrocytes differ from antigens on maternal erythrocytes. The antigenic properties of erythrocytes are determined genetically: they may be type A, B, or O and may or may not include Rh antigen D. Erythrocytes that express Rh antigen D are Rh positive; those that do not are Rh negative. The frequency of Rh negativity is higher in whites (15%) than in blacks (5%), and is rare in Asians. Maternal-fetal incompatibility exists if mother and fetus differ in ABO blood type or if the fetus is Rh positive and the mother is Rh negative. (The antigenic properties of erythrocytes are described in Chapter 8.)

ABO incompatibility occurs in about 20% to 25% of all pregnancies, but only 1 in 10 cases of ABO incompatibility results in HDN. Rh incompatibility occurs in fewer than 10% of pregnancies and rarely causes HDN in the first incompatible fetus. Even after five or more pregnancies, only 5% of women have babies with hemolytic disease. Usually erythrocytes from the first incompatible fetus cause the mother's immune system to produce antibodies that affect the fetuses of subsequent incompatible pregnancies. Only one in three cases of HDN is caused by Rh incompatibility; most cases are caused by ABO incompatibility.

PATHOPHYSIOLOGY   If the mother and fetus have antigenically incompatible erythrocytes, HDN will result (1) if the mother's blood contains preformed antibodies against fetal erythrocytes or produces them on exposure to fetal erythrocytes, (2) if sufficient amounts of antibody (usually immunoglobulin G [IgG]) cross the placenta and enter fetal blood, and (3) if IgG binds with sufficient numbers of fetal erythrocytes to cause widespread antibody-mediated hemolysis or splenic removal. (Antibody-mediated cellular destruction is discussed in Chapter 7.)

Maternal antibodies may be formed against type B erythrocytes if the mother is type A or against type A if the mother is type B. Usually, however, the mother is type O and the fetus is A or B. ABO incompatibility can cause HDN even if fetal erythrocytes do not escape into the maternal circulation during pregnancy. This occurs because the blood of most adults already contains anti-A or anti-B antibodies, which are produced on exposure to certain foods or infection by gram-negative bacteria. (Anti-O antibodies do not exist because type O erythrocytes are not antigenic.) Therefore IgG against type A or B erythrocytes usually is preformed in maternal blood and can enter the fetal circulation throughout the first incompatible pregnancy.

Anti-Rh antibodies, on the other hand, are formed *only* in response to the presence of incompatible (Rh-positive) erythrocytes in the blood of an Rh-negative mother. Sources of exposure include fetal blood that is mixed with the mother's blood at the time of delivery, transfused blood, and, rarely, previous sensitization of the mother by her own mother's incompatible blood.

The first Rh-incompatible pregnancy usually presents no difficulties because very few fetal erythrocytes cross the placental barrier during gestation. When the placenta detaches at birth, however, large numbers of fetal erythrocytes usually enter the mother's bloodstream. If the mother is Rh negative and the fetus is Rh positive, the mother produces anti-Rh antibodies. The capacity of the mother's immune system to produce anti-Rh antibodies depends on many factors, including her genetic capacity to make antibodies against the Rh antigen D, the amount of fetal-to-maternal bleeding, and the occurrence of any bleeding earlier in the pregnancy. Anti-Rh antibodies persist in the bloodstream for a very long time, and if the next offspring is Rh positive, the mother's anti-Rh antibodies can enter the fetus's bloodstream and destroy the erythrocytes. Antibodies against Rh antigen D are of the IgG class and easily cross the placenta.

IgG-coated fetal erythrocytes are destroyed extravascularly, primarily by mononuclear phagocytes in the spleen. As hemolysis proceeds, the fetus becomes anemic. Erythropoiesis accelerates, particularly in the liver and spleen, and immature nucleated cells (erythroblasts) are released into the bloodstream (hence the name *erythroblastosis fetalis*) (Figure 28-2). The degree of anemia depends on the length of time the antibody has been in the fetal circulation, antibody concentration, and the ability of the fetus to compensate for increased hemolysis. Unconjugated (indirect) bilirubin, which is formed during breakdown of hemoglobin, is transported across the placental barrier into the maternal circulation and is excreted by the mother. **Hyperbilirubinemia** occurs in the

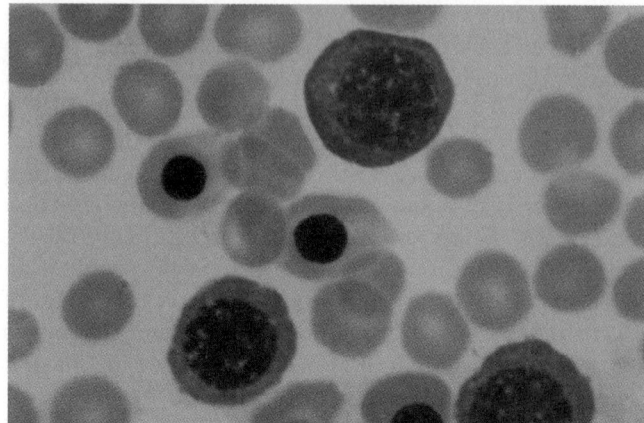

Figure 28-2 **Rh incompatibility in hemolytic disease of the newborn.** This micrograph shows immature red blood cells not normally found in blood. Large purple cells are erythroblasts; nucleated red blood cells are normoblasts. Normal red blood cells also shown (×500). (Copyright Ed Reschke.)

neonate after birth because excretion of lipid-soluble unconjugated bilirubin through the placenta no longer is possible.

The pathophysiologic effects of HDN are more severe in Rh incompatibility than in ABO incompatibility. ABO incompatibility may resolve after birth without life-threatening complications. Maternal-fetal incompatibility in which a mother with type O blood has a child with type A or B blood usually is so mild that it does not require treatment.

Rh incompatibility is more likely than ABO incompatibility to cause severe or even life-threatening anemia, death in utero, or damage to the central nervous system (CNS). Severe anemia alone can cause death as a result of cardiovascular complications (see Chapter 26). Extensive hemolysis also results in increased levels of unconjugated bilirubin in the neonate's circulation. If bilirubin levels exceed the liver's ability to conjugate and excrete bilirubin, some of it is deposited in the brain, causing cellular damage and eventually, if the neonate does not receive exchange transfusions, death.

Fetuses that do not survive anemia in utero usually are stillborn, with gross edema in the entire body, a condition called **hydrops fetalis.** Death can occur as early as 17 weeks of gestation and results in spontaneous abortion.

CLINICAL MANIFESTATIONS Neonates with mild HDN may appear healthy or slightly pale, with slight enlargement of the liver and spleen. Pronounced pallor, splenomegaly, and hepatomegaly indicate severe anemia, which predisposes the neonate to cardiovascular failure and shock. Life-threatening Rh incompatibility is rare today, largely because of the routine use of Rh immune globulin.

Because the maternal antibodies remain in the neonate's circulatory system after birth, erythrocyte destruction can continue. This causes hyperbilirubinemia and **icterus neonatorum (neonatal jaundice)** shortly after birth. Without replacement transfusions, in which the child receives Rh-negative erythrocytes, the bilirubin is deposited in the brain, a condition termed **kernicterus.** Kernicterus produces cerebral damage and usually causes death (**icterus gravis neonatorum**). Infants who do not die may have mental retardation, cerebral palsy, or high-frequency deafness.

EVALUATION AND TREATMENT Routine evaluation of fetuses at risk for HDN (i.e., fetuses resulting from Rh- or ABO-incompatible matings) include the Coombs test. The indirect Coombs test measures antibody in the mother's circulation and indicates whether the fetus is at risk for HDN. The direct Coombs test measures antibody already bound to the surfaces of fetal erythrocytes and is used primarily to confirm the diagnosis of antibody-mediated HDN. Determining prior history of fetal hemolytic disease, as well as diagnostic

tests, may help predict the severity of the disorder. Diagnostic measures include maternal antibody titers, fetal blood sampling, amniotic fluid spectrophotometry, and ultrasound fetal assessment.[12]

The key to treatment of HDN resulting from Rh incompatibility lies in prevention (immunoprophylaxis). One of the success stories of immunology has been the spectacular results obtained through the use of Rh immune globulin (RhoGAM), a preparation of antibody against Rh antigen D. If an Rh-negative woman is given Rh immune globulin within 72 hours of exposure to Rh-positive erythrocytes, she will not produce antibody against the D antigen and the next Rh-positive baby will be protected (Figure 28-3). The injected

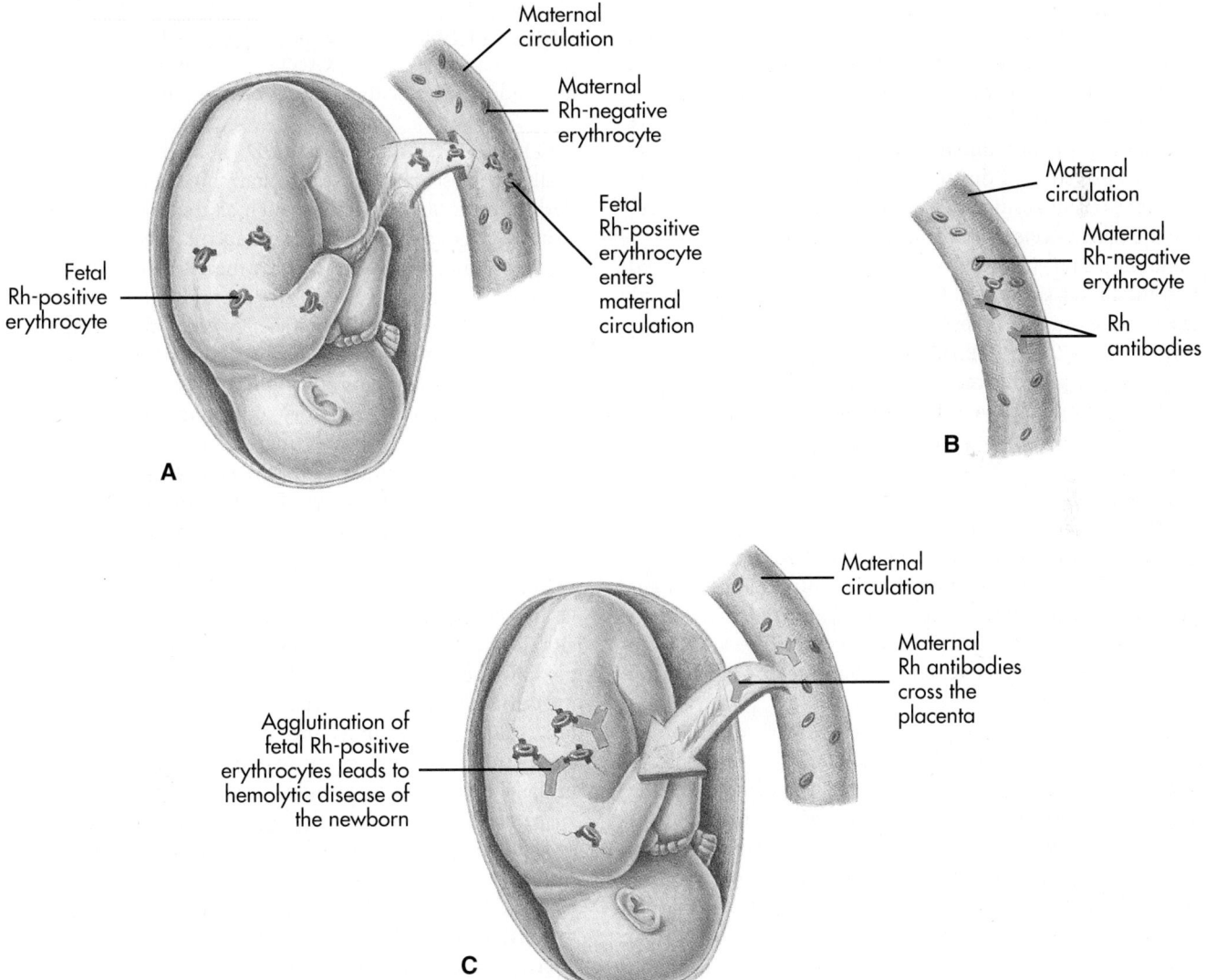

Figure 28-3 Hemolytic disease of the newborn (HDN). **A,** Before or during delivery, Rh-positive erythrocytes from the fetus enter the blood of an Rh-negative woman through a tear in the placenta. **B,** The mother is sensitized to the Rh antigen and produces Rh antibodies. Because this usually happens after delivery, there is no effect on the fetus in the first pregnancy. **C,** During a subsequent pregnancy with an Rh-positive fetus, Rh-positive erythrocytes cross the placenta, enter the maternal circulation, and stimulate the mother to produce antibodies against the Rh antigen. The Rh antibodies from the mother cross the placenta, using agglutination and hemolysis of fetal erythrocytes, and HDN develops. (Modified from Seeley RR, Stephens TD, Tate P: *Anatomy and physiology,* ed 3, St Louis, 1995, Mosby.)

antibodies remain in the mother's bloodstream long enough to prevent her immune system from producing its own anti-Rh antibodies but not long enough to affect subsequent offspring. The mother must be given Rh immune globulin injections after the birth of each Rh-positive baby and after an abortion. Also, the mother must be especially careful not to receive a transfusion containing Rh-positive blood, because this also would stimulate production of anti-Rh antibodies. In many hospitals, Rh immune globulin is given prophylactically at 28 weeks to all pregnant Rh-negative women with Rh-positive partners. Immunoprophylaxis with Rh immune globulin, unfortunately, appears to be underused in the United States. Failure to use immunoprophylaxis, such as in cases of unrecognized abortion, has led to a small increase in mothers who will require comprehensive treatment during subsequent pregnancies.[12,13]

If antigenic incompatibility of the mother's erythrocytes is not discovered in time to administer RhoGAM and a child is born with HDN, treatment consists of exchange transfusions in which the neonate's blood is replaced with new Rh-positive blood that is not contaminated with anti-Rh antibodies. This treatment is instituted during the first 24 hours of extrauterine life to prevent kernicterus. Phototherapy also is used to reduce the toxic effects of unconjugated bilirubin.

Jaundice and indirect hyperbilirubinemia are reduced when the infant is exposed to a high intensity of light in the visible spectrum, the most effective being the blue range (from 420 to 470 nm). Bilirubin in the skin absorbs light energy, which, by photoisomerization, converts the toxic unconjugated bilirubin into conjugated isomers that are excreted in the bile. Phototherapy also causes autosensitization that results in oxidation reactions. Breakdown products from the oxidation reactions are excreted by the liver and kidney without need for conjugation. The therapeutic effect of phototherapy depends on the light energy emitted in the effective wavelengths, the distance between the infant and the light source, and the amount of skin exposed; the rate of hemolysis and the infant's ability to excrete bilirubin also are factors in determining the effectiveness of phototherapy in lowering serum bilirubin levels.

Anemia of Infectious Disease

Infections of the newborn, often initially acquired by the mother and transmitted to the fetus, may result in a hemolytic anemia with clinical manifestations similar to those of HDN. Congenital syphilis, toxoplasmosis, cytomegalic inclusion disease, rubella, coxsackievirus B infection, herpesvirus infection, and bacterial sepsis all can cause hemolytic anemia in the neonate.

The exact mechanism of anemia caused by congenital infections is unclear. In some instances it is related to direct injury of erythrocyte membranes or erythrocyte precursors by the infectious organism. In other instances it results from traumatic destruction of erythrocytes during their passage through inflamed capillaries.

Inherited Disorders

A number of inherited and intrinsic erythrocyte defects are known to cause increased hemolysis (see Table 28-2). These defects may be associated with enzymatic abnormalities that disrupt metabolic processes and prevent normal biochemical balance within the cell, with alterations of hemoglobin structure or synthesis, or with plasma membrane defects accompanied by changes in erythrocyte size or shape.

Glucose-6-Phosphate Dehydrogenase Deficiency

Glucose-6-phosphate dehydrogenase (G6PD) deficiency is an inherited, X-linked, recessive disorder, most fully expressed in homozygous males, although partial expression and a carrier state are possible in heterozygous females. (X-linked inheritance is discussed in Chapter 4.) The deficiency is present in 10% of black Americans and also tends to occur in Sephardic Jews, Greeks, Iranians, Chinese, Filipinos, and Indonesians, with a frequency ranging from 5% to 40%.

PATHOPHYSIOLOGY   G6PD is an enzyme that normally enables erythrocytes to maintain metabolic processes despite injurious conditions, such as the presence of certain drugs (sulfonamides, antimalarial agents, salicylates, or naphthaquinolones); ingestion of fava beans (a dietary staple in some Mediterranean areas); hypoxemia; infection; fever; or acidosis. Therefore G6PD deficiency is usually asymptomatic unless one of these stressors is present. Erythrocyte damage in affected children begins after intense or prolonged exposure to one of these substances or conditions, and it ceases when they are removed. In black American males the G6PD defect becomes more pronounced as the erythrocyte ages; in other populations the defect is profound even in young erythrocytes. By ingesting a substance with oxidant properties, such as a salicylate (aspirin), a pregnant woman may precipitate an episode of hemolysis in a fetus with G6PD deficiency.

In the absence of G6PD, oxidative stressors damage hemoglobin and the plasma membranes of erythrocytes and they possibly interfere with the activities of other enzymes within the cell. Hemoglobin is oxidized progressively to methemoglobin, sulfmethemoglobin, and denatured globin-glutathione complexes. Eventually, exposure to oxidizing substances results in the precipitation of insoluble hemoglobin inclusions, called *Heinz bodies*, within the cell. Plasma damage and the presence of Heinz bodies cause hemolysis, chiefly in the spleen.

CLINICAL MANIFESTATIONS   In Asian and Mediterranean infants, G6PD deficiency is likely to be associated with icterus neonatorum. The most common clinical manifestation of G6PD deficiency is acute hemolytic anemia, usually after infections or the ingestion of certain oxidative drugs. The fava bean produces a severe hemolytic reaction called favism in infants with G6PD deficiency.[14]

Hemolytic episodes are characterized by pallor, icterus, dark urine, back pain, and, in severe cases, shock, cardiovascular collapse, and death. Between hemolytic episodes, anemia is absent and erythrocyte survival is normal.

EVALUATION AND TREATMENT Direct or indirect demonstration of reduced G6PD activity in erythrocytes is required for evaluation. Satisfactory screening test results are based on discoloration of methylene blue and reduction of methemoglobin. Immediately after a hemolytic episode, reticulocytes and young erythrocytes predominate. Because young erythrocytes have significantly higher enzyme activity than do older cells, testing should be performed a few weeks after a crisis so that a low level of enzyme activity can be demonstrated. G6PD activity that is within the low normal range in the presence of a high reticulocyte count suggests G6PD deficiency. G6PD deficiency also can be detected by electrophoretic analysis.

Prevention of hemolysis is the most important therapeutic measure. Males belonging to high-risk groups (Greeks, Southern Italians, Sephardic Jews, Filipinos, Chinese, Africans, Thais) should be tested for the defect before being given drugs known to be oxidant. When hemolysis has occurred, supportive treatment may include blood transfusions and oral iron therapy. Spontaneous recovery generally follows treatment.

Hereditary Spherocytosis

Hereditary spherocytosis, also known as *congenital hemolytic anemia* or *congenital acholuric jaundice,* is the most common of the hemolytic disorders in which there is no abnormality of hemoglobin.

PATHOPHYSIOLOGY Transmitted as an autosomal dominant trait, hereditary spherocytosis is presumed to represent new mutations in about 25% of cases. The defect is believed to be caused by an undefined abnormality of proteins or spectrins of the erythrocyte membrane. Affected cells are unduly permeable to sodium and acquire a particular characteristic structure (Figure 28-4). An increased concentration of intracellular sodium is believed to lead to increased use of adenosine triphosphate (ATP) to drive the so-called cation pump. Early aging and destruction of erythrocytes are believed to result from metabolic overwork and loss of erythrocyte membrane.[15]

Circulation of blood to the spleen creates a metabolic environment that is stressful to spherocyte cells, and repeated passages through this stressful environment result in their sequestration and destruction. The spherocyte is relatively rigid and passes with difficulty through the small openings between the splenic cords and sinuses. Thus the spleen is intimately involved in the hemolytic process.

CLINICAL MANIFESTATIONS With onset in the neonatal period or in early infancy, anemia and hyperbilirubinemia are severe enough to require phototherapy or exchange transfusions. During infancy and childhood, severity of the anemia varies widely but tends to be similar within families. Slight jaundice usually is present. Moderate expan-

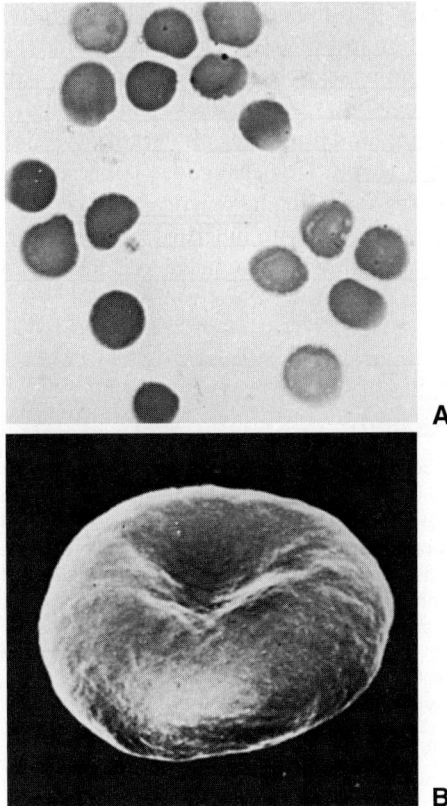

Figure 28-4 The microspherocyte. **A,** Blood smear from patient with hereditary spherocytosis (Wright stain). **B,** Scanning electron micrograph. (Courtesy Dr. M Bessis. From Miale JB: *Laboratory medicine: hematology,* ed 6, St Louis, 1982, Mosby.)

sion of the marrow cavity of the skull may occur because of compensatory mechanisms to overproduce cells. After infancy the spleen almost always is enlarged. Although gallstones have been reported to occur as early as 4 to 5 years of age, they usually do not develop until late childhood or early adolescence. If the spleen is not surgically removed, gallstones will form in approximately one half of cases. Aplastic crises are the most serious complications during childhood.[15]

EVALUATION AND TREATMENT It is important to evaluate the family history, blood smear, and studies of osmotic fragility and autohemolysis. As yet, however, no single test is specific for the diagnosis of hereditary spherocytosis.[16] Surgical removal of the spleen invariably produces a clinical cure and should be performed when the child is 5 years of age or older (see What's New? box). Since the use of total splenectomy for symptomatic children with various hemolytic anemias is associated with the risk of postsplenectomy sepsis, partial splenectomy is an alternative procedure that appears to control hemolysis while retaining splenic function.[17]

Sickle Cell Disease

Sickle cell disease is a group of disorders characterized by the presence of an abnormal form of hemoglobin—**hemoglobin**

S (**Hb S**)—within the erythrocytes. Hb S is formed by a genetic mutation in which one amino acid (valine) replaces another (glutamic acid) (Figure 28-5, *A*). Hb S, the so-called sickle hemoglobin, reacts to deoxygenation and dehydration by solidifying and stretching the erythrocyte into an elongated sickle shape. This change has a variety of pathologic consequences, including hemolytic anemia.

Sickle cell disease is an inherited, autosomal recessive disorder that is expressed as sickle cell anemia, sickle cell–

thalassemia disease, or sickle cell–hemoglobin C disease, depending on mode of inheritance (Table 28-3). (See Chapter 4 for a discussion of genetic inheritance of disease.) **Sickle cell anemia,** a homozygous form, is the most severe. **Sickle cell–thalassemia disease** and **sickle cell–Hb C disease** are heterozygous forms in which the child simultaneously inherits another type of abnormal hemoglobin from one parent. **Sickle cell trait,** in which the child inherits Hb S from one parent and normal hemoglobin (Hb A) from the other, is a heterozygous carrier state that rarely has clinical manifestations. All forms of sickle cell disease are lifelong conditions and have no known cure.

Sickle cell disease tends to occur in persons with origins in equatorial countries, particularly central Africa, the Near East, the Mediterranean area, and parts of India. In the United States, sickle cell disease is most common in blacks, with a reported incidence ranging from 1 in 400 to 1 in 500 live births. In the general population the risk of two black American parents having a child with sickle cell anemia is 0.7%. Sickle cell–hemoglobin C disease is less common (1 in 800 births), and sickle cell–thalassemia disease occurs in 1 in 1700 births.

Sickle cell trait occurs in 7% to 13% of black Americans, whereas its incidence among East Africans may be as high as 45%. The sickle cell trait may provide protection against lethal forms of malaria, a genetic advantage to carriers who

---

WHAT'S NEW? Laparoscopic Splenectomy

Laparoscopic splenectomy (LS) has been demonstrated to be safe and effective in children with hematologic disorders and is associated with minimal complications, zero mortality, and a short hospital stay. One hundred twelve children underwent LS at a single pediatric facility between August 1995 and February 2001. Three children required conversion to open splenectomy. Complications included ileus (4), acute chest syndrome (4), bleeding (2), pneumonia (1), and diaphragm perforation (1). None of the children died as a result of the procedure. Average length of stay was 1.51 days (range from 1 to 11 days).

Data from Rescorla FJ et al: *Am Surg* 68(3):297-301, 2002.

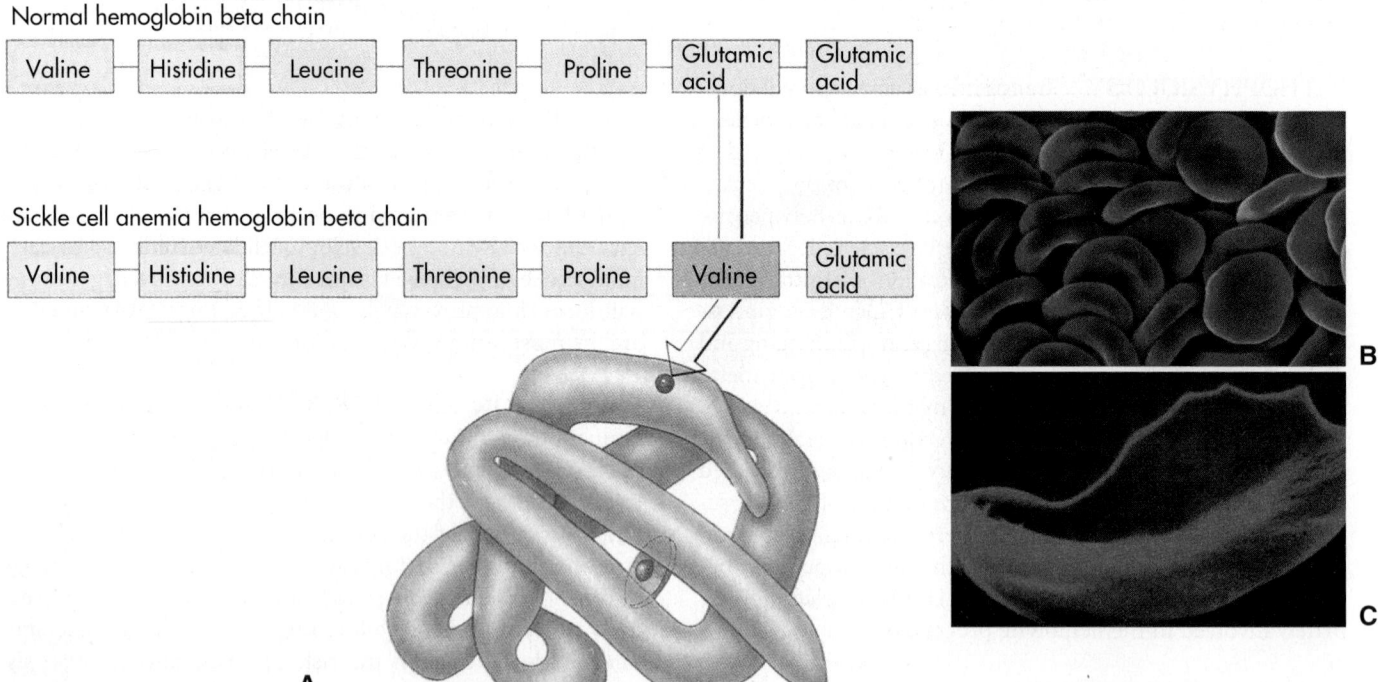

Figure 28-5 Sickle cell hemoglobin. **A,** Sickle cell hemoglobin is produced by a recessive allele of the gene encoding the beta chain of the protein hemoglobin. It represents a single amino acid change—from glutamic acid to valine at the sixth position on the chain. In this model of a hemoglobin molecule, the position of the mutation can be seen near the end of the upper arm. **B,** Color-enhanced electron micrograph shows normal erythrocytes. **C,** Illustration of the characteristic shape of a red blood cell containing the abnormal hemoglobin. (**A,** From Raven PH, Johnson GB: *Biology,* ed 3, St Louis, 1992, Mosby. **B,** Copyright Dennis Kunkel Microscopy, Inc. **C,** From Miale JB: *Laboratory medicine: hematology,* ed 6, St Louis, 1982, Mosby.)

Table 28-3   Inheritance of Sickle Cell Disease

Hemoglobin Inherited From First Parent	Hemoglobin Inherited From Second Parent	Form of Sickle Cell Disease in Child
Hb S (an abnormal hemoglobin)	Hb S	Sickle cell anemia: homozygous inheritance in which the child's hemoglobin is mostly Hb S, with the remainder Hb F (fetal hemoglobin)
Hb S	Defective or insufficient alpha or beta chains of Hb A (alpha- or beta-thalassemia)	Sickle cell: thalassemia disease (heterozygous inheritance of Hb S and alpha- or beta-thalassemia)
Hb S	Hb C or D (both abnormal hemoglobins)	Sickle cell: hemoglobin C (or D) disease (heterozygous inheritance of hemoglobin S and either C or D)
Hb S	Normal hemoglobins (mostly Hb A)	Sickle cell trait, the carrier state (heterozygous inheritance of Hb S and normal hemoglobin)

NOTE: See Chapter 25 for a description of normal fetal and adult hemoglobins.

reside in endemic regions for malaria (Mediterranean and African zones) but no advantage to carriers living in the United States.

PATHOPHYSIOLOGY   Deoxygenation is probably the most important variable in determining the occurrence of sickling.[18] The degree of deoxygenation required to produce sickling varies with the percentage of Hb S in the cells. Sickle trait cells will sickle at oxygen tensions of about 15 mmHg, whereas those from an individual with sickle cell disease will begin to sickle at about 40 mmHg. Hb S that is not bound with oxygen forms aggregates of semisolid gel that become stacked within the erythrocyte, stretching it into an elongated crescent (Figures 28-5, C, and 28-6). Sickled erythrocytes are stiff and cannot change shape as easily as normal cells when they pass through the microcirculation. (The reversible deformability of erythrocytes is described in Chapter 25.) As a result, sickled erythrocytes tend to plug the blood vessels, causing vascular occlusion, pain, and organ infarction. Sickled cells undergo hemolysis in the spleen or become sequestered there, causing blood pooling and infarction of splenic vessels. The anemia that follows triggers erythropoiesis in the marrow and, in extreme cases, in the liver.

Sickling usually is not permanent; most sickled erythrocytes regain a normal shape after reoxygenation and rehydration. Irreversible sickling is not caused by irreversible hemoglobin changes but rather by irreversible plasma membrane damage caused by sickling. The precise nature of the permanent membrane injury is not known, but it is known that, while in the sickled state, the plasma membrane loses some of its capacity for active transport, permitting an influx of calcium ions. (Membrane transport and the effects of calcium influx are described in Unit I.) In persons with sickle cell anemia, in which the erythrocytes contain a high percentage of Hb S (75% to 95%), up to 30% of the erythrocytes can become irreversibly sickled. Occasionally, irreversible sickling occurs in sickle cell disease but never in the carrier state (sickle cell trait).

Sickling is an occasional, intermittent phenomenon that can be triggered or sustained by one or more of the following stressors: decreased oxygen tension (P_{O_2}) of the blood (i.e., hy-

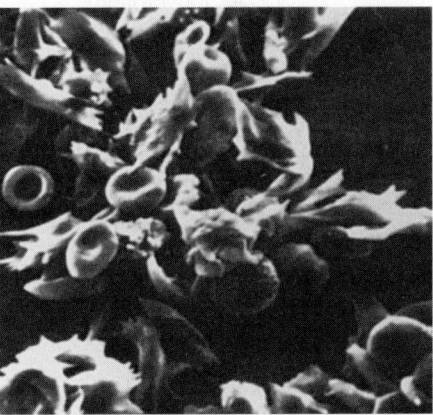

Figure 28-6   Normal and sickle-shaped blood cells. Scanning electron micrograph of normal and sickle-shaped red blood cells. The irregularly shaped cells are the sickle cells; the circular cells are the normal blood cells. (From Raven PH, Johnson GB: *Biology*, ed 3, St Louis, 1992, Mosby.)

poxemia), increased hydrogen ion concentration in the blood (decreased pH), increased plasma osmolality, decreased plasma volume, and low temperature (Figure 28-7). The same decrease in P_{O_2} will cause the most sickling in persons with sickle cell anemia (high concentrations of Hb S), the second most in children with sickle cell–thalassemia, the third most in those with sickle cell–hemoglobin C disease, and the least or none in those with sickle cell trait. The duration of the P_{O_2} decrease also is important, because sickling tends to occur only after the inciting stimulus has been present for some time.

The level of P_{O_2} in the microcirculation also affects sickling because hemoglobin releases whatever oxygen it is carrying to tissues. The P_{O_2} normally is lower in the microcirculation. The added reduction in P_{O_2} caused by persistent hypoxemia—induced by stressors—eventually results in sickling in the microcirculation of all cells that contain Hb S in that site (not throughout the body). Sickling within the microcirculation decreases blood flow as sickled cells clog the vessels. Slow blood flow promotes hypoxemia and perpetuates sickling. Finally, decreased blood pH decreases hemoglobin's affinity for oxygen. As less oxygen is taken up by hemoglobin in the lungs, P_{O_2} drops, promoting sickling further.

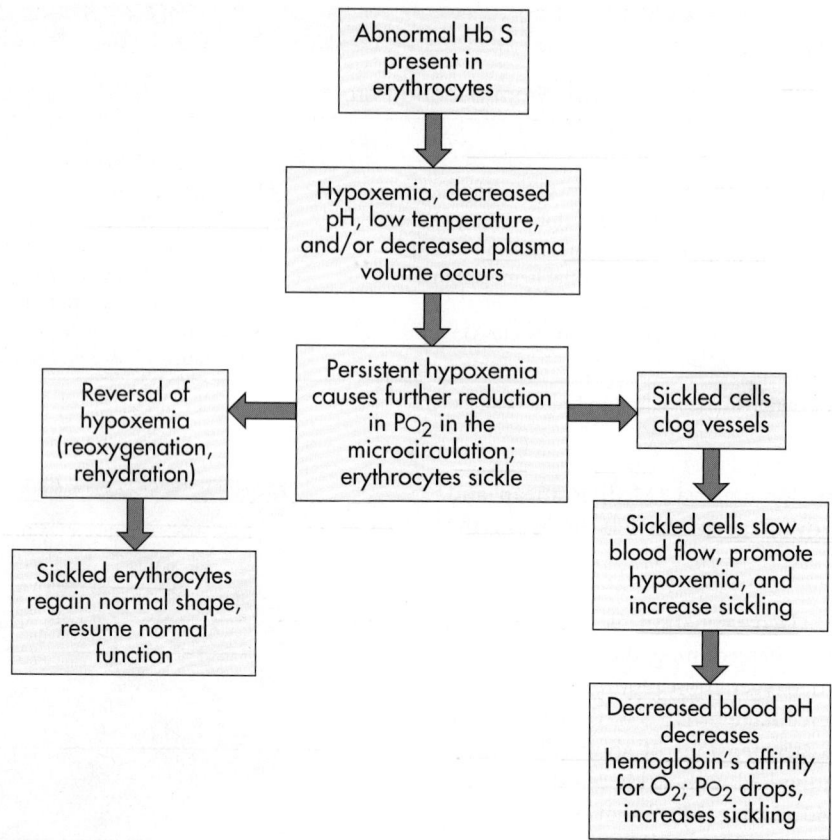

Figure 28-7 Sickling of erythrocytes.

Polymerization of sickle hemoglobin is central to the disorder. **Polymerization** stiffens the sickle erythrocyte, changing it from a flexible, nourishing cell to an inflexible obstacle that starves and damages tissues.

Increased osmolality of the plasma (increased concentration of solutes; see Chapters 1 and 3) draws water out of the erythrocytes. This promotes sickling by raising the relative Hb S content in erythrocytes. Decreased plasma volume, which occurs in states of dehydration, causes the blood to become viscous (thick and sticky). Increased viscosity of the blood is the final common pathway leading to many pathologic effects of sickle cell disease. Viscous blood flows slowly and promotes vascular obstruction by increasing opportunities for sickling while decreasing opportunities for reoxygenation in the lungs. This is an example of positive feedback in a vicious cycle of events. Low temperatures precipitate sickle crisis, presumably because of vasoconstriction.[18]

Once sickling begins, it tends to perpetuate itself until PO_2 returns to normal; then it ceases spontaneously. The extent, severity, and clinical manifestations of sickling depend to a great extent on the percentage of hemoglobin that is Hb S. That is why homozygous inheritance of Hb S produces the severest form of sickle cell disease—sickle cell anemia. Heterozygous inheritance of sickle cell disease results in less sickling because the individual's erythrocytes contain other forms of abnormal hemoglobin that, although defective, do not participate in sickling to any great degree. Heterozygous inheritance (sickle cell

trait), in which abnormal hemoglobin is inherited from one parent and normal hemoglobin from the other, rarely results in sickling because normal fetal hemoglobin (Hb F) and adult hemoglobin (Hb A) do not participate in sickling at all. Anemia persists because Hb F does not live 120 days.

CLINICAL MANIFESTATIONS   When sickling occurs, the general manifestations of hemolytic anemia—pallor, fatigue, jaundice, and irritability—sometimes are accompanied by acute manifestations called *crises*. Extensive sickling can precipitate four types of crises: (1) vasoocclusive (or thrombotic) crisis, (2) aplastic crisis, (3) sequestration crisis, or rarely (4) hyperhemolytic crisis. Sites of specific dysfunction are shown in Figure 28-8.

Vasoocclusive crisis (thrombotic crisis) begins with sickling in the microcirculation. As blood flow is obstructed by tangled masses of rigid, sickled cells, vasospasm occurs and a "logjam" effect brings all blood flow through the vessel to a halt. Unless the process is reversed, thrombosis and infarction (death caused by lack of oxygen) of local tissue follow. Vasoocclusive crisis is extremely painful and may last for days or even weeks, with an average duration of 4 to 6 days. The frequency of this type of crisis is variable and unpredictable.

Vasoocclusive crises may develop spontaneously or be precipitated by infection, exposure to cold, dehydration, low PO_2, acidosis (low pH), or localized hypoxemia. Symmetric, painful swelling of the hands and feet (hand-foot syndrome)

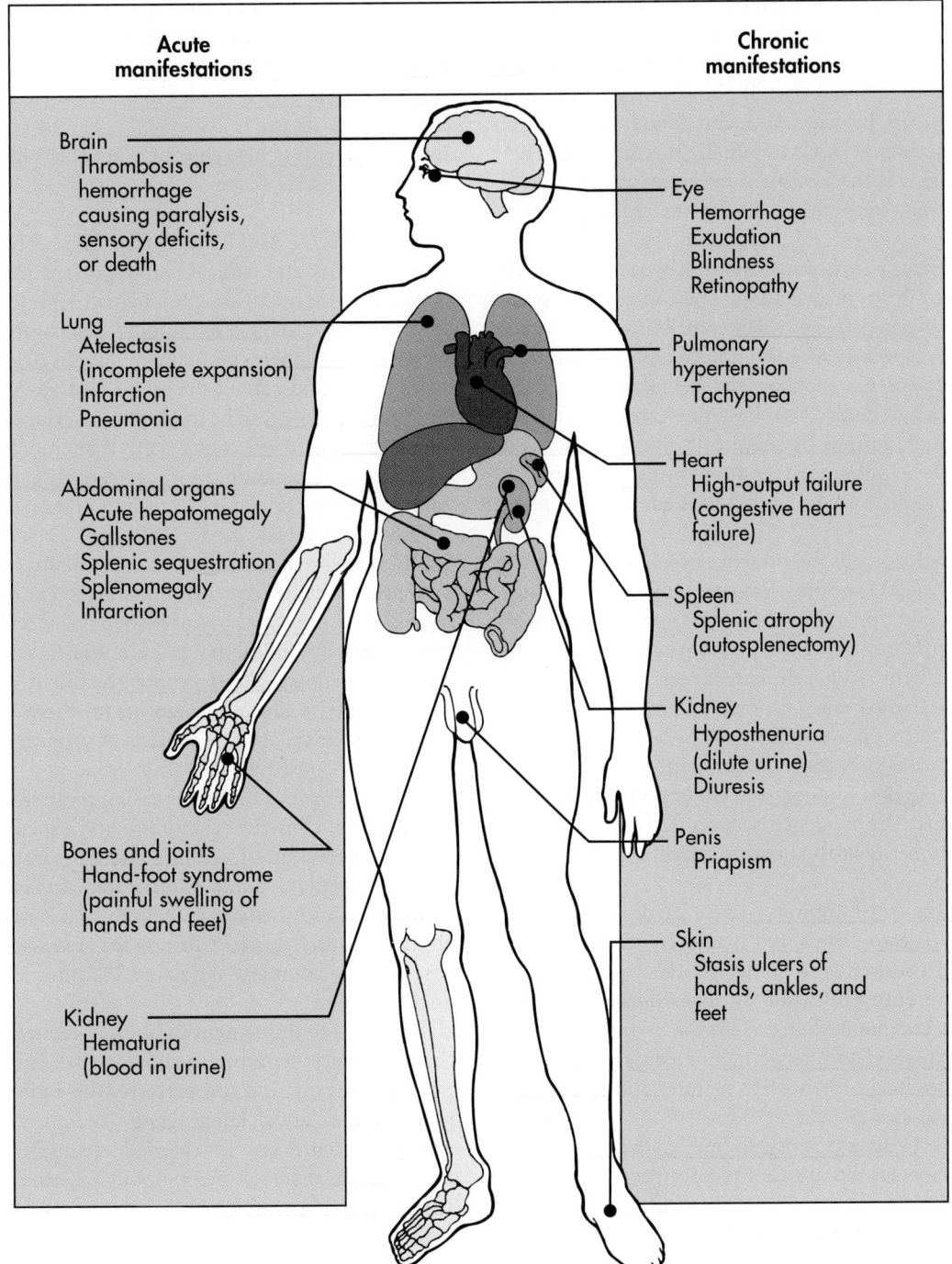

Figure 28-8 Clinical manifestations of sickle cell disease.

caused by infarction in the small vessels of the extremities often is the initial manifestation of sickle cell disease in infancy. In older children and adults the large joints and surrounding tissue become painful and swollen. Priapism (persistent erection of the penis) may occur if penile veins become obstructed. Severe abdominal pains often are caused by infarction in abdominal structures. Strokes resulting from cerebral occlusion may leave the child with paralysis (usually hemiplegia) or other CNS deficits.

Aplastic crisis consists of profound anemia caused by diminished erythropoiesis despite increased need for new erythrocytes. In sickle cell anemia, erythrocyte survival is only 10 to 20 days. Normally a compensatory increase in erythropoiesis (five to eight times normal) replaces the cells lost through premature hemolysis. If this compensatory response is compromised, aplastic crisis develops in a very short time.

In **sequestration crisis,** large amounts of blood become acutely pooled in the liver and spleen. This type of crisis is seen only in the young child. Because the spleen can hold as much as one fifth of the body's blood supply at one time, mortality rates up to 50% have been reported, with death caused by cardiovascular collapse. If blood volume and pressure are maintained by hydration and blood transfusion, much of the sequestered blood eventually is remobilized. Removal of the spleen is the treatment for recurrent sequestration crises and may be performed after the child reaches 5 years of age.[19]

Hyperhemolytic crisis is unusual but may occur in association with certain drugs or infections. The concomitant presence of G6PD deficiency (see p. 1006) contributes to hyperhemolytic episodes, especially when combined with infections.

Although intravascular sickling and hemolysis can begin by 6 to 8 weeks of age, clinical manifestations are not yet present. Clinical manifestations of sickle cell disease usually do not appear until the infant is at least 6 months old, at which time the postnatal decrease in Hb F causes concentrations of Hb S to rise.

Acute chest syndrome is the presence of a new pulmonary infiltrate (involving at least one complete lung segment—not atelectasis) with chest pain, a temperature of more than 38.5° C, increased respiratory rate (tachypnea), wheezing, or cough in an individual with sickle cell disease. An injured, underventilated, and inflamed lung becomes "spleenlike" as sickled red cells attach to its endothelium, fails to be reoxygenated, and eventually undergoes more inflammation and lung infarction. The prognosis is poor, and infarction is a leading cause of morbidity. The incidence is about 12.8 cases per 1000 patient-years and is the most common condition at the time of death.[20]

Infection is the most common cause of death resulting from sickle cell disease. Sepsis and meningitis develop in as many as 10% of children with sickle cell anemia during the first 5 years of life, with a mortality rate of 25%. Survival time is unpredictable, and many young adults die in their twenties.

Glomerular disease and renal failure cause substantial morbidity.[21] Proteinuria is an early manifestation of sickle nephrology.

Sickle cell–Hb C disease is usually milder than sickle cell anemia. The peripheral blood smear reveals many target cells resulting from the presence of Hb C. The main clinical problems are related to vasoocclusive crises and are believed to result from higher hematocrit values and viscosity. In older children, sickle cell retinopathy, renal necrosis, and aseptic necrosis of the femoral heads occur along with obstructive crises.

Sickle cell–thalassemia has the mildest clinical manifestations of all the sickle cell diseases. Even though most of the child's hemoglobin is Hb S (60% to 90%), normal hemoglobins (Hb A and Hb F) also are present. The normal hemoglobins, particularly Hb F, inhibit sickling. In addition, the erythrocytes tend to be small (microcytic) and to contain relatively little hemoglobin (hypochromic). Their small size makes them less likely than normal-size cells to clog the microcirculation, even when in a sickled state.

The sickle cell trait does not affect life expectancy or interfere with daily activities. However, on rare occasions, severe hypoxia caused by shock, vigorous exercising at high altitudes, flying at high altitudes in unpressurized aircraft, or undergoing anesthesia is associated with vasoocclusive episodes in persons with sickle cell trait. These cells form an ivy shape instead of a sickle shape.

EVALUATION AND TREATMENT   The parents' hematologic history and clinical manifestations may suggest that a child has sickle cell disease, but hematologic tests are necessary for diagnosis. If the sickle solubility test confirms the presence of Hb S in peripheral blood, hemoglobin electrophoresis provides information about the amount of Hb S in erythrocytes. Prenatal diagnosis can be made after chorionic villus sampling, as early as 8 to 10 weeks of gestation or amniotic fluid analysis at 15 weeks of gestation. Newborn screening for sickle cell disease should be performed according to state law.

Treatment advances over the past 25 years have significantly decreased morbidity and mortality in children with sickle cell disease.[22] Aggressive management of fever, early diagnosis of *acute chest syndrome* (hypoxia, decreased hemoglobin, progressive multilobar pneumonia, fat emboli), judicious use of transfusions, and proper treatment of pain can improve quality of life and prognosis for these children.[23] Treatment of sickle cell disease consists of supportive care aimed at preventing consequences of anemia and avoiding crises. Crises can be prevented by avoiding fever, infection, acidosis, dehydration, constricting clothes, and exposure to cold. Immediate correction of acidosis and dehydration with appropriate intravenous fluids is imperative. Infections require aggressive antibiotic therapy. Oxygen is not needed unless the child becomes hypoxic.[23] Pain associated with sickle cell disease is very complex, requiring continuous adjustment of analgesics.[24]

Protocols to implement individual-controlled analgesia in the emergency department shorten the time of initiation of narcotic therapy and are preferred by individuals.[25] Therapeutic use of antisickling agents (urea, cyanate, carbamoyl phosphate) currently is regarded as unsafe and ineffective. Hydroxyurea increases hemoglobin F synthesis in individuals with sickle cell anemia. One hundred twenty-two children with sickle cell disease who received hydroxyurea therapy from 1995 to 2002, led to significant increases in hemoglobin level, mean corpuscular volume, and fetal hemoglobin (HbF) level, whereas significant decreases occurred in reticulocyte, white blood cell, and platelet counts and serum bilirubin levels.[26] To avoid increased acidosis, acetaminophen is preferable to salicylates for antipyretic therapy. Immunization against influenza and pneumococcal organisms should be seriously considered. Blood transfusion, including hypertransfusion therapy (e.g., packed red blood cells to raise the hematocrit to a level of 35% for a period of time), can be effective but must be weighed against the risks of hemosiderosis and iron and splenic overload. Oral maintenance therapy with folic acid is needed to meet the increased demands of chronic hemolytic anemia. Splenectomy may be performed if sequestration crises recur. The most definitive approach to the treatment of sickle cell disease requires a permanent alteration in the hemoglobin phenotype. This can be accomplished through stem cell transplantation.

Genetic counseling and psychologic support are important for the child and family. Recently, a genetic technique called **preimplantation genetic diagnosis** has been performed on parents to diagnose whether their offspring will or will not carry the gene for sickle cell disease. Figure 28-9 summarizes this prepregnancy sickle cell test. Genetic counseling enables persons with sickle cell disease or trait to make informed decisions about transmitting this genetic disorder to their offspring, because there is a 25% chance with each pregnancy that a child born to two parents with sickle cell trait will have sickle cell disease.

Thalassemias

The alpha- and beta-thalassemias are inherited autosomal recessive disorders that cause an impaired rate of synthesis of one of the two chains—alpha or beta—of adult hemoglobin (Hb A). The disorder was named **thalassemia,** which is derived from the Greek word for *sea,* because it was defined initially in persons with origins near the Mediterranean Sea. Beta-thalassemia, in which synthesis of the beta globin chain is slowed or defective, is prevalent among Greeks, Italians, and some Arabs and Sephardic Jews. Alpha-thalassemia, in which the alpha chain is affected, is most common among Chinese, Vietnamese, Cambodians, and Laotians. Both alpha-thalassemia and beta-thalassemia are common among black Americans.

Alpha- and beta-thalassemia can be major or minor, depending on how many of the genes that control alpha or beta chain synthesis are defective and whether the defects are inherited homozygously (thalassemia major) or heterozygously (thalassemia minor). Pathophysiologic effects range from mild microcytosis to death in utero, depending on the number of defective genes and mode of inheritance. The anemic manifestation of thalassemia is microcytic-hypochromic hemolytic anemia.

PATHOPHYSIOLOGY   Normally two genes control beta chain synthesis and four genes control alpha chain synthesis. The number of genetic defects in the controlling genes determines the severity of the disorder. As in sickle cell disease the hemoglobin abnormality usually consists of the substitution of a single amino acid for another amino acid. Other molecular abnormalities that cause thalassemia are two amino acid substitutions, amino acid deletions or fusions, and synthesis of elongated chains.

The fundamental defect in beta-thalassemia is the uncoupling of alpha and beta chain synthesis. Beta chain production is depressed—moderately in the heterozygous form, **beta-thalassemia minor,** and severely in the homozygous form, **beta-thalassemia major** (also called **Cooley anemia**). Depression of beta chain synthesis results in erythrocytes having a reduced amount of hemoglobin and accumulations of free alpha chains. The free alpha chains are unstable and easily precipitate in the cell. Most erythroblasts that contain precipitates are destroyed by mononuclear phagocytes in the marrow, resulting in ineffective erythropoiesis and anemia. Some of the precipitate-carrying cells do mature and enter the bloodstream, but they are destroyed prematurely in the spleen, resulting in mild hemolytic anemia.

There are four forms of alpha-thalassemia:
1. **Alpha trait** (the carrier state), in which a single alpha chain–forming gene is defective.
2. **Alpha-thalassemia minor,** in which two genes are defective.
3. **Hemoglobin H disease,** in which three genes are defective.

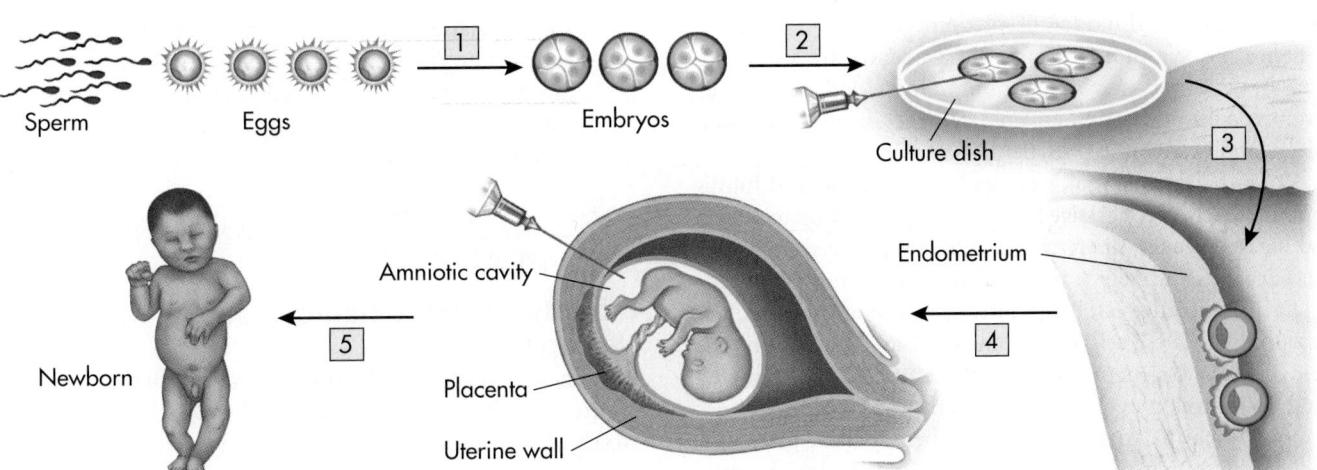

Figure 28-9 **Prepregnancy sickle cell test.** (This technique has potential for other inherited diseases.) *1,* Fertilization produces several embryos. *2,* The embryos are tested for the presence of the gene. *3,* The embryo(s) without the gene are implanted. *4,* Amniocentesis confirms whether the fetus (or fetuses) has the sickle cell gene. *5,* Woman has a normal child.

4. **Alpha-thalassemia major,** a fatal condition in which all four alpha-forming genes are defective; death is inevitable because alpha chains are absent and oxygen cannot be released to the tissues.

Beta-thalassemia occurs more commonly than does alpha-thalassemia. Occasionally synthesis of gamma or delta polypeptide chains is defective, resulting in gamma- or delta-thalassemia. (Hemoglobin chains are described in Chapter 25.)

CLINICAL MANIFESTATIONS Beta-thalassemia minor causes mild to moderate microcytic-hypochromic anemia, mild splenomegaly, bronze coloring of the skin, and hyperplasia of the bone marrow. The degree of reticulocytosis depends on the severity of the anemia, resulting in skeletal changes. Hemolysis of immature (and therefore fragile) erythrocytes may cause a slight elevation in serum iron and indirect bilirubin levels. Persons with beta-thalassemia minor usually are asymptomatic.

Persons with beta-thalassemia major may become quite ill. Anemia is severe and results in a significant cardiovascular burden, with high-output congestive heart failure. In the past, death resulted from cardiac failure. Today, blood transfusions can increase life span by one to two decades, and death usually is caused by hemochromatosis (from transfusions). (Hemosiderosis and hematochromatosis are described in Chapter 26.) Liver enlargement occurs as a result of progressive hemosiderosis, whereas enlargement of the spleen is caused by extramedullary hematopoiesis and increased destruction of red blood cells. Spinal impairment that starts in infancy retards linear growth.[27] Bone marrow hyperplasia causes a characteristic deformity of the facial bones, as the nasal bridge, mandible, and maxilla widen.

Persons who inherit the mildest form of alpha-thalassemia, the alpha trait, usually are symptom free, having, at most, mild microcytosis. Alpha-thalassemia minor has clinical manifestations that are virtually identical to those of beta-thalassemia minor: mild microcytic-hypochromic reticulocytosis, bone marrow hyperplasia, increased serum iron concentrations, and moderate splenomegaly.

Signs and symptoms of alpha-thalassemia are similar to those of beta-thalassemia major but milder. Moderate microcytic-hypochromic anemia, enlargement of the liver and spleen, and bone marrow hyperplasia are evident.

Alpha-thalassemia major causes hydrops fetalis and fulminant intrauterine congestive heart failure. In addition to edema and massive ascites, the fetus has a grossly enlarged heart and liver. Diagnosis usually is made postmortem. Prenatal screening for this disorder can be performed by use of chorionic villus sampling. These cells can be analyzed, and a deoxyribonucleic acid (DNA) genetic map can be constructed and evaluated for the abnormalities characteristic of hydrops fetalis.

Both alpha-thalassemia major and beta-thalassemia major are life threatening. Children with thalassemia major generally are weak, fail to thrive, show poor development, and experience cardiovascular compromise with high-output failure secondary to anemia. Untreated, they will die by 5 to 6 years of age.

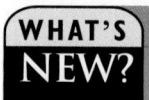

WHAT'S NEW? Bone Marrow Transplantation for Beta-Thalassemia Major

Stem cell transplantation (SCT) remains the only cure for thalassemia major. Fifty-five children underwent SCT for thalassemia major in the United Kingdom between 1991 and 2001. The median age at SCT was 6.4 years. Overall survival and thalassemia-free survival at 8 years following transplant were 94.5% and 81.8%, respectively. Transplant-related mortality was low (5.4%). The rejection rate was 4.6% of cases, acute graft-versus-host disease (GVHD) of grade II to IV occurred in 21%, and chronic GVHD occurred in 14.5%. These data suggest that allogeneic SCT is an important treatment option for children with beta-thalassemia major.

Data from Lawson SE et al:. *Br J Haematol* 120(2):289-295, 2003.

EVALUATION AND TREATMENT Evaluation of thalassemia is based on familial disease history, clinical manifestations, and blood tests. Peripheral blood smears that show microcytosis and hemoglobin electrophoresis that demonstrates diminished amounts of alpha or beta chains are used to make the diagnosis. Analysis of fetal DNA from withdrawn amniotic fluid is used as a screening test to detect hydrops fetalis (alpha-thalassemia major). Newborn screening for thalassemia should be done according to state law.

Persons who are "silent" carriers or have thalassemia minor generally have few if any symptoms and require no specific treatment. Therapies to support and prolong life are necessary, however, for thalassemia major. There is no cure for either condition. Prenatal diagnosis and genetic counseling may be the most important therapeutic measures offered.

At present, thalassemia major is treated with the following therapies:

1. Blood transfusions, which can return hemoglobin and hematocrit levels to normal, thus alleviating the anemia-induced cardiac failure; iron overload and hemochromatosis are complications of transfusion therapy.
2. Iron chelation therapy in combination with hyper-transfusion (transfusion to a hematocrit of 35 ml/dl).
3. Splenectomy, which can reduce the need for transfusions by eliminating the site of hemolysis, thus prolonging erythrocyte survival.

DISORDERS OF COAGULATION AND PLATELETS

Inherited Hemorrhagic Disease

Hemophilias

Awareness of a serious bleeding disorder in males was documented nearly 2000 years ago in the Babylonian Talmud, which exempted from the rite of circumcision those boys having male relatives prone to excessive bleeding. In 1803 the first description of this disorder appeared in the medical literature, where it was noted to be X linked in nature and associated with joint bleeding and crippling.

Table 28-4 lists the coagulation factors. Until 1952 the term *hemophilia* was reserved for deficiency of factor VIII (antihemophilic factor). Since that time two additional coagulation proteins, factor IX (plasma thromboplastin component [PTC]) and factor XI (plasma thromboplastin antecedent [PTA]), have been identified and their deficiency associated with similar clinical manifestations. Congenital deficiencies of these three plasma clotting factors—VIII, IX, XI—account for 90% to 95% of the hemorrhagic bleeding disorders collectively called *hemophilia*.

Types of Hemophilia

Hemophilia A (classic hemophilia) is caused by factor VIII deficiency. It is the most common of the hemophilias. Hemophilia A is inherited as an X-linked recessive disorder that affects males and is transmitted by females; its estimated incidence is 1 per 10,000 male births.

Hemophilia B (Christmas disease), caused by factor IX deficiency, also is transmitted as an X-linked recessive trait and is clinically indistinguishable from factor VIII deficiency. Approximately 15% of cases, or 1 in every 25,000 to 30,000 males born with hemophilia, are caused by factor IX.[28]

Hemophilia A and hemophilia B occur with varying degrees of clinical severity, depending on concentrations of clotting factor VIII or IX in the blood. Severe hemophilia (concentration of clotting factors less than 1% of normal) is associated with spontaneous bleeding. In moderate hemophilia (1% to 5% of normal), bleeding usually occurs only after trauma; in the mild form (5% to 35% of normal), bleeding occurs only after severe trauma or surgery. The severity of hemophilia is similar in all affected members of a family.

Hemophilia C (factor XI deficiency) occurs as an autosomal recessive disease and occurs equally in males and females. Bleeding usually is less severe than in hemophilia A or B.

von Willebrand disease results from an inherited autosomal dominant trait with variable clinical manifestations and hematologic findings. The factor VIII deficiency differs from that of hemophilia A in mode of inheritance and response to treatment. In hemophilia A the deficiency is inherited as an X-linked recessive trait, whereas in von Willebrand disease, it is inherited as an autosomal dominant trait. The most important difference, however, is in responses to the infusion of plasma. In von Willebrand disease, infusion of plasma causes factor VIII activity to increase for several days because infusion of factor VIII temporarily induces endogenous synthesis of factor VIII.

PATHOPHYSIOLOGY Two types of defects dominate the hereditary defects of hemophilia to date: gene deletions and point mutations. Both types of genetic defects are associated with severe hemophilia A, in which no factor VIII circulates in the blood. To date, about 50 deletion mutations in the gene for factor VIII have been identified at the molecular level, and about 34 independent deletion mutations in the factor IX gene have been found to be the cause of hemophilia B.[29] The molecular defect that leads to hemophilia is identical among members of a given family; however, the deletional mutation has been unique in each family studied.[30]

Point mutations, in which a single base in the DNA is mutated to another base, represent a second type of mutation that causes hemophilia. When a point mutation gives rise to a de novo stop codon (nonsense mutation), translation of the protein ceases and a shortened version of the protein is synthesized. Usually the protein is destroyed intracellularly and never reaches the plasma. This type of defect is associated with severe hemophilia, that is, with coagulant activity levels below 1%. Point mutations in which one amino acid is substituted for another can cause phenotypes of varying severity. The mutation of an important amino acid can destroy protein function, activation, or folding; inhibit intracellular processing; or cause protein clearance.[30] Unlike deletional mutations, point mutations at the same site have been recorded in different families with hemophilia.

Table 28-4 summarizes the types of coagulation disorders. Not all the disorders are discussed in this chapter because some are extremely rare (congenital dysfibrinogenemias) and others have no clinical significance (e.g., Hageman factor deficiency, a condition in which profound laboratory deficiency of factor XII is associated with absolutely no clinical defects).

CLINICAL MANIFESTATIONS Children with severe hemophilia start to bleed at different ages. In one study, 44% of children demonstrated their first bleeding episode before 1 year of age.[31] Although there is no transfer of maternal clotting factor to the fetus, many boys with hemophilia are cir-

Table 28-4	The Coagulation Factors	
Clotting Factors	**Synonym**	**Disorder**
I	Fibrinogen	Congenital deficiency (afibrinogenemia) and dysfunction (dysfibrinogenemia)
II	Prothrombin	Congenital deficiency or dysfunction
V	Labile factor, proaccelerin	Congenital deficiency (papahemophilia)
VII	Stable factor or proconvertin	Congenital deficiency
VIII	Antihemophilic factor (AHF)	Congenital deficiency is hemophilia A (classic hemophilia)
IX	Christmas factor	Congenital deficiency is hemophilia B
X	Stuart-Prower factor	Congenital deficiency
XI	Plasma thromboplastin antecedent	Congenital deficiency, sometimes referred to as hemophilia C
XII	Hageman factor	Congenital deficiency is *not* associated with clinical symptoms
XIII	Fibrin-stabilizing factor	Congenital deficiency

cumcised without excessive bleeding. Normal hemostasis is achieved in these infants because clotting is activated through the extrinsic coagulation cascade, which does not involve factors VII, IX, or XI.

During the first year, spontaneous bleeding often is minimal, but hematoma formation may result from injections and from firm holding (e.g., under the arms). Easy bruising or hemarthrosis (bleeding into joints) or both occur with ambulation. By 3 to 4 years of age, 90% of children with hemophilia have had episodes of persistent bleeding from relatively minor traumatic lacerations (e.g., to the lip or tongue). This usually is the first clinical manifestation of hemophilia. Hemorrhage into the elbows, knees, and ankles causes pain, limits joint movement, and predisposes the child to degenerative joint changes. Spontaneous hematuria and epistaxis are troublesome but minor complications.

Recurrent bleeding, both spontaneous and after minor trauma, is a lifelong problem. Many affected persons experience phases or cycles of spontaneous bleeding episodes. Mechanisms that cause this phenomenon are unknown. Intracranial hemorrhage and bleeding into the neck or abdomen constitute life-threatening emergencies.

EVALUATION AND TREATMENT Although laboratory tests are of primary value in the evaluation of hemorrhagic disorders, the history and physical assessment also should be given careful consideration. The three phases of coagulation can be assessed individually by simple, reliable tests. In any hemorrhagic condition, the adequacy of phase III should be determined first. Unless adequate fibrinogen is present, the blood is incapable of coagulation; thus other laboratory tests that require formation of a visible clot will be invalid. Phase III can be evaluated by the **thrombin time,** the time required for plasma to clot after the addition of bovine thrombin. Fibrinogen can be measured by chemical or immunologic methods.

Phase II is assessed by the **prothrombin time (PT),** the time required for plasma to clot after the addition of thromboplastin and calcium. If phase III is intact, a prolonged prothrombin time indicates a deficiency involving factors II, V, VII, or X, alone or in combination. Specific assays for each of the factors are available.

Phase I, the most complex part of coagulation, can be evaluated by several tests. The **activated partial thromboplastin time (PTT)** is the time required for clotting of plasma that has been activated by incubation with kaolin when calcium and platelets (or partial thromboplastin) are added. PTT assesses the adequacy of factors XII, XI, IX, and VII. The **prothrombin consumption time** is a standard prothrombin test of serum instead of plasma. Because prothrombin is used up during coagulation, the serum normally contains little prothrombin and the serum prothrombin time is prolonged. Deficiencies of the phase I factors are associated with poor use of prothrombin. If the serum and plasma prothrombin times are similar, deficiency of a phase I factor is likely. The **thromboplastin generation test** is the most sensitive of all phase I

tests. The test can precisely identify deficiencies of factors VIII and IX. If the PTT, prothrombin consumption, or thromboplastin generation test results are abnormal, the way in which they can be corrected identifies the specific deficiency.

The treatment of hemophilia has advanced during the past 50 years. Plasma first was used in the 1920s, and by the 1940s it was used routinely to treat persons with hemophilia. The disadvantages of fresh frozen plasma (FFP), which is low in factor VIII per volume of plasma, led to the development of cryoprecipitate. In 1964 cryoprecipitate (quick-frozen precipitate), which is rich in factor VIII per volume, was used to treat persons with hemophilia. Although cryoprecipitate advanced the treatment of hemophilia A, it has several disadvantages. The most notable complication is the possibility of transmission of viral diseases. Factor VIII concentrates were first introduced in 1965. In addition to the predictable factor VIII content, other advantages of the early factor VIII concentrates included greater purity than cryoprecipitate and less contamination with other plasma proteins.[32] The recent cloning of the factor VIII gene and the development of recombinant factor VIII have resulted in new factor VIII products that minimize the risk of transmission of viral infection (e.g., HIV and hepatitis) and are potentially less expensive than plasma-derived factor VIII. Transmission of viral diseases (e.g., hepatitis A, C, and G) in individuals receiving factor concentrates has historically been problematic.[33-36]

Recombinant antihemolytic factor plasma/albumin-free method (rAHF-PFM, Advate™) is a new product used for the prevention and control of bleeding episodes in individuals with hemophilia A, and in the perioperative management of those with hemophilia A. By excluding proteins or raw materials derived from human or animal sources in the final product, the risk of transmission of potentially infectious agents is removed.[37]

Continuous prophylaxis from ages 2 to 18 years reduces the incidence of joint damage and synovitis, which remain the primary causes of disability in people with hemophilia.[38]

Congenital Hypercoagulability and Thrombosis

Hereditary bleeding disorders, such as hemophilia, have been recognized and treated for centuries; however, the counterpart of these disorders, **thrombophilia,** has not been recognized until very recently. The inherited thrombophilic conditions generally are caused by defects in the clotting factors that inhibit clot formation; thus the balance between bleeding and clotting is directed toward the clotting aspects of hemostasis. Defects in specific proteins (C and S) and antithrombin (AT), as well as resistance to activated protein C (APC) and hyperhomocystinemia, are the major recognized causes of inherited thrombophilia.[39]

Both proteins C and S are inhibitors of coagulation and depend on vitamin K for synthesis in the hepatocytes of the liver. Decreased levels of either of these proteins interfere with the normal homeostatic balance of procoagulant and anticoagulant activity at the endothelial level. Protein C and S deficiency states predispose affected individuals to thrombosis, especially venous thrombosis of the lower extremities.

Inheritance of **protein C deficiency** is autosomal dominant. Heterozygotes have protein C levels 50% to 60% of normal and may develop superficial thrombophlebitis, deep venous thrombosis, or pulmonary embolism in their late teens and early twenties. The majority of these thrombotic events (75%) occur spontaneously, whereas only 25% are the result of predisposing conditions.[39] Homozygotes have less than 1% of normal levels of protein C and tend to develop thrombosis of the cutaneous vessels with large areas of skin necrosis. It is rare for individuals with protein C deficiency to develop arterial thrombosis.

Protein C deficiency exists in two forms: types I and II. Type I, the most common form, involves a reduction in both biologic and immunologic activity of protein C. Type I is caused by deletion of the entire gene. In type II, the less common form, there is a normal level of protein C antigen but decreased functional levels of activity.[40]

Neonatal purpura fulminans is a fatal syndrome found in infants who are homozygous or double heterozygous for types I and II protein deficiency. Manifestations of this syndrome are ecchymosis that becomes apparent on the first day of life and develops around the head, trunk, and extremities. These cutaneous manifestations often are accompanied by cerebral thrombosis and infarction. The lesions apparent on the skin often coalesce and demonstrate ulceration and necrosis. The condition is treated with fresh frozen plasma and heparinization, although the infant rarely survives.[41]

Treatment for protein C deficiency is heparin for acute episodes of thrombosis. Long-term therapy is required and consists of either oral warfarin sodium (Coumadin) or subcutaneous heparin (2500 to 5000 units) every 12 hours. Protein C concentrates have been developed; however, they have not yet been formally approved for treatment.

Protein S deficiency is similar to protein C deficiency, and the inheritance pattern (autosomal dominant) is also similar. Heterozygotes demonstrate a strong tendency for deep venous thrombosis, with the first incidence often occurring before age 25 years. Other manifestations include superficial thrombophlebitis and pulmonary emboli. There are predisposing conditions for thrombi development in some cases, with evidence of spontaneous thrombi development in most cases.

Protein S deficiency exists in two forms: type I and type II. Type I is identified as a quantitative deficiency and manifests as low levels of protein S antigen and activity, and type II is identified as a qualitative deficiency with low levels of free protein S and normal levels of free and total protein S antigen.[39]

Homozygotes demonstrate severe manifestations of the condition and may develop a form of purpura fulminans in the neonatal period. It also is possible that the homozygous state may lead to uterine death.[40] Treatment with heparin and Coumadin is similar to that of protein C deficiency.

Antithrombin III (AT III) deficiency is inherited as an autosomal dominant condition, with the heterozygote state being the most common. AT III also exists in two forms, type I and type II, with type I being a quantitative deficiency of the AT III antigen. Type II is characterized as a dysfunctional form: normal levels of AT III are present but with reduced activity.

Individuals with AT III deficiency are at risk for early development of venous thrombosis and pulmonary embolism. These events often occur in the middle to late teens, with the potential of occurring as early as 10 years of age. The deep veins of the lower extremities most commonly are involved, with the iliofemoral vein being the most common site of involvement. Other sites include the mesenteric veins, vena cava, renal veins, and retinal veins. Cerebral thromboses also have been described. Arterial thrombotic events are rare. In some cases, thrombosis is precipitated by predisposing conditions, such as surgery, trauma, pregnancy, oral contraceptives, and infection.

The treatment of choice for AT III deficiency is heparin. Antiplatelet agents (e.g., aspirin, dipyridamole) may be used, as well as AT III concentrates.

Antibody-Mediated Hemorrhagic Disease

The antibody-mediated hemorrhagic diseases are a group of disorders caused by the immune response. Antibody-mediated destruction of platelets or antibody-mediated inflammatory reactions to allergens damage blood vessels and cause seepage into tissues. The thrombocytopenic purpuras may be intrinsic or idiopathic, or they may be transient phenomena transmitted from mother to fetus. The inflammatory, or "allergic," purpuras occur in response to allergens in the blood. All these disorders first appear during infancy or childhood.

Idiopathic Thrombocytopenic Purpura

Acute **idiopathic thrombocytopenic purpura (ITP) (autoimmune or primary thrombocytopenic purpura)** is the most common of the thrombocytopenic purpuras of childhood. It is a disorder of platelet consumption in which antiplatelet antibodies bind to the plasma membranes of platelets, causing platelet sequestration and destruction by mononuclear phagocytes in the spleen and other lymphoid tissues at a rate that exceeds the ability of the bone marrow to produce them.

PATHOPHYSIOLOGY   Platelets have several tissue-specific antigens on their plasma markers that may be targets for antiplatelet antibody. In approximately 70% of cases of ITP, there is an antecedent viral disease (e.g., cytomegalovirus [CMV], Epstein-Barr virus [EBV], human immunodeficiency virus [HIV], parvovirus, or viral respiratory infection), thus suggesting that viral sensitization has occurred. The interval between infection and onset of purpura is 1 to 4 weeks. A comparison with purpura seen in adults has identified an immune mechanism as the basis for ITP. High levels of IgG have been found bound to platelets and may represent immune complexes on the platelet surface.[42]

CLINICAL MANIFESTATIONS   One to four weeks after a viral infection, bruising and a generalized petechial rash often occur with acute onset. Asymmetric bleeding is typical and is found most often on the legs and trunk. Hemorrhagic bullae of the gums, lips, and other mucous membranes may be prominent. Epistaxis (nose bleeding) may be severe and difficult to control. Except for the signs of bleeding, the child appears well. The acute phase of the disease associated with spontaneous hemorrhages lasts 1 to 2 weeks, but thrombocytopenia often persists. Although its incidence is less than 1%, intracranial hemorrhage is the most serious complication of ITP. In some cases the onset is more gradual and clinical manifestations consist of moderate bruising and a few petechiae.

EVALUATION AND TREATMENT   Laboratory examination reveals a reduced platelet count, and the few platelets observed on a peripheral blood smear are large in size, reflecting increased bone marrow production. The Ivy bleeding time is prolonged. Bone marrow aspiration reveals megakaryocytes in normal or increased numbers and normal erythrocytes and granulocytes.

Even without treatment, the prognosis for children with ITP is excellent. Seventy-five percent recover completely within 3 months. After the initial acute phase, spontaneous clinical manifestations subside. By 6 months after onset, 80% to 90% of affected children have regained normal platelet counts.[43]

Because of the short life span of platelets (10 days), fresh blood or platelets are of no value or of transient benefit; however, their use is indicated when life-threatening hemorrhage occurs. For many children, corticosteroid therapy reduces the severity and shortens the duration of the initial phase by suppressing the immune attack on platelets.[44,45]

Intravenous IgG has been demonstrated to increase the platelet count in some children with ITP, but it is quite costly.[46,47] A newer product, anti-D, is a gamma globulin fraction containing a high proportion of antibodies to the RhO (D) antigen of the red blood cells. Intravenous anti-D is a safe and effective treatment for Rh-positive, nonsplenectomized individuals with ITP, although it is expensive. Intravenous anti-D is an effective treatment for Rh-positive, nonsplenectomized children with ITP, although it is associated with side effects including chills, fever, headache, and a decrease in hemoglobin levels. Administration of steroids and antipyretics prior to the anti-D treatment may prevent side effects.[48]

Parents should be instructed to protect the child from falls or other trauma that might result in bleeding. Splenectomy should be reserved for chronic cases that fail to respond to nonsurgical intervention.[49]

Autoimmune Neonatal Thrombocytopenias
Antibody-mediated thrombocytopenic purpura occurs in neonates in either autoimmune or alloimmune form. Both forms are characterized by the immunologic destruction of platelets by antibodies (IgG) against tissue-specific antigens expressed by the platelets (i.e., platelet-specific antigens).

Autoimmune neonatal thrombocytopenia was first noted in the early 1950s when it was observed that mothers with ITP often delivered infants who were transiently thrombocytopenic. Neonatal thrombocytopenia was observed in approximately 50% of infants at risk and lasted an average of 1 month. As platelet counts returned to normal, a concomitant drop in the level of maternal antiplatelet antibody on the child's platelets occurred. The antibody is directed against antigens common to maternal and neonatal platelets.[50] The prognosis generally is favorable. The frequency of intracranial hemorrhage has been estimated to be 1% to 3% of cases. The principal aim of the management of affected infants is to prevent the deleterious consequences of severe thrombocytopenia by administering intravenous immunoglobulins.[50]

Neonatal alloimmune thrombocytopenic purpura (NATP) is less common, estimated to occur in 1 in 800 to 1000 live births.[50] NATP is suspected in thrombocytopenic infants of mothers with normal platelet counts and no history of purpura. The disorder is caused by the production of a maternal antibody against a fetal platelet-specific antigen inherited from the father and not shared by the mother. More than 50% of NATP cases are associated with the presence of the P1^{A}1 antigen on neonatal and paternal platelets but not on maternal platelets.

It is not known why NATP occurs in only half of the neonates genetically at risk for NATP. Because 98% of the population show P1^{A}1 positivity, approximately 1 in 50 pregnancies would be expected to show maternal-fetal incompatibility, but the incidence of NATP is 100 times less. NATP does not develop in neonates born to some mothers with high antiplatelet antibody levels.

The diagnosis of NATP is confirmed by detection in the maternal serum of antibody that reacts with platelets from the infant and father but not with platelets from the mother. In approximately 75% to 85% of cases, NATP recurs in subsequent pregnancies. Purpura usually develops in the affected infant shortly after delivery, and intracranial, renal, and gastrointestinal hemorrhages are possible. The mortality rate from intracranial hemorrhage has been estimated at 10% to 15%. Following birth, maternal platelet transfusion (mother to infant) is the treatment of choice.[50]

Most of the life-threatening clinical manifestations of both transient neonatal thrombocytopenia and NATP can be avoided through cesarean delivery. If the mother has antiplatelet disease, however, surgery can result in hemorrhage and serious maternal morbidity. Maternal morbidity resulting from NATP during pregnancy is low (less than 5%): the principal maternal risk is bleeding from surgical incisions during cesarean delivery. This poses a problem for the obstetrician. The incidence of transient thrombocytopenia in infants born to mothers with NATP is about 50%. If all deliveries were cesarean, half the mothers would undergo cesarean delivery unnecessarily. Conversely, if all deliveries were vaginal, half the infants—those with thrombocytopenia—would be at risk for intracranial bleeding.

A considerable amount of research has focused on methods of predicting whether the fetus is thrombocytopenic so that the route of delivery can be chosen to minimize the risks for both mother and child. No satisfactory method has been found, despite reports from many laboratories that fetal platelet counts correlate closely with levels of antiplatelet antibody on maternal platelets or in the maternal circulation. Equally unreliable are predictions of neonatal thrombocytopenia based on immunosuppression with corticosteroids. Research continues in areas such as the identification of specific subclasses of antiplatelet antibodies.

Autoimmune Vascular Purpura

Autoimmune vascular purpura (allergic purpura) is caused by antibody-mediated injury of blood vessel walls, typically arterioles and capillaries. The inflammatory reaction is to foreign proteins or chemicals in the blood (microorganisms, drugs, or other chemicals).

Autoimmune vascular purpura usually is seen in children, with the incidence decreasing in adolescents and adults and occurring only rarely in elderly persons. The average age at onset is 5 years, with a slightly higher proportion of males being affected. Purpura occurs as vessel integrity is disrupted by inflammatory processes, causing effusion of serosanguineous exudate to perivascular tissues.

Clinical manifestations vary and include headache, anorexia, fever, abdominal pain, arthralgias, and skin lesions (urticaria and erythema). The lesions usually are located symmetrically on the proximal portions of the extremities, particularly on the legs and buttocks, and may be accompanied by itching or paresthesias.[51] Abdominal pain results from hemorrhage into the bowel, which may lead to colic, nausea, and vomiting. These symptoms may precede the appearance of skin lesions. The pain usually is midabdominal but may radiate to other parts of the abdomen. Constipation may occur.

Some forms of autoimmune vascular purpura may produce joint pain and tenderness. Periarticular swelling and edema of the hands and feet are common, but hemarthrosis does not occur. These symptoms may precede the onset of symptoms associated with abdominal pain and purpura. Subacute glomerulonephritis occurs in some cases but usually is reversible.

The characteristic skin lesions (purpura and cutaneous manifestations of allergy), accompanied by a history of joint and abdominal pain, are clues for diagnosis. Laboratory test results often reveal no major abnormalities. Attacks may last several weeks and may recur at odd intervals and with changing manifestations with each episode. Treatment, if necessary, consists of the alleviation of symptoms.

LEUKEMIA AND LYMPHOMA

Leukemia, the most common malignancy of childhood, represents approximately 33% of all childhood cancers. Childhood lymphoma is the third most common malignant neoplasm of children in the United States, representing approximately 11% of all childhood cancers. (See Chapter 27 for a discussion of leukemia in adults.)

Leukemia

Of the varieties of childhood leukemia, 80% to 85% of leukemias in children are acute lymphoblastic leukemia (ALL) or acute undifferentiated leukemia (AUL). The remaining 15% to 20% are acute nonlymphocytic leukemias (ANLLs) (which include myeloblastic, promyelocytic, monocytic, and myelomonoblastic leukemias) and the very rare red blood cell leukemia, erythroleukemia. Because the vast majority of ANLLs involve the myeloblastic cell, many experts refer to the disease as acute myelogenous leukemia (AML). Leukemia accounts for 25% of cases of cancer in black children and 34% of cases of cancer in white children. Approximately 2200 new cases are diagnosed each year in the United States.[52] Of those 2200 children, 1700 are diagnosed with ALL. Both a juvenile form and an adult form of chronic granulocytic leukemia (CGL) can develop in children, but CGL is uncommon and accounts for only 2% of all leukemias in childhood. Chronic lymphocytic leukemia (CLL) is virtually nonexistent in children.

The peak incidence for childhood ALL is between 2 and 6 years of age. Although this peak is very evident in white children in the United States, it is not observed in black children. The reason for this difference is unknown, but it may be related to genetic susceptibility or to exposure to the environmental influences that might play a role in leukemia. Further, acute leukemia is nearly twice as common in white children as in nonwhite children (4.2:100,000 versus 2.4:100,000, respectively). For a white child the risk of acute leukemia developing before age 10 years is 1:2800.[52] Childhood ALL also is more common in boys than in girls (1.3:1.0).

Types of Leukemia

A number of different classifications are used for the leukemias. First, acute leukemia is differentiated from chronic leukemia. Second, the cell line determines whether lymphoid cells or myeloid cells are involved. In acute leukemia this difference separates ALL from ANLL and vice versa. Then, within each of these categories, further subdivisions have been developed. (See Chapter 27 for a discussion of leukemias in adults.)

Cytogenic studies of leukemic cells are performed routinely at most major treatment centers during the diagnostic process. Abnormal morphologic characteristics, as well as abnormalities in the number of copies of chromosomes, are found in leukemic cells. Hyperdiploidy (increased number of chromosome copies) is associated with a good prognosis. Other genetic abnormalities include chromosome translocations and fragility (break sites). Translocations are more common in children with a poor prognosis. Some oncogenes have been associated with various types of childhood leukemia, including *src, abl, N-ras*, and *c-myb*.[53-55]

Two additional classifications of ALL (morphologic and immunologic) have proved clinically useful because they have prognostic value. Although a number of different morphologic classifications have been developed, the accepted system was developed by a cooperative effort of French, American, and British scientists and is known as the French-American-British Cooperative Group (FAB) classification.[56,57] This system divides lymphoblasts into three categories—L1, L2, and L3—on the basis of histologic appearance of the abnormal lymphoblast. Approximately 85% of cases of ALL are of the L1 subtype; less than 15% are L2, a subtype more common in adults with ALL; and the L3 subtype, which is rare, occurs in fewer than 1% of children with ALL.

Flow cytometric immunophenotyping has made distinguishing between lymphoblastic and nonlymphoblastic leukemia much easier than in the past, when the degree of immaturity of the cell sometimes made such distinction difficult. In addition, immunologic classifications have assisted clinicians in determining the degree of aggressive therapy needed.[58]

Immunologic classification has been used on identification of various surface markers. Five categories of ALL have been identified on the basis of their presumed origin from thymic cells (T cells) and bursa-equivalent cells (B cells) of normal lymphocytes:

1. T cell ALL—characterized by the presence of abnormal T lymphocytes and found more commonly in older boys whose diagnosis includes mediastinal masses, high white blood cell counts, and hepatosplenomegaly (20% of ALL)
2. B cell ALL—characterized by the presence of abnormal B lymphoblasts and associated with a poor prognosis (5% of ALL)
3. Pre–B cell ALL—characterized by the presence of pre–B lymphoblasts (20% of ALL)
4. Unclassified ALL—also known as *null cell* (meaning neither T nor B lymphoblasts), and now classified as early B cell lineage (15% of ALL)
5. Common ALL—characterized by the presence of a specific antigen known as *common ALL antigen,* or common lymphocytic leukemia antigen (CALLA), recently designated cellular differentiation 10 or CD-10, in which the actual cell usually is considered to be of the B lineage (39% of ALL)

The identification of CALLA is important because this type of ALL has a more favorable prognosis.

Subtypes of ANLL also have been classified by the FAB system according to the morphologic and cytochemical characteristics of the leukemic cell. Seven categories have been established:

1. M1 involves cells that are myeloblastic without differentiation.
2. M2 involves cells that are myeloblastic with differentiation.
3. M3 involves the promyelocyte.
4. M4 involves the myeloblastic and monoblastic cell lines.
5. M5 involves monoblasts.

6. M6 involves precursors of erythrocytes.
7. M7 involves precursors of megakaryocytes.

Nearly half of all childhood ANLL is M1 or M2. Another one third is categorized as M4 or M5. ANLL subtypes M3, M6, and M7 are quite rare.[58]

PATHOGENESIS The exact cause of childhood leukemia is unclear. Investigations have focused on genetic susceptibility, environmental factors, and viral infections (see Chapter 13). Observations of a familial tendency and links with a number of inherited disorders have implicated genetic factors in the origin of leukemia. Analyses of leukemia in twins has revealed a frequent prenatal origin and an early or initiating role for chromosome translocations. In addition, twin studies also suggest that there is a protracted latency and the need in ALL and ANLL for postnatal exposures or genetic events to produce clinical disease.[59] A positive family history of hematopoietic malignancies among first- or second-degree relatives has been associated with a slight increase for risk for childhood ALL, although it is modest (odds ratio 2.06).[60]

Inherited diseases that predispose a child to leukemia (both ALL and ANLL) include Down syndrome (1:74 before age 10 years), Fanconi anemia (1:12 before age 21 years), Bloom syndrome (1:8 before age 26 years), and ataxia-telangiectasia (1:8 before age 25 years). Leukemia also has been associated with known genetic diseases, such as congenital agammaglobulinemia. ANLL in children sometimes is associated with loss or deletion of chromosome 7.[61] ANLL can develop from preexisting myeloproliferative disorders that also are preleukemia syndromes. When these disorders progress to ANLL, an insidious pattern of leukemic dysfunction usually is revealed.

Most research on environmental factors as etiologic agents has centered on exposure to ionizing radiation. Atomic bomb survivors have an increased risk for leukemia. The degree of risk depends on the distance from the epicenter. The peak incidence period is 4 to 8 years after exposure to the radiation.[62] Whereas ANLL most often develops in adults who are exposed to radiation, ALL is more likely to develop in children. The therapeutic use of x-rays for thymic enlargement in children also has been linked to subsequent development of ALL in children.[63] In a more recent study, no increased risk of childhood leukemia was found in children who had received small doses of radiation from diagnostic x-rays.[64] Some doubt remains concerning the relative risk of prenatal exposure to radiation. Although it is likely that in utero radiation presents a cancer risk to the fetus, the magnitude of the risk is uncertain.[65] Although most studies of radiation exposure have focused on artificial radiation sources, there is considerable interest in natural background radiation, particularly the possible role of radon exposure in subsequent childhood and adult cancers, although no association has been found.

Electromagnetic field (EMF) exposure from power poles and small appliances has been studied as a causative factor in acute leukemias. Some studies suggest an increased risk in malignant diseases with exposure to electromagnetic fields.[67-69]

Other studies, however, have not supported these findings, and further investigation is ongoing.[70]

Although chemicals such as benzene have been associated with the development of ANLL in adults, no evidence suggests a similar chemical or drug association in childhood leukemia. Leukemia (primarily ANLL) has been reported as a secondary malignancy (development of a second cancer after the first) in children treated for Hodgkin disease and Wilms tumor, although such cases are rare. In most cases the children received both chemotherapy (alkylating agents or dactinomycin) and radiation therapy for the primary cancer, perhaps accounting for the subsequent development of another cancer.

Leukemic "clusters" that represent a greater number of leukemia cases occurring in a particular geographic location have raised speculation about environmental factors or infectious patterns of transmission. Careful follow-up, however, has failed to document the abnormal clustering.[71] Explanations for this phenomenon therefore are statistical artifact and coincidence. However, one reported leukemic cluster in the town of Woburn, Massachusetts, has been linked to possible water supply contamination by chemicals from factory waste.[72]

Another area of interest has been the role of viruses in the development of leukemia. Viruses clearly have been shown to cause leukemia in a number of animals, including cats, fowl, and mice. Retroviruses are associated with the development of malignancies, including (1) human T cell leukemia/lymphoma virus (HTLV-I) with an unusual form of adult T cell leukemia, (2) HTLV-II with hairy cell leukemia, and (3) HIV with non-Hodgkin lymphoma and Kaposi sarcoma.[27] However, retroviruses have not been linked with childhood leukemia.

CLINICAL MANIFESTATIONS Few variations appear in the presenting symptoms of the various cell types of acute leukemias. The onset may be abrupt or insidious, but the most common symptoms reflect the consequence of bone marrow failure, which results in decreased red blood cells and platelets and changes in white blood cells. Pallor, fatigue, petechiae, purpura, bleeding, and fever generally are present. Approximately 45% of children have a hemoglobin level below 7 g/dl; in contrast to adults, children seem to demonstrate fewer symptoms. If acute blood loss occurs, however, characteristic symptoms of tachycardia, air hunger, restlessness, and thirst may be present. Epistaxis, excessive bruising, and hematuria often occur in children with severe thrombocytopenia. Three fourths of children with ALL have platelet counts below 100,000/mm³ at diagnosis, and 28% have platelet counts below 20,000/mm³. Half of all children newly diagnosed with ANLL have platelet counts below 50,000/mm³. Disseminated intravascular coagulation occurs more commonly with ANLL, particularly with promyelocytic leukemia. The granules in the leukemic promyelocytes may then indicate thromboplastin activity.

Fever usually is present as a result of two causes: (1) infection associated with the decrease in functional neutrophils

and (2) hypermetabolism associated with the ongoing rapid growth and destruction of leukemic cells. In most children with ALL, the total white blood count is less than 10,000/mm³, and with ANLL most have white cell counts below 50,000/mm³. In a few children, however, the peripheral white blood count can go well above 100,000/mm³. White blood cell counts greater than 200,000/mm³ can cause leukostasis, an intravascular clumping of cells that results in infarction and hemorrhage, usually in the brain and lung. An excessive leukocyte count at diagnosis is the most important predictor of prognosis in ALL.[73]

Renal failure as a result of hyperuremia (high uric acid levels) can be associated with ALL, particularly at diagnosis. Cell breakdown results as a natural process in the presence of a high white blood cell count or as a result of cellular breakdown caused by chemotherapy. Uric acid levels rise as an end product of purine metabolism from cellular destruction. Because the major excretory pathway is through the kidney, urates can precipitate in renal tubules or ureters and can lead to oliguria and acute renal failure. Renal failure is preventable if uric acid levels are monitored and treatment is aimed at optimal hydration, alkalinization of urine to assist with the excretion of soluble urates, and blockage of further uric acid formation by administration of the drug allopurinol.

Extramedullary invasion with leukemic cells can occur in nearly all body tissue. Most children with ALL have some extramedullary involvement at diagnosis. Leukemic invasion of tissue other than bone marrow is believed to represent metastatic infiltration. Hepatosplenomegaly and lymphadenopathy, resulting from extramedullary hematopoiesis, occur in nearly one half of children with ALL, but they are less common in children with ANLL.

The CNS is a common site of infiltration of extramedullary leukemias, although fewer than 10% of children with ALL have CNS involvement at diagnosis. CNS infiltration manifests later in the course of the disease. Because successful chemotherapy prolongs the time of remission, the incidence of CNS involvement has increased. The most common symptoms of CNS involvement relate to increased intracranial pressure, causing early-morning headaches, nausea, vomiting, irritability, and lethargy. Prophylactic CNS treatment therefore is necessary, because systemic treatment with chemotherapy does not cross the blood-brain barrier.

Gonadal involvement, with testicular and ovarian infiltration, has been demonstrated in postmortem examination in 57% and 35% of children, respectively. Clinical detection of gonadal involvement is much less frequent. The incidence of testicular involvement, like CNS involvement, has increased with lengthened duration of remission. Prophylactic treatment has not been successful and currently is not recommended.

Leukemic infiltration into bones and joints is common in children. Reports of bone or joint pain actually lead to the diagnosis of leukemia in some children. In most children, bone pain is characterized as migratory, vague, and without areas of swelling or inflammation. If joint pain is the primary symp-

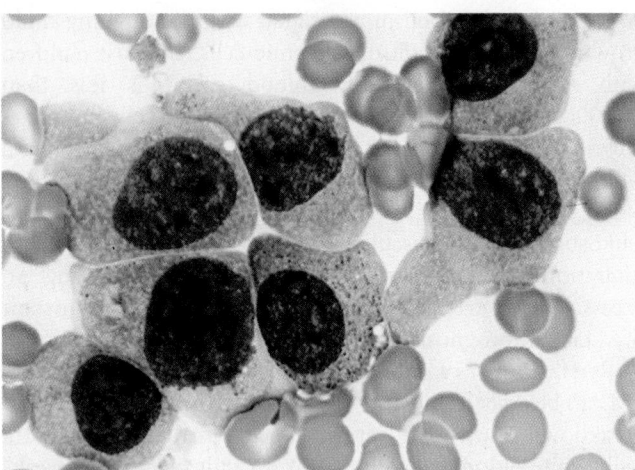

Figure 28-10 Monoblasts from acute monoblastic leukemia. Monoblasts in a marrow smear from a patient with acute monoblastic leukemia (M5A). The monoblasts are larger than myeloblasts and usually have abundant cytoplasm, often with delicate scattered azurophilic granules (an element that stains well with blue aniline dyes). (From Damjanov I, Linder J, editors: *Anderson's pathology,* ed 10, St Louis, 1996, Mosby.)

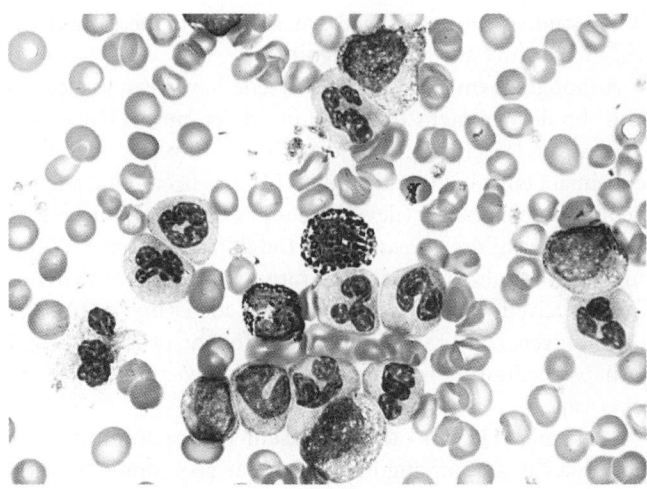

Figure 28-11 Leukocytosis and basophilia in chronic myeloid leukemia. Blood smear from child with chronic myeloid leukemia (blasts) showing marked leukocytosis and basophilia. Karyotype analysis identified a Philadelphia chromosome (Wright-Giemsa stain). (From Damjanov I, Linder J, editors: *Anderson's pathology,* ed 10, St Louis, 1996, Mosby.)

tom and some swelling is associated with the pain, however, misdiagnoses of rheumatoid arthritis and rheumatic fever may occur.

Other organs reported to be sites of leukemic invasion include the kidneys, heart, lungs, thymus, eyes, skin, and gastrointestinal tract. Of these, the kidneys, lungs, and gastrointestinal tract are the most frequently reported sites. Skin involvement is more common in ANLL than in ALL.

EVALUATION AND TREATMENT   Although blood test results can raise the clinician's suspicion of leukemia, a bone marrow aspiration is required to establish the diagnosis. The **blast cell** is the hallmark of acute leukemia (Figure 28-10). The blast cell is a relatively undifferentiated cell characterized by diffusely distributed nuclear chromatin, with one or more nucleoli and basophilic cytoplasm (Figure 28-11).

Healthy children have fewer than 5% blast cells in the bone marrow and none in the peripheral blood. The bone marrow is categorized on the basis of blast percentage. Normal bone marrow is called M1 marrow; M2 and M3 represent an increased percentage of blasts in the sample. This categorization system should not be confused with the similar terminology used to denote subtypes of ANLL. In ALL the bone marrow often is replaced by 80% to 100% blast cells, with a reduction in normally developing red blood cells and granulocytes. The marrow, which is considered hypercellular, is composed of a homogeneous population of cells. Occasionally, however, the marrow appears hypocellular, making the diagnosis difficult to differentiate from aplastic anemia. When this occurs, bone marrow biopsy or biopsy of extramedullary sites is necessary to confirm the diagnosis.

Combination chemotherapy, with or without radiation therapy to localized sites, such as the CNS, is the treatment of choice for acute leukemia. In ALL, identification of various

risk groups has led to the development of different intensities of drug protocols. Thus treatment is tailored specifically for a particular risk group. (Table 28-5 outlines the various prognostic factors for ALL that are considered in determining the degree of risk.)

Most ALL treatment programs have four distinct phases: (1) induction of remission, (2) preventive therapy for the CNS, (3) intensification (also called *consolidation*), and (4) maintenance. In remission induction, the goal is no clinical evidence of disease and a normal bone marrow biopsy result, which is achieved in 95% of children with ALL. Children with persistent leukemia at the end of 1 month of induction therapy have a dismal prognosis.[74] Prophylactic CNS treatment has included both chemotherapy and radiation in the past, but evidence increasingly has shown that this therapy, although effective in preventing CNS leukemia, adversely affects neurologic and intellectual function. A marked incidence of learning disabilities has been identified in children previously treated to prevent CNS disease.[75] New, less toxic treatment protocols are now being studied to deal with this problem.[76] Once remission is achieved, an intensification phase of treatment begins. This treatment is necessary because leukemic cells will continue to be present despite successful remission. Thus the goal of the intensification phase is to further decrease and eliminate the remaining leukemic cells. Intensification therapy often overlaps prophylactic CNS treatment. The final phase of initial treatment is called *maintenance therapy.* The goal of this phase is to maintain disease control. The optimal duration of maintenance therapy is not well defined, but it usually continues for 2.5 to 3 years. During maintenance therapy, intermittent "pulses" of new drugs may be given. Periods of intensified therapy are believed to minimize development of drug-resistant leukemic cells.

Table 28-5	Prognostic Factors in Acute Lymphoblastic Leukemia (ALL)	
Prognostic Factor	Better Prognosis	Worse Prognosis
Age*		
<2 yr or >10 yr		X
2–7 yr	X	
Gender*		
Male		X
Female	X	
Initial white blood count*		
>50,000/mm³		X
<10,000/mm³	X	
Race		
Black		X
White	X	
Morphology		
L₂ or L₃		X
L₁	X	
Immunology*		
T or B cell ALL		X
Early pre–B cell or common lymphocytic leukemia antigen (CALLA)	X	
Leukemic involvement		
Mediastinal mass		X
Central nervous system involvement at diagnosis		X
Splenic enlargement		X

*The four most reliable prognostic factors. Initial prognostic factors become less effective predictors with increasing length of remission. Age and gender are not significant after 15 months of continuous remission, and white blood cell count is not significant after 24 months of continuous remission.

ALL is a curable disease. This prognosis is a dramatic reversal of the outlook for a child diagnosed with this disease 30 years ago, when ALL was uniformly fatal and the average survival time was only 2 to 3 months. Today, with prompt and appropriate treatment, 70% to 80% of children with ALL are cured. Those children with the more favorable early pre–B cell or CALLA-positive ALL have a survival rate of 90%.[73]

Prognostic factors in ANLL are not as well defined as they are for ALL because of the small number of affected children and their overall poor prognosis. The goal of treatment for ANLL is similar to that of ALL except that much more aggressive chemotherapy is administered. With intensive chemotherapy, significant bone marrow suppression is necessary but predisposes children to infection, bleeding, and anemia. The use of colony-stimulating factor (CSF), which stimulates the rapid proliferation of specific blood cell lines, is a recent advance that now shortens this period of bone marrow aplasia (CSFs are discussed in Chapter 25). Although initial remission is achieved relatively easily in all cases of ALL, successful and lasting remission can be achieved in only 70% to 80% of children with ANLL.[73] If remission is achieved, further treatment, called *continuation therapy,* is required. The specific intensity, timing, and length of continuation therapy are

controversial. The use of either a stem cell or bone marrow transplantation (BMT) is an important treatment consideration in ANLL. Because long-term remission and cure of ANLL are difficult to achieve with chemotherapy alone, transplant often is recommended after the first remission is achieved. Transplant is the treatment of choice after relapse of ANLL. The long-term survival rate for children with ANLL, whether treated with chemotherapy or chemotherapy and BMT, is approximately 40%.[73]

Lymphomas

Non-Hodgkin lymphoma (NHL) and Hodgkin disease make up approximately 11% of all childhood cancer. Approximately 750 cases of childhood lymphoma are diagnosed in the United States annually.[52] Either group of diseases is rare before age 5 years, and the relative incidence increases throughout childhood. NHL is 1.5 times more common than Hodgkin disease in children. Boys are more likely to be diagnosed with a malignant lymphoma than are girls, and the high-risk groups have been identified. At particular risk are children with inherited or acquired immune deficiency syndromes. These children have been found to have increased rates of lymphoreticular cancers that range from 100 to 10,000 times the rate of normal children. The cancers are most commonly NHLs.[77] Children who are artificially immunosuppressed after organ transplantation, especially if cyclosporine is the immunosuppressive agent, also are at increased risk for lymphomas.

Non-Hodgkin Lymphoma

The classification of **non-Hodgkin lymphoma (NHL)** has been confusing because of the heterogeneity of this group of diseases. Generally, most classification systems divide NHL into two categories, nodular or diffuse, on the basis of cellular pattern. Whereas one half of all adults with NHL have a nodular form of the disease, children rarely demonstrate this pattern. Nodular disease represents a less aggressive form of lymphoma. Almost without exception, childhood NHL becomes evident as a diffuse disease and can be further subdivided into three groups: (1) large cell (histiocytic), (2) lymphoblastic, and (3) small noncleaved cell (Burkitt or non-Burkitt lymphoma). Large cell NHL often involves chromosomal translocations. Disease sites commonly involve extranodal sites, such as brain, lung, bone, and skin. Lymphoblastic NHL also shows chromosomal translocations, particularly chromosomes 7 and 14. Disease sites commonly include the mediastinum and peripheral lymph nodes. Small noncleaved cell NHL involves chromosome translocations of 8 and 14. It is believed that this translocation triggers the *c-myc* oncogene. Children with small noncleaved cell NHL commonly have intraabdominal disease at diagnosis.

An area of intensive study concerns the apparent biologic similarities of NHL and ALL in children. These two diseases are cytologically identical, and the histologic distinction between them is indicated by the degree of infiltration in the blood and bone marrow. The more bone marrow involvement and the less nodal and organ infiltration that are present, the more likely the disease is to be classified as ALL. Childhood NHL also is much more like ALL in its clinical manifestations and much less like Hodgkin disease or adult NHL.

As in ALL, immunophenotyping is an important part of the classification of childhood NHL. Almost 45% of the disease in children originates from T cells; an equal number originates from B cells. The remaining group, which represents 10% of childhood NHLs, is classified as non-T, non-B.

PATHOGENESIS   The origin of NHL in childhood is still elusive. Although defective host immunity is implicated in most children in whom NHL develops, an immune deficit cannot be identified. Viral etiology is suggested, but the role in development of human lymphoma is still unclear. The strongest correlation exists between EBV and African Burkitt lymphoma. This form of NHL is associated with a break point on chromosome 8 that is located near the *c-myc* oncogene.[78] The relationship between EBV infection and Burkitt lymphoma outside Africa is weak, however, even though the tumor is histopathologically and clinically indistinguishable. Chronic immunostimulation also has been suggested as a factor in the development of lymphomas because these diseases are seen more often when chronic persistent antigenic stimulation occurs from infection, such as malaria or intestinal parasites. Genetic susceptibility also may play a role in the process of malignant transformation. There is increased evidence of NHL in children with congenital immune deficiency syndromes, such as Wiskott-Aldrich syndrome, ataxia-telangiectasia, and Bloom syndrome. Children with acquired immunodeficiency syndrome (AIDS) also are at greater risk for NHL.[78,79] HIV-infected children who develop NHL may have already had a lymphoproliferative disorder such as lymphoid interstitial pneumonitis (LIP) or pulmonary lymphoid hyperplasia (PLH).

CLINICAL MANIFESTATIONS   In children, NHL has been found to arise from any lymphoid tissue. Signs and symptoms therefore are specific for the site involved. Some children have such widespread involvement that no original site can be determined. Because childhood NHL is a rapidly progressive disease, symptoms generally are present only a few weeks before diagnosis is made. Rapidly enlarging lymphoid tissue and painless lymphadenopathy are common in about one third of children with abdominal sites of involvement, usually representing a gastrointestinal origin for the disease. Symptoms often include abdominal pain and vomiting, but a palpable mass is not always present. Most children with abdominal symptoms have diffuse, small noncleaved cell NHL (Burkitt or non-Burkitt) of B cell origin. If the tumor recurs, it appears again in the abdomen before distant spread.

The other common site of childhood NHL is the chest region. An anterior mediastinal mass, with or without pleural effusion, often is present. If the mass is large enough, respiratory compromise, tracheal compression, and superior vena

cava syndrome may arise, which constitute a medical emergency. Children with anterior mediastinal involvement often are male adolescents and usually have diffuse lymphoblastic lymphoma of T cell origin. This form of diffuse lymphoblastic lymphoma often evolves into extensive bone marrow involvement and is considered to be an overt leukemic phase (Figure 28-12); therefore it is referred to as *leukemic transformation*. CNS involvement and testicular infiltration often then occur. CNS involvement occurs in about 30% of individuals with NHL, usually causing multiple deep-seated lesions within the brain parenchyma. In children with AIDS, NHL is the most common mass lesion found in the brain.[79]

Bone marrow involvement is less common than other primary sites, whereas CNS involvement is common. Relatively few children (10% to 20%) with NHL have lymphoid tissue involvement of the head and neck (Waldeyer ring, nasopharynx, sinuses). Signs and symptoms include tonsillitis, sinusitis, and a painless nasopharyngeal mass. In African Burkitt lymphoma, involvement of facial bones, particularly the jaw, is common, although this occurs infrequently in non-African cases.

EVALUATION AND TREATMENT   Diagnosis is made by biopsy of disease sites, usually the involved lymph nodes. Other sites of biopsy include the tonsils, bone marrow, spleen, liver, bowel, or skin. Advances in understanding the disease and progress in treatment strategies have meant that most children with NHL are cured of the disease. Optimal treatment is still being developed, but combination chemotherapy, with or without radiation therapy for prevention of CNS involvement, is being used successfully.[80] Treatment programs are based on the same four phases used in ALL. Radiation therapy may be combined with chemotherapy because lymphoma cells are easily destroyed by radiation. Because of the

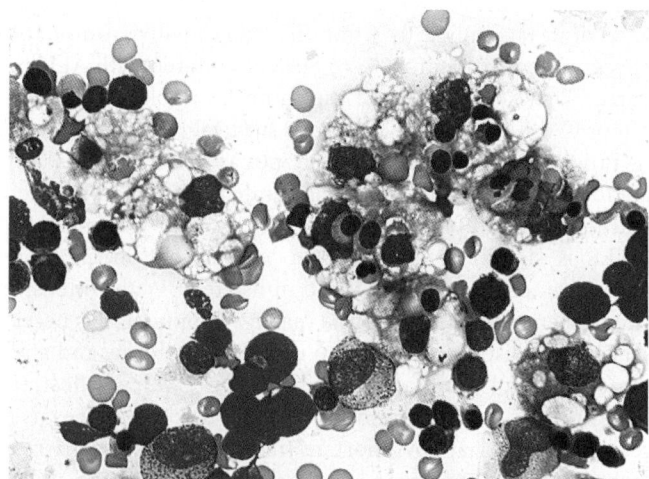

Figure 28-12   Bone marrow aspirate from a child with T cell lymphoma in a lymph node biopsy. There is marked histiocytic hyperplasia. Two of the histiocytes contain phagocytosed red cells. The histiocytic hyperplasia regressed with disease remission and recurred with relapse of the lymphoma (Wright-Giemsa stain). (From Damjanov I, Linder J, editors: *Anderson's pathology*, ed 10, St Louis, 1996, Mosby.)

delay in diagnosis, CNS lymphomas are difficult to treat successfully. Intrathecal chemotherapy is needed in addition to systemic chemotherapy to induce remission.

Children with advanced small noncleaved cell lymphoma of the abdomen have the poorest prognosis. Although remission occurs in more than 90% of these children, most experience subsequent relapses. Even in the presence of advanced lymphoblastic lymphoma, however, 60% to 80% of children can be cured. Children with localized disease in more easily treated sites are likely to be cured with prompt and appropriate treatment. Overall, children with localized diseases have a 90% survival rate and those with advanced disease have a 70% to 80% survival rate.[80]

Hodgkin Disease

Although the etiologic agent for **Hodgkin disease,** a lymphoma, has not been identified in children, an infectious mode of transmission has been implicated. Major interest currently concerns viral activity, particularly in light of the association between the Epstein-Barr virus and African Burkitt lymphoma.[81] Many persons with Hodgkin disease have high EBV titers. At this time, however, the evidence is not sufficient to link EBV infection to Hodgkin disease.

The interest in a viral cause of Hodgkin disease has been supported by epidemiologic studies. The evidence suggests that the risk of Hodgkin disease is associated in part with infectious diseases, immune deficits, and genetic susceptibility. Environmental factors do not seem to be related.[82]

Clustering of cases within families may suggest a genetic predisposition to the disease or common exposure to a causative agent.[83]

Hodgkin disease is rare in childhood. It occurs infrequently in children younger than 2 years, and few cases are observed before age 5 years. A gradual rise in incidence occurs through age 11 years, with a marked increase through adolescence that continues into the thirties. The annual incidence of Hodgkin disease in the United States is 4:1,000,000 in children younger than 15 years.

Individuals typically have painless supraclavicular or cervical adenopathy. These nodes are firm and rubbery and may be sensitive to palpation if they have grown rapidly. At least two thirds of individuals have mediastinal involvement that may cause symptoms ranging from a nonproductive cough to tracheal or bronchial compression leading to airway obstruction. Systemic symptoms may include fatigue, anorexia, weight loss, fever, drenching night sweats, and pruritis.

The Ann Arbor staging system considers extent and location of disease, as well as substage classifications that consider systemic symptoms (presence of fever of 38° C for three consecutive days, drenching night sweats, or unexplained loss of 10% or more of body weight in the 6 months preceding diagnosis). Combination chemotherapy used in conjunction with involved field low-dose radiation has been shown to be an effective treatment, with long-term cure rates reported from 70% to 90%.[84]

SUMMARY REVIEW

Fetal and Neonatal Hematopoiesis
1. After 2 weeks of gestation, circulating erythrocytes play a major role in delivering oxygen to the tissues.
2. Erythropoiesis in the liver and, to a lesser extent, in the spleen and lymph nodes reaches a peak at about 4 months.
3. By the fifth month of gestation, hematopoiesis begins to occur in the bone marrow, and by the time of delivery it is the only significant site of hematopoiesis.
4. A biochemically distinct type of hemoglobin is synthesized during fetal life, including Gower 1, Gower 2, and Portland.

Postnatal Changes in the Blood
1. Blood cell counts tend to rise above adult levels at birth and then decline gradually throughout childhood.
2. The immediate rise in blood cell counts is the result of increased hematopoiesis during fetal life, trauma of birth, and cutting of the umbilical cord.
3. The active rate of fetal erythropoiesis is observed in the large numbers of reticulocytes in the peripheral blood of the full term neonate.
4. Erythrocyte values are age-dependent, and values in males and females are apparent in adolescence.
5. The lymphocyte count is high at birth, and continues to rise in some healthy infants during the first year of life.
6. Platelet counts in full-term neonates are comparable to platelet counts in children and adults.

Disorders of Erythrocytes
1. Iron deficiency anemia is the most common blood disorder of infancy and childhood; the highest incidence occurs between 6 months and 2 years of age.

2. Hemolytic disease of the newborn (HDN) results from incompatibility between the maternal and the fetal blood, which may involve differences in Rh factors or blood type (ABO). Maternal antibodies enter the fetal circulation and cause hemolysis of fetal erythrocytes. Because the immature liver is unable to conjugate and excrete the excess bilirubin that results from the hemolysis, icterus neonatorum or kernicterus or both can develop.
3. Kernicterus, which may result from other causes as well, results in increased breakdown of red blood cells or decreased liver output of enzymes.
4. Infections of the newborn, often acquired by the mother and transmitted to the infant, may result in hemolytic anemia.
5. Glucose-6-phosphate dehydrogenase (G6PD) deficiency is an inherited enzyme deficiency in erythrocytes that results in a disruption of a common pathway of glycolysis, shortening erythrocyte life span.
6. Hereditary spherocytosis is the most common of the hereditary hemolytic states in which there is no abnormality of hemoglobin. The basic defect is an undefined abnormality of the proteins or spectrins of the erythrocyte membrane in which affected cells are unduly permeable to sodium and acquire a characteristic structure.
7. Sickle cell disease is a genetically determined defect of hemoglobin synthesis, inherited by an autosomal recessive transmission; it causes a change in the shape of a red blood cell that results in decreased oxygen or hydration. This disease is most common among Africans, black Americans, and those of Mediterranean descent.

Continued

8. The thalassemias are a heterogeneous group of hereditary hypochromic anemias of varying severity. Basic genetic defects include abnormalities of messenger ribonucleic acid (mRNA) processing or deletion of genetic materials, resulting in a decrease in the chains for hemoglobin.

Disorders of Coagulation and Platelets

1. Hemophilia is a condition characterized by impairment of the coagulation of blood and subsequent tendency to bleed. The classic disease is hereditary and limited to males, being transmitted through the female to the second generation. Many similar conditions attributable to the absence of various clotting factors are now recognized.
2. Von Willebrand disease is a dominantly inherited disease characterized by a vascular abnormality that produces a prolongation of bleeding time and by decreased levels of clotting factor VIII. The platelets in von Willebrand disease have decreased adhesiveness because the plasma factor is absent.
3. Disorders of congenital hypercoagulability and thrombosis include protein C deficiency, protein S deficiency, neonatal purpura fulminans, and antithrombin III deficiency.
4. The acquired antibody-mediated hemorrhagic diseases include idiopathic thrombocytopenic purpura (ITP), autoimmune neonatal thrombocytopenia, and autoimmune vascular purpura.
5. ITP, the most common of the childhood thrombocytopenic purpuras, is a disorder of platelet consumption in which antiplatelet antibodies bind to the plasma membranes of platelets. This results in platelet sequestration and destruction by mononuclear phagocytes at a rate that exceeds the ability of the bone marrow to produce them.

6. Autoimmune neonatal thrombocytopenia is an antibody-mediated disorder that occurs in either autoimmune or alloimmune form.
7. The autoimmune vascular purpuras (allergic purpuras) are caused by the body's responses to allergens in the blood.

Leukemia and Lymphoma

1. The childhood leukemias include, in order of their rate of incidence, acute lymphoblastic leukemia (ALL), acute nonlymphoblastic leukemia (ANLL), and the very rare chronic granulocytic leukemia (CGL).
2. Although the cause of childhood leukemia is not known, it is probably the result of multiple interactions between hereditary or genetic predisposition and environmental influences.
3. Acute lymphoblastic leukemia is a potentially curable disease, with more than 70% to 80% of cases cured.
4. The lymphomas of childhood are non-Hodgkin lymphoma and Hodgkin disease.
5. The origin of non-Hodgkin lymphoma is unknown. Factors that have been implicated include defective host immunity, a viral agent, chronic immunostimulation, and genetic predisposition.
6. Non-Hodgkin lymphoma has a favorable prognosis, with a 70% to 80% cure rate.
7. The risk of Hodgkin disease is associated in part with infectious diseases, immune deficits, and genetic susceptibility.
8. Hodgkin disease is a readily curable disease with survival statistics similar to those of adults.

KEY TERMS

Activated partial thromboplastin time (PTT), 1016
Alpha-thalassemia major, 1014
Alpha-thalassemia minor, 1013
Alpha trait, 1013
Antithrombin III (AT III) deficiency, 1017
Aplastic crisis, 1011
Autoimmune neonatal thrombocytopenia, 1018
Autoimmune vascular purpura (allergic purpura), 1019
Beta-thalassemia major (Cooley anemia), 1013
Beta-thalassemia minor, 1013
Blast cell, 1022
Embryonic hemoglobin (Gower 1, Gower 2, and Portland), 1000
Fetal hemoglobin (Hb F), 1000
Glucose-6-phosphate dehydrogenase (G6PD) deficiency, 1006
Hemoglobin H disease, 1013

Hemoglobin S (Hb S), 1007
Hemolytic disease of the newborn (HDN) (erythroblastosis fetalis), 1002
Hemophilia A (classic hemophilia), 1015
Hemophilia B (Christmas disease), 1015
Hemophilia C (factor XI deficiency), 1015
Hereditary spherocytosis, 1007
Hodgkin disease, 1025
Hydrops fetalis, 1004
Hyperbilirubinemia, 1004
Hyperhemolytic crisis, 1012
Icterus gravis neonatorum, 1005
Icterus neonatorum (neonatal jaundice), 1004
Idiopathic thrombocytopenic purpura (ITP) (autoimmune or primary thrombocytopenic purpura), 1017
Kernicterus, 1004
Neonatal alloimmune thrombocytopenic purpura (NATP), 1018
Neonatal purpura fulminans, 1017

Non-Hodgkin lymphoma (NHL), 1023
Polymerization, 1010
Preimplantation genetic diagnosis, 1013
Protein C deficiency, 1017
Protein S deficiency, 1017
Prothrombin consumption time, 1016
Prothrombin time (PT), 1016
Sequestration crisis, 1011
Sickle cell anemia, 1008
Sickle cell disease, 1007
Sickle cell trait, 1008
Sickle cell–Hb C disease, 1008
Sickle cell–thalassemia disease, 1008
Thalassemia, 1013
Thrombin time, 1016
Thrombophilia, 1016
Thromboplastin generation test, 1016
Vasoocclusive crisis (thrombotic crisis), 1010
von Willebrand disease, 1015

REFERENCES

1. Graham BS: Pathogenesis of respiratory syncytial virus vaccine-augmented pathology, *Am J Respir Crit Care Med* 152(4Pt2):S63-S66, 1995.
2. Schelonka RL et al: Differentiation of segmented and band neutrophils during the early newborn period, *J Pediatr* 127(2):298-300, 1995.
3. Bartlett JA et al: Immune function in healthy inner-city children, *Clin Diagn Lab Immunol* 8(4):740-746, 2001.
4. Cunningham AS: Eosinophil counts—age and sex differences, *J Pediatr* 87(3):426-427, 1975.
5. Kuhne T, Imbach P: Neonatal platelet physiology and pathophysiology, *Eur J Pediatr* 157(2):87-94, 1998.
6. Khan JL et al: Persistence and emergence of anemia in children during participation in the Special Supplemental Nutrition Program for Women, Infants, and Children, *Arch Pediatr Adolesc Med* 156(10): 1028-1032, 2002.
7. Centers for Disease Control and Prevention: Iron deficiency—United States, *MMWR* 51(40):897, 2002.
8. Farhi DC, Luebbers EL, Rosenthal NS: Bone marrow biopsy findings in childhood anemia: prevalence of transient erythroblastopenia of childhood, *Arch Pathol Lab Med* 122(7):638-641, 1998.
9. Shah M et al: Effects of orange and apple juice on iron absorption in children, *Arch Pediatr Adolesc Med* 157(12):1232-1236, 2003.
10. Mamula P et al: Total dose intravenous infusion of iron dextran for iron-deficiency anemia in children with inflammatory bowel disease, *J Pediatr Gastroenterol Nutr* 34(3):286-290, 2002.
11. Nickerson HJ: Treatment of iron deficiency anemia and associated protein-losing enteropathy in children, *J Pediatr Hematol Oncol* 22(1): 50-54, 2000.
12. Bowman J: The management of hemolytic disease in the fetus and newborn, *Semin Perinatol* 21(1):39-44, 1997.
13. Urbaniak SJ: The scientific basis of antenatal prophylaxis, *Br J Obstet Gynaecol* 105(suppl 18):11-18, 1998.
14. Hampl JS et al: Acute hemolysis related to consumption of fava beans: a case study and medical nutrition therapy approach, *J Am Diet Assoc* 97(2):182-183, 1997.
15. Iolascon A, Perrotta S, Stewart GW: Red blood cell membrane defects. *Rev Clin Exp Hematol* 7(1):22-56, 2003.
16. Delhommeau F et al: Natural history of hereditary spherocytosis during the first year of life, *Blood* 95(2):393-397, 2000.
17. Rice HE et al: Clinical and hematologic benefits of partial splenectomy for congenital hemolytic anemias in children, *Ann Surg* 237(2):281-288, 2003.
18. Gibson, JS, Ellory JC: Membrane transport in sickle cell disease, *Blood Cells Mol Dis* 28(3):303-314, 2002.
19. Gill FM et al: Clinical events in the first decade of a cohort of infants with sickle cell disease: Cooperative Study of Sickle Cell Disease, *Blood* 86(2):776-783, 1995.
20. Platt OS: The acute chest syndrome of sickle cell disease, *N Engl J Med* 342(25):1904 (editorial), 2000.
21. Wigfall DR et al: Prevalence and clinical correlates of glomerulopathy in children with sickle cell disease, *J Pediatr* 136(6):749-753, 2000.
22. Wethers DL: Sickle cell disease in childhood. Part I. Laboratory diagnosis, pathophysiology and health maintenance, *Am Fam Physician* 62(5):1013-1020, 1027-1028, 2000.
23. Wethers DL: Sickle cell disease in childhood. Part II. Diagnosis and treatment of major complications and recent advances in treatment, *Am Fam Physician* 62(6):1309-1314, 2000.
24. Beyer JE: Judging the effectiveness of analgesia for children and adolescents during vaso-occlusive events of sickle cell disease, *J Pain Symptom Manage* 19(1):63-72, 2000.
25. Melzer-Lange MD et al: Patient-controlled analgesia for sickle cell pain crisis in a pediatric emergency department, *Pediatr Emerg Care* 20(1): 2-4, 2004.
26. Zimmerman SA et al: Sustained long-term hematologic efficacy of hydroxyurea at maximum tolerated dose in children with sickle cell disease, *Blood* 103(6):2039-2045, 2004.
27. Caruso-Nicoletti M et al: Short stature and body proportion in thalassaemia, *J Pediatr Endocrinol Metab* 11(suppl 3):811-816, 1998.
28. Goldman RD, Blanchette V, Koren G: Hemophilia during pregnancy, *Can Fam Physician* 49:1601-1603, 2003.
29. O'Connell NM: Factor XI deficiency, *Semin Hematol* 41(1 Suppl 1): 76-81, 2004.
30. Bowen DJ: Haemophilia A and haemophilia B: molecular insights, *Mol Pathol* 55(2):127-144, 2002.
31. Pollmann H et al: When are children diagnosed as having severe haemophilia and when do they start to bleed? A 10-year single-centre PUP study, *Eur J Pediatr* 158(suppl 3):S166-S170, 1999.
32. Roberts HR: Factor VIII replacement therapy: issues and future prospects, *Ann N Y Acad Sci* 614:106-113, 1991.
33. Centers for Disease Control and Prevention: Transmission of hepatitis C virus infection associated with home infusion therapy for hemophilia, *MMWR* 46(26):597, 1997.
34. Chudy M et al: A new cluster of hepatitis A infection in hemophiliacs traced to a contaminated plasma pool, *J Med Virol* 57(2):91-99, 1999.
35. Soucie JM et al: Hepatitis A virus infections associated with clotting factor concentrate in the United States, *Transfusion* 38(6):573-579, 1998.
36. Woelflel J et al: GB virus C/hepatitis G virus infection in HIV infected patients with haemophilia despite treatment with inactivated clotting factor concentrates, *Arch Dis Child* 80(5):429-432, 1999.
37. Ananyeva N et al: Treating hemophilia A with recombinant blood factors: a comparison, *Expert Opin Pharmacother* 5(5):1061-1070, 2004.
38. Manco-Johnson MJ: Update on treatment regimens: prophylaxis versus on-demand therapy, *Semin Hematol* 40(3 Suppl 3):3-9, 2003.
39. Spencer FA: Key references: protein C, protein S and antithrombin deficiencies, *J Thromb Thrombolysis* 9(1):127, 2000.
40. Gomez K, Laffan MA: Hunting for the mutation in inherited thrombophilia, *Blood Coagul Fibrinolysis* 15(2):125-127, 2004.
41. Ezer U et al: Neonatal purpura fulminans due to homozygous protein C deficiency, *Pediatr Hematol Oncol* 18(7):453-458, 2001.
42. Kubota M et al: Serum immunoglobulin levels at onset: association with the prognosis of childhood idiopathic thrombocytopenic purpura, *Int J Hematol* 77(3):304-307, 2003.
43. Bussel JB, Corrigan JJ: Platelet and vascular disorders. In Miller DR, Baehner RL, Miller LP, editors: *Blood diseases of infancy and childhood*, ed 7, St Louis, 1995, Mosby.
44. Carcao MD et al: Short-course oral prednisone therapy in children presenting with acute immune thrombocytopenia (ITP), *Acta Paediatr Suppl* 424:71-74, 1998.
45. Vesely S et al: Self-reported diagnostic and management strategies in childhood idiopathic thrombocytopenic purpura: results of a survey of practicing pediatric hematology/oncology specialists, *J Pediatr Hematol Oncol* 22(1):55-61, 2000.
46. Blanchette V, Freeman J, Garvey B: Management of chronic immune thrombocytopenic purpura in children and adults, *Semin Hematol* 35(1Suppl 1):36-51, 1998.
47. Laosombat V, Wiriyasateinkul A, Wongchanchailert M: Intravenous gamma globulin for treatment of chronic idiopathic thrombocytopenic purpura in children, *J Med Assoc Thai* 83(2):160-168, 2000.
48. Moser AM, Shalev H, Kapelushnik J: Anti-D exerts a very early response in childhood acute idiopathic thrombocytopenic purpura, *Pediatr Hematol Oncol* 19(6):407-411, 2002.
49. Tarantino MD: Treatment options for chronic immune (idiopathic) thrombocytopenia purpura in children, *Semin Hematol* 37(1Suppl 1): 35-41, 2000.
50. Kaplan C: Immune thrombocytopenia in the fetus and the newborn: diagnosis and therapy, *Transfus Clin Biol* 8(3):311-314, 2001.
51. Hilgartner MW, Corrigan JJ Jr: Coagulation disorders. In Miller DR, Baehner RL, Miller LP, editors: *Blood diseases of infancy and childhood*, ed 6, St Louis, 1995, Mosby.
52. Wartenberg D, Schneider D, Brown S: Childhood leukaemia incidence and the population mixing hypothesis in US SEER data, *Br J Cancer* 90(9):1771-1776, 2004.
53. Biondi A, Masera G: Molecular pathogenesis of childhood acute lymphoblastic leukemia, *Haematologica* 83(7):651-659, 1998.
54. Ma SK, Wan TS, Chan LC: Cytogenetics and molecular genetics of childhood leukemia, *Hematol Oncol* 17(3):91-105, 1999.
55. Strout MP, Caligiuri MA: Developments in cytogenetics and oncogenes in acute leukemia, *Curr Opin Oncol* 9(1):8-17, 1997.

56. Bennett J et al: French-American-British (FAB) Cooperative Group: the morphological classification of acute lymphoblastic leukaemia—concordance among observers and clinical correlations, *Br J Haematol* 47(4):553-561, 1981.

57. Khalidi HS et al: Acute lymphoblastic leukemia. Survey of immunophenotype, French-American-British classification, frequency of myeloid antigen expression, and karyotypic abnormalities in 210 pediatric and adult cases, *Am J Clin Pathol* 111(4):467-476, 1999.

58. Orfao A et al: Clinically useful information provided by the flow cytometric immunophenotyping of hematological malignancies: current status and future directions, *Clin Chem* 45(10):1708-1717, 1999.

59. Greaves MF et al: Leukemia in twins: lessons on natural history, *Blood* 102(7):2321-2333, 2003.

60. Infante-Rivard C, Guiguet M: Family history of hematopoietic and other cancers in children with acute lymphoblastic leukemia, *Cancer Detect Prev* 28(2):83-87, 2004.

61. Golub TR, Weinstein HJ, Grier HE: Acute myelogenous leukemia. In Pizzo PA, Poplack DG, editors: *Principles and practices of pediatric oncology*, ed 3, Philadelphia, 1997, Lippincott-Raven.

62. Alexander FE, Greaves MF: Ionising radiation and leukaemia potential risks: review based on the workshop held during the 10th Symposium on Molecular Biology of Hematopoesis and Treatment of Leukemia and Lymphomas at Hamburg Germany on 5 July 1997, *Leukemia* 12(8):1319-1323, 1998.

63. Murray R, Heckel P, Hempelmann L: Leukemia in children exposed to ionizing radiation, *N Engl J Med* 261:585, 1959.

64. Doll R, Wakeford R: Risk of childhood cancer from fetal irradiation, *Br J Radiol* 70:130-139, 1997.

65. Boice JD Jr, Miller RW: Childhood and adult cancer after intrauterine exposure to ionizing radiation, *Teratology* 59(4):227-233, 1999.

66. UK Childhood Cancer Study Investigators: The United Kingdom Child Cancer Study of exposure to domestic sources of ionizing radiation: 1: radon gas, *Br J Cancer* 86(11):1721-1726, 2002.

67. Hardell L et al: Exposure to extremely low frequency electromagnetic fields and the risk of malignant diseases: an evaluation of epidemiological and experimental findings, *Eur J Cancer Prev* 4:3-107, 1995.

68. Levallois P: Do power frequency magnetic fields cause leukemia in children? *Am J Prev Med* 11(4):263-270, 1995.

69. Thomas DC et al: Residential magnetic fields predicted from wiring configurations: relationships to childhood leukemia, *Bioelectromagnetics* 20(7):414-422, 1999.

70. Habash RW et al: Health risks of electromagnetic fields. Part I: evaluation and assessment of electric and magnetic fields, *Crit Rev Biomed Eng* 31(3):141-195, 2003.

71. Waller LA et al: Detection and assessment of clusters of disease: an application to nuclear power plant facilities and childhood leukemia in Sweden, *Stat Med* 14(1):3-16, 1995.

72. Lagakos SW, Wessen BJ, Zelen M: An analysis of contaminated well water and health effects in Woburn, Massachusetts, *J Am Stat Assoc* 81: 583, 1986.

73. Margolin JF, Poplack DG: Acute lymphocytic leukemia. In Pizzo PA, Poplack DG, editors: *Principles and practice of pediatric oncology*, ed 3, Philadelphia, 1997, Lippincott-Raven.

74. Silverman LB et al: Induction failure in acute lymphoblastic leukemia of childhood, *Cancer* 85(6):1395-1404, 1999.

75. Koh S et al: Anterior lumbosacral radiculopathy after intrathecal methotrexate treatment, *Pediatr Neurol* 21(2):576-578, 1999.

76. Hodgson PS et al: The neurotoxicity of drugs given intrathecally (spinal), *Anesth Analg* 88(4):797-809, 1999.

77. Granovsky MO et al: Cancer in human immunodeficiency virus–infected children: a case series from the Children's Cancer Group and the National Cancer Institute, *J Clin Oncol* 16(5):1729-1735, 1998.

78. Magrath IT: Malignant non-Hodgkin's lymphoma in children, *Hematol Oncol Clin North Am* 1(4):577-602, 1987.

79. Mueller BU, Pizzo PA: Cancer in children with primary or secondary immunodeficiencies, *J Pediatr* 126(1):1-10, 1995.

80. Shad A, Mcgrath I: Malignant non-Hodgkin's lymphomas in children. In Pizzo PA, Poplack DG, editors: *Principles and practices of pediatric oncology*, ed 3, Philadelphia, 1997, Lippincott-Raven.

81. Goldenberg D et al: Epstein-Barr virus and cancers of the head and neck, *Am J Otolaryngol* 22(3):197-205, 2001.

82. Cartwright RA, Watkins G: Epidemiology of Hodgkin's disease: a review, *Hematol Oncol* 22(1):11-26, 2004.

83. Oliapuram Jose B et al: Pediatric Hodgkin's disease, *J Ky Med Assoc* 102(3):104-106, 2004.

84. Smith RS et al: Prognostic factors for children with Hodgkin's disease treated with combined-modality therapy, *J Clin Oncol* 21(10): 2026-2033, 2003.

STRUCTURE AND FUNCTION OF THE CARDIOVASCULAR AND LYMPHATIC SYSTEMS

KATHRYN L. McCANCE

CHAPTER OUTLINE

evolve

http://evolve.elsevier.com/McCance/

The function of the circulatory system is simple: to deliver oxygen, nutrients, and other substances to all the body's cells and to remove the waste products of cellular metabolism. Delivery and removal are achieved by a wonderfully complex array of tubing—the blood vessels—connected to a pump—the heart. The heart pumps blood continuously through the blood vessels with cooperation from other systems, particularly the nervous and endocrine systems, which are intrinsic regulators of the heart and blood vessels. Nutrients and oxygen are supplied by the digestive and respiratory systems; gaseous wastes of cellular metabolism are blown off by the lungs; and other wastes are removed by the kidneys.

Evolving is the role of the vascular endothelium. It is a multifunctional organ whose health is essential to normal vascular physiology and whose dysfunction is a critical factor in the pathogenesis of vascular disease.

CIRCULATORY SYSTEM

The heart pumps blood through two separate circulatory systems, one to the lungs and one to all other parts of the body. Structures on the right side of the heart, or **right heart,** pump blood through the lungs. (This system, termed the **pulmonary circulation,** is described in Chapter 32.) The left side of the heart, or **left heart,** sends blood throughout the

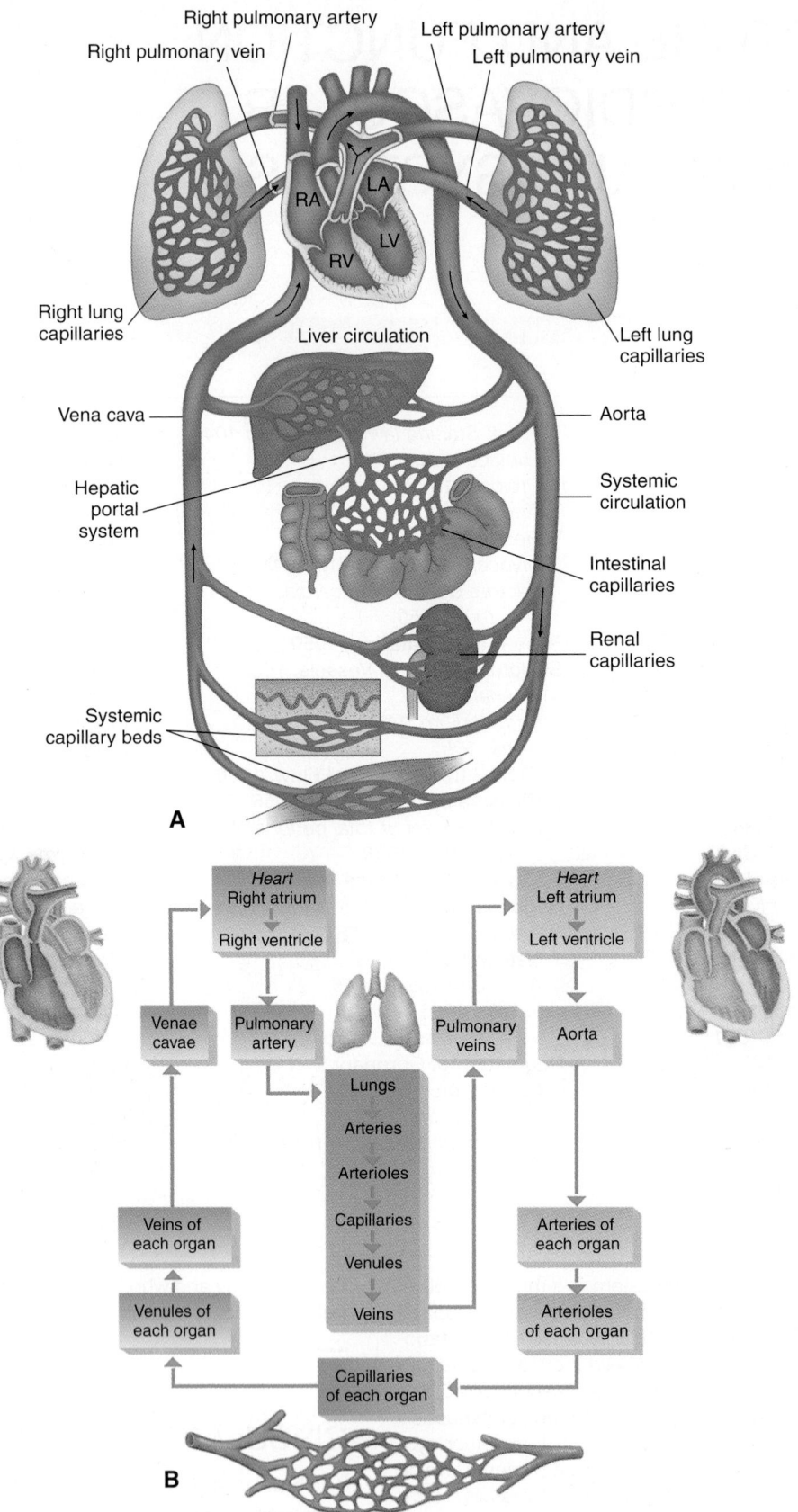

Figure 29-1 Diagram showing serially connected pulmonary and systemic circulatory systems and how to trace the flow of blood. **A,** Right heart chambers propel unoxygenated blood through the pulmonary circulation, and the left heart propels oxygenated blood through the systemic circulation. **B,** The direction of blood flow begins at the left ventricle of the heart, flows to arteries, arterioles, capillaries of each body organ, venules, veins, right atrium, right ventricle, pulmonary artery, lung capillaries, pulmonary veins, left atrium, and then goes back to left ventricle. *RA,* Right atrium; *RV,* right ventricle; *LA,* left atrium, *LV,* left ventricle. (**B** from Thibodeau GA, Patton KT: *Anatomy & physiology,* ed 5, St. Louis, 2003, Mosby.)

systemic circulation, which supplies all of the body except the lungs (Figure 29-1). These two systems are serially connected; thus the output of one becomes the input of the other.

Arteries carry blood from the heart to all parts of the body, where they branch into even smaller vessels until they become a fine meshwork of capillaries. Capillaries allow the closest contact and exchange between the blood and the interstitial space, or interstitium—the environment in which the cells live. Veins channel blood from capillaries in all parts of the body back to the heart. The plasma passes through the walls of the capillaries into the interstitial space. This fluid eventually is returned to the cardiovascular system by vessels of the lymphatic system.

THE HEART

The adult heart weighs less than 1 pound and is about the size of a fist. It lies obliquely (diagonally) in the **mediastinum,** an area above the diaphragm and between the lungs. The heart of a normal woman is smaller and lighter than that of a normal man.

Heart structures can be categorized by function:

1. *Structural support of heart tissues and circulation of pulmonary and systemic blood through the heart.* This category includes the heart wall and fibrous skeleton, which enclose and support the heart and divide it into four chambers; the valves that direct flow through the chambers; and the great vessels that conduct blood to and from the heart.
2. *Maintenance of heart cells.* This category comprises vessels of the coronary circulation—the arteries and veins that serve the metabolic needs of all the heart cells—and the lymphatic vessels of the heart.
3. *Stimulation and control of heart action.* Among these structures are the nerves and specialized muscle cells that direct the rhythmic contraction and relaxation of the heart muscles, propelling blood throughout the pulmonary and systemic circulatory system.

Structures that Direct Circulation Through the Heart

Heart Wall

The heart wall has three layers—the pericardium, myocardium, and endocardium. The pericardium is a double-walled membranous sac that encloses the heart (Figure 29-2). The **pericardium** has several functions. It (1) prevents displacement of the heart during gravitational acceleration or deceleration, (2) is a physical barrier that protects the heart against infection and inflammation from the lungs and pleural space, and (3) contains pain receptors and mechanoreceptors that can elicit reflex changes in blood pressure and heart rate. The outer layer of the pericardium, the **parietal pericardium,** is composed of a surface layer of mesothelium over a thin layer of connective tissue. The **visceral pericardium,** or **epicardium,** is the inner layer of the pericardium. At one point the visceral pericardium folds back and becomes con-

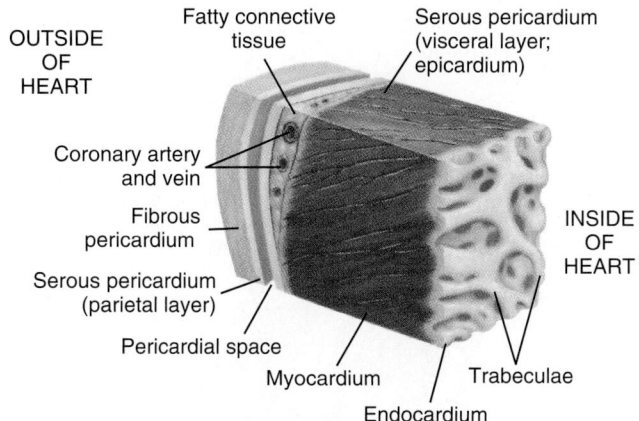

Figure 29-2 Wall of the heart. This section of the heart wall shows the fibrous pericardium, the parietal and visceral layers of the serous pericardium (with the pericardial space between them), the myocardium, and the endocardium. Note the fatty connective tissue between the visceral layer of the serous pericardium (epicardium) and the myocardium. Note also that the endocardium covers beamlike projections of myocardial muscle tissue, called *trabeculae.* (From Thibodeau GA, Patton KT: *Anatomy & physiology,* ed 5, St Louis, 2003, Mosby.)

tinuous with the parietal pericardium, allowing the large vessels to enter and leave the heart without breaching the pericardial layers.

The visceral and parietal pericardia are separated by a fluid-containing space called the **pericardial cavity.** The **pericardial fluid** (10 to 30 ml), which is secreted by cells of the mesothelium, lubricates the membranes that line the pericardial cavity, enabling them to slide over one another with a minimum of friction as the heart beats. The amount and character of the pericardial fluid are altered by inflammation of the pericardium (see Chapter 30).

The thickest layer of the heart wall, the **myocardium,** is composed of cardiac muscle and is anchored to the heart's fibrous skeleton. The thickness of the myocardium varies tremendously from one heart chamber to another. Thickness is related to the amount of resistance the muscle must overcome to pump blood from the different chambers. The internal lining of the myocardium is composed of connective tissue and a layer of squamous cells called the **endocardium** (see Figure 29-2). The endocardial lining of the heart is continuous with the endothelium that lines all the arteries, veins, and capillaries of the body, creating a continuous, closed circulatory system.

Chambers of the Heart

The heart has four chambers: the **right atrium, left atrium, right ventricle,** and **left ventricle.** (Blood flow through these chambers is illustrated in Figure 29-3.) The atria are smaller than the ventricles and have thinner walls. The wall of the right atrium is about 2 mm thick, and the wall of the left atrium is about 3 to 5 mm thick. The ventricles have a thicker myocardial layer and make up much of the bulk of the heart. The wall of the right ventricle is about 3 to 5 mm thick, and that of the left ventricle, the most muscular chamber, is about

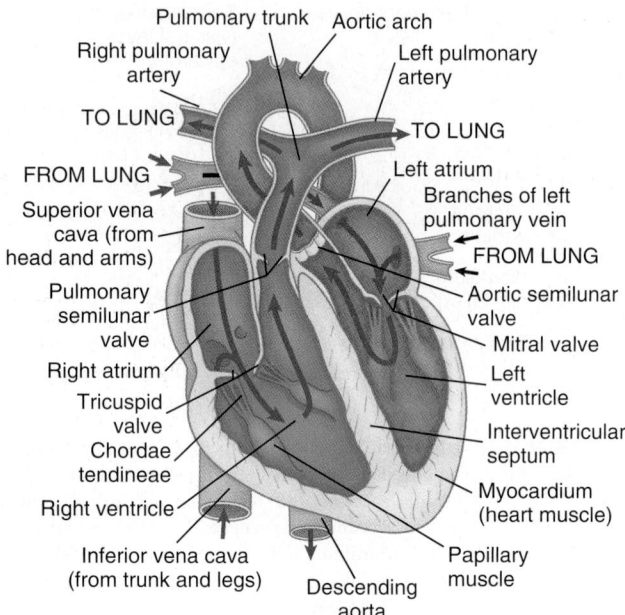

Figure 29-3 **Structures that direct blood flow through the heart.** Arrows indicate path of blood flow through chambers, valves, and major vessels.

13 to 15 mm. The ventricles are formed by a continuum of muscle fibers that take origin from the fibrous skeleton at the base of the heart (chiefly around the aortic orifice).

The myocardial thickness of each cardiac chamber depends on the amount of pressure or resistance it must overcome to eject blood. The two atria have the thinnest walls because they are low-pressure chambers that serve as storage units and conduits for blood that is emptied into the ventricles. Normally, there is little resistance to flow from the atria to the ventricles. The ventricles, on the other hand, must propel blood all the way through the pulmonary or systemic circulation. The ventricular myocardium also must be strong enough to pump against pressures in the pulmonary or systemic vessels. The mean pulmonary capillary pressure, which is the major force favoring movement of fluid out of the pulmonary capillaries into the interstitium, is only 15 mmHg. By comparison, the mean arterial pressure is about 92 mmHg. Pressure is greatest in the systemic circulation, driven by the left ventricle; the left ventricle's myocardium is several times thicker than that of the right ventricle.

The right ventricle is shaped like a crescent, or triangle, enabling it to function like a bellows and efficiently eject large volumes of blood through a very small valve into the low-pressure pulmonary system. The left ventricle is larger and bullet shaped, helping it to eject blood through a relatively large valve opening into the high-pressure systemic circulation.

The ventricles are structurally more complex than the atria. Each ventricle contains muscle fibers that divide it roughly into an **inflow tract,** which receives blood from the atrium, and an **outflow tract,** which sends blood to the circulation (see Figure 29-3).

Normally, blood does not flow between the chambers of the right side of the heart and the chambers of the left side of the heart. The adult right and left sides of the heart are separated by an intact septal membrane. The atria are separated by the interatrial septum, and the ventricles by the interventricular septum. The interventricular septum is an extension of the fibrous skeleton of the heart. Indentations of the endocardium form valves that separate the atria from the ventricles and the ventricles from the aorta and pulmonary arteries.

Fibrous Skeleton of the Heart

Four rings of dense fibrous connective tissue provide a firm anchorage for the attachments of the atrial and ventricular musculature, as well as the valvular tissue. The fibrous rings are adjacent and form a central, fibrous supporting structure collectively termed the anuli fibrosi cordis.

Valves of the Heart

One-way blood flow through the heart is ensured by the four heart valves. During ventricular relaxation the two **atrioventricular valves** open and blood flows from the higher-pressure atria to the relaxed ventricles. With increasing ventricular pressure these valves close and prevent backflow into the atria as the ventricles contract. The **semilunar valves** of the heart open when intraventricular pressure exceeds aortic and pulmonary pressures and blood flows out of the ventricles and into the pulmonary and systemic circulations. After ventricular contraction and ejection, intraventricular pressure falls and the **pulmonic** and **aortic semilunar valves** close, preventing backflow into the right and left ventricles (Figure 29-4; see also Figure 29-3).

The heart valve openings are guarded by flaps of tissue called *leaflets or cusps* that are attached to the papillary muscles by the **chordae tendineae** (see Figure 29-3). The **papillary muscles** are extensions of the myocardium that pull the cusps together and downward at the onset of ventricular contraction, thus preventing their backward expulsion into the atria. (See p. 1033 for a description of pressure changes and valvular function.)

The right atrioventricular valve is called the **tricuspid valve** because it has three cusps. The tricuspid opening (orifice) has the largest diameter of all the heart valves. The left atrioventricular valve is a bicuspid (two-cusp) valve called the **mitral valve.** The mitral valve resembles a cone-shaped funnel that extends into the cusps, which are connected by a fibrous tissue called the *commissure.* The anterior cusp of the mitral valve is continuous with supporting tissues of the aortic semilunar valve cusps and the left coronary valve cusps. (The coronary circulation is described on p. 1034.) Thus damage to this continuous tissue can alter function of both the aortic and mitral valves.

The tricuspid and mitral valves function as a unit because the atrium, fibrous rings, valvular tissue, chordae tendineae, papillary muscles, and ventricular walls are connected. Collectively, these six structures are known as the **mitral and tricuspid complex.** Damage to any one of the complex's six components can alter function significantly.

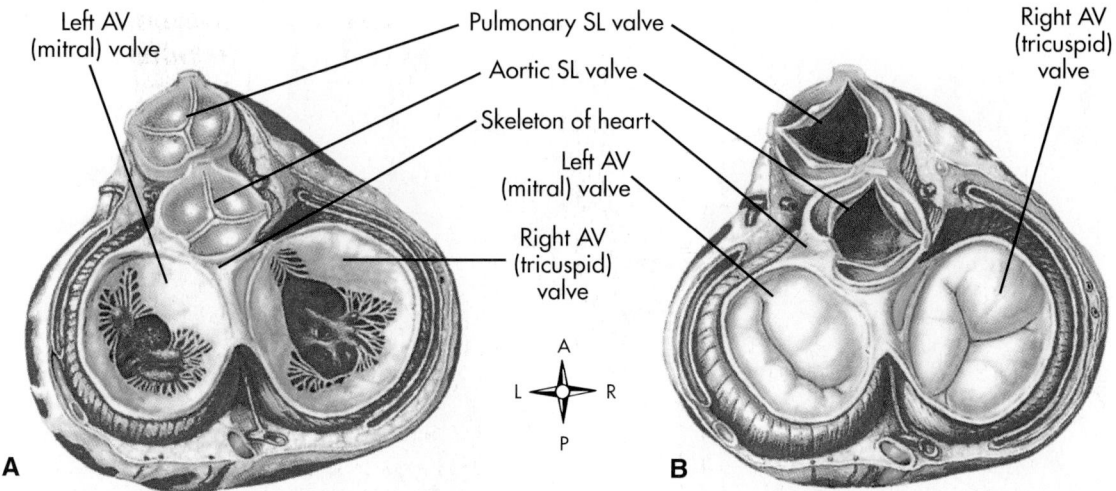

Figure 29-4 Structure of the heart valves. A, The heart valves in this drawing are depicted as viewed from above (looking down into the heart). Note that the semilunar (SL) valves are closed and the atrioventricular (AV) valves are open, as when the atria are contracting. **B,** Similar to **A** except that the semilunar valves are closed and the atrioventricular valves are open, as when the ventricles are contracting. (From Thibodeau GA, Patton KT: *Anatomy & physiology,* ed 5, St Louis, 2003, Mosby.)

Blood leaves the right ventricle through the pulmonic semilunar valve, and it leaves the left ventricle through the aortic semilunar valve (see Figures 29-3 and 29-4). Both the pulmonic and aortic semilunar valves have three cup-shaped cusps that arise from the fibrous skeleton. The pulmonic cusps are slightly thinner than the aortic cusps. The lower edges of each cusp are suspended from the root of the pulmonary artery or aorta, with the upper valve edges freely projecting into the vessel lumen. When the ventricles contract, the cusps behave like one-way swinging doors. The force of the blood propels the cusps outward against the vessel wall. When the ventricles relax, blood fills the cusps and causes their free edges to meet in the middle of the vessel, closing the valve and preventing any backflow.

Great Vessels

Blood moves in and out of the heart through several large vessels (see Figure 29-3). The right heart receives venous blood from the systemic circulation through the **superior** and **inferior venae cavae,** which enter the right atrium. Blood leaves the right ventricle and enters the pulmonary circulation through the pulmonary artery. The **pulmonary artery** divides into **right** and **left pulmonary arteries** to transport unoxygenated blood from the right heart to the right and left lungs. The pulmonary arteries branch further into the pulmonary capillary bed, where oxygen and carbon dioxide exchange occurs.

The four **pulmonary veins,** two from the right lung and two from the left lung, carry oxygenated blood from the lungs to the left side of the heart. The oxygenated blood moves through the left atrium and ventricle and out into the **aorta,** which delivers it to systemic vessels that supply the body.

Blood Flow During the Cardiac Cycle

The pumping action of the heart consists of contraction and relaxation of the myocardial layer of the heart wall. Each contraction and the relaxation that follows it constitute one **car-**

diac cycle. (Blood flow through the heart during a single cardiac cycle is illustrated in Figure 29-5.) During relaxation, termed **diastole,** blood fills the ventricles. The contraction that follows, termed **systole,** propels the blood out of the ventricles and into the circulation. Contraction of the left ventricle is slightly earlier than contraction of the right ventricle.

During diastole, blood from the veins of the systemic circulation enters the thin-walled right atrium from the superior vena cava and the inferior vena cava (see Figures 29-3 and 29-5). Venous blood from the coronary circulation enters the right atrium through the coronary sinus. The right atrium fills and distends, pushing open the right atrioventricular (tricuspid) valve. This permits blood to fill the right ventricle. The same sequence of events occurs a split second earlier in the left heart. The four pulmonary veins, two from the right lung and two from the left lung, carry blood from the pulmonary circulation to the left atrium. As the left atrium fills, it pushes the cusps of the mitral valve open and blood flows into the left ventricle. Left atrial contraction, "atrial kick," provides a significant increase of blood to the left ventricle. Filling of the right and left sides of the heart occurs during one period of diastole.

Four phases of the cardiac cycle can be identified on initiation of ventricular myocardial contraction (Figure 29-6):

Phase 1: Systole begins with "isovolumic contraction," so-called because ventricular volume is constant; that is, the lengths of the muscle fibers remain relatively constant. Isovolumic contraction is the first detectable rise in left ventricular pressure. Contraction pushes the atrioventricular valves shut. Their cusps bulge backward but are prevented from opening back into the atria by their anchors, the chordae tendineae (see Figure 29-3).

Phase 2: When left ventricular pressure reaches that of the aorta, the aortic valve opens and ventricular ejection occurs. Intraventricular pressure and ventricular volume decrease rapidly.

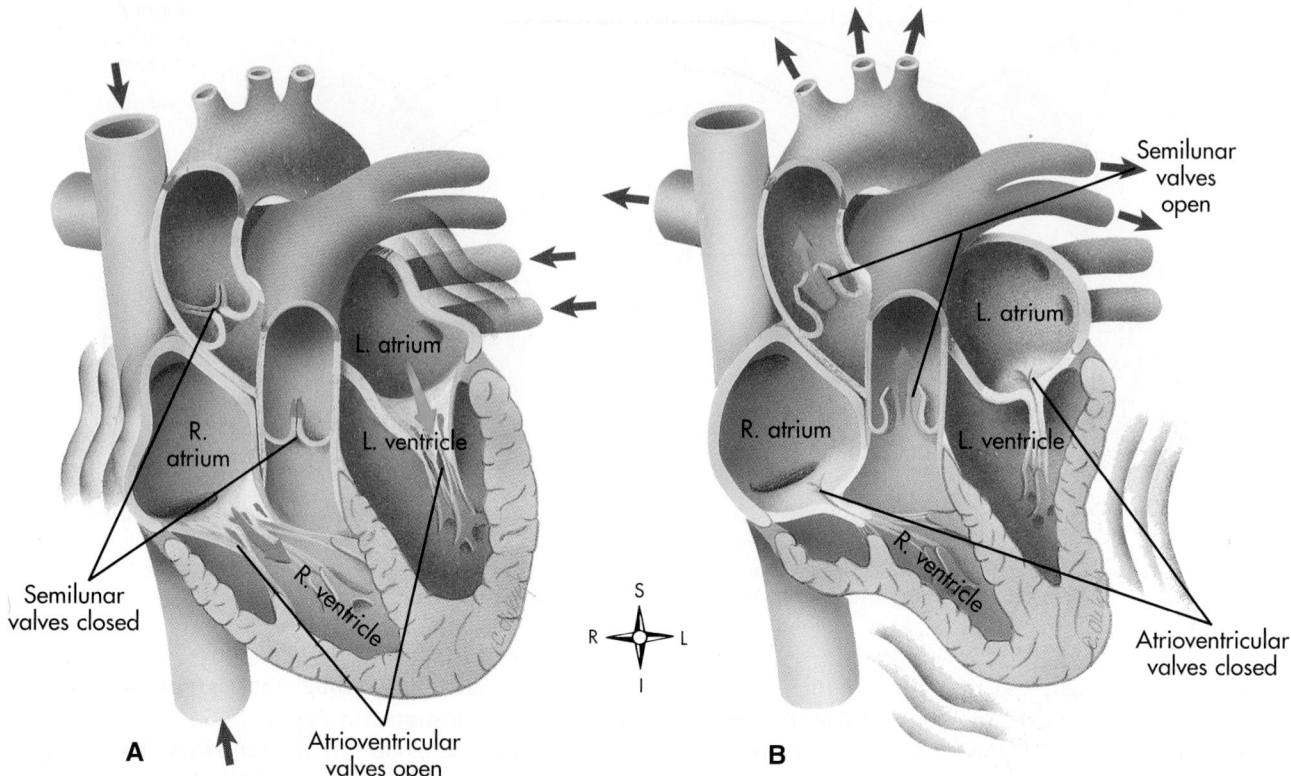

Figure 29-5 **Chambers and valves of the heart.** These illustrations depict the action of the heart chambers and valves when the atria contract (**A**) and when the ventricles contract (**B**). (From Thibodeau GA, Patton KT: *Anatomy & physiology,* ed 5, St Louis, 2003, Mosby.)

Phase 3: With left ventricular relaxation and decreased ventricular pressure, the aortic valve closes and "isovolumic relaxation" occurs.

Phase 4: When sufficient decreases exist in left ventricular pressure, the mitral valve opens and ventricular filling from the atrium occurs.

The ventricle fills rapidly in early diastole and again in late diastole when the atrium contracts. As blood is pushed through the inflow and outflow tracts of the ventricles, it flows around the **crista supraventricularis**—the muscle that separates the inflow from the outflow tracts—and is mixed by passing through the strands of the **trabeculae carneae.** Expulsion of blood from the ventricles marks the end of one cardiac cycle.

Normal Intracardiac Pressures

Normal intracardiac pressures are shown in Table 29-1 and Figures 29-6 and 29-7. Atrial pressure curves are composed of the **a wave,** which is generated by atrial contraction, and the **v wave,** which is an early diastolic peak caused by filling of the atrium from the peripheral veins. The **x descent** follows the a wave and is produced because of descent of the tricuspid valve ring and by the ejection of blood from both ventricles. The **y descent** follows the v wave and reflects the rapid flow of blood from the great veins and right atrium into the right ventricle. A small deflection, the **c wave,** occurs after the a wave in early systole and may represent bulging of the mitral

valve into the left atrium during early systole. Ventricular pressures are illustrated by a peak systolic pressure and an end-diastolic pressure, which is the ventricular pressure immediately before the onset of systole. The minimal left ventricular pressure occurs in early diastole.

Structures that Support Cardiac Metabolism: The Coronary Vessels

The blood within the heart chambers does not supply oxygen and other nutrients to the cells of the heart. Like all other organs, including the lungs, heart structures are nourished by vessels of the systemic circulation. The branch of the systemic circulation that supplies the heart is termed the *coronary circulation* and consists of coronary arteries, which receive blood through openings in the aorta, called the *coronary ostia,* and the cardiac veins, which empty into the right atrium through another ostium, the opening of a large vein called the *coronary sinus* (Figure 29-8). (Regulation of the coronary circulation, which is similar to regulation of flow through systemic and pulmonary vessels, is described elsewhere.)

Coronary Arteries

The major coronary arteries are the **right coronary artery** and the **left coronary artery** (see Figure 29-8). These arteries traverse the epicardium and branch several times. The pattern of branching through the visceral pericardium differs from heart to heart. The branches enter the myocardium and en-

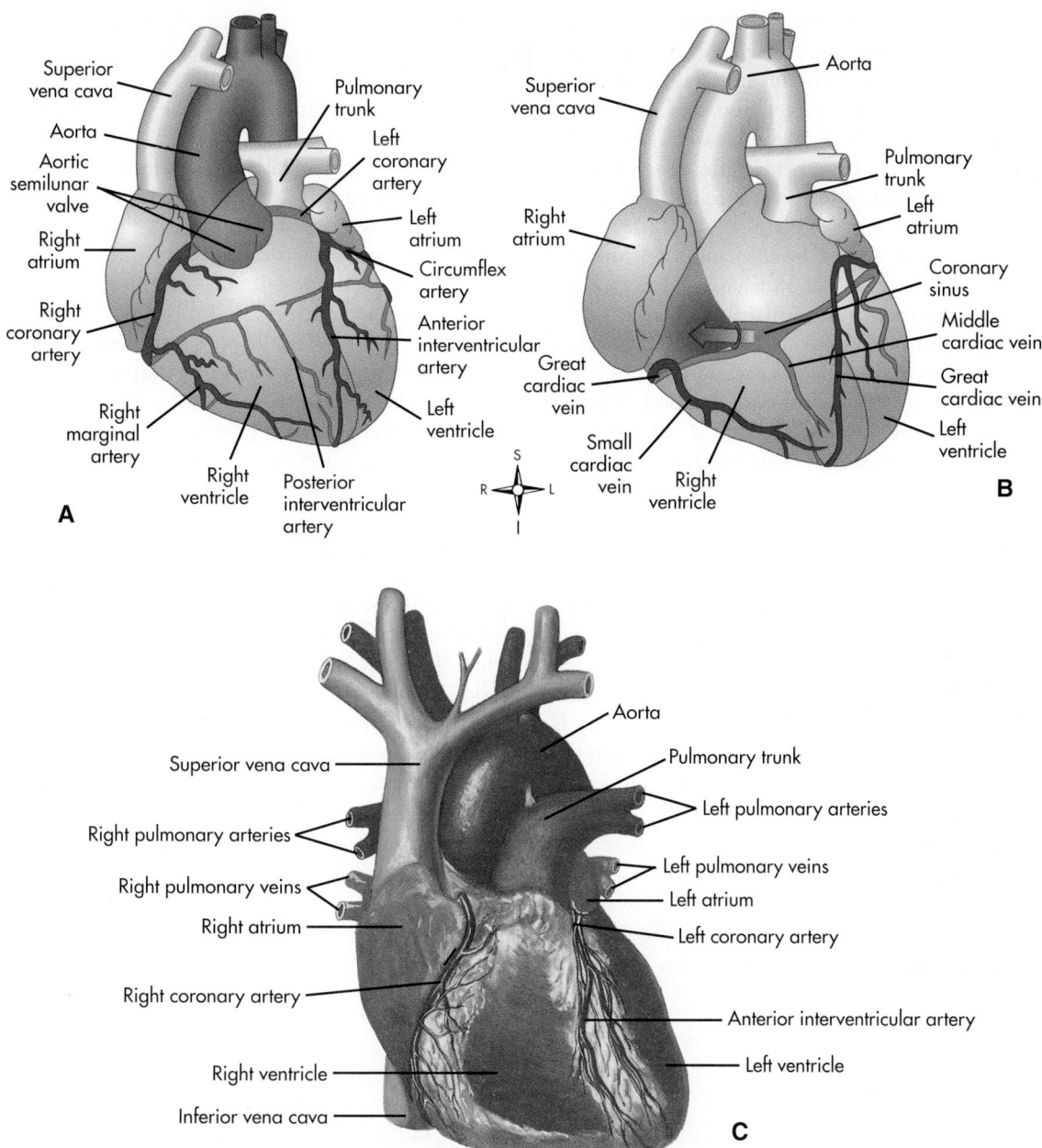

Figure 29-8 Coronary circulation. A, Arteries. **B,** Veins. Both **A** and **B** are anterior views of the heart. Vessels near the anterior surface are more darkly colored than vessels of the posterior surface seen through the heart. **C,** View of the anterior (sternocostal) surface. (**A** and **B,** Modified from Thibodeau GA, Patton KT: *Anatomy and physiology,* ed 5, St Louis, 2003, Mosby; **C,** From Seeley RR, Stephens TD, Tate P: *Anatomy and physiology,* ed 3, St Louis, 1995, Mosby.)

important for protecting the myocardium against injury. (The lymphatic vessels are described on p. 1067.)

Structures that Control Heart Action

The continuous, rhythmic repetition of the cardiac cycle (systole and diastole) depends on the transmission of electrical impulses, termed **cardiac action potentials,** through the myocardium. (Action potentials are described in Chapters 1 and 3.) As an electrical impulse passes from cell to cell (fiber to fiber) in the myocardium, it stimulates the fibers to shorten. Shortening causes muscular contraction, or systole. After the action potential passes, the fibers relax and return to

their resting length, causing diastole. The muscle fibers of the myocardium are uniquely joined so that action potentials pass from cell to cell very rapidly and efficiently. Therefore an action potential generated in one part of the myocardium passes almost simultaneously through all its contiguous fibers, causing rapid contraction.

The myocardium differs from other muscle tissues in that it contains its own **conduction system**—specialized cells that enable it to generate and transmit action potentials without stimulation from the nervous system. These cells are concentrated at certain sites in the myocardium called **nodes.** Although the heart is innervated by the autonomic nervous system (both sympathetic and parasympathetic fibers), neural impulses are not needed to maintain the cardiac cycle. Thus the heart will beat in the absence of any nervous connection. The cardiac cycle is stimulated by the nodes of specialized cells and "fine-tuned" as needed by the autonomic fibers. The sympathetic and parasympathetic nerves affect the speed of the cardiac cycle (**heart rate,** or beats per minute) and the diameter of the coronary vessels (see Figure 29-8, p. 1037).

Heart action is influenced also by substances delivered to the myocardium in coronary blood. Nutrients and oxygen are needed for cellular survival and normal function, and hormones and biochemicals affect the strength and duration of myocardial contraction and the degree and duration of myocardial relaxation. Normal or appropriate function depends on the availability of these substances, which is why coronary artery disease can seriously disrupt heart function.

Conduction System

Normally electrical impulses arise in the **sinoatrial node (SA node, sinus node),** which is often called the *pacemaker of the heart.* The SA node is located at the junction of the right atrium and superior vena cava, just above the tricuspid valve (Figure 29-9). The SA node lies only 1 mm or less beneath the visceral pericardium, making it vulnerable to injury and disease, especially pericardial inflammation.[6] The SA node is nourished by the sinus node artery, which passes through the center of the node. Numerous autonomic nerve endings are within the node. The SA node's **P cells,** so-called because they are pale and primitive appearing, are assumed to be the site of impulse formation.

In the resting adult the SA node generates about 75 action potentials per minute. Each one travels rapidly from cell to cell and through special pathways in the atrial myocardium, causing both atria to contract, beginning systole. Ventricular contraction is delayed because the fibrous skeleton of the heart interrupts cell-to-cell transmission of the electrical impulses. The action potential is transmitted from the atrial to the ventricular myocardium through fibers of the conduction system, traveling first to the **atrioventricular node (AV node),** then to the **bundle of His (atrioventricular bundle, common bundle),** and finally through the **bundle branches** of the interventricular septum to Purkinje fibers in the heart wall (see Figure 29-9).

The AV node is well situated for mediating conduction between the atria and ventricles. It is located in the right atrial wall above the tricuspid valve and anterior to the ostium of the coronary sinus. There is much variation from one heart to another in the size and length of the AV node fibers. Generally the AV node is thicker and shorter and has fewer P cells than the SA node. Behind the AV node are numerous autonomic ganglia, presumably vagal (parasympathetic).[7] (The nervous systems are described in Chapter 14.) These ganglia may serve as receptors for the vagus nerve and cause slowing of the cardiac cycle.

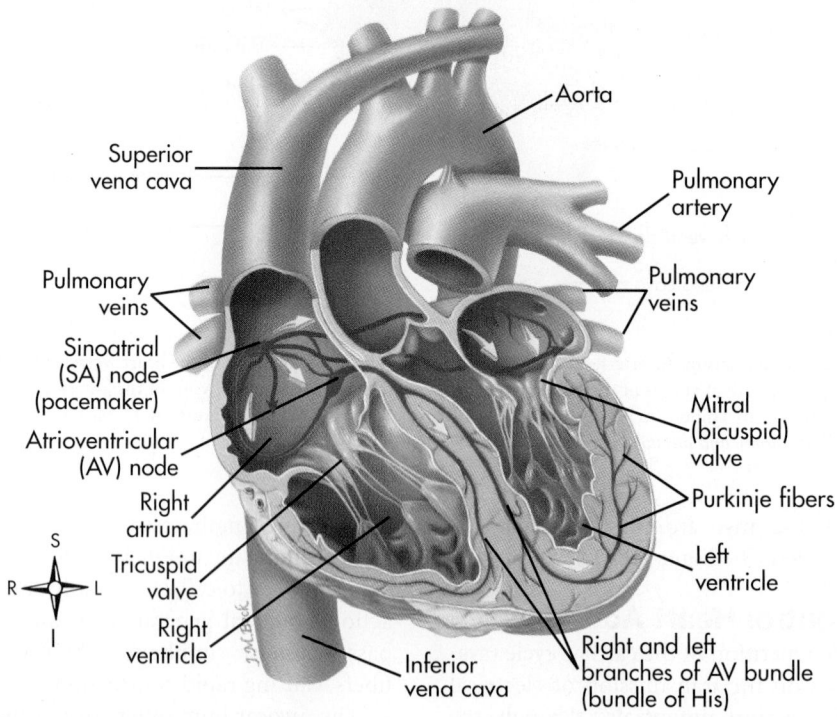

Figure 29-9 Conduction system of heart. Specialized cardiac muscle cells in the wall of the heart rapidly conduct an electrical impulse throughout the myocardium. The signal is initiated by the SA node (pacemaker) and spreads to the rest of the atrial myocardium and to the AV node. The AV node then initiates a signal that is conducted through the ventricular myocardium by way of the atrioventricular bundle (of His) and Purkinje fibers. (Modified from Thibodeau GA, Patton KT: *Anatomy & physiology,* ed 5, St Louis, 2003, Mosby.)

Conducting fibers from the AV node converge to form the bundle of His. The bundle of His, which is triangular in shape, lies within the posterior border of the interventricular septum. The two lower ends of the triangle give rise to the right and left bundle branches. The **right bundle branch (RBB)** is thin and travels without much branching to the right ventricular apex. Because of its thinness and relative lack of branches, the RBB is susceptible to interruption by damage to the endocardium.

The **left bundle branch (LBB)** arises perpendicularly from the bundle of His and, in some hearts, divides into two branches, or fascicles. The left anterior bundle branch (LABB) passes the left anterior papillary muscle and the base of the left ventricle and crosses the aortic outflow tract. Damage to the aortic valve or the left ventricle can interrupt this branch. The left posterior bundle branch (LPBB) travels posteriorly, crossing the left ventricular inflow tract to the base of the left posterior papillary muscle. This branch spreads diffusely through the posterior inferior left ventricular wall. Blood flow through this portion of the left ventricle is relatively nonturbulent, so the LPBB is somewhat protected from injury caused by wear and tear.

The **Purkinje fibers** are the terminal branches of the right and left bundle branches. They extend from the ventricular apices to the fibrous rings and penetrate the heart wall to the outer myocardium. P cells are found also among the Purkinje fibers.

Because impulses from the SA node arrive at the AV node extremely quickly, investigators have proposed that these nodes are connected by internodal pathways. A special pathway, the **anterior interatrial myocardial band** (or **Bachmann bundle**), conducts the impulse from the SA node to the left atrium. These pathways, the **anterior, middle,** and **posterior internodal pathways,** have been described thus. These pathways apparently consist of ordinary myocardial cells and specialized conducting fibers. The posterior internodal pathway apparently connects the right and left atria and the SA node and AV node for conduction from the SA to the AV node.

Cardiac Excitation

From the SA node the impulse that begins systole spreads throughout the right atrium at a conduction velocity of about 1 m/sec. The Bachmann bundle conducts the impulse from the SA node to the left atrium, and the posterior internodal pathway conducts the impulse from the SA node to the AV node.

The action potential is delayed in the region of the AV node, possibly because of electrophysiologic differences in the cells that make up the atrioventricular region.[2] The delay between atrial and ventricular excitation permits an additional boost to ventricular filling by atrial contraction (atrial kick). From the AV node the impulse travels from the atrioventricular bundle and through the bundle branches to the Purkinje fibers. Conduction velocities in the atrioventricular and Purkinje fibers are 2 to 4 m/sec, the most rapid in the heart.

Ventricular activation occurs sequentially in three phases: (1) septal activation, (2) apical activation, and (3) basal (upper) and posterior activation. The first areas of the ventricles to be excited are portions of the interventricular septum. The septum is activated from both the RBB and the LBB, although the impulse travels from left to right. The extensive network of Purkinje fibers promotes the rapid spread of the impulse to the ventricular apices. Activation traverses the heart wall from the inside outward (from the endocardium to the epicardium; see Figure 29-2). The basal and posterior portions of the ventricles are the last to be activated. Deactivation, which begins diastole, occurs in the opposite direction, spreading from the outside inward (epicardium to endocardium). All areas of the ventricle recover at about the same time.

Propagation of Cardiac Action Potentials

Electrical activation of the muscle cells, termed **depolarization,** is caused by the movement of electrically charged solutes (ions) across cardiac cell membranes. Deactivation, called **repolarization,** occurs the same way. (Movement of ions across cell membranes is described in Chapter 1; electrical activation of muscle cells is described in Chapter 41.)

Movement of ions into and out of the cell creates an electrical (voltage) difference across the cell membrane called the *membrane potential.* The resting membrane potential of myocardial cells is 280 to 290 millivolts (mV), and that of SA and AV node cells is 260 mV. During depolarization the inside of the cell becomes less negatively charged. In cardiac cells the difference between resting membrane potential (in millivolts) and the decreased negative charge caused by depolarization is the cardiac action potential. Table 29-2 summarizes the intracellular and extracellular ionic concentrations of cardiac muscle. The various phases of the cardiac action potential are related to changes in the permeability of the cell membrane, primarily to sodium and potassium. Threshold is the point at which the cell membrane's selective permeability to sodium and potassium is temporarily disrupted, leading to depolarization.

Normal myocardial cell depolarization and repolarization occur in five phases (Figure 29-10). Phase 0 consists of depolarization. This phase lasts 1 to 2 milliseconds (ms) and represents rapid sodium entry into the cell. Phase 1 is early repolarization, in which calcium slowly enters the cell. Phase 2, also called the *plateau,* is a continuation of repolarization, with slow entry of calcium and sodium into the cell. Potassium is moved out of the cell during phase 3, with a return to

Table 29-2	Intracellular and Extracellular Ion Concentrations in the Myocardium	
Ion	Intracellular Concentration	Extracellular Concentration
Sodium (Na$^+$)	15 mM	145 mM
Potassium (K$^+$)	150 mM	4 mM
Chloride (Cl$^-$)	5 mM	120 mM
Calcium (Ca^{++})	10^{-7} M	2 mM

mM, Millimoles per kilogram; *M,* moles.

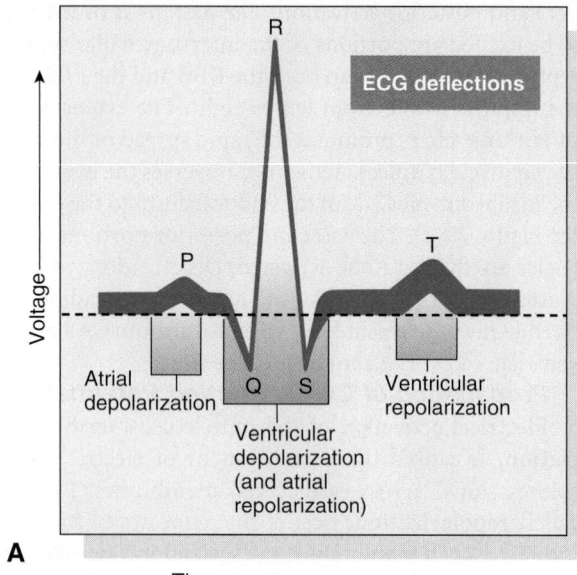

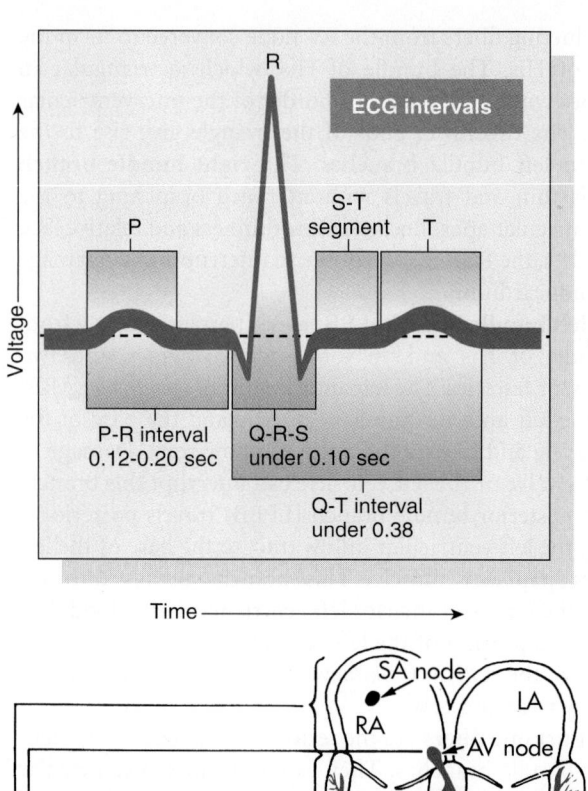

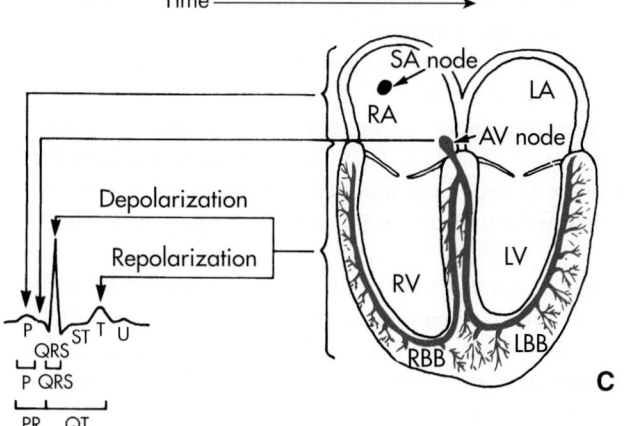

Figure 29-10 Electrocardiogram (ECG) and cardiac electrical activity. **A,** Normal ECG. Depolarization and repolarization. **B,** ECG intervals among P, QRS, and T waves. **C,** Schematic representation of ECG and its relationship to cardiac electrical activity. *RA,* right atrium; *LA,* left atrium; *AV,* atrioventricular; *RV,* right ventricle; *LV,* left ventricle; *LBB,* left bundle branch; *RBB,* right bundle branch. (**A** and **B,** From Thibodeau GA, Patton KT: *Anatomy & physiology,* ed 5, St Louis, 2003, Mosby. **C,** From Thibodeau GA: *Anatomy & physiology,* St Louis, 1987, Mosby.)

resting membrane potential in phase 4. This time between action potentials corresponds to diastole. If the resting membrane potential becomes more negative, for example, with a decrease in extracellular potassium concentration (hypokalemia), it is termed *hyperpolarization.*

The phases of depolarization and repolarization occur somewhat differently in the SA and AV node cells, a difference that enables these cells to generate cardiac action potentials independently. Although the cells of the Purkinje fibers, atria, and ventricles begin with a negative resting membrane potential and proceed to a rapid upstroke, or depolarization (phase 0), a rapid early repolarization (phase 1), a plateau (phase 2), and a rapid later repolarization (phase 3), cells of the SA and AV nodes begin with a less negative resting membrane potential, proceed to a slow upstroke (phase 0), and usually lack a plateau (phase 2) (see Figure 29-10, *B*). The fast inward current, mediated by sodium ions flowing through "fast channels" in the cell membrane, causes the rapid upstroke of the action potential in Purkinje fibers, atria, and ventricles (see Figure 29-10, *A*). The slow inward current, mediated by calcium (transient and long-lasting channels) and sodium ions flowing through "slow channels" of the cell

membrane, is responsible for the action potential of the SA node and the AV node. Hence, drugs that block calcium have profound effects on the slow inward current and can alter heart rate. Slow channel-blocking drugs, such as verapamil, are used to treat a variety of cardiovascular disorders.

A refractory period, during which no new cardiac action potential can be initiated by a stimulus, follows depolarization. This effective or absolute refractory period corresponds to the time needed for the reopening of channels that permit sodium and calcium influx (phase 0 through half of phase 3). A relative refractory period occurs near the end of repolarization, following the effective refractory period. During this time the membrane can be depolarized again but only by a greater-than-normal stimulus. Abnormal refractory periods as a result of disease can cause abnormal heart rhythms, or dysrhythmias, including ventricular fibrillation and cardiac arrest (see Chapter 30).

Normal Electrocardiogram. The genesis of the normal electrocardiogram is from electrical activity recorded by skin electrodes, that is, the sum of all cardiac action potentials (Figure 29-11). The **P wave** represents atrial depolarization. The **PR interval** is a measure of time from the onset of atrial

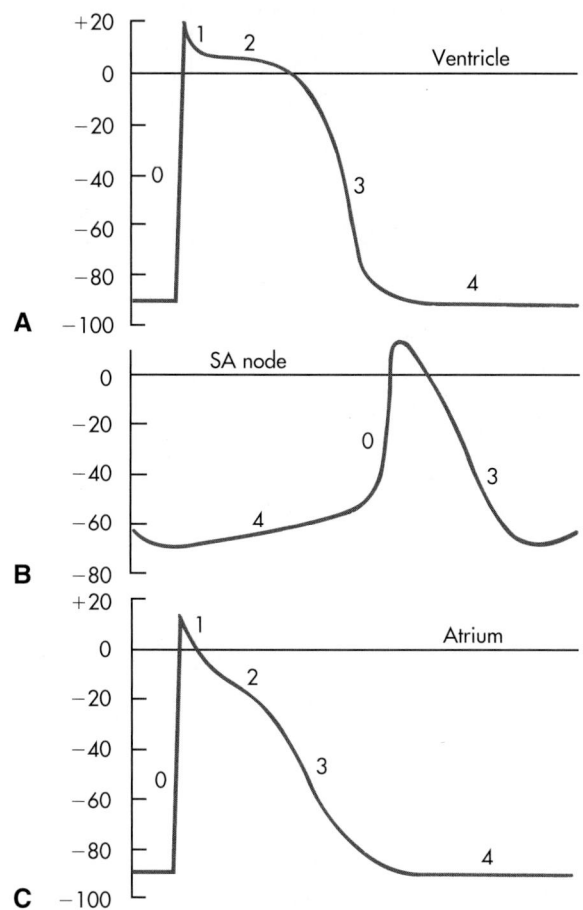

Figure 29-11 Cardiac action potentials. **A,** Ventricle. **B,** Sinoatrial (SA) node. **C,** Atrium. Sweep velocity in **B** is one half that in **A** or **C.** (Modified from Berne RM, Levy MN: *Cardiovascular physiology,* ed 8, St Louis, 2001, Mosby)

cle. Because threshold is approached during diastole, phase 4 in automatic cells is called **diastolic depolarization.** The electrical impulse normally begins in the SA node because its cells depolarize more rapidly than other automatic cells.

Rhythmicity. Rhythmicity is the regular generation of an action potential by the heart's conduction system. The SA node sets the pace because normally it has the fastest rate, which is why it is called the *natural pacemaker of the heart.* The SA node depolarizes spontaneously 60 to 100 times per minute. If the SA node is damaged, the AV node will become the heart's pacemaker at a rate of about 40 to 60 spontaneous depolarizations per minute. Eventually, however, conduction cells in the atria usually take over from the AV node. Purkinje fibers are capable of spontaneous depolarization but at a rate of only 30 to 40 beats/min.

Cardiac Innervation

Although the heart's nodes and conduction system generate cardiac action potentials independently, the autonomic nervous system influences the rate of impulse generation (firing), depolarization, and repolarization of the myocardium and the strength of atrial and ventricular contraction. Autonomic neural transmission produces changes in the heart and circulatory system faster than metabolic or humoral agents (Figure 29-12). Speed is important, for example, in stimulating the heart to increase its pumping action during times of stress or fear, the so-called *fight or flight response.* Although increased delivery of oxygen, glucose, hormones, and other blood-borne factors sustains increased cardiac activity, the rapid initiation of increased activity depends on the sympathetic and parasympathetic fibers of the autonomic nervous system. (The autonomic nervous system is described and illustrated in Chapter 14.)

Sympathetic and Parasympathetic Nerves

Sympathetic nerve fibers innervate all parts of the atria and ventricles. Parasympathetic fibers from the vagus nerve innervate these structures plus the SA and AV nodes. Strong vagal stimulation can block cardiac action potentials transmitted from the atria. Sympathetic nerves also can shorten the conduction time through the AV node and increase the rhythmicity of the atrioventricular pacemaker fibers.

Efferent sympathetic fibers originate in the thoracic spinal cord and branch into the superior middle and inferior cardiac nerves. The efferent parasympathetic fibers originate in the medulla oblongata and travel by way of the vagus nerves to join the sympathetic nerves in the **cardiac plexus,** a neural junction located at the root of the aorta, in front of the trachea.

Sympathetic nervous activity enhances myocardial performance. Neurally released norepinephrine or circulating catecholamines interact with β-adrenergic receptors on the cardiac cell membranes. The overall effect is an increased influx of Ca^{++} during the action potential plateau. The increased calcium increases the contractile strength of the heart. In addition, sympathetic nervous activity increases heart rate, whereas parasympathetic (vagal) activity decreases heart rate. The vagus nerve releases acetylcholine. In the heart, receptors

activation to the onset of ventricular activation; it normally ranges from 0.12 to 0.20 second. The PR interval represents the time necessary to travel from the sinus node through the atrium, AV node, and His-Purkinje system to activate ventricular myocardial cells. The **QRS complex** represents the sum of all ventricular muscle cell depolarizations. The configuration and amplitude of the QRS complex vary considerably among individuals. The duration is normally between 0.06 and 0.10 second. During the **ST interval** the entire ventricular myocardium is depolarized. The **QT interval** is sometimes called the "electrical systole" of the ventricles. It lasts about 0.4 second, but it varies inversely with the heart rate.

Automaticity. Automaticity, or the property of generating spontaneous depolarization to threshold, enables the SA and AV nodes to generate cardiac action potentials without any stimulus. Cells capable of spontaneous depolarization are called **automatic cells.** The automatic cells of the cardiac conduction system can stimulate the heart to beat even when the heart is removed from the body. Spontaneous depolarization is possible in automatic cells because the membrane potential does not "rest" during phase 4. Instead, it slowly creeps toward threshold during the diastolic phase of the cardiac cy-

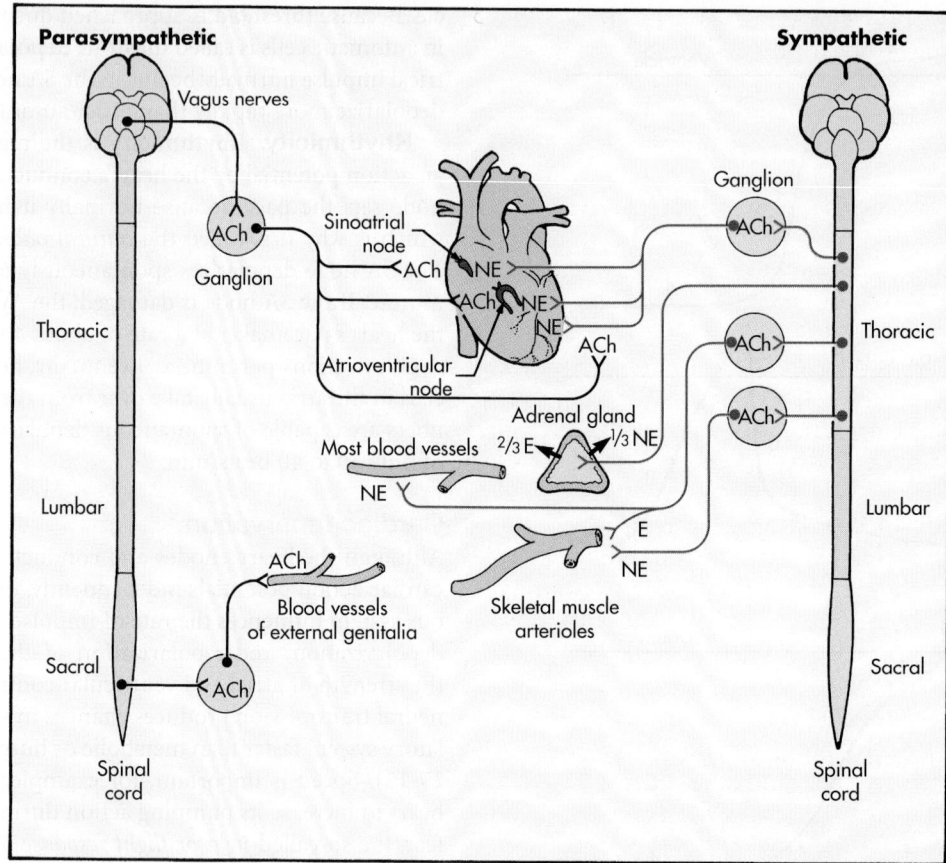

Figure 29-12 Autonomic innervation of cardiovascular system. *ACh*, Acetylcholine; *NE*, norepinephrine; *E*, epinephrine.

for these neurotransmitters are found in the myocardium and in the coronary vessels. When the autonomic nervous system is active, the vagal effects usually dominate.

Adrenergic Receptor Function

Sympathetic neural stimulation of the myocardium and coronary vessels depends on the presence of adrenergic receptors, which bind specifically with neurotransmitters of the sympathetic nervous system. (Receptor physiology is discussed in Chapter 1.) The effects of sympathetic stimulation depend on whether (1) α- or β-adrenergic receptors are most plentiful on cells of the effector tissue and (2) the neurotransmitter is norepinephrine or epinephrine.

Overall, cardiovascular structures have more β than α receptors; therefore effects mediated by the β receptors predominate. The β_1 receptors are found mostly in the heart, specifically the conduction system (AV and SA nodes, Purkinje fibers) and the atrial and ventricular myocardium. Norepinephrine binding with β_1 receptors increases the rate of impulse generation (firing) and conduction and also the strength of myocardial contraction during systole. These effects enable the heart to pump more blood. At the same time, epinephrine binds with β_2 receptors, which are most plentiful in the coronary arterioles. This causes the coronary arterioles to dilate, supplying the hard-working myocardium with more oxygen and nutrients (see Table 14-7).

α-Adrenergic receptors are also present in the coronary vessels but in fewer numbers than the β receptors. Norepinephrine binding with α_1 receptors in the coronary arteries causes vasoconstriction. The α_2 receptors are located mostly on the sympathetic ganglia and nerve terminals. The effect of norepinephrine on the α_2 receptors is to inhibit release of more norepinephrine, which promotes vasodilation.

Epinephrine stimulates all four types of receptors (β_1, β_2, α_1, α_2) strongly, whereas norepinephrine stimulates α_1, α_2, and β_1 receptors and certain β_2 receptors weakly or not at all. Thus both epinephrine and norepinephrine stimulate the heart (β_1) and constrict certain blood vessels (α_1), but only epinephrine dilates certain blood vessels (β_2).

Myocardial Cells

The cells of cardiac muscle (the myocardium) and of muscle that makes voluntary movement possible (skeletal muscle) are nearly identical in structure, function, and microscopic appearance. (The properties of skeletal muscle are described in detail in Chapter 41.) Both types of muscle tissue are composed of long, narrow cells, called *fibers*, which contain basically the same structures: bundles of longitudinally arranged myofibrils; a nucleus (cardiac muscle) or many nuclei (skeletal muscle); mitochondria; an internal membrane system (the sarcoplasmic reticulum); cytoplasm (sarcoplasm); and a plasma membrane (the sarcolemma), which encloses the cell. Cardiac and skeletal muscle cells also have an "external" membrane system made up of transverse tubules (T tubules) formed by invaginations of the sarcolemma. The sarcoplasmic reticulum forms a network of channels that surrounds the muscle fiber.

The microscopic appearance of cardiac and skeletal muscle is somewhat similar as well (see Chapter 1, Table 1-8). Because the myofibrils in both types of fibers are made up of alternating light and dark bands of protein, the fibers appear striped, or striated. The dark and light bands of the myofibrils make up longitudinal repeating units called *sarcomeres.* The length of the sarcomeres, normally between 1.6 to 2.2 mm, is important because it determines the limits of myocardial stretch at the end of diastole and subsequently the force of contraction during systole.

Cardiac muscle differs from skeletal muscle in several respects that reflect heart function. Cardiac cells are arranged in branching networks throughout the myocardium, whereas skeletal muscle cells tend to be arranged in parallel throughout the length of the muscle. Cardiac fibers have only one nucleus, whereas skeletal muscle cells have many nuclei. Other differences enable cardiac fibers to (1) transmit action potentials quickly from cell to cell, (2) maintain high levels of energy synthesis, and (3) gain access to more ions, particularly sodium and potassium, in the extracellular environment.

Rapid transmission of electrical impulses from cardiac fiber to cardiac fiber is possible because the network of fibers is connected at specialized intercellular junctions called *intercalated disks.* **Intercalated disks** are thickened portions of the sarcolemma that enable electrical impulses to spread quickly in a continuous cell-to-cell (syncytial) fashion. The intercalated disks contain two junctions: desmosomes, which attach one cell to another; and gap junctions, which allow the electrical impulse to spread from cell to cell (see Chapter 1). Together, these junctions provide a low-resistance pathway for impulse propagation.

Unlike skeletal muscle, the heart cannot rest and is in constant need of energy compounds, such as adenosine triphosphate (ATP). Therefore the cytoplasm surrounding the bundles of myofibrils in each cardiac muscle cell contains a superabundance of mitochondria (25% of the cellular volume). Cardiac muscle cells have more mitochondria than skeletal muscle cells. The large number of mitochondria provide the necessary respiratory enzymes for aerobic metabolism and supply quantities of ATP sufficient for the constant action of the myocardium.

The third major difference between cardiac and skeletal muscle cells has to do with the transverse tubule (T tubule) system. Cardiac fibers contain more T tubules than skeletal muscle fibers. This gives each myofibril in the myocardium ready access to molecules it needs for the continuous transmission of action potentials, a process that involves transport of sodium and potassium through the walls of the T tubules. (The mechanisms by which sodium and potassium transport

causes transmission of cardiac action potentials are described in Chapters 1 and 41.) Because the T tubule system is continuous with the extracellular space and the interstitial fluid, it facilitates the rapid transmission of electrical impulses from the surface of the sarcolemma to the myofibrils inside the fiber. This activates all the myofibrils of one fiber simultaneously. The sarcoplasmic reticulum is located around the myofibrils. When an action potential is transmitted through the T tubules, it induces the sarcoplasmic reticulum to release its stored calcium, which activates the contractile proteins, actin and myosin.

Actin, Myosin, and the Troponin-Tropomyosin Complex

The thick filaments of **myosin** constitute the central dark band called the **anisotropic, or A, bands** (Figure 29-13). The myosin molecule resembles a golf club with two large bulbous heads protruding from one end of a straight shaft (Figure 29-14). The bilobed heads contain an actin-binding site and a site of ATPase activity. A thick filament is composed of about 200 myosin molecules bundled together with the heads of the molecules (called *cross-bridges*) facing outward (see Figure 29-14). The actin molecules are part of the thin filaments (Figure 29-15). The light bands are called **isotropic, or I, bands** (see Figure 29-13). The thin filaments of actin appear light and extend from the **Z line,** a dense fibrous line that

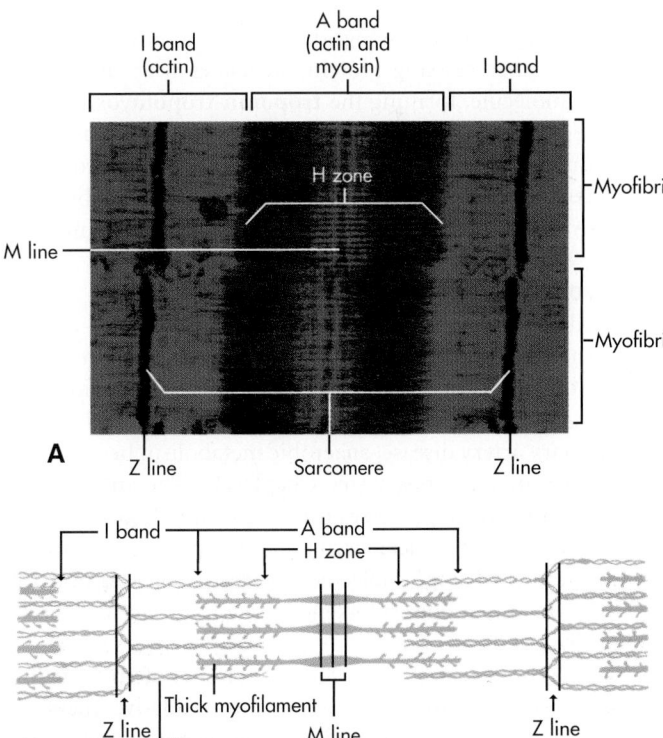

Figure 29-13 Sarcomere. **A,** Electron photomicrograph of sarcomere. **B,** Schematic of location and interaction of actin and myosin. (Modified from Thibodeau GA, Patton KT: *Anatomy & physiology,* ed 3, St Louis, 1996, Mosby.)

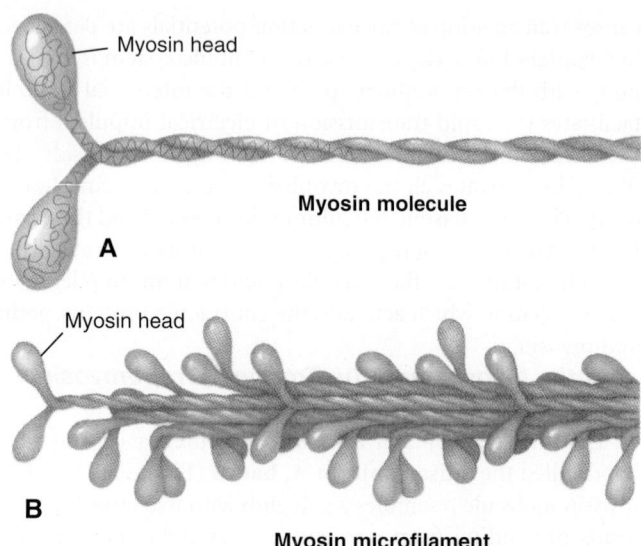

Figure 29-14 **Structure of myosin. A,** Each myosin molecule is a coil of two chains wrapped around one another. At the end of each chain is a globular region, much like a golf club, called the *head*. **B,** Myosin molecules usually are combined into filaments, which are stalks of myosin from which the heads protrude at regular intervals.

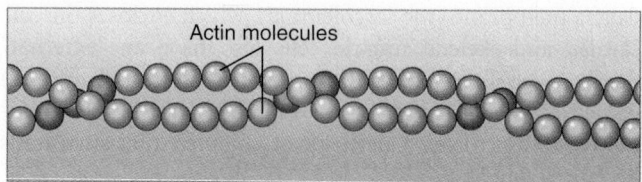

Figure 29-15 Actin microfilament. (From Raven RH, Johnson GB: *Understanding biology,* ed 3, Dubuque, Iowa, 1995, Brown.)

crosses the center of each I band. A sarcomere is the area from one dark Z line to an adjacent Z line with a length that varies from 1.6 to 2.2 mm. In the center of a sarcomere is the H zone, a somewhat less dense region. A thin, dark **M line** travels the center of the H zone. A single tropomyosin molecule (a relaxing protein) lies alongside seven actin molecules. **Troponin,** another relaxing protein, associates with the tropomyosin molecule, forming the **troponin-tropomyosin complex** (Figure 29-16). The troponin complex itself has three components. **Troponin T** aids in binding of the troponin complex to actin and tropomyosin; troponin I inhibits the ATPase of actomyosin; and **troponin C** contains binding sites for the calcium ions involved in contraction.

Myocardial Metabolism

Cardiac muscle, like other muscle tissue, depends on the constant production of ATP for energy. ATP is produced within the mitochondria mainly from glucose, fatty acids, and lactate. If the myocardium is inadequately perfused because of coronary artery disease, anaerobic metabolism becomes an essential source of energy (see Chapter 1). The energy produced by metabolic processes is used for muscle contraction and relaxation, electrical excitation, membrane transport, and synthesis of large molecules. Normally, the amount of ATP produced supplies sufficient energy to pump blood systemically.

Cardiac work often is expressed in terms of **myocardial oxygen consumption (MV̇O₂).** Because oxidative metabolism is the main process of cardiac energy generation, the rate of MV̇O₂ correlates closely with total cardiac energy requirements. MV̇O₂ is determined by three major factors: (1) the amount of wall stress during systole, which can be estimated by measuring the systolic blood pressure; (2) the duration of systolic wall tension, which is measured indirectly by the

heart rate; and (3) the contractile state of the myocardium, for which no clinical measurement exists.

The oxygen supply to the myocardium is delivered exclusively by the coronary arteries. From 70% to 75% of the oxygen from the coronary arteries is used immediately by cardiac muscle, leaving little oxygen in reserve. Therefore increased energy needs can be met only by increasing coronary blood flow. When oxygen content decreases, the local concentration of local metabolic factors increases. One of these, adenosine, dilates coronary arterioles, increasing coronary blood flow. Oxygen content of the blood cannot be increased under normal atmospheric conditions, nor can the amount of O_2 extracted from the blood be appreciably increased from the resting level (see Chapter 32). Myocardial O_2 consumption can increase severalfold with exercise and decrease moderately under conditions such as hypotension and hypothermia.[2]

Myocardial Contraction and Relaxation

Myocardial contractility is a change in developed tension at a given resting fiber length. In functional terms, contractility is the ability of the heart muscle to shorten. On a molecular basis, thin filaments of actin slide over thick filaments of myosin, called the **cross-bridge theory of muscle contraction.** Anatomically, contraction occurs when the sarcomere shortens causing adjacent Z lines to move closer together (Figure 29-17). The width of the A band, which contains the thick myosin filaments, is unchanged. The movement comes from the long sets of filaments. The degree of shortening of the muscle fibers depends on how much the thin filaments overlap the thick filaments. Maximal contraction occurs when the sarcomere length is 2.2 mm. At 2.2 mm the number of cross-bridge attachments between actin and myosin is maximal.

Cross-Bridge Theory

The globular head-end of the myosin contains a binding site for actin and a separate enzymatic site that catalyzes the breakdown of ATP to adenosine diphosphate (ADP) and inorganic phosphate (see Figure 29-17). This reaction releases the chemical energy stored in ATP. Magnesium is required for the binding of ATP to the myosin site. The splitting of ATP occurs on the myosin molecule before it attaches to actin, but the ADP and inorganic phosphate (P_i) released remain bound to the active site on myosin. The chemical energy released is transferred to myosin (m), producing a high-energy form of myosin (M):

$$M \cdot ATP \rightarrow M \cdot ADP + P_i$$

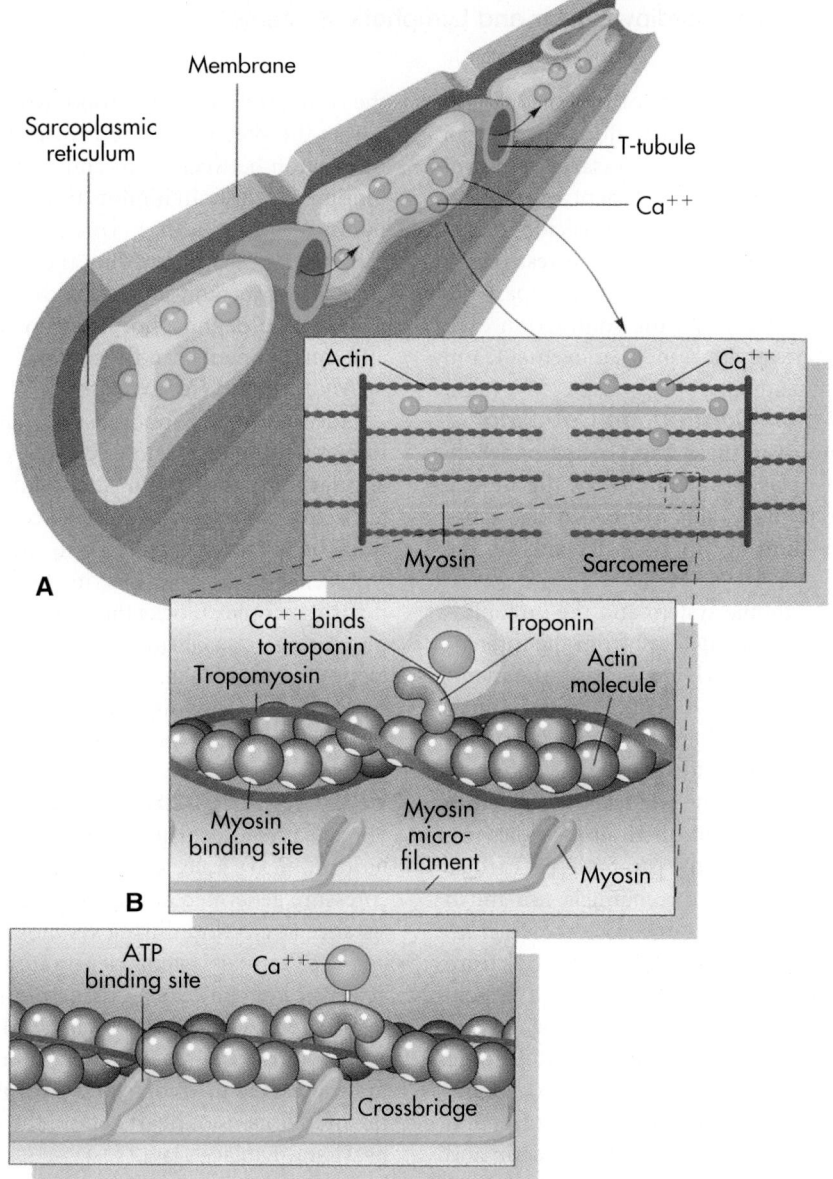

Membrane

Sarcoplasmic reticulum

T-tubule

Ca++

Actin

Ca++

Myosin

Sarcomere

A

Ca++ binds to troponin

Troponin

Tropomyosin

Actin molecule

Myosin binding site

Myosin microfilament

Myosin

B

ATP binding site

Ca++

Crossbridge

C

Figure 29-16 **Myofilaments and mechanisms of muscle contraction. A,** Thin and thick myofilaments. In resting muscle, calcium ions are stored in the sarcoplasmic reticulum. When an action potential reaches the muscle cell, the T tubules carry the action potential deep into the sarcoplasm. The action potential causes the sarcoplasmic reticulum to release the store of calcium ions. **B,** In resting muscle the myosin binding sites are covered by troponin and tropomyosin. The calcium ions released into the sarcoplasm as a result of action potential bind to the troponin. This binding causes the tropomyosin and troponin to move out of the way of the myosin binding sites, leaving the myosin heads free to bind to the actin microfilament. (From Raven PH, Johnson GB: *Understanding biology*, ed 3, Dubuque, Iowa, 1995, Brown.)

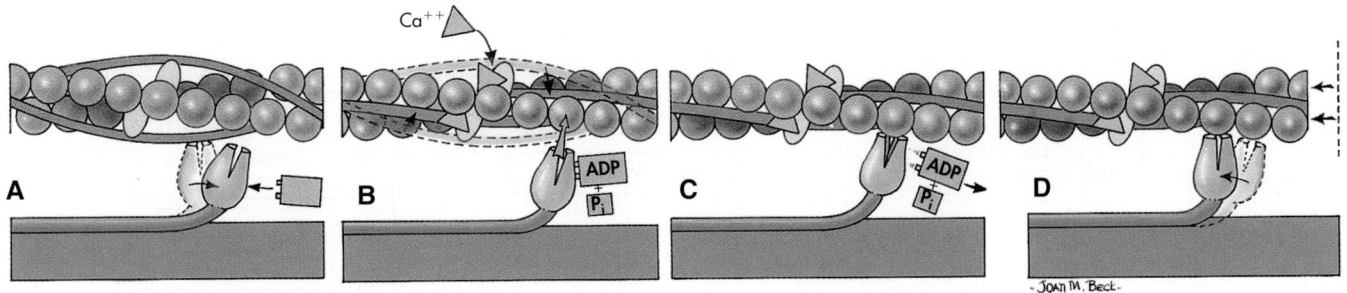

Ca++

ADP
P$_i$

ADP
P$_i$

A   **B**   **C**   **D**

- Joan M. Beck -

Figure 29-17 **Cross-bridge theory of muscle contraction. A,** Each myosin cross-bridge in the thick filament moves into a resting position after an adenosine triphosphate (ATP) molecule binds and transfers its energy. **B,** Calcium ions released from the sarcoplasmic reticulum bind to troponin in the thin filament, allowing tropomyosin to shift from its position blocking the active sites of actin molecules. **C,** Each myosin cross-bridge then binds to an active site on a thin filament, displacing the remnants of ATP hydrolysis— adenosine diphosphate (ADP) and inorganic phosphate (P$_i$). **D,** The release of stored energy from step *A* provides the force needed for each cross-bridge to move back to its original position, pulling actin along with it. Each cross-bridge will remain bound to actin until another ATP molecule binds to it and pulls it back into its resting position, *A*. (From Thibodeau GA, Patton KT: *Anatomy & physiology*, ed 4, St Louis, 1999, Mosby.)

The binding of this high-energy form of myosin to actin through a cross-bridge releases the energy stored in myosin (e.g., ADP and P_i), producing the force necessary for movement of the cross-bridge. With the attachment of actin to myosin at the cross-bridge, the myosin head molecule undergoes a position change, exerting traction on the rest of the myosin bridge, causing the thin filaments to slide past the thick filaments (see Figure 29-17). During contraction each cross-bridge undergoes cycles of attachment, movement, and dissociation from the thin filaments.

Calcium and Excitation-Contraction Coupling

Excitation-contraction coupling is the process by which an action potential in the plasma membrane of the muscle fiber triggers the cycle of events leading to cross-bridge activity and contraction. Activation of this cycle depends on the availability of calcium.

Calcium is stored in the tubule system and the sarcoplasmic reticulum. It enters the myocardial cell from the interstitial fluid after electrical excitation, which increases the membrane permeability to calcium. Two types of calcium channels (L-type and T-type) are identified in cardiac tissues. The L-type, or long-lasting, channels are the predominant type of calcium channels and are the channels blocked by **calcium channel–blocking drugs** (verapamil, nifedipine, diltiazem). Their major effect is to decrease the strength of cardiac contraction. The T-type, or transient, channels are much less abundant in the heart and are not blocked by calcium channel–blocking drugs.[2] Calcium that enters the cell from the interstitial fluid triggers release of calcium from the storage sites. The storage sites most important for contraction are from the sarcoplasmic reticulum. Calcium from these sites diffuses toward the myofibrils, where it binds with troponin.

The calcium-troponin complex facilitates the contraction process. In the resting state, troponin I is bound to actin and the configuration of the tropomyosin molecule is such that it covers the sites where the myosin heads bind to actin. Thus interaction between actin and myosin is prevented. Calcium binding to troponin inhibits troponin C (which enhances troponin I–actin binding). This in turn causes tropomyosin to move away, thus uncovering the binding sites on the myosin heads. Myosin and actin can then form cross-bridges, and ATP can be dephosphorylated to ADP. Sliding of the thick and thin filaments can then occur, and the muscle contracts.

Myocardial Relaxation

Adequate relaxation is just as vital to optimal cardiac function as contraction, and calcium, troponin, and tropomyosin also facilitate relaxation. After contraction, free calcium ions are actively pumped out of the cell back into the interstitial fluid or reaccumulated in the sarcoplasmic reticulum and stored. Troponin releases its bound calcium. The tropomyosin complex blocks the active sites on the actin molecule, preventing cross-bridges with the myosin heads. Each tropomyosin molecule is held in this blocking position by a molecule of troponin. Troponin is bound to both tropomyosin and actin (see Figures 29-16, *A*, and 29-17).

Factors Affecting Cardiac Performance

Four factors affect cardiac performance directly: preload, afterload, heart rate, and myocardial contractility. **Preload** (pressure generated at the end of diastole) and **afterload** (resistance to ejection during systole) depend on both the heart and the vascular system. Heart rate and contractility are characteristics of the cardiac tissue per se and are influenced by neural and humoral mechanisms (Figure 29-18). To understand the role of these factors in cardiac performance, it is first necessary to understand two physical laws that explain the mechanisms of heart action: the Frank-Starling law of the heart and Laplace's law.

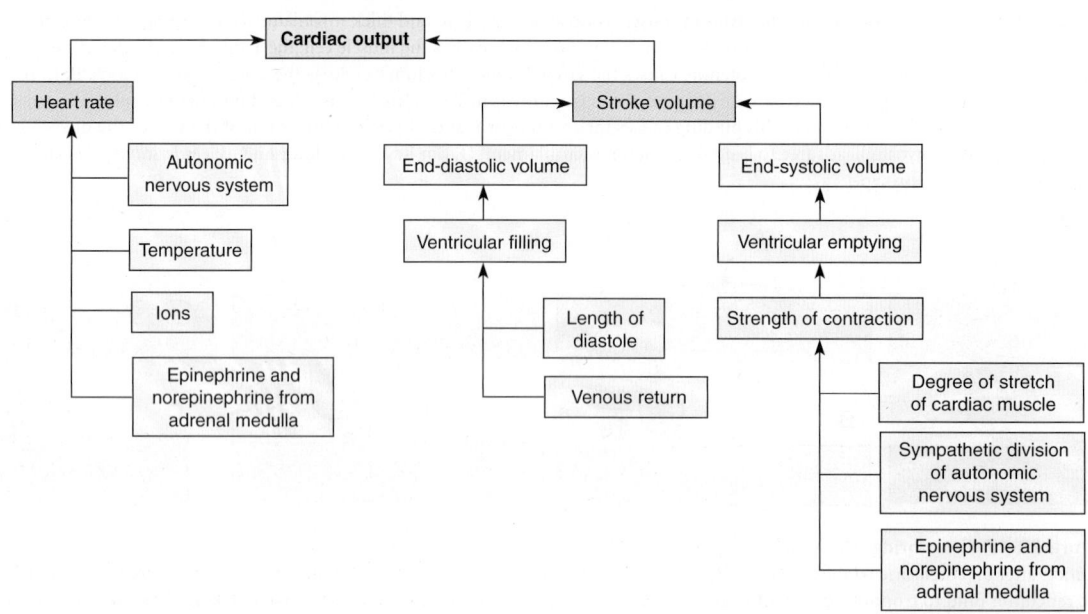

Figure 29-18 Factors affecting cardiac performance. Cardiac output, which is amount of blood (in liters) ejected by the heart per minute, depends on heart rate (beats per minute) and stroke volume (milliliters of blood ejected during ventricular systole).

Frank-Starling Law of the Heart

Cardiac muscle, like other muscle, increases its strength of contraction when it is stretched. This relationship was described in 1914 by a British physiologist, Ernest Starling, who based his studies on the earlier work of a German physiologist, Otto Frank. In 1914 Starling wrote that "the output of any heart can be varied within wide limits by alterations of the venous inflow, and that within these limits it varies directly as the venous inflow. So long as the functional condition of the heart remains constant, the amount put out at each beat depends directly on the diastolic filling."

The **Frank-Starling law of the heart,** or the length-tension relationship of cardiac muscle, relates resting sarcomere length, expressed as the volume of blood in the heart at the end of diastole, or **end-diastolic volume,** to tension generation, described as development of left ventricular pressure. Thus the volume of blood in the heart at the end of diastole (the length of its muscle fibers) is directly related to the force of contraction during the next systole. Although the change in pressure is related to volume of the ventricle and, consequently, to the length of the ventricular muscle fibers, it is common to use preload (i.e., filling pressure) as an index of ventricular volume. The length-tension mechanism is the major mechanism by which the normal right and left ventricles maintain equal minute outputs even though their stroke outputs may vary considerably during normal respiration. For example, changes in volume occur when an individual assumes a reclining position after being in a standing position; the volume of blood returning to the heart temporarily increases. The right ventricle stretches to accommodate this increase in volume and thereby increases its force of contraction. A larger stroke volume (i.e., the amount of blood ejected per beat) is pumped to the lungs, generating higher pressures. Pulmonary vascular pressure increases, causing a rise in the left ventricular filling pressure or preload. Left ventricular volume and pressure increase. The left ventricle pumps a larger stroke volume, and arterial vascular pressure rises.

The mechanical function of the heart is characterized by a number of length-tension curves (Figure 29-19). Factors that increase contractility (i.e., positive inotropic), such as sympathetic nerve stimulation, cause the heart to operate on a higher length-tension curve (curve *A* in Figure 29-19). A higher tension or increase in ventricular stroke volume is generated without a necessary change in left ventricular end-diastolic volume or fiber length. Heart failure (curve *C* in Figure 29-19) is characterized by a lower length-tension curve (see Chapter 30). The failing or dilated heart may not be able to use the Frank-Starling law of the heart because its fibers are lengthened maximally already. The failing heart is unable to respond significantly to increased filling or stretch with a greater force. Thus at the same left ventricular end-diastolic volume as curves *A* and *B* (see Figure 29-19), the force of contraction of stroke volume is decreased. The relationship between stretch and contraction can be compared to that of a rubber band. To a certain point, the more the rubber band is

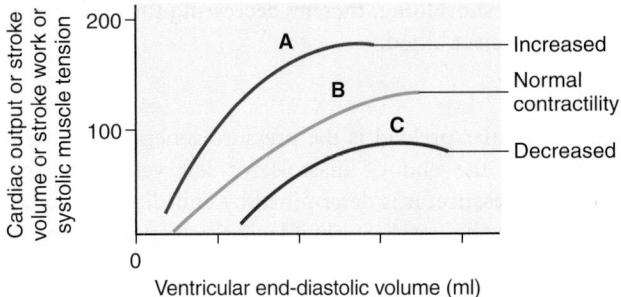

Figure 29-19 Frank-Starling law of the heart. Relationship between length and tension in heart. End-diastolic volume determines end-diastolic length of ventricular muscle fibers and is proportional to tension generated during systole, as well as to cardiac output, stroke volume, and stroke work. A change in myocardial contractility causes the heart to perform on a different length-tension curve. **A,** Increased contractility; **B,** normal contractility; **C,** heart failure or decreased contractility. (See text.)

stretched, the farther it will fly when one end is released. Beyond that point, however, the rubber band will break.

The cross-bridge theory partially accounts for the length-tension mechanism of cardiac muscle. According to the Frank-Starling law, the longer the initial resting length of the cardiac muscle fiber (optimal length is between 2.2 mm and 2.4 mm), the greater the strength of contraction. At 2.2 mm there is an optimal number of active cross-bridges between actin and myosin. If the fibers are stretched beyond 2.2 to 2.4 mm, the force of contraction decreases because actin and myosin become partially disengaged, disrupting many of the cross-bridges. Excessive stretching, to about 3.65 mm, causes actin and myosin to become completely disengaged and causes developed tension (force of contraction) to drop to zero. Heart failure occurs when it takes higher and higher filling pressures to accomplish normal contractile force.

Laplace's Law

In Laplace's law, wall tension is related directly to the product of intraventricular pressure and internal radius and inversely to the wall thickness. This relationship can be calculated by Laplace's equation:

$$T = (p \times v)/\mu m$$

where T = wall tension, p = intraventricular pressure, n = internal radius of the sphere, and μm = wall thickness. In other words, the amount of tension generated in the wall of the ventricle (or any chamber or vessel) to produce a given intraventricular pressure depends on the size (radius and wall thickness) of the ventricle.

The law of Laplace is useful for understanding aneurysm formation, distensibility in blood vessels, and the effects of ventricular dilation on myocardial contraction. Dilation is an important factor in heart failure (see Chapter 30). With a dilated ventricle, myocardial fibers in the wall must develop greater tension to produce a given pressure within the ventricle. The disadvantage of dilation is that the increased force, or tension, in the myocardial fibers required to develop a given pressure inside a dilated ventricle results in a decrease in the rate of fiber shortening, thereby decreasing the ability of the ventricle to eject blood.

Preload

Left ventricular preload is the pressure generated in the left ventricle at the end of diastole, or left ventricular **end-diastolic pressure.** It is determined by end-diastolic volume, according to the Frank-Starling law, which stretches the cardiac muscle fibers, which in turn develop tension, or force, for contraction. Within a physiologic range of muscle stretching (2.2 mm to 2.4 mm), increased preload increases cardiac output (volume of blood pumped per minute; see Figure 29-18). In monitoring preload the clinician measures indexes of left ventricular end-diastolic pressure. Pressure changes are important because increased left ventricular filling pressures "back up" into the pulmonary circulation, where they force plasma out through vessel walls, causing fluid to accumulate in lung tissues (pulmonary edema; see Chapter 33). Treatment goals are to maintain an end-diastolic volume that will maintain or increase cardiac output.

Afterload

Left ventricular afterload is the resistance or impedance to ejection of blood from the left ventricle. It is the load the muscle must move after it starts to contract. Aortic systolic pressure is a good index of afterload. Low aortic pressures (decreased afterload) enable the heart to contract more rapidly, whereas high aortic pressures (increased afterload) slow contraction and cause higher workloads against which the heart must function so it can eject less blood. Pressure in the ventricle must exceed aortic pressure before blood can be pumped out during systole. Afterload involves a force-velocity relationship; that is, the lighter the afterload, the faster the contraction, and the heavier the afterload, the slower the contraction.

In addition to influencing the speed of shortening, afterload is related to extent of shortening. Increases in aortic pressure, with a constant preload, result in decreased blood pumped by the left ventricle. Decreased aortic pressure allows the left ventricle to pump a larger volume.

Heart Rate

The average heart rate in normal adults is about 70 beats/min. The average heart rate is significantly greater in children. Heart rate diminishes by 10 to 20 beats/min during sleep and can accelerate to more than 100 beats/min during muscular activity or emotional excitement. In well-conditioned athletes at rest the heart rate is normally about 50 to 60 beats/min. In highly trained or elite athletes the resting heart rate can be below 50 beats/min. Highly trained athletes have a lower resting heart rate, greater stroke volume, and lower peripheral resistance in active muscles than they had before training. The low resting heart rate is the result of an increased vagal stimulation and lower sympathetic stimulation.[2] The lowered peripheral resistance is thought to be caused by an increase in the number of arterioles in skeletal muscle. The decrease in

peripheral resistance increases the venous return, causing the cardiac output to increase.[2] As the resting heart rate falls in individuals during physical training, the end-diastolic fiber length of the ventricles increases; this occurs because the longer duration of diastole results in greater filling. The increased end-diastolic fiber length increases stroke volume, which helps compensate for the decreased heart rate.

Neural factors, including neural reflexes, and hormonal and chemical factors influence the heart rate. Neural control is exerted by both the central and autonomic nervous systems. Hormonal factors include the catecholamines (norepinephrine and epinephrine), thyroid hormones, growth hormones, and pancreatic hormones. (Hormonal function is described in Unit VI.) Stimulation by the sympathetic nervous system increases the rhythmicity of the cardiac pacemaker (SA node), whereas the parasympathetic stimulation has an inhibiting effect.

Cardiovascular Control Centers in the Brain

The major **cardiovascular control center** is in the brain stem in the medulla with secondary areas in the hypothalamus, the cerebral cortex, the thalamus, and complex networks of exciting or inhibiting interneurons (connecting neurons) throughout the brain. The hypothalamic centers regulate cardiovascular responses to changes in temperature; the cerebral cortex centers adjust cardiac reaction to a variety of emotional states; and the medullary control center regulates heart rate and blood pressure (see p. 1061 for blood pressure regulation). The medullary neurons often are classified as cardiac and vasomotor (vasoconstrictor or vasodilator) centers; however, because these centers are not discrete anatomic areas and actually constitute diffuse networks of interneurons, it is preferable to call the entire area the cardiovascular control center.

The nerve fibers from the cardiovascular control center synapse with the autonomic neurons (see Chapter 14 and Table 14-7). When the parasympathetic nerves to the heart are stimulated, the sympathetic nerves to the heart, arterioles, and veins usually are inhibited. The opposite also is true: when the sympathetic nerves are stimulated, the parasympathetic nerves usually are inhibited. Because parasympathetic excitation and simultaneous sympathetic inhibition generally depress cardiac function (e.g., decrease the heart rate), these interneurons often are referred to as the **cardioinhibitory center.** Excitation occurs with parasympathetic inhibition and sympathetic stimulation, and these interneurons are collectively called the **cardioexcitatory center.** Therefore heart rate can be slowed by two simultaneous events that begin in the cardiovascular control center: (1) inhibition of sympathetic stimulation of the SA node and (2) activation of parasympathetic stimulation of the SA node. Heart rate can be increased by activation of sympathetic nerves and inhibition of parasympathetic nerves.

The resting heart rate in healthy individuals is primarily under the control of parasympathetic stimulation. While the individual is at rest, parasympathetic effects from the vagus nerves override sympathetic effects in the SA node. Interruption of the vagus nerves causes significant tachycardia (abnormally fast heart rate) because the inhibitory parasympathetic influence is lost.

Neural Reflexes

Two important neural reflexes that affect heart rate and rhythm are the Bainbridge reflex and the baroreceptor reflex. The **Bainbridge reflex** causes the heart rate to increase after intravenous infusions of blood or other fluid. The increased rate is thought to be caused by a reflex mediated by volume receptors in the atria that are innervated by the vagus nerves. (Volume receptors are thought to respond to increased plasma volume.) The magnitude of the change in heart rate depends on the initial heart rate. If the initial rate is slow, intravenous infusion usually accelerates it, but if the initial rate is rapid, infusions usually will slow it down.[2] Contractility usually is not affected by the Bainbridge reflex.

The **baroreceptor reflex** facilitates blood pressure changes and heart rate changes. The baroreceptor reflex is mediated by tissue pressure receptors (pressoreceptors) in the aortic arch and carotid arteries. (Because the receptors respond to mechanical factors, they are also called *aortic and carotid mechanoreceptors.*) The pressoreceptors increase their rate of discharge when stretched by blood pressure elevations. Neural impulses are then transmitted over the glossopharyngeal nerve (ninth cranial nerve) from the carotid artery and through the vagus nerve from the aorta to the cardiovascular control centers in the medulla. These centers initiate an increase in parasympathetic activity and a decrease in sympathetic activity, causing blood vessels to dilate and heart rate to decrease. In the heart the initial response is caused by a decrease in sympathetic stimulation, but most of the decrease in heart rate is probably the result of increased parasympathetic activity. Responses to the baroreceptor reflex return the blood pressure to its previous level, which may or may not be normal. The higher the blood pressure, the greater the reflexive decrease in heart rate.

If blood pressure is decreased, the baroreceptor reflex accelerates heart rate and causes vessels to constrict. These responses raise blood pressure back toward normal. The pressoreceptors are more effective in compensating for a decrease in arterial blood pressure than a rise in pressure.[8]

Neural receptors in the lungs cause heart rate to increase during inspiration and decrease during expiration. The increase in heart rate during inspiration is caused by the stretching (activation) of vagal fibers in the lungs that cause heart rate to speed up by inhibiting the cardioinhibitory center of the medulla. Inhibition of this center allows unopposed sympathetic acceleration of heart rate.

Atrial Receptors

Receptors that influence heart rate exist in both atria[2] (see Figure 29-20). They are located in the right atrium at its junctions with the vena cava and in the left atrium at its junctions with the pulmonary veins.[2] Distension of these atrial receptors sends impulses via C-fiber afferents. Stimulation of these atrial receptors also increases urine volume, presumably because of a neurally mediated reduction in antidiuretic hormone.[2] In addition, atrial natriuretic peptide (ANP) is released from atrial tissue in response to the increases in blood volume. ANP has powerful diuretic and natriuretic (salt excretion) properties resulting in decreased blood volume pressure.

Hormones and Biochemicals

Hormones and biochemicals affect the arteries, arterioles, venules, capillaries, and contractility of the myocardium. Norepinephrine increases heart rate, enhances myocardial contractility, and constricts blood vessels. Epinephrine dilates vessels of the liver and skeletal muscle and also causes an increase in myocardial contractility. Some adrenocortical hormones, such as hydrocortisone, potentiate the effects of the catecholamines.

Thyroid hormones enhance sympathetic activity, promoting an increase in cardiac output. The exact mechanism by which this occurs is not known. A decrease in growth hormone, as well as thyroid and adrenal hormones, results in bradycardia (heart rate below 60 beats/min), reduced cardiac output, and low blood pressure.

Myocardial Contractility

Stroke volume, or the volume of blood ejected during systole, depends on the force of contraction, which depends on myocardial contractility, or the degree of myocardial fiber shortening. Two major factors determine the force of contraction: (1) changes in the stretching of the ventricular myocardium caused by changes in ventricular volume (preload) and (2) alterations in the sympathetic activation of the ventricles. Increased flow of blood from the veins into the heart distends

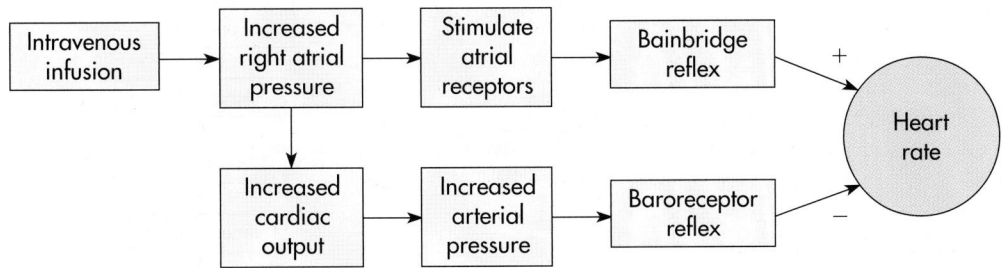

Figure 29-20 Heart rate and intravenous infusions. Intravenous infusions of blood or electrolyte solutions tend to increase heart rate through the Bainbridge reflex and to decrease heart rate through the baroreceptor reflex. The actual change in heart rate induced by such infusions is the result of these two opposing effects. (From Berne RM, Levy MN: *Cardiovascular physiology,* ed 8, St Louis, 2001, Mosby.)

the ventricle by increasing preload. Greater preload increases the stroke volume and, subsequently, cardiac output. Increased output then causes increased venous return, atrial volume and pressure, and eventually end-diastolic volume and stroke volume.

Myocardial contractility is difficult to measure because measurement requires keeping preload, afterload, and heart rate constant. Only when these factors are held constant can changes in cardiac performance be attributed to changes in the inotropic (contractile) state of the myocardium itself.

Factors affecting contractility are called **inotropic agents.** Positive inotropic agents increase the velocity of myocardial contraction (phase 0) and stroke volume. The positive inotropic agents are excess thyroid hormone, epinephrine, norepinephrine, dopamine or isoproterenol infusion, and calcium salt infusion. The negative inotropic agents decrease the velocity of myocardial contraction and the stroke volume. These agents include alcohol, procainamide, quinidine, and propranolol.

Myocardial contractility is affected also by oxygen and carbon dioxide levels (tensions) in the coronary blood. (Blood gases are discussed in Chapters 3 and 32.) Different degrees of arterial oxygen deficiency—termed *hypoxemia*—affect contractility differently. With severe hypoxemia (arterial oxygen saturation less than 50%), contractility is decreased. With less severe hypoxemia (saturation more than 50%), contractility is stimulated. Moderate degrees of hypoxemia may increase contractility by enhancing the myocardial response to circulating catecholamines.[2]

Factors Determining Cardiac Output

Cardiac output is the volume of blood flowing through either the systemic or the pulmonary circuit per minute and is expressed in liters per minute. Heart rate and stroke volume determine cardiac output. The volume to which the ventricle fills is determined by the ventricular filling pressure and the compliance of the ventricle. The filling pressure of the right ventricle is the **right atrial pressure,** and the filling pressure of the left ventricle is the **left atrial pressure.** The cardiac output is determined by multiplying the heart rate and the stroke volume. Normal cardiac output is about 5 L/min for a resting adult. A summary of the major factors that determine cardiac output is presented in Figure 29-21. (Also see discussion of heart rate and myocardial contractility [stroke volume], pp. 1049 and 1062.)

The ventricle does not eject all of the blood it contains; the amount ejected is called the *ejection fraction,* or the stroke volume divided by the end-diastolic volume. The end-diastolic volume of the normal ventricle is about 70 to 80 ml/m²; the normal ejection fraction of the resting heart is about 60% to 75%. The ejection fraction is increased by factors that increase contractility (e.g., sympathetic nervous system activity), and a decrease in ejection fraction is a hallmark of ventricular failure.

SYSTEMIC CIRCULATION

The arteries and veins of the systemic circulation are illustrated in Figure 29-22. Blood from the left side of the heart flows through the aorta and into the systemic arteries. The **arteries** branch into small **arterioles** that branch further into the smallest vessels, the **capillaries,** where nutrient exchange between the blood and tissues occurs. Blood from the capillaries then enters tiny **venules** that join together to form the larger **veins,** which return venous blood to the right heart. **Peripheral vascular system** is an imprecise term used to de-

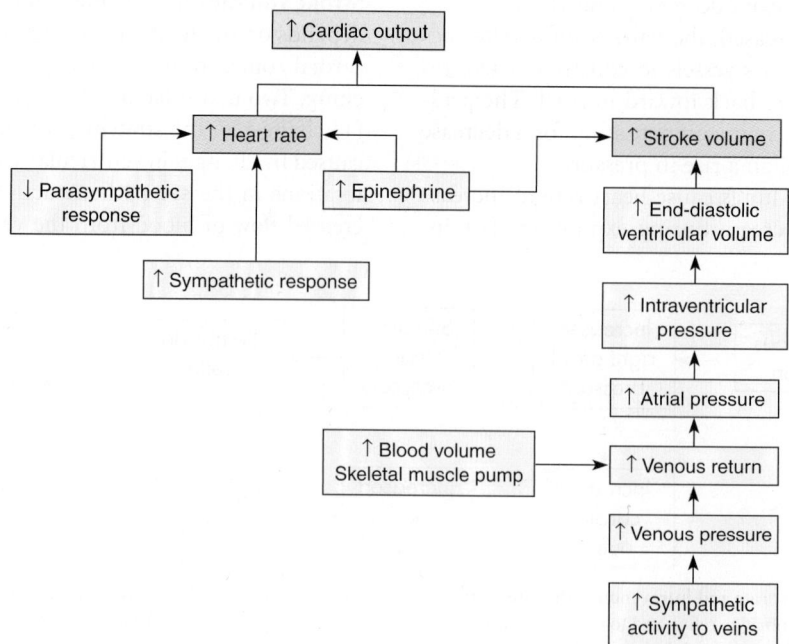

Figure 29-21 Major factors determining increased cardiac output.

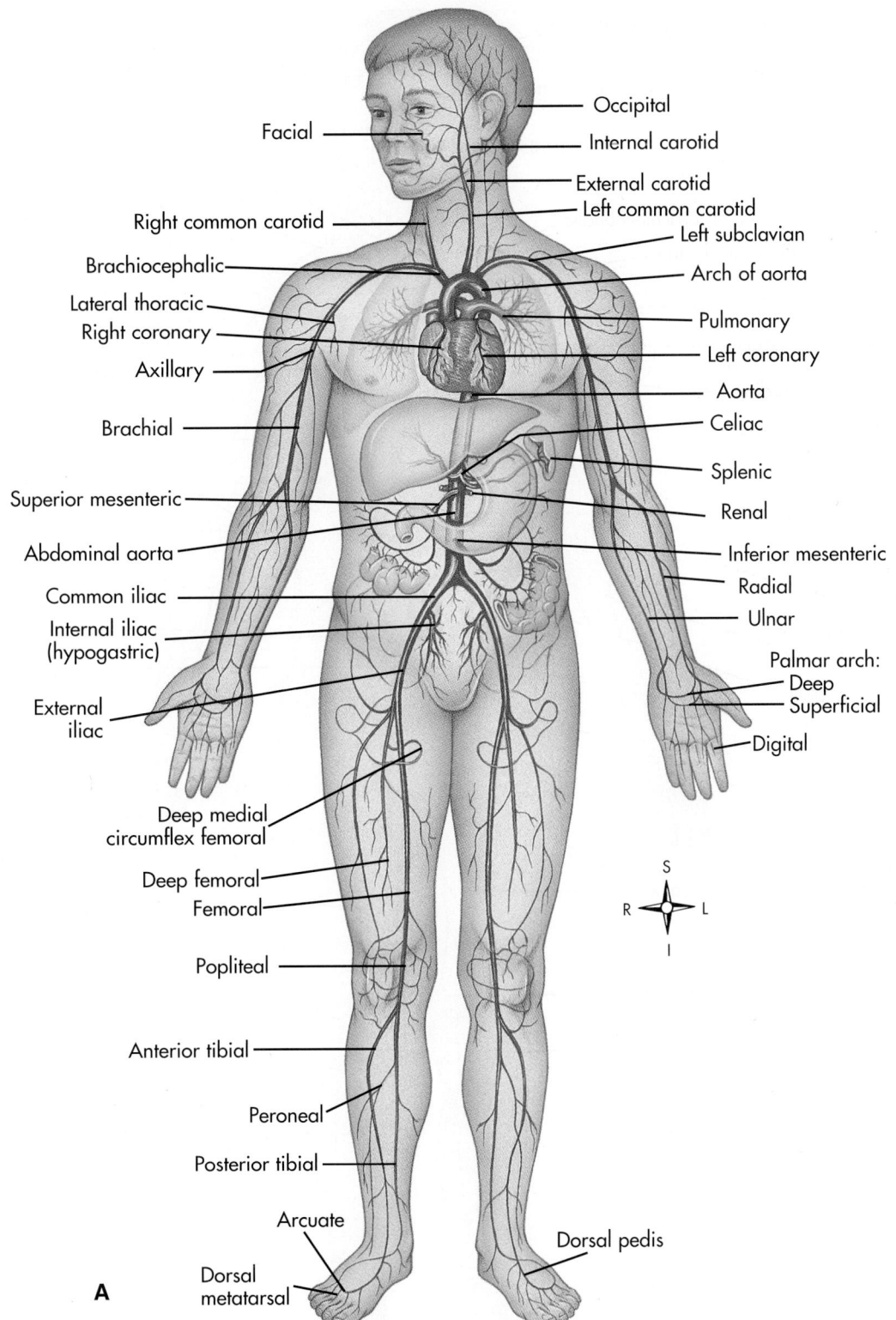

Figure 29-22 Circulatory system. **A,** Principal arteries of the body. . (From Thibodeau GA, Patton KT: *Anatomy & physiology,* ed 5, St Louis, 2003, Mosby.)

Continued

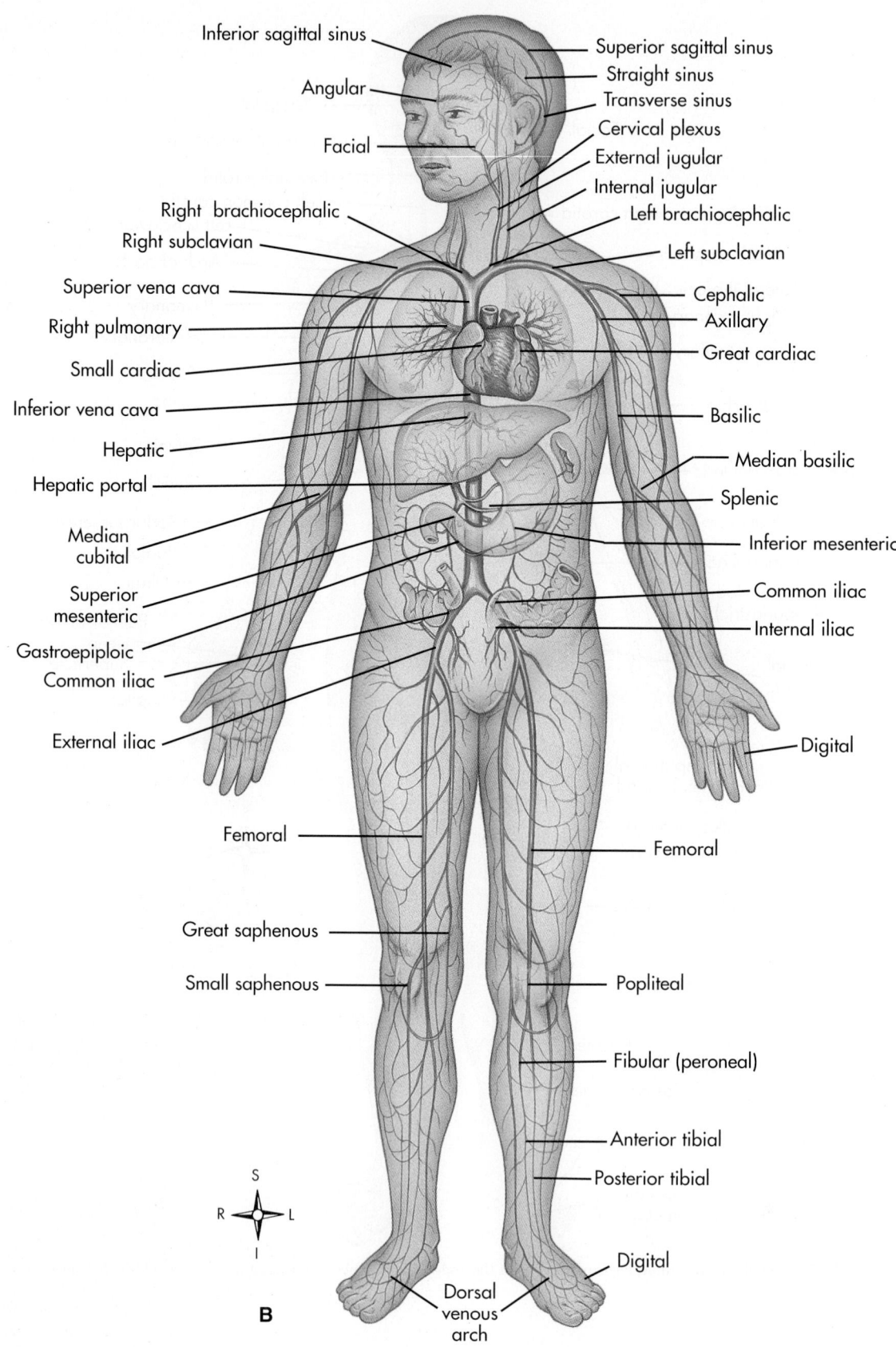

Figure 29-22, cont'd Circulatory system. **B,** Principal veins of the body. (From Thibodeau GA, Patton KT: *Anatomy & physiology,* ed 5, St Louis, 2003, Mosby.)

scribe the part of the systemic circulation that supplies the skin and the extremities, particularly the legs and feet.

Structure of Blood Vessels

Blood vessel walls are composed of three layers: the **tunica intima** (innermost or intimal layer), the tunica media (middle or medial layer), and the tunica externa or adventitia (outermost or external layer). These structures are illustrated in Figure 29-23 and 29-24. The tunica intima is composed of a layer of squamous epithelium or endothelium, a layer of connective tissue, and a basement membrane. (These cellular structures are described in Chapter 1.) The **tunica media** is composed of smooth muscle fibers mixed with elastic fibers. The **tunica externa**, or **adventitia**, has a thin layer of connective tissue containing elastic and collagenous fibers that run lengthwise in the vessel. Blood vessel walls vary in thickness depending on the thickness or absence of one or more of these three layers. Cells of the larger vessels are nourished by the **vasa vasorum**, small vessels located in the tunica externa. The vasa vasorum arise from the blood vessel itself or from other vessels nearby.

Arterial Vessels

Arterial walls are composed of elastic connective tissue, fibrous connective tissue, and smooth muscle. The two types of arteries are elastic and muscular. The **elastic arteries** have a

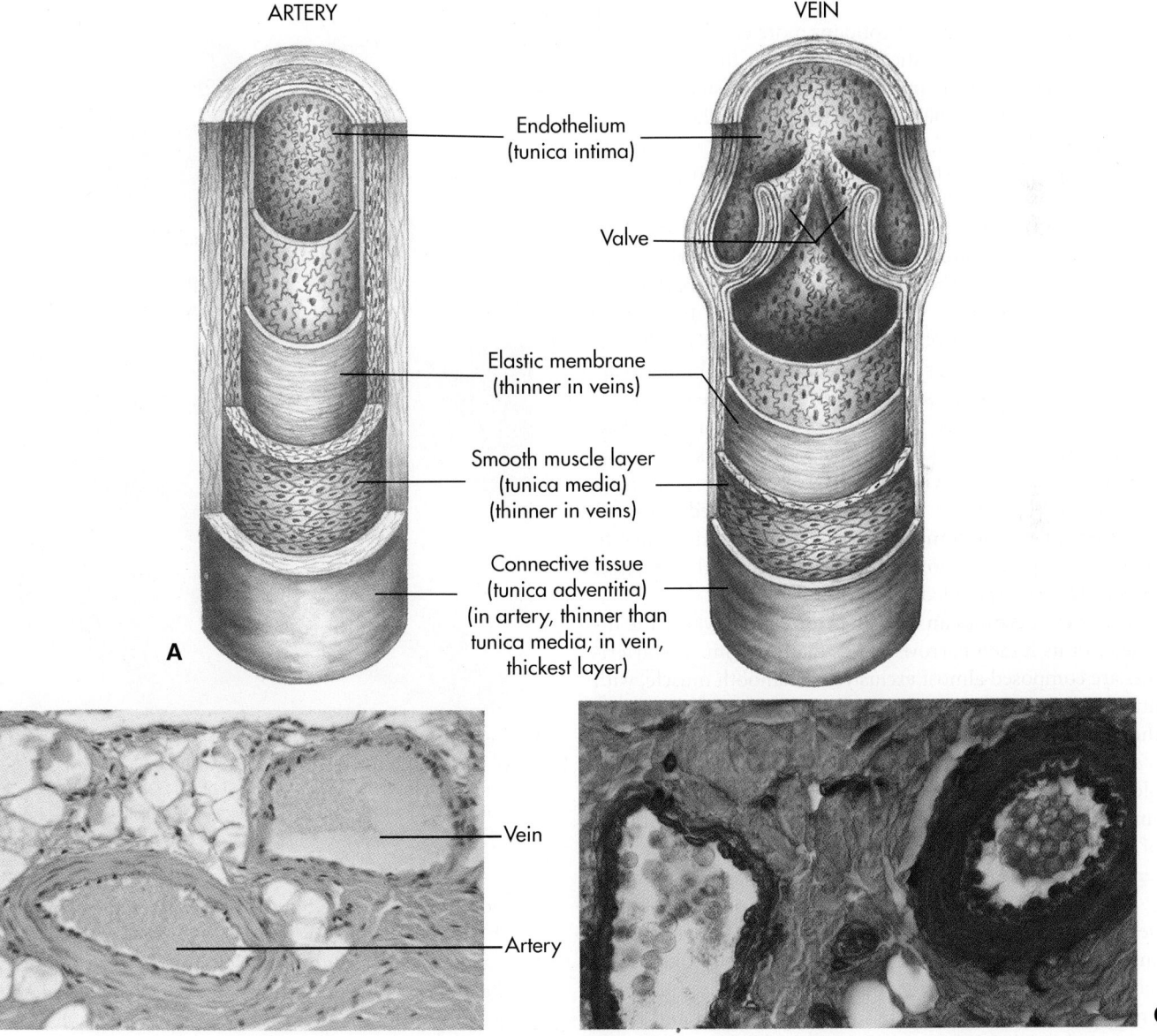

ARTERY   VEIN

Endothelium (tunica intima)

Valve

Elastic membrane (thinner in veins)

Smooth muscle layer (tunica media) (thinner in veins)

Connective tissue (tunica adventitia) (in artery, thinner than tunica media; in vein, thickest layer)

A

Vein

Artery

B   **C**

Figure 29-23 Schematic drawings and micrograph of artery and vein. **A,** Shown are the comparative thickness of three layers: outer layer (tunica adventitia), muscle layer (tunica media), and lining of endothelium (tunica intima). Note that muscle and outer coats are much thinner in veins than in arteries and that veins have valves. **B,** Micrograph (×250) of a cross section of tissue containing both an artery *(left)* and a vein *(right).* Note the thickness of the smooth muscle (tunica media) in the artery compared with the vein. **C,** Micrograph showing both an artery and vein. The tunica media is much thicker in the artery. (**A,** Modified from Thompson JM et al: *Mosby's clinical nursing,* ed 5, St Louis, 2002, Mosby. **B,** From Thibodeau GA, Patton KT: *Anatomy & physiology,* ed 5, St Louis, 2003, Mosby. **C,** Copyright Ed Reschke.)

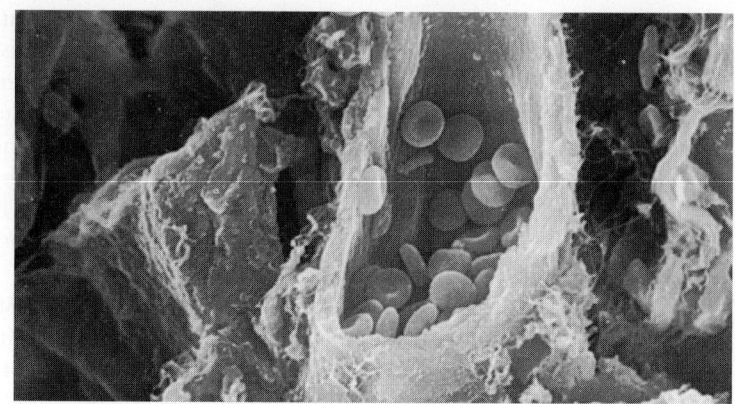

Figure 29-24 This ruptured tube is a blood vessel. It is full of red blood cells, which move through these blood vessels transporting oxygen and carbon dioxide from one place to another in the body. (From Raven RH, Johnson GB: *Biology,* ed 3, St Louis, 1992, Mosby)

very thick tunica media that contains more elastic fibers than smooth muscle fibers. Elastic arteries include the aorta and its major branches and the pulmonary trunk. Elasticity enables the vessel to stretch as blood is ejected from the heart during systole. During diastole, elasticity promotes recoil of the arteries, which is important for maintaining blood pressure within the vessels.

The **muscular arteries** are the medium-size and small arteries farther from the heart than the elastic arteries. They contain fewer elastic fibers and more muscle fibers than the elastic arteries because, being farther from the heart, they have less need of the properties of stretch and recoil. The function of the muscular arteries is to distribute blood to arterioles throughout the body. They also play a role in controlling blood flow because their smooth muscle can be stimulated to contract or relax. Contraction narrows the vessel **lumen** (the internal cavity of the vessel), which diminishes flow through the vessel. This condition is termed **vasoconstriction.** The smooth muscle layer also can be stimulated to relax, which permits more blood to flow through the vessel lumen. This state is called **vasodilation.**

An artery becomes an arteriole at the point where the diameter of its lumen narrows to less than 0.5 mm. The arterioles are composed almost exclusively of smooth muscle, with little elastic tissue. Arterioles regulate the flow of blood into the capillaries by vasoconstriction, which retards the flow of blood into the capillaries, and vasodilation, which permits blood to enter the capillaries freely (Figure 29-25). The thick, smooth muscle layer of the arterioles is a major determinant of the resistance blood encounters as it flows through the systemic circulation.

The capillary network is composed of connective channels, or thoroughfares, called **metarterioles,** and "true" capillaries (Figure 29-26). The capillaries branch from the metarterioles, meeting at a ring of smooth muscle called the **precapillary sphincter.** As the sphincters contract and relax, they regulate blood flow through the capillaries. Appropriately stimulated, the precapillary sphincters help maintain arterial pressure and regulate selective flow to vascular beds.

The capillary walls are very thin, making possible the rapid exchange of substrates, metabolites, and special products (e.g.,

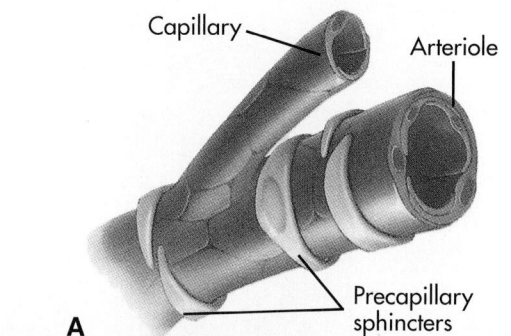

A

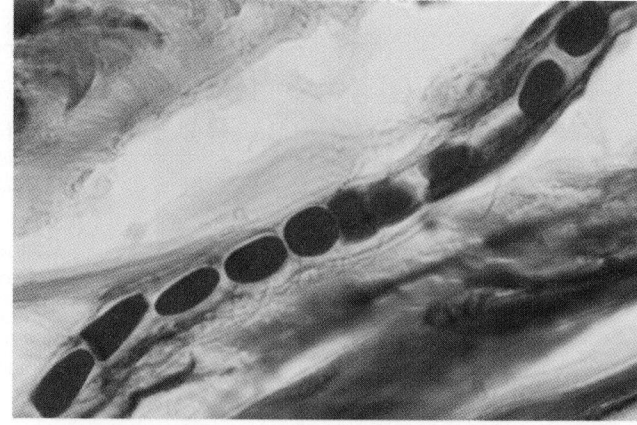

B

Figure 29-25 Capillary wall. **A,** Capillaries have a wall composed of only a single layer of flattened cells, whereas the walls of the larger vessels also have smooth muscle. **B,** Capillary with red blood cells in single file (×500). (**A,** From Thibodeau GA, Patton KT: *Anatomy & physiology,* ed 5, St Louis, 2003, Mosby. **B,** Copyright © Ed Reschke.)

hormones) between the blood and the interstitial fluid, from which they are taken up by the cells. The capillary wall consists of a single layer of endothelial cells surrounded by the thin basement membrane of the tunica intima. A single endothelial cell may form the entire vessel wall if the capillary has no tunica media or tunica externa. In some capillaries the endothelial cells contain oval windows or pores termed **fenestrations.** Fenestrations generally are covered by a thin diaphragm.

Substances pass between the capillary lumen and the interstitial fluid in several ways: (1) through junctions between

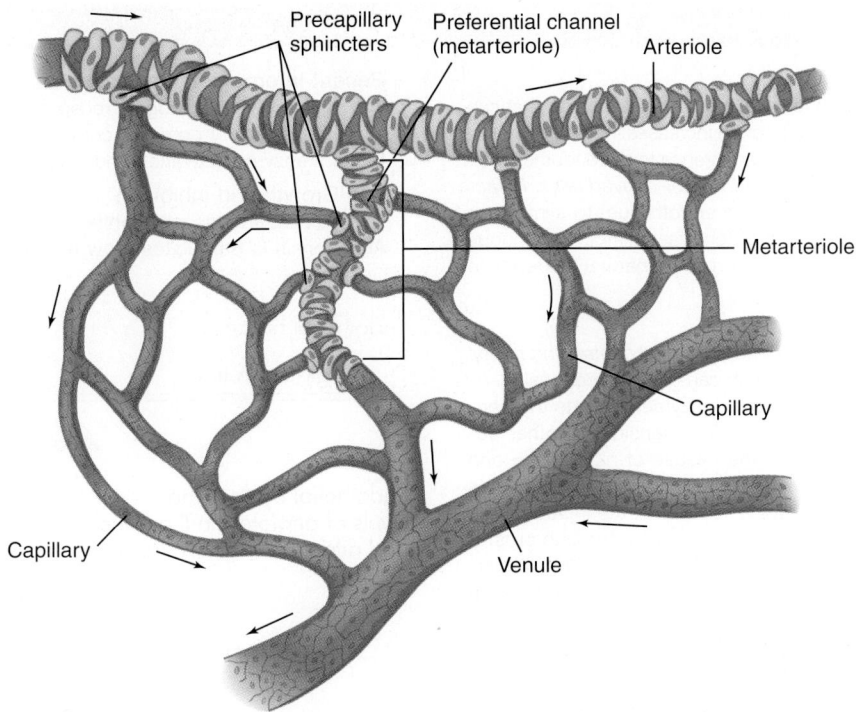

Figure 29-26 Capillary network. Blood enters network as arterial blood and exits as venous blood.

endothelial cells, (2) through fenestrations in endothelial cells, (3) in vesicles moved by active transport across the endothelial cell membrane, or (4) by diffusion through the endothelial cell membrane. (Movement across cell membranes is described in Chapter 1.) A single capillary may be only 0.5 to 1 mm in length and 0.01 mm in diameter, but the capillaries are so numerous that their total surface area may be more than 600 m², or larger than 100 football fields.

Endothelium

All tissues depend on a blood supply and the blood supply depends on **endothelial cells,** which form the lining, or **endothelium,** of the blood vessel (Figure 29-27) Endothelial cells are really quite remarkable in that they can adjust their number and arrangement to accommodate local requirements. Thus they are a life-support tissue extending and remodeling the network of blood vessels to enable tissue growth, promote contraction or relaxation or **vasomotion,** repair, antithrombogenesis, and fibrinolysis. The endothelium performs these vital functions via synthesis and release of vasoactive chemicals. Box 29-1 summarizes some of the more important functions.

Veins

The smallest venules closest to the capillaries have an inner lining, composed of the endothelium of the tunica intima and surrounded by fibrous tissue. The largest venules, those farthest from the capillaries, are surrounded by a few smooth muscle fibers comprising a thin tunica media.

Compared with arteries, veins are thin walled and fibrous with a larger diameter (see Figure 29-23). A given vein is

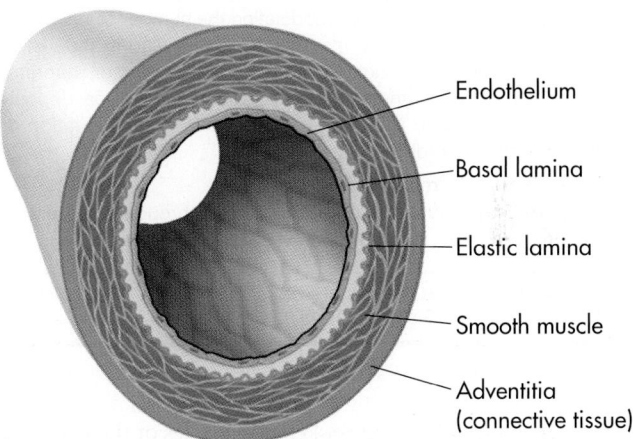

Figure 29-27 Endothelium. Practically imperceptible, the endothelial cells arrange themselves as a fine lining that has numerous life support functions.

larger than the artery that lies within the same sheath. Veins are more numerous than arteries. In veins the tunica externa has less elastic tissue than in arteries, so veins do not recoil after distention as quickly as arteries. Like arteries, veins receive nourishment from the tiny vasa vasorum. Some veins, most commonly in the lower limbs, contain valves that regulate the one-way flow of blood toward the heart (Figure 29-28). These valves are folds of the tunica intima and resemble the semilunar valves of the heart. Backflow in veins of the legs is stopped as the flaps of the valves fill with blood and block the vessel. The position of the valves also facilitates blood flow in the proper direction during venous compression. When a person

---

Box 29-1   Endothelium Functions and Vasoactive Substances

Dilators

Prostacyclin: A prostaglandin formed from arachidonic acid that can relax vascular smooth muscle through increases in cAMP. The primary function is to inhibit platelet adherence to the endothelium.

Nitric oxide (NO): Also known as *endothelial-derived relaxing factor (EDRG)*. Bradykinin prompts the endothelium to synthesize and release nitric oxide (NO), a potent vasodilator. Continuous small amounts of NO overcome the vessel's natural tendency to constrict.

Constrictors

Endothelin: Also known as *endothelium-derived contracting factor*, a potent constrictor. Overproduction can cause hypertension.

Angiotensin II: Angiotensin-converting enzyme converts the peptide angiotensin I to angiotensin II. Angiotensin II, another potent vasoconstrictor, can block the release of nitric oxide and prostacyclin. Angiotensin II has multiple functions beyond its hemodynamic effects and plays a key role in the inflammatory response. It (1) increases vascular permeability (through prostaglandins and vascular endothelial growth factor [VEGF]); (2) participates in the recruitment of infiltrating cells; (3) participates in the regulation of the expression of adhesion molecules by resident cells; and (4) contributes to tissue repair by regulation of cell growth and matrix synthesis. Thus angiotensin II is involved in both anti-inflammatory and proinflammatory reactions. Binding of angiotensin I to angiotensin II type 1 receptor is responsible for most of its physiologic reactions.

Platelet and Monocyte Adhesion

Monocytes and macrophages: The endothelium helps regulate clotting and inflammation by modulating the number of inflammatory cells (monocytes and macrophages) that bind to the vessel wall, von Willebrand factor, platelet-activating factor, heparan sulfate, t-PA, and others. Monocytes increase plaque deposition. A reduction in NO causes an increase in the oxidation of low-density lipoprotein.

Filtration and Permeability

Facilitates movement of large molecules through intercellular junctions and small molecules via vesicles and junctions.

Recent Information: Estrogen Receptors

The discovery of estrogen receptors (ERs) on endothelial cell membranes and a complex comprised of ER and other proteins triggers enzyme activation and release of NO.

Cell Growth and Inhibition

Nitric oxide, prostacyclin: **Inhibits cellular growth.**
Angiotensin II: **Stimulates growth.**

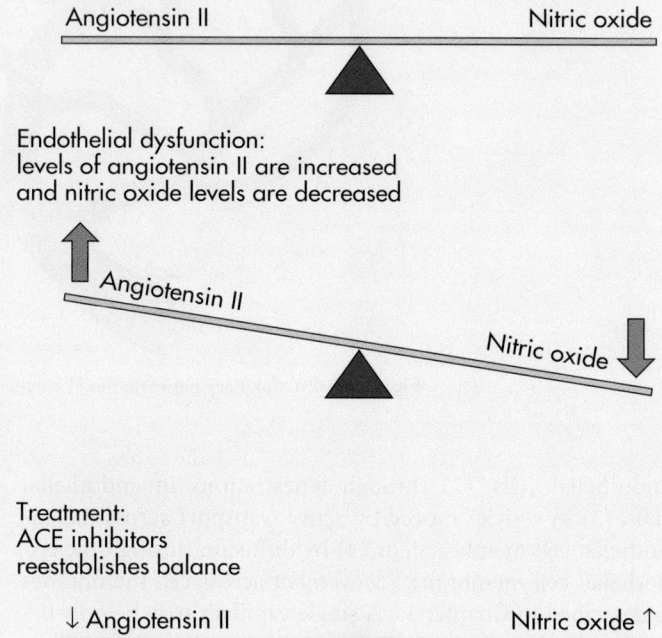

Endothelial balance

Endothelial dysfunction: levels of angiotensin II are increased and nitric oxide levels are decreased

Treatment: ACE inhibitors reestablishes balance

Data from Hisamoto K, Bender JR: *Steroids* 70(5-7):382-387, 2005; Suzuki Y, Ruiz-Ortega M, Egido J: *J Nephrol* 13(suppl 3):S101, 2000. Figure adapted from Rocket JL: *Am J Nurs* 99(10):44, 1999.

---

stands up, contraction of the skeletal muscles of the legs compresses the deep veins of the legs and assists the flow of blood toward the heart. This important mechanism of venous return is called the *muscle pump* (Figure 29-29).

Factors Affecting Blood Flow

Blood flow is the amount of fluid moved per unit of time and usually is expressed as liters or milliliters per minute (ml/min) or cubic centimeters per second (cm³/sec). Flow is regulated by the same physical properties that govern the movement of simple fluids in a closed, rigid system, that is, pressure, resistance, velocity, turbulent versus laminar flow, and compliance.

Pressure and Resistance

Blood flow is determined primarily by two factors: pressure and resistance. **Pressure** in a liquid system is the force exerted on the liquid per unit area and is expressed as dynes per square centimeter (dyn/cm²), millimeters of mercury (mmHg), or torr. Blood flow depends partly on the difference between pressures in the arterial and venous vessels supplying the organ. Fluid moves from the arterial "side" of the capillaries, a region of greater pressure, to the venous side, a region of lesser pressure.

Resistance is the opposition to force. In the cardiovascular system most opposition to blood flow is provided by the diameter and length of the blood vessels themselves. Therefore changes in blood flow through an organ result from changes in the vascular resistance within the organ. The major mechanisms causing changes in vascular resistance are an increase or a decrease in vessel diameter and the opening or closing of vascular channels. Resistance in a vessel is inversely related to blood flow; that is, increased resistance leads to decreased blood flow.

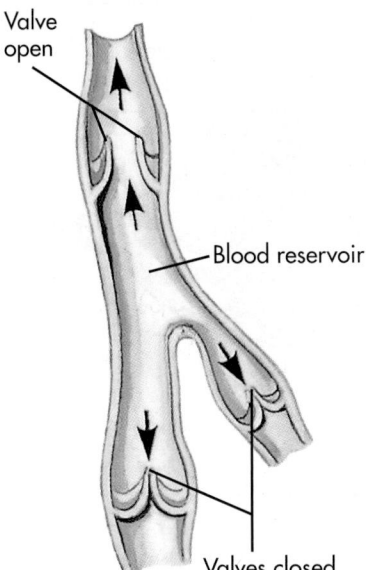

Figure 29-28 Valves of vein. Pooled blood is moved toward heart as valves are forced open by pressure from volume of blood downstream. (From Thibodeau GA, Patton KT: *Anatomy & physiology,* ed 5, St Louis, 2003, Mosby.)

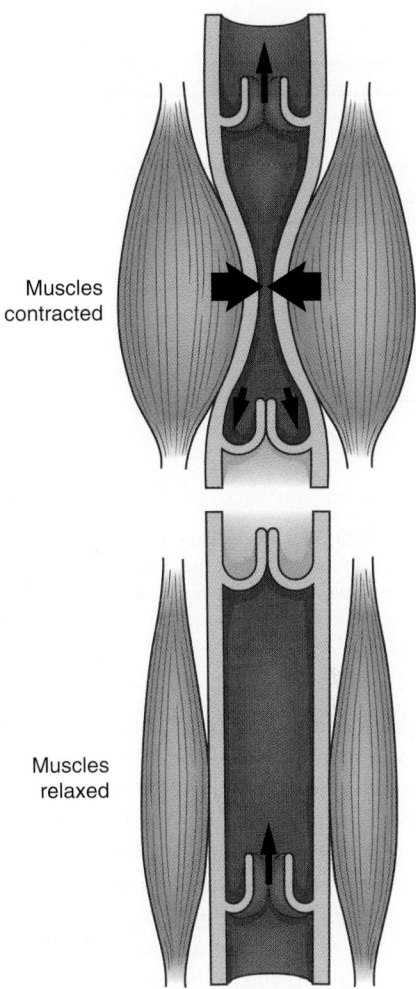

Figure 29-29 Muscle pump.

Blood flow *(Q)* through a vessel can be calculated from measurements of pressure at the inflow end of the vessel *(P_1)*, pressure at the outflow end of the vessel *(P_2)*, and resistance *(R)*. The difference between P_1 and P_2 often is referred to as the change in pressure and is expressed as δP. The following formula, which expresses Poiseuille's law, shows the relationship among blood flow, pressure, and resistance:

$$Q = \delta P/R$$

where *Q* = blood flow, *δP* = the pressure difference *($P_1 - P_2$)*, and *R* = resistance.

Resistance to flow cannot be measured directly, but it can be calculated if the pressure difference and flow volumes are known. To determine resistance, the equation for flow is re-arranged as follows:

Flow varies inversely with the viscosity of the fluid. Thick fluids move more slowly and cause greater resistance to flow than thin fluids. The viscosity of blood depends on its red cell content. The greater the percentage of red cells in the blood, the more viscous the blood. This relationship is expressed as the hematocrit—the ratio of the volume of red blood cells to the volume of whole blood (see Chapter 25). A high hematocrit reduces flow through the blood vessels, particularly the microcirculation (arterioles, capillaries, venules). Conditions in which the hematocrit is elevated, such as dehydration, cyanotic congenital heart disease (see Chapter 31), or polycythemia (see Chapter 26), can lead to increased cardiac work as a result of increased vascular resistance.

The viscosity of blood also increases if blood flow becomes very slow or stagnates (**anomalous viscosity**). Anomalous viscosity is generally not significant unless cardiac output is low. (Shock is described in Chapter 46.)

Poiseuille's formula for resistance to fluid flow through a tube takes into account the length of the tube, the viscosity of the fluid, and the radius of the tube's lumen. Resistance *(R)* is proportional to a constant 8/π, the viscosity of the blood (η), and the length of the vessel *(l)*, and it is inversely proportional to the fourth power of the lumen's radius *(v^4)*.[2] Thus

$$R = \frac{8\eta l}{\pi v 4}$$

Because this equation was derived using straight, rigid tubes with steady, streamlined flow, it cannot be applied directly to the vascular system. Nevertheless, it is a useful model of vascular resistance.

The most important factor determining resistance in a single vessel is the caliber of the vessel's lumen, expressed in Poiseuille's formula as its radius and in Figure 29-30 as its diameter. Small changes in the lumen's radius lead to large changes in vascular resistance. Because vessel length is relatively constant, length is not as important as lumen size in determining flow through a single vessel.

Generally, resistance to flow is greater in longer tubes because resistance increases with length. That resistance increases with increased length is demonstrated by comparing

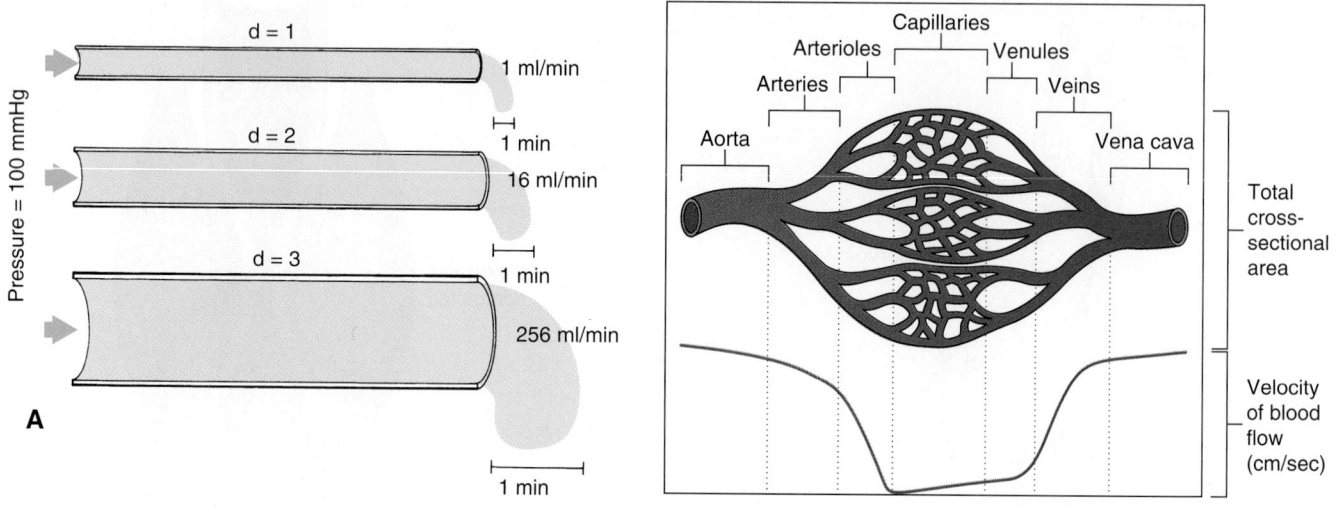

Figure 29-30 Lumen diameter, blood flow, and resistance. **A,** Effect of lumen diameter on flow through vessel. *d,* Diameter. **B,** Blood flows with great speed in the large arteries. However, branching of arterial vessels increases the total cross-sectional area of the arterioles and capillaries, reducing the flow rate. When capillaries merge into venules and venules merge into veins, the total cross-sectional area decreases, causing the flow rate to increase. (**B,** From Thibodeau GA, Patton KT: *Anatomy & physiology,* ed 5, St Louis, 2003, Mosby.)

flow of the same amount of blood under the same pressure through vessels arranged in different configurations. Blood flowing through the distributing arteries, beginning with branches off the aorta and ending at arterioles in the capillary bed, encounters more resistance than blood flowing through the capillary bed itself, where flow is distributed among many short, tiny branches arranged in parallel. This is because the distributing arteries comprise a long system of tubes connected in series (end to end), whereas the arterioles and capillaries comprise a short system of many vessels arranged in parallel (side by side) (Figure 29-31). Although the arterioles are arranged in series with the distributing arteries and the capillaries, they are arranged in parallel with other arterioles. Similarly, the capillaries are in series with the metarterioles, but they are in parallel with other capillaries.

Resistance to flow through a system of vessels, or **total resistance,** depends not only on characteristics of individual vessels but also on whether the vessels are arranged in series or in parallel (see Figure 29-31). For vessels arranged in series, total resistance equals the sum obtained by adding all the individual resistances calculated using Poiseuille's formula. For vessels arranged in parallel, total resistance equals the sum of the reciprocals *(I/R)* of the individual resistances.

Total resistance is related to the total cross-sectional area of a system of vessels in parallel and to the number of vessels in parallel that make up the total cross-sectional area. The larger the total cross-sectional area, as in the capillary system, the lower the resistance. However, if a cross-sectional area is made up of a very large number of parallel vessels, the overall resistance will be greater than it would be if the cross-sectional area were made up of only two or three parallel vessels. Therefore resistance is greater in smaller vessels than in larger vessels. The total cross-sectional area of the arteriolar system is greater than that of the arterial system (see Figure 29-30); the

greater number of arterioles arranged in parallel, however, leads to great resistance to flow in the arteriolar system. Because resistance reaches a maximal level in the arteries, they are sometimes called the "stopcocks" of the vascular system. The pressure drop is greatest across the arterioles. Many capillaries arise from each arteriole so that the total cross-sectional area of the capillary bed is very large and resistance is low, despite the fact that the cross-sectional area of each capillary is less (which normally increases resistance) than that of each arteriole. As a result, blood flow becomes quite slow in the capillaries, analogous to water flow in a river. A narrow river whose bed widens flows more slowly through the wide section than through the narrow section. The slow velocity of flow in each vessel promotes optimal capillary-tissue exchange.

Neural Control of Total Peripheral Resistance

Total resistance in the systemic circulation, sometimes called *total peripheral resistance,* is determined primarily by change in the diameter of the arterioles. Reflex control of total cardiac output and peripheral resistance includes (1) sympathetic stimulation of heart, arterioles, and veins and (2) parasympathetic stimulation of the heart only.

The autonomic nervous system is monitored by the cardiovascular control center in the brain (see p. 1048). The hypothalamic centers regulate vascular (and cardiac) responses to changes in temperature. When the body's core temperature exceeds normal, the hypothalamus reflex initiates dilation of arterioles and veins in the skin. This causes shunting of blood to the skin, where heat is lost from sweating, radiation, conduction, or convection. When body core temperature decreases below normal, surface vessels constrict, shunting blood to the vital organs. Vasoconstriction is regulated by an area of the brain stem that maintains a constant (tonic) out-

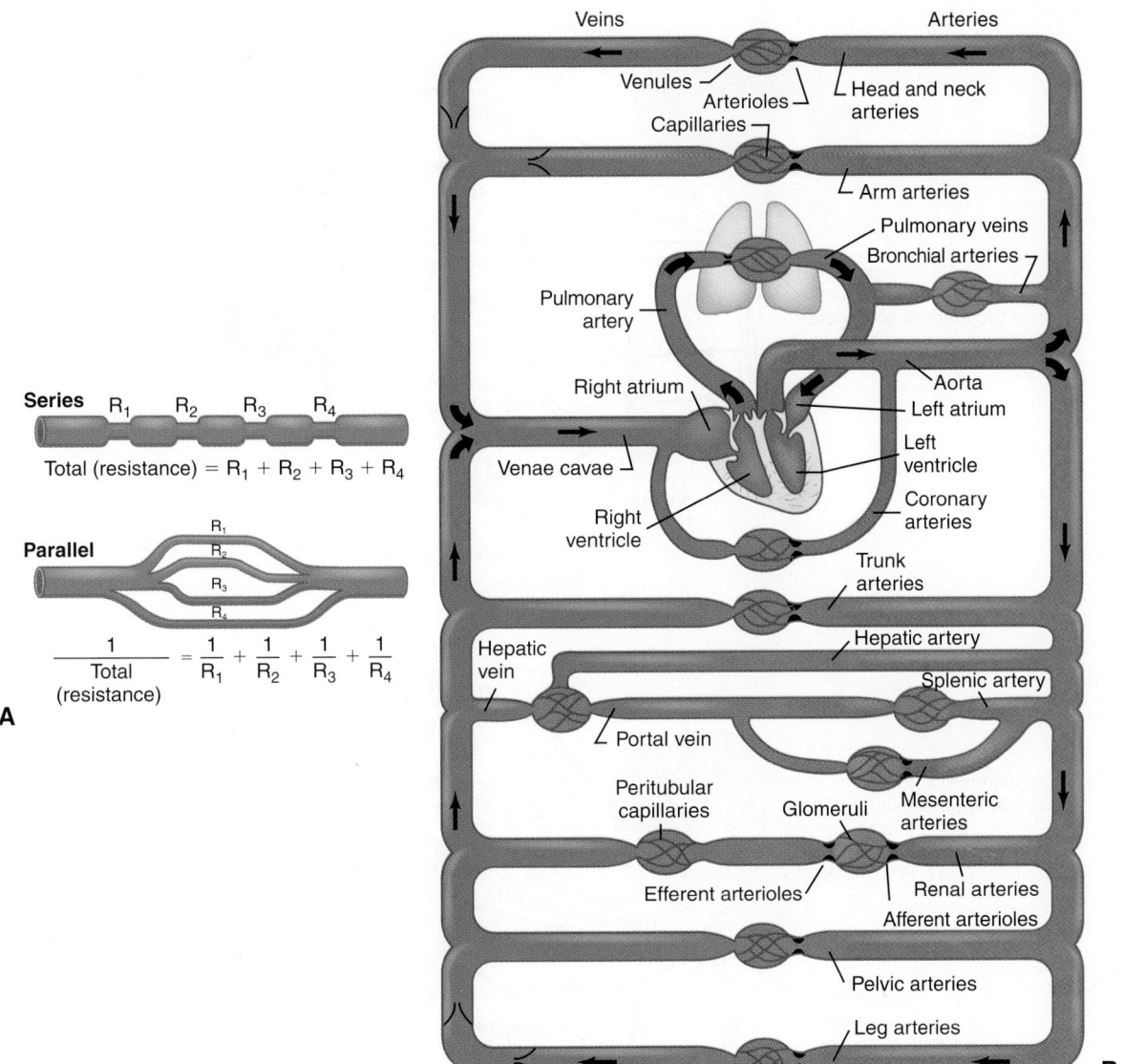

Figure 29-31 Schematic diagram of the parallel and series arrangement of the vessels composing the circulatory system. **A,** Resistance in blood vessels arranged in series or parallel. *R,* Resistance in an individual vessel. **B,** The capillary beds are represented by thin lines connecting the arterioles (on the right) and the veins (on the left). The crescent-shaped thickenings proximal to the capillary beds represent the arterioles (resistance vessels). (**B,** Modified from Berne RM, Levy MN: *Cardiovascular physiology,* ed 8, St Louis, 2001, Mosby.)

put of norepinephrine from sympathetic fibers in the peripheral arterioles. This tonic activity is essential for maintenance of blood pressure.

During exercise and stress, the sympathetic fibers that stimulate vasodilation of skeletal muscle arterioles are thought to be under the direct control of the cerebral cortex and hypothalamus and not the medullary centers.[9] Information about pressure and resistance is sensed by neural receptors (baroreceptors and chemoreceptors) in arterial walls and delivered to the medullary centers.

Baroreceptors

Major stretch receptors are located in the aorta and in the carotid sinus (Figure 29-32). These baroreceptors respond to changes in smooth muscle fiber length by altering their rate of discharge, and they supply sensory information to the cardio-

vascular center that regulates blood pressure. (Technically they are mechanoreceptors, but they usually are called *baroreceptors* or *pressoreceptors.*) The rate of firing of the baroreceptors increases and decreases with changes in blood pressure. An increase in arterial pressure increases the rate of firing of both the carotid sinus and aortic arch baroreceptors. These impulses travel up the afferent nerves to the medulla (e.g., the cardiac control center) and (1) slow heart rate by decreasing sympathetic discharge and increasing parasympathetic discharge (vagus nerve), (2) decrease myocardial contractility by inhibiting sympathetic discharge, and (3) increase arteriolar and venous dilation by decreasing sympathetic discharge to smooth muscle. The net effect of this major blood pressure–regulating reflex is to reduce blood pressure to normal by decreasing cardiac output (heart rate and stroke volume) and

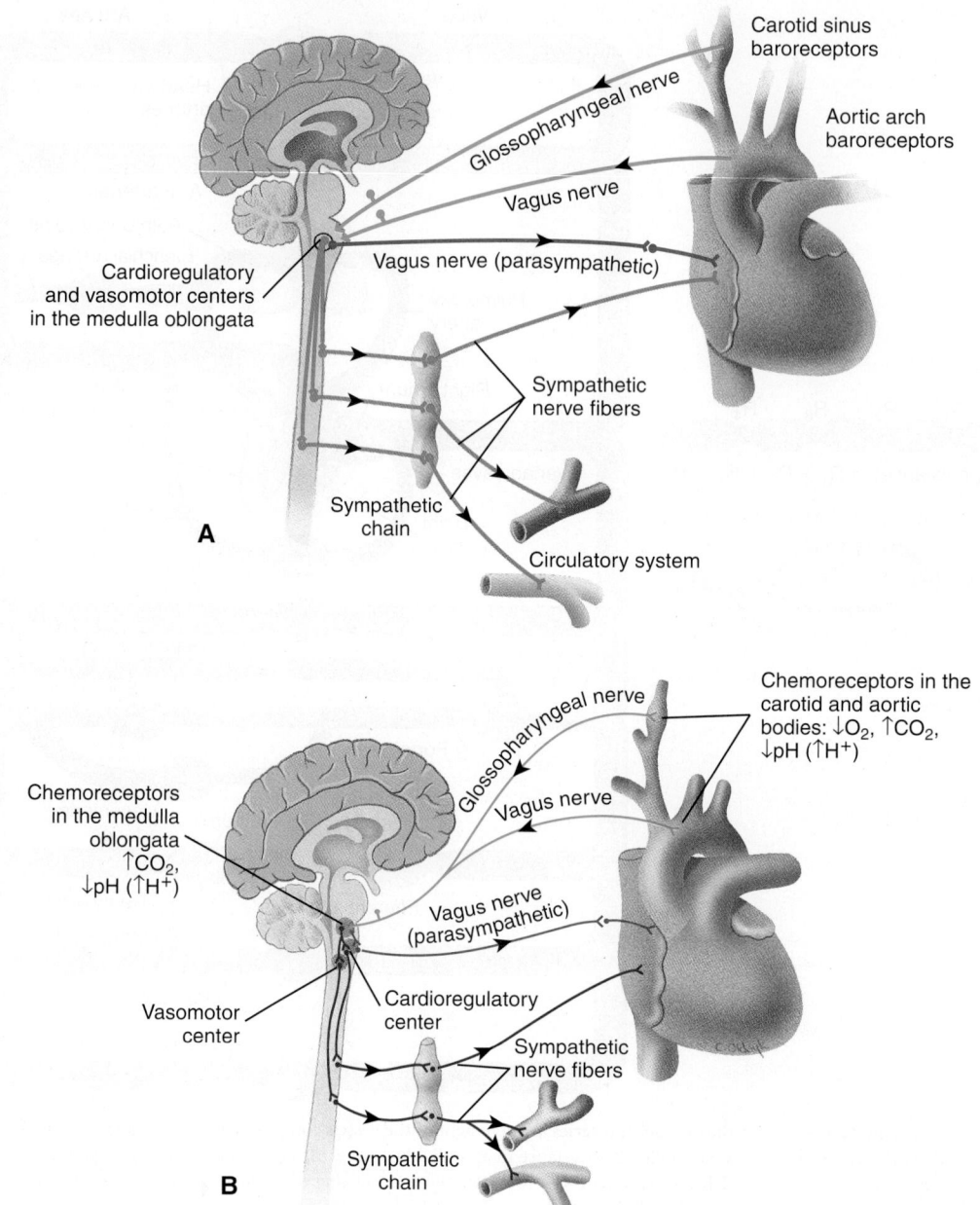

Figure 29-32 Baroreceptor and chemoreceptor reflex control of blood pressure. **A,** Baroreceptor reflexes. Baroreceptors located in the carotid sinuses and aortic arch detect changes in blood pressure. Action potentials are conducted to the cardioregulatory and vasomotor centers. The heart rate can be decreased by the parasympathetic system; the heart rate and stroke volume can be increased by the sympathetic system. The sympathetic system also can constrict or dilate blood vessels. **B,** Chemoreceptor reflexes. Chemoreceptors located in the medulla oblongata and in the carotid and aortic bodies detect changes in blood oxygen, carbon dioxide, or pH. Action potentials are conducted to the medulla oblongata. In response, the vasomotor center can cause vasoconstriction or dilation of blood vessels by the sympathetic system, and the cardioregulatory center can cause changes in the pumping activity of the heart through the parasympathetic and sympathetic systems. (From Seeley RR, Stephens TD, Tate P: *Anatomy & physiology,* ed 3, St Louis, 1995, Mosby.)

peripheral resistance. (Postural changes and the baroreceptor reflex are discussed in Chapter 30.)

Arterial Chemoreceptors

Specialized areas within the medulla oblongata and aortic and carotid arteries are sensitive to concentrations of oxygen, carbon dioxide, and hydrogen ions (pH) in the blood (see Figure 29-32, *B*). Although these receptors, called *chemorecep-*

tors, are more important for the control of respiration, they also transmit impulses to the medullary cardiovascular centers that regulate blood pressure. A decrease in arterial oxygen concentration or pH causes a reflexive increase in blood pressure, whereas an increase in carbon dioxide causes an increase in blood pressure. Blood pressure changes are carried out by smooth muscle layers in the vessels. Vasoconstriction raises blood pressure, and vasodilation lowers it. The major chemoreceptive reflex is caused by alterations in arterial oxygen concentration. The effects of altered pH or carbon dioxide levels are minor.

Velocity

Blood velocity is the distance blood travels in a unit of time, usually centimeters per second (cm/sec). Blood velocity is directly related to blood flow (amount of blood moved per unit of time) and inversely related to the cross-sectional area of the vessel in which the blood is flowing.

The relationship between velocity and flow can be understood by thinking of a river. The volume of water flowing in a river is the same whether the river is narrow or wide. Where the river narrows, the water flows quickly; where it widens, the water flows slowly. The volume of water moving between the river banks does not change. In the body, as blood moves from the aorta to the capillaries, the total cross-sectional area of the vessels increases and velocity of flow decreases.

Laminar versus Turbulent Flow

Flow through any tubular system is either laminar or turbulent. Normally, blood flow through the vessels is laminar. In **laminar flow,** concentric layers of molecules move "straight ahead." Each concentric layer flows at a different velocity (Figure 29-33). The cohesive attraction between the fluid and the vessel wall prevents the molecules of blood that are in contact with the wall from moving. The next thin layer of blood is able to slide slowly past the stationary layer and so

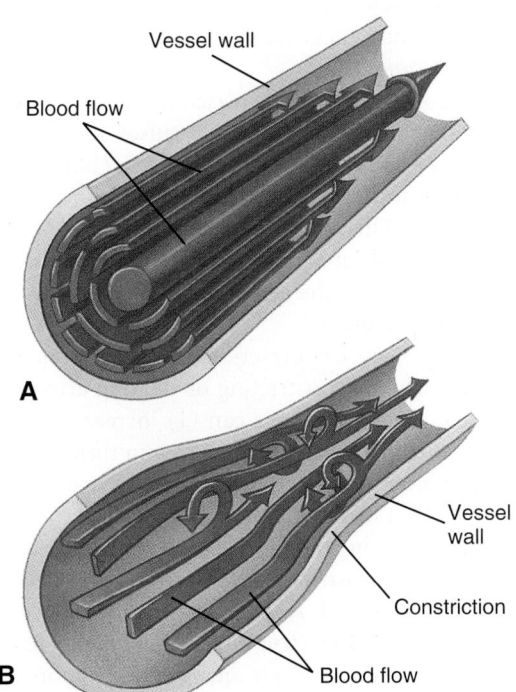

Figure 29-33 Laminar and turbulent flow. **A,** Laminar flow. Fluid flows in long, smooth-walled tubes as if it is composed of a large number of concentric layers. **B,** Turbulent flow. Turbulent flow is caused by numerous small currents flowing crosswise or oblique to the long axis of the vessel, resulting in flowing whorls and eddy currents. (From Seeley RR, Stephens TD, Tate P: *Anatomy and physiology,* ed 3, St Louis, 1995, Mosby.)

on until, at the center, the blood velocity is greatest. The centermost concentric layer of fluid is not slowed by friction against the vessel wall. Large vessels have room for a large center layer; therefore they have less resistance to flow and greater flow and velocity than smaller vessels.

Where flow is obstructed, the vessel turns, or blood flows over rough surfaces, it becomes **turbulent** with whorls or eddy currents that produce noise, causing a murmur to be heard on auscultation. Resistance increases with turbulence.

Vascular Compliance

Vascular compliance is the increase in volume a vessel is able to accommodate for a given increase in pressure (e.g., $C = VP$). Compliance depends on the ratio of elastic fibers to muscle fibers in the vessel wall. The elastic arteries are more compliant than the muscular arteries; the veins are more compliant than either type of artery and serve as storage areas for the circulatory system.

Compliance determines a vessel's response to pressure changes. For example, with a very small increase in pressure, a large volume of blood can be accommodated by the venous system. In the less compliant arterial system, where smaller volumes and higher pressures are normal, small variations in pressure cause little or no change in the volume of blood within the arterial vessels.

Stiffness is the opposite of compliance. Several conditions and disorders can cause stiffness, with the most common being arteriosclerosis (see Chapter 30). Arteriosclerosis increases the rigidity or stiffness of arterial walls, which in turn increases peak arterial pressure at a given volume of blood.

Regulation of Blood Pressure

Arterial Pressure

Arterial pressure is constantly regulated to maintain tissue **perfusion,** or blood supply to the capillary beds, during a wide range of physiologic conditions, including changes in body position, muscular activity, and circulating blood volume. The **mean arterial pressure (MAP),** which is the average pressure in the arteries throughout the cardiac cycle, depends on the elastic properties of the arterial walls and the mean volume of blood in the arterial system. MAP can be approximated from the measured values of the systolic (Ps) and diastolic (Pd) pressures by means of the following formula:

$$MAP = Pd + \frac{1}{3}(Ps - Pd, \text{ or pulse pressure})$$

The major factors and relationships that regulate arterial blood pressure are summarized in Figure 29-34.

Effects of Cardiac Output

The cardiac output (minute volume) of the heart can be changed by alterations in heart rate, stroke volume (volume of blood ejected during each ventricular contraction), or both. An increase in cardiac output without a decrease in peripheral resistance will cause both arterial volume and mean blood pressure to increase. The higher arterial pressure increases blood flow through the arterioles. On the other hand,

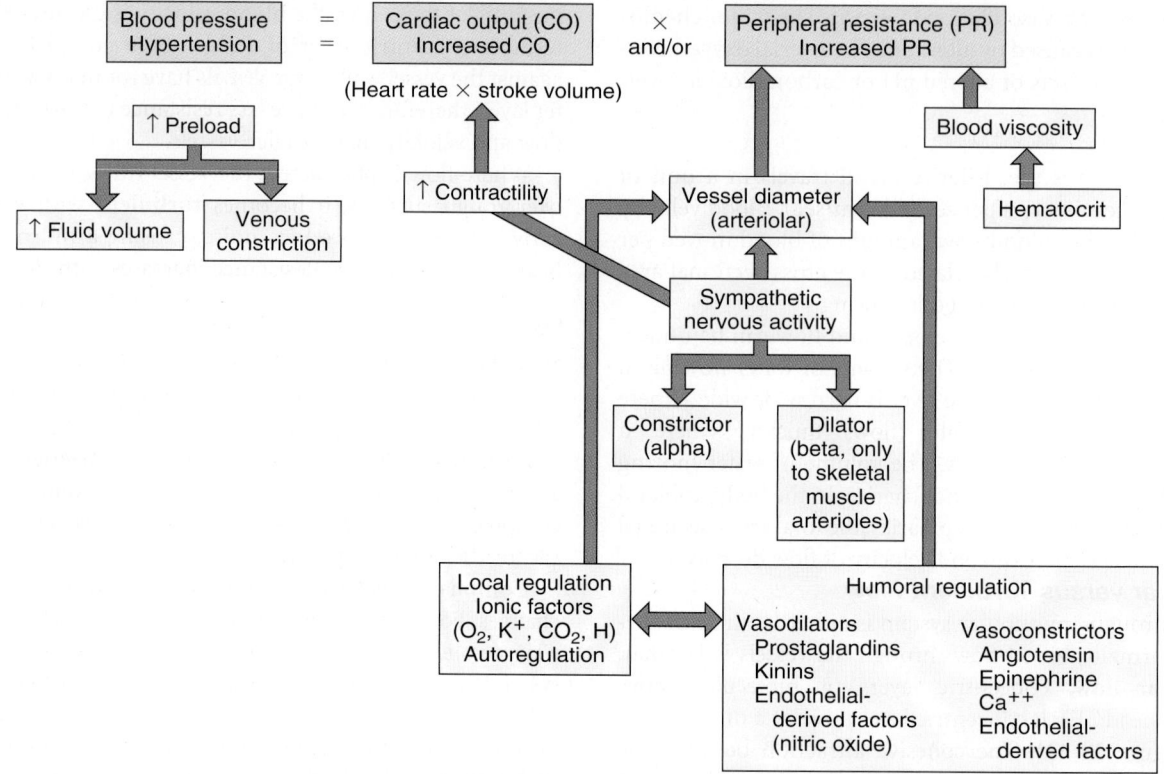

Figure 29-34 Factors regulating blood flow.

Table 29-3	Factors that Affect Mean Arterial Pressure and Capillary Flow	
	Mean Arterial Pressure	**Capillary Flow**
Peripheral Resistance*		
Increased	Increased	Decreased
Decreased	Decreased	Increased
Heart Rate†		
Increased	Increased	Increased
Decreased	Decreased	Decreased
Stroke Volume‡		
Increased	Increased	Increased
Decreased	Decreased	Decreased

From Little RC: *Physiology of the heart and circulation,* ed 3, St Louis, 1985, Mosby.
*Cardiac output maintained constant.
†Peripheral resistance and stroke volume constant.
‡Peripheral resistance and heart rate constant.

a decrease in the cardiac output causes an immediate drop in mean arterial blood pressure and arteriolar flow (Table 29-3).

Effects of Total Peripheral Resistance

Total peripheral resistance is determined primarily by a change in the diameter of the arterioles: arteriolar constriction raises mean arterial pressure by preventing the free flow of blood into the capillaries. Dilation has the opposite effect.

Reflex control of vasoconstriction and vasodilation is mediated by the sympathetic nervous system.

Effect of Hyperemia

When metabolic activity is increased in the heart, skeletal muscle, and other muscular organs, it causes an increase in blood flow termed **hyperemia.** For example, the blood flow to exercising skeletal muscle increases in proportion to the activity of the muscle. This condition, known as *active (exercise) hyperemia,* is the result of arteriolar dilation and autoregulation of blood flow within the active organ.

Effects of Hormones

Many hormones cause contraction or relaxation of arteriolar smooth muscle. By constricting or dilating arterioles in specific vascular beds, hormones can (1) increase the blood supply to vital organs requiring more flow in times of stress, (2) redistribute blood volume during hemorrhage or shock, and (3) regulate heat loss.

Epinephrine, the hormone released from the adrenal medulla, causes vasoconstriction in most vascular beds (exceptions are the liver and skeletal muscles). However, the effects of **norepinephrine** (from the sympathetic nervous system and adrenal medulla) are quantitatively more vasoconstrictive than the effects of epinephrine.

Antidiuretic hormone, renin-angiotensin system, natriuretic peptides, adrenomedullin and insulin. Blood pressure can be influenced by factors that change the total volume of blood in the circulatory system. Antidiuretic hormone (ADH) is released by the posterior pituitary and causes reabsorption of water by the kidney. With reabsorption the blood plasma volume will increase, increasing blood pressure (see Chapters 3 and 35 and Figure 29-37).

Renin is an enzyme synthesized and secreted by the juxtaglomerular cells of the kidney. It also has been found in the adrenal cortex, salivary gland, prolactin-producing and luteinizing hormone–producing cells of the pituitary, arterial smooth muscle cells in the vascular endothelium, brain, myocardium, and possibly other tissues.[10] The following factors control renin release:

1. A drop in blood pressure (e.g., the renal artery)
2. A decrease in the amount of sodium delivered to the kidney (although recent evidence indicates a role for chloride in regulating renin secretion)[10]
3. Stimulation of renin release by β-adrenergic stimuli and a decrease in renin release caused by β-adrenergic inhibitors
4. Reduced renin release caused by angiotensin II
5. Increased renin release caused by low potassium concentrations in plasma

Once in the circulation, renin splits off a polypeptide from angiotensinogen to generate **angiotensin I (Ang I)**. Angiotensin I appears to be physiologically inactive.[10] Angiotensin I, however, is converted by an enzyme to **angiotensin II (Ang II)**. Angiotensin-converting enzyme (ACE) is a powerful vasoconstrictor that stimulates the secretion of **aldosterone** from the adrenal gland (see Figures 20-20 and 29-37). Aldosterone causes reabsorption of sodium in the kidneys. Aldosterone plays an important role in the pathogenesis of cardiovascular and renal disease independent of Angiotensin II.[11] (See What's New: Emerging Roles of Aldosterone.)

In addition, Ang II causes some sodium retention in the kidneys and suppresses renin secretion from the juxtaglomerular cells.[10] In some tissues, Ang II is converted to Ang III, which is also biologically active.

This kidney-based renin-angiotensin system serves as an important regulatory loop. For example, decreases in blood pressure or sodium delivery to the kidneys (macula densa), as might occur after hemorrhage or extracellular volume deficits (dehydration), stimulate secretion of renin, which forms Ang I, which is converted to Ang II and restores blood pressure. Sodium retention also results from increased secretion of aldosterone. Overall, the renin-angiotensin system is activated after volume depletion or hypotension or both, and it is suppressed after volume repletion and hypertension. Basic knowledge of the renin-angiotensin system has advanced. Important is knowledge of a **tissue-based renin-angiotensin system** that can be regulated independently from the circulation. These new data are redefining our understanding of hypertension and other vascular disorders. The tissue renin-angiotensin system is activated in response to tissue injury. This system is involved in maladaptive alterations, such as ventricular and vascular remodeling, alterations in renal functions, and atherosclerosis, (see Chapter 30). Particularly significant is an increased recognition of the role of Ang II in these processes (Figure 29-35).

Ang II has two subtypes of receptors, **AT$_1$** and **AT$_2$** (Figure 29-36). Both subtypes are expressed in human hearts. AT$_1$ is also found on vascular smooth muscle and endothelial cells, nerve endings, conduction tissues, adrenal cortex, liver, kidney and brain.[12] AT$_2$ receptors are found in fetal mesenchymal tissue, adrenal medulla, uterus and ovarian follicles, renal tubules, and vasculature.[12] The majority of ang II actions are thought to occur via the AT$_1$ receptor, including growth promotion, vasoconstriction, antinatriuresis (save Na$^+$), aldosterone secretion, inhibition of renin synthesis and release, salt appetite, thirst, and sympathetic outflow.[13] (See What's New: AT$_1$ Signaling and Inflammation.)

Although the majority of Ang II actions are mediated via the AT$_1$ receptor, emerging is evidence that AT$_2$ receptor opposes the AT$_1$ receptor, especially by inducing vasodilation instead of vasoconstriction.[14] AT$_2$ dilator action is mediated by nitric oxide (NO) in a bradykinin-dependent or independent manner (see Figure 29-37). Vasodilation has now been shown in microarteries of the coronary, mesenteric, and uterine circulation. In addition, continuous use of compounds that stimulate AT$_2$ receptor (agonists) cause sustained vasodilation and hypotension.[15] Therapeutically, these data predict that AT$_2$ receptor stimulation would be a beneficial addition to AT$_1$ receptor blockage. Treatments such as angiotensin-converting enzyme (ACE) inhibitors and angiotensin receptor antagonists that inhibit AT$_1$ receptor are a main target in preventive and reparative strategies in cardiovascular disease.

Ang II is now considered to be a growth promoter in cardiovascular tissues, and the resultant vascular hypertrophy is a significant factor in the pathogenesis of hypertension. Ang II plays a role in the kidney, not only as a regulator of blood flow but also in the development of structural changes (i.e., hypertrophy). A central role for the renin-angiotensin system

---

WHAT'S NEW?   Emerging Roles of Aldosterone

Experimental data support a role for aldosterone in mediating cardiovascular injury. In these studies prolonged exposure to aldosterone was associated with the development of myocardial hypertrophy and fibrosis. Basically, aldosterone moves across the plasma membrane, binds to the epithelial mineralocorticoid receptor (MR), translocates to the nucleus, binds to hormone response elements in the nucleus, and stimulates protein synthesis that ultimately leads to the absorption of Na$^+$ ions and water intracellularly in the colon and kidney. Aldosterone can be synthesized locally in blood vessels, heart, and brain. These sites of synthesis appear to be regulated by the renin-angiotensin system. Other possibly paracrine/autocrine sites independent of renin, however, may exist in vascular smooth muscle cells. Peripheral infusion of aldosterone in rats with a high sodium intake causes cardiac hypertrophy and fibrosis independent of effects on blood pressure. The exact mechanisms of how aldosterone causes these effects is the focus of ongoing studies.

Data from Stier CT, Rocha R, Chander PN: *Heart Fail Rev* 10(1): 53-62, 2005; Magni P, Motta M: *Curr Hypertens Rep* 7(3):206, 2005; Brown NJ: *Curr Opin Nephrol Hypertens* 14(3):235-241, 2005.

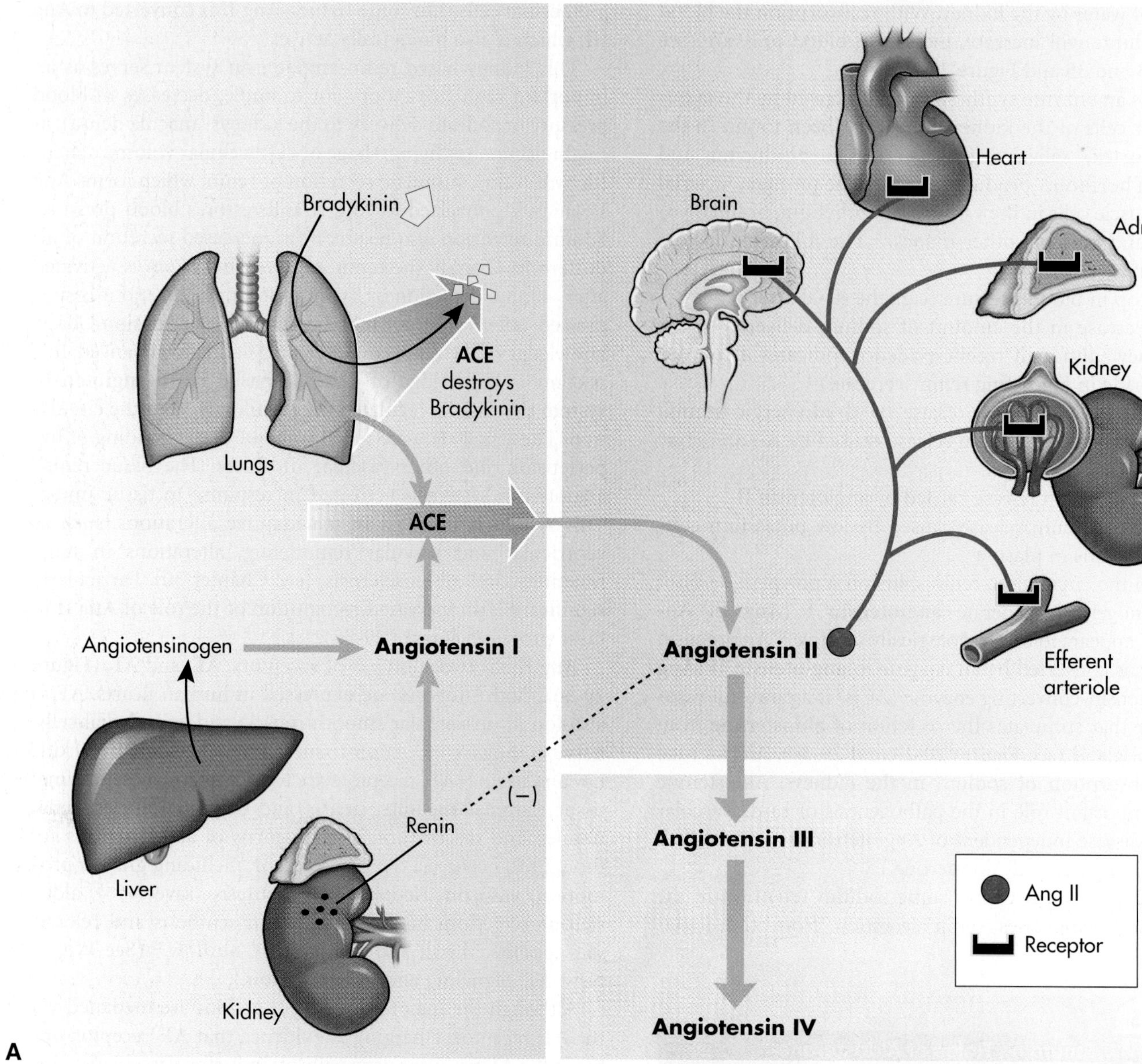

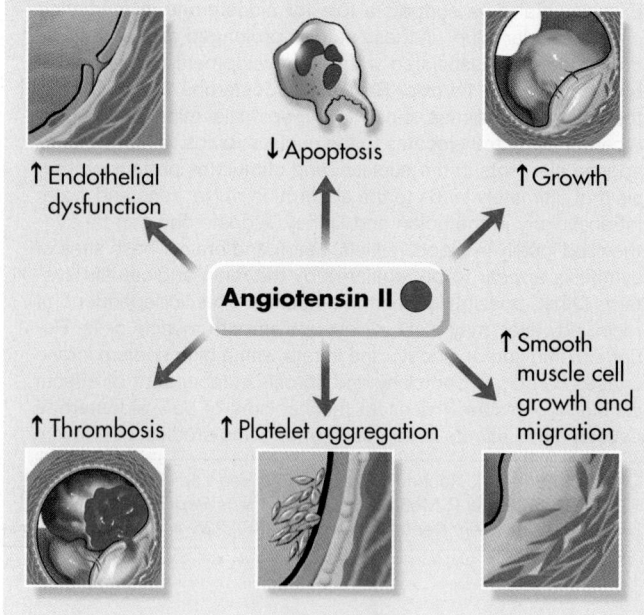

A

B

Figure 29-35 Angiotensins and the organs affected. A, The shaded blue area is the classical pathway of biosynthesis that generates the renin and angiotensin I. Angiotensinogen is synthesized in the liver and is released into the blood where it is cleaved to form angiotensin I by renin secreted by cells in the kidneys. Angiotensin-converting enzyme (ACE) in the lung catalyzes the formation of angiotensin II from angiotensin I, and destroys the potent vasodilator, bradykinin. Further cleavage generates the angiotensins III and IV. The reddish shading shows the organs affected by angiotensin II including brain, heart, adrenals, kidney, and the kidney's efferent arterioles. The *dashed arrow* (on the left) shows the inhibition of renin by angiotensin II. **B,** Summary of angiotensin II effects on blood vessel structure and function leading to arterosclerosis. (Redrawn from Goodfriend TL et al: *N Engl J Med* 334: 2649-2654, 1996.)

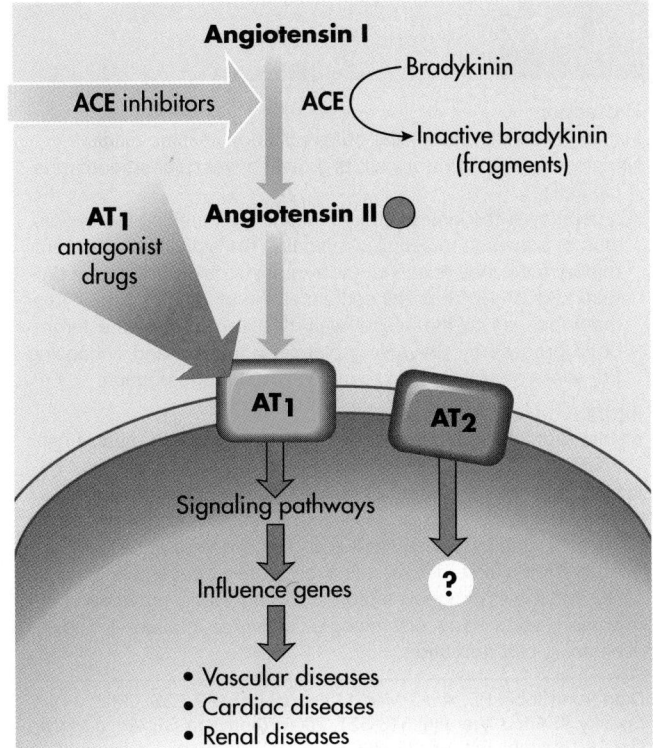

Figure 29-36 Angiotensins and their receptors, AT_1 and AT_2. Blocking the angiotensin-converting enzyme (ACE) with ACE inhibitors decreases the amount of angiotensin II. Blocking the receptor AT_1 with drugs (AT_1 antagonists) blocks the attachment of angiotensin II to the cell preventing the cellular effects and decreasing the vascular, cardiac, and renal effects.

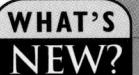

WHAT'S NEW? AT_1 Signaling and Inflammation

Activation of angiotensin 1 receptor (AT_1) has dramatic proinflammatory effects including production of many proinflammatory mediators, such as cytokines (e.g., IL-6, IL-2, TNF-α, etc), chemokines, and adhesion molecules through the activation of signaling pathways (e.g., MAPK NF-κB, etc). These effects promote the wound and repair response including vascular permeability, infiltration of inflammatory cells (macrophages) tissue repair and remodeling, angiogenesis, matrix synthesis, and eventually fibrosis. AT_1 activation increases vasoconstriction. The AT_1 receptor, therefore, may mediate inflammatory myocyte hypertrophy, fibroblast proliferation, collagen synthesis, smooth muscle cell growth, endothelial adhesion molecule expression, and catecholamine synthesis. Thus angiotensin II and its key receptor, AT_1 have been implicated in the progression of heart failure as well as other chronic diseases.

Data from Tsutamoto T et al: *J Am College Cardiology* 35:715-721, 2000.

---

is experimental vascular hypertension in the renal system. Ang II has been implicated in the progression of heart failure (see Chapter 30 and What's New?: AT_1 Signaling and Inflammation).

Natriuretic Peptides

Another mechanism that can change blood plasma volume and therefore blood pressure is the natriuretic peptides (NPs). The natriuretic peptides include atrial natriuretic peptide (ANP), brain natriuretic peptide (BNP), C-type natriuretic peptide (CNP), and urodilatin. These peptides help regulate sodium excretion or **natriuresis,** diuresis, vasodilation, and antagonism of the renin-angiotensin system. All of these effects lead to the formation of a large volume of dilute urine that decreases blood volume and blood pressure. **Atrial natriuretic peptide ([ANP] or factor)** is a peptide secreted from cells (monocytes) in the right atrium when right atrial blood pressure increases. In addition, under pathologic conditions, the left ventricle may secrete ANP. ANP inhibits antidiuretic hormone by increasing urine sodium loss, leading to the formation of a large volume of dilute urine that decreases blood volume and blood pressure. **Brain natriuretic peptide (BNP)** was originally isolated from paracrine brain and named *brain natriuretic peptide.* The name is misleading, however, because BNP is mostly synthesized, stored, and secreted from cardiac cells (i.e., atria). BNP is proposed to be a biochemical marker

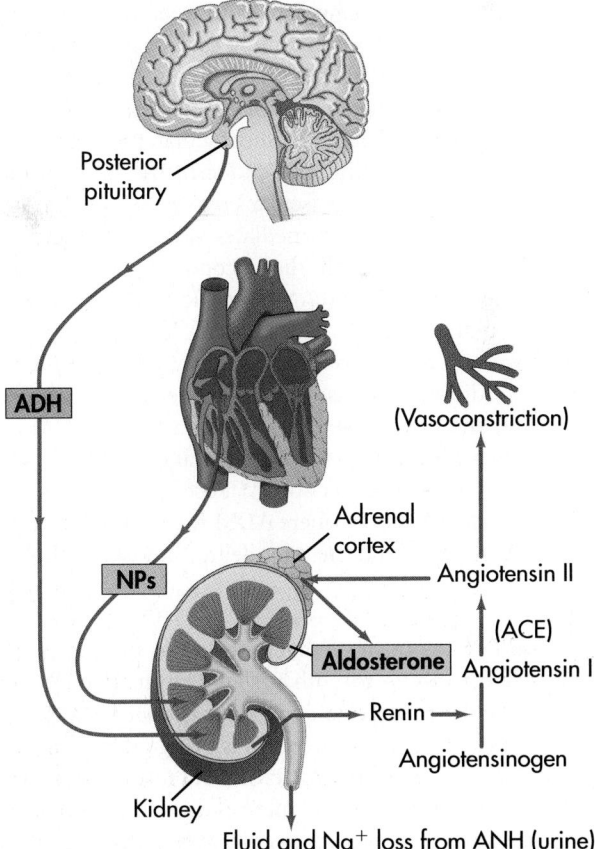

Figure 29-37 Three mechanisms that influence total plasma volume. The antidiuretic hormone (ADH) mechanism and renin-angiotensin and aldosterone mechanisms tend to increase water retention and thus increase total plasma volume. The natriuretic peptides antagonize these mechanisms by promoting water loss and sodium loss, thus promoting a decrease in total plasma volume. *NPs,* Natriuretic peptides; *ACE,* angiotensin-converting enzyme. (Modified from Thibodeau GA, Patton KT: *Anatomy & physiology,* ed 5, St Louis, 2003, Mosby.)

that may provide a screening test for left ventricular dysfunction.[16] **C-type natriuretic peptide (CNP)** is widely expressed throughout the vasculature and is found in very high concentrations in the endothelium.[17] Recent findings suggest that CNP complement nitric oxide (NO) and prostacyclin, mediators of vasodilation.[17] **Urodilatin** is a natriuretic peptide isolated from urine, is synthesized in kidney tubular cells, and is secreted into the kidney tubules. The function of urodilatin and the *renal urodilation system* is as a paracrine intrarenal regulator for Na^+ and water balance, thus a diuretic-natriuretic regulatory peptide.[18] Abnormal natriuretic peptide production and/or activity have been associated with several cardiovascular disorders and interventions that selectively target these peptides may be of therapeutic benefit.

Adrenomedullin

Adrenomedullin (ADM) is a recently discovered, widely dispersed peptide present in numerous tissues with powerful vasodilatory activity. Other functions of ADM included neurotransmission, growth, hormone secretion regulation, down-regulation of proinflammatory cytokines, such as tumor necrosis factor-α, and modulation of anticoagulant properties.[19] Therefore, changes in ADM levels have been correlated with several diseases including cardiovascular and renal sepsis, cancer, and diabetes. Originally isolated from human pheochromocytoma (tumor of the adrenal medulla), it is now known to be present in cardiovascular, pulmonary, renal, gastrointestinal, cerebral, and endocrine tissues. It is synthesized and secreted from vascular endothelial and smooth muscle cells. Adrenomedullin mediates vasodilatory and natriuretic properties through the second messenger cyclic adenosine monophosphate (cAMP), nitric oxide, and the renal prostaglandin system. ADM acts as a local autocrine or paracrine vasoactive hormone and is increased in the plasma in various cardiorenal diseases such as hypertension, chronic renal failure, and congestive heart failure. Overall, ADM appears to play an important role in fluid and electrolyte balance and cardiorenal regulation.[20-22] Recent studies in rats with myocardial infarction where ADM was administered revealed decreased left ventricle remodeling and heart failure.[19]

Insulin

In vitro studies demonstrate that **insulin** has direct vascular actions that contribute to both vascular protection and injury. The vascular protection and injury properties are summarized in Box 29-2. More attention is being given to insulin resistance as a cause of atherosclerosis because persons with type II diabetes have a threefold increased risk of coronary artery disease and persons with prediabetes, without chronic hyperglycemia, have a twofold increased risk.

Venous Pressure

The main determinants of venous blood pressure are (1) the volume of fluid within the veins and (2) the compliance (distensibility) of the vessel walls. Veins have much thinner walls than arteries and are more distensible than arteries. The ve-

---

Box 29-2	Vascular Protection and Injury Properties of Insulin

Protection

Insulin increases endothelial cell production of nitric oxide.

Nitric oxide (NO) (in vitro) inhibits growth of vascular smooth muscle cells.

NO decreases the inflammatory reaction by inhibiting the expression of adhesion molecules, inhibiting the activity of proinflammatory cytokines (e.g., TNF-α, monocyte chemoattractant protein-1 [MCP-1]). Thus NO decreases the binding of monocytes/macrophages to the vessel wall. NO also inhibits the thrombotic process by preventing platelet adhesion and enhancing the effect of prostacyclin to inhibit platelet aggregation.

Injury

Insulin slightly increases growth of vascular smooth muscle cells (VSMCs).

Insulin increases the effect of platelet-derived growth factor.

Insulin resistance is likely more important to the atherogenesis process than *hyperinsulinemia,* and insulin resistance likely disrupts the balance between vasoprotective effects mediated by NO and the atherogenic effects involving VSMC growth and migration, stimulating plasminogen activator inhibitor-1 and increasing clot formation.

Data from Sobel BE: *Am J Med* 113(suppl 6A):12S-22S, 2002; Sorisky A: *Am J Ther* 9(6):516-521, 2002; Tennyson GE: *Am J Manag Care* 8(16 suppl):5450-5429, 2002.

---

nous system accommodates approximately 60% of the total blood volume at any given moment, with venous pressure averaging less than 10 mmHg. Conversely, the arteries accommodate about 15% of the total blood volume, with an average arterial pressure (blood pressure) of about 100 mmHg.

The sympathetic nervous system controls compliance. The walls of the veins are highly innervated by sympathetic fibers that, when stimulated, cause venous smooth muscle to contract. This increases muscle tone (i.e., prevents distention) rather than causing vasoconstriction, as occurs in arterial vessels. The effect of increased muscle tone is to stiffen the wall of the vein, which reduces distensibility and increases blood pressure, forcing more blood through the veins and into the right heart.

Two other mechanisms that increase venous pressure and venous return to the heart are (1) the skeletal muscle pump and (2) the respiratory pump. During skeletal muscle contraction the veins within the muscles are partially compressed, causing a decrease in venous capacity and increased return to the heart. The respiratory pump acts during inspiration, when the veins of the abdomen are partially compressed by the downward movement of the diaphragm. Increased abdominal pressure moves blood toward the heart.

Regulation of Coronary Circulation

Flow of blood *(F)* in the coronary circulation, as in vascular beds, is directly proportional to the perfusion pressure *(P)* and inversely proportional to the vascular resistance *(R)* of the bed *(F = P/R)*. **Coronary perfusion pressure** is the difference between pressure in the aorta and pressure in the coronary vessels of the right atrium. Aortic pressure is the driving pressure that perfuses vessels of the myocardium. Mechanisms of vasodilation and vasoconstriction normally maintain coronary blood flow despite stresses imposed by the constant contraction and relaxation of the heart muscle and despite shifts (within a physiologic range) of coronary perfusion pressure.

Several anatomic factors influence coronary blood flow. Because of their location, the aortic valve cusps obstruct coronary blood flow by pushing against the openings of the coronary arteries during systole. Also during systole, the coronary arteries are compressed by ventricular contraction. These anatomic factors have a **systolic compressive effect,** which is particularly evident in the subendocardial layers of the left ventricular wall and can greatly decrease coronary blood flow. Therefore most coronary blood flow in the left ventricle occurs during diastole. During the period of systolic compression, when flow is slowed or stopped, oxygen is supplied by **myoglobin,** a protein that is present in heart muscle that binds oxygen during diastole and then releases it when blood levels of oxygen fall during systole.

Autoregulation

Autoregulation (automatic self-regulation) enables individual vessels to regulate blood flow by altering their own arteriolar resistances. Autoregulation in the coronary circulation maintains constant blood flow at perfusion pressures (mean arterial pressure) between 60 and 180 mmHg when other influencing factors are held constant. Thus autoregulation ensures constant coronary blood flow despite shifts in the perfusion pressure within the stated range.

The mechanism of autoregulation is not known, but two explanations have been proposed: the myogenic hypothesis and the metabolic hypothesis. The myogenic hypothesis proposes that autoregulation originates in vascular smooth muscle, presumably of the arterioles, as a response to an increase in arterial pressure. Smooth muscle stretches in response to an increase in perfusion pressure. The stretching eventually stimulates contraction of the smooth muscles, which increases vascular resistance. Initially, coronary blood flow increases with the abrupt distention of the blood vessels. The return of more normal flow follows constriction of the arterioles. This mechanism also works in the opposite direction; that is, vasodilation is stimulated by decreased arterial pressure. Because stretch of vascular smooth muscle increases intracellular Ca^{++}, it is proposed that an increase in transmural pressure activates membrane calcium channels.[2]

The myogenic hypothesis illustrates the law of Laplace (tension equals pressure times radius). Increased coronary perfusion pressure increases the pressure against the vessel wall, and the stretch increases the vessel's radius, resulting in an increase in wall tension. The increase in tension stimulates constriction of the vessel to a radius less than the original radius, so that the product of pressure (increased) times radius (decreased) is restored to normal.

The metabolic hypothesis of autoregulation, which is better documented, proposes that autoregulation of coronary vessels originates in the myocardium. The stimulus is a drop in coronary perfusion pressure or an increase in the metabolic needs of the myocardium (e.g., because of strenuous exercise). With an increased myocardial oxygen requirement, myocardial cells release substances that promote vasodilation. Substances implicated include CO_2, O_2 (reduced O_2 tension), hydrogen ions (lactic acid), potassium ions, and adenosine. The best known of these substances is adenosine, a potent vasodilator released in response to a decrease in myocardial oxygenation. Little evidence supports the concept that CO_2, hydrogen ions, or O_2 plays a significant direct role in regulating coronary flow.[2] Low coronary blood flow, hypoxemia, and increased metabolic activity of the heart can all increase the heart muscle's need for oxygen.[2] An increased concentration of adenosine in the interstitial fluid decreases the resistance of the coronary arterioles and increases blood flow. Perfusion strongly correlates with the amount of adenosine released. When coronary perfusion pressure is increased, the increased flow washes out the vasodilatory substances. As the dilators are washed out, vasoconstriction occurs and returns flow toward normal.

Autonomic Regulation

Stimulation of the sympathetic nerves to the heart causes a marked increase in coronary blood flow, even though it also causes vasoconstriction of the coronary vessels. Why? The increased coronary flow is caused by acceleration of heart rate and enhancement of myocardial contractility (more forceful systole). Although the longer, forceful myocardial contraction and the tachycardia (heart rate greater than 100 beats/min) tend to restrict coronary flow, the increase in myocardial metabolism tends to counteract these factors by dilating the coronary arterioles.[2] Therefore the net effect of sympathetic stimulation is to increase coronary blood flow.

Although the coronary vessels themselves contain sympathetic (α- and β-adrenergic) and parasympathetic neural receptors, coronary blood flow is regulated locally through metabolic autoregulation. Metabolic autoregulation overrides neurogenic influences.[2]

LYMPHATIC SYSTEM

The **lymphatic system** is a special vascular system that picks up excess tissue fluid and returns it to the bloodstream. Normally, fluid is forced out of the blood at the arterial end of the capillary bed and is reabsorbed into the bloodstream at the venous end (Figure 29-38), yet capillary outflow exceeds venous reabsorption by about 3 L/day so some fluid lags behind in the interstitium. To maintain sufficient blood volume in the cardiovascular system, this fluid must eventually rejoin the bloodstream, which is the function of the lymphatic system.

The lymphatic system consists of lymphatic vessels and the lymph nodes (Figure 29-39). (Lymph nodes and lymphoid tissues are described in Chapters 7 and 25.) In this pumpless

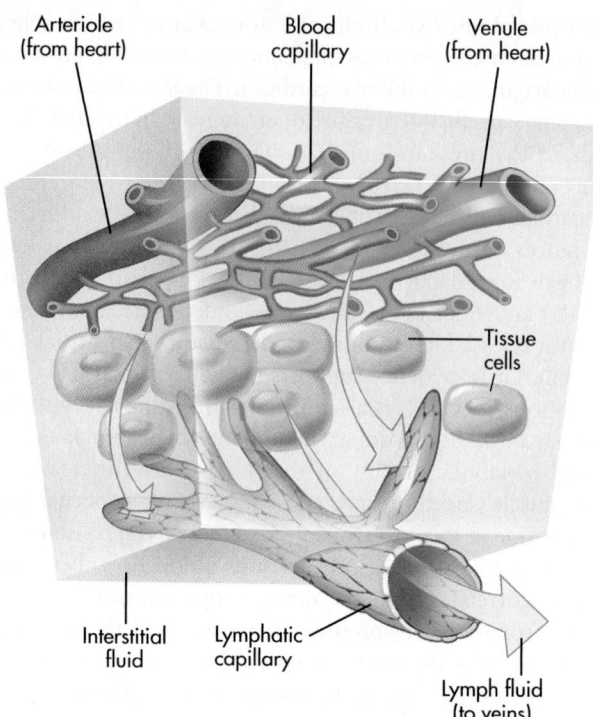

Figure 29-38 Role of the lymphatic system in fluid balance. Fluid from plasma flowing through the capillaries moves into interstitial spaces. Although much of this interstitial fluid is either absorbed by tissue cells or reabsorbed by capillaries, some of the fluid tends to accumulate in the interstitial spaces. As this fluid builds up, it tends to drain into lymphatic vessels that eventually return the fluid to the venous blood. (From Thibodeau GA, Patton KT: *Anatomy & physiology,* ed 5, St Louis, 2003, Mosby.)

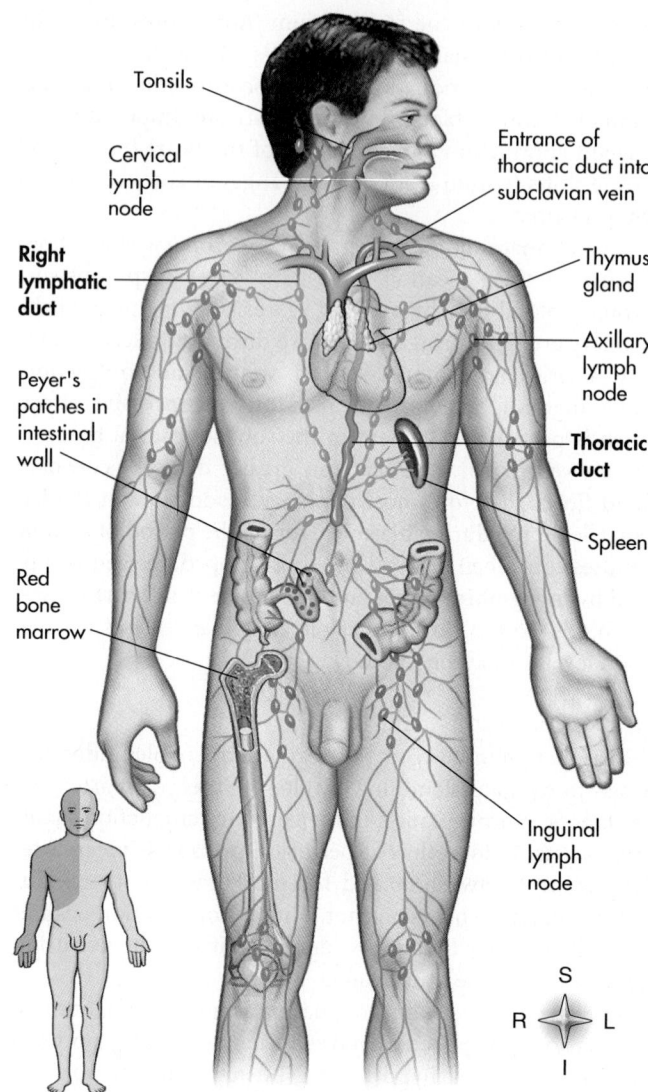

Figure 29-39 Principle organs of the lymphatic system. The inset shows the areas drained by the right lymphatic duct (green) and the thoracic duct (blue). (From Thibodeau GA, Patton KT: *Anatomy & physiology,* ed 5, St. Louis, 2003, Mosby.)

system a series of valves ensures one-way flow of the excess interstitial fluid (then called *lymph*) toward the heart. The lymphatic capillaries are closed at the ends (Figure 29-40).

Lymph consists primarily of water and small amounts of dissolved proteins, mostly albumin, that are too large to be reabsorbed into the less permeable blood capillaries. Once within the lymphatic system, lymph travels successively through larger and larger vessels called **lymphatic venules** and **lymphatic veins.** The lymphatic vessels run in the same sheaths with the arteries and veins and eventually drain into one of two large ducts in the thorax—the right lymphatic duct and the thoracic duct. The **right lymphatic duct** drains lymph from the right arm and the right side of the head and thorax, whereas the larger thoracic duct receives lymph from the rest of the body (see Figure 29-39). The right lymphatic duct and the **thoracic duct** drain lymph into the right and left subclavian veins, respectively.

The lymphatic veins are thin walled, like the veins of the cardiovascular system. In the larger lymphatic veins, endothelial flaps form valves similar to those in the circulatory veins (see Figure 29-26). The valves permit lymph to flow in only one direction because lymphatic vessels are compressed intermittently by contraction of skeletal muscles, pulsatile expansion of an artery in the same sheath, and contraction of the smooth muscles in the walls of the lymphatic vessel.

As lymph is transported toward the heart, it is filtered through thousands of bean-shaped lymph nodes clustered along the lymphatic vessels (see Figure 29-39). Lymph enters the node through several **afferent lymphatic vessels,** filters through the sinuses in the node, and leaves by way of **efferent lymphatic vessels.** Lymph flows slowly through the node, which facilitates the phagocytosis of foreign substances within the node and prevents them from reentering the bloodstream. (Phagocytosis is described in Chapter 6.)

TESTS OF CARDIOVASCULAR FUNCTION

Historically, cardiac function was first measured by subjective means and by simple objective observations that included the individual's sensorium, mucous membrane color, and a man-

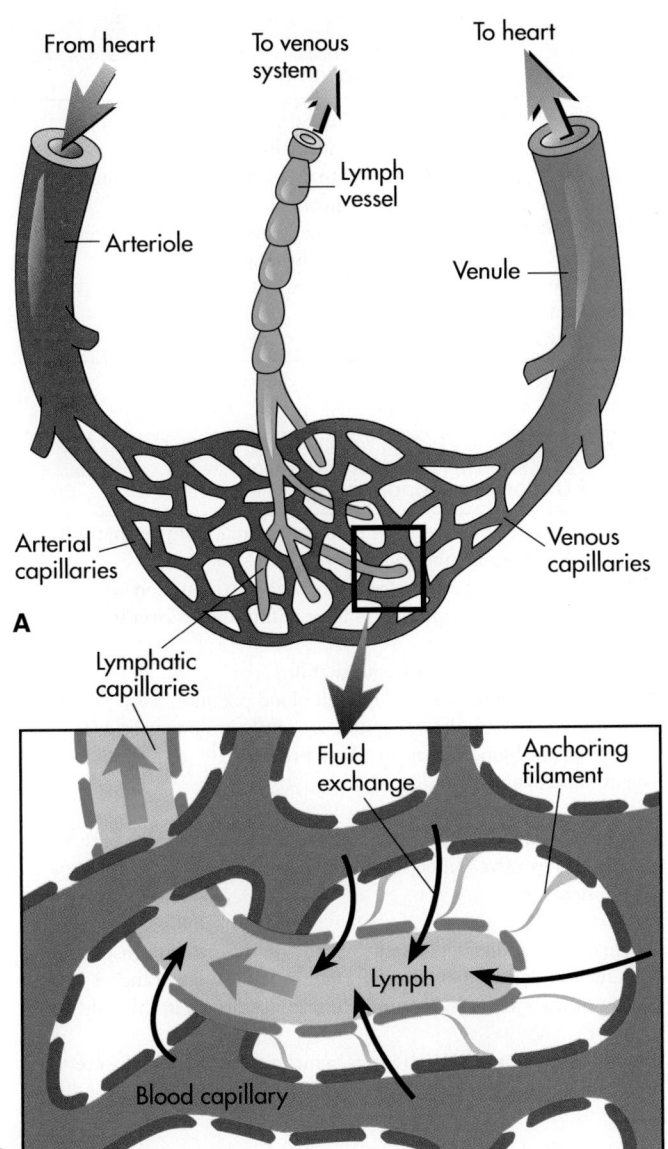

Figure 29-40 Lymphatic capillaries. A, Schematic representation of lymphatic capillaries. **B,** Anatomic components of microcirculation.

central nervous system. A decrease in cardiac pumping ability, if sufficiently severe, will almost immediately be followed by a decrease in neural efficiency, which includes impairment of mentation and such simple motor functions as conjugate gaze, enunciation, and pupillary reflexes (see Chapters 14 and 15).

Mucous Membrane Color

When lung, blood, and vessel structure and function are normal, a darkening or bluing of the mucous membranes, called *cyanosis,* signifies decreased cardiac function. Mucous membrane color is a reflection of hemoglobin saturation in the capillary blood (see Chapters 25 and 30). Hemoglobin that is well oxygenated and well saturated takes on a bright red color, whereas poorly oxygenated hemoglobin is dark red or purple. These colors are best observed in the mucous membranes of the conjunctivae, gums, nail beds, and genitalia, where the capillary network is dense and the epithelium is thin.

Cardiac function indirectly affects the affinity of hemoglobin for oxygen. If cardiac function decreases and blood flow slows in the capillary beds, two changes occur. First, hemoglobin will come in contact with tissues for an extended time, allowing more oxygen to diffuse into the tissues. The capillary blood will darken, as will mucous membranes. Second, a decrease in the amount of oxygen delivered per minute to the tissues will result in a metabolic acidosis, as cells switch from aerobic to anaerobic metabolism and produce lactic acid. Interstitial pH and capillary blood pH will drop. Acidosis causes more oxygen to dissociate from hemoglobin and diffuse out of the capillaries (see Chapter 32). Capillary blood in mucous membranes will darken further.

Manually Palpated Pulse

If cardiac function is impaired, the pulse will be affected. When palpated, changes in the radial, femoral, and carotid pulses offer information regarding heart rate, regularity of heart rhythm, the length and strength of ventricular systole, and peripheral artery patency. A decrease in cardiac function may be detected as a decrease in pulsatile strength. A bilateral comparison of pulses may reveal decreased pulsatile flow unilaterally, in which case arterial narrowing or occlusion would be suspected.

Irregular heartbeats (dysrhythmias) may be reflected in changes in pulse rhythmicity and pulse pressure per beat. Turbulent blood flow caused by valve or septal disease may be reflected in the carotid pulses and felt as a "thrill." A pulsatile thrill elsewhere may indicate a fistula, or an opening, between an artery and a nearby vein.

Auscultation of Heart Sounds

Auscultation (auditory examination) of the heart is done with a stethoscope placed over the valve, chamber, or great vessel being examined. Different sounds are normally heard over different heart structures during systole and diastole. The dominant sounds are made by the four heart valves as they close. The first sound, S_1, is made by atrioventricular valve closure. The second, S_2, is made by closure of the aortic and

ually palpated pulse. Currently, many sophisticated methods measure heart function, ranging from no-risk, noninvasive electrocardiography to relatively high-risk, invasive cardiac catheterization.

Noninvasive Assessment of Function
Sensorium of the Individual

Often, the first observation indicating an impairment of cardiac function is a decreased level of consciousness. Should the pumping ability of the heart decrease for any reason, the amount and pressure of blood ejected from the heart will decrease. Consequently, the amount and pressure of blood that reaches all body tissues will be insufficient to supply oxygen and nutrients to cells and remove waste products.

Perhaps no other system is more sensitive to a decrease in oxygen and nutrient supply, particularly of glucose, than the

Table 29-4	Normal Heart Sounds		
Sound	**Event in Cardiac Style**	**Cause of Sound**	**Comments**
First sound (S_1)	Beginning of ventricular systole	Closure of atrioventricular valves, particularly mitral valve	With S_2, the loudest heart sound normally heard
Second sound (S_2)	End of ventricular systole	Closure of semilunar valves, particularly aortic valves	With S_1, the loudest heart sound normally heard
Third sound (S_3)	Early ventricular diastole (filling)	Vibration of ventricular walls as blood rushes in	Normally heard only in children and young adults
Fourth sound (S_4)	Atrial systole during late ventricular diastole (filling)	Uncertain, but thought to be the result of a sudden change in filling rate (i.e., shudder of the left ventricle)	Rarely heard in the normal heart

Table 29-5	Abnormal Heart Sounds	
Sound	**Cause of Sound**	**Typical Underlying Abnormality**
Accentuated S_1	Forceful closure of mitral valve	Rapid heart rate resulting from exercise, anemia, or hyperthyroidism
		Mitral valve stenosis (narrowing)
Diminished S_1	Premature partial closure of the mitral valve before systole, so that systole causes only the completion of closure	Prolonged diastole resulting from blockage in conduction system that slows impulse conduction to or within the atrioventricular node
	Failure of the mitral valve to close completely	Mitral valve incompetence (regurgitation)
Accentuated S_2	Forceful closure of the aortic or pulmonic semilunar valve, which closes late and must close quickly	Prolonged systole resulting from high blood pressure in the systemic or pulmonary circulation; systole is slightly prolonged so as to force all the blood out against high pressure
	Valvular stiffness, which increases the impact of closure	Aortic valve syphilis
Diminished S_2	Gentle closure of aortic semilunar valve	Low blood pressure in the systemic arteries, which reduces pressure that pushes valve leaflets shut
	Gentle closure of aortic semilunar valve caused by incomplete opening	Aortic stenosis
Split heart sounds (S_1 and S_2)	Delayed closure of various heart valves, usually caused by late right ventricular systole	Normal increase in venous return to the right heart with inspiration
		Conduction defects involving the right or left bundle branches
		Defect of the interatrial septum that raises pressures in the right heart
		Pulmonic semilunar valve stenosis, which causes delayed closure
Gallop sounds S_3 (in adults)	Possibly the "thud" of blood hitting noncompliant ventricular walls at the start of ventricular filling	Myocardial damage that stiffens muscle and prevents relaxation during systole
S_4 (in children)	Ejection of blood into overfilled ventricle during atrial systole	Incomplete emptying of ventricle during systole of preceding cardiac cycle, causing overfilling and overdistention during next cycle; causes include myocardial damage or disease, aortic stenosis, high blood pressure, fluid overload (see Chapter 3)
Murmurs	Turbulent blood flow at high blood pressure	Irregularity, constriction, or dilation of any structure that blood flows through, such as valvular stenosis or incompetence, perforation or interatrial or interventricular septum
		Increased rate of flow (blood flow) through normal structures (e.g., during pregnancy)
Rub	Friction within the pericardium, usually caused by disruption of the pericardial fluid; loss of fluid causes the visceral and parietal pericardium to rub against one another	Surgery, infection, inflammation, or adhesion that damages the parietal or visceral pericardium
Click	Sudden, abnormal movement of an aortic or pulmonic semilunar valve leaflet	Valve prolapse, in which valve leaflets open backward as well as forward; usually resulting from increase in valve opening (anulus)
Snap	Opening of stenotic (stiff) atrioventricular valve (mitral or tricuspid)	Atrioventricular valve stenosis
Hum	Vibration of heart walls or vessel walls caused usually by movement during turbulent blood flow at low pressure	Irregularity of any structure that blood flows through; normal in jugular veins of children

pulmonic semilunar valves. The first two heart sounds provide information about heart rate, heart rhythm, and the length of ventricular systole.

Abnormal heart sounds indicate abnormalities of the heart valves or chamber walls. In healthy adults, only S_1 and S_2 can be heard. Abnormalities of these sounds or detection of the third and fourth heart sounds (S_3 and S_4) indicates disease. The mechanisms causing the normal heart sounds are listed in Table 29-4. Causes of abnormal heart sounds, or **adventitious sounds,** are listed in Table 29-5.

Cardiography

Electrocardiography, typically the 12-lead electrocardiogram (ECG), gives information about heart rate and rhythm, the effects of electrolytes or drugs on the heart, and the electrical orientation of the cardiac muscle. An ECG gives no direct information about the contractile state or mechanical performance of the heart.

Einthoven's triangle places the heart in the center of a triangle, with angles placed at the right shoulder, the left shoulder, and the pubic area. Body fluids conduct electrical potential differences that can be detected by bipolar or unipolar electrical leads placed on the skin. Einthoven's triangle gives a triaxial (three-axis) reference for the detection of cardiac electrical potentials.

Serial 12-lead ECGs are of primary importance in establishing the presence of myocardial infarction. This examination has become part of the routine hospital admission assessment, even when the admitting diagnosis is not cardiac in nature, because it establishes baseline information about the electrical function of the heart. Also, recent ECGs can be compared with ECGs obtained from the same individual in the past. Changes in the ECG over time assist in determining the cause, amount, or nature of changes in cardiac anatomy and physiology.

In conjunction with a 12-lead ECG, a vectorcardiogram can assist one to (1) precisely locate the site of a myocardial infarction, (2) diagnose conduction defects, and (3) diagnose chamber hypertrophy. Commonly, five electrodes are placed over the precordium, one electrode is placed on the left leg, and one is placed on the back of the neck. Recorded in conjunction with the ECG, the electrodes of the vectorcardiogram provide a series of dots over time that represent the vector of the heart in microseconds.

Pulse Tracing

The pulsation described by the flow of blood through an artery during the cardiac cycle can be drawn as a waveform plotting pressure against time (Figure 29-41). The waveform can be obtained noninvasively by placing a transducer on the skin over the carotid artery while the individual's head is turned slightly away from the transducer. In conjunction with phonocardiography and an ECG, the arterial pulse tracing gives a reference for the phonocardiograph and assists in the timing of the events of the cardiac cycle.

Like an arterial pulse tracing, a venous pulse tracing gives a reference for the phonocardiograph and assists in the timing of

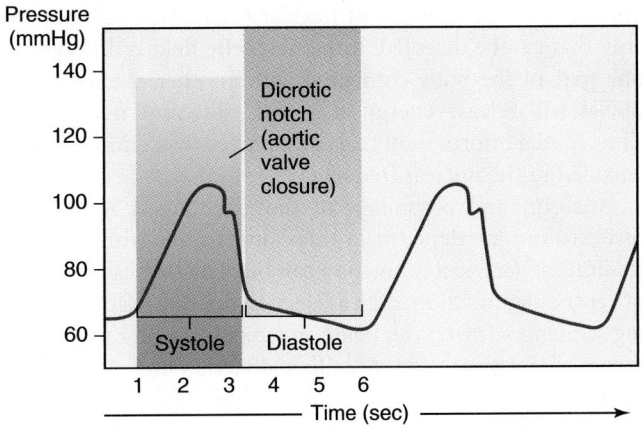

Figure 29-41 Arterial pulse waveforms.

the cardiac cycle. A venous pulse tracing is obtained by placing a transducer over the jugular vein at the supraclavicular area near the manubrium. A waveform is produced that reflects pressures in the vein over time during the cardiac cycle.

Vibrations at the apex of the heart during the cardiac cycle are recorded by placing a transducer at the point of maximal impulse. An apexcardiogram is used to assist in the timing of the cardiac cycle and is made along with a phonocardiogram and an ECG.

A **phonocardiogram** is made by placing microphones over the precordium. An ECG is recorded simultaneously as a reference point. By recording the sounds made during the cardiac cycle, the phonocardiogram can assist one to time the events and length of diastole and systole. Abnormal sounds also can be examined more closely for timing, characteristics, and sources of those sounds.

An **echocardiogram** is an ultrasonic examination. The skin is first prepared by applying a lubricating agent (usually cooking oil), and a piezoelectric crystal is placed against the chest. Ultrasonic sound waves are then generated and directed into the cardiac structures, which reflect the waves at different angles and lengths according to structure and density. The crystal picks up these deflected waves and passes them through a transducer, which transforms the waves into electrical impulses. The impulses are displayed on an oscilloscope and are viewed with a simultaneously recorded ECG.

Like an ECG, an echocardiogram is recorded continuously over time so that changes in the heart during the cardiac cycle (e.g., valve position, chamber size, myocardial wall position) can be examined. Information about cardiac anatomy and function, including stroke volume and cardiac output, is gained.

Magnetic Resonance Imaging

Magnetic resonance imaging (MRI) is based on the principle that the frequency of energy (resonant frequency) given up by a nucleus is exactly proportional to the surrounding magnetic field (see Chapter 14). Hydrogen nuclei present in high concentrations in body water and fat tend to align parallel to a magnetic field (the individual is placed on a magnet). This orientation can be disturbed by energy at the proper frequency, and the recovery of nuclear orientation releases energy that can be detected. If the magnetic field is different in one part of the body compared with another, the hydrogen nuclei will release energy at slightly different frequencies. Thus spatial information (e.g., different body sections) can be encoded in the nuclear frequency.[23]

Anatomy and physiology of the great blood vessels and myocardium are depicted in three dimensions with excellent resolution. Ventricular function can be evaluated using indices of ventricular function, such as ejection fraction. Rapidly moving sequences (MRI) can determine regional wall motion and myocardial deformation. Also, flow direction and velocity can be quantitatively determined. The clinical application of MRI for coronary artery angiography is unclear because of interference from cardiac and respiratory motion.

Doppler Studies

A Doppler study is made by using a handheld microphone placed on the skin over a lubricating gel. The microphone amplifies and can record sounds made by blood flowing in peripheral vessels. The Doppler microphone is placed over the vessel to be studied, and sounds related to obstructions to flow, vessel wall mobility, and heart murmurs are transmitted through the gel to the microphone. The microphone amplifies sound waves so that they are audible to the human ear.

Stress Testing

Cardiac activity during exercise is examined during a stress test. Stress testing elicits signs and symptoms of heart disease and coronary artery disease that may not appear at rest. A 12-lead ECG, blood pressure measurement, and bipolar ECG strip recording are done before the study and at regular intervals during and after the study. Cardiac stress from exercise is induced by having the individual walk on a treadmill. Other, less frequently used forms of exercise include stair climbing (the Stairmaster's double two-step) and bicycle ergometry. The individual exercises until the maximal heart rate for gender and age is reached or until other subjective or objective indicators of cardiac dysfunction or distress appear. Subjective indicators include chest pain, extreme fatigue, extreme dyspnea, leg pain, or the individual's request to stop the test. Objective criteria are ST segment elevation or depression, SA node or atrial dysrhythmias, AV node dysrhythmias, ventricular dysrhythmias, elevated or decreased blood pressure, signs of cerebral hypoxia, and signs of circulatory insufficiency.

A stress test is useful also in determining the rate or progress of recovery from a myocardial infarction or cardiac surgery. Recently, graded exercise in individuals with low-to-moderate-risk chest pain evaluated in an emergency department was shown to be a prognostic indicator of adverse cardiac events.[24] When a differential diagnosis for chest pain has been difficult to determine, stress testing may help distinguish coronary artery insufficiency from other causes of pain. There is some risk associated with stress testing. The mortality rate is about 1 per 10,000, and the morbidity rate is approximately 24 per 10,000.[25] The risk is greater when the test is performed soon after an acute ischemic event.

Chest X-Ray Examinations

In a chest x-ray examination the size and contour of the heart and related structures are visualized. A chest x-ray examination is a routine part of a cardiac examination. The most commonly obtained views are anteroposterior and lateral, with the individual upright and the lungs fully expanded.

Invasive Assessment of Function

Invasive studies generally carry a greater risk to the individual than noninvasive studies, with the possible exception of stress testing. Ingestion of substances is considered invasive.

X-Ray Films with Barium

The cardiac silhouette obtained with routine radiographic studies of the chest can be enhanced by ingestion of barium. The contrast medium causes the esophagus to appear white on the x-ray film, creating a bright background against which the heart is more distinctly outlined. X-ray films are taken using four different axes.

Nuclear Imaging with Radiolabeled Pharmaceuticals

Hot Spot Imaging

Technetium pyrophosphate (^{99m}TcPYP) is injected intravenously into a resting individual during a "hot spot" imaging examination. Two hours after injection, the distribution pattern of the radioactive solution is recorded by nuclear scan. During the 2-hour delay, the injected material will have been taken up by infarcted areas of the myocardium, particularly 1 to 3 days after the onset of symptoms. This study is not definitive during the first 12 hours after an infarct.

Hot spot imaging is used when (1) there is a conflicting history for myocardial infarction, (2) there are equivocal ECG abnormalities, or (3) an individual's cardiac enzymes have been elevated because of surgery or trauma. Such small amounts of the injected material are used in this examination that the risks associated with radioactive substances are not an issue.

Cold Spot Imaging

Thallium is the radioactive substance injected intravenously during a perfusion imaging examination. During stress testing and at the peak of exercise, thallium is injected intravenously. After a 1- or 2-minute delay the distribution of thallium within the myocardium is determined by nuclear scan, and it is again determined after a period of rest. Thallium typically is not taken up by areas of ischemic or infarcted myocardium, creating "cold spots." Cold spots disappear at rest if the ischemia is reversible and remain at rest if infarction has occurred. Perfusion imaging is useful to differentiate a myocardial infarction from reversible angina (cardiac pain) in the presence of conflicting or equivocal enzymatic and historical data. Risks associated with perfusion imaging are the same as for stress testing. No risk attributable to the small quantity of injected material has been documented.

Tomographic Studies

In the past 10 years, **single photon emission computed tomography (SPECT)** has been used increasingly in cardiac imaging. A series of planar images are obtained from an individual around 180 or 360 degrees. A computer creates a set of transaxial images from these planar images, allowing the radioisotope distribution to be displayed in three dimensions. SPECT, along with many other tomographic modalities (e.g., positron emission tomography [PET], x-ray computed tomography [CT]), uses a computer-based algorithm during reconstruction of the planar images, called *filtered back projection*. PET is believed to be more accurate than SPECT (see Chapter 14). The main disadvantages of the PET technology are its limited availability and high costs.

Atrioventricular Bundle Electrocardiography

Two electrode-tipped catheters are inserted percutaneously into the femoral vein, floated up the inferior vena cava, and positioned in or near the right atrium during atrioventricular bundle (His bundle) electrocardiography. The first electrode is quadripolar and is lodged against the right atrial wall. Two poles of this electrode record the difference in electrical potential between two points, and the other two poles are a pacing electrode and a ground (that allow for pacing of the right atrium). The second electrode is bipolar and is placed across the tricuspid valve, at the location of the bundle of His, and records the electrical potentials across the bundle. These recordings across the bundle divide the PR interval into two segments: the atrial-His interval and the His-ventricular interval. The atrial-His interval is the interval from the onset of atrial electrical activity to the arrival of the impulse at the bundle of His. The His-ventricular interval is the interval between the passage of the impulse through the His bundle and the passage of the impulse through the ventricular conduction system and muscle.

His bundle electrocardiography can detect secondary sites of impulse generation (ectopic foci), as well as accessory pathways of conduction. Other conduction defects and the effects of drugs on conduction also can be illuminated. Risks related to this procedure can be grave and include dysrhythmias, death, vessel or heart perforation, clot or plaque embolization, and kidney failure.

Cardiac Catheterization

One or both sides of the heart can be examined using **cardiac catheterization.** This procedure requires the use of fluoroscopy and strict sterile techniques and takes place in a specially equipped catheterization laboratory. Local anesthesia is given, and a catheter is introduced percutaneously into the vasculature and passed caudally into the atrium and ventricle. For a right-heart catheterization, the catheter is placed in the brachial or femoral vein. The femoral artery is commonly used for a left-heart study. Once the catheter has been guided into the atrium, pressures are recorded, blood samples are obtained to examine oxygen content, and a contrast medium is injected to visualize chamber function and valve patency. The catheter is then passed into the ventricles and the sequence is repeated.

Cardiac catheterization provides a means to visualize the chambers of the heart continuously, although for a short time. A great deal of information can be obtained about heart structure and function. Pressures in each chamber and across heart valves can be precisely measured, along with timing of events in the cardiac cycle. Of particular value is the ability to compare the oxygen content of blood in each heart chamber.

Risks for this procedure have decreased over time, and mortality rates range from 0.1% to 0.3%.[26] Morbidity rates, including serious and relatively minor complications, ranged from 3.1% to 10.1% in 1968,[27] but the morbidity rate currently is less than 0.5%.[28] One of the most serious complications of cardiac catheterization is the development of dysrhythmias and the possible sequelae of inflammation. Death usually is caused by cardiac arrest after ventricular fibrillation. The role of early cardiac catheterization in the management of acute coronary syndromes (see Chapter 30) remains controversial.[29]

Coronary Angiography

Fluoroscopic visualization of the coronary arteries and left heart structures using contrast dye (e.g., iodine) is called **coronary angiography** or arteriography. Like cardiac catheterization, this study takes place in a catheterization laboratory using local anesthesia and a sterile field. A catheter is threaded into the left ventricle through the femoral artery. A ventriculogram generally is performed first. Contrast dye is injected into the apex of the ventricle, and the next few cardiac cycles are visualized and filmed. The contrast dye used is 66% diatrizoate meglumine and 10% diatrizoate sodium, an iodine preparation that is not tolerated by individuals who are allergic to iodine. Like cardiac catheterization, coronary angiography is used to gain information about the structure and function of the ventricles and related valves.

After the ventriculogram, catheters are introduced individually into the ostia of the coronary arteries. When the catheter is in position, 5 to 10 ml of contrast dye is mechanically and rapidly injected into the artery and the results are visualized and filmed. Dye injection is repeated with the individual tilted at various angles to afford views of the artery other than the anteroposterior view. The catheter is then either moved to the next artery to be studied or withdrawn to conclude the study. Pressures in the left side of the heart are usually obtained, but blood samples are not. The right side of the heart is not studied.

The risks of this procedure are similar to those of cardiac catheterization, with exceptions. Because the blood supply to the cardiac muscle is briefly interrupted when dye is introduced into the coronary arteries, angina (chest pain) caused by ischemia (lack of oxygen) is much more common. Coronary artery spasms also can occur. Interrupted flow also causes decreased heart rate (bradycardia), as well as some tachydysrhythmias, hypotension, and ST segment depression.

The administration of nitroglycerin sublingually or directly into the coronary artery can dilate the artery sufficiently to alleviate ischemic complications. Persistent bradycardia is corrected by having the individual cough to stimulate the heart rate or, in severe cases, by the administration of atropine. Bradycardia is such a common complication that a temporary pacer often is introduced into the right ventricle through the femoral vein at the beginning of coronary angiography. Heparin is given to avoid thrombus formation. The effects of heparin may be reversed after the procedure by using protamine.

Combined Indicators of Cardiac Function

Cardiac function can be evaluated using indicators calculated from pressures and flow rates in the heart and vessels. Table 29-6 defines the indicators most often used in the clinical setting.

AGING AND THE CARDIOVASCULAR SYSTEM

Cardiovascular disease is the most common cause of hospitalization and death in the elderly population in Western society. The most common cardiovascular pathologic condition is coronary atherosclerosis. It is difficult to describe normal physiologic changes in cardiac function with aging because many pathologic changes are usually present as well. Studies of the effect of age on cardiovascular function must be rigorous in their distinction between persons who are free of disease and those who have disease that may be evident only during stress testing. A consistent finding is the large variation in the older population for nearly every cardiovascular variable. These variations are in part the result of a sharp increase in the prevalence of coronary disease with advancing age and

in part the result of major age-associated changes in life-style (e.g., fitness status).[30] The most relevant age associated changes in cardiovascular performance are myocardial and blood vessel stiffening, decreased beta-adrenoreceptor responsiveness, and impaired autonomic reflex control of heart rate. These changes pose considerable consequences with increased demand for flow, changes in posture, or with disease.

Arterial stiffening occurs with aging even in the absence of clinical hypertension[30] (Figure 29-42). Arterial stiffness is a growing epidemic associated with risk of cardiovascular events, dementia, and death.[31] These changes apparently result from alterations within the vascular media, including age-associated changes in cross linking of collagen, an increase in the amount of collagen, and changes in the nature of elastin, and extracellular matrix, inflammatory molecules, endothelial cell function, and reactive oxygen species.[31] Other influences include glucose regulation, chronic renal disease, salt, and changes in neurohormonal (e.g., renin-angiotensin-aldosterone) regulation.[31] Systolic arterial pressure increases (even in the absence of clinical hypertension) within the clinically "normal" range are considered to result from the age-associated increase in arterial stiffness (see Figure 29-42). The increased arterial stiffness may not be related strictly to an

Table 29-6	Indicators of Cardiac Function	
Indicator	**Definition***	**Common Cause of Abnormality**
Heart rate (HR)	Number of heartbeats (cardiac cycles) per min Normal adult value: 70 beats/min	Ischemia, electrolyte disturbances, drug toxicity
Cardiac output (CO)	Amount of blood (in liters) moved by the heart in 1 min Normal range: 4-8 L/min	Decrease indicates heart failure Increase indicates decreased systemic vascular resistance, common in sepsis
Cardiac index (CI)	Relationship between cardiac output and body surface area (BSA, in square meters) Normal range: 2.8-4.2 L/min/m²	Decrease indicates heart failure Increase indicates decreased systemic vascular resistance, common in sepsis
Stroke volume (SV)	Amount of blood (in milliliters) ejected by the left ventricle during systole, i.e., per beat Normal range: 60-100 ml/beat	Decrease indicates heart failure Increase indicates deceased systemic vascular resistance, common in sepsis
Stroke volume index (SVI)	Relationship between stroke volume and body surface area Normal range: 33-47 ml/beat/m²	Decrease indicates heart failure Increase indicates decreased systemic vascular resistance, common in sepsis
Oxygen consumption index (V̇O₂I)	Amount of oxygen (VO₂ in milliliters) consumed per minute in relation to BSA	Decrease: sedation, anesthesia, hypothermia Increase: elevated temperature, sepsis, seizures
Stroke work index (SWI)	Amount of work (expressed as done) by the left or right ventricle per systole per square meter of BSA Normal value: 35 g/m²	Decreases within specific ranges indicate cardiogenic or hypovolemic shock (see Chapter 46) Increase: elevated systemic vascular resistance
Systemic mean arterial pressure (MAP)	Mean blood pressure (in millimeters of mercury) in the systemic arteries Normal range: 70-100 mm Hg	Elevated: epinephrine release, diseases of arteries, primary hypertension Decreased: cardiac failure, decreased vascular resistance of sepsis
Pulmonary vascular resistance (PVR)	Relationship among cardiac output, preload, and afterload, expressed as units of force of resistance per second per centimeter of water Normal value: less than 250 dyn/sec/cm⁻⁵	Increased: acute respiratory distress syndrome (ARDS), pneumonia, primary pulmonary hypertension, congestive heart failure Decreased: late shock
Systemic vascular resistance (SVR)	Same definition as for PVR Normal range: 770-1500 dyn/sec/cm⁻⁵	Increased: epinephrine release Decreased: inflammatory response

*Values given are for adults at rest.

age-associated change in vascular structure but also may be caused by changes in baroreceptor activity. Baroreceptor activity may decrease with age, slowing physiologic adjustment to changes in blood pressure because of vasodilation or vasoconstriction. In addition, plasma catecholamines increase with aging, which may be a result of exaggerated central nervous system adrenergic flow, possibly associated with blunting of baroreceptor sensitivity,[30] yet elevated plasma catecholamine levels in older individuals are associated with a decreased postsynaptic β-adrenergic response of the heart vasculature. In addition, plasma catecholamine levels are not correlated or are inversely correlated with arterial pressure in elderly persons with normotension or hypertension. In populations in whom the increase in arterial stiffness with age is blunted, the arterial pressure increase with age is also blunted.[30] Recent observations indicate that arterial stiffening is reduced in older individuals who regularly engage in vigorous exercise.[32]

Stress testing is used to uncover changes in functional capacity that are not apparent at rest. In contrast to the subtle age effects on resting cardiac tests, more dramatic changes occur during exercise. Table 29-7 summarizes age-associated changes at rest and during exercise. Overall, long-term exercise conditioning in older individuals increases aerobic capacity and decreases arterial stiffness and left ventricular function.

In summary, age does not appear to significantly alter left ventricular performance except in the presence of a superimposed stress such as severe exercise or disease, particularly dysrhythmia or hypertension. In these instances, impaired diastolic relaxation and systolic emptying may occur. Recent research is focused on decreased endothelial vasoreactivity and prolonged diastolic relaxation. Impaired nitric oxide signaling may contribute to slowed ventricular relaxation.[33] Impaired systolic emptying may be related to a decreased responsiveness to catecholamine β-adrenoreceptor stimulation.[30,32]

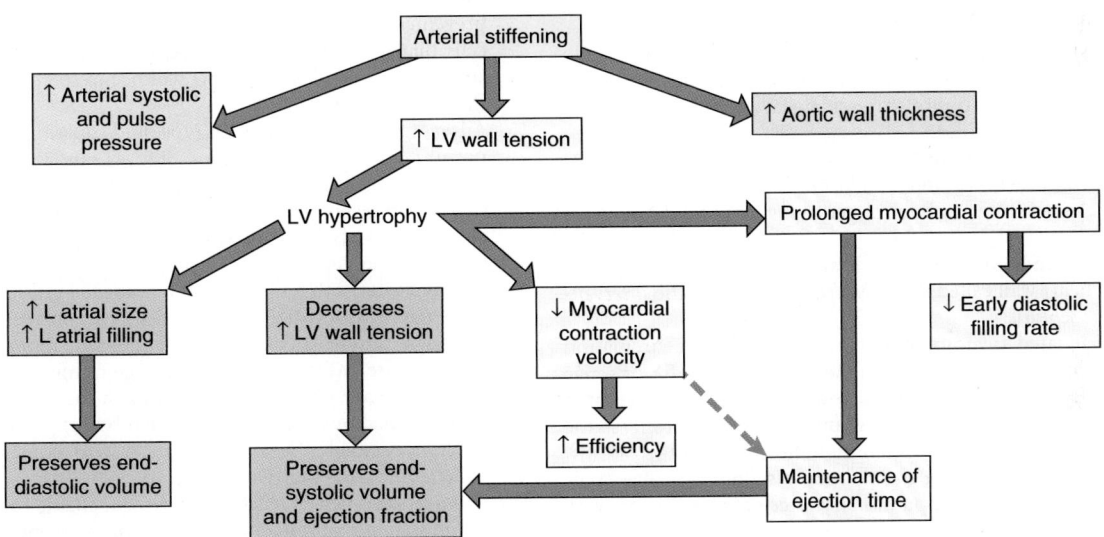

Figure 29-42 Cardiac consequences of age-associated increase in arterial (central) stiffness. *LV,* Left ventricular; *L,* left.

Table 29-7	Cardiovascular Function in Elderly Persons	
Determinant	**Resting Cardiac Performance**	**Exercise Cardiac Performance**
Cardiac output	Unchanged or slightly decreased in women only	Declines because of a decrease in heart rate and stroke volume
Heart rate	Slight decrease	Increases less than in younger people, possibly because of decreased cardiovascular response to catecholamines; overall slight decrease
Stroke volume	Slight increase	Slight increase
Ejection fraction	Unchanged	Increases more from rest to exercise in younger people than in older people
Afterload	Increased	Uncertain
End-diastolic volume	Unchanged	Smaller for women
End-systolic volume	Unchanged	Lesser increase
Contraction	Increased because of prolonged relaxation	Decreases with vigorous exercise*
Cardiac dilation	No change	Increases at end-diastole and end-systole
$\dot{V}O_2$ max	Not applicable	Declines because of a decline in skeletal muscle mass

Data from Gerstenblith G, Lakatta EG: Aging and the cardiovascular system. In Willerson JT, Cohn JN, editors: *Cardiovascular medicine,* New York, 1995, Churchill Livingstone.
*As measured by end-systolic volume/systolic blood pressure (ESV/SBP), an index of contractility.

SUMMARY REVIEW

Circulatory System

1. The circulatory system is the body's transport system. It delivers oxygen, nutrients, metabolites, hormones, neurochemicals, proteins, and blood cells throughout the body and carries metabolic wastes to the kidneys and lungs for excretion.
2. The circulatory system consists of the heart and blood vessels and is made up of two separate, serially connected systems: the pulmonary circulation and the systemic circulation.
3. The pulmonary circulation is driven by the right side of the heart. The function of the pulmonary circulation is to deliver blood to the lungs for oxygenation.
4. The systemic circulation is driven by the left side of the heart, and its function is to move oxygenated blood throughout the body.
5. The lymphatic vessels collect fluids from the interstitium and return the fluids to the circulatory system.

The Heart

1. The heart consists of four chambers (two atria and two ventricles), four valves (two atrioventricular valves and two semilunar valves), a muscular wall, a fibrous skeleton, a conduction system, nerve fibers, systemic vessels (the coronary circulation), and openings where the great vessels enter the atria and ventricles.
2. The heart wall, which encloses the heart and divides it into chambers, is made up of three layers: the pericardium (outer layer), the myocardium (muscular layer), and the endocardium (inner lining).
3. The myocardial layer of the two atria, which receive blood entering the heart, is thinner than the myocardial layer of the ventricles, which must be stronger to squeeze blood out of the heart.
4. The right and left sides of the heart are separated by portions of the heart wall called the *interatrial septum* and the *interventricular septum*.
5. Unoxygenated (venous) blood from the systemic circulation enters the right atrium through the superior and inferior venae cavae. From the atrium the blood passes through the right atrioventricular (tricuspid) valve into the right ventricle. In the ventricle the blood flows from the inflow tract to the outflow tract and then through the pulmonic semilunar valve (pulmonary valve) into the pulmonary artery, which delivers it to the lungs for oxygenation.
6. Oxygenated blood from the lungs enters the left atrium through the four pulmonary veins (two from the left lung and two from the right lung). From the left atrium the blood passes through the left atrioventricular valve (mitral valve) into the left ventricle. In the ventricle the blood flows from the inflow tract to the outflow tract and then through the aortic semilunar valve (aortic valve) into the aorta, which delivers it to systemic arteries of the entire body.
7. The heart valves ensure the one-way flow of blood from atrium to ventricle and from ventricle to artery.
8. Oxygenated blood enters the coronary arteries through an opening in the aorta, and unoxygenated blood from the coronary veins enters the right atrium through the coronary sinus.
9. The pumping action of the heart consists of two phases: diastole, during which the myocardium relaxes and the chambers fill with blood, and systole, during which the myocardium contracts, forcing blood out of the ventricles. A cardiac cycle consists of one systolic contraction and the diastolic relaxation that follows it. Each cardiac cycle makes up one heartbeat.
10. The conduction system of the heart generates and transmits electrical impulses (cardiac action potentials) that stimulate systolic contractions. The autonomic nerves (sympathetic and parasympathetic fibers) can adjust heart rate and systolic force, but they do not stimulate the heart to beat.
11. The normal electrocardiogram is the sum of all action potentials. The P wave represents atrial depolarization; the QRS complex is the sum of all ventricular cell depolarizations. The ST interval occurs when the entire ventricular myocardium is depolarized.
12. Cardiac action potentials are generated by the sinoatrial node at the rate of about 75 impulses per minute. The impulses can travel through the conduction system of the heart, stimulating myocardial contraction as they go.
13. Cells of the cardiac conduction system possess the properties of automaticity and rhythmicity. Automatic cells return to threshold and depolarize rhythmically without outside stimulus. The cells of the sinoatrial node depolarize faster than other automatic cells, making it the natural pacemaker of the heart. If the sinoatrial node is disabled, the next fastest pacemaker, the atrioventricular node, takes over.
14. Each cardiac action potential travels from the sinoatrial (SA) node to the atrioventricular (AV) node to the bundle of His (atrioventricular bundle), through the bundle branches, and finally to the Purkinje fibers. There the impulse is stopped. It is prevented from reversing its path by the refractory period of cells that have just been polarized. The refractory period ensures that diastole (relaxation) will occur, thereby completing the cardiac cycle.
15. Adrenergic receptor number, type, and function govern autonomic (sympathetic) regulation of heart rate, contractile force, and dilation or constriction of coronary arteries. The presence of specific receptors (α_1, α_2, β_1, β_2) in the myocardium and coronary vessels determines the effects of the neurotransmitters norepinephrine and epinephrine.
16. Unique features that distinguish myocardial cells from skeletal cells enable myocardial cells to transmit action potentials faster (through intercalated disks), synthesize more adenosine triphosphate (ATP) (because of a large number of mitochondria), and have readier access to ions in the interstitium (because of an abundance of transverse tubules). These combined differences enable the myocardium to work constantly, which skeletal muscle is not required to do.
17. Cross-bridges between actin and myosin enable contraction to occur. Calcium and its interaction with the troponin complex facilitate the contraction process. With troponin release of calcium, myocardial relaxation begins.
18. Cardiac performance is affected by preload, afterload, heart rate, and myocardial contractility.
19. Preload, or pressure generated in the ventricles at the end of diastole, depends on the amount of blood in the ventricle. Afterload is the resistance to ejection of the blood from the ventricle. Afterload depends on pressure in the aorta.
20. Heart rate is determined by the SA node and by components of the autonomic nervous system, including cardiovascular control centers in the brain, neuroreceptors in the atria and aorta, hormones, and catecholamines (epinephrine and norepinephrine).
21. Contractility is the potential for myocardial fiber shortening during systole. It is determined by the amount of stretch during diastole (i.e., preload) and by sympathetic stimulation of the ventricles.
22. The Frank-Starling law of the heart states that the myocardial stretch determines the force of myocardial contraction (the greater the stretch, the stronger the contraction).
23. Laplace's law states that the amount of contractile force generated within a chamber depends on the radius of the chamber

and the thickness of its wall (the smaller the radius and the thicker the wall, the greater the force of contraction).

Systemic Circulation

1. Blood flows from the left ventricle into the aorta and from the aorta into arteries that eventually branch into arterioles and capillaries, the smallest of the arterial vessels. Oxygen, nutrients, and other substances needed for cellular metabolism pass from the capillaries into the interstitium, where they are available for uptake by the cells. Capillaries also absorb products of cellular metabolism from the interstitium.
2. Venules, the smallest veins, receive capillary blood. From the venules the venous blood flows into larger and larger veins until it reaches the venae cavae, through which it enters the right atrium.
3. Vessel walls consist of three layers: the tunica intima (inner layer), the tunica media (middle layer), and the tunica externa (outer layer).
4. Layers of the vessel wall differ in thickness and composition from vessel to vessel, depending on the vessel's size and location within the circulatory system. In general, the tunica media of arteries close to the heart contains a greater proportion of elastic fibers because these arteries must be able to distend during systole and recoil during diastole. Distributing arteries farther from the heart contain a greater proportion of smooth muscle fibers because these arteries must be able to constrict and dilate to control blood pressure and volume within specific capillary beds.
5. Blood flow into the capillary beds is controlled by the contraction and relaxation of smooth muscle bands (precapillary sphincters) at junctions between metarterioles and capillaries. The endothelium is probably a source of prostaglandins that control vasomotion.
6. Blood flow through the veins is assisted by the contraction of skeletal muscles (the muscle pump), and backflow in the lower body is prevented by one-way valves, particularly in the deep veins of the legs.
7. Blood flow is affected by blood pressure; resistance to flow within the vessels; blood consistency (which affects velocity); anatomic features that may cause turbulent or laminar flow; and compliance (distensibility) of the vessels.
8. Poiseuille's law describes the relationship of blood flow, pressure, and resistance as the difference between pressure at the inflow end of the vessel and pressure at the outflow end divided by resistance within the vessel.
9. According to Poiseuille's formula, resistance depends on the vessel's length and radius and on the viscosity of the blood. The greater the vessel's length and the blood's viscosity and the narrower the radius of the vessel's lumen, the greater the resistance within the vessel.
10. Total peripheral resistance, or the resistance to flow within the entire systemic circulatory system, depends on the combined lengths and radii of all the vessels within the system and on whether the vessels are arranged in series (greater resistance) or in parallel (lesser resistance).
11. Poiseuille's law and Poiseuille's formula are based on physical laws governing the behavior of fluids in a straight tube. In the body, blood flow is influenced also by neural stimulation (of vasoconstriction or vasodilation) and by autonomic features that cause turbulence within the vascular lumen (e.g., protrusions from the vessel wall, twists and turns, bifurcations).
12. Arterial blood pressure is influenced and regulated by factors that affect cardiac output (heart rate and stroke volume), total resistance within the system, and blood volume.

13. Many hormones alter vasomotion including epinephrine, norepinephrine, antidiuretic hormone, renin-angiotensin system, natriuretic peptides, adrenomedullin and insulin.
14. Angiotensin II (Ang II) has two subtypes of receptors, AT_1 and AT_2. The majority of Ang II actions are thought to be mediated by AT_1 receptor.
15. Venous blood pressure is influenced by blood volume within the venous system and compliance of the venous walls.
16. Blood flow through the coronary circulation is governed not only by the same principles as flow through other vascular beds but also by adaptations dictated by cardiac dynamics. First, blood flows into the coronary arteries during diastole rather than systole because, during systole, the cusps of the aortic semilunar valve block the openings of the coronary arteries. Second, systolic contraction inhibits coronary artery flow by compressing the coronary arteries.
17. Autoregulation enables the coronary vessels to maintain optimal perfusion pressure despite systolic effects, and myoglobin in heart muscle stores oxygen for use during the systolic phase of the cardiac cycle.

Lymphatic System

1. The vessels of the lymphatic system run in the same sheaths in which the arteries and veins run.
2. Lymph (interstitial fluid) is absorbed by lymphatic venules in the capillary beds and travels through ever larger lymphatic veins until it is emptied through the right or left thoracic duct into the right or left subclavian vein.
3. As lymph travels toward the thoracic ducts, it is filtered by thousands of lymph nodes clustered around the lymphatic veins. The lymph nodes are sites of immune function.

Tests of Cardiovascular Function

1. Observable signs of cardiovascular disease include a decreased level of consciousness (caused by insufficient perfusion of brain tissue) and cyanosis, particularly mucous membrane color (caused by insufficient perfusion of vascular beds of the skin).
2. Palpable signs of cardiovascular disease include abnormal pulses of the radial, femoral, and carotid arteries.
3. Abnormal heart sounds, which are detected by auscultation with a stethoscope or by phonocardiography, are auditory signs of cardiovascular disease.
4. Stress tests elicit clinical manifestations of cardiovascular disease that might not be present at rest.
5. Noninvasive diagnostic tests include electrocardiography (ECG) and Holter monitoring, which detect disturbances of impulse generation or conduction; pulse tracings and Doppler studies, which detect abnormalities of blood flow; phonocardiography; ultrasound (echocardiography), which detects structural and functional abnormalities over time; and chest x-ray films, which detect cardiac enlargement and structural abnormalities. Recently, magnetic resonance imaging has been used to study the anatomy and physiology of the great vessels, flow, direction and velocity, and myocardial deformation.
6. Invasive diagnostic tests involve intravenous injection of radiolabeled substances (barium x-rays, nuclear imaging) or the introduction of a catheter that is threaded through the vascular system to the heart (atrioventricular bundle ECG, cardiac catheterization, coronary angiography).
7. Cardiac catheterization is used to measure the oxygen content and pressure of blood in the heart's chambers and to inject contrast media for x-ray examination of the size and shape of the chambers and valves. Injection of contrast medium in the coronary arteries (coronary angiography), on the other hand,

Continued

SUMMARY REVIEW—cont'd

permits visualization of the coronary circulation and every tissue perfused by the coronary arteries.

Aging and the Cardiovascular System

1. Much controversy exists regarding the effects of normal aging on the cardiovascular system. Separating the physiologic from the pathologic alterations is difficult because of the presence of arteriosclerosis in a majority of the elderly population.

2. Recent studies have documented no change in cardiac output, a slight decrease in heart rate, and a slight increase in stroke volume in healthy (lack of ischemic heart disease) elderly persons at rest. No changes were noted at rest in ejection fraction. A slight increase in afterload (e.g., as systolic blood pressure) and prolonged left ventricular relaxation were noted.

3. The most relevant age associated changes in cardiovascular performance are myocardial and blood vessel stiffening, decreased beta-adrenoreceptor response, and impaired autonomic reflex control of heart rate.

4. With exercise the healthy elderly subjects demonstrated a decrease in maximum oxygen consumption and no age-related changes in cardiac output but did demonstrate significant decreases in heart rate and increases in stroke volume. Thus the healthy elderly subjects maintained a normal cardiac output during exercise by dilating the ventricle and using the Frank-Starling mechanism to increase stroke volume.

5. Contrary to previous studies, recent studies have found no age-related increase with exercise for systolic blood pressure and systemic vascular resistance.

KEY TERMS

a wave, 1034
Adrenomedullin (ADM), 1066
Adventitious sounds, 1071
Afferent lymphatic vessel, 1068
Afterload, 1046
Aldosterone, 1063
Angiotensin I (Ang I), 1063
Angiotensin II (Ang II), 1063
Anisotropic (A) band, 1043
Anomalous viscosity, 1057
Anterior interatrial myocardial band (Bachmann bundle), 1039
Anterior, middle and posterior internodal pathways, 1039
Antidiuretic hormone, 1062
Aorta, 1033
Aortic semilunar valve, 1032
Arteriogenesis, 1036
Arterioles, 1050
Arteries, 1050
AT_1, 1063
AT_2, 1063
Atrial natriuretic peptide (ANP or factor), 1065
Atrioventricular node (AV node), 1038
Atrioventricular valves, 1032
Automatic cells, 1041
Automaticity, 1041
Bainbridge reflex, 1049
Baroreceptor reflex, 1049
Brain natriuretic peptide (BNP), 1065
Bundle branches, 1038
Bundle of His (atrioventricular bundle, common bundle), 1038
c-type natriuretic peptide (CNP), 1066
c wave, 1034
Calcium channel–blocking drugs, 1046
Capillaries, 1050
Cardiac action potentials, 1037
Cardiac catheterization, 1073
Cardiac cycle, 1033
Cardiac output, 1050
Cardiac plexus, 1041
Cardioexcitatory center, 1048

Cardioinhibitory center, 1048
Cardiovascular control center, 1048
Chordae tendineae, 1032
Circumflex artery, 1035
Collateral arteries, 1035
Conduction system, 1037
Coronary angiography, 1073
Coronary perfusion pressure, 1066
Coronary sulcus, 1035
Crista supraventricularis, 1034
Cross-bridge theory of muscle contraction, 1044
Depolarization, 1039
Diastole, 1033
Diastolic depolarization, 1041
Echocardiogram, 1071
Efferent lymphatic vessel, 1068
Elastic arteries, 1053
End-diastolic pressure, 1048
End-diastolic volume, 1047
Endocardium, 1031
Endothelial cells, 1055
Endothelium, 1055
Epinephrine, 1062
Excitation-contraction coupling, 1046
Fenestrations, 1054
Frank-Starling law of the heart, 1047
Great cardiac vein, 1036
Heart rate, 1038
Hyperemia, 1062
Inflow tract, 1032
Inotropic agents, 1050
Insulin, 1066
Intercalated disks, 1043
Isotropic (I) band, 1043
Laminar flow, 1061
Left anterior descending artery, 1035
Left atrial pressure, 1050
Left atrium, 1031
Left bundle branch (LBB), 1039
Left coronary artery, 1034
Left heart, 1029
Left pulmonary artery, 1033
Left ventricle, 1031

Lumen, 1054
Lymph, 1068
Lymphatic system, 1067
Lymphatic veins, 1068
Lymphatic venules, 1068
M line, 1044
Mean arterial pressure (MAP), 1061
Mediastinum, 1031
Metarterioles, 1054
Mitral and tricuspid complex, 1032
Mitral valve, 1032
Muscular arteries, 1054
Myocardial contractility, 1044
Myocardial oxygen consumption ($M\dot{V}O_2$), 1044
Myocardium, 1031
Myoglobin, 1067
Myosin, 1043
Natriuresis, 1065
Natriuretic peptides, 1062
Nodes, 1037
Norepinephine, 1062
Outflow tract, 1032
P cells, 1038
P wave, 1040
Papillary muscles, 1032
Parietal pericardium, 1031
Perfusion, 1061
Pericardial cavity, 1031
Pericardial fluid, 1031
Pericardium, 1031
Peripheral vascular system, 1050
Phonocardiogram, 1071
Poiseuille's formula, 1057
Posterior vein of the left ventricle, 1036
Precapillary sphincter, 1054
Preload, 1046
Pressure, 1056
PR interval, 1040
Pulmonary artery, 1033
Pulmonary circulation, 1029
Pulmonary veins, 1033
Pulmonic semilunar valve, 1032
Purkinje fibers, 1039

MEDIA RESOURCES 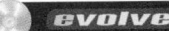 *evolve*

Review questions and answers for this chapter are available in the *CD Companion* included with this book.

WebLinks—links to Internet sites pertaining to this chapter—are available on Evolve at http://evolve.elsevier.com/McCance/.

REFERENCES

1. Werner GS et al: Immediate changes of collateral function after successful recanalization of chronic total coronary occlusion, *Circulation* 102(24):2959, 2000.
2. Berne RM, Levy MN, editors: *Cardiovascular physiology,* ed 8, St Louis, 2001, Mosby.
3. Matsunaga T et al: Ischemia-induced coronary collateral growth is dependent on vascular endothelial growth factor and nitric oxide, *Circulation* 102(25):3098, 2000.
4. Werner GS et al: Collaterals and the recovery of left ventricular function after recanalization of a chronic total coronary occlusion, *Am Heart J* 149(1):129-137, 2005.
5. Underhill SL et al, editors: *Cardiac nursing,* Philadelphia, 1982, Lippincott.
6. James TN: Pericarditis and the sinus nodes, *Arch Intern Med* 110:305, 1962.
7. James TN: The coronary circulation and conduction system in acute myocardial infarction, *Prog Cardiovasc Dis* 10:410, 1968.
8. Kirchheim HR: Systemic arterial baroreceptor reflexes, *Physiol Rev* 56(1):110, 1976.
9. Vander AJ, Sherman JH, Luciano DS: *Human physiology: the mechanisms of body function,* ed 6, New York, 1994, McGraw-Hill.
10. Kim SD: Measurement of the renin-angiotensin system in heart failure, *Biol Res Nurs* 1(3):210, 2000.
11. Takeda Y: Pleiotropic actions of aldosterone and the effects of eplerenone, a selective mineralocorticoid receptor antagonist, *Hypertens Res* 27(11):781-789, 2004.
12. Smith GR, Missailidis S: Cancer, inflammation, and the AT1 and AT2 receptors. *J Inflamm (Lond)* 1(1):3, 2004.
13. de Gasparo M et al: International union of pharmacology XXIIII. The angiotensin II receptors, *Pharmacol Rev* 52(3):415-472, 2000.
14. Cary RM: Update on the role of the AT$_2$ receptor, *Curr Opin Neph Hyperten* 14(1):66-71, 2005.
15. Widdop RE et al: AT2 receptor-mediated relaxation is preserved after long-term AT1 receptor blockade, *Hypertension* 40(4):516-520, 2002.

16. Doust JA, Pictrzak E: How well does B-type natriuretic peptide predict death and cardiac events in patients with heart failure: systematic review, *BMJ* 330(7492):625, 2005.
17. Scotland RS, Ahluwalia A, Hobbs AJ: C-type natriuretic peptide in vascular physiology and disease, *Pharmacol Ther* 105(2):85-93, 2005.
18. Forssmann W, Meyer M, Forssmann K: The renal urodilatin system: clinical implications, *Cardiovas Res* 51(3):450-462, 2001.
19. Nakamura R et al: Adrenomedullin administration immediately after myocardial infarction ameliorates progression of heart failure in rats, *Circulation* 110(4):426-431, 2004.
20. Jougasaki M, Burnett JC: Adrenomedullin: potential in physiology and pathophysiology, *Life Sci* 66(10):855, 2000.
21. Hinson JP, Kapas S, Smith DM: Adrenomedullin, a multifunctional regulatory peptide, *Endocr Rev* 21(2):138, 2000.
22. Ueta Y et al: A physiological role for adrenomedullin in rats; a potent hypotensive peptide in the hypothalamo-neurohypophysial system, *Exp Physiol* 85(spec):163S, 2000.
23. Duerinckx AJ: Imaging of coronary artery disease—MR, *J Thorac Imaging* 16(1):25-34, 2001.
24. Diercks DB et al: Identification of patients at risk by graded exercise testing in an emergency department chest pain center, *Am J Cardiol* 86(3):289, 2000.
25. Rochmis P, Blackburn H: Exercise tests: a survey of procedures, safety, and litigation experience in approximately 170,000 tests, *JAMA* 217(8):1061-1066, 1971.
26. Abrams HL: Complications of coronary arteriography. In Abrams HL, editor: *Angiography: vascular and interventional radiology,* ed 3, Boston, 1983, Little, Brown.
27. Braunwald E: Cooperative study on cardiac catheterization: Deaths related to cardiac catheterization, *Circulation* 37(5 Suppl:III):74-79, 1968.
28. Silverman BD, Neeld JB Jr: Evaluation of the cardiac patient for noncardiac surgery, *J Med Assoc Ga* 73(5):315-318, 1984.
29. Cantor WJ et al: Early cardiac catherization is associated with lower mortality only among high-risk patients with ST-and non–ST-elevation acute coronary syndromes: observations from the OPUS-TIMI 16 trial, *Am Heart J* 149(2):275-283, 2005.
30. Gerstenblith G: Consequences of vascular aging: concepts for the clinician, *Ital Heart J* 1(suppl 3):S103, 2000.
31. Zieman SJ, Melenovsky V, Kass DA: Mechanisms, pathophysiology, and therapy of arterial stiffness, *Arterioscler Thromb Vasc Biol* 25(5):932-943, 2005.
32. Vaitkevicius PV, Fleg JL: An abnormal exercise treadmill test in an asymptomatic older patient, *J Am Geriatr Soc* 44(1):83, 1996.
33. Zieman SJ et al: Upregulation of the nitric oxide–cGMP pathway in aged myocardium: physiological response to L-arginine, *Circ Res* 88(1):97, 2001.

ALTERATIONS OF CARDIOVASCULAR FUNCTION

VALENTINA L. BRASHERS

CHAPTER OUTLINE

The pathophysiology of heart disease is now known to be much more complicated than just structural and hemodynamic changes. Today the focus is on the genetic, neurohumoral, and inflammatory mechanisms that underlie tissue and cellular processes, such as endothelial injury, remodeling, stunning, reperfusion injury, and autoimmune disease.

DISEASES OF THE ARTERIES AND VEINS

Arteriosclerosis

Arteriosclerosis is a chronic disease of the arterial system characterized by abnormal thickening and hardening of the vessel walls. In arteriosclerosis the tunica intima undergoes a series of changes that decrease the artery's ability to change lumen size. Smooth muscle cells and collagen fibers migrate into the tunica intima, causing it to stiffen and thicken. This process gradually narrows the arterial lumen (Figure 30-1). Changes in lipid, cholesterol, and phospholipid metabolism within the tunica intima also contribute to arteriosclerosis. Although these structural changes may be part of the normal aging process, they can cause or worsen pathophysiologic conditions such as high blood pressure, insufficient perfusion of tissues, or weakening and outpouching of arterial walls.

Atherosclerosis

Atherosclerosis is a form of arteriosclerosis in which the thickening and hardening of the vessel is caused by the accumulation of lipid-laden macrophages within the arterial wall, which leads to the formation of a lesion called a **plaque.** Atherosclerosis is not a single disease entity but rather a pathologic process that can affect vascular systems throughout the body resulting in ischemic syndromes that can vary widely in their severity and clinical manifestations. It is the leading contributor to coronary artery and cerebrovascular disease. (Atherosclerosis of the coronary arteries is described on p. 1100; atherosclerosis of the cerebral arteries is discussed in Chapter 17.)

PATHOPHYSIOLOGY Atherosclerosis is an inflammatory disease.[1-5] Pathologically, the lesions progress from en-

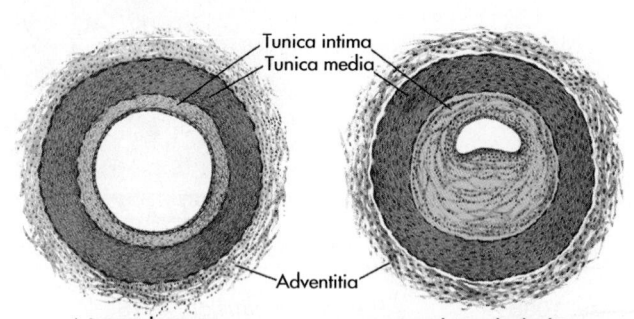
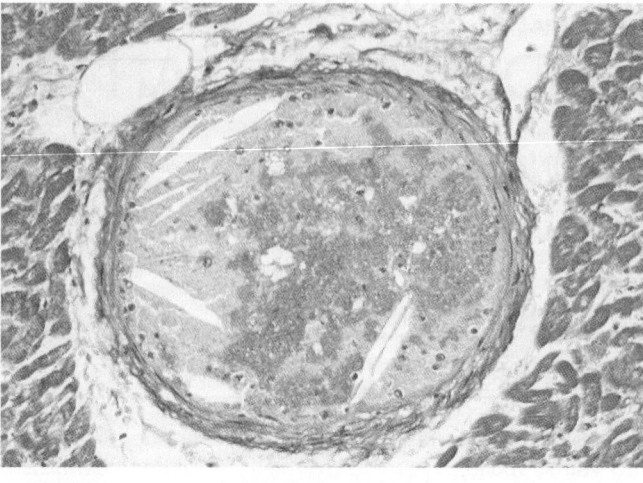

Figure 30-1 **Arteriosclerosis. A,** Cross section of a normal artery and an artery altered by disease. **B,** A small artery in the myocardium is occluded by a mass of blue-staining platelets, yellow-staining red cells, and cholesterol bodies. (**B** from Damjanov I, Linder J, editors: *Anderson's pathology*, ed 10, St Louis, 1996, Mosby.)

dothelial injury and dysfunction to fatty streak to fibrotic plaque to complicated lesion (Figures 30-2 and 30-3). Atherosclerosis begins with injury to the endothelial cells that line artery walls. Possible causes of endothelial injury include the common risk factors for atherosclerosis, such as smoking, hypertension, diabetes, increased levels of low-density lipoprotein (LDL), decreased levels of high-density lipoprotein (HDL), and hyperhomocystinemia. (See Nutrition box on Prevention of Cornary Heart Disease.) Other causes of endothelial injury are called the "novel" risk factors, such as elevated C-reactive protein, increased serum fibrinogen, insulin resistance, oxidative stress, infection, and peridontal disease.[6-11] Once injury has occurred, endothelial dysfunction and inflammation lead to the following pathophysiologic events:

1. Injured endothelial cells become inflamed and cannot make normal amounts of antithrombotic and vasodilating cytokines[6,12,13] (Figures 30-4 and 30-5).
2. Numerous inflammatory cytokines are released, including tumor necrosis factor-alpha (TNF-α), interferon-γ, interleukin-1, toxic oxygen radicals, and heat shock proteins.[4,5]
3. Growth factors are also released, including angiotensin II, fibroblast growth factor, and platelet-derived growth factor, which stimulate smooth muscle cell proliferation in the affected vessel.[4]
4. Macrophages adhere to injured endothelium by way of adhesion molecules, such as vascular cell adhesion molecule-1 (VCAM-1).[2,4]
5. These macrophages then release enzymes and toxic oxygen radicals that create oxidative stress, oxidize LDL, and further injure the vessel wall.[3,5]

The oxidation of LDL is an important step in atherogenesis. Inflammation with oxidative stress and activation of macrophages is the primary mechanism.[14,15] Diabetes, smoking, and hypertension are associated with increased LDL oxidation, and increased levels of angiotensin II have been linked to LDL oxidation through stimulation of the angiotensin re-

NUTRITION & DISEASE

Prevention of Coronary Heart Disease

Disease influences the risk of coronary heart disease (CHD). Disease mechanisms influenced by diet include lipid alterations, blood pressure, thrombotic tendency, endothelial function, oxidative stress, homocysteine level, and cardiac rhythm. Emerging evidence from epidemiologic studies, metabolic studies, and clinical trials indicate that at leat three dietary strategies are effective in preventing CHD: (1) substitute unsaturated fats—especially polyunsaturated fats for saturated and *trans* fats; (2) increase consumption of omega-3 fatty acids from fish oil or plant sources; and (3) eat a diet high in vegetables, fruits, nuts and whole grains and low in refined grains. These diets, together with no smoking, regular physical activity, and maintaining a healthy weight may prevent the majority of CHD in Western populations.

Data from Hu FB, Willet WC: *JAMA* 288(20):2569-2578, 2002.

ceptor AT$_1$[16] (see Chapter 29). Oxidized LDL is toxic to endothelial cells, causes smooth muscle proliferation, and activates further immune and inflammatory responses.[17-20] The oxidized LDL penetrates into the intima of the arterial wall and is engulfed by macrophages. Macrophages filled with oxidized LDL are called **foam cells.**

Once these lipid-laden foam cells accumulate in significant amounts, they form a lesion called a **fatty streak** (see Figure 30-2). These lesions can be found in the walls of arteries of most people, even young children. Once formed, fatty streaks produce more toxic oxygen radicals and cause immunologic and inflammatory changes, resulting in progressive damage to the vessel wall. Decreasing levels of LDL can cause regression of atherosclerotic lesions and can improve endothelial function.[21-24] Increasing attention is being given to the evaluation of children for dyslipidemia so that early dietary intervention to prevent atherosclerosis can be initiated.

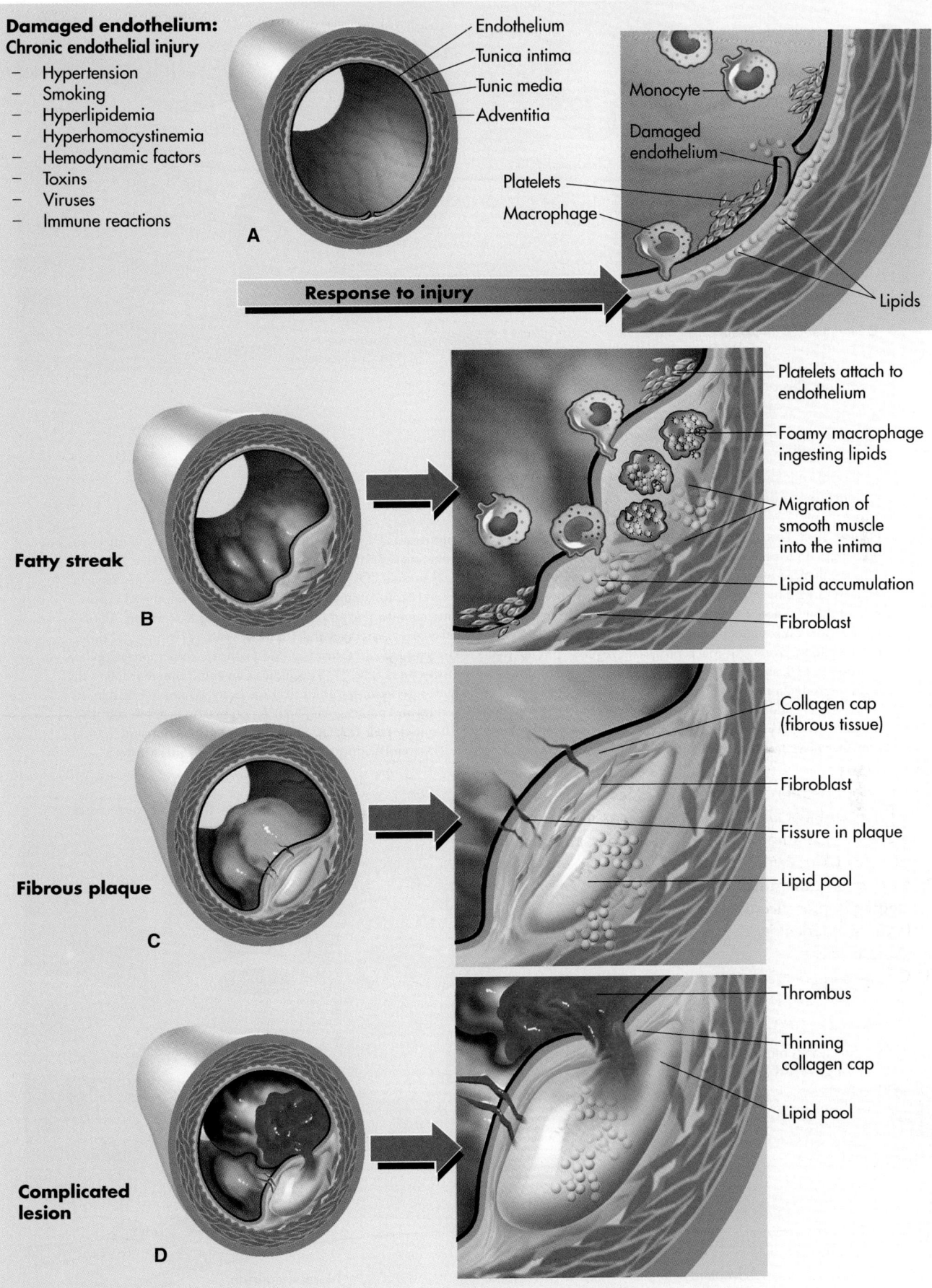

Damaged endothelium:
Chronic endothelial injury

- Hypertension
- Smoking
- Hyperlipidemia
- Hyperhomocystinemia
- Hemodynamic factors
- Toxins
- Viruses
- Immune reactions

Endothelium
Tunica intima
Tunic media
Adventitia

A

Monocyte

Damaged endothelium

Platelets

Macrophage

Lipids

Response to injury

Platelets attach to endothelium

Foamy macrophage ingesting lipids

Migration of smooth muscle into the intima

Lipid accumulation

Fibroblast

Fatty streak

B

Collagen cap (fibrous tissue)

Fibroblast

Fissure in plaque

Lipid pool

Fibrous plaque

C

Thrombus

Thinning collagen cap

Lipid pool

Complicated lesion

D

Figure 30-2 Progression of atherosclerosis. **A,** Damaged endothelium. **B,** Diagram of fatty streak and lipid core formation (see Figure 30-3 for a diagram of oxidized low-density lipoprotein [LDL]). **C,** Diagram of fibrous plaque. Raised plaques are visible: some are yellow; others are white. **D,** Diagram of complicated lesion; thrombus is red; collagen is blue. Plaque is complicated by red thrombus deposition.

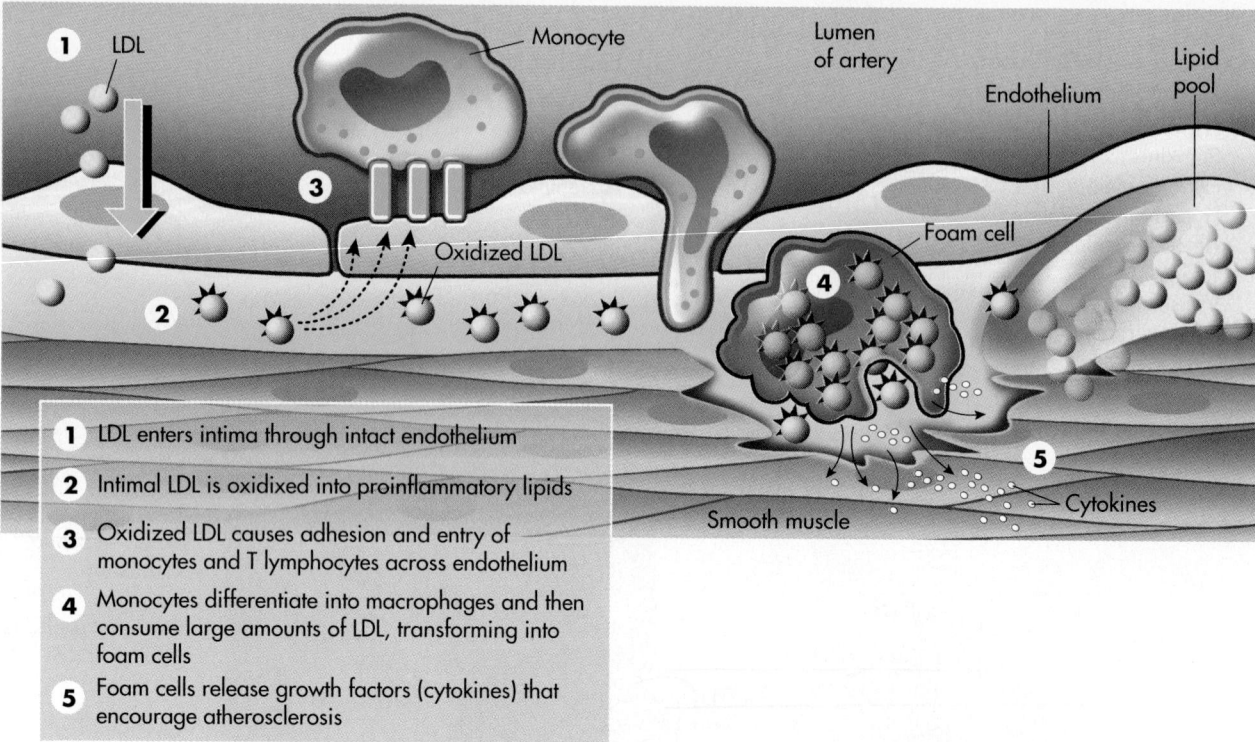

Figure 30-3 **Low-density lipoprotein oxidation.** (1) Low-density lipoprotein (LDL) enters the arterial intima through an intact endothelium. In hypercholesterolemia, the influx of LDL exceeds the eliminating capacity and an extracellular pool of LDL is formed. This is enhanced by association of LDL with the extracellular martrix. (2) Intimal LDL is oxidized through the action of free oxygen radicals formed by enzymatic or nonenzymatic reactions. (3) This generates proinflammatory lipids that induce endothelial expression of the adhesion molecule; vascular cell adhesion molecule-1 activates complement and stimulates chemokine secretion. All of these factors cause adhesion and entry of mononuclear leukocytes, particularly monocytes and T lymphocytes. (4) Monocytes differentiate into macrophages. Macrophages up-regulate and internalize oxidized LDL and transform into foam cells. Macrophage update of oxidized LDL also leads to presentation of fragments of it to antigen-specific T cells. (5) This induces an autoimmune reaction that leads to production of proinflammatory cytokines. Such cytokines include interferon-γ, tumor necrosis factor-α, and interleukin-1, which act on endothelial cells to stimulate expression of adhesion molecules and procoagulant activity; on macrophages to activate proteases, endocytosis, nitric oxide (NO), and cytokines; and on smooth muscle cells *(SMCs)* to include NO production and inhibit growth, collagen, and actin expression. (Modified from Crawford MH, DiMarco JP, editors: *Cardiology,* London, 2001, Mosby.)

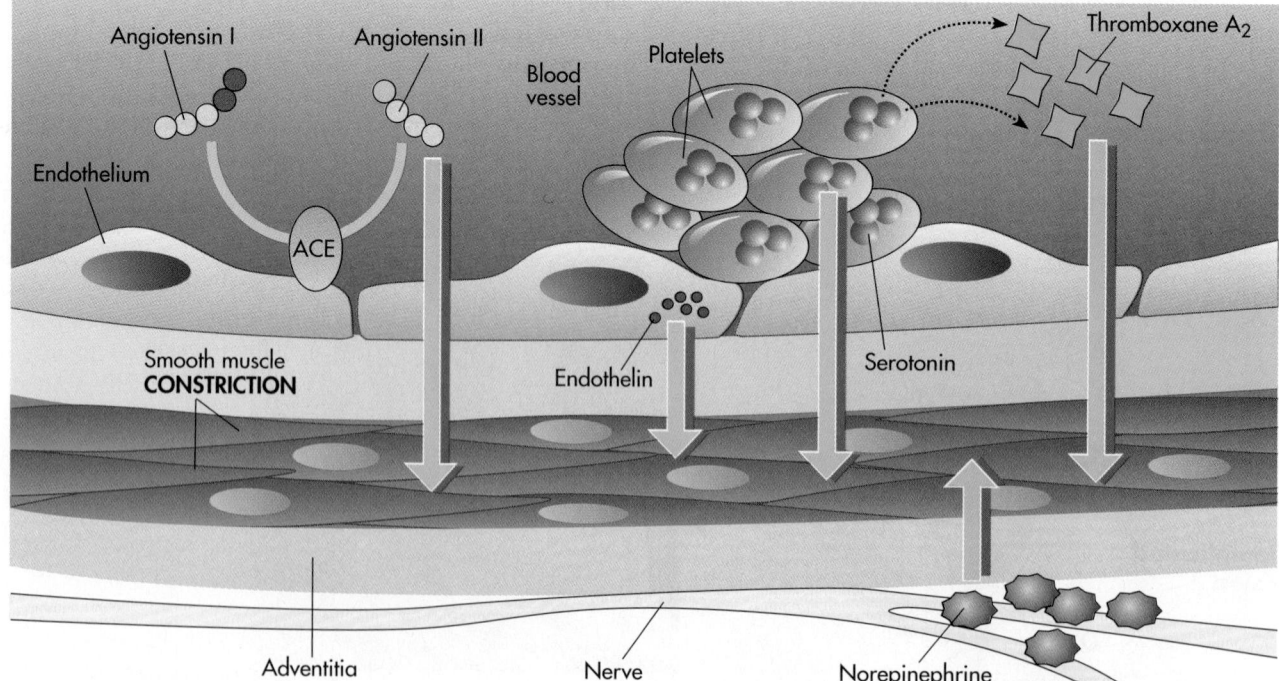

Figure 30-4 **Endothelium regulation of vasomotion (constriction and dilation) and platelet aggregation by release of a variety of constricting and dilating substances.** Constricting factors include arachidonic and metabolites, such as thromboxane A₂ (which aspirin inhibits), and a potent amino acid peptide called *endothelin.* The endothelium also converts angiotensin I into angiotensin II by the membrane-bound angiotensin-converting enzyme that also metabolizes the endogenous endothelium-dependent vasodilator, bradykinin. (Modified from Stern S, editor: *Silent myocardial ischemia,* St Louis, 1998, Mosby.)

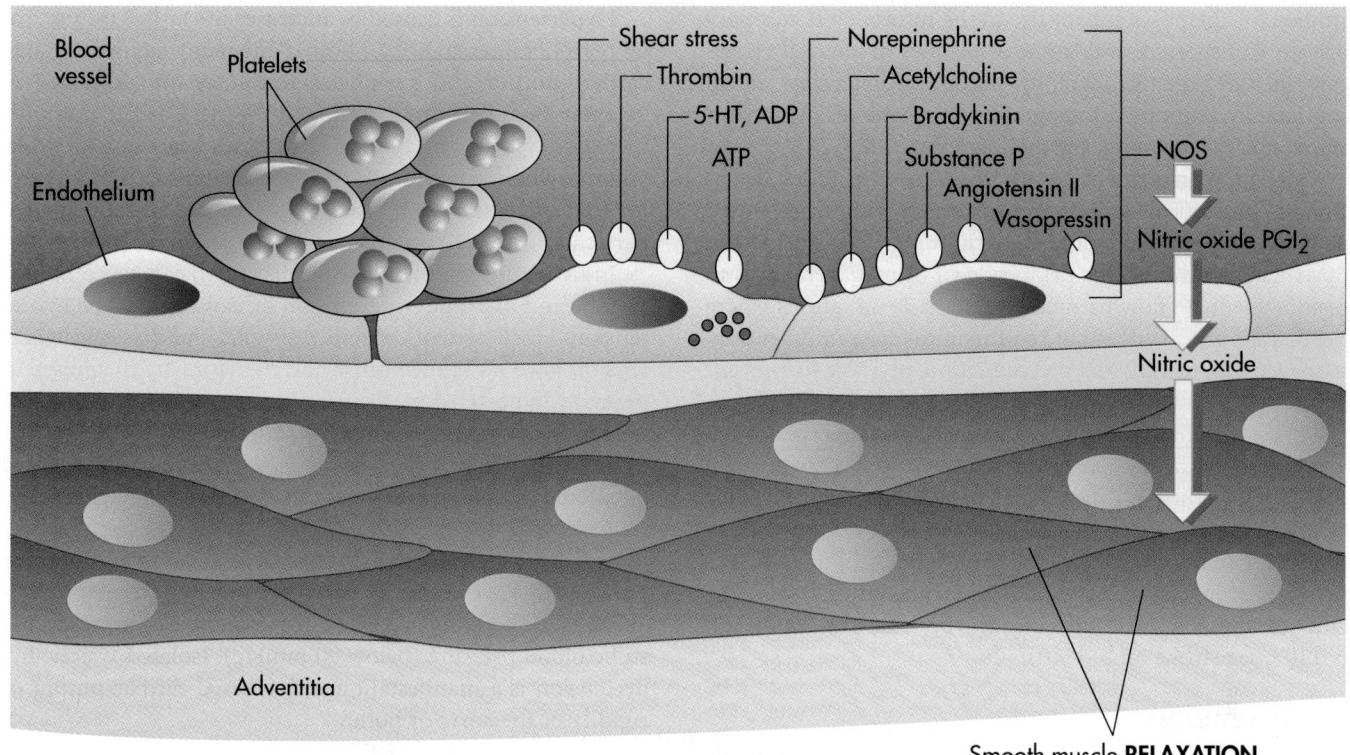

Figure 30-5 Factors causing endothelium-dependent vasodilation. A variety of exogenous pharmacologic substances, platelet-derived factors, and shear stress can promote release of nitric oxide by stimulating nitric oxide synthase (NOS). Prostacyclin (PGI₂) causes relaxation of vascular smooth muscle cells by cyclic adenosine monophosphate (cAMP)-dependent mechanism, and both nitric oxide and PGI₂ inhibit platelet aggregation. *5-HT,* Serotonin; *ADP,* adenosine diphosphate; *ATP,* adenosine triphosphate. (Modified from Stern S, editor: *Silent myocardial ischemia,* St Louis, 1998, Mosby.)

At this point, smooth muscle cells proliferate, produce collagen, and migrate over the fatty streak forming a **fibrous plaque** (see Figure 30-2). This process is mediated by many inflammatory cytokines, including growth factors (e.g., transforming growth factor–beta [TGF-β]). The fibrous plaque may calcify, protrude into the vessel lumen, and obstruct blood flow to distal tissues, especially during exercise, which may cause symptoms (e.g., angina or intermittent claudication).

Many plaques, however, are "unstable," meaning they are prone to rupture even before they affect blood flow significantly, and are clinically silent until they rupture. Plaque rupture occurs because of the inflammatory activation of proteinases, such as the matrix metalloproteinases and the cathepsins, and can be accelerated by bleeding within the lesion (plaque hemorrhage).[25] Atherosclerotic plaques can be classified according to their structure, which gives insight into their stability and proneness to rupture.[26,27] Plaques that have ruptured are called **complicated plaques** (see Figure 30-2). Once rupture occurs, exposure of underlying tissue results in platelet adhesion, initiation of the clotting cascade, and rapid thrombus formation. The thrombus may suddenly occlude the affected vessel resulting in ischemia and infarction. Aspirin or other antithrombotic agents are used to prevent this complication of atherosclerotic disease.[28,29]

CLINICAL MANIFESTATIONS Atherosclerosis presents with symptoms and signs that result from inadequate per-

fusion of tissues because of obstruction of the vessels that supply them. Partial vessel obstruction may lead to transient ischemic events, often associated with exercise or stress. Once the lesion becomes complicated, increasing obstruction with superimposed thrombosis may result in tissue infarction. Coronary artery disease (CAD) caused by atherosclerosis is the major cause of myocardial ischemia and is one of the most important health issues in the United States (see p. 1100). Atherosclerotic obstruction of the vessels supplying the brain is the major cause of stroke. Similarly, any part of the body may become ischemic when its blood supply is compromised by atherosclerotic lesions. Often more than one vessel will become involved with this disease process; consequently, an individual may present with symptoms from several ischemic tissues at the same time, and disease in one area may indicate that the individual is at risk for other ischemic complications elsewhere. Finally, diffuse atherosclerotic disease may elevate the total systemic vascular resistance and cause hypertension.

EVALUATION AND TREATMENT In evaluating individuals for the presence of atherosclerosis, a complete health history including the presence of risk factors and symptoms of cardiovascular disease is essential. Physical examination may detect arterial bruits and evidence of decreased blood flow to tissues. Serum should be tested for risk indicators, such as lipid profile and C-reactive protein. More recently, serum testing for the subclinical presence of atherosclerotic plaques has been studied for the possibility of use in the future.[30,31] If coronary disease is suspected, evaluation of plaques in affected vessels can include roentgenography, electrocardiography, ultrasonography, computed tomography, magnetic resonance imaging, nuclear scanning, and angiography.

Current management of atherosclerosis includes detection of "preclinical" lesions and treatment with drugs aimed at stabilizing plaques before they rupture.[32-34] Once a lesion obstructs blood flow, the primary goal of management is to restore adequate flow to affected tissues. In situations where the disease process does not require immediate intervention, management focuses on the reduction of risks to prevent continued endothelial injury and the prevention of plaque progression. Risk reduction includes smoking cessation, weight loss, and the control of hypertension, diabetes, and dyslipidemia through diet, exercise, and medication. Management of atherosclerotic risk factors is discussed further on p. 1100. If an individual presents with acute ischemia, such as myocardial infarction (MI) or stroke, interventions are specific to the diseased area (see myocardial infarction on p. 1107; see stroke on p. 1110).

Hypertension

Hypertension is defined as a sustained elevation of systemic arterial blood pressure. In many developed countries the risk of hypertension increases with aging. One in three adults in the United States has been diagnosed with hypertension. Of those with high blood pressure, it is estimated that up to 30% do not know they have it. Individuals are diagnosed as having hypertension when the average of two or more blood pressure measurements made on two or more consecutive clinical visits documents a diastolic pressure of 90 mmHg or greater *or* a systolic pressure of 140 mmHg or greater.[35] Systolic hypertension, even when not accompanied by an increase in diastolic pressure, is the most significant factor in causing target organ damage.[35,36] A new classification scheme was introduced in 2003 and is presented in Table 30-1. "Optimal" blood pressure is associated with the lowest cardiovascular risk, whereas those who fall into the "prehypertension" category are at risk for developing hypertension unless life-style modification is instituted. All stages of hypertension are associated with increased risk for target organ disease events, such as myocardial infarction, kidney disease, and stroke; thus both stage I and stage II hypertension need effective long-term therapy.[35,37]

Table 30-1	Classification of Blood Pressure for Adults Age 18 Years or Older	
Category	Systolic (mmHg)	Diastolic (mmHg)
Normal	<120	<80
Prehypertension	120-139	80-89
Stage 1 hypertension	140-159	90-99
Stage 2 hypertension	≥160	≥100

Data from the JNC 7 Report, *JAMA* 289(19):2560-2572, 2003.

Hypertension is caused by increases in cardiac output, total peripheral resistance, or both. (The many factors affecting cardiac output and peripheral resistance are described in Chapter 29 (see Figures 29-18 and 29-28). Cardiac output is increased by any condition that increases heart rate or stroke volume, whereas peripheral resistance is increased by any factor that increases blood viscosity or reduces vessel diameter, particularly arteriolar diameter.

Individuals with hypertensive disease may have combined systolic and diastolic hypertension or isolated systolic hypertension. Most cases of combined systolic and diastolic hypertension have no known cause and therefore are diagnosed as **primary hypertension**. Primary hypertension, also called *essential* or *idiopathic hypertension*, affects 90% to 95% of hypertensive individuals.[35,38] **Secondary hypertension** is caused by altered hemodynamics associated with a primary disease, such as renal disease. Although many diseases can cause secondary hypertension, this form of hypertension accounts for only 5% to 8% of cases. **Isolated systolic hypertension** is elevated systolic blood pressure accompanied by normal diastolic blood pressure (below 90 mmHg). Isolated systolic hypertension is a manifestation of increased cardiac output or rigidity of the aorta or both.

Factors Associated with Primary Hypertension

A specific cause for primary hypertension has not been identified, and a combination of genetic and environmental factors is thought to be responsible for its development. Genetic predisposition to hypertension is thought to be polygenic. The inherited defects are associated with renal sodium excretion, insulin and insulin sensitivity, activity of the renin-angiotensin-aldosterone system, cell membrane sodium or calcium transport, and sympathetic response to neurogenic hormones. Recently, a mutation in the adducin gene has been linked to changes in renal tubular sodium transport and hypertension[37,39-41] (see What's New? Gene Mutation Predicts Hypertension). Factors associated with primary hypertension include (1) family history of hypertension; (2) advancing age; (3) gender (men younger than 55 years and women older than 74 years); (4) black race; (5) high dietary sodium intake; (6) glucose intolerance (diabetes mellitus); (7) cigarette smoking; (8) obesity; (9) heavy alcohol consumption; and (10) low dietary intake of potassium, calcium, and magnesium. Many of these factors are also risk factors for other cardiovascular disorders. In fact, hypertension, dyslipidemia, and glucose intolerance often are found together.

Although populations with high dietary sodium intake have long been shown to have an increased incidence of hypertension, recent studies indicate that low dietary potassium, calcium, and magnesium intakes are also risk factors because without their intake sodium is retained[38,42] (see p. 1088). The nicotine in cigarette smoke is a vasoconstrictor that can elevate both systolic and diastolic blood pressure acutely. In habitual smokers an individual cigarette may not raise blood pressure, yet habitual smoking is associated with a high incidence of severe hypertension, myocardial hypertrophy, and

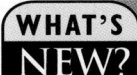
Adducin is a membrane-skeleton protein that plays an important role in the determination of cellular morphology and motility and in the regulation of membrane ion transport. It interacts with Na^+-K^+ ATPase and thus regulates the sodium-potassium pump. Mutations (e.g., *ADD1* Gly460Trp) of the gene that codes for adducin cause an increase in tubular renal reabsorption of sodium and are associated with an approximately 50% to 70% increase in risk for hypertension in whites. This risk increases to a ratio of 4:2 in older, heavier persons with higher triglycerides. No association between hypertension and adducin gene mutations are seen in blacks. Whites homozygous for the adducin gene mutation have a high risk of low-renin hypertension, and carriers of the mutation have a significant shift in their pressure-natriuresis curve, even if hypertension is not yet evident. The risk for hypertension is much greater if the adducin gene mutation is associated with other genetic abnormalities, especially those affecting the renin-angiotensin-aldosterone system. In addition to an increased risk for hypertension, individuals with these gene mutations are more likely to develop target organ affects including coronary artery disease and hypertensive renal disease. Finally, the presence of the adducin gene mutation indicates that the affected individual is more likely to be salt sensitive and to respond more effectively to diuretic treatment of his or her hypertension.

Data from Bianchi G, Tripodi G: *Ann N Y Acad Sci* 986:660-668, 2003. Hopkins PN, Hunt SC: *Genet Med* 5(6):413-429, 2003; Kosachunhanun N et al: *Hypertension* 42(5):901-908, 2003; Morrison AC et al: *Hypertension* 39(6):1053-1057, 2002; Nicod J et al: *Kidney Intern* 61(4):1270-1275, 2002; Sciarrone MT et al: *Hypertension* 41(3):398-403, 2003; Wang JG et al: *Kidney Intern* 62(6):2152-2159, 2002.

death resulting from CAD. The incidence of hypertension is higher among heavy drinkers of alcohol (more than three drinks per day) than among abstainers, but moderate drinkers (two to four drinks per week) appear to have lower blood pressures, as well as lower cardiovascular mortality, than either abstainers or heavy drinkers.[43] Obesity is recognized as an important risk factor for hypertension and contributes to many of the neurohumoral, metabolic, renal, and cardiovascular processes that cause hypertension, especially those factors that contribute to endothelial dysfunction and renal sodium retention.[44-46]

PATHOPHYSIOLOGY

Primary Hypertension. Primary hypertension is the result of a complicated interaction between genetics and the environment and their effects on vascular and renal function. Many gene polymorphisms have been implicated in the pathogenesis of primary hypertension (see What's New? Gene Mutation Predicts Hypertension). These genetic changes interact with the environment to increase vascular tone (increased peripheral resistance) and blood volume, thus causing sustained increases in blood pressure. Multiple pathophysiologic mechanisms mediate these effects including the sympathetic nervous system (SNS), the renin-angiotensin-aldosterone (RAA) system, adducin, and natriuretic peptides. Inflammation, endothelial dysfunction, and insulin resistance also contribute to both increased peripheral resistance and increased blood volume. Increased vascular volume is related to a decrease in renal excretion of salt, often referred to as a shift in the **pressure-natriuresis relationship**. This means that for a given blood pressure, individuals with hypertension tend to secrete less salt in their urine. The pathophysiology of primary hypertension is summarized in Figure 30-6.

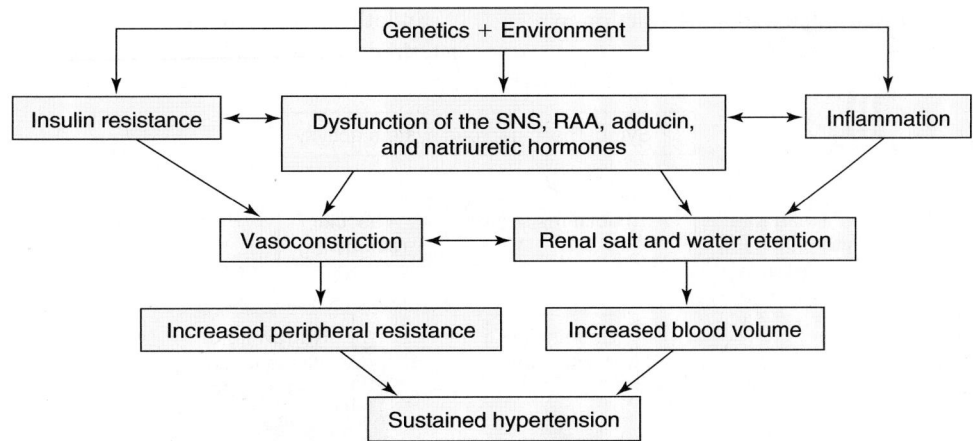

Figure 30-6 Pathophysiology of hypertension. Numerous genetic vulnerabilities have been linked to hypertension and these, in combination with environmental risks, cause neurohumoral dysfunction (sympathetic nervous system [SNS], renin-angiotensin-aldosterone [RAA] system, adducin, and natriuretic hormones) and promote inflammation and insulin resistance. Insulin resistance and neurohumoral dysfunction contribute to sustained systemic vasoconstriction and increased peripheral resistance. Inflammation contributes to renal dysfunction, which, in combination with the neurohumoral alterations, results in renal salt and water retention and increased blood volume. Increased peripheral resistance and increased blood volume are two primary causes of sustained hypertension.

The sympathetic nervous system (SNS) contributes to the pathogenesis of hypertension in many persons. In the healthy individual, the SNS contributes to the maintenance of adequate blood pressure and tissue perfusion by promoting cardiac contractility and heart rate (maintenance of adequate cardiac output) and by inducing arteriolar vasoconstriction (maintenance of adequate peripheral resistance). In individuals with hypertension, over-activity of the sympathetic nervous system can result from increased production of catecholamines (epinephrine and norepinephrine) or from increased receptor reactivity involving these neurotransmitters. Increased SNS activity causes increased heart rate and systemic vasoconstriction, thus raising the blood pressure. Additional mechanisms of SNS-induced hypertension include structural changes in blood vessels (vascular remodeling), renal sodium retention, insulin resistance, increased renin and angiotensin levels, and procoagulant effects.[38,47-49] The role of the SNS in the pathogenesis of cardiovascular disease is summarized in Figure 30-7.

In the healthy individual, the renin-angiotensin aldosterone (RAA) system provides an important homeostatic mechanism for maintaining adequate blood pressure and, therefore, tissue perfusion (see Chapter 29). Dysfunction of this system in the hypertensive individual can lead to persistent increases in peripheral resistance and renal salt retention. Angiotensin II also causes structural changes in blood vessels (remodeling) that contribute to permanent increases in peripheral resistance and make vessels more vulnerable to endothelial dysfunction and platelet aggregation.[38,50] Angiotensin II is also responsible for the hypertrophy of the myocardium associated with hypertension. Aldosterone not only contributes to sodium retention by the kidney but also has further deleterious effects on the cardiovascular system.[38,51,52] Drugs that block either angiotensin-converting enzyme (ACE inhibitors) or angiotensin and aldosterone receptors are used widely in the treatment of hypertension and have been shown to improve cardiac and renal function in select populations.[35,38,53-55]

Recent genetic analyses have found a strong link between the presence of a mutation in the gene for production of the protein **adducin** (*ADD1* Gly460Trp) and a 50% to 70% increased risk for essential hypertension in white adults. This mutation, in association with dysfunction of the RAA, results in a significant increase in salt retention by the kidney, an increased risk for cardiac and renal complications associated with hypertension, and an improved response to diuretic treatment.[56-60]

Natriuretic hormones modulate renal sodium (Na^+) excretion and include atrial natriuretic peptide (ANP), brain natriuretic peptide (BNP), C-type natriuretic peptide (CNP), and urodilanton. The function of these hormones can be affected by excessive sodium intake; inadequate dietary intake of potassium, magnesium, and calcium; and obesity.[61,62] Dysfunction of these hormones, along with alterations in the RAA system and the SNS, cause an increase in vascular tone and a shift in the pressure-natriuresis relationship.[63-65] Salt retention leads to water retention and increased blood volume, which contributes to an increase in blood pressure. Subtle renal injury results, with renal vasoconstriction and tissue ischemia. Tissue ischemia causes inflammation of the kidney and contributes to dysfunction of the glomeruli and tubules and promotes additional sodium retention. Drugs that increase the effectiveness of natriuretic peptides are now being used for the treatment of hypertension and heart failure.

Inflammation plays a role in the pathogenesis of hypertension. Endothelial injury and tissue ischemia result in the release of vasoactive inflammatory cytokines. Although many of these cytokines (e.g., histamine, prostaglandins) have vasodilatory actions in acute inflammatory injury, chronic inflammation contributes to vascular remodeling and smooth muscle contraction.[66] In the kidney, decreased renal perfusion leads to tubular ischemia and preglomerular arteriopathy leading to decreased sodium filtration and increased sodium retention, thus shifting the pressure-natriuresis curve and contributing to sustained hypertension.[38]

Endothelial dysfunction in primary hypertension is characterized by a decreased production of vasodilators, such as

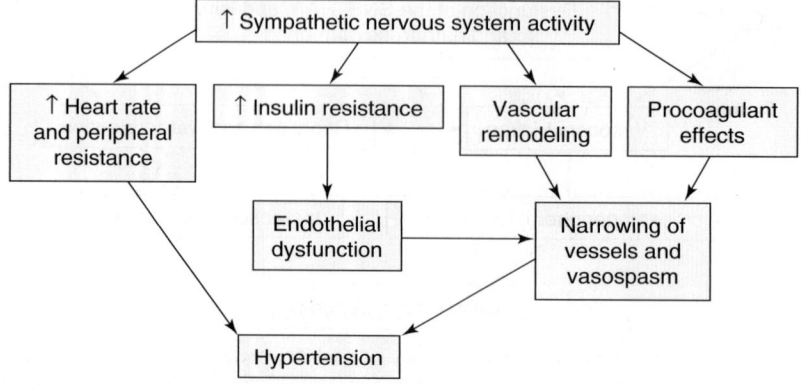

Figure 30-7 Role of the sympathetic nervous system in the pathogenesis of hypertension. Increased activity of the sympathetic nervous system (SNS) not only increases heart rate and peripheral resistance but also causes vascular remodeling with narrowing and vasospasm of arteries. The SNS contributes to insulin resistance, which is associated with endothelial dysfunction and decreased production of vasodilators, such as nitric oxide. The SNS also has procoagulant properties making vascular spasm and thrombosis more likely. All of these factors contribute to sustained increases in blood pressure.

nitric oxide, and increased production of vasoconstrictors, such as endothelin (see Chapter 29, Box 29-1). Dysfunction of the endothelium also contributes to vascular remodeling. Drugs that block the RAA system improve endothelial function.[38,67] Insulin resistance is associated with endothelial dysfunction in primary hypertension even without overt diabetes.[68,69] Insulin has several important roles in vascular protection including increased endothelial cell production of nitric oxide. Although hyperinsulinemia may serve as a growth factor and contribute to vascular remodeling, it is believed that it is the resistance to insulin that results in endothelial injury and dysfunction and contributes to the pathogenesis of hypertension and atherosclerosis. Diabetes and insulin resistance also cause changes in SNS and RAA activity, cause renal glomerular dysfunction, and contribute to the target organ effects of hypertension.[44,69-72] It is interesting to note that in many individuals with diabetes treated with drugs that increase insulin sensitivity, blood pressure often declines, even in the absence of antihypertensive drugs.[73]

Primary hypertension is the result of an interaction between many of the above-described processes. The majority of these factors influence renal sodium excretion and shift the pressure-natriuresis relationship as summarized in Figure 30-8. Other effects of this complex group of mechanisms include alterations in endothelial function, vasomotor tone, vascular remodeling, and target organ injury. While no single gene or discrete pathophysiologic process is likely responsible for the pathogenesis of primary hypertension, our understanding of these complex mechanisms contributes to the development of new and more effective treatments.

Secondary Hypertension. Secondary hypertension is caused by a systemic disease process that raises peripheral vascular resistance or cardiac output. If the cause is identified and removed before permanent structural changes occur,

blood pressure returns to normal. Table 30-2 summarizes the pathogenesis of major forms of secondary hypertension.

Isolated Systolic Hypertension. Elevations of systolic pressure are caused by increases in cardiac output or total peripheral vascular resistance or both. Isolated systolic hypertension caused by increased cardiac output can be secondary to dysfunction of the aortic semilunar valve (aortic valve insufficiency), any abnormal opening between heart chambers (arterioventricular fistula, patent ductus arteriosus; see Chapter 31), thyrotoxic crisis (thyroid storm), Paget disease of the bone, and beriberi.

Peripheral resistance can be increased by rigidity of the proximal large arteries, and is the chief vascular cause of isolated systolic hypertension in the elderly population. This rigidity most often is caused by arteriosclerosis. Isolated systolic hypertension is now recognized as an important risk factor for cardiovascular disease and stroke, and it should be treated aggressively.[32,36]

Complicated Hypertension. Chronic hypertension damages the walls of systemic blood vessels. Within the walls of arteries and arterioles, smooth muscle cells undergo hypertrophy and hyperplasia with associated fibrosis of the tunica intima and media in a process called *vascular "remodeling"* (see Figure 30-9). Endothelial dysfunction, angiotensin II, catecholamines, insulin resistance, and inflammation all contribute to this process. Once significant fibrosis has occurred, reduced blood flow and dysfunction of the organs perfused by these affected vessels is inevitable. Target organs for hypertension include the kidney, brain, heart, extremities and eyes—these effects are summarized in Table 30-3.

Cardiovascular complications include left ventricular hypertrophy, angina pectoris, congestive heart failure (left heart failure), coronary artery disease, myocardial infarction, and sudden death. Myocardial hypertrophy in response to hyper-

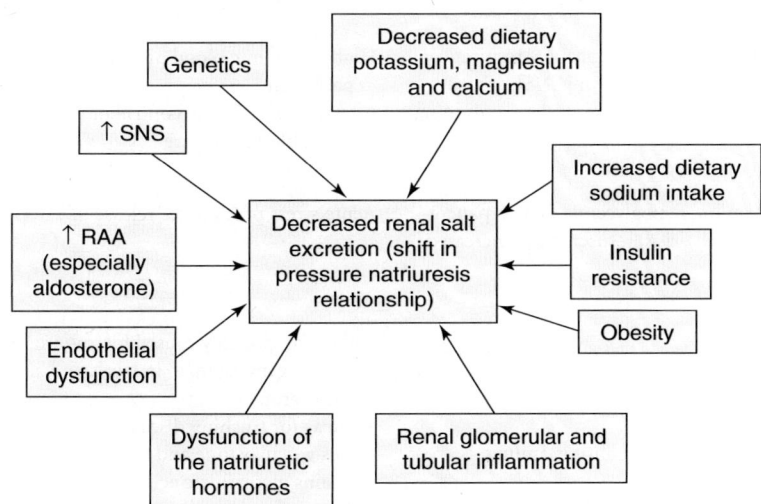

Figure 30-8 Shift in the pressure-natriuresis relationship. Numerous factors have been implicated in the pathogenesis of sodium retention in individuals with hypertension. These factors cause less renal excretion of salt than would normally occur with increased blood pressure. This is called a *shift in the pressure-natriuresis relationship* and is believed to be a central process in the pathogenesis of primary hypertension. *SNS,* Sympathetic nervous system; *RAA,* renin-angiotensin-aldosterone.

Table 30-2	Pathogenesis of Major Forms of Secondary Hypertension by Cause
Primary Disease	**Pathogenesis of Hypertension**
Renal Disorders	
Renal parenchymal disease	Disturbances in filtration and reabsorption of serum sodium, potassium, and calcium initiate the hemodynamics of early hypertension
Renovascular disease	Impaired blood flow and renal ischemia invoke the compensatory renin-angiotensin-aldosterone mechanism in an effort to raise the renal perfusion pressure
Renin-producing tumors	Elevated blood renin levels invoke elevations in angiotensin and aldosterone, which cause blood pressure to rise
Renal failure	Disturbances in filtration and reabsorption of serum sodium, potassium, and calcium initiate the hemodynamics of early hypertension
Primary sodium retention	Disturbance in filtration and/or reabsorption of serum sodium initiates the hemodynamics of early hypertension
Endocrine Disorders	
Acromegaly	Excess human growth hormone causes increased peripheral resistance
Hypothyroidism	Mucopolysaccharide deposits in vascular tissue increase resistance
Hypercalcemia	Calcium ion directly affects vascular tonicity; elevated serum calcium levels increase vascular tone and peripheral resistance
Hyperthyroidism	Increased inotropic effect on the heart elevates systolic pressure; diastolic pressure decreases as a result of decreased peripheral resistance

Adrenal disorders
  Cortical disturbances
  Cushing syndrome
	Glucocorticoids facilitate sodium and water retention, initiating the hemodynamics of early hypertension

Primary aldosteronism	Excess aldosterone promotes sodium retention and initiation of the hemodynamics of early hypertension
Congenital adrenal hyperplasia	Excess production of adrenocortical hormones promotes sodium and water retention
Medullary disturbance: pheochromocytoma	Excess catecholamines raise vascular tone and increase peripheral resistance
Extraadrenal chromaffin tumors	Excess catecholamines raise vascular tone and increase peripheral resistance
Vascular Disorders	
Coarctation of the aorta	Decreased blood flow in distal areas initiates maximum peripheral resistance as an autoregulatory effort to adjust perfusion pressure
Arteriosclerosis	Loss of elasticity in vessel walls results in increased peripheral resistance
Pregnancy-Induced Hypertension	Pathogenesis unclear
Neurologic Disorders	
Elevated intracranial pressure (brain tumor, encephalitis, respiratory acidosis of pulmonary or central nervous system [CNS] origin)	Higher systemic blood pressure required to maintain adequate cerebral perfusion
Quadriplegia, acute porphyria, familial dysautonomia, lead poisoning, Guillain-Barré syndrome	Interface with neural control of blood pressure initiates increased systemic blood pressure
Acute Stress	
Surgery, psychogenic hyperventilation, hypoglycemia, burns, pancreatitis, alcohol withdrawal, sickle cell crisis, resuscitation, increased intravascular volume	Acute stress precipitates release of catecholamines and glucocorticoids
Drugs and Other Substances	
Oral contraceptives and estrogen	Unknown; possibly caused by sodium retention, plasma retention, weight gain, changes in levels and actions of renin, angiotensin, and aldosterone
Corticosteroids	Same as for Cushing disease
Sympathetic stimulants, appetite suppressants, antihistamines	Raises vascular tone and increases vascular resistance
Licorice	Contains glycerrhizic acid, a mineralocorticoid that causes salt and water retention
Monoamine oxidase inhibitors	Hypertension may develop in an individual who routinely takes a monoamine oxidase (MAO) inhibitor with ingestion of a food containing tyramine, such as aged cheese

From Kaplan NM: *Clinical hypertension,* ed 8, Baltimore, 2002, Lippincott, Williams & Wilkins.

tension is mediated by several neurohormonal substances, including the SNS and angiotensin II.[74-77] This results in changes in the myocyte proteins, apoptosis of myocytes, and deposition of collagen into the heart muscle. In addition, the increased size of the heart muscle increases demand for coronary perfusion, such that, over time, contractility of the heart is impaired and the individual is at increased risk for heart failure. Vascular complications include the formation, dissection, and rupture of aneurysms (outpouchings in vessel walls); intermittent claudication; and gangrene resulting from vessel occlusion. Possible renal complications are parenchymal damage, nephrosclerosis, renal arteriosclerosis, and renal insufficiency or failure.[78,79] Microalbuminuria (small amounts of protein in the urine) occurs in 10% to 25% of individuals with essential hypertension and is now recognized as an early sign of impending renal dysfunction and significantly increased risk for cardiovascular events.[80-82]

Changes in the vascular beds can be estimated by viewing the arterioles of the retina. Complications specific to the retina include retinal vascular sclerosis, exudation, and hem-

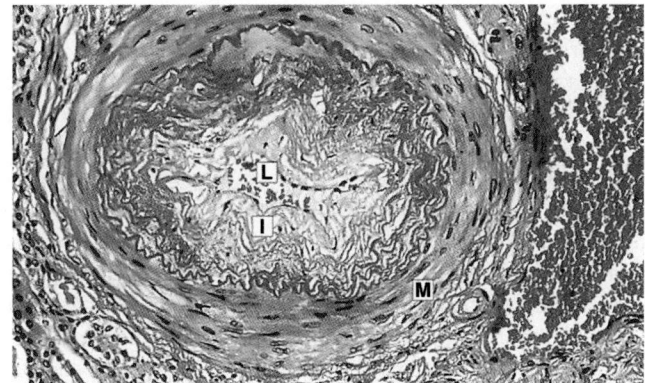

Figure 30-9 Dramatic hypertension change in small arterioles. Fibrous intimal proliferation *(I)* with reduction in lumen vessel caliber (radius) *(L)* and normal media *(M)*. (From Stevens A, Lowe J: *Pathology,* ed 2, St Louis, 2000, Mosby.)

orrhage. Cerebrovascular complications are similar to those of other arterial beds and include transient ischemia, stroke, cerebral thrombosis, aneurysm, and hemorrhage. Chronic hypertension also has been linked to cognitive decline in the elderly.[83,84]

Malignant hypertension (rapidly progressive hypertension in which diastolic pressure is usually above 140 mmHg) can cause encephalopathy, a profound cerebral edema that disrupts cerebral function and causes loss of consciousness. Encephalopathy occurs because high arterial pressure renders the cerebral arterioles incapable of regulating blood flow to the cerebral capillary beds. Capillary permeability is increased by high hydrostatic pressures in the capillaries, and vascular fluid exudes into the interstitial space. If blood pressure is not reduced, cerebral edema and cerebral dysfunction increase until death occurs. Organ damage resulting from malignant hypertension is life threatening. Besides encephalopathy, malignant hypertension can cause papilledema, cardiac failure, uremia, retinopathy, and cerebrovascular accident. This should be considered a hypertensive emergency and managed with rapid administration of parenteral vasodilators with the goal of lowering the blood pressure by 25% within minutes to 2 hours.[36,85]

CLINICAL MANIFESTATIONS   The early stages of hypertension have no clinical manifestations other than elevated blood pressure. Most important, no signs and symptoms cause the individual to seek health care; thus hypertension is called a **lanthanic (silent) disease.** Some hypertensive individuals never have signs, symptoms, or complications, whereas others become very ill, in which case hypertension can cause death. Still others have anatomic and physiologic damage caused by past hypertensive disease despite having current blood pressures within normal ranges.

The chance of developing primary hypertension increases with age, over and above the natural rise in blood pressure associated with aging. Although hypertension usually is thought to be an adult health problem, it is important to re-

Table 30-3	Pathologic Effects of Sustained, Complicated Primary Hypertension	
Site of Injury	**Mechanism of Injury**	**Potential Pathologic Effect**
Heart		
Myocardium	Increased workload combined with diminished blood flow through coronary arteries	Left ventricular hypertrophy, myocardial ischemia, left heart failure
Coronary arteries	Accelerated atherosclerosis (coronary artery disease)	Myocardial ischemia, myocardial infarction, sudden death
Kidneys	Renin and aldosterone secretion stimulated by reduced blood flow	Retention of sodium and water, leading to increased blood volume and perpetuation of hypertension
	Reduced oxygen supply	Tissue damage that compromises filtration
	High pressures in renal arterioles	Nephrosclerosis leading to renal failure
Brain	Reduced blood flow and oxygen supply; weakened vessel walls, accelerated atherosclerosis	Transient ischemic attacks, cerebral thrombosis, aneurysm, hemorrhage, acute brain infarction
Eyes (retinas)	Reduced blood flow	Retinal vascular sclerosis
	High arteriolar pressure	Exudation, hemorrhage
Aorta	Weakened vessel wall	Dissecting aneurysm (see p. 1094)
Arterial vessels of lower extremities	Reduced blood flow and high pressures in arterioles, accelerated atherosclerosis	Intermittent claudication, gangrene

member that hypertension does occur in children and is being diagnosed with increasing frequency. Usually, however, increased peripheral resistance and early hypertension develop in the second, third, and fourth decades of life. If elevated blood pressure is not detected and treated, it becomes established and may begin to accelerate atherosclerosis when the individual is 30 to 50 years of age. This sets the stage for the complications of hypertension that begin to appear during the fourth, fifth, and sixth decades of life.

Most clinical manifestations of hypertensive disease are caused by complications that damage organs and tissues outside the vascular system. Besides elevated blood pressure, the signs and symptoms therefore tend to be specific for the organs or tissues affected. Evidence of heart disease, renal insufficiency, central nervous system dysfunction, impaired vision, impaired mobility, vascular occlusion, or edema can all be caused by sustained hypertension. (See appropriate chapters for specific clinical manifestations of organ dysfunction.)

EVALUATION AND TREATMENT   A single elevated blood pressure reading does not mean that a person has hypertension; the diagnosis requires documenting increased blood pressure on two or more different occasions. Some people tend to have high readings whenever they visit a health care setting (sometimes called "white coat hypertension") or if they have had recent caffeine intake or have been smoking. Many clinicians use 24-hour ambulatory blood pressure monitoring in selected individuals to document the blood pressure during their daily activities and to determine whether a management modality is working throughout the day. Twenty-four–hour blood pressure measurement is better correlated than clinic measurements with the risk of target organ damage and is indicated in individuals who are suspected of white coat hypertension, hypotensive episodes, drug resistance, or autonomic dysfunction.[35,86] Evaluation of the hypertensive individual should include a complete medical history and assessment of life-style and other risk factors for hypertension and cardiovascular disease, as well as evidence of possible secondary causes of hypertension. Physical examination should include examination of the optic fundi; calculation of body mass index; auscultation for carotid, abdominal, and femoral bruits; examination of the heart and lungs; palpation of the abdomen; assessment of lower extremity pulses and edema; and neurologic examination.[35] Further routine diagnostic tests for the evaluation of hypertension include hematocrit, urinalysis, biochemical blood profile (fasting glucose, sodium, potassium, calcium, creatinine, total cholesterol, high-density cholesterol, triglycerides), and an electrocardiogram (ECG). Optional tests include urinary albumin excretion or albumin/creatinine ratio.[35] Individuals who have elevated blood pressure are assumed to have primary hypertension unless their history, physical examination, or initial diagnostic screening indicates secondary hypertension.

Hypertension usually is managed with both pharmacologic and nonpharmacologic methods. An overview of the current recommendations for the management of hypoten-

sion is illustrated in Figure 30-10. Treatment begins with reducing or eliminating risk factors. Life-style modification can prevent hypertension from developing in those individuals who fall into the "prehypertension" category, may control the blood pressure in stage I hypertension, and can enhance the effects of drug treatment for those with more significant blood pressure elevation. The usual dietary recommendations are to restrict sodium intake to 2.4 g/day, to increase potassium intake, to restrict saturated fat intake, and to adjust calorie intake as required to maintain optimum weight. The Dietary Approaches to Stop Hypertension (DASH) diet is recommended.[35,62] An exercise program that promotes endurance and relaxation usually is recommended. Physical training increases stroke volume, which has the effect of lowering heart rate and hence systolic blood pressure, and should consist of regular aerobic physical activity at least 30 minutes most days of the week.[35] Relaxation is expected to reduce levels of circulating catecholamines, which has the effect of reducing vascular tone and blood pressure. Individuals are counseled to stop smoking to eliminate vasoconstrictor effects of nicotine.

Pharmacologic treatment of hypertension reduces the risk of end-organ damage and prevents major diseases, such as myocardial ischemia and stroke.

Thiazide diuretics have been shown to be the safest and most effective medications for lowering blood pressure and preventing the cardiovascular complications of hypertension.[35,87] If the individual requires two drugs for blood pressure control, the recommendation is combinations of thiazide diuretics and other antihypertensives, such as beta blockers and ACE inhibitors. Some individuals will have "compelling indications" for choosing a particular antihypertensive as a first-line medication. For example, individuals with heart failure, chronic kidney disease, or who are post-myocardial infarction or have had recurrent stroke should begin antihypertensive treatment with an ACE inhibitor, angiotensin receptor blocker (ARB), or aldosterone antagonist.[35]

Orthostatic (Postural) Hypotension

The term **orthostatic (postural) hypotension** means a decrease in both systolic and diastolic arterial blood pressure on standing. The American Autonomic Society (AAS) and the American Academy of Neurology (AAN) define orthostatic hypertension as a systolic blood pressure decrease of at least 20 mmHg or a diastolic blood pressure decrease of at least 10 mmHg within 3 minutes of standing up.[88] When a normal individual stands up, the resultant gravitational changes on the circulation are compensated for by several mechanisms that include reflex arteriolar and venous constriction, increased heart rate, and mechanical factors, such as the closure of valves in the venous system, pumping of the leg muscles, and a decrease in intrathoracic pressure. The normally increased sympathetic activity during upright posture is mediated through stretch receptors (baroreceptors) in the carotid sinus and the aortic arch (see Chapter 29). Their reflex response to shifts in volume caused by postural changes leads to a prompt

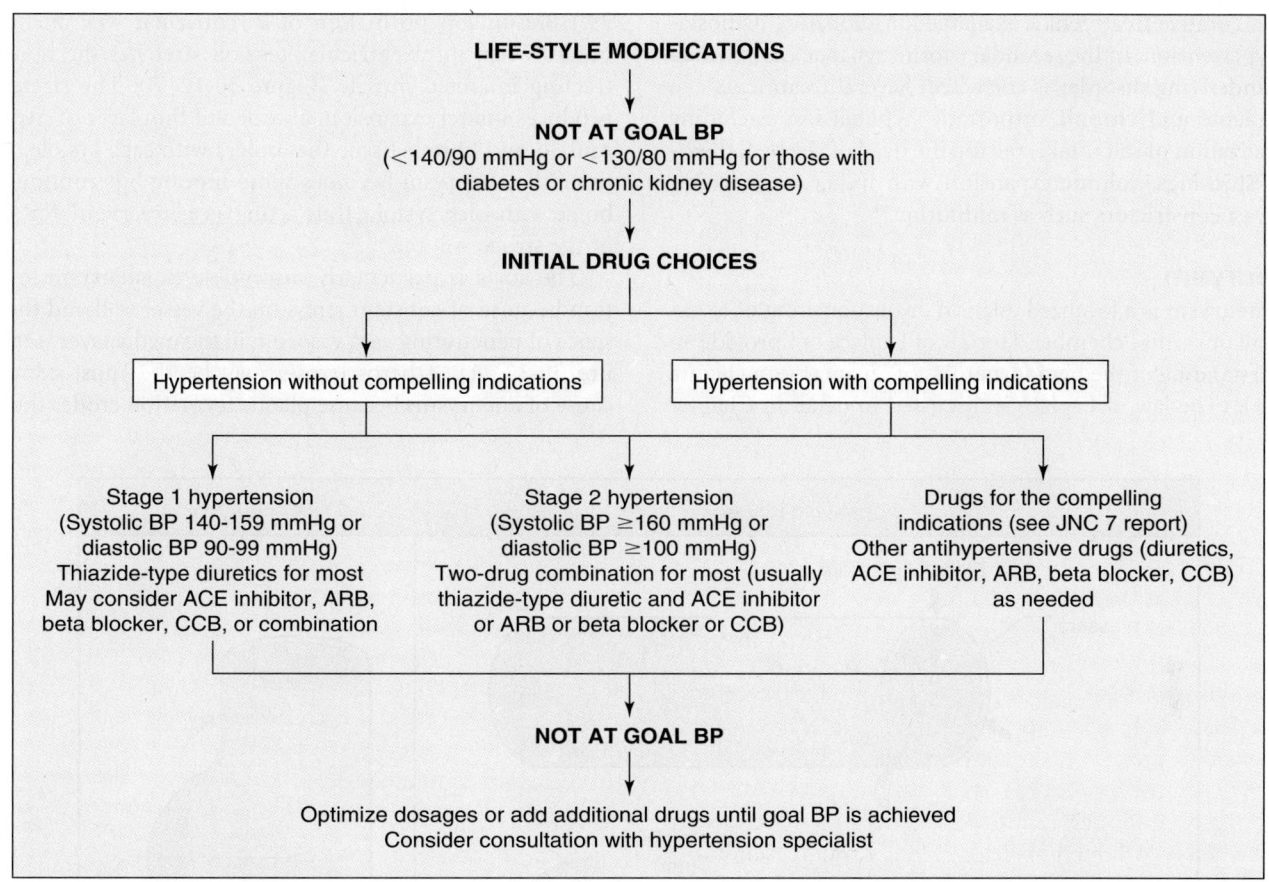

LIFE-STYLE MODIFICATIONS
↓
NOT AT GOAL BP
(<140/90 mmHg or <130/80 mmHg for those with
diabetes or chronic kidney disease)
↓
INITIAL DRUG CHOICES

| Hypertension without compelling indications | Hypertension with compelling indications |

Stage 1 hypertension
(Systolic BP 140-159 mmHg or
diastolic BP 90-99 mmHg)
Thiazide-type diuretics for most
May consider ACE inhibitor, ARB,
beta blocker, CCB, or combination

Stage 2 hypertension
(Systolic BP ≥160 mmHg or
diastolic BP ≥100 mmHg)
Two-drug combination for most (usually
thiazide-type diuretic and ACE inhibitor
or ARB or beta blocker or CCB)

Drugs for the compelling
indications (see JNC 7 report)
Other antihypertensive drugs (diuretics,
ACE inhibitor, ARB, beta blocker, CCB)
as needed

NOT AT GOAL BP
↓
Optimize dosages or add additional drugs until goal BP is achieved
Consider consultation with hypertension specialist

Figure 30-10 **Summary of treatment for hypertension.** *BP,* Blood pressure; *ACE,* angiotensin-converting enzyme; *ARB,* angiotensin-receptor blocker; *CCB,* calcium channel blocker. (Data from Chobanian AV et al: The seventh report of the Joint National National Committee on prevention, detection, evaluation, and treatment of high blood pressure, *JAMA* 289:2560-2572, 2003.)

increase in heart rate and constriction of the systemic arterioles. Thus despite a marked decrease in cardiac output, arterial blood pressure is maintained. These compensatory mechanisms are not effective in maintaining a stable blood pressure in individuals with orthostatic hypotension.

Orthostatic hypotension often is accompanied by dizziness, blurring or loss of vision, and syncope or fainting. Fainting is caused by insufficient vasomotor compensation and reduction of blood flow through the brain. The normal or compensatory vasoconstrictor response to standing is thus replaced by a marked vasodilation and blood pooling in the muscle vasculature, as well as in the splanchnic and renal beds.

Orthostatic hypotension may be acute and temporary or chronic. **Acute orthostatic hypotension,** or temporary type, is caused when the normal regulatory mechanisms are sluggish. This delay may be the result of (1) anatomic variation, (2) altered body chemistry, (3) drug action (e.g., antihypertensives or antidepressants), (4) prolonged immobility caused by illness, (5) starvation, (6) physical exhaustion, (7) any condition that produces volume depletion (e.g., massive diuresis, potassium or sodium depletion), and (8) venous pooling (e.g., pregnancy, extensive varicosities of the lower extremities). Elderly persons are susceptible to this type of orthostatic hypotension, in which postural reflexes apparently are slowed as part of the aging process. This is not a universal finding in the elderly population, however.

The two forms of **chronic orthostatic hypotension** are (1) secondary to a specific disease and (2) idiopathic or primary. The diseases that cause secondary orthostatic hypotension are endocrine disorders (e.g., adrenal insufficiency, diabetes mellitus), metabolic disorders (e.g., porphyria), or diseases of the central or peripheral nervous system (e.g., intracranial tumors, cerebral infarcts, Wernicke encephalopathy, peripheral neuropathies). Cardiovascular autonomic neuropathy is a common cause of orthostatic hypotension in diabetes and is a serious and often overlooked complication.

Idiopathic, or primary, orthostatic hypotension is the term for hypotension in which there is no known initial cause. It affects men more often than women and usually occurs between the ages of 40 and 70 years. Up to 30% to 49% of the elderly population may be affected by orthostatic hypotension. It is a significant risk factor for falls and associated injuries and has been associated with an increased risk for cardiovascular events.[89,90] In addition to cardiovascular symptoms, impotence and bowel and bladder dysfunction often are found in this type. Orthostatic hypotension is also a feature of multiple system atrophy (MSA), in which there are multiple central nervous system degenerative changes.

No curative treatment is available for idiopathic orthostatic hypertension. In the secondary form, syncope ceases when the underlying disorder is corrected. Several treatments can help acute and chronic orthostatic hypotension, including liberalization of salt intake, raising the head of the bed, thigh-high stockings, volume expansion with mineralocorticoids, and vasoconstrictors such as midodrine.[91]

Aneurysm

An **aneurysm** is a localized dilation or outpouching of a vessel wall or cardiac chamber. The law of Laplace can provide an understanding of the hemodynamics of an aneurysm (Figure 30-11). (The law of Laplace is discussed in detail in Chapter 29.) Presumably, formation of a ventricular wall aneurysm occurs when intraventricular tension stretches the noncontracting infarcted muscle (Figure 30-12, *B*). The stretching produces infarct expansion, a weak and thin layer of necrotic muscle, and fibrous tissue that bulges with each systole. With time, the aneurysm becomes more fibrotic but continues to bulge with each systole, thus acting as a "reservoir" for some of the stroke volume.

The aorta is particularly susceptible to aneurysm formation because of constant stress on the vessel wall and the absence of penetrating vasa vasorum in the media layer (see Figure 30-12, *A*). Atherosclerosis may be the most common cause of aneurysms because plaque formation erodes the ves-

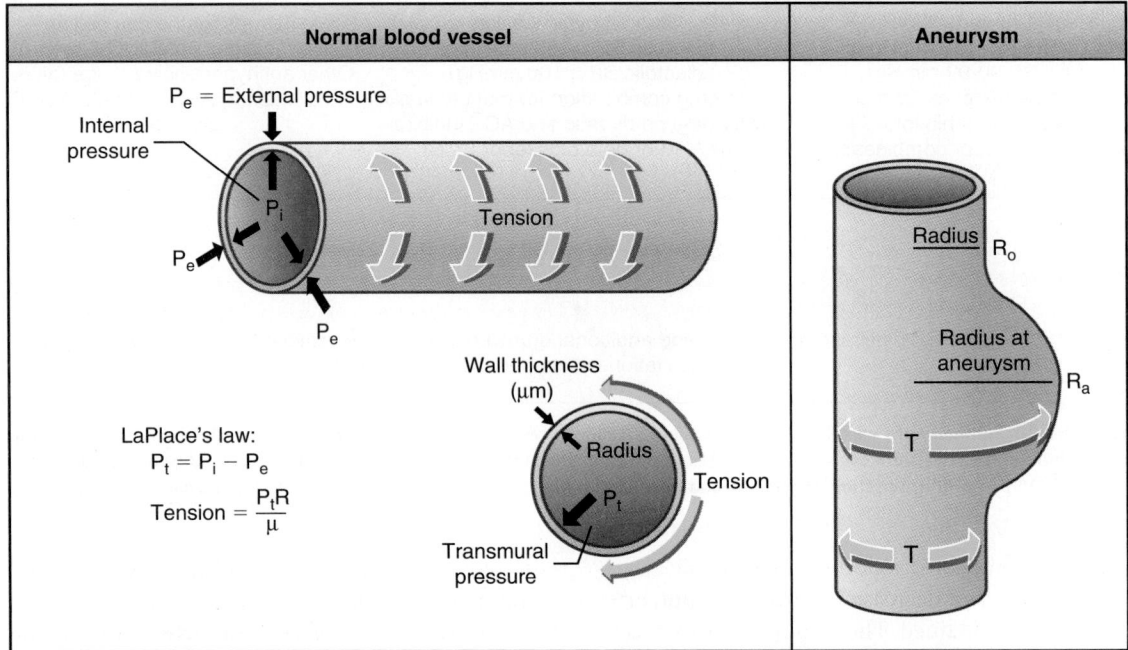

Figure 30-11 Pressure-tension and wall thickness relations in blood vessels or cardiac chambers (Laplace's law).

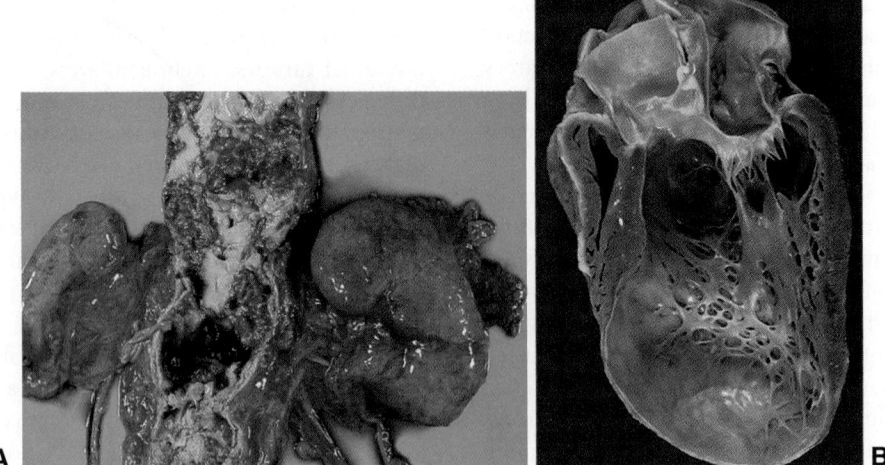

Figure 30-12 Aneurysms. **A,** Abdominal aortic atherosclerotic aneurysm. **B,** In a long-axis view of the left ventricle there is a large, thin-walled apical aneurysm that does not contain thrombus. (From Damjanov I, Linder J, editors: *Anderson's pathology,* ed 10, St Louis, 1996, Mosby.)

sel wall. Arteriosclerosis and hypertension are found in more than half of all individuals with aneurysms. Syphilis and other infections also can cause aortic aneurysms. A review of the literature suggests that for those aortic aneurysms not clearly related to atherosclerosis, contributing factors may include (1) the presence of a genetic marker, (2) deficiencies in wall collagen or collagen-elastin connections, (3) elastin failure from excessive protease activity or the production of nonfunctional elastin with aging, or (4) an increased turnover of aortic collagen. Inflammation, with the production of toxic oxygen radicals, activates matrix degrading proteins and smooth muscle cell apoptosis resulting in loss of medial elastic lamellae and thinning of the tunica media. Mechanical and shear forces, especially like those found in chronic hypertension, contribute to vessel wall remodeling. Aneurysm growth is supported by endothelial injury and development of atherosclerotic changes in the vessel wall.[92] Another important cause of aortic aneurysms of the thoracic aorta is Marfan syndrome. This inherited collagen-vascular disease carries a high mortality rate because of rupture of the ascending thoracic aorta unless surgical repair with graft placement is done.[93,94]

True aneurysms involve all three layers of the arterial wall and are best described as a weakening of the vessel wall. Most are fusiform and circumferential (Figure 30-13). **False aneurysm** is an extravascular hematoma that communicates with the intravascular space. A common cause of this type of lesion is a leak between a vascular graft and a natural artery. **Saccular aneurysms** are basically spherical in shape. Dissection of the layers of the arterial wall occurs when blood enters the wall of the artery, creating an opening in the vessel wall itself.

Clinical manifestations of aneurysm include a variety of symptoms. Aortic aneurysms often are asymptomatic until they rupture, when they become painful. Symptoms of dysphagia (difficulty in swallowing) and dyspnea (breathlessness) are caused by the pressure of a thoracic aneurysm on surrounding organs. An abdominal aneurysm can impair flow to an extremity and cause symptoms of ischemia. Cerebral aneurysms, which often occur in the circle of Willis, are associated with signs and symptoms of increased intracranial pressure. Signs and symptoms of stroke occur when cerebral aneurysms leak. (Cerebral aneurysms are described in Chapter 17.)

The diagnosis of an aneurysm is usually confirmed by ultrasonography, computed tomography, magnetic resonance imaging, or angiography. The goals of medical treatment of aneurysms are to maintain a low blood volume and low blood pressure to decrease mechanical forces thought to contribute to vessel wall dilation. Medical treatment is indicated for slow-growing aortic aneurysms, particularly in early stages, and includes smoking cessation, reducing blood pressure and blood volume, and beta-adrenergic blockage. For those

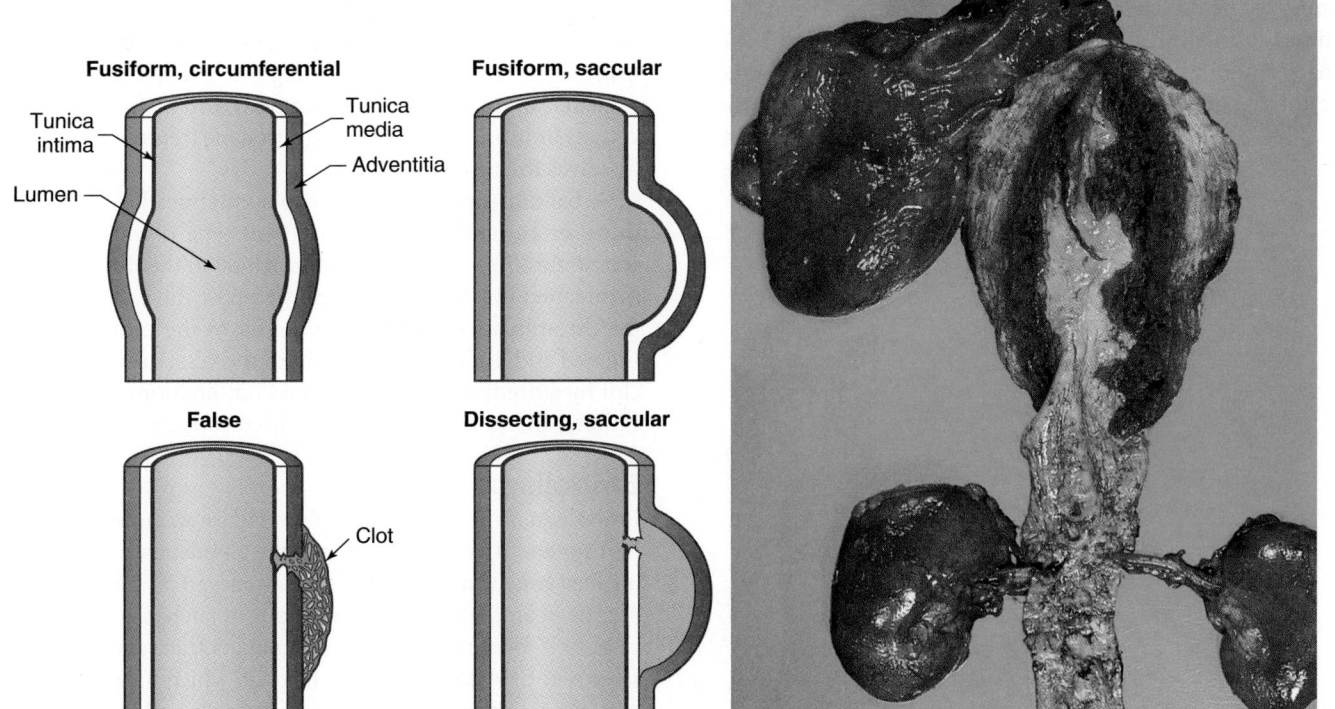

Figure 30-13 Longitudinal sections showing types of aneurysms. **A,** The fusiform circumferential and fusiform saccular aneurysms are true aneurysms, caused by weakening of the vessel wall. False and saccular aneurysms involve a break in the vessel wall, usually caused by trauma. **B,** Dissecting aneurysm of thoracic aorta. (**B** from Damjanov I, Linder J, editors: *Anderson's pathology,* ed 10, St Louis, 1996, Mosby.)

aneurysms that are dilating rapidly, surgical treatment often is indicated. Surgery should be done when aortic aneurysms reach 5 cm in diameter and usually includes replacement with a prosthetic graft. New endovascular surgical techniques make aneurysm repair possible for more individuals.[95,96]

Dissection of an aneurysm is a devastating complication (Figure 30-13, *B*). Persistent chronic hypertension and inflammation contribute to further degradation of the vessel wall with fibrotic obstruction of vessels that feed the arterial wall. Tissue ischemia and smooth muscle cell necrosis lead to intimal disruption, most often at the edges of atherosclerotic plaques.[94] Other individuals suffer aneurysmal dissection resulting from underlying conditions such as Marfan or Ehlers-Danlos syndromes. Iatrogenic aortic dissection can occur with invasive retrograde catheter interventions or after valve or aortic surgery. Emergent evaluation and surgical intervention are indicated.[97,98]

Thrombus Formation

A **thrombus** is a blood clot that remains attached to a vessel wall (see Figure 30-14). A detached thrombus is called a **thromboembolus.** Thrombi tend to develop wherever intravascular conditions promote activation of the coagulation, or clotting, cascade. These conditions include intimal irritation and roughening, inflammation, traumatic injury, infection, and low blood pressures or obstructions that cause blood stasis and pooling within the vessels. (Mechanisms of coagulation are described in Chapter 25.) In the arteries, activation of the coagulation cascade usually is caused by roughening of the tunica intima by atherosclerosis. Invasion of the tunica intima by an infectious agent also roughens the normally smooth lining of the artery, causing platelets to adhere readily. Anatomic changes of an artery can stimulate throm-

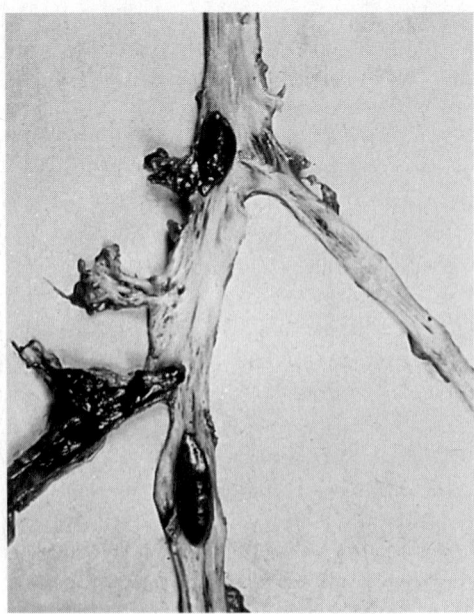

Figure 30-14 Multiple venous thrombi. (From Rosai J: *Ackerman's surgical pathology*, ed 8, vol 2, St Louis, 1996, Mosby.)

bus formation, particularly if the change results in pooling of arterial blood. This can occur, for example, in blood that is pooled within an aneurysm. In the veins, thrombus formation is associated more often with inflammation (phlebitis), a condition termed **thrombophlebitis.** Thrombi form also on heart valves altered by calcification or bacterial vegetation. Valvular thrombi are associated most commonly with inflammation of the endocardium (endocarditis) and rheumatic heart disease.

Shock (circulatory failure), particularly shock resulting from septicemia, can activate the intrinsic and extrinsic pathways of coagulation. The impaired cellular metabolism that occurs with all types of shock activates the extrinsic pathway of coagulation, whereas blood stasis caused by very low blood pressures activates the intrinsic pathway (see Chapter 25). Thrombus formation may be confined to one area or may progress to diffuse coagulopathy, such as disseminated intravascular coagulation (see Chapter 27).

Arterial thrombi pose two potential threats to the circulation. First, the thrombus may grow large enough to occlude the artery, causing ischemia in tissue supplied by the artery. Second, the thrombus may dislodge, becoming a thromboembolus that travels through the vascular system until it occludes flow into a distal systemic vascular bed. Venous thrombi can make it more difficult for blood to drain from distant venous beds (especially the legs), resulting in edema. Venous thrombi also can embolize and travel to the pulmonic vascular bed (see Chapter 33).

Pharmacologic treatment includes the administration of heparin and warfarin derivatives. These derivatives interfere with the clotting cascade by accelerating the activity of antithrombin III, thereby slowing or stopping thrombus growth. Pharmacologic treatment may also include the intravenous or intraarterial administration of streptokinase, which dissolves the thrombus.

A balloon-tipped catheter can sometimes be used to remove or compress a thrombus. This type of catheter is inserted into the vessel at a point proximal to the thrombus and is threaded into the vessel until the tip of the catheter is past the thrombus. The balloon on the tip of the catheter is then inflated and drawn backward out of the vessel, pulling out the clot by a dredging action. Various combinations of drug and catheter therapies are sometimes used concurrently.

Embolism

Embolism is the obstruction of a vessel by an **embolus**—a bolus of matter that is circulating in the bloodstream. The embolus may consist of a dislodged thrombus; an air bubble; an aggregate of amniotic fluid; an aggregate of fat, bacteria, or cancer cells; or a foreign substance. An embolus travels in the bloodstream until it reaches a vessel through which it cannot fit. No matter how tiny it is, an embolus eventually will lodge in a systemic or pulmonary vessel. The source of the embolus determines whether the embolus will lodge in a vessel of the pulmonary or systemic circulation. Pulmonary emboli originate on the venous side (mostly from the deep veins of the legs) of the systemic circulation or in the right heart; systemic (or arterial) emboli most commonly originate in the left heart and are associated with thrombi after myocardial infarction, valvular disease, left heart failure, endocarditis, and dysrhythmias.

Embolism causes ischemia or infarction in tissues distal to the obstruction. A limb that is ischemic because of arterial occlusion is characterized (1) by an almost waxy whiteness of the skin because the vasculature is devoid of erythrocytes, and (2) by numbness and pain resulting from neural ischemia.

Embolism of a central organ causes organic dysfunction and pain. For example, pulmonary artery embolism causes chest pain and dyspnea; renal artery embolism causes abdominal pain and oliguria; and mesenteric artery embolism causes abdominal pain and a paralytic, ischemic bowel. Infarction and subsequent necrosis of a central organ are life threatening, not only because of organ dysfunction but also because of sepsis. Necrotic tissue is a rich medium for the growth of bacteria from the lungs; bowel; and, occasionally, bladder. Necrosis of the bladder, in particular, can quickly lead to peritonitis or septicemia.

Embolism of a coronary or cerebral artery is an immediate threat to life if the embolus severely obstructs a major vessel. Occlusion of a coronary artery will cause a myocardial infarction (see p. 1110), whereas occlusion of a cerebral artery causes a stroke (see Chapter 17).

Thromboembolism

Thromboembolism is a vascular obstruction resulting from a dislodged thrombus. The most common source of arterial thromboemboli to the systemic circulation is the heart. Mitral or aortic valvular disease, especially that associated with abnormal heart rhythms (atrial fibrillation and flutter), causes thrombus formation on roughened vascular surfaces and in atrial blood as a result of stasis. More than half of these thromboemboli lodge in the lower extremities (in the femoral and popliteal arteries). Others lodge in the coronary arteries and the cerebral vasculature.

Heart failure is associated with an increased risk of thrombotic complications, although the mechanism for this increased risk is unclear. There is evidence that abnormalities of prothrombotic markers are associated with ischemic heart disease, independent of the presence of systolic or diastolic dysfunction.

Air Embolism

Room air that enters the circulation through intravenous lines is probably the most common cause of air embolism. Room air is about 70% nitrogen. Although nitrogen dissolves quickly in blood, large amounts of air cannot be dissolved rapidly enough to prevent the displacement of blood in the arterioles and capillary beds. Ischemia and necrosis occur when air totally blocks a vessel.

Air also can be introduced into the bloodstream if trauma to the chest causes air from the lungs to enter the vascular space. For example, gunshot wounds and puncture wounds of the thorax sometimes introduce air emboli. Treatment for air

embolism is supportive, including bed rest and supplemental oxygen, once the connection between the source of air and the vascular system is eliminated.

Amniotic Fluid Embolism

The great intraabdominal pressures generated during labor and delivery may force amniotic fluid into the bloodstream of the mother through the highly vascular uterine wall. Amniotic fluid not only displaces blood, reducing oxygen, nutrient, and waste exchange, but also introduces antigens, cells, and protein aggregates that trigger inflammation, coagulation, and the immune response within the bloodstream. Capillary beds usually are affected by amniotic fluid emboli, especially the capillary beds of the lungs and kidneys. Treatment is supportive and may include dialysis, particularly after a cesarean delivery or hysterectomy.

Bacterial Embolism

Isolated bacteria in the bloodstream do not cause embolism, but aggregates of bacteria may be large enough to do so. The most common cause of bacterial embolism is subacute bacterial endocarditis, during which clumps of vegetation are dislodged from infected cardiac valves and ejected into the pulmonary or systemic circulation. A less common cause is erosion of an artery or vein by bacteria at a source of infection, such as an abscess. Treatment for bacterial embolism includes bed rest, supplemental oxygen, and antibiotics to eradicate the source of infection.

Fat Embolism

Trauma to the long bones is associated with fat embolism, particularly in the lungs. Two mechanisms have been proposed to account for the generation of fat emboli after skeletal trauma. The first is that trauma to the bones initiates defective fat metabolism, causing globules of fat to form in the blood. Platelets adhere to these globules until the conglomerate is large enough to lodge in a capillary bed. The second possible explanation is that globules of fat are released from fatty bone marrow exposed by fracture. Again, platelets adhere to the fat globules and embolism occurs.

Treatment for fat embolism consists of prompt immobilization of fractures and supportive measures that include administration of supplemental oxygen, steroids, and glucose. Steroid administration may decrease the inflammation that occurs with vascular occlusion. Inflammation in the pulmonary bed is especially dangerous because it can cause the acute respiratory distress syndrome (ARDS) (see Chapter 33). Intravenous administration of glucose is thought to prevent inappropriate fat metabolism.

Foreign Matter

Foreign matter can enter the bloodstream during trauma or through an intravenous or intraarterial line. If the bolus of foreign matter is relatively large, it usually is removed surgically. Small particles, such as drug precipitates, small glass shards, or fibers from linen, are sometimes introduced unintentionally into a vessel through intravenous injections or manipulation of monitoring lines. Once in the blood, these small particles initiate the coagulation cascade. The thromboemboli that form around the particles are large enough to occlude a vessel and result in ischemia. Treatment is aimed at preventing thrombus formation around the particle, dissolution of the particle, and supportive measures to alleviate ischemia.

Peripheral Arterial Disease

Peripheral artery disease (PAD) refers to atherosclerotic disease of arteries that perfuse the limbs, especially the lower extremities. It is estimated that 12 million people in the United States have significant PAD. The risk factors for PAD are the same as those previously described for atherosclerotic disease, and it is especially prevalent in individuals with diabetes.[99]

Lower extremity ischemia resulting from arterial obstruction in PAD can be gradual or acute. In most individuals, gradually increasing obstruction to arterial blood flow to the legs caused by atherosclerosis in the iliofemoral vessels results in pain with ambulation called **intermittent claudication.** If a thrombus forms over the atherosclerotic lesion, perfusion can cease acutely with severe pain, loss of pulses, and skin color changes in the affected extremity.

PAD is often asymptomatic, therefore evaluation for PAD requires a careful history and physical examination that focuses on looking for evidence of atherosclerotic disease (e.g., bruits) and noninvasive doppler measurement of blood flow. Treatment includes risk factor reduction (smoking cessation and treatment of diabetes, hypertension, and dyslipidemia) and antiplatelet therapy.[100] Symptomatic PAD should be managed with vasodilators in combination with antiplatelet or antithrombotic medications (aspirin, cilostazol, ticlopidine, or clopidogrel) and exercise rehabilitation.[101,102] If acute or refractory symptoms occur, emergent percutaneous or surgical revascularization may be indicated.[103]

Thromboangiitis Obliterans (Buerger Disease)

Thromboangiitis obliterans (Buerger disease), which tends to occur in young men who are heavy cigarette smokers, is an inflammatory disease of the peripheral arteries. The inflammatory lesions are accompanied by thrombi and sometimes by vasospasm of arterial segments. Inflammation, thrombus formation, and vasospasm eventually can occlude and obliterate (render physiologically useless) portions of small and medium-size arteries in the feet and sometimes in the hands.[104] Typically affected are the digital, tibial, and plantar arteries of the feet and the digital, palmar, and ulnar arteries of the hands. The disease sometimes is associated with inflammation of adjacent veins and nerves. The pathogenesis of thromboangiitis obliterans is not known, although there is evidence of significant T cell activation and autoimmunity.[105] The incidence of Buerger disease has been steadily declining, presumably because of a decrease in cigarette smoking in men.

The chief symptoms of thromboangiitis obliterans are pain and tenderness of the affected part. Clinical manifestations are caused by sluggish blood flow and include rubor (redness of the skin), which is caused by dilated capillaries under the skin, and cyanosis, which is caused by blood that remains in the capillaries after its oxygen has diffused into the interstitium. Chronic ischemia causes the skin to thin and become shiny and the nails to become thickened and malformed. In advanced disease, ischemia resulting from vessel obliteration can cause gangrene. Buerger disease has been associated with cerebrovascular disease and rheumatic symptoms (joint pain).

The most important part of treatment is cessation of cigarette smoking.[106] All other measures are aimed at improving circulation to the foot or hand. Vasodilators are prescribed to alleviate vasospasm, and exercises are taught that use gravity to improve blood flow. If vasospasm persists, sympathectomy may be performed. Gangrene necessitates amputation.

Raynaud Phenomenon and Disease

Raynaud phenomenon and **Raynaud disease** are both characterized by attacks of vasospasm in the small arteries and arterioles of the fingers and, less commonly, the toes. Although the clinical manifestations of the phenomenon and the disease are the same, their causes differ. Raynaud phenomenon is secondary to systemic diseases, particularly collagen vascular disease (scleroderma), pulmonary hypertension, thoracic outlet syndrome, myxedema trauma, serum sickness, or long-term exposure to environmental conditions, such as cold or vibrating machinery in the workplace. (The effects of segmental vibration are described in Chapter 2.) There is some evidence that Raynaud phenomenon may be the presenting feature of an underlying malignancy. In these cases the vascular disease is characterized by sudden onset and rapid progression of severe digital ischemia. Raynaud disease, however, is a primary vasospastic disorder of unknown origin. Raynaud disease tends to affect young women and to consist of vasospastic attacks triggered by brief exposure to cold or by emotional stress. Blood vessels in these individuals demonstrate endothelial dysfunction with decreased nitric oxide production and increased endothelin-1 activity.[107] Genetic predisposition may play a role in its development.

The clinical manifestations of the vasospastic attacks of either disorder are changes in skin color and sensation caused by ischemia. Vasospasm occurs with varying frequency and severity and causes pallor, numbness, and the sensation of cold in the digits.[108] Attacks tend to be bilateral, and manifestations usually begin at the tips of the digits and progress to the proximal phalanges. Sluggish blood flow resulting in ischemia may cause the skin to appear cyanotic. Rubor follows as vasospasm ends and the capillaries become engorged with oxygenated blood. Rubor often is accompanied by throbbing and paresthesias. Skin color returns to normal after the attack, but frequent, prolonged attacks interfere with cellular metabolism, causing the skin of the fingertips to thicken and the nails to become brittle. In severe, chronic Raynaud phenomenon or disease, ischemia eventually can cause ulceration and gangrene. This outcome is rare, however.

Treatment for Raynaud phenomenon consists of removing the stimulus or treating the primary disease process. When Raynaud phenomenon is associated with malignancy, surgical removal of the tumor may resolve the ischemia. For Raynaud phenomenon not associated with malignancy, treatment is limited to amelioration of symptoms with medications such as nifedipine. Attacks of vasospasm sometimes can be alleviated at their onset by an exercise in which the arms are swung forward and backward. This maneuver increases hydrostatic pressure (and perfusion pressure) in the arteries by means of centrifugal force.

Treatment of Raynaud disease is limited to prevention or alleviation of vasospasm itself, because no underlying disorder has been identified Stimuli that trigger attacks (e.g., emotional stress, cold) are avoided, and cigarette smoking is stopped to eliminate the vasoconstricting effects of nicotine. Exercises that build centrifugal force in the extremities also are helpful in the early stages of vasospasm. If attacks of vasospasm become frequent or prolonged, vasodilators such as dibenzylchlorethamine, reserpine, or calcium channel blockers may be helpful. Angiotensin II receptor blockers also have been found to relieve the vasospasm. New treatments being explored include nitric oxide donors and endothelin-1 receptor antagonists.[109] Sympathectomy, which is not always effective, is the next line of treatment. If ischemia leads to ulceration and gangrene, amputation is necessary.

Diseases of the Veins

Varicose Veins and Chronic Venous Insufficiency

A **varicose vein** is a vein in which blood has pooled. Varicose veins typically involve the saphenous veins of the legs and are distended, tortuous, and palpable. Varicose veins are caused by (1) trauma to the saphenous veins that damages one or more valves; or (2) gradual venous distention caused by a combination of standing for long periods, which diminishes the action of the muscle pump, and the action of gravity on blood within the legs.

Veins are thin-walled, highly distensible vessels. Normally, valves prevent backflow and pooling of blood. If a valve is damaged, permitting backflow, a section of the vein is subjected to the pressure exerted by a larger volume of blood under the influence of gravity. The vein swells as it becomes engorged and surrounding tissue becomes edematous because increased hydrostatic pressure pushes plasma through the stretched vessel wall.

In individuals who habitually stand for long periods, wear constricting garments, or cross the legs at the knees, distention progresses until the pressure in the vein damages venous valves, rendering the valves incompetent. Damaged valves cannot maintain normal venous pressure, which causes hydrostatic pressure in the vein to increase. As the vein distends further, it becomes tortuous, and edema develops in the extremity.

Varicose veins and valvular incompetence can progress to **chronic venous insufficiency (CVI).** CVI is inadequate venous return over a long period. It causes pathologic changes as a result of ischemia in the vasculature, skin, and supporting tissues. CVI is marked by chronic pooling of blood in the veins of the lower extremities and leads to hyperpigmentation of the skin over the feet and ankles. Edema of the feet and ankles becomes marked and may progress proximally to the knees.

Circulation to the extremities becomes so sluggish that the metabolic demands of the cells for oxygen, nutrients, and waste removal are barely met. Any trauma or pressure can therefore lower the oxygen supply to injurious levels by further reducing blood flow into the area. Cell death occurs, and necrotic tissue develops into **venous stasis ulcers.** Persistent ulceration develops because the high metabolic demands of healing tissue—particularly an increased need for oxygen—cannot be met by the existing circulation. Venous stasis ulcers are susceptible to infection because poor circulation impairs the delivery of the cells and biochemicals of the immune and inflammatory responses. (The role of inflammation in processes of healing is described in Chapter 6.) Varicose veins and CVI may be associated with deep venous thrombosis in up to 15% of affected individuals.[110]

Treatment of varicose veins and CVI begins conservatively. The individual wears antiembolism stockings and avoids standing and other factors, such as constrictive clothing, that contribute to venous stasis. If conservative treatment is ineffective, saphenous vein stripping is performed.[98]

Thrombus Formation in Veins

Deep venous thrombosis (DVT) is a common condition that can occur in individuals in both outpatient and hospital settings. In those hospitalized for a general medical condition, it is estimated that up to 26% will develop DVT, although the risk is far higher in other conditions such as stroke, shock, myocardial infarction, congestive heart failure, and malignancy.[111,112] Orthopedic (trauma or surgery), spinal cord injury, and obstetric/gynecologic conditions can be associated with up to a 100% likelihood of DVT. In individuals not in the hospital, risks include inherited coagulation disorders (e.g., factor V Leiden mutation and deficiencies of protein C, protein S, and antithrombin) and prolonged limb dependency (e.g., plane travel).[111]

Deep venous thrombosis occurs primarily in the lower extremity. Three factors promote venous thrombosis: (1) venous stasis (e.g., immobility, age, congestive heart failure), (2) venous endothelial damage (e.g., trauma, medications), and (3) hypercoagulable states (e.g., inherited disorders, malignancy, pregnancy, oral contraceptives, hormone replacement). Accumulation of clotting factors and platelets leads to thrombus formation in the vein, often near a venous valve. Inflammation around the thrombus promotes further platelet aggregation and the thrombus propagates or grows proximally. This inflammation may cause local symptoms but because the vein is deep in the leg, it is usually not accompanied by clinical symptoms or signs. If the thrombus creates significant obstruction to venous blood flow, increased pressure in the vein behind the clot may lead to edema of the extremity. Most thrombi will eventually dissolve without treatment, but untreated DVT is associated with a high risk of embolization of a part of the clot (pulmonary embolism) and may lead to persistent venous outflow obstruction and post-thrombotic syndrome.

Post-thrombotic syndrome (PTS) is a frequent complication of deep venous thrombosis (DVT) and is characterized by chronic, persistent pain, swelling, and ulceration of the affected limb.[116] The most serious complication of DVT is pulmonary embolism (PE) (see Chapter 33).

Because DVT is usually asymptomatic and difficult to detect clinically, prevention in at-risk individuals is crucial. If possible, individuals should be mobilized as soon as possible after illness, injury, or surgery. Prophylactic treatment can include heparin, warfarin, or pneumatic devices. In individuals at high risk for pulmonary embolism but for whom anticoagulation is contraindicated, placement of an inferior vena caval filter may be necessary to prevent pulmonary embolism.[113]

Diagnosis is most often made by combining measurement of serum D-dimer concentration with lower extremity ultrasonography.[114] If noninvasive testing is nondiagnostic, a venogram may be indicated. DVT is treated with low-molecular-weight heparin, unfractionated intravenous heparin, or adjusted-dose subcutaneous heparin. Fibrinolytic therapy may be used in selected individuals to dissolve the clot more quickly but is associated with a greater risk for bleeding than heparin.[115]

Superior Vena Cava Syndrome

Superior vena cava syndrome (SVCS) is a progressive occlusion of the superior vena cava (SVC) that leads to venous distention in the upper extremities and head. The leading cause of SVCS is bronchogenic cancer (75% of cases), followed by lymphomas (15%) and metastasis of other cancers (7%). Benign causes of SVCS include histoplasmosis, tuberculosis, mediastinal fibrosis, cystic fibrosis, and benign tumors, such as retrosternal goiter. Invasive therapies, including pacemaker wires, central venous catheters, and pulmonary artery catheters, can lead to acute and chronic SVCS in about 0.3% to 4% of individuals undergoing these therapies. The SVC is a relatively low-pressure vessel that lies in the closed thoracic compartment; therefore tissue expansion within the thoracic compartment can easily compress the SVC. The right main stem bronchus abuts the SVC so that cancers occurring in this bronchus may press on the SVC. The SVC is surrounded by lymph nodes and lymph chains that commonly become involved in thoracic cancers and compress the SVC during tumor growth. In individuals with small cell lung cancers, the presence of SVCS is a favorable prognostic sign, possibly because mediastinal metastases to lymph nodes near the SVCS occur early in the disease. When these enlarged nodes lead to SVCS, the malignancy may be detected earlier than in those individuals without SVCS. When onset of SVCS is slow, collateral venous drainage to the azygous vein usually has time to develop.

Clinical manifestations of SVCS include edema and venous distention in the upper extremities and face, including the ocular beds. Individuals may complain of a feeling of fullness in the head, or tightness of shirt collars, necklaces, and rings. Cerebral and central nervous system edema may cause headache, visual disturbance, and impaired consciousness. The skin of the face and arms is purple and taut, and capillary refill time is prolonged. Respiratory distress may be present because of edema of bronchial structures or compression of the bronchus by a carcinoma.

Diagnosis is made by chest roentgenogram, Doppler studies, computed tomography (CT), magnetic resonance imaging (MRI), and ultrasound. Treatment of SVCS may be delayed for 24 hours to determine its cause. With slow onset and the development of collateral venous drainage, SVCS is generally not a vascular emergency but, rather, an oncologic emergency. Treatment includes radiation therapy and the administration of diuretics, steroids, and anticoagulants, as necessary.[117] Treatment also may include bypass surgery using various grafts; thrombolysis, both locally and systemically; balloon angioplasty; and placement of intravascular stents.[118]

Coronary Artery Disease, Myocardial Ischemia, and Myocardial Infarction

Coronary artery disease (CAD), myocardial ischemia, and myocardial infarction form a pathophysiologic continuum that impairs the pumping ability of the heart by depriving the heart muscle of blood-borne oxygen and nutrients. The earliest lesions of the continuum are those of **coronary artery disease**—virtually any vascular disorder that narrows or occludes the coronary arteries. By far the most common cause of coronary artery obstruction is atherosclerosis (Figure 30-15). CAD can diminish the myocardial blood supply until deprivation impairs myocardial metabolism enough to cause **ischemia,** a local state in which the cells are temporarily deprived of blood supply. They remain alive but cannot function normally. Persistent ischemia or the complete occlusion of a coronary artery causes **infarction,** or death, of the deprived myocardial tissue. Infarction constitutes the often-fatal event known as the "heart attack."

Development of Coronary Artery Disease

Until very recently CAD was the single largest killer of American males and females. Each year, an estimated 700,000 persons in the United States have a new myocardial infarction, and about 500,000 will suffer a recurrent event. This means that about every 26 seconds, an American suffers a coronary event, and about every minute someone will die from one.[119] In the 1960s researchers began to identify the risk factors that contribute to the onset and escalation of CAD. The primary cause of CAD is atherosclerosis of the coronary vessels; therefore those factors that contribute to the development of atherosclerosis also are risk factors for CAD.

Risk factors for CAD can be categorized as conventional (major) versus nontraditional (novel) and modifiable versus nonmodifiable. Much new information has been obtained

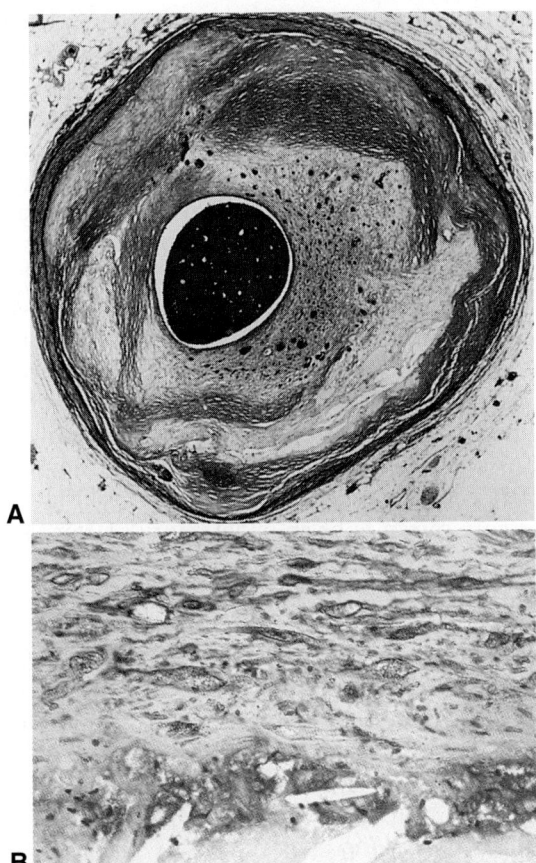

Figure 30-15 Atherosclerosis. **A,** Concentric coronary plaque. The lumen is central. Multiple new small blood vessels are shown within the plaque, the late result of disruption. **B,** Cell types in a fibrolipid plaque. The plaque cap (brownish) contains numerous elongated smooth muscle cells; some contain lipid. Macrophages are clustered on the edge of the core. (From Damjanov I, Linder J, editors: *Anderson's pathology,* ed 10, St Louis, 1996, Mosby.)

about the conventional risk factors that has markedly improved prevention and management of CAD. In addition, nontraditional risk factors have been identified in recent years that have provided insight in to the pathogenesis of CAD and may lead to future more effective interventions.

Conventional or major risk factors for CAD that are nonmodifiable include (1) advanced age, (2) male gender or women after menopause, and (3) family history (genetics; see What's New? Gene Mutation Predicts Hypertension, p. 1087). Modifiable major risks include (1) dyslipidemia, (2) hypertension, (3) cigarette smoking, (4) diabetes and insulin resistance, (5) obesity, (6) sedentary life-style, and (7) atherogenic diet.[120] In individuals with known CAD, 80% to 90% will have the risk factors of smoking, diabetes, dyslipidemia, or hypertension, and many persons will have several of these risks.[121] Fortunately, modification of these factors can dramatically reduce the risk for CAD.

Dyslipidemia

The strong link between CAD and elevated plasma lipoprotein concentrations is well documented.[122] The term **lipoprotein** refers to lipids, phospholipids, cholesterol, and triglycerides bound to carrier proteins. Lipids (cholesterol in particular) are required by most cells for the manufacture and repair of plasma membranes. Cholesterol is also a necessary component for the manufacture of such essential substances as bile acids and steroid hormones. Although cholesterol can easily be obtained from dietary fat intake, most body cells also can manufacture cholesterol.

The cycle of lipid metabolism is complex. Dietary fat is packaged into particles known as **chylomicrons** in the small intestine. Chylomicrons are required for absorption of fat; they function by transporting exogenous lipid from the intestine to the liver and peripheral cells. Chylomicrons are the least dense of the lipoproteins and primarily contain triglyceride. Some of the triglyceride may be removed and either stored by adipose tissue or used by muscle as an energy source. The chylomicron remnants, composed mainly of cholesterol, are taken up by the liver. A series of chemical reactions in the liver results in the production of several lipoproteins that vary in density and function. These include **very-low-density lipoproteins (VLDLs),** primarily triglyceride and protein; **low-density lipoproteins (LDLs),** mostly cholesterol and protein; and **high-density lipoproteins (HDLs),** mainly phospholipids and protein.

Dyslipidemia (or **dyslipoproteinemia**) refers to abnormal concentrations of serum lipoproteins as defined by the Third Report of the National Cholesterol Education Program[122] (Table 30-4). It is estimated that nearly half of the U.S. population has some form of dyslipidemia, especially among whites and Asian populations.[119] These abnormalities are the result of a combination of genetic and dietary factors. Primary or familial dyslipoproteinemias result from genetic defects that cause abnormalities in lipid-metabolizing enzymes and abnormal cellular lipid receptors (Table 30-5). Secondary causes of dyslipidemia include several common systemic disorders, such as diabetes, hypothyroidism, pancreatitis, and renal nephrosis.

An increased serum concentration of LDL is a strong indicator of coronary risk.[122] LDL is responsible for the delivery of cholesterol to the tissues. Serum levels of LDL are normally controlled by hepatic receptors for LDL that bind LDL and limit liver synthesis of this lipoprotein. High dietary intake of cholesterol and fats, often in combination with a genetic predisposition to accumulations of LDL in the serum (e.g., dysfunction of the hepatic LDL receptor), results in high levels of LDL in the bloodstream.[123] The term LDL actually describes several types of LDL molecules; the "small dense" LDL particles are the most atherogenic.[121,124] LDL oxidation, migration into the vessel wall, and phagocytosis by macrophages are key steps in the pathogenesis of atherosclerosis (see p. 1082 and Figure 30-2). LDL also plays a role in endothelial injury, inflammation, and immune responses that have been identified as being important in atherogenesis. Aggressive reduction of LDL with diet and cholesterol-lowering drugs, such as the statins and ezetimibe, is associated with a dramatic decrease in risk for CAD.[122,125-128]

Low levels of HDL cholesterol also are a strong indicator of coronary risk, and high levels of HDL may be more protective for the development of atherosclerosis than low levels of LDL.[129-133] HDL is responsible for "reverse cholesterol transport," which returns excess cholesterol from the tissues to the liver for metabolism.[130,131] HDL also participates in endothelial repair and decreases thrombosis. It can be fractionated into several particle sizes that have different effects on vascular function. Exercise, weight loss, fish oil consumption, and moderate alcohol use can result in modest increases in HDL.[134,135] Niacin, fibrates, and statins are drugs that can cause modest increases in HDL, but a new drug that is a variety of HDL (recombinant ApoA-I Milano) is currently being studied as a direct way to increase HDL activity.[128,129,133]

Other lipoproteins associated with increased cardiovascular risk include elevated serum VLDL (triglycerides) and increased lipoprotein (a) (Lp[a]). Triglycerides are associated with an increased risk for CAD, especially in combination with other risk factors such as diabetes. **Lipoprotein (a) (Lp[a])** is a genetically determined molecular complex between LDL and a serum glycoprotein called *apolipoprotein A* that has been shown to be an important risk factor for atherosclerosis, especially in women.[121,136]

Hypertension

Hypertension is responsible for a twofold to threefold increased risk of atherosclerotic cardiovascular disease.[120] A reduction in systolic blood pressure of only 12 to 13 mmHg can reduce the risk of CAD by as much as 21%. It contributes to endothelial injury, a key step in atherogenesis (see p. 1081), and causes myocardial hypertrophy, which increases myocardial demand for coronary flow.

Cigarette Smoking

Studies indicate that 20% of the annual mortality from CAD is traceable to cigarette smoking.[119] Passive (environmental) smoking also increases the risk of CAD. The mechanism by which smoking increases atherosclerosis is uncertain. Nicotine stimulates the release of catecholamines (epinephrine and norepinephrine), which increase heart rate and peripheral vascular constriction. As a result, blood pressure increases, as do cardiac workload and oxygen demand. Elevated catecholamines also stimulate release of free fatty acids. Cigarette smoking is associated with an increase in LDL, a decrease in HDL, and induction of a prothrombotic state, as well as increases in inflammatory markers of CAD such as C-reactive protein and fibrinogen[137] (see p. 1084). Further, the carbon monoxide in cigarette smoke reduces the oxygen content of arterial blood. Hypoxemia (insufficient oxygen in arterial blood) may promote atherosclerosis by decreasing the availability of oxygen to the vessel walls and increasing vessel wall permeability. The cadmium in cigarette smoke may be related to elevations in blood pressure. The risk of CAD increases with heavy smoking and decreases when smoking is

Table 30-4	Criteria for Dyslipidemia						
	Optimal	Near Optimal	Desirable	Low	Borderline	High	Very High
Total cholesterol			<200		200-239	≥240	
LDL	<100	100-129			130-159	160-189	≥190
Triglycerides			<150		150-199	200-499	≥500
HDL				<40		≥60	

Data from Expert Panel on Detection, Evaluation, and Treatment of High Blood Cholesterol in Adults, *JAMA* 285:2486-2497, 2001.

Table 30-5	Familial Dyslipoproteinemias		
Name	**Laboratory Findings[a]**	**Clinical Features**	**Therapy**
Type I: exogenous hyperlipidemia; fat-induced hypertriglyceridemia	Cholesterol normal Triglycerides increased 3 times Chylomicrons increased	Abdominal pain Hepatosplenomegaly Skin and retinal lipid deposits Usual onset: childhood	Low-fat diet
Type IIa: hypercholesterolemia	Triglycerides normal LDL increased Cholesterol increased	Premature vascular disease Xanthomas of tendons and bony prominences Common Onset: all ages	Low–saturated fat and low-cholesterol diet Cholestyramine[b] Colestipol[c] Lovastatin[d] Nicotinic acid[e] Neomycin[f] Intestinal bypass
Type IIb: combined hyperlipidemia; carbohydrate-induced hypertriglyceridemia	LDL, VLDL increased Cholesterol increased Triglycerides increased	Same as IIa	Same as IIa; *plus* carbohydrate restriction Clofibrate[g] Gemfibrozil[h] Lovastatin
Type III: dysbetalipoproteinemia	IDL or chylomicron remnants increased Cholesterol increased Triglycerides increased	Premature vascular disease Xanthomas of tendons and bony prominences Uncommon Onset: adulthood	Weight control Low-carbohydrate, low–saturated fat, and low-cholesterol diet Alcohol restriction Clofibrate Gemfibrozil Lovastatin Nicotinic acid Estrogens[i] Intestinal bypass
Type IV: endogenous hyperlipidemia; carbohydrate-induced hypertriglyceridemia	Glucose intolerance Hyperuricemia Cholesterol normal or increased VLDL increased Triglycerides increased	Premature vascular disease Skin lipid deposits Obesity Hepatomegaly Common onset: adulthood	Weight control Low-carbohydrate diet Alcohol restriction Clofibrate Nicotinic acid Intestinal bypass
Type V: mixed hyperlipidemia; carbohydrate and fat-induced hypertriglyceridemia	Glucose intolerance Hyperuricemia Chylomicrons increased VLDL increased LDL increased Cholesterol increased Triglycerides increased 3 times	Abdominal pain Hepatosplenomegaly Skin lipid deposits Retinal lipid deposits Onset: childhood	Weight control Low-carbohydrate and low-fat diet Clofibrate Lovastatin Nicotinic acid Progesterone[j] Intestinal bypass

[a]*LDL*, Low-density lipoprotein; *VLDL*, very-low-density lipoprotein; *IDL*, intermediate-density lipoprotein.
[b]*Cholestyramine* (Questran), anion exchange resin; binds bile acids; enhances cholesterol excretion.
[c]*Colestipol* (Colestid), same as cholestyramine.
[d]*Lovastatin*, 3-hydroxy-3-methylglutaryl-coenzyme A (HMG-CoA) reductase inhibitor; decreases cholesterol synthesis in the liver.
[e]*Nicotinic acid* (niacin), decreases release of free fatty acids from adipose tissue; increases lipogenesis in liver; decreases glucagon release; most effective for type V disorder.
[f]*Neomycin*, experimental medication; questionable mode of action; decreases LDLs.
[g]*Clofibrate* (Atromid-S), decreases release of free fatty acids from adipose tissue; decreases hepatic secretion of VLDL and increases catabolism of VLDL.
[h]*Gemfibrozil* (Lopid), similar to clofibrate but increases HDLs more.
[i]*Estrogens*, decrease IDL levels in type III disorders; experimental.
[j]*Progesterone*, decreases plasma triglycerides in type V disorders; experimental.

stopped. After smoking is discontinued, the risks associated with CAD may decrease as much as 50% in 1 year.

Diabetes Mellitus

Diabetes mellitus is an extremely important risk factor for CAD. Diabetes is associated with a two-fold increase in the risk for CAD death and up to a sixfold risk for stroke.[119,138] Diabetes and insulin resistance have multiple effects on the cardiovascular system through the production of toxic reactive oxygen species (ROS) that alter vascular cell function (also see Chapter 2). These effects can include endothelial damage, thickening of the vessel wall, increased inflammation and leukocyte adhesion, increased thrombosis, glycation of vascular proteins, and decreased production of endothelial-derived vasodilators such as nitric oxide.[139-141] Diabetes is also associated with dyslipidemia because of the resulting alteration of hepatic lipoprotein synthesis and increases in LDL oxidation. Aggressive management of this additional risk factor can significantly improve CAD risk in individuals with diabetes.[142]

Obesity/Sedentary Life-Style

It is estimated that 65% of the adult population in the United States is overweight or obese resulting in a much increased risk for CAD and stroke.[119] An estimated 47 million U.S. residents have a combination of obesity, dyslipidemia, and hypertension called the **metabolic syndrome,** which is associated with an even higher risk for CAD events.[119,122] Obesity is caused by genetics, diet, and inadequate physical exercise. Abdominal obesity has the strongest link with increased CAD risk and is related to insulin resistance, decreased HDL, increased blood pressure, and decreased levels of a recently described cardioprotective protein called *adiponectin*.[143] A sedentary life-style not only increases the risk of obesity but also has an independent effect on increasing CAD risk.[144,145] Physical activity and weight loss offer substantial reductions in risk factors for CAD.[144-146]

Nontraditional Risk Factors

Nontraditional, or novel, risk factors for CAD include (1) increased serum markers for inflammation and thrombosis, (2) hyperhomocysteinemia, and (3) infection. The amount of risk conferred by these relatively newly identified factors is still being explored.

Markers of Inflammation and Thrombosis. Of the numerous markers of inflammation that have been linked to an increase in CAD risk (C-reactive protein, fibrinogen, protein C, plasminogen activator inhibitor), serum levels of C-reactive protein has been explored in the greatest depth. **C-reactive protein (C-rp)** is an acute phase reactant or protein mostly synthesized in the liver whose plasma concentration increases shortly after infarction as part of the systemic inflammatory response. C-rp is an indirect measure of atherosclerotic plaque; related inflammation and is an important indicator of CAD risk.[147-150] Elevated levels of C-rp are associated with numerous other CAD risk factors including smoking, obesity, and diabetes. However, as a nonspecific serum marker for inflammation, its utility as a screening tool for cardiovascular risk continues to be debated.[151-153] Other markers of inflammation associated with CAD include the erythrocyte sedimentation rate, von Willebrand factor concentration, interleukin-6, interleukin-18, tumor necrosis factor, fibrinogen, and CD 40 ligand.[148,154-158]

Hyperhomocysteinemia. Hyperhomocysteinemia occurs because of a genetic lack of the enzyme that breaks down homocysteine (an amino acid) or because of a nutritional deficiency of folate, cobalamin (vitamin B_{12}), or pyridoxine (vitamin B_6). It has been identified as a risk factor for CAD, although its significance in CAD and stroke continues to be explored.[121,159,160] Mechanisms by which it contributes to coronary disease include associated increases in LDL, decreases in endogenous vasodilators, and an increased tendency for thrombosis. Routine serum measurement of homocysteine is not currently recommended and prevention and

management are focused on increasing the dietary intake of folate and B vitamins.

Infection. Emerging is evidence that infection may play a role in atherogenesis and CAD risk. Studies have found that several microorganisms, especially *Chlamydia pneumonae* and *Helicobacter pylori* are often present in atherosclerotic lesions.[161-163] Serum antibodies to microorganisms have been linked to an increased risk for CAD as has the presence of periodontal disease.[161] Although a few early studies suggested that antibiotics used to treat these infections are associated with a decrease in CAD events, recent studies have been less compelling[161,164-166] (see What's New? Atherosclerosis and Infectious Disease).

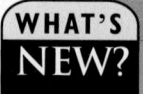 **WHAT'S NEW?** Inflammatory Markers for Cardiovascular Risk

Atherosclerosis is an inflammatory disease. In the past, markers for coronary atherosclerosis and cardiovascular risk included only the well-known factors such as cholesterol, diabetes, smoking, and hypertension. Recently a number of serum markers of inflammation have been found to be excellent predictors of cardiovascular risk, especially C-reactive protein (C-rp). Other inflammatory markers found to be predictive of cardiovascular risk include fibrinogen, erythrocyte sedimentation rate, von Willebrand factor, interleukin-6, interleukin-1, tumor necrosis factor–α, adhesion molecules (selectins, intercellular adhesion molecules [ICAMs]), and serum amyloid A. C-rp is made by the liver in response to inflammatory stimuli and has been demonstrated convincingly to be a good predictor of coronary artery disease. Some studies suggest that it is even more predictive than LDL cholesterol. However, several problems remain in determining its use in clinical practice. C-rp must be measured by a high-sensitivity technique (hs-C-rp), and it is a nonspecific marker of inflammation. It can therefore be elevated in many other inflammatory states; so measurement must include (1) evaluation of the individual for other inflammatory or infectious conditions and (2) must be an average of two measurements taken 2 weeks apart. The current guidelines for the use of hs-C-rp in clinical practice suggest that it should be used to (1) identify individuals without known coronary disease who may be at higher absolute risk than estimated by major risk factors and who might benefit from further evaluation (e.g., stress testing), and (2) estimate prognosis in patients who need secondary preventative care, such as those with stable coronary disease or who have undergone percutaneous coronary intervention (PCI). It should not be used to screen the general population.

Specific interventions for inflammation in atherosclerosis are being studied that could contribute to prevention and regression of plaques, as well as to plaque stabilization. To date, the only clinically useful intervention that has been evaluated for these purposes are the HMG-CoA reductase drugs (statins) that reduce cholesterol and decrease C-rp levels.

Data from Balk EM et al: *Ann Intern Med* 139(8):670-682, 2003; Blake GJ, Ridker PM: *J Am Coll Cardiol* 41(4Suppl S): 37S-42S, 2003; Danesh J et al: *N Engl J Med* 350(14):1387-1397, 2004; Hackam DG, Anand SS: *JAMA* 290(7):932-940, 2003; Linton MF, Fazio S: *Am J Cardiol* 92(1A):19i-26i, 2003; Pearson TA et al: *Circulation* 107(3):449-511, 2003; Ridker P: *Am J Cardiol* 92(4B):17K-22K, 2003; Rosenson RS, Koenig W: *Am J Cardiol* 92(1A):10i-8i, 2003; Van der Meer IM et al: *Arch Intern Med* 163(11):1323-1328, 2003.

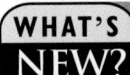

WHAT'S NEW?   Atherosclerosis—An Infectious Disease?

Endothelial injury has been implicated as the first step in the atherosclerotic process, and one of the hypothesized triggers for atherogenesis has been infection of the vessel by pathogenic microorganisms. Infectious agents have been linked to coronary artery disease (CAD) since the 1980s. Since then, a large body of research has found that the presence of serum antibodies to *Chlamydia pneumoniae* is highly correlated to CAD risk, and the bacterium has been cultured from atherosclerotic plaques. Approximately 50% of individuals with acute coronary syndromes have positive *C. pneumoniae* serology.

C. pneumoniae is known to cause endothelial dysfunction, decreased vascular nitric oxide production, increased thrombosis, and elevations in inflammatory markers such as C-reactive protein. Although this is suggestive of an etiologic effect of this bacterium, cause and effect has never been proved. In an effort to address this dilemma, many studies have begun to explore the protective and treatment effects of antibiotics in atherosclerotic disease. Of interest, the class of antibiotics most potent in the treatment of *C. pneumoniae*, the macrolides (e.g., erythromycin) also have potent anti-inflammatory and antioxidant effects. To date, several studies have found improvements in inflammatory markers in individuals with coronary disease, and a few have found a reduction in cardiovascular events. However, still other studies have found no effect of antibiotics on atherosclerotic disease or cardiovascular risk. Many criticisms of the studies so far have engendered further large-scale research efforts that are currently underway.

Data from Anderson JL et al:, *J Infect Dis* 181(suppl 3):S569-S571, 2000; Higgins JP: *Mayo Clinic Proc* 78:321-332, 2003; O'Connor CM et al: *JAMA* 290(11):1459-1466, 2003; Pislaru SV, Van de Werf F: *JAMA* 290(11):1515-1516, 2003; Spence JD, Norris J: *Stroke* 34(2):333-334, 2003; Stone AF et al: *Circulation* 106(10):1219-1223, 2002; Zebrack JS, Anderson JL: *Prog Cardiovas Nurs* 18(1):42-49, 2003.

Myocardial Ischemia

PATHOPHYSIOLOGY   The coronary arteries normally supply blood flow sufficient to meet the demands of the myocardium as it labors under varying workloads. Oxygen extraction from these vessels occurs with maximal efficiency. If efficient exchange does not meet myocardial oxygen needs, healthy coronary arteries are able to dilate to increase the flow of oxygenated blood to the myocardium. A variety of pathologic mechanisms can interfere with blood flow through the coronary arteries, giving rise to myocardial ischemia. Narrowing of a major coronary artery by more than 50% impairs blood flow sufficiently to hamper cellular metabolism under conditions of increased myocardial demand (see Figure 30-15).

Myocardial ischemia develops if the supply of coronary blood cannot meet the demand of the myocardium for oxygen and nutrients. Imbalances between coronary blood supply and myocardial demand can result from a number of conditions. The most common cause of decreased coronary blood flow and resultant myocardial ischemia is the formation of atherosclerotic plaques in the coronary circulation (see p. 1081). As the plaque increases in size, it may partially occlude the vessel lumina, thus limiting coronary flow and causing ischemia especially during exercise. Some plaques are "unstable," meaning they are prone to ulceration or rupture. When this occurs, underlying tissues of the vessel wall are exposed resulting in platelet adhesion and thrombus formation. This can suddenly cut off blood supply to the heart muscle resulting in acute myocardial ischemia and, if the vessel obstruction cannot be reversed rapidly, ischemia will progress to infarction. Myocardial ischemia also can result from other causes of decreased blood and oxygen delivery to the myocardium, such as coronary spasm, hypotension, arrhythmias, and decreased oxygen-carrying capacity of the blood (anemia, hypoxemia). Common causes of increased myocardial demand for blood include tachycardia, exercise, hypertension (hypertrophy), and valvular disease.

Myocardial cells become ischemic within 10 seconds of coronary occlusion. After several minutes the heart cells lose the ability to contract, and cardiac output decreases. Ischemia also causes conduction abnormalities that lead to changes in the electrocardiogram and may initiate dysrhythmias. Anaerobic processes take over, and lactic acid accumulates. Cardiac cells remain viable for approximately 20 minutes under ischemic conditions. If blood flow is restored, aerobic metabolism resumes, contractility is restored, and cellular repair begins. If the coronary arteries cannot compensate for lack of oxygen, myocardial infarction occurs (Figure 30-16).

CLINICAL MANIFESTATIONS   Individuals with reversible myocardial ischemia present clinically in several ways. Chronic coronary obstruction results in recurrent predictable chest pain called **stable angina.** Abnormal vasospasm of coronary vessels results in unpredictable chest pain called **Prinzmetal angina.** Myocardial ischemia that does not cause detectable symptoms is called **silent ischemia.**

Stable Angina.   Angina pectoris is chest pain caused by myocardial ischemia. The discomfort is usually transient, lasting approximately 3 to 5 minutes. If blood flow is restored, no permanent change or damage results. **Angina pectoris** is typically experienced as substernal chest discomfort, ranging from a sensation of heaviness or pressure to moderately severe pain. Individuals often describe the sensation by clenching a fist over the left sternal border. Discomfort may radiate to the neck, lower jaw, left arm, and left shoulder or, occasionally, to the back or down the right arm. Discomfort is commonly mistaken for indigestion. The pain is presumably caused by the buildup of lactic acid or abnormal stretching of the ischemic myocardium that irritates myocardial nerve fibers. These afferent sympathetic fibers enter the spinal cord from levels C3 to T4, accounting for the variety of locations and radiation patterns of anginal pain. Pallor, diaphoresis, and dyspnea may be associated with the pain. Stable angina is caused by gradual luminal narrowing and hardening of the arterial walls, so that affected vessels cannot dilate in response to increased myocardial demand associated with physical exertion or emotional stress. The pain is usually relieved by rest

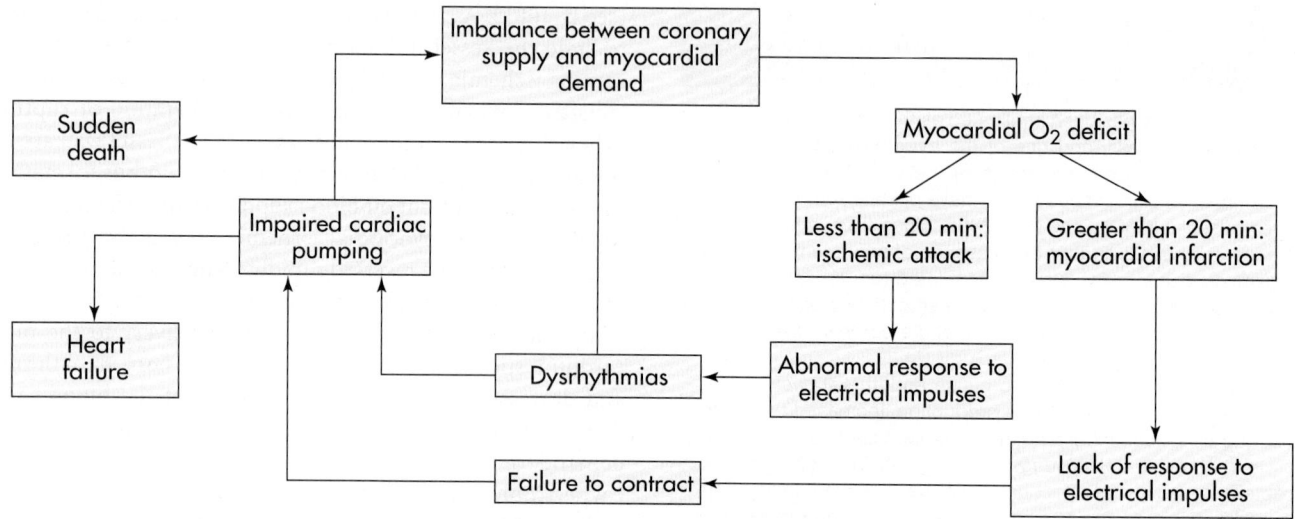

Figure 30-16 Cycle of ischemic events.

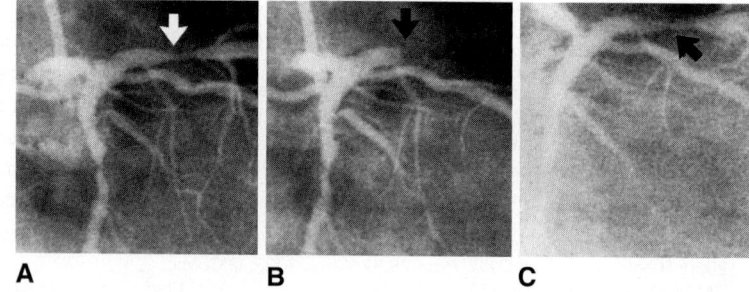

Figure 30-17 Angiogram. **A,** Baseline. **B,** Transient total occlusion of left anterior descending branch of the left coronary artery after mental stress. **C,** After administration of nitrates and nifedipine, artery reopened to same diameter as baseline. (From Stern S, editor: *Silent myocardial ischemia,* St Louis, 1998, Mosby.)

and nitrates; lack of relief indicates an individual may be developing infarction.

Prinzmetal Angina. Prinzmetal angina is chest pain attributable to transient ischemia of the myocardium that occurs unpredictably and almost exclusively at rest. Pain is caused by vasospasm of one or more major coronary arteries with or without associated atherosclerosis. The pain often occurs at night during rapid eye movement sleep and may have a cyclic pattern of occurrence. The angina may result from hyperactivity of the sympathetic nervous system, increased calcium reflux in arterial smooth muscle, or impaired production or release of prostaglandin or thromboxane. If the spasm persists long enough, infarction results.[167]

Silent Ischemia and Mental Stress (Induced Ischemia. Myocardial ischemia often does not cause detectable symptoms such as angina. Ischemia can be totally asymptomatic and referred to as silent ischemia. In addition, myocardial ischemia can be silent in the majority of episodes in individuals who also experience angina. Recent studies have addressed the pathophysiologic differences between silent and symptomatic ischemia. One proposed mechanism for the absence of angina in silent myocardial ischemia is the presence of a global or regional abnormality in left ventricular symptomatic afferent innervation. Such an abnormality might occur as part of a metabolic dysfunction in diabetes mellitus, following surgical denervation during coronary artery bypass grafting (CABG) or cardiac transplantation, or following ischemic local nerve injury by myocardial infarction. It also has been suggested that silent ischemia is associated with less local inflammation, suggesting that a high level of inflammatory cytokines may be necessary to induce anginal pain.[168]

Another area that is receiving renewed interest is the lack of angina, even though an artery is occluded, in some individuals during mental stress (Figures 30-17, 30-18, and 30-19). Rozanski and colleagues documented myocardial ischemia by radionuclide angiography (RNA) during mental stress; the majority of these cases (83%) were silent ischemias.[169] They also noted a smaller increase in heart rate during mental stress than during exercise, although the systolic blood response was comparable and the diastolic blood pressure response is even greater with mental stress. These observations confirmed in similar studies that the increases in blood pressure induced by mental stress and increases in myocardial oxygen demand may play a role in the pathophysiology of myocardial ischemia induced by mental stress. Chronic stress has been linked to a hypercoagulable state that may contribute to acute ischemic events.[170]

Silent myocardial ischemia is very prevalent in individuals with a variety of acute and chronic coronary syndromes. Silent ischemia is detected with greater sensitivity and specificity using stress radionucleotide imaging than by exercise

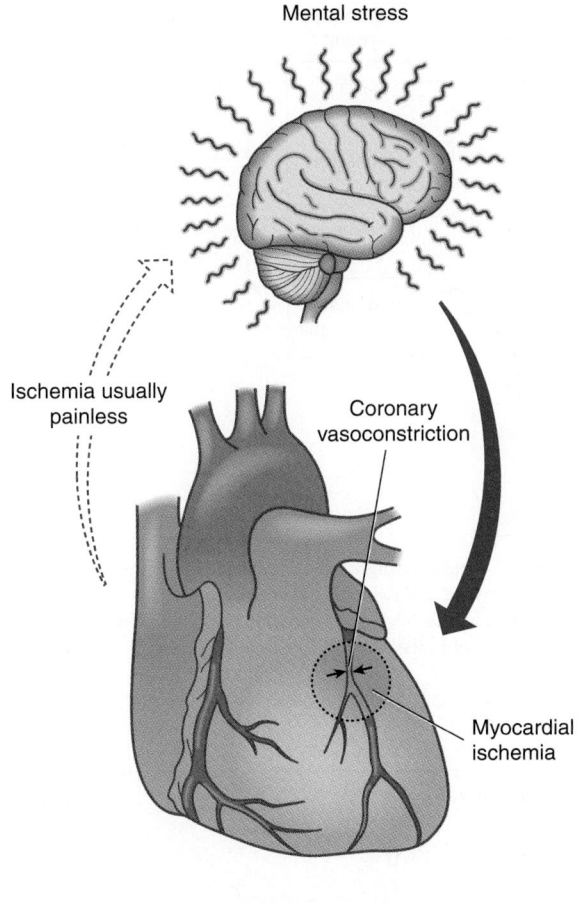

Mental stress

Ischemia usually painless

Coronary vasoconstriction

Myocardial ischemia

Electrocardiogram

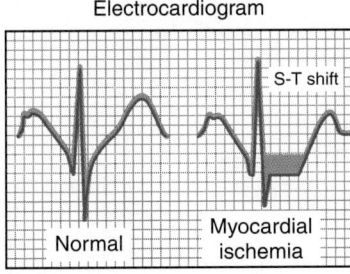

S-T shift

Normal   Myocardial ischemia

Figure 30-18 **The ischemic cost of aggravation.** Linkages among daily mental and emotional stimuli, brain activity, and coronary and myocardial physiology. (Modified from Papodemetrion V et al: *Am Heart J* 132:1299, 1996.)

electrocardiogram testing alone. Detection of silent ischemia is important because it is an indicator of a markedly increased risk for cardiovascular death.[171]

EVALUATION AND TREATMENT   Physical examination may disclose extra, rapid heart sounds (left ventricular gallop or S_3), indicating impaired left ventricular function during the ischemic attack. The presence of **xanthelasmas** (small fat deposits) around the eyelids or **arcus senilis** of the eyes (a yellow lipid ring around the cornea) suggests dyslipidemia and possible atherosclerosis. The presence of peripheral or carotid arterial bruits suggests probable atherosclerotic disease and increases the likelihood that CAD is present.

Electrocardiography is a critical tool for the diagnosis of myocardial ischemia. Because many individuals have normal electrocardiograms (ECGs) in the absence of pain, diagnosis requires that electrocardiography be performed during an attack of angina. Transient ST segment depression and T wave inversion are characteristic signs of subendocardial ischemia. ST elevation, indicative of transmural ischemia, is seen in individuals with variant angina (Figure 30-20). The ECG also can give some indication of which coronary artery is involved. Approximately 30% of individuals with angina will have nondiagnostic ECG tracings and require other diagnostic studies. Exercise stress testing is useful in differentiating angina from other types of chest pain, as well as detecting ischemic changes that occur in the absence of anginal pain (silent ischemia).

Radioisotope imaging with thallium-201 is another technique used to diagnose CAD. Active transport mechanisms (the Na^+, K^+ATPase system) cause thallium to enter myocardial cells. An area of myocardial infarction appears as a region of diminished activity or no activity (a "cold spot"). Defects that are absent at rest but can be induced by exercise represent ischemia. **SPECT (single-photon emission computed tomography)** is even more effective at identifying ischemia and estimating coronary risk.

Coronary angiography is useful in determining the anatomic extent of CAD. The procedure is expensive and carries some risk; thus it is used primarily to evaluate for possible percutaneous coronary intervention (PCI) or coronary artery bypass graft (CABG) surgery for individuals whose noninvasive studies suggest severe disease.

The primary aim of therapy for myocardial ischemia and angina is to reduce myocardial oxygen consumption by favorably altering its various determinants. The factors most amenable to pharmacologic manipulation are blood pressure, heart rate, contractility, and left ventricular volume.

Nitrates are often the drug of choice because they increase oxygen supply and reduce demand. Nitrates cause peripheral veins and, to a lesser extent, peripheral arteries to dilate. Dilation reduces both peripheral vascular resistance and venous return to the heart (preload) and thereby reduces left ventricular filling pressure and left ventricular volume. Reduced filling pressure and volume decrease workload (myocardial demand). Nitrates also improve coronary blood flow by reducing coronary artery spasm and thereby increase myocardial blood supply. These drugs cannot enhance vasodilation in coronary vessels altered by atherosclerosis or arteriosclerosis because these disorders impair the vessels' ability to change lumen size.

β-Adrenergic blocking agents have had great impact on therapy for ischemic heart disease in the past 20 years. By blocking β receptors, these medications can increase oxygen supply and reduce myocardial demand. Beta blockers diminish catecholamine-induced elevations of heart rate, myocardial contractility, and blood pressure. Coronary blood flow also can be augmented by beta blockade. Reduction in heart rate provides additional diastolic filling time for coronary perfusion, leading to enhanced oxygen delivery to the heart.

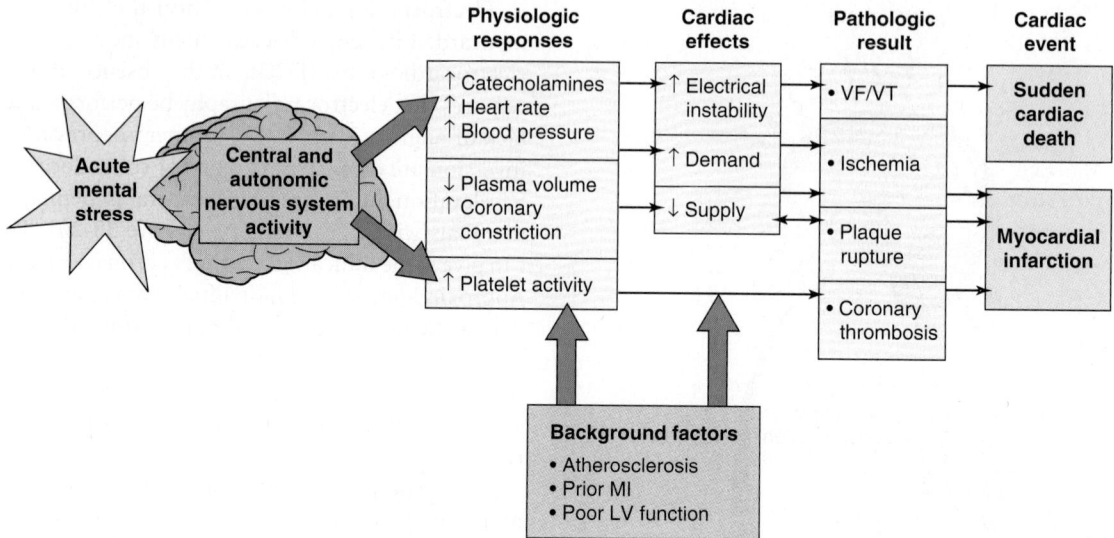

Figure 30-19 Pathophysiologic model of acute stress effects triggering cardiac clinical events. Acting via the central and autonomic nervous systems, stress can produce a cascade of physiologic responses that may lead to myocardial ischemia, potentially fatal dysrhythmia, plaque rupture, or coronary thrombosis. *VF,* Ventricular fibrillation; *VT,* ventricular tachycardia; *MI,* myocardial infarction; *LV,* left ventricular. (From Kranz DS et al: Mental stress as a trigger of myocardial ischemia and infarction. In Deedwania PC, Tofler GH, editors: *Triggers and timing of cardiac events,* ed 2, London, 1996, Saunders.)

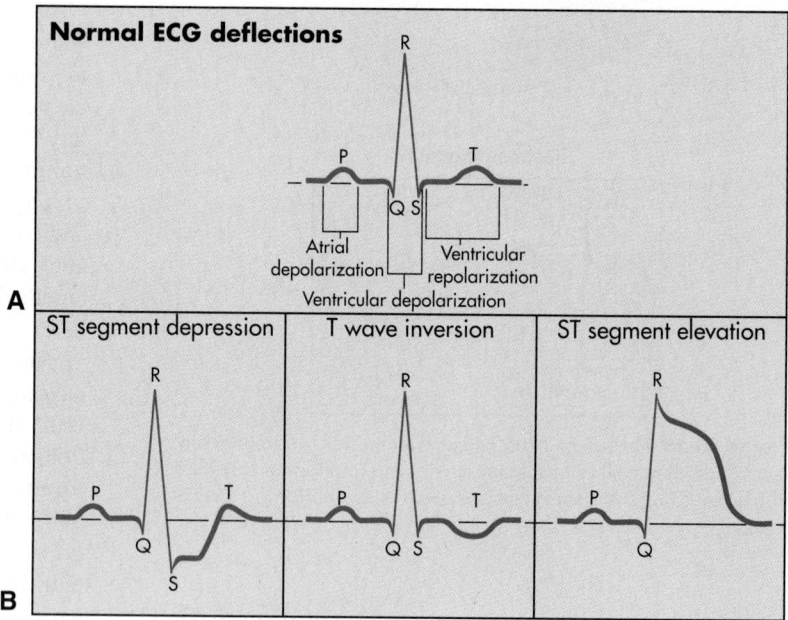

Figure 30-20 Electrocardiogram (ECG) and ischemia. **A,** Normal ECG. **B,** Electrocardiographic alterations associated with ischemia.

Calcium plays a key role in the electrical excitation of cardiac cells and in mechanical contraction of the myocardial and vascular smooth muscle cells (see Chapter 29). By blocking the influx of calcium into myocardial cells and vascular smooth muscle cells, the pacemaker activity of the sinoatrial (SA) node and conduction properties of the atrioventricular (AV) node can be modified. Combinations of nitrates, beta-blockers, and calcium antagonists may provide dramatic relief from clinical manifestations of ischemic heart disease and make more invasive interventions unnecessary.

Experimental evidence linking platelet aggregation with decreased coronary blood flow has led to the use of antiplatelet agents for individuals with ischemic heart disease. Effective antiplatelet agents include aspirin, clopidogrel, or dipyridamole.[172] Aggressive reversal of risk factors, especially lipid lowering therapy, can reverse disease progression and improve outcomes. This type of secondary prevention reduces the risk of subsequent myocardial infarction.[125,173,174]

Percutaneous coronary intervention (PCI) is a procedure whereby stenotic (narrowed) coronary vessels are dilated with a catheter. Several different types of catheters can be used to open the blocked vessel.[175] PCI is generally used to treat single-vessel disease, but it can be effective with multiple-vessel disease or restenosis of a coronary artery bypass graft. Restenosis of the artery is the major complication of the procedure; however, placement of a coronary stent can reduce this risk. Antithrombotic treatment with glycoprotein IIb/IIIa receptor antagonists after stenting also can greatly improve outcomes.[176]

Ischemic heart disease can be surgically treated by a **coronary artery bypass graft.** A saphenous vein from the lower leg is most commonly used to bypass the obstructed coronary artery. A technique using the left internal mammary artery (LIMA) rather than the saphenous vein has shown significant improvement in long-term graft patency. In selected individuals a procedure called **minimally invasive direct coronary artery bypass (MIDCAB)** can allow for effective bypass grafting of the heart, but with minimal disruption of the chest wall and without cardiopulmonary bypass or cardioplegia; thus recovery times are much shorter. One of the most common indications for bypass surgery is incapacitating angina in an individual who has good left ventricular function and technically operable coronary arteries but who has not responded to medical therapy. Although surgery has been shown to relieve angina, it does not halt the progress of atherosclerosis or prolong life except when multiple coronary vessels are obstructed or when the left main coronary artery is blocked. A successful coronary artery bypass graft can, however, diminish the probability of lethal insult to the coronary tissues and can markedly improve quality of life. Newer therapies for refractory angina include transmyocardial laser revascularization (TMR) and gene therapy for myocardial angiogenesis. A new class of drugs that inhibit fatty acid oxidation (e.g., ranolazien) also has shown promise for refractory angina.[177]

Acute Coronary Syndromes

The process of atherosclerotic plaque progression can be gradual. However, when there is sudden coronary obstruction caused by thrombus formation over a ruptured or ulcerated atherosclerotic plaque, the acute coronary syndromes result (Figure 30-21). **Unstable angina** is the result of reversible myocardial ischemia and is a harbinger of impending infarction (p. 1110). **Myocardial infarction** results when there is prolonged ischemia causing irreversible damage to the heart muscle. Sudden cardiac death can occur as a result of any of the acute coronary syndromes.

The American Heart Association Committee on Vascular Lesions provided criteria for subdividing coronary atherosclerotic plaque progression into five phases, with different lesion types corresponding to each phase.[178] The main point of this system is that some atherosclerotic lesions are "stable" and progress by gradually occluding the vessel lumen, whereas other lesions are "unstable" or complicated lesions and (even before there is any significant coronary occlusion) are prone to sudden plaque rupture and thrombus formation, resulting in the acute coronary syndromes of unstable angina,

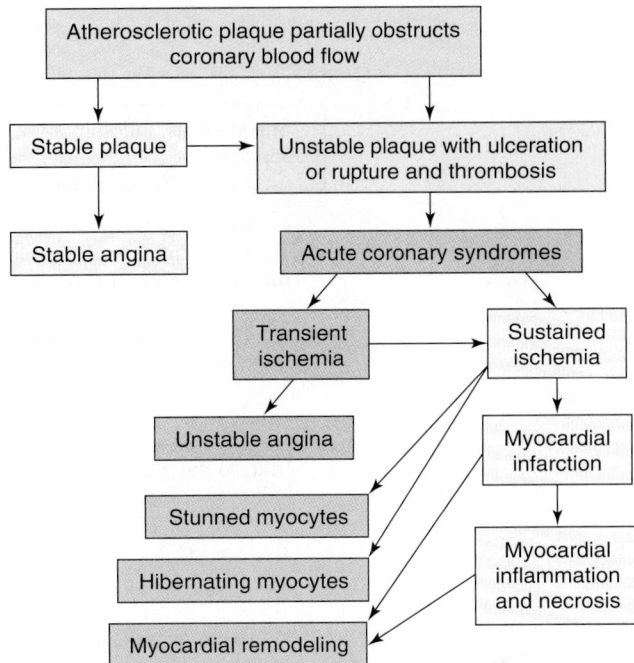

Figure 30-21 Pathophysiology of acute coronary syndromes. The atherosclerotic process can lead to stable plaque formation and stable angina or can result in unstable plaques that are prone to rupture and thrombosus. Thrombus formation on a ruptured plaque that disperses in less than 20 minutes leads to transient ischemia and unstable angina. If the vessel obstruction is sustained, myocardial infarction with inflammation and necrosis of the myocardium results. In addition, myocardial infarction is associated with other structural and functional changes, including myocyte stunning and hibernation and myocardial remodeling.

myocardial infarction, and even sudden death. Figure 30-22 provides an overview of the steps in the development of the acute coronary syndromes. Plaques that are unstable and prone to rupture are those with a core that is especially rich in deposited oxidized LDL and those with thin fibrous caps.[179] Plaque disruption (ulceration or rupture) occurs because of shear forces, inflammation with release of multiple inflammatory mediators, secretion of macrophage-derived degradative enzymes, and apoptosis of cells at the edges of the lesions.[180] Exposure of the plaque substrate activates the clotting cascade.[181] In addition, platelet activation results in the release of coagulants and exposure of platelet glycoprotein IIb/IIIa surface receptors, resulting in further platelet aggregation and adherence.[182] The resulting thrombus can form very quickly. Vessel obstruction is further exacerbated by the release of vasoconstrictors such as thromboxane A_2. The thrombus may break up before permanent myocyte damage has occurred (unstable angina), or it may cause prolonged ischemia with infarction of the heart muscle (myocardial infarction). Some individuals have sudden cardiac death without underlying histologic evidence of infarction. New therapies are being developed to help stabilize plaques and prevent them from rupturing.[183,184]

Unstable Angina

Unstable angina is a form of acute coronary syndrome that results in reversible myocardial ischemia. Important, how-

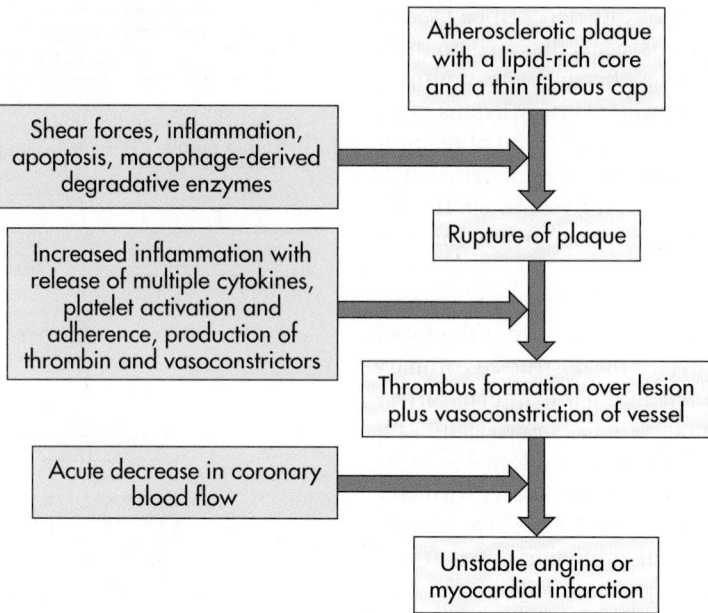

Figure 30-22 Pathogenesis of unstable plaques and thrombus formation.

ever, is that it signals that the atherosclerotic plaque has become complicated, and infarction may soon follow.

PATHOPHYSIOLOGY   A fairly small fissuring or superficial erosion of the plaque leads to transient episodes of thrombotic vessel occlusion and vasoconstriction at the site of plaque damage.[185] This thrombus is labile and occludes the vessel for no more than 10 to 20 minutes, with return of perfusion before significant myocardial necrosis occurs.

CLINICAL MANIFESTATIONS   Unstable angina presents as new onset angina, angina that is occurring at rest, or angina that is increasing in severity or frequency (Box 30-1). Individuals may experience increased dyspnea, diaphoresis, and anxiety as the angina worsens. Those with unstable angina at rest have the greatest risk of subsequent infarction or death.

Box 30-1	Three Principal Presentations of Unstable Angina

Rest angina*—Angina occurring at rest and prolonged, usually >20 minutes
New-onset angina—New-onset angina of at least CCS Class III severity
Increasing angina—Previously diagnosed angina that has become distinctly more frequent, longer in duration, or lower in threshold (i.e., increased by ≥1 CCS class to at least CCS Class III severity)

From Braunwald ET et al: *Management of patients with unstable angina and non–ST-segment elevation myocardial infarction*, update 2002. Available at www.acc.org/clinical/guidelines/unstable/update_index.htm.
Originally adapted from Braunwald E: *Circulation* 80:410-414, 1989.
*Patients with non–ST-elevation myocardial infarction (NSTEMI) usually present with angina at rest.

EVALUATION AND MANAGEMENT   Physical examination may reveal evidence of ischemic myocardial dysfunction such as tachycardia, S_3 gallop, or pulmonary congestion. The ECG most commonly reveals ST segment depression and T wave inversion during pain that resolves as the pain is relieved. The ECG may be inconclusive in up to one third of individuals with unstable angina, for whom further evaluation is necessary. The cardiac isoenzymes (creatine phosphokinase-myocardial bound [CPK-MB], lactate dehydrogenase [LDH_1]) remain normal. Sensitive markers of myocyte damage such as the troponins may increase transiently in some individuals diagnosed with unstable angina but remain clinically insignificant.[185] Emergency echocardiography may reveal abnormal cardiac contraction. Approximately 20% of individuals with unstable angina will progress to myocardial infarction or death within 30 days. Unfortunately, up to 4% of individuals with unstable angina are inadvertently discharged from the emergency room, resulting in considerable risk for subsequent infarction and death. Treatment of unstable angina usually includes antischemic medications such as nitrates, beta-blockers and calcium channel blockers, and antithrombotic medications such as aspirin, clopidogrel, or IIb/IIIa platelet receptor antagonists. Heparin, low-molecular-weight heparin, or bivaliruden and emergent PCI also may be indicated.[186,187]

Myocardial Infarction

When coronary blood flow is interrupted for an extended period of time, myocyte necrosis occurs. This results in myocardial infarction (MI). Pathologically there are two major types of myocardial infarction, subendocardial infarction and transmural infarction.

PATHOPHYSIOLOGY   Plaque progression, disruption, and subsequent clot formation is the same for myocardial infarction as it is for the other acute coronary syndromes (see Figures 30-21, 30-22, and 30-23). In this case, however, the thrombus is less labile and occludes the vessel for a prolonged period, such that myocardial ischemia progresses to myocyte necrosis and death. If the thrombus breaks up before complete distal tissue necrosis has occurred, the infarction will involve only the myocardium directly beneath the endocardium (subendocardial MI). It is especially important to recognize this form of acute coronary syndrome because recurrent clot formation on the disrupted atherosclerotic plaque is likely unless some intervention is undertaken as soon as possible. If the thrombus lodges permanently in the vessel, the infarction will extend through the myocardium all the way from endocardium to epicardium, resulting in severe cardiac dysfunction (transmural MI). Clinically, it is important to identify those individuals with transmural infarction who are at highest risk for serious complications and who should receive definitive intervention without delay. Those individuals usually have marked elevations in the ST segments on ECG and are categorized as having ST-elevation MI, or STEMI. Those without T segment elevation are said to have non-STEMI.

Cellular Injury. Cardiac cells can withstand ischemic conditions for about 20 minutes before cellular death takes place. After only 30 to 60 seconds of hypoxia, ECG changes are visible. Yet even if cells are metabolically altered and nonfunctional, they can remain viable if blood flow returns within 20 minutes. Reports suggest previous recurrent episodes of myocardial ischemia can result in myocyte adaptation to oxygen deprivation and preservation of myocardium. This process, termed **ischemic preconditioning,** is being studied to determine whether it has potential prophylactic or therapeutic uses. Although this phenomenon is now well described in other organs, such as the liver, its clinical utility in heart disease and surgery has yet to be determined.[188,189]

After 8 to 10 seconds of decreased blood flow, the affected myocardium becomes cyanotic and cooler. Myocardial oxygen reserves are used very quickly (within about 8 seconds) after complete cessation of coronary flow. Glycogen stores decrease as anaerobic metabolism begins. Unfortunately, glycolysis can supply only 65% to 70% of the total myocardial energy requirement and produces much less adenosine triphosphate (ATP) than aerobic processes. Hydrogen ions and lactic acid accumulate. Because myocardial tissues have poor buffering capabilities and myocardial cells are very sensitive to low cellular pH, accumulation of these products further compromises the myocardium. Acidosis may make the myocardium more vulnerable to the damaging effects of lysosomal enzymes and may suppress impulse conduction and contractile function, thereby leading to heart failure.

Oxygen deprivation also is accompanied by electrolyte disturbances—specifically, loss of potassium, calcium, and magnesium from cells. Myocardial cells deprived of necessary oxygen and nutrients lose contractility, thereby diminishing the pumping ability of the heart. Normally, the myocardium takes up varying quantities of catecholamines (epinephrine and norepinephrine). Significant arterial occlusion causes the myocardial cells to release catecholamines, predisposing the individual to serious imbalances of sympathetic and parasympathetic function, irregular heartbeats (dysrhythmia), and heart failure. Catecholamines mediate the release of glycogen, glucose, and stored fat from body cells. Therefore plasma concentrations of free fatty acids and glycerol rise within 1 hour after onset of acute myocardial infarction. Excessive levels of free fatty acids can have a harmful detergent effect on cell membranes. Norepinephrine elevates blood sugar levels through stimulation of liver and skeletal muscle cells. It also suppresses pancreatic B cell activity, which reduces insulin secretion and elevates blood glucose further. Not surprisingly, hyperglycemia is noted approximately 72 hours after an acute myocardial infarction.

Angiotensin II is released during myocardial ischemia and contributes to the pathogenesis of MI in several ways. First, it

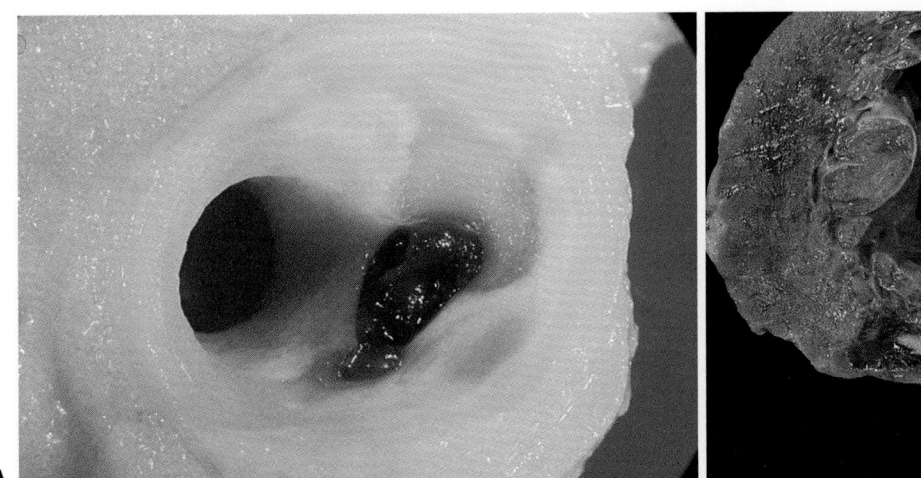
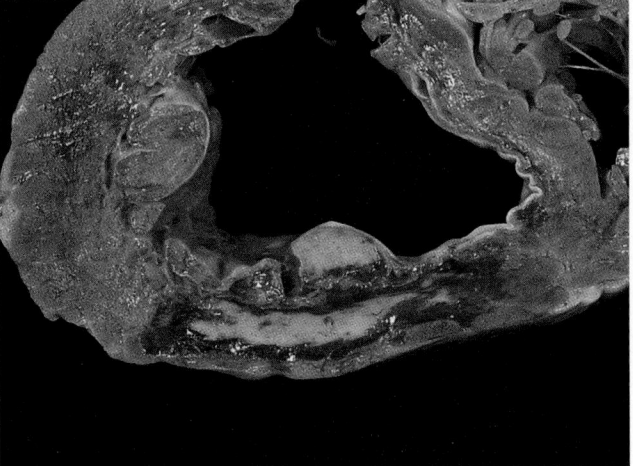

Figure 30-23 Plaque disruption and myocardial infarction. **A,** Plaque disruption. The cap of the lipid-rich plaque has become torn with the formation of a thrombus, mostly inside the plaque. **B,** Myocardial infarction. This infarct is 6 days old. The center is yellow and necrotic with a hemorrhagic red rim. The responsible coronary artery occlusion is probably in the right coronary artery. The infarct is on the posterior wall. (From Damjanov I, Linder J, editors: *Anderson's pathology,* ed 10, St Louis, 1996, Mosby.)

results in the systemic effects of peripheral vasoconstriction and fluid retention. These homeostatic responses are counterproductive in that they increase myocardial work and thus exacerbate the effects of the loss of myocyte contractility. Angiotensin II is also released locally, where it is a growth factor for vascular smooth muscle cells, myocytes, and cardiac fibroblasts; promotes catecholamine release; and causes coronary artery spasm.

Cellular Death. After about 20 minutes of myocardial ischemia, irreversible hypoxic injury causes cellular death and tissue necrosis. (Types of necrosis are described in Chapter 2.) Necrosis of myocardial tissue results in the release of certain intracellular enzymes through the damaged cell membranes into the interstitial spaces. The lymphatics pick up the enzymes and transport them into the bloodstream, where they can be detected by serologic tests.

Structural and Functional Changes. Myocardial infarction results in both structural and functional changes of cardiac tissues (Figure 30-24). Table 30-6 outlines the tissue changes that may follow myocardial infarction. Gross tissue changes in the area of infarction may not become apparent for several hours, despite almost immediate onset (within 30 to 60 seconds) of electrocardiographic changes. The infarcted myocardium is surrounded by a zone of hypoxic injury, which may progress to necrosis, undergo remodeling, or return to normal. Cardiac tissue surrounding the area of infarction also undergoes changes that can be categorized into (1) **myocardial stunning,** a temporary loss of contractile function that persists for hours to days after perfusion has been restored; (2) **hibernating myocardium,** tissue that is persistently ischemic and undergoes metabolic adaptation to prolong myocyte survival until perfusion can be restored; and (3) **myocardial remodeling,** a process mediated by angiotensin II, aldosterone, catecholamines, adenosine, and inflammatory cytokines which causes myocyte hypertrophy and loss of contractile function in the areas of the heart distant from the site of infarction.[190-195] All these changes can be limited through rapid restoration of coronary flow and the use of angiotensin-converting enzyme (ACE) inhibitors and beta blockers after MI.

Table 30-6	Tissue Changes After Myocardial Infarction	
Time After Myocardial Infarction	**Tissue Changes**	**Stage of Healing Process**
6-12 hours	No gross changes; subcellular cyanosis with decreased temperature	Not begun
18-24 hours	Pale to gray-brown; slight pallor	Inflammatory response; intercellular enzyme release
2-4 days	Visible necrosis: yellow-brown in center and hyperemic around edges	Proteolytic enzymes remove debris; catecholamines, lipolysis, and glycogenolysis elevate plasma glucose and increase free fatty acids to assist depleted myocardium recovery from anaerobic state
4-10 days	Area soft, with fatty changes in center, regions of hemorrhage in infarcted area	Debris cleared; collagen matrix laid down
10-14 days	Weak, fibrotic scar tissue with beginning revascularization	Healing continues but area very mushy, vulnerable to stress
6 weeks	Scarring usually complete	Tough inelastic scar replaces necrotic myocardium

NOTE: Processes of tissue healing are described and illustrated in Chapter 7.

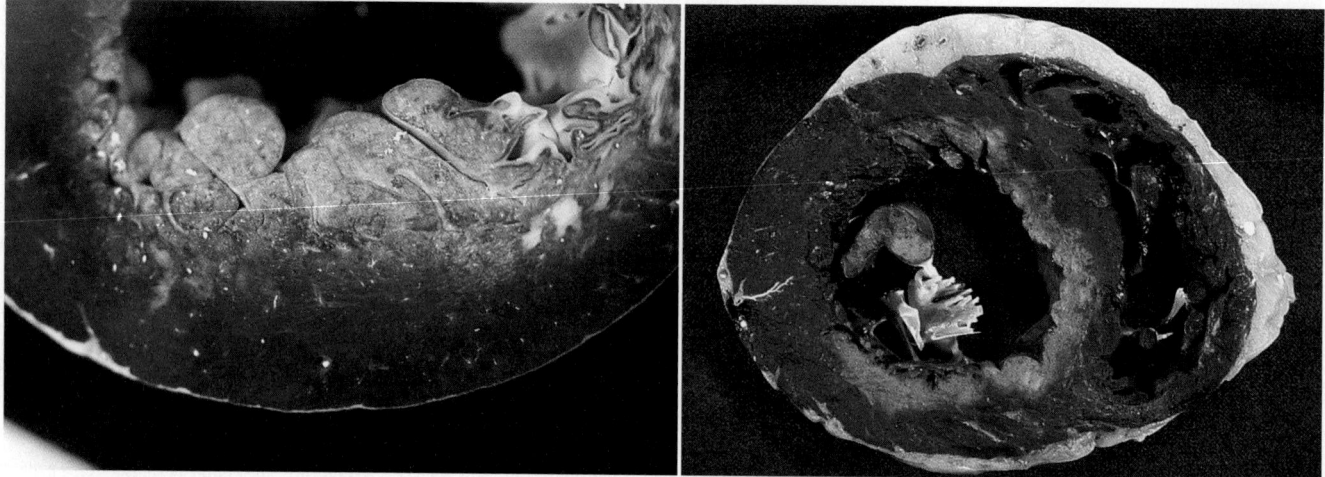

A   B

Figure 30-24 Myocardial infarction. A, Local infarct confined to one region. **B,** Massive large infarct caused by occlusion of three coronary arteries. (From Damjanov I, Linder J, editors: *Anderson's pathology,* ed 10, St Louis, 1996, Mosby.)

The severity of functional impairment depends on the size of the lesion and the site of infarction. Functional changes can include (1) decreased cardiac contractility with abnormal wall motion, (2) altered left ventricular compliance, (3) decreased stroke volume, (4) decreased ejection fraction, (5) increased left ventricular end-diastolic pressure, and (6) SA node malfunction. Life-threatening dysrhythmias and heart failure often follow MI.

Repair. Myocardial infarction causes a severe inflammatory response that ends with wound repair (see Chapter 6). Repair consists of degradation of damaged cells, proliferation of fibroblasts, and synthesis of scar tissue. Many cell types, hormones, and nutrient substrates must be available for optimal healing to proceed. Within 24 hours, leukocytes infiltrate the necrotic area and proteolytic enzymes from scavenger neutrophils degrade necrotic tissue. A pseudodiabetic state often develops as catecholamines released from damaged cells stimulate release of glucose and free fatty acids. By the second week, insulin secretion increases to mobilize glucose from the repair processes. The collagen matrix that is deposited is initially weak, mushy, and vulnerable to reinjury. Unfortunately, it is at this time in the recovery period (10 to 14 days after infarction) that individuals feel more capable of increasing activities and thus may stress the newly formed scar tissue. After 6 weeks the necrotic area is completely replaced by scar tissue, which is strong but unable to contract and relax like healthy myocardial tissue.

CLINICAL MANIFESTATIONS   The first symptom of acute myocardial infarction is usually sudden, severe chest pain. It is not possible to distinguish between angina and MI by symptoms alone, although the pain associated with MI tends to be more severe and prolonged. It may be described as heavy and crushing, such as a "truck sitting on my chest." Radiation to the neck, jaw, back, shoulder, or left arm is common. Some individuals (especially those who are elderly or diabetic) experience no pain, thereby having a "silent" infarction. Infarction often stimulates a sensation of unrelenting indigestion. Nausea and vomiting may occur because of reflex stimulation of vomiting centers by pain fibers. Vasovagal reflexes from the area of the infarcted myocardium also may affect the gastrointestinal tract. Catecholamine release results in sympathetic stimulation, producing diaphoresis and peripheral vasoconstriction that cause the skin to become cool and clammy.

A variety of cardiovascular changes may be found on physical examination. With an acute myocardial infarction, blood pressure may initially decrease. The drop in blood pressure reflexively activates the sympathetic nervous system to compensate and then causes a temporary increase in heart rate and blood pressure. Abnormal extra heart sounds (S_3, S_4) reflect left ventricular dysfunction. Inflammation can cause pericardial friction rub, along with a variety of cardiac murmurs.

Laboratory data reveal leukocytosis and elevated sedimentation rate, both of which indicate inflammation. The individual's blood sugar usually is elevated, and the glucose tolerance level may remain abnormal for several weeks.

The cardiac troponins (troponin I and troponin T) are the most specific indicators of MI. In addition, a transient rise in plasma enzyme levels can confirm the occurrence of MI and indicate its severity. The enzymes released by myocardial cells include creatine kinase (CK) and lactic dehydrogenase (LDH). These enzymes exist in several different active molecular forms called *isoenzymes,* which are present in different amounts within particular tissues. If serologic tests show abnormally high levels of troponin and isoenzymes associated with cardiac tissue (creatine kinase-myocardial bound [CK-MB], LDH_1), acute myocardial infarction probably has occurred. CK-MB is less specific than troponins and may increase in individuals with certain other conditions (e.g., muscular dystrophy, hypothermia, chronic obstructive pulmonary disease [COPD] associated with left heart failure and pulmonary embolism, extensive third-degree burns, small bowel infarction). Elevation of troponin, CK-MB and LDH_1 may be noted at characteristic times, and laboratory confirmation that an infarction has occurred may be delayed up to 12 hours. The amount of troponin and CK elevation may be correlated with severity of infarction. The higher the serum concentration of CK-MB and troponin is, the more extensive the tissue damage that has occurred.[196] Blood is drawn for troponin and isoenzyme determinations as soon as possible after the onset of symptoms, and serial serum levels of these markers are assessed for several days.

Myocardial infarction can occur in various regions of the heart wall and may be described as anterior, inferior, posterior, or lateral depending on the anatomic location (Figure 30-25). Twelve-lead ECGs help to localize the affected area through identification of Q waves and changes in ST segments and T waves (Figure 30-26).

TREATMENT   Acute myocardial infarction requires immediate admission to a hospital with a coronary care unit, if possible. Aspirin should be administered to all individuals immediately on recognition of MI and clopidogrel should be added if emergent surgery is not anticipated. Heparin should be begun and the addition of gpII$_b$IIIa receptor blockers should be considered. Pain relief is of utmost importance and involves the use of sublingual or topical nitroglycerine and morphine sulfate. Supplemental oxygen is administered to increase arterial oxygen content and deliver more oxygen to the ischemic myocardium. Continuous close monitoring of cardiac rhythms and enzymatic changes is especially important. The first 24 hours after onset of symptoms is the time of highest risk for sudden death. In complicated cases, invasive monitoring techniques (e.g., arterial, central venous pressure, and Swan-Ganz lines) may be required. If the infarction is diagnosed within a few hours of the onset of pain and the individual has no contraindications, thrombolytic therapy with tissue plasminogen activator (t-PA), or TNK-t-PA, should be administered. Alternatively, emergent PCI has been shown to be as or more effective than thrombolytics, especially in those suffering from shock. PCI with stent placement and antithrombotic medications is becoming the treat-

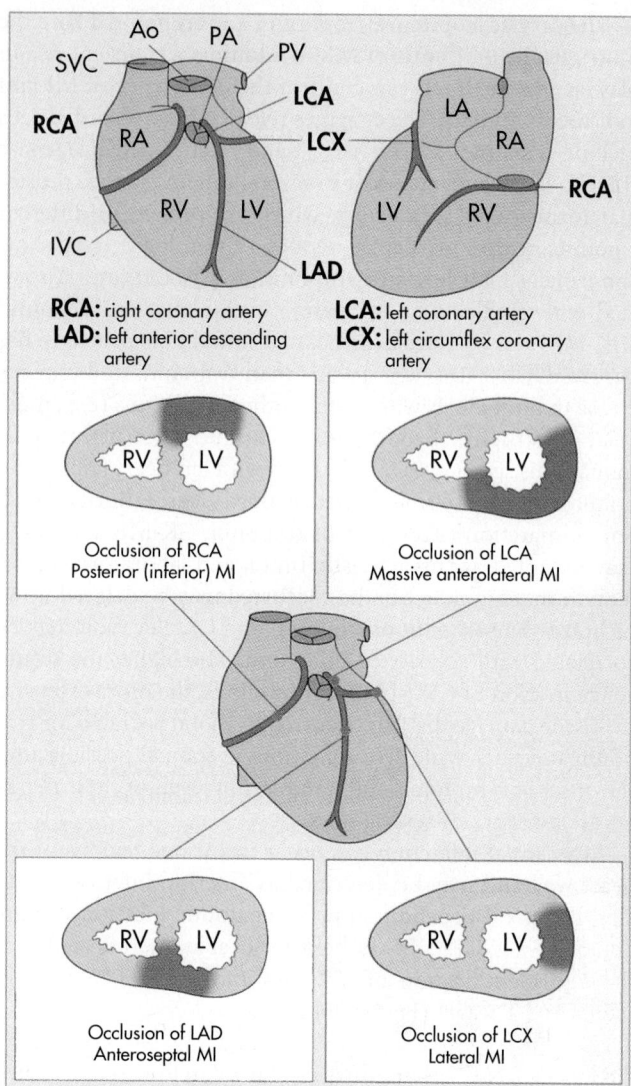

Figure 30-25 Site of myocardial infarction (MI) and vessel involvement. *Ao,* Aorta; *PA,* pulmonary artery; *PV,* pulmonary vein; *LV,* left ventricle; *RV,* right ventricle; *IVC,* inferior vena cava; *RA,* right atrium; *SVC,* superior vena cava; *LA,* left atrium. (Modified from Stevens A, Lowe J: *Pathology,* St Louis, 1995, Mosby.)

ment of choice for many individuals with acute myocardial infarction.[198,199]

Bed rest, followed by gradual return to activities of daily living, reduces the myocardial oxygen demands of the compromised heart. Dietary measures are aimed at preventing nausea and vomiting, and consumption of sodium, saturated fats, sugar, and caffeine is limited. Stool softeners are given to eliminate the need for straining, which can precipitate bradycardia (i.e., vasovagal response) and can be followed by increased venous return to the heart, causing possible cardiac overload.

Additional therapies that should be used in the management of acute myocardial infarction include ACE inhibitors, beta-blockers, and antiplatelet drugs, which have been shown to improve survival and cardiac function after MI.[200-202] Risk reduction, especially lipid-lowering therapy, is important to reduce the risk of future acute coronary events.[203,204] Education on diet, smoking cessation, exercise, and other aspects of risk factor reduction is crucial for secondary prevention of recurrent myocardial ischemia.

COMPLICATIONS The number and severity of postinfarction complications depend on the location and extent of necrosis, the individual's physiologic condition before the infarction, and the availability of swift therapeutic intervention.

Dysrhythmias (arrhythmias), which are disturbances of cardiac rhythm, are the most common complication of acute myocardial infarction, affecting more than 90% of individuals. Dysrhythmias can be caused by ischemia, hypoxia, autonomic nervous system imbalances, lactic acidosis, electrolyte abnormalities, alterations of impulse conduction pathways or conduction defects, drug toxicity, or hemodynamic abnormalities. Dysrhythmias may originate from the atria, ventricles, nodal regions, or conduction tissues. The seriousness of dysrhythmias depends on the hemodynamic consequences. For example, there is no ventricular contraction in ventricular fibrillation; consequently, there is no cardiac output. Atrial fibrillation, however, does not affect ventricular contraction and thus can be tolerated by most individuals. (Dysrhythmias are described on p. 1134.) Prophylactic use of antiarrhyth-

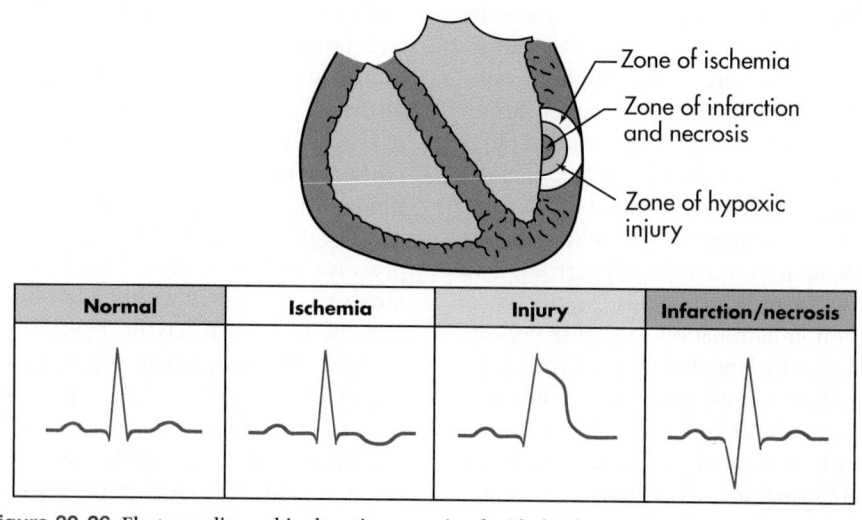

Figure 30-26 Electrocardiographic alterations associated with the three zones of myocardial infarction.

mics, such as lidocaine and amiodarone, do not improve mortality; however, individuals at high risk should be considered for implantable cardioverter-defibrillators (ICDs).

Acute myocardial infarction usually is accompanied by a reduction in cardiac output and some degree of left ventricular failure (congestive heart failure), which is characterized by pulmonary congestion, reduced myocardial contractility, and abnormal heart wall motion (see p. 1113). Anterior infarction is associated with more severe left heart failure than is inferior infarction. If cardiac output is insufficient to maintain normal arterial pressure and to perfuse the kidneys and other organs adequately, cardiogenic shock develops. Cardiogenic shock characteristically develops if 40% or more of the left ventricular myocardium is infarcted. (Cardiogenic shock is discussed in Chapter 46.)

Inflammation of the pericardium (pericarditis) is a common complication of acute myocardial infarction. Pericardial friction rubs often are noted 2 to 3 days after MI and are associated with anterior chest pain that worsens with respiratory effort. Specific treatment is not required; however, corticosteroids dramatically relieve symptoms.

Dressler postinfarction syndrome, which is essentially a delayed form of acute pericarditis, can occur from 1 week to several months after acute myocardial infarction. Although poorly understood, the syndrome is thought to be an immunologic (antigen-antibody) response to the necrotic myocardium. Pain, fever, friction rub, pleural effusion, and arthralgias may accompany this syndrome. Steroids may alleviate symptoms.

Organic brain syndrome may occur in acute or chronic form if blood flow to the brain is impaired secondary to MI. Transient ischemic attacks or an outright cerebrovascular accident may result from thromboemboli that have broken loose from the wall of the left ventricle or from cardiac valves.

Cardiac complications of MI can include rupture of heart structures. Necrosis of tissue in or around the papillary muscles can cause rupture of these muscles or of the chordae tendineae. Factors that lead to rupture of the free wall of the infarcted ventricle include thinning of the wall, poor collateral flow, shearing effect of muscular contraction against the stiffened necrotic area, marked necrosis at the terminal end of the blood supply, and aging of the myocardium with laceration of the myocardial microstructure.

Rupture of the wall of the infarcted ventricle may be a consequence of aneurysm formation. According to the law of Laplace, with decreased muscle mass at the infarcted site, the wall is weakened and tension stretches the noncontracting infarcted heart muscle, thus producing infarct expansion or aneurysm formation (see discussion of aneurysm, p. 1094). Decreased muscle mass causes an increase in the radius of the ventricle, and because the radius is directly proportional to pressure and tension, both increase with time. The wall of the aneurysm becomes more fibrotic but continues to bulge with systole. The bulge results in impaired pump function. Although rare, rupture may occur when the tension becomes too great. Death in individuals with a left ventricular aneurysm is usually related to ventricular tachydysrhythmias and not to ventricular

rupture. Left ventricular aneurysm is a late complication of MI, occurring months or years after the acute event.

Infarctions around septal structures that separate the heart chambers can lead to septal rupture. Ruptures are associated with audible, harsh cardiac murmurs, increased left ventricular end-diastolic pressure, and decreased systemic blood pressure.

Systemic thromboembolism is commonly found during postmortem examinations of individuals who have died of MI. Thromboemboli may disseminate from debris and clots that collect inside dilated aneurysmal sacs or from the infarcted endocardium. Pulmonary emboli are especially common, and result from the breaking loose of deep venous thrombi of the legs (see p. 991). Early mobilization and prophylactic anticoagulation therapy is essential to reduce the incidence of this complication.

Sudden death resulting from cardiac arrest is often caused by dysrhythmias, particularly ventricular fibrillation. Other dysrhythmias may be equally lethal. Widespread knowledge of cardiopulmonary resuscitation has increased the probability of survival during the first few hours after cardiac insult. Immediate intervention and careful monitoring also have reduced mortality and have improved chances for long-term survival. Several factors, however, contribute to the risk of death during acute infarction or reduce the chances of long-term survival, despite the best possible treatment. They are (1) degree of left ventricular dysfunction, (2) degree of left ventricular ischemia, (3) potential for ventricular dysrhythmias, and (4) age of the individual.

DISORDERS OF THE HEART WALL
Disorders of the Pericardium
Pericardial disease is often a localized manifestation of another disorder, such as infection (bacterial, viral, fungal, rickettsial, parasitic); trauma or surgery; neoplasm; or a metabolic, immunologic, or vascular disorder (uremia, rheumatoid arthritis, systemic lupus erythematosus, periarteritis nodosa). The pericardial response to injury from these diverse causes may consist of acute pericarditis, pericardial effusion, or constrictive pericarditis.

Acute Pericarditis
Although often idiopathic, **acute pericarditis** (acute inflammation of the pericardium) is also caused by surgery, infection, connective tissue disease, or radiation therapy. The pericardial membranes become inflamed and roughened, and an exudate may develop (Figure 30-27).

The primary symptom of acute pericarditis is the sudden onset of severe chest pain that worsens with respiratory movements and with lying down. Although the pain may radiate to the back, it is generally felt in the anterior chest and may be confused initially with the pain of acute myocardial infarction.[205,206] Individuals with acute pericarditis also may report dysphagia, restlessness, irritability, anxiety, weakness, and malaise.

Physical examination often discloses low-grade fever and sinus tachycardia. Friction rub—a short, scratchy, grating

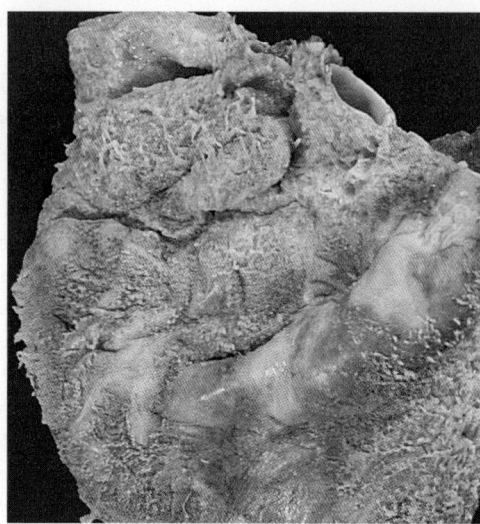

Figure 30-27 **Acute pericarditis.** Note shaggy coat of fibers covering surface of heart. (From Damjanov I, Linder J: *Pathology: a color atlas*, St Louis, 2000, Mosby.)

sensation similar to the sound of sandpaper—may be heard at the cardiac apex and left sternal border and is pathognomonic for pericarditis. The rub is caused by the roughened pericardial membranes rubbing against each other. Friction rubs are not always present and may be intermittently heard. ECG changes may reflect inflammatory processes through diffuse ST segment elevation without Q waves.[207] The ECG may remain abnormal for days or even weeks. Echocardiography may reveal a small pericardial effusion.

Treatment for uncomplicated acute pericarditis consists of relieving symptoms. Rest is helpful during episodes of acute pain. Salicylates and nonsteroidal antiinflammatory drugs reduce inflammation.[207] Combined nonsteroidals and colchicine (prevents fibrosis) is a highly effective regimen.[205,206] Additonal analgesics may be given to relieve pain, but doses or narcotics are limited to avoid excessive respiratory depression in individuals who are already limiting respiratory effort because of pain. Exploration of the underlying cause is important. If pericardial effusion develops, aspiration of the excessive fluid may be necessary. Acute pericarditis is usually self-limiting but occasionally may progress to chronic constrictive pericarditis.

Pericardial Effusion

Pericardial effusion—the accumulation of fluid in the pericardial cavity—can occur in all forms of pericarditis. The fluid may be a transudate, such as the serous effusion that develops with left heart failure, overhydration, or hypoproteinemia. More often, however, the fluid is an exudate, which reflects pericardial injury and inflammation. (Types of exudate are described in Chapter 6.) If the fluid is serosanguineous, the underlying cause is likely to be tuberculosis, neoplasm, uremia, or radiation. Idiopathic serosanguineous (cause unknown) effusion is possible, however. Effusions of frank blood are generally related to aneurysms, trauma, or coagulation defects. If chyle leaks from the thoracic duct, it may enter the pericardium and lead to cholesterol pericarditis.

Pericardial effusion, even in large amounts, is not necessarily clinically significant, except that it indicates an underlying disorder. The important consideration is whether the fluid creates sufficient pressure to cause cardiac compression, which is a serious condition known as **tamponade.** If an effusion develops gradually, the pericardium can stretch to accommodate large quantities of fluid without compressing the heart. If the fluid accumulates rapidly, however, even a small amount (50 to 100 ml) may cause serious tamponade. The danger is that pressure exerted by the pericardial fluid eventually will equal diastolic pressure within the heart chambers thus preventing chamber filling. The first structures to be affected by tamponade are the right atrium and ventricle, where diastolic pressures are normally lowest. Compression by pericardial fluid interferes with right atrial filling during diastole, resulting in increased venous pressure, systemic venous congestion, and signs and symptoms of right heart failure (distention of the jugular veins, edema, hepatomegaly). Decreased atrial filling leads to decreased ventricular filling, decreased stroke volume, and reduced cardiac output. Life-threatening circulatory collapse may occur.[206]

An important clinical finding in tamponade is pulsus paradoxus, in which arterial blood pressure during expiration exceeds arterial pressure during inspiration by more than 10 mmHg. This clinical finding reflects impairment of diastolic filling of the left ventricle plus reduction of blood volume within all four cardiac chambers. Presence of a large pericardial effusion or tamponade magnifies the normally insignificant effect of inspiration on intracardiac flow and volume.

Other clinical manifestations of pericardial effusion are distant or muffled heart sounds, poorly palpable apical pulse, dyspnea on exertion, and dull chest pain. A chest roentgenogram may disclose a "water-bottle" configuration of the cardiac silhouette. An echocardiogram can detect an effusion as small as 20 ml and is considered the most accurate and reliable method of diagnosis.

Treatment of pericardial effusion or tamponade generally consists of pericardiocentesis (aspiration of excessive pericardial fluid).[208] Pericardiocentesis is both diagnostic and therapeutic: the fluid is analyzed to identify the cause of the effusion, and its removal alone may bring dramatic relief from symptoms. Persistent pain may be treated with analgesics, antiinflammatory medications, or steroids. Surgery may be required if the underlying cause of tamponade is trauma or aneurysm.

Individuals with acute pericarditis secondary to certain underlying conditions may have pericardial effusion.[206] This manifestation is common in (1) individuals with uremia who are in need of dialysis and have fluid overload and left ventricular failure; (2) individuals who have lymphoma or breast cancer or who are receiving radiation therapy; (3) individuals who are taking drugs such as procainamide and minoxidil; and (4) individuals who have undergone surgery that involved an incision of the heart wall. If the effusion recurs, a pericardial "window" can be created or the individual may require pericardectomy.[206] If an effusion is neoplasm induced, chemotherapeutic agents may be injected into the pericardial space. Minocycline or mitoxantrone also may be injected into the pericardium to induce pericardial sclerosis and prevent further fluid accumulation.[209]

Constrictive Pericarditis

Constrictive pericarditis or **restrictive pericarditis** (**chronic pericarditis**) was synonymous with tuberculosis years ago (Figure 30-28). Currently in the United States, this form of pericardial disease is more often idiopathic or associated with radiation exposure, rheumatoid arthritis, uremia, or coronary artery bypass graft.[206] In constrictive pericarditis, fibrous scarring with occasional calcification of the pericardium causes the visceral and parietal pericardial layers to adhere, obliterating the pericardial cavity. The fibrotic lesions encase the heart in a rigid shell. Like tamponade, constrictive pericarditis compresses the heart and eventually reduces cardiac output. Unlike tamponade, however, constrictive pericarditis never develops suddenly.

Because the onset of constrictive pericarditis is gradual, clinical manifestations seldom include pulsus paradoxus. Symptoms tend to be exercise intolerance, dyspnea on exertion, fatigue, and anorexia. Clinical assessment shows weight loss, edema, distention of the jugular vein, and hepatic congestion. Restricted ventricular filling may cause a pericardial knock (early diastolic sound).

ECG findings include T wave inversions and atrial fibrillation. An echocardiogram may suggest evidence of nonspecific pericardial thickening. CT or MRI is best able to detect constrictive processes.[210] Chest roentgenograms often disclose prominent pulmonary vessels and calcification of the pericardium. Some individuals require diagnostic thoracotomy in order to make the diagnosis, especially in cases of postoperative restrictive pericarditis.

Initial treatment for constrictive pericarditis consists of dietary sodium restriction, digitalis glycosides and diuretics to improve cardiac output. If these modalities are not successful, surgical excision of the restrictive pericardium is indicated. After surgery, most individuals exhibit significant improvement. For individuals with severe restrictive disease, pericardiectomy may prevent untimely death from heart failure.[211]

Disorders of the Myocardium: The Cardiomyopathies

The **cardiomyopathies** are a diverse group of diseases that primarily affect the myocardium itself. Most are the result of underlying cardiovascular disorders, such as ischemic heart disease or hypertension. Cardiomyopathies also can be secondary to infectious disease, exposure to toxins, systemic connective tissue disease, infiltrative and proliferative disorders, or nutritional deficiencies. Despite this large number of possible causes, most cases of cardiomyopathy are idiopathic; that is, their cause is unknown. The cardiomyopathies are categorized as dilated, hypertrophic, restrictive, or obliterative, depending on their hemodynamic effects[212] (Figure 30-29 and

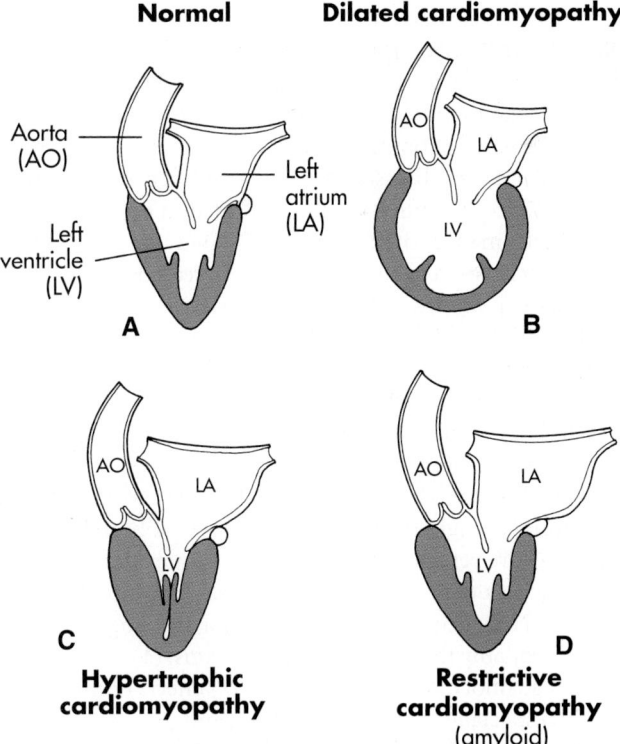

Figure 30-29 Diagram showing major distinguishing pathophysiologic features of the types of cardiomyopathy. **A,** The normal heart. **B,** In the dilated type of cardiomyopathy, the heart has a globular shape and the largest circumference of the left ventricle is not at its base but midway between apex and base. **C,** In the hypertrophic type the wall of the left ventricle is greatly thickened; the left ventricular cavity is small, but the left atrium may be dilated because of poor diastolic relaxation of the ventricle. **D,** In the restrictive type the left ventricular cavity is of normal size, but again, the left atrium is dilated because of the reduced diastolic compliance of the ventricle. (From Kissane JM, editor: *Anderson's pathology,* ed 9, St Louis, 1990, Mosby.)

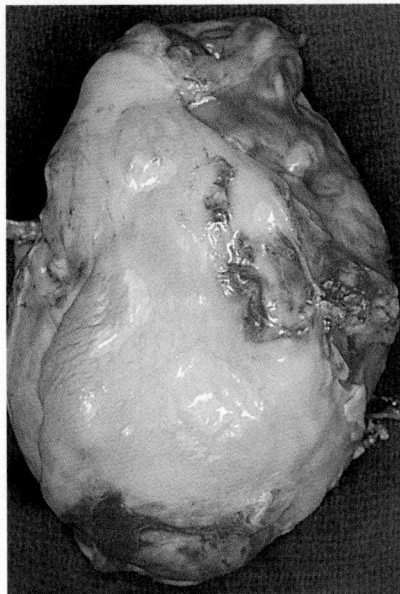

Figure 30-28 Constrictive pericarditis. The fibrotic pericardium encases the heart in a rigid shell. (From Damjanov I, Linder J: *Pathology: a color atlas,* St Louis, 2000, Mosby.)

Table 30-7	Effects of Cardiomyopathies on Circulation Through the Heart		
	Type of Cardiomyopathy		
Effect	**Dilated**	**Hypertrophic**	**Restrictive**
Hemodynamic			
Cardiac output	Decreased	Normal	Normal or decreased
Stroke volume	Decreased	Normal or increased	Decreased
Ventricular filling pressure	Increased	Normal or increased	Increased
Ejection fraction	Decreased	Increased	Normal or decreased
Inflow resistance	Normal	Increased	Increased
Outflow tract obstruction	None	Increased	None
Formation of intracardiac thrombi	Increased	None	Increased
Structural or Functional			
Chamber size	Increased	Normal or decreased	Decreased or normal
Myocardial mass	Increased	Increased	Normal or increased
Endocardial thickness	Normal or increased	Increased	Increased
Contractility	Decreased	Increased or decreased	Normal or decreased
Mitral valve competence	Decreased	Decreased	Decreased

Data from Wynne J, Braunwald E: The cardiomyopathies. In Zipes DP et al: *Braunwald's heart disease,* ed 7, Philadelphia, 2005, Saunders.

Table 30-7). An individual may display characteristics of more than one type.

Dilated Cardiomyopathy

Dilated cardiomyopathy (congestive cardiomyopathy) is characterized by ventricular dilation and grossly impaired systolic function, leading to dilated heart failure (Figure 30-30). The most common causes are ischemic heart disease or valvular heart disease. The basic problem is diminished myocardial contractility, which is reflected in diminished systolic performance of the heart. Dilated cardiomyopathy causes decreased ejection fractions, increased end-diastolic and residual volumes, decreased ventricular stroke volume, and biventricular failure.

About one half of the cases of dilated cardiomyopathy are idiopathic, and the remainder result from some known disease process. Secondary causes of dilated cardiomyopathy include ischemic heart disease, drug toxicity, hyperthyroidism, and valvular heart disease. Idiopathic dilated cardiomyopathy has a familial origin in 20% to 30% of cases, although the specific genes are yet to be identified. A disproportionate number of individuals with idiopathic dilated cardiomyopathy are alcoholics. Heavy consumption of alcohol is thought to cause cardiomyopathy through three mechanisms: (1) a direct toxic effect of alcohol or of its metabolites; (2) effects of nutritional deficits, especially thiamine deficiency; and (3) toxic effects of beverage additives such as cobalt. In addition, chronic alcoholic cardiomyopathy may be related to underlying viral infection. In contrast to other forms of cardiomyopathy, the progression of myocardial dysfunction may be stopped or reversed if alcohol consumption is reduced or stopped early in the course of the disease.[213]

Peripartum cardiomyopathy is another idiopathic form of dilated cardiomyopathy. The cardiomyopathy usually develops in the first 3 to 4 months after completion of a pregnancy,

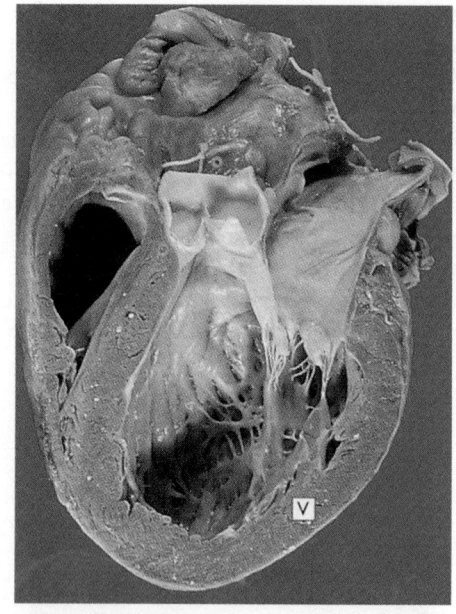

Figure 30-30 Dilated cardiomyopathy. The dilated left ventricle has a thin wall *(V).* (From Stevens A, Lowe J: *Pathology,* St Louis, 1995, Mosby.)

after the period of maximum physiologic stress is thought to have ended.[214] A few cases have resulted from acute myocardial inflammation (myocarditis).

Dilated cardiomyopathies also may be the late consequences of previous viral, bacterial, or parasitic infections or an autoimmune process. Inflammatory and immune responses include release of cytokines and interleukins resulting in significant myocarditis and contractile function.[215,216] This type of cardiomyopathy is classified as "inflammatory cardiomyopathy" by the World Health Organzation.[212] (Pathophysiologic effects of the cardiomyopathies are summarized in Table 30-8.)

Table 30-8	Pathophysiologic Effects of the Cardiomyopathies		
	Type of Cardiomyopathy		
Pathophysiology	**Dilated**	**Hypertrophic**	**Restrictive**
Major symptoms	Fatigue, weakness, palpitations	Dyspnea, angina pectoris, fatigue, dizziness (syncope), palpitations	Dyspnea, fatigue
Cardiomegaly	Moderate to marked	Mild to moderate	Mild
Hypertrophy	Left ventricular myocardium	Left ventricular myocardium and interventricular septum	Left ventricular myocardium
Alterations of chamber volume	Volume increased	Volume decreased, particularly in left ventricle	Volume normal to decreased
Alterations of chamber compliance	Compliance increased	Compliance decreased, particularly in left ventricle	Compliance decreased, particularly in left ventricle
Alterations of systolic function (myocardial contractility)	Contractility decreased in left ventricle	Contractility increased or vigorous	None
Valvular incompetence	Atrioventricular valves, particularly mitral	Mitral valve	Atrioventricular valve
Conduction defects	Intraventricular	Nonspecific	Atrioventricular
Dysrhythmias	Sinoatrial tachycardia; atrial and ventricular dysrhythmias	Atrial and ventricular dysrhythmias	Tachydysrhythmias
Thromboembolism	Systemic or pulmonary	Systemic or pulmonary	Systemic or pulmonary
Associated conditions	Alcoholism, pregnancy, infection, nutritional deficiency, exposure to toxins	Possible inherited defect of muscle growth and development	Infiltrative disease
Eventual cardiovascular event	Left heart failure	Left heart failure	Right heart failure

The most common symptoms of dilated cardiomyopathy are dyspnea and fatigue. Pulmonary congestion is expected, but acute pulmonary edema is not. Palpitations are common, and associated dysrhythmias may cause dizziness (syncope). Systemic and pulmonary emboli are common complications. Chest pain may be present, but it is unlike anginal pain.

In the presence of dilated heart failure, blood pressure is often elevated. Extra heart sounds and cardiac murmurs may be present as well. Dilated cardiomyopathy may be difficult to distinguish from acute myocarditis, valvular heart disease, CAD, and hypertensive heart disease. Echocardiography and MRI can confirm the diagnosis.

Treatment for dilated cardiomyopathy consists of salt restriction and the prescription of digitalis glycosides, vasodilators, and diuretics. Anticoagulants are given to prevent pulmonary and systemic embolism. Bed rest for extended periods can be used to reduce the workload of the weakened heart. Corticosteroids and immunosuppressants can benefit individuals with documented inflammatory disease, and vasodilators are administered to combat congestion. Venous dilation reduces preload by promoting peripheral venous pooling, thereby decreasing central blood volume and alleviating pulmonary congestion. Arterial dilation reduces afterload and aortic impedance, making it easier for the failing left ventricle to eject blood. Combinations of these drugs have been effective in improving symptoms, although there is no indication that they prolong life. Myocardial pacemakers (pacing) can improve cardiac output in many individuals.[217] Cardiac transplantation may be lifesaving.

The prognosis is variable and depends on the degree of ventricular dysfunction. Left heart failure is the cause of death in 75% of individuals. Sudden death caused by dysrhythmias also occurs. The majority of deaths occur within 5 years.

Hypertrophic Cardiomyopathy

Hypertrophic cardiomyopathy refers to two major categories of thickening of the myocardium: (1) asymmetrical setpal hypertrophic cardiomyopathy (subaortic stenosis) and (2) hypertensive or valvular hypertrophic cardiomyopathy. These two categories are very different in their etiology, pathophysiology, and clinical presentation.

Asymmetrical septal hypertrophy is often called "idiopathic hypertrophic cardiomyopathy." It is an autosomal dominant inherited disorder that results in thickening of the septal wall (Figure 30-31), which may cause outflow obstruction to the left ventricle.[218,219] Additional changes include abnormalities of collagen deposition and altered contractile proteins in the myocytes. The thickening of the septum results in a hyperdynamic state, especially with exercise. Diastolic relaxation also is impaired and ventricular compliance is decreased. Obstruction of left ventricular outflow can occur when heart rate is increased and intravascular volume is decreased.[218] Individuals complain of angina, syncope, palpitations, and symptoms of myocardial infarction and left heart failure. Examination may reveal extra heart sounds and murmurs. Echocardiography and cardiac catheterization can confirm the diagnosis. This type of hypertrophic cardiomyopathy is a significant risk for serious ventricular arrhythmias and sudden death. Management in-

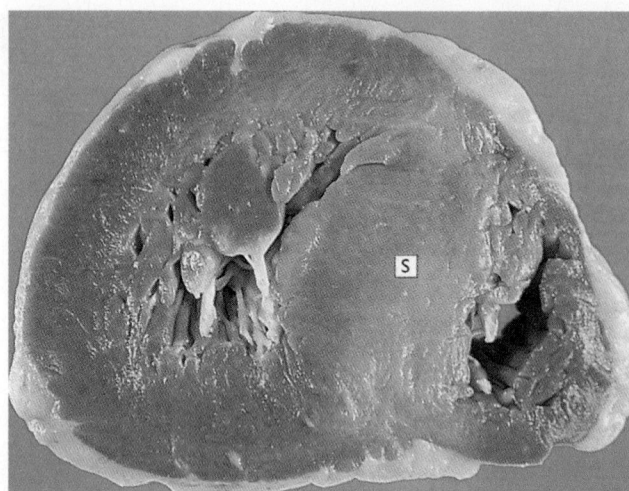

Figure 30-31 Hypertrophic cardiomyopathy. There is marked left ventricular hypertrophy. This often affects the septum *(S)*. (From Stevens A, Lowe J: *Pathology,* St Louis, 1995, Mosby.)

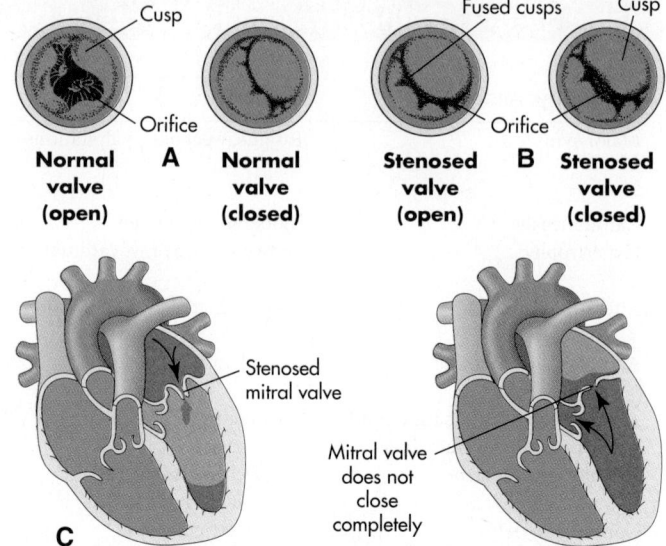

Figure 30-32 Valvular stenosis and regurgitation. **A,** Normal position of the valve leaflets, or cusps, when the valve is open and closed. **B,** Open position of a stenosed valve (left) and open position of a closed regurgitant valve (right). **C,** Hemodynamic effect of mitral stenosis. The stenosed valve is unable to open sufficiently during left atrial systole, inhibiting left ventricular filling. **D,** Hemodynamic effect of mitral regurgitation. The mitral valve does not close completely during left ventricular systole, permitting blood to reenter the left atrium.

cludes beta-blockers to slow the heart rate, surgical resection of the hypertrophied myocardium, and prophylactic placement of an implantable cardioverter-defibrillator in high-risk individuals.[219-222]

Hypertensive, or **valvular hypertrophic, cardiomyopathy** occurs because of increased resistance to ventricular ejection commonly seen in hypertension or in valvular stenosis (usually aortic). In this case, hypertrophy of the myocytes is an attempt to compensate for increased workload, however, long-term dysfunction of the myocytes develops over time, with diastolic dysfunction leading eventually to systolic dysfunction of the ventricle (see "Heart Failure," p. 1129).

Restrictive Cardiomyopathies

Restrictive cardiomyopathy usually is caused by an infiltrative disease of the myocardium, such as amyloidosis, hemochromatosis, or glycogen storage disease. The myocardium becomes rigid and noncompliant, impeding ventricular filling and raising filling pressures during diastole. The overall clinical and hemodynamic picture mimics and may be confused with that of constrictive pericarditis.

The most common clinical manifestation of restrictive cardiomyopathy is congestive heart failure, particularly right heart failure. Cardiomegaly and dysrhythmias are common. In most cases there is no therapy for restrictive cardiomyopathy other than treating the underlying disease process. Death occurs as a result of congestive failure or dysrhythmias.

Disorders of the Endocardium
Valvular Dysfunction
Disorders of the endocardium, the innermost lining of the heart wall, all damage the heart valves, which are made up of endocardial tissue. Endocardial damage can be either congenital or acquired. The acquired forms cause inflammatory, ischemic, traumatic, degenerative, or infectious alterations of valvular structure and function.

The usual cause of acquired valvular dysfunction is inflammation of the endocardium secondary to acute rheumatic fever or infective endocarditis (see p. 1124). Structural alterations of the heart valves lead to stenosis, incompetence, or both.

In **valvular stenosis** the valve orifice is constricted and narrowed, impeding the forward flow of blood and increasing the workload of the cardiac chamber "behind" the diseased valve (Figure 30-32). Intraventricular or atrial pressure increases in the chamber to overcome resistance to flow through the valve. Increased pressure causes the myocardium to work harder, causing myocardial hypertrophy. In **valvular regurgitation** (also called *insufficiency* or *incompetence*) the valve leaflets, or cusps, fail to shut completely, permitting blood flow to continue even when the valve is supposed to be closed (see Figure 30-32). During systole some blood leaks back into the chamber "upstream." Valvular regurgitation increases the volume of blood the heart must pump and increases the workload of the affected heart chamber. Increased volume leads to chamber dilation, and increased workload leads to hypertrophy. Although all four heart valves may be affected, those of the left heart (mitral and aortic semilunar valves) are far more commonly affected than those of the right heart (tricuspid and pulmonic semilunar valves).

Valvular dysfunction stimulates chamber dilation and myocardial hypertrophy, both of which are compensatory mechanisms intended to increase the pumping capability of the heart. Eventually, myocardial contractility is diminished, the ejection fraction is reduced, diastolic pressure increases, and the ventricles fail from overwork. Depending on the severity of the valvular dysfunction and the capacity of the heart to compensate, valvular alterations cause a range of symptoms and some degree of incapacitation (Table 30-9). The effects of valvular dysfunction are treated with cardiac glycosides, diuretics, dietary salt restriction, and antibiotics until prosthetic valve replacement becomes necessary.

Stenosis

Aortic Stenosis. **Aortic stenosis** has three common causes: (1) inflammatory damage caused by rheumatic heart disease, (2) congenital malformation (see Chapter 3), and (3) degeneration thickening and calcification (see Chapter 2). Evidence suggests that degenerative aortic stenosis is linked to hyperlipidemia and that its prevalence might be decreased by more aggressive lipid lowering in adults.[223] The orifice of the aortic semilunar valve narrows, causing diminished blood flow from the left ventricle into the aorta (see Figures 30-32 and 30-33). Outflow obstruction increases pressure within the left ventricle as it tries to eject blood through the narrowed opening.

Aortic stenosis tends to develop gradually. Clinical manifestations include decreased stroke volume, reduced systolic blood pressure, and narrowed pulse pressure (difference between systolic and diastolic pressure). Heart rate is often slow, and pulses are faint. Resistance to flow gives rise to a crescendo-decrescendo systolic heart murmur. Left ventricular hypertrophy develops to compensate for the increased workload. Eventually, hypertrophy increases myocardial oxygen demand, which the coronary arteries may not be able to

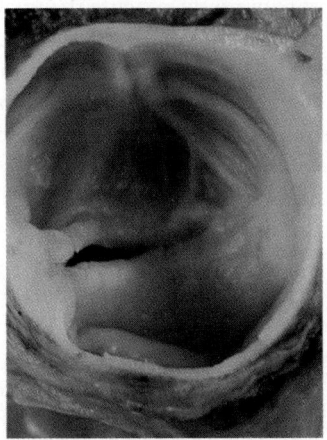

Figure 30-33 Aortic stenosis. Mild stenosis in valve leaflets of a young adult. (From Damjanov I, Linder J: *Pathophysiology: a color atlas*, St Louis, 2000, Mosby.)

Table 30-9	Clinical Manifestations of Valvular Stenosis and Regurgitation				
Manifestation	Aortic Stenosis	Mitral Stenosis	Aortic Regurgitation	Mitral Regurgitation	Tricuspid Regurgitation
Cardiovascular outcome*	Left ventricular failure	Right ventricular failure	Left heart failure	Left heart failure	Right heart failure
General symptoms	Fatigue	Fatigue, weakness		Fatigue, weakness	Peripheral edema (with heart failure)
Respiratory effects	Dyspnea on exertion	Dyspnea on exertion, orthopnea, paroxysmal nocturnal dyspnea, predisposition to respiratory infections, hemoptysis, pulmonary hypertension, edema	Dyspnea with effort	Dyspnea; occasional hemoptysis	Dyspnea
Central nervous system effects	Syncope, especially on exertion	Neural deficits only associated with emboli (e.g., hemiparesis)	Syncope	None	None
Gastrointestinal effects	None	Ascites; hepatic angina with hepatomegaly	None	None	Ascites, hepatomegaly (with heart failure)
Pain	Angina pectoris	Chest pain	Chest pain (anginal)	None	Palpitations
Heart rate, rhythm	Bradycardia, dysrhythmias (with heart failure)	Palpitations (atrial fibrillation)	Palpitations, water-hammer pulse	Palpitations	Atrial fibrillations
Heart sounds	Systolic murmur	Diastolic murmur, accentuated first heart sound, opening snap	Diastolic and systolic murmurs	Murmur throughout systole	Murmur throughout systole
Most common cause	Congenital, rheumatic fever	Rheumatic fever	Bacterial endocarditis; aortic root disease	Floppy valve; coronary artery disease	Congenital

Data from Zipes DP et al: *Braunwald's heart disease*, ed 7, Philadelphia, 2005, Saunders.
*Untreated disease.

supply. If this occurs, ischemia may cause attacks of angina. Untreated aortic stenosis can lead to dysrhythmias, myocardial infarction, and heart failure. Most symptoms of aortic stenosis are attributable to diminished stroke volume, which results in diminished tissue perfusion.

Mitral Stenosis. **Mitral stenosis** impairs the flow of blood from the left atrium to the left ventricle. Mitral stenosis is caused most commonly by acute rheumatic fever or bacterial endocarditis, although uncommonly it can be congenital. Narrowing of the orifice occurs as inflammatory lesions in the valvular leaflets heal (Figure 30-34). Scarring causes the leaflets to become fibrous and fused and the chordae tendineae to become shortened.

Clinical manifestations depend on the size of the valvular orifice. Impedance to blood flow results in incomplete emptying of the left atrium and elevated atrial pressure as the chamber tries to force blood through the stenotic valve. Continued increases in left atrial volume and pressure cause chamber dilation and hypertrophy. The risk of developing atrial dysrhythmias (especially fibrillation) and dysrhythmia-induced thrombi is high. As mitral stenosis progresses, symptoms of decreased cardiac output occur, especially during exertion. Continued elevation of left atrial pressure and volume causes pressure to rise in the pulmonary circulation. The outcomes of untreated chronic mitral stenosis are pulmonary hypertension, edema, and right ventricular failure.

Atrial enlargement is demonstrated by chest roentgenograms and electrocardiography. Blood flow through the stenotic valve gives rise to a rumbling decrescendo diastolic murmur. The first heart sound (S_1) is often accentuated and somewhat delayed because of increased left atrial pressure. If the valve snaps open during diastole, a sharp diastolic sound called an "opening snap" may be heard. Other signs and symptoms are generally those of pulmonary congestion and right heart failure.

Regurgitation
Aortic Regurgitation. **Aortic regurgitation** is caused by a variety of disorders that affect the valve cusps and aortic root, such as rheumatic fever, bacterial endocarditis, syphilis,

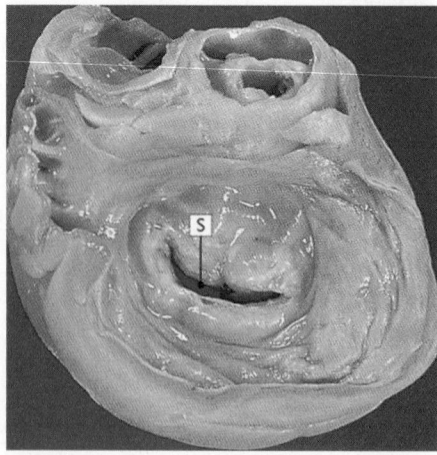

Figure 30-34 Mitral stenosis with classic "fish mouth" orifice. (From Stevens A, Lowe J: *Pathology*, ed 2, St Louis, 2000, Mosby.)

hypertension, connective tissue disorders (e.g., Marfan syndrome), and atherosclerosis. The hemodynamic repercussions depend on the size of the "leak." During systole, blood is ejected from the left ventricle into the aorta. If the aortic semilunar valve fails to close completely, some of the ejected blood flows back into the left ventricle. Volume overload occurs in the ventricle because it receives blood from the left atrium during diastole and blood from the aorta during systole. Over time, the end-diastolic volume of the left ventricle increases and myocardial fibers stretch to accommodate the extra fluid. Compensatory dilation permits the left ventricle to increase its stroke volume and maintain cardiac output. Ventricular dilation and hypertrophy eventually cease to compensate for aortic incompetence, and heart failure develops.

Clinical manifestations include widened pulse pressure resulting from increased stroke volume and diastolic backflow. Turbulence across the aortic valve during diastole produces a characteristic murmur. Large stroke volume and rapid runoff of blood from the aorta result in prominent carotid pulsations and throbbing peripheral pulses (water-hammer pulse). Other symptoms are usually associated with heart failure that occurs when the ventricle can no longer enlarge. Dysrhythmias and endocarditis are common complications of aortic regurgitation.

Mitral Regurgitation. **Mitral regurgitation**, unlike mitral stenosis, has a variety of causes. The most common are mitral valve prolapse and rheumatic heart disease. Other causes include infective endocarditis, CAD, connective tissue diseases (Marfan syndrome), and congestive cardiomyopathy. Mitral regurgitation permits backflow of blood from the left ventricle into the left atrium during ventricular systole, giving rise to a loud pansystolic (throughout systole) murmur that radiates into the back and axilla. The left ventricle becomes dilated and hypertrophied to maintain adequate cardiac output, despite increased volume from the left atrium. The volume of backflow reentering the left atrium gradually increases, causing atrial dilation. As the left atrium enlarges, the valve structures stretch and become deformed, leading to further backflow. As mitral valve regurgitation progresses, left ventricular function may become impaired to the point of failure. Eventually, increased atrial pressure also causes pulmonary hypertension and failure of the right ventricle. Mitral incompetence is usually well tolerated—often for years—until ventricular failure occurs. Most clinical manifestations are caused by heart failure.

Tricuspid Regurgitation. **Tricuspid regurgitation** is more common than tricuspid stenosis and usually is associated with cardiac failure and dilation of the right ventricle secondary to high pressures in the pulmonary circulation (usually due to hypoxic lung disease or pulmonary emboli). Rheumatic heart disease and infective endocarditis are less common causes. Tricuspid valve incompetence leads to volume overload in the right ventricle, increased systemic venous blood pressure, and right heart failure. Pulmonic semilunar valve dysfunction can have the same consequences as tricuspid valve dysfunction.

Mitral Valve Prolapse Syndrome

Mitral valve prolapse syndrome is a condition in which the anterior and posterior cusps of the mitral valve billow upward (prolapse) into the atrium during systole (Figure 30-35). The cusps are enlarged, thickened, and scalloped, possibly secondary to collagenous abnormalities, and the chordae tendineae may be elongated, permitting the valve cusps to stretch upward. Mitral regurgitation occurs if the ballooning valve permits blood to leak into the atrium.

Although previous studies have suggested that the prevalence of mitral valve prolapse may be as high as 5% to 35%, a recent estimate suggests it is much less common (less than 3%). Mitral valve prolapse tends to be most prevalent in young women. Studies suggest an autosomal dominant inheritance pattern. Because mitral valve prolapse often is associated with other inherited connective tissue disorders (Marfan syndrome, Ehlers-Danlos syndrome, osteogenesis imperfecta), it may result from a genetic or environmental disruption of valvular development during the fifth or sixth week of gestation. There may be a relationship between symptomatic mitral valve prolapse and hyperthyroidism. Other neuroendocrine abnormalities have been suggested, including polymorphisms of the Ang II type 1 (AT_1) receptor.

Many cases of mitral valve prolapse are completely asymptomatic. Cardiac auscultation on routine physical examination may disclose a regurgitant murmur or midsystolic click in an otherwise healthy individual, or echocardiography may demonstrate the condition in the absence of auscultatory findings. Symptomatic mitral valve prolapse can cause palpitations related to dysrhythmias, tachycardia, light-headedness, syncope, fatigue (especially in the morning), lethargy, weakness, dyspnea, chest tightness, hyperventilation, anxiety, depression, panic attacks, and atypical chest pain. Many symptoms are vague and puzzling and are unrelated to the degree of prolapse. Mitral valve prolapse was once considered a psychiatric malady. Research has suggested that individuals with mitral valve prolapse have an autonomic dysfunction in which inordinate quantities of catecholamines are produced, with or without adrenergic stimulation. This finding could

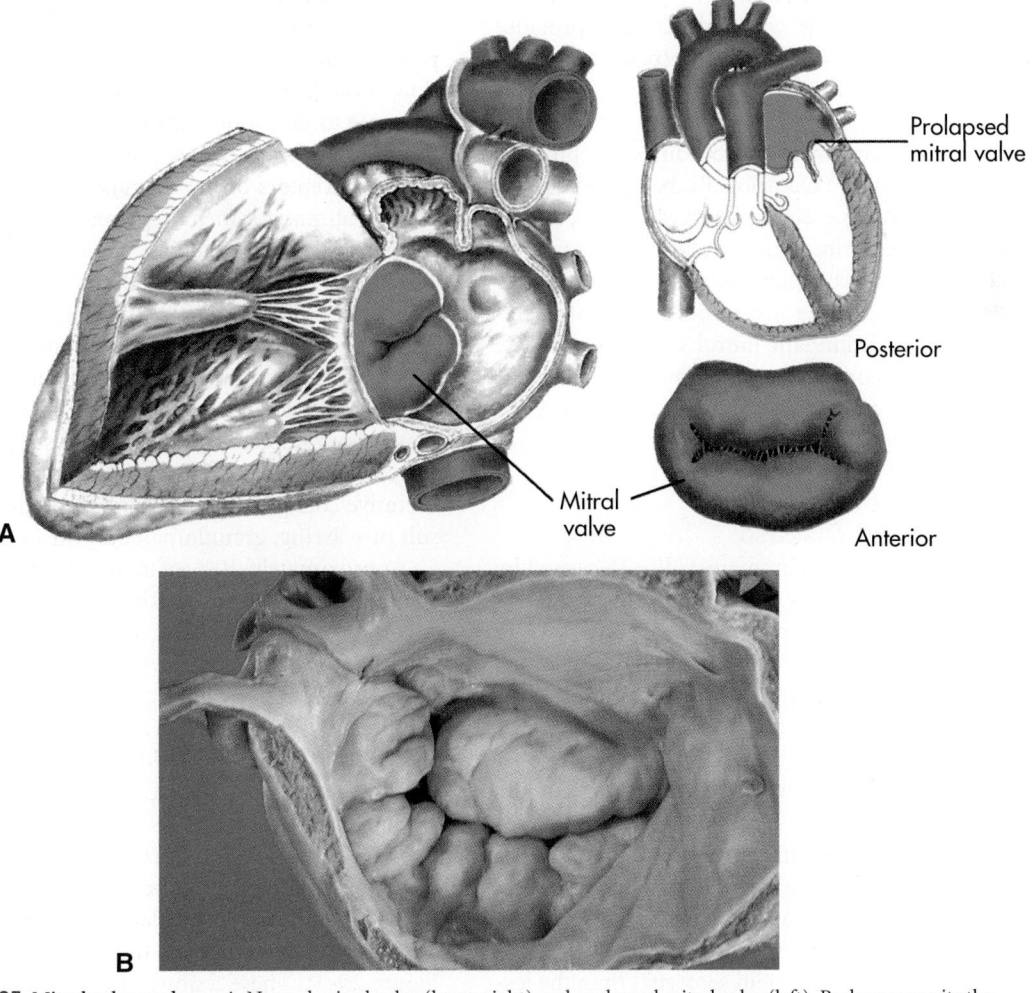

Figure 30-35 Mitral valve prolapse. **A,** Normal mitral valve (lower right) and prolapsed mitral valve (left). Prolapse permits the valve leaflets to billow back into the atrium during left ventricular systole. The billowing causes the leaflets to part slightly, permitting regurgitation into the atrium. **B,** Looking down on the mitral valve, the ballooning of the leaflets is seen. (**B** from Stevens A, Lowe J: *Pathology,* St Louis, 1995, Mosby.)

explain why mitral valve prolapse causes such a variety of subjective complaints. Although severe sequelae—such as chordae rupture, ventricular failure, systemic emboli, and sudden death—are possible, the disorder is actually associated with minimal mortality and morbidity. Most individuals experience no physical limitations. In fact, the psychologic effects of chest pain and knowledge of the diagnosis may be more disabling than the disease itself.

EVALUATION AND TREATMENT   The diagnosis of valvular heart disease is most often made by echocardiography. Cardiac catheterization is done prior to surgery to more directly evaluate valve structure and function as well as cardiac output. Valvular heart disease can often be managed temporarily with medications, such as diuretics and vasodilators. However, most significant valvular abnormalities eventually require surgical intervention either by repair of the valve or replacement with either a porcine or mechanical valve.[224,225] In the case of mechanical valve replacement, life-long antibiotic prophylaxis prior to invasive procedures is required, as is life-long anticoagulation to prevent clot formation on the valve with the possibility of embolization.

The majority of individuals with mitral valve prolapse have very few complications and require no treatment. Management is matched to the degree of mitral regurgitation. If regurgitation is present, antibiotic prophylaxis for infective endocarditis is given before invasive procedures but physical activities are not restricted.[228] Occasionally, beta-blockers are required to alleviate syncope, severe chest pain, or palpitations. Hypovolemia (resulting from diuretics or donating blood) is avoided because it can decrease ventricular volume, thereby increasing stress on the prolapsed mitral valve. Because surgical repair of redundant mitral valve tissue is safe and effective, some surgeons are now recommending operative treatment even in asymptomatic individuals to reduce the risk of stroke or sudden death.[226,227]

Acute Rheumatic Fever and Rheumatic Heart Disease

Rheumatic fever is a diffuse, inflammatory disease caused by a delayed immune response to infection by the group A β-hemolytic streptococcus. In its acute form, rheumatic fever is a febrile illness characterized by inflammation of the joints, skin, nervous system, and heart. If untreated, rheumatic fever can cause scarring and deformity of cardiac structures, resulting in **rheumatic heart disease.**

The incidence of acute rheumatic fever declined in the United States during the 1960s, 1970s, and early 1980s because of medical and socioeconomic improvements, as well as changes in the virulence of group A streptococci. Recent outbreaks in the United States and abroad corresponded to the reappearance of highly virulent strains. These virulent microorganisms have different M protein serotypes than the less pathogenic strains and can be identified as nephritogenic or rheumatogenic.[229] Because crowding and poor hygiene are environmental risk factors for acute rheumatic fever, the dis-

ease continues to be a major cause of death and disability for underprivileged populations.

The acute disease occurs most often in children between 5 and 15 years of age. Only 3% of those in whom pharyngeal streptococcal infection develops acquire acute rheumatic fever. Because the β-hemolytic streptococcus infection must persist for some time to cause acute rheumatic fever, appropriate antibiotic therapy given within the first 9 days of infection usually prevents rheumatic fever. Initiation of antibiotic therapy 2 weeks after the start of streptococcal infection does not prevent rheumatic fever in susceptible individuals.

The incidence of rheumatic fever tends to run in families, lending support to the concept of genetic predisposition, perhaps involving an abnormal immune response to antigens expressed by the bacterial membrane. Individuals who have experienced one attack of acute rheumatic fever are more susceptible than the general population to recurrent attacks.

PATHOPHYSIOLOGY   Acute rheumatic fever can develop *only* as a sequel to pharyngeal infection by group A β-hemolytic streptococcus. Streptococcal skin infections do not progress to acute rheumatic fever, although both skin and pharyngeal infections can cause acute glomerulonephritis. Acute rheumatic fever probably affects the heart, joints, central nervous system, and skin through an abnormal humoral and cell-mediated immune response to the M proteins on the microorgamisms that cross react with normal tissues (Figure 30-36). These antigens can bind to receptors on heart, muscle, and brain cells. They also have an affinity for membrane receptors within synovial joints, where they trigger an autoimmune response.

Diffuse, proliferative, and exudative inflammatory lesions develop in the connective tissues, especially in the heart, joints, and skin. The inflammation may subside before treatment, leaving behind damage to the heart valves and increasing the individual's susceptibility to recurrent acute rheumatic fever after any subsequent streptococcal infections. Repeated attacks of acute rheumatic fever cause chronic proliferative changes in the previously mentioned organs as a result of scarring, granulomas, and thromboses.

Approximately 10% of cases of rheumatic fever develop rheumatic heart disease. Rheumatic heart disease begins as **carditis,** or inflammation of the heart. Even mild cases of rheumatic fever can cause carditis in all three layers of the heart wall (endocardium, myocardium, pericardium; see Chapter 29, Figure 29-2). The primary lesion usually involves the endocardium, which lines the heart chambers and includes the heart valves. Endocardial inflammation causes swelling of the valve leaflets, with secondary erosion along the lines of leaflet contact. Small, beadlike clumps of vegetation containing platelets and fibrin are deposited on eroded valvular tissue and on the chordae tendineae (Figure 30-37). (The chordae tendineae anchor the valve leaflets; see Chapter 29, Figure 29-3). These lesions can become progressively adherent. Scarring and shortening of the involved structures occur over time. The valves lose their elasticity, and the leaflets may adhere to each other.

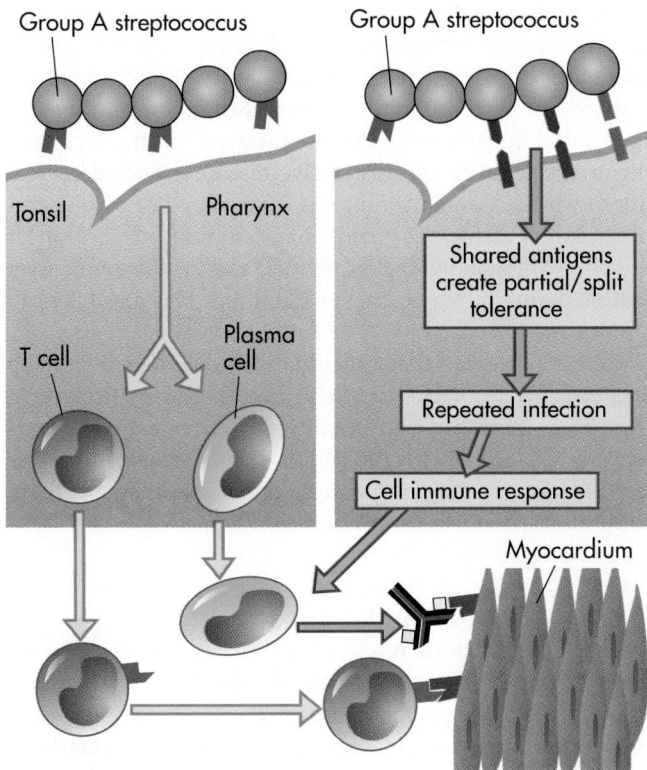

Figure 30-36 Possible mechanisms whereby molecular mimicry could help induce rheumatic fever. *Left,* Group A streptococci infecting the pharynx and sensitizing both B cells primed for humoral antibody response and T cells capable of cell-mediated immune response against streptococcal cross-reacting epitopes within autologous tissues, such as the heart. *Right,* An alternative pathologic mechanism whereby sharing of antigens between the streptococcus and various autologous human tissues allows a state of partial tolerance to exist. This in turn down-regulates an effective eliminative immune response by the host and sets the stage for a series of indolent repetitive group A streptococcal infections, eventually producing rheumatic heart disease through the direct cross-reactive mechanisms shown.

If inflammation penetrates the myocardium, localized fibrin deposits develop that are surrounded by areas of necrosis. These fibrinoid necrotic deposits are called *Aschoff bodies.* Pericardial inflammation is usually characterized by serofibrinous effusion within the pericardial cavity. Cardiomegaly and left heart failure may occur during episodes of untreated acute or recurrent rheumatic fever. Conduction defects and atrial fibrillation are often associated with rheumatic heart disease.

CLINICAL MANIFESTATIONS   Many common clinical manifestations of acute rheumatic fever—fever, lymphadenopathy, arthralgia, nausea, vomiting, epistaxis, abdominal pain, and tachycardia—are associated with other disorders as well and are by no means diagnostic of the disease. The major specific manifestations of acute rheumatic fever are carditis, acute migratory polyarthritis, chorea, and erythema marginatum, which may occur singly or in combination after a latent period of 1 to 5 weeks after streptococcal infection of the pharynx.

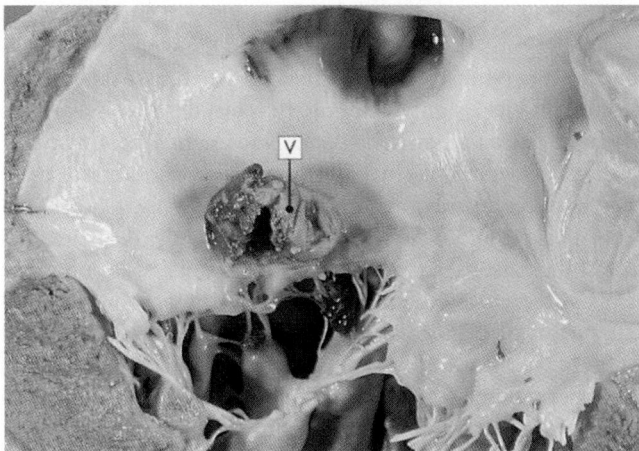

Figure 30-37 Mitral stenosis. Mitral stenosis and clumps of vegetation *(V)* containing platelets and fibrin. Mitral leaflets are thickened and fused and have clumps of vegetation containing platelets and fibrin. (From Stevens A, Lowe J: *Pathology,* St Louis, 1995, Mosby.)

Carditis. The earliest cardiac manifestation of acute rheumatic fever may be a previously undetected murmur caused by mitral or aortic semilunar valve dysfunction. Chest pain is caused by pericardial inflammation. Pericardial effusion produces an audible friction rub. Extra heart sounds, heart block (see p. 1134), atrial fibrillation, and a prolonged PR interval are often associated with chronic rheumatic heart disease.

Polyarthritis. The classic presenting manifestation of acute rheumatic fever is acute migratory polyarthritis (inflammation of more than one joint). Although all of the synovial joints may be involved, the large joints of the extremities are most often affected. Two or more joints are usually involved simultaneously or in succession. Exudative synovitis causes heat, redness, swelling, severe pain, and tenderness but no permanent disability. Palpable subcutaneous nodes often develop over bony prominences and along extensor tendons. They do not interfere with joint function and often go unnoticed.

Chorea. Sydenham chorea, or **St. Vitus dance,** is a disorder of the central nervous system characterized by sudden, aimless, irregular, involuntary movements. (Chorea is described in Chapter 16.) It is more common in girls than in boys and may occur several months after the streptococcal infection. The chorea is self-limiting. It runs its course within weeks or months and has no permanent neural sequelae.

Erythema Marginatum. Erythema marginatum is a distinctive truncal rash that often accompanies acute rheumatic fever. It consists of nonpruritic, pink, erythematous macules that never occur on the face or hands. The rash is transitory and may change in appearance within minutes or hours. Heat (e.g., bathing) darkens the rash. The macules may fade in the center and be mistaken for ringworm.

EVALUATION AND TREATMENT   When correlated with findings from physical assessment, laboratory values lend significant support to the diagnosis of acute rheumatic fever. A throat culture positive for group A β-hemolytic streptococci can be an important finding when associated with certain physical signs. Cultures may be negative when the rheumatic attack begins, however. Documented recent scarlet fever is another potentially strong diagnostic aid to acute rheumatic fever, but diagnosis of scarlet fever also depends on a positive throat culture and may be difficult to distinguish from other disorders associated with a similar rash. A high or rising antistreptolysin O (ASO) antibody titer is a more accurate means of diagnosing the presence of a streptococcal infection. Most strains of group A β-hemolytic streptococcus produces a hemolytic factor called *streptolysin O*. Antibodies against this hemolytic factor increase as the individual's immune system fights the disease. ASO antibody titers higher than 250 Todd units in adults and 333 Todd units in children are considered elevated. Several other antibody tests are sensitive prognosticators of streptococcal infection. These include antideoxyribonucleotidase (anti-DNase B), antihyaluronidase, and antistreptozyme (ASTZ).

Elevated white blood cell count, erythrocyte sedimentation rate, and C-reactive protein indicate inflammation. All three are usually increased at the time cardiac or joint symptoms begin to appear. They are more useful in identifying an acute inflammatory process and suggesting prognosis than in diagnosing acute rheumatic fever. The levels of these tests decrease as the inflammatory process resolves.

In 1944 the Jones criteria were established to assist in the diagnosis of acute rheumatic fever. The criteria have been modified several times by the American Heart Association, most recently in 1992[230] (Table 30-10). No single laboratory test, sign, or symptom is pathognomonic of acute rheumatic fever, but certain combinations of criteria indicate that acute disease is probably present.

Therapy for acute rheumatic fever is aimed at eradicating the streptococcal infection. This is accomplished by a 10-day regimen of oral penicillin or erythromycin administration. Salicylates are used as antiinflammatory agents for both rheumatic carditis and arthritis. Nonsteroidal antiinflammatory agents may be substituted for salicylates.[231,232] Serious carditis may require that cardiac glycosides, corticosteroids, diuretics, and bed rest be added to the regimen. Surgical repair of damaged valves may be necessary in cases of chronic recurrent rheumatic fever or carditis. Active disease is considered resolved when (1) the murmur has disappeared or cardiac status becomes stable, (2) major manifestations are no longer present, (3) the individual is afebrile, and (4) the erythrocyte sedimentation rate is normal or stabilized. This may take 1 to 6 months.

Research suggests that a rheumatic recurrence will develop in 50% to 65% of children with known rheumatic fever if they have another group A streptococcal infection. Recurrence rates decline with the length of time elapsed since the last infection. To prevent recurrence of acute rheumatic fever, continuous prophylactic antibiotic therapy is necessary for as long as 5 years.

Infective Endocarditis

Infective endocarditis is a general term used to describe inflammation of the endocardium—especially the cardiac valves. Causal agents include bacteria, viruses, fungi, rickettsiae, and parasites, but bacterial infection, particularly by streptococci or staphylococci, is most common.[233] Infective endocarditis was once a lethal disease, but morbidity and mortality diminished significantly with the advent of antibiotics and improved diagnostic techniques. This is still a lethal disease without treatment.

Risk factors for infective endocarditis include acquired valvular heart disease (especially mitral valve prolapse) and implantation of prosthetic heart valves. Congenital lesions associated with highly turbulent flow, such as ventricular septal defect, are also risk factors. (Congenital lesions are discussed in Chapter 31.) Other risk factors include a previous attack of infective endocarditis, male gender, intravenous drug abuse, long-term indwelling catheterization (e.g., for pressure monitoring, hyperalimentation, or hemodialysis), and recent cardiac surgery.[233]

PATHOPHYSIOLOGY The pathogenesis of infective endocarditis is a complex process that requires at least three critical elements (Figure 30-38). First, the endocardium (e.g., heart valve) must be "prepared," usually by endothelial damage, for microorganism colonization. Second, blood-borne microorganisms must adhere to the damaged endocardial surface. Third, the adherent microorganisms must proliferate and promote the propagation of infective endocardial vegetation.

The first critical element, endocardial damage, exposes the endothelial basement membrane. The basement membrane contains a type of collagen that attracts platelets and thereby stimulates thrombus formation on the membrane.[233] Platelet activation and thrombus formation can cause an inflammatory reaction termed **nonbacterial thrombotic endocarditis.** Infective endocarditis cannot develop unless microorganisms gain access to the bloodstream. Microorganisms may enter

Table 30-10	Jones Criteria (revised) for Diagnosis of Rheumatic Fever
Criteria	**Description**
Essential	Evidence of streptococcal infection (increased titer of streptococcal antibodies: antistreptolysin O [ASO]; positive throat culture for group A streptococcus; recent scarlet fever)
Major	Carditis, arthritis, chorea, erythema marginatum, subcutaneous nodules
Minor	*Clinical:* arthralgia, fever
	Laboratory: increased C-reactive protein, increased white blood cell count, increased erythrocyte sedimentation rate
	Electrocardiographic: prolonged PR interval

From Dajani AS, et al: Guidelines for the diagnosis of rheumatic fever: Jones criteria, updated 1992, *Circulation* 87: 302-307, 1993.

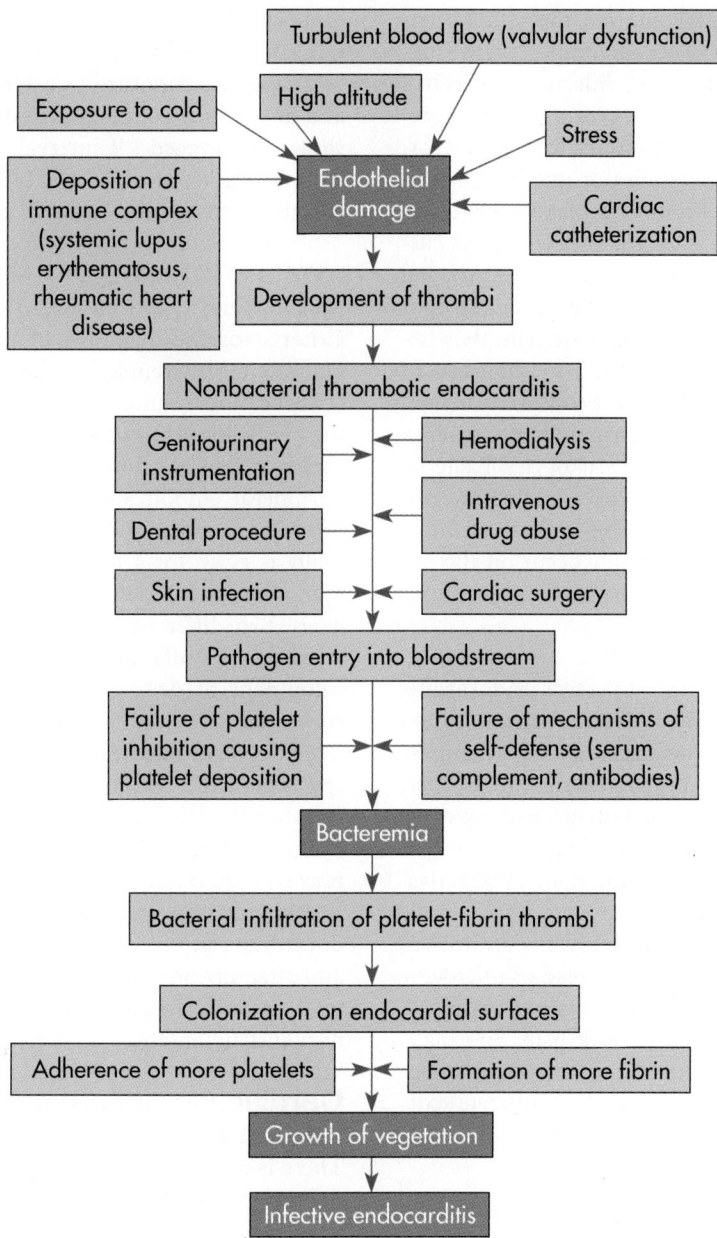

Figure 30-38 Pathogenesis of infective endocarditis.

the bloodstream as a result of minor procedures, such as dental cleaning or bladder catheterization, or they may spread from uncomplicated upper respiratory or skin infections. Any time pathogens gain access to the bloodstream, the potential for endocardial infection exists. Bacteremia and adherence constitute the second critical element. Adherence of microorganisms to the endocardial surface is facilitated by the coexistence of nonbacterial thrombotic endocarditis. It should be noted, however, that highly invasive organisms can cause infective endocarditis even on the healthy, intact endocardium. The third critical element, bacterial proliferation and vegetation formation, is also promoted by coexistent nonbacterial thrombotic endocarditis.

Not all microorganisms are capable of colonization. This capability, which determines the microorganism's pathogenicity, depends on the organism's ability to survive interactions with circulating serum complement, antibodies, and platelets aggregated on the endocardial surface. Complement, antibodies, and platelets may serve as effective inhibitors to bacterial colonization.

In addition to circumventing the host's defense mechanisms, the circulating microorganisms must adhere to the endocardial surface to initiate endocardial infection. Studies suggest that bacteria are able to synthesize extracellular polysaccharides, such as dextran or fibronectin, which promote stickiness on endocardial surfaces.

Once the endocardial surface is colonized, formation of infected vegetation proceeds by a series of complex steps (Figure 30-39). Within 3 to 6 hours after infection, microbial replication occurs and bacterial colonies form within aggregates of fibrin and platelets. Within 24 hours, infected vegetation has increased in size, with colonies of microorganisms sandwiched between layers of fibrin and platelets. Bacteria may accelerate fibrin formation by activating the clotting cascade in some as yet undetermined manner. As the growing bacterial colonies become progressively enmeshed in the tight fibrin network, which contains few phagocytic cells, they become less and less susceptible to the host's mechanisms of self-defense. Although endocardial tissue is constantly bathed in antibody-containing blood and is surrounded by scavenging monocytes and polymorphonuclear leukocytes, bacterial colonies are inaccessible to host defenses because they are embedded in the protective fibrin clots. The lesions can form anywhere on the endocardium but usually occur on the endocardial surfaces of heart valves and surrounding structures (see Figure 30-39).

CLINICAL MANIFESTATIONS   Infective endocarditis may be acute, subacute, or chronic. It causes varying degrees of valvular dysfunction and may be associated with manifestations involving any number of organ systems (lungs, eyes, kidneys, bones, joints, central nervous system), making diagnosis exceedingly difficult. The "classic" findings of fever; cardiac murmur; and petechial lesions of the skin, conjunctiva, and oral mucosa are not always present.

Signs and symptoms of infective endocarditis are caused by infection and inflammation, systemic spread of microemboli, and immune complex deposition in various organs. A history of fever, anorexia, weight loss, back pain, and night sweats; a new or significantly changed cardiac murmur; petechiae; positive blood cultures; an elevated erythrocyte sedimentation rate; and urine abnormalities make the diagnosis

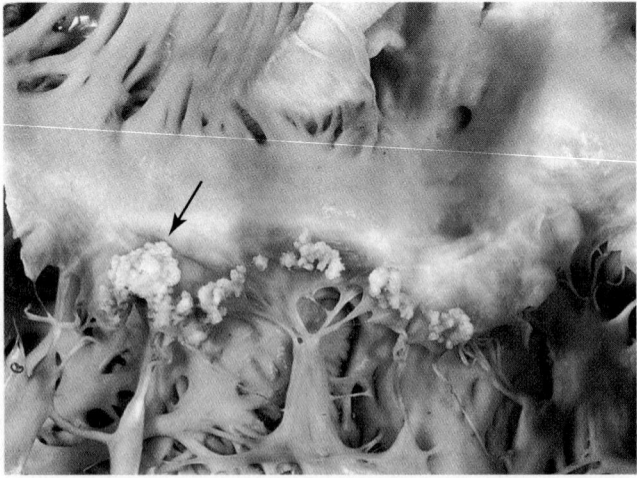

Figure 30-39 **Bacterial endocarditis of mitral valve.** Lesion (see *arrow*) in combination with old rheumatic valvulitis. (From Damjanov I, Linder J: *Pathology: a color atlas,* St Louis, 2000, Mosby.)

quite clear.[234] Sudden onset of severely debilitating symptoms indicates acute disease.

If infective endocarditis extends farther into the heart wall and invades the conduction system, electrocardiography may show a prolonged PR interval, left bundle branch block, or complete heart block (see p. 1134). Emboli may travel to the coronary arteries and cause an acute myocardial infarction.

EVALUATION AND TREATMENT   Diagnostic evaluation includes blood cultures to identify microorganisms.[235] Criteria for the diagnosis of infective endocarditis include persistent bacteremia, new regurgitant murmurs, vascular complications, and appropriate echocardiographic findings.[233] Echocardiography is used to identify the anatomic location of the infection and any intracardiac complications. If peripheral emboli are suggested, organ scans can be performed to confirm their presence. Antimicrobial therapy generally is given for 4 to 6 weeks, beginning with intravenous administration and ending with oral administration. In some cases, two different antibiotics are given simultaneously to eliminate the offending microorganism and prevent the development of drug resistance. Penicillin and streptomycin commonly are used to treat infective endocarditis, although many resistant microorganisms are found that require broad-spectrum antibiotic coverage.[235,236] Other drugs may be necessary to treat left heart failure secondary to valvular dysfunction, and surgical intervention to repair or replace the valve may be required.[237]

Individuals who are known to be at risk for infective endocarditis can avoid the disease by taking antibiotics before and after any procedure that carries the risk of transient bacteremia. Such procedures include dental cleaning, genitourinary instrumentation, and open cardiovascular surgery.

Cardiac Complications in Acquired Immunodeficiency Syndrome

There is growing evidence that up to 25% to 70% of individuals infected with the human immunodeficiency virus (HIV) have cardiac involvement consisting of myocarditis, endocarditis, pericarditis, or cardiomyopathy.[238,239] Myocarditis is the most common pathologic finding, followed by infective endocarditis and dilated cardiomyopathy.[239] Cardiac involvement can result from the HIV itself, inflammation, coinfections, malignancy, or drugs. Microorganisms that can cause cardiac complications in AIDS include bacterial, viral, protozoan, mycobacterial, and fungal pathogens. Malignancies, such as lymphoma and Kaposi sarcoma, often are seen in individuals with acquired immunodeficiency syndrome (AIDS) and can affect the heart. Anti-HIV drugs or drugs used to combat opportunistic infections may produce toxic lesions. Lipodystrophy (abnormality in metabolism or deposition of fats) associated with high active antiretroviral therapy (HAART) is associated with accelerated coronary artery disease and MI.[239,240]

Cardiac disease severe enough to cause clinical signs and symptoms is seen in about 10% of those with HIV. The symptoms of left heart failure are the most common cardiac manifestation and are related to dilated cardiomyopathy and dysfunction.[238] Pericardial effusion, ventricular dysrhythmias, ECG changes, pulmonary hypertension, and right ventricular dilation and hypertrophy are other less common findings.[239]

MANIFESTATIONS OF HEART DISEASE

Heart Failure

Types

Heart failure is a general term used to describe several types of cardiac dysfunction that result in inadequate perfusion of tissues with vital blood-borne nutrients. It is estimated that nearly 1% of Americans over the age of 65 have heart failure, and that 20% of all hospitalizations in that age group are the result of this disorder.[241] Most causes of heart failure result from dysfunction of the left ventricle (systolic and diastolic heart failure). The right ventricle also may be dysfunctional, especially in pulmonary disease (right ventricular failure). Finally, some conditions cause inadequate perfusion despite normal or elevated cardiac output (high-output failure).

Congestive Heart Failure (Left Heart Failure)

Congestive heart failure (left heart failure) is categorized as systolic heart failure or diastolic heart failure. Synonyms for these terms are systolic ventricular dysfunction and diastolic ventricular dysfunction. These two types of heart failure can occur together in one individual or singly.

Systolic Heart Failure. **Systolic heart failure** is defined as an inability of the heart to generate an adequate cardiac output to perfuse vital tissues. Cardiac output depends on the heart rate and stroke volume. Stroke volume is influenced by three major factors: contractility, preload, and afterload (see Chapter 29).

Contractility is reduced by diseases that disrupt myocyte activity. Myocardial infarction is the most common cause of decreased contractility; other causes include myocarditis and cardiomyopathies. Myocardial ischemia results in a process called **ventricular remodeling,** which causes progressive myocyte contractile dysfunction over time (Figure 30-40). When contractility is decreased, stroke volume falls and left ventricular end-diastolic volume (LVEDV) increases. This increase causes dilation of the heart and an increase in preload.

Preload, or LVEDV, increases with decreased contractility (see above) or when there is an excess of plasma volume (intravenous fluid administration, renal failure, mitral valvular disease). Increases in LVEDV can actually improve cardiac output to a certain point, but as preload continues to rise, it causes a stretching of the myocardium that eventually can lead to dysfunction of the sarcomeres and decreased contractility (Figure 30-41).

Increased afterload is most commonly a result of increased peripheral vascular resistance (PVR), such as that seen with hypertension (Figure 30-42); it also can be the result of aortic valvular disease. With increased PVR, there is resistance to ventricular emptying and more workload for the left ventricle, which responds with hypertrophy of the myocardium. Hypertrophy results in an increase in oxygen demand by the thickened myocardium and leads to changes in the myocytes themselves, also called *ventricular remodeling.*[241] In addition, hypertrophy results in the deposition of collagen between the myocytes; this can disrupt the integrity of the muscle, decrease contractility, and make the ventricle more likely to dilate and fail. Weakness of the cardiac muscle due to hypertension-induced hypertrophy is called hypertensive hypertrophic cardiomyopathy.

As cardiac output falls, renal perfusion diminishes with activation of the renin-angiotensin-aldosterone system, which acts to increase PVR and plasma volume, thus increasing afterload and preload further. In addition, baroreceptors in the central circulation detect the decrease in perfusion and stimulate the sympathetic nervous system to cause yet more vasoconstriction and to cause the hypothalamus to produce antidiuretic hormone. This vicious cycle of decreasing contractility, increasing preload, and increasing afterload causes progressive worsening of left heart failure (Figure 30-42, *B*).

In addition to these hemodynamic interactions, systolic congestive heart failure is characterized by a complex constellation of neurohumoral and inflammatory processes.[241-243] These processes involve a large number of important mediators:

1. *Catecholamines.* Sympathetic nervous system activation initially compensates for a decrease in cardiac output by increasing heart rate and peripheral vascular resistance. However, catecholamines cause numerous deleterious effects on the myocardium, including direct toxicity to myocytes, induction of myocyte apoptosis, myocardial remodeling, down-regulation of adrenergic receptors, facilitation of arrhythmias, and potentiation of autoimmune effects on the heart muscle.[241,244,245]

2. *Angiotensin II (Ang II).* Activation of the renin-angiotensin-aldosterone system not only causes increases in preload and afterload but also causes direct toxicity to the myocardium (see Figure 30-40). Ang II mediates remodeling of the ventricular wall, with associated loss of contractility. High circulating levels of Ang II are associated with an increased mortality in individuals with congestive heart failure (CHF).[241,242,244,246]

3. *Aldosterone.* Aldosterone not only causes salt and water retention by the kidney but also contributes to myocardial fibrosis, autonomic dysfunction, and dysrhythmias.[247,248]

4. *Arginine vasopressin.* Arginine vasopressin is also known as *antidiuretic hormone* and causes both peripheral vasoconstriction and renal fluid retention. These actions exacerbate hyponatremia and edema in CHF.[242,249]

5. *Natriuretic peptides.* Atrial and brain natriuretic peptides (BNPs) are increased in CHF and may have some protective effect by decreasing preload.[250,251]

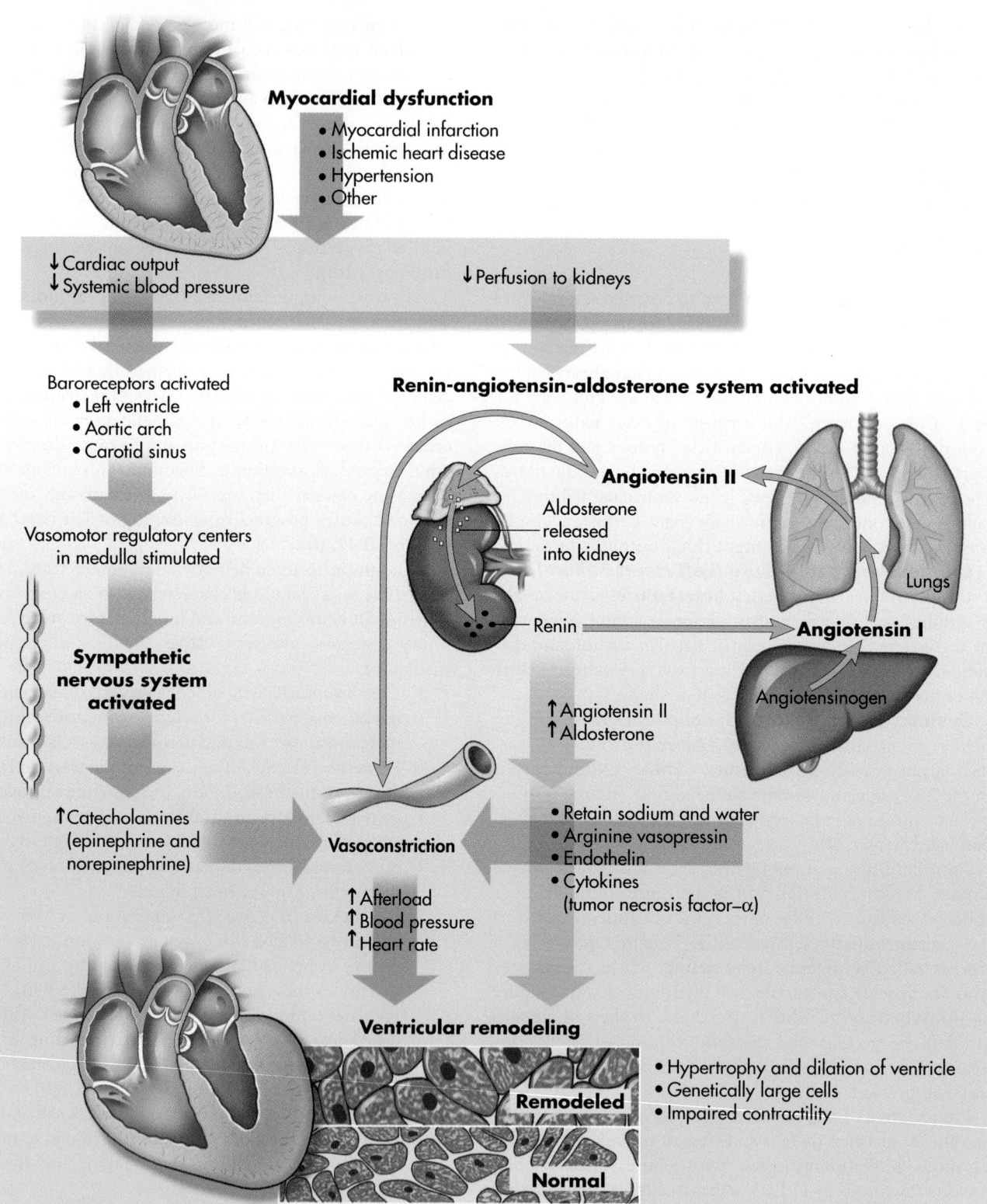

Figure 30-40 **Pathophysiology of ventricular remodeling.** Myocardial dysfunction activates the renin-aldosterone and sympathetic nervous systems releasing neurohormones (angiotensin II, aldosterone, catecholamines, and cytokines). These neurohormones contribute to ventricular remodeling. (Redrawn from Carelock J, Clark AP: *Am J Nurs* 101[12]:27, 2001.)

6. *Endothelial hormones.* Endothelin is a potent vasoconstrictor and is associated with a poor prognosis in individuals with CHF.[252]

7. *Endotoxin.* Increased serum levels of endotoxin have been found in many individuals with CHF, especially those with significant peripheral edema, and has been linked to myocyte apoptosis and release of tumor necrosis factor and interleukins.[253]

8. *Tumor necrosis factor–α (TNF-α) and interleukin-6 (IL-6).* TNF-α is elevated in CHF and contributes to myocardial remodeling, downregulates the synthesis of the vasodilator nitric oxide, induces myocyte apoptosis, and may contribute to weight loss and weakness in individuals with CHF (cardiac cachexia).[254] IL-6 is also high in individuals with severe CHF and cardiogenic shock and may contribute to further deleterious immune activation.[255]

The interaction of these neurohumoral and inflammatory processes results in a gradual decline in myocardial function.[241] Pathologically, the heart muscle exhibits progressive changes in myocyte myofilaments, decreased contractility, myocyte apoptosis and necrosis, abnormal fibrin deposition in the ventricle wall, myocardial hypertrophy, and changes in the ventricular chamber geometry. These changes reduce myocardial function and cardiac output and lead to increased morbidity and mortality. These discoveries have led to the routine use of ACE inhibitors or Ang II receptor blockers plus beta-blockers in the management of CHF, which has resulted in significant decreases in morbidity and mortality. In addition, aldosterone blockade with spironolactone is also used to improve myocardial function.[247]

The clinical manifestations of left heart failure are the result of pulmonary vascular congestion and inadequate perfusion of the systemic circulation. Individuals experience dyspnea, orthopnea, cough of frothy sputum, fatigue, decreased urine output, and edema. Physical examination often reveals pulmonary edema (cyanosis, rales, pleural effusions), hypotension or hypertension, an S_3 gallop, and evidence of underlying

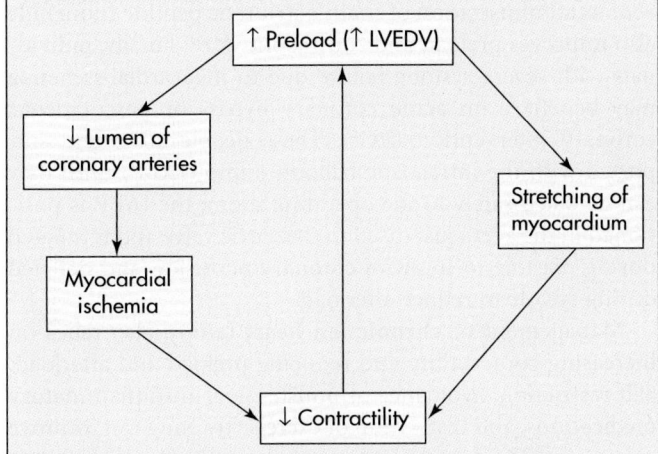

Figure 30-41 The effect of elevated preload on myocardial oxygen supply and demand. *LVEDV,* Left ventricular end-diastolic volume.

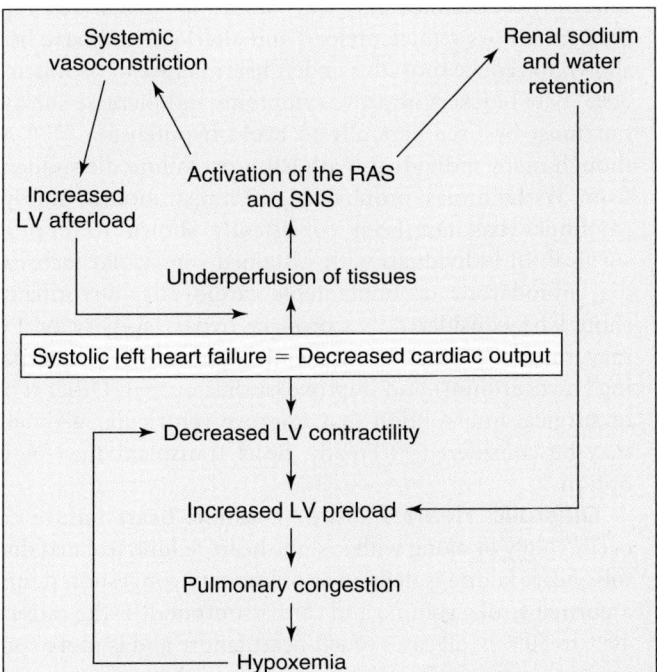

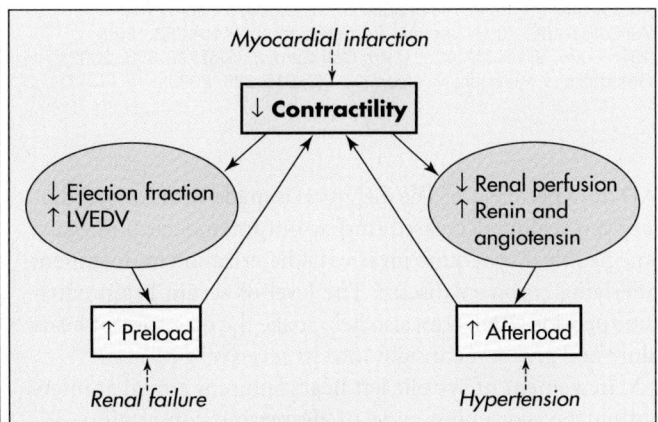

Figure 30-42 **Systolic heart failure.** **A,** The pathogenesis of systolic congestive heart failure is defined by an inability of the left ventricle *(LV)* to generate adequate cardiac output. This leads to tissue ischemia and release of renin, angiotensin II *(RAS),* and catecholamines *(SNS).* These neurohormones cause systemic vasoconstriction and increased resistance to LF ejection (afterload) and renal salt and water retention that contribute to increased preload. Preload is also increased by the inability of the LV to empty properly because of decreased contractility. Increased LV preload causes pulmonary congestion and hypoxemia, which further contributes to heart failure. **B,** The vicious cycle of systolic heart failure. Although the initial insult may be one of primary decreased contractility (e.g., myocardial infarction), increased preload (e.g., renal failure), or increased afterload (e.g., hypertension), all three factors play a role in the progression of left heart failure. *RAS,* Renin-angiotensin-aldosterone system; *SNS,* sympthetic nervous system; *LVEDV,* Left ventricular end-diastolic volume.

CAD or hypertension. The diagnosis is made with echocardiography, revealing decreased cardiac output and cardiomegaly; some people may require invasive catheterization to document underlying coronary disease. The level of serum brain natriuretic peptide (BNP) can also help make the diagnosis of heart failure and give some insight into its severity.[256,257]

Management of systolic left heart failure is aimed at interrupting the worsening cycle of decreasing contractility, increasing preload, and increasing afterload, as well as blocking the neurohormonal mediators of myocardial toxicity. The acute onset of left (congestive) heart failure is most often the result of acute myocardial ischemia and must be managed in conjunction with managing the underlying coronary disease (see p. 1105). Oxygen, nitrate, and morphine administration improve myocardial oxygenation and help relieve coronary spasm while lowering preload through systemic venodilation.

Intravenous inotropic drugs, such as dopamine or dobutamine, increase contractility and can help raise the blood pressure in hypotensive individuals.[258] A new class of inotropic drugs (e.g., levosimendan) has shown promise for acute heart failure.[259] Diuretics reduce preload, and ACE inhibitors reduce both preload and afterload by decreasing aldosterone levels and reducing PVR. Short-acting intravenous beta-blockers also have been found to reduce mortality.[258] Intravenous administration of brain natriuretic peptide (nesiritide also improves preload and contractility.[260,261] Finally, individuals with severe systolic failure due to myocardial ischemia may benefit from acute coronary bypass or percutaneous coronary intervention (PCI). These people are often supported with the intraaortic balloon pump (IABP) until they can be taken safely to the operating room; the IABP is positioned in the aorta just distal to the aortic valve and is inflated during diastole to improve coronary perfusion and deflated during systole to reduce afterload.

Management of **chronic left heart failure** also relies on increasing contractility and reducing preload and afterload. Salt restriction, avoidance of nonsteroidal antiinflammatory medications, and institution of exercise training can improve symptoms. The inotropic drug of choice in chronic systolic heart failure is digoxin but should be used only in selected individuals.[262] Salt restriction and diuretics are effective in reducing preload, and spironolactone has been shown to significantly reduce mortality when added to standard therapy. ACE inhibitors reduce preload and afterload and have been shown to reduce mortality in left heart failure by as much as 30%. Beta blockers improve symptoms and increase survival but must be used carefully to avoid hypotension.[258,263] Although many individuals with left heart failure die suddenly from dysrhythmias, prophylactic administration of antidysrhythmics has not been consistently shown to improve survival. In individuals with sustained ventricular tachycardia, amiodarone or implantable cardioverter-defibrillators should be considered.[244] Coronary bypass surgery or PCI may improve perfusion to ischemic myocardium ("hibernating" myocardium) and improve cardiac output. Other types of surgical intervention that improve ventricular geometry may be considered.[264] Finally, heart transplant may be an option.

Diastolic Heart Failure. **Diastolic heart failure** can occur singly or along with systolic heart failure. Isolated diastolic heart failure is defined as pulmonary congestion despite a normal stroke volume and cardiac output. It is the cause of 40% to 50% of all cases of left heart failure and is more common in women.[265] It results from decreased compliance of the left ventricle and abnormal diastolic relaxation such that a normal LVEDV results in an increased left ventricular end-diastolic pressure (LVEDP). This pressure is reflected back into the pulmonary circulation and results in pulmonary edema. The major causes of diastolic dysfunction include hypertension-induced myocardial hypertrophy, and myocardial ischemia with resultant ventricular remodeling. Hypertrophy and ischemia cause a decreased ability of the myocytes

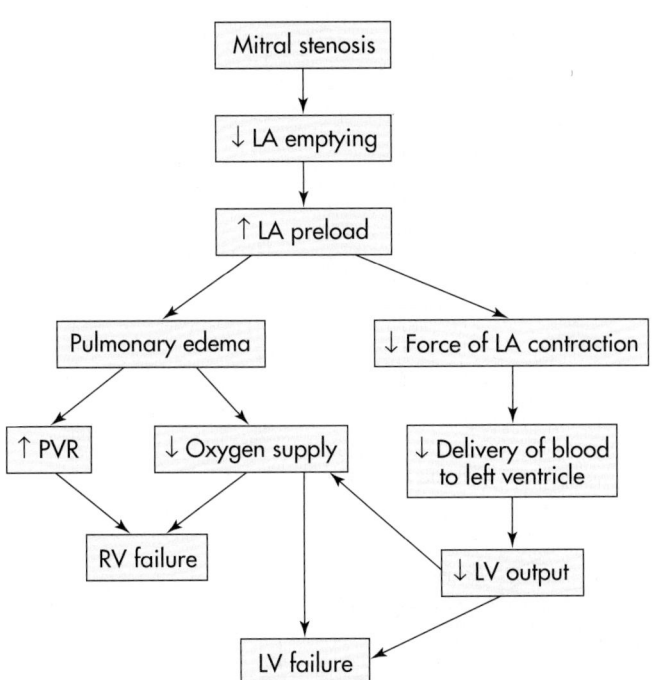

Figure 30-43 Left atrial failure caused by mitral stenosis. *LA,* Left atrial; *PVR,* pulmonary vascular resistance; *LV,* left ventricular.

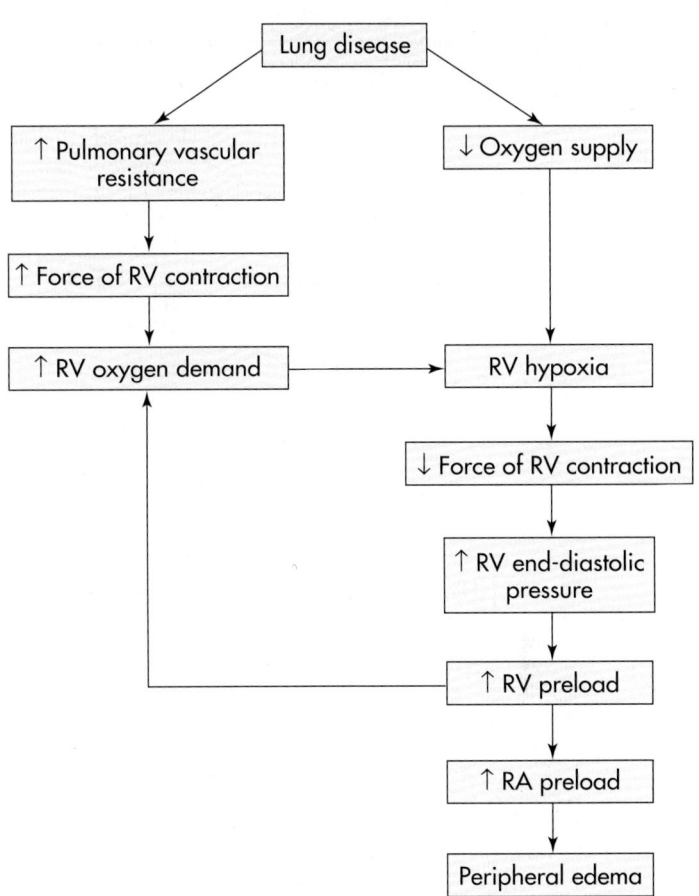

Figure 30-44 Right heart failure (cor pulmonale) caused by lung disease. *RV,* Right ventricular; *RA,* right atrial.

to actively pump calcium from the cytosol, resulting in impaired relaxation.[265] Other causes include aortic valvular disease, mitral valve disease (Figure 30-43), pericardial diseases, and cardiomyopathies. Diabetes also increases the risk for diastolic dysfunction.[266]

Individuals with diastolic dysfunction present with dyspnea on exertion; fatigue; evidence of pulmonary edema (rales on auscultation, pleural effusions). There also may be evidence of underlying coronary disease, hypertension, or valvular disease. Diagnosis is made initially by echocardiography, which demonstrates poor ventricular filling with normal ejection fractions. Management is aimed at improving ventricular relaxation and prolonging diastolic filling times to reduce diastolic pressure. Calcium channel blockers, beta-blockers, ACE inhibitors, and angiotensin receptor blockers (ARBs) have been used with varying success. Inotropic drugs are not indicated in isolated diastolic heart failure because contractility and ejection fraction are not affected; however, digoxin may be used to slow the heart rate in individuals with atrial fibrillation.[265] An innovative surgical technique that involves the transplantation of a portion of the latissimus dorsi muscle into the wall of the noncompliant left ventricle (dynamic cardiomyoplasty) is being tried, with some early success. Mortality is lower with diastolic failure than with systolic; however, risk of death is four times that of the population without heart failure.[267]

Right Heart Failure

Right heart failure can result from left heart failure when the increase in left ventricular filling pressure that is reflected back into the pulmonary circulation is severe enough. As pressure in the pulmonary circulation rises, the resistance to

right ventricular emptying increases (Figure 30-44). The right ventricle is poorly prepared to compensate for this increased workload and will dilate and fail. When this happens, pressure will rise in the systemic venous circulation, resulting in peripheral edema and hepatosplenomegaly. Treatment relies on management of the left ventricular dysfunction as just outlined. When right heart failure occurs in the absence of left heart failure, it is caused most commonly by diffuse hypoxic pulmonary disease such as COPD, cystic fibrosis, and ARDS. The mechanisms for this type of right ventricular dysfunction *(cor pulmonale)* are discussed in Chapter 33.

High-Output Failure

High-output failure is the inability of the heart to adequately supply the body with blood-borne nutrients, despite adequate blood volume and normal or elevated myocardial contractility. In high-output failure the heart increases its output but the body's metabolic needs are still not met. Common causes of high-output failure are anemia, septicemia, hyperthyroidism, and beriberi (Figure 30-45).

Anemia decreases the oxygen-carrying capacity of the blood (see Chapter 26). Metabolic acidosis occurs as the body's cells switch to anaerobic metabolism (see Chapter 3). In response to metabolic acidosis, heart rate and stroke volume increase in an attempt to circulate blood faster. If anemia

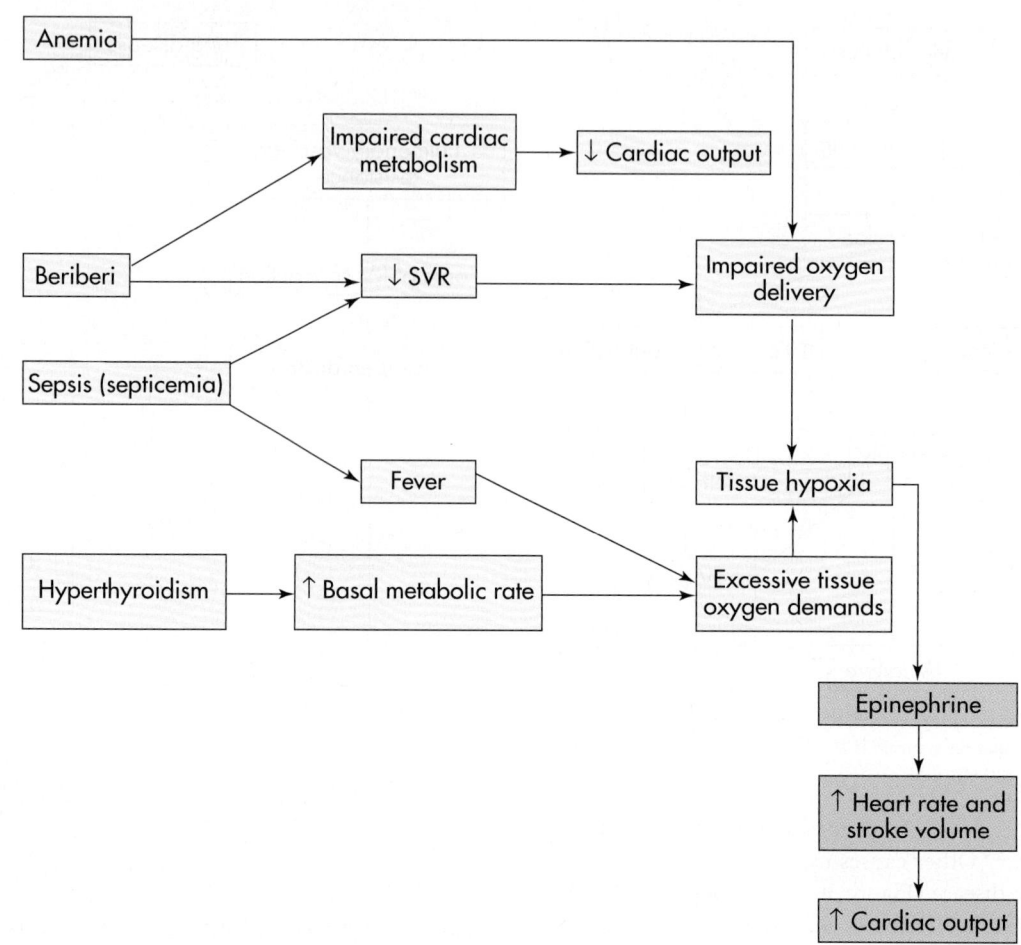

Figure 30-45 High-output failure. *SVR,* Systemic vascular resistance.

is severe, however, even maximum cardiac output does not supply the cells with enough oxygen for metabolism.

In septicemia, disturbed metabolism, bacterial toxins, and the inflammatory process cause systemic vasodilation and fever. Faced with a lowered systemic vascular resistance (SVR) and an elevated metabolic rate, cardiac output increases to maintain blood pressure and prevent metabolic acidosis. In overwhelming septicemia, however, the heart may not be able to raise its output enough to compensate for vasodilation. Body tissues show signs of inadequate blood supply despite a very high cardiac output.

Hyperthyroidism accelerates cellular metabolism through the actions of elevated levels of thyroxine from the thyroid gland. This may occur chronically (thyrotoxicosis) or acutely (thyroid storm). Because the body's demand for oxygen threatens to cause metabolic acidosis, cardiac output increases. If blood levels of thyroxine are high and the metabolic response to thyroxine is quite vigorous, even an abnormally elevated cardiac output may be inadequate.

In the United States, beriberi (thiamine deficiency) usually is caused by malnutrition secondary to chronic alcoholism. Beriberi actually causes a mixed type of heart failure. Thiamine deficiency impairs cellular metabolism in all tissues, including the myocardium. In the heart, im-

paired cardiac metabolism leads to insufficient contractile strength. In blood vessels, thiamine deficiency leads mainly to peripheral vasodilation, which decreases SVR. Heart failure ensues as decreased SVR triggers increased cardiac output, which the impaired myocardium is unable to deliver. The strain of demands for increased output in the face of impaired metabolism may deplete cardiac reserves until low-output failure begins.

Dysrhythmias

A dysrhythmia, or arrhythmia, is a disturbance of heart rhythm. Normal heart rhythms are generated by the SA node and travel through the heart's conduction system, causing the atrial and ventricular myocardium to contract and relax at a regular rate that is appropriate to maintain circulation at various levels of physical activity (see Chapter 29). Dysrhythmias range in severity from occasional "missed" or rapid beats to serious disturbances that impair the pumping ability of the heart, contributing to heart failure and death. Dysrhythmias can be caused by either an abnormal rate of impulse generation (Table 30-11) by the SA node or other pacemaker or the abnormal conduction of impulses (Table 30-12) through the heart's conduction system, including the myocardial cells themselves.

Table 30-11	Disorders of Impulse Formation			
Type	**Electrocardiogram**	**Effect**	**Pathophysiology**	**Treatment**
Sinus bradycardia	P rate 60 or less PR interval normal QRS for each P	Increased preload Decreased mean arterial pressure	Hyperkalemia: slows depolarization Vagal hyperactivity: unknown Digoxin toxicity common Late hypoxia: lack of adenosine triphosphate (ATP)	If hypotensive, treat cause and support Follow with sympathomimetics, cardiotonics, and pacer Vagolytics
Simple sinus tachycardia	P rate 100-150 PR interval normal QRS for each P	Decreased filling times Decreased mean arterial pressure Increased myocardial demand	Catecholamines; rise in resting potential, calcium influx Fever: unknown Early failure and lung disease: hypoxic cell metabolism Hypercalcemia	Oxygen, bed rest Calcium blockers
Premature atrial contractions (PACs) or beats*	Early P waves that may have changed morphology PR interval normal QRS for each P	Occasional decreased filling time and mean arterial pressure	Electrolyte disturbances: decrease all phases Hypoxia and elevated preload: cell membrane disturbances Hypercalcemia	Treat underlying cause Digoxin
Sinus dysrhythmias	Rate varies P-P regularly irregular, short with inspiration, long with exhalation PR interval normal QRS for each P	Variable filling times Variable mean arterial pressures Variable oxygen demand	Unknown Common in young children and young adults	None
Atrial tachycardia (includes premature atrial tachycardia if onset is abrupt)	P rate 151-250 P morphology may differ from sinus P PR interval normal P/QRS ratio variable	Decreased filling time Decreased mean arterial pressure Increased myocardial demand	Same as PACs: leads to increased atrial automaticity, atrial reentry Digoxin toxicity: common	Control ventricular rate Digoxin, calcium blockers, vagus stimulation Pace to override
Atrial flutter*	P rate 251-300, morphology may vary from sinus P PR interval usually not observable P/QRS ratio variable	Decreased filling time Decreased mean arterial pressure	Same as atrial tachycardia Aging	Same as atrial tachycardia Synchronous cardioversion
Atrial fibrillation*	P rate > 300 and usually not observable No PR interval QRS rate variable and rhythm irregular	Same as atrial flutter	Same as atrial tachycardia Aging	Same as atrial tachycardia
Idiojunctional rhythm	P absent or independent QRS normal, rate 41-59, regular	Decreased cardiac output from loss of atrial contribution to ventricular preload Decreased mean atrial pressure as a result of bradycardia	Atrial and sinus bradycardia, standstill, or block	Same as sinus bradycardia
Junctional bradycardia	P absent or independent QRS normal, rate 40 or less	Same as idiojunctional rhythm	Same as idiojunctional rhythm Vagal hyperactivity	Same as sinus bradycardia
Premature junctional contractions (PJCs) or beats	Early beats without P waves QRS morphology normal	Decreased cardiac output from loss of atrial contribution to ventricular preload for that beat	Hyperkalemia (6-5.4 mEq/L) Hypercalcemia, hypoxia, and elevated preload (see PACs)	Same as PAC

*Most common in adults.

Continued

Table 30-11	Disorders of Impulse Formation—cont'd			
Type	**Electrocardiogram**	**Effect**	**Pathophysiology**	**Treatment**
Accelerated junctional rhythm	P absent or independent QRS morphology normal, rate 60-99	Decreased cardiac output from loss of atrial contribution to ventricular preload	Same as PJCs	Same as PAC
Junctional tachycardia	P absent or independent QRS morphology normal, rate 100 or more	Decreased cardiac output from loss of atrial contribution to ventricular preload Increased myocardial demand because of tachycardia	Same as PJCs	Same as PAC
Idioventricular rhythm†	P absent or independent QRS >0.11 and rate 20-39	Same as idiojunctional rhythm	Sinus, atrial, and junctional bradycardia, standstill, or block	Same as sinus bradycardia
Ventricular bradycardia†	P absent or independent QRS >0.11 and rate 60-21	Same as idiojunctional rhythm	Same as idiojunctional rhythm	Same as sinus bradycardia
Agonal rhythm/ electromechanical dissociation†	P absent or independent QRS >0.11 and rate 20 or less	Absent or barely present cardiac output and pulse Not compatible with life	Depolarization and contraction not coupled: electrical activity present with little or no mechanical activity Usually caused by profound hypoxia	Vigorous pharmacology aimed at restoring rate and force Usually ineffective May attempt to pace
Ventricular standstill or asystole†	P absent or independent QRS absent	No cardiac output Not compatible with life	Profound ischemia, hyperkalemia, acidosis	Same as agonal rhythm, including electrical defibrillation
Premature ventricular contractions (PVCs) or depolarizations*	Early beats with P waves QRS occasionally opposite in deflection from usual QRS	Same as premature junctional contractions	Same as PJCs, including aging and induction of anesthesia Impulse originates in cell outside normal conduction system and spreads through intercalated disks	Pharmacology to change thresholds, refractory periods; reduce myocardial demand, increase supply Removal of cause
Accelerated ventricular rhythm	P absent or independent QRS >0.11 and rate 41-99	Same as accelerated junctional rhythm	Same as PVCs	Same as PVCs
Ventricular tachycardia†	P absent or independent QRS >0.11 and rate 100 or more	Same as junctional tachycardia	Same as PVCs	Same as PVCs, including electrical cardioversion
Ventricular fibrillation†	P absent QRS >300 and usually not observable	Same as ventricular standstill	Same as PVCs Rapid infusion of potassium	Same as PVCs including electrical defibrillation

*Most common in adults.
†Life threatening in adults.

Table 30-12   Disorders of Impulse Conduction

Type	Electrocardiogram	Effect	Pathophysiology	Treatment
Sinus block	Occasionally absent P, with loss of QRS for that beat	Occasional decrease in cardiac output Increase in preload for the following beat	Local hypoxia, scarring of intraatrial conduction pathways, electrolyte imbalances Increased atrial preload	Conservative Usually do not progress in severity Pharmacologic treatment includes vagolytics, sympathomimetics, pacing
First-degree block*	PR interval >0.2	None	Same as sinus block Hyperkalemia (>7 mEq/L) Hypokalemia (<3.5 mEq/L) Formation of myocardial abscesses in endocarditis	Conservative Discovery and correction of cause
Second-degree block, Mobitz I, or Wenckebach*	Progressive prolongation of PR interval until one QRS is dropped Pattern of prolongation resumes	Same as sinus block	Hypokalemia (<3.5 mEq/L) Faulty cell metabolism in atrioventricular (AV) node Severity increases as heart rate increases Supports theory that AV node is fatiguing Digoxin toxicity, β blockade Coronary artery disease (CAD), myocardial infarction (MI), hypoxia, increased preload, valvular surgery and disease, diabetes	Same as sinus block
Second-degree block or Mobitz II	Same as sinus block	Same as sinus block	Hypokalemia (<3.5 mEq/L) Faulty cell metabolism below AV node Antidysrhythmics, cyclic antidepressants CAD, MI, hypoxia, increased preload, valvular surgery and disease, diabetes	More aggressively than Mobitz I, since can progress to type III Pacemaker after pharmacologic treatment
Third-degree block†	P waves present and independent of QRS No observed relationship between P and QRS Always atrioventricular (AV) dissociation	Same as idiojunctional rhythm	Hypokalemia (<3.5 mEq/L) Faulty cell metabolism low in bundle of His MI, especially inferior wall, as nodal artery interrupted; results in ischemia of AV node	Pharmacologic until pacemaker inserted Temporary pacing if caused by inferior MI, since ischemia usually resolves
Atrioventricular dissociation	P waves present and independent of QRS, but not always because of block (e.g., ventricular tachycardia) AV dissociation not always third-degree block	Decreased cardiac output from loss of atrial contribution to ventricular preload Variable effect on myocardial demand, depending on ventricular rate	May result from third-degree block or accelerated junctional or ventricular rhythm, or be caused by sinus, atrial, and junctional bradycardias	Treat according to cause Pacemaker or reducing rate of AV or ventricular discharge, or increasing rate of sinus or AV node discharge

*Most common in adults.
†Life threatening in adults.

Continued

Table 30-12	Disorders of Impulse Conduction—cont'd			
Type	Electrocardiogram	Effect	Pathophysiology	Treatment
Ventricular block	QRS >0.11 R-S-R' in V$_1$, V$_2$, V$_5$, V$_6$	None	Faulty cell metabolism in right and left bundle branches RBBB more common than LBBB because of dual blood supply to left bundle branch Congestive heart failure, mitral regurgitation, especially anterior MI, because of infarct of fascicles Left anterior hemiblock more common than left posterior hemiblock, since posterior fascicles have dual blood supply	Isolated right bundle branch block (RBBB) or left bundle branch block (LBBB) or hemiblock not treated If acute and/or associated with acute anterior MI, treated with permanent pacer and vigorous pharmacology
Aberrant conduction	QRS >0.11	None unless ventricular rate abnormalities present	Conduction of impulse through intercalated disks, since conduction system transiently blocked because of hypoxia, electrolyte imbalances, digoxin toxicity, excessively rapid rates of discharge	Correct underlying cause
Preexcitation syndromes (Wolff-Parkinson-White and Lown-Ganong-Levine)	P present with QRS for each P PR interval >0.12 and QRS >0.11 because of presence of delta wave in PR interval	None	Congenital presence of accessory pathways (bundle of Kent and fiber of Mahaim) that conduct very rapidly and bypass the AV node, causing early ventricular depolarization in relation to atrial depolarization Prone (reason unknown) to tachycardias and atrial fibrillation that can result in very rapid ventricular rates	Aimed at lining up refractory periods of accessory pathway and AV node to prevent reentry May slow rate with pharmacology May surgically cut pathways

*Most common in adults.
†Life threatening in adults.

SUMMARY REVIEW

Diseases of the Arteries and Veins

1. Atherosclerosis is a form of arteriosclerosis and is the leading contributor to coronary artery and cerebrovascular disease.
2. Atherosclerosis is an inflammatory disease that begins with endothelial injury (smoking, hypertension, diabetes [insulin resistance], hyperhomocystinemia, dyslipidemia, etc.) and progresses through several stages to become a fibrotic plaque.
3. Novel risk factors include elevated C-reactive protein, increased serum fibrinogen, oxidative stress, infection, and periodontal disease.
4. Once a plaque has formed, it can rupture, resulting in thrombosis and vasoconstriction leading to obstruction of the lumen and inadequate perfusion of distal tissues.
5. Hypertension is a sustained elevation of the system arterial blood pressure resulting from increases in cardiac output or total peripheral resistance or both. Hypertension can be primary (without known cause) or secondary (caused by disease or drugs). Systolic hypertension is the most significant factor in causing target organ damage.

6. The risk factors for hypertension include a positive family history; male gender; advanced age; black race; obesity; high sodium intake; low potassium, calcium, and magnesium intake; diabetes mellitus; labile blood pressure; cigarette smoking; and heavy alcohol consumption.

7. Primary hypertension is the result of extremely complicated interactions of genetics and the environment mediated by a host of neurohumoral effects. These genes interact with diet, smoking, age, and the other risk factors to cause chronic changes in vasomotor tone and blood volume.

8. The most frequently cited theories of the pathogenesis of primary hypertension include (1) overactivity of the sympathetic nervous system; (2) overactivity of the renin-angiotensin-aldosterone system; (3) alterations in other neurohumoral mediators of blood volume and vasomotor tone such as atrial natriuretic peptide, brain natriuretic peptide, and adrenomedullin; and (4) a complex interaction involving insulin resistance and endothelial function.

9. Clinical manifestations of hypertension result from damage of organs and tissues outside the vascular system. These include heart disease, renal disease, central nervous system problems, and musculoskeletal dysfunction.

10. Hypertension is managed pharmacologically, using diuretics, adrenergic blockers, calcium channel blockers, angiotensin-converting enzyme (ACE) inhibitors, and angiotensin II receptor blockers (losartan). Nonpharmacologic methods include cessation of smoking, dietary modifications, and exercise.

11. Orthostatic hypotension is a drop in blood pressure that occurs on standing. The compensatory vasoconstriction response to standing is altered by a marked vasodilation and blood pooling in the muscle vasculature.

12. Orthostatic hypotension may be acute or chronic. The acute form is caused by a delay in the normal regulatory mechanisms. The chronic forms are secondary to a specific disease or are idiopathic in nature.

13. The clinical manifestations of orthostatic hypotension include fainting and may involve cardiovascular symptoms, as well as impotence and bowel and bladder dysfunction.

14. An aneurysm is a localized dilation of a vessel wall, to which the aorta is particularly susceptible.

15. A thrombus is a clot that remains attached to a vascular wall. Arteriosclerosis can generate thrombus formation through roughening of the intima that activates the clotting cascade. Thrombus formation may be discrete or diffuse.

16. An embolus is a mobile aggregate of a variety of substances that occludes the vasculature. Sources of emboli include clots, air, amniotic fluid, bacteria, fat, and foreign matter.

17. The most common cause of arterial thrombotic emboli is the heart, as a result of mitral and aortic valvular disease and atrial fibrillation, followed by myxomas. Tissues affected include the lower extremities, the brain, and the heart.

18. Emboli to the central organs cause tissue death in lungs, kidneys, and mesentery.

19. The generation of air emboli requires a connection between the vascular compartment and a source of air. These emboli cause ischemia and necrosis when a vessel is totally blocked.

20. Amniotic fluid may be forced into the bloodstream and generate an embolus during the labor and delivery of pregnancy.

21. Aggregates of bacteria in the vasculature may be large enough to form an embolus.

22. Fat emboli are caused mainly by trauma to the long bones, either through defective fat metabolism after trauma or through the release of fat globules from bone marrow exposed by fracture.

23. The introduction of foreign matter into the vasculature can occur with trauma and also can occur in a hospital setting in which intravenous and intraarterial lines are being used.

24. Peripheral artery disease (PAD) is atherosclerosis of arteries that perfuse the limbs, especially the lower extremities.

25. PAD is often asymptomatic. Treatment includes risk factor reduction and antiplatelet therapy.

26. Vasospastic disorders include Raynaud disease, involving arterioles of the extremities; variant angina, involving coronary arteries; and Buerger disease, involving arteries of the hands and feet.

27. Diabetic lesions of the arteries may be caused by a defect in glycoprotein metabolism that involves the capillary basement membranes in kidneys, retinas, and extremities.

28. Varicosities are areas of veins in which blood has pooled, usually in the saphenous veins. Varicosities may be caused by damaged valves as a result of trauma to the valve or by chronic venous distention involving gravity and venous constriction.

29. Chronic venous insufficiency is inadequate venous return over a long period that causes pathologic ischemic changes in the vasculature, skin, and supporting tissues.

30. Venous stasis ulcers follow the development of chronic venous insufficiency and probably develop as a result of the borderline metabolic state of the cells in the affected extremities.

31. Deep venous thrombosis occurs in individuals who have venous stasis (immobility, age, left heart failure), spinal cord injury, vein wall damage (trauma, intravenous medications), or hypercoagulable states (pregnancy, oral contraceptives, malignancy, genetic coagulopathies).

32. Deep venous thrombosis is often asymptomatic but may lead to potentially fatal pulmonary emboli; thus prevention and careful assessment in individuals at risk is crucial.

33. Coronary artery disease (CAD) is spasm or occlusion of the coronary arteries and is most often the result of atherosclerotic lesions that limit the flow of blood to the heart.

34. Many risk factors contribute to the onset and escalation of CAD, including advanced age, male gender (under the age of 60), hypertension, dyslipidemia (including elevated Lp[a]), hyperhomocysteinemia, diabetes mellitus, smoking, obesity, sedentary life-style, psychosocial factors, elevated fibrinogen, serum amyloid, C-reactive protein, and possibly infectious agents.

35. CAD results in an imbalance between coronary supply of blood and myocardial demand for oxygen and nutrients such that reversible myocardial ischemia or irreversible infarction may result.

36. Reversible myocardial ischemia presents clinically in several ways. Chronic coronary obstruction results in recurrent predictable chest pain called *stable angina*. Abnormal vasospasm of coronary vessels results in unpredictable chest pain called *Prinzmetal angina*. Myocardial ischemia that does not cause detectable symptoms is called *silent ischemia*.

37. Stable angina is evaluated by noninvasive techniques of assessing coronary flow with or without exercise (stress electrocardiogram [ECG], thallium, or single-photon emission computed tomography [SPECT]). Management may include life-style changes, vasodilators, antithrombotics percutaneous coronary intervention (PCI), or coronary bypass graft (CABG) surgery.

38. When there is sudden coronary obstruction because of thrombosis formation over a ruptured atherosclerotic plaque, the acute coronary syndromes result. Unstable angina causes reversible myocardial ischemia and is a harbinger of impending infarction. Myocardial infarction results when there is pro-

Continued

longed ischemia causing irreversible damage to the heart muscle. Sudden cardiac death can occur in any of the acute coronary syndromes.

39. Unstable angina occurs because of transient episodes of thrombotic vessel occlusion and vasoconstriction at the site of plaque damage, with return of perfusion before significant myocardial necrosis occurs. This must be managed aggressively with antithrombotic agents to prevent myocardial infarction.

40. When coronary blood flow is interrupted for an extended period of time, myocyte necrosis occurs; this is called myocardial infarction (MI). There are two major types of myocardial infarction: subendocardial infarction transmural infarction. In addition to myocyte necrosis, other changes in the heart with MI include hibernating, stunning, and remodeling of the myocardium.

41. Acute coronary syndromes are assessed by measuring serum enzymes, such as creatinine kinase and troponins, as well as looking for characteristic changes in the ECG. Those individuals at highest risk for complications present with ST segment elevations on the ECG (STEMI) and require immediate intervention. Smaller subendocardial infarctions are not associated with ST segment elevations (non-STEMI) but suggest that additional myocardium is still at risk for recurrent ischemia and infarction. Management may include thrombolytic drugs, antithrombotic drugs, vasodilators, PCI, or immediate surgery.

42. Dysrhythmias, congestive heart failure, and sudden death are the most common complications of the acute coronary syndromes.

Disorders of the Heart Wall

1. Inflammation of the pericardium (pericarditis) may result from innumerable sources (infection, drug therapy, tumors). Pericarditis presents with symptoms that are physically troublesome, but in and of themselves they are not life threatening.

2. Fluid may collect within the pericardial sac (pericardial effusion). Cardiac function may be severely impaired if a large volume of fluid accumulates rapidly.

3. Cardiomyopathies are a diverse group of primary myocardial disorders that are poorly understood. The cardiomyopathies are categorized as dilated (congestive), restrictive (rigid and noncompliant), and hypertrophic (asymmetric). Size of the cardiac muscle walls and chambers may increase or decrease, depending on the type of cardiomyopathy, thereby altering contractile activity.

4. Hemodynamic integrity of the cardiovascular system depends to a great extent on properly functioning cardiac valves. Congenital or acquired disorders that result in stenosis or incompetence or both can structurally alter the valves.

5. Characteristic heart sounds, cardiac murmurs, and systemic complaints assist in determination of which valve is abnormal. If severely compromised function exists, a prosthetic heart valve may be surgically implanted to replace the faulty one.

6. Mitral valve prolapse (MVP) is a common finding, especially in young women. Although not grossly abnormal, the mitral valve leaflets do not position themselves properly during systole. MVP may be a completely asymptomatic condition, or it may result in severe subjective symptoms. Afflicted valves may be at greater risk for developing infective endocarditis.

7. Rheumatic fever is an inflammatory disease that results from a delayed autoimmune response to a streptococcal infection. The disorder usually resolves without sequelae if treated early.

8. Severe or untreated cases of rheumatic fever may progress to rheumatic heart disease, a potentially disabling cardiovascular disorder.

9. Infective endocarditis is a general term for inflammation of the endocardium, especially the cardiac valves. A wide range of conditions predisposes one to the development of this disorder. In the mildest cases, valvular function may be slightly impaired by vegetations that collect on the valve leaflets. If infective endocarditis is left unchecked, severe valve abnormalities, chronic bacteremia, and systemic emboli may occur as vegetations break off the valve surface and travel through the bloodstream. Antibiotic therapy can limit the extent of this disease.

10. Human immunodeficiency virus is associated with cardiac abnormalities, including myocarditis, endocarditis, pericarditis, and cardiomyopathy. Left heart failure is the most common clinical manifestation.

Manifestations of Heart Disease

1. Heart failure is an inability of the heart to supply the metabolism with adequate circulatory volume and pressure.

2. Congestive heart failure can be categorized as systolic heart failure or diastolic heart failure.

3. Systolic heart failure is defined as an inability of the heart to generate an adequate cardiac output to perfuse vital tissue.

4. Cardiac output depends on the heart rate and stroke volume. Stroke volume is influenced by contractility, preload, and afterload. Myocardial infarction is the most common cause of decreased contractility. Myocardial ischemia results in ventricular remodeling that causes progressive myocyte contractile dysfunction over time.

5. Preload (left ventricular end-diastolic volume [LVEDV]) is increased when there is decreased contractility or an excess of plasma volume.

6. Increased afterload is most commonly the result of increased peripheral vascular resistance. This increase in resistance decreases ventricular emptying and makes more workload for the left ventricle, resulting in hypertrophy and ventricular remodeling. The vicious cycle of decreasing contractility, increasing preload, and increasing afterload causes progressive worsening.

7. Neurohumoral mechanisms of CHF include abnormalities in the sympathetic nervous system, the renin-angiotensin-aldosterone system, arginine vasopressin, natriuretic peptides, endothelial hormones, endotoxin, and inflammatory cytokines.

8. The clinical manifestations of left heart failure are the result of pulmonary vascular congestion and inadequate systemic perfusion.

9. Management of left heart failure relies on increasing contractility and reducing preload and afterload.

10. Diastolic heart failure can occur singly or together with systolic heart failure. The major causes of diastolic dysfunction include hypertension-induced myocardial hypertrophy and ischemia with resultant ventricular remodeling.

11. Right heart failure can result from left heart failure and/or diffuse hypoxic pulmonary disease, such as chronic obstructive pulmonary disease (COPD), cystic fibrosis, and adult respiratory distress syndrome (ARDS). These mechanisms are discussed in Chapter 33.

12. High output failure is the inability of the heart to adequately supply the body with blood-borne nutrients despite adequate volume and normal or elevated myocardial contractility. Common causes are anemia, septicemia, hyperthyroidism, and beriberi.

13. A dysrhythmia (arrhythmia) is a disturbance of heart rhythm. Dysrhythmias range in severity from occasional missed beats or rapid beats to disturbances that impair myocardial contractility and are life threatening.

14. Dysrhythmias can occur because of an abnormal rate of impulse generation or the abnormal conduction of impulses.

KEY TERMS

MEDIA RESOURCES   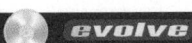 evolve

Review questions and answers for this chapter are available in the *CD Companion* included with this book. Also see the CD for animations of *myocardial infarction, angina, atherosclerosis,* and *hypertension.*

WebLinks—links to Internet sites pertaining to this chapter—are available on Evolve at http://evolve.elsevier.com/McCance/.

REFERENCES

1. Davidson J, Rotondo D: Lipid metabolism: inflammatory-immune responses in atherosclerosis, *Curr Opin Lipidol* 14(3):337-339, 2003.
2. Libby P: Vascular biology of atherosclerosis: overview and state of the art, *Am J Cardiol* 91(3A):3A-6A, 2003.
3. Libby P: Changing concepts of atherogenesis, *J Intern Med* 247(3): 349-358, 2000.
4. Libby P, Ridker PM, Maseri A: Inflammation and atherosclerosis, *Circulation* 105(9):1135-1143, 2002.
5. Ross R: Mechanisms of disease: Atherosclerosis—an inflammatory disease, *N Engl J Med* 340(2):115-126, 1999.
6. Bonetti PO, Lerman LO, Lerman A: Endothelial dysfunction: a marker of atherosclerotic risk, *Arterioscler Thromb Vasc Biol* 23(2):168-175, 2003.
7. Fernandez-Real JM, Ricard W: Insulin resistance and chronic cardiovascular inflammatory syndrome, *Endocr Rev* 24(3):278-301, 2003.
8. Prasad A et al: Predisposition to atherosclerosis by infections: role of endothelial dysfunction, *Circulation* 106(2):184-190, 2002.

9. Ridker PM, Morrow DA: C-reactive protein, inflammation, and coronary risk, *Cardiol Clin* 21(3):315-325, 2003.
10. Scannapieco FA, Bush RB, Paju S: Associations between periodontal disease and risk for atherosclerosis, cardiovascular disease, and stroke: a systematic review, *Ann Periodontol* 8(1):38-53, 2003.
11. Zebrack JS, Anderson JL: The role of infection in the pathogenesis of cardiovascular disease, *Prog Cardiovasc Nurs* 18(1):42-49, 2003.
12. Davignon J, Ganz P: Role of endothelial dysfunction in atherosclerosis, *Circulation* 109(23 Suppl 1):III27-III32, 2004.
13. John S, Schmieder RE: Impaired endothelial function in arterial hypertension and hypercholesterolemia: potential mechanisms and differences, *J Hypertens* 18(4):363-374, 2000.
14. Harrison D et al: Role of oxidative stress in atherosclerosis, *Am J Cardiol* 91(3A):7A-11A, 2003.
15. Cathcart MK: Regulation of superoxide anion production by NADPH oxidase in monocytes/macrophages: contributions to atherosclerosis, *Arterioscler Thromb Vasc Biol* 24(1):23-28, 2004.
16. Jacoby DS, Rader DJ: Renin-angiotensin system and atherothrombotic disease: from genes to treatment, *Arch Intern Med* 163(10):1155-1164, 2003.
17. Fredrikson GN et al: Identification of immune responses against aldehyde-modified peptide sequences in apoB associated with cardiovascular disease, *Arterioscler Thromb Vasc Biol* 23(5):872-878, 2003.
18. Hulthe J et al: Antibodies to oxidized LDL in relation to carotid atherosclerosis, cell adhesion molecules, and phospholipase A(2), *Arterioscler Thromb Vasc Biol* 21(2):269-274, 2001.
19. Kiechl S et al: Toll-like receptor 4 polymorphisms and atherogenesis, *N Engl J Med* 347(3):185-192, 2002.

20. Li D et al: LOX-1, an oxidized LDL endothelial receptor, induces CD40/CD40L signaling in human coronary artery endothelial cells, *Arterioscler Thromb Vasc Biol* 23(5):816-821, 2003.

21. Berenson GS et al: Association between multiple cardiovascular risk factors and atherosclerosis in children and young adults: the Bogalusa Heart Study, *N Engl J Med* 338(23):1650-1656, 1998.

22. McGill HC Jr et al: Associations of coronary heart disease risk factors with the intermediate lesion of atherosclerosis in youth: the Pathobiological Determinants of Atherosclerosis in Youth (PDAY) Research Group, *Arterioscler Thromb Vasc Biol* 20(8):1998-2004, 2000.

23. Millonig G, Malcom GT, Wick G: Early inflammatory-immunological lesions in juvenile atherosclerosis from the Pathobiological Determinants of Atherosclerosis in Youth (PDAY) study, *Atherosclerosis* 160(2):441-448, 2002.

24. Tuzcu EM et al: High prevalence of coronary atherosclerosis in asymptomatic teenagers and young adults: evidence from intravascular ultrasound, *Circulation* 103(22):2705-2710, 2001.

25. Lutgens E et al: Atherosclerotic plaque rupture: local or systemic process? *Arterioscler Thromb Vasc Biol* 23(12):2123-2130, 2003.

26. Stary HC: Natural and historical classification of atherosclerotic lesions: an update, *Arterioscler Thromb Vasc Biol* 20(5):1177-1178, 2000.

27. Virmani R et al: Lessons from sudden coronary death: a comprehensive morphological classification scheme for atherosclerotic lesions, *Arterioscler Thromb Vasc Biol* 20(5):1262-1275, 2000.

28. Hayden M et al: Aspirin for the primary prevention of cardiovascular events: a summary of the evidence for the US Preventive Services Task Force, *Ann Intern Med* 136(2):161-172, 2002.

29. Knight CJ: Antiplatelet treatment in stable coronary artery disease, *Heart* 89(10):1273-1278, 2003.

30. Greenland J et al: AHA Conference Proceedings: prevention conference V. Beyond secondary prevention: identifying the high-risk patient for primary prevention. Noninvasive tests of atherosclerotic burden, *Circulation* 101(1):111-116, 2000.

31. Hunziker PR et al: Bedside quantification of atherosclerosis severity for cardiovascular risk stratification: a prospective cohort study, *J Am Coll Cardiol* 39(4):702-709, 2002.

32. Chiong JR, Miller AB: Agents that stabilize atherosclerotic plaque, *Expert Opin Investig Drugs* 12(10):1681-1692, 2003.

33. Grobbee DE, Bots ML: Statin treatment and progression of atherosclerotic plaque burden, *Drugs* 63(9):893-911, 2003.

34. Kastelein JP, Stroes E, Groot E: Subclinical atherosclerosis as a target of therapy: potential role of statins, *Am J Cardiol* 93(6):737-740, 2004.

35. Chobanian A et al: The Seventh Report of the Joint National Committee on Prevention, Detection, Evaluation, and Treatment of High Blood Pressure: The JNC 7 report, *JAMA* 289(19):2560-2572, 2003.

36. 1999 World Health Organization–International Society of Hypertension guidelines for the management of hypertension: guidelines subcommittee, *J Hypertens* 17(2):151-183, 1999.

37. Staessen JA et al: Essential hypertension, *Lancet* 361(9369):1629-1641, 2003.

38. Oparil S, Zaman MA, Calhoun DA: Pathogenesis of hypertension, *Ann Intern Med* 139(9):761-776, 2003.

39. Hopkins PN, Hunt SC: Genetics of hypertension, *Genet Med* 5(6):413-429, 2003.

40. Luft FC: Present status of genetic mechanisms in hypertension, *Med Clin North Am* 88(1):1-18, vii, 2004.

41. Staessen JA et al: Effects of three candidate genes on prevalence and incidence of hypertension in a Caucasian population, *J Hypertens* 19(8):1349-1358, 2001.

42. Strazzullo P, Galletti F, Barba G: Altered renal handling of sodium in human hypertension: short review of the evidence, *Hypertension* 41:1000-1005, 2003.

43. Vriz O et al: The effects of alcohol consumption on ambulatory blood pressure and target organs in subjects with borderline to mild hypertension, *Am J Hypertens* 11(2):230-234, 1998.

44. Bloomgarden ZT: Obesity, hypertension and insulin resistance, *Diabetes Care* 25(11):2088-2097, 2002.

45. Coatmellec-Taglioni G, Ribiere C: Factors that influence the risk of hypertension in obese individuals, *Curr Opin Nephrol Hypertens* 12(3):305-308, 2003.

46. Hall JE: The kidney, hypertension, and obesity, *Hypertension* 41(3Pt2):625-633, 2003.

47. DiBona GF: The sympathetic nervous system and hypertension: recent developments, *Hypertension* 43(21):147-150, 2004.

48. Grassi G: Role of sympathetic nervous system in human hypertension, *J Hypertens* 16(12Pt2):1979-1987, 1998.

49. Schlaich MP et al: Sympathetic augmentation in hypertension: role of nerve firing, norepinephrine reuptake, and angiotensin neuromodulation, *Hypertension* 43(2):169-175, 2004.

50. Ruiz-Ortega M et al: Molecular mechanisms of angiotensin II-induced vascular injury, *Curr Hypertens Rep* 5(1):73-79, 2003.

51. Fritsch Neves M: Schiffrin EL: Aldosterone: a risk factor for vascular disease, *Curr Hypertens Rep* 5(1):59-65, 2003.

52. Lim PO: Role of aldosterone in the pathogenesis of hypertension, *Hypertension* 39(2):E14, 2002.

53. Conti CR: Aldosterone antagonism and hypertension, *Clin Cardiol* 26(5):209-210, 2003.

54. Liew D, Krum H: Aldosterone receptor antagonists for hypertension: what do they offer? *Drugs* 63(19):1963-1972, 2003.

55. Lip GY, Beevers DG: More evidence on blocking the renin-angiotensin-aldosterone system in cardiovascular disease and the long-term treatment of hypertension: data from recent clinical trials (CHARM, EUROPA, ValHEFT, HOPE-TOO and SYST-EUR2), *J Human Hypertens* 17(11):747-750, 2003.

56. Barlassina C et al: Synergistic effect of [alpha]-adducin and ACE genes causes blood pressure changes with body sodium and volume expansion, *Kidney Int* 57(3):1083-1090, 2000.

57. Grant FD et al: Low-renin hypertension, altered sodium homeostasis, and an alpha-adducin polymorphism, *Hypertension* 39(2):191-196, 2002.

58. Nicod J et al: Role of the alpha-adducin genotype on renal disease progression, *Kidney Int* 61(4):1270-1275, 2002.

59. Psaty BM et al: Diuretic therapy, the alpha-adducin gene variant, and the risk of myocardial infarction or stroke in persons with treated hypertension, *JAMA* 287(13):1680-1689, 2002.

60. Sciarrone MT et al: ACE and alpha-adducin polymorphism as markers of individual response to diuretic therapy, *Hypertension* 41(3):398-403, 2003.

61. McDonough AA, Leong PK, Yang LE: Mechanisms of pressure natriuresis: how blood pressure regulates renal sodium transport, *Ann N Y Acad Sci* 986:669-777, 2003.

62. Akita S et al: Effects of the Dietary Approaches to Stop Hypertension (DASH) diet on the pressure natriuresis relationship, *Hypertension* 42(1):8-13, 2003.

63. Bulut D et al: Impaired vasodilator responses to atrial natriuretic peptide in essential hypertension *Euro J Clin Invest* 33(7):567-573, 2003.

64. Semplicini A et al: Regulation of glomerular filtration in essential hypertension: role of abnormal Na+ transport and atrial natriuretic peptide, *J Nephrol* 15(5):489-496, 2002.

65. Suzuki M et al: Brain natriuretic peptide as a risk marker for incident hypertensive cardiovascular events, *Hyperten Res-Clin Exp* 25(5):669-776, 2002.

66. Suematsu M et al: The inflammatory aspect of the microcirculation in hypertension: oxidative stress, leukocytes/endothelial interaction, apoptosis, *Microcirc* 9(4):259-276, 2002.

67. Taddei S, Salvetti A: Endothelial dysfunction in essential hypertension: clinical implications, *J Hypertens* 20(9):1671-1674, 2002.

68. Brands MW, Fitzgerald SM: Blood pressure control early in diabetes: a balance between angiotensin II and nitric oxide, *Clin Exp Pharmacol Physiol* 29(1-2):127-131, 2002.

69. Hsueh WA, Quinones M: Role of endothelial dysfunction in insulin resistance, *Am J Cardiol* 92(suppl):10J-17J, 2003.

70. Andronico G et al: Insulin resistance and glomerular hemodynamics in essential hypertension, *Kidney Int* 62(3):1005-1009, 2002.

71. Reaven GM: Insulin resistance/compensatory hyperinsulinemia, essential hypertension, and cardiovascular disease, *J Clin Endocrinol Metab* 88(6):2399-2403, 2003.

72. Sowers JR, Frohlich ED: Insulin and insulin resistance: impact on blood pressure and cardiovascular disease, *Med Clin North Am* 88(1):63-82, 2004.

73. Fonseca VA: Management of diabetes mellitus and insulin resistance in patients with cardiovascular disease, *Am J Cardiol* 92(4A):50J-60J, 2003.

74. Hannan RD et al: Cardiac hypertrophy: a matter of translation, *Clin Exp Pharmacol Physiol* 30(8):517-527, 2003.

75. Schlaich MP et al: Relation between cardiac sympathetic activity and hypertensive left ventricular hypertrophy, *Circulation* 108(5):560-565, 2003.

76. Unger T:The role of the renin-angiotensin system in the development of cardiovascular disease, *Am J Cardiol* 89(2A):3A-9A, discussion 10A, 2002.

77. Varagic J, Frohlich ED: Local cardiac renin-angiotensin system: hypertension and cardiac failure, *J Molec Cell Cardiol* 34(11):1435-1442, 2002.

78. Fogo AB: Mechanisms in nephrosclerosis and hypertension-beyond hemodynamics, *J Nephrol* 14(Suppl 4):S63-S69, 2001.

79. Ljutic D, Kes P: The role of arterial hypertension in the progression of non-diabetic glomerular diseases, *Nephrol Dial Transplant* 18(Suppl 5):v28-v30, 2003.

80. Donnelly R, Yeung JM, Manning G: Microalbuminuria: a common, independent cardiovascular risk factor, especially but not exclusively in type 2 diabetes, *J Hypertens Suppl* (Suppl 1):S7-S12, 2003.

81. Leoncini G et al: Mild renal dysfunction and subclinical cardiovascular damage in primary hypertension, *Hypertension* 42(1):14-18, 2003.

82. Park HY et al: A structured review of the relationship between microalbuminuria and cardiovascular events in patients with diabetes mellitus and hypertension, *Pharmacotherapy* 23(12):1611-1616, 2003.

83. Manolio TA, Olson J, Longstreth WT: Hypertension and cognitive function: pathophysiologic effects of hypertension on the brain, *Curr Hypertens Rep* 5(3):255-261, 2003.

84. Sasaki R et al: Vascular remodeling of the carotid artery in patients with untreated essential hypertension increases with age, *Hypertens Res* 25(3):373-379, 2002.

85. Phillips RA, Greenblatt J, Krakoff LR: Hypertensive emergencies: diagnosis and management, *Prog Cardiovas Dis* 45(1):33-48, 2002.

86. O'Brien E: Ambulatory blood pressure monitoring in the management of hypertension, *Heart* 89(5):571-576, 2003.

87. The ALLHAT Officers and Coordinators, for the ALLHAT Collaborative Research Group: Major outcomes in high-risk hypertensive patients randomized to angiotensin-converting enzyme inhibitor or calcium channel blocker vs. diuretic: The Antihypertensive and Lipid-Lowering Treatment to Prevent Heart Attack Trial (ALLHAT), *JAMA* 288(23):2981-2997, 2002.

88. The Concensus Committee of the American Autonomic Society and the American Academy of Neurology: Consensus statement on the definition of orthostatic hypotension, pure autonomic failure, and multiple system atrophy, *Neurology* 46(5):1470, 1996.

89. Eigenbrodt ML et al: Orthostatic hypotension as a risk factor for stroke: the atherosclerosis risk in communities (ARIC) study, 1987-1996, *Stroke* 31(10):2307-2313, 2000.

90. Ooi WL, Hossain M, Lipsitz LA: The association between orthostatic hypotension and recurrent falls in nursing home residents, *Am J Med* 108(2):106-111, 2000.

91. Bradley JG, Davis KA: Orthostatic hypotension, *Am Fam Physician* 68(12):2393-2398, 2003.

92. Miller FJ Jr et al: Oxidative stress in human abdominal aortic aneurysms: a potential mediator of aneurysmal remodeling, *Arterioscler Thromb Vasc Biol* 22:560-565, 2002.

93. Devereux RB, Roman MJ: Aortic disease in Marfan's syndrome, *N Engl J Med* 340(17):1385-1359, 1999.

94. Nienaber CA, Eagle KA: Aortic dissection: new frontiers in diagnosis and management: Part I: from etiology to diagnostic strategies, *Circulation* 108(5):628-635, 2003.

95. Ouriel K, Greenberg RK, Clair DG: Endovascular treatment of aortic aneurysms, *Curr Prob Surg* 39(3):242-345, 2002.

96. Najibi S et al: Endovascular aortic aneurysm operations, *Arch Surg* 137(2):211-216, 2002.

97. Knaut AL, Cleveland JC Jr: Aortic emergencies, *Emerg Med Clin North Am* 21(4):817-845, 2003.

98. Nienaber CA, Eagle KA: Aortic dissection: new frontiers in diagnosis and management: Part II: therapeutic management and follow-up, *Circulation* 108(6):772-778, 2003.

99. American Diabetes Association Consensus Statement: Peripheral arterial disease in people with diabetes, *Diabetes Care* 26(12):3333-3341, 2003.

100. Peripheral Arterial Diseases Antiplatelet Consensus Group: Antiplatelet therapy in peripheral arterial disease. Consensus statement, *Eur J Vasc Endovas Surg* 26(1):1-16, 2003.

101. Drugs for intermittent claudication, *Med Lett Drugs Ther* 46(1176): 13-15, 2004.

102. Bradbury AW: The role of cilostazol (Pletal) in the management of intermittent claudication, *Int J Clin Pract* 57(5):405-409, 2003.

103. Cassar K, Bachoo P, Brittenden J: The effect of peripheral percutaneous transluminal angioplasty on quality of life in patients with intermittent claudication, *Eur J Vasc Endovasc Surg* 26(2):130-136, 2003.

104. Mills JL Sr: Buerger's disease in the 21st century: diagnosis, clinical features, and therapy, *Semin Vasc Surg* 16(3):179-189, 2003.

105. Lee T, Seo JW, Sumpio BE, Kim SJ: Immunobiologic analysis of arterial tissue in Buerger's disease, *Eur J Vasc Endovasc Surg* 25(5):451-457, 2003.

106. Ohta T, Ishioashi H, Hosaka M, Sugimoto I: Clinical and social consequences of Buerger disease, *J Vasc Surg* 39(1):176-180, 2004.

107. Charkoudian N: Skin blood flow in adult human thermoregulation: how it works, when it does not, and why, *Mayo Clin Proc* 78(5): 603-612, 2003.

108. Wigley FM: Clinical practice: Raynaud's phenomenon, *N Engl J Med* 347(13):1001-1008, 2002.

109. Herrick AL: Treatment of Raynaud's phenomenon: new insights and developments, *Curr Rheumatol Rep* 5(2):168-174, 2003.

110. Decousus H et al: Superficial vein thrombosis: risk factors, diagnosis, and treatment, *Curr Opin Pulm Med* 9(5):393-397, 2003.

111. Haas SK: Venous thromboembolic risk and its prevention in hospitalized medical patients, *Sem Thromb Hemost* 28(6):577-584, 2002.

112. Kroegel C, Reissig A: Principle mechanisms underlying venous thromboembolism: epidemiology, risk factors, pathophysiology and pathogenesis, *Respiration* 70(1):7-30, 2003.

113. Kinney TB: Update on inferior vena cava filters, *J Vasc Interv Radiol* 14(4):425-440, 2003.

114. Zierler BK: Ultrasonography and diagnosis of venous thromboembolism, *Circulation* 109(12 Suppl 1):I9-I14, 2004.

115. Lee AY, Hirsh J: Diagnosis and treatment of venous thromboembolism, *Annu Rev Med* 53:15-33, 2002.

116. Kahn SR, Ginsberg JS: Relationship between deep venous thrombosis and the postthrombotic syndrome, *Arch Intern Med* 164(1):17-26, 2004.

117. Rowell NP, Gleeson FV: Steroids, radiotherapy, chemotherapy and stents for superior vena caval obstruction in carcinoma of the bronchus: a systematic review, *Clin Oncol (R Coll Radiol)* 14(5): 338-351, 2002.

118. Sharafuddin MJ, Sun S, Hoballah JJ: Endovascular management of venous thrombotic diseases of the upper torso and extremities, *J Vasc Interv Radiol* 13(10):975-990, 2002.

119. American Heart Association: *Heart disease and stroke statistics—2004 update*, Dallas, Tex, 2003, Author.

120. Khot UN et al: Prevalence of conventional risk factors in patients with coronary heart disease, *JAMA* 290(7):898-904, 2003.

121. Linton MF, Fazio S: National Cholesterol Education Program (NCEP)—the third Adult Treatment Panel (ATP III). A practical approach to risk assessment to prevent coronary artery disease and its complications, *Am J Cardiol* 92(suppl):19i-26i, 2003.

122. Expert Panel on Detection, Evaluation, and Treatment of High Blood Cholesterol in Adults: Executive summary of the third report of the National Cholesterol Education Program (NCEP) expert panel on detection, evaluation, and treatment of high blood cholesterol in adults (Adult Treatment Panel III), *JAMA* 285(19): 2486-2497, 2001.

123. Kwiterovich PO Jr: Lipoprotein heterogeneity: diagnostic and therapeutic implications, *Am J Cardiol* 90(8A):1i-10i, 2002.

124. Kwiterovich PO Jr: Clinical relevance of the biochemical, metabolic, and genetic factors that influence low-density lipoprotein heterogeneity, *Am J Cardiol* 90(8A):30i-47i, 2002.

125. Heart Protection Study Collaborative Group: MRC/BHF Heart Protection Study of cholesterol lowering with simvastatin in 20,536 high-risk individual: a randomized placebo-controlled trial, *Lancet* 360(9326): 7-22, 2002.

126. Ballantyne CM: Current and future aims of lipid lowering therapy: changing paradigms and lessons from the heart protection study on standards of efficacy and safety, *Am J Cardiol* 92(suppl):3k-9k, 2003.

127. Ballantyne CM et al: Effect of ezetimibe coadministered with atorvastatin in 628 patients with primary hypercholesterolemia, *Circulation* 107(19):2409-2415, 2003.

128. Nissen SE et al: Effect of intensive compared with moderate lipid-lowering therapy on progression of coronary atherosclerosis: a randomized controlled trial, *JAMA* 291(9):1071-1080, 2004.

129. Brewer HB Jr: Increasing HDL cholesterol levels, *N Engl J Med* 350(15):1491-1494, 2004.

130. Brewer HB Jr, Santamarina-Fojo S: Clinical significance of high-density lipoproteins and the development of atherosclerosis, *Am J Cardiol* 92(suppl):10k-16k, 2003.

131. Rader DJ: High-density lipoproteins and atherosclerosis, *Am J Cardiol* 90(suppl):62i-70i, 2002.

132. Rader DJ: High-density lipoproteins as an emerging therapeutic target for atherosclerosis, *JAMA* 290(17):2322-2324, 2003.

133. Toth PP: High-density lipoprotein and cardiovascular risk, *Circulation* 109(15):1809-1812, 2004.

134. Kraus WE et al: Effects of the amount and intensity of exercise on plasma lipoproteins, *N Engl J Med* 347(19):1483-1492, 2002.

135. Rimm EB et al: Moderate alcohol intake and lower risk of coronary heart disease: meta-analysis of effects on lipids and hemostatic factors, *BMJ* 319(7224):1523-1528, 1999.

136. Scanu AM: Lipoprotein (a) and the atherothrombotic process: mechanistic insights and clinical applications, *Curr Atheroscler Rep* 5(2): 106-113, 2003.

137. Bazzano LA et al: Relationship between cigarette smoking and novel risk factors for cardiovascular disease in the United States, *Ann Intern Med* 138(11):891-897, 2003.

138. Mooradian AD: Cardiovascular disease in type 2 diabetes mellitus, *Arch Intern Med* 163(1):33-40, 2003.

139. Eckel RH et al: Prevention conference VI: diabetes and cardiovascular disease: Writing Group II: pathogenesis of atherosclerosis in diabetes, *Circulation* 105(18):e138-e143, 2002.

140. Haffner SM: Insulin resistance, inflammation, and the prediabetic state, *Am J Cardiol* 92(suppl):18J-26J, 2003.

141. Sheetz MJ, King G: Molecular understanding of hyperglycemia's adverse effects for diabetic complications, *JAMA* 288(20):2579-2588, 2002.

142. Knopp RH et al: Management of patients with diabetic hyperlipidemia, *Am J Cardiol* 91(7A):24E-28E, 2003.

143. Pischon T et al: Plasma adiponectin levels and risk of myocardial infarction in men, *JAMA* 291(14):1730-1737, 2004.

144. Carnethon M et al: Cardiorespiratory fitness in young adulthood and the development of cardiovascular disease risk factors, *JAMA* 290(23):3092-3100, 2003.

145. Manson JE et al: The escalating pandemics of obesity and sedentary lifestyle, *Arch Intern Med* 164(3):249-258, 2004.

146. Gregg EW: Relationship of changes in physical activity and mortality among older women *JAMA* 289(18):2379-2386, 2003.

147. Blake GJ, Ridker PM: C-reactive protein and other inflammatory risk markers in acute coronary syndromes, *J Am Coll Cardiol* 41(4Suppl S):37S-42S, 2003.

148. Danesh J et al: C reactive protein and other circulating markers of inflammation in the prediction of coronary heart disease, *N Engl J Med* 350(14):1387-1397, 2004.

149. Ridker P: High sensitivity C-reactive protein and cardiovascular risk: rationale for screening and primary prevention, *Am J Cardiol* 92(suppl):17K-22K, 2003.

150. Rosenson RS, Koenig W: Utility of inflammatory markers in the management of coronary artery disease, *Am J Cardiol* 92(1A):10i-18i, 2003.

151. Hackam DG, Anand SS: Emerging risk factors for atherosclerotic vascular disease: a critical review of the evidence, *JAMA* 290(7):932-940, 2003.

152. Pearson TA et al: Markers of inflammation and cardiovascular disease: application to clinical and public health practice [AHA/CDC Scientific Statement], *Circulation* 107(3):449-511, 2003.

153. Van der Meer I et al: The value of C-reactive protein in cardiovascular risk prediction, *Arch Inter Med* 163(11):1323-1328, 2003.

154. Blankenberg S et al: Interleukin-18 is a strong predictor of cardiovascular death in stable and unstable angina, *Circulation* 106(1):24-30, 2002.

155. Heeschen C et al: Soluble CD40 ligand in acute coronary syndromes, *N Engl J Med* 348(12):1104-1111, 2003.

156. Maresca G et al: Measuring plasma fibrinogen to predict stroke and myocardial infarction: an update, *Arterioscler Thromb Vasc Biol* 19(6):1368–1377, 1999.

157. Ridker PM, Rifai N, Stampfer MJ, Hennekens CH: Plasma concentration of interleukin-6 and the risk of future myocardial infarction among apparently healthy men, *Circulation* 101(15):1767-1572, 2000.

158. Ridker PM et al: Elevation of tumor necrosis factor-[alpha] and increased risk of recurrent coronary events after myocardial infarction, *Circulation* 101(18):2149-2153, 2000.

159. The Homocysteine Studies Collaboration: Homocysteine and risk of ischemic heart disease and stroke: a meta-analysis, *JAMA* 288(16):2015-2022, 2002.

160. Toole JF et al: Lowering homocysteine in patients with ischemic stroke to prevent recurrent stroke, myocardial infarction and death, *JAMA* 291(5):565-575, 2004.

161. Higgins JP: Chlamydia pneumoniae and coronary artery disease: the antibiotic trials, *Mayo Clin Proc* 78:321-332, 2003.

162. Spence JD, Norris J: Infection, inflammation, and atherosclerosis, *Stroke* 34(2):333-334, 2003.

163. Zebrack JS, Anderson JL: The role of infection in the pathogenesis of cardiovascular disease, *Prog Cardiovasc Nurs* 18(1):42-49, 2003.

164. Pislaru S, Van de Werf F: Antibiotic therapy for coronary artery disease: can a WIZARD change it all? *JAMA* 290(11):1515-1516, 2003.

165. O'Connor CM et al, for the investigators in the WIZARD study: Azithromycin for the secondary prevention of coronary heart disease events: the WIZARD study: a randomized controlled trial, *JAMA* 290(11):1459-1466, 2003.

166. Stone AF et al: Effect of treatment for *Chlamydia pneumoniae* and *Helicobacter pylori* on markers of inflammation and cardiac events in patients with acute coronary syndromes: South Thames Trial of Antibiotics in Myocardial Infarction and Unstable Angina (STAMINA), *Circulation* 106(10):1219-1223, 2002.

167. Wang K, Asinger RW, Marriott HJ: ST-segment elevation in conditions other than acute myocardial infarction, *N Engl J Med* 349(22): 2128-2135, 2003.

168. Mazzone A et al: Increased production of inflammatory cytokines in patients with silent myocardial ischemia, *J Am Coll Cardiol* 38(7): 1895-1901, 2001.

169. Rozanski A et al: Mental stress and the induction of silent myocardial ischemia in patients with coronary disease, *N Engl J Med* 318(16):1005-1012, 1988.

170. von Kanel R et al: Effects of psychological stress and psychiatric disorders on blood coagulation and fibrinolysis: a biobehavioral pathway to coronary artery disease, *Psychosom Med* 63(4):531-544, 2001.

171. Kurl S et al: Association of exercise-induced, silent ST-segment depression with the risk of stroke and cardiovascular diseases in men, *Stroke* 34(7):1760-1765, 2003.

172. Knight CJ: Antiplatelet treatment in stable coronary artery disease, *Heart* 89(10):1273-1278, 2003.

173. Corti R et al: Lipid lowering by simvastatin induces regression of human atherosclerotic lesions: two years' follow-up by high-resolution noninvasive magnetic resonance imaging, *Circulation* 106(23): 2884-2887, 2002.

174. Jabbour S et al: Long-term outcomes of optimized medical management of outpatients with stable coronary artery disease, *Am J Cardiol* 93(3):294-299, 2004.

175. Holmes DR: State of the art in coronary intervention, *Am J Cardiol* 91(suppl 1):50-53, 2003.

176. Dery JP, Harrington RA, Tcheng JE: GP IIb/IIIa blockade in elective percutaneous coronary intervention, *Curr Pharm Design* 10(4): 387-398, 2004.

177. Chaitman BR et al: Effects of ranolazine with atenolol, amlodipine, or diltiazem on exercise tolerance and angina frequency in patients with severe chronic angina: a randomized controlled trial, *JAMA* 291(3):309-316, 2004.

178. Stary HC et al: A definition of advanced types of atherosclerotic lesions and a histological classification of atherosclerosis: a report from the Committee on Bascular Lesions of the Council on Artriosclerosis, American Heart Association, *Arterioscler Thromb Vasc Biol* 15(9): 1512-1531, 1995.

179. Corti R, Fuster V, Badimon JJ: Pathogenetic concepts of acute coronary syndromes, *J Am Coll Cardiol* 41(4Suppl S):7S-14S, 2003.

180. Shah PK: Mechanisms of plaque vulnerability and rupture, *J Am Coll Cardiol* 41(4 Suppl S): 15S-22S, 2003.

181. Libby P: Current concepts of the pathogenesis of the acute coronary syndromes, *Circulation* 104(3):365-372, 2001.

182. Tousoulis D et al: Inflammatory and thrombotic mechanisms in coronary atherosclerosis, *Heart* 89(9):993-997, 2003.

183. Shah PK: Pathophysiology of plaque rupture and the concept of plaque stabilization, *Cardio Clin* 21(3):303-314, v, 2003.

184. Timmis AD: Plaque stabilisation in acute coronary syndromes: clinical considerations, *Heart* 89(10):1268-1272, 2003.

185. Grech ED, Ramsdale DR: Acute coronary syndrome: unstable angina and non-ST segment elevation myocardial infarction, *BMJ* 326(7401):1259-1261, 2003.

186. Braunwald E et al: ACC/AHA guideline update for the management of patients with unstable angina and non–ST-segment elevation myocardial infarction—2002: summary article: a report of the American College of Cardiology/American Heart Association Task Force on Practice Guidelines (Committee on the Management of Patients With Unstable Angina), *Circulation* 106(14):1893-1900, 2002.

187. Antman EM: Glycoprotein IIb/IIIa inhibitors in patients with unstable angina/non-ST-segment elevation myocardial infarction: appropriate interpretation of the guidelines, *Am Heart J* 146(4 Suppl):S18-S22, 2003.

188. Penttila HJ et al: Ischemic preconditioning does not improve myocardial preservation during off-pump multivessel coronary operation, *Ann Thorac Surg* 75(4):1246-1252, discussion 1252-1253, 2003.

189. Kosieradzki M: Mechanisms of ischemic preconditioning and its application in transplantation, *Ann Transplant* 7(3):12-20, 2002.

190. Camici PG: Hibernation and heart failure, *Heart (Br Cardiac Soc)* 90(2):141-143, 2004.

191. Frangogiannis NG: The pathological basis of myocardial hibernation, *Histol Histopathol* 18(2):647-655, 2003.

192. Luss H et al: Biochemical mechanisms of hibernation and stunning in the human heart, *Cardiovasc Res* 56(3):411-421, 2002.

193. Maytin M, Colucci WS: Molecular and cellular mechanisms of myocardial remodeling, *J Nucl Cardiol* 9(3):319-327, 2002.

194. Rozenberg VD, Nepomniashchikh LM: Pathomorphological characteristics of cardiac remodeling after myocardial infarction, *Bull Exp Biol Med* 135(1):96-100, 2003.

195. Sharpe N: Left ventricular remodeling: pathophysiology and treatment, *Heart Fail Monit* 4(2):55-61, 2003.

196. Collinson P et al: Multicentre evaluation of the diagnostic value of cardiac troponin T, CK-MB mass, and myoglobin for assessing patients with suspected acute coronary syndromes in routine clinical practice, *Heart* 89(3):280-286, 2003.

197. Zimetbaum P, Josephson M: Use of the electrocardiogram in acute myocardial infarction, *N Engl J Med* 348(10):933-940, 2003.

198. Keeley EC, Grines CL: Primary coronary intervention for acute myocardial infarction, *JAMA* 291(6):736-739, 2004.

199. Mehta RH et al: Effectiveness of primary percutaneous coronary intervention compared with that of thrombolytic therapy in elderly patients with acute myocardial infarction, *Am Heart J* 147(2):253-259, 2004.

200. Kandzari DE et al: Improved clinical outcomes with abciximab therapy in acute myocardial infarction: a systematic overview of randomized clinical trials, *Am Heart J* 147(3):457-462, 2004.

201. Moller JE et al: Effects of losartan and captopril on left ventricular systolic and diastolic function after acute myocardial infarction: results of the Optimal Trial in Myocardial Infarction with Angiotensin II Antagonist Losartan (OPTIMAAL) echocardiographic substudy, *Am Heart J* 147(3):494-501, 2004.

202. Hognestad A et al: Effect of combined statin and beta-blocker treatment on one-year morbidity and mortality after acute myocardial infarction associated with heart failure, *Am J Cardiol* 93(5):603-606, 2004.

203. Cannon CP et al: Intensive versus moderate lipid lowering with statins after acute coronary syndromes, *N Engl J Med* 350(15):1495-1504, 2004.

204. Newby LK et al: Early statin initiation and outcomes in patients with acute coronary syndromes, *JAMA* 287(23):3087-3095, 2002.

205. Spodick DH: Acute pericarditis: current concepts and practice, *JAMA* 289(9):1150-1153, 2003 .

206. Troughton RW, Asher CR, Klein AL: Pericarditis, *Lancet* 363(9410):717-727, 2004.

207. Schifferdecker B, Spodick DH: Nonsteroidal anti-inflammatory drugs in the treatment of pericarditis, *Cardiol Rev* 11(4):211-217, 2003.

208. Lindenberger M, Kjellberg M, Karlsson E, Wranne B: Pericardiocentesis guided by 2-D echocardiography: the method of choice for treatment of pericardial effusion, *J Intern Med* 253(4):411-417, 2003.

209. Musch E et al: Intrapericardial instillation of mitoxantrone in palliative therapy of malignant pericardial effusion, *Onkologie* 26(2):135-139, 2003.

210. Glockner JF: Imaging of pericardial disease, *Magn Reson Imaging Clin North Am* 11(1):149-162, vii, 2003.

211. Schofield RS et al: Left ventricular dysfunction after pericardiectomy for constrictive pericarditis, *Ann Thorac Surg* 77(4):1449-1451, 2004.

212. Richardson P et al: Report of the 1995 World Health Organization/International Society and Federation of Cardiology Task Force on the Definition and Classification of Cardiomyopathies, *Circulation* 93(5):841-842, 1996.

213. Noutsias M et al: Current insights into the pathogenesis, diagnosis and therapy of inflammatory cardiomyopathy, *Heart Fail Monit* 3(4):127-135, 2003.

214. Kozelj M, Novak-Antolic Z, Noc M, Antolic G: Idiopathic dilated cardiomyopathy in pregnancy, *Acta Obstet Gynecol Scand* 82(4):389-390, 2003.

215. Mason JW: Myocarditis and dilated cardiomyopathy: an inflammatory link, *Cardiovasc Res* 60(1):5-10, 2003.

216. Noutsias M et al: Immunomodulatory treatment strategies in inflammatory cardiomyopathy: current status and future perspectives, *Exp Rev Cardiovasc Ther* 2(1):37-51, 2004.

217. Linde C: Implantable cardioverter-defibrillator treatment and resynchronisation in heart failure, *Heart (Br Cardiac Soc)* 90(2):231-234, 2004.

218. Nishimura RA, Holmes DR Jr: Clinical practice. Hypertrophic obstructive cardiomyopathy, *N Engl J Med* 350(13):1320-1327, 2004.

219. Kovacic JC, Muller D: Hypertrophic cardiomyopathy: state-of-the-art review, with focus on the management of outflow obstruction, *Int Med J* 33(11):521-529, 2003.

220. Maron BJ et al: American College of Cardiology/European Society of Cardiology clinical expert consensus document on hypertrophic cardiomyopathy. A report of the American College of Cardiology Foundation Task Force on Clinical Expert Consensus Documents and the European Society of Cardiology Committee for Practice Guidelines, *J Am Coll Cardiol* 42(9):1687-1713, 2003.

221. Frenneaux MP: Assessing the risk of sudden cardiac death in a patient with hypertrophic cardiomyopathy, *Heart (Br Cardiac Soc)* 90(5):570-575, 2004.

222. Maron BJ et al: Primary prevention of sudden death as a novel treatment strategy in hypertrophic cardiomyopathy, *Circulation* 107(23):2872-2875, 2003.

223. Chan KL: Is aortic stenosis a preventable disease? *J Am Coll Cardiol* 42(4):593-599, 2003.

224. Aazami M, Schafers HJ: Advances in heart valve surgery, *J Intervent Cardiol* 16(6):535-541, 2003.

225. Wiegand DL: Advances in cardiac surgery: valve repair, *Crit Care Nurse* 23(2):72-91, 2003.

226. David TE et al: Late outcomes of mitral valve repair for floppy valves: implications for asymptomatic patients, *J Thor Cardiovasc Surg* 125(5):1143-1152, 2003.

227. Galloway AC et al: Evolving techniques for mitral valve reconstruction, *Ann Surg* 236(3): 288-294, 2002.

228. Triezenberg D, Helmen J, Pearson M: When should patients with mitral valve prolapse get endocarditis prophylaxis? *J Fam Pract* 53(3):223-228, discussion 228, 2004.

229. Miner LJ et al: Molecular characterization of Streptococcus pyogenes isolates collected during periods of increased acute rheumatic fever activity in Utah, *Pediatr Infect Dis J* 23(1):56-61, 2004.

230. Djani AS et al: Guidelines for the diagnosis of rheumatic fever. Jones criteria, updated 1993, *Circulation* 87:302, 1993.

231. Karademir S et al: Tolmetin and salicylate therapy in acute rheumatic fever: comparison of clinical efficacy and side-effects, *Pediatr Int* 45(6):676-679, 2003.

232. Hashkes PJ et al: Naproxen as an alternative to aspirin for the treatment of arthritis of rheumatic fever: a randomized trial, *J Pediatr* 143(3):399-401, 2003.

233. Moreillon P, Que YA: Infective endocarditis, *Lancet* 363(9403):139-149, 2004.

234. Crawford MH, Durack DT: Clinical presentation of infective endocarditis, *Cardiol Clin* 21(2):159-166, v, 2003.

235. Murtagh B, Frazier OH, Letsou GV: Diagnosis and management of bacterial endocarditis in 2003, *Curr Opin Cardiol* 18(2):106-110, 2003.

236. Furuya EY, Lowy FD: Antimicrobial strategies for the prevention and treatment of cardiovascular infections, *Curr Opin Pharmacol* 3(5):464-469, 2003.

237. Olaison L, Pettersson G: Current best practices and guidelines. Indications for surgical intervention in infective endocarditis, *Cardiol Clin* 21(2):235-251, vii, 2003.

238. Barbarini G, Barbaro G: Incidence of the involvement of the cardiovascular system in HIV infection, *AIDS* 17(Suppl 1):S46-S50, 2003.

239. Barbaro G: Pathogenesis of HIV-associated heart disease, *AIDS* 17(Suppl 1):S12-S20, 2003.

240. Murphy RL, Barbaro G: Clinical and biological insights in HIV-associated cardiovascular disease in the era of highly active antiretroviral therapy, *AIDS* 17(Suppl 1):S1-S3, 2003.

241. Jessup M, Brozena S: Heart failure, *N Engl J Med* 348:2007-2018, 2003.

242. Piano MR, Prasun M: Neurohormone activation, *Crit Care Nurs Clin North Am* 15(4):413-421, 2003.

243. Katz AM: Pathophysiology of heart failure: identifying targets for pharmacotherapy, *Med Clin North Am* 87(2):303-316, 2003.

244. Francis GS, Tang WH: Pathophysiology of congestive heart failure, *Rev Cardiovasc Med* 4(Suppl 2):S14-S20, 2003.

245. Lohse MJ, Engelhardt S, Eschenhagen T: What is the role of beta-adrenergic signaling in heart failure? *Circ Res* 93(10):896-906, 2003.

246. Manohar P, Pina IL: Therapeutic role of angiotensin II receptor blockers in the treatment of heart failure, *Mayo Clin Proc* 78(3):334-338, 2003.

247. Dawson A, Davies JI, Struthers AD: The role of aldosterone in heart failure and the clinical benefits of aldosterone blockade, *Exp Rev Cardiovasc Ther* 2(1):29-36, 2004.

248. Weber KT et al: Toward a broader understanding of aldosterone in congestive heart failure, *J Renin-Angiotensin-Aldosterone Sys* 4(3):155-163, 2003.

249. Krum H, Liew D: New and emerging drug therapies for the management of acute heart failure, *Intern Med J* 33(11):515-520, 2003.

250. Maisel AS, McCullough PA: Cardiac natriuretic peptides:a proteomic window to cardiac function and clinical management, *Rev Cardiovasc Med* 4(Suppl 4):S3-S12, 2003.

251. Stoupakis G, Klapholz M: Natriuretic peptides: biochemistry, physiology, and therapeutic role in heart failure, *Heart Dis* 5(3):215-223, 2003.

252. Moe GW et al: Role of endothelins in congestive heart failure, *Can J Physiol Pharmacol* 81(6):588-597, 2003.

253. Peschel T et al: Invasive assessment of bacterial endotoxin and inflammatory cytokines in patients with acute heart failure, *Eur J Heart Fail* 5(5):609-614, 2003.

254. Anker SD, von Haehling S: Inflammatory mediators in chronic heart failure: an overview, *Heart (Br Cardiac Soc)* 90(4):464-470, 2004.

255. Vasan RS et al: Framingham Heart Study. Inflammatory markers and risk of heart failure in elderly subjects without prior myocardial infarction: the Framingham Heart Study, *Circulation* 107(11):1486-1491, 2003.

256. Maisel AS: The diagnosis of acute congestive heart failure: role of BNP measurements, *Heart Fail Rev* 8(4):327-334, 2003.

257. Prahash A, Lynch T: B-type natriuretic peptide: a diagnostic, prognostic, and therapeutic tool in heart failure, *Am J Crit Care* 13(1):46-53, quiz 54-55, 2004.

258. Lowery SL, Massaro R, Yancy CW Jr: Advances in the management of acute and chronic decompensated heart failure, *Lippincott's Case Manag* 9(2 Suppl):S1-S15, quiz S1-S7, 2004.

259. Cleland JG, Nikitin N, McGowan J: Levosimendan: first in a new class of inodilator for acute and chronic severe heart failure, *Exp Rev Cardiovasc Ther* 2(1):9-19, 2004.

260. de Denus S, Pharand C, Williamson DR: Brain natriuretic peptide in the management of heart failure: the versatile neurohormone, *Chest* 125(2):652-668, 2004.

261. Fonarow GC: B-type natriuretic peptide: spectrum of application. Nesiritide (recombinant BNP) for heart failure, *Heart Fail Rev* 8(4):321-325, 2003.

262. Dec GW: Digoxin remains useful in the management of chronic heart failure, *Med Clin North Am* 87(2):317-337, 2003.

263. Sackner-Bernstein JD, Hart D: Neurohormonal antagonism in heart failure: what is the optimal strategy? *Mount Sinai J Med* 71(2):115-126, 2004.

264. Dec GW: Management of heart failure: crossing boundary over to the surgical country, *Surg Clin North Am* 84(1):1-25, 2004.

265. Angeja BG, Grossman W: Evaluation and management of diastolic heart failure, *Circulation* 107(5):659-663, 2003.

266. Piccini JP, Klein L, Gheorghiade M, Bonow RO: New insights into diastolic heart failure: role of diabetes mellitus, *Am J Med* 116(Suppl 5A):64S-75S, 2004.

267. Hogg K, Swedberg K, McMurray J: Heart failure with preserved left ventricular systolic function: epidemiology, clinical characteristics, and prognosis, *J Am Coll Cardiol* 43(3):317-327, 2004.

ALTERATIONS OF CARDIOVASCULAR FUNCTION IN CHILDREN

JEAN ANNE CONNOR

CHAPTER OUTLINE

Cardiovascular disease in children can be classified as congenital or acquired heart disease. Congenital heart disease is the most common. The diagnosis and management of congenital heart defects continue to improve with the use of fetal echocardiography, early interventional catheterization, and refined surgical repair. Acquired heart defects in children continue to present challenges to the practitioner; although guidelines for diagnosing acquired defects are available, work is needed in developing standards of treatment and long-term follow-up.

DEVELOPMENT OF THE CARDIOVASCULAR SYSTEM

Developmental Anatomy

Embryology

Cardiogenesis begins at approximately 3 weeks of gestation; however, most cardiovascular development occurs between the fourth and seventh weeks.[1] The heart arises from the mesenchyme and begins development as an enlarged blood vessel with a large lumen and a muscular wall (Figure 31-1, *A*). Initially, two lateral endocardial heart tubes fuse to form a single structure (Figure 31-1, *B*). During the fifth week of gestation, the midsection of this tube begins to grow faster than its ends. This single heart tube elongates and rotates to the right

(D-loop formation), creating a bulboventricular loop by approximately the twenty-eighth day[1] (Figure 31-1, *C*). Also at this time the first fetal heart contractions occur. At this stage the primitive heart structures include a common atrium; common ventricle; the sinus venosus, which eventually evolves into the superior and inferior venae cavae; the bulbus cordis, which eventually evolves into the ventricular outflow tracts; and the truncus arteriosus, which eventually yields the main pulmonary artery and aorta (Figure 31-1, *D*). By the fourth week of gestation, cardiovascular septation, ventricular development, aortic arch evolution, and circulation begin.

Cardiac Septation

Separation first begins when collections of mesenchymal cells cause the endocardial lining of the heart to bulge into the internal lumen. These changes, known as **endocardial cushions,** are instrumental in closing the atrial septum, dividing the atrioventricular (AV) canals into the right and left AV orifices, and closing the interventricular septum. Altered formation of the endocardial cushions can result in ostium primum atrial septal defects, ventricular septal defects (VSDs), malformation of the AV valves, or a complete AV defect.

Atrial separation begins when two thin membrane-like structures, known as the **septum primum** and the **septum secundum,** grow toward the area of the endocardial cushions (Figure 31-2). The septum primum forms along the posterior wall of the common atrium and grows downward toward the

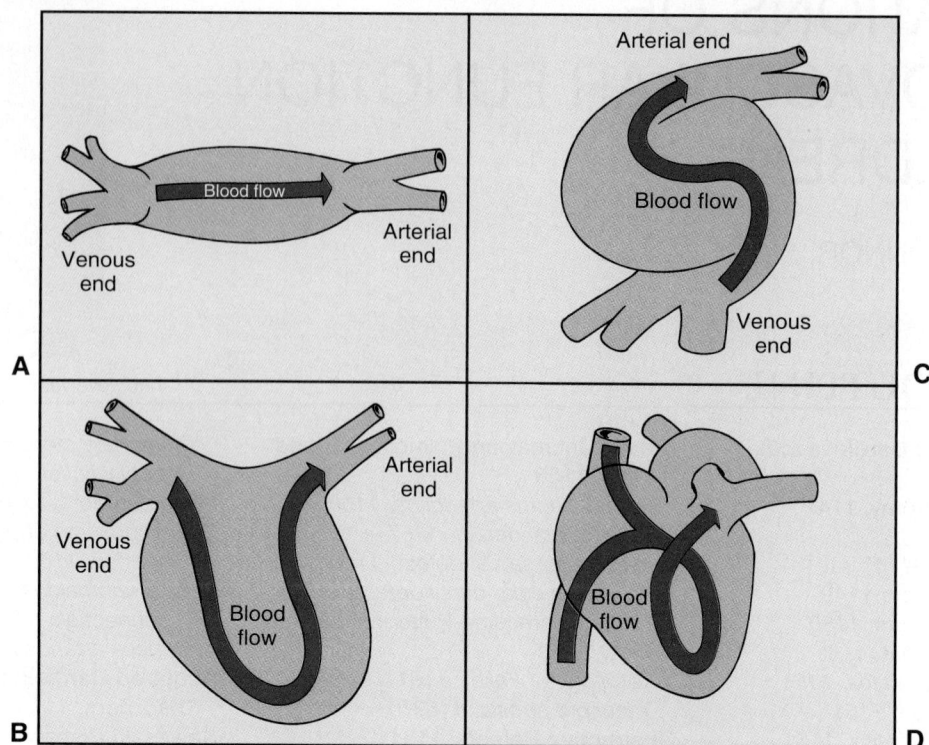

Figure 31-1 **Embryologic development of the heart. A,** The earliest heart structure consists of a muscular tube with a large lumen. About the fifth week of gestation, the tube, **B,** bulges and, **C,** twists until, **D,** the ends come together and fuse.

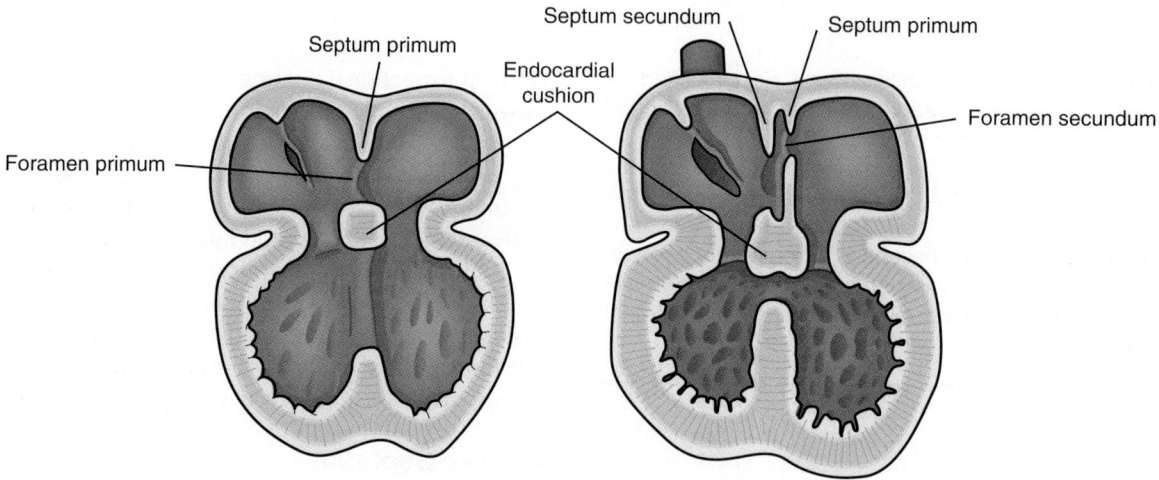

Figure 31-2 Development of the cardiac septa.

center portion of the heart. The gap between the two structures, known as the **ostium primum,** normally closes by extensions from the endocardial cushions. At the time of closure, fenestrations or openings develop in the superior portion of the septum primum, creating the **ostium secundum.** Failure of the septum primum to fuse with the endocardial cushions results in an ostium primum defect in the atrial septum near the atrioventricular valve area.

The septum secundum is also a fenestrated, membrane-like structure located anteriorly that grows toward the endocardial cushions. During fetal development this structure does not completely fuse with the endocardial cushions to achieve complete atrial septal closure. The nonfused septum secundum and ostium secundum result in the formation of a flapped orifice known as the **foramen ovale,** which allows the right-to-left shunting necessary for fetal circulation. Altered development in any of these structures can lead to an atrial septal defect.

Ventricular septation develops when the muscular ridge located at the apex, the endocardial tissue, and the bulbar ridges in the bulbus cordis fuse (Figure 31-3). Closure of the interventricular septum ensures communication between the

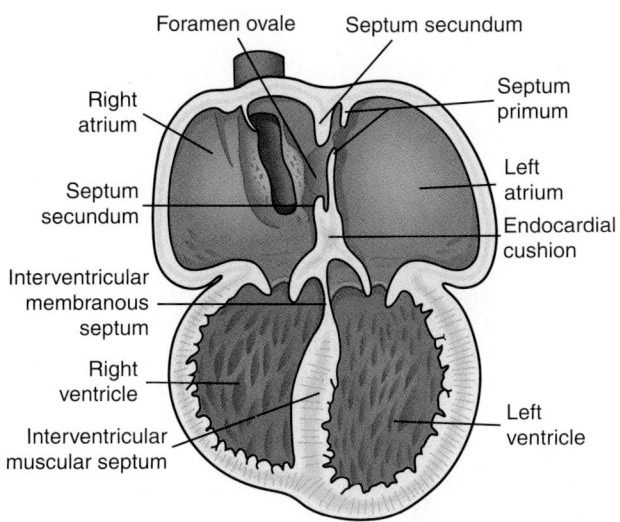

Figure 31-3 Septal development of the heart.

right ventricle (RV) and the pulmonary artery and between the left ventricle (LV) and the aorta. Further evolution of the endocardial tissue gives rise to the membranous ventricular septum and the AV valves. The conal portion of the ventricular septum that separates the aorta from the pulmonary artery forms from the **bulbus cordis.**

When the single primitive heart tube begins to form the D-loop, the venous and arterial poles of the heart are fixed, resulting in torsion within the anterosuperior region of the loop, known as the *truncus arteriosus*. This torsion creates a spiral, ridgelike structure or septum within the truncus arteriosus that divides it into the pulmonary artery and the aorta. The semilunar valves evolve from tubercles after this division is complete.

Before this division occurs, however, two large arteries form at the distal end of the truncus arteriosus. They give rise to the six aortic arches. By the fifth week of gestation, the first two pairs disappear and the third eventually evolves into the common carotid artery, the external carotid artery, and part of the internal carotid artery. The fourth pair of aortic arches will form part of the true aortic arch and the proximal segment of the right subclavian artery. The fifth pair disappears; however, the sixth pair yields the proximal and branch pulmonary arteries with lung parenchyma and the ductus arteriosus.

Swellings in the conal region at the base of the main trunk separate the right ventricular outflow (pulmonary outflow) tract from the left ventricular outflow (aortic outflow) tract. The conus also contributes to complete closure of the interventricular septum, and normal reabsorption of the subaortic conal region ensures rotation of the great arteries so that the aorta is posterior and to the right of the pulmonary artery and the pulmonary artery is anterior and to the left of the aorta. Despite division of the truncus arteriosus and separation of the right and left outflow tracts, a communication exists between the aorta and the pulmonary artery known as the **ductus arteriosus.**

Fetal circulation differs physiologically and anatomically from postnatal circulation because of the presence of fetal shunts and altered metabolic needs of the various organs (Figure 31-4). Fetal oxygenation occurs in the placenta instead of the fetal lungs because they are deflated and therefore nonfunctional. In addition, the fetal liver is only partially functional; therefore the majority of blood is diverted away from these areas through fetal shunts. Because the fetal brain requires maximum concentrations of oxygen and nutrients for growth, fetal circulation is streamlined to ensure optimal perfusion to the brain.

In utero the fetus receives blood carrying oxygen and nutrients from the placenta through the umbilical vein. Fetal arterial oxygen tension is much lower than that found in the postnatal period—approximately 20 to 30 torr (mmHg pressure). Yet, despite this hypoxemic state, tissue hypoxia does not occur because of high fetal cardiac output of approximately 400 ml/kg/min.[2] The blood travels to the liver, where a portion enters the portal and hepatic circulation; approximately half the flow is diverted away from the liver through the ductus venosus and into the inferior vena cava. Because the blood received from the inferior vena cava yields a higher pressure, blood entering the right atrium (RA) from the inferior vena cava is shunted through the foramen ovale and into the left atrium (LA) and is then pumped through the left ventricle (LV) and into the aorta. Approximately two thirds of the blood flows to the head and upper extremities. Because this blood is mainly from the placenta, the brain and coronary arteries receive the blood with the highest oxygen concentration. The remaining blood flows into the descending aorta.

Less-saturated blood, with an oxygen tension of 15 to 19 torr, returns from the upper body, head, neck, and arms and travels from the superior vena cava (SVC) into the RA. A small portion of this blood flows into the right ventricle (RV) and out the pulmonary artery (PA) and enters the nonfunctioning lungs. Most of the blood, however, bypasses the lungs by flowing through the ductus arteriosus and into the descending aorta. Blood from the descending aorta returns to the placenta through two umbilical arteries.[1]

The collapsed lungs and low oxygen tension induce vasoconstriction, creating high pulmonary vascular resistance. This is transmitted to the right side of the heart and the pulmonary arteries. Conversely, fetal systemic resistance is low because of the large-volume placenta and ductus arteriosus. Therefore, because blood flow follows the path of least resistance, high pulmonary resistance diverts most of the blood flow into the pulmonary artery, through the ductus arteriosus, and into the aorta. From there it travels into the low-resistance placenta.

Transitional Circulation

At birth a series of circulatory changes occur that affect blood flow, vascular resistance, and oxygen tension. The most important change that takes place in the circulation is the shift of gas exchange from the placenta to the lungs. In addition, alterations in pressure and volume of blood flowing through the heart chambers functionally close the ductus arteriosus, duc-

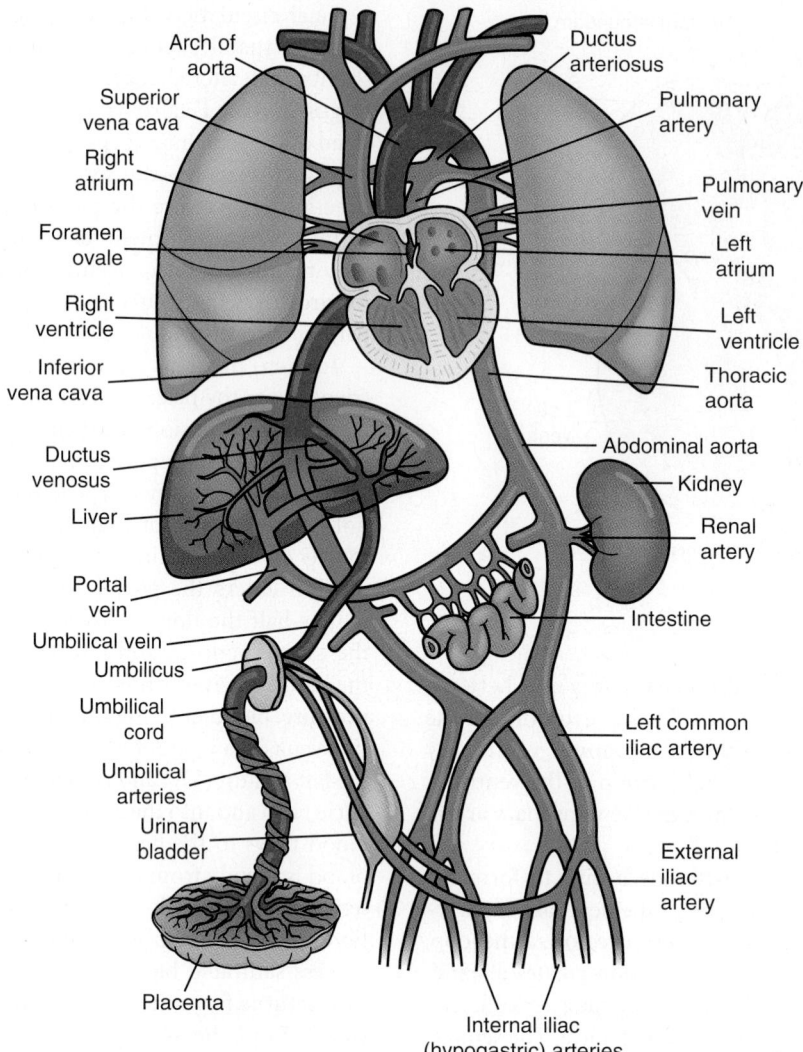

Figure 31-4 **Fetal circulation.** Circulation of the fetus reflects the fact that oxygenation of fetal blood does not take place in the lungs, but rather in the placenta. Therefore the pulmonary circulatory system is essentially "bypassed." Instead of traveling from the right heart to the lungs, as occurs after birth, most blood entering the right heart passes through the ductus arteriosus and into the systemic circulation.

tus venosus, and foramen ovale. A decrease of pulmonary vascular resistance and an increase of systemic vascular resistance lead to changes in the size and shape of the heart chambers.

Clamping of the umbilical cord and expansion of the lungs at birth shift gas exchange from the placenta to the lungs. Removal of the low-resistance placenta from circulation also causes an immediate increase in systemic vascular resistance to about twice that before birth. Conversely, pulmonary vascular resistance decreases because of expansion of the lungs that results from the infant's respirations and exposure to more oxygen-rich blood.

Closure of Fetal Shunts

Once the umbilical cord is tied, the umbilical arteries and vein, which comprise the cord, vasoconstrict and undergo fibrous changes. Therefore blood flow through the ductus venosus falls instantly; absence of fetal shunting through this vessel usually occurs within the first 7 days of life. The ductus venosus evolves into the **ligamentum venosum.**

Increased pulmonary venous return and decreased inferior vena cava return cause functional closure of the foramen ovale within the first month of life. In the fetus the foramen ovale is held open by the blood flow from the high-pressure right side, reflecting pulmonary vascular resistance, to the lower-pressure area on the left side of the heart, reflecting systemic vascular resistance. At birth the pressure gradients reverse, causing the valve flaps of the foramen ovale to close. Functional closure occurs by the adherence of these flaps to the atrial septum. Anatomic closure occurs within the first month of life after deposition of fibrin tissue and cell products permanently seals the flaps closed. Until this occurs, any condition that stimulates an increase in the right-sided pressures or causes dilation of the right atrium can reopen the foramen ovale. Conditions in which a patent foramen ovale may continue past the first month of life include pulmonary hypertension, RV failure, and tricuspid atresia.

The ductus arteriosus closes more gradually. Increased oxygen saturation in the systemic arterial blood is thought to be the major stimulus causing vasoconstriction of the ductus arteriosus. In addition, a decrease in the amount of endogenous prostaglandins promoting dilation and the release of vasoactive substances stimulate further ductal closure. Vasoconstriction of the ductal medial smooth muscle shortens and thickens the intima of the ductal wall within 15 to 18 hours after birth. Permanent closure is complete 10 to 21 days after birth. Fibrous tissue adheres to the remaining structure, and the ductus arteriosus eventually evolves into the ligamentum arteriosum. Conditions that involve low arterial oxygen saturations, such as cyanotic heart disease, decreased medial muscle layer within the ductus, or increased levels of circulating vasodilating substances in the blood, may delay or prevent ductal closure.[3]

Postnatal Development

The infant's cardiopulmonary system is proportionally larger in relation to body surface area than the adult's. The infant's heart points at a transverse angle, but as the lungs and heart mature, the heart shifts lower in the chest and is rotated at a more oblique angle. Unlike the adult heart, the newborn heart has RV dominance with a thickened RV wall. This is because of the high pulmonary vascular resistance in the fetal circulation that subjects the right ventricle to high afterload, which in turn causes the right ventricular myocardium to become as thick and strong as the left.

After birth the right ventricular myocardium begins to thin out as the pulmonary vascular resistance drops. As systemic vascular resistance increases, the left ventricular myocardium becomes thicker. By 1 month of age, the newborn's ventricles are approximately equal in weight. As the child grows, the heart size increases accordingly. The weight of the heart doubles during the first year of life and increases six times that by 9 years of age.[4]

Postnatal changes involve a rise in arterial oxygen tension and an increase in alveolar oxygenation that stimulates vasodilation, resulting in a decrease in pulmonary vascular resistance. During the first 2 to 9 weeks of life, the inner medial linings of the small pulmonary arterioles thin out in response to decreased pulmonary arterial pressure. This increased diameter of the pulmonary vessels, along with further development of the pulmonary bed in response to lung growth, results in a decrease in pulmonary vascular resistance. By 2 months of age, pulmonary resistance may approximate adult levels. During the neonatal period, however, care must be taken to maintain homeostasis because of hyperactivity of the pulmonary bed. Adverse conditions, such as alveolar hypoxia, acidosis, and hypothermia, may trigger pulmonary vasoconstriction and lead to pulmonary hypertension.

Postnatal Hemodynamics

As stated earlier, systemic vascular resistance begins to rise once the placenta is removed from the circulation. Normal levels in the infant range from approximately 10 to 15 Wood units × body surface area (in square meters) and gradually increase to 15 to 30 Wood units × body surface area (in square meters) by childhood.[5] Likewise, the systolic pressure is low in the full-term newborn (approximately 39 to 59 mmHg), reflecting the decreased LV strength. As the left ventricle becomes more developed, the systolic pressure rises steadily until it equals adult levels once the child reaches puberty.

The heart rate of the newborn ranges from 100 to 180 beats/min, which gradually decreases as the child grows. Similarly, the newborn's cardiac output is high, which is a reflection of the fetal circulation described earlier. Oxygen consumption doubles at birth; to maintain adequate oxygen delivery, the cardiac output also remains high. These changes, however, cause minimal cardiac reserve in the newborn. Additional stressors could increase oxygen demands and result in acute deterioration. By 2 months of age, oxygen consumption decreases by half. As the newborn grows, stroke volume steadily increases while the heart rate decreases.[3]

Postnatal Circulation

Postnatal circulation allows the lungs to oxygenate the venous blood and allows saturated blood to be delivered to the systemic circulation. Desaturated blood returning from the superior vena cava, inferior vena cava, and coronary veins enters the right atrium and is pumped to the right ventricle through the tricuspid valve. The right ventricle then pumps the blood through the pulmonic valve to the pulmonary artery; the blood flows to the lungs, where it is oxygenated. The oxygenated blood returns from the lungs through the pulmonary veins and enters the left atrium. The left atrium pumps blood to the left ventricle through the mitral valve. The left ventricle then pumps blood through the aortic valve and into the aorta. The coronary arteries receive the saturated blood along with delivery to the systemic circulation.

CONGENITAL HEART DEFECTS

Congenital heart disease is the leading cause of death, excluding prematurity, during the first year of life[6] (Table 31-1). It is estimated that as many as 35% of deaths caused by congenital heart defects occur in the first year of life and that one

Table 31-1	Critical Times in Fetal Heart Development Related to Specific Defects	
Defect	**Critical Time in Gestation**
Transposition of the great vessels	Third to fourth week
Patent ductus arteriosus	Third to eighth week
Anomalous pulmonary venous connection	Third to eighth week
Tricuspid or mitral atresia	Third to sixth week
Ventricular septal defect (muscular)	Fourth to sixth week
Coarctation of the aorta	Fourth week on
Truncus arteriosus	Sixth to seventh week
Ventricular septal defect (membranous)	Sixth to seventh week
Persistent foramen ovale	Eighth week on

Data from Keith JD, Rowe RD, Vlad P, editors: *Heart disease in infancy and childhood*, ed 3, New York, 1978, Macmillan.

third of children born with congenital heart disease will die as a result of their cardiac disease[7] (also see Box 31-1). Currently there are more than 35 documented types of congenital heart defects and the frequency of occurrence in the United States is on the rise. Although researchers have not determined the reason for this increase, one explanation is that it may be the result of improved methods of detection.

The underlying cause of congenital heart disease is known in only 10% of cases. Several factors place the fetus at risk for developing congenital heart disease, including prenatal, envi-

ronmental, and genetic factors. Among the prenatal factors are maternal rubella, maternal insulin-dependent diabetes, maternal alcoholism, maternal age (older than 40 years), maternal phenylketonuria, and maternal hypercalcemia (Table 31-2). The use of some drugs during pregnancy is associated with an above-average incidence of congenital heart disease. Examples of these drugs include thalidomide, lithium, phenytoin (Dilantin), warfarin, and dextroamphetamine sulfate. The incidence of heart defects also has been found to be higher in stillbirths, spontaneous abortions, and low-birth-weight or small-for-gestational-age infants.[3] In general, the likelihood of unaffected parents having a child with congenital heart disease ranges from 2% to 6%.[7]

Genetic factors also have been implicated in the development of congenital heart disease, although the mechanism of causation is often multifactorial. Recent progress, accelerated through the Human Genome Project, has resulted in the rapid identification of some genes causing congenital heart disease.[6]

ETIOLOGY The etiology of congenital heart disease is unknown. Early epidemiologic studies report a multifactorial influence to be the cause of up to 90% of cardiac anomalies, with a recurrence rate of 2% to 6%.[7] Associated risk factors include maternal, gestational, and familial conditions. Maternal risk factors are discussed in the previous section. Exposure to teratogens in utero also may be a risk factor. Likewise, fetal expo-

---

Box 31-1	Endocarditis Risk

Children with congenital heart disease are at risk for developing endocarditis. Although the risk is low, transient bacteria have been identified in children following dental and surgical procedures and instrumentation involving mucosal surfaces. A blood-borne pathogen can settle in areas of the heart where there is high turbulence, an abnormal valve or vessel, or an artificial material such as a valve or homograft. *Streptococcus viridians* (α-hemolytic streptococci) is the most common pathogen found after dental or oral procedures. *Enterococcus faecalis* (enterococci) is the most common bacterium found after genitourinary and gastrointestinal tract surgery or instrumentation. The American Heart Association has provided updated guidelines for the prevention of bacterial endocarditis. The type and dose of antibiotic prophylaxis recommended depend on the procedure and the cardiac classification of risk for endocarditis.

Table 31-2	Environmental Factors and Associated Congenital Heart Defects
Cause	**Type of Congenital Heart Defect**
Infection	
Intrauterine	Patent ductus arteriosus (PDA), pulmonary stenosis, coarctation of aorta
Systemic viral	PDA, pulmonary stenosis, coarctation of aorta
Rubella	PDA, pulmonary stenosis, coarctation of aorta
Coxsackie B5	Endocardial fibroelastosis
Herpesvirus	
Cytomegalovirus (HCMV)	Can infect endothelial cells and vascular endothelium
Radiation	Specific cardiovascular effect not known
Metabolic Disorders	
Diabetes	Ventricular septal defect (VSD), cardiomegaly, transposition of the great vessels
Phenylketonuria (PKU)	Coarctation of aorta, PDA
Hypercalcemia	Supravalvular aortic stenosis, pulmonic stenosis; aortic hyperplasia
Drugs	
Thalidomide	No specific lesion
Dextroamphetamine	One case of reported transposition
Alcohol	Tetralogy of Fallot, atrial septal defect, VSD
Lithium	Exact effect not known
Phenytoin	Embryonic arrhythmia and valvular heart disease?
Warfarin	Atrial septal defect (ASD) and patent ductus arteriosus
Dextroamphetamine sulfate	VSD?
Peripheral Conditions	
Increased maternal age	VSD, tetralogy of Fallot (relationship unclear)
Antepartal bleeding	Various defects (relationship unclear)
Prematurity	PDA, VSD
High altitude	PDA, atrial septal defect (increased incidence)

sure to active maternal infections, such as rubella, herpesvirus, coxsackievirus B5, and cytomegalovirus, may be a risk.

Chromosomal aberrations account for about 6% of all congenital heart defects (Table 31-3). Many genetic and hereditary diseases are associated with congenital heart defects, although the mechanism of causation is unknown (Table 31-4). As many as 50% of infants with trisomy 21 have a congenital heart defect, either an AV canal defect or a VSD. Extracardiac defects are noted in as many as 35% of infants with cardiac lesions. Prospective studies using chromosomal analysis have suggested that congenital cardiac malformations may be the result of a single gene defect.[5]

Because of improved screening methods, surgical interventions, and management, children with congenital heart defects are now surviving into adulthood and bearing children of their own. Studies report a 5% to 15% incidence of congenital heart disease in offspring of a parent having a congenital heart lesion. If two siblings have a congenital cardiac anomaly, the recurrence risk is 9%, and if three siblings have a congenital cardiac anomaly, the rate jumps to a 50% chance that the next child also will have a cardiovascular malformation.

CLASSIFICATION AND CLINICAL MANIFESTATIONS   There are more than 35 different types of congenital anomalies that can be classified into four categories based on blood flow pattern: (1) lesions increasing pulmonary blood flow; (2) lesions decreasing pulmonary blood flow; (3) obstructive lesions, where right- or left-sided outflow tract obstructions curtail or prohibit blood flow out of the heart; and (4) mixed lesions, where desaturated blood and saturated blood mix within the chambers or great arteries of the heart (Table 31-5). By classifying lesions in this way, the clinical manifestations, as well as associated sequelae, are more predictable.

Table 31-3	Genetic Factors and Congenital Heart Defects	
Chromosomal Aberrations or Syndrome	**Incidence of Defects**	**Type of Defect**
Trisomy 13	80%	Ventricular septal defect (VSD), atrial septal defect (ASD), patent ductus arteriosus (PDA), anomalous pulmonary venous connection, bicuspid aorta, overriding aorta
Trisomy 18	90%	VSD, PDA, patent foramen ovale, bicuspid aortic valve, dextrocardia
Down syndrome	12%-44%	Endocardial cushion defects, VSD, PDA, ASD, transposition of great vessels, tetralogy of Fallot, persistent truncus arteriosus, coarctation of aorta, endocardial fibroelastosis
Cri du chat syndrome	20%	PDA, mixed defects
Turner syndrome	20%-40%	Coarctation of aorta, pulmonary stenosis, subaortic and aortic stenosis, PDA, septal defects

Data from Doyle EF, Rutkowski M: Etiology of congenital heart disease, *Cardiovasc Clin* 2:1, 1970.

Table 31-4	Disorders Coexistent With Congenital Heart Defects
Disorder	**Associated Cardiovascular Defect**
Connective Tissue Disorders	
Marfan syndrome	Aortic or mitral regurgitation, aortic aneurysm
Hurler syndrome	Pseudoatherosclerosis
Hunter syndrome	Pseudoatherosclerosis, hypertension
Osteogenesis imperfecta	Incompetent aortic valve
Complex Syndromes	
Kartagener syndrome	Dextrocardia
Holt-Oram syndrome	Atrial septal defect (ASD), ventricular septal defect (VSD)
Ellis–van Creveld syndrome	Defect or absence of atrial septum
Laurence-Moon-Biedl syndrome	Tetralogy of Fallot, single ventricle, transposition of aorta
Inborn Errors of Metabolism	
Pompe disease	Cardiomegaly, left heart failure
Homocuptinuria	Thromboembolic episodes, pulmonic and aortic regurgitation
Phakomatosis	
Neurofibromatosis (von Recklinghausen disease)	Hypertension, pheochromocytoma
von Hippel–Lindau disease	Hypertension, pheochromocytoma
Sturge-Weber-Dimitri disease	Anomalies of carotid and meningeal arteries
Vascular Malformations	
Osler-Weber-Rendu disease (hereditary hemorrhagic telangiectasia)	Atrioventricular fistula, telangiectasia
Milroy disease (lymphedema)	Hypoplasia or lymphatic vessels

Data from Doyle EF, Rutkowski M: Etiology of congenital heart disease, *Cardiovasc Clin* 2:1, 1970.

Table 31-5	Classification of Congenital Heart Defects			
Classification	Shunt Direction	Newborn Presentation	Specific Defects
Lesions increasing pulmonary blood flow	Left to right	Acyanotic congestive heart failure	Patent ductus arteriosus, atrial septal defect, ventricular septal defect, complete atrioventricular canal defect
Lesions decreasing pulmonary blood flow	Right to left	Cyanotic	Tetralogy of Fallot, tricuspid atresia
Obstructive lesions*	None	Low cardiac output Shock	Coarctation of the aorta, hypoplastic left heart syndrome, aortic stenosis, pulmonary stenosis
Mixed lesions†	Variable	Variable	Transposition of the great arteries, total anomalous pulmonary venous connection, truncus arteriosus

*If patent ductus arteriosus closes, newborns with hypoplastic left heart syndrome, coarctation of the aorta, or critical aortic stenosis will present with shock. Newborns with aortic stenosis or pulmonary stenosis may have only mild symptoms depending on severity of stenosis.
†Transposition of the great arteries and truncus arteriosus will present with cyanosis as patent ductus arteriosus closes. Total anomalous pulmonary venous connection usually presents with congestive heart failure.

Clinical manifestations are lesion dependent. Lesions increasing pulmonary blood flow include defects that allow blood flow to shunt from the high-pressure left side to the lower-pressure right side, resulting in pulmonary congestion and right heart failure. Lesions that cause decreased pulmonary blood flow are generally complex and result in cyanosis. Obstructive lesions limit the amount of blood flow out of the ventricles. The two types of obstructive lesions are right-sided lesions that result in cyanosis and left-sided lesions that result in congestive heart failure. Mixed lesions result in a variable amount of mixing and pulmonary blood flow; the clinical manifestations usually consist of left heart failure and hypoxemia that may be associated with cyanosis.

Congestive Heart Failure

Congestive heart failure (CHF) is a common complication of many congenital heart defects. In addition, it can occur as the result of decreased myocardial function or excessive metabolic demands. The most common causes of CHF in infancy, however, are pressure and volume overloads secondary to congenital disease. (Table 31-6 lists the congenital heart defects that cause CHF by age.) Ninety percent of children who develop CHF do so within 12 months of age, often by the age of 6 months.

PATHOPHYSIOLOGY   In general, the pathophysiologic mechanisms of CHF in infants and children are very similar to those in adults. The same compensatory mechanisms are activated in the face of inadequate cardiac output. A decrease in blood pressure stimulates stretch receptors and baroreceptors in the aorta and carotid arteries, which in turn stimulate the sympathetic nervous system. With the release of catecholamines and the stimulation of β receptors, heart rate and the force of myocardial contraction increase. Venous smooth muscle tone also increases, which increases return of venous blood to the heart. Sympathetic stimulation also decreases

blood flow to the kidneys, skin, spleen, and extremities so that maximum flow to the brain, heart, and lungs can be maintained. Decreased blood flow to the kidneys causes the release of renin, angiotensin, and aldosterone. This cycle results in retention of sodium and fluid by the kidneys, which in turn increases volume in the circulatory system.

The myocardium hypertrophies in CHF, which increases ventricular pressure. The myocardial fibers also stretch to accommodate the increased volume. This increases contractility and hence the force of ventricular contraction. Both hypertrophy and increased stretch eventually fail to maintain cardiac output as CHF progresses. A review of the Frank-Starling law of the heart (see Chapter 29) is useful for an understanding of the cycle of compensation and decompensation that occurs in CHF.

CLINICAL MANIFESTATIONS   Although CHF in children has many causes, it is often difficult to determine right from left ventricular failure. When assessing a child with CHF, a combination of symptoms generally is present. Usually, both ventricles are involved by the time signs and symptoms are apparent.[4]

Left heart failure in infants is manifested as poor feeding and sucking, often leading to failure to thrive. In left heart failure, dyspnea, tachypnea, and diaphoresis may be accompanied by retractions, grunting, and nasal flaring, wheezing, coughing, and rales.[3] Common skin changes, such as pallor or mottling, are often present.

Hepatomegaly (enlargement of the liver) is atypically attributable to systemic venous congestion caused by right ventricular failure. In infants the normal liver is sharp-edged and palpable 1 to 2 cm below the costal margin. However, the absence of hepatomegaly does not rule out CHF.

Periorbital edema and weight gain without caloric increase are common manifestations of right ventricular failure in infants. Peripheral edema, which is a common finding in adults, is usually more difficult to detect in infants and young children.[3] The clinical manifestations of CHF are given in Box 31-2.

EVALUATION AND TREATMENT   A thorough physical examination with an emphasis on cardiac and pulmonary findings often will reveal the degree of CHF. Plotting the child's growth (height, weight, head circumference) is an important method of assessing failure to thrive. An electrocardiogram (ECG) should be performed to determine the presence of dysrhythmias or hypertrophy. A chest roentgenogram is useful in assessing the presence of cardiomegaly and signs of increased pulmonary circulation.

Treatment is aimed at decreasing cardiac workload and increasing the efficiency of the heart. Medical management initially consists of diuretics, such as furosemide. Depending on the degree of CHF, other diuretics can be used in combination with furosemide to counteract potassium losses. Afterload reducers have recently been employed to further manage severe CHF.[3,4] Medications, such as digoxin (Lanoxin), an inotropic agent, also are used to increase myocardial contractility.

Hypoxemia

Heart defects that allow desaturated blood to enter the systemic system without passing through the lungs result in hypoxemia and cyanosis. Hypoxemia occurs when arterial oxygen tension is below normal and results in low oxygen arterial saturations and cellular function alteration. **Cyanosis,** a blue discoloration of the mucous membranes and nail beds, results from deoxygenated hemoglobin in a concentration of at least 5 g/dl of blood or from arterial saturations less than 85%.[3,5] Anemia may mask the signs of hypoxemia, whereas children who are polycythemic with a normal arterial saturation may appear cyanotic. Older children who have an unrepaired septal defect with a left-to-right shunt may become cyanotic because of pulmonary vascular changes secondary to increased pulmonary blood flow. Because of these progressive pulmonary vascular changes, pulmonary vascular resistance increases to exceed or equal vascular resistance, resulting in a reversal of shunting known as **Eisenmenger syndrome.** Three types of defects cause hypoxemia and cyanosis:

1. Lesions that cause right ventricular outflow tract obstruction and shunting from the right side of the heart to the left side, as in tetralogy of Fallot (see p. 1161)
2. Defects involving the mixing of saturated and unsaturated blood within the heart chambers, as in a univentricular heart
3. Defects in children with transposition of the great arteries (see p. 1169), in which two parallel circulations

Table 31-6	Congenital Heart Defects Causing Congestive Heart Failure
Age	**Congenital Heart Defect**
Time of birth	Hypoplastic left heart syndrome
	Volume overload caused by tricuspid regurgitation
	Arterial venous fistula
Birth to 1 week	Hypoplastic left heart syndrome
	Aortic atresia
	Transposition of the great vessels
	Coarctation of the aorta
	Total anomalous pulmonary venous connection (TAPVC) with obstruction
	Patent ductus arteriosus (PDA) in premature infants
First 4 weeks	Coarctation of the aorta
	TAPVC
	Large left-to-right shunt caused by ventricular septal defect (VSD), PDA in premature infants
	Tricuspid atresia
	All previously mentioned defects
4 to 6 weeks	Transposition of the great vessels
	Large left-to-right shunt caused by endocardial cushion defect
6 weeks to 6 months	VSD
6 months	Endocardial fibroelastosis
	Persistent truncus arteriosus with large left-to-right shunt

Box 31-2	Clinical Manifestations of Congestive Heart Failure		

Impaired Myocardial Function	**Pulmonary Congestion**	**Systemic Venous Congestion**
Tachycardia	Tachypnea	Weight gain
Sweating (inappropriately)	Dyspnea	Hepatomegaly
Decreased urinary output	Retractions (infants)	Peripheral edema, especially periorbital
Fatigue	Flaring nares	Ascites
Weakness	Exercise intolerance	Neck vein distention (children)
Restlessness	Orthopnea	
Anorexia	Cough, hoarseness	
Pale, cool extremities	Cyanosis	
Weak peripheral pulses	Wheezing	
Decreased blood pressure	Grunting	
Gallop rhythm		
Cardiomegaly		

From Hockenberry MJ et al: *Wong's nursing care of infants and children,* ed 7, St Louis, 2003, Mosby.

exist and survival depends on the existence of a patent ductus arteriosus or septal shunt

CLINICAL MANIFESTATIONS Infants with mild hypoxemia may show signs of cyanosis only occasionally when stressed; otherwise they may exhibit near-normal age-projected growth and development. Infants with severe hypoxemia may display signs of feeding intolerance, poor weight gain, tachypnea, and dyspnea. Children with chronic hypoxemia are small for their age, display cognitive and motor skill delays, experience shortness of breath with exertion, fatigue easily, and have exercise intolerance. Severe hypoxemia will lead to tissue hypoxia, metabolic acidosis, hyperventilation, poor perfusion, and eventually shock.

In response to chronic hypoxemia, polycythemia occurs as the body generates additional red blood cells to increase the oxygen-carrying capacity of the blood. However, anemia may result because of limited stores of iron, and the increased velocity of the blood limits the amount of circulating platelets and other coagulation factors. Polycythemia also places children at risk for thromboembolic events, especially infants with severe cyanosis and iron deficiency anemia. In addition to the 2% risk of cerebrovascular accidents, there is a 2% chance that children with right-to-left shunting will develop a brain abscess.[5] Clubbing of the nail beds occurs because of chronic tissue hypoxemia and polycythemia.

Defects Increasing Pulmonary Blood Flow

Cardiac lesions that increase pulmonary blood flow include defects that involve septal abnormalities or communications between the great arteries. These allow the shunting of blood from the high-pressure left side to the lower-pressure right side. Infants with left-to-right shunts are acyanotic and, depending on the degree of shunting, will often develop signs and symptoms of congestive heart failure. Children with significant left-to-right shunts left untreated are at risk for development of irreversible pulmonary hypertension.

Patent Ductus Arteriosus

The **patent ductus arteriosus (PDA)** is a vessel located between the junction of the main and left pulmonary arteries and the lesser curvature of the descending aorta just distal to the left subclavian artery. During fetal circulation the PDA allows blood to shunt from the pulmonary artery to the aorta. At birth, once the placenta is removed and the lungs are expanded, the PDA will start to constrict within the first hours of life. Closure of the PDA in full-term infants is usually noted between 15 hours of life and 2 weeks of age.[8] As an isolated defect, PDA occurs in 5% to 10% of all congenital cardiac defects.[3] In premature infants, studies have shown that the incidence of PDA is as high as 20% in newborns less than 1750 g.[9]

PATHOPHYSIOLOGY Failure of the PDA to close results in persistent patency of the ductus arteriosus. The hemodynamic effects of PDA depend on the size of the lumen and the resistance in the pulmonary and systemic circulations.[6] At birth the pulmonary and systemic vascular resistances are almost equal and are reflected in the pulmonary artery and aorta, respectively. Therefore shunting is minimal. However, as pulmonary vascular resistance falls, a reversal of fetal shunting occurs. Blood now begins to shunt left to right, from the aorta to the pulmonary artery. The hemodynamic effect is increased pulmonary blood flow, resulting in an increased workload on the left side of the heart. The increased workload is caused by increased pulmonary venous return to the left atrium and, potentially, an increase in right ventricular pressure if pulmonary vascular changes occur in response to the increased blood flow, leading to an increase in pulmonary vascular pressure (Figure 31-5, C).

CLINICAL MANIFESTATIONS Once pulmonary vascular resistance has fallen, infants with PDA will characteristically have a continuous-machinery type murmur heard best at the left upper sternal border throughout systole and diastole. If the PDA is significant, the infant also will have bounding pulses, an active precordium, a thrill upon palpation, and signs and symptoms of CHF. Infants with a small PDA will usually remain asymptomatic.

EVALUATION AND TREATMENT Chest roentgenogram will reveal left atrial and ventricular enlargement and increased pulmonary vascular markings. An ECG may demonstrate ventricular enlargement, particularly on the left, but in most cases it is within normal ranges. Echocardiography and auscultation confirm the diagnosis based on the characteristic continuous-machinery type of murmur. Cardiac catheterization is not warranted if the results of all noninvasive studies are consistent with the diagnosis.

PDA closure in asymptomatic children is recommended by 2 years of age because of the risk of subacute bacterial endocarditis. Premature infants who develop respiratory distress are initially given indomethacin, a prostaglandin inhibitor, to close the duct.[9] If this is unsuccessful, more invasive measures are taken to close the duct.

Historically, the most widely used method for PDA closure is surgical closure involving ligation and division of the ductus. Cardiopulmonary bypass is not needed because of the extracardiac location of the lesion. The rate of successful closure is 100%. Mortality associated with surgical intervention nears 0%; however, there continues to be some morbidity caused by the approach through a left thoracotomy incision.

Several other options for PDA closure are currently available depending on the size of the child and the PDA. Many specialists perform coil embolization of the PDA during catheterization. The catheter is advanced into the ductal opening whereby multiple coils are ejected into the lumen that embolize and prohibit flow through the duct. The greatest advantages to this procedure are the avoidance of a surgi-

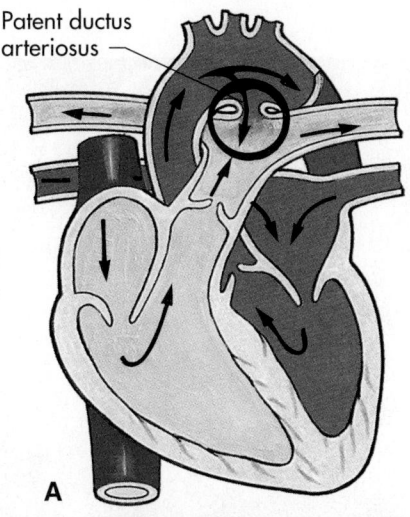

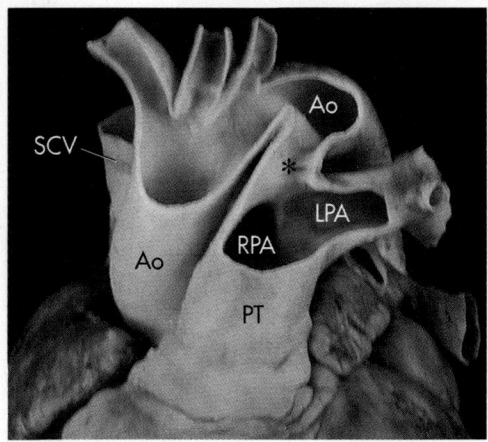

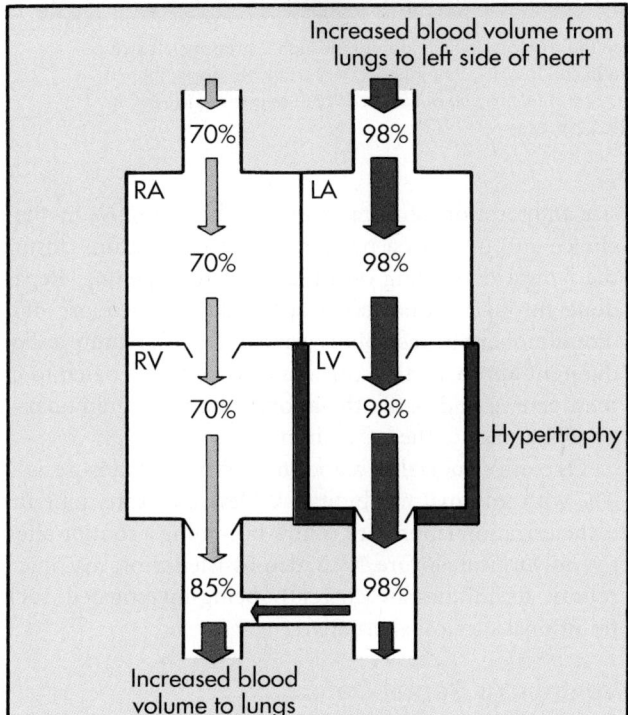

Figure 31-5 Patent ductus arteriosus (PDA). **A,** PDA with left-to-right shunt. **B,** PDA (*) in an adult with pulmonary hypertension. **C,** Changes in oxygen saturation, left ventricular volume, and the myocardium caused by left-to-right shunt through a PDA. *SCV,* Subclavian vein; *Ao,* aorta; *LPA,* left pulmonary artery; *RPA,* right pulmonary artery; *PT,* pulmonary trunk; *RA,* right atrium; *RV,* right ventricle; *LA,* left atrium; *LV,* left ventricle. (**A** from Hockenberry MJ et al: *Wong's nursing care of infants and children,* ed 7, St Louis, 2003, Mosby; **B** from Damjanov I, Linder J, editors: *Anderson's pathology,* ed 10, St Louis, 1996, Mosby.)

cal procedure and thoracotomy pain and a brief observation stay in the hospital.[10-12]

Another option is closure through video-assisted thoracoscopic surgery. This procedure involves making three small incisions in the left lateral wall, through which a probe is inserted. A clip is then placed around the vessel to occlude it. An advantage of this procedure is that there is less associated morbidity because of the avoidance of a thoracotomy incision.[13-15]

Atrial Septal Defect

An **atrial septal defect (ASD)** is an abnormal communication between the atria (Figure 31-6, *A* and *B*). Although it is an iso-

lated lesion, it is the fourth most common congenital heart defect, occurring in 5% to 10% of all congenital cardiac defects. The three major types are an ostium primum defect, an opening found low in the septum that may be associated with atrioventricular valve abnormalities, especially mitral insufficiency; an ostium secundum defect, an opening in the center of the septum (this is the most common type of atrial defect); and a sinus venosus defect, an opening that occurs high up in the atrial septum near the SVC and RA junction. This defect is often associated with partial anomalous pulmonary venous connection.

PATHOPHYSIOLOGY   Although the pressure difference between the two atria is minimal, the ASD allows blood to be

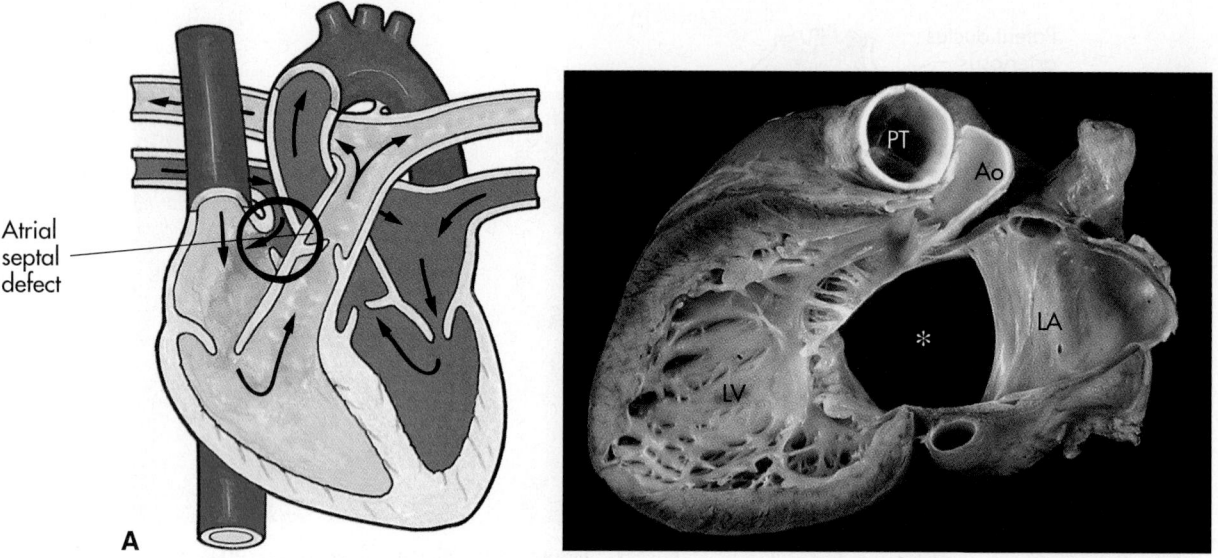

Figure 31-6 Atrial septal defect (ASD). **A,** Abnormal opening between the atria causing blood from the higher-pressure left atrium to flow into the lower-pressure right atrium. **B,** Complete ASD (*) form in children. *PT,* Pulmonary artery trunk; *Ao,* aorta; *LA,* left atrium; *LV,* left ventricle. (**A** from Hockenberry MJ et al: *Wong's nursing care of infants and children,* ed 7, St Louis, 2003, Mosby; **B** from Damjanov I, Linder J, editors: *Anderson's pathology,* ed 10, St Louis, 1996, Mosby.)

shunted from left to right because of the slightly higher pressure of the left atrial chamber. Right atrial and ventricular enlargement develops as a result of left-to-right shunting. Children with ASD are generally asymptomatic and rarely display signs of cardiac failure. Moderate to large ASDs allow an increase in pulmonary blood flow, and over time, pulmonary vascular changes can occur, eventually resulting in pulmonary hypertension.

CLINICAL MANIFESTATIONS   Because most children with ASD are asymptomatic, diagnosis usually is made during a routine physical examination by the auscultation of a crescendo-decrescendo systolic ejection murmur that reflects increased blood flow through the pulmonary valve. The location of the murmur is between the second and third intercostal spaces along the left sternal border. A wide fixed splitting of the second heart sound is also characteristic of ASD, reflecting volume overload to the right ventricle causing prolonged ejection time and delay of pulmonic valve closure.

EVALUATION AND TREATMENT   In most cases an echocardiogram is sufficient to confirm the diagnosis of an ASD. A chest roentgenogram may reveal cardiomegaly and increased pulmonary vascular markings in an asymptomatic child, although this is rare. An ECG often reflects right axis deviation and diastolic overload of the right ventricle.[3]

ASD closure generally is recommended before the child reaches school age, because if left unrepaired, pulmonary hypertension and right ventricular hypertrophy occurs, placing the child at risk for the development of CHF, atrial dysrhythmias, or embolic events by 20 years of age, depending on the

size and location. Surgical closure is the corrective method of choice and involves a pericardial patch or suture closure of the defect, depending on the size of the opening. Repair is done through a midsternal approach with the use of cardiopulmonary bypass. Sinus venosus defects require a slightly different approach that consists of a synthetic patch to close the opening and baffle the anomalous right pulmonary venous drainage to the left atrium.

Operative mortality associated with ASD closure is near 0%, with minimal morbidity.[16,17] Device closure done in the catheterization laboratory is now becoming a routine alternative to surgical closure.[18-23] Video-assisted thoracoscopic and robotic techniques are currently being investigated, such as traditional surgical alternatives.

Ventricular Septal Defect

A **ventricular septal defect (VSD)** is an abnormal communication between the ventricles (Figure 31-7, *A*). VSDs are the most common type of congenital heart lesion and account for 25% to 33% of all congenital heart defects. The four types of VSDs are based on location in the septum. The perimembranous type, which occurs in the outflow tract on the left ventricle immediately below the aortic valve, is the most common type, accounting for up to 80% of all VSDs. Muscular VSDs, which occur low in the ventricular septum between the trabeculae, are most likely to close spontaneously and are difficult to reach because of their location low in the apex. Supracristal VSDs occur in the infundibulum, below the pulmonary valve. AV canal VSDs occur posterior and inferior to the membranous system, beneath the septal cusp of the tricuspid valve and inferior to the papillary muscles of the conus.

PATHOPHYSIOLOGY The direction of shunting in a child with a VSD is from the high-pressure left side to the lower-pressure right side. The amount of shunting depends on the size of the defect and the degree of pulmonary vascular resistance. Small VSDs present increased resistance to shunting and limit blood flow through the defect; thus the degree of pulmonary vascular congestion and ventricular chamber enlargement is minimal (Figure 31-7, *C*).

After about 12 weeks of life, when pulmonary vascular resistance has decreased, moderate-size to large VSDs allow a large amount of shunting from left to right. However, it is the LV rather than the RV that is under pressure and volume overload because most of the shunting occurs during systole when the RV contracts. The shunted blood goes directly out the right ventricle and into the pulmonary artery rather than remaining in the RV cavity (Figure 31-7, *D*). Therefore the

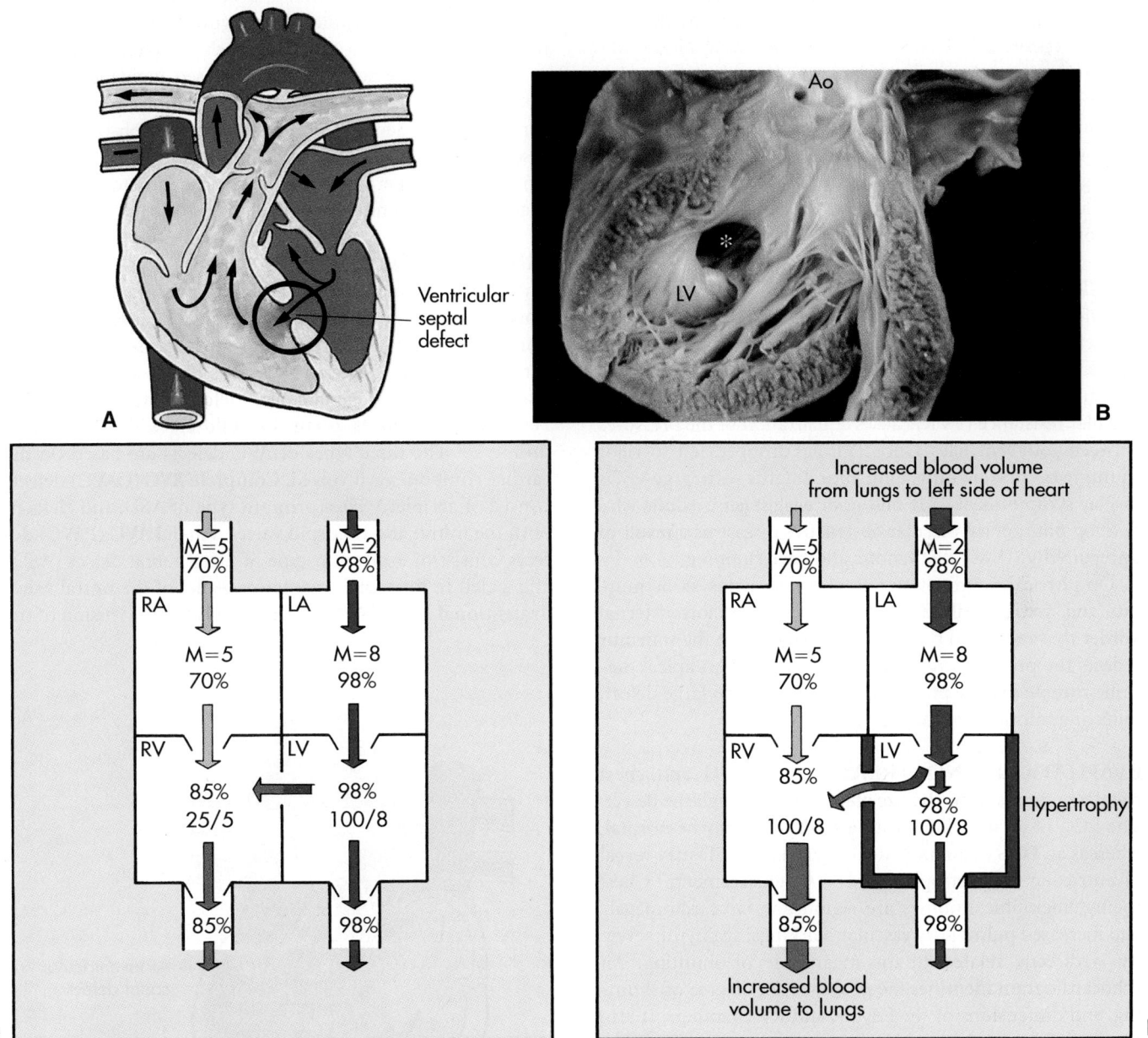

Figure 31-7 Ventricular septal defects (VSDs). **A,** VSD with left-to-right shunt. **B,** Muscular (*) defect (opened left ventricles). **C,** Hemodynamics of a small VSD with left-to-right shunt. Mean (M) indicates mean of pressure; systolic/diastolic pressures are in mmHg; and percentages indicate oxygen saturation. **D,** Hemodynamics of a large VSD with left-to-right shunt. Like the shunting that occurs in preductal coarctation of the aorta, the shunting pictured here causes left ventricular overload and hypertrophy. *Ao,* Aorta; *LV,* left ventricle; *RA,* right atrium; *RV,* right ventricle; *LA,* left atrium. (**A** from Hockenberry MJ et al: *Wong's nursing care of infants and children,* ed 7, St Louis, 2003, Mosby; **B** from Damjanov I, Linder J, editors: *Anderson's pathology,* ed 10, St Louis, 1996, Mosby.)

main pulmonary artery, LA, and LV all enlarge. LV hypertrophy occurs to effectively pump the additional volume. Eventually the heart is unable to handle the increased volume and CHF develops.

Over time the pulmonary bed also undergoes changes because of increased pulmonary blood flow caused by the left-to-right shunting. In an attempt to maintain normal blood volume, vessels undergo changes that increase their resistance to flow. The smooth muscle layer in the arteriolar walls enlarges, and proliferation of the intimal layer occurs. The effect of these changes is a decrease in the diameter of the pulmonary vessels, which increases the resistance to blood flow and produces a decrease in the amount of blood volume going to the lungs. These changes eventually become irreversible, and pulmonary vascular resistance continues to rise. In some cases it exceeds systemic vascular resistance, causing the shunt through the VSD to reverse direction. Deoxygenated blood now flows into the systemic circulation, and cyanosis occurs, a phenomenon known as *Eisenmenger syndrome.*

CLINICAL MANIFESTATIONS   Clinical manifestations in children with VSDs depend on the age of the child, size of the defect, and level of pulmonary vascular resistance. Newborns with small VSDs are relatively asymptomatic. Initially no murmur is present because the newborn's high pulmonary vascular resistance (PVR) causes equalization of the pressures between both ventricles. Once PVR has dropped, left-to-right shunting occurs, creating a murmur. Infants with large VSDs display symptoms of CHF and poor weight gain. Adults who develop pulmonary vascular obstructive disease as a result of unrepaired VSD will be cyanotic and have clubbing.

On physical examination a loud, harsh, holosystolic murmur and systolic thrill can be detected at the left lower sternal border that radiate to the neck. The intensity of the murmur reflects the pressure gradient across the VSD. An apical diastolic rumble may be present with a moderate to large defect, reflecting mitral regurgitation.

EVALUATION AND TREATMENT   ECG and chest roentgenograms show the size of shunting through the defect. The ECG of an individual with a small VSD may be normal, whereas an ECG of an individual with a large VSD may reveal biventricular hypertrophy and LA enlargement. Chest roentgenographic findings are significant for cardiomegaly and increased pulmonary vascular markings; again, the severity is directly related to the magnitude of shunting. An echocardiogram identifies the position, size, degree of shunting, and dimensions of the LA, LV, and RV chambers. It also can provide an estimate of pulmonary artery and RV pressures and pulmonary vascular resistance. Cardiac catheterization may be performed to determine hemodynamics and, in some instances, the location of other VSDs.

Many VSDs spontaneously close during the first year of life.[3] Infants with symptoms of CHF and poor weight gain despite medical management should have their VSD corrected

as soon as possible. Left-to-right shunting with a pulmonary flow–systemic flow (Qp:Qs) ratio of greater than 2:1 or evidence of elevated pulmonary vascular resistance is an indication for closure. Closure of the VSD at this time is to prevent the development of pulmonary vascular obstructive disease.

Placement of a pulmonary artery band to decrease the amount of pulmonary blood flow was initially used as a palliative procedure but is now rarely used unless the presence of an additional lesion makes complete repair impossible. Patch closure, using a synthetic material such as Dacron, is accomplished through a sternotomy and with the use of cardiopulmonary bypass. A transatrial approach is preferable to a right ventriculotomy because of the increased incidence of conduction disturbances.[14,20,21] Contraindications for VSD closure include evidence of pulmonary vascular obstructive disease or Eisenmenger syndrome. Occlusion devices for VSD closure that are performed in the cardiac catheterization laboratory are now under investigation.[24,25]

Atrioventricular Canal Defect

An **atrioventricular canal (AVC) defect** results from nonfusion of the endocardial cushions during fetal life, yielding abnormalities in both the atrial and ventricular septa and atrioventricular valves (Figure 31-8). This defect accounts for as many as 5% of all congenital heart defects, and approximately 30% of AVC defects occur in children with Down syndrome.[26-28] The three types of AVC defects are based on the cardiac components involved. **Complete AVC (CAVC)** defects consist of an inlet VSD, a primum type of ASD, and clefts in both the mitral and tricuspid valves. **Partial AVC (PAVC) defects** consist of a primum type of atrial septal defect (ASD) and a cleft in the septal or anterior leaflet of the mitral valve. **Transitional AVC (TAVC)** defects involve partial fusion of the

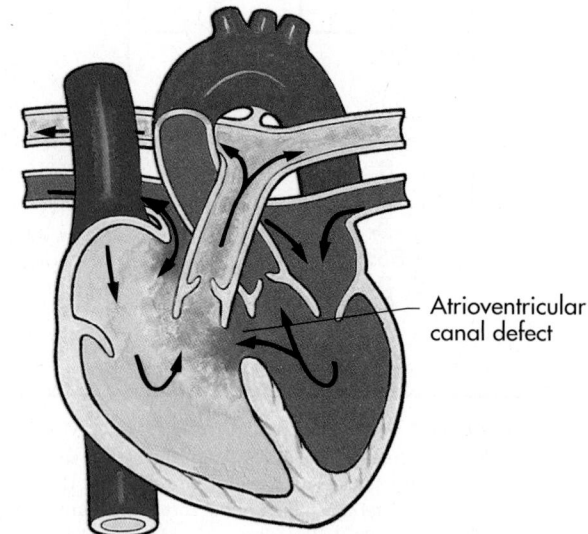

Figure 31-8 Atrioventricular canal defect. (From Hockenberry MJ et al: *Wong's nursing care of infants and children,* ed 7, St Louis, 2003, Mosby.)

endocardial cushions, resulting in variable atrioventricular valve abnormalities.

PATHOPHYSIOLOGY   Hemodynamic abnormalities seen in AVC defects depend on the components of the lesion and the level of pulmonary vascular resistance. Shunting is minimal during the neonatal period when pulmonary vascular resistance is high. However, once pulmonary vascular resistance drops, left-to-right shunting occurs through the septal defects, resulting in increased pulmonary blood flow and CHF.

PAVC defects mimic the hemodynamics of secundum ASD in which the left-to-right shunting through the primum ASD causes RA and RV dilation and increased pulmonary blood flow. The mitral regurgitation that occurs, caused by the cleft mitral valve, is not hemodynamically significant because blood that flows back into the LA from the LV is immediately shunted into the RA through the primum ASD, resulting in decompression of the LA.

CAVC defects reflect the hemodynamics of both an ASD and a VSD, resulting in biatrial and biventricular enlargement. RA and RV volume overload occurs because of shunting through the primum ASD and tricuspid regurgitation. Likewise, LA and LV volume overload occurs because of shunting through the VSD and mitral regurgitation.

CLINICAL MANIFESTATIONS   Children with PAVC defects are generally asymptomatic. Findings on physical examination are similar to those of secundum ASD except for the systolic regurgitant murmur of mitral regurgitation at the apex. At 4 to 12 weeks of age, when pulmonary vascular resistance drops, children with CAVC defects begin to show symptoms of CHF. Physical findings are similar to those found in individuals with VSDs in addition to the systolic murmur radiating to the back and apex, reflecting mitral regurgitation; a middiastolic rumble at the left lower sternal border or apex reflects stenosis of the mitral or tricuspid valve; and signs of CHF, especially frequent respiratory infections.

EVALUATION AND TREATMENT   The ECG generally demonstrates a superior left axis deviation, first-degree AV block, and RV hypertrophy or right bundle branch block. The ECG of CAVC defects also may have LV hypertrophy. Chest roentgenogram shows cardiomegaly of all four chambers in the presence of mitral regurgitation, increased pulmonary vascular changes, and a prominent main pulmonary artery. Echocardiography allows visualization of the components of the defect, including continuity between the AV valves, their sizes, and chordal attachments. Cardiac catheterization confirms the location of septal defects, AV valve abnormalities, degree of left-to-right shunting, and presence of pulmonary hypertension.

Timing of surgical repair depends on the severity of symptoms, degree of shunting, and level of pulmonary vascular resistance. The current trend is to perform complete repair between 6 and 12 months of life[26,29] to avoid the development of pulmonary vascular changes. Surgical repair is performed through a midsternotomy implementing a one- or two-patch repair to close the septal defects and repair the involved AV valves. Mortality has declined below 10% unless the child is a newborn, has severe AV valve incompetence, or has a small LV. Postoperative complications include heart block, dysrhythmias, or mitral regurgitation requiring further surgical intervention or valve replacement.[26,29]

Defects Decreasing Pulmonary Blood Flow

Defects decreasing pulmonary blood flow involve obstruction to pulmonary blood flow and septal communications. Because of RV outflow tract obstruction, right-sided pressures exceed left-sided pressures, resulting in right-to-left shunting. Children with these defects have hypoxemia and cyanosis.

Tetralogy of Fallot

Tetralogy of Fallot consists of four defects: a VSD that is high in the septum and usually large, an overriding aorta that straddles the VSD, pulmonary stenosis, and RV hypertrophy (Figure 31-9, *A*). It is the most common cyanotic congenital heart defect and accounts for 10% of all defects.[3]

PATHOPHYSIOLOGY   Tetralogy of Fallot develops during two phases of embryologic growth: (1) during the division of the truncus arteriosus by the spiral septum in the third or fourth week of gestation and (2) during the division of the ventricles between the fourth and eighth weeks of gestation. Normally, as these events progress, the truncal septum fuses with the bulbar ridges and, in turn, with the endocardial cushions. The membranous portion of the interventricular septum grows upward to meet the endocardial cushions, and ultimately all of these tissues come together to complete the interventricular septum.

The embryologic error that causes tetralogy of Fallot is not known for certain, but two theories have been proposed.[1] The first is that the truncus arteriosus divides unevenly, resulting in great vessels of unequal size. Because of this asymmetry, the part of the spiral septum that normally fuses with the AV septa is not where it should be, causing a VSD. Concomitantly, pulmonary stenosis develops because there is a larger than normal amount of tissue in the infundibulum of the right ventricle. (This infundibulum is on the ventricular side of the pulmonic valve.) The second theory proposes that infundibular overgrowth in the right ventricle is the major developmental anomaly. The extra tissue restricts the blood flow through the pulmonary artery, causing the artery to be smaller than normal at birth. Concomitantly, the aorta is subjected to greater than normal blood flow during fetal life, causing it to be larger than normal at birth. In addition, infundibular overgrowth in the right ventricle prevents normal closure of the ventricular septum, causing the VSD.

The pathophysiology associated with tetralogy of Fallot varies widely, depending primarily on the degree of pul-

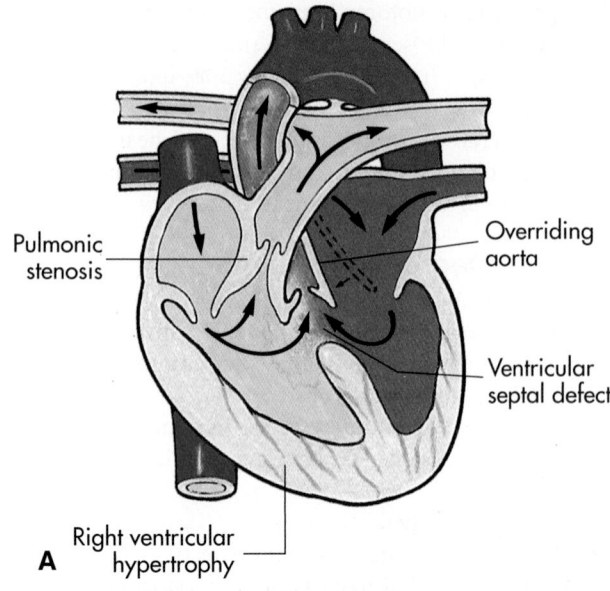

Pulmonic stenosis

Overriding aorta

Ventricular septal defect

Right ventricular hypertrophy

A

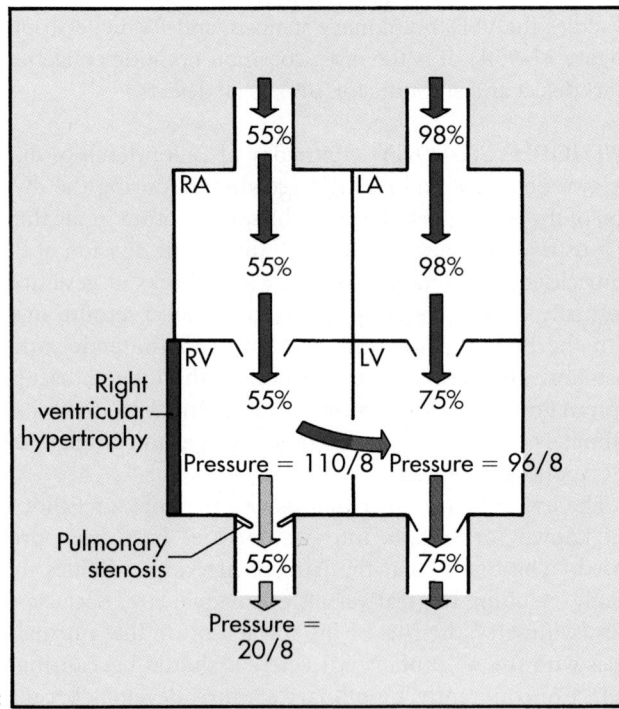

RA   LA

55%   98%

55%   98%

RV   LV

Right ventricular hypertrophy

55%   75%

Pressure = 110/8   Pressure = 96/8

Pulmonary stenosis

55%   75%

Pressure = 20/8

C

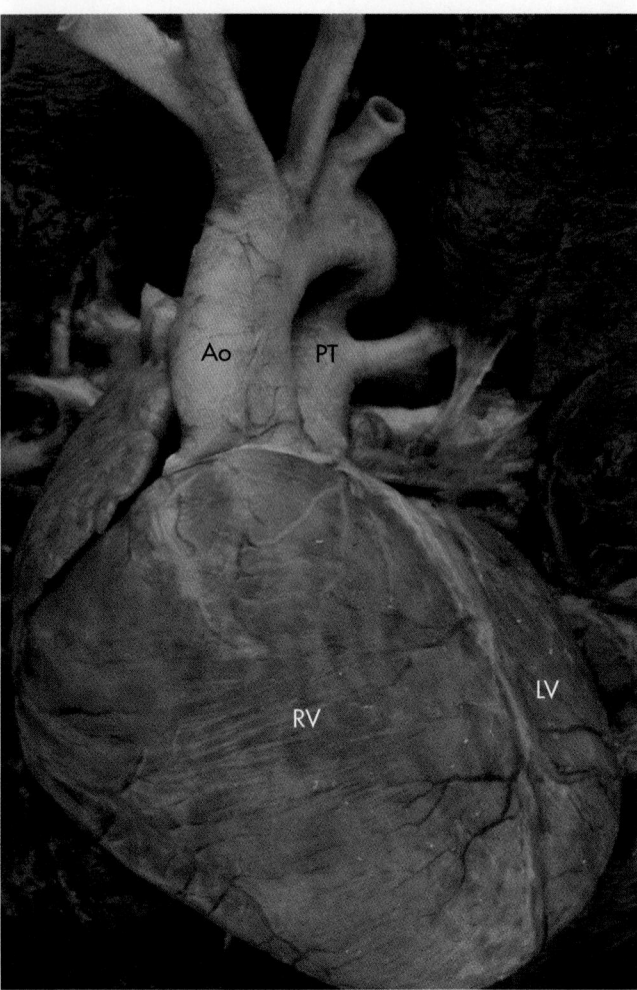

Ao   PT

LV

RV

B

Figure 31-9 Tetralogy of Fallot. **A,** Anatomic defects in tetralogy of Fallot. **B,** Complete transposition of the aorta and pulmonary artery. **C,** Hemodynamics of tetralogy of Fallot with right-to-left shunt. *Ao,* aorta; *PT,* pulmonary artery trunk; *RV,* right ventricle; *LV,* left ventricle; *RA,* right atrium; *LA,* left atrium. (**A** from Hockenberry MJ et al: *Wong's nursing care of infants and children,* ed 7, St Louis, 2003, Mosby; **B** from Damjanov I, Linder J, editors: *Anderson's pathology,* ed 10, St Louis, 1996, Mosby.)

monary stenosis but also on the size of the VSD and the pulmonary and systemic resistance to flow. Because the VSD is usually large, pressures may be equal in the right and left ventricles. Therefore the major determinant of shunt direction through the VSD is the difference between pulmonary and systemic vascular resistance (see Figure 31-9, *C*). Infants who have little or no shunting are acyanotic and are known as "pink tets." If pulmonary vascular resistance is higher than systemic resistance, the shunt is from right to left. If systemic resistance is higher than pulmonary resistance, the shunt is from left to right. Because many factors can alter the balance between pulmonary and systemic resistance, shunt direction is not necessarily constant.

Pulmonary stenosis decreases blood flow to the lungs and, consequently, the amount of oxygenated blood that returns to the left heart. If blood also shunts from right to left through the VSD, deoxygenated blood mixes with the small amount of relatively oxygenated blood returning from the lungs. The result is low O_2 saturation (hypoxemia) in the systemic circulation. The body attempts to compensate for hypoxemia by producing more red blood cells (thereby causing polycythemia) and by increasing blood flow to the lungs through collateral bronchial vessels.

CLINICAL MANIFESTATIONS   As long as the ductus arteriosus remains open, the newborn's pulmonary blood flow may be adequate. As the ductus closes, however, cyanosis becomes apparent. Chronic hypoxemia causes clubbing of the fingers and toes (see Chapter 33).

A common manifestation of tetralogy of Fallot is the sudden onset of dyspnea, cyanosis, and restlessness, sometimes called a *hypoxic spell* or a *"tet spell,"* that generally occurs with crying and exertion. The cause of these episodes is unknown, but it is theorized that the RV outflow tract goes into spasm or the systemic resistance drops suddenly.[7,30] In either case the relative or actual increase in pulmonary vascular resistance increases the right-to-left shunt and the cyanosis. Infants often have difficulty with feeding because the exertion required increases hypoxia, and therefore they experience slow growth and failure to thrive.

Squatting is a spontaneous compensatory mechanism used by older children to alleviate hypoxic spells. Squatting and its variants increase systemic resistance while decreasing venous return to the heart from the inferior vena cava. The decrease of systemic return makes relatively more oxygenated blood available to the body. The increase of systemic resistance also reverses the shunt through the VSD to a left-to-right shunt, which has the effect of increasing pulmonary blood flow. Through both of these mechanisms, squatting decreases the degree of hypoxemia temporarily.

The typical heart murmur of tetralogy is a pulmonary systolic ejection murmur caused by the obstruction in the outflow tract, which creates turbulence during systole. The smaller the obstruction, the louder the murmur is. This explains why the murmur often disappears during a hypoxic spell, when obstruction increases. The second heart sound seems to be single, but in fact it is not. The pulmonary component is very soft and delayed and usually is not heard, although it is present. The enlarged right ventricle may cause the left side of the chest to be more prominent, and a "heave" also may be palpated.

EVALUATION AND TREATMENT   The ECG indicates RV hypertrophy. Chest roentgenographic examination shows that the heart is shaped like a boot and that pulmonary vascular markings are decreased. Echocardiograms and angiograms enable the clinician to see the size and position of the VSD, the stenotic pulmonary infundibulum or valve, the smaller-than-normal pulmonary artery, and the overriding aorta. Measurements made during cardiac catheterization demonstrate normal systemic pressure in the right ventricle, decreased pressure in the RV outflow tract, and low oxygen saturation in the aorta.

The current trend is to repair tetralogy of Fallot before 1 year of life. Triggers for repair include increasing cyanosis and hypercyanotic spells. Palliative procedures include the placement of a pulmonary-to-systemic artery shunt known as the Blalock-Taussig shunt to increase pulmonary blood flow or a modification of the shunt using prosthetic graft material placed from either the subclavian or innominate artery to the pulmonary artery. These shunts may cause pulmonary artery distortion. Corrective repair involves patch closure of the VSD, resection of infundibular stenosis, and patch augmentation of the RV outflow tract. The procedure is done through a median sternotomy on cardiopulmonary bypass. The operative mortality is less than 5%. Complications include dysrhythmias and occasionally heart block.[30,31]

Tricuspid Atresia

Tricuspid atresia consists of an imperforate tricuspid valve, resulting in no communication between the right atrium and right ventricle (Figure 31-10). This defect accounts for 2% to 3% of congenital heart defects and is the third most common cyanotic heart defect.[3,14] Tricuspid atresia is a combination of defects, including the imperforate tricuspid valve as well as a septal defect, hypoplastic or absent right ventricle, enlarged mitral valve and left ventricle, and varying degrees of pul-

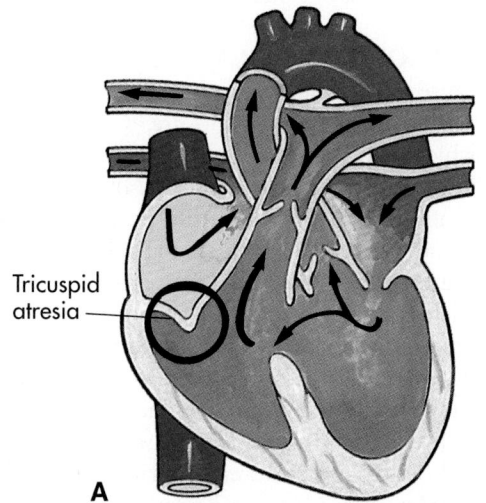

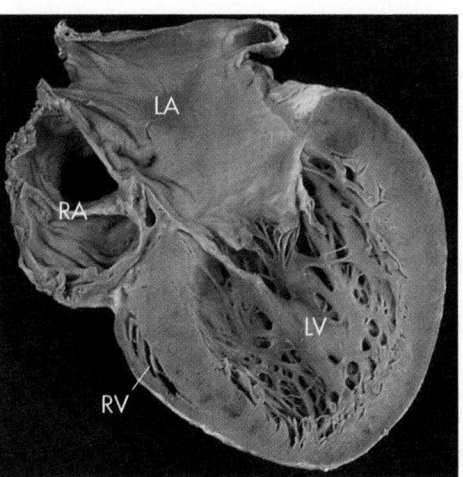

Figure 31-10 Tricuspid atresia. **A,** No communication from the right atrium to right ventricle. **B,** Tricuspid atresia with absent right atrioventricular connection with a hypoplastic right ventricle (four-chamber view). *LA,* Left atrium; *RA,* right atrium; *LV,* left ventricle; *RV,* right ventricle. (**A** from Hockenberry MJ et al: *Wong's nursing care of infants and children,* ed 7, St Louis, 2003, Mosby; **B** from Damjanov I, Linder J, editors: *Anderson's pathology,* ed 10, St Louis, 1996, Mosby.)

monic stenosis.[20] Tricuspid atresia also may be associated with transposition of the great vessels. The most common type of tricuspid atresia involves a hypoplastic right atrium with decreased pulmonary blood flow and a VSD and is not associated with transposition.[3]

PATHOPHYSIOLOGY   Systemic blood returns through the superior and inferior venae cavae to the right atrium. Because there is no opening between the right atrium and right ventricle, blood flows through the ASD into the left atrium, mixing with blood returning from the pulmonary circulation. The blood then enters the left ventricle. Most of this blood goes out into the systemic circulation through the aorta, but varying amounts pass through the VSD into the hypoplastic right ventricle and then out through the pulmonary valve to the lungs. Pulmonary circulation depends on the presence of a VSD and the presence of a functioning right ventricle of reasonable capacity. If the right ventricle is absent, the pulmonary valve is usually imperforate as well. If this is the case, a PDA is necessary to ensure that some blood flows into the pulmonary circulation.[28]

Pulmonary circulation also depends on the relationship between pulmonary and systemic vascular resistance. As long as pulmonary resistance is lower than systemic resistance, blood flows through the VSD from left to right, feeding the pulmonary circulation. If pulmonary resistance rises above systemic resistance, blood will not reach the pulmonary circulation through the VSD.

CLINICAL MANIFESTATIONS   Some degree of central cyanosis is common in tricuspid atresia, depending on the amount of pulmonary blood flow. Growth failure also is common. Children experience exertional dyspnea, tachypnea, and hypoxemia. Long-term effects of hypoxia are polycythemia and clubbing. These children also may display hypercyanotic spells. Hepatomegaly may be present if the ASD is restrictive or congestive heart failure occurs as a result of increased pulmonary blood flow.

The murmur heard with tricuspid atresia may have several components. The VSD causes a systolic regurgitant murmur; the larger the VSD, the softer and shorter the murmur is likely to be. A narrowly split second heart sound caused by decreased pulmonary blood flow may be present, or the pulmonic component may be absent when no VSD is involved.

EVALUATION AND TREATMENT   Chest roentgenographic examination shows a heart size that is normal or slightly increased. ECG shows RA, LA, and LV hypertrophy. Echocardiography and cardiac catheterization depict left-to-right shunting at the ventricular level, inability of blood flow to enter the right ventricle, and the presence of associated defects.

Newborns who are ductal dependent are immediately given prostaglandins to maintain adequate pulmonary blood flow. Initial surgical intervention involves the placement of a Blalock-Taussig shunt (or its modifications). If the ASD is restrictive, a Rashkind procedure may be performed during catheterization. Children who experience increased pulmonary blood flow may require the placement of a pulmonary artery band. Corrective repair involves closing the septal defects, taking down the previous shunts or band, and connecting the superior and inferior venae cavae to the pulmonary artery to separate the pulmonary systemic circulation (Fontan procedure and its modifications). Postoperative complications include pleural effusions, elevated pulmonary vascular resistance, LV dysfunction, and dysrhythmias.[29,30]

Obstructive Defects

Obstructive defects are conditions in which anatomic stenosis (narrowing) in either the right or left outflow tract causes obstruction to blood flow and results in a pressure load on the ventricles and decreased output. The difference between the obstruction is the gradient that reflects the severity of the narrowing; the higher the gradient is, the more obstruction to flow and increased afterload on the ventricle, with resultant decreased cardiac output. The location is classified according to the location of the narrowing in relation to the valve. Valvular stenosis refers to stenosis of the valve itself; subvalvular indicates that the stenotic area is below the valve or in the ventricular outflow tract; and supravalvular is the area above the valve in the great artery. The obstructive defects include coarctation of the aorta, aortic stenosis, pulmonary stenosis, and hypoplastic left heart syndrome. Symptoms associated with the defect depend on the site of stenosis.

Coarctation of the Aorta

Coarctation of the aorta (COA) is a narrowing of the lumen of the aorta that impedes blood flow. This defect accounts for 8% to 10% of all congenital heart defects.[30] COA is almost always in a juxtaductal position, although it can occur anywhere between the origin of the aortic arch and the bifurcation of the aorta in the lower abdomen. As many as 85% of individuals with COA have a bicuspid aortic valve (Figure 31-11).

PATHOPHYSIOLOGY   COA commonly develops because of an abnormal contractile ductal tissue that constricts at the time of ductal closure.[3] COA causes a condition in which there are higher pressures above the site of stenosis and lower pressures below the site. In preductal COA the right ventricle acts as a systemic pump, sending unoxygenated blood through the ductus into the descending aorta below the coarctation (Figure 31-12). In postductal COA the right ventricle cannot pump enough blood through the ductus to the descending aorta because of pressure caused by the narrowed aorta. Systolic pressures increase in the ascending aorta and left ventricle and decrease in the descending aorta beyond the COA (Figure 31-13). To bypass the COA, collateral circulation, which involves small arteries arising from the subclavian arteries, joins intercostal arteries that flow into the descending aorta. This bypasses the COA and supplies more oxygenated blood to the lower extremities. The direction of shunting through the ductus depends on the pressure differ-

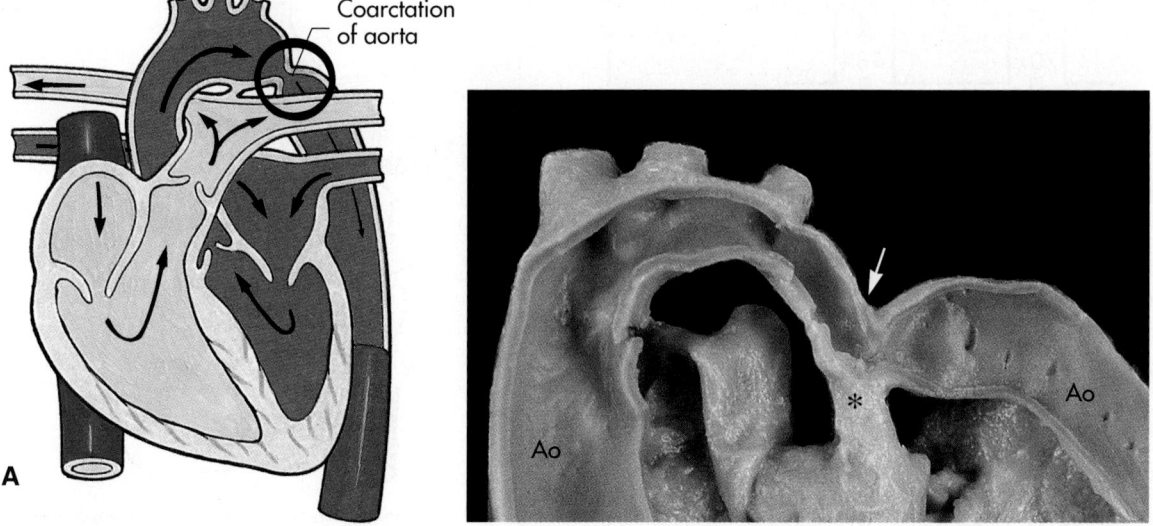

Figure 31-11 **Postductal and preductal coarctation of the aorta. A,** Postductal coarctation occurs distal to ("after") the insertion of the closed ductus arteriosus into the aortic arch. Preductal coarctation occurs proximal to ("before") insertion of the patent ductus arteriosus. The coarctation consists of a flap of tissue that protrudes from the tunica media of the aortic wall. **B,** Coarctation of the aorta with typical indentation of the aortic wall *(arrow)* opposite the ductal arterial ligament (*). *Ao,* Aorta. (**A** from Hockenberry MJ et al: *Wong's nursing care of infants and children,* ed 7, St Louis, 2003, Mosby; **B** from Damjanov I, Linder J, editors: *Anderson's pathology,* ed 10, St Louis, 1996, Mosby.)

ence between the pulmonary artery and aorta. When blood pressure is greater in the aorta than in the pulmonary artery, blood flow through the ductus will be left to right toward the lungs, resulting in increased pulmonary blood volume return to the left side of the heart. This places a strain on the left atrium and left ventricle, leading to congestive heart failure. LV hypertrophy develops because of increased afterload from the increased volume of the pulmonary circulation and obstruction to flow caused by the coarctation.

CLINICAL MANIFESTATIONS   Clinical manifestations vary depending on the severity of the coarctation and age of presentation. In newborns the onset of symptoms depends on the timing of ductal closure after a fall in pulmonary vascular resistance, the location of the COA, and the presence of associated defects. The newborn usually presents with congestive heart failure secondary to LV failure. Once the ductus closes, these infants will deteriorate rapidly from the development of hypotension, acidosis, and shock. Older children may not be diagnosed until hypertension is noted. Hypertension is noted in the upper extremities with decreased or absent pulses in the lower extremities, accompanied by cool mottled skin and, occasionally, leg cramps during exercise caused by tissue anoxia. Hypertension may cause dizziness, headache, fainting, or epistaxis. A systolic ejection murmur, heard best on the left interscapular area, is caused by rapid blood flow through the narrowed area.

EVALUATION AND TREATMENT   A chest roentgenogram shows an enlarged heart with congested lung fields in newborns. Rib notching between the fourth and eighth ribs may be seen in children older than 5 years, reflecting erosion of the

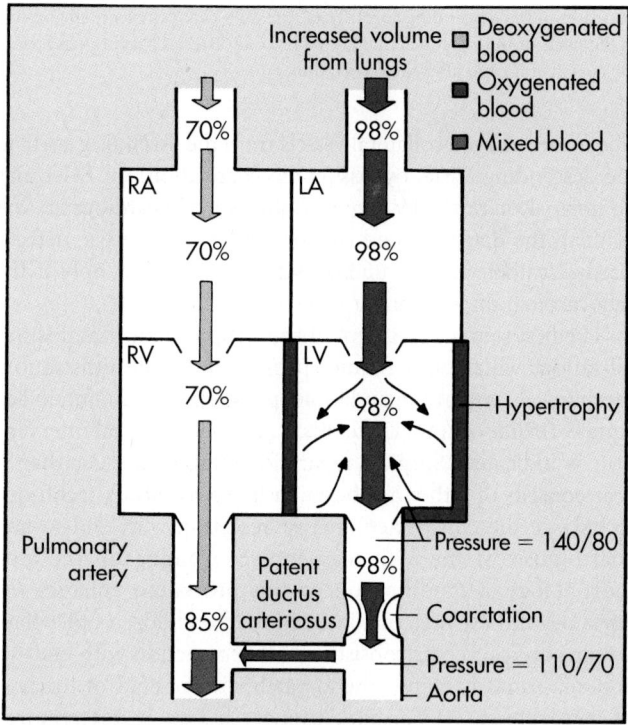

Figure 31-12 **Hemodynamics of preductal coarctation of the aorta with a patent ductus arteriosus.** The left-to-right shunt through the ductus arteriosus increases the volume of blood in the pulmonary circulation. Afterload (dashed arrows) is increased in the left heart by *(1)* increased return from the lungs and *(2)* decreased ventricular outflow caused by the coarctation. The outcome is left heart failure (congestive heart failure). *RA,* right atrium; *LA,* left atrium; *RV,* right ventricle; *LV,* left ventricle.

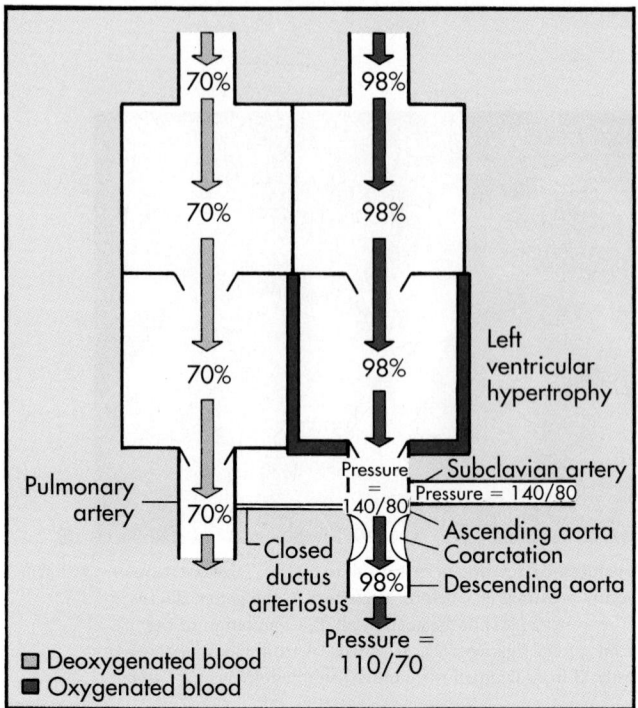

Figure 31-13 Hemodynamics of postductal coarctation of the aorta. Blood pressure increases in the ascending aorta and subclavian artery and decreases in the descending aorta. These pressure changes eventually occur in the parts of the systemic circulation served by arteries that branch from the aorta before and after the coarctation.

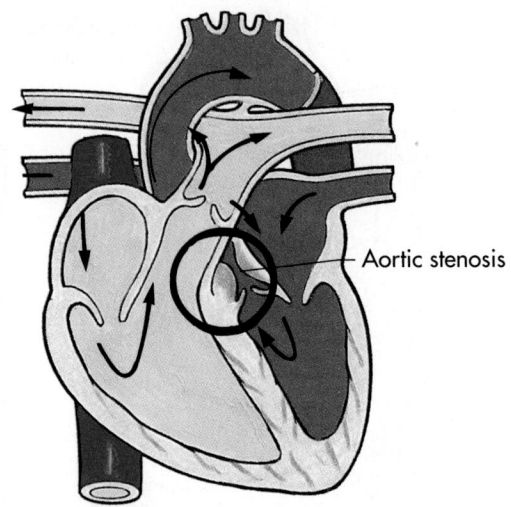

Figure 31-14 Aortic stenosis. Narrowing of the aortic valve causing resistance to blood flow in the left ventricle, decreased cardiac output, left ventricular hypertrophy, and pulmonary congestion. (From Hockenberry MJ et al: *Wong's nursing care of infants and children,* ed 6, St Louis, 1999, Mosby.)

ribs from enlarged collateral vessels from the ascending aorta to the descending aorta, bypassing the coarctation. An ECG may be normal or reveal LV hypertrophy. An echocardiogram will confirm the diagnosis and rule out other intracardiac defects. Cardiac catheterization and/or MRI is performed only if the echocardiogram is inconclusive.

The first step in treatment of the symptomatic infant is stabilization, which may require prostaglandin administration, mechanical ventilation, and inotropic support to maintain adequate cardiac output. Once this is achieved, surgical intervention is indicated. Surgical repair for infants younger than 1 year consists of either a subclavian flap aortoplasty technique to enlarge the constricted area or resection with end-to-end anastomosis of the arch segments. Depending on the arch morphology, a modification of this procedure enlarges the aorta beyond the area of constriction. For children older than 1 year, surgical repair consists of either resection with end-to-end anastomosis or prosthetic patch enlargement of the area of constriction.[29,30] Cardiopulmonary bypass is not required because of the extracardiac nature of the lesion, and the approach is accomplished through a left thoracotomy.

Postoperative complications include recoarctation and paradoxical postoperative hypertension. Residual permanent hypertension requiring continued medical therapy is related to age at repair; therefore surgical intervention is recommended at the time of diagnosis. Operative mortality for infants is less than 5%, and for children older than 1 year, it is less than 1%.[30] Balloon dilation angioplasty in newborns has

been successfully performed. However, aortic aneurysm formation and restenosis have been noted;[32-36] therefore surgical repair remains the correction of choice for the newborn.[37,38]

Aortic Stenosis

Aortic stenosis is a narrowing of the aortic outflow tract (Figure 31-14). The lesion accounts for 5% of all congenital heart defects.[3] Valvular stenosis is caused by malformation or fusion of the cusps. It is the most common type of aortic stenosis, tends to be progressive, and can lead to sudden death as a result of low cardiac output or myocardial infarction. For children with mild to moderate aortic stenosis, exercise restrictions are advised.[28] Less common forms of aortic stenosis are subvalvular stenosis caused by a constricting fibrous ring below the valve and supravalvular stenosis that occurs above the valve.

PATHOPHYSIOLOGY   Obstruction to blood flowing out the aorta causes an increased workload on the left ventricle, resulting in left ventricle hypertrophy (LVH). LV failure may develop, leading to an increase in LA pressure and a backup in the system, eventually resulting in pulmonary vascular congestion and pulmonary arterial hypertension. LVH can decrease coronary artery perfusion, resulting in myocardial infarction, or it can alter the LV papillary muscle, causing mitral insufficiency.

CLINICAL MANIFESTATIONS   Most children with mild to moderate aortic stenosis are asymptomatic. Signs of exercise intolerance may not appear until preadolescence. Syncopal episodes, epigastric pain, and exertional chest pain may occur in more severe forms of aortic stenosis. A systolic ejection murmur at the right upper sternal border that transmits to the neck and left lower sternal border is produced by blood flow through the stenotic area. An ejection click may be heard with valvular aortic stenosis. Severe forms of aortic stenosis, especially critical aortic stenosis in the newborn, result in shock and require immediate intervention.

EVALUATION AND TREATMENT   Diagnosis may be made based on previous medical history and physical findings. Chest roentgenographic examination may reveal a dilated ascending aorta or LV enlargement. Increased pulmonary vascular markings may be seen in severe forms. In mild cases the ECG is normal. LVH with strain pattern may be seen in severe forms. An echocardiogram may reveal a thickened and poorly functioning left ventricle with abnormal closure of the aortic valve. Cardiac catheterization will determine the location, cause, and severity of obstruction.

The presence of ST segment changes on ECG, severe congestive heart failure, and evidence of discrete stenosis at the aortic outflow tract are indications for intervention. Balloon aortic valvuloplasty is a palliative procedure that is performed for valvular aortic stenosis; however, it is associated with complications, including aortic insufficiency and dysrhythmia.[39,40] Aortic valvotomy, under inflow occlusion or cardiopulmonary bypass, is currently performed for valvular aortic stenosis. Operative mortality remains high in infants (up to 20%), although older children have a mortality close to 0%.[29] As many as 25% of individuals require a second surgery

within 10 years for restenosis, at which time valve replacement may be the procedure of choice.

Subvalvular aortic stenosis and supravalvular aortic stenosis require surgical repair involving excision of the area causing the constriction. For subvalvular aortic stenosis involving a small LV outflow tract and aortic annulus, a Konno procedure may be done to enlarge the LV outflow tract and aortic annulus with a patch.[41,42]

Pulmonary Stenosis

Pulmonary stenosis is the narrowing of the pulmonary outflow tract. This may be in the form of abnormal thickening of the valve leaflets or narrowing of the arterial (supravalvular) or ventricular (subvalvular) side of the valve (Figure 31-15, *A*). **Pulmonary atresia** is the severe form of pulmonary stenosis and involves complete fusion of the commissures, allowing no blood flow out of the pulmonary artery. Pulmonary stenosis accounts for 5% to 8% of all congenital heart defects.[3]

PATHOPHYSIOLOGY   Pulmonary stenosis creates resistance to blood flow from the right ventricle to the pulmonary artery. Less blood flow can pass through the pulmonary valve under normal systolic pressure, causing some

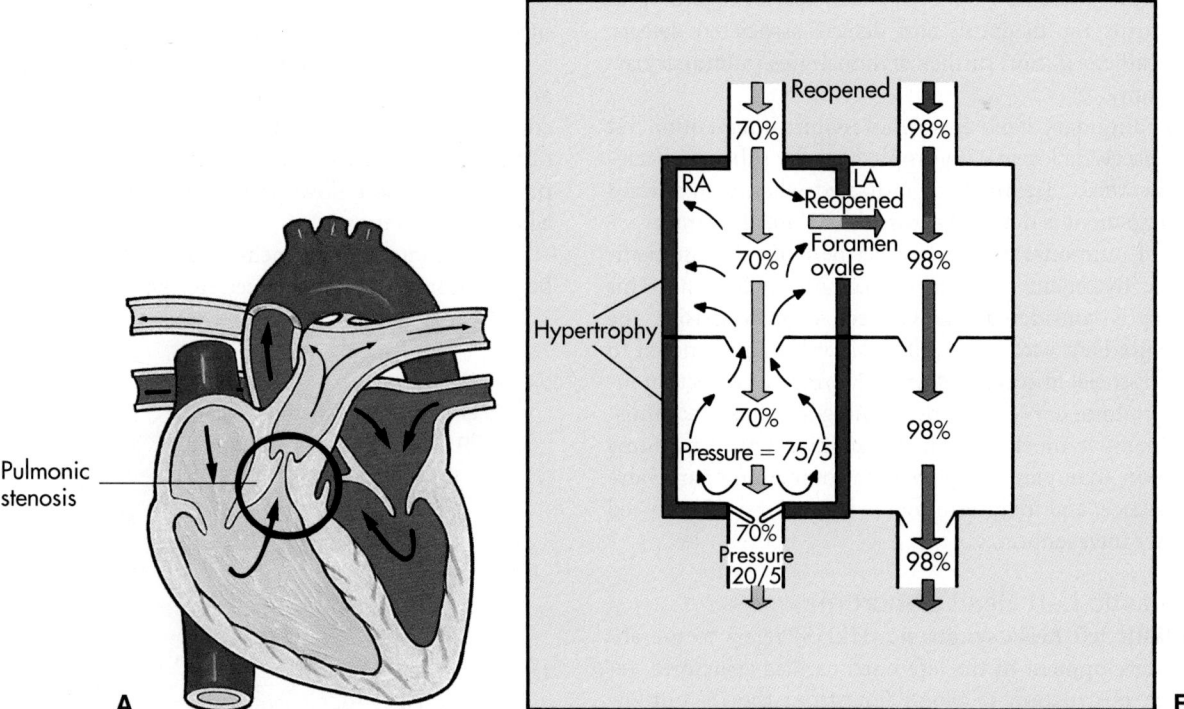

Figure 31-15 Pulmonary stenosis. A, Obstruction of right ventricular outflow caused by pulmonary stenosis. Pressure on the ventricular side of the pulmonic semilunar valve (pulmonary valve) is much greater than that on the pulmonary arterial side. This difference disrupts the normal pressure gradient across the valve. Pulmonary stenosis increases ventricular afterload by decreasing blood flow through the valve, which causes ventricular hypertrophy. **B,** The backup of ventricular afterload into the right atrium reopens the foramen ovale. Venous blood then flows from the area of higher pressure (the right atrium) to the area of lower pressure (the left atrium), causing a left-to-right shunt. Cyanosis occurs if enough venous blood shunts from right to left to reduce oxygen saturation in the systemic circulation by 3% to 5%. *RA,* Right atrium; *LA,* left atrium. (**A** from Hockenberry MJ et al: *Wong's nursing care of infants and children,* ed 7, St Louis, 2003, Mosby.)

blood to remain in the right ventricle, resulting in increased afterload. In order for the right ventricle to maintain adequate cardiac output, the myocardium hypertrophies. If the RV outflow tract obstruction is severe, blood will back up into the right atrium, causing dilation and hypertrophy. This may result in reopening of the foramen ovale with resultant unoxygenated blood shunting to the left atrium, causing cyanosis (see Figure 31-15, *B*).

CLINICAL MANIFESTATIONS   Clinical manifestations depend on the severity of pulmonary stenosis. A systolic ejection murmur at the left upper sternal border reflects obstruction to flow through the narrowed pulmonary valve. A systolic ejection click is present with valvular stenosis at the upper left sternal border. A thrill also may be palpated at the upper left sternal border. Children with moderate pulmonary stenosis have exertional dyspnea and fatigability because of the inability of the body to provide sufficient pulmonary blood flow to meet demands for increased cardiac output. Severe pulmonary stenosis will produce cyanosis and right-sided CHF.

EVALUATION AND TREATMENT   A chest roentgenogram shows a normal-size heart with a prominent main pulmonary artery caused by poststenotic dilation. An ECG is normal but may reveal right axis deviation and RV hypertrophy with moderate pulmonary stenosis. Echocardiography confirms the diagnosis and detects associated defects. Cardiac catheterization further demonstrates pulmonary artery anatomy.

Mild pulmonary stenosis may not require intervention but will be observed closely with prophylaxis for subacute bacterial endocarditis. Treatment is indicated when a significant pressure gradient is detected across the RV outflow tract.

Critical pulmonary stenosis must be addressed immediately. The treatment of choice is balloon angioplasty. This procedure is considered highly effective in decreasing the pressure gradient across the pulmonic valve and is noted to have few associated complications.[36,43] Surgical correction involves a pulmonary valvotomy incising the fused commissures. Operative mortality is less than 1%.[3] Both valvotomy and balloon angioplasty may result in some pulmonary valve incompetence, and long-term follow-up may reveal the need for further intervention.

Hypoplastic Left Heart Syndrome

Hypoplastic left heart syndrome (HLHS) refers to the abnormal development of the left-sided cardiac structures, resulting in obstruction to blood flow from the LV outflow tract. HLHS involves underdevelopment of the left ventricle, aorta, and aortic arch, as well as mitral atresia or stenosis (Figure 31-16). Therefore infants with HLHS depend on a well-functioning right ventricle and the presence of a PDA or atrial septal communication for survival. HLHS accounts for 1% of all congenital heart defects and is considered the most complex congenital defect.

PATHOPHYSIOLOGY   Because of the high pressures caused by LV outflow tract obstruction, saturated blood enters the left atrium and mixes with desaturated blood in the right atrium through an atrial septal communication. Blood flow follows the normal pathways through the right side of the heart. Exiting the pulmonary artery, the mixed-saturation blood flows through the ductus and to the descending aorta. The amount of blood flow that travels to the pulmonary and systemic circulations depends on vascular resistance in the respective systems. Retrograde blood flow through the hypoplastic ascending aorta provides coronary and cerebral blood flow.

CLINICAL MANIFESTATIONS   Newborn infants with HLHS generally are born full term and initially appear healthy. As the ductus closes, systemic perfusion is decreased, resulting in hypoxemia, acidosis, and shock. Usually no heart murmur is detected. The second heart sound is loud and single because of aortic atresia.

EVALUATION AND TREATMENT   A chest roentgenogram shows cardiomegaly and increased pulmonary venous congestion. ECG shows RV hypertrophy and diminished left-sided forces. Echocardiography reveals the components of the defect with a diminutive LV cavity, hypoplastic aortic valve and arch, and hypoplastic or absent mitral valve with a dilated RV cavity. Cardiac catheterization with balloon septostomy may be necessary if the atrial septum is inadequate.

Prostaglandin infusion to maintain patency of the ductus arteriosus is essential for newborn infant survival. Immediate correction of acidosis, inotropic support for adequate cardiac output, and ventilatory manipulation to balance systemic and pulmonary blood flow prevent further deterioration and achieve stabilization.

Surgical intervention includes a three-stage approach that begins with a Norwood procedure. The Norwood procedure

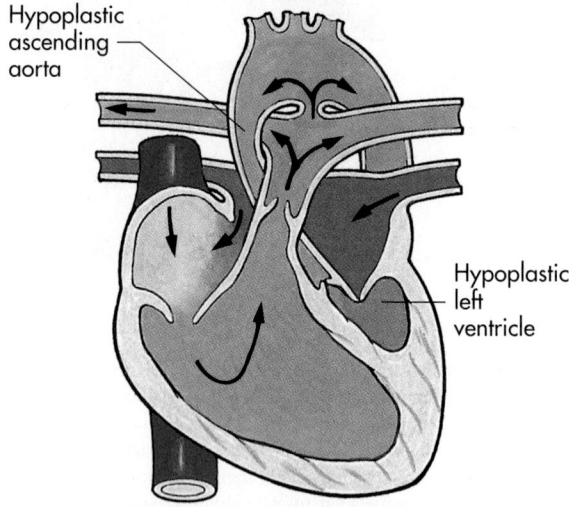

Figure 31-16 Hypoplastic left heart syndrome. (From Hockenberry MJ et al: *Wong's nursing care of infants and children,* ed 7, St Louis, 2003, Mosby.)

consists of an atrial septectomy, placement of a pulmonary-to-systemic artery shunt to maintain adequate pulmonary blood flow, creation of a permanent communication between the right ventricle and aorta, and patch augmentation of the aorta. Postoperative complications include imbalance of systemic and pulmonary blood flow, leading to inadequate cardiac output and persistent heart failure. In most centers, survival after the Norwood procedure is now averaging greater than 70%.

The second stage is the bidirectional Glenn procedure, which is performed between 2 and 9 months of age, depending on the child's clinical status, pulmonary vascular resistance, and ventricular function. This involves joining the superior vena cava to the pulmonary artery. Complications include superior vena cava syndrome, pleural effusion, and low cardiac output.

The third stage is the Fontan procedure, described earlier, which separates the systemic from the pulmonary circulation. Timing for surgical repair depends on the child's ventricular function, presence of atrioventricular valve regurgitation, and pulmonary vascular resistance. Most surgeons perform the Fontan procedure when the child is approximately 2 to 4 years of age.[44,45]

Cardiac transplant also may be an option for these newborns.[42,43] Most surgical centers offer the three-staged palliative surgeries as an initial approach, with an option for cardiac transplantation later in life.[45-48]

Mixed Defects

Many complex defects are classified as mixed defects because of their dependence on the mixing of pulmonary and systemic circulations for survival during the postnatal period. This mixing results in desaturated systemic blood flow and cyanosis. Pulmonary congestion occurs because of preferen-

tial pulmonary blood flow and decreased cardiac output caused by ventricular volume overload. Clinically, each defect has varying degrees of cyanosis and CHF depending on the various components of the lesion.

Transposition of the Great Arteries

Transposition of the great arteries (TGA) refers to a condition in which the aorta arises from the RV and the pulmonary artery from the LV (Figure 31-17, *A*). The result is two separate, parallel circuits in which unoxygenated blood circulates continuously through the systemic circulation and oxygenated blood circulates repeatedly through the pulmonary circulation. This condition is incompatible with extrauterine life unless a communication exists between the two circuits to provide the necessary oxygen to the body. Communication is accomplished through mixing of pulmonary and systemic circulations through a PDA, ASD, or VSD (see Figure 31-17, *B*). Dextro–transposition of the great arteries (D-TGA) is the most common cyanotic congenital heart defect and accounts for 10% of all congenital heart defects; "dextro" refers to the aorta remaining to the right of the pulmonary artery.

Two factors allow newborns with complete transposition to survive long enough to be treated. First, blood from the two closed systems can mix through the ductus arteriosus for a short time after birth if pulmonary vascular resistance remains high. Some mixing also may occur through the foramen ovale. If the child has a VSD, mixing occurs through that opening as well.

PATHOPHYSIOLOGY   It is not known precisely which embryologic events lead to transposition, but researchers have proposed that the fault lies in the development of conal tissue in the fibrous skeleton of the heart.[7] The **conus** is a seg-

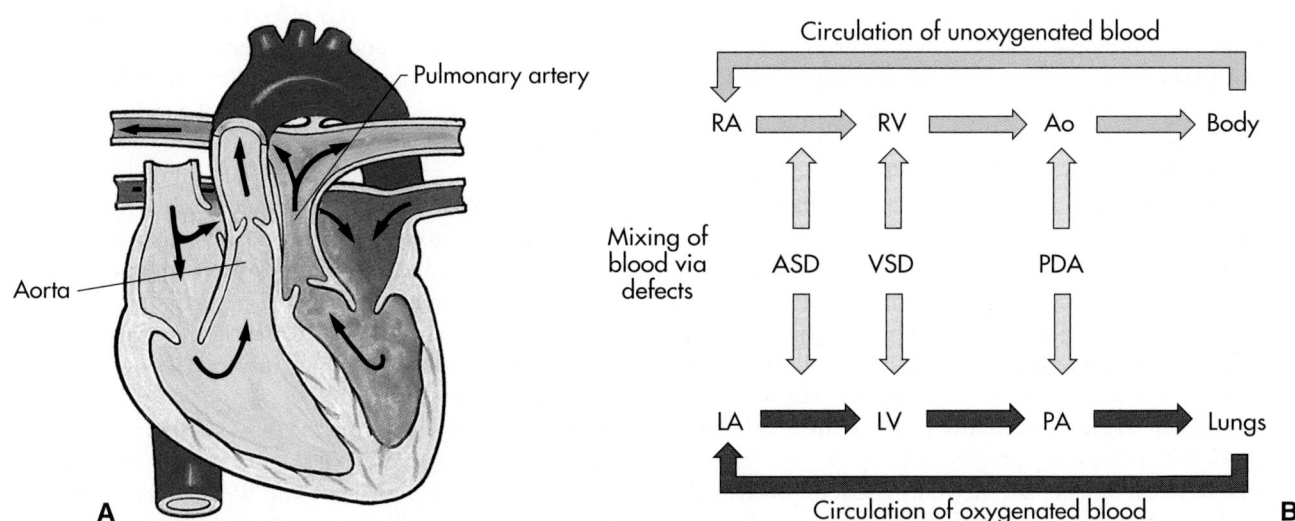

Figure 31-17   Hemodynamics in transposition of the great vessels (TGV). **A,** Complete transposition of the great vessels with an intact interventricular septum. The aorta arises from the right ventricle and the pulmonary artery from the left. **B,** Oxygen saturation in the two parallel circuits. *RA,* Right atrium; *RV,* right ventricle; *Ao,* aorta; *ASD,* atrial septal defect; *VSD,* ventricular septal defect; *PDA,* patent ductus arteriosus; *LA,* left atrium; *LV,* left ventricle; *PA,* pulmonary artery. (**A** from Hockenberry MJ et al: *Wong's nursing care of infants and children,* ed 7, St Louis, 2003, Mosby.)

ment of muscle that separates the atrioventricular (tricuspid and mitral) valves from the semilunar (aortic and pulmonic) valves. (The fibrous skeleton and heart valves are described and illustrated in Chapter 29; see Figure 29-4.) Normally, the conus grows more on the left side, under the pulmonic valve. This pushes the pulmonic valve anteriorly and to the left of the aortic valve. Some researchers believe that in transposition of the great vessels, nearly the opposite occurs; that is, the conus beneath the aortic valve grows more, pushing the aortic valve until it is anterior (forward) and superior to the pulmonic valve. This causes the aorta to rise anteriorly and to the right of the pulmonary artery.[1] Recent research indicates that looping and/or wedging of the outflow tract during embryogenesis is the cause of clonal malformation.[7] The interventricular septum is intact in about 60% of cases of transposition; a VSD is present in the remaining 40%. Pulmonary stenosis is associated with the transposition in about 4% to 6% of children with intact septums and in 28% to 31% of children with VSDs.[1]

The discussion that follows is limited to the pathophysiology of complete transposition with an intact interventricular septum.

CLINICAL MANIFESTATIONS   The degree of mixing permitted by fetal structures determines the type and severity of clinical manifestations. Cyanosis may be mild shortly after birth and worsen during the first day because of functional closure of the ductus arteriosus. Low oxygen levels in the blood (hypoxemia) cause metabolic acidosis, tachycardia, and tachypnea. The presence of a PDA or large septal defect allows for more mixing and results in only mild cyanosis, but the infant may develop congestive heart failure.

The first heart sound is normal, and the second sound may be heard as a single sound even though both the aortic and pulmonic valves are functioning. The single S_2 may occur because transposition places the aortic valve closer to the chest wall than the pulmonic valve. No murmur is noted with transposition of the great arteries with an intact ventricular septum.

EVALUATION AND TREATMENT   On chest roentgenogram the heart has a characteristic shape—like an egg on its side—and pulmonary vascular markings are increased. The heart may be enlarged if the infant is a few weeks old and has a VSD. ECG findings reveal a right-axis deviation and some RV hypertrophy. Echocardiography confirms the diagnosis of transposition of the great arteries. Cardiac catheterization is necessary to determine the coronary anatomy; measure ventricular ratios; and, if need be, perform a balloon septostomy.

Surgical repair during the newborn period involves the Jantene (arterial switch) operation that transposes the great arteries. The coronary arteries are removed from the aorta before the arterial switch is performed and reimplanted without torsion or kinking into the aorta. This establishes normal blood flow with the left ventricle as the systemic pump. Re-

sults are now approaching 100% survival. Complications include narrowing at the sites of the great artery anastomoses and coronary insufficiency.[29,30]

Mustard and Senning operations (the creation of an intraatrial tunnel to baffle the systemic venous blood flow to the mitral valve and the pulmonary venous blood flow to the tricuspid valve) are no longer the procedures of choice because the right ventricle must perform as the systemic pump. Long-term follow-up of children with Mustard and Senning operations revealed significant rates of RV failure and dysrhythmias.

The Rastelli procedure is used with children with transposition, VSD, and severe pulmonary stenosis. This procedure involves closing the VSD with a baffle by rerouting LV blood through the VSD to the aorta. The pulmonary valve is closed, and a right ventricle–to–pulmonary artery prosthetic or homograft valve conduit is placed. This procedure requires prosthetic conduit replacement as the child grows and is associated with ventricular failure and dysrhythmias in the postoperative period.

Total Anomalous Pulmonary Venous Connection

Total anomalous pulmonary venous connection (TAPVC), or total anomalous pulmonary venous return, occurs when the pulmonary veins abnormally connect to the right side of the heart either directly or through one or more systemic veins that drain into the right atrium (Figure 31-18). An ASD generally is present also. This defect is extremely rare, accounting for only 1% of all congenital heart defects. The four types of TAPVC are based on the site of drainage. Supracardiac TAPVCs are the most common form (50%) and drain to the SVC through the vertical or innominate vein. Cardiac TAPVCs (20%) drain directly into the right atrium or through the coronary sinus. Infracardiac TAPVCs (20%) traverse the diaphragm and drain into the portal or hepatic vein or the IVC. Mixed TAPVCs (10%) are a combination of the various types. Partial anomalous venous connection is a condition in which only one or a few of the pulmonary veins, usually the right-sided veins, drain to the right atrium or one of its tributaries.[3]

PATHOPHYSIOLOGY   Physiologically, TAPVC can be differentiated into two groups: nonobstructive and obstructive, depending on the absence or presence of obstruction to pulmonary venous drainage. The hemodynamics of the nonobstructive group involves the right atrium receiving the oxygenated blood that would normally flow into the left atrium. The amount of blood shunted into the left atrium versus the volume entering the right ventricle depends on the size of the ASD and compliance of the right ventricle. Therefore, if the ASD is restrictive and RV compliance approaches normal, more blood will enter the right ventricle than the left atrium, resulting in RA and RV enlargement, as well as increased pulmonary blood flow. This causes increased pulmonary venous blood return and larger amounts of saturated blood. If the ASD is unrestrictive and the right ventricle does

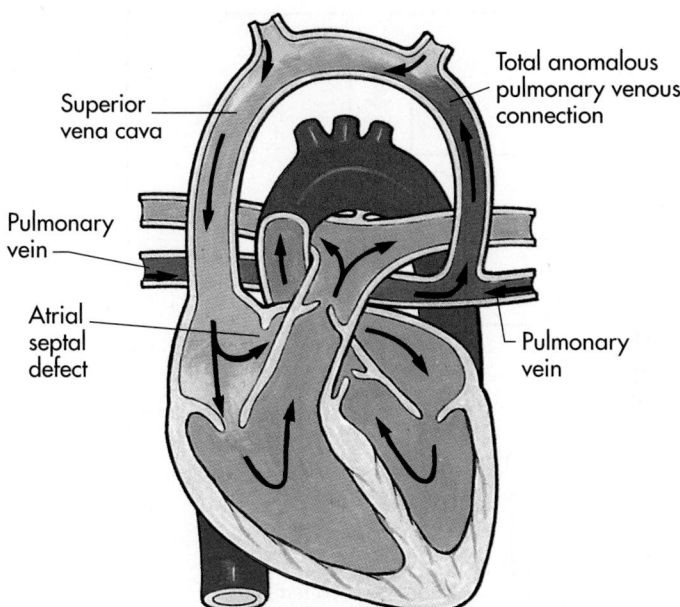

Figure 31-18 Hemodynamics of total anomalous pulmonary venous connection (TAPVC). In the form of TAPVC represented here, the pulmonary veins enter the left anomalous vertical vein instead of the left atrium. From the left anomalous vertical vein, the mixed blood from the lungs flows into the superior vena cava through an innominate vein (literally, a "vein without a name"). Oxygen saturation within the four heart chambers, the pulmonary artery, and the aorta is the same. Blood pressure in the right heart exceeds that in the left heart because the right heart is receiving blood from both the pulmonary and systemic circulatory systems. (Abnormal vessels are shaded.) (From Hockenberry MJ et al: *Wong's nursing care of infants and children,* ed 7, St Louis, 2003, Mosby.)

not thin out to increase compliance, the majority of mixed saturated blood is shunted from the higher pressure right atrium to the left atrium.

The hemodynamics of obstructed TAPVC cause pulmonary venous hypertension because of resistance caused by the obstruction resulting in an elevation in pulmonary vascular and RV pressures. Pulmonary edema occurs from hydrostatic capillary pressure exceeding the osmotic pressure of the blood and eventually contributing to the development of CHF. This group has a strong association with the infracardiac type of TAPVC and is a surgical emergency.

CLINICAL MANIFESTATIONS   The predominant clinical manifestation in infants with TAPVC is cyanosis caused by mixture of oxygenated and deoxygenated blood entering the systemic circulation. The degree of cyanosis is inversely related to the amount of pulmonary blood flow. Children with unobstructed TAPVC may be asymptomatic until pulmonary vascular resistance drops, at which time pulmonary blood flow will increase, resulting in signs of CHF, particularly growth retardation and frequent pulmonary infections, in addition to mild cyanosis. Obstructed TAPVC results in cyanosis and rapid deterioration necessitating immediate surgical correction, or death will occur.

The physical examination also may reveal a systolic murmur at the left upper sternal border and a middiastolic murmur at the left lower sternal border. Occasionally a venous hum may be detected. A murmur may be absent in obstructed TAPVC. A characteristic quadruple rhythm, consisting of S_1, widely split S_2, and S_3 or S_4, or a gallop rhythm is also present.

EVALUATION AND TREATMENT   The ECG shows a right-axis defect (RAD); RV hypertrophy; and occasionally, RA hypertrophy. The chest roentgenogram of unobstructed TAPVC reveals cardiomegaly, increased pulmonary vascular markings, and a snowman or figure-8 appearance in the supracardiac type. A chest roentgenogram of obstructed TAPVC shows a normal-size heart and a ground-glass appearance of the lung fields, reflecting pulmonary venous congestion or edema. The echocardiogram reveals the abnormal pulmonary venous connections. Cardiac catheterization confirms the site of anomalous connection, the degree of pulmonary blood flow, and the oxygen saturations in the various chambers. The aorta and pulmonary artery have nearly identical oxygen saturations caused by complete mixing of the pulmonary and systemic venous returns to the right atrium.

Surgical repair varies with the type of TAPVC and whether the defect is obstructed or unobstructed. Obstructed lesions are repaired at the time of diagnosis, whereas the unobstructed type generally is repaired during infancy. The procedure is performed on cardiopulmonary bypass and involves anastomosis of the common pulmonary vein to the left atrium; ligating the common pulmonary vein; and closing the ASD, as in the supracardiac and infracardiac types. Repair of the supracardiac type involves baffling the pulmonary venous drainage to the LA. This repair has the highest success rate because of the low technical difficulty, whereas infracardiac repair is associated with a high mortality (up to 25%) and morbidity. Potential complications include reobstruction; atrial dysrhythmias, including sick sinus syndrome; pulmonary artery hypertension; and LV dysfunction.[29,30,46]

Truncus Arteriosus

Truncus arteriosus is the failure of the large embryonic artery and the truncus arteriosus to divide into the pulmonary artery and the aorta. This results in a single vessel arising from both ventricles, providing blood flow to both the pulmonary and systemic circulations (Figure 31-19, *A*). This common trunk straddles the VSD (always present) and has a single valve with three or four leaflets, which may result in stenosis or regurgitation. The incidence is 2% of all congenital heart defects, and a right aortic arch is present 50% of the time. There are four types of truncus arteriosus. Type I is the most common (60%) and involves the main pulmonary artery arising from the truncus and then dividing into the right and left pulmonary arteries. Type II is less common (20%) and involves the pulmonary arteries arising from the posterior aspect of the truncus. Type III is the least common (10%) and involves the pulmonary arteries arising from the lateral aspect of the truncus. Type IV, also known as pseudotruncus, is now considered a severe form of tetralogy of Fallot with the

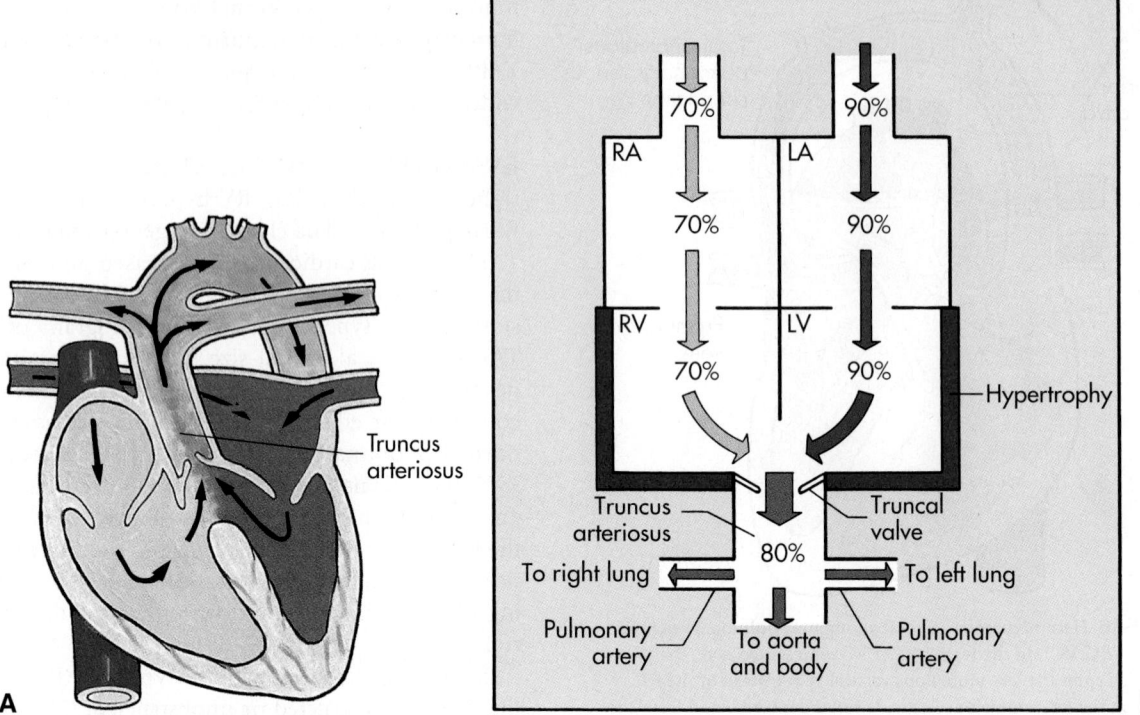

Figure 31-19 **Truncus arteriosus. A,** Persistent truncus arteriosus. The truncus arteriosus fails to divide into the pulmonary artery and aorta, and the interventricular septum fails to close at the top. Blood from both ventricles mixes in the truncus arteriosus and then enters the pulmonary and systemic circuits. **B,** Alterations of hemodynamics and oxygen saturation by persistent truncus arteriosus. *RA,* Right atrium; *LA,* left atrium; *RV,* right ventricle; *LV,* left ventricle. (**A** from Hockenberry MJ et al: *Wong's nursing care of infants and children,* ed 7, St Louis, 2003, Mosby.)

bronchial arteries arising from the descending aorta to supply the lungs.[3]

PATHOPHYSIOLOGY   Blood flow from both the right and left ventricles is pumped into the main truncus, resulting in mixing of the pulmonary and systemic circulations (see Figure 31-19, *B*). The differential flow out to either the pulmonary bed or the systemic circulation depends on the pulmonary and systemic vascular resistances. Generally the pulmonary vascular resistance is less than the systemic vascular resistance, resulting in the majority of blood flow traveling to the lungs. This may be altered, however, because of pulmonary stenosis, small pulmonary arteries, or increased pulmonary vascular resistance. Pulmonary vascular disease develops early with this defect because of increased pulmonary blood flow.

CLINICAL MANIFESTATIONS   Physical findings depend on the amount of pulmonary blood flow and the presence of other cardiac anomalies. If pulmonary stenosis is present, the newborn will present with cyanosis, caused by already elevated pulmonary vascular resistance, but no CHF. Conversely, if pulmonary stenosis is not present, the newborn initially will have mild to moderate cyanosis that worsens with activity. Once pulmonary vascular resistance drops, the pulmonary bed will receive preferential flow and the infant will have signs of CHF. A wide pulse pressure with bounding pulses also may be present, caused by increased pulmonary

blood flow. A harsh systolic regurgitant murmur is present along the left sternal border as a result of the VSD, and a systolic click at the apex and left upper sternal border may be present, reflecting opening of the truncal valve. An apical rumble with or without a gallop rhythm also may be present because of increased pulmonary blood flow. If truncal valve insufficiency exists, an early diastolic, high-pitched, decrescendo murmur may be present.

EVALUATION AND TREATMENT   An ECG generally reveals biventricular hypertrophy and occasionally LA hypertrophy. A chest roentgenogram reveals cardiomegaly with biventricular and LA enlargement, as well as increased pulmonary vascular markings. When pulmonary stenosis is present, the heart size is normal and the pulmonary vascular markings are decreased. Echocardiography and cardiac catheterization determine the type of truncal defect, competency of the truncal valve, and differential blood flow.

Surgical repair in early infancy is recommended to prevent the sequelae of severe CHF and pulmonary vascular disease. The definitive repair consists of a modified Rastelli procedure involving VSD patch closure to divert the blood flow from the LV outflow tract into the truncus. The pulmonary arteries are excised from the aorta and connected to the right ventricle through a valved homograft—namely, aortic and pulmonary artery segments or cadaver tissue that is specially preserved. Synthetic conduits may be used but tend to calcify and develop narrowing within the lumen, leading to obstruction and the need for early replacement. Mortality varies depending on the type of truncal anomaly (20% to 50%).[20] Postoperative complications include heart failure, residual VSD, dysrhythmias, and pulmonary hypertension. The right ventricle to pulmonary artery homograft requires replacement because it becomes inadequate for somatic growth.

ACQUIRED CARDIOVASCULAR DISORDERS

Acquired heart diseases are those disease processes or abnormalities that occur after birth. They result from various causes, such as infection, genetic disorders, autoimmune processes in response to infection, environment factors, or autoimmune diseases. Examples of acquired heart diseases include Kawasaki disease, myocarditis, rheumatic heart disease, cardiomyopathy, and systemic hypertension. This chapter discusses Kawasaki disease and systemic hypertension. Myocarditis, rheumatic heart disease, and cardiomyopathy are discussed in Chapter 30.

Kawasaki Disease

Kawasaki disease, otherwise known as mucocutaneous lymph node syndrome, is an acute, self-limiting systemic vasculitis that may result in cardiac sequelae. It was first described in 1967 by Dr. Thomisakyu Kawasaki. Although Kawasaki disease occurs throughout the world, the greatest number of cases are reported in Japan.[44]

Kawasaki disease is primarily a condition of young children. Eighty percent of cases are seen in children younger than 5 years of age, with the incidence peaking in the toddler age group. Males are affected slightly more than females. Its peak incidence is in winter and spring.[3,46]

The etiology of Kawasaki disease remains unknown. Current etiologic theories center on an immunologic response to an infectious, toxic, or antigenic substance (including superantigen).[3,48,49]

PATHOPHYSIOLOGY   Kawasaki disease progresses pathologically and clinically in the following stages:

Stage I (days 0 to 12): Small capillaries, arterioles, and venules become inflamed, as does the heart itself.

Stage II (days 12 to 25): Inflammation spreads to larger vessels, and aneurysms of the coronary arteries develop.

Stage III (days 26 to 40): Medium-size arteries begin granulation process, causing coronary artery thickening; inflammation resolves in the microcirculation; and there is increased formation of thrombi.

Stage IV (day 40 and beyond): Vessels develop scarring, intimal thickening, calcification, and stenosis of coronary arteries.

CLINICAL MANIFESTATIONS   The clinical course of the disease progresses in three stages: acute, subacute, and convalescent. In the acute phase the child has fever, conjunc-

tivitis, oral changes ("strawberry" tongue), rash, and lymphadenopathy and is often irritable. During this phase, myocarditis may develop. The subacute phase begins when the fever ends and continues until the clinical signs have resolved. It is at this time that the child is most at risk for coronary artery aneurysm development. Desquamation of the palms and soles occurs at this time, as well as marked thrombocytosis. The convalescent phase is marked by the continued elevation of the erythrocyte sedimentation rate and platelet count.[3,46] Arthritis still may be present. This phase continues until all laboratory values return to normal—usually about 6 to 8 weeks after onset.[3,4]

EVALUATION AND TREATMENT   The diagnosis is based on the diagnosis criteria for Kawasaki disease, which state that the child must exhibit five of six criteria, including fever (Box 31-3). These children usually have leukocytosis, increased erythrocyte sedimentation rates, marked thrombocytosis, and elevated liver enzymes. An echocardiogram is obtained at the time of diagnosis as a baseline to assess for coronary aneurysms or inflammation. Serial echocardiograms are obtained after treatment to assess for future development of coronary aneurysms.

The use of high-dose aspirin and intravenous immunoglobulin during the acute phase has decreased the mortality of Kawasaki disease and has reduced the incidence of coronary abnormalities from approximately 65% to less than 25% at 6 to 8 weeks after initiation of therapy.[48] Most children recover completely from Kawasaki disease, including the regression of aneurysms. The most common cardiovascular sequela is coronary thrombosis. Current studies are investigating long-term results of the disease.[47-49]

Systemic Hypertension

Hypertension (HTN) in children differs from adult hypertension in etiology and presentation. Children diagnosed with HTN are often found to have some underlying disease, such

---

Box 31-3	Diagnostic Criteria for Kawasaki Disease

The child must exhibit five of the following six criteria, including fever:

1. Fever for 5 or more days (often diagnosed with shorter duration of fever if other symptoms are present)
2. Bilateral conjunctival infection without exudation
3. Changes in the oral mucous membranes, such as erythema, dryness, and fissuring of the lips; oropharyngeal reddening; or "strawberry tongue"
4. Changes in the extremities, such as peripheral edema, peripheral erythema, and desquamation of palms and soles, particularly periungual peeling
5. Polymorphous rash, often accentuated in the perineal area
6. Cervical lymphadenopathy

Modified from Hockenberry MJ et al: *Wong's nursing care of infants and children,* ed 7, St Louis, 2003, Mosby.

Box 31-4	Conditions Associated with Secondary Hypertension in Children

Renal Disorders
Congenital defects
  Polycystic kidney, ectopic kidney, horseshoe kidney, etc.
  Obstructive anomalies
  Hydronephrosis
Renal tumor
  Wilms tumor
  Retrovascular
Abnormalities of renal arteries
Renal vein thrombosis
Acquired disorders
  Glomerulonephritis—acute or chronic
  Pyelonephritis
  Nephritis associated with collagen disease

Cardiovascular Disease
Coarctation of the aorta
Arteriovenous fistulae
Patent ductus arteriosus
Aortic or mitral insufficiency

Metabolic and Endocrine Diseases
Adrenal tumors
  Adenoma
  Pheochromocytoma
  Neuroblastoma

Cushing syndrome
Adrenogenital syndrome
Hyperthyroidism
Aldosteronism
Hypercalcemia
Diabetes mellitus

Neurologic Disorders
Space-occupying lesions of cranium (increased intracranial pressure)
  Tumors, cysts, hematoma
  Cerebral edema
  Encephalitis (including Guillain-Barré and Reye syndromes)

Miscellaneous Causes
Drugs (corticosteroids, oral contraceptives, pressor agents, amphetamines)
Burns
Genitourinary surgery
Trauma (e.g., stretching of femoral nerve with leg traction)
Insect bites (e.g., scorpion)
Intravascular overload (blood, fluid)
Hypernatremia
Toxemia of pregnancy
Heavy metal poisoning

From Hockenberry MJ et al: *Wong's nursing care of infants and children*, ed 7, St Louis, 2003, Mosby.

as renal disease or coarctation of the aorta (Box 31-4). In recent years an increased prevalence of primary HTN in older children has been noted. Researchers are now focusing on primary HTN in older children in relation to morbidity and mortality and the presence of early atherosclerotic disease.[3,31]

Systemic hypertension in children is defined as systolic and diastolic blood pressure levels greater than the ninety-fifth percentile for age and gender on at least three occasions.[3,28] The Second Task Force on Blood Pressure Control in Children has added height as an additional criterion to the blood pressure guide.[45]

PATHOPHYSIOLOGY   Hypertension is classified as (1) primary (or essential) hypertension, in which a specific cause cannot be identified; or (2) secondary hypertension, in which a cause is secondary to another alteration (see Box 31-4).[3] In infants and children a cause of HTN is almost always found. In general, the younger the child with significant hypertension, the more likely that a correctable cause can be found. Therefore a thorough evaluation needs to be done.[50-53]

The pathophysiology of primary HTN in children is not clearly understood but may result from a complex interaction of a strong disposing genetic component with disturbances in sympathetic vascular smooth muscle tone, humoral agents (angiotensin, catecholamines), renal sodium excretion, and cardiac output (Figure 31-20). Ultimately these factors impair the ability of the peripheral vascular bed to adjust its own resistance to meet tissue perfusion needs.

CLINICAL MANIFESTATIONS   Most children with systemic HTN are asymptomatic. It is necessary that a thorough history and physical examination be obtained. The examination should include an accurate blood pressure measurement on three separate occasions using a cuff of appropriate size[3,50,54] (Tables 31-7 and 31-8).

Certain factors influence blood pressure in children. Children who are overweight are often hypertensive.[52] Smoking is also associated with an increased risk for HTN. The gender or race of the child has not been an associated risk factor for primary HTN.[50,54] Recent data suggests that elevation of serum uric acid is related to the onset of essential hypertension in children (see What's New? Uric Acid and Childhood Hypertension). In addition, researchers have concluded that normalization of uric acid may improve new onset of essential hypertension.[55]

EVALUATION AND TREATMENT   In children the history and physical examination should be directed at determining the etiology of HTN, such as coarctation of the aorta or renal disease (Table 31-9). If coarctation of the aorta is found, surgical or interventional correction is initiated. A complete blood count, serum chemistry levels, urinalysis, urine culture, lipid profile, and renal ultrasound are part of the routine evaluation for renal disease (Table 31-10). If HTN is found to be essential, or primary, in nature, nonpharmacologic therapy is used initially. Moderate weight loss can decrease systolic and diastolic pressures in many children. Appropriate diet, regular physical activity, and avoidance of smoking have been shown to be effective in reducing blood pressure.[3,50,54]

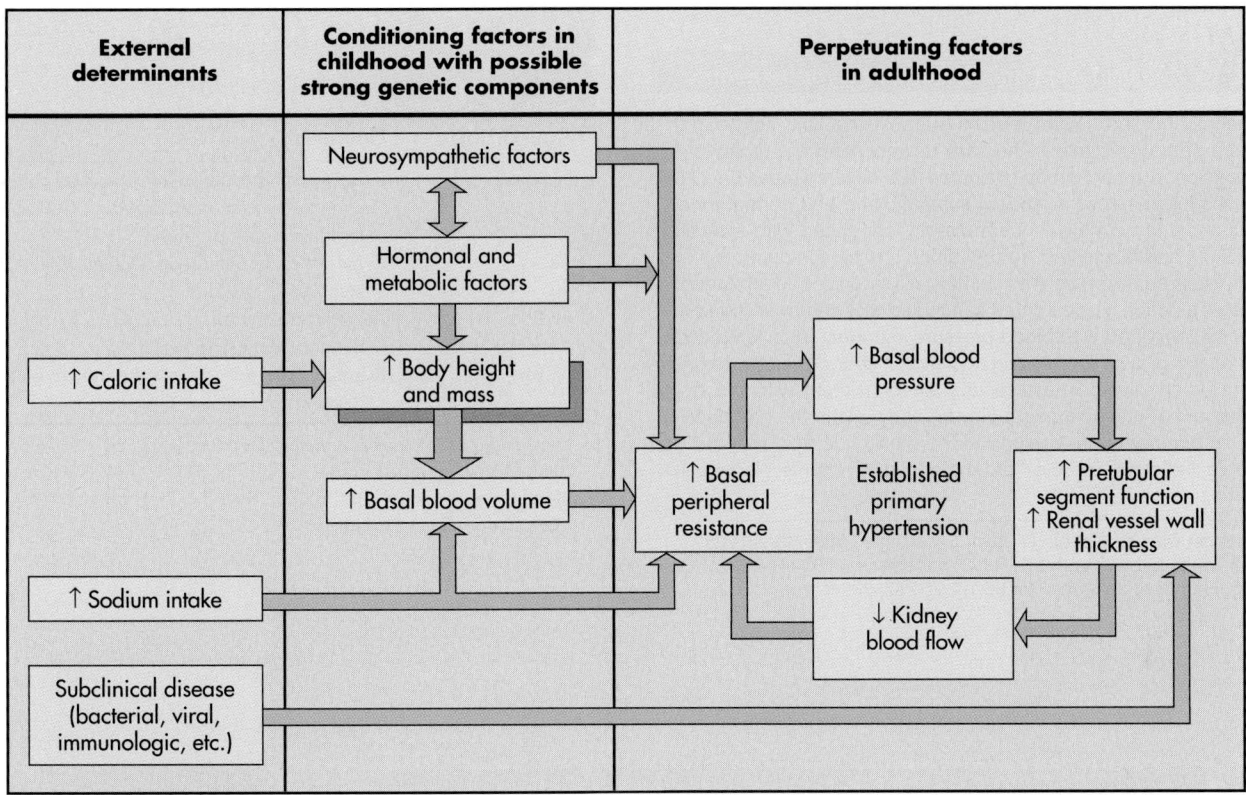

Figure 31-20 Mechanisms believed to influence blood pressure in children. According to this model, a critical factor in the development of hypertension is obesity during childhood. Increased body mass, coupled with excessive sodium intake, can cause primary hypertension in children or set the stage for its development later in life.

Table 31-7	Suggested Normal BP Values (mmHg) by Ausculatory Method (Systolic/Diastolic K5)		
Age (yrs)	Mean BP Levels	90th Percentile	95th Percentile
6-7	104/55	114/73	117/78
8-9	106/58	117/76	120/82
11-11*	108/60	120/77	124/82
12-13*	112/62	124/78	128/83
14-15			
Boys	116/66	132/80	138/86
Girls	112/68	126/80	130/83
16-18			
Boys	121/70	136/82	140/86
Girls	110/68	125/81	127/84

From Park MK: *Pediatric cardiology for practitioners,* ed 4, St. Louis, 2002, Mosby; modified from Goldring D et al: *Journal of Pediatrics* 91:884, 1977; Prineas RJ et al: *Hypertension* 1 (suppl):18, 1980.
BP, Blood pressure; *K5,* phase V of Korotkoff sound.
*Values for ages 10-13 yr have been extrapolated from these two studies using age-related increments from other studies.

Table 31-8	Normative BP Levels (Systolic/Diastolic [Mean]) by Dinamap Monitor in Children 5 Years Old and Younger		
Age	Mean BP Levels (in mmHg)	90th Percentile	95th Percentile
1-3 days	64/41 (50)	75/49 (50)	78/52 (62)
1 mo-2 yr	95/58 (72)	106/68 (83)	110/71 (86)
2-5 yr	101/57 (74)	112/66 (82)	115/68 (85)

From Park MK: *Pediatric cardiology for practitioners,* ed 4, St. Louis, 2002, Mosby; modified from Park MK, Menard SM: *American Journal of Diseases in Children* 143:860, 1989.
BP, Blood pressure.

Drug therapy is controversial in children with primary hypertension; however, when nonpharmacologic therapy fails, a staged approach with the use of diuretics and/or beta-blockers and vasodilators is indicated.[3,51-53] The current emphasis on preventive cardiology, especially for children, is significant because many investigators believe signs of atherosclerosis are present from childhood.[53]

Childhood Obesity

Childhood obesity is now considered an epidemic in not only the United States but also in other countries such as Australia.[56] Despite attention from U.S. federal and state initiatives, the prevalence of obesity in children and young adults has steadily increase over the last four decades with estimates as high as 16% of children considered obese.[57-60] Percentile of Body Mass Index (BMI), expressed as weight/height^2 (BMI; kg/m^2), is used

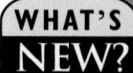

WHAT'S NEW? Uric Acid and Childhood Hypertension

Experimental and animal models suggest that uric acid might have a pathogenic role in the early development of primary hypertension. A recent study evaluated 125 children (ages 6 to 18 yrs; $\bar{X}$ 13.4 [mean of a random sample]) who had normal renal function. Uric acid levels were directly correlated with systolic (r = 0.80) and diastolic (r = 0.66) blood pressure in controls and in children/adolescents with primary hypertension independent of renal function. Researchers concluded that serum uric acid is directly correlated with blood pressure in untreated children and that a level of >5.5 mg/dl in an adolescent strongly suggests primary hypertension. These results are consistent with the hypothesis that uric acid might play an early role in the pathogenesis of primary hypertension. Furthermore, uric acid may be a reliable indicator for the "pre-metabolic syndrome" in obese youths.

Data from Denzer C et al: *J Pediatr Endocrinol Metab* 16(9):1225-1232, 2003; Feig DI, Johnson RJ: *Hypertension* 42(3):247-252, 2003; Feig DI et al: *Kidney Int* 66(1):281-287, 2004.

Table 31-9	Most Common Causes of Chronic Sustained Hypertension
Age-Group	**Causes**
Newborn	Renal artery thrombosis, renal artery stenosis, congenital renal malformation, COA, bronchopulmonary dysplasia
<6 yr	Renal parenchymal disease, COA, renal artery stenosis
6-10 yr	Renal artery stenosis, renal parenchymal disease, primary hypertension
>10 yr	Primary hypertension, renal parenchymal disease

From Park MK: *Pediatric cardiology for practitioners*, ed 4, St Louis, 2002, Mosby; modified from Report of the Second Task Force on Blood Pressure Control in Children. *Pediatrics* 79:1, 1987.
COA, Coarctation of the aorta.

Table 31-10	Routine and Special Laboratory Tests for Hypertension
Laboratory Tests	**Significance of Abnormal Results**
Urinalysis, urine culture, blood urea nitrogen, and creatinine levels	Renal parenchymal disease
Serum electrolyte levels (hypokalemia)	Hyperaldosteronism, primary or secondary
	Adrenogenital syndrome
	Renin-producing tumors
Serum uric acid level	Elevations associated with systolic and diastolic levels and premetabolic syndrome
ECG, chest roentgenogram	Cardiac cause of hypertension, also baseline function
Intravenous pyelography (or ultrasonography, radionuclide studies, computed tomography of the kidney)	Renal parenchymal disease
	Renovascular hypertension
	Tumors (neuroblastoma, Wilms tumor)
Plasma renin activity, peripheral	High-renin hypertension
	Renovascular hypertension
	Renin-producing tumors
	Some caused by Cushing syndrome
	Some caused by essential hypertension
	Low-renin hypertension
	Adrenogenital syndrome
	Primary hyperaldosteronism
24-hour urine collection for 17-ketosteroids and 17-hydroxycorticosteroids	Cushing syndrome
	Adrenogenital syndrome
24-hour urine collection for catecholamine levels and vanillylmandelic acid	Pheochromocytoma
	Neuroblastoma
Aldosterone	Hyperaldosteronism, primary or secondary
	Renovascular hypertension
	Renin-producing tumors
Renal vein plasma renin activity	Unilateral renal parenchymal disease
	Renovascular hypertension
Abdominal aortogram	Renovascular hypertension
	Abdominal COA
	Unilateral renal parenchymal diseases
	Pheochromocytoma

Adapted from Park MK: *Pediatric cardiology for practitioners*, ed 4, St Louis, 2002, Mosby.
ECG, Electrocardiogram; *COA,* coarctation of the aorta.

to identify overweight and obesity in children and adolescents. The Centers for Disease Control (CDC), the supplier of national growth charts and prevalence data, avoids characterizing children and adolescents as "obese;" instead, the CDC suggests two levels of overweight: (1) the 85th percentile, an "at risk" level; and (2) the 95th percentile, the more severe level.[61]

Causes of obesity in young children and adolescents are multivariable and multidimensional. Risk factors associated with developing childhood obesity include race, socioeconomic status, and lack of health insurance. Children of black and Hispanic race are at higher risk, as well as children with no insurance.[57] The presence of parental obesity also is associated with childhood obesity.[62] In addition, early childhood nutrition, level of physical activity, and engagement of sedentary activities, such as watching television and computer use, is associated with the development of overweight and obese children.[63-65]

Similar to obese adults, overweight and obese children are at risk for acquiring numerous other serious and potentially life-threatening illnesses such as asthma, sleep apnea, hypertension, type 2 diabetes, dyslipidemia, and cardiovascular disease.[66-68] Researchers also have reported a multitude of social and economic consequences in adolescents as a result of being overweight. Overweight adolescents were more likely to complete fewer years of education, are less likely to marry, and have a lower household income in adulthood, independent of familial socioeconomic status.[69]

As in other acquired diseases, efforts should be focused on prevention. The initial approach is a combined program of physical activity with nutritional improvements.[70] Health care professionals play a vital role in recognizing the need for intervention, immediate referral, and support. Successful outcomes for most overweight and obese children require support, change in life-style at home, and involvement of family members.[71] Researchers are involving school-based programs in promoting and preventing obesity in the young.[72]

SUMMARY REVIEW

Development of the Cardiovascular System

1. The heart arises from the mesenchyme and begins as an enlarged blood vessel with a large lumen and a muscular wall. By approximately the eighth week of gestation, all structures of the fetal heart and vascular system are present.
2. The endocardial cushions are instrumental in closing the atrial septum, dividing the atrioventricular canals into the right and left atrioventricular orifices, and closing the septum.
3. In the fetus the pulmonary and systemic circulatory systems are connected by the foramen ovale, an opening between the atria; by the ductus arteriosus, a fetal vessel that joins the pulmonary artery to the aorta; and by the ductus venosus, a fetal vessel that connects the inferior vena cava to the umbilical vein.
4. Fetal circulation is different from postnatal circulation because of the presence of fetal shunts and altered metabolic needs of the various organs.
5. Fetal blood flow depends on resistance for its distribution through the body. Resistance in the pulmonary circulation is higher than resistance in the systemic circulation, so myocardial thickness is about the same in the right heart and the left heart.
6. After birth, systemic resistance increases and pulmonary resistance decreases.
7. Pulmonary vascular resistance drops suddenly at birth because the lungs expand and the pulmonary vessels dilate. It continues to decrease gradually during the first 6 to 8 weeks after birth. Decreased resistance causes the right myocardium to thin out.
8. Systemic vascular resistance increases markedly at birth because severance of the umbilical cord removes the low-resistance placenta from the systemic circulation. Increased systemic resistance causes the left myocardium to thicken.
9. Changes in resistance cause the fetal connections between the pulmonary and systemic circulatory systems to disappear. The foramen ovale closes functionally at birth and anatomically several months later; the ductus arteriosus closes functionally 15 to 18 hours after birth and anatomically within 10 to 21 days; and the ductus venosus closes within 1 week after birth.
10. At birth a series of circulatory changes occur that affect blood flow, vascular resistance, and oxygen tension. The most important change is the shift of gas exchange from the placenta to the lungs.
11. After birth, significant postnatal changes occur, including thinning of the right ventricular myocardium as the pulmonary vascular resistance drops. As the systemic vascular resistance increases, the left ventricular myocardium becomes thicker.

Congenital Heart Defects

1. Most congenital cardiovascular defects have begun to develop by the eighth week of gestation, and most have many causes, both environmental and genetic.
2. Environmental risk factors associated with the incidence of congenital heart defects typically are maternal conditions. Among these are viral infections, diabetes, drug intake, alcohol intake, metabolic disorders, and advanced maternal age.
3. Genetic factors associated with congenital heart defects include but are not limited to Down syndrome, trisomy 13, trisomy 18, cri du chat syndrome, and Turner syndrome. It now appears, however, that most genetic mechanisms of causation are multifactorial.
4. Classification of congenital heart defects is based on whether they (a) cause blood flow to the lungs to increase or decrease, (b) obstruct ventricular blood flow patterns, or (c) cause mixing of unoxygenated and oxygenated blood.
5. Congestive heart failure is usually the result of congenital heart defects that increase blood volume and pressure in the pulmonary circulation. Clinical manifestations are almost the same as the manifestations of congestive heart failure in adults. Unique manifestations in children include failure to thrive and periorbital edema.
6. Cyanosis, a bluish discoloration of the skin, indicates that the tissues are not receiving adequate oxygenated blood. Cyanosis can be caused by defects that (a) restrict blood flow into the pulmonary circulation; (b) overload the pulmonary circulation, causing pulmonary hypertension, pulmonary edema, and respiratory difficulty; and (c) cause large amounts of unoxygenated blood to shunt from the pulmonary to the systemic circulation.
7. Congenital defects that maintain or create direct communication between the pulmonary and systemic circulatory systems cause blood to shunt from one system to another, mixing oxy-

Continued

SUMMARY REVIEW—cont'd

genated and unoxygenated blood and increasing blood volume and pressure on the receiving side of the shunt.

8. The direction of shunting through an abnormal communication depends on differences in pressure and resistance between the two systems. Flow is always from an area of high pressure to an area of low pressure.

9. Acyanotic congenital defects that increase pulmonary blood flow consist of abnormal openings (patent ductus arteriosus, atrial septal defect, ventricular septal defect, atrioventricular canal defect, or truncus arteriosus) that permit blood to shunt from left (systemic circulation) to right (pulmonary circulation). Cyanosis does not occur because the left-to-right shunt does not interfere with the flow of oxygenated blood through the systemic circulation.

10. If the abnormal communication between the left and right circuits is large, volume and pressure overload in the pulmonary circulation leads to congestive heart failure.

11. In truncus arteriosus the main trunk fails to divide longitudinally into the aorta and pulmonary artery. All blood from both ventricles enters the truncus, so that mixed blood is delivered by both circulatory systems, causing cyanosis and CHF.

12. In heart defects that decrease pulmonary blood flow (tetralogy of Fallot, tricuspid atresia), myocardial hypertrophy cannot compensate for restricted right ventricular outflow. Flow to the lungs decreases, and cyanosis is caused by an insufficient volume of oxygenated blood.

13. Obstruction of ventricular outflow commonly is caused by pulmonary stenosis, aortic stenosis, coarctation of the aorta, interrupted aortic arch, or hypoplastic left heart syndrome.

14. Despite obstruction, ventricular outflow remains normal because of compensatory ventricular hypertrophy stimulated by increased afterload and, in postductal coarctation of the aorta, development of collateral circulation around the coarctation.

15. Left heart failure can develop as a result of right ventricular obstruction if afterload backs up into the pulmonary circulation. Congestive heart failure can result from left ventricular obstruction in preductal coarctation of the aorta, in which left-to-right shunting through the patent ductus arteriosus greatly increases blood flow into the pulmonary circulation.

16. Complex congenital defects that depend on mixing of the pulmonary and systemic circulations for survival during the postnatal period include complete transposition of the great arteries, total anomalous pulmonary venous connection, and double-outlet right ventricle. This mixing results in desaturated systemic blood flow and cyanosis.

17. In complete transposition of the great vessels, the circulatory systems are not connected serially or through a shunt, so that oxygenated blood remains permanently in the pulmonary circulation and unoxygenated blood remains permanently in the systemic circulation. Survival depends on patency of the ductus arteriosus; after that, surgical intervention is mandatory.

18. Total anomalous pulmonary venous connection is caused by the persistence of the fetal common pulmonary artery and the lack of pulmonary venous return to the left atrium. All blood from the pulmonary and systemic circulations enters the right atrium. Mixed blood enters the left atrium through an atrial septal defect; it then flows into the systemic circulation and causes cyanosis. Obstruction in the common pulmonary vein causes pressure to back up into the lungs, leading to congestive heart failure.

19. Treatment for all congenital defects is surgical correction of the anomaly and management of cyanosis and left heart failure.

Acquired Cardiovascular Disorders

1. The most common acquired cardiovascular disorders of childhood are Kawasaki disease, rheumatic heart disease, and hypertension.

2. Kawasaki disease is an acute systemic vasculitis that also may result in the development of coronary artery aneurysms and thrombosis.

3. Primary hypertension in children is the same as that in adults, except that it is more likely to be in an early, asymptomatic stage.

4. Obesity in childhood is an epidemic in the United States and other countries.

5. Obese children are at risk for acquiring numerous other serious and potentially life-threatening illnesses, such as asthma, sleep apnea, hypertension, type 2 diabetes mellitus, and cardiovascular disease.

KEY TERMS

Aortic stenosis, 1166
Atrial septal defect (ASD), 1157
Atrioventricular canal (AVC) defect, 1160
Bulbus cordis, 1149
Coarctation of the aorta (COA), 1164
Complete AVC (CAVC) defect, 1160
Conus, 1169
Cyanosis, 1155
Ductus arteriosus, 1149
Eisenmenger syndrome, 1155
Endocardial cushion, 1147
Foramen ovale, 1148

Hypoplastic left heart syndrome (HLHS), 1168
Kawasaki disease, 1173
Ligamentum venosum, 1150
Ostium primum, 1148
Ostium secundum, 1148
Partial AVC (PAVC) defect, 1160
Patent ductus arteriosus (PDA), 1156
Pulmonary atresia, 1167
Pulmonary stenosis, 1167
Septum primum, 1147
Septum secundum, 1147

Systemic hypertension, 1174
Tetralogy of Fallot, 1161
Total anomalous pulmonary venous connection (TAPVC), 1170
Transitional AVC (TAVC) defect, 1160
Transposition of the great arteries (TGA), 1169
Tricuspid atresia, 1163
Truncus arteriosus, 1171
Ventricular septal defect (VSD), 1158

REFERENCES

1. Clark EB, Nakazawa M, Takao A, editors: *Etiology and morphogenesis of congenital heart disease: twenty years of progress in genetics and developmental biology,* Mount Kisco, NY, 2000, Future Publishing Company.
2. Thompson J, Moore P, Teitel DF: Pulmonary venous wedge pressures accurately predict pulmonary arterial pressures in children with single ventricle physiology, *Pediatr Cardiol* 24(6):531-537, 2003.
3. Park MK: *Pediatric cardiology for practitioners,* ed 4, St Louis, 2002, Mosby.
4. Hockenberry MJ: *Wong's nursing care of infants and children,* ed 7, St Louis, 2003, Mosby.
5. Hazinski MF: *Nursing care of the critically ill child,* ed 2, St Louis, 1991, Mosby.
6. Gelb DB: Genetic basis of congenital heart disease, *Curr Opin Cardiol* 19(2):110-115, 2004.
7. Yelbuz TM et al: Shortened outflow tract leads to altered cardiac looping after neural crest ablation, *Circulation* 106(4):504-510, 2002.
8. Moller JH, Neal WA: *Fetal, neonatal, and infant cardiac disease,* Norwalk, Conn, 1992, McGraw-Hill/Appleton & Lange.
9. Garson A et al: *The science and practice of pediatric cardiology,* ed 2, Baltimore, 1998, Williams & Wilkins.
10. LeBlanc JG et al: The evolution of ductus arteriosus treatment, *Int Surg* 85(1):1-5, 2000.
11. Hijazi ZM, Ruiz, CE, Hellenbrand WE: The Eighth Pediatric Interventional Cardiac Symposium (PICS-VIII) and Second Emerging New Technologies in Congenital Heart Surgery (ENTICHS-II), *Pediatr Cardiol* May 5, 2005. (Epub ahead of print: PMID:15868328, DOI: 10.1007/s00246-004-0951-7.)
12. Grifka RG: Transcatheter closure of the patent ductus arteriosus, *Catheter Cardiovasc Interv* 61(4):554-570, 2004.
13. Burke RP et al: Video-assisted throacoscopic surgery for patent ductus arteriosus in low birth weight neonates and infants, *Pediatrics* 104(2 Pt 1):227-230, 1999.
14. Hines MH et al: Video-assisted ductal ligation in premature infants. *Ann Thorac Surg* 76(5):1417-1420, 2003.
15. Villa E et al: Paediatric video-assisted thoracoscopic clipping of patent ductus arteriosus: experience in more than 700 cases, *Eur J Cardiothorac Surg* 25(3):387-393, 2004.
16. Bichell DP et al: Minimal access approach for the repair of atrial septal defect: the initial 135 patients, *Ann Thorac Surg* 70(1):115-118, 2000.
17. Moodie DS, Sterba R: Long-term outcomes excellent for atrial septal defect repair in adults, *Cleve Clin J Med* 67(8):591-597, 2000.
18. Preventza O et al: Late cardiac perforation following transcatheter atrial septal defect closure. *Ann Thorac Surg* 77(4):1435-1437, 2004.
19. Zanchetta M et al: Transcatheter atrial septal defect closure assisted by intracardiac echocardiography: 3-year follow-up, *J Interv Cardiol* 17(2):95-98, 2004.
20. Berger FM et al: Comparison of results and complications of surgical and Amplatzer device closure of atrial septal defects, *J Thorac Cardiovasc Surg* 118(4):674-678, 1999.
21. Cao Q et al: Transcatheter closure of multiple atrial septal defects. Initial results and value for two- and three-dimensional transoesophageal echocardiography, *Eur Heart J* 21(11):941-947, 2000.
22. Hausdorf GR et al: Transcatheter closure of atrial septal defect with a new flexible, self-centering device (the STARFlex Occluder), *Am J Cardiol* 84(9):1113-1116, 1999.
23. Pedra CA et al: Transcatheter closure of atrial septal defects using the Cardio-Seal implant, *Heart* 84(3):320-326, 2000.
24. Holtzer R et al: Device closure of muscular ventricular septal defects using the Amplatzer muscular ventricular septal defect occluder: immediate and mid-term results of a U.S. registry, *J Am Coll Cardiol* 43(7):1257-1263, 2004.
25. Holtzer R, Hijazi ZM: Interventional approach to congenital heart disease, *Curr Opin Cardiol* 19(2):84-90, 2004.
26. El-Najdawi EK et al: Operation for partial atrioventricular septal defect: a forty-year review, *J Thorac Cardiovasc Surg* 119(5):880-889, 2000.
27. Fukuda T et al: Complete atrioventricular septal defect and Ebstein's anomaly, *Pediatr Cardiol* 20(3):232-235, 1999.
28. Allen HD et al, editors: *Moss and Adams' heart disease in infants, children and adolescents,* ed 6, Baltimore, 2001, Williams & Wilkins.
29. Castaneda AR et al: *Cardiac surgery of the neonate and infant,* Philadelphia, 1994, Saunders.
30. Chang AC et al: *Pediatric cardiac intensive care,* Baltimore, 1998, Williams & Wilkins.
31. Mavroudis C, Backer CL, editors: *Pediatric cardiac surgery,* ed 3, St Louis, 2003, Mosby.
32. Fawzy MR et al: Long-term outcome (up to 15 years) of balloon angioplasty of discrete native coarctation of the aorta in adolescents and adults, *J Am Coll Cardiol* 43(6):1062-1067, 2004.
33. Walhout RJ et al: Comparison of surgical repair with balloon angioplasty for native coarctation in patients from 3 months to 16 years of age, *Eur J Cardiothorac Surg* 25(5):722-727, 2004.
34. Maheshwari S et al: Balloon angioplasty of postsurgical recoarctation in infants: the risk of restenosis and long-term follow-up, *J Am Coll Cardiol* 35(1):209-213, 2000.
35. Egito ES et al: Transvascular balloon dilation for neonatal critical aortic stenosis: early and midterm results, *J Am Coll Cardiol* 29(2):442-447, 1997.
36. Morgan-Hughes GJ et al: Dilation of the aorta in pure, severe, bicuspid aortic valve stenosis. *Am Heart J* 147(4):736-740, 2004.
37. Pearl JM et al: Risk of recoarctation should not be a deciding factor in the timing of coarctation repair. *Am J Cardiol* 93(6):803-805, 2004.
38. Ricci M: Repair of coarctation of the aorta, *J Thorac Cardiovasc Surg* 127(4):1224-1225, 2004.
39. Radtke WA: Vascular access and management of its complications, *Pediatr Cardiol* May 5, 2005. (Epub ahead of print, PMID:15868325.)
40. Hasaniya N et al: Outcome of aortic valve repair in children with congenital aortic valve insufficiency, *J Thorac Cardiovasc Surg* 127(4):970-974, 2004.
41. Hrasja V et al: Ross and Ross-Konno procedure in children and adolescents: mid-term results. *Eur J Cardiothorac Surg* 25(5):742-747, 2004.
42. Razzouk AJ et al: Transplantation as a primary treatment for hypoplastic left heart syndrome: intermediate-term results, *Ann Thorac Surg* 62(1): 1-7, 1996.
43. Poon LK, Menahem S: Pulmonary regurgitation after percutaneous balloon valvoplasty for isolated pulmonary valvar stenosis in childhood, *Cardiol Young* 13(5):444-450, 2003.
44. Ikle L et al: Developmental outcome of patients with hypoplastic left heart syndrome treated with heart transplantation, *J Pediatr* 142(1):20-25, 2003.
45. Dibardino DJ et al: Current expectations for newborns undergoing the arterial switch operation. *Ann Surg* 239(5):588-598, 2004.
46. Bove EL: Surgical treatment for hypoplastic left heart syndrome, *Jpn J Thorac Cardiovasc Surg* 47(2):47-56, 1999.
47. Daebritz SH et al: Results of Norwood stage I operation: comparison of hypoplastic left heart syndrome with other malformations, *J Thorac Cardiovasc Surg* 119(2):358-367, 2000.
48. Boger AJ et al: Early results and long-term follow-up after corrective surgery for total anomalous pulmonary venous return, *Eur J Cardiothorac Surg* 16(3):269-269, 1999.
49. Gutgesell HP, Massaro TA: Management of hypoplastic left heart syndrome in a consortium of university hospitals, *Am J Cardiol* 76(11):809-811, 2000.
50. Jenkins PC et al: Morbidities in patients with hypoplastic left heart syndrome. *Pediatr Cardiol* 25(1):3-10, 2004.
51. Goldberg CS, Gomez CA: Hypoplastic left heart syndrome: new developments and current controversies, *Semin Neonatal* 8(6):461-468, 2003.
52. Seymour JJ, Dickinson ET: Delayed cardiovascular sequelae from Kawasaki syndrome, *Am J Emerg Med* 16(6):579-581, 1998.
53. Park AH et al: Patterns of Kawasaki syndrome presentation, *Int J Pediatr Otorhinolaryngol* 40(1):41-50, 1997.
54. Dajani AS et al: Prevention of bacterial endocarditis: recommendations by the American Heart Association [see comments], *Circulation* 96(1):358-366, 1997.
55. Feig DI et al: Hypothesis: uric acid, nephron number, and the pathogenesis of essential hypertension, *Kidney Int* 66(1):281-287, 2004.
56. Proietto J, Baur LA: Management of obesity, *Med J Aust* 180(9):747-780, 2004.

57. Haas, JS et al: The association of race, socioeconomic status, and health insurance status with the prevalence of overweight among children and adolescents, *Am J Public Health* 93(12):2105-2110, 2003.

58. Hedley AA et al: Prevalence of overweight and obesity in US children, adolescents, and adults, 1999-2002, *JAMA* 291(23):2847-2850, 2004.

59. Nesbitt SD et al: Overweight as a risk factor in children: a focus on ethnicity, *Ethn Dis* 14(1):94-100, 2004.

60. Strauss RS, Pollack HA: Epidemic increase in childhood overweight, 1986-1998, *JAMA* 286(22):2845-2848, 2001.

61. Kuczmarski RJ et al: CDC growth charts: United States, *Adv Data* (314):1-27, 2000.

62. Whitaker RC et al: Predicting obesity in young adulthood from childhood and parental obesity, *N Engl J Med* 337(13):869-873, 1997.

63. Crespo CJ et al: Television watching, energy intake, and obesity in US children: results from the third National Health and Nutrition Examination Study, 1988-1994, *Arch Pediatr Adolesc Med* 155(3):360-365, 2001.

64. Gordon-Larsen P, McMurray RG, Popkin BM: Adolescent physical activity and inactivity vary by ethnicity: The National Longitudinal Study of Adolescent Health, *J Pediatr* 135(3):301-306, 1999.

65. Kimm SY et al: Racial divergence in adiposity during adolescence: the NHLBI Growth and Health Study, *Pediatrics* 107(3):E34, 2001.

66. Daniels SR: Cardiovascular disease risk factors and atherosclerosis in children and adolescents, *Curr Atheroscler Rep* 3(6):479-485, 2001.

67. Davis SP et al: Assessing cardiovascular risk in children: the Jackson, Mississippi CRRIC Study, *J Cult Divers* 9(3):67-72, 2002.

68. Sharma AM: Obesity and cardiovascular risk, *Growth Horm IGF Res* 13(Suppl A):S10-17, 2003.

69. Lugwig DS, Gortmaker SL: Programming obesity in childhood, *Lancet* 364(9430):226-227, 2004.

70. Rome ES et al: Children and adolescents with eating disorders: the state of the art, *Pediatrics* 111(1):e98-108, 2003.

71. Wardle J: Parental influences on children's diets, *Proc Nutr Soc* 54(3):747-758, 1995.

72. Centers for Disease Control: Guidelines for school health programs to promote lifelong healthy eating: Centers for Disease Control, *MMWR Recomm Rep* 45(RR-9):1-41, 1996.

STRUCTURE AND FUNCTION OF THE PULMONARY SYSTEM

VALENTINA L. BRASHERS

CHAPTER

32

evolve

http://evolve.elsevier.com/McCance/

The pulmonary system consists of upper and lower airways, the chest wall, and pulmonary circulation. In addition, the respiratory center of the central nervous system and the phrenic nerve participate in pulmonary function by providing the neurochemical control of breathing. The primary function of the pulmonary system is the exchange of gases between the environmental air and the blood. There are three steps in this process: (1) ventilation, the movement of air into and out of the lungs; (2) diffusion, the movement of gases between air spaces in the lungs and the bloodstream; and (3) perfusion, the movement of blood into and out of the capillary beds of the lungs to body organs and tissues. The first two functions are carried out by the pulmonary system and the third by the cardiovascular system (see Chapter 29). Normally the pulmonary system functions efficiently under a variety of conditions and with little energy expenditure.

STRUCTURES OF THE PULMONARY SYSTEM

The pulmonary system is made up of the upper airways, two lungs, the lower airways, and the blood vessels that serve them (Figure 32-1) and the chest wall, or thoracic cage. The lungs are divided into lobes, three in the right lung (upper, middle, lower) and two in the left lung (upper, lower). Each lobe is further divided into segments and lobules. The space between the lungs, which contains the heart, great vessels, and esophagus, is called the *mediastinum*. A set of tubes, or conducting airways, delivers air to each section of the lung. The lung tissue that surrounds the airways supports them, preventing their distortion or collapse as gas moves in and out during ventilation.

The lungs are protected from a variety of exogenous contaminants by a series of mechanical barriers (Table 32-1). These defense mechanisms are so effective that, in the healthy individual, contamination of the lung tissue itself is unusual. (Other mechanisms of self-defense are discussed in Chapters 6 and 7.)

Conducting Airways

The conducting airways are the portion of the pulmonary system that provides a passage for the movement of air into and out of the gas-exchange portions of the lung. They consist of upper and lower airways. The **nasopharynx, oropharynx,** and related structures often are called the *upper airway* (Figure 32-2). These structures are lined with a ciliated mucosa with a very rich vascular supply. The mucosal lining warms and humidifies inspired air and removes foreign particles from it as it passes into the lungs. During quiet breathing, gas usually flows through the nose, nasopharynx, and oropharynx to the lower airways. The mouth and oropharynx provide for ventilation when the nose is obstructed or when increased flow is required, such as during exercise. Filtering and humidifying are not, however, as efficient with mouth breathing.

The **larynx** connects the upper and lower airways. The structure of the larynx consists of the endolarynx and its surrounding triangular-shaped bony and cartilaginous structures. The endolarynx is formed by two pairs of folds that form the false vocal cords (supraglottis) and the true vocal cords. The slit-shaped space between the true cords forms the

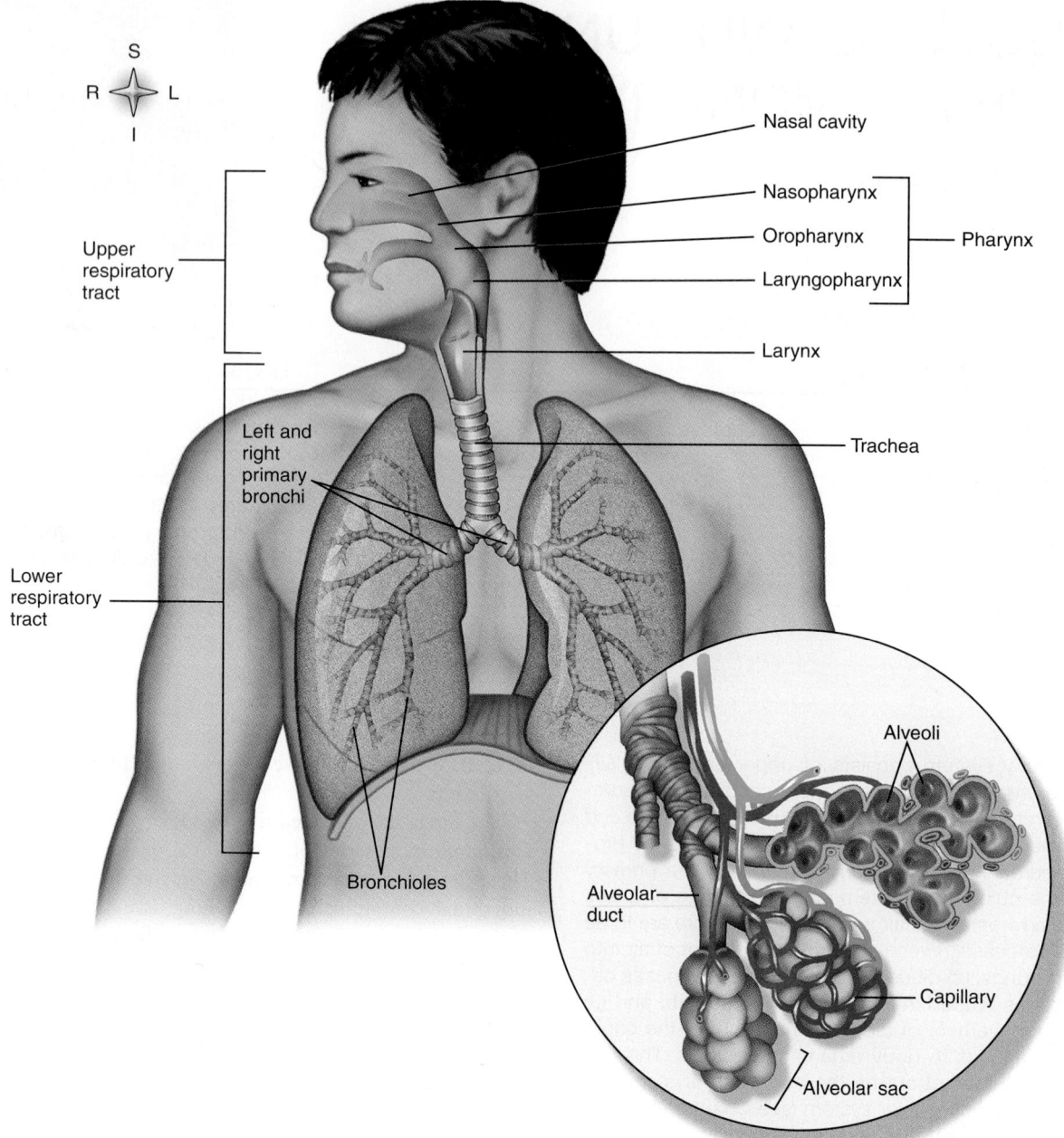

Figure 32-1 **Structural plan of the respiratory system.** *Inset* shows alveolar sacs where the interchange of oxygen and carbon dioxide takes place through the walls of the grapelike alveoli. Capillaries surround the alveoli. (From Thibodeau GA, Patton KT: *Anatomy & physiology*, ed 5, St Louis, 2003, Mosby.)

Table 32-1	Pulmonary Defense Mechanisms
Structure or Substance	**Mechanism of Defense**
Upper respiratory tract mucosa	Maintains constant temperature and humidification of gas entering the lungs; traps and removes foreign particles, some bacteria, and noxious gases from inspired air
Nasal hairs and turbinates	Trap and remove foreign particles, some bacteria, and noxious gases from inspired air
Mucous blanket	Protects trachea and bronchi from injury; traps most foreign particles and bacteria that reach the lower airways
Cilia	Propel mucous blanket and entrapped particles toward the oropharynx, where they can be swallowed or expectorated
Alveolar macrophages	Ingest and remove bacteria and other foreign material from alveoli by phagocytosis (see Chapters 7 and 8)
Irritant receptors in nares (nostrils)	Stimulation by chemical or mechanical irritants triggers sneeze reflex, which results in rapid removal of irritants from nasal passages
Irritant receptors in trachea and large airways	Stimulation by chemical or mechanical irritants triggers cough reflex, which results in removal of irritants from the trachea and large airways

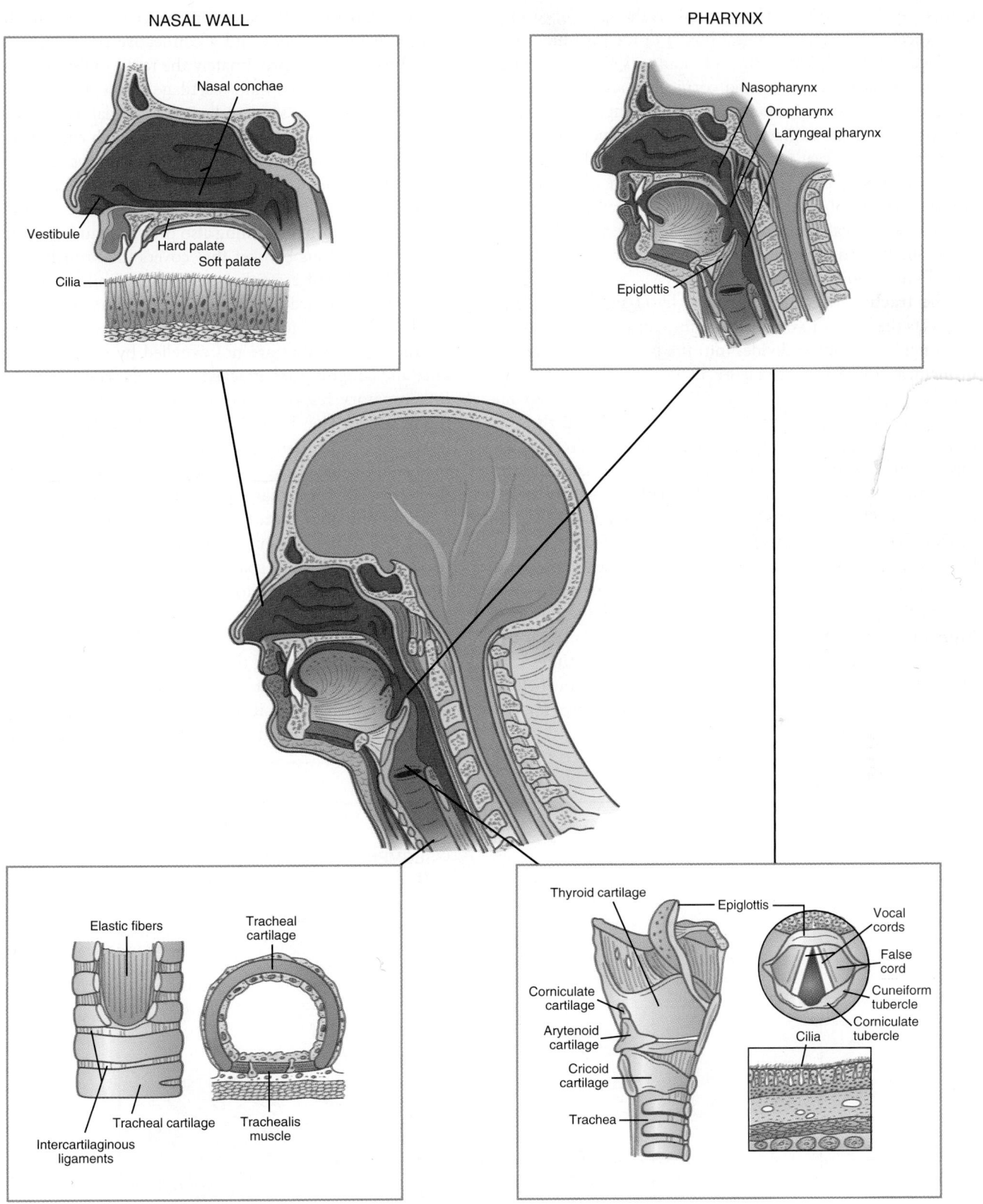

Figure 32-2 Structures of the upper airway. (Redrawn from Thompson JM et al: *Mosby's clinical nursing,* ed 5, St Louis, 2002, Mosby.)

glottis (see Figure 32-2). The vestibule is the space above the false vocal cords. The laryngeal box is formed of three large cartilages—the epiglottis, thyroid, and cricoid—and three smaller cartilages—the arytenoid, corniculate, and cuneiform—that are connected by ligaments. The supporting cartilages prevent collapse of the larynx during inspiration and swallowing. The internal laryngeal muscles control vocal cord length and tension, and the external laryngeal muscles move the larynx as a whole. Both sets of muscles are important to swallowing, respiration, and vocalization. The internal muscles contract during swallowing to prevent aspiration into the trachea and also contribute to voice pitch.

The **trachea,** which is supported by U-shaped cartilage, connects the larynx to the **bronchi,** the conducting airways of the lungs. The trachea divides into the two main airways, or bronchi, at the **carina** (see Figure 32-1). This area is very sensitive and when stimulated can cause coughing and airway narrowing. The right main bronchus extends from the trachea more vertically than the left main bronchus, so that aspirated fluids or foreign particles tend to enter the right lung rather than the left. The right and left main bronchi enter the lungs at the **hila,** or "roots" of the lungs, along with the pulmonary blood and lymphatic vessels. From the hila the main bronchi branch into lobar bronchi, then to segmental and subsegmental bronchi, and finally end at the sixteenth division in the smallest of the conducting airways, the terminal **bronchioles** (Figure 32-3). With these multiple divisions, the cross-sectional area of the airways increases to 20 times that of the trachea. This results in decreased velocity or airflow into the gas-exchange portion of the lung and allows for optimal gas diffusion.[1]

The bronchial walls have three layers: an epithelial lining, a smooth muscle layer, and a connective tissue layer. In the large bronchi (to approximately the tenth division), the connective tissue layer contains cartilage. The epithelial lining of the bronchi contains single-celled exocrine glands—the mucus-secreting **goblet cells**—and ciliated cells. High columnar pseudostratified epithelium lines the larger airways, changing to columnar cuboidal epithelium in the bronchioles (types of epithelium are illustrated in Chapter 1). The submucosal glands of the bronchial lining also produce mucus, contributing to the mucous blanket that covers the bronchial epithelium. The ciliated epithelial cells rhythmically beat this mucous blanket toward the trachea and pharynx, where it can be swallowed or expectorated by coughing. Foreign particles and microorganisms that are not expelled by mucociliary clearance and coughing are attacked by cellular components of the inflammatory response and antibodies of the secretory immune system (see Unit III). The biochemical mediators released early in inflammation also play a part in antibody-mediated hypersensitivity reactions, such as asthma, because they stimulate bronchial smooth muscles to constrict.

With branching, the layers of epithelium that line the bronchi become thinner (Figure 32-4). Ciliated cells and goblet cells become more sparse, and smooth muscle and connective tissue layers thin toward the terminal bronchioles.[2]

Gas-Exchange Airways

The conducting airways terminate in gas-exchange airways, where oxygen (O_2) enters the blood and carbon dioxide (CO_2) is removed from it. The gas-exchange airways are made up of **respiratory bronchioles, alveolar ducts,** and **alveoli.**

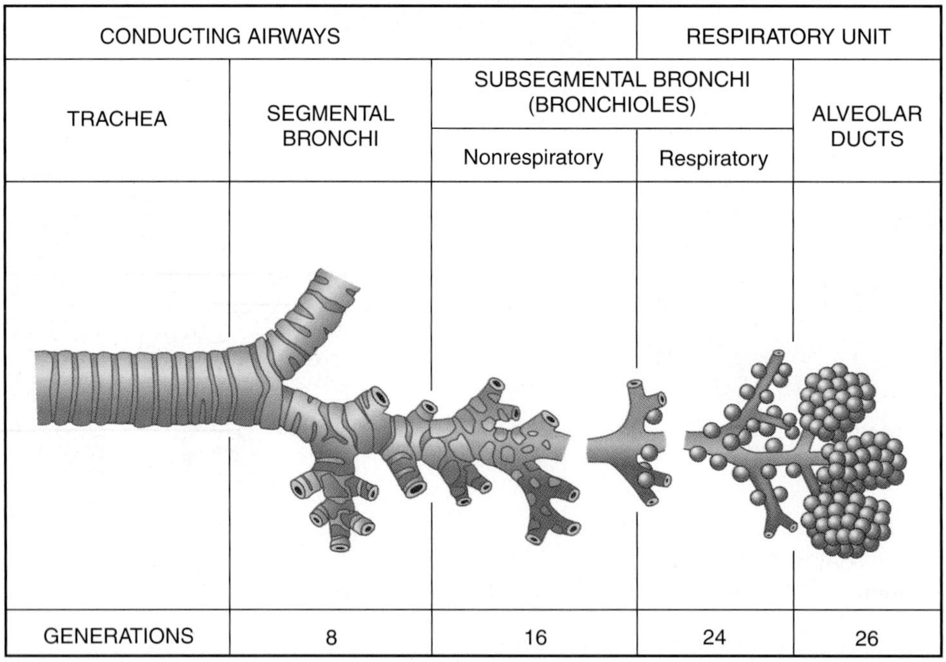

CONDUCTING AIRWAYS				RESPIRATORY UNIT
TRACHEA	SEGMENTAL BRONCHI	SUBSEGMENTAL BRONCHI (BRONCHIOLES)		ALVEOLAR DUCTS
		Nonrespiratory	Respiratory	
GENERATIONS	8	16	24	26

Figure 32-3 Structures of the lower airway. (Redrawn from Thompson JM et al: *Mosby's clinical nursing,* ed 5, St Louis, 2002, Mosby.)

Lower airways   **Cellular structures**

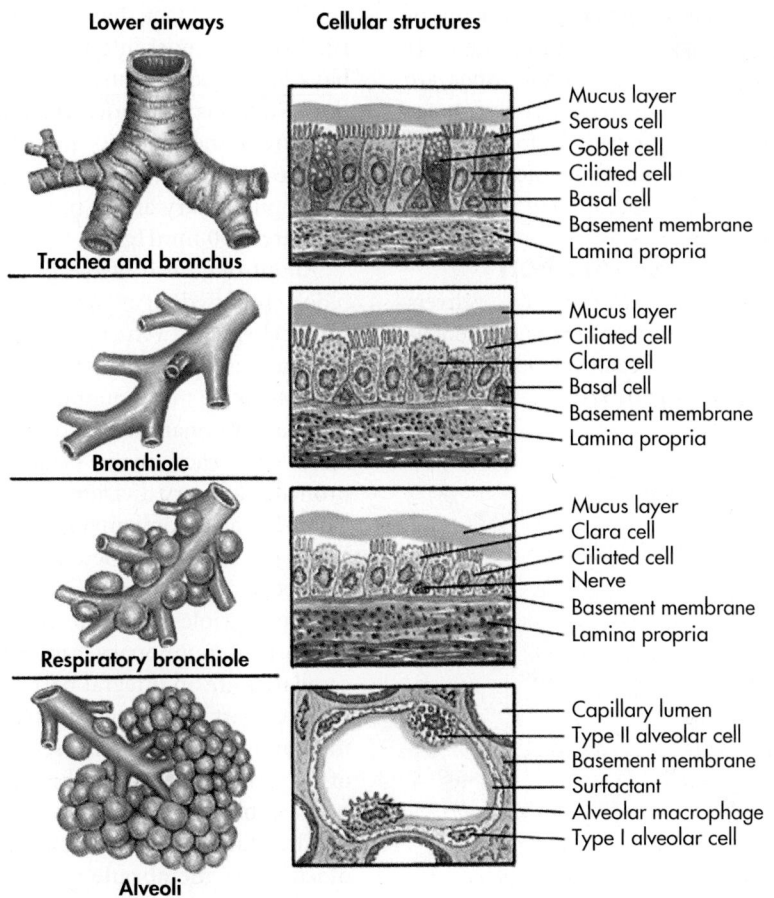

Trachea and bronchus
- Mucus layer
- Serous cell
- Goblet cell
- Ciliated cell
- Basal cell
- Basement membrane
- Lamina propria

Bronchiole
- Mucus layer
- Ciliated cell
- Clara cell
- Basal cell
- Basement membrane
- Lamina propria

Respiratory bronchiole
- Mucus layer
- Clara cell
- Ciliated cell
- Nerve
- Basement membrane
- Lamina propria

Alveoli
- Capillary lumen
- Type II alveolar cell
- Basement membrane
- Surfactant
- Alveolar macrophage
- Type I alveolar cell

Figure 32-4 Changes in the bronchial wall with progressive branching. (From Wilson SF, Thompson JM: *Respiratory disorders,* St Louis, 1990, Mosby.)

These structures together are sometimes called the **acinus** (see Figure 32-3), and all of them participate in gas exchange.

The bronchioles from the sixteenth through the twenty-third divisions contain increasing numbers of alveoli and are called *respiratory bronchioles.* The walls of the respiratory bronchioles are very thin, consisting of an epithelial layer devoid of cilia and goblet cells, very little smooth muscle fiber, and a very thin and elastic connective tissue layer. These bronchioles end in alveolar ducts, which lead to alveolar sacs made up of numerous alveoli.

The alveoli are the primary gas-exchange units of the lung, where oxygen enters the blood and carbon dioxide is removed (Figure 32-5). Tiny passages called *pores of Kohn* permit some air to pass through the septa from alveolus to alveolus, promoting collateral ventilation and even distribution of air among the alveoli. In cross sections, alveoli appear similar to common sponges. The lungs contain approximately 25 million alveoli at birth and 300 million by adulthood.

The alveolar septa consist of an epithelial layer and a thin, elastic basement membrane but no muscle layer (Figure 32-6). Two major types of epithelial cells appear in the alveolus. Type I alveolar cells provide structure, and type II alveolar cells secrete **surfactant,** a lipoprotein that coats the inner surface of the alveolus and facilitates its expansion during inspiration.[1]

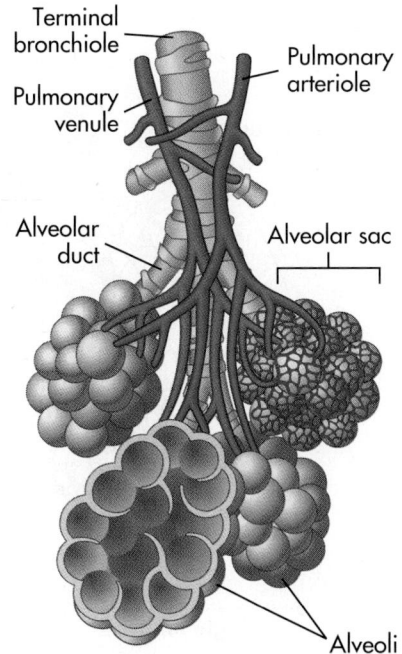

Terminal bronchiole
Pulmonary venule
Pulmonary arteriole
Alveolar duct
Alveolar sac
Alveoli

Figure 32-5 Alveoli. Bronchioles subdivide to form tiny tubes called *alveolar ducts,* which end in clusters of alveoli called *alveolar sacs.* (From Thibodeau GA, Patton KT: *Anatomy & physiology,* ed 5, St Louis, 2003, Mosby.)

Like the bronchi, alveoli contain cellular components of inflammation and immunity, particularly the mononuclear phagocytes. The mononuclear phagocytes of the lungs are called *alveolar macrophages.* These cells ingest foreign material that reaches the alveolus and prepare it for removal through the lymphatics. (Phagocytosis and the mononuclear phagocyte system are described in Chapters 6 and 7.)

Pulmonary and Bronchial Circulation

The pulmonary circulation facilitates gas exchange, delivers nutrients to lung tissues, acts as a reservoir for the left ventricle, and serves as a filtering system that removes clots, air, and other debris from the circulation (Figure 32-7).

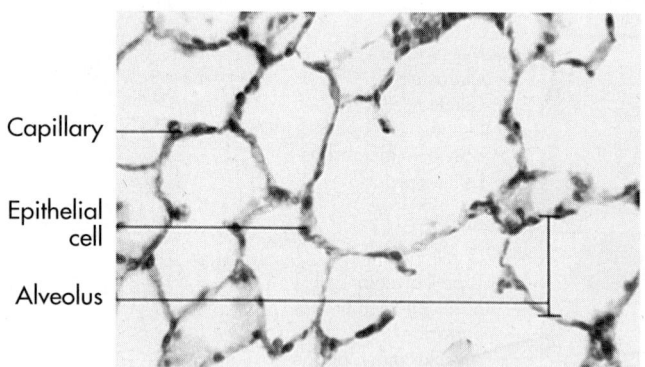

Figure 32-6 Photomicrograph of lung, showing several alveoli. Note the proximity of the capillary to the alveolar wall. (From Thibodeau GA: *Anatomy & physiology,* St Louis, 1987, Mosby.)

Despite the fact that the entire cardiac output from the right ventricle goes into the lungs, the pulmonary circulation has a lower pressure and resistance than the systemic circulation. Pulmonary arteries are exposed to about one fifth the pressure of the systemic circulation and have a much thinner muscle layer. (Systemic vessels are described in Chapter 29.) Mean pulmonary artery pressure is 18 mm Hg; mean aortic pressure is 90 mmHg.

About one third of the pulmonary vessels are filled with blood (perfused) at any given time. More vessels become perfused when right ventricular cardiac output increases. Therefore increased delivery of blood to the lungs does not normally increase mean pulmonary artery pressure.

The pulmonary artery divides and enters the lung at the hilus with each main bronchus and branches with the bronchus at every division, so that every bronchus and bronchiole has an accompanying artery or arteriole. The arterioles, less than 1 mm in diameter, regulate blood flow through their respective capillary beds.

The arterioles divide at the terminal bronchiole to form a network of pulmonary capillaries around the acinus. The capillaries are an integral part of the alveolar septa. Capillary walls consist of an endothelial layer and a thin basement membrane, which often fuses with the basement membrane of the alveolar septum. This results in very little separation between blood in the capillary and gas in the alveolus.

The shared alveolar and capillary walls compose the **alveolocapillary membrane,** a very thin membrane made up of the alveolar epithelium, the alveolar basement membrane, an

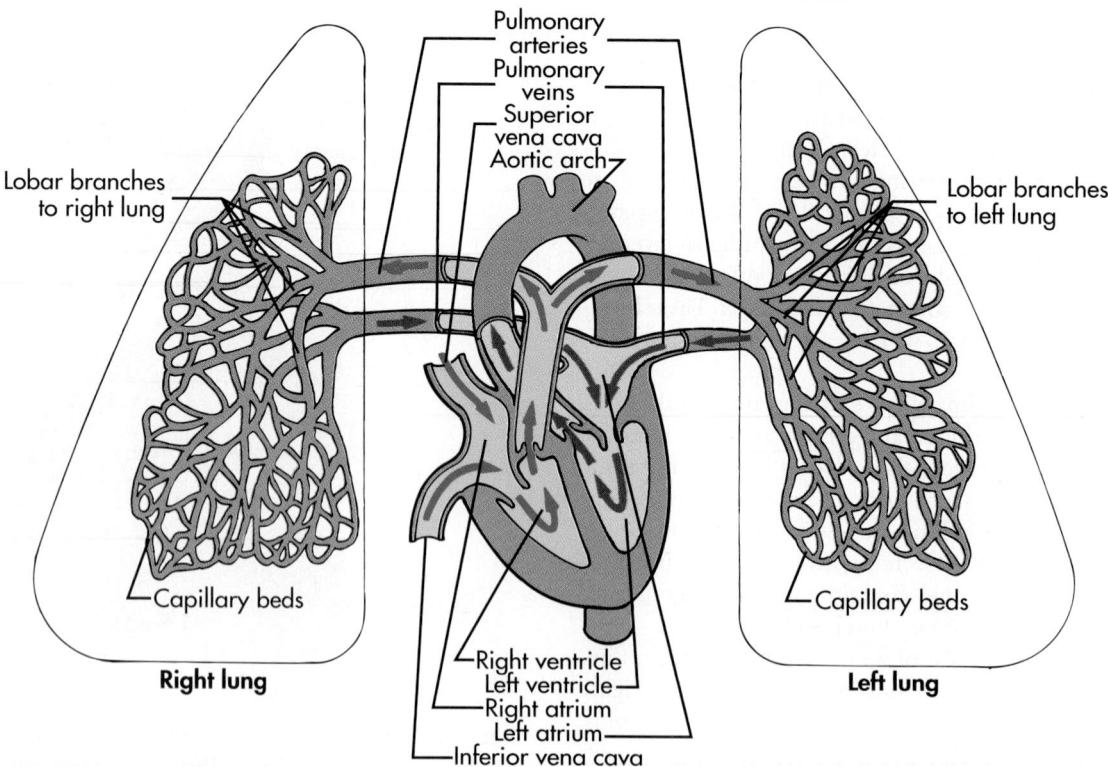

Figure 32-7 The pulmonary circulation. The right and left pulmonary veins and arteries and the branching capillaries are illustrated.

interstitial space, the capillary basement membrane, and the capillary endothelium (Figure 32-8). These extremely thin alveolar walls are easily damaged and can leak plasma and blood into the alveolar space. Gas exchange occurs across the alveolocapillary membrane. With normal perfusion, approximately 100 ml of blood in the pulmonary capillary bed is spread very thinly over 70 to 100 m^2 of alveolar surface area. The alveolocapillary membrane efficiently exposes large quantities of blood to gas in the alveoli. Any disorder that thickens the membrane impairs gas exchange.

Each pulmonary vein drains several pulmonary capillaries. Unlike the pulmonary arteries, which follow the branching bronchi, pulmonary veins are dispersed randomly throughout the lung and then leave the lung at the hila and enter the left atrium. They are similar to veins in the systemic circulation, but they have no valves.

The bronchial circulation is part of the systemic circulation. It supplies nutrients to the conducting airways, nerves, lymph nodes, large pulmonary vessels, and membranes (pleurae) that surround the lungs.[1] The bronchial circulation is unique in that not all of its capillaries drain into its own venous system. Some of the bronchial capillaries empty into the pulmonary vein and contribute to the normal venous admixture (mixing of oxygenated and deoxygenated blood) or right-to-left shunt (right-to-left shunts are described in Chapter 33). The bronchial circulation does not participate in gas exchange.

Lung vasculature also includes deep and superficial lymphatic capillaries. The deep lymphatic capillaries begin at the level of the terminal bronchioles; there are no lymphatic structures in the acinus. Fluid and alveolar macrophages migrate from the alveoli to the terminal bronchioles, where they enter the lymphatic system. The superficial lymphatic capillaries drain the membrane that surrounds the lungs. Both deep and superficial lymphatic vessels leave the lung at the hilus. The lymphatic system plays an important role in keeping the lung free of fluid. (The lymphatic system is described in Chapter 29.)

Chest Wall and Pleura

The chest wall (skin, ribs, intercostal muscles) protects the lungs from injury, and its muscles, in conjunction with the diaphragm, perform the muscular work of breathing. The **thoracic cavity** is contained by the chest wall and encases the lungs (Figure 32-9). A serous membrane called the **pleura** adheres firmly to the lungs. It then folds over itself and attaches firmly to the chest wall. The membrane covering the lungs is the visceral pleura; that lining the thoracic cavity is the parietal pleura. The area between the two pleurae is called the **pleural space,** or pleural cavity. Normally only a thin layer of fluid secreted by the pleura (pleural fluid) fills the pleural space. This lubricates the pleural surfaces, allowing the two layers to slide over each other without separating. Pressure in the pleural space is usually negative or subatmospheric (-4 to -10 mmHg).

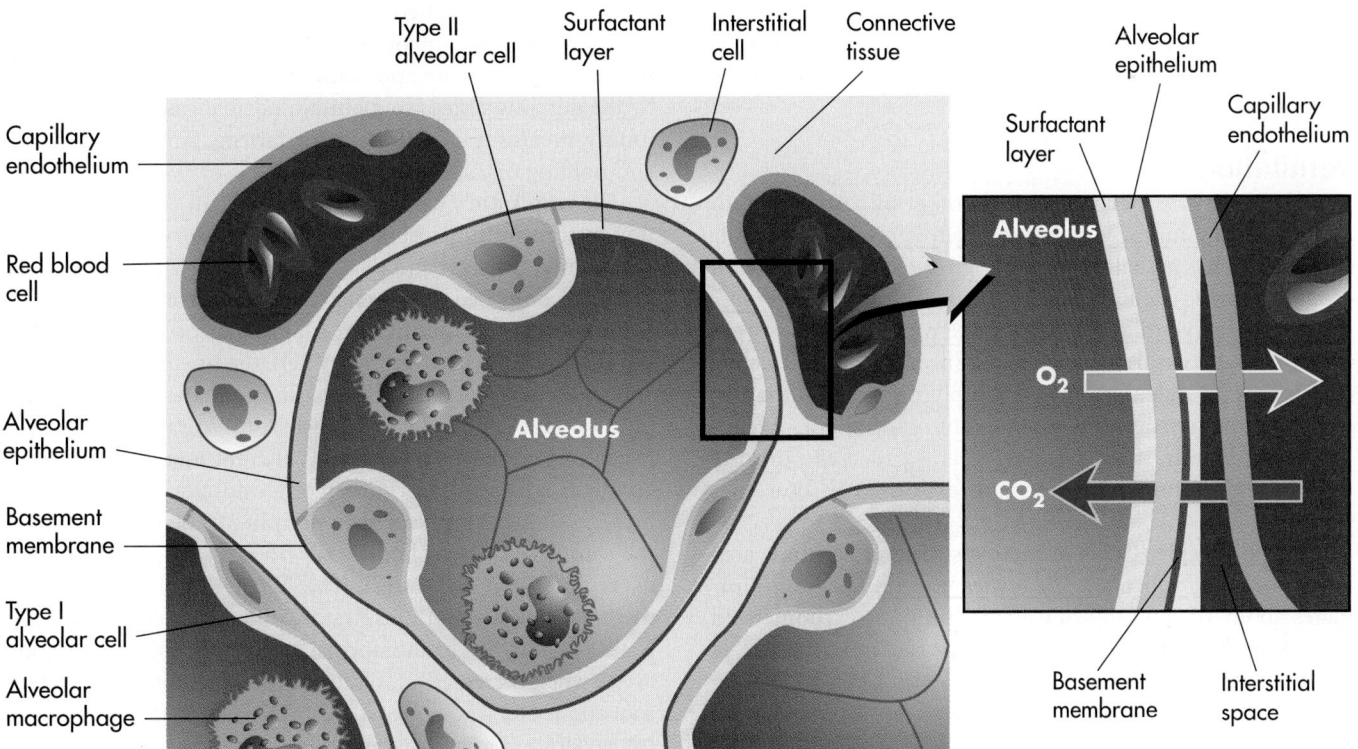

Figure 32-8 **Section through the alveolar septum (gas-exchange membrane).** *Inset* shows a magnified view of the respiratory membrane composed of the alveolar wall (fluid coating, epithelial cells, basement membrane), interstitial fluid, and wall of a pulmonary capillary (basement membrane, endothelial cells). The gases carbon dioxide (CO_2) and oxygen (O_2) diffuse across the respiratory membrane.

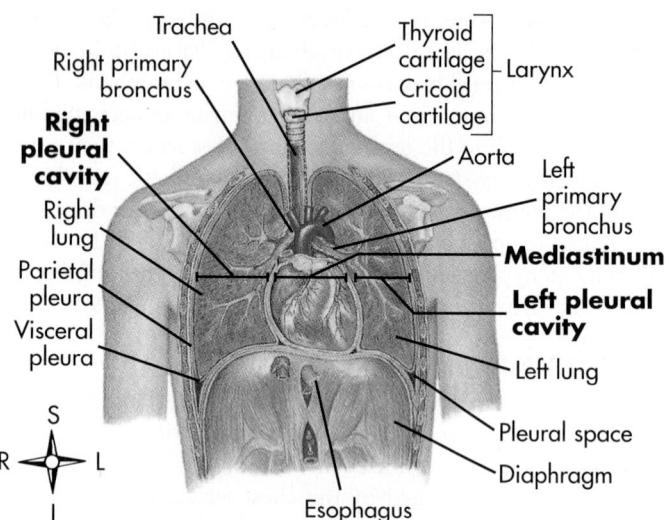

Figure 32-9 Thoracic (chest) cavity and related structures. The thoracic ("chest") cavity is divided into three subdivisions (left and right pleural divisions and mediastinum) by a partition formed by a serous membrane called the *pleura*. (From Thibodeau GA, Patton KT: *Anatomy & physiology,* ed 3, St Louis, 1996, Mosby.)

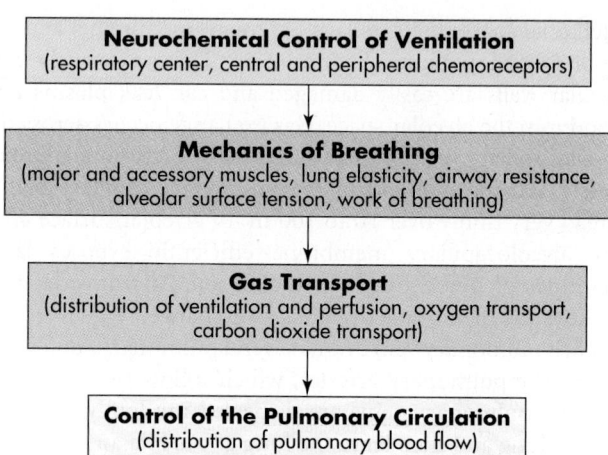

Figure 32-10 Functional components of the respiratory system. The central nervous system responds to neurochemical stimulation of ventilation and sends signals to the chest wall musculature. The response of the respiratory system to these impulses is influenced by several factors that affect the mechanisms of breathing and therefore affect the adequacy of ventilation. Gas transport between the alveoli and pulmonary capillary blood depends on a variety of physical and chemical activities. The control of the pulmonary circulation plays a role in the appropriate distribution of blood flow.

FUNCTION OF THE PULMONARY SYSTEM

The pulmonary system functions to (1) ventilate the alveoli, (2) diffuse gases into and out of the blood, and (3) perfuse the lungs so that the organs and tissues of the body receive blood that is rich in oxygen and low in carbon dioxide. Each component of the pulmonary system contributes to one or more of these functions (Figure 32-10).

Ventilation

Ventilation is the mechanical movement of gas or air into and out of the lungs. Ventilation often is misnamed **respiration,** which is actually the exchange of oxygen and carbon dioxide during cellular metabolism. "Respiratory rate" is actually the ventilatory rate, or the number of times gas is inspired and expired per minute. The amount of effective ventilation is calculated by multiplying the ventilatory rate (breaths per minute) by the volume of air per breath (liters per breath, tidal volume). This is called the **minute volume** or minute ventilation and expressed in liters per minute.

Carbon dioxide (CO_2), the gaseous form of carbonic acid (H_2CO_3), is a product of cellular metabolism. The lung eliminates about 10,000 milliequivalents (mEq) of carbonic acid per day in the form of CO_2, which is produced at the rate of approximately 200 ml/min. CO_2 elimination is necessary to maintain a normal arterial CO_2 (Pa_{CO_2}) of 40 mmHg and normal acid-base balance (see Chapter 3 for a discussion of acid-base regulation).

The adequacy of **alveolar ventilation** *cannot* be accurately determined by observation of ventilatory rate, pattern, or effort. If a health care professional needs to determine the ade-

quacy of ventilation, an arterial blood gas analysis must be performed to measure Pa_{CO_2}.

Neurochemical Control of Ventilation

The mechanisms that control respiration are very complex.[3,4] Breathing is usually involuntary because homeostatic changes in the ventilatory rate and volume are adjusted automatically by the nervous system to maintain normal gas exchange. Voluntary breathing is necessary for talking, singing, laughing, and holding one's breath.

The **respiratory center** in the brain stem controls respiration by transmitting impulses to the respiratory muscles, causing them to contract and relax (Figure 32-11). The respiratory center is composed of several groups of neurons located bilaterally in the brain stem: the dorsal respiratory group (DRG), the ventral respiratory group (VRG), the pneumotaxic center, and the apneustic center.[5] The basic automatic rhythm of respiration is set by the DRG, a cluster of inspiratory nerve cells located in the medulla that sends efferent impulses to the diaphragm and inspiratory intercostal muscles. The DRG also receives afferent impulses from **peripheral chemoreceptors** in the carotid and aortic bodies and from several different types of receptors in the lungs. The VRG, also located in the medulla, contains both inspiratory and expiratory neurons. It is almost inactive during normal, quiet respiration, becoming active when increased ventilatory effort is required. The pneumotaxic center and apneustic center, situated in the pons, do not generate primary rhythm but rather act as modifiers of the inspiratory depth and rate established by the medullary centers.[5] Breathing can be modified by input from the cortex, the limbic system, and the hypothalamus, and the pattern of breathing can be influenced by emotion and by disease.

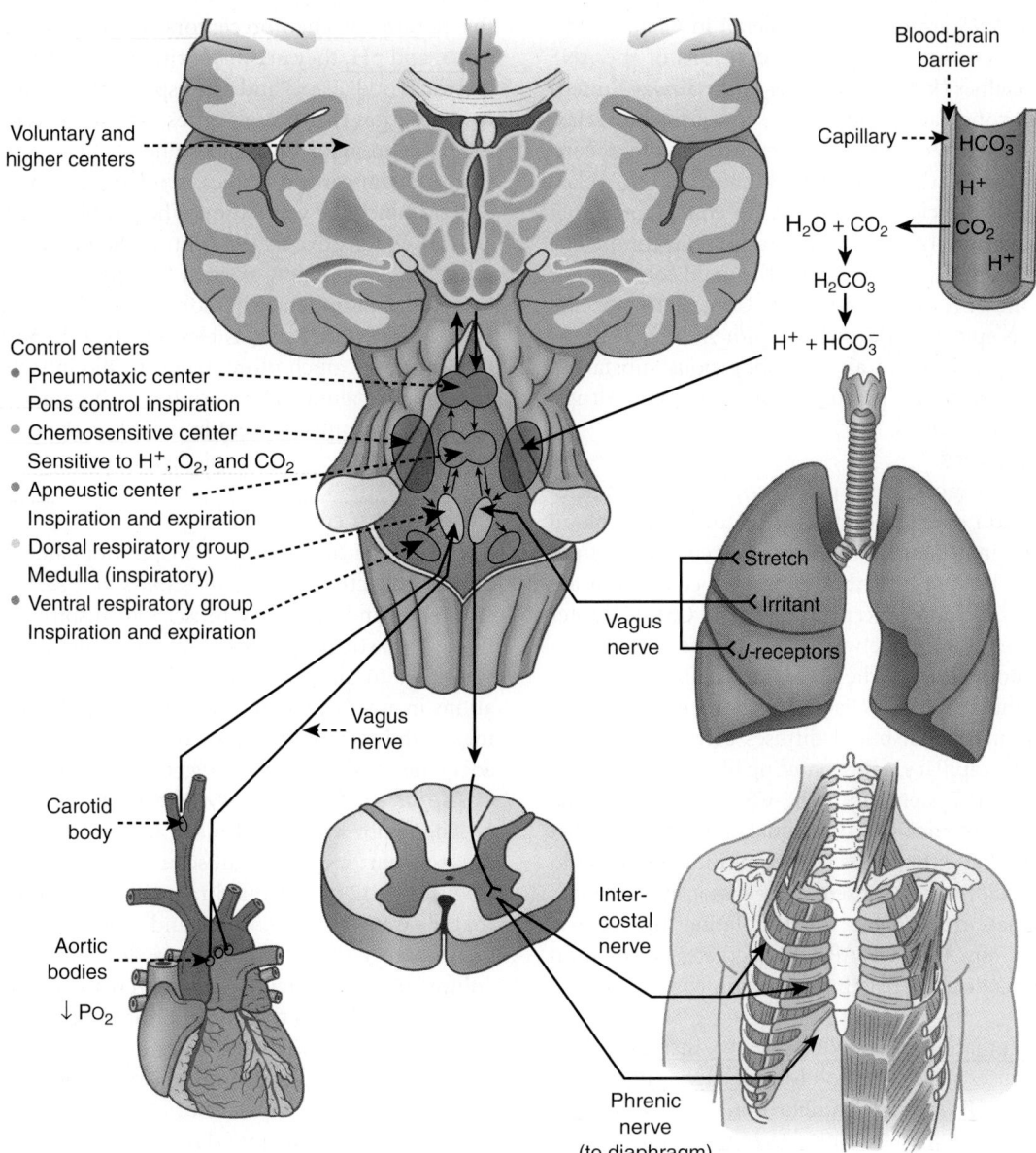

Figure 32-11 Neurochemical respiratory control system.

Lung Receptors

Three types of lung receptors send impulses from the lungs to the dorsal respiratory group:

1. **Irritant receptors** are found in the epithelium of the conducting airways. They are sensitive to noxious aerosols (vapors), gases, and particulate matter (e.g., inhaled dusts), which cause them to initiate the cough reflex. When stimulated, irritant receptors also cause bronchoconstriction and increased ventilatory rate. These receptors are located primarily in the proximal larger airways and are nearly absent in the distal airways; thus it is possible for secretions to accumulate in the distal respiratory tree without initiating cough.[6]

2. **Stretch receptors** are located in the smooth muscles of airways and are sensitive to increases in the size or volume of the lungs. They decrease ventilatory rate and volume when stimulated, an occurrence sometimes referred to as the *Hering-Breuer expiratory reflex*. This reflex is active in newborns and assists with ventilation. In adults, this reflex is active only at high tidal volumes (such as with exercise) and may play a role in protecting against excess lung inflation.[7]

3. **J-receptors** (juxtapulmonary capillary receptors) are located near the capillaries in the alveolar septa. They are sensitive to increased pulmonary capillary pressure, which stimulates them to initiate rapid, shallow breathing; hypotension; and bradycardia.[5]

The lung is innervated by the autonomic nervous system (ANS). Fibers of the sympathetic division of the ANS in the lung branch from the upper thoracic and cervical ganglia of the spinal cord. Fibers of the parasympathetic division of the ANS travel in the vagus nerve to the lung. (Structures and function of the ANS are discussed in detail in Chapter 14.) The parasympathetic and sympathetic divisions of the ANS control airway caliber (interior diameter of the airway lumen) by stimulating bronchial smooth muscle to contract or relax. The parasympathetic receptors cause smooth muscle to contract, whereas sympathetic receptors cause it to relax. Bronchial smooth muscle tone depends on equilibrium, that is, equal stimulation of contraction and relaxation. The parasympathetic division of the ANS is the main controller of airway caliber under normal conditions.[5] Constriction occurs if the irritant receptors in the airway epithelium are stimulated by irritants in inspired air, by endogenous substances (e.g., histamine, serotonin, prostaglandins), by many drugs, and by humoral substances.

Chemoreceptors

Chemoreceptors monitor the pH, $Paco_2$, and Pao_2 of arterial blood. **Central chemoreceptors** monitor arterial blood indirectly by sensing changes in the pH of cerebrospinal fluid (CSF). They are located near the respiratory center and are sensitive to hydrogen ion concentration in the CSF. (Chapter 3 describes the relationship between ions and the pH, or acid-base status, of body fluids.) The pH, or concentration of hydrogen ions in the CSF, reflects $Paco_2$ because, unlike H^+ ions, carbon dioxide in arterial blood diffuses across the blood-brain barrier (the capillary wall separating blood from cells of the central nervous system) into the CSF until the partial pressure of carbon dioxide (Pco_2) is equal on both sides. Carbon dioxide that has entered the CSF combines with H_2O to form carbonic acid, which subsequently dissociates into hydrogen ions that are capable of stimulating the central chemoreceptors. In this way $Paco_2$ regulates ventilation through its impact on the pH (hydrogen ion content) of the CSF.[5]

If alveolar ventilation is inadequate, $Paco_2$ increases. Carbon dioxide diffuses across the blood-brain barrier until Pco_2 in blood and CSF reaches equilibrium. As the central chemoreceptors sense the resulting decrease in pH (increase in hydrogen ion concentration), they stimulate the respiratory center to increase the depth and rate of ventilation. Increased ventilation causes the Pco_2 of arterial blood to decrease below that of the CSF, and carbon dioxide diffuses back out of the CSF, returning its pH to normal.

The central chemoreceptors are sensitive to very small changes in the pH of CSF (equivalent to a 1 to 2 mmHg change in Pco_2) and are able to maintain a normal $Paco_2$ under many different conditions, including strenuous exercise. If inadequate ventilation, or hypoventilation, is long term (e.g., in chronic obstructive pulmonary disease), these receptors become insensitive to small changes in $Paco_2$ and regulate ventilation poorly. In addition, prolonged increases in $Paco_2$ result in renal compensation through bicarbonate retention. This bicarbonate gradually diffuses into the CSF where it normalizes the pH and negates the effect on ventilatory drive.[1,5]

The peripheral chemoreceptors are located in aortic bodies, the aortic arch, and carotid bodies at the bifurcation of the carotids, near the baroreceptors (see Chapter 29). Although the peripheral chemoreceptors are sensitive to changes in $Paco_2$ and pH, they are primarily sensitive to oxygen levels in arterial blood (Pao_2) and are responsible for all of the increase in ventilation that occurs in response to arterial hypoxemia.[5] As Pao_2 and pH decrease, peripheral chemoreceptors, particularly in the carotid bodies, send signals to the respiratory center to increase ventilation. The peripheral chemoreceptors are not as sensitive as the central chemoreceptors. The Pao_2 must drop well below normal (to approximately 60 mmHg) before the peripheral chemoreceptors have much influence on ventilation. If $Paco_2$ is elevated as well, however, ventilation increases much more than it would in response to either abnormality alone. The peripheral chemoreceptors become the major stimulus to ventilation when the central chemoreceptors are "reset" by chronic hypoventilation.

Mechanics of Breathing

The mechanical aspects of inspiration and expiration are known collectively as the *mechanics of breathing* and involve (1) major and accessory muscles of inspiration and expiration, (2) elastic properties of the lungs and chest wall, and (3) resistance to airflow through the conducting airways. Alterations in any of these properties increase the work of breathing, or the metabolic energy that must be exerted to achieve adequate ventilation and oxygenation of the blood.

Major and Accessory Muscles

The major muscles of inspiration are the diaphragm and the external intercostal muscles (muscles between the ribs) (Figure 32-12). The diaphragm is a dome-shaped muscle that separates the abdominal and thoracic cavities. When the diaphragm contracts, it flattens downward, increasing the volume of the thoracic cavity, and creates a negative pressure that draws gas into the lungs. Contraction of external intercostal muscles elevates the anterior portion of the ribs. This increases the volume of thoracic cavity by increasing its front-to-back (anteroposterior [AP]) diameter. Although the external intercostal muscles may contract during quiet breathing, inspiration at rest usually is assisted by the diaphragm only.

The accessory muscles of inspiration are the sternocleidomastoid and scalene muscles. Like the external intercostal muscles, these muscles enlarge the thorax by increasing its AP diameter. The accessory muscles of inspiration assist inspiration when minute volume (volume of air inspired and expired per minute) is very high, such as during strenuous exercise, or when the work of breathing is increased because of disease. The accessory muscles do not increase the volume of the thorax as efficiently as the diaphragm does.

There are no major muscles of expiration because normal, relaxed expiration is passive and requires no muscular effort. The accessory muscles of expiration, the abdominal and internal intercostal muscles, assist expiration when minute volume is high, during coughing, or when airway obstruction is present. When the abdominal muscles contract, intraabdominal pressure increases, pushing up the diaphragm and decreasing the volume of the thorax. The internal intercostal

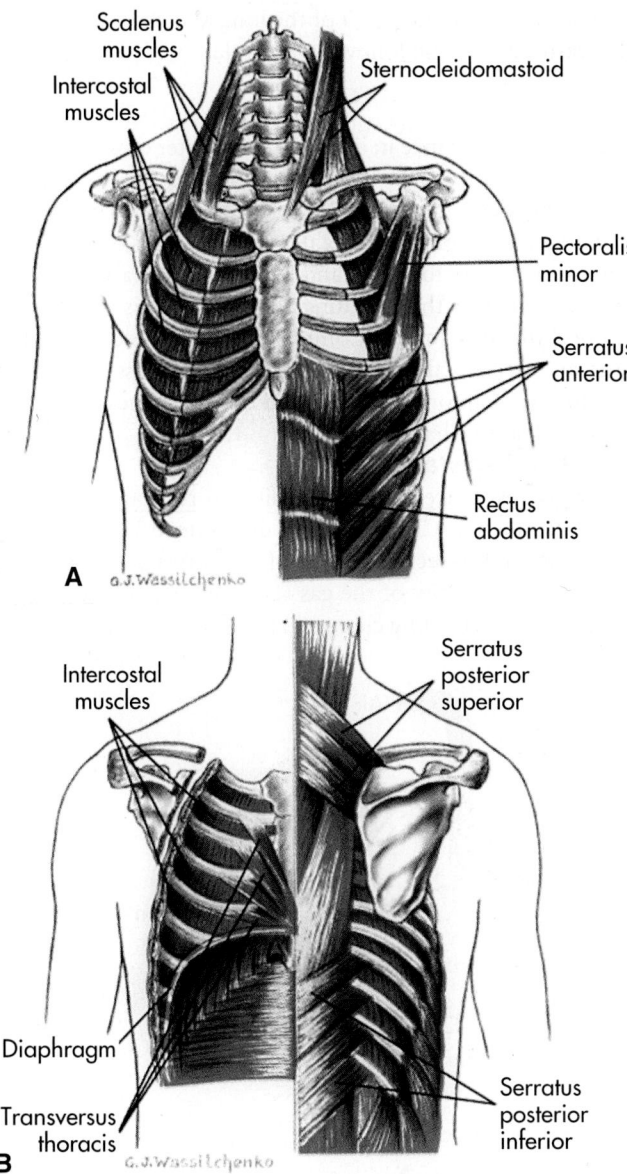

Scalenus
muscles

Intercostal
muscles

Sternocleidomastoid

Pectoralis
minor

Serratus
anterior

Rectus
abdominis

A a.J.Wassilchenko

Intercostal
muscles

Serratus
posterior
superior

Diaphragm

Transversus
thoracis

Serratus
posterior
inferior

B a.J.Wassilchenko

Figure 32-12 Muscles of ventilation. **A,** Anterior view. **B,** Posterior view. (From Wilson SF, Thompson JM: *Respiratory disorders,* St Louis, 1990, Mosby.)

muscles pull down the anterior ribs, decreasing the AP diameter of the thorax.

Alveolar Surface Tension

Surface tension occurs at any gas-liquid interface and refers to the tendency for liquid molecules that are exposed to air to adhere to one another. This phenomenon can be seen, for example, in a glass of liquid that is about to overflow or in the way liquids "bead" when splashed on a waterproof surface. In both examples this phenomenon decreases the surface area exposed to the air.

Within a sphere, such as an alveolus, surface tension tends to make expansion difficult. According to the law of Laplace, the pressure *(P)* required to inflate a sphere is equal to two times the surface tension *(2T)* divided by the radius (r) of the sphere, or P = *(2T/r)*. As the radius of the sphere (or alveo-

lus) becomes smaller, more and more pressure is required to inflate it. If the alveoli were lined with a water-like fluid, taking breaths would be extremely difficult.

Alveolar ventilation, or distention, is made possible by surfactant, which lowers the surface tension by coating the air-liquid interface in the alveoli. Surfactant, a lipoprotein produced by type II alveolar cells, has a detergent-like effect that separates the liquid molecules, thereby decreasing alveolar surface tension.

Surfactant lines the alveolar side of the alveolocapillary membrane and, in effect, reverses Laplace's law. As the radius of a surfactant-lined sphere (alveolus) grows smaller, the surface tension *decreases,* and as the radius grows larger, the surface tension *increases.* This occurs because the surfactant molecules have much weaker intermolecular attraction compared with the liquid molecules. The surfactant molecules occupy most of the air-fluid interface and disrupt the intermolecular forces that tend to collapse the alveoli. Therefore the alveoli are much easier to inflate at low lung volumes (i.e., after expiration) than at high volumes (i.e., after inspiration). If surfactant production is disrupted or surfactant is not produced in adequate quantities, alveolar surface tension increases and results in alveolar collapse, decreased lung expansion, increased work of breathing, and severe gas-exchange abnormalities.

The decrease in surface tension caused by surfactant is also responsible for keeping the alveoli free of fluid. In the absence of surfactant, the surface tension tends to attract fluid into the alveoli. In addition, surfactant participates in host defense against respiratory pathogens.[8]

Elastic Properties of the Lung and Chest Wall

The lung and chest wall have elastic properties that permit expansion during inspiration and return to resting volume during expiration. The elasticity of the lungs is caused both by elastin fibers in the alveolar walls and surrounding the small airways and pulmonary capillaries and by surface tension at the alveolar air-liquid interface. The elasticity of the chest wall is the result of the configuration of its bones and musculature.

Elastic recoil is the tendency of the lungs to return to the resting state after inspiration. Normal elastic recoil permits passive expiration, eliminating the need for major muscles of expiration. Passive elastic recoil may be insufficient during labored breathing (high minute volume), in which case the accessory muscles of expiration are used. The accessory muscles also are used if disease comprises elastic recoil (e.g., in emphysema) or blocks the conducting airways.

Normal elastic recoil depends on an equilibrium between opposing forces of recoil in the lungs and chest wall. Under normal conditions the chest wall tends to recoil by expanding outward. This can be observed readily during open heart surgery. When the sternum is split to open the thoracic cavity, the chest wall moves outward laterally. The tendency of the chest wall to recoil by expanding is balanced by the tendency of the lungs to recoil or collapse around the hila. The tendency of the lungs to collapse can be demonstrated if the chest is opened without mechanically ventilating the lungs (e.g., at postmortem examination). As the thorax is opened, the lungs immediately collapse, like inflated balloons that have been released. This reaction is caused by elastic recoil and surface tension in the alveoli. The opposing forces of the chest wall and lungs create, in part, the negative intrapleural pressure.

Balance between the outward recoil of the chest wall and inward recoil of the lungs occurs at the resting level, at the end of expiration. During inspiration, the diaphragm and intercostal muscles contract, air flows into the lungs, and the chest wall expands. Muscular effort is needed to overcome the resistance of the lungs to expansion. During expiration the muscles relax and the elastic recoil of the lungs causes the thorax to decrease in volume until, once again, balance between the chest wall and lung recoil forces is reached[1] (Figure 32-13).

Compliance is the measure of lung and chest wall distensibility. It represents the relative ease with which these structures can be stretched. Compliance is therefore the reciprocal of elasticity. Compliance is determined by alveolar surface

tension and the elastic recoil of the lung and chest wall. It can be measured with the following formula:

$$C = \frac{\Delta V}{\Delta P}$$

where C = compliance in liters per centimeter of water, ΔV = volume change (usually tidal volume), and ΔP = pressure change (airway or pleural pressure) in centimeters of water.[1,9]

Increased compliance indicates that the lungs or chest wall is abnormally easy to inflate and has lost some elastic recoil. A decrease indicates that the lungs or chest wall is abnormally stiff or difficult to inflate. Compliance is increased in emphysema and decreased in acute respiratory distress syndrome, pneumonia, pulmonary edema, and fibrosis. (These disorders are described in Chapter 33.)

Airway Resistance

Airway resistance, which is similar to resistance to blood flow (described in Chapter 29), is determined by the length, radius, and cross-sectional area of the airways and density, viscosity, and velocity of the gas (Poiseuille's law). Resistance is computed by dividing change in pressure (P) by rate of flow

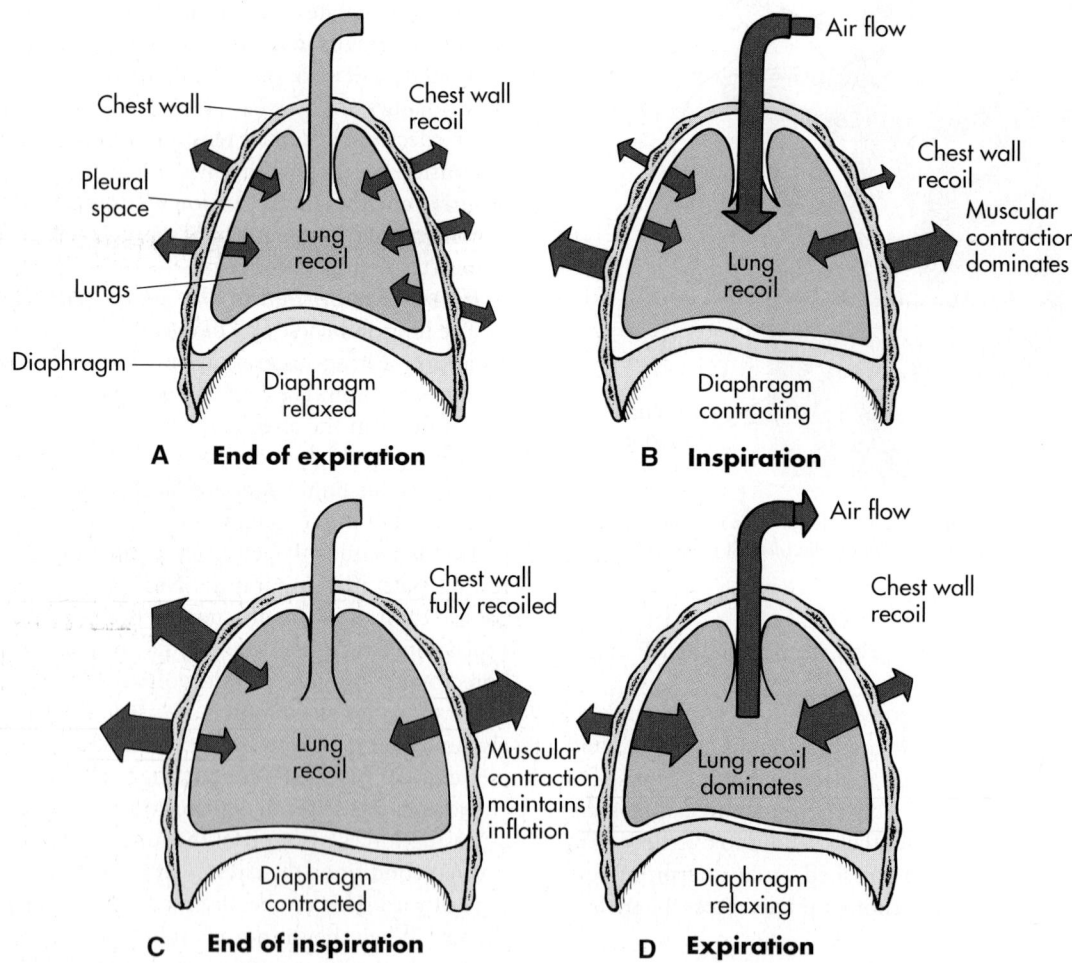

A   End of expiration

B   Inspiration

C   End of inspiration

D   Expiration

Figure 32-13 Interaction of forces during inspiration and expiration. **A,** Outward recoil of the chest wall equals inward recoil of the lungs at the end of expiration. **B,** During inspiration, contraction of respiratory muscles, assisted by chest wall recoil, overcomes tendency of lungs to recoil. **C,** At the end of inspiration, respiratory muscle contraction maintains lung expansion. **D,** During expiration, respiratory muscles relax, allowing elastic recoil of the lungs to deflate the lungs.

(F), or *R = {P/F}*(Ohm's law) and can easily be measured in the pulmonary function laboratory.[5] Airway resistance is normally very low. One half to two thirds of total airway resistance occurs in the nose. The next highest resistance is in the oropharynx and larynx. There is very little resistance in the conducting airways of the lungs because of their large cross-sectional area. The most common causes of increased airway resistance are swelling (edema), obstruction (i.e., mucous plugging), and spasm of bronchial smooth muscle (bronchospasm), all of which decrease the radius of the airways. Resistance increases as the diameter of the airways (total cross-sectional area) decreases.

Work of Breathing

The work of breathing is determined by the muscular effort (and therefore oxygen and energy) required for ventilation. The work of breathing is normally very low but may increase considerably in disease states that disrupt the equilibrium between forces exerted by the lung and chest wall. More muscular effort is required when lung compliance is decreased (e.g., in pulmonary edema), chest wall compliance is decreased (e.g., in spinal deformity or obesity), or airways are obstructed by bronchospasm or mucous plugging (e.g., in asthma or bronchitis). An increase in the work of breathing can result in a marked increase in oxygen consumption and metabolic demand, which can cause significant morbidity in individuals with severe lung disease.

Measurement of Gas Pressure

A gas is made up of millions of molecules moving randomly. As they move, they collide with each other and the wall of the space in which they are contained. These collisions exert pressure. If more molecules are present in the space, the pressure, or number of collisions, increases (Figure 32-14). If the same number of gas molecules is contained in a small and a large container, the pressure is greater in the small container because more collisions occur in the smaller space. Heat increases the speed of the molecules, which increases the number of collisions. Therefore pressure also increases at higher temperatures.

Barometric pressure (P_B) (atmospheric pressure) is the pressure exerted by gas molecules in air at specific altitudes. At sea level, barometric pressure is 760 mmHg. This number is the sum of the pressure exerted by each gas in the air at sea level. The portion of the total pressure exerted by any individual gas is its **partial pressure** (see Figure 32-14). At sea level the air is made up of oxygen (20.9%), nitrogen (78.1%), and a few other trace gases. The partial pressure of oxygen is equal to the percentage of oxygen in the air (20.9%) times the total pressure (760 mmHg), or 159 mmHg ($760 \times 0.209 = 158.84$). (Symbols used in the measurement of gas pressures and pulmonary ventilation are defined in Table 32-2.)

The amount of water vapor contained in a gas mixture is determined by the temperature of the gas and is unrelated to barometric pressure. Gas that enters the lungs becomes saturated with water vapor (humidified) as it passes through the upper airway. At body temperature (37° C), water vapor exerts a pressure of 47 mmHg. Because this is true regardless of total (barometric) pressure, the partial pressure of water vapor (always 47 mmHg) must be subtracted from the barometric pressure before the partial pressure of other gases in the mixture can be determined. In saturated air at sea level, the partial pressure of oxygen is therefore $(760 - 47) \times 0.209 = 149$. All pressure and volume measurements made in pulmonary function laboratories specify the temperature and humidity of a gas at the time of measurement.

Many pressure measurements are stated as variations from barometric pressure, rather than percentages of it. On such

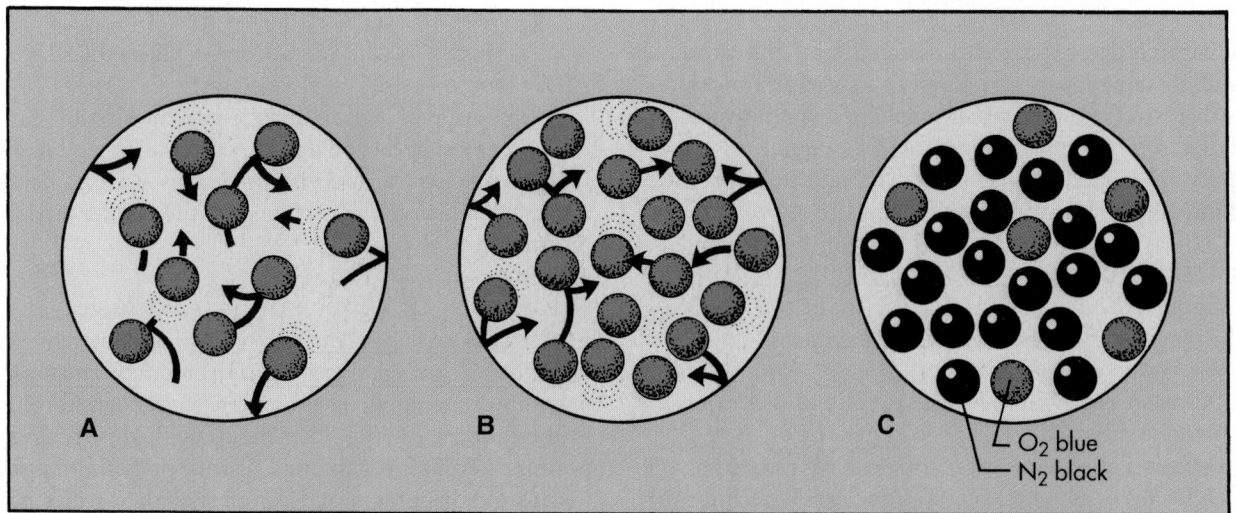

Figure 32-14 Relationship between number of gas molecules and pressure exerted by the gas in an enclosed space. **A,** Theoretically, 10 molecules of the same gas exert a total pressure of 10 within the space. **B,** If the number of molecules is increased to 20, total pressure is 20. **C,** If there are different gases in the space, each gas exerts a partial pressure: here the partial pressure of nitrogen (N_2) is 18, that of oxygen (O_2) is 6, and total pressure is 24.

	Table 32-2	Common Pulmonary Abbreviations
	Symbol	**Definition**
	V	Volume or amount of gas
	Q	Perfusion or blood flow
	P	Pressure (usually partial pressure) of a gas
	S	Percentage of hemoglobin saturation with a gas (usually oxygen)
	F	Fraction of gas, or gas flow (in a laboratory test)
	C	Content or amount of gas
	C_T	Thoracic compliance
	E	Expired gas
	i	Inspired gas
	A	Alveolar gas
	a	Arterial blood
	$\bar{v}$	Mixed venous or pulmonary artery blood
	D	Dead space
	Pa_{O_2}	Partial pressure of oxygen in arterial blood
	PA_{O_2}	Partial pressure of oxygen in alveolar gas
	Pa_{CO_2}	Partial pressure of carbon dioxide in arterial blood
	$P\bar{v}_{O_2}$	Partial pressure of oxygen in mixed venous or pulmonary artery blood
	$P(A - a)_{O_2}$	Difference between alveolar and arterial partial pressure of oxygen (A − a [gradient])
	P_B	Barometric or atmospheric pressure
	Sa_{O_2}	Saturation of hemoglobin (in arterial blood) with oxygen
	$S\bar{v}_{O_2}$	Saturation of hemoglobin (in mixed venous blood) with oxygen
	Ca_{O_2}	Content or amount (volume) of oxygen in arterial blood
	$C\bar{v}_{O_2}$	Content of oxygen in mixed venous blood
	$C(a - \bar{v})_{O_2}$	Oxygen content difference between arterial and mixed venous blood
	$\dot{V}_A$	Alveolar ventilation
	$\dot{V}_D$	Dead-space ventilation
	$\dot{V}_E$	Minute volume
	VC	Vital capacity
	V_T	Tidal volume or average breath
	$\dot{Q}T$	Total perfusion or blood flow (cardiac output)
	$\dot{V}/\dot{Q}$	Ratio of ventilation to perfusion
	Fi_{O_2}	Fraction of inspired oxygen
	FRC	Functional residual capacity
	IC	Inspiratory capacity

NOTE: Subscripts identify the particular gas, volume, or pressure being discussed. A dot (·) means measurement over time, usually 1 minute.

scales, barometric pressure is considered zero, and pressure varies up or down from zero. Physiologic pressure measurements that involve fluids, rather than gases, are measured as variations from barometric pressure. For example, a systolic blood pressure of 120 mmHg indicates that systolic pressure is 120 mmHg above barometric pressure.

Gas Transport

Gas transport, the delivery of oxygen to the cells of the body and the removal of carbon dioxide, has four steps:
1. Ventilation of the lungs
2. Diffusion of oxygen from the alveoli into the capillary blood
3. Perfusion of systemic capillaries with oxygenated blood
4. Diffusion of oxygen from systemic capillaries into the cells

Steps in the transport of carbon dioxide occur in reverse order:
1. Diffusion of carbon dioxide from the cells into the systemic capillaries

2. Perfusion of the pulmonary capillary bed by venous blood
3. Diffusion of carbon dioxide into the alveoli
4. Removal of carbon dioxide from the lung by ventilation

If any step in gas transport is impaired by a respiratory or cardiovascular disorder, gas exchange at the cellular level is compromised.

Distribution of Ventilation and Perfusion

Effective gas exchange depends on an approximately even distribution of gas (ventilation) and blood (perfusion) in all portions of the lungs. The lungs are suspended from the hila in the thoracic cavity. When the individual is in an upright position (sitting or standing), gravity pulls the lungs down toward the diaphragm and compresses their lower portions or bases. The alveoli in the upper portions, or apices, of the lungs contain a greater residual volume of gas and are larger and less numerous than those in the lower portions. Because surface tension increases as the alveoli become larger, the larger alveoli in the upper portions of the lung are more difficult to inflate (less compliant) than the smaller alveoli in the lower portions of the lung. Therefore during ventilation most of the tidal volume is distributed to the bases of the lungs, where compliance is greater.

The heart pumps against gravity to perfuse the pulmonary circulation. As blood is pumped into the lung apices of a sitting or standing individual, some blood pressure is dissipated in overcoming gravity. As a result, blood pressure at the apices is lower than that at the bases. Because greater pressure causes greater perfusion, the bases of the lungs are better perfused than the apices (Figure 32-15). Thus ventilation and perfusion are greatest in the same lung portions: the lower lobes. Ventilation and perfusion depend on body position. If a standing individual assumes a supine or side-lying position, the areas of the lungs that are then most dependent become the best ventilated and perfused.

Distribution of perfusion in the pulmonary circulation also is affected by alveolar pressure (gas pressure in the alveoli). The pulmonary capillary bed differs from the systemic capillary bed in that it is surrounded by gas-containing alveoli. If the gas pressure in the alveoli exceeds the blood pressure

in the capillary, the capillary collapses and flow ceases. This is most likely to occur in portions of the lung where blood pressure is lowest and alveolar gas volume and therefore pressure are greatest, that is, the apex of the lung.

The lungs are divided into three zones on the basis of the relationships among all the factors affecting pulmonary blood flow. Alveolar pressure plus the forces of gravity, arterial blood pressure, and venous blood pressure affect the distribution of perfusion (Figure 32-16).

Zone I is where alveolar pressure exceeds pulmonary arterial and venous pressures. The capillary bed collapses, and normal blood flow ceases. Normally zone I is a very small part of the lung at the apex. Zone II is the portion where alveolar pressure is greater than venous pressure but not greater than arterial pressure. Blood flows through zone II, but it is impeded to a certain extent by alveolar pressure. Zone II is normally above the level of the left atrium. In zone III both arterial and venous pressures are greater than alveolar pressure and blood flow is not affected by alveolar pressure. Zone III is in the base of the lung. Blood flow through the pulmonary capillary bed increases in regular increments from the apex to the base.

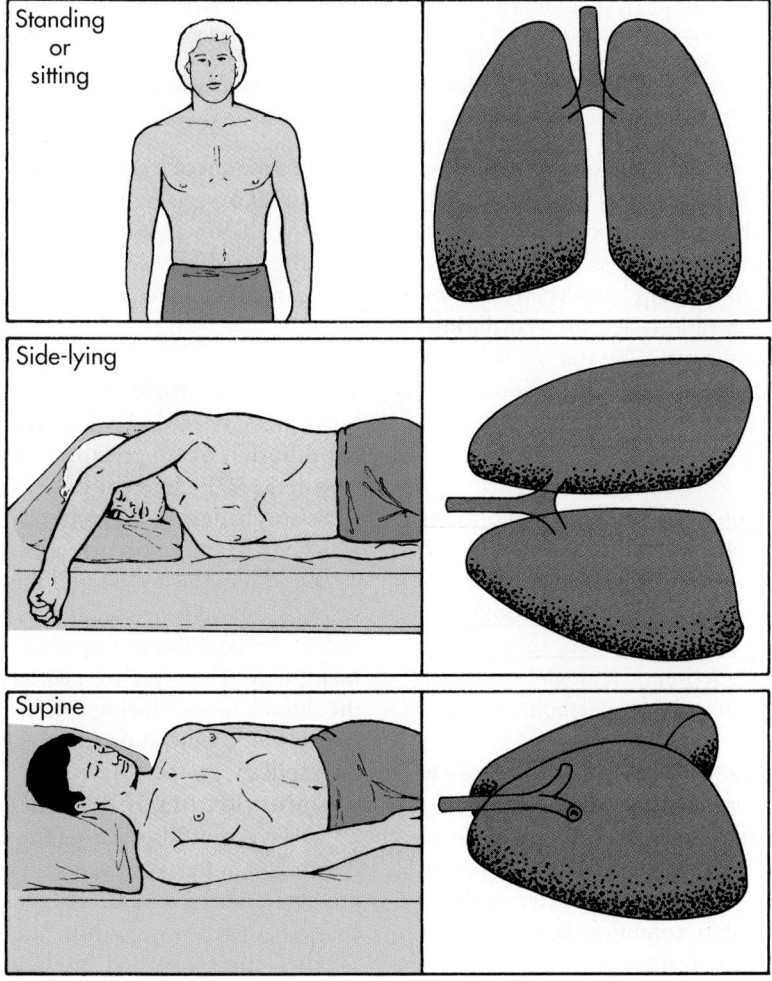

Figure 32-15 Pulmonary blood flow and gravity. The greatest volume of pulmonary blood flow will normally occur in the gravity-dependent areas of the lungs. Body position has a significant effect on the distribution of pulmonary blood flow.

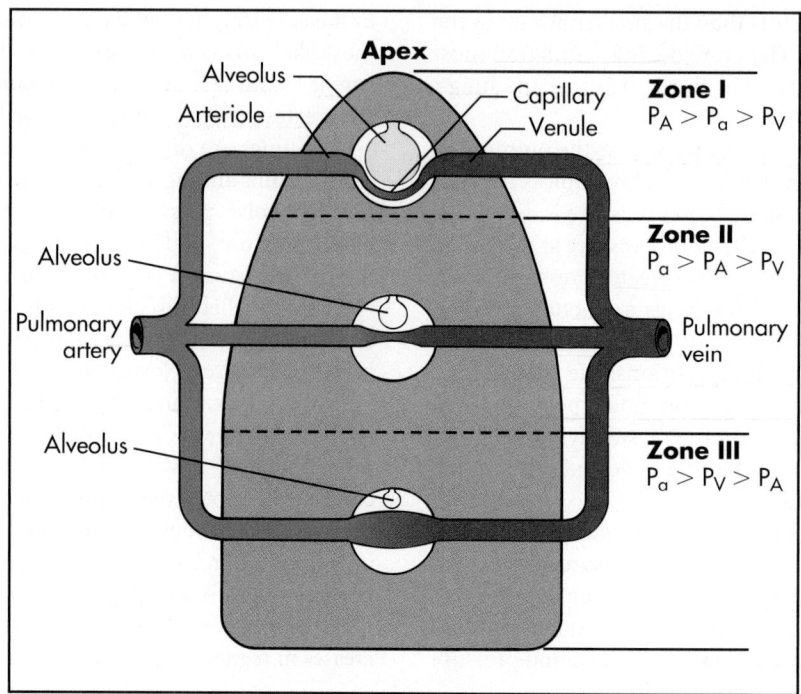

Figure 32-16 **Gravity and alveolar pressure.** Effects of gravity and alveolar pressure on pulmonary blood flow in the three lung zones. In zone I, alveolar pressure (P_A) is greater than arterial and venous pressure, and no blood flow occurs. In zone II, arterial pressure (P_a) exceeds alveolar pressure, but alveolar pressure exceeds venous pressure (P_V). Blood flow occurs in this zone, but alveolar pressure compresses the venules (venous ends of the capillaries). In zone III, both arterial and venous pressures are greater than alveolar pressure and blood flow fluctuates, depending on the difference between arterial and venous pressures.

Although both blood flow and ventilation are greater at the base of the lungs than at the apices, they are not perfectly matched in any of the zones. Perfusion exceeds ventilation in the bases of the lungs, and ventilation exceeds perfusion in the apices of the lung. The relationship between ventilation and perfusion is expressed as a ratio called the **ventilation-perfusion ratio,** or **V̇/Q̇.**[1,5] The normal V̇/Q̇ ratio is 0.8. This is the amount by which perfusion exceeds ventilation under normal conditions.

Oxygen Transport

Approximately 1000 ml (1 L) of oxygen is transported to the cells each minute. Oxygen is transported in the blood in two forms. A small amount dissolves in plasma, and the remainder binds to hemoglobin molecules. Without hemoglobin, oxygen would not reach the cells in amounts sufficient to maintain normal metabolic function. (Hemoglobin is discussed in detail in Chapter 25; cellular metabolism is discussed in Chapter 1.)

Diffusion Across the Alveolocapillary Membrane

The alveolocapillary membrane is the ideal medium for oxygen diffusion because it has a large total surface area (70 to 100 m^2) and is very thin (0.5 μm). In addition, the partial pressure of oxygen molecules (PO_2) is much greater in alveolar gas than in capillary blood, a condition that promotes rapid diffusion down the concentration gradient from the alveolus into the capillary.

The amount of oxygen in the alveoli (PAO_2) depends on the amount of oxygen in the inspired air (see p. 1193) and on the amount of air that remains in the alveoli and tracheobronchial tree between breaths (**physiologic dead space**).[1,5] This can be estimated by using the alveolar gas equation:

$$PAO_2 = 149 - PaCO_2/0.8 \text{ (the respiratory quotient)}$$

This value is approximately 104 with relaxed breathing; therefore a pressure gradient of approximately 60 mmHg facilitates the diffusion of oxygen from the alveolus into the capillary (Figure 32-17). Different values for PAO_2 can be calculated if there are changes in the inspired oxygen content or the $PaCO_2$, which are common occurrences in clinical settings.

Blood remains in the pulmonary capillary for about 0.75 seconds, but only 0.25 seconds is required for oxygen concentration to equilibrate (equalize) across the alveolocapillary membrane. Therefore oxygen has ample time to diffuse into the blood, even during increased cardiac output, which speeds blood flow, shortening the time the blood remains in the capillary.

Determinants of Arterial Oxygenation

As oxygen diffuses across the alveolocapillary membrane, it dissolves in the plasma, where it exerts pressure (the partial pressure of oxygen in arterial blood, or PaO_2). As the PaO_2 increases, oxygen moves from the plasma into the red blood cells (erythrocytes) and binds with hemoglobin molecules. Oxygen continues to bind with hemoglobin until the hemo-

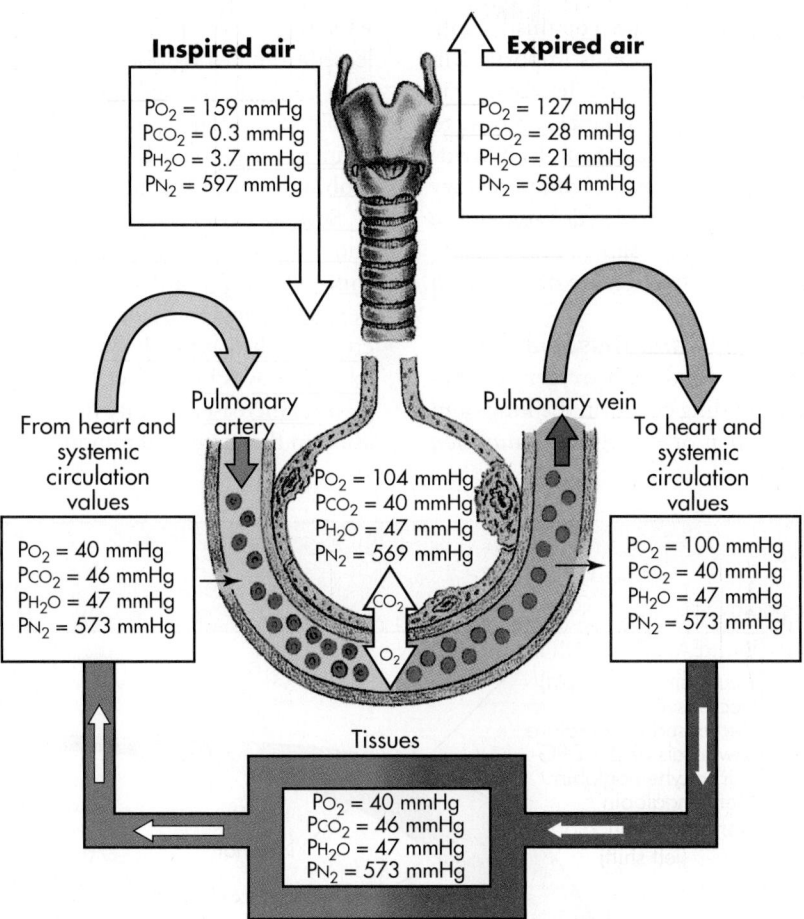

Figure 32-17 Partial pressure of respiratory gases in normal respiration. These are average values. The values of P_{O_2}, P_{CO_2}, and P_{N_2} fluctuate from breath to breath.

globin binding sites are filled or saturated. Oxygen then continues to diffuse across the alveolocapillary membrane until the P_{AO_2} (oxygen dissolved in plasma) and P_{aO_2} equilibrate, eliminating the pressure gradient across the alveolocapillary membrane. At this point diffusion ceases (see Figure 32-17).

Normally approximately 20 ml of oxygen is transported per 100 ml of blood. Because oxygen is not very soluble in plasma, most of the oxygen molecules bind with hemoglobin. Plasma carries only about 0.3 ml of oxygen per 100 ml of blood (at sea level). Although the remaining 19.7 ml is carried by hemoglobin, it is the small amount of oxygen dissolved in plasma that is responsible for oxygen's partial pressure (P_{aO_2}) in the blood.

Although P_{aO_2} is important in that it provides the driving pressure that loads the hemoglobin with oxygen, it gives little information about the *amount* of oxygen carried in the blood. This amount, which is measured in milliliters per deciliter (100 ml) of blood, is the **oxygen content** of the blood. The total oxygen content of the blood depends on the amount of oxygen chemically combined with hemoglobin, as well as that dissolved in the blood. To calculate the total arterial oxygen content, we must know (1) hemoglobin concentration, or the amount of hemoglobin that is available to bind with oxygen

(hemoglobin [Hb] in grams per deciliter); (2) the oxygen saturation or percentage of available hemoglobin that is bound to oxygen (S_{aO_2}); and (3) the partial pressure of oxygen (P_{aO_2}). The maximum amount of oxygen that can be transported by hemoglobin is 1.34 ml/g. The amount of oxygen that can be physically dissolved in blood is 0.003 ml/dl per mmHg P_{O_2}. If these specific values are known, the oxygen content of arterial blood can be calculated.[1]

$$O_2 \text{ content} = (Hb \times S_{aO_2} \times 1.34) + (P_{aO_2} \times 0.003)$$

To calculate the oxygen content of venous blood, the partial pressure of mixed venous blood ($P\dot{V}_{O_2}$) and venous oxygen saturation ($S\dot{V}_{O_2}$) are substituted for the arterial values in the basic formula. Normal venous oxygen content is 15 to 16 ml/dl.

Because hemoglobin transports all but a small fraction of the oxygen carried in arterial blood, increases in hemoglobin concentration affect the oxygen content of the blood. Decreases in hemoglobin concentration below the normal value of 15 ml/dl of blood reduce oxygen content, and increases in hemoglobin concentration may minimize the impact of impaired gas exchange. In fact, an increase in hemoglobin concentration is a major compensatory mechanism in pulmonary diseases that impair gas exchange. For this reason, measurement of hemoglobin concentration is important in the assessment of individuals with pulmonary disease. If cardiovascular function is normal, the body's initial response to low oxygen content is to speed up cardiac output. In individuals who also have cardiovascular disease, this compensatory mechanism does not work, making increased hemoglobin concentration an even more important compensatory mechanism. (Hemoglobin structure and function are described in Chapter 25.)

Oxyhemoglobin Association and Dissociation

When hemoglobin molecules bind with oxygen, **oxyhemoglobin (HbO$_2$)** is formed. Binding occurs in the lungs and is called *oxyhemoglobin association* or *hemoglobin saturation*

with oxygen (SaO$_2$). The reverse process, in which oxygen is released from hemoglobin, occurs in the body tissues at the cellular level and is called *hemoglobin desaturation*. When hemoglobin saturation and desaturation are plotted on a graph, the result is a distinctive S-shaped curve known as the **oxyhemoglobin dissociation curve** (Figure 32-18).

Several factors can change the relationship between PO$_2$ and SO$_2$, causing the oxyhemoglobin dissociation curve to shift to the right or left (see Figure 32-18). A shift to the right depicts hemoglobin's decreased affinity for oxygen or an increase in the ease with which oxyhemoglobin dissociates and oxygen moves into the cells. A shift to the left depicts hemoglobin's increased affinity for oxygen, which promotes association in the lungs and inhibits dissociation in the tissues.

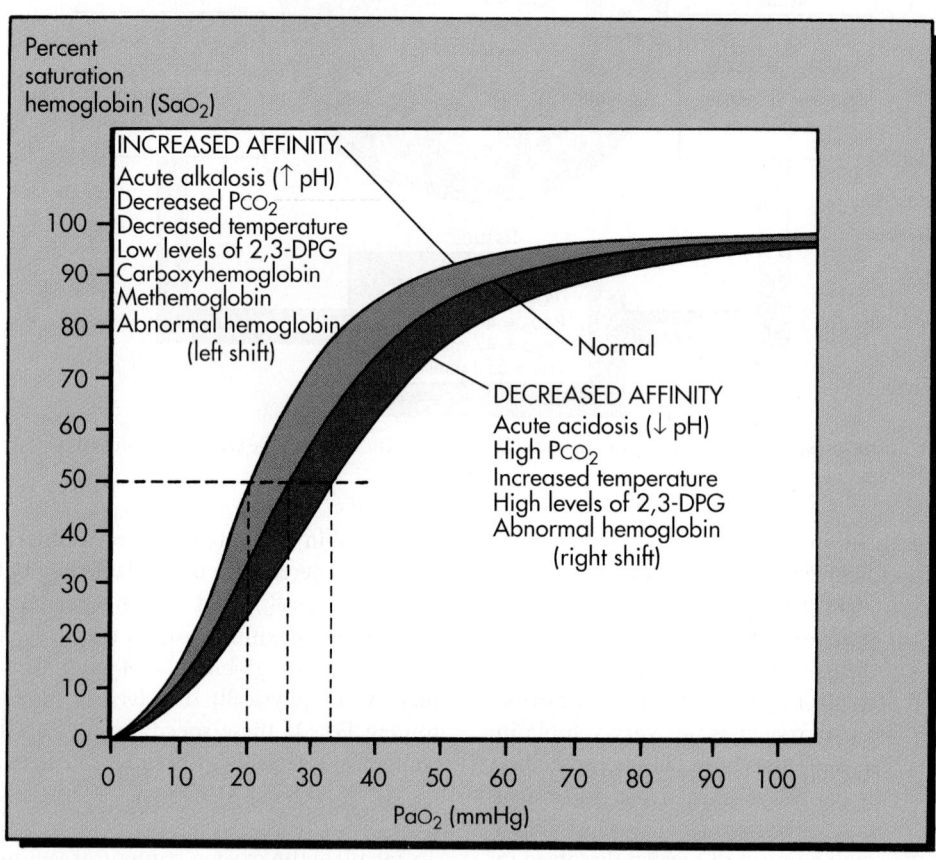

Figure 32-18 Oxyhemoglobin dissociation curve. The horizontal or flat segment of the curve at the top of the graph is sometimes called the *arterial portion*, or that part of the curve where oxygen is bound to hemoglobin. This portion of the curve is flat because partial pressure changes of oxygen between 60 and 100 mmHg do not significantly alter the percent saturation of hemoglobin with oxygen. The wide range of partial pressures of oxygen (PaO$_2$—60 to 100 mmHg, represented by the flat part of the curve—allows adequate hemoglobin saturation at a variety of altitudes. For example, a PaO$_2$ of 100 mmHg at sea level results in a hemoglobin saturation with oxygen of 98%. At an altitude of 5000 feet the PaO$_2$ is about 70 mmHg and hemoglobin saturation is 94%, only 4% less than at sea level. If the relationship between SaO$_2$ and PaO$_2$ were linear (in a downward-sloping straight line) instead of flat between 60 and 100 mmHg, there would be inadequate saturation of hemoglobin with oxygen. For example, with a PaO$_2$ of 70 mmHg the saturation would be only 70%, which is equivalent to normal venous oxygen saturation, and life could not be sustained at altitudes much above sea level. The steep part of the oxyhemoglobin dissociation curve occurs after the PaO$_2$ drops below 60 mmHg and represents the rapid dissociation of oxygen from hemoglobin. During this phase oxygen diffuses rapidly from the blood into tissue cells. Conditions associated with altered affinity of hemoglobin for O$_2$ are listed. P$_{50}$ is the PaO$_2$ at which hemoglobin is 50% saturated, normally 26.6 mmHg. A lower than normal P$_{50}$ represents increased affinity of hemoglobin for O$_2$; a high P$_{50}$ is seen with decreased affinity. Note that variation from the normal is associated with decreased (low P$_{50}$) or increased (high P$_{50}$) availability of O$_2$ to tissues *(dotted lines)*. The *shaded area* shows the entire oxyhemoglobin dissociation curve under the same circumstances. *2,3-DPG*, 2,3-diphosphatidylglycerate. (From Lane EE, Walker JF: *Clinical arterial blood gas analysis*, St Louis, 1987, Mosby.)

The oxyhemoglobin dissociation curve is shifted to the right by acidosis (low pH) and hypercapnia (increased $PaCO_2$). In the tissues the increased levels of carbon dioxide and hydrogen ions produced by metabolic activity decrease the affinity of hemoglobin for oxygen. The curve is shifted to the left by alkalosis (high pH) and hypocapnia (decreased $PaCO_2$). In the lungs, as carbon dioxide diffuses from the blood into the alveoli, the blood carbon dioxide level is reduced and the affinity of hemoglobin for oxygen is increased. The shift in the oxyhemoglobin dissociation curve caused by changes in carbon dioxide and hydrogen ion concentration in the blood is called the **Bohr effect.**

The oxyhemoglobin curve is shifted also by changes in body temperature and increased or decreased levels of 2,3-diphosphoglycerate (2,3-DPG), a substance normally present in erythrocytes. Hyperthermia and increased 2,3-DPG levels shift the curve to the right. Hypothermia and decreased 2,3-DPG levels shift the curve to the left.

Carbon Dioxide Transport

Approximately 200 ml of CO_2 is produced by the tissues per minute as a byproduct of cellular metabolism. This CO_2 equilibrates with carbonic acid ($H_2O + CO_2 \rightleftharpoons H_2CO_3 \rightleftharpoons H + HCO_3^-$) and must be eliminated continuously to prevent acidosis. The elimination of carbon dioxide by the lungs plays an important role in the regulation of acid-base balance (see Chapter 3).

CO_2 is carried in the blood in three ways: (1) dissolved in plasma (PCO_2), (2) as bicarbonate, and (3) as carbamino compounds. As CO_2 diffuses out of the cells into the blood, it dissolves in the plasma. Approximately 10% of the total CO_2 in venous blood and 5% of the CO_2 in arterial blood is carried dissolved in the plasma (PCO_2). As CO_2 moves into the blood, it diffuses into the red blood cells. Within the red blood cells, carbon dioxide, with the help of the enzyme carbonic anhydrase, combines with water to form carbonic acid and then quickly dissociates into H^+ and HCO_3^-. As carbonic acid dissociates, the H^+ binds to hemoglobin, where it is buffered, and the HCO_3^- moves out of the red blood cell into the plasma. Approximately 60% of the CO_2 in venous blood and 90% of the CO_2 in arterial blood are carried in the form of bicarbonate. The remainder combines with blood proteins, hemoglobin in particular, to form carbamino compounds. Approximately 30% of the CO_2 in venous blood and 5% of the CO_2 in arterial blood are carried as carbamino compounds (see Figure 3-9).

CO_2 is 20 times more soluble than O_2 and diffuses quickly from the tissue cells into the blood. The amount of CO_2 that is able to enter the blood is enhanced by diffusion of oxygen out of the blood and into the cells. Reduced hemoglobin (hemoglobin that is dissociated from oxygen) is able to carry more CO_2 than hemoglobin that is saturated with O_2. Therefore the drop in SO_2 at the tissue level increases the ability of hemoglobin to carry CO_2 back to the lung.

The diffusion gradient for CO_2 in the lung is only approximately 6 mmHg (venous $PCO_2 = 46$ mmHg; alveolar $PCO_2 = $ 40 mmHg), yet CO_2 is so soluble in the alveolocapillary membrane that the CO_2 in the blood quickly diffuses into the alveoli, where it is removed from the lung with each expiration. Diffusion of CO_2 in the lung is so efficient that diffusion defects that cause hypoxemia (low oxygen content of the blood) do not cause hypercapnia (excessive carbon dioxide in the blood).

The diffusion of CO_2 out of the blood also is enhanced by oxygen binding with hemoglobin in the lung. As hemoglobin binds with O_2, the amount of CO_2 carried by the blood is decreased. Thus, in the tissue capillaries, O_2 dissociation from hemoglobin facilitates the pickup of CO_2, and the binding of O_2 to hemoglobin in the lungs facilitates the release of CO_2 from the blood. This effect of oxygen on CO_2 transport is called the **Haldane effect** and can have significant clinical implications for the management of lung disease.[10-12]

Control of the Pulmonary Circulation

The caliber of pulmonary artery lumina decreases as smooth muscle in arterial walls contracts. Contraction increases pulmonary artery pressure. Caliber increases as these muscles relax, decreasing blood pressure. Contraction (vasoconstriction) and relaxation (vasodilation) apparently occur in response to local humoral conditions, even though the pulmonary circulation is innervated by the ANS in the same manner as the systemic circulation.

The most important cause of pulmonary artery constriction is a low alveolar PO_2 (PAO_2). Vasoconstriction caused by alveolar hypoxia, often termed **hypoxic vasoconstriction,** can affect only one portion of the lung (i.e., one lobe that is obstructed, decreasing the PAO_2) or the entire lung. If only one segment of the lung is involved, the arterioles to that segment constrict, shunting blood to other, well-ventilated portions of the lung. This reflex improves the lung's efficiency by better matching ventilation and perfusion. If alveolar hypoxia affects all segments of the lung, however, pulmonary hypertension (elevated pulmonary artery pressure) can result. The pulmonary vasoconstriction caused by low alveolar PO_2 is reversible if the alveolar PO_2 is corrected. Chronic alveolar hypoxia can result in permanent pulmonary artery hypertension, which eventually leads to cor pulmonale and heart failure.

Acidemia also causes pulmonary artery constriction. If the acidemia is corrected, the vasoconstriction is reversed. (Respiratory acidosis and metabolic acidosis are described in Chapter 3.) It is important to note that an elevated $PaCO_2$ without a drop in pH does not cause pulmonary artery constriction. Other biochemical factors that affect the caliber of vessels in pulmonary circulation are histamine, prostaglandins, endothelin, serotonin, nitric oxide, and bradykinin.[13]

TESTS OF PULMONARY FUNCTION

Several laboratory tests aid in the diagnosis and evaluation of pulmonary system abnormalities. Most of them are easy to perform at hospitals and clinics. They provide valuable information as to the possible cause of a respiratory abnormality and evaluate the progression or resolution of disease.

Spirometry is used to measure forced expiration, which often is affected by diffuse pulmonary disease. Because the pulmonary system has remarkable reserves, disease may become well established before clinical manifestations appear. Spirometry enables clinicians to detect restrictive or obstructive deficits early in the course of disease. Restrictive lung diseases restrict the lung's volume: the lungs are unable to expand normally, diminishing the amount of gas that can be inspired. Obstructive diseases affect gas flow: airflow into and out of the lungs is obstructed.

Spirometry measures both volume and flow. The test is performed with a spirometer, which is a water-filled cylinder into which an inverted cylinder or bell has been inserted. A length of tubing runs from the inverted bell to a mouthpiece through which a person breathes during testing. The bell is attached to a pen that writes on calibrated paper rotating at a constant speed. As a person performs various breathing maneuvers, the inverted bell moves up and down, causing the pen to move on the calibrated paper. This produces a spirogram, which is a record of the individual's ventilation in relation to time (Figure 32-19). Clinically, the most important spirometric tests are the forced vital capacity (FVC), and the forced expiratory volume in one second (FEV_1). (These tests and other important measures are described in Table 32-3.)

Lung capacities, such as vital capacity and total lung capacity, are always the sum of two or more volumes. Norms for volumes and capacities are based on age, gender, and height and are referred to as *predicted values.* Changes from predicted or baseline values are taken into account in diagnosing and assessing respiratory disorders.

Diffusing capacity is a measure of the rate of gas diffusion across the alveolocapillary membrane. Oxygen, or more commonly carbon monoxide, is used to measure diffusing capacity. The measurement is made by determining how much carbon monoxide is taken up by the blood and dividing this amount by the pressure gradient across the alveolocapillary membrane. Helium often is added to the gas mixture to obtain a simultaneous measurement of **residual volume (RV)**, **functional reserve capacity (FRC)**, and **total lung capacity (TLC)**. Individuals are asked to perform ventilatory maneuvers similar to those of spirometry. A decreased diffusing capacity can be the result of an abnormal ventilation-perfusion

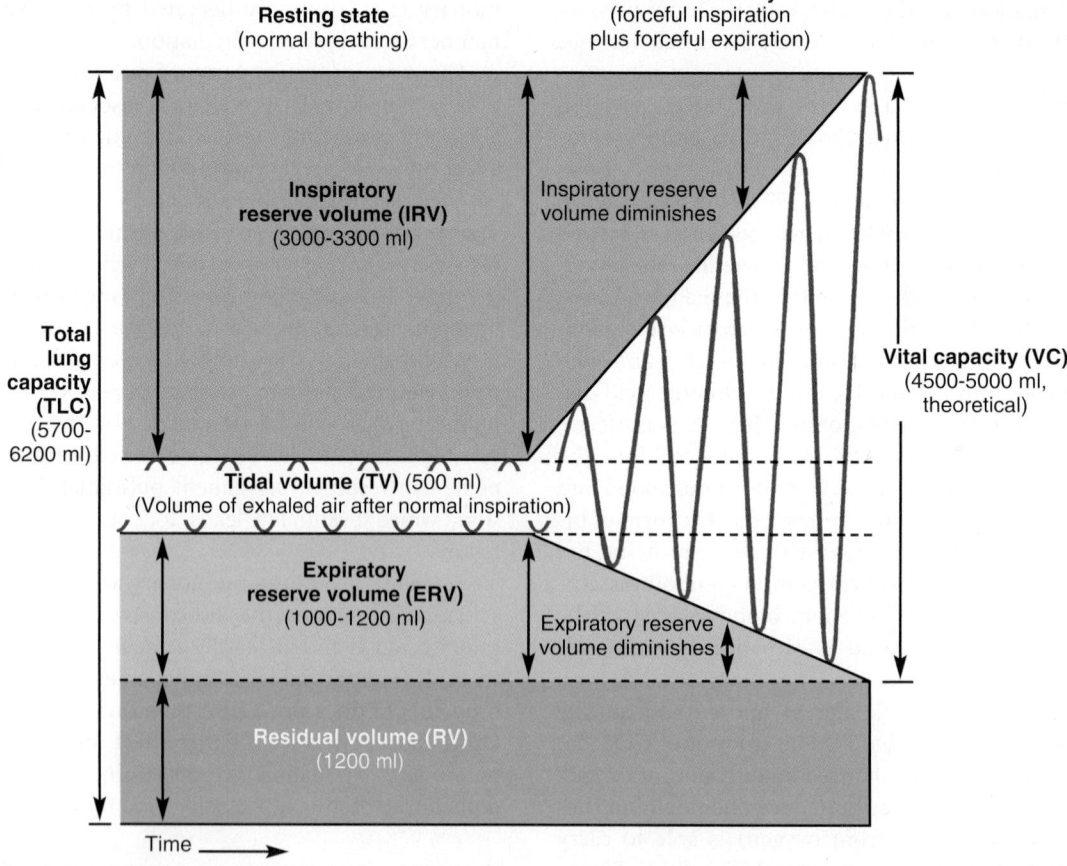

Figure 32-19 Spirogram. During normal, quiet respirations the atmosphere and lungs exchange about 500 ml of air *(TV).* With a forcible inspiration, about 3300 ml more air can be inhaled *(IRV).* After a normal inspiration and normal expiration, approximately 1000 ml more air can be forcibly expired *(ERV).* Vital capacity is the amount of air that can be forcibly expired after a maximal inspiration and indicates, therefore, the largest amount of air that can enter and leave the lungs during respiration. Residual volume is the air that remains trapped in the alveoli. (From Thibodeau GA, Patton KT: *Anatomy & physiology,* ed 5, St Louis, 2003, Mosby.)

Table 32-3	Values Measured by Spirometry
Symbol	Ventilatory Property Measured
FVC	Forced vital capacity: maximum amount of gas that can be displaced from the lung during a forced expiration
FEV_1	Forced expiratory volume in 1 sec: maximum amount of air that can be expired from the lung in 1 sec
FEV_1/FVC	Percentage of maximum inspiration that is expired in 1 sec, usually 80% of FVC
FEV_3	Forced expiratory volume in 3 sec; maximum amount of gas that can be expired in 3 sec
FEV_3/FVC	Percentage of FVC that is expired in 3 sec; usually 95% of FVC
$FEF_{25\%-75\%}$	Forced expiratory flow rate during the middle 50% of expiration; sometimes reported as maximum midexpiratory flow rate (MMFR)

Table 32-4	Normal Ranges for Arterial and Mixed Venous Blood Gases		
Measurement	Arterial Blood	Mixed Venous Blood*	Clinical Notes
Acid-base status (pH)	7.35-7.45	7.33-7.43	Most important acid-base value; detects acidosis or alkalosis
Partial pressure of carbon dioxide (PCO_2)	35-45 mmHg	41-57 mmHg	Measures adequacy of ventilation and respiratory contribution of acid-base abnormality (respiratory acidosis)
Bicarbonate (HCO_3^-)	22-26 mEq/L	24-28 mEq/L	Measures metabolic contribution to acid-base abnormality (metabolic acidosis); calculated from pH and PCO_2
Base excess (BE)	-2 to $+2$	0 to $+4$	Reflects deviation of bicarbonate concentration from normal
Partial pressure of oxygen (PO_2) (sea level)	80-100 mmHg	35-40 mmHg	Indicates driving pressure that causes oxygen-hemoglobin binding; varies with age and barometric pressure
Saturation of hemoglobin with oxygen (SO_2)	96%-98%	70%-75%	Indicates abnormalities of oxyhemoglobin association and dissociation; may be measured directly or calculated from PO_2, pH, and body temperature
Concentration of hemoglobin in the blood	15 g/dl	15 g/dl	Detects alterations of gas transport caused by anemia

*Mixed venous (pulmonary artery) blood is analyzed for critically ill individuals and those undergoing cardiac catheterization (it is not practical to withdraw samples except from a pulmonary artery catheter). Mixed venous blood gas analysis, in conjunction with arterial analysis, provides important information about the adequacy of cardiac output and tissue oxygenation.

ratio or an actual diffusion defect. Diffusing capacity is decreased in individuals with emphysema.

Arterial blood gas analysis commonly is performed for individuals with suggested or diagnosed pulmonary disease. Direct analysis of the pH and gas concentrations in arterial blood provides valuable information about an individual's gas exchange and acid-base status. Acidosis (low pH), alkalosis (high pH), ventilatory alterations, and decreased PaO_2 can be diagnosed accurately only by arterial blood gas analysis. A blood gas report may be divided into an acid-base/ventilation portion and an oxygenation portion. (Normal values for arterial blood gases are given in Table 32-4.) (Acid-base alterations are described in Chapter 3.) Oximetry can be used to monitor oxygen saturation once the arterial blood gas analysis has accurately measured the PaO_2, but it does not measure $PaCO_2$ or pH.

Signs and symptoms of most respiratory abnormalities first appear when the system is stressed during exercise. Therefore, if pulmonary disease is suspected, the individual is evaluated at rest and during exercise. During exercise the usual procedures are spirometry and withdrawal of arterial blood for gas analysis. The exercise usually consists of riding a stationary bicycle or walking on a treadmill. Exercise testing enables clinicians to detect early changes in respiratory function and thus begin treatment. Exercise tests also are used in planning and evaluating exercise and rehabilitation programs.

Chest radiographs are among the most common examinations of the pulmonary system. A few of the abnormalities detected in chest radiographs are air trapping in the alveoli and airways (e.g., in asthma or emphysema), consolidation of lung tissue (in pneumonia or pulmonary edema), cavities (abscesses or tuberculosis), and nodules (lung cancer). Often pulmonary abnormalities are detected in routine chest radiographs of asymptomatic individuals. Various radiographic techniques are available for the diagnosis and evaluation of respiratory disorders.

AGING AND THE PULMONARY SYSTEM

Most knowledge about pulmonary structure and function is based on norms for the middle years. Less is known about structure and function in very young (see Chapter 34) and elderly persons, but a few normal physiologic (developmental and degenerative) changes are known to occur from birth to old age. An understanding of these changes is needed to provide appropriate care and to differentiate between normal alterations and disease. Normal alterations include (1) loss of elastic recoil, (2) stiffening of the chest wall, (3) alterations in gas exchange, and (4) increases in flow resistance (Figure 32-20). These changes are influenced by environmental factors, respiratory disease, body size, and race.[14]

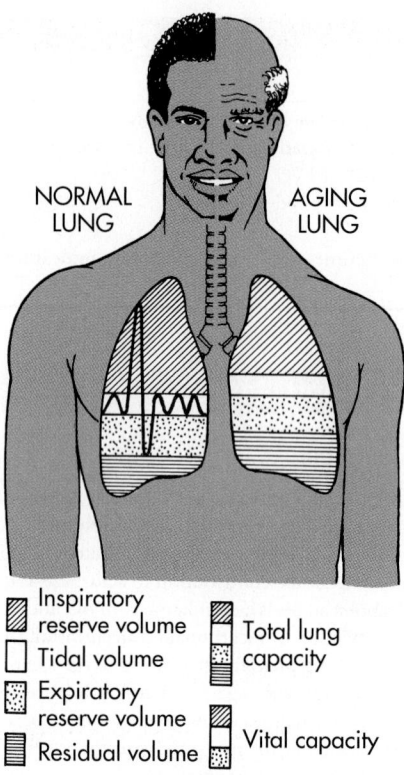

Inspiratory
reserve volume

Tidal volume

Total lung
capacity

Expiratory
reserve volume

Residual volume

Vital capacity

Figure 32-20 Changes in lung volumes with aging. With aging, note particularly the decrease in vital capacity and the increase in residual volume.

During adulthood and as age advances, the alveoli tend to lose alveoli wall tissue and capillaries. This process diminishes alveolar surface area available for gas diffusion and decreases airway support provided by normal lung tissues. Mechanical changes involve elastic properties of the lungs and chest wall. Chest wall compliance decreases with age because the ribs become ossified (less flexible) and joints become stiffer. As a result the chest wall loses some of its ability to expand. In addi-

tion, respiratory muscle strength and endurance decrease by up to 20% by age 70.[14,15] These mechanical changes in the lung and chest wall, along with structural changes in the alveoli, reduce ventilatory capacity in old age. Vital capacity decreases and residual volume increases; however, total lung capacity remains unchanged. These changes decrease ventilatory reserves and lead to decreased ventilation-perfusion ratios.[14] With advancing age, there is also increased immune dysregulation, asymptomatic low-grade inflammation, and increased risk of infection.

Alterations in gas exchange are reflected by blood gas analysis. With advancing age, pH and Pco_2 do not change much, even though it has been documented that the chemoreceptors become less sensitive to gas partial pressures with age. The elderly have a decreased compensatory response to hypercapnia and hypoxemia; however, the perception of dyspnea remains intact and is even enhanced.[14] Po_2 declines with age as a result of structural and mechanical changes, such as loss of alveolar surface area and increased ventilation-perfusion mismatch.[16] The maximum Pao_2 in an elderly individual at sea level can be estimated by multiplying the person's age by 0.3 and subtracting the product from 100. For example, an 80-year-old individual would have an estimated maximum Po_2 of 76 mmHg ($0.3 \times 80 = 24$; $100 - 24 = 76$). There is also a decrease in the capillary network.

The decrease in Pao_2 and diminished ventilatory reserve in the elderly person lead to a decrease in exercise tolerance. Furthermore, the elderly are at greater risk for respiratory depression caused by medications. Changes in respiratory function can vary considerably from person to person, however.[17] Changes also are affected by activity and fitness earlier in life. A very active, physically fit individual will, all else being equal, have fewer changes in function at any age than one who has been sedentary. Respiratory muscle strength and endurance decrease with age but can be enhanced with exercise.[18]

SUMMARY REVIEW

Structures of the Pulmonary System

1. The pulmonary system consists of the lungs, airways, chest wall, and pulmonary and bronchial circulation.
2. Air is inspired and expired through the conducting airways, which include the nasopharynx, oropharynx, trachea, bronchi, and bronchioles to the sixteenth division.
3. Gas exchange occurs in structures beyond the sixteenth division: the respiratory bronchioles, alveolar ducts, and alveoli. Together these structures compose the acinus.
4. The chief gas-exchange units of the lungs are the alveoli. The membrane that surrounds each alveolus and contains the pulmonary capillaries is called the *alveolocapillary membrane.*
5. The gas-exchange airways are served by the pulmonary circulation, a separate division of the circulatory system. The bronchi and other lung structures are served by a branch of the systemic circulation called the *bronchial circulation.*
6. The chest wall, which contains and protects the contents of the thoracic cavity, consists of the skin, ribs, and intercostal muscles, which lie between the ribs.

7. The chest wall is lined by a serous membrane called the *parietal pleura;* the lungs are encased in a separate membrane called the *visceral pleura.* The area where these two pleurae come into contact and slide over one another is called the *pleural space.*

Function of the Pulmonary System

1. The pulmonary system enables oxygen to diffuse into the blood and carbon dioxide to diffuse out of the blood.
2. Ventilation is the process by which air flows into and out of the gas-exchange airways.
3. Successful ventilation involves the mechanics of breathing: the interaction of forces and counterforces involving the muscles of inspiration and expiration, alveolar surface tension, elastic properties of the lungs and chest wall, and resistance to airflow.
4. The major muscle of inspiration is the diaphragm. When the diaphragm contracts, it moves downward in the thoracic cavity, creating a vacuum that causes air to flow into the lungs.
5. The alveoli produce surfactant, a lipoprotein that lines the alveoli. Surfactant reduces alveolar surface tension and permits the alveoli to expand more easily as air flows in.

6. Compliance is the ability of the lungs and chest wall to expand during inspiration. Lung compliance is ensured by adequate production of surfactant; chest wall expansion depends on flexibility.

7. Elastic recoil is the tendency of the lungs and chest wall to return to their resting state after inspiration. The elastic recoil forces of the lungs and chest wall are in opposition and pull on each other, creating the normally negative pressure of the pleural space.

8. Most of the time ventilation is involuntary. It is controlled by the sympathetic and parasympathetic divisions of the autonomic nervous system, which adjust airway caliber (by causing bronchial smooth muscle to contract or relax) and control the rate and depth of ventilation.

9. Neuroreceptors in the lungs (lung receptors) monitor the mechanical aspects of ventilation. Irritant receptors sense the need to expel unwanted substances, stretch receptors sense lung volume (lung expansion), and J-receptors sense alveolar size.

10. Chemoreceptors in the circulatory system and brain stem sense the effectiveness of ventilation by monitoring the pH status of cerebrospinal fluid and the oxygen content (P_{O_2}) of arterial blood.

11. The pulmonary circulation is innervated by the autonomic nervous system, but vasodilation and vasoconstriction are controlled mainly by local and humoral factors, particularly arterial oxygenation and acid-base status.

12. Gas transport depends on ventilation of the alveoli, diffusion across the alveolocapillary membrane, perfusion of the pulmonary and systemic capillaries, and diffusion between systemic capillaries and tissue cells.

13. Efficient gas exchange depends on an even distribution of ventilation and perfusion within the lungs. Both ventilation and perfusion are greatest in the bases of the lungs because the alveoli in the bases are more compliant (their resting volume is low) and perfusion is greater in the bases as a result of gravity.

14. Almost all of the oxygen that diffuses into pulmonary capillary blood is transported by hemoglobin, a protein contained within red blood cells. The remainder of the oxygen is transported dissolved in plasma.

15. Oxygen enters the body by diffusing down the concentration gradient, from high concentrations in the alveoli to lower concentrations in the capillaries. Diffusion ceases when alveolar and capillary oxygen pressures equilibrate.

16. Oxygen is loaded onto hemoglobin by the driving pressure exerted by P_{aO_2} in the plasma. As pressure decreases at tissue level, oxygen dissociates from hemoglobin and enters tissue cells by diffusion, again down the concentration gradient.

17. Carbon dioxide is more soluble in plasma than oxygen is and diffuses readily from tissue cells into plasma. Carbon dioxide returns to the lungs dissolved in plasma, as bicarbonate, or in carbamino compounds (e.g., bound to hemoglobin).

18. Vasoconstriction of the pulmonary arterial system is caused by alveolar hypoxia, acidemia, and inflammatory mediators—histamine, serotonin, prostaglandins, and bradykinin.

Tests of Pulmonary Function

1. Spirometry measures both volume and flow rate during forced expiration.

2. The alveolar-arterial oxygen gradient is used to evaluate the cause of hypoxia.

3. Diffusing capacity is a measure of the gas diffusion rate at the alveolocapillary membrane.

4. Arterial blood gas analysis can be used to determine pH and oxygen and carbon dioxide concentrations.

5. Radiographic examination of the chest evaluates air trapping, consolidation, cavity formation, or presence of tumors.

Aging and the Pulmonary System

1. Aging affects the mechanical aspects of ventilation by decreasing chest wall compliance and elastic recoil of the lungs. Changes in these elastic properties reduce ventilatory reserve.

2. Aging causes the P_{aO_2} to decrease but does not affect the P_{aCO_2}.

Acinus, 1185
Alveolar ducts, 1184
Alveolar ventilation, 1188
Alveolocapillary membrane, 1186
Alveolus (pl., alveoli), 1184
Arterial blood gas analysis, 1201
Bohr effect, 1199
Bronchioles, 1184
Bronchus (pl., bronchi), 1184
Carina, 1184
Central chemoreceptors, 1190
Chest radiographs, 1201
Compliance, 1192
Diffusing capacity, 1200
Elastic recoil, 1191
Functional reserve capacity (FRC), 1200

Goblet cells, 1184
Haldane effect, 1199
Hilus (pl., hila), 1184
Hypoxic vasoconstriction, 1199
Irritant receptors, 1189
J-receptors, 1189
Larynx, 1181
Minute volume, 1188
Nasopharynx, 1181
Oropharynx, 1181
Oxygen content, 1197
Oxyhemoglobin (HbO_2), 1198
Oxyhemoglobin dissociation curve, 1198
Partial pressure (tension) of a gas, 1193
Peripheral chemoreceptors, 1188
Physiologic dead space, 1196

Pleura (pl., pleurae), 1187
Pleural space (pleural cavity), 1187
Residual volume (RV), 1200
Respiration, 1188
Respiratory bronchioles, 1184
Respiratory center, 1188
Spirometry, 1200
Stretch receptors, 1189
Surface tension, 1191
Surfactant, 1185
Thoracic cavity, 1187
Total lung capacity (TLC), 1200
Trachea, 1184
Ventilation, 1188
Ventilation-perfusion ratio (mismatch) ($\dot{V}/\dot{Q}$), 1196

MEDIA RESOURCES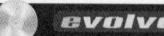

Review questions and answers for this chapter are available in the *CD Companion* included with this book.

WebLinks—links to Internet sites pertaining to this chapter—are available on Evolve at http://evolve.elsevier.com/McCance/.

REFERENCES

1. Clouter M, Thrall R: The respiratory system. In Berne R et al, editors: *Physiology,* ed 5, St Louis, 2004, Mosby.
2. Corrin B: *Pathology of the lungs,* London, 2000, Churchill Livingstone.
3. Hilaire G, Pasaro R: Genesis and control of the respiratory rhythm in adult mammals, *New Physiol Sci* 19:23-28, 2003.
4. Richter DW et al: Serotonin receptors: guardians of stable breathing, *Tends Mol Med* 9(12):542-548, 2003.
5. West JB: *Respiratory physiology: the essentials,* ed 6, Philadelphia, 2000, Lippincott, Williams, & Wilkins.
6. Widdicombe JG: Sensory neurophysiology of the cough reflex, *J Allergy Clin Immunol* 98(5 Pt2):S84-S89, 1996.
7. Caruana-Montaldo B, Gleeson K, Zwillich CW: The control of breathing in clinical practice, *Chest* 117(1):205-225 2000.
8. Lawson PR, Reid KB: The roles of surfactant proteins A and D in innate immunity, *Immunol Rev* 173:66-78, 2000.
9. Ward ME, Roussos C, Macklem PT: Respiratory mechanisms. In Murray JF, Nadel JA, editors: *Textbook of respiratory medicine,* ed 3, Philadelphia, 2000, Saunders.
10. Giovannini I et al: Quantitative assessment of changes in blood CO_2 tension mediated by the Haldane effect, *J Appl Physiol* 87(2):862, 1999.
11. Rigg CD, Cruickshank S: Carbon dioxide during and after the apnoea test—an illustration of the Haldane effect, *Anaesthesia* 56(4):377, 2001.
12. Chien JW et al: Uncontrolled oxygen administration and respiratory failure in acute asthma, *Chest* 117(3):728-733, 2000.
13. Johnson W et al: Contribution of endothelin to pulmonary vascular tone under normoxic and hypoxic conditions, *Am J Physiol Heart Circ Physiol* 283(2):H568-H575, 2002.
14. Gold W: Pulmonary function testing. In Murray JF, Nadel JA, editors: *Textbook of respiratory medicine,* ed 3, Philadelphia, 2000, Saunders.
15. McClaran SR et al: Longitudinal effects of aging on lung function at rest and exercise in healthy active fit elderly adults, *J Appl Physiol* 78(5):1957-1968, 1995.
16. Hardie JA et al: Reference values for arterial blood gases in the elderly, *Chest* 125(6):2053-2060, 2004.
17. Zeleznik J: Normative aging of the respiratory system, *Clin Geriatr Med* 19(1):1-18, 2003.
18. Meyer KC: The role of immunity in susceptibility to respiratory infection in the aging lung, *Respir Physiol* 128(1):23-31, 2001.

ALTERATIONS OF PULMONARY FUNCTION

VALENTINA L. BRASHERS

CHAPTER OUTLINE

Pulmonary disease is often classified as acute or chronic, obstructive or restrictive, and infectious or noninfectious. Because skillful and knowledgeable clinical care plays a major role in decreasing respiratory mortality and morbidity, the clinician with a clear understanding of the pathophysiology of common respiratory problems can greatly affect the outcome for each individual.

CLINICAL MANIFESTATIONS OF PULMONARY ALTERATIONS

Signs and Symptoms of Pulmonary Disease

Pulmonary disease is associated with many signs and symptoms. The most common of these are cough and dyspnea. Other manifestations include chest pain, abnormal sputum, hemoptysis, altered breathing patterns, cyanosis, and fever. The signs and symptoms present and their specific characteristics often help in identifying the underlying disorder.

Dyspnea

Dyspnea is the subjective sensation of uncomfortable breathing, the feeling of being unable to get enough air. It is often described as breathlessness, air hunger, shortness of breath, labored breathing, and preoccupation with breathing. Dyspnea is a common symptom of respiratory disease.

Dyspnea is usually caused by diffuse and extensive pulmonary disease but can be caused by focal pulmonary disorders as well. Disturbances of ventilation, gas exchange, or ventilation-perfusion relationships can cause dyspnea, as can increased work of breathing or diseases that damage lung tissue (lung parenchyma).

Many mechanisms have been proposed to explain the complex sensation of dyspnea, but no single mechanism has been found to be responsible in all situations. The most commonly accepted explanation is the *length/tension inappropriateness theory*, which involves stimulation of receptors in respiratory muscles. According to this theory, the perception of dyspnea develops when muscle spindles in intercostal muscles are stimulated by a disparity between the tension generated by the muscles and the tidal volume (change in muscle fiber length) that results. This can occur if increased airway resistance or decreased compliance results in respiratory effort that is greater than appropriate for the ventilation achieved.

A second explanation involves the stimulation of central and peripheral chemoreceptors. It has long been known that decreased pH, hypercapnia, and hypoxemia can cause dyspnea. Stimulation of chemoreceptors causes dyspnea in many lung diseases in which oxygenation and gas exchange are impaired.

A third explanation is stimulation of the afferent receptors in the lung (the stretch receptors, irritant receptors, and J-receptors), which send impulses to the central nervous system through the vagus nerve. Stretch receptors are stimulated in asthma and may be the primary cause of the sensation of dyspnea and chest tightness in that disorder.[1] J-receptors also trigger dyspnea in individuals with pulmonary edema and pulmonary microemboli. (The neurochemical control of ventilation is described in Chapter 32.) Other receptors in the face, upper airway, and chest wall can contribute to the sensation of dyspnea. Finally, the sensation of dyspnea also can be caused by increased work of breathing, respiratory muscle fatigue, decreased breathing reserve, and strong emotions, particularly anxiety and anger. There is general agreement that neurologic control and function of respiratory muscles are the common elements in most clinical experiences of dyspnea and that the sensation perceived is that of increased respiratory effort.

The signs of dyspnea include flaring of the nostrils, use of accessory muscles of respiration, and retraction (pulling back) of the intercostal spaces. In dyspnea caused by parenchymal disease (e.g., pneumonia), retractions of tissue between the ribs (subcostal and intercostal retractions) are observed more often than supercostal retractions (retractions of tissues above the ribs), which predominate in upper airway obstruction. Retractions of any type are more commonly seen in children or in adults who are thin and have poorly developed thoracic musculature. Dyspnea can be quantified by the use of both ordinal rating scales or visual analog scales.[2]

Dyspnea can occur suddenly or can progress over time. The first episode commonly occurs with exercise and is called *dyspnea on exertion*. Dyspnea also can be associated with body positioning. Pulmonary congestion tends to cause dyspnea when the individual is lying down. This type is called **orthopnea**. Orthopnea is caused by the horizontal position, which redistributes body water, causes the abdominal contents to exert pressure on the diaphragm, and decreases the efficiency of the respiratory muscles. Orthopnea is generally relieved by sitting up in a forward-leaning posture or supporting the upper body on several pillows. Some individuals with left ventricular failure wake up at night gasping for air and must sit up or stand to relieve the dyspnea. This type of positional dyspnea is termed **paroxysmal nocturnal dyspnea (PND)**. PND results from fluid in the lungs caused by the redistribution of body water while the individual is recumbent.

Abnormal Breathing Patterns

Normal breathing (eupnea) is rhythmic and effortless. Ventilatory rate is 8 to 16 breaths per minute, and tidal volume ranges from 400 to 800 ml. A short expiratory pause occurs with each breath, and the individual takes an occasional deeper breath or sigh. Sigh breaths, which help maintain normal lung function, are usually 1.5 to 2 times the normal tidal volume and occur approximately 10 to 12 times per hour.

The rate, depth, regularity, and effort of breathing undergo characteristic alterations in response to physiologic and pathophysiologic conditions. Patterns of breathing automatically adjust to minimize the work of respiratory muscles. Strenuous exercise or metabolic acidosis induces **Kussmaul respiration (hyperpnea)**. Kussmaul respiration is characterized by a slightly increased ventilatory rate, very large tidal volume, and no expiratory pause.

Labored, or obstructed, breathing occurs if the airways are obstructed, as in chronic obstructive pulmonary disease (COPD). Obstructed breathing consists of slow ventilatory rate, large tidal volume, increased effort, and prolonged inspiration or expiration, depending on the site of obstruction. Audible wheezing (whistling sounds) or stridor (high-pitched sounds made during inspiration) is often present.

Restricted breathing is commonly caused by disorders such as pulmonary fibrosis that stiffen the lungs or chest wall and decrease compliance. Restricted breathing is characterized by small tidal volumes and rapid ventilatory rate (tachypnea).

Panting occurs with exercise. Shock and severe cerebral hypoxia (insufficient oxygen in the brain) contribute to gasping respirations that consist of irregular, quick inspirations with an expiratory pause. Sighing respirations consist of irregular breathing characterized by frequent, deep sighing inspirations. Sighing respirations are caused by anxiety.

Cheyne-Stokes respirations are characterized by alternating periods of deep and shallow breathing. Apnea lasting 15 to 60 seconds is followed by ventilations that increase in volume until a peak is reached, after which ventilation (tidal volume) decreases again to apnea. Cheyne-Stokes respirations result from any condition that slows the blood flow to the brain stem, which in turn slows impulses sending information to the respiratory centers of the brain stem. Neurologic impairment above the brain stem is also a contributing factor.

Hypoventilation and Hyperventilation

Hypoventilation is inadequate alveolar ventilation in relation to metabolic demands. It is caused by alterations in pulmonary mechanics or in the neurologic control of breathing. When alveolar ventilation is normal, CO_2 is removed from the lungs at the same rate at which it is produced by cellular metabolism. This maintains arterial and alveolar P_{CO_2} at normal levels (40 mmHg). With hypoventilation, CO_2 removal does not keep up with CO_2 production and Pa_{CO_2} increases, causing hypercapnia (Pa_{CO_2} greater than 44 mmHg). (Table 32-2 contains the definition of gas partial pressure and other pulmonary abbreviations.) This results in respiratory acidosis, which can affect the function of many tissues throughout the body. Hypoventilation and hypercapnia occur when minute volume (tidal volume (respiratory rate) is reduced.

Hypoventilation is often overlooked until it is severe because breathing pattern and ventilatory rate may appear normal.

Blood gas analysis (i.e., measurement of the $PaCO_2$ of arterial blood) reveals the hypercapnia. Pronounced hypoventilation can cause somnolence or disorientation. In addition, hypoventilation with hypercapnia results in secondary hypoxemia.

Hyperventilation is alveolar ventilation that exceeds metabolic demands. The lungs remove CO_2 at a faster rate than it is produced by cellular metabolism, resulting in decreased $PaCO_2$ or **hypocapnia** ($PaCO_2$ less than 36 mmHg). Hypocapnia results in a respiratory alkalosis that also can interfere with tissue function. Like hypoventilation, hyperventilation can be determined only by arterial blood gas analysis. Hyperventilation commonly occurs with severe anxiety, acute head injury, and conditions that cause insufficient oxygenation of the blood.

Cough

Cough is an important reflex that helps clear the airways of large amounts of inhaled material, excessive secretions, or abnormal substances, such as edema or pus. Individuals with an inability to cough normally are at greater risk for pneumonia.[3] Most coughs are initiated in the larynx and in the tracheobronchial tree by both mechanical and chemical "irritant" receptor stimulation. There are few such receptors in the most distal bronchi and the alveoli; thus it is possible for significant amounts of secretions to accumulate in the distal respiratory tree without cough being initiated. Other cough receptors are located in the external auditory canal, diaphragm, pericardium, pleura, and stomach. Stimulation of cough receptors is transmitted centrally through the vagus nerve, and central modulation of the cough reflex can be influenced by opiates and serotoninergic agents.[4]

Acute cough is cough that resolves within 2 to 3 weeks of the onset of illness or resolves with treatment of the underlying condition. It is most commonly the result of upper respiratory infections, allergic rhinitis, acute bronchitis, pneumonia, congestive heart failure, pulmonary embolus, or aspiration.[5] **Chronic cough** is defined as cough that has persisted for more than 3 weeks, although some authors have suggested that 7 or 8 weeks is a more appropriate timeframe because acute cough and bronchial hyperreactivity can be prolonged in some cases of viral infection. In nonsmokers, chronic cough is almost always caused by postnasal drainage syndrome, asthma, or gastroesophageal reflux disease.[5] In smokers, chronic bronchitis is the most common cause of chronic cough, although lung cancer must always be considered. Up to 33% of individuals taking angiotensin-converting enzyme inhibitors for cardiovascular disease develop chronic cough that resolves with discontinuation of the drug.

Hemoptysis

Hemoptysis is the coughing up of blood or bloody secretions. Hemoptysis is sometimes confused with hematemesis, which is the vomiting of blood. Blood that is coughed up is usually bright red, has an alkaline pH, and is mixed with frothy sputum, whereas blood that is vomited is dark, has an acidic pH, and is mixed with food particles.

The most common causes of hemoptysis are bronchiectasis, lung cancer, bronchitis, and pneumonia. Tuberculosis remains an important cause of hemoptysis but is less common in the United States than in many other parts of the world. Hemoptysis results from damage to the lung parenchyma with rupture of pulmonary vessels or from inflammation, injury, or cancer of the bronchial tree. The amount and duration of bleeding (i.e., a sudden large amount versus a persistent slight amount) provide important clues about the source of the bleeding.[6] Bronchoscopy combined with chest computed tomography (CT) can identify the cause in the majority of cases of hemoptysis.

Cyanosis

Cyanosis is a bluish discoloration of the skin and mucous membranes caused by increasing amounts of desaturated or reduced hemoglobin (which is bluish) in the blood. Cyanosis generally develops when 5 g of hemoglobin is desaturated, regardless of hemoglobin concentration. For example, if total hemoglobin concentration is 15 g/dl of blood, 5 g/dl must be desaturated to cause cyanosis. If total hemoglobin (Hb) is 11 g/dl, 5 g/dl must still be desaturated for cyanosis to occur.

Cyanosis can be caused by decreased arterial oxygenation (low PaO_2), pulmonary or cardiac right-to-left shunts, decreased cardiac output, cold environments, or anxiety. In adults, cyanosis is not evident until severe hypoxemia is present and therefore is an insensitive indicator of respiratory distress. Lack of cyanosis does not necessarily indicate that oxygenation is normal. For example, severe anemia (inadequate hemoglobin concentration) and carbon monoxide poisoning (in which hemoglobin binds to carbon monoxide instead of to oxygen) can cause inadequate oxygenation of tissues without causing cyanosis. Individuals with polycythemia (an abnormal increase in numbers of red blood cells), however, may have cyanosis when oxygenation is adequate. Because polycythemia causes hemoglobin concentration to be greater than normal, 5 g/dl can be desaturated, causing cyanosis, without having much effect on oxygenation. Therefore the significance of cyanosis as a clinical finding must be interpreted in relation to the underlying pathophysiology. If cyanosis is suggested, the PaO_2 should be measured. Central cyanosis (decreased oxygen saturation of hemoglobin in arterial blood) is best seen in buccal mucous membranes and lips. Peripheral cyanosis (slow blood circulation in fingers and toes) is best seen in nail beds.

Pain

Pain caused by pulmonary disorders originates in the pleurae, airways, or chest wall. Pleural pain is the most common pain caused by pulmonary disease and is usually sharp or stabbing in character. Infection and inflammation of the parietal pleura cause pain when the pleura stretches during inspiration. The pain is usually localized to a portion of the chest wall, where a unique breath sound called a *pleural friction rub* may be heard over the painful area. Laughing or coughing makes pleural pain worse. Pleural pain is also common with pulmonary infarction (tissue death) caused by pulmonary embolism. In the case of infarction the pain emanates from the area around the infarction.

Pulmonary pain is central chest pain that is pronounced after coughing and occurs in individuals with infection and inflammation of the trachea or bronchi (tracheitis or tracheobronchitis). Central chest pain must be differentiated from cardiac pain (see Chapter 30). High blood pressure in the pulmonary circulation (pulmonary hypertension) can cause pain during exercise that is often mistaken for cardiac pain (angina pectoris).

Pain in the chest wall is muscle pain or rib pain. The common causes of chest wall pain are excessive coughing, which makes the muscles sore, and rib fractures. Inflammation of the costochondral junction (costochondritis) also can cause chest wall pain. Chest wall pain often mimics pleural pain.

Clubbing

Clubbing is the selective bulbous enlargement of the end (distal segment) of a digit (finger or toe) (Figure 33-1) whose severity can be graded from 1 to 5 based on the extent of nail bed hypertrophy and the amount of changes in the nails themselves. Usually it is painless. Clubbing is commonly associated with diseases that interfere with oxygenation, such as bronchiectasis, cystic fibrosis, pulmonary fibrosis, lung abscess, and congenital heart disease. It is usually reversible with treatment of the underlying pulmonary condition.[7] Lung cancer is sometimes associated with clubbing even in the absence of significant hypoxemia. This syndrome is called *hypertrophic osteoarthropathy (HOA)* and its pathogenesis is unknown, although tumor-associated production of inflammatory cytokines and growth factors have been implicated.[8]

Clubbing—early

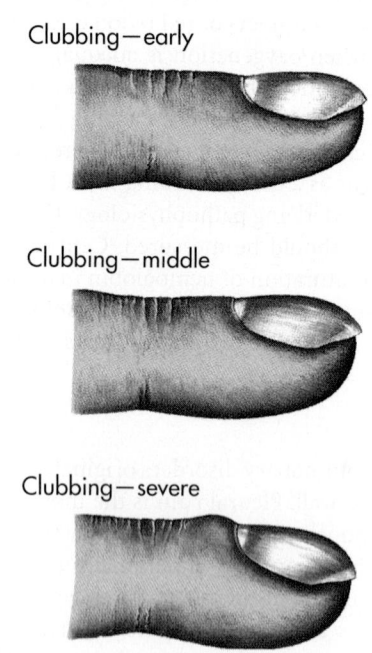

Clubbing—middle

Clubbing—severe

Figure 33-1 Clubbing of fingers caused by chronic hypoxemia. (From Seidel HM et al: *Mosby's guide to physical examination*, ed 5, St Louis, 2003, Mosby.)

Abnormal Sputum

The color, consistency, odor, and amount of sputum vary with different pulmonary disorders. A distinctive color or odor may suggest infection by a specific microorganism. Changes in the amount and consistency of sputum provide information about progression of disease and effectiveness of therapy. The gross and microscopic appearances of sputum enable the clinician to identify cellular debris or microorganisms that aid in diagnosis and choice of therapy.

Conditions Caused by Pulmonary Disease or Injury
Hypercapnia

Hypercapnia, or increased carbon dioxide in the arterial blood (increased $PaCO_2$), is caused by hypoventilation of the alveoli. As discussed in Chapter 32, carbon dioxide is easily diffused from the blood into the alveolar space; thus minute volume (respiratory rate × tidal volume) determines not only alveolar ventilation but also $PaCO_2$. Hypoventilation is often overlooked because breathing pattern and ventilatory rate may appear normal; it is important to obtain blood gas analysis to determine the severity of hypercapnia and resultant respiratory acidosis (acid-base balance is described in Chapter 3).

There are many causes of hypercapnia. Most are a result of decreased drive to breathe or an inadequate ability to respond to ventilatory stimulation. Causes include (1) depression of the respiratory center by drugs; (2) diseases of the medulla, including infections of the central nervous system or trauma; (3) abnormalities of the spinal conducting pathways, as in spinal cord disruption or poliomyelitis; (4) diseases of the neuromuscular junction or of the respiratory muscles themselves, as in myasthenia gravis or muscular dystrophy; (5) thoracic cage abnormalities, as in chest injury or congenital deformity; (6) large airway obstruction, as in tumors or sleep apnea; and (7) increased work of breathing or physiologic dead space, as in emphysema.

Hypercapnia and the associated respiratory acidosis can result in several important clinical manifestations. Of greatest concern are electrolyte abnormalities that occur in response to the low pH that may cause dysrhythmias. Individuals also may have somnolence and even be in coma because of changes in intracranial pressure associated with high levels of arterial carbon dioxide, which causes cerebral vasodilation. Alveolar hyperventilation with increased alveolar carbon dioxide limits the amount of oxygen available for diffusion into the blood, leading to hypoxemia.

Hypoxemia

Hypoxemia, or reduced oxygenation of arterial blood (reduced PaO_2), is caused by respiratory alterations, whereas **hypoxia,** or reduced oxygenation of cells in tissues, may be caused by alterations of other systems as well. (Hypoxia can occur anywhere in the body; if it occurs in arterial blood, it is correctly called *hypoxemia*.) Although hypoxemia can lead to tissue hypoxia, tissue hypoxia can result from other abnormalities, such as low cardiac output or cyanide poisoning, that have no relation to alterations of pulmonary function.

The five causes of hypoxemia are (1) decreased oxygen content (PO_2) of inspired gas, (2) hypoventilation, (3) diffusion abnormalities, (4) abnormal ventilation-perfusion ratios, and (5) pulmonary right-to-left shunt (Table 33-1). The physiologic mechanisms for each cause of hypoxemia are different, and each requires different clinical management.

The PaO_2 of arterial blood depends on the fraction of inspired oxygen (FiO_2) of inspired gas. If the FiO_2 of inspired gas is below normal, less oxygen is available to diffuse into the blood. The most common cause of a decrease in inspired oxygen is the drop in atmospheric pressure that occurs at high altitudes. FiO_2 drops proportionately with atmospheric pressure, resulting in a decrease in PaO_2. Hypoxemia caused by high altitude is prevented by the use of supplemental oxygen.

Hypoventilation of the alveoli causes elevated $PaCO_2$ (hypercapnia). If oxygen-rich gas is not delivered to the alveoli, the oxygen content of alveolar gas (PAO_2) decreases as $PaCO_2$ increases. As PAO_2 decreases, less oxygen diffuses into the blood, causing hypoxemia. This type of hypoxemia can be completely corrected if alveolar ventilation is improved by increases in the rate and depth of breathing. Hypoventilation is a common cause of hypoxemia in unconscious persons, individuals receiving extensive sedation, and individuals who have COPD.

Diffusion of oxygen through the alveolocapillary membrane is impaired if the alveolocapillary membrane is thickened or the surface area available for diffusion is decreased. Abnormal thickness, as occurs with edema (tissue swelling) and fibrosis (formation of fibrous lesions), increases the time required for diffusion across the alveolocapillary membrane. If diffusion is slowed enough, the PO_2 of alveolar gas (PAO_2) and capillary blood does not have time to equilibrate during the fraction of a second that blood remains in the capillary. Destruction of alveoli, such as that which occurs in emphy-

sema, decreases the surface area available for diffusion. Hypercapnia is rarely produced by impaired diffusion because carbon dioxide diffuses so easily from capillary to alveolus that the individual with impaired diffusion would die from hypoxemia before hypercapnia could occur.

An abnormal ventilation-perfusion ratio ($\dot{V}/\dot{Q}$) is the most common cause of hypoxemia (Figure 33-2). Normally, alveolocapillary lung units receive almost equal amounts of ventilation and perfusion. The normal $\dot{V}/\dot{Q}$ is 0.8 to 0.9 because perfusion is somewhat greater than ventilation in the lung bases. $\dot{V}/\dot{Q}$ mismatch refers to an abnormal distribution of ventilation and perfusion. Hypoxemia can be caused by inadequate ventilation of well-perfused areas of the lung (low $\dot{V}/\dot{Q}$). Blood passing through pulmonary capillaries is exposed to less oxygen than normal. Mismatching of this type is called *shunting* and occurs in those with asthma as a result of bronchoconstriction and in those with pulmonary edema and pneumonia when alveoli are filled with fluid. A pulmonary right-to-left shunt exists when blood passes through portions of the pulmonary capillary bed that receive no ventilation, either because the airway leading to the alveoli is completely obstructed or because the alveoli are collapsed or filled with fluid and cellular debris. Blood flows through the pulmonary circulation without being oxygenated. This results in decreased systemic PaO_2 and hypoxemia. $PaCO_2$ is usually not affected except by severe shunting. Hypoxemia resulting from shunting does not respond to increases in supplemental inspired oxygen concentration because a portion of the pulmonary capillary bed is never exposed to the oxygen-rich gas. This makes hypoxemia produced by shunting very difficult to treat. Shunting is the cause of hypoxemia in adult respiratory distress syndrome (ARDS) and respiratory distress syndrome of the newborn.

Hypoxemia also can be caused by poor perfusion of well-ventilated portions of the lung (high $\dot{V}/\dot{Q}$), resulting in wasted ventilation. In this case, oxygen in the alveoli is not exposed to

Table 33-1	Causes of Hypoxemia
Mechanism	**Common Clinical Cause**
Decrease in inspired oxygen (decreased FiO_2)	High altitude
	Low oxygen content of gas mixture
	Enclosed breathing spaces (suffocation)
Hypoventilation	Lack of neurologic stimulation of the respiratory center (oversedation, drug overdose, neurologic damage)
Alveolocapillary diffusion abnormality	Emphysema
	Fibrosis
	Edema
Ventilation-perfusion mismatch	Asthma
	Chronic bronchitis
	Pneumonia
	Acute respiratory distress syndrome
	Respiratory distress syndrome of the newborn (hyaline membrane disease)
	Atelectasis
	Shunting
	Arteriovenous malformations
	Congenital heart defects

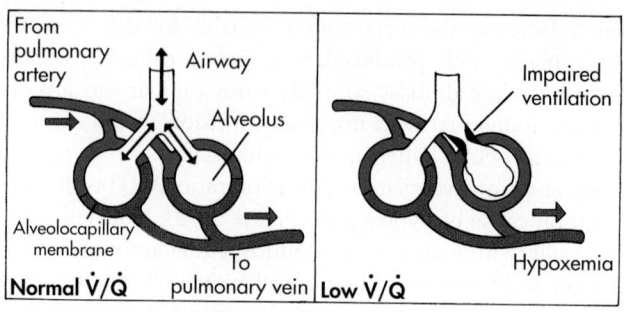

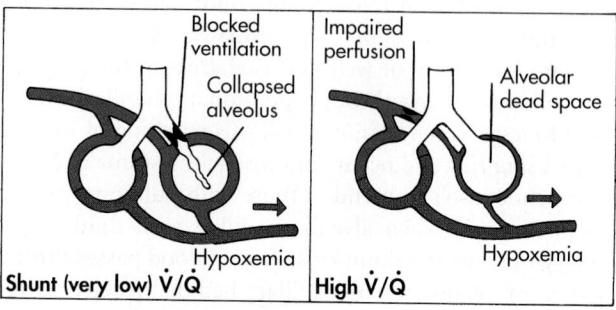

Figure 33-2 Ventilation-perfusion abnormalities.

circulating blood. The result is a decrease in PaO_2. The most common cause of high $\dot{V}/\dot{Q}$ is a pulmonary embolus that impairs blood flow to a segment of the lung. An area where alveoli are ventilated but not perfused is termed *alveolar dead space.*

Hypoxemia is often associated with a compensatory hyperventilation and resultant respiratory alkalosis (i.e., decreased $PaCO_2$ and increased pH). However, in individuals with associated ventilatory difficulties, hypoxemia may be complicated by hypercapnia and respiratory acidosis. Hypoxemia results in widespread tissue dysfunction and, when severe, can lead to organ infarction. In addition, hypoxic pulmonary vasoconstriction can contribute to increased pressures in the pulmonary artery and lead to right heart failure and cor pulmonale[9] (see p. 1236). Clinical manifestations of acute hypoxemia may include cyanosis, confusion, tachycardia, edema, and decreased renal output.

Acute Respiratory Failure

Respiratory failure is defined as inadequate gas exchange, that is, hypoxemia, where PaO_2 is ≤ 50 mmHg, or hypercapnia, where $PaCO_2$ is ≥ 50 mmHg with a pH of ≤ 7.25. Respiratory failure can result from direct injury to the lungs, airways, or chest wall or indirectly because of injury to another body system such as the brain. It can occur in individuals who have an otherwise normal respiratory system or in those with underlying chronic pulmonary disease. Most pulmonary diseases can cause episodes of acute respiratory failure. If the respiratory failure is primarily hypercapnic, it is the result of inadequate alveolar ventilation and the individual must receive ventilatory support, such as with a bag-valve mask or mechanical ventilator. If the respiratory failure is primarily hypoxemic, it is the result of inadequate exchange of oxygen be-

tween the alveoli and the capillaries (see Hypoxemia, earlier in this chapter) and the individual must receive supplemental oxygen therapy. Many individuals have a combined hypercapnic and hypoxemic respiratory failure and require both kinds of support.

Pulmonary Edema

Pulmonary edema is excess water in the lung. The normal lung contains very little water or fluid. It is kept dry by lymphatic drainage and a balance among capillary hydrostatic pressure, capillary oncotic pressure, and capillary permeability. In addition, surfactant lining the alveoli repels water, keeping fluid from entering the alveoli. Predisposing factors for pulmonary edema include heart disease, ARDS, and inhalation of toxic gases. The pathogenesis of pulmonary edema is shown in Figure 33-3.

The most common cause of pulmonary edema is heart disease (see Chapter 30). When the left ventricle fails, filling pressures on the left side of the heart increase and cause a concomitant increase in pulmonary capillary hydrostatic pressure. When the hydrostatic pressure exceeds oncotic pressure, fluid moves out into the interstitium, or interstitial space (the space within the alveolar septum between alveolus and capillary). Initially fluid is picked up by lymphatic vessels and removed from the lung. When the flow of fluid out of the capillaries exceeds the lymphatic system's ability to remove it, pulmonary edema develops.

Pulmonary edema usually begins to develop at a pulmonary capillary wedge pressure or left atrial pressure of 20 mmHg. If the capillary oncotic pressure is decreased for any reason (e.g., anemia or decreased plasma proteins), pulmonary edema develops at a lower hydrostatic pressure. Individuals with chronically elevated hydrostatic pressure tend to develop pulmonary edema at higher left atrial pressures.

Another cause of pulmonary edema is capillary injury that increases capillary permeability. Capillary injury causes edema in cases of acute respiratory distress syndrome (ARDS) or inhalation of toxic gases, such as ammonia. Capillary injury causes water and plasma proteins to leak out of the capillary and move into the interstitium. When plasma proteins move into the lung interstitium, they increase the interstitial oncotic pressure, which is usually very low. As the interstitial oncotic pressure begins to equal capillary oncotic pressure, water moves out of the capillary and into the lung. (This phenomenon is discussed in Chapter 3, Figure 3-1.)

Pulmonary edema also can result from obstruction of the lymphatic system. Drainage can be blocked by compression of lymphatic vessels caused by edema, tumors and fibrotic tissue, or by increased systemic venous pressure that elevates hydrostatic pressure of the large pulmonary veins into which the pulmonary lymphatic system drains. This can happen in left-sided heart failure.

Clinical manifestations of pulmonary edema include dyspnea, orthopnea, hypoxemia, and increased work of breathing. Physical examination may reveal inspiratory crackles (rales), dullness to percussion over the lung bases, and evi-

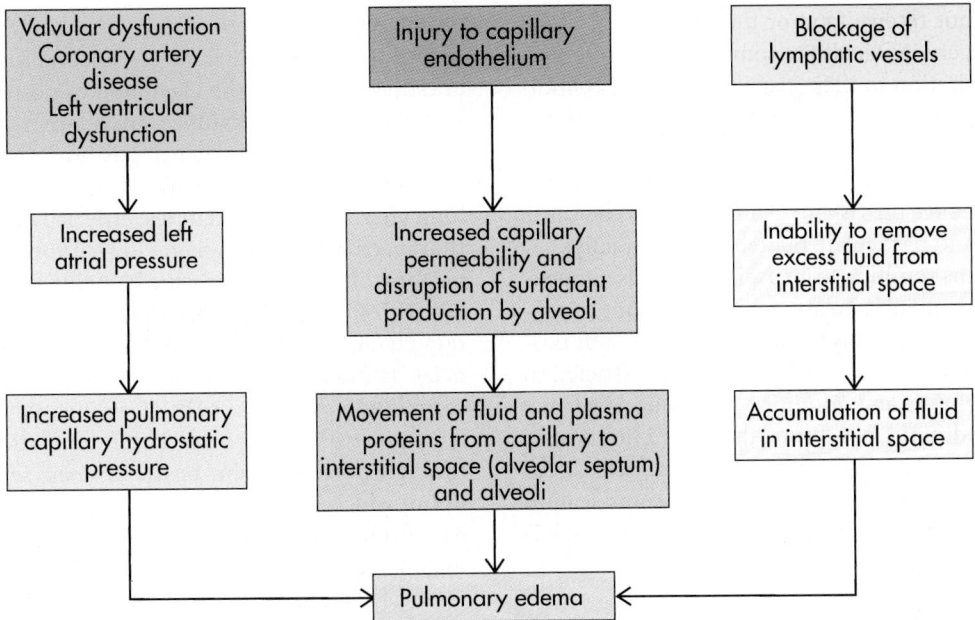

Figure 33-3 Pathogenesis of pulmonary edema.

dence of ventricular dilation (S_3 gallop and cardiomegaly). In severe edema, pink, frothy sputum is expectorated and PCO_2 increases.

The treatment of pulmonary edema depends on its cause. If the edema is caused by increased hydrostatic pressure, therapy is geared toward improving volume status with diuretics, vasodilators, and drugs that improve the contraction of the heart muscle. If edema is the result of increased capillary permeability resulting from injury, the treatment is focused on removing the offending agent and supportive therapy to maintain adequate ventilation and circulation. Individuals with either type of pulmonary edema require supplemental oxygen. Mechanical ventilation also is used if edema significantly impairs ventilation and oxygenation.

Aspiration

Aspiration is the passage of fluid and solid particles into the lung. It tends to occur in individuals whose normal swallowing mechanism and cough reflex are impaired by a decreased level of consciousness or central nervous system abnormalities. Predisposing factors include altered level of consciousness caused by substance abuse, sedation, or anesthesia; seizure disorders; cerebrovascular accident; myasthenia gravis (a neuromuscular disorder); and Guillain-Barré syndrome (inflammation of the nerves). In individuals who require enteral feeding (through a nasogastric feeding tube), aspiration is common and leads to bacterial pneumonia.[10] Aspiration is also common in children with tracheoesophageal fistula (a congenital abnormality in which the trachea and esophagus communicate; see Chapter 40). The right lung, particularly the right lower lobe, is more susceptible to aspiration than the left lung because the branching angle of the right main stem bronchus is straighter than the branching angle of the left main stem bronchus.

The effects of aspiration depend on the material aspirated. The aspiration of large food particles or gastric fluid with pH of less than 2.5 has serious consequences. Solid food particles can obstruct a bronchus, resulting in bronchial inflammation and collapse of airways distal to the obstruction. If the aspirated solid is not identified and removed by bronchoscopy, a chronic, local inflammation develops that may lead to recurrent infection and bronchiectasis (permanent dilation of the bronchus). Once the pathologic process has progressed to bronchiectasis, surgical resection of the affected area is usually required.

Aspiration of oral or pharyngeal secretions can lead to aspiration pneumonia, especially if the oral cavity is colonized with bacteria (e.g., individuals with poor dentition).[11] Intubation of the trachea also can cause aspiration and bacterial pneumonia.

Aspiration of acidic gastric fluid may cause severe pneumonitis (localized lung inflammation). Bronchial damage includes inflammation, loss of ciliary function, and bronchospasm. In the alveoli, acidic fluid damages the alveolocapillary membrane. This allows plasma and blood cells to move from capillaries into the alveoli, resulting in hemorrhagic pneumonitis. The lung becomes stiff and noncompliant as surfactant production is disrupted, leading to further edema and collapse. Hypoventilation may develop as this progresses, and systematic complications, such as hypotension, may occur.

The clinical manifestations of aspiration include the sudden onset of choking and intractable cough with or without vomiting, fever, dyspnea, and wheezing. Some individuals have no symptoms acutely; instead they have recurrent lung infections, chronic cough, or persistent wheezing over months and even years.

Preventive measures for individuals at risk are more effective than treatment of known aspiration. Individuals undergoing surgery do not receive food or fluid for several hours before or after surgery. Antacids are sometimes given to persons at risk for aspiration to keep gastric pH above 2.5. Individuals who have difficulty swallowing are fed with extreme caution and positioned to minimize the likelihood of aspiration. Nasogastric tubes, which often are used to remove stomach contents and reduce the risk for aspiration, also can cause aspiration if fluid and particulate matter are regurgitated.

The rate of deaths resulting from aspiration-caused pneumonitis is greater than 50%. Treatment includes supplemental oxygen and may require mechanical ventilation with positive end-expiratory pressure (PEEP). Fluids are restricted to decrease blood volume and minimize pulmonary edema. Steroids often are administered during the first 72 hours after aspiration, although their effectiveness is not well documented. Bacterial pneumonia may develop as a complication of aspiration pneumonitis. If bacterial pneumonia occurs, it is treated with organism-specific antibiotics.

Atelectasis

Atelectasis is the collapse of lung tissue. The two types of atelectasis are compression and absorption:

1. **Compression atelectasis** is caused by the external pressure exerted by a tumor in the lung, or by fluid or air in the pleural space. Atelectasis at the base of the lungs can be caused by abdominal distention pressing on a portion of the lung, causing the alveoli to collapse.
2. **Absorption atelectasis** results from gradual absorption of air from obstructed or hypoventilated alveoli or from inhalation of concentrated oxygen or anesthetic agents.

Clinical manifestations of atelectasis are similar to those of pulmonary infection: dyspnea, cough, fever, and leukocytosis.

Atelectasis tends to occur after surgery. Intraoperative high-dose supplemental oxygen in combination with general anesthesia increases the likelihood of postoperative atelectasis.[12] In addition, individuals are often in pain, breathe shallowly, are reluctant to change position, and produce viscous secretions that tend to pool in dependent portions of the lung after surgical procedures, especially those involving the thorax or upper abdomen. Prevention and treatment of postoperative atelectasis usually include deep breathing (often with the aid of an incentive spirometer), frequent position changes, and early ambulation. Deep breathing is beneficial because it (1) promotes the ciliary clearance of secretions, (2) stabilizes the alveoli by redistributing surfactant, and (3) permits collateral ventilation of the alveoli through pores of Kohn in the alveolar septa. The pores of Kohn, which open only during deep breathing, allow air to pass from well-ventilated alveoli to obstructed alveoli, minimizing their tendency to collapse and facilitating obstruction removal (Figure 33-4).

Bronchiectasis

Bronchiectasis is persistent abnormal dilation of the bronchi. It usually occurs in conjunction with other respiratory conditions and can be caused by obstruction of an airway with mucous plugs, atelectasis, aspiration of a foreign body, infection, cystic fibrosis, tuberculosis, congenital weakness of the bronchial wall, or impaired defense mechanisms. Bronchiectasis is also associated with a number of systemic disorders such as rheumatologic disease, inflammatory bowel disease, and acquired immunodeficiency syndrome (AIDS). The underlying cause of bronchiectasis is found in less than 40% of cases. Bronchiectasis is often associated with inflammation of the bronchi (**bronchitis**) and has similar symptoms (see p. 1226).

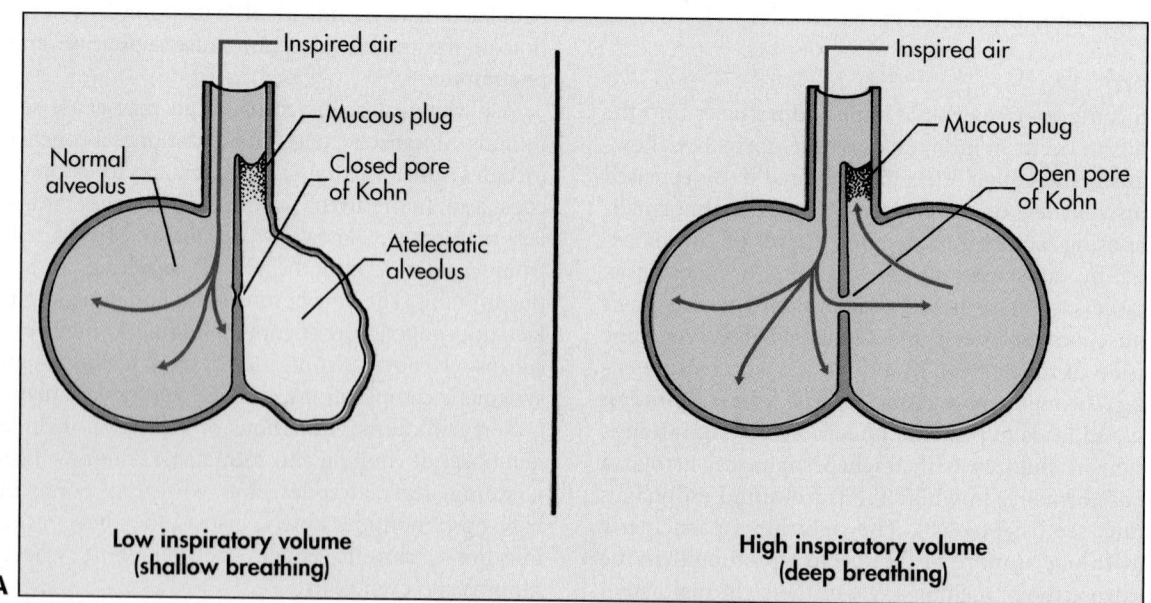

Figure 33-4 Pores of Kohn. **A,** Absorption atelectasis caused by lack of collateral ventilation through pores of Kohn. **B,** Restoration of collateral ventilation during deep breathing.

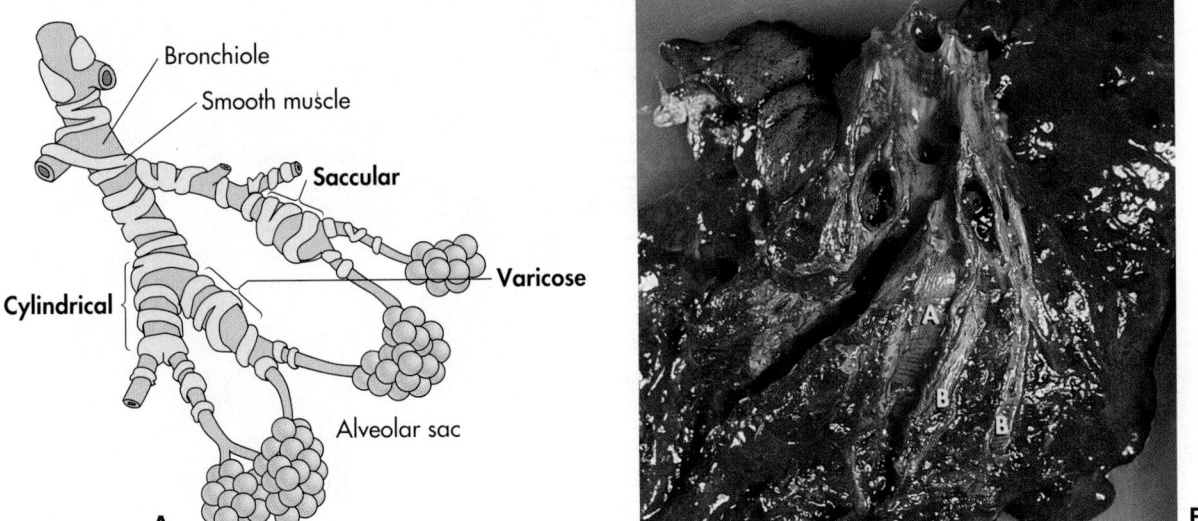

Figure 33-5 Bronchiectasis. **A,** Types of bronchiectasis. **B,** Cylindrical bronchiectasis. The dilated bronchi *(A)* and bronchioles *(B)* can be dissected almost to the pleural surface. (**B,** From Damjanov I, Linder J, editors: *Anderson's pathology,* ed 10, St Louis, 1996, Mosby.)

Bronchial dilation (Figure 33-5) may be *cylindrical* (**cylindrical bronchiectasis**), with symmetrically dilated airways as is commonly seen after pneumonia and is reversible; *saccular* (**saccular bronchiectasis**), in which the bronchi become large and balloon-like; or *varicose* (**varicose bronchiectasis**), in which constrictions and dilations deform the bronchi. In both varicose and saccular bronchiectasis, the smaller bronchial divisions are plugged with secretions or obliterated by fibrosis. Large anastomoses (connections) develop between the bronchial and pulmonary blood vessels, increasing blood flow through the bronchial circulation. These anastomoses are thought to cause the hemoptysis experienced by individuals with bronchiectasis. Airway damage leads to bronchospasm and copious production of purulent mucus. Ventilation-perfusion abnormalities develop and result in hypoxemia. In severe cases, $PaCO_2$ also may be elevated.

The symptoms of bronchiectasis may date back to a childhood illness or infection. The disease is commonly associated with recurrent lower respiratory tract infections and expectoration of voluminous amounts of purulent sputum (measured in cupfuls). If the individual is not receiving antibiotics, the sputum has a foul odor. Hemoptysis and clubbing of the fingers are common. Pulmonary function studies show decreases in vital capacity (VC) and expiratory flow rates. Bronchiectasis is often associated with bronchitis and atelectasis. Hypoxemia eventually leads to cor pulmonale (see p. 1236). Bronchiectasis is treated with antibiotics, bronchodilators, chest physiology, and supplemental oxygen.[13]

Bronchiolitis

Bronchiolitis is an inflammatory obstruction of the small airways or bronchioles. It is most common in children (see Chapter 34). In adults it usually occurs with chronic bronchitis but can occur in otherwise healthy individuals in association with a viral infection, such as respiratory syncytial virus (RSV), or inhalation of toxic gases. Atelectasis or emphysematous destruction of the alveoli may develop distal to the inflammatory lesion. Bronchiolitis is usually diffuse. A decrease in the ventilation-perfusion ratio results in hypoxemia and carbon dioxide retention.

Bronchiolitis is often preceded by an upper respiratory infection. Manifestations include a rapid ventilatory rate; marked use of accessory muscles; low-grade fever; dry, nonproductive cough; and hyperinflated chest. If bronchiolitis is caused by an inhalation injury, pulmonary edema occurs rapidly and then quickly clears. One to two weeks later, respiratory distress develops, and infiltrates are seen on chest radiographs.[14] Bronchiolitis is treated with appropriate antibiotics, steroids, and chest physical therapy (humidified air, coughing and deep breathing, postural drainage).

Bronchiolitis obliterans is a late-stage fibrotic process that occludes the airways and causes permanent scarring of the lungs. This process can occur in all causes of bronchiolitis but is most common after lung transplantation, where it affects almost 50% of recipients.[15] Diagnosis is made by spirometry and bronchoscopy with biopsy. Treatment includes corticosteroids and other immunosuppressive agents.[16]

Pleural Abnormalities

Pneumothorax

Pneumothorax is the presence of air or gas in the pleural space caused by a rupture in the visceral pleura (which surrounds the lungs) or the parietal pleura and chest wall (see Chapter 32). As air separates the visceral and parietal pleurae, it destroys the negative pressure of the pleural space. This disrupts the state of equilibrium that normally exists between elastic recoil forces of the lung and chest wall. No longer held in check by the recoil forces of the chest wall, the lung fulfills its tendency to recoil by collapsing toward the hilus (Figure 33-6).

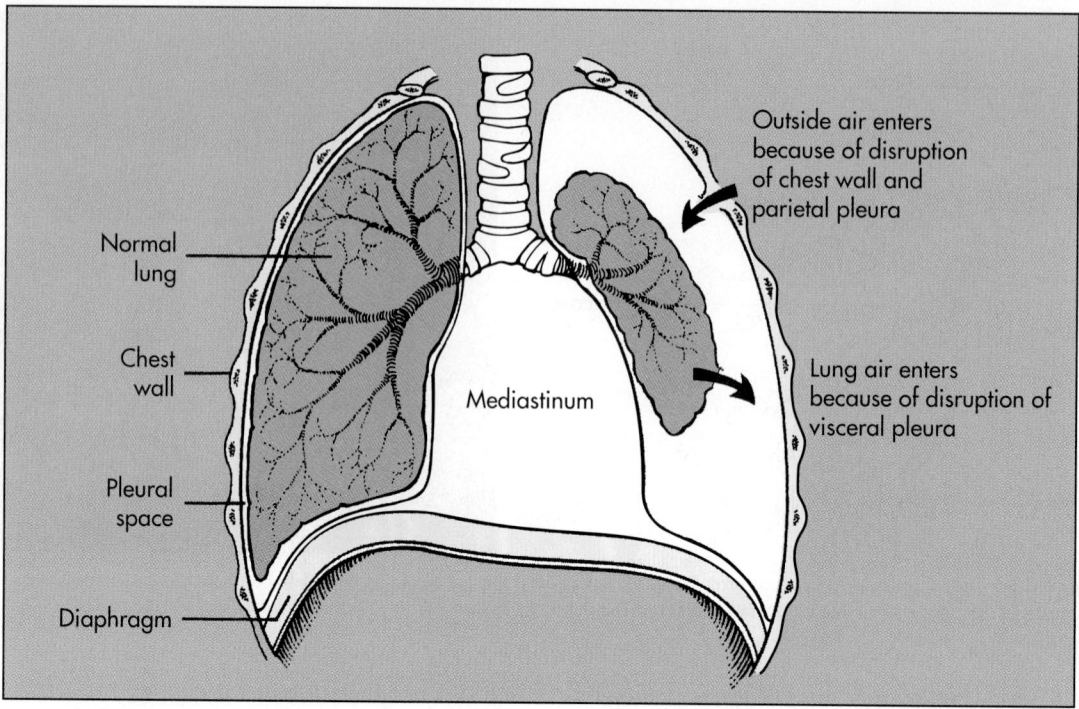

Figure 33-6 Pneumothorax. Air in the pleural space causes the lung to collapse around the hilus and may push mediastinal contents (heart and great vessels) toward the other lung.

In **open pneumothorax (communicating pneumothorax),** air pressure in the pleural space equals barometric pressure because air that is drawn into the pleural space during inspiration (through the damaged chest wall and parietal pleura or through the lungs and damaged visceral pleura) is forced back out during expiration. In **tension pneumothorax,** however, the site of pleural rupture acts as a one-way valve, permitting air to enter on inspiration but preventing its escape by closing up during expiration. As more and more air enters the pleural space, air pressure in the pneumothorax begins to exceed barometric pressure. The pathophysiologic effects of tension pneumothorax are life threatening. Air pressure in the pleural space pushes against the already recoiled lung, causing compression atelectasis, and against the mediastinum, compressing and displacing the heart and great vessels.

Spontaneous pneumothorax, which occurs unexpectedly in healthy individuals (usually men) between ages 20 and 40 years, is most often caused by the spontaneous rupture of blebs (blister-like formations) on the visceral pleura.[17,18] Bleb rupture can occur during sleep, rest, or exercise. The ruptured bleb or blebs are usually located in the apexes of the lungs. The cause of bleb formation is not known, although more than 80% of these individuals have been found to have emphysema-like changes in their lungs even if they have never smoked or have no known genetic disorder. Tension pneumothorax can develop with bleb rupture.

Clinical manifestations of spontaneous pneumothorax begin with sudden pleural pain, tachypnea, and possibly mild dyspnea. The manifestations depend on the size of the pneumothorax. If the pneumothorax is large or if there is a tension pneumothorax, it may push the mediastinum toward the un-

affected lung, causing the chest to appear asymmetric. Hypoxemia may develop. Lung collapse causes diminished breath sounds over the affected lung. Diagnosis is made with chest radiographs. CT scanning is used after the individual is stabilized to determine the risk of recurrence. Small open pneumothorax can be managed with observation and supplemental oxygen or with simple aspiration using a small catheter.[19] Larger pneumothoraces require the placement of a chest tube that is connected to a water-seal drainage system with suction. After the pneumothorax is evacuated and the plural rupture healed, the chest tube is removed.

A **secondary pneumothorax** can be caused by chest trauma, such as a rib fracture or stab and bullet wounds that tear the pleura; rupture of a bleb or bulla (larger vesicle), as occurs in COPD; or mechanical ventilation, particularly if it includes PEEP. The pathophysiology and clinical manifestations of secondary pneumothorax are similar to those of spontaneous pneumothorax. Occasionally air enters the mediastinum. Secondary pneumothorax is managed in the same way as spontaneous pneumothorax, although surgical repair of the chest wall may be required in more severe injuries before the pleura can heal.

Tension pneumothorax, in which air in the pleural space cannot escape through the rupture, is a life-threatening emergency. As increasing positive pressure in the pleural space compresses lung tissue and thoracic blood vessels, venous return and cardiac output decrease. Clinical manifestations of tension pneumothorax include severe hypoxemia, dyspnea, and hypotension (low blood pressure), as well as other signs and symptoms of pneumothorax. Severe pressure on the mediastinum can cause the trachea to deviate away from the side of the pneumothorax. Deterioration occurs rapidly, and shock and bradycardia (reduced heart rate) may develop.

Tension pneumothorax requires immediate treatment. A chest tube is placed quickly, usually after physical examination alone. If a chest tube is not readily available, a large-bore needle is inserted into the pleural space to decompress it until a chest tube can be placed. An outward gush of air as the needle or chest tube is inserted confirms the presence of tension pneumothorax. The chest tube is connected to a water-seal drainage and suction until the damaged pleura is healed.[20]

In some situations, the pleural tear does not heal spontaneously, and it is necessary to prevent recurrence of the pneumothorax by a process called *pleurodesis*. This procedure uses the chest tube to instill a caustic substance, such as talc, into the pleural space. The resultant inflammation and scarring as the pleura heals result in closure of the pleural tear. Some individuals require thoracotomy with pleurectomy.

Pleural Effusion

Pleural effusion is the presence of fluid in the pleural space. The source of the fluid is usually blood vessels or lymphatic vessels lying beneath either pleura, but occasionally the source is an abscess or other lesion that drains into the pleural space. Because the pleura is a relatively permeable membrane, fluids that accumulate in the lung can cross into the pleural space.

Like pneumothorax, pleural effusion can cause compression atelectasis and displace mediastinal contents. Unlike pneumothorax, however, pleural effusion does not cause the lung to collapse as a result of elastic recoil. Because there is no communication between the pleural space and environmental air, pressure in the pleural space remains negative and atelectasis is caused solely by pressure exerted by the effusion.

The most common mechanism of pleural effusion is migration of fluids and other blood components through the walls of intact capillaries bordering the pleura. Pleural effusions that enter the pleural space from the intact blood vessels can be transudative or exudative. In **transudative effusion,** the fluid, or transudate, is watery and diffuses out of the capillaries as a result of disorders that increase intravascular hydrostatic pressure or decrease capillary oncotic pressure. Examples are congestive heart failure, in which venous and left atrial pressures are increased, and liver or kidney disorders that cause hypoproteinemia. Hypoproteinemia decreases capillary oncotic pressure, which promotes diffusion of water out of the capillaries. (This mechanism is discussed in Chapter 3.)

Exudative effusion is less watery and contains high concentrations of white blood cells and plasma proteins. Exudative effusion occurs in response to inflammation, infection, or malignancy and involves inflammatory processes that increase capillary permeability (see Chapter 6). When stimulated by biochemical mediators of inflammation, junctions in the capillary endothelium separate slightly, enabling leukocytes and plasma proteins to migrate out into affected tissues. Mechanisms of pleural effusion are summarized in Table 33-2. Inflammation of the pleura with associated exudative effusion can lead to the clinical symptom known as **pleurisy** in which the individual may complain of pain with inspiration and a pleural friction rub may be heard on examination.

Small collections of fluid normally can be drained away by the lymphatics. Large effusions cause clinical manifestations related to their volume and the rate at which they accumulate in the pleural space. Dyspnea, compression atelectasis with impaired ventilation, and mediastinal shift occur with large effusions. Pleural pain is present if the pleura is inflamed, and cardiovascular manifestations occur in a large, rapidly developing **hemothorax** (hemorrhage into the pleural space). A pleural friction rub can be heard over areas of extensive effusion.

The type of effusion, and its potential underlying cause, can frequently be determined by thoracentesis (needle aspira-

Table 33-2	Mechanisms of Pleural Effusion	
Type of Fluid/Effusion	**Source of Accumulation**	**Primary or Associated Disorder**
Transudate (hydrothorax)	Watery fluid that diffuses out of capillaries beneath the pleurae (i.e., capillaries in lung or chest wall)	Cardiovascular disease that causes high blood pressure; liver or kidney disease that disrupts plasma protein production, causing hypoproteinemia (decreased oncotic pressure in the blood vessels)
Exudate	Fluid rich in proteins (leukocytes, plasma proteins of all kinds; see Chapter 7) that migrates out of the capillaries	Infection, inflammation, or malignancy of the pleurae that stimulates mast cells to release biochemical mediators that increase capillary permeability
Empyema (pus)	Detritus of infection (microorganisms, leukocytes, cellular debris) dumped into the pleural space by blocked lymphatic vessels	Pulmonary infections, such as pneumonia; lung abscesses; infected wounds
Hemothorax (blood)	Hemorrhage into the pleural space	Traumatic injury, surgery, rupture, or malignancy that damages blood vessels
Chylothorax (chyle)	Chyle (milky fluid containing lymph and fat droplets) that is dumped by lymphatic vessels into the pleural space instead of passing from the gastrointestinal tract to the thoracic duct	Traumatic injury, infection, or disorder that disrupts lymphatic transport

NOTE: The principles of diffusion are discussed in Chapter 1; mechanisms that increase capillary permeability and cause exudation of cells and proteins are discussed in Chapter 7.

tion) of the fluid with examination in the laboratory. If the effusion is causing considerable impairment of pulmonary function, then a chest tube is placed to allow for complete drainage of the fluid. A pleural effusion can contain several liters of fluid. Correction of the underlying condition usually leads to resolution of the pleural effusion, however, pleurodesis occasionally may be necessary.

Empyema

Empyema (infected pleural effusion), or the presence of pus in the pleural space, is a complication of respiratory infection, usually pneumonia caused by *Staphylococcus aureus, Escherichia coli,* anaerobic bacteria, or *Klebsiella pneumoniae* (*Staphylococcus* is responsible for more than 90% of empyemas in children). Empyema is thought to develop when the pulmonary lymphatics become blocked, leading to an outpouring of contaminated lymphatic fluid into the pleural space.[21] They often occur adjacent to a pneumonia (parapneumonic) when the effusion becomes infected. Empyemas can occur also after thoracic surgery or in association with intraabdominal infection.

Individuals with empyema have clinical manifestations of toxicity, including cyanosis, fever, tachycardia (rapid heart rate), cough, and pleural pain. Breath sounds are decreased directly over the empyema. Diagnosis is made by chest radiographs and thoracentesis, although positive cultures from fluids are obtained only about 50% of the time. Therefore the offending microorganism is usually identified by its preponderance in a sputum culture.[22]

The treatment for empyema is similar to that for pneumonia (see p. 1230). Antibiotics are given, and thoracentesis is performed to drain the pleural space. Chest tube placement with continuous drainage is often required. In severe cases, surgical debridement of the pleural space is performed to prevent reaccumulation.[21,22]

Abscess Formation and Cavitation

An **abscess** is a circumscribed area of suppuration and destruction of lung parenchyma. Abscess formation follows **consolidation** of lung tissue, in which inflammation causes alveoli to fill with fluid, pus, and microorganisms. Necrosis (death and decay) of consolidated tissue may progress proximally until it communicates with a bronchus. If this occurs, the abscess empties into the bronchus, leaving a cavity that has a radiographic appearance similar to that of a lesion of tuberculosis. **Cavitation** is the process of abscess emptying and cavity formation. The diagnosis is made by radiography.

Pneumonia caused by aspiration, *Klebsiella,* or *Staphylococcus* is the most common cause of abscess formation. Aspiration abscess is usually associated with alcohol abuse, seizure disorders, general anesthesia, and swallowing disorders. Immunocompromised individuals are also at greater risk for lung abscesses and may be infected with opportunistic microorganisms, such as fungi and mycobacteria.[23] The clinical manifestations of abscess formation are similar to those of pneumonitis: fever, cough, chills, sputum production, and pleural pain. Abscess communication with a bronchus causes

a severe cough, copious amounts of often foul-smelling sputum, and occasionally hemoptysis.

Treatment includes the administration of appropriate antibiotics and chest physical therapy, including chest percussion and postural drainage. Sometimes bronchoscopy is performed to drain the abscess. Mortality rates are influenced by the severity of the primary disease that initially caused consolidation and by the virulence of the causative microorganism. Overall, the mortality rate for lung abscess remains at about 20%.[23]

Pulmonary Fibrosis

Pulmonary fibrosis is an excessive amount of fibrous or connective tissue in the lung. It can be caused by healing (formation of scar tissue) after active disease (e.g., ARDS, tuberculosis) or by inhalation of harmful substances (e.g., coal dust, asbestos). When no specific cause for the development of fibrosis is known, it is called *idiopathic pulmonary fibrosis.* The fibrotic process results from dysregulated repair processes resulting in chronic inflammation, alveolar epithelialization, and myofibroblast proliferation.[24]

Fibrosis causes a marked loss of lung compliance. The lung becomes stiff and difficult to ventilate, and the diffusing capacity of the alveolocapillary membrane may decrease, causing hypoxemia. Diffuse pulmonary fibrosis is treated with oral corticosteroids but response rates are poor. Additional therapies include cytotoxic agents and colchicine. Newer agents under study include interferon and cyclosporin.[25]

Chest Wall Restriction

If the chest wall is deformed, immobilized, or made heavy by fat, the work of breathing is increased and ventilation may be compromised because of a decrease in tidal volume. The degree of ventilatory impairment depends on the severity of the chest wall abnormality. Grossly obese individuals are often dyspneic on exertion or when recumbent. Individuals with severe kyphoscoliosis (lateral bending and rotation of the spinal column, with distortion of the thoracic cage) often have dyspnea on exertion that can progress to respiratory failure. Such individuals are also susceptible to lower respiratory tract infections. Both obesity and kyphoscoliosis are risk factors for respiratory disease in individuals admitted to a hospital for other problems, particularly those who require surgery. Other musculoskeletal abnormalities that can impair ventilation are ankylosing spondylitis (see Chapters 42 and 43) and pectus excavatum (a deformity characterized by depression of the sternum).

Impairment of respiratory muscle function caused by neuromuscular disease also can restrict the chest wall or impair pulmonary function. Muscle weakness can result in hypoventilation and hypercapnia, inability to remove secretions, and hypoxemia. The most common cause of hospital admission for individuals with neuromuscular diseases such as poliomyelitis, muscular dystrophy, myasthenia gravis, and Guillain-Barré syndrome is respiratory difficulty. (See Unit V for a more complete discussion of these disorders.)

Flail Chest

Flail chest results from the fracture of several consecutive ribs in more than one place, or the fracture of the sternum plus several consecutive ribs. These multiple fractures result in instability of a portion of the chest wall, causing paradoxic movement of the chest with breathing. During inspiration the unstable portion of the chest wall moves inward, and during expiration it moves outward, impairing movement of gas in and out of the lungs (Figure 33-7). Flail chest is usually associated with significant underlying lung contusion.

The clinical manifestations of flail chest are pain, dyspnea, unequal chest expansion, hypoventilation, and hypoxemia. Treatment is internal fixation by controlled mechanical ventilation until the chest wall has stabilized.

Inhalation Disorders

Exposure to Toxic Gases

Inhalation of gaseous irritants can cause significant respiratory dysfunction. Commonly encountered toxic gases include smoke, ammonia, hydrogen chloride, sulfur dioxide, chlorine, phosgene, and nitrogen dioxide. Inhalation of a toxic gas results in severe inflammation of the airways, alveolar and capillary damage, and pulmonary edema. (The cellular effects of toxic gases are described in Chapter 2.) Initial symptoms include burning of the eyes, nose, and throat; coughing; chest tightness; and dyspnea. Hypoxemia is common. Treatment includes supplemental oxygen, mechanical ventilation with PEEP, and support of the cardiovascular system. Steroids sometimes are used, although their effectiveness has not been well documented. Most individuals respond quickly to therapy. Some, however, may improve initially and then deteriorate as a result of bronchiectasis or bronchiolitis (inflammation of the bronchioles).

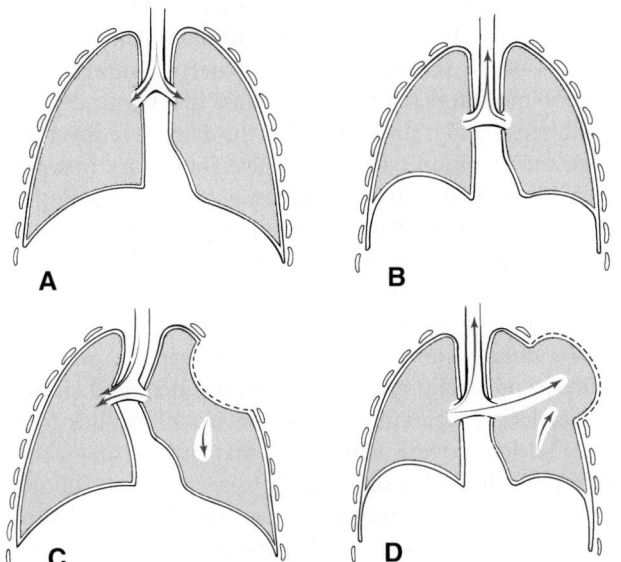

Figure 33-7 Flail chest. Normal respiration: **A,** inspiration; **B,** expiration. Paradoxic motion: **C,** inspiration, area of lung underlying unstable chest wall sucks in on inspiration; **D,** expiration, unstable area balloons out. Note movement of mediastinum toward opposite lung during inspiration.

Prolonged exposure to high concentrations of supplemental oxygen can result in a relatively rare iatrogenic condition known as **oxygen toxicity.** Although there is great individual variation in susceptibility to oxygen toxicity, generally the higher the concentration and longer the exposure, the more likely the occurrence of toxicity. Oxygen concentrations of 50% to 75% for greater than 24 to 48 hours have been associated with injury to cells of the lungs. The basic underlying mechanism of injury is a severe inflammatory response mediated primarily by oxygen radicals. The result is damage to alveolocapillary membranes, disruption of surfactant production, interstitial and alveolar edema, and decrease in compliance. Toxicity is often undetected because it occurs in individuals who are already in acute respiratory failure. Clinical manifestations are indistinguishable from those of ARDS. Treatment involves ventilatory support and reduction of inspired oxygen concentration to less than 60% as soon as tolerated by the individual.

Pneumoconiosis

Pneumoconiosis represents any change in the lung caused by inhalation of inorganic dust particles, which usually occurs in the workplace. As in all cases of environmentally acquired lung disease, the individual's history of exposure is important in determining the diagnosis. Pneumoconiosis often occurs after years of exposure to the offending dust, and manifestations are often difficult to differentiate from those resulting from smoking.

The dusts of silica, asbestos, and coal are the most common causes of pneumoconiosis. Others include talc, fiberglass, clays, mica, slate, cement, cadmium, beryllium, tungsten, cobalt, aluminum, and iron. No matter what the substance, the dust deposits are permanent. In most cases, diagnosis is made by chest x-ray and careful occupational history.[26] Treatment, therefore, is palliative and focuses on preventing further exposure and improving working conditions, along with pulmonary rehabilitation and management of associated hypoxemia and bronchospasm.[27]

Silicosis is a type of pneumoconiosis resulting from the inhalation of free silica (silicon dioxide) and silica-containing compounds. Silica exposure occurs in mining and other industries involved with the extraction and processing of ores; preparation and use of sand; and manufacture of pipe, building, and roofing materials. Silica exposure causes acute inflammation and chronic fibrosis of the lung tissue and has been shown to result in apoptosis of lung cells.[27,28] The silica produces fibrous nodules within the lung. Exposed individuals usually remain asymptomatic long after the nodules are visible on chest radiography. When clinical manifestations do appear, they include cough and dyspnea. Silicosis is also a predisposing factor for lower respiratory tract infection and bronchospasm with wheezing. There is no specific treatment for the disease, although corticosteroids may produce some improvement.

Coal worker pneumoconiosis (coal miner lung, black lung) is caused by coal dust deposits in the lung. Although coal dust, itself, is relatively well tolerated by the lung, it is frequently inhaled as a mixture of coal, silica, and quartz, which is strongly inflammatory.[27,29] Its mild form is asymptomatic, except for possible chronic bronchitis. Its advanced form consists of severe pulmonary fibrosis. Individuals usually are seen with a productive cough and wheezing. Symptoms are more severe with advanced disease and mimic those of chronic bronchitis (see p. 1224). Diagnosis is made by history of exposure and characteristic chest radiographs. There is no specific treatment for coal worker pneumoconiosis. Individuals with the mild form of the disease usually do well. Those with more complicated forms often develop marked cardiopulmonary dysfunction.

Asbestos exposure affects not only factory workers but also individuals who live in areas of asbestos emission. Asbestos exposure can result in a type of pulmonary fibrosis called **asbestosis** or in tumor formation, depending on the amount of exposure and other risk factors such as smoking. It is caused by inhalation of hydrous silicates of various metals in fibrous form. Asbestos fibers cause inflammation, release of toxic oxygen radicals, and cellular apoptosis leading to both fibrosis and cancers such as mesothelioma.[30-32] The most prominent clinical manifestations of fibrosis are dyspnea on exertion, a nonproductive cough, hypoxemia, and decreased lung volume. Progressive disease may lead to respiratory failure and cardiac complications. Asbestos workers who smoke have a marked increase in risk for developing bronchogenic cancer (see p. 1237).

Allergic Alveolitis

Inhalation of organic dusts can result in an allergic inflammatory response called **extrinsic allergic alveolitis (hypersensitivity pneumonitis).** Many allergens can cause this disorder, including grains, silage, bird droppings or feathers, wood dust (particularly redwood and maple), cork dust, animal pelts, coffee beans, fish meal, mushroom compost, and molds that grow on sugar cane, barley, and straw. The immune response to these allergens results in antibody production and initiation of the inflammatory response. The lung inflammation, or pneumonitis, occurs after repeated, prolonged exposure to the allergen.

Allergic alveolitis can be acute, subacute, or chronic. The acute form causes a fever, cough, dyspnea, and chills a few hours after exposure that resolve without treatment in 1 to 3 days. With continued exposure, the disease becomes chronic and pulmonary fibrosis develops. (The mechanisms of hypersensitivity reactions are discussed in Chapter 7.) Chronic allergic alveolitis causes weight loss, fever, fatigue, and gradually progressive respiratory failure. Diagnosis is made by obtaining a history of allergen exposure and by serum antibody testing, chest x-ray, bronchoscopy, and CT.[33]

Systemic Disorders

Several systemic diseases affect the airways, pleurae, or lung parenchyma, causing fibrosis, vasculitis, pulmonary hemorrhage, or granuloma formation. Clinical manifestations of lung involvement are usually nonspecific, and the diagnosis is based on involvement of other organs. There is usually no

specific treatment, although corticosteroids often are used. Some of the systemic diseases affecting the lung are granulomatous disorders such as sarcoidosis, Wegener granulomatosis, lymphomatoid granulomatosis, and eosinophilic granuloma; connective tissue diseases such as rheumatoid disease, systemic lupus erythematosus, scleroderma, polymyositis or dermatomyositis, Sjögren syndrome, and polyarteritis nodosa; angioimmunoblastic or immunoblastic lymphadenopathy, a disease of the lymph nodes; cystic fibrosis (see Chapter 34); and Goodpasture syndrome, a renal disorder.

PULMONARY DISORDERS

Acute Respiratory Distress Syndrome

Acute respiratory distress syndrome (ARDS) is a fulminant form of respiratory failure characterized by acute lung inflammation and diffuse alveolocapillary injury. The syndrome affects an estimated 200,000 to 250,000 people per year in the United States and complicates over 30% of all ICU admissions.[34] Advances in therapy have decreased the overall mortality rate to less than 40%, although older people and those with severe infections continue to have a much higher mortality rate.[34] Most survivors, however, have almost normal lung function 1 year after the acute illness. ARDS is the result of injury to the lung by numerous unrelated causes. The most common predisposing factors are sepsis and multiple trauma (especially when multiple transfusions are received); however, there are many other causes, including pneumonia, burns, aspiration, cardiopulmonary bypass surgery, pancreatitis, drug overdose, smoke or noxious gas inhalation, oxygen toxicity, radiation therapy, and disseminated intravascular coagulation.

PATHOPHYSIOLOGY All disorders that result in ARDS acutely injure the alveolocapillary membrane and cause severe pulmonary edema (Figure 33-8). The alveolocapillary damage can occur directly, as with the aspiration of highly acidic gastric contents or inhalation of toxic gases, or indirectly from chemical mediators released in response to systemic disorders, as with sepsis and trauma. Whether the damage is direct or indirect, the common pathway for alveolocapillary membrane injury is a massive inflammatory response by the lungs. Several cell types and inflammatory mediators play key roles in the lung injury. The most important of these are neutrophils, macrophages, complement, endotoxin, interleukin-1 (IL-1), and tumor necrosis factor (TNF).[35]

The initial injury to the lungs damages the pulmonary capillary endothelium, activating complement and stimulating platelet aggregation and intravascular thrombus formation. Platelets release substances that attract and activate neutrophils. In ARDS caused by sepsis, endotoxin (lipopolysaccharide [LPS]) is recognized by the CD14 receptor on macrophages and results in chemotaxis of large numbers of neutrophils to the lungs. A cascade of inflammatory mediators is released by the macrophages, including tumor necrosis factor (TNF), interleukin-1 (IL-1), alpha and beta chemokines, and other interleukins.[35]

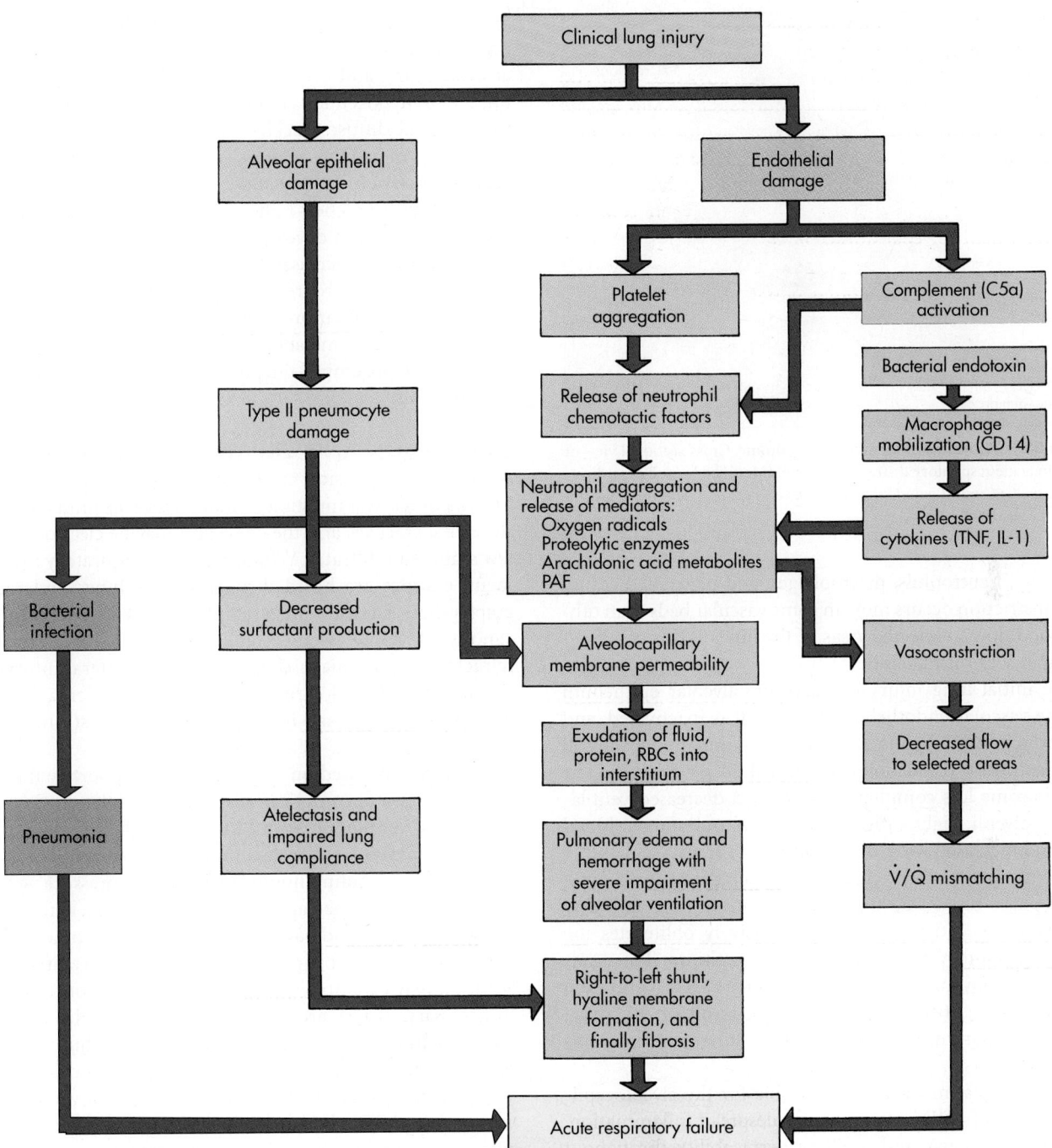

Figure 33-8 Pathogenesis of adult respiratory distress syndrome (ARDS). *TNF,* Tumor necrosis factor; *IL-1,* interleukin-1; *PAF,* platelet-activating factor; *RBCs,* red blood cells.

The role of neutrophils is central to the development of ARDS. Activated neutrophils release a battery of inflammatory mediators, among them proteolytic enzymes, oxygen free radicals (superoxide radicals, hydrogen peroxide, hydroxyl radicals), arachidonic acid metabolites (prostaglandins, thromboxanes, leukotrienes), and platelet-activating factor. These mediators cause extensive damage of the alveolocapillary membrane and greatly increase capillary membrane permeability.[36]

Increased capillary permeability, a hallmark of ARDS, allows fluids, proteins, and blood cells to leak from the capillary bed into the pulmonary interstitium and alveoli. The resulting pulmonary edema and hemorrhage severely reduce lung compliance and impair alveolar ventilation (Figure 33-9).

Mediators released by neutrophils, and to a certain extent by macrophages, also cause pulmonary vasoconstriction. Pulmonary hypertension occurs early in the course of the disease secondary to vasoconstriction and to vascular occlusion by

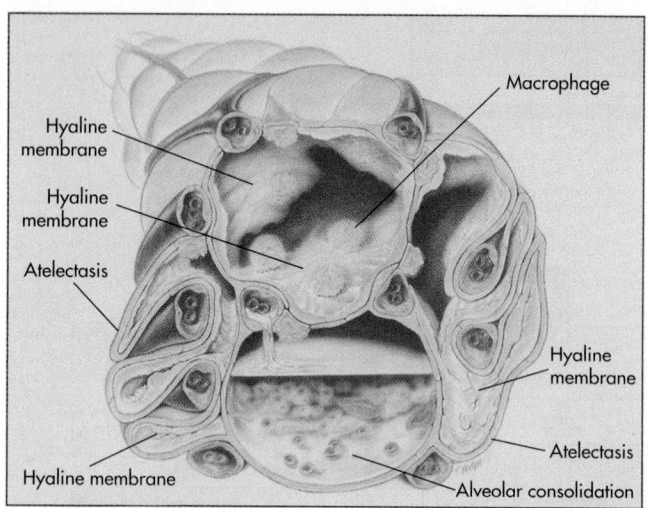

Figure 33-9 Acute respiratory distress syndrome. Cross-sectional view of alveoli in acute respiratory distress syndrome. (Modified from Des Jardins T, Burton GG: *Clinical manifestations and assessment of respiratory disease,* ed 3, St Louis, 1995, Mosby.)

aggregated neutrophils, macrophages, and platelets. Because vasoconstriction occurs more in some vascular beds than others, blood flow to selected areas of the lungs is decreased, resulting in $\dot{V}/\dot{Q}$ mismatching.

The initial lung injury damages the alveolar epithelium and the vascular endothelium. Surfactant is inactivated, and its production by type II alveolar cells is impaired as alveoli and respiratory bronchioles fill with fluid or collapse. The lungs become less compliant, resulting in decreased ventilation of alveoli, right-to-left shunting of pulmonary blood flow, and increased work of breathing.

Twenty-four to forty-eight hours after the acute hemorrhagic phase of ARDS, hyaline membranes form, and after approximately 7 days, fibrosis progressively obliterates the alveoli, respiratory bronchioles, and interstitium. This leads to a decrease in functional residual capacity (FRC) and even more severe right-to-left shunting. The result of this overwhelming inflammatory response by the lungs is acute respiratory failure.

The chemical mediators responsible for the alveolocapillary damage of ARDS often cause widespread inflammation, endothelial damage, and capillary permeability throughout the body resulting in the systemic inflammatory response syndrome (SIRS), which then leads to multiple organ dysfunction syndrome (MODS). In fact, death may not be caused by respiratory failure alone but by MODS associated with ARDS. (MODS is discussed in Chapter 46.)

CLINICAL MANIFESTATIONS   The classic signs and symptoms of ARDS are rapid, shallow breathing; respiratory alkalosis; marked dyspnea; decreased lung compliance; hypoxemia unresponsive to oxygen therapy (refractory hypoxemia); and diffuse alveolar infiltrates seen on chest radiographs, without evidence of cardiac disease. Symptoms develop as the disease progresses. Initially individuals hyper-

ventilate, causing respiratory alkalosis. As the work of breathing increases because of the decrease in compliance caused by alveolar filling and collapse, the individual experiences dyspnea and hypoxemia. Hypoxemia worsens despite oxygen therapy, and diffuse crackles can be heard on auscultation. Eventually metabolic acidosis develops because of the increased work of breathing and cellular hypoxia, and fluffy infiltrates appear on chest radiographs. If ARDS is not reversed, respiratory acidosis develops and further hypoxemia results in hypotension, decreased cardiac output, and death. The clinical course of progressive ARDS can be summarized as follows: hyperventilation → respiratory alkalosis → dyspnea and hypoxemia → metabolic acidosis → respiratory acidosis → further hypoxemia → hypotension, decreased cardiac output → death.

EVALUATION AND TREATMENT   Diagnosis is made on the basis of physical examination, analysis of blood gases, and radiologic examination. Initial physical examination may show fine crackles, and the chest film may be clear or show a few scattered infiltrates. With progressive respiratory involvement, crackles are heard throughout the lungs and radiographs show extensive bilateral infiltrates. The criteria for diagnosis of ARDS were established in 1994 and include refractory hypoxemia, a chest x-ray with bilateral infiltrates, and the exclusion of cardiogenic pulmonary edema. Further diagnostic testing may include CT of the chest and bronchoscopy.

Treatment is based on early detection, supportive therapy, and prevention of complications. Traditional therapy involves mechanical ventilation with PEEP and high oxygen concentrations. Numerous alternative modalities of ventilation are being tested, including noninvasive positive pressure ventilation, permissive hypercapnia, prone positioning, extracorporeal gas exchange, and partial liquid ventilation; some of these methods have shown apparent reductions in mortality rates.[37] Sedation may be employed to decrease oxygen consumption. If necessary, drugs are given to increase cardiac output. Steroid administration remains controversial but may improve overall outcomes when given in physiologic doses.[38,39]

Many studies are underway investigating new ways to prevent or treat ARDS. Prophylactic immunotherapy, antibodies against endotoxin, antioxidants, surfactant replacement, nitric oxide inhalation, and inhibition of various inflammatory mediators are among the possibilities being tested.[40] Recently, anticoagulant therapy with recombinant human activated protein C has shown positive results in ARDS.[41]

Postoperative Respiratory Failure

Respiratory failure is an important potential complication of any major surgical procedure, especially those that involve the central nervous system, thorax, or upper abdomen. Smokers are at risk, particularly if they have preexisting lung disease. Limited cardiac reserve, chronic renal failure, chronic hepatic disease, and infection also increase the tendency to develop postoperative respiratory failure.

The most common postoperative pulmonary problems are atelectasis, pneumonia, pulmonary edema, and pulmonary emboli. These problems usually result in reduced FRC, decreased compliance, and ventilation-perfusion mismatch. Individuals in whom respiratory failure develops usually have had a period of hypotension during surgery, and many have sepsis.

Prevention of postoperative respiratory failure includes frequent turning, deep breathing, and early ambulation to prevent atelectasis and accumulation of secretions. Humidification of inspired air can help loosen secretions. Incentive spirometry gives individuals immediate feedback about tidal volumes, which encourages them to breathe deeply. Supplemental oxygen is given for hypoxemia, and antibiotics are given as appropriate to treat infection. If respiratory failure develops, the individual may require mechanical ventilation for a time.

Obstructive Pulmonary Disease

Obstructive pulmonary disease is characterized by airway obstruction that is worse with expiration. Either more force (i.e., use of accessory muscles of expiration) is required to expire a given volume of air or emptying of the lungs is slowed or both. The unifying symptom of obstructive pulmonary disease is dyspnea; the unifying sign is wheezing. Individuals have an increased work of breathing, ventilation-perfusion mismatching, and a decreased forced expiratory volume in one second (FEV_1). The most common obstructive diseases are asthma, chronic bronchitis, and emphysema. Because many individuals have both chronic bronchitis and emphysema, these diseases together are often called *chronic obstructive pulmonary disease (COPD)*. Asthma is more acute and intermittent than COPD, even though it can be chronic (Figure 33-10).

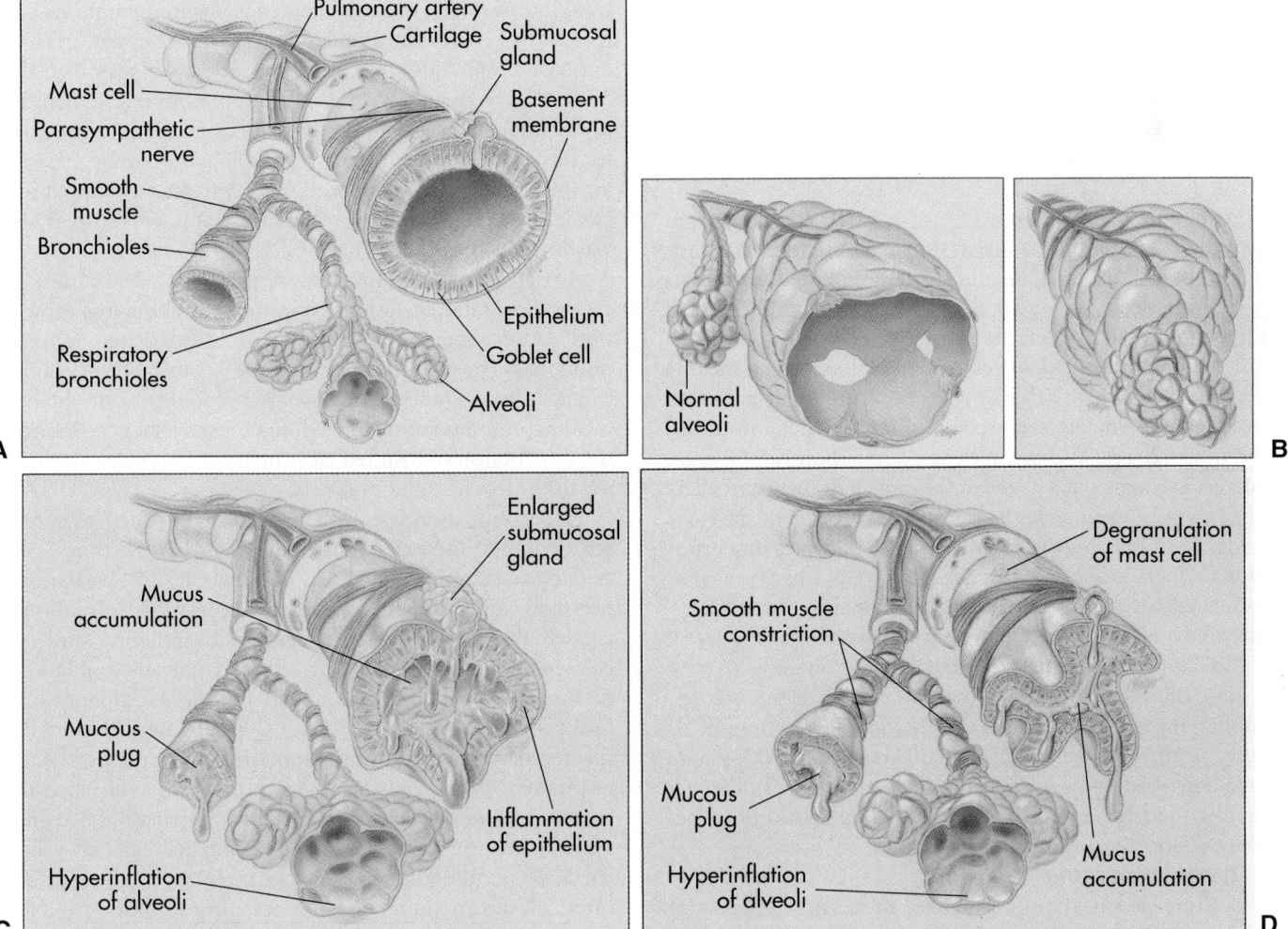

Figure 33-10 Airway obstruction caused by emphysema, chronic bronchitis, and asthma. **A,** The normal lung. **B,** Emphysema: enlargement and destruction of alveolar walls with loss of elasticity and trapping of air; *(left)* panlobular emphysema showing abnormal weakening and enlargement of all air spaces distal to the terminal bronchioles (normal alveoli shown for comparison only); *(right)* centrilobular emphysema showing abnormal weakening and enlargement of the respiratory bronchioles in the proximal portion of the acinus. **C,** Chronic bronchitis: inflammation and thickening of mucous membrane with accumulation of mucus and pus leading to obstruction; characterized by cough. **D,** Bronchial asthma: thick mucus, mucosal edema, and smooth muscle spasm causing obstruction of small airways; breathing becomes labored and expiration is difficult. (Modified from Des Jardins T, Burton GG: *Clinical manifestations and assessment of respiratory disease,* ed 3, St Louis, 1995, Mosby.)

Asthma

Asthma is defined[42] as

> "a chronic inflammatory disorder of the airways in which many cells and cellular elements play a role, in particular, mast cells, eosinophils, T lymphocytes, macrophages, neutrophils, and epithelial cells. In susceptible individuals, this inflammation causes recurrent episodes of wheezing, breathlessness, chest tightness, and coughing, particularly at night or in the early morning. These episodes are usually associated with widespread but variable airflow obstruction that is often reversible, either spontaneously or with treatment. The inflammation also causes an associated increase in the existing bronchial hyperresponsiveness to a variety of stimuli. Subbasement membrane fibrosis may occur in some patients with asthma and these changes contribute to persistent abnormalities of lung function."[42, p. 8]

Most attacks of asthmatic bronchospasm are short lived, with freedom from symptoms between episodes. However, airway inflammation is present even in asymptomatic individuals.

Asthma occurs at all ages, with approximately half of all cases developing during childhood and another third before age 40. In the United States, more than 11 million persons reported having an asthma attack in 2000, and more than 5% of children under the age of 18 report having asthma attacks.[42] Mortality rates have declined since 1995, but the incidence of asthma has increased over the past two decades, especially in urban areas.[42]

Asthma is a familial disorder and over 20 genes have been identified that may play a role in the susceptibility and pathogenesis of asthma, including those that influence the production of interleukins 4 and 5, IgE, eosinophils, mast cells, beta adrenergic receptors, and bronchial hyperresponsiveness.[43,44] Risk factors for asthma, in addition to family history, include allergen exposure, urban residence, exposure to air pollution and cigarette smoke, recurrent respiratory viral infections, and other allergic diseases, such as allergic rhinitis.[45] Of great interest in recent years has been the impact of recurrent allergen exposure during childhood on the subsequent development of asthma. A great deal of evidence indicates that exposure to high levels of most allergens (e.g., dust mites) is correlated with an increased risk of asthma; however, exposure to cat allergens does not seem to have the same effect.[46] It also has been noted that children who live on farms or have certain childhood infections may have a decreased risk for asthma, theoretically because they become less immunologically "primed" to be allergic.[43,47,48] These relationships have been described as the *hygiene hypothesis* and many studies are being conducted to further elucidate this relationship between allergen exposure and asthma risk.

Types of Asthma

Asthma classification has changed in recent years. A consensus was reached for a system of asthma classification based on clinical severity rather than on underlying pathophysiologic differences; this scheme correlates with management choices and clinical outcomes.[42,43]

PATHOPHYSIOLOGY Inflammation resulting in hyperresponsiveness of the airways is the major pathologic feature of asthma. IgE and irritant-mediated mast cell degranu-

lation (see Chapter 7) causes the release of a large number of inflammatory mediators, such as histamine, prostaglandins, and leukotrienes[43,49-51] (Figure 33-11). In addition, chemotactic factors are produced that result in bronchial infiltration by neutrophils, eosinophils, and lymphocytes.[52,53] The resulting inflammatory process produces bronchial smooth muscle spasm, vascular congestion, increased vascular permeability, edema formation, production of thick tenacious mucus, impaired mucociliary function (see Figure 33-10), thickening of airway walls, and increased contractile response of bronchial smooth muscle.[49,52] Other inflammatory cytokines, such as TNF and IL-1, have been found to alter muscarinic receptor function leading to increased levels of acetylcholine, which causes bronchial smooth muscle contraction and mucus secretion.[49,54] These changes, combined with the epithelial cell damage caused by eosinophil infiltration, produce acute airway hyperreponsiveness and obstruction. In cases of significant allergen exposure, symptoms can recur 4 to 12 hours after the initial attack because of persistent eosinophil and lymphocyte activation. This is called the *late asthma response,* and it can be even more severe than the initial attack. Recent studies have identified important roles for nitric oxide and reduced airway pH in the pathogenesis of asthma and airway inflammation.[55] Untreated inflammation can lead to long-term airway damage that is irreversible (airway remodeling).[49,56]

Airway obstruction increases resistance to airflow and decreases flow rates, including expiratory flow. Impaired expiration causes hyperinflation distal to obstructions, altered pulmonary mechanics, and increased work of breathing. Changes in resistance to airflow are not uniform throughout the lungs. Because of regional differences in airway resistance, the distribution of inspired air is uneven, with more air flowing to the less resistant portions.

Hyperventilation is eventually triggered by lung receptors responding to increased lung volume and obstruction. Continued air trapping increases intrapleural and alveolar gas pressures and causes decreased perfusion of the alveoli. Increased alveolar gas pressure, decreased ventilation, and decreased perfusion lead to variable and uneven ventilation-perfusion relationships within different lung segments. The result is early hypoxemia without CO_2 retention. Hypoxemia further increases hyperventilation through stimulation of the respiratory center, causing $PaCO_2$ to decrease and pH to increase (respiratory alkalosis). As the obstruction becomes more severe, the number of alveoli being inadequately ventilated and perfused increases. As air trapping in the lungs because of obstruction of expiratory airflow progresses, the lungs and thorax become hyperexpanded putting the respiratory muscles at a mechanical disadvantage. This leads to CO_2 retention and respiratory acidosis. Respiratory acidosis signals respiratory failure.[57]

CLINICAL MANIFESTATIONS During full remission, individuals are asymptomatic and pulmonary function tests are normal. During partial remission, no clinical symptoms

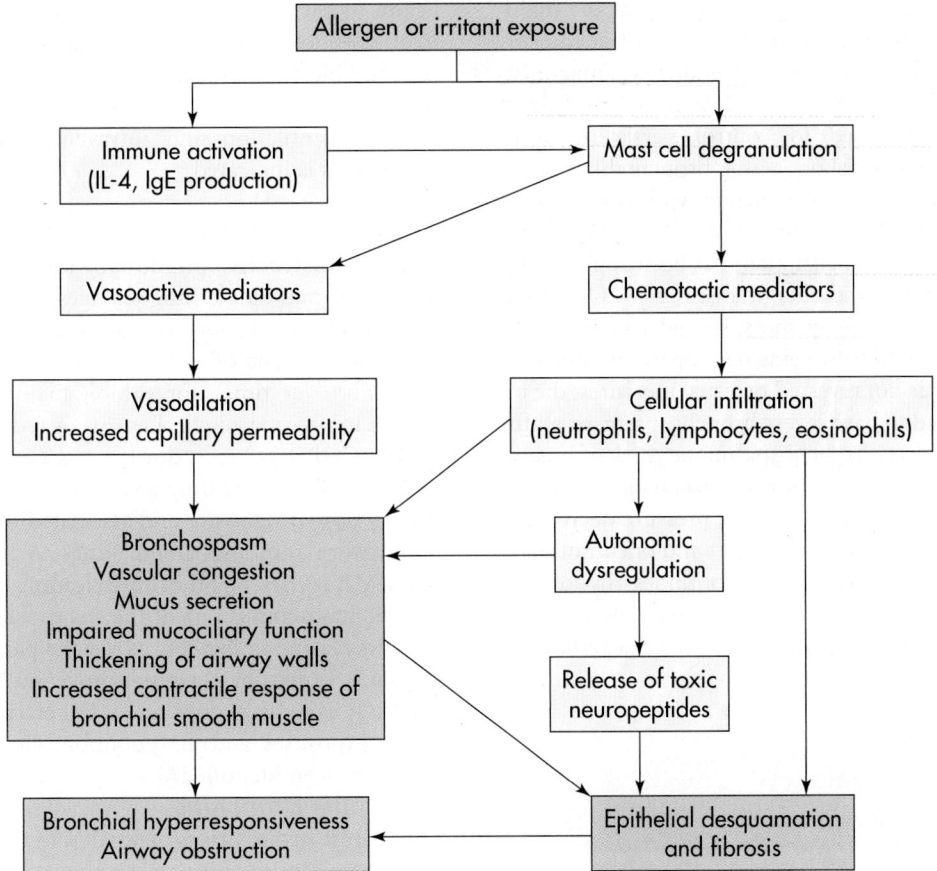

Figure 33-11 **Pathophysiology of asthma.** Allergen or irritant exposure results in a cascade of inflammatory events leading to acute and chronic airway dysfunction.

are observed but pulmonary function tests are abnormal. Asthma attacks can present in two primary ways. Most develop over hours or days with slowly progressive clinical deterioration (slow-onset acute asthma). These often follow upper respiratory infection and are characterized by widespread airway inflammation. Hyperacute asthma attacks develop over minutes to hours with rapid progression of symptoms. This type of attack is most commonly triggered by allergens, exercise, or stress.[57]

During attacks, individuals are dyspneic and respiratory effort is marked. Breath sounds are decreased except for considerable wheezing. Because the severity of alterations in blood gases is difficult to evaluate by clinical signs alone, arterial blood gas tensions should be measured if oxygen saturation falls below 90%. Similarly, a peak flow measurement should be obtained early in an acute attack because it is common for the clinical examination to underestimate the degree of airway obstruction, often leading to inadequate intervention.

A sensation of chest constriction, inspiratory and expiratory wheezing, dyspnea, nonproductive coughing, prolonged expiration, tachycardia, and tachypnea occur at the beginning of an attack. With severe attacks the accessory muscles of respiration are prominent. As the episode resolves, coughing produces a thick, stringy mucus with casts of the small airways that can be seen microscopically.

EVALUATION AND TREATMENT During an attack of asthma, spirometry shows decreases in expiratory flow rate, forced expiratory volume (FEV), and forced vital capacity (FVC) (see Chapter 32). FRC and total lung capacity (TLC) are increased. Blood gas analysis shows hypoxemia with early respiratory alkalosis or late respiratory acidosis.

The most successful treatment of asthma is elimination of the causative agents. Acute episodes are treated with drugs that are geared toward reversing bronchospasm and airway inflammation. Management of the acute asthma attack requires immediate administration of oxygen and inhaled bronchodilators. In addition, oral corticosteroids should be administered early in the course of management.[43,57] Careful monitoring of gas exchange and airway obstruction in response to therapy provides information necessary to determine whether hospitalization is necessary. Antibiotics are not indicated for acute asthma unless there is a documented bacterial infection.[43]

Chronic management of asthma begins with avoidance of allergens and other triggers. Individuals tend to underestimate the severity of their asthma and should receive extensive patient education, including the use of a peak flowmeter and the adherence to an action plan should symptoms worsen.[43] Pharmacologic management of chronic asthma is based on asthma severity (see Table 33-3) and includes antiinflammatories such as inhaled corticosteroids as the mainstay of therapy.[43,50,58] In individuals who are not adequately controlled on inhaled corticosteroids, leukotriene antagonists can be considered. Long-acting beta agonists and ipratropium also can be used to control persistent bronchospasm.[43,52] Quick relief, short-acting bronchodilators can be prescribed as well. Long-term therapy with oral corticosteroids should be avoided if possible. Recently, monoclonal antibody that blocks IgE (omalizumab) has been approved for the treatment of asthma and allergic diseases.[43,59] Other immune therapies, such as allergy shots, should be considered. New treatments are continually being developed and tested.[43,60]

If bronchospasm is not reversed by usual measures, the individual is considered to have severe bronchospasm, or **status asthmaticus.** With severe bronchospasm, the work of breathing can be 5 to 10 times that of normal. When air trapping is severe, paradoxic pulse (a systolic blood pressure decrease of more than 10 mmHg during inspiration) and pneumothorax are common. If status asthmaticus continues, hypoxemia worsens, expiratory flows and volumes decrease further, and the individual begins to tire. Acidosis develops as arterial P_{CO_2}

begins to rise. Asthma becomes life threatening at this point if treatment does not reverse this process quickly. A silent chest (no audible air movement) and a P_{CO_2} of more than 70 mmHg are ominous signs. Immediate intervention with mechanical ventilation and intravenous steroids and bronchodilators is indicated.[57,61]

Chronic Obstructive Pulmonary Disease

Chronic obstructive pulmonary disease (COPD) has been defined as pathologic lung changes consistent with emphysema or chronic bronchitis and is a syndrome characterized by abnormal tests of expiratory airflow that do not change markedly over time, nor exhibit major reversibility in response to pharmacological agents. A recent consensus report defines COPD as " . . . a disease state characterized by airflow limitation that is not fully reversible. The airflow limitation is usually both progressive and associated with an abnormal inflammatory response of the lungs to noxious particles or gases."[62] It is currently the fourth leading cause of death in the United States and is one of the few causes of death that have been increasing in incidence over the past 30 years. COPD is primarily caused by cigarette smoke; both active and passive smoking have been implicated. Other risks include occupational exposures and air pollution. Genetic susceptibilities also have been identified.[63]

Chronic Bronchitis
Chronic bronchitis is defined as hypersecretion of mucus and chronic productive cough that continues for at least 3

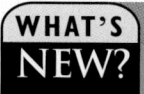

WHAT'S NEW? New Anti-IgE Drug Omalizumab for the Treatment of Asthma

In genetically predisposed individuals, exposure to inhaled allergens can lead to an allergic response that is manifested clinically as asthma. This immunologic response is a type I hypersensitivity reaction (see Chapter 7) and results from a complex interaction of macrophages, T lymphocytes, antibodies, mast cells, and eosinophils. The immune response leads to a profound inflammatory response, with resultant bronchospasm, mucus formation, and mucosal edema in the airways. At first, asthma treatments were confined to relieving the symptomatic effects of this process, that is, bronchodilators and expectorants. In 1997, new guidelines emphasized the importance of anti-inflammatory drugs in the treatment of asthma. Now attention is focused on preventing or limiting the immune response. Allergen avoidance is the first step in preventing this type I hypersensitivity reaction and immunotherapy (allergy shots) can be effective. New therapies are being introduced that help in limiting the severity of this response. Recently, the FDA approved a drug that blocks IgE, the antibody responsible for allergy and asthma. This drug, called omalizumab (Xolair), is humanized monoclonal anti-immunoglobulin E (IgE) antibody. It is currently indicated for individuals with moderate or severe asthma who do not respond adequately to inhaled corticosteroids alone. The addition of this new drug to more standard asthma therapies has been shown to improve symptoms, reduce hospitalizations, and limit the need for systemic corticosteroid therapy. It is well tolerated by both children and adults, although long-term safety studies are still underway.

Data from Ames SA, Gleeson CD, Kirkpatrick P: *Nat Rev Drug Discov* 3(3):199-200, 2004; Boushey HA: *Chest* 123(3 Suppl): 439S-445S, 2003; Bousquet J et al: *Chest* 125(4):1378-1386, 2004; Finn A et al: *J Allergy Clin Immunol* 111(2):278-284, 2003; Lanier BQ et al: *Ann Allergy Asthma Immunol* 91(2):154-159, 2003; Rambasek TE, Lang DM, Kavuru MS: *Clev Clin J Med* 71(3):251-261, 2004.

NUTRITION & DISEASE

Chronic Obstructive Pulmonary Disease

Malnutrition is a major concern for individuals with chronic obstructive pulmonary disease (COPD) because they have increased energy expenditure, decreased energy intake, and impaired oxygenation. The disproportionate muscle wasting is similar to what occurs with other chronic diseases, such as cancer, heart failure, and AIDS. Systemic inflammatory mediators may impair appetite and contribute to hypermetabolism. Malnutrition (1) adversely affects exercise tolerance by limiting skeletal and respiratory muscle strength and aerobic capacity, (2) limits surfactant production, (3) reduces cell-mediated immune responses, (4) reduces protein synthesis, and (5) increases morbidity and mortality. The medical nutrition therapy goal is to maintain an acceptable and stable weight for the person. This can be accomplished by including foods of high energy density, frequent snacking, soft foods and beverages, assistance with shopping and meal preparation. Increasing omega-3 fatty acids and antioxidant intake may modulate the effects of systemic inflammation. Protein intake should be maintained at 1.0 to 1.5 g/kg of body weight, and a daily vitamin C supplement should be added to the diet if the individual is still smoking.

Data from Calikoglu M et al: *Respiration* 71(1):45-50, 2004; Godoy I et al: *Eur Respir J* 22(6):920-925, 2003; Thomas DR: *Clin Geriatr Med* 18(4):835-839, viii, 2002.

months of the year (usually the winter months) for at least 2 consecutive years. Incidence is increased in smokers (up to twentyfold) and even more so in workers exposed to air pollution. It is a major health problem for the elderly population. Repeated infections are common.

PATHOPHYSIOLOGY Inspired irritants not only increase mucus production but also increase the size and number of mucous glands and goblet cells in airway epithelium. The mucus produced is thicker and more tenacious than normal. This sticky mucus coating makes it much more likely that bacteria, such as *Haemophilus influenzae* and *Streptococcus pneumoniae*, will become embedded in the airway secre-

tions, where they reproduce rapidly. Ciliary function is impaired, reducing mucus clearance further. The lung's defense mechanisms are therefore compromised, increasing susceptibility to pulmonary infection and injury. As infection and injury increase mucus production further, the bronchial walls become inflamed and thickened from edema and accumulation of inflammatory cells.[64] Persistent inflammation and recurrent infection leads to bronchospasm and eventual permanent narrowing of the airways. (The pathogenesis of chronic bronchitis is shown in Figure 33-12.)

Initially chronic bronchitis affects only the larger bronchi, but eventually all airways are involved. The thick mucus and hypertrophied bronchial smooth muscle obstruct the airways

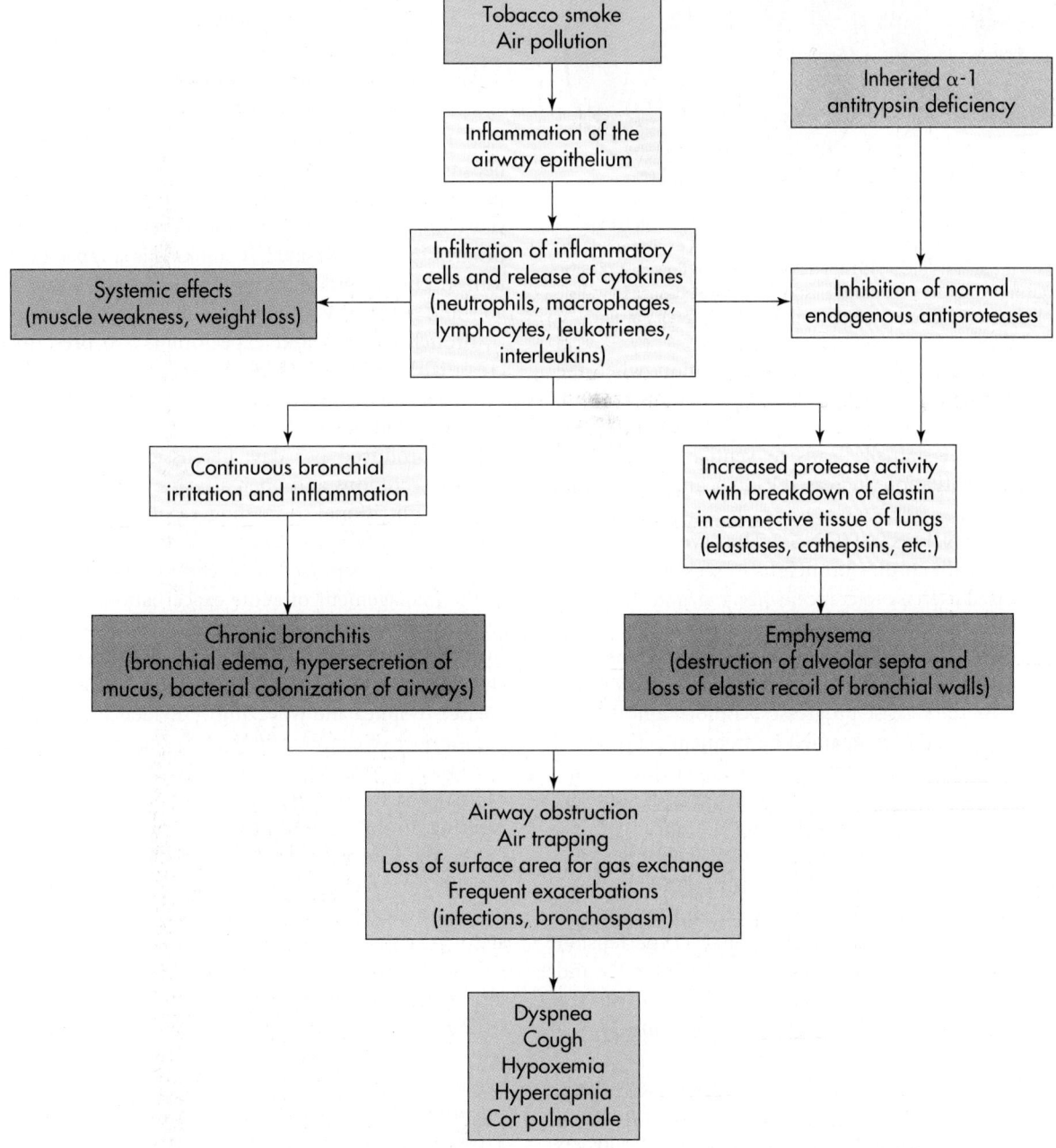

Figure 33-12 Pathogenesis of chronic bronchitis and emphysema (chronic obstructive pulmonary disease [COPD]).

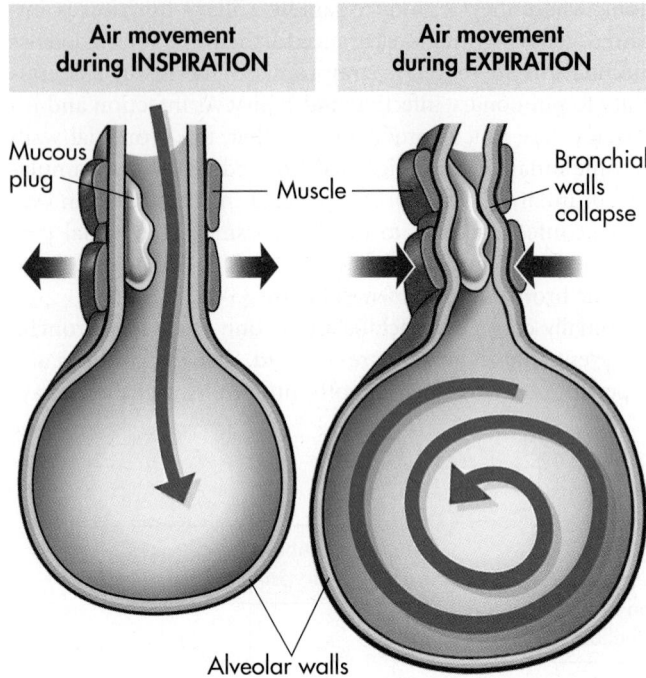

Air movement during INSPIRATION

Air movement during EXPIRATION

Mucous plug — Muscle — Bronchial walls collapse

Alveolar walls

Figure 33-13 Mechanisms of air trapping in COPD. Mucous plugs and narrowed airways cause air trapping and hyperinflation on expiration. During inspiration the airways are pulled open allowing gas to flow past the obstruction. During expiration, decreased elastic recoil of the bronchial walls results in collapse of the airways and prevents normal expiratory airflow.

Table 33-3	Clinical Manifestations of Chronic Pulmonary Disease	
Clinical Manifestations	**Chronic Bronchitis**	**Emphysema**
Productive cough	Classic sign	Late in course with infection
Dyspnea	Late in course	Common
Wheezing	Intermittent	Minimal
History of smoking	Common	Common
Barrel chest	Occasionally	Classic
Prolonged expiration	Always present	Always present
Cyanosis	Common	Uncommon
Chronic hypoventilation	Common	Late in course
Polycythemia	Common	Late in course
Cor pulmonale	Common	Late in course

and lead to closure, particularly during expiration, when the airways are narrowed (Figure 33-13). The airways collapse early in expiration, trapping gas in the distal portions of the lung. Obstruction eventually leads to ventilation-perfusion mismatch, hypoventilation (increased $PaCO_2$), and hypoxemia.

CLINICAL MANIFESTATIONS The symptoms that lead individuals with chronic bronchitis to seek medical care include decreased exercise tolerance, wheezing, and shortness of breath. Individuals usually have a productive cough ("smoker's cough"), and evidence of airway obstruction (decreased FEV_1) is shown by spirometry. Hypoxemia may occur with exercise. As the disease progresses, copious amounts of sputum are produced, accompanied by frequent pulmonary infections. FVC and FEV_1 become markedly reduced, and FRC and residual volume (RV) are increased as airway obstruction and air trapping become more pronounced.

Airway obstruction results in decreased alveolar ventilation and increased $PaCO_2$. Marked hypoxemia leads to polycythemia (overproduction of erythrocytes) and cyanosis. If not reversed, hypoxemia leads to pulmonary hypertension and eventually results in cor pulmonale (see Chapter 32) and can lead to severe disability or death. (Table 33-3 lists the common clinical manifestations of chronic bronchitis.)

EVALUATION AND TREATMENT Diagnosis is made on the basis of history of symptoms, physical examination, chest radiograph, pulmonary function tests, and blood gas analyses; these tests reflect the progressive nature of the dis-

ease. The best "treatment" for chronic bronchitis is prevention, because pathologic changes are not reversible. By the time an individual seeks medical care for symptoms, considerable airway damage is present. If the individual stops smoking, disease progression can be halted. If smoking is stopped before symptoms occur, the risk of chronic bronchitis decreases considerably and eventually reaches that of nonsmokers.

Bronchodilators and expectorants are prescribed to increase airway caliber, improve secretion removal, and maximize gas exchange. Chest physical therapy includes deep breathing and postural drainage when 30 ml or more of sputum is produced per day; percussion also is employed to remove secretions and open airways. Teaching of individuals includes nutritional counseling, respiratory hygiene, recognition of the early signs of infection, and techniques that relieve dyspnea, such as pursed-lip breathing. The role of antibiotics in the management of acute exacerbations of chronic bronchitis has been controversial. Good evidence now indicates that antibiotics should be used for all acute exacerbations of chronic bronchitis (change in sputum amount or color, increased dyspnea and wheezing).[65] Evidence also indicates that the number of exacerbations of chronic bronchitis can be reduced using prophylactic antibiotics; however, this is not recommended for routine care because of the concern for increasing antibiotic resistance.[66] Steroids sometimes are used late in the course of the disease but should be reserved only for those people in whom less toxic therapies are inadequate and who demonstrate some improvement after a trial of steroid therapy.

Individuals with severe hypoxemia require oxygen therapy to prevent cor pulmonale. Low-flow oxygen is administered with care to individuals with severe hypoxemia and CO_2 retention. Because of the chronic elevation of $PaCO_2$, the central chemoreceptors no longer act as the primary stimulus for breathing. (Chemoreceptors are described in Chapter 32.) This role is taken over by the peripheral chemoreceptors, which are sensitive to changes in PaO_2. Peripheral chemoreceptors do not stimulate breathing if the PaO_2 is much more than 60 mmHg. Therefore, if oxygen therapy causes PaO_2 to exceed 60 mmHg, the stimulus to breathe is lost, $PaCO_2$ increases, and apnea results. If adequate oxygenation cannot be achieved without resulting in respiratory depression, the individual must be mechanically ventilated.

Emphysema

Emphysema is abnormal permanent enlargement of gas-exchange airways (acini) accompanied by destruction of alveolar walls without obvious fibrosis. In emphysema, obstruction results from changes in lung tissues, rather than mucus production and inflammation, as in chronic bronchitis. The major mechanism of airflow limitation in emphysema is loss of elastic recoil. Some degree of emphysema is considered normal in elderly individuals but results in a slow and predictable decline in lung function with aging. When it occurs earlier in life, however, it is usually secondary to cigarette smoking, although in rare cases it may be primary emphysema.

Primary emphysema, which accounts for 1% to 2% of all cases of emphysema, is commonly linked to an inherited deficiency of the enzyme α_1-antitrypsin. α_1-Antitrypsin is a major component of α_1-globulin, a plasma protein. Normally α_1-antitrypsin inhibits the action of many proteolytic enzymes (enzymes that break down proteins). Individuals who have α_1-antitrypsin deficiency (an autosomal recessive trait) have an increased likelihood of developing emphysema because proteolysis in lung tissues is not inhibited. Homozygous individuals have a 70% to 80% likelihood of developing lung disease. (Mechanisms of genetic inheritance are described in Chapter 4.) Persons with α_1-antitrypsin deficiency who smoke are even more susceptible to emphysema than those with the deficiency alone. α_1-Antitrypsin deficiency is suggested in individuals who develop emphysema before age 40 years (or in their early forties) and in nonsmokers who develop emphysema. (The principles of risk factor analysis are discussed in Chapter 5.)

Secondary emphysema also is caused by an inability of the body to inhibit proteolytic enzymes in the lung. It results from an insult to the lungs from inhaled toxins, such as cigarette smoke and air pollution. Not all smokers develop emphysema, but approximately 20% are especially susceptible and develop significant lung damage if they continue to smoke.

PATHOPHYSIOLOGY Emphysema is characterized by destruction of alveoli through the breakdown of elastin within the septa by proteases. In most individuals, this process is initiated through the inhalation of inflammatory oxidants such as cigarette smoke. Toxins in smoke lead to airway epithelial inflammation with infiltration of numerous cells such as neutrophils, macrophages, and lymphocytes (see Figure 32-12). Inflammatory cytokines are released that increase protease activity and inhibit the normal endogenous antiproteases in the lung. Some of the most important proteases activated in emphysema are elastases, cathepsins, and matrix metalloproteases.[67,68] α-1 Antitrypsin is an important antiprotease that is inhibited by cigarette smoke and is absent or reduced in individuals with inherited emphysema. The imbalance between proteases and antiproteases leads to breakdown of elastin in the alveolar septa.[67,68] Septal destruction eliminates portions of the pulmonary capillary bed and increases the volume of air in the acinus. In addition, destruction of elastin in the bronchial walls reduces elastic recoil of the airways. Expiration becomes difficult because loss of elastic recoil reduces the volume of air that can be expired passively. Hyperinflation of alveoli causes large air spaces (bullae) and air spaces adjacent to pleura (blebs) to develop. Septal destruction also affects airway caliber because the force that normal alveoli exert on bronchiolar walls is diminished. The combination of increased RV in the alveoli and diminished caliber of the bronchioles causes part of each inspiration to be trapped in the acinus. Additional airway narrowing can result from inflammatory hyperreactivity of the bronchi with bronchoconstriction, which may be partially reversible with bronchodilators.

Emphysema can be centriacinar (centrilobular) or panacinar (panlobular), depending on the site of involvement (Figure 33-14). In **centriacinar emphysema,** septal destruction occurs in the respiratory bronchioles and alveolar ducts, usually in the upper lobes of the lung. The alveolar sac (alveoli distal to the respiratory bronchiole) remains intact. It tends to occur in smokers with chronic bronchitis. **Panacinar emphysema** involves the entire acinus, with damage more randomly distributed and involving the lower lobes of the lung. It tends to occur in elderly persons and in those with α_1-antitrypsin deficiency.

CLINICAL MANIFESTATIONS Individuals with emphysema usually have dyspnea on exertion that later progresses to marked dyspnea, even at rest (see Table 33-4). Little coughing and very little sputum are produced. The individual often is thin, has tachypnea with prolonged expiration, and must use accessory muscles for ventilation. The anteroposterior diameter of the chest is increased, and the chest has a hyperresonant sound with percussion. To increase lung capacity, the individual often leans forward with arms extended and braced on knees when sitting.

EVALUATION AND TREATMENT Emphysema is usually diagnosed by pulmonary function measures. Pulmonary function tests indicate obstruction to gas flow during expiration. Airway collapse and air trapping in distal portions of the lung lead to a decrease in FVC and FEV_1 and an increase in FRC, RV, and TLC. TLC can increase to twice the normal value.[65] Diffusing capacity is decreased because of destruction of the alveolocapillary membrane. On radiographs the diaphragm appears flattened and the lung fields appear translucent. Marked and persistent overdistention of the lungs is suggestive of emphysema. Some centers are now using computed tomography to assess lung changes in emphysema but the clinical utility of this testing has yet to be deter-

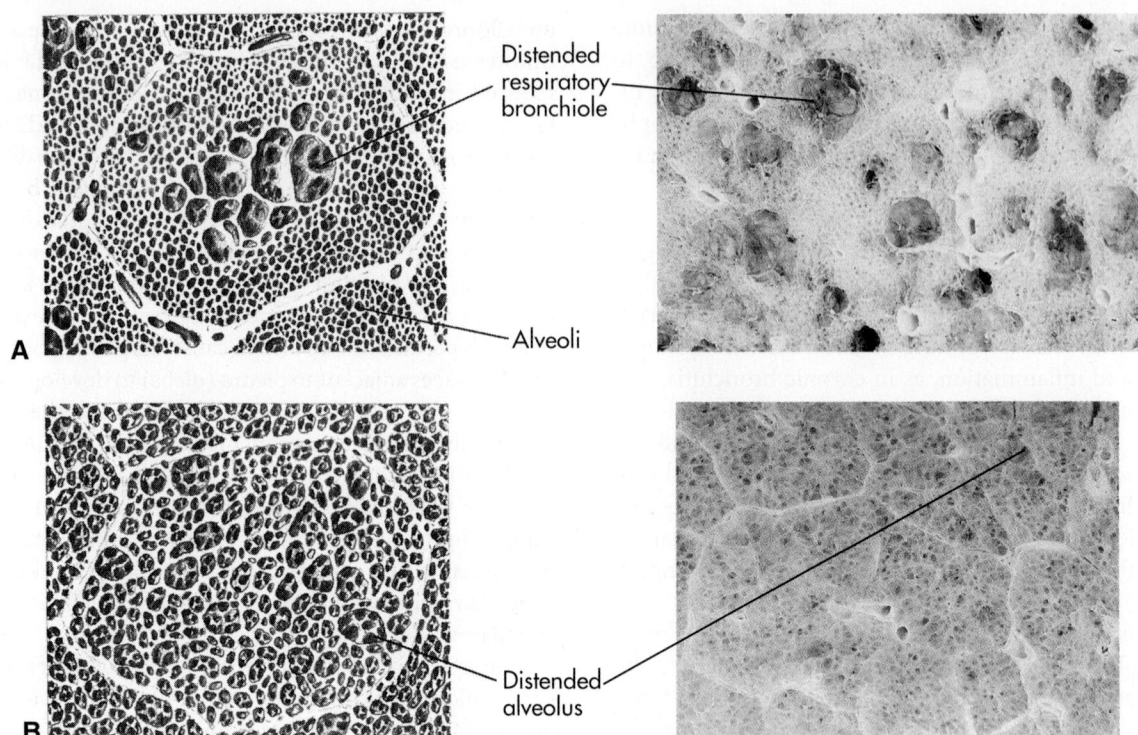

Figure 33-14 Types of emphysema. **A,** Centriacinar emphysema. **B,** Panacinar emphysema. (Micrographs from Damjanov I, Linder J, editors: *Anderson's pathology,* ed 10, St Louis, 1996, Mosby.)

mined. Arterial blood gas measurements reveal varying degrees of hypoxemia and/or hypercapnia. The disease course is usually prolonged, with increasing dyspnea and intermittent bouts of infection that culminate in failure of the right side of the heart (cor pulmonale) and death.

Management of acute exacerbations of emphysema requires obtaining a chest radiograph, serum white blood count, arterial blood gas, and sputum sample.[65,69] Individuals should receive oxygen and may require noninvasive positive pressure ventilation or mechanical ventilation. Inhaled bronchodilators should be administered by either inhaler or nebulizer. Oral corticosteroids and antibiotics should be begun immediately.[65,69] Chronic management of emphysema begins with smoking cessation. Inhaled anticholinergic agents and beta agonists should be prescribed.[65,70,71] A trial of inhaled corticosteroids also can be undertaken, although long-term therapy with oral steroids should be avoided if possible.[65,70] Pulmonary rehabilitation, improved nutrition, and breathing techniques all can improve symptoms. Oxygen therapy is indicated in chronic hypoxemia but must be administered with care. Progressive pulmonary dysfunction with hypoxemia and hypercapnia may require long-term oxygen therapy and ventilation if indicated.[72] In selected patients, lung reduction surgery or transplantation can be considered.[65,70]

Respiratory Tract Infections

Respiratory tract infections are the most common cause of short-term disability in the United States. Most of these infections—the common cold, pharyngitis (sore throat), and laryngitis—involve only the upper airways. Although the lungs have direct contact with the atmosphere, they remain sterile under most circumstances. Infections of the lower respiratory tract occur most often in the very young, the very old, or individuals with impaired immunity or underlying disease. In all cases the body's normal defense mechanisms are impaired.

Pneumonia

Pneumonia is infection of the lower respiratory tract caused by bacteria, viruses, fungi, protozoa, or parasites. It is the sixth leading cause of death in the United States. The incidence and mortality of pneumonia are highest in the elderly.[73] Risk factors for pneumonia include advanced age, immunocompromise, underlying lung disease, alcoholism, altered consciousness, smoking, endotracheal intubation, malnutrition, immobilization, underlying cardiac or liver disease, and residence in a nursing home.[74] The causative microorganism influences the symptoms and signs with which the patient presents, how the pneumonia should be treated, and the prognosis.[74,75] Community-acquired pneumonia tends to be caused by different microorganisms than those infections acquired in the hospital (nosocomial). In addition, the characteristics of the individual are important in determining which etiologic microorganism is likely; for example, immunocompromised persons tend to be susceptible to opportunistic infections that are uncommon in normal adults. In general, nosocomial infections and those affecting immunocompromised individuals have a higher mortality rate than community-acquired pneumonias. Some of the most common causal microorganisms include the following:[74-78]

Community Acquired	Nosocomial Pneumonia	Immunocompromised Individuals
Streptococcus pneumoniae	*Pseudomonas aeruginosa*	*Pneumocystis jerovici (formerly carinii)*
Mycoplasma pneumoniae	*Staphylococcus aureus*	*Mycobacterium tuberculosis*
Haemophilus influenzae	*Klebsiella pneumoniae*	Atypical mycobacteria
Oral anaerobic bacteria	*Escherichia coli*	Fungi
Influenza virus		Respiratory viruses
Legionella pneumophila		Protozoa
Chlamydia pneumoniae		Parasites
Moraxella catarrhalis		

The most common community-acquired pneumonia is caused by *Streptococcus pneumoniae* (also known as the *pneumococcus*), which has a relatively low overall mortality rate, although the rate is higher in the elderly and smokers. *Mycoplasma pneumoniae* is a common cause of pneumonia in young people, especially those living in group housing such as dormitories and army barracks. Influenza is the most common viral community-acquired pneumonia in adults. *Legionella* species can contaminate cooling systems and water supplies, thereby leading to outbreaks of disease such as the 1976 incident at the American Legion Convention in Philadelphia.[79] *Pseudomonas aeruginosa*, other gram-negative organisms, and *Staphylococcus aureus* are the most common etiologic agents in nosocomial pneumonia.[80] Immunocompromised (human immunodeficiency virus, transplant) individuals are especially susceptible to *Pneumocystis jerovici* (formerly *carinii*), mycobacterial infections, and fungal infections of the respiratory tract. These infections can be difficult to treat and have a high mortality rate.[81]

PATHOPHYSIOLOGY   Aspiration of oropharyngeal secretions is the most common route of lower respiratory tract infection; thus the nasopharynx and oropharynx constitute the first line of defense for most infectious agents. Another route of infection is through the inhalation of microorganisms that have been released into the air when an infected individual coughs, sneezes, or talks, or from aerosolized water, such as that from contaminated respiratory therapy equipment. This route of infection is most important in viral and mycobacterial pneumonias and in *Legionella* outbreaks. Pneumonia also can occur when bacteria are spread to the lungs in the blood from bacteremia that can result from infection elsewhere in the body or from intravenous drug abuse.

In healthy individuals, pathogens that reach the lungs are expelled or held in check by mechanisms of self-defense (see Chapters 6, 7, and 32). If a microorganism gets past the upper airway defense mechanisms, such as the cough reflex and mucociliary clearance, the next line of defense is the alveolar macrophage. This phagocyte is capable of removing most infectious agents without setting off significant inflammatory or immune responses. However, if the microorganism is virulent or present in large enough numbers, it can overwhelm the alveolar macrophage and result in a full-scale activation of the body's defense mechanisms, including the release of multiple inflammatory mediators, cellular infiltration, and immune activation.[82] These inflammatory mediators and immune complexes can damage bronchial mucous membranes and alveolocapillary membranes, causing the acini and terminal bronchioles to fill with infectious debris and exudate. In addition, some microorganisms release toxins from their cell walls that can cause further lung damage. The accumulation of exudate in the acinus leads to dyspnea and to $\dot{V}/\dot{Q}$ mismatching and hypoxemia.

Pneumococcal Pneumonia

The pathogenesis of pneumococcal pneumonia *(Streptococcus pneumoniae)* has been well documented and serves as a model for understanding other forms of bacterial pneumonia (Figure 33-15). *Streptococcus pneumoniae* microorganisms initiate the inflammatory and immune responses (see Chapters 6 and 7). The immune response includes complement activation and the production of antibodies, which are crucial for opsonizing the encapsulated bacterium.[83] Inflammatory cytokines and cells are released that cause alveolar edema.[84] Edema creates a medium for the multiplication of bacteria and aids in the spread of infection into adjacent portions of the lung. The involved lobe undergoes consolidation (solidification of the tissue caused by filling with exudate). A stage of red hepatization follows in which alveoli fill with blood cells, fibrin, edematous fluid, and pneumococci, giving lung tissue a red appearance. This passes into the stage of gray hepatization, in which affected tissues become gray because of fibrin deposition over the pleural surfaces and the presence of fibrin and leukocytes (neutrophils) in the consolidated alveoli, where phagocytosis is rapidly taking place.[84] With resolution, increasing numbers of macrophages appear in the alveolar spaces, the neutrophils degenerate, and the fibrin threads and remaining bacteria are digested by macrophages and removed by lymphatic vessels. Usually infection is limited to one or two lobes. Rapid lysis of pneumococcal bacteria (as occurs with antibiotic treatment) results in the release of intracellular bacterial proteins that can be toxic. The best known of these proteins is pneumolysin, which is cytotoxic to virtually every cell in the lung and is partially responsible for the worsening in clinical symptoms sometimes seen in individuals immediately after they begin antibiotic treatment.

Viral Pneumonia

Viral pneumonia is usually mild and self-limiting, but it can set the stage for a secondary bacterial infection by providing an ideal environment for bacterial growth and by damaging ciliated epithelial cells, which normally prevent pathogens from reaching the lower airways.[85] Viral pneumonia can be a primary infection (e.g., influenza pneumonia) or a complication of another viral illness (e.g., chickenpox, measles). The virus not only destroys the ciliated epithelial

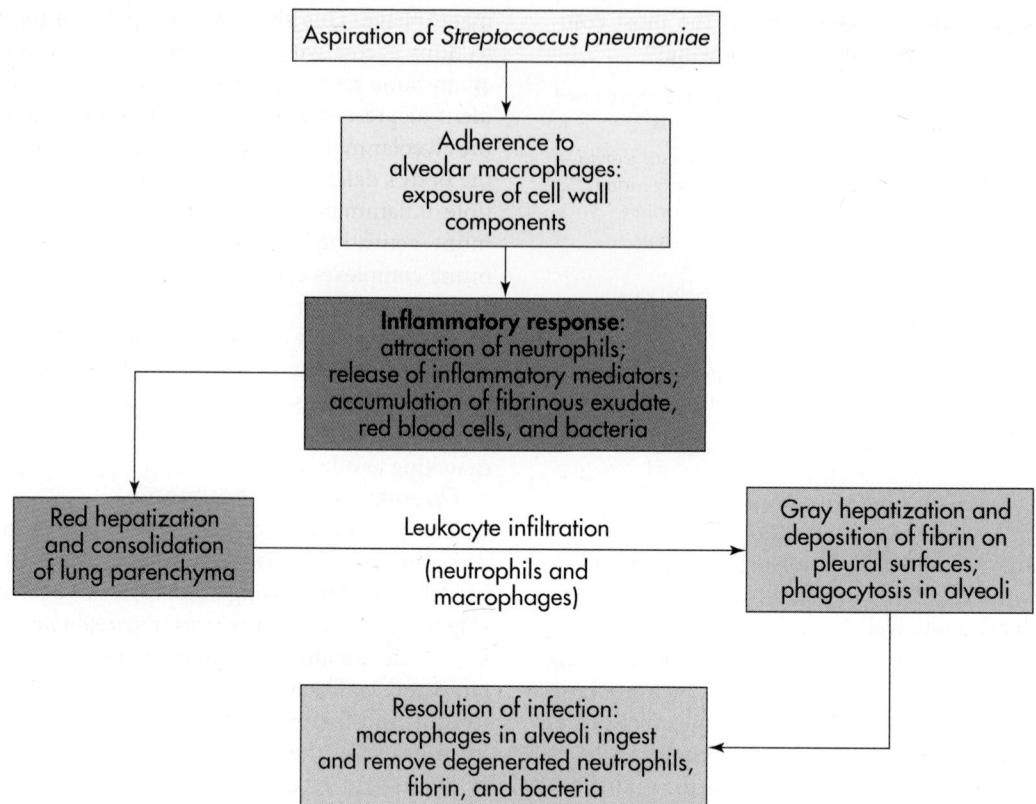

Figure 33-15 Pathophysiologic course of pneumococcal pneumonia.

cells but also invades the goblet cells and bronchial mucous glands. Sloughing of destroyed bronchial epithelium occurs throughout the respiratory tract, preventing mucociliary clearance. Bronchial walls become edematous and infiltrated with leukocytes.

CLINICAL MANIFESTATIONS   Most cases of pneumonia are preceded by an upper respiratory infection, which is usually viral. This is then followed by the onset of cough, dyspnea, and fever. The cough is often productive but may be nonproductive, especially in viral pneumonia. Other symptoms include chills, malaise, and pleuritic chest pain. Physical examination may reveal signs of pulmonary consolidation, such as inspiratory crackles, increased tactile fremitus, egophony, and whispered pectoriloquy. Individuals also may demonstrate symptoms and signs of underlying systemic disease or sepsis.

EVALUATION AND TREATMENT   The diagnosis of pneumonia is confirmed by finding infiltrates on chest x-ray.[86] These infiltrates may be patchy, lobar, or diffuse. The white blood cell count is usually elevated and, in the case of bacterial pneumonia, displays a preponderance of polymorphonucleocytes on differential. Sputum Gram stain is indicated in all patients with pneumonia, and sputum and blood cultures should be done in all hospitalized persons.[74,87] In immunocompromised or severely ill individuals, further diagnostic testing, such as transtracheal aspiration, bronchoscopy, or lung biopsy, may be necessary to identify the etiologic microorganism.[76-78,88]

The first step in the management of pneumonia is establishing adequate ventilation and oxygenation. Most individuals have hypoxemia and a respiratory alkalosis, although persons with underlying lung disease may require ventilation. Adequate hydration and good pulmonary hygiene (e.g., deep breathing, coughing, chest physical therapy) are also important.

Antibiotics are used to treat bacterial infections and should be chosen based on the likely causative microorganism (community acquired versus nosocomial) and the underlying condition of the individual.[74,75,87] Empiric therapy with broad-spectrum antibiotics should be initiated.[87,89,90] If a specific causative microorganism is identified, the choice of antimicrobial often can be simplified, however, resistant microorganisms are increasingly common.[91,92] Viral pneumonia is usually treated with supportive therapy, although antivirals may be indicated in severe infection. Infections with opportunistic organisms may be polymicrobial and require multiple drugs, including antifungals.

Tuberculosis

Tuberculosis (TB) is an infection caused by *Mycobacterium tuberculosis*, an acid-fast bacillus that usually affects the lungs but may invade other body systems.[93] The World Health Organization 2005 Global Tuberculosis Report indicates that although the global TB prevalence has declined by over 20% since 1990, there has been an alarming increase in TB cases in

Africa, where incidence has tripled since 1990 in areas where there is a high prevalence of HIV infection. In 2002, the Centers for Disease Control announced that the prevalence of TB had dropped to 5.2 cases per 100,000 people in the United States, the lowest rate ever recorded.[94] In the United States, the incidence of TB decreased during the years 1950 to 1980, increased from 1985 to 1992, and has decreased once again since 1992. The largest increases have occurred in men age 25 to 44 years; in children younger than age 15 years; and in Hispanic, black, and Asian populations. The major reason for this trend is the epidemic of acquired immunodeficiency syndrome (AIDS).[95] Individuals with AIDS are highly susceptible to respiratory infections, including multidrug-resistant TB. Emigration of infected individuals from high-prevalence countries, transmission in crowded institutional settings, homelessness, substance abuse, and lack of access to medical care have contributed to the spread of TB.[96]

PATHOPHYSIOLOGY   Like some types of pneumonia, tuberculosis is transmitted from person to person in airborne droplets. It is highly contagious; individuals living with an infected person have a 33% risk of developing the infection.[97] In immunocompetent individuals, the microorganism is contained by the inflammatory and immune response systems and no clinical disease develops.[93,98] Microorganisms lodge in the lung periphery, usually in the upper lobe. Once the bacilli are inspired into the lung, they multiply and cause nonspecific pneumonitis (lung inflammation). Some bacilli migrate through the lymphatics and become lodged in the lymph nodes, where they encounter lymphocytes and initiate the immune response.

Inflammation in the lung causes neutrophils and then alveolar macrophages to migrate to the area. These cells are phagocytes that engulf the bacilli and begin the process by which the body's defense mechanisms isolate the bacilli, preventing their spread. However, the bacteria is successful as a pathogen because it can survive within macrophages, resist lysosomal killing, and multiply within the cell.[99] In defense, macrophages and lymphocytes release interferon, which inhibits the replication of the microorganism and stimulates more macrophages to attack the bacterium.[93,100] Apoptotic infected macrophages also can activate cytotoxic T cells (CD8).[101] Neutrophils, lymphocytes, and macrophages seal off the colonies of bacilli, forming a granulomatous lesion called a *tubercle*[100,102] (see Chapter 6). Infected tissues within the tubercle die, forming cheeselike material called *caseation necrosis*. (Necrosis is described in Chapter 2.) Collagenous scar tissue then grows around the tubercle, completing isolation of the bacilli. The immune response is complete after 10 days or so, preventing further multiplication of the bacilli.[102]

Once the bacilli are isolated in tubercles and immunity develops, tuberculosis may remain dormant for life. If the immune system is impaired, however, or if live bacilli escape into the bronchi, active disease occurs and may spread through the blood and lymphatics to other organs. Infection with human immunodeficiency virus (HIV) is the single greatest risk factor for reactivation of tuberculosis infection. Other medical conditions that can cause reactivation include cancer, immunosuppressive medications, and renal failure.[93] Endogenous reactivation of dormant bacilli in elderly persons may be caused by poor nutritional status, insulin-dependent diabetes, long-term corticosteroid therapy, and other debilitating diseases.

CLINICAL MANIFESTATIONS   In many infected individuals, tuberculosis is asymptomatic. In others, symptoms develop so gradually that they are not noticed until the disease is advanced. However, symptoms can appear in immunosuppressed individuals within weeks of exposure to the bacillus. Common clinical manifestations include fatigue, weight loss, lethargy, anorexia (loss of appetite), and a low-grade fever that usually occurs in the afternoon. (These are common signs and symptoms of all chronic infections.) A cough that produces purulent sputum develops slowly and becomes more frequent over several weeks or months. Night

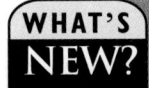
WHAT'S NEW?   Multi-Drug Resistant Tuberculosis in HIV Infection

It is estimated that in the year 2000, 11 million people worldwide were coinfected with tuberculosis (TB) and human immunodeficiency virus (HIV), and in that same year, there were over 500,000 new cases of active TB in individuals with HIV infection. In the United States, the estimated rate of HIV coinfection among reported TB cases decreased from approximately 15% to 9% between 1993 and 2000, although rates are declining much slower in high-risk populations such as minorities, intravenous drug abusers, and the homeless. The interaction between these two infections leads to an acceleration in the progression of HIV disease; TB remains the leading cause of HIV-related morbidity and mortality in most of the world. In turn, HIV infection is the most common identifiable risk factor for progression from latent TB to active disease. Treatment of TB in HIV-infected persons is characterized by relatively good short-term responses (especially if rifampicin is used as a primary drug) but becomes more difficult as both diseases progress and is associated with more adverse reactions to the antituberculous medications. This scenario is made even more challenging by the increasing prevalence of multi-drug resistant TB microorganisms. Management of these resistant infections requires taking a minimum of four drugs for at least 3 to 6 months, with reduction to three drugs for an additional 15 to 18 months. This 2-year regimen often requires the use of alternative pharmacologic agents that generally are less effective and more toxic than standard therapy; some of these medications need to be taken several times a day, which can make adherence difficult. The World Health Organization and the Centers for Disease Prevention and Control are developing improved prevention and treatment programs throughout the world; however, it is estimated that current public health systems may fail to reach 50% of the reported cases of TB in remote areas.

Data from Centers for Disease Control: *Reported tuberculosis in the United States, 2002,* Atlanta, Ga, 2003, U.S. Department of Health and Human Services; Corbett EL et al: *Arch Intern Med* 163(9):1009-1021, 2003; Davies PD: *Ann Med* 35(4):235-243, 2003; de Jong BC et al: *Ann Rev Med* 55:283-301, 2004; Frieden TR et al: *Lancet* 362(9387):887-899, 2003.

sweats and general anxiety are often present. Dyspnea, chest pain, and hemoptysis may also occur as the disease progresses. Extrapulmonary TB disease is common in HIV infected individuals and may cause neurologic deficits, meningitis symptoms, bone pain, and urinary symptoms.[93]

EVALUATION AND TREATMENT Tuberculosis is diagnosed by a positive tuberculin skin test (purified protein derivative [PPD]), sputum culture, and chest radiographs.[93,103,104] A positive tuberculin skin test indicates that an individual has been infected and has produced antibodies against the bacillus. By itself the positive skin test does not indicate the presence of active disease. It is important that the material used for skin testing be standardized to minimize the number of false-positive and false-negative results. Those who have received the tuberculosis vaccine with bacille Calmette-Guérin (BCG) also will have a positive PPD.

When active pulmonary disease is present, the tubercle bacillus can be cultured from the sputum and may be seen with an acid-fast stain. However, sputum culture can take up to 6 weeks to become positive.[93,103] Chest radiographs of individuals with current or previous active disease demonstrate characteristic changes. Nodules, calcifications, cavities, and hilar enlargement (enlarged mediastinal lymph nodes) commonly are seen in the upper lobes. A positive skin test indicates the need for yearly chest radiographs to detect active disease.

Tuberculosis is classified as follows to aid in evaluation and determination of appropriate therapy:[104]

0—No tuberculosis, no exposure, no infection
1—Exposure to tuberculosis, no infection
2—Latent tuberculosis infection, no disease
3—Tuberculosis, clinically active disease
4—Tuberculosis, not clinically active
5—Tuberculosis suspected (diagnosis pending)

Treatment consists of antibiotic therapy to control active or dormant tuberculosis and prevent transmission. The choice of drugs and the duration of treatment depend on the individual's health history, the likelihood of bacterial resistance to certain drugs, and the presence of active disease.[93,105] The waxy coat of *M. tuberculosis* renders it impermeable to many common drugs. Before the increase in tuberculosis incidence during the past decade, treatment with two effective drugs generally was sufficient. Today, with the increased numbers of immunosuppressed and susceptible individuals and drug-resistant bacilli, the recommended treatment for those at high risk is a combination of four drugs: isoniazid, rifampin, pyrazinamide, and ethambutol or streptomycin.[93,105,106] Newer drugs being tested include rifapentine and immune amplifiers.

In the past, individuals with active tuberculosis were isolated from the community and their families in sanitariums. Today individuals remain at home or, rarely, in the hospital, until sputum cultures show that the active bacilli have been eliminated. This usually takes a few weeks to 2 months if the antibiotics are taken conscientiously. If the individual's cooperation is in question, it is advisable for the administration of the drugs to be supervised by health care workers.[93,105,107]

Acute Bronchitis

Acute bronchitis is acute infection or inflammation of the airways or bronchi. Acute bronchitis commonly follows a viral illness and is usually self-limiting. Many of the clinical manifestations are similar to those of pneumonia (i.e., fever, cough, chills, malaise), but physical examination does not reveal signs of pulmonary consolidation, and chest radiographs show no infiltrates. Individuals with viral bronchitis have a nonproductive cough that frequently occurs in paroxysms and is aggravated by cold, dry, or dusty air. Purulent sputum may be produced. Chest pain often develops from the effort of coughing. Treatment consists of rest, aspirin, humidity, and a cough suppressant, such as codeine.

Individuals with bacterial bronchitis have a productive cough, fever, and pain behind the sternum (breast bone) that is aggravated by coughing. It is rare in previously healthy adults except after viral infection but is common in those with COPD. Bacterial bronchitis is treated with rest, aspirin, humidity, and antibiotics (usually a penicillinase-resistant penicillin). If the cough is nonproductive, a cough suppressant is given, because a dry cough can cause bronchial irritation and damage. Acute bronchitis may progress to pneumonia.

Pulmonary Vascular Disease

Blood flow through the lungs can be disrupted by a number of disorders that result in occlusion of the vessels, an increase in pulmonary vascular resistance, or destruction of the vascular bed. The consequences of altered pulmonary blood flow may be of no functional significance or can result in severe and life-threatening changes in ventilation-perfusion ratios. Major disorders include pulmonary embolism, pulmonary hypertension, and cor pulmonale.

Pulmonary Embolism

Pulmonary embolism (**PE**) is occlusion of a portion of the pulmonary vascular bed by an embolus: a thrombus (blood clot), a tissue fragment, lipids (fats), or an air bubble (Figure 33-16). The most common emboli are thrombi dislodged from deep veins in the thigh. This is termed *venous thromboembolism*. PE has an estimated incidence of 100,000 to 300,000 cases per year in the United States and 14% to 25% of those individuals will die.[108-110] Emboli also can originate in the pelvis, particularly in pregnant women. Symptomatic pulmonary embolism occurs in approximately 30% of cases of untreated deep venous thrombosis.[109]

Risk factors for **pulmonary thromboembolism,** the obstruction of a pulmonary vessel by a thrombus, include many conditions and disorders that promote blood clotting (see Chapter 25). The three categories of pathologic risks are called the *Virchow triad* and include (1) venous stasis (slowing or stagnation of blood flow through the veins), (2) hypercoagulability (increased tendency of the blood to form clots), and (3) injuries to the endothelial cells that line the vessels. Venous stasis is usually caused by immobility associated with prolonged bed rest or sitting, obesity, neurologic disease, or old age, but it also can be caused by pregnancy, congestive heart failure, sickle

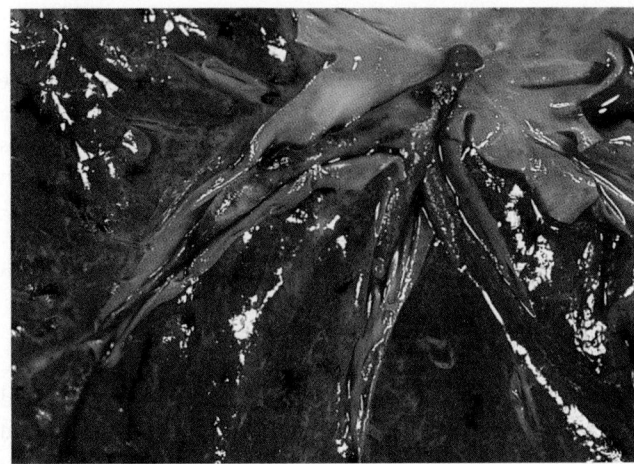

Figure 33-16 Pulmonary embolus. The embolus extends into major branches of the pulmonary artery. (From Damjanov I, Linder J, editors: *Anderson's pathology,* ed 10, St Louis, 1996, Mosby.)

cell disease, and systemic lupus erythematosus. Hypercoagulability can result from inherited or acquired coagulation disorders of the blood, malignancy, or oral contraceptive use. Some of the most common inherited clotting disorders include Factor V Leiden mutation, thrombin mutation, and deficiencies of antithrombin III, protein C, or protein S.[107] Clot formation also proceeds if vessel damage occurs, as in traumatic injury, surgery, or spontaneous rupture (e.g., cerebrovascular accident). Deep venous thrombosis and pulmonary embolism are frequent complications of hospitalization, especially in individuals who undergo obstetric or orthopedic procedures.[111] No matter what its source, a blood clot becomes an embolus when all or part of it breaks away from the site of formation and begins to travel in the bloodstream. (Thromboembolism is described further in Chapter 25.)

Although the overall incidence of pulmonary embolism has declined in recent years, it remains an important cause of death, especially in elderly and hospitalized persons. Approximately 10% of individuals with deep vein thrombosis (DVT) die suddenly before medical intervention can be initiated and another 5% even with appropriate care.[112] It is estimated that many cases of PE go undiagnosed.

PATHOPHYSIOLOGY   The impact or effect of the embolus depends on the extent of pulmonary blood flow obstruction, the size of the affected vessels, the nature of the embolus, and the secondary effects. Pulmonary emboli can occur as any of the following:

1. *Massive occlusion:* an embolus that occludes a major portion of the pulmonary circulation (i.e., main pulmonary artery embolus)
2. *Embolus with infarction:* an embolus that is large enough to cause infarction (death) of a portion of lung tissue
3. *Embolus without infarction:* an embolus that is not severe enough to cause permanent lung injury
4. *Multiple pulmonary emboli:* multiple emboli may be chronic or recurrent

As a result of the thrombus lodging in the pulmonary circulation, there is a release of neurohumoral substances, such as serotonin, histamine, catecholamines and angiotensin II, and inflammatory mediators, such as endothelin, leukotrienes, thromboxanes, and toxic oxygen radicals.[113] This causes widespread vasoconstriction that further impedes blood flow to the lung. Hemodynamically, this results in increased pulmonary artery pressures and can lead to right heart failure.[107,108] Absent blood flow to a lung segment causes a ventilation/perfusion mismatch (increased dead space) and a decrease in surfactant production. The resulting atelectasis of the affected lung segments further contributes to hypoxemia. If the thrombus is large enough, infarction of lung tissue, arrhythmias, decreased cardiac output, shock, and death are possible outcomes. The pathogenesis of venous thromboembolism is summarized in Figure 33-17.

If the embolus does not cause infarction, eventual dissolution of the clot by the fibrinolytic system (see Chapter 25) is likely, and about two-thirds of affected individuals have a re-

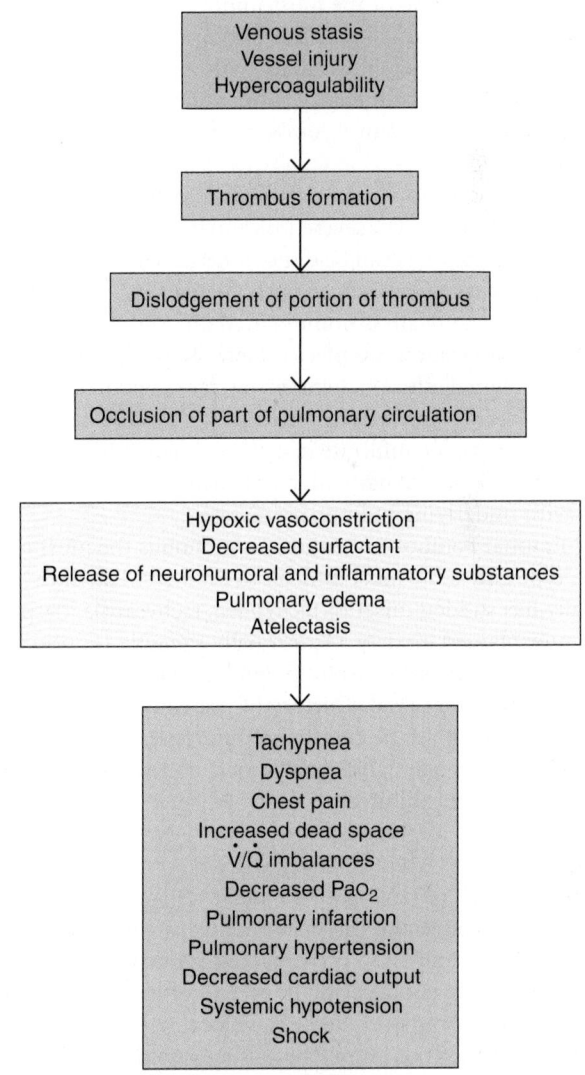

Figure 33-17 Pathogenesis of massive pulmonary embolism caused by a thrombus (pulmonary thromboembolism).

turn to normal lung perfusion over the next few months.[112] If pulmonary infarction occurs, shrinking and scarring develop in the affected area of the lung (infarction is described in detail in Chapter 2). The risk of recurrent venous thromboembolism is 10% per year, and is much higher in those individuals that have irreversible risk factors for the disease.[112]

CLINICAL MANIFESTATIONS In most cases the clinical manifestations of pulmonary embolism are nonspecific; therefore evaluation of risk factors and predisposing factors is an important aspect of diagnosis. More than 90% of pulmonary emboli are the consequence of clots that were initially formed in the veins of the legs and pelvis. Although characteristic symptoms and signs of DVT are leg pain and leg swelling, DVT is usually asymptomatic and the physical findings can be subtle. Consequently, the recognition of individuals at high risk for PE is crucial to assessing the clinical presentation.[108] Sometimes the thrombus is palpable, but often the legs appear normal or signs are masked by superficial thrombophlebitis. Calf asymmetry, when documented with a tape measure, is one of the most important findings in deep venous thrombosis. This clinical finding is often overlooked in the assessment of individuals with suspected deep vein thrombosis; calf asymmetry of more than 1 cm increases the likelihood of a deep vein thrombosis from 27% to 56% in an at-risk individual.

Massive occlusion causes profound shock, hypotension, tachypnea, tachycardia, severe pulmonary hypertension, and chest pain. Diagnosis can be difficult because the signs mimic those of other cardiopulmonary problems. Once these manifestations occur, death is imminent. Manifestations of emboli that cause infarction are pleural pain, dyspnea, pleural friction rub, pleural effusion, hemoptysis, fever, and leukocytosis. On chest radiographs the infarcted portion of the lung shows up as a nonspecific infiltrate in a classic wedge shape bordering the pleura. Pulmonary infarction is most likely in individuals with underlying pulmonary disease.

Pulmonary embolism without infarction is the most common type and is the most difficult to evaluate. The individual usually has sudden onset of tachypnea, tachycardia, dyspnea, and unexplained anxiety. Occasionally syncope (fainting) or pleural pain occurs. Recurrent pulmonary emboli occur in individuals who have had a history of previous emboli. Recurrent emboli may not be detected until progressive incapacitation, precordial pain, anxiety, dyspnea, and right ventricular enlargement are exhibited.

EVALUATION AND TREATMENT When an individual is suspected of having a PE based on the presence of risk factors, symptoms, and physical findings, a chest x-ray, arterial blood gas, and ECG are obtained immediately.[108] Chest x-ray findings are nonspecific in PE and often can be normal for the first 24 hours until atelectasis occurs in the lung. The arterial blood gas commonly reveals hypoxemia with a respiratory alkalosis (most individuals will hyperventilate in response to PE). The ECG may show evidence of strain on the right heart. A serum D-dimer measures a product of thrombus degradation by the fibrinolytic system and, if normal, makes the presence of a PE highly unlikely.[114,115] If the D-dimer is elevated, further evaluation is conducted using a spiral CT scan.[116,117] This highly sensitive and specific test has replaced the radionucleotide ventilation/perfusion scan in most hospitals. In rare cases, a pulmonary angiogram is necessary to confirm the diagnosis of PE. Recently, the measurement of elevated serum troponin levels has been useful in stratifying the risk and severity of PE.[118,119]

The ideal treatment of PE is prevention through risk factor recognition and elimination of predisposing factors. Venous stasis in hospitalized individuals is minimized by bed exercises, frequent position changes, early ambulation, and pneumatic calf compression. Most at-risk individuals also will receive prophylactic anticoagulation with low-molecular weight heparin or warfarin.[120] In individuals who have contraindications to anticoagulation, the placement of a filter in the inferior vena cava can prevent emboli from reaching the lungs.[121,122]

Pulmonary embolism is treated with the rapid administration of anticoagulation, usually unfractionated or low-molecular weight heparin.[120] This is usually followed by weeks or months of outpatient warfarin. If massive life-threatening embolism occurs, a fibrinolytic agent, such as streptokinase, can be used, and some individuals require emergent surgical embolectomy. Reversal of the underlying cause of the thrombus is important to preventing future venous thromboembolism.

Pulmonary Hypertension

Pulmonary hypertension is defined as a mean pulmonary artery pressure 5 to 10 mmHg above normal or above 20 mmHg.[123-125] Pulmonary artery pressure is lower than systemic arterial pressure and is normally 15 to 18 mmHg. Pulmonary hypertension is classified as (1) pulmonary arterial hypertension, (2) pulmonary venous hypertension, (3) pulmonary hypertension caused by diseases of the respiratory system or hypoxemia, (4) pulmonary hypertension resulting from chronic thrombotic and/or embolic disease, and (5) pulmonary hypertension resulting from disorders directly affecting the pulmonary vasculature.[125]

Primary pulmonary hypertension (PPH) is an idiopathic form of pulmonary artery hypertension and is characterized by pathologic changes in precapillary pulmonary arteries. Pulmonary artery pressures are elevated to more than 25 mmHg at rest and 30 mmHg with exercise.[123] PPH is relatively rare with only 1 to 2 cases per million people. It is more common in women than in men and presents in women in the third decade of life and in men in the fourth decade. There is a familial tendency to develop PPH, although only 10% to 20% of those with a genetic predisposition actually develop the disease. Risk factors for PPH include HIV infection, collagen vascular diseases, and the use of appetite suppressants.[123,126]

Diseases of the respiratory system and hypoxemia are much more common causes of pulmonary artery hypertension and are characterized by pulmonary arteriolar vasoconstriction and arterial remodeling. In some cases, pulmonary hypertension is the result of recurrent pulmonary emboli, however, this is relatively uncommon. Pulmonary venous hypertension is caused by congestive heart failure and is discussed in Chapter 30.

PATHOPHYSIOLOGY   Although PPH is still considered an idiopathic disorder, much has been discovered about the complex interaction between genes and environment that leads to this disease. Mutation in the *BMPR2* gene with an autosomal pattern of inheritance has been identified in approximately half of all individuals with PPH. This, in combination with environmental risk factors, results in endothelial dysfunction with overproduction of vasoconstrictors, such as thromboxane and endothelin, and decreased production of vasodilators, such as prostacyclin.[123,126-128] Vascular growth factors are released that cause changes in the vascular smooth wall called *remodeling*. Angiotensin II, serotonin, electrolyte transporter mechanisms, and nitric oxide also play a role in the pathogenesis of this disorder. Together, this results in pathologic changes in the pulmonary vasculature characterized by fibrosis and thickening of the vessel wall with luminal narrowing and abnormal vasoconstriction.[123,126] These changes cause resistance to pulmonary artery blood flow, thus increasing the pressure in the pulmonary arteries. As resistance and pressure increase, the workload of the right ventricle increases and subsequent right ventricular hypertrophy, followed by failure, may occur (cor pulmonale). This eventually results in the death of most individuals with PPH.

Pulmonary hypertension caused by disease of the respiratory system or hypoxia is much more common than PPH. Common etiologic disorders include COPD, interstitial lung disease, and obesity-hypoventilation syndrome. Prolonged exposure to high altitude with low levels of inspired oxygen can also cause pulmonary hypertension. The degree of pulmonary hypertension in these disorders is usually mild to moderate; however, resultant cor pulmonale is a significant cause of morbidity and mortality in late-stage chronic lung disease.[129,130] Chronic hypoxemia, especially in association with respiratory acidosis, results in vasoconstriction and in vascular remodeling with significant smooth muscle hypertrophy, fibrosis, and luminal narrowing.[129,130] The pathogenesis of pulmonary hypertension and cor pulmonale, resulting from disease of the respiratory system or hypoxia, is shown in Figure 33-18.

CLINICAL MANIFESTATIONS   Pulmonary hypertension may not be detected until it is quite severe. The symptoms are often masked by primary pulmonary or cardiovascular disease. The first indication of pulmonary hypertension is often an abnormality seen on a chest radiograph (enlarged pulmonary arteries and right heart border) or an electrocardiogram that shows right ventricular hypertrophy. Symptoms of fatigue, chest discomfort, tachypnea, and dyspnea, particularly with exercise, are common. Examination may reveal pe-

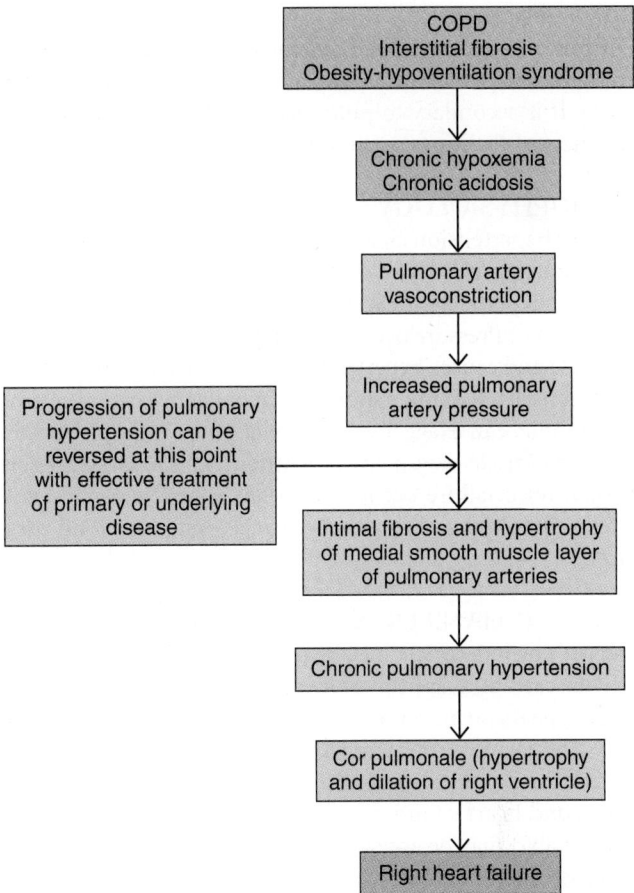

Figure 33-18 Pathogenesis of pulmonary hypertension and cor pulmonale caused by disease of the respiratory system or hypoxia.

ripheral edema, jugular venous distension, a precordial heave, and accentuation of the pulmonary compartment of the second heart sound.[123,130]

EVALUATION AND TREATMENT   Definitive diagnosis and accurate assessment of pulmonary artery pressure can be made only with right-sided heart catheterization. The diagnosis of primary pulmonary hypertension is made when all other causes of hypertension have been ruled out.

There is no curative treatment for primary pulmonary hypertension except lung transplantation. Other standard therapies include anticoagulants, calcium channel blockers, and prostacyclin (epoprostenol).[123,131,132] Epoprostenol improves survival but must be given as a continuous intravenous infusion. Emerging therapies include vasodilators, such as prostacyclin analogues that can be inhaled (iloprost), endothelin antagonists (bosentan), and nitric oxide (NO).[123,133]

The most effective treatment for secondary pulmonary hypertension is treatment of the primary disorder. However, once pulmonary hypertension has persisted long enough for hypertrophy of the medial smooth muscle layer to develop, as it does with chronic hypoxemia, it is no longer reversible. Treatment relies upon the use of supplemental oxygen to reverse hypoxic vasoconstriction.[129,130]

Cor Pulmonale

Cor pulmonale, also called *pulmonary heart disease,* consists of right ventricular enlargement (hypertrophy, dilation, or both). It is secondary to pulmonary hypertension caused by disorders of the lungs or chest wall.

PATHOPHYSIOLOGY   Cor pulmonale develops as pulmonary hypertension creates chronic pressure overload in the right ventricle similar to that created in the left ventricle by systemic hypertension. (Systemic hypertension is discussed in Chapter 30.) Pressure overload increases the work of the right ventricle and causes hypertrophy of the normally thin-walled heart muscle.[130] Acute hypoxemia, such as might occur with pneumonia, can exaggerate pulmonary hypertension and dilate the ventricle as well. Right ventricular filling pressures are normal until failure occurs. The right ventricle usually fails when pulmonary artery pressure equals systemic blood pressure.

CLINICAL MANIFESTATIONS   The clinical manifestations of cor pulmonale may be obscured by primary respiratory disease and appear only during exercise testing. The heart appears normal at rest, but with exercise, cardiac output falls. The electrocardiogram shows right ventricular hypertrophy. Chest pain is common. The pulmonary component of the second heart sound, which represents closure of the pulmonic valve, may be accentuated, and a pulmonic valve murmur also may be present. Tricuspid valve murmur may accompany the development of right ventricular failure. Peripheral edema, hepatic congestion, and jugular venous distention often may be detected.

EVALUATION AND TREATMENT   Diagnosis is made on the basis of physical examination, radiologic examination, and electrocardiogram or echocardiogram or both. Physical examination findings are often similar to those of chronic lung disease with dyspnea and distended neck veins. The goal of treatment for cor pulmonale is to decrease the workload of the right ventricle by lowering pulmonary artery pressure. Treatment is the same as for pulmonary hypertension, and its success depends on reversal of the underlying lung disease.[130]

Lip Cancer

Cancer of the lip is more prevalent in men, with 3100 new cases per year accounting for about 1% of all cancers in men.[134] Long-term exposure to sun, wind, and cold over a period of years results in dryness, chapping, hyperkeratosis, and predisposition to malignancy. The lower lip is the most common site.

PATHOPHYSIOLOGY   The most common form of lower lip cancer is termed *exophytic.* The lesion usually develops in the outer part of the lip along the vermilion border. The lesion becomes thickened and evolves to an ulcerated center with a raised border (Figure 33-19). Verrucous-type lesions are less common. They have an irregular surface, follow cracks in the lip, and tend to extend toward the inner surface. Squamous cell carcinoma is the most common cell type. Basal cell carcinoma does not develop unless there is extension beyond the mucous membrane or vermilion border of the lip.

CLINICAL MANIFESTATIONS   Malignant lesions often are preceded by the development of a blister that evolves into a superficial ulceration. In some cases there is a history of recurrent scales that precede development of a bleeding ulceration. Metastases to the cervical lymph nodes have a low rate of occurrence (2% to 8%) and are more likely when the primary lesion is thicker and exists for a longer period.[135]

EVALUATION AND TREATMENT   Diagnosis is commonly made by clinical history and presentation of the lesion. Biopsy confirms the presence of malignant cells. The staging for lip cancer is summarized in Box 33-1. Surgical excision is effective for smaller lesions. Larger lesions that require extensive resection may need subsequent cosmetic surgeries. Interstitial irradiation and radioactive implants have proved effective for control of primary lesions.[136,137] The prognosis for recovery is excellent, and deaths are usually the result of inadequate treatment. The overall recurrence rate is approximately 40% and 5-year survival role is 73%.[136]

Laryngeal Cancer

Cancer of the larynx represents approximately 2% to 3% of all cancers in the United States. There are approximately 10,300 new cases per year, 8000 of them in men.[134] The risk of

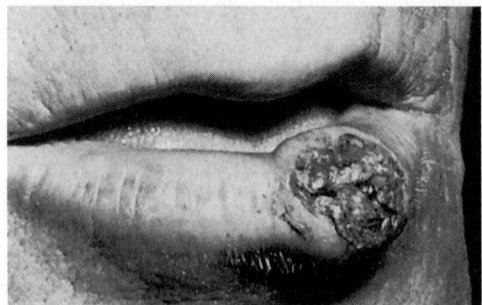

Figure 33-19 Lip cancer. Carcinoma of the lower lip with central ulceration and raised, rolled borders. (From del Regato JA, Spjut HJ, Cox JD: *Ackerman and del Regato's cancer,* ed 2, St Louis, 1985, Mosby.)

Box 33-1	Staging of Lip Cancer

Stage I
Primary tumor less than 2 cm; no palpable nodes

Stage II
Primary tumor 2 to 4 cm; no palpable nodes

Stage III
Primary tumor larger than 4 cm; metastatic lymph nodes

Stage IV
Large primary tumors; nodes fixed to mandible or distant metastases

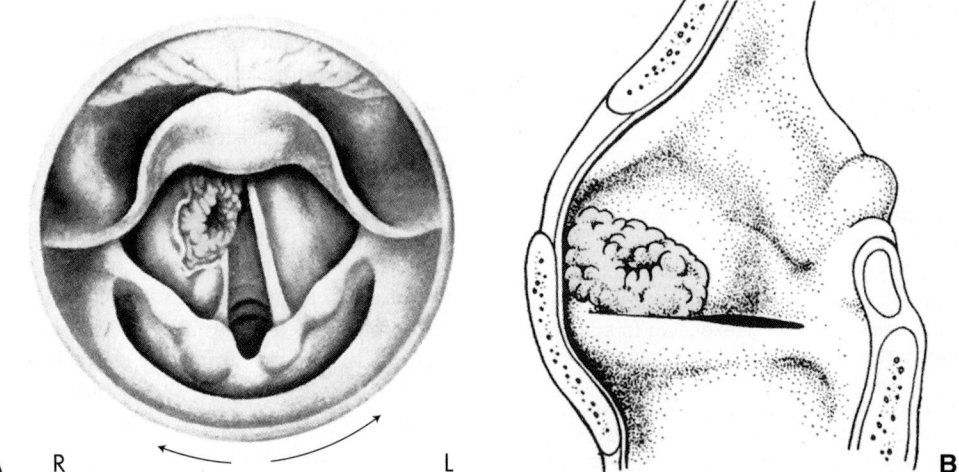

Figure 33-20 Laryngeal cancer. **A,** Mirror view of carcinoma of right false cord partially hiding true cord. **B,** Lateral view. (From del Regato JA, Spjut HJ, Cox JD: *Ackerman and del Regato's cancer,* ed 2, St Louis, 1985, Mosby.)

laryngeal cancer is increased by the amount of tobacco smoked; risk is further heightened with the combination of smoking and alcohol consumption. Gastroesophageal reflux disease is also a risk factor.[138,139] The highest incidence is in men between 50 and 75 years of age.

PATHOPHYSIOLOGY Carcinoma of the true vocal cords (glottis) is more common than that of the supraglottic structures (epiglottis, aryepiglottic folds, arytenoids, and false cords). Tumors of the subglottic area are rare. Squamous cell carcinoma is the most common cell type, although small cell carcinomas also occur[140] (Figure 33-20). Metastasis develops by spread to the draining lymph nodes, and distant metastasis, usually to the lung, is rare.

CLINICAL MANIFESTATIONS The presenting symptoms of laryngeal cancer include hoarseness, dyspnea, and cough. Progressive hoarseness is the most significant symptom and can result in voice loss. Dyspnea is rare in the case of supraglottic tumors but can be severe in subglottic tumors. Cough occurs less commonly and may follow swallowing. Laryngeal pain or a sore throat is likely to be present with supraglottic lesions.

EVALUATION AND TREATMENT Evaluation of the larynx includes external inspection and palpation of the larynx and the lymph nodes in the neck. Indirect laryngoscopy provides a stereoscopic view of the structure and movement of the larynx. A biopsy also can be obtained during this procedure. Direct laryngoscopy provides specific visualization of the tumor. Plain films of the larynx and CT facilitate the identification of tumor boundaries and the degree of extension to surrounding tissue. Magnetic resonance imaging (MRI) and positron emission tomography (PET) can be used for staging.[141]

Radiation therapy has shown good results for early carcinoma of the vocal cords.[142,143] Chemotherapy may be useful as an adjunct to surgery and in some cases allows for organ spar-ing and retained speech.[144] Partial laryngectomies are the preferred treatment for small supraglottic and subglottic malignancies. Total laryngectomy is required when lesions are extensive and involve the cartilage. Swallowing and speech therapy after treatment can significantly improve recovery.[145]

Lung Cancer

Lung cancers (bronchogenic carcinomas) arise from the epithelium of the respiratory tract. As such, the term *lung cancer* excludes other pulmonary tumors, including sarcomas, lymphomas, blastomas, hematomas, and mesotheliomas. Lung cancer is an epidemic in the United States, with an estimated 174,000 new cases in 2004.[134,146] It accounts for 13% of all cancers in both men and women but is responsible for 31% of all cancer deaths in men and 25% of all cancer deaths in women[134] (Box 33-2). Lung cancer is more common in African Americans and survival rates for them are lower.[147] Although the mortality rate for lung cancer has leveled off in men, it is still rising in women. The lung cancer death rate for women is higher than that of any other cancer, including breast cancer, because of increased cigarette smoking by women.[148] Deaths from lung cancer appear at 35 to 44 years of age; a sharp increase occurs between ages 45 and 55 years; and the incidence continues to increase through ages 65 to 74 years, after which it levels off and decreases among the very old.[134]

The most common cause of lung cancer is cigarette smoking. Heavy smokers have about a 20 times greater chance of developing lung cancer than nonsmokers.[146] Passive smoking at home and in the workplace is associated with as much as a 30% increase in the risk for lung cancer.[146] Cigarette smoke contains several organ-specific carcinogens, and smoking has been causally related to carcinogenesis at several sites, including the larynx, oral cavity, esophagus, and urinary bladder. Genetic predisposition to developing lung cancer, which is evident in analysis of pedigrees, also plays a role in its pathophysiology[146] (see Chapter 5). The incidence of lung cancer decreases among people who stop smoking, however, the risk of lung cancer among former smokers remains higher than among those who have never smoked, even after 40 years of abstinence.[146] Theories of carcinogenesis are discussed in Chapter 12.

Environmental or occupational risk factors associated with lung cancer include benzopyrene and radon particles associated with uranium mining, radiation, and nuclear bombs. Others are polycyclic aromatic hydrocarbons and arsenicals, asbestos fibers, diesel exhaust, nitrogen mustard gases, nickel, silica, vinyl chloride, and chloromethyl methyl ether. Air pollution, coal, and iron mining are also considered risk factors.[146]

Types

Primary lung cancers arise from the bronchi within the lungs and are therefore called *bronchogenic carcinomas*. Although there are many types of lung cancer, in 1999 the World Health Organization reclassified lung cancer into two major categories, non–small cell lung carcinoma (NSCLC, 75% of all lung cancers) and small cell lung carcinoma (SCLC, 25% of all lung cancers).[149] The category of non–small cell carcinoma can be subdivided into three common types of lung cancer: squamous cell carcinoma, adenocarcinoma, and large cell undifferentiated carcinoma.[149,150] The clinical and pathologic features that most commonly characterize these cancer types are illustrated in Figure 33-21 and described in Table 33-4. Many cancers that arise in other organs of the body metastasize to the lungs; however, these are not considered lung cancers and are categorized by their primary site of origin.

Non–Small Cell Lung Cancer

Squamous cell carcinoma. Squamous cell carcinoma accounts for about 30% of bronchogenic carcinomas, representing a sharp decline in incidence in the past two decades. These tumors are typically located near the hilus and project into bronchi.

Because of the location in the central bronchi, obstructive manifestations are nonspecific and include nonproductive cough or hemoptysis. Pneumonia and atelectasis are often associated with squamous cell carcinoma (Figure 33-22, *A*). Chest pain is a late symptom associated with large tumors. These tumors can remain fairly well localized and tend not to metastasize until late in the course of the disease. The preferred treatment is surgical resection, although once metastasis has taken place, total surgical resection is difficult and survival rates dramatically decrease. Although chemotherapy has limited effectiveness, adjuvant treatment with newer agents has been shown to improve survival and quality of life.[151,152]

Adenocarcinoma. Adenocarcinoma (tumor arising from glands) of the lung constitutes 35% to 40% of all bronchogenic carcinomas (Figure 33-22, *B*). The recent increase in incidence of adenocarcinoma has been ascribed to the increasing frequency of lung cancer in women, environmental and occupational carcinogens, and changes in the histologic criteria for diagnosis. These tumors, which are usually smaller than 4 cm, more commonly arise in the peripheral regions of the pulmonary parenchyma. They may be asymptomatic and discovered by routine chest roentgenogram in the early stages, or the individual may seek treatment for pleuritic chest pain and shortness of breath from pleural involvement by the tumor.

Included in the category of adenocarcinoma is bronchioloalveolar cell carcinoma. These tumors tend to arise from the terminal bronchioles and alveoli. They are slow-growing tumors with an unpredictable pattern of metastasis. Metastasis occurs through the pulmonary arterial system and mediastinal lymph nodes. This cell type has the weakest association with smoking.

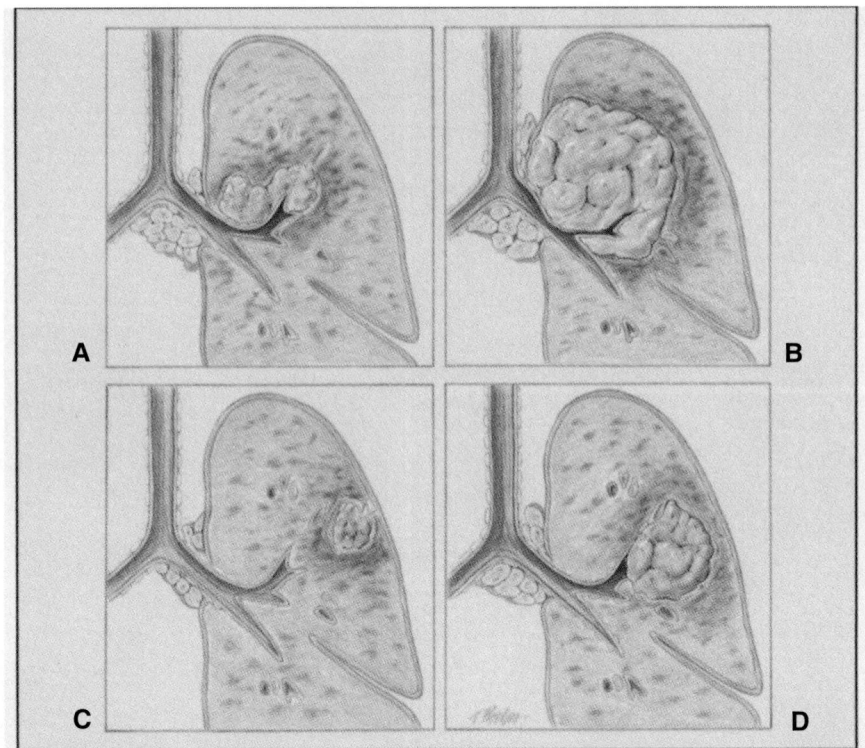

Figure 33-21 Cancer of the lung. **A,** Squamous (epidermoid) cell carcinoma. **B,** Small cell (oat cell) carcinoma. **C,** Adenocarcinoma. **D,** Large cell carcinoma. (Tumor characteristics are summarized in Table 33-5.) (From Des Jardins T, Burton GG: *Clinical manifestations and assessment of respiratory disease,* ed 3, St Louis, 1995, Mosby.)

Table 33-4	Characteristics of Lung Cancers			
Tumor Type	Growth Rate	Metastasis	Means of Diagnosis	Clinical Manifestations and Treatment
Squamous cell carcinoma	Slow	Late; mostly to hilar lymph nodes	Biopsy, sputum analysis, bronchoscopy, electron microscopy, immunohistochemistry	Cough, sputum production, airway obstruction; treated surgically, chemotherapy adjunctive
Adenocarcinoma	Moderate	Early	Radiography, fiber-optic bronchoscopy, electron microscopy	Pleural effusion; treated surgically, chemotherapy adjunctive
Large cell carcinoma	Rapid	Early and widespread	Sputum analysis, bronchoscopy, electron microscopy (by exclusion of other cell types)	Chest wall pain, pleural effusion, cough, sputum production, hemoptysis, airway obstruction resulting in pneumonia (if airways involved); treated surgically
Small cell (oat cell) carcinoma	Very rapid	Very early; to mediastinum or distally in lung	Radiography, sputum analysis, bronchoscopy, electron microscopy, immunohistochemistry, and clinical manifestations (cough, chest pain, dyspnea, hemoptysis, localized wheezing)	Airway obstruction, signs and symptoms of excessive hormone secretion; treated by chemotherapy and ionizing radiation to thorax and central nervous system

Surgical resection is possible in a high proportion of cases, but because metastasis occurs early, the 5-year survival rate remains below 15%. Newer chemotherapeutic agents are resulting in increased survival rates.[151,152]

Large Cell Carcinoma (Undifferentiated)

Undifferentiated large cell carcinomas constitute 10% to 15% of bronchogenic carcinomas. This cell type has lost all evidence of differentiation and is therefore commonly referred to as **undifferentiated large cell anaplastic cancer.** Because large cell carcinomas show none of the histologic findings of squamous cell carcinoma or adenocarcinoma, they are diagnosed by a process of exclusion. The cells are generally larger than leukocytes and contain large, darkly stained nuclei. These tumors commonly arise peripherally but are found

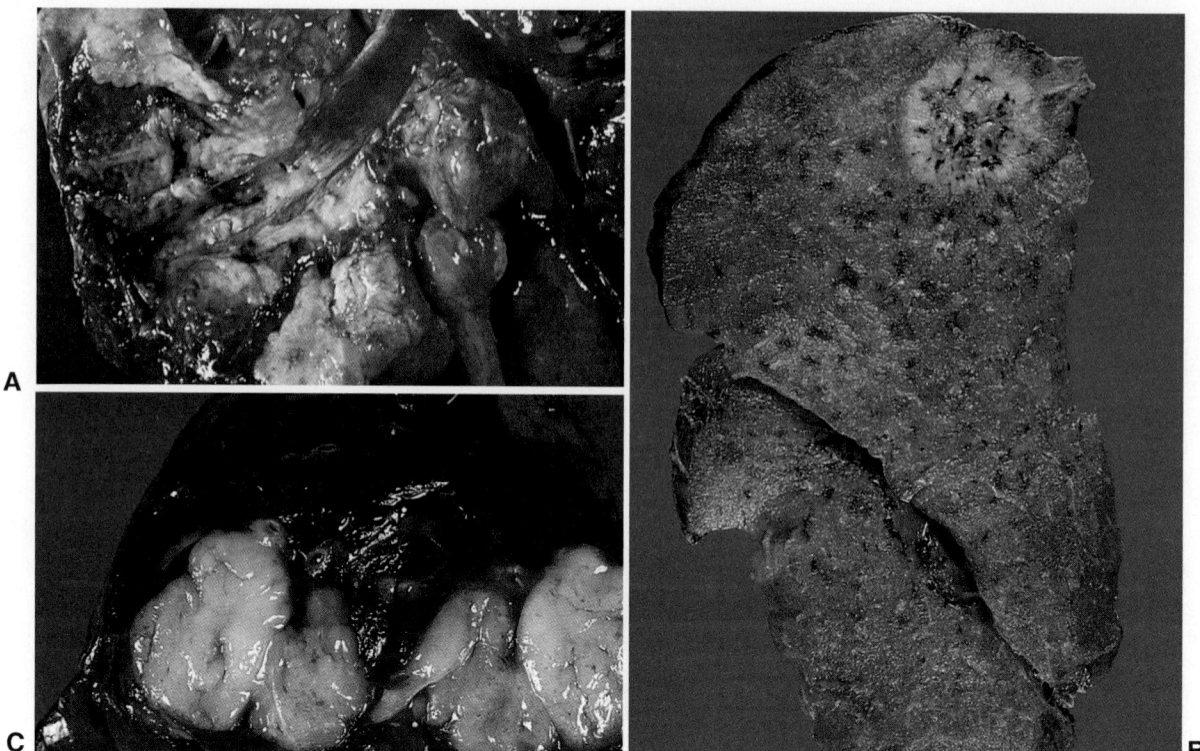

Figure 33-22 Lung cancer. **A,** Squamous cell carcinoma. This hilar tumor originates from the main bronchus. **B,** Peripheral adeno-carcinoma. The tumor shows prominent black pigmentation, suggestive of having evolved in an anthracotic scar. **C,** Small cell carci-noma. The tumor forms confluent nodules. On cross sectioning, the nodules have an encephalid appearance. (From Damjanov I, Linder J, editors: *Anderson's pathology,* ed 10, St Louis, 1996, Mosby.)

centrally and can grow to distort the trachea and cause widening of the carina.

Once metastasis has occurred, surgical therapy is limited to palliative procedures (comfort measures) designed to relieve obstructive pneumonitis or prevent recurrence of pleural effusion. Neither radiation therapy nor chemotherapy has been successful in increasing survival.

Small Cell Carcinoma

Small cell carcinomas constitute 14% of bronchogenic carcinomas.[153] It is estimated that most of these tumors are central in origin (see Figures 33-21 and 33-22, *C*). Cell sizes range from 6 to 8 μm. This cell type has the strongest correlation with cigarette smoking. Because these tumors show a rapid rate of growth and tend to metastasize early and widely, small cell carcinomas have the worst prognosis. Staging for small cell carcinoma is divided into only two categories: limited disease (20% to 30%) versus extensive disease (70% to 80%).[153] Survival time for untreated small cell carcinoma is usually 1 to 3 months; with treatment, however, approximately 10% of individuals are alive at 2 years.[153]

Small cell carcinoma is most often associated with ectopic hormone production, production of hormones by tumors of nonendocrine origin, or production of an inappropriate hormone by an endocrine gland. Neuroendocrine cells containing neurosecretory granules exist throughout the tracheo-bronchial tree. Ectopic hormone production is important to

the clinician because resulting signs and symptoms (called *paraneoplastic syndromes*) may be the first manifestation of the underlying cancer. The most common paraneoplastic syndrome associated with small cell lung cancer is the syndrome of inappropriate antidiuretic hormone secretion, which occurs in up to 40% of individuals. Small cell carcinomas also commonly produce gastrin-releasing peptide, calcitonin, arginine vasopressin, and adrenocorticotropic hormone (ACTH). As a result of ACTH secretion, individuals with lung cancer secrete large quantities of 17-hydroxysteroids and 17-ketosteroids, leading to the development of an atypical Cushing syndrome. Signs and symptoms related to this condition include muscular weakness, facial edema, hypokalemia, alkalosis, hyperglycemia, hypertension, and increased pigmentation. They are treated primarily with chemotherapy and radiation therapy, resulting in temporary remission.

PATHOGENESIS   Tobacco smoke contains as many as 20 documented lung carcinogens and is responsible for causing 80% to 90% of lung cancers.[146] These carcinogens, along with probable inherited genetic predisposition to cancers, result in multiple genetic abnormalities in bronchial cells, including deletions of chromosomes, activation of oncogenes, and inactivation of tumor-suppressor genes[154] (see What's New? The Genetics of Lung Cancer). Further, cellular damage is caused by smoke-induced toxic oxygen radical production. The most

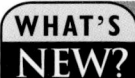

The Genetics of Lung Cancer

Lung cancer is caused by repetitive insults to the bronchial mucosa that result in multiple mutations in the genome of susceptible cells. By far the most important causes of these changes are the carcinogens in cigarette smoke, although air pollution and occupational exposures also are culprits. Genetic studies can help determine which individuals are at greatest risk for the development of cancer and identify the common mutations that occur during tumor development. The sequential accumulation of genetic mutations includes formation of oncogenes that secrete tumor growth–supporting factors, the loss of activity of tumor suppressor genes, the reordering of chromosomal sequences that lead to unregulated cell division, and the increased production of angiogenesis and tumor invasion factors. The expanded understanding of the genetics of lung cancer and the effect genetic mutations have on bronchial cell function and morphology are leading toward more effective means of detection and treatment of this deadly disease. Examples of how genetics can help with lung cancer management include (1) identification of genetically high-risk individuals who are critical candidates for focused intensive smoking cessation interventions, (2) screening for early tumor formation through examination of sputum DNA changes, (3) determination of those steps in carcinogenesis that would likely be most responsive to chemoprevention therapies, (4) better determination of treatment and prognosis through molecular examination of individual tumors, and (5) gene-directed therapies. Examples of gene therapies being developed for the treatment of lung cancer include administration of antisense molecules and angiogenesis blockers, induction of tumor cell "suicide" genes, promotion of the immune response to the cancer cells (cancer vaccines and immunogene therapy), and intratumoral gene replacement therapy (e.g., replacement of the tumor suppressor gene *p53*).

Data from Fong KM et al: *Thorax* 58(10):892-900, 2003; Hege K, Carbone D: *Lung Cancer* 41(suppl 1):S103-S113, 2003; Roth JA, Grammer SF: *Hematol-Oncol Clin North Am* 18(1):215-229, 2004; Sattler M, Salgia R:, *Semin Oncol* 30(1):57-71, 2003; Schrump DS: *J Surg Res* 117(1):107-113, 2004; Sekido Y et al: *Annu Rev Med* 54:73-87, 2003; Toyooka S, Tsuda T, Gazdar AF:, *Hum Mutat* 21(3):229-239, 2003.

common genetic abnormality associated with lung cancer is loss of the tumor-suppressor gene *p53;* mutations in this gene have been found in 45% to 55% of non–small cell lung cancers and 75% to 100% of small cell cancers.[154] Once lung cancer is initiated by these carcinogen-induced mutations, further tumor development is promoted by growth factors, such as epidermal growth factor.

The bronchial mucosa suffers multiple carcinogenic "hits" because of repetitive exposure to cigarette smoke, and eventually epithelial cell changes begin to be visible on biopsy. These changes progress from metaplasia to carcinoma in situ, and finally to invasive carcinoma. Further, tumor progression includes invasion of surrounding tissues and, finally, metastasis to distant sites, including the brain, bone marrow, and liver.

CLINICAL MANIFESTATIONS   Symptoms of early-stage, localized disease are nonspecific and are likely to be attributed by the individual to the effects of smoking. The clinical manifestations are ambiguous and insidious; they include coughing, chest pain, sputum production, hemoptysis, pneumonia, airway obstruction, and pleural effusions. Table 33-5 summarizes the common clinical manifestations according to tumor type. By the time manifestations are severe enough to motivate the individual to seek medical advice, the disease is usually advanced and symptoms and signs of metastatic disease (e.g., neurologic deficits, bone pain) or paraneoplastic syndromes may be evident.[155]

EVALUATION AND TREATMENT   While it is clear that diagnosing and treating lung cancer early in its development is crucial for long-term survival, screening for the presence of asymptomatic tumors in high-risk individuals remains controversial. The latest guidelines state that the evidence remains insufficient to recommend for or against screening asymptomatic individuals with sputum cytology, chest x-ray, or low-dose computed tomography (LDCT).[156] However, many clinicians and researchers continue to examine these and other modalities in an effort to find more effective ways of catching this deadly disease when it is still curable.[157,158] The diagnosis of lung cancer relies on the history of risk factors and symptoms, a careful physical examination, and a constellation of diagnostic tests including sputum cytology, chest x-ray, CT scanning, PET scanning bronchoscopy, biopsy, and search for potential metastatic disease.[159] The goal of these evaluations is to (1) establish the presence of a primary lung cancer, (2) determine its cell type, and (3) stage the tumor. As stated above, small cell lung cancer (SCLC) is staged as either limited or extensive. The staging of non–small cell lung cancer (NSCLC) uses the **TNM classification system** in which *T* denotes the extent of the primary tumor, *N* indicates nodal involvement, and *M* describes the extent of metastasis. This system as it applies to NSCLC was revised in 1997[160] and is described in Table 33-5 and is illustrated in Figure 33-23.

The choice of treatment for lung cancer relies on an accurate description of the type of cancer cell and the stage of the tumor. In general, surgical removal of the entire tumor is the only certain cure. NSCLC is less responsive to chemotherapy than is small cell carcinoma, but chemotherapy and radiation are commonly used as adjuvant or palliative care.[152,161,162] Small cell carcinoma is usually widely metastasized by the time of diagnosis, and treatment, while palliative, can markedly extend survival. Small cell carcinoma is most often treated with chemotherapy or radiation.[153,163] Other therapies for lung cancer that can be used in selected individuals are laser phototherapy, photodynamic therapy, cryotherapy, and brachytherapy.[164] New and exciting treatments for lung cancer are under investigation, including tumor sensitizing agents, gene therapy, and immunotherapy.[165-168]

Prevention of lung cancer relies primarily on reduction of exposure to carcinogens. For most individuals, this means smoking cessation, and numerous governmental and private organizations are working toward the complete end of cigarette smoking.[169] Other forms of prevention[170-172] are also being explored (see What's New?).

Table 33-5	1997 Revised International System for Staging Lung Cancer
Symbol	**Definition**
Primary Tumor (T)	
T0	No evidence of tumor
Tx	Tumor that cannot be assessed or is not apparent radiologically or bronchoscopically (malignant cells in broncho-pulmonary secretions)
Tis	Carcinoma in situ
T1	Tumor with the following characteristics:
a	Size: ≤3 cm
b	Airway location: in lobar bronchus or distal airways
c	Local invasion: none, surrounded by lung or visceral pleura
T2	Tumor with any of the following characteristics:
a	Size: >3 cm
b	Airway location: involvement of the main bronchus (distance to the carina is 2 cm or more) or presence of atelectasis or obstructive pneumonitis that extends to hilar region but does not involve the entire lung
c	Local invasion: involvement of the visceral pleura
T3	Tumor with the following location or invasion:
a	Size: any
b	Airway location: tumor in the main bronchus (within 2 cm of the carina) or tumor with atelectasis or obstructive pneumonitis of the entire lung
c	Local invasion: invasion of chest wall (including superior sulcus tumors), diaphragm, mediastinal pleura, or parietal pericardium
T4	Tumor with the following location or invasion:
a	Size: any
b	Airway location: satellite tumor nodule(s) within the ipsilateral primary-tumor lobe of the lung
c	Local invasion: invasion of the mediastinum, heart, great vessels, trachea, esophagus, vertebral body, or carina; or presence of malignant pleural/pericardial effusion
Lymph Nodes (N)	
Nx	Regional lymph nodes cannot be assessed
N0	Absence of regional lymph node involvement
N1	Presence of metastasis to ipsilateral peribronchial or ipsilateral hilar lymph nodes or both (including direct extension to intrapulmonary nodes)
N2	Presence of metastasis to ipsilateral mediastinal or subcarinal lymph nodes or both
N3	Presence of metastasis to any of the following lymph node groups: contralateral mediastinal, contralateral hilar, ipsilateral or contralateral scalene, or supraclavicular
Distant Metastasis (M)	
Mx	Metastasis cannot be assessed
M0	Absence of distant metastasis
M1	Presence of distant metastasis (separate metastatic tumor nodule[s] in the ipsilateral nonprimary-tumor lobe[s] of the lung also are grouped as MI)
Stage Grouping—TNM Subsets	
Stage 0	TisN0M0
Stage 1A	T1N0M0
Stage 1B	T2N0M0
Stage IIA	T1N1M0
Stage IIB	T2N1N0;T3N0M0
Stage IIIA	T3N1M0;T(1-3)N2M0
Stage IIIB	T4, any N, M0; any T, N3M0
Stage IV	Any T; any N; M1

From Mountain CF: *Chest* 111(6):1710, 1997.

NOTE: The uncommon superficial tumor of any size with its invasive component limited to bronchial wall is classified T1 even in the case of extension to main bronchus.

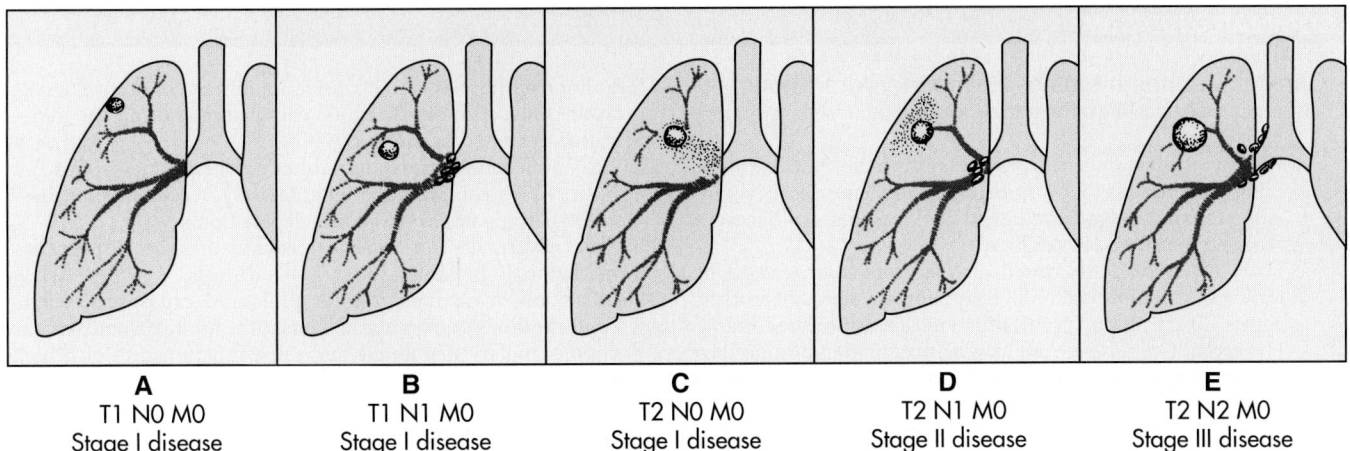

A T1 N0 M0 Stage I disease	**B** T1 N1 M0 Stage I disease	**C** T2 N0 M0 Stage I disease	**D** T2 N1 M0 Stage II disease	**E** T2 N2 M0 Stage III disease

Figure 33-23 Staging of lung cancer by the TNM classification system. **A, B,** Stage I disease includes tumors classified as T1, with or without metastasis to the lymph nodes in the ipsilateral hilar region. **C,** Also included in stage I are tumors classified as T2 but having no nodal or distant metastases. **D,** Stage II disease includes those tumors classified as T2, with metastasis only to the ipsilateral hilar lymph nodes. **E,** Stage III includes all tumors more extensive than T2 or any tumor with metastasis to the lymph nodes in the mediastinum or with distant metastasis.

Other Lung Cancers

Bronchial carcinoid tumors represent about 1% of all lung tumors. The tumor cells have dense granules containing neuroendocrine-like hormones, but they rarely produce endocrine symptoms (carcinoid syndrome).

Carcinoid tumors tend to occur earlier in life than bronchogenic carcinoma, although they can occur through the seventh decade of life. The average age at diagnosis is about 45 years, and carcinoid tumors are not related to smoking. The tumors arise more commonly in the main or segmental bronchi, are easily visualized bronchoscopically, and are found on routine chest radiographs. Cells are not recovered from bronchial washings because the tumor is covered with normal mucosa. These tumors are slow-growing cancers, and 50% of individuals with bronchial carcinoid tumors are asymptomatic. Local surgical resection is curative if metastasis has not occurred; this can often be done by bronchoscopic laser electrocautery.[173,174]

Adenocystic tumors (cylindromas) and **mucoepidermoid carcinomas** are rare bronchial gland tumors. They arise predominantly in the trachea or large airways and cause obstruction. They can be malignant and metastasize early, although distal pulmonary metastases are usually slow growing. Thus it is not unusual for an individual to survive 10 to 15 years after diagnosis.

Mesotheliomas can be benign but most often are aggressive malignant tumors arising from the epithelium covering the serous membranes. Most arise from the pleural surface (80%). Benign pleural mesotheliomas have a slow clinical onset and are usually asymptomatic, but over a period of years they can cause dyspnea and mild pleuritic pain. These tumors can grow to be very large and fill the entire pleural cavity. Mesotheliomas are more likely to be malignant than benign. The incidence of malignant mesothelioma is steadily increasing, with a projected 1300 cases per year by 2020.[175]

There is a clear association between asbestos exposure and malignant mesothelioma, especially in asbestos workers, although the minimum amount of exposure that constitutes risk has not been determined. A long latent interval between exposure to asbestos and appearance of mesothelioma usually occurs, and onset of symptoms may take 20 to 40 years.[176] Clinical manifestations include dyspnea and chest pain that result from tumor-derived pleural fluid and invasion of the chest wall. Diagnosis is made by chest x-ray, CT scan, and thoracentesis with cytologic examination of the pleural fluid. Thoracoscopy also may be used for biopsy.[175] Current management of malignant mesothelioma includes a combination of pleuropneumonectomy, chemotherapy, radiation, and hyperthermia.[175,177]

Clinical Manifestations of Pulmonary Alterations

1. Dyspnea is a feeling of breathlessness and increased respiratory effort.
2. Abnormal breathing patterns are adjustments made by the body to minimize the work of respiratory muscles. They include Kussmaul, obstructed, restricted, gasping, and Cheyne-Stokes respirations, and sighing.
3. Hypoventilation is decreased alveolar ventilation caused by airway obstruction, chest wall restriction, or altered neurologic control of breathing. Hypoventilation causes increased Pa_{CO_2}.
4. Hyperventilation is increased alveolar ventilation produced by anxiety, head injury, or severe hypoxemia. Hyperventilation causes decreased Pa_{CO_2}.
5. Coughing is a protective reflex that expels secretions and irritants from the lower airways.
6. Hemoptysis is expectoration of bloody mucus, which can be caused by bronchitis, tuberculosis, abscess, neoplasms, and other conditions that cause hemorrhage from damaged vessels.
7. Cyanosis is a bluish discoloration of the skin caused by desaturation of hemoglobin, polycythemia, or peripheral vasoconstriction.
8. Chest pain can result from inflamed pleurae, trachea, bronchi, or respiratory muscles.
9. Clubbing of the fingertips is associated with diseases that interfere with oxygenation of the tissues.
10. Hypercapnia is increased Pa_{CO_2} caused by a decrease in minute volume (respiratory rate X tidal volume).
11. Hypoxemia is a reduced Pa_{O_2} caused by (a) decreased oxygen content of inspired gas, (b) hypoventilation, (c) diffusion abnormality, (d) ventilation-perfusion mismatch, or (e) shunting.
12. Acute respiratory failure is caused by inadequate gas exchange or ventilation ($Pa_{O_2} \leq 50$ mmHg or $Pa_{CO_2} \geq 50$ mmHg and pH ≤ 7.25).
13. Pulmonary edema is excess water in the lung caused by disturbances of capillary hydrostatic pressure, capillary oncotic pressure, or capillary permeability. A common cause is left-sided heart failure that increases the hydrostatic pressure in the pulmonary circulation.
14. Aspiration is passage of fluid and solid particles into the lung, usually from impaired swallowing and coughing. It frequently results in pneumonitis and pulmonary infection.
15. Atelectasis is the collapse of alveoli resulting from compression of the lung tissue or absorption of gas from obstructed alveoli.
16. Bronchiectasis is abnormal dilation of the bronchi secondary to another pulmonary disorder, usually infection or inflammation.
17. Bronchiolitis is the inflammatory obstruction of small airways. It is most common in children.
18. Pneumothorax is the accumulation of air in the pleural space. It can be caused by spontaneous rupture of weakened areas of a pleura or can be secondary to pleural damage caused by disease, trauma, or mechanical ventilation.
17. Pleural effusion is the accumulation of fluid in the pleural space, usually resulting from disorders that promote transudation or exudation from capillaries underlying the pleura but occasionally resulting from blockage or injury that causes lymphatic vessels to drain into the pleural space.
18. Pleurisy is inflammation of the pleura.
19. Empyema is the presence of pus in the pleural space (infected pleural effusion). The source of the pus is usually lymphatic drainage from sites of bacterial pneumonia.
20. Abscesses are circumscribed areas of destruction of lung parenchyma with suppuration usually resulting from aspiration pneumonia.

21. Pulmonary fibrosis is an excessive amount of connective tissue in the lung. It diminishes lung compliance and may be idiopathic or caused by disease.
22. Chest wall compliance is diminished by obesity and kyphoscoliosis, which compress the lungs, and by neuromuscular diseases that impair chest wall muscle function.
23. Flail chest results from rib or sternal fractures that disrupt the mechanics of breathing.
24. Inhalation of noxious gases or prolonged exposure to high concentrations of oxygen can damage the bronchial mucosa or alveolocapillary membrane and cause inflammation or acute respiratory failure.
25. Pneumoconiosis, which is caused by inhalation of dust particles in the workplace, including coal dust, can cause pulmonary fibrosis, susceptibility to lower airway infection, and tumor formation.
26. Silicosis is a type of pneumoconiosis caused by inhalation of silica.
27. Allergic alveolitis is an allergic or hypersensitivity reaction to many allergens.

Pulmonary Disorders

1. Adult respiratory distress syndrome (ARDS) results from an acute, diffuse injury to the alveolocapillary membrane and decreased surfactant production, which increases membrane permeability and causes edema and atelectasis.
2. Postoperative respiratory failure is most common in individuals undergoing surgery who smoke or have chronic disease.
3. Obstructive pulmonary disease is characterized by airway obstruction that causes difficult expiration. Obstructive disease can be acute or chronic and includes asthma, chronic bronchitis, and emphysema.
4. In asthma, obstruction is caused by episodic attacks of bronchospasm, bronchial inflammation, mucosal edema, and increased mucus production.
5. Chronic obstructive pulmonary disease (COPD) is the coexistence of chronic bronchitis and emphysema.
6. Chronic bronchitis causes airway obstruction resulting from bronchial smooth muscle hypertrophy and production of thick, tenacious mucus.
7. In emphysema, destruction of the alveolar septa and loss of passive elastic recoil lead to airway collapse and obstruct gas flow during expiration.
8. Emphysema in which septal deterioration is caused by α_1-antitrypsin deficiency or old age tends to be panacinar.
9. Emphysema in which septal deterioration results from smoking tends to be centriacinar.
10. Upper respiratory tract infections, which are the most common cause of short-term disability in the United States, include rhinitis (the common cold), pharyngitis, and laryngitis.
11. Serious lower respiratory tract infections, which occur most often in very old persons and individuals with impaired immunity or underlying disease, include pneumonia and tuberculosis.
12. Pneumococcal pneumonia is an acute lung infection resulting in an inflammatory response with four phases: (a) consolidation, (b) red hepatization, (c) gray hepatization, and (d) resolution.
14. Viral pneumonia is an acute, self-limiting lung infection usually caused by the influenza virus.
15. Tuberculosis is a lung infection caused by *Mycobacterium tuberculosis* (tubercle bacillus).
16. In tuberculosis the inflammatory response isolates colonies of bacilli by enclosing them in tubercles and surrounding the tubercles with scar tissue.

SUMMARY REVIEW—cont'd

17. Bacilli may remain dormant within the tubercles for life or, if the immune system breaks down, cause recurrence of active disease.
18. Pulmonary vascular diseases are caused by embolism or hypertension in the pulmonary circulation.
19. Pulmonary embolism is occlusion of a portion of the pulmonary vascular bed by a thrombus (most common), a tissue fragment, or an air bubble. Depending on its size and location, the embolus can cause hypoxic vasoconstriction, pulmonary edema, atelectasis, pulmonary hypertension, shock, and even death.
20. Pulmonary hypertension (pulmonary artery pressure 5 to 10 mmHg above normal) is caused by (a) elevated left ventricular pressure, (b) increased blood flow through the pulmonary circulation, (c) obliteration or obstruction of the vascular bed, or (d) active constriction of the vascular bed produced by hypoxemia or acidosis.
21. Cor pulmonale is right ventricular enlargement caused by chronic pulmonary hypertension. Cor pulmonale progresses to right ventricular failure if the pulmonary hypertension is not reversed.
22. Lip cancer is most common in men and represents about 1% of all cancers. In the most common cell type, squamous cell, metastasis is rare when lesions are diagnosed and treated early.
23. Laryngeal cancer occurs primarily in men and represents 2% to 3% of all cancers. Squamous cell carcinoma of the true vocal cords is most common and manifests with a clinical symptom of progressive hoarseness.
24. Lung cancer, the most frequent cause of cancer death in the United States, is commonly caused by cigarette smoking.
25. Cancer cell types include squamous cell carcinoma, small cell (oat cell) carcinoma, adenocarcinoma, large cell carcinoma, bronchial adenoma, and mesothelioma. Each type arises in a characteristic site or type of tissue, causes distinctive clinical manifestations, and differs in likelihood of metastasis and prognosis.
26. Bronchial carcinoid and adenocystic tumors are rare tumors of the bronchial airways.

KEY TERMS

Abscess, 1216
Absorption atelectasis, 1212
Acute cough, 1207
Acute respiratory distress syndrome (ARDS), 1218
Adenocarcinoma, 1238
Adenocystic tumors (cylindromas), 1243
Asbestosis, 1218
Aspiration, 1211
Asthma, 1222
Atelectasis, 1212
Bronchial carcinoid tumors, 1243
Bronchiectasis, 1212
Bronchiolitis, 1213
Bronchiolitis obliterans, 1213
Bronchitis, 1212
Cavitation, 1216
Centriacinar emphysema, 1227
Cheyne-Stokes respirations, 1206
Chronic bronchitis, 1224
Chronic cough, 1207
Chronic obstructive pulmonary disease (COPD), 1224
Clubbing, 1208
Coal worker pneumoconiosis (coal miner lung, black lung), 1217
Compression atelectasis, 1212

Consolidation, 1216
Cor pulmonale, 1236
Cough, 1207
Cyanosis, 1207
Cylindrical bronchiectasis, 1213
Dyspnea, 1205
Emphysema, 1227
Empyema (infected pleural effusion), 1216
Extrinsic allergic alveolitis (hypersensitivity pneumonitis), 1218
Exudative effusion, 1215
Flail chest, 1217
Hemoptysis, 1207
Hemothorax, 1215
Hypercapnia, 1208
Hyperventilation, 1207
Hypocapnia, 1207
Hypoventilation, 1206
Hypoxemia, 1208
Hypoxia, 1208
Kussmaul respiration (hyperpnea), 1206
Mesothelioma, 1243
Mucoepidermoid carcinoma, 1243
Open pneumothorax (communicating pneumothorax), 1214
Orthopnea (positional dyspnea), 1206
Oxygen toxicity, 1217

Panacinar emphysema, 1227
Paroxysmal nocturnal dyspnea (PND), 1206
Pleural effusion, 1215
Pleurisy, 1215
Pneumoconiosis, 1217
Pneumonia, 1228
Pneumothorax, 1213
Pulmonary edema, 1210
Pulmonary embolism (PE), 1232
Pulmonary fibrosis, 1216
Pulmonary thromboembolism, 1232
Saccular bronchiectasis, 1213
Secondary pneumothorax, 1214
Silicosis, 1217
Small cell carcinomas, 1240
Spontaneous pneumothorax, 1214
Status asthmaticus, 1224
Tension pneumothorax, 1214
TNM classification system, 1241
Transudative effusion, 1215
Tuberculosis (TB), 1230
Undifferentiated large cell carcinoma (undifferentiated large cell anaplastic cancer), 1239
Varicose bronchiectasis, 1213

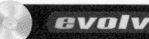
REFERENCES

1. Binks AP et al: "Tightness" sensation of asthma does not arise from the work of breathing, *Am J Respir Crit Care Med* 165(1):78-82, 2002.
2. Lansing RW, Moosavi SH, Banzett RB: Measurement of dyspnea: word labeled visual analog scale vs. verbal ordinal scale, *Respir Physiol Neurobiol* 134(2):77-83, 2003.
3. Niimi A et al: Impaired cough reflex in patients with recurrent pneumonia, *Thorax* 58(2):152-153, 2003.
4. Widdicombe J: Neuroregulation of cough: implications for drug therapy, *Curr Opin Pharmacol* 2(3):256-263, 2002.
5. Brashers VL, Haden K: Differential diagnosis of cough: focus on lung malignancy, *Lippincotts Prim Care Pract* 4(4):374-389, 2000.
6. Corder R: Hemoptysis, *Emerg Med Clin North Am* 21(2):421-435, 2003.
7. Augarten A et al: Reversal of digital clubbing after lung transplantation in cystic fibrosis patients: a clue to the pathogenesis of clubbing, *Pediatr Pulmonol* 34(5):378-380, 2002.
8. Nagasawa K: Rheumatic manifestations in paraneoplastic syndrome, *Intern Med* 39(9):685-686, 2000.
9. Dumas JP et al: Hypoxic pulmonary vasoconstriction, *Gen Pharmacol* 33(4):289-297, 1999.
10. Gomes GF et al: The nasogastric feeding tube as a risk factor for aspiration and aspiration pneumonia, *Curr Opin Clin Nut Metab Care* 6(3):327-333, 2003.
11. Mojon P, Bourbeau J: Respiratory infection: how important is oral health? *Curr Opin Pulmon Med* 9(3):166-170, 2003.
12. Dahan LJ, Teppema LJ: Influence of anaesthesia and analgesia on the control of breathing, *Br J Anaesthesia* 91(1): 40-49, 2003.
13. Silverman E et al: Current management of bronchiectasis: review and 3 case studies, *Heart Lung: J Acute Crit Care* 32(1):59-64, 2003.
14. Bordley WC et al: Diagnosis and testing in bronchiolitis: a systematic review, *Arch Pediatr Adolesc Med* 158(2):119-126, 2004.
15. Boehler A, Estenne M: Post-transplant bronchiolitis obliterans, *Eur Respir J* 22(6):1007-1018, 2003.
16. Corris PA: Lung transplantation. Bronchiolitis obliterans syndrome, *Chest Surg Clin North Am* 13(3):543-557, 2003.
17. Noppen M, Baumann MH: Pathogenesis and treatment of primary spontaneous pneumothorax: an overview, *Respir* 70(4):431-438, 2003.
18. Roman M, Weinstein A, Macaluso S: Primary spontaneous pneumothorax, *Medsurg Nurs* 12(3):161-169, 2003.
19. Morimoto T et al: Optimal strategy for the first episode of primary spontaneous pneumothorax in young men: a decision analysis, *J Gen Intern Med* 17(3):193-202, 2002.
20. Miller A: Management of pneumothorax, *Practitioner* 246(1631):108, 111-112, 2002.
21. de Hoyos A, Sundaresan S: Thoracic empyema, *Surg Clin North Am* 82(3):643-671, viii, 2002.
22. Vikram HR, Quagliarello VJ: Diagnosis and management of empyema, *Curr Clin Top Infect Dis* 22:196-213, 2002.
23. Mansharamani NG, Koziel H: Chronic lung sepsis: lung abscess, bronchiectasis, and empyema, *Curr Opin Pulmon Med* 9(3):181-185, 2003.
24. Thannickal VJ et al: Mechanisms of pulmonary fibrosis, *Annu Rev Med* 55:395-417, 2004.
25. Davies HR, Richeldi L: Idiopathic pulmonary fibrosis: current and future treatment options, *Am J Respir Med* 1(3):211-224, 2002.
26. Kuschner WG, Stark P: Occupational lung disease. Part 2. Discovering the cause of diffuse parenchymal lung disease, *Postgrad Med* 113(4):81-88, 2003.
27. Cohen R, Velho V: Update on respiratory disease from coal mine and silica dust, *Clin Chest Med* 23(4):811-826, 2002.
28. Ding M et al: Diseases caused by silica: mechanisms of injury and disease development, *Int Immunopharmacol* 2(2-3):173-182, 2002.
29. Borm PJ, Tran L: From quartz hazard to quartz risk: the coal mines revisited, *Ann Occup Hyg* 46(1):25-32, 2002.
30. Cugell DW, Kamp DW: Asbestos and the pleura: a review, *Chest* 125(3):1103-1117, 2004.
31. Manning CB, Vallyathan V, Mossman BT: Diseases caused by asbestos: mechanisms of injury and disease development, *Int Immunopharmacol* 2(2-3):191-200, 2002.
32. Upadhyay D, Kamp DW: Asbestos-induced pulmonary toxicity: role of DNA damage and apoptosis, *Exp Biol Med* 228(6):650-659, 2003.
33. Lacasse Y et al: Clinical diagnosis of hypersensitivity pneumonitis, *Am J Respir Crit Care Med* 168(8):952–958, 2003.
34. Rubenfeld GD: Epidemiology of acute lung injury, *Crit Care Med* 31(4Suppl):S276-S284, 2003.
35. Bhatia M, Moochhala S: Role of inflammatory mediators in the pathophysiology of acute respiratory distress syndrome, *J Pathol* 202(2): 145-156, 2004.
36. Abraham E: Neutrophils and acute lung injury, *Crit Care Med* 31(4Suppl): S195-S199, 2003.
37. Brower RG, Rubenfeld GD: Lung-protective ventilation strategies in acute lung injury, *Crit Care Med* 31(4Suppl):S312-S316, 2003.
38. Chadda K, Annane D: The use of corticosteroids in severe sepsis and acute respiratory distress syndrome, *Ann Med* 34(7-8):582-589, 2002.
39. Thompson BT: Glucocorticoids and acute lung injury, *Crit Care Med* 31(4Suppl): S253S25-7, 2003.
40. Rodriguez RJ: Management of respiratory distress syndrome: an update, *Respir Care* 48(3): 279-286, 2003.
41. Laterre PF, Wittebole X, Dhainaut JF: Anticoagulant therapy in acute lung injury, *Crit Care Med* 31(4Suppl): S329-S336, 2003.
42. Second Expert Panel on the Management of Asthma, National Heart, Lung, and Blood Institute: *Highlights of the expert panel report 2: guidelines for the diagnosis and management of asthma*, Bethesda, Md, 1997, National Institutes of Health (pub no NIH 97-4051A).
43. NAEPP Expert Panel Report Guidelines for the Diagnosis and Management of Asthma: *Update on selected topics*, Bethesda, Md, 2002, National Institutes of Health.
44. Cookson WO: Asthma genetics, *Chest* 121(3 Suppl):7S-13S, 2002.
45. Kaiser HB: Risk factors in allergy/asthma, *Allergy Asthma Proc* 25(1): 7-10, 2004.
46. Arshad SH: Indoor allergen exposure in the development of allergy and asthma, *Curr Allergy Asthma Rep* 3:115-120, 2003.
47. Custovic A, Murray CS: The effect of allergen exposure in early childhood on the development of atopy, *Curr Allergy Asthma Rep* 2(5): 417-423, 2002.
48. Tantisira K, Weiss S: Childhood infections and asthma: at the crossroads of the hygiene and Barker hypotheses, *Respir Res* 2 (6):324–327, 2001.
49. Busse WW, Rosenwasser LJ: Mechanisms of asthma, *J Allergy Clin Immunol* 11(3Suppl)1:S799-S804, 2003.
50. Barnes PJ: The role of inflammation and anti-inflammatory medication in asthma, *Respir Med* 96(Suppl A):S9-S15, 2002.
51. Fireman P: Understanding asthma pathophysiology, *Allergy Asthma Proc* 24:79-83, 2003.
52. Lemanske RF Jr, Busse WW: 6. Asthma, *J Allergy Clin Immunol* 111(2Suppl): S502-S519, 2003.
53. Hamid Q et al: Inflammatory cells in asthma: mechanisms and implications for therapy, *J Allergy Clin Immunol* 111(1Suppl): S5-S12, 2003.
54. Coulson FR, Fryer AD: Muscarinic acetylcholine receptors and airway diseases, *Pharmacol Ther* 98(1): 59-69, 2003.
55. Kharitonov SA, Barnes PJ: Nitric oxide, nitrotyrosine, and nitric oxide modulators in asthma and chronic obstructive pulmonary disease, *Curr Allergy Asthma Rep* 3(2):121-129, 2003.
56. Davies DE et al: Airway remodeling in asthma: new insights, *J Allergy Clin Immunol* 111(2): 215-225, 2003.
57. Rodrigo GJ, Rodrigo C, Hall JB: Acute asthma in adults: a review, *Chest* 125(3):1081-1102, 2004.
58. Rowe BH et al: Corticosteroid therapy for acute asthma, *Respir Med* 98(4):275-284, 2004.
59. Rambasek TE, Lang DM, Kavuru MS: Omalizumab: where does it fit into current asthma management? *Clev Clin J Med* 71(3):251-261, 2004.
60. Boushey HA: New and exploratory therapies for asthma, *Chest* 123(3Suppl): 439S-445S, 2003.

61. Kenyon NJ, Jarjour NN: Severe asthma, *Clin Review Allergy Immunol* 25(2):131-149, 2003.

62. Gomez FP, Rodriguez-Roisin R: Global initiative for chronic obstructive lung disease (GOLD) guidelines for chronic obstructive pulmonary disease, *Curr Opin Pulmon Med* 8(2):81-86, 2002.

63. Sandford AJ, Joos L, Pare PD: Genetic risk factors for chronic obstructive pulmonary disease, *Curr Opin Pulmon Med* 8(2):87-94, 2002.

64. White AJ et al: Resolution of bronchial inflammation is related to bacterial eradication following treatment of exacerbations of chronic bronchitis, *Thorax* 58(8):680-685, 2003.

65. National Collaborating Centre for Chronic Conditions: Chronic obstructive pulmonary disease. National clinical guideline on management of chronic obstructive pulmonary disease in adults in primary and secondary care, *Thorax* 59(Suppl 1):1-232, 2004.

66. Black P et al: Prophylactic antibiotic therapy for chronic bronchitis, *Cocharane Database Syst Rev* (1):CD004105, 2003.

67. Suki B, Lutchen KR, Ingenito EP: On the progressive nature of emphysema: roles of proteases, inflammation, and mechanical forces, *Am J Respir Crit Care Med* 168(5):516-521, 2003.

68. Tuder RM et al: Apoptosis and emphysema: the missing link, *Am J Respir Cell Molec Biol* 28(5):551-554, 2003.

69. Wedzicha JA, Donaldson GC: Exacerbations of chronic obstructive pulmonary disease, *Respir Care* 48(12):1204-1213, discussion 1213-1215, 2003.

70. Man SF et al: Contemporary management of chronic obstructive pulmonary disease: clinical applications, *JAMA* 290(17):2313-2316, 2003.

71. Faulkner MA, Hilleman DE: Pharmacologic treatment of chronic obstructive pulmonary disease: past, present, and future, *Pharmacol* 23(10):1300-1315, 2003.

72. Calverley PM: Respiratory failure in chronic obstructive pulmonary disease, *Eur Respir J Suppl* 47:26s-30s, 2003.

73. Loeb M: Pneumonia in the elderly, *Curr Opin Infect Dis* 38(9):1292-1297, 2004.

74. Andrews J et al: Community-acquired pneumonia, *Curr Opin Pulmon Med* 9(3):175-180, 2003.

75. File TM: Community-acquired pneumonia, *Lancet* 362(9400):1991-2001, 2003.

76. Agusti C et al: Nosocomial pneumonia in immunosuppressed patients, *Infect Dis Clin North Am* 17(4):785-800, 2003.

77. Alcon A, Fabregas N, Torres A: Hospital-acquired pneumonia: etiologic considerations, *Infect Dis Clin North Am* 17(4):679-695, 2003.

78. Hubmayr RD et al: Statement of the 4th international consensus conference in critical care on ICU-acquired pneumonia, *Intensive Care Med* 28(11):1521-1536, 2002.

79. Roig J, Sabria M, Pedro-Botet ML: Legionella spp: community acquired and nosocomial infections, *Curr Opin Infect Dis* 16(2):145-151, 2003.

80. Garau J, Gomez L: Pseudomonas aeruginosa pneumonia, *Curr Opin Infect Dis* 16(2):135-143, 2003.

81. Morris A et al: Prevalence and clinical predictors of pneumocystis colonization among HIV-infected men, *AIDS* 18(5):793-798, 2004.

82. Delclaux C, Azoulay E: Inflammatory response to infectious pulmonary injury, *Eur Respir J Suppl* 42:10s-14s, 2003.

83. Kadioglu A, Andrew PW: The innate immune response to pneumococcal lung infection: the untold story, *Trends Immunol* 25(3):143-149, 2004.

84. Mizgerd JP: Molecular mechanisms of neutrophil recruitment elicited by bacteria in the lungs, *Semin Immunol* 14(2):123-132, 2002.

85. Sethi S: Bacterial pneumonia. Managing a deadly complication of influenza in older adults with comorbid disease, *Geriatrics* 57(3):56-61, 2002.

86. Mabie M, Wunderink RG: Use and limitations of clinical and radiologic diagnosis of pneumonia, *Semin Respir Infect* 18(2):72-79, 2003.

87. American Thoracic Society: guidelines for the management of adults with community-acquired pneumonia, *Am J Respir Crit Care Med* 163:1730-1754, 2001.

88. Baughman RP: Diagnosis of ventilator-associated pneumonia, *Curr Opin Crit Care* 9(5):397-402, 2003.

89. de Castro FR, Torres A: Optimizing treatment outcomes in severe community-acquired pneumonia, *Am J Respir Med* 2(1):39-54, 2003.

90. Chastre J: Antimicrobial treatment of hospital-acquired pneumonia, *Infect Dis Clin North Am* 17(4):727-737, vi, 2003.

91. Feldman C: Clinical relevance of antimicrobial resistance in the management of pneumococcal community-acquired pneumonia, *J Lab Clin Med* 143(5):269-283, 2004.

92. Kollef M: Appropriate empirical antibacterial therapy for nosocomial infections: getting it right the first time, *Drugs* 63(20):2157-2168, 2003.

93. Frieden TR et al: Tuberculosis, *Lancet* 362(9387):887-899, 2003.

94. Centers for Disease Control: *Reported tuberculosis in the United States, 2002.* Atlanta, Ga, 2003, US Department of Health and Human Services, CDC.

95. Corbett EL et al: The growing burden of tuberculosis: global trends and interactions with the HIV epidemic, *Arch Intern Med* 163(9):1009-1021, 2003.

96. Davies PD: The world-wide increase in tuberculosis: how demographic changes, HIV infection and increasing numbers in poverty are increasing tuberculosis, *Ann Med* 35(4):235-243, 2003.

97. Musher DM: How contagious are common respiratory tract infections? *New Engl J Med* 348(13):1256-1266, 2003.

98. Maartens G: Advances in adult pulmonary tuberculosis, *Curr Opin Pulmon Med* 8(3):173-177, 2002.

99. Chan J, Flynn J: The immunological aspects of latency in tuberculosis, *Clin Immunol* 110(1):2-12, 2004.

100. Zhang Y: Persistent and dormant tubercle bacilli and latent tuberculosis, *Frontiers Biosci* 9:1136-1156, 2004.

101. Drobniewski FA et al: Modern laboratory diagnosis of tuberculosis, *Lancet Infect Dis* 3(3):141-147, 2003.

102. American Thoracic Society: Diagnostic standards and classification of tuberculosis in adults and children, *Am J Respir Care Med* 161:1376-1395, 2000.

103. Centers for Disease Control and Prevention, Morbidity and Mortality Weekly Recommendations and Reports: treatment of tuberculosis, *MMWR* 52(RR11):1-77, 2003, American Thoracic Society and Infectious Disease Society of America. Available at www.cdc.gov/mmwr/pdf/rr/rr5211.pdf.

104. de Jong BC et al: Clinical management of tuberculosis in the context of HIV infection, *Annu Rev Med* 55:283-301, 2004.

105. Mitchison DA: The search for new sterilizing anti-tuberculosis drugs, *Frontiers Biosci* 9:1059-1072, 2004.

106. Goldhaber SZ: Pulmonary embolism, *Lancet* 363(9417):1295-1305, 2004.

107. Goldhaber SZ, Elliott CG: Acute pulmonary embolism. Part I. Epidemiology, pathophysiology, and diagnosis, *Circulation* 108(22):2726-2729, 2003.

108. White RH: The epidemiology of venous thromboembolism, *Circulation* 107(23 Suppl 1):I4-I8, 2003.

109. Anderson FA Jr, Spencer FA: Risk factors for venous thromboembolism, *Circulation* 107(23Suppl 1):I9-I16, 2003.

110. Kearon C: Natural history of venous thromboembolism, *Circulation* 107(23 Suppl 1):I22-I30, 2003.

111. Stratmann G, Gregory GA: Neurogenic and humoral vasoconstriction in acute pulmonary thromboembolism, *Anesth Analg* 97(2):341-354, 2003.

112. Bockenstedt P: D-dimer in venous thromboembolism, *New Engl J Med* 349(13):1203-1204, 2003.

113. Stein PD et al: D-dimer for the exclusion of acute venous thrombosis and pulmonary embolism: a systematic review, *Ann Intern Med* 140(8):589-602, 2004.

114. Fedullo PF, Tapson VF: Clinical practice. The evaluation of suspected pulmonary embolism, *New Engl J Med* 349(13):1247-1256, 2003.

115. Kanne JP, Lalani TA: Role of computed tomography and magnetic resonance imaging for deep venous thrombosis and pulmonary embolism, *Circulation* 109(12 Suppl 1):I15-I21, 2004.

116. Horlander KT, Leeper KV: Troponin levels as a guide to treatment of pulmonary embolism, *Curr Opin Pulmon Med* 9(5):374-377, 2003.

117. Kucher N, Goldhaber SZ: Cardiac biomarkers for risk stratification of patients with acute pulmonary embolism, *Circulation* 108(18):2191-2194, 2003.

118. Goldhaber SZ, Elliott CG: Acute pulmonary embolism: part II: risk stratification, treatment, and prevention, *Circulation* 108(23):2834-2388, 2003.

119. Jacobs DG, Sing RF: The role of vena caval filters in the management of venous thromboembolism, *Am Surgeon* 69(8):635-642, 2003.

120. Kinney TB: Update on inferior vena cava filters, *J Vasc Intervent Radiol* 14(4):425-440, 2003.

121. Runo JR, Loyd JE: Primary pulmonary hypertension, *Lancet* 361(9368):1533-1544, 2003.

122. Ghamra ZW, Dweik RA: Primary pulmonary hypertension: an overview of epidemiology and pathogenesis, *Clev Clin J Med* 70(Suppl 1):S2-S8, 2003.

123. Rich S, editor: *Executive summary from the world symposium: primary pulmonary hypertension,* Geneva, 1998, World Health Organization.

124. Blaise G, Langleben D, Hubert B: Pulmonary arterial hypertension: pathophysiology and anesthetic approach, *Anesthesiology* 99(6): 1415-1432, 2003.

125. Budhiraja R, Tuder RM, Hassoun PM: Endothelial dysfunction in pulmonary hypertension, *Circulation* 109(2):159-165, 2004.

126. Galie N, Manes A, Branzi A: The endothelin system in pulmonary arterial hypertension, *Cardiovasc Res* 61(2):227-237, 2004.

127. Presberg KW, Dincer HE: Pathophysiology of pulmonary hypertension due to lung disease, *Curr Opin Pulmon Med* 9(2):131-138, 2003.

128. Weitzenblum E: Chronic cor pulmonale, *Heart* 89(2):225-230, 2003.

129. Paramothayan NS et al: Prostacyclin for pulmonary hypertension, *Cochrane Database Syst Rev* (2):CD002994, 2003.

130. Sulica R, Poon M: Current medical treatment of pulmonary arterial hypertension, *Mt Sinai J Med* 71(2):103-114, 2004.

131. Clozel M: Effects of bosentan on cellular processes involved in pulmonary arterial hypertension: do they explain the long-term benefit? *Ann Med* 35(8):605-613, 2003.

132. Jemal A et al: Cancer statistics 2004, *CA Cancer J Clin* 54:8-29, 2004.

133. Vartanian JG et al: Predictive factors and distribution of lymph node metastasis in lip cancer patients and their implications on the treatment of the neck, *Oral Oncol* 40(2):223-227, 2004.

134. Bilkay U et al: Management of lower lip cancer: a retrospective analysis of 118 patients and review of the literature, *Ann Plast Surg* 50(1):43-50, 2003.

135. Guinot JL et al: Lip cancer treatment with high dose rate brachytherapy, *Radiotherapy Oncol* 69(1):113-115, 2003.

136. Wight R, Paleri V, Arullendran P: Current theories for the development of nonsmoking and nondrinking laryngeal carcinoma, *Curr Opin Otolaryngol Head Neck Surg* 11(2):73-77, 2003.

137. Assimakopoulos D, Patrikakos G: The role of gastroesophageal reflux in the pathogenesis of laryngeal carcinoma, *Am J Otolaryngol* 23(6):351-357, 2002.

138. Nadal A, Cardesa A: Molecular biology of laryngeal squamous cell carcinoma, *Virchows Arch* 442(1):1-7, 2003.

139. Zinreich SJ: Imaging in laryngeal cancer: computed tomography, magnetic resonance imaging, positron emission tomography, *Otolaryngol Clin North Am* 35(5):971-991, v, 2002.

140. Hinerman RW et al: Early laryngeal cancer, *Curr Trends Options Oncol* 3(1):3-9, 2002.

141. Lee DJ: Definitive radiotherapy for squamous carcinoma of the larynx, *Otolaryngol Clin North Am* 35(5):1013-1033, 2002.

142. Gilbert J, Forastiere AA: Organ preservation trials for laryngeal cancer, *Otolaryngologic Clin North Am* 35(5):1035-1054, vi, 2002.

143. Samlan RA, Webster KT: Swallowing and speech therapy after definitive treatment for laryngeal cancer, *Otolaryngol Clin North Am* 35(5):1115-1133, 2002.

144. Alberg AJ, Samet JM: Epidemiology of lung cancer, *Chest* 123(1 Suppl):21S-49S, 2003.

145. Gadgeel S, Kalemkerian G: Racial differences in lung cancer, *Cancer Metastasis Rev* 22(1):39-46, 2003.

146. Patel J, Bach P, Kris M: Lung cancer in US women: a contemporary epidemic, *JAMA* 291(14):1763-1768, 2004.

147. Travis WD et al: Histological typing of tumours of lung and pleura. In Sobin LH: *World Health Organization International Classification of Tumours,* ed 3, Berlin, 1999, Springer-Verlag.

148. Franklin WA: Pathology of lung cancer, *J Thoracic Imaging* 15(1):3-12, 2000.

149. Smith W, Khuri F: The care of the lung cancer patient in the 21st century, a new age, *Semin Oncol* 31(2 suppl 4):11-15, 2004.

150. Blum R: Adjuvant chemotherapy for lung cancer—a new standard of care, *New Engl J Med* 350(4):404-405, 2004.

151. Simon GR, Wagner H, American College of Chest Physicians: Small cell lung cancer, *Chest* 123(1 Suppl):259S-271S, 2003.

152. Sekido Y, Fong KM, Minna JD: Molecular genetics of lung cancer, *Annu Rev Med* 54:73-87, 2003.

153. Beckles MA et al: Initial evaluation of the patient with lung cancer: symptoms, signs, laboratory tests, and paraneoplastic syndromes, *Chest* 123(1 Suppl):97S-104S, 2003.

154. Humphrey LL et al: Lung cancer screening with sputum cytologic examination, chest radiography, and computed tomography: an update for the U.S. Preventive Services Task Force, *Ann Intern Med* 140(9):740-753, 2004.

155. Petty TL: Sputum cytology for the detection of early lung cancer, *Curr Opin Pulmon Med* 9(4):309-312, 2003.

156. Henschke CI et al: Guidelines for the use of spiral computed tomography in screening for lung cancer, *Eur Respir J Suppl* 39:45s-51s, 2003.

157. Rivera MP, et al: Diagnosis of lung cancer: the guidelines, *Chest* 123(1Suppl):129S-136S, 2003.

158. Mountain C: Revisions in the international system for staging lung cancer, *Chest* (6):1710, 1997.

159. Cullen M: Lung cancer. 4: chemotherapy for non-small cell lung cancer: the end of the beginning, *Thorax* 58(4):352-356, 2003.

160. Spira A, Ettinger DS: Multidisciplinary management of lung cancer, *New Engl J Med* 350(4):379-392, 2004.

161. Sandler AB: Chemotherapy for small cell lung cancer, *Semin Oncol* 30(1):9-25, 2003.

162. Chan AL et al: Advances in the management of endobronchial lung malignancies, *Curr Opin Pulmon Med* 9(4):301-308, 2003.

163. Fong KM et al: Lung cancer. 9: Molecular biology of lung cancer: clinical implications, *Thorax* 58(10):892-900, 2003.

164. Hege K, Carbone D: Lung cancer vaccines and gene therapy, *Lung Cancer* 41(Suppl 1):S103-S113, 2003.

165. Saha D, Pyo H, Choy H: COX-2 inhibitor as a radiation enhancer: new strategies for the treatment of lung cancer, *Am J Clin Oncol* 26(4): S70-S74, 2003.

166. Schrump DS: Genomic surgery for lung cancer, *J Surg Res* 117(1): 107-113, 2004.

167. American Society of Clinical Oncology: American Society of Clinical Oncology policy statement update: tobacco control—reducing cancer incidence and saving lives, 2003, *J Clin Oncol* 21(14):2777-2786, 2003.

168. Dragnev K, Stover D, Dmitrovsky E: Lung cancer prevention: the guidelines, *Chest* 123: 60S-71S, 2003.

169. Kelley MJ, McCrory DC: Prevention of lung cancer: summary of published evidence, *Chest* 123(1Suppl):50S-59S, 2003.

170. Winterhalder RC et al: Chemoprevention of lung cancer—from biology to clinical reality, *Annals Oncol* 15(2):185-196, 2004.

171. McMullan DM, Wood DE: Pulmonary carcinoid tumors, *Semin Thorac Cadiovasc Surg* 15(3):289-300, 2003.

172. Mezzetti M et al: Assessment of outcomes in typical and atypical carcinoids according to latest WHO classification, *Ann Thorac Surg* 76(6):1838-1842, 2003.

173. Parker C, Neville E: Lung cancer * 8: management of malignant mesothelioma, *Thorax* 58(9):809-813, 2003.

174. Cugell DW, Kamp DW: Asbestos and the pleura: a review, *Chest* 125(3):1103-1117, 2004.

175. Janne PA: Chemotherapy for malignant pleural mesothelioma, *Clin Lung Cancer* 5(2):98-106, 2003.

ALTERATIONS OF PULMONARY FUNCTION IN CHILDREN

DEBORAH K. FROH

Alterations of respiratory function in children are influenced by age, development, gender, race, genetic dominance, and environmental conditions. Newborns are especially vulnerable to a variety of upper and lower airway infections caused by immunologic immaturity. Structural differences in infants and children also render them less competent to tolerate conditions causing increased work of breathing. Access to health care and timeliness of immunizations influence the incidence and severity of pulmonary disorders.

STRUCTURE AND FUNCTION

A number of structural characteristics of the pulmonary system influence the way in which infants and children respond to respiratory disturbances. These include structural characteristics of the upper and lower respiratory tracts, chest wall and lung dynamics, metabolic requirements, immunologic immaturity, and physiologic control of respiration.

Upper Airway

All conducting airways (the portions of airway that do not conduct gas exchange) are present at birth and change only in size throughout childhood. Branching of the bronchial tree is, in fact, complete by the sixteenth week of fetal life.

Because infants and children naturally have smaller-diameter airways than do adults, they suffer exponentially more obstruction for a given degree of mucosal edema or se-

cretion accumulation. The relative sizes of tonsils, adenoids, and epiglottis, likewise, are proportionately greater in the young child and, with swelling, can impose a significant site of obstruction. Infants up to 2 to 3 months of age are "obligatory nose breathers" and are unable to breathe in through their mouths. Nasal congestion is therefore a serious threat to the young infant.

Lower Airways and Lung Parenchyma

During fetal development, the lung is transformed from a somewhat dense organ to one that is more delicately structured to facilitate air exchange. Beginning in the second trimester, there is loss of interstitial (mesenchymal) tissue with concomitant expansion of the future airspaces. Capillaries grow into the distal respiratory units, which keep subdividing (alveolarization) to maximize surface area for gas exchange. In fact, the number of alveoli continues to increase during the first 5 to 8 years of life, after which the alveoli increase in size and complexity. In addition to the structural development of the lung *in utero,* there is accompanying functional maturation, and specialized cell types, such as type II cells, become manifest (Figure 34-1).

Surfactant is a lipid-protein mix that is produced by type II cells and is critical for maintaining alveolar expansion (and thus allowing normal gas exchange). It lines alveoli and reduces surface tension, preventing alveolar collapse at the end of each exhalation. Without surfactant the alveoli tend to stay closed, demanding greater inspiratory force and work of breathing to reexpand the alveoli on the next breath. Defi-

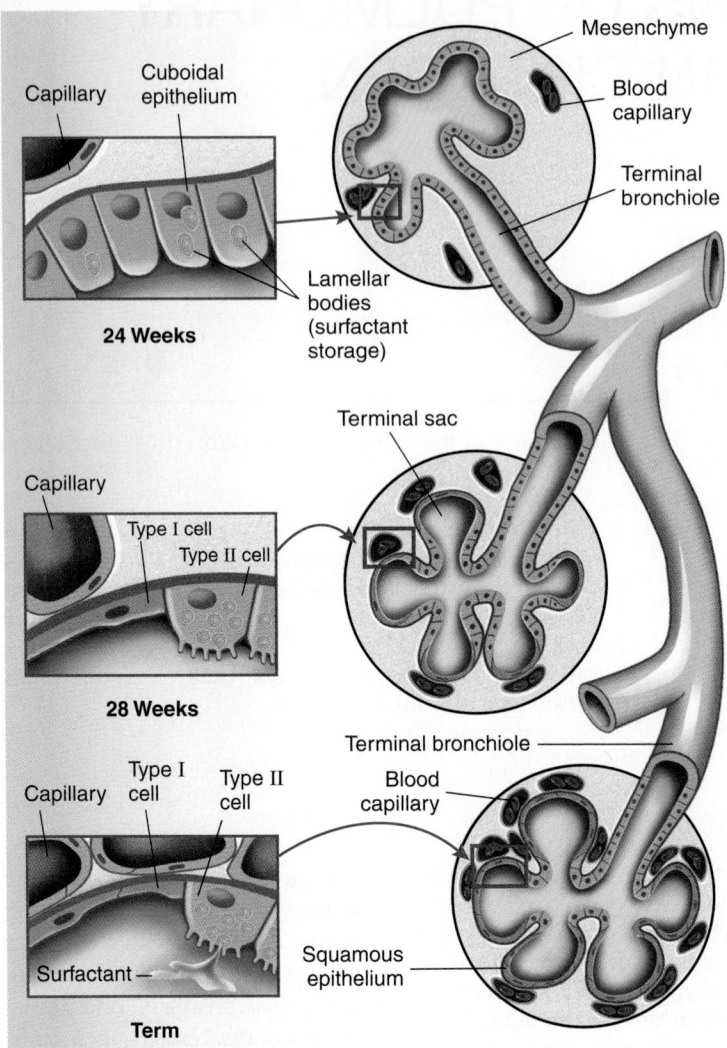

Figure 34-1 **Prenatal development of the alveolar unit.** Epithelial cells differentiate into type II and type I cells. Mature type II cells are cuboidal, have apical microvilli, and contain lamellar bodies for surfactant storage and secretion. Type I cells are derived from type II cells and consist of flattened epithelium overlying capillaries, thus forming part of the desired thin air-blood barrier. During fetal development the pulmonary capillaries initially are randomly distributed in mesenchyme. They progressively arrange around the epithelial tubes and establish close contacts to the lining epithelium. Overall, the volume of mesenchyme decreases and that of the potential airspace increases.

ciency of surfactant is often seen in premature infants and causes respiratory distress syndrome (RDS), also known as hyaline membrane disease. Thus surfactant deficiency reflects developmental immaturity. Surfactant lipid is being produced by 20 to 24 weeks of gestation and is secreted into the fetal airways by 30 weeks. The more premature the infant, the higher the risk of RDS.

Chest Wall Dynamics

Chest wall compliance is high in infants, particularly premature infants. The cartilaginous structures of the thoracic cage are not yet well ossified (ossification continues to occur throughout childhood), and the chest wall is easily collapsible. During inspiration in the young child, air is drawn in by the downward movement of the diaphragm, but the resulting negative pressure causes the "soft" chest wall to be drawn *inward* (Figure 34-2); this produces so-called *paradoxic breathing*, or *diaphragmatic breathing*. Paradoxic breathing is especially seen during rapid eye movement (REM) sleep of premature infants. With pulmonary compromise the accessory muscles also are drawn inward, creating retraction of the intercostal and supraclavicular spaces (Figure 34-3).

Resting lung volume, or **functional residual capacity (FRC)**, represents the balance point between the natural elastic recoil of the lungs (to collapse) and the elastic recoil of the chest wall (to expand). In the face of an overly compliant chest wall, infants up to about 1 year of age are thought to maintain their FRC and avoid atelectasis by muscular "braking" of their expi-

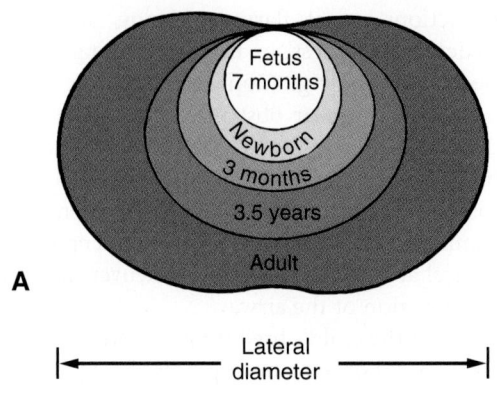

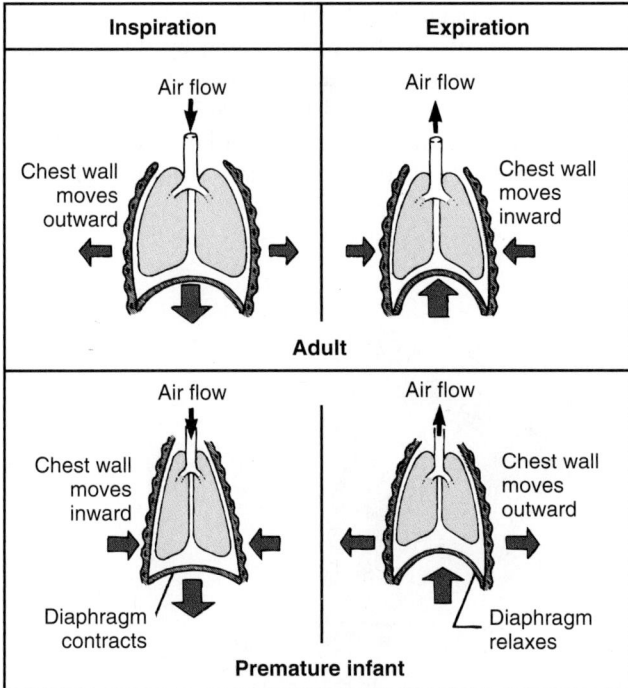

Figure 34-2 Developmental differences in the chest wall and lung mechanics. **A,** Changes in chest wall shape with age. **B,** Differences in lung mechanics caused by differences in chest wall compliance (degree of rigidity) in premature infants and adults. (*Arrows* indicate direction of airflow, chest wall movement, and diaphragm movement.)

ration. This may occur either by active glottic narrowing or by increased activity of the inspiratory intercostal muscles.

Metabolic Characteristics
The basal metabolic rate of a child is greater than that of an adult, and thus oxygen consumption ($\dot{V}O_2$) is greater per unit of body weight. The $\dot{V}O_2$ of the child's normal pulmonary state accounts for up to 25% of the total $\dot{V}O_2$. The work of breathing increases $\dot{V}O_2$ exponentially with respiratory distress. Less muscle glycogen reserve limits the efficiency of accessory muscles, and consequently fatigue, with lactic acidosis, occurs quickly. Children also have a high proportion of extracellular fluid; they more quickly lose fluid as a result of fever, environmental heat, or in association with tachypnea

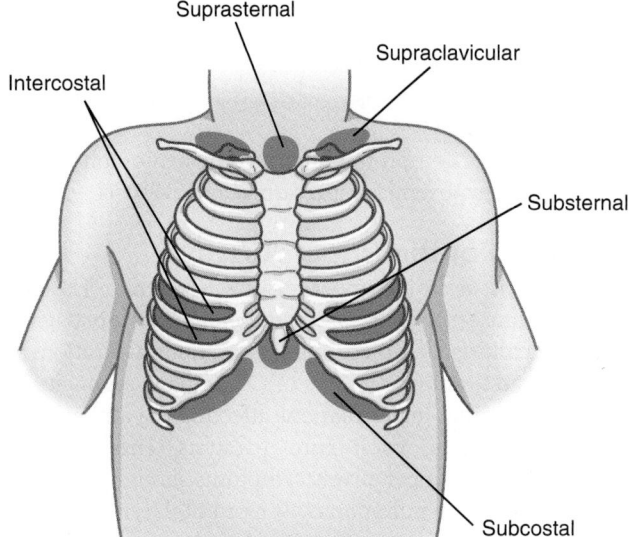

Figure 34-3 Areas of chest muscle retraction.

(which causes evaporation from the respiratory tract) and thereby become dehydrated.

Immunologic Incompetence
Passive immunity with immunoglobulin G (IgG) is normally conveyed transplacentally from the mother to the fetus beginning at 20 weeks of gestation; thus levels are lower in preterm than term infants. Breast-feeding allows further transfer of IgG after birth. Because IgG has a half-life of approximately 21 days, the placentally transferred antibodies are gone after just a few months. Babies are able to make IgG, IgM, and IgA, and levels of these increase slowly with age. Cell-mediated immunity is also not fully developed in the neonate, which creates a situation of enhanced susceptibility to viral and fungal infections.

Physiologic Control of Respiration
The newborn, for up to 3 weeks, has a blunted ventilatory response to hypoxia compared with older children and adults. The mechanisms for this are not well understood but may reflect reduced activity of the peripheral chemoreceptors (in the carotid body) and nonadaptive responses in the respiratory center (in the brain stem). Ventilatory response to hypercarbia is normal in term infants but may be reduced in premature infants. Congenital or acquired lesions of the central nervous system may cause hypoventilation or apnea.

PULMONARY DISORDERS
Pulmonary dysfunction can be categorized into disorders of either the upper airway or lower airway. Signs of acute respiratory failure, however, are the same regardless of etiology. These include the following:
- Increased respiratory effort with retractions (see Figure 34-3) or gasping; apnea in some conditions

- Cyanosis or pallor
- Agitation
- Decreased level of consciousness
- Cardiovascular signs: tachycardia, mottled color, or bradycardia
- Physiologic compromise reflected by hemoglobin desaturation, hypoxemia, hypercarbia, and acidosis

Disorders of the Upper Airway

The crucial issue in the upper airways is patency. The most common causes of *acute-onset* **upper airway obstruction (UAO)** in children are infections, foreign body aspiration, angioedema, and trauma. *Chronic UAO* has many etiologies, including congenital malformations affecting the airway, cartilaginous weakness, vocal cord paralysis, and subglottic stenosis. Chronic upper airway symptoms should prompt referral to a pediatric pulmonologist or an otolaryngologist because specialized diagnostic studies may be needed. A list of causes of pediatric UAO can be found in Box 34-1.

The site and nature of the obstruction are often discernible by assessing the noise associated with breathing, the quality of the voice or cry, and presence of feeding difficulties.[1,2] This assessment can often be made without even touching the patient. Likewise, the severity of the problem can to a great extent be judged by simple visual observation of signs, in-

cluding retractions, nasal flaring, gasping or obstructed breaths, anxiety, restlessness, or need to maintain a specific head or body position. Agitation should be regarded as a likely sign of hypoxemia or obstruction. In acute UAO, increasing the child's anxiety, as by excessive examination, can worsen the condition further. The child should be kept as calm as possible. The clinician should never attempt a pharyngeal examination if there is any suspicion of epiglottitis or retropharyngeal abscess, because this maneuver may precipitate acute obstruction of the airway.

The sounds of the child's breathing can provide key clues (Figure 34-4). A sonorous, snoring noise is typical for nasopharyngeal obstruction, such as adenotonsillar hypertrophy. A common sign of pediatric UAO is **stridor,** a harsh, vibratory sound of variable pitch caused by turbulent flow through the partially obstructed airway. A diagnostic approach to stridor is outlined in Figure 34-5. Whether it is present in inspiration or expiration, or both, reflects the site of the problem. In general, *inspiratory* stridor is generated

Box 34-1	Causes of Upper Airway Obstruction in Children According to Site of Obstruction

Nose and Pharynx
Choanal atresia
Lingual thyroid or thyroglossal cyst
Macroglossia
Micrognathia
Hypertrophic tonsils/adenoids
Retropharyngeal or peritonsillar abscess

Larynx
Laryngomalacia
Laryngeal web, cyst, or laryngocele
Laryngotracheobronchitis (viral croup)
Acute spasmodic laryngitis (spasmodic croup)
Epiglottitis
Vocal cord paralysis
Laryngotracheal stenosis
Intubation
Foreign body
Cystic hygroma
Subglottic hemangioma
Laryngeal papilloma
Angioneurotic edema
Laryngospasm (hypocalcemic tetany)
Psychogenic stridor

Trachea
Tracheomalacia
Bacterial tracheitis
External compression

From Leung AKC, Cho H: *Am Fam Physician* 60(8):2289, 1999.

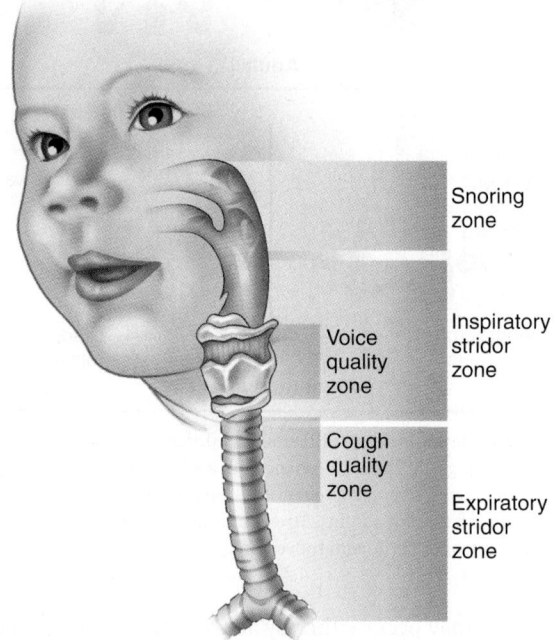

Figure 34-4 Listening can help locate the site of airway obstruction. A loud, gasping snore suggests enlarged tonsils or adenoids. Stridor during inspiration suggests the airway is compromised at the level of the supralaryngeal structures (epiglottis and arytenoid cartilages), vocal cords, subglottic region, or upper trachea. With forced inspiration, intrathoracic pressure becomes quite negative and is less than atmospheric pressure, promoting collapse at or just above the site of obstruction. Expiratory stridor or central wheeze results from narrowing or collapse of the lower trachea or bronchi. During forced exhalation, rising pleural pressure may exceed intratracheal pressure. Airway noise during both inspiration and expiration often represents a fixed obstruction of the vocal cords or subglottic space. Hoarseness or a weak cry is a by-product of obstruction at the vocal cords. If a cough is croupy or low pitched, suspect tracheal pathology. (Redrawn from Eavey RD: A sound workup for evaluating airway obstructions, *Contemp Pediatr* 3(6):78, 1986; used with permission; original illustration by Paul Singh-Roy.)

The image labels (top to bottom): Snoring zone; Voice quality zone; Inspiratory stridor zone; Cough quality zone; Expiratory stridor zone.

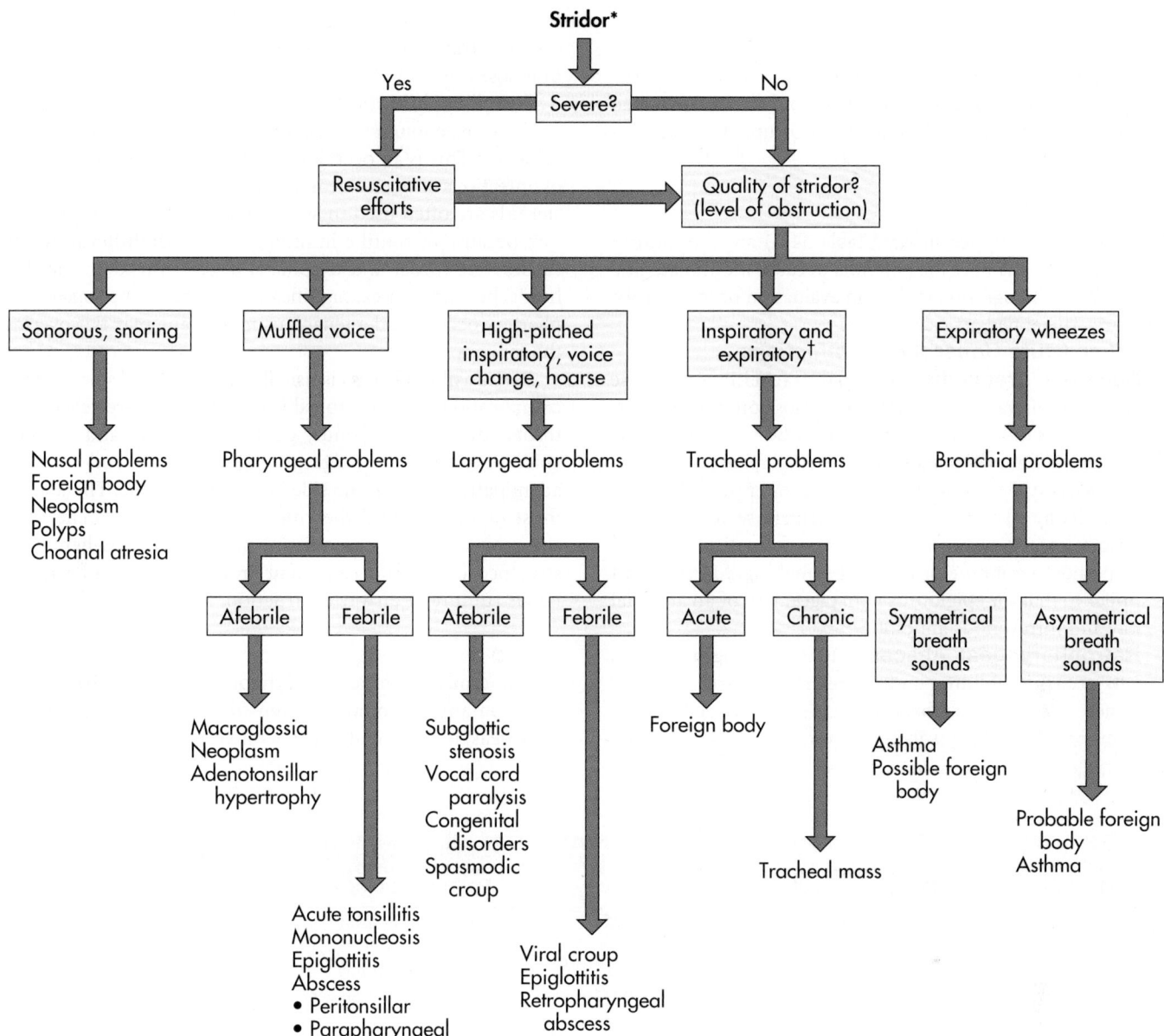

Figure 34-5 **Diagnostic approach to stridor.** (Adapted from Handler SD: Stridor. In Fleisher GR, Ludwig S, editors: *Textbook of pediatric emergency medicine,* Baltimore, 1993, Williams & Wilkins.)

with obstruction of the *extrathoracic* airway (above the thoracic inlet), which includes the supraglottic structures, the larynx, the subglottic space, and the upper trachea. *Expiratory* stridor or a monophonic wheeze may be generated by an obstruction in the *intrathoracic* airway (the mid to lower trachea and central bronchi). Biphasic stridor typically reflects obstruction at the glottis (e.g., vocal cord paralysis) itself or a *fixed* rather than a *dynamic* lesion in the subglottic space (e.g., hemangioma or subglottic stenosis). Biphasic noise may sometimes mean abnormalities of both extrathoracic and intrathoracic trachea (long-segment stenosis or malacia).

Abnormalities of voice or cry (weak or hoarse) suggest problems at the larynx, such as vocal cord paralysis. Muffling of the voice, especially in an acute condition, suggests supralaryngeal obstruction, such as epiglottitis or retropharyngeal abscess. Pronounced cough may be an irritative symptom, such as that produced by an aspirated foreign body, or may be a sign of tracheal obstruction. The cough associated with croup or tracheal foreign body is usually harsh and barking.

Airway obstruction occurs sooner in infants than in older children. Obviously, airway luminal size is smaller in accordance with smaller body size, but any decrease in luminal diameter will be much more significant. This is because airway resistance is proportional to the inverse of the *fourth* power of the radius; thus a decrease to half the original diameter increases resistance sixteenfold. Furthermore, an infant's cartilaginous structures are more collapsible and thus are prone to creating or contributing to a situation of upper airway obstruction.

Infections

Infections of the upper airway (Table 34-1) are common in children, and some have the potential to cause life-threatening emergencies. Recognition and rapid evaluation of these problems are crucial pediatric care skills.

Other Acute Upper Airway Infections

Bacterial Tracheitis. Bacterial tracheitis can cause rapidly fatal airway obstruction. It is most often caused by *Staphylococcus aureus* or *Haemophilus influenzae.* Onset may be sudden and mimic epiglottitis, or it may complicate a preexisting viral upper respiratory infection or croup. The presence of airway edema and copious purulent secretions leads to obstruction; sometimes there is even formation of a tracheal pseudomembrane or mucosal sloughing. Management is similar to that for epiglottitis with placement of an artificial airway and intravenous antibiotics.

Retropharyngeal Abscess. Retropharyngeal abscess usually occurs in children under 2 years of age and as a consequence of either nasopharyngeal infection or penetrating local injury. Clinical signs include fever, dysphagia, drooling, stridor, respiratory distress, and stiff neck. This condition requires intravenous antibiotics and sometimes incision and drainage.

Tonsillar Infections. Tonsillar infections occasionally are severe enough to cause upper airway obstruction (UAO).[3,4] This is an occasional but well known complication of infectious mononucleosis, especially in a young child— steroids are often used in such cases. A classic example, now rare because of routine immunization, is **diphtheria,** which causes sore throat and dysphagia along with fever, malaise, headache, and nausea. Significant swelling of the tonsils and pharynx occurs, and a tenacious membrane may be covering the mucosa.

Peritonsillar abscess is usually unilateral and sometimes a complication of acute tonsillitis.[4] Children have fever, sore throat, dysphagia, trismus, pooling of saliva, and muffled voice. Peritonsillar bulging (Figure 34-6) and cervical adenopathy on the same side are usually visible. The abscess must be drained and the child given antibiotics. The most common causative microorganism is group A β-hemolytic streptococcus. Death can occur from aspiration of spontaneous rupture or airway obstruction.[5]

Croup

Classic **croup** is an acute **laryngotracheobronchitis** and is common among young children from 6 months to 5 years, with peak incidence at age 1 to 2 years.[6,7] In 85% of cases,

Table 34-1	Comparison of Upper Airway Infections				
Condition	**Age**	**Onset**	**Etiology**	**Pathophysiology**	**Symptoms**
Acute laryngo-tracheobronchitis	6 mo-3 yr	Usually gradual	Viral	Inflammation from vocal cords to bronchial lumina	Harsh cough; stridor; low-grade fever; may have nasal discharge, conjunctivitis
Acute tracheitis	1-12 yr	Abrupt or following viral illness	*Staphylococcus aureus*	Inflammation of upper trachea	High fever; toxic appearance; thick harsh cough; purulent secretions; may prefer head elevation
Epiglottitis	2-6 yr	Abrupt	*Haemophilus influenzae* Group A streptococcus	Inflammation of supraglottic structures	Severe sore throat; high fever; toxic appearance; muffled voice; may drool; sits erect and quietly
Retropharyngeal abscess	>6 yr	Gradual, 2-5 days; may follow oral trauma	*Staphylococcus aureus* *Streptococcus pyogenes* Anaerobes Group A β-hemolytic streptococcus	Abscess in posterior pharyngeal wall	Similar to epiglottitis
Peritonsillar abscess	>9 yr	May be abrupt	Group A β-hemolytic streptococcus *Staphylococcus aureus*	Abscess within or around tonsil	Similar to epiglottitis; may have trismus

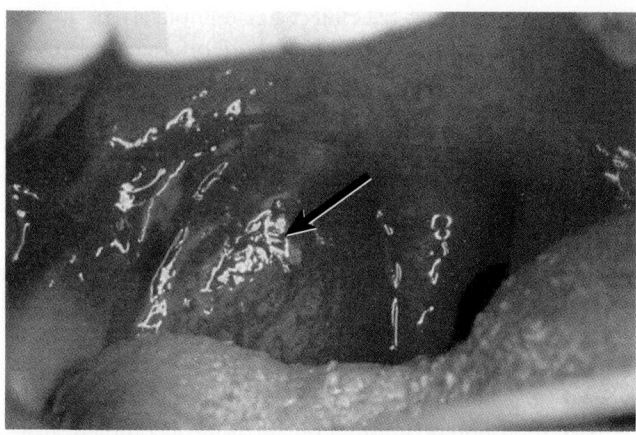

Figure 34-6 Peritonsillar abscess. Unilateral bulging of the tonsillar region is evident. (From Whiting JL, Chow AW: Life-threatening infections of the mouth and throat, *J Crit Illness* 2(7):36, 1987.)

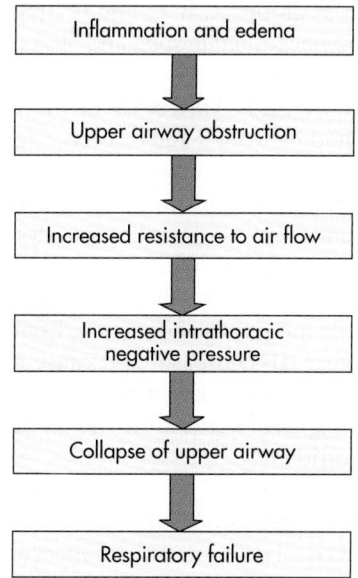

Figure 34-7 Upper airway obstruction with croup.

croup is caused by a virus, most commonly parainfluenza but sometimes others such as influenza A or respiratory syncytial virus.[8] The incidence of croup is highest in late autumn and winter, corresponding to parainfluenza season. Croup is more common in boys than girls. In a significant portion of affected children, croup is a recurrent problem during childhood, and in about 15% of cases there is a family history of croup.

PATHOPHYSIOLOGY   The pathophysiology of viral croup is due primarily to subglottic edema from the infection. The mucous membranes of the larynx are tightly adherent to the underlying cartilage, whereas those of the subglottic space are looser and thus allow accumulation of mucosal and submucosal edema. Furthermore, the cricoid cartilage is structurally the narrowest point of the airway, making edema in this area critical. As depicted in Figure 34-7, increased resistance to airflow leads to increased work of breathing, which generates more negative intrathoracic pressure, which, in turn, may exacerbate dynamic collapse of the upper airway.

CLINICAL MANIFESTATIONS   Typically there is a prodrome of rhinorrhea, sore throat, and low-grade fever for a few days. The child then develops the characteristic seal-like barking cough and, in severe cases, inspiratory stridor. Most cases are mild and resolve spontaneously after several more days. Occasionally, however, upper airway obstruction becomes severe and requires urgent management.[6]

Spasmodic croup is another clinical entity that is characterized by similar hoarseness, barking cough, and stridor but is of sudden onset, usually at night and without viral prodrome. It often resolves as quickly as it develops. The etiology is unknown.

EVALUATION AND TREATMENT   The degree of symptoms determines the level of treatment. Most children have just a barking cough and viral symptoms and may need no specific treatment. However, the presence of stridor (especially at rest), retractions, or agitation suggests a sicker child.

Croup therapy has been the subject of debate for years, particularly the role of glucocorticoids. The consensus from numerous controlled studies is that there is a demonstrable benefit by 6 hours after a single dose of either dexamethasone (0.15 to 0.6 mg/kg) or nebulized budesonide (2 mg) for moderate to severe croup.[9,10] Dexamethasone has a biologic half-life of 36 to 72 hours, long enough to carry the child through the acute phase of the illness before it naturally subsides. The use of steroids in outpatient management of croup is expected to have a huge impact on related hospitalizations and health care costs.

Traditional therapy for croup has included mist. However, scientific studies have neither supported nor refuted its benefit. Acute use of nebulized epinephrine is extremely helpful when significant respiratory distress is present. Epinephrine is usually given as either 5 ml of a 1:1000 solution of L-epinephrine or as 0.5 ml of racemic epinephrine (2.25%) mixed with 2.5 ml of normal saline. It stimulates α- and β-adrenergic receptors and is thought to decrease airway secretions and mucosal edema. However, its effect lasts only 2 hours and should be considered a temporizing measure until concomitantly given steroids begin to take effect. Thus children who are given nebulized epinephrine should be observed for 2 to 3 hours to ensure that they will remain stable if released, and close follow-up is mandatory.

Acute Epiglottitis

Acute epiglottitis is a severe, life-threatening, rapidly progressive infection of the epiglottis and surrounding area. Historically, cases were nearly always caused by *H. influenzae type B*. However, since the advent of *H. influenzae type B* immunization, acute epiglottitis incidence has decreased to only 10% to 20% of previous levels and has become an adult as well as a pediatric disease.[11-14] Current pediatric cases usually represent vaccine failures or are caused by alternative pathogens such as groups A, B, C, and G streptococci, *Streptococcus pneumoniae*, *Candida* spp., and viral pathogens.[14,15]

CLINICAL MANIFESTATIONS   In the classic form of the disease, a child between 2 and 6 years of age suddenly develops high fever, sore throat, inspiratory stridor, and severe respiratory distress. The child appears ill and anxious and has a voice that sounds muffled. Drooling and dysphagia (inability to swallow) are common. Death may occur in a few hours. Nasotracheal intubation or tracheotomy is mandatory in instances of rapidly increasing obstruction. Examination of the throat may trigger laryngospasm and cause respiratory collapse. Pneumonia, cervical lymph node inflammation, otitis, and rarely, meningitis or septic arthritis may occur during the course of epiglottitis.

EVALUATION AND TREATMENT   Despite its decreasing incidence, all pediatric practitioners must be familiar with epiglottitis and understand it is a life-threatening emergency. The essentials are recognition, avoiding disturbing the child (which could worsen the obstruction), securing of the airway by the most experienced personnel (usually an anesthesiologist and otolaryngologist), and intravenous antibiotics. Despite the severe presentation of epiglottitis, resolution with treatment is usually rapid, with intubation rarely needed for more than a couple of days.

When caused by microorganisms other than *H. influenzae*, as is now the usual situation, epiglottis may present in ages outside the typical range and with more gradual rather than fulminant onset, thus making diagnosis less obvious. Such cases also may respond more slowly to treatment. Mean duration of intubation associated with beta-hemolytic streptococcal epiglottis is 6 days.[14]

Aspiration of Foreign Bodies

Most children who aspirate a foreign object (**foreign body aspiration**) are between 1 and 3 years of age. Often the aspiration either is not witnessed or does not seem significant to the parent, so during the first 24 hours, medical care is sought for fewer than one third of children who aspirate an object.[16,17] At the time of the aspiration event, the child may cough, choke, gag, or wheeze; occasionally stridor or cyanosis occurs. There may then be a quiescent interval of minutes to even weeks or months before symptoms reappear from resulting local irritation, granulation, bronchial obstruction, or infection (pneumonia or bronchiectasis). Pronounced inspiratory stridor, cough, and wheezing are typical symptoms that prompt the parents to seek medical attention. Examples of common objects that are aspirated include nuts, sunflower seeds, hot dog chunks, popcorn, coins, and small toys.[16-19]

Symptoms are determined by the size of the object and the site in which it is located (see Figure 34-4). Foreign bodies lodged in the upper trachea typically produce inspiratory stridor, whereas those located in the lower intrathoracic airways more commonly produce wheezing. About 75% of aspirated foreign bodies lodge in a bronchus. Many objects are not radiopaque; however, if the object has completely occluded a lung segment, atelectasis will be visible on a chest x-ray examination or air will accumulate distal to the obstruction if the object is causing a ball-valve effect. This effect can sometimes be documented by inspiratory and expiratory chest films (Figure 34-8). In a younger child, bilateral decubitus films may show failure to compress the obstructed lung when in the "down" position.

Most foreign bodies can be removed by bronchoscopy; rarely is a pulmonary lobectomy required. Food particles, which are soft, must be removed, as well as hard objects, because infection will occur otherwise. Objects lodged in the laryngeal or subglottic regions are particularly dangerous because of their potential for complete or near-complete airway occlusion.[19,20]

Other Causes of Upper Airway Compromise
Angioedema

Angioedema is a localized edema involving the deep, subcutaneous layers of skin or mucous membranes. Generally, angioedema causes facial swelling first, particularly around the eyes and lips, and may progress to airway swelling.[21] Angioedema is usually secondary to allergic phenomena, and standard treatment includes epinephrine (subcutaneous), antihistamines, and steroids if airway compromise is apparent. An occasional cause of pediatric angioedema is use of angiotensin-converting enzyme inhibitors for treatment of hypertension or heart disease. Increased levels of bradykinin appear to mediate this adverse effect by causing vasodilation, increased vascular permeability, and histamine release.[22] Deficiency of C-1 inhibitor (C-1 INH), a rare problem in children, may cause recurring attacks of angioedema involving subcutaneous tissues (especially limbs, genitalia, and face), and much less often, the airway. Laryngeal attacks in these individuals may be life-threatening and do not respond reliably to standard measures for airway edema. Concentrates of C-1 INH appear to produce rapid improvement (within 30 to 60

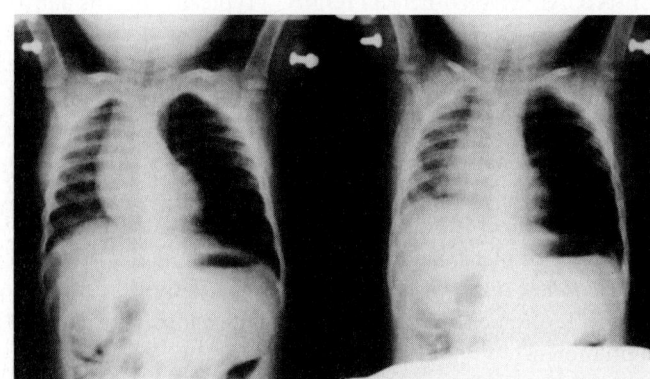

Figure 34-8 Foreign body aspiration. Inspiratory *(left)* and expiratory *(right)* chest radiographs of a child who aspirated a portion of a potato into the left main stem bronchus. Left lung field is hyperaerated and the mediastinum is shifted to the right on expiration because of left-sided obstructive emphysema. (From Kenna MA, Bluestone CD: Foreign bodies in the air and food passages, *Pediatr Rev* 10(1):25, 1988.)

minutes) but are not yet licensed for use in the United States.[23]

Subglottic Stenosis

Traumatic injury to the upper airway with development of **subglottic stenosis** is a well-described complication of endotracheal intubation.[24] Factors that contribute to subglottic stenosis include long-term assisted ventilation, use of an endotracheal tube that is too large, excessive movement of the tube, and individual susceptibility.[25] The occurrence of subglottic stenosis can be minimized by ensuring that the tube size allows a small air leak during inspiration (at a peak inspiratory force of approximately 25 mmHg) and that the tube is securely taped. Sedation is generally required to reduce head movement for children who are intubated. For significant subglottic stenosis, tracheostomy or tracheal reconstructive surgery may be needed.[26,27]

Laryngomalacia and Tracheomalacia

Laryngomalacia is the most common cause of chronic stridor in babies, but it is usually mild and improves spontaneously over the first year of life as the supralaryngeal cartilage structures stiffen. In laryngomalacia, the epiglottis or arytenoids or both fold inward with inspiration, partially covering the glottis (Figure 34-9). Typical signs of laryngomalacia include inspiratory stridor beginning in the first days or weeks of life, accentuated with activity, and sometimes with positional changes (worse in supine or head-flexed positions). Feeding difficulties may be noted, but they are usually mild. Cry is normal.

In **tracheomalacia,** the tracheal cartilages tend to collapse during the respiratory cycle. Symptoms are more subtle than in laryngomalacia. Low-pitched inspiratory stridor may be a sign of malacia of the upper trachea or centrally located, single-pitch (monophonic) wheeze may be present in malacia

of the mid to distal trachea. Both laryngomalacia and tracheomalacia can be suspected clinically and confirmed by bronchoscopy.

Vocal Cord Paralysis

The vocal cords should move apart to facilitate inspiration and move together to facilitate vocalization. Paralysis of one or both vocal cords may affect both breathing and speech. In infants and children, vocal cord dysfunction is usually a consequence of other problems, such as surgical trauma to the recurrent laryngeal nerve during cardiac surgery or Arnold-Chiari malformation of the brain stem, the region in which the nucleus ambiguus acts as the "relay station" for laryngeal function. **Vocal cord paralysis** sometimes resolves spontaneously or with correction of the underlying problem, such as decompression of hydrocephalus. However, tracheostomy is sometimes required for bilateral vocal cord paralysis as a temporary or permanent measure.[28]

Congenital Malformations

Congenital malformations of the trachea and bronchial tree cause airway obstruction. Affected infants develop obvious airway symptoms or feeding difficulties or both. Many children are first thought to have gastroesophageal reflux as the principal problem. Lesions include laryngeal webs, cysts, clefts, subglottic hemangiomas, and abnormalities involving the great vessels that result in tracheal compression (vascular rings).[29] Surgical management is usually required for these conditions.[30,31]

Obstructive Sleep Apnea

Obstructive sleep apnea syndrome (OSAS) is defined by partial or complete UAO during sleep, with disruption of normal ventilation and normal sleep patterns. Childhood OSAS is common, with an estimated prevalence of 3% to 12%.[32,33] In children, unlike adults, OSAS occurs equally among males and females.

PATHOPHYSIOLOGY   The pathophysiology of childhood OSAS may be multifactorial in origin. In otherwise healthy children, the most common predisposing factor is adenotonsillar hypertrophy, which causes physical impingement on the nasopharyngeal airway. OSAS also may occur in obese children and in those with craniofacial anomalies or neurologic disorders. In addition to physical narrowing, other mechanisms have been suggested, such as abnormalities in the motor tone of the upper airways (frequently an issue in neurologically impaired children) or abnormal arousal mechanisms.[34]

CLINICAL MANIFESTATIONS   Usually a history of snoring and labored breathing during sleep, which may be continuous or intermittent, is reported. There may be episodes of increased respiratory effort but no audible airflow, often terminated by snorting, gasping, repositioning, or arousal. Sleep is often described as restless. Occasionally, daytime sleepiness is reported. The child is often a chronic mouth breather and has large tonsils.

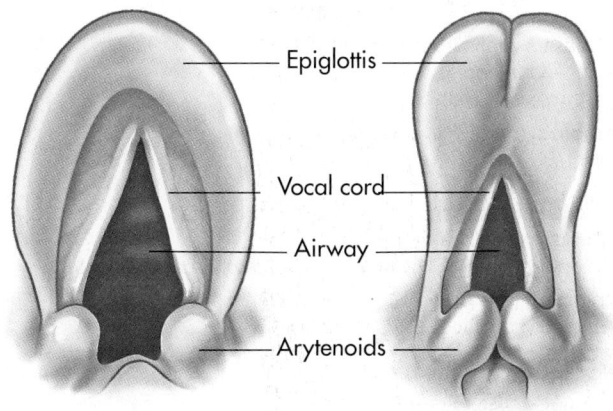

Epiglottis

Vocal cord

Airway

Arytenoids

Normal   **Laryngomalacia**

Figure 34-9 Laryngomalacia. In the normal larynx *(left)*, supralaryngeal structures maintain their upright orientation during inspiration. In contrast, in infants with laryngomalacia *(right)*, there is inward prolapse of the arytenoid masses, which include the prominent cuneiform tubercles and the arytenoid cartilages. The glottis becomes partially covered, and airflow is impeded. Sometimes the edges of the epiglottis curl inward, further exacerbating the obstruction. In expiration, these structures are "blown" aside passively.

EVALUATION AND TREATMENT   All parents should be asked if their child exhibits snoring, a symptom that is often not spontaneously reported to the pediatrician.[35] The most definitive evaluation is the polysomnographic sleep study, which documents obstructed breathing and physiologic impairment. If obstructive sleep apnea is documented or strongly suspected clinically, children are most often referred for tonsillectomy and adenoidectomy (T & A) on the basis of described symptoms and physical findings, such as enlarged tonsils, "adenoidal facies," and mouth breathing. For severely affected children who do not respond to T & A or who have different problems, such as obesity, that cannot be remedied rapidly, continuous positive airway pressure (CPAP) delivered through a tight-fitting nasal mask may be used during sleep.[36] Treatment is important to prevent associated morbidities that may occur, including pulmonary and systemic hypertension, nocturnal enuresis, learning and cognitive deficits, and reduced somatic growth.[37-39]

Disorders of the Lower Airways

Lower airway disease is one of the leading causes of morbidity in the first year of life and continues to be an important component of other illnesses. Pulmonary conditions commonly observed include perinatal conditions, such as newborn respiratory distress syndrome; congenital malformations; asthma; cystic fibrosis; infections; aspiration syndrome; and acute respiratory distress syndrome.

Neonatal Respiratory Distress Syndrome

Respiratory distress syndrome (RDS) of the newborn, also known as **hyaline membrane disease (HMD),** is a major cause of morbidity and mortality in premature newborns.[40] RDS is outlined in Box 34-2. The major predisposing factor is prematurity because the immature lung is not well structured for gas exchange and has not yet developed adequate surfactant production and secretion. Occasionally RDS is seen in other situations, most notably infants of diabetic mothers. An additional factor that increases risk is cesarean delivery. It is more common in boys than girls and in whites than nonwhites. The incidence of RDS (in the absence of preventive treatment) is approximately 50% to 60% at 29 weeks of gestation and decreases significantly by 36 weeks. Antenatal stress on the fetus may accelerate lung maturation and decrease RDS risk. In special circumstances, such as elective early delivery (e.g., for maternal health reasons), RDS risk is assessed by sampling amniotic fluid for quantification of se-

---

Box 34-2	**Respiratory Distress Syndrome**

Epidemiology
Worldwide
Prematurity predisposes
Cesarean section without labor predisposes
Perinatal asphyxia predisposes
Male > female
White > black
Second-born twin at greater risk
PROM spares
IUGR spares
Maternal stress spares
Maternal diabetes predisposes if <37 weeks
Maternal hemorrhage predisposes

Clinical Signs
Onset near the time of birth
Retractions and tachypnea
Expiratory grunt
Cyanosis
Systemic hypotension
Characteristic chest film
Course to death or improvement in 3 to 5 days
Fine inspiratory rales
Hypothermia
Peripheral edema
Pulmonary edema

Pathophysiology
Reduced lung compliance
Reduced FRC
Poor lung distensibility

Poor alveolar stability
Right-to-left shunts
Reduced effective pulmonary blood flow
If hypotensive and hypoxic, poor peripheral perfusion, poor renal perfusion, myocardial malfunction
Patent ductus arteriosus contributes

Pathobiochemistry
Respiratory acidosis
Decreased saturated phospholipids
Low amniotic fluid L/S ratio
Low surfactant-associated proteins
Decreased total serum proteins
Decreased fibrinolysis
Low thyroxine levels

Pathology
Atelectasis
Injury to epithelial cells, edema
Membrane contains fibrin and cellular products
No tubular myelin
Osmiophilic lamellar bodies decreased early, increased later

Etiology
Surfactant deficiency during disease
Probable inadequate hormonal (corticoid) stimulus in utero
DPL synthesis impaired and/or destruction increased
Autonomic dysfunction

Prevention
Prenatal glucocorticoids for >24 hours
Surfactant replacement before 1-2 hours

From Welty S, Hansen TN, Corbet A: Respiratory distress in the preterm infant. In Taeusch HW, Ballard RA, Gleason CA, editors: *Avery's diseases of the newborn*, ed 8, Philadelphia, 2005, Saunders.
DPL, dipalmitoyl lecithin; *FRC,* functional residual capacity; *IUGR,* intrauterine growth retardation/restriction; *L/S,* lecithin/sphingomyelin; *PROM,* prolonged rupture of membranes (>16 hours).

creted surfactant lipids, the basis of the lecithin/sphingomyelin (L/S) ratio (value of 2.0 or greater predicts low risk). Another common test looks for presence of the lipid phosphatidylglycerol, which also reflects lung maturity.

PATHOPHYSIOLOGY   RDS is caused primarily by surfactant deficiency and, secondarily, by a deficiency in alveolar surface area for gas exchange. Premature infants are born with many underdeveloped and small alveoli that are difficult to inflate. Those that are available for gas exchange do not have adequate surfactant, which is necessary at the air interface to maintain alveolar distention at end expiration. The chest wall is weak and highly compliant.[41] The net effect is *atelectasis* (Figure 34-10), which is difficult for the neonate to overcome because it requires a significant negative inspiratory pressure to open the alveoli with each breath. The infant uses more oxygen to sustain the work of breathing and becomes hypoxemic and hypercapnic. Hypoxia and atelectasis cause pulmonary vasoconstriction and increase intrapulmonary resistance and shunting (Figure 34-11). This results in hypoperfusion of the lung and a decrease in effective pulmonary blood flow. Increased pulmonary vascular resistance causes a partial return to fetal circulation, with right-to-left shunting of blood through the ductus arteriosus and foramen ovale.

Capillary permeability increases and epithelium may be damaged because of ventilation-induced injury, together resulting in the leakage of plasma proteins. Fibrin deposits in the airspaces create the appearance of *hyaline membranes* for which the disorder is named. The plasma proteins leaked into the airspace have the additional adverse effect of interfering with the function of surfactant that may be present.

To make the situation more complex, prolonged hypoxemia activates anaerobic glycolysis, which produces increased amounts of lactic acid and promotes metabolic acidosis. Because the collapsed alveoli are unable to get rid of excess carbon dioxide, respiratory acidosis also develops. Lowered pH causes

further vasoconstriction. With inadequate pulmonary circulation and alveolar perfusion, the oxygen content of the blood continues to decrease, pH decreases, and materials needed for surfactant production are not circulated to the alveoli. The pathogenesis of RDS is summarized in Figure 34-11.

CLINICAL MANIFESTATIONS   Signs of RDS appear within minutes of birth. Some neonates require resuscitation at birth because of asphyxia or initial severe respiratory distress. Tachypnea (respiratory rate over 60 breaths per minute), expiratory grunting or whining, intercostal and subcostal retractions, nasal flaring, and poor color are the most striking clinical manifestations of RDS. The natural course is characterized by progressive hypoxemia and dyspnea. Apnea and irregular respirations occur as the infant tires. The typical chest radiograph shows diffuse, fine granular densities within the first 6 hours of life. RDS can progress to death in severe cases, but in most cases the clinical manifestations reach a peak within 3 days, after which there is gradual improvement with appropriate treatment.

EVALUATION AND TREATMENT   Diagnosis is made on the basis of clinical manifestations, chest radiographs, and, occasionally, confirmatory analysis (e.g., L/S ratio) of amniotic fluid or tracheal aspirates. The ultimate treatment for RDS would be prevention of premature birth, but in the meantime other significant advances in treatment have been made.

The first is *antenatal treatment with glucocorticoids* for women in preterm labor. Glucocorticoids induce a significant and rapid acceleration of lung maturation, and there is extensive evidence that maternal steroid therapy significantly reduces the incidence of RDS, intraventricular hemorrhage, and death.[42,43] This treatment is currently recommended in the setting of preterm labor at 24 to 34 weeks of gestation unless delivery is imminent; ideally, dosing continues for 48 hours while attempts are made to halt labor.

The second major advance in RDS treatment has been *exogenous surfactant*, either synthetic or purified from animal sources and instilled down an endotracheal tube.[44] Many current protocols recommend prophylactic administration to infants weighing less than 1000 g beginning within 15 to 30 minutes of birth, after the infant is stabilized. Repeat dosing is usually given every 12 hours during the first few days. There is usually a dramatic improvement in oxygenation. For infants weighing more than 1000 g, surfactant replacement is based on clinical need. Recently, because of concerns about intervention-induced lung injury, guidelines for surfactant administration are being reconsidered (see What's New? box on p. 1261). Therapy with surfactant should be considered complementary to antenatal glucocorticoids, which promote not only accelerated surfactant synthesis but also enhanced structural development of the lung and beneficial effects on mechanisms of fluid clearance from the lung. In preterm infants, supplemental inositol may promote maturation of surfactant and prevent adverse neonatal outcomes.[45]

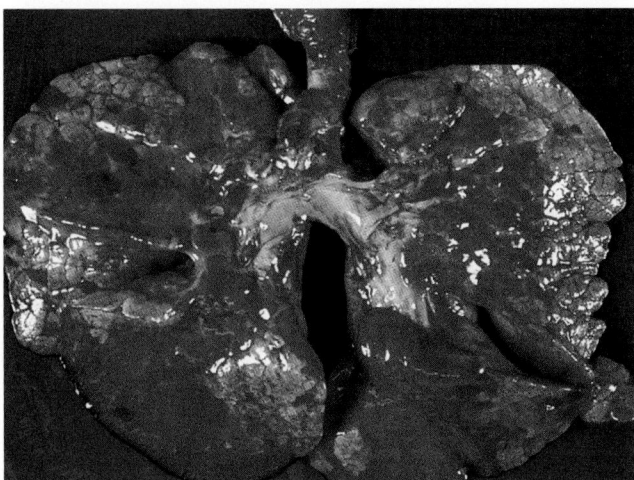

Figure 34-10 Patchy atelectasis of neonatal lungs with respiratory distress syndrome (RDS). (From Damjanov I, Linder J, editors: *Anderson's pathology,* ed 10, St Louis, 1996, Mosby.)

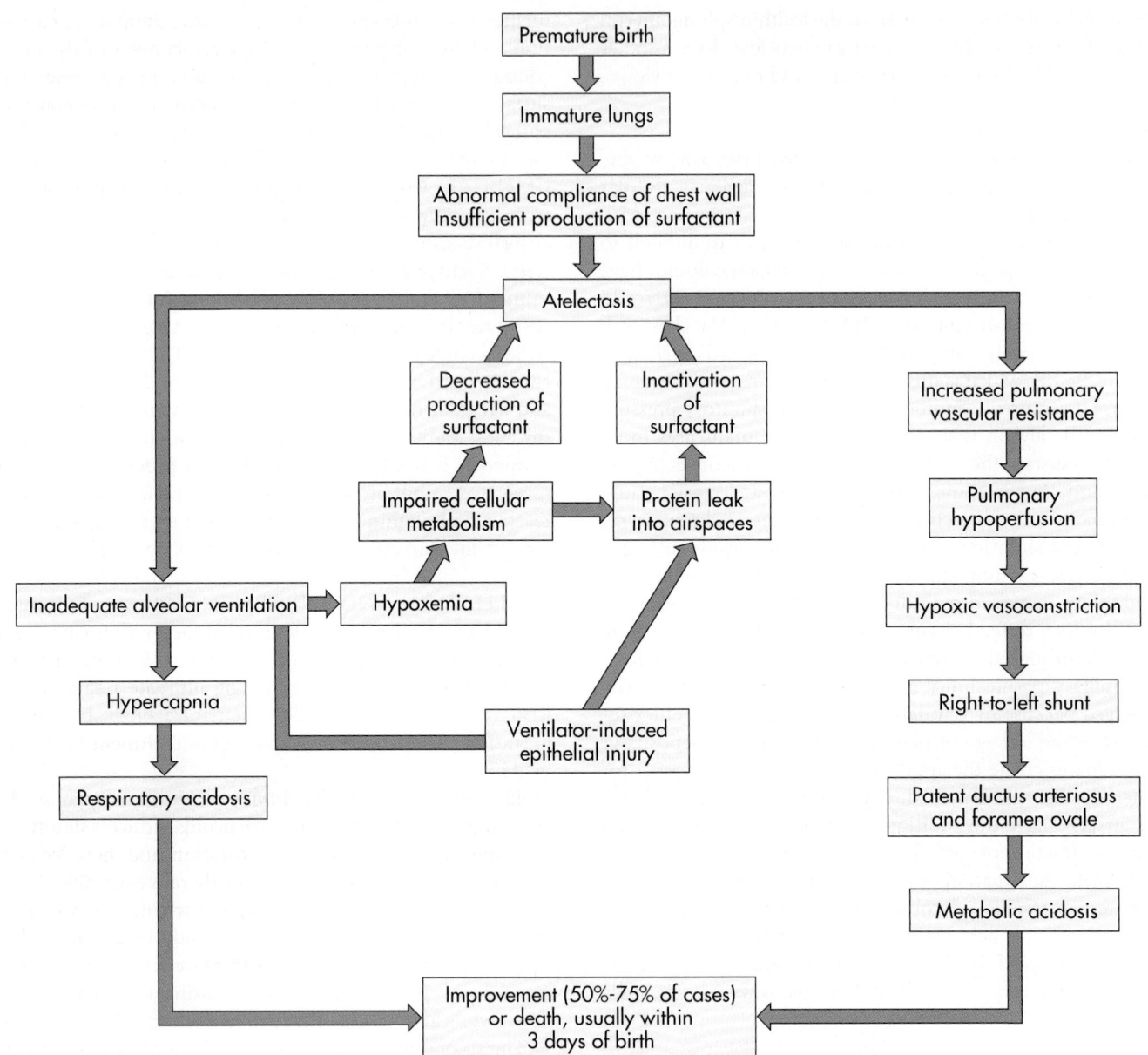

Figure 34-11 Pathogenesis of respiratory distress syndrome (RDS) of the newborn. RDS is also known as hyaline membrane disease.

The third advance in RDS treatment has been in *supportive care*. Newborns with RDS need oxygen and often support such as continuous positive airway pressure (CPAP) or mechanical ventilation. A great deal of interest has been shown recently in establishing which strategies are the most lung protective, such as greater reliance on nasal CPAP, permissive hypercapnia and lower oxygen saturation targets, choice of tidal volume, use of nitric oxide, and use of high-frequency oscillation.[46-50] Nitric oxide has found acceptance for treatment of persistent pulmonary hypertension of the newborn and for hypoxic respiratory failure in term and near-term infants.[51] However, its use in preterm infants remains controversial.[52,53] The extremely preterm lung is particularly vulnerable to injury. Mechanical ventilation may interfere with alveolarization and surfactant metabolism and may aggravate the proinflammatory state that

is believed to accompany premature birth and RDS, as reflected by abnormal cytokine profiles that have been documented in this scenario. Injury from oxygen toxicity is mediated through reactive oxygen species.[54] A combination of factors may lead to subsequent development of chronic lung disease or bronchopulmonary dysplasia.[54-56]

Most infants with RDS survive with treatment. However, the incidence of subsequent chronic lung disease is significant among very low-birth-weight infants.

Bronchopulmonary Dysplasia

Bronchopulmonary dysplasia (BPD), often used synonymously with *chronic lung disease of infancy,* is the term used for persisting lung disease following premature birth and perinatal respiratory support. When originally described by

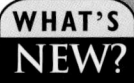

WHAT'S NEW? Pulmonary Resuscitation of the Newborn—Setting the Stage for Injury?

Newborns, especially those born prematurely, appear to be exceptionally susceptible to harm from therapies intended to help them, starting as early as the delivery room resuscitation and the early hours afterward. For example, oxygen has known toxicities, and the standard use of 100% oxygen to resuscitate asphyxiated newborns (term or preterm), has come into question. Data from animal studies and from limited human studies suggests that initial resuscitation with room air appears to be similarly effective as 100% oxygen, and may carry reduced risk. Although current data has not been considered conclusive, even brief resuscitation with 100% oxygen has been reported to be associated with delayed initiation of breathing, increased mortality, and persistence of systemic markers of oxidative stress for as long as 28 days postpartum. The potential for oxygen-induced brain injury exists theoretically but so far this has not been substantiated in clinical studies.

Similarly, excessively large inflations, perhaps even just a few breaths given after birth, may be sufficient to damage the immature lung. Commonly used self-inflating bags do not allow monitoring of tidal volume or inspiratory pressure, nor can they deliver PEEP (positive end-expiratory pressure) or prolonged inflation (useful for establishing the baby's functional residual capacity). Other devices incorporate these features but require more expertise to use. Finally, use of nasal CPAP (continuous positive airway pressure) in the delivery room for spontaneously breathing premature infants has been reported to significantly reduce the need for subsequent mechanical ventilation. One group has reported a dramatic drop in their incidence of chronic lung disease, to less than 5% of infants under 1500 g, associated with use of nasal CPAP (with permissive hypercapnia) instead of intubation and mechanical ventilation.

Data from Finer NN, Rich WD: *Curr Opin Pediatr* 16(2):157-162, 2004; Polin RA, Sahni R: *Semin Neonatol* 7(5):379-382, 2002; Saugstad OD: *Semin Neonatol* 6(3):233-239, 2001; Kirchner L et al: *J Perinat Med* 33(1):60-66, 2005; Vento M et al: *J Pediatr* 142(3):240-246, 2003.

Northway and colleagues in 1967, the term was applied to premature infants (30 to 37 weeks gestation) who had survived acute RDS but had continued to have pulmonary dysfunction and oxygen dependence, which was attributed to injury from postnatal mechanical ventilation and oxygen therapy.[57] The characteristic pathologic findings were those of severe airway injury and fibrosis, alternating areas of atelectasis and overinflation, and pulmonary hypertensive vascular lesions.

In the current era of neonatology, the widespread use of antenatal glucocorticoids and postnatal surfactant has lessened the incidence and severity of RDS, and BPD is occurring almost exclusively in the smallest premature infants (24 to 28 weeks gestation) who have received mechanical ventilation. Surprisingly, some of these tiny infants who develop BPD have had few or no clinical signs of RDS at birth or have initially received only low levels of supplemental oxygen or ventilatory support, sometimes for other reasons such as apnea.[58] Nevertheless, a highly significant predictor of subsequent

BPD seems to be ventilation on the day of birth.[59] The presence of antenatal chorioamnionitis, postnatal sepsis, or a patent ductus arteriosus may confer additive risk of developing BPD.[60-62] Interestingly, the predominant histopathologic findings of the so-called "new BPD" are those of arrested lung development with poor formation of alveolar architecture.[63]

The reported incidence of BPD is widely variable because of the lack of consistent diagnostic criteria, but is certainly inversely proportional to birth weight. Definitions of BPD have traditionally been based on persistence of an oxygen requirement for 28 days, or at a postgestational age of 36 weeks, but the changing clinical picture has introduced new complexities as to appropriate criteria.

PATHOPHYSIOLOGY   Most infants currently developing BPD are born at less than or equal to 28 weeks gestation. At this time the fetal lung is in the *canalicular stage* of development (16 to 26-28 weeks), a critical period during which type II epithelial cells appear, capillaries grow into the future distal alveolar regions, and the interstitium begins to condense. Ultimately, the alveoli must have a very thin interface between the airspace and the capillary for appropriate gas exchange. The extensive network of alveoli develops by septation within the terminal respiratory unit, beginning in the *saccular stage*, which starts at approximately 26 to 28 weeks.

The characteristic pathologic changes seen in *new BPD* are fewer and larger alveoli, with less functional surface area, and reduced and dysplastic capillary ingrowth to the alveolar region. There may be accompanying pulmonary hypertensive changes, interstitial fibrosis, and smooth muscle hyperplasia, but certainly to a much lesser degree than that associated with *classic BPD*. Airway epithelial lesions are negligible.[64] The pathophysiology of BPD is diagrammed in Figure 34-12. To a significant extent, cytokines may mediate the abnormal alveolarization and injury response that lead to BPD, although this has not been directly proven. In the case of intrauterine infection, inflammatory mediators may prime the lung for an exaggerated path of injury after birth.[65] Cytokines, such as TNF-α, IL-1, IL-6, and IL-8 have been found to be elevated in the amniotic fluid or tracheal aspirates of preterm infants who later develop BPD.[66-68]

Ventilation-perfusion matching is compromised as a result of structural underdevelopment, pulmonary hypertension, increased lung fluid content, airway injury, and smooth muscle hypertrophy, as well as adverse chest well dynamics. Thus infants with BPD exhibit an increased oxygen requirement, increased work of breathing, and in the most severe cases, right-sided heart failure.

CLINICAL MANIFESTATIONS   Clinically, the affected infant exhibits hypoxemia and hypercapnia caused by ventilation-perfusion mismatch and diffusion defects. Work of breathing is elevated, and ability to feed may be impaired. Intermittent bronchospasm, mucus plugging, and pulmonary hypertension characterize the clinical course of the most severely affected babies. Dusky spells may occur with agitation

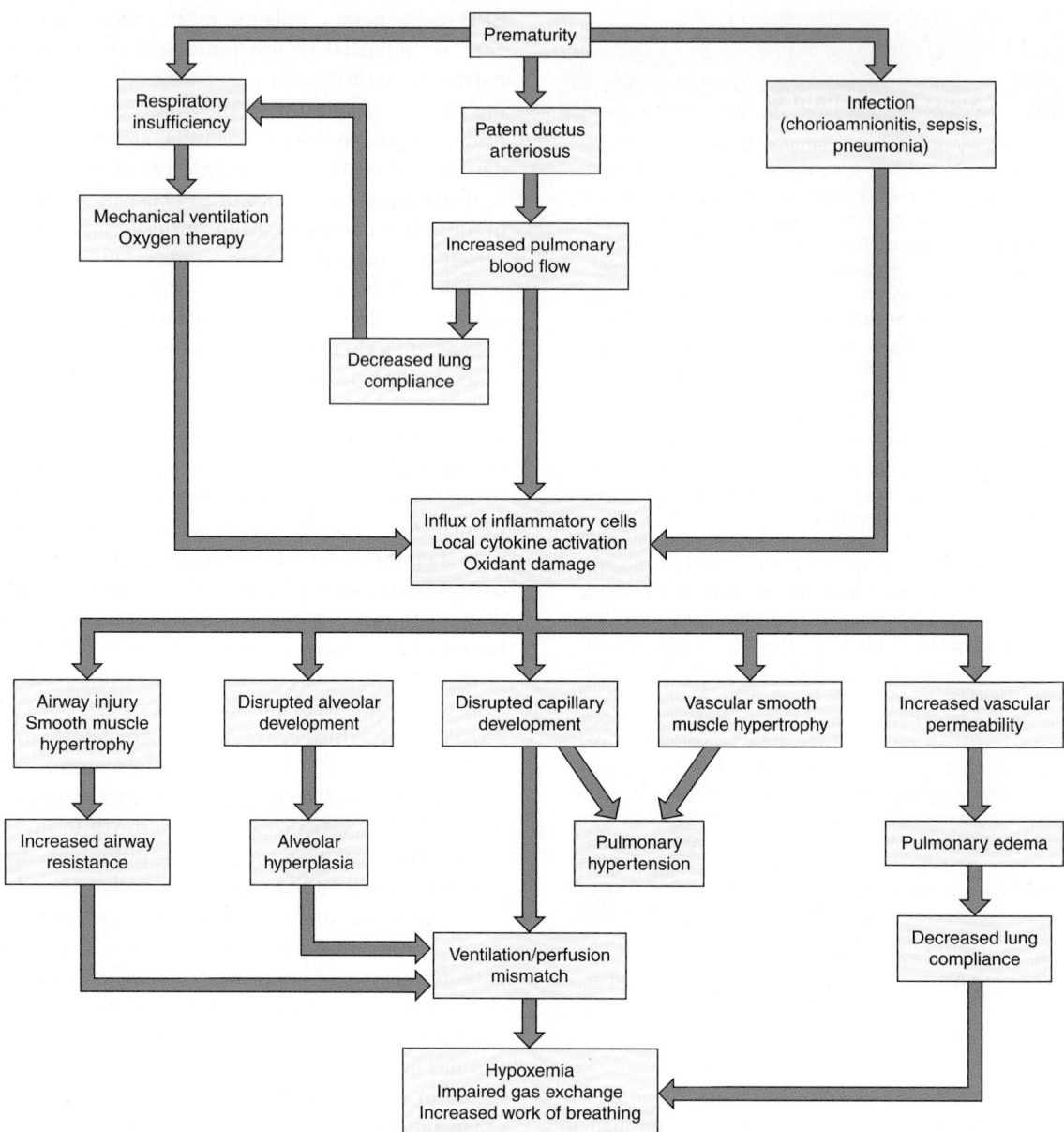

Figure 34-12 Pathophysiology of bronchopulmonary dysplasia (BPD).

or reflux because of several contributing factors, including nonhomogeneous ventilation, air trapping, bronchospasm, laryngospasm, sudden increases in pulmonary vascular resistance, or occasionally, pneumothorax.

Infants with severe BPD require prolonged, assisted ventilation with cautious weaning. Diuretics are used to control pulmonary edema. Bronchodilators are employed to reduce airway resistance. Early anti-inflammatory therapies, such as steroids, may facilitate weaning but introduce significant risks, such as abnormal neurodevelopment.[69] Nutritional needs are high and must be met to promote growth and healing; the infant usually can be fed enterally. Early supplemental vitamin A, which plays a role in normal lung development, may be required in low-birth-weight infants, although the ef-

fectiveness of this therapy for preventing BPD remains unclear.[70,71] Infection is a constant threat because of invasive lines, the endotracheal tube, and a compromised immune system.

Death from BPD is usually caused by infection or respiratory failure. Often, infants who survive are discharged with home oxygen therapy (some on ventilators). In addition to respiratory management, growth and nutrition are essential to recovery. Gradual improvement is usually noted in the first 2 years, but pulmonary function may remain abnormal for many years, and there is an increased incidence of asthma during childhood. Characteristic abnormalities on pulmonary function testing include expiratory airflow obstruction and air trapping.[63,72-74]

Respiratory Infections

Infections may be localized to the bronchioles and bronchi, alveoli, interstitium, or pleura. The cause and site of infections are related to the age of the child, seasonal variables, and environmental exposures. Infants and young children tend to have more viral infections, especially during late autumn to early spring. Environmental factors may include presence of siblings, day-care exposure, and other variables.

Bronchiolitis

Bronchiolitis is a rather common, viral-induced lower respiratory tract infection that occurs almost exclusively in infants and young toddlers. The most common associated pathogen is respiratory syncytial virus (RSV), but it also may be associated with adenovirus, influenza, parainfluenza, and mycoplasma. RSV infects nearly 100% of children in the United States by 2 to 3 years of age. This infection is restricted to the respiratory mucosa.[75] It has a peak incidence during winter and spring and is a major reason for hospital admission of children younger than 1 year, particularly children of lower socioeconomic status. Healthy infants usually make a full recovery from RSV bronchiolitis, but infants who are premature or who have underlying lung disease, heart disease, or immune deficiency may have a much more severe or even deadly course.

PATHOPHYSIOLOGY   Viral infection causes necrosis of the bronchial epithelium and destruction of ciliated epithelial cells. There is infiltration with lymphocytes around the bronchioles and a cell-mediated hypersensitivity to viral antigens with release of lymphokines causing inflammation, as well as activation of eosinophils, neutrophils, and monocytes.[75] The submucosa becomes edematous, and cellular debris and fibrin form plugs within the bronchioles. Edema of the bronchiolar wall, accumulation of mucus and cellular debris, and possibly bronchospasm narrow many peripheral airways. Other airways become partially or completely occluded. Atelectasis occurs in some areas of the lung and hyperinflation in others.

The mechanics of breathing are disrupted by bronchiolitis. There is air trapping, and FRC is greatly increased. Compliance is decreased because the lungs are already hyperinflated and because airway resistance within the lung is uneven and increased. The decrease in compliance and the increase in airway resistance result in a substantial increase in the work of breathing. Serious alterations in gas exchange occur because of airway obstruction and patchy atelectasis. Hypoxemia develops because of ventilation-perfusion mismatch, and hypercapnia may occur in severe cases.

CLINICAL MANIFESTATIONS   Children with bronchiolitis have tachypnea, expiratory wheezing, cough, rhinorrhea, mild fever, and varying grades of respiratory distress. Chest radiographs often reveal hyperexpanded lungs, patchy or peribronchial infiltrates, and sometimes, atelectasis of the right upper lobe. Severely affected infants appear anxious and distressed because of dyspnea or hypoxemia. The thoracic cage is overexpanded, particularly in its anteroposterior diameter. The infant takes rapid, short breaths, and wheezing and rales are often heard on auscultation. With overexpansion of the lungs, the diaphragm is flattened, causing downward displacement of the liver and spleen. Abdominal distention results from air swallowing. Some individuals have persistent high airway resistance and airway hyperresponsiveness, including increased risk for asthma, long after resolution of the viral process.[76-78]

EVALUATION AND TREATMENT   Diagnosis is made by review of signs and symptoms (e.g., rhinitis, cough, wheezing, chest retractions, tachypnea) and radiologic examination. Nasal washings may be tested for specific viral agents, such as RSV. Treatment is determined by the severity of the disease and age of the child. Infants younger than 1 year are most at risk for acute respiratory failure and may require assisted ventilation. Supplemental oxygen is given as needed, and adequate hydration should be maintained. Bronchodilators have not been scientifically validated as consistently providing significant benefit, but are widely tried on an empiric basis.[79] Likewise, steroids are not of proven benefit.[80] Antiviral agents (ribavirin) for RSV are no longer widely used because of high cost and unclear efficacy. Prophylactic treatment with RSV-specific monoclonal antibody is recommended for high-risk infants under 2 years old, although high cost is sometimes a barrier.[81]

Pneumonia

Pneumonia involves inflammation and infection in the terminal airways and alveoli. It is a major cause of morbidity and mortality, particularly in developing countries. The most common agents are viral, followed by bacteria and mycoplasma. In children, fungal pneumonia is rare. Opportunistic infections occur only in the immunocompromised child and are not discussed further in this chapter. Widespread childhood vaccination has decreased the incidence of *Haemophilus influenza* type b and *Streptococcus pneumonia* infections.[82,83]

PATHOPHYSIOLOGY   **Bacterial pneumonia** usually results from inhalation of microbes dispersed in ambient air or in secretion droplets (person-to-person spread) or by aspiration of one's own nasopharyngeal bacteria. Once in the alveolar region, bacteria encounter local host defenses, such as opsonins and IgG, which prepare bacteria for ingestion by alveolar macrophages. If these mechanisms fail, neutrophils will be recruited and an intense, cytokine-mediated inflammation will ensue. Vascular engorgement, edema, and a fibrinopurulent exudate occur. Alveolar filling precludes gas exchange and, if extensive, could lead to respiratory failure.[84] If sepsis occurs at the same time, shock and end-organ hypoperfusion will cause metabolic acidosis. A spreading viral infection of the lower respiratory tract sometimes sets the stage for bacterial infection by causing epithelial damage and reduced mucociliary clearance.

The most common bacterial pathogens for young children beyond the neonatal period are pneumococcal, staphylococcal, and streptococcal organisms (Table 34-2). Pneumococcal pneumonia is the most common and manifests acutely and with variable severity. It is usually lobar in pattern. Staphylococcal and group A streptococcal pneumonia can be particularly fulminant and necrotizing, with a high incidence of accompanying empyema, pneumatoceles, and sepsis. Empyema is increasingly associated with methicillin-resistant *Staphylococcus aureus*.[85,86]

Viral pneumonia is more common than bacterial pneumonia and is acquired by direct contact, droplet transmission, or aerosol. There is initial destruction of ciliated epithelium of the distal airway, with sloughing of cellular material. A mononuclear-predominant inflammatory response occurs, in the interstitium initially, and may later involve the alveoli as well.

The most common cause of viral pneumonia in infants is RSV,[87] usually in the winter to early spring. A number of other viruses are important, including parainfluenza, influenza, and adenoviruses. Certain serotypes of adenovirus can cause necrotizing disease, sometimes leading to obliterative bronchiolitis and significant lung disability.

Atypical pneumonia (*Mycoplasma pneumoniae, Chlamydia pneumoniae*) is the most common cause of community-acquired pneumonia for school-age children and young adults. ***Chlamydia pneumoniae*** is clinically indistinguishable from and is typically grouped with ***Mycoplasma pneumoniae*** as "atypical" pneumonia.[88,89] Transmission is person to person, with a 2- to 3-week incubation period.

Mycoplasma microorganisms lack cell walls but have a limiting membrane and a specialized tip for attaching to ciliated respiratory epithelial cells. Local sloughing of cells occurs. Peribronchial lymphocytic infiltration develops, along with neutrophil recruitment to the airway lumen. The pattern resembles bronchitis or bronchopneumonia.

Onset is usually gradual, resembling a typical upper respiratory infection with low-grade fever and prominent cough. There may be accompanying sore throat, myalgia, and headache. Cases are not usually clinically severe, and full recovery should be expected.

EVALUATION AND TREATMENT Diagnosis of pneumonia is based on clinical findings and chest radiograph confirmation. A bacterial pneumonia will initially produce a

Table 34-2	Common Types of Pneumonia in Children				
Type	**Causal Agent**	**Age**	**Onset**	**Signs/Symptoms**	**Pathophysiology**
Viral pneumonia	Respiratory syncytial virus (RSV), influenza, adenovirus, others	Infants for RSV All ages for others	Acute or gradual, winter and early spring	Mild to high fever, cough, rhinorrhea, malaise, rales, rhonchi, or wheezing, variable radiographic pattern	Edema, increased mucus, and interstitial pneumonia
Pneumococcal pneumonia	Pneumococci (*Streptococcus pneumoniae*)	1-4 yr	Acute, follows an upper respiratory infection, winter and early spring	High fever, productive cough, pleuritic pain, increased respiratory rate, decreased breath sounds in area of consolidation; lobar pattern or "round pneumonia" on radiograph	Inflammation of bronchial mucosa, alveolar exudate *Early:* red hepatization with WBCs, RBCs, and fibrin consolidation *Late:* gray hepatization with fibrin and neutrophils in alveoli *Resolution:* many phagocytic macrophages
Staphylococcal pneumonia	*Staphylococcus aureus* Methicillin-resistant *Staphylococcus aureus*	1 wk-2 yr	Acute, winter months	High fever, cough, respiratory distress; toxic appearance; sepsis, empyema, pneumatoceles common; multilobar consolidation	Necrotizing patterns may occur in severe cases
Streptococcal pneumonia	Group A streptococci	All ages	Acute, any season	High fever, chills, respiratory distress; sepsis or shock; empyema, pneumatoceles	Tracheobronchitis, and interstitial pneumonia with ulcers, exudate, edema, and localized hemorrhage
Mycoplasma and chlamydia pneumonia	*Mycoplasma pneumoniae, Chlamydia pneumoniae*	School-age and adolescents	Gradual	Low grade fever; cough	Inflammation of bronchi with lymphocyte and neutrophil recruitment

WBCs, White blood cells; *RBCs,* red blood cells.

patchy infiltration and later cause a segmental or lobar disease. Pleural effusion or empyema is an occasional complication that often requires tube drainage or thoracoscopic debridement.[86] Aspiration pneumonia characteristically produces perihilar or lower lobe infiltrates.

Most pneumonias may be treated on an outpatient basis; however, many children require oxygen supplementation and, occasionally, assisted ventilation. This is particularly true with infants who have a viral interstitial pneumonia, such as RSV. In addition, adequate hydration, nutrition, and supportive pulmonary therapy are required to reduce the duration and severity of illness. Many hospitalized infants are markedly tachypneic and unable to coordinate their breathing with swallowing; they may require enteral feeding. Aspiration is always a risk with infants in respiratory distress.

Appropriate antibiotic administration for bacterial pneumonias is usually instituted for a minimum of 10 days, and longer for S. aureus or group A streptococci. Local patterns of drug resistance must be considered, and new antibacterials are being developed for treatment of antibiotic-resistant pathogens.[90,91] Use of the heptavalent pneumococcal vaccine has led to a decrease in invasive infections.[92]

Aspiration Pneumonitis

Aspiration pneumonitis is caused by a foreign substance, such as food, secretions, or chemical compounds, entering the lung and causing inflammation. The aspiration of meconium from amniotic fluid can occur at birth. Meconium contains bile salts from the fetal intestinal tract that cause inflammation. Neurologically compromised children or children undergoing sedation or anesthesia may aspirate oral secretions (containing anaerobic bacteria) or stomach contents. The severity of lung injury after an aspiration incident is determined by the amount of material aspirated, the pH of the aspirated material, and the presence of pathogenic bacteria. Very low pH or very high pH will cause a significant inflammatory response. With hydrocarbon ingestions, lung injury is determined by the volatility and viscosity of the aspirated substance. A low-viscosity substance, such as gasoline or lighter fluid, is the most toxic; high-viscosity hydrocarbons, such as petroleum jelly or mineral oil, are much less likely to cause pneumonitis. Treatment for aspiration pneumonitis depends on the material aspirated. Strategies for prevention of aspiration are an important part of the therapeutic plan for every person and are important at every well-child visit. Children at highest risk are toddlers, children with poor airway reflexes or gastroesophageal reflux, or both.

Bronchiolitis Obliterans

Bronchiolitis obliterans is fibrotic obstruction of the respiratory bronchioles and alveolar ducts secondary to intense inflammation. Most cases of bronchiolitis obliterans in children are associated with viral pulmonary infections (e.g., influenza, adenoviral infection, pertussis [whooping cough]), or measles. It also may occur after lung transplantation.[93] Cough, respiratory distress, and cyanosis occur initially, followed by a brief period of improvement. The progression of disease is then reflected by increasing dyspnea, cough, sputum production, and wheezing and is related to airway obstruction.[94]

There is no specific treatment for bronchiolitis obliterans. Some children deteriorate rapidly and die within weeks, while others follow a more chronic course.

Asthma

Asthma is an obstructive airway disease characterized by reversible airflow obstruction, bronchial hyperreactivity, and inflammation. It is the most prevalent chronic disease in childhood, affecting 5% to 10% of all children, and has become more prevalent in the past two decades. In the prepubertal years, more boys than girls are affected. Inner-city black and Hispanic children have higher morbidity and mortality rates than white children.[95] The mortality rate rose among children with asthma from 1980 to 1993[96] but may be leveling off.[97] Severity and persistence of asthma is influenced by age at disease onset, genetics, atopy, air pollution, level of allergen exposure, environmental tobacco smoke, gastroesophageal reflux, and respiratory infections.[98,99] Asthma-related deaths almost always occur outside the hospital setting.

There are currently many theories regarding the mechanisms of disease in childhood asthma. The wide spectrum of clinical disease probably reflects a complex interaction between genetic susceptibility and environmental factors, including allergens and infections, particularly viral respiratory infections.[100-104] A number of experts postulate that a key determinant of asthma is the T-lymphocyte phenotype being tipped toward a "Th$_2$ response" in which CD4 T-helper (Th) cells produce specific cytokines, such as IL-4, IL-5, and IL-13, that promote an atopic/allergic response in the airways as opposed to a "Th$_1$ response" characteristic of delayed-type hypersensitivity and phagocyte-mediated host defense.[105,106] IL-4 and IL-13 are particularly important for B cell switching to favor IgE production; IL-5 is crucial for local differentiation and enhanced survival of eosinophils within the airways.

It is possible that certain early childhood respiratory viral infections could favor the Th$_2$-predominant phenotype and contribute to inducing asthma in susceptible individuals. It also has been suggested that lack of sufficient early exposure to viruses and aeroallergens could favor the Th$_2$ phenotype in the airways and permit induction of asthma. This so-called "hygiene hypothesis"[107-110] has been offered as an explanation for the higher prevalence of asthma in Westernized countries than in less developed countries, and for the inverse relationship between number of siblings and incidence of atopy. These theories about the origins of asthma are interesting although not proven.[111,112]

Allergen sensitization is associated with risk for asthma.[113] There is significant evidence that asthma has a strong familial and genetic component, but asthma clearly involves a number of genes rather than a single "asthma gene."[114] Population genomic screening has led to the proposal of a number of candidate genes or chromosomal regions that are associated with asthma. In addition, genes may impart associated phenotypes, such as bronchial hyperresponsiveness, high levels of serum IgE, sensitization to allergens, and responsiveness to asthma therapies. For example, a specific polymorphism in the gene for the β-adrenergic receptor appears to be associated with poor response to β-adrenergic inhaled medication.[115]

PATHOPHYSIOLOGY   For acute allergen-induced asthma, the paradigm of the *early asthmatic response* remains useful

(Figure 34-13, *A*). This begins immediately after exposure and lasts up to 2 hours. The allergen binds to preformed IgE on the surface of mucosal mast cells, and crosslinking of these IgE molecules triggers degranulation of the mast cell, releasing mediators such as histamine, leukotrienes, prostaglandin D_2, platelet-activating factor, chemotactic chemokines, and certain cytokines (i.e., IL-1 beta)[116] (see Figure 6-8, p. 187). These mediators cause airway smooth muscle constriction (bronchospasm),

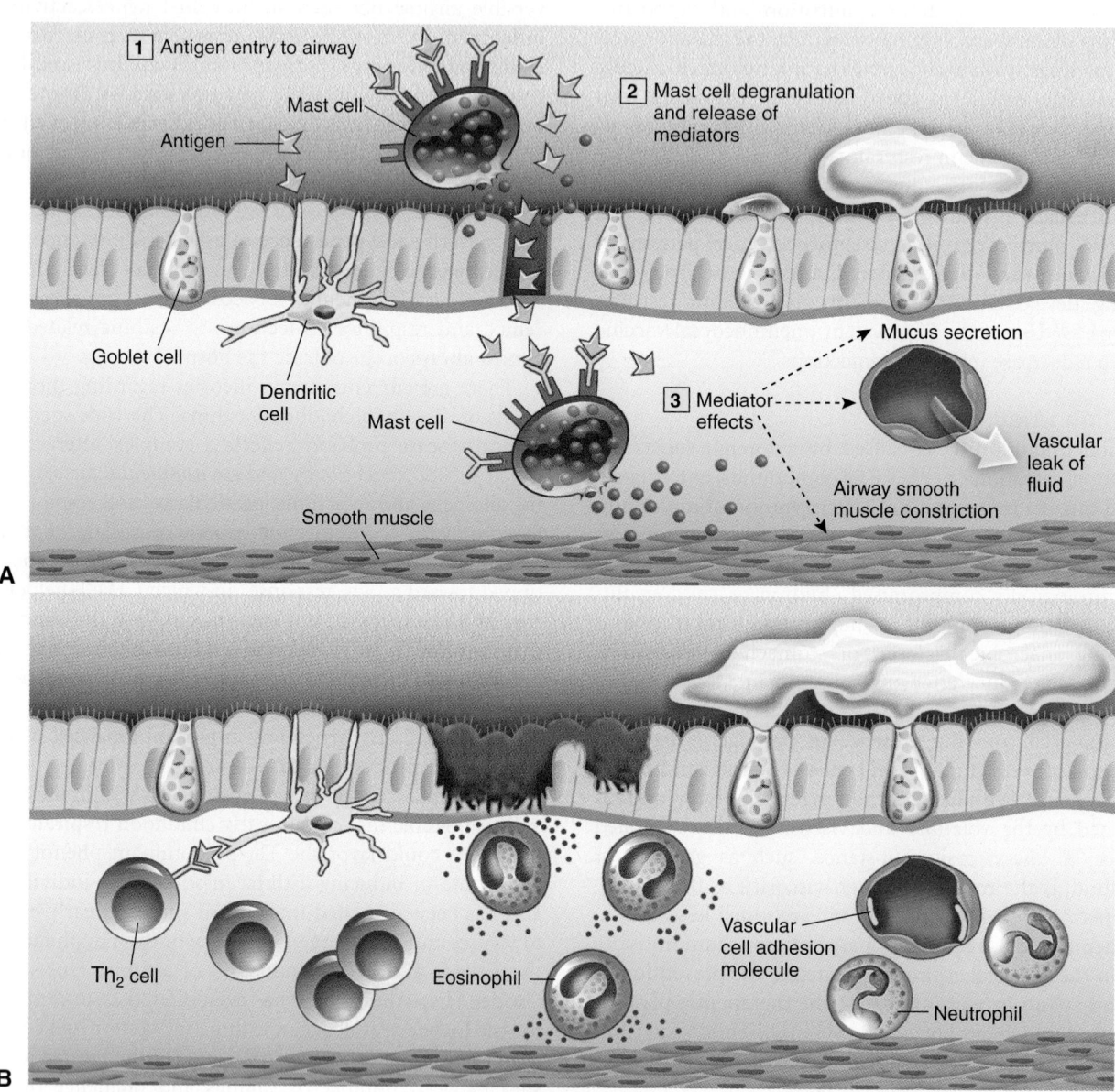

Fig 34-13 Asthmatic responses. A, In the early asthmatic response, inhaled antigen *(1)* binds to preformed IgE on mast cells. Mast cells degranulate *(2)* and release mediators such as histamine, leukotrienes, prostaglandin D_2, platelet-activating factor, and others. Acute inflammation opens intercellular tight junctions, allowing antigen to penetrate and activate submucosal mast cells. Secreted mediators *(3)* induce active bronchospasm, edema, and mucus secretion. Inflammatory responses are set in motion by chemotactic factors and upregulation of adhesion molecules *(not shown)*. At the same time, as shown on the left, antigen may be received by dendritic cells that process and later present it, either in regional lymph nodes to naive (Th₀) T lymphocytes or locally to memory Th₂ cells in the airway mucosa (see **B**). **B,** In the late asthmatic response, there are areas of epithelial damage caused at least in part by toxicity of eosinophil products (major basic protein, eosinophilic cationic protein, eosinophil-derived neurotoxin, and eosinophil peroxidase). Many inflammatory cells have been recruited by chemokines and upregulation of vascular cell adhesion molecules. Local T lymphocytes display a predominant Th₂ cytokine profile. They produce IL-4 and IL-13, which promote switching of B cells to favor IgE production, and IL-3, IL-5, and granulocyte-macrophage colony–stimulating factor, which encourage eosinophil differentiation and survival.

increased vascular permeability (mucosal edema), and mucus secretion. The *late asthmatic response* starts 4 to 8 hours after exposure and may persist up to 24 hours (Figure 34-13, *B*). The response is characterized by inflammatory cell recruitment (neutrophils, eosinophils, basophils, and T lymphocytes) that was triggered earlier by chemotactic factors and upregulation of endothelial adhesion molecules. Another wave of mediator release occurs, again inciting bronchospasm, edema, and mucus secretion. Epithelial damage and impaired mucociliary function may be seen because of direct toxic effects of products such as major basic protein from eosinophils. This local injury stimulates local nerve endings, which may aggravate bronchoconstriction and mucus secretion through autonomic pathways (Figure 34-14).

In a full-blown asthma attack (**status asthmaticus**), there are components of bronchospasm, as well as acute airway inflammation directed by a number of cells and the mediators they secrete. Mucous plugging, edema, and cellular infiltration lead to further airway narrowing. A partial obstruction is present that creates a "ball-valve" effect leading to segmental hyperinflation, which may become extreme and compromise effective tidal volume. Measures of expiratory flow rates, such as FEV_1 and peak flow, are markedly reduced.

Examination of postmortem lung specimens of individuals who died from asthma reveals abnormalities consistent with both acute and chronic changes in the airways. These include extensive mucous plugging, mucosal edema, and denudation of bronchial and bronchiolar epithelium. Eosinophilia is present in the submucosa, and a multicellular inflammatory infiltrate accumulates in the airways. Thickening of the basement membrane, airway smooth muscle hypertrophy, and mucous gland hypertrophy are often noted, sometimes even in pathology specimens from mild asthmatics, providing evidence that there may be long-term airway structural changes associated with asthma. In chronic asthma, chronically increased numbers of inflammatory cells may lead to long-term changes, such as goblet cell hyperplasia and

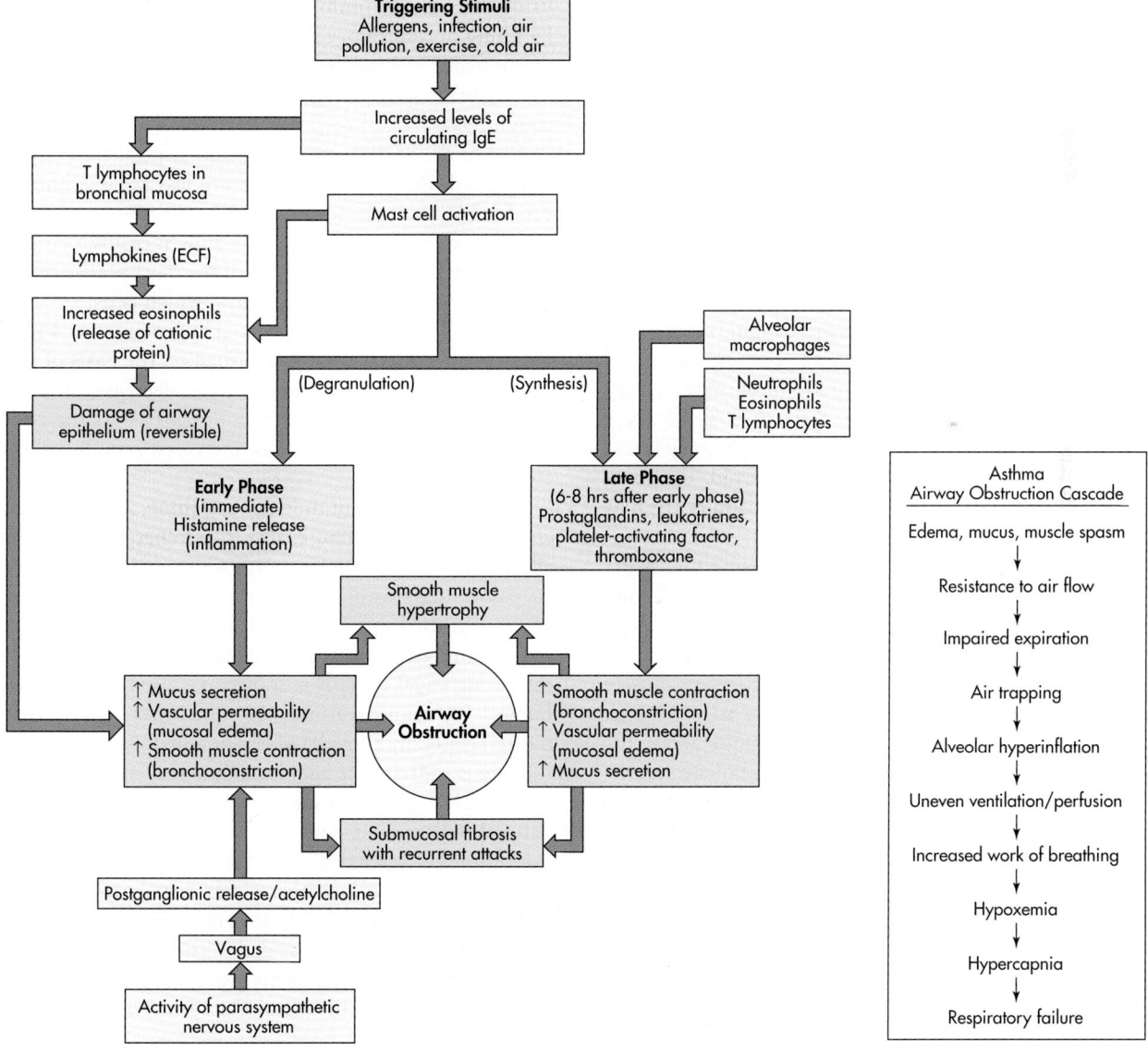

Figure 34-14 Pathophysiology of childhood asthma. *IgE,* Immunoglobulin E; *ECF,* eosinophil chemotactic factor.

airway wall remodeling (subepithelial fibrosis, smooth muscle hypertrophy).

The typical arterial blood gas abnormalities in acute asthma are hypoxemia, hypocarbia, and respiratory alkalosis. Because bronchial obstruction is nonuniform, ventilation is likewise uneven, causing ventilation mismatch and hypoxemia. The degree of hypoxemia is usually mild, however, and arterial saturations of less than 90% indicate severe airway obstruction. Pulmonary circulation may be altered by regional hypoxic vasoconstriction, as well as the effect of increased intra-alveolar pressure (caused by expiratory airway obstruction and alveolar hyperinflation) to decrease perfusion of alveolar capillaries. Typically, respiratory rate is elevated to compensate for hypoxemia, with reduced minute ventilation because of increased airway resistance and lung hyperinflation. The hypoxemic hyperventilation reduces arterial P_{CO_2} (usually 30 to 35 mmHg), and even a normal value should be of concern if respiratory distress is significant. Retention of CO_2 is a late finding, usually occurring only if FEV_1 falls to around 15% to 20% of predicted values, and reflects inadequate alveolar ventilation and increased functional dead space. Alterations of pH homeostasis usually start with respiratory alkalosis caused by the hyperventilation. With severe airway obstruction, the end result of the pathophysiologic processes may be respiratory failure with acute CO_2 retention and respiratory acidosis. Metabolic acidosis may accompany life-threatening asthma, especially when left ventricular filling and thus cardiac output become compromised because of severe hyperinflation.

CLINICAL MANIFESTATIONS In a typical acute asthma attack, the major complaints are cough, wheeze, and shortness of breath. Signs of a preceding upper respiratory infection, such as rhinorrhea or low-grade fever, may or may not have been present. In children, 70% to 80% of acute wheezing episodes are associated with viral respiratory infections. In infants and toddlers under 2 years old, the most common of these is RSV. In older children and adults, the major viral trigger is rhinovirus.[117]

On physical examination, expiratory wheezing that is often described as high-pitched and musical is found, along with prolongation of the expiratory phase of the respiratory cycle. Sometimes hyperinflation is visible. Respiratory rate is elevated, as is heart rate. Nasal flaring and accessory muscle use are evident, with retractions in the substernal, subcostal, intercostal, suprasternal, or sternocleidomastoid areas. Infants may appear to be "head bobbing" because of sternocleidomastoid muscle use. Pulsus paradoxus may be present. The child may appear anxious or diaphoretic, important signs of respiratory compromise.

Findings in chronic asthma may include hyperinflation of the thorax (barrel chest) or pectus excavatum. Clubbing should not be seen in those with asthma and, if present, should trigger evaluation for other conditions, such as cystic fibrosis.

EVALUATION AND TREATMENT For objective evaluation of asthma, including both diagnosis and chronic management, the widely used indicators are measures of pulmonary function typically obtained through spirometry. Characteristic abnormalities would be reduced expiratory flow rates, namely forced expiratory volume in 1 second (FEV_1) and to an even greater extent, the midexpiratory flow rate ($FEF_{25\%-75\%}$, or forced expiratory flow rate between 25% and 75% of total exhaled volume); also the ratio of FEV_1 to forced vital capacity (FVC) would be typically decreased. Unlike asthmatic adults, however, asthmatic children often have normal or near-normal spirometry when they are at baseline. Other potentially useful supportive diagnostic findings would include evidence of air trapping on lung volume measurement (by plethysmography), documentation of bronchial hyperreactivity (in response to challenge such as exercise or inhaling methacholine) or increased expiratory flow rates in response to an inhaled bronchodilator. Often it is not feasible to obtain the above tests on children, so in practice an empiric trial of asthma-directed medications is commonly initiated, using clinical symptoms (wheeze, cough, exercise tolerance, handling of respiratory infections, etc.) as a guideline. During a significant asthma attack, individuals may be too dyspneic to perform spirometry, and it may precipitate excessive coughing.

For home management of asthma, peak flow meters are often used. Peak flow measures are less reliable and less reproducible than those obtained by spirometry but can be helpful. For serial tracking, peak flow measurements should be obtained at consistent times of the day because of the natural diurnal variation in peak flow, which is usually lowest at approximately 4 AM and highest at approximately 4 PM. Once a baseline value has been established on the basis of repeated measurements over a period of time, decreases in peak flow can be interpreted meaningfully to help assess the child and modify treatment in the face of increased symptoms or intercurrent illness.

For management of mild acute asthma, rapid-acting bronchodilators, such as albuterol (a β_2-adrenergic agonist) or levalbuterol, may be sufficient, with addition of systemic steroids for more significant attacks to decrease inflammatory responses in the lung.[118-120] Inhaled ipratropium bromide is an anticholinergic agent that contributes to bronchodilation by inhibiting vagal tone; it is sometimes used together with albuterol for acute treatment or sometimes as an alternative, though generally considered less potent, for those who cannot tolerate β_2-adrenergic agonists because of side effects.[121]

There is a growing number of options for management of chronic asthma depending on chronicity and severity of symptoms, as well as on individual compliance issues. Guidelines have been outlined and widely distributed by a National Institutes of Health (NIH) expert panel.[122] For individuals with persistent symptoms, daily "controller" medication is recommended. The most widely preferred controller therapy remains inhaled corticosteroids. However, montelukast (an oral leukotriene receptor antagonist) is frequently used as supplemental therapy or, for milder or exercise-induced asthma, as monotherapy.[123,124] Inhaled cromolyn and nedocromil remain available anti-inflammatory therapies but their use has declined, in favor of other therapies, at least in the United States.[125-127] Long-acting β₂-adrenergic agonists, such as salmeterol, also may be applied to pediatric asthma except in the youngest children. For allergic asthma, anti-IgE therapy has recently become available for select individuals (see What's New? Box in Chapter 33, p. 1224).

Acute Respiratory Distress Syndrome

Acute respiratory distress syndrome (ARDS) is a condition resulting from a direct pulmonary insult (such as pneumonia, aspiration, near-drowning, or smoke inhalation) or a systemic insult (such as sepsis or multiple trauma), either of which activates an inflammatory response that causes alveolocapillary injury. *Adult respiratory distress syndrome* is the historical term for this condition, but its recognition in children has led to renaming it *acute respiratory distress syndrome.* Clinically, ARDS is characterized by severe hypoxemia, decreased pulmonary compliance, and diffuse densities on chest radiograph. ARDS accounts for approximately 10% of total patient days and one third of all deaths in pediatric intensive care units.[128] The mortality rate in pediatric ARDS remains high, at approximately 50%.[129,130]

PATHOPHYSIOLOGY   The hallmark of ARDS is lung inflammation. There is activation of a number of systems and mediators (Figure 34-15), including complement, cytokines, arachidonic acid metabolites, platelet-activating factor, reactive oxygen species, and others. Sources of these mediators include neutrophils, activated platelets, macrophages, and injured endothelium. Early, during the *inflammatory* or *exudative phase* of ARDS, there is pulmonary neutrophil influx along with intraluminal fibrin and platelet aggregation. Injury to the endothelial barriers results in capillary leak and noncardiogenic pulmonary edema. Edema fluid contains plasma proteins that can inactivate surfactant, contributing further to alveolar collapse. This fluid also has procoagulant activity, leading to fibrin clotting within airspaces. Similarly, the pulmonary microcirculation is compromised by the formation of thrombi composed of fibrin, platelets, and leukocytes.

The early accumulation of edema fluid in the airspaces results in decreased lung compliance, decreased functional residual volume, and increased dead space. Ventilation-perfusion mismatching, intrapulmonary shunting, and hypoxemia occur. Diffuse pulmonary thrombosis contributes further to the

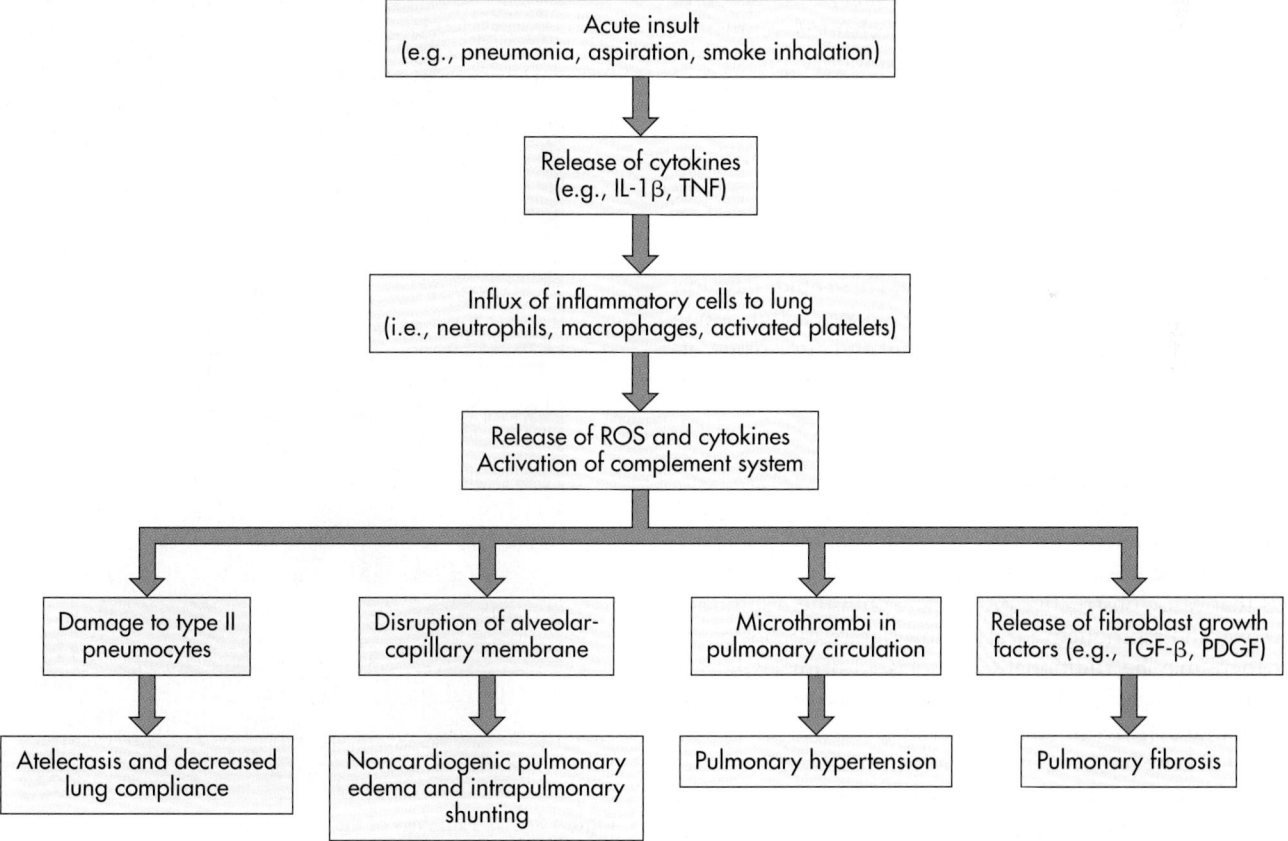

Figure 34-15 Proposed mechanisms for the pathogenesis of acute respiratory distress syndrome (ARDS). *IL-1β,* Interleukin-1β; *TNF,* tumor necrosis factor; *ROS,* reactive oxygen species; *TGF-β,* transforming growth factor–β; *PDGF,* platelet-derived growth factor. (From Soubani AO, Pieroni R: Acute respiratory distress syndrome: a clinical update, *South Med J* 92(5):452, 1999.)

formation of pulmonary edema by increasing capillary hydrostatic pressure and may lead to pulmonary hypertension.

In the *fibroproliferative phase,* type II alveolar cells proliferate, and there is alveolar septal thickening and collagen deposition. Interstitial fibrosis can be evident as early as 10 days after the initial insult. Similarly, vascular changes may occur, including obliteration of the microcirculation and thickening of the walls of pulmonary arterioles and arteries, which can lead to chronic pulmonary hypertension in survivors.

CLINICAL MANIFESTATIONS   ARDS develops acutely after the initial insult, usually within 24 hours (although occasionally it is delayed up to a few days). There is progressive respiratory distress and severe hypoxemia with poor response to oxygen supplementation. Initially, hyperventilation occurs, but CO_2 retention may ultimately occur because of inadequate functional airspace and respiratory muscle fatigue. Severity of the overall picture is modified by comorbid factors, such as the presence of sepsis or multiorgan failure and whether complications develop, such as nosocomial pneumonia.

EVALUATION AND TREATMENT   Treatment of ARDS remains supportive in nature. Of course, any underlying condition, such as sepsis, must be treated. Beyond that, the goals are maintaining adequate tissue oxygenation, minimizing acute lung injury, and avoiding iatrogenic pulmonary complications. Most individuals with ARDS require mechanical ventilation and often high levels of positive end-expiratory pressure to promote alveolar recruitment and stabilization and redistribution of alveolar edema fluid into the interstitium. Various ventilation strategies may be used for ARDS, such as low tidal volumes, permissive hypercapnia, prone positioning, inverse inspiratory/expiratory ratio, and high-frequency oscillatory ventilation.[131-133] Liquid ventilation through perfluorocarbons instilled in the lungs is being investigated. These fluids have low surface tension and are efficient carriers of oxygen and carbon dioxide. Other therapies, such as surfactant and nitric oxide, offer theoretic promise, but their efficacy in pediatric ARDS has not yet been validated.[134]

Cystic Fibrosis

Cystic fibrosis (CF) is an autosomal recessive inherited disorder that is associated with defective epithelial ion transport. On a simplistic level, CF is characterized by abnormal secretions that cause obstructive problems within the respiratory, digestive, and reproductive tracts. However, research suggests that there may be additional CF-associated primary defects, such as an intrinsic proinflammatory state and abnormal local immune defenses in the lungs.

The CF gene has been located on chromosome 7. Its mutation results in the abnormal expression of the protein **cystic fibrosis transmembrane conductance regulator (CFTR),** which is a cAMP-activated chloride channel present on the surface of many types of epithelial cells, including those lining airways, bile ducts, pancreas, sweat ducts, and vas deferens. Despite knowing that chloride transport is a fundamen-

tal abnormality, the exact disease mechanisms in CF have still not been clearly defined at the cellular and end-organ levels. CF affects primarily whites (approximately 1 in 3500) but is seen in other groups as well.[135] Estimated carrier frequency is high (1 in 29 whites in the United States), and carriers are healthy.

PATHOPHYSIOLOGY   Although CF is a multiorgan disease, the lungs are the most critical site of involvement, and respiratory failure is almost always the cause of death. The typical features of CF lung disease are mucus plugging, chronic inflammation, and infection. The abnormalities primarily involve the airways, with progressive bronchiectasis that becomes widespread. Parenchymal involvement occurs much later and includes microabscess formation, patchy consolidation and pneumonia, peribronchial fibrosis, and cyst formation (Figure 34-16). The pathophysiology for these changes is outlined in a simplified form in Figure 34-17. Peripheral bullae may develop because of obstruction and airway wall weakening, and pneumothorax may occur. Hemoptysis, sometimes life threatening, may occur because of erosion of enlarged bronchial arteries that develop in response to the inflammation associated with bronchiectasis.

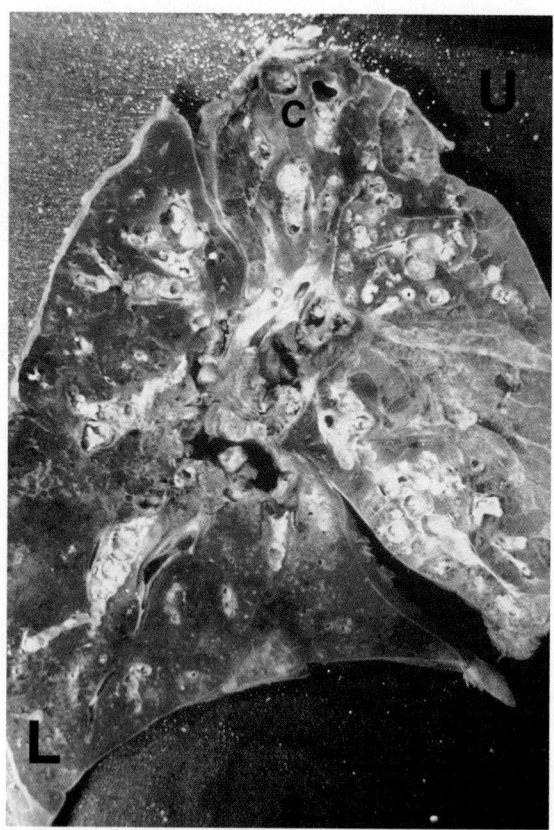

Figure 34-16 Pathology of the lung in end-stage cystic fibrosis. Key features are widespread mucus impaction of airways and bronchiectasis (especially in upper lobe, *U*), with hemorrhagic pneumonia in the lower lobe *(L)*. Small cysts *(C)* are present at the apex of the lung. (From Kleinerman J, Vauthy P: *Pathology of the lung in cystic fibrosis,* Atlanta, 1976, Cystic Fibrosis Foundation.)

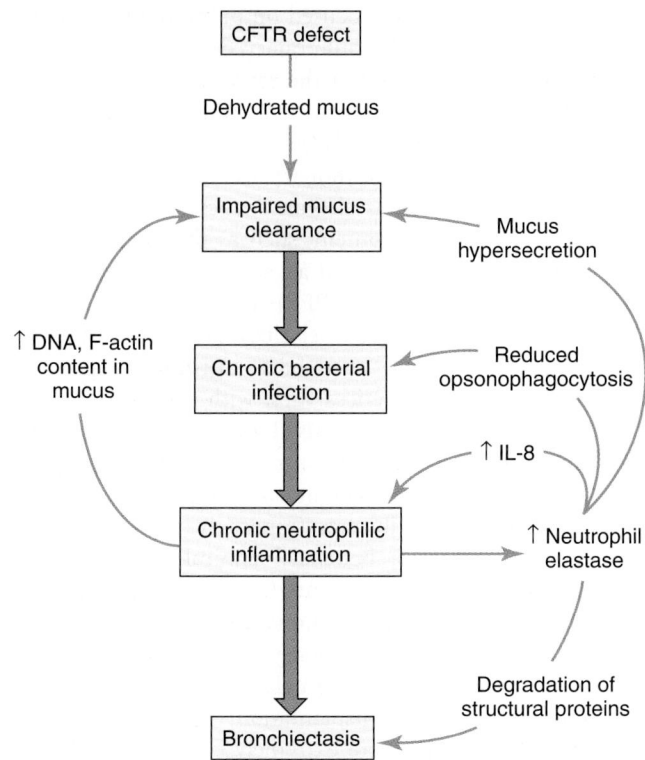

Figure 34-17 Pathogenesis of cystic fibrosis lung disease. *CFTR*, Cystic fibrosis transmembrane conductance regulator; *Il-8*, interleukin-8.

Over a long period of time, pulmonary vascular remodeling occurs because of localized hypoxia and arteriolar vasoconstriction; pulmonary hypertension and cor pulmonale may develop with end-stage disease.

The mucus plugging seen in CF probably results from the combination of increased production of mucus, altered physicochemical properties of the mucus, and reduced mucociliary clearance.[136-138] Mucus-secreting airway cells (goblet cells and submucosal glands) are increased in number and size. CF mucus is dehydrated and viscous because of abnormal chloride secretion and exaggerated sodium absorption, resulting in depletion of the airway surface liquid volume. This appears to facilitate mucus adherence to the epithelium, impairment of ciliary mobility, and retention of bacteria that can then form biofilms. Finally, after secretion, CF mucus becomes even more viscous because of DNA and filamentous (F) actin released from degraded neutrophils, which are present in very high numbers in CF airways.

Chronic, intense neutrophil-dominated inflammation occurs in CF airways, and plays a critical role in long-term damage.[139] Evidence indicates that excess inflammation may even begin in infancy, and may be at least initially independent of bacterial colonization.[140] Abnormal cytokine profiles have been documented in CF airway fluids, including deficient interleukin-10 (IL-10) and excessive IL-1, IL-8, and TNF-α, all changes conducive to promoting inflammation.[137,141] Neutrophils are present in great excess in CF airways and release damaging oxidants, such as myeloperoxidase[142] and proteases in massive amounts that overwhelm local antiprotease de-

fenses. One protease in particular, neutrophil elastase, has the following detrimental effects: (1) direct damage to lung structural proteins, such as elastin; (2) induction of airway cells to produce IL-8, a strong attractant for neutrophils and thus a means for augmenting a local "vicious cycle" of inflammation; (3) cleavage of IgG and complement components important for opsonization and phagocytosis of pathogens; and (4) direct stimulation of mucus secretion by mucus-producing cells.

Children with CF have a propensity for chronic endobronchial infection that remains poorly understood. It is likely that local factors in the CF airway microenvironment favor bacterial colonization, because no systemic immune defect has been found. *Staphylococcus aureus* is common, and *Pseudomonas aeruginosa* ultimately colonizes airways in 75% of children with CF. Infecting colonies of *Pseudomonas* appear to adopt a mucoid phenotype and organize themselves into adherent biofilms, making it difficult for antibiotics and local defenses to reach them. *Pseudomonas* acquisition has been linked with more rapid decline in pulmonary function.[137,143,144] Persistence of infection incites chronic local inflammation, airway damage, bronchiectasis, microabscess formation, and foci of hemorrhagic pneumonia.

CLINICAL MANIFESTATIONS   The median age at diagnosis is 6 months; nearly 75% of cases are diagnosed by 1 year. Approximately 10% of cases are not diagnosed until after age 10, however, and these cases usually have milder symptoms. The most common manifestations are respiratory and gastrointestinal, including the pancreas and biliary tract. Respiratory symptoms at presentation may include persistent (but not necessarily severe) cough or wheeze, sputum production, and recurrent or severe pneumonia. More subtle respiratory tract presentations of CF include chronic sinusitis and nasal polyps. With appropriate treatment, the level of cough, sputum production, and exercise limitation does not usually reach debilitating levels during childhood. Physical signs include digital clubbing, which may appear quite early, and in the absence of significant pulmonary impairment. Development of barrel chest or persistent rales occurs much later.

Classic gastrointestinal manifestations include meconium ileus at birth, which is almost pathognomonic for CF, and approximately 15% to 20% of individuals with CF present with this. Another classic presentation is failure to thrive and malabsorptive symptoms, such as frequent loose and oily stools. Rectal prolapse is an occasional presenting sign that should always prompt testing for CF. About 10% of CF patients do not experience gastrointestinal problems and are termed "pancreatic sufficient." Several specific CFTR mutations are predictive of this milder digestive and nutritional phenotype. Males with CF are typically infertile (98%). Other complications of CF may include liver disease (approximately 5%) and diabetes mellitus (10% to 25%). Overall severity of CF lung disease is highly variable and has not proven predictable on the basis of CFTR genotype. Even affected siblings may have disparate courses despite identical CFTR mutations, environment, and treatment strategy. Researchers are trying to identify "gene modifiers," which are genes other than CFTR that may serve to lessen or aggravate the degree of CF lung disease and increase or decrease the risk of developing other CF complications such as severe liver disease.[145]

EVALUATION AND TREATMENT The standard method of diagnosis has been the sweat test, which will reveal sweat chloride concentration in excess of 60 mEq/L. Genotyping for CFTR mutations is also available as an alternative or supplemental method but may fail to confirm up to 10% of cases because of a lack of ability to screen for every described CF-associated mutation. There are more than 1100 mutations, but most standard laboratory panels include fewer than 100 mutations. Newborn screening for CF is currently mandated in several states in the United States and will soon be widely expanded, on a voluntary state-by-state basis, subsequent to recent recommendations developed by the Centers for Disease Control and Prevention (CDC) and an advisory panel of CF experts[146] (see What's New?).

WHAT'S NEW? Newborn Screening for Cystic Fibrosis

Unfortunately, the diagnosis of cystic fibrosis is still frequently missed or significantly delayed, after perplexing and frustrating struggles for the child and family. Often there have been hospitalizations, unexplained recurrent respiratory symptoms, and failure to thrive. Several states piloted newborn screening for CF starting in the 1980s (Colorado, Wisconsin, and Wyoming) and several others have added programs since then. Long-term data shows that patients with CF identified by newborn screening have better nutritional status and growth than those identified by symptomatic presentation, not only at diagnosis but persisting for at least 7 years. This has important implications because poor nutritional status has been linked to poor clinical outcome over the long term. There has been less overwhelming evidence for pulmonary benefit related to neonatal screening for CF than for the nutritional benefits, although several studies support the presence of an advantage in pulmonary function and, possibly, delayed colonization with *Pseudomonas aeruginosa*. Based on available evidence, the Centers for Disease Control and Prevention issued a recommendation in 2004 supporting neonatal screening for CF. However, the methodologies involved in screening are rather cumbersome. They require more than one step of testing, a high level of support from CF centers and genetic counseling professionals, as well as education of primary physicians and the community. Difficult problems include handling initial false positives, appropriate information for those with select "mild" mutations that are not well understood, and making sure that the many CF gene carriers that will be identified do not misunderstand their status. States choosing to adopt screening will have to tailor the details of their programs to match available resources statewide.

Data from Castellani C: *Paediatric Resp Rev* 4(4):278-284, 2003; Centers for Disease Control and Prevention: *MMWR* 53(RR-13), 2004; Farrell PM et al: *Am J Respir Crit Care Med* 168(9):1100-1108, 2003; Farrell PM et al: *Pediatrics* 107(1):1-13, 2001; Lai HJ et al: *Am J Epidemiol* 159(6):537-546, 2004; Wang SS et al: *J Pediatr* 141(6):804-810, 2002.

Treatment is primarily focused on pulmonary health and on nutrition. Because the pulmonary decline in CF is slow and insidious, and because of the early onset of chronic inflammation and infection, treatment strategies begin immediately at diagnosis and are layered on over time as disease progresses. Universally, pulmonary therapies include techniques to promote mucus clearance, such as chest physical therapy and related equipment, such as the high-frequency chest wall oscillation vest, and an assortment of hand-held positive expiratory pressure (PEP) devices. Aerosol therapy includes bronchodilators and nebulized DNase, which acts to liquefy mucus and may even have anti-inflammatory effects.[147,148] Antibiotic practices vary, with both prophylactic and treatment strategies being used. Increasing emphasis has been placed on delaying and controlling *Pseudomonas* colonization.[137,149] *Pseudomonas aeruginosa* suppression using inhaled maintenance antibiotics (especially tobramycin) has been shown to have a beneficial clinical impact.[150] Oral macrolide antibiotics were recently reported to improve pulmonary function.[151,152] Intravenous antibiotics are used to treat major flare-ups of pulmonary infection, which may be either subacute or acute. Individuals with end-stage lung disease may consider lung transplantation.

Nutritional problems are extremely common in CF, and poor nutrition is correlated with worse outcomes including progression of lung disease and onset of additional complications such as decreased bone mineral density. Elements of aggressive nutritional support include meticulous monitoring of growth parameters, controlling fat malabsorption, ensuring adequate intake, and keeping overall health stable. Approximately 90% of children with CF have pancreatic insufficiency. This is the result of abnormal ion transport causing decreased fluid and bicarbonate secretion from the pancreatic acinar cells, which leads to thickened secretions plugging the smaller pancreatic ducts, and eventual autodigestion or atrophy of the acinar cells. Therefore, patients must take exogenous pancreatic enzymes with meals and snacks in order to absorb nutrients and control malabsorptive symptoms. Fat-soluble vitamins (A, D, E, and K) must be supplemented. Caloric needs are high, especially with advancing lung disease, and high-calorie supplements or even gastrostomy feeding may be warranted.

There is in fact a growing contingent of adults with CF living into their 40s and 50s. Gene therapy for this disease appears to be more complex than anticipated and is not close at hand, but trials are in progress;[153] meanwhile, aggressive care and a continuing stream of new therapies aimed at the triad of mucus, inflammation, and infection are continuing to improve the outlook for these individuals.

SUDDEN INFANT DEATH SYNDROME

Sudden infant death syndrome (SIDS) remains a disease of unknown cause and is the most common cause of unexplained infant death in Western countries.[154-156] It is defined as "sudden death of an infant under 1 year of age which remains unexplained after a thorough case investigation, including performance of a complete autopsy, examination of the death scene, and review of the clinical history."[157]

The incidence of SIDS is low during the first month of life but sharply increases in the second month of life, peaks at 3 to 4 months old, and is unusual after 6 months of age. It is more common in male (60%) than female (40%) infants. It almost always occurs during nighttime sleep, when infants are least likely to be observed. A seasonal variation has been noted, with higher frequencies during the winter months. This has been related to a higher rate of respiratory tract infection during those months, and such infections are often reported to have preceded the death, an association that has led to speculation regarding etiology.

Clinical risk groups include babies who were preterm or low birth weight, multiple births, and siblings of prior SIDS victims (fourfold to sixfold increased risk). The occurrence of an apparent life-threatening event seems to predict increased SIDS risk. Nevertheless, about three quarters of all SIDS victims have no known predisposing clinical risk factor.

Additional risk factors fall into the categories of socioeconomic or maternal factors, and factors in the baby's sleeping situation.[158-162] SIDS is more prevalent among infants of low or adverse socioeconomic status.[163-165] Maternal factors that predict increased SIDS risk are maternal smoking,[158] young maternal age (under 20 years), unmarried mother, less prenatal care, poverty, and illicit drug use. Risk factors that relate to the baby's sleeping situation are prone positioning (and to a lesser extent, side sleeping), sleeping on soft bedding, and overheating. Prone sleeping was concluded to be a major and modifiable risk factor. Young babies cannot yet roll over and reposition themselves. Epidemiologic studies have shown that SIDS rates decreased by 40% to 70% in countries, including the United States, where massive public campaigns warned against prone sleeping for infants.[154,156,166] Infants should sleep on their backs. Other avoidable risk factors include loose bedding materials and sleeping on top of any soft surface (such as sheepskins, quilts, comforters, pillows, adult-type mattresses, or waterbeds). Bed sharing with parents increases risk in some situations.[161,162,167] Overwrapping the infant or overheating the room also appear to increase risk, particularly if the infant is sleeping prone.

The etiology of SIDS remains unknown, but probably involves a combination of predisposing factors along with external stressors.[154,155] There has been longstanding interest in hypotheses involving impaired autonomic regulation, and failure of cardiovascular, ventilatory, and arousal responses to hypoxemia or hypercarbia, or to airway obstruction events.[168-171] This blunted responsiveness could be related to developmental immaturity, or as was suggested by recent studies, may be inducible by external factors such as exposure to maternal smoking or recent infection.[172,173] In fact, there is evidence that arousability from quiet sleep is depressed in infants after recent illness.[172] Others speculate that infection may be linked to SIDS on the basis of exaggerated inflammation, eosinophil degranulation, and massive cytokine release causing pulmonary or airway edema in response to either bacterial pathogens from the nasopharynx or viral respiratory tract infections. A number of investigators have noted various neuropathologic findings in SIDS victims.[174,175] Finally, there is growing evidence that genetic factors may predispose certain individuals to SIDS[176]; a number of candidate gene polymorphisms have been proposed based on epidemiologic evidence, including genes for the serotonin transporter, the complement component C4, and IL-10, an anti-inflammatory cytokine.[176-178]

Currently, the best strategy to reduce SIDS is avoidance of all the controllable risk factors, particularly unsafe sleeping practices and maternal smoking. Parents of infants with clinical risk should be taught cardiopulmonary resuscitation as a precaution. Although home monitoring has not been proven to decrease the incidence of SIDS, some at-risk infants may warrant cardiorespiratory monitoring after careful consideration of the individual situation.[179,180]

SUMMARY REVIEW

Structure and Function

1. The airways of infants and children are narrower than those of adults, thus making them more prone to obstruction.
2. Infants and young children continue to form new alveoli for several years after birth.
3. Surfactant production is an important marker of developmental maturity of the fetal lung.
4. The immature chest wall is soft and compliant, contributing to inefficient mechanisms of breathing.
5. Children have greater oxygen consumption than adults.
6. Immune mechanisms are not fully developed at birth, making young infants more susceptible to infection.
7. Physiologic control of breathing may be impaired during the first few weeks of life.

Pulmonary Disorders

1. Physical examination can provide important clues in assessing the location and nature of upper airway obstruction.
2. Upper airway infections can pose serious threats; these include bacterial tracheitis, retropharyngeal abscess, and peritonsillar infections. Recognition and rapid evaluation are crucial.
3. Viral croup (laryngotracheobronchitis) is the most common cause of acute upper airway obstruction in children and usually affects children ages 6 months to 5 years. Subglottic edema may be mild to severe. Parainfluenza is the most common cause.
4. Acute epiglottitis is a life-threatening emergency that is now rarely seen because of vaccination against *Haemophilus influenzae*, which had been the primary causative microorganism. Current cases usually represent vaccine failure or are caused by other bacteria, such as group A streptococci.
5. Aspiration of a foreign body should be considered whenever there is a sudden onset of stridor, coughing, wheezing, or hoarseness. This usually occurs in 1- to 3-year-olds. Occasionally, diagnosis is delayed and symptoms may be attributed to

Continued

asthma, bronchitis, or pneumonia without recognition of the underlying cause.

6. Chronic upper airway obstruction may be manifested by stridor, abnormal cry, wheezing, or dyspnea. The most common cause of stridor in infants is laryngomalacia. Other causes include subglottic stenosis, vocal cord paralysis, and vascular rings.

7. Obstructive sleep apnea usually occurs in older children rather than infants and is underdiagnosed. Typical symptoms are snoring, gasping, and restless sleep. The most common cause in children is adenotonsillar hypertrophy.

8. Respiratory distress syndrome (RDS) of the newborn usually occurs in premature infants who are born before surfactant production and alveolocapillary development are complete. Atelectasis and hypoventilation cause shunting, hypoxemia, and hypercapnia.

9. Bronchopulmonary dysplasia is a chronic lung disease of infancy that is usually the consequence of acute respiratory disease in the newborn period. Almost always this occurs in infants who were premature and required ventilatory support. Contributing factors include structural immaturity, inflammation, and disordered lung repair processes.

10. Bronchiolitis occurs in infants and toddlers, usually in the winter and early spring. It is caused by viruses, most commonly respiratory syncytial virus (RSV). There is extensive edema, inflammation, and damage to the bronchiolar epithelium. Injections of monoclonal antibody against RSV are recommended as a preventive measure for high-risk infants.

11. Childhood pneumonia can be caused by viruses, bacteria, or *Mycoplasma*. Lobar pneumonia is usually bacterial. Certain bacteria, such as *Staphylococcus aureus* and group A streptococci, can cause particularly fulminant disease, as well as abscesses and empyema.

12. Aspiration pneumonitis can occur because of lung inflammation from entry of any foreign substance, including food, drink, or chemicals. Aspiration of oropharyngeal bacteria can occur because of loss of protective reflexes in neurologically impaired children, or during anesthesia.

13. Acute respiratory distress syndrome (ARDS) is an acute, life-threatening condition characterized by severe hypoxemia, poor lung compliance, and diffuse densities on chest radiograph. It can be triggered by acute pulmonary insults or major systemic illness (e.g., sepsis) or trauma. High level ventilatory support is required, and mortality is significant.

14. Asthma is an obstructive airway disease with episodes of acute respiratory symptoms (cough, wheeze, dyspnea) and intermittent or chronic subacute symptoms. It is the most common chronic condition in children. It is a disease of local airway inflammation, with exacerbation in response to triggers, such as infections or allergens. Inflammatory cell infiltration, mucosal edema, mucous plugging of airways, and epithelial damage are seen, and there is evidence of long-term remodeling of airways.

15. Cystic fibrosis (CF) is an autosomal recessive disease characterized by thick, tenacious mucus, plugging of airways, chronic pulmonary infection, and bronchiectasis. The other major manifestations are digestive and nutritional, related to pancreatic insufficiency. Median survival is currently 32 years, with mortality primarily related to lung disease.

Sudden Infant Death Syndrome

1. Sudden infant death syndrome (SIDS) is a diagnosis of exclusion after thorough investigation and autopsy following sudden death of an infant under 6 months of age. Usually the event occurs during nighttime sleep.

2. The cause is unknown. However, some known risk factors are avoidable, such as maternal smoking, prone sleeping, soft bedding surfaces, and overheating. The incidence of SIDS has decreased significantly since public health campaigns have encouraged the supine sleeping position for babies.

Acute epiglottitis, 1255
Acute respiratory distress syndrome (ARDS), 1269
Angioedema, 1256
Aspiration pneumonitis, 1265
Asthma, 1265
Atypical pneumonia, 1264
Bacterial pneumonia, 1263
Bacterial tracheitis, 1254
Bronchiolitis, 1263
Bronchiolitis obliterans, 1265
Bronchopulmonary dysplasia (BPD), 1260
Chlamydia pneumoniae, 1264
Croup, 1254

Cystic fibrosis (CF), 1270
Cystic fibrosis transmembrane conductance regulator (CFTR), 1270
Diphtheria, 1254
Foreign body aspiration, 1256
Functional residual capacity (FRC), 1250
Hyaline membrane disease (HMD), 1258
Laryngomalacia, 1257
Laryngotracheobronchitis, 1254
Mycoplasma pneumoniae, 1264
Obstructive sleep apnea syndrome (OSAS), 1257
Peritonsillar abscess, 1254
Pneumonia, 1263

Respiratory distress syndrome (RDS) of the newborn, 1258
Spasmodic croup, 1255
Status asthmaticus, 1267
Stridor, 1252
Subglottic stenosis, 1257
Sudden infant death syndrome (SIDS), 1272
Surfactant, 1249
Tracheomalacia, 1257
Upper airway obstruction (UAO), 1252
Viral pneumonia, 1264
Vocal cord paralysis, 1257

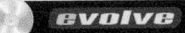
REFERENCES

1. Eavey RD: A sound workup for evaluating airway obstruction, *Contemp Pediatr* 3(6):78, 1986.
2. Leung AKC, Cho H: Diagnosis of stridor in children, *Am Fam Physician* 60(8):2289-2296, 1999.
3. Hammer J: Acquired upper airway obstruction, *Paediatr Respir Rev* 5(1):25-33, 2004.
4. Whiting JL, Chow AW: Life-threatening infections of the mouth and throat, *J Crit Illness* 2(7):36, 1987.
5. Brooke I: Microbiology and management of peritonsillar, retropharyngeal, and parapharyngeal abscesses, *J Oral Maxillofac Surg* 62(12):1545-1550, 2004.
6. Fitzgerald DA, Kilham HA: Croup: assessment and evidence based management, *Med J Aust* 179(7):372-377, 2003.
7. Knutson D, Aring A: Viral croup, *Am Fam Physician* 69(3):535-540, 2004.
8. Leung AK, Kellner JD, Johnson DW: Viral croup: a current perspective, *J Pediatr Health Care* 18(6):297-301, 2004.
9. Rittichier KK: The role of corticosteroids in the treatment of croup, *Treat Respir Med* 3(3):139-145, 2004.
10. Russell K et al: Glucocorticoids for croup, *Cochrane Database Syst Rev* (1):CD001955, 2004.
11. Hickerson SL et al: Epiglottitis: a 9-year case review, *South Med J* 89(5):487, 1996.
12. Carey MJ: Epiglottitis in adults, *Am J Emerg Med* 14(4):421-424, 1996.
13. Gonzalez-Valdapena H et al: Epiglottitis and Haemophilus influenzae immunization: the Pittsburgh experience—a five-year review, *Pediatrics* 96(3 pt 1):424, 1995.
14. Isaacson G, Isaacson DM: Pediatric epiglottitis caused by group G beta-hemolytic streptococcus, *Pediatr Infect Dis J* 22(9):846-847, 2003.
15. Wenger JK: Supraglottitis and group A *Streptococcus*, *Pediatr Infect Dis J* 16(10):1005-1007, 1997.
16. Blazer S, Naveh Y, Friedman A: Foreign body in the airway, a review of 200 cases, *Am J Dis Child* 134:68, 1980.
17. Kenna MA, Bluestone CD: Foreign bodies in the air and food passages, *Pediatr Rev* 10(1):25-31, 1988.
18. Fitzpatrick PC, Guarisco JL: Pediatric airway foreign bodies, *J La State Med Soc* 150(4):138-141, 1998.
19. Morley RE et al: Foreign body aspiration in infants and toddlers: recent trends in British Columbia, *J Otolaryngol* 33(1):37-41, 2004.
20. Halvorson DJ et al: Management of subglottic foreign bodies, *Ann Otol Rhinol Laryngol* 105(7):541-544, 1996.
21. Nielsen EW et al: C1 inhibitor and diagnosis of hereditary angioedema in newborns, *Pediatr Res* 35(2):184-187, 1994.
22. Quintana E, Attia MW: Angiotensin-converting enzyme inhibitor angioedema in a pediatric patient: a case report and discussion, *Pediatr Emerg Care* 17(6):438-440, 2001.
23. Zuran BL: Current and future therapy for hereditary angioedema, *Clin Immunol* 114(1):10-16, 2005.
24. Shinkwin CA, Gibbin KP: Tracheostomy in children, *J R Soc Med* 89(4):188-192, 1996.
25. Othersen HB Jr: Subglottic tracheal stenosis, *Semin Thorac Cardiovasc Surg* 6(4):200-205, 1994.
26. Brodner DC, Guarisco JL: Subglottic stenosis: evaluation and management, *J La State Med Soc* 151(4):159-164, 1999.
27. Cotton RT: Management of subglottic stenosis, *Otolaryngol Clin North Am* 33(1):111-130, 2000.
28. de Jong AL et al: Vocal cord paralysis in infants and children, *Otolaryngol Clin North Am* 33(1):131-149, 2000.
29. Gormley PK et al: Congenital vascular anomalies and persistent respiratory symptoms in children, *Int J Pediatr Otorhinolaryngol* 51(1):23-31, 1999.
30. Dennie CJ, Coblentz CL: The trachea: pathologic conditions and trauma, *Can Assoc Radiol* 44(3):157, 1993.
31. Dunham ME et al: Management of severe congenital tracheal stenosis, *Ann Otol Rhinol Laryngol* 103(5 Pt 1):351, 1994.
32. Chan J, Edman JC, Koltai PJ: Obstructive sleep apnea in children, *Am Fam Physician* 69(5):1147-1154, 2004.
33. Erler T, Paditz E: Obstructive sleep apnea syndrome in children: a state-of-the-art review, *Treat Respir Med* 3(2):107-122, 2004.
34. Arens R, Marcus CL: Pathophysiology of upper airway obstruction: a developmental perspective, *Sleep* 27(5):997-1019, 2004.
35. Schechter MS: Technical report: diagnosis and management of childhood obstructive sleep apnea syndrome, *Pediatrics* 109(4):e69, comment 704-712, 2002.
36. Massa F et al: The use of nasal continuous positive airway pressure to treat obstructive sleep apnoea, *Arch Dis Child* 87(5):438-443, 2002.
37. American Academy of Pediatrics: Clinical practice guidelines: diagnosis and management of childhood obstructive sleep apnea, *Pediatrics* 109(4):704-712, 2002.
38. Gozal D, O'Brien LM: Snoring and obstructive sleep apnoea in children: why should we treat? *Paediatr Respir Rev* 5(suppl A):S371-376, 2004.
39. Rosen CL: Obstructive sleep apnea syndrome in children: controversies in diagnosis and treatment, *Pediatr Clin North Am* 51(1):153-167, vii, 2004.
40. Fraser J, Walls M, McGuire W: Respiratory complications of preterm birth, *Br Med J* 329:962-965, 2004.
41. Verma RP: Respiratory distress syndrome of the newborn infant, *Obstet Gynecol Surv* 50(7):542-555, 1995.
42. Crowley P, Chalmers I, Keirse MJ: The effects of corticosteroid administration before preterm delivery: an overview of the evidence from controlled trials, *Br J Obstet Gynaecol* 97(1):11-25, 1990.
43. NIH Consensus Development Conference Statement: Effect of corticosteroids for fetal maturation on perinatal outcomes, *Am J Obstet Gynecol* 173:246, 1995.
44. Lacaze-Masmonteil T: Exogenous surfactant therapy: newer developments, *Semin Neonatol* 8(6):433-440, 2003.
45. Howlett A, Ohlsson A: Inositol for respiratory distress syndrome in preterm infants, *Cochrane Database Syst Rev* (4):CD000366, 2004.
46. Askie LM et al: Oxygen-saturation targets and outcomes in extremely preterm infants, *N Engl J Med* 349(10):959-967, 2003.
47. Donn SM, Sinha SK: Can mechanical ventilation strategies reduce chronic lung disease? *Sem Neonatol* 8(6):441-448, 2003.
48. Jobe AH, Ikegami M: Lung development and function in preterm infants in the surfactant treatment era, *Annu Rev Physiol* 62:825-846, 2000.
49. Shah S: Is elective high frequency oscillatory ventilation better than conventional mechanical ventilation in very low birth weight infants? *Arch Dis Child* 88(9):833-834, 2003.
50. Thome UH, Carlo WA: Permissive hypercapnia, *Semin Neonatol* 7(5):409-419, 2002.
51. Firer NN, Barrington KJ: Nitric oxide for respiratory failure in infants born at or near term, *Cochrane Database Syst Rev* CD000399(1), 2005.
52. Schreiber MD et al: Inhaled nitric oxide in premature infants with the respiratory distress syndrome, *N Engl J Med* 349(22):2099-2107, 2003.
53. Martin RJ: Nitric oxide for premies—not so fast, *N Engl J Med* 349(22):2157-2159, 2003.
54. Asikainen TM, White CW: Pulmonary antioxidant defenses in the preterm newborn with respiratory distress and bronchopulmonary dysplasia in evolution: implications for antioxidant therapy, *Antioxid Redox Signal* 6(1):155-167, 2004.
55. Baier RJ et al: CC chemokine concentrations increase in respiratory distress syndrome and correlate with development of bronchopulmonary dysplasia, *Pediatr Pulmonol* 37(2):137-148, 2004.
56. Jobe AH: Antenatal factors and the development of bronchopulmonary dysplasia, *Semin Neonatol* 8(1):9-17, 2003.
57. Northway WH Jr, Rosan RC, Porter DY: Pulmonary disease following respiratory therapy of hyaline-membrane disease: bronchopulmonary dysplasia, *N Engl J Med* 276(7):357-368, 1967.
58. Bancalari E, Claure N, Sosenko IRS: Bronchopulmonary dysplasia: changes in pathogenesis, epidemiology, and definition, *Semin Neonatol* 8(1):63-71, 2003.
59. Van Marter LJ et al: Do clinical markers of barotrauma and oxygen toxicity explain interhospital variation in rates of chronic lung disease? *Pediatrics* 105(6):1194-1201, 2000.

60. Gonzalez A et al: Influence of infection on patent ductus arteriosus and chronic lung disease in premature infants weighing 1000 grams or less, *J Pediatr* 128(4):470-478, 1996.

61. Jobe AH, Ikegami M: Mechanisms initiating lung injury in the preterm, *Early Hum Dev* 53(1):81-94, 1998.

62. Van Marter LJ et al: Chorioamnionitis, mechanical ventilation, and postnatal sepsis as modulators of chronic lung disease in preterm infants, *J Pediatr* 140(2):171-176, 2002.

63. Eber E, Zach MS: Long term sequelae of bronchopulmonary dysplasia (chronic lung diseases of infancy), *Thorax* 56(4):317-323, 2001.

64. Coalson JJ: Pathology of new bronchopulmonary dysplasia, *Semin Neonatol* 8(1):73-81, 2003.

65. Speer CP: Inflammation and bronchopulmonary dysplasia, *Semin Neonatol* 9(1):20-38, 2003.

66. Groneck P et al: Bronchoalveolar inflammation following airway infection in preterm infants with chronic lung disease, *Pediatr Pulmonol* 31(5):331-338, 2001.

67. Jonsson B et al: Early increase of TNF-α and IL-6 in tracheobronchial aspirate fluid indicator of subsequent chronic lung disease in preterm infants, *Arch Dis Child Fetal Neonatal Ed* 77(3):F198-F201, 1997.

68. Yoon BH et al: Amniotic fluid cytokines (interleukin-6, tumor necrosis factor-alpha, interleukin-1 beta, and interleukin-8) and the risk for the development of bronchopulmonary dysplasia, *Am J Obstet Gynecol* 177(4):825-830, 1997.

69. Grier DG, Halliday HL: Corticosteroids in the prevention and maintenance of bronchopulmonary dysplasia, *Semin Neonatol* 8(1):83-91, 2003.

70. Ambalavanan N et al: A comparison of three vitamin A dosing regimens in extremely-low-birthweight infants, *J Pediatr* 142(6):656-661, 2003.

71. Mentro AM: Vitamin A and bronchopulmonary dysplasia: research, issues and related clinical practice, *Neonatal Netw* 23(4):19-21, 2004.

72. Bhandari A, Bhandari V: Pathogenesis, pathology, and pathophysiology of pulmonary sequelae of bronchoppulmonary dysplasia in premature infants, *Front Biosci* 8:e370-e380, 2003.

73. Doyle LW et al: Bronchopulmonary dysplasia and very low birth weight: lung function at 11 years of age, *J Paediatrics Child Health* 32(4):339-343, 1996.

74. Mai XM et al: Asthma, lung function and allergy in 12-year-old children with very low birth weight: a prospective study, *Ped Allergy Immunol* 14(3):184-192, 2003.

75. Ogra PL: Respiratory syncytial virus, the disease and the immune response, *Paediatr Respir Rev* 5(Suppl A):S119-S126, 2004.

76. Castleman WL et al: Viral bronchiolitis during early life induces increased numbers of bronchiolar mast cells and airway hyperresponsiveness, *Am J Pathol* 137(4):821-831, 1990.

77. Martinez FD: Respiratory syncytial virus bronchiolitis and the pathogenesis of childhood asthma, *Pediatr Infect Dis J* 22(2 Suppl):S76-S82, 2003.

78. Piedimonte G: Contribution of neuroimmune mechanisms to airway inflammation and remodeling during and after respiratory syncytial virus infection, *Pediatr Infect Dis J* 22(2 Suppl):S66-S74, 2003.

79. Plint AC et al: Practice variation among pediatric emergency departments in the treatment of bronchiolitis, *Acad Emerg Med* 11(4):353-360, 2004.

80. Patel H et al: Glucocorticoids for acute viral bronchiolitis in infants and young children, *Cochrane Database Syst Rev* (3):CD004878, 2004.

81. Steiner RW: Treating acute bronchiolitis associated with RSV, *Am Fam Physician* 15(69):325-330, 2004.

82. Ostapchuk M, Roberts, DM, Haddy R: Community-acquired pneumonia in infants and children, *Am Fam Physician* 70(5):899-908, 2004.

83. Schuchat A, Dowell SF: Pneumonia in children in the developing world: new challenes, new solutions, *Semin Pediatr Infect Dis* 15(3):181-189, 2004.

84. Light RB: Pulmonary pathophysiology of pneumococcal pneumonia, *Semin Respir Infect* 14(3):218-226, 1999.

85. Ozcelik C et al: Management of postpneumonic empyemas in children, *Eur J Cardiothorac Surg* 25(6):1072-1078, 2004.

86. Schultz KD et al: The changing face of pleural empyemas in children: epidemiology and management, *Pediatrics* 113(6):1735-1740, 2004.

87. Sinaniotis CA: Viral pneumoniae in children: incidence and aetiology, *Paediatr Respir Rev* 5(Suppl A):S197-S200, 2004.

88. Hammerschlag MR: Pneumonia due to *Chlamydia pneumoniae* in children: epidemiology, diagnosis, and treatment, *Pediatr Pulmonol* 36(5):384-390, 2003.

89. Waites KB: New concepts of *Mycoplasma pneumoniae* infections in children, *Pediatr Pulmonol* 36(4):267-278, 2003.

90. Low DE, Pichichero ME, Schaad UB: Optimizing antibacterial therapy for community-acquired respiratory tract infections in children in an era of bacterial resistance, *Clin Pediatr (Phil)* 43(2):135-151, 2004.

91. Marcinak & Frank AL: Treatment of community-acquired methicillin-resistant *Staphylococcus aureus* in children, *Curr Opin Infect Dis* 16(3):265-269, 2003.

92. Posfay-Barbe KM, Wald ER: Pneumococcal vaccines: do they prevent infection and how? *Curr Opin Infect Dis* 17(3):177-184, 2004.

93. Vilchez RA, Dauber J, Kusne S: Infectious etiology of bronchiolitis obliterans: the respiratory viruses connections—myth or reality? *Am J Transplant* 3(3):245-249, 2003.

94. Chan PW, Muridan R, Debruyne JA: Bronchiolitis obliterans in children: clinical profile and diagnosis, *Respirology* 5(4):269-275, 2000.

95. Weiss KB, Gergen PJ, Crain EE: Inner-city asthma: the epidemiology of an emerging US public health concern, *Chest* 101(6 Suppl):362S, 1992.

96. Asthma mortality and hospitalization among children and young adults—United States, 1980-1993, *MMWR* 45(17):350, 1996.

97. Sly RM: Decreases in asthma mortality in the United States, *Ann Allergy, Asthma, Immunol* 85(2):121-127, 2000.

98. Chipps BE: Determinants of asthma and its clinical course, *Ann Allergy, Asthma, Immunol* 93(4):309-315, 2004.

99. Jacoby DB: Virus-induced asthma attacks, *J Aerosol Med* 17(2):169-173, 2004.

100. Gern JE: Viral and bacterial infections in the development and progression of asthma, *J Allergy Clin Immunol* 105(2 Pt 2):S497, 2000.

101. Nafstad P, Magnus P, Jaakkola JJK: Early respiratory infections and childhood asthma, *Pediatrics* 106(3):E38, 2000.

102. Holt PG et al: Microbial stimulation as an aetiologic factor in atopic disease, *Allergy* 54(Suppl 49):12-16, 1999.

103. Martinez FD et al: Asthma and wheezing in the first six years of life, *N Engl J Med* 332(3):133-138, 1995.

104. Platts-Mills TA, Rakes G, Heymann PW: The relevance of allergen exposure to the development of asthma in childhood, *J Allergy Clin Immunol* 105(2 Pt 2):S503-S508, 2000.

105. Colavita AM, Reinach AJ, Peters SP: Contributing factors to the pathobiology of asthma: the Th1/Th2 paradigm, *Clin Chest Med* 21(2):263-277, 2000.

106. Fahy JV: Reducing IgE levels as a strategy for the treatment of asthma, *Clin Exp Allergy* 30(suppl 1):16-21, 2000.

107. Romagnani S: The increased prevalence of allergy and hygiene hypothesis: missing immune deviation, reduced immune suppression, or both? *Immunol* 112(3):352-363, 2004.

108. Sheikh A, Strachan DP: The hygiene theory: fact or fiction? *Curr Opin Otolaryngol Neck Head Surg* 12(3):232-236, 2004.

109. Von Hertzen LF, Haahtela T: Asthma and atopy—the price of affluence? *Allergy* 59(2):124-137, 2004.

110. Braun-Fahrlander C: Environmental exposure to endotoxin and other microbial products and the decreased risk of childhood atopy: evaluating developments since April 2002, *Curr Opin Allergy Clin Immunol* 3(5):325-329, 2003.

111. Platts-Mills TA, Carter MC, Heymann PW: Specific and nonspecific obstructive lung disease in childhood: causes of changes in the prevalence of asthma, *Environ Health Perspect* 108(Suppl 4):725-731, 2000.

112. Kemp A, Bjorksten B: Immune deviation and the hygiene hypothesis: a review of the epidemiological evidence, *Pediatr Allergy Immunol* 14(2):74-80, 2003.

113. Platts-Mills TA, Rakes G, Heymann PW: The relevance of allergen exposure to the development of asthma in childhood, *J Allergy Clin Immunol* 105(2 Pt 2):S503-S508, 2000.

114. Howard TD, Meyers DA, Bleecker ER: Mapping susceptibility genes for asthma and allergy, *J Allergy Clin Immunol* 105(2 Pt 2):S477-S481, 2000.

115. Pelaia G et al: Potential genetic influences on the response to asthma treatment, *Pulmon Pharmacol Ther* 17(5):253-261, 2004.

116. Hakonarson H, Grunstein MM: Autocrine regulation of airway smooth muscle responsiveness, *Respir Physiol Neurobiol* 137(2-3):263-276, 2003.

117. Heymann PW et al: Viral infections in relation to age, atopy, and season of admission among children hospitalized for wheezing, *J Allergy Clin Immunol* 114(2):239-247, 2004.

118. Berger WE: Levalbuterol: pharmacologic properties and use in the treatment of pediatric and adult asthma, *Ann Allergy, Asthma, Immunol* 90(6):583-591, 2003.

119. Scarfone RJ, Friedlaender EY: Beta2-agonists in acute asthma: the evolving state of the art, *Pediatr Emerg Care* 18(6):442-447, 2002.

120. Streetman DD, Bhatt-Mehta V, Johnson CE: Management of acute, severe asthma in children, *Ann Pharmacother* 36(7-8):1249-1260, 2002.

121. Plotnick LH, Ducharme FM: Acute asthma in children and adolescents: should inhaled anticholinergics be added to beta(2)-agonists? *Am J Respir Med* 2(2):109-115, 2003.

122. National Institutes of Health, National Heart, Lung, and Blood Institute: *Expert panel report 2: guidelines for the diagnosis and management of asthma*, NIH Pub. No. 97-4051A, 1997.

123. Bisgaard H: Leukotriene modifiers in pediatric asthma management, *Pediatrics* 107(2):381-390, 2001.

124. Szefler SJ: Current concepts in asthma treatment for children, *Curr Opin Pediatrics* 16(3):299-304, 2004.

125. Andersson F et al: Comparison or the cost-effectiveness of budesonide and sodium cromoglycate in the management of childhood asthma in everyday clinical practice, *Ann Allergy, Asthma, Immunol* 86(5): 537-544, 2001.

126. van der Wouden JC et al: Inhaled sodium cromoglycate for asthma in children, *Cochrane Database Syst Rev* (3):CD002173, 2003.

127. Zimmermann T et al: Salmeterol versus sodium cromoglycate for the protection of exercise-induced asthma in children—a randomised cross-over study, *Euro J Med Res* 8(9):428-434, 2003.

128. Schears GJ, Costarino AT: Complexity of inflammatory mediators in acute respiratory distress syndrome (ARDS), *J Pediatr* 135(2 Pt 1): 144-146, 1999.

129. Soubani AO, Pieroni R: Acute respiratory distress syndrome: a clinical update, *South Med J* 92(5):450-457, 1999.

130. Moloney-Harmon PA: When the lung fails. Acute respiratory distress syndrome in children, *Crit Care Nursing Clin North Am* 11(4):519-528, 1999.

131. Mehta NM, Arnold JH: Mechanical ventilation in children with acute respiratory failure, *Curr Opin Crit Care*, 10(1):7-12, 2004.

132. Priestley MA, Helfaer MA: Approaches to the management of acute respiratory failure in children, *Curr Opin Pediatr* 16(3):293-298, 2004.

133. Prodhan P, Noviski N: Pediatric acute hypoxemic respiratory failure: management of oxygenation, *J Intensive Care Med* 19(3):140-153, 2004.

134. Sokol J, Jacobs SE, Bohn D: Inhaled nitric oxide for acute hypoxemic respiratory failure in children and adults, *Cochrane Database Syst Rev* (1):CD002787, 2003.

135. Kosorok MR, Wei WH, Farrell PM: The incidence of cystic fibrosis, *Stat Med* 15(5):449, 1996.

136. Boucher RC: New concepts of the pathogenesis of cystic fibrosis lung disease, *Eur Respir J* 23(1):156-158, 2004.

137. Gibson RL, Burns JL, Ramsey BW: Pathophysiology and management of pulmonary infections in cystic fibrosis, *Am J Respir Crit Care Med* 168(8):918-951, 2003.

138. Verkman AS, Song Y, Thiagarajah JR: Role of airway surface liquid and submucosal glands in cystic fibrosis lung disease, *Am J Physiol Cell Physiol* 284(1):C2-C15, 2003.

139. Koehler DR et al: Lung inflammation as a therapeutic target in cystic fibrosis, *Am J Respir Cell Mol Biol* 31(4):377-381, 2004.

140. Khan TZ et al: Early pulmonary inflammation in infants with cystic fibrosis, *Am J Respir Crit Care Med* 151(4):1075-1082, 1995.

141. Bonfield TL, Konstan MW, Berger M: Altered respiratory epithelial cell cytokine production in cystic fibrosis, *J Allergy Clin Immunol* 104(1):72-78, 1999.

142. Conese M et al: Neutrophil recruitment and airway epithelial cell involvement in chronic cystic fibrosis lung disease, *J Cyst Fibros* 2(3):129-135, 2003.

143. Elkin S, Geddes D: Pseudomonal infection in cystic fibrosis: the battle continues, *Expert Rev Anti Infect Ther* 1(4):609-618, 2003.

144. Emerson J et al: *Pseudomonas aeruginosa* and other predictors of mortality and morbidity in young children with cystic fibrosis, *Pediatr Pulmonol* 34(23):91-100, 2002.

145. Sontag MK, Accurso FJ: Gene modifiers in pediatrics: application to cystic fibrosis, *Adv Pediatr* 51:5-36, 2004.

146. Grosse SD et al: Newborn screening for cystic fibrosis: evaluation of benefits and risks and recommendations for state newborn screening programs, *MMWR* 53(RR-13):1-36, 2004.

147. Paul K et al: Effect of treatment with dornase alpha on airway inflammation in patients with cystic fibrosis, *Am J Respir Crit Care Med* 169(6):719-725, 2004.

148. Robinson PJ: Dornase alfa in early cystic fibrosis lung disease, *Pediatr Pulmonol* 34(3):237-341, 2002.

149. Rosenfeld M, Ramsey BW, Gibson RL: *Pseudomonas* acquisition in young patients with cystic fibrosis: Pathophysiology, diagnosis, and management, *Curr Opin Pulmon Med* 9(6):492-497, 2003.

150. Burns JL et al: Effect of chronic intermittent administration of inhaled tobramycin on respiratory microbial flora in patients with cystic fibrosis, *J Infect Dis* 179(5):1190-1196, 1999.

151. Equi A et al: Long term azithromycin in children with cystic fibrosis: a randomized, placebo–controlled crossover trial, *Lancet* 360(9338): 978-984, 2002.

152. Saiman L et al: Azithromycin in patients with cystic fibrosis chronically infected with *Pseudomonas aeruginosa*: a randomized controlled trial, *JAMA* 290(13):1749-1756, 2003.

153. Klink D et al: Gene delivery systems—gene therapy vectors for cystic fibrosis, *J Cyst Fibros* 3(Suppl 2):203-212, 2004.

154. Daley KC: Update on sudden infant death syndrome, *Curr Opin Pediatr* 16(2):227-232, 2004.

155. Byard RW, Krous HF: Sudden infant death syndrome: overview and update, *Perspect Pediatr Pathol* 6:112-127, 2003.

156. American Academy of Pediatrics Task Force on Infant Sleep Position and Sudden Infant Death Syndrome: Changing concepts of sudden infant death syndrome: implications for infant sleeping environment and sleep position, *Pediatrics* 105(3 Pt 1):650-656, 2000.

157. Willinger M, James LS, Catz C: Defining the sudden infant death syndrome: deliberations of an expert panel convened by the National Institute of Child Health and Human Development, *Pediatr Pathol* 11:677-684, 1991.

158. Alm B et al: A case-control study of smoking and sudden infant death syndrome in the Scandinavian countries, 1992 to 1995. The Nordic Epidemiological SIDS Study, *Arch Dis Child* 78(4):329-334, 1998.

159. Daltveit AK et al: Sociodemographic risk factors for sudden infant death syndrome: associations with other risk factors. The Nordic Epidemiological SIDS Study, *Acta Paediatr* 87(3):284-290, 1998.

160. Leach CE et al: Epidemiology of SIDS and explained sudden infant deaths. CESDI SUDI Research Group, *Pediatrics* 104(4):e43, 1999.

161. Mitchell EA et al: Risk factors for sudden infant death syndrome following the prevention campaign in New Zealand: a prospective study, *Pediatrics* 100(5):835-840, 1997.

162. Kemp JS et al: Unsafe sleep practices and an analysis of bedsharing among infants dying suddenly and unexpectedly: results of a four-year, population-based, Death-Scene Investigation Study of Sudden Infant Death Syndrome and Related Deaths, *Pediatrics* 106(3):E41, 2000.

163. Hauck FR et al: Sleep environment and the risk of sudden infant death in an urban population: the Chicago Infant Mortality Study, *Pediatrics* 111(5 Pt 2):1207-1214, 2003.

164. Samuels M: Virsues and sudden infant death, *Paediatr Respir Rev* 4(3):178-183, 2003.

165. Spencer N, Logan S: Sudden unexpected death in infancy and socioeconomic status: a systematic review, *J Epidemiol Community Health* 58(5):366-374, 2004.

166. de Jonge GA et al: Sleeping position for infants and cot death in the Netherlands 1985-1991, *Arch Dis Child* 69(6):660-663, 1993.

167. Berkowitz CD: Cosleeping: benefits, risks, and cautions, *Adv Pediatr* 51:329-349,2004.

168. Givan DC: Physiology of breathing and related pathological processes in infants, *Semin Pediatr Neurol* 10(4):271-280, 2003.

169. Horne RS, Parslow PM, Harding R: Respiratory control and arousal in sleeping infants, *Paediatr Respir Rev* 5(3):190-198, 2004.

170. Kahn A et al: Sudden infant deaths: stress, arousal and SIDS, *Early Hum Dev* 75(Suppl)S147-S166, 2003.

171. Franco P, Szliwowski H, Dramix M et al: Decreased autonomic responses to obstructive sleep events in future victims of sudden infant death syndrome, *Pediatr Res* 46:33-39, 1999.

172. Horne RS et al: Influences of maternal cigarette smoking on infant arousability, *Early Hum Dev* 79(1):49-58, 2004.

173. Horne R, Osborne A, Vitkovic J et al: Arousal from sleep in infants is impaired following an infection, *Early Hum Dev* 66:89-100, 2002.

174. Valdes-Dapena M: The sudden infant death syndrome: pathologic findings, *Clin Perinatol* 19:701-716, 1992.

175. Matturri L, Biondo B, Suarez-Mier MP: Brain stem lesions in the sudden infant death syndrome: variability in the hypoplasia of the arcuate nucleus, *Acta Neuropathol* 104: 12-20, 2002.

176. Hunt CE: Gene-environment interactions: implications for sudden unexpected deaths in infancy, *Arch Dis Child* 90(1):48-53, 2005.

177. Narita N, Narita M, Takashima S et al: Serotonin transporter gene variation is a risk factor for sudden infant death syndrome in the Japanese population, *Pediatr* 107:690-692, 2001.

178. Opdal SH, Vege A, Stave AK et al: The complement component C4 in sudden infant death, *Eur J Pediatr* 158:210-212, 1999.

179. Summers AM, Summers CW, Drucker DB et al: Association of IL-10 genotype with sudden infant death syndrome, *Hum Immunol* 61: 1270-1273, 2000.

180. Committee on Fetus and Newborn, American Academy of Pediatrics: Apnea, sudden infant death syndrome, and home monitoring, *Pediatrics* 111(4 Pt 1):914-917, 2003.

STRUCTURE AND FUNCTION OF THE RENAL AND UROLOGIC SYSTEMS

SUE E. HUETHER

CHAPTER OUTLINE

The primary function of the kidney is to maintain a stable internal environment for optimal cell and tissue metabolism. The kidneys accomplish these life-sustaining tasks by balancing solute and water transport, excreting metabolic waste products, conserving nutrients, and regulating acids and bases. The kidney also has an endocrine function, secreting the hormones renin, erythropoietin, and 1,25-dihydroxyvitamin D_3 for regulation of blood pressure, erythrocyte production, and calcium metabolism, respectively. In times of severe fasting the kidney also can synthesize glucose from amino acids, performing the process of gluconeogenesis. The formation of urine is achieved through the processes of filtration, reabsorption, and secretion by the glomeruli and tubules within the kidney. The bladder stores the urine that it receives from the kidney by way of the ureters. Urine is then removed from the body through the urethra.

STRUCTURES OF THE RENAL SYSTEM

Structures of the Kidney

The **kidneys** are paired organs located on the posterior abdominal wall outside the peritoneal cavity. They lie on either side of the vertebral column with their upper and lower poles extending from the twelfth thoracic to the third lumbar vertebrae (Figure 35-1). Each kidney is approximately 11 cm long, 5 to 6 cm wide, and 3 to 4 cm thick. A tightly adhering capsule (the **renal capsule**) surrounds each kidney, and the kidney then is embedded in a mass of fat. The capsule and fatty layer are covered with a double layer of **renal fascia,** fibrous tissue that attaches the kidney to the posterior abdominal wall.

The cushion of fat and the position of the kidney between the abdominal organs and muscles of the back protect it from trauma. The right kidney is slightly lower than the left; it is displaced downward by the overlying liver. A medial indentation (the **hilum**) contains the entry and exit for the renal blood vessels, nerves, lymphatic vessels, and ureter.

The gross structure of the kidney can be identified when it is divided from top to bottom in a coronal plane (Figure 35-2). The major components are the outer **renal cortex** and the inner **renal medulla.** The cortex contains all the glomeruli and portions of the tubules. The medulla is formed by the straight segments of the proximal and distal tubules and the collecting ducts. It consists of a series of wedges, called **renal pyramids,** with an outer zone close to the cortex and an inner zone. **Renal columns** extend from the cortex down between the renal pyramids. The apexes of the pyramids project into a **minor calyx** (a cup-shaped cavity), which joins together to form a **major calyx.** The major calyces join to form the **renal pelvis,** an extension of the upper end of the ureter. The walls of the calyces and ureters contain smooth muscles that contract to move urine to the bladder.

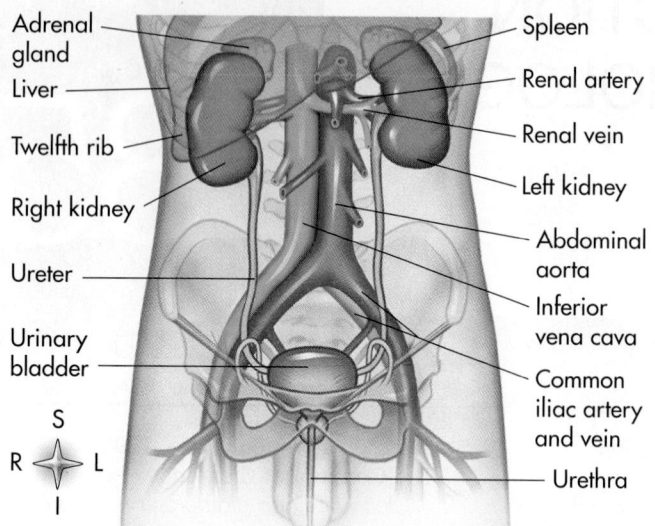

Figure 35-1 Organs of the urinary system. (From Thibodeau GA, Patton KT: *Anatomy & physiology,* ed 5, St Louis, 2003, Mosby.)

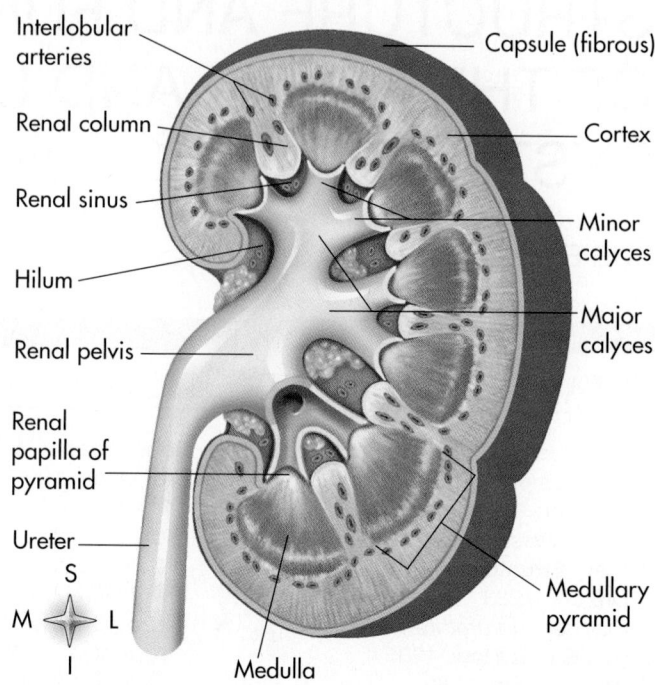

Figure 35-2 Kidney structure. (From Thibodeau GA, Patton KT: *Anatomy & physiology,* ed 5, St Louis, 2003, Mosby.)

The structural unit of the kidney is the lobe. Each lobe is composed of a pyramid and the overlying cortex. There are about 14 lobes in each kidney.

Nephron

The **nephron** is the functional unit of the kidney. Approximately 1.2 million nephrons are contained in each kidney. The nephron is a tubular structure with subunits that include the renal corpuscle, proximal convoluted tubule, loop of Henle, distal convoluted tubule, and collecting duct, all of which contribute to the formation of final urine (Figure 35-3). The different structures of the epithelial cells lining various segments of the tubule facilitate the special functions of secretion and reabsorption (Figure 35-4).

The kidney has three kinds of nephrons: (1) **superficial cortical nephrons** (85% of all nephrons), which extend only partially into the medulla; (2) **midcortical nephrons** with short or long loops; and (3) **juxtamedullary nephrons,** which lie close to and extend deep into the medulla and are important for the process of concentrating urine (Figure 35-5). The **glomerulus** (Figure 35-6; see also Figure 35-3) is a tuft of capillaries, the glomerular capillaries, that loop into a circular capsule, the **Bowman capsule,** like fingers pushed into bread dough. **Mesangial cells** (shaped like smooth muscle cells) and the mesangial matrix lie between and support the glomerular capillaries.[1] They have contractile and phagocytic properties, similar to monocytes, and produce vasoactive substances that may influence the glomerular filtration rate (GFR) by regulating glomerular capillary blood flow. The space inside the Bowman capsule is called the **Bowman space.** Together, the glomerulus, Bowman capsule, and mesangial cells are called the **renal corpuscle.**

The wall of the glomerular capillary serves as a filtration membrane (the **glomerular filtration membrane**) and has

three layers: (1) an inner capillary endothelium, (2) a middle basement membrane, and (3) an outer layer of capillary epithelium (also called *podocytes* or *visceral epithelium*). Each layer has unique structural properties that allow all components of the blood to filter through, with the exception of blood cells and plasma proteins with a molecular weight greater than 70,000 (Figure 35-7; see also Figure 35-6). The **glomerular endothelium** is composed of cells in continuous contact with the basement membrane. Glomerular endothelial cells synthesize both nitric oxide (a vasodilator) and endothelin-1 (a vasoconstrictor important to regulating glomerular blood flow). The glomerular endothelium is perforated by many small openings or windows, called *fenestrae.* The fenestra are maintained by vascular epithelial growth factor (VEGF) produced by visceral epithelium. The middle basement membrane is a negatively charged, selectively permeable network of glycoproteins and mucopolysaccharides and may be secreted and maintained by the epithelial cells.[2] The **visceral epithelium,** also called **podocytes,**[3] have footlike processes that radiate and adhere to the basement membrane covering the glomerular capillaries. The visceral epithelium is reflected back at the vascular pole to become the **parietal epithelium.** The space between the visceral and parietal epithelium is the Bowman space, which continues to become the proximal tubule. The foot processes of one podocyte interlock with the foot processes of adjacent podocytes, forming an elaborate network of intercellular clefts. These clefts are called **filtration slits,** or slit membranes, and modulate filtration. *Nephrin, podocin,* and *CD2-associated protein* are proteins that are exclusively located in the slit membrane and are

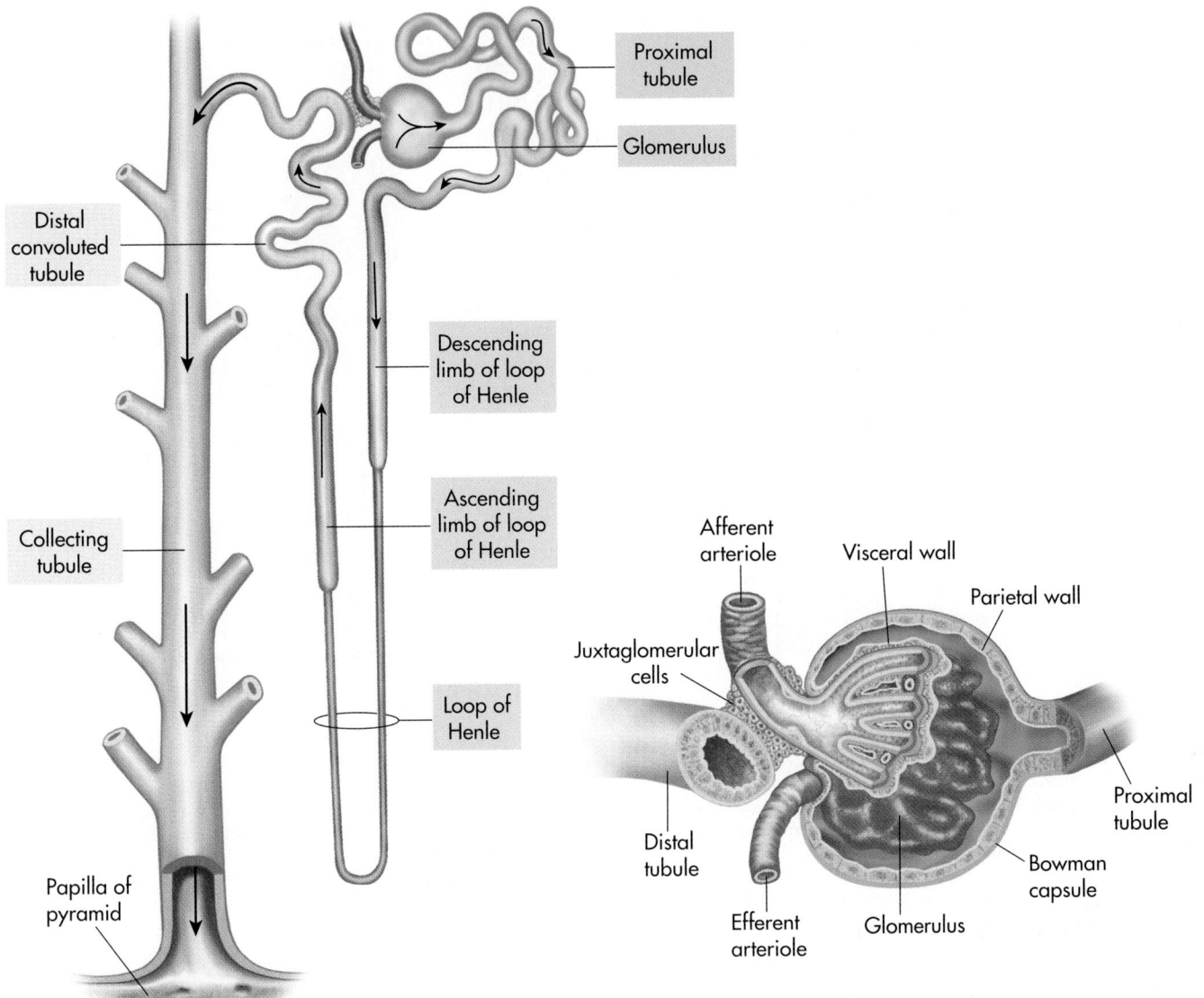

Figure 35-3 Components of the nephron. (From Thibodeau GA, Patton KT: *Anatomy & physiology,* ed 5, St Louis, 2003, Mosby.)

required for normal filtration.[4] The podocytes are endocytic, which allows molecules to enter the cell without passing through the cell membrane.

The glomerular filtration membrane separates the blood of the glomerular capillaries from the fluid in the Bowman space. The glomerular filtrate passes through the three layers of the glomerular membrane and forms the primary urine. The endothelial cells and basement membrane of the filtration membrane express negatively charged glycoproteins and form a filtration barrier to anionic proteins.

The glomerulus is supplied by the afferent arteriole and drained by the efferent arteriole. A group of specialized cells known as **juxtaglomerular cells** are located around the afferent arteriole where it enters the renal corpuscle (see Figure 35-3). Between the afferent and efferent arterioles is a portion of the distal convoluted tubule with specialized sodium and chloride-sensing cells known as **macula densa** (see Figure 35-6). Together the juxtaglomerular cells and macula densa cells form the **juxtaglomerular apparatus (JGA)** (see Figure 35-3). Control of renal blood flow, glomerular filtration, and renin secretion occurs at this site.

The **proximal tubule** continues from the Bowman space and has an initial convoluted segment (pars convoluta) and then a straight segment (pars recta) that descends toward the medulla (see Figure 35-3). The proximal tubular lumen consists of one layer of cuboidal cells with a surface layer of microvilli that increases reabsorptive surface area. This is the only surface inside the nephron where the cells are covered with microvilli (a brush border) (see Figure 35-4). The proximal tubule joins the **loop of Henle,** a hairpin-shaped loop composed of thick and thin portions of a descending segment that goes into the medulla. The tube then loops and becomes

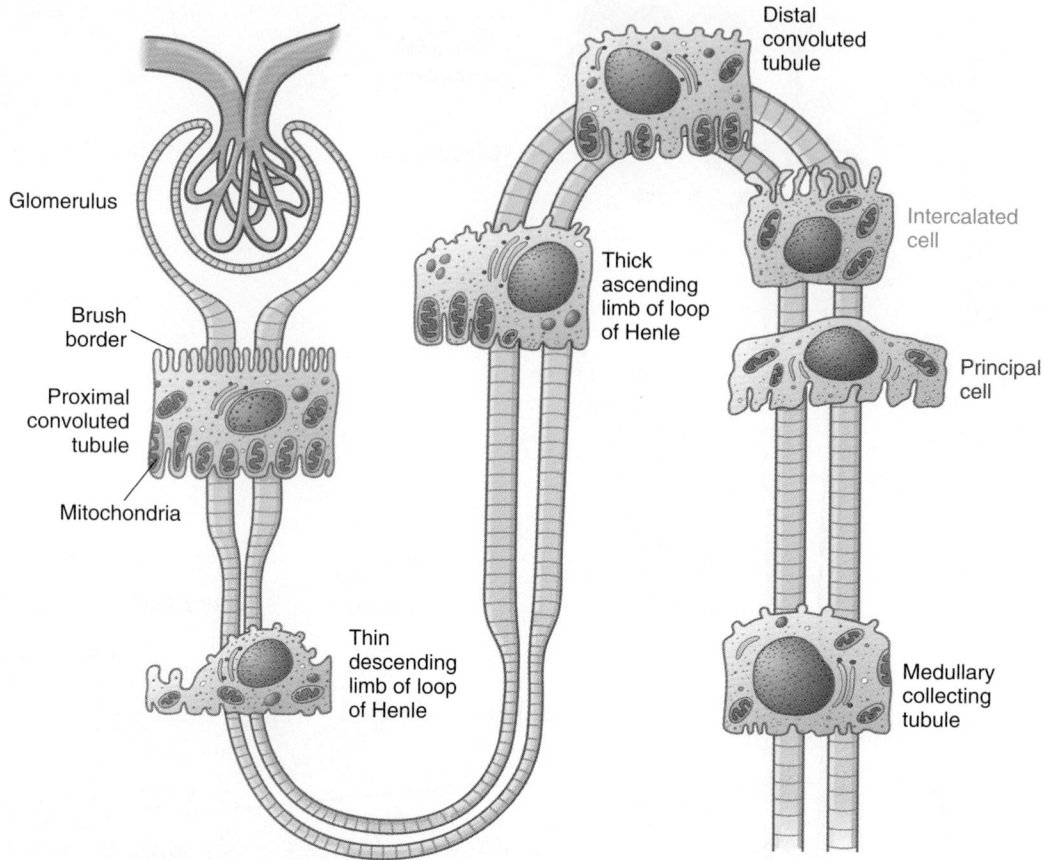

Figure 35-4 Epithelial cells of the various segments of nephron tubules. The brush border and high number of mitochondria in the cells of the proximal convoluted tubule permit reabsorption of 60% of the glomerular filtrate. *Intercalated cells* (blue) secrete either H^+ (reabsorb HCO_3^-) or HCO_3^- and reabsorb K^+. *Principal cells* (magenta) reabsorb Na^+ and water and secrete K^+.

the thickening ascending segment that extends toward the cortex. The thin segment is composed of thin squamous cells with no active transport function. The cells of the thick segment are cuboidal and actively transport several solutes.

The more numerous cortical nephrons have glomeruli originating close to the surface of the cortex or in the mid-cortex, unlike the juxtamedullary nephrons, whose glomeruli are located deep in the cortex close to the medulla. The major structural difference between the glomeruli in the two types of nephrons is the length of the loop of Henle. In cortical nephrons the loop is short and may not extend into the medulla. The loops of Henle for the juxtamedullary nephrons, however, may extend the whole length of the medulla (40 mm). Juxtamedullary nephrons represent about 12% of the total number of nephrons.

The **distal tubule** has convoluted and straight segments. It extends from the macula densa to the **collecting duct.** The collecting duct is a large tubule that descends down the cortex, through the renal pyramids of the inner and outer medullae, and into the minor calyx. The collecting duct is composed of two cell types: principle cells and intercalated cells (see Figure 34-4). **Principle cells** resorb sodium and water and secrete potassium. **Intercalated cells** secrete either hydrogen or bicarbonate and reabsorb potassium.

Blood Vessels

The blood vessels of the kidney closely parallel nephron structure. The **renal arteries** arise as the fifth branches of the abdominal aorta. At the renal hilum they divide into anterior and posterior branches and then subdivide into lobar arteries that supply blood to the lower, middle, and upper thirds of the kidney. The **interlobar arteries** are further subdivisions that travel down the renal columns and between the pyramids. At the cortical medullary junction, interlobar arteries branch into the **arcuate arteries**, which arch over the base of the pyramids and run parallel to the surface of the kidney.

The interlobular arteries arise from the arcuate arteries and extend through the cortex toward the periphery and form the afferent glomerular arterioles (see Figure 35-5). The afferent arteriole subdivides into a fistlike structure of four to eight **glomerular capillaries** (see Figure 35-6). The glomerular capillaries empty into the efferent arteriole, which conveys blood to a second capillary bed, the peritubular capillaries. This is the only place in the body where an arteriole is positioned between two capillary beds. Increases or decreases in the resistance of the afferent and efferent arterioles increase or decrease glomerular filtration.

The **peritubular capillaries** surround the convoluted portions of the proximal and distal tubules and the loop of Henle

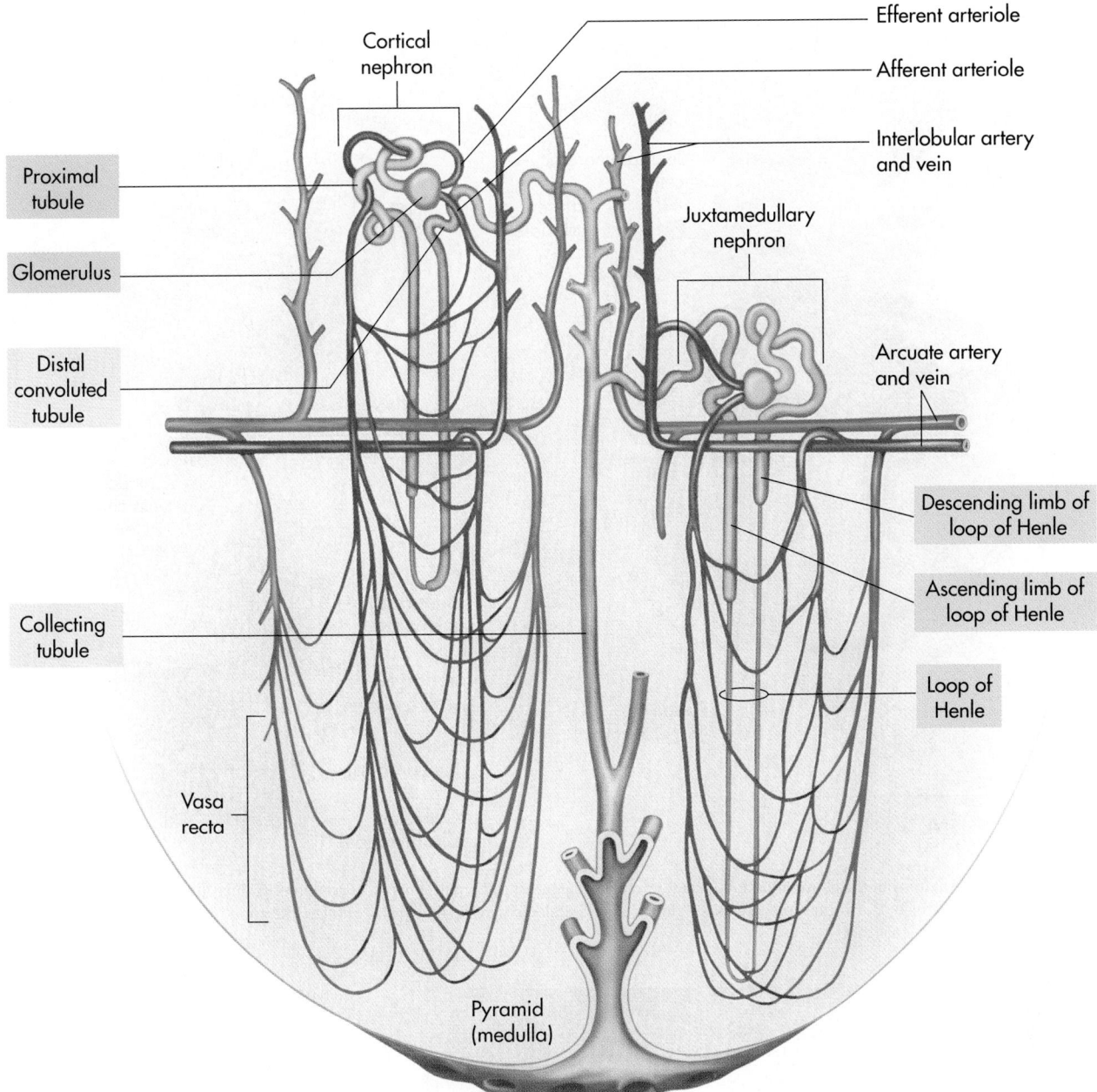

Figure 35-5 **The nephron unit with its blood vessels.** Blood flows through nephron vessels as follows: interlobular artery, afferent arteriole, glomerulus, efferent arteriole, peritubular capillaries (around the tubules), venules, interlobular vein. (From Thibodeau GA, Patton KT: *Anatomy & physiology,* ed 5, St Louis, 2003, Mosby.)

(see Figure 35-5). The peritubular capillaries are adapted differently for the cortical and juxtamedullary nephrons. The peritubular capillaries surrounding the tubules of the cortical nephrons are similar to capillaries in other tissues. For the juxtamedullary nephrons a network of capillaries called the **vasa recta** forms loops and closely follows the loops of Henle. The capillaries of the vasa recta are the only blood supply to the medulla. They influence the osmolar concentration of the medullary extracellular fluid, which is important to the formation of a concentrated urine. All capillaries then drain into the venous system. The renal veins follow the arterial path in a reverse direction and have the same names as the arteries. The renal vein empties into the inferior vena cava. The lymphatic vessels tend also to follow the distribution of the blood vessels.

Urinary Structures
Ureters
The urine formed by the nephrons flows from the distal tubules and collecting ducts through the duct of Bellini, the **renal papillae** (projections of the ducts), and into the calyces and is collected in the renal pelvis (see Figure 35-2). From the

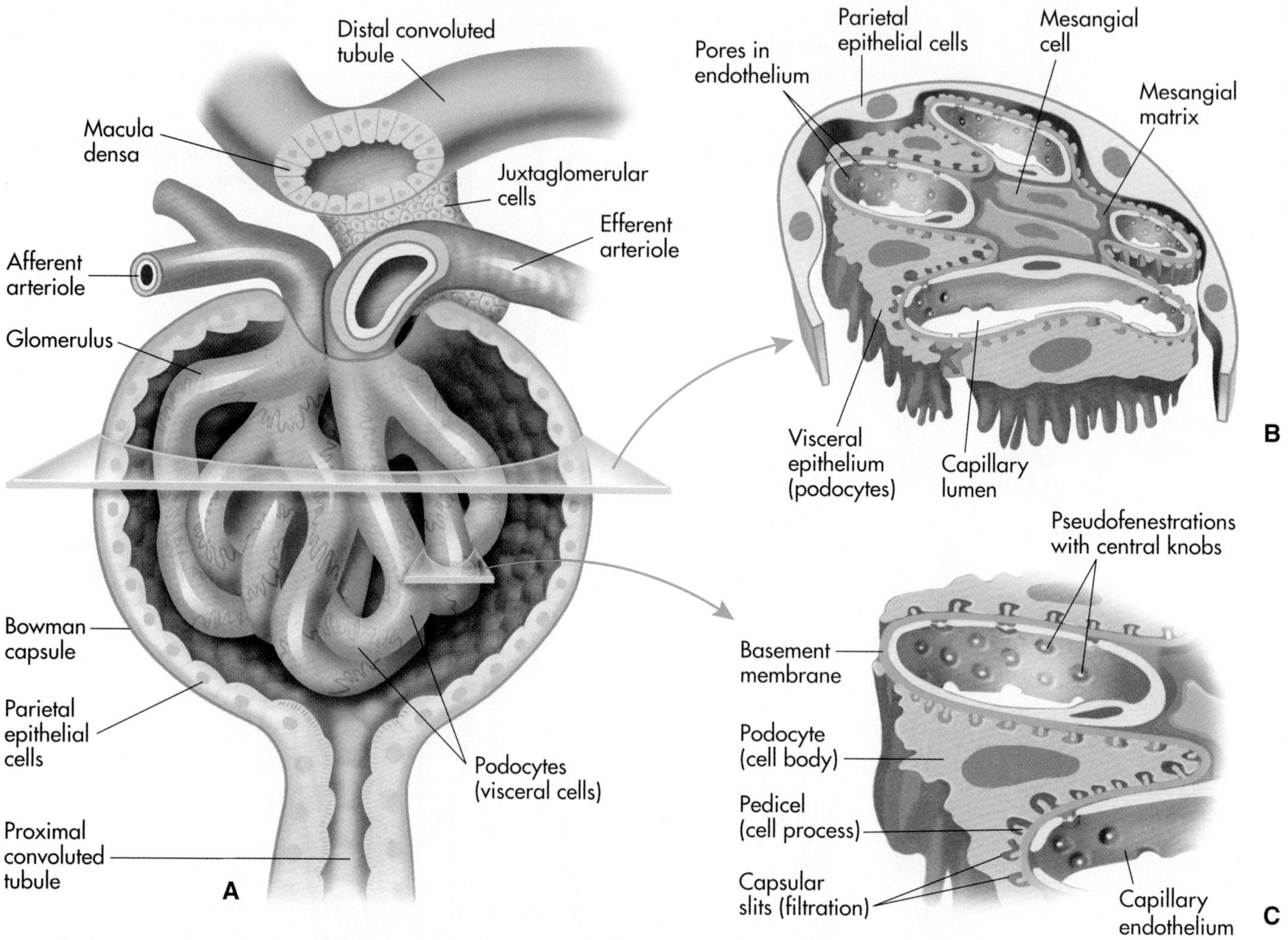

Distal convoluted tubule

Macula densa

Juxtaglomerular cells

Afferent arteriole

Efferent arteriole

Glomerulus

Bowman capsule

Parietal epithelial cells

Proximal convoluted tubule

Podocytes (visceral cells)

A

Pores in endothelium

Parietal epithelial cells

Mesangial cell

Mesangial matrix

Visceral epithelium (podocytes)

Capillary lumen

B

Pseudofenestrations with central knobs

Basement membrane

Podocyte (cell body)

Pedicel (cell process)

Capsular slits (filtration)

Capillary endothelium

C

Figure 35-6 **Anatomy of the glomerulus and juxtaglomerular apparatus. A,** Longitudinal cross section of glomerulus and juxta-glomerular apparatus **B,** Horizontal cross section of glomerulus. **C,** Enlargement of glomerular capillary filtration membrane.

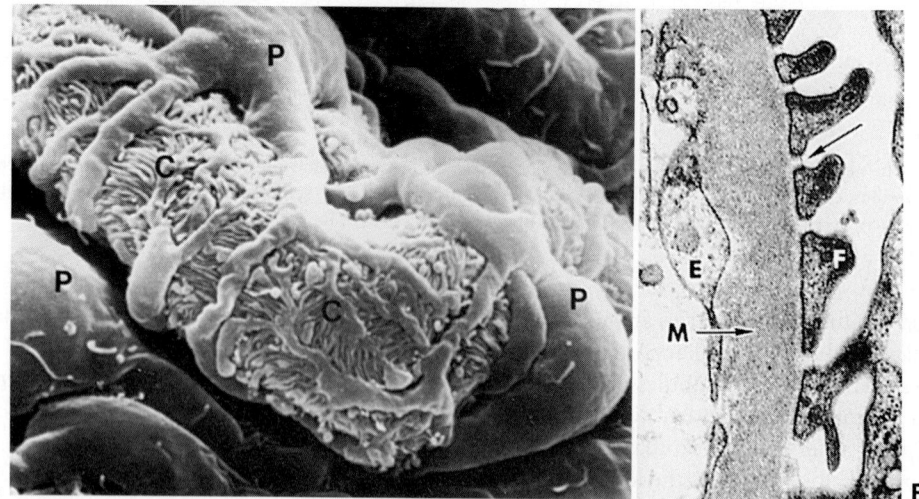

Figure 35-7 **Glomerular capillary. A,** Scanning electron micrograph of normal glomerular capillary *(C)* enclosed by podocytes *(P)* with primary processes and interdigitating foot processes. **B,** Glomerular capillary wall showing foot processes of endothelial podocytes *(F),* filtration slit membrane *(arrow),* basement membrane *(M),* and fenestrated endothelium *(E).* (×40,000.) (From Kissane JM, editor: *Anderson's pathology,* ed 9, St Louis, 1990, Mosby.)

renal pelvis, urine is funneled into the **ureters.** Each adult ureter is approximately 30 cm long and is composed of long, intertwining muscle bundles. The lower ends of the ureters pass obliquely through the posterior aspect of the bladder wall. The close approximation of muscle cells permits the direct transmission of electrical stimulation, and the resulting peristaltic activity propels urine into the bladder. Peristaltic activity is affected by urine volume. When urine flow is slow, the contraction is segmented, with downward propulsion of urine. Increasing flow rates increase peristalsis. Peristalsis is maintained even when the ureter is denervated, so ureters can be transplanted.

Sensory innervation for the upper part of the ureter arises from the tenth thoracic nerve roots, with referred pain to the umbilicus. The innervation of lower segments arises from the sacral nerves with referred pain to the vulva or penis. The ureters have a rich blood supply. The primary arteries come from the kidney with contributions from the lumbar and superior vesical arteries. Contraction of the bladder during **micturition** (urination) compresses the lower end of the ureter, preventing reflux.

Bladder and Urethra

The **bladder** is a bag composed of a basket weave of smooth muscle fibers that forms the **detrusor muscle** and its smooth lining of transitional epithelium (uroepithelium). As the bladder fills with urine, it distends and the layers of transitional epithelium slide past each other and become thinner as the volume of the bladder increases. The uroepithelium maintains an important barrier function to prevent movement of water and solutes between the urine and blood.[5] The **trigone** is a smooth triangular area lying between the openings of the two ureters and the urethra (Figure 35-8). The position of the bladder varies with age and gender. In infants and young children the bladder rises above the symphysis pubis, providing easy access for percutaneous aspiration. In adults it lies in the true pelvis, in front of the rectum and in front of the uterus in women. Inferiorly, the bladder sits on the prostate in men and on the anterior vagina in women. The bladder has a profuse blood supply, accounting for the bleeding that readily occurs with trauma, surgery, or inflammation.

The **urethra** extends from the inferior side of the bladder to the outside of the body. Two muscles called *sphincters* control excretion of urine from the bladder through the urethra. A ring of smooth muscle forms the **internal urethral sphincter** at the junction of the urethra and bladder. The **external urethral sphincter** is composed of striated muscles and is under voluntary control. The entire urethra is lined with mucus-secreting glands. The female urethra is short (3 to 4 cm). The male urethra is long (18 to 20 cm) and has three segments: prostatic, membranous, and cavernous. The prostatic urethra is closest to the bladder. It passes through the prostate gland and contains the openings of the ejaculatory ducts. The membranous urethra is the segment that passes through the floor of the pelvis. The cavernous segment forms the remainder of the tube. The cavernous segment is surrounded by erectile tis-

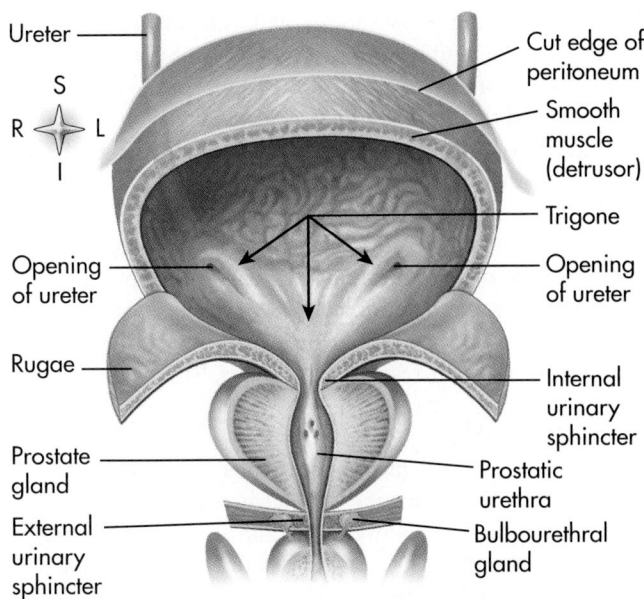

Figure 35-8 Structure and location of the urinary bladder. Frontal view of a dissected urinary bladder (male) in a fully distended position. (From Thibodeau GA, Patton KT: *Anatomy & physiology,* ed 5, St Louis, 2003, Mosby.)

sue and contains the openings of the bulbourethral mucous glands.

The innervation of the bladder and internal urethral sphincter is supplied by parasympathetic fibers of the autonomic nervous system. They primarily pass with the arteries to and from the sacral levels of the spinal cord. Sensory fibers may extend as high as the T6 portion of the spinal cord. Motor fibers from the pudendal nerve supply the external urethral sphincter. The reflex arc required for micturition is stimulated by mechanoreceptors, which respond to stretching of tissue. The mechanoreceptors sense bladder fullness and send impulses to the sacral level of the cord with bladder filling. When the bladder accumulates 250 to 300 ml of urine, the bladder contracts and the internal urethral sphincter relaxes through activation of the spinal reflex arc (known as the *micturition reflex*). At this time a person feels the urge to void. In older children and adults, the reflex can be inhibited or facilitated by impulses coming from the brain, resulting in voluntary control of micturition.

RENAL BLOOD FLOW

The kidneys are highly vascular organs and usually receive 1000 to 1200 ml of blood per minute, or about 20% to 25% of the cardiac output. With a normal hematocrit of 45%, about 600 to 700 ml of blood flowing through the kidney per minute is plasma. From the renal plasma flow (RPF), 20% (approximately 120 to 140 ml/min) is filtered at the glomerulus and passes into the Bowman capsule. The filtration of the plasma per unit of time is known as the **glomerular filtration rate (GFR),** and the GFR is directly related to the perfusion pressure in the glomerular capillaries.

The remaining 80% (about 480 ml) of plasma flows through the efferent arterioles to the peritubular capillaries. The ratio of glomerular filtrate to RPF per minute (120/600 = 0.20) is called the *filtration fraction.* Normally all but 1 to 2 ml of the glomerular filtrate is reabsorbed and returned to the circulation by the peritubular capillaries.

The GFR is directly related to renal blood flow (RBF), which is regulated by intrinsic autoregulatory mechanisms, neural regulation, and hormonal regulation. In general, blood flow to any organ is determined by the arteriovenous pressure differences across the vascular bed. If mean arterial pressure decreases or vascular resistance increases, RBF decreases.

Autoregulation

In the kidney a local mechanism tends to keep the rate of blood flow and therefore the GFR fairly constant over a range of arterial pressures between 80 and 180 mmHg (Figure 35-9). This means that changes in afferent arteriolar resistance and arteriolar pressure occur in the same direction. For example, as systemic blood pressure increases, the afferent arterioles constrict, preventing an increase in glomerular blood flow and filtration pressure. Opposite processes occur with a decrease in systemic blood pressure. Therefore RBF and GFR are relatively constant. This "constant" state is maintained by intrinsic autoregulatory mechanism mediating the arteriolar resistance changes. The purpose of renal autoregulation is to prevent wide fluctuations in systemic arterial pressure from being transmitted to the glomerular capillaries. In this way, large fluctuations in GFR are prevented and solute and water excretion is constantly maintained when arterial pressure changes.[6]

One mechanism responsible for the autoregulatory response in the kidney is probably a **myogenic mechanism.** As

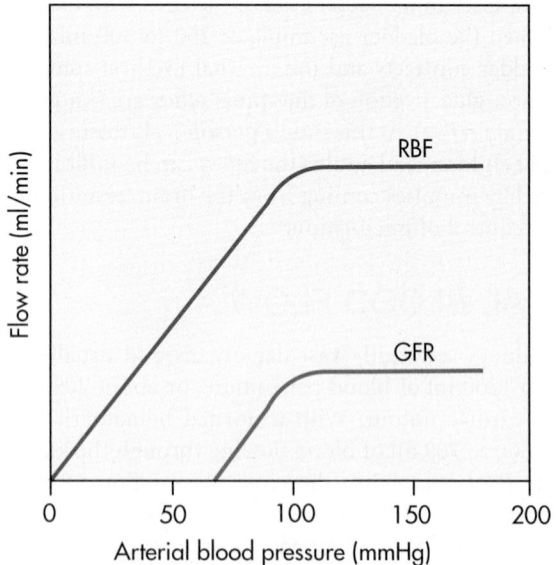

Figure 35-9 Renal autoregulation. Blood flow and glomerular filtration rate are stabilized in the face of changes in perfusion pressure. (From Berne RM, Levy MN, editors: *Principles of physiology,* ed 3, St Louis, 2000, Mosby.)

arterial pressure declines, the stretch on the afferent arteriolar smooth muscle decreases and the arteriole relaxes, with an increase in RBF; an increase in arteriolar pressure causes the arteriole smooth muscle to contract and decreases RBF. **Tubuloglomerular feedback** is a second mechanism for autoregulation of RBF and GFR. The macula densa cells of the distal tubule in the JGA sense changes in flow rate and sodium chloride content of the lumenal fluid. This information initiates a signal causing compensatory changes in afferent arteriolar resistance and GFR.[7]

Neural Regulation

The blood vessels of the kidney are innervated by the sympathetic noradrenergic fibers that cause arteriolar vasoconstriction and reduces renal blood flow. The innervation of the kidney comes primarily from the celiac ganglion and greater splanchnic nerve (see Figure 14-25). The afferent and efferent arterioles are richly innervated, but nerves have not been observed in the glomerular capillaries.

The RBF is reflexly related to the systemic arterial pressure. When systemic arterial pressure decreases, increased renal sympathetic nerve activity is mediated reflexively through the carotid sinus and the baroreceptors of the aortic arch. This stimulates renal arteriolar vasoconstriction and decreases both RBF and GFR. Thus RBF still changes when systemic arterial pressure is significantly reduced, although autoregulatory processes dampen the response. The decreased RBF decreases the GFR and diminishes excretion of sodium and water, promoting an increase in blood volume and thus an increase in systemic pressure. The afferent and efferent arterioles are innervated by sympathetic nerves. Norepinephrine causes vasoconstriction by activation of α_1-adrenoreceptors on afferent arterioles. The nerves are stimulated by decreased blood volume and cause vasoconstriction and decreased glomerular filtration.

Exercise, body position, and hypoxia also influence RBF. Exercise and change of body position activate renal sympathetic neurons and cause mild vasoconstriction. Severe hypoxia stimulates the chemoreceptors of the carotid and aortic bodies and decreases RBF by means of sympathetic stimulation. Hemorrhage induces intense sympathetic stimulation and vasoconstriction, and both GFR and blood flow are reduced.

Hormones and Other Factors

Hormonal factors and many mediators can alter the resistance of the renal vasculature by stimulating vasodilation or vasoconstriction. A major hormonal regulator of RBF is the **renin-angiotensin system,** which can increase systemic arterial pressure and change RBF. Renin is an enzyme formed and stored in the cells of the arterioles of the JGA (see Figure 35-3). Several complex physiologic mechanisms stimulate the release of renin. These mechanisms are principally decreased blood pressure in the afferent arterioles, which reduces stretch of the juxtaglomerular cells; decreased sodium chloride concentration in the distal convoluted tubule; and sympathetic nerve stimulation of β-adrenergic receptors on the juxta-glomerular cells.[8]

When renin is released, it cleaves an α-globulin (angiotensinogen) in the plasma to form angiotensin I, which is physiologically inactive. In the presence of a converting enzyme, angiotensin I is converted to angiotensin II and angiotensin III. Angiotensin II stimulates secretion of aldosterone by the adrenal cortex (see Chapter 20), is also a potent vasopressor, and inhibits renin release. Vitamin D$_3$ is a potent negative endocrine regulator of renin gene expression.[9] Angiotensin III has less of an effect than angiotensin II. Numer-ous physiologic effects of the renin-angiotensin system serve the purpose of stabilizing systemic blood pressure and preserving the extracellular fluid volume during hypotension or hypovolemia, including sodium reabsorption, systemic vasoconstriction, sympathetic nerve stimulation, thirst stimulation, and drinking. (The combined effects of the renin-angiotensin system and antidiuretic hormone [ADH] are summarized in Figure 35-10.) Angiotensin II is also produced within the kidney.

Natriuretic peptides are a group of peptide hormones with atrial natriuretic peptide (ANP) secreted from cells in

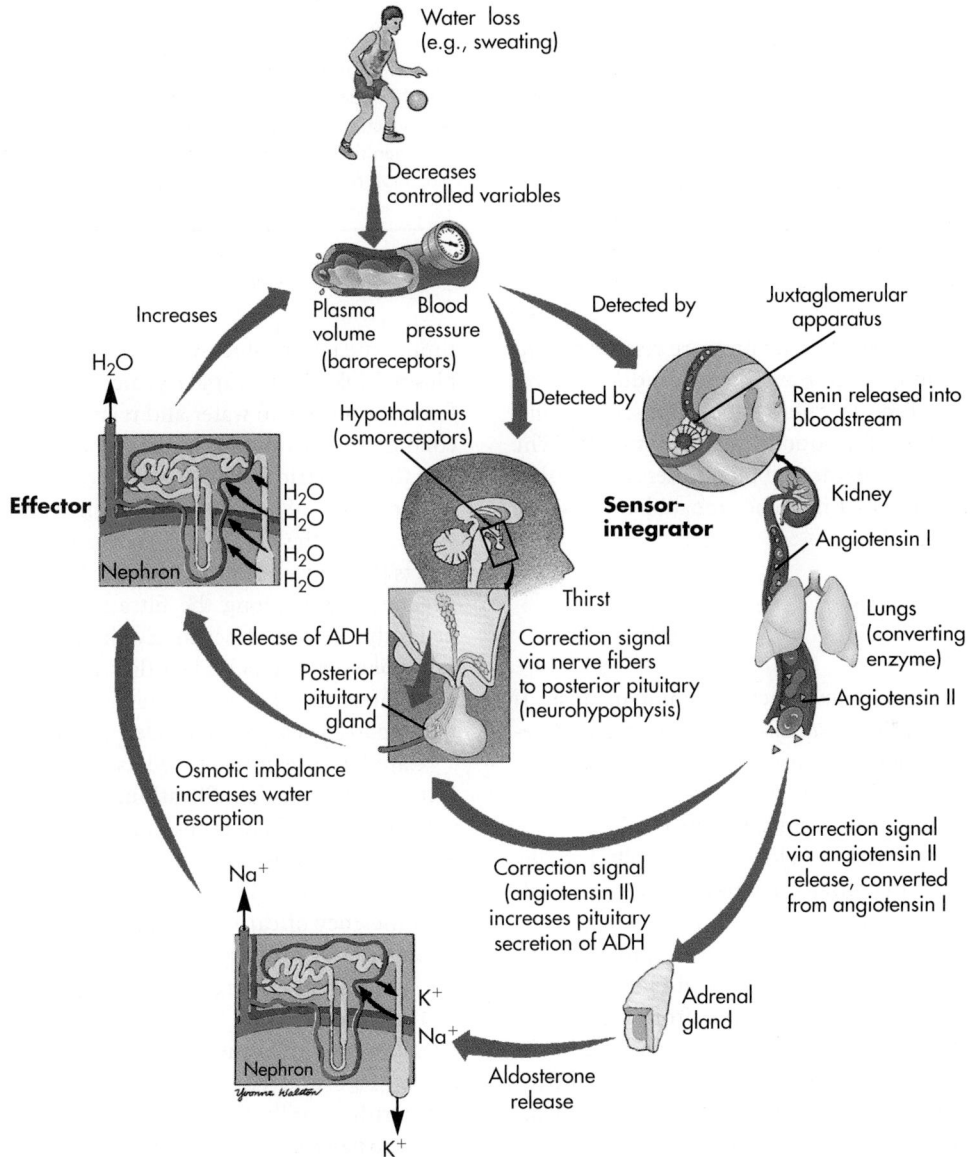

Figure 35-10 Cooperative roles of antidiuretic hormone (ADH) and aldosterone in regulating urine and plasma volume. The drop in blood pressure that accompanies loss of fluid from the internal environment triggers the hypothalamus to rapidly release ADH from the posterior pituitary gland. ADH increases water reabsorption by the kidney by increasing water permeability of the distal tubules and collecting ducts. The drop in blood pressure is also detected by the juxtaglomerular apparatus of each nephron, which responds by secreting renin. Renin triggers the formation of angiotensin II, which stimulates release of aldosterone from the adrenal cortex. Aldosterone then slowly boosts water reabsorption by the kidneys by increasing reabsorption of NaCl. Because angiotensin II also stimulates secretion of ADH, it serves as an additional link between the ADH and aldosterone mechanisms. (From Thibodeau GA, Patton KT: *Anatomy & physiology,* ed 5, St Louis, 2003, Mosby.)

Table 35-1	Hormones, Mediators, and Renal Blood Flow
Hormone or Mediator	**Effect on Renal Blood Flow**
Adenosine	Produced within kidney; causes vasoconstriction of afferent arteriole; decreases RBF and GFR
Angiotensin II	Produced systemically and within kidneys; constricts afferent and efferent arterioles; decreases RGF and GFR
Atrial natriuretic peptide	Produced by atria of the heart with hypertension and increased blood volume; causes vasodilation of afferent arteriole and vasoconstriction of efferent arteriole; modest increase in GFR with little change in RBF
Bradykinin	Produced in kidney from kininogen and causes vasodilation by release of nitric oxide and prostaglandins; increases RBF and GFR
Dopamine	Produced by the proximal tubule; increases RBF; inhibits renin secretion
Endothelin	Produced by renal vessel endothelial cells, mesangial cells, and distal tubule cells in response to bradykinin, angiotensin II, epinephrine, and stretch; most active with renal disease; profound vasoconstriction of afferent and efferent arterioles; decreases RBF and GFR
Histamine	Produced locally within the kidney; modulates RBF in basal state and during inflammation; increases RBF by decreasing afferent and efferent arteriolar resistance and does not decrease GFR
Nitric oxide	Produced by renal vessel endothelial cells with increased stretch and by stimulation of acetylcholine, histamine, bradykinin, ATP; increases vasodilation of afferent and efferent arterioles
Prostaglandins PGI_2, PGE_2	Produced locally within kidney with decreased RBF; dampen vasoconstriction caused by sympathetic nerves and angiotensin II; prevent harmful vasoconstriction and renal ischemia
Urodilatin	Produced by distal tubule and collecting duct when there is increased circulating volume and increased blood pressure; inhibits sodium and water reabsorption from medullary part of collecting duct, thereby producing diuresis

RBF, Renal blood flow; *GFR*, glomerular filtration rate; *ATP*, adenosine triphosphate.

the right atrium.[10] When right atrial pressure rises, ANP inhibits secretion of renin, inhibits angiotensin-induced secretion of aldosterone, relaxes vascular smooth muscle, and inhibits sodium and water absorption by kidney tubules. The result is decreased blood volume and blood pressure.[11] Other hormones and mediators that influence renal blood flow are summarized in Table 35-1.

KIDNEY FUNCTION

Nephron Function

The nephron can perform many functions simultaneously. It filters the plasma at the glomerulus and reabsorbs and secretes different substances at various parts of its tubular structure (Figure 35-11). The function of the nephron is to form a filtrate of protein-free plasma. This process, known as **ultrafiltration,** occurs across the glomerular capillaries. The nephron then regulates the filtrate to maintain body fluid volume, electrolyte composition, and pH within narrow limits.

Regulation of the filtrate occurs through two processes: tubular reabsorption and tubular secretion. **Tubular reabsorption** is the movement of fluids and solutes from the tubular lumen to the peritubular capillary plasma. Transfer of substances from the plasma of the peritubular capillary to the tubular lumen is **tubular secretion.** The transport mechanisms are both active and passive (processes defined in Chapter 1). The elimination of a substance in the final urine is known as **excretion** (Figure 35-12).

Glomerular Filtration

The fluid filtered by the glomerular capillary filtration membrane is protein free but contains electrolytes such as sodium, chloride, and potassium and organic molecules such as crea-

tinine, urea, and glucose in the same concentrations as in plasma. Like other capillary membranes, the glomerulus is freely permeable to water and relatively impermeable to large colloids such as plasma proteins. The size of the molecules and their electrical charge are important factors affecting the permeability of substances crossing the glomerulus. The small size of the filtration slits or pores in the membrane restricts the passage of proteins and other macromolecules. The negative charge along the filtration membrane further impedes the passage of negatively charged macromolecules (because like forces repel each other). Positively charged macromolecules therefore permeate the membrane more readily than neutrally charged particles.

Capillary pressure, as well as electrical charge, has an effect on glomerular filtration. The hydrostatic pressure within the capillary is the major force for inducing water and solutes across the filtration membrane and into the Bowman capsule. This pressure is determined indirectly by the efficiency of cardiac contraction and directly by the systemic arterial pressure and the resistances to blood flow in the afferent and efferent arterioles. Two forces oppose the filtration effects of the glomerular capillary hydrostatic pressure (P_{GC}): (1) the hydrostatic pressure in the Bowman space (P_{BC}) and (2) the effective oncotic pressure of the glomerular capillary blood (π_{GC}). (As explained in Chapter 3, hydrostatic pressure is a pushing force in relation to water, and oncotic pressure is a pulling force.) Because the fluid in the Bowman space normally contains only minute amounts of protein, it normally does not have an oncotic influence on the plasma of the glomerular capillary (Figure 35-13).

The combined effect of forces favoring and forces opposing filtration determines the filtration pressure. The **net fil-**

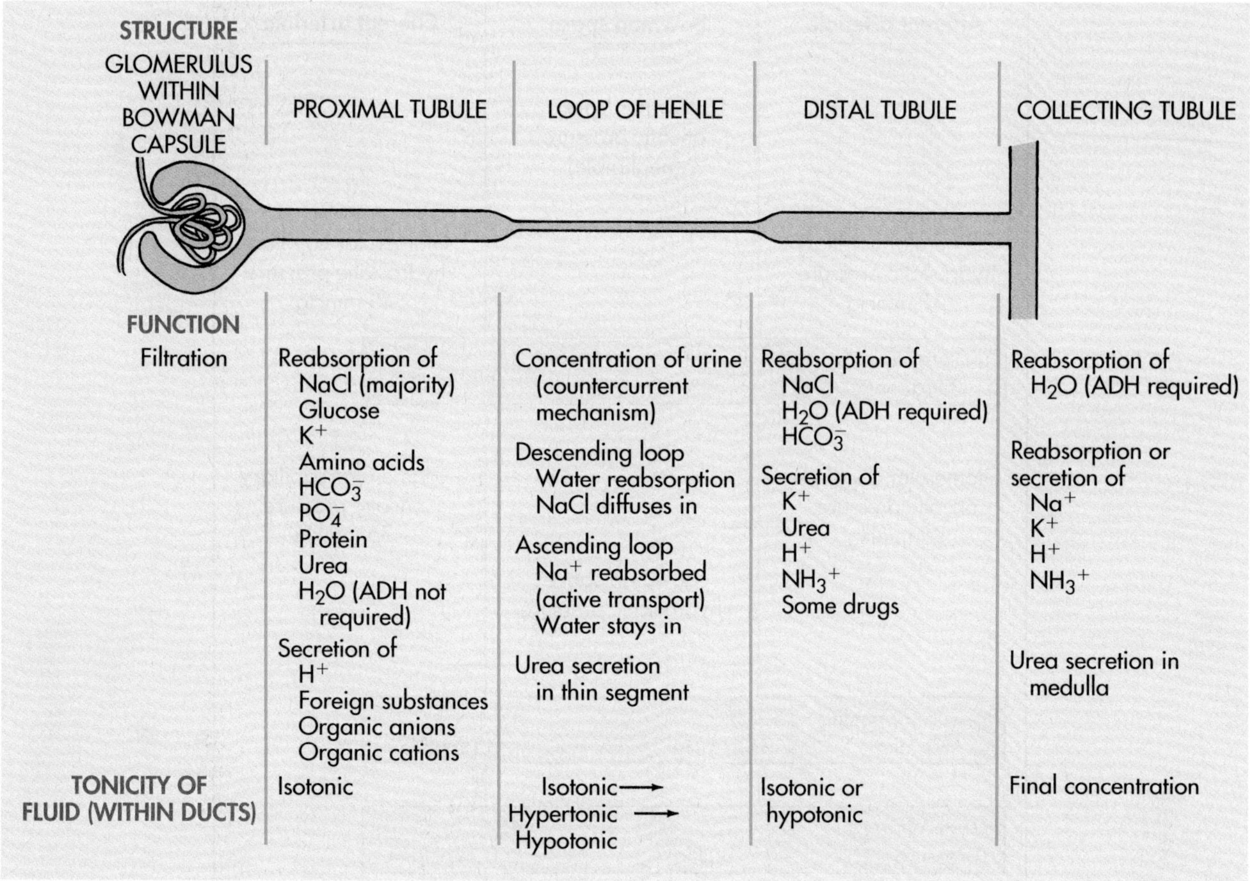

STRUCTURE GLOMERULUS WITHIN BOWMAN CAPSULE	PROXIMAL TUBULE	LOOP OF HENLE	DISTAL TUBULE	COLLECTING TUBULE
FUNCTION Filtration	Reabsorption of NaCl (majority) Glucose K^+ Amino acids HCO_3^- PO_4^- Protein Urea H_2O (ADH not required) Secretion of H^+ Foreign substances Organic anions Organic cations	Concentration of urine (countercurrent mechanism) Descending loop Water reabsorption NaCl diffuses in Ascending loop Na^+ reabsorbed (active transport) Water stays in Urea secretion in thin segment	Reabsorption of NaCl H_2O (ADH required) HCO_3^- Secretion of K^+ Urea H^+ NH_3^+ Some drugs	Reabsorption of H_2O (ADH required) Reabsorption or secretion of Na^+ K^+ H^+ NH_3^+ Urea secretion in medulla
TONICITY OF FLUID (WITHIN DUCTS)	Isotonic	Isotonic $\longrightarrow$ Hypertonic $\longrightarrow$ Hypotonic	Isotonic or hypotonic	Final concentration

Figure 35-11 Major functions of nephron segments. *ADH,* Antidiuretic hormone. (Modified from Hockenberry MJ: *Wong's nursing care of infants and children,* ed 7, St Louis, 2003, Mosby.)

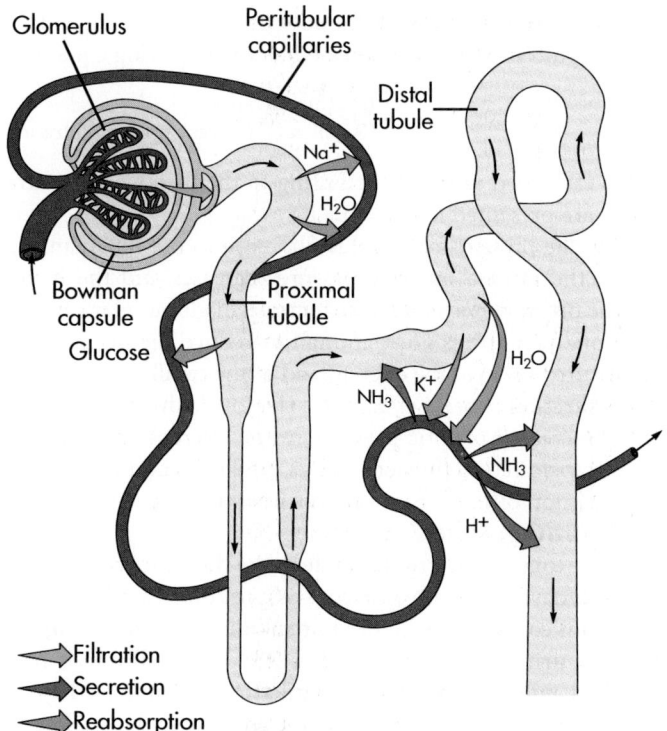

Figure 35-12 Glomerular filtration, tubular reabsorption, and tubular secretion. The three processes by which the kidneys excrete urine. From proximal convoluted tubules, sodium and glucose are reabsorbed into peritubular capillaries by active transport. Water reabsorption by osmosis follows. From distal convoluted tubules, sodium is reabsorbed by active transport. Osmotic reabsorption of water from them occurs when ADH is present. Secretion of ammonia and hydrogen occurs from peritubular capillaries into distal tubules by active transport. (From Thibodeau GA, Patton KT: *Anatomy & physiology,* ed 5, St Louis, 2003, Mosby.)

Glomerulus
Peritubular capillaries
Distal tubule
Na^+
H_2O
Bowman capsule
Proximal tubule
Glucose
NH_3
K^+
H_2O
NH_3
H^+

Filtration
Secretion
Reabsorption

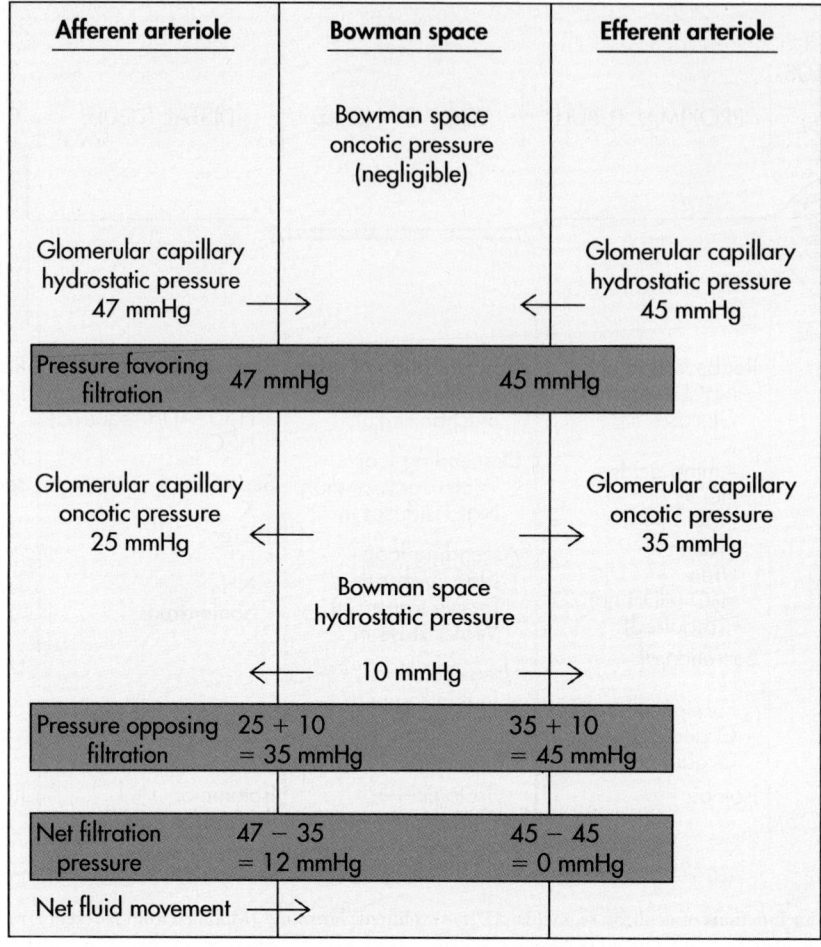

Figure 35-13 Glomerular filtration pressures.

Table 35-2	Glomerular Filtration Pressures		
		Pressures (mmHg)	
Forces	Pressures	Beginning of Capillary	End of Capillary
Promoting Filtration			
Glomerular capillary hydrostatic pressure	P_{GC}	47	45
Bowman capsule oncotic pressure	π_{BC}	Negligible effect	Negligible effect
Opposing Filtration			
Bowman capsule hydrostatic pressure	P_{BC}	10	10
Glomerular capillary oncotic pressure	π_{GC}	25	35
NET FILTRATION PRESSURE		12	0

tration pressure **(NFP)** is the sum of forces favoring and opposing filtration and is expressed by the following equation:

$$\text{NFP} = (P_{GC} + \pi_{BC}) \text{ (forces favoring filtration)} -$$
$$(P_{BC} + \pi_{GC}) \text{ (forces opposing filtration)}$$

The estimated values contributing to the forces of net filtration are presented in Table 35-2.

As the protein-free fluid is filtered into the Bowman capsule, the plasma oncotic pressure increases and the hydrostatic pressure decreases. The increase in glomerular capillary oncotic pressure is great enough to reduce the net filtration pressure to zero at the efferent end of the capillary and to stop the filtration process effectively. The low hydrostatic pressure and increased oncotic pressure in the efferent arteriole then are transferred to the peritubular capillaries and facilitate reabsorption of fluid from the proximal tubules.

Filtration Rate

The total volume of fluid filtered by the glomeruli averages 180 L/day, or approximately 120 ml/min, a phenomenal amount considering the size of the kidneys. Because only 1 to 2 L of urine is excreted per day, 99% of the filtrate is reabsorbed into the peritubular capillaries and returned to the blood. The factors determining the GFR are directly related to the pressures that favor or oppose filtration. Any changes in afferent or efferent arteriolar resistance will alter glomerular capillary hydrostatic pressure and GFR. Vasoconstriction of one or the other of these two arterioles produces opposite effects on glomerular pressure. For example, if the afferent arteriole constricts, blood flow decreases, with a corresponding drop in glomerular pressure. The GFR then decreases, and body fluids are conserved. Conversely, constriction of the efferent arteriole increases the net filtration pressure and the GFR increases. When both afferent and efferent arterioles constrict, little change occurs in filtration pressure, but RBF is reduced and so is the GFR.

Obstruction to the outflow of urine (caused by strictures, stones, or tumors along the urinary tract) can cause a retrograde increase in pressure at the Bowman capsule and a decrease in GFR. Excessive loss of protein-free fluid from vomiting, diarrhea, use of diuretics, or excessive sweating can increase glomerular capillary oncotic pressure and decrease the GFR. Renal disease also can cause changes in pressure relationships by altering capillary permeability and the surface area available for filtration (see Chapter 36).

Tubular Transport

By the time fluid reaches the end of the proximal tubule, approximately 60% to 70% of filtered sodium and water and about 50% of urea have been reabsorbed, along with 90% or more of potassium, glucose, bicarbonate, calcium, phosphate, amino acids, and uric acid. All this occurs by active transport. Chloride, water, and urea are reabsorbed passively but are linked to the active transport of sodium (cotransport). Active transport in the renal tubules can be limited as the carrier molecules become saturated, a phenomenon known as **transport maximum (T_m)**. Transport maximums exist for most substances actively transported by the tubular epithelium. The reabsorption of glucose is a significant example. Glucose is coupled to sodium transport and is almost completely reabsorbed in the proximal tubule. Like other actively transported substances, glucose has a maximal transport capacity, or renal threshold. This means that when the carrier molecules for glucose become saturated, the excess will be excreted in the urine. Normally, the plasma level and filtered glucose load are not high enough to saturate the carrier mechanism. When the plasma glucose reaches 180 mg/dl, however, as occurs in the individual with uncontrolled diabetes mellitus, the threshold for glucose is achieved. Any further increase in the plasma level causes loss of glucose in the urine.

Proximal Tubule. Active reabsorption of sodium is the primary function of the proximal tubule. Water, most electrolytes, and organic substances are cotransported with sodium. The osmotic force generated by active sodium transport promotes the passive diffusion of water out of the tubular lumen and into the peritubular capillaries. Passive transport of water is further enhanced by the elevated oncotic pressure of the blood in the peritubular capillaries. The reabsorption of water leaves an increased concentration of urea within the tubular lumen, creating a gradient for its passive diffusion to the peritubular plasma.

As the positively charged sodium ions leave the tubular lumen, negatively charged chloride ions passively follow to maintain electroneutrality. Because the luminal membrane (the inside of the tubule) of the proximal tubular cell has a limited permeability to chloride, however, chloride reabsorption lags behind sodium.

Hydrogen ions are actively exchanged for sodium ions. The hydrogen ions (H^+) then combine with bicarbonate (HCO_3^-). Bicarbonate is completely filtered at the glomerulus, and approximately 90% is reabsorbed in the proximal tubule. This process also occurs to a lesser extent in the ascending loop of Henle and the distal tubule.

In the tubular lumen, hydrogen and bicarbonate ions form carbonic acid (H_2CO_3). The carbonic acid rapidly breaks down, or dissociates, to carbon dioxide (CO_2) and water (H_2O) in the presence of the enzyme carbonic anhydrase, which is in the luminal membrane. The CO_2 and H_2O then diffuse into the tubular cell, where carbonic anhydrase again catalyzes the CO_2 and H_2O to form HCO_3^- and H^+. The H_2CO_3 thus produces H^+ and HCO_3^-. The H^+ is secreted again, and HCO_3^- combines with sodium and is transported to the peritubular capillary blood.

Thus, because bicarbonate is not highly permeable at the peritubular capillary membrane, it is reabsorbed as CO_2 and H_2O, which are readily diffusible. One of the unusual aspects of this process is that the bicarbonate molecule filtered at the glomerulus is not the same molecule that is reabsorbed (because it dissociates) and the hydrogen ion secreted by the proximal tubule is not excreted in the urine. Bicarbonate is thus conserved, and the hydrogen is reabsorbed as water. Therefore these ions normally do not contribute to the urinary excretion of acid or the addition of acid to the blood (Figure 35-14).

In addition to the proximal tubular secretion of hydrogen ions, secretory transport mechanisms exist for creatinine, other organic bases, and endogenous and exogenous organic acids, including para-aminohippurate and penicillin (Box 35-1). These secretory mechanisms are important for eliminating drugs and other exogenous chemical products from the body. Frequently, exogenous substances are conjugated with sulfate and glucuronic acid by the liver and then actively secreted by the renal tubules. This has important clinical implications because many drugs and their metabolites are eliminated from the body in this way. When the renal tubules are damaged, metabolic by-products and drugs may accumulate, causing toxic levels in the body.

Loop of Henle and Distal Tubule. The filtrate entering and leaving the proximal tubule is essentially isoosmotic with the plasma and has a concentration of about 285 mOsm. Although approximately 65% of salt and water is reabsorbed along the proximal tubule, they are reabsorbed in equal amounts, causing only minor changes in the osmotic and electrolyte concentrations of the fluid flowing into the loop of Henle. Therefore any concentration or dilution of urine occurs at more distal sites of the nephron, principally in the loop of Henle and collecting ducts. Near the top of the renal pyramids, the interstitial osmolality reaches 1200 mOsm/L.

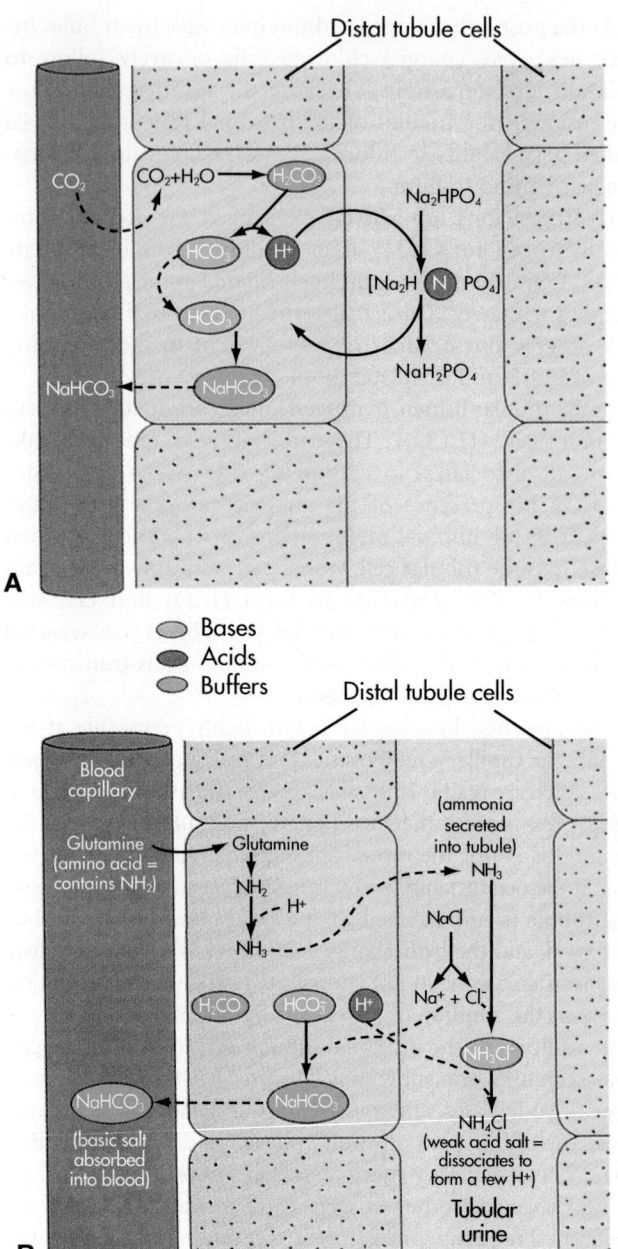

Distal tubule cells

A,

Bases
Acids
Buffers

Distal tubule cells

B,

Figure 35-14 Acidification of urine by tubule excretion of ammonia (NH_3). **A,** Acidification of urine and conservation of base by distal renal tubule excretion of H^+. **B,** An amino acid (glutamine) moves into the tubule cell and loses an amino group (NH_2) to form ammonia, which is secreted into the urine. In exchange, the tubule cell absorbs a basic salt (mainly $NaHCO_3$) into blood from urine. (From Thibodeau GA, Patton KT: *Anatomy & physiology*, ed 4, St Louis, 1999, Mosby.)

Box 35-1	Substances Transported by Renal Tubules

Reabsorption	Secretion
Albumin	Choline
Ascorbate	Creatinine
Fructose	Histamine
Galactose	Methyl guanidine
Glucose	Para-aminohippurate
Glutamate	Penicillin
Phosphate	Steroid glucuronides
Sulfate	Thiamine
Xylose	

The primary function of the loop of Henle is to establish a hyperosmotic state within the medullary interstitial fluid. This is achieved by reabsorbing more solute than water into the interstitium. The fluid leaving the ascending limb of the loop is therefore hypoosmotic, or more dilute than the fluid that entered. This dilution allows the distal tubule and collecting duct to make final adjustments in the concentration or dilution of the excreted urine according to body needs. The vasa recta act to maintain the high osmotic gradient established by the loop of Henle.

Different transport or permeability functions of the loop of Henle are important for dilution and concentration of urine. The thin, descending segment of the loop of Henle is highly permeable to water and moderately permeable to sodium, urea, and other solutes. The thin, ascending segment is more permeable to solutes and almost impermeable to water. The thick portion of the ascending segment is highly permeable to sodium, potassium, and chloride and significantly less permeable to water and urea. *Tamm-Horsfall glycoprotein,* also known as uromodulin, is formed on the epithelial surface of the thick ascending segment and first segment of the distal tubule. It is the most abundant urinary protein and protects against urolithiasis and is a ligand for lymphokines.[12]

The convoluted portion of the distal tubule is poorly permeable to water but readily absorbs ions and contributes to the dilution of the tubular fluid. The later, straight segment of the distal tubule and the collecting duct are permeable to water as controlled by ADH. Sodium is readily absorbed by the later segment of the distal tubule and collecting duct under the regulation of the hormone aldosterone (see Chapter 20). Potassium is actively secreted in these segments and is also controlled by aldosterone and other factors related to the concentration of potassium in body fluids.[13]

Hydrogen is also secreted by the distal tubule and combines with nonbicarbonate buffers for the elimination of acids in the urine. (See Chapter 3 for further discussion of renal regulation of acid-base balance.) The distal tubule thus contributes to the regulation of acid-base balance by excreting hydrogen ions into the urine and by adding new bicarbonate to the plasma. The mechanism is similar to the conservation of bicarbonate by the proximal tubule, except that

These quantitative changes taking place in the loop of Henle are related to the length of the loop and its depth of penetration into the medulla. The structural features of the medullary hairpin loops provide the kidney with the ability to concentrate urine and conserve water for the body. The transition of the filtrate into urine is a function of the concentrating ability of the loops and final adjustments in urine composition made by the distal tubule and collecting duct.

the hydrogen ion is excreted in the urine. (The specific mechanisms of acid-base balance and acid excretion are described in Chapter 3.)

Glomerulotubular Balance

To regulate body fluid balance, the kidney must not reabsorb or excrete too much sodium or water. Normally, 99% of the glomerular filtrate is reabsorbed. When the GFR spontaneously decreases or increases, the renal tubules, primarily the proximal tubules, automatically adjust their rate of reabsorption of sodium and water to balance the change in GFR. Thus a constant fraction of filtered sodium and water is reabsorbed from the proximal tubule. This prevents wide fluctuations in sodium and water excretion into the urine and maintains sodium and water balance.[14]

Concentration and Dilution of Urine

The production of a concentrated urine involves a **countercurrent exchange system,** in which fluid flows in opposite directions through parallel tubes. A concentration gradient causes fluid to be exchanged across the parallel pathways. In the nephron the fluid moves up and down the parallel sides of the hairpin loop of Henle in the medulla. The longer the loop, the greater the concentration gradient because the concentration gradient increases from the cortex to the tip of the medulla. The loops of Henle serve as multipliers of the concentration gradient, and the vasa recta act as a countercurrent exchanger for maintaining the gradient.[15]

Water, Sodium, and Chloride

The process is initiated in the thick ascending limb of the loop of Henle with the active transport of chloride and sodium out of the tubular lumen and into the medullary interstitium (Figure 35-15). Because the lumen of the ascending limb is impermeable to water, water cannot follow the sodium/chloride transport. This lack of luminal permeability causes

the ascending tubular fluid to become hypoosmotic and the medullary interstitium to become hyperosmotic. The descending limb of the loop, which receives fluid from the proximal tubule, is highly permeable to water, but it is the only place in the nephron that does not actively transport either sodium or chloride. Sodium and chloride may, however, diffuse into the descending tubule from the interstitium. The hyperosmotic interstitium causes water to move out of the descending limb, and the remaining fluid in the descending tubule becomes increasingly concentrated as it flows toward the tip of the medulla. As the tubular fluid rounds the loop and enters the ascending limb, sodium and chloride are removed and water is retained. The fluid then becomes more and more dilute as it encounters the distal tubule.

The slow rate of blood flow and the hairpin structure of the vasa recta allow blood to flow through the medullary tissue without disturbing the osmotic gradient. As blood flows into the descending limb of the vasa recta, it encounters the increasing osmotic concentration gradient of the medullary interstitium. Water moves out, and sodium and chloride diffuse into the descending vasa recta. The plasma becomes increasingly concentrated as it flows toward the tip of the medulla.

As the blood flow passes into the ascending limb and back toward the cortex, the surrounding interstitial fluid becomes comparatively more dilute. Water then moves back into the vasa recta, and sodium and chloride diffuse out. The net result is a preservation of the medullary osmotic gradient. If blood were to flow rapidly through the vasa recta, as occurs in some renal diseases, the medullary concentration gradient would be washed away and the ability to concentrate urine and conserve water would be lost. The efficiency of water conservation is related to the length of the loops: the longer the loops, the greater the ability to concentrate the urine. Many desert animals have very long loops and can reabsorb water so efficiently that they rarely need to drink.

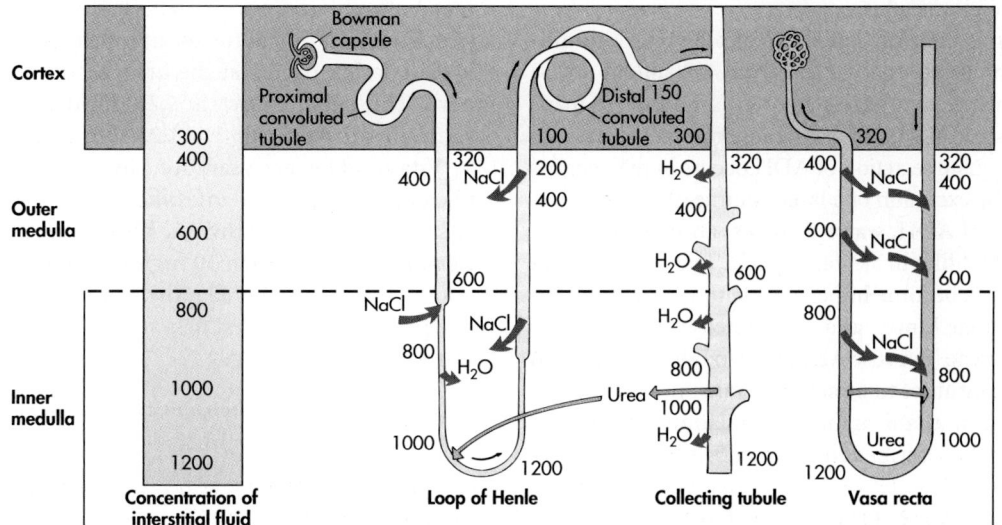

Figure 35-15 **Countercurrent mechanism for concentrating and diluting urine.** (NOTE: numbers on illustration represent milliosmoles [mOsm].)

Urea

Urea is an end product of protein metabolism and is the major constituent of urine along with water. The glomerulus freely filters urea, and tubular reabsorption of urea depends on urine flow rate with less reabsorption at higher flow rates. Approximately 50% of urea is excreted in the urine, and 50% is recycled within the kidney. The recycling of urea from the tubules and collecting ducts contributes to the osmotic gradient within the medulla and is necessary for the concentration and dilution of urine. Because urea is an end product of protein metabolism, individuals with protein deprivation cannot maximally concentrate their urine.

Catecholamines

With hemorrhage or extracellular fluid depletion, sympathetic nerves are activated to release norepinephrine and the adrenal medulla releases epinephrine. Sodium and water are reabsorbed by the proximal tubule, the thick ascending limb of the loop of Henle, the distal tubule, and the collecting duct.[14]

Antidiuretic Hormone

The distal tubule in the cortex receives the hypoosmotic urine from the ascending limb of the loop of Henle. The concentration of the final urine is controlled by antidiuretic hormone (ADH), which is secreted from the posterior pituitary, or neurohypophysis. ADH increases water permeability in the last segment of the distal tubule and along the entire length of the collecting ducts, which pass through the inner and outer zones of the medulla.

In the presence of ADH, water reabsorption is high. Most of the water is reabsorbed in the medullary collecting ducts because of the high osmotic gradient in the medullary interstitium. The water diffuses into the ascending limb of the vasa recta and returns to the systemic circulation. The excreted urine can have a high osmotic concentration, up to 1400 mOsm. The volume is normally reduced to about 1% of what was filtered at the glomerulus.

ADH secretion is therefore one cause of **oliguria,** or diminished excretion of urine, that is, less than 400 ml/day or 30 ml/hr. Fluid imbalance may be related to the syndrome of inappropriate secretion of ADH, which is a cause of water excess (see Chapter 3). Inadequate secretion of ADH occurs in diabetes insipidus, causing the excretion of a large volume of dilute urine.

In the absence of ADH, **water diuresis,** an increase in excretion of a highly dilute urine, takes place. The distal tubules and collecting ducts become impermeable to water. Water remains in the tubular lumen and is excreted as a dilute and large volume of urine. Because ADH has no effect on sodium reabsorption, it continues to be actively transported from the distal tubule. (The mechanism for the regulation of ADH and plasma osmolality is described in Chapter 3.)

Urodilantin and Atrial Natriuretic Peptide

Urodilantin and atrial natriuretic peptide are encoded by the same gene and have a similar structure. **Atrial natriuretic peptide (ANP)** is secreted by the cardiac atria, and **urodilantin** is secreted by the distal tubules and collecting ducts and functions only in the kidney. Both are stimulated by a rise in blood pressure and an increase in extracellular fluid volume. ANP inhibits ADH secretion, and ADH regulates water reabsorption and promotes water excretion. Urodilantin inhibits sodium chloride (NaCl) and water reabsorption in the medullary part of the collecting duct, thereby producing diuresis.[16]

Diuretics as a Factor in Urine Flow

A **diuretic** is any agent that enhances the flow of urine. Clinically, diuretics interfere with renal sodium reabsorption and reduce extracellular fluid volume. Diuretics are commonly used to treat hypertension and edema caused by heart failure, cirrhosis, and nephrotic syndrome.

Different diuretics affect different sites of tubular function and may produce side effects that alter acid-base and electrolyte balance. Therefore health professionals need to understand their indications for use, mechanisms of action, and toxic side effects. Diuretics are divided into four general categories: (1) osmotic diuretics, (2) carbonic anhydrase inhibitors (inhibitors of urinary acidification), (3) inhibitors of loop sodium or chloride transport, and (4) aldosterone antagonists. (The physiologic mechanism related to each category is summarized in Table 35-3).

Renal Hormones

Certain hormones are either activated or synthesized by the kidney. These hormones have significant systemic effects and include the active form of vitamin D, erythropoietin, and natriuretic hormone (see p. 1287).

Vitamin D

Vitamin D is a hormone that can be obtained in the diet or synthesized by the action of ultraviolet radiation on cholesterol in the skin. These forms of vitamin D_3 (cholecalciferol) are inactive and require two hydroxylations to establish a metabolically active form. The first step occurs in the liver with hydroxylation at the twenty-fifth carbon, and the second hydroxylation occurs at the first carbon position in the kidneys. The end product is 1,25-dihydroxycholecalciferol, or 1,25-dihydroxyvitamin D_3 (1,25-OH$_2$D$_3$).

Vitamin D is necessary for the absorption of calcium and phosphate by the small intestine. The renal hydroxylation step is stimulated by parathyroid hormone. A decreased plasma calcium level (less than 10 mg/dl) stimulates the secretion of parathyroid hormone. Parathyroid hormone then stimulates a sequence of events that help restore plasma calcium back toward normal:

Calcium mobilization from bone
Synthesis of 1,25-dihydroxyvitamin D_3
↓
Absorption of calcium from the intestine
↓
Increased renal calcium reabsorption
↓
Decreased renal phosphate reabsorption

Table 35-3	Action of Diuretics		
Diuretic	**Site of Action**	**Action**	**Side Effects**
Osmotic Diuretic			
Mannitol Glycerol Urea	Proximal tubule	Freely filtered but not reabsorbed; osmotically attracts water and diminishes sodium reabsorption	Hypokalemia, dehydration
Carbonic Anhydrase Inhibitors			
Acetazolamide	Proximal tubule	Inhibits carbonic anhydrase; blocks hydrogen ion secretion and reabsorption of sodium and bicarbonate	Hypokalemia, systemic acidosis, alkaline urine
Inhibitors of Sodium/Chloride Reabsorption			
Thiazides	Between end of ascending loop and beginning of distal tubule	Blocks sodium and chloride reabsorption; mildly suppresses carbonic anhydrase	Hypokalemia, metabolic alkalosis
Furosemide Ethacrynic acid Torsemide	Thick ascending limb of Henle loop	Blocks active transport of chloride, sodium, and potassium	Hypokalemia, uric acid retention
Bumetanide	Cortical vasodilation	Increased rate of urine formation	Hypokalemia, uric acid retention
Potassium Sparing			
Spironolactone	Distal tubule	Inhibits aldosterone, blocks sodium reabsorption, and results in potassium retention	Hyperkalemia, nausea, confusion, gynecomastia
Triamterene and amiloride	Distal tubule	Blocks sodium reabsorption and inhibits potassium excretion	Nausea, vomiting, headache, granulocytopenia, skin rash

Serum phosphate fluctuations also influence the renal hydroxylation of vitamin D. Decreased levels stimulate active $1,25\text{-}OH_2D_3$ formation, and increased levels inhibit formation. This results in compensatory changes in phosphate absorption from bone and the intestine. The clinical significance of the role of the kidney in calcium and phosphate metabolism is evident in renal disease. Patients with renal disease have a deficiency of $1,25\text{-}OH_2D_3$ and manifest symptoms of disturbed calcium and phosphate balance (see Chapter 3).

Erythropoietin

Erythropoietin (Epo) is produced by the fetal liver and in the adult kidney and is essential for normal erythropoiesis. Epo stimulates the bone marrow to produce red blood cells in response to tissue hypoxia. (Erythrocyte production is discussed in Chapter 25.) The stimulus for erythropoietin release is decreased oxygen delivery in the kidneys. The anemia of chronic renal failure, in which kidney cells have become nonfunctional, may be related to the lack of this hormone. Epo also affects endothelium and promotes angiogenesis, mitogenesis, and antipoptosis.[17]

TESTS OF RENAL FUNCTION

The Concept of Clearance

A number of specific renal functions can be measured by renal clearance. Renal clearance techniques determine how much of a substance can be cleared from the blood by the kidneys per given unit of time. The application of this principle permits an indirect measure of GFR, tubular secretion, tubular reabsorption, and renal blood flow.

Clearance and Glomerular Filtration Rate

The GFR provides the best estimate of functioning renal tissue. Loss or damage to nephrons leads to a corresponding decrease in GFR. The measurement of GFR requires use of a substance that has a stable plasma concentration; is not protein bound; is freely filtered at the glomerulus; does not influence GFR; and is not secreted, reabsorbed, or metabolized by the tubules. *Inulin* (a fructose polysaccharide) is one substance that meets the criteria for measurement of GFR.

The kidney "clears" inulin from the plasma by filtering it at the glomerulus, reabsorbing nearly all of the fluid, and excreting the inulin left behind in the urine. The amount of inulin filtered is equal to the volume of plasma filtered (GFR) multiplied by the plasma concentration of inulin (P_{IN}). The amount of inulin in the urine is equal to a volume of urine per unit of time ($\dot{V}$) (usually 24 hours) multiplied by the inulin concentration of urine (U_{IN}). Because all the inulin filtered is excreted in the urine,

$$GFR \times P_{IN} = U_{IN} = \dot{V}$$

GFR can be calculated by rearranging the formula:

$$GFR \ (ml/min) = \frac{U_{IN} \times \dot{V}}{P_{IN}}$$

The accurate determination of inulin clearance requires constant infusion to maintain a stable plasma level. This is time consuming, inconvenient, and at risk for error. Therefore the clearance of *creatinine*, a natural substance produced by muscle and released into the blood at a relatively constant rate, is commonly used clinically. It is freely filtered at the glomerulus, but a small amount is secreted by the renal tubules.

Therefore creatinine clearance overestimates the GFR but within tolerable limits. Creatinine clearance provides a good measure of GFR because only one blood sample is required in addition to a 24-hour volume of urine. The GFR estimated by creatinine clearance is calculated as follows:

$$\text{GFR (ml/min)} = \frac{U_{CR} \times \dot{V}}{P_{CR}}$$

Similar calculations can be made for all solutes excreted in the urine per unit of time. Substances freely filtered at the glomerulus but with a clearance less than inulin or creatinine have been reabsorbed along the tubules. For example, glucose is completely reabsorbed and has a clearance rate of nearly zero. Conversely, substances secreted by the tubules have a clearance rate greater than inulin or creatinine (i.e., greater than 1.0). Numerous formulas have been developed for estimating GFR using creatine and other indicators.[18]

Clearance and Renal Blood Flow

The standard clearance formula also can be used to estimate RPF and RBF. The substance used for this evaluation is para-aminohippurate (PAH). Some PAH is filtered at the glomerulus, and most of the remainder is secreted into the tubules in one circulation through the kidney. If all the PAH were removed from the plasma during a single pass through the kidney, total RPF could be determined. Because the supporting and nonsecreting structures of the kidney receive 10% to 15% of effective renal blood flow (ERBF), clearance of PAH measures only what is known as the **effective renal plasma flow (ERPF),** which is 85% to 90% of the true renal plasma flow:

$$ERBF = \frac{ERPF}{1 - Hematocrit}$$
$$(1.0 - 0.45)$$

The estimation of ERBF can then be calculated by considering the hematocrit in the following formula:

$$EPRG = \frac{U_{PAH}\dot{V}}{P_{PAH}}$$

where C_{PAH} = renal clearance of PAH, U_{PAH} = PAH in urine, and P_{PAH} = PAH in plasma.

Blood Tests

Plasma Creatinine Concentration

A long-term decline in GFR over weeks or months is reflected in the **plasma creatinine (P_{CR}) concentration** (normal value = 0.7 to 1.2 mg/dl). The P_{CR} concentration has a stable value when the GFR is stable because creatinine has a constant rate of production as a product of muscle metabolism. The amount filtered is approximately equal to the amount excreted, and a small amount is secreted by kidney tubules. When the GFR declines, the P_{CR} increases proportionately. Thus the GFR and P_{CR} are inversely related. If the GFR were to decrease by 50%, the filtration and excretion of creatinine would be reduced by 50% and creatinine would accumulate in plasma to twice the normal value. Therefore elevated P_{CR}

values represent decreasing GFR. In the new steady state, however, the total amount of creatinine excreted in the urine would remain the same because of the proportionate decrease in GFR and increase in P_{CR}.

The application of this principle is simple and useful for monitoring progressive changes in renal function. The test is most valuable for monitoring the progress of chronic rather than acute renal disease because it takes 7 to 10 days for the plasma creatinine level to stabilize when GFR declines. Serial measures can be obtained over a long time and plotted as a curve of glomerular function. The P_{CR} also becomes elevated during trauma or breakdown of muscle tissue. In such instances the value is then not useful for estimating GFR.

Plasma Cystatin C Concentration

Serum concentrations of *cystantin C* (see What's New? box) also can be used for estimations of GFR. The reciprocal of the serum concentrations of cystatin C can be used as estimates of changes in GFR similar to measures of plasma creatinine concentration. The National Kidney Foundation publishes guidelines for estimating GFR for monitoring renal failure.[19]

Blood Urea Nitrogen

The concentration of urea nitrogen in the blood reflects glomerular filtration and urine-concentrating capacity. Because urea is filtered at the glomerulus, blood urea nitrogen (BUN) levels increase as glomerular filtration drops. Because urea is reabsorbed by the blood through the permeable tubules, the BUN rises in states of dehydration and acute and chronic renal failure when passage of fluid through the

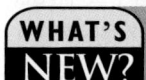
WHAT'S NEW?   Cystatin C and Glomerular Filtration Rate

Cystatin C (CysC) is a low molecular weight protein produced at a constant rate by all nucleated cells. Serum concentrations are independent of age, weight, height, gender, and body composition. The protein is freely filtered by the glomerulus and is almost completely reabsorbed and catabolized by proximal tubular cells, thus making measures of plasma concentration an effective measure of glomerular filtration rate (GFR). Several studies have reported that the reciprocal of the serum CysC concentration is a more sensitive estimate of GFR than the reciprocal of the serum creatinine concentration or creatinine clearance. Formulas also have been proposed for calculating GFR in ml/min from plasma CysC values in mg/L. The measure may be more sensitive for early and minimal decreases in GFR and superior to measures of serum creatinine for those in intensive care units, older persons, monitoring of renal function in those with diabetes mellitus or chronic renal failure, and after kidney transplant. One study reported that subclinical changes in thyroid function can significantly alter CysC levels and should be considered when using CysC as a measure of GFR.

Data from Delanaye P et al: *Intensive Care Med* 30(5):980-983, 2004; Gokkusu CA et al: *Clin Biochem* 37(2):94-97, 2004; Hoek FJ, Kemperman FA, Krediet RT: *Nephrol Dial Transplant* 18(10):2024-2031, 2003; Larsson A et al: *Scand J Clin Lab Invest* 64(1):25-30, 2004; Filler G et al: *Clin Biochem* 38(1):1-8, 2005.

tubules is slowed. BUN also varies as a result of altered protein intake and protein catabolism and therefore is a poor measure of GFR. The normal range for BUN in the adult is 10 to 20 mg/dl of blood.

Urinalysis

Urinalysis is a noninvasive and relatively inexpensive diagnostic procedure. The best results are obtained from a fresh, cleanly voided specimen, because decay permits changes in the composition of urine. Urinalysis includes evaluation of color, turbidity, protein, pH, specific gravity, sediment, and supernatant.

Urine color is normally a clear, light yellow color because of urochrome and other pigments. When formed substances (crystals, blood cells, or casts) are in the urine, it appears turbid. Protein in the urine creates marked foaming when shaken, and the foam is yellow or orange when the urine contains bile pigments. Urine does not normally contain protein or bile.

Urine pH normally ranges between 5.0 and 6.5, but it may vary from 4.5 to 8.0. Urine is more alkaline after eating and then declines, becoming less alkaline, before the next meal. Because sleep is accompanied by intermittent hypoventilation, urine is more acidic upon awakening.

Specific gravity is an estimated measure of the solute concentration of the urine. Specific gravity of any solution is measured by comparing the weight of the solution with an equal volume of distilled water. Hence, specific gravity is not a true measure of the number or concentration of particles, but it correlates well with osmolality and is a useful clinical tool. Specific gravity usually is measured with a hydrometer in a cylinder of urine; the normal value is 1.016 to 1.022. Dipstick evaluations may be falsely high when urine pH is less than 6 and falsely low when the pH is more than 7.

The final urine osmolality is primarily a function of ADH, which controls water reabsorption in the collecting ducts. If the kidney is unable to concentrate or dilute urine, given a stimulus, the cause is usually a malfunction of the renal tubules or inappropriate ADH secretion by the posterior pituitary gland. The state of hydration also affects the urine specific gravity, so hydration status should be evaluated before making a diagnosis. This determination is helpful for differentiating oliguria caused by intrinsic renal disease from hypovolemia as a result of dehydration.

Urine Sediment

The urine sediment is examined microscopically and may contain cells, casts, crystals, and bacteria. Epithelial cells may be seen in the microscopic field because they are shed naturally throughout the urinary tract.

Red Blood Cells

Normal urine contains few or no red blood cells. If a large number of red cells are present, this is known as **hematuria** and the sediment may be red. An alkaline or hypotonic urine causes lysis of red cells, however, so that the cells will not be seen. Urine then will be positive for hemoglobin, and the spe-

cific gravity will be elevated. Hematuria can occur with the administration of anticoagulants and with several renal diseases.

Casts

Casts (accumulations of cellular precipitates) originate in the renal tubules, from which they take their shape. They are cylindrical with distinct borders. All casts have a precipitated microprotein matrix and arise primarily from the ascending limb of the distal tubule. Red cell casts indicate bleeding into the tubules; white cell casts are associated with an inflammatory process. Epithelial cell casts indicate degeneration of the tubular lumen or necrosis of the renal tubules. The type of cast identified suggests the disease process occurring in the kidney.

Crystals

Numerous kinds of **crystals** can be observed in the urine. They may be composed of cystine, uric acid, calcium oxalate, or phosphate. They may not be initially observable, but as the urine cools, crystals will form. Crystals tend to form in a concentrated acidic or alkaline urine. Generally, they are not clinically significant. Crystal formation is diagnostically significant, usually indicating inflammation, infection, or a metabolic disorder.

White Blood Cells

White blood cells (WBCs) in the urine (a condition termed **pyuria**) are primarily indicative of urinary tract infection, particularly when bacteria are present. Glomerulonephritis and nephrotic syndrome also may demonstrate pyuria, but usually in combination with proteinuria, red cells, and casts. The finding of WBC casts reflects a kidney infection, because these casts are not formed in the bladder or prostate. If WBCs are present in the urine, a culture should be done for specific identification of bacteria and sensitivity of bacteria to antibiotics.

Other Measures

Dipsticks and reagent strips are available for detecting other substances in the urine, including glucose, bilirubin, urobilinogen, leukocyte esterase and nitrates, ketones, proteins, hemoglobin, and myoglobin.[2]

AGING AND RENAL FUNCTION

Throughout life the kidney responds to an increased workload by compensatory hypertrophy. This hypertrophy is marked in individuals who have donated a kidney for transplant or have lost functioning nephrons from trauma or disease. The glomeruli increase in diameter, and the tubules enlarge effectively to maintain the regulatory functions of the kidney. Hypertrophy occurs more rapidly and with a larger size increase in younger individuals and in those with high protein intake.

Changes in the kidneys occur throughout life, with decrease in size and a linear decrease in renal blood flow and GFR.[20,21] With aging the number of nephrons decreases.[22] The primary mechanism appears to be a change in the renal vasculature and perfusion pattern, which leads to a reduction in numbers of nephrons. The rate of nephron loss accelerates between 40 and 80 years of age. By 75 years of age the nephron population is reduced by 30% to 50%, with loss of renal mass occurring primarily in the cortex.[2] Degenerative changes within nephrons also occur with aging. The glomerular capillaries atrophy, with a reduction in the branching vessels. The glomeruli then may disappear completely. The arcuate and interlobular arteries become tortuous, contributing to ischemia. The loss of the glomerular tuft may cause a shunt between the afferent and efferent arterioles. Although loss of juxtaglomerular nephrons still allows the vasa recta to be perfused, the combination of events contributes to a decreasing ability to excrete a concentrated urine. Thus the specific gravity of the urine in older individuals tends to be on the low side of normal.

Tubular transport changes with aging although under normal conditions the tubules function adequately. Adaptation to stressful conditions is more difficult. Glucose, bicarbonate, and sodium are not as efficiently reabsorbed, and hyperkalemia is more common because of decreased secretion. Response to acid or base loads is delayed and prolonged. Sudden or large changes in pH or fluid load may lead to serious imbalances with increased risk of hypervolemia or hypovolemia. Acute losses or chronic fluid deficits can lead to renal insuffi-

ciency in the elderly person. Administration of drugs eliminated by renal processes may require dose modifications and more astute observations for toxic side effects.[23] The T_m for glucose reabsorption decreases with age, contributing to a greater amount of glucose in the urine. This is an important consideration when glycosuria is used for screening or monitoring the process of diabetes mellitus in elderly persons. These changes occur independently of disease, however, indicating a normal process of aging. An age-related decline in renal activation of vitamin D decreases intestinal absorption of calcium and older adults need more vitamin D to overcome diminishing renal function.[24] Previous or concurrent renal disease or urinary tract obstruction may amplify age-related changes in function.

Bladder symptoms are common among elderly individuals and include frequency, urgency, and nocturia. Age-related changes in bladder structure and function may contribute to some symptoms as well as influences outside the urinary tract. Changes in neurotransmission influence the micturition reflex and may lead to overactive bladder.[25] Obstruction related to prostate hypertrophy may lead to urine retention with frequency, urgency, nocturia, and slow or intermittent urinary stream.

SUMMARY REVIEW

Structures of the Renal System

1. The kidneys are paired structures lying bilaterally between the twelfth thoracic and third lumbar vertebrae.
2. The kidney is composed of an outer cortex and an inner medulla.
3. The calyces join to form the renal pelvis, which is continuous with the upper end of the ureter.
4. The nephron is the urine-forming unit of the kidney and is composed of the glomerulus, proximal tubule, hairpin loops of Henle, distal tubule, and collecting duct.
5. The glomerulus contains loops of capillaries. The capillary walls serve as a filtration membrane for the formation of the primary urine. The layers of the glomerular capillary include the endothelium, basement membrane, and epithelium.
6. The Bowman space is the space between the visceral and parietal epithelium.
7. The proximal tubule is lined with microvilli to increase surface area and enhance reabsorption.
8. The hairpin-shaped loops of Henle transport solutes and water, contributing to the hypertonic state of the medulla.
9. The distal tubule adjusts acid-base balance by excreting acid into the urine and forming new bicarbonate ions.
10. The collecting duct contains principle cells and intercalated cells.
11. The ureters extend from the renal pelvis to the posterior wall of the bladder. Urine flows through the ureters by means of peristaltic contraction of the ureteral muscles.
12. The bladder is a bag composed of the detrusor and trigone muscles and innervated by parasympathetic fibers. When accumulation of urine reaches 250 to 300 ml, mechanoreceptors, which respond to stretching of tissue, stimulate the micturition reflex.

Renal Blood Flow

1. Renal blood flows at about 1000 to 1200 ml/min, or 20% to 25% of the cardiac output.

2. Blood flow through the glomerular capillaries is maintained at a constant rate in spite of a wide range of arterial pressures (autoregulation).
3. The glomerular filtration rate (GFR) is the filtration of plasma per unit of time and is directly related to the perfusion pressure of renal blood flow.
4. Autoregulation of renal blood flow and sympathetic neural regulation of vasoconstriction maintain a constant GFR.
5. The renal blood vessels are innervated by the sympathetic noradrenergic nerves that regulate vasoconstriction.
6. Renin is an enzyme secreted from the juxtaglomerular apparatus; it causes the generation of angiotensin, a potent vasoconstrictor. The renin-angiotensin system is thus a regulator of renal blood flow.
7. Natriuretic hormone from the right atrium of the heart promotes sodium and water loss by inhibiting aldosterone.

Kidney Function

1. The major function of the nephron is urine formation, which involves the processes of glomerular filtration, tubular reabsorption, and tubular secretion and excretion.
2. Glomerular filtration is favored by capillary hydrostatic pressure and opposed by oncotic pressure in the capillary and hydrostatic pressure in the Bowman capsule. The balance of favoring and opposing filtration forces is known as net filtration pressure (NFP).
3. The GFR is approximately 120 ml/min, and 99% of the filtrate is reabsorbed.
4. The proximal tubule reabsorbs about 60% to 70% of the filtered sodium and water and 90% of other electrolytes.
5. Because most molecules are reabsorbed by active transport, the carrier mechanism can become saturated at a point known as the transport maximum (T_m). Molecules not reabsorbed are excreted with the urine.

6. The distal tubules actively reabsorb sodium and secrete potassium and hydrogen for the regulation of electrolyte and acid-base balance.
7. The concentration of the final urine is a function of the level of antidiuretic hormone (ADH) that stimulates the distal tubules and collecting ducts to reabsorb water. The countercurrent exchange system of the long loops of Henle and their accompanying capillaries establishes a concentration gradient within the renal medulla to facilitate the reabsorption of water from the collecting duct.
8. The distal nephron regulates acid-base balance by excreting hydrogen ions and forming new bicarbonate.
9. The kidney secretes or activates a number of hormones that have systemic effects, including vitamin D_3 (1,25-OH_2D_3) and erythropoietin, which stimulates erythropoiesis when there is hypoxia.

Tests of Renal Function

1. Tests that measure renal clearance indicate how much of a substance can be cleared from the blood by the kidneys per given amount of time.
2. Creatinine, a substance produced by muscle, is measured in both plasma and urine to calculate a commonly used clinical measurement of GFR (creatinine clearance).
3. The plasma creatinine concentration, cystatin C plasma concentration, and the blood urea nitrogen (BUN) levels indicate glomerular function. Plasma creatinine and cystatin C are measured to monitor progressive renal dysfunction; BUN is an indicator of hydration status.
4. Urinalysis involves evaluation of color, turbidity, protein, pH, specific gravity, sediment, and supernatant.
5. Presence of bacteria, red blood cells, white blood cells, casts, or crystals in the urine sediment may indicate a renal disorder.

Aging and Renal Function

1. As a person grows older, a decrease occurs in the number of nephrons. Both renal blood flow and glomerular filtration rate decline.
2. Tubular transport and reabsorption decrease with age. Response to acid-base changes and reabsorption of glucose are delayed. Drugs eliminated by the kidney can accumulate in the plasma, causing toxic reactions.

KEY TERMS

Arcuate arteries, 1282
Atrial natriuretic peptide (ANP), 1294
Bladder, 1285
Bowman capsule, 1280
Bowman space, 1280
Casts, 1297
Collecting duct, 1282
Countercurrent exchange system, 1293
Crystals, 1297
Detrusor muscle, 1285
Distal tubule, 1282
Diuretic, 1294
Effective renal plasma flow (ERPF), 1296
Excretion, 1288
External urethral sphincter, 1285
Filtration slits, 1280
Glomerular capillaries, 1282
Glomerular endothelium, 1280
Glomerular filtration membrane, 1280
Glomerular filtration rate (GFR), 1285
Glomerulus, 1280
Hematuria, 1297
Hilum, 1279
Interlobar arteries, 1282
Intercalated cells, 1282
Internal urethral sphincter, 1285
Juxtaglomerular apparatus (JGA), 1281

Juxtaglomerular cells, 1281
Juxtamedullary nephrons, 1280
Kidneys, 1279
Loop of Henle, 1281
Macula densa, 1281
Major calyx, 1279
Mesangial cells, 1280
Micturition, 1285
Midcortical nephrons, 1280
Minor calyx, 1279
Myogenic mechanism, 1286
Natriuretic peptide, 1287
Nephron, 1280
Net filtration pressure (NFP), 1288
Oliguria, 1294
Parietal epithelium, 1280
Peritubular capillaries, 1282
Plasma creatinine (P_{CR}) concentration, 1296
Podocytes, 1280
Principle cells, 1282
Proximal tubule, 1281
Pyuria, 1297
Renal arteries, 1282
Renal capsule, 1279
Renal columns, 1279
Renal corpuscle, 1280

Renal cortex, 1279
Renal fascia, 1279
Renal medulla, 1279
Renal papillae, 1283
Renal pelvis, 1279
Renal pyramids, 1279
Renin-angiotensin system, 1286
Specific gravity, 1297
Superficial cortical nephrons, 1280
Transport maximum (T_m), 1291
Trigone, 1285
Tubular reabsorption, 1288
Tubular secretion, 1288
Tubuloglomerular feedback, 1286
Ultrafiltration, 1288
Urea, 1294
Ureters, 1285
Urethra, 1285
Urinalysis, 1297
Urine color, 1297
Urine pH, 1297
Urodilantin, 1294
Vasa recta, 1283
Visceral epithelium, 1280
Water diuresis, 1294

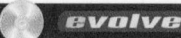
REFERENCES

1. Haas CS et al: Regulatory mechanism in glomerular mesangial cell proliferation, *J Nephrol* 12(6):405-415, 1999.
2. Brenner BM: *Brenner and Rector's the kidney*, vol 1, ed 6, Philadelphia, 2000, Saunders.
3. Pavenstadt H: Roles of the podocyte in glomerular function, *Am J Physiol Renal Physiol* 278(2):F173-F179, 2000.
4. Pavenstadt H, Kriz W, Kretzler M: Cell biology of the glomerular podocyte, *Physiol Rev* 83(1):253-307, 2003.
5. Lewis SA: Everything you wanted to know about the bladder epithelium but were afraid to ask, *Am J Physiol Renal Physiol* 278(6):F967-F974, 2000.
6. Persson PB: Renal blood flow autoregulation in blood pressure control, *Curr Opin Nephrol Hypertens* 11(1):67-72, 2002.
7. Persson AE et al: Mechanisms for macula densa cell release of renin, *Acta Physiol Scand* 181(4):471-474, 2004.
8. Bie P, Wamberg S, Kjolby M: Volume natriuresis vs. pressure natriuresis, *Acta Physiol Scand* 181(4):495-503, 2004.
9. Li YC: Vitamin D regulation of the renin-angiotensin system, *J Cell Biochem* 88(2):327-331, 2003.
10. Kramer HS: Atrial natriuretic peptides and the natriuretic hormone(s): regulatory roles and therapeutic applications. In Gronick HC, editor: *Concepts of nephrology*, vol 19, St Louis, 1996, Mosby.
11. Vesely DL: Natriuretic peptides and acute renal failure, *Am J Physiol Renal Physiol* 285(2):F167-F177, 2003.
12. Serafini-Cessi F, Malagolini N, Cavallone D: Tamm-Horsfall glycoprotein: biology and clinical relevance, *Am J Kidney Dis* 42(4):658-676, 2003.
13. Palmer LG: Potassium secretion and the regulation of distal nephron K channels, *Am J Physiol* 277(6 Pt 2):F821-F825, 1999.
14. Koeppen BM, Stanton BA: *Renal physiology*, ed 3, St Louis, 2001, Mosby.
15. Knepper MA, Chou CL, Layton HB: How is urine concentrated by the renal inner medulla? In Bourke E, Mallick NP, Pollak VE, editors: *Moving points in nephrology*, vol 12, Basel, 1993, Karger.
16. Tremblay J et al: Biochemistry and physiology of the natriuretic peptide receptor guanylyl cyclases, *Mol Cell Biochem* 230(1-2):31-47, 2002.
17. Ribatti D et al: Erythropoietin as an angiogenic factor, *Eur J Clin Invest* 33(10):891-896, 2003.
18. Silkensen JR, Kasiske BL: Laboratory assessment of kidney disease: clearance, urinalysis, and kidney biopsy. In Brenner BM, editor: *Brenner & Rector's: the kidney*, ed 7, Philadelphia, 2004, Saunders.
19. National Kidney Foundation: K/DOQI clinical practice guidelines for chronic kidney disease: evaluation, classification, stratification, *Am J Kidney Dis* 39(Suppl 1):S1-S266, 2002.
20. Beck LH: The aging kidney. Defending a delicate balance of fluid and electrolytes, *Geriatrics* 55(4):26-28, 31-32, 2000.
21. Fehrman-Ekholm I, Skeppholm L: Renal function in the elderly (>70 years old) measured by means of iohexol clearance, serum creatinine, serum urea and estimated clearance, *Scand J Urol* Hephrol 38(1):73-77, 2004.
22. Hoang K et al: Determinants of glomerular hypofiltration in aging humans, *Kidney Int* 64(4):1417-1424, 2003.
23. Crome P: What's different about older people, *Toxicology* 192(1):49-54, 2003.
24. Vieth R, Ladak Y, Walfish PG: Age-related changes in the 25-hydroxyvitamin D versus parathyroid hormone relationship suggest a different reason why older adults require more vitamin D, *J Clin Endocrinol Metab* 88(1):185-191, 2003.
25. Yoshida M et al: Management of detrusor dysfunction in the elderly: changes in acetylcholine and adenosine triphosphate release during aging, *Urology* 63(3 Suppl 1):17-23, 2004.

ALTERATIONS OF RENAL AND URINARY TRACT FUNCTION

MIKEL GRAY • SUE E. HUETHER • BETH A. FORSHEE

CHAPTER

36

CHAPTER OUTLINE

Renal and urinary tract function can be altered by a variety of disorders. The most common type of urinary dysfunction is infection of the bladder. The urinary tract also can be obstructed by stones or tumors. Renal function can be impaired by disorders within the kidney or by many systemic diseases. Because the kidney filters the blood and regulates fluid, electrolyte, acid base, and red blood cell volume, it is directly linked to every other organ system. Renal failure, whether acute or chronic, is therefore a life-threatening condition.

URINARY TRACT OBSTRUCTION

Urinary tract obstruction is defined as a blockage of urine flow within the urinary tract (Figure 36-1). Blockage may be caused by an anatomic or functional defect. Regardless of its cause, the consequence is an impedance to flow that leads to urinary stasis, dilates the urinary system, increases the risk for infection, and compromises urinary system function. Anatomic and functional changes in the urinary system arising from obstruction are referred to as *obstructive uropathy*. Treatment focuses on relief of the obstruction, but prolonged or possibly permanent impairment occurs when complete or partial obstruction exists over a period of weeks to months or longer.

PATHOPHYSIOLOGY   The severity of an **obstructive uropathy** is determined by (1) the location of the blockage, (2) the completeness of the blockage, (3) involvement of one or both upper urinary tracts, (4) duration, and (5) the cause

of the lesion.[1,2] Most research into the pathophysiology of obstruction is based on models of complete blockage of urinary flow in animal models. Complete obstruction of the upper urinary tract causes dilation of the ureter (hydroureter), and renal pelvis and calyces (hydronephrosis) proximal to the site of urinary blockage. Dilation is attributable to smooth muscle hypertrophy in combination with accumulation of urine above (proximal to) the site of obstruction. Within days two deleterious processes, tubulointerstitial fibrosis and apoptosis, begin and ultimately lead to irreversible renal damage unless the underlying obstruction is relieved.[3] **Tubulointerstitial fibrosis** is the deposition of excessive amounts of extracellular matrix (collagen and other proteins). Deposition of extracellular matrix is a normal process of organ repair and maintenance, and the deposition of extracellular matrix is balanced by its breakdown under the influence of metalloproteinases. Multiple cytokines and growth factors have been implicated in the process of tubulointerstitial fibrosis, including transforming growth factor β-1, angiotensin II, and various tumor necrosis factors. **Apoptosis** is a normal process that the body uses to replace damaged or senescent cells with new ones, but the imbalance in growth factors provoked by obstruction leads to excess cellular destruction and death, ultimately resulting in loss of functioning nephrons and kidney damage.

Tubulointerstitial fibrosis and apoptosis result in detectable damage to the distal renal tubules between 7 and 14 days after obstruction is initiated, and glomerular damage is present by the end of the 4th week. Despite the damage wrought by these processes, partial renal function may be restored provided the obstruction is relieved within 56 to 69 days, although the recovery process usually requires up to 4

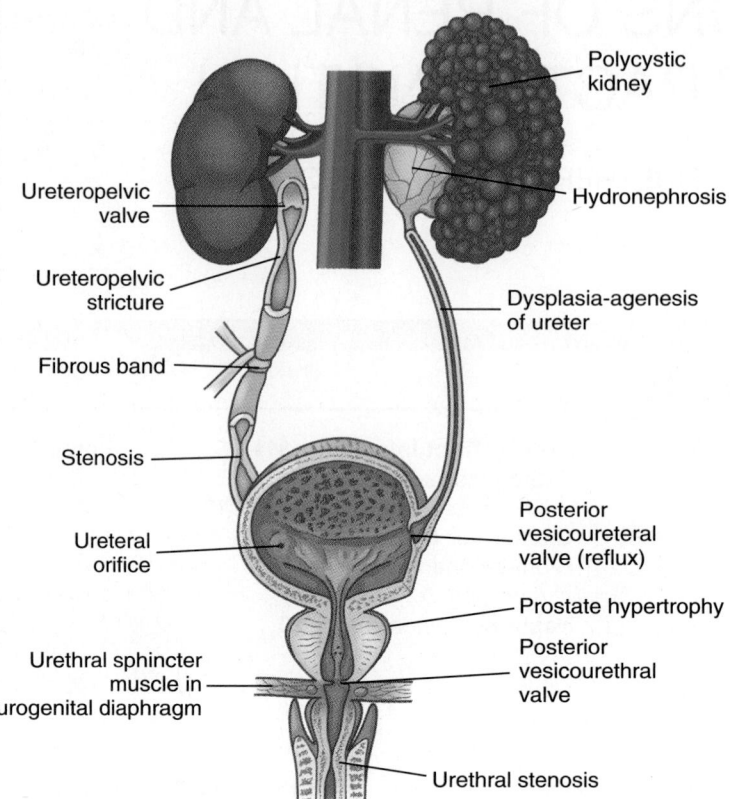

Figure 36-1 Major sites of urinary tract obstruction.

months.[1] Unfortunately, both the severity and rapidity of damage are amplified in the presence of infection.

Partial obstruction, provided it occurs in the *absence* of infection, produces less severe damage and is more readily alleviated when the obstruction is removed. Nevertheless, permanent impairment of renal function, including impairment of the ability to concentrate urine, reabsorb bicarbonate, excrete ammonia or regulate metabolic acid-base balance occurs when obstruction persists over a prolonged period.

Compensatory hypertrophy is essential to the recovery of renal function after an obstruction has occurred.[1] It is the result of two physiologic processes: **obligatory growth** of nephrons under the influence of somatostatin (human growth hormone) and **compensatory growth** of nephrons under the influence of a yet unidentified hormone or hormones. As a result, nephrons in the unaffected kidney increase in size, leading to visible changes in the volume of functioning renal parenchyma. Although this increase in parenchymal volume reflects growth and increase in function of individual glomeruli and tubules, it does not reflect increases in the total number of functioning nephrons. Compensatory hypertrophy is reversible when relief of obstruction results in recovery of function by the obstructed kidney. Recovery diminishes with aging.

Relief of bilateral, partial urinary tract obstruction or complete obstruction of a single kidney provokes a transient period of brisk urine production (postobstructive diuresis) as

the body restores fluid and electrolyte imbalances caused by obstruction.[1,2] **Postobstructive diuresis** is typically mild, but it occasionally results in rapid excretion of as much as 10 liters of urine within a 24-hour period. Diuresis on this level may cause dehydration and dangerous electrolyte imbalances that must be promptly corrected. Risk factors for severe postobstructive diuresis include bilateral obstruction, *nephrogenic diabetes insipidus* (inability to concentrate urine because of damage to the renal parenchyma), hypertension, edema, congestive heart failure, and uremic encephalopathy.

Obstruction of the lower urinary tract affects the entire urinary system, especially when it occurs in infants and children (see Chapter 37). Partial obstruction of the bladder outlet or urethra initially causes an increase in the force of detrusor contraction. If the blockage persists, afferent nerves within the bladder wall are adversely affected, leading to urinary urgency and (in some cases) overactive detrusor contractions, a condition referred to as *overactive bladder*. Depending on the severity of the obstruction and the contractility (strength) of the detrusor muscle, an individual may be unable to completely evacuate urine during micturition. A postvoid residual volume that is at least 150 ml to 200 ml increases the risk for urinary tract infections and may exacerbate bothersome lower urinary tract symptoms. When obstruction persists, excess deposition of extracellular matrix occurs that is expressed as trabeculation of the bladder wall. This process has been postulated to be an attempt by the body to increase the force of its contraction strength, but the process may paradoxically result in a loss of detrusor contractility and a sharp rise in postvoid residual volume.[4]

In some individuals, excessive deposition of extracellular matrix in the bladder wall and detrusor muscle decompensation results in an inability to accommodate urine at low pressures, a condition called **low bladder wall compliance.** Low bladder wall compliance creates pressures within the bladder that reduces or blocks the transport of urine from the upper to the lower urinary tract and greatly increases the risk of hydrourter, hydronephrosis, vesicoureteral reflux, impaired renal function, and urinary tract infection.[5]

Urinary tract obstruction also predisposes individuals to hypertension and recurring urinary tract infection.[6,7] During acute unilateral renal obstruction, hypertension occurs because the renin-angiotensin-aldosterone cascade is activated.[8] Blood pressure increases in chronic, bilateral partial obstruction because of retention of water, sodium, and urea, but it is typically reversible.[6,8] The risk for urinary tract infection is greatest in the lower urinary tract because of incomplete bladder emptying and urine turbulence in the urethra. Nevertheless, infection tends to be more severe and more difficult to eradicate when the upper urinary tract is obstructed, and pyelonephritis poses a serious risk for systemic sepsis and shock unless infection is controlled before invasive treatment of the obstructive lesion begins.

Upper Urinary Tract Obstruction

Obstruction of the upper urinary tracts arises from congenital, inflammatory, malignant or metabolic conditions. The most common disorder in adults is related to kidney stones. (Disorders in children are presented in Chapter 37.)

Kidney Stones

Calculi, or **urinary stones,** are masses of crystals, protein, or other substances that form within and may obstruct the urinary tract. The prevalence of stones in the United States is approximately 2% to 3%, and the incidence of recurrent stone formation once a person experiences an initial calculus is approximately 50% within 10 years.[9] Risk factors include gender, race, geographic location, seasonal factors, fluid intake, diet, and occupation. Men have a higher incidence than do women, and gender also influences the character of stones. The greatest risk for forming an obstructive stone occurs between the second and fourth decades of life. Geographic location influences the risk of stone formation via indirect factors such as average temperature, humidity, as well as regional differences in fluid and dietary intake. For example, persons who live in desert or warm tropical areas tend to have a higher incidence of urinary stones than do persons living in cooler regions. Protective factors against stone formation include regular consumption of an adequate volume of water combined with physical activity.

Urinary calculi are classified according to the primary minerals (salts) comprising the stones.[9] The most common salts include calcium oxalate or calcium phosphate, which collectively account for approximately 70% to 80% of all calculi. Struvite (magnesium, ammonium, and phosphate) stones comprise about 15%, and uric acid stones account for about 7%. Less common stone elements include cystine, 2,8-dihydroxyadenine (DHA), triamterene, indinavir, and ammonium acid urate.

PATHOPHYSIOLOGY   Three factors are required before a stone is formed in the urine: (1) supersaturation of one or more salts in the urine, (2) precipitation of that salt from a liquid to solid state, and (3) growth into a stone via crystallization or agglomeration (sometimes called *aggregation*).[9] *Supersaturation* is the presence of a higher concentration of a salt within a fluid (urine) than the volume is able to dissolve in equilibrium. Within the urine, the potential for supersaturation of various salts is determined by their effective concentration. The effective concentration is determined by the ionic strength of individual salts within the solution, and the influence of other ions. Ionic strength derives from the electrical fields formed when ions combine to salts (common salts in the urine include calcium oxalate and calcium phosphate). Because the urine contains high concentrations of positively and negatively charged ions, multiple salts may form and *precipitate* into a small crystal, capable of forming a nidus (nucleus) of a urinary calculus.

Temperature and pH of the urine also influence the risk of precipitation and calculus formation. However, since the temperature of urine is relatively constant, the influence of pH is most important. An alkaline urinary pH significantly increases the risk of a calcium phosphate stone formation whereas acidic urine increases the risk of a uric acid stone. Cystine and xanthine precipitates more readily in acidic urine, but the influence of pH is less profound than that associated with uric acid or calcium phosphate stones.

Precipitation leads to the formation of crystals in the urine. Stone formation requires an additional step, *growth*, into a structure with adequate mass to obstruct the urinary tract. In a chemical solution containing distilled water and a precise quantity of a salt, under the condition of tightly controlled temperature and pH, it is possible to predict crystal formation and growth with great accuracy. In the clinical setting, however, clinicians are faced with the considerable challenge of predicting which individuals will experience an initial stone and whether they are likely to develop recurring calculi. Unlike the chemical solution, urine contains many different ions that are capable of combining into a large number of salts that may or may not form crystals or larger calculi. In addition, the volume of diluent (water) in the urine changes frequently and rapidly depending on the person's hydration, intake of fluids, and water loss via sweat, stool, or breathing. Although the temperature of urine is relatively constant, the pH also varies significantly, according to metabolic needs, as well as dietary and fluid intake. Further complexity emerges from the multiple surfaces within the urinary tract, such as the renal tubules and papillae that may attract a crystal that clings to other similar crystals or to biologic material (matrix) also found within the urinary tract. As a result of these and other factors, it is not possible to accurately measure the risk of calculus formation within an individual.

Nevertheless, the two main processes that promote or inhibit stone growth have been identified. *Crystallization* is the process by which crystals cling together into complex and geometrically elegant lattices to grow larger structures in the presences of a supersaturated urine. Growth occurs at identifiable surfaces within the nidus (imperfections within the lattice of the crystal called *screw dislocations*) and the stone ultimately forms a spiral. *Agglomeration* is a more random process that occurs when smaller crystals collide within the supersaturated urine and adhere to one another, or when crystals combine with matrix to form stones. Crystallization tends to produce a dense calculus with elegant geometric surfaces whereas stones formed by agglomeration are less dense and amorphous. Although supersaturation is essential for stone formation, the urine need not remain continuously supersaturated for a calculus to grow once its nidus has precipitated from solution. Instead, intermittent periods of supersaturation after the ingestion of a meal or during times of dehydration are sufficient for stone growth in many individuals.

The likelihood of stone formation and growth is further influenced by three endogenous factors: (1) crystal growth-inhibiting factors, (2) particle retention, and (3) matrix.[9] The presence of these factors are particularly important from a clinical perspective because they are thought to explain why some individuals form large, recurring stones whereas others with similar risk profiles remain free of urinary stones. **Crystal growth-inhibiting substances,** such as pyrophosphate, potassium citrate, and magnesium, are capable of reducing the risk of calcium phosphate or calcium oxalate precipitation in the urine and subsequent stone formation.

Particle retention occurs primarily at the papillary collecting ducts. Although most crystals are flushed from the tract via antegrade urine flow, urinary stasis, anatomic abnormalities, or urothelial inflammation within the urinary tract may prevent prompt flushing of crystals from the system, thus increasing the risk of calculus formation.

Matrix is defined as the organic material contained in a urinary calculus. Although urinary stones primarily contain mineralized crystals (97%), some contain significant proportions of organic matrix, usually caused by tissue damage present when urea-splitting pathogens promote growth of infection calculi.

The size of a stone is the principal determinant of the risk for subsequent obstruction.[10] A stone that is less than 5 mm in size has about a 50% chance of spontaneous passage, but a 1-cm stone has almost no chance of spontaneous passage. Nevertheless, persons with ureteral dilation from previous stone passage may be able to excrete larger stones when compared to the person experiencing an initial obstructing calculus.

Calculi containing calcium (calcium phosphate or calcium oxalate) account for up to 80% of all obstructive stones requiring treatment. The majority have **idiopathic calcium urolithiasis (ICU),** a condition whose exact etiology has not yet been defined. However, it is known that most persons with ICU have hypercalciuria, hyperoxaluria, hyperuricosuria, hypocitraturia, mild renal tubular acidosis, and/or crystal growth inhibitor deficiencies. Hypercalciuria is usually attributable to intestinal hyper-absorption of dietary calcium, hyperthyroidism, and bone demineralization caused by prolonged immobility. In contrast, primary hyperoxaluria is a rare, inherited disorder, and it is rarely found in individuals whose stones contain oxalates. Instead, individuals with stones containing oxalates are more likely to have ICU.

Struvite stones contain magnesium-ammonium-phosphate, often mixed with significant amounts of matrix. They are closely associated with urinary tract infection caused by a urease-producing bacteria such as *Proteus, Klebsiella,* or *Pseudomonas.* Struvite calculi may grow quite large and branch into a staghorn configuration that approximates the pelvicaliceal collecting system. Although women have an overall reduced risk for stone formation when compared to men, they are at greater risk for struvite stone formation.

Cystinuric stones are associated with a genetic disorder of amino acid metabolism. It leads to excretion of large volumes of cystine in the urine which, when combined with a urinary pH of 5.5 or less, often leads to cystine stone formation. Uric acid is primarily a product of biosynthesis of endogenous purines, and it is also influenced by the consumption of purines in the diet. Persons who excrete excessive uric acid in the urine and have a low urinary pH, are at particular risk for **uric acid stones. 2,8-Dihyhydroxyadeninuria** is a rare genetic disorder characterized by abnormal purine reabsorption and an increased risk of xanthiuria and xanthine stone formation. Similar to uric acid, its solubility is adversely influenced by a low urinary pH. **Indinavir** is a protease inhibitor used in the management of HIV infection. Approximately 20% of those who use this drug will experience precipitation of indinavir crystals and an increased risk for stone formation. Ammonium acid urate stones are associated with chronic laxative abuse in women. It is postulated to arise from loss of fluids through the gastrointestinal tract with subsequent depletion of urinary citrate and potassium.

EVALUATION AND TREATMENT   The evaluation and diagnosis of urinary calculi is based on presenting symptoms and history, combined with a focused physical assessment, imaging studies, and possibly a functional study of renal pelvic and ureteral pressures.[11] The principal symptom is called **renal colic.** Renal colic is typically described as moderate to exquisitely intense pain characterized by a gradual crescendo, intense peak, and gradual decline thought to correlate with peristaltic waves proximal to the obstruction. If the stone is located in the renal pelvic or proximal ureter, the pain tends to originate in the flank and radiate to the groin.[12] Colic that radiates to lateral flank or lower abdomen typically indicates obstruction in the mid-ureter, and bothersome lower urinary tract symptoms (bothersome urgency, frequent voiding, urge incontinence) may indicate obstruction of the lower ureter or ureterovesical junction with irritation of the lower urinary tract. The history also should include the age of the first stone episode, stone analysis, and presence of complicating factors including hyperparathyroidism or recent gastrointestinal or genitourinary surgery. Urinalysis (including pH) is obtained and a 24-hour urine is typically completed to identify calcium oxalate, citrate, and other significant constituents. In addition, every effort is made to retrieve and analyze calculi that are passed spontaneously or retrieved via aggressive intervention. Additional testing is indicated when a metabolic or endocrine disorder is suspected. A plain abdominal film is obtained to evaluate radiopaque stones (comprising more than 90% of all stones), and an ultrasound, intravenous pyelogram (IVP) or computerized tomographic (CT) scan are obtained to determine the location of the calculi, the severity of obstruction, and associated obstructive uropathy. Traditionally, the IVP was considered the primary method for locating obstructive urinary calculi and assessing related obstructive uropathy, but the spiral abdominal CT provides a rapid and accurate means of completing this task and is now preferred over the IVP in most cases.[13]

Management is directed at removal of the obstructive stone and prevention of recurrence. Smaller stones may be managed conservatively with analgesia and a normal volume of fluid intake. All voided urine is strained and any stone fragments carefully preserved for subsequent analysis. Larger stones are removed by extracorporeal or percutaneous lithotripsy or surgery. Individuals can be counseled to drink a substantial volume of fluids (primarily water) to ensure a urine output of greater than 2 and (ideally) 3 liters per day.[11] Increasing dietary fiber is recommended because it binds calcium in the bowel and reduces its absorption and excretion in the urine. Reduction in dietary intake of calcium is *contraindicated* because it paradoxically increases the concentration of calcium and calcium salts in the urine and raises the risk of stone formation. This effect is hypothesized to occur because calcium is needed to bind oxalate in the bowel rather than relying on its excretion in the urine.[14]

Lower Urinary Tract Obstruction

A number of disorders may cause obstruction in the lower urinary tract. **Bladder neck dyssynergia** occurs when the smooth muscle of the urethrovesical junction fails to funnel during micturition obstructing the bladder outlet. This condition typically occurs in men,[15] but it also has been observed in women.[16] **Prostate enlargement** is caused by acute inflammation, benign prostatic hyperplasia, or prostate cancer. Obstruction is caused by impingement of the urethra as it courses through the inflamed or enlarged prostate and secondarily by pelvic floor muscle guarding and increased striated sphincter tone (see Chapter 23).

A **urethral stricture** is a scar that narrows the urethral lumen. It occurs when infection, injury, or surgical manipulation injures the urethra, leading to wound repair and subsequent scarring.[17] Although the vast majority of urethral strictures occur in men, they are occasionally seen in women as well.[18] The severity of obstruction seen with a urethral stricture is influenced by its location within the urethra, its length, and the minimum caliber of urethral lumen within the stricture.

Severe pelvic organ prolapse in a woman causes bladder outlet obstruction when a cystocele descends below the level of the urethral outlet. Cystoceles that reach or protrude beyond the vaginal introitus are at greatest risk for obstruction, particularly if the bladder neck has been surgically repaired without simultaneous repair of the cystocele. Rarely, the bladder may herniate into the scrotum causing a similar type of obstruction in men.

Neurogenic bladder dysfunction disrupts normal bladder filling and emptying, leading to urinary incontinence (UI) or urinary retention.[19] Neurologic lesions of the brain, spinal cord, or peripheral nervous system cause neurogenic bladder dysfunction. Lesions affecting the brain produce neurogenic detrusor overactivity and urge UI, with preservation of coordination between detrusor contraction and urethral sphincter response. However, although lesions affecting spinal cord segments C2 to S1 produce neurogenic detrusor overactivity, they also cause a condition called *vesicosphincter dyssynergia*. The term *dyssynergia* means lack of harmonious coordination. In the case of the neurogenic bladder, coordination between the detrusor and urethral sphincter muscles is regulated by the pons, and neurologic lesions that affect spinal segments below the pons causes incoordination between these muscles. As a result, the urethral sphincter paradoxically closes during micturition, functionally obstructing the bladder outlet and increasing the risk for obstructive uropathy. Lesions affecting sacral segments S2-S4 or the cauda equina are associated with loss of the detrusor contraction reflex and denervation of the sphincter mechanism. The result is stress UI (activity-induced urinary leakage) because the urethral sphincter mechanism is unable to contract and prevent urine loss during physical exertion, and urinary retention occurs because the detrusor is unable to contract with enough force to effectively evacuate urine from the bladder.

Several factors are associated with low bladder wall compliance including (1) neurologic lesions affecting the lumbosacral spinal segments, (2) chronic urinary tract infection with subsequent bladder wall fibrosis, (3) chronic obstruction associated with severe bladder trabeculation, and (4) pelvic radiation therapy. Low bladder wall compliance places the individual at high risk for obstructive uropathy because it produces chronically elevated intravesical pressures that interfere with ureteral, pelvicaliceal, and ultimately, renal tubular function.

EVALUATION AND TREATMENT   No symptom, or cluster of symptoms, has been identified that accurately differentiates obstruction from urinary retention caused by nonobstructive disorders or other associated conditions such as the overactive bladder.[20] Lower urinary tract symptoms often seen in individuals who have obstruction include (1) daytime voiding frequency (urination more than every 2 hours while awake); (2) nocturia (awakening three or more times at night because of an urge to urinate); (3) weak or intermittent urinary stream; (4) bothersome urinary urgency, often combined with hesitancy; (5) a perception of incomplete bladder emptying following micturition; and (6) a history of acute urinary retention (incomplete inability to urinate that requires catheterization). Physical examination is often unrevealing in adults (and obese adults in particular).

Lower urinary tract obstruction may or may not be associated with incomplete bladder emptying. The postvoid residual volume is measured by catheterization within 5 to 15 minutes of urination, or through a bladder ultrasound machine that measures bladder height and width to approximate the volume of urine within the bladder. This measurement may be combined with uroflowmetry, a graphic representation of the force of the urinary stream expressed as milliliters voided per second. Each of these measurements assesses the efficiency of the lower urinary tract in evacuating urine via micturition, but neither differentiates poor detrusor contraction strength from obstruction as a cause of urinary retention. Multichannel urodynamic testing (a voiding pressure flow study) identifies obstruction, quantifies its severity, and evaluates detrusor contraction strength (Figure 36-2). An evaluation of renal function, including functional imaging studies and serum creatinine is completed, particularly when obstruction is severe and associated with elevated residuals or urinary tract infection.

Because the bladder neck consists of circular smooth muscle with adrenergic innervation, bladder neck dyssynergia may be managed by alpha-adrenergic blocking medications. Obstruction that is not adequately managed by pharmacotherapy may require bladder neck incision.

Urethral strictures are initially managed by dilation. However, the risk for recurrence is significant and longer or particularly dense strictures may be initially treated surgically.[21]

Severe pelvic organ prolapse may be managed conservatively or surgically. A pessary (rubber or silicone device designed to compensate for vaginal wall prolapse) may be inserted to provide support for the vaginal walls. Intravaginal hormone replacement therapy and regular follow up are essential to the long-term success of a pessary.

Detrusor sphincter dyssynergia may be managed by intermittent catheterization and antimuscarinic drugs in order to prevent overactive detrusor contractions and associated vesicosphincter dyssynergia while ensuring regular, complete bladder evacuation via catheterization. Males with dyssynergia may be managed by condom catheter containment, and sphincter resistance may be reduced by supplementation with an alpha-adrenergic blocking drug or transurethral sphincterotomy (surgical incision of the striated sphincter). Low bladder wall compliance may be managed by antimuscarinic drugs and intermittent catheterization, but more severe cases may require augmentation enterocystoplasty (enlargement of the bladder using a detubularized bowel segment), urinary diversion, or long-term indwelling catheterization.

Neurogenic Bladder

Neurogenic bladder is a broad term that describes a variety of lower urinary tract disorders caused by a neurologic lesion or disease. Multiple classification schemas have been devel-

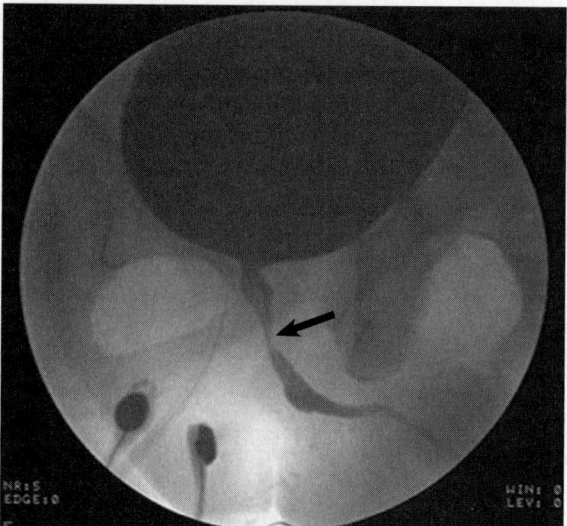

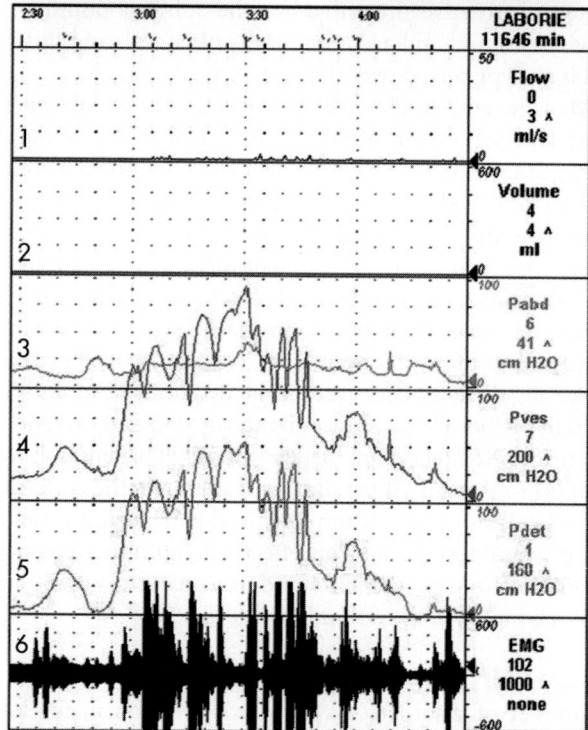

Figure 36-2 Neurogenic detrusor overactivity with vesicosphincter. The *arrow* indicates narrowing of the striated sphincter consistent with electromyographic activity *(Line 6)* noted on the urodynamic tracing. Note the characteristic poor flow pattern *(Line 1)* with elevated voiding pressures *(Lines 4 and 5)* indicating obstruction. *Line 1* = Urine flow rate; *Line 2* = urine volume; *Line 3* = abdominal pressure (Pabd); *Line 4* = intravesicular (inside) bladder) pressure (Pves); *Line 5* = detrusor muscle pressure (Pdet); *Line 6* = bladder electromyelogram (EMG).

oped to describe neurogenic bladder dysfunction,[22-25] but none has gained prominence primarily because all fail to account for the evolution of dysfunction over time or the variable influence of the underlying disorder. This discussion focuses on the common disorders that characterize neurogenic bladder dysfunction, and the nomenclature is limited to that promulgated by the International Continence Society.[26] Causes of neurogenic bladder are presented in Figure 36-3.

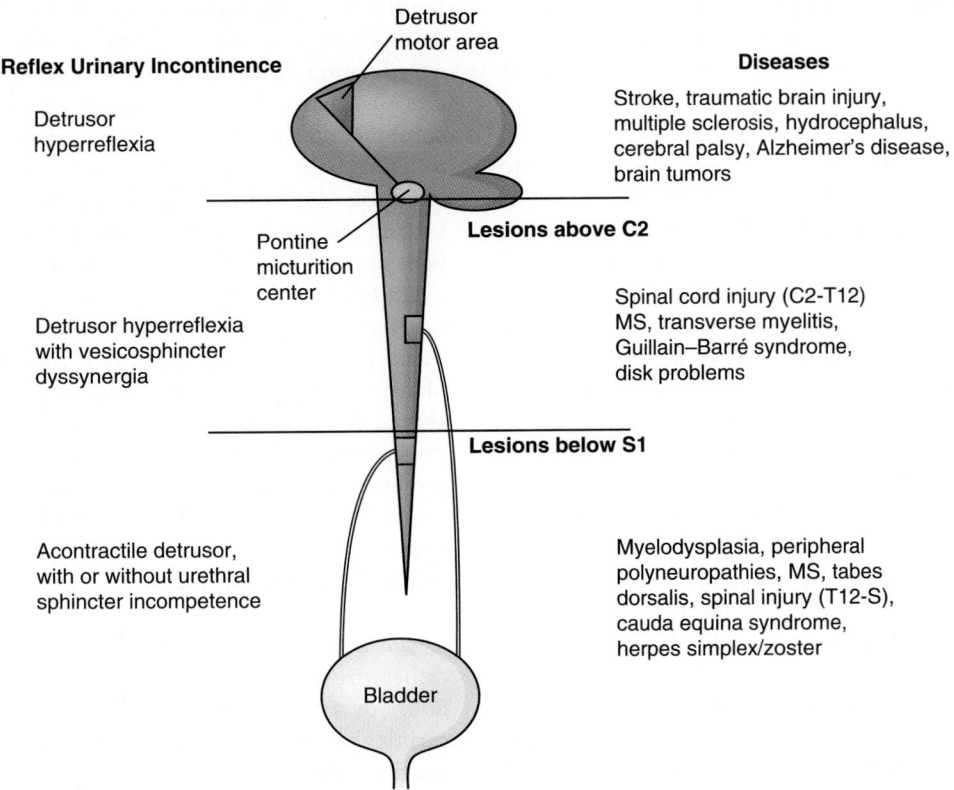

Figure 36-3 Causes of neurogenic bladder and reflex incontinence. (Adapted from Doughty DB: Urinary and fecal incontinence. In Doughty DB, editor: *Urinary and fecal incontinence: nursing management*, ed 2, St Louis, 2000, Mosby.)

PATHOPHYSIOLOGY   Neurogenic detrusor overactivity is defined as uncontrolled or premature contractions of the detrusor muscle associated with a neurologic disorder in the person. Overactive detrusor contractions cause bothersome urgency, urinary leakage, or a combination of these symptoms in those with neurologic disorders primarily affecting the brain, such as a cerebrovascular accident, traumatic brain injury, or brain tumor. In contrast, lesions affecting the spinal cord are usually associated with loss of sensations of bladder filling and loss of coordination between detrusor and urethral sphincter muscles. Therefore, in addition to neurogenic detrusor overactivity, persons with a spinal cord injury, transverse myelitis, or Guillain-Barré syndrome experience *detrusor sphincter dyssynergia* resulting in a functional obstruction of the bladder outlet.

An acontractile detrusor cannot contract despite bladder filling or the desire to urinate. It is typically associated with neurologic disorders affecting the lumbosacral spinal segments or the cauda equina, such as myelomeningocele or a low spinal cord injury. Depending on whether the neurons of Onuf's nucleus are involved with the neurologic disorder, an acontractile detrusor is often seen with urethral sphincter incompetence, caused by denervation of the striated muscle of the urethra and resulting in stress urinary incontinence.

Although recognition of these dysfunctions is critical to treatment, successful management indicates accurate diagnosis of the underlying dysfunction at the time of diagnosis combined with knowledge that a neurogenic bladder evolves over time in response to complex interactions among three principal factors: (1) presence and severity of associated obstruction, (2) low bladder wall compliance, and (3) the natural history of the underlying neurologic disorder.[27]

Obstruction

The reader should refer to the previous section for a detailed description of lower urinary tract obstruction. Obstruction associated with neurogenic bladder dysfunction is typically the result of detrusor sphincter dyssynergia (incoordination between the striated urethral sphincter and detrusor muscles) or bladder neck dyssynergia (incoordination between urethral and detrusor smooth muscle). As noted previously, obstruction of the bladder outlet leads to obstructive uropathy, adversely affecting both the lower and upper urinary tracts.

Low Bladder Wall Compliance

A hostile neurogenic bladder is one whose function threatens the upper urinary tracts it serves. Two aspects of neurogenic bladder dysfunction are associated with a risk of upper urinary tract distress, low bladder wall compliance, and obstruction. Compliance of the bladder wall is defined as its ability to distend and accommodate increasing urine volumes while maintaining low intravesical pressures.[27] Low bladder wall compliance is associated with chronic obstruction, nerve damage affecting lumbosacral spinal segments; radiation therapy; and recurring urinary tract infection. Its presence is clinically relevant because it greatly increases the risk that the individual will experience upper urinary tract distress characterized by ureterohydronephrosis, recurring febrile urinary tract infections, renal scarring, and/or compromised renal function.

EVALUATION AND TREATMENT   Routine diagnostic procedures include a focused history and physical examination and a urinalysis (followed by a urine culture and sensitivities when indicated). Frequently performed tests also include measurement of postvoid residual volume, serum creatinine and BUN, imaging of the upper urinary tracts, and urodynamic testing in selected cases. The history focuses on the bladder management program. Although the majority of persons with neurogenic bladders void spontaneously, many others use an alterative strategy to manage their bladder including (1) clean intermittent catheterization, (2) condom catheter containment (often referred to as reflex, trigger, or kick off voiding), (3) micturition into an adult containment brief or infant's diaper, and (4) indwelling catheterization. The urinalysis is used to identify evidence of clinically relevant urinary tract infection. For many individuals with a neurogenic bladder, particularly those managed by indwelling or intermittent catheterization, asymptomatic bacteriuria does not indicate a clinically significant infection, and it does not justify completion of a culture or treatment with antibiotics.[28] However, when an individual has a symptomatic infection (associated with urinary incontinence, fever, hematuria, autonomic dysreflexia, or an exacerbation of spasticity that interferes with activities of daily living), a urine culture is completed and sensitivity guided antibiotics are used to eradicate the infection. The serum creatinine and creatinine levels are obtained to evaluate renal function. However, because they usually remain within normal ranges until renal function is significantly impaired, upper urinary tract function is often assessed with an ultrasound, radionuclide study, or IVP. Urodynamic testing accomplishes three goals: (1) it characterizes urinary incontinence type, (2) it identifies the cause of urinary retention, and (3) it predicts hostile neurogenic bladder function before the onset of upper urinary tract distress.[27,29]

In addition to providing clues to renal function, upper urinary tract imaging is used to diagnose upper urinary tract distress, urinary stones, and preexisting anatomic defects. An ultrasound is usually preferred when establishing a baseline of renal anatomy or when following individuals with serial images over time. An intravenous pyelogram or computerized tomographic (CT) scan may be used when more detailed anatomic images are needed. The use of intravenous contrast also allows evaluation of renal function. When a detailed analysis of renal function is indicated, a radionuclide study is preferred.

Treatment of neurogenic bladder dysfunction must address existing lower urinary tract dysfunction, ensure regular and complete evacuation of urine from the bladder, protect upper urinary tract function, and correct or contain urinary incontinence. *Spontaneous voiding* is maintained whenever feasible. Individuals with neurologic lesions affecting the brain usually experience neurogenic detrusor overactivity resulting in urge urinary incontinence (UI), and preservation of coordination between detrusor and urethral sphincter muscles. Overactive detrusor contractions may be managed by a combination of antimuscarinic medications and scheduled toileting, with adequate assistance to ensure that the person can successfully move to the toilet, stand at or sit on the toilet, and remove and restore clothing. Individuals with incomplete spinal lesions also may experience neurogenic detrusor overactivity and urge UI, but their bladder dysfunction is usually complicated by detrusor sphincter dyssynergia. Treatment for these individuals may comprise antimuscarinic pharmacotherapy combined with scheduled toileting, or an alpha-adrenergic blocking drug if dyssynergia causes significant obstruction or elevated urinary residuals. Despite the presence of dyssynergia, those with incomplete spinal cord lesions and preservation of sensations of bladder filling are able to maintain a spontaneous voiding program with a moderate risk for urinary incontinence and very low risk of upper urinary tract distress.[30]

Clean intermittent catheterization requires a person to catheterize the urethra on a regular basis, usually every 4 to 6 hours or 4 times daily. It is often combined with antimuscarinic therapy, in order to prevent overactive detrusor contractions and urge or reflex urinary incontinence between catheterizations. The risk for urinary incontinence approaches 50%, but the risk for upper urinary tract risk is less than 10%.[30]

Voiding into a *condom catheter* is a viable option for men who are unable or unwilling to perform self catheterization. Condom containment does not remove the risk of obstructive uropathy associated with vesicosphincter dyssynergia, and individuals may require surgery to transect striated urethral sphincter muscles or an alpha-adrenergic-blocking drug to reduce urethral resistance to micturition. Urinary leakage (incomplete containment within the condom catheter system) occurs in approximately 30% and upper urinary tract distress is seen in 29%.[30]

An *indwelling catheter* provides an attractive alternative for managing neurogenic bladder dysfunction on initial consideration, but they are outweighed by adverse long-term consequences.[30-33] They include (1) urethral erosion causing leakage (bypassing) around the catheter; (2) high risk for upper urinary tract distress and urinary calculi, particularly when the catheter has been in place for 15 years or longer; and (3) an elevated risk for bladder cancer.

Tumors
Renal Tumors

Renal adenomas (benign tumors) are solid, rarely detected small tumors.[34] The tumors are encapsulated and are usually located near the cortex of the kidney. Because they can become malignant, they are usually surgically removed. **Renal cell carcinoma (RCC)**, the most common renal neoplasm (85% of all renal neoplasms), arises from proximal tubule epithelial cells and represents about 2% of cancer deaths.[35] Re-

Overactive bladder (OAB) syndrome is a constellation of symptoms including urgency with or without urge incontinence and usually accompanied by frequency and nocturia in the absence of other disease. Incontinence occurs in over 50% of women with OAB. The problem is more prevalent after menopause and in the elderly.

The pathophysiology of OAB syndrome is complex and involves both the peripheral and central nervous systems. Voluntary or involuntary contraction of the bladder results from stimulation of muscarinic receptors on the detrusor muscle by acetylcholine (ACh). Studies of human detrusor muscle function among the elderly indicate there are changes in cholinergic and purinergic neurotransmission, as well as in the release and actions of ACh from non-neuronal bladder uroepithelial cells. Purinergic transmission increases and cholinergic transmission decreases. These effects are related to decreased ACh release and increased release of adenosine triphosphate (ATP) from postganglionic parasympathetic nerves innervating the bladder. Non-neuronal ACh release increases with age and detrusor stretch. The age-related increase in purinergic transmission and ATP release result in detrusor overactivity.

Oral antimuscarinic drugs are the mainstay of treatment for OAB, although not everyone responds favorably. A transdermal delivery system is showing favorable response with less side effects. Anticholinergics also have been used with some success. Adverse effects of both agents include dry mouth and constipation, and they should be used with caution in men because they may cause urinary retention. Intravesicular vanilloid substances (capsacin and resiniferatoxin-2) and botulinum-A toxin are newer therapies for OAB. Vanilloids increase bladder capacity and reduce bladder pain. Botulinium-A toxin blocks release of acetylcholine from cholinergic nerve endings and relaxes detrusor smooth muscle.

Data from Abrams P: *Urology* 62(5 Suppl 2):28-37, 2003; Burgard EC et al: *Curr Opin Investig Drugs* 6(1):81-9, 2005; Davila GW: *Expert Opin Pharmacother* 4(12):2315-2324, 2003; Gonzalez RR, Te AE: *Curr Urol Rep* 4(6):429-435, 2003; Hegde SS, Mammen M, Jasper JR: *Curr Opin Investig Drugs* 5(1):40-49, 2004; Serels S: *Curr Med Res Opin* 20(6):791-801, 2004; Smith CP, Chancellor MB: *J Urol* 171(6 Pt 1): 2128-2137, 2004; Yoshida M et al: *Urology* 63(3 Suppl 1):17-23, 2004; Zobrist RH et al: *Pharm Res* 20(1):103-109, 2003.

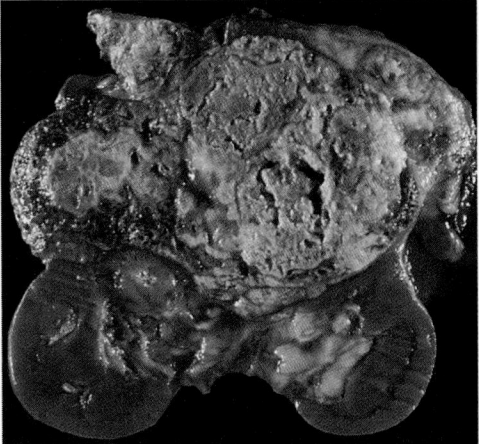

Figure 36-4 Renal cell carcinoma. Renal cell carcinomas usually are spheroidal masses composed of yellow tissue mottled with hemorrhage, necrosis, and fibrosis. (From Damjanov I, Linder J, editors: *Anderson's pathology,* ed 10, St Louis, 1996, Mosby.)

Table 36-1	Staging of Renal Cell Carcinoma	
Stage	**Metastasis**	
I	Tumor confined within kidney capsule	
II	Invasion through renal capsule and renal vein but within surrounding fascia	
III	Involvement of regional lymph nodes and vena cava	
IV	Distant metastases	

nal cell carcinoma occurs in men (22,080 new cases in 2004) more often than in women (13,630 new cases in 2004) and is sporadic in children.[35] The 5-year survival rate is about 60%.[35]

PATHOGENESIS   An association has been identified between tobacco use, obesity, long-term analgesic use, and the incidence of renal cell carcinoma.[36,37] Work is in progress to identify the relationship between environmental exposures and molecular and genetic processes involved in RCC. RCCs are adenocarcinomas and are classified according to cell type and extent of metastasis. *Clear cell tumors* are the most common and have a better prognosis than *granular cell* or *spindle tumors.* Confinement within the renal capsule, together with treatment, is associated with a better survival rate. The tumors usually occur unilaterally, and in about 33% of cases

spread through the lymph nodes and blood vessels to the lungs, liver, lymph nodes, adrenal glands, brain, and bone[38] (Figure 36-4).

CLINICAL MANIFESTATIONS   The classic clinical manifestations of renal cell carcinoma are hematuria, flank pain, and palpable flank or abdomen mass. Early stages are often silent. Hematuria is the most common presenting symptom.[39] The flank pain is usually dull and aching. Tumor palpation is generally difficult but easier in thin people. Systemic manifestations usually represent an advanced stage of disease and include weight loss and fatigue; intermittent fever from tumor toxins; anemia from hematuria and lack of erythropoietin or polycythemia from secretion of erythropoietin factor; liver function with elevated serum alkaline phosphatase, prothrombin, and bilirubin; and hypertension from elevated renin levels.

EVALUATION AND TREATMENT   Diagnosis is based on the clinical symptoms, plain x-ray films of the abdomen, ultrasonography, intravenous pyelography, CT scan or magnetic resonance imagery (MRI), and in special cases, renal angiography. Staging of renal cell carcinoma is assisted with the use of MRI[40] (Table 36-1). The biologic diversity of RCCs present a challenge for targeted, specific therapies.[41] Treatment is usually surgical removal of the affected kidney (radical nephrectomy) with combined use of chemotherapeutic agents and the immunomodulating cytokines interferon-alpha and interleukins, particularly for metastatic disease.[42] Hormonal agents (antiestrogen drugs) are less effective. Radiation therapy also may be used, and new techniques, using radiofrequency ablation and laparoscopic and percutaneous nephron sparing surgery, are promising.[43,44] Immediate relief of obstruction caused by invading tumors can be obtained by placing ureteral catheters past the obstruction or by inserting a nephrostomy tube percutaneously into the renal pelvis. If the obstruction is not treatable, urinary diversion procedures may be required to prevent chronic infection. Survival is related to tumor grade, tumor cell type, and extent of metastasis.

Bladder Tumors

Bladder tumors represent about 3% of all malignant tumors and are the fifth most common malignancy.[35] Approximately 60,240 people develop bladder cancer each year, and 15,600 die of it.[35] Seventy percent of tumors are superficial bladder tumors.[45] The development of bladder cancer is highest in men older than age 60 years.

PATHOGENESIS   The risk of bladder cancer is greater for men who smoke cigarettes or are exposed to metabolites of aniline dyes or other aeromatic amines and among women who take large amounts of phenacitin.[46,47] Bladder cancer is associated with mutations in the tumor-suppressor gene *p53* with overexpression of the *p53* protein product; other genes are under study.[48] The tumor is usually composed of transitional cells (the cells lining the bladder) and may have a papillary growth pattern (a tuftlike lesion attached to a stalk) (Figure 36-5). Nonpapillary tumors (representing 10% of bladder tumors) are not as common as papillary tumors, but they tend to be more invasive and have a poorer prognosis. Metastasis is usually to lymph nodes, liver, bones, and lungs. Staging for bladder carcinoma is presented in Table 36-2. Secondary bladder cancer develops by invasion of cancer from bordering organs, such as cervical carcinoma in women or prostatic carcinoma in men.

CLINICAL MANIFESTATIONS   Bladder tumors may be asymptomatic or accompanied by hematuria. Advanced cancers are associated with pelvic pain and frequent urination.

EVALUATION AND TREATMENT   Diagnosis is made by cystoscopy (visual examination of the urinary tract through a cystoscope,[49] including fluorescence cystocopy,[50] cell studies, biologic markers,[51] urograms (x-ray examinations), and transurethral biopsy. Advances are being made in the development of urine and serum markers that are specific and sensitive.[52] Treatment is related to the type and size of the lesion. Transurethral resection is the treatment of choice for superficial tumors because of the high propensity for bladder tumors to recur. Endoscopic treatment with the neodymium: yttrium-aluminum-garnet (Nd:YAG) laser also has proven effective.[53] Carcinoma in situ is treated with intravesicular (inside the bladder) bacille Calmette-Guérin (BCG) or interferon, which induces a local immune response.[54] Chemotherapeutic agents also have been used with some success to prevent recurrence. Radiation therapy is not as effective, and candidates for radiation must be carefully selected based on tumor type. Chemotherapy may be combined with radiation and surgical resection. Gene therapy for bladder cancer is be-

Table 36-2	Staging of Bladder Carcinoma
Stages	**Metastasis**
0	Limited to mucosal involvement
A	Submucosal involvement
B	Involvement of the muscularis layer
C	Invasion of the perivesical fat
D_1	Spread to regional lymph nodes
D_2	Spread to distant sites, bone, and visceral organs

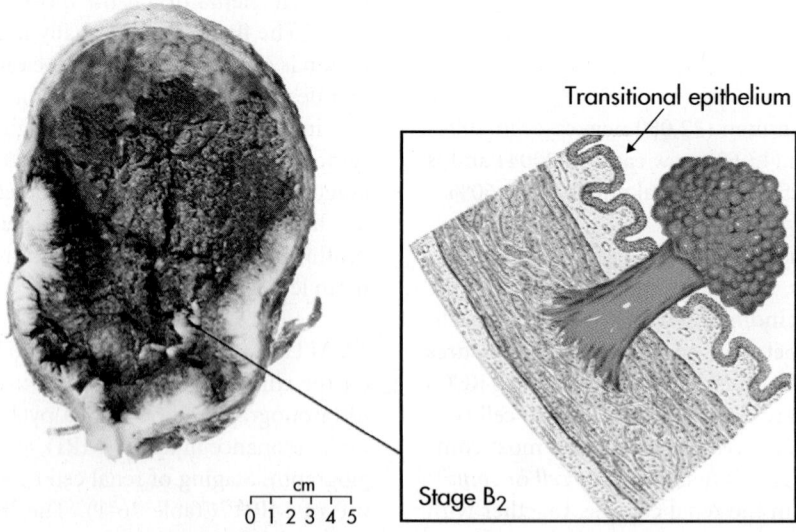

Figure 36-5 Cystectomy specimen. Multiple papillary tumors cover greater part of bladder wall. (From Kissane JM, editor: *Anderson's pathology*, ed 9, St Louis, 1990, Mosby.)

ing developed.[55] Cystectomy is standard for invasive bladder cancer and orthotopic bladder substitution is demonstrating effective functional outcomes.[56] Because of the risk of recurrence, cystoscopic evaluations are performed every 3 to 6 months after initial treatment.

URINARY TRACT INFECTION

A **urinary tract infection (UTI)** is an inflammation of the urinary epithelium following invasion and colonization by some pathogen.[57] The most common cause is bacterial, but fungi or parasites also may provoke a UTI. Infections are classified according to their location within the urinary system or their association with complicating factors. **Cystitis** is an inflammation of the bladder causing urinary frequency, dysuria, urgency, and/or lower abdominal, lower back, or suprapubic pain, and *pyelonephritis* is an inflammation of the upper urinary tracts. An *uncomplicated UTI* occurs in an individual who is otherwise healthy and has a functionally normal urinary system, and a *complicated UTI* occurs in those with defects of the urinary system or other health problems that compromise their resistance to colonization with a pathogen or their ability to fight an existing infection.

An uncomplicated UTI is termed *isolated* when it is a first infection or occurs at least 1 year after any prior UTI. A *recurring UTI* occurs after an initial infection that was successfully eradicated, but recurred no sooner than 5 to 10 days after resolution of the original episode. In contrast, a *persistent UTI* is characterized by ongoing infection despite at least 3 days of treatment with an appropriate antimicrobial agent. These distinctions are clinically relevant to both treatment and preventive strategies. Bacterial persistence is caused by resurgence of the same microorganism after incomplete suppression caused by insufficient administration of antibiotics. Reinfections are usually caused by different species. Causes of bacterial persistence include (1) bacterial resistance to the antibiotic; (2) emergence of a resistant, secondary bacterial strain after the primary organism is eradicated; (3) renal insufficiency causing poor excretion of the antibiotic in the urine; (4) a foreign body (such as a stone) acting as a harbor for bacteria; and (5) papillary necrosis from analgesic abuse.

The lifetime risk of a UTI in a woman is approximately 30%. The risk in young adult men is under 1%, although it rises to approximately 10% among men aged 65 years or older. Groups at elevated risk for UTI include (1) premature infants, (2) sexually active women, (3) women using a diaphragm and spermacide, (4) persons with diabetes mellitus, (5) individuals with an immunosuppressive disorder such as AIDS, (6) persons undergoing instrumentation of the urinary system or those managed with an indwelling catheter, and (7) those with obstruction of the lower urinary tract.[58]

Pathogenesis

The most common pathogens associated with uncomplicated UTI are the gram-negative bacterial species common to the intestinal tract of all humans. *Escherichia coli* infections comprise approximately 80% of UTI found in community-dwelling women. *Staphylococcus saprophyticus* accounts for 10% to 20% and other *Enterobacter* species (*Klebsiella* and *Proteus*) account for the remaining 5%. *E. coli* is not as prominent among complicated UTI and accounts for only 20% of complicated UTI, and pseudomonas or gram-positive microorganisms are relatively common.

Fungal infections are comparatively uncommon. The most common pathogen is *Candida*, but multiple fungal species may colonize the urinary tract, produce symptomatic UTI, and rarely form an obstructive fungal ball, particularly in those who are significantly immunosuppressed.[59-61]

Schistosomiasis is the most common cause of parasitic invasion of the urinary tract on a global basis; it infects over 200 million people.[62] Although rare among people living in the United States, the parasite dwells in waters of the various rivers of fresh water bodies in Africa, South America, and Pacific Rim countries. It usually enters the human by swimming up the urethra while the host swims or is partly submerged in an infected body of water. The parasite burrows into the walls of the urinary tract causing inflammation and scarring of the urinary tract and an increased risk for urothelial malignancies.

PATHOPHYSIOLOGY   Two factors account for the presence of a UTI: the efficiency of defense mechanisms within the host (individual) and the virulence of the pathogen (bacteria, fungus, or parasite). In the healthy individual, host defense mechanisms maintain a sterile posterior urethra and bladder. Even if bacteria manage to enter the bladder, these

---

WHAT'S NEW?   Women and Urinary Tract Infections

Cystitis occurs in approximately 30% of women during their lifetime, and about one third of them will have upper urinary tract infection (UTI) (pyelonephritis). *E. coli* is the most common causative microorganism for uncomplicated UTI. Asymptomatic bacteriuria is common and is a particular complication of pregnancy. All pregnant women should be screened, and infection should be treated promptly to prevent maternal and infant complications. Women at greatest risk for recurrent UTI include first UTI at an early age; maternal history of UTI; frequent sexual intercourse, particularly in women with vaginal epithelial cells that adhere uropathogens; and use of spermicidal products. Young women may have a familial genetic predisposition. Three-day antibiotic treatment is standard for uncomplicated UTI, although a single dose with some newer drugs is proving effective. Treatment for 10 to 14 days is common for uncomplicated pyelonephritis. Vaginal estrogen in postmenopausal women may reduce recurrent infections. Cranberry products reduce the incidence of UTI within 12 months of treatment. The use of probiotics and vaccines to prevent UTI are being evaluated. Antibiotic resistance is a concern for recurrent infections.

Data from Finer G, Landau D: *Lancet Infect Dis* 4(10):631-635, 2004; Jepson RG, Mihaljevic L, Craig J: *Cochrane Database Syst Rev* (1):CD001321, 2004; Nicolle L: *Expert Opin Pharmacother* 4(5):693-704, 2003; Ronald A: *Dis Mon* 49(2):71-82, 2003; Rozenberg S et al: *Int J Fertil Womens Med* 49(2):71-74, 2004.

defense mechanisms prevent it from clinging to the walls of the bladder or ascending to the upper urinary tracts.[57] Most people are able to rapidly rid the urinary tract of invading bacteria, but some show evidence of bacteria in the urine that does not provoke an infection. This condition is called **asymptomatic bacteriuria** and does not harm urinary function or require intervention. A UTI occurs when a pathogen circumvents or overwhelms the host's defense mechanisms and reproduces so avidly that the host must mount a localized or systemic response in order to rid itself of the pathogen and minimize its adverse effects.

Virulence of Uropathogens

Virulence is defined as a potential pathogen's ability to evade or overwhelm the host defense mechanisms and cause disease in a host (see Chapter 9). Several factors contribute to bacterial virulence within the urinary tract. The first is the ability of bacteria to adhere (attach) to the uroepithelium.[63] Most of the research has focused on *E. coli*. Virulent strains of *E. coli* have been shown to form **pili** (threadlike structures) that allow the bacterium to cling to the epithelium of the urinary tract or enter the epithelial cell and resist flushing during normal micturition. Certain bacterial species also enhance their virulence by acting together to form a biofilm.[64] A biofilm consists of three main components: (1) a polysaccharide edifice that adheres to the bladder wall or catheter, (2) a basal layer of bacteria that live in a state of near starvation, and (3) numerous free floating or loosely adherent bacteria that live near the surface of the biofilm that avidly consume nutrients and reproduce rapidly. Biofilms contain a primitive circulatory system that transports nutrients to bacteria deep within the polysaccharide edifice and removes waste products. The presence of a biofilm reduces the efficiency of both innate host defense mechanisms and antimicrobial therapy. Specifically, some bacteria live in a state of near starvation at the base of the biofilm and they are resistant to both flushing from the urinary system through micturition or eradication during antibiotic therapy.[65]

Host Defense Mechanisms

Opposing bacterial virulence are multiple host defense mechanisms.[57,63] For example, periurethral mucous-secreting glands surround the distal two-thirds of the female urethra. Mucus from these glands traps bacteria before it can ascend from proximal urethra to the bladder. In men, the length of the male urethra and secretions from the prostate and accessory periurethral glands combine to form a protective barrier against infection. In addition, the urethral sphincter mechanism acts as a mechanical barrier to bacterial ascent from the distal urethra.

Bacteria that successfully ascend the urethra face detection and destruction by components of the body's immune system provided they come into contact with the bladder wall. Unfortunately, time is required for the immune system to respond to the potential threat, and this period may provide adequate time for bacteria or other pathogens to reproduce several times.

The efficiency of the bladder's defenses is also influenced by the person's Lewis blood group.[66] This taxonomy is based on recognition of inherited antigens associated with the ABO blood factors. Individuals with certain Lewis blood groups are more prone to UTI because they secrete fewer antigens capable of resisting bacterial adherence by pili formation.

The urine itself may contain components that enhance resistance to UTI. These include hydrogen ion concentration (pH), osmolarity (concentration of salts within the urine), glucose content, urea, and glycoproteins. Ideally, the urine should have a slightly acidic pH (6.0 or less), moderate to high urea concentration, and abundant glycoproteins (slimy substances that interfere with bacterial adherence). Dilute urine washes out bacteria, and urine with higher urea concentrations (high osmolarity) is more bacteriostatic. In contrast, glucose in the urine, a higher (alkaline) pH, or urine with high osmolarity but low urea concentration is less bacteriostatic.

CLINICAL MANIFESTATIONS   The clinical manifestations of a UTI differ based on the person's age and urinary tract function.[57] The classic presentation (that seen in young adult women), produces dysuria (pain on urination) frequent urination, and suprapubic or lower back discomfort. The urine may be cloudy and foul smelling. However, symptoms are nonspecific in younger children or older adults. Adults in the 8th decade of life or older may experience confusion and poorly localized abdominal discomfort whereas young children may experience failure to thrive and generalized symptoms of a systemic illness.

EVALUATION AND TREATMENT   A focused history and physical examination document lower urinary tract symptoms such as dysuria, and related findings including suprapubic, flank, abdominal or lower back pain. Information is obtained regarding the character of urine (odor, turbidity, presence of bright or darker blood, etc.), prior UTI, and relevant risk factors.[67] Physical assessment includes temperature and associated vital signs and the presence of flank pain or signs and symptoms of systemic illness indicating possible pyelonephritis. A clean catch urine specimen is obtained whenever feasible[68] and a catheterized specimen is obtained in selected cases. Dipstick urinalysis and microscopy are adequate to diagnose an uncomplicated UTI, but urine culture is critical for complicated infections.

Treatment of cystitis focuses on antimicrobial therapy to eradicate the underlying pathogen. Strategies to relieve lower urinary tract symptoms and pain include increased fluid intake and avoidance of bladder irritants (including caffeine) and urinary analgesics.[58] Empiric selection of an antibiotic is often adequate for management of an uncomplicated UTI, and for initial treatment of a complicated UTI. Antibiotic choice for a complicated UTI is confirmed or adjusted based on results of culture and sensitivity testing. Acute pyelonephritis requires more aggressive treatment, including hospitalization if the person is unable to tolerate fluids or oral antibiotic therapy. Urosepsis and septic shock are medical emergencies that usually demand parenteral, broad spectrum antibiotic therapy and may necessitate management in a critical care setting. UTI caused by *Schistosomiasis* is treated with praziquantel.[69]

Acute Pyelonephritis

Pyelonephritis is an infection of one or both upper urinary tracts (ureters, renal pelvis, and renal parenchyma) (Table 36-3). **Acute pyelonephritis** is defined as an acute infection involving the ureter, renal pelvis, and/or parenchyma. **Chronic pyelonephritis** is persistent or recurring episodes of acute pyelonephritis that leads to a shrunken, fibrotic kidney seen on an x-ray or other imaging study. It indicates a kidney whose parenchyma has been severely damaged and mostly replaced by fibrotic tissue.

Approximately 250,000 cases of pyelonephritis are diagnosed annually in the United States. Women are five times more likely to experience pyelonephritis than men, but men are 30% more likely to die from associated complications.[70] The severity tends to increase with age, and up to 2% of pregnant women will experience an episode of pyelonephritis, with a subsequent increased risk for miscarriage.[71]

PATHOPHYSIOLOGY   The infection probably is spread by ascending microorganisms along the ureters, but spread may occur also by way of the bloodstream. The inflammatory process is usually focal and irregular, affecting primarily the pelvis, calyces, and medulla. The infection causes medullary infiltration of white blood cells with renal inflammation, renal edema, and purulent urine. The release of phagocytic lysozymes and oxygen radicals and the presence of other inflammatory mediators may damage tubular cells.[72] In severe infections, localized abscesses may form in the medulla and extend to the cortex. The tubules are primarily affected, but the glomeruli are usually spared. Necrosis of renal papillae can develop (Figure 36-6). After the acute phase, healing occurs with deposition of scar tissue and atrophy of affected tubules. The number of bacteria decreases until the urine again becomes sterile. Acute pyelonephritis rarely causes renal failure.[73,74]

CLINICAL MANIFESTATIONS   The most common clinical manifestations are a rapid onset of a fever, chills, malaise, and flank pain. Bothersome lower urinary tract symptoms characteristic of a UTI (dysuria, frequent urination, suprapubic discomfort) may have existed prior to the onset of systemic signs and symptoms or they may present at roughly the same time.[75] It is important to remember that not all individuals will exhibit these classic symptoms. Frail elders tend to experience only a small increased in body temperature, or they may have a slight decline in temperature (approximately 1° F). Infants may not develop a high fever, whereas toddlers and young children may experience very high fevers, frequently exceeding 102° F.

EVALUATION AND TREATMENT   Differentiating cystitis from pyelonephritis by clinical symptoms alone is difficult.[75] Rather, diagnosis usually relies on a combination of

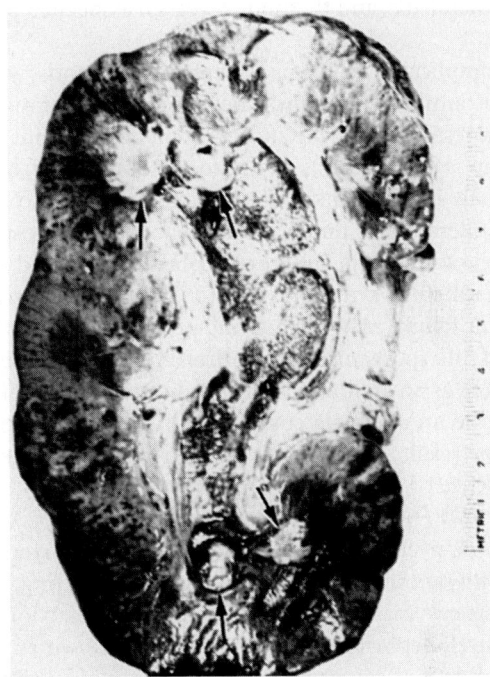

Figure 36-6 Acute pyelonephritis. Papillary necrosis resulting from acute pyelonephritis and obstruction. Note necrotic papillae (arrows); mottled patchy cortical infiltrate of acute pyelonephritis; and congested, dilated renal pelvis. (From Kissane JM, editor: *Anderson's pathology,* ed 9, St Louis, 1990, Mosby.)

Table 36-3	Common Causes of Pyelonephritis	
Predisposing Factors	**Pathologic Mechanisms**
Kidney stones	Obstruction and stasis of urine contributing to bacteriuria and hydronephrosis; irritation of epithelial lining with entrapment of bacteria
Vesicoureteral reflux	Chronic reflux of urine up the ureter and into kidney during micturition contributing to bacterial infection
Pregnancy	Dilation and relaxation of ureter with hydroureter and hydronephrosis; partly caused by obstruction from enlarged uterus and partly from ureteral relaxation caused by higher progesterone levels
Neurogenic bladder	Neurologic impairment interfering with normal bladder contraction with residual urine and ascending infection
Instrumentation	Introduction of organisms into urethra and bladder by catheters and endoscopes introduced into the urinary tract for diagnostic purposes
Female sexual trauma	Movement of organisms from the urethra into the bladder with infection and retrograde spread to kidney

clinical signs and symptoms (particularly flank pain and fever) combined with laboratory tests or the results of imaging studies in selected cases. Urinalysis will reveal evidence of a UTI, including pyuria and bacteriuria. Urine culture may or may not be positive, depending on the causative agent, any history of antibiotic administration prior to obtaining a specimen for culture, and the presence of urinary tract obstruction. The presence of antibody-coated bacteria has been associated with acute pyelonephritis,[76] but this testing is not routinely performed in those with clinical signs and symptoms of pyelonephritis. Blood cultures may be obtained and the results matched to the pathogen obtained from the urine. Positive results indicating the same pathogen in blood and urine provide strong evidence that systemic illness is caused by pyelonephritis, but negative cultures do not necessarily exclude this possibility. Imaging studies may assist the diagnosis of pyelonephritis, and they may reveal an associated perirenal abscess.

Uncomplicated acute pyelonephritis responds well to 2 weeks of antibiotic therapy. The choice of antibiotic ideally relies on results of a urine and/or blood cultures, but a broad spectrum agent such as a fluoroquinolone may be given empirically in the community-dwelling person who remains able to tolerate oral fluids and does not require hospitalization. Follow-up urine cultures are obtained at 1 and 4 weeks after treatment if symptoms recur.[77] Symptom recurrence or treatment failure may indicate the presence of an antibiotic-resistant microorganism or perirenal abscess. An imaging study such as an abdominal CT is indicated if symptoms persist despite an adequate course of antibiotic treatment supported by results of culture and sensitivity testing to rule out the presence of an abscess.

Chronic Pyelonephritis

Chronic pyelonephritis is a persistent or recurrent infection of the kidney with inflammation and scarring. One or both kidneys may be involved. Recurrent infections from acute pyelonephritis may be associated with chronic pyelonephritis. The urine in chronic pyelonephritis may, however, contain only a few white cells and bacteria.[78] Generally, chronic pyelonephritis is more likely to occur in those who have renal infections associated with some type of obstructive pathologic condition. This includes renal stones and vesicoureteral reflux.

PATHOPHYSIOLOGY Chronic urinary tract obstruction prevents elimination of bacteria in the normal flow of urine, resulting in progressive inflammation that causes fibrosis and scarring. The renal pelvis and calyces become dilated and blunted. Gradual destruction of the tubules occurs, with areas of atrophy or dilation and diffuse scarring. Impairment of function may affect urine-concentrating ability, with the excretion of a dilute urine, and can lead to chronic renal failure.

The lesions of chronic pyelonephritis are sometimes termed chronic interstitial nephritis because the inflammation and fibrosis are located in the interstitial spaces between the tubules. Chronic interstitial nephritis occurs from causes other than chronic pyelonephritis, including drug toxicity from analgesics such as phenacetin, aspirin, and acetaminophen; ischemia; irradiation; and immune complex diseases.

CLINICAL MANIFESTATIONS The clinical manifestations associated with chronic pyelonephritis are similar to those seen with end stage renal disease when both kidneys are affected. Recurring episodes of acute pyelonephritis is also common. Nevertheless, definitive diagnosis is based on an imaging study such as a x-ray, ultrasound, or CT scan rather than a characteristic combination of physical signs or symptoms.[57]

EVALUATION AND TREATMENT The urinalysis usually shows white blood cells and less commonly white blood cell casts. Bacteriuria may be associated with the presenting symptoms. Intravenous pyelogram and ultrasound reveal a small kidney with a characteristic "clubbing" of the affected calyces. Treatment is related to the underlying cause. When obstruction occurs, it must be relieved. Antibiotics may be given, and recurrent infection requires prolonged antibiotic therapy.

GLOMERULAR DISORDERS

Glomerulopathies are disorders that affect the glomerulus. Immunologic mechanisms are primarily responsible for glomerular disease, with the exception of hereditary disorders, nephritis associated with systemic diseases, and vascular pathologic conditions. Glomerular disease may be classified by distribution and characteristics of lesions (Table 36-4). Different diseases may have more than one type of lesion so lesions are not necessarily disease-specific. Different types of glomerular disease may be associated with patterns of urinary sediment. Diseases associated with a **nephrotic sediment** have massive proteinuria, lipiduria, and microscopic or no hematuria. Urine in diseases associated with a **nephritic sediment** is characterized by hematuria with red blood cell casts, white blood cell casts, and varying degrees of proteinuria, which is usually not severe. The **sediment of chronic glomerular disease** has waxy casts, granular casts, and less proteinuria and hematuria than nephrotic or nephritic sediment.

The onset of glomerular disease may be sudden or insidious, with hypertension, edema, and an elevated blood urea nitrogen (BUN). Low levels of serum complement are associated with acute poststreptococcal glomerulonephritis (APSGN) and normal levels associated with immunoglobulin A (IgA) nephropathy and cresentic or idiopathic rapidly progressive glomerulonephritis (RPGN).[79] Some individuals are asymptomatic, and disease is detected through the presence of microscopic hematuria from a routine urinalysis. The most definitive indication of glomerular disease is microscopic evaluation of tissue obtained by renal biopsy. The presence of clinical symptoms such as edema, hypertension, urinary

Table 36-4	Classification of Glomerular Lesions
Lesion	**Distribution When Many Glomeruli Considered**
Diffuse	Relatively uniform involvement of most (>50%) or all glomeruli; most common form of glomerulonephritis
Focal	Changes in only some glomeruli (>50%), whereas others are normal
Lesion	**Distribution When Single Glomeruli Considered**
Global	A lesion involving the entire glomerulus
Segmental-local	Changes in one part of the glomerulus with other parts unaffected
Lesion	**Lesion Characteristics**
Mesangial	Deposits of immunoglobulins in the mesangial matrix; mesangial cell proliferation
Membranous	Thickening of the glomerular capillary wall with immune deposits (i.e., IgG and C3)
Proliferative	Increase in the number of glomerular cells: endothelial, epithelial, mesangial
Sclerotic	Glomerular scarring from previous glomerular injury
Crescentic	Accumulation of proliferating cells within Bowman space, making the appearance of a crescent
Interstitial fibrosis	Scarring between the glomerulus and the tubules

changes, or systemic diseases associated with glomerular injury provides supporting evidence for the diagnosis.

Reduced GFR during glomerular disease is evidenced by elevated plasma creatinine and urea concentration or reduced creatinine clearance (see Chapter 35). Glomerular damage causes a decrease in glomerular membrane surface area, glomerular capillary blood flow, and driving hydrostatic pressure. An increasing glomerular capillary permeability may be accompanied by a loss of the negative ionic charge barrier and loss of plasma proteins into the urine (nephrotic syndrome). In the presence of hypoalbuminemia, plasma fluid tends to move to the interstitial spaces, contributing to decreased blood volume, decreased renal blood flow, and decreased glomerular capillary hydrostatic pressure with a decline in GFR.

Edema is commonly associated with the proteinuria of nephrotic syndrome (see p. 1320) or it may be caused by salt and water retention from reduced GFR. Excessive fluid retention may cause systemic and pulmonary edema, requiring the use of diuretics or dialysis. The volume expansion that accompanies salt and water retention leads to hypertension. Excessive renin production is usually not a cause of hypertension in glomerular diseases unless it is associated with ischemia, as in uremia (see p. 1331), or when there is profound hypovolemia.

Death occurs in 2% to 5% of all persons during acute glomerular disease. During the first few weeks, the major life-threatening problems are acute renal insufficiency with fluid, electrolyte, and acid-base imbalances; acute hypertension that may cause hypertensive encephalopathy; circulatory failure; and pulmonary edema.

Glomerulonephritis

Glomerulonephritis is an inflammation of the glomerulus. The inflammation can be caused by a variety of factors, including immunologic abnormalities; effects of drugs or toxins; vascular disorders; systemic diseases, including diabetes mellitus and lupus erythematosus; and viral causes related to hepatitis B and C viruses and human immunodeficiency virus (HIV). In most cases the exact cause of glomerular injury may be unknown. Immunologic alterations are most commonly responsible for glomerular injury (Figure 36-7) and glomerulonephritis.[80,81] Glomerular disease is the most common cause of chronic renal disease and end-stage renal failure.

Types

The classification of glomerulonephritis is arbitrary and can be described according to cause, pathologic lesions, disease progression, or clinical presentation.[82] Features of different types of glomerulonephritis are summarized in Table 36-5.

Acute Glomerulonephritis

Acute glomerulonephritis is an inflammation of the glomerulus. It is often associated with a group A (nephritogenic strain) poststreptococcal infection (acute poststreptococcal glomerulonephritis). The disease has an abrupt onset and usually occurs 7 to 10 days after a streptococcal infection of the throat (5% to 10% incidence) or skin (25% incidence), commonly in children (see Chapter 37). Sporadic occurrences have been observed after bacterial endocarditis, which may be associated with streptococcal or staphylococcal microorganisms, or after viral diseases such as varicella, hepatitis B, and hepatitis C.

Symptoms usually occur 10 to 21 days after infection and include hematuria, red blood cell casts, proteinuria, decreased GFR, oliguria, edema, and hypertension. The edema of acute glomerulonephritis tends to be around the eyes but may involve dependent areas such as the feet and ankles. Occasionally, ascites or pleural effusions develop. Serum complement levels are usually low because they are consumed by the initial infection. Immunofluorescent findings from renal biopsy indicate the presence of immune complex deposits or formation in the glomerulus (complement C3 and IgG) and neutrophil and macrophage recruitment and activation, with diffuse mesangial cell and capillary endothelial cell proliferation of the entire glomeruli[83] (Figure 36-8). The thickening of the glomerular membrane contributes to the decreased GFR. Activated complement, inflammatory cytokines, oxidants, proteases, and growth factors attack epithelial cells, altering membrane permeability and leading to proteinuria. More severe renal disease is observed after a prolonged infection and before antibiotic therapy, but there is no specific treatment for the glomerulonephritis. Most individuals, especially children, recover without significant loss of renal function or recurrence of the disease.

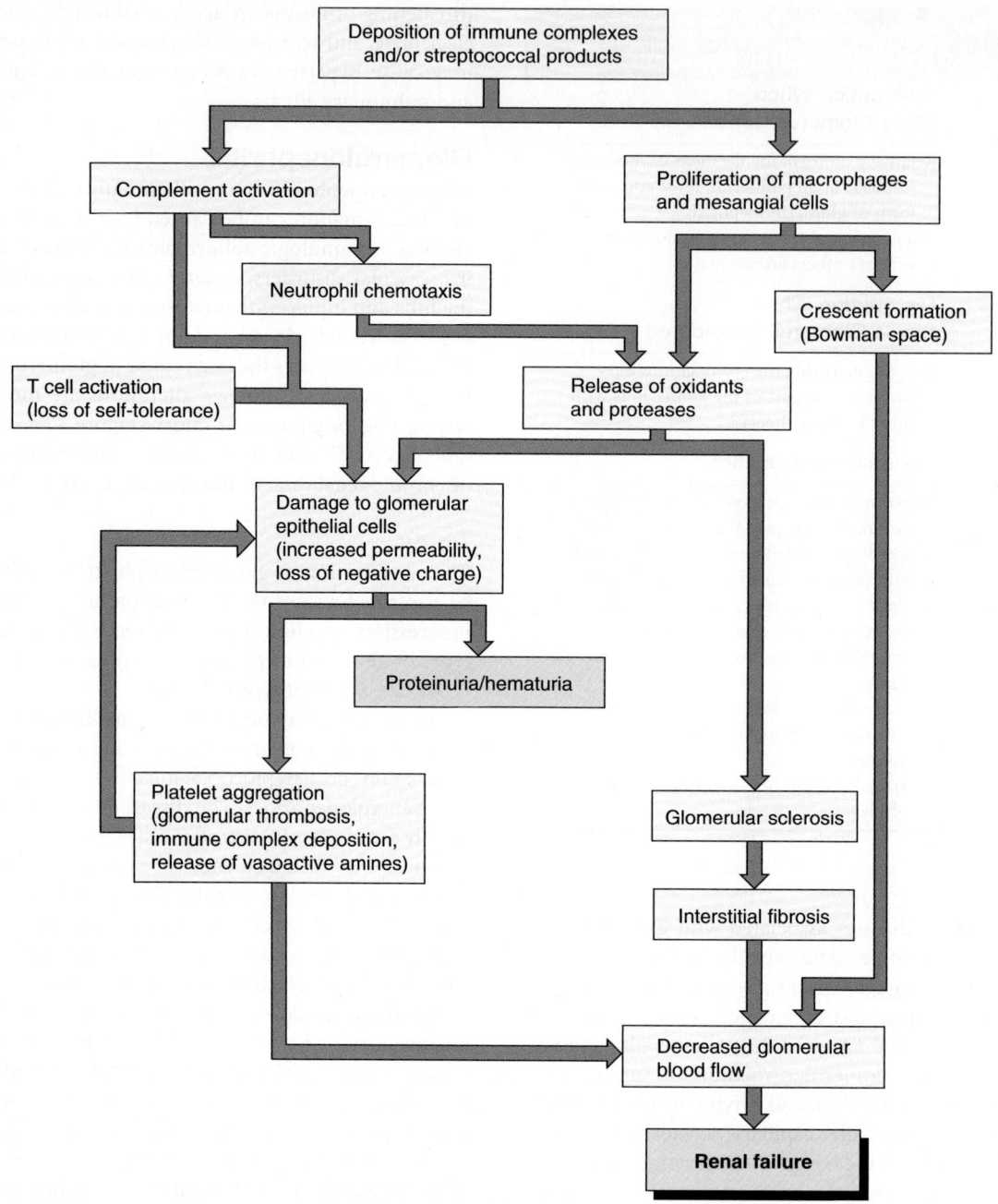

Figure 36-7 **Mechanisms of glomerular injury.** (Adapted from Couser WG: Rapidly progressive glomerulonephritis: classification, pathogenetic mechanisms, and therapy, *Am J Kidney Dis* 11(6):449, 1988.)

IgA Nephropathy

IgA nephropathy (Berger disease) is the most common form of acute glomerulonephritis in developed countries, especially Asia. The cause is unknown and more commonly affects adults ages 20 to 30 years. The disease manifests with gross or microscopic (30% to 40%) hematuria 24 to 48 hours after an upper respiratory or gastrointestinal viral infection. Proteinuria, edema, and hypertension are less common. Abnormal glycosylated IgA (galactose-deficient IgA-1) produced by the bone marrow and complement molecules bind to glomerular mesangial cells, stimulating them to proliferate and release oxidants and proteases, thereby contributing to diffuse mesangioproliferative glomerular injury and

glomerulosclerosis. Treatment may include angiotensin-converting enzyme (ACE) inhibitors, glucocorticoids, and cyclophosphamide. The prognosis is variable, with 20% to 50% of cases progressing to renal failure.[84,85]

Crescentic Glomerulonephritis

Crescentic glomerulonephritis is also known as subacute, rapidly progressive, or extracapillary glomerulonephritis and develops over a period of days to weeks.[86] The term crescentic refers to cellular proliferation, primarily in the Bowman space, that creates lesions appearing as crescents. The disease affects primarily adults in their fifties and sixties and may be idiopathic or associated with a number of proliferative glomerular diseases (with diffuse proliferation of extracapil-

Table 36-5	Features of the Common Types of Glomerulonephritis
Type and Cause	**Pathophysiology**
Diffuse proliferative Group A β-hemolytic streptococcus	Usually diffuse lesions; subepithelial deposits of IgG and complement complexes; infiltration of neutrophils and monocytes; proliferation of mesangial and epithelial cells with occlusion of glomerular capillary blood flow and decreased glomerular filtration
Rapidly progressive or crescentic Nonspecific response to glomerular injury; can occur in any severe glomerular disease	Diffuse lesions; accumulation of fibrin, macrophages, and epithelial cell proliferation into the Bowman space forms crescents and occludes glomerular capillary blood flow decreasing glomerular filtration; antiglomerular basement membrane antibodies lead to necrotizing, proliferative glomerulonephritis, and renal failure
Membranoproliferative Usually idiopathic; associated with hypocomplementemia Type I: activation of classical complement pathway with nephrotic syndrome Type II: activation of alternate complement pathway with hematuria	Diffuse lesions; mesangial cell proliferation; thickening of basement membrane; subendothelial deposits of immune complex occlude glomerular capillary blood flow and decrease glomerular filtration
Mesangial proliferative; usually associated with IgA nephropathy	Deposits of immune complexes in the mesangium with mesangial cell proliferation; results in decreased glomerular blood flow and filtration
IgA nephropathy (Berger disease) Usually idiopathic; elevated IgA plasma levels	Usually focal, some diffuse lesions; mesangial cell proliferation with IgA deposits; release of inflammatory mediators with crescent formation, sclerosis, interstitial fibrosis, and decreased GFR
Minimal change disease (lipoid nephrosis) Usually idiopathic	Diffuse fusion of epithelial foot processes; loss of negative charge in basement membrane and increased permeability lead to severe proteinuria and nephrotic syndrome
Focal segmental glomerulosclerosis Usually idiopathic	Similar to minimal change disease with focal glomerulosclerosis from hyaline deposits in the glomerular membrane resulting in proteinuria and nephrotic syndrome
Membranous nephropathy Usually idiopathic; can be associated with systemic diseases, i.e., hepatitis B virus, systemic lupus erythematosus, solid malignant tumors	Diffuse thickening of glomerular basement membrane and capillary wall from deposits of antibody and complement; increased permeability with proteinuria and nephrotic syndrome

IgG, Immunoglobulin G; *IgA,* immunoglobulin A; *GFR,* glomerular filtration rate.

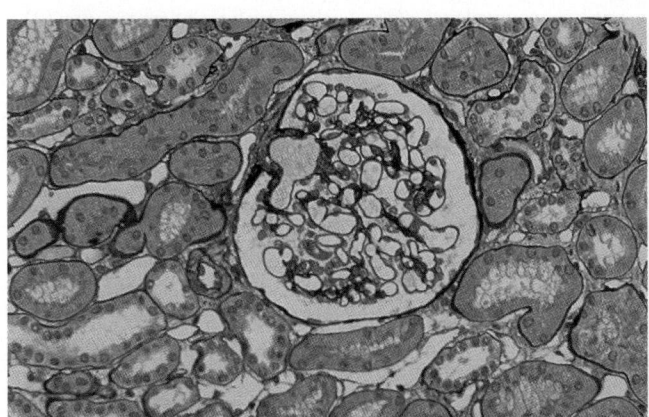

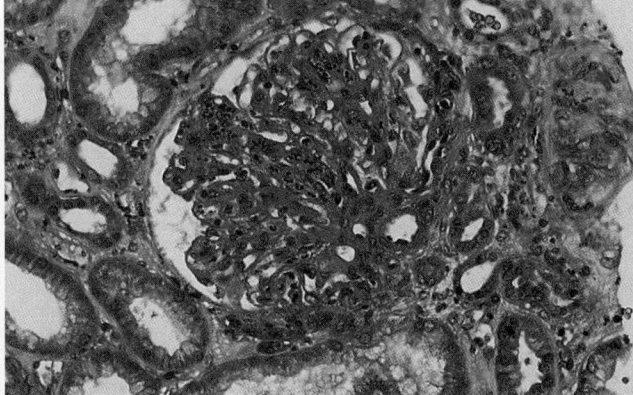

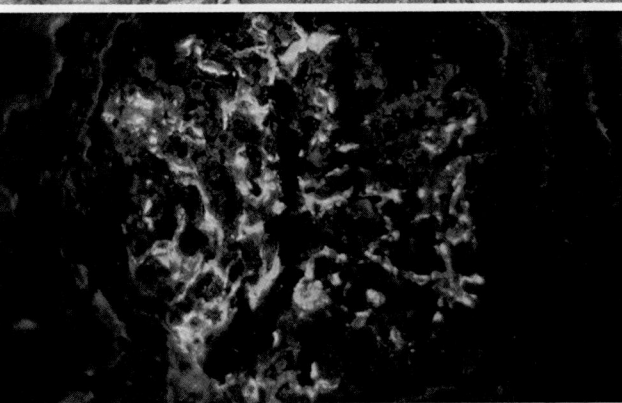

Figure 36-8 Glomerulonephritis. A, Normal glomerulus; note single-contoured walls, patent capillaries, inconspicuous mesangium, and degree of cellularity. (Periodic acid–methenamine silver stain.) **B,** Acute postinfectious glomerulonephritis. There is considerable increase in cellularity, mainly because of accumulation of numerous polymorphonuclear leukocytes in capillary lumina. Note numerous subepithelial hump-shaped fuchsinophilic deposits in many capillary walls. Protein precipitates (hyalinization) are in the arteriole. (Masson trichrome stain.) **C,** Postinfectious glomerulonephritis. Irregular mesangial and capillary wall immunostaining for C3. (From Damjanov I, Linder J, editors: *Anderson's pathology,* ed 10, St Louis, 1996, Mosby.)

lary cells), such as poststreptococcal glomerulonephritis and Goodpasture syndrome. Antineutrophil cytoplasmic antibodies with associated vasculitis are common in this disease.[87]

Anti-glomerular basement membrane disease (Goodpasture syndrome) is an example of crescentic glomerulonephritis. The disease is associated with antibody formation against both pulmonary capillary and glomerular basement membranes with pulmonary hemorrhage and glomerulonephritis. The disease is rare but occurs most commonly in men 20 to 30 years of age (lung hemorrhage) and older adults (renal disease).[88]

By the time crescentic glomerulonephritis is diagnosed, renal insufficiency is apparent. There is extensive proliferation of epithelial cells into the Bowman space with macrophage infiltration. The cells become mixed with fibrin and form crescent-shaped deposits (Figure 36-9). Podocytes may become detached. Typically, the glomerular injury is accompanied by a rapid decline in glomerular function progressing to renal failure in a few weeks or months. Hematuria is common and may be accompanied by proteinuria, edema, or hypertension.

Crescentic glomerulonephritis has a relatively poor prognosis if not diagnosed and treated early. Plasma exchange (plasmapheresis) combined with immunosuppression and steroids improves renal function.[89,90] Antiviral therapy reduces severity related to hepatitis C virus.[89-91] Anticoagulants, such as heparin or warfarin, may be of some benefit in reducing the fibrin component of crescent formation. Dialysis or transplantation is required when failure is irreversible.

Chronic Glomerulonephritis

Chronic glomerulonephritis encompasses several glomerular diseases with a progressive course that leads to chronic renal failure. There may be no history of renal disease before the diagnosis, although several years of proteinuria and hematuria may have preceded the diagnosis. Various pathologic changes are evident in the glomerulus. Proliferation of mesangial cells (cells in connective tissue supporting the glomerular capillaries) may be focal or diffuse with segmental fibrosis and glomerular deterioration. Secondary tubular dilation and atrophy may develop. Tubulointerstitial injury contributes to the progression to renal failure and occurs from activated complement fragments, damage from exposure to filtered macromolecules, and chronic tubulointerstitial hypoxia.[92] Hypercholesterolemia and proteinuria also have been associated with progressive glomerular and tubular injury. The proposed mechanism is related to glomerulosclerosis and interstitial injury.[93,94] The primary cause may be difficult to establish because advanced pathologic changes may obscure specific disease characteristics (Figure 36-10). Insulin-dependent diabetes mellitus and lupus erythematosus are examples of secondary causes of chronic glomerular injury.[95]

PATHOPHYSIOLOGY Patterns of antigen-antibody complex deposition or formation within the glomerular capillary filtration membrane have been established using light, electron, and immunofluorescent microscopy for different disease processes (Table 36-6). Electron microscopy differentiates morphologic changes within the glomerular capillary wall. Staining with fluorescein identifies different antibodies (i.e., IgG or IgA) and their configurations when viewed under ultraviolet light with a microscope (see Figure 36-8, C).

Three types of immune mechanisms contribute to acute glomerular injury: (1) deposition of circulating soluble antigen-antibody complexes, often with complement fragments; (2) formation of antibodies specific against the glomerular basement membrane; and (3) streptococcal release of neuraminidase, which alters IgG with binding of anti-IgG to the glomerulus.[96]

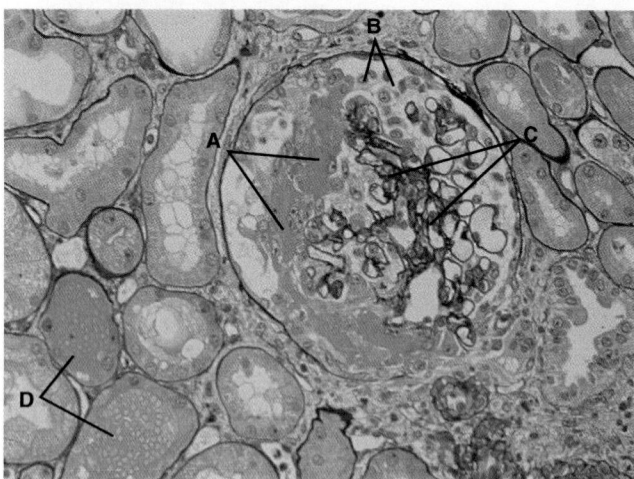

Figure 36-9 **Anti-glomerular basement membrane nephritis.** Glomerulus with a fresh crescent consisting of fibrin and cells in the Bowman space *(A)*. There is disruption of the basement membrane of the Bowman capsule, with migration of cells from the interstitium into the Bowman space *(B)*. The capillary tufts *(C)* are distorted and compressed because of the crescent. Note the free erythrocytes in tubular lumina *(D)*. The interstitium is mildly edematous. (Periodic acid–methenamine silver stain.) (Modified from Damjanov I, Linder J, editors: *Anderson's pathology*, ed 10, St Louis, 1996, Mosby.)

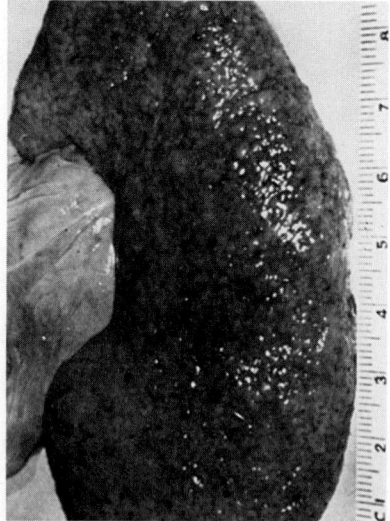

Figure 36-10 **End-stage chronic glomerulonephritis.** Pebbly surface corresponds to surviving hypertrophied nephrons amid atrophy. (From Kissane JM, editor: *Anderson's pathology*, ed 9, St Louis, 1990, Mosby.)

Table 36-6	Immunologic Pathogenesis of Glomerulonephritis
Glomerular Injury	**Mechanism**
Soluble immune-complex glomerulonephritis (90%)	Formation of antibodies stimulated by the presence of endogenous or exogenous antigens results in circulating soluble antigen-antibody complexes, which are deposited in glomerular capillaries; glomerular injury occurring with complement deposition and activation and release of immunologic substances that lyse cells and increase membrane permeability; immune deposits with a microscopic appearance that fluoresce in a *granular pattern* when stained with fluorescein and viewed under ultraviolet light; severity of glomerular injury related to the number of complexes formed; a type III hypersensitivity
Anti-glomerular basement membrane glomerulonephritis (5%)	Antibodies are formed and act directly against the glomerular basement membrane; immune response that causes crescent formation and a *linear pattern* of immunofluorescence; generally associated with rapidly progressive renal failure such as Goodpasture syndrome
Alternative complement pathway	A relatively obscure mechanism associated with low levels of complement and membranoproliferative glomerulonephritis
Cell-mediated immunity	A delayed hypersensitivity response that damages the glomerulus; actual cellular mechanism not clearly understood

The response of glomerular cells to inflammatory mediators leads to cell proliferation, sclerosis, and chronic impaired renal function. The severity of glomerular damage and renal insufficiency is related to the size, number, location (focal or diffuse), duration of exposure, and type of antigen-antibody complexes.

Glomerular damage generally occurs as a result of activation of biochemical mediators of inflammation (complement, leukocytes, fibrin), which begins after the antibody or antigen-antibody complexes have localized in the glomerular capillary wall. Complement is deposited with the antibodies, followed by a sequence of metabolic events that initiate an attack on the glomerular membrane. Complement activation can serve as a chemotactic stimulus for attraction of neutrophils and monocytes.[97] The neutrophils and monocytes further the inflammatory reaction by releasing lysosomal enzymes and reactive oxygen species, which damage glomerular cell walls.[98]

These processes alter membrane permeability and may cause loss of the negative electrical charge across the glomerular filtration membrane. Membrane damage can lead to platelet aggregation and degranulation, whereby platelets release vasoactive amines such as serotonin or histamine. These substances then increase glomerular permeability. Changes in membrane permeability and electrical charge permit the passage of protein molecules and/or red blood cells into the urine, causing proteinuria or hematuria or both. The coagulation system also may be activated and lead to fibrin deposition in the Bowman space, contributing to crescent formation (deposition of substances in the Bowman space). (Coagulation is discussed in Chapter 25.) Membrane proliferation, deposits in the membrane, mesangial proliferation, and swelling reduce renal blood flow and depress glomerular filtration and contribute to hypoxic injury.

CLINICAL MANIFESTATIONS Two major changes in the urine distinguish glomerulonephritis: (1) hematuria with red blood cell casts and (2) proteinuria exceeding 3 to 5 g/day, with albumin as the major protein. Several disorders may produce hematuria because bleeding can occur anywhere along the urinary tract. However, the characteristics of hematuria from red blood cells escaping through the glomerular membrane include a smoky brown-tinged urine, red blood cell casts, and an accompanying proteinuria. Bleeding from sites lower in the urinary tract may produce a pink- or red-colored urine. Glomerular bleeding provides prolonged contact with the acidic urine and transforms hemoglobin to methemoglobin, which has a brownish color and no blood clots. The immune-mediated inflammatory response with cellular infiltration decreases GFR, which leads to fluid retention. Salt and water are reabsorbed, contributing to fluid volume expansion and hypertension. The history and physical examination may disclose findings that differentiate glomerular disease from another source of urinary tract bleeding. Gross proteinuria is associated with nephrotic syndrome; a decrease in urine output accompanies a decreased GFR.

Mild proteinuria and hematuria may occur during the early years of the disease. Blood pressure may be normal. After 10 or 20 years, renal insufficiency begins to develop, followed by nephrotic syndrome and an accelerated progression to end-stage renal failure. Symptom patterns vary depending on the underlying cause. Steroids usually do not change the course of the disease, and dialysis or kidney transplantation ultimately may be necessary.

EVALUATION AND TREATMENT The diagnosis of glomerular disease is confirmed by the progressive development of clinical manifestations and laboratory findings of abnormal urinalysis with proteinuria, red blood cells, white blood cells, and casts. In APSGN the streptococcal exoenzymes are elevated, such as antistreptolysin O and antistreptokinase. Serum complement is decreased, and serum creatinine concentration is elevated. Creatinine clearance evaluates the extent of glomerular damage. Microscopic evaluation from renal biopsy provides a specific determination of renal injury and type of pathology.

Management principles for treating glomerulonephritis are related to treating the primary disease, preventing or minimizing immune responses, and correcting accompanying problems such as edema, hypertension, hyperkalemia, and hyperlipidemia. Specific treatment regimens are necessary for particular types of glomerulonephritis.

Nephrotic Syndrome

Nephrotic syndrome is the excretion of 3.5 g or more of protein in the urine per day. The large amount of urine protein is characteristic of glomerular injury. Other findings include hypoalbuminemia, edema, hyperlipidemia, and lipiduria (Table 36-7). Lipoid nephrosis (minimal change disease [see Chapter 37]), membranous nephropathy, and focal glomerulosclerosis are directly related to nephrotic syndrome, although these conditions can occur with other types of glomerular disease.[99] Familial forms of nephrotic syndrome result from genetic defects that affect the function and composition of the glomerular capillary wall (i.e., Alport syndrome with alterations in basement membrane type IV collagen).[100]

Secondary forms of nephrotic syndrome occur as a result of other organic pathologic processes. Systemic diseases often implicated in secondary nephrotic syndrome include diabetes mellitus, amyloidosis, systemic lupus erythematosus, and Henoch-Schönlein purpura (syndrome). Nephrotic syndrome also is seen in association with certain drugs, infections, malignancies, and vascular disorders. When present as a secondary complication with renal diseases, nephrotic syndrome often signifies a more serious prognosis. The more common forms of idiopathic nephrotic syndrome include membranous glomerulonephritis, focal and segmental glomerulosclerosis, and minimal change disease.

Membranous glomerulonephritis (membranous nephropathy) is the most common form of idiopathic nephrotic syndrome in whites and is associated with hyperlipidemia and hypercoaguability.[102] Serum complement levels are normal although there is complement in the glomerular immune deposits. Hypercoagulability increases risk for pulmonary emboli and renal vein thrombosis. Immune deposits result in thickening of the glomerular capillary wall and basement membrane proliferation. Spontaneous remissions occur in 50% of cases.[103]

Focal and **segmental glomerulosclerosis** are the most common forms of idiopathic nephrotic syndrome in blacks. Glomeruli show progressive segmental sclerosing lesions with deposits of IgM and C3.[104,105]

Minimal change disease (lipoid nephrosis) is the most common form of nephrotic syndrome in children (see Chapter 37). No glomerular abnormalities are seen with light microscopy.

PATHOPHYSIOLOGY   Disturbances in the glomerular basement membrane, which may be metabolic, biochemical, or physiochemical, lead to increased permeability to protein. Loss of plasma proteins, particularly albumin and some immunoglobulins, occurs across the injured glomerular filtration membrane[106] (Figure 36-11). Hypoalbuminemia results from urinary loss of albumin combined with a diminished synthesis of replacement albumin by the liver. Albumin is lost in the greatest quantity because of its high plasma concentration and low molecular weight. Hyperlipidemia is primarily related to increased lipid synthesis of both low-density lipoproteins (LDLs) and very-low-density lipoproteins (VLDLs) by the liver, decreased lipoprotein catabolism,[107] reduced plasma oncotic pressure from hypoalbuminemia, and increased hepatic delivery of cholesterol precursors.[108]

Increased synthesis of plasma proteins may be insufficient to compensate for losses. Factors such as decreased dietary intake of protein from anorexia or malnutrition, or accompanying liver disease, may contribute to lower levels of plasma albumin. Loss of immunoglobulins may increase susceptibility to infections.

CLINICAL MANIFESTATIONS   **Proteinuria** is an excessive amount of protein in the urine (up to 10 g/24 hr).[109]

Table 36-7	Clinical Manifestations of Nephrotic Syndrome	
Manifestations	**Contributing Factors**	**Result**
Proteinuria	Increased glomerular permeability, decreased proximal tubule reabsorption	Edema, increased susceptibility to infection from loss of immunoglobulins
Hypoalbuminemia	Increased urinary losses of protein	Edema
Edema	Hypoalbuminemia (decreased oncotic pressure, sodium and water retention, increased aldosterone and antidiuretic hormone [ADH] secretion), unresponsiveness to atrial natriuretic peptides	Soft, pitting, generalized edema
Hyperlipidemia	Decreased serum albumin; increased hepatic synthesis of very-low-density lipoproteins; increased cholesterol, phospholipids, triglycerides	Increase atherogenesis
Lipiduria	Sloughing of tubular cells containing fat (oval fat bodies); free fat from hyperlipidemia	Fat droplets that may float in urine
Decreased vitamin D	The globulin to which 1,25-vitamin D is attached for transport passes through the glomerulus and is lost in the urine	Decreased absorption of calcium from gut

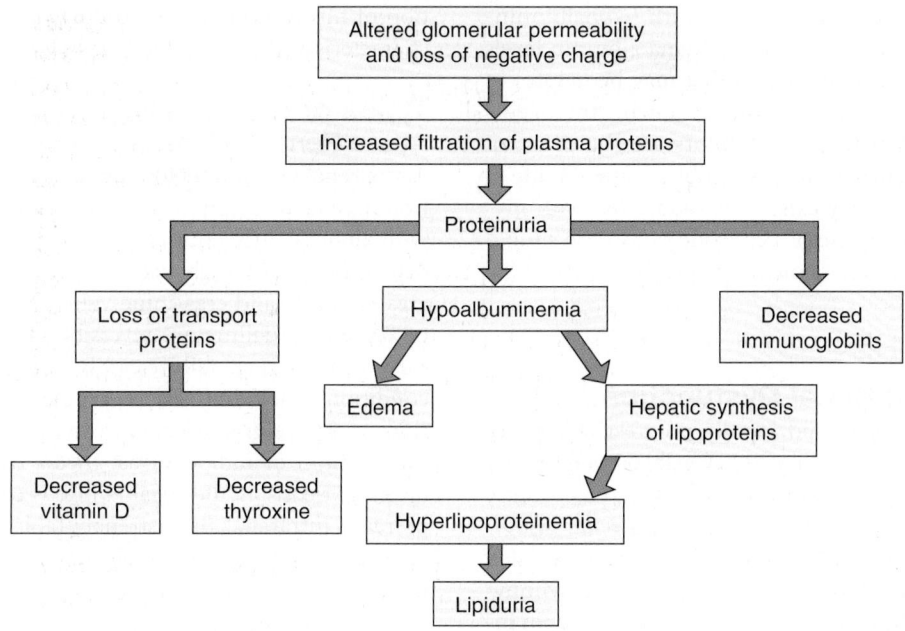

Figure 36-11 Pathophysiology of nephrotic syndrome.

Many of the clinical manifestations of nephrotic syndrome are related to loss of serum proteins[110] (see Table 36-7).

Edema may be the first symptom (see Chapter 3). Renal edema is associated with hypoalbuminemia and is soft, pitting, and in areas of low tissue pressure, such as the periorbital regions. According to Starling's law, hydrostatic pressure acts to force fluid into the interstitial space at the arterial end of the capillaries. The hydrostatic pressure is balanced by the oncotic pressure of the plasma proteins, which tends to draw the fluid back into the capillaries at the venous end (see Chapter 3). Plasma albumin concentration in nephrotic syndrome is often reduced to 20% of normal, with a considerable decrease in the plasma oncotic pressure. The threat of decreased plasma volume from the accumulation of fluid in the tissues stimulates compensatory mechanisms. Among these mechanisms are activation of the renin-angiotensin-aldosterone system and antidiuretic hormone (ADH), which together lead to excessive sodium and water retention. The nephrotic kidney is also unresponsive to atrial natriuretic peptide with increased sodium and water retention.[111,112] Increased lymph flow may allow some compensation. Edema in the interstitial space may facilitate lymph flow by elevating tissue pressure, facilitating the return of interstitial fluid into the plasma compartment.

Levels of all the plasma lipids (triglycerides, phospholipids, cholesterol) are elevated, producing a hyperlipidemia. **Lipiduria** is manifested by lipid casts or free fat droplets that leak across the glomerular capillary walls and into the urine. Tubular epithelial cells that reabsorb lipoprotein also may be shed and appear in the urine as "oval fat bodies."

The hormone 25-hydroxycholecalciferol (vitamin D_3) and thyroxine are normally bound to a circulating globulin. If the globulin is lost in the urine, both circulating vitamin D_3 and absorption of intestinal calcium will be decreased resulting in **hypocalcemia** (see Chapter 3). Symptoms of vitamin D deficiency will develop, including low plasma levels of ionized calcium, secondary hyperparathyroidism, and osteomalacia. Losses of thyroid-binding globulin result in reduced circulating levels of total thyroxine. Free thyroxine and TSH remain in normal ranges. Most individuals remain euthyroid but can develop hypothyroidism that improves with resolution of nephrotic syndrome.

Hypercoagulability occurs in nephrotic syndrome.[102,113] Although the exact causes are uncertain, increased platelet aggregation, increases in fibrinogen and coagulation factors, decreased antithrombin levels, and fibrinolysis are present. Risk of thromboembolic complications increase with dehydration.

EVALUATION AND TREATMENT Nephrotic syndrome is diagnosed when the protein level in a 24-hour urine collection is greater than 3.5 g. Serum albumin decreases (to less than 3 g/dl), and serum cholesterol, phospholipids, and triglycerides increase. Fat bodies may be present in the urine. The specific pathology is identified by renal biopsy.

Nephrotic syndrome is commonly treated with a normal-protein, low-fat diet; salt restriction; diuretics; anticoagulants; removal of glomerular toxic factors;[114] steroids; and occasionally albumin replacement.[115] Because the nephrotic state is caused primarily by protein depletion, dietary protein supplements (up to 100 g) are essential, unless renal failure has occurred. Diuretics may be used, particularly loop diuretics such as furosemide or ethacrynic acid, to control edema or hypertension. Care must be taken to observe for hypovolemia and hypokalemia or potassium toxicity in the presence of renal insufficiency. Aldactone may be combined with loop diuretics to suppress aldosterone activity and conserve potassium.

Because hyperlipidemia is associated with hypoalbuminemia, correction occurs when normal plasma albumin levels are reestablished. A low–saturated fat diet may be helpful in chronic nephrosis as a way of slowing down atherogenic processes. HMG-CoA reductase inhibitors are the drugs of choice. Lipid lowering drugs, such as clofibrate, are not safe to use when renal insufficiency exists; it is associated with myopathy. The underlying cause of nephrotic syndrome should be treated specifically if it is known.

RENAL FAILURE

Classification of Renal Dysfunction

Renal failure may be acute and rapidly progressive (within hours), although the process may be reversible. Renal failure also can be chronic, progressing to end-stage renal failure over a period of months or years.[116] The terms *renal insufficiency, renal failure, uremia,* and *azotemia* are all associated with decreasing renal function. Often they are used synonymously, although with some distinctions. Generally, **renal insufficiency** refers to a decline in renal function to about 25% of normal or a GFR of 25 to 30 ml/min. Levels of serum creatinine and urea are mildly elevated. **Renal failure** often refers to significant loss of renal function. When less than 10% of renal function remains, this is termed **end-stage renal failure (ESRF)**. **Uremia** is a syndrome of renal failure and includes elevated blood urea and creatinine levels accompanied by fatigue, anorexia, nausea, vomiting, pruritus, and neurologic changes. Uremia represents the numerous consequences related to renal failure, including retention of toxic wastes, deficiency states, and electrolyte disorders. **Azotemia** means increased serum urea levels and frequently increased creatinine levels as well. Renal insufficiency or renal failure causes azotemia. Both azotemia and uremia indicate an accumulation of nitrogenous waste products in the blood, a common characteristic that explains the overlap in definitions of terms.

Types of Renal Failure
Acute Renal Failure

Acute renal failure (ARF) is an abrupt (within hours) reduction in renal function. Acute renal failure is usually associated with oliguria (urine output of less than 30 ml/hr or less than 400 ml/day), although urine output may be normal or increased. BUN and creatinine values are elevated. Most types of acute renal failure are reversible if diagnosed and treated early.[117] Acute renal failure can be caused by different clinical conditions, including severe hypotension, vascular obstruction, or severe glomerular disease, or it can occur after administration of radiocontrast media or exposure to certain drugs or toxins. Acute renal failure is commonly classified as prerenal, intrarenal, or postrenal (Table 36-8). A combination of ischemic or hepatotoxic factors may produce acute renal failure.[118]

PATHOPHYSIOLOGY   **Prerenal acute renal failure** (prerenal azotemia) is the most common cause of ARF and is caused by impaired renal blood flow. The GFR declines because of the decrease in filtration pressure. Poor perfusion can result from renal vasoconstriction, hypotension, hypovolemia, hemorrhage, or inadequate cardiac output (heart failure). Acute prerenal failure may occur when chronic renal failure exists if a sudden stress is imposed on already marginally functioning kidneys. Failure to restore blood volume or blood pressure may cause acute tubular necrosis or acute cortical necrosis.[119]

Intrarenal acute renal failure (intrinsic renal azotemia) may result from acute tubular necrosis, cortical necrosis, acute glomerulonephritis, vascular disease (malignant hyper-

Table 36-8	Classification of Acute Renal Failure
Area of Dysfunction	**Possible Causes**
Prerenal	Hypovolemia
	Hemorrhagic blood loss (trauma, gastrointestinal bleeding, complications of childbirth)
	Loss of plasma volume (burns, peritonitis)
	Water and electrolyte losses (severe vomiting or diarrhea, intestinal obstruction, uncontrolled diabetes mellitus, inappropriate use of diuretics)
	Hypotension or hypoperfusion
	Septic shock
	Cardiac failure or shock
	Massive pulmonary embolism
	Stenosis or clamping of renal artery
Intrarenal	Acute tubular necrosis (postischemic or nephrotoxic)
	Glomerulopathies
	Malignant hypertension
	Coagulation defects
	Bilateral acute pyelonephritis
	Renal artery/vein occlusion
Postrenal	Obstructive uropathies (usually bilateral)
	Ureteral obstruction (edema, tumors, stones, clots)
	Bladder neck obstruction (enlarged prostate)

tension, disseminated intravascular coagulation, and renal vasculitis), allograft rejection, or interstitial disease (drug allergy, infection, tumor growth). A combination of events and predisposing factors leads to the greatest risk for acute renal failure. **Acute tubular necrosis (ATN)** is the most common cause of intrarenal acute renal failure.[120] The terms *acute tubular necrosis* and *acute renal failure* are sometimes used interchangeably, but the conditions are not the same because acute renal failure can occur without ATN. ATN is generally described as postischemic or nephrotoxic.

ATN caused by ischemia occurs most often after surgery (40% to 50% of cases), but ATN is also associated with sepsis, obstetric complications, severe burns, or trauma. A severe episode of hypotension often associated with hypovolemia is a significant contributing event. The ischemia generates toxic oxygen free radicals and inflammatory mediators that cause cell swelling, injury, and necrosis, a form of reperfusion injury.[121,123] Injury is most severe in the outer medulla with scattered necrosis in the cortex and loss of cells along the tubular epithelium. Vasoconstriction and congestion of peritubular capillaries contributes to hypoxia and injury. Ischemic necrosis tends to be patchy and may be distributed along any part of the nephron.

Nephrotoxic ATN can be produced by numerous antibiotics, but the aminoglycosides (neomycin, gentamicin, tobramycin) are the major culprits. The drugs tend to accumulate in the renal cortex and may not cause renal failure until after treatment is complete. Radiocontrast media (x-ray media) and cisplatin also may be nephrotoxic. Dehydration, advanced age, concurrent renal insufficiency, and diabetes mellitus tend to enhance nephrotoxicity from either aminoglycosides or radiocontrast media. Other substances such as excessive myoglobin (oxygen-transporting substance in muscles), carbon tetrachloride, heavy metals (mercury, arsenic), methoxyflurane anesthesia, or bacterial toxins may promote renal failure. Necrosis and tubular cell apoptosis caused by nephrotoxins is usually uniform and limited to the proximal tubules. The high surface area of the brush border of the proximal tubular cells makes them more vulnerable to toxic injury.[124]

Three pathophysiologic explanations have been proposed to account for the significant reduction in GFR and oliguria associated with ARF: tubular obstruction, tubular back-leak, and alterations in renal blood flow.[125] All three mechanisms probably contribute to oliguria in varying degrees throughout the course of the disease (Figure 36-12). *Tubular obstruction* occurs when ischemia of the tubules causes sloughing of cells, cast formation (composed of granular and epithelial cells), or ischemic edema, resulting in tubular obstruction. Obstruction then causes a retrograde increase in pressure and reduces the GFR. Renal failure can occur within 24 hours.

Back-leak is the unregulated movement of glomerular filtrate from the tubular lumen to the interstitium and into the renal arteries and veins. The movement of filtration is accelerated because of changes in permeability caused by ischemia and loss of epithelial cells. Most studies of renal function in ATN, however, indicate a decrease in glomerular filtration, and back-leak may be only a minor aspect of acute failure (Figure 36-13).

Alterations in renal blood flow are a major cause of decreased glomerular filtration and decreased intrarenal blood flow. Intrarenal vasoconstriction is caused by activation of renin-angiotensin, release of endothelin from injured endothelial cells, and decreased vasodilators, including nitric

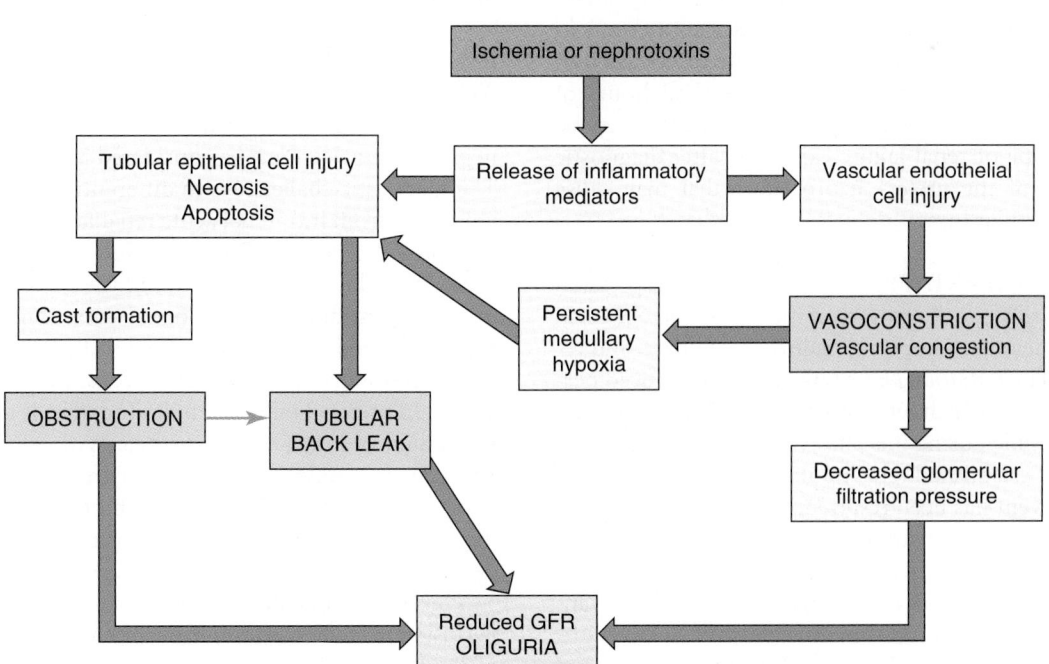

Figure 36-12 Mechanisms of oliguria in acute renal failure. *GFR,* Glomerular filtration rate.

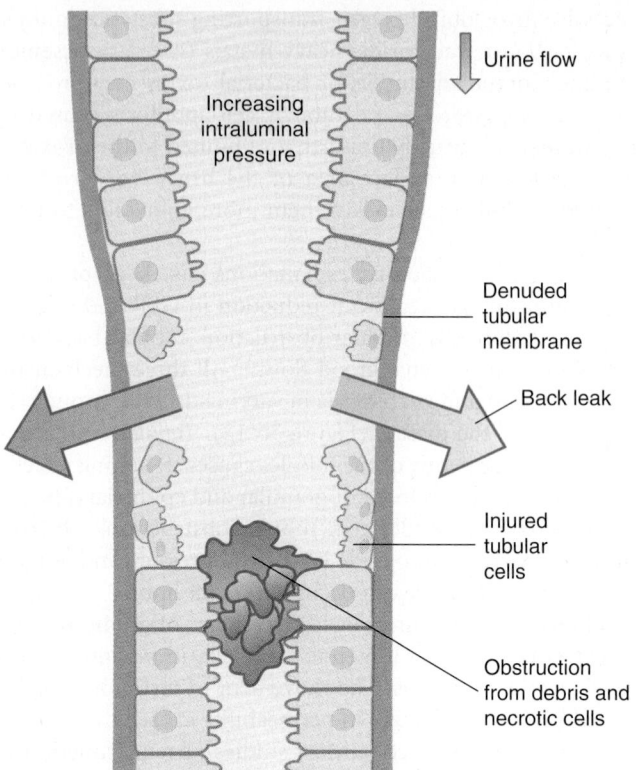

Figure 36-13 **Theories of oliguria.** Diagram representing the back leak and obstruction theories of oliguria in acute renal failure.

oxide and prostaglandin I_2. Activation of platelets and congestion with red and white blood cells contribute to obstruction of blood flow.[126]

Postrenal acute renal failure is rare and occurs with urinary tract obstruction that affects the kidneys bilaterally (e.g., bladder outlet obstruction, prostatic hypertrophy, or bilateral ureteral obstruction). The obstruction causes an increase in intraluminal pressure upstream from the site of obstruction with a gradual fall in GFR. A pattern of several hours of anuria with flank pain followed by polyuria is a characteristic finding. This type of renal failure can occur after diagnostic catheterization of the ureters, a procedure that may cause edema of the tubular lumen.

CLINICAL MANIFESTATIONS   The clinical progression of acute renal failure with recovery of renal function occurs in three phases: the initiation phase, maintenance phase, and recovery phase. The *initiation phase* is the phase of reduced perfusion or toxicity in which renal injury is evolving. Prevention of injury is possible during this phase. The *maintenance phase* is the period of established renal injury and dysfunction after the initiating event has been resolved. Urine output is lowest during this phase, and serum creatinine and blood urea nitrogen both increase. The *recovery phase* is the interval when renal injury is repaired and normal renal function is reestablished. Diuresis is common during this phase.

Oliguria begins within 1 day after a hypotensive event and lasts for 1 to 3 weeks, but it may regress in several hours or ex-

tend for several weeks, depending on the duration of ischemia or severity of toxic injury. Anuria (urine output less than 50 ml/day) is uncommon in ATN, and 10% to 20% of cases have nonoliguric failure (decreased urine output but greater than 30 ml per hour). Anuria suggests bilateral renal artery occlusion, obstructive uropathy, or acute cortical necrosis. Nonoliguric failure usually represents less severe injury. The urine output may vary in volume, but the BUN and plasma creatinine concentrations increase (plasma creatinine is inversely proportional to the GFR). Urine sediment should be evaluated for casts, cells, and crystals.

Other early manifestations depend on the underlying cause of renal failure. Individuals who have experienced trauma or surgery or persons in a catabolic state may have more rapid elevations in BUN. They are prone to hyperkalemia and hyperphosphatemia from cellular breakdown. Fluid retention may cause edema. Symptoms of congestive heart failure develop in persons with cardiac disease. Nausea, vomiting, and fatigue accompany uremia and electrolyte imbalances. Wound healing is delayed, and the risk of infection, particularly pneumonia, is greater. Nonoliguric renal failure generally has a better prognosis because of fewer complications. Oliguric patients may require maintenance dialysis to attenuate symptoms of renal failure.

As renal function improves during the recovery phase, increase in urine volume (diuresis) is progressive. During the early diuretic phase the tubules are still damaged. Sodium and potassium are lost in the urine, and the risk for hypokalemia is greater. Volume depletion may ensue, with fluid losses of 3 to 4 L/day. Fluid and electrolyte balance must be carefully monitored and excessive urinary losses replaced. Return to normal status may take 3 to 12 months, and approximately 30% of individuals do not have full recovery of a normal GFR or tubular function.

EVALUATION AND TREATMENT   The diagnosis of ATN is related to the cause of the disease. A history of surgery, trauma, or cardiovascular disorders is common. Exposure to nephrotoxins also must be considered and carefully explored. The diagnostic challenge is to differentiate prerenal acute renal failure from intrarenal acute renal failure. Urine composition provides helpful diagnostic clues to changes in tubular function (Table 36-9). The ratios of the BUN to plasma creatinine concentration and fractional excretion of sodium (the ratio of filtered sodium to excreted sodium) are helpful diagnostic indicators. The tests reflect renal tubular reabsorption ability. In prerenal failure, tubular function is maintained and salt, water, and urea are reabsorbed. With ATN, reabsorption and urinary concentration abilities are compromised. Other causes of renal failure also may exhibit similar clinical findings. Serial measurements of plasma creatinine provide an index of renal function during the recovery phase.

Prevention of acute renal failure and maintenance of renal perfusion is a major treatment factor and involves maintenance of fluid volume before and after surgery or diagnostic procedures or when nephrotoxic drugs or contrast agents are in use.

Table 36-9	Urine Characteristics of Prerenal and Intrinsic Renal Failure	
Diagnostic Index	Prerenal	Intrinsic
Urine volume	<400 ml	<400 ml
Urine specificity	1.016-1.020	1.010-1.012
Urine osmolality	>500 mOsm	<300 mOsm
Urine sodium	<10 mEq/L	>30 mEq/L
BUN/plasma creatinine	>15:1	<15:1
FE_{Na}	<1% (also seen in acute glomerulonephritis	>1% (also seen in urinary tract obstruction and renal parenchymal disease)
Urine sediment	Usually no cells, some hyaline casts	Brown granular casts, epithelial cells

BUN, Blood urea nitrogen; FE_{Na}, fraction excretion of sodium.

The primary goal of therapy is to maintain the individual's life until renal function has recovered. There is no specific treatment for acute renal failure. Management principles directly related to physiologic alterations generally include (1) correcting fluid and electrolyte disturbances, (2) managing blood pressure, (3) treating infections, (4) maintaining nutrition, and (5) remembering that drugs or their metabolites are not excreted. Fluid and electrolyte replacement must be carefully calculated with consideration of urine losses, insensible losses (up to 1000 ml/day), and production of endogenous water by oxidation (450 ml/day). Overhydration of patients dilutes their plasma sodium concentration. Metabolic acidosis is usually not treated until serum HCO_3^- is less than 15 mEq/L.[127]

Hyperkalemia can be managed by restricting dietary sources of potassium, using nonpotassium-sparing diuretics, or using cation-ion exchange resins, which may be administered orally or rectally. These resins exchange potassium for another cation, such as sodium in the bowel, and the potassium then is excreted attached to the resin. With severe hyperkalemia (>6.5 mEq/L), dialysis may be required or potassium can be driven back temporarily into the cells by administering glucose and insulin or by infusing sodium bicarbonate or albuterol. Glucose metabolism causes potassium to move to the intracellular fluid, and insulin infusions therefore can be effective in shifting potassium from the extracellular to intracellular space, along with the transport of glucose, within 30 minutes. (Glucose metabolism is discussed in Chapter 21.) Causing alkalemia with sodium bicarbonate also shifts potassium into cells in exchange for hydrogen ions.

Careful monitoring of the electrocardiogram for peaking T waves is essential for patients with hyperkalemia. Intravenous infusion of calcium is the most rapid method of treating cardiac effects of hyperkalemia. Calcium decreases the threshold potential and reduces the membrane excitability

caused by hyperkalemia (see Chapter 3). Calcium should be used only in emergencies, however, because hypercalcemia also may cause cardiac arrest.

Azotemia is generally controlled and nutrition maintained with a low-protein, high-carbohydrate diet. Essential amino acid replacement can be given orally or parenterally. Adequate carbohydrate intake slows protein catabolism and helps prevent hyperkalemia. Because sepsis is a common serious or fatal complication of renal failure, observation for signs of infection and early treatment with antibiotics are necessary. Drug dosage levels may require adjustment if they are metabolized or excreted by the kidneys. Recovery may take up to 1 year.

Dialysis (mechanical removal of water, electrolytes, and toxins from the blood) is indicated for uncontrollable hyperkalemia or acidosis or severe fluid overload. Continuous renal replacement therapy is particularly promising in critically ill patients with multiple organ dysfunction.[128]

Chronic Renal Failure

Chronic renal failure is the irreversible loss of renal function and affects nearly all organ systems. Individuals with chronic renal disease progress steadily toward end stage renal disease (ESRD). The most common causes of chronic renal failure are diabetes mellitus and hypertension. The kidneys, however, exhibit remarkable adaptive abilities, and symptomatic changes resulting from increased creatinine, urea, and potas-

---

WHAT'S NEW?　Continuous Renal Replacement Therapy

Continuous renal replacement therapy (CRRT) is a treatment that provides a form of continuous dialysis for acute renal failure. It is replacing intermittent hemodialysis (IHD) or peritoneal dialysis, particularly for critically ill individuals. Generally, there are two forms of CRRT, hemofiltration and hemodiafiltration. Each may be further subdivided into arteriovenous or venovenous, depending on the site of vascular access. Hemofiltration removes excess fluid and solutes (urea, creatinine, sodium, potassium) by pumping blood through the semipermeable membranes of a hemofilter in a compartment of ultrafiltrate. Individuals must be carefully monitored for either volume excess or deficit and electrolyte imbalance. Hemodiafiltration is a combination of hemofiltration and hemodialysis with the removal of solutes by diffusion gradients from the blood across semipermeable membranes to a dialysis solution. In clinical trials comparing CRRT and IHD in critically ill patients, CRRT proved to be a better treatment and resulted in better outcomes. Fluids, wastes, and inflammatory mediators are removed in a controlled manner, and metabolic control, hemodynamic stability, and tissue oxygenation are better. There are opportunities for early and aggressive nutritional support, decreased duration of acute renal failure, and prevention of multiple organ failure. CRRT dosing requirements are still being determined; they are complicated by critical illness.

Data from Hansard PC et al: *Crit Care Med* 32(4):1075-1077, 2004; Salvatori G et al: *Int J Artif Organs* 27(5):404-408, 2004; Schiffl H: *Minerva Urol Nefrol* 56(3):265-277, 2004.

NUTRITION & DISEASE

Acute and Chronic Renal Failure

Malnutrition-inflammation-complex syndrome is a common condition associated with renal failure and leads to accelerated atherosclerosis and cardiovascular disease. Inflammatory cytokines including interleukin-6, tumor necrosis factor-alpha, and interferon suppress appetite and cause muscle proteolysis, decreased protein assimilation, and hypoalbuminemia. Reduced renal function, oxidative stress, decreased levels of antioxidants, infection, exposure to dialysis tubing and membranes during hemodialysis, and back-filtration of contaminants during hemodialysis contribute to inflammation. Acidosis also acts synergistically with inflammatory cytokines and insulin to promote protein catabolism. The provision of nutrients including adequate calories along with protein supplementation that includes amino acids in the form of intradialytic parenteral nutrition or enteral feeding during dialysis assists a person to meet the metabolic requirement. Dietary supplements of antioxidants such as vitamins A and C and carotinoids are required. Adequate nutrition support promotes renal recovery and may prevent consequences of muscle weakness and immune dysfunction.

Data from Bammens B et al: *Am J Clin Nutr* 80(6):1536-1543, 2004; Druml W: *J Ren Nutr* 15(1):63-70, 2005; Ikizler TA: *Adv Chronic Kidney Dis* 11(2):162-171, 2004; Kalantar-Zadeh D et al: *Semin Dial* 17(6):455-465, 2004; Pupim LB, Flakoll PH, Ikizler TA: *Curr Opin Clin Nutr Metab Care* 7(1):89-95, 2004.

sium and alterations in salt and water balance usually do not become apparent until renal function declines to less than 25% of normal.

PATHOPHYSIOLOGY   The progression of chronic renal failure occurs in stages that correlate with specific signs and symptoms. The first stage is *reduced renal reserve,* during which GFR is reduced to about 50%. Although clinical symptoms may not be present, BUN may be elevated. The second stage is *renal insufficiency.* This stage occurs when GFR is severely reduced and mild clinical symptoms of renal dysfunction are apparent. The remaining functional nephrons attempt to compensate for the loss, but the individual may experience mild azotemia (accumulation of nitrogenous wastes in the blood) with a normal diet. Impaired urine concentration with nocturia, mild anemia, and impaired renal function during stress are common during this stage. *Renal failure* is the third stage and is characterized by azotemia, acidosis, impaired urine dilution, severe anemia, and a number of electrolyte imbalances such as hypernatremia, hyperkalemia, and hyperphosphatemia. GFR is reduced below 20%, and the disease begins to affect nonrenal organ systems. The final stage is *en- stage renal disease (ESRD)* and is characterized by near complete absence of GFR. During this stage excretory and reabsorptive capacities are also severely impaired resulting in severe alterations in electrolyte and water regulation and in acid-base balance. Cardiovascular, hematologic, neurologic, gastrointestinal, endocrine, and metabolic symptoms are apparent, as are integumentary and bone and mineral disorders.

Different theories have been proposed to account for the adaptation to loss of renal function. One view suggests that the adaptive response depends on the *particular location of kidney damage.* For example, tubular interstitial diseases damage primarily the tubular or medullary parts of the nephron, producing problems such as renal tubular acidosis, salt wasting, and difficulty diluting or concentrating the urine. When the damage is primarily vascular or glomerular, proteinuria, hematuria, and nephrotic syndrome are more prominent. This theory is useful for planning treatment in early stages of renal failure when symptomatic differences in renal disease may be distinct.

A second theory, the *intact nephron hypothesis,* proposes that loss of nephron mass with progressive kidney damage causes the remaining nephrons to sustain normal or increased function. These nephrons are capable of a compensatory expansion in their rates of filtration, reabsorption, and secretion. They also can maintain a constant rate of excretion in the presence of a declining GFR. The increased workload is achieved primarily by hypertrophy and hyperfunction of the remaining nephrons. As a result, as the rate of remaining nephron loss increases, disease progression occurs more quickly.

The intact nephron hypothesis explains adaptive changes in solute and water regulation that occur with advancing renal failure. Although the urine of an individual with chronic renal failure may contain abnormal amounts of protein and red and white blood cells or casts, the major end products of excretion will be similar to normally functioning kidneys until advanced stages of renal failure, when there is a significant reduction of functioning nephrons.[129]

The *hyperfiltration hypothesis* provides an explanation for progressive failure of intact nephrons. Continued long-term exposure to increased capillary pressure and blood flow velocity leads to glomerulosclerosis and loss of GFR.[130,131] This pathology is common to diabetic and hypertensive nephropathy. Use of angiotensin-converting enzyme inhibitors combined with other drugs (calcium channel blockers or beta blockers) slows this process.[132,133]

Several alterations in electrolyte and acid-base balance occur with chronic renal failure. They are summarized in Table 36-10.

Creatinine and Urea Clearance

Creatinine is constantly released from muscle and excreted primarily by glomerular filtration with relatively no reabsorption and some secretion. In a steady state, the amount produced approximates the amount filtered and excreted. If either the rate of production or the GFR changes, the plasma concentration of creatinine changes until the amount excreted again equals the amount produced. Therefore, if the GFR falls, as in chronic renal failure, the plasma creatinine level increases by a reciprocal amount to maintain a constant rate of excretion. Because no significant tubular adjustment occurs for creatinine (i.e., tubular secretion), the plasma levels continue to increase as the GFR decreases. This relationship allows the plasma creatinine concentration to serve as an

Table 13-10	Electrolyte and Acid-Base Alterations of Chronic Renal Failure
Factor	**Characteristics**
Creatinine and urea clearance	In chronic renal failure, the GFR falls and the plasma creatinine concentration increases by a reciprocal amount; because there is no regulatory adjustment for creatinine, plasma levels continue to rise and serve as an index of changing glomerular function.
	As GFR declines, urea clearance increases. (NOTE: Urea is both filtered and absorbed and varies with the state of hydration.)
Sodium and water balance	In chronic renal failure, sodium load delivered to nephrons exceeds normal, so excretion must increase; thus less is reabsorbed. Obligatory loss occurs, leading to sodium deficits and volume depletion. As GFR is reduced, ability to concentrate and dilute urine diminishes.
Phosphate and calcium balance	Changes in acid-base balance affect phosphate and calcium balance.
	The major disorders associated with chronic renal failure are reduced renal phosphate excretion, decreased renal synthesis of 1,25-(OH)$_2$ vitamin D$_3$, and hypocalcemia.
	Hypocalcemia leads to secondary hyperparathyroidism, GFR falls, and progressive hyperphosphatemia, hypocalcemia, and dissolution of bone result.
Potassium balance	In chronic renal failure, tubular secretion of potassium increases until oliguria develops. Use of potassium-sparing diuretics also may precipitate elevated serum potassium levels. As disease progresses, total body potassium levels can rise to life-threatening levels and dialysis is required.
Acid-base balance	In early renal insufficiency, acid excretion and bicarbonate reabsorption are increased to maintain normal pH.
	Metabolic acidosis begins to develop when GFR decreases to 30% to 40% of normal. When end-stage renal failure develops, the metabolic acidosis may be severe enough to require dialysis.

GFR, Glomerular filtration rate.

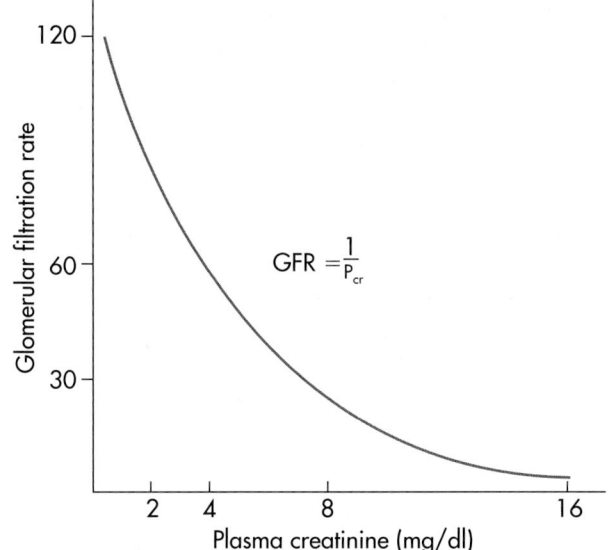

Figure 36-14 Plasma creatinine (P$_{CR}$) and glomerular filtration rate (GFR).

estimate of changing glomerular function.[134] (This relationship is represented in Figure 36-14.)

The clearance of urea is similar, although urea is both filtered and reabsorbed and varies with the state of hydration and diet. Urea clearance therefore is less than the GFR. If protein intake and metabolism are constant, however, plasma levels increase as the GFR declines. Thus no tubular adaptation modifies urea levels because urea is excreted primarily by glomerular filtration.

Sodium and Water Balance

Levels of sodium must be regulated within narrow limits, because sodium is the major extracellular solute. In chronic renal failure the kidneys lose their regulatory capacity for sodium and water. The sodium load delivered to each remaining nephron is greater than normal, so the fractional excretion of sodium (the ratio of excreted to filtered sodium) must increase to maintain normal sodium balance. Although the tubules exhibit a compensatory increased reabsorption, a large obligatory loss remains.[135]

Although the nephron is highly efficient at excreting sodium, it has difficulty conserving sodium when GFR decreases to 25% (approximately 25 ml/min) of normal. At this GFR an obligatory loss of 20 to 40 mEq of sodium per day occurs. If dietary intake is less than this amount, sodium deficits and volume depletion occur. These may be caused by osmotic diuresis from loss of urea or by an inability to inhibit natriuretic hormone after a sudden decrease in sodium intake.

The regulation of water balance and osmolality is normally achieved by urinary concentration mediated by ADH. As GFR is reduced, ability to concentrate and dilute the urine diminishes. In earlier stages of renal failure, this may be caused by osmotic diuresis produced by increased fractional excretion of solutes by the remaining nephrons or by a decreased tubular response to ADH. Individual nephrons can maintain water balance until severe renal failure occurs and GFR declines to 15% to 20% of normal with extensive loss of nephron and tubular function. At this stage the urinary concentration becomes fixed and approaches that of the plasma at 285 mOsm/L with a specific gravity of about 1.010.

Phosphate and Calcium Balance

The metabolism of calcium and phosphate is mediated by parathyroid hormone (PTH) and vitamin D. Changes in acid-base balance also influence the status of calcium and phosphate (see Chapter 3). The major calcium and phosphate disorders associated with chronic renal failure are reduced renal phosphate excretion, decreased renal synthesis of 1,25-(OH)$_2$

Table 36-11	Calcium and Phosphate Metabolism in Chronic Renal Failure	
Kidney	**Plasma**	**Bone**
Decreased renal production of vitamin D₃	Decreased calcium absorption from gut Decreased ionized calcium Increased PTH section (secondary hyperparathyroidism)	Decreased calcium deposition
Decreased phosphate excretion	Elevated phosphate Formation of CaHPO₄	Release of calcium and phosphate Osteitis fibrosa, osteomalacia, calcium deposits in soft tissue (occurs when kidney fails to respond to PTH secretion because of loss of renal mass and calcium and phosphate continues to be absorbed from bone)

PTH, Parathyroid hormone.

vitamin D_3 (the active form of vitamin D), and hypocalcemia (Table 36-11).

In early chronic renal failure, excreted phosphate levels decrease and the plasma phosphate concentration increases because of the decrease in GFR. The elevated plasma phosphate binds calcium ($CaHPO_4$) thereby reducing the free calcium levels and causing hypocalcemia. The decreased calcium stimulates the secretion of PTH. PTH causes release of calcium from bone and enhanced urinary excretion of phosphate. The adaptive effect is a secondary hyperparathyroidism with return of phosphate and calcium levels toward normal (see Chapter 21). With each incremental loss of GFR, however, the effectiveness of PTH in maintaining phosphate balance diminishes. Reducing the dietary intake of phosphate and providing calcium supplementation are helpful at this early stage of failure. When the GFR declines to 25% of normal, however, PTH is no longer effective in maintaining serum phosphate levels. The persistent decreased GFR and hyperparathyroidism cause progressive hyperphosphatemia, hypocalcemia, and dissolution of bone (e.g., osteitis fibrosa, osteomalacia).[136,137] Other consequences of secondary hyperparathyroidism include soft tissue and vascular calcification, cardiovascular disease, and less commonly, calcific uremic arteriolopathy.[138]

Potassium Balance

Urinary excretion of potassium is related primarily to distal tubular secretion mediated by aldosterone and sodium-potassium adenosine triphosphatase (see Chapter 3). In renal failure there is increased tubular secretion that provides effective regulation until the onset of oliguria. Larger amounts of potassium are also lost through the bowel.[139] Although nonoliguric patients can maintain potassium excretion with normal dietary intake, they are more prone to develop hyperkalemia with increased loading (i.e., use of salt substitutes). Use of potassium-sparing diuretics, such as spironolactone (Aldactone), volume depletion, acute infection, severe acidosis, or marked hyperglycemia also may precipitate elevated levels of serum potassium. With progression of disease to end-stage renal failure, total body potassium can increase to life-threatening levels and must be controlled by dialysis.[140]

Acid-Base Balance

The intake of a normal diet produces 50 to 100 mEq of hydrogen per day. These ions are secreted from the renal tubules and excreted in the urine combined with phosphate and ammonia buffers (buffering is described in Chapter 3). During early stages of renal insufficiency, normal pH is maintained by an increased rate of acid excretion and bicarbonate reabsorption by individual nephrons. Metabolic acidosis begins to develop when the GFR decreases by 30% to 40%, primarily because of decreased ammonia synthesis and decreased bicarbonate reabsorption. Phosphate buffers remain effective until late stages of chronic renal failure. When end-stage renal failure develops, serum bicarbonate levels stabilize at 15 to 20 mEq/L, partly because the excess hydrogen is buffered by anions in bone. Individuals with end-stage renal failure develop metabolic acidosis, which may be severe enough to require dialysis.

Nearly every organ system is affected by the consequences of chronic renal failure. The consequences are summarized in Table 36-12.

Skeletal and Bone Alterations

Hypocalcemia and *bone disease* are accelerated by impaired synthesis of 1,25-vitamin D_3 when loss of functioning nephrons is significant and GFR is less than 25% of normal. Lack of the active form of vitamin D reduces intestinal absorption of calcium and impairs the effectiveness of calcium and phosphate resorption from bone by PTH. The toxicity of uremia also may suppress vitamin D action in the gut. This depletion can be treated with vitamin D supplements, but larger than normal doses are required. A negative calcium balance also occurs when acidosis is present, which is common in chronic renal failure. Generally, patients with advanced chronic renal failure have high phosphate and low serum calcium concentrations. The secondary hyperparathyroidism, however, may cause calcium levels to approach normal, and in a small percentage of cases they may be elevated.

Cardiovascular System Function

Cardiovascular morbidity and mortality is high among individuals with CRF. *Hypertension* is a common complication of chronic renal failure that can lead to congestive heart failure if left untreated. The rise in blood pressure is usually the

Table 36-12   Systemic Effects of Chronic Renal Failure

System	Manifestations	Mechanisms	Treatment
Skeletal	Osteitis fibrosa (bone inflammation with fibrous degeneration); bone demineralization (principally subperiosteal loss of cortical bone in the fibers, lateral ends of the clavicles, and lamina dura of the teeth); spontaneous fractures, bone pain; osteomalacia (rickets) with end-stage renal failure	Bone resorption associated with hyperparathyroidism, vitamin D deficiency, and demineralization; lowered calcium and raised phosphate levels	Control of hyperphosphatemia to reduce hyperparathyroidism; administration of calcium and aluminum hydroxide antacids, which bind phosphate in the gut, together with a phosphate-restricted diet; vitamin D replacement; avoidance of magnesium antacids because of impaired magnesium excretion
Cardiopulmonary	Hypertension, pericarditis with fever, chest pain, and pericardial friction rub, pulmonary edema, Kussmaul respirations	Extracellular volume expansion as cause of hypertension; hypersecretion of renin also associated with hypertension; fluid overload associated with pulmonary edema and acidosis leading to Kussmaul respirations	Volume reduction with diuretics that are not potassium sparing (to avoid hyperkalemia); angiotensin-converting enzyme (ACE) inhibitors; combination of propranolol, hydralazine, and minoxidil for those with high levels of renin; bilateral nephrectomy with dialysis or transplantation
Neurologic	Encephalopathy (fatigue, loss of attention, difficulty problem solving); peripheral neuropathy (pain and burning in the legs and feet, loss of vibration sense and deep tendon reflexes); loss of motor coordination, twitching, fasciculations, stupor, and coma with advanced uremia	Uremic toxins associated with end-stage renal disease	Dialysis
Endocrine and reproductive	Retarded growth in children	Decreased growth hormone	Exogenous recombinant human growth hormone
	Osteomalacia	Elevated parathyroid hormone levels	Same as for Skeletal above
	Higher incidence of goiter	Decreased thyroid hormone	Replacement when indicated
	Sexual dysfunction: menorrhagia, amenorrhea, infertility, and decreased libido in women; decreased testosterone levels, infertility, and decreased libido in men	Elevated hormones: luteinizing hormone (LH), follicle-stimulating hormone (FSH), prolactin, and LH-releasing hormone; decreased testosterone, estrogen, and progesterone	No specific treatment
Hematologic	Anemia, usually normochromic normocytic; platelet disorders with prolonged bleeding times	Reduced erythropoietin secretion associated with loss of renal mass, leading to reduced red cell production in the bone marrow; uremic toxins associated with shortened red cell survival	Dialysis; recombinant human erythropoietin and iron supplementation; conjugated estrogens; DDAVP (1-desamino-8-D-arginine vasopressin); transfusion
Gastrointestinal	Anorexia, nausea, vomiting; mouth ulcers, stomatitis, urinous breath (uremic fetor), hiccups, peptic ulcers, gastrointestinal bleeding, and pancreatitis associated with end-stage renal failure	Retention of urea, metabolic acids, and other metabolic waste products, including methylguanidine	Protein-restricted diet for relief of nausea and vomiting
Integumentary	Abnormal pigmentation and pruritus	Retention of urochromes, contributing to sallow, yellow color; high plasma calcium levels associated with pruritus	Dialysis with control of serum calcium levels
Immunologic	Increased risk of infection that can cause death; decreased response to vaccination	Suppression of cell-mediated immunity; reduction in number and function of lymphocytes, diminished phagocytosis	Routine dialysis

result of excess fluid volume and sodium levels associated with renal failure. However, hypertension also may be caused by hyperreninemia secondary to a decrease in renal perfusion or sympathetic hyperactivity.[141] Elevated renin triggers the renin-angiotensin-aldosterone system to increase sodium reabsorption (see Chapter 35).

Dyslipidemia occurs early in chronic renal failure. Arterial wall thickness increases with decreased elastic fibers and increased extracellular matrix. Atheromatous plaque and calcium deposits contribute to loss of vessel elasticity and obstruction.[142] Macrovascular disease is responsible for increased risk for ischemic heart disease, left ventricular hypertrophy, congestive heart failure, stroke, and peripheral vascular disease in individuals with uremia. The anemia of CRF contributes to increased demands for cardiac output, adding to cardiac workload.

In the presence of uremia, individuals with chronic renal failure may develop *pericarditis* resulting from inflammation of the pericardium. These individuals may present with chest pain that may or may not radiate to the left shoulder and may be relieved by leaning forward. A pericardial friction rub may be heard near the left sternal edge. Signs of right ventricular failure, such as dependent edema, also may be present.

Neural Function

Neurologic symptoms are progressive and many are nonspecific to chronic renal disease. Mild sleep disorders, impaired concentration, memory loss, and impaired judgment may occur in some individuals. Some may experience frequent hiccups, muscle cramps and twitching, and other symptoms of neuromuscular irritation. In more advanced stages, asterixis, seizures, and coma may occur. Asterixis is an involuntary flapping motion of the fingers when the arm is hyperextended and is caused by altered nerve conduction secondary to encephalopathy.

Peripheral neuropathy of the sensory systems and, less commonly, motor systems also may be present in individuals with chronic renal failure. This disorder manifests in the lower limbs more than the upper limbs and may present as impairment in localizing sensory stimuli or the perception of sensations when sensory stimuli is not present. Motor manifestations may include involuntary movements of the lower limbs (restless legs syndrome).

Individuals who receive dialysis are susceptible to a host of additional neurologic symptoms. Hemodialysis may result in an aluminum toxicity that can manifest as the inability to repeat words (speech dyspraxia), dementia, and seizures. Dialysis also may rapidly change pH or osmolality in the extracellular fluid resulting in cerebral edema. Clinical symptoms vary but may include nausea, vomiting, headache, drowsiness, and seizures.

Endocrine Function and Reproduction

Uremic males and females experience a decrease in circulating sex steroids. Females have reduced estrogen levels resulting in amenorrhea and the inability to maintain a pregnancy to term. Menses may return with dialysis treatment, but a majority of pregnancies are still unsuccessful. Uremic males often experience a reduction in testosterone levels and may be impotent. Oligospermia and germinal cell dysplasia also may result in infertility. A decrease in libido in both genders is commonly observed.

A failure in kidney function also may result in hyperinsulinemia. As chronic renal failure progresses, the ability of the kidney to degrade insulin is reduced. As a result, the half-life of insulin is prolonged, which may be beneficial to those persons experiencing chronic renal failure secondary to diabetes mellitus.

Hematologic Alterations

Normochromic-normocytic anemia accompanies chronic renal failure because of inadequate production of erythropoietin, decreased red blood cell life span, and blood loss related to diseased kidneys and the uremic state. Lethargy, dizziness, and low hematocrit are common findings.[143] Anemia in these individuals also may be caused by scarring of the bone marrow secondary to hyperparathyroidism. The anemia is commonly associated with left ventricular hypertrophy. However, evidence indicates that treatment normalizes hemoglobin and may result in regression of left ventricular hypertrophy.[144]

Defective platelet aggregation and alterations in vascular endothelial cells leads to an increased bleeding tendency in the instance of uremia.[145] Altered platelet function may be related to the L-arginine-nitric oxide signaling pathway, which is stimulated by high nitric oxide levels.[146,147] Coexisting thrombotic tendencies may be a function of procoagulant platelet-derived microparticles from activated platelets.[148] Bruising and epitaxis are common, and susceptibility to gastrointestinal tract and cerebrovascular hemorrhage is increased.

Immunologic Dysregulation

Immune system dysregulation is a consequence of uremia and chronic renal failure. Chemotaxis, phagocytosis, antibody production, and cell-mediated immune responses are suppressed.[149] Immunosuppression may be amplified because of acidosis, hyperglycemia, gastrointestinal malabsorption, or effects of hemodialysis, or it may be related to a separate underlying cause of renal failure. Susceptibility to infection is increased and there is a deficient response to vaccination, particularly to hepatitis B.[150,151] Dialysis generally improves the immune response.

Gastrointestinal Function

Approximately 25% of individuals with chronic renal failure develop gastrointestinal complications. Uremic gastroenteritis and uremic fetor can occur in chronic renal failure. Uremic gastroenteritis is characterized by bleeding ulcerations along the mucosa that results in significant blood loss. Uremic fetor is a form of bad breath caused by urea breakdown by salivary enzymes. Other gastrointestinal complications are relatively nonspecific, including anorexia, nausea, and vomiting. Many of these symptoms can be relieved by dialysis. Malnutrition is a common problem.

Integument Alterations

Most dermatologic effects associated with chronic renal failure are the result of other complications. For example, anemia may cause pallor whereas dialysis-mediated hemochromatosis may cause gray coloration of the skin. The accumulation of pigmented metabolites also may result in alterations in skin color. Clotting disorders may cause bleeding into the skin (ecchymoses) and hematomas. Calcification secondary to hyperparathyroidism may result in itching (pruritus) and excoriations from scratching. When urinary excretion of urea declines and serum urea concentrations rise, a residue may be left on the skin after the evaporation of sweat, a condition known as "uremic frost."

Alterations in Proteins, Carbohydrates, and Lipids

Proteinuria and a catabolic state contribute to the negative nitrogen balance of chronic renal failure. Muscle protein diminishes, and serum levels of albumin, complement, and transferrin are often low. Proteinuria may independently cause renal damage by promoting inflammation and fibrosis.[152] The amount of proteinuria is also related to the extent of renal injury and predicts disease progression.[153] Restricting dietary protein intake slows the decline in GFR in chronic renal failure, particularly in the case of diabetic nephropathy.[154]

Glucose intolerance because of insulin resistance is common in chronic renal failure. A protein molecule found in uremic serum may interfere with insulin action at a postreceptor site. Secondary parahyperthyroidism and vitamin D deficiency may be contributing factors.[155]

Hypertriglyceridemia occurs in 30% to 70% of individuals with chronic renal failure. There is a high ratio of high-density lipoprotein (HDL) to low-density lipoprotein (LDL) with accelerated atherosclerosis.[156] Uremia produces a deficiency of lipoprotein lipase in capillary endothelium of muscle and fat tissue and decreased hepatic triglyceride lipase. Decreased lipolytic activity results in a reduction of HDL. Apolipoprotein B is also elevated, thereby accelerating atherogenesis.

CLINICAL MANIFESTATIONS   The clinical manifestations of chronic renal failure are often described using the term *uremia*. Uremia refers to a number of symptoms caused by a decline in renal function with the accumulation of toxins in the plasma. The specific mechanisms contributing to toxic symptoms are unknown, although studies have shown that urea and creatinine are only minimally responsible. A combination of other end products of metabolism is associated with toxic symptoms and accompanies accumulations of urea and creatinine. Generally, the symptoms include anorexia, nausea, vomiting, diarrhea, weight loss, pruritus, edema, and neurologic changes.

EVALUATION AND TREATMENT   Evaluation of chronic renal failure is based on the history and presenting signs and symptoms. Elevated serum creatinine concentrations and urea nitrogen are consistent with chronic renal failure. Ultrasound, intravenous pyelogram, or plain x-ray films show small kidney size. Renal biopsy confirms the diagnosis.

Dietary Management

The management of nutrition is essential for the person with chronic renal failure (see Nutrition & Disease box, p. 1326). Generally, nutritional management requires limiting the intake of some nutrients. Loss of renal function causes retention of end products of protein metabolism and alterations in the ability to maintain fluid and electrolyte balance. Regulation of food and fluid intake may delay the need for dialysis. Diet therapy is planned according to individual needs by considering the type and severity of renal disease. The major objective is to maintain adequate nutrition while preventing the accumulation of metabolic waste products.[157]

Sodium and Fluids

Sodium requirements for individuals with renal failure vary widely depending on the type of renal disease and use of diuretics. Glomerular disease tends to cause sodium retention, whereas tubulointerstitial diseases lead to sodium wasting. Sodium requirements can be evaluated by determining 24-hour urinary sodium levels. Usually sodium and fluids are restricted in patients with renal failure.

Fluid intake is usually limited to the amount of urine output, plus an additional amount for insensible water losses. Higher insensible losses occur with fever, excessive sweating, and environment elevations greater than 5000 feet.

Potassium Management

Potassium is usually retained in chronic renal failure and requires dietary restriction. In the presence of anuria or oliguria, potassium is restricted to 0.5 mEq/kg of body weight per day (i.e., 50 mEq/day, or about 2 g/day). Many individuals with renal failure can control serum potassium levels if foods high in potassium are avoided.

Erythropoietin

Anemia of renal failure can be successfully treated with recombinant human erythropoietin. Individuals are significantly less lethargic and experience an increased sense of well-being, increased appetite, and improved sleeping patterns. Supplemental iron and vitamin B_{12} are also given.[158]

SUMMARY REVIEW

Urinary Tract Obstruction

1. Obstructive uropathy can occur anywhere in the urinary tract and is usually caused by renal stones or tumors. The most serious complications are hydronephrosis, hydroureter, and infection caused by an accumulation of urine behind the obstruction.

2. The most common kidney stone is formed from supersaturation, precipitation, and crystallization of urinary calcium. Obstruction is caused by the stone lodging in the ureter.

3. Lower urinary tract obstruction can be caused by bladder neck dyssynergia, prostate enlargement, urethral stricture, pelvic organ prolapse, or a neural lesion that interrupts innervation of the bladder (neurogenic bladder).

Continued

4. Neurogenic bladder can result from brain, spinal cord, or peripheral nerve injuries or lesions.
5. Renal cell carcinoma is the most common renal neoplasm. The larger neoplasms tend to metastasize to the lung, liver, and bone.
6. Bladder tumors are commonly composed of transitional cells with a papillary appearance and a high rate of recurrence.

Urinary Tract Infection

1. Urinary tract infections (UTIs) are usually caused by bacteria, commonly from the retrograde movement of bacteria into the urethra and bladder.
2. Cystitis is an inflammation of the bladder commonly caused by bacteria, although types of "nonbacterial" cystitis may be caused by other conditions or by an autoimmune reaction.
3. The most common pathogens associated with uncomplicated UTI are the gram-negative bacterial species common to the intestinal tract of all humans. *Escherichia coli* infections comprise approximately 80% of UTI found in community-dwelling women.
4. Virulent strains of *E. coli* form pili that cling to the uroepithelium and form biofilms that promote survival and resist antibiotics.
5. Host defenses against uropathogens include protective periurethral mucous production, immune responses, urine acid pH, high urine osmolarity and the presence of glycoproteins.
6. Pyelonephritis is an acute or a chronic inflammation of the renal pelvis that may cause abscess formation and scarring with an alteration in renal function. Pyelonephritis may be acute or chronic.

Glomerular Disorders

1. Glomerulonephritis is a group of related diseases of the glomerulus that can be caused by infection, immune responses, toxins or drugs, vascular disorders, and other systemic diseases.
2. Acute glomerulonephritis commonly results from inflammatory damage to the glomerulus as a consequence of immune reactions after a streptococcal infection.

3. IgA nephropathy is a common cause of glomerulonephritis with deposition of abnormal serum IgA and complement, which causes glomerular injury and sclerosis.
4. Crescentic glomerulonephritis is associated with injury that results in proliferation of glomerular capillary endothelial cells and rapid loss of renal function.
5. Chronic glomerulonephritis is related to a variety of diseases that cause deterioration of the glomerulus and progressive loss of renal function.
6. Immune mechanisms in glomerulonephritis include complement activation, deposition of antigen-antibody complexes, and the formation of antibodies specific for the glomerular basement membrane.
7. Nephrotic syndrome is the excretion of at least 3.5 g of protein in the urine per day. Its principal symptoms are proteinuria, hypoproteinemia, hyperlipidemia, and edema.
8. Nephrotic syndrome is caused by a loss of plasma proteins, principally albumin and some immunoglobulins, across the injured glomerular filtration membrane.

Renal Failure

1. Acute renal failure is classified as prerenal, intrarenal, or postrenal and is usually accompanied by oliguria with elevated plasma blood urea nitrogen (BUN) and plasma creatinine levels.
2. Prerenal acute failure is caused by decreased renal perfusion with a decreased glomerular filtration rate (GFR), ischemia, and tubular necrosis.
3. Intrarenal acute renal failure is associated with several systemic diseases but is commonly related to acute tubular necrosis (ATN).
4. Postrenal failure is associated with diseases that obstruct the flow of urine from the kidneys.
5. Chronic renal failure represents a progressive loss of renal function. Plasma creatinine and urea levels gradually become elevated as GFR declines, sodium is lost in the urine, potassium is retained, acidosis develops, calcium and phosphate metabolism are altered, hematocrit drops, and serum lipids increase.
6. All organ systems are affected by the consequences of renal failure.

KEY TERMS

MEDIA RESOURCES  *evolve*

Review questions and answers for this chapter are available in the *CD Companion* included with this book.

WebLinks—links to Internet sites pertaining to this chapter—are available on Evolve at http://evolve.elsevier.com/McCance/.

REFERENCES

1. Gillenwater JY: Hydronephrosis. In Gillenwater JY et al, editors: *Adult and pediatric urology,* ed 3, Philadelphia, 2002, Lipincott Williams & Wilkins.
2. Gulmi FA, Felsen D, Vauchan ED: Pathophysiology of urinary tract obstruction. In Walsh PC et al, editors: *Campbell's urology,* ed 8, Philadelphia, 2002, Saunders.
3. Misseri R et al: Inflammatory mediators and growth factors in obstructive renal injury, *J Surg Res* 119(2):149-159, 2004.
4. Sullivan MP, Yalla SV: Detrusor contractility and compliance characteristics in adult male patients with obstructive and nonobstructive voiding dysfunction, *J Urol* 155(6):1995-2000, 1996.
5. Ghoniem GM et al: The value of leak pressure and bladder compliance in the urodynamic evaluation of meningomyelocele patients, *J Urol* 144(6):1440-1442, 1990.
6. Galla JH, Luke RG: Hypertension in renal parenchyma disease. In Brenner BM, editor: *The kidney,* Philadelphia, 2000, Saunders.
7. Stern JA, Hsieh YC, Schaeffer AJ: Residual urine in an elderly female population: novel implications for oral estrogen replacement and impact on recurrent urinary tract infection, *J Urol* 171(2 Pt 1):768-770, 2004.
8. Ishidoya S et al: Chronic unilateral ureteral obstruction represented as renin-dependent hypertension, *Nephron* 85(2):175-177, 2000.
9. Jenkins AD: Calculus formation. In Gillenwater JY et al, editors: *Adult and pediatric urology,* ed 4, Philadelphia, 2002, Lipincott Williams & Wilkins.
10. Lingeman JE, Lifshitz DA, Evan AP: Surgical management of urinary lithiasis. In Walsh PC et al, editors: *Campbell's urology,* ed 8, Philadelphia, 2002, Saunders.
11. Rivers K, Shetty S, Menon M: When and how to evaluate a patient with nephrolithiasis, *Urol Clin North Am* 27(2):203-213, 2000.
12. Gray M, Brown KC: Genitourinary system. In Thompson JM et al, editors: *Clinical Nursing,* ed 5, St Louis, 2002, Mosby.
13. Older RA, Jenkins AD: Stone disease, *Urol Clin North Am* 27(2):215-229, 2000.
14. Curhan GC et al: A prospective study of dietary calcium and other nutrients and the risk of symptomatic kidney stones, *N Engl J Med* 328(12):833-838, 1993.
15. Yamanishi T et al: The nature of detrusor bladder neck dyssynergia in non-neurogenic bladder dysfunction, *J Auton Nerv Syts* 66(3):163-168, 1997.
16. Coblentz T, Gray M: Bladder neck obstruction in the female, *Urol Nurs* 21(4):265-272, 2001.
17. Andrich DE, Mundy AR: Urethral strictures and their surgical treatment, *BJU Int* 86(5):571-580, 2000.
18. Valchanov K et al: An unusual cause of acute renal failure: urethral stricture in a female, *Nephron* 87(1):89-90, 2001.
19. Gray M: Neurogenic bladder. In George-Gay B, Chernecky CC, editors: *Clinical medical surgical nursing: a decision making reference,* Philadelphia, 2002, Saunders.
20. Gray M: Psychometric evaluation of the international prostate symptom score, *Urol Nurs* 18(3): 175-183, 1998.
21. Zinman L: Muscular, myocutaneous, and fasciocutaneous flaps in complex urethral reconstruction, *Urol Clin North Am* 29(2):443-466, 2002.
22. Bors E, Comarr AE: *Neurological urology,* Baltimore, Md, 1971, University Park Press.
23. Gibbon NO: Nomenclature of neurogenic bladder, *Urol* 8(5):423-431, 1976.
24. Krane, RJ, Siroky MB: Classification of neurourologic disorders. In Krane RJ, Siroky MB, editors: *Clinical neurourology,* Boston, Mass, 1979, Little-Brown.
25. Lapides J: Neuromuscular, vesical and ureteral dysfunction. In Campbell MF, Harrison JH, editors: *Urology,* Philadelphia, 1970, Saunders.

26. Abrams P: Describing bladder storage function: overactive bladder syndrome and detrusor overactivity, *Urology* 62(5 Suppl 2):28-37, 2003.
27. Gray M: Reflex urinary incontinence. In Doughty DB, editor: *Urinary and fecal incontinence: nursing management,* St. Louis, 2000, Mosby.
28. Bakke A: Clean intermittent catheterization—physical and psychological complications, *Scand J Urol Nephrol Suppl* 150:1-69, 1993.
29. Bauer SB: Neuropathic dysfunction of the lower urinary tract. In: Walsh PC et al, editors: *Campbell's urology,* ed 8, Philadelphia, 2002, Saunders.
30. Anson C, Gray M: Secondary urologic complications of spinal injury, *Urol Nurs* 13(4):107-112, 1993.
31. Stonehill WH et al: Risk factors for bladder tumors in spinal cord injury patients, *J Urol* 155(4):1248-1250, 1996.
32. Weld KJ, Dmochowski RR: Effect of bladder management on urological complications in spinal cord injured patients, *J Urol* 163(3):768-772, 2000.
33. Weld KJ et al: Influences on renal function in chronic spinal cord injured patients, *J Urol* 164(5):1490-1493, 2000.
34. Licht MR: Renal adenoma and oncocytoma, *Semin Urol Oncol* 13(4):262, 1995.
35. American Cancer Society: *Cancer facts and figures, 2004,* Atlanta, 2004, Author. Available online at www.cancer.org/cancerinfo.
36. Dhote R et al: Risk factors for adult renal cell carcinoma, *Urol Clin North Am* 31(2):327-347, 2004.
37. Lindblad P: Epidemiology of renal cell carcinoma, *Scand J Surg* 93(2):88-96, 2004.
38. Flanigan RC et al: Metastatic renal cell carcinoma, *Curr Threat Options Oncol* 4(5):385-390, 2003.
39. Smith JA: Genitourinary tumors. In Jacobson HR, Striker GE, Klahr S, editors: *The principles and practice of nephrology,* St Louis, 1995, Mosby.
40. Ho VB, Choyke PL: MR evaluation of solid renal masses, *Magn Reson Imaging Clin N Am* 12(3):413-427, 2004.
41. Uzzo RG et al: The basic biology and immunobiology of renal cell carcinoma: considerations for the clinician, *Urol Clin North Am* 30(3):423-436, 2003.
42. Pyrhonen SO: Systemic therapy in metastatic renal cell carcinoma, *Scand J Surg* 93(2):156-161, 2004.
43. Lam JS, Shvarts O, Pantuck AJ: Changing concepts in the surgical management of renal cell carcinoma, *Eur Urol* 45(6):692-705, 2004.
44. Matlaga BR et al: Radiofrequency ablation of renal tumors, *Curr Urol Rep* 5(1):39-44, 2004.
45. Kamat AM: Chemoprevention of superficial bladder cancer, *Expert Rev Anticancer Ther* 3(6):799-808, 2003.
46. de Braud F et al: Bladder cancer, *Crit Rev Oncol/Hematol* 41(1):89-106, 2002.
47. Zeegers MP et al: The association between smoking, beverage consumption, diet and bladder cancer: a systematic literature review, *World J Urol* 21(6):392-401, 2004.
48. Algaba F et al: TP53 in urologic tumors, *Anal Quant Cytol Histol* 25(3):123-130, 2003.
49. Han KR et al: Tumor markers for the early detection of bladder cancer, *Front Biosci* 7:e19-26, 2002.
50. Jichlinski P: New diagnostic strategies in the detection and staging of bladder cancer, *Curr Opin Urol* 13(5):351-355, 2003.
51. Tiguert R, Fradet Y: New diagnostic and prognostic tools in bladder cancer, *Curr Opin Urol* 12(3):239-243, 2002.
52. Little B: Non-invasive methods of bladder cancer detection, *Int Urol Nephrol* 35(3):331-343, 2003.
53. Frimberger D, Zaak D, Hofstetter A: Endoscopic fluorescence diagnosis and laser treatment of transitional cell carcinoma of the bladder, *Semin Urol Oncol* 18(4):264-272, 2000.
54. Witjes JA: Bladder carcinoma in situ in 2003: state of the art, *Eur Urol* 45(2):142-146, 2004.
55. Irie A: Advances in gene therapy for bladder cancer, *Curr Gene Ther* 3(1):1-11, 2003.
56. Gschwend JE: Bladder substitution, *Curr Opin Urol* 13(5):477-482, 2003.
57. Schaeffer AJ. Urinary tract infections. In Gillenwater JY et al, editors: *Adult and pediatric urology,* ed 4, Philadelphia, 2002, Lippincott Williams & Wilkins.
58. Gray, M: Urinary tract infection. In Brashers VL, editor: *Clinical applications of pathophysiology,* ed 2, St Louis, 2002, Mosby.
59. Boedeker KS, Kilzer WJ: Fluconazole dose recommendation in urinary tract infection, *Ann Pharmacother* 35(3):369-372, 2001.

60. Burgues Gasion JP et al: Pyeloureteral fungus ball in patients with urinary lithiasis: treatment with ureterorenoscopy, *Acta Urologicas Espanolas* 27(1):60-64, 2003.

61. Kale H, Narlawar RS, Rathod K. Renal fungal ball: an unusual sonographic finding, *J Clin Ultrasound* 30(3):178-180, 2002.

62. Barsoum RS: Schistosomiasis and the kidney, *Semin Nephrol* 23(1): 24-46, 2003.

63. Mulvey MA et al: Bad bugs and beleaguered bladders: interplay between uropathogenic *Escherichia coli* and innate host defenses, *Proc Natl Acad Sci U S A* 97(16):8829-8835, 2000.

64. Costerton JW: Introduction to biofilm, *Int J Antimicrob Agents* 11 (3-4):217-221, 1999.

65. Gray M: Managing urinary encrustation in the indwelling catheter, *J Wound, Ostomy Continence Nurs* 28(5):226-229, 2001.

66. Funfstuck R, Jacobsohn N, Stein G: Interrelationship between virulence properties of uropathogenic *E. coli* and blood group phenotype of patients with chronic urinary tract infection, *Adv Exp Med Biol* 485: 201-212, 2000.

67. Bent S, Saint S: The optimal use of diagnostic testing in women with acute uncomplicated cystitis, *Dis Mon* 49(2):83-98, 2003.

68. Lifshitz E, Kramer L. Outpatient urine culture: does collection technique matter? *Arch Intern Med* 160(16):2537-2540, 2000.

69. Nsowah-Nuamah NN et al: Predicting the timing of second praziquantel treatment and its effect on reduction of egg counts in southern Ghana, *Acta Trop* 90(3):263-270, 2004.

70. Foxman B, Klemstine KL, Brown PD: Acute pyelonephritis in US hospitals in 1997: hospitalization and in-hospital mortality, *Ann Epidemiol* 13(2):144-150, 2003.

71. Papanicolaou N, Pfister RC: Acute renal infections, *Radiol Clin North Am* 34(5):965-995, 1996.

72. Roberts JA: Management of pyelonephritis and upper urinary tract infections, *Urol Clin North Am* 26(4):753, 1999.

73. Kooman JP et al: Acute pyelonephritis: a cause of acute renal failure? *Neth J Med* 57(5):185, 2000.

74. Talner LB et al: Acute pyelonephritis: can we agree on terminology? *Radiology* 192(2):297, 1994.

75. Rollino C et al: Acute pyelonephritis: analysis of 52 cases, *Renal Failure* 24(5): 601-608, 2002.

76. Ratner JJ et al: Bacteria-specific antibody in the urine of patients with acute pyelonephritis and cystitis, *J Infect Dis* 143(3):404-412, 1981.

77. Korman TM, Grayson ML: Treatment of urinary tract infections, *Aust Fam Physician* 24(12):2205, 1995.

78. Rubin RH, Cotran RS, Tolkoff-Rubin NE: Urinary tract infection, pyelonephritis, and reflux nephropathy. In Brenner BM, Rector RC, editors: *The kidney*, ed 5, Philadelphia, 1996, Saunders.

79. Couser WG: Glomerulonephritis, *Lancet* 353(9163):1509-1515 1999.

80. Yoshizawa N: Acute glomerulonephritis, *Intern Med* 39(9):687, 2000.

81. Hricik DE, Chung-Park M, Sedor UR: Glomerulonephritis, *N Engl J Med* 339(13):888, 1998.

82. Glassock RJ, Cohen AH: The primary glomerulopathies, *Dis Mon* 42(6):329, 1996.

83. Nikolic-Paterson DJ, Atkins RC: The role of macrophages in glomerulonephritis, *Nephrol Dial Transplant* 16(Suppl 5):3-7, 2001.

84. Barratt J, Feehally J, Smith AC: Pathogenesis of IgA nephropathy, *Semin Nephrol* 24(3):197-217, 2004.

85. Julian BA, Novak J: IgA nephropathy: an update, *Curr Opin Nephrol Hypertens* 13(2):171-179, 2004.

86. Erwig LP, Rees AJ: Rapidly progressive glomerulonephritis, *J Nephrol* 112(suppl 2):S111, 1999.

87. Hagen EC et al: Diagnostic value of standardized assays for anti-neutrophil cytoplasmic antibodies in idiopathic systemic vasculitis. EC/BCR Project for ANCA Assay Standardization, *Kidney Int* 53(3): 743, 1998.

88. Borza DB, Neilson EG, Hudson BG: Pathogenesis of Goodpasture syndrome: a molecular perspective, *Semin Nephrol* 23(6):522-531, 2003.

89. Kluth DC, Rees AJ: New approaches to modify glomerular inflammation, *J Nephrol* 12(2):66, 1999.

90. Stegmayr BC et al: Plasma exchange or immunoadsorption in patients with rapidly progressive crescentic glomerulonephritis: a Swedish multi-center study, *Int J Artif Organs* 22(2):81-87, 1999.

91. Levy JB et al: Long-term outcome of anti-glomerular basement membrane antibody disease treated with plasma exchange and immunosuppression, *Ann Intern Med* 134(11):1033-1042, 2001.

92. Nangaku M: Mechanisms of tubulointerstitial injury I the kidney: final common pathways to end-stage renal failure, *Intern Med* 43(1):9-17, 2004.

93. Remuzzi G, Ruggenenti P, Perico N: Chronic renal disease: renoprotective benefits of renin-angiotensin system, *Ann Intern Med* 126(8): 604-615, 2002.

94. Shoji T et al: Atherogenic lipoproteins in end-stage renal disease, *Am J Kidney Dis* 38(4 Suppl 1):S30-33, 2001.

95. Ordóñez NG, Rosai J: The urinary track. In Rosai J, editor: *Ackerman's surgical pathology*, ed 9, St Louis, 2004, Mosby.

96. Madaio MP: Postinfectious glomerulonephritis. In Jacobson HR, Striker GE, Klahr S: *The principles and practice of nephrology*, St Louis, 1995, Mosby.

97. Welch TR: The complement system in renal diseases, *Nephron* 88(3):199-204, 2001.

98. Daha MR: Mechanisms of mesangial injury in glomerular diseases, *J Nephrol* 13(Suppl 3):S89-95, 2000.

99. Schena FP: Primary glomerulonephritides with nephrotic syndrome. Limitations of therapy in adult patients, *J Nephrol* 12(suppl 2):S125, 1999.

100. van den Berg JG, Weening JJ: Role of the immune system in the pathogenesis of idiopathic nephrotic syndrome, *Clin Sci (Lond)* 107(2): 125-136, 2004.

102. Nickolas TL, Radhakrishnan J, Appel GB: Hyperlipidemia and thrombotic complications in patients with membranous nephropathy, *Semin Nephrol* 23(4):406-411, 2003.

103. Glassock RJ: Diagnosis and natural course of membranous nephropathy, *Semin Nephrol* 23(4):324-332, 2003.

104. Kitiyakara C, Kopp JB, Eggers P: Trends in the epidemiology of focal segmental glomerulosclerosis, *Semin Nephrol* 23(2):172-182, 2003.

105. Schnaper HW: Idiopathic focal segmental glomerulosclerosis, *Semin Nephrol* 23(2):183-193, 2003.

106. Fogo A: Nephrotic syndrome: molecular and genetic basis, *Nephron* 85(1):8-13, 2000.

107. de Sain-van der Velden MG: Increased VLDL in nephrotic patients results from a decreased catabolism while increased LDL results from increased synthesis, *Kidney Int* 53(4):994, 1998.

108. Kaysen GA, de Sain–van der Velden MG: New insights into lipid metabolism in the nephrotic syndrome, *Kidney Int* 71:S18, 1999.

109. Bergstein JM: A practical approach to proteinuria, *Pediatr Nephrol* 13(8):697, 1999.

110. Kaysen GA: Nonrenal complications of nephrotic syndrome, *Annu Rev Med* 45:201-210, 1994.

111. Coe FL et al, editors: *The yearbook of nephrology*, St Louis, 1992, Mosby.

112. Koomans HA: Pathophysiology of oedema in idiopathic nephrotic syndrome, *Nephrol Dial Transplant* 18(Suppl 6):vi30-32, 2003.

113. Sirolli V et al: Platelet activation markers in patients with nephrotic syndrome: a comparative study of different platelet function tests, *Nephron* 91(3):424-430, 2002.

114. Schwartz A: New aspects of the treatment of nephrotic syndrome, *J Am Soc Nephrol* 12(Suppl 17):S44-S47, 2001.

115. Kuhn K et al: Treatment of severe nephrotic syndrome, *Kidney Int* 64:S50, 1998.

116. Schrierer RW: *Diseases of the kidney*, New York, 1997, Little, Brown.

117. Alkhunaizi AM, Schrier RW: Management of acute renal failure: new perspectives, *Am J Kidney Dis* 28(3):315, 1996.

118. Agmon Y, Brezis M: Acute renal failure: a multifactorial syndrome. In Bourke E, Mallick NP, Pollak BE, editors: *Moving points in nephrology*, Basel, 1993, Karger.

119. Nissenson AR: Acute renal failure: definition and pathogenesis, *Kidney Int* 66:S7, 1998.

120. Mandal AK, Lightfoot BO, Treat RC: Mechanisms of protection in acute renal failure, *Circ Shock* 11(3):245, 1983.

121. Lameire NH, Vanholder R: Pathophysiology of ischaemic acute renal failure, *Best Pract Res Clin Anaesthesiol* 18(1):21-36, 2004.

122. Nath KA, Norby SM: Reactive oxygen species and acute renal failure, *Am J Med* 109(8):665, 2000.

123. Johnson KS, Weinberg JM: Postischemic renal injury due to oxygen radicals, *Curr Opin Nephrol Hypertens* 2(4):625, 1993.

124. Ortiz A et al: Targeting apoptosis in acute tubular injury, *Biochem Pharmacol* 66(8):1589-1594, 2003.

125. Agrawal M, Swartz R: Acute renal failure, *Am Fam Physician* 61(7):2077-2088, 2000.

126. Thijs A, Thijs LG: Pathogenesis of renal failure in sepsis, *Kidney Int* 53(Suppl):S34-S37, 1998.

127. Brady HR, Clarkson MR, Lieberthal W: Acute renal failure. In Brenner BM, editor: *Brenner & Rector's the kidney*, ed 7, Philadelphia, 2004, Saunders.

128. Ronco C et al: Future technology for continuous renal replacement therapies, *Am J Kidney Dis* 28(5 Suppl 3):S121, 1996.

129. Bricker NS, Morrin PA, Kime SW Jr: The pathologic physiology of chronic Bright's disease. An exposition of the "intact nephron hypothesis," *J Am Soc Nephrol* 8(9):1470, 1997.

130. Sackman H et al: Contrasting renal functional reserve in very long-term type I diabetic patients with and without nephropathy, *Diabetologia* 43(2):177, 2000.

131. Schmieder RE et al: Glomerular hyperfiltration during sympathetic nervous system activation in early essential hypertension, *J Am Soc Nephrol* 8(6):893, 1997.

132. Bakis GL et al: Preserving renal function in adults with hypertension and diabetes: a consensus approach. National Kidney Foundation Hypertension and Diabetes Executive Committees Working Group, *Am J Kidney Dis* 36(3):646, 2000.

133. Chantrel F, Moulin B, Hannedouche T: Blood pressure, diabetes and diabetic nephropathy, *Diabetes Metab* 26(suppl 4):37, 2000.

134. Walser M: Assessing renal function from creatinine measurements in adults with chronic renal failure, *Am J Kidney Dis* 32(1):23, 1998.

135. Andreucci M et al: Diuretics in renal failure, *Miner Electrolyte Metab* 25(1-2):32, 1999.

136. Hoyland JA, Picton ML: Cellular mechanisms of renal osteodystrophy, *Kidney Int Suppl* 73:S8, 1999.

137. Stehman-Breen C: Osteoporosis and chronic kidney disease, *Semin Nephrol* 24(1):78-81, 2004.

138. Moe SM, Drueke TB: Management of secondary hyperparathyroidism: the importance and the challenge of controlling parathyroid hormone levels without elevating calcium, phosphorus, and calcium-phosphorus product, *Am J Nephrol* 23(6):369-379, 2003.

139. Kupin WL, Narins RG: The hyperkalemia of renal failure: pathophysiology, diagnosis, and therapy. In Bourke E, Mallick NP, Pollak BE, editors: *Moving points in nephrology*, Basel, 1993, Karger.

140. Giovannetti S, Cupisti A, Barsotti G: The metabolic acidosis of chronic renal failure: pathophysiology and treatment. In Berlyn GM, editor: *The kidney today*, Basel, 1992, Karger.

141. Amann K, Veelken R: Mechanisms and consequences of sympathetic hyperactivity in renal disease, *Clin Nephrol* 60(Suppl 1):S81-S92, 2003.

142. Amann K et al: Special characteristics of atherosclerosis in chronic renal failure, *Clin Nephrol* 60(Suppl 1):S13-S21, 2003.

143. Eckhardt KY: Pathophysiology of renal anemia, *Clin Nephrol* 53 (1 suppl):S2, 2000.

144. Blacher J et al: Impact of aortic stiffness on survival in end-stage renal disease, *Circulation* 99(18):2434-2439, 1999.

145. Moal V et al: Impaired expression of glycoproteins on resting and stimulated platelets in uraemic patients, *Nephrol Dial Transplant* 18(9):1834-1841, 2003.

146. Brunini TM et al: Increased nitric oxide synthesis in uraemic platelets is dependent on L-arginine transport via system y(+)L, *Pflugers Arch* 445(5):547-550, 2003.

147. Fayed HM et al: Nitric oxide generation by peripheral blood cells in chronic renal failure, *Br J Biomed Sci* 49(1):24-29, 2002.

148. Ando M et al: Circulating platelet-derived microparticles with procoagulant activity may be a potential cause of thrombosis in uremic patients, *Kidney Int* 62(5):1757-1763, 2002.

149. Girndt M et al: Molecular aspects of T- and B-cell function in uremia, *Kidney Int Suppl* 78:S206-S211, 2001.

150. Descamps-Latscha B, Jungers P, Witko-Sarsat V: Immune system dysregulation in uremia: role of oxidative stress, *Blood Purif* 20(5):481-484, 2002.

151. Girndt M: Humoral immune responses in uremia and the role of IL-10, *Blood Purif* 20(5):485-488, 2002.

152. Burton C, Harris KP: The role of proteinuria in the progression of chronic renal failure, *Am J Kidney Dis* 27(6):765, 1996.

153. Klahr S: Mechanisms of progression of chronic renal damage, *J Nephrol* 12(suppl 1):S53, 1999.

154. Fouque D et al: Low protein diets delay end-stage renal disease in non-diabetic adults with chronic renal failure, *Cochrane Database Syst Rev* (2):CD001892, 2000.

155. Mak RH: 1,25-Dihydroxyvitamin D3 corrects insulin and lipid abnormalities in uremia, *Kidney Int* 53(5):1353-1357, 1998.

156. Kaysen GA, de Sain-van der Velden MG: New insights into lipid metabolism in the nephrotic syndrome, *Kidney Int Suppl* 71:S18, 1999.

157. Mitch WE, Maroni BJ: Factors causing malnutrition in patients with chronic uremia, *Am J Kidney Dis* 33(1):176, 1999.

158. Macdougall IC: Strategies for iron supplementation: oral versus intravenous, *Kidney Int Suppl* 69:S61, 1999.

ALTERATIONS OF RENAL AND URINARY TRACT FUNCTION IN CHILDREN

SUE E. HUETHER

evolve

http://evolve.elsevier.com/McCance/

CHAPTER OUTLINE

Some renal and urinary disorders occur in both children and adults. In childhood, however, the kidney and genitourinary structures are continuing to develop, so renal dysfunction may be associated with mechanisms and manifestations that are different from those in adults. In addition, some renal and urinary disorders are congenital; many of these involve structural anomalies of the renal system.

STRUCTURE AND FUNCTION OF THE URINARY SYSTEM IN CHILDREN

Development of the Urinary System

The embryonic urinary system develops as three sets of sequentially replaced organs (Figure 37-1). The Wilms tumor 1 (*WT1*) gene plays an important role at all stages of kidney development and maintenance of kidney function.[1] Wingless type signaling (WNT signaling) transduction pathway also is important for secreted growth and differentiation factors.[2] First, the **pronephros** is a nonfunctional structure that arises at the level of the cervical and upper thoracic regions during the third fetal week. The **mesonephros** begins development more caudally about the fourth fetal week and begins excretory function in the sixth week. Most of the mesonephros degenerates and disappears by the end of the embryonic period. The **metanephros,** the permanent kidney, arises distal to the bifurcation of the aorta and develops from two different sources. The *ureteric bud* (metanephric duct) grows dorsocranially and starts subdividing to become the collecting system for the kidneys by forming the ureter, renal pelvis, and calyces. By the fifth fetal month, it will have progressively branched into the collecting ducts. The *metanephrogenic blastema* sits atop the terminal branches of the collecting ducts and develops into primitive glomeruli and uriniferous tubules. Establishing the connection between the uriniferous tubules and the collecting ducts is a vital part of kidney development; errors in this stage can result in polycystic kidneys. As the embryo grows, the definitive kidneys migrate from the caudal position to the lumbar region.

After glomeruli and tubules form, the tissues organize and progressively differentiate over approximately 30 days. Initial glomerular development is staggered, so there are glomeruli in various stages. In fact, a few of the first glomeruli formed degenerate and disappear during the later stages of pregnancy. Progressive development continues into the ninth fetal month, when all metanephrogenic tissue then disappears.

As the embryo develops and the vertebral column straightens, the kidneys appear to ascend to the sacral area at about 6 weeks, to the third lumbar area by the third month, and to the first lumbar area at term. The kidneys rotate 90 degrees as they ascend so that renal tissue is lateral and the collecting system is medial.

While the kidneys mature, the cloaca becomes the urogenital sinus. It then differentiates into the vesicourethral canal, which forms the bladder and the upper urethra, and the urogenital sinus, which forms the main part of the urethra.

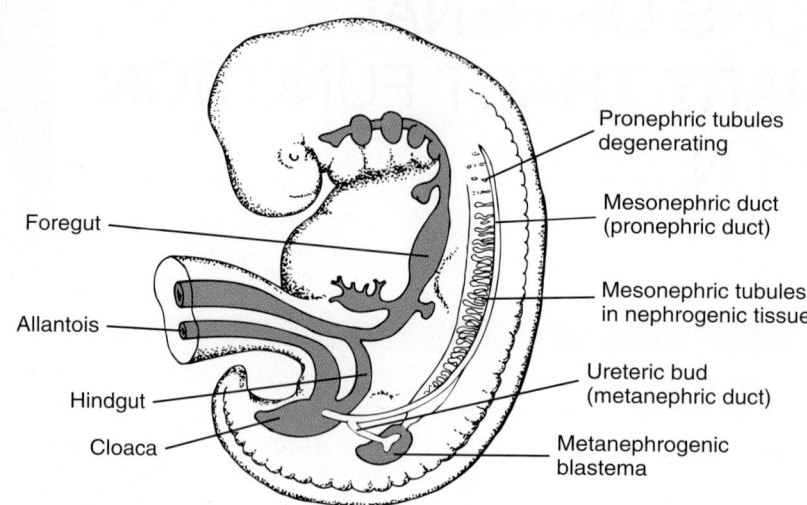

Figure 37-1 Topography of the pronephros, mesonephros, and metanephric primordium. (From Netter F, Shapter R, Yonkman F, editors: *The ciba collection of medical illustrations,* vol 6, *Kidneys, ureters, and urinary bladder,* Summit, NJ, 1973, Ciba Pharmaceutical Corporation.)

Table 37-1	Average Daily Urine Output in Children
Age	**Output (ml/day)**
1 and 2 days	15-50
3-10 days	50-300
10 days-2 months	250-400
2 months-1 year	400-500
1-3 years	500-600
5-8 years	700-1000
8-14 years	700-1500

From Kempe CH, Silver KH, O'Brien D: *Current pediatric diagnosis and treatment,* Los Altos, Calif, 1982, Lange Medical Publishers.

At birth the kidneys occupy a large portion of the posterior abdominal wall, and the ureters are proportionately shorter than those of an adult. All the nephrons are present at birth, and their number does not increase as the kidney grows and matures. The kidney reaches adult size by adolescence and, because of maturation of the tubular system, increases in weight tenfold from the time of birth.

Urine formation and excretion begin by the third month of gestation, contributing to the amniotic fluid. In infancy the bladder lies close to the abdominal wall, making urinary bladder aspiration for diagnostic purposes a relatively simple procedure. The bladder descends into the pelvis with growth, changing from a cylindric organ to the adult pyramidal shape. Although small amounts of urine are found in the bladder at birth, the newborn may not void for 12 to 24 hours. (The average daily urine output is shown in Table 37-1.)

Immediately upon birth the renal blood flow and glomerular filtration rate (GFR) increase because of a decrease in vascular resistance and the need to perform excretory functions no longer performed by the placenta. Renal vascular resistance remains higher in newborns and infants, however, which may be attributed to increased levels of circulating renin. The resistance progressively declines during the first year of development, with an increasing fraction of the cardiac output going to the kidney. The GFR continues to increase, becoming stable at 1 or 2 years, but retaining only 30% to 50% of adult levels until the end of the first year. Although glomerular filtration is important in removing nitrogenous and other wastes, the amount of urea to be removed is small.

Fluid and Electrolyte Balance in Children

Because the kidney develops from the center toward the periphery, renal distribution of blood flow during the newborn period is primarily to the renal medulla. The result is a preferential flow to the medullary nephrons, which have comparatively short loops at this stage of development. The combination of higher blood flow and shorter loops produces a more dilute urine—approximately 600 to 700 mOsm. The dilute urine is accentuated by a low rate of urea excretion because urea is necessary to establish the concentration gradient in the medulla. Urea excretion is low primarily because infants are in a high anabolic state and use their protein for growth.

Because of a high hydrogen ion concentration, limited ability to regulate the internal environment, and lowered osmotic pressure, the infant's renal system has a narrow chemical safety margin. The immaturity and smaller surface area of the tubules also may diminish the water reabsorption response to antidiuretic hormone (ADH). An immature tubular transport capacity means that the ability to excrete a potassium load, reabsorb bicarbonate, or buffer hydrogen with ammonia does not become efficient until approximately 2 years of age. Consequently, any disturbance such as diarrhea, infection, fasting for diagnostic tests, or improper feeding can rapidly lead to severe acidosis and fluid imbalance because the infant can rapidly develop overhydration, or edema.[3]

After birth the proportion of total body water to body weight does not change markedly. Considerable change occurs, however, in the location of that body water as the child matures (see Chapter 3). The percentage of extracellular fluid volume of the newborn infant is nearly double that of the adult. Decrease in extracellular fluid volume occurs in two different periods of rapid growth—infancy and adolescence.

Not only does the infant have a greater content of extracellular fluid but also a greater rate of fluid exchange. The adult takes in and excretes approximately 2000 ml of water daily, representing 5% of the total body fluid and 14% of the extracellular fluid. In contrast, the infant's daily exchange of 600 to 700 ml represents 290% of the total or nearly 50% of the extracellular volume, making control of dehydration and overhydration more difficult.

The composition of body fluids differs slightly with age. The total electrolyte concentration in extracellular fluids is greater in the newborn than in the adult. The concentration of sodium, chloride, phosphates, and organic acids is also greater. The concentration of bicarbonate ions is lower in the infant than in the older child, with a mild acidosis evidenced by a lowered pH. These variations, combined with a lowered plasma protein level, cause a reduced oncotic pressure of the vascular compartment and favor accumulation of fluid in the tissue spaces and an increased GFR. In the healthy child, these differences remain for a few weeks or months. The premature infant and the normal newborn infant are usually in a state of well-compensated acidosis and potential edema.

ALTERATIONS IN RENAL FUNCTION IN CHILDREN

Structural Abnormalities

Variations from the normal anatomic structure of the urinary tract occur in 10% to 15% of the total population. The structural abnormalities range from minor, nonpathologic, or easily correctable anomalies to those that are incompatible with life. For example, the kidneys may fail to ascend from the pelvis to the abdomen, causing ectopic kidneys—which usually function normally. The kidneys also may fuse in the midline as they ascend, causing a single U-shaped **horseshoe kidney** with an incidence of 1 per 600 births.[4] Approximately one third of individuals with horseshoe kidneys are asymptomatic, and the most common problems are hydronephrosis, infection, and stone formation.[5] Collectively, structural anomalies of the renal system account for approximately 45% of cases of renal failure in children.

Some anomalies are obvious at birth, whereas others remain latent. The following structural anomalies are commonly associated with urinary tract malformations:[6]

Low-set, malformed ears
Chromosomal disorders, especially trisomy 13 (Patau syndrome) and trisomy 18
Absent abdominal muscles (prune-belly syndrome)
Anomalies of the spinal cord and lower extremities
Imperforate anus or genital deviation
Wilms tumor
Congenital ascites
Cystic disease of the liver
Positive family history of renal disease (hereditary nephritis or cystic disease)

Hypospadias

Hypospadias is a congenital condition in which the urethral meatus is located on the ventral side or undersurface of the penis. The meatus can be located anywhere on the glans, the penile shaft, the base of the penis, the penoscrotal junction, or the perineum (Figure 37-2). This is the most common anomaly of the penis and occurs in about 1 in 300 infant boys. The etiology is multifactorial and related to disruptions in male hormones, including testosterone biosynthesis defects, 5a-reductase mutations, hormones administered for in vitro fertilization, and other environmental factors.[7] **Chordee,** or penile torsion, may accompany hypospadias. In chordee a shortage of skin on the ventral surface causes the penis to bend or to "bow" ventrally (Figure 37-3). Penile torsion is a counterclockwise twist of the penile shaft. Partial absence of the foreskin and cryptorchidism (undescended testes, see Chapter 23) are associated with the anomaly.[8]

The goal for corrective surgery on the child with hypospadias is a cosmetically acceptable, straight penis with the urinary meatus at the tip. Formerly performed in two or more stages, hypospadias repairs are now done in one stage. Improvements in microsurgical techniques have improved outcomes and decreased complications. Surgery is usually performed between 6 and 12 months of age. Surgery is most effective between 8 and 12 months of age.[9]

Epispadias

Epispadias and exstrophy of the bladder are the same congenital defect but expressed to a different degree. In male epispadias the urethral opening is on the dorsal surface of the penis. In females a cleft along the ventral urethra usually extends to the bladder neck. The incidence of epispadias is about 1 in 40,000 to 118,000 births. Twice as many boys as girls present with this defect.

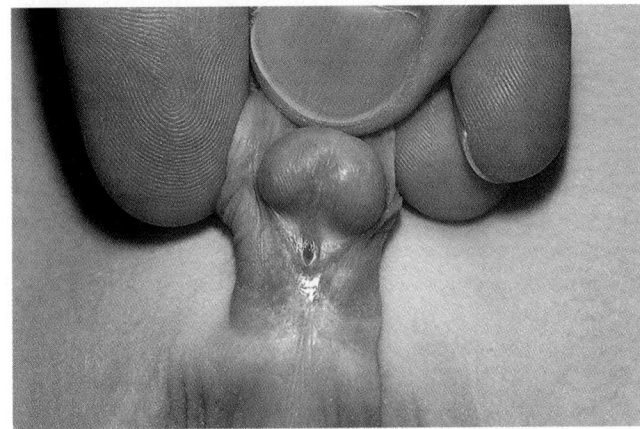

Figure 37-2 Hypospadias. (Courtesy H. Gil Rushton, MD, Children's National Medical Center, Washington, DC; from Hockenberry MJ: *Wong's nursing care of infants and children,* ed 7, St Louis, 2003, Mosby.)

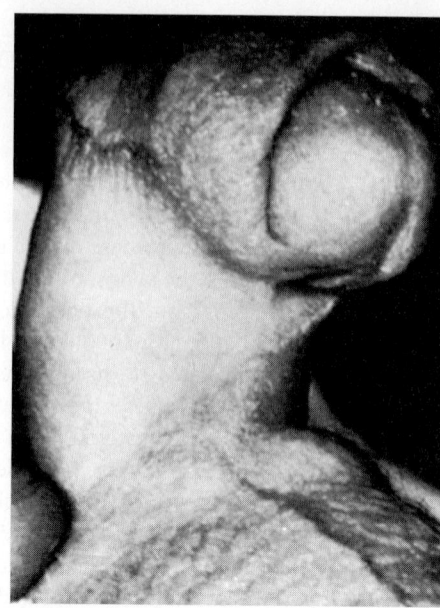

Figure 37-3 Hypospadias with significant chordee. (From Shirkey HC, editor: *Pediatric therapy,* ed 6, St Louis, 1980, Mosby.)

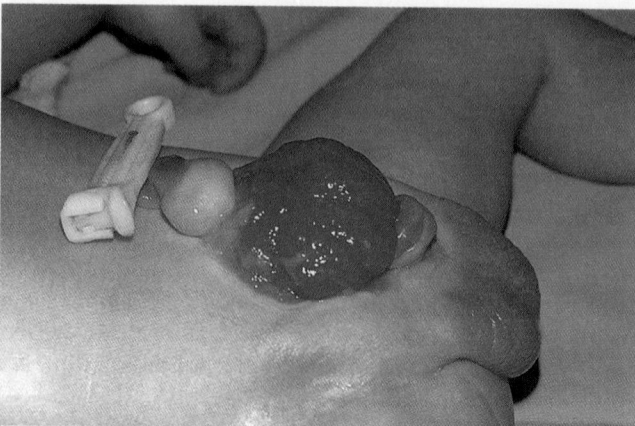

Figure 37-4 Exstrophy of bladder. (Courtesy H. Gil Rushton, MD, Children's National Medical Center, Washington, DC; from Hockenberry MJ: *Wong's nursing care of infants and children,* ed 7, St Louis, 2003, Mosby.)

In boys the urethral opening may be small and situated behind the glans (anterior epispadias) or a fissure may extend the entire length of the penis and into the bladder neck (posterior epispadias). Children with anterior epispadias can be continent with perhaps only stress incontinence, but those with posterior epispadias will experience constant dribbling of urine.[10]

Exstrophy of the Bladder

Exstrophy of the bladder is an extensive congenital anomaly in which the lower urinary tract is exposed directly to the surface of the body (Figure 37-4). The posterior portion of the bladder mucosa is exposed and appears bright red through a fissure in the abdominal wall. The incidence of exstrophy of the bladder is about 1 in 400,000 live births. Boys are predominant by a ratio of 5:1.[11]

Exstrophy of the bladder is caused by intrauterine failure of the abdominal wall and the mesoderm of the anterior bladder to fuse. The rectus muscles below the umbilicus are separated, and the pubic rami (bony projections of the pubic bone) are not joined. In addition, the posterior aspect of the pelvis is externally rotated, which retroverts the acetabula and causes external rotation of the feet.[12] This causes a waddling gait when the child first learns to walk, but most children quickly learn to compensate. Urine seeps onto the abdominal wall from the ureters, causing a constant odor of urine and excoriation of the surrounding skin. Because the exposed bladder mucosa becomes hyperemic and edematous, it bleeds easily and is painful. It should be covered with Silastic or a plastic dressing (Glad Wrap or Saran Wrap) for protection from diaper irritation while permitting urine drainage.

The unrepaired exstrophic bladder is cosmetically unacceptable and prone to cancerous changes as soon as 1 year after birth. Ideally, the bladder and pubic defect should be closed before the infant is 48 hours old. Reconstruction of the internal and external genitalia can be done when girls reach their late teens. Epispadias repair in boys is better done at 2 to 3 years of age as are bladder neck reconstruction, ureteral implantation, and bladder augmentation. Objectives of management include preservation of renal function, attainment of urinary control, prevention of infection, reconstructive repair of the defect, and improvement of sexual function and quality of life.

Ureteropelvic Junction Obstruction

Ureteropelvic junction (UPJ) obstruction is a blockage of the tapered point where the renal pelvis transitions into the ureter.[13] It is the most common cause of hydronephrosis in neonates. An intrinsic malformation of smooth muscle or urothelial development produces obstruction in 90% of cases, and approximately 10% are caused by extrinsic compression.[13,14] Treatment is a surgical pyeloplasty or endopyelotomy.[15] During infancy or childhood, **secondary ureteropelvic junction (UPJ) obstruction** is caused by kinking of secondary scarring in the presence of high-grade vesicoureteral reflux. An increased risk of vesicoureteral reflux in children with UPJ affects both the obstructed and contralateral kidneys; whether this represents a sequela of the embryonic defect leading to the UPJ defect is not known. Other defects are sometimes associated with ureteral duplication including complete ureteral duplication (abnormal growth of two ureters and ureteral orifices draining a single kidney), incomplete duplication (bifurcation of the ureter terminates into one ureteral orifice and serves a single kidney), and ureterocele (cystic dilation of the intravesical ureter). Obstruction of the distant ureter causes dilation of the entire ureter, renal pelvis, and caliceal system.[16] It occurs when a short acontractile segment of the ureter develops just above the ureterovesical junction.

Bladder Outlet Obstruction

Congenital causes of bladder outlet obstruction include urethral valves and polyps. A urethral valve is a thin membrane of tissue that occludes the urethral lumen and obstructs urinary outflow in males.[17] Most valves occur in the posterior

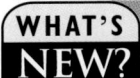

WHAT'S NEW?   Pediatric Ureteroscopy

Endoscopic diagnosis and treatment of upper urinary tract conditions in children is new, safe, and efficacious. Technological advances in fiber optics—including both rigid and flexible ureteroscopes—has led to success with few complications for treatment of renal calculi, tumor excision, incising strictures, coagulation of bleeding lesions, and repair of ureteropelvic junction obstructions.

Data from Johnson WK III, Low RK, Das S: *Urol Clin North Am* 31(1):5-13, 2004; Reddy PP: *Urol Clin North Am* 31(1):145-156, 2004; Satar N et al: *J Urol* 172(1):298-300, 2004.

urethra, although a few arise from the embryologically distinct anterior urethra. Polyps rarely arise from the prostatic urethra. They often cause relatively severe obstruction and may impair renal embryogenesis and lead to urinary tract infection, vesicoureteric reflux, and renal failure.[18]

Congenital abnormalities (valves or polyps) must be resected as soon as possible, ideally during the first days of life. These structures can be resected using a small cystoscope. Infants with significant renal (and pulmonary) hypoplasia who are unable to undergo primary resection may be managed with a vesicostomy, a small opening created by pulling the bladder wall to the abdomen.[19]

Hypoplastic or Dysplastic Kidneys

During embryologic development the ureteric duct grows into the metanephric tissue, triggering the formation of the kidneys. If this growth does not occur, the kidney is absent—a condition called **renal aplasia.** Occasionally a **hypoplastic kidney,** a very small normal kidney, may develop. These aberrations may be unilateral or bilateral; the occurrence may be incidental or familial. Bilateral hypoplastic kidneys are a common cause of chronic renal failure in children. Segmental hypoplasia (the Ask-Upmark kidney) is not the result of developmental abnormalities but instead a deformity acquired secondary to intrarenal reflux.[20]

Renal dysplasia usually results from abnormal differentiation of the renal tissues; for example, primitive glomeruli and tubules, cysts, and nonrenal tissue (such as cartilage) are found in the dysplastic kidney. Dysplasia usually is associated also with a functional or organic obstruction of the collecting system. The obstruction may begin before birth, as in prune-belly syndrome (absent abdominal muscles), posterior urethral valves, or ureteroceles.

Renal Agenesis

Renal agenesis (the absence of one or both kidneys) may be unilateral or bilateral, and it may occur randomly or be clearly hereditary. Bilateral agenesis is usually fatal. The condition may occur as an isolated entity or as a problem associated with other unrelated disorders.[21]

Unilateral renal agenesis occurs in approximately 1 of 1000 live births. Males are more often affected, and it is usually the left kidney that is absent. The single kidney is often completely normal so that the child can expect a normal, healthy life. The normal solitary kidney grows because of compensatory hypertrophy before and after birth, and by the time the child is several years older, the volume of this kidney may approach twice the normal size.[22]

In some instances, the single kidney is abnormally formed and associated with abnormalities of its collecting system.[23] Extrarenal congenital abnormalities are relatively more common with unilateral renal agenesis.

Bilateral renal agenesis (also called **Potter syndrome**) occurs in about 1 to 4 in 10,000 live births,[24] and 75% of affected infants are male. Bilateral renal agenesis results from either an abnormal development of the normal progression from pronephros to mesonephros to metanephros or an isolated bilateral failure of development of the ureteral buds. The term *Potter syndrome* refers to the association with a specific group of facial anomalies (wide-set eyes, parrot-beak nose, low-set ears, and receding chin). Affected infants rarely live more than a few hours. Most die of respiratory distress caused by associated pulmonary hypoplasia rather than from renal failure. Approximately 40% of affected infants are stillborn. Renal agenesis can be detected prenatally by ultrasound.

Polycystic Kidneys

Polycystic kidney disease (PKD) is an autosomal dominant inherited disorder that occurs in about 1 in 1000 live births. Mutations of two genes, *PKD-1* (chromosome 16) and *PKD-2* (chromosome 4) account for the disease most often found in adults. In children, there is an autosomal recessive form of PKD (ARPKD) that has been localized to the short arm of chromosome 6. The gene products regulate epithelial growth and differentiation.[25] It is proposed that the tubular epithelium proliferates with a transition to transepithelial fluid transport causing cyst formation and obstruction.[26] Individuals may live for decades before developing symptoms, and PKD is often an adult disease. Other organs also may have cysts, including the liver and pancreas. Hypertension, heart valve defects, and cerebral and aortic aneurysms may develop. Other signs include urinary tract infection, hematuria, and flank pain. Diagnosis is usually confirmed by ultrasound.

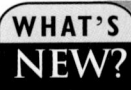

WHAT'S NEW?   Prenatal Diagnosis of Congenital Genitourinary Anomalies

Prenatal ultrasound can detect an infant's gender (important in diagnosing gender-linked hereditary disorders) and possibly genital epispadias, unilateral renal agenesis, pelvic kidney, and double collecting system. In addition, color Doppler ultrasound can detect the lack of renal arteries and renal agenesis and magnetic resonance imaging (MRI) can detect the anatomy of fetal genitourinary anomalies.

Data from Caire JT et al: *AJR Am J Roentgenol* 181(5):1381-1385, 2003; Isaksen CV et al: *Ultrasound Obstet Gynecol* 15(3):177, 2000.

Infundibular stenosis (stenosis of the calyx infundibulum), often associated with multicystic or polycystic renal dysplasia, may cause obstruction and dilation of one or more calyces (megacalycosis). **Megacalycosis** is congenital, nonobstructive dilation of the calyces without pelvic or ureteric dilation that typically affects both kidneys and is associated with glomerulosclerosis and an increased risk of end-stage renal disease throughout the infant's lifespan.

Glomerular Disorders

Glomerular disease can manifest in different ways, including glomerulonephritis, nephrotic syndrome, and hemolytic uremic syndrome. These are the most common diseases in children and are the focus of this chapter. Most glomerular diseases are acquired and immunologically mediated. The disease can be acute or chronic; renal failure is rare.

Glomerulonephritis

Glomerulonephritis includes a number of renal disorders in which proliferation and inflammation of the glomeruli are secondary to an immune mechanism (Table 37-2). (The major glomerulopathies are described in Chapter 36.) Chronic glomerulonephritis is the causative factor for 53% of renal failure in children and is the condition responsible for most school-age and teenage children requiring dialysis and kidney transplantation.

Acute Poststreptococcal Glomerulonephritis

Acute poststreptococcal glomerulonephritis (PSGN) is one of the most common postinfectious renal diseases in children ages 5 to 15 years. It occurs after a throat (pharyngitis) or skin (impetigo) infection with certain strains of group A β-hemolytic streptococci and is characterized by a sudden onset of gross hematuria, edema, hypertension, and renal insufficiency.

Table 37-2	Primary Glomerulonephritis in Children	
Classification	**Findings**
Cause	Poststreptococcal infection
	Related to other bacterial or viral infection
	Unknown
Immunologic mechanism	Antigen-antibody complex
	Anti-glomerular basement membrane disease
	No immunologic cause established
Histopathology	No lesion
	Diffuse, focal, or segmented
	Membranous, proliferative, or combination of types
	Lobular, exudative, necrotizing, and other types
	Chronic with glomerular proliferation
Clinical manifestations of disease	Acute glomerulonephritis
	Persistent (chronic) glomerulonephritis
	Idiopathic nephrotic syndrome

Pharyngeal infections are most common during cold weather. Skin infections from impetigo, infected insect bites, or varicella sores usually occur during warm weather. The pathophysiology of PSGN in children is similar to that occurring in adults (see Chapter 36). Antigen-antibody complexes of IgG, IgA, and C_3 complement are deposited in the glomerulus or the antigen may be trapped within the glomerulus and immune complexes formed in situ. The immune complexes initiate inflammation and glomerular injury. Immunofluorescence microscopy shows lumpy deposits of immunoglobulin and complement on the glomerular basement membrane. The exact mechanism of immune complex formation is unknown. Increased vascular permeability and loss of negative charge, along the glomerular vascular membrane, leads to hematuria and proteinuria. Hypertension occurs with increased blood volume and release of endothelin-1, a potent vasoconstrictor, as a result of endothelial injury and platelet activation.[27] The most severely affected children develop acute renal failure with oliguria. Other children may be asymptomatic.

Typically a child is in good health until the onset of an upper respiratory or skin infection. One to two weeks later, mild proteinuria (less than 2 g per 4 hours), hematuria, and periorbital edema appear. The urine is usually smoky brown or cola colored because of the presence of red blood cells, and the volume is reduced. The onset of symptoms in the child is abrupt and consists of flank or midabdominal pain, irritability, general malaise, and fever. Acute hypertension may cause headache; vomiting; somnolence; and other central nervous system (CNS) manifestations, including seizures. Cardiovascular symptoms are related to circulatory overload and are compounded by hypertension. These include dyspnea; tachypnea; and an enlarged, tender liver. As many as half the children affected are asymptomatic.

The disease is usually mild and runs its course in 1 month, but urine abnormalities may be found up to 1 year after the onset. Some children (less than 1%) become oliguric and develop rapidly progressive glomerulonephritis, whereas others slowly progress to chronic glomerulonephritis. Prolonged proteinuria and abnormal GFR indicate an unfavorable prognosis. More than 95% recover completely.

Acute glomerulonephritis (AGN) may be accompanied by a positive throat or skin culture for *Streptococcus*. The urine usually contains red blood cells and proteins. Treatment is symptom specific. Because oliguria and hypertension are common, fluid, sodium, and potassium intakes are restricted. Antihypertensive medication and diuretic agents are indicated during the acute phase.

As a precautionary measure, penicillin is given in therapeutic doses for 10 to 14 days to eradicate residual streptococci. Early treatment of streptococcal infections with antibiotics does not preclude the development of the disease. Family members of the affected child should have throat or skin cultures and be treated with penicillin if a culture is positive.[28]

Immunoglobulin A Nephropathy

Immunoglobulin A (IgA) nephropathy (Berger nephropathy) is one of the most common types of glomerulonephritis, occurs almost twice as often in males as in females, and is rare in African Americans. It is characterized by deposition mainly of IgA, but also some immunoglobulin M (IgM) and complement proteins, in the mesangium of the glomerular capillaries, even though there is no evidence of systemic immunologic disease such as systemic lupus erythematosus or anaphylactoid purpura. IgA may show decreased glycosylation that favors mesangial deposition.[29] Binding of the IgA to mesangial cells stimulates them to proliferate, secrete extracellular matrix proteins, and release cytokines and chemokines (interleukin-6, tumor necrosis factor-alpha, and transforming growth factor beta 1) that cause injury. The damage to the glomerulus can progress to glomerulosclerosis and tubular interstitial involvement, which is usually reversible.[30]

The classic presentation of the disease is recurrent gross hematuria, often after a respiratory infection. Most continue to have microscopic hematuria between the attacks of gross hematuria. Many children also have a mild proteinuria in spite of otherwise normal renal function and may report flank pain caused by renal swelling. Treatment is supportive. Long-term follow-up should consist of checking blood pressure, urinalysis, proteinuria levels, and renal function every 6 to 12 months.[31] However, approximately 20% of affected children develop the progressive form of the disease, with hypertension and decreasing renal function that extends into adulthood. Hypertriglyceridemia and hyperuricemia are predictors of poor outcome.[32] These children eventually require dialysis and transplantation.

Henoch-Schönlein Purpura Nephritis— IgA Nephropathy

Henoch-Schönlein purpura nephritis, also known as *anaphylactoid purpura*, is an IgA nephropathy that affects the glomerular blood vessels causing inflammation and damage to the vessel wall. The disease also involves small vessels in the skin and gut. The most typical renal lesion is segmental focal glomerulonephritis with IgA deposits in the mesangium. Transient hematuria and mild proteinuria without functional impairment is more common in children. Children also may exhibit signs of intestinal colic and arthralgia.[33] The development of interstitial fibrosis and crescent formation from subepithelial immune deposits along the glomeruli increases the risk of chronic renal failure.[34] No definitive treatment is known and most children recover with supportive care.

Hemolytic-Uremic Syndrome

Hemolytic-uremic syndrome is an acute disorder characterized by hemolytic anemia originating in the microcirculation with thrombocytopenia. It is the most common cause of acute renal failure in young children.[35] The etiology remains unknown, although an association between hemolytic-uremic syndrome and both bacterial and viral agents has been established. *Escherichia coli* O157:H7, a shiga toxin-producing bacteria, is the most common associated microorganism in the United States, usually found in undercooked meat and unpasteurized milk.[36] The disease occurs in infants and children younger than 4 years. The prognosis has improved dra-

matically in recent years, with more than 90% of children surviving and most regaining normal renal function.

PATHOPHYSIOLOGY   In hemolytic-uremic syndrome, verotoxin from *E. coli* is absorbed from the intestines and damages red blood cells and endothelial cells. The endothelial lining of the glomerular arterioles becomes swollen and occluded with platelets and fibrin clots. There is decreased glomerular filtration with hematuria and proteinuria. Oliguria with renal failure occurs in up to 50% of children. Narrowed vessels damage erythrocytes as they pass through. These damaged burr cells, helmet cells, and fragmented red blood cells are removed by the spleen, causing acute hemolytic anemia. Fibrinolysis, the process of dissolution of a clot, acts on precipitated fibrin, causing the fibrin split products to appear in serum and urine. The platelet clustering within damaged vessels, combined with the damage and removal of platelets, produces thrombocytopenia. Fibrin-rich thrombi can be found throughout the microcirculation. Other tissues, including the brain, liver, heart, and intestines, are often involved and portends a poorer prognosis.

CLINICAL MANIFESTATIONS   A prodromal gastrointestinal illness (fever, vomiting, diarrhea) or, less frequently, an upper respiratory infection often precedes the onset of hemolytic-uremic syndrome by 1 to 2 weeks. After a symptom-free 1- to 5-day period, the sudden onset of pallor, bruising or purpura, irritability, and oliguria heralds the onset of the disease. Slight fever, anorexia, vomiting, diarrhea (with the stool characteristically watery and blood stained), abdominal pain, mild jaundice, and circulatory overload are accompanying symptoms. Seizures and lethargy indicate CNS involvement. Renal failure is apparent within 2 days to 2 weeks of onset. The renal failure causes metabolic acidosis, azotemia, hyperkalemia, and often hypertension.

EVALUATION AND TREATMENT   Clinical evaluation includes history of preexisting illness, presenting symptoms, and urine and blood analysis. Management consists of maintaining nutrition and fluid and electrolyte balance and controlling hypertension and seizures.[37] When renal failure occurs, early and frequent dialysis is indicated. Blood transfusions with packed red blood cells are needed to maintain reasonable hemoglobin levels. The response to treatment is usually good.

Nephrotic Syndrome

In children with nephrotic syndrome the kidney is usually the only or principal organ involved. This condition is termed **primary nephrotic syndrome** when no other identifiable causes are found. If it results from a systemic disease or other causes (e.g., drugs, toxins), it is called **secondary nephrotic syndrome** (see Chapter 36).

Approximately 95% of cases of nephrotic syndrome in children occur in the absence of systemic or preexisting renal disease. Primary nephrotic syndrome is found predominantly in preschool children, with a peak incidence of onset between 2 and 3 years of age. It is rare after 8 years of age. Boys are affected more often than girls. No prevalent racial or geographic distributions are evident. The incidence is approximately 3 per 100,000 children per year.

PATHOPHYSIOLOGY   **Nephrotic syndrome** is a term used to describe a symptom complex characterized by proteinuria, hypoproteinemia, hyperlipidemia, and edema. The syndrome is more common in children than in adults, and the cause is usually idiopathic (minimal change neuropathy 85%, focal glomerulosclerosis 10%, and mesangial proliferation 5%).[28] Transient hematuria or hypertension may occur. Nephrotic syndrome may develop during the course of several different renal or systemic diseases. (The pathophysiology and common clinical manifestations of nephrotic syndrome in adults are described in Chapter 36, and are similar in children.) The most common causes of idiopathic nephrotic syndrome in children are minimal change nephropathy and focal segmental glomerulosclerosis.

Minimal change nephropathy (MCN), also known as *lipoid nephrosis*, is characterized by fusion of the glomerular podocyte foot processes. There are few other renal structural abnormalities. A systemic immune mechanism is a likely cause of the disease, but the true etiology is unknown. MCN is found in 85% of children with idiopathic nephrosis. The mechanism of increased glomerular permeability is unknown but is related, in part, to release of permeability factors from abnormal circulating T cells and loss of negative charge within the glomerular capillary wall.[38,39] The glomeruli appear normal, and immunoglobulin deposition is usually absent. The only change is fusion of epithelial cell podocytes.[28] The increased permeability permits protein to leak from the blood into the urine. The hyperlipidemia results from increased hepatic synthesis, decreased plasma catabolism, treatment with corticosteroids, diet, or obesity.[40] In nephrotic syndrome not due to minimal change disease, the distal tubules are unable to excrete salt. This may be related to vascular hyperpermeability in primary nephrotic syndrome. The severe edema may lead to hypovolemia.[41,42]

Focal segmental glomerulosclerosis (FSGS) is present in approximately 15% of children with nephrotic syndrome and is more common in blacks. There is segmental loss of glomerular capillaries with proliferation of the mesangial matrix and adhesion of the capillaries to the Bowman capsule. In both MCN and FSGS there is loss of the glomerular basement membrane negative charge and an increase in glomerular capillary permeability, which leads to proteinuria and the symptoms of nephrotic syndrome. Sodium retention also contributes to the edema.[43] The more severe the proteinuria, the more likely that end stage renal disease will occur.[44] There is an increase in mesangial cells and mesangial matrix, and effacement of epithelial cell foot processes in **mesangial proliferation.**

CLINICAL MANIFESTATIONS   Onset of nephrotic syndrome is insidious, with periorbital edema as the first sign. The edema is most noticeable in the morning but subsides

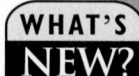

WHAT'S NEW?   **Allergy and Minimal Change Nephropathy**

Minimal change nephropathy (MCN) in children has been associated with allergy to cow's milk, eggs, pork, inhaled pollen, and house dust. Children with MCN have increased type Th-2 lymphocytes and increased type II immunoglobulin E (IgE) receptors on B cells. The Th-2 subset of lymphocytes produces interleukins (IL-4, IL-5, and IL-6) with long-lasting production of IgE and immunoglobulin G (IgG). Children with MCN who go into remission in response to steroid therapy have decreased IL-4-induced type II IgE receptors. Although the cause of this disease remains unknown, alterations in the IL-4 and STAT 6 genes and changes in mRNA transcription levels may be implicated.

Data from Ashizawa M et al: *Am J Kidney Dis* 42(1):76-86, 2003; Cho BS et al: *Pediatr Nephrol* 13(3):199, 1999; Waga I et al: *Kidney Int* 64(4):1253-1264, 2003.

during the day as fluid shifts to the abdomen and lower extremities (Figure 37-5). Because toddlers have picky eating habits, parents are often pleased with the weight gain associated with edema. Parents become alerted to an abnormality when they notice diminished, "frothy," or "foamy" urine and when edema becomes pronounced with ascites, respiratory difficulty from pleural effusion, and labial or scrotal swelling.

Edema of the intestinal mucosa may cause diarrhea, anorexia, and poor absorption. Edema often masks the malnutrition caused by malabsorption and protein loss. Because of protein deficiency, changes in the quality of hair indicate a malnourished state. Pallor, with shiny skin and prominent veins, is also common. Blood pressure is usually normal or slightly decreased. The child has an increased susceptibility to infection, especially pneumonia, peritonitis, cellulitis, and septicemia. Irritability, fatigue, and lethargy are common. Infants born with congenital nephrotic syndrome have large fontanelles, have separated cranial sutures, and may show gingival hyperplasia[45] (see Box 37-1).

EVALUATION AND TREATMENT   The diagnosis of nephrotic syndrome is evident from the finding of proteinuria, hyperlipidemia, and lipiduria. Several diagnostic tests,

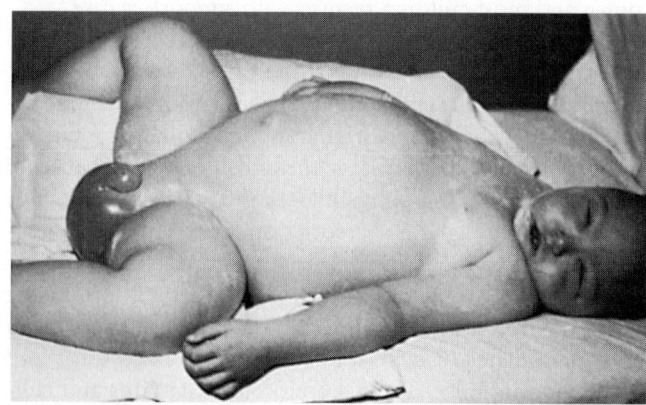

Figure 37-5 Child with nephrotic syndrome. (From Shirkey HC, editor: *Pediatric therapy,* ed 6, St Louis, 1980, Mosby.)

including kidney biopsy, may be required to determine whether the cause is an intrinsic renal disease or a consequence of systemic disease.

The goals of treatment are to reduce the excretion of protein and to maintain a protein-free urine. Prevention or treatment of infection, control of edema, establishment of a balanced nutritional state, and restoration of normal metabolic processes are also important in managing the disorder. Corticosteroids are the primary therapeutic agents,[46] and outcomes in children are often described according to their response to steroid therapy (Table 37-3). Basic management of nephrotic syndrome includes activity as tolerated; a low-sodium, well-balanced diet; glucocorticosteroids (prednisone), diuretics (furosemide [Lasix]), ACE-inhibitors, and immunosuppressive agents (cyclophosphamide [Cytoxan], azathioprine [Imuran]); paracentesis (for ascites); and skin care. Children who fail to respond to prednisone within 8 weeks are termed *steroid resistant.*[47]

Adults and children respond differently to management. Most children have complete remission; few adults do. Most children have minimal or no pathologic renal changes. The prognosis for ultimate recovery is quite good. Although relapses are common, usually after respiratory infections or live-virus immunizations, most children can look forward to a healthy future. Even those with frequent relapses usually have a spontaneous resolution before 30 years of age.[48] Renal transplant is performed for those children who progress to renal failure.[49]

Box 37-1	Congenital Nephrotic Syndrome

Congenital nephrotic syndrome is the development of nephrotic syndrome sometime during the first 3 months of life. The disease is an autosomal recessive disorder, is most common in individuals of Scandinavian descent, and is known as *Finnish-type nephrotic syndrome.* The most common cause is the mutation of the *NPHSI* gene on chromosome 19, which encodes the protein nephrin. Nephrin is a structural protein of the glomerular podocyte slit diaphragm and is important for normal glomerular filtration. Pathologic characteristics include glomerular sclerosis, mesangial hypercellularity, and proximal tubule dilation. The disease may be detected in utero by increased α fetoprotein and a large placenta. Infants present with severe proteinuria, edema, prematurity, respiratory distress, and separation of cranial sutures. Treatment includes ACE inhibitors, indomethacin, unilateral nephrectomy, bilateral nephrectomy, chronic dialysis, and kidney transplantation.

Data from Gubler MC: *J Am Soc Nephrol* 14(Suppl 1):S22-S26, 2003; Papez KE, Smoyer WE: *Curr Opin Pediatr* 26(2):165-170, 2004; Rivera M et al: *Pediatr Pathol Mol Med* 22(2):105-116, 2003. *ACE,* Angiotensin-converting enzyme.

Renal Failure

Renal failure, either acute or chronic, is rare in children. The pathophysiology and management is similar to renal failure in adults (see Chapter 36). The most common causes of *prerenal acute renal failure* are dehydration, hemorrhage, and sepsis. Glomerulonephritis, hemolytic uremic syndrome, and hypersensitivity reactions to drugs or infectious agents are the most common causes of *intrinsic renal failure.* Obstructive uropathies, such as posterior urethral valves and obstruction of the ureteropelvic junction, are associated with *postrenal failure.*[50] Chronic renal failure in very young children is commonly associated with renal structural abnormalities. In older children the most common cause is glomerulonephropathies.[51,52] Renal transplants are successful in children.[53,54] The use of growth hormone before and after transplant has contributed to normal growth and development.[55]

Obstructive Disorders
Urinary Tract Infections

Urinary tract infection (UTI) is one of the most common bacterial infections in infants. UTIs are most common in 7- to 11-year-old girls as a result of bacteria. Usually, a pathogenic strain of *E. coli* ascends the urethra in cystitis or the ureter to the kidney in pyelonephritis. Individual susceptibility, bacterial virulence, and the host's anatomy (presence of reflux, obstruction, stasis, stones, or structural anomalies of the urinary tract) affect the severity of the disease. The recurrence rate is approximately 30% to 40%[56] and is highest in females. Similar to adult women, susceptibility is increased when genetically controlled blood group antigens (P1 and Lewis blood group nonsecretor) are present on surface uroepithelial cells and act as receptors for bacterial attachment.[57]

Cystitis, or infection of the bladder, results in mucosal inflammation and congestion. This causes detrusor muscle hyperactivity and a resulting decrease in the bladder capacity. It also can lead to reflux of urine up the ureters. Transient reflux caused by the cystitis, or chronic vesicoureteral reflux, can send bacteria all the way to the kidney, causing acute or chronic pyelonephritis. Either of these can cause renal abscesses or scarring.

Differentiating whether an infection is in the bladder or the kidneys is difficult based on symptoms alone. Infants usually develop nausea, vomiting, diarrhea, or jaundice. Young children may present only with fever of undetermined origin and others may present with urinary tract symptoms of frequency; urgency; enuresis or incontinence in a previously dry child; abdominal, flank, or back pain; foul-smelling urine; and sometimes hematuria. *Acute pyelonephritis* usually causes chills, fever, and flank or abdominal pain along with enlarged

---

Table 37-3	Corticosteroid Treatment in Children with Nephrotic Syndrome	
Response to Corticosteroid	**Incidence (%)**	**Outcomes**
Steroid responsive	93	Single course of therapy, low recurrence rate
Steroid dependent (frequently relapsing)	7	Intermittent exacerbations with remissions for several years
Steroid resistant	Rare	Resistance to steroids, eventual development of chronic renal failure

kidney(s) caused by edema. *Chronic pyelonephritis* may be asymptomatic.

Diagnosis of UTIs is by urine culture. An accompanying urinalysis can show pyuria and microscopic hematuria.[58] The presence of casts in the urine can indicate pyelonephritis. Ultrasound, cortical scintigraphy, computed tomography (CT) scan, or voiding cystourethrogram may be necessary to rule out obstructions, abscesses, or reflux. Sexually active female adolescents are more likely to have UTI.[59]

With treatment, UTI symptoms are usually relieved in 1 to 2 days and the urine becomes sterile. A 2- to 4-day course of oral antibiotics is effective for uncomplicated UTI.[60] More potent medications may be required if the child has been previously treated for a UTI or has a complicated UTI including congenital abnormalities of the urinary tract. About 3 to 6 weeks after treatment is completed, all children with a first UTI should have a voiding cystourethrogram done to rule out reflux.[61] It is important not to rush this test because the UTI can cause mild to severe reflux, and there may be concern because the test involves catheterization and gonadal radiation.[62] If reflux is found, an intravenous pyelogram may be done to check for renal damage or scarring. Follow-up urine cultures should be done 2 to 3 weeks after the medication is completed and every 3 months for the next 1 to 2 years to monitor for recurrence and for normal renal development and function, even if the child is asymptomatic.

Surgical correction of reflux or obstruction is necessary before the urinary tract can be sterilized. Children who develop frequent recurrences and who do not have surgically correctable anomalies may need prophylactic antibiotic therapy. These children also require regular cultures to rule out asymptomatic infections with resistant microorganisms.

Vesicoureteral Reflux

Vesicoureteral reflux (VUR) is the retrograde flow of bladder urine into the ureters. Reflux allows infected urine from the bladder to be repeatedly swept up into the kidneys. The reflux perpetuates infection by preventing complete emptying of the bladder, because infected, refluxed urine drains back into the bladder at the end of each voiding. In addition, the reflux allows the maximal intravesical pressure to be transmitted to the renal calyces and pyramids. The combination of reflux and infection is an important cause of pyelonephritis, especially in children younger than 5 years.

Vesicoureteral reflux occurs more often in girls by a ratio of 10:1 and is uncommon in blacks. Its incidence is approximately 1 in 1000 children, and siblings of those affected have up to a 50% chance of developing reflux.[63] Although reflux is considered abnormal at any age, the shortness of the submucosal segment of the ureter during infancy and childhood renders the antireflux mechanism relatively inefficient and delicate. Thus reflux is seen commonly in association with infections during early childhood but rarely in older children and adults. (Among adults with UTIs, the incidence of reflux is approximately 5%.)

Reflux may be unilateral or bilateral, and it can be classified or graded (Figure 37-6) for comparative purposes:

Grade I—Reflux into a nondilated distal ureter

Grade II—Reflux into the upper collecting system without dilation

Grade III—Reflux into dilated ureter or blunting of calyceal fornices

Grade IV—Reflux into a grossly dilated ureter

Grade V—Massive reflux with ureteral dilation and tortuosity and effacement of the calyceal details; occurs almost exclusively in male infants[64]

PATHOPHYSIOLOGY Primary reflux results from a congenitally abnormal or ectopic insertion of the ureter into the bladder. In some infants, VUR may be related to inadequate relaxation of the external urethral sphincter.[65] Occasionally the condition is hereditary. Secondary reflux is more serious and may be transient or persistent. It develops in association with infection, malformations of the ureterovesical (UV) junction, increased intravesical pressures, and surgery on the UV junction (Figure 37-7). Urinary tract infection associated with VUR may lead to renal scarring, particularly when there is pyelonephritis.[66]

CLINICAL MANIFESTATIONS Children with reflux have recurrent UTIs or unexplained fever, poor growth and development, irritability, and feeding problems. Both children and adults may have a family history of reflux or UTI, pain with voiding, and signs of urinary obstruction or nephropathy.

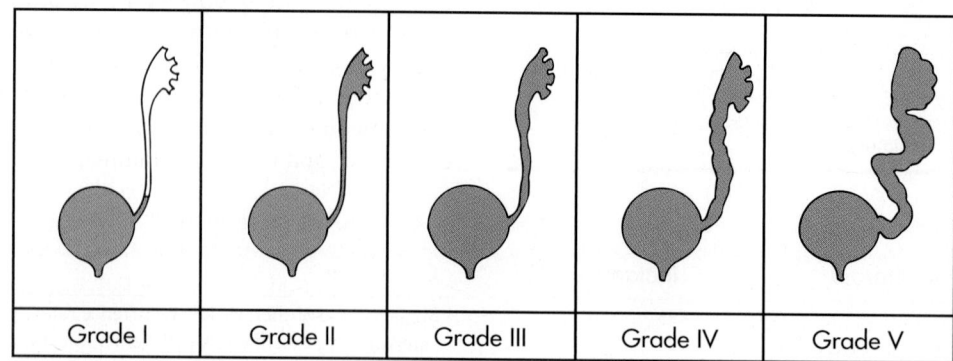

Figure 37-6 Grades of reflux. (From Retik A, Cukier J, editors: *Pediatric urology*, Baltimore, 1987, Williams & Wilkins.)

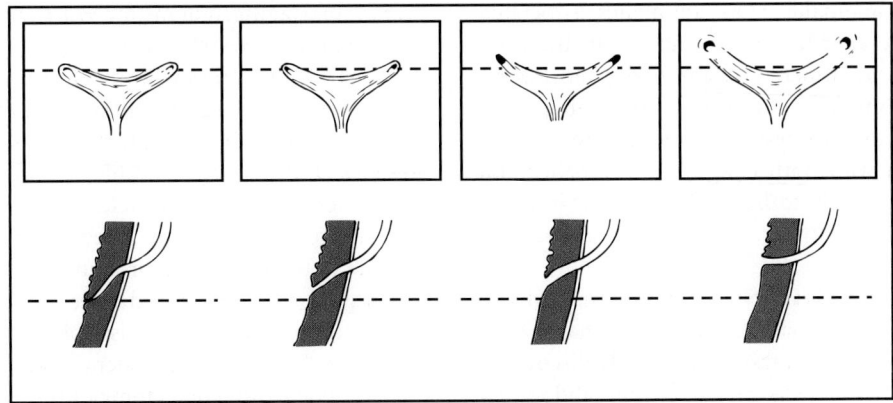

Figure 37-7 Normal and abnormal configuration of the ureteral orifices. *Left to right,* Progressive lateral displacement of the ureteral orifices and shortening of the intramural tunnels. *Top row,* Endoscopic appearance. *Bottom row,* Sagittal view through the intramural ureter. (From Behrman R et al, editors: *Nelson textbook of pediatrics,* ed 16, Philadelphia, 2000, Saunders.)

EVALUATION AND TREATMENT Early diagnosis of VUR in infants is critical to preventing renal scarring. Some infants may have renal scarring at birth from intrauterine damage caused by destruction or reflux.

In addition to the history of recurrent UTIs and other symptoms, a voiding cystourethrogram (VCUG) and an intravenous pyelogram may be required for diagnosis. Radionuclide and sonographic cystography allow assessment of structural change, scarring, and urinary tract function.[67] Most children with vesicoureteral reflux respond to nonoperative management aimed at prevention and treatment of infection. Spontaneous remission of grades I and II reflux may occur in 30% to 60% of children younger than 5 years. Children with grades III and IV reflux need long-term monitoring and prophylactic antibiotics.[68] Recurrent infection may require surgical intervention. In cases of grade V reflux, early surgical intervention is indicated to prevent renal scarring, although spontaneous resolution can occur during the first year.[64] Siblings of children with vesicoureteral reflux should have a screening VCUG performed. Up to 50% have been found to have asymptomatic vesicoureteral reflux.[69,70]

Wilms Tumor

Wilms tumor is an embryonal tumor of the kidney arising from epigenetic and genetic changes that lead to abnormal proliferation of renal stem cells (metanephric blastema). It is also known by the histologic name of **nephroblastoma** and is the most common solid tumor occurring in children.

The incidence of Wilms tumor remains constant in the United States, with approximately 500 children diagnosed each year in the United States. Most children are between 1 and 5 years of age when they are diagnosed. The peak incidence occurs between 2 and 3 years of age. Wilms tumor is the most common childhood cancer of the urinary tract. There are no associations between frequency and gender; however, Wilms tumor is slightly more common in females and in black children than in white children.[71]

Microscopically, Wilms tumor is composed of three cellular components: stromal, epithelial, and blastemic. This occurs because blastemic cells, which are primitive and undifferentiated, may have partially developed into epithelial or stromal tissue. With each of these three cellular components, varying stages of differentiation may be evident.

PATHOGENESIS Wilms tumor has both sporadic and inherited origins. The sporadic form occurs in children with no known genetic predisposition. Inherited cases, which are relatively rare (1% to 2% of cases), are transmitted in an autosomal dominant fashion.

One Wilms tumor suppressor gene *(WT1)* has been located at chromosome 11p13. Other chromosomal regions have been located and include 7p, 11p15, 16q, and 17q.[72,73] The deletion or inactivation of these genes demonstrated that the mechanism for development of Wilms tumor involved tumor-suppressor genes.

The pathogenesis of both the sporadic and inherited forms of Wilms tumor is similar to retinoblastoma. In the inherited form of the disease, the child inherits the loss of one copy of the Wilms tumor-suppressor gene *(WT3)* in all of the primitive metanephric blastemic (fetal renal) cells that normally differentiate into the renal tubules and glomeruli. All that is needed is the loss of the other copy of the gene for a Wilms tumor to develop. Because many cells are vulnerable to the loss of this second copy of the gene, bilateral presentation of Wilms tumor (tumor in both kidneys) occurs occasionally in the inherited form of the disease. In the sporadic form of Wilms tumor, both copies of the gene are lost during fetal development. Because normal renal development occurs during the eighth to the thirty-fourth week of gestation, gene loss likely occurs during this time.[74]

Approximately 10% of children who have Wilms tumor also have a number of congenital anomalies. Children with these abnormalities are usually found to have large deletions of the short arm of chromosome 11. Besides loss of the Wilms tumor–suppressor genes, several other important genes are lost, resulting in the anomalies. The anomalies associated with Wilms tumor are aniridia (lack of an iris in the eye), hemihypertrophy (an asymmetry of the body), and genitourinary malformations (i.e., horseshoe kidneys, hypospadias, ureteral duplication, polycystic kidneys, uterine abnormalities).[75,76] Children with both congenital anomalies and Wilms tumor are more likely to have the inherited bilateral form of the disease.

CLINICAL MANIFESTATIONS Most Wilms tumors (90%) are enlarging asymptomatic upper abdominal masses at the time of diagnosis. Many tumors are actually discovered by the child's parent, who feels or notices an abdominal swelling, usually while dressing or bathing the child. The child appears healthy and thriving. Other presenting complaints include vague abdominal pain (37%), hematuria (21%), and fever (23%).[77] Hypertension also may be present. The reported frequency is quite variable, from 25% to as high as 63% in one report.[78] Hypertension is probably caused by either encroachment by the tumor on the blood supply or secretion of renin by the tumor.

Wilms tumor may occur in any part of the kidney and varies greatly in size at the time of diagnosis. The tumor generally appears as a solitary mass surrounded by a smooth, fibrous external capsule and may contain cystic or hemorrhagic areas. A pseudocapsule generally separates the tumor from the renal parenchyma.

EVALUATION AND TREATMENT On physical examination the tumor feels firm, nontender, and smooth. The mass is generally confined to one side of the abdomen. Should the tumor be palpable past the midline of the abdomen, it may be very large or may be arising from a horseshoe or ectopic kidney. Once an abdominal mass is detected, an abdominal ultrasound may be the initial study and may demonstrate a solid intrarenal mass. Abdominal CT scan or magnetic resonance imaging also may be obtained before biopsy and surgical removal of the tumor.

Diagnosis is based on surgical biopsy. Additional laboratory and radiologic studies are used to evaluate the presence or absence of metastasis. The most common sites of metastasis are regional lymph nodes and the lungs. Metastases also occur in the liver, brain, and bone.

Several staging systems for Wilms tumor have been developed. The most widely accepted system was developed by the National Wilms Tumor Study Group (Table 37-4). The system is based on surgical findings and the extent of disease at diagnosis.[75] Children are further classified as either high or low risk according to favorable or unfavorable histology. Unfavorable histology is characterized by anaplasia and may be resistant to chemotherapy. The staging classifications provide a guide to treatment and prognosis.

Surgical exploration and resection begin the treatment of Wilms tumor. The abdomen is explored to determine the extent of disease. In the case of bilateral disease, surgical intervention may include heminephrectomy of the less involved kidney and nephrectomy of the other. Wilms tumor is considered radiosensitive, and radiation therapy has been found to be most effective if begun 1 to 3 days after surgery. Radiation is not needed for stages I or II disease; it may be used in stages III and IV disease. Radiation therapy also is used for lung, nonresectable liver, brain, bone, and lymph node metastases should they be present. Chemotherapy is recommended for children with favorable histology with different regimens for different stages.[79]

Tremendous advances have been made in the treatment and cure of Wilms tumor. Before the 1930s, 90% of children died of Wilms tumor. Today, with modern treatment, the overall cure rate is as high as 95% for children with stage I through stage III disease. Prognosis is improving for children with metastases, and this is one of the few tumors for which lung metastases have been cured.

Various factors affect the child's prognosis. These include tumor weight at diagnosis, the age of the child, lymph node invasion, and histologic category. The most important prognostic factors, however, appear to be the histologic category and regional lymph node involvement (Table 37-5). Children with a favorable history and no metastatic sites have a 90% survival rate. Even those children with less favorable results do very well, with up to an 80% survival rate.[80]

Recurrent disease is treated aggressively in children with favorable histology. The lung is the most common site of recurrence. Chemotherapy is the usual treatment; degree of success varies.[81]

Enuresis

Enuresis refers to the involuntary passage of urine by a child who is beyond the age when voluntary bladder control should have been acquired. Bladder control is accomplished by most

Table 37-4	Staging of Wilms Tumor
Stage	**Tumor Characteristics**
Stage I	Tumor limited to the kidney, completely resected
Stage II	Tumor ascending beyond the kidney or into vessels of renal sinus, but appearing to be totally resected
Stage III	Residual nonhematogenous tumor confined to the abdomen, positive lymph nodes in renal hilas
Stage IV	Hematogenous metastases, e.g., lung, liver, bone, brain
Stage V	Bilateral disease either at diagnosis or later, but need to stage each kidney

NOTE: Staging system of the Third National Wilms Tumor Study Group (NWTS-3).

Table 37-5	National Wilms Tumor Study-3 Survival Rates	
Stage	**Relapse-Free Survival, 4 Years (%)**	**Four-Year Survival (%)**
Stage I/FH	89	95.6
Stage II/FH	87.4	91.1
Stage III/FH	82.0	90.9
Stage IV/FH	70.0	80.9

From Green DM et al: *CA Cancer J Clin* 46(1):56, 1996.
FH, Favorable histology.

children before the age of 4 years. Five years of age is more accurate and widely accepted, however, and is determined largely by cultural beliefs and practices of parents regarding toilet training. In 80% of children, enuresis occurs at night only and is called **nocturnal enuresis.** Wetting during the day is called **diurnal enuresis.**

Types

Primary enuresis refers to a condition in which the child has never been continent. Secondary enuresis, or acquired enuresis, occurs when a child who has experienced a period of dryness of at least 3 to 6 months after toilet training becomes incontinent again. **Secondary enuresis** may be diurnal, nocturnal, or a combination of both. (Types of incontinence are defined in Table 37-6.)

The incidence of enuresis is difficult to determine because it is not a problem that parents readily share with others and because definitions vary according to cultural norms and family practices. Some families start toilet training before 1 year of age and expect continence by the age of 1 to 1½ years, whereas other families do not expect dryness earlier than 5 years. According to research data, the incidence of enuresis in children older than 5 years ranges from 15% to 20%. Boys are more enuretic than girls by a ratio of 3:2. Teenage enuresis is usually a continuation of childhood bed-wetting and is in the rage of 2%.[82,83]

Theories

Theories about the cause of enuresis abound. A combination of factors is likely to be responsible for enuresis. All or part of each one might be operating in a given child. A reasonable approach is to eliminate organic or physiologic causes for enuresis before exploring the psychologic ones.

Organic causes of enuresis account for 2% to 10% of cases. The causes include urinary tract infections; neurologic disturbances; congenital defects of the meatus, urethra, and bladder neck; allergies; or alteration in renal tubular ion and water transport related to prostaglandin secretion.[84] Disorders that increase the normal output of urine, such as diabetes mellitus and diabetes insipidus, or disorders that impair the concentrating ability of the kidney, such as chronic renal failure or sickle cell disease, must be considered in the evaluation of enuresis.

Enuresis in children is possibly caused by a maturational lag. Studies have demonstrated that the child with enuresis has a smaller functional bladder capacity than a nonenuretic child.[85] A number of children show a general developmental delay along with elevated intravesical pressure and spikelike detrusor contractions during bladder filling. Enuresis may spontaneously disappear in these children as they get older. Other studies have shown that children with enuresis completely fill and empty their bladder several times each night because of a constant urine output and a stable level of antidiuretic hormone (ADH). Children who remain dry usually have elevated levels of ADH and thus a decreased urine output at night.[86] Still other studies indicated loss of diurnal variation in ADH.[87]

Genetic factors as a cause of enuresis are being investigated. Linkages have been proposed between nocturnal enuresis and chromosomes 8, 12, 13, and 22.[88] Bed-wetting does occur with high frequency among parents, siblings, and other near relatives of symptomatic children. These observations are further supported by a high concordance rate in enuretic monozygotic twins.

Recent research studying sleep and nocturnal enuresis indicate that enuresis may be related to non–rapid eye movement (non-REM) sleep, and that those with enuresis may spend more time in stage 3 sleep and have a greater depth of sleep.[89,90] Enuresis may be a symptom of obstructive sleep apnea. Inspiratory effort against a closed airway increases intrathoracic negative pressure causing cardiac distention and release or atrial natriuretic hormone and decreased vasopressin and renin-angiotensin-aldosterone complex. Children with nocturnal polyuria and enuresis should be evaluated for sleep disordered breathing.[91]

A variety of psychosocial theories also have been postulated as explanations of enuresis. Enuresis has been associated with temper tantrums, fear reactions, excitability, low birth weight, and minimal brain dysfunction.[92,93]

Behavioral interventions—such as self-awakening techniques, enuresis alarms, and motivational therapy—have the best results in treating enuresis.[82,83] Treatment with desmopressin and tricyclics have similar beneficial effects, but most children relapse when treatment is stopped.[94] Desmopressin acetate nasal spray, a synthetic ADH, is best used when other treatments have not worked. Psychotherapy and behavior modification are recommended when enuresis is associated with psychologic stress.

Table 37-6	Classification of Incontinence	
Types of Incontinence	**Definition**
Total incontinence	Inability to store any urine; indicates an anatomic or functional absence of urinary sphincters (e.g., epispadias, myelomeningocele) or a bypassing of urinary sphincters (e.g., vesicovaginal fistula)
Overflow incontinence	Frequent dribbling that relieves a constantly full bladder; occurs when urinary outlet is obstructed
Urge incontinence	Sudden and uncontrollable need to void that cannot be suppressed; suggests bladder irritation
Precipitate voiding	Voiding without a preceding urge to void; suggests neurologic origin
Stress incontinence	Uncontrollable voiding that occurs when intravesical pressure momentarily exceeds intravesical resistance, as in "giggle incontinence"
Paradoxic incontinence	Incontinence in spite of normal voiding; suggests an ectopic ureteral orifice outside the urinary sphincter mechanism (e.g., a girl who is constantly wet, yet voids normally)

Structure and Function of the Urinary System in Children

1. The WT1 gene and WNT signaling are important for kidney development, growth, and differentiation.
2. The kidney develops from three sets of structures: the pronephros (nonfunctional by end of embroynic period), mesonephros (nonfunctional), and metanephros (the functional kidney).
3. All nephrons are present at birth, and the number does not increase with maturation but they nephrons do increase in weight and function.
4. Urine formation begins by the third gestational month and contributes to the amniotic fluid.
5. Because of high hydrogen ion concentration, limited ability to regulate the internal environment, and lowered osmotic pressure, infants have a narrow chemical safety margin.
6. Any disturbance, such as diarrhea, infection, fasting, or feeding alterations, can lead rapidly to severe acidosis and fluid imbalance in infants.
7. The composition of body fluids differs with age, thus making children more vulnerable to pathophysiologic changes.
8. Because the kidney develops from the medulla to the cortex, blood flow to the medullary nephrons is limited in infancy and infants thus have limited urine-concentrating capacity.

Alterations in Renal Function in Children

1. Congenital renal disorders affect 10% to 15% of the population. These disorders range in severity from minor, easily correctable anomalies to those incompatible with life.
2. Horseshoe kidney is a U-shaped malformation of the kidney that may be asymptomatic or associated with hydronephrosis, stone formation, or infection.
3. Hypospadias is a congenital condition in which the urethral meatus is located on the undersurface of the penis; epispadias is a congenital condition in which the urethral opening is located on the dorsal surface of the penis.
4. Epispadias is a mild form of exstrophy—a congenital condition that affects the urethra and bladder neck. The urethral opening in boys is on the dorsal surface of the penis.
5. Exstrophy of the bladder is a congenital malformation in which the pubic bones are separated, the lower portion of the abdominal wall and anterior wall of the bladder are missing, and the back wall of the bladder is everted through the opening.
6. Ureteropelvic junction obstruction is blockage where the renal pelvis joins the ureter and is often caused by smooth muscle or urothelial malformation or scarring that leads to hydronephrosis.
7. Bladder outlet obstruction is usually caused by urethral valves or polyps.

8. A dysplastic kidney is the result of abnormal differentiation of renal tissues. The hypoplastic kidney is a very small but otherwise normal kidney.
9. Renal agenesis is the failure of a kidney to grow or develop. The condition may be unilateral or bilateral and may occur as an isolated entity or in association with other disorders.
10. Polycystic kidney disease is an autosomal dominant disorder in which the renal tubule or epithelium proliferates; excessive fluid transport causes cyst formation and obstruction.
11. Glomerulonephritis is an inflammation of the glomeruli characterized by hematuria, edema, and hypertension. The cause is unknown, but poststreptococcal glomerulonephritis may occur after infections, especially those of the upper respiratory tract.
12. Deposition of IgA immunoglobulins in the mesangium of the glomerular capillaries leads to immunoglobulin A nephropathies.
13. Henoch-Schönlein nephritis is an IgA nephropathy that affects glomerular blood vessels.
14. Hemolytic-uremic syndrome is an acute disorder characterized by hemolytic anemia, acute renal failure, and thrombocytopenia and can be associated with *E. coli* verotoxin.
15. Nephrotic syndrome is a term used to describe a symptom complex characterized by proteinuria, hypoproteinemia, hyperlipidemia, and edema. Metabolic, biochemical, or physiochemical disturbance in the glomerular basement membrane leads to increased permeability to protein. The most common form is minimal change nephropathy.
16. Renal failure is rare in children and the most common cause is prerenal acute renal failure related to dehydration, sepsis, or hemorrhage.
17. Urinary tract infections can result from general sepsis in the newborn but are caused by bacteria ascending the urethra in older children. The bladder alone is infected in cystitis. The infection ascends to the kidney or kidneys in pyelonephritis. Urinary tract anomalies must be surgically corrected to prevent frequent recurrent infections.
18. Vesicoureteral reflux, which refers to the retrograde flow of bladder urine into the ureters, provides mechanisms for bladder infection in children, whose ureters are shorter than those of adults.
19. Wilms tumor is an embryonal tumor of the kidney that usually presents between birth and 5 years of age. The tumor can be successfully treated by surgery, with a combination of drugs and, sometimes, radiation therapy.
20. Enuresis refers to the involuntary passage of urine. Enuresis may occur during the day (diurnally) or night (nocturnally). The disorder tends to occur during non–rapid eye movement (non-REM) sleep and can have a variety of organic and psychologic causes.

KEY TERMS

Acute poststreptococcal glomerulonephritis (PSGN), 1342
Chordee, 1339
Congenital nephrotic syndrome, 1345
Cystitis, 1345
Diurnal enuresis, 1349
Enuresis, 1348
Epispadias, 1339
Exstrophy of the bladder, 1340

Focal segmental glomerulosclerosis (FSGS), 1344
Glomerulonephritis, 1342
Hemolytic-uremic syndrome, 1343
Henoch-Schönlein purpura nephritis, 1343
Horseshoe kidney, 1339
Hypoplastic kidney, 1341
Hypospadias, 1339
Infundibular stenosis, 1342

Megacalycosis, 1342
Mesangial proliferation, 1344
Mesonephros, 1337
Metanephros, 1337
Minimal change nephropathy (MCN), 1344
Nephroblastoma, 1347
Nephrotic syndrome, 1344
Nocturnal enuresis, 1349
Polycystic kidney disease (PKD), 1341

KEY TERMS—cont'd

MEDIA RESOURCES *evolve*

Review questions and answers for this chapter are available in the *CD Companion* included with this book.

WebLinks—links to Internet sites pertaining to this chapter—are available on Evolve at http://evolve.elsevier.com/McCance/.

REFERENCES

1. Menke AI, Schedl A: WT1 and glomerular function, *Semin Cell Dev Biol* 14(4):233-240, 2003.
2. Vainio SJ: Nephrogenesis regulated by Wnt signaling, *J Neprhol* 16(2):279-285, 2003.
3. Hartnoll G: Basic principles and practical steps in the management of fluid balance in the newborn, *Semin Neonatol* 8(4):307-313, 2003.
4. Weizer AZ et al: Determining the incidence of horseshoe kidney from radiographic data at a single institution, *J Urol* 170(5):1722-1726, 2003.
5. McAninch JW: Disorders of the kidneys. In Taragho EA, McAninch JW, editors: *Smith's general urology,* Norwalk, Conn, 1995, Appleton & Lange.
6. Kelalis PP, Lowell RK, Bellmam BA: *Clinical pediatric oncology,* ed 3, Philadelphia, 1992, Saunders.
7. Silver RI: Endocrine abnormalities in boys with hypospadias, *Adv Exp Med Biol* 545:45-72, 2004.
8. Mingin G, Baskin LS: Management of chordee in children and young adults, *Urol Clin North Am* 29(2):277-284, 2002.
9. Morrocco G et al: Hypospadias surgery: a 10-year review, *Pediatr Surg Int* 20(3):200-203, 2004.
10. Grady RW, Mitchell ME: Management of epispadias, *Urol Clin North Am* 29(2):349-360, vi, 2002.
11. Frimberger D, Gearhart JP, Mathews R: Female exstrophy: failure of initial reconstruction and its implications for continence, *J Urol* 170(6 PT 1):2428-2431, 2003.
12. Sponseller PD et al: The anatomy of the pelvis in the exstrophy complex, *J Bone Joint Surg Am* 77(2):177, 1995.
13. Zhang PL, Peters CA, Rosen S: Ureteropelvic junction obstruction: morphological and clinical studies, *Pediatr Nephrol* 14(8-9):820-826, 2000.
14. Rooks VJ, Lebowitz RL: Extrinsic ureteropelvic obstruction from a crossing renal vessel: demography and imaging, *Pediatr Radiol* 31(2):120-124, 2001.
15. Tan BJ, Smith AD: Ureteropelvic junction obstruction repair: when, how, what? *Curr Opin Urol* 14(2):55-59, 2004.
16. Shokier AA, Nijman RJ: Primary megaureter: current trends in diagnosis and treatment, *BJU Int* 86(7):861-868, 2000.
17. Close CE: The valve bladder. In Gillenwater JY et al, editors: *Adult and pediatric urology,* ed 4, Philadelphia, 2002, Lippincott, Williams, & Wilkins.
18. Lopez Pereira P et al: Posterior urethral valves: prognostic factors, *BJU Int* 91(7):687-690, 2003.
19. Narasimhan KL et al: Does mode of treatment affect the outcome of neonatal posterior urethral valves? *J Urol* 171(6 Pt 1):2423-2426, 2004.
20. Holliday MA, Barratt TM, Avner ED: *Pediatric nephrology,* ed 2, Baltimore, 1994, Williams & Wilkins.
21. Hitchcock T, Burge DM: Renal agenesis: an acquired condition? *J Pediatr Surg* 29(3):454, 1994.
22. Glazebrook KN, McGrath FP, Steele BT: Prenatal compensatory renal growth: documentation with US, *Radiology* 189(3):733, 1993.
23. Cascio S, Paran S, Puri P: Associated urological anomalies in children with unilateral renal agenesis, *J Urol* 162(3 Pt 2):1081, 1999.
24. Parikh CR et al: Congenital renal agenesis: case-control analysis of birth characteristics, *Am J Kidney Dis* 39:689-694, 2002.
25. Pei Y: Molecular genetics of autosomal dominant polycystic kidney disease, *Clin Invest Med* 26(5):252-258, 2003.
26. Sutters M, Germino GG: Autosomal dominant polycystic kidney disease: molecular genetics and pathophysiology, *J Lab Clin Med* 141(2):91-101, 2003.
27. Nicolaidou P et al: Endothelin-1 in children with acute poststreptococcal glomerulonephritis and hypertension, *Pediatr Int* 45(1):35-38, 2003.
28. Behrman RE, Kliegman RM, Jenson HB, editors: *Nelson textbook of pediatrics,* ed 17, Philadelphia, 2004, Saunders.
29. Wada J, Sugiyama H, Makino H: Pathogenesis of IgA nephropathy, *Semin Nephrol* 23(6):5560-5563, 2003.
30. Julian BA, Novak J: IgA nephropathy: an update, *Curr Opin Nephrol Hypertens* 13(2):171-179, 2004.
31. Andreoli SP: Chronic glomerulonephritis in childhood, *Pediatr Clin North Am* 42(6):1487, 1995.
32. Syrhanen J, Mustonen J, Pasternack A: Hypertriglyceridaemia and hyperuricaemia are risk factors for progression of IgA nephropathy, *Nephrol Dial Transplant* 15(1):34, 2000.
33. Delos Santos NM, Wyatt RS: Pediatric IgA nephropathies: clinical aspects and therapeutic approaches, *Semin Nephrol* 24(3):269-286, 2004.
34. Rieu P, Noel LH: Henoch-Schonlein nephritis in children and adults. Morphological features and clinicopathological correlations, *Ann Med Interne (Paris)* 150(2):151, 1999.
35. Miller DP et al: Incidence of thrombotic thrombocytopenic purpura/hemolytic uremic syndrome, *Epidemiology* 15(2):208-215, 2004.
36. Blackall DP, Marques MB: Hemolytic urenic syndrome revisited: shiga toxin, factor H, and fibrin generation, *Am J Clin Pathol* 121(Suppl):S81-S88, 2004.
37. Trachtman H, Christen E: Pathogenesis, treatment, and therapeutic trials in hemolytic uremic syndrome, *Curr Opin Pediatr* 11(2):162, 1999.
38. Salomon R et al: NF-kappa B p65 antagonizes IL-4 induction by c-maf in minimal change nephrotic syndrome, *J Immunol* 172(1):688-698, 2004.
39. Tain YL, Chen TY, Yang KD: Implications of serum TNF-beta and IL-13 in the treatment response of childhood nephrotic syndrome, *Cytokine* 21(3):155-159, 2003.
40. Saland JM, Ginsberg H, Fisher EA: Dyslipidemia in pediatric renal disease: epidemiology, pathophysiology, and management, *Curr Opin Pediatr* 14(2):197-204, 2002.
41. Rostoker G, Behar A, Lagrue G: Vascular permeability in nephrotic edema, *Nephron* 85(3):194, 2000.
42. Vande Walle JG, Donckerwolcke RA, Koomans HA: Pathophysiology of edema formation in children with nephrotic syndrome not due to minimal change disease, *J Am Soc Nephrol* 10(2):323, 1999.
43. Vande Walle JG, Donckerwolcke RA: Pathogenesis of edema formation in the nephrotic syndrome, *Pediatr Nephrol* 16(3):283-293, 2001.
44. Korbet SM: Clinical picture and outcome of primary focal segmental glomerulosclerosis, *Nephrol Dial Transplant* 14(suppl 3):68, 1999.
45. Mattoo TK: Gingival hyperplasia in congenital and infantile nephrotic syndrome, *Pediatr Nephrol* 11(3):388, 1997.
46. Hodson EM et al: Corticosteroid therapy for nephrotic syndrome in children, *Cochrane Database Syst Rev* (2):CD001533, 2004.
47. Habashy D, Hodson E, Craig J: Interventions for idiopathic steroid-resistant nephrotic syndrome in children, *Cochrane Database Syst Rev* (2):CD003594, 2004.
48. Warshaw BL: Nephrotic syndrome in children, *Pediatr Ann* 23(9):495, 1994.
49. Wyhl E et al: Impact of recurrent nephrotic syndrome after renal transplantation in young patients, *Pediatr Nephrol* 12(7):529, 1998.

50. Andreoli SP: Acute renal failure in the newborn, *Semin Perinatol* 28(2):112-123, 2004.

51. Hari P et al: Chronic renal failure in children, *Indian Pediatr* 40(11):1035-1042, 2003.

52. Seikaly MG et al: Acute renal failure in the newborn, *Semin Perinatol* 28(2):112-123, 2004.

53. Adedoyin O et al: Outcome after renal transplantation in children: results of follow-up by nephrologists in a primary referral center, *Pediatr Transplant* 7(6):479-483, 2003.

54. Benfield MR: Current status of kidney transplant: update 2003, *Pediatr Clin North Am* 50(6):1301-1334, 2003.

55. Acott PD, Pernica JM: Growth hormone therapy before and after pediatric renal transplant, *Pediatr Transplant* 7(6):426-440, 2003.

56. Le Saux N, Pham B., Moher D: Evaluating the benefits of antimicrobial prophylaxis to prevent urinary tract infections in children: a systemic review, *CMAJ* 163(5):523, 2000.

57. Schlager TA: Urinary tract infection in infants and children, *Infect Dis Clin North Am* 17(2):353-365, 2003.

58. Doley A, Nelligan M: Is a negative dipstick urinalysis good enough to exclude urinary tract infection in paediatric emergency department patients? *Emerg Med (Fremantle)* 15(1):77-80, 2003.

59. Nguyen H, Weir M: Urinary tract infection as a possible marker for teenage sex, *South Med J* 95(8):867-869, 2002.

60. Michael M et al: Short versus standard duration oral antibiotic therapy for acute urinary tract infection in children, *Cochrane Database Syst Rev* (1):CD003966, 2003.

61. Kass EJ, Kernen KM, Carey JM: Paediatric urinary tract infection and the necessity of complete urological imaging, *BJU Int* 86(1):94, 2000.

62. Ahmed SM, Swelund SK: Evaluation and treatment of urinary tract infections in children, *Am Fam Physician* 57(7):1573-1580, 1998.

63. Mak RH, Kuo HJ: Primary urethral reflux: emerging insights from molecular and genetic studies, *Curr Opin Pediatr* 15(2):181-185, 2003.

64. Sillen U: Viscoureteral reflux in infants, *Pediatr Nephrol* 13(4):355, 1999.

65. Chandra M, Maddix H: Urodynamic dysfunction in infants with viscoureteral reflux, *J Pediatr* 136(6):754, 2000.

66. Jakobsson G, Jacobson SH, Hjalmas K: Vesico-ureteric reflux and other risk factors for renal damage: identification of high- and low-risk children, *Acta Pediatr Suppl* 88(431):31, 1999.

67. Riccabona M: Cystography in infants and children: a critical appraisal of the many forms with special regard to voiding cystourethrography, *Eur Radiol* 12(12):2910-2919, 2002.

68. Wheeler D et al: Antibiotics and surgery for vesicoureteric reflux: a meta-analysis of randomised controlled trials, *Arch Dis Child* 88(8):688-694, 2003.

69. Chertin B, Puri P: Familial vesicoureteral reflux, *J Urol* 269(5):1804-1808, 2003.

70. Peeden JN, Noe HN: Is it practical to screen for familial vesicoureteral reflux within a private pediatric practice? *Pediatrics* 89(4):758, 1992.

71. National Cancer Institute: Wilm's tumor and other childhood kidney tumors (PDQ®): treatment, 2004. Available from http://www.nih.gov/cancertopics/pdq/treatment/wilms/health professional.

72. Brown KW, Malik KTA: The molecular biology of Wilm's tumour, *Exp Rev Mol Med*. Available from http://www.expertreviews.org/010030227h.htm.

73. Peres EM et al: Chromosome analyses of 16 cases of Wilms tumor: different pattern in unfavorable histology, *Cancer Cenet Cytogenet* 148(1):66-70, 2004.

74. Belasco J, Chatten J, D'Angio G: Wilms tumor. In Sutow W, Fernbach D, Vietti T, editors: *Clinical pediatric oncology*, ed 3, St Louis, 1984, Mosby.

75. Neville HL, Ritchey ML: Wilms' tumor: overview of National Wilms' Tumor Study Group results, *Urol Clin North Am* 27(3):435, 2000.

76. Nicholson HS et al: Uterine anomalies in Wilms' tumor survivors, *Cancer* 78(4):887, 1996.

77. Green DM: The diagnosis and management of Wilms' tumor, *Pediatr Clin North Am* 32:735, 1985.

78. Sukarochana K, Tolentino W, Kiesewetter WB: Wilms' tumor and hypertension, *J Pediatr Surg* 7:573, 1972.

79. Neville HL, Richey ML: Wilm's tumor. Overview of National Wilm's Tumor Study group results, *Urol Clin North Am* 27:435-442, 2000.

80. Pritchard-Jones K: Controversies and advances in the management of Wilm's tumor, *Arch Dis Child* 87(3):241-244, 2002.

81. Firoozi F, Kogan BA: Follow-up and management of recurrent Wilm's tumor, *Urol Clin North Am* 30:869-879, 2003.

82. Glazener CM, Evans JH: Simple behavioral and physical interventions for nocturnal enuresis in children, *Cocharane Database Syst Rev* (2):CD003637, 2004.

83. Glazener CM, Evans JH, Peto RE: Alarm interventions for nocturnal enuresis in children, *Cochrane Database Syst Rev* (2):CD002911, 2003.

84. Kuznetsova AA et al: Possible role of prostaglandins in pathogenesis of nocturnal enuresis in children, *Scand J Urol Nephrol* 34(1):27, 2000.

85. Troup CW, Hodgson NB: Nocturnal functional bladder capacity in enuretic children, *J Urol* 105:129, 1971.

86. Stark M: Assessment and management of the care of children with nocturnal enuresis: guidelines for primary care, *Nurs Practit Forum* 5(3):170, 1994.

87. Uygur MC, Ergen A, Remzi D: Enuresis nocturna: new concepts in pathophysiology, *Int Urol Nephrol* 27(4):439, 1995.

88. Gontard A et al: Molecular genetics of nocturnal enuresis: linkage to a locus on chromosome 22, *Scand J Urol Nephrol Suppl* 202:76, 1999.

89. Neveus T: The role of sleep and arousal in nocturnal enuresis, *Acta Pediatr* 92(10):1118-1123, 2003.

90. Neveus T et al: Sleep of children with enuresis: a polysomnographic study, *Pediatrics* 103(6 part 1):1193, 1999.

91. Umlauf MG, Chasens ER: Sleep disordered breathing and nocturnal polyuria: nocturia and enuresis, *Sleep Med Rev* 7(5):403-411, 2003.

92. Backes M et al: Cognitive and behavioral profile of fragile X boys: correlations to molecular data, *Am J Med Genet* 95(2):150-156, 2000.

93. Von Gontard A, Hollmann E: Comorbidity of functional urinary incontinence and meet: somatic and behavioral associations, *J Urol* 171(6 Pt 2):2644-2647, 2004.

94. Glazener CM, Evans JH, Peto RE: Trycyclic and related drugs for nocturnal enuresis in children, *Cochrane Database Syst Rev* (3):CD002117, 2003.

STRUCTURE AND FUNCTION OF THE DIGESTIVE SYSTEM

SUE E. HUETHER

CHAPTER OUTLINE

The digestive system breaks down ingested food, prepares it for uptake by the body's cells, provides body water, and eliminates wastes. This system consists of the gastrointestinal tract and accessory organs of digestion: the liver, gallbladder, and exocrine pancreas.

Food breakdown begins in the mouth with chewing and continues in the stomach, where food is churned and mixed with acid, mucus, enzymes, and other secretions. From the stomach, the fluid and partially digested food pass into the small intestine, where biochemicals and enzymes secreted by the liver and exocrine pancreas break the food down into absorbable components of proteins, carbohydrates, and fats. These nutrients pass through the walls of the small intestine into blood vessels and lymphatics that carry them to the liver for storage or further processing.

Ingested substances and secretions that are not absorbed in the small intestine pass into the large intestine, where fluid continues to be absorbed. Fluid wastes travel to the kidneys and are eliminated in the urine. Solid wastes pass into the rectum and are eliminated from the body through the anus.

Except for chewing, swallowing, and defecation of solid wastes, the movements of the digestive system (gastrointestinal motility) are all controlled by hormones and the autonomic nervous system. As ingested substances move through the gastrointestinal tract, they trigger the release of hormones that stimulate or inhibit (1) the muscular contractions that mix and propel food from the esophagus to the anus and (2) the timely secretion of substances that aid in digestion. The autonomic innervation, both sympathetic and parasympathetic, is controlled by centers in the brain and by local stimuli that are mediated at plexuses (networks of nerve fibers) within the gastrointestinal walls.

THE GASTROINTESTINAL TRACT

The **gastrointestinal tract (alimentary canal)** consists of the mouth, esophagus, stomach, small intestine, large intestine, rectum, and anus (Figure 38-1). It carries out the following digestive processes:

1. Ingestion of food
2. Propulsion of food and wastes from the mouth to the anus
3. Secretion of mucus, water, and enzymes
4. Mechanical digestion of food particles
5. Chemical digestion of food particles
6. Absorption of digested food
7. Elimination of waste products by defecation

Histologically, the gastrointestinal tract consists of four layers. From the inside out they are the mucosa, submucosa, muscularis, and serosa or adventitia. These concentric layers vary in thickness, and each layer has sublayers (Figure 38-2). Intrinsic nerves are located solely within the gastrointestinal tract and are controlled by local and autonomic nervous system stimuli through the **enteric plexus,** which comprises three nerve plexuses located in different layers of the gastrointestinal walls. The **submucosal plexus (Meissner plexus)** is located in the muscularis mucosae, the **myenteric plexus (Auerbach plexus)** in the muscle layers (tunica muscularis), and the **subserosal plexus** just beneath the serosa. These enteric nerve circuits regulate motility, blood flow, and secretions.[1]

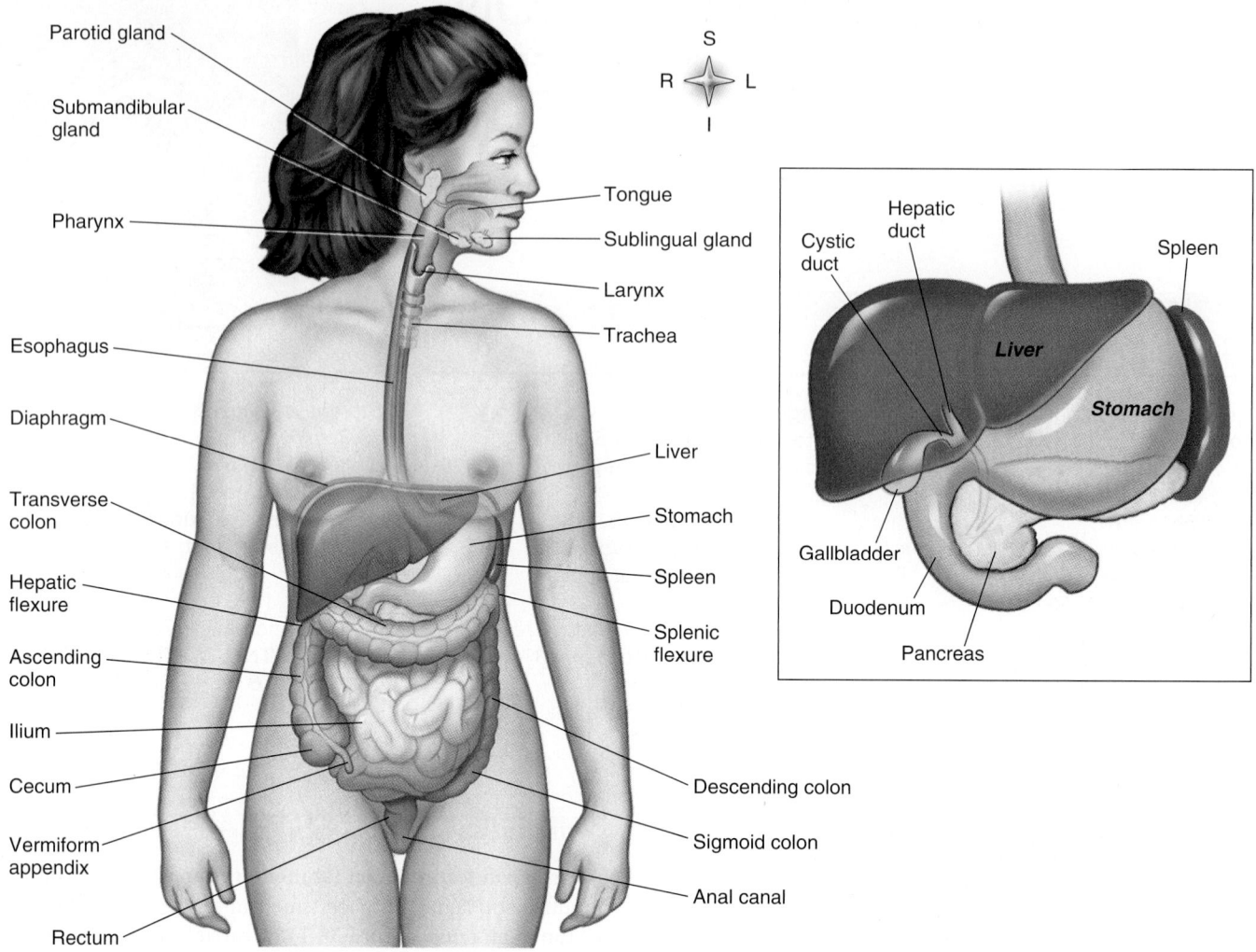

Figure 38-1 **Structure and function of the digestive system.** Digestion begins in the mouth with chewing, which breaks down food mechanically and mixes it with saliva. Swallowing propels chewed food through the esophagus to the stomach, where acids and stomach motility liquefy it further. Next the liquefied food enters the small intestine, where secretions of the intestinal walls, liver, gallbladder, and pancreas digest it into absorbable nutrients. Nutrients are absorbed through intestinal walls, and unabsorbed wastes enter the large intestine (colon), where fluids are removed. Solid wastes then enter the rectum and leave the body through the anus. (From Thibodeau GA, Patton KT: *Anatomy & physiology,* ed 5, St Louis, 2003, Mosby.)

Mouth and Esophagus

The **mouth** is a reservoir for the chewing and mixing of food with saliva. As food particles become smaller and move around in the mouth, the taste buds and olfactory nerves are continuously stimulated, adding to the satisfaction of eating. The tongue's surface contains thousands of chemoreceptors, or taste buds, that can distinguish salty, sour, bitter, and sweet tastes. Tastes and food odors help to initiate salivation and the secretion of gastric juice in the stomach. There are 32 permanent teeth in the adult mouth, and they are important for speech and mastication.

Salivation

The three pairs of **salivary glands** (the submandibular, sublingual, and parotid glands) (Figure 38-3) secrete about 1 L of saliva per day. **Saliva** consists mostly of water that contains varying amounts of mucus; sodium; bicarbonate; chloride; potassium; and **salivary α-amylase (ptyalin),** an en-

zyme that initiates carbohydrate digestion in the mouth and stomach.

Both sympathetic and parasympathetic divisions of the autonomic nervous system control salivation. Because cholinergic parasympathetic fibers stimulate the salivary glands, atropine (an anticholinergic agent) inhibits salivation and makes the mouth dry. β-Adrenergic stimulation from sympathetic fibers also increases salivary secretion. The salivary glands are not regulated by hormones.

The composition of saliva depends on the rate of secretion (Figure 38-4). Aldosterone can increase an exchange of sodium for potassium, increasing sodium conservation and potassium excretion. The bicarbonate concentration of saliva sustains a pH of about 7.4, which neutralizes bacterial acids and prevents tooth decay. Saliva also contains immunoglobulin A (IgA), which helps to prevent infection. Exogenous fluoride (e.g., fluoride in drinking water) is absorbed and then secreted in the saliva, providing additional protection against tooth decay.

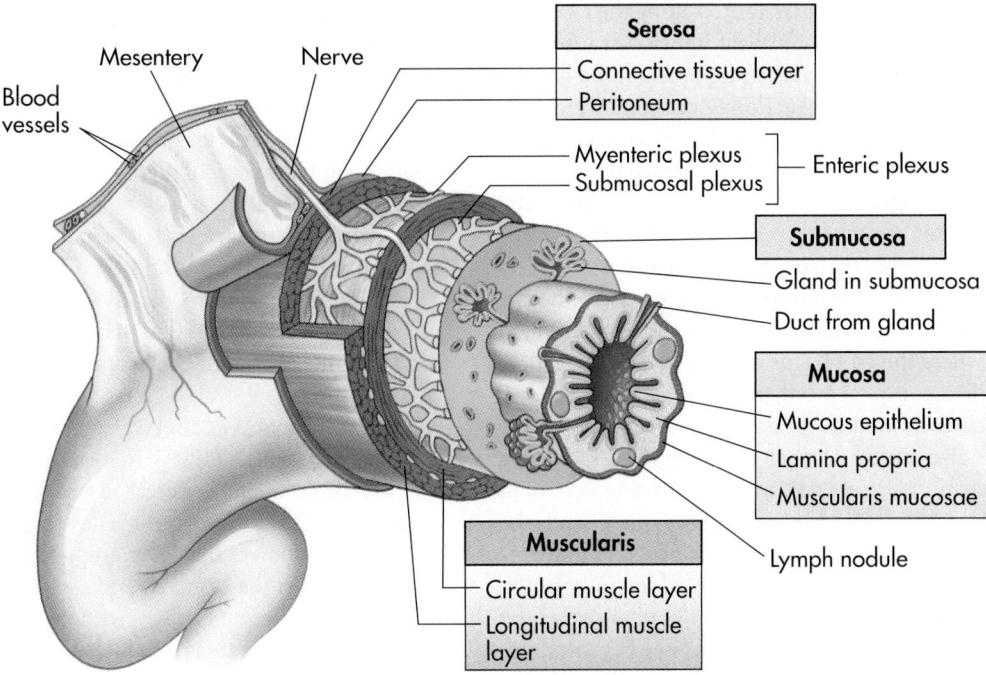

Figure 38-2 **Wall of the gastrointestinal (GI) tract.** The wall of the GI tract is made up of four layers with a network of nerves between the layers. Shown here in a generalized diagram of a segment of the GI tract. Note that the serosa is continuous with a fold of serous membrane called a *mesentery.* Note also that digestive glands may empty their products into the lumen of the GI tract by way of ducts. (From Thibodeau GA, Patton KT: *Anatomy & physiology,* ed 5, St Louis, 2003, Mosby.)

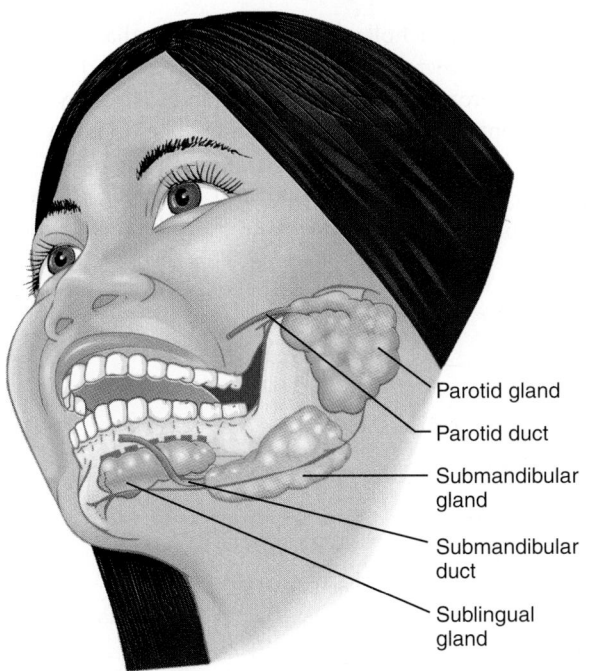

Figure 38-3 **Salivary glands.** (From Thibodeau GA, Patton KT: *Anatomy & physiology,* ed 5, St Louis, 2003, Mosby.)

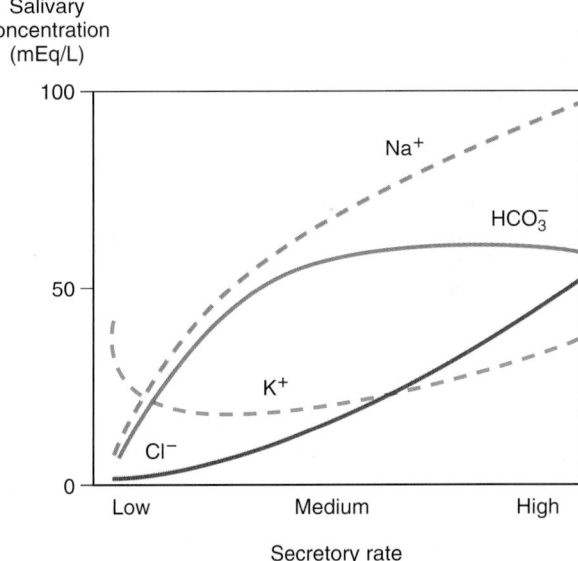

Figure 38-4 **Salivary electrolyte concentrations and flow rate.** Changes in concentration of sodium (Na^+), potassium (K^+), chloride (Cl^{++}), and bicarbonate (HCO_3^-) with increases in flow rate of saliva. *Green line,* Sodium; *orange line,* bicarbonate; *red line,* chloride; *blue line,* potassium.

Swallowing

The **esophagus** is a hollow muscular tube approximately 25 cm long that conducts substances from the oropharynx to the stomach (see Figure 38-1). Swallowed food is moved to the stomach by **peristalsis,** the coordinated sequential contraction and relaxation of outer longitudinal and inner circular layers of muscles. The upper third of the esophagus contains striated muscle that is directly innervated by motor neurons. The middle third contains a mix of striated and smooth muscle, and the lower third is smooth muscle that is innervated by preganglionic cholinergic fibers from the vagus nerve. The muscles are activated in a downward sequence. Peristalsis is stimulated when afferent fibers distributed along the length of the esophagus sense changes in wall tension caused by stretching as food passes. The greater the tension, the greater the intensity of esophageal contraction. Occasionally, intense contractions cause pain similar to "heartburn" or angina.

Each end of the esophagus is opened and closed by a sphincter. The **upper esophageal sphincter (cricopharyngeal muscle)** prevents entry of air into the esophagus during respiration.[2] The **lower esophageal sphincter (cardiac sphincter)** prevents regurgitation from the stomach. The lower esophageal sphincter is located near the esophageal hiatus—the opening in the diaphragm where the esophagus ends at the stomach.

Swallowing is a complex event mediated by the swallowing center, which is located in the reticular formation of the brain stem and also involves other brain regions, including the insula/claustrum and cerebellum.[3,4] Swallowing occurs in two phases: the oropharyngeal (voluntary) phase and the esophageal (involuntary) phase. During the **oral and pharyngeal phases of swallowing,** food is segmented into a bolus by the tongue and forced posteriorly toward the pharynx as the tongue pushes upward against the hard palate. The swallowing center and respiratory center provide the coordinating innervation. The superior constrictor muscle of the pharynx contracts, preventing movement of food into the nasopharynx. At the same time, respiration is inhibited and the epiglottis slides downward to prevent the bolus from entering the larynx and trachea. The movements of the tongue and pharyngeal constrictors propel the food into the esophagus in a series of coordinated events taking less than 1 second.[5]

The **esophageal phase of swallowing** begins as the bolus of food enters the esophagus. The bolus is transported by peristalsis—the sequential waves of muscular contractions that travel down the esophagus and are preceded by receptive waves of relaxations.[6] The wave of relaxation reduces resistance and allows food to pass, after which the wave of contraction pushes food farther along. The lower esophageal sphincter relaxes just before the arrival of a peristaltic wave. The sphincter muscles return to their resting tone after the bolus of food passes into the stomach. The esophageal phase of swallowing takes 5 to 10 seconds, with the bolus moving 2 to 6 cm/sec. Throughout swallowing, the sphincters and esophagus work in concert with the peristaltic wave that moves food from the mouth to the stomach.

Peristalsis that immediately follows the oropharyngeal phase of swallowing is called **primary peristalsis.** If a bolus of food becomes stuck in the esophageal lumen, the distention of the esophageal wall stimulates **secondary peristalsis,** a wave of contraction and relaxation that is independent of voluntary swallowing. This is in response to stretch receptors that are stimulated by increased wall tension, causing an increase in impulses from the swallowing center of the brain.

When it is closed, the lower esophageal sphincter serves as a barrier between the stomach and esophagus. The muscle tone of the lower sphincter changes with neural and hormonal stimulation. Cholinergic vagal input and the digestive hormone gastrin increase sphincter tone. Nonadrenergic, noncholinergic vagal impulses relax the lower esophageal sphincter, as do the hormones progesterone, secretin, and glucagon. Relaxation during swallowing is mediated by the vagus.[7]

Stomach

The **stomach** is a hollow, muscular organ that stores food during eating, secretes digestive juices; mixes food with these juices; and propels partially digested food, called **chyme,** into the duodenum of the small intestine. The anatomy of the stomach is presented in Figure 38-5. Its major anatomic boundaries are the lower esophageal sphincter, where food passes through the **cardiac orifice** (gastroduodenal junction)

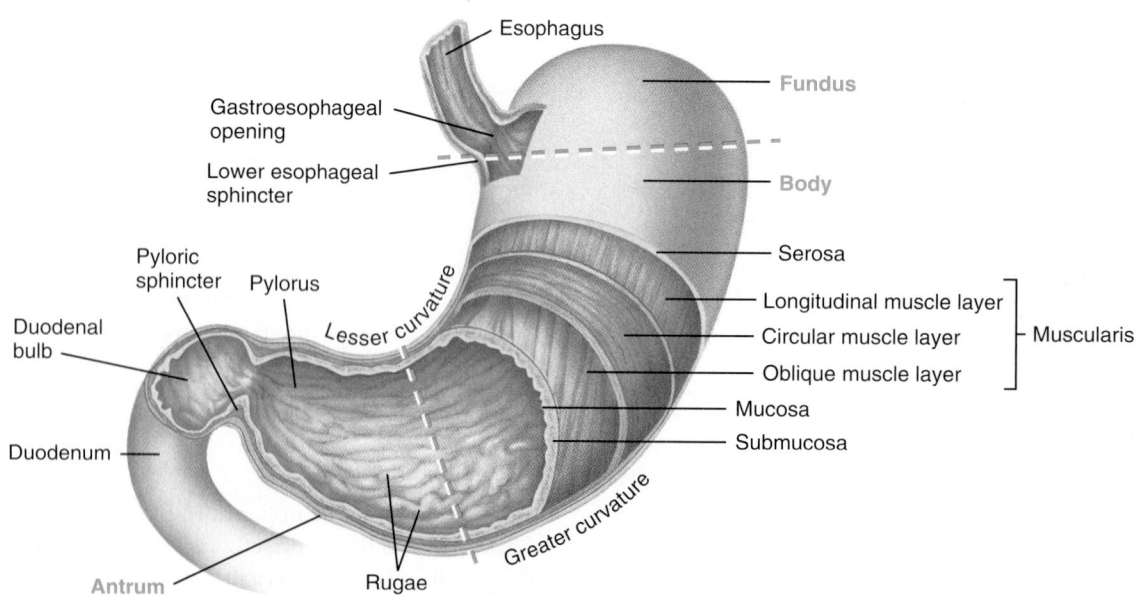

Figure 38-5 Stomach. A portion of the anterior wall has been cut away to reveal the muscle layers of the stomach wall. Note that the mucosa lining the stomach forms folds called *rugae.* The dotted lines distinguish the fundus, body, and antrum of the stomach. (Modified from Thibodeau GA, Patton KT: *Anatomy & physiology,* ed 5, St Louis, 2003, Mosby.)

into the stomach; the greater and lesser curvatures; and the **pyloric sphincter,** which relaxes as food is propelled through the **pylorus** into the duodenum. Functional areas of the stomach are the **fundus** (upper portion), **body** (middle portion), and **antrum** (lower portion).

The stomach has three layers of smooth muscle: an outer, longitudinal layer; a middle, circular layer; and an inner, oblique layer (see Figure 38-5). These layers become progressively thicker in the body and antrum, where food is mixed, churned, and pushed out into the duodenum. The circular layer is most prominent and the oblique layer is the least complete. The glandular epithelium is discussed in the section about secretory functions of the stomach (see p. 1358).

Blood is supplied to the stomach by a branch of the celiac artery. The blood supply is so abundant that nearly all arterial vessels must be occluded before ischemic changes occur in the stomach wall. The splenic vein drains the right side of the stomach, and the gastric vein drains the left side.

The stomach is innervated by sympathetic and parasympathetic divisions of the autonomic nervous system. Some of the autonomic fibers are extrinsic; that is, they originate outside the stomach and are controlled by nerve centers in the brain: the vagus nerve and branches of the celiac plexus. Others are intrinsic; that is, they originate within the stomach and also respond to local stimuli, that is, the myenteric plexus, which lies between the longitudinal and circular muscle layer and within the circular layer. Extrinsic sympathetic fibers reach the stomach through the celiac plexus (solar plexus), whereas extrinsic parasympathetic fibers enter through the gastric branch of the vagus nerve.

Few substances are absorbed in the stomach. The stomach mucosa is impermeable to water, but the stomach can absorb alcohol and aspirin.

Gastric Motility

In its resting state the stomach is small and contains about 50 ml of fluid. There is little wall tension, and the muscle layers in the fundus contract very little. Swallowing causes the fundus to relax (receptive relaxation) to receive a bolus of food from the esophagus. Relaxation is coordinated by efferent, nonadrenergic, noncholinergic vagal fibers and is facilitated by **gastrin** and **cholecystokinin,** two polypeptide hormones secreted by the gastrointestinal mucosa. (The actions of digestive hormones are summarized in Table 38-1.) Food is stored in vertical or oblique layers as it arrives in the fundus, whereas fluids flow relatively quickly down to the antrum.

Table 38-1	Selected Hormones and Neurotransmitters of the Digestive System		
Source	**Hormone**	**Stimulus for Secretion**	**Action**
Mucosa of the stomach	Gastrin	Presence of partially digested proteins in the stomach	Stimulates gastric glands to secrete hydrochloric acid and pepsinogen; growth of gastric mucosa
	Histamine	Gastrin	Stimulates acid secretion
	Somatostatin	Acid in the stomach	Inhibits acid and pepsinogen secretion and release of gastrin
	Acetylcholine	Vagus and local nerves in stomach	Stimulates release of pepsinogen and acid secretion
	Gastrin-releasing peptide (bombesin)	Vagus and local nerves in stomach	Stimulates release of pepsinogen and acid secretion
Mucosa of the small intestine	Motilin	Presence of acid and fat in the duodenum	Increases gastrointestinal motility
	Secretin	Presence of chime (acid, partially digested proteins, fats) in the duodenum	Stimulates pancreas to secrete alkaline pancreatic juice and liver to secrete bile; decreases gastrointestinal motility; inhibits gastrin and gastric acid secretion
	Cholecystokinin	Presence of chime (acid, partially digested proteins, fats) in the duodenum	Stimulates gallbladder to eject bile and pancreas to secrete alkaline fluid; decreases gastric motility; constricts pyloric sphincter; inhibits gastrin
	Enteroglucagon	Intraluminal fats and carbohydrates	Weakly inhibits gastric and pancreatic secretion and enhances insulin release, lipolysis, ketogenesis, and glycogenolysis
	Gastric inhibitory peptide (GIP)	Fat and glucose in small intestine	Inhibits gastric secretion, stimulates insulin release
	Peptide YY	Intraluminal fat and bile acids	Inhibits postprandial gastric acid and pancreatic secretion and delays gastric and small bowel emptying
	Pancreatic polypeptide	Protein, fat and glucose in small intestine	Decreases pancreatic HCO_3^- and enzyme secretion
	Vasoactive intestinal peptide	Intestinal mucosa and muscle	Relaxes intestinal smooth muscle

Modified from Johnson LR: *Gastrointestinal physiology,* ed 6, St. Louis, 2001, Mosby.
Data from Rehfeld JF: *Horm Metab Res* 36(11-12):735-741, 2004; Small CJ, Bloom SR: *Trends Endocrinol Metab* 5(6):259-263, 2004; Druce MR, Bloom SR: *Endocrinology* 145(6):2660-2665, 2004.
NOTE: The digestive hormones are not secreted into the gastrointestinal lumen but rather into the bloodstream, in which they travel to target tissues. There are more than 30 peptide hormone genes expressed in the gastrointestinal tract and more than 100 hormonally active peptides.

Gastric (stomach) motility increases with the initiation of peristaltic waves, which sweep over the body of the stomach toward the antrum. The rate of peristaltic contractions is approximately three per minute and is influenced by neural and hormonal activity. Gastrin, **motilin** (an intestinal hormone), and the vagus nerve increase contraction by lowering the threshold potential of muscle fibers. (The neural and biochemical mechanisms of muscle contraction are described in Chapter 41.) Sympathetic activity and **secretin** (another intestinal hormone) are inhibitory and raise the threshold potential. The rate of peristalsis is mediated by pacemaker cells that initiate a wave of depolarization (basic electrical rhythm), which moves from the upper part of the stomach to the pylorus.

The mixing and emptying of food (chyme) from the stomach take several hours. Mixing occurs as food is propelled toward the antrum. As food approaches the pylorus, the velocity of the peristaltic wave increases, forcing the contents back toward the body of the stomach. This **retropulsion** effectively mixes food with digestive juices, and the oscillating motion breaks down large food particles. With each peristaltic wave a small portion of the gastric contents (chyme) passes through the pylorus and into the duodenum. The pylorus is about 1.5 cm long and is always open about 2.0 mm. It opens wider during antral contraction. Normally there is no regurgitation from the duodenum into the antrum.

The rate of **gastric emptying** (movement of gastric contents into the duodenum) depends on the volume, osmotic pressure, and chemical composition of the gastric contents. Larger volumes of food increase gastric pressure, peristalsis, and rate of emptying. Solids, fats, and nonisotonic solutions delay gastric emptying. (Osmotic pressure and tonicity are described in Chapters 1 and 3.) Products of fat digestion, which are formed in the duodenum by the action of bile from the liver and enzymes from the pancreas, stimulate the secretion of cholecystokinin. This hormone inhibits gastric motility and decreases gastric emptying so that fats are not emptied into the duodenum at a rate that exceeds the rate of bile and enzyme secretion. Osmoreceptors in the wall of the duodenum are sensitive to the osmotic pressure of duodenal contents. The arrival of hypertonic or hypotonic gastric contents activates the osmoreceptors, which delay gastric emptying to facilitate formation of an isoosmotic duodenal environment. The rate at which acid enters the duodenum also influences gastric emptying. Secretions from the pancreas, liver, and duodenal mucosa neutralize gastric acid in the duodenum. The rate of emptying is adjusted to the duodenum's ability to neutralize the incoming acidity.[8] Peristaltic activity in the stomach is also effected by blood glucose levels. Low blood glucose levels stimulate the vagus nerve and gastric smooth muscles. There is an increase in peristalsis but not gastric emptying, stimulating the sensation of "hunger pains."[9]

Gastric Secretion

Stimulated by eating, the stomach secretes large volumes of gastric juices or gastric secretions. Specialized cells located throughout the gastric mucosa produce mucus, acid, en-zymes, hormones, intrinsic factor, and gastroferrin. Intrinsic factor is necessary for the intestinal absorption of vitamin B_{12} and gastroferrin facilitates the absorption of iron in the small intestine. The hormones are secreted into the blood and travel to target tissues in the bloodstream. The other gastric secretions are released directly into the stomach lumen under neural and hormonal regulation.[10] Mucus covers the entire mucosa, forming a protective barrier against acid and proteolytic enzymes, which otherwise would damage the gastric lining.[11]

In the fundus and body of the stomach the **gastric glands** of the mucosa are the primary secretory units (Figure 38-6). Several of these glands (three to seven) empty into a common duct known as the **gastric pit.** The **parietal cells (oxyntic cells)** within the glands secrete hydrochloric acid and intrinsic factor. The **chief cells** within the glands secrete **pepsinogen,** an enzyme precursor that is readily converted to **pepsin** (a proteolytic enzyme) in the gastric juice. The pyloric gland mucosa in the antrum synthesizes and releases the hormone gastrin from **G cells. Enterochromaffin-like cells** secrete **histamine** and **D cells** secrete **somatostatin.**

The composition of gastric juice depends on volume and flow rate (Figure 38-7). Potassium remains relatively constant, but its concentration is greater in gastric juice than in plasma. The rate of secretion varies with the time of day. Generally the rate and volume of secretion are lowest in the morning and highest in the afternoon and evening. Loss of

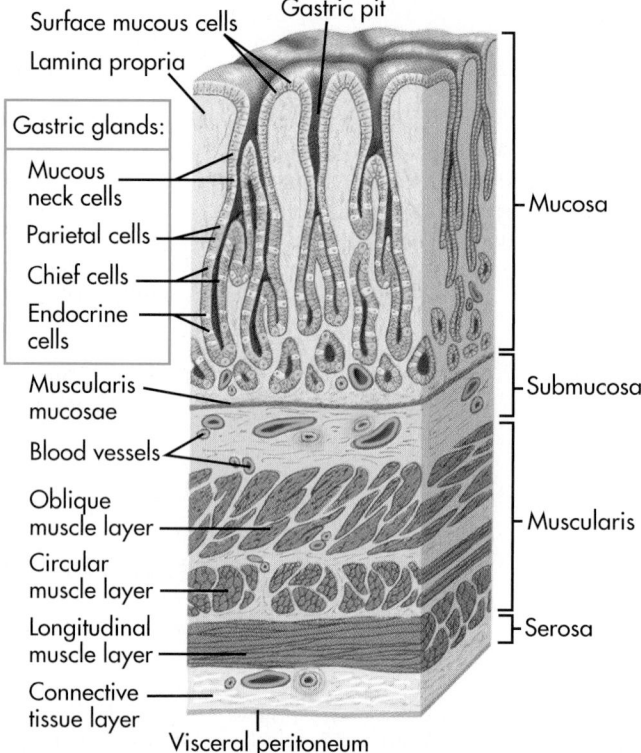

Figure 38-6 Gastric pits and gastric glands. Gastric pits are depressions in the epithelial lining of the stomach. At the bottom of each pit is one or more tubular gastric glands. Chief cells produce the enzymes of gastric juice, and parietal cells produce stomach acid. (From Thibodeau GA, Patton KT: *Anatomy & physiology,* ed 5, St Louis, 2003, Mosby.)

Concentration in
gastric juice
(mEq/L)

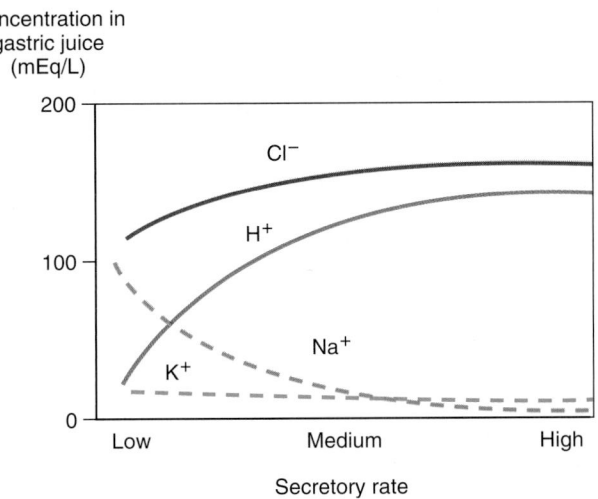

Secretory rate

Figure 38-7 Relationship between secretory rate and electrolyte composition of the gastric juice. Sodium (Na^+) concentration is lower in the gastric juice than in the plasma, whereas hydrogen (H^+), potassium (K^+), and chloride (Cl^{++}) concentrations are higher. *Red line,* Chloride; *orange line,* hydrogen; *green line,* sodium; *blue line,* potassium.

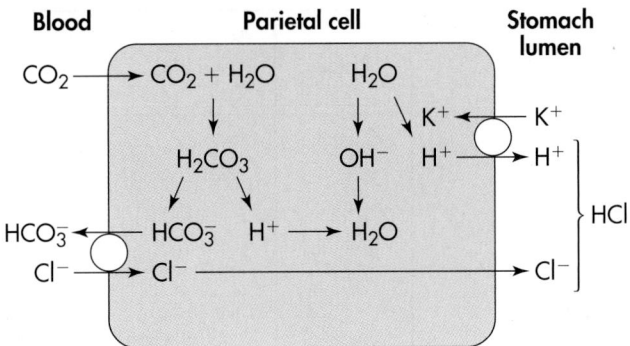

Figure 38-8 Hydrochloric acid secretion by parietal cell.

gastric juices through vomiting, drainage, or suction may decrease body stores of sodium and potassium.

Gastric secretion is inhibited by unpleasant odors and tastes and by rage, fear, or pain. These sensations and emotions cause a discharge of sympathetic impulses and inhibit parasympathetic impulses. Increased secretions may be associated with feelings of aggression or hostility and may contribute to some forms of gastric pathology.

Acid

The major functions of gastric acid are to dissolve food fibers, act as bactericide against swallowed organisms, and convert pepsinogen to pepsin. The production of acid by the parietal cells requires the transport of hydrogen and chloride from the parietal cells to the stomach lumen. Acid is formed in the parietal cells, primarily through the hydrolysis of water (Figure 38-8). At a high rate of gastric secretion, bicarbonate moves into the plasma, producing an "alkaline tide" in the venous blood, which also may result in a more alkaline urine.[12]

Acid secretion by parietal cells is stimulated by acetylcholine (a neurotransmitter), gastrin (a hormone), and histamine (a biochemical mediator) and is inhibited by somatostatin (a hormone). The vagus nerve also releases acetylcholine and stimulates the secretion of histamine.[13] Histamine secretion is also stimulated by gastrin. Histamine is stored in enterochromaffin cells (mast cells; see Chapter 6) in the gastric mucosa. Histamine receptors in the gastric mucosa are H2 receptors (unlike those in the bronchial mucosa, which are H1 receptors). Gastric lipase is produced by glands in the fundus of the stomach and is most effective in an acid environment. Prostaglandins, enterogastrones, such as gastric inhibitory peptide, somatostatin and secretin, inhibit acid secretion.[14]

Pepsin

Acetylcholine, gastrin, and secretin stimulate the chief cells to release pepsinogen during eating. Gastrin indirectly stimulates pepsinogen secretion through a cholinergic reflex that it causes while stimulating acid secretion. Pepsinogen is quickly converted to pepsin at any pH below 5.0, but the optimum pH for pepsin activation is 2.0. Pepsin is a proteolytic enzyme that breaks down protein-forming polypeptides in the stomach. Once chyme has entered the duodenum, the alkaline environment of the duodenum inactivates pepsin.

Mucus

The gastric mucosa is protected from the digestive actions of acid and pepsin by a coating of mucus called the **mucosal barrier.** Gastric mucosal blood flow is important to maintaining mucosal barrier function.[15] The quality and quantity of mucus and the tight junctions between epithelial cells make gastric mucosa relatively impermeable to acid. Prostaglandins and nitric oxide protect the mucosal barrier by stimulating the secretion of mucus and bicarbonate and by inhibiting secretion of acid. A break in the protective barrier may occur because of exposure to aspirin, Helicobacter pylori, ethanol, regurgitated bile, or ischemia. Breaks cause inflammation and ulceration.

Phases

The secretion of gastric juice is influenced by numerous stimuli that together facilitate the process of digestion. The phases of gastric secretion are the cephalic phase, the gastric phase, and the intestinal phase (Figure 38-9).

Cephalic Phase. The anticipatory and sensory experiences of smelling, seeing, tasting, chewing, and swallowing food contribute to the **cephalic phase of secretion.**[16] The cephalic phase of gastric secretion is mediated by the vagus nerve through the myenteric plexus. Acetylcholine (ACh) is liberated and stimulates the parietal and chief cells to secrete acid and pepsinogen, respectively. The G cells in the antrum release gastrin into the bloodstream, through which it travels to the gastric glands and stimulates acid secretion.

Insulin secretion by the endocrine pancreas, which is stimulated by hyperglycemia, is also a strong stimulus for gastric secretion and is mediated by the vagus through sensors located in the hypothalamus. Maintenance of steady serum glucose levels suppresses the gastric response to insulin.

Gastric Phase. The **gastric phase of secretion** begins with the arrival of food in the stomach. Two major stimuli have a secretory effect: (1) distention of the stomach and (2) the

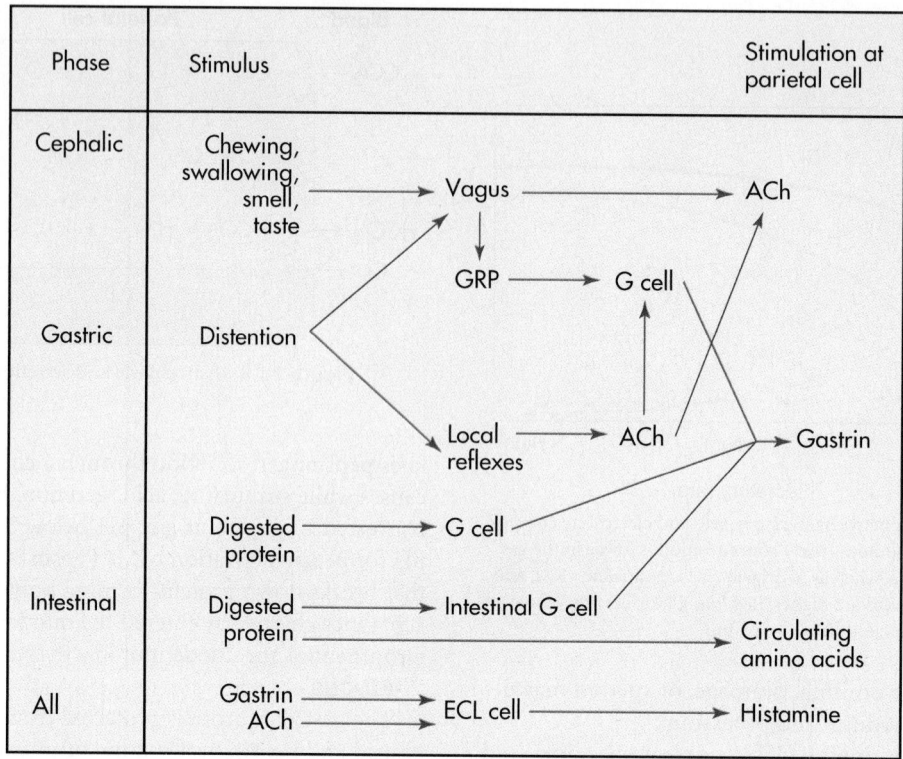

Phase	Stimulus	Stimulation at parietal cell
Cephalic	Chewing, swallowing, smell, taste	
Gastric	Distention	
Intestinal	Digested protein Digested protein	
All	Gastrin ACh	

Figure 38-9 Mechanisms for stimulating acid secretion. *ACh,* Acetylcholine; *GRP,* gastrin-releasing peptide; *ECL,* enterochromaffin-like cell. (From Johnson LR: *Gastrointestinal physiology,* ed 6, St Louis, 2001, Mosby.)

presence of digested protein. The vagus and enteric nerve plexuses are stimulated by distention and contribute to gastric secretion through a local reflex. Both neural reflexes are mediated by acetylcholine and can be blocked by atropine. As digestion proceeds, products of protein break down, stimulating the release of gastrin from G cells in the antrum. Proteins in the stomach buffer the acid gastric juice and increase the gastric pH. Caffeine stimulates acid secretion, as does calcium.

Intestinal Phase. The movement of chyme from the stomach into the duodenum initiates the **intestinal phase of secretion.** This phase represents a slowdown of the gastric secretory response and appears to be hormonally mediated by a hormone called *entero-oxyntin.* Gastric inhibitory peptide decreases gastric motility and the secretion of acid and pepsin when chyme enters the duodenum. The intestinal absorption of some amino acids (products of protein breakdown) also stimulates gastric secretion. The intestinal phase of gastric secretion is limited by the fact that acidic chyme in the duodenum tends to inhibit both gastric acid secretion and gastric motility. Acid in the duodenum stimulates the release of hormones that inhibit acid secretion while stimulating pepsinogen secretion. One of these hormones, cholecystokinin-pancreozymin, inhibits gastrin-stimulated acid production. Other intestinal hormones probably also act synergistically to regulate gastric secretion.

Small Intestine

The **small intestine** is about 5 to 6 meters long and is functionally divided into three segments: the **duodenum, jejunum,** and **ileum** (Figure 38-10). The duodenum begins at the pylorus and ends where it joins the jejunum at a suspensory ligament called the *Treitz ligament.* The end of the jejunum and beginning of the ileum are not distinguished by an anatomic marker. These structures are not grossly different, but the jejunum has a slightly larger lumen. The **ileocecal valve (sphincter)** controls the flow of digested material from the ileum into the large intestine and prevents reflux into the small intestine.[17]

The **peritoneum** is the serous membrane surrounding the organs of the abdomen and pelvic cavity. It is analogous to the pericardium and pleura that surround the heart and lungs, respectively. The visceral peritoneum lies over the organs, and the parietal peritoneum lines the wall of the abdominal cavity. The space between these two layers is called the **peritoneal cavity.** This cavity normally contains just enough fluid to lubricate the two layers and prevent friction during organ movement. Inflammation of the peritoneum, called *peritonitis,* may occur with perforation of the large intestine or after abdominal surgery. As the inflammatory process resolves, adhesions may form and cause colonic obstruction.

The duodenum lies behind the peritoneum, or retroperitoneally, and is attached to the posterior abdominal wall and has an essential role in mixing food with digestive juices from the liver and pancreas. The ileum and jejunum are suspended in loose folds from the posterior abdominal wall by a peritoneal membrane called the **mesentery.** The mesentery facilitates intestinal motility and supports blood vessels, nerves, and lymphatics.

The arterial supply to the duodenum arises primarily from the gastroduodenal artery. The jejunum and ileum are

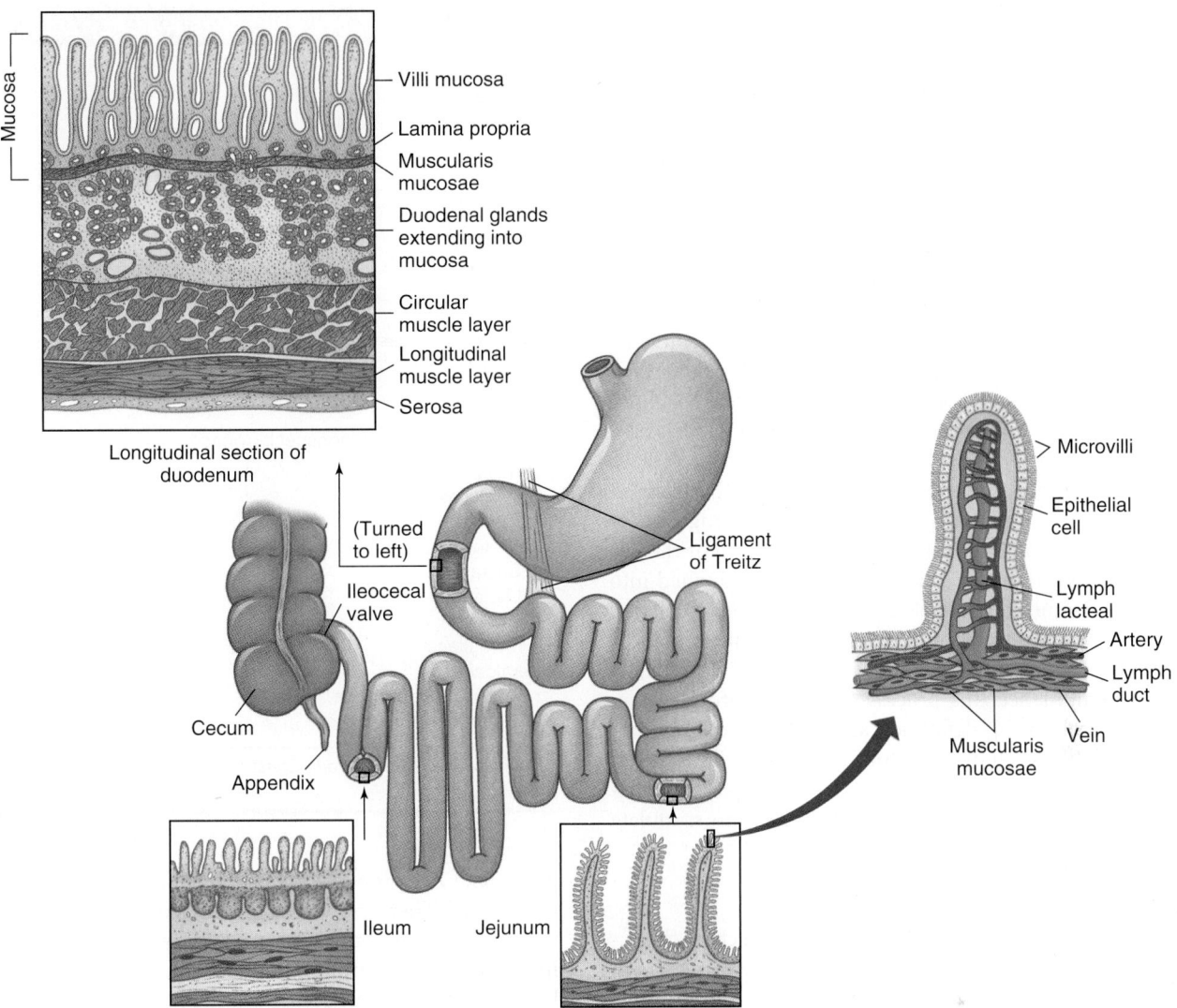

Figure 38-10 Small intestine.

supplied by branches of the superior mesenteric artery. Blood flow increases significantly during digestion. The superior mesenteric vein joins the splenic vein and empties into the portal circulation to the liver. The regional lymph nodes and lymphatics drain into the thoracic duct. Both divisions of the autonomic nervous system innervate the small intestine. Secretion, motility, pain sensation, and intestinal reflexes (e.g., relaxation of the lower esophageal sphincter) are mediated by parasympathetic nerves. Sympathetic activity inhibits motility and produces vasoconstriction. Intrinsic motor innervation is mediated by the myenteric plexus (Auerbach plexus) and the submucosal plexus (Meissner plexus).

The smooth muscles of the small intestine are arranged in two layers: a longitudinal, outer layer; and a thicker, inner circular layer (see Figure 38-10). Mucosal folds (plica) within the small intestine slow the passage of food, thereby providing more time for digestion and absorption. The folds are most numerous and prominent in the jejunum and upper ileum (see Figure 38-10).

Absorption occurs through **villi,** which cover the mucosal folds and are the functional units of the intestine (see Figure 38-10). Each villus secretes some of the enzymes necessary for digestion and absorbs nutrients. A villus is composed of absorptive columnar cells and mucus-secreting goblet cells of the mucosal epithelium. Near the surface, columnar cells closely adhere to each other at sites called *tight junctions.* Water and electrolytes are absorbed through these intercellular spaces. The surface of each columnar epithelial cell contains tiny projections called **microvilli** (see Figure 38-10). Together the microvilli create a mucosal surface known as the **brush border.** The villi and microvilli greatly increase the surface area available for absorption. Coating the brush border is an "unstirred" layer of fluid that is important for the absorption of substances other than water and electrolytes. The **lamina propria** (a connective tissue layer of the mucous membrane) lies beneath the epithelial cells of the villi and contains lymphocytes; plasma cells, which produce immunoglobulins; and macrophages.

Central arterioles ascend within each villus and branch into a capillary array that extends around the base of the columnar cells and cascades down to the venules that lead to the portal circulation. The opposing ascending and descending blood flow provide a countercurrent exchange system for absorbed substances and blood gases. A central **lacteal,** or lymphatic channel, is also contained within each villus and is important for the absorption and transport of fat molecules. Contents of the lacteals flow to regional nodes and channels that eventually drain into the thoracic duct[18] (see Figure 38-10).

Between the bases of the villi are the crypts of Lieberkühn, which extend to the submucosal layer. Undifferentiated and secretory cells and Paneth epithelial cells are located here. The undifferentiated cells are precursors of columnar epithelial cells. These premature cells produce alkaline fluids containing electrolytes, mucus, and water. The Paneth cells produce lysozyme, which is antibacterial, and other secretory cells produce digestive enzymes.[19] These cells arise from the base of the crypt and move toward the tip of the villus, maturing in shape and function as they progress. After becoming columnar cells and completing their migration to the tip of the villus, they function for a few days and then are sloughed into the intestinal lumen and digested. Sloughed epithelial cells are an important source of endogenous protein. The entire epithelial population is replaced about every 4 to 7 days. Many factors can influence this process of cellular proliferation. Starvation, vitamin B_{12} deficiency, and cytotoxic drugs or irradiation suppress cell division and shorten the villi. The decreased absorption that results can cause diarrhea and malnutrition. Nutrient intake and intestinal resection stimulate cell production.

Intestinal Digestion and Absorption

The process of digestion is initiated in the stomach by the actions of hydrochloric acid and pepsin, which break down food fibers and proteins. The chyme that passes into the duodenum is a liquid that contains small particles of undigested food. Digestion is continued in the proximal portion of the small intestine by the action of pancreatic enzymes, intestinal enzymes, and bile salts (Box 38-1). Here carbohydrates are broken down to monosaccharides and disaccharides; proteins are degraded further to amino acids and peptides; and fats are emulsified and reduced to fatty acids and monoglycerides (Figure 38-11). These nutrients, along with water, vitamins, and electrolytes, are absorbed across the intestinal mucosa and into the blood by active transport, diffusion, or facilitated diffusion. Products of carbohydrate and protein breakdown move into villus capillaries and then to the liver through the portal vein. Digested fats move into the lacteals and eventually reach the liver through the systemic circulation. Intestinal motility exposes nutrients to a large mucosal surface area by mixing chyme and moving it through the lumen. Different segments of the gastrointestinal tract absorb different nutrients. Sites of absorption are shown in Figure 38-12.

Water and Electrolytes

The epithelial cell membranes of the small intestine are formed of lipids and therefore are hydrophobic, or tend to re-

Box 38-1	Sources of Digestive Enzymes

Salivary Glands
Amylase
Lingual lipase

Stomach
Pepsin
Gastric lipase

Pancreas
Amylase
Trypsin
Chymotrypsin
Carboxypeptidase
Elastase
Lipase-colipase
Phospholipase A_2
Cholesterol esterase-nonspecific lipase

Small Intestine
Enterokinase
Disaccharidases
  Maltase
  Sucrase
  Lactase
  α, α-Trehalase
  Isomaltase
Peptidases
  Aminooligopeptidase
  Dipeptidase

From Johnson LR: *Gastrointestinal physiology,* ed 6, St Louis, 2001, Mosby.

pel water. (The properties of cell membranes are described in Chapter 1.) Therefore water and electrolytes are transported in both directions (toward the capillary blood or toward the intestinal lumen) through the tight junctions and intercellular spaces rather than across cell membranes. Water diffuses passively according to hydrostatic pressure and in relation to osmotic gradients established by the active transport of sodium and other substances. Approximately 85% to 90% of the water that enters the gastrointestinal tract each day is absorbed in the small intestine. The remaining water and electrolytes are absorbed at a constant rate in the colon.[20] Sodium passes through the tight junctions and is actively transported across cell membranes. The proximal part of the small intestine is more permeable to sodium than the distal part. Sodium is transported into the intestinal cells in exchange for hydrogen at the brush border, and chloride actively enters the cell in exchange for bicarbonate to maintain electroneutrality in the ileum. There is also a sodium pump at the basolateral membrane. Sodium and glucose share a common carrier mechanism, so that sodium absorption is enhanced by glucose transport (Figure 38-13). Potassium moves passively across the tight junctions with changes in the electrochemical gradient. Net potassium secretion occurs in the colon. Because of potassium secretion in the colon and the exchange of chloride for bicarbonate, prolonged diarrhea results in hypokalemic metabolic acidosis.

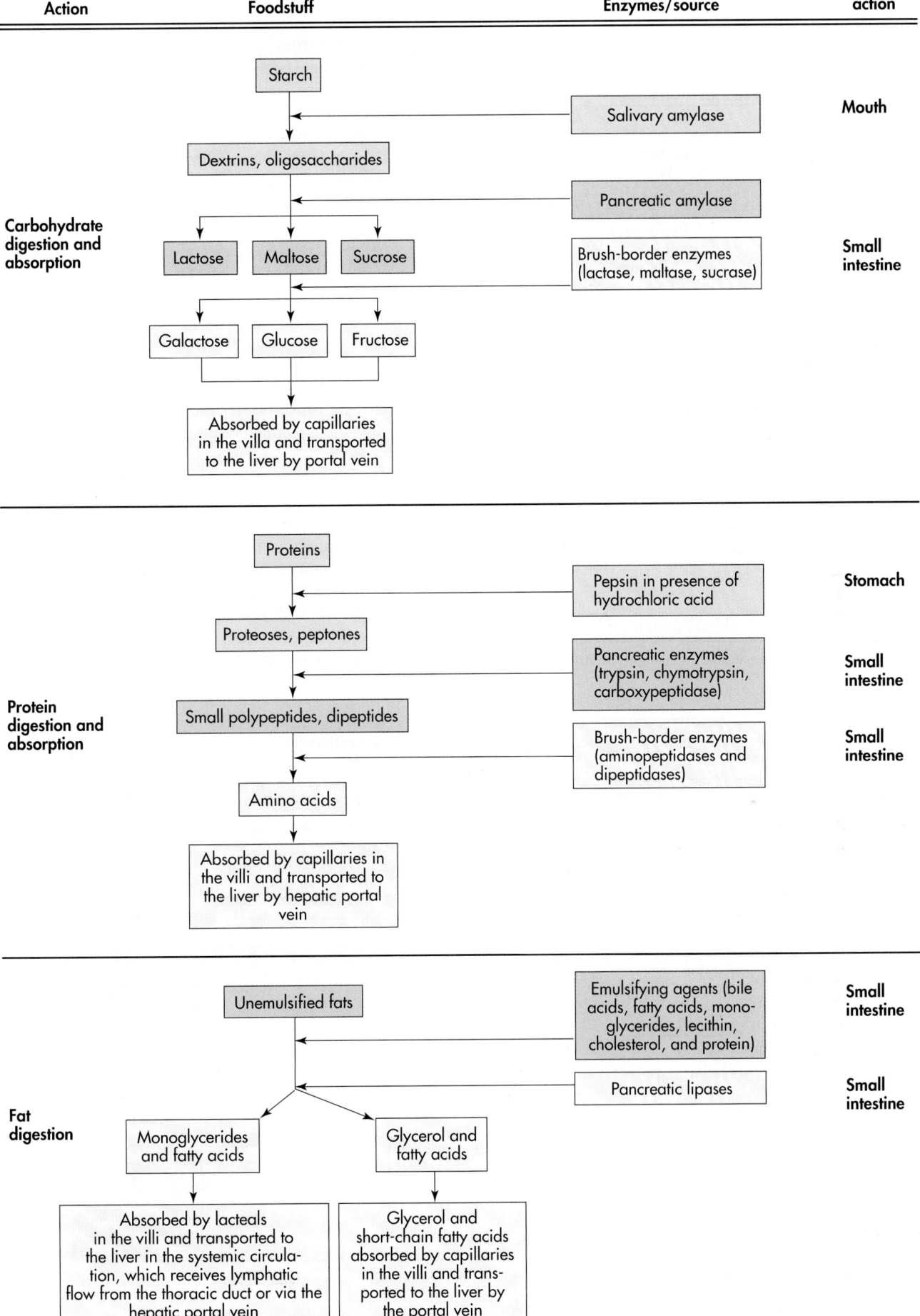

Figure 38-11 Digestion and absorption of foodstuffs.

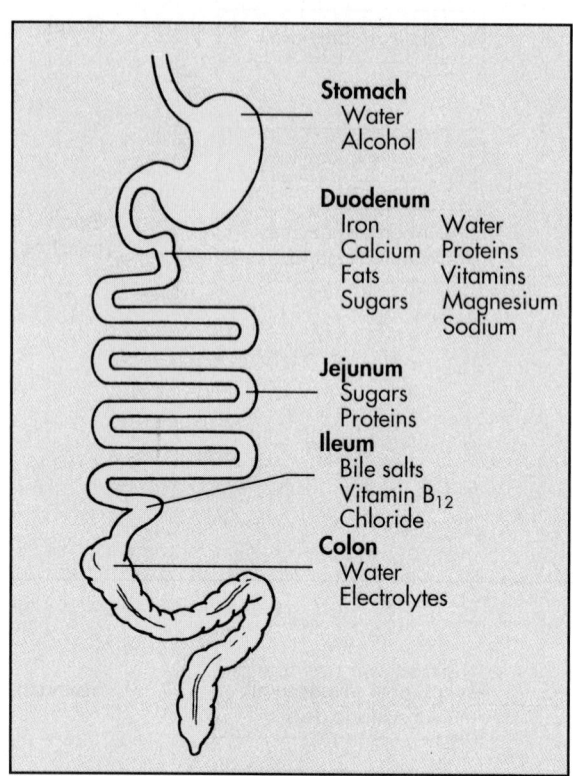

Figure 38-12 Sites of absorption of major nutrients.

Carbohydrates

Carbohydrate (starch, table sugar, milk, sugar, maltose) accounts for at least 50% of the American diet. Because only monosaccharides (galactose, glucose, fructose) are absorbed by the intestinal mucosa, the complex carbohydrates (polysaccharides and oligosaccharides) must be hydrolyzed to their simplest form (see Figure 38-10). Ribose, a 5-carbon sugar that forms part of ribonucleic acid (RNA), adenosine triphosphate (ATP), and deoxyribonucleic acid (DNA), is an important part of the diet. Salivary and pancreatic amylases break down starches to oligosaccharides by splitting α-1,4-glucosidic linkages of long-chain molecules. The major oligosaccharides are sucrose (glucose-fructose), maltose (glucose-glucose), and lactose (glucose-galactose). Approximately half of starch hydrolysis occurs in the stomach and about half in the duodenum. In the small intestine the oligosaccharides are hydrolyzed by brush-border enzymes, mainly sucrase, maltase, and lactase, to their respective monosaccharides (fructose, glucose, galactose). The sugars then pass through the unstirred layer by diffusion. At the cell membrane, glucose and galactose are actively transported with a sodium carrier (sodium-glucose transporter [SGLT]) and fructose is absorbed Absorption is facilitated by a glucose transporter. Consequently, glucose and galactose are absorbed more rapidly than fructose. Insulin is not required for the intestinal absorption of carbohydrates. Fructose passes by facilitated diffusion into the bloodstream, and glucose and galactose enter by diffusion or active transport. The sugars are absorbed pri-

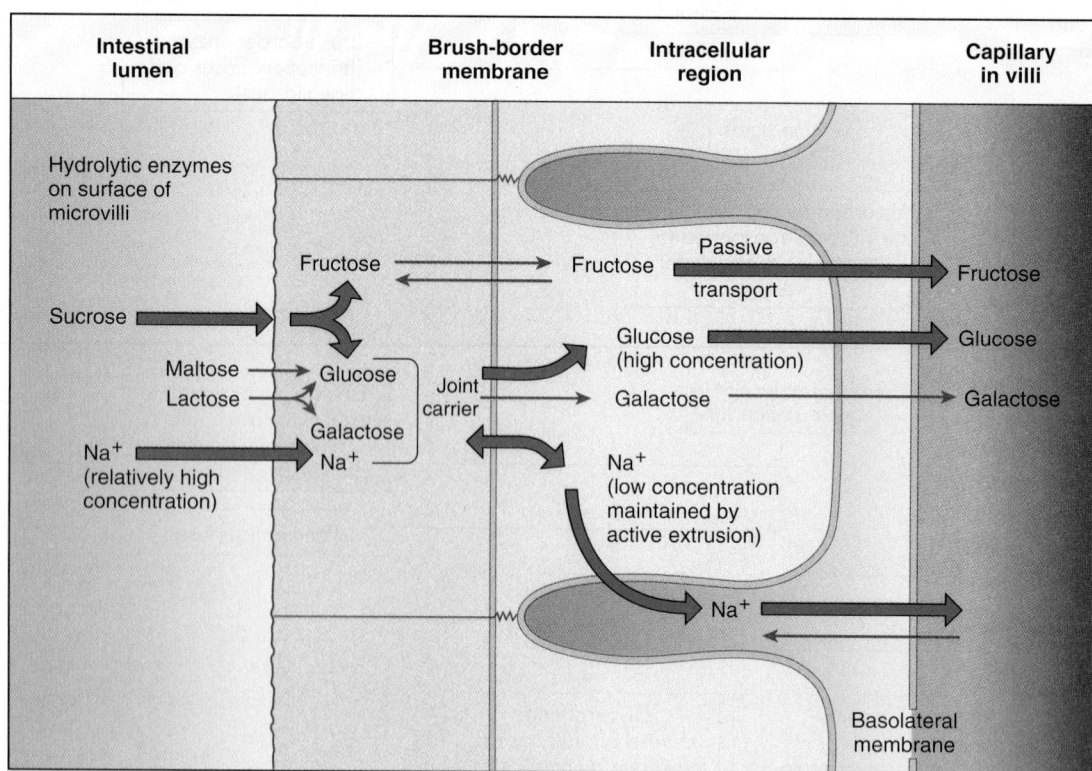

Figure 38-13 Glucose and sodium transport. Schematic showing glucose and sodium (Na^+) transport through the intestinal epithelium. Glucose and sodium are transported into the epithelial cell by a joint carrier.

marily in the duodenum and upper jejunum. Cellulose is a glucose polysaccharide found in plants. Humans do not have enzymes to digest cellulose, but the undigested material contributes to volume and stimulates large intestine motility. In addition to Na^+/glucose transporters, five facilitative glucose transporters (**GLUT**) facilitate hexose transport in mammalian cells: GLUT1, GLUT2, GLUT3, GLUT4, and GLUT5. GLUT1, GLUT2, and GLUT5 are present in enterocytes. GLUT4 is insulin sensitive and present in muscle and adipose tissue.[21]

Proteins

Protein intake varies among different populations. Adults require 44 to 56 g of protein per day. Approximately 20 to 30 g of protein is derived endogenously from shed epithelial cells and small amounts of plasma proteins. Most protein is absorbed; only 5% to 10% is eliminated in the stool.

Gastric digestion of protein by pepsin and acid is not essential. Major protein hydrolysis is accomplished in the small intestine by the pancreatic enzymes: trypsin, chymotrypsin, and carboxypeptidase (see Figure 38-10). **Trypsin** and **chymotrypsin** (endopeptidase) hydrolyze the interior bonds of the large molecules, and **carboxypeptidases** break away the end amino acids (exopeptidase). Hydrolysis of proteins is also carried out by the brush-border enzymes and enzymes in the epithelial cytosol (intracellular fluid). The brush-border enzymes hydrolyze the large oligopeptides (proteins composed of three to six amino acids) into smaller peptides, which can cross cell membranes. The cytosol then breaks them down to amino acids. Amino acids are actively transported by a carrier at the basal membrane. Protein absorption is directly linked to the active transport of sodium. There are three groups of free amino acids:

1. Neutral amino acids (methionine, glycine, phenylalanine, tryptophan)
2. Basic amino acids (arginine, ornithine, lysine, cystine)
3. Proline and hydroxyproline

Each group enters the circulation through a specific mechanism of transport. A small amount of protein may be taken into the cells by pinocytosis (see Chapter 1).

Like the sugars, proteins are absorbed primarily in the proximal area of the small intestine. Protein absorption is impaired if inadequate amounts of proteolytic enzymes are secreted from the pancreas, as occurs with cystic fibrosis.

Fats

Approximately 90 to 100 g of fat is consumed daily by the average American. Fat is an important source of calories and is a primary structural component of cell membranes and organelles. Sources of dietary fat are reviewed in Box 38-2. Although triglycerides are the major dietary lipids, cholesterol, phospholipids, and fat-soluble vitamins also have nutritional importance. The digestion and absorption of fat occur in four phases: (1) emulsification and lipolysis, (2) micelle formation, (3) fat absorption, and (4) resynthesis of triglycerides and phospholipids.

The mechanical action of the stomach and small intestine disperses the triglyceride droplets into small particles. **Emul-**

Box 38-2   Dietary Fat

Saturated Fatty Acid (Palmitic Acid [$C_{16}H_{32}O_2$])
Each carbon atom in the chain is linked by single bonds to adjacent carbon and hydrogen atoms; atoms are solid at room temperature and found in animal fat and tropical oils (coconut and palm oil); they increase low-density lipoprotein (LDL) cholesterol ("bad" cholesterol) blood levels and increase the risk of coronary artery disease

Unsaturated Fatty Acid
Unsaturated fatty acids are soft or liquid at room temperature; omega 6 fatty acids are found in plants and vegetables (olive, canola, and peanut oils), and omega 3 fatty acids are found in fish and shellfish
1. Monounsaturated fatty acids (oleic acid [$C_{18}H_{34}O_2$])
   Contain one double bond in the carbon chain and are found in both plants and animals; may be beneficial in reducing blood cholesterol, glucose levels, and systolic blood pressure; do not lower high-density lipoprotein (HDL) cholesterol ("good" cholesterol) level; low HDL levels have been associated with coronary heart disease
2. Polyunsaturated fatty acids (linoleic acid [$C_{18}H_{32}O_2$])
   Contain two or more double bonds in the carbon chain and are found in plants and fish oils; omega 6 fatty acids lower total and LDL cholesterol blood levels; high levels of polyunsaturated fatty acids may lower LDL; omega 3 fatty acids lower blood triglycerides levels and reduce platelet aggregation and reduce blood clotting tendency; are necessary for growth and development and may prevent coronary artery disease, hypertension, cancer, inflammatory and immune disorders

---

sification is the process by which emulsifying agents (fatty acids, monoglycerides, lecithin, cholesterol, protein, bile salts) in the intestinal lumen cover the small fat particles and prevent them from re-forming into fat droplets (decrease their surface tension). Emulsified fat is then ready for **lipolysis** (lipid hydrolysis) by pancreatic lipase, phospholipase, and hydrolase. **Lipase** breaks down triglycerides to diglycerides, monoglycerides, free fatty acids, and glycerol (see Figure 38-11). The action of lipase requires the presence of colipase, a pancreatic enzyme that allows lipase to penetrate the triglyceride molecule. **Phospholipase** cleaves fatty acids from phospholipids, and **hydrolase** breaks cholesterol esters into fatty acids and cholesterol.

The products of lipid hydrolysis must be made water soluble if they are to be absorbed efficiently from the intestinal lumen. This is accomplished by the formation of water-soluble molecules known as **micelles** (Figure 38-14). Micelles are formed of bile salts, the products of fat hydrolysis, fat-soluble vitamins, and cholesterol. The fats form the core of the micelle, and the polar bile salts form an outer shell, with the hydrophobic ("water-hating") side facing the interior and the hydrophilic ("water-loving") side facing the aqueous (water-like) content of the intestinal lumen. Because the unstirred layer of the brush border is aqueous, the micelles readily diffuse through it. The micelles maintain the fat molecules in the dissolved or solubilized form, which allows them to move more rapidly from the micelle toward the absorbing surface of the intestinal epithelium. The fat products of the micelle then readily diffuse through the epithelial cell membrane, while the bile salts remain in the lumen and proceed to the ileum, where they are absorbed into the circulation and returned to the liver (Figure 38-15). Almost all of the bile salts are recycled in this way.

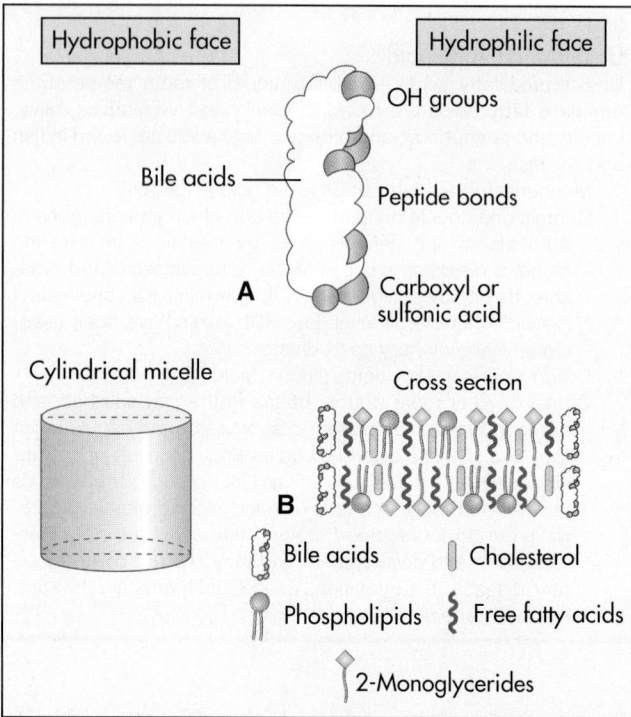

Figure 38-14 Structure of bile acid and micelle. **A,** A bile acid molecule in solution. The molecule is amphipathic in that it has a hydrophilic face and a hydrophobic face. The amphipathic structure is key in the ability of the bile acids to emulsify lipids and form micelles. **B,** A model of the structure of a bile acid–lipid mixed micelle, an emulsified fat. (From Berne RM, Levy MN, editors: *Principles of physiology,* ed 3, St Louis, 2000, Mosby.)

When the fat products reach the inside of the epithelial cell, they are resynthesized into triglycerides and phospholipids. The triglycerides are covered with phospholipids, lipoproteins, and cholesterol to become particles called **chylomicrons.** The chylomicrons travel to the basolateral membrane of the columnar epithelial cells, where they are extruded into the intercellular spaces of the villus. From here they enter the lacteals and lymphatic channels and, eventually, the systemic circulation.

Minerals and Vitamins

The recommended intake of calcium ranges from 1000 to 1500 mg/day. Between 500 and 600 mg is secreted or shed into the lumen with desquamated epithelial cells. Not all of this calcium is absorbed. Daily absorption of **calcium** is approximately 600 mg. This amount increases with increased intake. When its concentration in the lumen is greater than 5 mmol/L, calcium is absorbed by passive diffusion. At concentrations less than 5 mmol/L, calcium is transported actively across cell membranes, bound to a carrier protein. The carrier formation requires the presence of the active form of vitamin D_3 (1,25-dihydroxyvitamin D). The calcium-protein complex moves into the epithelial cell, where the calcium binds to proteins or other substances. Then these complexes move through the basolateral membrane to the interstitial fluid by diffusion or active transport. Calcium is absorbed throughout the small intestine, but primarily in the ileum.

Increased demand for calcium results in increased uptake, as evidenced by the fact that calcium is absorbed more rapidly in children and pregnant or lactating women. Bile salts enhance calcium absorption indirectly by facilitating the absorption of vitamin D. In addition, bile salts promote the absorption of free fatty acids, which, at high concentrations, bind calcium and form soaps in the intestinal lumen. In older individuals, calcium is absorbed less readily because of inadequate amounts of the active form of vitamin D.

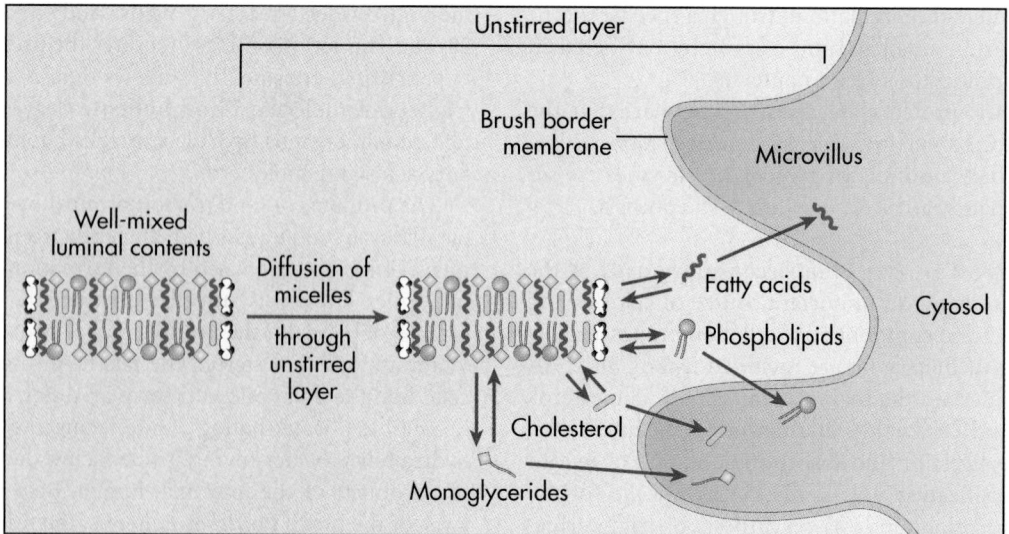

Figure 38-15 Lipid absorption in the small intestine. Micelles of bile salts and products of lipid digestion diffuse through the unstirred layer and among the microvilli. As digestive products are absorbed from free solution by epithelial cells of the villi, more digestive products dissociate from the micelles. (From Berne RM, Levy MN, editors: *Principles of physiology,* ed 3, St Louis, 2000, Mosby.)

The recommended intake of **magnesium** for adults is 300 to 350 mg/day. Approximately 50% of it is absorbed by active transport or passive diffusion in the jejunum and ileum. Phosphate is also absorbed in the small intestine by passive diffusion and active transport.

The levels of **iron** in the body are regulated primarily by intestinal absorption and secretion. The average intake ranges from 15 to 30 mg/day. Of this amount, menstruating women absorb 1.0 to 1.5 mg and men absorb 0.15 to 1.0 mg. Generally the amount of iron absorbed is equal to the amount required. Iron is absorbed more rapidly if a deficiency exists. The primary sources of iron are heme from hemoglobin and myoglobin from animal protein. This iron is rapidly absorbed by the epithelial cells of the duodenum and jejunum. Inorganic iron (e.g., iron in fruits, cereals, eggs, vegetables) is also readily absorbed. The presence of vitamin C reduces ferric iron to ferrous iron, which is the form more easily absorbed. Calcium phosphate and phosphoproteins (milk and antacids) in the intestinal lumen bind iron and reduce absorption. Tea also binds iron by forming iron tannate complexes.

Iron is bound to *intestinal transferrin* in the small bowel and is absorbed and bound to the protein *ferritin* and to amino acid chelates in the cytosol of epithelial cells. Transport of iron across the basolateral membrane is determined by the amount of iron in the circulation. It is transported in the blood by *plasma transferrin* and is carried to body tissues. During hemorrhage, pregnancy, or growth, iron is actively transported from the epithelial cell to the plasma, where it is carried by the globulin protein transferrin (see Chapter 25). When there is less need for iron, it remains in the cell and is carried into the lumen when the cell is sloughed from the end of the villus. The intestinal cells require 3 days to increase their rate of iron absorption after hemorrhage. This is because the need for iron is perceived by the precursor cells in the crypts of Lieberkühn, and they take 3 days to mature and migrate to the tips of the villi, where they absorb more iron.

The absorption of **vitamins** is summarized in Table 38-2. Most of the water-soluble vitamins are absorbed passively or by sodium-dependent active transport. Most vitamin B_{12} (cobalamin) is bound to intrinsic factor (making it resistant to digestion) and absorbed in the terminal ileum, although a small amount of the vitamin is absorbed in its free (unbound) form. Because intrinsic factor is secreted by gastric cells of the stomach, gastric resection and gastric atrophy with achlorhydria diminish the secretion of intrinsic factor and hence the absorption of vitamin B_{12}. Lack of vitamin B_{12} prevents normal erythrocyte maturation and causes pernicious (macrocytic) anemia. (Anemias are discussed in Chapter 26.)

Vitamin B_{12} is present in animal protein and is particularly abundant in liver and kidney. Normally the liver can store vitamin B_{12} for years. Gastric and pancreatic enzymes release vitamin B_{12} from food, after which the vitamin binds to intrinsic factor through an intermediary transport protein. The intrinsic factor–vitamin B_{12} complex then attaches to specific receptor sites on epithelial cells of the terminal ileum, where it is absorbed. After several hours the vitamin enters the plasma, attaches to the carrier protein transcobalamin, and is transported to tissues.

Intestinal Motility

The movements of the small intestine facilitate both digestion and absorption. Chyme coming from the stomach stimulates intestinal movements that mix in secretions from the liver, pancreas, and intestinal glands. A churning motion brings the luminal content into contact with the absorbing cells of the villi. Propulsive movements then advance the chyme toward the large intestine.

Intestinal motility is regulated by the enteric nervous system and is affected by two movements: segmentation and peristalsis.[22] **Segmentation,** which occurs more frequently than peristalsis, consists of localized rhythmic contractions of the circular smooth muscles.[23] The contractions occur at different rates in different parts of the small intestine. Frequency is greatest

Table 38-2	Intestinal Absorption of Vitamins	
Vitamin	**Mechanisms of Absorption**	**State of Absorption**
Fat-Soluble Vitamins		
A (retinal)	Micelle formation with bile salts	Upper small intestine
D (1,25 dihydroxycalciferol)		
E (tocopherol)		
K		
Water-Soluble Vitamins		
B_1 (thiamine)	Active transport (sodium dependent)	Duodenum and jejunum
B_2 (riboflavin)	Unknown	Duodenum and jejunum
Niacin (nicotinic acid)	Passive diffusion	Jejunum
C (ascorbic acid)	Active transport (sodium dependent)	Ileum
Folic acid	Active transport (sodium dependent)	Jejunum
B_{12} (cobalamin)	Active transport (intrinsic factor dependent)	Terminal ileum
B_6 (pyridoxine, pyridoxamine, pyridoxal)	Passive diffusion	Jejunum
Pantothenic acid	Passive diffusion	Duodenum and jejunum
Biotin	Unknown	Unknown

(12 per minute) in the upper small intestine and least (8 per minute) in the distal part of the ileum. Segmentation divides and mixes the chyme, bringing it into contact with the absorbent mucosal surface. It also helps to propel the chyme toward the large intestine. The frequency of the segmentation is regulated intrinsically by the frequency of the basic electrical rhythm (BER), which arises in the myenteric plexus of longitudinal smooth muscle. Although the basic rate of contraction is controlled intrinsically, the force of contraction can be enhanced by vagal stimulation (i.e., extrinsically).

Peristalsis involves short segments (about 10 cm) of longitudinal smooth muscle and propels chime through the intestine. The wave of contraction moves slowly (1 to 2 cm/sec) to allow time for digestion and absorption.

The intestinal villi move with contractions of the muscularis mucosae, a very thin layer of muscle that separates the mucosa and submucosa. Absorption is promoted by the swaying of villi in the luminal contents. Contractile activity also helps to empty the central lacteals, which contain products of fat digestion.

Peptide hormones, including motilin, gastrin, secretin, and cholecystokinin, facilitate intestinal motility. Neural reflexes along the length of the small intestine facilitate motility, digestion, and absorption. Through reflex action, receptors in one part of the intestine transmit signals that influence the function of another part. The **ileogastric reflex** inhibits gastric motility when the ileum becomes distended. This prevents the continued movement of chyme into an already distended intestine. The **intestinointestinal reflex** inhibits intestinal motility when one part of the intestine is overdis-

tended. Both of these reflexes require extrinsic innervation. The **gastroileal reflex,** which is activated by an increase in gastric motility and secretion, stimulates an increase in ileal motility and relaxation of the ileocecal sphincter. This empties the ileum and prepares it to receive more chyme. The gastroileal reflex is probably regulated by the hormone gastrin or through the autonomic nerves.

During prolonged fasting or between meals, particularly overnight, slow waves sweep along the entire length of the intestinal tract from the stomach to the terminal ileum. This is known as the *interdigestive myoelectric complex,* and it appears to propel residual gastric and intestinal contents into the colon.

The ileocecal valve (sphincter) marks the junction between the terminal ileum and the large intestine. This valve is intrinsically regulated and is normally closed. The arrival of peristaltic waves from the last few centimeters of the ileum causes the ileocecal valve to open, allowing a small amount of chyme to pass through. Distention of the upper large intestine causes the sphincter to constrict, preventing further distention or retrograde flow of intestinal contents.

Large Intestine

The **large intestine** is approximately 1.5 m long and consists of the cecum, appendix, colon (ascending, transverse, descending, and sigmoid), rectum, and anal canal (Figure 38-16). The **cecum** is a pouch that receives chyme from the ileum. Attached to the cecum is the **vermiform appendix,** an appendage having little or no physiologic function. From the cecum, chyme enters the **colon,** a four-part length of intestine that loops upward, traverses the abdominal cavity, and de-

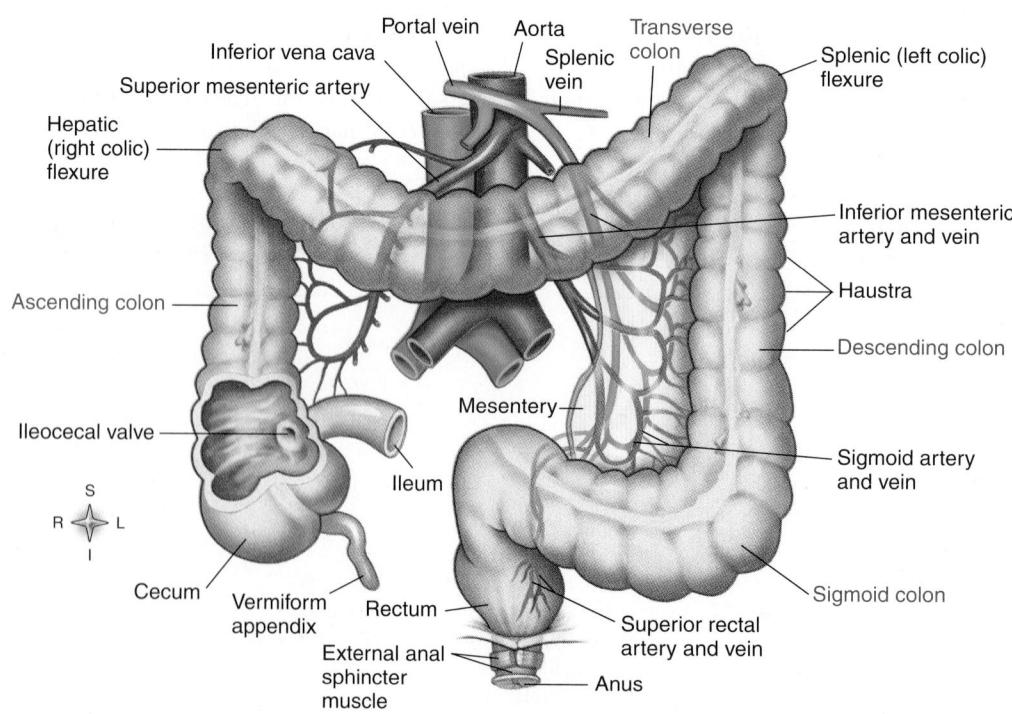

Figure 38-16 Large intestine. (Modified from Thibodeau GA, Patton KT: *Anatomy & physiology,* ed 5, St Louis, 2003, Mosby.)

scends to the anal canal. The four parts of the colon are the **ascending colon, transverse colon, descending colon,** and **sigmoid colon.** Two sphincters control the flow of intestinal contents through the cecum and colon: the ileocecal valve, which admits chyme from the ileum to the cecum, and the **O'Beirne sphincter,** which controls the movement of wastes from the sigmoid colon into the rectum. A thick (2.5 to 3 cm) portion of smooth muscle surrounds the anal canal, forming the **internal anal sphincter.** Overlapping it distally is the striated muscle of the **external anal sphincter.**

In the cecum and colon the longitudinal muscle layer consists of three longitudinal bands called **teniae coli** (see Figure 38-17). The teniae coli are shorter than the colon, giving the colon its "gathered" appearance. The circular muscles of the colon separate the gathers into outpouchings called **haustra.** The haustra become more or less prominent with the contractions and relaxations of the circular muscles. The mucosal surface of the colon has rugae (folds), particularly between the haustra, and **Lieberkühn crypts** but no villi. Columnar epithelial cells and mucus-secreting goblet cells form the mucosa throughout the large intestine. The columnar epithelium absorbs fluid and electrolytes, and the mucus-secreting cells lubricate the mucosa.

The myenteric plexus regulates motor and secretory activity independently of the extrinsic system. Extrinsic parasympathetic innervation occurs through the vagus and extends from the cecum up to the first part of the transverse colon. Vagal stimulation increases rhythmic contraction of the proximal colon. Extrinsic parasympathetic fibers reach the distal colon through the pelvic nerves and can increase motility throughout the colon. The internal anal sphincter is usually in a state of contraction, and its reflex response is to relax when the rectum is distended. The intrinsic nerve plexuses provide the major innervation of the internal anal sphincter, which also receives sympathetic innervation to maintain contraction and parasympathetic innervation that facilitates relaxation when the rectum is full. The external anal sphincter is innervated by branches of the sacral division of the spinal cord. Sympathetic innervation of this sphincter arises from the celiac and superior mesenteric ganglia and the sphincter nerve. The external anal sphincter is paralyzed after destruction of the lower spinal cord, but the internal sphincter is not. Sympathetic activity in the entire large intestine modulates intestinal reflexes, conveys somatic sensations of fullness and pain, participates in the defecation reflex, and constricts blood vessels. The blood supply of the large intestine and rectum is derived primarily from branches of the superior and inferior mesenteric artery.[24]

The primary type of colonic movement is segmental. The circular muscles contract and relax at different sites, shuttling the intestinal contents back and forth between the contracting and relaxing haustra, most commonly during fasting. The movements massage the intestinal contents, then called the **fecal mass,** and facilitate the absorption of water. Propulsive movement occurs with the proximal-to-distal contraction of several haustral units. **Peristaltic movements** also occur and promote the emptying of the colon. The **gastrocolic reflex** initiates propulsion in the entire colon, usually during or immediately after eating, when chyme enters from the ileum. The gastrocolic reflex causes the fecal mass to pass rapidly into the sigmoid colon and rectum, stimulating defecation. Gastrin and cholecystokinin participate in stimulating this reflex. Epinephrine inhibits contractile activity.

Approximately 500 to 700 ml of chyme flows from the ileum to the cecum per day. Most of the water is absorbed in the colon by diffusion and active transport. The electrochemical gradient established by sodium movement enhances the diffusion of serum potassium from the capillaries in the lumen. Aldosterone increases membrane permeability to sodium, thereby increasing both the diffusion of sodium into the cell and its active transport across the basolateral membrane to the interstitial fluid. (See Chapter 20 for a discussion of aldosterone secretion.) This increases the cell-to-lumen diffusion gradient for potassium. Potassium moves outward, and chloride is absorbed with sodium as the complementary anion. Chloride also enters the cell in exchange for bicarbonate.

Absorption and epithelial transport occur in the cecum, ascending colon, transverse colon, and descending colon. By the time the fecal mass enters the sigmoid colon, the mass consists entirely of wastes and is called the feces. **Feces,** or excrement, consists of food residue, unabsorbed gastrointestinal secretions, shed epithelial cells, and bacteria.

The movement of feces into the sigmoid colon and rectum stimulates the **defecation reflex (rectal reflex).** The rectal wall stretches and the tonically constricted internal anal sphincter (smooth muscle with autonomic nervous system control) relaxes, creating the urge to defecate. The defecation reflex can be overridden voluntarily by contraction of the external anal sphincter and muscles of the pelvic floor. The rectal wall gradually relaxes, reducing tension, and the urge to defecate passes. Retrograde contraction of the rectum may displace the feces out of the rectal vault until a more convenient time for evacuation. Pain or fear of pain associated with defecation (e.g., rectal fissures or hemorrhoids) can inhibit the defecation reflex. The defecation reflex is regulated by parasympathetic and cholinergic fibers. Voluntary inhibition or facilitation of defecation is mediated from cortical projections onto the medulla and down to sacral segments of the cord.

Defecation is facilitated by squatting or sitting because these positions straighten the angle between the rectum and anal canal and increase the efficiency of straining (increasing intraabdominal pressure). Intraabdominal pressure is increased by initiating the Valsalva maneuver. This maneuver consists of inhaling and forcing the diaphragm and chest muscles against the closed glottis. This increases both intrathoracic and intraabdominal pressure, which is transmitted to the rectum.

Intestinal Bacteria

The type and number of bacteria vary greatly throughout the normal gastrointestinal tract, with an increasing number of bacteria from the stomach to the distal colon. The stomach is relatively sterile because of the secretion of acid that kills ingested pathogens or inhibits bacterial growth. Bile acid secretion, intestinal motility, and antibody production suppress bacterial growth in the duodenum, and in the duodenum and jejunum there is a low concentration of aerobes (10^{-1} per ml to 10^{-4} per ml), primarily streptococci, lactobacilli, staphylococci, enterobacteria, and *Bacteroides*.[25] There are no anaerobes proximal to the ileum. Anaerobes are found distal to the ileocecal valve. They constitute about 95% of the fecal flora in the colon and contribute one third of the solid bulk of feces. *Bacteroides*, clostridia, anaerobic lactobacilli, and coliforms are the most common microorganisms from the ileum to the cecum.

The intestinal tract is sterile at birth but becomes colonized with *Escherichia coli, Clostridium welchii,* and *Streptococcus* within a few hours. Within 3 to 4 weeks after birth, the normal flora is established. The intestinal bacteria do not have major digestive or absorptive functions. They do play a role in the metabolism of bile salts (contributing to the intestinal reabsorption of bile and the elimination of toxic bile metabolites); the metabolism of estrogens, androgens, and lipids and conversion of unabsorbed carbohydrates to absorbable organic acids; metabolism of various nitrogenous substances and drugs; and protection against exogenous infection.[26]

ACCESSORY ORGANS OF DIGESTION

The liver, gallbladder, and exocrine pancreas all secrete substances necessary for the digestion of chyme. These secretions are delivered to the duodenum through ducts (Figure 38-17). The liver produces bile, which contains salts necessary for fat digestion and absorption. Between meals, bile is stored in the gallbladder. The exocrine pancreas produces enzymes needed for the complete digestion of carbohydrates, proteins, and fats. The exocrine pancreas also produces an alkaline fluid that neutralizes chyme, creating a duodenal pH that supports enzymatic action. The liver receives nutrients absorbed by the small intestine and metabolizes or synthesizes these nutrients into forms that can be absorbed by the body's cells. It then releases the nutrients into the bloodstream or stores them for later use.

Liver

The **liver,** which weighs 1200 to 1600 g, is the largest single organ in the body. It is located under the right diaphragm and is divided into right and left lobes. The larger, right lobe is divided further into the caudate and quadrate lobes (Figure 38-18). The falciform ligament separates the right and left lobes and attaches the liver to the anterior abdominal wall. A fibrous cord called the *round ligament (ligamentum teres)* extends along the free edge of the falciform ligament. The round ligament is the remnant of the umbilical vein and extends from the umbilicus to the inferior surface of the liver. The coronary ligament branches from the falciform ligament and extends over the superior surface of the right and left lobes, adhering the liver to the inferior surface of the diaphragm. The liver is covered by a fibroelastic capsule called the *Glisson capsule.* The **Glisson capsule** contains blood vessels, lymphatics, and nerves. When the liver is diseased or swollen, distention of the capsule causes pain and the lymphatics may ooze fluid into the peritoneal space.

The metabolic functions of the liver require a large amount of blood. The liver receives blood from both arterial and venous sources. The hepatic artery branches from the abdominal aorta and provides oxygenated blood at the rate of 400 to 500 ml/min (about 25% of the cardiac output). The hepatic portal vein, which receives deoxygenated blood from the inferior and superior mesenteric veins and the splenic vein, delivers about 1000 to 1200 ml/min to the liver. Portal venous blood constitutes 70% of the blood supply to the liver. This blood carries some oxygen and is rich in nutrients that have been absorbed from the digestive tract. (Figure 38-19)

Within the liver lobes are multiple, smaller anatomic units called **liver lobules** (Figure 38-20). The lobules are formed of cords or plates of **hepatocytes,** which are the functional cells of the liver. These cells are capable of regeneration; therefore damaged or resected liver tissue can regrow. Hepatocytes secrete electrolytes, lipids, lecithin, bile acids and cholesterol into the canaliculi. Plasma proteins are also synthesized and released into the blood stream. **Lipocytes** are star-shaped cells that store lipids, including vitamin A. Small capillaries, or **sinusoids,** are located between the plates of hepatocytes. The sinusoids receive a mixture of venous and arterial blood from branches of the hepatic artery and portal vein. Blood from the sinusoids drains to a central vein in the middle of each liver lobule. Venous blood from all the lobules then flows into the hepatic vein, which empties into the inferior vena cava. Small channels known as **bile canaliculi** are adjacent to hepatocytes and conduct bile, which is produced by the hepatocytes, outward to bile ducts and eventually drain into the **common bile duct** (see Figure 38-20). The common bile duct empties bile

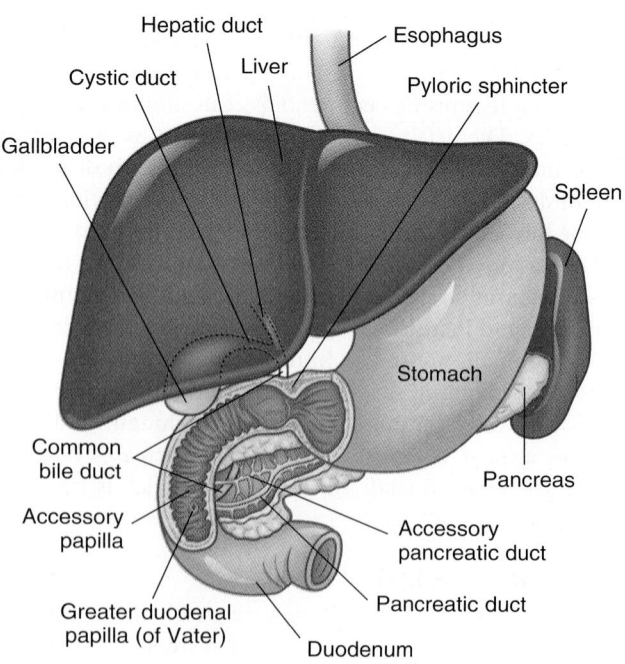

Figure 38-17 Location of the liver, gallbladder, and exocrine pancreas, which are the accessory organs of digestion.

Labels on figure: Hepatic duct; Cystic duct; Liver; Esophagus; Pyloric sphincter; Gallbladder; Spleen; Stomach; Common bile duct; Pancreas; Accessory papilla; Accessory pancreatic duct; Greater duodenal papilla (of Vater); Pancreatic duct; Duodenum

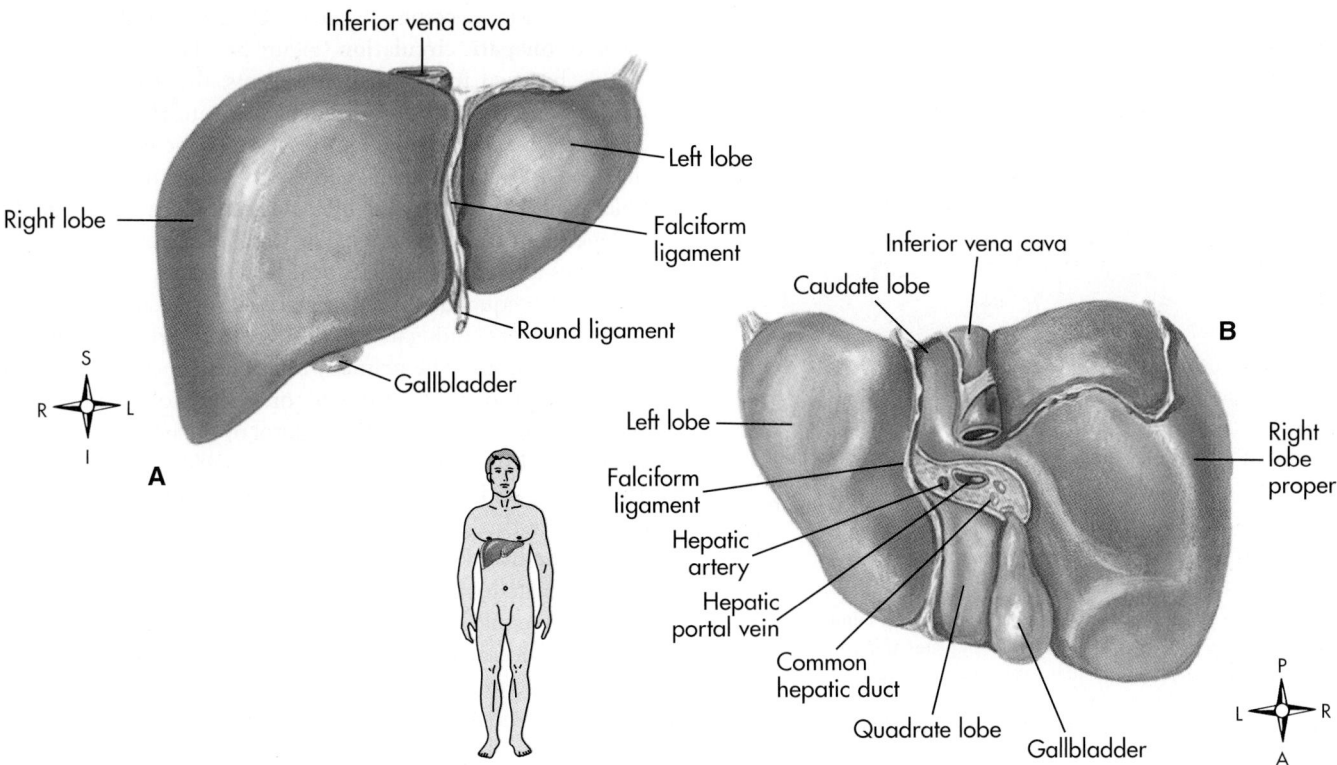

Figure 38-18 Gross structure of the liver. **A,** Anterior view. **B,** Inferior view. (From Thibodeau GA, Patton KT: *Anatomy & physiology,* ed 5, St Louis, 2003, Mosby.)

into the duodenum through an opening called the **major duodenal papilla** (sphincter of Oddi).[27]

The sinusoids of the liver lobules are lined with highly permeable endothelium. This permeability enhances the transport of nutrients from the sinusoids into the hepatocytes, where they are metabolized. The sinusoids are also lined with phagocytic cells known as **Kupffer cells.** Kupffer cells are part of the mononuclear phagocyte system (see Chapter 25) and are the largest population of tissue macrophages. They are bacteriocidal and are important for bilirubin production and lipid metabolism.[28] **Stellate cells** contain retinoids (vitamin A) and are contractile and may regulate sinusoidal blood flow. They remove foreign substances from the blood and trap bacteria. **Pit cells** are natural killer cells found in the sinusoidal lumen; they produce interferon-gamma and are important in tumor defense.[29] Between the endothelial lining of the sinusoid and the hepatocyte is the **Disse space,** which drains interstitial fluid into the hepatic lymph system.

Secretion of Bile

The liver assists intestinal digestion by secreting 700 to 1200 ml of bile per day. **Bile** is an alkaline, bitter-tasting, yellowish green fluid that contains bile salts (conjugated bile acids), cholesterol, bilirubin (a pigment), electrolytes, and water. It is formed by hepatocytes and secreted into the canaliculi. **Bile salts,** which are conjugated bile acids, are required for the intestinal emulsification and absorption of fats. Having facilitated fat emulsification and absorption, most bile salts are actively absorbed in the terminal ileum and returned to the liver through the portal

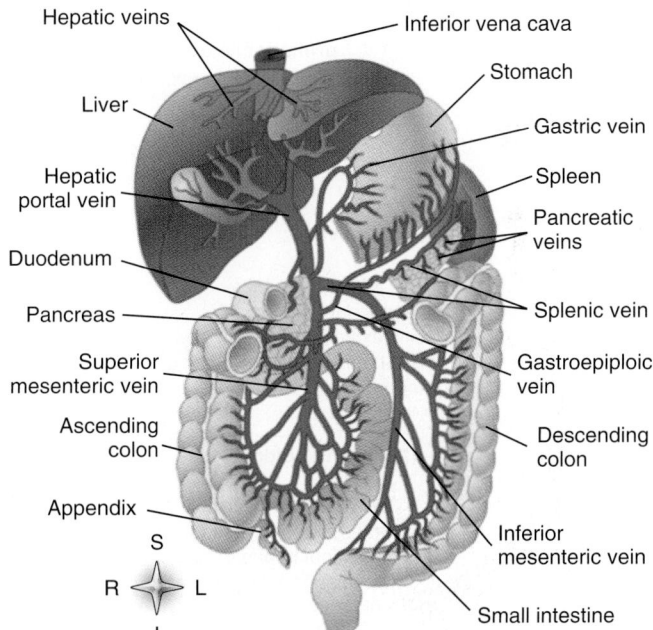

Figure 38-19 Hepatic portal circulation. In this unusual circulatory route, a vein is located between two capillary beds. The hepatic portal vein collects blood from capillaries in visceral structures located in the abdomen and empties into the liver. Hepatic veins return blood to the inferior vena cava. (Organs are not drawn to scale.) (From Thibodeau GA, Patton KT: *Anatomy & physiology,* ed 5, St Louis, 2003, Mosby.)

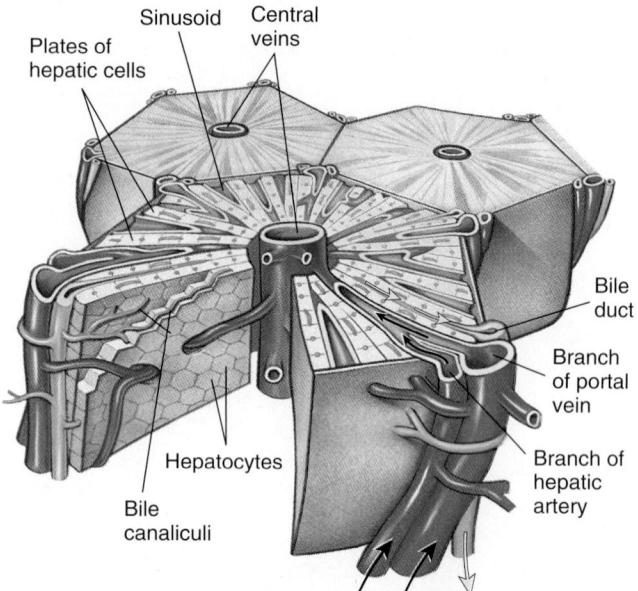

Figure 38-20 Diagrammatic representation of a liver lobule. A central vein is located in the center of the lobule with plates of hepatic cells disposed radially. Branches of the portal vein and hepatic artery are located on the periphery of the lobule, and blood from both perfuse the sinusoids. Peripherally located bile ducts drain the bile canaliculi that run between the hepatocytes. (Modified from Thibodeau GA, Patton KT: *Anatomy & physiology,* ed 5, St Louis, 2003, Mosby.)

circulation for resection.[30] The recycling of bile salts is termed the **enterohepatic circulation** (Figure 38-21).

Bile has two fractional components: the acid-dependent fraction and the acid-independent fraction. Hepatocytes secrete the **bile acid–dependent fraction** of the bile. This fraction consists of bile acids, cholesterol, lecithin (a phospholipid), and bilirubin (a bile pigment). The **bile acid–independent fraction** of the bile, which is secreted by the hepatocytes and epithelial cells of the bile canaliculi, is a bicarbonate-rich aqueous fluid that gives bile its alkaline pH.

Bile salts are conjugated in the liver from primary and secondary bile acids. The **primary bile acids** are cholic acid and chenodeoxycholic (chenic acid or chenodiol) acid. These acids are synthesized from cholesterol by the hepatocytes. The **secondary bile acids** are deoxycholic acid and lithocholic acid. These acids are formed in the small intestine by the action of intestinal bacteria, after which they are absorbed and flow to the liver (see Figure 38-21). Both forms of bile acids are conjugated with amino acids (glycine or taurine) in the liver to form bile salts. Conjugation makes the bile acids more water soluble, thus restricting their diffusion from the duodenum and ileum. The primary and secondary bile acids together form the **bile acid pool.** Other components of bile include phospholipids and cholesterol.

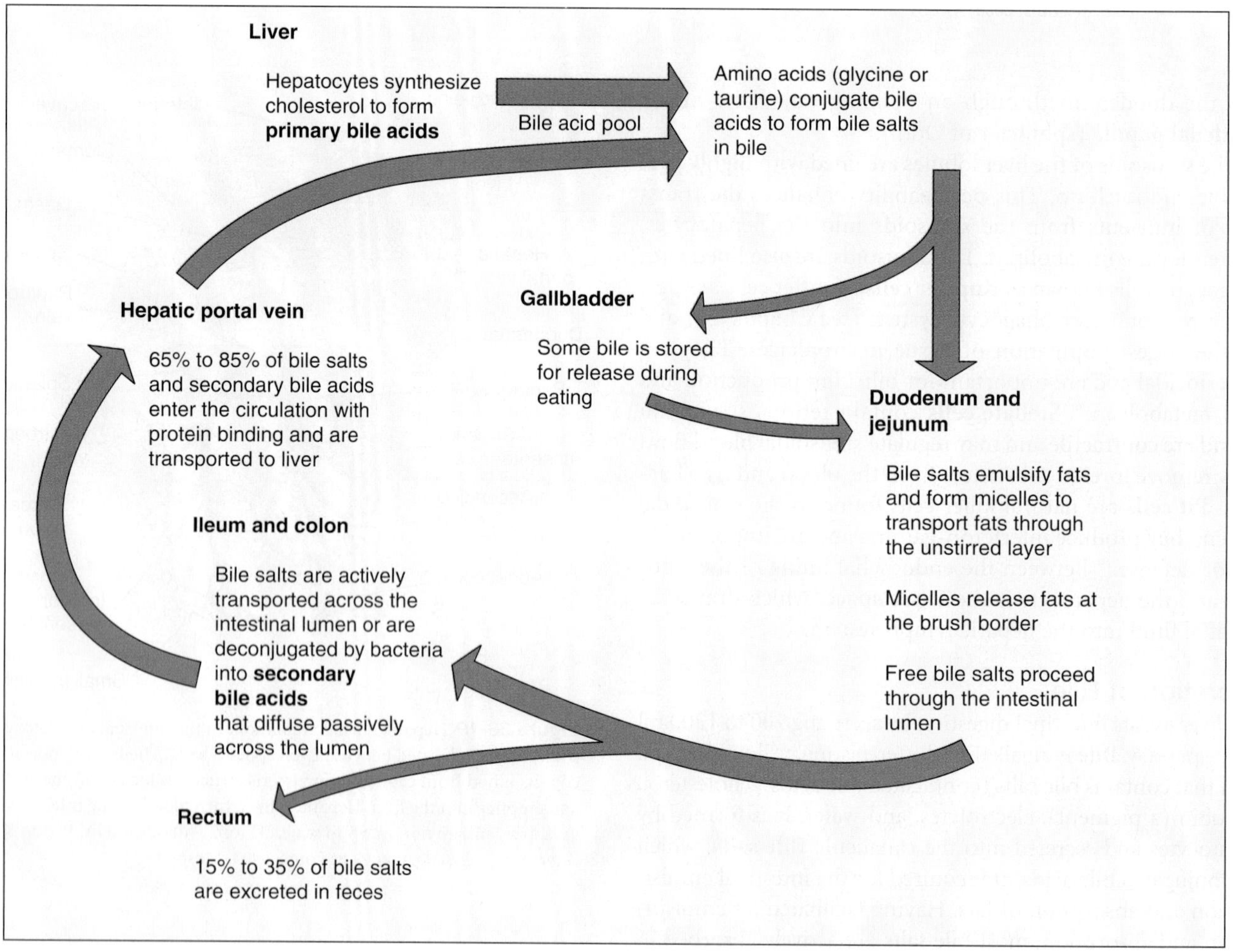

Liver

Hepatocytes synthesize cholesterol to form **primary bile acids**

Bile acid pool

Amino acids (glycine or taurine) conjugate bile acids to form bile salts in bile

Hepatic portal vein

65% to 85% of bile salts and secondary bile acids enter the circulation with protein binding and are transported to liver

Gallbladder

Some bile is stored for release during eating

Duodenum and jejunum

Bile salts emulsify fats and form micelles to transport fats through the unstirred layer

Micelles release fats at the brush border

Free bile salts proceed through the intestinal lumen

Ileum and colon

Bile salts are actively transported across the intestinal lumen or are deconjugated by bacteria into **secondary bile acids** that diffuse passively across the lumen

Rectum

15% to 35% of bile salts are excreted in feces

Figure 38-21 The enterohepatic circulation of bile salts.

Bile salts are planar molecules; that is, they are hydrophobic on one end and hydrophilic on the other. When the concentration of bile salts is adequate or has reached the **critical micelle concentration,** the molecules form micelles with their hydrophilic side toward the watery chyme of the intestine and their hydrophobic side surrounding fat molecules such as cholesterol, free fatty acids, and phospholipids (see Figure 38-14). Micelle formation facilitates the absorption of fat by the intestinal mucosa.

Bile secretion is called **choleresis.** A **choleretic agent** is a substance that stimulates the liver to secrete bile. One strong stimulus is a high concentration of bile salts. Other choleretics include secretin, which increases the rate of bile flow by promoting the secretion of bicarbonate from canaliculi and other intrahepatic bile ducts; cholecystokinin; and vagal stimulation.

Metabolism of Bilirubin

Bilirubin is a byproduct of destruction of aged red blood cells. It gives bile a greenish black color and produces the yellow tinge of jaundice. Aged red blood cells are taken up and destroyed by macrophages of the mononuclear phagocyte system, primarily in the spleen and liver. (In the liver these macrophages are Kupffer cells.) Within these cells, hemoglobin is separated into its component parts—heme and globin (Figure 38-22). The globin component is further degraded into its constituent amino acids, which are recycled to form new protein. The heme moiety is converted to biliverdin by the enzymatic cleavage of iron. The iron attaches to transferrin in the plasma and can be stored in the liver or used by the bone marrow to make new red blood cells. The biliverdin is enzymatically converted to bilirubin in the macrophage of the mononuclear phagocytic system

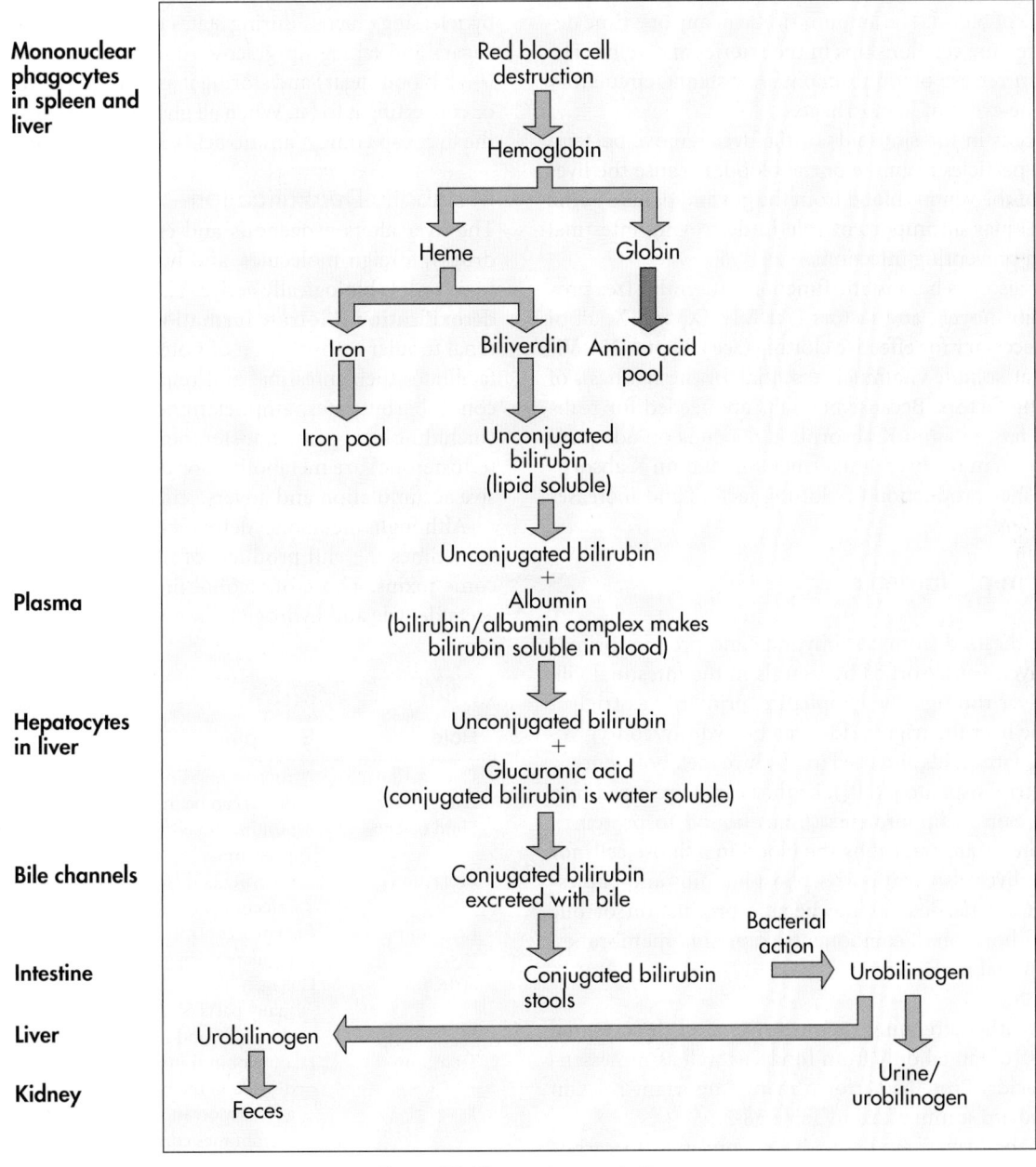

Figure 38-22 Bilirubin metabolism.

and then is released into the plasma. In the plasma, bilirubin binds to albumin and is known as **unconjugated bilirubin,** or free bilirubin, which is lipid soluble. Bilirubin also may have a role as an antioxidant and provide cytoprotection.[31,32]

In the liver, unconjugated bilirubin moves from plasma in the sinusoids into the hepatocyte. Within hepatocytes it joins with glucuronic acid to form **conjugated bilirubin,** which is water soluble. Conjugation transforms bilirubin from a lipid-soluble substance that can cross biologic membranes to a water-soluble substance that can be excreted in the bile. When conjugated bilirubin reaches the distal ileum and colon, it is deconjugated by bacteria and converted to **urobilinogen.** Most of the urobilinogen is then excreted in the urine, and a small amount is eliminated in feces.

Vascular and Hematologic Functions

Because of its extensive vascular network, the liver can store a large volume of blood. The amount stored at any one time depends on pressure relationships in the arteries and veins. The liver also can release blood to maintain systemic circulatory volume in the event of hemorrhage.

Kupffer cells in the sinusoids of the liver remove bacteria and foreign particles from the portal blood. Because the liver receives all of the venous blood from the gut and pancreas, the Kupffer cells play an important role in destroying intestinal bacteria and preventing infections.

The liver also has hemostatic functions. It synthesizes prothrombin; fibrinogen; and factors I, II, VII, IX, and X, all of which are necessary for effective clotting (see Chapter 25). Vitamin K, a fat-soluble vitamin, is essential for the synthesis of other clotting factors. Because bile salts are needed for reabsorption of fats, vitamin K absorption depends on adequate bile production in the liver. Impairment of vitamin K absorption diminishes production of clotting factors and increases risk of bleeding.

Metabolism of Nutrients

Fats

Fat is synthesized from carbohydrate and protein, primarily in the liver. Fat absorbed by lacteals in the intestinal villi enters the liver through the lymphatics, primarily as triglycerides. In the liver the triglycerides can be hydrolyzed to glycerol and free fatty acids and used to produce metabolic energy (adenosine triphosphate [ATP]), or they can be released into the bloodstream as lipoproteins (lipids bound to proteins). The lipoproteins are carried by the blood to adipose cells for storage. The liver also synthesizes phospholipids and cholesterol, which are needed for the hepatic production of bile salts, steroid hormones, components of plasma membranes, and other special molecules.

Proteins

Protein synthesis requires the presence of all the essential amino acids (obtained only from food), as well as nonessential amino acids. Proteins perform many important roles in the body and are summarized in Table 38-3.

Within hepatocytes, amino acids are converted to carbohydrates by the removal of ammonia (NH_3), a process known as **deamination.** The ammonia is converted to urea by the liver and passes into the blood to be excreted by the kidneys. Depending on need, the ketoacids are converted to fatty acids for fat synthesis and storage or are oxidized by the Krebs tricarboxylic acid cycle (see Chapter 1) to provide energy for the liver cells.

The plasma proteins, including albumins and globulins (with the exception of γ-globulin, which is formed in lymph nodes and lymphoid tissue), are synthesized by the liver. The liver also synthesizes several nonessential amino acids and serum enzymes, including aspartate aminotransferase (AST; previously serum glutamate oxaloacetate transaminase [SGOT]), alanine aminotransferase (ALT; previously serum glutamate pyruvate transaminase [SGPT]), lactate dehydrogenase (LDH), and alkaline phosphatase.

Carbohydrates

The liver contributes to the stability of blood glucose levels by releasing glucose during states of hypoglycemia (low blood sugar) and taking up glucose during states of hyperglycemia (high blood sugar) and storing it as glycogen (glyconeogenesis) or converting it to fat. When all glycogen stores have been used, the liver can convert amino acids and glycerol to glucose.

Metabolic Detoxification

The liver alters exogenous and endogenous chemicals (e.g., drugs), foreign molecules, and hormones to make them less toxic or less biologically active. This process, called **metabolic detoxification (biotransformation),** diminishes intestinal or renal tubular reabsorption of potentially toxic substances and facilitates their intestinal and renal excretion. In this way alcohol, barbiturates, amphetamines, steroids, and hormones (including estrogens, aldosterone, antidiuretic hormone, and testosterone) are metabolized or detoxified, preventing excessive accumulation and adverse effects.

Although metabolic detoxification is usually protective, sometimes the end products of metabolic detoxification become toxins. Those of alcohol metabolism, for example, are acetaldehyde and hydrogen. Excessive intake of alcohol over a

Table 38-3	Proteins in the Body	
Role	**Example**
Contraction	Actin and myosin enable muscle contraction
Energy	Proteins can be metabolized for energy
Fluid balance	Albumin, a major source of plasma oncotic pressure
Protection	Antibodies and complement protect against infection and foreign substances
Regulation	Enzymes control chemical reactions; hormones regulate many physiologic processes
Structure	Collagen fibers provide structural support to many parts of the body; keratin strengthens skin, hair, and nails
Transport	Hemoglobin transports oxygen and carbon dioxide in the blood; plasma proteins serve as transport molecules; proteins in cell membranes control movement of materials into and out of cells

prolonged period causes these end products to damage hepatocytes. Acetaldehyde damages cellular mitochondria, and the excess hydrogen promotes fat accumulation. This is how alcohol impairs the liver's ability to function.

Storage of Minerals and Vitamins

The liver stores certain vitamins and minerals, including iron and copper, in times of excessive intake and releases them in times of need. The liver can store vitamins B_{12} and D for several months and vitamin A for several years. The liver also stores vitamins E and K. Iron is stored in the liver as ferritin, an iron-protein complex, and is released as needed for red blood cell production.

Gallbladder

The **gallbladder** is a saclike organ that lies on the inferior surface of the liver (Figure 38-23). The wall of the gallbladder is composed of the mucous membrane, muscularis, and serosa or adventitia. The primary function of the gallbladder is to store and concentrate bile between meals. During the interdi-

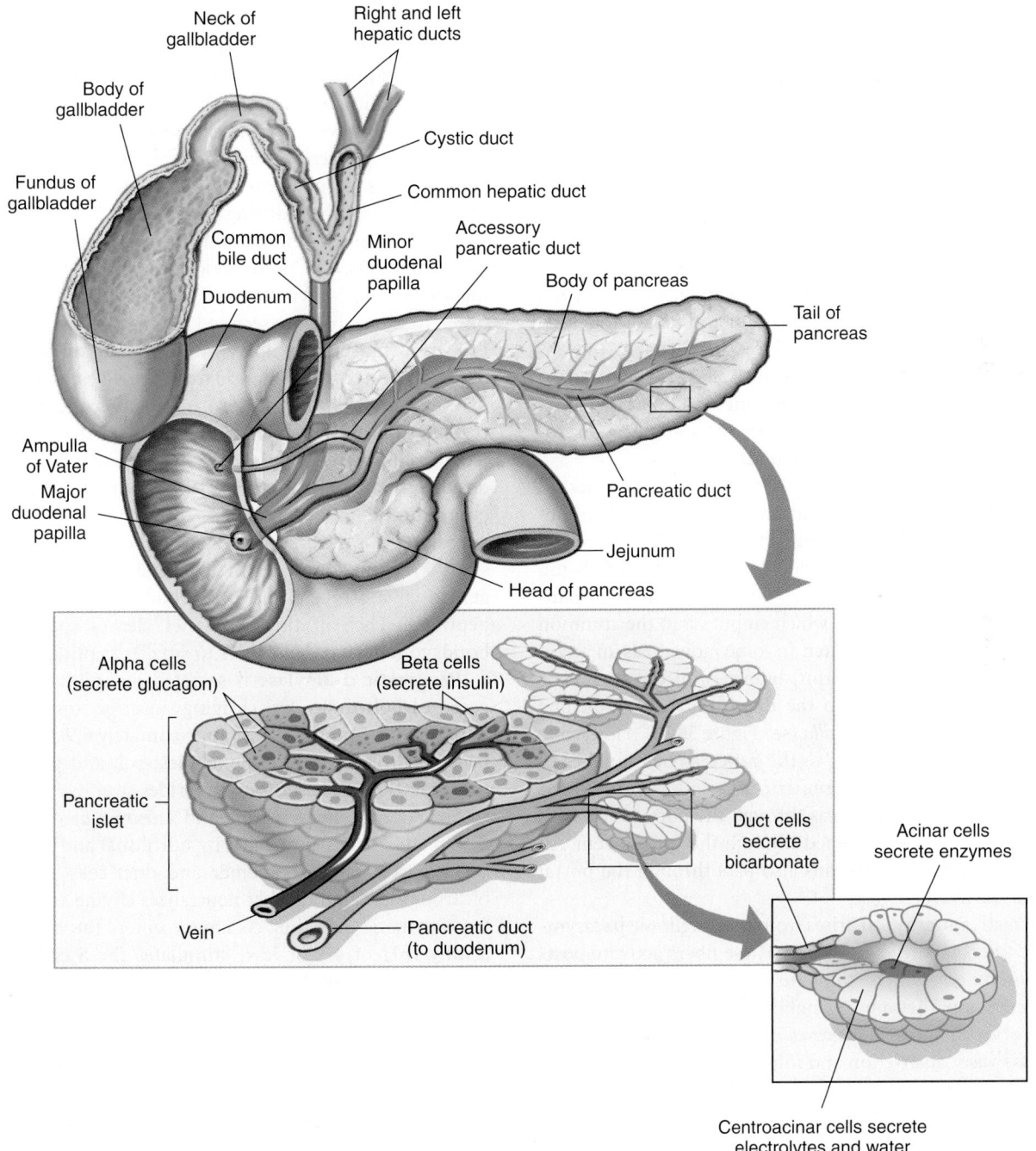

Figure 38-23 Associated structures of the gallbladder, pancreas, and pancreatic acinar cells and duct. (Modified from Thibodeau GA, Patton KT: *Anatomy & physiology*, ed 5, St Louis, 2003, Mosby.)

gestive period, bile flows from the liver through the right or left hepatic duct into the common hepatic duct and meets resistance at the closed **sphincter of Oddi,** which controls flow into the duodenum and prevents reflux of duodenal contents into the pancreatobiliary system.[33] Bile then flows to the **cystic duct** into the gallbladder, where it is concentrated and stored. The mucosa of the gallbladder wall readily absorbs water and electrolytes, leaving a high concentration of bile salts, bile pigments, and cholesterol. The gallbladder holds about 90 ml of bile.

Within 30 minutes after eating, the gallbladder begins to contract and the sphincter of Oddi relaxes, forcing bile into the duodenum through the major duodenal papilla. During the cephalic and gastric phases of digestion, gallbladder contraction is mediated by cholinergic branches of the vagus nerve. Hormonal regulation of gallbladder contraction is derived from the release of *cholecystokinin* and *motilin* secreted by the duodenal mucosa in the presence of fat. Vasoactive intestinal peptide, pancreatic polypeptide, and sympathetic nerve stimulation relax the gallbladder.

Exocrine Pancreas

The **pancreas** is approximately 20 cm long, with its head tucked into the curve of the duodenum and its tail touching the spleen. The body of the pancreas lies deep in the abdomen, behind the stomach (see Figure 38-23). The pancreas is unique in that it has both endocrine and exocrine functions. The endocrine pancreas secretes insulin, glucagon, somatostatin, and pancreatic polypeptide.[8]

The **exocrine pancreas** is composed of acini and networks of ducts that secrete enzymes and alkaline fluids with important digestive functions. The acinar cells are organized into spherical lobules around small secretory ducts (see Figure 38-23, *B* and *C*). Secretions drain into a system of ducts that leads to the **pancreatic duct (Wirsung duct),** which empties into the common bile duct at the **ampulla of Vater.** In some individuals an accessory duct (the duct of Santorini) branches off the pancreatic duct and drains directly into the duodenum at an opening called the *minor duodenal papilla* (see Figure 38-23, *A*).

Arterial blood is supplied to the pancreas by branches of the celiac and superior mesenteric arteries. Venous blood leaves the head of the pancreas through the portal vein, with the body and tail being drained through the splenic vein. All hormonal pancreatic secretions also pass through the portal vein into the liver.

Pancreatic innervation arises from preganglionic parasympathetic fibers of the vagus nerve. These fibers activate postganglionic fibers, which stimulate enzymatic and hormonal secretion. Sympathetic postganglionic fibers from the celiac and superior mesenteric plexuses innervate the blood vessels and cause vasoconstriction and inhibit pancreatic secretion.

The aqueous secretions of the exocrine pancreas are isotonic and contain potassium, sodium, bicarbonate, magnesium, calcium, and chloride. Sodium and potassium concentrations are about equal to those in the plasma. The concentration of bicarbonate in pancreatic juice varies directly with the secretory flow rate. As bicarbonate secretion increases, chloride secretion decreases to maintain a constant anionic concentration. The highly alkaline pancreatic juice neutralizes the acidic chyme that enters the duodenum from the stomach and provides the alkaline medium needed for the actions of digestive enzymes and the absorption of fat in the intestine.

In the pancreas, transport of water and electrolytes through the ductal epithelium involves both active and passive mechanisms. The secretory cells of the acini actively transport hydrogen into the blood and bicarbonate into the duct lumen. Potassium and chloride are secreted by diffusion according to changes in electrochemical potential gradients. As the secretion flows down the duct, water is osmotically transported into the juice until it becomes isoosmotic. At low flow rates, bicarbonate is exchanged passively for chloride, but at higher flow rates there is less time for this exchange and bicarbonate concentration increases. Because eating stimulates the flow of pancreatic juice, the juice is most alkaline when it needs to be—during digestion.

The pancreatic enzymes hydrolyze proteins, carbohydrates, and fats. The proteolytic (protein-digesting) enzymes include trypsin, chymotrypsin, carboxypeptidase and elastase. These enzymes are secreted in their inactive forms—that is, as trypsinogen, chymotrypsinogen, and procarboxypeptidase—to protect the pancreas from the digestive effects of its own enzymes. For further protection the pancreas produces **trypsin inhibitor,** which prevents the activation of proteolytic enzymes while they are in the pancreas. Once in the duodenum, the inactive forms (proenzymes) are activated by **enterokinase,** an enzyme secreted by the duodenal mucosa. Trypsinogen is the first proenzyme to be activated. Its conversion to trypsin stimulates the conversion of chymotrypsinogen to chymotrypsin and procarboxypeptidase to carboxypeptidase. Each of these enzymes cleaves specific peptide bonds to reduce polypeptides to smaller peptides.

Pancreatic α-amylase is secreted in active form and digests carbohydrate by cleaving interior α-1,4-glucosidic bonds at an optimum pH of approximately 6.9. **Pancreatic lipases** hydrolyze triglyceride, cholesterol, and phospholipids to free fatty acids and uronoglycerides.

Secretion of the aqueous and enzymatic components of pancreatic juice is controlled by hormonal and vagal stimuli. Secretin stimulates the acinar and duct cells to secrete the bicarbonate-rich fluid that neutralizes chyme and prepares it for enzymatic digestion. As chyme enters the duodenum, its acidity (pH of 4.5 or less) stimulates the **S cells** (secretin-producing cells) of the duodenum to release secretin, which is absorbed by the intestine and delivered to the pancreas in the bloodstream. In the pancreas, secretin causes ductal and acinar cells to release alkaline fluid. Secretin also inhibits the actions of gastrin, thereby decreasing gastric acid secretion and motility. The overall effect is to neutralize contents of the duodenum.

Enzymatic secretion follows, stimulated by cholecystokinin and acetylcholine. Cholecystokinin is released in the duodenum in response to the essential amino acids and fatty acids already present in chyme. Cholecystokinin and acetylcholine both act on the acinar cells, causing enzyme release. Once in the small intestine, activated pancreatic enzymes inhibit the release of more cholecystokinin and acetylcholine. This feedback mechanism inhibits the secretion of more pancreatic enzymes. Acetylcholine is liberated from pancreatic branches of the vagus nerve during the cephalic phase of digestion. Pancreatic polypeptide is released after eating and inhibits postprandial pancreatic exocrine secretion. (Table 38-1 summarizes hormonal stimulation of pancreatic secretions.)

TESTS OF DIGESTIVE FUNCTION

Gastrointestinal Tract

Although important diagnostic information can be obtained from the patient's medical history and presenting symptoms, numerous disease-specific tests must be performed to evaluate the structure and function of the gastrointestinal tract. A description of selected studies is presented in Tables 38-4 and 38-5. Radiography and imaging techniques, including ultrasound and radionuclide and computed tomography (CT) scanning, are common procedures for evaluating structure and function. Plain roentgenograms using contrast media such as barium- or iodine-containing compounds can be used to outline the gastrointestinal lumen, biliary tree and pancreatic ducts, fistulae, and arteriovenous systems. CT scanning is particularly useful for diagnosis of pancreatic or hepatic tumors or cysts. Ultrasonic scanning is a safe, simple, and relatively inexpensive technique used to detect liver-related jaundice and intraabdominal masses, particularly abscesses.

Fiberoptic endoscopy, using flexible endoscopes, allows direct visualization of the gastrointestinal tract. A biopsy channel allows tissue sampling, and suction can be applied to remove gastrointestinal secretions or blood. Analysis of stool, gastric secretions, and plasma provides important clues to infection, malabsorption syndromes, ulcerative lesions, and tumor growth.

Liver

A variety of diagnostic tests can be performed to evaluate liver function[34,35] (Table 38-6). Imaging techniques similar to those described for the gastrointestinal tract are also useful for evaluating liver structure and function. Plasma chemistry findings are also altered with many liver diseases because of release of cytoplasmic enzymes into the circulation when there is damage to the hepatocyte. Of particular importance are elevations of aminotransferases and LDH. Obstruction of bile canaliculi or ducts results in regurgitation of bile back into the hepatic sinusoids and into the circulation, with elevation of bilirubin levels. Prothrombin times are often prolonged with both hepatitis and chronic liver disease. In severe disease, other plasma proteins, such as albumin and globulins, may be diminished as a result of hepatocyte damage. Liver biopsies are often performed to evaluate the extent of liver involvement or degeneration with cirrhosis or hepatitis.

Table 38-4	Selected Studies of Gastrointestinal Structure	
Test	**Description**	**Application**
Plain roentgenograms	Use of high-energy electromagnetic radiation to evaluate tissue structure by radiopacity or radiolucency	Visualization of the position, size, and structure of abdominal contents
Air or barium contrast roentgenograms	Introduction of radiopaque substances into the upper or lower gastrointestinal tract	Enhanced visualization of the contours, position, and size of the gastrointestinal tract to detect umbilical hernia, ulcers, diverticula, congenital anomalies, polyps, tumors, strictures, obstructions
Endoscopy Esophagoscopy (esophagus) Gastroscopy (stomach) Duodenoscopy (duodenum) Colonoscopy (large intestine) Sigmoidoscopy (sigmoid colon)	Passage of rigid or flexible (fiberoptic) endoscope into the gastrointestinal tract for visualization or biopsy	Visualization or biopsy of inflamed hernias, polyps, ulcers, strictures, varices, tumors, sites of bleeding, mucosal or neoplastic lesions and for culture of *Helicobacter pylori* from stomach
Ultrasound	Use of piezoelectric crystal to generate sound waves that are reflected from tissue interfaces to provide an image	Imaging of abdominal organs (gallbladder, liver, pancreas, spleen), masses, stones, abscesses, structural abnormalities
Computed tomography (CT)	Use of a computer to integrate differences in absorption of a large number of x-rays to produce a cross-sectional image; may be done with contrast agents	Imaging of gallbladder, liver, pancreas, spleen, cysts, hematomas, abscesses, stones, extrahepatic bile ducts, and portal vein
Magnetic resonance imaging (MRI)	Projection of differences in magnetic properties of molecules within different cells and tissues, using the field of a large magnet	Same applications as CT scan; also can detect blood flow and vessel patency

Table 38-5	Selected Tests of Gastrointestinal Function	
Test	Normal Findings	Clinical Significance of Abnormal Findings
Stool studies	Resident microorganisms: clostridia, enterococci, *Pseudomona*, a few yeasts	Detection of *Salmonella typhi* (typhoid fever), *Shigella* (dysentery), *Vibrio cholerae* (cholera), *Yersinia* (enterocolitis), *Escherichia coli* (gastroenteritis), *Staphylococcus aureus* (food poisoning), *Clostridium botulinum* (food poisoning), *Clostridium perfringens* (food poisoning), *Aeromonas* (gastroenteritis)
	Fat: 2-6 g/24 hr	Steatorrhea (increased values) can result from intestinal malabsorption or pancreatic insufficiency
	Pus: none	Large amounts of pus are associated with chronic ulcerative colitis, abscesses, and anal-rectal fistula
	Occult blood: none (OrthoTolidin or guaiac test)	Positive tests associated with bleeding
	Ova and parasites: none	Detection of *Entamoeba histolytica* (amebiasis), *Giardia lamblia* (giardiasis), and worms
D-Xylose absorption	5-Hr urinary excretion: 4.5 g/L Peak blood level: >30 mg/dl	Differentiation of pancreatic steatorrhea (normal D-xylose absorption) from intestinal steatorrhea (impaired D-xylose absorption)
Gastric acid stimulation	11-20 mEq/hr after stimulation	Detection of duodenal ulcers, Zollinger-Ellison syndrome (increased values), gastric atrophy, gastric carcinoma (decreased values)
Manometry (use of water-filled catheters connected to pressure transducers passed into the esophagus, stomach, colon, or rectum to evaluate contractility)	Values vary at different levels of the intestine	Inadequate swallowing, motility, sphincter function
Culture and sensitivity of duodenal contents	No pathogens	Detection of *Salmonella typhi* (typhoid fever)
Breath tests		
Glucose breath test or D-xylose	Negative for hydrogen or CO_2	May indicate intestinal bacterial overgrowth
Urea breath test	Negative for isotopically labeled CO_2	Presence of *Helicobacter pylori* infection

Gallbladder

Evaluation of structural alterations in the gallbladder may be achieved by the use of various imaging techniques. Table 38-7 summarizes these techniques. Obstruction of the common ducts from stones, tumors, or inflammation prevents the flow of bile from the liver and gallbladder from reaching the gastrointestinal tract. Both the conjugated and total serum bilirubin values are elevated, urine urobilinogen is increased, stools are clay colored, and jaundice develops. Fat absorption can be impaired and the prothrombin time prolonged if vitamin K is not absorbed. With inflammation of the gallbladder, the white cell count is elevated.

Exocrine Pancreas

Tests of pancreatic function are summarized in Table 38-8. Evaluation of plasma and urinary amylase provides particularly significant measures of pancreatic function. Inflammation or obstruction of the pancreas results in an increase in serum amylase levels. Decreased renal absorption of amylase results in increased urine amylase levels. Increased stool fat can reflect pancreatic insufficiency caused by decreased lipase secretion when biliary function is normal.

AGING AND THE GASTROINTESTINAL SYSTEM

Age-related changes in gastrointestinal function begin to occur before 50 years of age. Tooth enamel and dentin wear down, making the teeth vulnerable to cavities. Teeth are lost, often as a result of periodontal (gum) disease, recession of the gums, osteoporotic bone changes and more brittle roots that fracture easily. Taste buds decline in number, and the sense of smell diminishes. Together these losses decrease the sense of taste. Salivary secretion decreases and contributes to dry mouth. In very old persons, these oral and sensory changes make eating less pleasurable and reduce appetite. Food may not be chewed or lubricated sufficiently, making swallowing difficult. The esophagus develops decreased motility and there are changes in the upper esophageal sphincter that may effect swallowing.[36]

Age also diminishes gastric motility and volume, including secretion of bicarbonate and gastric mucus.[37] Acid content of gastric juice is related to gastric atrophy, which results in hypochlorhydria (insufficient hydrochloric acid) and delayed gastric emptying, best managed with frequent and small meals. Decreased production of intrinsic factor leads to pernicious anemia. Aging is also associated with a greater frequency of *Helicobacter pylori* infection[38] and compromise of

Table 38-6   Common Liver Function Tests

Test	Normal Value	Interpretation
Serum Enzymes		
Alkaline phosphatase	13-39 U/L	Increases with biliary obstruction and cholestatic hepatitis
γ-Glutanyltransferase	Male 12-38 U/L	Increases with biliary obstruction and cholestatic hepatitis
	Female 9-31 U/L	
Aspartate amino transferase (AST; previously serum glutamate oxaloacetate transaminase [SGOT])	5-40 U/L	Increases with hepatocellular injury
Alanine amino transferase (ALT; previously serum glutamate pyruvate transaminase [SGPT])	5-35 U/L	Increases with hepatocellular injury
LDH (lactate dehydrogenase)	90-220 U/L	Isoenzyme LD_5 is elevated with hypoxic and primary liver injury
5'-Nucleotidase	2-11 U/L	Increases with increase in alkaline phosphatase and cholestatic disorders
Bilirubin Metabolism		
Serum bilirubin		
Indirect (unconjugated)	<0.8 mg/dl	Increases with hemolysis (lysis of red blood cells)
Direct (conjugated)	0.2-0.4 mg/dl	Increases wit hepatocellular injury or obstruction
Total	<1.0 mg/dl	Increases with biliary obstruction
Urine bilirubin	0	Decreases with biliary obstruction
Urine urobilinogen	0-4 mg/24 hr	Increases with hemolysis or shunting or portal blood flow
Serum Proteins		
Albumin	3.5-5.5 g/dl	Reduced with hepatocellular injury
Globulin	2.5-3.5 g/dl	Increases with hepatitis
Total	6-7 g/dl	
Albumin/globulin (A/G) ratio	1.5:1 to 2.5:1	Ratio reverses with chronic hepatitis or other chronic liver disease
Transferrin	250-300 mcg/dl	Liver damage with decreased values, iron deficiency with increased values
α-Fetoprotein	6-20 ng/ml	Elevated values in primary hepatocellular carcinoma
Blood Clotting Functions		
Prothrombin time (PT)	11.5-14 sec or 90%-100% of control	Increases with chronic liver disease (cirrhosis) or vitamin K deficiency
Partial thromboplastin time (PTT)	25-40 sec	Increases with severe liver disease or heparin therapy
BSP (bromsulphalein) excretion	<6% retention in 45 min	Increased retention with hepatocellular injury

Table 38-7   Diagnostic Evaluation of the Gallbladder

Test	Application
Plain roentgenogram of the abdomen	Visualization of calcified gallstones
Oral cholecystogram (use of an oral contrast medium such as iodopanoic acid, which is excreted with bile and concentrated in the gallbladder for visualization by radiography; may be administered as a double dose)	Visualization of gallstones; evaluation of filling and emptying of gallbladder
Intravenous cholangiography (use of intravenous contrast agents for visualization of gallbladder and bile ducts)	Diagnosis of acute gallbladder inflammation (cholecystitis) or disease of bile ducts
Cholecystonography (ultrasound imaging of gallbladder and bile ducts)	Preferred method for detecting gallstones; differentiation of hepatic disease from biliary obstruction; diagnosis of chronic cholecystitis
Cholescintigraphy (radioisotope imaging of gallbladder)	Diagnosis of cholecystitis in individuals allergic to iodine-containing contrast agents; diagnosis of cystic duct obstruction
Endoscopic retrograde cholangiography (instillation of contrast medium through cannulation of ampulla of Vater with a duodenoscope)	Differentiation of intrahepatic or extrahepatic obstructive jaundice
Computed tomography (CT)	Diagnosis of biliary obstruction or malignancy when ultrasound is not successful

Table 38-8	Selected Tests of Pancreatic Function	
Test	Normal Value	Clinical Significance
Serum amylase	60-180 Somogyi units/ml	Elevated levels with pancreatic inflammation
Serum lipase	1.5 Somogyi units/ml	Elevated levels with pancreatic inflammation (may be elevated with other conditions; differentiates with amylase isoenzyme study)
Urine amylase	35-260 Somogyi units/hr	Elevated levels with pancreatic inflammation
Secretin test	Volume 1.8 ml/kg/hr	Decreased volume with pancreatic disease as secretin stimulates pancreatic secretion
	Bicarbonate concentration: >80 mEq/L	
	Bicarbonate output: >10 mEq/L/30 sec	
Stool fat	2-5 g/24 hr	Measures fatty acids; decreased pancreatic lipase increases stool fat

the gastric mucosal barrier. The villi of the small intestine become broader and shorter, perhaps because of a decrease in cell turnover. Intestinal absorption, motility, and blood flow decrease, impairing nutrient absorption.[39] Proteins, fats, minerals (including iron and calcium), and vitamins are absorbed more slowly and in lesser amounts, and absorption of carbohydrates, particularly lactose, is decreased.[40,41] Constipation is often described as a condition of old age, but it is probably caused by life-style factors rather than physiologic decline although recent studies demonstrate there can be alterations in myenteric innervation.[42] Lifelong bowel habits, current diet, lack of fluid intake, and immobility contribute to constipation in elderly persons.[43]

The liver decreases in size and weight with advancing age. Cell numbers and their regeneration decrease.[44] However, liver function test results often remain within relatively normal ranges. Alterations in liver function in older individuals are usually a sign of a pathologic condition. Liver blood flow decreases with age and can influence efficiency of drug metabolism. Oxidative metabolism of drugs may be decreased.[45] The pancreas undergoes structural changes, such as fibrosis, fatty acid deposits, and atrophy. Pancreatic secretion decreases, but there is usually no observable dysfunction.[41,46] Aging does not cause apparent changes in the structure and function of the gallbladder and bile ducts, but incidence of gallstones increases.

SUMMARY REVIEW

The Gastrointestinal Tract

1. The major functions of the gastrointestinal tract are the mechanical and chemical breakdown of food and the absorption of digested nutrients.
2. The gastrointestinal tract is a hollow tube that extends from the mouth to the anus.
3. The walls of the gastrointestinal tract have several layers: mucosa, muscularis mucosae, submucosa, tunica muscularis (circular muscle and longitudinal muscle), and serosa.
4. The peritoneum is a double layer of membranous tissue. The visceral layer covers the abdominal organs, and the parietal layer extends along the abdominal wall.
5. Except for swallowing and defecation, which are controlled voluntarily, the functions of the gastrointestinal tract are controlled by extrinsic and intrinsic autonomic nerves and intestinal hormones.
6. Digestion begins in the mouth, with chewing and salivation. The digestive component of saliva is α-amylase, which initiates carbohydrate digestion.
7. The esophagus is a muscular tube that transports food from the mouth to the stomach. The tunica muscularis in the upper part of the esophagus is striated muscle, and that in the lower part is smooth muscle.
8. Swallowing is controlled by the swallowing center in the reticular formation of the brain. The two phases of swallowing are the oropharyngeal phase (voluntary swallowing) and the esophageal phase (involuntary swallowing).
9. Food is propelled through the gastrointestinal tract by peristalsis: waves of sequential relaxations and contractions of the tunica muscularis.
10. The lower esophageal sphincter opens to admit swallowed food into the stomach and then closes to prevent regurgitation of food back into the esophagus.

11. The stomach is a baglike structure that secretes digestive juices, mixes and stores food, and propels partially digested food (chyme) into the duodenum.
12. The vagus nerve stimulates gastric (stomach) secretion and motility.
13. The hormones gastrin and motilin stimulate gastric emptying; the hormones secretin and cholecystokinin delay gastric emptying.
14. Gastric glands in the fundus and body of the stomach secrete intrinsic factor, which is needed for vitamin B_{12} absorption, and hydrochloric acid, which dissolves food fibers, kills microorganisms, and activates the enzyme pepsin.
15. Chief cells in the stomach secrete pepsinogen, which is converted to pepsin in the acid environment created by hydrochloric acid.
16. Acid secretion is stimulated by the vagus nerve, gastrin, and histamine and inhibited by sympathetic stimulation and cholecystokinin.
17. Mucus is secreted throughout the stomach and protects the stomach wall from acid and digestive enzymes.
18. The three phases of acid secretion by the stomach are the cephalic phase (anticipation and swallowing), the gastric phase (food in the stomach), and the intestinal phase (chyme in the intestine).
19. The small intestine is 5 m long and has three segments: the duodenum, jejunum, and ileum.
20. The duodenum receives chyme from the stomach through the pyloric valve. The presence of chyme stimulates the liver and gallbladder to deliver bile and the pancreas to deliver digestive enzymes. Bile and enzymes flow through an opening guarded by the sphincter of Oddi.
21. Bile is produced by the liver and is necessary for fat digestion and absorption. Bile's alkalinity helps to neutralize chyme,

thereby creating a pH that enables the pancreatic enzymes to digest proteins, carbohydrates, and sugars.

22. Enzymes secreted by the small intestine (maltase, sucrose, lactase), pancreatic enzymes, and bile salts act in the small intestine to digest proteins, carbohydrates, and fats.

23. Digested substances are absorbed across the intestinal wall and then transported to the liver, where they are metabolized further.

24. The ileocecal valve connects the small and large intestines and prevents reflux into the small intestine.

25. Villi are small finger-like projections that extend from the small intestinal mucosa and increase its absorptive surface area.

26. Sugars, amino acids, and fats are absorbed primarily by the duodenum and jejunum; bile salts and vitamin B_{12} are absorbed by the ileum. Vitamin B_{12} absorption requires the presence of intrinsic factor.

27. Bile salts emulsify and hydrolyze fats and incorporate them into water-soluble micelles, which transport them through the unstirred layer to the brush border of the intestinal mucosa. The fat content of the micelles readily diffuses through the epithelium into lacteals (lymphatic ducts) in the villi. From there fats flow into lymphatics and into the systemic circulation, which delivers them to the liver.

28. Minerals and water-soluble vitamins are absorbed by both active and passive transport throughout the small intestine.

29. Peristaltic movements created by longitudinal muscles propel the chyme along the intestinal tract, while contractions of the circular muscles (segmentation) mix the chyme.

30. The ileogastric reflex inhibits gastric motility when the ileum is distended.

31. The intestinointestinal reflex inhibits intestinal motility when one intestinal segment is overdistended.

32. The gastroileal reflex increases intestinal motility when gastric motility increases.

33. The large intestine consists of the cecum, appendix, colon (ascending, transverse, descending, and sigmoid), rectum, and anal canal.

34. The teniae coli are three bands of longitudinal muscle that extend the length of the colon.

35. Haustra are pouches of colon that are formed with alternating contraction and relaxation of the circular muscles.

36. The mucosa of the large intestine contains mucus-secreting cells and mucosal folds, but no villi.

37. The large intestine massages the fecal mass and absorbs water and electrolytes.

38. Distention of the ileum with chyme causes the gastrocolic reflex, or the mass propulsion of feces to the rectum.

39. Defecation is stimulated when the rectum is distended with feces. The conically contracted internal anal sphincter relaxes, and if the voluntarily regulated external sphincter relaxes, defecation occurs.

40. The largest number of intestinal bacteria are in the colon. They are anaerobes consisting of *Bacteroides*, clostridia, coliforms, and lactobacilli.

41. The intestinal tract is sterile at birth and becomes totally colonized within 3 to 4 weeks.

42. Endogenous infections of the gastrointestinal tract occur by excessive proliferation of bacteria, perforation of the intestine, or contamination from neighboring structures.

Accessory Organs of Digestion

1. The liver is the largest organ in the body. It has digestive, metabolic, hematologic, vascular, and immunologic functions.

2. The liver is divided into the right and left lobes and is supported by the falciform, round, and coronary ligaments.

3. Liver lobules consist of plates of hepatocytes, which are the functional cells of the liver.

4. The hepatocytes synthesize 700 to 1200 ml of bile per day and secrete it into the bile canaliculi, which are small channels between the hepatocytes. The bile canaliculi drain bile into the common bile duct and then into the duodenum through an opening called the *major duodenal papilla (sphincter of Oddi)*.

5. Sinusoids are capillaries located between the plates of hepatocytes. Blood from the portal vein and hepatic artery flows through the sinusoids to a central vein in each lobule and then to the hepatic vein and inferior vena cava.

6. Kupffer cells, which are part of the mononuclear phagocyte system, line the sinusoids and destroy microorganisms in sinusoidal blood.

7. The primary bile acids are synthesized from cholesterol by the hepatocytes. The primary acids are then conjugated to form bile salts. The secondary bile acids are the product of bile salt deconjugation by bacteria in the intestinal lumen.

8. Most bile salts and acids are recycled. The absorption of bile salts and acids from the terminal ileum and their return to the liver are known as the enterohepatic circulation of bile.

9. Bilirubin is a pigment liberated by the lysis of aged red blood cells in the liver and spleen. Unconjugated bilirubin is fat soluble and can cross cell membranes. Unconjugated bilirubin is converted to water-soluble, conjugated bilirubin by hepatocytes and is secreted with bile.

10. The gallbladder is a saclike organ located in the inferior surface of the liver. The gallbladder stores bile between meals and ejects it when chyme enters the duodenum.

11. Stimulated by cholecystokinin, the gallbladder contracts and forces bile through the cystic duct and into the common bile duct. The sphincter of Oddi relaxes, enabling bile to flow through the major duodenal papilla into the duodenum.

12. The pancreas is a gland located behind the stomach. The endocrine pancreas produces hormones (glucagon and insulin) that facilitate the formation and cellular uptake of glucose. The exocrine pancreas secretes an alkaline solution and the enzymes (trypsin, chymotrypsin, carboxypeptidase, α-amylase, lipase) that digest proteins, carbohydrates, and fats.

13. Secretin stimulates pancreatic secretion of alkaline fluid, and cholecystokinin and acetylcholine stimulate secretion of enzymes. Pancreatic secretions originate in acini and ducts of the pancreas and empty into the duodenum through the common bile duct or an accessory duct that opens directly into the duodenum.

Tests of Digestive Function

1. Numerous diagnostic tests are performed to evaluate structure and function (digestion, secretion, absorption) of the gastrointestinal tract. Roentgenograms and scans are most commonly used to evaluate structure, in addition to direct observation by endoscopy. Gastric and stool analysis and blood studies provide important information about digestion, absorption, and secretion.

2. Plasma chemistry levels and imaging procedures are commonly used to diagnose alterations in liver function. Of particular importance are the enzymes lactate dehydrogenase (LDH), aspartate aminotransferase (AST), and alanine aminotransferase (ALT). Plasma bilirubin levels reflect alterations in bilirubin and bile metabolism, and prothrombin times are prolonged in hepatitis and chronic liver disease.

3. Obstructive diseases of the gallbladder are evident by elevated serum bilirubin, elevated urine urobilinogen, and increased stool fat. The serum leukocytes become elevated with inflammation of the gallbladder.

Continued

SUMMARY REVIEW—cont'd

4. The most significant indicators of pancreatic dysfunction are serum amylase and stool fat. Both values are increased with diseases of the pancreas.

Aging and the Gastrointestinal System

1. Advancing age is often associated with the loss or wearing down of teeth, diminished senses of taste and smell, and diminished salivary secretions, all of which may make eating difficult and reduce appetite.

2. Aging reduces gastric motility and secretions, particularly of hydrochloric acid. These changes slow gastric digestion and emptying.

3. Intestinal motility and absorption of carbohydrates, proteins, fats, and minerals decrease with age.

KEY TERMS

Ampulla of Vater, 1376
Antrum of stomach, 1357
Ascending colon, 1369
Bile, 1371
Bile acid pool, 1372
Bile acid–dependent fraction, 1372
Bile acid–independent fraction, 1372
Bile canaliculi, 1370
Bile salts, 1371
Bilirubin, 1373
Body of stomach, 1357
Brush border, 1361
Calcium, 1366
Carboxypeptidase, 1365
Cardiac orifice, 1356
Cecum, 1368
Cephalic phase of secretion, 1359
Chief cells, 1358
Cholecystokinin, 1357
Choleresis, 1373
Choleretic agent, 1373
Chylomicrons, 1366
Chyme, 1356
Chymotrypsin, 1365
Colon, 1368
Common bile duct, 1370
Conjugated bilirubin, 1374
Critical micelle concentration, 1373
Cystic duct, 1376
D cells, 1358
Deamination, 1374
Defecation reflex (rectal reflex), 1369
Descending colon, 1369
Disse space, 1371
Duodenum, 1360
Emulsification, 1365
Enteric plexus, 1353
Enterochromaffin-like cells, 1358
Enterohepatic circulation, 1372
Enterokinase, 1376
Esophageal phase of swallowing, 1356
Esophagus, 1355
Exocrine pancreas, 1376
External anal sphincter, 1369
Fecal mass, 1369
Feces, 1369
Fundus of stomach, 1357
G cells, 1358
Gallbladder, 1375

Gastric emptying, 1358
Gastric glands, 1358
Gastric phase of secretion, 1359
Gastric pit, 1358
Gastrin, 1357
Gastrocolic reflex, 1369
Gastroileal reflex, 1368
Gastrointestinal tract (alimentary canal), 1353
Glisson capsule, 1370
GLUT, 1365
Haustrum (pl., haustra), 1369
Hepatocytes, 1370
Histamine, 1358
Hydrolase, 1365
Ileocecal valve (sphincter), 1360
Ileogastric reflex, 1368
Ileum, 1360
Internal anal sphincter, 1369
Intestinal phase of secretion, 1360
Intestinointestinal reflex, 1368
Iron, 1367
Jejunum, 1360
Kupffer cells, 1371
Lacteal, 1362
Lamina propria, 1361
Large intestine, 1368
Lieberkühn crypts, 1369
Lipase, 1365
Lipocytes, 1370
Lipolysis, 1365
Liver, 1370
Liver lobule, 1370
Lower esophageal sphincter (cardiac sphincter), 1356
Magnesium, 1367
Major duodenal papilla, 1371
Mesentery, 1360
Metabolic detoxification (biotransformation), 1374
Micelles, 1365
Microvilli, 1361
Motilin, 1358
Mouth, 1354
Mucosal barrier, 1359
Myenteric plexus (Auerbach plexus), 1353
O'Beirne sphincter, 1369
Oral phase of swallowing, 1356
Pancreas, 1376

Pancreatic α-amylase, 1376
Pancreatic duct (Wirsung duct), 1376
Pancreatic lipases, 1376
Parietal cells (oxyntic cells), 1358
Pepsin, 1358
Pepsinogen, 1358
Peristalsis, 1355
Peristaltic movements, 1369
Peritoneal cavity, 1360
Peritoneum, 1360
Pharyngeal phase of swallowing, 1356
Phospholipase, 1365
Pit cells, 1371
Primary bile acids, 1372
Primary peristalsis, 1356
Pyloric sphincter, 1357
Pylorus, 1357
Retropulsion, 1358
S cells, 1376
Saliva, 1354
Salivary α-amylase (ptyalin), 1354
Salivary glands, 1354
Secondary bile acids, 1372
Secondary peristalsis, 1356
Secretin, 1358
Segmentation, 1367
Sigmoid colon, 1369
Sinusoids, 1370
Small intestine, 1360
Somatostatin, 1358
Sphincter of Oddi, 1376
Stellate cells, 1371
Stomach, 1356
Submucosal plexus (Meissner plexus), 1353
Subserosal plexus, 1353
Swallowing, 1356
Teniae coli, 1369
Transverse colon, 1369
Trypsin, 1365
Trypsin inhibitor, 1376
Unconjugated bilirubin, 1374
Upper esophageal sphincter (cricopharyngeal muscle), 1356
Urobilinogen, 1374
Vermiform appendix, 1368
Villus (pl., villi), 1361
Vitamins, 1367

REFERENCES

1. Furness JB: Types of neurons in the enteric nervous system, *J Auton Nerv Syst* 81(1-3):87-96, 2000.
2. Lang IM, Shaker R: An overview of the upper esophageal sphincter, *Curr Gastroenterol Rep* 2(3):185-190, 2000.
3. Zald DH, Pardo JV: The functional neuroanatomy of voluntary swallowing, *Ann Neurol* 46(3):281-286, 1999.
4. Ertekin C, Aydogdu I: Neurophysiology of swallowing, *Clin Neurophysiol* 114(2):2226-2244, 2003.
5. Aly YA, Abdel-Aty H: Normal oesophageal transit time on digital radiography, *Clin Radiol* 54(8):545-549, 1999.
6. Ludlow CL: Sensorimotor control for voice, speech and swallowing, *Curr Opin Otolaryngol Head Neck Surg* 12(3):160-165, 2004.
7. Diamant NE: Neuromuscular mechanisms of primary perstalsis, *Am J Med* 103(5A):40S-43S, 1997.
8. Johnson LR: *Gastrointestinal physiology,* ed 7, St Louis, 2001, Mosby.
9. Smith ME, Morton DG: *The digestive system,* St Louis, 2001, Mosby
10. Schubert ML: Gastric secretion, *Curr Opin Gastroentero* 20(6):519-525, 2004.
11. Pabst MA, Wachter C, Holzer P: Morphologic basis of the functional gastric acid barrier, *Lab Invest* 74(1):78-85, 1996.
12. Helander HF, Keeling DJ: Cell biology of gastric acid secretion, *Baillieres Clin Gastroenterol* 7(1):1-21, 1993.
13. Schubert ML: Gastric secretion, *Curr Opin Gastroenterol* 19(6):519-525, 2003.
14. Wolfe MM, Soll AH: The physiology of gastric acid secretion, *N Engl J Med* 319(26):1707-1715, 1988.
15. Kawano S, Tsuji S: Role of mucosal blood flow: a conceptional review in gastric mucosal injury and protection, *J Gastroenterol Hepatol* 15(suppl): D1-D6, 2000.
16. Nederkoorn C, Smulders FT, Jansen A: Cephalic phase responses, craving, and food intake in normal subjects, *Appetite* 35(1):45-55, 2000.
17. Thompson AB et al: Small bowel review: part 1, *Can-S-Gastroentrol* 12(7):487, 1998.
18. Kvietys PR, Barrowman JA, Granger ND: *Pathophysiology of the splanchnic circulation,* Boca Raton, Fla, 1987, CRC Press.
19. Bevins CL: The Paneth cell and the innate immune response, *Curr Opin Gastroenterol* 20(6):572-580, 2004.
20. Ashton KA et al: Basal and meal-stimulated colonic absorption, *Dis Colon Rectum* 39(8):865-870, 1996.
21. Wright EM et al: Intestine absorption in health and disease-sugars, *Best Pract Res Clin Gastroenterol* 17(6):943-956, 2003.
22. Bornstein JC, Costa M, Grider JR: Enteric motor and interneuronal circuits controlling motility, *Neurogastroenterol Motil* 16(Suppl 1):34-38, 2004.
23. Husebye E: The patterns of small bowel motility: physiology and implications in organic disease and functional disorders, *Neurogastroenterol Motil* 11(3):141-161, 1999.
24. Rosenblum JD, Boyle CM, Schwartz LB: The mesenteric circulation. Anatomy and physiology, *Surg Clin North Am* 77(2):289-306, 1997.
25. Mims CA et al: *Medical microbiology,* ed 2, St Louis, 1998, Mosby.
26. Guarner F, Malagelada JR: Gut flora in health and disease, *Lancet* 361(9356):512-519, 2003
27. Zakim D, Bayer TD: Hepatology: *A textbook of liver disease,* ed 3, Philadelphia, 1996, Saunders.
28. Naito M, Hasegawa G, Ebe Y, Yamamoto T: Differentiation and function of Kupffer cells, *Med Electron Microsc* 37(1):16-28, 2004.
29. Nakatani K et al: Pit cells as liver-associated natural killer cells: morphology and function, *Med Electron Microsc* 37(1):29-36, 2004.
30. Wolkoff AM, Cohen DE: Bile acid regulation of hepatic physiology: I. Hepatocyte transport of bile acids, *Am J Physiol Gastrointest Liver Physiol* 284(2):G175-G179, 2003.
31. Stocker R: Antioxidant activites of bile pigments, *Antioxid Redox Signal* 6(5):841-849, 2004.
32. McGeary RP, Szyczew AJ, Toth I: Biological properties and therapeutic potential of bilirubin, *Mini Rev Med Chem* 3(3):253-256, 2003.
33. Tooouli J, Craig A: Sphincter of Oddi function and dysfunction, *Can J Gastroenterol* 14(5):411-419, 2000.
34. Johnston DE: Special considerations in interpreting liver function tests, *Am Fam Physician* 59(8):2223-2230, 1999.
35. Aranda-Michel J, Sherman KE: Tests of the liver: use and misuse, *Gastroenterologist* 6(1):34-43, 1998.
36. Achem SR, Devault KR: Dysphagia in aging, *J Clin Gastroenterol* 39(5):357-371, 2005.
37. Guslandi M, Pellegrini A, Sorghi M: Gastric mucosal defences in the elderly, *Gerontology* 45(4):206-208, 1999.
38. Pilotto A: Aging and upper gastrointestinal disorders, *Best Pract Res Clin Gastroenterol* 18(Suppl):73-81, 2004.
39. Madsen JL, Graff J: Effects of ageing on gastrointestinal motor function, *Age Agein* 33(2):154-159, 2004.
40. Timiras PS: *Physiological basis of aging and geriatrics,* ed 3, Boca Raton, Fla, 2003, CRC Press.
41. Saltzman JR, Russell RM: The aging gut. Nutritional issues, *Gastroenterol Clin North Am* 27(2):309-324, 1998.
42. Hananai M et al: Age-related changes in the morphology of the myenteric plexus of the human colon, *Auton Neurosci* 113(1-2):71-78, 2004.
43. Wilson JA: Constipation in the elderly, *Clin Geriatr Med* 15(3):499-510, 1999.
44. Wakabayashi H et al: Evaluation of the effect of age on functioning hepatocyte mass and liver blood flow using liver scintigraphy in preoperative estimations for surgical patients: comparison with CT volumetry, *J Surg Res* 106(2):246-253, 2002.
45. Kinirons MT, O'Mahony MS: Drug metabolism and ageing, *Br J Clin Pharmacol* 57(5):540-544, 2004 May.
46. Glaser J, Stienecker K: Pancreas and aging: a study using ultrasonography, *Gerontology* 46(2):93, 2000.

ALTERATIONS OF DIGESTIVE FUNCTION

SUE E. HUETHER

CHAPTER OUTLINE

The gastrointestinal tract is a continuous, hollow organ that extends from the mouth to the anus. It includes the esophagus, stomach, small intestine (duodenum, jejunum, ileum), large intestine (ascending, transverse, descending, and sigmoid colon), and rectum.

Disorders of the gastrointestinal tract disrupt one or more of its functions. Structural and neural abnormalities can slow, obstruct, or accelerate the movement of chyme at any level of the gastrointestinal tract. Inflammatory and ulcerative conditions of the gastrointestinal wall disrupt secretion, motility, and absorption. Many clinical manifestations of gastrointestinal tract disorders are nonspecific: that is, they can be caused by a variety of impairments. These manifestations are described in the next section.

DISORDERS OF THE GASTROINTESTINAL TRACT

Clinical Manifestations of Gastrointestinal Dysfunction

Anorexia

Anorexia is lack of a desire to eat despite physiologic stimuli that would normally produce hunger. Anorexia is a nonspecific symptom that is often associated with nausea, abdominal pain, and diarrhea. Disorders of other organ systems, including cancer, heart disease, and renal disease, are often accompanied by anorexia (see p. 1412 for a discussion of anorexia nervosa).

Vomiting

Vomiting is the forceful emptying of stomach and intestinal contents (chyme) through the mouth. Several types of intestinal, vagal, or sympathetic stimuli initiate the vomiting reflex, including the presence of ipecac or copper salts in the duodenum; severe pain; distention of the stomach or duodenum; torsion or trauma affecting the ovaries, testes, uterus, bladder, or kidney; and activation of the chemoreceptor trigger zone in the medulla. 5-Hydroxytryptamine (5-HT, i.e., serotonin) stimulates the emetic center and appears to be released from enterochromaffin cells in the intestinal wall and possibly from neurons in the brain stem.[1-3] 5-HT receptor antagonists are effective antiemetics and have been used to treat nausea and vomiting associated with chemotherapy (i.e., ondansetron and granisetron). Dopamine (D_2) receptors also play a role in mediating vomiting. Apomorphine, levodopa, and bromocriptine are domamine D_2 agonists and cause nausea and vomiting. Metoclopramide, domperidone, and haloperidol are dopamine D_2 antagonists and are effective antiemetics.

Nausea and retching usually precede vomiting. **Nausea** is a subjective experience that is associated with many different conditions, including visceral pain, labyrinthine stimulation (i.e., motion). Specific neural pathways have not been identified for nausea. Hypersalivation and tachycardia are common associated symptoms. **Retching** begins with deep inspiration. The glottis closes, intrathoracic pressure falls, and the esophagus becomes distended. Simultaneously the abdominal muscles contract, creating a pressure gradient from abdomen to thorax. The lower esophageal sphincter and body of the stomach relax, but the duodenum and antrum of the stomach go into spasm. The reverse peristalsis and pressure gradient force chyme from the stomach and duodenum up into the esophagus. Because the upper esophageal sphincter is closed, chyme does not enter the mouth. As the abdominal muscles relax, the contents of the esophagus drop back into the stomach. This process may be repeated several times before vomiting occurs. A diffuse sympathetic discharge causes the tachycardia, tachypnea, and sweating that accompany retching and vomiting. The parasympathetic system mediates copious salivation, increased gastric motility, and relaxation of the upper and lower esophageal sphincters.

Vomiting usually follows retching. The duodenum and antrum of the stomach produce retrograde peristalsis while the body of the stomach and esophagus relax. When the stomach is full of gastric contents, the diaphragm is forced high into the thoracic cavity by strong contractions of the abdominal muscles. The higher intrathoracic pressure forces the upper esophageal sphincter to open, and chyme is expelled from the mouth. Then the stomach relaxes and the upper part of the esophagus contracts, forcing the remaining chyme back into the stomach. The lower esophageal sphincter then closes. The cycle is repeated if there is a volume of chyme remaining in the stomach.

Spontaneous vomiting that is not preceded by nausea or retching is called **projectile vomiting.** Projectile vomiting is caused by direct stimulation of the vomiting center by neurologic lesions (e.g., tumors, aneurysms) involving the brain stem. The metabolic consequences of vomiting are fluid, electrolyte, and acid-base disturbances (see Chapter 3).

Constipation

Constipation is difficult or infrequent defecation and is estimated to affect 2% to 28% of the population.[4] Constipation must be individually defined because patterns of bowel evacuation differ greatly among individuals. Constipation usually means a decrease in the number of bowel movements per week, hard stools, and difficult evacuation. Normal bowel habits range from two or three evacuations per day to one per week. Constipation is not significant until it causes health risks or impairs quality of life.

PATHOPHYSIOLOGY Constipation can be caused by neurogenic disorders of the large intestine in which neurotransmitters are altered or neural pathways are absent or degenerated.[5] An example is Hirschsprung disease (congenital megacolon)—the absence of ganglion cells in the myenteric plexus of the large intestine. Constipation is usually evident from birth, because the colon is incapable of the propulsive movements that move feces into the rectum (see Chapter 40). Other disorders associated with constipation include acquired megacolon (enlarged or dilated colon), pelvic hiatal hernia, multiple sclerosis, spinal cord trauma, and cerebrovascular disease (Box 39-1).

Many functional or mechanical conditions can slow intestinal transit time. Muscle weakness or pain caused by abdominal surgery can impair or inhibit defecation. Normally the abdominal muscles are used to create the intraabdominal pressure required to evacuate the rectum. Weakness or pain can interfere with the generation of adequate intraabdominal pressure. Lesions of the anus, such as inflamed hemorrhoids, fissures, or fistulae, make defecation painful because of stretching. With the urge to defecate, the sphincter becomes hypertonic, and the stool is not eliminated.

A low-residue diet (the habitual consumption of highly refined foods) decreases the volume and number of stools and causes constipation. Increased consumption of cereals, fruits, and vegetables adds nonabsorbable fiber to the feces and is conducive to regular and easy evacuations.

Box 39-1	Causes of Constipation

Megacolon (enlarged or dilated colon)
Pelvic floor dyssynergia
Abdominal muscle weakness
Painful anal lesions
Low-residue diet
Sedentary life-style
Delayed spontaneous defecation
Emotional depression
Selected drugs
   Opiates
   Anticholinergics
   Antacids (calcium carbonate, aluminum hydroxide)
Systemic diseases
   Hypothyroidism
   Diabetic neuropathy

A sedentary life-style and lack of regular exercise are common causes of constipation. Lack of access to toilet facilities and consistent suppression of the urge to empty the bowel are other causes. Depression often impairs bowel evacuation, partly because depressed individuals tend to be sedentary and lack the motivation to eat a healthy diet. The problem is made worse if antidepressant drugs (e.g., anticholinergics) are used to treat the depression. Anticholinergics block parasympathetic impulses in the gastrointestinal tract, thereby impairing motility.

Excessive use of antacids containing calcium carbonate or aluminum hydroxide often results in constipation. Opiates, particularly codeine, tend to inhibit bowel motility.

CLINICAL MANIFESTATIONS   Changes in bowel evacuation patterns—such as less frequent defecation, smaller stool volume, difficulty in evacuating the rectum, or a feeling of bowel fullness and discomfort—require investigation.

EVALUATION AND TREATMENT   The individual's medical history, physical examination, and stool diaries provide precise clues regarding the nature of constipation. Functional constipation (i.e., constipation resulting from life-style or bowel habits) usually has a long history. Dysfunctional constipation is more likely to be sudden. Sudden-onset constipation can accompany the development of organic lesions and requires careful evaluation.

The Rome 2 criteria for constipation includes two of the following criteria occurring for 12 weeks (consecutive not required) in the previous 12 months:[4]

1. Straining
2. Lumpy or hard stool
3. Sensation of incomplete evacuation
4. Sensation of anorectal blockage/obstruction
5. Less than three bowel movements per week

The individual's description of frequency, stool consistency, associated pain, and presence of blood is significant. Blood may be present as a result of bleeding hemorrhoids or a neoplastic lesion of the colon. Cramping abdominal pain may be symptomatic of partial bowel obstruction. In assessing frequency, it is important to discover whether evacuation was stimulated by enemas or cathartics (laxatives). Palpation discloses colonic distention, masses, and tenderness. Stool transit time is evaluated. Digital examination of the rectum is performed to assess sphincter tone and detect anal lesions. Proctosigmoidoscopy is used to visualize the lumen directly. A barium enema may be required if no lesions are directly visualized and symptoms continue after simple treatment. Colonic transit studies and anal manometry may be useful.

The treatment for dysfunctional constipation is to manage the underlying lesion or disease. Management of functional constipation likewise depends on its cause. Treatment usually consists of bowel retraining, in which the individual establishes a satisfactory bowel evacuation routine without becoming preoccupied with bowel movements. Biofeedback training can be effective for dyssynergic defecation.[6] Moderate exercise, increased fluid and fiber intake, bulk supplements (e.g., Metamucil, Konsyl), stool softeners, and laxative agents are useful for some individuals. Enemas can be used to establish bowel routine, but they should not be used habitually.

Diarrhea

Diarrhea is an increase in the frequency of defecation and the fluidity, volume, and weight of feces and is often a protective response. Three or more stools per day are considered abnormal. Many factors determine stool volume and consistency, including water content of the colon and the presence of unabsorbed food, unabsorbable material, and intestinal secretions. Stool volume in the normal adult averages less than 200 g/day. Stool volume in children depends on age and size. An infant may pass up to 100 g/day. The adult intestine processes approximately 9 L of luminal content per day; 2 L is ingested, and the remaining 7 L consists of intestinal secretions. Of this volume, 99% of the fluid is absorbed—90% (7 to 8 L) in the small intestine and 9% (1 to 2 L) in the colon. Normally, approximately 150 ml of water is excreted daily in the stool.

PATHOPHYSIOLOGY   Diarrhea in which the volume of feces is increased is called *large-volume diarrhea*. Large-volume diarrhea generally is caused by excessive amounts of water or secretions or both in the intestines. Small-volume diarrhea, in which the volume of feces is not increased, usually results from excessive intestinal motility. The three major mechanisms of diarrhea are osmotic, secretory, and motile.[7] (Specific mechanisms of diarrhea in children are described in Chapter 40.)

In **osmotic diarrhea** a nonabsorbable substance in the intestine draws water into the lumen by osmosis. The excess water and the nonabsorbable substance cause large-volume diarrhea. Magnesium, sulfate, and phosphate are poorly absorbed ions. *Lactase deficiency* is the most common cause of osmotic diarrhea and loss of pancreatic enzymes can be a contributing factor. In this condition the nonabsorbable substance is milk sugar, or lactose. Lactose remains in the intestinal lumen because it is not digested or absorbed (see p. 1403). Excessive ingestion of synthetic, nonabsorbable sug-

---

WHAT'S NEW?   Opioids and Constipation

Opioids can induce constipation because many of the same opioid neurotransmitters located in the brain also are located in the enteric nervous system. There are three classes of opioid receptors: mu, delta, and kappa. They mediate the central analgesic and peripheral actions of opioids. The mu opioid receptors specifically inhibit gut motility. *Methylnaltrexone* and *alvimopan* are specific to mu receptors and can reverse opioid-induced bowel dysfunction without reversing analgesia or cause symptoms of withdrawal.

Data from Holzer P: *Neurosci Lett* 361(1-3):192-195, 2004; Kurz A, Sessler DI: *Drugs* 63(7):649-671, 2003.

ars (e.g., sorbitol) has a similar effect. Osmotic diarrhea disappears when ingestion of the osmotic substance stops.

Secretory diarrhea is a form of large-volume diarrhea caused by excessive mucosal secretion of chloride- or bicarbonate-rich fluid or inhibition of net sodium absorption. Primary causes are bacterial enterotoxins (particularly those released by cholera or strains of *Escherichia coli*) and neoplasms (such as gastrinoma or thyroid carcinoma). These tumors produce hormones that stimulate intestinal secretion.

Large-volume diarrhea also can result from excessive motility of the intestine. The cause is usually a lesion that impairs autonomic control of motility, such as diabetic neuropathy. Excessive motility decreases transit time, mucosal surface contact, and opportunities for fluid absorption. Therefore a larger volume of stool reaches the rectum, producing urgency and frequency of elimination.

Small-volume diarrhea usually is caused by an inflammatory disorder of the intestine, such as ulcerative colitis or Crohn disease. Inflammation of the colon causes cramping pain, urgency, and frequency. Small-volume diarrhea also can be caused by fecal impaction, a severe form of constipation. In that case the diarrhea consists of secretions (mucus and fluid) produced by the colon to lubricate the impacted feces and move it toward the anal canal. These secretions flow around the impaction and cause low-volume, secretory diarrhea.

Motility diarrhea is caused by resection of the small intestine, surgical bypass of an area of the intestine, or fistula formation between loops of intestine. Food is not mixed properly, and there is impaired digestion and increased motility.

CLINICAL MANIFESTATIONS   Diarrhea can be acute or chronic, depending on its cause. Systemic effects of prolonged diarrhea are dehydration, electrolyte imbalance, metabolic acidosis, and weight loss. Manifestations of acute bacterial or viral infection include fever, with or without cramping pain. Fever, cramping pain, and bloody stools accompany diarrhea caused by inflammatory bowel disease. Steatorrhea (fat in the stools) and diarrhea are common signs of malabsorption syndromes.

EVALUATION AND TREATMENT   A thorough history is taken to document the onset and frequency of diarrhea. Exposure to contaminated food or water is indicated if the individual has traveled in foreign countries or areas where drinking water might be contaminated. Iatrogenic diarrhea is suggested if the individual has undergone abdominal radiation therapy, intestinal resection, or treatment with selected drugs (e.g., antibiotics, diuretics, antihypertensives, laxatives).[8] Physical examination helps the clinician to identify underlying systemic disease. Stool culture, examination of stool specimens for blood, abdominal roentgenograms, and intestinal biopsies provide more specific data.

Treatment for diarrhea includes restoration of fluid and electrolyte balance, management of distressing symptoms, and treatment of causal factors. In older adults and children, dehydration and electrolyte imbalance may be severe and re-

quire intravenous fluid therapy. Nutritional deficiencies need to be corrected in cases of chronic diarrhea or malabsorption. Substances that solidify stools decrease frequency and water content. Natural bran and commercial preparations of psyllium, such as Konsyl and Metamucil, are inexpensive and effective treatments for mild diarrhea. Opium alkaloids such as Lomotil suppress motility, relieve cramping, and reduce stool volume and frequency.

Abdominal Pain

Abdominal pain is the presenting symptom of a number of gastrointestinal diseases and is usually associated with tissue injury. (The physiology of pain is described in Chapter 15.) The causal mechanisms of abdominal pain are mechanical, chemical mediators of inflammation, or ischemic. Generally the abdominal organs are not sensitive to mechanical stimuli, such as cutting, tearing, or crushing. These organs are, however, sensitive to stretching and distention, which activate nerve endings in both hollow and solid structures. The onset of pain is associated with rapid distention; gradual distention causes little pain. Traction on the peritoneum caused by adhesions, distention of the common bile duct, or forceful peristalsis resulting from intestinal obstruction causes pain because of increased tension. Capsules that surround solid organs, such as the liver and gallbladder, contain pain fibers that are stimulated by stretching if these organs swell.

Biochemical mediators of the inflammatory response, such as histamine, bradykinin, and serotonin, stimulate organic nerve endings and produce abdominal pain. The edema and vascular congestion that accompany chemical, bacterial, or viral inflammation also cause painful stretching. Obstruction of blood flow from the distention of bowel obstruction or mesenteric vessel thrombosis produces the pain of ischemia, and increased concentrations of tissue metabolites stimulate pain receptors.

Abdominal pain can be parietal (somatic), visceral, or referred. **Parietal pain** arises from the parietal peritoneum. This pain is more localized and intense than visceral pain, which arises from the organs themselves. Nerve fibers from the parietal peritoneum travel with peripheral nerves to the spinal cord, and the sensation of pain corresponds to skin dermatomes T6 and L1. Parietal pain lateralizes because, at any particular point, the parietal peritoneum is innervated from only one side of the nervous system.

Visceral pain arises from a stimulus acting on an abdominal organ. It is usually felt near the midline in the epigastrium (upper midabdomen), midabdomen, or lower abdomen. The pain is poorly localized, is dull rather than sharp, and is difficult to describe. Its location is generally related to the corresponding skin dermatomes of the affected organ. Visceral pain is diffuse and vague because nerve endings in abdominal organs are sparse and multisegmented. Pain arising from the stomach, for example, is experienced as a sensation of fullness, cramping, or gnawing in the midepigastric area.

Referred pain is visceral pain felt at some distance from a diseased or an affected organ. Referred pain is usually well localized and is felt in skin or deeper tissues that share a central afferent pathway with the affected organ. Generally, referred pain develops as the intensity of a visceral pain stimulus increases. Intense gallbladder pain is, for example, referred to the back between the scapulae (shoulder blades). The pain may begin as a vague discomfort in the right epigastric region and then, as inflammation worsens, progress to a sharp, localized, referred pain between the shoulder blades.

Gastrointestinal Bleeding

Numerous disorders cause bleeding in the gastrointestinal tract, and the bleeding can occur from more than one site. **Upper gastrointestinal bleeding,** which is defined as bleeding in the esophagus, stomach, or duodenum, is commonly caused by bleeding peptic ulcers. Other causes include esophageal or gastric varices, a Mallory-Weiss tear at the esophageal gastric junction from severe retching, or cancer. **Lower gastrointestinal bleeding**—bleeding below the ligament of Trietz or bleeding from the jejunum, ileum, colon, or rectum—can be caused by polyps, inflammatory disease, diverticulosis, cancer, vascular ectasias, or hemorrhoids. Acute, severe gastrointestinal bleeding is life threatening. Mortality depends on the volume and rate of blood loss, associated disease, age, and effectiveness of treatment.[9,10]

The signs of gastrointestinal bleeding are defined in Table 39-1. Acute blood loss is usually characterized by **hematemesis** (the presence of blood in the vomitus), **hematochezia** (bright red or burgundy blood from the rectum), or **melena** (dark, tarry stools). **Occult bleeding** is usually caused by slow, chronic blood loss that is not obvious and results in iron deficiency anemia as iron stores in the bone marrow are slowly depleted. Physiologic response to gastrointestinal bleeding depends on the amount and rate of the loss (Figure 39-1). Changes in blood pressure and heart rate are the best indicators of massive blood loss in the gastrointestinal tract. Blood losses of 1000 ml or more over a short time cause a decrease in cardiac output, a decrease in systolic and diastolic blood pressure, and an increase in pulse rate. With losses of 1000 ml or more, the heart rate is greater than 100 beats/min and systolic blood pressure is less than 100 mmHg. During the early

stages of blood volume depletion, the peripheral vascular compartment constricts to shunt blood to vital organs, including the brain (see Chapter 29). Signs that this is happening are postural hypotension (a drop in blood pressure that occurs with a change from the recumbent position to a sitting or upright position), light-headedness, and loss of vision. If blood loss continues, hypovolemic shock progresses. Diminished blood flow to the kidneys causes decreased urine output and may lead to oliguria (low urine output), tubular necrosis, and renal failure. Ultimately, insufficient cerebral and coronary blood flow causes irreversible anoxia and death.

The accumulation of blood in the gastrointestinal tract is irritating and increases peristalsis, causing diarrhea. If bleeding is from the lower gastrointestinal tract, the diarrhea is frankly bloody. Bleeding from the upper gastrointestinal tract also can be rapid enough to produce bright red stools, but generally some digestion of the blood components will have occurred, producing melena. The digestion of blood proteins originating from massive upper gastrointestinal bleeding is reflected by an increase in blood urea nitrogen (BUN) levels (see Figure 39-1).

The hematocrit and hemoglobin values are not the best indicators of acute gastrointestinal bleeding because plasma and red cell volume are lost proportionately. As the plasma volume is replaced, the hematocrit and hemoglobin values begin to reflect the extent of blood loss. The interpretation of these values is modified to account for exogenous replacement of fluids and the hydration status of the tissues.

Disorders of Motility
Dysphagia
PATHOPHYSIOLOGY   **Dysphagia** is difficulty swallowing. It can result from mechanical obstruction of the esophagus or a disorder that impairs esophageal motility. *Mechanical obstructions* can be intrinsic or extrinsic. Intrinsic obstructions originate in the wall of the esophageal lumen. Tumors, strictures, and diverticular herniations (outpouchings) are all causes of intrinsic mechanical obstruction. Extrinsic mechanical obstructions originate outside the esophageal lumen and narrow the esophagus by pressing inward on the esophageal

---

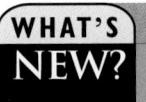

WHAT'S NEW?

Video Capsule Endoscopy and the Small Intestine

The wireless video capsule is an imaging unit that is swallowed and allows noninvasive direct visualization of the complete small intestine. It is particularly effective for diagnosing occult bleeding and lesions of Crohn disease. It is safe and well tolerated by individuals undergoing the procedure. The major limitations are the taking of biopsies, obstructions caused by strictures, and the performance of therapeutic interventions.

Data from Buchman AL et al: *Am J Gastroenterol* 99(11):2171-2177, 2004; Moreno C et al: *Acta Gastroenterol Belg* 68(1):10-14, 2005; Keuchel M, Hagenmuller F: *Endoscopy* 37(2):122-32, 2005

Table 39-1	Presentations of Gastrointestinal Bleeding	
Presentation	**Definition**
Acute bleeding	
Hematemesis	Bloody vomitus; either fresh, bright red blood or dark, grainy, digested blood with "coffee grounds" appearance
Melena	Black, sticky, tarry, foul-smelling stools caused by digestion of blood in the gastrointestinal tract
Hematochezia	Fresh, bright red blood passed from the rectum
Occult bleeding	Trace amounts of blood in normal-appearing stools or gastric secretions; detectable only with a guaiac test

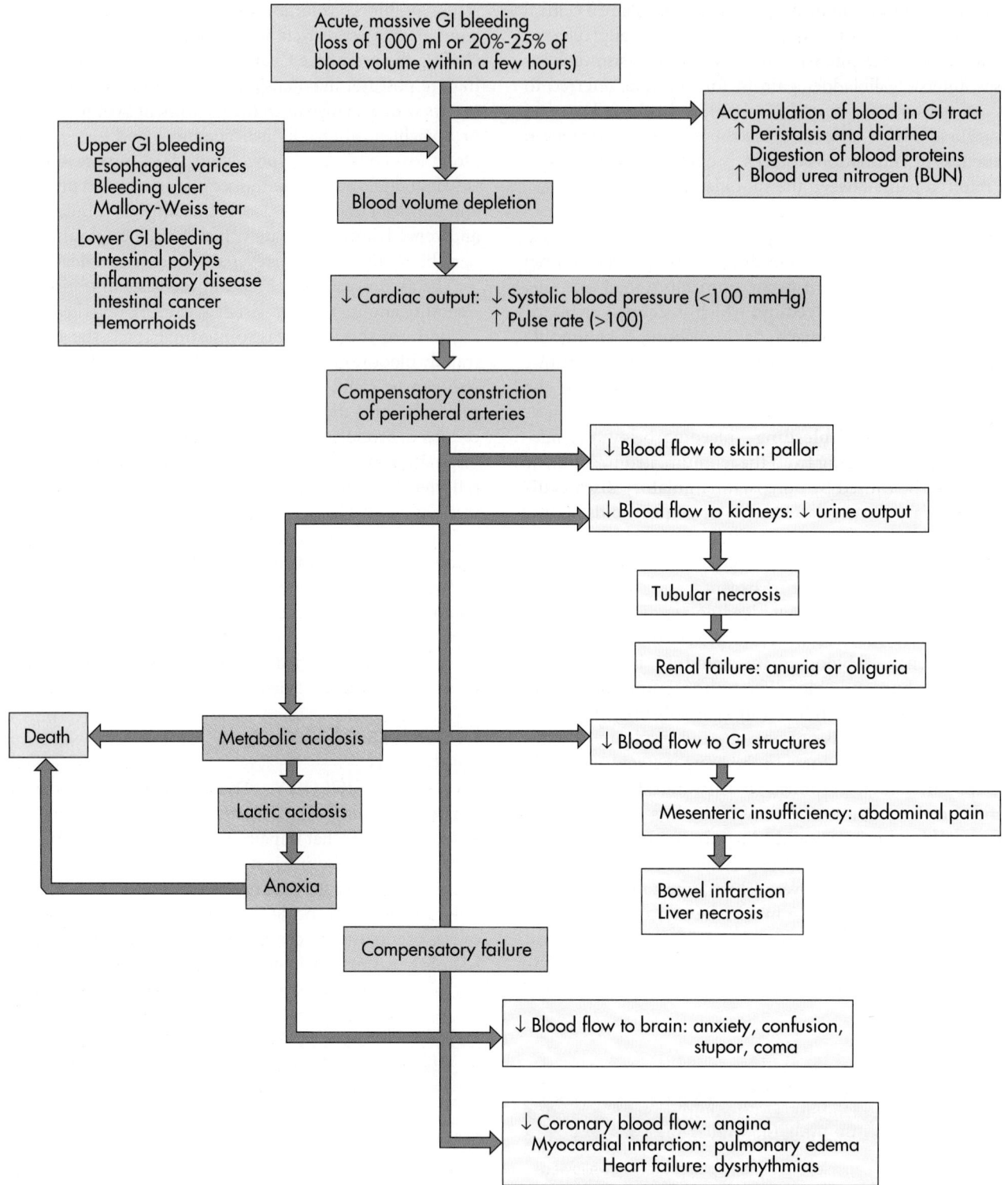

Figure 39-1 Pathophysiology of gastrointestinal (GI) bleeding.

wall. The most common cause of extrinsic mechanical obstruction is tumor.

Functional dysphagia is caused by neural or muscular disorders that interfere with voluntary swallowing or peristalsis. Disorders that affect the striated muscles of the upper esophagus interfere with the oropharyngeal (voluntary) phase of swallowing. Typical causes of functional dysphagia in the upper esophagus are dermatomyositis (a muscle disease) and neurologic impairments caused by cerebrovascular accidents, Parkinson disease, or achalasia.[11]

Achalasia is a rare disorder related to (1) denervation of smooth muscle in the middle and lower portions of the esophagus, and (2) lower esophageal sphincter (LES) relaxation.[12] Achalasia results from neural dysfunction, probably a decrease in the number of myenteric ganglion cells and atrophy of smooth muscle cells. Disrupted innervation results in loss of neuromuscular coordination and muscle tone at the lower end of the esophagus. The three mechanisms that impair swallowing are decreased peristalsis of the middle esophagus, loss of tone in the LES, and decreased relaxation of the LES after swallowing. Food accumulates above the obstruction and distends the esophagus (Figure 39-2). As hydrostatic pressure increases, food is slowly forced past the obstruction into the stomach.

CLINICAL MANIFESTATIONS   Clinical manifestations of dysphagia vary according to the cause and location of the obstruction. Distention and spasm of the esophageal muscles during eating or drinking may cause a mild or severe stabbing pain at the level of obstruction. Discomfort occurring 2 to 4 seconds after swallowing is associated with upper esophageal obstruction. Discomfort occurring 10 to 15 seconds after swallowing is more common in obstructions of the lower esophagus. If the cause of obstruction is a growing tumor, dysphagia begins with difficulty swallowing solids and advances to difficulty swallowing semisolids and liquids.[13] Dysphagia is experienced with both solids and liquids if the cause is loss of motor function. Regurgitation of undigested food, unpleasant taste, vomiting, and weight loss are common manifestations of all types of dysphagia. Aspiration of esophageal contents can lead to pneumonia.

EVALUATION AND TREATMENT   Knowledge of the individual's history and clinical manifestations contributes significantly to a diagnosis of dysphagia. A barium swallow is used to visualize the contours of the esophagus and identify structural defects. Manometry documents the duration and amplitude of abnormal pressure changes associated with obstruction or loss of neural regulation. Esophageal endoscopy is performed to examine the esophageal mucosa and obtain biopsy specimens.

The individual is taught to manage symptoms by eating slowly, eating small meals, taking fluid with meals, and sleeping with the head elevated to prevent regurgitation and aspiration. Anticholinergic drugs, such as dicyclomine (Bentyl), or botulinum toxin (inhibits acetylcholine) may alleviate achalasia.[14] Definitive treatments include mechanical dilation of the esophageal sphincter and surgical separation of the lower esophageal muscles with a longitudinal incision (myotomy). Myotomy widens the passage into the stomach.

Gastroesophageal Reflux Disease (GERD)

Gastroesophageal reflux is the reflux of chyme from the stomach to the esophagus. The LES may relax spontaneously and transiently 1 to 2 hours after eating, permitting gastric contents to regurgitate into the esophagus. The acid is usually neutralized and cleared from the esophagus by peristaltic action within 1 to 3 minutes, and sphincter tone is restored. Gastroesophageal reflux that does not cause symptoms is known as *physiologic reflux*. In some individuals, however, a combination of factors causes injury and an inflammatory response to reflux called **reflux esophagitis**.

PATHOPHYSIOLOGY   Normally the resting tone of the LES maintains a zone of high pressure that prevents gastroesophageal reflux. In individuals who develop reflux esophagitis, this pressure tends to be lower than normal from either transient relaxation or weakness of the sphincter. Vomiting, coughing, lifting, or bending that increases abdominal pressure can contribute to the development of reflux esophagitis. The severity of the esophagitis depends on the composition of the gastric contents, the length of time they are in contact with the esophageal mucosa, and epithelial resistance to acid.[15] If the chyme is highly acidic or contains bile salts and pancreatic enzymes, reflux esophagitis can be severe. In individuals with weak esophageal peristalsis, refluxed chyme remains in the esophagus longer than usual. This increases the amount of time the esophageal mucosa is exposed to acids, pepsin, bile, and enzymes. The presence of *H. pylori* in lowering the prevalence of reflux disease is controversial, with some studies reporting that cagA strains lower risk of GERD.[16] However, there is uncertainty about the possible negative effect of eradicating *H. pylori* infection on gastroesophageal reflux disease and esophageal adenocarcinoma and in relation to treatment with proton pump inhibitors.[17-19] The presence of hiatal hernia contributes to reflux. Finally, delayed gastric emptying contributes to reflux esophagitis by (1) lengthening the period during which reflux is possible, and (2) increasing the acid content of chyme. Disorders that delay emptying include gastric or duodenal ulcers, which can cause pyloric edema; strictures that narrow the pylorus; and hiatal hernia, which can weaken the LES.[20]

Reflux esophagitis causes inflammatory responses in the esophageal wall, such as hyperemia, increased capillary per-

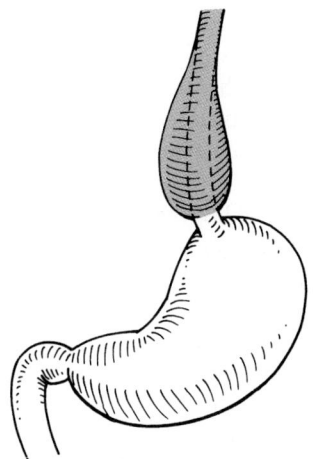

Figure 39-2 Achalasia. Decreased muscle tone and peristaltic function prevent food from entering the stomach, causing esophageal distention. (From Phipps WP et al: *Medical-surgical nursing: concepts and clinical practice*, ed 4, St Louis, 1991, Mosby.)

meability, edema, tissue fragility, erosion, and ulcerations (Figure 39-3). Fibrosis, basal cell hyperplasia, and elongation of papillae are common.[21] Precancerous lesions (Barrett esophagus) can be a long-term consequence.[22]

CLINICAL MANIFESTATIONS   The clinical manifestations of reflux esophagitis are heartburn, regurgitation of acidic chyme, and upper abdominal pain within 1 hour of eating. The symptoms worsen if the individual lies down or if intraabdominal pressure increases (e.g., as a result of coughing, vomiting, or straining at stool). Symptoms may be present when no acid is in the esophagus.[21] Heartburn also may be experienced as chest pain, which requires ruling-out cardiac ischemia. Edema, fibrosis (strictures), esophageal spasm, or decreased esophageal motility may result in dysphagia. Alcohol or acid-containing foods, such as citrus fruits, can cause discomfort during swallowing. There also is an association between acid reflux, laryngitis, asthma, and chronic cough.[23,24]

EVALUATION AND TREATMENT   Diagnosis of reflux esophagitis is based on the history and clinical manifestations, which are usually chronic and relapsing. Esophageal endoscopy shows edema and erosion, and allows for evaluation of dysplastic changes (Barrett esophagus) and the development of esophageal carcinoma. Ambulatory pH monitoring evaluates acidity near the LES. A barium swallow may be used to identify associated conditions, such as hiatal hernia, gastric ulcers, and abnormal contours of the esophageal lumen.

Antacids relieve symptoms by neutralizing gastric contents. Elevation of the head of the bed 6 inches prevents reflux. Weight reduction and cessation of smoking also help to alleviate symptoms. Proton pump inhibitors are more effective than H_2 receptor antagonists or prokinetics for severe dis-

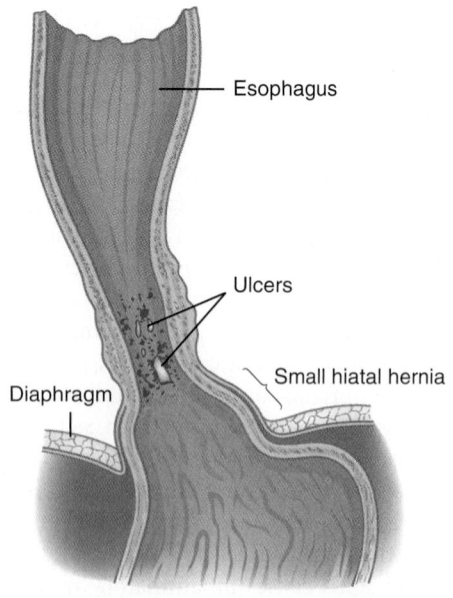

Figure 39-3 Esophagitis with esophageal ulcerations.

(Image labels: Esophagus; Ulcers; Small hiatal hernia; Diaphragm)

ease.[25] Laparoscopic fundoplication is the most common surgical treatment.[26]

Hiatal Hernia

PATHOPHYSIOLOGY   **Hiatal hernia,** a type of diaphragmatic hernia, is the protrusion (herniation) of the upper part of the stomach through the diaphragm and into the thorax. The two types of hiatal hernia are (1) sliding (direct) hiatal hernia, and (2) paraesophageal (rolling) hiatal hernia (Figure 39-4). In **sliding hiatal hernia** (the most common type, 90%) the stomach slides or moves into the thoracic cavity through the esophageal hiatus, an opening in the diaphragm for the esophagus and vagus nerves. A congenitally short esophagus, trauma, or weakening of the diaphragmatic muscles at the gastroesophageal junction contributes to the hernia. While the individual is in the supine position, the lower esophagus and stomach are pulled into the thorax. Standing causes the stomach to "slide" back into the abdomen. Sliding hiatal hernia is exacerbated by factors that increase intraabdominal pressure. Therefore coughing, bending, tight clothing, ascites, obesity, or pregnancy accentuates the hernia. This type of hernia is associated with gastroesophageal reflux and esophagitis because the hernia diminishes the resting pressure of the LES. In pregnant women with sliding hiatal hernia, progesterone and estrogen may lower the resting pressure of the LES further.

Paraesophageal hiatal hernia (rolling hiatal hernia) is herniation of the greater curvature of the stomach through a secondary opening in the diaphragm (see Figure 39-4). The entire stomach can pass into the thorax. As the stomach protrudes through the opening into the thorax, it lies alongside the esophagus. The gastroesophageal junction remains below the diaphragm. With paraesophageal hernia, reflux is uncommon. The position of a portion of the stomach above the diaphragm, however, causes congestion of mucosal blood flow and can lead to gastritis and ulcer formation. A mechanical strangulation of the hernia is a major complication, and surgical correction is required. Strangulation occludes blood vessels and causes vascular engorgement, edema, ischemia, and hemorrhage. Hiatal hernias of both types tend to occur in conjunction with several other diseases, including reflux, peptic ulcer, cholecystitis (gallbladder inflammation), cholelithiasis (gallstones), chronic pancreatitis, and diverticulosis.

CLINICAL MANIFESTATIONS   Hiatal hernias are often asymptomatic. Generally a wide variety of symptoms develop later in life and are associated with other gastrointestinal disorders as well. Manifestations of the various types of hiatal hernia are difficult to distinguish and include gastroesophageal reflux, dysphagia, heartburn, and epigastric pain.[27] Regurgitation and substernal discomfort after eating are common.

EVALUATION AND TREATMENT   Diagnostic procedures include barium roentgenogram and endoscopy. A chest roentgenogram often will show the protrusion of the stomach into the thorax, indicating paraesophageal hiatal hernia.

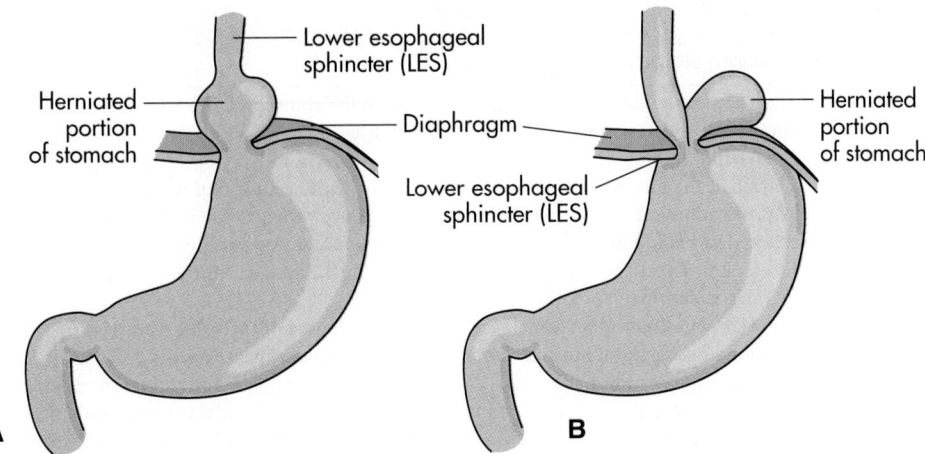

Figure 39-4 Types of hiatal hernia. **A,** In sliding hiatal hernia the visceral peritoneum remains intact and restrains the size of the hernia. **B,** In paraesophageal hernia the membrane becomes thinned out or defective, allowing a true peritoneal sac to protrude into the posterior mediastinum, where negative intrathoracic pressure causes it to enlarge. (From Phipps WP et al: *Medical-surgical nursing: concepts and clinical practice,* ed 7, St Louis, 2003, Mosby.)

Treatment for sliding hiatal hernia is usually conservative. The individual can diminish reflux by eating small, frequent meals and avoiding the recumbent position after eating. Abdominal supports and tight clothing are avoided, and weight control is recommended for obese individuals. Antacids alleviate reflux esophagitis. Anticholinergic drugs are contraindicated because they relax the LES and delay gastric emptying. Individuals who are uncomfortable at night benefit from sleeping in a semi-Fowler position. Surgery (fundoplication) may be performed for paraesophageal hiatal hernia or if medical management fails to control symptoms.[28]

Pyloric Obstruction

PATHOPHYSIOLOGY   **Pyloric obstruction** is the narrowing or blocking of the opening between the stomach and the duodenum. This condition can be congenital (see Chapter 40) or acquired. Acquired obstruction is caused by peptic ulcer disease or carcinoma near the pylorus. Duodenal ulcers are more likely than gastric ulcers to obstruct the pylorus. Ulceration causes obstruction resulting from inflammation, edema, spasm, fibrosis, or scarring. Tumors cause obstruction by growing into the pylorus.

CLINICAL MANIFESTATIONS   Early in the course of pyloric obstruction, the individual experiences vague epigastric fullness, which becomes more distressing after eating and later in the day. Nausea and epigastric pain may occur as the muscles of the stomach contract in attempts to force chyme past the obstruction. These symptoms disappear when the chyme finally moves into the duodenum. As obstruction progresses, anorexia develops, sometimes accompanied by weight loss. Severe obstruction causes gastric distention and atony (lack of muscle tone and gastric motility). Gastric distention stimulates gastric secretion, which increases the feeling of fullness. Rolling or jarring of the abdomen produces a sloshing sound called the *succussion splash.* At this stage, vomiting is a cardinal sign of obstruction. It is usually copious and occurs several hours after eating. The vomitus contains undigested food but no bile. Prolonged vomiting leads to dehydration, which is accompanied by a hypokalemic and hypochloremic metabolic alkalosis caused by loss of potassium and gastric acid. Because food does not enter the intestine, stools are infrequent and small. Prolonged pyloric obstruction causes malnutrition, dehydration, and extreme debilitation.

EVALUATION AND TREATMENT   Diagnosis is based on clinical manifestations, a history of ulcer disease, and examination of residual gastric contents. Endoscopy is performed if gastric carcinoma is the suggested cause of pyloric obstruction. Barium studies are contraindicated because the barium may harden and be retained in the stomach.

Obstructions resulting from ulceration often resolve with conservative management. Gastric drainage is used to decompress the stomach and restore normal motility. Gastric secretions that contribute to inflammation and edema can be suppressed with omeprazole or cimetidine. Fluids and electrolytes (saline and potassium) are given intravenously to effect rehydration and correct hypokalemia and alkalosis (see Chapter 3). Severely malnourished individuals may require parenteral hyperalimentation (intravenous nutrition). Surgery may be required to treat gastric carcinoma or persistent obstruction caused by fibrosis and scarring.[29]

Intestinal Obstruction and Ileus

Intestinal obstruction can be caused by any condition that prevents the normal flow of chyme through the intestinal lumen or failure of normal intestinal motility in the absence of an obstructing lesion (ileus). Common causes of intestinal obstruction are summarized in Table 39-2. More specific causes of small and large bowel obstruction are summarized in Table 39-3. Criteria for classifying intestinal obstruction are summarized in Table 39-4. Intestinal obstruction is classified by cause as simple or functional. *Simple obstruction* is mechanical blockage of the lumen by a lesion; *functional obstruction* is a

Table 39-2	Common Causes of Intestinal Obstruction
Cause	**Pathophysiology**
Herniation	Protrusion of the intestine through a weakness in the abdominal muscles or through the inguinal ring
Intussusception	Telescoping of one part of the intestine into another; this usually causes strangulation of the blood supply; more common in the ileocecal area in infants 10-15 months of age than in adults
Torsion(volvulus)	Twisting of the intestine on its mesenteric pedicle, with occlusion of the blood supply; often associated with fibrous adhesions in the small intestine; occurs most often in the large intestine in the elderly
Diverticulosis	Inflamed saccular herniations (diverticuli) of the mucosa and submucosa through the tunica muscularis of the colon; diverticuli are interspersed between thick, circular, fibrous bands; most common in obese individuals older than 60 years
Tumor	Tumor growth into the intestinal lumen; adenocarcinoma of the colon and rectum is the most common tumoral obstruction; most common in individuals older than 60 years
Paralytic (adynamic) ileus	Loss of peristaltic motor activity in the intestine; associated with abdominal surgery, peritonitis, hypokalemia, ischemic bowel, spinal trauma, or pneumonia; affects both small and large intestine
Fibrous adhesions	Peritoneal irritation from surgery or trauma leads to formation of fibrin and adhesions that attach to intestine, omentum, or peritoneum and can cause obstruction; most common in small intestine

Table 39-3	Large and Small Bowel Obstruction
Cause	**Pathophysiology**
Small bowel obstruction	Adhesions: secondary to previous abdominal surgeries—50%-70%
	Hernia: inguinal, ventral, or femoral—20%-25%
	Tumors: may be associated with intussception—10%
	Mesenteric ischemia 3%-5%
Large bowel obstruction	Colon/rectal cancer—90%
	Volvulus—4%-5%
	Diverticular disease—3%
	Other causes (inflammatory bowel disease, adhesions, hernia)

From Feldman M et al: *Sleisenger & Fordtran's gastrointestinal liver disease*, ed 7, Philadelphia, 2003, Saunders; Moses BV: Surgical corrections of the small intestine.

failure of motility (paralytic ileus). Simple obstruction of the small intestine from fibrous adhesions is the most common type of intestinal obstruction. Acute obstructions usually have mechanical causes, such as adhesions or hernias. Chronic or partial obstructions are more often associated with tumors or inflammatory disorders, particularly of the large intestine. Intussusception is rare in adults compared to the more frequent occurrence in infants. Common causes of intestinal obstruction in children are presented in Chapter 40.

PATHOPHYSIOLOGY The consequences of intestinal obstruction are related to its onset and location, the length of intestinal tract proximal to the obstruction, and the presence and severity of ischemia. The major pathophysiologic alterations are presented in Figure 39-5. *Small intestinal obstruction* leads to accumulation of fluid and gas inside the lumen proximal to the obstruction. Fluids accumulate from impaired water and electrolyte absorption and enhanced secretion with net movement of fluid from the vascular space to

the intestinal lumen. Gas from swallowed air, and to a lesser extent from bacterial overgrowth, contribute to the distention. Distention begins almost immediately, as gases and fluids accumulate proximal to the obstruction. Distention decreases the intestine's ability to absorb water and electrolytes and increases the net secretion of these substances into the lumen. Within 24 hours, up to 8 L of fluid and electrolytes enters the lumen in the form of saliva, gastric juice, bile, pancreatic juice, and intestinal secretions. Copious vomiting or sequestration of fluids in the intestinal lumen prevents their reabsorption and produces severe fluid and electrolyte disturbances. Extracellular fluid volume and plasma volume decrease, causing dehydration. Hemoconcentration (decreased plasma volume) elevates hematocrit, decreases central venous pressure, and causes tachycardia. Severe dehydration leads to hypovolemic shock.

If the obstruction is at the pylorus or high in the small intestine, metabolic alkalosis develops initially as a result of excessive loss of hydrogen ions that normally would be reabsorbed from the gastric juice. With prolonged obstruction or obstruction lower in the intestine, metabolic acidosis is more likely to occur because bicarbonate from pancreatic secretions and bile cannot be reabsorbed. Hypokalemia can be extreme, promoting acidosis and atony of the intestinal wall. Metabolic acidosis also may be accentuated by ketosis, the result of declining carbohydrate stores caused by starvation. If pressure from the distention is severe enough, it occludes the arterial circulation and causes ischemia, necrosis, perforation, and peritonitis. Fever and leukocytosis are often associated with strangulation. Lack of circulation permits the buildup of significant amounts of lactic acid, which worsen the metabolic acidosis. Bacterial proliferation and translocation across the mucosa to the mesenteric lymph nodes or systemic circulation causes peritonitis or sepsis.

Consequences of colonic or *large bowel obstruction* are related to the competence of the ileocecal valve, which normally prevents reflux of colonic contents into the small intestine. When the ileocecal valve is competent, the cecum cannot decompress into the small intestine resulting in distention.

Table 39-4	Classification of Intestinal Obstruction	
Criteria for Classification	**Definition**	

Onset

Acute	Sudden onset; often caused by torsion, intussusception, or herniation
Chronic	Protracted onset; more commonly from tumor growth or progressive formation of strictures

Extent of Obstruction

Partial	Incomplete obstruction of intestinal lumen
Complete	Complete obstruction of intestinal lumen

Location of Obstructing Lesion

Intrinsic	Obstruction develops within intestinal lumen; examples: luminal edema or hemorrhage, foreign bodies (gallstones), tumors, or intraluminal fibrosis
Extrinsic	Obstruction originates outside the intestine; examples: tumors, torsion, fibrosis, hernia, intussusception

Effects on Intestinal Wall

Simple	Luminal obstruction without impairment of blood supply
Strangulated	Luminal obstruction with occlusion of blood supply
Closed loop	Obstruction at each end of a segment of the intestine

Causal Factors

Mechanical	Blockage of the intestinal lumen by intrinsic or extrinsic lesions; usually treated surgically
Functional (paralytic ileus)	Paralysis of the intestinal musculature as a result of trauma, peritonitis, electrolyte imbalances, or spasmolytic agents; usually treated surgically

Ischemia occurs when the intraluminal pressure exceeds capillary pressure in the lumen.

CLINICAL MANIFESTATIONS   Signs and symptoms of small intestinal obstruction are consistent with the pathophysiology. Colicky pains caused by distention followed by vomiting are the cardinal symptoms. Typically the pain occurs intermittently. Pain intensifies for seconds or minutes as a peristaltic wave of muscle contraction meets the obstruction. The passing of the wave is followed by a pain-free interval. With severe distention the pain may diminish in intensity. If strangulation occurs, the pain loses its colicky character, becoming more constant and severe as ischemia progresses to necrosis or perforation. Sweating, nausea, and hypotension occur as an autonomic nervous system response.

Vomiting and distention vary, depending on the level and completion of the obstruction. Obstruction at the pylorus causes early, profuse vomiting of clear gastric fluid. Obstruction in the proximal small intestine causes mild distention and vomiting of bile-stained fluid. Obstruction lower in the small intestine causes more pronounced distention because a greater length of intestine is proximal to the obstruction. In this case, vomiting may not occur or may occur later and contain fecal material. Partial obstruction can cause diarrhea or constipation, but complete obstruction usually causes constipation only. Complete obstruction increases the number of bowel sounds, which may be tinkly and accompanied by peristaltic rushes and crampy, abdominal pain. Signs of dehydration, hypovolemia, and metabolic acidosis may be observed as early as 24 hours after the occurrence of complete obstruction. Distention may be severe enough to push against the diaphragm and decrease lung volume. This can lead to atelectasis and pneumonia, particularly in debilitated individuals.

Colonic obstruction usually presents as hypogastric pain and abdominal distention. Pain can vary from vague to excruciating, depending on the degree of ischemia and the development of peritonitis.

EVALUATION AND TREATMENT   Evaluation is based on clinical manifestations and includes ultrasound and radiography.[30,31] Successful management requires early identification of the site and type of obstruction. Replacement of fluid and electrolytes and decompression of the lumen with gastric or intestinal suction are essential forms of therapy. Immediate surgical intervention is required for strangulation and complete obstruction.

Gastritis

Gastritis is an inflammatory disorder of the gastric mucosa. It can be acute or chronic and can affect the fundus or antrum or both. Acute gastritis erodes the surface epithelium in a diffuse or localized pattern. The erosions are usually superficial.

Acute gastritis is usually injury of the protective mucosal barrier by drugs, chemicals, or *Helicobacter pylori* infection. Nonsteroidal antiinflammatory drugs, such as aspirin, ibuprofen, naproxen, and indomethacin, are known to cause erosive gastritis, perhaps because they inhibit prostaglandins, which normally stimulate the secretion of mucus[32,33] (Figure 39-6). Alcohol, histamine, digitalis, and metabolic disorders such as uremia are contributing factors. *H. pylori* infection causes inflammation, pain, nausea, and vomiting.[34] The clinical manifestations of acute gastritis can include vague abdominal discomfort, epigastric tenderness, and bleeding. Healing usually occurs spontaneously within a few days. Discontinuing injurious drugs, using antacids, or decreasing acid

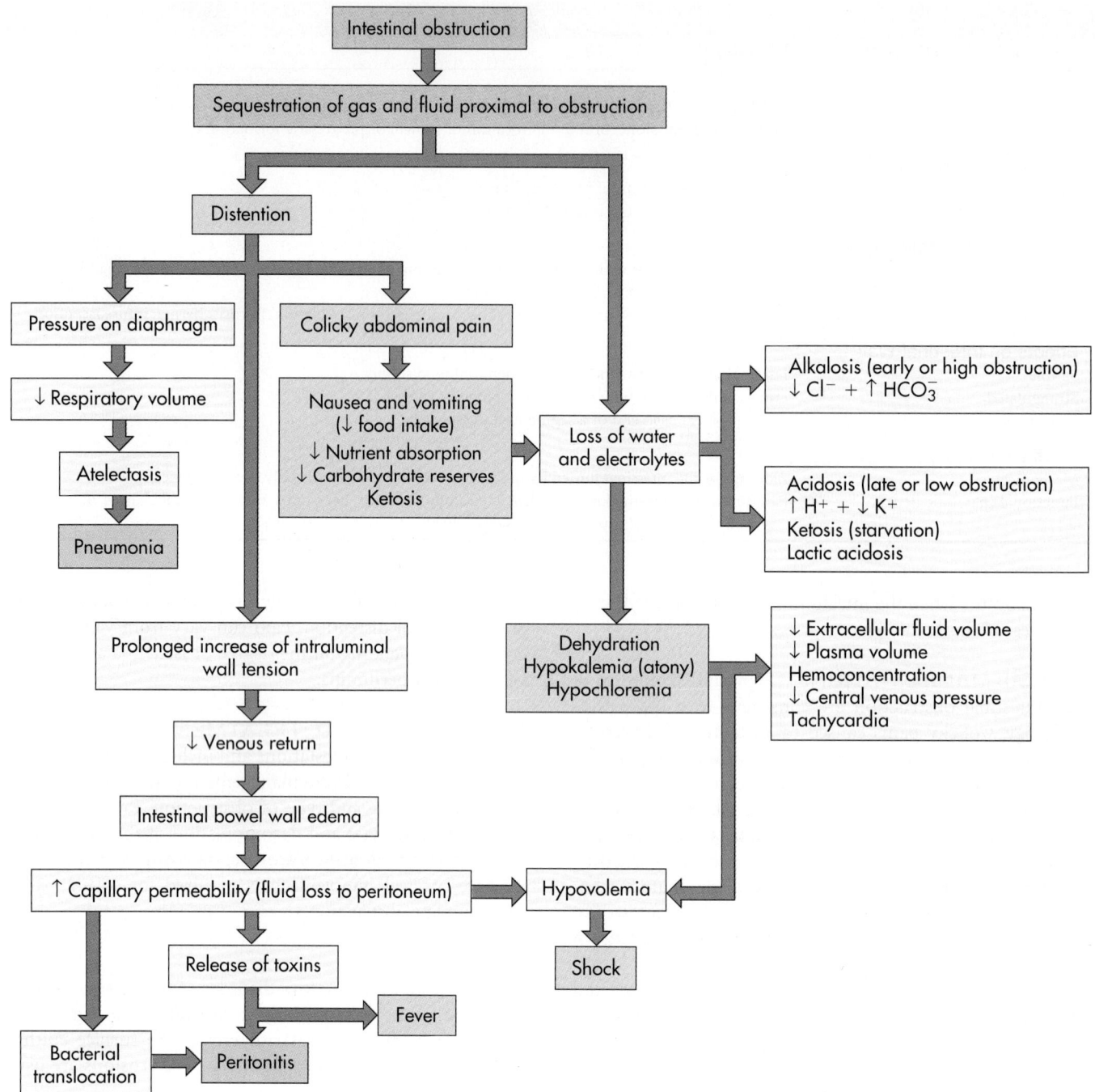

Figure 39-5 Pathophysiology of intestinal obstruction.

secretion with a histamine H_2 receptor antagonist and proton pump inhibitor also promote healing.

Chronic gastritis tends to occur in elderly individuals and causes thinning and degeneration of the stomach wall with atrophy of the gastric epithelium. Chronic gastritis usually is classified as type A, or immune (fundal), or type B, nonimmune (antral), depending on the pathogenesis and location of the lesions. Chronic fundal gastritis is the most rare and severe type. The gastric mucosa degenerates extensively in the body and fundus of the stomach, leading to gastric atrophy. Loss of chief cells and parietal cells diminishes secretion of

pepsinogen, hydrochloric acid, and intrinsic factor. Because acid secretion is insufficient, the feedback mechanism that normally inhibits gastrin secretion is impaired, causing elevated plasma levels of gastrin. Pernicious anemia can develop because intrinsic factor is less available to facilitate vitamin B_{12} absorption.

A significant number of individuals with chronic fundal gastritis have antibodies to parietal cells, intrinsic factor, and gastric cells in their sera, suggesting that an autoimmune mechanism is involved in the pathogenesis of the disease. The fact that chronic fundal gastritis occurs in association with

WHAT'S NEW?   Abdominal Compartment Syndrome

Abdominal compartment syndrome (ACS), also known as *intra-abdominal hypertension*, develops when there is abnormally high intra-abdominal pressure associated with organ dysfunction. ACS is associated with abdominal injury, including trauma, ruptured aortic aneurysm, acute pancreatitis, and massive fluid volume replacement. Increased intra-abdominal pressure increases intrathoracic, intracardiac, and intracranial filling pressures and results in decreased cardiac output, atelectasis, pulmonary edema, oliguria, compromise of spanchnic and hepatic blood flow, and translocation of bacteria from the gut. The end consequence is multiple organ failure.

Normally intra-abdominal pressure is slightly greater than atmospheric pressure. Organ dysfunction begins to develop at pressures greater than 20 mmHg. Automated monitoring of pressure inside the bladder provides an estimate of intra-abdominal pressure. New techniques of measurement, identification of risk factors, and standards of care are emerging. Treatment is decompressive laparotomy, which may be performed at the bedside if the individual is too unstable to move.

Data from Diaz JJ Jr et al: *Surg Infect (Larchmt)* 5(1):15-20, 2004; Malbrain ML: *Intensive Care Med* 30(3):357-371, 2004; Malbrain ML: *Curr Opin Crit Care* 10(2):132-145, 2004; Malbrain ML et al:, *Intensive Care Med* 30(5):822-829, 2004; Moore AF et al: *Br J Surg* 91(9):1102-1110, 2004.

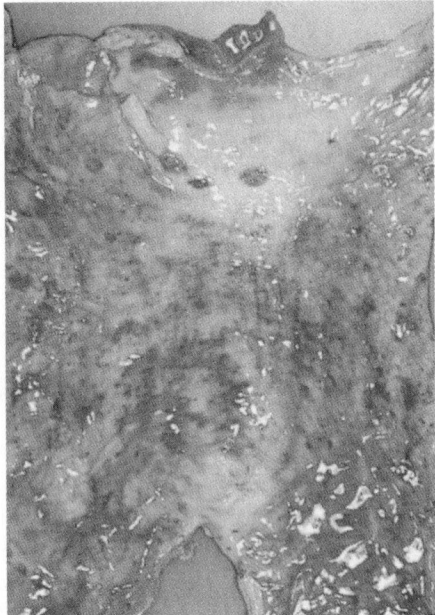

Figure 39-6 **Acute erosive gastritis.** Acute erosive gastritis is shown in the opened stomach. The mucosa appears hyperemic, and the foci of superficial ulceration are manifest as scattered, small, red areas termed erosions. (From Stevens A, Lowe J: *Pathology,* ed 2, London, 2000, Mosby.)

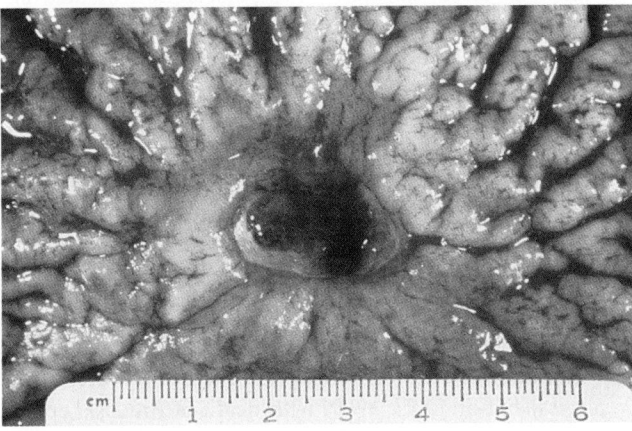

Figure 39-7 **Chronic peptic ulcer.** Gross photograph of a chronic peptic ulcer located in the lesser curvature, straddling the antrum and corpus of the stomach. (From Damjanov I, Linder J, editors: *Anderson's pathology,* ed 10, vol 2, St Louis, 1996, Mosby.)

other autoimmune diseases, such as diabetes, Addison disease, and thyroid disease, strengthens this association. Chronic fundal gastritis is a risk factor for gastric carcinoma, particularly in individuals who develop pernicious anemia.[35,36]

Chronic antral gastritis generally involves the antrum only and is approximately four times more common than fundal gastritis. It is not associated with decreased hydrochloric acid secretion, pernicious anemia, or presence of parietal cell antibodies. Several factors are associated with chronic antral gastritis, including use of alcohol, tobacco, and nonsteroidal anti-inflammatory drugs. *H. pylori* is a major causative factor associated with chronic atrophic antral gastritis. The host response to *H. pylori* infection is activation of T and B lymphocytes with infiltration of neutrophils. Release of inflammatory cytokines (e.g., tumor necrosis factor-α; IL-6. IL-8, and IL-10; and leukotrienes) damage the gastric epithelium.[37-39] In approximately 10% of cases, antibodies to gastrin-secreting cells are found in the serum. Chronic reflux of bile may contribute to the gastritis by persistently disrupting the mucosal barrier.

Signs and symptoms of chronic gastritis often do not correlate with the severity of the disease. Gastroscopic examination and biopsy may show a long-standing inflammatory process and gastric atrophy in an individual with no history of abdominal distress. *H. pylori* infection is evidence for *H. pylori* gastritis. Failure to stimulate acid secretion confirms achlorhydria (diminished secretion of hydrochloric acid). The gastric secretions also can be evaluated for the presence of intrinsic factor. Individuals may report vague symptoms, including anorexia, fullness, nausea, vomiting, and epigastric pain. Gastric bleeding may be the only clinical manifestation of gastritis.

Symptoms usually can be managed with smaller meals; a soft, bland diet; and avoidance of alcohol, aspirin, or other nonsteroidal inflammatory drugs. Antibiotics are used to treat *H. pylori*. Vitamin B_{12} is administered to correct pernicious anemia[40] (see Chapter 26).

Peptic Ulcer Disease

A **peptic ulcer** is a break, or an ulceration, in the protective mucosal lining of the lower esophagus, stomach, or duodenum. Such breaks expose submucosal areas to gastric secretions and autodigestion. Peptic ulcers can be acute or chronic, and superficial or deep. Superficial ulcerations are called *erosions* because they erode the mucosa but do not penetrate the muscularis mucosae (Figure 39-7). True ulcers extend through the muscularis mucosae and damage blood vessels, causing hemorrhage, or perforate the gastrointestinal wall.

Approximately 5 million people in the United States have peptic ulcer disease.[41] Risk factors for peptic ulcer disease are smoking, *H. pylori* infection, and habitual use of nonsteroidal antiinflammatory drugs (NSAIDs) or alcohol. Some chronic diseases, such as emphysema, rheumatoid arthritis, and cirrhosis, are associated with the development of peptic ulcers. Psychologic stress may be a risk factor for peptic ulcer disease, although studies of life stress and ulcer disease are inconclusive.[42] Individuals with multiple stressors, poor coping skills, and persistent anxiety and depression in the presence of recurrent peptic ulcers may require psychiatric management.[43] The exact mechanism of causation is not known.

Duodenal Ulcers

Duodenal ulcers occur with greater frequency than other types of peptic ulcers and affect 10% to 15% of the population.[44] The incidence of duodenal ulcers is approximately the same among men and women in the United States.[45] Duodenal ulcers tend to develop in younger persons and in individuals with type O blood.

PATHOPHYSIOLOGY   Infection with *H. pylori* is a major cause of duodenal ulcers.[46] Hypersecretion of acid and pepsin is a contributing cause, and inadequate secretion of bicarbonate by the duodenal mucosa also may be a factor. Other factors that contribute to ulcer formation are as follows:

1. A greater than usual number of parietal (acid-secreting) cells in the gastric mucosa
2. High serum gastrin levels that remain high longer than normal after eating and continue to stimulate secretion of acid and pepsin (may be caused by *H. pylori*)
3. Failure of the feedback mechanism whereby acid in the gastric antrum inhibits gastrin release
4. Rapid gastric emptying, which overwhelms the buffering capacity of the bicarbonate-rich pancreatic secretions
5. Association of *H. pylori* with death of mucosal epithelial cells and elevated levels of gastrin and pepsinogen
6. *H. pylori* release of toxins and enzymes that promote inflammation and ulceration
7. Use of NSAIDs, which inhibit prostaglandins
8. Acid production stimulated by cigarette smoking
9. Decreased mucosal bicarbonate secretion

All these factors, singly or in combination, cause acid and pepsin concentrations in the duodenum to penetrate the mucosal barrier and cause ulceration[47,48] (Figure 39-8).

CLINICAL MANIFESTATIONS   The characteristic manifestation of a duodenal ulcer is chronic intermittent pain in the epigastric area. The pain begins 30 minutes to 2 hours after eating, when the stomach is empty. It is not unusual for pain to occur in the middle of the night and disappear by morning. The pain results from sensorineural stimulation by acid, muscle spasm, or both. Pain is relieved rapidly by ingestion of food or antacids, creating a typical "pain-food-relief"

pattern. Some individuals with duodenal ulcer have no symptoms, particularly elderly persons; the first manifestation may be hemorrhage or perforation, particularly with a history of NSAID or anticoagulant use.

Duodenal ulcers often heal spontaneously but recur within months. Exacerbations tend to develop in the spring and fall. Healing is accompanied by relief of pain. Constant, unremitting pain may be caused by complications, such as intestinal obstruction or perforation. Bleeding from duodenal ulcers causes hematemesis or melena.

EVALUATION AND TREATMENT   Several diagnostic approaches are used to differentiate duodenal ulcers from gastric ulcers or gastric carcinoma. Barium roentgenograms may show an anatomic deformity created by the ulcer crater. If the roentgenographic examination is inconclusive, flexible endoscopic evaluations may be performed. Radioimmune assays of gastrin levels are evaluated to identify ulcers associated with gastric carcinomas. The urea breath test, stool antigen, and positive findings from gastric biopsy detect *H. pylori* infection.[49]

Management of duodenal ulcers is aimed at relieving the causes and effects of hyperacidity. Antacids neutralize gastric contents, elevate pH, inactivate pepsin, and relieve pain. Acid secretion can be suppressed with drugs (e.g., cimetidine) that block histamine (H2) receptors and inhibit the secretion of acid. Proton pump inhibitors (Omeprazole) inhibit acid production. Therapy with bismuth, metronidazole or clarithromycin, and either amoxicillin or tetracycline for *H. pylori* usually prevents relapse.[50,51] Ulcer-coating agents, such as sucralfate and colloidal bismuth, promote healing. Anticholinergic drugs may be used to inhibit gastric secretion, suppress gastric motility, and delay gastric emptying. Surgical resection may be required for bleeding or perforating ulcers or obstruction.[52] Risk of duodenal ulcer may be reduced with a diet high in vitamin A and fiber.[53] Clinical trials are in progress for a vaccine against *H. pylori*.[54]

Gastric Ulcers

Gastric ulcers are ulcers of the stomach. They occur with about equal frequency in males and females, usually between the ages of 55 and 65 years, and are about one fourth as common as duodenal ulcers (Table 39-5 and Figure 39-9).

PATHOPHYSIOLOGY   Generally gastric ulcers develop in the antral region, adjacent to the acid-secreting mucosa of the body. The primary defect is an abnormality that increases the mucosal barrier's permeability to hydrogen ions. Gastric secretion may be normal or less than normal.

Chronic gastritis is often associated with development of gastric ulcers and may precipitate ulcer formation by limiting the mucosa's ability to secrete a protective layer of mucus (Figure 39-10). Decreased mucosal synthesis of prostaglandin may be one factor causing decreased mucus secretion.[55]

Other factors associated with gastric ulcer development include duodenal reflux of bile and use of ulcerogenic drugs (aspirin and indomethacin). Reflux of bile is caused by loss of

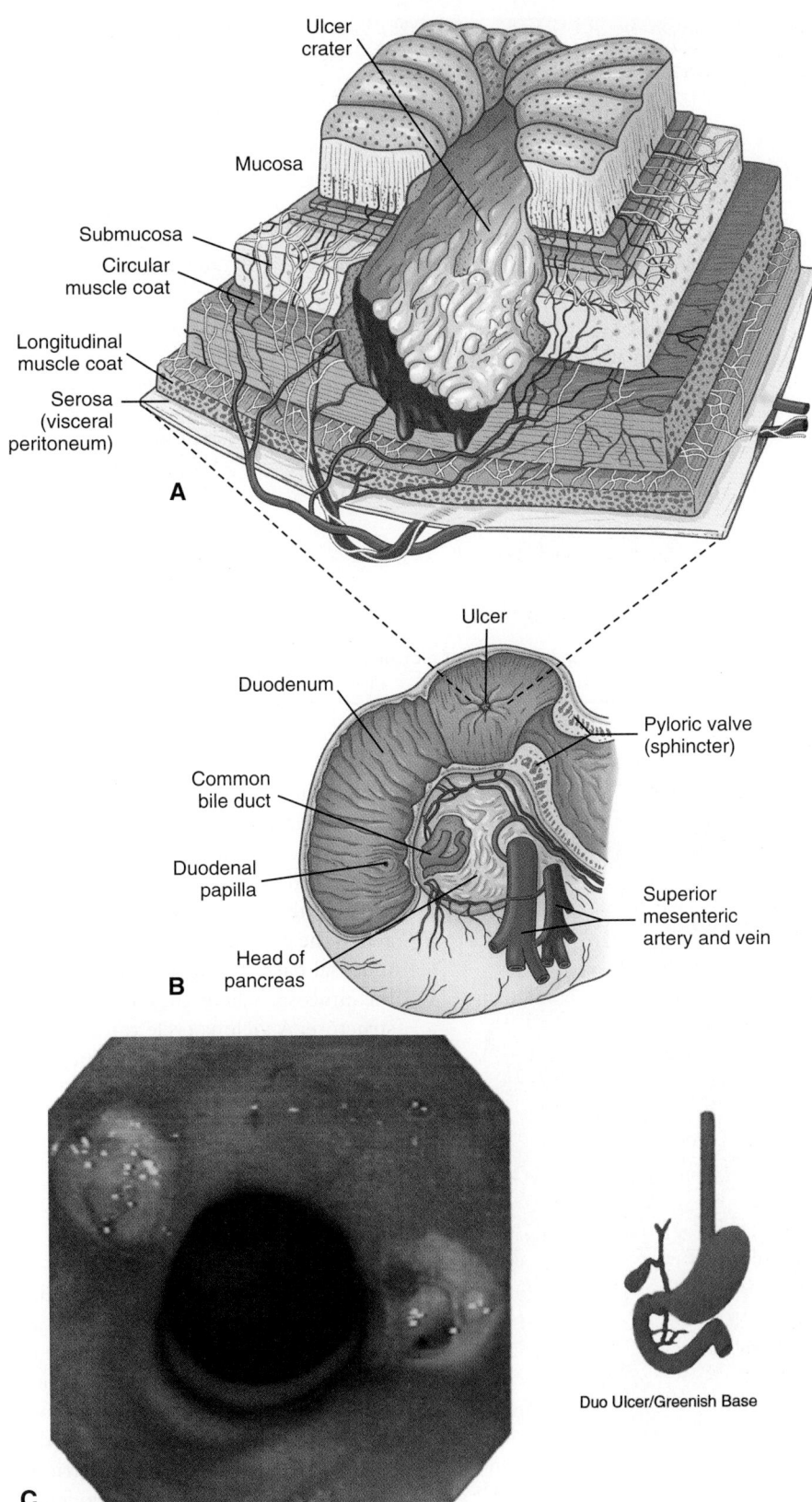

Figure 39-8 Duodenal ulcer. A, A deep ulceration in the duodenal wall extending as a crater through the entire mucosa and into the muscle layers. **B,** Duodenal ulcer. **C,** Bilateral (kissing) duodenal ulcers in a person using nonsteroidal antiinflammatory drugs (NSAIDs). (**C,** Courtesy David Bjorkman, M.D., University of Utah School of Medicine, Department of Gastroenterology.)

Table 39-5	Characteristics of Gastric and Duodenal Ulcers	
Characteristics	**Gastric Ulcer**	**Duodenal Ulcer**
Incidence		
Age at onset	50-70 years	20-50 years
Family history	Usually negative	Positive
Gender (prevalence)	Equal in women and men	Equal in women and men
Stress factors	Increased	Average
Ulcerogenic drugs	Normal use	Increased use
Cancer risk	Increased	Not increased
Pathophysiology		
Abnormal mucus	May be present	May be present
Parietal cell mass	Normal or decreased	Increased
Acid production	Normal or decreased	Increased
Serum gastrin	Increased	Normal
Serum pepsinogen	Normal	Increased
Associated gastritis	More common	Usually not present
Helicobacter pylori	May be present (60%-80%)	Often present (95%-100%)
Clinical Manifestations		
Pain	Located in upper abdomen	Located in upper abdomen
	Intermittent	Intermittent
	Pain-antacid-relief pattern	Pain-antacid or food-relief pattern
	Food-pain pattern	Nocturnal pain common
Clinical course	Chronic ulcer without pattern of remission and exacerbation	Pattern of remissions and exacerbations for years

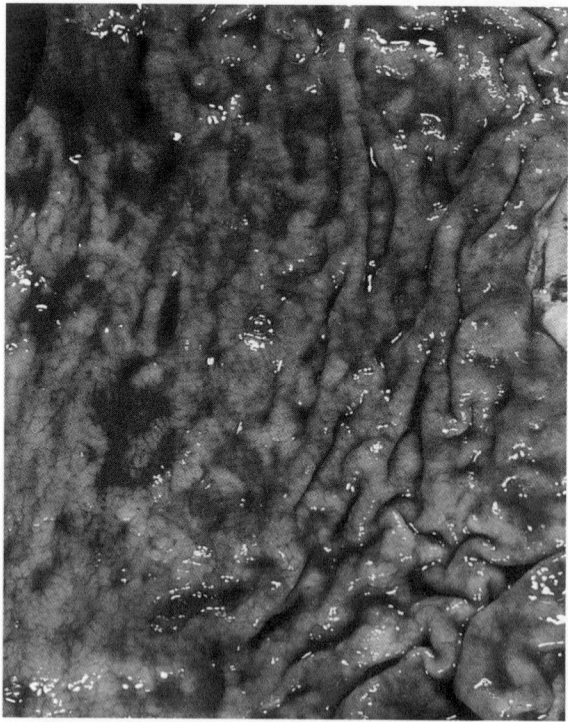

Figure 39-9 Macroscopic appearance of benign gastric ulcers. (From Damjanov I, Linder J, editors: *Anderson's pathology,* vol 2, ed 10, St Louis, 1996, Mosby.)

tone at the pyloric sphincter. The pyloric sphincter may fail to respond to stimuli that normally increase resting tone, such as entry of acid, protein, and fat into the duodenum.

An increased concentration of bile salts disrupts the gastric mucosa; this disruption may decrease the electrical potential across the gastric mucosal membrane. The break damages the mucosal barrier by permitting hydrogen ions to diffuse into the mucosa, where they disrupt permeability and cellular structure. A vicious cycle can be established as the damaged mucosa liberates histamine, which stimulates the increase of acid and pepsinogen production, blood flow, and capillary permeability. The disrupted mucosa becomes edematous and loses plasma proteins. Destruction of small vessels causes bleeding.

CLINICAL MANIFESTATIONS   The clinical manifestations of gastric ulcers are similar to those of duodenal ulcers (see Table 39-5). The pattern of pain, food, and relief is common, but the pain of gastric ulcers also may occur immediately after eating. Another difference is that gastric ulcers tend to be chronic rather than alternate between periods of remission and exacerbation. Gastric ulcers also cause more anorexia, vomiting, and weight loss than duodenal ulcers. The evaluation and treatment of gastric ulcers are similar to the evaluation and treatment of duodenal ulcers.

Stress-Related Mucosal Disease

A **stress ulcer** is an acute form of peptic ulcer that tends to accompany severe illness, systemic trauma, or neural injury. Mental stress may be associated with stress ulcer.[56] Usually,

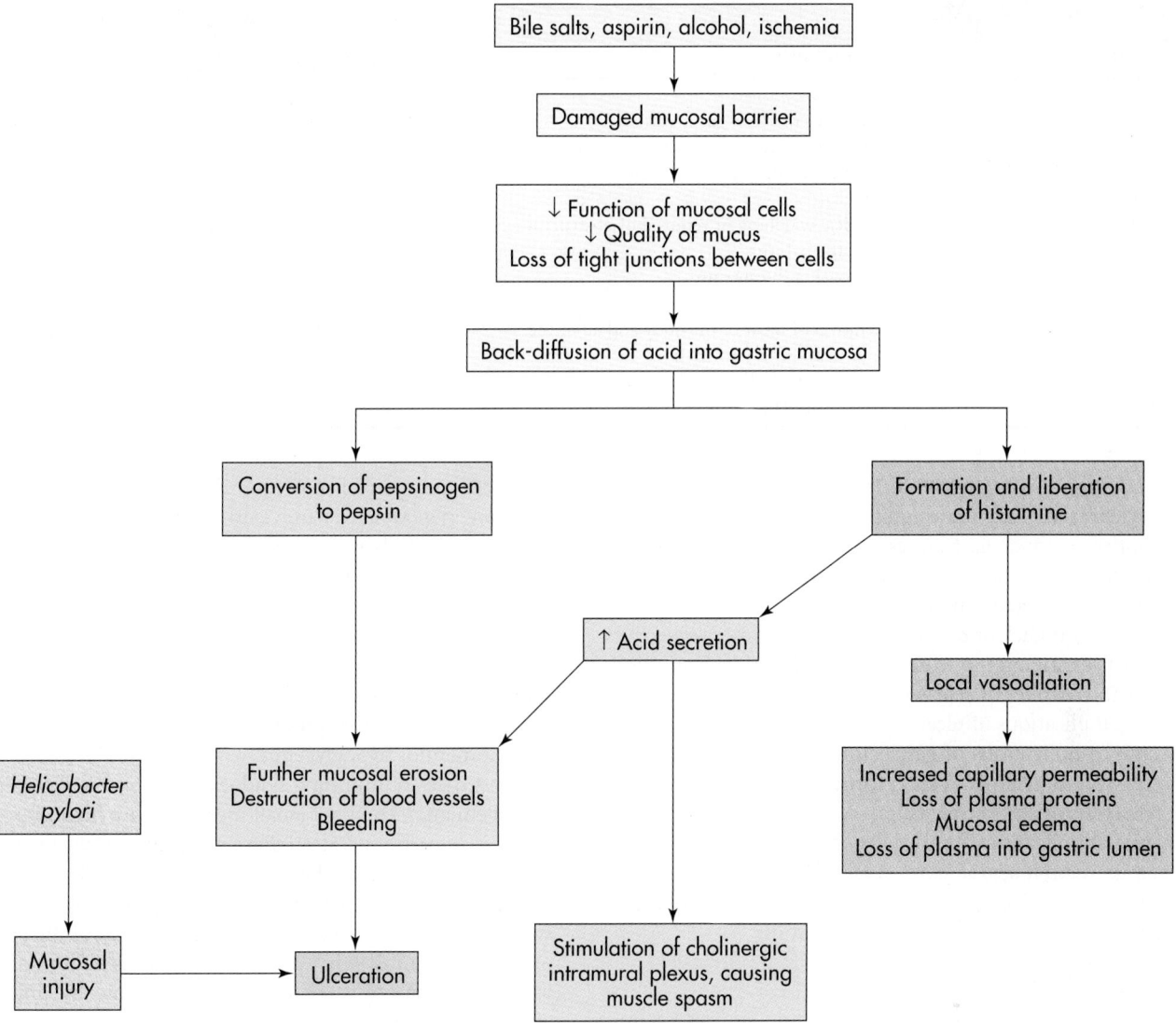

Figure 39-10 Pathophysiology of gastric ulcer formation.

multiple sites of ulceration are distributed within the stomach or duodenum. Decreased mucosal blood flow is an important contributing event in stress ulcer formation.[57] Stress ulcers may be classified as ischemic ulcers or Cushing ulcers.

Ischemic ulcers develop within hours of an event—such as hemorrhage, multisystem trauma, severe burns, heart failure, or sepsis—that causes ischemia of the stomach and duodenal mucosa. Stress ulcers that develop as a result of burn injury are often called **Curling ulcer**.

The shock, anoxia, and sympathetic responses produced by the precipitating event decrease mucosal blood flow, leading to ischemia. In intensive care units, use of positive-pressure mechanical ventilation can induce splanchnic hypoperfusion and contribute to stress-related mucosal injury.[58] Because the metabolism of the mucosal cells declines as a result of lack of arterial blood, the mucosal lining degenerates. Acid diffuses back into the mucosa, causing inflammation, ulceration, hemorrhage, and necrosis. The ulcerative process is accelerated if bile or pancreatic enzymes are regurgitated

from the duodenum. Bleeding occurs more readily with the presence of coagulopathy.[59]

Cushing ulcer is a stress ulcer associated with severe head trauma or brain surgery. This ulcer results from decreased mucosal blood flow and hypersecretion of acid caused by overstimulation of the vagal nuclei. Excessive acid damages the mucosal barrier, initiating the processes summarized in Figure 39-10.

The primary clinical manifestation of stress ulcers is bleeding. Other symptoms may not be present. The bleeding may be slight or, if a small vessel is perforated, amount to hundreds of milliliters. Use of prophylactic antacids and H_2 receptor blockers and suppression of vagal stimulation with anticholinergic drugs are effective forms of therapy. Stress ulcers seldom become chronic.

Surgical Treatment of Ulcer

Advances in the medical treatment of peptic ulcer disease and laparoscopic repair techniques have reduced the number of

Table 39-6	Surgical Management of Peptic Ulcer Disease	
Procedure	**Definition**	**Purpose**
Neural surgery		
Vagotomy	Severance of the vagus nerve	Eliminate neural stimulus of acid secretion
Selective vagotomy	Severance of vagal branches supplying acid-secreting (parietal) cells	Eliminate neural stimulus of acid secretion
Gastric surgery		
Pyloroplasty	Surgical widening or removal of obstruction of the pylorus	Facilitate gastric emptying
Antrectomy (partial gastrectomy)	Removal of the antrum	Eliminate hormonal stimulus of acid secretion—that is, the gastrin-secreting cells of the antral mucosa
Subtotal gastrectomy	Removal of most of the body and all of the antrum of the stomach	Remove acid-secreting and gastrin-secreting mucosa
Anastomosis (Billroth operation)	Reattachment of stomach to duodenum (Billroth I) or jejunum (Billroth II)	Restore continuity of the gastrointestinal tract after resection

cases requiring surgery to 10% to 15%.[60] Despite this small percentage, clinicians care for a significant number of individuals who undergo upper gastrointestinal surgery and experience long-term complications. The most common indications for ulcer surgery are recurrent or uncontrolled bleeding and perforation of the stomach or duodenum.[61,62] The primary objectives of surgical treatment are to reduce stimuli for acid secretion, decrease the number of acid-secreting cells in the stomach, and correct complications of ulcer disease (Table 39-6).

Acute complications of gastrectomy or anastomosis, such as poor wound healing, abscess formation, or suture failure, are relatively uncommon except in the debilitated person. Chronic complications, however, occur more often and are likely to develop if a large portion of the stomach has been removed. These complications and their pathophysiologic mechanisms are described in the next section.

Postgastrectomy Syndromes
Postgastrectomy syndromes are a group of signs and symptoms that occur after gastric resection. They are caused by changes in motor and control functions of the stomach and upper small intestine.[63]

Dumping Syndrome
Dumping syndrome is the rapid emptying of hypertonic chyme from the surgically created, residual stomach into the small intestine 10 to 20 minutes after eating. It occurs with varying severity in 5% to 10% of individuals who have undergone partial gastrectomy or pyloroplasty. It is not common in individuals who have undergone a Billroth II anastomosis (gastrojejunostomy) accompanied by vagotomy. Factors that promote dumping syndrome include (1) loss of gastric capacity, (2) loss of emptying control when the pylorus is removed, and (3) loss of feedback control by the duodenum when it is removed. Rapid gastric emptying and creation of a high osmotic gradient within the small intestine cause a sudden shift of fluid from the vascular compartment to the intestinal lumen. Plasma volume decreases, causing vasomotor responses, such as increased pulse rate, hypotension, weakness, pallor, sweating, and dizziness. Rapid distention of the intestine produces a feeling of epigastric fullness, cramping, nausea, vomiting, and diarrhea.[64]

A less common form of dumping syndrome, termed *late dumping syndrome,* occurs 1 to 2 hours after eating. The symptoms include weakness, diaphoresis, and confusion, but they cannot be explained by rapid gastric emptying. After a high-carbohydrate meal, individuals who have undergone gastrectomy may develop hypoglycemia, which causes the symptoms. The hypoglycemia is caused by an increase in insulin secretion stimulated by the hyperglycemia that follows eating. Other hormonal responses may also participate in the development of hypoglycemia.

Most cases of dumping syndrome respond well to dietary management.[65] Frequent small meals that are high in protein and low in carbohydrates relieve symptoms. Other measures include drinking fluids between meals instead of at mealtime and reclining on the left side after eating. Some cases require surgical intervention, including reconstruction of the pylorus or a gastrojejunostomy.[63] Octreotide reduces abdominal and vasomotor symptoms of dumping syndrome by unknown mechanisms.[66]

Alkaline Reflux Gastritis
Alkaline reflux gastritis is a stomach inflammation caused by reflux of bile and alkaline pancreatic secretions that contain proteolytic enzymes and disrupt the mucosal barrier. This form of gastritis occurs in 5% to 20% of individuals who have undergone gastrectomy or pyloroplasty. Clinical manifestations include nausea, bilious vomiting (vomiting in which the vomitus contains bile), and sustained epigastric pain that worsens after eating and is not relieved by antacids.[67] Endoscopy shows a hemorrhagic and friable gastric mucosa. Conservative management is often difficult because antacids do not consistently improve symptoms. Avoidance of aspirin and alcohol may decrease gastric irritation, and a low-fat diet may limit bile secretion. Surgical correction may ultimately be required.

Afferent Loop Obstruction
Afferent loop obstruction is a rare problem that may occur after gastrojejunostomy (Billroth II; see Table 39-6). The problem is caused by recurring tumor growth, volvulus, hernia, adhesion, or stenosis in the duodenal stump on the proximal side of the gastrojejunostomy.[68] Partial obstruction causes bile and pancreatic secretions to accumulate and dis-

tend the loop. Obstruction also causes delayed emptying. The symptoms of afferent loop obstruction include intermittent severe pain and epigastric fullness after eating. Vomiting usually relieves symptoms. Conservative management consists of a low-fat diet. Surgical correction is required for complete obstruction.

Diarrhea

Diarrhea is one of the most common long-term alterations caused by gastric surgery. Diarrhea can accompany dumping syndrome or occur as a solitary symptom. Diarrhea can occur as frequent, persistent elimination of liquid stool or as intermittent, precipitous, and unpredictable elimination of a large volume of stool. Both types can be either mild or severe. Postgastrectomy diarrhea appears to be related to rapid gastric emptying, particularly after intake of large amounts of high-carbohydrate liquids, which increase the osmotic gradient and attract water into the intestinal lumen. Small, dry meals and anticholinergic drugs are effective control measures.

Weight Loss

Weight loss often follows gastric resection. Inadequate food intake is a common cause, because many individuals cannot tolerate the osmotic effect of carbohydrates or a normal-size meal. Foods may be poorly absorbed because the stomach is less able to mix, churn, and break down food particles. Vomiting, diarrhea, and malabsorption of fats also contribute to weight loss.

Anemia

Anemia after gastrectomy results from iron, vitamin B_{12}, or folate deficiency. Iron malabsorption may be caused by decreased acid secretion. Acid changes iron from a trivalent to a divalent molecule, making it easier to absorb. Iron absorption is also compromised in individuals who have undergone a Billroth II procedure because the duodenum is no longer available to absorb iron.

Vitamin B_{12} deficiency may occur several years after gastrectomy. Contributing factors include loss of parietal cells, which secrete intrinsic factor. (Intrinsic factor facilitates absorption of vitamin B_{12}; see Chapter 38.) Vitamin B_{12} absorption is also compromised if gastric contents are not mixed adequately with pancreatic enzymes, such as may occur after a Billroth II anastomosis.

Folate deficiency is related to poor intake or malabsorption. Management of deficiencies consists of replacement of iron and folate with supplements. Vitamin B_{12} can be administered monthly by injection or oral supplements.[40]

Malabsorption Syndromes

Malabsorption syndromes interfere with nutrient absorption in the small intestine. Historically malabsorption disorders have been classified as maldigestion or malabsorption. **Maldigestion** is failure of the chemical processes of digestion that take place in the intestinal lumen or at the brush border of the intestinal mucosa. **Malabsorption** is the failure of the intestinal mucosa to absorb (transport) the digested nutrients. Often maldigestion and malabsorption are interrelated or occur together, making classification difficult. Generally, however, maldigestion is caused by deficiencies of enzymes,

such as pancreatic lipase or intestinal lactase, which are necessary for digestion. Inadequate secretion of bile salts and inadequate reabsorption of bile in the ileum also contribute to maldigestion. Malabsorption is the result of mucosal disruption caused by gastric or intestinal resection, vascular disorders, or intestinal disease.

Pancreatic Insufficiency

The pancreatic enzymes (lipase, amylase, trypsin, chymotrypsin) are required for the digestion of proteins, carbohydrates, and fats. **Pancreatic insufficiency** is the deficient production of these enzymes by the pancreas. Causes of pancreatic insufficiency include chronic pancreatitis, pancreatic carcinoma, pancreatic resection, and cystic fibrosis. Significant damage to or loss of pancreatic tissue must occur before enzyme levels decrease sufficiently to cause maldigestion. Although pancreatic insufficiency causes poor digestion of all nutrients, fat maldigestion is the chief problem. Salivary amylase and enzymes secreted by the intestinal brush border assist in carbohydrate and protein digestion, but these enzymes do not digest fats. Absence of pancreatic bicarbonate in the duodenum and jejunum causes an acidic pH that worsens maldigestion by preventing activation of pancreatic enzymes that are present. Maldigestion, a large amount of fat in the stool (steatorrhea), and weight loss are the most common signs of pancreatic insufficiency.[69] Lipase supplementation is usually successful.[70]

Lactase Deficiency

Deficiency of disaccharidase at the villus brush border of the small intestine is caused by a congenital defect in which a single enzyme, usually lactase, is lacking.[71] **Lactase deficiency** inhibits the breakdown of lactose (milk sugar) into monosaccharides and therefore prevents lactose digestion and absorption across the intestinal wall. Lactase deficiency is most common in blacks. The deficiency usually does not develop until adulthood. Secondary (acquired) lactase deficiency can be caused by several diseases of the intestine, including gluten-sensitive enteropathy (see Chapter 40), enteritis, and bacterial overgrowth.

The undigested lactose remains in the intestine, where bacterial fermentation causes gases to form. Undigested lactose also increases the osmotic gradient in the intestine, causing irritation and osmotic diarrhea. Clinical manifestations of lactase deficiency are bloating, crampy pain, diarrhea, and flatulence. The disorder is diagnosed by a lactose-tolerance test.[72] Avoiding milk products and adhering to a lactose-free diet relieve symptoms. Maintaining an adequate calcium intake with restricted intake of milk products decreases risk of osteoporosis.[73]

Bile Salt Deficiency

Conjugated bile acids (bile salts) are necessary for the digestion and absorption of fats. Bile salts are conjugated in the bile that is synthesized from cholesterol and secreted from the liver.[74] When bile enters the duodenum, the bile salts aggregate with fatty acids and monoglycerides to form micelles.

Micelle formation solubilizes fat molecules and allows them to pass through the unstirred layer at the brush border (see Chapter 38). A minimum concentration of bile salts, termed the *critical micelle concentration,* is required to allow micelles to form. Therefore conditions that decrease the production or secretion of bile result in decreased micelle formation and fat malabsorption. These conditions include advanced liver disease, which decreases production of bile salts; obstruction of the common bile duct, which decreases flow of bile into the duodenum; intestinal stasis (lack of motility), which permits overgrowth of intestinal bacteria that deconjugate bile salts; and diseases of the ileum, which prevent the reabsorption and recycling of bile salts (enterohepatic circulation).

Clinical manifestations of bile salt deficiency are related to poor intestinal absorption of fat and fat-soluble vitamins (A, D, E, K). Increased fat in the stools (steatorrhea) leads to diarrhea and decreased plasma proteins. The losses of fat-soluble vitamins and their effects include the following:

1. Vitamin A deficiency results in night blindness.
2. Vitamin D deficiency results in decreased calcium absorption with bone demineralization (osteoporosis), bone pain, and fractures.
3. Vitamin K deficiency prolongs prothrombin time, leading to spontaneous development of purpura (bruising) and petechiae.
4. Vitamin E deficiency has uncertain effects but may cause testicular atrophy and neurologic defects in children.

The most effective treatment for fat-soluble vitamin deficiency is to increase medium-chain triglycerides in the diet, for example, by using coconut oil for cooking. Vitamins A, D, and K are given parenterally.

Inflammatory Bowel Disease

Ulcerative colitis and Crohn disease are chronic relapsing inflammatory bowel diseases of unknown origin. Both diseases are associated with genetic factors, alterations in epithelial cell barrier functions, immune reactions to intestinal bacteria, and abnormal T-cell reactions. Ulcerative colitis is limited to the mucosa of the colon. Crohn disease can involve any part of the gastrointestinal tract from the mouth to the anus and involves transmural granulomatous inflammatory lesions (Figure 39-11).

Ulcerative Colitis

Ulcerative colitis (UC) is a chronic inflammatory disease that causes ulceration of the colonic mucosa and extends proximally from the rectum into the colon. The lesions appear in susceptible individuals between 20 and 40 years of age. Risk factors include family history of disease and Jewish descent, and the disease is more prevalent among white populations and northern Europeans. The disease affects up to 2 million people in the United States.

Although the cause of UC is unknown, dietary, infectious, genetic, and immunologic factors are all suggested causes.[75,76] The hypothesis that inflammation is caused by infectious

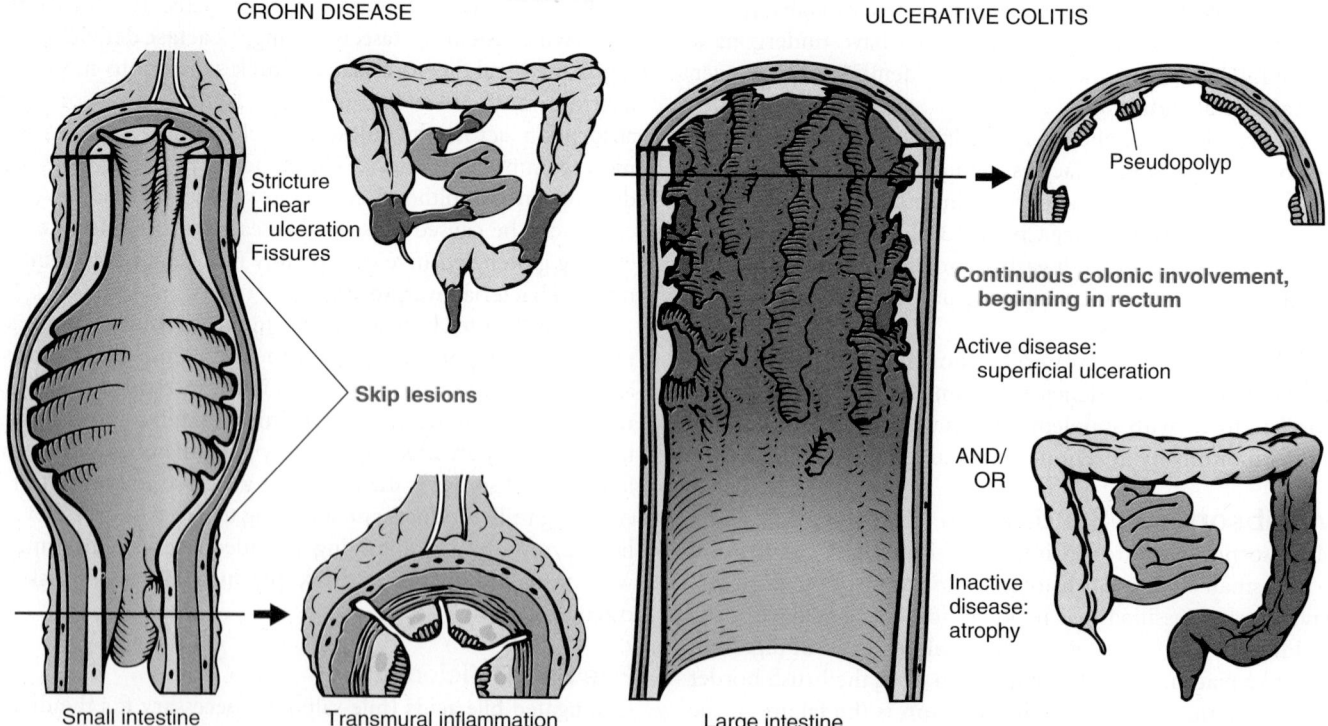

CROHN DISEASE   ULCERATIVE COLITIS

Stricture
Linear
ulceration
Fissures

Pseudopolyp

Skip lesions

Continuous colonic involvement, beginning in rectum

Active disease: superficial ulceration

AND/ OR

Inactive disease: atrophy

Small intestine   Transmural inflammation   Large intestine

Figure 39-11 Distribution patterns of Crohn disease and ulcerative colitis. Comparison of distribution patterns the Crohn disease and ulcerative colitis as well as different conformations of ulcers and wall thickenings. (From Kumar V, Cotran RS, Robbins SL: *Robbins basic pathology,* ed 7, St Louis, 2003, Mosby.)

agents is not supported by consistent identification of specific viruses or bacteria in affected individuals. The familial tendency to develop ulcerative colitis and the occurrence of disease in identical twins support a genetic theory of causation. Perhaps most significant are the humoral and cellular immunologic factors associated with the disease. Colonic epithelial antibodies of the IgG class have been identified in the sera of individuals with ulcerative colitis and a large number of plasma cells are found in the inflamed colon. Lymphocytes (T-cells) in individuals with ulcerative colitis may have cytotoxic effects on the epithelial cells of the colon, as well as damage caused by inflammatory cytokines (interleukins [IL-1, IL-2, IL-6, IL-8] and tumor necrosis factor-α [TNF-α]), toxic oxygen radicals, interferon-gamma (IFN-γ), and IL-10.[77] Activated macrophages also contribute cytokines that cause fever and the acute phase response. Furthermore, autoimmune disorders, such as systemic lupus erythematosus and erythema nodosum, may accompany ulcerative colitis.

PATHOPHYSIOLOGY   The primary lesions of UC are limited to the mucosa. Inflammation begins at the base of the crypt of Lieberkühn in the large intestine, primarily the left colon, with infiltration of neutrophils, lymphocytes, plasma cells, macrophages, eosinophils, and mast cells. The disease is most severe in the rectum and sigmoid colon. The mucous layer is thinner than normal. With milder inflammation, the mucosa is hyperemic, edematous, and may appear dark red and velvety (Figure 39-12). Inflammatory cytokines released from lymphocytes, macrophages, and neutrophils cause tissue damage.[77] In more severe inflammation, the mucosa becomes hemorrhagic and small erosions form and coalesce into ulcers. Abscess formation occurs in the crypts. Necrosis and ragged ulceration of the mucosa ensue. Edema and thickening of the muscularis mucosae may narrow the lumen of the involved colon. In chronic disease, inflammatory polyps (pseudopolyps) develop in the colon from rapidly regenerating epithelium.

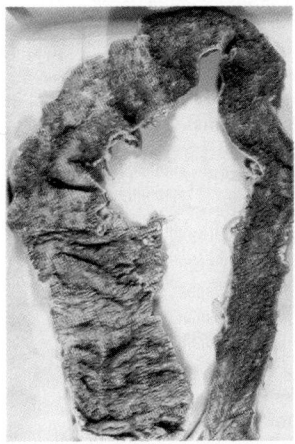

Figure 39-12 **Acute ulcerative colitis.** Colitis with extensive mucosal ulceration involving the entire colon. (From Damjanov I, Linder J, editors: *Anderson's pathology,* ed 10, St. Louis, 1996, Mosby.)

CLINICAL MANIFESTATIONS   The course of UC consists of intermittent periods of remission and exacerbation. Clinical manifestations vary with the severity and extent of disease. Loss of the absorptive mucosal surface and decreased colonic transit time can cause large volumes of watery diarrhea. Mucosal destruction causes bleeding, cramping pain, and an urge to defecate.[78] Frequent diarrhea, with passage of small amounts of blood and purulent mucus, is common.

Mild UC involves less mucosa, so that frequency of bowel movements, bleeding, and pain are minimal. Severe forms may involve the entire colon and are characterized by fever; elevated pulse rate; frequent diarrhea (10 to 20 movements per day); urgency; obviously bloody stools; and continuous, crampy pain. Dehydration, weight loss, anemia, and fever result from fluid loss, bleeding, and inflammation. Complications include toxic megacolon, anal fissures, hemorrhoids, and perirectal abscess. Severe hemorrhage is rare, but chronic blood loss may precipitate hypotension and shock. Edema, strictures, or fibrosis can obstruct the colon. Perforation is an unusual but possible complication. The risk of left-sided colon cancer increases significantly after many years of ulcerative colitis.[79]

Extraintestinal manifestations of UC occur in 5% to 15% of cases and include migratory polyarthritis and sacroilitis, osteopenia and osteoporosis, mouth ulcers, episcleritis or anterior uveitis in the eye, and primary sclerosing colangitis in the liver.[80] Gallstones are common. Alterations in coagulation can cause life-threatening microthrombi and deep vein thrombosis.[81,82]

EVALUATION AND TREATMENT   Diagnosis of ulcerative colitis is based on the medical history, clinical manifestations, and imaging procedures. Endoscopic evaluation shows an inflamed and hemorrhagic mucosa. Radiologic assessment may show loss of haustra, ulceration, and irregular mucosa. The laboratory data include low hemoglobin values, hypoalbuminemia, and low serum potassium levels. Infectious causes are ruled out by stool culture. The symptoms of ulcerative colitis are very similar to those of Crohn disease, making differential diagnosis difficult.[83]

Treatment depends on the severity of symptoms and the extent of mucosal involvement. The disease is often treated with sulfasalazine (a combination of a sulfa drug and aminosalicylates). Steroids and salicylates suppress the inflammatory response and help to alleviate the cramping pain.[83] Immunosuppressive agents (e.g., 6-mercaptopurine and cyclosporine) are used for chronic active disease. Broad-spectrum antibiotics may be prescribed if bacterial infection is suggested. For unknown reasons, nicotine may have a protective effect in ulcerative colitis but not in Crohn disease.[84] Severe, unremitting disease can require hospital admission and administration of intravenous fluids. Extreme malnutrition may require intravenous hyperalimentation. Surgical resection of the colon or a colostomy may be performed if other forms of therapy are unsuccessful.[85]

Crohn Disease

Crohn disease (CD) (granulomatous colitis, ileocolitis, or regional enteritis) is an idiopathic inflammatory disorder that affects any part of the gastrointestinal track from the mouth to the anus. The distal small intestine and proximal large colon are most commonly affected by the disease. In a small percentage of cases, CD is difficult to differentiate from ulcerative colitis (Table 39-7). Risk factors and theories of causation are the same as those for ulcerative colitis. Like ulcerative colitis, CD tends to run in families. Ten to twenty percent of affected individuals have a positive family history. The discovery of the NOD2/CARD15 gene on chromosome 16 as a determinant in the susceptibility to CD is providing insights into the pathophysiology of the disease.[86] This gene regulates macrophage activation in response to bacterial lipopolysaccharide. The colony-stimulating factor IR gene, which is involved in monocyte to macrophage differentiation, also may be a susceptibility gene for CD.[87] The pathogenesis of CD may be associated with an overly aggressive response to normal flora bacteria in genetically predisposed individuals.[88,89] Th-1 mediated inflammation with activation of macrophages and cytokines (TNF-α, INF-γ, and interleukins) causes injury and alterations in immunoglobulin A (IgA) production. Recruited leukocytes release proinflammatory substances, including prostaglandins, leukotrienes, proteases, reactive oxygen species, and nitric oxide, which cause further injury and inflammation. Smoking, dietary substances, and bacteria not part of the normal flora also may be precipitating factors.

PATHOPHYSIOLOGY The inflammatory process of CD begins in the intestinal submucosa and spreads across the intestinal wall to involve the mucosa and serosa. The most common site of the disease is the ileocolon, but both the large and small intestines may be involved. The inflammation can affect some haustral segments but not others, creating a pattern called *skip lesions.* One side of the intestinal wall may be affected but not the other.

The ulcerations of CD produce longitudinal and transverse fissures that extend inflammation into lymphoid tissue. The typical lesion is a granuloma having cobblestone projections of inflamed tissue surrounded by areas of ulceration (Figure 39-13). (Granulomas are described in Chapter 6.) Fistulae may form in the perianal area between loops of intestine or extend into the bladder.

CLINICAL MANIFESTATIONS Individuals with CD may have no specific symptoms other than an "irritable bowel" for several years. Diarrhea is the most common sign, with passage of blood and mucus. Diarrhea can result from decreased colonic absorption, bypass fistulae, bacterial overgrowth, and the presence of bile in the colon that inhibits water absorption.[90] Other manifestations are related to the location and extent of intestinal involvement. Inflammation of the ileum, for example, causes tenderness in the lower right side of the abdomen. Weight loss and lower abdominal pain accompany CD. If the ileum is involved, the individual may be anemic as a result of malabsorption of vitamin B_{12}. There also may be deficiencies in folic acid, vitamin D absorption, and calcium leading to bone disease. Proteins may be lost, leading to hypoalbuminemia. Anal manifestations occur in about 30% of cases, including anal fissure, perianal abscess, and fistula.[75] Individuals with CD of long duration are also at risk

Table 39-7	Features of Ulcerative Colitis and Crohn Disease	
Feature	**Ulcerative Colitis**	**Crohn Disease**
Incidence		
Age at onset	Any age; 10-40 years most common	Any age; 10-30 years most common
Family history	Less common	More common
Gender (prevalence)	Equal in women and men	About equal in women and men
Cancer risk	Increased	Increased
Pathophysiology		
Location of lesions	Colon and rectum, no "skip" lesions	All of GI tract: mouth to anus, "skip" lesions common
Inflammation and ulceration	Mucosal layer involved	Entire intestinal wall involved
Granulomas	Rare	Common
Friable mucosa	Common	Less common
Fistuale and abscesses	Rare	Common
Strictures and possible obstruction	Rare	Common
Clinical Manifestations		
Abdominal pain	Occasional	Common
Diarrhea	Common	Common
Bloody stools	Common	Less common
Abdominal mass	Rare	Common
Small intestinal malabsorption	Rare	Common
Steatorrhea	Rare	Common
Potential for malignancy	Common	Common
Clinical course	Remissions and exacerbations	Remissions and exacerbations

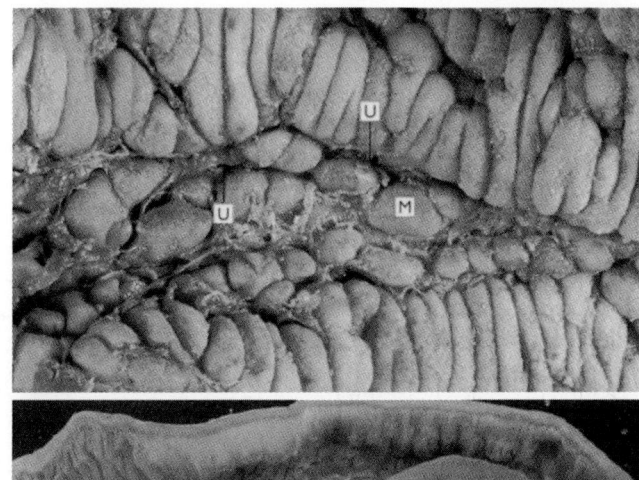

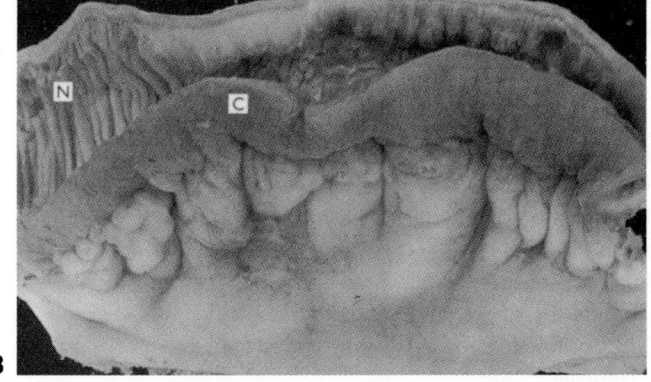

Figure 39-13 **Crohn disease. A,** The mucosa in Crohn disease demonstrates a cobblestone pattern as a result of fissured ulcers *(U)* with intervening areas of edematous mucosa *(M).* **B,** Compared with normal small bowel wall *(N),* the Crohn segment *(C)* shows wall thickening that has caused a stenosis. (From Stevens A, Lowe J: *Pathology,* ed 2, London, 2000, Mosby.)

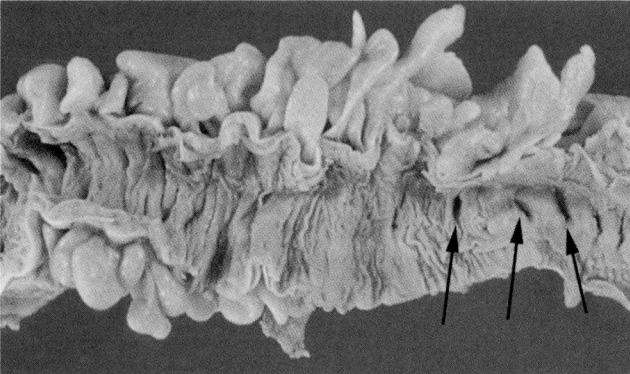

Figure 39-14 **Diverticular disease.** In diverticular disease, the outpouches (arrows) of mucosa seen in the sigmoid colon appear as slitlike openings from the mucosal surface of the opened bowel. (Modified from Stevens A, Lowe J: *Pathology,* ed 2, London, 2000, Mosby.)

for intestinal adenocarcinoma, particularly in the small intestine.[91] Complications include obstruction, fistulae, abscess formation, and chronic blood loss. Extraintestinal manifestations are similar to those described for UC.

EVALUATION AND TREATMENT   The diagnosis and treatment of CD are similar to the diagnosis and treatment of ulcerative colitis. Treatment with immunomodulatory agents can be effective. Antibody to TNF-α (Infliximab) is used for treatment of fistulas.[92] Surgery is generally performed to manage complications such as strictures, fistula, abscess, and perforation, or to relieve obstruction.[93]

Diverticular Disease of the Colon

Diverticula are herniations or saclike outpouchings of mucosa through the muscle layers of the colon wall. **Diverticulosis** is asymptomatic diverticular disease. The cause is unknown but is associated with decreased dietary fiber and increased intracolonic pressure. **Diverticulitis** represents inflammation. Diverticular disease is most common in individuals over 60 years of age, particularly those who live in developed countries where much of the diet consists of refined foods.

PATHOPHYSIOLOGY   Although diverticula can occur anywhere in the gastrointestinal tract, the most common site

is the sigmoid colon.[94] The diverticula form at weak points in the colon wall, usually where arteries penetrate the tunica muscularis to nourish the mucosal layer. Abnormal colonic motility with intraluminal hypertension also may be contributing factors. The colonic mucosa herniates through the smooth muscle layers (Figure 39-14). A common associated finding is thickening of the circular and longitudinal (teniae coli) muscles surrounding the diverticula. Hypertrophy and contraction of these muscles increase intraluminal pressure and degree of herniation. Habitual consumption of a low-residue diet reduces fecal bulk, thus reducing the diameter of the colon. According to the law of Laplace (see Chapter 29), wall pressure increases as the diameter of a cylindrical structure decreases. Therefore pressure within the narrow lumen can increase enough to rupture the diverticula. Dietary fiber deficiency also may change the intestinal microflora, decreasing the immune response in the colon and permitting low grade inflammation.[95,96] Diverticulitis can cause abscess formation or peritonitis.[97]

CLINICAL MANIFESTATIONS   Symptoms of diverticular disease are usually vague or absent. Cramping pain of the lower abdomen can accompany constriction of the hypertrophied colonic muscles. Diarrhea, constipation, distention, or flatulence may occur. Diverticula with an obstructed opening become inflamed or abscesses form, and the individual develops fever, leukocytosis (increased white blood cell count), and tenderness of the lower left quadrant. Right lower quadrant pain and severe complications, such as hemorrhage, perforation with peritonitis, bowel obstruction, and fistula formation, are rare.

EVALUATION AND TREATMENT   Diverticula are often discovered during diagnostic procedures performed for other problems. Ultrasound, sigmoidoscopy, or barium enema are used for diagnosis of uncomplicated diverticuli. Abdominal computed tomography (CT) is used for complicated cases.

Diverticulitis and Diet

Daily consumption of fiber-enriched foods is recommended for the prevention of diverticula. A high-fiber diet increases fecal bulk, decreases transit time, lowers intracolonic pressures, and eases stool elimination. The recommendation for fiber is 20 to 35 g/day. Some examples of high-fiber choices are whole wheat bread and other grain products, baked potato with skin, fresh fruit with skins, raw vegetables, beans, peas, legumes, wheat bran, and brown rice. Side effects may include flatulence, intestinal rumbling, cramps, and diarrhea. A gradual increase in dietary fiber over a month or two helps to avoid these problems. Other potential problems with an excessively high fiber diet (greater than 40 to 45 g) might include a decrease in nutrient absorption because of the increased volume of intestinal contents, which in turn decreases the ability of the digestive enzymes to come in contact with the food. An increase of water (eight 8-oz glasses) is important so intestinal blockage will not occur. For small children and elderly persons a high-fiber diet increases the volume of food needed to meet energy requirements, and that increase may be difficult to obtain. Although some doctors recommend restricting nuts; seeds; and foods containing seeds such as berries, kiwi, and tomatoes that might lodge in the pouches, there is no evidence that this happens. If the diverticula become inflamed, a low-fiber, low-residue (no milk products), or elemental diet, or in complicated cases, total parenteral nutrition (TPN), is required to prevent continued irritation of the inflamed tissue.

Data from Floch MH, Bina I: *J Clin Gastroenterol* 38(5 Suppl):S2-7, 2004; Steel M: *Aust Fam Physician* 33(12):983-986, 2004; Kang JY, Melville D, Maxwell JD: *Drugs Aging* 21(4):211-228, 2004.

An increase of dietary fiber intake increases stool weight, lowers colonic pressures, improves transit times, and often relieves symptoms. Probiotics combined with salicylates are effective in arresting infection. Uncomplicated diverticulitis is treated with antibiotics.[98] Surgical resection may be required if there are severe complications.[99]

Appendicitis

Appendicitis is an inflammation of the vermiform appendix, which is a projection from the apex of the cecum. It is the most common surgical emergency of the abdomen and affects 7% to 12% of the population. The most common occurrence is between 20 and 30 years of age, although it may develop at any age.[100]

PATHOPHYSIOLOGY The exact cause of appendicitis is controversial. Obstruction of the lumen with stool, tumors, or foreign bodies with consequent, increased, intraluminal pressure, ischemia, bacterial infection, and inflammation[101] is a common theory. The obstructed lumen does not allow drainage of the appendix, and as mucosal secretion continues, intraluminal pressure increases. The resultant increased pressure decreases mucosal blood flow, and the appendix becomes hypoxic. The mucosa ulcerates, promoting bacterial or other microbial invasion with further inflammation and edema. In-flammation may involve the distal or entire appendix. Gangrene develops from thrombosis of the luminal blood vessels, followed by perforation.

CLINICAL MANIFESTATIONS Epigastric or periumbilical pain is the typical symptom of an inflamed appendix. The pain may be vague at first, increasing in intensity over 3 to 4 hours. It may subside and then recur with a shift of location to the right lower quadrant. Right lower quadrant pain is associated with extension of the inflammation to the surrounding tissues. Nausea, vomiting, and anorexia follow the onset of pain, and fever is common. Diarrhea occurs in some individuals, particularly children; others have a sensation of constipation. Perforation, peritonitis, and abscess formation are the most serious complications of appendicitis.

EVALUATION AND TREATMENT In addition to clinical manifestations, the clinician can usually locate the painful site with one finger. Rebound tenderness is usually referred to the right lower quadrant. The white blood cell count ranges from 10,000 to 16,000 cells/mm³, with increased neutrophils. C-reactive protein is elevated.[102] Roentgenograms of the abdomen, CT scans, and ultrasound assist diagnostic accuracy. The combined information provides the best discriminating diagnosis.[103]

Antibiotics and appendectomy is the treatment for simple or perforated appendicitis. Laparoscopic surgery provides quick recovery for simple appendicitis. Recovery is more complicated in cases of perforation or abscess formation.[104]

Vascular Insufficiency

The stomach and intestines are supplied by three branches of the abdominal aorta: the celiac axis and the superior and inferior mesenteric arteries. Because of the rich collateral circulation, at least two of the supplying vessels must be compromised to cause ischemia.[105] Atherosclerotic lesions, thrombi, and emboli can develop in these vessels, occluding blood flow and causing ischemia or necrosis in the gastrointestinal tract.

Mesenteric venous thrombosis is the least common of the causes of mesenteric vascular insufficiency. Malignancies, right-sided heart failure, and deep vein thrombosis are risk factors.

Acute occlusion of mesenteric artery blood flow results from dissecting aortic aneurysms or emboli. Embolic obstruction is associated with atrial fibrillation, mitral valve disease, and heart valve prostheses. The superior mesenteric artery has a more direct line of flow from the aorta; therefore emboli enter it more readily than the inferior branch, causing ischemia and necrosis of the small intestine.[106] Ischemia and necrosis alter membrane permeability. There is initially increased motility, nausea and vomiting, urgent bowel evacuation, and severe abdominal pain. The damaged intestinal mucosa cannot produce enough mucus to protect itself from digestive enzymes.[107] Ischemia leads to decreased motility and distention. Mucosal alteration causes fluid to move from the blood vessels into the bowel wall and peritoneum. Fluid loss causes hypovolemia and further decreases in intestinal blood flow. As intestinal infarction progresses, shock, fever, bloody diarrhea, and leukocytosis develop. Abdominal pain may be severe. Bacteria invade the necrotic intestinal wall, causing gangrene and peritonitis.

Chronic mesenteric insufficiency can develop secondary to congestive heart failure, acute myocardial infarction, dysrhythmias, hemorrhage, stenosis, thrombus formation, aortic aneurysm, or any condition that decreases arterial blood flow. Elderly individuals with arteriosclerosis are particularly susceptible. Chronic occlusion is often accompanied by formation of collateral circulation that may be able to nourish the resting intestine. After eating, however, when the intestine requires more blood, the arterial supply may be insufficient. Ischemia develops, causing a cramping abdominal pain, called *abdominal angina*, after meals. Progressive vascular obstruction eventually causes continuous abdominal pain and necrosis of the intestinal tissue. Reperfusion injury related to reactive oxygen metabolites and inflammatory mediators contributes to further tissue damage.

Colicky abdominal pain after eating is a cardinal symptom of chronic mesenteric insufficiency. Some individuals suffer significant weight loss because they stop eating to control the pain. Chronic segmental ischemia may lead to strictures and destruction.

Diagnosis of mesenteric artery occlusion is based on clinical manifestations, laboratory findings, mesenteric artery angiography, and abdominal radiography. Bruit often can be heard over the occluded artery. After angiography a vasodilating agent may be injected into the vessels to improve the circulation. Heparin may be used if there are no contraindictions. Surgery is required to remove necrotic tissue or repair sclerosed vessels. Mortality is high (60% to 80%) for individuals with acute occlusion and compromised cardiac output.[108] Early diagnosis and aggressive treatment result in the best survival rates.[109]

Disorders of Nutrition

Obesity

Obesity is an increase in body fat mass and a metabolic disorder that has increased in rate of incidence significantly over the past two decades. Obesity is defined as a body mass index (BMI) greater than 30.[110] It is a major cause of morbidity, death, and high health care cost in the United States and the Western World.[111,112] Three leading causes of death in the United States are associated with obesity: cardiovascular disease, type 2 diabetes mellitus, and cancer (colon, breast in postmenopausal women, endometrium, prostate, kidney and esophagus[113] (see Chapter 11 and Figures 11-28 and 11-29). Obesity is also a risk factor for hypertension, stroke, hepatobiliary disease (gallstones and nonalcoholic steatohepatitis), osteoarthritis, and sleep apnea. Visceral obesity is associated with a higher incidence of cardiovascular disease.

The causes and consequences of obesity are multiple and complex with rapidly advancing research regarding causal mechanisms and complications. Genotype and gene-environment interactions are important predisposing factors, and both single gene syndromes and numerous susceptibility

genes influence the development of obesity.[114,115] Single gene defects are rare and obesity is usually polygenic and associated with other phenotypes such as endocrine disorders (i.e., diabetes and hypothyroidism) and mental retardation (i.e., Down and Prader-Willi syndromes). Single gene defects include the melanocortin-receptor gene, leptin gene (also known as the *obesity gene*) and leptin receptor gene. All single gene defects are directly or indirectly related to leptin. Metabolic abnormalities contributing to obesity include Cushing syndrome, Cushing disease, polycystic ovarian syndrome, hypothyroidism, and hypothalamic injury. Environmental factors include culture, socioeconomic status, food intake, and exercise. Obesity is associated with adverse social and psychological consequences.[116-118]

PATHOPHYSIOLOGY   Adipocytes secrete a number of hormones and cytokines known as adipokines (Box 39-2). These adipokines participate in regulation of food intake, lipid storage and metabolism, insulin sensitivity, the alterna-

---

Box 39-2	Hormones and Adipokines Secreted by Adipose Tissue

Hormones (Adipokines)
Leptin
  Satiety (hunger/appetite suppression) and regulation of eating behavior by hypothalamus
  Sympathoactivation
  Insulin sensitizing
Adiponectin
  Insulin sensitizing
  Anti-inflammatory
  Anti-athrogenic
Resistin
  Promotes insulin resistance and increased blood glucose levels
  Inhibits adipocyte differentiation and may function as a feedback regulator of adipogenesis
Visfatin (from visceral fat)
  Mimics insulin and binds to insulin receptor in rats

Regulators of Lipoprotein Metabolism
Lipoprotein lipase
Apolipoprotein E
Cholesterol ester transfer protein

Inflammatory Cytokines
Tumor necrosis factor-alpha
Interleukins (IL-6, IL-8, IL-10)
Plasminogen activator inhibitor-1

Other Hormones and Cytokines
Estrogen
Angiotensinogen
Tissue factor
Nitric oxide synthase
Acylation stimulating protein
Adipophilin
AdipoQ
Monobutyrin
Agouti protein

Data from Fasshauer M, Paschke R, Stumvoll M: *Biochimie* 86(11):779-784, 2004; Fukuhara A et al: *Science* 307(5708):426-430, 2005.

tive complement system, vascular homeostasis, blood pressure regulation, angiogenesis, the inflammatory and immune responses, female reproduction, and regulation of energy metabolism.[119] Visceral fat accumulation causes dysfunction of adipocytes and results in alterations in the regulation and interaction of these hormones and cytokines contributing to the causes and complications of obesity.[120]

Neuroendocrine regulation of eating behavior, energy metabolism, and body fat mass is controlled by a dynamic circuit of signaling molecules from the periphery acting on the hypothalamus. An imbalance in this system is usually associated with excessive caloric intake in relation to exercise with the consequence of weight gain and obesity.

Many different hormones control appetite and body weight. The sources of them include insulin from the beta cells of the pancreas, ghrelin from the stomach, peptide YY from the intestines, and leptin, adiponectin and resistin from adipose tissue. These hormones circulate in the blood at concentrations proportional to body fat mass, and serve as peripheral signals to the arcuate nucleus (ARC) in the hypothalamus where appetite and metabolism is regulated (Figure 39-15). The ARC has two sets of neurons with opposing effects that interact to regulate food intake and energy metabo-

lism. One set of neurons produce the molecules neuropeptide Y (NPY) and agouti-related protein (AGRP), which stimulate eating and decrease metabolism (i.e., promote catabolism). Another set of neurons synthesize proopiomelanocortin (POMC)-producing peptide, which is then processed to alpha-melanocyte stimulating hormone (α-MSH) and cocaine- and amphetamine-regulated transcript (CART), collectively known as α-MSH/CART neurons, which inhibit eating. Both sets of neurons express their effects by activating second order neurons in the hypothalamus, which increase or decrease appetite and energy metabolism. Leptin and insulin decrease appetite by inhibiting NPY/AGRP neurons and stimulating POMC-α-MSH/CART neurons. Ghrelin stimulates appetite by activating NPY/AGRP–expressing neurons. Peptide YY (PYY) inhibits these neurons and decreases appetite. Other peripheral hormones and neurotransmitters also can influence the hypothalamus and effect appetite and energy expenditure (see Figure 39-15). Molecules that stimulate eating are called *orexins* (i.e., hypocretins [from the hypothalamus] are a peptide family that acts as neurotransmitters for stimulating eating), and molecules that inhibit eating are called *anorexins* (Box 39-3). Peripheral effects of these signaling pathways are transmitted via the autonomic nervous

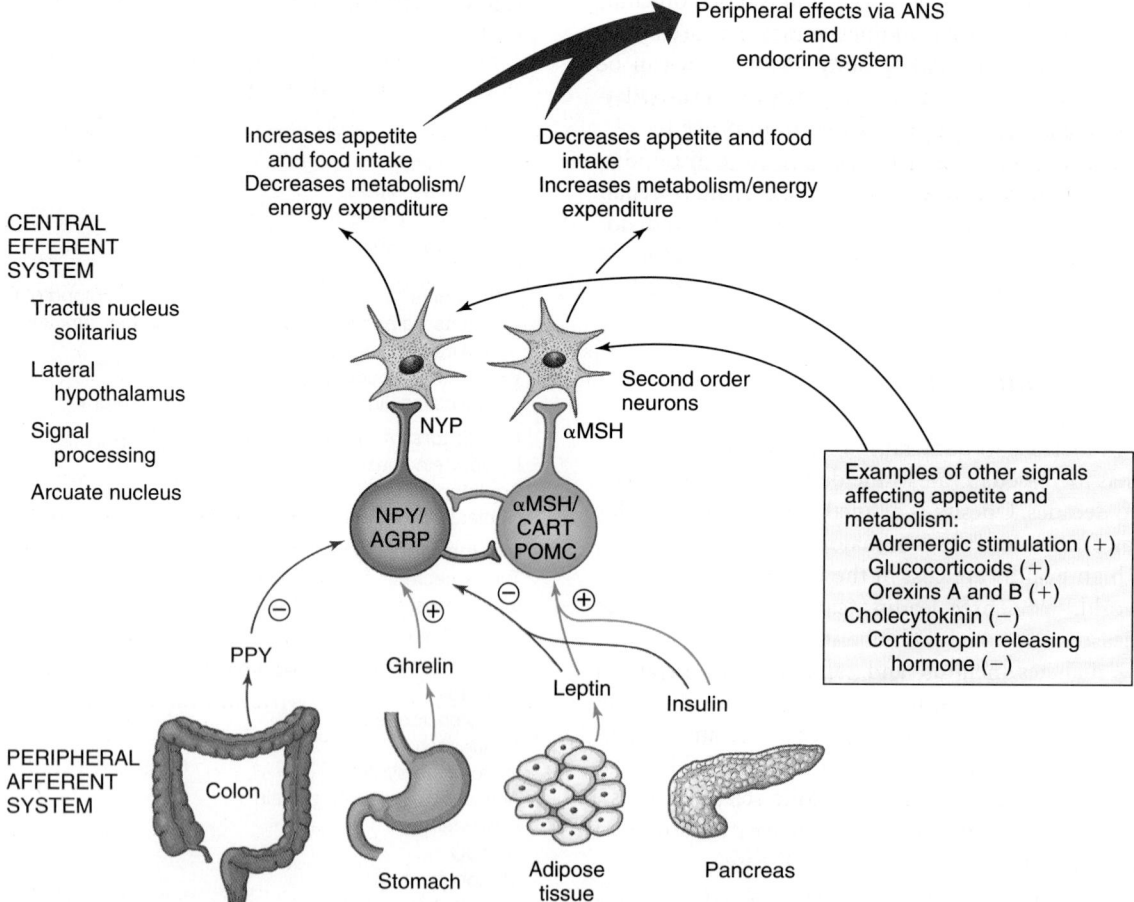

Figure 39-15 Actions of afferent signaling in central control of food intake and energy expenditure. *NPY,* Neuropeptide Y; *AGRP,* agouti-related protein; *POMC,* proopiomelanocortin; *α-MSH,* alpha-melanocyte-stimulating hormone; *CART,* cocaine- and amphetamine-regulated transcript; *PYY,* peptide YY; *ANS,* autonomic nervous system.

Orexins (appetite stimulants)
Neuropeptide Y
Melanin-concentrating hormone
Agouti-related protein
Ghrelin
Galanin
Orexins A and B
Peptide YY

Anorexins (appetite suppressants)
Leptin
Insulin
Cholecystokinin
Corticotropin-releasing hormone (CRF)
Urocortin (a CRF satiety signaling hormone)
Cocaine- and amphetamine-regulated transcript (CART)
Alpha-melanocyte-stimulating hormone (α-MSH)
Bombesin

system and endocrine system to regulate appetite, food intake, and energy metabolism.

Obesity is associated with increased circulating plasma levels of leptin, insulin, ghrelin, and peptide YY. Interaction among these hormones at the level of the hypothalamus may be an important determinant of excessive fat mass. Leptin receptors in the hypothalamus function to regulate body weight within a fairly narrow range or set point. The leptin signal may serve as an anorexin by altering secretion of orexins and anorexins. Leptin secretion increases as adipocytes increase in size or number and decreases during fasting (hyperleptinemia). The high levels of leptin are ineffective at decreasing appetite and increasing energy expenditure—this is known as **leptin resistance.** Leptin resistance disrupts hypothalamic satiety signaling and promotes overeating and excessive weight gain.

The cause of leptin resistance is unknown. It may be related to a defect in leptin transport,[121] an inability of leptin to cross the blood brain barrier,[122] an alteration in the permissive effect of leptin on urocortin,[123] or a defect in the leptin receptor.[124] *Hyperleptinemia* also stimulates the sympathetic nervous system, vascular inflammation, oxidative stress, and ventricular hypertrophy and may contribute to the pathogenesis of hypertension, atherosclerosis, and left ventricular hypertrophy associated with obesity.[125,126]

Ghrelin is an endogenous ligand for growth-hormone-secretagogue-receptor (GHS-R) and stimulates release of growth hormone (GH) from anterior pituitary cells. Ghrelin stimulates food intake and induces metabolic changes leading to an increase in body weight and body fat mass. Ghrelin also stimulates the release of gastric acid and gastric motility and affects pancreatic functions. It has vasodilatory, cardioprotective, and antiproliferative effects.[127,128] Leptin and ghrelin are complementary, yet antagonistic signals reflecting acute and chronic changes in energy balance the effects of which are mediated by hypothalamic neuropeptides, such as neuropep-

tide Y (NPY) and agouti-related peptide (AGRP). Plasma ghrelin levels are decreased in obesity, and it's role in contributing to obesity is yet to be defined. Leptin may regulate ghrelin levels.[129] Endocrine and vagal afferent pathways are also involved in the actions of ghrelin, and leptin adding to the complexity of mechanisms that can affect obesity.

Adiponectin has insulin sensitizing properties and is inversely related to obesity and insulin resistance in adults and children.[130-133] Obese individuals, particularly those with expansion of visceral adipose tissue, are at increased risk for coronary artery disease resulting from hyperlipidemia, hypertension, and factors that promote thrombosis and inflammation (see Chapter 30). It has recently been demonstrated that adiponectin levels decrease with obesity resulting in increased levels of inflammatory markers such as IL-6 and C-reactive protein. Decreases in adiponectin are related to increased risk for cardiovascular disease and type 2 diabetes mellitus.[134] Adiponectin may serve as an anti-inflammatory and anti-atherogenic plasma protein and may have an important role in vascular remodeling that is limited with obesity.[135,136]

Obesity is associated with insulin resistance, and insulin resistance predisposes an individual to type 2 diabetes mellitus (see Chapter 21). The insulin resistance may be related to an insulin receptor defect or to postreceptor effects with alteration in glucose transporter functions. Excess insulin also may be a response to excessive caloric intake.[137] Resistin is found in the serum of mice and humans and is antagonistic to insulin action. Resistin also inhibits adipocyte differentiation and may function as a feedback regulator of adipogenesis. It is greatly increased in those with obesity.[138,139]

CLINICAL MANIFESTATIONS   Increased visceral fat is associated with *metabolic syndrome* (hypertriglyceridemia, reduced high-density lipoprotein, and increased low-density lipoproteins), a complex of traits that increase risk for ischemic heart disease and insulin resistance (type 2 diabetes mellitus).[140,141] Metabolic syndrome is discussed in Chapters 21 and 30.

Obesity is a major modifiable risk factor for cardiovascular disease, including hypertension, coronary artery disease (CAD), and congestive heart failure. The presence of metabolic syndrome and type 2 diabetes mellitus promotes high risk for CAD.[142,143] The release of atherogenic and inflammatory cytokines from visceral fat also may contribute to cardiovascular complications.[144,145]

The *hypertension* of obesity is complex and may be related to insulin resistance, activation of the sympathetic nervous system, activation of renin-angiotensin, leptin resistance, physical compression of the kidneys, and alterations in vascular structure and function.[146,147]

Pulmonary function can be compromised by a large amount of adipose tissue overlying the chest cage. Work of breathing increases, and gas exchange, vital capacity, and expiratory volume all decrease causing low oxygen tension and high carbon dioxide tension. The hypoventilation and hypoxemia cause pulmonary hypertension contributing to right ventricular hypertrophy and heart failure. Asthma is also associated with obesity, particularly among females, but the exact mechanisms of airway hyper-responsiveness are unknown.[148,149]

Obstructive sleep apnea syndrome (OSAS) is also a consequence of obesity; it involves episodic partial or complete obstruction of the upper airway, hypoventilation, and hypercapnia (see Chapters 15, 33, and 34). The hypoventilation also may be caused by insensitivity to leptin, which has respiratory stimulant effects independent of the amount of visceral fat mass.[150] OSAS results in fragmentation of sleep with daytime sleepiness and further complications of hypoxia and heart disease.

The development of *osteoarthritis* occurs as a function of mechanical stress and limb malalignment on weight-bearing joints. Exercise intolerance and pain in the weight-bearing joints, particularly the hips and knees, are common. Inflammation may cause erosion of cartilage.[151,152]

EVALUATION AND TREATMENT There are several methods for measuring or estimating body fat mass, including computerized tomography (CT) and magnet resonance imaging (MRI) techniques; bioimpedance analysis; underwater weighing; and anthropometric measurements, such as skinfold thickness, circumferences, and various body diameters (i.e., waist-to-hip ratios and waist circumference, and body mass index [BMI—kg/m²] tables).[153,154] The BMI and waist-to-hip ratios are most commonly used because they are the easiest to measure. Overweight is defined as a BMI greater than 25 and obesity is a BMI greater than 30. BMI charts are available for children ages 2 to 20 years; these can be used for comparison during adulthood because obese children generally become obese adults.[110,155] No specific diagnostic criteria for obesity have been established.

Obesity is a chronic disease for which various approaches to treatment have been used; these include correction of metabolic abnormalities, individually tailored weight reduction diets, and exercise programs.[156-161] A combination of weight reduction and exercise are the most effective treatments.[162] Self-motivation and support systems are critical aspects of treatment. Additional treatments, such as psychotherapy, behavioral modification, medications, and bariatric surgery (i.e., the Roux-en-Y gastric bypass or gastric banding) are also prescribed and when successful result in a significant reduction in comorbidities and a decrease in insulin resistance.[163-165] Unraveling the causes of obesity will lead to more specific pharmacotherapies.

Anorexia Nervosa and Bulimia Nervosa

Anorexia nervosa and bulemia nervosa are characterized by aberrant eating behavior and weight regulation and disturbed attitudes toward body weight and shape.[166] Many young adults and adolescents—as many as 1% of women and adolescent girls in the United States—are affected by these two complex and related eating disorders. They occur rarely in black women, and only 5% to 10% of cases are men.[167] Risk

factors include genetic, familial, biologic, psychologic, and social factors.[168] There is an association between sexual assault history and eating disorders.[169] An increasing number of children, young men, and elderly women are experiencing eating disorders, often with an associated depression, anxiety, or personality disorder.[170]

Alterations in hypothalamic and gut-related neuropeptides that effect eating behavior and neuroendocrine disturbances are associated with weight loss and malnutrition.[171,172] Understanding these alterations may contribute to an explanation of the difficulty of reversing behaviors associated with these diseases.[173]

Anorexia nervosa (AN) is a psychiatric disorder and physiologic syndrome that affects 1% to 3% of women in the United States and is characterized by the following:[174,175]

1. A fear of becoming obese despite progressive weight loss
2. A distorted body image: the perception that the body is fat when it is actually underweight
3. Body weight 15% less than normal for age and height because of refusal to eat
4. In women and girls, absence of three consecutive menstrual periods

Persons with AN frequently deny they have any eating problem. Two types of eating behavior are distinguished in AN and both involve subnormal body weight and ongoing malnutrition. *Restrictive AN* entails unremitting food avoidance. *Binge eating/purging AN* includes binge eating followed by self-induced vomiting or laxative abuse. AN usually emerges during adolescence and in females who have a history of childhood abuse.[176]

As the disease progresses, muscle and fat depletion give the individual a skeleton-like appearance. Iron deficiency anemia promotes fatigue, and low white blood cell count increases risk of infection. Reproductive functioning is affected, including ovarian function, menstruation, fertility, and pregnancy. Postural hypotension, edema, bradycardia, hypothermia, low total body potassium, constipation, and sleep disturbances may ensue. The loss of 25% to 30% of ideal body weight can eventually lead to death caused by starvation-induced cardiac failure.[177] Most organ systems are affected by progressive starvation. Diagnosis of anorexia nervosa involves a thorough medical history, physical and psychologic examination, and ruling out other causes of anorexia and malnutrition.[178]

There are no universally accepted treatments. Treatment objectives for anorexia nervosa include reversing the compromised physical state, promoting insights and knowledge about the disorder, mutual goals, interaction with family members, restoring development growth, and modifying food habits.[179,180] Correction of nutritional status may require intensive treatment, including total parenteral nutrition. When the individual demonstrates the willingness to eat food for nourishment, dietary protein, carbohydrate, and fat are introduced in tolerable amounts. Care must be taken to prevent refeeding syndrome, which can result in fluid and electrolyte, cardiac, neurologic, and hematologic complications during nutritional rehabilitation.[181] Psychotherapy begins as soon as the physical symptoms are stabilized and may continue for several years. Fluoxetine administration may improve weight gain and reduction in obsessions.[182] Formal genetic studies are in progress and results may advance specificity of treatment.[183]

Bulimia nervosa is more common than anorexia, and body weight remains near normal but with aspirations for weight loss. The group at risk is the same as that for anorexia nervosa, except that bulimia tends to occur in slightly older, less affluent women. Diagnosis of bulimia is based on the following findings:[184]

1. Recurrent episodes of binge eating during which the individual fears not being able to stop
2. Self-induced vomiting, use of laxatives (purging type)
3. Two binge-eating episodes per week for at least 3 months (purging type)
4. Fasting to oppose the effect of binge eating or excessive exercise (nonpurging type)

Because of negative connotations associated with self-stimulated vomiting and purging, individuals who have bulimia binge and purge secretly. Bulimic individuals may binge and purge as often as 20 times each day. Weight will fluctuate by about 10 pounds. Continual vomiting of acidic chyme can cause pitted teeth, pharyngeal and esophageal inflammation, and tracheoesophageal fistulae. Overuse of laxatives can cause rectal bleeding. Secret binging isolates the bulimic individual and leads to depression and anger that is turned inward. A vicious cycle of depression, overeating to try to feel better, vomiting and purging to maintain a normal weight, and returning depression perpetuates this eating disorder. Mood symptoms are often worse in the winter.[185]

Because persons with bulimia are usually older than individuals with anorexia nervosa and usually have separated from a family core, individual or group cognitive behavior change is the treatment focus. Antidepressants may be of some benefit.[186] Individuals with bulimia rarely have physical problems requiring hospital care and respond to treatment more readily than those with anorexia nervosa.[187]

Starvation

Starvation is a reduction in energy intake leading to weight loss. Short-term starvation and long-term starvation have different effects. Therapeutic short-term starvation is part of many weight-reduction programs because it causes an initial rapid weight loss that reinforces the individual's motivation to diet. Therapeutic long-term starvation is used in medically controlled environments to facilitate rapid weight loss in morbidly obese individuals. Pathologic long-term starvation can be caused by poverty; chronic diseases of the cardiovascular, pulmonary, hepatic, and digestive systems; malabsorption syndromes; HIV infection; and cancer. In-hospital starvation primarily affects individuals with functional and cognitive deficits and inadequate caloric intake.[188]

Short-term starvation, or extended fasting, consists of several days of total dietary abstinence or deprivation. The body responds with protective mechanisms. For 4 to 6 hours after the last meal, the body is in a well-fed state and its energy requirements are supplied by glucose from recently ingested carbohydrates. Once all available energy has been absorbed from the intestine, glycogen in the liver is converted to glucose through **glycogenolysis,** the splitting of glycogen into glucose. This process peaks within 4 to 8 hours, and gluconeogenesis begins. **Gluconeogenesis** is the formation of glucose from noncarbohydrate molecules: lactate, pyruvate, amino acids, and the glycerol portion of fats. Like glycogenolysis, gluconeogenesis takes place within the liver. Both of these processes deplete stored nutrients and thus cannot meet the body's energy needs indefinitely. Proteins continue to be catabolized to a minimal degree, providing carbon for the synthesis of glucose.

Long-term starvation begins after several days of dietary abstinence and eventually causes death. Absolute deprivation of food causes **marasmus** or protein energy malnutrition. Protein deprivation in the presence of carbohydrate intake is called **kwashiokor.** Marasmic kwashiokor is a combination of chronic energy deficiency and chronic or acute protein deficiency.[189,190] The major characteristic of long-term starvation is a decreased dependence on gluconeogenesis and an increased use of ketone bodies (products of lipid and pyruvate metabolism) as a cellular energy source. During long-term starvation, depressed insulin levels and increased glucagon, cortisone, epinephrine, and growth hormones promote lipolysis in adipose tissue. Lipolysis liberates fatty acids, which supply energy to cardiac and skeletal muscle cells, and ketone bodies, which sustain brain tissue. Fatty acid, or ketone body, oxidation meets most of the energy needs of the cells. (Some glucose is still needed as fuel for brain tissue.) Once the supply of adipose tissue is depleted, proteolysis begins. The breakdown of muscle and visceral protein is the last process the body engages to supply energy for life. Death results from severe alterations in electrolyte balance and loss of renal, pulmonary, and cardiac function.[191]

Adequate ingestion of appropriate nutrients is the obvious treatment for starvation. In medically induced starvation the body is maintained in a ketotic state until the desired amount of adipose tissue has been lysed. Starvation imposed by chronic disease, long-term illness, or malabsorption is treated with enteral or parenteral nutrition. Perioperative management of nutrition is necessary to prevent unnecessary starvation.[192]

DISORDERS OF THE ACCESSORY ORGANS OF DIGESTION

The accessory organs of digestion (liver, gallbladder, pancreas) secrete substances necessary for digestion and, in the case of the liver, carry out metabolic functions needed to maintain life. Inflammatory disease is a common cause of accessory organ dysfunction. Inflammation disrupts secretory function and prevents secretions from flowing into the duodenum. Lack of accessory organ secretions is a major cause of maldigestion and malabsorption in the small intestine. Other causes of accessory organ dysfunction are obstruction of ducts by aggregates in the secretions themselves (e.g., obstruction of bile flow by gallstones) or by tumors. (Cancers of the digestive tract are described at the end of this chapter.)

Clinical Manifestations of Liver Disorders

Of all the accessory organ disorders, acute or chronic liver disease leads to the most systemic, life-threatening complications. These complications include portal hypertension, ascites, hepatic encephalopathy, jaundice, and hepatorenal syndrome.

Portal Hypertension

Portal hypertension is abnormally high blood pressure in the portal venous system primarily caused by resistance to portal blood flow. Pressure in this system is normally 3 mmHg; portal hypertension is an increase to at least 10 mmHg. The portal veins carry blood from the gastrointestinal tract, pancreas, and spleen to the liver. In the liver the blood flows through the sinusoids and empties into the hepatic veins, which carry it into the inferior vena cava. The inferior vena cava delivers blood to the right atrium. The portal veins, sinusoids, and hepatic veins compose the portal venous system.

PATHOPHYSIOLOGY   Portal hypertension is caused by disorders that obstruct or impede blood flow through any component of the portal venous system or vena cava. *Intrahepatic* causes result from thrombosis, inflammation, or fibrosis of the sinusoids, as occurs in cirrhosis of the liver, viral hepatitis, or schistosomiasis (a parasitic infection). *Posthepatic* causes occur from hepatic vein thrombosis or cardiac disorders—such as failure of the right side of the heart or constrictive pericarditis—that impair the pumping ability of the right heart. This causes blood to back up and increase pressure in the portal system. Thrombosis or narrowing of the portal vein is the major *prehepatic* cause. The most common cause of portal hypertension is obstruction caused by cirrhosis of the liver (see p. 1423), and increased portal blood flow from anterior splanchnic vasodilation.[193]

High pressure in the portal veins causes collateral vessels to open between the portal veins and the systemic veins, in which blood pressure is considerably lower (Figure 39-16). This enables blood to bypass the obstructed portal vessels. The collateral veins develop in the esophagus, anterior abdominal wall, and rectum. High pressure and increased flow volume are transmitted through these veins from the portal to the systemic venous circulation.

Long-term portal hypertension causes several problems that are difficult to treat and can be fatal:[194]

1. *Varices* (distended, tortuous, collateral veins): prolonged elevation of pressure in collateral veins causes their transformation into varices, particularly in the lower esophagus and stomach but also in the rectum.
2. *Splenomegaly* (enlargement of the spleen): caused by increased pressure in the splenic vein, which branches from the portal vein.

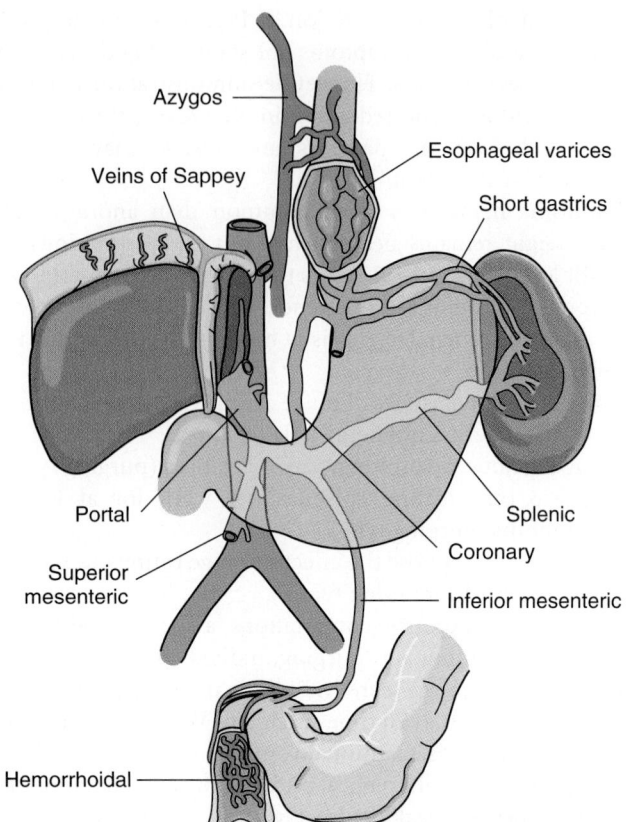

Figure 39-16 Varices related to portal hypertension. Portal vein, its major tributaries, and the most important shunts (collateral veins) between the portal and caval systems. (From Phipps WJ et al: *Medical-surgical nursing: concepts and clinical practice,* ed 7, St Louis, 2003, Mosby.)

3. *Ascites* (the accumulation of fluid in the peritoneal cavity, which is the space between the visceral peritoneum and the parietal peritoneum): caused in part by increased pressure in the mesenteric tributaries of the portal vein. Hydrostatic pressure forces water out of these vessels and into the peritoneal cavity. (This process, termed *transudative effusion,* is described in Chapter 33.)
4. *Hepatic encephalopathy* (also called *portosystemic encephalopathy*): characterized by central nervous system disturbances with astrocyte changes that lead to alterations of consciousness.

CLINICAL MANIFESTATIONS   The vomiting of blood from bleeding **esophageal varices** is the most common clinical manifestation of portal hypertension.[195] Slow, chronic bleeding from varices causes anemia or melena. Usually the bleeding is from varices that have developed slowly over a period of years.

Rupture of esophageal varices causes hemorrhage and voluminous vomiting of dark-colored blood. The ruptured varices are usually painless. Rupture is caused by a combination of erosion by gastric acid and elevated venous pressure. Mortality from ruptured esophageal varices ranges from 30% to 60%. Recurrent bleeding of esophageal or gastric varices indicates a poor prognosis. Most individuals die within 1 year.

EVALUATION AND TREATMENT   Diagnosis of portal hypertension is often made at the time of variceal bleeding and confirmed by endoscopy and evaluation of portal venous pressure. Distended collateral veins may radiate over the abdomen, giving rise to caput medusae (Medusa's head). The individual usually has a history of jaundice, hepatitis, or alcoholism.

Beta-blockers can be effective in preventing variceal bleeding. Emergency management of bleeding varices includes compression of the varices with an inflatable tube or balloon, band ligation, and injection of a sclerosing agent.[195] Surgical construction of a portacaval shunt (anastomosis of the portal vein to the inferior vena cava) may decompress the varices, but this treatment can precipitate encephalopathy or liver failure resulting from reduced hepatic blood flow. There is no effective, definitive treatment for portal hypertension. Liver transplant is an option for liver failure.

Splenomegaly

Splenomegaly is an enlargement of the spleen. Portal hypertension contributes to congestive splenomegaly by increasing intrasplenic blood pressure. Thrombocytopenia (decreased platelet count) is the most common manifestation of congestive splenomegaly and can contribute to an increased bleeding tendency. Splenomegaly also can be predictive of severity of esophageal varices.[196,197]

Ascites

Ascites is the accumulation of fluid in the peritoneal cavity. Ascites traps body fluid in a "third space" from which it cannot escape. The effect is to reduce the amount of fluid available for normal physiologic functions. Cirrhosis is the most common cause of ascites. Other diseases associated with ascites include heart failure, constrictive pericarditis, abdominal malignancies, nephrotic syndrome, and malnutrition. Twenty-five percent of individuals who develop ascites caused by cirrhosis die within 1 year. Continued heavy drinking of alcohol is associated with this mortality rate.

PATHOPHYSIOLOGY   Several factors contribute to the development of ascites. Impaired excretion of sodium by the kidneys promotes water retention, but the initiating event is not clear. The *overflow theory* proposes that renal sodium retention is stimulated by portal hypertension with intravascular hypervolemia and overflow into the peritoneal cavity. This imbalance tends to push water into the peritoneal cavity. Portal hypertension also increases the production of hepatic lymph, which "weeps" into the peritoneal cavity. The *underfill theory* proposes an increase in hepatic sinusoidal hydrostatic pressure and decreased oncotic pressure with weeping of lymph fluid from the surface of the liver. There is a decrease in effective circulating plasma volume, stimulating the kidney to retain more sodium and water, leading to intravascular volume overload.[198] The *arterial vasodilation theory* proposes that circulating nitric oxide triggers peripheral vasodilation early in the course of cirrhosis and stimulates renal sodium

retention through renin-angiotensin-aldosterone, increased sympathetic tone, and changes in the intrarenal blood flow.[199,200]

In cases of cirrhosis, both portal hypertension and decreased production of albumin by hepatocytes contribute to the ascites. Besides reducing albumin synthesis, deranged liver metabolism permits the accumulation of hormones that regulate sodium and water balance. Excessive amounts of aldosterone and antidiuretic hormone remain in the blood, stimulating the kidneys to retain sodium and water. High aldosterone levels can be attributed also to increased secretion mediated by excessive plasma renin activity. The increased plasma renin activity may develop because of decreased metabolic function of the liver, increased renal secretion stimulated by low blood flow, or both.

As ascites sequesters more and more body fluid, the kidneys respond by retaining sodium and water in amounts exceeding intake. Retention of sodium and water expands plasma volume, thereby accelerating portal hypertension and ascites formation.

Ascites can be complicated by bacterial peritonitis. Peritonitis involves an inflammatory response that worsens ascites by increasing mesenteric capillary permeability. As plasma seeps out of the permeable mesenteric capillaries, it adds to the volume of ascitic fluid. Figure 39-17 summarizes the mechanisms by which cirrhosis of the liver causes ascites.

CLINICAL MANIFESTATIONS   The accumulation of ascitic fluid causes weight gain, abdominal distention, and increased abdominal girth (Figure 39-18). Large volumes of fluid (10 to 20 L) displace the diaphragm and cause dyspnea by decreasing lung capacity. Respiratory rate increases, and the individual assumes a semi-Fowler position to relieve the dyspnea. Some peripheral edema is usually present. Approximately 10% of individuals with ascites develop bacterial peritonitis, either spontaneously or as a result of paracentesis (needle aspiration of ascitic fluid). Peritonitis causes fever, chills, abdominal pain, decreased bowel sounds, and cloudy ascitic fluid.

EVALUATION AND TREATMENT   Diagnosis of ascites is usually based on clinical manifestations and identification of liver disease. Paracentesis is used to aspirate ascitic fluid for bacterial culture, biochemical analysis, and microscopic examination. The goal of treatment is to relieve discomfort. If the restoration of liver function is possible (e.g., in ascites caused by viral hepatitis), the ascites diminishes spontaneously. In the meantime, dietary salt restriction and potassium-sparing diuretics can reduce ascites. Strong diuretics, such as furosemide or ethacrynic acid, may be used. Albumin may be given.[201] Serum electrolytes are monitored carefully because the individual is at risk for hyponatremia and hypokalemia.

Palliative measures include paracentesis to remove 1 or 2 L of ascitic fluid and relieve respiratory distress. This procedure

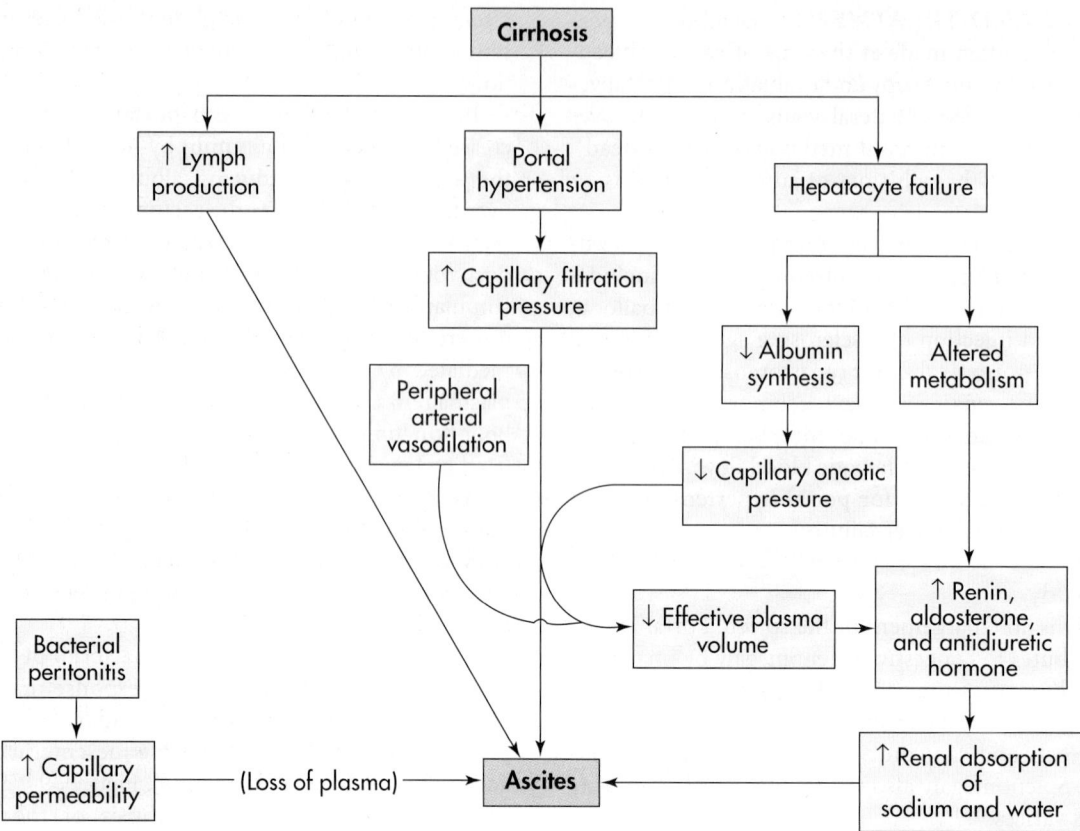

Figure 39-17 Mechanisms of ascites caused by cirrhosis.

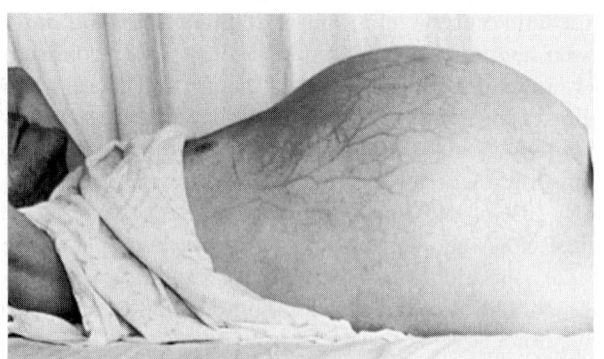

Figure 39-18 Massive ascites in an individual with cirrhosis. Distended abdomen, dilated upper abdominal veins, and inverted umbilicus are classic manifestations. (From Prior JA, Silberstein JS, Stang JM: *Physical diagnosis: the history and examination of the patient,* ed 6, St Louis, 1981, Mosby.)

can have serious complications, however. The removal of too much fluid too fast relieves pressure on blood vessels causing arteriolar vasodilation and carries the risk of hypotension, shock, or death.[202] Despite repeated paracenteses, ascitic fluid reaccumulates in individuals with irreversible disease, drawing more albumin and electrolytes out of the vascular compartment. Paracentesis is also likely to cause peritonitis. A peritoneovenous shunt may alleviate the need for frequent paracentesis.[203] Individuals with ascites and portal hypertension have a poor prognosis.

Hepatic Encephalopathy

Hepatic encephalopathy (portosystemic encephalopathy) is a complex neurologic syndrome characterized by impaired cognitive function, flapping tremor (asterixis), and electroencephalogram (EEG) changes. The syndrome may develop rapidly during acute fulminant hepatitis or slowly during the course of chronic liver disease. Risk factors in the presence of advanced liver disease include gastrointestinal bleeding, increased dietary protein, electrolyte imbalance, and hypoxia.

Blood that is shunted through collateral vessels to the systemic veins bypasses the liver, where toxins, hormones, and other harmful substances normally are removed. Hepatic encephalopathy results from the presence of these substances, particularly ammonia, in blood that reaches the brain.[204]

PATHOPHYSIOLOGY Hepatic encephalopathy probably results from a combination of biochemical alterations that affect neurotransmission. The astrocyte is the most vulnerable.[205] Liver dysfunction and collateral vessels that shunt blood around the liver to the systemic circulation permit neurotoxins absorbed from the gastrointestinal tract to circulate freely to the brain. Also, permeability of the blood-brain barrier may be increased. The most hazardous substances are end products of intestinal protein digestion, particularly ammonia.[206] The digestion of blood from leaking or ruptured varices adds to the amount of ammonia present in systemic blood, as does the action of ammonia-forming bacteria in the colon. Ammonia that reaches the brain may alter cerebral energy metabolism, interfere with neurotransmitters, or cause edema, which can result in brain herniation and death.[207,208]

Blood levels of ammonia do not account for all symptoms associated with hepatic encephalopathy. The accumulation of short-chain fatty acids, serotonin, tryptophan, and false neurotransmitters probably contributes to neural derangement.[209] Excessive γ-aminobutyric acid (GABA), an inhibitory neurotransmitter, may contribute to reduced levels of consciousness. Infection, hemorrhage, electrolyte imbalance, sedatives, and analgesics also can precipitate stupor and coma in the presence of liver disease.

CLINICAL MANIFESTATIONS   Subtle changes in personality, memory loss, irritability, lethargy, and sleep disturbances are common initial manifestations of hepatic encephalopathy. Symptoms then can progress to confusion, flapping tremor of the hands, stupor, convulsions, and coma. Coma is usually a sign of liver failure and ultimately results in death.

EVALUATION AND TREATMENT   Diagnosis of hepatic encephalopathy is based on a history of liver disease and clinical manifestations. Electroencephalography and blood chemistry tests, including blood ammonia levels, provide supportive data. There is no specific diagnostic test.

Correction of fluid and electrolyte imbalances and withdrawal of depressant drugs metabolized by the liver are the first steps in the treatment of hepatic encephalopathy. Reduction of blood ammonia levels is a major objective. This is accomplished by restricting dietary protein intake and eliminating intestinal bacteria. Neomycin is effective in sterilizing the bowel, but it can be nephrotoxic. Lactulose may be administered to prevent ammonia absorption in the colon.[210] Antibiotics appear superior to nonabsorbable disaccharides in improving hepatic encephalopathy.[210] Sodium benzoate and L-ornithine-Láspartate also detoxify ammonia.

Jaundice

Jaundice (icterus) is a yellow or greenish pigmentation of the skin caused by **hyperbilirubinemia** (total plasma bilirubin concentrations above 2.5 to 3 mg/dl). Hyperbilirubinemia and jaundice can result from excessive hemolysis of red blood cells or obstructive disorders of the bile ducts or liver cells (Figure 39-19). Jaundice in newborns is caused by impaired bilirubin uptake and conjugation (see Chapter 40).

PATHOPHYSIOLOGY   **Obstructive jaundice** can result from extrahepatic or intrahepatic obstruction.[211] *Extrahepatic obstructive jaundice* develops if the common bile duct is occluded by a gallstone, tumor, or compression from edema of

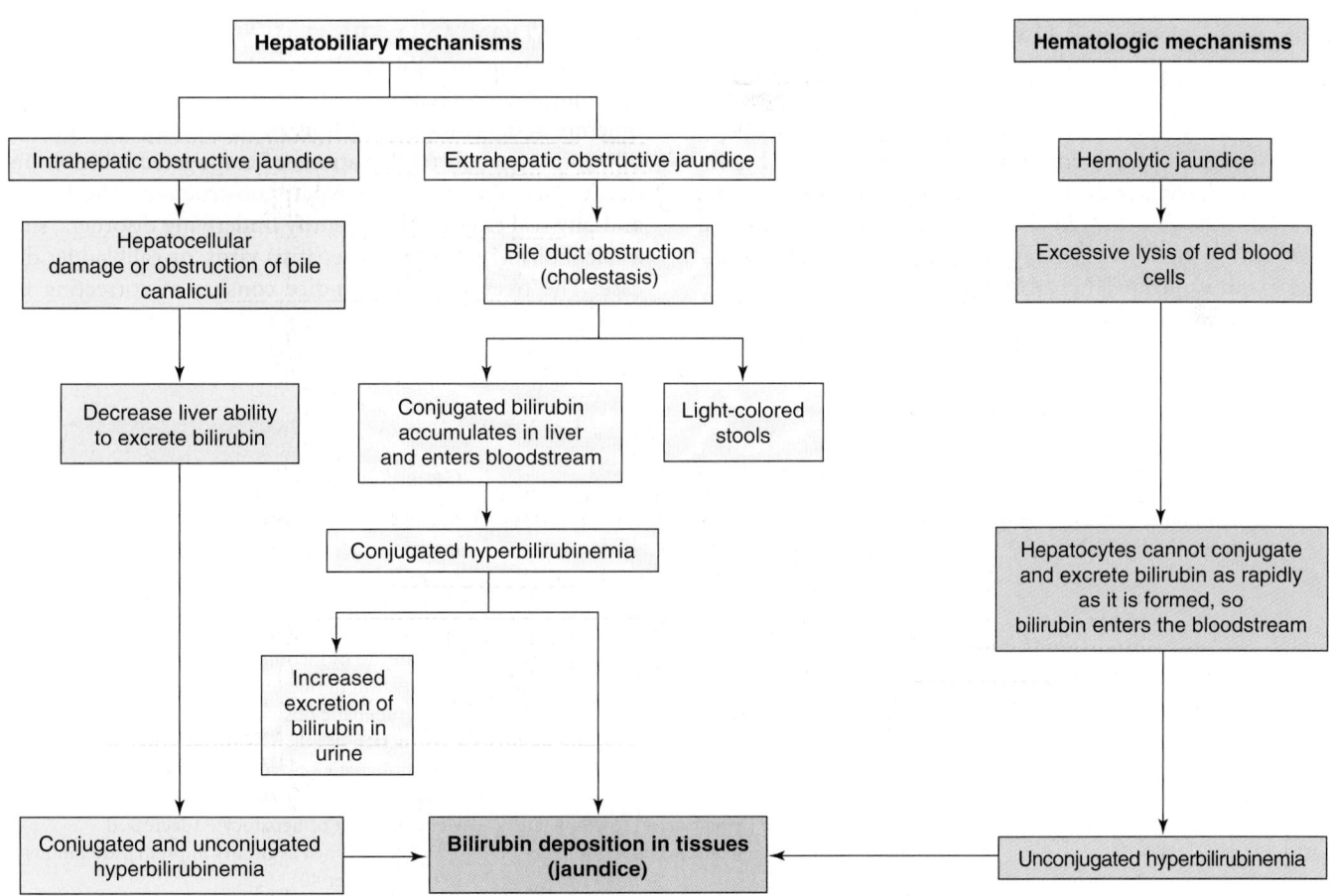

Figure 39-19 Mechanisms of jaundice.

pancreatitis. Because the bile duct is obstructed, bilirubin is conjugated by the hepatocytes but cannot flow into the duodenum. (Conjugated bilirubin is soluble in water and is then soluble in acqueous bile.) Therefore it accumulates in the liver and enters the bloodstream, causing hyperbilirubinemia. Because conjugated bilirubin is water soluble, it appears in the urine. The stools may be light colored or clay colored because they lack bile pigments. The stools also lack urobilinogen because bile is not available for conversion to urobilinogen.

Intrahepatic obstructive jaundice involves disturbances in hepatocyte function and obstruction of bile canaliculi. The uptake, conjugation, and excretion of bilirubin are affected with elevated levels of both conjugated and unconjugated bilirubin. Hepatocellular damage increases plasma concentrations of unconjugated bilirubin. The major disorder, however, is obstruction of bile canaliculi, which diminishes flow of conjugated bilirubin into the common bile duct with elevations in the plasma. In mild cases, some of the bile canaliculi open. Consequently, the amount of bilirubin in the intestinal tract may be only slightly decreased. The stools may appear normal or light colored.

Excessive hemolysis (breakdown) of red blood cells or absorption of hematoma can cause **hemolytic jaundice (prehepatic jaundice).** An increased amount of unconjugated (indirect) bilirubin is formed through metabolism of the heme component of destroyed red blood cells. The extra amount of unconjugated bilirubin exceeds the conjugation ability of the liver, causing blood levels of unconjugated bilirubin to rise. Unconjugated bilirubinemia is the major cause of hemolytic jaundice. Because unconjugated bilirubin is not water soluble, it is not excreted in the urine. The reserve conjugation ability of the liver usually prevents long-term unconjugated hyperbilirubinemia greater than 4 to 5 mg/dl. Severe hemolytic crisis, as occurs with sickle cell disease (see Chapter 28), is a cause of hemolytic jaundice. Hemolytic drugs also can cause jaundice. If unconjugated hyperbilirubinemia exceeds 5 mg/dl, both hemolytic and liver disorders are indicated.

Hyperbilirubinemia and jaundice can be caused also by metabolic defects that impair the uptake or conjugation of unconjugated bilirubin in the liver. Gilbert disease, for example, causes an elevation of unconjugated bilirubin in the plasma but no other symptoms of liver disease. Gilbert disease is probably caused by an inherited deficiency of glucuronyl transferase enzyme, which is required for the hepatic uptake of unconjugated bilirubin. The causes of jaundice are summarized in Table 39-8.

CLINICAL MANIFESTATIONS   The clinical manifestations of jaundice vary and are related to the underlying pathology. Conjugated hyperbilirubinemia may cause the urine to darken several days before the onset of jaundice. The complete obstruction of bile flow from the liver to the duodenum causes light-colored stools. With partial obstruction the stools are normal in color and bilirubin is present in the urine.

Fever, chills, and pain often accompany jaundice resulting from viral or bacterial inflammation of the liver (e.g., viral hepatitis). Manifestations of liver injury from any cause commonly include anorexia, malaise, and fatigue. Yellow discoloration may first occur in the sclera of the eye and then progress to the skin. Pruritus commonly accompanies jaundice with an elevation of serum alkaline phosphatase and bilirubin accumulation in the skin.[212]

EVALUATION AND TREATMENT   Laboratory evaluation of serum establishes whether elevated plasma bilirubin is conjugated or unconjugated or both. Unconjugated bilirubinemia results from hemolysis or hereditary disorders of bilirubin metabolism. Elevations of conjugated bilirubin indicate liver injury or extrahepatic obstruction. The history and physical examination identify underlying disorders, such as alcoholism, exposure to hepatitis virus, or gallbladder disease. The treatment for jaundice consists of correcting the cause.

Table 39-8	Three Common Types of Jaundice	
Type	**Mechanism**	**Causes**
Hemolytic jaundice (predominately unconjugated bilirubin)	Destruction of erythrocytes	Membrane defect of erythrocytes Immune reaction Severe infection Toxic substances in the circulation (e.g., snake venom) Transfusion of incompatible blood
Obstructive jaundice (predominately conjugated bilirubin)	Obstruction of passage of conjugated bilirubin from liver to intestine	Obstruction of bile duct by gallstones or tumor (extrahepatic obstructive jaundice) Obstruction of bile flow through the liver (intrahepatic obstructive jaundice) Drugs
Hepatocellular jaundice	Failure of liver cells (hepatocytes) to conjugate bilirubin and of bilirubin to pass from liver to intestine	Genetic defect of hepatocyte (decreased enzymes), such as occurs in premature infants (see Chapter 40) Severe infections

Hepatorenal Syndrome

Hepatorenal syndrome (HRS) is a complication of advanced liver disease characterized by functional renal failure with oliguria, sodium and water retention (with or without ascites and peripheral edema), hypotension, and peripheral vasodilation. Renal disorders associated with liver disease can have numerous causes, but HRS is usually associated with alcoholic cirrhosis and fulminant hepatitis. The renal failure is not caused by primary renal disease or other extrinsic factors, but rather by arterial vasodilation of the splanchnic vasculature and vasoconstriction of the renal circulation (prerenal renal failure).[213]

PATHOPHYSIOLOGY   Oliguric hepatic failure generally accompanies a sudden decrease in blood volume secondary to massive gastrointestinal bleeding or hypotension caused by failing liver function. Hypotension also can be caused by the excessive use of diuretics to treat ascites with decreased renal blood flow, glomerular filtration rate, and oliguria. The hypotension results in decreased glomerular filtration and ischemia with tubular necrosis. A significant number of individuals with advanced liver disease develop oliguria unrelated to any precipitating event. Inappropriate constriction of renal arterioles is proposed as the causative mechanism. Intrarenal vasoconstriction may result from the selective effects of vasoactive substances that accumulate in the blood because of liver failure. The diseased liver fails to remove excessive angiotensin, vasopressin, prostaglandins, and catecholamines from the blood. These substances travel to the kidneys and cause vasoconstriction. Vasoconstriction also may be a compensatory response to portal hypotension and the pooling of blood in the splanchnic circulation. The exact reason for the vasoconstriction is unknown[214] but is related to vasoconstrictive mediators[215] and sympathetic nerve stimulation. Systemic vasodilation caused by increases in nitric oxide and other substances also may contribute to vascular alterations and renal failure in advanced liver disease.[216]

CLINICAL MANIFESTATIONS   The onset of hepatorenal manifestations may be gradual or acute. Oliguria and complications of advanced liver disease, including jaundice, ascites, and gastrointestinal bleeding, are usually present. Systolic blood pressure is usually below 100 mmHg. Nonspecific symptoms of hepatorenal syndrome include anorexia, weakness, and fatigue.

EVALUATION AND TREATMENT   Diagnosis of HRS is made by excluding all other causes of renal failure. Despite oliguria, serum potassium levels do not become dangerously elevated until the terminal stages of the hepatorenal syndrome. Blood urea increases, followed by an increase in creatinine concentration. Urine osmolality is increased, but urine sodium concentrations are below normal. Urine specific gravity is above 1.015. The prognosis for hepatorenal syndrome is usually poor and is related to liver function. Secondary problems, including fluid and electrolyte disorders, bleeding, in-fections, and encephalopathy, are vigorously treated. Treatment may include systemic vasoconstrictors (alpha adrenergic agonists). Pentoxifylline is used to treat HRS in severe alcoholic hepatitis.[217] Liver transplant reverses symptoms.[218]

Disorders of the Liver
Viral Hepatitis

Viral hepatitis is a relatively common systemic disease that affects primarily the liver. Six strains of viruses cause various types of hepatitis: hepatitis A virus (HAV), hepatitis B virus (HBV), hepatitis D virus (HDV), hepatitis C virus (HCV), and hepatitis E virus (HEV). Hepatitis A was previously known as infectious hepatitis, and hepatitis B as serum hepatitis. Coinfection of HBV, HCV, HDV, and the human immunodeficiency virus (HIV) occurs because these viruses share the same routes of transmission with more rapid progression of liver disease.[219] Hepatitis G virus is usually not a significant cause of liver disease, but it may be associated with fulminant hepatitis.[220,221] Characteristics of the various types are presented in Table 39-9.

Types

Hepatitis A.   The hepatitis A virus can be recovered from the feces, bile, and sera of infected individuals. The usual mode of transmission is the fecal-oral route (contaminated food or water), but the virus can be spread also by the transfusion of infected blood. Approximately 45% of adults in urban areas have HAV antibodies in their blood. The disease spreads readily in crowded, unsanitary conditions, usually through contaminated food or water. Person-to-person spread is more likely to occur in settings such as day care centers or institutions for the mentally retarded, where there is close contact between clients and caregivers.[222]

The incubation period (the time between exposure and onset of symptoms) for hepatitis A is 4 to 6 weeks (Figure 39-20). Fecal shedding of the virus is greatest for 10 to 14 days before the onset of symptoms and during the first week of symptoms and up to 3 months after onset of symptoms. The disease is most contagious during this time. Antibodies to HAV (anti-HAV) develop about 4 weeks after infection. The serum immunoglobulin M (IgM) concentration increases initially and is followed by an increase of serum immunoglobulin G (IgG). IgG levels remain elevated for several years after infection, creating immunity to the disease. (See Chapters 6 and 7 for a description of immune functions.) Immunization is effective in preventing the disease and confers long-term immunity.[223] A combined HAV and HBV vaccine is available and effective.[224]

Hepatitis B.   Hepatitis B is transmitted through contact with infected blood, body fluids, or contaminated needles. Hepatitis B is also a sexually transmitted disease (see Chapter 24). Transmission among homosexual men may be by oral or genital contact with bleeding lesions in the rectal mucosa. People receiving hemodialysis, multiple blood transfusions, or immunosuppressive drugs have a greater risk of exposure or less resistance to HBV. Co-infection with HCV, HDV, and human immunodeficiency virus (HIV) is not uncommon be-

Table 39-9	Characteristics of Viral Hepatitis					
Characteristic	Hepatitis A	Hepatitis B	Hepatitis D	Hepatitis C	Hepatitis E	Hepatitis G
Size of virus	27 nm RNA virus	47 nm DNA virus	36 nm RNA virus, defective virus with HbsAg coat	30-60 nm RNA virus	32 nm RNA virus	30-60 nm RNA virus
Incubation period	30 days	60-180 days	30-180 days	35-60 days	15-60 days	Unknown
Route of transmission	Fecal-oral, parenteral, sexual	Parenteral, sexual	Parenteral, ? fecal-oral, sexual	Parenteral	Fecal-oral	Parenteral, sexual
Onset	Acute with fever	Insidious	Insidious	Insidious	Acute	Unknown
Carrier state	Negative	Positive	Positive	Positive	Negative	Positive
Severity	Mild	Severe; may be prolonged or chronic	Severe	Mild to severe	Severe in pregnant women	Unknown
Chronic hepatitis	No	Yes	Yes	Yes	No	Unknown
Age-group affected	Children and young adults	Any	Any	Any	Children and young adults	Any
Prophylaxis	Hygiene, immune serum globulin HAV vaccine	Hygiene, HBV vaccine	Hygiene, HBV vaccine	Hygiene, screening blood, interferon-alpha	Hygiene, safe water	

RNA, Ribonucleic acid; *DNA,* deoxyribonucleic acid; *HbsAg,* hepatitis B surface antigen; *HBV,* hepatitis B virus.

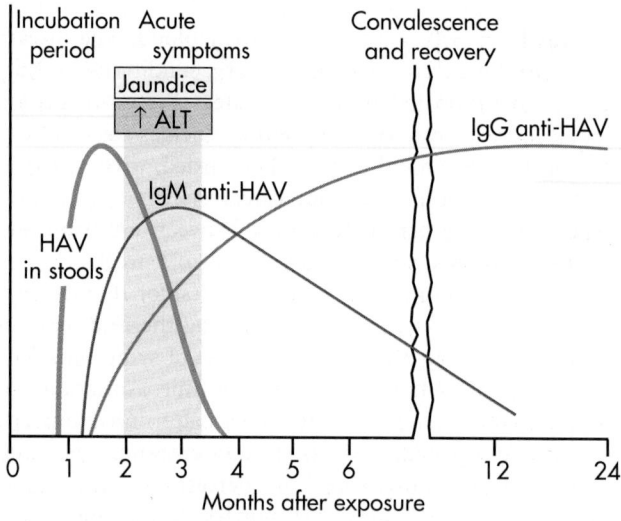

Figure 39-20 Course of infection with the hepatitis A virus (HAV). *IgM,* Immunoglobulin M; *IgG,* immunoglobulin G.

cause these viruses share the same routes of transmission.[225] Mother-infant transmission of HBV occurs if the mother becomes infected during the third trimester of pregnancy. Approximately 0.3% of adults in the United States carry the hepatitis B surface antigen (HBsAg) marker for active HBV and up to 400 million worldwide.[226,227]

Three types of viral particles are involved in HBV infection. The larger (47 nm) Dane particle probably represents the intact HBV. The Dane particle has a double-layered outer coat and carries the hepatitis B surface antigen (HBsAg), which was originally called the *Australia antigen.* HBsAg can

be identified in the serum by radioimmunoassay. Hepatitis B core antigen (HBcAg) usually is not detected in the serum. The HBeAg is a derivative of HBcAg and is a marker of HBV replication. The HBV has an incubation period of 6 to 8 weeks. The initial serologic change is a transient increase in IgM. Levels of IgG antibodies to HBsAg rise more slowly and remain elevated for years (Figure 39-21). Chronic infection develops in 15% to 30% of those with acute infection with increased risk for cirrhosis and hepatocellular carcinoma.[227,228] Antiviral treatment for chronic hepatitis B includes interferon alpha, lamivadine, and adefovir dipivoxil.[228] Vaccine prevents transmission of hepatitis B and the development of acute or chronic hepatitis B.[229]

Hepatitis C. Hepatitis C virus (non-A, non-B hepatitis) causes most cases of posttransfusion hepatitis. Hepatitis C antibody is present in 1.8% of the United States population, with new infections originating from intravenous drug use.[230] The risk for developing hepatitis C is greater with large volumes of blood replacement and among intravenous drug users. Persistent infection may result from weak T-cell response during acute infection. The U.S. Food and Drug Administration (FDA) has approved an assay for screening hepatitis C antibodies in blood products. Chronic hepatitis occurs in 50% to 80% of cases and is a risk factor for chronic liver disease, cirrhosis, and hepatocellular carcinoma.[231] Pegylated interferon and ribavirin are used to prevent progressive hepatic fibrosis.[232]

Hepatitis D. The hepatitis D virus (HDV) occurs in individuals with hepatitis B. The delta virus depends on the hepatitis B virus for its replication because the coat of the delta virus consists of HBsAg molecules that are on the sur-

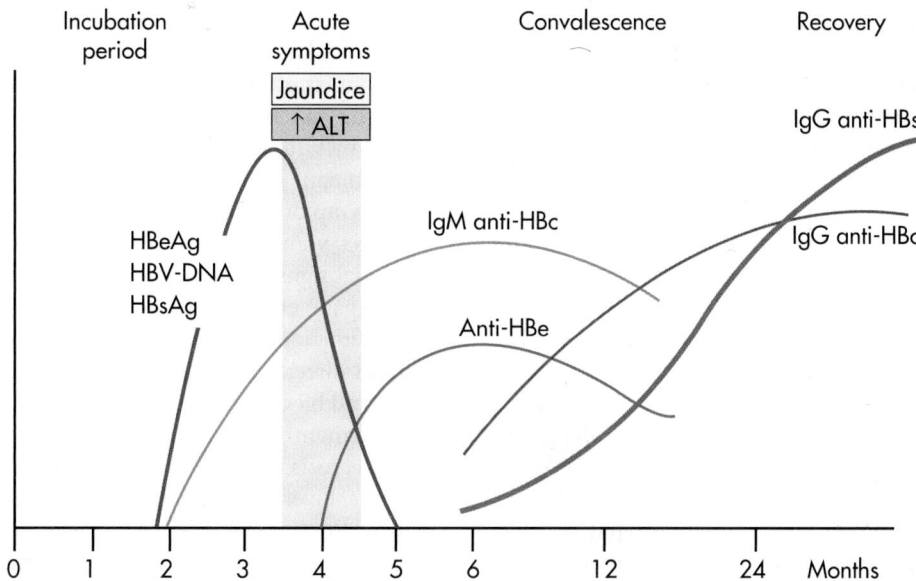

Figure 39-21 Course of infection with the hepatitis B virus (HBV). *HbsAg,* Hepatitis B surface antigen; *anti-HBs,* antibody to HBsAg; *HbeAg,* hepatitis B e antigen; *anti-Hbe,* antibody to HBeAg; *anti-HBc,* antibody to hepatitis B core antigen. The antibody to HBs (anti-HBs) is IgG, the immunoglobulin that creates immunity. *DNA,* Deoxyribonucleic acid; *IgM,* immunoglobulin M; *IgG,* immunoglobulin G.

face of the HBV virus. Parenteral drug users have a high incidence of HDV infection. Hepatitis D has been shown to suppress replication of hepatitis B virus.[233] The clinical course of HDV is similar to that of hepatitis A and B, although it is sometimes more severe.

Hepatitis E. Hepatitis E is most common in developing countries and is transmitted by the fecal-oral route,[234] usually by way of contaminated water. It is more prevalent among adults and has the highest mortality in pregnant women. Clinically, it resembles HAV. Currently no vaccine for HEV is available but development is in progress.[235]

Hepatitis G. Hepatitis G virus is a recently discovered parenterally and sexually transmitted virus. Currently much about this virus is still unknown, and it is uncertain whether it is associated with post-transfusion hepatitis.[236] No association with hepatocellular carcinoma has been reported.[237,238]

PATHOPHYSIOLOGY   The pathologic lesions of hepatitis are similar to those caused by other viral infection. Hepatic cell necrosis, scarring, Kupffer cell hyperplasia, and infiltration by mononuclear phagocytes occur with varying severity. Cellular injury is promoted by cell-mediated immune mechanisms (i.e., cytotoxic T cells and natural killer cells). Regeneration of hepatic cells begins within 48 hours of injury. The inflammatory process can damage and obstruct bile canaliculi, leading to cholestasis and obstructive jaundice. In milder cases the liver parenchyma is not damaged. Damage tends to be most severe in cases of hepatitis B and hepatitis C. Hepatitis B is also associated with *acute fulminating hepatitis,* a rare form of the disease that is characterized by massive hepatic necrosis. Acute fulminating hepatitis causes severe encephalopathy, which is manifested as confusion, stupor, and coma. Liver failure can occur, leading to intestinal bleeding,

cardiorespiratory insufficiency, and renal failure. Mortality is high, but recovery can be complete.

CLINICAL MANIFESTATIONS   The clinical manifestations of the various types of hepatitis are very similar. The spectrum of manifestations ranges from absence of symptoms to fulminating hepatitis, with rapid onset of liver failure and coma. Acute viral hepatitis causes abnormal liver function test results. The serum aminotransferase values, aspartate transaminase (AST) and alanine transaminase (ALT), are elevated, but their elevation may not be consistent with the extent of cellular damage. The clinical course of hepatitis usually consists of four phases: incubation, prodromal, icteric, and recovery phases. The **incubation phase** is reviewed in Table 39-9 (p. 1420).

Prodromal Phase. The **prodromal (preicteric) phase** of hepatitis begins about 2 weeks after exposure and ends with the appearance of jaundice. Fatigue, anorexia, malaise, nausea, vomiting, headache, hyperalgia, cough, and low-grade fever are prodromal symptoms that precede the onset of jaundice. About 10% of individuals may develop extrahepatic symptoms including rash, arthralgias, and purpura. HBV may cause nephritis.[239] Food odors often cause nausea, and changes in taste suppress the desire to smoke and drink alcohol. Right upper abdominal pain is common, and a weight loss of 2 to 4 kg is not unusual. The infection is highly transmissible during this phase.

Icteric Phase (Jaundice). The **icteric phase** begins about 1 to 2 weeks after the prodromal phase and lasts 2 to 6 weeks. Hepatocellular destruction and intrahepatic bile stasis cause jaundice (icterus). The urine may be dark and the stools clay colored before the onset of jaundice from conjugated hyperbilirubinemia. The icteric phase is the actual phase of illness. The liver is enlarged, smooth, and tender, and percussion over the liver causes pain. During the icteric phase, gastrointestinal and respiratory symptoms subside, but fatigue and abdominal pain may persist or become more severe. The stools may be lighter in color as a result of cholestasis. Serum bilirubin levels range from 5 to 10 mg/dl, with conjugated bilirubin fraction increasing. The jaundice may last 2 to 6 weeks or longer. Mild and transient itching often accompanies jaundice. The prothrombin time may be prolonged in individuals with more serious forms of the disease.

Recovery Phase. The posticteric or **recovery phase** begins with resolution of jaundice, about 6 to 8 weeks after exposure. Although the liver may still be enlarged and tender, symptoms diminish. In most cases, liver function test results return to normal within 2 to 12 weeks after the onset of jaundice.

Chronic hepatitis may begin at this point and is associated with HBV and HCV infection. **Chronic active hepatitis** is the persistence of clinical manifestations and liver inflammation after acute hepatitis B, hepatitis C, and hepatitis D. Liver function tests remain abnormal for longer than 6 months, and HBsAg persists. Chronic, active hepatitis B is a predisposition to cirrhosis and primary hepatocellular carcinoma. Chronic active hepatitis constitutes a carrier state and hepatitis C can be transmitted from mothers to infants.[240]

EVALUATION AND TREATMENT   The most specific diagnostic test for viral hepatitis is serologic analysis for HBsAg, which is the marker for HBV. Diagnosis of type A hepatitis is based on the presence of anti-HAV, as is the diagnosis of HCV. The assay for HDV is the total antibody to hepatitis D and antigen (anti-HDV). A test for HEV has not been developed. Liver function tests also can indicate other viral liver diseases, drug toxicity, or alcoholic hepatitis.

Specific treatments are previously described for the different types of hepatitis viruses. Physical activity may be restricted. A low-fat, high-carbohydrate diet is beneficial if bile flow is obstructed.

To prevent transmission of hepatitis A, hand washing and use of gloves for disposing of bedpans and fecal matter are imperative. There should be no direct contact with blood or body fluids of individuals with hepatitis B or hepatitis C. The administration of immune globulin before exposure or early in the incubation period can prevent hepatitis A. A combined vaccine for HAV and HBV is now available. Prophylactic immune globulin administered before exposure can prevent hepatitis B. Prophylaxis is recommended for health care workers and others who are at risk for contact with infected body fluids.[241]

Fulminant Hepatitis

Fulminant hepatitis is a clinical syndrome resulting in severe impairment or necrosis of liver cells and potential liver failure. The disorder may occur as a complication of hepatitis C or hepatitis B, particularly HBV infection compounded by infection with the delta virus. Toxic reactions to drugs and congenital metabolic disorders also can cause fulminant hepatitis.[242,243]

Causative mechanisms of fulminant hepatic failure are poorly understood. Hepatocytes become edematous, and patchy areas of necrosis and inflammatory cell infiltrates disrupt the parenchyma. The death of hepatocytes may be caused by viral or immunologic damage.

Fulminant hepatitis usually develops 6 to 8 weeks after the initial symptoms of viral hepatitis or a metabolic liver disorder. Anorexia, vomiting, abdominal pain, and progressive jaundice are initial signs, followed by ascites and gastrointestinal bleeding. Hepatic encephalopathy is manifested as lethargy, altered motor functions, and coma. Liver function tests show elevations of both direct and indirect serum bilirubin, serum transaminases, and blood ammonia. Prothrombin time is prolonged.

Treatment of fulminant hepatitis is supportive. The hepatic necrosis is irreversible, and 60% to 90% of affected children die. Liver transplantation may be life saving.[244] Survivors usually do not develop cirrhosis or chronic liver disease. Bioartificial liver support systems promote survival and may be used as a bridge to transplant.[245]

Cirrhosis

Cirrhosis is an irreversible inflammatory disease that disrupts liver structure and function and is a leading cause of death in the United States. Disorganization of hepatic tissues

---

WHAT'S NEW? **Artificial Liver Support**

During the past several years, advances have been made in the development of materials and methods to artificially support liver function. Because of the shortage of donor organs there is a high incidence of mortality related to acute or chronic liver failure. Bioartificial liver devices have demonstrated temporary support of liver function in animal studies and are encouraging in early clinical trials in humans. Bioartificial livers can serve as a bridge to liver transplantation or support liver function long enough to allow regeneration of normal liver function. One type of bioartificial liver (BAL) circulates the individual's blood around the outside of a system of hollow fibers packed with pig hepatocytes. The fiber membrane allows toxins to be removed and nutrients to be replaced but does not allow cells to be exchanged. Another type of liver support is the Molecular Absorbents Recirculating System (MARS), an extracorporeal albumin dialysis technique that uses an albumin-impregnated membrane to remove both protein-bound and water-soluble toxins from the blood. Clinical trials are in progress for the development of internal devices, strategies that promote hepatic regeneration, and ways to enhance replacement of pig hepatocytes with human hepatocytes, including stem cell research, with continuing evaluation of safety and biochemical outcomes.

Data from Auth MK et al: *J Pediatr Gastroenterol Nutr* 40(1):54-59, 2005; Boyle M et al: *Crit Care* 8(4):280-286, 2004; Demetriou AA et al: *Ann Surg* 239(5):660-667, 2004; Ding YT et al: *Hepatobiliary Pancreat Dis Int* 3(4):508-510, 2004; Khuroo MS, Khuroo MS, Farahat KL: *Liver Transpl* 10(9):1099-1106, 2004; Lahdenpera A et al: *Transpl Int*, 17(11):717-723, 2005; Li LJ et al: *World J Gastroenterol* 10(20):2984-2988, 2004; Liu JP et al:, *Cochrane Database Syst Rev* (1):CD003628, 2004; Liu Q et al: *World J Gastroenterol* 10(9):1379-1381, 2004; Sen S et al: *Liver Transpl* 10(9):1109-1119, 2004.

Table 39-10	Cirrhosis of the Liver	
Type and Disease Name	**Causal Mechanisms**	**Pathophysiology**
Alcoholic cirrhosis, Laennec cirrhosis, portal cirrhosis, fatty cirrhosis	Toxic effects of chronic, excessive alcohol intake; acetylaldehyde formed by alcohol metabolism damages hepatocytes	Fatty liver, inflammation (alcoholic hepatitis), and derangement of the lobular architecture by necrosis and fibrosis (cirrhosis) with obstruction of biliary and vascular channels
Biliary cirrhosis (intrahepatic or extra-hepatic obstruction of bile flow)		
Primary biliary cirrhosis	Unknown; possible an autoimmune mechanism	Inflammation and scarring of lobular bile ducts
Secondary biliary cirrhosis	Obstruction by neoplasms, strictures, or gallstones	Inflammation and scarring of bile ducts proximal to the obstruction
Postnecrotic cirrhosis	Viral hepatitis caused by hepatitis A, B, or C virus; drugs or other toxins; autoimmune destruction	Replacement of necrotic tissue with cirrhotic tissue, particularly fibrous, nodular scar tissue
Metabolic cirrhosis	Metabolic defects and storage disease, such as α1-antitrypsin deficiency, glycogen storage disease, hemochromatosis, Wilson disease, galactosemia	Inflammation and scarring with specific morphologic changes related to cause

is caused by diffuse fibrosis and nodular regeneration. Nodules of regenerated tissue form between fibrous bands, giving the liver a cobbly appearance. The liver may be larger or smaller than normal, and usually it is firm or hard when palpated. A variety of disorders can cause cirrhosis. Therefore it is often classified by cause (Table 39-10).

The precise process of cellular injury depends on the cause of cirrhosis, and the causes are not all clearly understood. Structural changes result from fibrosis, which is a consequence of inflammation. The parenchyma of the liver becomes distorted, and biliary channels may be altered or obstructed, producing jaundice. Obstruction caused by cirrhosis can cause portal hypertension (see p. 1414). New vascular channels can form shunts, and blood from the portal vein bypasses the liver. These vascular changes compromise liver function further, and the process of regeneration is replaced by hypoxia; necrosis; atrophy; and, ultimately, liver failure.

Cirrhosis develops slowly over a period of years. Its severity and rate of progression depend on the cause. If toxins, such as alcohol, are involved, the rate of cell death and the severity of inflammation depend on the amount of toxin present.[246]

Alcoholic Liver Disease

Alcoholic hepatitis is a precursor of cirrhosis characterized by inflammation, degeneration, and necrosis of hepatocytes, infiltration of polymorphonuclear leukocytes and lymphocytes, immunologic alterations, and lipid peroxidation. The injured hepatocytes contain Mallory bodies (hyaline endoplasmic reticulum). The presence of Mallory bodies indicates the onset of fibrosis. Neutrophils infiltrate and surround degenerating hepatocytes. The mechanism of hepatocyte injury is not clearly understood, but inflammatory mediators, acetaldehyde, reactive oxygen and nitrogen species, and genetic factors are involved.[247,248] Serum IgA is often elevated in individuals with alcoholic hepatitis, and liver antigens and antibodies have been identified in persons with progressive alcoholic liver disease. The inflammation and necrosis caused by alcoholic hepatitis stimulate the fibrosis characteristic of the cirrhotic stage of disease.[249]

Deaths from alcohol-related liver disease have increased over the past decade. The incidence of alcoholic cirrhosis is greatest in middle-age men. In the United States, mortality resulting from cirrhosis is highest among nonwhites. Although alcoholic cirrhosis is the most prevalent of the various types of cirrhosis, the occurrence of cirrhosis among persons with alcoholism is relatively low (approximately 25%). The amount and duration of alcohol consumption are positively related to the extent of liver damage. Abuse of any type of alcoholic beverage can cause cirrhosis. Malnutrition may add to the risk of cirrhosis in alcohol abusers.

PATHOPHYSIOLOGY   **Alcoholic cirrhosis** is a complex process that begins with fatty infiltration (hepatic steatosis). Fatty infiltration can occur without subsequent hepatitis or cirrhosis. Fat deposition (deposition of triglycerides) within the liver hepatocytes is caused primarily by increased lipogenesis and decreased fatty acid oxidation by hepatocytes. Lipids mobilized from adipose tissue or dietary fat intake may contribute to fat accumulation. Cessation of alcohol intake reverses the fatty accumulation.

Alcoholic cirrhosis is caused by the toxic effects of alcohol on the liver, immunologic alterations, and lipid peroxidation.[250] Alcoholic cirrhosis is also associated with HCV.[251] The oxidative metabolism of alcohol occurs primarily in the liver (see Chapter 2). Alcohol is transformed to acetaldehyde. Excessive amounts of acetaldehyde induce lipid peroxidation and disrupt cytoskeleton and membrane function. Mitochondrial function is impaired, decreasing oxidation of fatty acid. Enzyme and protein synthesis may be depressed or altered, and hormone and ammonia degradation is diminished. Acetaldehyde inhibits export of proteins from the liver, alters metabolism of vitamins and minerals, promotes liver fibrosis, and induces malnutrition.[252] Alcohol also may stimulate the formation of autoantibodies specific to hepatic cells. Bacterial endotoxin from the intestine contributes to progressive injury and inflammation.[253,254] Cellular damage initiates an inflammatory response. Inflammatory cytokines, including tumor necrosis factor-alpha and IL-6, -8, and -18, are associated with alcoholic liver disease. Inflammation and necrosis result in excessive collagen formation. Transforming growth factor-beta contributes to fibrosis.[255] Dense bands of fibrosis surround regenerative hepatocellular nodules. Fibrosis and scarring alter the structure of the liver and obstruct biliary and vascular channels.[256] Examples of liver damage are shown in Figure 39-22.

CLINICAL MANIFESTATIONS

Fatty infiltration causes no specific symptoms or abnormal liver function test results. The liver is usually enlarged, however, and the individual has a history of continuous alcohol intake during the previous weeks or months. Anorexia, nausea, jaundice, and edema develop with advanced fatty infiltration or the onset of alcoholic hepatitis (Figure 39-23).

The clinical manifestations of alcoholic hepatitis can be mild or severe. Nonspecific symptoms include fatigue, weight loss, and anorexia.[257] Manifestations of acute illness include nausea, anorexia, fever, abdominal pain, and jaundice. Toxic effects of alcohol also can cause testicular atrophy, reduced libido, azoospermia, and decreased testosterone in men.[258] Cirrhosis is a multiple-system disease and causes hepatomegaly, splenomegaly, ascites, gastrointestinal hemorrhage, portal hypertension, hepatic encephalopathy, and esophageal varices. Anemia results from blood loss, poor nutrition, and hypersplenism. Risk for infection is greater, in part because of altered macrophage function.[259] The presence of numerous and severe manifestations increases the risk of death. The clinical features of alcoholic cirrhosis depend on the duration of the disease and the severity of liver damage.

EVALUATION AND TREATMENT

The diagnosis of alcoholic hepatitis is based on the individual's history and clinical manifestations. The results of liver function tests are abnormal, and serologic studies show elevated serum enzymes and bilirubin, decreased serum albumin, and prolonged prothrombin time.

Liver biopsy can confirm the diagnosis of cirrhosis, but biopsy is not necessary if clinical manifestations of cirrhosis are evident. Liver function test results are usually abnormal and reflect the severity of liver damage, including the consequences of portal hypertension. In severe disease with a poor prognosis, the serum albumin concentration is very low, prolonged prothrombin times cannot easily be corrected with vitamin K therapy, and serum bilirubin levels are high.

There is no specific treatment for alcoholic cirrhosis, but many of the complications are treatable. Rest; a nutritious diet; corticosteroids; antioxidants; drugs that slow fibrosis; and management of complications, such as ascites, gastrointestinal bleeding, infection, and encephalopathy slow disease progression. Cessation of alcohol consumption slows the progression of liver damage, improves clinical symptoms, and prolongs life. Although the liver damage is irreversible, measures that halt the inflammation and destruction of liver cells prolong life. Liver transplant is the treatment for liver failure.[260]

Biliary Cirrhosis

Biliary cirrhosis differs from alcoholic cirrhosis in that the damage and inflammation leading to cirrhosis begin in bile canaliculi and bile ducts, rather than in the hepatocytes. The two types of biliary cirrhosis are *primary* and *secondary*. Although both involve bile duct pathology, they differ with respect to cause, risk factors, and mechanisms of obstruction and inflammation.

Primary Biliary Cirrhosis. Primary biliary cirrhosis is an autoimmune disease of unknown etiology leading to destruction of small intrahepatic bile ducts. Mitochondrial autoantibodies are a hallmark of the disease and may be triggered by xenobiotics of infectious agents in genetically susceptible individuals.[261,262] The disease is characterized by inflammation and destruction of small intrahepatic bile ducts with portal inflammation and, ultimately, fibrosis. Women are affected more commonly than men. Symptoms rarely develop before the age of 30 years. Primary biliary cirrhosis often accompanies the autoimmune diseases.[263]

Primary biliary cirrhosis develops insidiously. It begins with inflammation, destruction, fibrosis, and obstruction of the intrahepatic bile ducts. Nodular regeneration and cirrho-

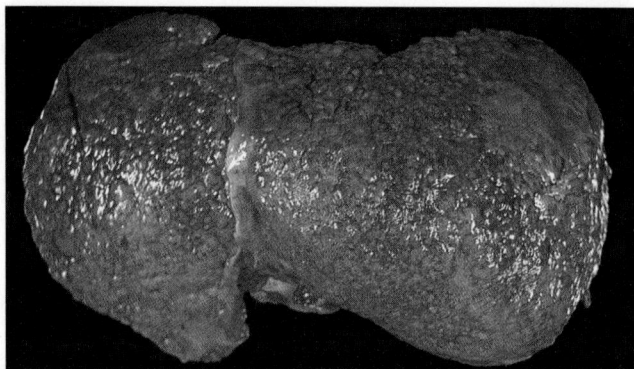

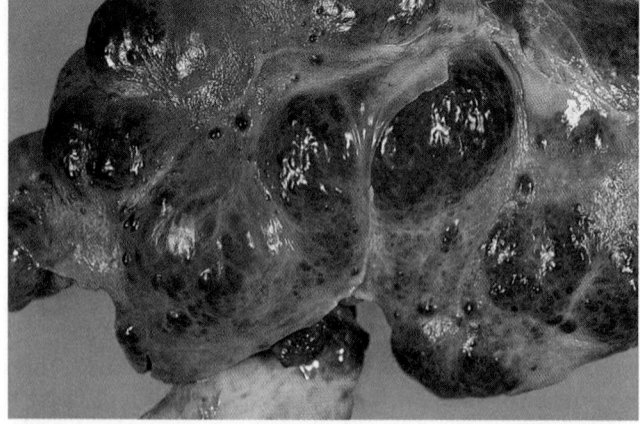

Figure 39-22 Cirrhosis. **A,** Micronodular cirrhosis. The nodular appearance develops from regeneration of hepatocytes projecting through fibrous bands of tissue. **B,** Macronodular cirrhosis. (From Damjanov I, Linder J, editors: *Anderson's pathology,* ed 10, St Louis, 1996, Mosby.)

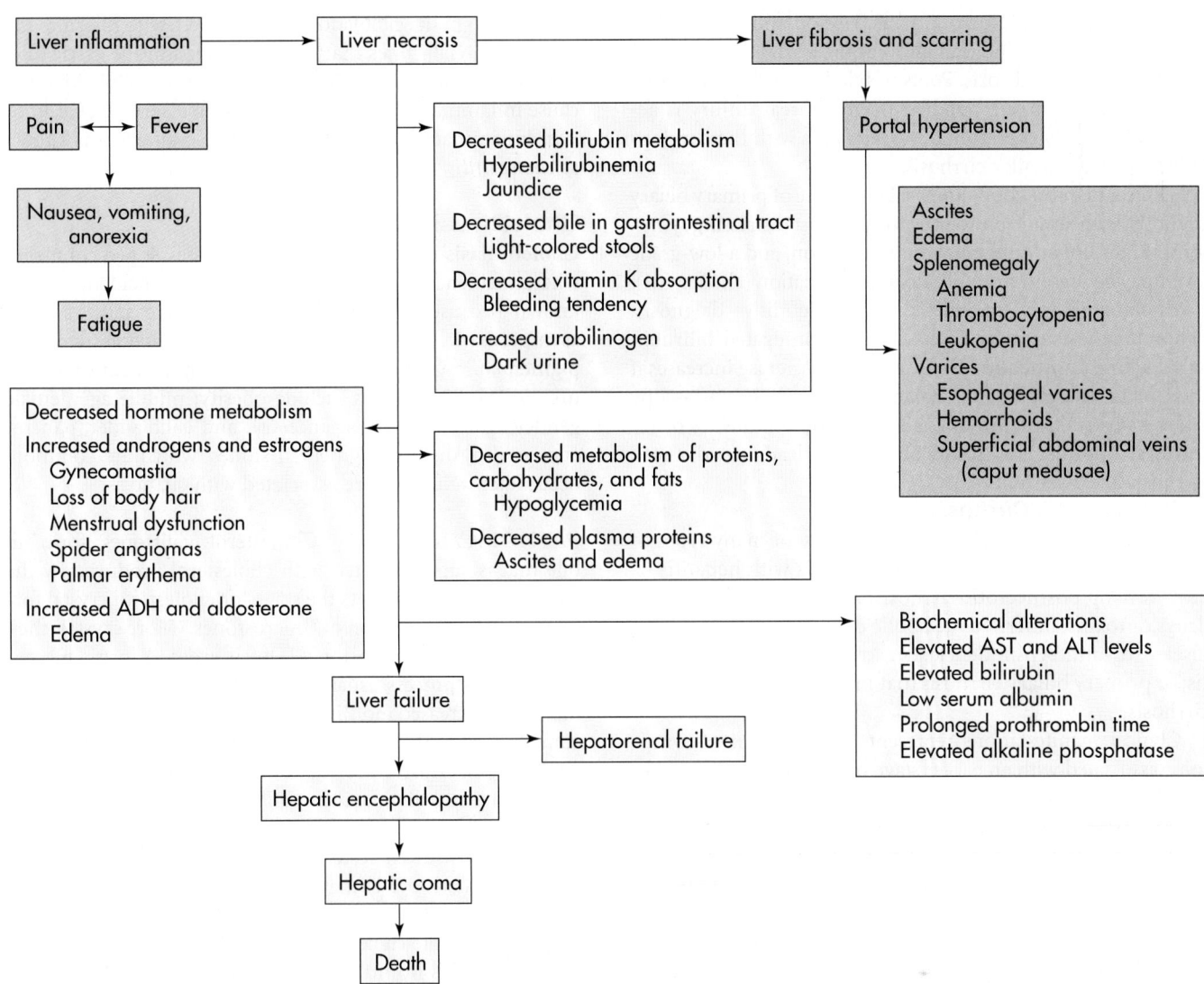

Figure 39-23 Clinical manifestations of cirrhosis. *ADH,* Antidiuretic hormone; *AST,* aspartate transaminase; *ALT,* alanine transaminase.

sis follow. Portal hypertension develops during the later stages of the disease.[264]

Individuals with primary biliary cirrhosis may be asymptomatic or symptomatic.[265] The earliest manifestations are pruritus, fatigue, and abdominal pain. Jaundice and light-colored stools are later symptoms. These symptoms are caused by intrahepatic obstruction of bile flow. Steatorrhea and fat-soluble vitamin deficiencies are present in some cases. The malabsorption can lead to osteomalacia and osteoporosis. Cirrhosis, symptoms of portal hypertension and encephalopathy, and ultimately liver failure develop. Life expectancy is approximately 8 to 10 years after onset of symptoms.[266]

Serologic tests show elevated alkaline phosphatase levels, hyperbilirubinemia, and hyperlipidemia, with or without other clinical manifestations. Most individuals have a circulating IgG antimitochondrial antibody that is not found in other types of liver disease. Evaluation involves ruling out biliary obstruction caused by gallstones, tumor, or inflammation

of the common bile duct (i.e., secondary biliary cirrhosis). Liver biopsy usually confirms the diagnosis of primary biliary cirrhosis.

Corticosteroids or azathioprine may be used to suppress the immune response. No specific treatment is available. The distressing pruritus may be relieved by cholestyramine, which binds bile salts in the intestine. Intramuscular injections of vitamins D and K alleviate the vitamin deficiency. The other symptoms of cirrhosis are managed as they develop. Long-term treatment with ursodeoxycholic acid slows disease progression.[267] Liver transplant is the only definitive therapy.

Secondary Biliary Cirrhosis. **Secondary biliary cirrhosis** develops when there is prolonged partial or complete obstruction of the common bile duct or its branches. The obstruction may be caused by gallstones, tumors, fibrotic strictures, or chronic pancreatitis. Biliary atresia and cystic fibrosis cause secondary biliary cirrhosis in children.

Chronic obstruction to bile flow increases pressure in the hepatic bile duct and results in the accumulation of bile in the centrilobular spaces. Necrotic areas develop and are followed by proliferation and inflammation of the portal ducts that result in edema and fibrosis. Pools of bile form when the portal ducts rupture into surrounding necrotic areas. Injury is accompanied by regeneration of hepatic cells with the development of finely nodular cirrhosis.

Clinical manifestations are similar to those of primary biliary cirrhosis, with jaundice and pruritus the most distressing symptoms. Right upper quadrant pain is common, and a low-grade fever may be present from bile duct inflammation (cholangitis).

Cholangiography provides the most definitive diagnosis. Laboratory tests usually show elevated conjugated bilirubin and alkaline phosphatase levels. Aminotransferase increases if there is an accompanying cholangitis. Surgery or endoscopy relieves obstruction, prolongs survival, and diminishes or resolves symptoms. Continued obstruction leads to advanced cirrhosis and liver failure.

Postnecrotic Cirrhosis

Postnecrotic cirrhosis is a consequence of many types of chronic, severe liver disease. Of individuals with hepatitis C, 25% develop postnecrotic cirrhosis. Liver injury results from drugs or toxins; inherited metabolic disorders, such as Wilson disease; α_1-antitrypsin deficiency; advanced alcoholic cirrhosis; or primary biliary cirrhosis that progresses to postnecrotic cirrhosis.

Clinical manifestations represent a progression of symptoms associated with an earlier stage of liver disease. Portal hypertension with ascites, bleeding varices, hypersplenism, and encephalopathy are the most prominent symptoms. As a consequence of progressive liver injury, broad and dense bands of fibrosis separate islands of liver cells, giving the liver a nodular appearance. The liver is small in size and distorted in shape.

Diagnosis is confirmed by needle biopsy, and treatment is directed toward relief of symptoms. Death usually occurs as a result of bleeding or encephalopathy.

Disorders of the Gallbladder

Obstruction and inflammation are the most common disorders of the gallbladder. Obstruction is caused by **gallstones,** which are aggregates of substances in the bile. The gallstones may remain in the gallbladder or be ejected, with bile, into the cystic duct. Gallstones that become lodged in the cystic duct obstruct the flow of bile into and out of the gallbladder and cause inflammation. Gallstone formation is termed *cholelithiasis.* Inflammation of the gallbladder or cystic duct is known as *cholecystitis.*

Cholelithiasis

Cholelithiasis is a prevalent disorder in developed countries, where incidence is 10% to 20%. The actual incidence is unknown because many individuals who have gallstones are asymptomatic. Gallstones are of two types: cholesterol and pigmented.[268] Cholesterol stones are the most common (Figure 39-24). Risk factors include obesity; middle age; female gender; American Indian ancestry; and gallbladder, pancreatic, or ileal disease. Pigmented stones, which are common, occur later in life and are associated with cirrhosis.

PATHOPHYSIOLOGY   Cholesterol gallstones form in bile that is supersaturated with cholesterol produced by the liver. Supersaturation sets the stage for cholesterol crystal formation, or the formation of "microstones." More crystals then aggregate on the microstones, which grow to form "macrostones." This process usually occurs in the gallbladder, which may have decreased motility. The stones may lie "silent" or become lodged in the cystic or common duct, causing pain and cholecystitis. Gallstone formation may be such that the stones accumulate and fill the entire gallbladder (Figure 39-25).

It is not known why the hepatocytes secrete bile that is supersaturated with cholesterol. Proposed mechanisms include (1) an enzymatic defect that increases the hepatocytes' synthesis of cholesterol; (2) diminished secretion of bile acids, which normally promote cholesterol solubility; (3) decreased resorption of bile salts from the ileum, which decrease the bile acid pool; (4) gallbladder smooth muscle hypomotility and stasis; (5) genetic predisposition; and (6) some combination of these mechanisms.[269,270] In obese individuals the mechanism appears to involve cholesterol synthesis, whereas in nonobese individuals, it appears to involve decreased secretion of bile acids.

Pigmented stones are created by cholesterol, calcium bilirubinate, or pigmented polymers. The formation of pigmented stones is associated with biliary tract obstruction and bacterial degradation and precipitation of biliary lipids.[271]

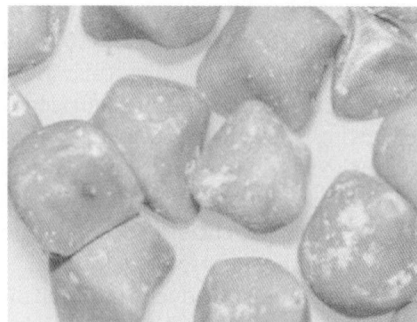

Figure 39-24 Cholesterol stones. Stones are round and faceted; they can be 0.5 to 3 cm in size but are typically large. Biochemical analysis reveals over 50% cholesterol composition with lesser amounts of calcium salts so, strictly, most such stones are of mixed composition. (From Stevens A, Lowe J: *Pathology,* ed 2, London, 2000, Mosby.)

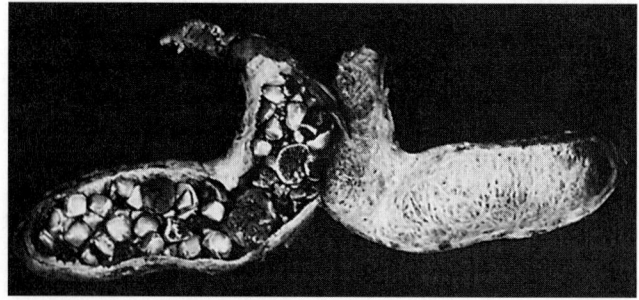

Figure 39-25 Resected gallbladder containing mixed gallstones. (From Kissane JM, editor: *Anderson's pathology,* ed 9, St Louis, 1990, Mosby.)

CLINICAL MANIFESTATIONS Epigastric and right hypochondrium pain and intolerance to fatty foods are the cardinal manifestations of cholelithiasis. Vague symptoms include heartburn; flatulence; epigastric discomfort; and food intolerances, particularly to fats and cabbage, pruritus, and jaundice. The pain, often called *biliary colic* is most characteristic and is caused by the lodging of one or more gallstones in the cystic or common duct.[272] The pain can be intermittent or steady. It usually is located in the right upper quadrant and radiates to the mid-upper back. Jaundice indicates that the stone is located in the common bile duct. Abdominal tenderness and fever indicate cholecystitis. Complications can also include pancreatitis.

EVALUATION AND TREATMENT Diagnosis is based on the patient's medical history, physical examination, and radiographic evaluation. An oral cholecystogram usually outlines the stones. Intravenous cholangiography is used to differentiate cholelithiasis from other causes of extrahepatic biliary obstruction if the cholecystogram is negative. Endoscopic or percutaneous cholangiography and endoscopy or transabdominal ultrasonography are diagnostic options.[273]

Laparoscopic cholecystectomy is the preferred treatment for gallstones that cause obstruction or inflammation. Large stones may be managed with lithotripsy.[274] An alternative treatment is the administration of drugs that dissolve the stones. For example, the bile acid chenodeoxycholic acid (CDCA) can completely or partially dissolve cholesterol gallstones. Ursodeoxycholic acid (UDCA), which is structurally similar to CDCA, is also effective; is less toxic to hepatocytes; and does not cause fatty diarrhea, as does CDCA.

Cholecystitis
Cholecystitis can be acute or chronic. Both forms are almost always caused by the lodging of a gallstone in the cystic duct. Obstruction causes the gallbladder to become distended and inflamed. The pain is similar to that caused by gallstones. Pressure against the distended wall of the gallbladder decreases blood flow. Ischemia, necrosis, and perforation of the gallbladder are possible. Fever, leukocytosis, rebound tenderness, and abdominal muscle guarding are common findings. Serum bilirubin and alkaline phosphatase levels may be elevated. Nevertheless, the acute abdominal pain of cholecystitis must be differentiated from the pain caused by other disorders, such as pancreatitis, myocardial infarction, and acute pyelonephritis of the right kidney. Cholangiography or radioactive scan can confirm a diagnosis of cholecystitis.

Narcotics may be required to control pain, and antibiotics (e.g., gentamicin and clindamycin) are often prescribed to manage bacterial infection in severe cases. Persistent symptoms or development of chronic cholecystitis punctuated by recurrent acute attacks usually requires gallbladder resection (cholecystectomy). If pancreatic abscesses develop, they usually are resected.[275]

Disorders of the Pancreas
Pancreatitis, or inflammation of the pancreas, is a relatively rare and potentially serious disorder. Incidence is about equal in men and women and is more common between 50 and 60 years of age. Pancreatitis can be acute or chronic. It is associated with several other clinical conditions, including alcoholism, obstructive biliary tract disease (particularly cholelithiasis), peptic ulcers, trauma, and hyperlipidemia; and with certain drugs.[276] The cause is unknown in 10% to 20% of cases.[277] The risk of mortality increases with the development of infection or pulmonary, cardiac, and renal complications.

Acute Pancreatitis
PATHOPHYSIOLOGY **Acute pancreatitis (acute hemorrhagic pancreatitis)** is usually a mild disease, but about 20% of those afflicted develop a severe pancreatic inflammation requiring hospital care. Although the precise pathogenic mechanism or sequence of events often is unknown, alcoholism and biliary tract obstruction are commonly associated. The pancreatic acinar cell metabolizes ethanol with the generation of toxic metabolites.[278] The most common theory is that pancreatitis develops because of an injury or disruption of pancreatic acinar cells, which permit leakage of pancreatic enzymes (trypsin, chymotrypsin, and elastase) into pancreatic tissue.[279] The leaked enzymes become activated in the tissue, initiating autodigestion and acute pancreatitis (Figure 39-26). Bile reflux into the pancreas occurs if gallstones obstruct the common bile duct and bile contributes to attacks of acute pancreatitis.[280] The activated proteolases (trypsin and elastase) and lipases break down tissue and cell membranes, causing edema, vascular damage, hemorrhage, necrosis, and fibrosis.[281] (Fatty necrosis is described in Chapter 2.) Toxic enzymes and inflammatory mediators (TNF-α, IL-1β, IL-6, IL-8, IL-10, C5a, ICAM, and substance P) are released into the bloodstream and cause injury to vessels and other organs, such as the lungs and kidneys.[282] Myocardial depression and shock can develop secondary to release of vasoactive peptides. These systemic effects are major causes of multiple-organ dysfunction and mortality.

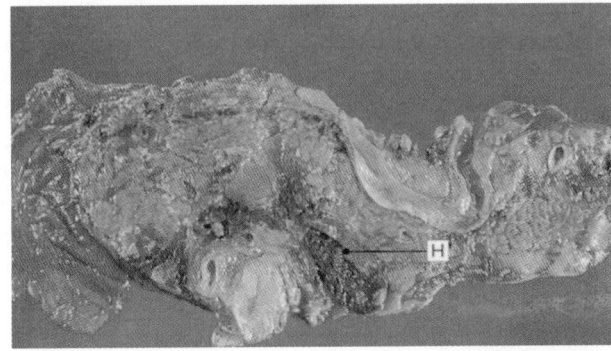

Figure 39-26 **Acute pancreatitis.** The pancreas appears edematous and is commonly hemorrhagic. (From Stevens A, Lowe J: *Pathology,* ed 2, London, 2000, Mosby.)

CLINICAL MANIFESTATIONS Epigastric or midabdominal pain is the cardinal symptom of acute pancreatitis. The pain may radiate to the back because of the retroperitoneal location of the pancreas. The pain is caused by edema, which distends the pancreatic ducts and capsule; chemical irritation and inflammation of the peritoneum; and irritation or obstruction of the biliary tract. Fever and leukocytosis accompany the inflammatory response. Nausea and vomiting are caused by hypermotility or paralytic ileus secondary to the pancreatitis or peritonitis.

Abdominal distention accompanies bowel hypermotility and the accumulation of fluids in the peritoneal cavity. Hypotension and shock occur frequently because plasma volume is lost because enzymes and kinins released into the circulation increase vascular permeability and dilate vessels. Hypovolemia, hypotension, and myocardial insufficiency result. A small percentage of individuals develop tachypnea and hypoxemia secondary to pulmonary edema, atelectasis, or pleural effusions caused by circulating pancreatic enzymes and inflammatory mediators.[283] In severe cases, hypovolemia decreases renal blood flow sufficiently to impair renal function. Tetany may develop as a result of deposition of calcium in areas of fat necrosis or as a decreased response to parathormone. Transient hyperglycemia also can occur if glucagon is released from damaged A cells in the pancreatic islets. A systemic inflammatory response and multiple organ failure accounts for most deaths with severe pancreatitis.[283] In hemorrhagic pancreatitis, some individuals develop flank or periumbilical ecchymosis, a sign of poor prognosis.

EVALUATION AND TREATMENT Diagnosis of pancreatitis is based on clinical findings, identification of associated disorders, and laboratory studies. Elevated serum amylase is a characteristic diagnostic feature. The amylase level usually rises within 12 hours after the onset of symptoms and returns to normal within 3 to 5 days in most cases. Serum lipase levels increase within 4 to 8 hours of clinical symptom onset and decrease within 8 to 14 days. Serum trysin levels are very specific for pancreatitis but may not be readily available. Urine trypsinogen-2 and urine amylase also are elevated. C-reactive protein elevates within 48 hours and is a marker of severity.[284,285] The ratio of amylase clearance to creatinine clearance by the kidney can be diagnostic because, in cases of pancreatitis, amylase clearance increases significantly compared with creatinine clearance. Acute pancreatitis is difficult to diagnose because several other disorders can cause similar clinical and laboratory findings. These disorders include perforating duodenal ulcer, acute cholecystitis, small-bowel obstruction, and kidney stones. Ultrasound and computed tomography (CT) scan are used in more severe cases to evaluate extent of involvement and complications.

The goal of treatment for acute pancreatitis is to stop the process of autodigestion and prevent systemic complications. Narcotic medications may be needed to relieve pain. Meperidine hydrochloride (Demerol) is used instead of morphine because it causes less spasm of the sphincter of Oddi than morphine. Nasogastric suction may not be necessary with mild pancreatitis but may help relieve pain and prevent paralytic ileus in individuals who are nauseated and vomiting. Enteral nutrition with use of jejunal tube feedings is often effective, but an effort is made to maintain normal enteral nutrition.[286] Parenteral fluids are essential to restore blood volume and prevent hypotension and shock. Parenteral hyperalimentation should be initiated when enteral feeding is not tolerated.[287] Drugs that decrease gastric acid production (e.g., cimetidine) can decrease stimulation of the pancreas by secretin. Antibiotics may control infection. The risk of mortality increases significantly with the development of pulmonary, cardiac, and renal complications.

Chronic Pancreatitis

Structural or functional impairment of the pancreas leads to **chronic pancreatitis.** Chronic alcohol abuse is the most common cause.[288] Chronic pancreatitis causes continuous or intermittent abdominal pain, which usually intensifies after a meal. Pain is associated with increased intraductal pressure, increased tissue pressure, ischemia, neuritis, or ongoing injury.[289] Occasionally manifestations of pancreatic enzyme deficiency, such as steatorrhea or a malabsorption syndrome, are present. To correct enzyme deficiencies and prevent malabsorption, oral enzyme replacements are taken before and during meals. Loss of islet cell function can cause insulin-dependent diabetes. Cessation of alcohol intake is essential for the management of chronic pancreatitis.

Fibrosis, strictures, continued inflammation, and pancreatic cysts are common lesions of chronic pancreatitis. The cysts are walled-off areas or pockets of pancreatic juice, necrotic debris, or blood within or adjacent to the pancreas. Surgical drainage or partial resection of the pancreas may be required to relieve pain and prevent cystic rupture.[290] Chronic pancreatitis is a risk factor for pancreatic cancer.[291]

CANCER OF THE DIGESTIVE SYSTEM

Cancer of the Gastrointestinal Tract

Cancer of the Esophagus

Carcinoma of the esophagus is a rare disease but adenocarcinoma is increasing, particularly in white men.[292] The incidence in the United States and Europe is less than 1% of new cancers per year.[293] The incidence in the United States is higher in blacks than in whites and peaks at about 60 years of age.

Esophageal cancer is strongly associated with malnutrition caused by poor economic conditions, special dietary habits, or alcoholism.[294] Alcohol use and tobacco use have long been established as risk factors for esophageal cancer. Obesity is also a risk factor.[295] The risk of esophageal cancer increases with the amount of alcohol consumed. Alcohol abuse, in combination with dietary zinc deficiency, renders the esophageal mucosa susceptible to carcinogens. Although heavy cigarette smoking is known to increase the risk of esophageal cancer, esophageal cancer is found more often in pipe and cigar smokers than cigarette smokers.

Reflux esophagitis is associated with carcinomas of the esophagus, as is sliding hiatal hernia. Both of these conditions can cause erosive esophagitis and ulceration that can eventually lead to metaplasia (Barrett esophagus) and neoplastic changes.

PATHOGENESIS   Carcinoma of the esophagus is usually squamous cell carcinoma or, less commonly, adenocarcinoma. Adenocarcinomas of the esophagus are often secondary to infiltration by a gastric carcinoma or to the presence of Barrett (dysplastic) epithelium (columnar rather than squamous epithelium in the lower esophagus), which is associated with chronic gastroesophageal reflux. Carcinomas can occur at any level of the esophageal tract but are most common where the esophagus joins the stomach (the gastroesophageal junction).[296-298]

The pathogenesis of esophageal carcinoma is facilitated by (1) alterations of esophageal structure and function that permit food and drink to remain in the esophagus for prolonged periods; (2) ulceration and metaplasia caused by esophageal reflux; and (3) long-term exposure to irritants, such as alcohol and tobacco, that cause neoplastic transformation (see Chapter 11). *Helicobacter pylori* do not colonize the intestinal epithelium of Barrett esophagus, and *H. pylori* may be a protection against esophageal adenocarcinoma.[299] Chronic inadequate nutrition can impair both structure and function of the esophagus. Nutritional deprivation, particularly deficiencies of vitamin A and zinc, results in mucosal changes that make the esophageal mucosa vulnerable to neoplastic changes. Mutation of the TP53 gene is an early event in Barrett adenocarcinoma.[300]

CLINICAL MANIFESTATIONS   The two main manifestations of esophageal carcinoma are chest pain and dysphagia. The most common type of pain is heartburn (pyrosis). It is initiated by eating spicy or highly seasoned foods and by lying down. Dysphagia (pain on swallowing), another common symptom, is usually pressure-like and may radiate posteriorly between the scapulae. Odynophagia may be initiated by the swallowing of cold liquids. Spontaneous chest pain is more difficult to diagnose positively. Some individuals with esophageal cancer complain of a constant retrosternal pain that radiates to the back. Dysphagia usually progresses rapidly. It is mostly painless during the early stages of esophageal carcinoma.

EVALUATION AND TREATMENT   Individuals who present with dysphagia undergo endoscopy so that specimens can be obtained and examined for neoplastic change. CT studies of the thorax also are used for diagnosis. Prevention of gastroesophageal reflux is essential to the management of Barrett esophagus. Untreated esophageal cancer metastasizes rapidly and therefore has a poor prognosis. The lymphatic vessels of the esophagus are continuous with vital mediastinal structures and drain to the lymph nodes from the neck of the celiac axis, making it impossible to remove all the lymph nodes with the tumor. Removal of the primary lesion and the local lymph nodes, however, can benefit the individual with esophageal cancer. If the malignancy has not spread beyond these sites, cure is likely. If spread has occurred, however, an incomplete resection is of little benefit and treatment is combined radiation and chemotherapy.[301]

Cancer of the Stomach

Although the incidence of gastric cancer has declined in the United States, it still represents about 2% (21,860 cases) of all new cancer cases annually.[293] In countries such as Japan, the British Isles, and Iceland, the incidence of stomach cancer has remained high consistently. The incidence rate in Japan is one of the highest in the world. Studies of Japanese immigrants to the United States show that offspring who are born and raised in the United States have an incidence rate comparable to that of other Americans. These data illustrate the importance of environmental factors, such as diet, to carcinogenesis.

The most important risk factors in causing gastric cancer are (1) infection with *Helicobacter pylori* that carries the cytotoxin-associated antigen A (CagA) gene; (2) salt added to food; (3) food additives (e.g., nitrates) in pickled or salted foods (e.g., bacon); and (4) low intake of fruits and vegetables. Vitamin C and carotenoids are possible protective factors. Dietary salt enhances the conversion of nitrates to carcinogenic nitrosamines in the stomach. Salt is also caustic to the stomach and can cause chronic atrophic gastritis. Finally, hypertonic salt solutions delay gastric emptying. Delayed emptying increases the time during which carcinogenic nitrosamines can exert their effects on the stomach mucosa. Infection with *H. pylori* and severe chronic gastritis change the mucosal cell proliferation pattern, increasing the risk for gastric and duodenal carcinoma.[302,303]

The metabolism of nitrates and nitrites is very complex. Nitrates interact with amino acids in the stomach to form nitrosamines. The conversion of these carcinogenic nitrosamines is enhanced at a low pH by iodides and thiocyanates. Nitrates are thought to be active only when converted to nitrites and to cause stomach cancer once atrophic gastritis has occurred.

The incidence of gastric cancer is greater in males than in females. Other nonenvironmental risk factors are a family history of gastric adenocarcinoma; blood type (blood group A); and pernicious anemia, which causes atrophy of the gastric mucosa in the same locations where gastric tumors arise.

PATHOGENESIS   Gastric cancer usually begins in the glands of the stomach mucosa. Approximately 50% of all gastric cancers develop in the prepyloric antrum (Figure 39-27). Atrophic gastritis and intestinal metaplasia are strongly linked to the development of gastric cancer.[304] Insufficient acid secretion by the atrophic mucosa creates a relatively alkaline environment that permits bacteria to multiply and act on nitrates. The resulting increase in nitrosoamines damages

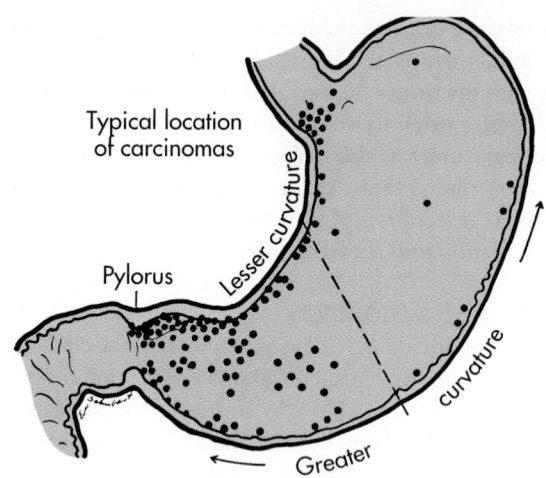

Figure 39-27 Typical sites of stomach cancer. (From del Regato JA, Spjut HJ, Cox JD: *Cancer: diagnosis, treatment, and prognosis*, ed 2, St Louis, 1985, Mosby.)

the deoxyribonucleic acid (DNA) of mucosal cells further, promoting metaplasia and neoplasia. Duodenal reflux also may contribute to intestinal metaplasia. The reflux contains caustic bile salts that destroy the mucosal barrier that normally protects the stomach.

Alterations in *p53* gene occur in gastric carcinomas. Other genetic events, including alterations in tumor suppressor genes, cell cycle regulators, cell adhesion molecules, and DNA repair genes, contribute to the development of carcinoma.[305,306] COX-2 prostanoids (COX-2) may promote aggressive growth of gastric adenocarcinomas.[307]

CLINICAL MANIFESTATIONS The early stages of gastric cancer are generally asymptomatic or produce vague symptoms such as loss of appetite (especially for meat), malaise, and "indigestion." Later manifestations of gastric cancer include unexplained weight loss, upper abdominal pain, vomiting, change in bowel habits, and anemia caused by persistent occult bleeding. The prognosis is poor because symptoms do not occur until the tumor has penetrated the muscle layers of the stomach; spread to surrounding tissues; and entered the draining lymph nodes and veins, causing distant metastases. Generally the first manifestations of carcinoma are caused by distant metastases.

EVALUATION AND TREATMENT The choice of diagnostic tests depends on the clinical manifestations at the time of presentation. Most symptoms suggest a problem in the upper gastrointestinal tract. Direct endoscopic visualization and biopsy usually establish the diagnosis, or microscopic examination of exfoliated cells obtained by lavage during endoscopy.

Surgery is the treatment for gastric cancer. Staging is determined by pathologic findings after resection. Chemotherapy combined with chemoradiotherapy may provide the best postoperative outcomes.[308] Screening and treatment for *H. pylori* infection is a preventive approach to gastric cancer.[309]

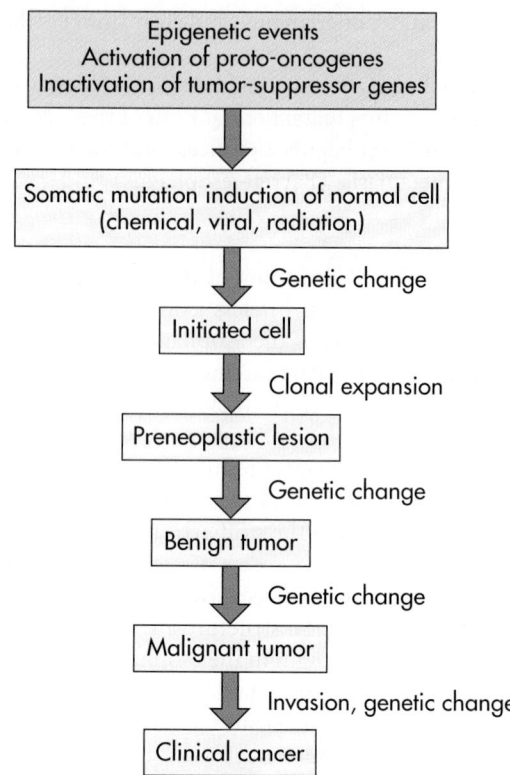

Figure 39-28 Multistage development of colonic cancer.

Cancer of the Colon and Rectum

Cancer of the lower intestinal tract (colorectal cancer) is the second most common cause of cancer death in the United States for both men and women. Colorectal cancer accounts for 10% to 15% of all cancer deaths; 56,290 deaths in 2005.[293] Cancer of the colon tends to occur in individuals older than 50 years. It is rare in children. Worldwide, the prevalence of colorectal cancer is highest in populations with high socioeconomic standards, possibly because of dietary and lifestyle habits.[310,311] *Cancer of the small intestine is rare and represents less than 1% of gastrointestinal cancers.*[312]

PATHOGENESIS Both genetic and environmental factors are associated with the development of colonic cancer (Figure 39-28). Alterations in the tumor-suppressor *p53* gene are present in 85% of colorectal cancers.[313,314] Allelic deletion on chromosomes 5, 17, and 18 appears to promote transition from normal to malignant colon mucosa. Familial polyposis carries a very high risk for colorectal carcinoma. Dietary factors, including high fat, low fiber, and low calcium, may promote somatic mutations. Promoting mechanisms are related to prolonged contact of the fecal mass with colon mucosa[315] and substances produced by microflora of the sigmoid colon.[315,316] Lower risk for colon cancer may be associated with diets high in cereal grains, vegetables, folic acid, and calcium and/or vitamin D; hormone replacement therapy; physical activity; nitric oxide donating; and use of nonsteroidal antiinflammatory drugs.[317-320]

Many colorectal cancers develop from adenomatous polyps (chromosome 5 mutation). A polyp, or papilloma, is a finger-like projection arising from the mucosal epithelium. Most polyps are benign. The adenomatous polyposis coli (APC) gene was first identified as the gene mutated in an inherited syndrome of colon cancer known as *familial adenomatous polyposis coli (FAP)*.[321] The two major types of neoplastic polyps are pedunculated (stalk) adenomatous polyps and sessile (papillary or villous) adenomas (Figure 39-29). Once the adenoma traverses the muscularis mucosae, it becomes invasive and highly malignant. Adenomas can be detected early, however, and the submucosa may not be penetrated for several years. The larger the polyp is, the greater the risk of colorectal cancer. Although lesions larger than 1.5 cm occur less often, they are more likely to be malignant than those smaller than 1.0 cm. The adenomatous polyp forms in an area of epithelial cell hyperproliferation and crypt dysplasia. Table 39-11 gives other conditions commonly confused with colorectal cancer. Cyclooxygenase-2 (COX-2) expression is variably expressed in right-sided and left-sided colorectal cancer, and COX-2 may participate in regulation of apoptosis, angiogenesis, and invasiveness.[322,323]

Most colorectal cancers are moderately differentiated adenocarcinomas. Progression to cancer is a multistep process and involves several suppressor genes that result in cell regulation abnormalities.[324] These tumors have a long preinvasive phase, and when they invade they tend to grow slowly. Because the lymphatic channels are located underneath the muscularis mucosae, the lesions must traverse this layer before metastasis can occur.

CLINICAL MANIFESTATIONS   Tumors of the right (ascending) and left (descending) colon evolve into two distinct tumor types. On the right side the lesions are polypoid and extend along one wall of the cecum and ascending colon. Clinical manifestations include pain, a palpable mass in the lower right quadrant, anemia, and dark red or mahogany-colored blood mixed with the stool (Figure 39-30). These large, bulky tumors become necrotic and ulcerated, con-

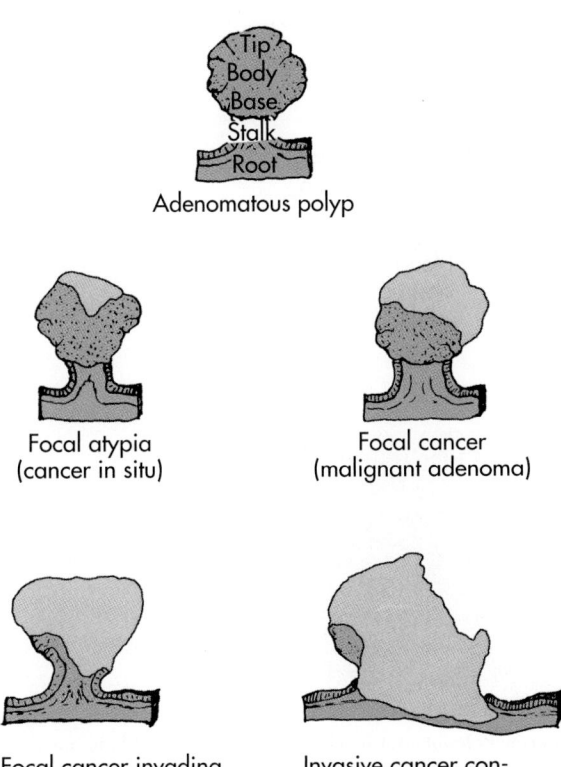

Adenomatous polyp

Focal atypia (cancer in situ)

Focal cancer (malignant adenoma)

Focal cancer invading stalk with some "benign" polyp still in body

Invasive cancer containing piece of polyp

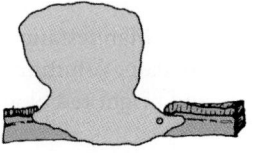

Polypoid invasive cancer without polyp remnant

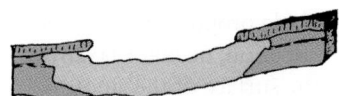

Ulcerated invasive cancer without polyp remnant

A

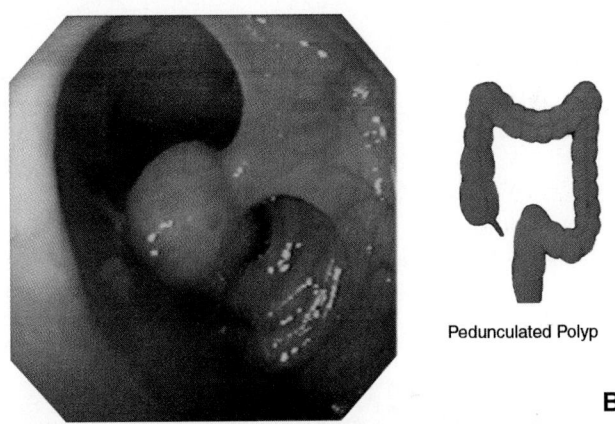

Pedunculated Polyp

B

Figure 39-29 Development of cancer of the colon from adenomatous polyps. **A,** The tumor becomes invasive if it penetrates the muscularis mucosae and enters the submucosal layer. **B,** Endoscopic image of pedunculated polyp in descending colon. (**A** from del Regato JA, Spjut HJ, Cox JD: *Cancer: diagnosis, treatment, and prognosis,* ed 2, St Louis, 1985, Mosby; **B** courtesy David Bjorkman, M.D., University of Utah School of Medicine, Department of Gastroenterology.)

Table 39-11	Conditions Commonly Confused with Colorectal Cancer
Condition	Significant Characteristics
Diverticulitis	Left-sided pain similar to that of appendicitis; tender lower left quadrant. Associated findings: nausea, vomiting, fever, obstruction, anorexia, and leukocytosis; mucosa is intact, and perforation, peritonitis, and abscesses occur more often than in cancer; proctosigmoidoscopy or barium enema used to distinguish from cancer
Chronic ulcerative colitis	Younger people with chronic attacks of bloody diarrhea, crampy abdominal pain, fever, malnutrition, and dehydration; usually involves the left colon and rectum; endoscopy, barium enema, and biopsy performed for definitive diagnosis
Crohn disease (granulomatous colitis)	Generally involves the right colon; chronic diarrhea with abdominal cramps, fever, weight loss, and often a palpable abdominal mass; difficult at times to distinguish Crohn disease from ulcerative colitis; endoscopic examination and barium enema used to distinguish from cancer
Appendicitis	Vague abdominal symptoms, often with a tender or nontender mass in the lower right quadrant; associated symptoms: mild fever and leukycytosis; barium enema used to distinguish cancer of the cecum from appendiceal abscess
Thrombosed hemorrhoids	Examination shows a tender, swollen, bluish painful mass in the anus; patient will have a history of hemorrhoids

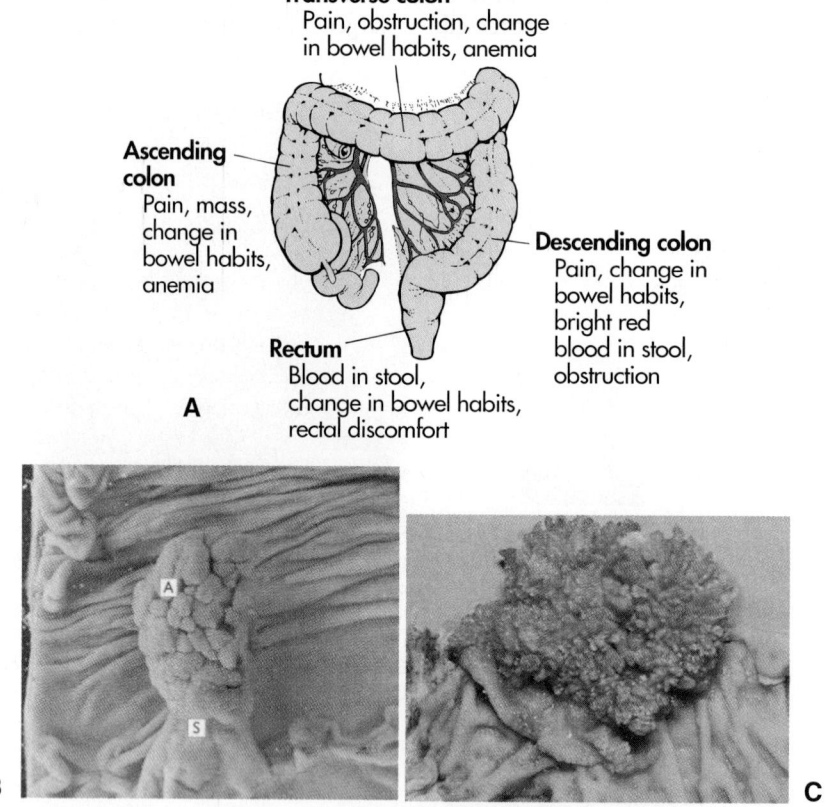

Figure 39-30 Signs and symptoms of colorectal cancer by location of primary lesion. **A,** Clinical manifestations are listed in order of frequency for each region (lymphatics of colon also shown). **B,** Tubular adenomata *(A)* are rounded lesions 0.5 to 2 cm in size that are generally red and sit on a stalk *(S)* of normal mucosa that has been dragged up by traction of the polyp in the bowel lumen. **C,** Villous adenomata are frondlike lesions about 0.6 cm thick that occupy a broad area of mucosa generally 1 to 5 cm in diameter. (**B** and **C** from Stevens A, Lowe J: *Pathology,* ed 2, London, 2000, Mosby.)

tributing to persistent blood loss and anemia. Obstruction is unusual because the feces are more liquid.

Tumors of the left, or descending, colon start as small, elevated, button-like masses. This type grows circumferentially and spreads along the entire bowel wall, eventually ulcerating in the middle as the tumor penetrates the blood supply. Ob-

struction is common but occurs slowly. Manifestations include progressive abdominal distention, pain, vomiting, constipation, need for laxatives, cramps, and bright red blood on the surface of the stool.

Systemic lymphatic spread occurs along the aorta to the mesenteric and pancreatic lymph nodes. Liver metastasis follows invasion of the mesenteric veins (left colon) or superior veins (right colon), which drain into the portal circulation.

Rectal carcinomas are defined as tumors occurring up to 15 cm from the anal opening. Tumors of the rectum can spread through the rectal wall to nearby structures: the prostate in men and the vagina in women. Penetration occurs more readily in the lower third of the rectum because it has no serosal covering. Systemic and pulmonary metastases occur through the hemorrhoidal plexus, which drains into the vena cava.

EVALUATION AND TREATMENT   Individuals with a family history of polyps should be screened using colonoscopy, with removal of polyps when polyps are found. Screening asymptomatic at-risk individuals over age 50 includes fecal occult blood tests and sigmoidoscopy or colonoscopy.[325,326] A diet rich in vegetables, grains, fruit, and calcium and low in fat can modify cancer risk.[317-320] Genetic markers have been developed to identify inherited forms of colorectal cancer.[327,328] In 8% to 29% of cases, bowel obstruction is the primary symptom at diagnosis.[329]

The staging of colorectal cancer involves preoperative testing and operative exploration. Preoperative testing begins with physical examination of the abdomen to detect liver enlargement and ascites and palpation of appropriate lymph nodes. Elevations of carcinoembryonic antigen (CEA) are often detected in the sera of individuals with colorectal carcinoma. The amount of CEA in the serum is a function of the stage of the disease and the type of tumor. Operative staging consists of careful exploration during surgery and biopsy of possible metastases. The Dukes classification is widely used for staging of colorectal cancer and is as follows:

Stage A: Cancer limited to the bowel wall
Stage B: Cancer extending through the bowel wall
Stage C: Nodal metastases regardless of extension into bowel wall
Stage D: Distant metastases regardless of primary size

Treatment for cancer of the colon is always surgical. The location and amount of colon resected depend on the site of the cancer. Resection and anastomosis can be performed for cancer of the ascending, transverse, descending, or sigmoid colon and upper rectum. These surgeries are performed through abdominal incisions, and natural defecation is preserved.

Growths in the lower portion of the rectum require removal of the entire rectum. The proximal end of the descending colon is brought out through a small incision in the abdominal wall and becomes a permanent colostomy. Prognosis after surgery depends on the stage and location of the tumor.

Radiation therapy is often given before surgery in the hope that it will shrink the tumor, alter the malignant cells, or do both, so that these cells will not survive after surgery. Adjuvant chemotherapy is used to treat metastatic disease and cases with a high risk of recurrence. New chemotherapeutic agents are improving first line treatment.[330] Immunotherapy can boost the immune response.[331] Recombinant vaccines for colon cancer are in clinical trials.[332,333]

Cancer of the Accessory Organs of Digestion
Cancer of the Liver

Cancer in the liver is usually caused by metastatic spread from a primary site elsewhere in the body. Primary liver cancer is relatively rare in the United States but is common in densely populated parts of the Far East, southern Africa, China, and Greece. The number of deaths in the United States from liver cancer is greatest among Asians and Pacific Islanders (third leading cause of cancer deaths) and is higher in African Americans and Hispanics compared to whites.[334] For reasons not understood, incidence is higher in males than in females. Primary liver cancer is rare before the age of 40 years and most common during the sixth decade. Together, primary and secondary liver cancer accounts for less than 2% of all cancer deaths in the United States.[293] The incidence of hepatocellular carcinoma is increasing from dissemination of hepatitis B and C infection.[335,336]

Risk factors for primary liver cancer include the following:
1. Infection with hepatitis B virus (HBV), hepatitis C virus (HCV), and hepatitis D virus (HDV), particularly in conjunction with cirrhosis, acts either as a carcinogen or as a cocarcinogen in chronically infected hepatocytes.[336]
2. Chronic liver disease, especially cirrhosis.[337]
3. Exposure to mycotoxins. The most significant mycotoxins are the aflatoxins, particularly those produced by *Aspergillus flavus*, a mold found on spoiled corn, peanuts, and grain. Aflatoxins cause mutation of the *p53* suppressor gene.[338]
4. Heavy smoking and heavy drinking of alcohol.[337]
5. The presence of liver flukes in Southeast Asia.[338]

PATHOGENESIS   Primary carcinomas of the liver are hepatocellular or cholangiocellular. **Hepatocellular carcinoma (hepatocarcinoma) (HCC)** develops in the hepatocytes, whereas **cholangiocellular carcinoma (cholangiocarcinoma)** develops in the bile ducts. Hepatocellular carcinoma can be nodular (consisting of multiple, discrete nodules), massive (consisting of a large tumor mass having satellite nodules), or diffuse (consisting of very small nodules distributed throughout most of the liver). Hepatocellular carcinoma is the type of primary liver cancer that is closely associated with cirrhosis (Figure 39-31). Chronic hepatitis and cirrhosis gives rise to HCC repetitive cellular proliferation that occurs in the inflamed liver in response to growth factor and cytokine stimulation. Numerous genetic and epigenetic alterations, including failure of tumor-suppressor genes, combine to promote carcinogenesis.[337] Because carcinoma of the liver invades the hepatic and portal veins, it often spreads to the heart and lungs. Other sites of metastases are the brain, kidney, and spleen.

Cholangiocellular carcinomas occur less often than hepatocellular carcinomas in the United States. This type of primary liver cancer is most common in areas where liver fluke infestation is prevalent, such as southeast China and Thai-

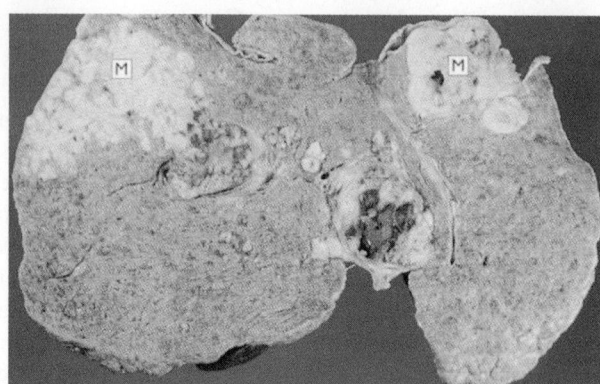

Figure 39-31 Hepatocellular carcinoma. Macroscopically, hepatocellular carcinomas may be single or multifocal. They usually develop in a liver already affected by cirrhosis. Tumor appears as an abnormal mass *(M)* within the liver. (From Stevens A, Lowe J: *Pathology,* ed 2, London, 2000, Mosby.)

land.[338] The mechanism by which fluke infestation causes cholangiocellular carcinoma is unknown. Cholangiocellular carcinoma can occur anywhere along the bile duct and extend directly into the liver, usually as a solitary lesion. It is difficult to distinguish an invasion of cholangiocellular carcinoma from a metastatic adenocarcinoma except by neoplastic changes found in nearby ducts.

CLINICAL MANIFESTATIONS   The clinical presentation of liver cancer in adults is characterized by vague abdominal symptoms, such as nausea and vomiting, fullness, pressure, and dull ache in the right hypochondrium. Manifestations of hepatocellular carcinoma can occur slowly or abruptly. In individuals with cirrhosis, deepening jaundice or abrupt lack of appetite is a sign of hepatocellular carcinoma. Obstruction by the tumor can cause sudden worsening of portal hypertension and development of ascites. As the tumor enlarges, it causes pain. Cholangiocellular carcinoma more commonly presents insidiously as pain, loss of appetite, weight loss, and gradual onset of jaundice. Some carcinomas of the liver rupture spontaneously, causing hemorrhage. Others are discovered accidentally during evaluation of a bone fracture or surgical exploration.

EVALUATION AND TREATMENT   There is no specific test for the diagnosis of liver cancer. The diagnosis is based on biopsy findings, laboratory findings, radiologic examination, and exploratory laparotomy. Increased surveillance and improved imaging is leading to earlier diagnosis.[339,340]

Levels of alkaline phosphatase, serum glutamic oxaloacetic transaminase (AST), and serum glutamic pyruvic transaminase (ALT) are commonly elevated in individuals with hepatocellular carcinoma. α-Fetoprotein is elevated (in excess of 400 ng/ml) in individuals with advanced hepatocellular carcinoma. Excessive levels of α-fetoprotein have been correlated with hepatitis B antigen, rapid tumor growth, and poor tumor differentiation. Erythrocytosis is secondary to erythropoietin production.

In individuals without cirrhosis, liver scans can document filling defects. CT or ultrasonography is used to detect solid tumors, but neither can distinguish benign from malignant tumors. A liver biopsy can be diagnostic unless scattered nodules are missed by the examiner. Hepatitis B vaccination and antiviral treatment of hepatitis C will advance prevention of HCC.[341]

Staging of the tumor is important to guiding treatment.[342] Surgical resection is possible only if the tumor is localized to a removable lobe of the liver. Tumors of the posterior segment of the right lobe are not resectable, because this segment contains the right hepatic vein. Chemotherapeutic agents are administered systemically or locally. Radiation is not part of the treatment regimen, because the dosages needed for effectiveness exceed the tolerance of liver tissue. Liver transplant is the only alternative for cure.[343] Gene therapy, immunotherapy, signal transduction inhibition, and antiangiogenic treatments are being explored.[344]

The overall median survival rate for those with symptomatic liver cancer is only 3 to 4 months. Surgery is hazardous and usually not undertaken if the individual has cirrhosis. Most individuals develop metastases after surgical resection, but long-term survival is possible.

Cancer of the Gallbladder

Cancer of the gallbladder is more common in women than in men by a ratio of about 4 to 3.[293] It occurs rarely before the age of 40 years and is most common between the ages of 50 and 60 years. Obesity is a risk factor. Native populations in North and South America have greater risk of gallbladder cancer, and it is more common in Chile, Poland, India, Japan, and Israel.[345,346] Most gallbladder cancer is caused by metastasis. Primary carcinoma of the gallbladder is rare and is usually associated with chronic cholecystitis and cholelithiasis.

PATHOGENESIS   Most primary carcinomas of the gallbladder are adenocarcinomas. A few are squamous cell carcinomas; *p53* gene mutation, altered expression of P-glycoprotein, COX-2, epidermal growth factor receptor, and *K-ras* gene mutation occur.[347] Invasion of the liver occurs early. Spreading progresses to the cystic and periportal lymph nodes with invasion of the pancreas and retroperitoneal lymph nodes. Direct invasion of the stomach and the duodenum can cause pyloric obstruction. Infection often accompanies cancer of the gallbladder. Generalized peritonitis, gangrene, perforation, and liver abscesses are potential complications of infection.

CLINICAL MANIFESTATIONS   A typical presentation of carcinoma of the gallbladder is steady, upper-right-quadrant pain for about 2 months. Other manifestations include diarrhea, belching, weakness, loss of appetite, weight loss, and vomiting. Obstructive jaundice can occur if an enlarging tumor presses on the extrahepatic ducts.

EVALUATION AND TREATMENT   Early diagnosis of cancer of the gallbladder is not possible because of lack of symptoms, and individuals present with an advanced stage of disease. Individuals with gallstones, especially older women, are evaluated carefully. Inflammatory disorders, such as cholangitis (bile duct inflammation) and peritonitis, often obscure an underlying malignancy. The most specific diagnostic procedures include ultrasonography, CT, and magnetic resonance imaging (MRI).

Complete surgical resection of the gallbladder is the only effective treatment. Because advanced malignancies cannot be resected, gallbladders containing stones are removed as a preventive measure. Palliative chemotherapy provides symptom improvement.[348] The prognosis of gallbladder cancer is extremely poor; most individuals die within 1 year after surgery.[349]

Cancer of the Pancreas

Pancreatic cancer now ranks fourth in men and fifth in women as a cause of cancer deaths in the United States. The incidence of pancreatic cancer rises steadily with age. Males are affected slightly more often than females and blacks more often than whites. Pancreatic cancer accounts for about 31,800 deaths annually in the United States.[293] Mortality is nearly 100%. The cause of pancreatic cancer is not known, and with the exception of an association of risk with cigarette smoking, no external risk factors have been identified.[350] Pancreatitis is associated with 50% of pancreatic cancers.[351]

PATHOGENESIS   Cancer of the pancreas can arise from exocrine or endocrine cells. Most pancreatic tumors arise from exocrine cells in the ducts and are called *ductal adenocarcinomas.* Tumors arising in small ducts invade nearby glandular tissue, penetrate the covering of the pancreas, and extend into surrounding tissues.[352] A K-ras mutation is the most common genetic alteration; tumor suppressor gene alterations are also found, including *p53, p16,* and *DCC.* Growth factors may be overexpressed.[353,354]

Ductal adenocarcinomas can occur in the head, body, or tail of the pancreas. Tumors of the head quickly spread to obstruct the common bile duct and portal vein (Figure 39-32). These tumors can then infiltrate the superior mesenteric artery, the vena cava, and the aorta. Cancer cells that enter the blood vessels can form emboli. Tumors of the body and tail infiltrate the posterior abdominal wall. Lymphatic invasion occurs early and rapidly and involves local and regional lymph nodes. Venous invasion causes metastases to the liver.

Tumor implants on the peritoneal surface can obstruct veins and promote development of ascites.

Ductal adenocarcinomas arising in the head of the pancreas cause biliary obstruction somewhat early in the disease. Individuals with such tumors survive slightly longer than those with cancer of the body and tail, presumably because they seek medical attention earlier.

Tumors of the endocrine pancreas are rare neoplasms of the islets of Langerhans known as *apudomas.* The first four letters in *apudoma* derive from *amine precursor uptake* and *decarboxylation.* The apudomas are so named because they contain neurosecretory granules. Endocrine neoplasms are fatal because they secrete abnormal amounts of hormones, such as insulin.

CLINICAL MANIFESTATIONS   Cancer of the body and tail of the pancreas is generally asymptomatic until there is intraductal obstruction or the tumor invades adjacent tissue. Often vague back pain is an initial symptom. Jaundice develops in most cases, usually caused by obstruction of the bile duct.[355] Because obstruction impairs enzyme secretion and flow to the duodenum, pancreatic cancer causes fat and protein malabsorption, resulting in weight loss. Distant metastases are found in the neck nodes, the lungs, and the brain. Most individuals die of hepatic failure, malnutrition, or systemic diseases.

EVALUATION AND TREATMENT   Pancreatic cancer is usually at an advanced stage at the time of diagnosis and has a poor prognosis. A laparotomy is often performed, particularly if jaundice is present. Ultrasonography and CT may be needed to confirm the need for a laparotomy, especially in individuals without jaundice. Laparotomy is used to establish a definitive diagnosis, evaluate the extent of disease, and determine whether palliative bypass surgery (i.e., cholecystojejunostomy and gastrojejunostomy) is needed. Most individuals require palliative double bypass of the blocked bile ducts, as well as gastrojejunostomy to prevent duodenal obstruction.

Many surgeons recommend a total pancreatectomy because cancer of the pancreas seldom consists of a single lesion.[356] Adjuvant chemotherapy and new systemic agents are improving survival.[357] Radiation therapy is seldom beneficial except as a palliative measure. Because almost all pancreatic cancers are advanced at the time of diagnosis, staging has little relevance in determining treatment. Cancers of the gastrointestinal tract are summarized in Table 39-12.

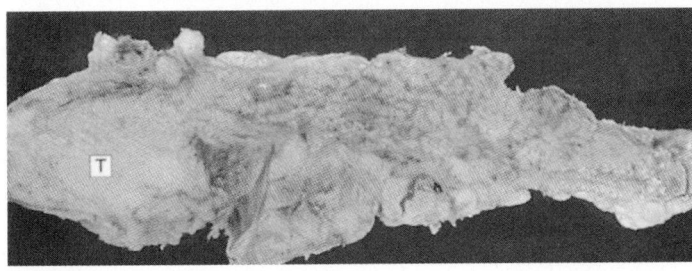

Figure 39-32 Hepatocellular carcinoma. Tumors appear as gritty, gray, hard nodules (*T*) irregularly invading the adjacent gland and local structures. (From Stevens A, Lowe J: *Pathology,* ed 2, London, 2000, Mosby.)

Table 39-12   Cancer of the Gut, Liver, and Pancreas

Organ	Percentage of Deaths of All Cancers	Risks	Cell Type	Common Manifestations
Esophagus	2%	Malnutrition Alcohol Tobacco Chronic reflux	Squamous cell Adenocarcinoma	Chest pain Dysphagia
Stomach	2%	Salty food Nitrates and nitrosamines Gastric atrophy	Adenocarcinoma Squamous cell	Anorexia Malaise Weight loss Upper abdominal pain Vomiting Occult blood
Colorectal	10%	Polyps Ulcerative colitis Diverticulitis High–refined carbohydrate, low-fiber, high-fat diet	Adenocarcinoma (left colon grows in ring; right colon grows as mass)	Pain Mass Anemia Bloody stool Obstruction Distention
Liver	3%	Hepatitis B, C, and D viruses Cirrhosis Intestinal parasite Aflatoxin from moldy peanuts	Hepatomas Cholangiomas	Pain Anorexia Bloating Weight loss Portal hypertension Ascites ± jaundice
Pancreas	5%	Chronic pancreatitis Cigarette smoking Alcohol (?) Diabetic women	Adenocarcinoma (exocrine part of gland, ductal epithelium)	Weight loss Weakness Nausea Vomiting Abdominal pain Depression ± jaundice May have insulin-secreting tumors with symptoms of hypoglycemia

From American Cancer Society: *Estimated new cancer cases and deaths by sex, United States, 2005.* Available at http://www.cancer.org/docroot/MED/content/downloads/MED11xCFF2005 Estimated New Cases Deaths by Sex US.asp
All of the above cancers are within the top 10 causes of death from cancer.

SUMMARY REVIEW

Disorders of the Gastrointestinal Tract

1. Anorexia (loss of appetite), vomiting, constipation, diarrhea, abdominal pain, and evidence of gastrointestinal bleeding are clinical manifestations of many disorders of the gastrointestinal tract.
2. Vomiting is the forceful emptying of the stomach effected by gastrointestinal contraction and reverse peristalsis of the esophagus. It is usually preceded by nausea and retching, with the exception of projectile vomiting, which is associated with direct stimulation of the vomiting center in the brain.
3. Constipation is often caused by unhealthy dietary and bowel habits combined with lack of exercise. Constipation also can result from a neurogenic disorder or a disorder that impairs intestinal motility or obstructs the intestinal lumen.
4. Diarrhea can be caused by excessive fluid drawn into the intestinal lumen by osmosis (osmotic diarrhea), excessive secretion of fluids by the intestinal mucosa (secretory diarrhea), or excessive gastrointestinal motility.
5. Abdominal pain is caused by stretching, inflammation, or ischemia (insufficient blood supply). Abdominal pain originates in the organs themselves (visceral pain) or in the peritoneum (parietal pain). Visceral pain is often referred to the back.

6. Gastrointestinal bleeding can occur in the upper or lower gastrointestinal (GI) tract. Obvious manifestations of GI bleeding are hematemesis (vomiting of blood), melena (dark, tarry stools), and hematochezia (frank bleeding from the rectum). Occult bleeding can be detected only by testing stools or vomitus for the presence of blood.
7. Dysphagia is difficulty in swallowing. It can be caused by a mechanical or functional obstruction of the esophagus. Functional obstruction is an impairment of esophageal motility.
8. Achalasia is a form of functional dysphagia caused by loss of esophageal innervation or relaxation of the lower esophageal sphincter.
9. Gastroesophageal reflux is the regurgitation of chyme from the stomach into the esophagus. An inflammatory response (reflux esophagitis) ensues if the esophageal mucosa is repeatedly exposed to acids and enzymes in the regurgitated chyme.
10. Hiatal hernia is the protrusion of the upper part of the stomach through the hiatus (esophageal opening in the diaphragm) at the gastroesophageal junction. Hiatal hernia can be sliding or paraesophageal.
11. Pyloric obstruction is the narrowing or blockage of the pylorus, which is the opening between the stomach and the duo-

denum. It can be caused by a congenital defect, inflammation and scarring secondary to a gastric ulcer, or tumor growth.

12. Intestinal obstruction prevents the normal movement of chyme through the intestinal tract. It is usually mechanical—that is, caused by torsion, herniation, or tumor. Functional obstruction is caused by paralytic ileus.

13. The most severe consequences of intestinal obstruction are fluid and electrolyte losses, hypovolemia, shock, intestinal necrosis, and perforation of the intestinal wall.

14. Gastritis is an acute or a chronic inflammation of the gastric mucosa.

15. Regurgitation of bile, use of antiinflammatory drugs or alcohol, *H. pylori* infection, and some systemic diseases are associated with gastritis.

16. Chronic gastritis of the fundus and body is the most severe form of gastritis. It can result in gastric atrophy and decreased secretion of hydrochloric acid, pepsinogen, and intrinsic factor.

17. Chronic gastritis of the antrum, the most common type, is not usually associated with impaired secretion or gastric atrophy.

18. A peptic ulcer is a circumscribed area of mucosal inflammation and ulceration caused by excessive secretion of gastric acid, disruption of the protective mucosal barrier, or both.

19. The three types of peptic ulcers are duodenal, gastric, and stress ulcers and they are usually caused by *H. pylori* infection or NSAIDs.

20. Duodenal ulcers, the most common peptic ulcers, are associated with increased numbers of parietal (acid-secreting) cells in the stomach, elevated gastrin levels, and rapid gastric emptying. Pain occurs when the stomach is empty, and pain is relieved with food or antacids. Duodenal ulcers tend to heal spontaneously and recur frequently.

21. Gastric ulcers develop near parietal cells, generally in the antrum, and tend to become chronic. Gastric secretions may be normal or decreased, and pain may occur after eating.

22. Ischemic stress ulcers develop suddenly after severe illness, systemic trauma, or neural injury. Ulceration follows mucosal damage caused by ischemia (decreased blood flow to the gastric mucosa).

23. Cushing ulcer is a stress ulcer caused by head trauma. Ulceration follows hypersecretion of hydrochloric acid caused by overstimulation of the vagal nuclei.

24. Postgastrectomy syndromes are long-term complications that follow gastrectomy—the resection of all or part of the stomach. The postgastrectomy syndromes include dumping syndrome, alkaline reflux gastritis, afferent loop obstruction, diarrhea, weight loss, and anemia.

25. Dumping syndrome is the rapid emptying of hypertonic chyme from the surgically created residual stomach into the small intestine. It causes an osmotic shift of fluid from the vascular compartment to the intestinal lumen, which decreases plasma volume.

26. Alkaline reflux gastritis is stomach inflammation caused by the reflux of bile and pancreatic secretions from the duodenum into the stomach. These substances disrupt the mucosal barrier and cause inflammation.

27. Afferent loop obstruction is an obstruction of the duodenal stump on the proximal side of a gastrojejunostomy. Biliary and pancreatic secretions accumulate in the stump, causing distention, intermittent pain, and vomiting.

28. Malabsorption syndromes result in impaired digestion or absorption of nutrients.

29. Pancreatic insufficiency causes malabsorption associated with insufficient amounts of the enzymes that digest protein, car-

bohydrates, and fats into components that can be absorbed by the intestine.

30. Deficient lactase production in the brush border of the small intestine inhibits the breakdown of lactose. This prevents lactose absorption and causes osmotic diarrhea.

31. Bile salt deficiency causes fat malabsorption, including fat soluble vitamins, and steatorrhea (fatty stools). Bile salt deficiency can result from inadequate secretion of bile, excessive bacterial deconjugation of bile, or impaired reabsorption of bile salts caused by ileal disease.

32. Ulcerative colitis is an inflammatory disease that causes ulceration, abscess formation, and necrosis of the colonic and rectal mucosa. Cramping pain, bleeding, frequent diarrhea, dehydration, and weight loss accompany severe forms of the disease. A course of frequent remissions and exacerbations is common.

33. Crohn disease is similar to ulcerative colitis, but it affects both the large and small intestines, and ulceration tends to involve all the layers of the lumen. "Skip lesion" fissures and granulomas are characteristic of Crohn disease. Abdominal tenderness, nonbloody diarrhea, and weight loss are the usual symptoms.

34. Diverticula are outpouchings of colonic mucosa through the muscle layers of the colon wall. Diverticulosis is the presence of these outpouchings; diverticulitis is inflammation of the diverticula.

35. Appendicitis is the most common surgical emergency of the abdomen. Obstruction of the lumen leads to increased pressure, ischemia, and inflammation of the appendix. Without surgical resection, inflammation may progress to gangrene, perforation, and peritonitis.

36. Vascular insufficiency in the intestine is associated most often with acute or chronic occlusion or obstruction of the mesenteric vessels or insufficient arterial blood flow. The resulting ischemia and necrosis produce abdominal pain, fever, bloody diarrhea, hypovolemia, and shock.

37. Obesity is defined as a body mass index greater than 30 and is a major cause of cardiovascular disease, type 2 diabetes mellitus, and cancer.

38. Both single gene and polygenetic disorders are associated with obesity, as well as social, cultural, economic, exercise, and metabolic factors.

39. Increases in body fat mass are associated with increases in the adipokines leptin and resistin, as well as other hormones including insulin, ghrelin, and peptide YY. Adiponectin is decreased. Obesity may be associated with alterations in the expression and action of peripheral hormones and neurotransmitters that affect appetite and metabolic rate at the level of the hypothalamus.

40. Anorexia nervosa, or self-imposed starvation, is a psychogenic disorder primarily of adolescent and young women. It causes significant weight loss and developmental delays and can be fatal.

41. Bulimia nervosa (binging and purging) involves eating normal or large amounts of food and then purging by inducing vomiting or abusing laxatives. Severe weight loss is rare, but frequent vomiting causes tooth decay, pharyngitis, and esophagitis.

42. Short-term starvation, or lack of dietary intake for 3 or 4 days, stimulates mobilization of stored glucose by two metabolic processes: glycogenolysis (splitting of glycogen into glucose) and gluconeogenesis (formation of glucose from noncarbohydrate molecules).

43. Long-term starvation triggers the breakdown of ketone bodies and fatty acids. Eventually proteolysis (protein breakdown) begins, and death ensues if nutrition is not restored.

Continued

Disorders of the Accessory Organs of Digestion

1. Portal hypertension, ascites, hepatic encephalopathy, jaundice, and hepatorenal syndrome are complications of many liver disorders.

2. Portal hypertension is an elevation of portal venous pressure to at least 10 mmHg. It is caused by increased resistance to venous flow in the portal vein and its tributaries, including the sinusoids and hepatic vein.

3. Portal hypertension is the most serious complication of liver disease because it can cause potentially fatal complications, such as bleeding varices, ascites, hepatic encephalopathy, and renal failure.

4. Splenomegaly is an enlargement of the spleen caused by increased splenic vein pressure caused by portal hypertension.

5. Ascites is the accumulation and sequestration of fluid in the peritoneal cavity, often as a result of portal hypertension and decreased concentrations of plasma proteins.

6. Hepatic encephalopathy (portal systemic encephalopathy) is impaired cerebral function caused by blood-borne toxins (particularly ammonia) not metabolized by the liver. Toxin-bearing blood may bypass the liver in collateral vessels opened as a result of portal hypertension, or diseased hepatocytes may be unable to carry out their metabolic functions.

7. Manifestations of hepatic encephalopathy range from confusion and asterixis (flapping tremor of the hands) to loss of consciousness, coma, and death.

8. Jaundice (icterus) is a yellow or greenish pigmentation of the skin or sclera of the eyes caused by increases in plasma bilirubin concentration (hyperbilirubinemia).

9. Obstructive jaundice is caused by obstructed bile canaliculi (intrahepatic obstructive jaundice) or obstructed bile ducts outside the liver (extrahepatic obstructive jaundice). Bilirubin accumulates proximal to sites of obstruction, enters the bloodstream, and is deposited in the skin and other connective tissues.

10. Hemolytic jaundice is caused by destruction of red blood cells at a rate that exceeds the liver's ability to metabolize unconjugated bilirubin.

11. Hepatorenal syndrome is functional kidney failure caused by advanced liver disease, particularly cirrhosis with portal hypertension. Renal failure is caused by a sudden decrease in blood flow to the kidneys, usually as a result of massive gastrointestinal hemorrhage or liver failure. Its chief clinical manifestation is oliguria.

12. Viral hepatitis is an infection of the liver caused by strains of the hepatitis virus (i.e., hepatitis A virus (HAV), hepatitis B virus (HBV), or hepatitis C virus (HCV). Although they differ with respect to modes of transmission and severity of acute illness, all types cause hepatic cell necrosis, Kupffer cell hyperplasia, and infiltration of liver tissue by mononuclear phagocytes. These changes obstruct bile flow and impair hepatocyte function.

13. The clinical manifestations of viral hepatitis depend on the stage of infection. Fever, malaise, anorexia, and liver enlargement and tenderness characterize the prodromal phase (stage 1). Jaundice and hyperbilirubinemia mark the icteric phase (stage 2). During the recovery phase (stage 3), symptoms resolve. Recovery takes several weeks.

14. Chronic active hepatitis can occur with HBV and HCV with predisposition to cirrhosis and hepatocellular carcinoma.

15. Fulminant hepatitis is a complication of hepatitis B (with or without hepatitis D infection) or hepatitis C. It causes widespread hepatic necrosis and is often fatal.

16. Cirrhosis is an inflammatory disease of the liver that causes disorganization of lobular structure, fibrosis, and nodular regeneration. Cirrhosis can result from hepatitis or exposure to toxins, such as acetaldehyde (a product of alcohol metabolism). The disease causes progressive irreversible liver damage, usually over a period of years.

17. Alcoholic cirrhosis impairs the hepatocytes' ability to oxidize fatty acids, synthesize enzymes and proteins, degrade hormones, and clear portal blood of ammonia and toxins. The inflammatory response includes excessive collagen formation, fibrosis, and scarring, which obstruct bile canaliculi and sinusoids. Bile obstruction causes jaundice. Vascular obstruction causes portal hypertension, shunting, and varices.

18. Primary biliary cirrhosis is an autoimmune disease with inflammatory destruction of intrahepatic bile ducts. Mitochondrial autoantibodies are found in this disease.

19. Secondary biliary cirrhosis develops from prolonged obstruction of bile flow with increased pressure in the hepatic bile ducts that causes pooling of bile and necrosis of tissue. Relief of obstruction relieves symptoms of jaundice and pruritus. Continued obstruction causes cirrhosis and liver failure.

20. Postnecrotic cirrhosis is the consequence of many severe, chronic liver diseases. Fibrosis, atrophy, and nodular regeneration are characteristic of liver structure with severely altered liver function and manifestations, including portal hypertension, ascites, bleeding varices, and encephalopathy.

21. Cholelithiasis (the formation of gallstones) is a common disorder of the gallbladder. Gallstones form in the bile as a result of the aggregation of cholesterol crystals (cholesterol stones) or precipitates of unconjugated bilirubin (pigmented stones). Gallstones that fill the gallbladder or obstruct the cystic or common bile duct cause abdominal pain and jaundice.

22. Cholecystitis is an inflammation of the gallbladder. It is usually associated with obstruction of the cystic duct by gallstones.

23. Acute pancreatitis (pancreatic inflammation) is a serious but relatively rare disorder associated with biliary obstruction and alcoholism. Injury permits leakage of digestive enzymes into pancreatic tissue, where they become activated and begin the process of autodigestion, inflammation, and destruction of tissues. Release of pancreatic enzymes into the bloodstream or abdominal cavity causes damage to other organs.

24. Chronic pancreatitis results from structural or functional impairment of the pancreas related to alcoholism. It causes recurrent abdominal pain and digestive disorders.

Cancer of the Digestive System

1. Cancer of the esophagus is rare and tends to occur in people older than 60 years. Alcohol and tobacco use, reflux esophagitis, and nutritional deficiencies are associated with esophageal carcinoma.

2. Dysphagia and chest pain are the primary manifestations of esophageal cancer. Early treatment of tumors that have not spread into the mediastinum or lymph nodes results in a good prognosis.

3. Gastric carcinoma is associated with *H. pylori* (CagA) high salt intake, food preservatives (nitrates and nitrites), and atrophic gastritis.

4. Approximately 50% of all gastric cancers are located in the prepyloric antrum. Clinical manifestations (weight loss, upper abdominal pain, vomiting, hematemesis, anemia) develop only after the tumor has penetrated the wall of the stomach.

5. Cancer of the colon and rectum (colorectal cancer) is the second most common cancer death in the United States. Preexisting polyps are highly associated with adenocarcinoma of the colon.

SUMMARY REVIEW—CONT'D

6. Tumors of the right (ascending) colon are usually large and bulky; tumors of the left (descending, sigmoid) colon develop as small, button-like masses. Manifestations of colon tumors include pain, bloody stools, and change in bowel habits.

7. Rectal carcinoma is located up to 15 cm from the opening of the anus. The tumor spreads transmurally to the vagina in women or to the prostate in men.

8. Metastatic invasion of the liver is more common than primary cancer of the liver.

9. Primary liver cancers are associated with chronic liver disease (cirrhosis and hepatitis B and C). Hepatocellular carcinomas arise from the hepatocytes, whereas cholangiocellular carcinomas arise from the bile ducts. Primary liver cancer spreads to the heart, lungs, brain, kidney, and spleen through the circulation.

10. Cancer of the gallbladder is relatively rare and tends to occur in women older than 50 years. Adenocarcinoma is most common. Because clinical manifestations occur late in the disease, metastases to lymph channels have usually occurred by the time of diagnosis, and the prognosis is poor.

11. Cancer of the pancreas ranks fifth as a cause of cancer deaths. The one known risk factor is heavy cigarette smoking. Most tumors are adenocarcinomas that arise in the exocrine cells of ducts in the head, body, or tail of the pancreas. Symptoms may not be evident until the tumor has spread to surrounding tissues. Treatment is palliative, and mortality is nearly 100%.

KEY TERMS

MEDIA RESOURCES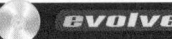

Review questions and answers for this chapter are available in the *CD Companion* included with this book. Also see the CD for an animation of *gastrointestinal obstruction*.

WebLinks—links to Internet sites pertaining to this chapter—are available on Evolve at http://evolve.elsevier.com/McCance/.

REFERENCES

1. Bountra C et al: Towards understanding the aetiology and pathophysiology of the emetic reflex: novel approaches to antiemetic drugs, *Oncology* 53(suppl 1):102-109, 1996.
2. Gale JD: Serotonergic mediation of vomiting, *J Pediatr Gastroenterol Nutr* 21(suppl 1):S22-28, 1995.
3. Meadows N: The central control of vomiting, *J Pediatr Gastroenterol Nutr* 21(suppl 1):S20-S21, 1995.

4. Talley NJ: Definitions, epidemiology, and impact of chronic constipation, *Rev Gastroenterol Disord* 4(Suppl 2):S3-S10, 2004.

5. Mitolo-Chieppa D et al: Cholinergic stimulation and nonadrenergic, noncholinergic relaxation of human colonic circular muscle in idiopathic chronic constipation, *Dig Dis Sci* 43(12):2719-2726, 1998.

6. Rao SS: Constipation: evaluation and treatment, *Gastroenterol Clin North Am* 32(2):659-683, 2003.

7. Haubrich WS, Schaffner F, Berk JE: *Bockus gastroenterology,* vol 1, ed 5, Philadelphia, 1995, Saunders.

8. Ratnaike RN, Jones TE: Mechanisms of drug-induced diarrhoea in the elderly, *Drugs Aging* 13(3):245-253, 1998.

9. Bounds BC, Friedman LS: Lower gastrointestinal bleeding, *Gastroenterol Clin North Am* 32(4):1107-1125, 2003.

10. Huang CS, Lichtenstein DR: Nonvariceal upper gastrointestinal bleeding, *Gastroenterol Clin North Am* 32(4):1053-1078, 2003.

11. Vela MF, Vaezi MF: Cost-assessment of alternative management strategies for achalasia, *Expert Opin Pharmacother* 4(11):2019-2025, 2003.

12. Podas T et al: Achalasia: a critical review of epidemiological studies, *Am J Gastroenterol* 93(12):2345-2347, 1998.

13. Nellemann H, et al: Bread and barium: diagnostic value in patients with suspected primary esophageal motility disorders, *Acta Radiol* 41(2):145-150, 2000.

14. Bittinger M, Wienbeck M: Pneumatic dilation in achalasia, *Can J Gastroenterol* 15(3):195, 2001.

15. Orlando RC: Mechanisms of reflux-induced epithelial injuries in the esophagus, *Am J Med* 108(suppl 4a):104S, 2000.

16. Ishiki K et al: *Helicobacter pylori* eradication improves pre-existing esophagitis in patients with duodenal ulcer disease, *Clin Gastroenterol Hepatol* 2(6):474-479, 2004.

17. Loffeld RJ, van der Putten AB: *Helicobacter pylori* and gastro-oesophageal reflux disease: a cross-sectional epidemiological study, *Neth J Med* 62(6):188-191, 2004.

18. Pandolfino JE, Howden CW, Kahrilas PJ: *H. pylori* and GERD: is less more? *Am J Gastroenterol* 99(7):1213-1221, 2004.

19. Queiroz DM et al: ILIB and ILIRN polymorphic genes and *Helicobacter pylori* cagA strains decrease the risk of reflux esophagitis, *Gastroenterology* 127(1):73-79, 2004.

20. Johanson JF: Epidemiology of esophageal and supraesophageal reflux injuries, *Am J Med* 108(suppl 41):99S, 2000.

21. Haggitt RC: Histopathology of reflux-induced esophageal and supraesophageal injuries, *Am J Med* 108(suppl 4a):109S, 2000.

22. Koop H: Reflux disease and Barrett's esophagus, *Endoscopy* 32(2):101, 2000.

23. Holmes RL, Fadden CT: Evaluation of the patient with chronic cough, *Am Fam Physician* 69(9):2159-2166, 2004.

24. Vaezi MF: Extraesophageal manifestations of gastroesophageal reflux disease, *Clin Cornerstone* 5(4):32-38; discussion 39-40, 2003.

25. DeVault KR: Overview of medical therapy for gastroesophageal reflux disease, *Gastroenterol Clin N Am* 28(4):831, 1999.

26. Hogan WJ, Shaker R: Life after antireflux surgery, *Am J Med* 108 (suppl 4a):181S, 2000.

27. Hashemi M, Sillin LF, Peters JH: Current concepts in the management of paraesophageal hiatal hernia, *J Clin Gasterol* 29(1):8, 1999.

28. Andujar JJ et al: Laparoscopic repair of large paraesophageal hernia is associated with a low incidence of recurrence and reoperation, *Surg Endosc* 18(3):444-447, 2004.

29. Mittal A et al: Match study of three methods for palliation of malignant pyloroduodenal obstruction, *Br J Surg* 91(2):205-209, 2004.

30. Cerro P et al: Sonographic diagnosis of intussusceptions in adults, *Abdom Imaging* 25(1):45, 2000.

31. Sandrasegaran K et al: The multifaceted role of radiology in small bowel obstruction, *Semin Ultrasound CT MR* 24(5):319-335, 2003.

32. Chan FK, Graham DY: Review article: prevention of non-steroidal anti-inflammatory drug gastrointestinal complications—review and recommendations based on risk assessment, *Aliment Pharmacol Ther* 19(10)1051-1061, 2004.

33. Kashiwagi H: Ulcers and gastritis, *Endoscopy* 35(1):9-14, 2003

34. Yardley JH, Hendrix TR: Gastritis and gastropathy. In Yamada T, Alpers DH, Laine L, editors: *Atlas of gastroenterology,* ed 3, Philadelphia, 1999, Lippincott Williams & Wilkins.

35. Genta RM: The gastritis connection: prevention and early detection of gastric neoplasms, *J Clin Gastroenterol* 36(5 Suppl):S44-S49, discussion S62-S62, 2003.

36. Kapadia CR: Gastric atrophy, metaplasia, and dysplasia: a clinical perspective, *J Clin Gastroentrol* 36(5 Suppl):S29-S36, discussion S61-S62, 2003.

37. D'Elios MM et al: Gastric autoimmunity: the role of *Helicobacter pylori* and molecular mimicry, *Trends Mol Med* 10(7):316-323, 2004.

38. Oksanen A et al: Atrophic gastritis and *Helicobacter pylori* infection in outpatients referred for gastroscopy, *Gut* 46(4):460, 2000.

39. Presotto F et al: *Helicobacter pylori* infection and gastric autoimmune disease: is there a link? *Helicobacter* 8(6):578-584, 2003.

40. Nyholm E et al: Oral vitamin B12 can change our practice, *Postgrad Med J* 79(930):218-220, 2003.

41. Vakil N, Fennerty B: The economics of eradicating *Helicobacter pylori* infection in duodenal ulcer disease, *Am J Med* 100(5A):605, 1996.

42. Shigemi J, Mino Y, Tsuda T: The role of perceived job stress in the relationship between smoking and the development of peptic ulcers, *J Epidemiol* 9(5):320, 1999.

43. Levenstein S: The very model of a modern etiology: a biopsychosocial view of peptic ulcer [review], *Psychosom Med* 62(2):176, 2000.

44. Kurata JH: Epidemiology of peptic ulcer disease. In Swabb EA, Szabo S, editors: *Investigation and basis for therapy,* New York, 1991, Marcel Dekker.

45. Schineller BA, Ramchandani D: Psychologic factors associated with peptic ulcer disease, *Med Clin North Am* 75(4):865, 1991.

46. Qureshi WA, Graham DY: Diagnosis and management of *Helicobacter pylori* infection, *Clin Cornerstone* 1(5):18, 1999.

47. Gisbert JP et al: *H. pylori*-negative duodenal ulcer prevalence and causes in 774 patients, *Dig Dis Sci* 44(11):2295, 1999.

48. Tovey FI, Hobsley M: Is *Helicobacter pylori* the primary cause of duodenal ulceration? *J Gastroenterol Hepatol* 14(11):1053, 1999.

49. Freston JW: Management of peptic ulcers: emerging issues, *World J Surg* 24(3):250, 2000.

50. Frazer AG et al: An audit of low dose triple therapy for eradication of *Helicobacter pylori,* *NZ Med J* 109(1027):290, 1996.

51. Megraud F, Marshall BJ: How to treat *Helicobacter pylori:* first-line, second-line, and future therapies, *Gastroenterol Clin North Am* 29(4): 759, 2000.

52. Dubois F: New surgical strategy for gastroduodenal ulcer: laparoscopic approach, *World J Surg* 24(3):270, 2000.

53. Aldoori WH et al: Prospective study of diet and the risk of duodenal ulcer in men, *Am J Epidemiol* 145(1):42, 1997.

54. Lee CK: Vaccination against *Helicobacter pylori* in non-human primate models and humans, *Scand J Immunol* 53(5):437, 2001.

55. Tatsuguchi A et al: Localization of cyclooxygenase 1 and cyclooxygenase 2 in *Helicobacter pylori*–related gastritis and gastric ulcer tissues in humans, *Gut* 46(6):782, 2000.

56. Aoyma N et al: Peptic ulcer after the Hanshin-Awaji earthquake: increased incidence of bleeding gastric ulcer, *Am J Gastroenterol* 93(3):311, 1998.

57. van der Voort PH, Zandstra DF: Pathogenesis, risk factors, and incidence of upper gastrointestinal bleeding after cardiac surgery: is specific prophylaxis in routine bypass procedures needed? *J Cardiothorac Vasc Anesth* 14(3):293, 2000.

58. Mutlu GM, Mutlu EA, Factor P: Prevention and treatment of gastrointestinal complications in patients on mechanical ventilation, *Am J Respir Med* 2(5):395-411, 2003.

59. Yang YX, Lewis JD: Prevention and treatment of stress ulcers in critically ill patients, *Semin Gastroentest Dis* 14(1):11-19, 2003.

60. Kleeff J, Friess H, Buchler MW: How *Helicobacter pylori* changed the life of surgeons, *Dig Surg* 20(2):93-102, 2003.

61. Lee KH, Chang HC, Lo CJ: Endoscope-assisted laparoscopic repair of perforated peptic ulcers, *Am Surg* 70(4):352-356, 2004.

62. Siu WT et al: Routine use of laparoscopic repair for perforated peptic ulcers, *Br J Surg* 91(4):4891-484, 2004.

63. Mehagnoul-Schipper DJ et al: Sympathoadrenal activation and the dumping syndrome after gastric surgery, *Clin Auton Res* 10(5):301, 2000.

64. Carvajal SH, Mulvihill SJ: Postgastrectomy syndromes: dumping and diarrhea, *Gastroenterol Clin North Am* 23(2):261, 1994.

65. Khoshoo V et al: Nutritional management of dumping syndrome associated with antireflux surgery, *J Pediatr Surg* 29(11):1452, 1994.

66. Hasler WL, Soudah HC, Owyang C: Mechanisms by which octreotide ameliorates symptoms in the dumping syndrome, *J Pharmacol Exp Ther* 277(3):1359, 1996.

67. Klingler PJ et al: Indications, technical modalities and results of the duodenal switch operation for pathologic duodenogastric reflux, *Hepatogastroenterology* 46(25):97, 1999.

68. Kim HC et al: Afferent loop obstruction after gastric cancer surgery: helical CT findings, *Abdom Imaging* 28(5):624-630, 2003.

69. Bruno MJ et al: Maldigestion associated with exocrine pancreatic insufficiency: implications of gastrointestinal physiology and properties of enzyme preparations for a cause-related and patient-tailored treatment, *Am J Gastroenterol* 90(9):1383, 1995.

70. Layer P, Keller J: Lipase supplementation therapy: standards, alternatives, and perspectives, *Pancreas* 26(1):1-7, 2003.

71. Swallow DM: Genetics of lactase persistence and lactose intolerance, *Annu Rev Genet* 37:197-219, 2003.

72. Shaw AD, Davies GJ: Lactose intolerance: problems in diagnosis and treatment, *J Clin Gastroenterol* 28(3):208, 1999.

73. Savaiano D: Lactose intolerance: a self-fulfilling prophecy leading to osteoporosis? *Nutr Rev* 61(6 Pt 1):221-223, 2003.

74. Russell DW: The enzymes, regulation, and genetics of bile acid synthesis, *Annu Rev Biochem* 72:37-74, 2003.

75. Allison MC et al: *Inflammatory bowel disease,* St Louis, 1998, Mosby.

76. Geerling BJ et al: Diet as a risk factor for the development of ulcerative colitis, *Am J Gastroenterol* 95(4):1108, 2000.

77. Murata Y et al: The role of proinflammatory and immunoregulatory cytokines in the pathogenesis of ulcerative colitis, *J Gastroenterol* 30 (suppl 8):56, 1995.

78. Kirsner JB: *Inflammatory bowel disease,* ed 5, Philadelphia, 2000, Saunders.

79. Gasche C: Complications of inflammatory bowel disease, *Hepatogastroenterology* 47(31):49, 2000.

80. Bernstein CN et al: The prevalence of extraintestinal diseases in inflammatory bowel disease: a population-based study, *Am J Gastroenterol* 96(4):116-122, 2001.

81. Michsler W et al: Is inflammatory bowel disease an independent and disease-specific risk factor for thromboembolism? *Gut* 53(4):542-548, 2004.

82. Solem CE et al: Venous thromboembolism in inflammatory bowel disease, *Am J Gastroenterol* 99(1):97-101, 2004.

83. Karlinger K et al: The epidemiology and the pathogenesis of inflammatory bowel disease, *Eur J Radiol* 35(3):154, 2000.

84. Cosnes J: Tobacco and IBD: relevance in the understanding of disease mechanisms and clinical practice, *Best Pract Res Clin Gastroenterol* 18(3):481-496, 2004.

85. Hanover SB: Ulcerative colitis. In Lichtenstein LM, Fauci AS, editors: *Current therapy in allergy, immunology, and rheumatology,* ed 5, St Louis, 1996, Mosby.

86. Russell RK, Wilson DC, Satsangi J: Unravelling the complex genetics of inflammatory bowel disease, *Arch Dis Child* 89(7):5989-5603, 2004.

87. Ng AZ-VS-S et al: Associate of the T allele of an intronic single nucleotide polymorphism in the colony stimulating factor 1 receptor with Crohn's disease: a case-control study, *J Immune Based Ther Vaccines* 2:6, 2004.

88. Bruzzese E et al: Microflora in inflammatory bowel diseases: a pediatric perspective, *J Clin Gastroenterol* 38(6 Suppl):S91-93, 2004.

89. Darfeuille-Michaud A et al: High prevalence of adherent-invasive *Escherichia coli* associated with ileal mucosa in Crohn's disease, *Gastroenterology* 127(2):412-421, 2004.

90. Winar SJ, editor: *Management of gastrointestinal diseases,* vol 2, New York, 1992, Gower Medical Publishing.

91. Itzkowitz SH, Yio X: Inflammation and cancer IV. Colorectal cancer in inflammatory bowel disease: the role of inflammation, *Am J Physiol Gastrointest Liver Physiol* 287(1):G7-17, 2004.

92. Rutgeerts P, Van Assche G, Vermeire S: Optimizing anti-TNF treatment in inflammatory bowel disease, *Gastroenterology* 126(6): 1593-1610, 2004.

93. Krupnick AS, Morris JB: The long-term results of resection and multiple resections in Crohn's disease, *Sem Gastrointest Dis* 11(1):41, 2000.

94. Steel M: Colonic diverticular disease, *Aust Fam Physician* 33(12): 983-986, 2004.

95. Colecchia A et al: Diverticular disease of the colon: new perspectives in symptom development and treatment, *World J Gastroenterol* 9(7):1385-1389, 2003.

96. Floch MH, Bina O: The natural history of diverticulitis: fact and theory, *J Clin Gastroenterol* 38(5 Suppl):S2-7, 2004.

97. Stollman NH, Raskin JB: Diverticular disease of the colon, *Lancet* 363(9409):631-639, 2004.

98. Tursi A: Acute diverticulitis of the colon—current medical therapeutic management, *Expert Opin Pharmacolther* 5(1):55-59, 2004.

99. Aydin HN, Remzi FH: Diverticulitis: when and how to oeprate, *Dig Liver Dis* 36(7):435-445, 2004.

100. Addiss DG et al: The epidemiology of appendicitis and appendectomy in the United States, *Am J Epidemiol* 132(5):910-925, 1990.

101. Carr NJ: The pathology of acute appendicitis, *Ann Diagn Pathol* 4(1):46-58, 2000.

102. Andersson et al: Repeated clinical and laboratory examinations in patients with an equivocal diagnosis of appendicitis, *World J Surg* 24(4):479, 2000.

103. Andersson RE: Meta-analysis of the clinical and laboratory diagnosis of appendicitis, *Br J Surg* 91(1):28-37, 2004.

104. Guller U et al: Laparoscopic versus open appendectomy: outcomes comparison based on a large administrative database, *Ann Surg* 239(1):43-52, 2004.

105. Patel A, Kaleya RN, Sammartano JR: Pathophysiology of mesenteric ischemia, *Surg Clin North Am* 72(1):31, 1992.

106. Oldenburg WA et al: Acute mesenteric ischemia, *Arch Intern Med* 164(10):1054-1062, 2004.

107. Kvietys PR, Barrowmand A, Granger ND: *Pathophysiology of the splanchnic circulation,* vol 1, Boca Raton, Fla, 1987, CRC Press.

108. Lock G: Acute intestinal ischaemia, *Best Pract Res Clin Gastroenterol* 15(1):83-98, 2001.

109. Char DJ et al: Intestinal ischemia: experience in a community teaching hospital, *Vasc Endovascular Surg* 37(4):245-252, 2003.

110. National Heart, Lung, and Blood Institute, National Institutes of Health: *Clinical guidelines on the identification, evaluation, and treatment of overweight and obesity in adults—executive summary,* 1998. Available at www.nhlbi.nih.gov/guidelines/obesity/sum_intr.htm.

111. Bray GA: Medical consequences of obesity, *J Clin Endocrinol Metab* 89(6):2583-2589, 2004.

112. Stein CJ, Colditz GA: The epidemic of obesity, *J Clin Endocrinol Metab* 89(6): 2522-2525, 2004.

113. Calle EE, Thun MJ: Obesity and cancer, *Oncogene* 23(38):6365-6378, 2004.

114. Bouchard C, Peerusse L, Rice R, Rao DC: Genetics of human obesity. In Bray GA, Brouchard C, editors: Handbook of obesity: etiology and pathophysiology, ed 2, New York, 2004, Marcel Dekker Inc.

115. Speakman JR: Obesity: the integrated roles of environment and genetics, *J Nutr* 134(8 Suppl):2090S-2105S), 2004.

116. Puhl RM, Brownell KD: Psychosocial origins of obesity stigma: toward changing a powerful and pervasive bias, *Obes Rev* 4(4):213-227, 2003.

117. Ruser CB, Federman DG, Kashaf SS: Whittling away at obesity and overweight: small lifestyle changes can have the biggest impact, *Postgrad Med* 117(1):31-34, 37-40 review, 2005.

118. van Hout GC, van Oudheusden I, van Heck GL: Psychological profile of the morbidly obeses, *Obes Surg* 14(5):579-588, 2004.

119. Fruhbeck G: The adipose tissue as a source of vasoactive factors, *Curr Med Chem Cardiovasc Hematol Agents* 2(3):197-208, 2004.

120. Matsuzawa Y: Adipocytokines: emerging therapeutic targets, *Curr Atheroscler Rep* 7(1):58-62, 2005.

121. Levin BE, Dunn-Meynell AA, Banks WA: Obesity-prone rats have normal blood-brain barrier transport but defective central leptin signaling before obesity onset, *Am J Physiol Regul Integr Comp Physiol* 286(1):R143-R150, 2004.

122. Banks WA: The many lives of leptin, *Peptides* 25(3):331-318, 2004.

123. Pan W: Modulation of feeding-related peptide/protein signals by the blood-brain barrier, *J Neurochem* 90(2):455-461, 2004.

124. Sahu A: Leptin signaling in the hypothalamus: emphasis on energy homeostasis and leptin resistance, *Front Neuroendocrinol* 24(4): 225-253, 2003.

125. Correia ML, Haynes, WG: Leptin, obesity and cardiovascular disease, *Curr Opin Nephrol Hypertens* 13(2):215-223, 2004.

126. Rahmouni K, Haynes, WG: Leptin and the cardiovascular system, *Recent Prog Horm Res* 59:255-244, 2004.

127. Small CJ, Bloom SR: Gut hormones and the control of appetite, *Trends Endocrinol Metab* 15(6):59-63, 2004.

128. Wu JT, Kral JG: Ghrelin: integrative neuroendocrine peptide in health and disease, *Ann Surg* 239(4):464-474, 2004.

129. Williams J, Mobarhan S: A critical interaction: leptin and ghrelin, *Nutr Rev* 61(11):391-393, 2003.

130. Iniguez G et al: Adiponectin levels in the first two years of life in a prospective cohort: relations with weight gain, leptin levels and insulin sensitivity, *J Clin Endocrinol Metab* 89(11):5500-5503, 2004.

131. Matsuzawa Y et al: Importance of adipocytokines in obesity-related diseases, *Horm Res* 60(Suppl 3):56-59, 2003.

132. Reinehr T et al: Adiponectin before and after weight loss in obese children, *J Clin Endocrinol Metab* 89(8):3790-3794, 2004.

133. Steffes MW et al: Serum adiponectin in young adults—interactions with central adiposity, circulating levels of glucose, and insulin resistance: the CARDIA Study, *Ann Epidemiol* 14(7):492-498, 2004.

134. Schulze MB et al: Adiponectin and future coronary heart disease events among men with type 2 diabetes, *Diabetes,* 54(2):534-539, 2005.

135. Haluzik M, Parizkova J, Haluzik MM: Adiponectin and its role in the obesity-induced insulin resistance and related complications, *Physiol Res* 53(2):123-129, 2004.

136. Ouchi N et al: Obesity, adiponectin and vascular inflammatory disease, *Curr Opin Lipidol* 14(6):561-566, 2003.

137. Zick Y: Molecular basis of insulin action, *Novartis Found Symp* 262: 36-50; discussion 50-55, 265-268, 2004.

138. Jarkovska Z et al: Endocrine and metabolic activities of a recently isolated peptide hormone ghrelin, an endogenous ligand of the growth hormone secretagogue receptor, *Endocr Regul* 38(2):80-86, 2004.

139. Wolf G: Insulin resistance and obesity: resistin, a hormone secreted by adipose tissue, *Nutr Rev* 62(10):389-394, 2004.

140. Doelle GC: The clinical picture of metabolic syndrome: an update on this complex of conditions and risk factors, *Postgrad Med* 116(1): 30-32, 35-38, 2004.

141. Moller DE, Kaufman KD: Metabolic syndrome: a clinical and molecular perspective, *Annu Rev Med* 56:45-62, 2005.

142. Carr MC, Brunzell JD: Abdominal obesity and dyslipidemia in the metabolic syndrome: importance of type 2 diabetes and familial combined hyperlipidemia in coronary artery disease risk, *J Cin Endocrinol Metab* 89(60):2601-2607, 2004.

143. Sharma AM: Obesity and cardiovascular risk, *Growth Horm IGF Res* 13(Suppl A):S10-S17, 2003.

144. Toni R et al: New paradigms in neuroendocrinology: relationships between obesity, systemic inflammation and the neuroendocrine system, *J Endocrinol Invest* 27(2):182-186, 2004.

145. Vega GL: Obesity and the metabolic syndrome, *Minerva Endocrinol* 29(2):47-54, 2004.

146. Rahmouni K et al: Obesity-associated hypertension: new insights into mechanisms, *Hypertension* 45(1):9-14, 2005.

147. Wofford MR, Hall JE: Pathophysiology and treatment of obesity hypertension, *Curr Pharm Des* 10(29):3621-3637. 2004.

148. Aaron SD et al: Effect of weight reduction on respiratory function and airway reactivity in obese women, *Chest* 125(6):2046-2052, 2004.

149. Akerman MJ, Calacanis CM, Madsen MK: Relationship between asthma severity and obesity, *J Asthma* 41(5):521-526, 2004.

150. Shimura R et al: Fat accumulation, leptin, and hypercapnia in obstructive sleep apnea-hypopnea syndrome, *Chest* 127(2):543-549, 2005.

151. Felson DT et al: The effect of body weight on progression of knee osteoarthritis is dependent on alignment, *Arthritis Rheum* 50(12): 3904-3909, 2004.

152. Powell A et al: Obesity: a preventable risk factor for large joint osteoarthritis which may act through biomechanical factors, *Br J Sports Med* 39(1):4-5, 2005.

153. Dagenais GR et al: Prognostic impact of body weight and abdominal obesity in women and men with cardiovascular disease, *Am Heart J* 149(1):54-60, 2005.

154. Hoffman DJ et al: Human body composition. In Eckel RH, editor: *Obesity: mechanisms and clinical management,*. Philadelphia, 2003, Lippincott, Williams & Wilkins.

155. Centers for Disease Control and Prevention: *BMI—Body Mass Index: BMI calculator for children and teens, 2004.* Available at www.cdc.gov/growthcharts/

156. Hensrud DD: Diet and obesity, *Curr Opin Gastroenterol* 20(2):119-124, 2004.

157. Ruser CB, Federman DG, Kashaf SS: Whittling away at obesity and overweight: small lifestyle changes can have the biggest impact, *Postgrad Med* 117(1):31-34, 37-40, 2005.

158. Teixeira PJ et al: A review of psychosocial pre-treatment predictors of weight control, *Obes Rev* 6(1):43-65, 2005.

159. Tsai AG, Wadden TA: Systematic review: an evaluation of major commercial weight loss programs in the United States, *Ann Intern Med* 142(1):56-66, 2005.

160. Volek JS, Vanheest JL, Forsythe CE: Diet and exercise for weight loss: a review of current issues, *Sports Med* 35(1):1-9, 2005.

161. Wynne K, Stanley S, McGowan B, Bloom S: Appetite control, *J Endocrinol* 184(2):291-318, 2005.

162. Orzano AJ, Scott JG: Diagnosis and treatment of obesity in adults: an applied evidence based review, *J Am Board Fam Pract* 17(5):359-369, 2004.

163. Buchwald H et al: Bariatric surgery: a systematic review and meta-analysis, *JAMA* 292(14):1724-1737, 2004.

164. Fujioka K: Follow-up of nutritional and metabolic problems after bariatric surgery, *Diabetes Care* 28(2):481-484, 2005.

165. Profumo RJ: Bariatric surgery: review of common procedures and mortality analysis, *J Insur Med* 36(3):187-193, 2004.

166. Kaye WH et al: Anorexia and bulimia nervosa, *Ann Rev Med* 51: 299-313, 2000.

167. National Institute of Mental Health: *Eating disorders,* NIH Pub 93-3477, Washington, DC, 1993, US Government Printing Office.

168. Kaye WH et al: Genetic analysis of bulimia nervosa: methods and sample description, *Int J Eat Disord* 35(4):556-570, 2004.

169. Law SA, Golding JM: Sexual assault history and eating disorder among White, Hispanic, and African-American women and men, *Am J Public Health* 86(14):579, 1996.

170. Emous SJ: Eating disorders in adolescent girls, *Pediatr Int* 42(1):107, 2000.

171. Jimerson DC, Wolfe BE: Neuropeptides and eating disorders, *CNS Spectr* 9(7):516-522, 2004.

172. Klein DA, Walsh BT: Eating disorders: clinical features and pathophysiology, *Physiol Behav* 81(2):359-374, 2004.

173. Mantzoros C et al: Cerebrospinal fluid leptin in anorexia nervosa: correlation with nutritional status and potential role in resistance to weight gain, *J Clin Endocrinol Metab* 82(6):1845-1851, 1997.

174. American Psychiatric Association: *Diagnostic and statistical manual of mental disorders,* ed 4, Washington, DC, 1994, Academic Press.

175. Seidenfeld ME, Sosin E, Rickert VI: Nutrition and eating disorders in adolescents, *Mt Sinai J Med* 71(3):155-161, 2004.

176. Rayworth BB, Wise LA, Harlow BL: Childhood abuse and risk of eating disorders in women, *Epidemiology* 15(3):271-278, 2004.

177. Hartman D: Anorexia nervosa: diagnosis, aetiology, and treatment, *Postgrad Med* 71(842):712, 1995.

178. Kohn M, Golden NH: Eating disorders in children and adolescents: epidemiology, diagnosis, and treatment, *Paediatr Drugs* 3(2):91-99, 2001.

179. Fassino S et al: Psychological treatment of eating disorders. A review of the literature, *Panminerva Med* 46(3):189-198, 2004.

180. Hsu LK: Eating disorders: practical interventions, *J Am Med Womens Assoc* 59(2):113-124, 2004.

181. Golden NH, Meyer W: Nutritional rehabilitation of anorexia nervosa. Goals and dangers, *Int J Adolesc Med Health* 15(2):131-144, 2004.

182. Attia E et al: Does fluoxetine augment inpatient treatment of anorexia nervosa? *Am J Psychiatry* 155(4):548-551, 1998.

183. Hinney A et al: Genetic risk factors in eating disorders, *Am J Pharmacogenomics* 4(4):209-223, 2004.

184. Mehler PA: Eating disorders: bulimia nervosa, *Hosp Pract (Off Ed)* 31(2):107, 1996.

185. Lam RW, Golder EM, Gerwal A: Seasonality of symptoms in anorexia and bulimia nervosa, *Int J Eat Disord* 19(1):35, 1996.

186. Jimerson DC et al: Medications in the treatment of eating disorders, *Psychiatr Clin North Am* 19(4):739-754, 1996.

187. Williamson DA, Martin CK, Stewart T: Psychological aspects of eating disorders, *Best Pract Res Clin Gastroentrol* 18(6):1073-1088, 2004.

188. Incalzi RA et al: Energy intake and in-hospital starvation, *Arch Intern Med* 156(4):425, 1996.

189. Mahan LK, Escott-Stump S, editors: *Krause's food, nutrition and diet therapy,* ed 10, Philadelphia, 2000, Saunders.

190. Stipanuk MH: *Biochemical and physiological aspects of human nutrition,* Philadelphia, 2000, Saunders.

191. Berkley JA et al: Prognostic indicators of early and late death in children admitted to district hospital in Kenya: cohort study, *BMJ* 326(7385):361, 2003.

192. Lidder PG, Lewis S: Perioperative and postoperative nutrition, *Hosp Med* 65(12):717-720, 2004.

193. Bosch J, Garcia-Pagan JC: Complications of cirrhosis. I. Portal hypertension, *J Hepatol* 32(suppl 2):141, 2000.

194. Bosch J: The sixth Carlos E. Rubio Memorial Lecture: prevention and treatment of variceal hemorrhage, *P R Health Sci J* 19(1):57-67, 2000.

195. Binmoeller KF, Borsatto R: Variceal bleeding and portal hypertension, *Endoscopy* 32(3):189, 2000.

196. Liangpunsakul S, Ulmer, BJ, Chalasani N: Predictors and implications of severe hypersplenism in patients with cirrhosis, *Am J Med Sci* 326(3):111-116, 2003.

197. Thomopoulos KC et al: Non-invasive predictors of the presence of large oesophageal varices in patients with cirrhosis, *Dig Liver Dis* 35(7):473-478, 2003.

198. Blendis L, Wong F: The natural history and management of hepatorenal disorders: from pre-ascites to hepatorenal syndrome, *Clin Med* 3(2):154-159, 2003.
199. Cardenas A, Arroyo V: Mechanisms of water and sodium retention in cirrhosis and the pathogenesis of ascites, *Best Pract Res Clin Endocrinol Metab* 17(4):607-622, 2003.
200. Palmer BF: Pathogenesis of ascites and renal salt retention in cirrhosis, *J Investig Med* 47(5):183, 1999.
201. Gentilini P et al: Albumin improves the response to diuretics in patients with cirrhosis and ascites: results of a randomized, controlled trial, *J Hepatol* 30(4):639, 1999.
202. Coll S et al: Mechanisms of early decrease in systemic vascular resistance after total paracentesis: influence of flow rate of ascites extraction, *Eur J Gastroenterol Hepatol* 16(3):347-353, 2004.
203. Sanyal AJ et al: The North American study for the treatment of refractory ascites, *Gastroenterology* 124(3):634-641, 2004.
204. Butterworth KF, Borsatto R: Complications of cirrhosis III: hepatic encephalopathy, *J Hepatol* 32(suppl 1):171, 2000.
205. Lizardi-Cervera J et al: Hepatic encephalopathy: a review, *Ann Hepatol* 2(3):122-130, 2003.
206. Shimamoto C, Hirata I, Katsu K: Breath and blood ammonia in liver cirrhosis, *Hepatogastroenterology* 47(32):443, 2000.
207. Clemmeson JO et al: Cerebral herniation in patients with acute liver failure is correlated with arterial ammonia concentration, *Hepatology* 29(3):648, 1999.
208. Jalan R, Shawcross D, Davies N: The molecular pathogenesis of hepatic encephalopathy, *Int J Biochem Cell Biol* 35(8):1175-1181, 2003.
209. Schafer DF, Jones EA: Hepatic encephalopathy. In Zakim D, Boyer TD, editors: *Hepatology: a textbook of liver disease*, vol 1, ed 2, Philadelphia, 1990, Saunders.
210. Als-Nielsen B, Gluud LL, Gluud C: Nonabsorbable disaccharides for hepatic encephalopathy, *Cochrane Database Syst Rev* (2):CD003044.
211. Roche SP, Kobos R: Jaundice in the adult patient, *Am Fam Physician* 69(2):299-304, 2004.
212. Raiford DS: Pruritus of chronic cholestasis, *QJM* 88(9):603, 1995.
213. Moreau R, Lebrec D: Acute renal failure in patients with cirrhosis: perspective of the age of MELD, *Hepatology* 37(2):233-243, 2003.
214. Bataller R et al: Hepatorenal syndrome, *Forum (Genova)* 8(1):62, 1998.
215. Moore K: Renal failure is acute liver failure, *Eur J Gastroenterol Hepatol* 11(9):967, 1999.
216. Gines P, Arroyo V, Rodes J: Ascites and hepatorenal syndrome: Pathogenesis and treatment strategies. In Schrier RW et al, editors: *Advances in internal medicine*, vol 3, St Louis, 1998, Mosby.
217. Gines P et al: Hepatorenal syndrome, *Lancet* 362(9398):1819-1827, 2003.
218. Cardenas A. Arroyo V: Hepatorenal syndrome, *Ann Hepatol* 2(1): 23-29, 2003.
219. Shukla NB, Poles MA: Hepatitis B virus infection: co-infection with hepatitis C virus, hepatitis D virus, and human immunodeficiency virus, *Clin Liver Dis* 8(2):445-460, 2004.
220. Sheng L et al: Hepatitis G virus infection in acute fulminant hepatitis: prevalence of HGV infection and sequence analysis of a specific viral strain, *J Viral Hepat* 5(5):301, 1998.
221. Stapleton JT: GB virus type C/hepatitis G virus, *Semin Liver Dis* 23(2):137-148, 2003.
222. Ciocca M: Clinical course and consequences of hepatitis A infection, *Vaccine* 18(suppl 1):S71, 2000.
223. Vidor E et al: Aventis Pasteur vaccines containing inactivated hepatitis A virus: a compilation of immunogenicity data, *Eur J Clin Microbiol Infect Dis* 23(4):300-309, 2004.
224. Van Damme P, Van Herck K: A review of the efficacy, immunogenicity and tolerability of a combined hepatitis A and B vaccine, *Expert Rev Vaccines* 3(3):249-267, 2004.
225. Shukla NB, Poles MA: Hepatitis B virus infection: co-infection with hepatitis C virus, hepatitis D virus, and human immunodeficiency virus, *Clin Liver Dis* 8(2):445-460, viii, 2004.
226. Kumar R, Agrawal B: Novel treatment options for hepatitis B virus infection, *Curr Opin Investig Drugs* 5(2):171-178, 2004.
227. Lin KW, Kirchner JT: Hepatitis B, *Am Fam Physician* 69(1):75-82, 2004.
228. Karayiannis P: Current therapies for chronic hepatitis B virus infection, *Expert Rev Anti Infect Ther* 2(5):745-760, 2004.
229. Yu AS, Cheung RC, Keeffe EB: Hepatitis B vaccines, *Clin Liv Dis* 8(2):283-300, 2004.
230. Lawence SP: Advances in the treatment of hepatitis C. In Schrier RW, editor: *Advances in internal medicine*, vol 45, St Louis, 2000, Mosby.
231. Pawlotsky JM: Pathophysiology of hepatitis C virus infection and related liver disease, *Trends Microbiol* 12(2):96-102, 2004.
232. Pearlman BL: Hepatitis C treatment update, *Am J Med* 117(5): 344-352, 2004.
233. Tong MJ, Terrault NA, Klintmalm G: Hepatitis B transplantation: special conditions, *Semin Liver Dis* 20(suppl 1):25, 2000.
234. Wang L, Zhuang H: Hepatitis E: an overview and recent advanced in vaccine research, *World J Gastroenterol* 10(15):2157-2152, 2004.
235. Worm HC, Wirnsberger G: Hepatitis E vaccines: progress and prospects, *Drugs* 64(14):1517-1531, 2004.
236. Hitzler WE, Funkel S: Prevalence, persistence and liver enzyme levels of HGV RNA-positive blood donors determined by large-scale screening and transmission by blood components, *Clin Lab* 50(1-2):25-31, 2004.
237. Karayiannis P et al: Natural history and molecular biology of hepatitis G virus/GB virus C, *Clin Diagn Virol* 10(2-3):103, 1998.
238. Mandell GL, Bennett JE, Dolin R: *Principles and practice of infectious diseases*, vol 2, Philadelphia, 2000, Churchill Livingstone.
239. Han SH: Extrahepatic manifestations of chronic hepatitis B, *Clin Liver Dis* 8(2):403-418, 2004.
240. Ohto H et al: Transmission of hepatitis C from mothers to infants, *N Engl J Med* 330(11):744, 1994.
241. Jackson SH, Cheung EC: Hepatitis B and hepatitis C: occupational considerations for the anesthesiologist, *Anesthesiol Clin North Am* 22(3):357-377, v, 2004.
242. Garfein RS et al: Factors associated with fulminant liver failure during an outbreak among injection drug users with acute hepatitis B, *Hepathology* 40(4):865-873, 2004.
243. Kessler WR et al: Fulminant hepatic failure as the initial presentation of acute autoimmune hepatitis, *Clin Gastroentrol Hepatol* 2(7): 625-631, 2004.
244. Shakil AO, Mazariegos GV, Kramer DJ: Fulminant hepatic failure, *Surg Clin North Am* 79(1):77, 1999.
245. van de Kerkhove MP et al: Clinical application of bioartificial liver support systems, *Ann Surg* 240(2):216-230, 2004.
246. Hill DB, Kugelmas M: Alcoholic liver disease: treatment strategies for the potentially reversible stages, *Postgrad Med* 103(4):261, 1998.
247. Arteel G et al: Advances in alcoholic liver disease, *Best Pract Res Clin Gastroenterol* 17(4):625-647, 2003.
248. Bradbury MW, Berk PD: Lipid metabolism in hepatic steatosis, *Clin Liver Dis* 8(3):639-671, 2004.
249. Savolainen V et al: Early perivenular fibrosis—precirrhotic lesions among moderate alcohol consumers and chronic alcoholics, *J Hepatol* 23(5):524, 1995.
250. Zetterman RZ: Alcoholic liver disease. In Gitnick G, editor: *Current hepatology*, vol 16, St Louis, 1996, Mosby.
251. Lieber CS: Alcoholic liver disease: new insights in pathogenesis lead to new treatments, *J Hepatol* 32(suppl 1):113, 2000.
252. Greenwel P: Acetaldehyde-mediated collagen regulation in hepatic stellate cells, *Alcohol Clin Exp Res* 23(5):930, 1999.
253. Abillos A et al: Increased lipopolysaccharide binding protein in cirrhotic patients with marked immune and hemodynamic derangement, *Hepatology* 37(1):208-217, 2003.
254. Paik YH et al: Toll-like receptor 4 mediates inflammatory signaling by bacterial lipopolysaccharide in human hepatic stellate cells, *Hepatology* 37(5):1043-1055, 2003.
255. McClain CJ et al: Recent advances in alcoholic liver disease. IV. Dysregulated cytokine metabolism in alcoholic liver disease, *Am J Physiol Gastrointest Liver Physiol* 287(3):G497-502, 2004.
256. Lefkowitch JH: Morphology of alcoholic liver disease, *Clin Liver Dis* 9(1):37-53, 2005.
257. O'Shea RS, McCullough AJ: Treatment of alcoholic hepatitis, *Clin Liver Dis* 9(1):103-134, 2005.
258. Gavaler JS, van Thiel DH: Ethanol: its adverse effects upon the hypothalamic pituitary-gonadal axis, *J Lab Clin Med* 101:21, 1983.
259. Gomez F, Ruiz P, Schreiber AD: Impaired function of macrophage Fc gamma receptors and bacterial infection in alcoholic cirrhosis, *N Engl J Med* 331(17):1122-1128, 1994.
260. Tome S, Lucey MR: Review article: current management of alcoholic liver disease, *Aliment Pharmacol Ther* 19(7):707-714, 2004.
261. Kita H, He XS, Gershwin ME: Autoimmunity and environmental factors in the pathogenesis of primary biliary cirrhosis, *Ann Med* 36(1):72-80, 2004.

262. Selmi C et al: Epidemiology and pathogenesis of primary biliary cirrhosis, *J Clin Gastroenterol* 38(3):264-271, 2004.

263. Leuschner U: Primary biliary cirrhosis—presentation and diagnosis, *Clin Liver Dis* 7(4):741-758, 2003.

264. Heathcote EJ: Management of primary biliary cirrhosis. The American Association of the Study of Liver Disease practice guidelines, *Hepatology* 31(4):1005, 2000.

265. Pares A, Rodes J: Natural history of primary biliary cirrhosis, *Clin Liver Dis* 7(4):779-794, 2003.

266. Prince MI et al: Asymptomatic primary biliary cirrhosis: clinical features, prognosis, and symptom progression in a large population based cohort, *Gut* 53(6):865-870, 2004.

267. Van Den Bogaert E et al: The use of ursodeoxycholic acid in patients with primary biliary cirrhosis: sense of nonsense, *Acta Gastroenterol Belg* 66(4):283-287, 2003.

268. Carey MC: Pathogenesis of gallstones, *Am J Surg* 165(4):410, 1993.

269. Portincasa P et al: Pathobiology of cholesterol gallstone disease: from equilibrium ternary phase diagram to agents preventing cholesterol crystallization and stone formation, *Curr Drug Targets Immune Endocr Metabol Discord* 3(1):67-81, 2003.

270. Tomer G, Shneider BL: Disorders of bile formation and biliary transport, *Gastroenterol Clin North Am* 32(3):839-855, 2003.

271. Donovan JM: Physical and metabolic factors in gallstone pathogenesis, *Gastroenterol Clin North Am* 28(1):75, 1999.

272. Berger MY et al: Abdominal symptoms: do they predict gallstones? A systemic review, *Scand J Gastroenterol* 35(1):70, 2000.

273. Thorboll J et al: Endoscopic ultrasonography in detection of cholelithiasis in patients with biliary pain and negative transabdominal ultrasonography, *Scand J Gastroenterol* 39(3):267-269, 2004.

274. Hochberger J et al: Management of difficult common bile duct stones, *Gastrointest Endosc Clin North Am* 13(4):623-634, 2003.

275. Venu RP et al: Endoscopic transpapillary drainage of pancreatic abscess: technique and results, *Gastrointest Endosc* 51(4 Pt 1):391, 2000.

276. van Brummelen SE et al: Acute idiopathic pancreatitis: does it really exist or is it a myth? *Scand J Gastroenterol Suppl* (239):117-122, 2003.

277. Kim HJ et al: Idiopathic acute pancreatitis, *J Clin Gastroenterol* 37(3):238-250, 2003.

278. Wilson JS, Apte MV: Role of alcohol metabolism in alcoholic pancreatitis, *Pancreas* 27(4):311-315, 2003.

279. Bhatia M: Apoptosis versus necrosis in acute pancreatitis, *Am J Physiol Gastrointest Liver Physiol* 286(2):G189, 2004.

280. Arendt T et al: Gallstones, the choledochoduodenal junction and initiation of acute pancreatitis: are two stones the culprit rather than one stone? *Med Hypothesis* 54(4):570, 2000.

281. Apte MV, Wilson JS: Alcohol-induced pancreatic injury, *Best Pract Res Clin Gastroenterol* 17(4):593-612, 2003.

282. Bhatia M et al: Inflammatory mediators in acute pancreatitis, *J Pathol* 190(2):117, 2000.

283. Raraty MG et al: Acute pancreatitis and organ failure: pathophysiology, natural history, and management strategies, *Curr Gastroenterol Rep* 6(2):99-103, 2004.

284. Kemppainen EA et al: Advances in the laboratory diagnostics of acute pancreatitis, *Ann Med* 30(2):169, 1998.

285. Papachristou GI, Whitcomb DC: Predictors of severity and necrosis in acute pancreatitis, *Gastroenterol Clin North Am* 33(4):871-890, 2004.

286. Avgerinos C et al: Nutritional support in acute pancreatitis, *Dig Dis* 21(3):214-219, 2003.

287. Erstad BL: Enteral nutrition support in acute pancreatitis, *Ann Pharmacother* 34(4):514, 2000.

288. Layer P, DiMagno EP: Early and late onset in idiopathic and alcoholic chronic pancreatitis: different clinical courses, *Surg Clin North Am* 79 (4):847, 1999.

289. Owyang C: Chronic pancreatitis. In Yamada T, Alpers DH, Laine L, editors: *Atlas of gastroenterology*, ed 3, Phialdelphia, 1999, Lippincott Williams & Wilkins.

290. Olah A et al: Long-term follow-up results of surgery for chronic pancreatitis, *Hepatogastroenterology* 51(58):1170-1182, 2004.

291. Whitcomb DC: Inflammation and cancer V. Chronic pancreatitis and pancreatic cancer, *Am J Physiol Gastrointest Liver Physiol* 287(2): G315-G319, 2004.

292. Wei JT, Shaheen N: The changing epidemiology of esophageal adenocarcinoma, *Semin Gastrointest Dis* 14(3):112-127, 2003.

293. American Cancer Society: *Estimated new cancer cases and deaths by sex for all sites, United States, 2005*, Atlanta, 2005, The Society. Available at www3.cancer.org/cancerinfo/sitecenter

294. Heath EI et al: Adenocarcinoma of the esophagus: risk factors and prevention, *Oncology (Huntingt)* 14(4):507, 2000.

295. Tytgat GN et al: Cancer of the esophagus and gastric cardia: recent advances, *Dis Esophagus* 17(1):10-26, 2004.

296. Blot WJ, McLaughlin JK: The changing epidemiology of esophageal cancer, *Semin Oncol* 33(3):71, 2000.

297. Lam AK: Molecular biology of esophageal squamous cell carcinoma, *Crit Rev Oncol Hematol* 33(2):71, 2000.

298. Lambert R, Hainaut P, Parkin DM: Premalignant lesions of the esophagogastric mucosa, *Semin Oncol* 31(4):498-512, 2004.

299. Clark GW: Effect of Helicobacter pylori infection in Barrett's esophagus and the genesis of esophageal adenocarcinoma, *World J Surg* 27(9):994-998, 2003.

300. Lin J, Beerm DC: Molecular biology of upper gastrointestinal malignancies, *Semin Oncol* 31(4):476-486, 2004.

301. Brenner B, Ilson DH, Minsky BD: Treatment of localized esophageal cancer, *Semin Oncol* 31(4):554-565, 2004.

302. Hatakeyama M: Oncogenic mechanisms of the Helicobacter pylori CagA protein, *Nat Rev Cancer* 4(9):688-694, 2004.

303. Kelley JR, Duggan JM: Gastric cancer epidemiology and risk factors, *J Clin Epidemiol* 56(1):1-9, 2003.

304. Houben GM, Stockbrugger RW: Bacteria in the aetio-pathogenesis of gastric cancer: a review, *Scand J Gastroenterol* 212(suppl):13, 1995.

305. Fenoglio-Preiser CM et al: TP53 and gastric carcinoma: a review, *Hum Mutat* 21(3):258-270, 2003.

306. Tahara E: Genetic pathways of two types of gastric cancer, *IARC Sci Publ* (157):327-349, 2004.

307. Saukkonen K et al: Cyclooxygenase-2 and gastric carcinogenesis, *APMIS* 111(10):915-925, 2003.

308. Yao JC et al: Combined-modality therapy for gastric cancer, *Semin Surg Oncol* 21(4):223-227, 2003.

309. Sullivan T et al: Helicobacter pylori and the prevention of gastric cancer, *Can J Gastroenterol* 18(5):295-302, 2004.

310. Lipkin M et al: Dietary factors in human colorectal cancer, *Annu Rev Nutr* 19:545-586, 1999.

311. Slattery ML et al: Lifestyle and colon cancer: an assessment of factors associated with risk, *Am J Epidemiol* 150(8):869, 1999.

312. Kam MH et al: Small bowel malignancies: a review of 20 patients at a single centre, *Colorectal Dis* 6(3):195-197, 2004.

313. Ahnen JD: The genetic basis of colorectal cancer risk, *Adv Intern Med* 41:531-532, 1996.

314. Jen J et al: Allelic loss of chromosome 18q and prognosis in colorectal cancer, *N Engl J Med* 331(4):213-221, 1994.

315. Huycke MM, Gaskins HR: Commensal bacteria, redox stress, and colorectal cancer: mechanisms and models, *Exp Biol Med (Maywood)*, 229(7):586-597, 2004.

316. Cross AJ, Sinha R: Meat-related mutagens/carcinogens in the etiology of colorectal cancer, *Environ Mol Mutagen* 44(1):44-55, 2004.

317. Asano TK, McLeon RS: Non steroidal anti-inflammatory drugs (NSAID) and aspirin for preventing colorectal adenomas and carcinomas, *Cochrane Database Syst Rev* (2):CD004079, 2004.

318. Chia V, Newcomb PA: Calcium and colorectal cancer: some questions remain, *Nutr Rev* 62(3):115-120, 2004.

319. Weingarten MA, Zalmanovici A, Yaphe J: Dietary calcium supplementation for preventing colorectal cancer and adenomatous polyps, *Cochrane Database Syst Rev* (1):CD003548, 2004.

320. Yeh RK et al: NO-donating nonsteroidal antiinflammatory drugs (NSAIDs) inhibit colon cancer cell growth more potentially than traditional NSAIDs: a general pharmacological property? *Biochem Pharmacol* 67(12):2197-2205, 2004.

321. Baglioni S, Genuardi M: Simple and complex genetics of colorectal cancer susceptibility, *Am J Med Genet* 129C(1):35-43, 2004.

322. Nasir A et al: Cyclooxygenase-2 expression in right- and left-sided colon cancer: a rationale for optimization of cyclooxygenase-2 inhibitor therapy, *Clin Colorectal Cancer* 3(4):243-247, 2004.

323. Sinicrope FA, Gill S: Role of cyclooxygenase-2 in colorectal cancer, *Cancer Metastasis Rev* 23(1-2):63-75, 2004.

324. Winawer SJ: Natural history of colorectal cancer, *Am J Med* 106(1A):3S, 1999.

325. Bendardaf R, Lamlum H, Pyrhonen S: Prognostic and predictive molecular markers in colorectal carcinoma, *Anticancer Res* 24(4): 2519-2530, 2004.

326. Mak T et al: Molecylar stool screening for colorectal cancer, *Br J Surg* 91(7):790-800, 2004.

327. Annie Yu HJ et al: Hereditary nonpolyposis colorectal cancer: preventive management, *Cancer Treat Rev* 29(6):461-470, 2003.

328. Petersen GM et al: Genetic testing and counseling for hereditary forms of colorectal cancer, *Cancer* 86(suppl 11):2540-2550, 1999.

329. De Salvo GL et al: Curative surgery for obstruction from primary left colorectal carcinoma: primary or staged resection? *Cochrane Database Syst Rev* (2):CD002101, 2004.

330. Braun AH et al: New systemic frontline treatment for metastatic colorectal carcinoma, *Cancer* 100(8):1558-1577, 2004.

331. Midgley RS, Kerr DJ: Immunotherapy for colorectal cancer, *Expert Rev Anticancer Ther* 3(1):63-78, 2003.

332. Schlom J et al: Strategies in the development of recombinant vaccines for colon cancer, *Semin Oncol* 26(6):672-682, 1999.

333. Sobrero A et al: New directions in the treatment of colon cancer: a look to the future, *Eur J Cancer* 36(5):559-566, 2000.

334. Harrison LE et al: Racial discrepancies in the outcome of patients with hepatocellular carcinoma, *Arch Surg* 139(9):992-996, 2004.

335. Llovet T, Burroughs A, Bruix J: Hepatocellular carcinoma, *Lancet* 362(9399):1907-1917, 2004.

336. O'Brien TR, Kirk G, Zhang M: Hepatocellular carcinoma: paradigm of preventive oncology, *Cancer J* 10(2):67-73, 2004.

337 Coleman WB: Mechanisms of human hepatocarcinogenesis, *Curr Mol Med* 3(6):573-588, 2003.

338. Srivatanakul P, Sriplung H, Deerasamee S: Epidemiology of liver cancer: an overview, *Asian Pac J Cancer Prev* 5(2):118-124, 2004.

339. Sherman M, Takayama Y: Screening and treatment for hepatocellular carcinoma, *Gastroenterol Clin North Am* 33(3):671-691, 2004.

340. Talwalkar JA, Gores GJ: Diagnosis and staging of hepatocellular carcinoma, *Gastroenterology* 127(5 Suppl):S126-S132, 2004.

341. Fecht WJ Jr, Befeler AS: Hepatocellular carcinoma: updates in primary prevention, *Curr Gastroenterol Rep* 6(1):37-43, 2004.

342. Yan P, Yan LN: Staging of hepatocellular carcinoma, *Hepatobiliary Pancreat Dis Int* 2(4):491-495, 2003.

343. Nissen NN et al: Emerging role of transplantation for primary liver cancers, *Cancer J* 10(2):88-96, 2004.

344. Hu S, Keeffe EB: Management of hepatocellular carcinoma, *Rev Gastroenterol Disord* 3(1):8-24, 2003.

345. Lowenfels AB et al: Epidemiology of gallbladder cancer, *Hepatogastroenterology* 46(27):1529, 1999.

346. Pandy M: Risk factors for gallbladder cancer: a reappraisal, *Eur J Cancer Prev* 12(1):15-24, 2003.

347. Malik IA: Gallbladder cancer: current status, *Expert Opin Pharmacother* 5(6):1271-1277, 2004.

348. Misra S et al: Carcinoma of the gallbladder, *Lancet Oncol* 4(3):167-176, 2003.

349. Sheth S, Bedford A, Chopra S: Primary gallbladder cancer: recognition of risk factors and the role of prophylactic cholecystectomy, *Am J Gastroenterol* 95(6):1402-1410, 2000.

350. Li D, Jiao L: Molecular epidemiology of pancreatic cancer, *Int J Gastrointest Cancer* 33(1):3-124, 2003.

351. Lowenfels AB, Maisonneuve P, Lankisch PG: Chronic pancreatitis and other risk factors for pancreatic cancer, *Gastroenterol Clin North Am* 28(3):673-685, 1999.

352. Kloppel. G, Luttges J: The pathology of ductal-type pancreatic carcinomas and pancreatic intraepithelial neoplasia: insights for clinicians, *Curr Gastroenterol Rep* 6(2):111-118, 2004.

353. Li D et al: Pancreatic cancer, *Lancet* 363(9414):1049-1057, 2004.

354. Sakorafas GH, Tsiotou AG, Tsiotos GG: Molecular biology of pancreatic cancer; oncogenes, tumour suppressor genes, growth factors, and their receptors from a clinical perspective, *Cancer Treat Rev* 26(1):29, 2000.

355. Krech RL, Walsh D: Symptoms of pancreatic cancer, *J Pain Symptom Manage* 6(6):360-367, 1991.

356. Alexakis N et al: Current standards of surgery for pancreatic cancer, *Br J Surg* 91(11):1410-1427, 2004.

357. Raut CP et al: Neoadjuvant therapy for resectable pancreatic cancer, *Surg Oncol Clin North Am* 13(4):639-661, ix, 2004.

ALTERATIONS OF DIGESTIVE FUNCTION IN CHILDREN

DEBORAH B. EVERS

CHAPTER OUTLINE

D isorders of the gastrointestinal tract in children include anomalies with structural and functional alterations, as well as enzyme deficiencies. Structural alterations can occur throughout the gastrointestinal tract and include cleft lip and palate, esophageal atresia, tracheoesophageal fistula, pyloric stenosis, aganglionic megacolon, and imperforate anus. Gastroesophageal reflux, hepatic and pancreatic enzyme deficiencies, and bacterial or viral invasions of the gastrointestinal tract also contribute to the diseases and gastrointestinal clinical manifestations in children.

DISORDERS OF THE GASTROINTESTINAL TRACT

Congenital Impairment of Motility

Cleft Lip and Cleft Palate

Cleft lip (harelip) and **cleft palate,** developmental anomalies of the first branchial arch, are the fourth most common congenital disability in the United States[1] (Figure 40-1). In whites the incidence of cleft lip or cleft palate ranges from 1 in 600 to 1 in 1250 births. The incidence of cleft lip, with or without cleft palate, is 1 in 600 births, whereas the incidence of cleft palate alone is about 1 in 1000 births. Incidence is lower in

black populations and higher in Asian populations.[2] Cleft lip, with or without cleft palate, is more common in females. Both anomalies can be unilateral or bilateral, and both anomalies can be partial or complete.

In most cases, cleft lip and cleft palate are caused by multiple gene-environment interactions, including maternal tobacco and alcohol use, maternal diabetes mellitus, and genetic variations of the transforming growth factor–alpha gene.[3-11] Preliminary data offer evidence that maternal hyperhomocysteinemia also may be a factor associated with having offspring with nonsyndromic orofacial clefts.[12,13] (This phenomenon, called *multifactorial inheritance,* is discussed in Chapter 4.) Together, these factors reduce the amount of neural crest mesenchyme that migrates into the area that will develop into the face of the embryo. If the amount is sufficiently reduced, clefting occurs. The cleft can be part of a syndrome determined by single mutant genes or part of a chromosomal defect, usually trisomy 13.[14] Rarely, the cleft is caused by a teratogenic agent, such as an anticonvulsant drug.[15]

PATHOPHYSIOLOGY

Cleft Lip

Cleft lip is caused by the incomplete fusion of the nasomedial or intermaxillary process during the second month of embryonic development. The deformity develops during a

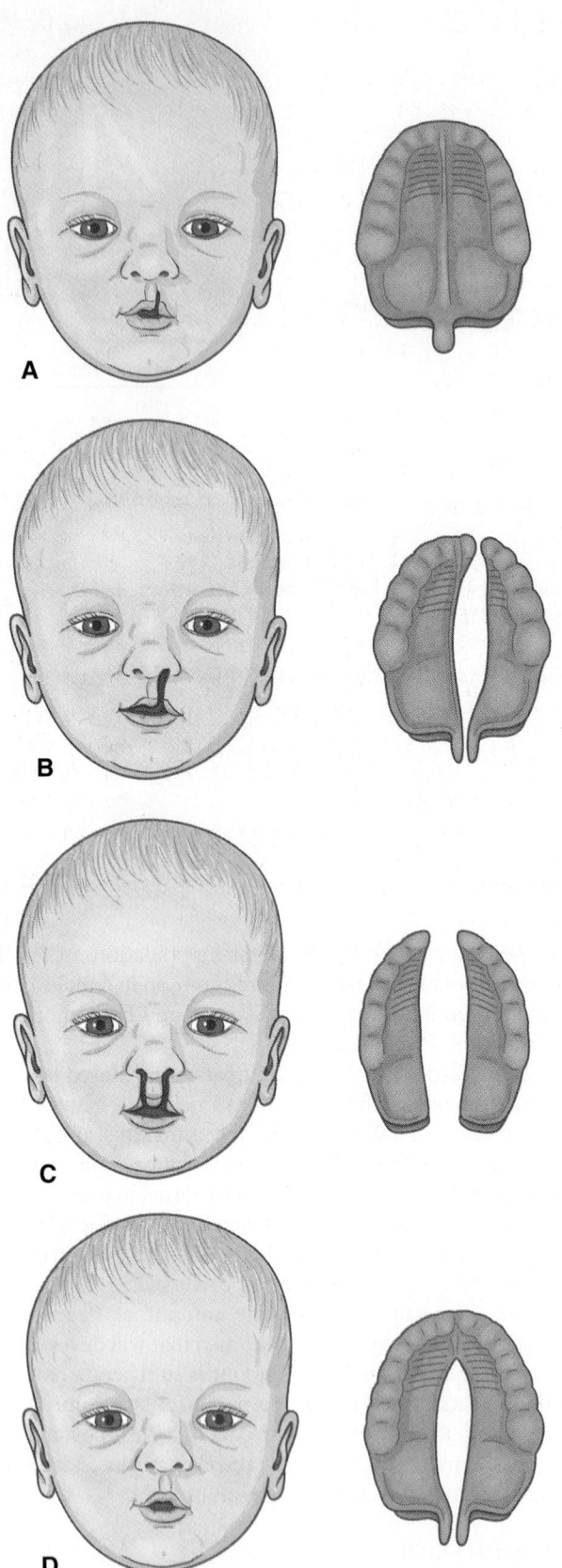

Figure 40-1 Variations in clefts of the lip and palate. **A,** Notch in vermilion border. **B,** Unilateral cleft lip and palate. **C,** Bilateral cleft lip and cleft palate. **D,** Cleft palate.

period of very rapid fetal growth. The cleft causes structures of the face and mouth to develop without the normal restraints of encircling lip muscles. A characteristic depression or flattening of the infant's midfacial contour may occur because normal antagonistic forces across the midline are absent, and growth of the involved facial segments is disturbed. The facial cleft may affect not only the lip but also the external nose, the nasal cartilages, the nasal septum, and the alveolar processes.

The cleft is usually just beneath the center of one nostril. The defect may occur bilaterally and may be symmetric or asymmetric. The cleft can range in severity from a slight indentation of the lip to a fissure that extends to the nostril, causing a sagging and flattening of the nose. The failure of lip fusion by 35 days of gestation may impair closure of the palatal shelves. The more complete the cleft lip, the greater the chance that teeth in the line of the cleft will be missing or malformed.

Cleft Palate

Cleft palate is often associated with cleft lip but may occur without it. Cleft palate results from the failure of the primary palatal shelves, or processes, to fuse during the third month of gestation. The fissure may affect only the uvula and soft palate, or it may extend forward to the nostril and involve the hard palate and the maxillary alveolar ridge. It may be unilateral or bilateral, with the cleft occupying the midline posteriorly and as far forward as the alveolar process, where it deviates to the involved side. Clefts involving the palate only are usually but not necessarily in the midline. In some cases the vomer and nasal septum are partly or completely undeveloped. When these facial bones are involved, the nasal cavity may freely communicate with the oral cavity.

CLINICAL MANIFESTATIONS   Feeding the infant with cleft lip usually presents no difficulty if the cleft lip is simple and the palate intact. Nursing at breast or bottle depends on suction developed by pressing the nipple against the hard palate with the tongue. Closure of the lips is not necessary, but the tongue must work harder if the infant cannot purse his or her lips. A baby with cleft palate usually requires large, soft nipples with cross-cut openings. Although most infants with cleft palate can be successfully breast-fed, it may be impossible for some because of an unproductive suck.[16,17] An orthodontic prosthesis for the roof of the mouth may facilitate sucking for some infants.[18]

EVALUATION AND TREATMENT   Facial x-ray films confirm the extent of bone deformity. Soft tissue alterations are evaluated by history and physical examination. Prenatal ultrasound has aided early diagnosis of orofacial clefting.[19]

The nature and extent of the cleft, the infant's condition, and the method of surgical correction proposed determine the course of treatment.[20] Surgical correction is often planned in stages. The lip is united first. Although this can be done within a few weeks of birth, most surgeons prefer to wait until the infant is 2 to 3 months old to allow sufficient growth to occur. The initial repair may be revised when the child is 4 to 5 years old.

Repair of a cleft lip that is accompanied by bilateral cleft palate is technically more difficult, so the procedure is often performed in two steps. The lip is repaired when the infant is a few weeks old. The palate is closed after the child is weaned from the nipple but before he or she has begun to talk, usually at about 12 to 18 months of age.[21] The aim of surgery is to obtain an airtight closure of the palatal cleft and to preserve the mobility and length of the soft palate. Even with early closure, the child may experience difficulty sealing off the nasopharynx from the buccal cavity during swallowing and while pronouncing certain consonants. Speech training and special attention by a prosthodontist and orthodontist are almost always required.

Both before and after surgery, children with cleft lip and palate tend to have recurrent infections of the paranasal sinuses and middle ear. Parents should be alerted to this increased risk so that otitis media can be detected and treated earlier to decrease the chance of long-term scarring and subsequent hearing loss.[22] Breast-milk feedings have been found to be associated with a lower incidence of otitis media in these infants.[23] Hypertrophy of the tonsils and adenoids is common. Children with an orofacial cleft are at an increased risk of being infected by *Streptococcus mutans* and *Lactobacillus* at a very early age. Such colonization indicates a high risk for caries in the primary dentition.[24,25] Displacement of the maxillary arches and malposition of the teeth usually require orthodontic correction.

Esophageal Malformations

Congenital malformations of the esophagus occur in 1 of 3000 to 4500 live births. **Esophageal atresia** is a condition in which the esophagus ends in a blind pouch. Esophageal atre-sia is usually accompanied by a fistula between the esophagus and the trachea. This connection is called a **tracheo-esophageal fistula (TEF)**. Either defect can occur alone, however (Figure 40-2).

PATHOPHYSIOLOGY   The esophageal abnormalities are thought to arise from defective differentiation as the trachea separates from the esophagus during the fourth to sixth weeks of embryonic development. Defective growth of endodermal cells leads to atresia. Incomplete fusion of the lateral walls of the foregut leads to incomplete closure of the laryngotracheal tube and fistula formation.

CLINICAL MANIFESTATIONS   Polyhydramnios is reported to occur in 14% to 90% of mothers of affected infants.[26] The blind end of the proximal esophagus has a capacity of only a few milliliters. As the infant with esophageal atresia swallows oral secretions, the pouch fills and overflows into the pharynx, resulting in drooling and occasionally in aspiration (see Figure 40-2, *A* and *C*).

If a fistula connects the trachea with the distal esophagus, the abdomen fills with air and becomes distended. The distention may be great enough to interfere with breathing (see Figure 40-2, *C* to *E*). If the fistula connects the proximal esophagus to the trachea, the first feeding after birth will be problematic (see Figure 40-2, *B, D,* and *E*). As the infant drinks, the blind end of the esophagus and the mouth fill with fluid. When the infant tries to take a breath, the fluid is aspirated into the lungs, which triggers protective cough and choke reflexes. Intermittent cyanosis may result. Plain water or glucose is recommended for the initial feeding to minimize the dangers associated with aspiration. If an abnormality of the esophagus is indicated, oral feedings are withheld until a diagnosis is confirmed.

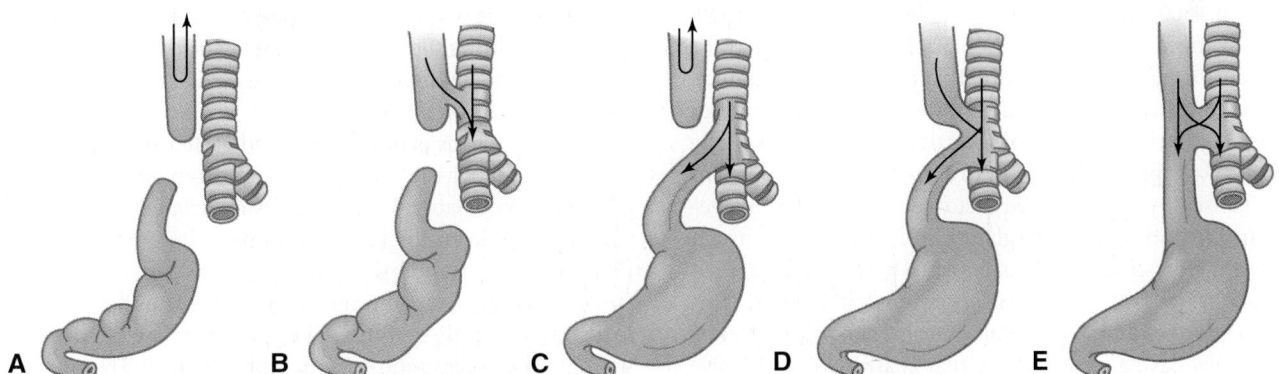

Figure 40-2 Five types of esophageal atresia and tracheoesophageal fistulas. **A,** Simple esophageal atresia. Proximal esophagus and distal esophagus end in blind pouches, and there is no tracheal communication. Nothing enters the stomach; regurgitated food and fluid may enter the lungs. **B,** Proximal and distal esophageal segments end in blind pouches, and a fistula connects the proximal esophagus to the trachea. Nothing enters the stomach; food and fluid enter the lungs. **C,** Proximal esophagus ends in a blind pouch, and a fistula connects the trachea to the distal esophagus. Air enters the stomach; regurgitated gastric secretions enter the lungs through the fistula. **D,** Fistula connects both proximal and distal esophageal segments to the trachea. Air, food, and fluid enter the stomach and the lungs. **E,** Simple tracheoesophageal fistula between otherwise normal esophagus and trachea. Air, food, and fluid enter the stomach and the lungs. Between 85% and 90% of esophageal anomalies are type C; 6% to 8% are type A; 3% to 5% are type E; and fewer than 1% are type B or D.

Pulmonary complications are compounded by reflux of air and gastric secretions into the tracheobronchial tree through the fistula (see Figure 40-2, *D* and *E*), causing severe chemical irritation. The upper lobe of the right lung is most commonly involved because of its proximity to the tracheoesophageal fistula. Infants with esophageal atresia but no fistula have a scaphoid (boat-shaped), gasless abdomen. In fistula without atresia (Figure 40-2, *E*), the usual symptoms are recurrent aspiration, pneumonia, and atelectasis that remains "silent" for days or even months. Late complication of esophageal atresia or tracheal esophageal fistula include stricture, reflux and dysphagia.[27]

In at least 50% of infants with esophageal defects, other congenital anomalies are present as well. Cardiovascular anomalies are the most common, but other digestive tract, urinary, vertebral, and central nervous system defects can accompany esophageal atresia and tracheoesophageal fistula.

EVALUATION AND TREATMENT   Esophageal atresia is usually diagnosed at birth, when attempts to pass a small-bore orogastric or nasogastric tube into the stomach fail.[28] X-ray films show the catheter coiled in the upper esophageal pouch. Barium x-ray examinations are used by some investigators.

Treatment is surgical. Esophageal continuity is restored, and the fistula is eliminated. Surgery is usually undertaken after birth, sometimes in stages. The child may continue to have problems with aspiration, gastroesophageal reflux, and esophagitis after surgical repair.[27,29,30] The overall survival rate for infants with esophageal defects is approximately 75%.[31]

Pyloric Stenosis

Pyloric stenosis is an obstruction of the pyloric sphincter caused by hypertrophy of the sphincter muscle. It is one of the most common disorders of early infancy and affects infants between the ages of either 1 and 2 weeks or 3 and 4 months.[32] The incidence of pyloric stenosis among males is approximately 5 in 1000, whereas among females it is only 1 in 1000. Whites are affected more often than blacks or Asians, and full-term infants are affected more often than premature infants.[33] Increased gastrin secretion by the mother in the last trimester of pregnancy increases the likelihood of pyloric stenosis in the infant. The overproduction of gastric secretions in the infant may be caused by stress-related factors in the mother. Exogenous administration of prostaglandin E is associated with an increased incidence of pyloric stenosis. There is an increased incidence of pyloric stenosis in children with Down syndrome; 6.9% of children have a parent who had pyloric stenosis, and 4.9% have a close relative that is affected.[34,35] Pyloric stenosis occurs in approximately 20% of male and 10% of female descendants of mothers who had pyloric stenosis.[2]

PATHOPHYSIOLOGY   The circular muscle of the pylorus is grossly enlarged because of an increase in cell size (hypertrophy) and an increase in cell number (hyperplasia).[36] Research has shown that transforming growth factor–alpha plays a role in stimulating this increase in muscle mass.[37] The

mucosal lining of the pyloric opening is folded and the lumen is narrowed by the encroaching muscle. Because of the extra peristaltic effort necessary to force the gastric contents through the narrow pylorus, the muscle layers of the stomach may become hypertrophied as well.

CLINICAL MANIFESTATIONS   Between 2 and 3 weeks after birth, an infant who has fed well and gained weight begins to vomit without apparent reason. The vomiting gradually becomes more forceful. In some cases, stomach contents may shoot out 3 or 4 feet. Food is often regurgitated through the nose. The forceful, or projectile, vomiting usually occurs immediately after eating, and the vomitus consists of the bulk of the feeding plus some food retained from previous feedings but is almost always free of bile. Usually infants are hungry and want to eat again after vomiting.[38]

Prolonged retention of food in the stomach is a characteristic feature of pyloric stenosis. In infants with pyloric stenosis, food is present after 4 hours unless vomiting has occurred. Constipation is the rule because not much food reaches the intestine.

In severe untreated cases, increased gastric peristalsis and vomiting lead to severe fluid and electrolyte imbalances (hypochloremic metabolic alkalosis), chronic malnutrition, and weight loss that can be fatal within 4 to 6 weeks. Infants with pyloric stenosis are irritable because of hunger, and they may have esophageal discomfort caused by repeated vomiting and esophagitis. The vomitus may be blood streaked because of rupture of gastric and esophageal vessels.

EVALUATION AND TREATMENT   Diagnosis is based on the history of clinical manifestations. Occasionally, gastric peristalsis is observable over the abdomen. A firm, small, movable mass, approximately the size of an olive, is felt in the right upper quadrant in 70% to 90% of infants with pyloric stenosis. A visible gastric peristaltic wave after eating is observed in some infants. Sonography is routinely done because this clearly shows the hypertrophied pyloric muscles and narrowed pyloric channel. This technique is replacing contrast x-ray examinations.[39]

Pyloric stenosis is now recognized earlier than in previous decades; the "classic" metabolic derangements (water and electrolyte imbalances) traditionally associated with this condition have been highly uncommon for the past three decades.[40] The standard treatment for hypertrophic pyloric stenosis is a pyloromyotomy, in which the muscles of the pylorus are split and separated. The procedure can be completed with an open technique or with laparoscopy.[41] The mortality rate associated with surgical correction is less than 0.5%.

Some infants respond to medical and nutritional management, which is based on the theory that the pylorus will open spontaneously by 6 to 8 months of age if nutrition can be maintained. To maintain nutrition, antispasmodic drugs are given to relax the pylorospasm and the infant is refed after vomiting. Medical management is associated with slow improvement and a higher mortality rate. Endoscopic balloon dilation and treatment with oral or intravenous atropine sulfate have been successful.[42, 42a]

Malrotation

During the tenth week of embryonic development, the emerging ileum and cecum normally rotate, so that the cecum moves into the lower right quadrant of the abdomen and is fixed there by the mesentery. **Malrotation** is a condition in which rotation does not occur and the colon remains in the upper right quadrant, where an abnormal membrane may press on and obstruct the duodenum. The obstructing band over the duodenum, called a **periduodenal band,** is one of the most significant findings in malrotation. Associated abnormalities are seen in 30% to 62% of children in a reported series; 50% of children with duodenal atresia and 33% of those with jejunal atresia have associated malrotation.[43]

PATHOPHYSIOLOGY   The small intestine lacks a normal posterior fixation in malrotation because it has only a rudimentary attachment near the origin of the superior mesenteric artery. Therefore the entire mass can twist when the mobile loops of intestine from the duodenojejunal junction to the middle of the transverse colon twist on themselves. The twisting is termed *volvulus.* Intestinal twisting around the rudimentary mesentery angulates and obstructs the intestinal lumen and partly or completely occludes the superior mesenteric artery, causing infarction and necrosis of the entire midgut.

CLINICAL MANIFESTATIONS   Although most cases of malrotation-associated volvulus and infarction develop during the neonatal period (50%) or infancy (85% are younger than 1 year), some develop during childhood or even adulthood.[44] In infants the obstruction causes intermittent or persistent bile-stained vomiting after feedings. Abdominal distention is limited initially to the epigastrium because only the stomach and duodenum are dilated. The degree of distention depends on the pressure of swallowed air and the degree of obstruction caused by the volvulus. Dehydration and electrolyte imbalance may occur rapidly because large amounts of pancreatic juice, bile, and gastric secretions are lost through vomiting. Fever usually ensues. Pain, scanty stools, diarrhea, and bloody stools are associated with progressive volvulus, vascular compression, and infarction of the intestine in infants. Intermittent or partial volvulus may be seen in older children and adults. This may be asymptomatic (25% to 50% of the time) and discovered during unrelated abdominal surgery, or it may cause minor abdominal complaints, such as nausea after meals, recurrent episodes of vomiting, or abdominal pain.[45]

EVALUATION AND TREATMENT   Diagnosis of malrotation with volvulus and infarction is based on a review of the clinical manifestations. X-ray films of the abdomen show gas bubbles and distention proximal to the site of obstruction.

Treatment consists of opening the abdomen and reducing the volvulus manually. The surgeon takes the entire intestinal mass in hand and rotates it counterclockwise. Necrotic bowel may be resected and a primary anastomosis performed. When there is gangrene and question of viability of the bowel ends, an enterostomy may be performed. Second-look operations may be done to avoid resection of viable bowel. In cases of malrotation without duodenal obstruction, the operative survival rate is 80%. The operative survival rate is 40% to 50% in cases of malrotation complicated by obstruction caused by periduodenal bands or other intraabdominal anomalies. Resection of large segments of the small intestine results in short-bowel syndrome and its long-term sequelae. Persistence of symptoms after surgical correction suggests pseudoobstructive motility disorders as the underlying problem.

Meconium Ileus

Meconium is a substance that fills the entire intestine before birth. It consists of intestinal gland secretions and some amniotic fluid. Normally, meconium is passed from the rectum during the first 12 to 72 hours after birth.

Meconium ileus is intestinal obstruction caused by meconium formed in utero that is abnormally sticky and adheres firmly to the mucosa of the small intestine, resisting passage beyond the terminal ileum. The cause is usually a lack of digestive enzymes during fetal life. This meconium is also found to contain albumin, which is not normally found in meconium. The detection of albumin in meconium has been used as a screening test for cystic fibrosis.[46] Neonatal meconium ileus occurs in 10% to 15% of newborns with cystic fibrosis.[47] Partial aplasia of the pancreas is an associated factor, however, and one fifth of infants with meconium ileus are premature or have a history of maternal hydramnios (excessive amniotic fluid). After intestinal atresia and malrotation with volvulus, meconium ileus is the most common cause of small intestinal obstruction in newborns.

PATHOPHYSIOLOGY   The terminal ileum is plugged with thick, viscous meconium resulting from the formation of an insoluble, calcium-glycoprotein compound in abnormal mucus. The segment of the ileum proximal to the obstruction is distended with liquid contents, and its walls may be hypertrophied. The segment distal to the obstruction is collapsed and filled with small pellets of pale-colored stool. Meconium in the obstructed segment has the consistency of thick syrup or glue. Peristalsis fails to propel this viscous material through the ileum, so it becomes impacted. Volvulus, atresia, or perforation of the bowel sometimes accompanies meconium ileus.

CLINICAL MANIFESTATIONS   Abdominal distention usually develops during the first few days after birth. The infant does not pass meconium and begins to vomit within hours or days of birth. Infants with cystic fibrosis may have signs of pulmonary involvement, such as tachypnea, intercostal retractions, and grunting respirations. The distended abdomen shows patterns of dilated intestinal loops that feel doughlike when palpated. Some of the loops contain scattered, firm, movable masses. Despite hyperactive peristalsis, the rectal ampulla is empty.

EVALUATION AND TREATMENT Radiologic examination is used to confirm the presence of meconium ileus.[48] The sweat test, which is accurate in 90% of infants, is performed to detect or rule out cystic fibrosis. The treatment of choice for cases not complicated by volvulus or perforation is a hyperosmolar enema done using fluoroscopy to evacuate the meconium. Although the success of this technique has not correlated with osmolality of the enema, the overall success rate is higher when meglumine diatrizoate (Gastrografin) is used than when it is not used. Also, the success rate is better when additives, such as polysorbate 80 (Tween 80) and acetylcysteine (Mucomyst), are used.[49] Enterotomy and irrigation are reserved for complicated cases and enema failures.

Survival of infants with meconium ileus is improving, with a 97% to 98% survival rate at 1 year.[50] The mortality rate increases to 70% if obstruction is complicated by peritonitis. After recovery from neonatal meconium ileus, the long-term outlook depends on the severity and progression of pulmonary disease. Recent research demonstrates a clear association of meconium ileus with poor long-term nutritional outcomes in children with cystic fibrosis related to surgical treatment for the ileus and poor essential fatty-acid status.[51]

Distal Intestinal Obstruction Syndrome

Distal intestinal obstruction syndrome (DIOS), formerly called *meconium ileus equivalent,* affects approximately 15% of children and adults with cystic fibrosis.[52] Intestinal contents may become abnormally thick and impact the intestinal lumen, particularly after episodes of dehydration or lack of pancreatic enzymes. Use of high-strength pancreatic enzymes has been implicated in formation of strictures of the ascending colon in children with cystic fibrosis and resultant chronic DIOS.[53] The child displays signs and symptoms of intestinal obstruction. In most cases the obstruction is relieved by hypertonic enemas. Meconium ileus and DIOS have been shown to be risk factors for the development of liver disease in those with cystic fibrosis.[54-56]

Obstructions of the Duodenum, Jejunum, and Ileum

Congenital obstruction of the duodenum can be caused by intrinsic malformations or external pressure. Intrinsic obstruction is caused by failure of the duodenum to become patent. The obstruction may be partial or complete and usually is located at or near the major duodenal papilla. Extrinsic obstructions can be caused by peritoneal bands that constrict the duodenum. The duodenum can be obstructed by an annular pancreas—a defect in which the head of the pancreas surrounds part of the duodenum. Congenital obstructions of the jejunum and ileum can be attributable to atresia, stenosis, meconium ileus, megacolon (Hirschsprung disease), intussusception, Meckel diverticulum, intestinal duplication, or strangulated hernia.

In ileal atresia or jejunal atresia, the intestine ends blindly proximal and distal to an interruption in its continuity, with or without a gap in the mesentery. Stenosis (narrowing of the lumen) causes dilation proximal to the obstruction and luminal collapse distal to it.

Congenital Aganglionic Megacolon

Congenital aganglionic megacolon (Hirschsprung disease) is a functional obstruction of the colon caused by inadequate motility. The exact cause is unknown but appears to involve multiple interacting factors and a complex inheritance pattern that involves the RET proto-oncogene.[57] There is an increased incidence in males (3.9:1) and increased incidence in the siblings of children with Hirschsprung disease (4%) as compared with the general population incidence of 0.02% (1:5000).[58] There is an increased incidence in children with Down syndrome.[59] The inheritance pattern seems to change with extension of the aganglionic portion of the colon. Aganglionosis beyond the sigmoid colon appears to be more compatible with a dominant gene pattern with incomplete penetrance. With short-segment Hirschsprung disease (involving the rectum up to the sigmoid colon), the inheritance patterns appear multifactorial with the recessive gene pattern of low penetrance.[60] Interaction of endothelin-3 with endothelin-B receptors has been found to be essential for the development of epidermal melanocytes and enteric neurons. Disruption of the endothelin-B receptor gene has been found to cause aganglionic megacolon in mice, and defects in this receptor gene have been mapped to human chromosome 13. It is postulated that this defect may be the cause of hereditary Hirschsprung disease.[61]

PATHOPHYSIOLOGY Congenital aganglionic megacolon is caused by a malformation of the parasympathetic nervous system. It is characterized by abnormalities of the basement membrane and extracellular matrix and absence of the intramural ganglion cells in the enteric nerve plexuses (Meissner and Auerbach plexuses) along variable lengths of the colon.[62] Lacking neural stimulation, the muscle layers of the colon wall fail to propel feces through the colon, leading to obstruction. In 80% of cases the aganglionic segment is limited to the rectal end of the sigmoid colon. In 3% of cases the entire colon lacks ganglion cells. The abnormally innervated colon obstructs fecal movements, causing the proximal colon to become distended; hence the term *megacolon* (Figure 40-3).

The ganglia normally develop from an advancing neural crest between the muscle layers (tunica muscularis) in the submucosal area (muscularis mucosae) of the intestinal wall. In cases of congenital megacolon, neurologic development is blocked and large, nonmyelinated fibers develop in place of these ganglion cells.[62] The segment of colon that lacks ganglion cells has a relatively normal lumen caliber and wall thickness. In the segment of the colon proximal to it, the lumen is dilated and the muscle hypertrophied. Therefore the abnormal portion of the colon appears to be normal and the normal portion appears to be diseased.

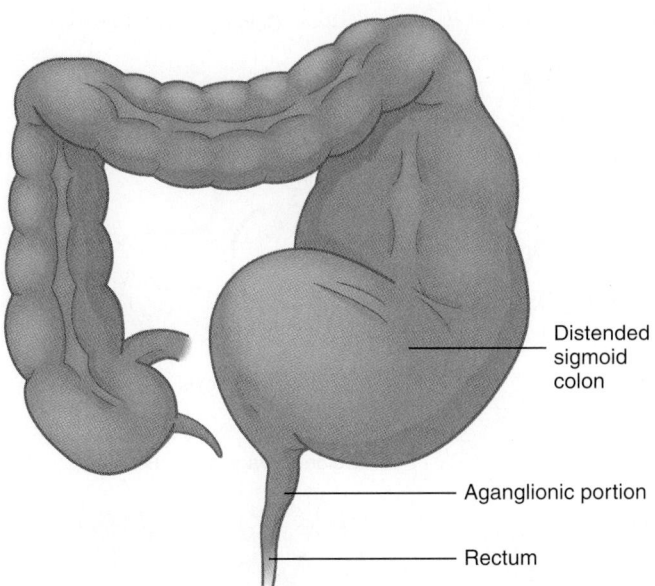

Distended sigmoid colon

Aganglionic portion

Rectum

Figure 40-3 Congenital aganglionic megacolon (Hirschsprung disease).

CLINICAL MANIFESTATIONS   The extent of the aganglionic portion of the colon determines the severity of the symptoms of congenital aganglionic megacolon. The most distal part of the rectum is always involved. This is the extent of the aganglionic portion in some children, and the child is said to have "ultrashort-segment" Hirschsprung disease and generally has only mild constipation as a symptom. These individuals may not be diagnosed until adulthood.[63] Symptoms of constipation increase in severity as the aganglionic portion extends proximally. Diarrhea may be the first sign, however, because only water can travel around the impacted feces.

The most serious complication in the neonatal period is enterocolitis related to fecal impaction. Bowel dilation stretches and partly occludes the encircling blood and lymphatic vessels, causing edema, ischemia, infarction of the mucosa, and significant outflow of fluid into the bowel lumen. Copious, liquid stools result. Infarction and destruction of the mucosa enable enteric microorganisms to penetrate the bowel wall. Frequently, gram-negative sepsis occurs, accompanied by fever and vomiting. Severe and rapid electrolyte changes may take place, causing collapse and rapid death.

EVALUATION AND TREATMENT   Anorectal manometry is a reliable screening tool for the diagnosis of Hirschsprung disease.[64] Serial manometry measurements may be required in neonates.[65] This test has uncovered ultrashort-segment Hirschsprung disease in older children with a history of constipation.[66] The definitive diagnosis is made by rectal biopsy showing an absence of ganglion cells in the submucosa of the colon. X-ray films show dilated loops of colon, and contrast films show aganglionic areas. The infant usually cannot expel the barium.

The involved segment is resected within the first few months of life. For children with short-segment Hirschsprung

disease, enemas are given to relieve impaction and laxatives with a dietary and bowel training program are used in preference to surgical intervention.[66] The child is not treated for diarrhea.

After surgery, enterocolitis sometimes recurs. If the postoperative enterocolitis is allowed to persist, pseudopolyps may appear. Because these are essentially identical to the lesions of ulcerative colitis, they have malignant potential. Therefore a colectomy is indicated if pseudopolyps develop.

In general, the prognosis of congenital megacolon is satisfactory for children who undergo surgical treatment. Bowel training may be prolonged, but most children achieve bowel continence before puberty.[67]

Anorectal Malformations

Several congenital malformations of anorectal structures can obstruct the passage of feces. The incidence of minor abnormalities is approximately 1 in 500, and that of major anomalies is approximately 1 in 5000.

Congenital anorectal malformations range from mild anal stenosis, which is corrected by simple dilation, to complex deformities, such as anal or rectal agenesis, atresia, and fistula (Figure 40-4). Deformities that cause complete obstruction are known collectively as **imperforate anus.**

Approximately 40% of infants with anorectal malformations have other developmental anomalies as well. The most commonly associated major anomalies are Down syndrome, congenital heart disease, renal abnormalities, cryptorchidism, esophageal atresia, and malformations of the spine.[34,68]

Imperforate anus may not be obvious. It can be detected by gentle insertion of a rectal tube. X-ray films show dilations throughout the intestinal tract. Anal stenosis can be treated by dilations, but all other anorectal malformations require surgical correction. The overall mortality rate is approximately 10%. More than 90% of children with a low (anal) anomaly achieve bowel continence; however, fewer than 30% of those with very high anomalies or anomalies associated with genitourinary fistulae achieve continence.[69]

Acquired Impairment of Motility
Intussusception

The most common cause of acquired intestinal obstruction in infants is intussusception. **Intussusception** is the telescoping or invagination of one portion of the intestine into another. Usually, the ileum invaginates the cecum and part of the ascending colon by collapsing through the ileocecal valve. Intussusception involving the ileum and colon (ileocolic intussusception) accounts for 80% to 90% of intestinal obstructions in infants and is two to three times more common in males than in females.[70] Nearly 75% of intussusceptions occur before age 2 years; 70% occur before age 1 year. Intussusception is rare in infants younger than 3 months and is infrequent after 36 months. Intussusception has occurred in children of all ages recovering from abdominal surgery; intussusception has been found in children with cystic fibrosis and symptoms of bowel obstruction that were initially misdi-

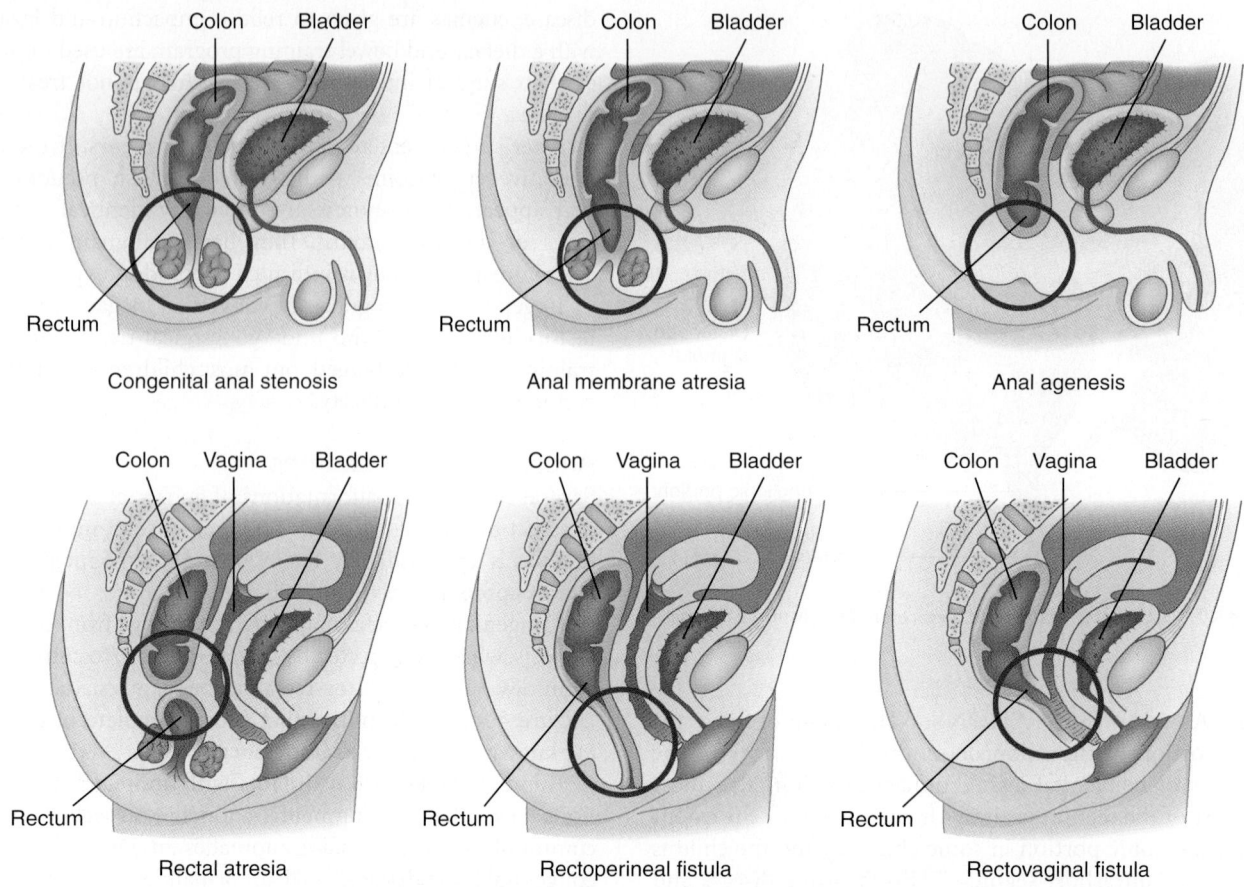

Figure 40-4 Anorectal stenosis and imperforate anus.

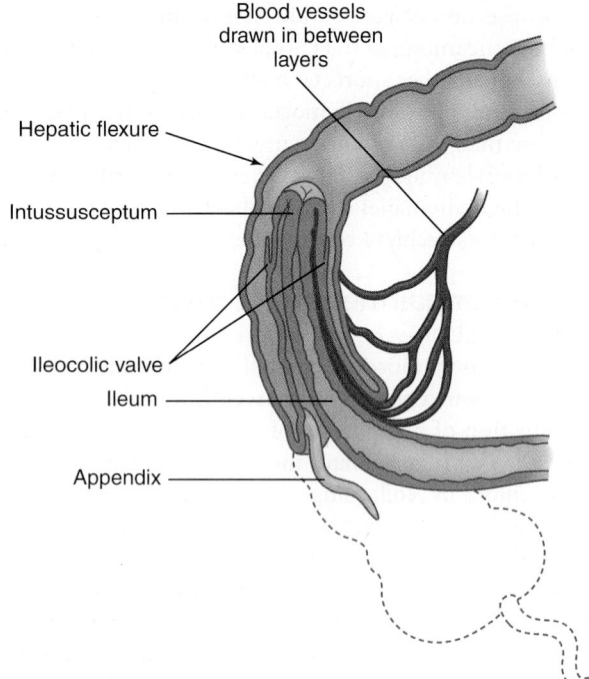

Figure 40-5 Ileocolic intussusception.

agnosed as having distal intestinal obstruction syndrome (meconium ileus equivalent).[71,72]

PATHOPHYSIOLOGY   Most commonly, the proximal portion of the intestine, the intussusceptum, collapses into the distal portion, the intussuscipiens, in the direction of peristaltic flow (Figure 40-5). As it does so, the intussusceptum drags its mesentery into the enveloping lumen. Initially, the mesentery is constricted, obstructing venous return. Compression of the mesenteric vessels between the two layers of intestinal wall and at the U-shaped angle at either end of the intussusceptum leads within hours to venous stasis, engorgement, edema, exudation, and further vascular compression. Unless the intussusception is treated, bleeding and gangrene ensue. The tension of the mesentery on the intussusceptum tends to arch the bowel in a curve with its center at the mesenteric root. Edema and compression obstruct the flow of chyme through the intestine.

CLINICAL MANIFESTATIONS   The affected infant suddenly develops abdominal pain, becomes irritable (colicky), and draws up the knees. Vomiting occurs soon afterward. A single normal stool may be passed, evacuating the colon distal to the apex of the intussusception. After that, 60% of infants pass "currant jelly" stools, which appear dark and gelatinous because of their blood and mucus content. In one study, less than one third of children had this clinical triad of vomiting, colicky abdominal pain, and bloody stools.[73] Most infants have a tender, sausage-shaped abdominal mass. Abdominal tenderness and distention develop as intestinal obstruction becomes more acute.[74]

EVALUATION AND TREATMENT   Diagnosis is based on clinical manifestations and onset of symptoms. Ultrasound of the abdomen, computed tomography (CT) and magnetic resonance imaging (MRI) are commonly completed for diagnosis.[75] More than 82% of children have positive ultrasound results in both ileocolic and jejunointestinal intussusception. Reduction is an emergency procedure involving hydrostatic pressure generated by an air or a barium enema given using fluoroscopic guidance.[76,77] This technique is successful 45% to 70% of the time. A potential complication of enema reduction is bowel perforation, and for this reason the use of air rather than barium is favored.[78] Surgical reduction is done on children who fail or are not candidates for hydrostatic reduction. Untreated intussusception in infants is nearly always fatal. Most infants recover if the intussusception is reduced within 24 hours.[79] Spontaneous reduction of intussusception may occur in symptomatic or asymptomatic children and occurs more commonly than previously reported. These intussusceptions are usually short-segment, small-bowel intussusceptions with no recognizable lead point.[80] Recurrent intussusception is more common after nonsurgical reduction than after surgical reduction. Risk of recurrence cannot be predicted by initial features or symptoms, and children with recurrent intussusception may exhibit fewer symptoms with a shorter interval to bowel necrosis and perforation.[81]

Gastroesophageal Reflux

Gastroesophageal reflux (GER) involves dilation of the esophagus and intrusion of acid contents into it; GER is believed to be related to relaxation or incompetence of the lower esophageal sphincter (see Chapter 39). In newborns, reflux is normal because neuromuscular control of the gastroesophageal sphincter is not fully developed. The frequency of reflux is highest in premature infants and decreases during the first 6 to 12 months of life.

There is an increased incidence of symptomatic reflux in children with neurologic impairment and cerebral palsy.[82,83] It is thought to be a factor in the stimulation of apnea and reactive airway disease in some children.[84-86] Reflux is thought to be a contributing cause in infant deaths and sudden infant death syndrome.[87] Increasingly, GER has been recognized as a significant problem for children with cystic fibrosis.[88]

PATHOPHYSIOLOGY   Delayed maturation of the lower esophageal sphincter or impaired hormonal or neurotransmitter response mechanisms (i.e., vasoactive intestinal peptide and nitric oxide) are possible causes of inappropriate sphincter relaxation. Factors that maintain lower esophageal sphincter integrity in children include location of the gastroesophageal junction in a high-pressure zone within the abdomen, mucosal gathering within the sphincter, and the angle at which the esophagus is inserted into the stomach. Reflux persists if any of these pressure-maintaining factors is altered. Irritation of the mucosa by acidic gastric contents results in deterioration of the esophageal epithelium and stimulation of the vomiting reflex.[89,90]

CLINICAL MANIFESTATIONS   The signs and symptoms of GER are caused by exposure of the esophageal epithelium to refluxed gastric contents. Eighty-five percent of affected infants vomit excessively during the first week of life and usually have other symptoms by 6 weeks.

Vomiting may be forceful and must be differentiated from pyloric stenosis. Aspiration pneumonia develops in one third of infants with GER. In cases that persist into childhood, chronic cough, wheezing, and recurrent pneumonia are common.[91,92] Repeated vomiting leads to inadequate retention of nutrients, adversely affecting growth and weight gain. Esophagitis from exposure of the esophageal mucosa to acidic gastric contents is manifested by pain, bleeding, and eventually stricture formation and abnormal motility. Approximately 25% of children with GER also have iron deficiency anemia caused by frank or occult blood loss.

EVALUATION AND TREATMENT   The clinical manifestations are often adequate to confirm a diagnosis of GER. A barium swallow, endoscopy, and esophageal pH monitoring with a probe are useful diagnostic procedures in complex cases.[76,93-95]

Mild GER resolves without treatment. Maintaining infants in a flat prone or a left lateral position, particularly during and for the first hour after a feeding, results in fewer or shorter episodes of GER.[96] Infants with GER are excepted from the Academy of Pediatrics' recommended sleep position for healthy infants to decrease the risk of SIDS.[97] Older infants and children achieve better results in an upright (sitting or standing) position while awake, with prone positioning used for sleeping.[96] Thickened feedings may help some infants;[98] however, this has not been shown to be consistently helpful. For some infants, thickened feedings may actually worsen reflux by causing a delay in gastric emptying time. Small, frequent feedings and frequent burping are generally universally accepted strategies for managing reflux.[35] Medications to increase motility, increase lower esophageal sphincter pressure, or decrease gastric acid production have been used to treat GER. If no improvement is seen with medical management or the child has life-threatening events with reflux, an antireflux surgical procedure, including gastropexy and fundoplication, is performed. A fundoplication recreates a valve by wrapping the fundus of the stomach around the lower esophagus.[99,100]

Impairment of Digestion, Absorption, and Nutrition
Cystic Fibrosis

Cystic fibrosis (CF) of the pancreas, which is also called *mucoviscidosis* or *fibrocystic disease* of the pancreas, is a genetically transmitted disease (mutation of the long arm of chromosome 7) that involves many organs and systems and usually causes death in childhood or young adulthood. It is the most common cause of chronic suppurative lung disease in children and is the most common life-threatening inherited disease in the white population. This section focuses on the deficiency of pancreatic enzymes. (Chapter 34 discusses the pulmonary consequences of cystic fibrosis.)

PATHOPHYSIOLOGY   The pathophysiologic triad that is the hallmark of CF includes (1) pancreatic enzyme deficiency, which causes maldigestion; (2) overproduction of mucus in the respiratory tract and inability to clear secretions, which cause progressive chronic obstructive pulmonary disease; and (3) abnormally elevated sodium and chloride concentrations in sweat. Exocrine secretions tend to be abnormally thick and to precipitate in the glandular ducts, obstructing flow. Almost all clinical manifestations of CF are a result of overproduction of extremely viscous mucus and pancreatic enzyme deficiency. The full spectrum of involvement is evident from Table 40-1.

Pancreatic function may range from normal to completely ablated. Approximately 85% of patients have pancreatic insufficiency. Obstruction of the pancreatic ducts with thick mucus blocks the flow of pancreatic enzymes and causes degenerative and fibrotic changes in the pancreas. Pancreatic damage eventually can affect the beta cells, resulting in diabetes mellitus in some children. The incidence of diabetes mellitus and cirrhosis in this population has increased as larger numbers of people with cystic fibrosis have moved into young and middle adulthood. Severe problems with maldigestion of proteins, carbohydrates, and fats occur because of insufficient secretion of pancreatic enzymes.[101]

CLINICAL MANIFESTATIONS   Clinical manifestations are presented in Table 40-1.

Table 40-1	Pathophysiology, Clinical Manifestations, and Complications of Cystic Fibrosis		
Organ Involved	**Secretory Dysfunction**	**Clinical Manifestations**	**Complications**
Sweat glands	Elevated concentration of sodium and chloride in sweat	Hyponatremia; hypochloremia	Heat prostration; shock
Intestine			
Newborn	Viscid meconium	Meconium ileus with intestinal obstruction	Meconium peritonitis
Older child and adult	Inspissated (dried out) mucofecal masses (intestinal sludging)	Partial intestinal obstruction with severe cramping pains	Volvulus (obstruction), intussusception (prolapse)
Pancreas (enzyme deficiency)	Inspissation and precipitation of pancreatic secretions, causing obstruction of pancreatic ducts	Absence of pancreatic enzymes, causing malabsorption of food and fatty, bulky stools	Hypoproteinemia; iron deficiency anemia; malnutrition
		Decreased vitamins A, D, E, and K absorption	Vitamins A, D, E, and K deficiency and rectal prolapse
	Insulin deficiency	Glucose intolerance	Diabetes mellitus
Liver	Inspissation and precipitation of bile in biliary system	Focal biliary cirrhosis; shrunken, "hob-nail" liver	Portal hypertension with esophageal varices and hematemesis
Salivary glands	Inspissation and precipitation of secretions in small ducts of submaxillary and sublingual salivary glands	Mild patchy fibrosis of salivary glands	None
Paranasal structures	Viscid mucus	Retention of mucus; clouding seen on sinus roentgenograms	Mucopyoceles (pus accumulations) with nasal deformity or orbital cavity extension
Nose	Nasal polyps	Obstruction of nasal air flow	None
Lungs	Viscid mucus in bronchioles and bronchi	Obstruction of bronchioles causing bronchiolectasis, bronchiectasis, and chronic lung infection	Hemoptysis; pneumothroaxl cor pulmonale; respiratory failure
Reproductive tract			
Male	Viscid genital tract secretions during embryologic development, causing failure of formation of normal vas deferens	Sterility	None
Female	Distention of endocervical epithelial cells with cytoplasmic mucin	Decreased fertility	Polypoid cervicitis (cervical inflammation) while taking oral contraceptives

Data from Rudolph CD et al: *Rudolph's pediatrics,* ed 21, New York, 2003, McGraw-Hill.

EVALUATION AND TREATMENT   Seventy-two–hour stool fat measurements are used to determine the extent of pancreatic function. Stools also may be examined for absence of pancreatic enzymes, particularly trypsin and chymotrypsin. To optimize treatment, the ^{13}C (carbon-13) mixed triglyceride breath test offers a simple, noninvasive way of assessing the need for pancreatic enzyme supplementation in children with cystic fibrosis.[102] Pancreatic replacement enzymes are administered before or with meals. However, even with enzyme replacement, the improvement in digestion is not complete or consistent.[103] High-calorie, high-protein diets with frequent snacks and vitamin supplements are used to treat the malnutrition; however, anorexia is not uncommon in this group secondary to pulmonary disease and frequently large sputum output. To combat the worsening problem of growth failure in children with cystic fibrosis, an increasing number of persons are using nasogastric or gastrostomy tube feedings to supplement oral intake.[85,104]

Gluten-Sensitive Enteropathy

Gluten-sensitive enteropathy, formerly called *celiac sprue* or *celiac disease,* is the loss of mature villous epithelium caused by ingestion of gluten, the protein component of cereal grains. The gluten in wheat, rye, barley, and oats is toxic to the intestinal epithelial cells of genetically susceptible individuals.[105] The disease occurs largely in whites and has been documented in Asians from India and Pakistan, but it is almost nonexistent in native Africans, Japanese, and Chinese. Prevalence rates in Europe range from 1 in 1000 to 1 in 3000. Recent data suggest that gluten-sensitive enteropathy, traditionally considered rare in the United States, may be as common as in Europe.[106,107] Other autoimmune diseases have been associated with gluten-sensitive enteropathy including diabetes mellitus and thyroid diseases.[108]

The pathogenesis appears to require interaction between a number of intrinsic factors (genetic susceptibility, activation of the immune system) and extrinsic factors (gluten and possibly other environmental factors). Both cellular immunity and humoral immunity are implicated. There are increases in the percentages of T cells, immunoglobulin, and complement in the mucosa of active celiac disease. Immunoglobulin A (IgA) and immunoglobulin M (IgM) antigliadin antibodies have been found in jejunal fluid of persons with untreated disease.[109] Although gluten-sensitive enteropathy is widely perceived as a malabsorption syndrome of childhood, the diagnosis is increasingly being made for the first time in adult life.[110]

PATHOPHYSIOLOGY   The mucosa of the upper small intestine appears shiny, cobble-stoned, and thin in children with gluten-sensitive enteropathy. The major pathophysiologic characteristics of the disease are atrophy of villi in the upper small intestine and malabsorption of most nutrients in the presence of cereal gluten (Figure 40-6). The atrophy is caused by accelerated shedding of epithelial cells from the villi. To compensate for this loss, epithelial cell production increases, causing hypertrophy of the crypts of Lieberkühn.[111] Increased cell production is not sufficient to keep pace with cell loss, however. Inflammation and edema develop around the enlarged cysts. The villi shorten and atrophy, and their

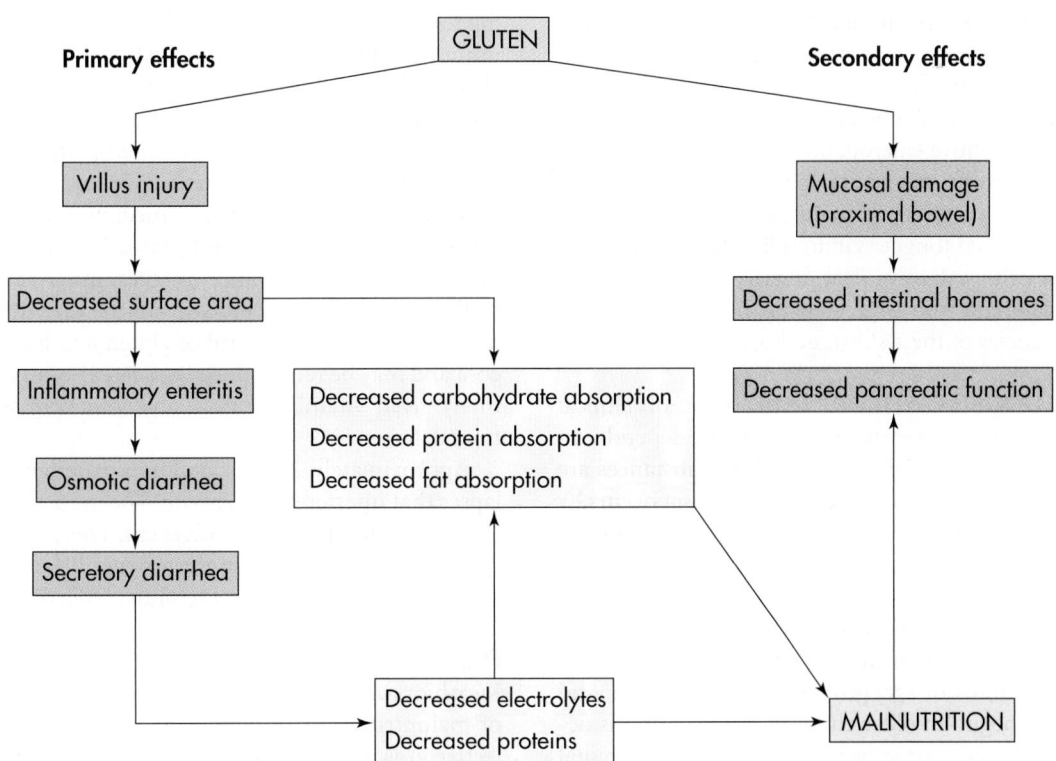

Figure 40-6 Pathophysiology of gluten-sensitive enteropathy.

surface cells are not mature enough to sustain absorptive functions. The microvilli and brush border disappear, leaving patches of bald mucosa. The loss of mucosal surface area and brush-border enzymes leads to severe malabsorption. The pathologic process is most pronounced in the duodenum and jejunum. The ileum may be spared. The severity of disease correlates with the length of the small intestinal mucosa involved.

Damage to the mucosa of the duodenum and jejunum has secondary effects that exacerbate malabsorption. The secretion of intestinal hormones, such as secretin and cholecystokinin-pancreozymin, may be diminished. Because these chemical messengers are scarce, secretion of pancreatic enzymes and expulsion of bile from the gallbladder decrease.

Destruction of mucosal cells causes inflammation, and water and electrolytes are secreted, leading to watery diarrhea. In addition, absorption that normally occurs by sodium-dependent active transport or facilitated diffusion is impaired. Carbohydrates, amino acids, dipeptides, water-soluble vitamins, bile salts, and cations are not absorbed from the intestinal lumen. Potassium loss, which is more severe than sodium loss, leads to muscle weakness. Magnesium and calcium malabsorption can cause seizures or tetany. Unabsorbed fatty acids combine with calcium, and secondary hyperparathyroidism increases phosphorus excretion, resulting in bone reabsorption. Calcium is no longer available to bind oxalate in the intestine and is absorbed, which causes hyperoxaluria. Gallbladder function may be abnormal, and bile salt conjugation may be decreased.

Fat malabsorption in the jejunum is the major cause of steatorrhea (fatty stools). Malabsorption may be mild early in the disease. Fecal nitrogen is elevated because peptidase deficiencies impair protein absorption. Pancreatic function is decreased, not only because of decreased hormonal levels but also because of malnutrition.

Deficiencies of fat-soluble vitamins are common in children with gluten-sensitive enteropathy. Vitamin K malabsorption leads to hypoprothrombinemia. In one third of cases, iron and folic acid malabsorption are manifested as cheilosis; anemia; and a smooth, red tongue. Vitamin B_{12} absorption is impaired in those with extensive ileal disease. Because the absorption of folate and iron is greatest in the proximal small intestine, deficiencies of these substances are common.

CLINICAL MANIFESTATIONS   The onset of clinical manifestations of gluten-sensitive enteropathy depends on the age of the infant when gluten-containing substances are added to the diet. In 50% of affected children, onset occurs by 18 months of age, with latent intervals varying from months to years. Severity of symptoms can vary tremendously.

Diarrhea is an early sign in most infants. The stools are pale, bulky, greasy, and foul smelling, and they may contain oil droplets. Three to five such movements occur daily. As early as 3 or 4 months of age, growth failure, anorexia, and constipation can begin. In older children, constipation is occasionally seen despite steatorrhea. Vomiting and abdominal pain are prominent in infants but unusual in older children. Anorexia is prevalent. The classic physical manifestations of organic failure to thrive, such as abdominal protuberance, wasted buttocks and limbs, and hypotonia, occur in fewer than 50% of infants with gluten-sensitive enteropathy. Growth is usually diminished.[112]

Manifestations of malabsorption, such as rickets, tetany, frank or occult bleeding, or anemia, may be obvious. Some children urinate more at night. The tongue is smooth and red, and the child may bruise and bleed easily. Hypomagnesemia and hypocalcemia cause irritability, tremor, convulsions, tetany, bone pain, osteomalacia, and dental abnormalities. If vitamin D deficiency is prolonged, rickets and clubbing of the terminal phalanges are likely. Eighty-six percent of older children have fingerprint changes (ridge atrophy). In older children, delayed puberty and infertility may be a manifestation of otherwise subtle gluten-sensitive enteropathy.[113] Osteomalacia may be severe.[114] Small intestinal lymphoma is also associated with gluten-sensitive enteropathy.[115]

An unusual complication of gluten-sensitive enteropathy in infancy is celiac crisis. Celiac crisis is characterized by severe diarrhea, dehydration, and hypoproteinemia as a result of malabsorption and protein loss.

EVALUATION AND TREATMENT   An intestinal biopsy is mandatory to detect the classic mucosal changes caused by gluten-sensitive enteropathy. The initial biopsy generally is followed by a second intestinal biopsy to demonstrate regeneration of intestinal villi after treatment with a gluten-free diet. Occasionally, the child will be rechallenged with gluten at a later point and a biopsy performed a third time to demonstrate return of intestinal mucosal damage. A wide variety of screening tests for malabsorption also may be useful. Serum IgA and immunoglobulin G (IgG) antigliadin (from gluten) antibodies also are measured. Urinary assay to determine the ratio of lactose to mannitol has been successfully used to differentiate children with active gluten-sensitive enteropathy from healthy children or children with inactive disease.[116]

Treatment consists of the immediate and permanent institution of a diet free of cereal grains (wheat, rye, barley, oats, malt). Lactose intolerance is presumed; therefore lactose (milk sugar) also is excluded from the diet. Tolerance to lactose improves with removal of gluten and healing of the mucosa and may be reintroduced at a later point. Infants are routinely given vitamin D, iron, and folic acid supplements to treat deficiencies.

Approximately 25% of children experience recurrent relapses that interfere with growth. For most children, however, the long-term prognosis is excellent. There is an increased incidence of malignant disease, particularly lymphoma, in individuals who fail to respond to gluten-free diets.

Protein Energy Malnutrition

Kwashiorkor and marasmus are the two most common types of malnutrition in children. These disorders are known collectively as **protein energy malnutrition (PEM).** Both are states of long-term starvation (see Chapter 39). **Kwashiorkor** is a severe protein deficiency, and **marasmus** is a severe deficiency of all nutrients. Kwashiorkor is a widespread nutritional problem among children in developing countries and economically destitute populations. The disease usually occurs in infants or children from 1 to 4 years of age who have been weaned from breast milk to a high-starch, protein-deficient diet.

Marasmus can occur at any age, but it is common in children younger than 1 year. In marasmus, starvation is attributable to lack of protein and carbohydrates. One third of the world's children suffer from PEM, with the highest concentrations in Latin America, Asia, and Africa.[117] The mortality risk for children in developing countries has been found to be inversely related to anthropometric indicators (height, weight, head circumference, skinfold thickness, midarm muscle circumference). There is elevated risk even in the mild to moderate range of malnutrition.[118] Poor sanitation and early weaning of breast-fed infants to overdiluted commercial formulas are major risk factors for PEM.

PEM is a complication of some diseases, such as chronic fever, tuberculosis, malignancy, digestive and malabsorptive disorders, and psychogenic illness. Radiation therapy and chemotherapy also can contribute to PEM. Acute and chronic malnutrition is common in hospitalized individuals in the United States. One study found that 25% of hospitalized children had PEM (5.1% severe, 7.7% moderate, and 14.5% mild). Although these results were significantly less than those obtained at the same institution in 1976, they are still alarming.[119]

PATHOPHYSIOLOGY   In kwashiorkor, the deficit of dietary amino acids reduces protein synthesis in all tissues. Physical growth and mental growth are stunted, and maintenance of minimal life processes is in jeopardy. The lack of sufficient plasma proteins, particularly albumin, causes systemic pressure changes that result in generalized edema. The volume of total body water and extracellular fluid increases, causing a substantial loss of potassium. The liver swells with stored fat because no hepatic proteins are synthesized to form and release lipoproteins. Pancreatic atrophy and fibrosis may be present. Kwashiorkor also causes malabsorption, reduced bone density, and impaired renal function. If the condition is not reversed, the prognosis is very poor.

Because the intake of all dietary nutrients is reduced to a minimum in marasmus, metabolic processes, including liver function, are preserved but growth is severely retarded. Caloric intake is too low to support protein synthesis for growth or the storage of fat. If more protein is needed than is ingested, muscle wasting occurs. Fat wasting and anemia are common and can be severe. The volume of total body water is high. Serum triglyceride and phospholipid levels increase with increasing severity of malnutrition, but other serum values, such as cholesterol, are normal or slightly reduced. High fasting phospholipid and triglyceride concentrations are predictive of a poor prognosis for these children.[120] Severe vitamin A deficiency commonly results in blindness.[121]

CLINICAL MANIFESTATIONS   Retarded physical, mental, and psychologic development; muscle wasting; diarrhea; dermatosis; low hemoglobin and infection characterize marasmus. The presence of subcutaneous fat, hepatomegaly, and fatty liver distinguishes kwashiorkor from marasmus. These manifestations are missing in marasmus because caloric intake is not sufficient to support fat synthesis and storage.[122]

EVALUATION AND TREATMENT   Evaluation of PEM is based on nutritional history and clinical manifestations. The provision of deficient nutrients will resolve clinical symptoms in 4 to 6 weeks. Physical and mental retardation may not be reversible, however. Nutritional rehabilitation with appropriate environmental stimulation for infants and young children has been shown to resolve or improve cerebral shrinkage, physical growth, and psychomotor development.[123,124]

Failure to Thrive

Failure to thrive (FTT) is the inadequate physical development of an infant or a child. It is manifested as a deceleration in weight gain, a low weight/height ratio, or a low weight/height/head circumference ratio. In the United States, FTT usually affects infants and young children. FTT is a nutritional disorder having organic or nonorganic causes. Nonorganic FTT is most common among psychosocially and economically deprived populations, whereas organic FTT occurs equally in all populations. The incidence of nonorganic FTT is greater than that of organic FTT.[125]

PATHOPHYSIOLOGY   **Organic FTT** has a pathophysiologic cause, such as gastroesophageal reflux, pyloric stenosis, gastroenteritis, infection by intestinal parasites, or congenital anomalies or chronic diseases of major body systems. All these factors reduce the availability of nutrients for maintenance and growth. Psychosocial problems can develop as a result of organic FTT.[126] A chronic disease or congenital anomaly that causes weakness or reduced stature can create developmental, psychosocial, and emotional problems for the child.

Nonorganic FTT occurs in the absence of any gastrointestinal, endocrine, or other chronic diseases. It is usually associated with psychosocial deprivation, although behavior problems also may contribute to its occurrence in the absence of maternal pathologic findings. Behavioral and psychosocial problems may be compounded by inadequate economic resources and lack of knowledge. Generally, the problem in nonorganic FTT is ineffective nurturing by primary caregivers. Infants and children are at risk for nonorganic FTT if their parents or primary caregivers are unable to provide nurturance. A variety of parental stressors may be involved and include the following:

Lack of nurturance in the parents' own childhood
Unwanted pregnancy
Inability to bond with the infant because of health or other problems
Postpartum depression

Family crisis, such as a death or marital problems
Stress caused by single parenthood or social isolation
Mental, emotional, or physical illness

The first few postnatal months appear to be a sensitive period in the relationship between growth and mental development, suggesting a critical need for early diagnosis and aggressive interventions.[127,128]

CLINICAL MANIFESTATIONS Clinical manifestations of organic FTT are retarded growth accompanied by manifestations of the underlying disease. Manifestations of nonorganic FTT are retarded growth plus reduced energy level, reduced responsiveness and interaction with the environment, social isolation, spasticity or rigidity when held or touched, inability to make eye contact or smile, refusal to eat, and rejection of foods. Weight loss and decelerated growth are accompanied by developmental retardation in many areas. Nonorganic FTT is a complex syndrome involving psychosocial, emotional, and parent-child problems that compound the pathophysiologic abnormalities.[129,130] Children with primarily organic FTT have been found to have lower developmental skills, and their parents have been found to have higher emotional distress. Infant stress, vomiting, and feeding disorders have been noted in children with both organic and inorganic FTT.[131]

EVALUATION AND TREATMENT Failure to thrive is suggested if a child falls below the third percentile on the growth curve or is falling off a previously established growth curve. Organic FTT is manifested in infancy by weight, height, and head circumference growth that may be parallel to but below the normal ranges. If no genetic, endocrine, or other systemic disorder is identified and if the physical and laboratory examinations show no abnormalities other than delayed growth, an environmental cause is indicated.

Hospital admission is recommended if the diagnosis is unclear or the child is in nutritional or emotional jeopardy. Eating patterns, food preferences, caloric intake, and family interactions can be assessed during the hospital stay. If the cause is environmental, the hospitalized child with FTT usually begins to gain weight.

If an organic problem has been identified, management of FTT consists of treating the cause. Management of nonorganic FTT involves the immediate total care of the child and measures to address (1) the psychosocial and emotional problems of the caregivers and (2) parent-child interactions. Counseling, parental modeling, and long-term family support are sometimes required.[132,133] Clinical manifestations of organic FTT have inorganic components in the majority of children, and the most successful interventions not only treat the underlying organic cause but also address the psychosocial symptoms.

Necrotizing Enterocolitis

Necrotizing enterocolitis (NEC) is the most common gastrointestinal emergency in the newborn. If left untreated, NEC can result in bowel necrosis, perforation, and death. The overall mortality rate is between 20% and 40%.[134] The exact etiology is unclear. The incidence of NEC is increasing, causing 1500 to 2000 infant deaths every year in the United States.[135] Premature babies are the most likely victims, but it also occurs in full-term infants.[136-138] Affected infants have a mean gestational age of 31 weeks and weigh about 1500 g.[139] The risk of NEC decreases as the gastrointestinal tract matures.

PATHOPHYSIOLOGY Factors contributing to the development of NEC include infections, immature immunity, maternal age greater than 35 years, perinatal stress, and the effects of medications and feeding practices. Reduced mucosal blood flow leading to hypoxic injury to intestinal mucosa is thought to be a cause. This injury allows bacterial invasion of the bowel wall and release of inflammatory mediators. Accumulation of gas in the mucosa and submucosa leads to ischemia inflammation and necrosis of intestinal segments. The terminal ileum and proximal colon are most often involved.[140] Premature infants have decreased secretory IgA and decreased intestinal T cells. The intestinal mucosal barrier is scanty and motility is slower, increasing the risk for infection.

CLINICAL MANIFESTATIONS Manifestations of NEC usually appear within 2 weeks of birth, with earlier symptoms in full-term infants (5.3 days compared with 15.3 days in premature infants).[141] They range from mild abdominal distention to bowel perforation, sepsis, and death. Abdominal pain, unstable temperature, bradycardia, and apnea are nonspecific signs. Affected infants have abdominal distention, occult or grossly bloody stools, retained gastric contents, and septicemia with elevated white blood cell and falling platelet counts. The more premature the infant, the greater the incidence of NEC and related diseases of prematurity, such as respiratory distress syndrome and immune compromise.

EVALUATION AND TREATMENT Diagnosis is based on clinical manifestations, laboratory results, and plain films of the abdomen that show gas accumulation in the intestine. Treatments include cessation of feeding, gastric suction to decompress the intestines, fluid and electrolyte maintenance, and administration of antibiotics to control sepsis. Surgical resection is the treatment of choice for intestinal perforation; however, for very ill infants weighing less than 1000 g, peritoneal drainage without laparotomy may improve survival.[134,142] Following treatment of NEC, infants treated by both medical and surgical management are at risk for intestinal obstruction related to the development of strictures.[143] Infants who have extensive resection of necrotic bowel may develop short-bowel syndrome, requiring chronic total parenteral nutrition. Intestinal transplantation is available as a lifesaving option for these children.[144] Low-birth-weight infants are at greatest risk of death from NEC. Prophylaxis with antibiotics, feeding with human milk, and stopping the inflammatory response are helpful treatments.[145,146]

Diarrhea

Diarrhea is a common gastrointestinal problem during infancy and early childhood. Severe diarrhea occurs one to three times during the first 3 years of life. Most episodes are self-limiting and resolve within 72 hours.

The pathophysiologic mechanisms of diarrhea in children are similar to those for adults described in Chapter 39. Prolonged diarrhea is more dangerous in children, however, because they have much smaller fluid reserves than adults. Therefore dehydration can develop rapidly if any disturbance increases fluid secretion into the gastrointestinal lumen (secretory diarrhea), draws fluid into the lumen by osmosis (osmotic diarrhea), or prevents fluid absorption in the intestine.

Infant diarrhea is of special concern because its cause may be a congenital or metabolic anomaly. Infants have low fluid reserves and relatively rapid peristalsis and metabolism. Therefore the danger of dehydration is great.

Common causes of acute diarrhea in infants include congenital aganglionic megacolon, infections, milk-protein allergies, and NEC. Less common causes are adrenogenital syndrome, impaired chloride-bicarbonate exchange, congenital lactase deficiency, glucose-galactose malabsorption, and sucrase-isomaltase deficiency.

Infectious diarrhea in newborns is usually associated with nursery epidemics involving such pathogens as *Escherichia coli*, *Klebsiella*, staphylococci, *Salmonella*, and *Shigella*. Diarrhea caused by these agents has a rapid onset, and acidosis and shock can occur quickly. *Clostridium difficile*, often associated with previous antibiotic therapy, can cause acute, profuse, watery diarrhea and symptoms of colitis.[147] True milk-protein allergy, which is uncommon, causes bloody, explosive stools after the introduction of milk into the diet.

Acute Diarrhea in Children

Acute diarrhea in children is almost synonymous with acute viral or bacterial gastroenteritis. Viral gastroenteritis tends to be self-limiting. Bacterial gastroenteritis is treated with antibiotics if the causal pathogen can be identified. Other causes of acute diarrhea in the older child include antibiotic therapy, appendicitis, chemotherapy, inflammatory bowel disease, parasitic infestation, parenteral infections, and ingestion of toxic substances.

Rotavirus, the leading cause of severe diarrhea in infants and young children, invades the cells of the intestinal mucosa and, by its presence (even without replicating), damages these cells. Damage decreases viable absorptive surface, causing an imbalance of secretion and absorption that results in diarrhea. This is consistent with a viral toxin–like effect that can take several weeks for recovery of mucosal damage.

Chronic Diarrhea in Children

Children with acute gastroenteritis often remain mildly symptomatic for up to 4 weeks; therefore diarrhea that persists longer than 4 weeks is considered to be chronic. Children with **chronic diarrhea** can be divided into two groups: (1) otherwise well children whose growth is normal and (2) ill children whose growth is retarded. Causes of chronic diarrhea in the first group include abnormal colonic motility, lactose intolerance, encopresis, parasitic infestation, and antibiotic use.[148,149] Chronic diarrhea in the second group is usually caused by a disease that impairs absorption.

Chronic Nonspecific Diarrhea

Chronic nonspecific diarrhea is a condition in which uncoordinated colonic motility causes forceful expulsion of feces. It affects children between 1 and 5 years of age. Apparently, the lower sigmoid colon remains in a tonically contracted state. Defecation occurs when pressure in the upper sigmoid colon and distal descending colon becomes great enough to force feces through the nonmotile, contracted segment. Prostaglandin synthesis is increased in the jejunum, and there are bile salts in the stools that may act as secretagogues.

In some instances, there is a family history of bowel complaints. As an infant, the child is likely to have experienced colic and diarrhea associated with teething and immunizations. In more than 90% of cases, chronic nonspecific diarrhea resolves by 40 to 50 months of age. The cure often accompanies toilet training. Many children with chronic nonspecific diarrhea develop irritable bowel syndrome (which is also called *mucous colitis*) as adults.[150] Children with chronic nonspecific diarrhea usually do well with normal food and fluid intake with a balance of fluid, fiber, fat, and fruit juices.

Primary Lactose Intolerance

Lactose intolerance is the inability to digest milk sugar. It is caused by inadequate production of lactase and is a common cause of diarrhea in children, particularly nonwhite children, under 7 years of age. The malabsorption of lactose results in osmotic diarrhea, in which fluids move by osmosis from the vascular compartment into the intestinal lumen. The undigested sugar is acted on by the colonic bacteria, and intestinal gas is produced. The diarrhea is accompanied by abdominal pain, bloating, and flatulence. Treatment consists of reducing milk consumption. Some children can tolerate lactose in fermented forms, such as cheese and yogurt. Complete restriction of lactose-containing foods is rarely necessary in young infants.[151]

DISORDERS OF THE LIVER

Disorders of Biliary Metabolism and Transport

Physiologic Jaundice of the Newborn

Physiologic jaundice of the newborn is usually a transient, benign icterus that occurs during the first week of life in otherwise healthy, full-term infants; 6.8% of all newborns have physiologic jaundice, with an increased frequency in breast-fed infants. In one study, 49% of full-term breast-fed infants had jaundice with a total bilirubin greater than 10 mg/dl by the third day of life.[152] Physiologic jaundice is caused by mild unconjugated (indirect-reacting) hyperbilirubinemia. A high level of indirect hyperbilirubinemia (greater than 15 mg/dl) is considered pathologic. There is a risk of brain damage (kernicterus) with persistent high indirect hyperbilirubinemia. The mechanism by which bilirubin crosses the blood-brain barrier and precipitates into brain cells is unknown.

PATHOPHYSIOLOGY   Physiologic jaundice results from the complex interaction of factors that cause (1) increased bilirubin production, (2) impaired hepatic uptake and excretion of bilirubin, and (3) reabsorption of bilirubin in the small intestine. Serum bilirubin values increase to 5 to 6 mg/dl by the second to fourth day after birth in full-term infants and 10 to 15 mg/dl by the fifth to seventh day in premature infants.

CLINICAL MANIFESTATIONS   Physiologic jaundice develops during the second or third day after birth and usually subsides in 1 to 2 weeks in full-term infants and 2 to 4 weeks in premature infants. After this, increasing bilirubin values and persistent jaundice indicate pathologic hyperbilirubinemia. A late rising bilirubin level also may be a manifestation of glucose-6-phosphate dehydrogenase deficiency.[153,154] Bilirubin encephalopathy (kernicterus), is caused by the deposition of toxic, unconjugated bilirubin in brain cells, and usually does not occur in healthy, full-term infants. Premature infants with respiratory distress, acidosis, or sepsis are at greater risk for encephalopathy. The resulting disabilities include athetoid cerebral palsy, and speech and hearing impairment.[155,156]

EVALUATION AND TREATMENT   Both total and direct (conjugated) bilirubin levels are measured; the direct bilirubin should not exceed 1 mg/dl.[2] Other causes of jaundice must be eliminated to confirm physiologic jaundice. Treatment depends on the degree of hyperbilirubinemia. Physiologic jaundice is usually treated by phototherapy (ultraviolet light).[157] Pathologic jaundice requires an exchange transfusion and treatment of the underlying cause.

Biliary Atresia
Biliary atresia is a rare congenital malformation characterized by the absence or obstruction of intrahepatic or extrahepatic bile ducts. Extrahepatic ducts may end in a blind pouch. The cause of the intrauterine injury to the ducts is not clear but is thought to be related to a chromosomal abnormality or active agents, such as infection or drugs or immune responses.[158] The disease expression is a continuum in which the principal process is one of bile duct destruction. The points of destruction are influenced by the stage of intrauterine development in which injury occurs.[2]

The atresia or obstruction of the bile ducts leads to plugging, inflammation, and fibrosis of the bile canaliculi and extrahepatic biliary tree. Progressive obstruction may lead to biliary cirrhosis (see Chapter 39), portal hypertension, or liver failure.[35]

Jaundice is the primary clinical manifestation of biliary atresia. Other signs are hepatomegaly and acholic (clay-colored) stools. Fat absorption is impaired for lack of bile salts, and the infant may fail to gain weight. Cirrhosis and liver failure lead to death within 2 years if untreated.

Early diagnosis of biliary atresia is mandatory and is based on clinical manifestations and liver biopsy. Liver function test results are abnormal. Serum transaminase and alkaline phosphatase values are elevated, and conjugated (direct) serum bilirubin levels rise progressively.

Extrahepatic atresia can be relieved by surgical drainage and correction in approximately 10% of cases. Some infants benefit from the Kasai procedure, in which a hepatic duct remnant is anastomosed to the jejunum or a jejunal segment is anastomosed to the porta hepatis if the patent hepatic duct remnant is not available (Figure 40-7). Even with initial restoration of bile flow, however, fibrosis and obliteration of intrahepatic bile ducts continues and cirrhosis results. Liver transplantation is the long-term therapy for biliary atresia. Approximately 40% of children with biliary atresia are immediate candidates for transplantation. Approximately 80% of children transplanted for biliary atresia will become long-term survivors with good physical and mental development.[159] The use of reduced and split livers from living, related donors has increased the number of children who survive after receiving transplantation.[160]

Inflammatory Disorders
Hepatitis
The pathophysiology of viral and fulminant hepatitis is described in Chapter 39.

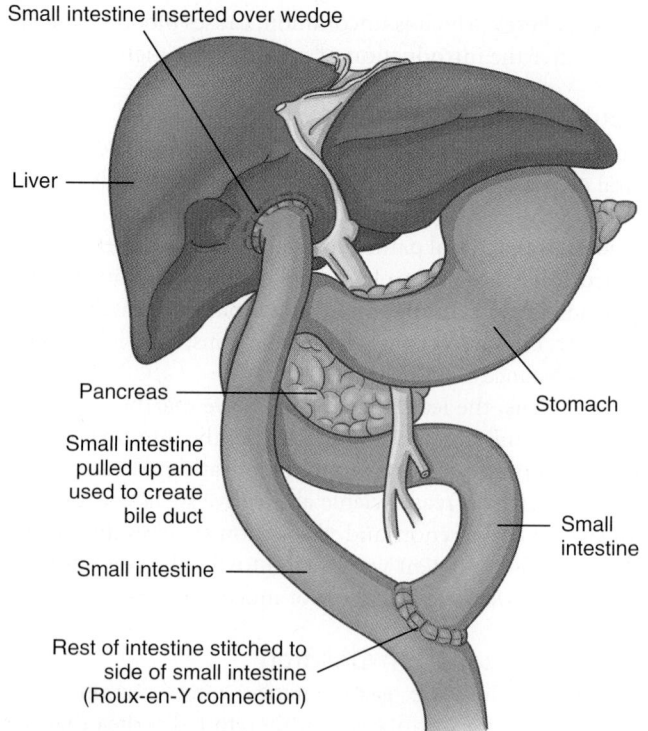

Small intestine inserted over wedge

Liver

Pancreas

Stomach

Small intestine pulled up and used to create bile duct

Small intestine

Small intestine

Rest of intestine stitched to side of small intestine (Roux-en-Y connection)

Figure 40-7 Kasai procedure. Surgical correction for extrahepatic biliary atresia. The jejunal segment between the liver and the bowel may be externalized, creating a double-barrel portoenterostomy.

Hepatitis A

Approximately one third to one half of the reported cases of **hepatitis A** occur in children.[161] Incidence is highest among young children of preschool age. Outbreaks tend to occur in day-care centers with large numbers of children who are not toilet trained and staff members who practice poor hand-washing techniques.[162] Hepatitis A in children is usually mild and asymptomatic. Clinical manifestations, however, may include nausea, vomiting, and diarrhea. Because jaundice is absent, infected children appear to have the "flu." Almost all children recover from hepatitis A without residual liver damage.[163]

Hepatitis B

Infants of mothers who are chronic **hepatitis B surface antigen (HBsAg)** carriers, hemophiliacs who receive frequent blood transfusions, children who abuse parenteral drugs, and children who live in institutions for the mentally retarded are all at risk for **hepatitis B virus (HBV)** infection. Of newborns infected by their mothers, 90% develop chronic hepatitis and become carriers. The risk of chronic hepatitis is more than 30% for children younger than 6 years who contract hepatitis B; hepatitis B leads to chronic hepatitis in only 5% of cases among populations of all ages.[164] Chronic hepatitis may develop more often in young children because of immaturity of the immune system. Infected infants and children are at risk for cirrhosis and hepatocellular carcinoma. The most serious consequence of HBV infection is fulminant hepatitis, which occurs in 1% of cases. Hepatitis D infection (HDV) depends on active infection with HBV. There is evidence that the risk of fulminant hepatitis is higher in individuals with combined infection of HBV and HDV than in those with HBV infection alone.[165] The most effective approach to the treatment of hepatitis B is prevention. The American Academy of Pediatrics has added immunization for hepatitis B to those immunizations recommended for infants. Efforts are underway to immunize children and adolescents who did not receive this series as infants.

Hepatitis C

Hepatitis C in children is associated primarily with blood transfusions. Children who receive frequent transfusions are at highest risk. Between 10% and 50% of affected children develop chronic liver disease. Interferon-α is effective in the treatment of both hepatitis B and hepatitis C.[166]

Chronic Hepatitis

The cause of **chronic hepatitis** is unknown in most cases, but an autoimmune mechanism is suggested because inflammatory findings are commonly seen in biopsy specimens of the liver. Manifestations of chronic hepatitis include malaise, anorexia, fever, gastrointestinal bleeding, hepatomegaly, edema, and transient joint pain. Serum transaminase and bilirubin levels are elevated. There may be evidence of impairment of synthetic functions of the liver: prolonged prothrombin time and hypoalbuminemia. Diagnosis is based on the clinical manifestations and liver biopsy.

Treatment has variable efficacy and differs by the causative pathogen. Treatment with ribavirin and interferon-α has been effective in managing persons coinfected with chronic hepatitis and human immunodeficiency virus (HIV).[167,168] Interferon-α has been most effective in young children with chronic hepatitis following hepatitis B and C.[169,170] Young children may respond to alternate-day treatment with steroids.[2]

Cirrhosis

Cirrhosis is the excessive formation of fibrous tissue in response to inflammation and tissue damage (see Chapter 39). Most forms of chronic liver diseases in children can progress to cirrhosis, but they seldom do so. The complications of cirrhosis in children are the same as those in adults: portal hypertension, the opening of collateral vessels between the portal and systemic veins, and varices. In addition, children with cirrhosis experience growth failure caused by nutritional deficits and developmental delay, particularly in gross motor function because of ascites and weakness. The cause of cirrhosis may influence its severity and course. Some types of cirrhosis can be stabilized if the cause is identified and treated early.

Portal Hypertension

The two basic causes of **portal hypertension** in children are (1) increased resistance to blood flow within the portal system and (2) increased volume of portal blood flow. Increased resistance to flow can occur anywhere in the portal circulatory system. Portal hypertension can accompany cirrhosis, intraabdominal infections, portal vein thrombosis, congenital anomalies of the portal vein, and congenital hepatic fibrosis.

Types

Extrahepatic Portal Hypertension

Extrahepatic (prehepatic) portal venous obstruction causes 50% to 70% of extrahepatic portal hypertension in children. For at least half of these children, no specific cause can be found. Obstruction is almost always in the portal vein and is usually caused by thrombosis. Umbilical infection with or without a history of catheterization of the umbilical vein may be a cause in neonates. Portal vein thrombosis can occur as a complication of intraabdominal infections, pancreatitis, and blunt abdominal trauma. It also has been associated with neonatal dehydration, inflammatory bowel disease, and hypercoagulable states, such as protein C and protein S deficiencies.[2] The liver is usually normal in cases of extrahepatic portal hypertension.

Intrahepatic Portal Hypertension

Cirrhosis is the primary cause of **intrahepatic portal hypertension.** The most common finding is fibrosis, which increases resistance to portal blood flow by constricting and reducing the compliance of the hepatic sinusoids.

Course of the Disease

The important consequence of portal hypertension in children is the development of collateral circulation, with portosystemic shunting, hypersplenism, and ascites.

CLINICAL MANIFESTATIONS   The clinical manifestations of portal hypertension are splenomegaly, upper gastrointestinal bleeding, ascites, and hepatic encephalopathy. **Splenomegaly** is the most common sign of portal hypertension in children. The spleen may be firm or hard, depending on the duration of portal hypertension. Hematemesis, possibly associated with abdominal pain, often accompanies sudden pallor. Melena is observed, either at the time of hematemesis or soon afterward. In children, most episodes of gastrointestinal bleeding are caused by rupture of esophageal varices. Clotting abnormalities caused by altered liver function promote the bleeding. If plasma volume is increased, esophageal varices readily rupture during activities, such as coughing, that increase blood pressure. Acetylsalicylic acid (aspirin), which should not be administered to children, can trigger bleeding, but its exact mechanisms of action are not known. Severe bleeding episodes can cause hypovolemic shock and death. Symptoms of ascites include weight gain, protruding abdomen, and reduced tidal volumes if the ascites is severe. Severe liver disease is characterized by hypoalbuminemia, prolonged prothrombin times, hyperbilirubinemia, electrolyte imbalance, and hypoglycemia.

Hepatic encephalopathy in children can be acute or chronic. Acute encephalopathy is characterized by major disorders of consciousness, which may progress to coma. This may follow an acute episode of variceal bleeding as the impaired liver attempts to metabolize the large protein (nitrogenous) load from the blood. Chronic, or minimal, encephalopathy is characterized by emotional or psychiatric disorders, decreased intellectual functioning, personality disorders caused by minimal brain dysfunction, and spatial disorientation.

EVALUATION AND TREATMENT Assessment of portal hypertension in children must be thorough because the cause dictates the management. The objectives of the clinical investigation are to locate the site of the venous block and identify the disease responsible for the portal hypertension. Thorough physical examination, laboratory tests of liver function, imaging procedures, and biopsy may be included in the diagnostic evaluation (see Chapter 38). Sclerotherapy is the initial treatment of choice for severe esophageal varices in children.[171]

The indications for surgical shunting include gastrointestinal hemorrhage not responsive to sclerotherapy. Surgical venous shunts rarely have been performed on small children because of the high failure rate secondary to vessel occlusion, but they may be an alternative in older children, with some success.[2,172] Surgical shunts had been a contraindication for subsequent liver transplantation but are no longer considered a contraindication, although the shunt does make the transplantation technically more difficult. The transjugular intrahepatic portosystemic shunt (TIPS) procedure is performed for some children. This is a therapeutic option in which a stent is placed between the right hepatic vein and the right or left portal vein to allow shunting of blood without surgical intervention.[173]

The outcome of portal hypertension depends almost entirely on its cause. Children with extrahepatic disease are expected to recover with little morbidity. For children with intrahepatic disease, the prognosis varies.

Metabolic Disorders

More than 5000 genetically determined metabolic pathways have been identified in liver tissue. The earliest possible identification of metabolic disorders is essential because (1) early treatment may prevent permanent damage to vital organs, such as the liver or brain; (2) precise genetic counseling may be possible with prenatal diagnosis; and (3) complications can be minimized, even if cure is not possible. Galactosemia,[174] fructosemia, and Wilson disease are rare treatable metabolic disorders that have hepatic clinical manifestations. These disorders are presented in Table 40-2.

Wilson Disease

Wilson disease (hepatolenticular degeneration) is an autosomal recessive defect of copper metabolism that causes toxic amounts of copper to accumulate in the liver, brain, kidneys, and corneas. The gene *ATP7B* is localized on chromosome 13 and encodes copper-transporting P-type adenosine triphosphatase (ATPase) membrane-spanning protein. It is highly expressed in the liver, kidney, and placenta and is expressed in lower levels in the brain, heart, muscle, and pancreas.[175] This defect in the uptake and excretion of copper by hepatocytes is an important cause of progressive liver disease in children and young adults. Wilson disease is very rare, with an incidence of 1 in 30,000 live births.[176] Between 1 in 200 and 1 in 500 persons are carriers.[2]

PATHOPHYSIOLOGY Two major abnormalities in copper metabolism have been identified: (1) diminished biliary excretion of copper and (2) failure to insert copper into ceruloplasmin (a glycoprotein that transports copper in the blood). A positive copper balance is present from birth in children with Wilson disease, despite increased excretion of copper in the urine. Copper toxicity with accumulation in the liver and brain is the major abnormality. Excesses of copper generate free radicals that disrupt cellular organelles, deoxyribonucleic acids (DNA), microtubules, enzymes, and proteins. Copper overload is related to impaired biliary excretion of copper and may be related to failure of hepatocyte lysosomes to eliminate copper by exocytosis.[177]

Early in the disease, intestinal absorption of copper is normal, as is hepatic clearance of albumin-bound, absorbed copper. As copper-binding proteins in the liver become saturated, hepatic uptake of copper diminishes, with elevated serum copper levels and biochemical and clinical evidence of liver damage caused by copper accumulation. In later stages of the disease, copper accumulates in extrahepatic tissues, including the eyes, brain, and kidneys.

When cerebral copper-binding proteins become saturated, a characteristic pattern of brain damage develops, particularly

Table 40-2   Galactosemia, Fructosemia, and Wilson Disease

	Galactosemia	Fructosemia	Wilson Disease
Mechanism of disease	Deficiency of galactose and phosphate, uridyl transferase An autosomal recessive trait Cannot convert galactose to glucose Toxic accumulation of galactose in body tissues, liver, and brain	Deficiency of fructose-1-phosphate aldolase An autosomal recessive trait Cannot metabolize fructose, sucrose, or honey; occurs when breast milk is replaced with cow's milk Toxic accumulation of fructose in body tissues	Probably autosomal recessive: defect on chromosome 13 Defect in copper excretion by liver Impaired transport of copper in blood caused by diminished transport protein (ceruloplasmin) Toxic accumulations of copper in liver, brain, kidney, corneas
Clinical manifestations	High levels of blood galactose Vomiting Hypoglycemia May have failure to thrive Symptoms of cirrhosis at 2 to 6 months—jaundice Mental retardation if not treated Cataracts if not treated	High levels of blood fructose Vomiting Hypoglycemia May have failure to thrive Hepatomegaly Jaundice Seizures	Intention tremors Indistinct speech Dystonia Greenish-yellow rings in cornea Hepatomegaly Jaundice Anorexia Renal tubular defects
Evaluation	Presence of reducing substances in urine when infant is receiving lactose	Detailed dietary history Liver or intestinal mucosa biopsy	Low plasma ceruloplasmin
Treatment	Galactose-free diet	Fructose-, sucrose-, honey-free diet Vitamin C supplementation	Chelation therapy to remove copper from body Decreased dietary intake of copper Liver transplant

in the basal ganglia. Neural effects include intention tremor, unsteady gait, dystonia, and behavioral changes. Manifestations of renal tubular injury usually appear simultaneously. The uptake of copper by red blood cells is thought to cause hemolytic anemia, a condition sometimes seen early in the clinical course of Wilson disease.

CLINICAL MANIFESTATIONS   The clinical manifestations of Wilson disease may begin as young as 4 years of age, when control mechanisms responsible for copper homeostasis and biliary excretion should have matured. The mean age at diagnosis in one large study was 15.5 years.[178]

The classic clinical presentation of Wilson disease is a triad of neuromuscular abnormalities, intention tremors, dysarthria (indistinct speech), and dystonia (disordered muscular tonicity): (1) Kayser-Fleischer rings (accumulation of copper in the limbus of the cornea, causing a greenish yellow ring), (2) cirrhosis associated with elevated serum copper, and (3) low ceruloplasmin levels. Initial symptoms vary from malaise and abdominal pain to jaundice. Changes in mental and motor performance may develop at age 6 years or into adult life. The earliest signs of liver involvement include enlargement of the liver and spleen, jaundice, and anorexia. Edema and ascites may develop suddenly, or gastrointestinal hemorrhage may be the initial sign of the disease. Occasion-

ally, Wilson disease begins with a hemolytic crisis caused by the toxic effects of copper on the red blood cells. Cirrhosis develops in all untreated cases. Copper deposition in the kidneys causes a proximal renal tubular defect that results in losses of glucose, amino acids, phosphate, and uric acid in the urine and renal tubular acidosis. All untreated individuals will develop behavioral or psychiatric disorders.

EVALUATION AND TREATMENT   Because Wilson disease is rare, it may not be diagnosed until clinical manifestations develop. Laboratory tests detect a serum ceruloplasmin concentration less than 30 mg/dl. Serum copper values may be normal or high, and urine copper values are elevated. Liver biopsy is used to assess structural changes and measure copper concentrations. Although D-penicillamine has traditionally been the drug of choice for Wilson disease, zinc, which has low toxicity, has demonstrated effectiveness.[179] Copper intake is reduced by eliminating organ meats, nuts, legumes, shellfish, and chocolate from the diet. Physiotherapy may accelerate the recovery of gait and muscular coordination. Liver transplantation is the sole resolutive therapy for Wilson disease and is the treatment of choice for persons who develop fulminant hepatic failure or end-stage cirrhosis.[180] Children with untreated Wilson disease die of neural, hepatic, renal, or hematologic complications.

Disorders of the Gastrointestinal Tract

1. Most alterations of digestive function in children are caused by congenital obstructions of the intestinal tract; disorders of digestion, absorption, or nutrition; or liver disease.
2. Cleft lip (harelip) and cleft palate (failure of the bony palate to fuse in the midline) may occur separately or together. The fissure may affect the uvula, soft palate, hard palate, nostril, and maxillary alveolar ridge.
3. Esophageal atresia, a condition in which the esophagus ends in a blind pouch, may occur with or without tracheoesophageal fistula, a connection between the esophagus and the trachea. As the infant swallows oral secretions or ingests milk, the pouch fills, causing either drooling or aspiration into the lungs.
4. Pyloric stenosis, one of the most common disorders requiring surgery in early infancy, is an obstruction of the pyloric outlet caused by hypertrophy and hyperplasia of circular muscles in the pyloric sphincter.
5. Malrotation of the intestine, with an obstructing band and volvulus (twisting of the bowel on itself), may partly or completely occlude the gastrointestinal tract and its blood vessels.
6. Meconium ileus is a condition in the newborn in which intestinal secretions and amniotic waste products produce a thick, tarry plug that obstructs the intestine. From 10% to 15% of children with cystic fibrosis have meconium ileus as neonates.
7. Duodenal, jejunal, and ileal obstructions can be caused by meconium ileus, atresia, congenital aganglionic megacolon, or acquired obstructive disorders.
8. Distal intestinal obstruction syndrome (DIOS), formerly called *meconium ileus equivalent,* can occur when intestinal contents become abnormally thick and impact the intestinal lumen. Cystic fibrosis and dehydration are common causes.
9. Congenital aganglionic megacolon (Hirschsprung disease) is caused by a malformation of the parasympathetic nervous system in a segment of the colon. It is characterized by the absence of nerves needed for peristalsis.
10. Malformations of the anus and rectum range from mild congenital stenosis of the anus to complex deformities, all of which are classified as imperforate anus.
11. The most common cause of acquired intestinal obstruction in infants is intussusception, a condition in which one portion of the bowel telescopes, or invaginates, into another, most commonly in the area of the ileocecal junction.
12. Gastroesophageal reflux is caused by the relaxation or incompetence of the lower esophageal sphincter. Infants are susceptible to reflux because the sphincter is not fully mature, their diet consists of liquids, and they are seldom in an upright position.
13. The pathophysiologic triad that is the hallmark of cystic fibrosis includes pancreatic enzyme deficiency (which causes maldigestion), overproduction of mucus in the respiratory tract, and abnormally elevated sodium and chloride concentrations in sweat. Older children with cystic fibrosis also may have diabetes mellitus caused by damage to endocrine function of the pancreas and chronic liver disease. Affected individuals seldom survive beyond their thirties.
14. Gluten-sensitive enteropathy is a lifelong disease characterized by the loss of mature villous epithelium in the presence of a gluten-containing diet. It results in malabsorption and growth failure.
15. Protein energy malnutrition is a group of disorders resulting from a severe dietary deficiency of proteins (kwashiorkor), carbohydrates, or both (marasmus). Starvation causes stunted mental and physical development. Kwashiorkor occurs most often in young toddlers who have stopped breast-feeding and subsist on a high-carbohydrate diet.
16. Failure to thrive is inadequate physical growth of a child. Organic failure to thrive is caused by genetic, anatomic, or pathophysiologic factors that retard normal growth and development. Nonorganic failure to thrive is caused by nutritional deficits associated with inadequate nurturing.
17. Necrotizing enterocolitis is a disorder in neonates, particularly premature infants, thought to result from stress and anoxia of the bowel wall. Bacteria invade the mucosa and submucosa, resulting in colitis, necrosis, and even perforation of the intestinal wall.
18. Diarrhea in infants and children can rapidly cause dehydration and electrolyte imbalances because fluid reserves are relatively small.
19. The most common cause of acute diarrhea in children is bacterial or viral enterocolitis (infection of the gastrointestinal tract).
20. Chronic diarrhea (diarrhea persisting longer than 4 weeks) can be caused by a wide variety of underlying conditions and often leads to growth failure and slow development.

Disorders of the Liver

1. Physiologic jaundice of the newborn is caused by mild hyperbilirubinemia that subsides in 1 to 2 weeks. Pathologic jaundice is caused by severe hyperbilirubinemia and can cause brain damage.
2. Biliary atresia is a congenital malformation of the bile ducts that obstructs bile flow. Atresia causes jaundice, cirrhosis, and liver failure. Biliary atresia is the most common reason for liver transplantation in children.
3. Acute hepatitis has the same clinical course in children and adults, but children have milder cases of the disease. Hepatitis A is the most common form of childhood hepatitis.
4. Cirrhosis is rare in children, but it can develop from most forms of chronic liver disease.
5. Portal hypertension in children usually is caused by extrahepatic obstruction. Thrombosis of the portal vein is the most common cause of portal hypertension in children, and splenomegaly is the most common sign.
6. The three most common metabolic disorders that cause liver damage in children are galactosemia, fructosemia, and Wilson disease. All three are inherited as genetic traits and permit the accumulation of toxins in the liver.
7. Wilson disease causes defective copper uptake and metabolism. Unexcreted copper accumulates in the liver, brain, kidney, and corneal cells. Damage from accumulated copper is gradual; the disease is usually not diagnosed before age 4 or 5 years.

KEY TERMS

Acute diarrhea, 1461
Biliary atresia, 1462
Chronic diarrhea, 1461
Chronic hepatitis, 1463

Chronic nonspecific diarrhea, 1461
Cirrhosis, 1463
Cleft lip (harelip), 1447
Cleft palate, 1447

Congenital aganglionic megacolon
(Hirschsprung disease), 1452
Cystic fibrosis (CF), 1456
Diarrhea, 1461

KEY TERMS—cont'd

MEDIA RESOURCES  *evolve*

Review questions and answers for this chapter are available in the *CD Companion* included with this book.

WebLinks—links to Internet sites pertaining to this chapter—are available on Evolve at http://evolve.elsevier.com/McCance/.

REFERENCES

1. Carinci F et al: Recent developments in orofacial cleft genetics, *J Craniofac Surg* 14(2):130-143, 2003.
2. Behrman RE, Kliegman R, Jenson HB: *Nelson textbook of pediatrics,* ed. 17, Philadelphia, 2003, Saunders.
3. Cobourne MT: The complex genetics of cleft lip and palate, *Eur J Orthod* 26(1):7-16, 2004.
4. Little J et al: Smoking and orofacial clefts: a United Kingdom-based case-controlled study, *Cleft Palate Craniofac J* 41(4):381-386, 2004.
5. Little J, Candy A, Munger RG: Tobacco smoking and oral clefts: a meta-analysis, *Bull World Health Organ* 82(3):213-218, 2004.
6. Marazita ML, Mooney MP: Current concepts in the embryology and genetics of cleft lip and cleft palate, *Clin Plast Surg* 31(2):125-140, 2004.
7. Stanier P, Moore GE: Genetics of cleft lip and palate: syndromic genes contributing to the incidence of non-syndromic clefts, *Hum Mol Genet* 13(1):73-81, 2004.
8. Zucchero TM et al: Interferon regulating factor 6 (IRF6) gene variants and the risk of isolated cleft lip or palate, *N Eng J Med* 351(8):769-780, 2004.
9. Abramowicz S et al: Demographic and prenatal factors of patients with cleft lip and palate: a pilot study, *J Am Dent Assoc* 134(10):1374-1376, 2003.
10. Batra P, Duggal R, Parkash H: Genetics of cleft lip and palate revisited, *J Clin Pediatr Dent* 27(4):311-320, 2003.
11. Spilson SV, Kim HJ, Chung KC: Association between maternal diabetes mellitus and newborn oral clefts, *Ann Plast Surg* 47(5):477-481, 2001.
12. Knott L et al: Homocysteine oxidation and apoptosis: a potential cause of cleft palate, *In Vitro Cell Dev Biol Anim* 39(1-2):98-105, 2003.
13. Van Rooij IA et al: Vitamin and homocysteine status of mothers and infants and the risk of nonsyndromic orofacial clefts, *Am J Obstet Gynecol* 189(4):1155-1160, 2003.
14. Perrotin F et al: Chromosomal defects and associated malformations in fetal cleft lip with or without cleft palate, *Euro J Obstet Reprod Biol* 99(1):19-24, 2001.
15. Holmes LB: The teratogenicity of anticonvulsant drugs: a progress report, *J Med Genet* 39(4):245-247, 2002.
16. da Silva Dalben G et al: Breastfeeding and sugar intake in babies with cleft lip and palate, *Cleft Palate Craniofac J* 40(1):84-87, 2003.
17. Redford-Badwal DA, Mabry K, Frassinelli JD: Impact of cleft lip and/or palate on nutritional health and oral-motor development, *Dent Clin North Am* 47(2):305-317, 2003.
18. Turner L et al: The effects of lactation education and a prosthetic obturator appliance of feeding efficiency in infants with cleft lip and palate, *Cleft Palate Craniofac J* 38(5):519-524, 2001.
19. Johnson N, R Sandy J: Prenatal diagnosis of cleft lip and palate, *Cleft Palate Craniofac J* 40(2):186-189, 2003.
20. Weinfeld AB et al: International trends in the treatment of cleft lip and palate, *Clin Plas Surg* 32(1):19-23, 2005.
21. Sadove AM, van Aalst JA, Culp JA: Cleft palate repair: art and issues, *Clin Plast Surg* 31(2):231-241, 2005.
22. Sheahan P et al: Incidence and outcome of middle ear disease in cleft lip and/or cleft palate, *Int J Pediatr Otorhinolaryngol* 67(7):785-793, 2003.
23. Aniansson G et al: Otitis media and feeding with breast milk of children with cleft palate, *Scan J Plast Reconstr Surg Hand Surg* 36(1):9-15, 2002.
24. Ahluwalia M et al: Dental caries, oral hygiene, and oral clearance in children with craniofacial disorders, *J Dent Res* 83(2):175-179, 2004.
25. Kirchberg A, Treide A, Hemprich A: Investigation of caries prevelance in children with cleft lip, alveolus, and palate, *J Craniomaxillofac Surg* 32(4):216-219, 2004.
26. Langer JC et al: Prenatal diagnosis of esophageal atresia using sonography and magnetic resonance imaging, *J Pediatr Surg* 36(5):804-807, 2001.
27. Kovesi T, Rubin S: Long-term complications of congenital esophageal atreasia and/or tracheoesophageal fistula, *Chest* 126(3):915-925, 2004.
28. Celayir AC, Erdogan E: An infrequent cause of misdiagnosis in esophageal atresia, *J Pediatr Surg* 38(9):1389, 2003.
29. Lin YC, Ni YH, Chang MH: Gastroesophageal disease beyond infancy, *Pediatr Int* 46(5):516-520, 2004.
30. Little DC et al: Long-term analysis of children with esophageal atresia and tracheoesophageal fistula, *J Pediatr Surg* 38(6):852-856, 2003.
31. Sparey C et al: Esophageal atresia in the Northern Region Congenital Anomaly Survey, *Am J Obstet Gyn* 182(2):427-431, 2000.
32. Hernanz-Schulman M: Infantile hypertrophic pyloric stenosis, *Radiology* 227(2):319-331, 2003.
33. Phillips JD: Abdominal surgical emergencies. In Wyllie R, Hyams J, editors: *Pediatric gastrointestinal diseases,* ed 2, Philadelphia, 1999, Saunders.
34. Armstrong M: The child with a cognitive deficit. In McKinney ES et al, editors: *Maternal-child nursing,* ed 2, St. Louis, 2005, Saunders.
35. Sams CA: The child with a gastrointestinal alteration. In McKinney ES et al, editors: *Maternal-child nursing,* ed 2, St. Louis, 2005, Saunders.
36. Spinelli C et al: Muscle thickness in infantile hypertrophic pyloric stenosis, *Pediatr Med Chir* 25(2):148-150, 2003.
37. Shima H, Puri P: Increased expression of transforming growth factor-alpha in hypertrophic pyloric stenosis, *Pediatr Surg Intern* 15(3-4):198-200, 1999.
38. Blumer SL et al: The vomiting neonate: a review of the ACR appropriateness criteria and ultrasound's role in the work-up of such patients, *Ultrasound Q* 20(3):78-89, 2004.
39. Vasavada P: Ultrasound evaluation of acute abdominal emergencies in infants and children, *Radiol Clin North Am* 42(2):445-456, 2004.
40. Papadakis K et al: The changing presentation of pyloric stenosis, *Am J Emerg Med* 17(1):67-69, 1999.
41. van der Bilt JD et al: Laparoscopic pyloromyotomy for hypertrophic pyloric stenosis: impact of experience on the results in 182 cases, *Surg Endosc* 18(6):907-909, 2004.
42. Kawahara H et al: Intravenous atropine treatment in infantile hypertrophic pyloric stenosis, *Arch Dis Child* 87(1):71-74, 2002.

42a. Singh UK, Kumar R: Congenital hypertrophic pyloric stenosis, *Indian J Pediatr* 69(8):713-715, 2002.

43. Sweeney B, Surana R, Puri P: Jejunoileal atresia and associated malformations: correlation with the timing of in utero insult, *J Pediatr Surg* 36(5):774-776, 2001.

44. Millar AJ, Rode H, Cywes S: Malrotation and volvulus in infancy and childhood, *Semin Pediatr Surg* 12(4):229-236, 2003.

45. Cohen Z et al: How much of a misnomer is "asymptomatic" intestinal malrotation? *Israel Med Assoc J* 5(3):172-174, 2003.

46. Lai HC: Nutritional status of patients with cystic fibrosis with meconium ileus: a comparison with patients without meconium ileus and diagnosed early through neonatal screening, *Pediatrics* 105(1 Pt 1):53, 2000.

47. Li Z et al: Longitudinal pulmonary status of cystic fibrosis children with meconium ileus, *Pediatr Pulmonol* 38(4):277-284, 2004.

48. McAlister WH, Kronemer KA: Emergency gastrointestinal radiology of the newborn, *Radiol Clin North Am* 34(4):819-844, 1996.

49. Kao SC, Franken EA Jr: Nonoperative treatment of simple meconium ileus: a survey of the Society for Pediatric Radiology, *Pediatr Radiol* 25(2):97-100, 1995.

50. Evans AK, Fitzgerald DA, McKay KO: The impact of meconium ileus on the clinical course of children with cystic fibrosis, *Eur Respir J* 18(5):784-789, 2001.

51. Oliveira MC et al: Effect of meconium ileus on the clinical prognosis of patients with cystic fibrosis, *Braz J Med Biol Res* 35(1):31-38, 2002.

52. Dray X et al: Distal intestinal obstruction syndrome in adults with cystic fibrosis, *Clin Gastroenterol Hepatol* 2(6):498-502, 2004.

53. Schibli S, Dune PR, Tullis ED: Proper usage of pancreatic enzymes, *Curr Opin Pulm Med* 8(6):542-546, 2002.

54. Corbett K et al: Cystic fibrosis-associated liver disease: a population-based study, *J Pediatr* 145(3):327-332, 2004.

55. Efrati O et al: Liver cirrhosis and portal hypertension in cystic fibrosis, *Eur J Gastroenterol Hepatol* 15(10):1073-1078, 2003.

56. Fridell JA et al: Liver and intestinal transplantation in a child with cystic fibrosis: a case report, *Pediatr Transplant* 7(3):240-242, 2003.

57. Fitz G et al: Functional haplotypes of the RET proto-oncogene promoter are associated with Hirschsprung disease, *Hum Mol Genet* 12(24):3207-3214, 2003.

58. Seri M et al: Frequency of RET mutation in long- and short-segment Hirschsprung disease, *Hum Mutat* 9(3):243-249, 1997.

59. Hackam DJ et al: The influence of Down syndrome in the management and outcome of children with Hirschsprung disease, *J Pediatr Surg* 38(6):946-949, 2003.

60. Puri P, Shinkai T: Pathogenesis of Hirschsprung disease and its variants: recent progress, *Semin Pediatr Surg* 13(1):18-24, 2004.

61. Amiel J, Lyonnet S: Hirschsprung disease, associated syndromes and genetics: a review, *J Med Genet* 38(11):729-739, 2001.

62. Dasgupta R, Langer JC: Hirschsprung disease, *Curr Probl Surg* 41(12):942-988, 2004.

63. Hackam DJ et al: Diagnosis and outcome of Hirschsprung's disease: does age really matter, *Pediatr Surg Int* 20(5):319-322, 2004.

64. Osatakul S, Patrapinyokul S, Osatakul N: The diagnostic value of anorectal manometry as a screening test for Hirschsprung disease, *J Med Assoc Thai* 82(11):1100-1105, 1999.

65. Emir H et al: Anorectal mamometry during the neonatal period: its specificity in the diagnosis of Hirschsprung disease, *Eur J Pediatr Surg* 9(2):101-103, 1999.

66. Khan AR, Vujanic GM, Huddart S: The constipated child: how likely is Hirschsprung disease? *Pediatr Surg Int* 19(6):439-442, 2003.

67. Bai Y et al: Long-term outcome and quality of life after the Swenson procedure for Hirschsprung disease, *J Pediatr Surg* 37(4):639-642, 2002.

68. Mittal A et al: Associated anomalies with anorectal malformation, *Indian J Pediatr* 71(6):509-514, 2004.

69. Rintala RJ: Fecal incontinence in anorectal malformations, neuropathy, and miscellaneous conditions, *Semin Pediatr Surg* 11(2):75-82, 2002.

70. Winslow BT, Westfall JM, Nicholas RA: Intussusception, *Am Fam Physician* 54(1):213, 1996.

71. de Vries S, Sleeboom C, Aronson DC: Postoperative intussusception in children, *Br J Surg* 13(4):81-83, 1999.

72. Eggermont E, De Boeck K: Small-intestinal anomalies in cystic fibrosis patients, *Eur J Pediatr* 150(12):824-828, 1991.

73. Chung JL: Intussusception in infants and children: risk factors leading to surgical reduction, *J Formos Med Assoc* 93(6):481-485, 1994.

74. Klein EJ, Kapoor D, Shugerman RP: The diagnosis of intussusception, *Clin Pediatr* 43(4):343-347, 2004.

75. Byrne AT et al: The imaging of intussusception, *Clin Radiol* 60(3):412, 2005.

76. Daneman A, Navarro O: Intussusception Part 2: an update on the evolution of management, *Pediatr Radiol* 34(2):97-108, 2004.

77. Crystal P et al: Sonographically guided hydrostatic reduction of intussusception in children, *J Clin Ultrasound* 30(6):343-348, 2002.

78. Navarro OM, Daneman A, Chae A: Intussusception: the use of delayed, repeated reduction attempts and the management of intussusception due to pathological lead points in pediatric patients, *Am J Roentgenol* 182(5):1169-1176, 2004.

79. Daneman A, Navarro O: Intussusception Part 1: a review of diagnostic approaches, *Pediatr Radiol* 33(2):79-85, 2003.

80. Kim JH: Ultrasound features of transient small bowel intussusception in pediatric patients, *Korean J Radiol* 5(3):178-184, 2004.

81. Bajaj L, Roback MG: Postreduction management of intussusception in a children's hospital emergency department, *Pediatrics* 112(6 Pt 1):1302-1307, 2003.

82. Harrington JW, Brand DA, Edwards KS: Seizure disorders as a risk factor for gastroesophageal reflux in children with neurodevelopmental disturbances, *Clin Pediatr* 43(6):557-562, 2004.

83. Spiroglou K et al: Gastric emptying in children with cerebral palsy and gastroesophageal reflux, *Pediatr Neurol* 31(3):177-182, 2004.

84. Ay M et al: Association of asthma with gastroesophageal reflux disease in children, *J Chinese Med Assoc (JCMA)* 67(2):63-66, 2004.

85. Chipps BE: Determinants of asthma and its clinical course, *Ann Allergy, Asthma, Immunol* 93(4):309-315, 2004.

86. Harding SM: Recent clinical investigations examining the association of asthma and gastroesophageal reflux, *Am J Med* 115 (3A Suppl): 39S-44S, 2003.

87. Thach BT: Sudden infant death syndrome: can gastroesophageal reflux cause sudden infant death? *Am J Med* 108(4a suppl):144S, 2000.

88. Brodzicki J, Trawinska-Bartnicka M, Korzon M: Frequency, consequences and pharmacological treatment of gastroesophageal reflux in children with cystic fibrosis, *Med Sci Monit* 8(7):529-537, 2002.

89. Simanovsky N, Buonomo C, Nurko S: The infant with chronic vomiting: the value of the upper GI series, *Pediatr Radiol* 32(8):549-550, 2002.

90. Spitz L, McLeod E: Gastroesophageal reflux, *Semin Pediatr Surg* 12(4):237-240, 2003.

91. Rohen R, Nurko S: The importance of multichannel intraluminal impedence in the evaluation of children with persistent respiratory symptoms, *Am J Gastroenterol* 99(12):2452-2458, 2004.

92. Foroutan HR, Ghafani M: Gastroesophageal reflux as a cause of chronic respiratory symptoms, *Indian J Pediatr* 69(2):137-139, 2002.

93. Pan JJ et al: Gastroesophageal reflux: comparison of barium studies with 24-h pH monitoring, *Eur J Radiol* 47(2):149-153, 2003.

94. El Mouzan MI, Abdullah AM: The diagnosis of gastroesophageal reflux disease in children, *Saudi Med J* 23(2):164-167, 2002.

95. Patwari AK et al: Diagnostic modalities for gastroesophageal reflux, *Indian J Pediatr* 69(2):133-136, 2002.

96. Arguin AL, Swartz MK: Gastroesophageal refux in infants: a primary care perspective, *Pediatr Nurs* 30(1):45-51, 71, 2004.

97. Rudolph C et al: Guidelines for the evaluation and treatment of gastroesophageal reflux in infants and children, *J Pediatr Gastroenterol Nutr* 32(2 suppl):1S-31S, 2001.

98. Craig WR et al: Metoclopramide, thickened feedings, and positioning for gastro-oesophageal reflux in children under two years, *Cochrane Database Syst Rev* (4):CDC003502, 2004.

99. Gilger MA et al: Outcomes of surgical fundoplication in children, *Clin Gastroenterol Hepatol* 2(11):978-984, 2004.

100. Zeid M et al: Nissan fundoplication in infants and children: a long-term clinical study, *Hepatogastroenterology* 51(57):697-700, 2004.

101. Konstan MW et al: Ultrase MT12 and Ultrase MT20 in the treatment of exocrine pancreatic insufficiency in cystic fibrosis: safety and efficiency, *Aliment Pharmacol Ther* 20(11-12):1365-1371, 2004.

102. Slater C et al: Bulk and compound specific analysis of stool lipid confirm that the "missing" 13C in the mixed triacylglycerol breath test is not in the stool, *Food Nutr Bull* 23(3 suppl):48-52, 2002.

103. Baker SS et al: Pancreatic enzyme therapy and clinical outcomes in patients with cystic fibrosis, *J Pediatr* 146(2):189-193, 2005.

104. Van Biervliet S et al: Percutaneous endoscopic gastrostomy in cystic fibrosis: patient acceptance and effect of overnight tube feedings on nutritional status, *Acta Gastroenterol Belg* 67(3):241-244, 2004.

105. Treem WR: Emerging concepts in celiac disease, *Curr Opin Pediatr* 16(5):552-559, 2004.

106. Fasano A et al: Prevalence of celiac disease in at-risk and non-at-risk groups in the United States: a large multi-center study, *Arch Int Med* 163(3):286-292, 2003.
107. Murray JA: Trends in the identification and clinical features of celiac disease in a North American community, *Clin Gastroenterol Hepatol* 1(1):19-27, 2003.
108. Iughetti L et al: Endocrine aspects of coeliac disease, *Pediatr Endocrinol Metab* 16(6):805-818, 2003.
109. Abdulkarim AS, Murray JA: Review article: the diagnosis of celiac disease, *Aliment Pharmacol Ther* 17(8):987-995, 2003.
110. Green PHR et al: Characteristics of adult celiac disease in the USA: results of a national survey, *Am J Gastroenterol* 96(1):126, 2001.
111. Rossi T: Celiac disease, *Adolesc Med Clin* 15(1):91-103, 2004.
112. Catassi C, Fasano A: Celiac disease as a cause of growth retardation in children, *Curr Opin Pediatr* 16(4):445-449, 2004.
113. Eliakim R, Sherer DM: Celiac disease: fertility and pregnancy, *Gynecol Obtset Invest* 51(1):3-7, 2001.
114. Kavak US et al: Bone mineral density in children with untreated and treated celiac disease, *J Pediatr Gastroenterol Nutr* 37(4):434-436, 2003.
115. Freeman HJ: Free perforation due to intestinal lymphoma in biopsy-defined or suspected celiac disease, *J Clin Gastroenterol* 37(4):299-302, 2003.
116. Celli M et al: Rapid gas-chromatographic assay of lactulose and mannitol for estimating intestinal permeability, *Clin Chem* 42(5):752-756, 1995.
117. Bern C et al: Assessment of potential indicators for protein-energy malnutrition in the algorithm for integrated management of childhood illness, *Bull WHO* 75(1 suppl):87-96, 1997.
118. Pelletier DL: The relationship between child anthropometry and mortality in developing countries: implications for policy, programs and future research, *J Nutr* 123(10 suppl):2047S-2081S, 1994.
119. Hendricks KM et al: Malnutrition in hospitalized pediatric patients: current prevalence, *Arch Pediatr Adolesc Med* 149(10):1118-1122, 1995.
120. Ogumkeye OO, Ighogboja IS: Increase in total serum triglyceride and phospholipids in kwashiorkor, *Ann Trop Pediatr* 12(4):463-466, 1992.
121. Kello AB, Gilbert C: Causes of severe visual impairment and blindness in children in schools for the blind in Ethiopia, *Br J Opthalmol* 87(5):526-530, 2003.
122. Latham MC: The dermatosis of kwashiorkor in young children, *Semin Dermatol* 10(4):270-272, 1991.
123. Ahmed T et al: Management of severe malnutrition and diarrhea, *Indian J Pediatr* 68(1):45-51, 2001.
124. Kalra V et al: Vitamin E administration and reversal of neurological deficits in protein-energy malnutrition, *J Trop Pediatr* 47(1):39-45, 2001.
125. Shah MD: Failure to thrive in children, *J Clin Gastroenterol* 35(5):371-374, 2002.
126. Steward DK, Moser DK, Ryan-Wenger NA: Behavioral characteristics of infants with failure to thrive, *J Pediatr Nurs* 16(3):162-171, 2003.
127. Feldman R et al: Mother-child touch patterns in infant feeding disorders: relation to maternal, child, and environmental factors, *J Am Acad Child Adolesc Psychiatry* 43(9):1089-1097, 2004.
128. Krugman SD, Dubowitz H: Failure to thrive, *Am Fam Physician* 68(5):879-884, 2003.
129. Piazza CC et al: Functional analysis of inappropriate mealtime behaviors, *J Appl Behav Anal* 36(2):187-204, 2003.
130. Steward DK: Behavioral characteristics of infants with nonorganic failure to thrive during a play interaction, *MCN Am J Matern Child Nurs* 26(2):79-85, 2001.
131. Chatoor I: Feeding disorders in infants and toddlers: diagnosis and treatment, *Child Adolesc Psychiatr Clin North Am* 11(2):163-183, 2004.
132. Marino R, Weinman ML, Soudelier K: Social work intervention and failure to thrive in infants and children, *Health Soc Work* 26(2):90-97, 2001.
133. Robinson JR, Drotar D, Boutry M: Problem-solving abilities among mothers of infants with failure to thrive, *J Pediatr Psychol* 26(1):21-32, 2001.
134. Pierro A, Hall N: Surgical treatment of infants with necrotizing enterocolitis, *Semin Neonatol* 8(3):223-232, 2003.
135. Lee JS, Polin RA: Treatment and prevention of necrotizing enterocolitis, *Semin Neonatol* 8(6):449-459, 2003.
136. Maayan-Metzger A et al: Necrotizing enterocolitis in full-term infants: a case-control study and review of the literature, *J Perinatol* 24(8):494-499, 2004.
137. Noerr B: Current controversies in the understanding of necrotizing enterocolitis, *Adv Neonatal Care* 3(3):107-120, 2003.
138. Ostlie DJ: Necrotizing enterocolitis in full-term infants, *J Pediatr Surg* 38(7):1039-1042, 2003.
139. Caplan MS, Jilling T: New concepts in necrotizing enterocolitis, *Curr Opin Pediatr* 13(2):111-115, 2001.
140. Chardot C et al: Surgical necrotizing enterocolitis: are intestinal lesions more severe in infants with low birth weight? *J Pediatr Surg* 38(2):167-172, 2003.
141. Kabeer A, Gunnlaugsson S, Coren C: Neonatal necrotizing enterocolitis: a 12-year review at a county hospital, *Dis Colon Rectum* 38(8):866-872, 1995.
142. Sato TT, Oldham KT: Abdominal drain placement versus laparoscopy for necrotizing enterocolitis with perforation, *Clin Perinatol* 31(3):577-589, 2004.
143. Butter A, Flageole H, Laberge JM: The changing face of surgical indications for necrotizing enterocolitis, *J Pediatr Surg* 37(3):496-499, 2002.
144. Kato T et al: The role of intestinal transplantation in the management of babies with extensive gut resections, *J Pediatr Surg* 38(2):145-149, 2003.
145. Henry MC, Moss RL: Current issues in the management of necrotizing enterocolitis, *Semin Perinatol* 28(3):221-233, 2004.
146. Updegrove K: Necrotizing enterocolitis: the evidence for use of human milk in prevention and treatment, *J Hum Lact* 20(3):335-339, 2004.
147. Oldfield EC: *Clostridium difficile*-associated diarrhea: risk factors, diagnostic methods, and treatment, *Rev Gastroenterol Disord* 4(4):186-195, 2004.
148. Turck D et al: Incidence and risk factors of oral antibiotic-associated diarrhea in an outpatient pediatric population, *J Pediatr Gastroenterol Nutr* 37(1):22-26, 2003.
149. Lee SD, Surawicz CM: Infectious causes of chronic diarrhea, *Gastroenterol Clin North Am* 30(3):679-692, 2001.
150. Besedovsky A, Li BU: Across the developmental continuum of irritable bowel syndrome: clinical and pathophysiologic considerations, *Curr Gastroenterol Rep* 6(3):247-253, 2004.
151. Swagerty DL, Walling AD, Klein RM: Lactose intolerance, *Am Fam Physician* 65(9):1845-1850, 2002.
152. Gourley GR et al: Neonatal jaundice and diet, *Arch PediatrAdolesc Med* 153(2):184-188, 1999.
153. Iranpour R, Akbar MR, Haghshenas I: Glucose-6-phosphate dehydrogenase deficiency in neonates, *Indian J Pediatr* 70(1):855-857, 2003.
154. Wong YH, Chou YH, Lien RI: Hyperbilirubinemia in healthy neonate with glucose-6-phosphate dehydrogenase deficiency, *Early Hum Dev* 71(2):129-136, 2003.
155. Blackmon LR, Fanaroff AA, Raju TN: Research on prevention of bilirubin-induced brain injury and kernicterus: National Institute of Child Health and Human Development conference executive summary, *Pediatrics* 114(1):229-233, 2004.
156. Bhutani VK, Johnson LH: Newborn jaundice and kernicterus-health and societal perspectives, *Indian J Pediatr* 70(5)407-416, 2003.
157. Boyd S: Treatment of physiological and pathological neonatal jaundice, *Nurs Times* 100(13):40-43, 2004.
158. Kahn E: Biliary atresia revisited, *Pediatr Dev Pathol* 7(2):109-124, 2004.
159. Hendrickson RJ et al: Pediatric liver transplantation, *Curr Opin Pediatr* 16(3):309-313, 2004.
160. Lopez-Santamaria M et al: Pediatric living donor liver transplantation, *Transplant Proc* 35(5):1808-1809, 2003.
161. Armstrong GL, Bell BP: Hepatitis A virus infections in the United States: model-based estimates and implications for childhood immunizations, *Pediatrics* 109(5):839-845, 2002.
162. Muecke CJ et al: Hepatitis A seroprevalence and risk factors among day care educators, *Clin Invest Med* 27(5):259-264, 2004.
163. Jenson HB: The changing picture of hepatitis A, *Curr Opin Pediatr* 16(1):89-93, 2004.
164. Hyams KC: Risks of chronicity following acute hepatitis B virus infection: a review, *Clin Infect Dis* 20(4):992-1000, 1995.
165. Shukla NB, Poles MA: Hepatitis B virus infection: co-infection with hepatitis C virus, hepatitis D virus, and human immunodeficiency virus, *Clin Liver Dis* 8(2):445-460, 2004.
166. Myers RP, Thibault V, Poynard T: The impact of prior hepatitis B virus infection on liver histology and the response to interferon therapy on chronic hepatitis C, *J Viral Hepat* 10(2):103-110, 2003.

167. Soriano V et al: Long-term follow-up of HIV-infected persons with chronic hepatitis C virus infection treated with interferon-based therapies, *Antivir Ther* 9(6):987-992, 2004.

168. Brau N: Update on chronic hepatitis C in HIV/HCV-coinfected patients: viral interactions and therapy, *AIDS* 17(16):2279, 2003.

169. Kobak GE et al: Interferon treatment for chronic hepatitis B: enhanced response in children 5 years old or younger, *J Pediatr* 145(3):340-345, 2004.

170. Jacobson KR et al: An analysis of published trials of interferon monotherapy in children with chronic hepatitis C, *J Pediatr Gastroenterol Nutr* 34(1):52-58, 2001.

171. Sokucu S et al: Long-term outcomes after sclerotherapy with or without a beta blocker for variceal bleeding in children, *Pediatr Int* 45(4):388-394, 2003.

172. Ryckman FC, Alonso MH: Causes and management of portal hypertension in the pediatric population, *Clin Liver Dis* 5(3):789-818, 2001.

173. Rossle M, Grandt D: TIPS: an update, *Best Pract Res Clin Gastroenterol* 18(1):99-123, 2004.

174. Schweitzer-Krantz S: Early diagnosis of inherited metabolic disorders towards improving outcome: the controversial issue of galactosaemia, *Eur J Pediatr* 162(Supp 1):S50-S53, 2003.

175. El-Youssef M: Wilson disease, *Mayo Clin Proc* 78(9):1126-1136, 2003.

176. Brewer GJ: Recognition, diagnosis, and management of Wilson disease, *Proc Soc Exp Biol Med* 233(1):39-46, 2000.

177. Ferenci P: Pathophysiology and clinical features of Wilson disease, *Metab Brain Dis* 19(3-4):229-239, 2004.

178. Stremmel W et al: Wilson disease: clinical presentation, treatment, and survival, *Ann Intern Med* 115(9):720-726, 1991.

179. Ala A, Schilsky ML: Wilson disease: pathophysiology, diagnosis, treatment, and screening, *Clin Liver Dis* 8(4):787-805, 2004.

180. Leggio L et al: Wilson disease: clinical, genetic and pharmacological findings, *Int J Immunopathol Pharmacol* 18(1):7-14, 2005.

STRUCTURE AND FUNCTION OF THE MUSCULOSKELETAL SYSTEM

CHRISTY L. CROWTHER

The way an individual functions in daily life, moves about, or manipulates objects physically depends on the integrity of the musculoskeletal system. The musculoskeletal system is actually composed of two systems: (1) the skeleton proper, which is composed of bones and joints, and (2) skeletal muscles. Each of the systems contributes to mobility. The skeleton supports the body and provides leverage to the skeletal muscles so that movement of various parts of the body is possible. Movement of the various body parts is accomplished by contraction of the skeletal muscles and bending or rotation at the joints.

STRUCTURE AND FUNCTION OF BONES

Bones give form to the body, support tissues, and permit movement by providing points of attachment for muscles. Many bones meet in movable joints that determine the type and extent of movement possible. Bones also protect many of the body's vital organs. For example, the bones of the skull, thorax, and pelvis are hard exterior shields that protect the brain, heart, lungs, and reproductive and urinary organs.

The marrow cavities within certain bones serve as sites of blood cell formation. In adults, blood cells originate exclu-

sively in the marrow cavities of the skull, vertebrae, ribs, sternum, shoulders, and pelvis. Bones also have a crucial role in mineral homeostasis, storing minerals (i.e., calcium, phosphate, carbonate, magnesium) that are essential for the proper working of many delicate cellular mechanisms.

Elements of Bone Tissue

Mature bone is a rigid connective tissue consisting of cells, fibers, a gelatinous material termed **ground substance,** and large amounts of crystallized minerals, mainly calcium, that give bone its rigidity. The structural elements of bone are summarized in Table 41-1.

Bone cells enable bone to grow, repair itself, change shape, and continuously synthesize new bone tissue and resorb (dissolve or digest) old tissue. The fibers in bone are made of collagen, which gives bone its tensile strength (the ability to hold itself together). Ground substance acts as a medium for the diffusion of nutrients, oxygen, metabolic wastes, biochemicals, and minerals between bone tissue and blood vessels.

Bone formation begins during fetal life as mesenchymal cells differentiate into chondrocytes (cartilage) or osteoblasts (bone). In mature bone the formation of new tissue begins with the production of an organic matrix by the bone cells. This **bone matrix** consists of ground substances, collagen, and other proteins (see Table 41-1) that take part in bone formation and maintenance.

Table 41-1	Structural Elements of Bone
Structural Element	**Function**
Bone Cells	
Osteoblasts	Synthesize collagen and proteoglycans; stimulate bone formation and are also involved in some osteoclast resorptive activity
Osteocytes	Maintain bone matrix
Osteoclasts	Resorb bone; assist with mineral homeostasis
Bone Matrix	
Collagen fibers	Lend support and tensile strength
Proteoglycans	Control transport of ionized materials through matrix
Bone morphogenic proteins*	Induce cartilage and bone formation
BMP-2	Induces osteoblast differentiation in mesenchymal stem cells
BMP-6	Accelerates bone repair
BMP-9	Induces osteogenesis in mature osteoblasts
Glycoproteins	
Sialoprotein	Promotes calcification
Osteocalcin	Inhibit calcium-phosphate precipitation; promotes bone resorption
Laminin	Stabilizes basement membranes in bones
Osteonectin	Binds calcium in bones
Albumin	Transports essential elements to matrix; maintains osmotic pressure of bone fluid
α-Glycoprotein	Promotes calcification
Minerals (elements)	
Calcium	Crystallizes to lend rigidity and compressive strength
Phosphate	Regulates vitamin D and thereby promotes mineralizaton

*Data from Cheng H et al: *J Bone Joint Surg Am* 85-A(8):1544-1552, 2003.

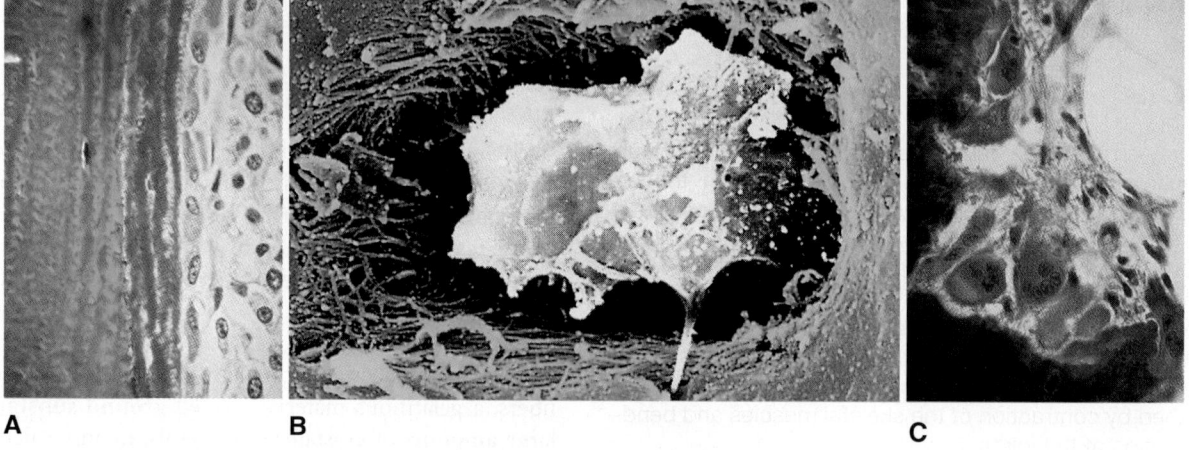

A   B   C

Figure 41-1 **Bone cells. A,** Osteoblasts are responsible for the production of collagenous and noncollagenous proteins that compose osteoid. Active osteoblasts are lined up on the osteoid. Note the eccentrically located nuclei. **B,** Osteocyte. Scanning electron micrograph showing an osteocyte within a lacuna. The cell is surrounded by collagen fibers and mineralized bone. **C,** Osteoclasts actively resorb mineralized tissue. The scalloped surface in which the multinucleated osteoclasts rest is termed the *Howship lacuna.* (**A** and **C,** From Damjanov I, Linder J, editors: *Anderson's pathology,* ed 10, St Louis, 1996, Mosby. **B** From Erlandsen S, Magney J: *Color atlas of histology,* St Louis, 1992, Mosby.)

The next step in bone formation is **calcification,** when minerals are deposited and crystallize. Minerals bind tightly to collagen fibers, producing tensile and compressional strength in bone, and withstand pressure and weight bearing to bone.

Bone Cells

Bone contains three types of cells: osteoblasts, osteocytes, and osteoclasts (Figure 41-1). Osteoblasts are the bone-forming cells. Their primary function is to lay down new bone. Once this function is complete, osteoblasts become osteocytes. Osteocytes are osteoblasts that have become imprisoned within the mineralized bone matrix. They help maintain bone by synthesizing new bone matrix molecules.[1] Osteoclasts function primarily to resorb (remove) bone during the process of growth and repair.

Osteoblasts

Osteoblasts are cells derived from mesenchymal stem cells that produce type I collagen, are responsive to parathyroid hormone (PTH) and produce osteocalcin when stimulated by 1,25-dihydroxyvitamin D. Osteoblasts are active on the outer surface of bones, where they form a single layer of cells. They bring about the formation of new bone by their synthesis of **osteoid** (nonmineralized bone matrix). The mechanism of osteoblast stimulation is reported to be the production of so-called coupling factors generated during the resorption process. Osteoblasts bring about the formation of new bone and the orderly mineralization of bone matrix by concentrating some of the plasma proteins (growth factors) found in the bone matrix and by facilitating the deposit and exchange of calcium and other ions at the site. Osteoblasts alter levels of receptor activator of nuclear factor κB-ligand (**RANKL**) and osteoprotegrin (OPG). The balance of these two cytokines determines overall osteoclast formation[2] (see Figure 42-11). RANKL is part of a ligand-receptor system that assists in regulating osteoclastic bone remodeling. As new bone is formed, it is shaped and remodeled through the effects of transforming growth factor-beta (TGF-β), as well as other plasma proteins (growth factors) found in the bone marrow (Table 41-2).

The concept of coupling bone formation with bone resorption has been extensively studied yet is still not entirely clear. Studies have shown that osteoblasts release factors that induce osteoclastic activity by stimulating osteoclasts to remove nonmineralized organic material from bone surfaces, exposing resorption-inducing bone mineral to osteoclastic contact. In contact with bone mineral, osteoclasts can be further stimulated by colony-stimulating factor and interleukins-1, -11, -15, -17, and tumor necrosis factor-alpha (TNF-α) produced by macrophage cells in the presence of PTH. Thus the cells of the osteoblastic lineage (osteoblasts and osteocytes) form a network of cells in bone that sense the shape and structure of bone and determine where it is appropriate that bone be formed or resorbed, according to Wolfe's law (bone is shaped according to its function).

Osteoblasts have an active state and a resting state. When active, osteoblasts synthesize and secrete osteoid. When in the resting state, they appear dormant. If appropriately stimulated, however, the resting osteoblasts are capable of resuming activity.

Osteocytes

An **osteocyte** is a transformed osteoblast that is trapped or surrounded in osteoid as it hardens from minerals that enter during calcification (see Figure 41-1, *B*). It is the final differentiation stage for an osteoblast. The osteocyte is within a space in the hardened bone matrix called a **lacuna.** Each osteocyte has a higher nucleus/cytoplasm ratio with a thin layer of nonmineralized osteoid around it, similar to the egg white surrounding an egg yolk.

The function of osteocytes is not fully known, but they do synthesize certain matrix molecules assisting bone calcification. They also help concentrate nutrients in the matrix. Osteocytes obtain nutrients from capillaries in the canaliculi, which contain nutrient-rich fluids. Osteocytes also may help synthesize and replace needed elements of the matrix, thus helping to maintain mineral homeostasis with the help of the PTH and osteoblast cells. Through exchanges between these cells, hormone catalysts, and minerals, optimal levels of calcium, phosphorus, and other minerals are maintained in blood plasma. The osteocyte also aids in modifying bone matrix through release of enzymes to dissolve the mineralized walls of the lacunae to prepare the bone for remodeling. Remodeling is described on p. 1477.

Osteoclasts

Osteoclasts are the major resorptive cells of bone. They are large, multinucleated cells with a short life span. Osteoclasts develop from the hematopoietic stem cell in the bone marrow stroma[2] and adjacent vessels and from mononuclear phagocytic cells. Osteoclasts contain lysosomes (digestive vacuoles) filled with hydrolytic enzymes. Fine projections, or mi-

Table 41-2	Effects of Selected Cytokines (Growth Factors) on Skeletal Tissues			
Cytokine (Growth Factor)		Target Tissue	Formation	Resorption
Transforming growth factor–beta		Bone	+, −	+, −
		Cartilage	+, −	−
Transforming growth factor–alpha or epidermal growth factor		Bone	+, −	+
		Cartilage	+	
Insulin-like growth factor		Bone	−	0
		Cartilage	−	?
Fibroblast growth factor		Bone	+, −	0
		Cartilage		?
Platelet-derived growth factor		Bone	+	0
Colony-stimulating factors		Bone	0	+
		Cartilage	?	?
Interferon-gamma		Bone	−	−
		Cartilage	−	?
Tumor necrosis factor		Bone	−	+
		Cartilage	−	+
Interleukin-1, -3, and -6		Bone	+, −	+
		Cartilage	−	+

+, −: Both stimulatory and inhibitory properties on the specific cell listed; 0: no effects presently known; ?: possible effects on cell listed.

crovilli, fan out from the osteoclast cell's surface and are known as **ruffled borders;** these projections result from extensive infoldings of the cell membrane adjacent to the resorptive surface.[3] Osteoclasts in regions of bone resorption lie in pits called *Howship lacunae*, where the infolded, ruffled borders of the osteoclasts greatly increase the surface area of the plasma membrane. The infolds end in numerous channels and vesicles in the cell cytoplasm, permitting them to resorb the bone under their ruffled, infolded borders.

Osteoclasts bind to the bone surface of cell attachment proteins called **integrins.**[3] They bring about resorption of bone by secretion of citric and lactic acids, which help dissolve bone minerals, and collagenase, which aids in digesting collagen, along with the action of cytokines (see Table 41-2). Matrix metalloproteinases (MMPs), a group of proteolytic enzymes, help control osteoclast-matrix interactions necessary for bone resorption.[4] Once resorption is completed, the osteoclast disappears by degeneration, either by reverting back to its parent cell or by leaving the site through the process of cell mobility, wherein the osteoclast then becomes an inactive, or "resting," osteoclast.

Bone Matrix

Bone matrix is made of the extracellular elements of bone tissue, composed of about 35% organic and 65% inorganic materials. The major organic components are collagen fibers, and the major inorganic components are the calcium and phosphate minerals. Other parts of the bone matrix are the proteins, carbohydrate-protein complexes, and ground substances. Water makes up 5% to 8% of the matrix.

Collagen Fibers

Collagen fibers make up the major organic component of bone matrix. The fibers are approximately 90% type I collagen, which is synthesized and secreted by osteoblasts. Once secreted, the collagen molecules assemble into thin chains called *alpha chains,* which combine in threes to form **fibrils.** The fibrils form a staggered pattern, overlapping nearby fibrils by approximately one fourth their length. This staggered, overlapping pattern creates regular gaps, called *hole zones,* into which mineral crystals are deposited. After mineral deposition the fibrils link together and twist to form ropelike fibers. Collagen fibers then join to form a framework that gives bone its tensile strength and enables it to bear weight.

Collagen is the most abundant macromolecule in the body, accounting for approximately one third of all protein and providing the structural framework for nearly all tissues. Collagen is one of the extracellular components, along with proteoglycans and noncollagenous matrix proteins, of articular cartilage. To date, 14 different types of collagen have been identified. Cartilage-specific collagens include types II (the principal component), VI, IX, X, and XI. Type IX collagen is thought to be the "glue" that holds together the type II collagen scaffold of articular cartilage, helps maintain the structural integrity of cartilage, and resists tensile forces on the joint cartilage. Type XI regulates the fibril diameter of type II cartilage. Degradation of type IX collagen by proteolytic enzymes has been seen in the early stages of osteoarthritis and rheumatoid arthritis. Researchers have proposed that this degradation, or "unplugging," may be the mechanism for the degenerative changes seen in osteoarthritic and rheumatoid cartilage. Table 41-3 gives the musculoskeletal distribution of other types of collagen.

Proteoglycans

Proteoglycans are large complexes of numerous polysaccharides attached to a common protein core. Hyaline cartilage is primarily composed of the glycosaminoglycans chondroitin sulfate and keratin sulfate.[5] They strengthen bone by forming compression-resistant networks between the collagen fibrils. Proteoglycans also control the transport and distribution of electrically charged particles (ions), particularly calcium, through the bone matrix, thereby playing a role in bone calcium deposition and calcification.

Glycoproteins

Glycoproteins are also carbohydrate-protein complexes of bone. Glycoproteins control the collagen interactions that lead to fibril formation. They also may play a role in calcification.

Some of the glycoproteins in bone matrix include bone sialoprotein, osteocalcin, osteonectin, laminin, albumin, and α-glycoprotein. Other proteins recently found in bone matrix are the compounds currently called **bone morphogenic proteins (BMPs)** (see Table 41-1). **Sialoprotein (osteopontin)** makes up about 8% of the noncollagenous matrix of bone and easily binds with calcium.

Osteocalcin is also a calcium-binding protein that binds preferentially to calcium that has already crystallized. The roles of osteocalcin may be to inhibit calcium phosphate precipitation and play a part in bone resorption by recruiting osteoclasts.

Osteonectin is also thought to bind calcium in bones, and laminin stabilizes basement membranes in bones. **Laminin** is an abundant bone matrix protein in humans that is most effective in neurite and axon growth.[3]

Table 41-3	Types of Collagen in Musculoskeletal Tissues
Type of Collagen*	**Distribution in Musculoskeletal Tissues**
I	Bone, tendon, ligament, intervertebral disk
II	Cartilage, intervertebral disk
IV	Basement cell membrane
V	Codistributed with type I
VI	Ubiquitous
IX	Codistributed with type II
X	Cartilage growth plate
XI	Cartilage
XII	Codistributed with type I
XIII	Molecule has not been isolated in connective tissues to date
XIV	Codistributed with type I

*To date, 14 different types of collagen have been identified.

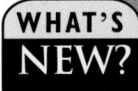

WHAT'S NEW?

Growth Factors: New Management Tools for Bones

Bone morphogenic proteins (BMPs), part of the transforming growth factor-beta (TGF-β) cytokines, are powerful inducers of bone formation. Use of BMPs is becoming more important in treating and filling in bone defects resulting from fracture, surgery, and periodontal disease and may aid in preventing osteoporosis.

Data from Cheng H et al:, *J Bone Joint Surg-Am* 85-A(8):1544, 2003; Sykaras N, Opperman LA: *J Oral Sci* 45(2):57-73, 2003.

Table 41-4	Sequence of Calcium and Phosphate Compound Formation and Crystallization	
Formula	Name	Abbreviation
$Ca(HPO_4) \cdot 2H_2O$	Dicalcium phosphate dihydrate	DCPD
$Ca_4H(PO_4)_3$	Octacalcium phosphate	OCP
$Ca_9(PO_4)_6$ (var.)	Amorphous calcium phosphate	ACP
$Ca_3(PO_4)_2$	Tricalcium phosphate	TCP
$Ca_5(PO_4)_3OH$	Hydroxyapatite	HAP

NOTE: Compounds are listed in the order in which precipitation and crystal formation occur.

Bone albumin is identical to serum albumin (see Chapter 25). In calcified matrix, bone albumin is permanently fixed to bone mineral crystals and remains so until the bone is resorbed. Researchers believe bone albumin transports essential elements such as hormones, ions, and other metabolites to and from the bone cells and maintains the osmotic pressure of **bone fluid** (fluid surrounding mineral crystals and osteoblasts).

α-Glycoprotein is thought to be synthesized in the liver, to be released into blood plasma, and to circulate to bone matrix, where it accumulates. α-Glycoprotein's affinity for calcium is 40 times greater than that of albumin. Therefore it probably plays an important role in the calcification of growing bone. α-Glycoprotein also may facilitate bone resorption by activating osteoclasts.

Bone Minerals

Mineralization is the final step in bone formation, after collagen synthesis and fiber formation. Mineralization has two distinct phases: (1) formation of the initial mineral deposit (initiation), and (2) proliferation or accretion of additional mineral crystals on the initial mineral deposits (growth).[3] The majority of the mineral content in the body is an analog of the naturally occurring mineral *hydroxyapatite.*

Table 41-4 lists the sequence in which calcium and phosphate form amorphous (fluid) calcium phosphate compounds that are converted, in stages, to solid hexagonal crystals of **hydroxyapatite (HAP).** As the calcium and phosphorus concentrations increase in the bone matrix, the first precipitate to form is dicalcium phosphate dihydrate (DCPD). Once DCPD precipitation begins, the remaining phases of bone crystal formation proceed until insoluble HAP is produced, with approximately 80% to 90% of the HAP being incorporated into the collagen fibers. Amorphous calcium phosphate is distributed throughout the bone matrix.

Types of Bone Tissue

Bone is made up of two types of bony (osseous) tissue: **compact bone (cortical bone)** and **spongy bone (cancellous bone)** (Figure 41-2). Compact bone makes up approximately 85% of the skeleton; spongy bone makes up the remaining 15%. Both types of bone tissue contain the same structural elements, and,

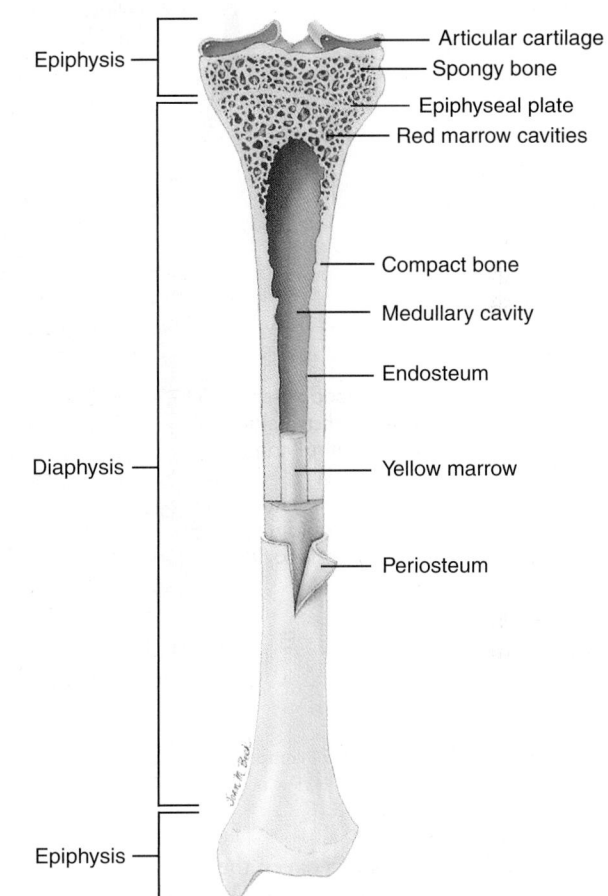

Figure 41-2 Cross section of bone. Longitudinal section of long bone (tibia) showing cancellous and compact bone. (From Thibodeau GA, Patton KT: *Anatomy & physiology,* ed 5, St Louis, 2003, Mosby.)

with a few exceptions, both compact tissue and spongy tissue are present in every bone. The major difference between the two types of tissue is the organization of the elements.

Compact bone is highly organized, solid, and extremely strong. The basic structural unit in compact bone is the haversian system (Figure 41-3). Each **haversian system** is made up of the following:

1. A central canal called the **haversian canal**
2. Concentric layers of bone matrix called **lamellae**

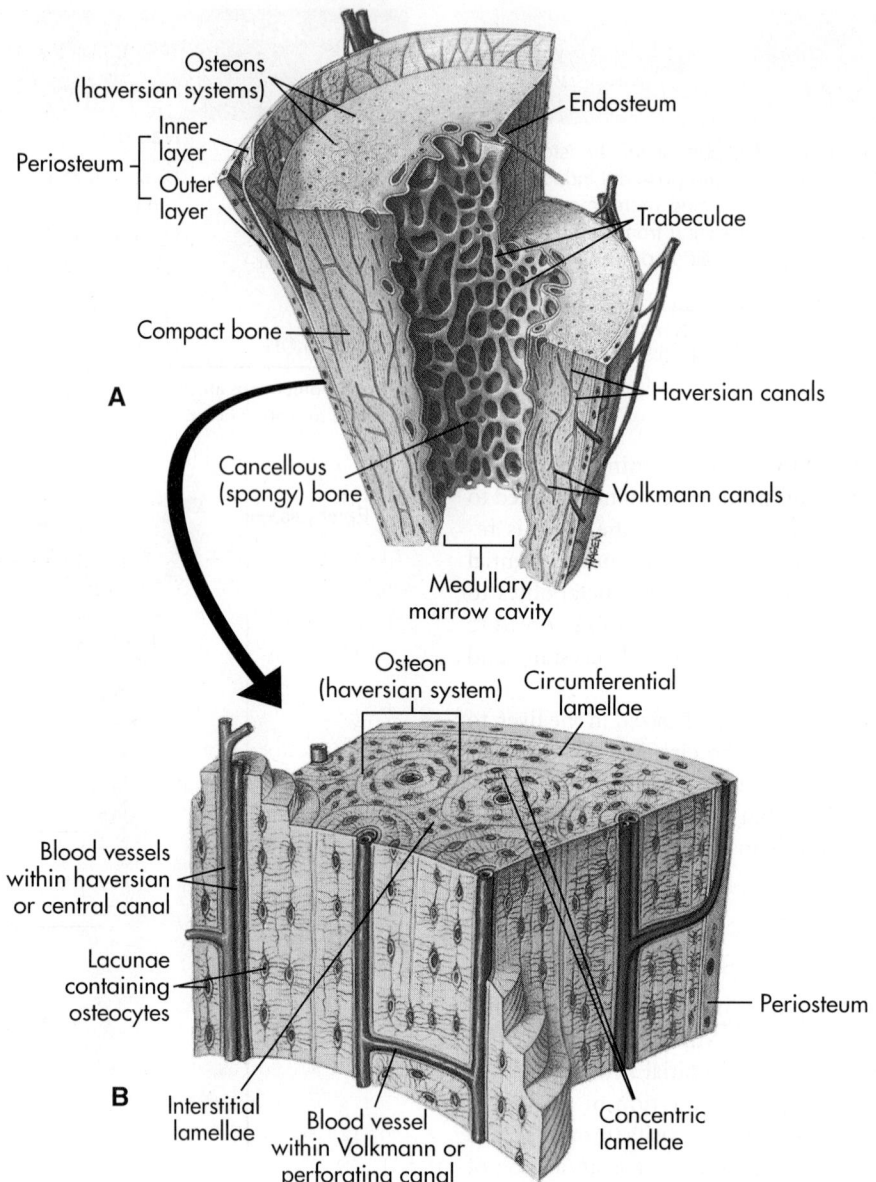

Figure 41-3 Structure of compact and cancellous bone. **A,** Longitudinal section of a long bone showing both cancellous and compact bone. **B,** A magnified view of compact bone. (From Thibodeau GA, Patton KT: *Anatomy & physiology,* ed 5, St Louis, 2003, Mosby.)

3. Tiny spaces (lacunae) between the lamellae
4. Bone cells (osteocytes) within the lacunae
5. Small channels or canals called **canaliculi**

Each haversian system is a separate cylindrical entity that looks like a set of concentric rings. In the center of the haversian system is the haversian canal. The haversian canal runs through the long axis of bone and contains one or two blood vessels and nerve fibers. The blood vessels in the canal communicate with blood vessels in the periosteum (surface cover) and marrow cavity to transport nutrients and wastes to and from the osteocytes contained within the lacunae. Surrounding each haversian canal are the concentric lamellae. Between the lamellae are the lacunae, each of which contains one osteocyte. The lacunae are connected to each other and to the haversian canal by the canaliculi, which run parallel to the

horizontal axis of the bone. Each canaliculus encloses a small extension (cytoplasmic process) from the osteocyte contained in the lacuna.

Spongy bone is less complex and lacks haversian systems. In spongy bone the lamellae are not arranged in concentric layers but in plates or bars termed **trabeculae** that branch and unite with one another to form an irregular meshwork. The pattern of the meshwork is determined by the direction of stress on the particular bone. The spaces between the trabeculae are filled with red bone marrow. The osteocyte-containing lacunae are distributed between the trabeculae and interconnected by canaliculi. Capillaries pass through the marrow to nourish the osteocytes.

All bones are covered with a double-layered connective tissue called the **periosteum.** The outer layer of the periosteum contains blood vessels and nerves, some of which penetrate to the inner structures of the bone through channels called Volkmann canals (see Figure 41-3). The inner layer of the periosteum is anchored to the bone by collagenous fibers (Sharpey fibers) that penetrate the bone. Sharpey fibers also help hold or attach tendons and ligaments to the periosteum of bones.[3]

Characteristics of Bone

The human skeleton consists of 206 bones, which constitute the axial skeleton and the appendicular skeleton (Figure 41-4). The **axial skeleton** consists of 80 bones that make up

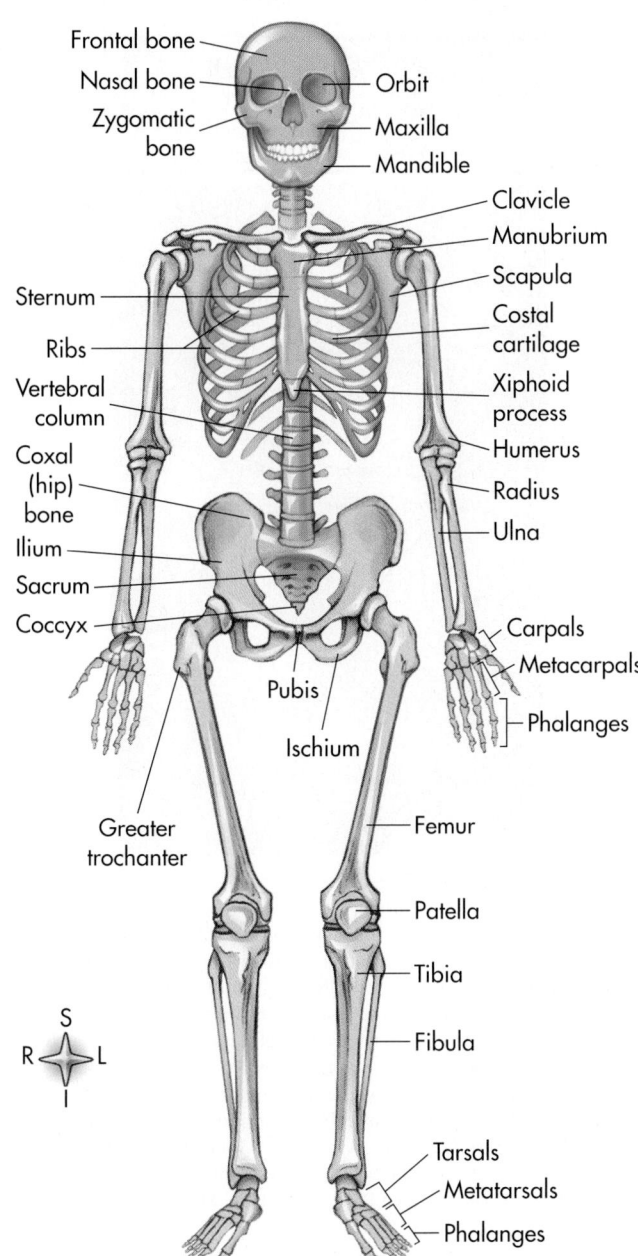

Frontal bone
Nasal bone
Zygomatic bone
Orbit
Maxilla
Mandible
Clavicle
Manubrium
Scapula
Costal cartilage
Xiphoid process
Humerus
Radius
Ulna
Carpals
Metacarpals
Phalanges
Sternum
Ribs
Vertebral column
Coxal (hip) bone
Ilium
Sacrum
Coccyx
Pubis
Ischium
Greater trochanter
Femur
Patella
Tibia
Fibula
Tarsals
Metatarsals
Phalanges

S
R   L
I

Figure 41-4 **Anterior view of skeleton.** Axial skeleton in blue; appendicular skeleton in tan. (From Thibodeau GA, Patton KT: *Anatomy & physiology,* ed 5, St. Louis, 2003, Mosby.)

the skull, vertebral column, and thorax. The **appendicular skeleton** consists of 126 bones that make up the upper and lower extremities, the shoulder girdle (pectoral girdle), and the pelvic girdle. The skeleton contributes about 14% of the weight of the adult body.

Bones can be classified by shape as long, flat, short (cuboidal), or irregular. **Long bones** are longer than they are wide and consist of a narrow tubular midportion (**diaphysis**) that merges into a broader neck (**metaphysis**) and a broad end (**epiphysis**) (see Figure 41-2).

The diaphysis consists of a shaft of thick, rigid compact bone that can tolerate bending forces. Contained within the diaphysis is the elongated marrow (medullary) cavity. The marrow cavity of the diaphysis contains primarily fatty tissue, which is referred to as *yellow marrow.* The yellow marrow assists red bone marrow in hematopoiesis only during times of stress. The yellow marrow cavity of the diaphysis is continuous with marrow cavities in the spongy bone of the metaphysis and diaphysis. The marrow contained within the epiphysis is red because it contains primarily blood-forming tissue (see Chapter 25). A layer of connective tissue, the **endosteum,** lines the outer surfaces of both types of marrow cavity.

The broadness of the epiphysis allows weight bearing to be distributed over a wide area. The epiphysis is made up of spongy bone covered by a very thin layer of compact bone. In a child the epiphysis is separated from the metaphysis by a cartilaginous **growth plate,** the **epiphyseal plate.** After puberty the epiphyseal plate calcifies and the epiphysis and metaphysis merge. By adulthood the line of demarcation between the epiphysis and metaphysis is undetectable.

In **flat bones,** such as the ribs or scapulae, two plates of compact bone are roughly parallel to each other. Between the compact bone plates is a layer of spongy bone. **Short bones (cuboidal bones),** such as the bones of the wrist or ankle, are often cuboidal in shape. They consist of spongy bone covered by a thin layer of compact bone.

Irregular bones, such as the vertebrae, mandibles, or other facial bones, have various shapes that include thin and thick segments. The thin part of an irregular bone consists of two plates of compact bone with spongy bone between the plates. The thick part consists of spongy bone surrounded by a layer of compact bone.

Maintenance of Bone Integrity
Remodeling

The internal structure of bone is maintained by **remodeling,** a three-phase process in which existing bone is resorbed and new bone is laid down to replace it. Remodeling is carried out by clusters of bone cells termed **bone-remodeling units.** The bone remodeling units are made up of bone precursor cells that differentiate into osteoclasts and osteoblasts. Precursor cells are located on the free surfaces of bones and along the vascular channels (especially the marrow cavities).

In phase 1 (activation) of the remodeling cycle, a stimulus (e.g., hormone, drug, vitamin, physical stressor) activates the bone cell precursors in a localized area of bone to form osteoclasts. In phase 2 (resorption), the osteoclasts form a "cutting cone," which gradually resorbs bone, leaving behind an elongated cavity termed a *resorption cavity.* The resorption cavity in compact bone follows the longitudinal axis of the haversian system, and the resorption cavity in spongy bone parallels the surface of the trabeculae.

Phase 3 (formation) is the laying down of new bone, termed *secondary bone,* by osteoblasts lining the walls of the resorption cavity. Successive layers (lamellae) in compact bone are laid down until the resorption cavity is reduced to a narrow haversian canal around a blood vessel. In this way, old haversian systems are destroyed and new haversian systems are formed. New trabeculae are formed in spongy bone. The entire process of remodeling takes about 3 to 4 months.

Repair

The remodeling process can repair microscopic bone injuries, but gross injuries, such as fractures and surgical wounds (osteotomies), heal by the same stages as soft tissue injuries, except that new bone, instead of scar tissue, is the final result (see Chapter 6). In bone the stages of wound healing are as follows:

1. *Hematoma formation:* occurs if vessels have been damaged, causing hemorrhage. Fibrin and platelets within the hematoma form a meshwork that is the initial framework for healing with the help of hematopoietic growth factors such as platelet-derived growth factor and TGF-β (see Table 41-2).

2. *Procallus formation:* fibroblasts, capillary buds, and osteoblasts move into the wound to produce granulation tissue called **procallus.** Cartilage is formed as a precursor of bone, and types I, II, and III collagen are formed. Enzymes and growth factors, such as insulin and insulin-like growth factors, plus bone morphogenic protein and osteogenin, aid in this stage of healing.

3. *Callus formation:* osteoblasts in the procallus form membranous or **woven bone (callus).** Enzymes increase the phosphate content and permit the phosphate to join with calcium to be deposited as mineral to harden the callus.

4. *Callus replacement:* osteoblasts continue to replace the callus with lamellar bone or trabecular bone (Figure 41-5).

5. *Remodeling:* the periosteal and endosteal surfaces of the bone are remodeled to the size and shape of the bone before injury. Synthesis of other types of collagen recedes in favor of type I, which is the collagen found in bone. This final stage of healing, or remodeling, is vital because bone that has not been remodeled does not have good mechanical properties for weight bearing and mobility.

The speed with which bone heals depends on the severity of the bone disruption; the type and amount of bone tissue that must be replaced (spongy bone heals faster); blood supply and oxygen to the site; presence of growth and thyroid hormones, insulin, vitamins, and other nutrients; presence of systemic disease; effects of aging; and effective treatment, including immobilization and the prevention of complications

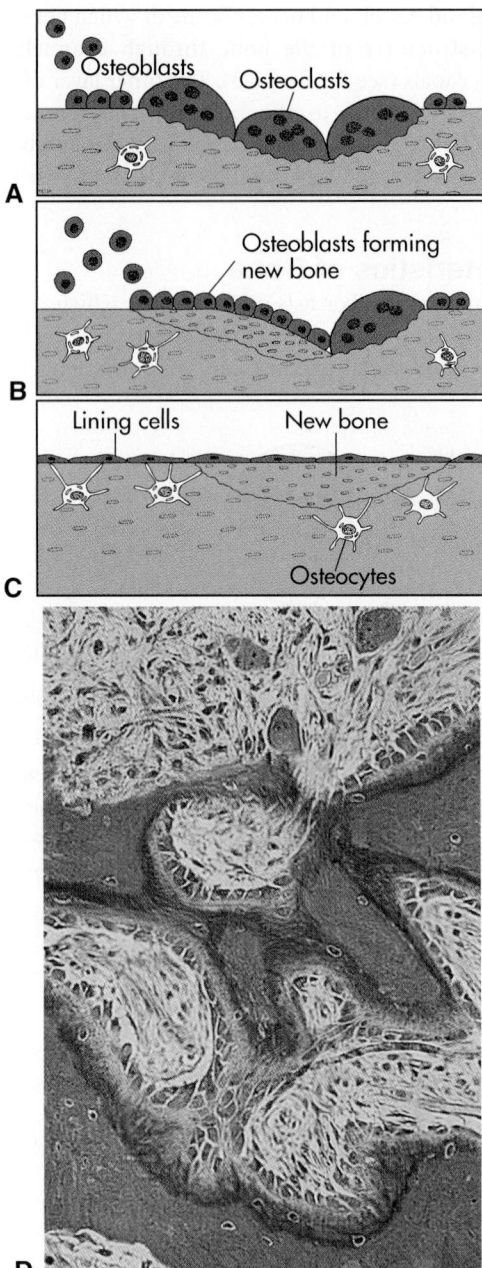

Figure 41-5 Bone remodeling. In the remodeling sequence, bone sections are removed by the bone-resorbing cells (osteoclasts) and replaced with a new section laid down by bone-forming cells (osteoblasts). The cells work in response to signals generated in that environment. The first phase of remodeling is mediated only by the multinucleated osteoclastic cells. They are activated, scoop out bone (**A**), and resorb it; then the work of the osteoblasts begins (**B**). They form new bone that replaces bone removed by the resorption process (**C**). The sequence takes 4 to 5 months. **D,** Active bone remodeling seen in the settings of primary or secondary hyperparathyroidism. Note the active osteoblasts surmounted on red-stained osteoid. Marrow fibrosis is present. (**A** to **C,** From Mundy GR: *Bone remodeling and its disorders,* St Louis, 1995, Mosby. **D,** From Damjanov I, Linder J, editors: *Anderson's pathology,* ed 10, St Louis, 1996, Mosby.)

such as infection. In general, however, hematoma formation occurs within hours of fracture or surgery; formation of pro-callus by osteoblasts occurs within days; callus formation occurs within weeks; and replacement and contour modeling occur within years—up to 4 years in some cases.

STRUCTURE AND FUNCTION OF JOINTS

The site where two or more bones meet is called a **joint (articulation)** (Figure 41-6). The primary function of joints is to provide stability and mobility to the skeleton. Whether a joint provides stability or mobility depends on its location and its structure. Generally, joints that stabilize the skeleton have a simpler structure than those that enable the skeleton to move. Most joints provide both stability and mobility to some degree (Figure 41-7).

Joints are classified based on the degree of movement they permit or on the connecting tissues that hold them together. Based on movement, a joint is classified as a **synarthrosis (immovable joint),** an **amphiarthrosis (slightly movable joint),** or a **diarthrosis (freely movable joint).** On the basis of connective structures, joints are classified broadly as fibrous, cartilaginous, and synovial. Each of these three structural classifications can be subdivided according to the shape and contour of the articulating surfaces (ends) of the bones and the type of motion the joint permits.

Fibrous Joints

A joint in which bone is united directly to bone by fibrous connective tissue is called a **fibrous joint.** Generally, fibrous joints are synarthroses (immovable), but many fibrous joints

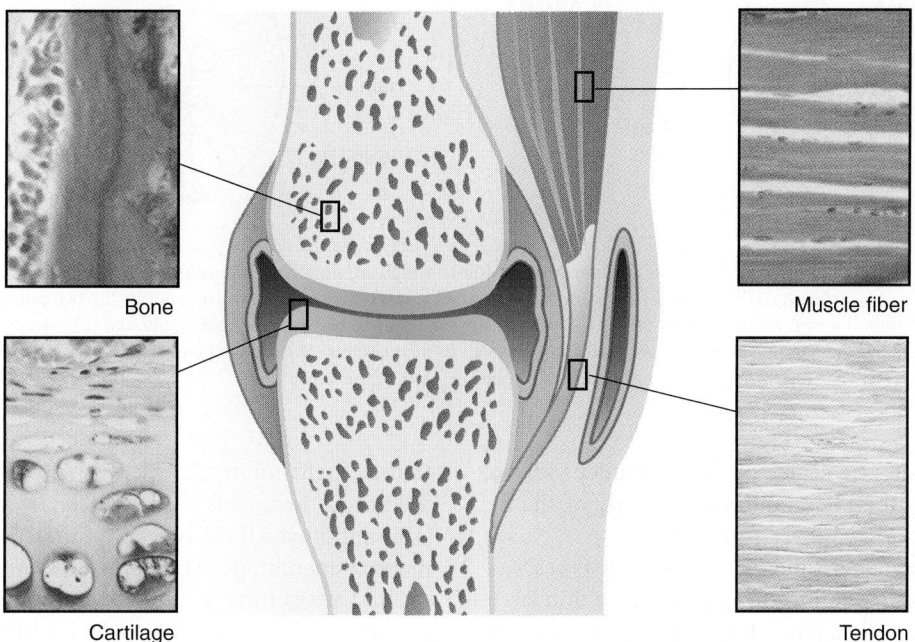

Bone

Cartilage

Muscle fiber

Tendon

Figure 41-6 **Main tissues of a joint.** (Micrographs from Erlandsen SL, Magney JE: *Color atlas of histology,* St Louis, 1992, Mosby.)

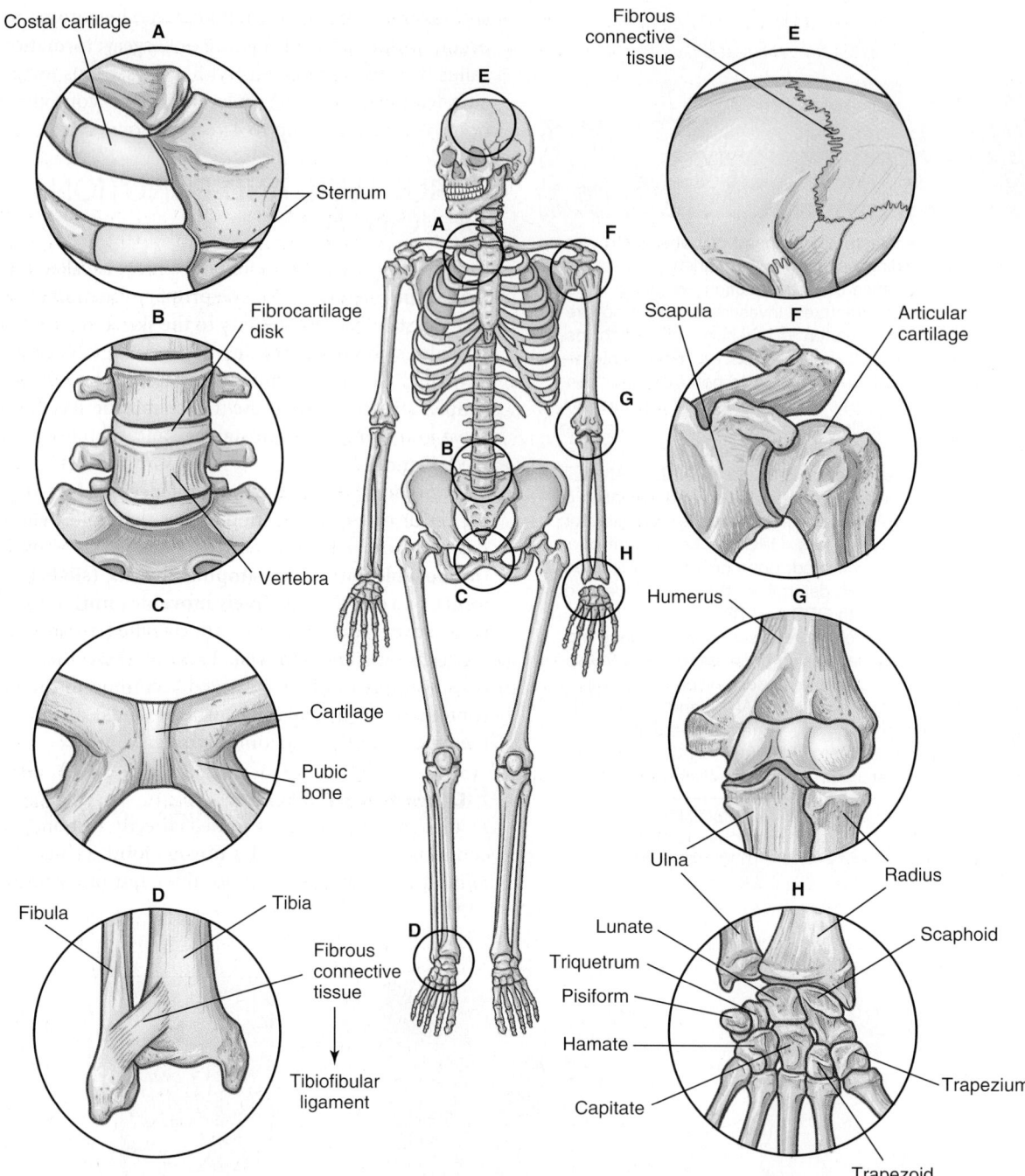

Figure 41-7 Types of joints. Cartilaginous (amphiarthrodial) joints, which are slightly movable, include (**A**) a synchondrosis that attaches ribs to costal cartilage; (**B**) a symphysis that connects vertebrae; and (**C**) the symphysis that connects the two pubic bones. Fibrous (synarthrodial) joints, which are immovable, include (**D**) the syndesmosis between the tibia and fibula; (**E**) sutures that connect the skull bones; and the gomphosis (not shown), which holds teeth in their sockets. The synovial joints include (**F**) the spheroid type at the shoulder; (**G**) the hinge type at the elbow; and (**H**) the gliding joints of the hand.

allow some movement. The degree of movement depends on the distance between the bones and the flexibility of the fibrous connective tissue.

Fibrous joints are further subdivided into three types: sutures, syndesmoses, and gomphoses. A **suture** has a thin layer of dense fibrous tissue that binds together interlocking flat bones in the skulls of young children. Sutures form an ex-

tremely tight union that permits no motion. By adulthood the fibrous tissue has been replaced by bone. A **syndesmosis** is a joint in which the two bony surfaces are united by a ligament or membrane. The fibers of ligaments are flexible and stretch, permitting a limited amount of movement. The paired bones of the lower arm (radius and ulna) and the lower leg (tibia and fibula) and their ligaments are syndesmotic joints. A **gomphosis** is a special type of fibrous joint in which a conical projection fits into a complementary socket and is held there by a ligament. The teeth held in the maxilla or mandible are gomphosis joints.

Cartilaginous Joints

The two types of cartilaginous joints are symphyses and synchondroses. A **symphysis** is a cartilaginous joint in which bones are united by a pad or disk of fibrocartilage. The articulating surfaces of the two bones are usually covered by a thin layer of hyaline cartilage, and the thick pad of fibrocartilage acts as a shock absorber and stabilizer. Examples of symphyses are the symphysis pubis, which joins the two pubic bones, and the intervertebral disks, which join the bodies of the vertebrae. A **synchondrosis** is a joint in which hyaline cartilage, rather than fibrocartilage, connects the two bones. The joints between the ribs and the sternum are synchondroses. The hyaline cartilage of these joints is called *costal cartilage.* Slight movement at the synchondroses between the ribs and the sternum allows the chest to move outward and upward during breathing.

Synovial Joints
Structure

Synovial joints (diarthroses) are the most movable and the most complex joints in the body (Figure 41-8). A synovial joint consists of the following parts:
1. A fibrous joint capsule (articular capsule)
2. A synovial membrane that lines the inner surface of the joint capsule

3. A joint cavity (synovial cavity), a space formed by the capsule
4. Synovial fluid, which fills the joint cavity and lubricates the joint surface
5. Articular cartilage, which covers and pads the articulating bony surfaces

Joint Capsule

The fibrous **joint capsule (articular capsule)** is connective tissue that covers the ends of the bones where they meet in the joint. Sharpey fibers firmly attach the proximal and distal capsule to the periosteum and ligaments and tendons, which also reinforce the capsule. The joint capsule is made up of parallel, interlacing bundles of dense, white fibrous tissue. It is richly supplied with nerves, blood vessels, and lymphatic vessels. The nerves in and around the joint capsule are sensitive to the rate and direction of motion, compression, tension, vibration, and pain.

Synovial Membrane

The **synovial membrane (synovium)** is the smooth, delicate inner lining of the joint capsule (Figure 41-9). It lines the nonarticular portion of the synovial joint and any ligaments or tendons that traverse the joint cavity. The synovial membrane is made up of two layers—a vascular layer called the **subintima** and a thin cellular layer called the **intima.** The vascular subintima merges with the fibrous joint capsule and is composed of loose fibrous connective tissue, elastin fibers, fat cells, fibroblasts, macrophages, and mast cells. The intima consists of rows of synovial cells embedded in a fiber-free intercellular matrix. The intima contains two

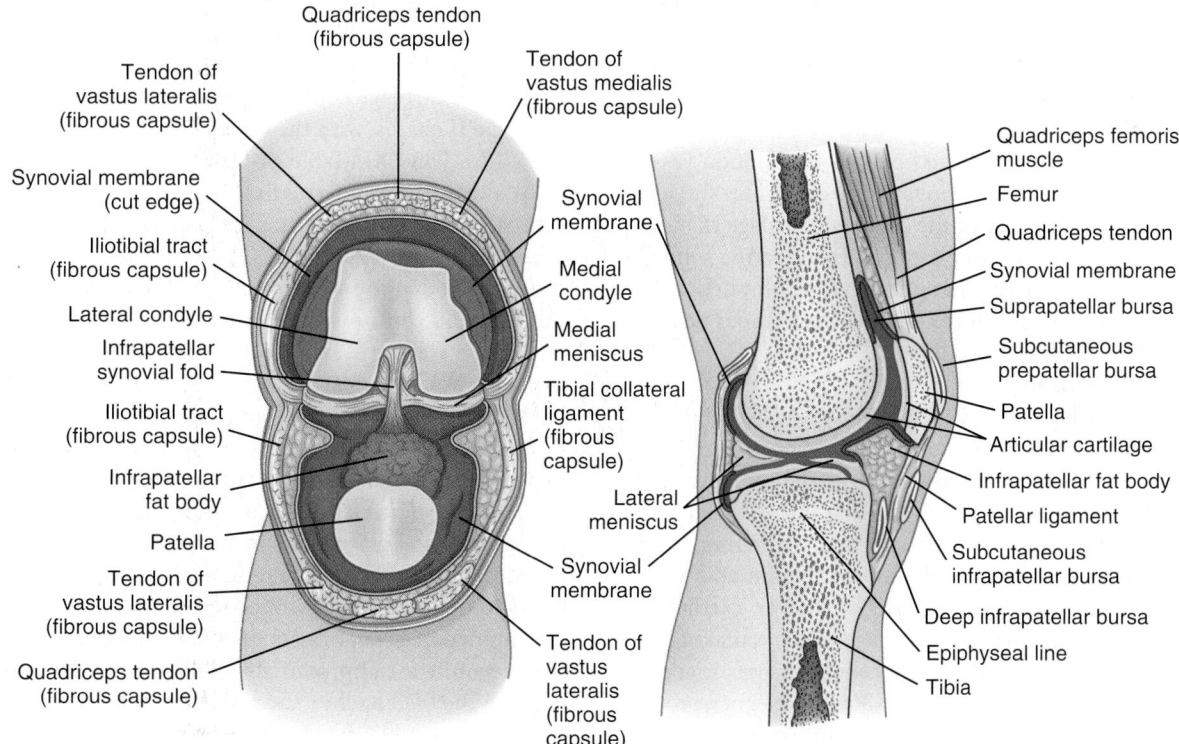

Figure 41-8 Knee joint (synovial joint).

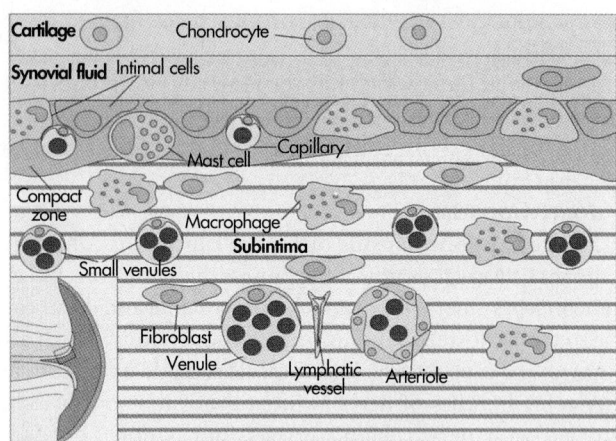

Figure 41-9 Synovium. Note the delicate synovial lining resting on a fibroadipose subintimal lining rich in capillaries, lymphatics, and nerve endings. (Modified from Klippel JH, Dieppe PA: *Rheumatology,* ed 2, London, 1998, Mosby.)

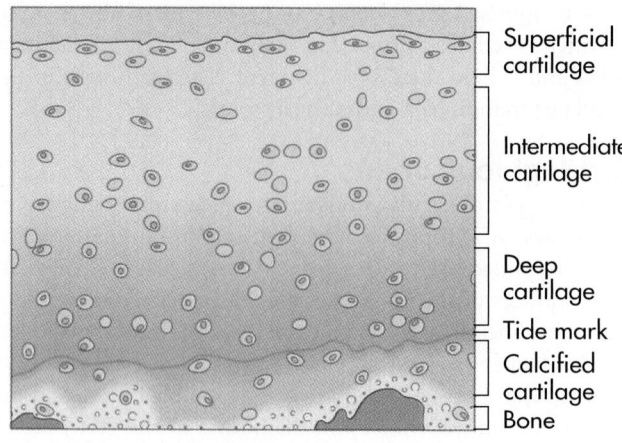

Figure 41-10 Articular cartilage. Note the different zones within the cartilage. (Modified from Klippel JH, Dieppe PA: *Rheumatology,* ed 2, London, 1998, Mosby.)

types of synovial cells: type A cells and type B cells. The **type A cells** ingest and remove bacteria and particles of debris by phagocytosis in the joint cavity. (Phagocytosis is described in Chapter 6.) The **type B cells** secrete **hyaluronate,** a binding agent that gives synovial fluid its viscous quality. The synovial membrane is richly supplied with blood and lymphatic vessels; therefore it is capable of rapid repair and regeneration.

Joint Cavity

The **joint cavity (synovial cavity)** is an enclosed, fluid-filled space between the articulating surfaces of the two bones. This small cavity, often called the *joint space,* enables the two bones to move "against" one another. The synovial cavity is surrounded by the synovial membrane and filled with a clear, viscous, slick fluid called the *synovial fluid.*

Synovial Fluid

Synovial fluid is superfiltrated plasma from blood vessels in the synovial membrane. Synovial fluid lubricates the joint surfaces, nourishes the pad of the articular cartilage that covers the ends of the bones, and contains free-floating synovial cells and various leukocytes that phagocytose joint debris and microorganisms. Loss of synovial fluid leads to rapid deterioration of articular cartilage.

Articular Cartilage

Articular cartilage is a layer of hyaline cartilage that covers the end of each bone (Figure 41-10). It ranges from 2 to 5 millimeters in thickness, depending on the size of the joint, the fit of the two bone ends, and the amount of weight and shearing force the joint normally withstands. The function of articular cartilage is to reduce friction in the joint and to distribute the forces of weight bearing. Articular cartilage is composed of **chondrocytes** (cartilage cells) (making up about 2% of the tissue) and an intercellular matrix made up of collagen (making up about 10% to 30% of weight), protein polysaccharides (making up 5% to 10% of weight), and water. The water content ranges from 60% to almost 80% of the

net weight of the cartilage,[5] and individual molecules rapidly enter or exit the articular cartilage to contribute to the resiliency of the tissue.[5]

The intercellular matrix is produced by the chondrocytes, which synthesize and extrude collagen, which, like the collagen produced by bone cells, is distributed throughout the cartilage in a highly organized system of fibers. Collagen fibers in cartilage are made up of many fine fibrils that, like bone fibrils, are assembled in an orderly fashion that makes them resistant to physical, metabolic, or chemical breakdown. The main differences between bone collagen and cartilage collagen are the amino acid content of the alpha chains and the composition of the fibrils. Bone collagen fibrils are made up of two type I chains and one type II chain. Approximately 90% of the cartilage collagen fibrils is made up of three identical type II chains, with the remaining 10% made up of types V, VI, IX, X, and XI (Table 41-5).

At the surface of articular cartilage, the collagen fibers run parallel to the joint surface and are closely compacted into a dense, protective mat.[5] (Loss of this dense, compacted configuration at the surface subjects the underlying fibers to splitting and thinning, in which case the cartilage is unable to tolerate weight bearing.) In the middle layer (the proliferative zone) of the cartilage, the fibers are arranged tangential to the surface, which allows them to deform and absorb some of the force of weight bearing. In the bottom layer (the hypertrophic zone) of the cartilage, the fibers are perpendicular to the joint surface, allowing them to resist shear forces, and are embedded in a calcified layer of cartilage called the **tidemark.** The tidemark anchors the collagen fibers to the underlying (subchondral) bone. Collagen fibers are important components of the cartilage matrix because they account for approximately 60% of the dry weight and because they (1) anchor the cartilage securely to underlying bone, (2) provide a taut framework for the cartilage, (3) control the loss of fluid from the cartilage, and (4) prevent

Table 41-5	Characteristics of Muscle Fibers	
Characteristic	Type I (Red)	Type II (White)
Anatomic location	Deep axial portion of surface muscle	Surface portion of surface muscle
Contraction speed	Slow	Fast
Motor neuron type	Type I, small alpha	Type II, large alpha
Firing frequency	Low, long duration	Rapid, short duration
Resistance to fatigue	High	Low
Myoglobin	High	Low
Capillary supply	Profuse	Intermediate to sparse
Metabolism	Oxidative	Glycolysis
Mitochondria	Many	Few
Enzymes	Lactate dehydrogenase, types 1–3	Lactate dehydrogenase, types 4 and 5
Creatine kinase	Cardiac type	Fast, skeletal
Example (most muscles are mixed)	Greater proportion of slow-contracting fibers in soleus	Greater proportion of fast-contracting fibers in laryngeal and ocular muscles
Glycogen content	Low	High
Intensity of contraction	Low	High
Aerobic metabolic capacity	High	Low
Fiber diameter	Small	Large
Myosin-adenosine triphosphatase (ATPase) activity	Low	High

From Spence AP, Mason EE: *Human anatomy and physiology,* ed 4, St Paul, Minn, 1992, West Publishing Co.

the escape of protein polysaccharides (proteoglycans) from the cartilage.

The proteoglycans are macromolecules consisting of proteins, carbohydrates (**glycosaminoglycans),** and hyaluronic acid. The glycosaminoglycans (keratan sulfate and chondroitin sulfate) are attached to the **protein core,** and several protein cores (with their attached glycosaminoglycans) are bound to a hyaluronic acid chain by a special protein called **link protein.** The proteoglycans give articular cartilage its stiff quality and regulate the movement of synovial fluid through the cartilage. Without proteoglycans, normal weight bearing would rapidly and completely press all the synovial fluid out of the cartilage. The proteoglycans act as a pump, permitting enough fluid to be pressed out to ensure that a fluid film is always present on the surface of the cartilage, even after hours of weight bearing. The pumping action of proteoglycans also draws synovial fluid back into the cartilage after a weight-bearing load is released. Mobility and weight bearing are necessary for the pumping action of proteoglycans to occur. Nonuse of a joint quickly reduces the pumping action, which changes the composition of the matrix and interferes with the nutrition of the chondrocytes.

Articular cartilage has no blood vessels, lymph vessels, or nerves. Therefore it is insensitive to pain and regenerates slowly and minimally after injury. Regeneration occurs primarily at sites where the articular cartilage meets the synovial membrane, where blood vessels and nutrients are available.

Movement

Synovial joints are described as uniaxial, biaxial, or multiaxial according to the shapes of the bone ends and the type of movement occurring at the joint (Figure 41-11). Usually one of the

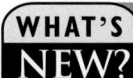
WHAT'S NEW?   New Cartilage Repair Treatments

In the past finding a treatment to facilitate cartilage repair has been a difficult task because of the unique, relatively avascular structure of cartilage. New treatments have now been developed that are showing promise. Some new therapies include (1) administration of matrix metalloproteinases inhibitors to prevent collagen degradation, (2) transplantation of osteochondral autografts or allografts, (3) use of resorbable collagen scaffolds, and (4) gene therapy.

These new techniques show promise in treating articular cartilage defects from osteoarthritis or trauma and are beneficial in improving surgical outcomes in cartilage repair. They may eventually even prevent degenerative cartilage damage from occurring.

Data from Janusz MJ et al: *Osteoarthritis Cartilage* 9(8):751-760, 2001; Kang R et al: *Clin Orthoped* 375:324-337, 2000; Lee CR et al: *J Orthoped Res* 21(2):272-281, 2003.

bones is stable and serves as an axis for the motion of the other bone. The body movements made possible by various synovial joints are either circular or angular (Figure 41-12).

STRUCTURE AND FUNCTION OF SKELETAL MUSCLES

The skeletal muscles are made up of millions of individual fibers that, by the process of contraction and relaxation, do the work necessary to complete movements as varied as a ballerina's pirouette or an artist's deft stroke (Figure 41-13). Muscle constitutes 40% of adults' body weight and 50% of children's body weight. Muscle is 75% water, 20% protein,

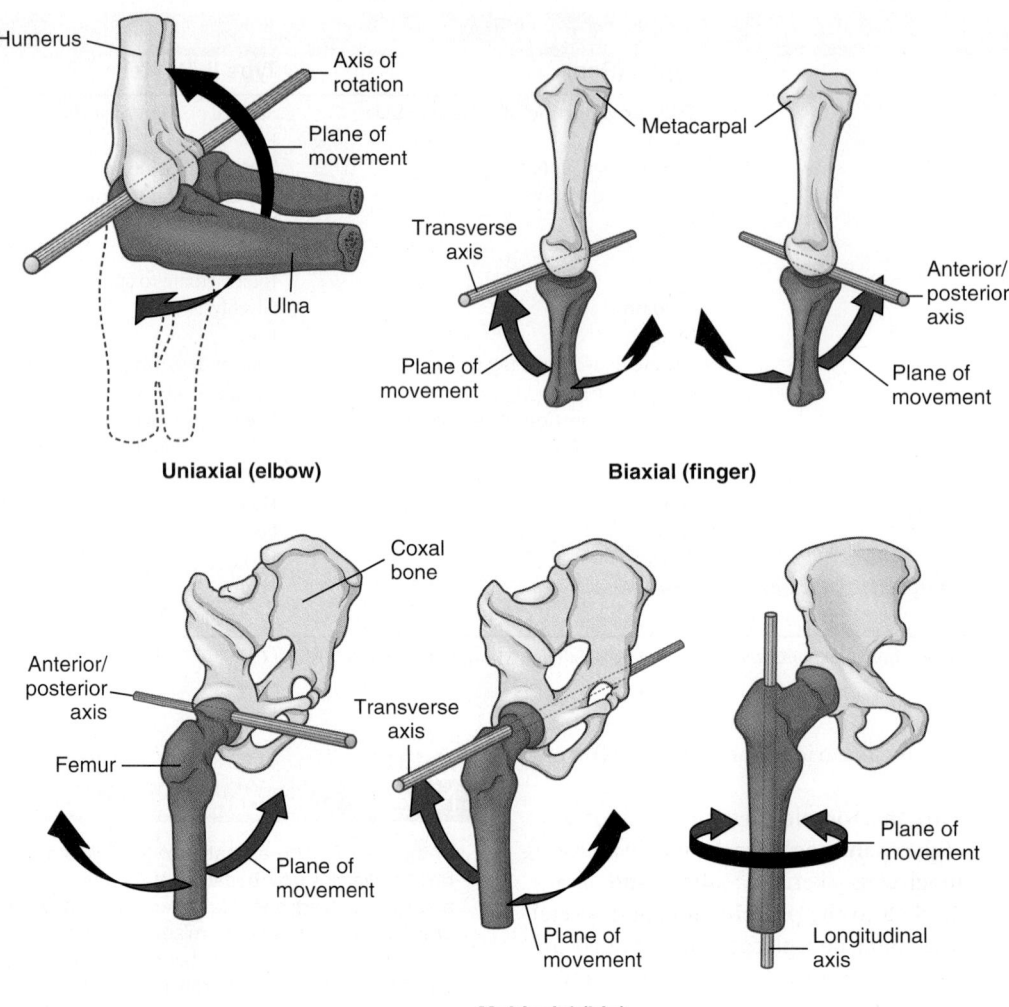

Uniaxial (elbow)

Biaxial (finger)

Multiaxial (hip)

Figure 41-11 Movements of synovial (diarthrodial) joints.

and 5% organic and inorganic compounds. Thirty-two percent of all protein stores for energy and metabolism is contained in muscle.

Whole Muscle

There are more than 350 named muscles; almost all are paired. The body's muscles vary dramatically in size and shape. They range from 2 to 60 cm in length and are shaped according to function. **Fusiform muscles** are elongated muscles shaped like straps and can run from one joint to another. **Pennate muscles** are broad, flat, and slightly fan shaped, with fibers running obliquely to the muscle's long axis. The multipennate deltoid muscle, which flexes and extends the arm, is a good example of a muscle shaped according to its function.

Each skeletal muscle is a separate organ encased in a three-part connective tissue framework called **fascia.** The layers of connective tissue protect the muscle fibers, attach the muscle to bony prominences, and provide a structure for a network of nerve fibers, blood vessels, and lymphatic channels.

The outermost layer, the **epimysium,** is located on the surface of the muscle and tapers at each end to form the **tendon** (Figure 41-14). Tendons allow a short muscle to exert power on a distant joint whereas a thick muscle would interfere with joint mobility. The next layer, the **perimysium,** further subdivides the muscle fibers into bundles of connective tissue, or **fascicles.** The **endomysium** surrounds the muscle fascicles, the smallest unit of muscle fibers visible without a microscope. The ligaments, tendons, and fascia are made up of connective tissue that also serves to buffer the limbs from the effects of sudden strains or changes in speed. The rapid recovery necessary for strenuous exercise is supported by the elastic property of muscle and its connective tissue.

Skeletal muscle is described, almost interchangeably, as **voluntary, striated,** or **extrafusal.** "Voluntary" indicates that the muscle is controlled directly by the central nervous system. "Striated" describes the striated, or striped, pattern of skeletal muscle viewed under a light microscope. The striations result from the organization of the muscle fibers into the contractile units called *sarcomeres.* "Extrafusal" distin-

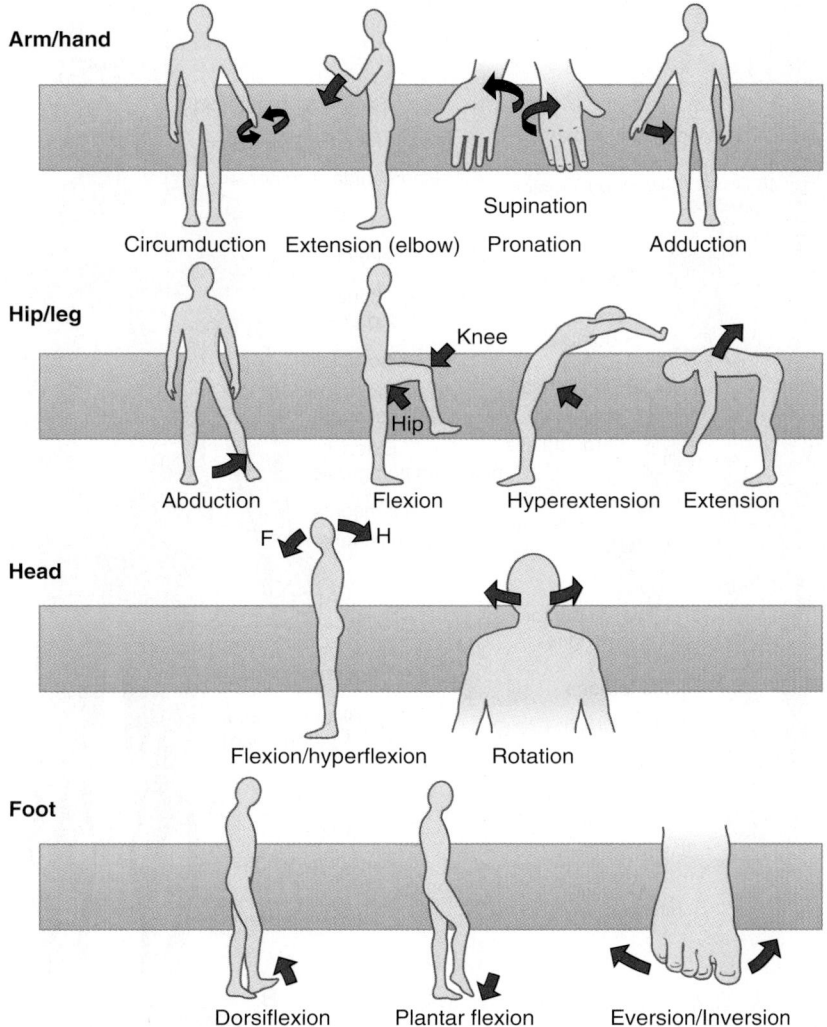

Figure 41-12 Body movements provided by synovial (diarthrodial) joints.

guishes the skeletal muscle fibers from other contractile fibers located within the sensory organs of the muscle.

Other components that are visible on gross inspection of the whole muscle include the motor and sensory nerve fibers. These function together with the muscle, innervating portions of it and providing the electrical impulses needed for motor function.

Motor Unit

From the anterior horn cell of the spinal cord, the axons of motor nerves branch out to innervate a specific group of muscle fibers. Each anterior horn cell, its axon (part of a lower motor neuron; see Chapter 14), and the muscle fibers innervated by it are called a **motor unit** (Figure 41-15). The motor units are composed of lower motor neurons, which extend to skeletal muscles. Often termed the *functional unit* of the neuromuscular system, the motor unit behaves as a single entity and contracts as a whole when it receives an electrical impulse.

The whole muscle may be controlled by several motor nerve axons. These branch to innervate many motor units within the muscle. The whole muscle then may be made up of many motor units. The number of motor units per individual muscle varies greatly. In the calf, for example, one motor axon will innervate approximately 2000 muscle fibers, out of a total of 1,200,000 muscle fibers. This is a high innervation ratio of muscle fibers to axons, and it contrasts markedly with the low innervation ratio in the laryngeal muscles. There, two to three muscle fibers constitute each motor unit, and the innervation ratio can be of great functional significance. The greater the innervation ratio of a particular organ, the greater its endurance. Higher innervation ratios prevent fatigue, and lower innervation ratios allow for precision of movement.

Sensory Receptors

Although muscles function as effector organs, they also contain sensory receptors and are involved in sending different signals to the central nervous system. Among these are the muscle spindles and Golgi tendon organs. **Spindles** are mechanoreceptors that lie parallel to muscle fibers and respond to muscle stretching. **Golgi tendon organs** are dendrites that terminate and branch to tendons near the neuro-

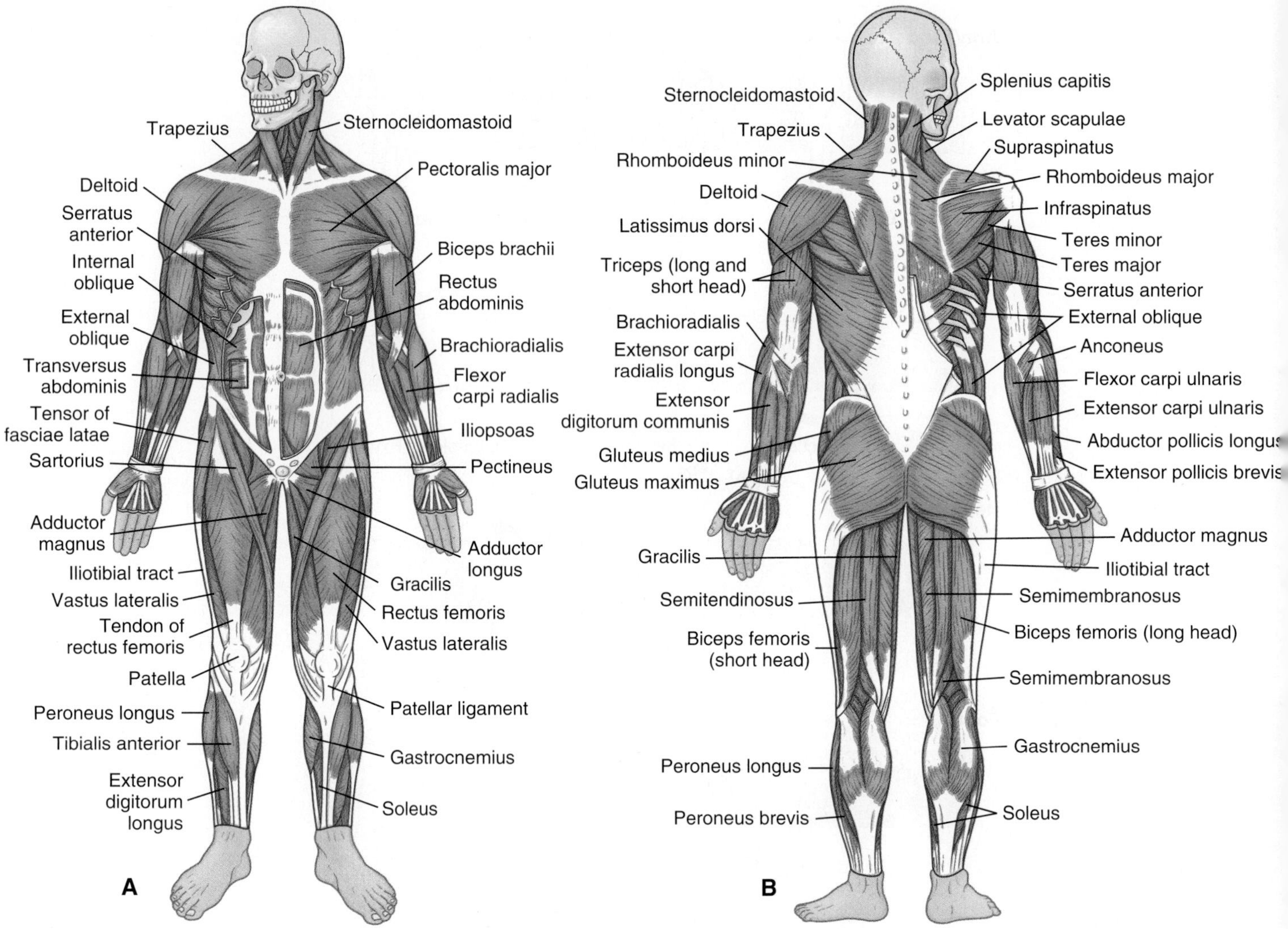

Trapezius

Sternocleidomastoid

Deltoid

Serratus anterior

Internal oblique

External oblique

Transversus abdominis

Tensor of fasciae latae

Sartorius

Adductor magnus

Iliotibial tract

Vastus lateralis

Tendon of rectus femoris

Patella

Peroneus longus

Tibialis anterior

Extensor digitorum longus

Sternocleidomastoid

Pectoralis major

Biceps brachii

Rectus abdominis

Brachioradialis

Flexor carpi radialis

Iliopsoas

Pectineus

Adductor longus

Gracilis

Rectus femoris

Vastus lateralis

Patellar ligament

Gastrocnemius

Soleus

A

Sternocleidomastoid

Trapezius

Rhomboideus minor

Deltoid

Latissimus dorsi

Triceps (long and short head)

Brachioradialis

Extensor carpi radialis longus

Extensor digitorum communis

Gluteus medius

Gluteus maximus

Gracilis

Semitendinosus

Biceps femoris (short head)

Peroneus longus

Peroneus brevis

Splenius capitis

Levator scapulae

Supraspinatus

Rhomboideus major

Infraspinatus

Teres minor

Teres major

Serratus anterior

External oblique

Anconeus

Flexor carpi ulnaris

Extensor carpi ulnaris

Abductor pollicis longus

Extensor pollicis brevis

Adductor magnus

Iliotibial tract

Semimembranosus

Biceps femoris (long head)

Semimembranosus

Gastrocnemius

Soleus

B

Figure 41-13 Skeletal muscles of body. **A,** Anterior view. **B,** Posterior view.

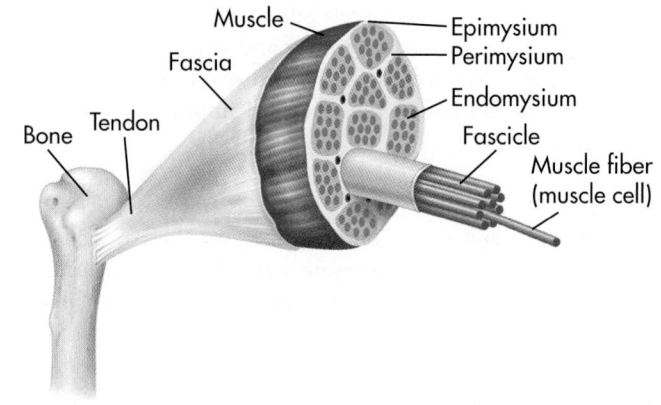

Figure 41-14 Cross section of skeletal muscle showing muscle fibers and their coverings. (From Thibodeau GA, Patton KT: *Anatomy & physiology,* ed 5, St Louis, 2003, Mosby.)

Muscle

Fascia

Tendon

Bone

Epimysium

Perimysium

Endomysium

Fascicle

Muscle fiber (muscle cell)

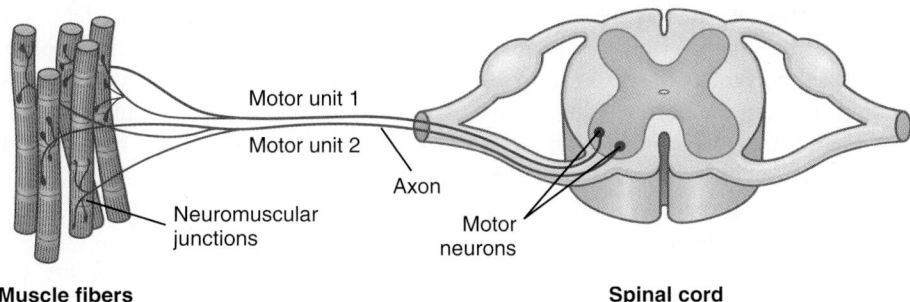

Figure 41-15 **Motor units of a muscle.** Each motor unit consists of a somatic motor neuron and all the muscle fibers (cells) supplied by the neuron and its axon branches.

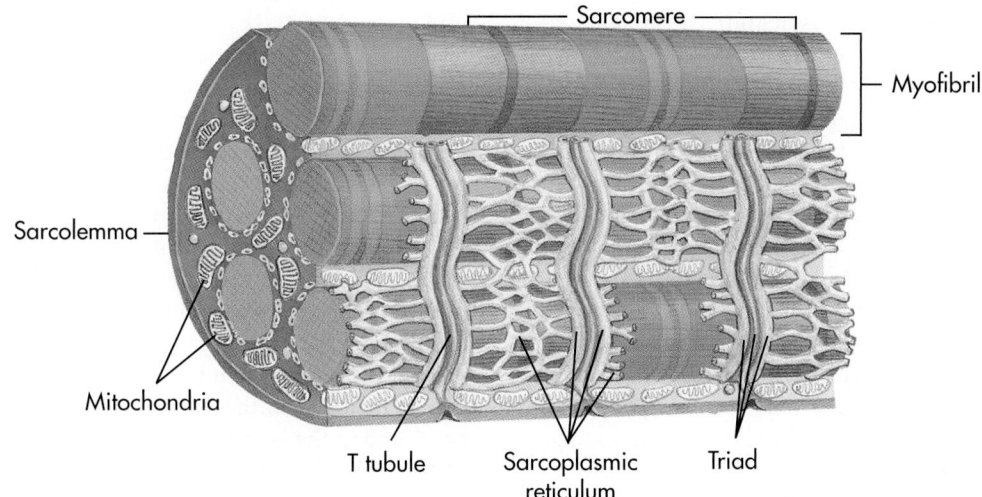

Figure 41-16 **Myofibrils of a skeletal muscle fiber (cell) and overall organization of skeletal muscle.** (From Thibodeau GA, Patton KT: *Anatomy & physiology,* ed 5, St Louis, 2003, Mosby.)

muscular junction. Motor and sensory neurons secrete a proteoglycan called *neuroregulin (NRG)* that increase acetylcholine receptors and helps in the formation of muscle spindle fibers.[6] The muscle spindles, Golgi tendon organs, and free nerve endings provide a means of reporting changes in length, tension, velocity, and tone in the muscle. This system of afferent signals is responsible for the muscle stretch response and maintenance of normal muscle tone.

Muscle Fibers

Each **muscle fiber** is a single **muscle cell.** This long cell is cylindrical in structure and is surrounded by a membrane capable of excitation and impulse propagation. The muscle fiber contains bundles of **myofibrils,** the fiber's functional subunits, in a parallel arrangement along the longitudinal axis of the muscle (Figure 41-16). At birth the muscle fibers have completed development from precursor cells called **myoblasts.** All voluntary muscles are derived from the mesodermal layer of the embryo.

The type of peripheral nerve influences the muscle fiber and motor unit considerably. Whether motor nerves are fast or slow determines the type of muscle fibers in the motor unit. Type II fibers, also called *white fast-motor fibers,* are innervated by relatively large type II alpha motor neurons with

fast conduction velocities. These fibers rely on a short-term anaerobic glycolytic system for rapid energy transfer, whereas type I fibers depend on aerobic oxidative metabolism. Histochemical stains are now routinely used to describe the structure of muscle fibers and contractile elements of muscle biopsy specimens. White muscle (**type II fibers**) stains dark in the enzyme stain adenosine triphosphatase (ATPase) at a pH of 9.4. Red muscle (**type I fibers**) appears lightly stained.

The overlap of muscle fibers that appear with staining gives the checkerboard appearance of muscle biopsy specimens and provides an equal distribution of fiber types throughout the muscle. This overlap also helps compensate for muscle fiber loss and fatigue of individual motor units during activity. In spite of this, some muscles contain proportionally more of one fiber type than another. The postural muscles have more type I fibers, allowing them the high resistance to fatigue that is necessary to maintain the same position for extended periods. The ocular muscles have more type II muscle fibers, allowing them to respond rapidly to visual changes. (Table 41-5 describes the specific characteristics of type I and type II fibers.)

The number of muscle fibers varies according to location. Large muscles, such as the gastrocnemius, have more fibers

(1,200,000) than the smaller muscles, such as the lumbrical muscles in the hand (10,000). The diameter of muscle fibers also varies. The closely packed polygons are small (10 to 20 μm) until puberty, when they attain the normal adult diameter of 40 to 80 μm. Women usually have smaller-diameter fibers than men. Small muscles, such as the ocular muscles, are 15 μm in diameter; larger, more proximal muscles are 40 μm. Fiber size can have functional significance. Studies have shown that larger fiber diameter is associated with generation of greater forces. Fiber diameter can be increased by activities that cause hypertrophied muscle, such as exercise or occupational overuse.

The major components of the muscle fiber include the muscle membrane, myofibrils, sarcotubular system, sarcoplasm, and mitochondria (see Figure 41-16). The **muscle membrane** is a two-part membrane. It includes the **sarcolemma,** which contains the plasma membrane of the muscle cell, and the cell's **basement membrane.** The sarcolemma is 7.5 nm thick and is capable of propagating electrical impulses to initiate contraction. At the motor nerve end-plate, where the nerve impulse is transmitted, the sarcolemma forms the highly convoluted synaptic cleft. The sarcolemma is made up of lipid molecules and protein systems. The protein systems perform special functions, such as transport of nutrients and protein synthesis. They also provide the sodium-potassium pump and include the cell's cholinergic receptor. The basement membrane is 50 nm thick and is composed primarily of proteins and polysaccharides. It serves as the cell's microskeleton and maintains the shape of the muscle cell. The basement membrane also may function in some way to restrict further diffusion of electrolytes once they have crossed the sarcolemma.

The **sarcoplasm** is the cytoplasm of the muscle cell and contains the intracellular components that are common to all cells (see Chapter 1). The sarcoplasm is an aqueous substance that provides a matrix that surrounds the myofibrils. It contains numerous enzymes and proteins that are responsible for the cell's energy production, protein synthesis, and oxygen storage. The mitochondria house enzyme systems for energy production, particularly those that regulate such processes as the citric acid cycle and adenosine triphosphate (ATP) formation. Many other structures are present in the sarcoplasm. The ribosomes are composed primarily of ribonucleic acid (RNA) and participate in the process of protein synthesis. The cell nucleus, satellite cells, glycogen granules, and lipid droplets are suspended in the sarcoplasmic matrix. Blood vessels, nerve endings, muscle spindles, and Golgi tendon organs are also directly located within this structure.

Unique to the muscle is the **sarcotubular system,** a network that includes the transverse tubules and the sarcoplasmic reticulum, which crosses the interior of the cell. The **sarcoplasmic reticulum** is made in the same manner as the endoplasmic reticulum in other cells. In the muscle cells the sarcoplasmic reticulum is involved in calcium transport, which initiates muscle contraction at the **sarcomere,** a portion of the myofibril. The sarcoplasmic reticulum is composed of tubules that run parallel to the myofibrils. The longitudinal tubules are termed **sarcotubules.** The **transverse tubules,** which are closely associated with the sarcotubules, run across the sarcoplasm and communicate with the extracellular space. Together, the tubules of this membrane system allow for intracellular calcium uptake, regulation, release during muscle contraction, and storage of calcium during muscle relaxation.

Myofibrils. The myofibrils are the functional units of muscle contraction. Each myofibril contains sarcomeres, which appear at intervals (see Figure 41-16). The sarcomeres are composed of two contractile proteins, **actin** and **myosin.** The sarcomere is responsible for converting chemical energy into movement.

The myofibrils are the most abundant subcellular muscle component, equaling 85% to 90% of the total volume. On cross section they are irregular polygons with a mean diameter of less than 1 μm. Each myofibril is composed of serially repeating sarcomeres, separated by Z lines, which give the muscle its striped, cross-striated appearance. Each sarcomere has a dark A band and is flanked by two light I bands (Figure 41-17). Within the sarcomere is the giant muscle protein, titin. Titin functions as a molecular spring that plays a significant role in determining muscle stiffness and elasticity.[7] The A band is 1.5 to 1.6 μm long and contains thick myosin filaments. Included in the A band is a lighter zone called the H band, and in the center of the H band is the dark M band, or M line. The I band, which contains actin, is divided at the midpoint of each sarcomere by the Z line. Its length varies with the start of muscle contraction.

Myofibrils are composed of myofilaments. Each myofilament is structured in a closely packed hexagonal arrangement, with two thin filaments for every thick filament. The thick filament, along with C protein and M line protein, is made up of myosin. Myosin has two subunits, heavy and light meromyosin, which resemble twisted golf club shafts. The thin filaments are twisted double strands made up of actin, troponin, and tropomyosin (see Chapter 28 and Figure 28-16).

Muscle Proteins. At present, 12 proteins have been identified in the muscle fibers.[3] (Table 41-6 outlines their distribution, location, and possible functional significance.) The contractile and regulatory functions of actin, myosin, and the troponin-tropomyosin complex (associated with actin) are the most commonly known. They also account for most of the protein found in the myofibril. The structural and regulatory processes of muscle proteins are less well understood. Alpha actin and beta actin are known to link the filaments. M protein contains the enzyme creatine kinase (CK). Creatine is released when muscle cells are damaged, making serum creatine an important test of pathologic conditions of muscles.

The most abundant proteins, actin and myosin, are also found in other cells, particularly motile cells such as platelets. The complete amino acid sequences of both actin and myosin have been identified. Noteworthy is the presence of the amino 3-methylhistidine, which is found only in the thin filament, actin. Eight-five to ninety percent of 3-methylhistidine is

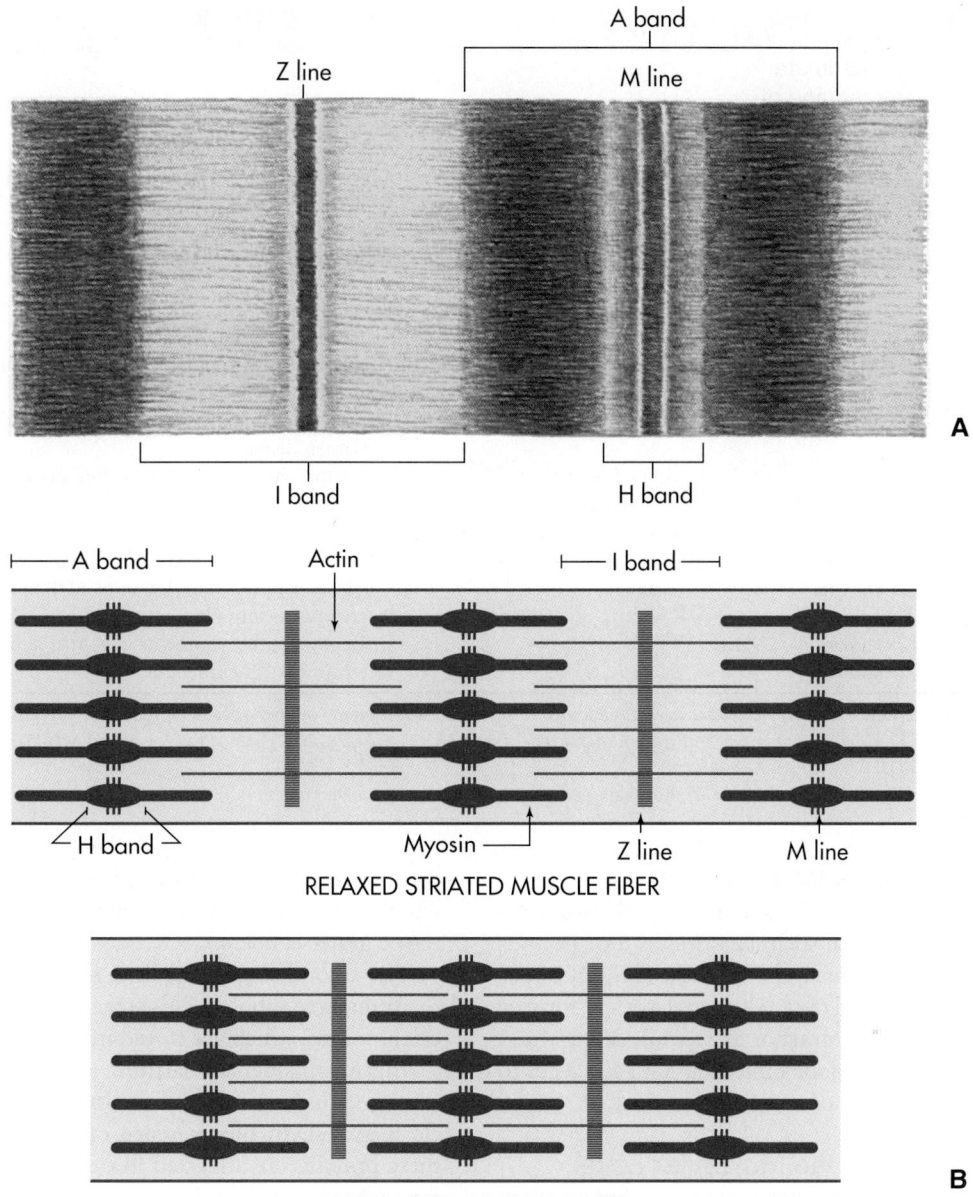

Figure 41-17 Muscle fibers. **A,** Lines and bands in striated muscle. **B,** Relationships of bands, actin, myosin, and lines in relaxed and contracted muscle fibers. (**A** modified from Thompson JM et al: *Mosby's clinical nursing,* ed 5, St Louis, 2002, Mosby.)

found in skeletal muscle. Because it is excreted unchanged (in the urine) after release from muscle and other tissue, 3-methylhistidine has been used to gauge muscle protein degradation. The amino acids lysine and histidine, in addition to leucine, have been used to study protein synthesis by means of stable isotope infusion and muscle biopsy analysis.

Nonprotein Constituents of Muscle. Substances such as nitrogen, creatine, creatinine, phosphocreatine, purines, uric acid, and amino acids all serve in the complex process of muscle metabolism. Glycogen and its derivatives are present as energy sources.

Creatine and creatinine metabolism have been used to measure muscle mass. Plasma creatine is taken up by muscle and converted into the high-energy phosphate compound *phosphocreatine* by the enzyme **creatine kinase.** Creatinine is formed in muscle from creatine at a constant rate of 2% per day. (Tests for plasma creatine are discussed in Chapter 35.) Creatine excretion is increased in muscle wasting. This change reflects the reduction in total body creatine stores and loss of muscle mass.

Inorganic compounds, anions (phosphate, chloride), and cations (calcium, magnesium, sodium, potassium) are important in the regulation of protein synthesis, muscle contraction, enzyme systems, and membrane stabilization. Total body potassium (TBK), measured by the K_{40} method, has been used to measure muscle mass, also called *lean body mass.* TBK levels reflect changes in muscle mass seen during growth, malnutrition, and muscle wasting.

Table 41-6	Contractile Proteins of Skeletal Muscle Fibrils		
Name	Approximate Percentage of Myofibrillar Protein	Location	Function
Myosin	55	A band (thick filament)	Contraction; hydrolyzes ATP and develops tension
Actin	20	I band (thin filament)	Contraction; activates myosin ATPase and interacts with myosin
Troponin	7	Thin filament	Regulatory protein; in presence of Ca^{++}, promotes actin-myosin activation
Tropomyosin	5-7	Thin filament	Regulatory and structural function; links filaments, controls filament length
Alpha (α) actin	10	Z band	Regulatory and structural function; links filaments, controls filament length
Beta (β) actin	2	Z band	Regulatory and structural function; links filaments, controls filament length
M protein	2	M line (center of thick filaments)	Regulatory and structural function; provides enzyme creatine kinase
C protein	2	A band (thick filaments)	Possible structural role
Titin	Unknown	Z line (thick filament)	Interconnects thin filaments in Z line
Creatine kinase	Unknown	M line	Catalyzes the phosphorylation of ADP to form ATP
Desmin	Unknown	Z line	Interconnects thin filaments in Z line
*Filamin	Unknown	Z line	Interconnects thin filaments in Z line; stabilizes membrane
*Nebulin	Unknown	Z line	Determines filament length

Modified from Simon SR, editor: *Orthopaedic basic science,* Chicago, 1994, American Academy of Orthopaedic Surgeons.
*Data from Ma K, Wang K: *Federation of European Biochemical Societies Letter* 532(3):273-278, 2002; Sampson LJ, Leyland ML, Dart D: *J Biol Chem* 278(43):41988-41997, 2003.
ATP, Adenosine triphosphate; *ATPase,* adenosine triphosphatase; *ADP,* adenosine diphosphate.

Components of Muscle Function

The ultimate function of muscle is to accomplish work. Although variously expressed in such measures as foot-pounds or kilogram-meters, work usually refers to the amount of energy liberated or force exerted over a distance (work = force × distance). Muscles usually contract or tense while doing work. Muscle contraction occurs on the molecular level and leads to the observable phenomenon of muscle movement.

Muscle Contraction at the Molecular Level

Muscle contraction is a four-step process that includes activation, coupling, contraction, and relaxation. The process involves the electrical properties of all cells and the movement of ions across the plasma membrane (see Chapter 1). The muscle fiber is an excitable tissue. At rest an electric charge of −90 mV is continually maintained across the sarcolemma. This resting potential, generated by the separation of positive and negative charges on either side of the membrane, creates an electrochemical equilibrium caused by the selective permeability of the sarcolemma to electrolytes in the intracellular and extracellular fluids, particularly potassium and sodium.

Activation, the first step of muscle contraction, begins with the spread of an action potential from the nerve terminal to the neuromuscular junction. The rapid depolarization of the membrane initiates an electrical impulse in the muscle fiber membrane called the **muscle fiber action potential.** As the action potential advances along the sarcolemmal membrane, it spreads to the transverse tubules. (The velocity of conduction is much slower in muscle fibers than in myelinated nerve fibers—only 3 to 5 m/sec compared with 54 to 90 m/sec in nerve fibers.)

The second stage, **coupling,** follows the depolarization of the transverse tubules. This stage consists of the migration of calcium ions, which are stored in the sarcoplasmic reticulum, to the myofilaments. Calcium affects troponin and tropomyosin, muscle proteins that bind with actin when the muscle is at rest. In the presence of calcium, however, both of these proteins are attracted to calcium ions, leaving the actin free to bind with myosin.

Contraction begins as the calcium ions combine with troponin, a reaction that overcomes the inhibitory function of the troponin-tropomyosin system. The thin filament *actin* then slides toward the thick filament, myosin. The two ends of the myofibril shorten after contraction when the myosin heads attach to the actin molecules, forming a cross-bridge that constitutes an actin-myosin complex. ATP, located on the actin-myosin complex, is released when the cross-bridges attach. This is the **sliding filament theory** described by A.F. Huxley in the 1950s, but it is now called the **cross-bridge theory** because of the formation of the actin-myosin cross-bridges.[8,9] The process is so named because the actin actually slides onto the myosin, causing the sarcomere to shorten. The useful distance of contraction of a skeletal muscle is approximately 25% to 35% of the muscle's length.

The last step, **relaxation,** begins as the sarcoplasmic reticulum absorbs the calcium molecules, removing them from interaction with troponin. Calcium is pumped back into the sarcoplasmic reticulum by means of an active transport process. The cross-bridges detach, and the sarcomere lengthens. (The cross-bridge theory of muscle contraction is discussed in Chapter 29.)

Muscle Metabolism

Skeletal muscle requires a constant supply of ATP and phosphocreatine. These substances are necessary to fuel the complex processes of muscle contraction, driving the cross-bridges of actin and myosin together and transporting calcium from the sarcoplasmic reticulum to the myofibril. Other internal processes of the muscular system that require ATP include protein synthesis, which replenishes muscle constituents and accommodates growth and repair. The rate of protein synthesis is related to hormone levels (particularly insulin), amino acid substrates, and overall nutritional status. At rest the rate of ATP formation by oxidation of glucose or acetoacetate is sufficient to maintain internal processes, given normal nutritional status. During activity the need for ATP increases 100-fold. The metabolic pathways for muscle activity in Table 41-7 show reactions to the immediate need for increased ATP caused by contraction. Activity lasting longer than 5 seconds expends the available stored ATP and phosphocreatine.

Stored glycogen and blood glucose are converted anaerobically to sustain brief activity without increasing the demand for oxygen.[10] Anaerobic glycolysis is much less efficient than aerobic glycolysis, using six to eight times more glycogen to produce the same amount of ATP. With increased activity, such as intense exercise, or ischemia, an increase in lactic acid occurs because of the breakdown of glycogen, thus causing a shift in muscle pH (see Table 41-7). This short-term mechanism "buys time" by allowing ATP formation in spite of inadequate energy stores or oxygen supply. When the anaerobic threshold is reached and more oxygen is required, physiologic changes occur, including an increase in lactic acid and increases in oxygen consumption, heart rate, respiratory rate, and muscle blood flow.

Strenuous exercise requires oxygen, which activates the aerobic glycogen pathway for ATP formation. During maximal exercise, free fatty acid mobilization and the aerobic glycogen pathways provide ATP over an extended time. These pathways require oxygen both to maintain maximal activity and to return the muscle to the resting state. Maximal exercise increases oxygen uptake 15 to 30 times over the resting state.[11] When this system becomes exhausted or inadequate to respond to the need for ATP, fatigue and weakness finally force the muscle to reduce activity, with a resultant buildup of lactic acid in muscle fibers.

The ability to sustain maximal muscular activity leads to the accumulation of oxygen debt. **Oxygen debt** is the amount of oxygen needed to convert the buildup of lactic acid to glucose and replenish ATP and phosphocreatine stores. For example, after running at maximal speed for 10 seconds, the average person has consumed 1 L of oxygen. At rest, oxygen consumption for the same period is approximately 40 ml. As the person recovers, the measured oxygen debt is 4 L greater than the amount used during activity.

Oxygen consumption is measured to calculate the metabolic cost of activity in normal and diseased muscle. It is an indirect measure of energy expenditure, along with timed tests of activity, heart rate, and respiratory quotient (ratio of carbon dioxide to expired oxygen consumed). Energy expenditure is measured directly by heat production because heat is released whenever work is accomplished.

Another factor that changes energy requirements is muscle fiber type. Type II fibers rely on anaerobic glycolytic metabolism and fatigue readily. Type I fibers can resist fatigue for longer periods because of their capacity for oxidative metabolism.

Muscle Mechanics

Muscle contraction cannot be viewed in isolation. Several factors determine how force is transmitted from the cross-bridges on individual muscle fibers to accomplish whole-muscle contraction. First, when a motor unit responds to a single nerve stimulus, it develops a phasic contraction, also called *twitch*. Because the motor unit contracts in an "all or nothing" manner, the contraction that is generated will be a maximal contraction. The central nervous system smoothly grades the force generated by "recruiting" additional motor units and varying the discharge frequency of each active motor unit. This adding of motor units within the muscle is called **repetitive discharge.**

Recruitment and repetitive discharge of motor units allow the muscle to activate the number of motor units needed to generate the desired force. The total force developed is the

Table 41-7	Energy Sources for Muscular Activity
Sources	Reactions
Short-term (anaerobic) sources	Adenosine triphosphate (ATP) $\rightarrow$ Adenosine diphosphate (ADP) + Inorganic phosphate (P_i) + Energy
	Phosphocreatine + ADP $\rightleftharpoons$ Creatine + ATP
	Glycogen/glucose + P_i + ADP $\rightarrow$ Lactate + ATP
Long-term (aerobic) sources	Glycogen/glucose + ADP + P_i + O_2 $\rightarrow$ H_2O + CO_2 + ATP
	Free fatty acids + ADP + P_i + O_2 $\rightarrow$ H_2O + CO_2 + ATP
	Creatine kinase catalyzes the reversible reaction of ATP to ADP: Creatine phosphate + ADP $\xrightarrow[\text{kinase}]{\text{Creatine}}$ Creatine + ATP

From Spence AP, Mason EE: *Human anatomy and physiology,* ed 4, St Paul, Minn, 1992, West Publishing Co.

sum of the force generated by each motor unit. As the strength, speed, and duration of stimuli increase, the summation of contractions reaches a critical frequency called **tetanus.** When tetanus is reached, no further increase in force can be achieved.

Other variables, such as fiber type, innervation ratio, muscle temperature, and muscle shape, influence the efficiency of muscular contraction. The two muscle fiber types differ in their responses to electrical activity. Tetanus and duration of phasic contractions, which take microseconds to accomplish, are achieved more rapidly in type II than in type I muscle fibers. Low innervation ratios promote control and coordination, whereas high ratios promote strength and endurance. Muscles work best at normal body temperature, 98.6° F (37° C). Finally, muscles with a large cross-sectional area, such as the fan-shaped pennate muscles, develop greater contractile forces than smaller-diameter muscles. The initial length of a muscle and the range of shortening that occur when the muscle contracts also determine the forces it can generate. The long fusiform muscles have a greater range of shortening and can contract up to 57% of their resting length. A certain amount of elongation is necessary to generate sufficient tension and muscular force. The elongation that occurs during the swing of a golf club or tennis racquet is an example of how stretch improves contractile force.

Types of Muscle Contraction

During **isometric contraction (static or holding contraction),** the muscle maintains constant length as tension is increased. Isometric contraction occurs, for example, when the arm or leg is pushed against an immovable object. The muscle contracts, but the limb does not move.

During **isotonic contraction** the muscle maintains a constant tension as it moves. Isotonic contractions can be **lengthening** or **shortening.** The terms "eccentric" for lengthening and "concentric" for shortening are technically inaccurate descriptions of muscle movement, and "lengthening" and "shortening" are more precise.[12] Positive work is accomplished during shortening and energy is released to exert force or lift a weight. In contrast, during lengthening the muscle lengthens and absorbs energy. Negative work is accomplished on the muscle by the load. Lengthening requires less energy to accomplish and may result in the development of pain and stiffness after unaccustomed exercise.

Movement of Muscle Groups

Muscles do not act alone but rather in groups, often under automatic control. When a muscle contracts and acts as a "prime mover," or **agonist,** its reciprocal muscle, or **antagonist,** relaxes. This is easily tested by holding the right arm in the horizontal position in front of the body and then bending the elbow while feeling the biceps in the front and the triceps in the back with the other hand. The biceps is firm, and the triceps is soft. As the arm is extended, the muscles change. When the elbow is completely extended, the biceps is soft and the triceps firm. Completing this movement causes the agonist and antagonist to change automatically; only the movement is commanded, not the alternate contraction and relaxation of the specific muscle groups.

Other associated actions may be seen during walking; as the foot leaves the ground, the paravertebral and gluteal muscles on the opposite sides of the body contract to maintain balance. One notices the loss of the associated muscle's action when paralysis offsets this process and decreases balance. If a person is paralyzed, difficulty in maintaining balance is noticeable.

TESTS OF MUSCULOSKELETAL FUNCTION

Tests of Bone Function

Diagnostic procedures to evaluate bone function include gait analysis, serum calcium and phosphorus, x-ray films, angiography, and bone scanning. Roentgenograms visualize bone structure, because bone absorbs x-ray beams better than soft tissue. Angiography is used to observe bone circulation. Bone scanning is the most frequently used procedure to evaluate bone function and can detect malignancy, trauma, necrosis, infection, metabolic bone disease, and osteoarthritis. Single- or dual-photon absorptiometry is often used to measure density of bones in the extremities (single-photon absorptiometry) and fracture risk of vertebral bodies and the femoral neck (dual-photon absorptiometry). Dual-photon absorptiometry allows the soft tissue component to be subtracted.

Tests of Joint Function

Procedures used to diagnose joint function include arthrography, arthroscopy, magnetic resonance imaging, and synovial fluid analysis. **Arthrography** (the injection of dye into the joint) is particularly useful to diagnose tears in the fibrocartilage of the knee (meniscus) and the rotator cuff of the shoulder. **Arthroscopy** is the direct visualization of a joint through an arthroscope. **Magnetic resonance imaging** (MRI) produces images of body tissues through the use of electromagnetic (radio) waves that alter the atoms (hydrogen ions) in the nuclei of cells being examined. When the radio waves are stopped, the nuclear atoms return to their original positions, emitting energy as signals as they move back. The signals produce visible images for examination and diagnosis. MRI produces excellent contrast of soft tissues for evaluation of musculoskeletal conditions.

Analysis of synovial fluid may reveal inflammatory, septic, and noninflammatory joint diseases, which cause characteristic changes in the color, clarity, viscosity, and cellular elements of the fluid. The presence of blood in the joint fluid (hemarthrosis) usually indicates joint trauma. Normal synovial fluid is sterile, so the presence of bacteria in the fluid always indicates disease. Cell fragments and fibrous tissue in the fluid are the result of inflammation or wear and tear on the articular surfaces.

Tests of Muscular Function

When the individual's history and physical examination disclose abnormalities, such as weakness, atrophy, muscle tenderness, cramps, and stiffness, specific tests of muscle function are in order. One of the most useful tests is the serum CK concentration. CK is found in large quantities in the muscle fibers, and when these are diseased or damaged, CK leaks into the serum. Myoglobin is also detectable in the urine after acute muscle damage caused by crush injury, ischemic disorders, extreme exertion, and some inherited diseases.

Because the muscle membrane tissue is excitable and carries an electrical charge, its capacity to function can be assessed by electromyography. Using sensitive needle electrodes, the **electromyogram (EMG)** records the summation of action potentials of the muscle fibers in each motor unit. The EMG is often compared with the electrocardiogram (ECG), but the activity recorded on the EMG is on a much smaller scale. The amplitude of the ECG is measured in volts, the duration of impulse is recorded in seconds, and both are recorded as the heart rate (e.g., 80 V/60 sec). EMG amplitude is recorded in millivolts and the duration is measured in milliseconds, with a frequency of about 5 to 50 action potentials per second. Motor unit potentials are measured to determine rate of firing, duration, and amplitude. Abnormalities in EMG and nerve conduction velocities help differentiate muscle diseases (myopathy) from peripheral nerve (neuropathy) and neuromuscular junction disorders. The muscle biopsy (using histologic, histochemical, and electron microscopic studies) is used to further define the presence of myopathic and neuropathic disorders, many of which can be diagnosed only by muscle biopsy.

Although manual muscle testing of strength and range of motion is still the most common way to detect changes, myometers are becoming increasingly popular. These handheld devices measure strength of contraction in several muscle groups, namely, the neck flexors, shoulder abductors, wrist extensors, hip flexors, knee extensors, and foot dorsiflexors.

A new area of evaluation is genetics. Recent advances in molecular genetics, deoxyribonucleic acid (DNA) libraries, genetic probes, and gene localization techniques have enhanced our knowledge of neuromuscular diseases, including types of muscular dystrophy, Charcot-Marie-Tooth disease, and familial amyotrophic lateral sclerosis.

AGING AND THE MUSCULOSKELETAL SYSTEM
Aging of Bones

Aging is accompanied by the loss of bone tissue. Bones become less stiff, less strong, and more brittle with aging. The bone remodeling cycle takes longer to complete, and the rate of mineralization also slows down. With aging, women experience loss of bone density, accelerated by rapid bone loss during early menopause from increased osteoclastic bone resorption. By age 70, susceptible women have lost an average of 50% of their peripheral cortical bone mass. Bone mass losses to such an extent lead to deformity, pain, stiffness, and a high risk for fractures. Men also experience bone loss but at later ages and much slower rates than women. Also, initial bone masses in men are approximately 30% higher than in women; therefore bone loss in men causes less risk of disability than for women. Men's peak bone mass is related to their race, heredity, hormonal factors (testosterone and estradiol), physical activity, and calcium intake during childhood. Bone loss in both sexes is related to smoking, calcium deficiency, magnesium deficiency, vitamin D deficiency, high protein intake, excess phosphorus intake, overly vigorous exercise, certain prescription and over-the-counter drug use, alcohol intake, and physical inactivity.[13]

Bone mass can be gained in healthy young women up to the third decade through physical activity, intake of dietary calcium, and magnesium. Exercise in the elderly does little to increase bone mineral density, but exercise has been shown to improve balance, coordination, muscle strength, lean body mass, and mobility.[13] The use of oral contraceptives and gaining of bone mass is controversial. Height is also lost with aging because of increased spinal curvature.

Aging of Joints

With aging, cartilage becomes more rigid, fragile, and susceptible to fibrillation because of more cross-linking of collagen and elastin, decreasing water content in the cartilage ground substance, and decreasing concentrations of glycosaminoglycans. Decreased range of motion of the joint is related to the changes in ligaments and muscles. Bones in joints develop evidence of osteoporosis with fewer trabeculae and thinner, less dense bones, making them prone to fractures. Intervertebral disk spaces decrease in height.

Aging of Muscles

The function of skeletal muscle depends on many factors that are affected by aging, including the nervous, vascular, and endocrine systems. In the young child the development of muscle tissue is highly dependent on continuing neurodevelopmental maturation. Muscle function remains trainable even into advanced age. Muscle diseases have a definite association with specific age groups. Muscular dystrophies occur in children, and muscle disabilities related to rheumatic diseases usually occur in advancing age.

Age-related loss in skeletal muscle is referred to as **sarcopenia** and is a direct cause of the age-related decrease in muscle strength. As the body ages, muscle bulk and strength decline slowly; thus strength is maintained into the fifties, with a slow decline in dynamic and isometric strength evident after age 70. Type II fibers decrease to a greater extent than the slower-acting type I fibers. There is reduced RNA synthesis, loss of mitochondrial volume, and reduction in the size of motor units. The regenerative function of muscle tissue remains normal in aging persons. As much as 30% to 40% of skeletal muscle mass and strength may be lost from the third to ninth decades.[14]

Maximal oxygen intake decreases with age. Reduced basal metabolic rate and decreased lean body mass are also seen in the elderly population. However, strength training can reduce sarcopenia in older women.[14]

Structure and Function of Bones

1. Bones provide support and protection for the body's tissues and organs and are important sources of minerals and blood cells.
2. Bone formation begins with the production of an inorganic matrix by bone cells. Bone minerals crystallize in and around collagen fibers in the matrix, giving bone its characteristic hardness and strength.
3. Bone tissue is continuously being resorbed and synthesized by bone-remodeling units of osteoclasts and osteoblasts.
4. Receptor activator of NF-κB ligand (RANKL) induces osteoclast activation and bone resorption. Osteoprotegrin (OPG), a protein, binds to a protein called OPG-ligand. This attachment serves as a decoy receptor for RANKL and blocks. The balance between RANKL and OPG determines the quality of bone.
5. Bones in the body are made up of compact bone tissue and spongy bone tissue. Compact bone is highly organized into haversian systems that consist of concentric layers of crystallized matrix surrounding a central canal that contains blood vessels and nerves. Dispersed throughout the concentric layers of crystallized matrix are small spaces containing osteocytes. Smaller canals, called *canaliculi*, interconnect the osteocyte-containing spaces. The crystallized matrix in spongy bone is arranged in bars or plates. Spaces containing osteocytes are dispersed between the bars or plates and interconnected by canaliculi.
6. Bone morphogenic proteins (BMPs) are members of the transforming growth factor-beta (TGF-β) superfamily that are involved in nearly all aspects of bone formation.
7. There are 206 bones in the body, divided into the axial skeleton and the appendicular skeleton. Bones are classified by shape as long, short, flat, or irregular. Long bones have a broad end (epiphysis), broad neck (metaphysis), and narrow midportion (diaphysis) that contains the medullary cavity.
8. Bone injuries are repaired in stages. Hematoma formation provides the fibrin framework for formation and organization of granulation tissue. The granulation tissue provides a cartilage model for the formation and crystallization of bone matrix. Remodeling restores the original shape and size to the injured bone.

Structure and Function of Joints

1. A joint is the site where two or more bones attach. Joints provide stability and mobility to the skeleton.
2. Joints are classified as synarthroses, amphiarthroses, or diarthroses, depending on the degree of movement they allow. Joints are classified also by the type of connecting tissue holding them together. Fibrous joints are connected by dense fibrous tissue, ligaments, or membranes. Cartilaginous joints are connected by fibrocartilage or hyaline cartilage. Synovial joints are connected by a fibrous joint capsule. Within the capsule is a small, fluid-filled space. The fluid in the space nourishes the articular cartilage that covers the ends of the bones meeting in the synovial joint.
3. Articular cartilage is a highly organized system of collagen fibers and proteoglycans. The fibers firmly anchor the cartilage to the bone, and the proteoglycans control the loss of fluid from the cartilage.
4. Joints help move bones and muscle.

Structure and Function of Skeletal Muscles

1. Skeletal muscle is the largest organ in the body and is made up of millions of individual fibers.

2. Whole muscles vary in size (2 to 60 cm) and shape (fusiform and pennate). They are encased in a three-part connective tissue framework. The fundamental concept of muscle function is the *motor unit*, defined as all muscle fibers innervated by a single motor nerve.
3. Muscle fibers contain bundles of myofibrils arranged in parallel along the longitudinal axis and include the muscle membrane, myofibrils, sarcotubular system, aqueous sarcoplasm, and mitochondria. There are two types of muscle fibers, type I and type II, determined by motor nerve innervation.
4. Myofibrils and myofilaments contain the major muscle proteins, actin and myosin, which interact to form cross-bridges during muscle contraction. The nonprotein muscle constituents provide an energy source for contraction and regulate protein synthesis, enzyme systems, and membrane stabilization.
5. Muscle contraction includes excitation, coupling, contraction, and relaxation.
6. Muscle strength is graded by the "all or nothing" phenomenon and recruitment. Speed of contraction is affected by several factors: muscle fiber type, temperature, stretch, and weight of the load.
7. The two types of muscle contraction are isometric and isotonic. Muscle shortening occurs during contraction but can be seen also during pathologic and physiologic contracture.
8. Actin and myosin filaments form cross-bridges that cause the sarcomere to shorten, a process now known as the *cross-bridge theory of muscle contraction*.
9. Skeletal muscle requires a constant supply of adenosine triphosphate (ATP) and phosphocreatine to fuel muscle contraction and for growth and repair. ATP and phosphocreatine can be generated aerobically or anaerobically.
10. Several factors determine how force is transmitted from the actin-myosin cross-bridges on individual muscle fibers to accomplish whole-muscle contraction. When a motor unit responds to a single nerve stimulus, it develops a phasic contraction. The central nervous system smoothly grades the force generated by "recruiting" additional motor units and varying the discharge frequency of each active motor unit.

Tests of Musculoskeletal Function

1. Various diagnostic procedures are used to evaluate bone function, including gait analysis, serum calcium and phosphorus, x-ray films, angiography, bone scanning, and magnetic resonance imaging.
2. Procedures used to evaluate joint function include arthrography, arthroscopy, magnetic resonance imaging, and synovial fluid analysis.
3. Tests of muscular function include physical examination, serum creatine kinase, myoglobin, electromyogram, muscle biopsy, myometers, and the forearm ischemic exercise test.
4. Genetic evaluation is useful in detecting, diagnosing, and developing specific treatment for certain inheritable muscle diseases such as muscular dystrophy.

Aging and the Musculoskeletal System

1. Muscle bulk and strength slowly decline with aging, although not to a pathologic degree. The bone remodeling cycle takes longer to complete, and the rate of mineralization also slows down.
2. Exercise in the elderly does little to increase bone mineral density, but exercise has been shown to improve balance, coordination, muscle strength, lean body mass, and mobility.
3. Age-related loss in skeletal muscle is referred to sarcopenia.

KEY TERMS

α-Glycoprotein, 1475
Actin, 1488
Activation, 1490
Agonist, 1492
Amphiarthrosis (slightly movable
 joint), 1479
Antagonist, 1492
Appendicular skeleton, 1477
Arthrography, 1492
Arthroscopy, 1492
Articular cartilage, 1482
Axial skeleton, 1477
Basement membrane, 1488
Bone albumin, 1475
Bone fluid, 1475
Bone matrix, 1471
Bone morphogenic protein (BMP), 1474
Bone-remodeling unit, 1477
Calcification, 1472
Canaliculus (*pl.,* canaliculi), 1476
Chondrocytes, 1482
Collagen fibers, 1474
Compact bone (cortical bone), 1475
Contraction, 1490
Coupling, 1490
Creatine kinase, 1489
Creatine, 1489
Cross-bridge theory, 1490
Diaphysis, 1477
Diarthrosis (freely movable joint), 1479
Electromyogram (EMG), 1493
Endomysium, 1484
Endosteum, 1477
Epimysium, 1484
Epiphyseal plate (growth plate), 1477
Epiphysis, 1477
Fascia, 1484
Fascicles, 1484
Fibrils, 1474
Fibrous joint, 1479
Flat bones, 1477
Fusiform muscle, 1484
Glycoproteins, 1474

Glycosaminoglycans, 1483
Golgi tendon organs, 1485
Gomphosis, 1481
Ground substance, 1471
Haversian canal, 1475
Haversian system, 1475
Hyaluronate, 1482
Hydroxyapatite (HAP), 1475
Integrins, 1474
Intima, 1481
Irregular bones, 1477
Isometric contraction (static or holding
 contraction), 1492
Isotonic contraction (lengthening or
 shortening), 1492
Joint (articulation), 1479
Joint capsule (articular capsule), 1481
Joint cavity (synovial cavity), 1482
Lacuna, 1473
Lamellae, 1475
Laminin, 1474
Link protein, 1483
Long bone, 1477
Magnetic resonance imaging (MRI), 1492
Metaphysis, 1477
Motor unit, 1485
Muscle cell, 1487
Muscle fiber action potential, 1490
Muscle fiber, 1487
Muscle membrane, 1488
Myoblasts, 1487
Myofibrils, 1487
Myosin, 1488
Osteoblasts, 1472
Osteocalcin, 1474
Osteoclasts, 1473
Osteocyte, 1473
Osteoid, 1473
Osteonectin, 1474
Osteoprotegerin, 1479
Oxygen debt, 1491
Pennate muscles, 1484
Perimysium, 1484

Periosteum, 1476
Procallus, 1478
Protein core, 1483
Proteoglycans, 1474
RANKL, 1473
Relaxation, 1490
Remodeling, 1477
Repetitive discharge, 1491
Ruffled borders, 1474
Sarcolemma, 1488
Sarcomere, 1488
Sarcopenia, 1493
Sarcoplasm, 1488
Sarcoplasmic reticulum, 1488
Sarcotubular system, 1488
Sarcotubules, 1488
Short bones (cuboidal bones), 1477
Sialoprotein (osteopontin), 1474
Skeletal (voluntary, striated, or extrafusal)
 muscle, 1484
Sliding filament theory, 1490
Spindles, 1485
Spongy bone (cancellous bone), 1475
Subintima, 1481
Suture, 1480
Symphysis, 1481
Synarthrosis (immovable joint), 1479
Synchondrosis, 1481
Syndesmosis, 1480
Synovial fluid, 1482
Synovial joints (diarthroses), 1481
Synovial membrane (synovium), 1481
Tendon, 1484
Tetanus, 1492
Tidemark, 1482
Trabecula (*pl.,* trabeculae), 1476
Transverse tubules, 1488
Type A synovial cells, 1482
Type B synovial cells, 1482
Type I fiber, 1487
Type II fiber, 1487
Woven bone (callus), 1478

MEDIA RESOURCES *evolve*

Review questions and answers for this chapter are available in the *CD Companion* included with this book.

WebLinks—links to Internet sites pertaining to this chapter—are available on Evolve at http://evolve.elsevier.com/McCance/.

REFERENCES

1. Baron R: Anatomy and ultrastructure of bone. In Favus MJ, Christakos S, editors: *Primer on the metabolic bone diseases and disorders of mineral metabolism,* ed 4, Philadelphia, 1999, Lippincott Williams & Wilkins.
2. Zaudi M et al: Osteoclastogenesis, bone resorption, and osteoclast-based therapeutics, *J Bone Mineral Res* 18(4):599-609, 2003.
3. Buckwalter JA, Einhorn TA, Simon SR, editors: *Orthopaedic basic science,* Rosemont, Ill, 1999, American Academy of Orthopaedic Surgeons.
4. Delaisse JM et al: Matrix metalloproteinases (MMPs) and cathepsin K contribute differently to osteoclastic activities, *Mircosci Res Tech* 61(6):504-513, 2003.
5. Ulrich-Vinther M et al: Articular cartilage biology, *J Am Acad Orthoped Surg* 11(6):421-430, 2003.
6. Jacobson C, Duggan D, Fishbach G: Neuregulin induces the expression of transcription factors and myosin heavy chains typical of muscle spindles in cultured human muscle, *Proc Natl Acad Sci U S A* 101(33):12218-12223, 2004.
7. Labiet D et al: Calcium-dependent molecular spring elements in the giant protein titin, *Proc Natl Acad Sci U S A* 100(23):13716-13721, 2003.
8. Huxley AF: Muscle contraction. Cross-bridge titling confirmed, *Nature* 375(6533):631, 1995.
9. Huxley AF: Cross-bridge action: present views, prospects, and unknowns, *J Biomechanics* 33(10):1189-1195, 2000.
10. De Feo P et al: Metabolic response to exercise, *J Endocrinol Invest* 26(9):851-854, 2003.
11. Richardson RS: Oxygen transport and utilization: an integration of the muscle systems, *Adv Physiol Educ* 27(1-4):183-191, 2003.
12. Faulkner JA: Terminology for contractions of muscle during shortening, while isometric, and during lengthening, *J Appl Physiol* 95(2):455-459, 2003.
13. Karlsson M: Does exercise reduce the burden of fractures? *Acta Orthop Scand* 73(6):691-705, 2002.
14. Curl WW: Aging and exercise: are they compatible in women? *Clin Orthop Relat Res* Mar(372):151-158, 2000.

ALTERATIONS OF MUSCULOSKELETAL FUNCTION

CHRISTY L. CROWTHER • KATHRYN L. McCANCE

CHAPTER OUTLINE

http://evolve.elsevier.com/McCance/

Musculoskeletal injuries include fractures, dislocations, sprains, and strains. Fractures are the most serious. Alterations in bones, joints, and muscles may be caused by metabolic disorders, infections, inflammatory or noninflammatory diseases, or tumors. Trauma is the leading cause of death of people ages 1 to 44 years of all races and socioeconomic levels.

MUSCULOSKELETAL INJURIES

Skeletal muscles can withstand many penetrating injuries without permanent loss of function. For example, studies of soldiers with severe combat injuries showed that muscle function was preserved after the removal of large portions of muscle tissue. Successful regeneration of skeletal muscle fibers depends primarily on the extent of injury, preservation of vascular supply (and source of nutrition), and the availability of terminal axons for reinnervation.

Skeletal Trauma
Fractures

A **fracture** is a break in the continuity of a bone. A break occurs when force is applied that exceeds the tensile or compressive strength of the bone. The incidence of fractures varies for individual bones according to age and gender. The highest incidence of fractures occurs in young males (between ages 15 and 24 years) and in adults 65 years of age and older. Fractures of healthy bones, particularly the tibia, clavicle, and lower humerus, tend to occur in young persons and tend to be the result of trauma. Fractures of the hands and feet are usually caused by accidents in the workplace. The incidence of fractures of the upper femur, upper humerus, vertebrae, and pelvis is highest in older or elderly adults and is often associated with osteoporosis (see p. 1507). In 1990, an estimated 1.66 million hip fractures occurred worldwide; that number is expected to increase to 6.3 million by the year 2050.[1]

Classification

Fractures can be classified as complete or incomplete and open or closed (Figure 42-1). In a **complete fracture** the bone

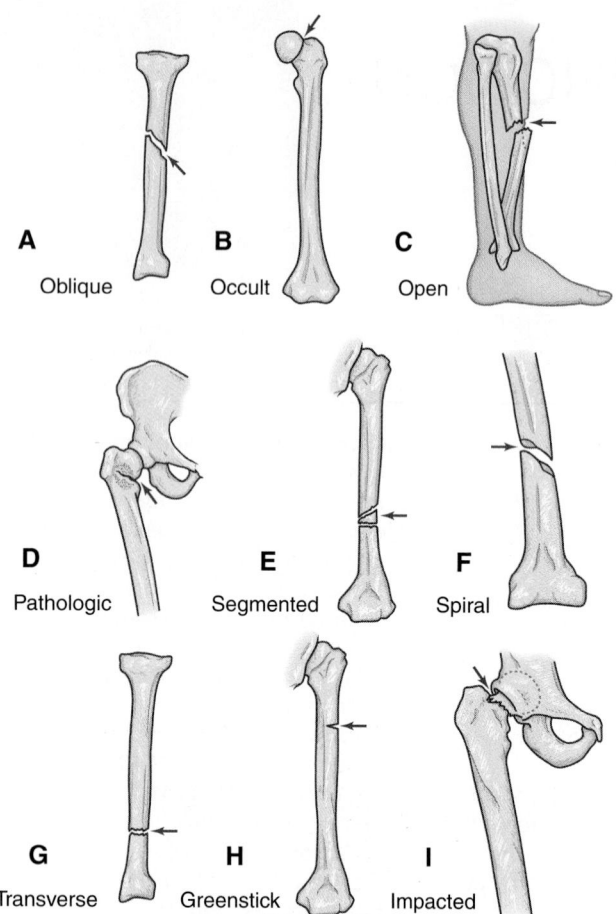

Figure 42-1 Examples of types of bone fractures. **A,** Oblique: fracture at oblique angle across both cortices. *Cause:* direct or indirect energy, with angulation and some compression. **B,** Occult: fracture that is hidden or not readily discernible. *Cause:* minor force or energy. **C,** Open: skin broken over fracture; possible soft tissue trauma. *Cause:* moderate to severe energy that is continuous and exceeds tissue tolerances. **D,** Pathologic: transverse, oblique, or spiral fracture of bone weakened by tumor pressure or presence. *Cause:* minor energy or force, which may be direct or indirect. **E,** Segmented: fracture with two or more pieces or segments. *Cause:* direct or indirect moderate to severe force. **F,** Spiral: fracture that curves around cortices and may become displaced by twist. *Cause:* direct or indirect twisting energy or force with distal part held or unable to move. **G,** Transverse: horizontal break through bone. *Cause:* direct or indirect energy toward bone. **H,** Greenstick: break in only one cortex of bone. *Cause:* minor direct or indirect energy. **I,** Impacted: fracture with one end wedged into opposite end of inside fractured fragment. *Cause:* compressive axial energy or force directly to distal fragment. (Redrawn from Mourad L: Musculoskeletal system. In Thompson JM et al, editors: *Mosby's clinical nursing,* ed 7, St Louis, 2002, Mosby.)

is broken all the way through, whereas in an **incomplete fracture** the bone is damaged but is still in one piece. Complete or incomplete fractures also can be classified as **open** (formerly referred to as *compound*) if the skin is broken or as **closed** (formerly called *simple*) if it is not. A fracture in which a bone breaks into two or more fragments is termed a **comminuted fracture**. Fractures are classified also according to the direction of the fracture line. A **linear fracture** runs parallel to the long axis of the bone. An **oblique fracture** is a slanted fracture

of the shaft of the bone. A **spiral fracture** encircles the bone, and a **transverse fracture** occurs straight across the bone.

Incomplete fractures tend to occur in the more flexible, growing bones of children. The three main types of incomplete fractures are greenstick, torus, and bowing. A **greenstick fracture** perforates one cortex and splinters the spongy bone. The name is derived from the damage sustained by a young tree branch (a green stick) when it is bent sharply. The outer surface is disrupted, but the inner surface remains intact. Greenstick fractures typically occur in the metaphysis or diaphysis of the tibia, radius, and ulna. In a **torus fracture** the cortex buckles but does not break. **Bowing fractures** usually occur when longitudinal force is applied to bone. This type of fracture is common in children and usually involves the paired radius-ulna or fibula-tibia. A complete diaphyseal fracture occurs in one of the bones of the pair, which disperses the stress sufficiently to prevent a complete fracture of the second bone, which bows. A bowing fracture resists correction (reduction) because the force necessary to reduce it must be equal to the force that bowed it. Treatment of bowing fractures is difficult also because the bowed bone interferes with reduction of the fractured bone. Types of fractures are summarized in Table 42-1.

Fractures may be further classified by cause as pathologic, stress, or transchondral. A **pathologic fracture** is a break at the site of a preexisting abnormality, usually by force that would not fracture a normal bone. Any disease process that weakens a bone (especially the cortex) predisposes the bone to pathologic fracture, commonly associated with tumors, osteoporosis, infections, and metabolic bone disorders.

Stress fractures occur in normal or abnormal bone that is subjected to repeated stress, such as occurs during athletics. The stress is less than the stress that usually causes a fracture. Two types of stress fractures are **fatigue fractures,** caused by abnormal stress or torque applied to a bone with normal ability to deform and recover (e.g., joggers, dancers, military recruits), and **insufficiency fractures,** stress fractures that occur in bones lacking normal ability to deform and recover (i.e., normal weight bearing or activity fractures the bone).

A **transchondral fracture** consists of fragmentation and separation of a portion of the articular cartilage that covers the end of a bone at a joint. (Joint structures are defined in Chapter 41.) The fragments may consist of cartilage alone or cartilage and bone. Typical sites of transchondral fracture are the distal femur, the ankle, the kneecap, the elbow, and the wrist. Transchondral fractures are most prevalent in adolescents.

PATHOPHYSIOLOGY When a bone is broken, the periosteum and blood vessels in the cortex, marrow, and surrounding soft tissues are disrupted. Bleeding occurs from the damaged ends of the bone and from the neighboring soft tissue. A clot (hematoma) forms within the medullary canal, between the fractured ends of the bone, and beneath the periosteum. Bone tissue immediately adjacent to the fracture dies. This necrotic tissue (along with any debris in the fracture area) stimulates an intense inflammatory response character-

Table 42-1	Types of Fractures
Type	**Definition**
Typical Complete Fractures	
Closed fracture	The skin overlying the bone is intact
Open fracture	Communicating wound between bone and skin
Comminuted fracture	Multiple bone fragments
Linear fracture	Fracture line parallel to long axis of bone
Oblique fracture	Fracture line at 45-degree angle to long axis of bone
Spiral fracture	Fracture line encircling bone (as a spiral staircase)
Transverse fracture	Fracture line perpendicular to long axis of bone
Impacted	Fracture fragments are pushed into each other
Pathologic	Fracture occurs at a point in the bone weakened by disease, for example, bones with tumors or osteoporosis
Avulsion	A fragment of bone connected to a ligament or tendon breaks off from the main bone
Compression	Fracture is wedged or squeezed together on one side of bone
Displaced	Fracture with one, both, or all fragments out of normal alignment
Extracapsular	Fragment is close to the joint but remains outside the joint capsule
Intracapsular	Fragment extends into or is within the joint capsule
Typical Incomplete Fractures	
Greenstick fracture	Break on one cortex of bone with splintering of inner bone surface, commonly occurs in children and elderly persons
Torus fracture	Buckling of cortex
Bowing fracture	Bending of the bone
Stress fracture	Microfracture
Transchondral fracture	Separation of cartilaginous joint surface (articular cartilage) from main shaft of bone

ized by vasodilation, exudation of plasma and leukocytes, and infiltration by inflammatory leukocytes and mast cells. Within 48 hours after the injury, vascular tissue invades the fracture area from surrounding soft tissue and the marrow cavity, and blood flow to the entire bone is increased. Bone-forming cells in the periosteum, endosteum, and marrow are activated to produce subperiosteal procallus along the outer surface of the shaft and over the broken ends of the bone (Figure 42-2). Osteoblasts within the procallus synthesize collagen and matrix, which becomes mineralized to form callus. As the repair process continues, remodeling occurs, during which unnecessary callus is resorbed and trabeculae are formed along lines of stress. Except for the liver, bone is unique among all body tissues in that it will form new bone, not scar tissue, when it heals after a fracture.

CLINICAL MANIFESTATIONS   The clinical manifestations of a fracture vary according to the type of fracture, site of the fracture, and associated soft tissue injury. In general, the signs and symptoms of a fracture include impaired function, unnatural alignment (deformity), swelling, muscle spasm, tenderness, pain, and impaired sensation. The position of the bone segments is determined by the pull of attached muscles, gravity, and the direction and magnitude of the force that caused the fracture. One or both segments may be rotated inward or outward on the bone's long axis (rotation), be misaligned at an angle (angulation), slide over the other segment (overriding), or be out of normal position (displaced).

The immediate pain of a fracture is severe and usually caused by the trauma. Subsequent pain may be produced by

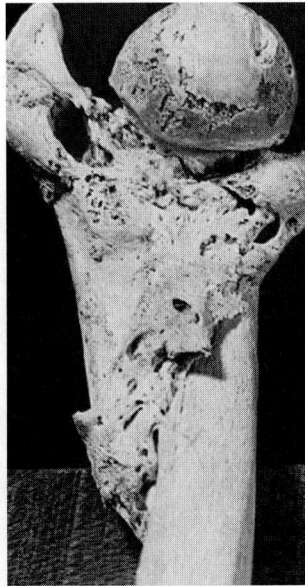

Figure 42-2 Exuberant callus formation following fracture. (From Rosai J: *Ackerman's surgical pathology,* ed 8, St Louis, 1996, Mosby.)

muscle spasm, overriding of the fracture segments, or damage to adjacent soft tissues. Numbness is common and is caused by swelling, by the pinching or severing of a nerve, by the trauma, or by bone fragments. Pathologic fractures usually cause angular deformity, painless swelling, or generalized bone pain. Pathologic fractures are not usually associated with trauma or trauma-related pain. Stress fractures are painful, not because of trauma, but because of accelerated remodeling. The pain occurs during activity and is usually relieved by rest. Stress fractures also cause local tenderness and soft tissue swelling. Transchondral fractures may be entirely asymptomatic or painful during movement. Range of motion in the joint is limited, and movement may evoke audible clicking sounds (crepitus).

EVALUATION AND TREATMENT   Treatment of a displaced fracture involves realigning the bone fragments (reduction) close to their normal or anatomic position and holding the fragments in place (immobilization) so that bone union can occur. Several methods are available to reduce a fracture: closed manipulation, traction, and open reduction. Many fractures heal without manipulation—they require only adequate immobilization. A fracture that is malaligned, however, requires more aggressive treatment.

Most fractures can be reduced by closed manipulation: the skin is not opened, and the bone is moved or manipulated into place. Closed manipulation is used when the contour of the bone is in fair alignment and can be maintained well with immobilization.

Traction is used to accomplish or maintain reduction. When bone fragments are displaced (not in their anatomic position), weights are used to apply firm, steady traction (pull) and countertraction to the long axis of the bone. Traction stretches and fatigues muscles that pull the bone fragments out of place, allowing the distal fragment to align with the proximal fragment. Traction can be applied to the skin (skin traction) (Figure 42-3), directly to the involved bone, or distal to the involved bone (skeletal traction). Skin traction is

used when only a few pounds of pulling force are needed to realign the fragments or when the traction will be used for brief times only, such as before surgery or, for children with femoral fractures, for 3 to 7 days before applying a cast. A traction boot is applied to the skin and is closed with self-adhering straps, with weights attached to the foot area of the traction boot. In skeletal traction, a pin or wire is drilled through the bone below the fracture site, and a traction bow, rope, and weights are attached to the pin or wire to apply tension and to provide the pulling force needed to overcome the muscle spasm and help realign the fracture fragments.

External fixation is used to reduce and immobilize significantly displaced open fractures. Pins are placed in the bone proximal and distal to the break and then stabilized by an external frame of clamps and rods (Figure 42-4).

Open reduction is a surgical procedure that exposes the fracture site; the fragments are brought into alignment under direct visualization. Some form of prosthesis, screw, plate, nail, or wire usually is used to maintain the reduction (internal fixation).

Splints and casts are used to immobilize and hold a reduction in place. Improper reduction or immobilization of a fractured bone may result in nonunion, delayed union, or malunion. **Nonunion** is failure of the bone ends to grow together (Figure 42-5). The gap between the broken ends of the bone fills with dense fibrous and fibrocartilaginous tissue instead of new bone. Occasionally, the fibrous tissue contains a fluid-filled space that resembles a joint and is termed a *false joint,* or *pseudoarthrosis.* **Delayed union** is union that does

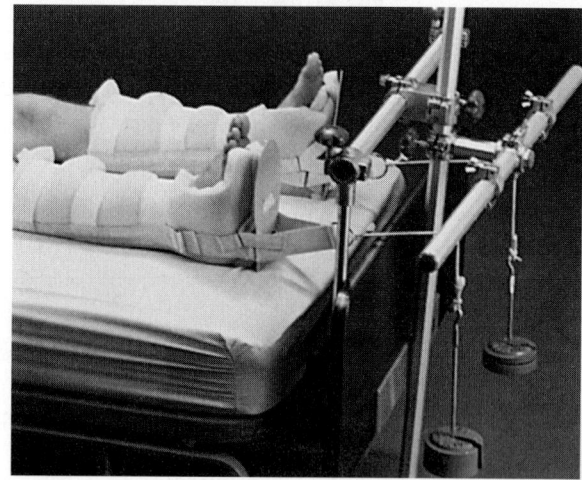

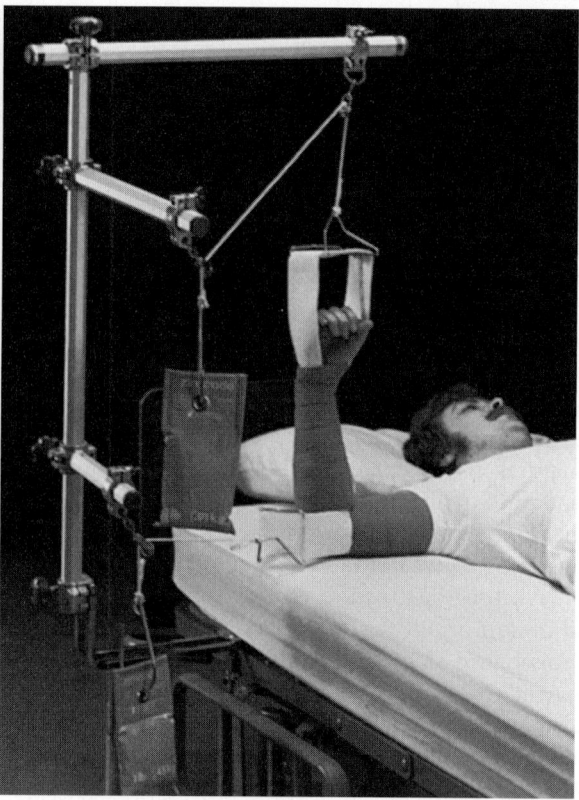

Figure 42-3 Two types of skin traction. **A,** Buck extension traction. **B,** Dunlop traction. (From Mourad L: *Orthopedic disorders,* St Louis, 1991, Mosby.)

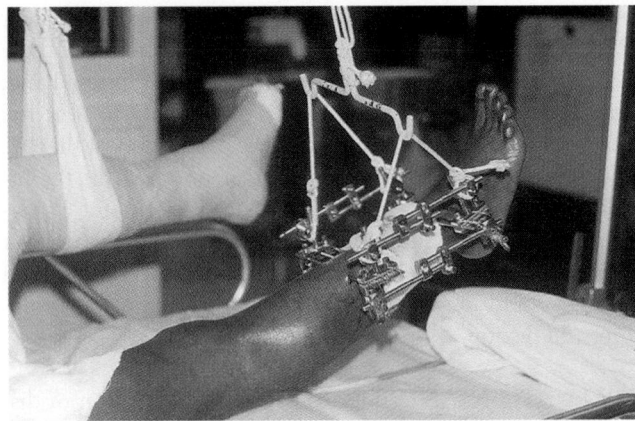

Figure 42-4 Example of an external fixation device on the right leg. The left leg is in a splint.

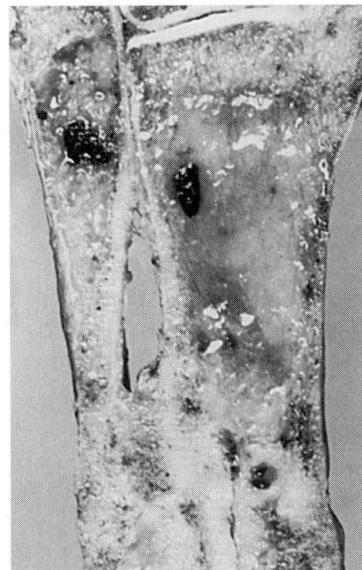

Figure 42-5 Nonunion of old fracture of tibia and fibula in 53-year-old white man. Multiple fractures had occurred in 2 years previous and necessitated bone grafting. (From Rosai J: *Ackerman's surgical pathology,* ed 8, St Louis, 1996, Mosby.)

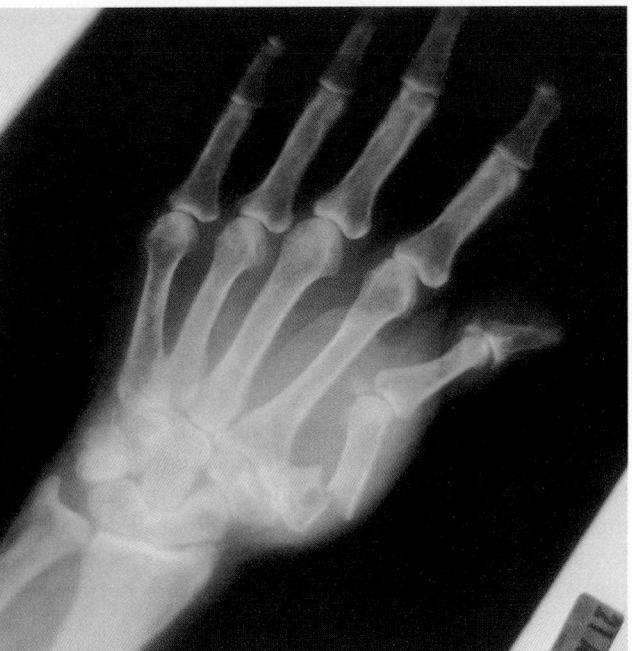

Figure 42-6 Displaced fracture. X-ray showing a displaced fracture of the base of the first metacarpal, also known as a *Bennett fracture.*

not occur until approximately 8 to 9 months after a fracture. **Malunion** is the healing of a bone in a nonanatomic position. Treatment of delayed union and nonunion includes use of various modalities designed to stimulate new bone formation. Physical modalities, such as implantable or external electric current devices, electromagnetic field generations, and low-density ultrasound, have all been effective in stimulating bone formation.[2] Gene therapy also shows promise in promoting formation of new bone.[3]

Dislocation and Subluxation

Dislocation and subluxation are usually caused by trauma. **Dislocation** is the temporary displacement of a bone from its normal position in a joint. If the contact between the two surfaces is only partially lost, the injury is called a **subluxation.**

Dislocation and subluxation are most common in persons younger than 20 years and are generally associated with frac-

tures. Dislocation and subluxation, however, may result from congenital or acquired disorders that cause (1) muscular imbalance, as occurs with congenital dislocation of the hip or neurologic disorders; (2) incongruities in the articulating surfaces of the bones, as occurs with rheumatoid arthritis (see p. 1525); or (3) joint instability.

The joints most often dislocated or subluxed are the joints of the shoulder, elbow, wrist, finger, hip, and knee (Figure 42-6). The shoulder's glenohumeral joint is a relatively unstable joint because the articular surface of the glenoid cavity is only one third as large as the surface of the humeral head. As a result, the glenohumeral joint is often injured. Physical trauma to the shoulder can cause anterior, posterior, superior, or inferior dislocation. Anterior dislocation is the most common and is usually the result of an indirect force that places the shoulder in extreme external rotation.[4] Posterior dislocations usually occur as a result of trauma. A superior dislocation is rare and usually the result of an extreme forward and upward force on an adducted arm. Inferior displacement is often seen in persons with neurologic injuries of the brachial plexus and is believed to be caused by stretching of the supporting muscles or by joint effusion.

Traumatic dislocation of the elbow joint is common in the immature skeleton. In adults an elbow dislocation is usually associated with a fracture of the ulna or head of the radius. Posterior dislocations occur when the individual falls on an outstretched hand with the elbow extended. Anterior dislocations are usually the result of a direct blow to the flexed elbow.

Traumatic dislocation of the wrist usually involves the distal ulna and carpal bones. Any one of the eight carpal bones can be dislocated after an injury. The most common cause is a fall on the hyperextended hand.

Dislocation in the hand usually involves the metacarpophalangeal and interphalangeal joints. Dislocation of the metacarpophalangeal joint is often the result of a fall on the outstretched hand that forces the joint into hyperextension. Dislocation of the interphalangeal joint occurs as a result of injury to the fingers in a hyperextended position.

Considerable trauma is needed to dislocate the hip. Anterior hip dislocation is rather rare and is caused by forced abduction, for example, when an individual lands on the feet from a high fall. Posterior dislocation of the hip can occur in an automobile accident in which the flexed knee strikes the dashboard.

The knee is an unstable joint that depends heavily on the soft tissue structures around it for support. Because the knee is an unstable weight-bearing joint exposed to many different types of motion (flexion, extension, rotation), it is one of the most commonly injured joints. A knee dislocation can be anterior, posterior, lateral, medial, or rotary. It is usually the result of a hyperextension injury that occurs during sports activities.

PATHOPHYSIOLOGY Dislocations and subluxations are often accompanied by fracture because stress is placed on areas of bone not normally subjected to stress. In addition, as the bone separates from the joint, it may bruise or tear adjacent nerves, blood vessels, ligaments, supporting structures, and soft tissue. Dislocation of the shoulder may damage the shoulder capsule and the axillary nerve. Damage to the axillary nerve causes anesthesia in the sensory distribution of the nerve and paralysis of the deltoid muscle. Elbow dislocations are accompanied by torn periosteum, ligaments, and muscle. Bleeding from the damaged periosteum and muscle puts pressure on adjacent arteries that shuts off circulation to and from the forearm and hand. If the pressure is not promptly relieved, ischemic paralysis develops. Dislocations of the hand often result in permanent disability because of damage to the tendons and intricate mechanisms that allow smooth gliding in the joints. Avascular necrosis of the femoral head is a complication seen in hip dislocations. Knee dislocation usually tears both the collateral and cruciate ligaments.

CLINICAL MANIFESTATIONS Signs and symptoms of dislocations or subluxations include pain, swelling, limitation of motion, and joint deformity. Pain may be caused by effusion of inflammatory exudate into the joint or associated tension and ligament injury. Joint deformity is usually caused by muscle contractions that exert pull on the dislocated or subluxed joint or fluid within the joint. Limitation of motion may be a result of effusion into the joint or the displacement of bones.

Tenderness and deformity are prominent in dislocations of the fingers. Unusual muscle pull and pain often result in abnormal posturing of the fingers; for example, the fingers or thumb may be abnormally flexed. A dislocated elbow is often held in a flexed position, and the joint resists active or passive movement. Pain is the key symptom of shoulder injuries. Attempts to lift the arm aggravate the pain. In most shoulder dislocations, the ability to elevate the arm is minimal and the individual supports the injured arm with the opposite hand. Pain and an abnormal gait or limp or inability to bear full weight usually accompanies traumatic dislocation of the hip. The pain is constant and severe and is often felt in the inguinal region or thigh. The thigh and leg may assume a position of inward rotation, adduction, or flexion and appear shortened. In a rare anterior dislocation, the limb is not shortened and the joint is fixed in abduction, outward rotation, and flexion.

EVALUATION AND TREATMENT Evaluation of dislocations and subluxations is based on clinical manifestations and roentgenograms. Treatment consists of reduction and immobilization for 2 to 6 weeks and exercises to maintain normal range of motion in the joint. Depending on the joint, healing is usually complete within months to years.

Support Structures
Sprains and Strains of Tendons and Ligaments

Tendon and ligament injuries can accompany fractures and dislocations. A **tendon** is fibrous connective tissue that attaches skeletal muscle to bone. A **ligament** is a band of fibrous connective tissue that connects bones where they meet at a joint. Tendons and ligaments support the bones and joints and either facilitate or limit motion. Tendons and ligaments can be torn, ruptured, or completely separated from bone at their points of attachment.

A tear in a tendon is commonly known as a **strain.** Major trauma can tear or rupture a tendon at any site in the body. Most often injured are the tendons of the hands and feet, the knee (patellar), the upper arm (biceps and triceps), the thigh (quadriceps), the ankle, and the heel (Achilles). Lifting excessive weight with the arms can cause traumatic rupture of the biceps tendon. Rupture of the Achilles tendon occurs when forced dorsiflexion is applied to the foot when it is in plantar flexion.[5] Spontaneous tendon ruptures can occur in individuals receiving local corticosteroid injections, fluoroquinolones, and persons with rheumatoid arthritis or systemic lupus erythematosus.[6]

Ligament tears are commonly known as **sprains.** Ligament tears and ruptures can occur at any joint but are most common in the wrist, ankle, elbow, and knee joints. A complete separation of a tendon or ligament from its bony attachment site is known as an **avulsion.** An avulsion is the result of abnormal stress on the ligament or tendon and is commonly seen in young athletes, especially sprinters, hurdlers, and runners.

Strains and sprains are classified as first degree (least severe), second degree, and third degree (most severe).

PATHOPHYSIOLOGY When a tendon or ligament is torn, an extensive cascade of inflammatory processes begins.[7] An inflammatory exudate develops between the torn ends. Later, granulation tissue containing macrophages, fibroblasts, and capillary buds grows inward from the surrounding soft tissue and cartilage to begin the repair process. Within 4 to 5 days after the injury, collagen formation begins. At first, collagen formation is random and disorganized. As the collagen fibers interweave and connect with preexisting tendon fibers, they become organized parallel to the lines of stress. Eventually vascular fibrous tissue fuses the new and surrounding tissues into a single mass. As reorganization takes place, the healing tendon or ligament separates from the surrounding soft tissue. Usually a healing tendon or ligament lacks sufficient strength to withstand strong pull for 4 to 5 weeks after the injury. If strong muscle pull does occur during this time, the tendon or ligament ends may separate again, which causes the tendon or ligament to heal in a lengthened shape with an excessive amount of scar tissue that renders the tendon or ligament functionless. Scar remodeling may take months to years before it is complete.[8]

CLINICAL MANIFESTATIONS   Tendon and ligament injuries are painful and are usually accompanied by soft tissue swelling, changes in tendon or ligament contour, and dislocation or subluxation of bones. The pain is generally sharp and localized, and tenderness persists over the distribution of the tendon or ligament. Painful joint swelling can usually be seen in finger and elbow sprains. Flexion deformities of the fingers and thumb occur in injuries to the extensor tendons. Crepitus may accompany tendon injury in the wrist. Pain in the elbow may be accentuated by flexion, supination, and extension of the elbow or by extension of the wrist. Lifting small objects requires extension of the wrist and therefore aggravates the pain. Tendon injuries in the upper arm cause weakness when the individual tries to flex the forearm. Pain is often the key symptom of shoulder injuries. It may be referred to the deltoid muscle or extend down the arm. The pain is usually aggravated by attempts to lift the arms. Depending on the ligament or tendon involved, tendon and ligament injuries in the knee may produce pronounced immobility, lost lateral movement, instability when walking down stairs, semiflexion, crepitus, or an upward shift of the patella.

EVALUATION AND TREATMENT   Evaluation is based on clinical manifestations, stress radiography, arthroscopy, or arthrography. When possible, treatment consists of protecting the involved structures (splinting), early motion, and rehabilitation. Suturing the tendon or ligament ends in close approximation may be necessary to treat complete rupture. If this is not possible because of the extent of damage, tendon or ligament grafting may be necessary. Prolonged rehabilitation exercises help ensure that the patient regains nearly normal functions.

Tendinopathy and Bursitis

Trauma and repetitive stress can cause painful degradation of collagen fibers (**tendinosis**), inflammation of tendons (**tendinitis**), or inflammation in bursal sacs (**bursitis**). Other causes of tendinopathy include crystal deposits, postural misalignment, and hypermobility in a joint. Table 42-2 summarizes classes of tendinopathies.

Epicondylitis is inflammation of a tendon where it attaches to a bone (at its origin). Epicondylar areas of the humerus, radius, or ulna and the area around the knee are most often inflamed. **Lateral epicondylitis,** commonly called **tennis elbow,** is probably the result of tissue degeneration or irritation of the extensor carpi radialis brevis tendon at its origin. **Medial epicondylitis,** referred to as **golfer's elbow,** is a degenerative process of the pronator teres, flexor carpi radialis, and palmaris longus tendons at the medial humeral condyle[9] (Figure 42-7). Epicondylitis is also related to work activities that involve repetitive cyclic flexion and extension of the elbow, or cyclic pronation, supination, extension, and flexion of the wrist that generates loads to the elbow and forearm region. Three sets of risk factors affect the incidence of epicondylitis related to work and include biomechanical con-

Table 42-2	Histopathological Classification of Tendon Disorders	
Pathologic Diagnosis	**Macroscopic Pathology**	**Histopathologic Findings**
Tendinosis	Intratendinous degeneration (commonly due to ageing, microtrauma, mascular compromise)	Collagen disorientation, disorganization and fiber separation by an increase in mucoid ground substance, increased preponderance of cells and vascular spaces with or without neovascularization and focal necrosis or calcification
Tendinitis	Symptomatic degeneration of the tendon with vascular disruption and inflammatory repair response	Degenerative changes as noted above with superimposed evidence of tear, including fibroblastic and myofibroblastic proliferation, hemorrhage and organizing granulation tissue.
Paratenonitis	"Inflammation" of the outer layer of the tendon (paratenon) alone, whether or not the paratenon is lined by synovium	Mucoid degeneration if the areolar tissue is seen. A scattered mild mononuclear infiltrate with or without focal fibrin deposition and fibrinous exudate
Paratenonitis with tendinosis	Paratenonitis associated with intratendinous degeneration	Degenerative changes as noted in tendinosis with mucoid degeneration with or without fibrous and scattered inflammatory cells in the paratenon alveolar tissue

From Maffulli N, Wong J, Almekinders LC: *Clin Sports Med* 22(4):675-692, 2003.

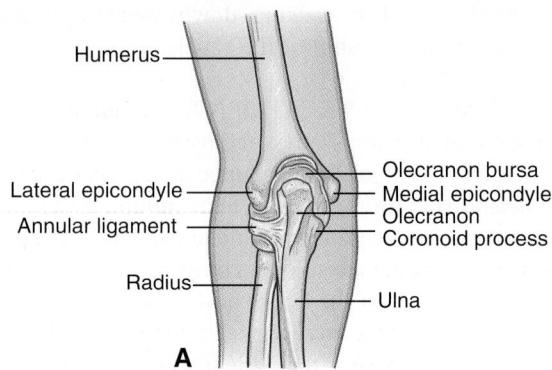

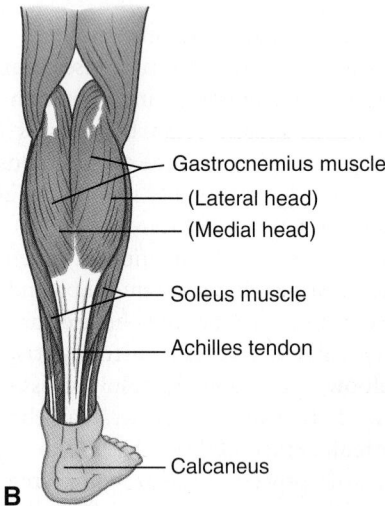

Figure 42-7 Tendinitis and epicondylitis. **A,** Medial or lateral epicondyles of humerus, site of epicondylitis. **B,** Achilles tendon, site of commonly occurring tendinitis.

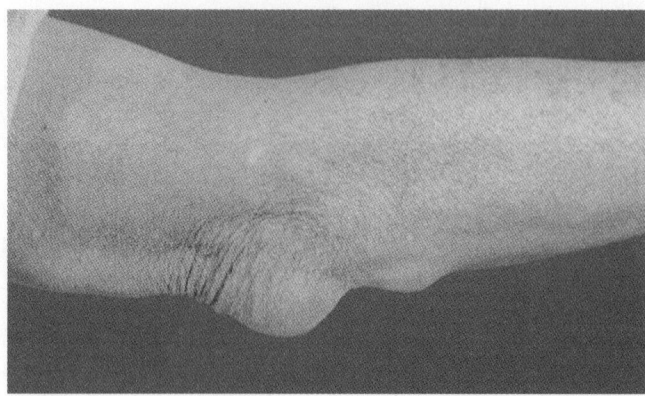

Figure 42-8 Olecranon bursa. A case of olecranon bursitis in a patient with rheumatoid arthritis. A rheumatoid nodule is also shown. (From Klippel JH, Deippe PA, editors: *Rheumatology,* ed 2, London, 1998, Mosby.)

straints, psychosocial factors, and personal factors—including social support at work.[10,11]

Bursae are small sacs lined with synovial membrane and filled with synovial fluid; they are located between tendons, muscles, and bony prominences. Their primary function is to separate, lubricate, and cushion these structures. Acute bursitis occurs primarily in the middle years and is caused by trauma. Chronic bursitis can result from repeated trauma. Septic bursitis is caused by wound infection or bacterial infection of the skin overlying the bursae. Bursitis commonly occurs in the shoulder, hip, knee, and elbow.

PATHOPHYSIOLOGY   In tendinitis, fluid from inflammation accumulates, causing swelling of the tendon and its enclosing sheath. Inflammatory changes cause thickening of the sheath, which limits movements and causes pain. Microtears cause bleeding, edema, and pain in the involved tendons or surrounding structures. At times, after repeated inflammations, calcium may be deposited in the tendon origin area, causing a calcific tendinitis.

The usual bursitis is an inflammation that is reactive to overuse or excessive pressure. The inflamed bursal sac becomes engorged, and the inflammation can spread to adjacent tissues (Figure 42-8). The inflammation may decrease with rest, heat, and aspiration of the fluid. (Inflammation is discussed in Chapter 6.)

CLINICAL MANIFESTATIONS   Tendinopathy may be asymptomatic but, generally, there is localized pain that worsens with active more than passive motion. With symptomatic tendinopathy, the pain is localized over the involved tendon and movement in the affected joint is limited. In bursitis, onset of pain may be gradual or sudden, and movement in the joint is not mechanically limited. Shoulder bursitis impairs arm abduction because of pain and swelling of the bursa. Bursitis in the knee produces pain when climbing stairs, and crossing the legs is painful in bursitis of the hip. Lying on the side of the inflamed trochanteric bursa is also very painful. Signs of infectious bursitis may include the presence of a puncture site, prior corticosteroid injection, severe inflammation, or an adjacent source of infection.

EVALUATION AND TREATMENT   Evaluation of tendinopathy, epicondylitis, and bursitis is based on clinical manifestations, physical examination, arthroscopy, arthrography, ultrasound, and possibly magnetic resonance imaging (MRI). Treatment includes immobilization of the joint with a sling, splint, or cast; systemic analgesics; ice or heat applications; or local injection of an anesthetic and a corticosteroid to reduce inflammation. Physical therapy to prevent loss of function begins after acute symptoms subside.

Muscle Strains

Mild injury such as **muscle strain** is usually seen after traumatic or sports injuries. *Muscle strain* is a general term for local muscle damage. It is often the result of sudden, forced motion causing the muscle to become stretched beyond normal capacity. Knife and gunshot wounds also cause traumatic rupture. Strains often involve the tendon as well. Muscles are ruptured more often than tendons in young people; the opposite is true in the older population. Muscle strain may be chronic when the muscle is repeatedly stretched beyond its usual capacity. There is evidence of tissue disruption with subsequent signs of muscle regeneration and connective tissue repair when a biopsy is performed. Hemorrhage into the surrounding tissue and signs of inflammation also may be present. Regardless of the cause of trauma, muscle cells usually can regenerate. Regeneration may take up to 6 weeks, and the affected muscle should be protected during this time. Types of muscle strain, together with their manifestations and treatment, are summarized in Table 42-3.

A late complication of localized muscle injury is **myositis ossificans.** Its true etiology is usually unknown.[12] This condition is thought to be caused by scar tissue calcification and subsequent ossification. Examples include "rider's bone," in which the adductor muscle of the thigh of equestrians becomes calcified, and "drill bone," in which the same complication is seen in the deltoid and pectoral muscles of fencers and infantry soldiers, as well as in football players after muscle injury to thigh muscles.

Rhabdomyolysis

Rhabdomyolysis, or **myoglobinuria,** can be a life-threatening complication of severe muscle trauma with muscle cell loss. Myoglobinuria is named for the principal manifestation of the condition—an excess of **myoglobin** (an intracellular muscle protein) in the urine. Muscle cell damage releases the myoglobin. The most severe form is often called *crush syndrome.* Less severe and more localized forms are called **compartment syndromes,** which can lead to **Volkmann ischemic contracture** in the forearm or leg. Crush syndrome first gained notoriety in the reports of injuries seen after the London air raids in World War II. More recently it has been reported in individuals found unresponsive and immobile for long periods, usually after a drug or alcohol overdose.[13] Rhabdomyolysis also can be seen after viral infections, administration of certain anesthetic agents, or some cholesterol-lowering agents known as "statins," strychnine poisoning, tetanus, heat stroke, electrolyte disturbances, and fractures. Excessive muscular activity also has been implicated in reports of myoglobinuria in athletes, such as long-distance runners, ice skaters, skiers, military recruits, and those subjected to fraternity hazing. Status epilepticus, electroconvulsive therapy, and high-voltage electrical shock are also associated with severe and sometimes fatal myoglobinuria. Box 42-1 summarizes some of these risk factors for rhabdomyolysis.

If the myoglobinuria is caused by fulminant malignant hyperthermia, severe muscle spasm and rhabdomyolysis can lead to renal failure. Other complications include intraoperative rigidity, tachycardia, cardiac dysrhythmias, metabolic and respiratory acidosis, and temperature elevations up to 43° C, which can occur very rapidly. Cerebral edema, cardiogenic and hypovolemic shock, pulmonary edema, and disseminated intravascular clotting can contribute to the death of an individual with malignant hyperthermia.

PATHOPHYSIOLOGY   The weight of a limp extremity can generate enough pressure to produce muscle ischemia (Figure 42-9). This causes edema, rising compartment pressure, and tamponade that leads to muscle infarction and neural injury and, finally, results in cell loss. Physical interruptions in the sarcolemmal membrane, called *holes* or *delta lesions,* suggest that the sarcolemmal membrane may be the route by which muscle constituents are released. (The sarcolemmal membrane, the plasma membrane [including creatine kinase, myoglobin, and phosphate] of the muscle cell, is described in Chapter 41.)

CLINICAL MANIFESTATIONS   When myoglobin is released from the muscle cells into the circulation, it can cause a visible, dark reddish brown pigmentation of the urine. The renal threshold for myoglobin is low, approximately 0.5 mg/dl of urine, so that only 200 g of muscle need be damaged to cause visible changes in the urine. Along with the release of myoglobin, creatine kinase (CK) and other serum enzymes are released in massive quantities. The CK level is often 100 times greater than normal (5 to 25 U/ml for women and 5 to 35 U/ml for men). The efflux of proteins and enzymes also includes loss of potassium, phosphate, nucleotides, creatinine, and creatine. Serum hypocalcemia is seen early in the course of myoglobinuria and is followed by late hypercalcemia.

EVALUATION AND TREATMENT   Careful and thorough preoperative assessment should alert the anesthesiologist to the possibility of a susceptible individual. A family history of anesthetic problems and previous untoward anesthetic experiences (muscle cramping, unexplained fevers, dark urine) are criteria that require further clarification before administration of a volatile anesthetic.

Table 42-3	Muscle Strain	
Type	**Manifestations**	**Treatment**
First degree (e.g., bench press in untrained athlete)	Muscle overstretched, painful	Ice should be applied 5 or 6 times in the first 24-48 hours; complete rest for up to 2 weeks, followed by weight bearing 3 times per week and range of motion daily
Second degree (e.g., any muscle strain with bruising and pain)	Muscle intact with some tearing pain, mild bruising, fascia is intact	Treatment similar to that for first-degree strains, with added mild analgesia; cryokinetics (a treatment system of alternating applications of heat and cold with progressive exercise)
Third degree (e.g., traumatic injury)	Caused by tearing of fascia, muscle rupture palpable, bleeding present	Surgery to approximate ruptured edges; immobilization and rest for 6 weeks, followed by an individualized rehabilitation regimen of strengthening exercises

Box 42-1	Causes of Rhabdomyolysis

Medications and Toxic Substances That Increase the Risk of Rhabdomyolysis

Direct myotoxicity
HMG-CoA reductase inhibitors, (statins), especially in combination with fibrate-derived lipid-lowering agents such as niacin (nicotinic acid; Nicolar)
Cyclosporine (Sandimmune)
Itraconazole (Sporanox)
Erythromycin
Colchicine
Zidovudine (Retrovir)
Corticosteroids

Indirect muscle damage
Alcohol
Central nervous system depressants
Cocaine
Amphetamine
Ecstasy (MDMA)
LSD
Neuromuscular blocking agents

Traumatic, Heat-Related, Ischemic and Exertional Causes

Traumatic causes
Lightning strike
Immobilization
Extensive third-degree burn
Crush injury

Heat-related causes
Heatstroke
Malignant hyperthermia
Neuroleptic malignant syndrome

Ischemic causes
Ischemic limb injury

Exertional causes
Marathon running
Physical overexertion in untrained athletes
Pathologic muscle exertion
Heat dissipation impairment
Physical overexertion in persons with sickle cell disease

Genetic Causes

Lipid metabolism
Carnitine palmitoyltransferase deficiency
Carnitine deficiency
Short-chain and long-chain acyl-coenzyme A dehydrogenase deficiency

Carbohydrate metabolism
Myophosphorylase deficiency (McArdle's disease)
Phosphorylase kinase deficiency
Phosphofructokinase deficiency
Phosphoglycerate mutase deficiency
Lactate dehydrogenase deficiency (characteristic elevation of creatine kinase level with normal lactate dehydrogenase level)

Purine metabolism
Myoadenylate deaminase deficiency
Duchenne's muscular dystrophy

Infectious, Inflammatory, Metabolic and Endocrinologic Causes

Infectious causes
Viruses: influenza virus B, parainfluenza virus, adenovirus, coxsackievirus, echovirus, herpes simplex virus, cytomegalovirus, Epstein-Barr virus, human immunodeficiency virus
Bacteria: Streptococcus, Salmonella, Legionella, Staphylococcus and Listeria species

Inflammatory causes
Polymyositis
Dermatomyositis
Capillary leak syndrome
Snake bites (mostly in South America, Asia and Africa)

Metabolic and endocrinologic causes
Electrolyte imbalances: hyponatremia, hypernatremia, hypokalemia, hypophosphatemia, hypocalcemia
Hypothyroidism
Thyrotoxicosis
Diabetic ketoacidosis
Nonketotic hyperosmolar syndrome

HMG-CoA = 3-hydroxy-3-methylglutaryl coenzyme A; *LSD* = lysergic acid diethylamide; *MDMA* = 3,4-methylene dioxymethamphetamine.
From Sauret JM, Marinides G, Want GK: Rhabdomyolysis, *Am Fam Physician* 65(3):907, 2002.

Priorities in treatment of myoglobinuria include identifying and treating the underlying disorder and preventing life-threatening renal failure. Malignant hyperthermia and myoglobinuria caused by succinylcholine or volatile anesthetic agents can be treated by halting the anesthetic administration and infusing dantrolene sodium (Dantrium). Diluting myoglobin using intravenous fluids and administration of mannitol, sodium bicarbonate, and furosemide (Lasix) to "flush" the kidney have been advocated to prevent renal failure. Other secondary problems include electrolyte imbalance, volume depletion, acidosis, hyperuricemia, hyperkalemia, and calcium imbalance. These require specific treatment. Short-term dialysis also may be necessary.

Compartment syndromes may require emergency treatment when blood flow to the affected extremity is compromised because of increased venous pressure, leading to decreased arterial inflow, ischemia, and edema.[14] When clinical evaluation is inconclusive, the rising compartment pressure can be directly measured by inserting a wick catheter, needle, or slit catheter into the muscle. Immediate fasciotomy and debridement have been advocated for pressures of more than 30 mmHg.[15] Compartments frequently affected are the anterior tibial, deep posterior tibial, volar, hand, and gluteal.

DISORDERS OF BONES

Metabolic Bone Diseases

Metabolic bone disease is characterized by abnormal bone structure that is caused by altered or inadequate biochemical reactions. The altered or inadequate biochemical reactions may be attributable to genetics, diet, or hormones.

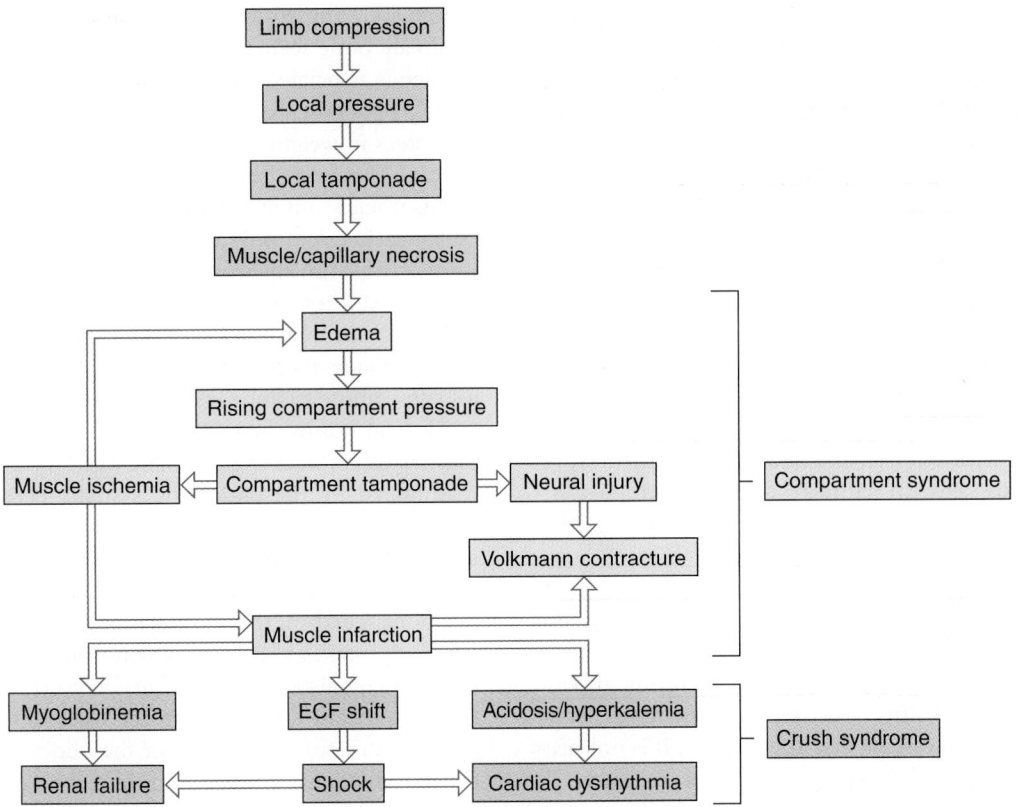

Figure 42-9 Pathogenesis of compartment syndrome and crush syndrome caused by prolonged muscle compression. *ECF,* Extracellular fluid.

Osteoporosis

Osteoporosis, or porous bone, is a disease in which bone tissue is normally mineralized but the mass—*density of bone*—is decreased and the structural integrity of trabecular bone is impaired. Cortical bone becomes more porous and thinner, making bone weaker and prone to fractures (Figures 42-10). The World Health Organization (WHO) has defined osteoporosis based on the bone density:

1. Normal bone is greater than 833 mg/cm^2
2. **Osteopenia,** or decreased bone mass, is 833 to 648 mg/cm^2
3. Osteoporosis is below 648 mg/cm^2

Severe or established osteoporosis is identified when there has been a fragility fracture. The disease can be (1) generalized, involving major portions of the axial skeleton, or (2) regional, involving one segment of the appendicular skeleton.

Throughout a lifetime, old bone is removed (resorption) and new bone is added (formation) to the skeleton. During childhood and teenage years, new bone is added faster than old bone is removed. Consequently, bones become larger, heavier, and denser. Bone formation continues at a pace faster than resorption until **peak bone mass,** or maximum bone density and strength, is reached, around age 30. After age 30, bone resorption slowly exceeds bone formation. In women, bone loss is most rapid in the first years after menopause but persists throughout the postmenopausal years. An estimated 10 million Americans over age 50 have osteoporosis and 34 million are at risk.[16] The major risks for persons with osteo-

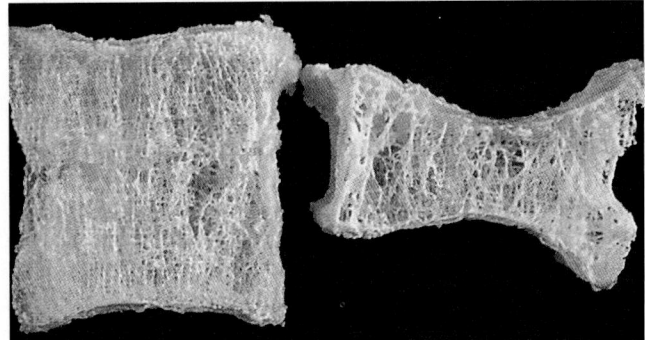

Figure 42-10 Vertebral body. Osteoporotic vertebra *(right)* shortened by compression fractures compared with normal vertebral body *(left).* Note that the osteoporotic vertebra has characteristic loss of horizontal trabeculae and thickened vertebral trabeculae. (From Cotran RS, Kumar V, Collins T: *Robbin's pathologic basis of disease,* ed 7, Philadelphia, 2005, Saunders.)

porosis are fractures. Men lose bone density with aging but because they begin with a higher bone density, they reach osteoporotic levels at an older age than do females. By the age of 90, about 17% of males have had a hip fracture, compared to 32% of females. Over half of all adults hospitalized for hip fracture do not return to their former level of functioning.[17]

Vertebral fractures also occur in the later years of life; however, they are more difficult to ascertain because people are unaware of the fracture.[18] The degree of compression necessary to define a vertebral fracture has not been standardized.[18] Thus the true prevalence is unknown, but fractures do increase in frequency by the sixth and seventh decades. Vertebral fracture prevalence in men is close to that in women.[18]

Osteoporosis is more common than it should be. A recent study in Britain revealed that the prevalence of osteoporosis was substantially lower in British subjects of both sexes that in U.S. subjects.[19] Osteoporosis is most common in whites and Asian woman, but affects all races. Whites are more susceptible than other races to osteoporosis caused by loss of bone density with age. Blacks have only about half the fracture of whites, probably related to their higher peak bone mass.[20] The cause of generalized osteoporosis remains uncertain but is probably multifactorial (see below).

Bone quality is not just bone mass (as measured by bone density) but also the microarchitecture of the bone. Thus other variables include crystal size and shape, brittleness, vitality of the bone cells, structure of the bone proteins, integrity of the trabecular network, and the ability to repair tiny cracks.[18] Because bone density relates to *quantity* of bone, *quality* of the bone is not accurately identified by bone density testing. Therefore, bone density testing may or may not accurately identify those who will go on to develop a fracture.

Osteoporosis is a complex, multifactorial, chronic disease that often progresses silently for decades until fractures occur. It is the most common disease that affects bone. It is not necessarily a consequence of the aging process because some elderly people retain strong, relatively dense bones.[21] In osteoporosis, the old bone is being reabsorbed faster than new bone is being made, causing the bones to lose density, becoming thinner and more porous. A progressive loss of bone mass may continue until the skeleton is no longer strong enough to support itself. Eventually, bones can fracture spontaneously. As bone becomes more fragile, falls or bumps that would not have caused fracture previously at that point do cause a fracture. Osteoporosis appears to be most severe in the spine, wrists, and hip.

Postmenopausal osteoporosis—which occurs in middle-aged and older women is probably caused by changes in osteoprotegerin (see Pathophysiology) insulin-like growth factor (IGF), a combination of inadequate dietary calcium intake and lack of vitamin D, possibly decreased magnesium, lack of exercise, decreased levels of estrogen, and family history.[22] IGF is known to help in fracture healing and collagen synthesis and improves conditions for bone mineralization. IGF levels significantly decline by age 60. Excessive phosphorus intake, chiefly through the intake of sodas and junk foods interferes with the calcium/phosphorus balance, resulting in an increased risk of brittle bones.

Estrogen replacement can slow bone loss around the time of menopause; however, osteoporosis and fractures are still common in older women who have used estrogen (studies with Premarin) continuously since menopause.[23] Estrogens are significant in premenopausal bone maintenance; however, when estrogen levels drop after menopause, it is possible that circulating androgens may become significant effectors on bone metabolism. In clinical studies of women, data have suggested that serum androgens may influence bone density in pre-, peri-, and postmenopausal women.[24-29] Androgens (i.e., testosterone and dihydrotestosterone have long been recognized to stimulate bone formation.[27] Increasing age in both men and women is associated with declining levels of estrogen. In addition, progesterone deficiency may be related to osteoporosis. Decreases in weight-bearing exercise is associated with osteoporosis. Other risk factors are identified in Box 42-2.

Insufficient intake or malabsorption of dietary minerals, particularly calcium, is a factor in the development of osteoporosis. Calcium absorption from the intestine decreases with age, and studies of individuals with osteoporosis show that their calcium intake is lower than that of age-matched controls. Deficiencies of vitamins, particularly vitamins C and D, also contribute to bone loss (see What's New box, p. 1513).

Skeletal homeostasis depends on a very narrow range of plasma calcium and phosphate concentrations, which are maintained by the endocrine system. Therefore endocrine dysfunction ultimately can cause metabolic bone disease. In addition to declining levels of sex steroids, the hormones most commonly associated with osteoporosis are parathyroid hormone, cortisol, thyroid hormone, and growth hormone. Excessive intakes of caffeine, alcohol, and nicotine along with low body fat also have been considered risk factors. In addition, significant differences in the trace elements (zinc, copper, manganese) were noted in the bones and hair of unaffected individuals compared to those with osteoporosis[30] (see Nutrition & Disease Box).

Iatrogenic osteoporosis sometimes develops temporarily in individuals receiving large doses of heparin, perhaps because heparin promotes bone resorption by decreasing collagen synthesis or by increasing collagen breakdown. Osteoporosis caused by heparin therapy usually resolves when therapy ceases. Treatment with other medications may lead to development of osteoporosis, such as the use of glucocorticoid treatment for rheumatoid arthritis. Other medications increasing risk of osteoporosis include lithium, methotrexate, anticonvulsants, cyclophosphamide, and cyclosporine.

Regional osteoporosis—osteoporosis confined to a region or segment of the appendicular skeleton—usually has a known cause. Classic regional osteoporosis is associated with disuse or immobilization of a limb because of fractures, motor paralysis, or bone or joint inflammation (see Figure 42-11). A negative calcium balance develops early and continues throughout the period of immobilization. After 8 weeks of immobilization, significant osteoporosis is present, although it may develop earlier in persons younger than 20 years or older than 50 years. A uniform distribution of osteoporosis also has been observed in astronauts and in individuals treated with air suspension therapy as a result of weightlessness and lack of mechanical strain.

PATHOPHYSIOLOGY   Whatever the cause, osteoporosis develops when the remodeling cycle—the process of bone resorption and bone formation—is disrupted, leading to an imbalance n the coupling process. Osteoclasts are differentiated cells that function to resorb bone. The explosion of new information in the field of bone biology has lead to new understanding of osteoclast biology and bone patho-

Box 42-2	Risk Factors for Osteoporosis

Genetic
Family history of osteoporosis
White race
Increased age
Female sex

Anthropometric
Small stature
Fair or pale skinned
Thin build

Hormonal and Metabolic
Early menopause (natural or surgical)
Late menarche
Nulliparity
Obesity
Hypogonadism
Gaucher disease
Cushing syndrome
Weight below healthy range
Acidosis

Dietary
Low dietary calcium and vitamin D
Low endogenous magnesium
Excessive protein*
Excessive sodium intake
High caffeine intake
Anorexia
Malabsorption

Life-style
Sedentary
Smoker
Alcohol consumption (excessive)

Concurrent
Hyperparathyroidism

Illness and Trauma
Renal insufficiency, hypocalciuria
Rheumatoid arthritis
Spinal cord injury
Systemic lupus

Liver Disease
Marrow disease (myeloma, mastocytosis, thalassemia)

Drugs
Corticosteroids
Dilantin
Gonadotropin-releasing hormone agonists
Loop diuretics
Methotrexate
Thyroid
Heparin
Cyclosporin
Depo-medroxyprogesterone acetate
Refinoids

*Low levels of protein intake also have been reported.

physiology. The osteoclast differentiation pathway is directed by a series of processes that include proliferation, differentiation, fusion, and activation.[31] These processes are controlled by hormones and cytokines and paracrine stromal-cell microenvironment interactions. Thus the intercellular communication in bone and the key molecular regulators are necessary for bone homeostasis. Interleukins (IL-1, IL-4, IL-6, IL-7, IL-11, IL-17), tumor necrosis factor (TNF), transforming growth factor-beta (TGF-β), prostaglandin E_2, and hormones interact to control osteoclasts[31] (see Figure 42-11). Staggering in its importance is the recent identification of the cytokine **receptor activator of nuclear factor κβ ligand (RANKL),** its receptor **RANK,** and its decoy receptor **osteoprotegerin (OPG);** this has led to a tremendously increased understanding of osteoclast biology and pathogenesis of bone diseases.

RANKL, a member of the TNF family, is expressed by osteoblasts and their immature precursors and is necessary for osteoclast development. RANKL activates the receptor RANK, which is expressed on osteoclasts and their precursors and suppresses apoptosis, which leads to activation and prolongation of osteoclast survival.[31] The effects of RANKL are blocked by osteoprotegerin (OPG), which is a glycoprotein that acts as a decoy or soluble receptor antagonist for RANKL that prevents it from binding and activating RANK (see Figure 42-11). The balance between RANKL and OPG is regulated by cytokines and hormones, and alterations of the RANKL/RANK/OPG system can lead to dysregulation

NUTRITION & DISEASE

Trace Elements and Their Effects on Skeletal Tissue*

Fluoride accumulates in new bone formation sites and results in a net gain in bone mass; however, at higher doses the new bone may be structurally abnormal.

Magnesium enhances bone turnover by stimulating osteoclastic function and may help with regulation of calcium.

Zinc regulates secretion of calcitonin from the thyroid gland and influences bone turnover; it is essential for enzymes in osteoblasts responsible for collagen synthesis and alkaline phosphatase and also is required for osteoblasts.

Iodine enhances bone turnover, as hormonal forms of thyroxine and triiodothyronine.

Aluminum induces impairment of bone formation by inhibiting osteoblastic function.

Copper induces low bone turnover by suppressing both osteoblastic and osteoclastic function.

Boron may be used by osteoblasts for bone formation and may be related to magnesium in its effect on bone.

Iron functions in mitochondrial oxidative phosphorylation in osteoblasts and osteoclasts.

Manganese is required for biosynthesis of mucopolysaccharides in bone matrix formation.

Data from Mahan LK, Escott-Stump S: *Krause's food, nutrition, and diet therapy,* ed 10, Philadelphia, 2000, Saunders; Okano T: *Nippon Rinsho* 54(1):148, 1996 (non-English).
*The exact involvement of these trace elements in osteoporosis has not been clarified.

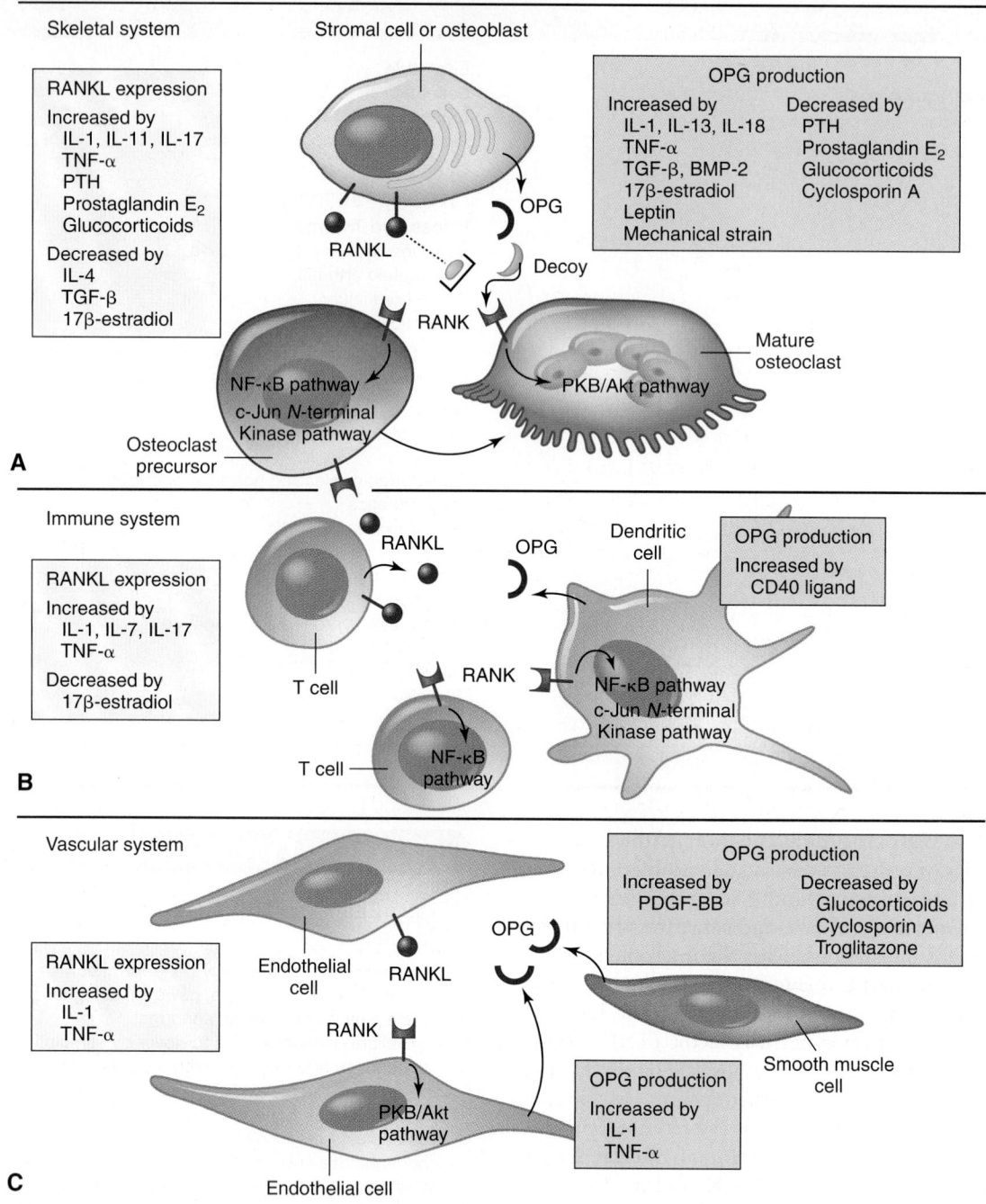

Figure 42-11 **OPG/RANKL/RANK system.** RANKL, receptor activator of nuclear factor κβ ligand, a cytokine and part of the tumor necrosis factor (TNF) family, expression and OPG, a glycoprotein receptor antagonist, are modulated by various cytokines, hormones, drugs, and mechanical strains *(see inserts).* **A,** In bone, RANKL is expressed by both stromal cells and osteoblasts. RANKL stimulates the receptor RANK on osteoclast precursor cells and mature osteoclasts, activates intracellular signaling pathways to promote osteoclast differentiation and activation, and cytoskeletal reorganization and survival (PKB/Akt pathway) that increases resorption and bone loss. OPG, secreted by stromal cells and osteoblasts, acts as a "decoy" receptor and blocks RANKL binding to and activating RANK. **B,** In the immune system, RANKL is expressed and secreted by T cells. T-cell–derived RANKL also can activate RANK on osteoclasts, T cells, and dendritic cells (antigen-presenting cells), which enhances bone loss that occurs in inflammatory bone diseases such as rheumatoid arthritis. Dendritic cells may regulate these processes by secreting OPG. **C,** In the vascular system, endothelial cells express RANKL and the RANK receptor. RANKL/RANK interactions contribute to endothelial and smooth muscle cells and can block RANKL binding. The physiologic significance of the OPG/RANKL/RANK system in endothelial and smooth muscle cells is currently being studied. *Il,* Interleukin, *TGF-κ,* transforming growth factor beta, *BMP-2,* bone morphogenic protein 2, *PTH,* parathyroid hormone, *PDGF-B,* platelet-derived growth factor B. (Adapted from Hofbauer LC, Schoppet M: *JAMA* 292(4):490-495, 2004.)

and pathologic conditions including osteoporosis, immune-mediated bone diseases, malignant bone disorders, and inherited skeletal diseases[32,33] (see Figure 42-11).

Postmenopausal osteoporosis is characterized by increased bone resorption, more than the rate of bone formation, leading to sustained bone loss, resulting from estrogen deficiency. Bone loss resulting from estrogen deficiency also contributes to osteoporosis in men.[33] The increase in bone resorption results from both increased development of osteoclasts and decreased osteoclast apoptosis.[32,34] Evidence involving the OPG/RANKL/RANK system is emerging (Figure 42-11). OPG production is stimulated by both estrogens and the drug referred to as selective estrogen receptor modulator—raloxifene.[31] Unlike normal bone remodeling whereby osteoblast development is stimulated by factors released from bone marrow stromal cells during osteoclastic resorption, estrogen deficiency unleashes signals capable of stimulating osteoblast progenitor cells that are different from those needed to stimulate bone resorption and thus are pathologic. Postmenopausal women express higher levels of RANKL on bone marrow stromal cells, T cells, and B cells than premenopausal women.[35] Importantly, RANKL expression is inversely correlated with serum level of 17 β-estradiol, that is, with estradiol deficiency, RANKL is increased.[35] Despite numerous studies, it is still unclear which paracrine mediators of the increased osteoclastogenic activity are induced by estrogen deficiency.

Recently, data revealed that sex steroids (e.g., estrogens) exert antiapoptotic effects on osteoblasts but exert proapoptotic effects on osteoclasts; in both scenarios this is accomplished by activating the **extracellular signal regulated kinases (ERKs)**. Estrogen activates ERKS outside the nucleus; ERKs then accumulate in the nucleus and activate downstream transcription factors.[36] This confusing and complicated data eventually revealed that the important determinant of whether proapoptosis or antiapoptosis was exhibited was the *length of time* that the phosphorylated ERKs remained in the nucleus. Prolonged nuclear accumulation of activated ERKs converted the antiapoptotic effect of estradiol to proapoptotic. In addition to ERKs, RANKL is required for the antiapoptotic and thus longer life span of osteoclasts.[37] These effects increase the life span of osteoclasts (i.e., longer bone resorbing) and shorten the life span of the bone-forming cells, or osteoblasts. These alterations account for critical pathophysiologic changes in most acquired metabolic bone diseases including postmenopausal osteoporosis, aging effects, and glucocorticoid (i.e., cortisone) excess.[37] In addition agents such as parathyroid hormone and bisphosphonates, used for treatment of bone loss, exert their positive effects by altering the rate of birth of new osteoblasts or osteoclasts or their apoptosis.[36]

Glucocorticoid (e.g., cortisone)-induced osteoporosis—is characterized by increased bone resorption and decreased bone formation. Glucocorticoids increase RANKL expression and inhibit OPG production by osteoblasts (see Figure 42-11). The use of immunosuppressive drugs (i.e., cyclosporine A) to reduce rejection of transplanted organs also alters the OPG/RANKL/RANK system and can lead to post-transplant osteoporosis. Other conditions affected by OPG/RANKL/RANK include rheumatoid arthritis, myeloma, and skeletal metastases from neoplastic disorders, vascular diseases, and others.

Age-related bone loss begins in the fourth decade. The cause remains unclear, but it is known that decreased serum growth hormone (GH) and insulin-like growth factor (IGF) levels along with increased binding of RANKL and decreased OPG affect osteoblast and osteoclast function. Loss of trabecular bone in men proceeds in a linear fashion, with thinning of trabecular bone rather than complete loss as is noted in women[17] (Figure 42-12). Men have approximately 30% more bone mass than women, which may be a factor in their later involvement with osteoporosis (Figure 42-13). In addition, men have a more gradual decrease in testosterone and estradiol (and possibly progesterone), thereby maintaining their bone mass longer than women[38] (Figure 42-14). Reduction in physical activity in older persons also may be a major factor in the degree of bone loss because preservation of bone mass

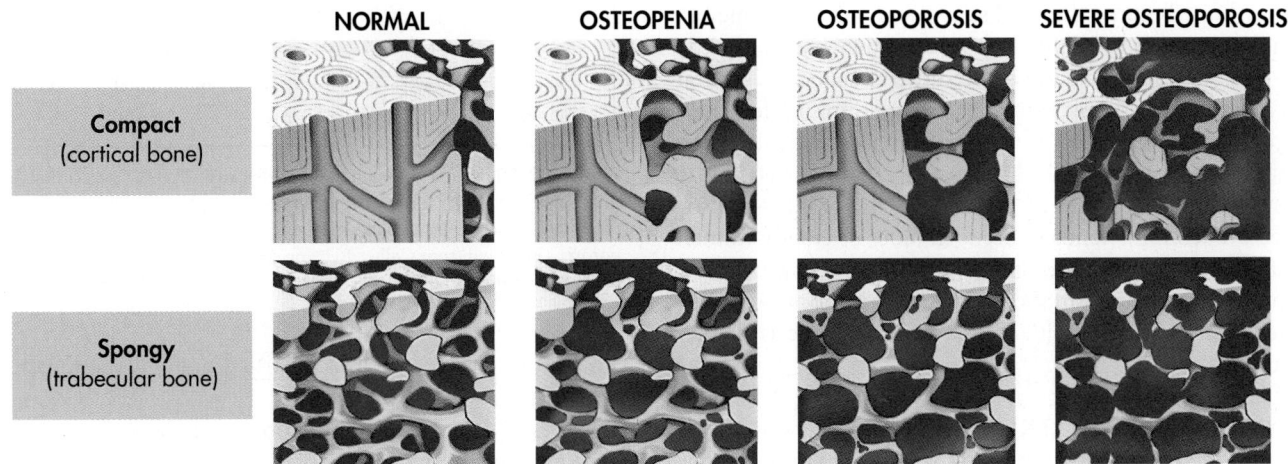

NORMAL   **OSTEOPENIA**   **OSTEOPOROSIS**   **SEVERE OSTEOPOROSIS**

Compact (cortical bone)

Spongy (trabecular bone)

Figure 42-12 Osteoporosis in cortical and trabecular bone.

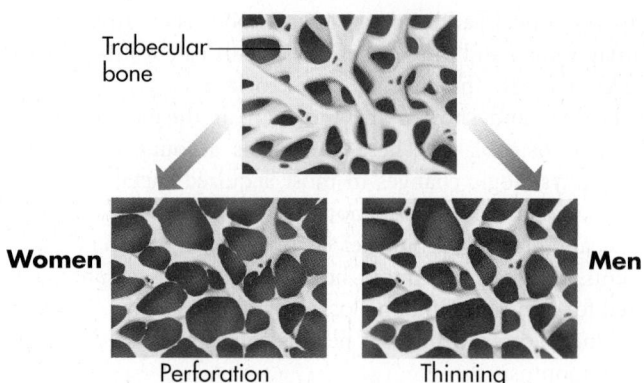

Figure 42-13 Mechanism of loss of trabecular bone in women and trabecular thinning in men. Bone thinning predominates in men because of reduced bone formation. Loss of connectivity and complete trabeculae predominates in women.

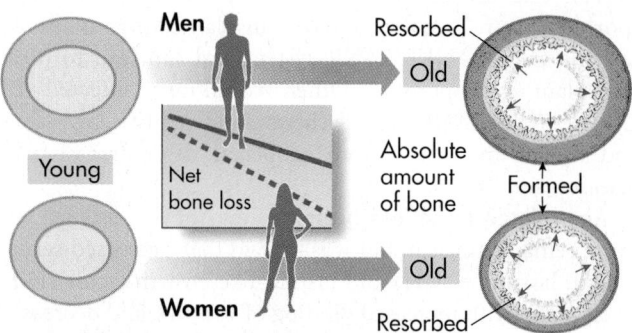

Figure 42-14 Bone loss in men and women. Absolute amount of bone resorbed on the inner bone surface and formed on the outer bone surface is more in men than women during aging.

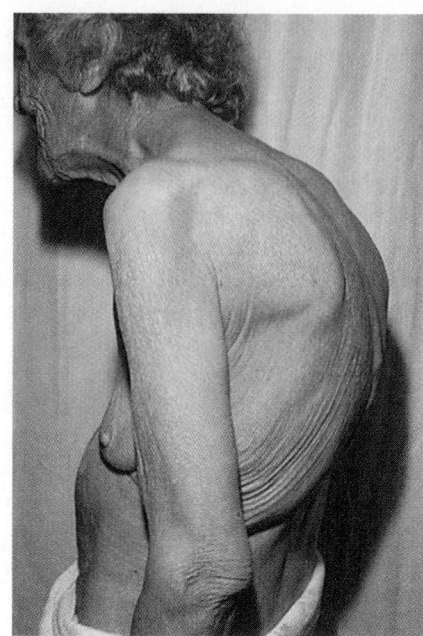

Figure 42-15 Kyphosis. This elderly woman's condition was caused by a combination of spinal osteoporotic vertebral collapse and chronic degenerative changes in the vertebral column. (From Kamal A, Brocklehurst JC: *Color atlas of geriatric medicine*, ed 2, St Louis, 1992, Mosby.)

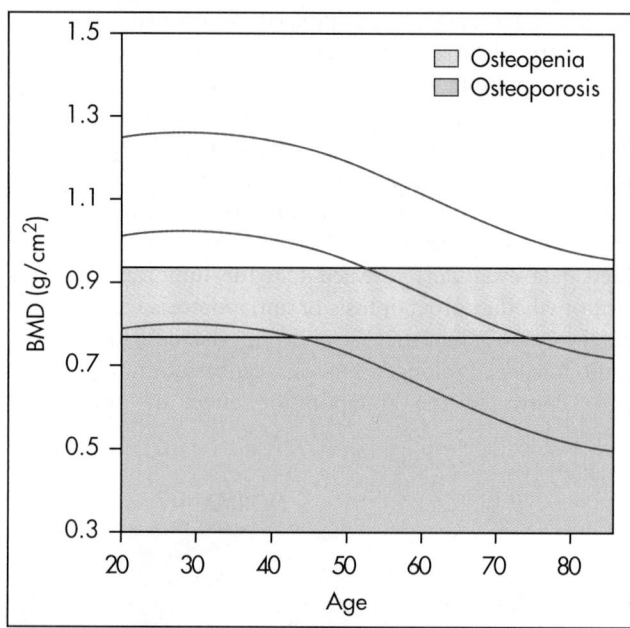

Figure 42-16 Lumbar spine bone mass density (BMD). The normal female reference curves for lumbar spine BMD are plotted in this graph to include the World Health Organization definitions of osteopenia and osteoporosis. (Redrawn from Collier BD, Fogelman I, Rosenthall L: *Skeletal nuclear medicine*, St Louis, 1996, Mosby.)

depends on skeletal stress (mechanical) through muscle contraction and weight bearing.[20]

CLINICAL MANIFESTATIONS The specific clinical manifestations of osteoporosis depend on the bones involved. The most common manifestation, however, is bone deformity. Pain tends to occur only when there is a fragility fracture. Fractures are likely to occur because the trabeculae of spongy bone become thin and sparse and compact bone becomes porous. As the bones lose volume, they become brittle and weak and may collapse or become misshapen. Vertebral collapse causes kyphosis (hunchback) and diminished height (Figure 42-15). Fractures of the long bones (particularly the femur and humerus), distal radius, ribs, and vertebrae are most common. Fracture of the neck of the femur—the so-called broken hip—tends to occur in older or elderly women with osteoporosis. Fatal complications of fractures include fat or pulmonary embolism, hemorrhage, and shock. Approximately 20% of persons with a hip fracture may die as a result of surgical complications.

EVALUATION AND TREATMENT Generally, osteoporosis is detected radiographically as increased radiolucency of bone. By the time abnormalities are detected by x-ray examination, as much as 25% to 30% of bone tissue may have been lost.

Types of radiologic examinations include single- or dual-photon absorptiometry (SXA, DXA) and computed tomography (CT) scans (Figure 42-16). Other evaluation procedures include tests for levels of serum calcium, phosphorus, and alkaline phosphatase and protein electrophoresis. Body calcium levels also can be measured by neuron activation analysis, a procedure involving use of radioactive calcium-49, whose gamma activity can be measured with a whole-body counter.

The goals of osteoporosis treatment are to slow down the rate of calcium and bone loss and to stop the disease before it progresses too far. Controversial is the role of calcium intake to both prevent and treat osteoporosis. It is well accepted that oral calcium intake sufficient to maintain normal calcium balance is necessary during adolescence to ensure development of peak bone mass, and that calcium-deficient diets can aggravate bone loss associated with menopause and aging. Although recommendations have been established for young women of 1000 mg of calcium daily and for postmenopausal women of 1500 mg daily (with vitamin D) if receiving sex hormone replacement therapy, it has been difficult to translate these recommendations into clear-cut clinical outcomes. A number of investigations lack an association between current calcium intake and bone mineral density.[39] A significant relationship has been observed between an individual's lifetime history of calcium intake and peak bone mineral density. Clinical trials must be done to test the effects of dietary calcium or supplements on bone loss that accounts for potential confounding factors, such as menopausal status, estrogen levels, vitamin D levels (see Nutrition and Disease Box), magnesium levels, smoking, contraceptive use, usual calcium intake, and level of physical activity.

Magnesium (Mg^{++}), another mineral important for skeletal development, is at risk of being deficient in the diet. It is an essential mineral in many biochemical and physiologic functions, including activation of enzymes, involvement in ATP synthesis, protein synthesis, regulation of membrane channels, and muscle contraction. New evidence suggests that large fluxes of magnesium can cross the cell plasma membrane in either direction following a variety of stimuli, resulting in a modification of activity for several cellular enzymes.[23] Magnesium is important to bone quality because it controls hydroxyapatite crystal growth and thereby prevents formation of brittle bones.[40] It seems reasonable that Mg^{++} is required for normal calcium (Ca^{++}) absorption because severe Mg^{++} deficiency results in hypocalcemia. Elevation of plasma Mg^{++} or Ca^{++} concentration inhibits Mg^{++} and Ca^{++} resorption, leading to hypermagnesiuria and hypercalciuria. An extracellular Ca^{++}/Mg^{++} sensing receptor has been found located on distal tubule cells. Also, recent data have shown a relationship between Mg^{++} and Ca^{++} signaling in pancreatic and other secretory epithelia.[41] Significant extrusion of Mg^{++} from these cells is related to mobilization of intracellular Ca^{++}.[41]

Regular, moderate weight-bearing exercise can slow down the bone loss and, in some cases, reverse demineralization because the mechanical stress of exercise stimulates bone formation. Although hormone treatment is controversial, postmenopausal women are sometimes prescribed estrogen and progestins in addition to exercise and dietary supplements of calcium and vitamin D. Magnesium also may be recommended. It is important to reduce the risk of falls and enhance bone quality. Therefore an exercise program to enhance rehabilitation is advised. Important new findings suggest that estrogen may prevent excessive bone loss before and after menopause by limiting osteoclast life span through promotion of apoptosis. Hormone replacement therapy helps maintain bone density but it is not routinely recommended because of the increased risk of stroke and breast cancer and no significant cardioprotective effects.[42]

Selective estrogen receptor modulators (SERMs) have been developed to provide the positive effects of estrogen on bone but minimize estrogen's negative effect on breast and endometrial tissues. Raloxifene and tamoxifen are examples of SERMs.

Other treatments include intranasal calcitonin given daily and sodium fluoride given orally. The bisphosphonates alendronate and risedronate have been effective in reducing hip and vertebral fractures in glucocorticoid-induced osteoporosis and in women with osteoporosis by inhibiting bone resorption. Recent evidence reveals the bisphosphonates activate a previously unknown signaling pathway that is triggered by the opening of connexin 43, a protein that forms a gap junction important for intercellular communication.[36] After opening of connexin 43, activation of ERKs (see p. 1511) occurs, which mediates osteocyte survival. Osteocyte viability possibly maintains the effectiveness of bisphosphonates as well as other agents (e.g., estrogen, and daily parathyroid injections) by preventing apoptosis of osteocytes and osteoblasts.[36] Teriparatide, a new biotech drug of parathormone, is injected subcutaneously. Several side effects including nausea, headache, cramps, hypercalcemia and hyperuricemia, however, have been reported. Men with osteo-

---

NUTRITION & DISEASE

Vitamin D and Fracture Risk

The beneficial effects of vitamin D on fracture risk are attributed to two explanations: (1) the decrease in bone loss in older persons and (2) the increase in muscle strength and balance mediated through Vitamin D receptors in muscle tissue.

In addition, vitamin D has been correlated with a significant (22%) reduction in the risk of falling in older people. Pooled analyses reveal that higher doses (700 to 800 IU/day) is better for reducing fractures than 400 IU/day. Previously the recommendations for vitamin D in middle-aged and older adults was 400 to 600 IU/day. With new data and the uncertainty of intake recommendations, higher doses may be more effective (i.e., 700 to 800 IU/day).

Because calcium was administered in combination with vitamin D in all but one of the higher-dose vitamin D trials, the independent effects of vitamin D alone could not be determined. Still needing further research is whether and in what dose calcium adds value to fracture prevention with vitamin D.

Data from Bischoff-Ferrari HA, et al: *JAMA* 293:2257-2264, 2005.

porosis are treated with bisphosphonates and testosterone. Controversial is testosterone treatment for women. Restoration of a balanced RANKL/OPG ratio (see p. 1509) or inhibiting RANK responsiveness is known to prevent osteoclast activation and bone resorption, which may lead to promising new therapies.[31]

Osteomalacia

Osteomalacia is a metabolic disease characterized by inadequate and delayed mineralization of osteoid in mature compact and spongy bone. In osteomalacia the remodeling cycle proceeds normally through osteoid formation, but mineral calcification and deposition do not occur. Bone volume remains unchanged, but the replaced bone consists of soft osteoid instead of rigid bone. Rickets is similar to osteomalacia in pathogenesis, but it occurs in the growing bones of children, whereas osteomalacia occurs in adult bone. (Rickets is described in Chapter 43.)

Both osteomalacia and rickets are rare in the United States and Western Europe but are significant health problems in Great Britain, Ethiopia, Pakistan, Iran, and India. In the United States these diseases occur in elderly persons, in premature infants of very low birth weight, and in individuals adhering to rigid macrobiotic vegetarian diets.

Many factors contribute to the development of osteomalacia, but the most important is a deficiency of vitamin D. The major risk factors in vitamin D deficiency are diets deficient in vitamin D, decreased endogenous production of vitamin D, intestinal malabsorption of vitamin D, renal tubular diseases, and anticonvulsant therapy. Classic vitamin D deficiency is rare in the United States because of the addition of synthetic vitamin D to dairy products and bread.

However, disorders of the small bowel, hepatobiliary system, and pancreas are common causes of vitamin D deficiency in the United States. In malabsorptive disease of the small bowel, vitamin D and calcium absorption are decreased, so that vitamin D is lost in feces. Liver disease interferes with the metabolism of vitamin D to its more active form, and diseases of the pancreas and biliary system cause a deficiency of bile salts, which are necessary for normal intestinal absorption of vitamin D.

The mechanism by which anticonvulsant drug therapy results in vitamin D deficiency is not completely understood, but researchers think that the anticonvulsants phenobarbital and phenytoin interfere with calcium absorption and increase degradation of vitamin D metabolism in the liver. Renal osteodystrophy is a common cause of osteomalacia.

PATHOPHYSIOLOGY Crystallization of minerals in osteoid requires adequate concentrations of calcium and phosphate. When the concentrations are too low, crystallization (and hence ossification) does not proceed normally.

Vitamin D deficiency disrupts mineralization because vitamin D normally regulates and enhances the absorption of calcium ions from the intestine. A lack of vitamin D causes the plasma calcium concentrations to fall. Low plasma cal-

cium levels stimulate increased synthesis and secretion of PTH. Although the increase in circulating PTH raises the plasma calcium concentration, it also stimulates increased renal clearance of phosphate. When the concentration of phosphate in the bone decreases below a critical level, mineralization cannot proceed normally.

Abnormalities occur in both spongy and compact bone. Trabeculae in spongy bone become thinner and fewer, whereas haversian systems in compact bone develop large channels and become irregular. Because osteoid continues to be produced but not mineralized, abnormal quantities of osteoid build up, coating the trabeculae and the linings of the haversian canals. Excessive osteoid also can accumulate in areas beneath the periosteum. The excess of osteoid leads to gross deformities of the long bones, spine, pelvis, and skull.

CLINICAL MANIFESTATIONS Osteomalacia causes varying degrees of diffuse skeletal pain and tenderness. Pain is noted particularly in the hips, and the individual may be hesitant to walk. Muscular weakness is common and may contribute to a waddling gait. Bone fractures and vertebral collapse occur with minimal trauma. Low back pain may be an early complaint, but pain also may involve ribs, feet, other areas of the vertebral column, and other sites. Uremia may be present in renal osteodystrophy.

EVALUATION AND TREATMENT Laboratory data may include elevated blood urea nitrogen (BUN) and creatinine levels, normal or low serum calcium levels, and a serum inorganic phosphate level that is usually higher than 5.5 mg. Alkaline phosphatase and PTH levels are usually elevated. Radiographic findings show pseudofractures and radiolucent bands perpendicular to the surface of involved bones. A bone biopsy is used to evaluate presence of renal osteodystrophy to determine bone aluminum deposits.

Treatment of osteomalacia includes the following:
1. Adjusting serum calcium and phosphorus levels to normal
2. Suppressing secondary hyperthyroidism
3. Chelating bone aluminum if needed
4. Administering calcium carbonate to decrease hyperphosphatemia
5. Dietary supplements of vitamin D
6. Renal dialysis
7. Renal transplant for renal osteodystrophy

Paget Disease

Paget disease (osteitis deformans) is a state of increased metabolic activity in bone characterized by abnormal and excessive bone remodeling, both resorption and formation. Chronic accelerated remodeling eventually enlarges and softens the affected bones.

Paget disease most often affects the axial skeleton, especially the vertebrae, skull, sacrum, sternum, pelvis, and femur. The disease process may occur in one or more bones without causing significant clinical manifestations.

The disease is seldom found before age 40 years, but its incidence almost doubles each decade from age 50. It affects men more than women in a proportion of 1.8:1.[43] Because it is often symptomless and can be diagnosed only by invasive procedures, few epidemiologic data are available. Autopsy data from England and Germany indicate that approximately 3% to 4% of persons older than 40 years have Paget disease. It is most prevalent in Australia, Great Britain, New Zealand, and the United States. Paget disease affects several members of the same family in 15% to 30% of individuals.[44]

The cause of Paget disease is unknown, but there appears to be a strong genetic component. A viral connection (slow virus infection) to Paget disease also has been proposed.[44] Classic Paget disease arises as a consequence of disorderly bone resorption and formation. Sporadic Paget disease involves localized areas of increased osteoclastic activity.

PATHOPHYSIOLOGY Paget disease begins with excessive resorption of spongy bone. The trabeculae diminish, and bone marrow is replaced by extremely vascular fibrous tissue.

The resorption phase of Paget disease is followed by the formation of abnormal new bone at an accelerated rate. The collagen fibers are disorganized, and glycoprotein levels in the matrix decrease. Mineralization may extend into the bone marrow. Bone formation is excessive around partially resorbed trabeculae, causing them to thicken and enlarge. Eventually, Paget disease progresses to an inactive phase, in which abnormal remodeling is minimal or absent. Sporadic Paget disease involves overexpression of RANKL (see p. 1509), and osteoclasts of individuals with Paget disease have increased responses to RANKL.[45]

CLINICAL MANIFESTATIONS In the skull, abnormal remodeling is first evident in the frontal or occipital regions; then it encroaches on the outer and inner surfaces of the entire skull. The skull thickens and assumes an asymmetric shape (Figure 42-17). Thickened segments of the skull may compress areas of the brain, producing altered mentality and dementia. Impingement of new bone on cranial nerves causes sensory abnormalities, impaired motor function, deafness, atrophy of the optic nerve, and obstruction of the lacrimal duct. Headache is commonly noted.

Extensive alterations of the facial bones are rare except in the jaw, where sclerosis and thickening of the maxilla and mandible displace teeth and produce malocclusion. In long bones, resorption begins in the subchondral regions of the epiphysis and extends into the metaphysis and diaphysis. Occasionally, Paget disease affects both ends of a tubular bone. In the femur, Paget disease produces an exaggerated lateral curvature. In the tibia, anterior curvature is also exaggerated. Stress fractures are common in the lower extremities

Clinical manifestations of Paget disease in the vertebral column depend on the level of involvement and are caused by compression of adjacent structures. In the cervical spine, cord compression can lead to spastic quadriplegia. Approximately 1% of persons with Paget disease develop osteogenic sarcoma.

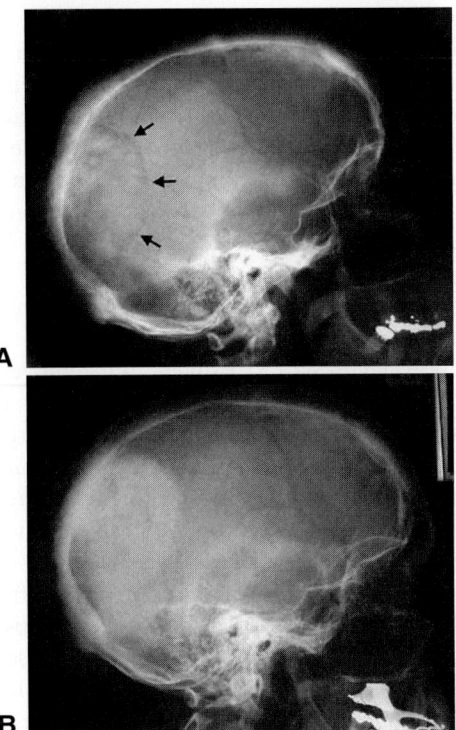

Figure 42-17 Paget disease of the skull. **A,** Active Paget disease of the skull, with marked cortical thickening and an area of osteoporosis circumscripta *(arrows)*. **B,** The same individual some years later (after bisphosphonate treatment), with the lytic lesion largely replaced by sclerotic bone. (From Walsh JP: *Med J Aust* 181(5):263, 2004.)

EVALUATION AND TREATMENT Evaluation of Paget disease is made on the basis of radiographic findings of irregular bone trabeculae with a thickened and disorganized pattern. Early disease is detected by bone scanning that shows increased uptake of bone radionuclides. Alkaline phosphatase and urinary hydroxyproline are elevated.

Most individuals require no treatment because the disease is localized and does not cause symptoms. Treatment during active disease is for pain relief, prevention of deformity, or fracture. Bisphosphonates (alendronate, risedronate, and pamidronate) and calcitonin (salmon and human) are the mainstays of treatment. Surgery is indicated if there are neurologic complications.[44]

Infectious Bone Disease: Osteomyelitis

Infectious bone disease is expensive and difficult to treat and often culminates in extensive physical disability. Several factors contribute to the difficulty in treating bone infection:

1. Bone contains multiple microscopic channels that are impermeable to the cells and biochemicals of the body's natural defenses. Once bacteria gain access to these channels, they are able to proliferate unimpeded.
2. The microcirculation of bone is highly vulnerable to damage and destruction by bacterial toxins. Vessel damage causes local thrombosis (blockage) of the small vessels, which leads to ischemic necrosis (death) of bone.

3. Bone cells have a limited capacity to replace bone destroyed by infections. Initially, osteoclasts are stimulated by infection to resorb bone, which opens up isolated bone channels so that cells of the inflammatory and immune system can gain access to the infected bone. At the same time, however, resorption weakens the structural integrity of the bone. New bone formation usually lags behind resorption, and the haversian systems in the new bone are incomplete.

Osteomyelitis is a bone infection most often caused by bacteria; however, fungi, parasites, and viruses also can cause bone infection (Figure 42-18). **Exogenous osteomyelitis** is an infection that enters from outside the body, for example, through open fractures, penetrating wounds, or surgical procedures. In exogenous osteomyelitis, the infection spreads from soft tissues into adjacent bone. **Endogenous (hematogenous) osteomyelitis** is caused by pathogens carried in the blood from sites of infection elsewhere in the body. In hematogenous osteomyelitis, the infection spreads from bone to adjacent soft tissues. Hematogenous osteomyelitis is commonly found in infants, children, and elderly persons. (Osteomyelitis in children is discussed in Chapter 43.) In infants, incidence rates among males and females are approximately equal. In children and older adults, however, males are most commonly affected. Osteomyelitis is a common complication of sickle cell anemia and low oxygen tension.

Staphylococcus aureus is the usual cause of hematogenous osteomyelitis. Other microorganisms include group B streptococci, *Haemophilus influenzae*, *Salmonella*, and gram-negative bacteria. Group B streptococci and *H. influenzae* tend to infect young children; *Salmonella* infection is associated with sickle cell anemia; and gram-negative infections are most common in older adults and individuals with impaired immunity. Mycobacterial and fungal infections occur in immunocompromised individuals.

Cutaneous, sinus, ear, and dental infections are the primary sources of bacteria in hematogenous bone infections. Soft tissue infections, disorders of the gastrointestinal tract, infections of the genitourinary system, and respiratory infections are also sources of bacterial contamination. In addition, infections contracted after total joint replacements can be causes of osteomyelitis. The vulnerability of specific bone depends on the anatomy of its vascular supply.

In adults, hematogenous osteomyelitis is more common in the spine, pelvis, and small bones. Microorganisms reach the vertebrae through arteries, veins, or lymphatic vessels. The spread of infection from pelvic organs to the vertebrae is well documented. Vaginal, uterine, ovarian, bladder, and intestinal infections can lead to iliac or sacral osteomyelitis.

Exogenous osteomyelitis can be caused by human bites or fist blows to the mouth. Superficial animal or human bites inoculate local soft tissue with bacteria that later spread to underlying bone. Deep bites can introduce microorganisms directly onto bone. The most common infecting organism in human bites is *S. aureus*. In animal bites the most common infecting organism is *Pasteurella multocida*, which is part of the normal mouth flora of cats and dogs.

Direct contamination of bones with bacteria also can occur in open fractures or dislocations with an overlying skin wound. Intervertebral disk surgery and operative procedures involving implantation of large foreign objects, such as metallic plates or artificial joints, are associated with exogenous osteomyelitis. Local injections and venous punctures are significant causes of exogenous osteomyelitis. Exogenous osteomyelitis of the arm and hand bones tends to occur in drug abusers. *S. aureus* is the most common pathogen. In general, persons who are chronically ill, have diabetes or alcoholism, or are receiving large doses of steroids or immunosuppressive drugs are particularly susceptible to exogenous osteomyelitis or recurring episodes of this disease.

PATHOPHYSIOLOGY   Regardless of the source of the pathogen, the pathologic features of bone infection are similar to those in any other body tissue (see Chapter 9). First, the invading pathogen provokes an intense inflammatory response. Inflammation in bone is characterized by vascular engorgement, edema, leukocyte activity, and abscess formation. Once inflammation is initiated, the small terminal vessels thrombose and exudate seals the bone's canaliculi. Inflammatory exudate extends into the metaphysis and the marrow cavity and through small metaphyseal openings into the cortex. In children, exudate that reaches the outer surface of the

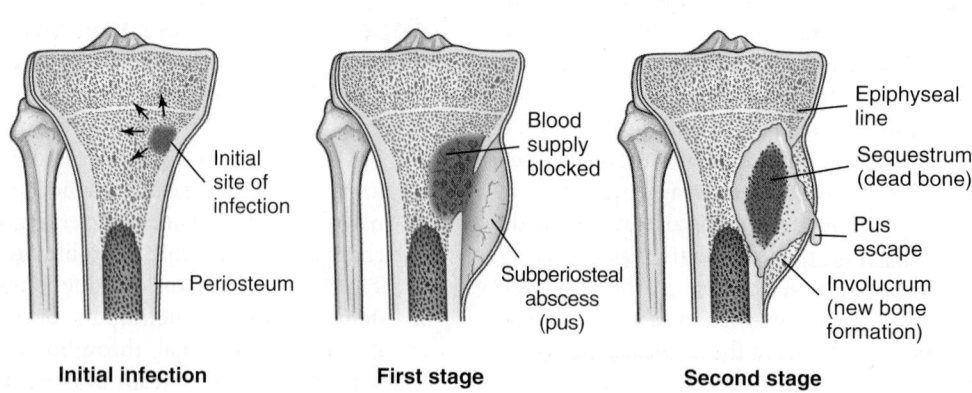

Initial infection   **First stage**   **Second stage**

Figure 42-18 Osteomyelitis showing sequestration and involucrum.

cortex forms abscesses that lift the periosteum off underlying bone. Lifting of the periosteum disrupts blood vessels that enter bone through the periosteum, which deprives underlying bone of its blood supply; this leads to necrosis and death of the area of bone infected, producing **sequestrum,** an area of devitalized bone (see Figure 42-18). Lifting of the periosteum also stimulates an intense osteoblastic response. Osteoblasts lay down new bone that can partially or completely surround the infected bone. This layer of new bone surrounding the infected bone is called an **involucrum.** Openings in the involucrum allow the exudate to escape into surrounding soft tissue and ultimately through the skin by way of sinus tracts.

In adults, this complication is rare because the periosteum is firmly attached to the cortex and resists displacement. Instead, infection disrupts and weakens the cortex, which predisposes the bone to pathologic fracture.

CLINICAL MANIFESTATIONS   Clinical manifestations of osteomyelitis vary with the age of the individual, the site of involvement, the initiating event, the infecting organism, and whether the infection is acute, subacute, or chronic. Acute osteomyelitis causes an abrupt onset of inflammation. If an acute infection is not completely eliminated, the disease may become subacute or chronic. In subacute osteomyelitis, signs and symptoms are usually vague. In the chronic stage, infection is indolent or silent between exacerbations. The microorganisms persist in small abscesses or fragments of necrotic bone and produce occasional flare-ups of acute osteomyelitis. The progression from acute to subacute osteomyelitis may be the result of inadequate or inappropriate therapy or the development of drug-resistant microorganisms.

In the adult, hematogenous osteomyelitis has an insidious onset. The symptoms are usually vague and include fever, malaise, anorexia, and weight loss. Recent infection (urinary, respiratory, skin) or instrumentation (catheterization, cystoscopy, myelography, diskography) usually precedes onset of symptoms.

The primary symptom of acute osteomyelitis in the spine is back pain. The pain may be intermittent or constant, aggravated by motion, and throbbing at rest. It may radiate in a radicular distribution and is commonly accompanied by spinal tenderness and rigidity. Hip contracture can occur in the presence of soft tissue inflammation as a result of irritation of the psoas muscle.

The signs and symptoms of sacroiliac osteomyelitis are generally severe and include local pain, tenderness, and a limp. The pain may radiate to the buttock or the abdomen.

Single or multiple abscesses (Brodie abscesses) characterize subacute or chronic osteomyelitis. Brodie abscesses are circumscribed lesions 1 to 4 cm in diameter, usually in the ends of long bones and surrounded by dense ossified bone matrix. The abscesses are thought to develop when the infectious microorganism has become less virulent or the individual's immune system is resisting the infection somewhat successfully.

In exogenous osteomyelitis, signs and symptoms of soft tissue infection predominate. Inflammatory exudate in the soft tissues disrupts muscles and supporting structures and forms abscesses. Low-grade fever, lymphadenopathy, local pain, and swelling usually occur within days of contamination by a puncture wound. Osteomyelitis in the hand causes exquisite tenderness over the course of tendon sheaths. The fingers are usually in a semiflexed position, and extension usually causes severe pain. Palmar swelling or symmetric swelling of the fingers may be present.

EVALUATION AND TREATMENT   Laboratory data show an elevated white cell count. Radiographic studies include radionuclide bone scanning, CT, and MRI. Treatment of osteomyelitis includes antibiotics and debridement with bone biopsy and culture. Initial antibiotic therapy should be intravenous. Chronic conditions may require surgical removal of the inflammatory exudate followed by continuous wound irrigation with antibiotic solutions in addition to systemic treatment with antibiotics. **Hyperbaric oxygen therapy** of 100% oxygen, given at 2 atmospheres of pressure for 2 hours' duration per day for 30 treatments, is also beneficial for chronic refractory osteomyelitis. Implants for total joint replacements may be removed to treat the infected joint more thoroughly.

Bone Tumors

Many different types of tumors involve the skeleton. Bone tumors may originate from bone cells, cartilage, fibrous tissue, marrow, or vascular tissue. Based on the tissue of origin, bone tumors are classified as osteogenic, chondrogenic, collagenic, and myelogenic. Each of the four types arises from one of the four stem cells that are ultimately derived from the primitive mesoderm (Figure 42-19). In addition, bone tumors may be classified as being of histiocytic, notochordal, lipogenic, and neurogenic origins.

The mesoderm contributes the primitive fibroblast and reticulum cells. The fibroblast is the progenitor of the osteoblast and the chondroblast. Each cell synthesizes a specific type of intercellular ground substance, and the tumor derived from the cell is generally characterized by the type of ground substance produced by the cell. For example, osteogenic tumors usually contain cells that have the appearance of osteoblasts and produce an intercellular substance that can be recognized as osteoid. Chondrogenic tumors contain chondroblasts and produce an intercellular substance similar to chondroid (cartilage). Collagenic tumors contain fibrous tissue cells and produce an intercellular substance similar to the type of collagen found in fibrous connective tissue.

Tumors are also classified as benign or malignant. The criteria used to identify tumor cells as malignant are (1) an increased nuclear/cytoplasmic ratio, (2) an irregular nuclear border, (3) excess chromatin, (4) a prominent nucleolus, and (5) an increase in the number of cells undergoing mitosis. However, many young, rapidly growing, normal cells and cells subjected to inflammation and change in their blood supply also exhibit many of these same characteristics. (Tumor characteristics in general are described in Chapter 11.)

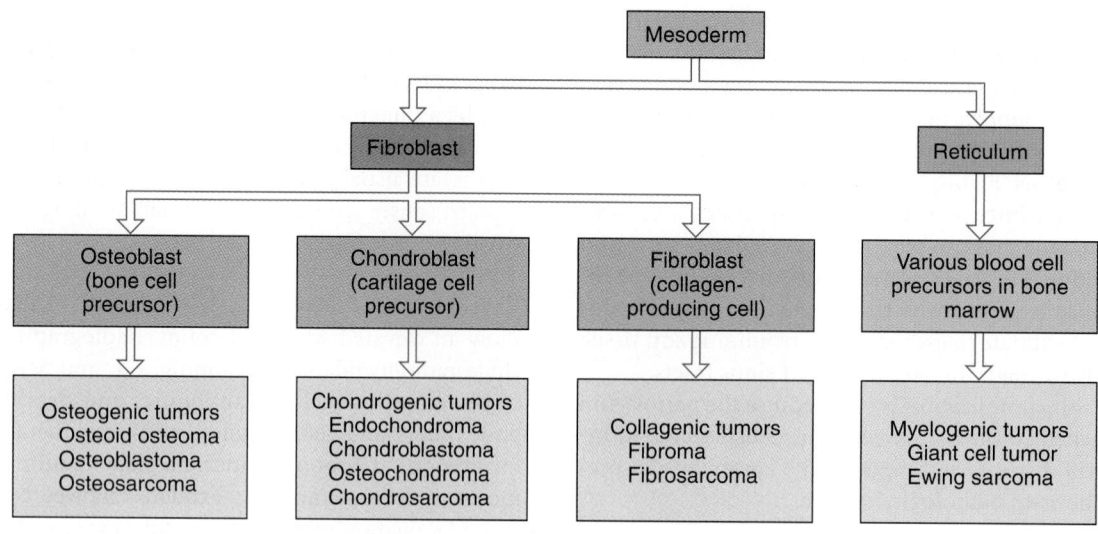

Figure 42-19 Derivation of bone tumors.

Epidemiology

The incidence of bone tumors varies with age. In children younger than 15 years, the rate of bone tumors is relatively low, constituting approximately 3% of all malignancies. Adolescents have the highest incidence of bone tumors, and adults between 30 and 35 years of age have the lowest incidence. After age 35, the incidence slowly increases until, at age 60, it equals the incidence in adolescents, primarily related to metastatic tumors.

Patterns of Bone Destruction

The general pathologic features of bone tumors include bone destruction, erosion or expansion of the cortex, and periosteal response to changes in underlying bone. The least amount of pathologic damage occurs with benign bone tumors, which push against neighboring tissue. Because they usually have a symmetric, controlled growth pattern, benign bone tumors tend to compress and displace neighboring normal bone tissue, which weakens the bone's structure until it is incapable of withstanding the stress of ordinary use, leading to pathologic fracture. Other tumors invade and destroy adjacent normal bone tissue by producing substances that promote resorption by increasing osteoclast activity or by interfering with a bone's blood supply.

Three patterns of bone destruction by bone tumors have been identified: (1) the geographic pattern, (2) the moth-eaten pattern, and (3) the permeative pattern (Table 42-4).

Tumors that erode the cortex of the bone usually stimulate a periosteal response, that is, new bone formation at the interface between the surface of the bone and the periosteum. Slow erosion of the cortex usually stimulates a uniform periosteal response. Additional layers of bone are added to the exterior surface of the bone to buttress the cortex. Eventually, the additional layers expand the bone's contour. Aggressive penetration of the cortex usually elevates the periosteum and stimulates erratic patterns of new bone formation. Examples

Table 42-4	Patterns of Bone Destruction by Bone Tumors
Type of Destruction	**Pattern Seen**
Geographic	Well-defined margins separated from surrounding normal bone; well-defined lytic area in affected bone
Moth eaten	Less-defined margin not easily separated from normal bone; areas of partially destroyed bone adjacent to completely lytic areas
Permeative	Poorly demarcated margins; abnormal lytic bone merges imperceptibly with surrounding normal bone

of erratic patterns include concentric layers of new bone; a sunburst pattern, in which delicate rays of new bone radiate toward the periosteum from a single focus on the underlying surface; and rays of new bone that grow perpendicularly, creating a brush or bristle pattern.

Diagnosis

A malignant bone tumor must be identified early to allow the survival of the individual and the preservation of the affected limb. However, individuals often have only vague symptoms that may be attributed to minor trauma, degenerative changes, or inflammatory conditions. In addition, other conditions may obscure the diagnosis.

Thorough diagnostic studies are needed to determine the exact type and extent of bone tumor present, which also helps determine the optimal treatment regimen. Staging of any bone tumor is critical to determine future treatment and results. The Enneking Staging System is the most commonly used arrangement (Table 42-5). This system classifies tumors

Table 42-5	The Ennenking Surgical Staging System for Malignant Bone Tumors		
Stage	Grade	Site (T)	Metastasis (M)
IA	Low (G_1)	Intracompartmental (T_1)	None (M_0)
IB	Low (G_1)	Extracompartmental (T_2)	None (M_0)
IIA	High (G_2)	Intracompartmental (T_1)	None (M_0)
IIB	High (G_2)	Extracompartmental (T_2)	None (M_0)
IIIA	Low (G_1)	Intracompartmental or extracompartmental (T_1 or T_2)	Regional or distant (M_1)
IIIB	High (G_2)	Intracompartmental or extracompartmental (T_1 or T_2)	Regional or distant (M_1)

Data from Rosen G et al: Bone tumors. In Bast RC et al, editors: *Cancer medicine*, ed 5, Hamilton, Ontario, 2000, B.D. Decker.

as to grade (G), tumor site (T), and metastasis (M). Benign tumors are given a numeric value of zero, whereas malignant tumors are low grade (G1) or high grade (G2).

Serum alkaline phosphatase levels are elevated in bone lytic tumors, and they are significantly elevated in osteosarcoma and Ewing sarcoma. Radiologic studies include plain radiologic films, technetium-99 bone scan, CT scan, and MRI, which has become the examination of choice for the local staging of bone tumors, especially the staging of peripheral osteosarcomas (see Table 42-6). MRI is also used to monitor the response of osteosarcomas to radiation or chemotherapy and to detect recurrent disease. A CT scan can evaluate involvement of osteosarcoma in flat bones when the tumor is not well defined on a plain film, can assist in differentiating the tumor, and can locate pulmonary metastases. Radionucleotide bone scans show an increased uptake at the tumor site.

Additional diagnostic studies done for specific bone tumors include a complete blood count and erythrocyte sedimentation rate (to rule out infection, myeloma, or Ewing sarcoma) and serum levels of calcium and phosphorus to detect hypercalcemia. Serum glucose levels may be elevated in chondrosarcoma. Acid phosphatase may show moderate elevations in bone metastases, multiple myeloma, and advanced Paget disease. Serum protein electrophoresis and immunoelectrophoresis are done to rule out multiple myeloma. Fineneedle biopsy is done, usually at the time of surgery, to determine the exact tumor type.

Types

A very large number of lesions are classified as bone tumors. The bone tumors most representative of the four derivative types (see Figure 42-19)—osteogenic, chondrogenic, collagenic, and myelogenic tumors—are described here.

Osteogenic Tumors: Osteosarcoma

Osteogenic (bone-forming) tumors are characterized by the formation of bone or osteoid tissue with a sarcomatous tissue. The tissue can have the appearance of compact or spongy bone. The most common malignant bone-forming tumor is the osteosarcoma. **Osteosarcomas** account for 38% of bone tumors. The male/female ratio is 3:2, and osteosarcoma occurs predominantly in adolescents and young adults. Sixty percent of osteosarcomas occur in persons younger than 20 years. A secondary peak incidence for osteosarcoma occurs

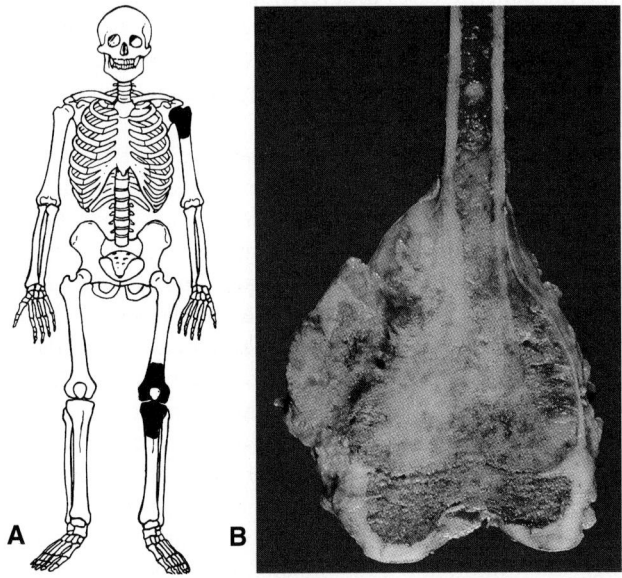

Figure 42-20 Osteosarcoma. **A,** Common locations of osteosarcoma. **B,** Femur has a large mass involving the metaphysis of the bone; the tumor has destroyed the cortex, forming a soft tissue component. (From Damjanov I, Linder J, editors: *Anderson's pathology*, ed 10, St Louis, 1996, Mosby.)

in the 50- to 60-year-old age group, primarily in individuals with a history of radiation therapy several years previously for pelvic or other malignancies (Figure 42-20).

An osteosarcoma is a malignant bone-forming tumor. It is aggressive and most often found in bone marrow; it has a moth-eaten pattern of bone destruction. The borders of the tumor are indistinct and merge into adjacent normal bone. Osteosarcomas always contain osteoid and callus (osteoblastic sarcoma), produced by anaplastic stromal cells, which are atypical, abnormal cells not seen in normal developing bone; they are neither normal nor embryonal. The osteosarcoma also may contain chondroid (cartilage) (chondroblastic sarcoma) and fibrinoid tissue (fibroblastic sarcoma) that may form the bulk of the tumor. The osteoid is deposited in thick masses or "streamers" between the trabeculae of callus, which infiltrate the normal compact bone, destroy it, and replace it with dense callus and masses of osteoid. Demonstrating the presence of osteoid aids in the diagnosis of osteosarcoma. Bone tissue produced by osteosarcomas never matures to compact bone.

Ninety percent of osteosarcomas are located in the metaphyses of long bones, especially the distal femur and proximal tibia, with 50% around the knee area.[46] The tumor typically breaks through the cortex, lifts the periosteum, and forms a soft tissue mass that is *not* covered by a smooth shell of new bone. Lifting of the periosteum stimulates bizarre patterns of new bone formation called a *periosteal reaction.* Distinct osteosarcomas occur on the surface of long bones, called parosteal, periosteal, or high-grade surface osteosarcomas; dedifferentiated parosteal and central osteosarcomas also occur.

The most common initial symptoms are pain and swelling. Initially, the pain is slight and intermittent, but within a short time the pain increases in severity and duration. Pain is usually worse at night and gradually requires medication. Systemic symptoms are uncommon. Usually, a coincidental history of trauma is noted. Occasionally, the individual may have a pathologic fracture.

Systemic chemotherapy and surgery are the treatments of choice, with the location of the tumor, its size, malignancy grade, and evidence of metastasis dictating the type and extent of surgery. Preoperative chemotherapy has greatly increased the number of individuals qualifying for limb salvage surgery. Limb salvaging procedures have been made possible by advances in reconstructive techniques and endoprosthetics. Limb salvage ultimately may be successful in as many as 80% of persons. Individuals must have achieved most of their bone growth to be candidates for limb salvage procedures—limb salvage procedures are preferred to amputation. Skeletally immature individuals may have a limb salvage operation, referred to as a *rotationplasty,* in which the major portions of the thigh, the tumor, and contaminated knee are resected while preserving the nerve supply (sciatic) to the leg and foot. The proximal tibia is internally fixed to the stump of the proximal femur after it has been rotated 180 degrees. The foot is positioned at a desired spot or direction, allowing the ankle joint to function as a knee joint with the foot supplying the traditional role of the tibial stump in a below-knee amputation.

If an amputation is done, individuals are monitored closely with chest roentgenograms and CT. Pulmonary metastases are surgically resected, and chemotherapy is now a common therapy given both before and after operation, using combinations of chemotherapeutic agents. New, promising agents under investigation include monoclonal antibodies, hormone antagonists, gene therapy, and other biologic agents that may dramatically improve survival.[46]

Chondrogenic Tumors: Chondrosarcoma

Chondrogenic (cartilage-forming) tumors produce cartilage or **chondroid,** a primitive cartilage or cartilage-like substance. The most common chondrogenic tumor is chondrosarcoma, accounting for 20% of bone tumors.

Chondrosarcoma, the second most common primary malignant bone tumor, is a tumor of middle-age and older adults. Most cases of primary chondrosarcoma are found in persons between 50 and 70 years of age. Secondary chondrosarcoma (a chondrosarcoma derived from an **endochondroma**) occurs most often in young adults between 20 and 30 years of age. The tumor is found more commonly in men than in women.

A chondrosarcoma is a large, ill-defined malignant tumor that infiltrates trabeculae in spongy bone. It occurs most often in the metaphysis or diaphysis of long bones, especially the femur, and in the bones of the pelvis (Figure 42-21). The tumor contains large lobules of hyaline cartilage that are separated by bands of fibrous tissue and anaplastic cells. Chondrosarcomas typically implant in surrounding tissue ("seeding").

Symptoms associated with chondrosarcoma have an insidious onset. Local swelling and pain are the usual symptoms that cause the individual to seek treatment. At first the pain is dull and intermittent, and then it gradually intensifies and becomes constant. It may waken the person at night.

Diagnostic studies include radiographs, which must be reviewed carefully for an accurate diagnosis. Biopsy is done at the time of surgery. (If biopsy is done before scheduled surgical incision, seeding of tumor cells could occur.) Sufficient tumor material must be obtained to facilitate an accurate diagnosis.

Surgical excision is generally regarded as the treatment of choice because chemotherapy and radiation seem to have little effect. Many surgically treated individuals demonstrate recurrences, however, so amputation is becoming one treatment of choice. Therefore individuals with tumors located in the limbs have a better prognosis than those with pelvic lesions.

Collagenic Tumors: Fibrosarcoma

Collagenic (collagen-forming) tumors produce fibrous connective tissue. The most typical collagenic tumor is the fibrosarcoma.

Fibrosarcomas represent 4% of primary malignant bone tumors, with a broad age distribution. They may occur at any age but are most common in adults between 30 and 50 years of age. The incidence is slightly greater in females. Fibrosar-

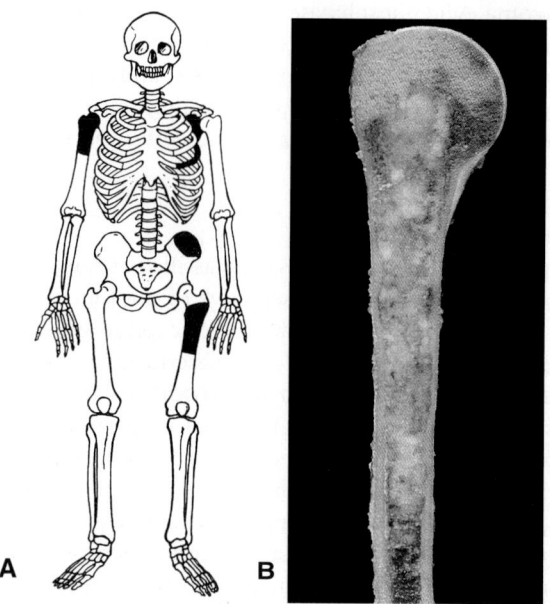

Figure 42-21 Chondrosarcoma. **A,** Common locations of chondrosarcoma. **B,** Chondrosarcoma of humerus. (From Damjanov I, Linder J, editors: *Anderson's pathology,* ed 10, St Louis, 1996, Mosby.)

coma also may be a secondary complication of radiation therapy, Paget disease, and long-standing osteomyelitis.

Fibrosarcoma is a solitary tumor that most often affects the metaphyseal region of the femur or tibia. The tumor is composed of a firm fibrous mass of tissue that contains collagen, malignant fibroblasts, and occasional osteoclast-like giant cells.

The tumor begins in the marrow cavity of the bone and infiltrates the trabeculae. It demonstrates a permeative growth pattern, destroys the cortex, and extends into the soft tissue. Metastasis to the lung is common.

Symptoms associated with the tumor have an insidious onset, which delays diagnosis. Pain and swelling, the usual symptoms that cause the individual to seek treatment, usually indicate that the tumor has broken through the cortex. Local tenderness, a palpable mass, and limitation of motion also may be present. A pathologic fracture in the affected bone is often the reason for seeking medical help. Diagnostic studies include radiographs and MRI.

Radical surgery and amputation are the treatments of choice for fibrosarcoma. Radiation therapy is generally considered ineffective treatment for this tumor.

Myelogenic Tumors

Myelogenic tumors originate from various bone marrow cells. Two types of myelogenic tumors are giant cell tumor and myeloma.

Giant Cell Tumor. Giant cell tumor is the sixth most common of the primary bone tumors, accounting for 4% to 5% of bone tumors. Giant cell tumors have a wide age distribution; however, they are rare in persons younger than 10 years or older than 70 years. Most giant cell tumors are found in persons between 20 and 40 years of age. Unlike most other bone tumors, giant cell tumors affect females more often than males.

The giant cell tumor is a benign, solitary, circumscribed tumor that causes extensive bone resorption because of its osteoclastic origin (Figure 42-22). The tumor is rich in osteoclast-like giant cells and anaplastic stromal cells. It also may contain osteoid, callus, and collagen. Overexpression of several genes, including osteoprotegerin ligand (OPGL), occurs in giant cell tumors.[47] The giant cell tumor is typically located in the center of the epiphysis in the femur, tibia, radius, or humerus. The tumor has a slow, relentless growth rate and is usually contained within the original contour of the affected bone. It may, however, extend into the articular cartilage. When the tumor extends, it is usually covered by periosteum or periosteal bone growth. The tumor also may extend into local soft tissue, but it has a low rate of metastasis to other organs or tissues, although it has a high recurrence rate.

The most common symptoms associated with giant cell tumor are pain, local swelling, and limitation of movement. Diagnostic studies include radiographs, CT, and MRI. Cryosurgery and resection of the tumor with the use of adjuvant polymethylmethacrylate (PMMA) for bone grafts decrease recurrence and are more successful treatments than curettage and radiation. Amputation may be necessary but is not common.

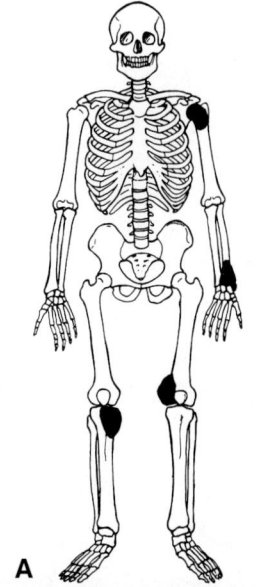

A

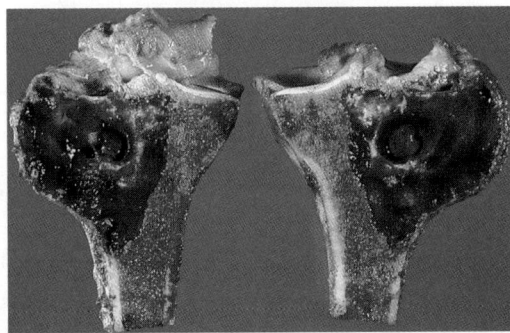

B

Figure 42-22 Giant cell tumor of bone. A, Common skeletal locations. **B,** Gross picture of cell tumor of bone (epimetaphysis). (From Damjanov I, Linder J, editors: *Anderson's pathology,* ed 10, St Louis, 1996, Mosby.)

DISORDERS OF JOINTS

The American College of Rheumatology (ACR) recognizes 13 groups of joint disease—**arthropathies.** Most of these disorders can be placed into two major categories: noninflammatory joint disease and inflammatory joint disease. With recent improvements in detection methods, conditions such as osteoarthritis that were previously classified as noninflammatory have now had inflammatory pathways identified.

Osteoarthritis

Traditionally, **noninflammatory joint disease** was differentiated from inflammatory joint disease by (1) the absence of synovial membrane inflammation, (2) the lack of systemic signs and symptoms, and (3) normal synovial fluid. **Degenerative joint disease—osteoarthritis—**was the most prevalent noninflammatory joint disease.[48,49] Recently, discovery of inflammation in the joints has emerged as an important feature of osteoarthritis. The use of MRI and arthroscopy have made it clear that osteoarthritic changes are not defined by changes noted on x-ray films alone.[50] Consequently osteoarthritis has been reclassified as inflammatory joint disease (Figure 42-23).

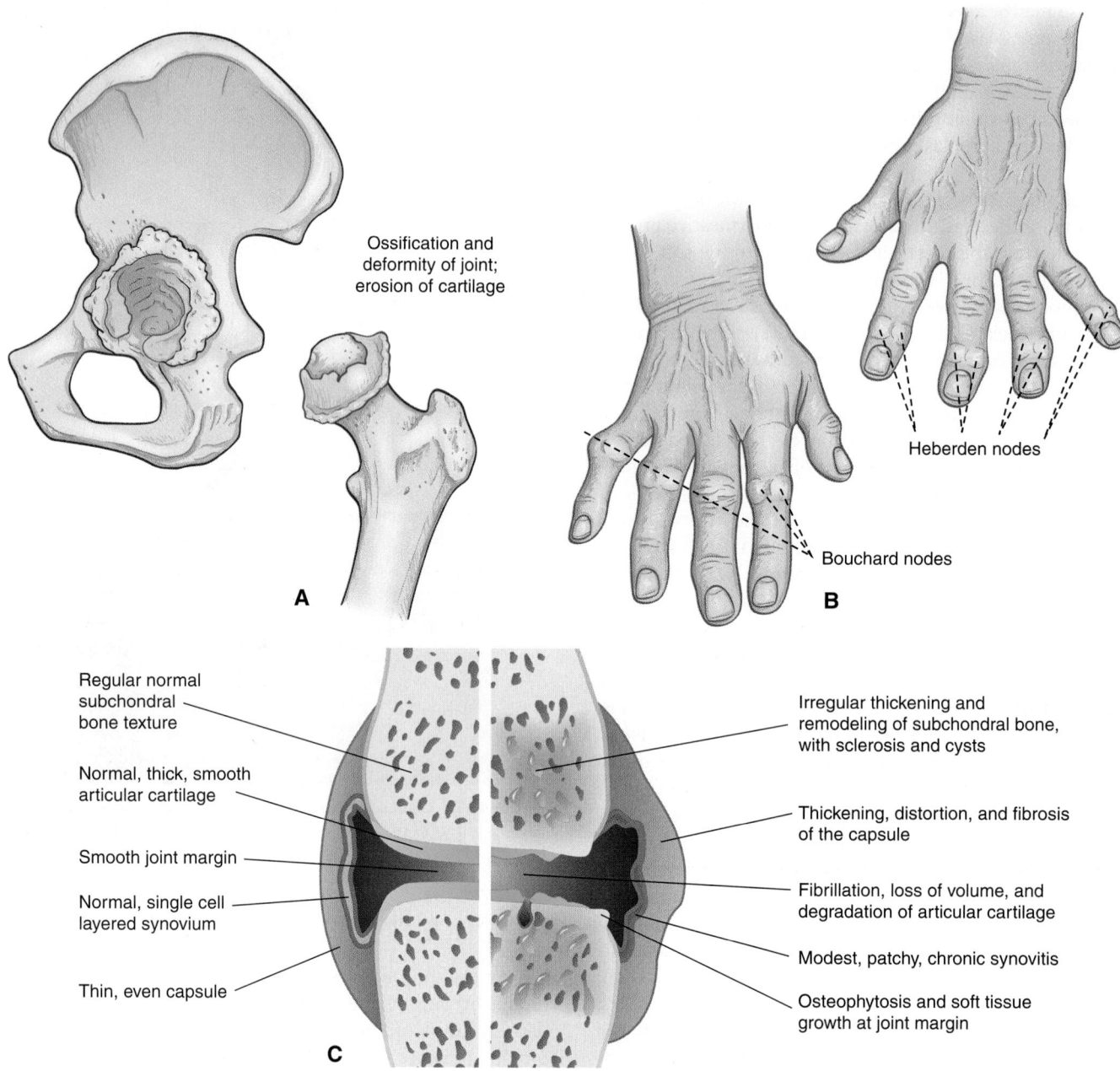

Figure 42-23 Osteoarthritis (OA). **A,** Cartilage and degeneration of the hip joint resulting from osteoarthritis. **B,** Heberden nodes and Bouchard nodes. **C,** Characteristics of OA. Normal versus osteoarthritic synovial joint.

Medical clinicians are somewhat divided about use of the terms *degenerative joint disease* and *osteoarthritis.* The term *osteoarthritis* has been used in most recent communications and appears to be the more accepted term in the European literature.

Osteoarthritis (OA)—is a common, age-related disorder of synovial joints. It is characterized by local areas of loss and damage of articular cartilage, new bone formation of joint margins (osteophytosis), subchondral bone changes, variable degrees of mild synovitis and thickening of the joint capsule (Figure 42-23). Pathology centers on load-bearing areas. Advancing disease reveals narrowing of the joint space because

cartilage loss, bone spurs (**osteophytes**) and sometimes changes in the subchondral bone. OA can arise in any synovial joint but is commonly found in the hands, knees, hips, and spine. It is less common in people less than 40 years but rises in incidence with age. With improved understanding of OA the previously common classification into primary and secondary no longer seems viable.[50] Osteoarthritis is a multifactorial disease involving environmental–life-style factors and genetics.

OA is generally distributed throughout the peripheral and central joints of the body and affects adult men more than women until after age 55. Although the exact causes of OA are unclear, they involve low-grade inflammation, calcification of articular cartilage, genetic alterations, and metabolic disorders.[50]

With aging the quality and quantity of the proteoglycans in cartilage decrease in direct proportion to the severity of OA. Evidence also suggests that OA involves a complex inter-action of cytokines, growth factors, matrix metallopro-teinases, and enzymes[30] (see pathophysiology).

OA can be caused by any condition that damages cartilage directly; subjects the joint surfaces or underlying bone to chronic, excessive, or abnormal forces; or causes instability in the joint. Specific risk factors include the following:

1. Trauma, particularly sprains, strains, joint dislocations, and fractures
2. Long-term mechanical stress associated with athletics, ballet dancing, or repetitive physical tasks worsened by obesity.
3. The presence of inflammation in joint structures, dur-ing which inflammatory cells release enzymes capable of digesting cartilage cells
4. Joint instability caused by damage to supporting struc-tures, such as the joint capsule, ligaments, or tendons
5. Neurologic disorders (e.g., diabetic neuropathy, Char-cot neuropathic joint) in which pain and propriocep-tive reflexes are diminished or lost, increasing the ten-dency for abnormal movement, positioning, or weight bearing
6. Congenital or acquired skeletal deformities
7. Hematologic or endocrine disorders, such as hemo-philia, which causes chronic bleeding into the joints, or hyperparathyroidism, which causes bone to lose cal-cium
8. Drugs (e.g., colchicine, indomethacin, steroids) that stimulate the activity of collagen-digesting enzymes in the synovial membrane
9. Obesity

All of these factors alter articular cartilage in some way and accelerate the rate of cartilage loss.

PATHOPHYSIOLOGY   The primary defect in OA is loss of articular cartilage. Early in the disease, the articular carti-lage loses its glistening appearance, becoming yellow-gray or brownish gray. As the disease progresses, surface areas of the articular cartilage flake off and deeper layers develop longitu-dinal fissures (fibrillation). The cartilage becomes thin and may be absent over some areas, leaving the underlying bone (subchondral bone) unprotected. Consequently, the unpro-tected subchondral bone becomes sclerotic (dense and hard). Cysts sometimes develop within the subchondral bone and communicate with the longitudinal fissures in the cartilage. Pressure builds in the cysts until the cystic contents are forced into the synovial cavity, breaking through the articular carti-lage on the way. As the articular cartilage erodes, cartilage-coated osteophytes may grow outward from the underlying bone and alter the bone contours and joint anatomy. These spur-like bony projections enlarge until small pieces, called *joint mice,* break off into the synovial cavity. If osteophyte

fragments irritate the synovial membrane, synovitis and joint effusion result. The joint capsule also becomes thickened and at times adheres to the deformed underlying bone, which may contribute to the limitation of movement (see Figure 42-23).

Articular cartilage is probably lost through enzymatic breakdown of the cartilage matrix—the proteoglycans, gly-cosaminoglycans, and collagen. First, the enzymes break down the macromolecules of proteoglycans, glycosaminogly-cans, and collagen into large, diffusible fragments. Then the fragments are taken up by the cartilage cells (chondrocytes) and digested by the cell's own lysosomal enzymes. (Processes of cellular uptake and lysosomal digestion are described in Chapter 1.) The loss of proteoglycans from articular cartilage is a hallmark of the osteoarthritic process.

Enzymatic destruction of articular cartilage begins in the matrix, with destruction of proteoglycans and collagen fibers. Enzymes, particularly stromelysin and acid metallopro-teinase, affect proteoglycans by interfering with assembly of the proteoglycan subunit or the proteoglycan aggregate (see Chapter 41); these enzymes are markedly elevated in OA. Changes in the conformation of proteoglycans disrupt the pumping action that regulates movement of water and sy-novial fluid into and out of the cartilage. Without the regula-tory action of the proteoglycan pump, cartilage imbibes too much fluid and becomes less able to withstand the stresses of weight bearing. Also with aging, the proteoglycan content is decreased and water content in cartilage can be increased by as much as 8%, affecting the strength of the cartilage. Persons with OA, even those with fairly extensive cartilage destruc-tion, have elevated levels of proteoglycans or fragments of proteoglycans in their synovial fluid, perhaps indicative of a more pronounced reparative phase. Other studies indicate that inflammatory cytokines, such as interleukin-1 (see Chap-ter 41 for discussion of cytokines), play a major role in carti-lage degradation in part through induction of nitric oxide synthase (iNOS) and nitric oxide (NO) increased generation. Cytokines release and activate proteolytic and collagenolytic enzymes causing an imbalance of cell responses to growth factor activity.

Enzymes that degrade collagen (i.e., collagenases) proba-bly originate in the chondrocytes or in leukocytes. With com-parisons to atherosclerotic lesions, cartilage calcification also appears to involve apoptosis. Chondrocyte apoptosis is in-creased in OA cartilage and is directly correlated with hy-droxyapatite crystal deposition.[51] NO stimulates apoptosis in chrondocytes.[50,52] Inflammatory mediators that promote degradation of the cartilage matrix possibly are an important factor for calcification. Genetic deficiencies of inhibitors of calcification also may contribute to "run away" calcification (see Figure 42-24). Recent animal studies have illustrated that calcification in the artery (and cartilage) is actively inhibited by surrounding local cells. Deficient expression of these in-hibitors (e.g., pyrophosphate [PPi]), as well as procalcifying mediators (e.g., inorganic phosphate [Pi]) may trigger the calcification process.[53-55] Collagen breakdown destroys the fibrils that give articular cartilage its tensile strength and ex-

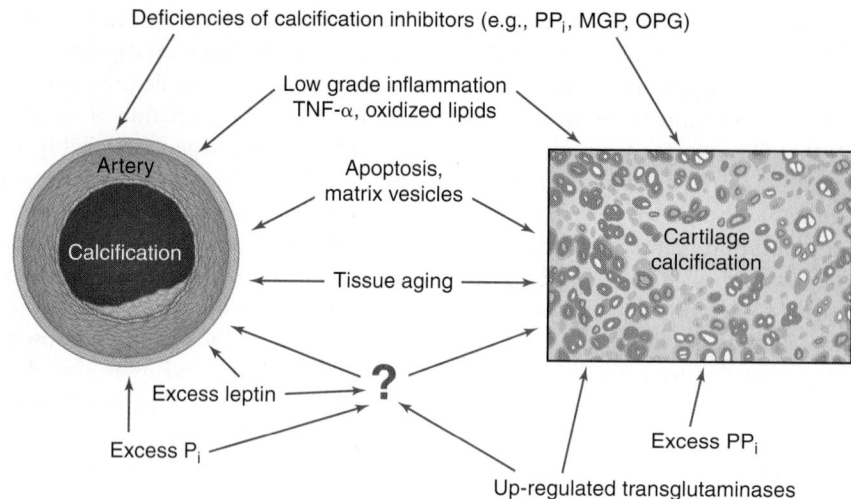

Figure 42-24 Mechanisms driving artery and cartilage calcification. All specified factors have been demonstrated to promote calcification in either arteries and/or cartilage (see text). (From Rutsch F, Terkeltaub R: *Joint Bone Spine* 72:110-118, 2005.)

poses the chondrocytes to mechanical stress and enzyme attack. Thus a cycle of destruction begins that involves all the components of articular cartilage—proteoglycans, collagen fibers, and chondrocytes.

CLINICAL MANIFESTATIONS   Clinical manifestations of OA typically appear during the fifth or sixth decade of life, although asymptomatic, articular surface changes are common after age 40 years. Pain and stiffness in one or more joints, usually weight-bearing or load-bearing joints, are the first symptoms of the disease. Use-related joint pain relieved by rest is a key feature. Examination usually shows general involvement of both peripheral and central joints. Peripheral joints most often involved are in the hands, wrists, knees, and feet. Central joints most often affected are in the lower cervical spine, lumbosacral spine, shoulders, and hips.

Joint structures are capable of generating a limited number of signs and symptoms. The primary signs and symptoms of joint disease are pain, stiffness, enlargement or swelling, tenderness, limited range of motion, muscle wasting, partial dislocation, and deformity.

Pain and stiffness are the predominant symptoms of OA. They are usually aggravated by weight bearing or use of the joint and relieved by resting the joint. Nocturnal pain is usually not relieved by rest and may be accompanied by paresthesias (numbness, tingling, prickling). Sometimes pain is referred to another part of the body. For example, osteoarthritis of the lumbosacral spine may mimic sciatica, causing severe pain in the back of the thigh along the course of the sciatic nerve. OA in the lower cervical spine may cause brachial neuralgia (pain in the arm) aggravated by movement of the neck. Osteoarthritic conditions in the hip cause pain that may be referred to the lower thigh and knee area.

The actual mechanisms of joint pain are complex and poorly understood, but several explanations are possible. The

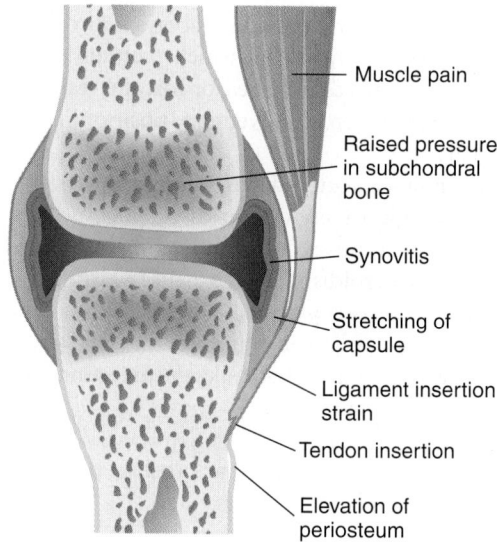

Figure 42-25 Possible causes of pain in osteoarthritis.

pain could be caused by articular distention and stretching of the fibrous joint capsule, which has an abundant nerve supply. In addition, inflammation of the joint capsule causes fibrous shrinking, so that movement of the joint in any direction causes painful stretching. Pain also can arise from the subchondral or periarticular bone (Figure 42-25).

The origin of joint stiffness is unknown. **Joint stiffness** is generally defined as difficulty in initiating joint movement, immobility, or a loss of range of motion. The stiffness usually occurs as joint movement begins, and it dissipates within 30 minutes. Enlargement and bulging of joint contour, commonly described as swelling, may be caused by bone enlargement or the proliferation of osteophytes around the margins of the joint. Swelling also occurs if inflammatory exudate or blood enters the joint cavity, thereby increasing the volume of synovial fluid. This condition, termed **joint effusion,** is caused by (1) the presence of osteophyte fragments in the synovial cavity, (2) drainage of cysts from diseased subchondral bone, or (3) acute trauma to joint structures, resulting in hemorrhage and inflammatory exudation into the synovial cavity.

Range of motion is limited to some degree, depending on the extent of cartilage degeneration. Frequently, joint motion is accompanied by sounds of crepitus, creaking, or grating. Hypermobility and subluxation of joints occur in OA secondary to a neurologic disorder.

As OA of the lower extremity progresses, the person may begin to limp noticeably. Having a limp is distressing because it affects the person's independence and ability to do activities of daily living. The affected joint is also more symptomatic after use, such as at the end of the day.

EVALUATION AND TREATMENT   Evaluation consists of clinical assessment and radiologic studies, CT scan, arthroscopy, and MRI. Treatment is based on severity of symptoms.[50] Conservative treatment includes rest of the involved joint until inflammation, if present, subsides; range-of-motion exercise to prevent joint capsule contraction; use of a cane, crutches, or walker to decrease weight bearing; weight loss if obesity is present; and analgesic and antiinflammatory drug therapy to reduce swelling and pain. Glucosamine, a nutraceutical, has shown some success in reducing the pain and progression of OA. Other alternative therapies, including magnetic bracelets and acupuncture, seem to improve symptoms in some people. Intraarticular injection of high-molecular-weight viscosupplements, particularly hyaluronic acid, also has been successful in decreasing knee pain with OA.[56] Surgery is used to improve joint movement, correct deformity or malalignment, or create a new joint with artificial implants. There are nearly 250,000 total hip replacements yearly in the United States, most of which are related to OA.

Classic Inflammatory Joint Disease

Inflammatory joint disease commonly is called *arthritis.* Inflammatory joint disease is characterized by inflammatory damage or destruction in the synovial membrane or articular cartilage and by systemic signs of inflammation (fever, leukocytosis, malaise, anorexia, hyperfibrinogenemia). See discussion on osteoarthritis, which now is considered part of inflammatory joint disease.

Inflammatory joint disease can be infectious or noninfectious. In infectious inflammatory joint disease, inflammation is caused by invasion of the joint by bacteria, mycoplasmas, viruses, fungi, or protozoa. These agents can invade the joint through a traumatic wound, surgical incision, or contaminated needle, or they can be delivered by the bloodstream from sites of infection elsewhere in the body, typically bones, heart valves, or blood vessels. In noninfectious inflammatory joint disease, which is the most common form, inflammation is caused by immune reactions or the deposition of crystals of

monosodium urate in and around the joint. Rheumatoid arthritis and ankylosing spondylitis are noninfectious inflammatory diseases caused by immune reactions and possibly hypersensitivity reactions[57]; gouty arthritis is a noninfectious inflammatory disease caused by crystal deposition.

Rheumatoid Arthritis

Rheumatoid arthritis (RA) is a systemic inflammatory autoimmune disease associated with swelling and pain in multiple joints. (Autoimmune disease is described in Chapter 8.) The first joint tissue to be affected is the synovial membrane, which lines the joint cavity (see Chapter 41, Figure 41-9). Eventually, inflammation may spread to the articular cartilage, fibrous joint capsule, and surrounding ligaments and tendons, causing pain, joint deformity, and loss of function (Figure 42-26). The joints most commonly affected are in the fingers, feet, wrists, elbows, ankles, and knees, but the shoulders, hips, and cervical spine also may be involved, as well as the tissues of the lungs, heart, kidneys, and skin.

RA affects 1% to 2% of adults and, like most autoimmune diseases, develops most often in women, with a female/male ratio of 3:1. The frequency of RA increases from the third decade on, affecting 5% or more of the population ages 70 years and older. Besides inflammation of the joints, RA can cause fever, malaise, rash, lymph node or spleen enlargement,

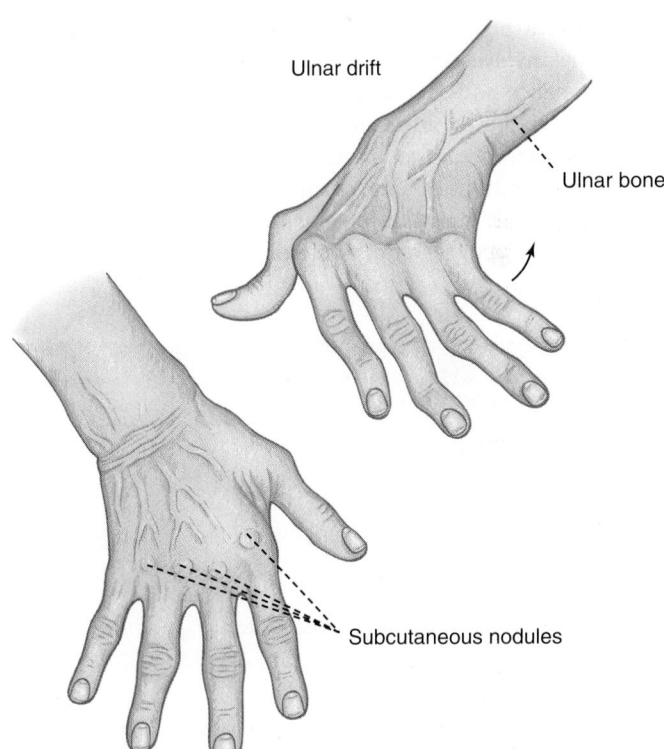

Figure 42-26 Rheumatoid arthritis of the hand. Note swelling from chronic synovitis of metacarpophalangeal joints, marked ulnar drift, subcutaneous nodules, and subluxation of metacarpophalangeal joints with extension of proximal interphalangeal joints and flexion of distal joints. Note also deformed position of thumb. Hand has wasted appearance. (From Mourad L: *Orthopedic disorders,* St Louis, 1991, Mosby.)

and Raynaud phenomenon (transient lack of circulation to the fingertips and toes).

Despite intensive research, the cause of RA remains obscure. Proposals of the initiating event include an infectious agent or other environmental exposure but genetic, hormonal, and reproductive factors may all contribute to developing RA. The initiating event unleashes an immune response that results in inflammation of the lining of the joint—the synovial membrane. RA probably occurs in a genetically susceptible person because of an aberrant immune response to an unidentified antigen. A key genetic element has been localized to the HLA-DR4, HLA-DRB1, and HLA-DP areas of the major histocompatibility complex. Infectious microorganisms that may play a role in the cause of RA include bacteria, mycoplasmas, and viruses (especially Epstein-Barr virus) (Table 42-6). With long-term or intensive exposure to the antigen, normal antibodies (immunoglobulins [Ig]) become autoantibodies—antibodies that attack host tissues (self-antigens). Because they are usually present in individuals with rheumatoid arthritis, the transformed antibodies are termed **rheumatoid factors (RFs).** The RFs usually consist of two classes of immunoglobulin antibodies (antibodies for IgM and IgG) but occasionally involve antibodies for IgA. Their main antigenic targets are portions of the immunoglobulin molecules. RFs bind with their target self-antigens in blood and synovial membrane, forming immune complexes (antigen-antibody complexes) (see Chapter 7).

RA has a higher incidence in women, with evidence of hormonal involvement because disease symptoms lessen during pregnancy and exacerbate in the postpartal period. Evidence for endocrine involvement in RA tissues and cells include (1) presence of androgen and estrogen receptors, (2) high concentrations of biologically active steroids, (3) key enzymes of steroid metabolism, and (4) significant changes of estrogen to androgen ratio. These data strongly suggest that individual immune cells, including synovial macrophages, may behave as steroid-sensitive cells. Most studies on the influence of exogenous hormones and risk of RA have focused on oral contraceptive pills, with inconsistent findings. Fewer studies have been done with hormone replacement; however, new interest has emerged on the role of estrogen and autoimmunity. RA also has seasonal variations, being worse in winter months.

PATHOPHYSIOLOGY The pathogenesis of rheumatoid arthritis is summarized in Figure 42-27.

Cartilage damage in RA is the result of several processes:
1. CD4 T helper cells, and other cells in the synovial fluid become activated, promoting cytokine release and activating B lymphocytes.
2. Recruitment and retention of inflammatory cells in the joint sublining region.
3. Viscous cycle of altered cytokine and signal transduction pathways.
4. Possible immune complex deposition and resultant inflammatory molecule release.
5. RANKL release and osteoclast activation.
6. Angiogenesis, or growth of new blood vessels in the synovium.

Several types of leukocytes are attracted out of the circulation and into the synovial membrane. The phagocytes of inflammation (neutrophils and macrophages) ingest the immune complexes and, in the process of doing so, release powerful enzymes that degrade synovial tissue and articular cartilage (Figure 42-28). The immune system's B and T lymphocytes are also activated. The B lymphocytes are stimulated to produce more RFs, and the T lymphocytes eventually cause release of enzymes that amplify and perpetuate the inflammatory response. Destruction of the extracellular matrix possibly leads to significant disability in individuals with

Table 42-6	Types of Infectious Arthritis	
Type and Microorganism	**Comments**
Lyme arthritis Spirochete *Borrelia burgdorferi* Transmitted via ticks (*Ixodes ricinus*)	Initial infection of skin followed by spreading to other sites including joints in days or weeks Arthritis is a predominant feature involving mainly large joints; possibly caused by immune reactions against Borrelia antigens (such as Osp A) that cross-react with tissue antigens in joints
Tuberculosis arthritis Complication of osteomyelitis or visceral, usually pulmonary, infection	Weight-bearing joints most susceptible Fibrous ankylosis and destruction of joint space; onset is insidious and gradual.
Suppurative arthritis Bacterial infections with *Gonococcus, Staphylococcus, Streptococcus, Haemophilus influenzae,* and gram-negative bacilli; *H. influenzae* arthritis more common in children under 2 years; *S. aureus* in older children and adults	Classic is a sudden onset of symptoms—painful, hot, swollen joint with decreased range of motion Prompt therapy prevents joint destruction
Viral arthritis Many viruses including parvovirus B19, rubella, hepatitis C virus, HIV	Symptoms vary from acute to subacute Unclear if effects are from direct invasion of the virus or an autoimmune reaction

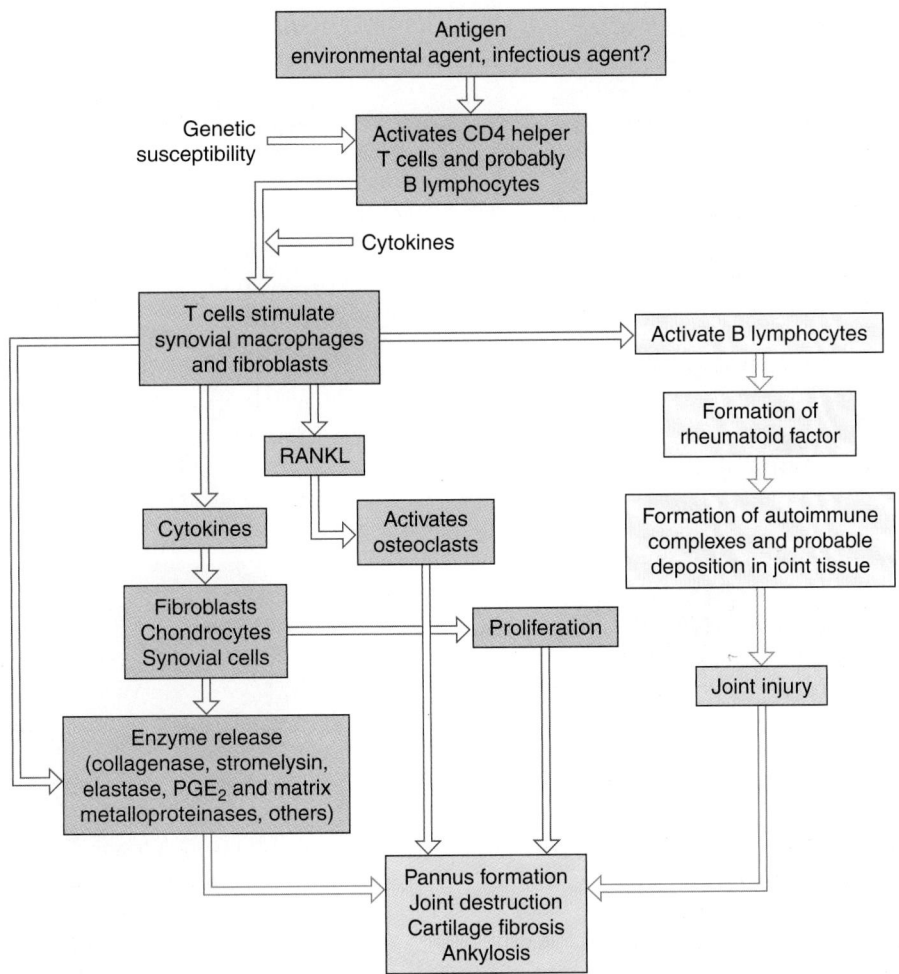

Figure 42-27 **Emerging Model of Pathogenesis of Rheumatoid Arthritis:** Rheumatoid arthritis is an autoimmune disease of a genetically susceptible host triggered by an unknown antigenic agent. Chronic autoimmune reaction with activation of CD4+ helper T cells and possibly other lymphocytes and the local release of inflammatory cytokines and mediators that eventually destroys the joint. T cells stimulate cells in the joint to produce cytokines that are key mediators of synovial damage. Apparently immune complex deposition also plays a role. Tumor necrosis factor (TNF) and interleukin-1 (IL-1), as well as some other cytokines, stimulate synovial cells to proliferate and produce other mediators of inflammation, such as prostaglandins (PGE$_2$) matrix metalloproteinases, and enzymes that all contribute to destruction of cartilage. Activated T cells and synovial fibroblasts also produce receptor activator of nuclear factor κβ ligand (RANKL) which activates the osteoclasts and promotes bone destruction. Pannus is a mass of synovium and synovial stroma with inflammatory cells, granulation tissue and fibroblasts that grows over the articular surface and causes its destruction.

rheumatoid arthritis.[58] Cartilage destruction is mediated by processes from the synovium and cellular invasion into the matrix. These processes may be facilitated by oxidative stress and alterations in DNA repair mechanisms, causing mutation in key genes.[58] In addition RANKL is expressed by various cells in the synovium and induces osteoclast maturation and activation (see p. 1509).

Inflammatory and immune processes have several damaging effects on the synovial membrane. Along with the swelling caused by leukocyte infiltration, the synovial membrane undergoes hyperplastic thickening as its cells proliferate and enlarge abnormally. As synovial inflammation progresses to involve its blood vessels, small venules become occluded by the hypertrophied endothelial cells, fibrin, platelets, and inflammatory cells, which decrease vascular flow to the synovial tissue. Compromised circulation, coupled with increased metabolic needs because of hypertrophy and hyperplasia, causes

hypoxia and metabolic acidosis. Acidosis stimulates the release of hydrolytic enzymes from synovial cells into the surrounding tissue, initiating erosion of the articular cartilage and inflammation in the supporting ligaments and tendons.

Inflammation causes hemorrhage, coagulation, and fibrin deposition on the synovial membrane, in the intracellular matrix, and in the synovial fluid. Over denuded areas of the synovial membrane, fibrin develops into granulation tissue called **pannus.** (Granulation tissue is the tissue produced earliest in the process of healing; see Chapter 6.) Researchers disagree about whether pannus is a cause or an effect of articular cartilage involvement in RA. Some believe that, as RA progresses, pannus extends from the synovial membrane into adjacent articular cartilage and destroys the cartilage. Other researchers think that pannus forms on articular cartilage after the cartilage has been destroyed by inflammation. In any case, pannus formation does not lead to synovial or articular

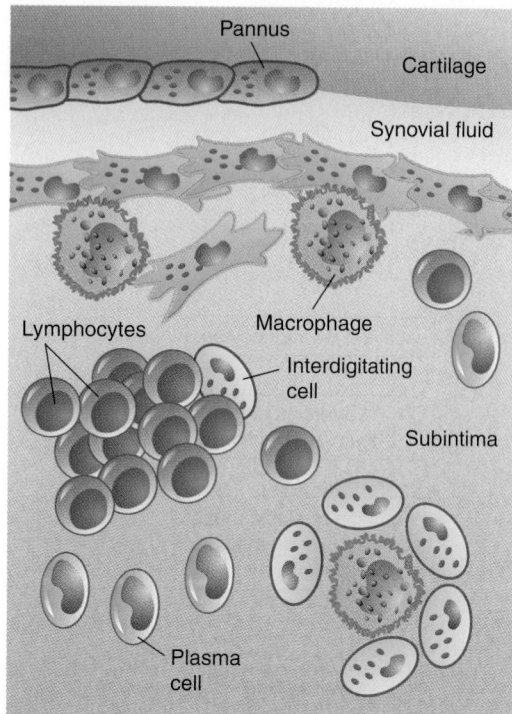

Figure 42-28 *Synovitis.* Inflamed synovium showing typical arrangements of macrophages *(red)* and fibroblastic cells.

regeneration but rather to formation of scar tissue that immobilizes the joint (Figure 42-29, *B*).

CLINICAL MANIFESTATIONS   The onset of RA is usually insidious, although as many as 15% of cases have an acute onset. RA begins with general systemic manifestations of inflammation, including fever, fatigue, weakness, anorexia, weight loss, and generalized aching and stiffness. Local manifestations also appear gradually over a period of weeks or months. Typically, the joints become painful, tender, and stiff. Pain early in the disease is caused by pressure from swelling. Later on, the disease pain is caused by sclerosis of subchondral bone and new bone formation. Stiffness usually lasts for about 1 hour after arising in the morning and is thought to be related to synovitis. Initially the joints most commonly involved are the metacarpophalangeal (MCP) joints, proximal interphalangeal (PIP) joints, and wrists, with later involvement of larger weight-bearing joints.

Joint swelling, which is widespread and symmetric, is caused by increasing amounts of inflammatory exudate (leukocytes, plasma, plasma proteins) in the synovial membrane, hyperplasia of inflamed tissues, and formation of new bone. On palpation, the swollen joint feels warm and the synovial membrane feels "boggy." The skin over the joint may have a ruddy, cyanotic hue and may look thin and shiny.

An inflamed joint may lose some of its mobility. Even mild synovitis can lead to loss of range of motion, which becomes evident after inflammation subsides. Extension becomes limited and is eventually lost if flexion contractures form. Loss of range of motion can progress to permanent deformities of the

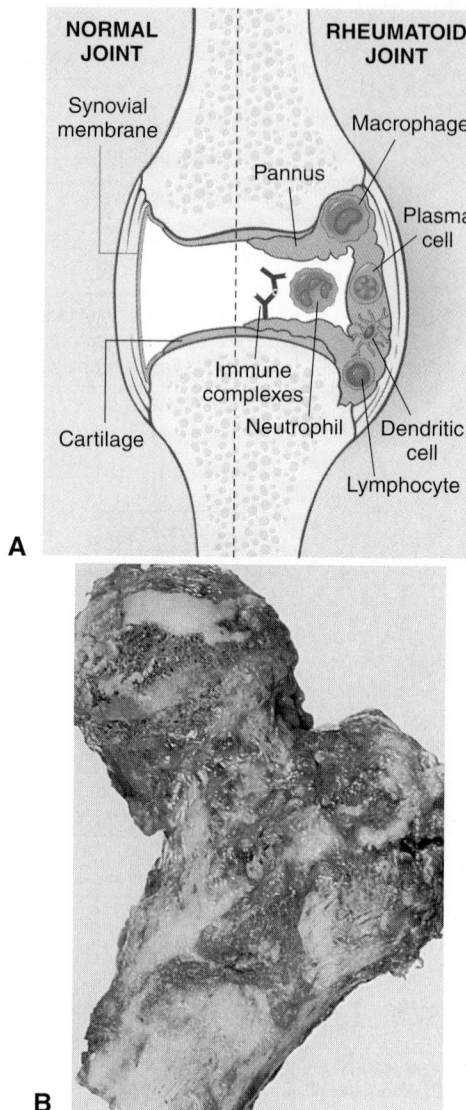

Figure 42-29 *Rheumatoid arthritis.* **A,** Schematic view of the joint lesion. **B,** Advanced rheumatoid arthritis involving femur. There is prominent proliferation of synovium and almost complete destruction of overlying articular cartilage. (**A,** Modified from Feldmann M: *Nat Rev Immunol* 2:364, 2002. **B,** From Rosai J: *Ackerman's surgical pathology,* ed 8, St Louis, 1996, Mosby.)

fingers, toes, and limbs, including ulnar deviation of the hands, boutonnière and swan-neck deformities of the finger joints, plantar subluxation of the metatarsal heads of the foot, and hallux valgus (angulation of the great toe toward the other toes). Flexion contractures of the knees and hips are also common.

Joint deformities cause the physical limitations experienced by persons with RA. Loss of joint motion is quickly followed by secondary atrophy of the surrounding muscles. With secondary muscle atrophy the joint becomes unstable, which further aggravates joint pathology.

Two complications of chronic RA are caused by an excessive amount of inflammatory exudate in the synovial cavity. One complication is the formation of cysts in the articular cartilage or subchondral bone. Occasionally, these cysts communicate with the skin surface (usually the sole of the foot) and can drain through passages called fistulae. The second complication is rupture of a cyst or of the synovial joint itself, usually caused by strenuous physical activity that places excessive pressure on the joint. Rupture releases inflammatory exudate into adjacent tissues, thereby spreading inflammation.

Extrasynovial **rheumatoid nodules,** or swellings, are observed in areas of pressure or trauma in 20% of individuals with RA. Each nodule is an aggregate of inflammatory cells surrounding a central core of fibrinoid and cellular debris. T lymphocytes are the predominant leukocytes in the nodule. B lymphocytes, plasma cells, and phagocytes are found around the periphery. Nodules are found most often in subcutaneous tissue over the extensor surfaces of elbows and fingers. Less common sites are the scalp, back, feet, hands, buttocks, and knees.

Rheumatoid nodules also may invade the skin, cardiac valves, pericardium, pleura, lung parenchyma, and spleen. These nodules are identical to those encountered in some individuals with rheumatic fever and are characterized by central tissue necrosis surrounded by proliferating connective tissue. Also noted are large numbers of lymphocytes and occasional plasma cells. Acute glaucoma may result, with nodules forming on the sclera. Pulmonary involvement may result in diffuse pleuritis or multiple intraparenchymal nodules. Together, the occurrence of pulmonary nodules and pneumoconiosis (chronic inflammation of the lungs from inhalation of dust) creates the syndrome called **Caplan syndrome.** Diffuse pulmonary fibrosis may occur because of immunologically mediated immune complex deposition.

Rheumatoid nodules within the heart may cause valvular deformities, particularly of the aortic valve leaflets Pericardial effusion or other pericardial problems occur in almost 50% of RA patients. Lymphadenopathy of the nodes close to the affected joints may develop. Rheumatoid nodules within the spleen result in splenomegaly. Involvement of blood vessels results in an acute necrotizing vasculitis, characteristic of that noted in other immunologic/inflammatory states. Thromboses of such involved vessels may give rise to myocardial infarctions, cerebrovascular occlusions, mesenteric infarction, kidney damage, and vascular insufficiency in the hands and fingers (Raynaud phenomenon). Vascular changes are noted primarily in individuals receiving steroid therapy; thus there is some concern that the therapy may play a role in initiating these lesions. Changes in skeletal muscle are often noted in the form of nonspecific atrophy secondary to joint dysfunction.

EVALUATION AND TREATMENT   Evaluation of RA is by physical examination, roentgenography of the joint, and serologic tests for rheumatoid factor and circulating immune complexes. The American College of Rheumatology lists the following diagnostic criteria for rheumatoid arthritis:

1. Morning stiffness for longer than 1 hour
2. Arthritis of three or more joint areas
3. Arthritis of hand joints
4. Symmetric arthritis
5. Rheumatoid nodules over extensor surfaces or bony prominences
6. Serum rheumatoid factor present in abnormal amounts
7. Radiographic changes

The presence of four or more of the criteria is diagnostic of RA. Criteria 1 through 4 with joint signs or symptoms must be present for 6 weeks.

Treatment is conservative or surgical. Conservative treatment includes rest of the inflamed joint and whole-body rest for several hours daily, use of hot and cold packs, physical therapy, antineoplastic medications, a diet high in calories and vitamins, corticosteroids, antiinflammatory drugs, immunosuppressants, and disease-modifying antirheumatic drugs (DMARDs) taken orally or by injection. Biologic agents that target cytokines have demonstrated significant improvement in outcomes for both adult and juvenile rheumatoid arthritis.[59] Surgical synovectomy may be done early in the disease to decrease inflammatory effusion and remove pannus. Surgery is used to correct deformity or mechanical deficiency in intermediate or late stages of the disease and includes arthrodesis, arthroplasty, or total joint replacement. Interestingly, total fasting induces a substantial reduction in joint pain, swelling, morning stiffness, and other symptoms in individuals with RA.

Ankylosing Spondylitis

Ankylosing spondylitis (AS) **(spondyloarthritis)** is a chronic, inflammatory joint disease characterized by stiffening and fusion (ankylosis) of the spine and sacroiliac joints. Although inflammation is the primary pathologic process in both RA and ankylosing spondylitis, the two diseases possibly differ in the primary site of inflammation and the end result. In RA the primary site of inflammation is the synovial membrane, resulting in the destruction and instability of synovial joints. In ankylosing spondylitis, the primary pathologic site has classically been proposed as the **enthesis** (the point at which ligaments, tendons, and the joint capsule are inserted into bone) and the end results are fibrosis, ossification, and fusion of the joint, primarily the sacroiliac joints and the vertebral column.[60] Recent data from MRI studies, however, show that synovitis and bone marrow inflammation, rather than enthesis, explain the alteration of AS in the sacroiliac joints.[61,62]

The prevalence of ankylosing spondylitis in the United States is approximately 0.5% to 1% among whites, 3% to 4% among blacks, and 18% to 50% in various nations of American Indians. Worldwide, the disease appears to be most prevalent in whites. The prevalence of ankylosing spondylitis in males is at least 10 times greater than previously considered. It affects men three times as often as women. In women, ankylosing spondylitis may affect the peripheral joints of the appendicular skeleton rather than the axial skeleton, progress less rapidly, and cause less dramatic spinal changes. Many individuals with ankylosing spondylitis remain undiagnosed.

Primary ankylosing spondylitis usually develops in late adolescence or young adulthood, with peak incidence at about 20 years of age. Secondary ankylosing spondylitis affects older age groups and is often associated with other inflammatory diseases (e.g., psoriatic arthropathy, inflammatory bowel disease, Reiter syndrome).

The cause of ankylosing spondylitis is unknown, but the disease is strongly associated with the presence of histocompatibility antigen HLA-B27 on the chromosomes of affected individuals, suggesting a genetic predisposition to the disease. Not all HLA-B27 subtypes, however, are associated with AS. *Klebsiella,* or chlamydia-delivered peptides, or other "triggers" may perpetuate the inflammatory response.[63]

PATHOPHYSIOLOGY   Ankylosing spondylitis has a strong association with HLA-B27. Several hypotheses have been proposed to explain this association including the arthritogenic peptide theory that proposes that certain B-27 alleles bind certain arthritogenic peptides because of their specific anchoring proteins.[64] Cartilage antigens are proposed as the targets for the immune response and the presentation of such antigens to CD8+ T cells.[65] In the early phases of AS, T cells and macrophages invade and cause erosion of the cartilage at different sites.[66] Based on these observations, it has recently been proposed that the cartilage is the primary target for the immune response.[64] **Aggrecan,** a proteoglycan, forms a major part of the extracellular matrix of cartilage and helps to maintain its stability. A specific CD4+ T cell response to proteins derived from aggrecan has been found in both animal and humans. Although these T cells have been found in AS, their role as a causative agent in AS remains unclear and necessitates future study.

Ankylosing spondylitis involves inflammation of fibrocartilage in cartilaginous joints, primarily in the vertebrae. The fibrous tissue of the joint capsule, the cartilage that surrounds intervertebral disks, the entheses, and periosteum are infiltrated by inflammatory cells. As inflammatory cells (chiefly macrophages) and lymphocytes infiltrate and erode bone and fibrocartilage in joint structures, repair begins. Repair of cartilaginous structures begins with the proliferation of fibroblasts. Fibroblasts synthesize and secrete collagen. The collagen becomes organized into fibrous scar tissue that eventually undergoes calcification and ossification. With time, all the cartilaginous structures of the joint are replaced by ossified scar tissue, causing the joint to fuse, or lose flexibility.

Repair of eroded bone begins with osteoblast activation and proliferation. Osteoblasts lay down new bone (callus), which is remodeled and replaced by compact, lamellar bone. Bone repair changes the contour of the bone's surface because the new bone grows outward to form a new enthesis with the end of the eroded ligament. The new enthesis, which forms on top of the old one, is called a **syndesmophyte.** As calcification of the spinal ligaments progresses, the vertebral bodies lose their concave anterior contour and appear square. On radiographs the spine assumes the classic "bamboo spine" appearance of ankylosing spondylitis.

CLINICAL MANIFESTATIONS   The most common signs and symptoms of early ankylosing spondylitis are low back

pain and stiffness. Typically, the individual with primary disease develops low back pain during the early twenties. The pain is at first insidious but progressively becomes persistent. It is often worse after prolonged rest and is alleviated by physical activity. Early morning stiffness usually accompanies the low back pain, and the individual typically has difficulty sitting up or twisting the spine. Forward flexion, rotation, and lateral flexion of the spine are restricted and painful. Early pain and resultant loss of motion are caused by the underlying inflammation and reflex muscle spasm rather than by soft tissue or bony fusion.

As the disease progresses, the normal convex curve of the lower spine (lumbar lordosis) diminishes and concavity of the upper spine (kyphosis) increases. The individual becomes increasingly stooped. The thoracic spine becomes rounded, the head and neck are held forward on the shoulders, and the hips are flexed (Figure 42-30).

Inflammation in the tendon insertions of the many costosternal and costovertebral muscles can cause pleuritic chest pain and restricted chest movement. The pain is usually worse on inspiration. Movement in the diaphragm is normal and full. Pressure on the anterior chest wall over the sternum, ribs, and costal cartilages may cause tenderness. Tenderness over the pelvic brim may cause discomfort at night and interfere with sleep because turning onto the iliac crests causes pain. Tenderness over the ischial tuberosities may make sitting on hard seats unbearable. Tenderness in the heels may contribute to a limp or the cautious placement of the feet during walking.

Along with low back pain, many individuals have peripheral joint involvement, uveitis, fibrotic changes in the lungs, cardiomegaly, aortic incompetence, amyloidosis, and Achilles tendinitis. Symptoms may include fatigue, weight loss, low-

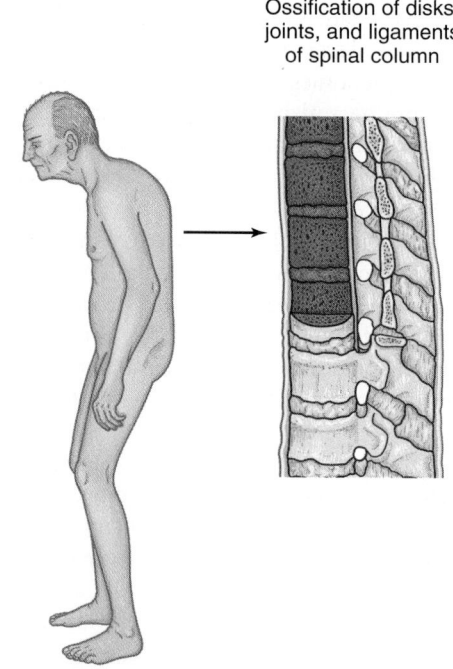

Ossification of disks, joints, and ligaments of spinal column

Figure 42-30 Ankylosing spondylitis. Characteristic posture and primary pathologic sites of inflammation and resulting damage.

grade fever, hypochromic anemia, and an increased erythrocyte sedimentation rate.[60]

EVALUATION AND TREATMENT   Diagnosis of ankylosing spondylitis is made from the history and physical examination, roentgenograms, MRI, and serum analysis for the presence of the histocompatibility antigen HLA-B27. Erythrocyte sedimentation rate is elevated throughout the disease to 10 to 15 mm/hr in males and 10 to 15 mm/hr in females (normal is 0 to 9 mm/hr in males and 0 to 2 mm/hr in females). Alkaline phosphatase levels often are elevated. Treatment of individuals with ankylosing spondylitis consists of physical therapy to maintain skeletal mobility and prevent the natural progression of contractures. Prevention of deformity and maintenance of mobility require a continuous program of physical therapy. Exercises are performed several times each day to maintain chest expansion, full extension of the spine, and complete range of motion in the proximal joints. The long term morbidity of AS has been previously underestimated.[67]

Nonsteroidal antiinflammatory drugs (NSAIDs) will often provide relief of symptoms within 48 hours. Analgesic medications are prescribed to suppress some of the pain and stiffness and to facilitate exercise. The medications do not prevent disease progression, but they do provide relief from symptoms (see What's New: Cox II Inhibitors and Side Effects). Disease-modifying antirheumatic drugs (DMARDs) such as gold, methotrexate, and sulfasalazine, have little or no effect in AS. Two drugs which do block the inflammatory effects (antagonists) of TNF, etanercept and infliximab, are now licensed for use by those with severe AS. The effect of anti-TNF therapy has been associated with lymphoma; however, it is unknown whether this association reflects a selection bias whereby individuals with the highest risk of lymphoma preferentially receive anti-TNF therapy or whether anti-TNF therapy actually increases the incidence of lymphoma.[68]

A combination of antibiotics also may be more effective that a single antibiotic. Potential therapeutic targets include IL-1, IL-12, B cells, accessory molecules on T cells, and angiogenic factors.[67] Surgical procedures, such as osteotomy, total hip replacement, and cervical spinal fusion, and radiation therapy are sometimes used to provide relief for individuals with end-stage disease or intolerable deformity. Persons should stop smoking to lessen pulmonary problems.

Gout

Gout is a syndrome caused by an inflammatory response to uric acid production or excretion resulting in high levels of uric acid in the blood (hyperuricemia) and in other body fluids, including synovial fluid. Although hyperuricemia is essential for the development of gout, it is not the only factor. Other factors include age (rare before 20 to 30 years), genetic predisposition (X-linked alteration of enzyme hypoxanthine guanine phosphoribosyl transferase [HGPRT]), excessive alcohol consumption, obesity, certain drugs (especially thiazides), and lead toxicity. When the uric acid reaches a certain concentration in fluids, it crystallizes, forming insoluble precipitates that are deposited in connective tissues throughout the body. Crystallization in synovial fluid causes acute, painful inflammation of the joint, a condition known as **gouty arthritis.** With time, crystal deposition in subcutaneous tissues causes the formation of small, white nodules, or **tophi,** that are visible through the skin. Crystal aggregates deposited in the kidneys can form urate renal stones and lead to renal failure.

In classic gouty arthritis, monosodium urate crystals form and cause joint inflammation. **Pseudogout** is caused by the formation of calcium pyrophosphate dihydrate (CPPD) crystals. The effect of either crystal is the same—the onset of a cytokine-mediated acute inflammatory response (see Chapter 6).

Gout is rare in children and premenopausal women and is uncommon in males younger than 30 years. The peak age of onset in males is between 40 and 50 years, whereas it is somewhat later in females. The risk of developing gouty arthritis is similar in males and females for a particular urate concentration. The plasma urate concentration is an important determinant of the risk of developing gout (Table 42-7).

Uric acid is a weak acid that is ionized at normal body pH and thus occurs in the blood or tissues in the form of urate ion. When ionized, uric acid can form salts with various cations, but 98% of extracellular uric acid is in the form of monosodium urate (uric acid salt). At any time the proportion of uric acid or urate is pH dependent, so the ratio of these two forms varies considerably in urine (Figure 42-31).

The solubility of urate and uric acid is critical to the development of crystals. Urate is more soluble in plasma, synovial fluid, and urine than in aqueous solutions. The solubility of uric acid in urine rises dramatically as the pH increases above 4. There is little change, however, in the solubility of urate within the normal pH range that exists in the plasma, synovial fluid, and other tissues. Decreasing temperatures cause both urate and uric acid solubility to fall. The pathways of production of uric acid are shown in Figure 42-32.

PATHOPHYSIOLOGY   The pathophysiology of gout is closely linked to purine metabolism (or cellular metabolism of purines) and kidney function. At the cellular level, purines are synthesized to purine nucleotides, which are used in the synthesis of nucleic acids, adenosine triphosphate, cyclic adenosine monophosphate (cAMP), and cyclic guanosine monophosphate (GMP). Uric acid is a breakdown product of

Table 42-7	Mean Urate Concentrations by Age and Gender
Characteristic	**Mean Urate Levels**
Prepuberty	3.5 mg/dl
Males (at puberty)	Steep rise to 5.2 mg/dl
Females (puberty to premenopause)	Slow rise to ≈ 4.0 mg/dl
Females (after menopause)	4.7 mg/dl
Hyperuricemia	
Males	7.0 mg/dl
Females	6.0 mg/dl

purine nucleotides (uric acid synthesis and elimination are illustrated in Figure 42-33). Some individuals with gout have an accelerated rate of purine synthesis accompanied by an overproduction of uric acid. Other individuals break down purine nucleotides at an accelerated rate that also results in an overproduction of uric acid. Production of uric acid can be

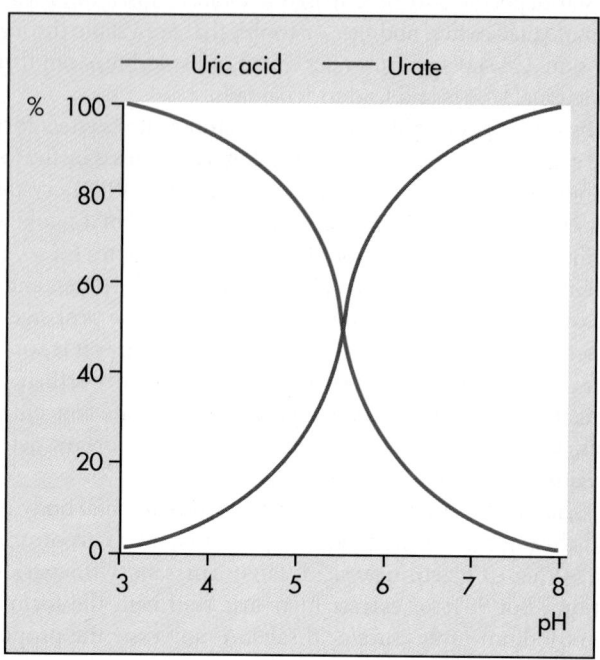

Figure 42-31 **Effect of pH on uric acid and urate equilibrium.** At pH 5.7, equal amounts of uric acid and urate are present in the solution. (Redrawn from Klippel JH, Dieppe PA, editors: *Rheumatology,* ed 2, London, 1998, Mosby.)

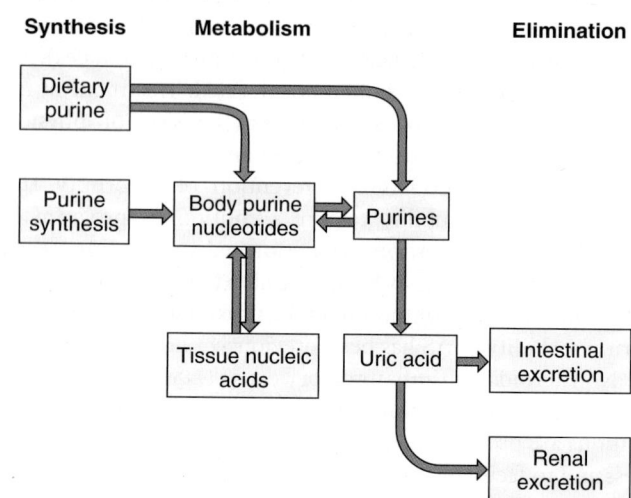

Figure 42-33 **Uric acid synthesis and elimination.** Uric acid is derived from purines ingested or synthesized from ingested foods, as well as being recycled following cell breakdown. Uric acid is then eliminated through the kidneys and gastrointestinal tract. (Redrawn from Klippel JH, Dieppe PA, editors: *Rheumatology,* ed 2, London, 1998, Mosby.)

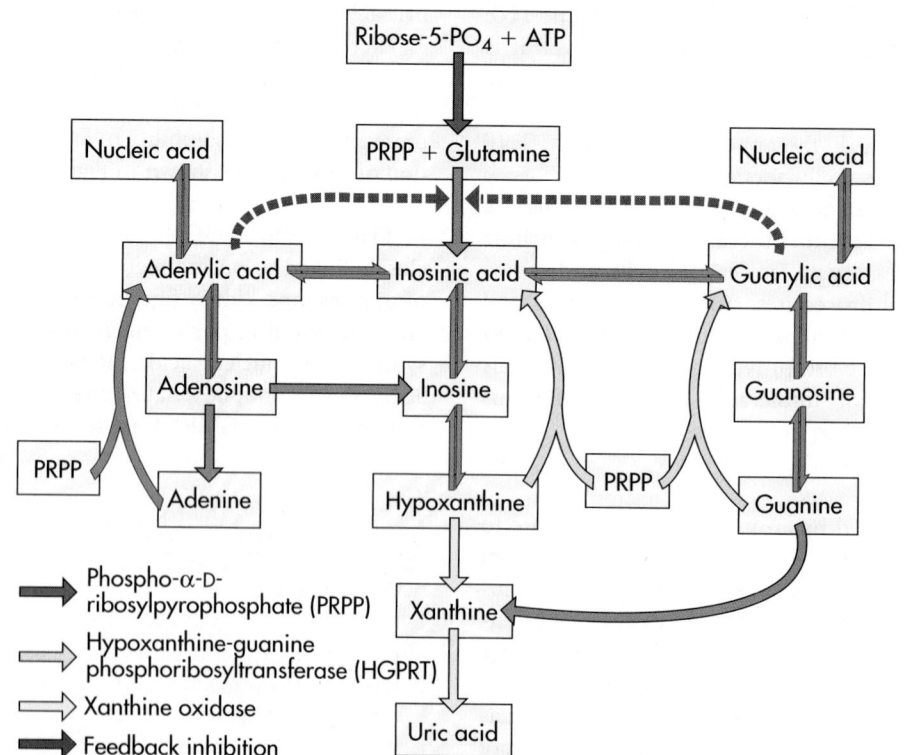

Figure 42-32 **Production of uric acid.** The major pathways involved in purine nucleotide synthesis. (Redrawn from Klippel JH, Dieppe PA, editors: *Rheumatology,* ed 2, London, 1998, Mosby.)

the result of an increased turnover of nucleic acids, which is associated with an increased turnover of cells at other body sites. The increased turnover of nucleic acids leads to increased levels of uric acid with a compensatory increase in purine synthesis. A deficiency of the enzyme HGPRT (see above) can lead to an increased production of uric acid. A complete absence of HGPRT is uncommon but can occur in the X-linked Lesch-Nyhan syndrome, with males at risk for hyperuricemia, neurologic alterations, and sometimes gouty arthritis.[69] The majority of individuals with gout, however, have an unknown metabolic defect, which is referred to as **primary gout.** When the etiology is known, it is referred to as **secondary gout.**

Most uric acid is eliminated from the body through the kidneys. Urate is filtered at the glomerulus and undergoes both reabsorption and excretion within the renal tubules. In primary gout, urate excretion by the kidneys is sluggish. The sluggish excretion may be the result of a decrease in glomerular filtration of urate or an acceleration in urate reabsorption. In addition, monosodium urate crystals are deposited in renal interstitial tissues, causing impaired urine flow. (Kidney function is described in Chapter 35.)

The exact process by which crystals of monosodium urate are deposited in joints and induce gouty arthritis is unknown. However, several mechanisms may be involved, including the following:

1. Monosodium urate precipitates at the periphery of the body, where lower body temperatures may reduce the solubility of monosodium urate
2. Decreased albumin or glycosaminoglycan levels, which cause decreased urate solubility
3. Changes in ion concentration and decreases of pH that enhance urate deposition
4. Trauma that promotes urate crystal precipitation

The monosodium urate crystals may form in the synovial fluid or in the synovial membrane, cartilage, or other connective tissues in joints and elsewhere, such as in the heart, earlobes, and kidneys. Evidence suggests that an acute attack of gout is the result of the *formation* of crystals rather than the *releasing* of the crystals from connective tissues into the synovial fluid.

Monosodium urate crystals can stimulate and perpetuate the inflammatory response (Figure 42-34). The presence of the crystals triggers the acute inflammatory response, during which neutrophils and macrophages are attracted out of the circulation and begin to phagocytize (ingest) the crystals.

Crystals coated with IgG are thought to react with crystallizable fragment (Fc) receptors on the surface of the responding cell (see Figure 42-34), thereby promoting phagocytosis with the formation of a phagolysosome. When the phagolysosomal enzymes strip the IgG from the surface of the crystal, the hydrogen bands on the surface of the crystal can induce membrane breakdown of the phagolysosome and cause rupture of the cell within. Recent evidence indicates that apolipoprotein-E coating of urate crystals will inhibit phagocytosis and the cellular response (see Figure 42-34, A).

A variety of inflammatory mediators are released during the crystal/cell response, including chemotactic factors, lysosomal enzymes, eicosanoids, prostaglandin E (PGE_2), interleukins (IL-1 and IL-6), reactive oxygen species, and collagenase (see Figure 42-34, B). Some of these mediators stimulate the influx of neutrophils, monocytes, and lymphocytes. (Acute inflammation and phagocytosis are described in Chapter 6.)

Within the joint fluid, urate crystals react particularly with neutrophils and monocytes. Tissue damage begins to occur, principally when the neutrophils release the contents of their phagolysosomes. These contents also perpetuate inflammation. At an early phase of an acute gouty attack, synovial microtophi have been demonstrated. As the process continues, numerous microtophi may be present on the synovial membrane (see Figure 42-34, C).

CLINICAL MANIFESTATIONS Gout is manifested by (1) an increase in serum urate concentration (hyperuricemia), (2) recurrent attacks of monoarticular arthritis (inflammation of a single joint), (3) deposits of monosodium urate monohydrate (tophi) in and around the joints, (4) renal disease involving glomerular, tubular, and interstitial tissues and blood vessels, and (5) the formation of renal stones. These manifestations appear in three clinical stages:

1. **Asymptomatic hyperuricemia:** the serum urate level is elevated but arthritic symptoms, tophi, and renal stones are not present; may persist throughout life.
2. **Acute gouty arthritis:** attacks develop with increased serum urate concentrations; tends to occur with sudden or sustained increases of hyperuricemia but also can be triggered by trauma, drugs, and alcohol.
3. **Tophaceous gout:** the third and chronic stage of disease; can begin as early as 3 years or as late as 40 years after the initial attack of gouty arthritis. Progressive inability to excrete uric acid expands the urate pool until urate crystal deposits (tophi) appear in cartilage, synovial membranes, tendons, and soft tissue.

Trauma is the most common aggravating factor. The great toe is subject to chronic strain in walking, and subsequently an acute gout attack may follow long walks. Trauma associated with occupations, such as truck driving, also may precipitate an attack.

Attacks of gouty arthritis occur abruptly, usually in a peripheral joint. The primary symptom is severe pain. Approximately 50% of the initial attacks occur in the metatarsophalangeal joint of the great toe. The other 50% involve the heel, ankle, instep of the foot, knee, wrist, or elbow. The pain is usually noticed at night. Within a few hours the affected joint becomes hot, red, and extremely tender and may be slightly swollen. Lymphangitis and systemic signs of inflammation (leukocytosis, fever, elevated sedimentation rate) are occasionally present. Untreated, mild attacks usually subside in

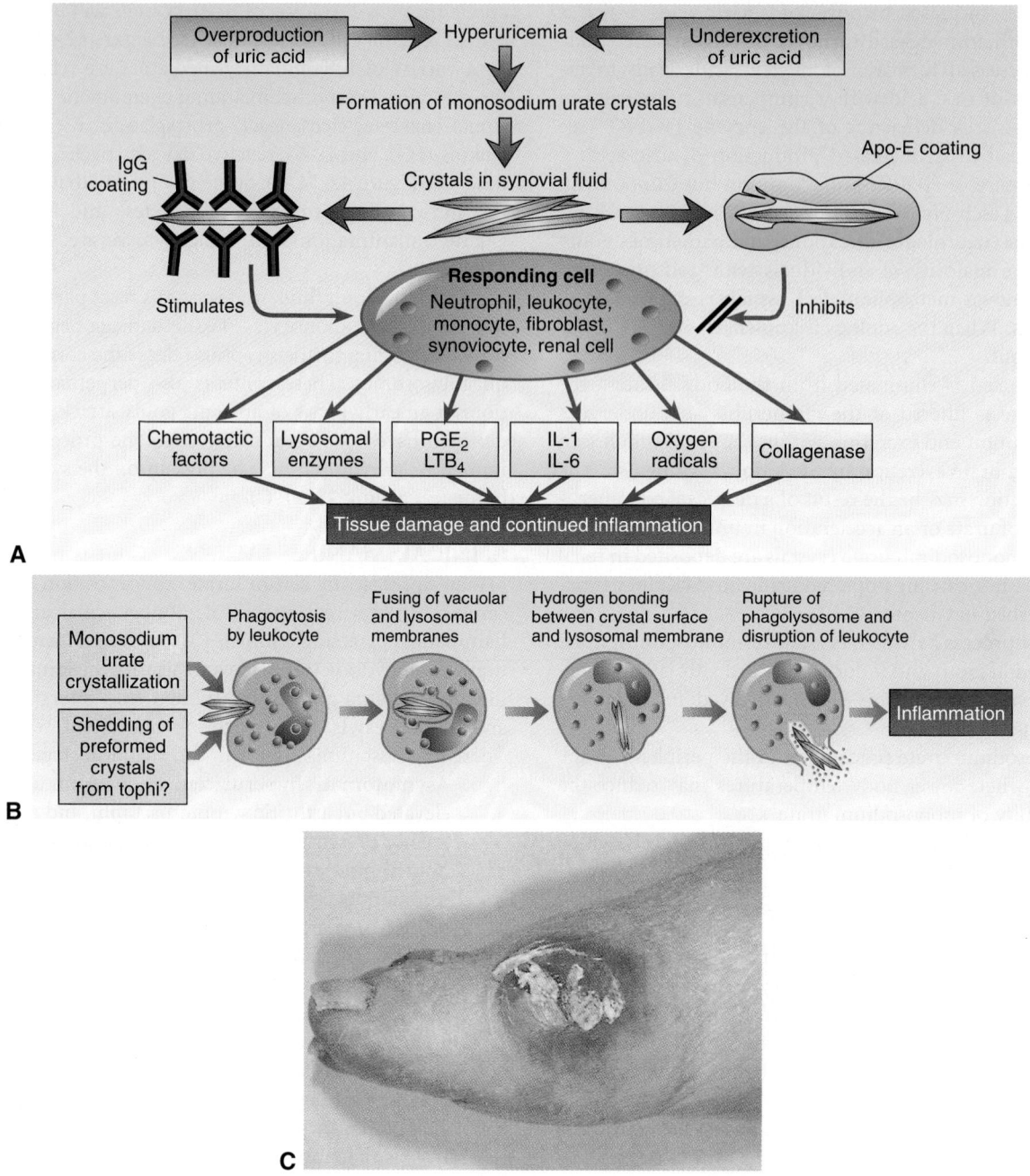

Figure 42-34 Pathogenesis of acute gouty arthritis. **A,** Depending on the urate crystal coating, a variety of cells may be stimulated to produce a wide range of inflammatory mediators. **B,** Sequence of events in the production of inflammation response to urate crystals. **C,** Gouty tophus on right foot. (**C,** From Dieppe P et al: *Arthritis and rheumatism in practice,* London, 1991, Gower.)

several hours but may persist for 1 or 2 days. Severe attacks may persist for several days or weeks. When the patient recovers, the symptoms resolve completely. Intervals between acute attacks of gouty arthritis are called *intercritical periods.* Some individuals never have a second attack; others experience subsequent attacks within days to as long as 5 to 10 years after the first.

The helix of the ear is the most common site of tophi, which are the characteristic diagnostic lesions of chronic gout. Each tophus consists of a deposit of urate crystals, sur-

rounded by a granuloma made up of mononuclear phagocytes (macrophages) that have developed into epithelial and giant cells. (Granuloma formation is described in and illustrated in Chapter 6.)

Tophaceous deposits produce irregular swellings of the fingers, hands, knees, and feet. Tophi commonly form lumps along the ulnar surface of the forearm, the tibial surface of the leg, the Achilles tendon, and the olecranon bursa. Tophi may produce marked limitation of joint movement and eventually cause grotesque deformities of the hands and feet. Although the tophi themselves are painless, they often cause progressive stiffness and persistent aching of the affected joint. Tophi in the upper extremities may cause nerve compressions such as carpal tunnel syndrome. Tophi in the lower extremities may cause tarsal tunnel syndrome. They also may erode and drain through the skin.

Renal stones are 1000 times more prevalent in individuals with primary gout than in the general population. The stones can be the size of a grain of sand or a piece of gravel, or they can accumulate in massive deposits called *staghorn calculi.* They range in color from pale yellow to brown to reddish black, depending on their composition. Some stones consist of pure monosodium urate; others consist of calcium oxalate or calcium phosphate. Renal stones can form in the collecting tubules, pelvis, or ureters, causing obstruction, dilation, and atrophy of the more proximal tubules and leading eventually to acute renal failure. Stones deposited directly in renal interstitial tissue initiate an inflammatory reaction that leads to chronic renal disease and progressive renal failure.

TREATMENT   The aims of gout treatment are to terminate the acute gouty attack as promptly as possible, prevent recurring attacks, prevent or reverse complications associated with urate deposits in the joints and kidneys, and prevent formation of kidney stones. Acute gouty arthritis is treated with antiinflammatory drugs. The drugs of choice are nonsteroidal antiinflammatory agents (NSAIDs) and allopurinol. Colchicine is used in individuals unable to tolerate NSAIDs. Hydrocortisone may be injected into the joint to relieve pain. Drugs that block TNF-α are controversial and costly (i.e., etanercept).[70] Ice also may relieve some of the inflammation of the joint. Weight bearing on the involved joint is avoided until the acute attack subsides. The individual is put on a low-purine diet, with high fluid intake to increase urinary output. Antihyperuricemic drugs are given to reduce serum urate concentrations.

DISORDERS OF SKELETAL MUSCLE

Muscle weakness and fatigue are common symptoms. In many cases, neural, traumatic, and psychogenic causes provide an adequate explanation for the failure to generate force (weakness) or sustain force (fatigue) seen in myopathies. The pathophysiologic mechanisms in some of the metabolic and inflammatory muscle diseases have been explored, but the cause of many of the myopathies remains obscure. The complex interaction between muscles and nerves affects muscular function as well. Only inherited and acquired disorders of skeletal muscles are discussed here.

Secondary Muscular Dysfunction

Muscular symptoms arise from a variety of causes unrelated to the muscle itself. Secondary muscular phenomena (contracture, stress-related muscle tension, immobility) are common disorders that influence muscular function.

Contractures

Contractures can be pathologic or physiologic. A physiologic muscle contracture occurs in the absence of a muscle action potential in the sarcolemma. Muscle shortening is explained on the basis of failure of the calcium pump in the presence of adenosine triphosphate (ATP). A physiologic contracture is seen in McArdle disease (muscle myophosphorylase deficiency) and malignant hyperthermia. The contracture is usually temporary if the underlying pathology is reversed.

A pathologic contracture is a permanent muscle shortening caused by muscle spasm or weakness. Heel cord (Achilles tendon) contractures are examples of pathologic contractures. They are associated with plentiful ATP and occur in spite of a normal action potential. The most common form of contracture is seen in such conditions as muscular dystrophy (see Chapter 43) and central nervous system (CNS) injury. Contractures also may develop secondary to scar tissue contraction in the flexor tissues of a joint, for example, contracture of burned tissues in the antecubital area of the forearm leading to a flexion contracture.

Stress-Induced Muscle Tension

Abnormally increased muscle tension has been associated with chronic anxiety, as well as a variety of stress-related muscular symptoms, including neck stiffness, back pain, and headache.[71,72] Abnormalities in the CNS, reticular activating system, and autonomic nervous system (ANS) have been implicated. For example, as an individual progressively relaxes, the amplitude of the knee-jerk reflex diminishes. Conversely, individuals with absent reflexes increase tension by such maneuvers as clenching the teeth or hand grip. The underlying pathophysiology may be related to the fact that as a muscle contracts, the muscle spindle is activated. This gamma-feedback system produces a series of impulses that are transmitted to the brain by the sensitive 1A afferent fibers. Unconscious tension is thought to increase the activity of the reticular activating system as well. This influences increasing firing of the efferent loop of the gamma fibers and produces further muscle contraction and increases muscle tension. ANS function that regulates increased blood flow to the muscle during sympathetic activity may be related to increased muscle contraction tension.

Various forms of treatment have been used to reduce the muscle tension associated with stress. Progressive relaxation training, yoga, meditation, and biofeedback are examples of stress reduction therapies. **Biofeedback** uses an integrated electromyogram (EMG) to make recordings from the skin surface. The goal is to teach the individual to control tension that has been functioning maladaptively. It is particularly useful in individuals who have a connection between skeletal muscle tension and pain.[73] **Progressive relaxation training** emphasizes the individual's ability to perceive the difference between tension and relaxation. This technique involves sequential tensing and a relaxing environment. The individual is taught to practice this routine daily, often with the use of audiotaped instructions. By teaching the individual to recognize excessive contraction of skeletal muscle, one hopes to enhance the ability to relax specific muscle groups to relieve tension and thus reduce CNS arousal, as well as ANS arousal.

Fibromyalgia

Fibromyalgia is a chronic musculoskeletal syndrome characterized by widespread joint and muscle pain, fatigue, and tender points. Increased sensitivity to touch (i.e., tender points), the absence of systemic or localized inflammation, and fatigue and sleep disturbances are common. Because the symptoms are vague, and the etiology unknown, fibromyalgia is primarily diagnosed by exclusion. A common misdiagnosis has been chronic fatigue syndrome. From 80% to 90% of individuals affected are women, and the peak age is 30 to 50 years. Although the incidence is unknown, the prevalence is reported to be 2% to almost 6% and increases with age.[74] The American College of Rheumatology classification criteria include diffuse soft tissue pain of at least 3 months duration and pain on palpation of at least 11 of 18 tender points (see Figure 42-35). It is more common than RA, but its cause is still unknown.

The etiology of fibromyalgia has been debated for more than a century. It is unlikely that it is caused by a single factor. The most common precipitating factors include the following:
- Flu-like viral illness
- Chronic fatigue syndrome
- Human immunodeficiency virus (HIV) infection
- Lyme disease
- Usually unspecified
- Physical trauma
- Emotional trauma
- Medications, especially steroid withdrawal

Certain rheumatic diseases, such as RA or systemic lupus erythematosus, may coexist if not initially manifest with fibromyalgia. In addition, fibromyalgia may overlap with myofascial pain syndromes[75] (Table 42-8).

PATHOPHYSIOLOGY   Fibromyalgia as a chronic pain syndrome is defined by subjective symptoms and not unique pathophysiologic characteristics. Individuals with fibromyalgia have lowered mechanical and thermal pain thresholds, high pain ratings for provoking stimuli, and altered temporal

Table 42-8	Comparison of Fibromyalgia and Myofascial Pain Syndromes	
Variable	Fibromyalgia	Myofascial Pain
Location	Generalized	Regional
Examination	Tender points	Trigger points
Response to local therapy	Not sustained	Curative
Gender	Female/male ratio: 10:1	Equal or unknown
Systemic features	Characteristic	Unknown

summation of pain stimuli.[76-78] These data provide some evidence of altered pain processing. Aggregation of fibromyalgia within families and other co-existing conditions such as irritable bowel syndrome, chronic fatigue, and mood disorders suggest a major role for neuroendocrine and stress-response alterations (see Chapter 10). Altered circadian activity of several neuroendocrine axes and autonomic nervous system dysfunction have been reported.[79] Corticotrophin-releasing hormone (CRH) locus ceruleus—norepinephrine (LC/NE), their peripheral effectors as well as the hypothalamus-pituitary-adrenal axis (HPA) are the main components of the stress system. Low HPA axis and LC/NE may be associated with fibromyalgia[80] (also see Chapter 10).

CLINICAL MANIFESTATIONS   The prominent symptom of fibromyalgia is diffuse, chronic pain. The locations of nine pairs of tender points for diagnostic classification of fibromyalgia are shown in Figure 42-35. The pain often begins in one location, especially the neck and shoulders, but then becomes more generalized. People describe the pain as *burning* or *gnawing*. Fatigue is profound. The effect on everyday life is considerable.[81] Some investigators have found that the majority of women experienced pain and fatigue for more than 90% of their time awake.[81] Fatigue is most notable when arising from sleep and during the midafternoon. Headaches, symptoms of irritable bowel syndrome, and excess sensitivity to cold (Raynaud-like) are reported in 50% of individuals.

Almost 25% of individuals seek psychologic support for depression. Anxiety, particularly in regard to their diagnosis and future, is almost universal.[82] Again, the only reliable finding on examination is the presence of multiple tender points.

EVALUATION AND TREATMENT   Because the manifestations of chronic, generalized pain and fatigue are present in many musculoskeletal (e.g., rheumatic) disorders, these disorders should be considered in the diagnosis of fibromyalgia (Tables 42-9 and 42-10).

No one regimen of medication has proved successful for fibromyalgia. Medications that improve sleep may be helpful. Antiinflammatory medications have been used despite the fact there is no evidence of tissue inflammation. These medications have not been effective. Certain CNS-active medications, most notably tricyclics, amitriptyline, and cyclobenzaprine, were significantly better than placebos in controlled trials. Amitriptyline significantly improved pain, morning stiffness, and sleep but not tender points. However, these successes occurred in only 25% to 45% of individuals. Treatment consists of a combination of patient education, medication, exercise, and cognitive therapy.[83] Box 42-3 illustrates some of these modalities.

Disuse Atrophy

The term **disuse atrophy** describes the pathologic reduction in normal size of muscle fibers after prolonged inactivity from bed rest, trauma (casting), or local nerve damage. The effects of muscular deconditioning associated with lack of

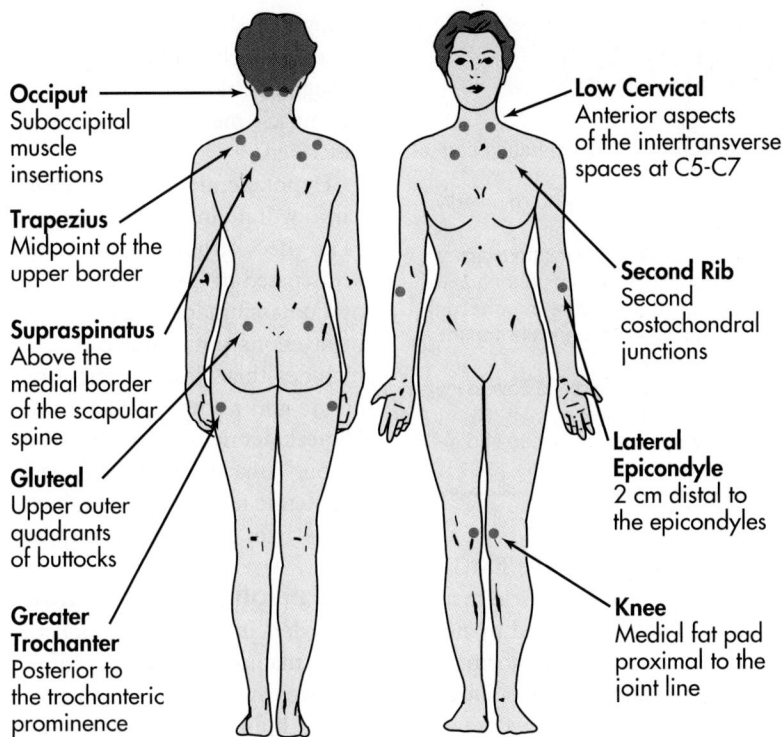

Occiput
Suboccipital
muscle
insertions

Trapezius
Midpoint of the
upper border

Supraspinatus
Above the
medial border
of the scapular
spine

Gluteal
Upper outer
quadrants
of buttocks

**Greater
Trochanter**
Posterior to
the trochanteric
prominence

Low Cervical
Anterior aspects
of the intertransverse
spaces at C5-C7

Second Rib
Second
costochondral
junctions

**Lateral
Epicondyle**
2 cm distal to
the epicondyles

Knee
Medial fat pad
proximal to the
joint line

Figure 42-35 Location of specific tender points for diagnostic classification of fibromyalgia. (Redrawn from Freundlich B, Leventhal L: The fibromyalgia syndrome. In Schumacher HR Jr, Klippel JH, Koopman WJ, editors: *Primer on the rheumatic diseases*, ed 11, Atlanta, 1997, Arthritis Foundation. Copyright 1997. Reprinted with permission of the Arthritis Foundation, 1330 W. Peachtree St., Atlanta, GA 30309.)

Table 42-9	Differential Diagnosis of Fibromyalgia
Differential Diagnosis	**Helpful Differential Features**
Rheumatoid arthritis*	Synovitis, serologic tests, elevated erythrocyte sedimentation rate (ESR)
Systemic lupus erythematosus*	Dermatitis, serositis (renal, central nervous system, etc.)
Polymyalgia rheumatica*	Elevated ESR, elderly persons, response to corticosteroids
Myositis	Increased muscle enzymes, weakness more than pain
Hypothyroidism*	Abnormal thyroid function tests
Neuropathies	Clinical and electrophysiologic evidence of neuropathy

Data from Klippel JH, Dieppe PA, editors: *Rheumatology*, ed 2, London, 1998, Mosby.
*Fibromyalgia may also more commonly coexist with these conditions.

Table 42-10	Concomitant Conditions With Fibromyalgia
Concomitant Condition	**Relationship to Fibromyalgia**
Depression	Present in 25%-60% of fibromyalgia cases
Irritable bowel	Present in 50%-80% of fibromyalgia cases
Migraine	Present in 50% of fibromyalgia cases
Chronic fatigue syndrome (CFS)	70% of CFS cases meet criteria for fibromyalgia
Myofascial pain	May be a localized form of fibromyalgia

Data from Klippel JH, Dieppe PA, editors: *Rheumatology*, ed 2, London, 1998, Mosby.

physical activity may be apparent in a matter of days. The normal individual on bed rest loses muscle strength from baseline levels at a rate of 3% per day. Bed rest also is associated with cardiovascular, skeletal, and other organ system changes.

Measures to prevent atrophy include frequent forceful isometric muscle contractions and passive lengthening exercises. If reuse is not restored within 1 year, regeneration of muscle fibers becomes impaired.

Muscle Membrane Abnormalities

Two defects of the muscle membrane (plasma membrane of the muscle fiber) have been linked to clinical syndromes: the hyperexcitable membrane seen in the myotonic disorders and the intermittently unresponsive membrane seen in the periodic paralyses. Although these are infrequent disorders, research into the pathologic processes has led to an improved understanding of the cell membrane.

Myotonia

Myotonia is a delayed relaxation after such voluntary muscle contractions as grip, eye closure, or muscle percussion. The distinctive "dive-bomber" noise, audible on needle EMG, is caused by the prolonged depolarization of the muscle membrane. Because the depolarization is not terminated by neuromuscular blocking agents, such as curare, the abnormality has been localized at the muscle membrane; the basic defect is due to ion channel dysfunction.[84] (These structures are described in Chapter 41.)

Myotonia can be reproduced by removing extracellular chloride, thus reducing chloride conductance across the plasma membrane. The delicate balance in which sodium diffuses into the intracellular fluid, potassium diffuses out of the intracellular fluid, and chloride is in flux is thus interrupted. Because the normal diffusion processes (described in Chapter 3) stabilize the membrane, the shift in chloride ions is thought to increase membrane excitability. The chloride abnormality may explain the resting membrane hyperexcitability, but it does not explain the delayed relaxation present in myotonia and has not been detected in human myotonia.

Myotonia is seen in several disorders: myotonia congenita, paramyotonia congenita, myotonic muscular dystrophy, and some forms of periodic paralysis. Most are inherited disorders and are mild in symptomatology, with the exception of myotonic muscular dystrophy (see p. 1562). Myotonia is treated by drugs that reduce muscle fiber excitability, such as procaine, procainamide, phenytoin, and quinine preparations. Recent treatments include acetazolamide, a carbonic anhydrase inhibitor, and verapamil, a calcium channel blocker.

Periodic Paralysis

During an attack of **periodic paralysis,** the muscle membrane is unresponsive to neural stimuli and the resting membrane potential is reduced from −90 to −45 mV. Periodic paralysis is triggered by exercise and any process or medication that increases serum potassium. The disorder is often inherited in an autosomal dominant pattern, although it can be seen in hyperthyroidism.

The paralysis, which leaves the individual flaccid and weak, does not affect the respiratory muscles. Many individuals have myotonia present on examination. In most cases the weakness is accompanied by a change in serum potassium, al-

though in some individuals the change may be negligible. Cardiac dysrhythmias have been present during attacks. Although the biochemical defect remains unknown, changes in the muscle membrane and sarcoplasmic reticulum have been described.

Hypokalemic periodic paralysis is triggered by high-carbohydrate meals, prolonged bed rest, or emotional stress. (The effect of potassium on the resting membrane potential is discussed in Chapter 3.) Glucose and insulin infusions and oral potassium loading are used as provocative tests; oral and intravenous potassium can relieve acute attacks. Treatment includes thiazides, diuretics, and a high-salt diet. Acetazolamide and a low-salt diet are useful for long-term therapy. **Hyperkalemic periodic paralysis** is caused by a genetic mutation. Attacks are usually less severe than with the hypokalemic form. Treatment includes small carbohydrate-rich meals, light exercise, and intravenous calcium gluconate.

Metabolic Muscle Diseases

Disorders in muscle metabolism can be caused by endocrine abnormalities or diseases of energy metabolism, such as glycogen storage disease, enzyme deficiencies, and abnormalities in lipid metabolism and mitochondrial function.

Endocrine Disorders

Often the systemic effects of hormonal imbalance overshadow the individual's muscular symptoms. For example, individuals with thyrotoxicosis may have signs of proximal weakness, paresis of the extraocular muscles (exophthalmic ophthalmoplegia), and rarely, hypokalemic periodic paralysis. Hypothyroidism is often associated with a decrease in muscle mass and strength, with weak, flabby skeletal muscles and sluggish movements.

Thyroid hormone is believed to regulate muscle protein synthesis and electrolyte balance. Changes in muscle protein synthesis and electrolyte balance may therefore explain the changes in muscle mass and contractility seen in endocrine disorders. The muscle symptoms subside with appropriate treatment of the primary hormonal disorder.

Diseases of Energy Metabolism

Muscle relies on carbohydrates, such as glycogen and lipids (free fatty acids), for energy. When stored glycogen or lipids cannot be used because of a lack of the enzyme necessary to convert energy for contraction, the individual experiences cramps, fatigue, and exercise intolerance. Disorders of muscle metabolism can be self-limiting, such as is seen in McArdle disease and some lipid disorders, or cause widespread irreparable muscle destruction, as in acid maltase deficiency.

McArdle Disease

McArdle disease, or myophosphorylase deficiency, was the first myopathy in which a single enzyme defect was identified (Figure 42-36). Although it is rare, more than 110 cases have been reported from one clinic alone. Individuals with McArdle disease lack muscle phosphorylase, which is responsible for the breakdown of glycogen in muscle. Normally, after the body uses the short-term ATP and phosphocreatine

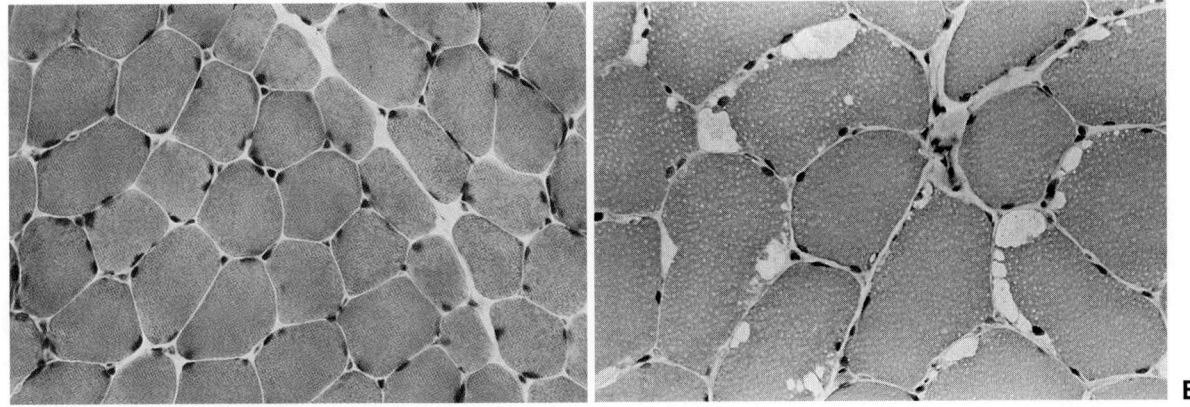

Figure 42-36 McArdle disease. **A,** Normal muscle fibers. **B,** McArdle disease. Note the *(white)* peripheral vacuoles. (From Damjanov I, Linder J, editors: *Anderson's pathology,* ed 10, St Louis, 1996, Mosby.)

stores, intramuscular lactic acid accumulates as glycogen is used (see Chapter 41). The individual with McArdle disease is not able to break down glycogen or produce lactic acid.

The altered energy production manifests itself in exercise intolerance, fatigue, and painful muscle cramps. When exercise is carried to an extreme, painful muscle contracture and myoglobinuria develop. Some individuals describe a "second wind" phenomenon, in which exercise tolerance increases if they slow their pace once the initial sensation of fatigue commences. This may be caused by the use of free fatty acids as a secondary source of energy. As the disease progresses, some individuals have pronounced muscle weakness and wasting. Other organs are not involved because the absence of phosphorylase is limited to muscle. Generally, individuals with McArdle disease learn to adapt their daily routine to avoid muscle symptoms. Usually the diagnosis of McArdle disease is made by the histochemical evaluation of myophosphorylase activity in frozen sections. There is no staining of myofibrils in affected individuals.

Acid Maltase Deficiency

Acid maltase deficiency is an uncommon glycogen storage disease associated with an accumulation of glycogen in the lysosomes of muscle cells and the cells of other tissues. The usual pathways of glycogen degradation are preserved. The absence of the enzyme acid maltase is responsible for the abnormality in glycogen metabolism, although the exact mechanism is unknown. It is an autosomal recessive disorder, with the gene located on the long arm of chromosome 17.

The infantile form is called **Pompe disease** and is recognized shortly after birth by hypotonia; dysreflexia; and an enlarged heart, tongue, and liver. Hypertrophy of these tissues is thought to be the result of glycogen deposition. Children die of cardiac or respiratory failure within 1 year of diagnosis. The adult variety becomes evident subacutely. The muscular symptoms resemble those of muscular dystrophy or polymyositis (see p. 1540). A distinguishing feature in adults may be the presence of severe respiratory muscle weakness.

Myoadenylate Deaminase Deficiency

An enzyme deficiency that produces changes in skeletal muscle and is associated with exercise intolerance is **myoad-**

enylate deaminase deficiency (MDD). Because these individuals lack myoadenylate deaminase, they have a poor capacity for sustained energy production. Myoadenylate deaminase is the catalytic enzyme that forms phosphocreatine and ATP during exercise through a metabolic pathway that binds the purine and phosphate molecules that constitute ATP. Persons with MDD differ from those with McArdle disease in that, during the ischemic exercise test, lactate production is normal when ATP and phosphocreatine are synthesized. The enzyme defect has been reported to be common, but in practice it may rarely be recognized as a cause of exercise intolerance.

Lipid Deficiencies

Disorders of lipid metabolism are uncommon but account for severe changes in muscle metabolism. The lipid content of muscle cells consists of the free fatty acids, which are oxidized in the mitochondria. These acids require carnitine and the enzyme carnitine palmityl transferase (CPT) to transport metabolic by-products and energy to the myofibrils. Individuals with CPT deficiency have mild muscular symptoms but can experience bouts of renal failure caused by myoglobinuria. Individuals with a deficiency of carnitine alone have progressive muscle weakness and can experience sudden exacerbations.

Measuring the CPT and carnitine content in muscle aids in the diagnosis. Cells in the muscle biopsy show vacuoles and lipid deposits. Treatments with riboflavin, medium-chain triglycerides, oral carnitine, and prednisone have been suggested.

Inflammatory Muscle Diseases: Myositis
Viral, Bacterial, and Parasitic Myositis

Viral, bacterial, and parasitic infections of varying severity are known to produce inflammatory changes in skeletal muscle, a group of conditions collectively described by the term **myositis.** In tuberculosis and sarcoidosis, chronic inflammatory changes and granulomas are found in muscle, as well as in other affected tissues. In trichinosis, *Trichinella* larvae reside in infected pork and, after ingestion, migrate to the intestinal mucosa and from there to the lymphatics. Symptoms include severe pain, rash, and muscle stiffness. Treatment includes administration of corticosteroids, prednisone, and the antiparasitic agent thiabendazole. Toxoplasmosis, a common parasitic infection, is also associated with a generalized polymyositis that responds rapidly to therapy.

In the tropics, more prevalent disorders include bacterial infections with *Staphylococcus aureus* and parasites such as cysticercus, the larva of the tapeworm *Taenia solium*. Viral infections can be associated with an acute myositis. Muscle pain, tenderness, signs of inflammation, and CK elevation are common manifestations of viral myositis. The self-limiting symptoms of muscle aches and pains during a bout of influenza may actually be a subacute form of viral myopathy.

Polymyositis and Dermatomyositis

Polymyositis (generalized muscle inflammation) and **dermatomyositis** (polymyositis accompanied by skin lesions) are the most common inflammatory muscle diseases requiring long-term care. Prevalence rates may be about 6 per 1,000,000 persons.

PATHOPHYSIOLOGY   Polymyositis and dermatomyositis are characterized by inflammation of connective tissue and muscle fibers that presumably causes the extensive necrosis and destruction of muscle fibers. The agent that causes the muscle inflammation has not been identified, but abnormalities in the immune system have been implicated (Figure 42-37). Both innate and adaptive immune responses are activated in these myopathies. Cytokines appear to play a key role in symptom manifestation.[85] This family of diseases is now designated as autoimmune because of the presence of autoantibodies in the serum of many individuals. Studies have shown that the inflammatory cells that surround the perimysial and perivascular sites are selectively enriched in B cells and helper T cells in those with dermatomyositis.[86] There is less vascular involvement in polymyositis, and most of the inflammatory cells, including B cells, T cells, and macrophages, surround the muscle fibers and fascicles.

CLINICAL MANIFESTATIONS   The acute symptoms include many of those seen in any inflammatory process: malaise, fever, muscle swelling, pain and tenderness, lethargy, and listlessness. In adults, weakness of the shoulder and pelvic girdle muscles is a primary manifestation of polymyositis.[87] Both illnesses are usually associated with a symmetric proximal muscle weakness and initially can be confused with other myopathies. A thorough evaluation is required to exclude other disorders. Clinical features common in both polymyositis and dermatomyositis are dysphagia, reduced esophageal motility, vasculitis, Raynaud phenomenon, cardiomyopathy, and interstitial pulmonary fibrosis. Some patients have other coexisting collagen vascular disorders, such as rheumatoid arthritis, systemic lupus erythematosus, and progressive systemic sclerosis (formerly called *scleroderma*).

The presence of skin rash, calcinosis, and eyelid edema most often suggests dermatomyositis (Figure 42-38). The skin rash is a purple (heliotrope) color and involves the eyelids, face, chest, and extensor surfaces of the extremities. Dermatomyositis is slightly more common in children and older adults, with an onset before age 15 years or after age 50 years. The adult with

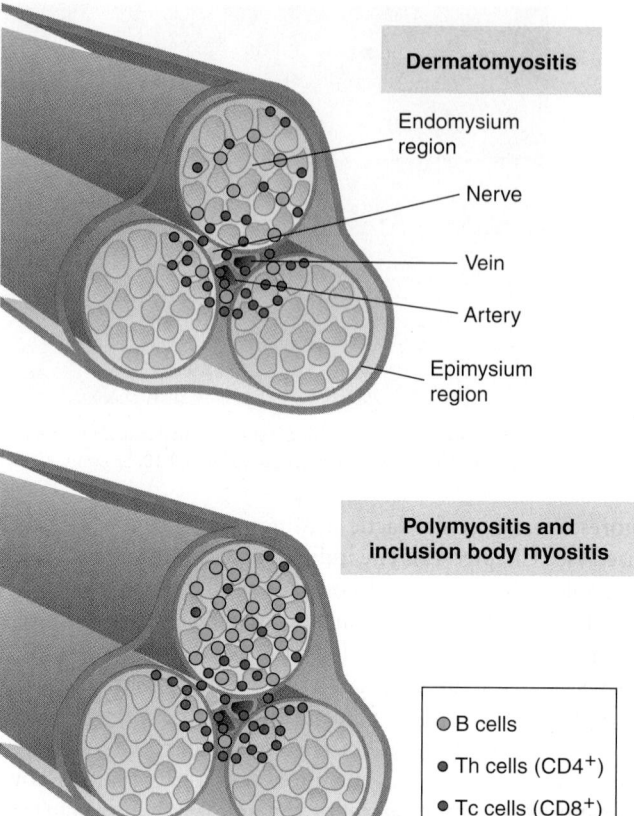

Figure 42-37 **Distribution of CD4 and CD8 lymphocytes in different clinical forms of myositis.** Dermatomyositis shows perivascular and CD4 T cells. Polymyositis shows mostly CD8 T cells.

dermatomyositis occasionally has underlying malignancies. Calcinosis, with calcium deposition in the subcutaneous tissue, can be a severe long-term complication of dermatomyositis.

EVALUATION AND TREATMENT   The muscle biopsy is striking in dermatomyositis, with most individuals showing inflammatory cells grouped around blood vessels and atrophy of cells in muscle fascicles. This change, perifascicular atrophy, is absent in polymyositis. CK and sedimentation rate are often extremely elevated in both disorders. EMG abnormalities include signs of muscle irritability and myopathic changes—usually large numbers of low-amplitude action potentials of brief duration. The EMG also shows a typical "myopathic" pattern, with short, low-amplitude polyphasic potentials, as well as signs of marked muscle irritability. Muscle biopsy is indispensable for determining a diagnosis of polymyositis or dermatomyositis as opposed to other myotonic diseases. MRI reveals inflammation and edema of the muscles.

Treatment primarily includes immunosuppressive drugs, although they are not always successful if uniformly applied. Most clinicians choose corticosteroids initially, usually prednisone on a daily or alternating-day schedule, tapering the dosage as the symptoms subside. Successful treatment with azathioprine, methotrexate, and cyclophosphamide also has been reported. Individuals with muscle weakness require

SUMMARY REVIEW—cont'd

inflammation. These are usually treatable and self-limiting disorders.

8. Polymyositis (generalized muscle inflammation) and dermatomyositis (polymyositis accompanied with skin rash) are characterized by inflammation of connective tissue and muscle fibers, and muscle fiber necrosis. Cell-mediated and humoral immune factors have been implicated. Treatment with immunosuppressive agents is effective in many cases.

9. The most common toxic myopathy is caused by alcohol abuse. Direct toxic effects of alcohol-producing necrosis of muscle fibers and nutritional deficiency have been suggested. The only treatment is abstinence and improved nutrition. The toxic effects of many drugs on muscle fibers cause local trauma to the muscle fibers from direct effects of the needle, secondary infection, and changes caused by nonphysiologic acidity and alkalinity in the fibers.

10. Sarcomas of muscle tissue are rare. Rhabdomyosarcoma has a uniformly poor prognosis because of an aggressive invasion and early, widespread dissemination. The usual treatment includes surgical excision, radiation therapy, and systemic chemotherapy.

KEY TERMS

Acid maltase deficiency, 1539
Acute gouty arthritis, 1533
Age-related bone loss, 1511
Aggrecan, 1530
Ankylosing spondylitis (AS) (spondyloarthritis), 1529
Asymptomatic hyperuricemia, 1533
Avulsion, 1502
Biofeedback, 1535
Bowing fracture, 1498
Bursae, 1504
Bursitis, 1503
Caplan syndrome, 1529
Chondrogenic (cartilage-forming) tumor, 1520
Chondroid, 1520
Chondrosarcoma, 1520
Closed (simple) fracture, 1498
Collagenic (collagen-forming) tumor, 1520
Comminuted fracture, 1498
Compartment syndrome, 1505
Complete fracture, 1497
Contractures, 1535
Degenerative joint disease (osteoarthritis), 1521
Delayed union, 1500
Dermatomyositis, 1540
Dislocation, 1501
Disuse atrophy, 1536
Enchondroma, 1520
Endogenous (hematogenous) osteomyelitis, 1516
Enthesis, 1529
Epicondylitis, 1503
Exogenous osteomyelitis, 1516
Extracellular signal regulated kinases (ERKS), 1511
Fatigue fractures, 1498
Fibromyalgia, 1536
Fibrosarcoma, 1521
Fracture, 1497
Giant cell tumor, 1521

Glucocorticoid (e.g., cortisone)-induced osteoporosis, 1511
Gout, 1531
Gouty arthritis, 1531
Greenstick fracture, 1498
Hyperbaric oxygen therapy, 1517
Hyperkalemic periodic paralysis, 1538
Hypokalemic periodic paralysis, 1538
Iatrogenic osteoporosis, 1508
Incomplete fracture, 1498
Inflammatory joint disease (arthritis), 1525
Insufficiency fractures, 1498
Involucrum, 1517
Joint effusion, 1525
Joint stiffness, 1524
Lateral epicondylitis (tennis elbow), 1503
Ligament, 1502
Linear fracture, 1498
Malunion, 1501
McArdle disease, 1538
Medial epicondylitis (golfer's elbow), 1503
Muscle strain, 1504
Myelogenic tumor, 1521
Myoadenylate deaminase deficiency (MDD), 1539
Myoglobin, 1505
Myoglobinuria, 1505
Myositis ossificans, 1505
Myositis, 1539
Myotonia, 1537
Noninflammatory joint disease, 1521
Nonunion, 1500
Oblique fracture, 1498
Open (compound) fracture, 1498
Osteoarthritis (OA), 1522
Osteogenic (bone-forming) tumor, 1519
Osteomalacia, 1514
Osteomyelitis, 1516
Osteopenia, 1507
Osteophyte, 1522
Osteoporosis, 1507
Osteoprotegerin (OPG), 1509

Osteosarcoma, 1519
Paget disease (osteitis deformans), 1514
Pannus, 1527
Pathologic fracture, 1498
Peak bone mass, 1507
Periodic paralysis, 1538
Polymyositis, 1540
Pompe disease, 1539
Postmenopausal osteoporosis, 1508
Primary gout, 1533
Progressive relaxation training, 1535
Pseudogout, 1531
RANK, 1509
Receptor activator of nuclear factor κβ ligand (RANKL), 1509
Regional osteoporosis, 1508
Rhabdomyolysis, 1505
Rhabdomyosarcoma, 1541
Rheumatoid arthritis (RA), 1525
Rheumatoid factors (RFs), 1526
Rheumatoid nodules, 1529
Secondary gout, 1533
Sequestrum, 1517
Spiral fracture, 1498
Sprains, 1502
Strain, 1502
Stress fractures, 1498
Subluxation, 1501
Syndesmophyte, 1530
Tendinitis, 1503
Tendinosis, 1503
Tendon, 1502
Tophaceous gout, 1533
Tophus (pl., tophi), 1531
Torus fracture, 1498
Toxic myopathy, 1541
Transchondral fracture, 1498
Transverse fracture, 1498
Volkmann ischemic contracture, 1505

MEDIA RESOURCES

Review questions and answers for this chapter are available in the *CD Companion* included with this book.

WebLinks—links to Internet sites pertaining to this chapter—are available on Evolve at http://evolve.elsevier.com/McCance/.

REFERENCES

1. Woolf AD, Pfleger B: Burden of major musculoskeletal conditions, *Bull World Health Organ* 81(9):646-656, 2003.
2. Bolander M, Selig J: Use of physical forces in bone healing, *J Am Acad Orthop Surg* 11(4):344, 2003.
3. Rundle CH et al: In vivo bone formation in fracture repair induced by direct retroviral-based gene therapy with bone morphogenic protein-4, *Bone* 32(6):591, 2003.
4. Cole BJ, Warner JJP: Arthroscopic versus open Bankart repair for traumatic anterior shoulder instability, *Clin Sports Med* 19(1):19, 2000.
5. Maffulli N, Wong J: Rupture of the Achilles and patellar tendons, *Clin Sports Med* 22(4):761-776, 2003.
6. van der Linden PD et al: Increased risk of Achilles tendon rupture with quinolone antibacterial use, especially in elderly patients taking oral corticosteroids, *Arch Intern Med* 163(15):1801, 2003.
7. Molloy T, Wang Y, Murrell G: The roles of growth factors in tendon and ligament healing, *Sports Med* 33(5):381, 2003.
8. Frank CB: Ligament healing: current knowledge and clinical applications, *J Am Acad Orthop Surg* 4(2):74, 1996.
9. Nirschl RP, Ashman ES: Elbow tendinopathy: tennis elbow, *Clin Sports Med* 22(4):813-836, 2003.
10. Leclerc A et al: Upper limb disorders in repetitive work, *Scand J Work Enviorn Health* 27(4):268-278, 2001.
11. Leclerc A: Exposure assessment in ergonomic epidemiology: is there something specific to the assessment of biomechanical exposures? *Occup Enviorn Med* 62(3):143-144, 2005.
12. Sirvanci M et al: Myositis ossificans of psoas muscle: magnetic resonance imaging findings, *Acta Radiol* 45(5):523-525, 2004.
13. Sauret JM, Marinides G, Want GK: Rhabdomyolysis, *Am Fam Physician* 65(3):907, 2002.
14. Allan D & Jones B: Compartment syndromw: a forgotten diagnosis, *Lancet* 359(9325):2248, 2002.
15. Blackman PG: A review of chronic exertional compartment syndrome in the leg, *Med Sci Sports Exerc* 32(3 suppl):S4, 2000.
16. *Bone Health and Osteoporosis: A report of the surgeon general 2004.* Available online at: www.surgeongeneral.gov/library/bonehealth/.
17. Stevens JA, Olson S: Reducing falls and resulting hip fractures among older women, *MMWR Recomm Rep* 49(RR-2):3-12, 2000.
18. Ott S: *Osteoporosis.* Available online at:http://courses.washington.edu/bonephys/oprisk.html.
19. Holt G et al: Prevalence of osteoporotic bone mineral density at the hip in Britain differs substantially from the US over 50 years of age: implications for clinical densitometry, *Br J Radiol* 75(897):736-742, 2002.
20. Moffett JD, Einhorn TA: General orthopedic principles. In Rosen CJ, Glowicki J, Bilezikian JP, editors: *The aging skeleton,* San Diego, 1999, Academic Press.
21. Ngyuen TV et al: Bone loss, physical activity, and weight change in elderly women: the Dubbo Osteoporosis Epidemiology Study, *J Bone Miner Res* 13(9):1458-1467, 1998.
22. Ueland T et al: Age-related changes in cortical bone contents of insulin-like growth factor binding protein (IGCBP)-3, osteoprotegerin, and calcium in postmenopausal osteoporosis: a cross-sectional study, *J Clin Indocrinol Metab* 85(3):1014, 2003.
23. Romani AM, Scarpa A: Regulation of cellular magnesium, *Front Biosci* 5:D720-D734, 2000.
24. Buchanan JR et al: Effect of excess endogenous androgens on bone density in young women, *J Clin Endocrinol Metab* 67(5):937-943, 1988.
25. Davidson BJ et al: Endogenous cortisol and sex steroids in patients with osteoporotic spinal fractures, *Obstet Gynecol* 61(3):275-278, 1983.
26. Ohta H et al: Differences in axial bone mineral density, serum levels of sex steroids, and bone metabolism between post-menopausal and age- and body-size-matched premenopausal subjects, *Bone* 14(2):111-116, 1993.
27. Pederson L et al: Androgens regulate bone resorption activity of isolated osteoclasts in vitro, *Proc Natl Acad Sci* 96(2):505-510, 1999.
28. Riggs BL et al: Short- and long-term effects of estrogen and synthetic anabolic hormone in postmenopausal osteoporosis, *J Clin Invest* 51(7):1659-1663, 1972.
29. Steinberg KK et al: Sex steroids and bone density in premenopausal and perimenopausal women, *J Clin Endocrinol Metab* 69(3):533-539, 1998.
30. Moskowitz RW, Kelly MA, Lewallen DG: Understanding osteoarthritis of the knee—causes and effects, *Am J Orthop* 33(2 Suppl):5-9, 2004.
31. Hofbauer LC, Schoppet, M: Clinical implications of the osteoprotegerin/RANKL/RANK System for bone and vascular diseases, *JAMA* 292(4):490-495, 2004.
32. Riggs BL, Khosla S, Melton LJ III : Sex steroids and the construction and conservation of the adult skeleton, *Endocr Rev* 23(3): 279-302, 2002.
33. Khosla S, Melton LJ, Riggs BL: Clinical review 144: estrogen and the male skeleton, *J Clin Endocrinol Metab* 87(4):1443-1450, 2002.
34. Manolagas SC: Birth and death of bone cells: basic regulatory mechanisms and implications for the pathogenesis and treatment of osteoporosis. *Endocr Rev* 21(2):115-137, 2000.
35. Eghboli-Fatourechi G et al: Role of RANK ligand in mediating increased bone resorption in early postmenopausal women, *J Clin Invest* 111(8):1221-1230, 2003.
36. Plotkin LI et al: Biphosphonates and estrogens inhibit osteocyte apoptosis via distinct molecular mechanisms downstream of extracellular signol-regulated kinase activation, *J Biol Chem* 280(8):7317-7325, 2005.
37. Chen JR et al: Transient versus sustained phosphorylation and nuclear accumulation of ERKS underlie anti-versus pro-apoptotic effects of estrogens, *J Biol Chem* 280(6):4632-4638, 2005.
38. Stuck H, Schneider A, Strauss E: Osteoporosis: a disease in men, *Clin Orthop Aug* (425):143, 2004.
39. McCabe LD et al: Diary intakes affect bone density in the elderly, *Am J Clin Nutr* 80(4):1066, 2004.
40. Weaver CM: Calcium and magnesium requirements of children and adolescents and peak bone mass, *Nutrition* 26(7-8):514, 2000.
41. Yago MD et al: Intracellular magnesium: transport and regulation in epithelial secretory cells, *Front Biosci* 5:D602, 2000.
42. Anderson GL et al: Effects of conjugated equine estrogen in postmenopausal women with hysterectomy: the Women's Health Initiative randomized controlled trial, *JAMA* 291(14):1701, 2004.
43. Walsh JP: Paget's disease of bone, *Med J Aust* 181(5):262, 2004.
44. Siris ES: Paget's disease of bone. In Flavus JM, editor: *Primer on the metabolic bone diseases and disorders of bone metabolism,* ed 4, Philadelphia, 1999, Lippincott Williams & Wilkins.
45. Menaa C et al: Enhanced RANK ligand expression and responsivy of bone marrow cells in Paget's disease of bone, *J Clin Invest* 105(12):1833-1838, 2000.
46. Marina N et al: Biology and therapeutic advances for pediatric osteosarcoma, *Oncologist* 9(4):422-441, 2004.
47. Skubitz KM et al: Gene expression in giant-cell tumors, *J Lab Clin Med* 144(4):193-200, 2004.
48. Abramson SB: Inflammation in osteoarthritis, *J Rhematol Suppl* 70: 70-76, 2004.
49. Dieppe PA, Lohmander LS: pathogenesis and management of pain in osteoarthritis, *Lancet* 365(9463):965-973, 2005.
50. Rutsch F, Terkeltaub R: Deficiencies of physiologic calcification inhibitors and low grade inflammation in arterial calcification: lessons for cartilage calcification, *Joint Bone Spine* 72(2):110-118, 2005.
51. Hashimoto S et al: Chondrocyte-derived apoptotic bodies and calcification of articular cartilage, *Proc Natl Acad Sci* 95(6):3094-3099, 1998.
52. Lotz M: The role of nitric oxide in articular cartilage damage, *Rheum Dis Clin North Am* 25(2):269-282, 1999.
53. Proudfoot D, Shanahan CM, Weissberg PL: Vascular calcification: New insights into an old problem, *J Pathol* 185(1):1-3, 1998.
54. Tintut Y et al: Monocyte/macrophage regulation of vascular calcification in vitro, *Circulation* 105(5):650-655, 2002.
55. Rutsch F et al: PC-1 nucleoside triphosphate pyrophosphohydrolase deficiency in idiopathic infantile arterial calcification, *Am J Pathol* 158(2):543-554, 2001.
56. McAlindon TE et al: Glucosamine and chondroitin for treatment of osteoarthritis: a systemic quality assessment and meta-analysis, *JAMA* 283(11):1469, 2000.
57. Behar SM, Porcelli SA: The immunology of inflammatory arthritis, *Sci Med* 3(6):12, 1996.
58. Sweeney SE, Firestein GS: Rheumatoid arthritis: regulation of synovial inflammation, *Int J Biochem Cell Biol* 36(3):372-378, 2004.

59. Lovell D: Biologic agents for the treatment of juvenile rheumatoid arthritis: current status, *Paediatr Drugs* 6(3):137, 2004.

60. Katana RK, Brent LJ: Spondyloarthropathies, *Am Fam Physican* 60(12):3853, 2004.

61. Francois RJ et al: Histopathologic evidence that sacroiliitis in ankylosing spondylitis is not merely enthesitis, *Arthritis Rheum* 43(9): 2011-2014, 2000.

62. Muche B et al: Anatomic structures involved in early- and late-stage sacroiliitis in spondylarthritis, *Arthritis Rheum* 48(5):1374-1384, 2003.

63. Ikbal M et al: Association of chromatid exchange frequencies in patients with ankylosing spondylitis with and without HLA-B27, *Ann Rheum Dis* 62(8):775, 2003.

64. Atagunduz P: HLA-B27-restricted CD8+ T cell response to cartilage-derived self peptides in ankylosing spondylitis, *Arthritis Rheum* 52(3) 892-901, 2005.

65. Zou J et al: analysis of the CD8 + T cell response to the G1 domain of aggrecan in ankylosing spondylitis, *Annals Rheum Dis* 64(5):722-729, 2005.

66. Bollow M et al: Quantitative analyses of sacroiliac biopsies in spondyloarthropathies: T cells and macrophages predominate in early and active sacroiliitis—cellularity correlates with the degree of enhancement detected by magnetic resonance imaging, *Ann Rheum Dis* 59(2): 135-140, 2000.

67. Anandarajah A, Ritchlin CT: Treatment update on spondyloarthropathy, *Curr Opin Rheumatol* 17(3):247-256, 2005.

68. Wolfe F, Michaud K: Lymphoma in rheumatoid arthritis: the effect of methotrexate and anti-tumor necrosis factor therapy in 18,572 patients, *Arthritis Rheum* 50(6):1740-1751, 2004.

69. Nyhan WL: Lesch-Nyhan disease, *J Hist Neurosci* 14(1):1-10, 2005.

70. Reinders MK et al: A costly therapeutic dilemma in tophaceous gout: is etanercept or rasburicase preferable? *Ann Rheum Diseases* 64(3):516, 2005.

71. Larsson R, Oberg PA, Larsson SE: Changes of trapezius muscle blood flow and electromyography in chronic neck pain due to trapezius myalgia, *Pain* 79(1):45, 1999.

72. Westgaard RH: Muscle activity as a releasing factor for pain in the shoulder and neck, *Cephalgia* 19(suppl 25):1, 1999.

73. Gandevia SC: Mind, muscles, and motoneurones, *J Sci Med Sport* 2(3):167, 1999.

74. Shaver JL: Fibromyalgia syndrome in women, *Nurs Clin North Am* 39(1):195-204, 2004.

75. Millea, PJ, Holloway RL: Treating fibromyalgia, *Am Fam Physician* 62(7):1575, 2000.

76. Gracely RH et al: Functional magnetic resonance imaging evidence of augmented pain processing in fibromyalgia, *Arthritis Rheum* 46(5):1333-1343, 2002.

77. Geisser ME et al: Perception of noxious and innocuous heat stimulation among healthy women and women with fibromyalgia: association with mood, somatic focus, and catastrophizing, *Pain* 102(3):243-250, 2003.

78. Staud R, Cannon RC: Temporal summation of pain from mechanical stimulation of muscle tissue in normal controls and subjects with fibromyalgia syndrome, *Pain* 102(1-2):87-95, 2003.

79. Goldenberg DL, Burckhardt C, Crofford L: Management of fibromyalgia syndrome, *JAMA* 292(19):2388-2395, 2004.

80. Tsigos C, Chrousos GP: Hypothalamic-pituitary-adrenal axis, neuroendocrine factors and stress, *J Psychosom Res* 53(4):865-871, 2002.

81. Buckwalter JA, Lappin DR: The disproportionate impact of chronic arthralgia and arthritis among women, *Clin Orthop* (372):159, 2000.

82. Van Houdenhove B, Egle UT: Fibromyalgia: a stress disorder? Piecing the biopsychosocial puzzle together, *Psychother Psychosom* 73(5):267-275, 2004.

83. Goldenberg DL, Burckhardt C, Crofford L: Management of fibromyalgia syndrome, *JAMA* 292(19):2388-2395, 2004.

84. Davies NP, Hanna MG: Neurologic channelopathies: diagnosis and therapy in the new millennium, *Ann Med* 31(6):406, 1999.

85. Lundberg IE, Dastmalchi M: Possible pathologic mechanisms in inflammatory myopathies, *Rheum Dis Clin North Am* 28(4):799-822, 2002.

86. Dalakas MC, Hohfeld R: Polymyositis and dermatomyositis, *Lancet* 362(9388):971-982, 2003.

87. Wortman RL: Inflammatory and metabolic diseases of muscle. In *Primer on the rheumatic diseases,* ed. 12, Atlanta, 2001, The Arthritis Foundation.

88. Adachi J et al: Alcoholic muscle disease and biomembrane perturbations (review), *J Nutr Biochem* 14(11):616-625, 2003.

89. Urbano-Marquez A, Fernandez-Sola J: Effects of alcohol on skeletal and cardiac muscle, *Muscle Nerve* 30(6):689-707, 2004.

90. Andrassy RJ: Advances in the surgical management of sarcomas in children, *Am J Surg* 184(6):484-491, 2002.

91. Ferrari A et al: Rhabdomyosarcoma in adults. A retrospective analysis of 171 treated patients at a single institution, *Cancer* 98(3):571-580, 2003.

ALTERATIONS OF MUSCULOSKELETAL FUNCTION IN CHILDREN

KRISTEN LEE CARROLL

CHAPTER OUTLINE

Musculoskeletal alterations in children are very common. They may be congenital, such as clubfoot; hereditary, such as muscular dystrophy; or acquired, such as Legg-Calvé-Perthes disease. Some of these disorders are acute, and the child will recover completely; other disorders are chronic or, in some cases, terminal. An understanding of the pathophysiology of these alterations will aid in providing the best care possible for these children.

MUSCULOSKELETAL DEVELOPMENT IN CHILDREN

Bone Formation

Bone formation, which begins at about the eighth week of gestation, involves two phases: (1) the delivery of bone cell precursors to sites of bone formation and (2) the aggregation of these cells at **primary centers of ossification,** where they mature and begin to secrete osteoid (see Chapter 41). Some of the bone cell precursors are present in fetal connective tissues, whereas others migrate in blood to sites of bone formation after blood vessels have grown into the tissue.

Cellular aggregation and maturation occur in two types of fetal tissue, depending on which bones are being formed. The cranium, facial bones, clavicles, and parts of the jawbone arise from a fetal membrane termed the *mesenchyme.* Bones that

develop on or within the mesenchyme grow by the process of **intramembranous formation.** As the mesenchyme becomes vascularized, the immature bone cells aggregate and mature into osteoblasts, which form the centers of ossification. Osteoblasts secrete osteoid, which surrounds them and quickly ossifies, forming the lacunae and canaliculi of compact bone. Spicules of bone radiate from the ossification centers to form the primary trabeculae characteristic of spongy bone. Later, some of the spongy bone is replaced by compact bone.

Endochondral formation is the development of new bone from cartilage (Figure 43-1). First, mesenchymal tissue forms a **cartilage anlage,** which defines the shape of the bone. This is usually found by 6 weeks of gestation. Vascular invasion of the anlage brings osteoprogenator cells leading to primary centers of calcification inside by 8 weeks. Endochondral bone formation begins in the outer layer of the cartilage model, which consists of a layer of dense connective tissue called **perichondrium.** The perichondrium contains cells that develop into osteoblasts, forming a collar of bone, termed the **periosteal collar,** around the cartilage model. Cartilage enclosed within the periosteal collar degenerates, and capillaries from outside the perichondrium invade the degenerating cartilage cells, carrying with them osteoblast precursors from the inner layer of the perichondrium and osteoclast precursors from the blood itself.

Endochondral bone formation progresses at the primary center of ossification in the middle of the cartilage model and

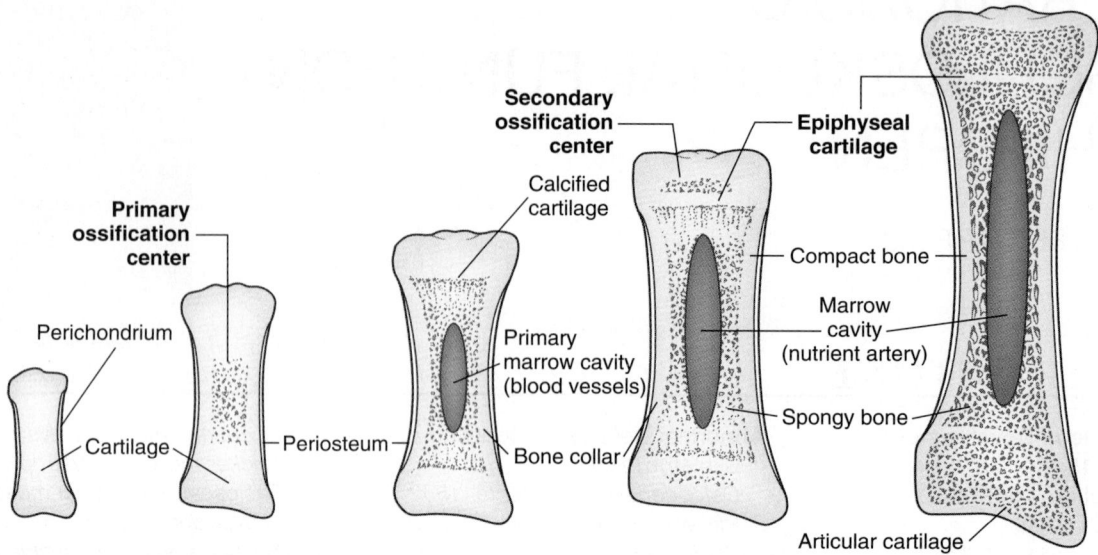

Figure 43-1 Stages of endochondral bone formation and centers of ossification in long bone.

extends toward either end of the developing bone. At the same time, the periosteal collar thickens and becomes wider toward the epiphyses. By the end of gestation, **secondary centers of ossification** (i.e., the epiphyseal centers) begin to lay down bone at both ends of the cartilage model. Here, too, cartilage within the periosteal collar degenerates, and blood vessels grow inward, delivering bone cell precursors. Once the osteoblasts begin to secrete osteoid, ossification spreads from the secondary centers in all directions until all the cartilage within the model is replaced by bone.

Two regions of cartilage remain at the ends of long bones: (1) articular cartilage over the free ends of the bone and (2) the physeal plate, a layer of cartilage between the metaphysis and epiphysis. (These structures are described and illustrated in Chapter 41; see Figure 41-2.) The physeal plate retains the ability to form and calcify new cartilage and deposit bone until the skeleton matures roughly 1 year after sexual maturity (11 to 15 years of age in females, 15 to 18 in males).

Bone Growth

Until adult stature is reached, growth in the length of bone occurs at the physeal plate through endochondral ossification. Cartilage cells at the epiphyseal side of the physeal plate multiply and enlarge. As rapidly as new cartilage cells form, cartilage cells at the metaphyseal side of the plate are destroyed and replaced by bone.

In the shaft of new bone, where growth is relatively slow, the bone produced by accretion is compact and dense. The compact bone is thickest where it has to withstand the maximal stresses, which generally occur in the middle of the shaft.

The two physeas of the long bone can have varying strengths. The more active of the two has more power to remodel deformity but also can be more sensitive to injury. The architecture of the physis also dictates its sensitivity to injury. The distal femur, for example, has an undulating pattern that increases its resistance to sheer force; when injured, however, growth disturbance is highly likely.

Growth in the diameter of bone occurs by deposition of new bone on an existing bone surface. Bone matrix is laid down by osteoblasts on the periosteal surface and subsequently becomes calcified. At the same time, bone resorption occurs on the endosteal surface. Endosteal resorption increases the diameter of the medullary cavity, which contains marrow and spongy bone.

Many factors affect the development, physiology, and rate of growth of the epiphyseal plate. Growth hormone must be secreted by the pituitary gland at a constant rate to stimulate the growth plate consistently. Other known factors affecting growth include peptide regulatory factors (e.g., fibroblast growth factor [FGF]); changes in cell-to-cell interactions through cell adhesion molecules (CAMs) and cell junctions; and complex interactions or changes in extracellular matrix (ECM), nutrition, general health, and other hormones (e.g., thyroid hormone, adrenal and gonadal androgens, estrogens). These factors influence both the rate of bone growth and the time of appearance of the secondary ossification centers. When the skeleton is mature, the epiphyseal plate is replaced by bone. This process, termed **physeal closure,** unites the metaphysis and the epiphysis. Physeal closure occurs earlier in females than males because of earlier puberty in females.

Throughout life, bone is constantly being destroyed and re-formed (see Chapter 41), but the process is at its maximum in children approximately $2\frac{1}{2}$ years of age. By young adulthood, bone turnover, or remodeling, occurs at a relatively slow rate. Peak bone mass is achieved by the mid to late 20s and slowly decreases throughout life; therefore, calcium intake, weight-bearing exercise, minimizing caffeine, and phosphorus are especially important for the young female if she is to avoid osteoporosis in later life.

Skeletal Development

The axial skeleton changes shape with growth. (The axial skeleton and appendicular skeleton are described and illustrated in Chapter 41; see Figure 41-4). In a newborn the entire spine is concave anteriorly, or **kyphosed.** In the first 3 months of life, with the infant's ability to control the head, the upper (cervical) spine begins to arch, or become **lordotic.** The normal lordotic curve of the lower (lumbar) spine begins to develop with sitting.

The appendicular skeleton (the extremities) grows faster during childhood than does the axial skeleton (see Figure 41-4). The newborn has a relatively large head and long spine with disproportionately shorter limbs than an adult. By 1 year of age, 50% of the total growth of the spine has occurred and is over 70% complete by age 8.[1] Therefore, failure of the spine to grow (e.g., spinal fusion) does not limit eventual height as much as the premature fusion of the growth plates of the lower extremities. In children with congenital curvature of the spine, growth tends to worsen the deformity rather than to increase the length of the spine.

Besides getting longer, growing bones of the extremities undergo changes in rotation and alignment. In the newborn the proximal femur is rotated forward up to 40 degrees and the tibia is rotated inward. With growth the femur assumes its normal alignment (by 8 years of age) and tibial rotation neutralizes at 5 years of age. Bowlegs and knock knees are normal at certain stages of growth. At birth the newborn's legs are bowed because of stresses in utero. **Genu varum (bowleg)** reaches a peak by 2½ years of age, whereas **genu valgum (knock knee)** maximizes by 5 to 6 years of age. If genu varum or genu valgum persists past these ages, a pathologic process rather than a physiologic phase may be present. Pathologic causes of genu varum are Blount disease, rickets, skeletal dysplasias (such as achondroplastic dwarfism), and traumatic injury. Genu valgum may persist also as a result of skeletal dysplasia.

Muscle Growth

The composition and size of muscles vary with age. In the fetus, muscle tissue contains a large amount of water and much intercellular matrix. After birth, both are reduced considerably as the muscle fibers (cells) enlarge by accumulating cytoplasm. Little information is available about the numbers of fibers in a given muscle at various ages, but the total mass of muscle in the body can be estimated from the amount of creatinine excreted in the urine, because the conversion of creatine to creatinine takes place only in muscle (see Chapter 41). Between birth and maturity, the number of muscle nuclei in the body increases 14 times in boys and 10 times in girls. Muscle fibers reach their maximal size in girls at approximately 10 years of age and in boys by 14 years. Growth in length occurs at the ends of muscles, and the increase in length is accompanied by an increase in number of nuclei in the fibers. Muscle fibers increase in diameter as the fibrils become more numerous. The fibrils themselves do not increase in diameter. Connective tissue components of muscle grow where the tendon and muscle meet.

A potent stimulus to the growth of a muscle is the separation of its attachments as the skeleton grows. The length of a muscle fiber is the direct consequence of the range of movement it is called on to perform. The stimulus for the formation of a tendon is probably the pull of the muscle rudiment

on undifferentiated connective tissue. The repair of a tendon from which a segment has been removed does not occur if the muscle is prevented from exercising tension on the damaged tendon. Replacement of muscle by tendon (tendinification) sometimes is the result of limitation of movement. If the normal opponents of a muscle are paralyzed, the muscle fails to grow properly, and it may be that the full development of a muscle depends on the progressive rise in the tension exerted on it by its antagonists.

Muscle growth during adolescence is a major factor in weight gain. Gender differences in muscle size and weight are minor in childhood but become considerable with the onset of puberty.

In the infant, muscle accounts for approximately 25% of total body weight, compared with 40% in the adult. In the adult, approximately 55% of muscle weight is in the lower limb muscles, whereas in the infant the majority of the weight is axial musculature. The respiratory and facial muscles are well developed at birth so that the infant can perform the vital functions of breathing and sucking. Other muscle groups, such as the pelvic muscles, take several years to develop fully. Throughout life the weight of the skeletal muscles can be increased by exercise. Less is known about the development of visceral and cardiac muscle. Visceral muscle fibers increase in both number and size, but the increase in fiber size is most important. Fiber enlargement alone can increase the bulk of visceral muscle by as many as eight times. Cardiac muscle also grows mainly by enlargement of existing fibers.

MUSCULOSKELETAL ALTERATIONS IN CHILDREN

Congenital Defects

Syndactyly

The most common congenital defect of the upper extremity is **syndactyly,** or webbing of the fingers (Figure 43-2). Simple webbing involves the soft-tissue envelope alone and is best released surgically when the child is 1 to 2 years of age. True syndactyly involves fusion of the bones and nails as well as the soft tissues; it may be associated with absence or anomaly of bony or neurovascular units. The primary goal in surgical

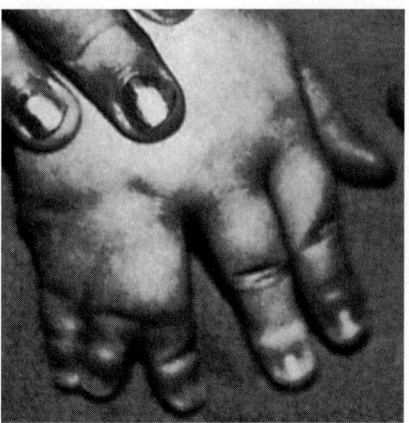

Figure 43-2 Syndactyly.

correction of these defects is to achieve maximal function and appearance. Ideally, corrective surgery is deferred until the child is 6 to 12 months of age and completed before the child enters school. **Vestigial tabs,** such as an extra digit, however are best removed during the immediate neonatal period. Anomalies on the medial or radial aspect of the arm are often associated with abnormalities of blood, heart, or kidneys. Lateral or ulnar-sided defects are less often associated with systemic anomalies and are far more rare.

Developmental Dysplasia of the Hip

Developmental dysplasia of the hip (DDH), formerly known as congenital dislocation of the hip, is an abnormality in the development of the proximal femur, acetabulum, or both. Although most often present at birth, it may occur at any time in the newborn or infant period.

The incidence of true dislocation of the hip or a dislocatable hip is 1 in 1000 live births. Some degree of instability of the hip is present in approximately 10 per 1000 live births. The left hip is affected in 60% of cases, whereas the right hip alone is affected only 20% of the time. Bilateral DDH occurs 20% of the time.

Risk factors for DDH include family history, female sex (6:1), metatarsus adductus (20%), torticollis (10%), oligohydramnios, first pregnancy, and breech presentation. First pregnancies and oligohydramnios (deficient volume of amniotic fluid) are thought to limit fetal movement, and breech presentation not only limits movement but places the hips in a position of flexion and adduction, although only 2% of births have breech history, as many as 40% of infants with DDH had a breech birth. Maternal hormones that reportedly increase joint laxity also have an effect on DDH, although the exact mechanism is unknown. DDH also is more common in whites and those cultures that swaddle infants with the hips in extension and adduction.

PATHOPHYSIOLOGY   The hip can be described as subluxated, dislocatable, or dislocated (Figure 43-3). The subluxated hip maintains contact with the acetabulum but is not well seated within the hip joint. The dislocatable hip is sometimes located but can be dislocated easily. The dislocated hip has no contact between the femoral head and the acetabulum. Some degree of acetabular dysplasia is present in almost all cases. Typically the acetabulum is shallow or sloping rather than cup shaped.

By approximately 10 weeks of gestation, the femur, acetabulum, and hip joint capsule are well developed. It appears that most dysplasias occur within the second and third trimesters and are often the result of positioning factors. Experimentally, DDH can be produced in laboratory animals by placing the developing hip in adduction and extension, replicating the breech position. There is, however, a genetic component that is poorly understood. In addition, 2% of DDH cases are teratologic or caused by a systemic syndrome, such as arthrogryposis or spina bifida, in which muscle contracture or imbalance leads to DDH.

If the DDH is left untreated in the growing child, secondary changes occur. If the hip is left subluxated or dislocated, the acetabulum becomes increasingly shallow and the soft tissues shorten about the proximal femur. If the hip is dislocated, the bone acetabulum fills with soft tissue and a false acetabulum forms where the femoral head contacts the iliac crest. An apparent limb length inequity and hip muscle weakness occurs, leading to a waddling gait. The subluxation leads to early osteoarthritis (OA), and it is now estimated that at least 60% of all OA of the hip is related to DDH.[2]

CLINICAL MANIFESTATIONS
The clinical manifestations of DDH vary with the severity of the condition and the age of the child. Signs and symptoms that should be noted include the following:

1. Asymmetry of gluteal or thigh folds
2. Limb length discrepancy (Galeazzi sign)
3. Limitation of hip abduction
4. Positive Ortolani sign (clunk of dislocation)
5. Positive Barlow test (clunk of reduction)
6. Positive Trendelenburg gait (waddling)
7. Pain (very late)

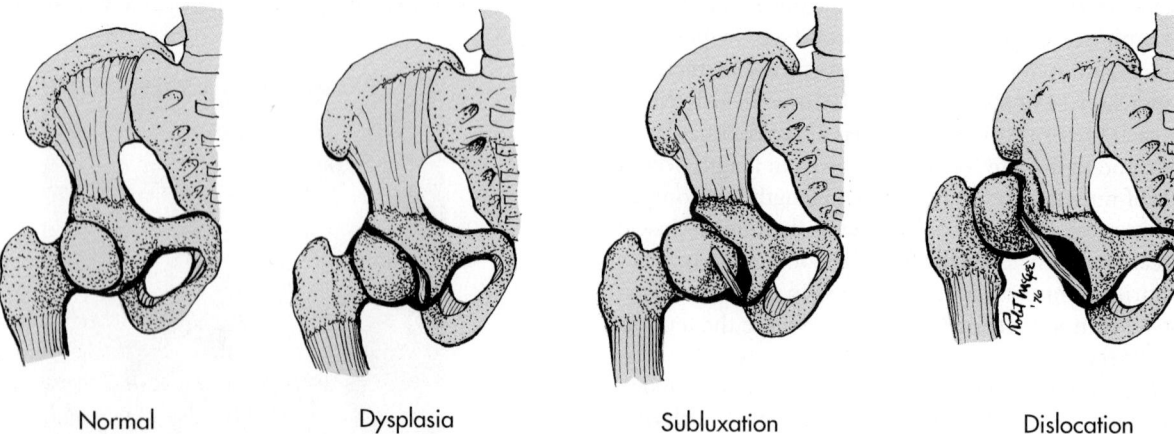

Normal   Dysplasia   Subluxation   Dislocation

Figure 43-3 Configuration and relationship of structures in developmental dysplasia of the hip. (From Hockenberry MJ: *Wong's nursing care of infants and children,* ed 7, St Louis, 2003, Mosby.)

The child also should be examined for other anomalies, such as torticollis or metatarsus adductus, which can be associated with DDH.

EVALUATION AND TREATMENT
In the newborn period, clinical examination is the most important diagnostic tool. Real-time ultrasound, in which the hip is examined while the ultrasound is performed, also is extremely valuable in the newborn period, especially in high-risk infants. The use of ultrasound allows visualization of the cartilaginous structures of the hip (the femoral head and the outer lip of the acetabulum), which are not seen on plain roentgenogram. Radiographs are used after age 6 months.[3]

Treatment depends on the age of the child, severity of dysplasia, and duration of dysplasia. The earlier that treatment is begun, the better the result. In children less that 4 months of age, a Pavlik harness can brace the hip in abduction and flexion and the acetabulum will remodel as the femoral head rests centered in the socket. With this treatment, up to 98% of children will have an excellent result. A "closed" reduction (without opening the joint) followed by spica or body casting for up to 3 months can be done in children up to 12 months of age. After 12 months, surgical intervention—including opening the joint and cutting and realigning the femur and/or acetabulum—may be required. In teratologic dislocations, bracing often is unsuccessful and therefore surgery is needed.

Deformities of the Foot
Congenital Deformity
Congenital foot deformity is found in approximately 4% of all newborns, and metatarsus adductus accounts for 75% of these (Table 43-1). **Metatarsus adductus** is a forefoot adduction deformity associated with a normal, plantigrade hindfoot and is believed to be secondary to intrauterine positioning. Metatarsus adductus is usually classified by two criteria: flexibility (passively correctable or rigid) and degree of deformity. The degree of deformity (mild, moderate, severe) is ascertained by the heel bisection line. A mild deformity is one in which the heel bisection line passes medial to the third toe; moderate, through the third or fourth toes; and severe, lateral to the fourth toes. It should be emphasized that a majority of children are well served by expectant treatment rather than early surgical intervention. Serial casts during the first 6 months of life are suggested for moderate to severe deformities and those deformities that appear less flexible. Casts are usually left in place for 6 to 12 weeks. Eighty-seven percent of children usually correct spontaneously by 6 years of age and 95% by 15 years of age. Even in those children with some residual deformity and an oblique medial cuneiform, few sequelae in adult life occur.

Equinovarus Deformity
There are three types of equinovarus (clubfoot): positional equinovarus, idiopathic congenital equinovarus, and teratologic equinovarus (Figure 43-4). The true positional equinovarus lends itself to rapid correction by application of serial casts. The idiopathic variety is treated by attempting cast cor-

Table 43-1	Terms Used to Describe Foot Abnormalities
Term	**Definition**
Position	
Abduction	Lateral deviation away from the midline of the body
Adduction	Lateral deviation toward the midline of the body
Eversion	Twisting of the foot outward along its long axis
Inversion	Twisting of the foot inward on its long axis
Dorsiflexion	Bending the foot upward and backward
Plantar flexion	Bending of the foot downward and forward
Abnormality	
Talipes	Congenital abnormality of the foot (clubfoot)
Pes	Acquired deformity of the foot
Varus	Inversion and adduction of the heel and the forefoot
Valgus	Eversion and abduction of the heel and forefoot
Equinus	Plantar flexion of the foot in which the heel is lower than the toes
Calcaneus	Dorsiflexion of the foot in which the heel is lower than the toes
Planus	Flattening of the medial longitudinal arch of the foot (flatfoot)
Cavus	Elevation of the medial longitudinal arch of the foot (high arch)
Equinovarus	Coexistent equinus and varus deformities
Calcaneovarus	Coexistent calcaneus and varus deformities
Equinovalgus	Coexistent equines and valgus deformities
Calcaneovalgus	Coexistent calcaneus and valgus deformities

NOTE: The position listed can all be achieved by voluntary movement of the normal foot; an abnormality exists if the foot is fixed in one or more of the positions while at rest.

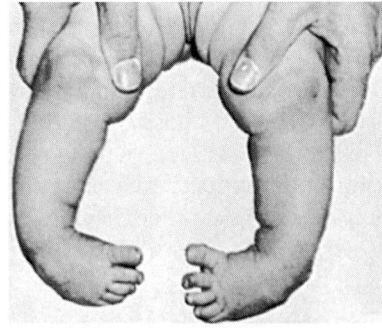

Figure 43-4 Infant with bilateral congenital talipes equinovarus. (From Brashear HR, Raney RB: *Shand's handbook of orthopedic surgery,* ed 9, St Louis, 1978, Mosby.)

rection, followed by surgical intervention of resistant deformities. Teratologic equinovarus nearly always requires surgical correction and/or muscle balancing procedures.

Positional Equinovarus. **Positional equinovarus** is a deformity in which the infant's foot is in equinovarus position but does not have a deep posterior or plantar medial crease. It appears to be secondary only to intrauterine position. The foot can be passively brought to a plantigrade position and is amenable to casting. In general, 1 to 3 months of above-knee casting corrects this foot without the need for surgical intervention.

Idiopathic Congenital Equinovarus. The etiology of idiopathic equinovarus (clubfoot) is unknown. In one human fetal study, all clubfeet were associated with identifiable anterior horn cell changes in L5 and S1. Enterovirus infection, known to potentially cause anterior horn cell damage if present intrauterinely, reaches a peak prevalence in the summer or fall of temperate climates. These two seasons correlate with the peaks of conception in children with clubfeet. Muscle biopsies of both the anterior tibialis long flexors and peroneus brevis muscles in clubfoot reveal that at least 50% of cases show a decreased number of muscle fibers and/or abnormal fiber histology. The soleus often has an increase in type 1 fibers, whereas the brevis has a fiber type disproportion. The more abnormal the histopathology is, the more severe the deformity, and the greater the chance of recurrent deformity after treatment. In addition to neurologic causes, positional abnormalities (e.g., oligohydramnios) have been implicated. The genetic component is unclear and studies are ongoing.

Idiopathic equinovarus occurs in approximately 1 of every 1000 live births, with males being affected twice as often as females. Although these deformities have been historically treated nonoperatively, surgical intervention became much more common after 1950. Over the past 10 years, nonoperative management has again become the mainstay. Inago Ponseti developed a casting technique that has been used for over 50 years now. Although used in Iowa since 1950, it was not well accepted nationally until recently. The technique involves 6 casts, left on for 5 to 7 days each, followed by a percutaneous tendoachilles lengthening procedure performed with local anesthesia in the clinic. The child then uses braces until 3 years of age. Noncompliance with braces leads to increased recurrence. Nearly 20% of children may need an anterior tibialis transfer around age 3.[4] Studies comparing operative posteriomedial release with Ponseti techniques show better long-term results with the less invasive Ponseti method[5] (see What's New box: Ponseti Casting).

Teratologic Equinovarus. The most common causes of **teratologic equinovarus** are either neuromuscular (such as

---

WHAT'S NEW?   Ponseti Casting

Ponseti casting implements toe-to-groin casts changed weekly for 6 weeks. Casting begins as early as possible after birth and culminates in a percutaneous tendoachilles lengthening in the clinic, followed by a final cast worn for 3 weeks. In recalcitrant cases, a full surgical posteriomedial release (PMR) still may be required. The need for PMR in idiopathic clubfoot has decreased from 90% to less than 20% of infants when this casting technique is used. Long-term results, presumably because of less scarring and more long-term flexibility, are better with Ponseti casting than the PMR method.

---

spina bifida) or syndromic, as in arthrogryposis or osteochondrodysplasia (such as diastrophic dwarfism). The teratologic clubfoot, unlike the idiopathic type, usually fails to be corrected with casting protocols and requires operative intervention. The surgery is often more extensive than that for an idiopathic clubfoot, and revision surgery is also more common.

Pes Planus (Flatfoot) Deformity. Pes planus (flatfoot) commonly raises parental concern. Despite medical evidence to the contrary, it can be very difficult to convince families that a flexible flatfoot is as functional as the one with a "normal" arch. The majority of babies are born with flat (or "fat") feet, with the arch becoming more apparent with age. The relatively benign natural history, however, should not overshadow the importance of accurate diagnosis. Significant ankle valgus, vertical talus, tarsal coalition, and skewfoot must be accurately differentiated from flexible pes planus.

Flexible flatfoot deformity appears to be familial, with occasional association of generalized ligamentous laxity. Careful evaluation of possible occult Achilles contracture is done by holding the hindfoot in varus position and dorsiflexing the ankle. Achilles contracture can signify a more severe flatfoot variant. The flexibility of the hindfoot is evaluated by having the child stand on his or her toes or by dorsiflexing the first toe passively with the child in a non–weight-bearing position. This "windlass mechanism" tightens the plantar fascia, thereby reconstituting an arch and hindfoot varus if the foot is indeed flexible. If hindfoot flexibility and an "underlying" arch are present, then flexible flatfoot is diagnosed.

By all recent data, the surgical or orthotic treatment of *asymptomatic* flexible pes planus is unnecessary. Custom orthotics, Helfet heel cups, and corrective orthopedic shoes may relieve discomfort but will have no influence over the natural history (clinically or radiographically) of flat feet. Adult studies on army recruits have shown that soldiers with flat feet perform just as well as their counterparts without "fallen" arches.

There is a small subset of children with painful flexible flat feet. For these children, careful attention to the possibility of Achilles contracture or tarsal coalition (congenital union of the hindfoot bones) must be made. This small group of children are best treated with inexpensive shoe inserts and then expectantly watched. If pain continues into adolescence, requiring more aggressive treatment, calcaneal lengthening will correct the pes planus without decreasing hindfoot motion. In rigid flat feet, a computed tomographic (CT) scan often will reveal coalition—if painful, this can be resected. Heel cord contractures can be surgically lengthened because stretching alone is often inadequate. All surgery carries risk; if a foot is flat but nonpainful, treatment is not required. The painless flatfoot should be viewed as a variation of normal feet.

Abnormal Density or Modeling of the Skeleton

Osteogenesis Imperfecta

Osteogenesis imperfecta (brittle bone disease) is an inherited disorder of connective tissues that affects primarily bone. The disorder was first described in 1840 as a syndrome in newborns that consisted of osteoporosis with fractures and skeletal deformities. The Sillence classification is based on both models of inheritance and clinical findings (Table 43-2). In the most severe form of this disorder, the child is usually stillborn or dies soon after birth, although some survive into childhood. Osteogenesis imperfecta (OI) in its more severe forms is evident at birth because fractures and deformity have occurred in utero. The less severe forms may not become evident until the child begins to walk. Some children with this milder form then experience numerous fractures and can be mistaken for battered children until the diagnosis is made.

Table 43-2	Sillence Classification of Osteogenesis Imperfecta Syndromes	
Type	Genetics	Description
I	Autosomal dominant	Mildest form of osteogenesis imperfecta Mild to moderate bone fragility without deformity Associated with blue sclerae, early hearing loss, easy bruising May have mild to moderate short stature Type 1A: dentinogenesis imperfecta absent Type 1B: dentinogenesis imperfecta present
II	Autosomal dominant or recessive	Perinatal lethal or recessive Extreme fragility of connective tissue, multiple in utero fractures, usually intrauterine growth retardation Soft, large cranium Micromelia, long bones bowed, ribs beaded
III	Autosomal recessive	Progressive deforming phenotype Sever fragility of bones, usually have in utero fractures Severe osteoporosis Relative macrocephaly with triangular facies Fractures heal with deformity and bowing Associated with white sclerae and extreme short stature, scoliosis
IV	Autosomal dominant	Skeletal fragility and osteoporosis more severe than type I Associated with bowing of long bones; light sclerae, ± moderate short statue, ± moderate joint hyperextensibility Type IVA: dentinogenesis imperfecta absent Type IVB: dentinogenesis imperfecta present

From Klippel JH, Dieppe PA, editors: *Rheumatology,* ed 2, London, 1998, Mosby.

The prevalence rate of the most common form is about 1 in 30,000. Inheritance is usually autosomal dominant but can be autosomal recessive. At least four syndromes have been identified that have various clinical manifestations and prognoses (see Table 43-2).

PATHOPHYSIOLOGY   The major errors in osteogenesis imperfecta lie in the synthesis of collagen. Genetic studies have shown that the gene responsible for the encoding of collagen easily mutates. These mutations cause osteogenesis imperfecta. The large range of phenotypes includes all mutants of the two collagen structural genes. (Genes are discussed in Chapter 4.) Abnormalities in collagen include (1) an increase in collagen hydroxylysine residue in bones; (2) a decrease in hydroxylysine-norleucine in skin collagen; and (3) absence of α-polypeptide production in cultured skin fibroblasts.[6]

A number of metabolic abnormalities have been reported. Some individuals have increased serum thyroxine levels, suggesting hyperthyroidism. This is consistent with the findings of increased sweating, heat intolerance, increased body temperature, a resting tachycardia, and tachypnea. The hyperthyroid findings, however, are not consistent in all individuals with osteogenesis imperfecta. Studies of leukocyte metabolism suggest an uncoupling of oxidative phosphorylation. Reports of alterations of platelet function with defects in adhesion and clot retraction also exist.

CLINICAL MANIFESTATIONS   The classic clinical manifestations of osteogenesis imperfecta are osteoporosis and increased rate of fractures, possible bony deformation, triangular facies, possible vascular weakness (i.e., aortic aneurysm), possible blue sclera, and poor dentition. The Sillence classification designated types I through IV based on severity. The most severe, types II and III, are comparable to osteogenesis imperfecta congenita. These two types are characterized by autosomal recessive inheritance and early onset of manifestations. Both can cause stillbirth or severe neonatal deformity and a short life expectancy. Less severe are types I and IV, which are comparable to osteogenesis imperfecta tarda. Type I is slightly more common than types II and III, and type IV is quite rare. Types I and IV are inherited as autosomal dominant traits and vary in age of onset from birth to adulthood. Type IV, especially when the sclera are white, is the least deforming type and is often confused with nonaccidental trauma (child abuse).

EVALUATION AND TREATMENT   Evaluation of osteogenesis imperfecta is based on clinical manifestations and serologic tests. Serum alkaline phosphatase is elevated in all forms of the disease. Osteogenesis imperfecta can be diagnosed prenatally by ultrasound or chorionic villi sampling. Quantitative analysis of cultured skin fibroblast collagen by electrophoresis shows a decreased quantity of collagen in the affected individual.

For osteogenesis imperfecta type II, no therapeutic intervention will be effective. For other types of osteogenesis imperfecta, careful positioning and handling of the newborn may prevent fractures. Beyond the neonatal period, various orthopedic measures are applied, such as prompt splinting of fractures and correction of deformities arising from the progressive bowing or bending of the skeleton by intermedullary rodding of the bones (Figure 43-5). These are sequentially replaced as the child grows. There presently is a multicenter study of bisphosphonate therapy showing promising results in type III, with marked improvements of bone density (up to 30%). Two recent studies of OI in children after 4 years of pamidronate use reveal significant improvements in height, bone mineral content (154%), bone volume (44%), and bone mineral density (65%). Genetic counseling for affected families should aim at primary prevention. Pamidronate has been used for OI types I, III, and IV.[7,8] Genetic counseling for affected families should aim at primary prevention.

Rickets

Rickets is a disorder in which growing bone fails to become mineralized (ossified), resulting in "soft" bones and skeletal deformity. Rickets results from either insufficient vitamin D, insensitivity to vitamin D, wasting of vitamin D by the kidney, or inability to absorb vitamin D and calcium in the gut. In industrialized nations the most common X-linked dominant form is hypophosphotemic rickets. Although in the past few years, as exclusive breast feeding for a lengthy period has been encouraged, vitamin D deficiency has been increasing. This is

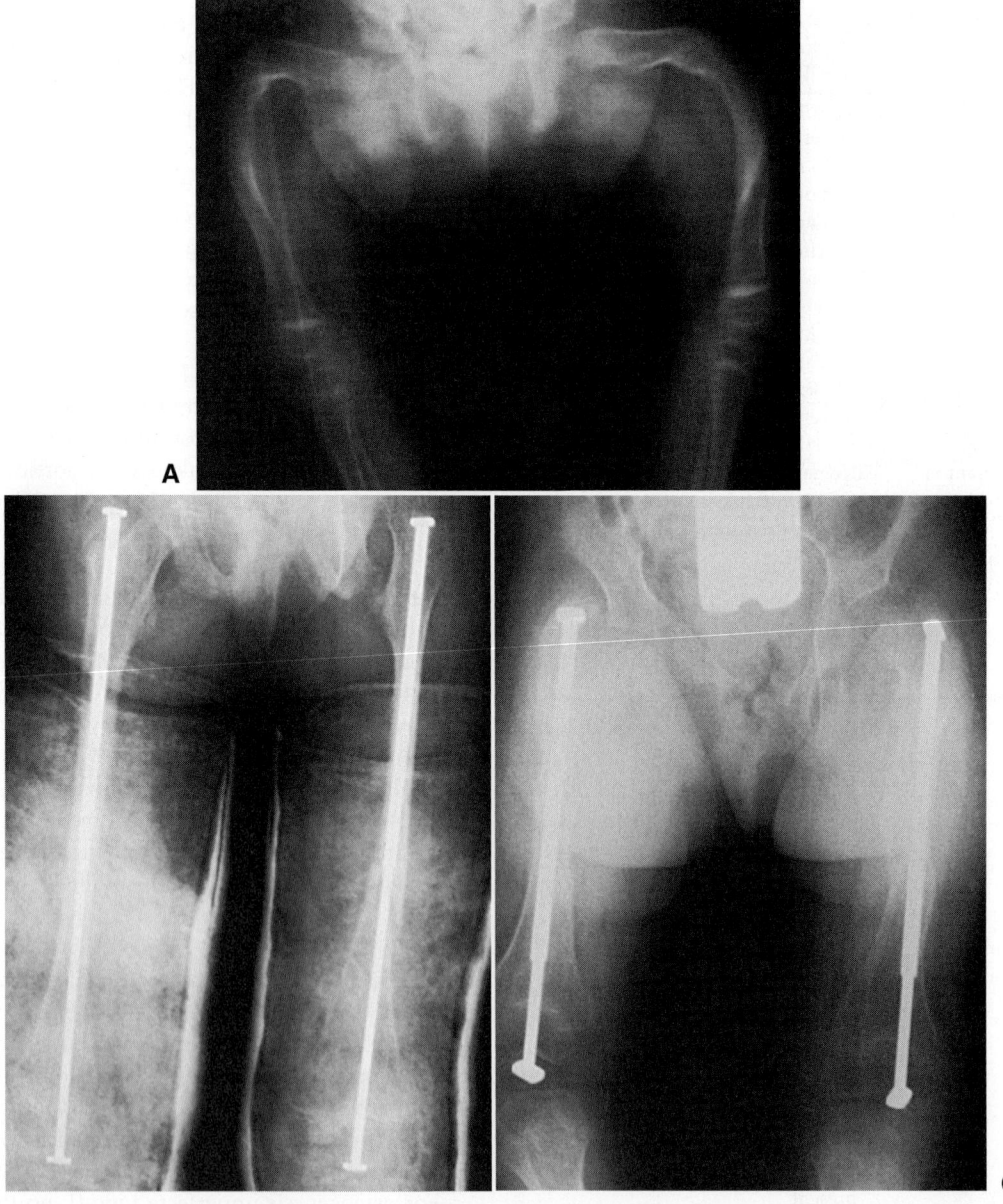

Figure 43-5 Osteogenesis imperfecta treated with osteotomies and telescoping medullary rods. **A,** Severe deformity of both femurs. **B,** Same individual after multiple osteotomies with telescoping medullary rod fixation. **C,** Same individual 4 years later demonstrating growth of femurs, no recurrence of deformity, and elongation of rods. (Plaster casts are in place for immobilization of tibial osteotomies.) (From Crenshaw AH, editor: *Campbell's operative orthopaedics*, ed 8, vol 3, St Louis, 1992, Mosby.)

especially problematic when the mother is vitamin D deficient.[9] Vitamin D is the mineral necessary for absorption and metabolism of calcium and phosphate. Rickets in the immature skeleton leads to broad, irregular growth plates because the rows of cells in the growth plate that are intended to ossify fail to do so as they reach the metaphysis (Figure 43-6).

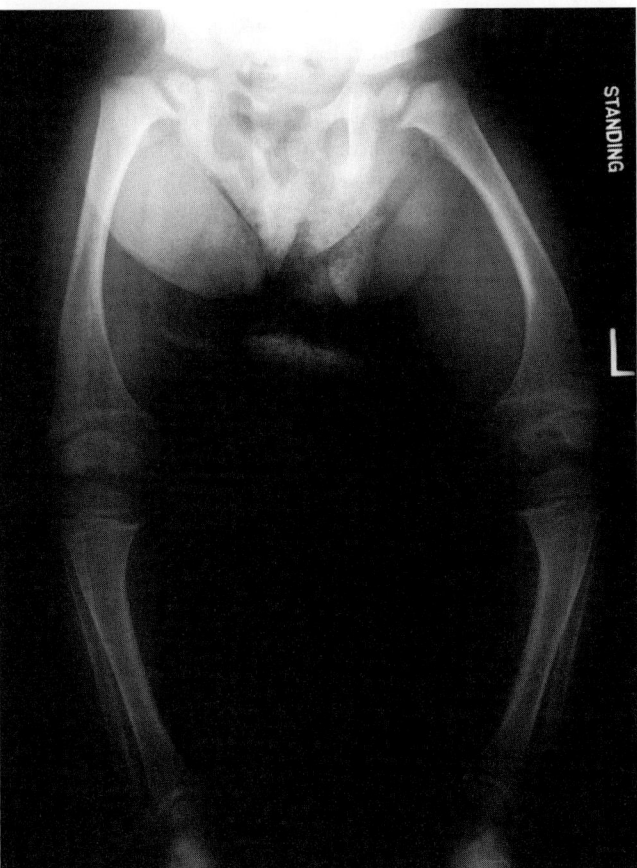

Figure 43-6 Rickets. This standing radiograph of an 8-year-old female with hypophosphotemic rickets shows cupping and widening of the growth plates throughout the lower extremities. Also note the bowing femoral deformity and hip deformity.

Children with rickets are often listless and irritable. They have hypotonia and muscle weakness and may be unable to walk without support. Abnormal parietal flattening and frontal bossing occur in the skull. The calvaria become soft, and the sutures may widen. Cartilaginous attachments of the ribs become prominent, and the long bones of the extremities (tibia, femur, radius, ulna) may be bowed. Growth is retarded, and fractures are common.

Like osteogenesis imperfecta, surgical treatment of bony deformity is often required. However, medical management of calcium, phosphorus, and vitamin D levels must be optimized before surgical intervention. Deformity often improves with normalization of bone metabolism.

Scoliosis

Scoliosis is a rotational curvature of the spine most obvious in the anterior-posterior plane (Figure 43-7). It can be classified as nonstructural or structural. **Nonstructural scoliosis** results from a cause other than the spine itself, such as posture, leg length discrepancy, or pain. **Structural scoliosis** is curvature of the spine associated with vertebral rotation. Nonstructural scoliosis can become structural if the underlying cause is not found and treated.

Structural scoliosis can be caused by a great variety of conditions. It can result from congenital skeletal abnormalities (15%), neuromuscular diseases (15%), trauma, extraspinal contractures, bone infections that involve the vertebrae, metabolic bone disorders (e.g., rickets, osteoporosis, osteogenesis imperfecta), joint disease, and tumors. Most cases of structural scoliosis, however, have no known cause, although genetic factors are suggested. Structural scoliosis with no known cause, termed **idiopathic scoliosis**, accounts for at least 65% of cases.

Idiopathic scoliosis is classified as infantile, juvenile, or adolescent, depending on the child's age at the time of onset. In infantile scoliosis, spinal curvature develops during the first 3 years of life; in juvenile scoliosis, curvature develops between the skeletal age of 4 years and the onset of adolescence;

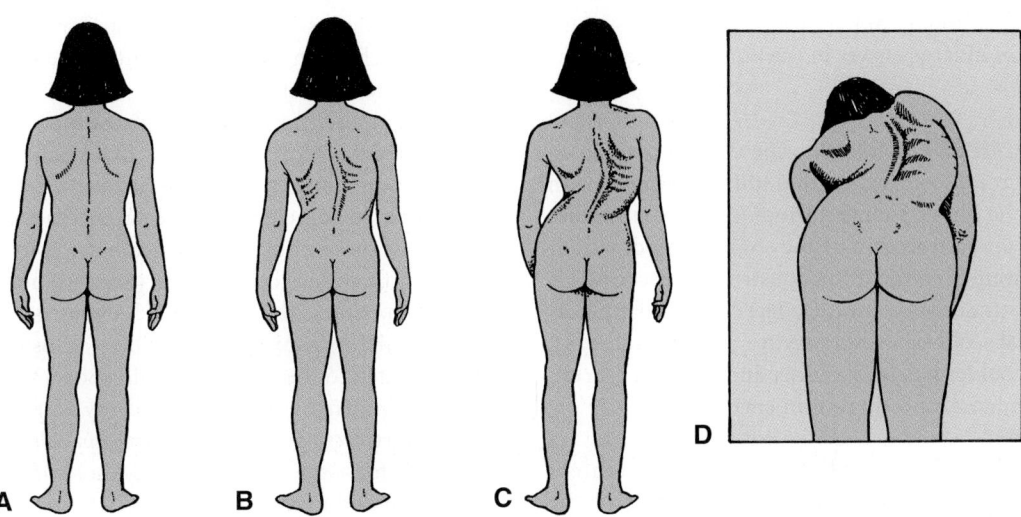

Figure 43-7 Scoliosis in children. Normal spinal alignment and abnormal spinal curvatures associated with scoliosis. **A,** Normal. **B,** Mild. **C,** Severe. **D,** Rotation and curvature of scoliosis.

and in adolescent scoliosis, it develops after the skeletal age of 10. Adolescent idiopathic scoliosis is the most common. Scoliosis in its milder forms occurs equally in boys and girls once curves measure more than 15 degrees; however, girls are 5 times as likely to have scoliosis than boys.

PATHOPHYSIOLOGY   It has been hypothesized that in individuals with adolescent scoliosis, there is an abnormality of the central nervous system involving the balance mechanism (reticular system) in the midbrain. A genetic component is also suggested because 30% occur within families. A recent study is making exciting gains in this area.

Experimentally, it also has been shown that individuals with adolescent idiopathic scoliosis have an abnormality in the function of the posterior columns of the spinal cord. This results in abnormal proprioception and is not evident clinically except in the presence of scoliosis. The exact cause of scoliosis, however, remains elusive.[10,11]

The earliest pathologic changes, which are probably secondary changes, occur in the soft tissues. The muscles, ligaments, and other soft tissues become shortened on the concave side of the curve. With time, progressive deformities of the vertebral column and ribs develop. In growing children, lateral deviation of the spinal column ceases and one-sided compression of the vertebral bodies on the concave side of the curve begins. Vertebral deformity occurs as asymmetric forces are applied to the epiphyseal center of the ossification by shortened and tight soft tissues on the concave side of the curve. The degree of compression and twisting varies according to the position of the vertebrae in the curve. The compressive force is greatest on the vertebrae in the apex of the concavity, so that the apical vertebrae become most deformed.

The curves increase most rapidly during periods of rapid skeletal growth. If the curve is less than 40 degrees at skeletal maturity, the risk of progression is quite small. In curves greater than 50 degrees, the spine is biomechanically unstable, and the curve will in all likelihood continue to progress even after the cessation of growth at an average rate of 1 degree per year. Curves in the thoracic spine greater than 60 degrees result in decreased pulmonary function, whereas the most common complication of large curves in the lumbar spine is back pain.

CLINICAL MANIFESTATIONS   The clinical manifestations of nonstructural scoliosis are mild spinal curvature with prominence of one hip or rounded shoulders. The curvature disappears with forward flexion of the spine, lying down, or traction of the head. Treatment for nonstructural scoliosis is correction of the underlying disorder. The clinical manifestations of structural scoliosis include asymmetry of hip height, asymmetry of shoulder height, shoulder and scapular (shoulder blade) prominence, and rib prominence.

EVALUATION AND TREATMENT   Spinal curvature is usually visible or palpable, and muscles on one side of the lower back (the convex side) may be prominent or bulging. Most cases of idiopathic scoliosis are noticed during school screening programs. In girls the deformity may be noticed because clothing does not "hang" properly on the body. Diagnosis is made by roentgenographic examinations.

Treatment of curves between 25 and 35 degrees in the skeletally immature child is with bracing. In most cases the low-profile brace is used. A brace used only at night, the Charleston bending brace, has shown it to be less effective than the traditional low-profile braces in preventing progression of curves. Occasionally a Milwaukee brace, which has a metal upper structure and neck ring, is needed for curves with an apex higher than midthoracic level. Low-profile and Milwaukee braces are worn for 23 hours daily until skeletal maturity. Bracing will only prevent progression of the curve; it will not correct the curvature. Bracing is not effective in curves greater than 40 degrees or in skeletally mature individuals; the most effective time for bracing is in a young child (less than 12 years of age) with a small curve.[12] Extensive chiropractic manipulations and electrical stimulation have not been shown to change natural history. Surgical treatment with spinal fusion with instrumentation is recommended for curves greater than 40 to 50 degrees. If surgery is indicated, it is better performed during the adolescent years while there is greater flexibility of the curves and less risk of complications.

One dilemma in the treatment of scoliosis is predicting which curves will progress and which will not. Currently, researchers are evaluating platelet calmodulin as a predictor for the severity and progression of adolescent idiopathic scoliosis.[13] Early results have shown a higher platelet calmodulin level in individuals with a progressive curve. If these early results are corroborated in future studies, these levels could be used to avoid unnecessary radiography in individuals with a low risk of progression and more accurately predict which individuals would benefit from brace or surgical treatment.[13]

Bone Infection: Osteomyelitis

Osteomyelitis is an infection of the bone. Occurring twice as often in males as females, acute osteomyelitis may affect infants and children of any age, but it occurs most often between 3 and 12 years of age.

Bacteria enter the bone through the bloodstream and lodge in the medullary cavity, where a rich phagocytic mechanism often prevents most of the bacteria from establishing an infectious state. In some cases, however, the bacteria may lodge at the end of the venous loops beneath the epiphyseal plate, and infection then develops because there are no phagocytic cells present to remove the bacteria[14-16] (Figure 43-8).

The microorganism responsible for osteomyelitis varies and is related to the age of the child (Box 43-1). Osteomyelitis in the newborn is caused primarily by *Staphylococcus aureus*. Group B streptococcus and *Escherichia coli* infections are responsible for some cases, especially those of multiple bone involvement and in high-risk infants.[16]

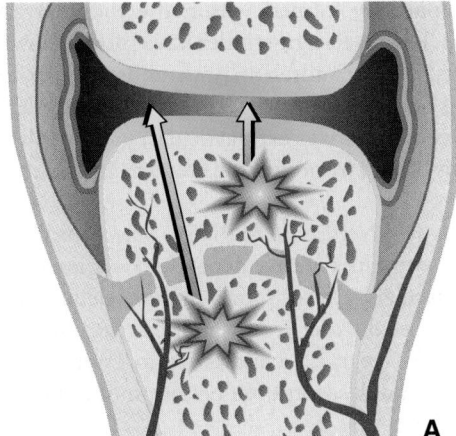

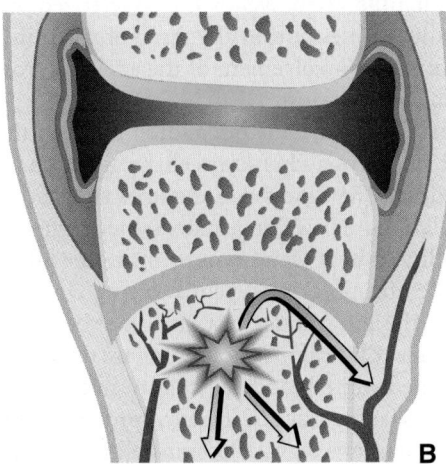

Figure 43-8 Pathogenesis of acute osteomyelitis differs with age. **A,** In infants younger than 1 year the epiphysis is nourished by penetrating arteries through the physis, allowing development of the condition within the epiphysis. **B,** In children up to 15 years of age the infection is restricted to below the physis because of interruption of the vessels.

Box 43-1	Causative Microorganisms of Osteomyelitis According to Age

Newborns	**Older Children**
Staphylococcus aureus	*Staphylococcus aureus*
Group B streptococcus	*Pseudomonas*
Gram-negative enteric rods	*Salmonella*
Infants	*Neisseria gonorrhoeae*
Staphylococcus aureus	**Adolescents and Adults**
Haemophilus influenzae	*Pseudomonas*
	Mycobacterium tuberculosis

Staphylococcus aureus is the responsible microorganism in 80% to 90% of osteomyelitis cases in older children. *Haemophilus influenzae,* a previously common cause of osteomyelitis in children less than 5 years of age, has now become rare with the improvements in immunization. Gram-negative microorganisms account for an increasing number of infections of the vertebrae,[17,18] whereas *Salmonella* infections are associated with sickle cell disease.

Factors that predispose an individual to the development of osteomyelitis include impetigo, furunculosis, infected lesions of varicella (chickenpox), infected burns, cerebral abscesses, immunization with bacille Calmette-Guérin (BCG) vaccine, prolonged intravenous or central parenteral alimentation, drug addiction, and direct trauma to the area adjacent to the site of osteomyelitis.

PATHOPHYSIOLOGY   Osteomyelitis usually begins as a bloody abscess in the metaphysis of the bone. The abscess ruptures under the periosteum and spreads along the bone shaft or into the bone marrow cavity if untreated. Infection rarely spreads down the medullary cavity of the bone but rather first gains entrance to the subperiosteal space in the metaphysis. This is the path of least resistance because the cortex of the bone in this area is porous or mazelike and the inflammatory response blocks spread within the bone.[19] Because of the accumulation of debris caused by the infection, the periosteum may separate and form a shell of new bone around the infected portion of the shaft. Because the periosteum is separated from an adequate blood supply, sections of the bone die; these pieces of dead bone are called **sequestra.** The periosteum that maintains a blood supply generates new bone and is responsible for the appearance of the periosteal new bone, or **involucrum.** The presence of the sequestra and involucrum indicates that the disease has progressed to subperiosteal abscess formation.

In cases where the infection in the metaphysis occurs near the joint, the accumulating pus (bacteria, white blood cells, fluid) creates increasing pressure that may cause a rupture into the joint cavity. If rupture into the joint occurs, the pus causes inflammation and a condition called **secondary septic arthritis.**[16] Although thought uncommon, a recent study shows 40% of children will have adjacent joint involvement with osteomyelitis. The most common joint to be affected is the knee. Osteomyelitis is most commonly caused by bacteria that reach the metaphysis through the bloodstream but may occur through secondary inoculation of microorganisms caused by trauma or contagious spread of infection from cellulitis in adjacent soft tissue.

Osteomyelitis in infants is often associated with septic arthritis because the infant's bone has blood vessels that perforate the growth plate. Because of the unique nature of blood supply to an infant's bones, osteomyelitis and septic arthritis commonly occur together. Normal anatomic variations in infants allow infection to spread directly to the epiphysis, which causes both joint disease and permanent epiphyseal disease. Multiple sites of osteomyelitis are also more common in children younger than 2 years, necessitating bone scan to check other bones when infants are infected. This can then lead to other areas of osteomyelitis and possibly septic arthritis.[20]

Children are susceptible to joint involvement for several reasons (Figure 43-9). In the immature infant, there is no epiphyseal plate or an ossific nucleus at the end of the bone and the cartilage precursor of bone is penetrated by vascular channels. In these infants the infection begins in the vulnerable cartilage precursor of the end bone itself and results in rapid destruction of the joint and arrested growth of the bone. For this reason the early detection and treatment of osteomyelitis are crucial if the infant's joint is to be saved from later destruction. As the child matures and the epiphyseal plate forms, a temporary barrier is established against infection because the arterioles end beneath the epiphyseal plate.[19]

In children older than 2 years, the epiphyseal plate prevents the spread of a metaphyseal abscess into the epiphysis and the cortex of the metaphysis is thicker. These anatomic differences increase the likelihood that the metaphyseal abscess will extend into the diaphysis and the blood supply of the bone will be disrupted. The periosteum is also more difficult to perforate in older children; this may lead to a larger subperiosteal abscess that could endanger the periosteal blood supply as well. This process commonly results in extensive sequestrum formation and chronic osteomyelitis.[19]

Osteomyelitis is much less common after the physeal plates are closed, except in the vertebral body. Infection may develop in any part of a bone, and abscesses spread slowly. Destruction of the cortex in a localized area may result in a pathologic fracture.[17,18]

Spread of infection to contiguous joints is related to the child's age. Infection may spread to adjacent joints because the epiphyseal plate of the proximal femur is located within the hip joint capsule; the distal femoral plate is partially located within the knee; and the proximal and distal humeral

plates are partially located within the shoulder and elbow joints, respectively. Recent studies have shown, however, that, like infants, older children may demonstrate up to 42% of contiguous joint involvement. Even in areas where the involved osteomyelitis was extraarticular, joint involvement occurred; this differs from previous reports in the literature.[20]

CLINICAL MANIFESTATIONS   The clinical manifestations of osteomyelitis are age dependent and are related to the differing vascular patterns found in the skeletal system at various ages. Three distinct groups may be identified: (1) infants younger than 1 year, (2) children from 1 year of age to puberty, and (3) adolescents after cessation of bone growth and adults.

Infants. Osteomyelitis may be an acute illness characterized by fever and failure to move the affected limb (pseudoparalysis). Infantile osteomyelitis is characterized by involvement of multiple sites within the same bone or in multiple bones. If untreated, involvement of the adjacent growth plate can result in growth arrest.

Children. Osteomyelitis in children between the ages of 1 year and puberty is characterized by fever and systemic signs of toxicity. The illness is sometimes subacute, with the child complaining of swelling, redness, tenderness, and decreasing ability to bear weight on or move the affected area. Onset can be abrupt. Osteomyelitis during childhood most often affects the long bones but also may be found in the pelvis and spine. Clinical manifestations are usually accompanied by elevated white blood cell counts and elevated erythrocyte sedimentation rates. C-reactive protein (CRP), when elevated, is a sensitive sign of osteomyelitis and can rapidly decrease with appropriate treatment. Evidence of infection using roentgenograms can be delayed but bone scan is positive within 48 hours.

Adolescents and Adults. In addition to the sites previously mentioned, osteomyelitis in adolescents and adults may involve the vertebrae. Back pain, with a duration of several weeks, may be the only clinical complaint. This age group is less often affected than younger populations.

EVALUATION AND TREATMENT   White blood cell counts and erythrocyte sedimentation rates are sometimes elevated, but this is not a consistent finding. Monitoring of erythrocyte sedimentation rates is an indication of response to management but can be delayed. C-reactive protein is more quickly responsive to appropriate treatment. Blood cultures (positive in 30% to 40%) and aspiration of the soft tissue or bone, or both, should be done to identify the causative microorganism. Appropriate antibiotics should be prescribed after culture and sensitivity studies have been completed. A tuberculin test also is administered because *Mycobacterium tuberculosis* is sometimes the responsible microorganism and has recently had a slight resurgence in incidence. Bone scans can be quite helpful with diagnosis and in children younger than 1 year are absolutely required to define whether multiple sites are involved.

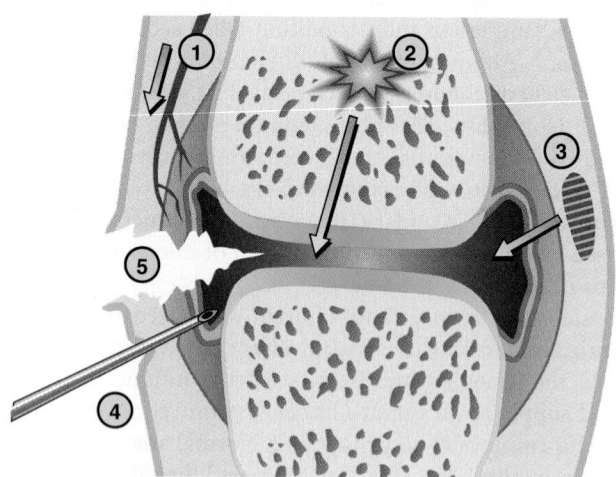

1. The hematogenous route
2. Dissemination from osteomyelitis
3. Spread from an adjacent soft tissue infection
4. Diagnostic or therapeutic measures
5. Penetrating damage by puncture or cutting

Figure 43-9 Routes of infection to the joint.

Treatment includes intravenous (IV) antibiotics or, in highly reliable children and families, a combination of IV and oral antibiotics for 6 weeks. Drainage and margination of bone is required if changes are present on radiographs signifying abscess. Immobilization may help with pain control. If a joint is also infected, the situation becomes a *surgical emergency;* surgery on the affected joint can help prevent damage to the articular cartilage by lysozymes released from the involved neutrophils.

Death is rare, but serious sequelae may occur. The course of the disease and prognosis depend on the age of the child, the rapidity with which the diagnosis is established, the initiation of early treatment, and maintenance of the treatment for an adequate time. The most serious complications are growth arrest, osseous necrosis, and recurrence. Recurrence with presently available antibiotic regimens is less than 10%.

Juvenile Rheumatoid Arthritis

The rheumatic diseases are a group of diverse conditions having in common the inflammation of connective tissues. They include rheumatoid arthritis, systemic lupus erythematosus, dermatomyositis, scleroderma, and polyarthritis. Incidence of these disorders in children is estimated in Table 43-3.

Juvenile rheumatoid arthritis (JRA) is the childhood form of rheumatoid arthritis (see Chapter 42). Like adult-onset rheumatoid arthritis, JRA is a syndrome that is often accompanied by systemic manifestations. Approximately 5% of all cases of rheumatoid arthritis begin in childhood. An estimated quarter of a million children in the United States have JRA.

The basic pathophysiology of JRA is the same as that of adult rheumatoid arthritis. The clinical manifestations of JRA may differ, however, beginning with mode of onset. Unlike adult rheumatoid arthritis, which begins insidiously with systemic signs of inflammation and generalized aches, JRA has three distinct modes of onset: arthritis in fewer than five joints (pauciarticular arthritis), arthritis in more than five joints (polyarticular arthritis), and systemic disease. Onset is less gradual in JRA than in adult rheumatoid arthritis. Juvenile rheumatoid arthritis also differs from the adult form in the following respects:[21,22]

1. Predominantly the large joints are affected.
2. Subluxation and ankylosis of the cervical spine are common if the disease progresses.

3. Joint pain is not as severe as in the adult type.
4. Serologic tests often detect antinuclear antibody (ANA).
5. Chronic uveitis is common, especially if ANA positive.
6. Serologic tests seldom detect rheumatoid factor.
7. Rheumatoid nodules are not limited to subcutaneous tissue but are found in the heart, lungs, eyes, and other organs.

Treatment for children with JRA is supportive but not curative. Many children with pauciarticular arthritis who are seronegative for ANA will resolve their symptoms over time. However, with systemic onset (Stills disease) or seropositivity, JRA may progress to true adult RA. The aims of treatment are to control inflammation and other clinical manifestations of the disease and to minimize deformity.

Avascular Diseases of the Bone: Osteochondrosis

The avascular diseases of the bone, collectively termed **osteochondroses,** are caused by insufficient blood supply to growing bones. Disturbances of blood supply to primary and secondary centers of ossification during periods of rapid bone growth result in a variety of skeletal abnormalities.

The cause of the osteochondroses remains obscure. In the past, infection, nutritional deficiencies, and hormonal imbalances were blamed, but these causes have been largely disproved. Currently, vascular impairment and trauma, coupled with an underlying developmental or genetic predisposition, have been identified as probable causes of osteochondroses. The most common osteochondroses are Osgood-Schlatter disease (tibial tubercle), distal patellar pole (Sinding-Larsen-Johansson syndrome), radial head (Panner disease), the navicular bone of the foot (Kohler disease), and calcaneus (Sever disease). All are associated with activity-related pain of the affected region that improves with rest. All are more common in boys than girls and in athletes more than nonathletes.

The osteochondroses involve areas of significant tensile or compressing stress that undergo partial osseous necrosis, progressive bony weakness, and then microfracture. Most of these are associated with trauma and overuse and improve with rest. Anti-inflammatories, modification of activities, and even immobilization are used during active disease. Reparative correction by revascularization is the rule, although this may be a lengthy process.

Table 43-3	Incidence of Connective Tissue Diseases in Children				
Disease	**Annual Rate/10⁵**	**Gender Ratio (Female/Male)**	**Race Ratio (White/Black)**	**Peak Age-Group at Risk (yr)**	**Childhood Onset (%)**
Rheumatoid arthritis	40	3:1	Equal	Increases with age (20-50)	5
Systemic lupus erythematosus	6	8:1	1:4	15-45	18
Dermatomyositis	0.8	2:1	1:3	45-65	20
Scleroderma	0.4	3:1	Equal	Increases with age (30-50)	3
Polyarteritis	0.2	1:3	Equal	Midadult	Rare

Data from Hollingworth P. In Klippel JH, Dieppe PA, editors: *Rheumatology,* St Louis, 1994, Mosby.

Legg-Calvé-Perthes Disease

Legg-Calvé-Perthes disease, commonly called Perthes disease, is classically thought to be an osteochondroses like those previously described. This self-limited disease of the hip is presumably produced by recurrent interruption of the blood supply to the femoral head. The ossification center first becomes necrotic, collapses, and then is gradually remodeled by live bone.

Legg-Calvé-Perthes disease is relatively common (1 in 5000 children), usually occurring in children between 3 and 10 years of age, with a peak incidence at 6 years. It is more common in boys than in girls by a ratio of about 5:1. The condition is bilateral in approximately 10% of affected children; in 80% of these children, the effect on the second side is less severe.[23]

The cause of decreased blood supply to the head of the femur is unknown. Several theories have been proposed, including trauma; infection; and protein C and S deficiencies, which cause a hypercoagulable state or vascular anamolies.[24] A plausible theory is that acute synovitis (infection of the synovial membrane) and increased hydrostatic pressure in the hip joint compress blood vessels that supply the femoral head.

Constitutional factors definitely play a role. Skeletal maturation is delayed an average of 2 years in children with Legg-Calvé-Perthes disease, and affected children are between 2.5 and 7 cm shorter than unaffected children of the same age. Familial occurrence is 30% to 40%. The disease is rare in blacks, and it is frequent in children of Japanese and central European ancestry.

PATHOPHYSIOLOGY Legg-Calvé-Perthes disease runs its natural course in 2 to 5 years. In the incipient stage the soft tissues of the hip (synovial membrane and joint capsule) are swollen, edematous, and hyperemic, often with fluid present in the joint (Figure 43-10). The joint space widens, and the joint capsule bulges. The first stage lasts only a few weeks. In the second (or active avascular necrotic) stage, the entire epiphysis or the anterior half of the epiphysis of the femoral head loses blood supply and the metaphyseal bone at the junction of the femoral neck and capital epiphyseal plate is softened because of decalcification. Soon granulation tissue (procallus) and blood vessels invade the dead bone. This stage lasts several months to 1 year.

The third (or regenerative healing) stage ordinarily lasts 2 to 4 years. The dead femoral head is replaced by procallus, and new bone is laid down. Collapse and flattening of the femoral head occur, and the femoral neck becomes short and wide (see Figure 43-10).

In the fourth (or residual) stage, remodeling takes place and the newly formed bone is organized into a live spongy bone. Children less than 6 years of age at onset have more time to remodel the damage Perthes has caused and have the best outcome.[25] Recent multicenter studies, using the "lateral pillar" classification,[25] have shown that hips younger than 6 years with *no* involvement of the lateral femoral head (type A) do better than those with involvement of the lateral femoral head. Those children with complete collapse of not only the lateral but also the entire femoral head (type C) have the worst prognosis. Long-term studies of type C hips show that without treatment 70% to 90% progress to osteoarthritis by 40 years of age.[26]

CLINICAL MANIFESTATIONS Injury or trauma precedes the onset of clinical manifestations in approximately one third of children with Legg-Calvé-Perthes disease. Onset of symptoms is insidious unless trauma aggravates the disease process. The child often complains of a limp or pain for several months. The pain usually is referred to the knee, inner thigh, and groin, following the path of the obturator nerve. In some children, pain may be absent or minimal. If pain is present, it is usually aggravated by activity and relieved by rest.

The typical physical findings include spasm on inward rotation of the hip and a limitation of both internal rotation flexion and adduction. If the child is walking, an abnormal gait, termed a Trendelenburg gait or abductor lurch, is apparent. The child moves his or her trunk toward the affected side with stance to compensate for weak abductor musculature. If the hip pain or limp has been present for a prolonged period, muscles of the hip and thigh atrophy. A limb length inequity may be present if the proximal femoral physis is involved

EVALUATION AND TREATMENT Diagnosis is confirmed by radiographic examination. Principles of treatment are "containment" (keeping the ball completely in the socket) and motion to maintain the articular cartilage. In the past, children were treated with bed rest and a variety of braces,

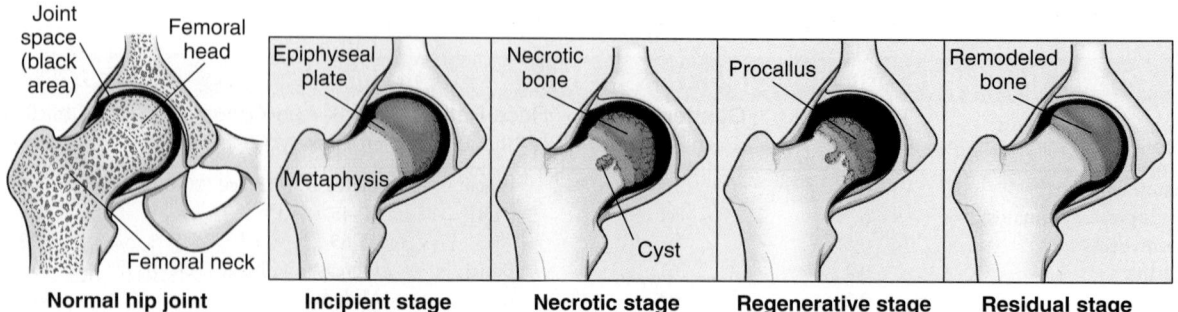

Figure 43-10 Stages of Legg-Calvé-Perthes disease, a form of osteochondrosis.

which have now been shown to be ineffective.[27] Currently, most children can be managed with antiinflammatory medications and crutches for episodes of synovitis and activity modification (avoidance of jumping activities that place increased stress on the hip) during the active phase of the disease. Serial roentgenograms to monitor the progress of the disease and to ensure that the hip remains congruent are done. Surgery may be necessary if the femoral head becomes subluxated or incongruent with the acetabulum before the reparative process. The ball must be congruent to take on the shape of the socket as remodeling occurs.

Factors affecting the outcome of Legg-Calvé-Perthes disease are the age of the child, the extent of necrosis, and the stage of disease at the time treatment is begun and congruence of the joint with skeletal maturity. Recent studies have shown that girls, despite earlier skeletal maturity, do as well as boys. Outcome is 70% satisfactory with Herring stage A; for Herring stages B and C or age greater than 8 years, outcome is guarded. Present prospective studies are evaluating more aggressive early treatment (i.e., osteotomy of the femur or pelvis) on the more involved hips to change long-term outcome.

Osgood-Schlatter Disease

Osgood-Schlatter disease consists of tendinitis of the anterior patellar tendon, within which the patella (kneecap) is embedded, and associated osteochondrosis of the tubercle of the tibia. Osgood-Schlatter disease occurs most often in preadolescents and adolescents who participate in sports. The incidence is higher in boys than in girls, many of whom have increased outward tibial fusion compared to controls.[28]

PATHOPHYSIOLOGY   The severity of the lesion varies from mild tendinitis to a complete separation of the anterior extension of the tibial epiphysis, which is the part of the epiphysis that contributes to growth of the tibial tubercle. The underlying pathologic alterations also vary. The mildest form of Osgood-Schlatter disease causes ischemic (avascular) necrosis in the region of the bony tibial tubercle, with hypertrophic cartilage formation during the stages of repair. In more severe cases the abnormality involves a true epiphyseal separation of the tibial tubercle, with the characteristics of avascular necrosis that are described in the section on Legg-Calvé-Perthes disease.

CLINICAL MANIFESTATIONS   The child experiences pain and swelling in the region of the patellar tendon and tibial tubercle, which becomes prominent and is tender to direct pressure. The pain is most severe after physical activity that involves vigorous quadriceps contraction or direct local trauma to the tibial tubercle area. Often the child experiences sudden acute discomfort referable to the affected region. Sudden onset of pain is caused by a pathologic fracture through an area of ischemic necrosis.

EVALUATION AND TREATMENT   Diagnosis is confirmed by roentgenographic examination. The goal of treatment for Osgood-Schlatter disease is to decrease the stress at the tubercle. Often a period of 4 to 8 weeks of restriction from strenuous physical activity, especially activities requiring deep knee bending, is sufficient. If pain relief is not achieved, a cast or brace is required to immobilize the knee, a situation that is particularly difficult if the condition is bilateral.

Gradual resumption of activity is permitted after 8 weeks, but return to unrestricted athletic participation requires an additional 8 weeks to allow for revascularization, healing, and ossification of the tibial tubercle.

Cerebral Palsy

Cerebral palsy (CP) is a static disorder of muscle tone and balance caused by an ischemic insult to the brain, usually perinatally. The incidence is presently 3% to 5% but is increasing with successful resuscitation of premature infants.

EVALUATION AND DIAGNOSIS   The diagnosis of cerebral palsy can be quite subtle but is often made when gross motor milestones are not met by predicted ages. In some infants, diagnosis can be made as early as 4 months.[29] Cognitive involvement is widely variable and is dependent on the amount of CNS involvement. There are classic patterns: hemiplegia involves one side of the body, diplegia usually involves the lower extremities only, and quadriplegia involves all four extremities. Quadraplegic involvement is most often associated with cognitive involvement, seizure disorder, and aphasia. Many quadriplegics, however, are of normal intelligence and are "trapped" within aphasia. When given communication devices, these children are sometimes "discovered," as is their normal intelligence.

TREATMENT   Treatment of cerebral palsy is multifaceted and undergoing constant evolution. The use of physical and occupational treatments, orthotics, spasticity reduction (by selected dorsal rhizotomy, oral, or intrathecal Baclofen), botulinum-A ("Botox") toxin injections, and surgery are often all used to maximize a child's function. In many centers, a multispecialty approach at "CP clinics" occurs so that a family may, within one clinic visit, see neurology, pediatrics, orthotics, orthopedic surgery, and rehabilitation clinicians.

Children with CP should be carefully followed and given all possible opportunities to flourish. Although CP is a static disorder, progressive deformity of ongoing muscle tone can occur. Monitoring these children as they grow with a multispecialty approach is essential to their optimal outcome.

Muscular Dystrophy

The **muscular dystrophies** are a group of familial disorders that cause degeneration of skeletal muscle fibers. The muscular dystrophies are the most prevalent of the muscle diseases in childhood and are characterized by progressive, symmetric weakness and wasting of skeletal muscle groups, with increasing disability and deformity.

Classification of the muscular dystrophies is based on age of onset, rate of progression, distribution of muscular involvement, and inheritance patterns. The major clinically and genetically distinct types are the pseudohypertrophic (Duchenne),

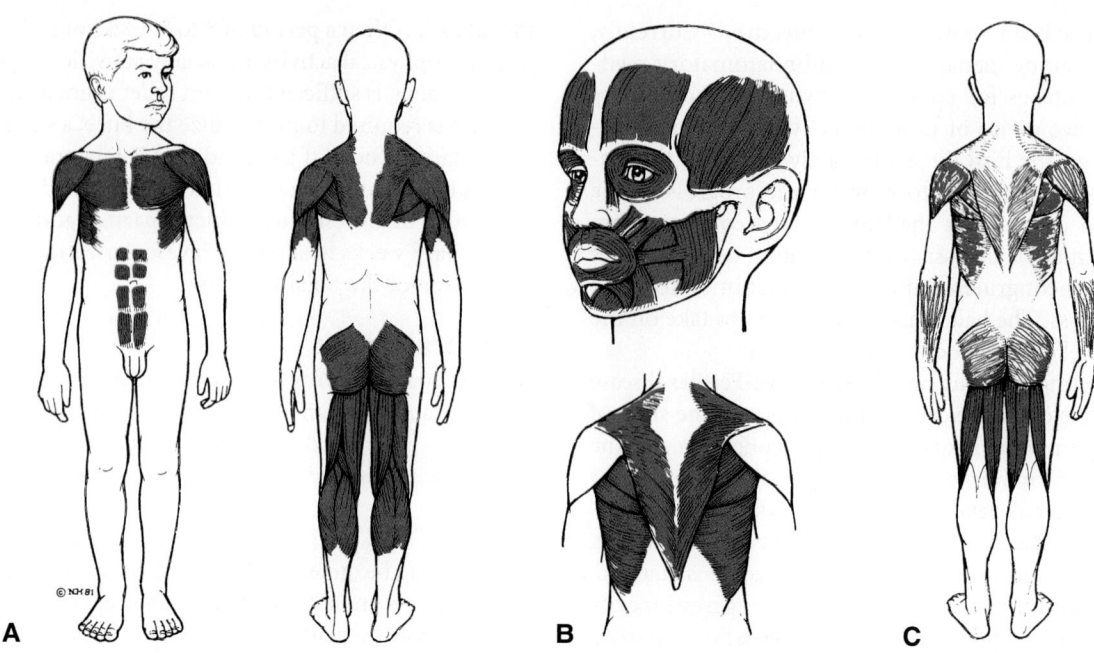

Figure 43-11 Initial muscle groups involved in three types of muscular dystrophy. **A,** Pseudohypertrophic. **B,** Facioscapulo-humeral. **C,** Limb girdle. (From Hockenberry MJ: *Wong's nursing care of infants and children,* ed 7, St Louis, 2003, Mosby.)

Table 43-4	Major Muscular Dystrophy Syndromes					
Disease	**Mode of Inheritance**	**Age at Clinical Onset**	**Usual Distribution**	**Rate of Progression**	**Mental Retardation**	**Distinguishing Findings**
Duchenne muscular dystrophy (DMD)	X-linked recessive	About 3 years	Hips and shoulders, quadriceps femoris, gastroc-nemius (pseudo-hypertrophy)	Rapid	Frequent	Elevated serum enzymes (CPK, LDH, SGOT, aldolase)
Facioscapulo-humeral dystrophy	Autosomal dominant	In first or second decade	Shoulder girdle, neck, face, pelvic girdle (late)	Moderate	Occasional	Several distinct muscle pathologic findings
Limb girdle (LG) dystrophy	Poorly defined or recessive	Variable	Pelvic and shoulder girdles	Variable	Variable	Collection of several diseases
Myotonic dystrophy (MyD)	Autosomal dominant	Variable—birth to fifth decade	Distal extensor muscle, eyelids, face, neck, hands, pharynx	Slow, related to age at clinical onset, faster with younger patients	Frequent	Percussion myotonia, cataracts, diabetic GTT despite increased insulin, testicular atropy, decreased IgG

CPK, Creatine phosphokinase; *LDH,* lactate dehydrogenase; *SGOT,* serum glutamic oxaloacetic transaminase; *GTT,* glucose tolerance test; *IgG,* immunoglobulin G.

facioscapulohumeral, limb girdle, and oculopharyngeal dystrophies (Figure 43-11). Because the clinical findings and genetic inheritance patterns are consistent for each type, some researchers believe that each involves a separate biochemical defect. Genetic research has focused on identifying the site of abnormal gene function for each defect. This will permit more accurate carrier detection and, eventually, description of the biochemical aberration. (Table 43-4 summarizes the types of muscular dystrophy.)

Duchenne Muscular Dystrophy

In 1868 the French neurologist G.B.A. Duchenne described a pseudohypertrophic muscular paralysis associated with large amounts of fat and connective tissue. Today this form of muscular dystrophy, called **Duchenne muscular dystrophy,** is the most common of the muscular dystrophies. Its incidence is approximately 1 in 3500 male births.[30] Classic Duchenne muscular dystrophy occurs only in boys and has a history of X-linked inheritance in half of the cases.

PATHOPHYSIOLOGY   The X-linked inherited type of Duchenne muscular dystrophy is thought to be caused by a deletion of a segment of deoxyribonucleic acid (DNA)[30] or a single-gene defect on the short arm of the X chromosome. A protein encoded by the Duchenne muscular dystrophy gene, called **dystrophin,** has been identified.

Dystrophin is present in normal muscle cells and absent in Duchenne muscular dystrophy. Dystrophin mediates anchorage of the actin cytoskeleton of skeletal muscle fibers to the basement membrane through a membrane glycoprotein complex. The complete lack of dystrophin in severe Duchenne dystrophy means that poorly anchored fibers tear themselves apart under the repeated stress of contraction. Free calcium then enters the muscle cells, causing cell death and fiber necrosis[31] (Figure 43-12).

There is increased endomysial connective tissue and fat; loss of striations; and concomitant hyaline, granular, and fatty degeneration of fibers. Disorganization of tendinous insertions is associated with fat accumulation in these areas. Although fibers regenerate in the younger child, they are abnormal in many ways and become nonfunctional with time.

CLINICAL MANIFESTATIONS   Duchenne muscular dystrophy is usually identified in children at approximately 3 years of age, when the parents first notice slow motor development with progressive weakness and muscle wasting. Sitting, standing, and walking are delayed, and the child is clumsy, falls frequently, and has difficulty climbing stairs.

Muscular weakness always begins in the pelvic girdle, causing a "waddling" gait. Hypertrophy of the calf muscles is apparent in 80% of cases. The method of rising from the floor by "climbing up the legs" (Gower sign) is characteristic and is caused by weakness of the lumbar and gluteal muscles. The foot assumes an equinovarus position (see Figure 43-4), and the child tends to walk on the toes because of weakness of the anterior tibial and peroneal muscles. Within 3 to 5 years, muscles of the shoulder girdle become involved. Contractures and wasting of the muscles contribute to muscular atrophy and deformity of the skeleton.

Duchenne muscular dystrophy has serious complications. Pulmonary function is compromised greatly because of marked kyphoscoliosis ("humped" upper spine combined with scoliosis), which usually develops after the child is confined to a wheelchair (Figure 43-13). The incidence of cardiac involvement in Duchenne muscular dystrophy is as high as 95%. Chronic heart failure may occur in 50% of children. A moderate degree of mental retardation causes these children to have a mean IQ of approximately 80. Smooth muscle dysfunction may cause megacolon, volvulus, cramping pain, and malabsorption in the gastrointestinal tract. The children usually succumb to other pulmonary or cardiac causes and death ensues by the late teens. Only 25% live to age 21.

EVALUATION AND TREATMENT   Diagnosis is confirmed by measurement of serum enzymes, electromyography (EMG), and muscle biopsy. The serum enzymes, especially creatine phosphokinase (CPK), are increased to more than 10 times normal, even during infancy and before the onset of weakness. Histologic changes in muscle include degeneration of muscle fibers, with variation in fiber size and central nuclei. Fat and connective tissue replace muscle fibers.

Although intrauterine diagnosis is not yet possible, work is being done in this area.[32] Elevated CPK levels at birth are diagnostic indicators of Duchenne muscular dystrophy. Identification of female carriers of the disease cannot be achieved with certainty, but serum CPK is elevated in 60% to 80% of carriers.

There is no effective treatment for Duchenne muscular dystrophy but, with characterization of the genetic deficit for Duchenne, gene therapy of Duchenne muscular dystrophy

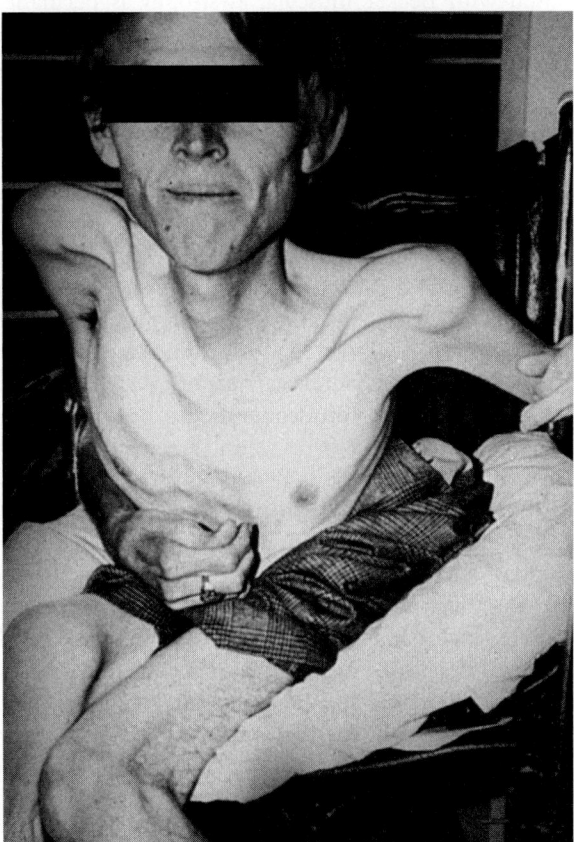

Figure 43-13 Duchenne muscular dystrophy. An individual with late-stage Duchenne muscular dystrophy, showing severe muscle loss. (From Jorde LB et al: *Medical genetics,* ed 2, St Louis, 1999, Mosby.)

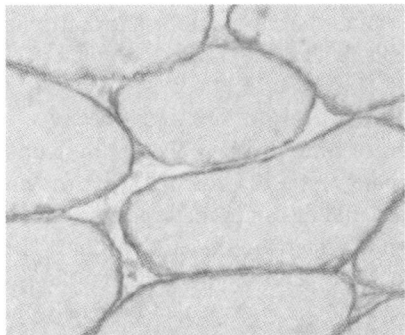

Figure 43-12 Dystrophin abnormalities. This shows staining of muscle for dystrophin (reddish brown). In Duchenne dystrophy this staining would be absent because no protein is produced. In Becker dystrophy, staining is reduced or patchy. (From Stevens A, Lowe J: *Pathology,* ed 2, St Louis, 2000, Mosby.)

now may be possible.[33] Maintaining function in unaffected muscle groups for as long as possible is the primary goal. Although activity fosters maintenance of muscle function, strenuous exercise may hasten the breakdown of muscle fibers. Range-of-motion exercises, bracing, and surgical release of contracture deformities are used to maintain normal function as long as possible. Scoliotic surgery is suggested when curves reach greater than 20 degrees to prolong respiratory function or walking ability or both. Genetic counseling is recommended. With X-linked inheritance, male siblings of an affected child have a 50% chance of being affected and female siblings have a 50% chance of being carriers.

Becker Muscular Dystrophy

Becker muscular dystrophy is often called *benign Duchenne muscular dystrophy* because it shares the X-linked inheritance pattern and similar but milder clinical features. The incidence of Becker dystrophy is one tenth that of Duchenne dystrophy. In Becker dystrophy, mutations in the middle rod region of dystrophin still allow anchorage of muscle to basement membrane. Clinical symptoms often begin between 5 and 15 years of age. Children with Becker muscular dystrophy remain ambulatory into their teens and early 20s; in one study the average age at the time of necessity for a wheelchair was 25 years.

The pattern of muscle weakness for both dystrophies is almost identical, but scoliosis and contractures are rare until the child with Becker muscular dystrophy is permanently wheelchair bound. The changes in creatine kinase levels and EMG and electrocardiogram (ECG) readings are the same as those seen in Duchenne muscular dystrophy. Many individuals live well into middle age. Heart failure is infrequent but can be a cause of premature death and disability.

Maintaining ambulation and careful follow-up for evidence of cardiopulmonary complications are essential measures for long-term care. Children with Becker muscular dystrophy rarely show the mental changes seen in Duchenne dystrophy. The accurate diagnosis of Becker muscular dystrophy is important. If the affected individual marries and has children, all daughters will be carriers of this X-linked recessive disorder. Genetic counseling should be offered to the mother, female siblings, offspring, and any maternal relatives.

Facioscapulohumeral Muscular Dystrophy

Facioscapulohumeral muscular dystrophy is a mild form of progressive, autosomal dominant muscular dystrophy. Age at onset varies from early childhood to adulthood, and the disease affects males and females equally. As the name implies, clinical manifestations begin with weakness and atrophy of facial and shoulder girdle (scapulohumeral) muscles. The illness progresses slowly. Inability to close the eyes completely may be noted from early childhood. The face is expressionless, and pouting of the lips makes whistling impossible. The first symptoms usually include drooping of the shoulders with difficulty in raising the arms above the head. Onset of weakness in the lower limbs often is delayed for 20 to 30 years, and pseudohypertrophy of muscles is rare. Contractures and

skeletal deformities develop less often and are less prominent than in Duchenne muscular dystrophy.

Treatment includes supportive physiotherapy to prevent contractures and prolong ambulation. Lightweight plastic ankle-foot orthoses (AFOs) for footdrop are extremely helpful. Surgery to stabilize the shoulder is sometimes advised.

Some individuals with facioscapulohumeral muscular dystrophy improve with steroid therapy, particularly if the clinical picture includes rapidly progressive weakness. The disease may be arrested for prolonged periods; however, most individuals remain active and have a normal life expectancy. Vocational training and genetic counseling are important to provide them with the information necessary to plan their future.

Scapuloperoneal Muscular Dystrophy

Scapuloperoneal muscular dystrophy is considered a variant of facioscapulohumeral muscular dystrophy, but distal muscles in the lower extremity are involved early instead of the facial and shoulder muscle weakness that is the early sign in facioscapulohumeral dystrophy. Many individuals seek initial treatment for troublesome footdrop and shoulder weakness. Analysis of inheritance patterns shows that the disease can be inherited either as an autosomal dominant trait or as an X-linked recessive trait.

The initial symptoms may resemble those of several other illnesses, including nemaline myopathy (a congenital muscle disease) and early hypertrophic peripheral neuropathy. A careful diagnostic evaluation therefore is in order. Other clinical findings include hypertrophy of the muscle that extends the toes, brought about by a futile attempt to overcome footdrop, and depressed or absent muscle stretch reflexes. Creatine kinase is elevated 2 to 20 times the normal level; EMG readings show myopathy.

Treatment is directed toward relieving symptoms and preserving ambulation and functional ability. Footdrop is easily treated with AFOs. Individuals with scapuloperoneal muscular dystrophy remain ambulatory for 40 or more years. Occasionally, walking may be hampered by paraspinal muscle contractures; in that case a wheelchair may assist the individual when it is necessary to cover long distances. The life span in this disorder is normal. It is important that genetic counseling be available to all persons affected.

Limb Girdle Muscular Dystrophy

The diagnosis of **limb girdle muscular dystrophy** is considered when acute causes of proximal weakness are eliminated and the clinical findings and genetic pattern exclude Duchenne and facioscapulohumeral muscular dystrophy. The diagnosis is often determined by exclusion because few consistent clinical features make this type of muscular dystrophy unique. In fact, some researchers think that limb girdle dystrophy actually may be several separate diseases awaiting more sophisticated methods of evaluation to give them precise labels. Most individuals have a negative family history, making sporadic disease or an autosomal recessive pattern of inheritance likely.

The prevalence rate for limb girdle muscular dystrophy is set at 20 per million.

The initial symptoms include shoulder and pelvic girdle weakness, which are usually noted in the early 20s but can be seen as late as the 40s. The muscle weakness is often asymmetric and progresses at a much slower pace than in Duchenne muscular dystrophy. The biceps and deltoid muscles can be extremely atrophic and weak. Individuals can remain ambulatory for extended periods, often up to 20 years after initial diagnosis. When confined to wheelchairs, they show few of the severe effects of other dystrophies, such as contractures and scoliosis. Heart involvement and mental retardation also are rare.

The individual will have mild elevation in creatine kinase levels and a myopathic pattern on EMG. Muscle biopsy is often more characteristic, with fiber splitting and fibers that appear profusely "moth-eaten" and whorled. Treatment includes supportive measures to maintain ambulation and functional ability and frequent follow-up to eliminate secondary complications such as cardiopulmonary disease.

Musculoskeletal Tumors in Children
Bone Tumors
Bone tumors are uncommon childhood tumors and comprise less than 5% of all childhood malignancies. Of the malignant tumors, osteosarcoma and Ewing sarcoma are the most common. Fortunately, the majority of pediatric tumors are benign, most commonly nonossifying fibroma, chondroma, simple bone cyst, aneurysmal bone cyst, osteoid osteoma, and fibrous dysplasia.

Benign Bone Tumors
Nonossifying Fibroma. The **nonossifying fibroma (fibrous cortical deficit),** which is believed to be a defect in ossification rather than a true tumor, makes up approximately 50% of benign bone tumors. Most fibrous cortical defects resolve spontaneously or are obliterated by reparative ossification or remodeling. In some cases, however, the fibrous cortical defect persists and proliferates, becoming a fibroma. Fibromas are found primarily in children and adolescents. Ninety percent of these tumors occur in persons younger than 20 years.

The nonossifying fibroma is a sharply demarcated, cortical-based tumor surrounded by a dense border of hardened bone. The tumor itself consists of fibrocytes arranged in whorled bundles, fibroblastic tissue, and osteoclast-like giant cells. As the tumor evolves, the fibrocytes imbibe lipids and assume a foamy appearance; thus they are known as *foam cells.* The tumor also contains extensive deposits of hemosiderin pigment. The long axis of the tumor parallels the long axis of the bone.

The nonossifying fibroma is usually asymptomatic and is found incidentally on radiographs. In the 1950s, as fluoride was added to drinking water, random skeletal surveys were done on hundreds of children. Nonossifying fribromas were discovered in 20% to 30% of all children. The fibroma is generally not treated until it occupies more than 50% of the diameter of the bone or extends more than 3 to 4 cm into the cortex. When the tumor grows to this size, a pathologic fracture may occur and, therefore, curettage and bone grafting of the defect is undertaken.

Simple Bone Cyst. **Simple bone cysts (SBCs)** are cystic lesions of the central region of the metaphysical region in skeletally mature children. With growth, these lesions may appear within the diaphysis. These children are usually asymptomatic until pathologic fracture or incidental discovery occur. Lesions often heal after a fracture, but large lesions may require treatment. Presently a large prospective, randomized study is comparing steroid injection (the classical treatment for these lesions) versus bone marrow injection for treatment. Very large lesions in weight-bearing areas may require internal fixation and bone grafting.

Aneurysmal Bone Cyst. **Aneurysmal bone cysts (ABCs)** are typically eccentric, metaphysical lesions that occur in a slightly older population than SBCs. The etiology remains controversial; many consider ABC a lesion secondary to another process, such as giant cell tumor. This lesion must be differentiated from telangestatic sarcoma and, therefore, biopsy is necessary. Once diagnosed, curettage with complete removal of the "pseudolining" must be done with chemical or electrocautery to minimize recurrence. Bone graft is placed in the defect. Even with modern techniques, recurrence can be as high as 21%.[34]

Osteoid Oteoma. **Osteoid osteoma,** or the larger counterpart osteoblastoma, present as painful lesions of the diaphysis or metadiaphysis of long bones. Involvement of the posterior elements of the spine—with resultant "splinting" scoliosis—can occur. Night pain is common, as is relief from symptoms with NSAIDs, because these tumors release prostaglandins. When pain is too extreme to be controlled medically, resection of the "nidus," or central portion, of the lesion is uniformly successful. Computed tomographic (CT) guidance to the lesion is often used and, if possible, CT-guided laser ablation can be done.

Fibrous Dysplasia. **Fibrous dysplasia (FD)** can occur in one bone (monostotic) or in multiple bones (polyostotic). Polyostotic fibrous dysplasia can occur with a triad Albright syndrome that also includes precocious puberty and cutaneous pigmentation. Although any bone can be affected, the long bones, ribs, and skull are the most common. A radiographic "ground glass" appearance is present primarily in the metaphyseal or metadiaphyseal areas. Deformity can be marked and necessitate operative intervention. When allograft is used to replace fibrous dysplasia bone, it can become involved in the fibrous dysplasia as well. The majority of individuals are simply observed; however; endocrinology management also will be involved if Albright syndrome is present.

Malignant Bone Tumors
Osteosarcoma. **Osteosarcoma** is the most common bone tumor that occurs during childhood; it originates from bone-producing mesenchymal cells. Osteosarcoma occurs most commonly in the metaphysis of long bones, especially near active physes, such as distal femur and proximal tibia. It

accounts for 60% of all malignant bone tumors and strikes between the ages of 10 to 18.

Molecular analysis has demonstrated deletion of genetic material on the long arm of chromosome 13, leading to the identification of a tumor suppressor gene as part of the mechanism for tumor development. The oncogene *src* also has been associated with osteosarcoma.

PATHOPHYSIOLOGY Osteosarcoma occurs mainly in the metaphyses of long bones. Most tumors arise in bones involved with the knee joint at the distal end of the femur or proximal end of the tibia. As a tumor of mesenchymal cells, osteosarcoma demonstrates production of osteoid tissue.

Osteosarcoma is a bulky tumor that extends beyond the bone into a soft-tissue mass. It may encircle the bone and destroy the trabeculae of the diseased bone. Osteosarcoma disseminates through the bloodstream, usually to the lung. As many as 25% of children diagnosed with osteosarcoma exhibit lung metastases at diagnosis. Other sites of metastatic spread include other bones and visceral organs.

CLINICAL MANIFESTATIONS The most common presenting complaint is pain. There may be swelling, warmth, and redness caused by the vascularity of the tumor. Symptoms also may include cough, dyspnea, and chest pain if lung metastasis is present. If a lower extremity is involved, a limp or even pathologic fracture may be present.

Initial evaluation includes roentgenographic examination that shows the osteosarcoma's characteristic osteoblastic and osteolytic changes. "Staging" studies to determine not only local extent of the tumor but also possible metastatic spread must be done. These include bone scan (to assess boney spread), magnetic resonance imaging (MRI) of the lesion (to plan surgical resection and to compare to postchemotherapy studies), and chest roentgenograms or CT or both. The chest roentgenogram must be done *before* biopsy because the general anesthetic required for biopsy can give false/positive results on the roentgenogram.

EVALUATION AND TREATMENT Tissue biopsy confirms the diagnosis, although needle biopsy is often sufficient to establish the diagnosis. There are five histologic types of osteosarcoma. The histologic type is determined by the predominant cell type. The tumor is then graded according to degree of malignancy; the higher the number is, the worse the prognosis.

Surgery and chemotherapy are the primary treatments for osteosarcoma. Radiation is occasionally used. The 5-year survival rate with modern protocols is 70%.[35]

Chemotherapy is an important component of treatment because as many as 80% of children treated with surgery alone eventually develop metastatic disease. Chemotherapy is used preoperatively to shrink the size of the tumor and minimize metastatic growth. Following chemotherapy, the child is given a short "rest period" to regain strength for surgery. Following adjunctive chemotherapy, the majority of children

now undergo "limb salvage" rather than amputation procedures. Using preoperative MRI, the extent of the lesion is mapped and a tumor-free margin is left and reconstructed either with allograft bone or arthroplasty (artificial joint). The long-term survival rates of children treated with limb salvage and chemotherapy is now near equal to amputation in 5- and 10-year survival.[36]

A number of approaches have been used to treat pulmonary metastases. Because pulmonary metastases are generally solitary, thoracotomy with wedge resection has proved the most effective treatment. Investigators have searched for adjuvant treatment to prevent pulmonary metastases, but nothing has proved useful.

Ewing Sarcoma. **Ewing sarcoma** is a malignant round cell tumor of bone and soft tissue that has a poor prognosis. It is the second most common and most lethal malignant bone tumor that can occur during childhood. This tumor is named after James Ewing, who first identified it as a separate clinical diagnosis in 1921. The most common period of diagnosis is between 5 and 15 years of age, and diagnosis is rare after 30 years of age; however, it may be seen in children younger than 3 years. Like osteosarcoma, Ewing sarcoma is slightly more common in males than females and is linked with periods of rapid bone growth. The incidence of Ewing sarcoma is less than 2% in blacks.[37]

PATHOPHYSIOLOGY Ewing sarcoma commonly occurs in the midshaft or diaphysis of long bones or in flat bones. The most common sites include the pelvis, femur, and tibia (Figure 43-14). The femur is involved in most cases, with the pelvis being the second most common site. It can occur in any bone.

Arising from bone marrow, Ewing sarcoma can break through the cortex of the bone to form a soft-tissue mass. It does not form bone, but abundant reactive bone may be present in an attempt to contain this quickly growing lesion. Metastasis occurs early and is usually apparent at diagnosis or within 1 year. The most common sites are the lung, other bones, lymph nodes, bone marrow, liver, spleen, and central nervous system, although invasion of any organ is possible.

CLINICAL MANIFESTATIONS Like osteosarcoma, the most common complaint is pain about the diaphysis that increases in severity. A soft-tissue mass is often present. Additional symptoms may include fever, malaise, and anorexia. Known as "the great imitator," Ewing sarcoma can appear radiographically identical to infection or even benign lesions such as Langerhans cell granulomatosis. Any pervasive diaphyseal or rib lesion must be regarded with a high index of suspicion.

EVALUATION AND TREATMENT In addition to plain roentgenogram, CT and MRI are needed to help establish the diagnosis and extent of the tumor. Bone scan, chest roentgenogram, and chest CT scan are also used to detect metastases. No specific laboratory test is diagnostic; however,

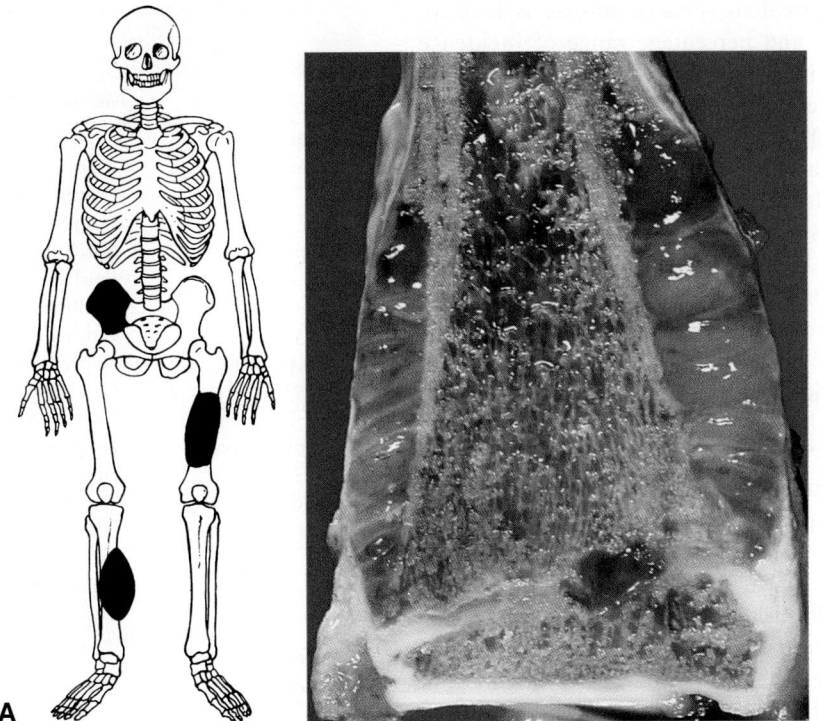

Figure 43-14 Ewing sarcoma. **A,** Most common anatomic sites. **B,** Close-up view of Ewing sarcoma of the distal end of the tibia. Tumor extends into the soft tissue. (From Damjanov I, Linder J, editors: *Anderson's pathology,* ed 10, St Louis, 1996, Mosby.)

the sedimentation rate will be elevated and lactic dehydrogenase (LDH) often is elevated. An elevated LDH level is a poor prognostic sign. Biopsy is used to conclusively establish the diagnosis. The identification of an 11:22 chromosomal translocation within the tumor cells will confirm the diagnosis of Ewing sarcoma.

The use of multidrug chemotherapy has improved survival rates. Recent treatment protocols call for preoperative chemotherapy followed by radiation or surgical resection or both, with continuation of chemotherapy for 12 to 18 months afterwards. Amputation is avoided when possible but may be considered in lower limb tumors of children younger than 8 years because of the serious discrepancy in bone growth that results if the primary treatment used is radiation, which can damage the physis. Secondary malignancies caused by high-dose radiation are also a concern.[38]

Ewing sarcoma has had a dismal prognosis, with 5-year survival rates no better than 5% to 10%. Combinations of aggressive radiation, chemotherapy, and surgical resection have, however, improved the survival rate for localized disease to more than 60%.[39] The major predictor of prognosis appears to be the location of the primary tumor and whether metastases are present at diagnosis. The most favorable sites of involvement are the extremities; the worst prognosis involves tumors of the trunk, particularly the pelvis.

Muscle Tumors

Most soft-tissue tumors in children are benign. Only two malignant soft-tissue tumors occur with any frequency—rhabdomyosarcoma in the younger child and synovial cell

Table 43-5	Classification of Tumors by Origin
Tissue	**Tumor**
Muscle	
Striated	Rhabdomyosarcoma
Smooth	Leiomyosarcoma
Adipose	Liposarcoma
Fibrous	Fibrosarcoma
Synovial mesothelium	Synovial sarcoma
Lymphatic structures	Lymphangiosarcoma
Blood vessels	Hemangiopericytoma
Nerve sheath	Neurogenic sarcoma

sarcoma in the teenager. Both of these occur rarely. The annual incidence is 8.0 per million for white children and 7.7 per million for black children. About 230 children are diagnosed with a soft-tissue tumor each year in the United States. Soft-tissue tumors originate from the primitive mesenchymal cells that normally give rise to muscle, tendons, blood vessels, lymphatic structures, fibrous and connective tissue, and bursa and fascia. Table 43-5 identifies the classification of soft-tissue tumors according to origin. All malignant soft-tissue tumors are characterized as highly aggressive tumors that invade surrounding structures and metastasize early.

Rhabdomyosarcoma (RMS) is the most common soft-tissue sarcoma of childhood and accounts for more than 50% of soft-tissue tumors but less than 3% of all childhood cancers. RMS arises from embryonal rhabdomyoblasts that normally differentiate into mature striated muscle.

RMS can develop anywhere striated muscle is located. The primary locations and percentage range of incidence are the head and neck (including the orbit), 36% to 61%; the trunk, 8% to 33%; the extremities, 14% to 24%; and the genitourinary tract, 10% to 17%. Two age ranges (2 to 6 years and 15 to 19 years) are associated with RMS. More than two thirds of children with RMS are diagnosed by 10 years of age, and RMS is slightly more common in males than females.

Recent studies demonstrate an association between *p53* (a tumor-suppressor gene) mutations and sporadic rhabdomyosarcoma.[40] Three oncogenes (*src*, H/K-*ras*, and *c-myb*) have been associated with this tumor.[41]

PATHOPHYSIOLOGY RMS generally appears as a firm, fleshy, grayish white mass. It sometimes exhibits variations that appear as a cystic polypoid mass. RMS has various appearances, depending on the phase of differentiation of the rhabdomyoblast. The cells may be round, spindle-shaped, tadpole-shaped, or multinucleated giant cells.

At least 20% of children with RMS have metastatic disease at diagnosis. The preferred sites of metastases include the lungs, lymph nodes, bone marrow, liver, brain, and bone. Another 30% have disease that is unresectable, although not widely spread. This also becomes a grave prognosis.

CLINICAL MANIFESTATIONS The signs and symptoms of RMS depend on the anatomic location of the primary tumor and presence of symptomatic metastases. The tumors are usually painless, and early detection of RMS is facilitated by the presence of a palpable or visible mass. Deep-seated tumors may cause functional impairment but can be silent until they are very large. The clinical manifestations of RMS are outlined in Table 43-6.

EVALUATION AND TREATMENT Diagnostic studies during the pretreatment phase are used to determine the extent of the primary tumor and presence or absence of distant metastases. Specific diagnostic studies depend on the primary site, but a combination of radiographic, nuclear, and CT scanning or MRI technology and blood studies is used. A biopsy of the primary tumor is necessary to confirm the diagnosis. Currently, chromosomal abnormalities are being investigated for RMS. Although not widely incorporated into clinical management at this time, identification of the DNA content has value as both a prognostic factor and a determinant of treatment.

RMS is treated by a combination of surgery, radiation, and chemotherapy. Complete surgical resection provides the greatest assurance that cure can be achieved; however, cure occurs in only 16% of children. If surgical resection leads to serious disfigurement or functional disability (e.g., enucleation for orbital tumors or cystectomy for bladder tumors), chemotherapy and radiation serve as the primary treatment and surgery is avoided or minimized. For all tumors except stage I disease, local radiation therapy is given. A variety of

Table 43-6	Clinical Manifestations of Rhabdomyosarcoma
Location	**Manifestation**
Head and Neck	
Orbit	Ptosis
	Exophthalmos
	Proptosis
Paranasal sinuses	Nasal obstruction
	Epistaxis
	Swelling
	Chronic sinusitis
Nasopharnx	Hypernasal speech
	Nasal discharge
	Visible polypoid mass
Oropharyngeal	Dysphagia
	Painful mastication
Middle ear	Chronic serous otitis media
	Discharge from affected ear
	Facial nerve palsy
	Conduction hearing loss
	Visible polypoid mass
Extremities	
All locations	Deep-seated, fixed palpable mass
Retroperitoneal	
All locations	Usually asymptomatic
	May have vague abdominal pain
	Bowel or genitourinary obstruction (late)
	Possible palpable mass
Genitourinary	
Vaginal	Abnormal vaginal bleeding
	Protruding polypoid mass
Prostate	Urinary tract obstruction
Bladder	Urinary retention
	Straining to void
	Hematuria
Paratesticular	Mass in scrotum that may be painful

combination chemotherapies are used for RMS. Chemotherapy for stage I or II disease is given for 1 year if disease does not recur. For stage III or IV, treatment (combined with radiation therapy) continues an additional year. Intrathecal chemotherapy is given to children whose tumor locations favor central nervous system spread.

The primary prognostic factor in RMS is the degree of residual disease after surgical resection. Children with localized disease (stages I and II) have long-term survival rates of 70% to 80%. If widespread disease is present, long-term survival rates drop to 20%. Orbital tumors have an overall favorable prognosis, probably because of the lack of lymphatics in the area and early physical signs of disease.

NONACCIDENTAL TRAUMA

Abuse is estimated to occur in over 1.5 million children per year in the United States. The maltreatment may be psychological, sexual, and/or physical. Of children who suffer physical abuse, 30% are initially seen by an orthopedist. Accurate and appropriate referrals to child protection are not only legally mandated but also essential for the well-being of the child; an abused child who returns unmonitored to an abusive situation has a 15% chance of mortality.

ETIOLOGY   Children who are not yet ambulatory and present with a long bone fracture have over a 75% chance of that fracture being caused by **nonaccidental trauma.** "Corner" metaphyseal fractures, caused by a twisting force, are nearly pathognomonic of abuse but occur only 25% of the time (Figure 43-15). Fractures at multiple stages of healing are also suggestive; however, osteogenesis imperfecta must be ruled out. The most common presentation is a transverse tibia fracture.[42] After walking age, only 2% of long bone fractures are the result of nonaccidental trauma.[43]

EVALUATION   If suspected, nonaccidental trauma necessitates early consultation with child protective services. The child should undergo skeletal radiographic survey, especially if less than 2 years of age, and have a complete physical examination to evaluate for patterned bruising, burns, or multiple soft tissue injuries. Ophthalmologic examination should be used to evaluate for retinal hemorrhage caused by shaking. A thorough history must be obtained for all identified injuries. It is important to remember that social isolation can lead to increased likelihood of abuse, but no social strata is immune.

When cause is unclear, bone scan can be helpful in diagnosing subtle injuries, especially rib fractures. Posterior rib fractures are especially likely to be caused by abuse. MRI and CT of the brain can help diagnose injuries caused by shaking.

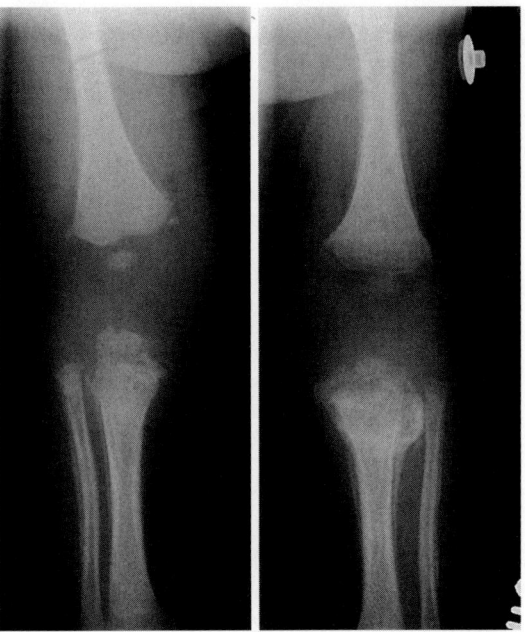

Figure 43-15 Corner fracture. Bilateral knee radiograph showing healing corner fractures of bilateral proximal tibias and distal femurs. Note the varying amount of callus formation signifying fractures at different stages of healing.

TREATMENT   A nonjudgmental attitude on the part of the treating health care provider is essential. The child and family involved in nonaccidental trauma are delicate and require not only physical but emotional care. Social workers need to be involved early to ensure appropriate medical care to the child. Fortunately, fractures heal quickly in young children; neurologic injury and social disease, however, are much more difficult to cure.

SUMMARY REVIEW

Musculoskeletal Development in Children

1. Skeletal growth and development consists of two phases: (a) delivery of bone cell precursors to sites of bone formation and (b) the aggregation of these cells at primary centers of ossification where they mature to secrete osteoid.
2. Ossification takes place in two centers in long bones: (a) the primary center, or the diaphysis (the long, central portion of the bone); and (b) the secondary center, or the epiphysis (the end portions of the bone).
3. Peak bone mass is achieved by mid to late 20s.
4. Fifty percent of the total growth of the spine has occurred by 1 year of age, and most children have achieved 50% of their adult height by 2 years of age.
5. The appendicular skeleton (extremities) grows faster during childhood than does the axial skeleton.
6. Muscle fibers reach their maximal size in females at 10 years of age and at 14 years of age in males.

Musculoskeletal Alterations in Children

1. The most common congenital defect of the upper extremities is syndactyly (webbing of the fingers).
2. Developmental dysplasia of the hip is a serious and disabling condition in children if not diagnosed and treated.

3. Congenital muscle disorders (myopathies) include absence of muscles, hypoplasia, hyperplasia, and faulty intrinsic development.
4. Osteogenesis imperfecta (brittle bone disease) is an inherited disorder of collagen that affects primarily bones and results in serious fractures of many bones.
5. Rickets is a condition caused by deficiencies in vitamin D, calcium, and usually phosphorus that is characterized by the failure of bones to become mineralized (ossified) and results in skeletal deformity.
6. Scoliosis is a lateral curvature of the spinal column that can be caused by congenital malformations of the spine, neuromuscular disease, trauma, extraspinal contractures, bone infections, metabolic bone disorders, joint disease and tumors.
7. Osteomyelitis is a local or generalized bacterial infection of bone and bone marrow. Bacteria are usually introduced by direct extension from a nearby infection, through the bloodstream, or by trauma.
8. Juvenile rheumatoid arthritis is an inflammatory joint disorder characterized by pain and swelling.
9. Avascular diseases of the bone are collectively referred to as osteochondroses and are caused by an insufficient blood supply to growing bones.

Continued

10. Legg-Calvé-Perthes disease is one of the most common osteo-chondroses. This disorder is characterized by epiphyseal necrosis or degeneration of the head of the femur followed by regeneration or recalcification.
11. Osgood-Schlatter disease is characterized by inflammation or partial separation of the tibial tubercle caused by chronic irritation, usually as a result of overuse of the quadriceps muscles. The condition is seen primarily in muscular, athletic adolescent males.
12. The muscular dystrophies are a group of genetically transmitted diseases characterized by progressive atrophy of symmetric groups of skeletal muscles without evidence of involvement or degeneration of neural tissue. There is an insidious loss of strength in all forms of the disorder with increasing disability and deformity.
13. Benign bone tumors include nonossifying fibroma, simple bone cysts, aneursysmal bone cysts, osteoid osteoma, and fibrous dysplasia.
14. The two main types of malignant childhood bone tumors are osteosarcoma and Ewing sarcoma.
15. Osteosarcoma, the most common malignant childhood bone tumor, originates in bone-producing mesenchymal cells and is most often located in the distal end of the femur or proximal end of the tibia.
16. Most childhood osteosarcoma tumors occur between the ages of 10 and 18 years of age.
17. Ewing sarcoma originates from cells within the bone marrow space and is located most often in the midshaft of long bones or in flat bones.
18. Ewing sarcoma is more common in males and is diagnosed most often between the ages of 5 and 15 years.
19. Pain is the usual presenting symptom for either osteosarcoma or Ewing sarcoma.
20. The primary treatments for osteosarcoma are surgery and chemotherapy. The primary treatment for Ewing sarcoma is a combination of chemotherapy, radiation, and surgery.
21. The most common type of childhood soft-tissue tumor is rhabdomyosarcoma.
22. Rhabdomyosarcoma originates from embryonal rhabdomyoblasts that normally differentiate into mature striated muscle.
23. Clinical manifestations of rhabdomyosarcoma depend on the anatomic location; superficial tumors exhibit a painless palpable mass, whereas deep-seated tumors cause functional impairment.
24. Rhabdomyosarcoma is treated with a combination of surgery, radiation, and chemotherapy.

Nonaccidental Trauma

1. Nonaccidental trauma must be considered with any long bone injury in a preambulatory child.
2. Evidence of soft tissue injury, corner fractures, and fractures at different stages of healing are extremely helpful in making a diagnosis of nonaccidental trauma.
3. When nonaccidental trauma is suspected, a child must be evaluated radiographically for other fractures, head trauma, and retinal hemorrhage.
4. All social strata are at risk.
5. The health care provider is legally responsible to report suspected nonaccidental trauma.

KEY TERMS

Aneurysmal bone cysts (ABCs), 1565
Becker muscular dystrophy, 1564
Cartilage anlage, 1547
Cerebral palsy (CP), 1561
"Corner" metaphyseal fracture, 1569
Developmental dysplasia of the hip (DDH), 1550
Duchenne muscular dystrophy, 1562
Dystrophin, 1562
Endochondral formation of bone, 1547
Ewing sarcoma, 1566
Facioscapulohumeral muscular dystrophy, 1564
Fibrous dysplasia (FD), 1565
Genu valgum (knock knee), 1549
Genu varum (bowleg), 1549
Idiopathic equinovarus, 1552
Idiopathic scoliosis, 1555
Intramembranous formation of bone, 1547

Involucrum, 1557
Juvenile rheumatoid arthritis (JRA), 1559
Kyphosed, 1549
Legg-Calvé-Perthes disease, 1560
Limb girdle muscular dystrophy, 1564
Lordotic, 1549
Metatarsus adductus, 1551
Muscular dystrophies, 1561
Nonaccidental trauma, 1569
Nonossifying fibroma (fibrous cortical deficit), 1565
Nonstructural scoliosis, 1555
Osgood-Schlatter disease, 1561
Osteochondrosis, 1559
Osteogenesis imperfecta (brittle bone disease), 1552
Osteoid osteoma, 1565
Osteomyelitis, 1556
Osteosarcoma, 1565

Perichondrium, 1547
Periosteal collar, 1547
Pes planus (flatfoot), 1552
Physeal closure, 1548
Positional equinovarus, 1551
Primary centers of ossification, 1547
Rhabdomyosarcoma (RMS), 1567
Rickets, 1554
Scapuloperoneal muscular dystrophy, 1564
Scoliosis, 1555
Secondary center of ossification, 1548
Secondary septic arthritis, 1557
Sequestrum (*pl.,* sequestra), 1557
Simple bone cysts (SBCs), 1565
Structural scoliosis, 1555
Syndactyly, 1549
Teratologic equinovarus, 1552
Vestigial tabs, 1550

MEDIA RESOURCES

Review questions and answers for this chapter are available in the *CD Companion* included with this book.

WebLinks—links to Internet sites pertaining to this chapter—are available on Evolve at http://evolve.elsevier.com/McCance/.

REFERENCES

1. Simkin P: The musculoskeletal system. In Klippel JH, Dieppe PA, editors: *Rheumatology,* ed 2, London, 1998, Mosby.
2. Weinstein SL: Congenital hip dislocation: long range problems, residual signs, and symptoms after successful treatments, *Clin Orthop Relat Res* Aug(281):69-74, 1992.
3. Weintraub S, Grill F: Ultrasonography in developmental dysplasia of the hip, *J Bone Joint Surg Am* 82-A(7):1004, 2000.

4. Ippolito E et al: Long-term comparative results in patients with congenital clubfoot treated with two different protocols, *Arch Gynecol Obstet* 268(4):331-332, 2003.

5. Dobbs MB et al: Factors predictive of outcome after use of the Ponseti method for the treatment of idiopathic clubfeet, *J Bone Joint Surg Am* 86-A(1):22-27, 2004.

6. Zaleske DJ, Doppelt SH, Mankin HJ: Endocrine abnormalities of the immature skeleton. In Lovell WW, Winter RB, editors: *Pediatric orthopedics*, ed 2, Philadelphia, 1986, Lippincott.

7. Rauch F et al: Bone mass, size, and density in children and adolescents with osteogensis imperfecta: effect of intravenous pamidronate therapy, *Bone Miner Res* 18(4):610-614, 2003.

8. Zeitlin L et al: Modern approach to children with osteogenesis imperfecta, *J Pediatr Orthop B* 12(2):77-87, 2003.

9. Wharton B, Bishop N: Rickets, *Lancet* 362(9393):1389-1400, 2003.

10. Barrack R et al: Vibratory hypersensitivity in idiopathic sclerosis, *J Pediatr Orthop* 8(4):389, 1988.

11. Byrd JA III: Current theories on the etiology of idiopathic scoliosis, *Clin Orthop Relat Res* Apr(299):114-119, 1988.

12. Vijermans V et al: Factors determining the final outcome of treatment of idiopathic scoliosis with the Boston brace: a longitudinal study, *J Pediatr Orthop B* 13(3):143-149, 2004.

13. Kindsfater K et al: Levels of platelet calmodulin for the prediction of progression and severity of adolescent idiopathic scoliosis, *J Bone Joint Surg Am* 76(8):1186, 1994.

14. Caksen H et al: Septic arthritis in childhood, *Pediatr Int* 42(5):534, 2000.

15. Gillespie WJ et al: Aspects of the microbe: host relationship in staphylococcal hematogenous osteomyelitis, *Orthopedics* 10(3):475, 1987.

16. Hedström SA, Lidgren L: Septic arthritis and osteomyelitis. In Klippel JH, Dieppe PA, editors: *Rheumatology*, ed 2, London, 1998, Mosby.

17. Przybylski GJ, Sharan AD: Single-stage autogenous bone grafting and internal fixation in the surgical management of pyogenic discitis and vertebral osteomyelitis, *J Neurosurg* 94(1 suppl):1, 2001.

18. Ray NJ, Basset RL: Pyogenic vertebral osteomyelitis, *Orthopedics* 8(4):504, 1985.

19. Mader JT et al: The host and skeletal infection: classification and pathogenesis of acute bacterial bone and joint sepsis, *Baillieres Best Pract Res Clin Rheumatol* 13(1):1, 1999.

20. Perlman M et al: The incidence of joint involvement of adjacent osteomyelitis in pediatric patients, *J Pediatr Orthop* 20(1):40, 2000.

21. Cassidy JT: *Textbook of pediatric rheumatology,* New York, 1982, Wiley & Sons.

22. Hollingworth P: Juvenile chronic arthritis. In Klippel JH, Dieppe PA, editors: *Rheumatology*, ed 2, London, 1998, Mosby.

23. Guille JT et al: Bilateral Legg-Calvé-Perthes disease: presentation and outcome, *J Pediatr Orthop* 22(4):458-463, 2002.

24. Glueck CJ et al: Association of antithrombotic factor deficiencies and hypofibrinolysis with Legg-Perthes disease, *J Bone Joint Surg Am* 78(1):3-13, 1996.

25. Herring JA et al: The lateral pillar classification of Legg-Calvé-Perthes disease, *J Pediatr Orthop* 12(2):143-150, 1992.

26. Schoenecker PL et al: Legg-Perthes disease in children under 6 years old, *Orthop Rev* 22:201, 1993.

27. Askoy MC et al: Comparison between braced and non-braced Legg-Calvé-Perthes-disease: a radiological outcome study, *J Pediatr Orthop B* 13(3):153-157, 2004.

28. Gigante A et al: What is the best treatment for Osgood-Schlatter disease? *J Fam Pract* 53(2):153-156, 2004.

29. Swanson MW et al: Identification of neurodevelopmental abnormality at 4 and 8 months by the movement assessment of infants, *Dev Med Child Neurol* 34(4):321-337, 1992.

30. Scott MO et al: Duchenne muscular dystrophy gene expression in normal and diseased human muscle, *Science* 239:1418, 1988.

31. Stevens A, Lowe J: *Pathology,* London, 1995, Mosby.

32. Nevo Y et al: Fetal muscle biopsy as a diagnostic tool in Duchenne muscular dystrophy, *Prenat Diag* 19(10):921, 1999.

33. Kapsa R et al: Novel therapies for Duchenne muscular dystrophy, *Lancet Neurol* 2(5):299-310, 2003.

34. Campanacci M, Capanna R, Picci P: Unicameral and aneurysmal bone cysts, *Clin Ortho Relat Res* Mar(204):25-36, 1986.

35. Glasser DB et al: Survival, prognosis, and therapeutic response in osteogenic sarcoma: the Memorial Hospital experience, *Cancer* 69(3):698-708, 1992.

36. Rougraff BT et al: Limb salvage compared with amputation for osteocarcoma of the distal end of the femur, *J Bone Joint Surg Am* 76(5):649-656, 1994.

37. Ayala AG, Ro JY, Raymond AK: Bone tumors. In Damjanov I, Linder J, editors: *Anderson's pathology,* ed 10, St Louis, 1996, Mosby.

38. Smith LM, Cox RS, Donaldson SS: Second cancers in long term survivors of Ewing's sarcoma, *Clin Orthop Relat Res* Jan(274):275-281, 1992.

39. Ruyman FB, Grovas AC: Progress in the diagnosis and treatment of rhabdomyosarcoma and related soft tissue sarcomas, *Cancer Invest* 18(3):223, 2000.

40. Lugo-Vicente H: Molecular biology and genetics affecting pediatric solid tumors, *Bol Asoc Med P R* 92(4-8):72-82, 2000.

41. Israel MA: Molecular and cellular biology in pediatric malignancies. In Pizzo PA, editor: *Principles and practices of pediatric oncology,* Philadelphia, 1989, Lippincott.

42. King J et al: Analysis of 429 fractures in 189 battered children, *J Pediatr Orthop* 8(5):585-589, 1988.

43. Thomas SA et al: Long-bone fracture in young children: distinguishing accidental injuries from child abuse, *Pediatrics* 88(3):471-476, 1991.

STRUCTURE, FUNCTION, AND DISORDERS OF THE INTEGUMENT

NOREEN HEER NICOL • SUE E. HUETHER • ROBIN WEBER

CHAPTER OUTLINE

The skin covers the entire body and is the largest body organ accounting for approximately 20% of the body's weight. Combined with the accessory structures of hair, nails, and glands, it forms the *integumentary system.* The primary function of the skin is to protect the body from the environment by serving as a barrier against microorganisms, ultraviolet radiation, loss of body fluids, and the stress of mechanical forces. The skin also regulates body temperature within a very narrow range and is involved in the production of vitamin D. Touch and pressure receptors provide important protective functions and pleasurable sensations.

STRUCTURE AND FUNCTION OF THE SKIN

Layers of the Skin
The skin consists of three layers: the outer layer of epidermis, a deeper layer of dermis, and the subcutaneous layer (Figure 44-1 and Table 44-1). This underlying subcutaneous layer of connective tissue contains macrophages, fibroblasts, and fat cells.

Epidermis
The **epidermis** grows continually by shedding the superficial layer of **stratum corneum,** which is formed primarily of keratinocytes and melanocytes. These cells are named for the substances they produce. **Keratinocytes** produce **keratin,** a scleroprotein. Keratin is the main constituent of skin, hair, and nail cells. The thickness of the epidermis varies from 0.3 mm on the eyelids to 1.5 mm on the palms of the hands and soles of the feet. New cells (keratinocytes) formed in the **basal layer (stratum basale)** move upward and differentiate, forming the **spinous layer (stratum spinosum).** Together they form the **germinative layer (stratum germinativum).** The cells enlarge and then become flattened, stacked, and cornified (stratum corneum) as they ascend to the skin surface. Cornification, or keratinization, prevents dehydration of

deeper skin layers. The average turnover of the epidermis is about 30 days.

The epidermis has three additional types of cells that facilitate its functional characteristics: melanocytes, Langerhans cells, and Merkel cells. The **melanocytes** are usually located near the base of the epidermis. They synthesize and secrete the pigment melanin with exposure to ultraviolet light in response to melanocyte-stimulating hormone (MSH). Melanin in the epidermis provides a shield against ultraviolet radiation and determines skin color. **Langerhans cells** migrate to the epidermis from the bone marrow. The Langerhans cells (a type of dendritic cell) initiate an immune response and provide a defense against environmental antigens. **Merkel cells** are associated with touch receptors, and they function as slowly adapting mechanoreceptors when stimulated by deformation of the epidermis.

Dermis

The **dermis** varies from 1 to 4 mm in thickness and is composed of three types of connective tissue: (1) collagen, (2) elastin and reticulin, and (3) a gel-like ground substance. The haphazard arrangement of connective tissue allows the skin to be mobile and to stretch and contract with body movement. Hair follicles, sebaceous glands, sweat glands, blood vessels, lymphatic vessels, and nerves are contained in the dermis. The conelike projections of the papillary dermis interface with the epidermis. The papillae provide texture to the surface of the skin by forming what are known as *rete pegs*.

The cells of the dermis include fibroblasts, mast cells, and macrophages. Fibroblasts secrete the connective tissue matrix. Mast cells release histamine and play a role in hypersensitivity reactions in the skin. Macrophages are phagocytic and participate in immune responses. Histiocytes are macrophages that reside in loose connective tissue and phagocytize pigments and the debris of inflammation.

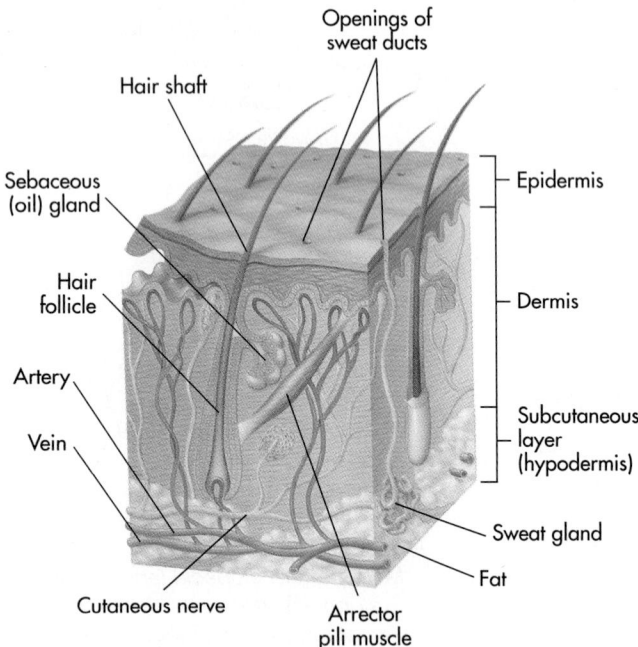

Figure 44-1 Structure of the skin. (From Thibodeau GA, Patton KT: *Anatomy and physiology*, ed 5, St Louis, 2003, Mosby.)

Table 44-1	Layers of the Skin	
Structure	**Cell Types**	**Characteristics**
Epidermis	Keratinocytes	Most important layer of skin; normally very thin (0.12 mm) but can thicken and form corns or calluses with constant pressure or friction
	Melanocytes	
	Merkel cells	
	Langerhans cells	Cells with dendrite process and immune functions
Stratum corneum	Keratinocytes	Tough superficial layer covering the body
Stratum lucidum	Keratinocytes	Clear layers of cells containing eleidin, which becomes keratin as cells move up to corneum layer
	Melanocytes	Melanocytes synthesize the pigment melanin
Stratum granulosum	Keratinocytes	
	Melanocytes	Keratohyalin gives a granular appearance to this layer
Stratum spinosum	New keratinocytes	Polygonal-shaped with spinous processes projecting between adjacent keratinocytes
Stratum basale (germinativum)	Keratinocytes	
	Melanocytes	Basal layer where keratinocytes divide and move upward to replace cells shed from the surface
	Merkel cells	The function of Merkel cells is not clearly known
Dermis	Macrophages	Irregular connective tissue layer with rich blood, lymphatic, and nerve supply; contains sensory receptors and special glands
Papillary layer (thin)	Mast cells	
Reticular layer (thick)	Histiocytes	Histiocytes are wandering macrophages that collect pigments and inflammatory debris
Subcutaneous		Subcutaneous tissue or superficial fascia of varying thickness that connects the overlying dermis to underlying muscle

Subcutaneous Layer

The third layer of the skin is subcutaneous tissue and consists of fat cells or adipocytes. The lobules are separated by fibrous walls (septa) of collagen and large blood vessels. Dermal collagen is continuous with the collagen found in the subcutaneous tissue.[1]

Dermal Appendages

The **dermal appendages** include the nails, hair, sebaceous glands, and the eccrine and apocrine sweat glands. The **nails** are protective keratinized plates that appear at the ends of fingers and toes. Each nail is composed of four structural units: (1) the proximal nail fold, (2) the matrix from which the nail grows, (3) the hyponychium (nail bed), and (4) the nail plate (Figure 44-2). Nail growth is continuous throughout life at a rate of 1 mm or less per day.

Hair follicles and sebaceous glands are integrated units (see Figure 44-1). Hair color, density, grain, and pattern of distribution have considerable variability and depend on age, gender, and race. **Hair follicles** arise from the matrix (or bulb) located deep in the dermis. They extend from the dermis at an angle and have an erector pili muscle attached near the middermis that straightens the follicle when contracted, causing the hair to stand up. Hair growth begins in the bulb, with cellular differentiation of stem cells occurring as the hair progresses up the follicle.[2] Hair is fully hardened, or cornified, by the time it emerges at the skin surface. Hair growth is cyclic, with periods of growth and rest that vary over different body surfaces.

The **sebaceous glands** open onto the surface of the skin through a canal. They are found in greatest numbers on the face, chest, and back; modified glands are found on the eyelids, lips, nipple, glans penis, and prepuce. Sebaceous glands secrete sebum that is composed primarily of lipids; sebum oils the skin and hair and prevents drying. Growth of sebaceous glands is stimulated by androgens, and their enlargement is one of the early signs of puberty.

The **eccrine sweat glands** are distributed over the body, with the greatest numbers in the palms of the hands, soles of the feet, and forehead. These secretions are important in thermoregulation and cooling of the body through evaporation. The **apocrine sweat glands** are fewer in number and are located in the axillae, scalp, face, abdomen, and genital area and have very limited proven function.

Blood Supply and Innervation

The blood supply to the skin is limited to the **papillary capillaries,** or plexus, of the dermis. These capillary loops arise from a subpapillary plexus that is supplied by a deeper horizontal cutaneous arterial plexus. Branches from the deep plexus supply hair follicles and sweat glands. A subpapillary network of veins drains the capillary loops. Arteriovenous anastomoses in the dermis facilitate the regulation of body temperature. Heat loss can be regulated by varying blood flow through the skin by opening and closing the arteriovenous anastomoses in conjunction with evaporative heat loss of sweat. The sympathetic nervous system regulates both vasoconstriction and vasodilation through the α-adrenergic receptors. The lymphatic vessels of the skin arise in the papillary dermis and drain into larger subcutaneous trunks, removing cells, proteins, and immunologic mediators.

AGING AND SKIN INTEGRITY

Many age-associated changes in the skin are readily observable and appear over the body surface. Both genetic and environmental factors, particularly ultraviolet radiation from sun exposure (photoaging), contribute to cutaneous changes with aging.[3,4] Structurally the skin becomes thinner, drier, and wrinkled with a change in pigmentation.[5,6] The cellular alterations contributing to the changes include a flattening of the dermoepidermal junction with a shortening and decrease in the number of capillary loops. There are fewer melanocytes, resulting in decreased protection against ultraviolet radiation. A significant decrease in the number of Langerhans cells decreases the skin's immune response with aging. The thickness of the dermis also decreases and accounts for the translucent, paper-thin quality of the skin. Loss of the rete pegs gives the skin a smooth, shiny appearance.[7]

The decreased vasculature and lymphatic drainage contribute to loss of barrier protection and the atrophy of eccrine, apocrine, and sebaceous glands that causes dry skin.[8] Loss of elastin fibers is associated with wrinkling. The collagen fibers become less flexible and decrease the ability of the skin to stretch and regain shape. Decreased cell proliferation,[9] decreased blood supply, and depressed immune responses also delay wound healing in aging skin. Changes in hair color and distribution also occur. Graying is caused by loss of melanocytes from hair bulbs, and thinning occurs from a gradual decline in the number of hair follicles and growth of finer hair.

The epidermal cells change shape, and the barrier function of the stratum corneum is reduced. There is increased permeability and decreased clearance of substances from the dermis. The accumulation of such substances is related to decreased vascularity and can cause skin irritation. Temperature

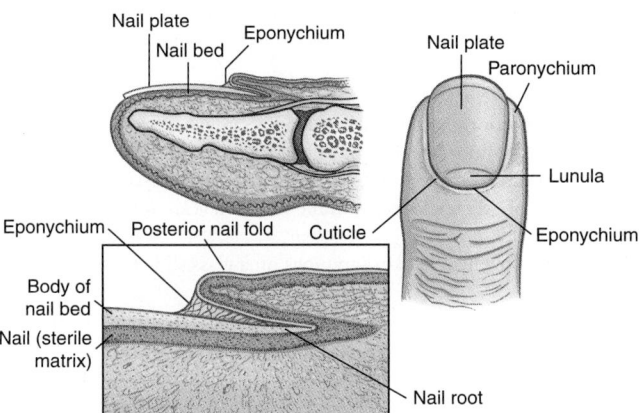

Figure 44-2 Structures of the nail. (Redrawn from Thompson JM et al: *Mosby's clinical nursing,* ed 5, St Louis, 2002, Mosby.)

regulation is compromised in elderly persons, and there is an increased risk for both heat stroke and hypothermia. Loss of cutaneous vasomotion and subcutaneous fat, decreased vascularity, and decreased eccrine sweat production are contributing factors. The pressure and touch receptors and free nerve endings all decrease in number and reduce sensory perception. Many of the protective functions of the skin are decreased with aging,[10] and there is increased risk of infection and delay in wound healing.[11,12]

Tests of Skin Function

Diagnostic evaluations of skin disorders often can be completed by gathering historical information, performing a physical examination, and observing the distribution and characteristics of the presenting lesions. Additional diagnostic studies are summarized in Table 44-2.

Clinical Manifestations of Skin Dysfunction
Lesions

Lesions of the skin are readily observable and easily assessed for distribution and structure. Identification of the morphologic structure and appearance of the skin in combination with a health history is necessary to identify the underlying pathophysiology. Table 44-3 describes and illustrates the basic lesions of the skin. Special skin lesions are described in Table 44-4.

Pressure Ulcers

Pressure ulcers are any lesions caused by unrelieved pressure resulting in damage of underlying tissue. Four factors contribute to the development of pressure ulcers: pressure, shearing forces, friction, and moisture. Pressure that consistently interrupts blood flow to the skin is the most significant causative factor.[13,14] The term *decubitus ulcer* refers to an ulcer or pressure sore that results when an individual lies in the re-

cumbent position for a long time. The more general terms of *pressure sore* or *ulcer* are used here. Factors associated with greatest risk are as follows:[15]

1. Elderly in hospitals and nursing homes
2. Neurologic disorders that result in loss of mobility and/or sensation (spinal cord injuries, dementia, or cerebrovascular disease)
3. Immobilization
4. Incontinence
5. Debilitation
6. Lying in bed without changing position or relieving pressure over an extended period
7. Lying for hours on hard imaging and operating tables
8. Chronic diseases accompanied by anemia, edema, renal failure, malnutrition, sepsis, and urinary or fecal incontinence
9. Coarse bed sheets used for turning by dragging, which produces a shearing force

Risk factors for the critically ill include the following:[16]

1. Norepinephrine infusion
2. APACHE II score
3. Fecal incontinence
4. Anemia
5. Length of hospital stay

Most individuals with darkly pigmented skin are at greater risk for the development of pressure ulcers because early signs of skin damage may not be clearly visible.[17,18] Pressure sores usually develop over bony prominences. The sacrum, heels, ischia, and greater trochanters are the most common sites. Continuous pressure on tissue between the bony prominence and a resistant outside surface distorts capillaries and occludes the blood flow and oxygen supply. If the pressure is relieved within a few hours, a brief period of reactive hyperemia (redness) occurs with no lasting tissue damage. If the pressure continues

Table 44-2	Summary of Skin Diagnostic Procedures
Test	**Purpose**
Skin biopsy	Histologic examination of tissue to determine differential diagnosis of cellular structure (i.e., benign growths vs. carcinoma, chronic infections, blistering diseases, and vasculitis)
Microscopic immunofluorescence	Identification of antibodies, immunoglobulins, and complement components for diseases such as pemphigus, vasculitis, and discoid lupus erythematosus using fluorescent light on slide-mounted biopsy specimens
Gram stain	Differentiation of gram-positive from gram-negative bacteria according to stain absorption
Culture	Identification of chronic bacterial and fungal infections by incubating skin specimens in culture media
Wood lamp examination	Examination of skin or hair to identify fungus that fluoresces bright yellow-green under ultraviolet light
Patch and scratch tests	Application of suspected allergens to skin by patch or scratch for evaluation of immune system responses to known allergens and evaluation of cell-mediated immune function (*Candida albicans*, skin fungus, chemicals, aeroallergens, and foods)
Skin scrapings	Application of potassium hydroxide (KOH) and low heat to skin scrapings on a glass slide to identify dermatophytes and *Candida albicans*
Side lighting	Indirect lighting of the skin using light to the side of the lesions to evaluate patterns of depression and elevation of skin lesions
Diascopy	Use of glass or clear plastic pressed on the skin to differentiate erythema caused by dilated capillaries (blanching) from extravasation of blood (no blanching)
Tzanck	A microscopic examination of cellular material from skin lesions to help diagnose vesicular diseases, including herpes simplex virus and varicella zoster

Table 44-3   Primary and Secondary Skin Lesions

Primary Skin Lesions	Examples		

Macule
A flat, circumscribed area that is a change in the color of the skin; less than 1 cm in diameter

Freckles, flat moles (nevi), petechiae, measles, scarlet fever

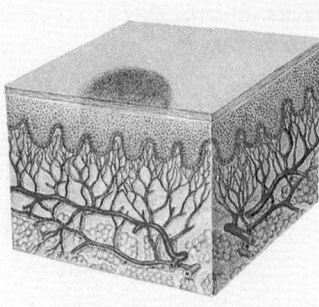 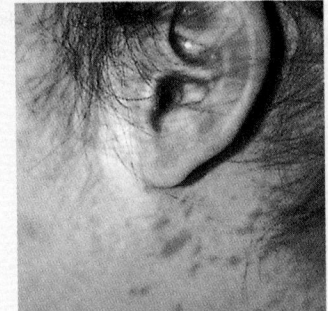

Macules[c]

Papule
An elevated, firm, circumscribed area less than 1 cm in diameter

Wart (verruca), elevated moles, lichen planus

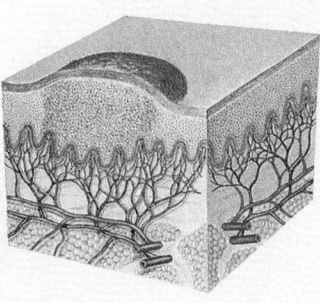 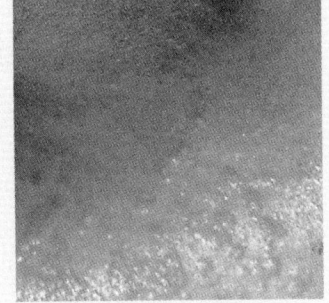

Flat warts[c]
(Courtesy Dr. E Sahn.)

Patch
A flat, nonpalpable, irregular-shaped macule more than 1 cm in diameter

Vitiligo, port-wine stains, mongolian spots, café au lait spot

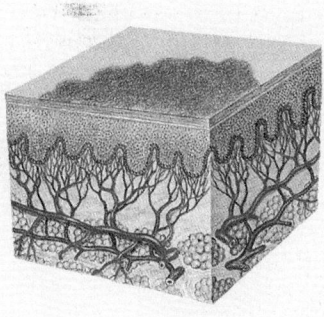 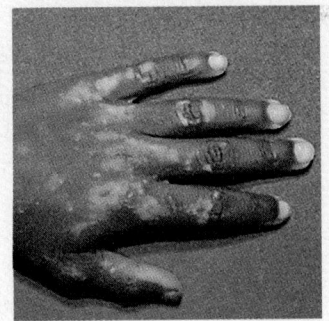

Vitiligo[h]

Plaque
Elevated, firm, and rough lesion with flat top surface greater than 1 cm in diameter

Psoriasis, seborrheic and actinic keratoses

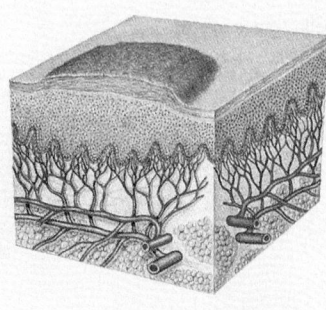 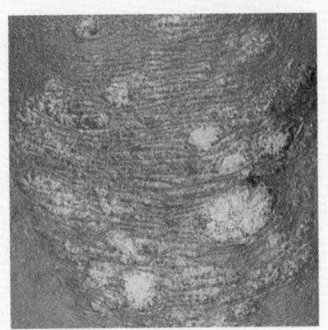

Plaque[e]

From Thompson JM, Wilson SF: *Health assessment for nursing practice,* St Louis, 2002, Mosby.
[c]Farrar WE et al: *Infectious diseases,* ed 2, London, 1992, Gower.
[e]Habif TP: *Clinical dermatology,* ed 4, St Louis, 2004, Mosby.
[h]Weston WL, Lane AT: *Color textbook of pediatric dermatology,* ed 3, St Louis, 2002, Mosby.

Continued

Table 44-3   Primary and Secondary Skin Lesions—cont'd

Primary Skin Lesions	Examples		
Wheal Elevated, irregular-shaped area of cutaneous edema; solid, transient; variable diameter	Insect bites, urticaria, allergic reaction	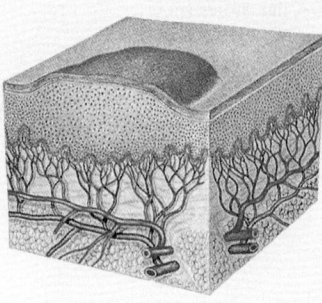	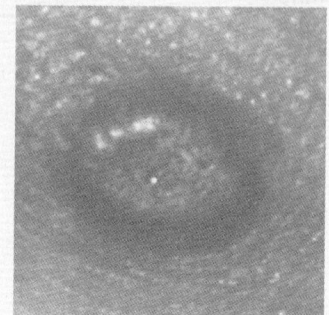 **Wheal**[c]
Nodule Elevated, firm, circumscribed lesion; deeper in dermis than a papule; 1-2 cm in diameter	Erythema nodosum, lipomas	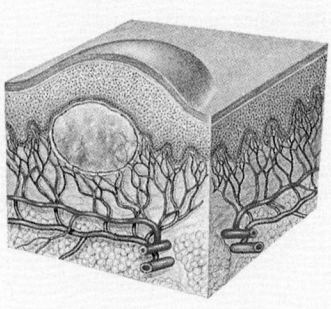	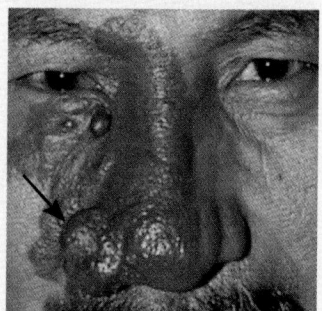 **Hypertrophic nodule**[d]
Tumor Elevated, solid lesion; may be clearly demarcated; deeper in dermis; greater than 2 cm in diameter	Neoplasms, benign tumor, lipoma, hemangioma	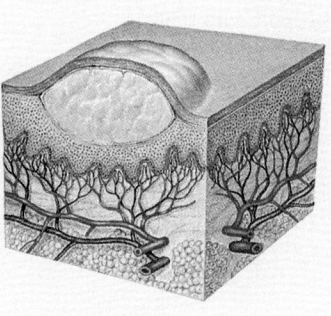	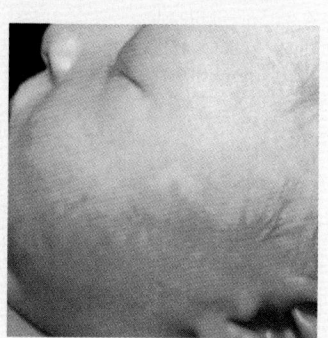 **Hemangioma**[h]
Vesicle Elevated, circumscribed, superficial, not into dermis; filled with serous fluid; less than 1 cm in diameter	Varicella (chickenpox), herpes zoster (shingles)	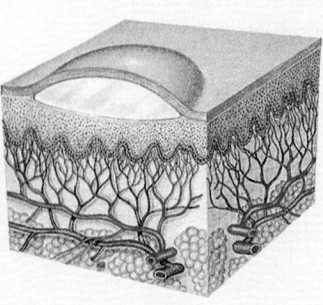	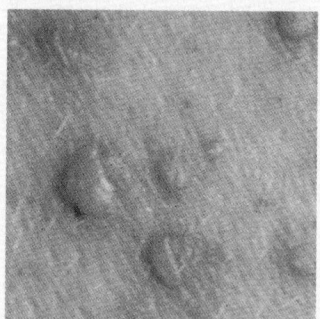 **Vesicles**[c]

From Thompson JM, Wilson SF: *Health assessment for nursing practice,* St Louis, 2002, Mosby.
[c]Farrar WE et al: *Infectious diseases,* ed 2, London, 1992, Gower.
[d]Goldman MP, Fitzpatrick RE: *Cutaneous laser surgery: the art and science of selective photo thermolysis,* ed 2, St Louis, 1998, Mosby.
[h]Weston WL, Lane AT: *Color textbook of pediatric dermatology,* ed 3, St Louis, 2002, Mosby.

Table 44-3	Primary and Secondary Skin Lesions—cont'd		
Primary Skin Lesions	**Examples**		

Bulla
Vesicle greater than 1 cm in diameter

Blister, pemphigus vulgaris

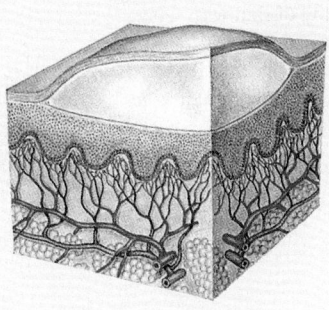

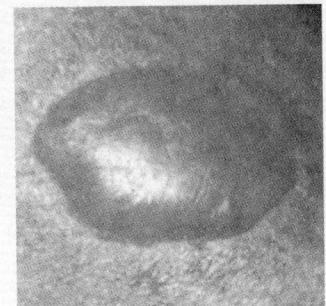

Bulla[c]
(Courtesy Dr. KA Riley)

Pustule
Elevated, superficial lesion; similar to a vesicle but filled with purulent fluid

Impetigo, acne

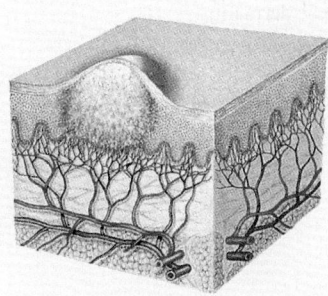

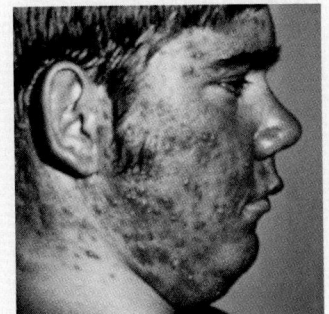

Acne[h]

Cyst
Elevated, circumscribed, encapsulated lesion; in dermis or subcutaneous layer; filled with liquid or semisolid material

Sebaceous cyst, cystic acne

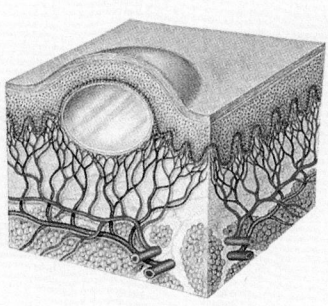

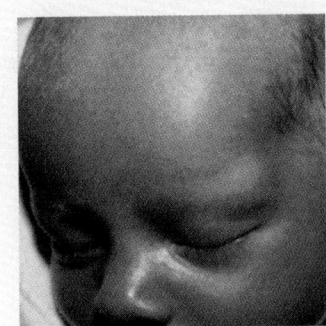

Sebaceous cyst[h]

Telangiectasia
Fine, irregular red lines produced by capillary dilation

Telangiectasia in rosacea

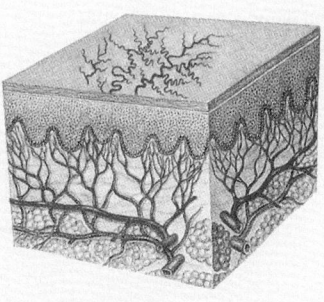

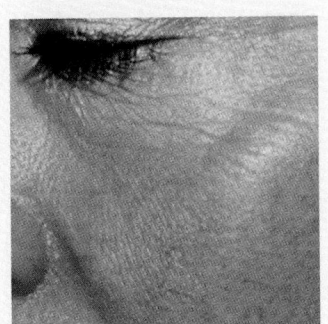

Telangiectasia[d]

Continued

[c]Farrar WE et al: *Infectious diseases,* ed 2, London, 1992, Gower.
[d]Goldman MP, Fitzpatrick RE: *Cutaneous laser surgery: the art and science of selective photo thermolysis,* ed 2, St Louis, 1998, Mosby.
[h]Weston WL, Lane AT: *Color textbook of pediatric dermatology,* ed 3, St Louis, 2002, Mosby.

Table 44-3   Primary and Secondary Skin Lesions—cont'd

Secondary Skin Lesions	Examples		
Scale Heaped-up, keratinized cells; flaky skin; irregular; thick or thin; dry or oily; variation in size	Flaking of skin with seborrheic dermatitis following scarlet fever, or flaking of skin following a drug reaction; dry skin	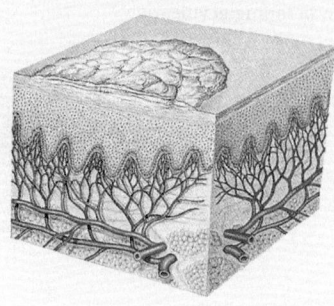	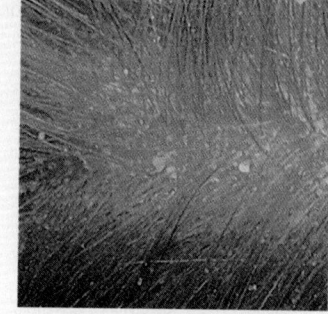 **Fine scaling**[a]
Lichenification Rough, thickened epidermis secondary to persistent rubbing, itching, or skin irritation; often involves flexor surface of extremity	Chronic dermatitis	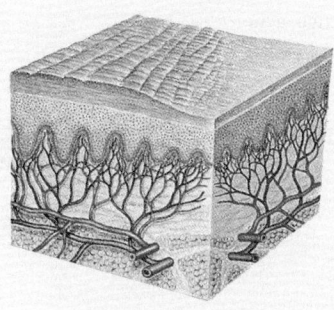	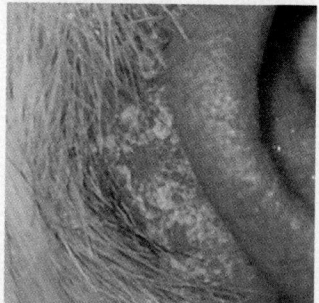 **Stasis dermatitis in early stage**[f]
Keloid Irregular-shaped, elevated, progressively enlarging scar; grows beyond the boundaries of the wound; caused by excessive collagen formation during healing	Keloid formation following surgery	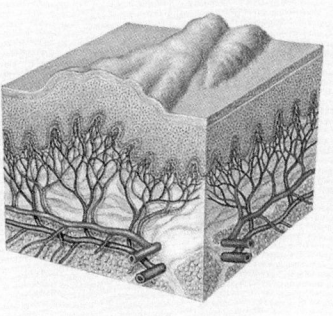	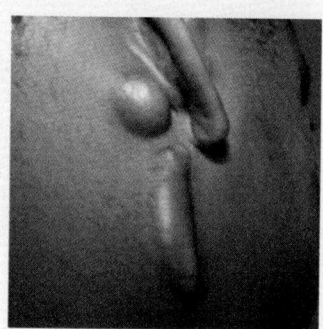 **Keloid**[h]
Scar Thin to thick fibrous tissue that replaces normal skin following injury or laceration to the dermis	Healed wound or surgical incision	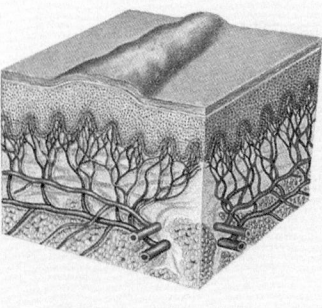	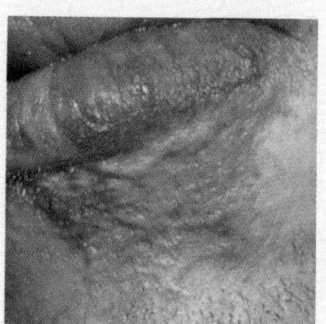 **Hypertrophic scar**[d]

[a]Baran R, Dawber RR, Levene GM: *Color atlas of the hair, scalp, and nails*, St Louis, 1991, Mosby.
[d]Goldman MP, Fitzpatrick RE: *Cutaneous laser surgery: the art and science of selective photo thermolysis*, ed 2, St Louis, 1998, Mosby.
[f]Marks JG Jr, DeLeo VA: *Contact and occupational dermatitis*, St Louis, 1991, Mosby.
[h]Weston WL, Lane AT: *Color textbook of pediatric dermatology*, ed 3, St Louis, 2002, Mosby.

Table 44-3	Primary and Secondary Skin Lesions—cont'd

Secondary Skin Lesions	Examples		
Excoriation Loss of the epidermis; linear, hollowed-out, crusted area	Abrasion or scratch, scabies	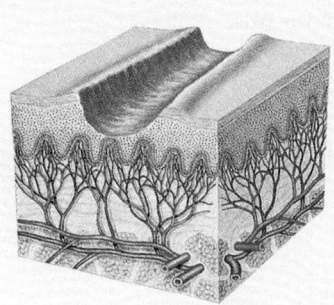	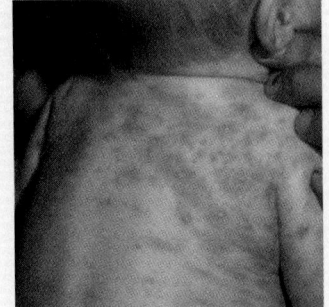 Scabies[h]
Fissure Linear crack or break from the epidermis to the dermis; may be moist or dry	Athlete's foot, cracks at the corner of the mouth	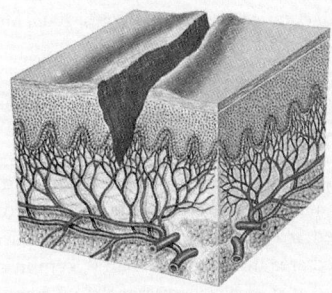	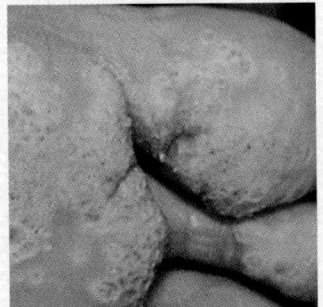 Fissures[d]
Erosion Loss of part of the epidermis; depressed, moist, glistening; follows rupture of a vesicle or bulla	Varicella, variola after rupture	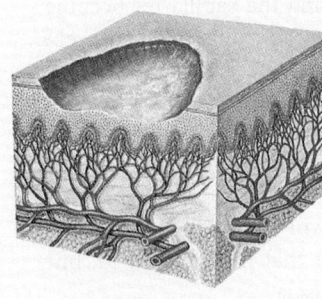	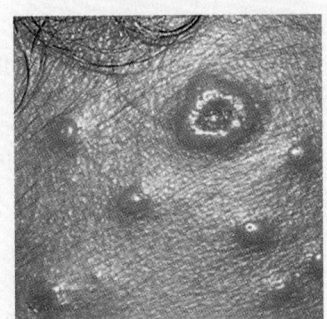 Erosion[b]
Ulcer Loss of epidermis and dermis; concave; varies in size	Decubiti, stasis ulcers	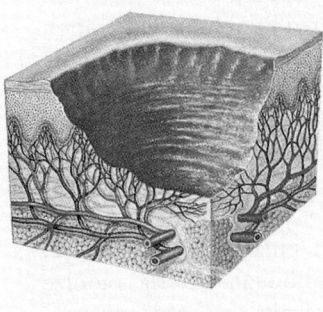	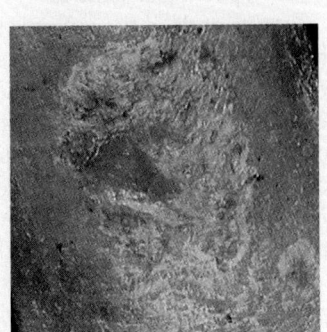 Stasis ulcer[e]

[b]Cohen BA: *Pediatric dermatology,* London, 1993, Wolfe.
[d]Goldman MP, Fitzpatrick RE: *Cutaneous laser surgery: the art and science of selective photo thermolysis,* ed 2, St Louis, 1998, Mosby.
[e]Habif TP: *Clinical dermatology,* ed 4, St Louis, 2004, Mosby.
[h]Weston WL, Lane AT: *Color textbook of pediatric dermatology,* ed 3, St Louis, 2002, Mosby.

Continued

Table 44-3	Primary and Secondary Skin Lesions—cont'd	
Secndary Skin Lesions	**Examples**	
Atrophy Thinning of the skin surface and loss of skin markings	Aged skin, striae	 **Aged skin[g]**

From Thompson JM, Wilson SF: *Health assessment for nursing practice,* St Louis, 2002, Mosby.
[g]Seidel HM et al: *Mosby's guide to physical examination,* ed 5, St Louis, 2003, Mosby.

Table 44-4	Special Skin Lesions
Type	**Clinical Manifestations**
Comedone	A plug of sebaceous and keratin material lodged in the opening of a hair follicle; an open comedone has a dilated orifice (blackhead), and a closed comedone has a narrow opening (whitehead)
Burrow	A narrow, raised, irregular channel caused by a parasite
Petechiae	A circumscribed area of blood less than 0.5 cm in diameter
Purpura	A circumscribed area of blood greater than 0.5 cm in diameter
Telangiectasia	Dilated, superficial blood vessels

unrelieved, the endothelial cells lining the capillaries become disrupted with platelet aggregation, forming microthrombi that block blood flow and cause anoxic necrosis of surrounding tissues. Pressure ulcers can be classified by stages:

I. Nonblanchable erythema of intact skin
II. Partial-thickness skin loss involving epidermis or dermis
III. Full-thickness skin loss involving damage or necrosis of subcutaneous tissue that may extend to, but not through, underlying fascia
IV. Full-thickness skin loss with extensive destruction, tissue necrosis, or damage to muscle, bone, or supporting structures[19]

A layer of dead tissue forms that appears as a blister when there is superficial damage or as a reddish blue discoloration when there is deeper tissue damage. Superficial sores are more common on the sacrum as a result of shearing or friction forces (forces parallel to the skin). Deep sores develop closer to the bone as a result of tissue distortion and vascular occlusion from pressure that is perpendicular to the tissue (over the heels, trochanter, and ischia).

The necrotic tissue initiates an inflammatory response, with pain, fever, and leukocytosis. Although bacteria colonize the dead tissue, the infection is usually localized and self-limiting. Proteolytic enzymes from bacteria and macrophages dissolve necrotic tissues and cause a foul-smelling discharge that resembles, but is not, pus.

Pressure sores are often painful in individuals who do not have loss of sensation from spinal cord trauma or neuropathy. The presence of necrotic tissue produces an inflammatory response with hyperemia, fever, and increased white blood cell count. If the ulceration is large, toxicity and pain lead to loss of appetite, debility, and renal insufficiency. Individuals who are immunosuppressed or have diabetes mellitus may develop infection and inflammation of adjacent tissues (cellulitis) or septicemia.

The primary goal for those at risk for pressure ulcers is prevention.[14,20] Pressure sores are not prevented by topical agents because they do not relieve the pressure. Frequent skin assessment and turning; use of pressure reduction surfaces; elimination of incontinence, moisture, and drainage; and maintenance of fluid, protein, and caloric intake are effective preventive techniques.[21,22] Nutrition, oxygenation, and fluid balance must be maintained.

Superficial ulcers should be covered with flat, nonbulky dressings that cannot wrinkle and cause increased pressure or friction. Spontaneous healing will occur more quickly when the ulcer is kept moist with an occlusive dressing.[23] Antibiotics are seldom required. Antiseptics, such as hydrogen peroxide or iodine, are damaging to granulation tissue and should not be used.[24] Successful healing requires continued adequate relief of pressure and débridement of dead tissue.

Large, deep pressure ulcers may require surgical débridement of necrotic tissue, opening of deep pockets for drainage, and skin grafting for wound closure and successful healing. The myocutaneous flap, a single unit of skin with its underlying muscle and vasculature, has been an effective treatment in large avascular areas over bony prominences.[25,26] Application of wound tension by range of motion may also promote healing.[25,26]

Keloids

Keloids are elevated, rounded, and firm with irregular clawlike margins that extend beyond the original site of injury. They are caused by excessive collagen formation during dermal connective tissue repair and many genes are involved.[27] Keloids are most common in darkly-pigmented skin types and burn scars. Burns incite this reaction more commonly than other types of injury (see Chapter 46).

Excessive or poorly aligned tension on a wound, introduction of foreign material into the skin, and certain types of trauma (e.g., burns) are all provocative factors. Those parts of the body at risk include shoulders, back, chin, ears, and lower legs. Most keloids appear within 1 year of trauma. Individuals 10 to 30 years of age develop lesions much more commonly than do children before puberty or older adults.

Type III collagen is increased with keloids. The increased synthesis of collagen is associated with IL-6 and dermal fibroblasts that have high metabolic and mitotic rates.[28] **Myofibroblasts,** cells with characteristics of both fibroblasts and smooth muscle cells, have been identified as the principal cells in keloids. Collagenase activity in keloids has been found to be normal or increased, but the collagen may be protected from degradation by **proteoglycan,** a glycoprotein present in connective tissue that serves as a binding (cementing) material, and by specific inhibitors of proteolytic enzymes. Genes regulating fibroblast apoptosis may be down-regulated in keloid tissue.[29] A familial tendency for keloid formation has been found, with both autosomal recessive and autosomal dominant inheritance patterns reported.[30]

Keloids start as pink or red, firm, well-defined, rubbery plaques that persist for several months after trauma. Later, uncontrolled overgrowth causes extension beyond the site of the original wound and the tumor becomes smoother, irregularly shaped, hyperpigmented, harder, and more symptomatic. The tendency to send out **clawlike prolongations** is typical of keloids (Figure 44-3).

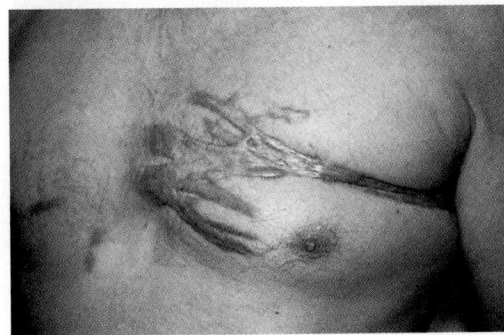

Figure 44-3 Keloid. (Courtesy Department of Dermatology, School of Medicine, University of Utah.)

Keloids are the most extreme example of cutaneous scarring and are the most difficult to treat. Preventive measures such as avoiding unnecessary, elective surgeries are of paramount importance. When surgery is necessary for cosmetic reasons, having it done in early childhood is best. Scalpel surgery with strict aseptic technique and avoidance of wound tension is imperative. Many keloids are unresponsive to silicone gel sheeting or steroids. Radiation therapy (1200 to 2000 gy in five doses) has been successful, as have local chemotrophic agents such as Bleomycin, 5-flurouracil, and imiquimod.[31-33]

Pruritus

Pruritus, or itching, is the most common symptom associated with many primary skin disorders, such as eczema, psoriasis, or lice infestations, or it can be a manifestation of systemic disease (e.g., xerosis, chronic renal failure, cholestatic liver disease, thyroid disorders, iron deficiency) or drug reactions. Pruritus may be localized or generalized and may move from one location to another.[34] Both central and peripheral nerve pathways are activated.[35]

Significant progress has been made recently in understanding the pathophysiology of itch. Studies have shown that peripheral itch mediators include neuropeptides, serotonin, prostaglandins, bradykinin, or acetylcholine and that the itch sensation is carried by specific unmyelinated C-nerve fibers.[36,37]

Itching also has been linked to pain, because many stimuli that induce pain produce itching at lower intensities. Central nervous system mechanisms also can modulate itching, and itching is less perceptible when the mind is concentrating on other things. How the central nervous system influences the itch sensation is unclear.

Chronic itching is an unpleasant sensation relieved by scratching—often done so intensely that trauma to the skin occurs, resulting in infection and scarring. Some individuals become so distraught with the constant irritation that they apply heat with enough intensity and duration to produce burns.

Management of localized itching depends on the cause, and the primary condition must be treated. Symptomatic relief may be obtained from antihistamines, which also have a sedative effect. Minor tranquilizers, such as promethazine, may be effective for some causes of pruritus. Itching related to dry, rough skin (xerosis) can be managed with applications of emollients and increased environmental humidity. Topical steroids are immediately effective with some occurrences of pruritus; however, in some instances, pruritus is resistant to any type of therapy. New topical treatment therapies are being developed, as are the use of phototherapy treatment with narrow band UVB and vagal nerve stimulation[38] and cutaneous field stimulation.[39]

DISORDERS OF THE SKIN

Disruptions in skin integrity may be precipitated by trauma, abnormal cellular function, infection and inflammation, and systemic diseases. Many skin disorders are benign and self-limiting, whereas others are severe and life threatening.

Inflammatory Disorders

The most common inflammatory disorder of the skin is **eczema,** or dermatitis. Eczema and dermatitis are both general terms that describe a particular type of inflammatory response in the skin—the terms can be used interchangeably. Diseases considered eczematous are generally characterized by pruritis, lesions with indistinct borders, and epidermal changes. These lesions can appear as either erythema, papules, or scales, and they can present in an acute, subacute, or chronic phase. Atopic dermatitis, contact dermatitis (whether nonallergic [irritant] or allergic), lichen simplex chronicus, nummular eczema, and seborrheic dermatitis are all examples of specific types of eczema or dermatitis.[40] Edema, serous discharge, and crusting occur with continued irritation and scratching. In chronic eczema the skin becomes thickened, leathery, and hyperpigmented from recurrent irritation and scratching. The location of eczema is related to the underlying cause. Eczematous inflammations need to be differentiated from other rashes and dermatoses, particularly psoriasis.

Allergic Contact Dermatitis

Allergic contact dermatitis is a common form of cell-mediated or delayed hypersensitivity.[41] (See Chapter 8 for various types of allergic responses.) Various allergens (e.g., microorganisms, chemicals, foreign proteins, drugs, metals, latex) can form the sensitizing antigen. The response is an interaction of skin barrier function; reaction to irritants; and neuronal response, such as itching.[42] Contact with poison ivy is a common example (Figure 44-4). As the allergen comes in contact with the skin, the allergen is bound to a carrier protein, forming a

sensitizing antigen. Langerhans (dendritic cells) process the antigen and carry it to T cells that then become sensitized to the antigen.[43] Keratinocytes also may activate lymphocytes and endothelial cells in allergic contact dermatitis.[44] IgE antibodies are recovered in latex allergy and are associated with an immediate allergic response to latex rubber protein.[45]

In delayed hypersensitivity, several hours pass before an immunologic response is apparent. The T cells play an important role because they differentiate and secrete lymphokines that affect macrophage movement and aggregation, coagulation, and other inflammatory responses (see Chapter 2). Sensitization usually develops with first exposure to the antigen, and symptoms of dermatitis occur with reexposure.

The manifestations of allergic contact dermatitis include erythema and swelling with pruritic (itching) vesicular lesions in the areas of allergen contact. The pattern of distribution provides clues to the source of the antigen (e.g., hands exposed to chemical solutions or boundaries from rings and bracelets). Patch tests with specific antigens may assist with diagnosis. Removal of the allergen is necessary for resolution of the inflammatory response and tissue repair.[46] Topical or systemic steroids, as well as other symptomatic treatment, may be required for treatment, depending on the severity of the lesion.

Atopic Dermatitis

Atopic dermatitis is more common in infancy and childhood; however, some individuals are affected throughout life. A family history of asthma, allergic rhinitis, dry skin, food allergy, and eczema often accompanies this disorder. During adolescence and childhood the lesions are usually localized to the hands and feet or flexor surfaces (i.e., antecubital fossa, popliteal space) of the arms and legs (Figure 44-5). The ery-

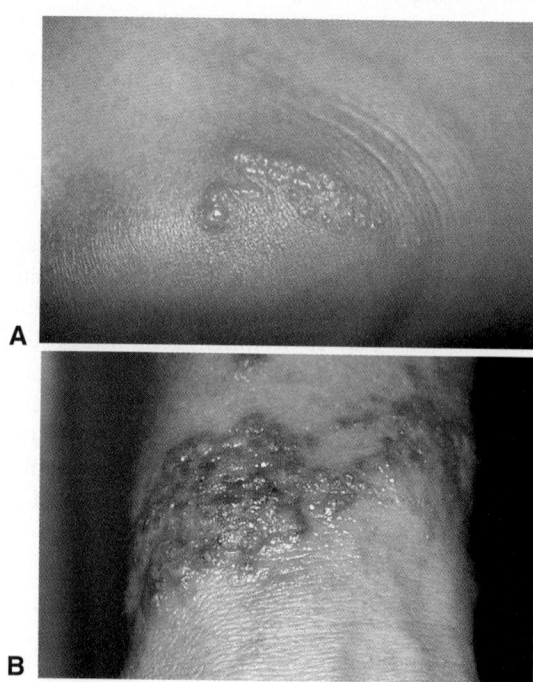

Figure 44-4 Poison ivy. **A,** Poison ivy on knee. **B,** Poison ivy dermatitis. (Courtesy Department of Dermatology, School of Medicine, University of Utah.)

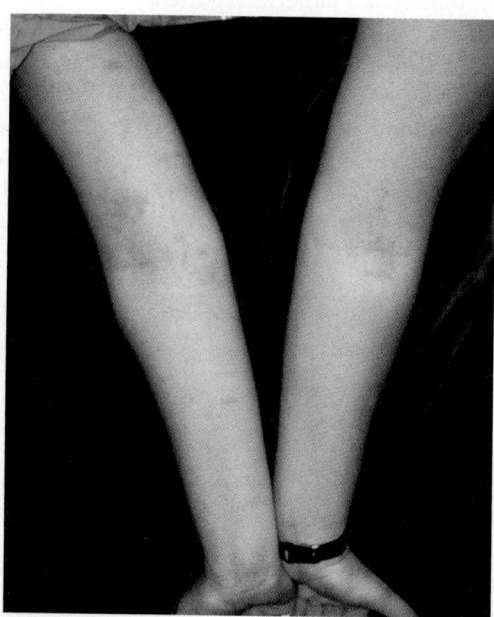

Figure 44-5 Atopic dermatitis. (Courtesy Department of Dermatology, School of Medicine, University of Utah.)

thema, scaling, and lichenification (thickened and leather-like skin) are exacerbated by scratching because the lesions are manifest by itching.[47] The scratching increases susceptibility to infections from *Staphylococcus aureus* and predisposition to cutaneous dissemination of viruses, particular herpes simplex. The immunopathogenesis and treatment of atopic dermatitis in adults is similar to that in children[48] and is discussed in detail in Chapter 45.

Stasis Dermatitis

Stasis dermatitis usually occurs on the legs as a result of venous stasis and edema. The disorder is associated with varicosities, phlebitis, and vascular trauma. First, erythema and pruritus develop and then scaling, petechiae, and hyperpigmentation. Progressive lesions become ulcerated, particularly around the ankles and tibia (Figure 44-6).

Treatment includes elevating the legs as often as possible, not wearing tight clothes around the legs, and not standing for long periods. Acute inflammations are treated with antibiotics. Chronic lesions with ulceration are treated with wet dressings of Burow solution or silver nitrate. Edema is controlled with external compression.

Irritant Contact Dermatitis

Irritant contact dermatitis is a nonimmunologically mediated inflammation of the skin. The intensity of the inflammation is related to the concentration of the irritant and exposure time. Irritation can occur from almost anything, especially if the epidermal barrier is compromised in any way (Box 44-1). Irritant contact dermatitis accounts for 80% of all contact dermatitis and allergic contact dermatitis for 20%.[49] The skin lesions are similar in appearance to allergic contact dermatitis. Removing the source of irritation and use of topical agents constitute effective treatment.

Seborrheic Dermatitis

Seborrheic dermatitis is a common chronic inflammation of the skin involving the scalp, eyebrows, eyelids, ear canals, nasolabial folds, axillae, chest, and back (Figure 44-7). In infants it is known as *cradle cap*. The cause is unknown, but an immunologic response to yeasts from the genus *Malassezia* have been implicated.[50] The lesions appear from infancy to old age, with periods of remission and exacerbation. The lesions appear as scaly, white, or yellowish inflammatory plaques with mild pruritus. Mild cases are treated with shampoos containing sulfur, salicylic acid, or tar. Ciclopirox 1% shampoo has antifungal and anti-inflammatory effects and has been used with some success.[51] Corticosteroid applications are useful for suppression of severe symptoms but should not be used for maintenance therapy.

Papulosquamous Disorders

Psoriasis, pityriasis rosea, and lichen planus are disorders characterized by inflammatory processes associated with papules, scales, plaques, and erythema. Collectively they are described as **papulosquamous disorders.**

Box 44-1	Substances Known to Cause Contact Dermatitis

Alkalis
  Soaps
  Detergents
  Ammonia preparations
  Lye
  Drainpipe cleaners
  Toilet bowl cleaners
  Oven cleaners
Acids
Metal salts
  Cyanides of calcium, copper, mercury, nickel, silver, zinc
  Chlorides of calcium and zinc
Bromine, chlorine, iodine, fluorine
Insecticides
Dusts of lime, zinc, arsenic
Dyes and fragrances
Wood dust from teak, cinchona bark, quinine, pyrethrum
Tobacco dust from cigars
Explosive powders
Hydrocarbons
  Crude petroleum, lubricating oil, cutting oil
  Paraffins, mineral oils
  Asphalt, other tar products
Soot, peat
Perservatives

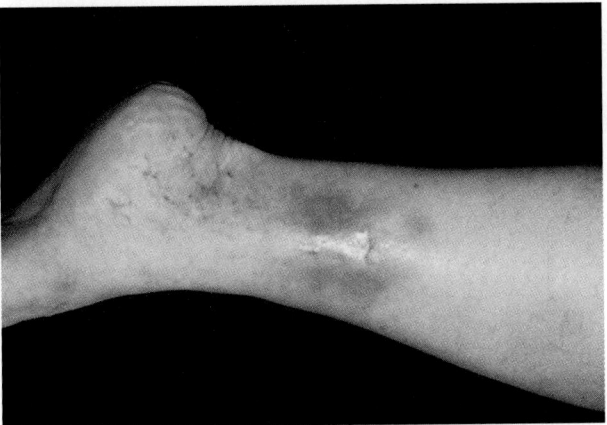

Figure 44-6 Stasis ulcer. (Courtesy Department of Dermatology, School of Medicine, University of Utah.)

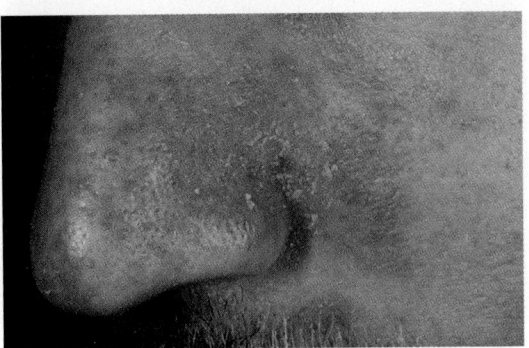

Figure 44-7 Seborrheic dermatitis. (Courtesy Department of Dermatology, School of Medicine, University of Utah.)

Psoriasis

Psoriasis is a chronic, relapsing, proliferative skin disorder that can occur at any age and affects 1% to 3% of the population.[52] The onset is generally established by 20 years of age. Psoriasis is a T-cell mediated autoimmune disease. Inflammatory cytokines from activated T-cells cause the skin changes seen in psoriasis.[53,54] A family history of psoriasis often is established, and an human leukocyte antigen (HLA)–associated inheritance is likely.[55]

Both the dermis and epidermis are thickened, with cellular hyperproliferation, altered differentiation, and inflammation.[56,57] The turnover time for shedding the epidermis is decreased from the normal 26 to 30 days to 3 to 4 days. There are increased numbers of germinative cells and an increase in transit time of cells through the dermis. The rapid cellular proliferation does not allow time for cell maturation and keratinization to occur, resulting in a thickened epidermis and plaque formation. The loosely cohesive keratin gives the lesion a silvery, scaly appearance. There is often capillary dilation and increased vascularization to accommodate the increased cell metabolism. The increased vascularity causes erythema.

The types of psoriasis include plaque (psoriasis vulgaris), inverse, guttate, pustular, and erythrodermic. *Plaque psoriasis* is the most common. The disease can be mild, moderate, or severe, depending on the size, distribution, and inflammation of the lesions. Early-onset psoriasis is an inflammatory lesion with epidermal hyperproliferation and the presence of activated T lymphocytes.[58] The progress of psoriasis is characterized by remissions and exacerbations. Antimalarial drugs, lithium, nonsteroidal anti-inflammatory drugs, and beta blockers, tend to exacerbate existing psoriasis Arthritis develops in approximately 30% of individuals with moderate to severe psoriasis.

The typical lesion of plaque psoriasis is a well-demarcated, thick, silvery, scaly, erythematous plaque surrounded by normal skin (Figure 44-8). Initial lesions usually develop insidiously as small erythematous papules that enlarge and coalesce into larger inflammatory lesions. The lesions are commonly located on the scalp, elbows, and knees and at sites of trauma. The scales are usually loosely adherent and may cause small bleeding points when removed. **Inverse psoriasis** involves lesions that develop in the axilla or groin. They are large, smooth, dry, and have a deep red color.

In **guttate psoriasis,** small papules appear suddenly on the trunk and extremities (Figure 44-9). The lesions may appear a few weeks after a streptococcal respiratory infection, and children with psoriasis reflect a tendency to develop guttate psoriasis. Guttate psoriasis may resolve spontaneously in weeks or months. **Pustular psoriasis** appears as blisters of noninfectious pus and show genetic susceptibility and a strong association with major histocompatibility complex (MHC) class 1 and alteration in T cell–mediated cytokines and growth factors.[59] **Erythrodermic (exfoliative) psoriasis** is often accompanied by itching or pain with widespread red, scaling lesions. Psoriatic arthritis is associated with the skin lesions and involves joints of the hands, feet, knees, and ankles,[60] and may affect up to 25% of individuals with psoriasis.[61]

Treatment is individualized and related to reducing epidermal cell turnover. Mild lesions are usually treated with emollients, keratolytic agents, and corticosteroids. Moderate lesions may respond to ultraviolet light, tar preparations, or a combination of both, and to methotrexate, cyclosporine, and acetretin. Vitamin D_1 (calcitriol) is used to reduce epidermal proliferation.[62,63] Moderate to severe disease is the indication for one of the new biologics (see What's New? box). Only the most severe disease may require hospitalization with a combination of topical agents and antimetabolites, such as methotrexate or cyclosporine.

Pityriasis Rosea

Pityriasis rosea is a benign, self-limiting inflammatory disorder that occurs more often in young adults, usually during the winter months. The cause is unknown but is thought to be associated with a virus because of the timing and clustering of the outbreaks.[64] Pityriasis rosea begins as a single lesion known

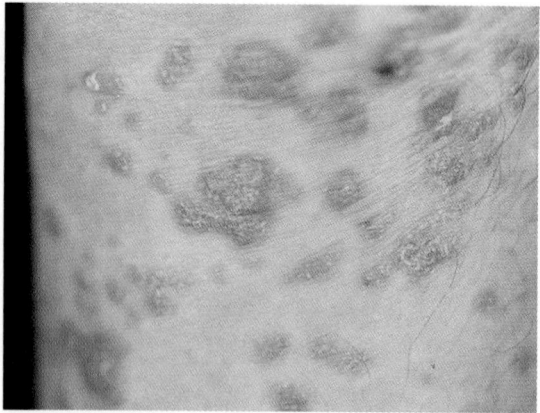

Figure 44-8 Psoriasis. Typical oval plaque with well-defined borders and silvery scale. (Courtesy Department of Dermatology, School of Medicine, University of Utah.)

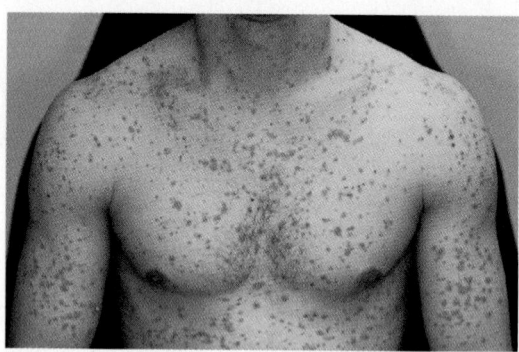

Figure 44-9 Guttate psoriasis after streptococcal infection. Numerous uniformly small lesions may abruptly occur after streptococcal pharyngitis. (Courtesy Department of Dermatology, School of Medicine, University of Utah.)

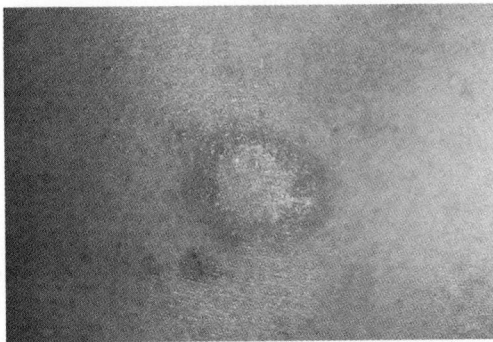

Figure 44-10 Pityriasis rosea herald patch. A collarette pattern has formed around the margins. (Courtesy Department of Dermatology, School of Medicine, University of Utah.)

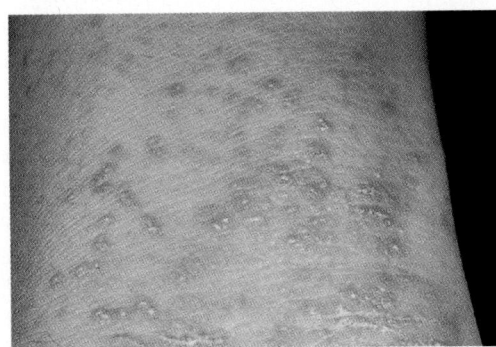

Figure 44-11 Hypertrophic lichen planus on arms. (Courtesy Department of Dermatology, School of Medicine, University of Utah.)

as a **herald patch** (Figure 44-10) that is circular, demarcated, salmon-pink, approximately 3 to 4 cm in diameter, and usually located on the trunk. Early lesions are macular and papular. Secondary lesions develop within 14 to 21 days and extend over the trunk and upper part of the extremities. Lesions are rarely located on the face. The lesions emerge as small erythematous papules that expand into characteristic oval lesions. There may be few or hundreds of lesions. The pattern of distribution follows the skin lines around the trunk and resembles a drooping pine tree. As scales flake off from the margin of the lesions, a collarette pattern is formed. Itching is the most common symptom. Occasionally headache, fatigue, or sore throat precedes the development of the lesions.[65]

The diagnosis of pityriasis rosea is made by the clinical appearance of the lesion. It can be confused with secondary syphilis, psoriasis, or seborrheic dermatitis. The disorder is usually self-limiting and resolves in a few months with symptomatic treatment for pruritus. Ultraviolet light, antihistamines, or topical corticosteroids may be used to control itching. Sun exposure facilitates resolution of the lesions.

Lichen Planus

Lichen planus is a benign, inflammatory disorder of the skin and mucous membranes. The cause is unknown, but T cells, adhesion molecules, inflammatory cytokines, perforin, and antigen-presenting cells are involved.[66] The infiltrate of T cells mediates immunoreactivity against basal layer keratinocytes, which have altered surface antigens and adhesion molecules.[67] More recently, lichen planus has been linked to hepatitis C virus.[68] Some individuals develop lichenoid lesions after exposure to drugs or film-processing chemicals. The age of onset is usually between 30 and 70 years. The disorder begins

with nonscaling, violet-colored pruritic papules, 2 to 4 mm in size, usually located on the wrists, ankles, lower legs, and genitalia (Figure 44-11). The papules are flat topped and have a polygonal shape. New lesions are pale pink and evolve into a dark violet color. Persistent lesions may be thickened and red, forming hypertrophic lichen planus. The lesions often involve the oral mucous membranes, appearing as lacy white rings that must be differentiated from leukoplakia or oral candidiasis.[69] Fine white lines, known as Wickham striae, can be seen throughout the oral lesions on magnification. These lesions also can develop on the penis and vulvovaginal area. More commonly, oral lesions do not ulcerate, but localized or extensive painful ulcerations do and frequently occur. Chronic ulcerated lesions become malignant in 1% of individuals with the disease. Thinning and splitting of nails are common, and part or all of the nail may be shed.

Pruritus is the most distressing symptom. The lesions are self-limiting and may last for months or years, with an average duration of 6 to 18 months. Postinflammatory hyperpigmentation is a common consequence of the lesion. Approximately 20% of individuals have a recurrence. Diagnosis is commonly made by the clinical appearance of the lesion. Treatment is individualized. Antihistamines are given for itching, and topical or systemic corticosteroids may be used to control inflammation. Mucous membrane lesions are treated with topical steroids or with injection into a single lesion.

Acne Vulgaris

Acne vulgaris is an inflammatory disorder of the pilosebaceous follicle (the sebaceous gland contiguous with a hair follicle). It occurs most commonly during adolescence. Details of this disorder are presented in Chapter 45.

Acne Rosacea

Acne rosacea is an inflammation of the skin that develops in middle-age adults. The disease is chronic with episodes of exacerbation.[70] The most common lesion types are erythematotelangiectatic, papulopustular, phymatous, and ocular.[71] They occur in the middle third of the face, including the forehead, nose, cheeks, and chin (Figure 44-12). The cause is unknown, but immune-mediated inflammation may be a factor.[72] The lesions are associated with chronic, inappropriate vasodilation resulting in flushing and sensitivity to the sun. Hypertrophy of the sebaceous glands may be severe enough to produce an irreversible bulbous appearance of the nose, known as *rhinophyma*. Disorders of the eye often accompany rosacea, particularly conjunctivitis and, more rarely, keratitis, which can result in visual impairment.[73] Facial application of fluorinated topical steroids may precipitate rosacea-like lesions that are difficult to treat. There is controversy regarding the association between *Demodex folliculorum, H. pylori* infection, and rosacea.[74,75]

Hot drinks or alcohol should be taken cautiously because the heat and vasodilation accentuate erythema. Tetracycline, though photosensitizing, continues to be the drug of choice for treatment, and a low maintenance dose may be required after the most severe lesions are controlled. Daily use of photoprotection, including sunscreens, is recommended. One percent topical metronidazole may be effective.[76] Surgical excision of excessive tissue may be required for rhinophyma.

Lupus Erythematosus

Lupus erythematosus is an inflammatory, autoimmune, systemic, disease with cutaneous manifestations. Discoid (or cutaneous) lupus erythematosus (DLE) is limited to the skin and can lead to systemic lupus erythematosus in approximately 5% of individuals. (Systemic lupus erythematosus [SLE], a diffuse, multisystem disease, is discussed in Chapter 8.)

Discoid Lupus Erythematosus

Discoid lupus erythematosus (DLE) usually occurs in adults, particularly in women in their late 30s or early 40s. The lesions may be single or multiple and of various sizes. Often the lesions are located on light-exposed areas of the skin, and photosensitivity is common. The face is the most common site of lesion involvement; a butterfly pattern of distribution is found over the nose and cheeks.[77]

The cause is thought to be an altered immune response to an unknown antigen. DLE may be described as a subset of SLE, with cutaneous manifestations being the only symptom[78] (Figure 44-13). Skin biopsy with immunofluorescent observation reveals lumpy deposits of immunoglobulins, especially IgM.

The early lesion is asymmetric, with a 1- to 2-cm raised red plaque with a brownish scale. The scale penetrates the hair follicle and leaves a carpet-tack appearance when removed. The lesions persist for months and then resolve spontaneously or atrophy. Healing progresses from the center of the lesion, with a residual telangiectasia (prominent skin capillaries) and scarring that is usually hypopigmented. Atrophy of the dermis and epidermis that results in a depressed scar can occur. Other symptoms of cutaneous lupus erythematosus include alopecia (hair loss), telangiectasia, urticaria, and Raynaud phenomenon. Scarring or atrophic alopecia is a com-

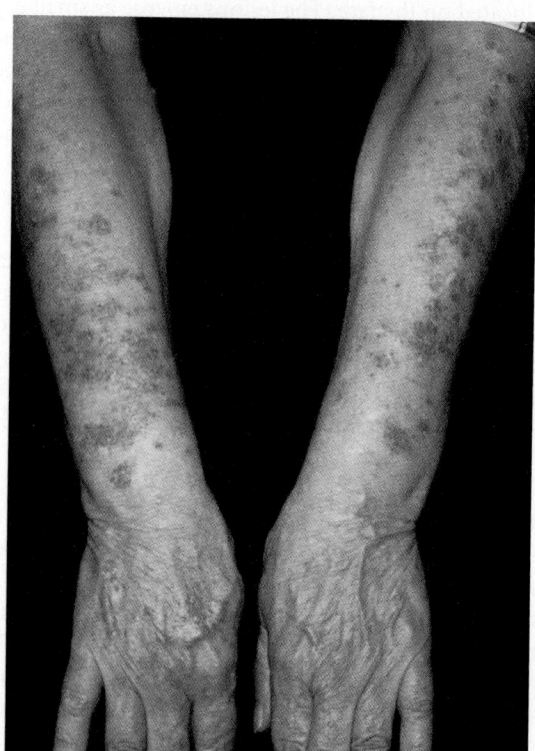

Figure 44-13 Subacute cutaneous lupus (discoid lupus erythematosus). (Courtesy Department of Dermatology, School of Medicine, University of Utah.)

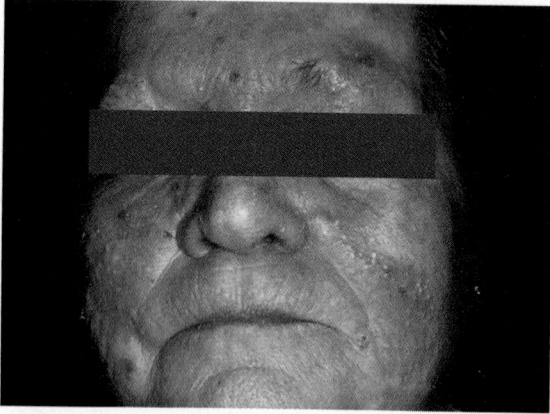

Figure 44-12 Granulomatous rosacea. Pustules and erythema occur on the forehead, cheeks, and nose. (Courtesy Department of Dermatology, School of Medicine, University of Utah.)

mon problem of DLE. Scaling and inflammation lead to destruction of hair follicles, followed by skin that is smooth and white with telangiectasia. Hair loss is random in distribution. Telangiectasia are distributed primarily over the palms and fingers in association with erythema. Urticaria of DLE may appear as typical hives, but they usually stay localized in a photo-distribution, are not pruritic, and last for greater than 24 hours. They probably result from immune complex deposition rather than an allergic response. Raynaud phenomenon with a history of episodic vasospasm of the arterioles of the fingers and toes with stress or exposure to cold often precedes the onset of DLE by several years. Raynaud phenomenon is characterized by an initial stage of vasospasm that leads to white, numb, and cold digits followed by cyanosis and then a reactive hyperemia as the vasospasm relaxes.

Diagnosis of DLE is made from the presenting symptoms, biopsy of skin lesions with direct immunofluorescence, as well as histology. Individuals with DLE must use sunscreen and limit direct exposure to the sun because this exacerbates lesions. Initial treatment with potent topical steroids relieves symptoms. Pimecrolimus 1% cream and tacrolimus 0.1% ointment also have been used with some success.[79,80] Antimalarial drugs (e.g., hydroxychloroquine sulfate) provide first-line systemic therapy and usually lead to clinical improvement within 1 to 3 months.[81] These medications must be used with caution to prevent serious side effects.

Vesiculobullous Disorders

Vesiculobullous skin disorders represent a group of diseases that have different causes and clinical courses but share a common characteristic of vesicle, or blister, formation. Two such diseases are pemphigus and erythema multiforme.

Pemphigus

Pemphigus (meaning to blister of bubble) is a rare autoimmune blistering disease of the skin and oral mucous membranes caused by circulating autoantibodies directed against the cell surface adhesion molecule, desmoglein, at the desmosomal cell junction in the suprabasal layer of the epidermis. Immunoglobulin G autoantibodies and C3 complement bind to the desmoglein adhesion molecules resulting in the destruction of cell-to-cell adhesion (acantholysis) in the epidermis with fluid accumulation and the resulting symptom of blister formation.[82] IgA autoantibodies have been found in some individuals.[83] Pemphigus can occur in all age groups but is more prevalent between 40 and 50 years of age.

Pemphigus presents in varying forms. *Pemphigus vulgaris* is the most common form with acantholysis at the suprabasal level. Oral lesions precede the onset of skin blistering, which is more prominent on the face, scalp, and axilla. The blisters rupture easily because of the thin, fragile overlying portion of epidermis. *Pemphigus vegetans* is a variant of pemphigus vulgaris with large blisters occurring in tissue folds of the axilla and groin. *Pemphigus foliaceus* is a milder form of the disease and involves acantholysis at the subcorneal level with blistering, erosions, scaling, crusting, and erythema usually of the

face and chest. Oral mucous membranes are rarely involved. *Pemphigus erythematosus* is a subset of pemphigus foliaceus often associated with systemic lupus erythematosus with positive antinuclear antibodies. The lesions are generally less widely distributed.

The diagnosis of pemphigus is made from the clinical manifestations and histologic examination of the skin. Immunofluorescence demonstrates the presence of antibodies at the site of blister formation. The clinical course of the disease may range from rapidly fatal to relatively benign. The primary treatment for pemphigus is systemic corticosteroids, usually in high doses during acute episodes or when there is widespread involvement. Adjuvant immunosuppressive therapy also may be used and decreases the steroid dosage requirement. Newer methods of treatment and a clearer understanding of the pathogenesis have improved the prognosis and decreased mortality.[84]

Bullous Pemphigoid

Bullous pemphigoid is a more benign disease than pemphigus vulgaris, with the presence of serum and bound IgG and blistering of the subepidermal skin layer.[85] It occurs more commonly after 60 years of age. The lesions of pemphigoid begin with localized erythema or as pruritic plaques that extend and become edematous. The plaques turn reddish purple by 2 to 3 weeks, with vesicles and bullae emerging on the surface (Figure 44-14). The bullae do not extend with pressure. The blisters rupture within 1 week and heal rapidly.

Diagnosis is by skin biopsy and immunofluorescent examination. The presence of subepidermal blistering and eosinophils distinguishes pemphigoid from pemphigus. Treatment usually includes hydroxyzine (Atarax) for itching and prednisone with an immunosuppressive drug to control blistering. Individuals who respond to treatment with sulfapyridine or dapsone do not require prednisone.

Erythema Multiforme

Erythema multiforme is not a single disease but rather a syndrome characterized by inflammation of skin and mucous membranes, which is often associated with an immunologic

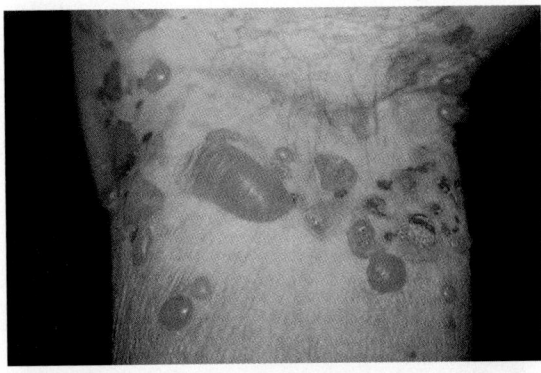

Figure 44-14 Bullous pemphigoid. Generalized eruption with blisters arising from an edematous, erythematous annular base. (Courtesy Department of Dermatology, School of Medicine, University of Utah.)

or toxic reaction to drugs or microorganisms (e.g., *Mycoplasma pneumoniae,* herpes simplex).[86] Overall, it is relatively rare and can occur at any age but is more common between 20 and 40 years of age. Immune complex formation and deposition of complement (C3), IgM, and fibrinogen around the superficial dermal blood vessels, basement membrane, and keratinocytes are found in most individuals with erythema multiforme. Edema develops in the superficial dermis, leading to the formation of vesicles and bullae. The lesions vary in clinical presentation and may involve the skin or mucous membranes or both. The characteristic "bull's-eye" or "target" lesions occur on the skin surface with a central dusky region surrounded by concentric rings or alternating edema and inflammation.[87] The lesions usually occur suddenly in groups over 2 to 3 weeks. Urticarial plaques, 1 to 2 cm in diameter, can develop without the target lesion. A vesiculobullous form is characterized by mucous membrane lesions and erythematous plaques over elbows and knees. Single or multiple vesicles or bullae may arise on a part of the plaque, accompanied by pruritus and burning. In the minor form there may be ten to hundreds of lesions.[88] The lesions heal within 3 to 4 weeks (Figure 44-15).

The most common severe forms in children and young adults are **Stevens-Johnson syndrome** (severe bullous form) and **toxic epidermal necrolysis,** in which there are numerous erythematous bullous lesions on both the skin and mucous membranes. These diseases may have a different etiology than erythema multiforme.[89] The cause is unknown, but an immune mechanism related to drug administration is involved.[90] Bursts of nitric oxide formation have been proposed as the cause of epidermal apoptosis and necrosis.[91] Prodromal symptoms of fever, headache, malaise, sore throat, and cough develop in approximately one third of the cases. The bullous lesions form erosions and crusts when they rupture. The mouth, air passages, esophagus, urethra, and conjunctiva may be involved. Blindness can result from corneal ulcerations. Difficulty with eating, breathing, and urinating may develop with severe manifestations. The disease can involve the kidneys and extend from the upper respiratory passages into the lungs. Severe forms of the disease can be fatal.

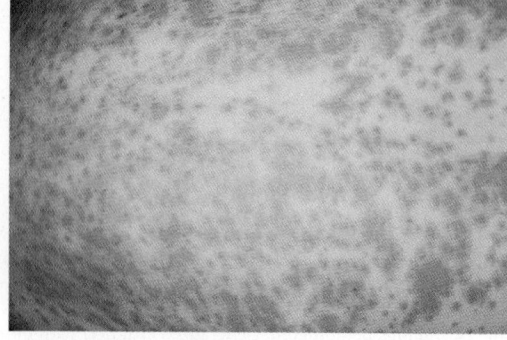

Figure 44-15 Erythema multiforme caused by doxepin. (Courtesy Department of Dermatology, School of Medicine, University of Utah.)

In toxic epidermal necrolysis there is destruction of the epidermis. Both cytotoxic lymphocytes (early) and monocytes-macrophages (late) are involved in this severe blistering disease.[92]

Diagnosis is made by medication history, recognition of the target lesion, or by skin biopsy if the target lesion is absent. Mild acute forms of the disease last 10 to 14 days. Mild forms of the disease, usually self-limiting, require no treatment. Any ongoing drug therapy should be withdrawn or reevaluated and underlying infections treated. Fluid and electrolyte balance should be monitored in severe forms of the disease, and mucous membranes must be carefully managed with a bland diet, warm saline eyewashes, topical anesthetics, or corticosteroids to maintain comfort and prevent infection. High-dose steroids have been used successfully in serious cases.[93] Cutaneous blisters can be treated with wet compresses of Burow solution. Ophthalmic, kidney, and lung involvement require special care. Resolution occurs in 8 to 10 days, usually without scarring. Mucosal lesions may take 6 weeks to heal.

Infections

Cutaneous infections are common forms of skin disease. They generally remain localized; however, serious complications can develop with systemic involvement. The types of skin infection include bacterial, viral, and fungal. Most infections occur superficially; however, systemic signs and symptoms occasionally develop and rarely become life threatening. Aerobes, yeast, and anaerobes comprise the normal flora of the skin and often provide protection against pathogens that cause skin infections, including *Staphylococcus* and *Streptococcus.*[94]

Bacterial Infections

Most bacterial infections of the skin are caused by local invasion of pathogens. Coagulase-positive S. *aureus* and, less often, α-hemolytic streptococci are the common causative organisms.[95] Community acquired methicillin resistant staphylococcus aureus (C-MRSA) is also a cause of serious skin infection (see Box 44-2).

Folliculitis

Folliculitis is usually caused by a bacterial infection of the hair follicle.[96] *Staphylococcus aureus* is the common causative organism. The infection develops from proliferation of the organism around the opening of the follicle and then spreads into the follicle. Inflammation is caused by the release of chemotactic factors and enzymes from the bacteria. The lesions appear as pustules with a surrounding area of erythema. They are most prominent on the scalp and extremities and rarely cause systemic symptoms. Prolonged skin moisture, skin trauma, and poor hygiene are associated contributing factors to the development of folliculitis. Cleaning with soap and water and topical application of antibiotics are effective forms of treatment.

Furuncles and Carbuncles

Furuncles, or "boils," are an inflammation of the hair follicles. They may develop from a preceding folliculitis and spread through the follicular wall into the surrounding der-

Community acquired methicillin resistant *Staphylococcus aureus* (C-MRSA) is emerging as a serious skin and soft tissue infection that includes abscesses, cellulitis, and necrotizing fasciitis. Infections are being documented among healthy individuals who have no known risk factors, that is, no recent hospitalization, surgical procedures, or prolonged antibiotic treatment. C-MRSA strains are epidemiologically and clonally unrelated to hospital or nursing home acquired MRSA. Genotyping for the staphylococcal chromosomal cassette mec (SCCmec) type IV and Panton-Valentine leukocidin genes are the most common tests. C-MRSA are more sensitive to antibiotic treatment and there is a wider choice of antibiotic treatment options for C-MRSA compared with hospital-acquired MRSA. Currently the most effective antibiotics are clindamycin, trimethoprim/sulfamethoxazole in combination with rifampin, and linezolid. There is some concern that resistance to clindamycin could develop during therapy, and clinicians should be aware of this complication. Daptomycin has been approved for treatment, and newer generation carbapenems and fluoroquinolones are under clinical investigation, but rapidly developing resistance is a concern. Mupirocin is used to clear MRSA from nasal secretions, if cultures show contamination in the nose. Preventive measures include good hand hygiene, applying antiseptics and covering cuts and abrasions, use of antibacterial soaps for showers after contact sports, avoidance of sharing towels and razors, and frequent towel washing.

Data from Fridkin SK et al: *N Engl J Med* 352(14):1436-1444, 2005; Robinson DA et al: *Lancet* 365(9466):1256-1258, 2005; Miller LG et al: *N Engl J Med* 352(14): 1445-1453, 2005; Raghavan M, Linden PK: *Drugs* 64(15):1621-1642, 2004.

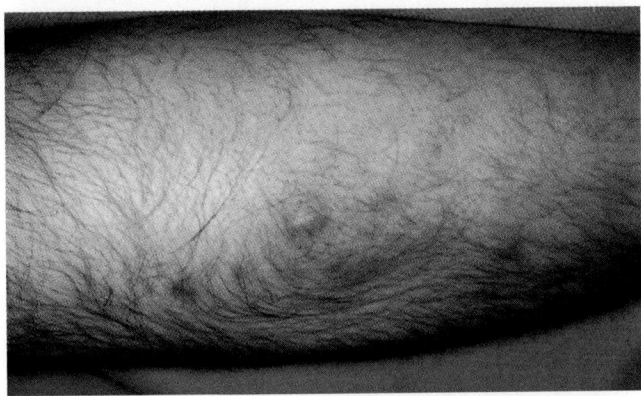

Figure 44-16 Furuncle of the forearm. (Courtesy Department of Dermatology, School of Medicine, University of Utah.)

mis. The invading organism is usually *S. aureus*. The infecting strain may spread to the skin from the anterior nares. Any skin area with hair can be infected, and one or several lesions may be present. The precipitating events are similar to folliculitis. The initial lesion is a deep, firm, red, painful nodule 1 to 5 cm in diameter (Figure 44-16). Within a few days the initial erythematous nodules change to a large fluctuant and tender cystic nodule that may be accompanied by cellulitis. No systemic symptoms are present, and the lesion may drain large amounts of pus and necrotic tissue.

Carbuncles are a collection of infected hair follicles. The lesion occurs most often on the back of the neck, the upper back, and the lateral thighs. The lesion begins in the subcutaneous tissue and lower dermis as a firm mass that evolves into an erythematous, painful, swollen mass that drains through many openings. Abscesses may develop. Chills, fever, and malaise are systemic symptoms that can occur during the early stages of lesion development.

Furuncles and carbuncles are treated with warm compresses to provide comfort and promote localization and spontaneous drainage. Abscess formation requires incision and drainage, and recurrent infections are treated with systemic antibiotics.

Cellulitis

Cellulitis is an infection of the dermis and subcutaneous tissue usually caused by *Staphylococcus* or group B streptococci.[97] Cellulitis can occur as an extension of a skin wound, an ulcer, or from furuncles or carbuncles. Risk factors include diabetes mellitus, edema, peripheral vascular disease, and tinea pedis.[98] The infected area is erythematous, warm, swollen, and painful. The infection responds to systemic antibiotics, and Burow soaks can be used to relieve pain.

Erysipelas

Erysipelas is an acute superficial infection of the upper dermis (a superficial form of cellulitis) most often caused by group A streptococci. The face, ears, and lower legs are common sites of involvement, and the site of initial infection may not be identified. Chills, fever, and malaise precede the onset of lesions by 4 hours to 20 days. The initial lesions appear as firm, red spots that then enlarge and coalesce to form a clearly circumscribed, advancing, bright red, hot lesion with a raised border. Vesicles may appear over the lesion and at the border, producing a bullous form of the disease.[99] Itching, burning, and tenderness accompany the development of the lesion. Cold compresses provide symptomatic relief, and systemic antibiotics are required to arrest the infection.

Impetigo

Impetigo is a superficial lesion of the skin caused by coagulase-positive *Staphylococcus* or α-hemolytic streptococci.[100] It may complicate atopic dermatitis. The disease occurs in adults but is more common in children (see Chapter 45).

Viral Infections

Herpes Simplex Virus

There are eight types of **herpes simplex virus (HSV),** a group of DNA viruses: HSV-1 (type 1), HSV-2 (type 2), cytomegalovirus (CMV), varicella-zoster virus (type 3), Epstein-Barr virus, and human herpesvirus 6, 7, and 8 (Kaposi sarcoma–associated herpesvirus) cause substantial neurologic morbidity among infants and children.[101,102] A "cold sore" or "fever blister" is a type of HSV-1 infection and is the most common manifestation of the herpes simplex virus.[103] HSV-1 usually occurs in nongenital sites and causes infection of the cornea (herpes keratitis), mouth (gingivostomatitis), and labia (labialis). Individuals receiving cytotoxic therapy for cancer are at risk.

The lesions of HSV-1 appear as a rash or clusters of inflamed and painful vesicles within the mouth, over the tongue, or on the lips and around the nose (Figure 44-17). Increased sensitivity, paresthesias, and mild burning may occur before onset of the lesion. The vesicles rupture, forming a crust. Lesions may last 2 to 6 weeks. Occasionally, there is an associated upper respiratory infection. HSV-1 is transmitted by contact with infected saliva. Treatment is symptomatic, and the lesions usually resolve within 2 weeks.

Genital infections are more commonly caused by HSV-2. The virus is spread by skin-to-skin mucous membrane contact during viral shedding. Risk of infection is high after sexual contact with infected individuals. Vertical transmission from mother to neonate is associated with significant neonatal morbidity and mortality.[104] After penetrating the skin, HSV is established in the sensory nerve ganglion innervating the primary site. Infection in one area does not protect other areas from subsequent infection. The primary infection is asymptomatic and can be determined only by a rising antibody titer.[105]

The incubation period ranges from 2 to 14 days, and clinical symptoms last 1 to 3 weeks. An individual then continues to shed the virus for 2 to 6 weeks. The virus remains dormant within sensory or autonomic nerve ganglia and can lead to recurrence of the disease. A number of factors stimulate recurrence, including sun exposure, fever, or stress, and lesions are usually located at or near the primary site. Because anti-HSV antibodies develop in response to infection, recurrence is also related to the titer or amount of antibodies present.

Genital herpes (HSV-2) also may occur in primary or recurrent forms, and a large number of infections are sexually transmitted, usually within 3 to 14 days after exposure (see Chapter 24). The lesions begin as small vesicles that progress to ulceration within 3 to 4 days with pain, itching, and weeping. Treatment includes oral or topical administration of an antiviral drug that decreases new lesion formation and promotes healing. A vaccine has been effective in controlling recurrent infection, and progress is being made with prophylactic vaccines.[106]

Herpes Zoster and Varicella

Herpes zoster (shingles) and **varicella** (chickenpox) are caused by the same herpesvirus, varicella-zoster virus (VZV). Varicella occurs as a primary infection followed years later by herpes zoster, particularly among those who are immune suppressed.[107] Chickenpox usually occurs in children (see Chapter 45).

Herpes zoster, or shingles, has initial symptoms of pain and paresthesia localized to the affected dermatome (the cutaneous area innervated by a single spinal nerve; see Chapter 14), followed by vesicular eruptions along a facial, cervical, or thoracic lumbar dermatome (Figure 44-18). Some individuals have vesicles scattered outside the area of the dermatome. Local symptoms are alleviated with compresses, calamine lotion, or baking soda. Persistent pain is a debilitating complication, particularly in the elderly and requires treatment.[108] Antiviral drugs are useful.[109,110] Approximately 20% of individuals experience postherpetic neuralgias.[111] The varicella vaccine is safe and effective and may boost humoral and cellular immunity in the elderly.[112] Treatment includes a topical lidocaine patch, gabapentin, controlled-release oxycodone, and tricyclic antidepressants.[113]

Warts

Warts (verrucae) are benign lesions of the skin caused by the human papillomavirus (HPV). There are many different types of HPV, and specific viruses are associated with specific kinds and locations of lesions. An oncoprotein expressed by HPV is thought to inactivate growth controls regulated by *p53* tumor-suppressor protein.[114] The lesions are round and elevated with a rough, grayish surface; can occur anywhere on

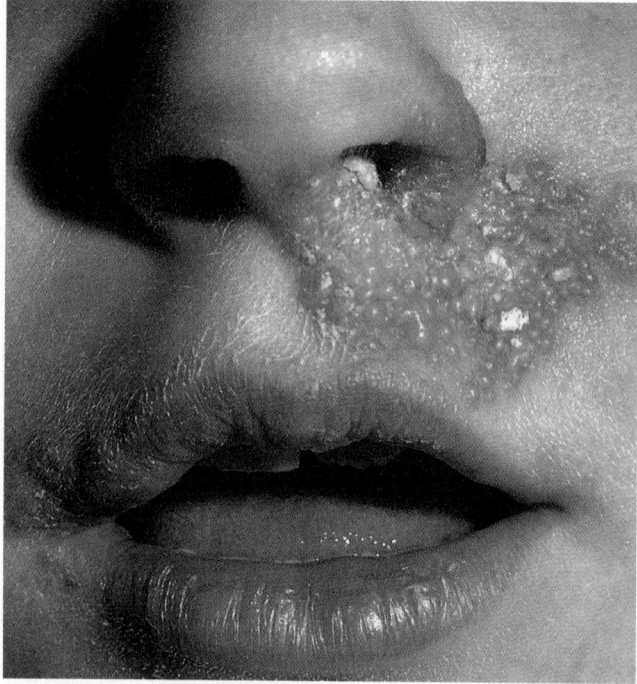

Figure 44-17 Herpes simplex labialis. Typical presentation with tense vesicles appearing on the lips and extending onto the skin. (From Habif TP: *Clinical dermatology: a color guide to diagnosis and therapy,* ed 4, St Louis, 2004, Mosby.)

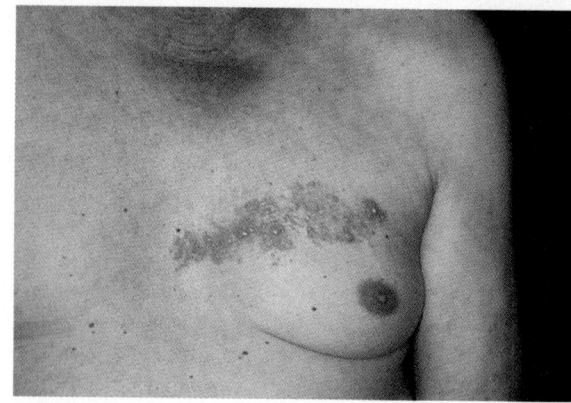

Figure 44-18 Herpes zoster. Diffuse involvement of a dermatome. (Courtesy Department of Dermatology, School of Medicine, University of Utah.)

the skin[115]; and are transmitted by touch. Common warts (verrucae vulgaris) occur most often in children and are usually on the fingers, although they may be located on any skin surface or mucous membrane. Warts vary in shape, size (flat, round, or fusiform), and location (Figure 44-19). Plantar warts are usually located at pressure points on the bottom of the feet.

Diagnosis of warts is by visualization. Treatment considers age of the individual and size and location of the lesion. Warts can be removed by freezing with liquid nitrogen; electrocautery; vaporization with lasers; application of keratolytics; or application of irritants and corrosives, such as salicylic acid, formaldehyde, interferons, or podophyllum.[116-118] Many warts resolve spontaneously, but there is often recurrence.

Condylomata acuminata (venereal warts) are a highly contagious, sexually transmitted disease.[119] The cauliflower-like lesions occur in moist areas, along the glans of the penis, vulva, and anus (see Chapter 24). Oncogenic HPV is a primary cause of cervical cancer[120,121] (see Chapter 23).

Fungal Infections

The fungi causing superficial skin infections are called *dermatophytes,* and they thrive on keratin (stratum corneum, hair, nails). Fungal disorders are known as *mycoses;* when caused by dermatophytes, the mycoses are termed *tinea* (dermatophytosis or ringworm).

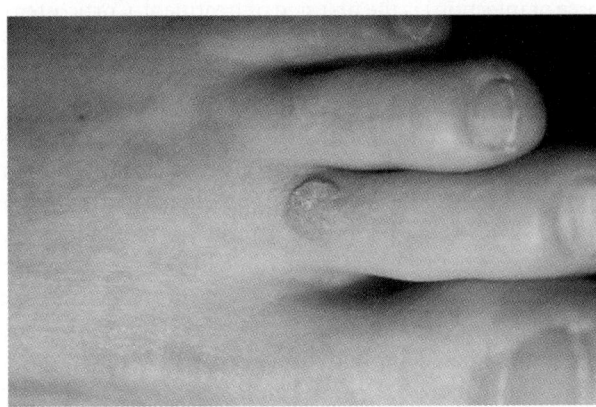

Figure 44-19 Verruca vulgaris. (Courtesy Department of Dermatology, School of Medicine, University of Utah.)

Tinea Infections

Tinea infections are fungal infections of the skin and are classified according to their location on the body.[122] The most common sites are summarized in Table 44-5. These infections are common in children (see Chapter 45). **Tinea pedis** is a chronic, superficial fungal infection of the skin of the foot common in adults (Figure 44-20). In prepubertal children, most scaling disorders of the toes and feet are eczema. **Tinea corporis** **(ringworm)** and **tinea capitis** (a fungal infection of the scalp) are much more common in children than adults. (See Chapter 45 for a discussion of fungal infections in children.)

Tinea is diagnosed by culture, microscopic examination of skin scrapings prepared with potassium hydroxide wet mount, or observation of the skin with an ultraviolet light (Wood lamp). Cultures establish the particular type of fungus and are necessary for hair and nail infections. Fungi have characteristic spores and filaments known as **hyphae** that are

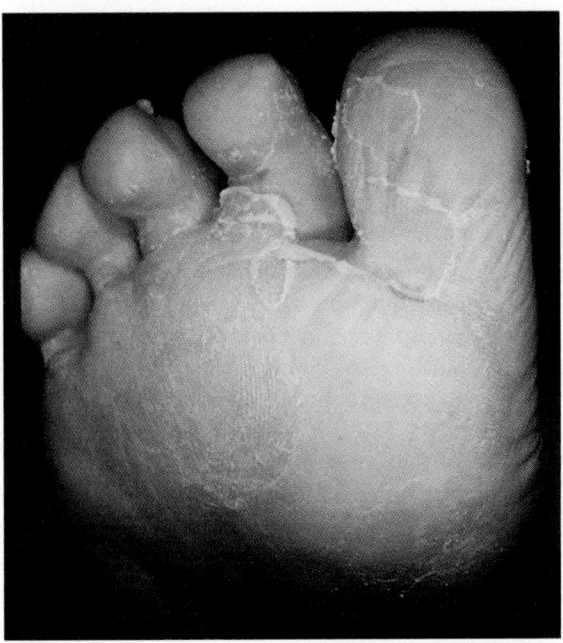

Figure 44-20 Tinea pedis. Inflammation has extended from the web area onto the dorsum of the foot. (Courtesy Department of Dermatology, School of Medicine, University of Utah.)

Table 44-5	Common Sites of Tinea Infections
Site	**Clinical Manifestations**
Tinea capitis (scalp)	Scaly, pruritic scalp with bald areas; hair breaks easily
Tinea corporis (skin areas, excluding scalp, face, hands, feet, groin)	Circular, clearly circumscribed, mildly erythematosus scaly patches with a slightly elevated ringlike border; some forms are dry and macular, and other forms are moist and vesicular
Tinea cruris (groin, also known as "jock itch")	Small erythematous and scaling vesicular patches with a well-defined border that spreads over the inner and upper surfaces of the thighs; occurs with heat and high humidity
Tinea pedis (foot, also known as "athlete's foot")	Occurs between the toes and may spread to the soles of the feet, nails, and skin of toes; slight scaling, macerated painful skin, occasionally with fissures and vesiculation
Tinea manus (hand)	Dry, scaly, erythematosus lesions, or moist vesicular lesions that begin with clusters of intensely itching, clear vesicles; often associated with fungal infection of the feet
Tinea unguium or onychomycosis (nails)	A superficial or deep inflammation of the nail that develops yellow-brown accumulations of brittle keratin over all or portions of the nail

more prominent when prepared in potassium hydroxide. The spores fluoresce blue-green when exposed to ultraviolet light. Treatment is related to the type of fungi and includes both topical and systemic antifungal medication.

Candidiasis

Candidiasis is caused by the yeastlike fungus *Candida albicans* and normally can be found on mucous membranes, on the skin, in the gastrointestinal tract, and in the vagina. *C. albicans* can, under certain circumstances, change from a commensal organism to a pathogen, particularly when the immune system is depressed.[123] Factors that predispose to infection include (1) a local environment of moisture, warmth, maceration, or occlusion; (2) the systemic administration of antibiotics; (3) pregnancy; (4) diabetes mellitus; (5) Cushing disease; (6) debilitated states; (7) age younger than 6 months (more likely to get an infection because of decreased immune reactivity); (8) immunosuppression; and (9) certain neoplastic diseases of the blood and monocyte/macrophage system. The resident bacteria on the skin, mainly cocci, inhibit proliferation of *C. albicans*. Cell-mediated immunity plays a major role in the defense against monilial infections. *C. albicans* can activate the complement system by the alternative pathway and can include small abscesses. Candidiasis affects only the outer layers of mucous membranes and skin and occurs in the mouth, vagina, uncircumcised penis, and large skinfolds. Table 44-6 lists the different sites of candidiasis. Depressed phagocytic function has been observed in individuals with extensive lesions.[124]

The initial lesion is a thin-walled pustule that extends under the stratum corneum with an inflammatory base that may burn or itch. The accumulation of inflammatory cells and scale produces a whitish yellow, curdlike substance over the infected area. The lesion ceases to spread when it reaches dry skin.[125]

Vascular Disorders

Vascular abnormalities are commonly associated with skin diseases, or they may be present as congenital vascular malformations (see Chapter 45) or as vascular responses to local or systemic vasoactive substances. Blood vessels may increase in number, dilate, constrict, or become obliterated by disease processes.

Cutaneous Vasculitis

Vasculitis (angiitis) is an inflammation of the blood vessels. The initiating site of inflammation may be the blood, the vessel wall, or the adjacent tissue. Small vessels are usually affected. Immune complexes, which initiate an uncontrolled inflammatory response, are often the cause of damage, and the lesions are often polymorphic.

Cutaneous vasculitis develops from the deposit of immune complexes in small blood vessels as a toxic response to drugs (phenothiazines, barbiturates, sulfonamides) or allergens or as a response to streptococcal or viral infection. The precise mechanism is not known, but the deposit of immune complex activates complement, which is chemotactic for polymorphonuclear leukocytes. The cutaneous form usually resolves in a few weeks and is treated with steroids.

The disorder is also known as *allergic vasculitis* and occurs primarily in adults. A systemic form (cutaneous systemic vasculitis) can involve other organs, including the kidneys, lungs, and gastrointestinal tract.[126] The extremities are the chief sites, primarily the lower legs and feet. The lesions appear as palpable purpuras (from the leakage of blood from damaged vessels) and progress to hemorrhagic bullae with necrosis and ulceration from occlusion of the vessel (Figure 44-21). Lesions appear in clusters and remain from 1 to 4 weeks. Recurrences are common. Biopsy may disclose the presence of complement or immunoglobulins in the vessel walls.

Identifying and removing the antigen (chemical, drug, or source of infection) is the first step of treatment. Corticosteroids and other drugs may be used when symptoms are severe.[127,128]

Urticaria

Urticaria (hives) is a circumscribed area of raised erythema and edema of the superficial dermis. **Urticarial lesions** are most commonly associated with type I hypersensitivity reactions to drugs (e.g., penicillin, aspirin), certain foods (e.g., strawberries, shellfish), systemic diseases (e.g., intestinal parasites, lupus erythematosus), physical agents (e.g., heat, cold), or complement mediated reactions (see Chapter 8). The lesions are mediated by IgE-stimulated release of histamine, bradykinin, kallikrein, or acetylcholine from mast cells or ba-

Table 44-6	Sites of Candidiasis		
Site	**Risk Factors**	**Clinical Manifestations**	**Treatment**
Vagina (vulvovaginitis)	Heat, moisture, occlusive clothing Pregnancy Systemic antibiotic therapy Diabetes mellitus Sexual intercourse with infected male	Vaginal itching; white, watery, or creamy discharge Red and swollen vaginal and labial membranes with erosions Lesions may spread to anus and groin	Miconazole cream Clotrimazole tablets or cream Nystatin tablets Ketoconazole cream Loose cotton clothing
Penis (balanitis)	Uncircumcised Sexual intercourse with infected female	Pinpoint, red, tender papules and pustules on glans and shaft of penis	Any of creams listed above Topical steroids for severe inflammation
Mouth	Diabetes mellitus Immunosuppressive therapy Inhaled steroids	Red, swollen, painful tongue and oral mucous membranes Localized erosions and plaques appear with chronic infection	Nystatin oral suspension Clotrimazole troches Ketoconazole

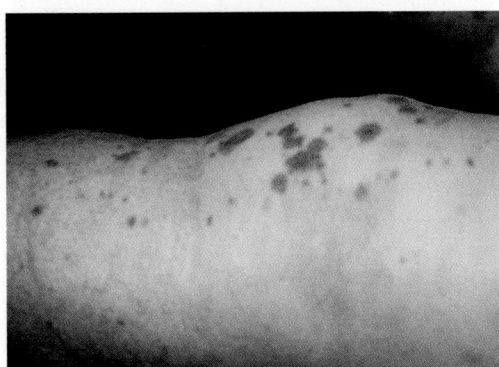

Figure 44-21 Vasculitis of the leg. (Courtesy Department of Dermatology, School of Medicine, University of Utah.)

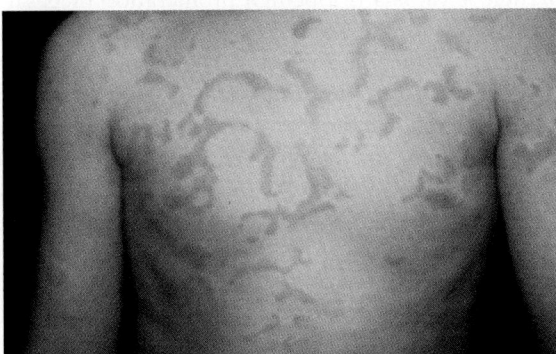

Figure 44-22 Urticaria. (Courtesy Department of Dermatology, School of Medicine, University of Utah.)

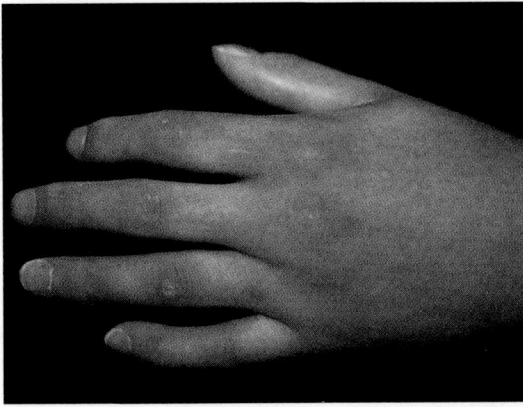

Figure 44-23 Scleroderma (acrosclerosis). Note inflammation and shiny skin. (Courtesy Department of Dermatology, School of Medicine, University of Utah.)

sophils, or both, which causes the endothelial cells of skin blood vessels to contract.[129] The leakage of fluid from the vessel appear as wheals, welts, or hives and may be a few leaks or many leaks distributed over the entire body (Figure 44-22). Most lesions resolve spontaneously within 24 hours, but new lesions may appear. All possible causes should be removed. Antihistamines (H1 antagonists) usually reduce hives and provide relief of itching. Epinephrine or corticosteroids and α-adrenergic agonists may be required for treatment of severe attacks (i.e., angioderma). Chronic urticaria is either an autoimmune or idiopathic disease.[130,131]

Scleroderma

Scleroderma means sclerosis of the skin, and the disease is associated with several autoantibodies.[132] The disease is more prominent in women. It may affect the visceral organs or remain localized to the skin. *Systemic scleroderma* involves the connective tissues of many organs, including the kidney, heart, peripheral nervous system, gastrointestinal tract, and lungs.[133] Only a few organs are involved in some individuals. The cutaneous lesions are most often on the face and hands, neck, and upper chest. The entire skin can be involved, however.

There are massive deposits of collagen with fibrosis, accompanied by inflammatory reactions, vascular changes in the capillary network with a decrease in the number of capillary loops, dilation of the remaining capillaries, enhanced expression of adhesion molecules, and perivascular infiltrates.[134] Fi-

brosis occurs in the papillary and reticular dermis and in the subcutaneous tissue and deep fascia. Autoimmunity and an immune reaction to a toxic substance are both possible initiating mechanisms of the disease, and autoantibodies are often recovered from the skin and serum of individuals with scleroderma.[135] Impaired regulation of collagen gene expression by fibroblasts probably underlies the persistent fibrosis.[136]

The skin is hard, hypopigmented, taut, shiny, and tightly connected to the underlying tissue. The tightness of the facial skin projects an immobile masklike appearance, and the mouth may not open completely. The nose may assume a beaklike appearance. The hands are shiny and sometimes red and edematous (Figure 44-23). The fingers become tapered and flexed, often with depressed scars and loss of fingertips from atrophy. Raynaud phenomenon with episodic arteriolar vasoconstriction of the fingers contributes to ulcer formation.[137] The nails may be shed. Calcium deposits develop in the subcutaneous tissue and erupt through the skin. Progression to body organs may occur, and death is caused by subsequent respiratory failure, renal failure, cardiac dysrhythmias, or esophageal or intestinal obstruction or perforation. There is no specific treatment, and progression of the disease is variable. Fifty percent of individuals die within 5 years of the onset of scleroderma.

Suitable clothing and a warm environment are essential to protecting the hands. Trauma and smoking should be avoided. Vasodilator drugs (i.e., angiotensin-converting enzyme inhibitors) or sympathectomy rarely has lasting effects. Symptomatic treatment is required for involved organs (e.g., intestinal resection for obstruction, antibiotics for pneumonitis, and regulation of hypertension).[138]

Insect Bites

Ticks

Ticks are significant vectors of transmitted diseases, including Rocky Mountain spotted fever and other rickettsial diseases, tularemia, and Lyme disease.[139] Ticks vary in size from 1 cm to about the size of a comma on this printed page. They embed their heads in the skin to obtain blood. As they gorge themselves on blood, they enlarge to many times their normal size and may release toxins or transmit microorganisms during feeding. In most instances, there is no consequence from a tick bite, with the exception of a papular urticaria at the site of the bite. If mouthparts remain in the skin when the tick is removed, a persistent nodule remains that may require excision; ideally the tick should be removed completely intact. Irritant substances, such as camphor, gasoline, soft wax, or heat from a match, may stimulate the tick to withdraw its head. Applying tick repellant, such as diethyltoluamide (DEET), butopyronoxyl (Indalone), or benzylbenzoate, helps to prevent tick bites.

Lyme disease is a multisystem inflammatory disease caused by the spirochete *Borrelia burgdorferi* transmitted by tick bites and is the most frequently reported vector-borne illness.[140] The highest incidence is among children, and 50% of infected individuals are symptom free. Symptoms of the disease occur in stages. Soon after the bite, there is localized infection (erythema migrans [rash] with or without flulike illness). Within weeks to months after the onset of the illness, there is disseminated infection (secondary erythema migrans, arthralgias, meningitis, neuritis, carditis). Late persistent infection can continue for years (arthritis, encephalopathy, polyneuropathy). An immune response to *B. burgdorferi* may contribute to the pathogenesis of the disease.[141] The microorganism is difficult to culture, and it escapes immunodefenses through antigenetic diversity.[142]

The diagnosis of Lyme disease is based on the clinical presentation and history of tick bite, if known. Serologic tests often are used to confirm the diagnosis.[143] Antibiotics (i.e., doxycycline) are used for treatment.[144] Vaccines are available for prevention in persons 15 to 70 years of age.[145]

Mosquitoes and Flies

There are thousands of species of **mosquitoes** throughout the world. Species from the Culicidae family are responsible for malaria, yellow fever, dengue fever, filariasis, and St. Louis encephalitis. Mosquitoes can bite through thin, loose clothing and are attracted by warmth and sweat. The edema, pruritus, and papular lesions of the mosquito bite are caused by the disruption of the skin from the insertion of a blood tube by a female mosquito. Irritating salivary secretions also contain anticoagulants. Reactions vary depending on the sensitivity of the victim.

Several species of flies are blood suckers. The black fly (Simuliidae) is usually found in swarms—near moving bodies of water in the late spring and early summer—and is a vicious biter. The initial bite is painless because the fly injects an anesthetic with the bite. Subsequent lesions are painful and accompanied by significant swelling of surrounding tissues. Systemic reactions, such as fever, headache, and nausea, are common.

Very small flies of the Ceratopogonidae family, also known as "no-see-ums," "midges," "punkies," or sand fleas, are also blood suckers. The bite of the female is particularly miserable and produces immediate pain, erythema, and vesicles. Itching and vesicular reactions may persist for weeks.

The fiercest blood-sucking flies are the Tabanidae, or horseflies, deer flies, gadflies, greenheads, and clegs. These flies vary in size from 1 to 5 cm and produce painful, bleeding bites because of their large mouthparts. The bites produce urticaria that may be accompanied by weakness, dizziness, and wheezing.

Wounds produced by biting insects should be cleansed with soap and water, and a local antiseptic should be applied. Local applications of steroid creams or antihistamine will reduce symptoms. Systemic reactions may require more specific medical care.

Benign Tumors

Most benign tumors of the skin are associated with aging. Benign tumors include seborrheic keratosis, keratoacanthoma, actinic keratosis, and moles.

Seborrheic Keratosis

Seborrheic keratosis is a benign proliferation of basal cells that produces smooth or warty elevated lesions. They are usually seen in older people and occur as multiple lesions on the chest, back, and face. The color varies from tan to waxy yellow, flesh colored, or dark brown-black. Lesion size varies from a few millimeters to several centimeters, and they are often oval and greasy appearing with a hyperkeratotic stuck-on scaly appearance (Figure 44-24). Cryotherapy with liquid nitrogen is effective treatment, and the lesions usually slough 2 to 3 weeks after treatment.

Keratoacanthoma

A **keratoacanthoma** is a benign, self-limiting tumor of squamous cell differentiation arising from hair follicles. It usually occurs on sun-damaged skin of elderly individuals and smokers; the incidence is high in males. The most commonly affected sites are the face, back of the hands, forearms, neck, and legs (Figure 44-25). The lesion develops over a period of 1 to 2 months and has a histology resembling a well-differentiated squamous cell carcinoma[146]:

Proliferative stage. Lesion develops as a rapidly growing, dome-shaped nodule with central crust.

Mature stage. Lesion fills with whitish keratin and requires differentiation from squamous cell carcinoma.[147]

Involution stage. This stage occurs over a 3- to 4-month period with regression of the lesion.

Although the lesions will resolve spontaneously, they can be removed by curettage or excision to improve cosmetic appearance.

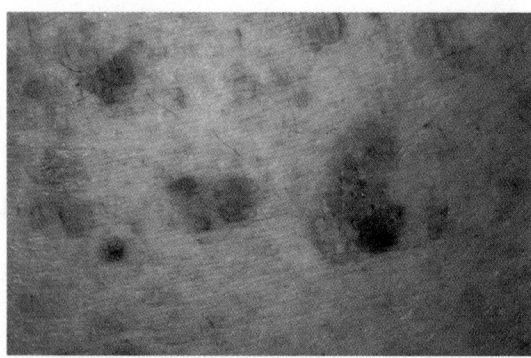

Figure 44-24 Seborrheic keratosis. Typical lesion that is broad, flat, and comparatively smooth surfaced. (Courtesy Department of Dermatology, School of Medicine, University of Utah.)

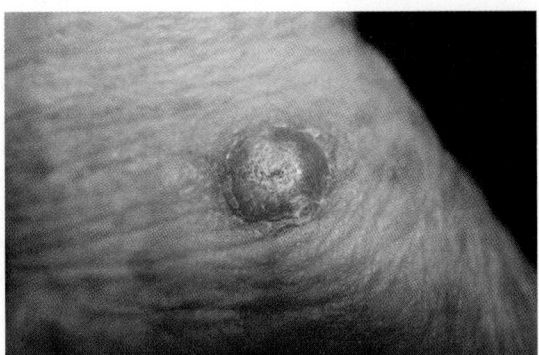

Figure 44-25 Keratoacanthoma. Classic presentation of a fully developed tumor. Round, smooth, dome-shaped mass with a central keratin-filled crater. (Courtesy Department of Dermatology, School of Medicine, University of Utah.)

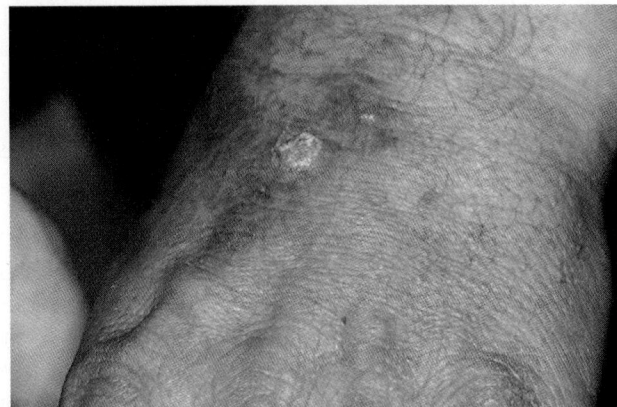

Figure 44-26 Actinic keratosis. (Courtesy Department of Dermatology, School of Medicine, University of Utah.)

Actinic Keratosis

Actinic keratosis is a premalignant lesion found on skin surfaces exposed to the ultraviolet radiation of the sun. The prevalence is highest in individuals with unprotected, light-colored skin. Actinic keratosis is rare in black skin. The lesions appear as rough, poorly defined papules that are felt more than seen (Figure 44-26). Surrounding areas may have telangiectasias. Freezing with liquid nitrogen provides quick, effective treatment. Application of topical modulators, including 5-fluorouracil, diclofenac sodium gel, or imiquimod cream, as well as excision, which provides tissue for histopathology, may be used for treatment.[148] The lesions should continue to be evaluated for progression to squamous cell carcinoma.[149] Protection from the sun with clothing or a sun-blocking agent to prevent lesions from developing elsewhere is advised.

Nevi

Nevi (moles) are pigmented or nonpigmented lesions that form from melanocytes beginning at ages 3 to 5 years. During the early stages of development, the cells accumulate at the junction of the dermis and epidermis and are macular lesions. Over time the cells move down into the dermis and the nevi become nodular and palpable. Nevi may appear on any part of the skin, and they vary in size. They occur singly or in groups and are not considered disfiguring. Nevi may undergo transition to malignant melanomas (see p. 1599). Nevi irritated by clothing can be excised.

Cancer

Skin cancers account for about 40% of all cancers, and the incidence of skin cancer is increasing.[150] Basal cell carcinoma and squamous cell carcinoma are the most common skin cancers. Incidence of these carcinomas is greater in men than in women, and incidence increases steadily with age. Malignant melanoma is the most serious skin cancer. An estimated 10,500 people die of skin cancer each year; 7700 of these deaths are from malignant melanoma.[150] Important trends related to skin cancer are presented in Box 44-3.

Ultraviolet solar radiation causes most skin cancers by inducing mutations in the *p53* tumor-suppressor gene.[151,152] Protection from the sun during the first 10 to 20 years of life

Box 44-3	Important Trends for Skin Cancer Incidence*

Over 1 million cases per year with likely under-reporting because of lack of a nonmelanoma skin cancer registry.

The majority are highly curable **basal** or **squamous** cell cancers accounting for more than 50% of all cancers; not as common is the most serious **malignant melanoma** with an estimated 59,580 cases in 2005, it represents 4% of all skin cancer cases but causes about 79% of all skin cancer deaths.

Mortality
Total estimated deaths in 2005 were 7770 from melanoma and approximately 10,500 from all other types of skin cancer.

Risk Factors
- Excessive exposure to ultraviolet radiation from the sun
- Fair complexion
- Occupational exposure to coal tar, pitch, creosote, arsenic compounds, and radium
- Exposure to human papillomavirus and human immunodeficiency virus
- Skin cancer is negligible in blacks because of heavy skin pigmentation

Warning Signals*
Any change on the skin, especially a change in the size or color of a mole or other darkly pigmented growth or spot.

Prevention and Early Detection
Avoidance of sun when ultraviolet light is strongest (e.g., 10:00 AM to 3:00 PM); use sunscreen preparations, especially those containing ingredients such as PABA (para-aminobenzoic acid); basal and squamous cell cancers often form a pale, waxlike, pearly nodule or a red, scaly, sharply outlined patch; melanomas are usually dark brown or black pigmentation; they start as small molelike growths that increase in size, change color, become ulcerated, and bleed easily from a slight injury.

Treatment
There are four methods of treatment: surgery, electrodesiccation (tissue destruction by heat), radiation therapy, or cryosurgery (tissue destruction by freezing); for malignant melanomas, wide and often deep excisions and removal of nearby lymph nodes are required.

Survival*
For basal cell and squamous cell cancers, cure is highly likely with early detection and treatment; malignant melanoma, however, metastasizes quickly; this accounts for a lower 5-year survival rate, particularly for white patients with this disease.

*Data from American Cancer Society: *Cancer facts and figures 2005,* Atlanta, 2005, The Society.

significantly reduces the risk of skin cancer.[153] Areas widely exposed to the sun's rays—the face, neck, and hands—are highly vulnerable for such lesions. Outdoor workers (farmers, sailors, fishermen) are high-risk skin cancer populations. Like other cancers, skin cancers progress through stages of initiation, progression, and metastasis.

Basal Cell Carcinoma

Basal cell carcinoma is a surface epithelial tumor of the skin originating from undifferentiated basal or germinative cells. The tumors grow upward and laterally or downward to the dermal epidermal junction (Figure 44-27). They usually have depressed centers and rolled borders. Early tumors are so small that they are not clinically apparent. Generally these tumors do not invade blood or lymph vessels; thus they do not metastasize beyond the skin. Basal cell carcinoma can cause severe local destruction, however.

Basal cell carcinoma is the most common type of skin cancer in whites and is thought to be caused by ultraviolet radiation exposure.[154] Lesions are seen most often on people who live in regions with intense sunlight and on those areas of the skin most exposed—namely, the face and neck. Dark-skinned persons and those avoiding sunlight are significantly less likely to develop these malignant tumors. In dark-skinned persons, basal cells contain the pigment melanin, a protective factor against sun exposure. Although ultraviolet radiation seems to be the primary causative agent, other factors are implicated: arsenic and genetic factors (i.e., an environmentally induced alteration on chromosome 9 that has tumor-suppressor activity and down-regulation of *TP53* gene).[154,155] The use of arsenic in insecticides has recently diminished; however, arsenic is still found in drinking water from ground wells.[156] Genetic factors are displayed in the less common nevoid basal cell carcinoma syndrome.

These tumors arise as a consequence of a defect that prevents the cells from being shed by the normal keratinization process. The maturing process of epidermal cells is called *keratinization;* however, the process of keratinization specifically means the synthesis of fibrous protein or keratin. Basal cell tumors lack the normal keratin proteins, but this condition

may be reversible. Transplantation of basal cell and in vitro cultures shows the property of keratinization can be restored.

The growth rate for these tumors is quite slow. The lesion starts as a nodule (greater than 5 mm across) that is pearly or ivory in appearance and slightly elevated above the skin surface; it has small blood vessels on the surface. As the lesion grows, it often ulcerates, develops crusting, and is firm to the touch. If left untreated, basal cell lesions invade surrounding tissues and, over months or years, can destroy a nose, an eyelid, or an ear (for treatment, see Box 44-3). Metastatic spread is rare.[157]

Squamous Cell Carcinoma

Squamous cell carcinoma is a tumor of the epidermis characterized by two types: in situ and invasive. Because of the invasive nature of some tumors, squamous cell carcinoma becomes significantly more malignant if left untreated.[158]

Ultraviolet exposure causes squamous cell carcinoma.[159] Areas affected are the head and neck (75%) and the hands (15%), with 10% of squamous cell carcinomas occurring elsewhere on the body. These tumors are more predominant in countries where arsenic is found in higher rates in drinking water. Gamma rays and x-rays are also associated with squamous cell carcinoma. In addition, patients who are immunosuppressed experience a greater occurrence of this carcinoma.

The exact mechanism for producing squamous cell carcinoma is unknown. Again, the initiator-promoter model can be applied to explain the cancer process (see Chapter 12), particularly with mutation of the *p53* gene.[160] It is unclear whether ultraviolet light produces its harmful effects because of problems in DNA synthesis, repair, or replication.

Invasive squamous cell carcinoma can arise from premalignant lesions of the skin. It rarely arises from normal-appearing skin or "de novo." The premalignant lesions include sun-damaged skin or dysplasias (actinic dermatitis); leukoplasia, or whitish, discolored areas; scars; radiation-induced keratosis; tar and oil keratosis; and chronic ulcers and sinuses. The invasive type grows more rapidly than basal cell carcinomas and can spread to regional lymph nodes. These tumors are firm and increase in both elevation and diameter. The surface may be granular and bleed easily (Figure 44-28).

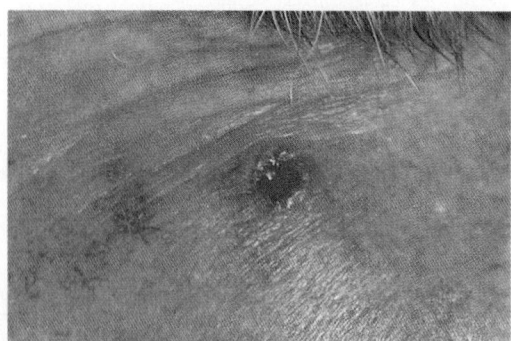

Figure 44-27 **Basal cell carcinoma.** Center has ulcerated. (Courtesy Department of Dermatology, School of Medicine, University of Utah.)

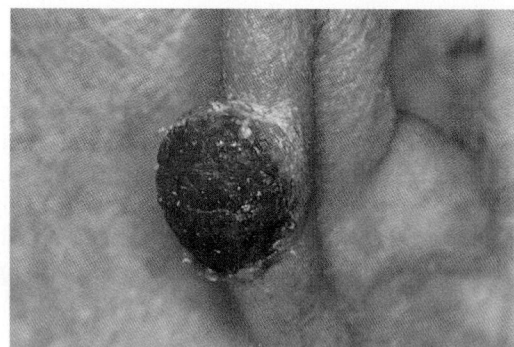

Figure 44-28 **Squamous cell carcinoma.** The sun-exposed ear is a common site for squamous cell carcinoma. (Courtesy Department of Dermatology, School of Medicine, University of Utah.)

In situ squamous cell carcinoma is usually confined to the epidermis (intraepidermal) but may extend into the dermis. Common premalignant skin lesions associated with in situ squamous cell carcinomas are actinic (solar) keratosis and Bowen disease. Actinic keratosis is a white, scaly, keratotic (horny) lesion on the exposed areas of the body. Bowen disease is a dysplasia of the basal layer of the dermis or carcinoma in situ. It often is found on unexposed areas of the body and is demonstrated by flat, reddish, scaly patches. These lesions may enlarge to more than 1 cm in diameter, rarely invading surrounding tissue and almost never metastasizing. Other cellular components in the skin (sweat glands, hair follicles, etc.) can give rise to skin cancer, but these cancers are relatively uncommon.

Malignant Melanoma

Melanoma is a malignant tumor of the skin originating from melanocytes, or cells that synthesize the pigment melanin. The incidence of melanoma is increasing, and young to middle-age adults are at highest risk.[161] Early recognition of cutaneous melanomas can have a major impact on surgically curing this disease. The ABCDE rule is used as a guide: **A**symmetry, **B**order irregularity, **C**olor variation, **D**iameter larger than 6 mm, and **E**levation, which includes raised appearance or rapid enlargement.[162]

Risk factors implicated in melanoma induction include genetic predisposition, exposure to ultraviolet light (solar and artificial), steroid hormone activity, fair hair, light skin with a propensity to sunburn, and freckles.[163,164] Melanomas arise as a result of malignant degeneration of melanocytes located either along the basal layer of the epidermis or in a benign melanocytic nevus. A number of proto-oncogenes have been identified in human malignant melanoma.[165] A nevus, or mole, is an aggregation of melanocytes (Figure 44-29). These clusters of cells may not be apparent until puberty, when the pigmentation process is initiated by steroid hormones. The relationship between nevi and melanoma makes it important for the clinician to understand the various neval forms (Table 44-7). Most nevi never become suspicious; however, suspicious pigmented nevi should be removed.[166] Indications for biopsy include color change, size change, irregular notched margin, itching, bleeding or oozing, nodularity, scab formation, and ulceration. Staging of melanoma is determined from tissue biopsy, by assessing the thickness of the lesion using the Breslow microstage, and the Clark levels of tumor invasion[167] (Figure 44-30). The clinical varieties of cutaneous melanoma include lentigo malignant melanoma (LMM) (Figure 44-31), superficial spreading melanoma (SSM) (Figure 44-32), primary nodular melanoma (PNM), and acral lentiginous melanoma. A melanotic melanoma is the most

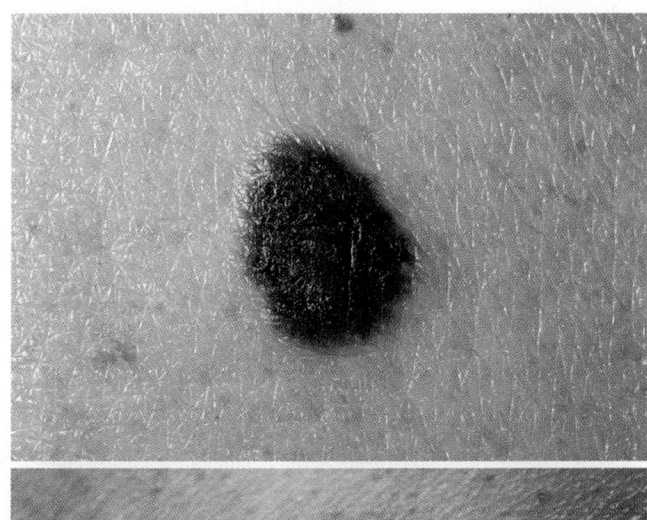

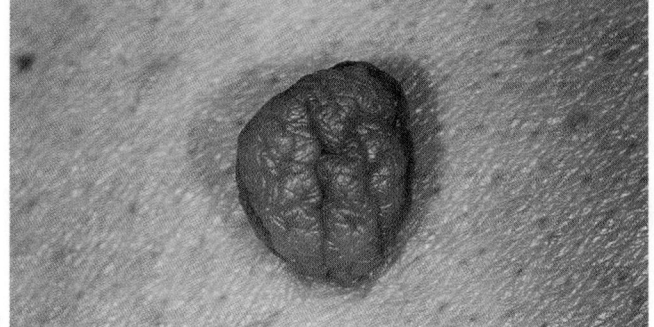

Figure 44-29 Nevi. **A,** Junction nevus: slightly raised, dark, and uniform. **B,** Dermal nevus: pedunculated with a soft, flabby, wrinkled surface. (From Habif TP: *Clinical dermatology: a color guide to diagnosis and therapy,* ed 4, St Louis, 2004, Mosby.)

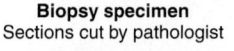

Biopsy specimen
Sections cut by pathologist

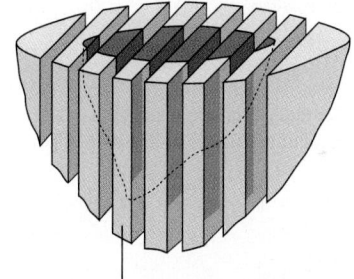

Section with deepest penetration of tumor; this section used to report Breslow microstage and Clark level

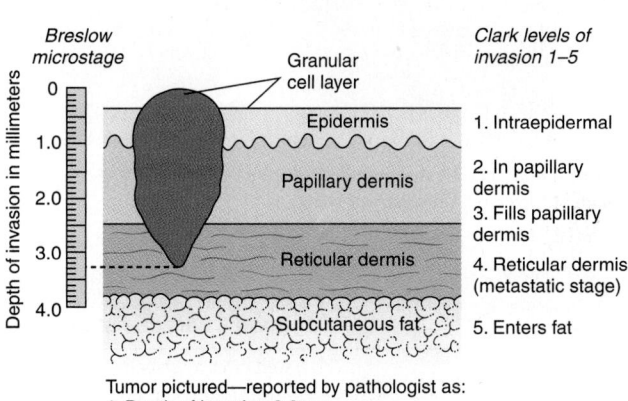

Figure 44-30 Melanoma staging using Breslow and Clark levels of invasion. (From Habif TP: *Clinical dermatology: a color guide to diagnosis and therapy,* ed 4, St. Louis, 2004, Mosby.)

rare subtype and is a nonpigmented melanoma. Clinical characteristics are summarized in Table 44-8.

Treatment of melanoma with no evidence of metastatic disease involves surgical excision to the primary site and regional lymph nodes. The extent of surgery is determined by the staging of disease. Lesions of the extremities have the best prognosis; head and neck lesions and trunk lesions have the poorest prognosis. Only 20% to 40% of patients with regional lymph node involvement are alive and cured at 5 years. Immune response modifiers, vaccines, and gene therapy are under investigation.[168,169]

Kaposi Sarcoma

Kaposi sarcoma (KS) is a vascular malignancy with four different presentations:

1. In association with drug-induced immunosuppressions, for example, after kidney transplant
2. An endemic form in equatorial Africa

3. A form presenting on the lower legs of elderly men
4. In association with acquired immunodeficiency syndrome (AIDS)

Kaposi-associated herpesvirus 8 is found in all four forms of KS.[170,171]

Individuals with AIDS are immunosuppressed, and this allows for opportunistic infections and malignancy. Proliferation of the tumor depends on the presence of platelet-derived growth factors.[172]

The human immunodeficiency virus and cytomegalovirus have been proposed as cofactors in the development of KS.[173] The herpesvirus may be a common etiology for all types of KS.[174] The endothelial cell is thought to be the progenitor of KS. The lesions emerge as purplish brown macules and develop into plaques and nodules. They tend to be multifocal rather than spreading by metastasis. The lesions initially appear over the lower extremities in the classic form (Figure 44-33). The rapidly progressive form associated with AIDS tends to spread symmetrically over the upper body, particularly the face and oral mucosa. The lesions are often pruritic and painful. About 75% of individuals with epidemic KS have involvement of lymph nodes, particularly in the gastrointestinal tract and lungs. Organ involvement is much less common in the classic form. The rapidly progressive form has a poor prognosis and shorter survival rates than the classic form. (See Chapter 24 for a further discussion on AIDS.)

Diagnosis is by skin biopsy, with a high index of suspicion for those with immune deficiency. Local lesions can be ex-

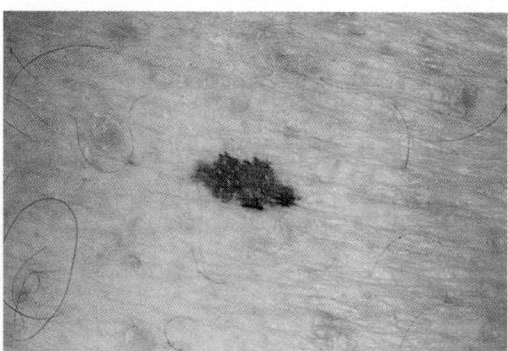

Figure 44-31 **Lentigo malignant melanoma.** (Courtesy Department of Dermatology, School of Medicine, University of Utah.)

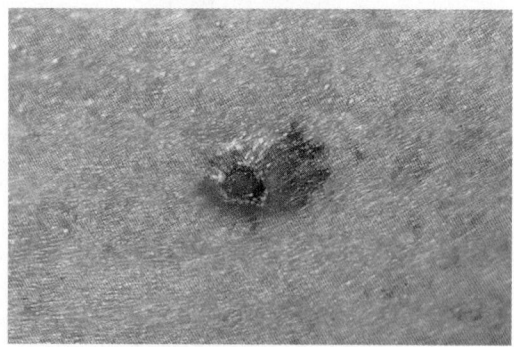

Figure 44-32 **Level 4 melanoma.** (Courtesy Department of Dermatology, School of Medicine, University of Utah.)

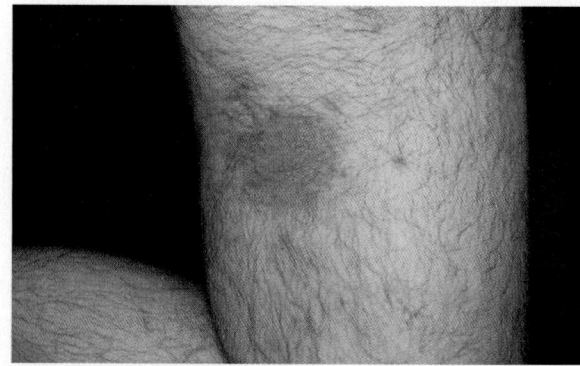

Figure 44-33 **Kaposi sarcoma.** The purple lesion commonly seen on the skin. (Courtesy Department of Dermatology, School of Medicine, University of Utah.)

Table 44-7	Classification of Nevi
Nevi	**Common Characteristics**
Junctional nevus	Flat, well circumscribed, vary in size up to 2 cm, dark color, hairs may be present; originate in basal layer of epidermis and can eventually reach the cutaneous surface; rarely develop into a melanoma
Compound nevus	Most common in adolescents; the majority of pigmented lesions in children; rarely does this lesion develop to melanoma; usually 1 cm in size; hairs may be present; surface is elevated and smooth
Intradermal nevus	Small (less than 1 cm) with regular edges and bristle-like hairs; color ranges from skin tone to light brown; has a slight likelihood of developing into a melanoma

Table 44-8	Clinical Characteristics of Varieties of Cutaneous Melanoma	
Characteristic	**Description**	
Lentigo Malignant Melanoma		
Frequency	10% to 15% of cutaneous melanomas	
Age at diagnosis	50 to 80 years old	
Primary location	Head, neck, dorsum of hands	
Pigmentation according to thickness		
<1.5 mm (levels I and II)	Tan and brown	
>1.5 mm (level III)	Tan, brown, and blue-black	
>1.5 mm (levels IV and V)	Nodule formation	
Superficial Spreading Melanomas		
Frequency	70% of cutaneous melanomas	
Age at diagnosis	20 to 60 years old	
Primary location	Legs of females; upper back of both genders	
Pigmentation according to thickness		
<1.5 mm (levels I and II)	Tan and brown	
>1.5 mm (level III)	Tan, brown, and blue-black	
>1.5 mm (levels IV and V)	Nodule formation	
Primary Nodular Melanoma		
Frequency	12% of cutaneous melanomas	
Age at diagnosis	20 to 60 years old	
Primary location	No specific site preference	
Pigmentation according to thickness		
>1.5 mm (level III)	Small nodule (any hue)	
>1.5 mm (levels IV and V)	Large nodule (any hue)	
Acral-Lentiginous Melanoma		
Frequency	2% to 8% in whites; 30% to75% in African-Americans, Hispanics, Asians	
Age at diagnosis	20 to 60 years old	
Primary location	Palms, soles of feet, mucous membranes	
Pigmentation at any thickness	Blue-black	

cised. Multiple disseminated lesions may be treated with a combination of interferon-α; radiation therapy; and cytotoxic drugs, particularly PEGylated liposomal doxorubicin, liposomal daunorubicin, and paclitaxel.[175] The new, highly active antiretroviral therapies for AIDS treatment is decreasing the incidence of KS. Experimental treatments include angiogenesis inhibitors; hormonal therapies; retinoic acid derivatives; and immune modulators, such as interleukin-12[175-177] and RNA-interference and gene therapy.[178]

Frostbite

Frostbite is injury to the skin caused by exposure to extreme cold. The areas most commonly affected are fingers, toes, ears, nose, and cheeks. Initially the body responds with alternating cycles of vasoconstriction and vasodilation—"the burning re-

action." The mechanism of injury is complex but appears to be related to direct cold injury to cells, indirect injury and cell death from extracellular and intracellular ice crystal formation, and impaired circulation with anoxia because of thrombosis in the exposed area.[179] The inflammatory mediators of frostbite are similar to burns and include prostaglandins, thromboxanes, bradykinin, and histamine. Reperfusion injury is part of the pathophysiology.[180] Frozen skin becomes white or yellowish and is waxy. There is numbness and no sensation of pain.

Skin damage can range from mild to severe. With mild frostbite, redness and discomfort occur during rewarming, followed by a return to normal in a few hours. In more severe cases, cyanosis and mottling develop, followed by redness, swelling, and burning pain on rewarming. Within 24 to 48 hours, vesicles and bullae appear that resolve into crusts that eventually slough off, leaving thin, newly formed skin. The most severe cases result in gangrene with loss of the affected part. Frostbite may be classified by depth of injury after rewarming[181]:

First degree. Superficial, characterized by a numb central white area surrounded by erythema and edema and including partial skin freezing without blistering

Second degree. Full-thickness skin freezing with blistering surrounded by edema and hyperemia

Third degree. Deep, characterized by full-thickness skin and subcutaneous freezing with tissue necrosis and hemorrhagic vesicles

Fourth degree. Deep tissue freezing with full-thickness necrosis and gangrene

Immediate treatment of frostbite is to cover affected areas with other body surfaces and warm clothing. The area should not be rubbed or massaged. Local, dry heat should be avoided. Immersion in a warm water bath (40° to 42° C) until frozen tissue is thawed is the best treatment. Aspirin is used to inhibit prostaglandins, and aloe vera is a topical inhibitor of thromboxane.[182] Pain during the thawing period is severe and should be treated with potent analgesics. Gentle cleansing and no pressure on the skin should be maintained during healing. Amputation of necrotic tissue is delayed until a clear line of demarcation is established.

DISORDERS OF THE HAIR

Alopecia

Male-Pattern Alopecia (Androcentric Alopecia)

Alopecia means loss of hair. Localized hair loss in men is not a disease but rather a genetically predisposed response to androgens. The mechanism of inheritance is unknown. Within the distribution of hair over the scalp, androgen-sensitive hair follicles are on top and androgen-insensitive follicles are on the sides and back. In genetically predisposed men, the androgen-sensitive follicles are transformed into vellus follicles. The normal hair is shed and replaced by fine, light, short hair. Male-pattern baldness begins with frontotemporal recession and progresses to loss of hair over the top of the scalp. Minoxidil may be used to stimulate hair growth and finasteride may decrease the effect of androgens on hair follicles.[183] Affected men may choose to wear wigs or have hair transplants.

Female-Pattern Alopecia

Some women in their 20s and 30s experience progressive thinning and loss of hair over the central part of the scalp.[184] Contrary to male-pattern baldness, no loss of hair occurs along the frontal hairline. Many of these women have elevated levels of serum adrenal androgen dehydroepiandrosterone sulfate (DHEAS).[185] In rare instances a male-pattern baldness develops. Laboratory evaluation of serum androgenic hormones shows elevations, and some women have decreased hair loss when treated with daily doses of spironolactone.

Alopecia Areata

Alopecia areata is an autoimmune T cell–mediated chronic inflammatory disease directed at hair follicles that results in baldness.[186] Hair loss occurs in multiple areas of the scalp, usually in round patches.[187] The eyebrows, eyelashes, beard, and other areas of the body are rarely involved. The cause is unknown, but stressful events, cell-mediated immune factors (including IL-1),[188] and genetic susceptibility are linked to hair loss. Metabolic disorders, such as Addison disease, thyroid disease, and lupus erythematosus, also are associated with alopecia areata.[189-191]

The affected areas of skin are smooth or may have short shafts of hair. The hair shaft is poorly developed and breaks at the surface. Regrowth occurs within 1 to 3 months, but hair loss may recur at the same site. Permanent regrowth of hair usually occurs. Total loss of hair (alopecia totalis) occurs in some young people; the long-term prognosis for total hair regrowth is poor.

Diagnosis is made by observation of the pattern of hair loss. Biopsy may show a lymphocytic infiltrate around the follicle. There are several treatments for alopecia areata. Intralesional steroids may be used to stimulate hair growth when there are a few small areas of hair loss. Systemic steroids are used for larger areas of alopecia. Topical applications of anthralin also are used to stimulate hair growth. Minoxidil has been tested for use in resistant cases and has been found effective in some cases, and topical immunotherapy is effective for extensive areas.[192]

Hirsutism

Hirsutism is the abnormal growth and distribution of hair on the face, body, and pubic area in a male pattern that occurs in women. There is also frontotemporal hair recession. These areas of hair growth are androgen sensitive.[193] Variations of hair growth in women are great, and a male pattern can be normal. Women who develop hirsutism may be secreting hormones associated with ovarian or adrenal disease, and such women should be evaluated for polycystic ovaries, adrenal hyperplasia, or adrenal tumors.[194] If no hormonal pathologic conditions exist, treatment may include cosmetic removal of hair, oral contraceptives, glucocorticoids, cimetidine, finasteride or flutamide, and insulin sensitizers.[195-197]

DISORDERS OF THE NAIL

Paronychia

Paronychia is an acute or chronic infection of the cuticle. Acute paronychia is manifest by the rapid onset of painful inflammation of the cuticle, usually after minor trauma. An abscess may develop, requiring incision and drainage for relief of pain. The most common causative organisms are staphylococci and streptococci. Occasionally *Candida* will be present.

Chronic paronychia develops slowly, with tenderness and swelling around the proximal or lateral nail folds. One or more fingers or toes may be involved. Individuals whose hands are frequently exposed to moisture are at greatest risk. Manipulation of the cuticle can be predisposing because it opens the space between the proximal nail fold and nail plate, leaving a moist, warm medium for the incubation of pathogenic organisms. The skin around the nail becomes more edematous and painful with progressive infection. Pus may be expressed from the proximal nail fold. The nail plate is usually not affected, although it can become discolored and develop ridges.

Treatment includes keeping the hands dry. Oral antibiotics are not very effective because they do not penetrate the affected tissues. Topical application of thymol is usually effective.

Onychomycosis

Onychomycosis is a fungal or dermatophyte infection of the nail plate that occurs in 2% to 18% of the population.[198] The most common pattern is a nail plate that turns yellow or white and becomes elevated as a result of the accumulation of hyperkeratotic debris within the plate. Fungal infections of the nail may require culture and microscopy. In psoriasis, pitting often is found on the nail surface.[199] Treatment is difficult because topical or systemic antifungal agents do not penetrate the nail plate readily. New oral and topical antifungals are proving effective.[200,201] Surgical excision of the nail may be required.

SUMMARY REVIEW

Structure and Function of the Skin

1. Skin is the largest organ of the body and equals about 20% of body weight.
2. The skin has three layers: the dermis, epidermis, and the subcutaneous layer.
3. The underlying epidermis contains a basal and a spinous layer with melanocytes, Langerhans cells, and Merkel cells.
4. The dermis is composed of connective tissue elements, hair follicles, sweat glands, sebaceous glands, blood vessels, nerves, and lymphatic vessels.
5. The subcutaneous layer contains fat cells and connective tissue.
6. The papillary capillaries provide the major blood supply to the skin, arising from deeper arterial plexuses.
7. Heat loss and heat conservation are regulated by arteriovenous anastomoses that lead to the papillary capillaries.

Aging and Skin Integrity

1. Older skin is thinner and drier and has fewer capillary loops and changes in pigmentation.
2. Loss of melanocytes and hair follicles leads to gray and thinner hair.
3. The skin of older persons is more permeable; there is decreased sweating and loss of thermal regulation and decreased protective functions.
4. Pressure ulcers develop from continuous pressure and shearing forces that occlude capillary blood flow, with resulting ischemia and necrosis. Areas at greatest risk are pressure points over bony prominences, such as the greater trochanter, sacrum, ischia, and heels. Immobilized individuals with fractures and neurologic deficits are most likely to develop pressure ulcers.
5. Pruritus is itching and is associated with many skin disorders. Itch mediators, peripheral polymodal-C nerve fibers and central processes contribute to itching. Scratching that causes skin trauma, potential infection, and scarring are associated with itching.

Disorders of the Skin

1. Allergic contact dermatitis is a form of delayed hypersensitivity that develops with sensitization to allergies, such as metals, chemicals, or poison ivy.
2. Atopic or allergic dermatitis is associated with a family history of allergies, hay fever, elevated immunoglobulin E (IgE) levels, and increased histamine sensitivity. Pruritus and scratching predispose the skin to infection, scaling, and thickening.
3. Stasis dermatitis occurs on the legs and results from venous stasis and edema.
4. Irritant contact dermatitis develops from prolonged exposure to chemicals, such as acids or soaps.
5. Seborrheic dermatitis involves scaly, yellowish, inflammatory plaques of the scalp, eyebrows, eyelids, ear canals, chest, axillae, and back. The cause is unknown.
6. Papulosquamous disorders are characterized by papules, scales, plaques, and erythema.
7. Psoriasis is a chronic autoimmune T-cell mediated skin disease with thickening of both the epidermis and dermis, characterized by scaly, erythematous, pruritic plaques.
8. Pityriasis rosea is a self-limiting disease characterized by oval lesions with scales around the edges located along skin lines of the trunk.
9. Lichen planus is a papular, violet-colored inflammatory lesion involving T cells and inflammatory cytokines manifest by severe pruritus.
10. Acne vulgaris is an inflammation of the pilosebaceous follicle.
11. Acne rosacea develops on the middle third of the face with hypertrophy and inflammation of the sebaceous glands that may be the result of infection or immune-mediated inflammation.
12. Lupus erythematosus can affect only the skin (discoid) or have a systemic presentation. The inflammatory lesions usually occur in sun-exposed areas, with a butterfly distribution over the nose and cheeks.
13. Pemphigus is a chronic, autoimmune, blistering disease that begins in the mouth or on the scalp and spreads to other parts of the body, often with a fatal outcome. There are two major forms: pemphigus vulgaris and pemphigus foliaceus. Bullous pemphigoid is a blistering disease that resolves rapidly.
14. Erythema multiforme is an acute inflammation of the skin and mucous membranes with lesions that appear target-like with alternating rings of edema and inflammation; it is often associated with allergic reactions to drugs. Stevens-Johnson syndrome and toxic epidermal necrolysis are severe forms that also involve the mucous membranes.

15. Folliculitis is a bacterial infection of the hair follicle.
16. A furuncle is an infection of the hair follicle that extends to the surrounding tissue.
17. A carbuncle is a collection of infected hair follicles that forms a draining abscess.
18. Cellulitis is a diffuse infection of the dermis and subcutaneous tissue.
19. Erysipelas is a superficial streptococcal infection of the skin commonly affecting the face, ears, and lower legs.
20. Impetigo may have a bullous or an ulcerative form and is caused by *Staphylococcus* or *Streptococcus*.
21. Herpes simplex virus type 1 (HSV-1) causes cold sores but can infect the cornea, mouth, and labia. HSV-2 causes genital lesions and is usually spread by sexual contact.
22. Herpes zoster and varicella are both caused by the same herpesvirus with herpes zoster manifesting years after the initial infection.
23. Warts are benign, rough, elevated lesions caused by papillomavirus. *Condylomata acuminata,* or venereal warts, are spread by sexual contact.
24. Tinea infections (fungal infections) can occur anywhere on the body and are classified by location (i.e., tinea pedis, tinea corporis, tinea capitis).
25. Candidiasis is a yeastlike fungal infection caused by *Candida albicans* occurring on skin, on mucous membranes, and in the gastrointestinal tract.
26. Cutaneous vasculitis is an immune-mediated inflammation of skin blood vessels with purpura, ischemia, and necrosis resulting from vessel necrosis.
27. Urticarial lesions are associated with hypersensitivity responses and appear as wheals, welts, or hives.
28. Scleroderma is an immune-mediated sclerosis of the skin that also may affect systemic organs and cause renal failure, bowel obstruction, or cardiac dysrhythmias.
29. Ticks cause a local reaction on the skin of humans and can cause systemic disease when mouthparts pierce the skin and remain embedded in the tissue.
30. Lyme disease is a multisystem inflammatory disease caused by *Borrelia burgdorferi* transmitted by tick bites. Complications may persist for years.
31. Mosquitoes can transmit infectious diseases, and the saliva from their bite produces the characteristic itching and wheal formation.
32. Blood-sucking flies are represented by many species, including Ceratopogonidae ("no-see-ums"), Tabanidae (horseflies), or Simuliidae (black flies). Their bites are usually painful and produce bleeding; the itching and local reactions may last for days and systemic symptoms of fever and malaise may develop.
33. Seborrheic keratosis is a proliferation of squamous cells that produce elevated, smooth, or warty lesions of varying size usually in sun-damaged skin. They are most common among the elderly population.
34. Keratoacanthoma arises from hair follicles on sun-exposed areas. There are three stages of development, which result in a dome-shaped, crusty lesion filled with keratin that resolves in 3 to 4 months.
35. Actinic keratosis is a pigmented scaly lesion that develops in sun-exposed individuals with fair skin. The lesion may become malignant in the form of squamous cell carcinoma.
36. Nevi arise from melanocytes and may be pigmented or fleshy pink. They occur singly or in groups and may undergo transition to malignant melanoma.
37. Basal cell carcinoma is the most common skin cancer and occurs most often on sun-exposed areas.

Continued

38. Squamous cell carcinoma is a tumor of the epidermis associated with sun exposure and can be localized (in situ) or invasive.
39. Malignant melanoma arises from melanocytes; if it is not excised early, metastasis occurs through the lymph nodes.
40. Kaposi sarcoma is a vascular malignancy associated with immune deficiency states.
41. Frostbite usually occurs on cheeks and digits, causing direct injury to cells and impaired circulation.

Disorders of the Hair

1. Male-pattern alopecia is an inherited form of irreversible baldness with hair loss in the central scalp and recession of the temporofrontal hairline.
2. Female-pattern alopecia is a thinning of the central hair of the scalp beginning in women at 20 to 30 years of age.
3. Alopecia areata is patchy loss of hair associated with an autoimmune process and triggered by stress or metabolic diseases; it is usually reversible.
4. Hirsutism is a male pattern of hair growth in women that may be normal or the result of excessive secretion of androgenic hormones.

Disorders of the Nail

1. Paronychia is an inflammation of the cuticle that can be acute or chronic and is usually caused by staphylococci or streptococci.
2. Onychomycosis is a fungal infection of the nail plate.

KEY TERMS

Acne rosacea, 1588
Acne vulgaris, 1588
Actinic keratosis, 1597
Allergic contact dermatitis, 1584
Alopecia, 1601
Alopecia areata, 1602
Apocrine sweat glands, 1575
Atopic dermatitis, 1584
Basal cell carcinoma, 1598
Basal layer (stratum basale), 1573
Bullous pemphigoid, 1589
Candidiasis, 1594
Carbuncles, 1591
Cellulitis, 1591
Clawlike prolongations, 1583
Condylomata acuminata, 1593
Cutaneous vasculitis, 1594
Dermal appendages, 1575
Dermis, 1574
Discoid lupus erythematosus (DLE), 1588
Eccrine sweat glands, 1575
Eczema, 1584
Epidermis, 1573
Erysipelas, 1591
Erythema multiforme, 1589
Erythrodermic (exfoliative) psoriasis, 1586
Folliculitis, 1590
Frostbite, 1601
Furuncles, 1590

Germinative layer (stratum germinativum), 1573
Guttate psoriasis, 1586
Hair follicles, 1575
Herald patch, 1587
Herpes simplex virus (HSV), 1591
Herpes zoster, 1592
Hirsutism, 1602
Hyphae, 1593
Impetigo, 1591
Inverse psoriasis, 1586
Irritant contact dermatitis, 1585
Kaposi sarcoma (KS), 1600
Keloids, 1583
Keratin, 1573
Keratinocytes, 1573
Keratoacanthoma, 1596
Langerhans cells, 1574
Lichen planus, 1587
Lupus erythematosus, 1588
Lyme disease, 1596
Melanocytes, 1574
Melanoma, 1599
Merkel cells, 1574
Mosquitoes, 1596
Myofibroblasts, 1583
Nails, 1575
Nevus (pl., nevi; also known as a mole), 1597

Onychomycosis, 1602
Papillary capillaries, 1575
Papulosquamous disorders, 1585
Paronychia, 1602
Pemphigus, 1589
Pityriasis rosea, 1586
Proteoglycan, 1583
Pruritus, 1583
Psoriasis, 1586
Pustular psoriasis, 1586
Scleroderma, 1595
Sebaceous glands, 1575
Seborrheic dermatitis, 1585
Seborrheic keratosis, 1596
Spinous layer (stratum spinosum), 1573
Squamous cell carcinoma, 1598
Stasis dermatitis, 1585
Stevens-Johnson syndrome, 1590
Stratum corneum, 1573
Tinea capitis, 1593
Tinea corporis (ringworm), 1593
Tinea infections, 1593
Tinea pedis, 1593
Toxic epidermal necrolysis, 1590
Urticaria, 1594
Urticarial lesions, 1594
Varicella, 1592
Warts, 1592

MEDIA RESOURCES *evolve*

Review questions and answers for this chapter are available in the *CD Companion* included with this book.

WebLinks—links to Internet sites pertaining to this chapter—are available on Evolve at http://evolve.elsevier.com/McCance/.

REFERENCES

1. Nicol NH: Anatomy and physiology of the skin. In Hill MJ, editor, *Dermatologic nursing essentials: a core curriculum,* ed 2, Pitman, NJ, 2003, Anthony J. Jannette, Inc.
2. Jankovic SM, Jankovic SV: The control of hair growth, *Dermatol Online J* 4(1):2, 1998.
3. Hadshiew IM, Eller MS, Gilchrest BA: Skin aging and photoaging: the role of DNA damage and repair, *Am J Contact Dermat* 11(1):19, 2000.
4. Wulf HC et al: Skin aging and natural photoprotection, *Micron* 34(3):185-191, 2004.
5. Hashizume H: Skin aging and dry skin, *Dermatol* 31(8):603-609, 2004.
6. Timiras PS: *Physiologic basis of aging and geriatrics,* ed 3, Boca Raton, Fla, 2002, CRC Press.
7. Gilchrist BA: *Skin and aging processes,* Boca Raton, Fla, 1984, CRC Press.
8. Ryan T: The ageing of the blood supply and the lymphatic drainage of the skin, *Micron* 35(3):161-171, 2004.
9. Yaar M: Molecular mechanisms of skin aging, *Adv Dermatol* 10:63-75, 1995.
10. Gilchrist BA: A review of skin ageing and its medical therapy, *Br J Dermatol* 135(6):867, 1996.
11. Laube S: Skin infections and ageing, *Ageing Res Rev* 3(1):69-89, 2004.

12. Normal D: The effects of age-related skin changes on wound healing rates, *J Wound Care* 13(5):199-201, 2004.

13. Cannon BC, Cannon JP: Management of pressure ulcers, *Am J Health Syst Pharm* 61(18):1895-1905, 2004.

14. Edlich RF et al: Pressure ulcer prevention, *J Long Term Eff Med Implants* 14(4):285-304, 2004.

15. Berlowitz DR et al: Predictors of pressure ulcer healing among long-term care residents, *J Am Geriatric Soc* 45(1):30-34, 1997.

16. Theaker C et al: Risk factors for pressure sores in the critically ill, *Anesthesia* 55(3):221, 2000.

17. Baumgarten M et al: Black/white differences in pressure ulcer incidence in nursing home residents, *J Am Geriatr Soc* 19(6):339-341, 2004.

18. Scanlon E, Stubbs N: Pressure ulcer risk assessment in patients with darkly pigmented skin, *Prof Nurse* 19(5):339-341, 2004.

19. Clinical guidelines: how to predict and prevent pressure ulcers, *Am J Nurs* 92(7):52, 1992.

20. Xakellis GC, Frantz RA: The cost effectiveness of interventions for preventing pressure ulcers, *J Am Board Fam Pract* 9(2):79, 1996.

21. AGS Clinical Practice Committee: Pressure ulcers in adults: prediction and prevention, *J Am Geriatr Soc* 44(9):1118, 1996.

22. Brem H, Lyder C: Protocol for the successful treatment of pressure ulcers, *Am J Surg* 188(1A Suppl):9-17, 2004.

23. Smith DM: Pressure ulcers in the nursing home, *Ann Intern Med* 123 (6):433, 1995.

24. Fine NA, Mustoe TA: Wound healing. In Greenfield LJ et al, editors: *Surgery: scientific principles and practice,* ed 2, Philadelphia, 1997, Lippincott-Raven.

25. Goldstein B, Saunders JE, Benson B: Pressure ulcers in SCI: does tension stimulate wound healing? *Am J Phys Med Rehabil* 75(2):130, 1996.

26. Sorenson JL, Jorgensen B, Gottrup F: Surgical treatment of pressure ulcers, *Am J Surg* 188(1A Suppl):42-51, 2004.

27. Chen W et al: Development of tene microarray in screening differently expressed genes in keloid and normal-control skin, *Chin Med J (Engl)* 117(6):877-881, 2004.

28. Xue H, McCauley RL, Zhang W: Elevated interleukin-6 expression in keloid fibroblasts, *J Surg Res* 89(1):74, 2000.

29. Sayah DN et al: Downregulation of apoptosis-related genes in keloid tissues, *J Surg Res* 87(2):209, 1999.

30. Bayat A et al: Genetic susceptibility to keloid disease: transforming growth factor beta receptor gene polymorphisms are not associated with keloid disease, *Exp Dermatol* 13(2):120-124, 2004.

31. Kelly AP: Medical and surgical therapies for keloids, 17(2):212-218, 2004.

32. Malaker K et al: Retrospective analysis of treatment of unresectable keoids with primary radiation over 25 years, *Clin Oncol (R Coll Radiol)* 16(4):290-298, 2004.

33. Mustoe TA: Scars and keloids, *Br Med J* 328(7452):1329-1330, 2004.

34. Greaves MW, Wall PD: Pathophysiology of itching, *Lancet* 348(9032): 938, 1996.

35. Heyer GR, Hornstein OP: Recent studies of cutaneous nicoception in atopic and non-atopic subjects, *J Dermatol* 26(2):77, 1999.

36. Schmeltz M et al: Active "itch fibers" in chronic pruritus, *Neurology* 61(4):564-566, 2003.

37. Stander S et al: Neurophysiology of pruritis: cutaneous elicitation of itch, *Arch Dermatol* 139(11):1463-1470, 2003.

38. Yosipovitch G, Fleischer A: Itch associated with skin disease: advances in pathophysiology and evolving treatment, *Am J Clin Dermatol* 4(9): 617-622, 2003.

39. Nilsson HJ et al: Profound inhibition of chronic itch induced by stimulation of thin cutaneous nerve fibres, *J Eur Acad Dermatol Venereol* 18(1):37-43, 2004.

40. Nicol NH: Dermatitis/eczema. In Hill MJ, editor: *Dermatologic nursing essentials: a core curriculum,* 2nd ed, Pitman, NJ, 2003, Anthony J Jannetti, Inc.

41. Saint-Mezard P et al: The role of CD4+ and CD8+ T cells in contact hypersensitivity and allergic contact dermatitis, *Eur J Dermatol* 14(3):131-138, 2004.

42. Mizzuddin N, Marenus KD, Maes DH: Factors defining sensitive skin and its treatment, *Am J Contact Dermat* 9(3):107, 1998.

43. Saint-Mezard P et al: Allergic contact dermatitis, *Eur J Dermatol* 14(4):284-295, 2004.

44. Barker JN: Role of keratinocytes in allergic contact dermatitis, *Contact Dermatol* 26(3):145, 1992.

45. Moussadeh N et al: A new quantitative in vitro for the detection of latex-specific IgE antibodies, *Allerg Immunol* 31(10):343, 1999.

46. Li LY, Cruz PD Jr: Allertic contact dermatitis: pathophysiology applied to future therapy, *Dermatol Ther* 17(3):219-223, 2004.

47. Wahlgren CF: Itch and atopic dermatitis: an overview, *J Dermatol* 26(11):770, 1999.

48. Leung DY et al: Disease management of atopic dermatitis: an updated practice parameter. Joint Task Force on Practice Parameters, *Ann Allergy, Asthma, Immunol* 93(3 Suppl 2):S1-S21, 2004.

49. Deleo VA, Elsner P, Marks JG Jr: *Contact and occupational dermatology,* ed 3, St. Louis, 2000, Mosby.

50. Gupta AK et al: Skin diseases associated with Malassezia species, *J Am Acad Dermatol* 51(5):785-798, 2004.

51. Shuster S et al: Treatment and prophylaxis of seborrheic dermatitis of the scalp with antipityrosporal 1% ciclopirox shampoo, *Arch Dermatol* 141(1):47-52, 2005.

52. Gottlieb AB: Psoriasis: emerging therapeutic strategies, *Nat Rev Drug Discov* 4(1):19-34, 2005.

53. Barry J, Kirby: Novel biological therapies for psoriasis, *Expert Opin Biol Ther* 4(6):975-987, 2004.

54. Lowes MA, Lew W, Krueger JG: Current concepts in the immunopathogenesis of psoriasis, *Dermatol Clin* 22(4):349-369, vii, 2004.

55. Asumalahti K et al: A candidate gene for psoriasis near HLS-C, HCR (Pg8) is highly polymorphic with a disease-associated susceptibility allele, *Hum Mol Genet* 9(10):1533, 2000.

56. Krueger JG, Bowcock A: Psoriasis pathophysiology: current concepts of pathogenesis, *Ann Rheum Dis* 64(Suppl 2):ii30-36, 2005.

57. Peters BP, Weissman FG, Gill MA: Pathophysiology and treatment of psoriasis, *Am J Health Syst Pharm* 57(7):645, 2000.

58. Prinz JC: Which T cells cause psoriasis? *Clin Exp Dermatol* 24(4):291, 1999.

59. Christophers E: The immunopathology of psoriasis, *Int Arch Allergy Immunol* 110(3):199, 1996.

60. Veale DJ, Richtlin C, FitzGerald O: Immunopathology of psoriasis and psoriatic arthritis, *Ann Rheum Dis* 64(Suppl 2):ii26-ii29, 2005.

61. Ruderman EM, Tambar S: Psoriatic arthritis: prevalence, diagnosis, and review of therapy for the dermatologist, *Dermatol Clin* 22(4):477-486, 2004.

62. Ashcroft DM et al: Systemic review of comparative efficacy and tolerability of calcipotriol in treating chronic plaque psoriasis, *Br Med J* 320(7240):963, 2000.

63. Harrison PV: Topical tacalcitol treatment for psoriasis, *Hosp Med* 61(6):402, 2000.

64. Chuh A, Chan H, Zawar V: Pityriasis rosea—evidence for and against an infectious aetiology, *Epidemiol Infect* 132(32):381-390, 2004.

65. Stulberg DL, Wolfrey J: Pityriasis rosea, *Am Fam Physician* 69(1):87-91, 2004.

66. Prpic Massari L et al: Perforin expression in peripheral blood lymphocytes and skin-infiltrating cells in patients with lichen planus, *Br J Dermatol* 151(2):433-439, 2005.

67. Porter SR et al: Immunologic aspects of dermal and oral lichen planus: a review, *Oral Surg Oral Med Oral Pathol Oral Radiol Endod* 83(3): 358-366, 1997.

68. Lodi G et al: Lichen planus and hepatitis C virus: a multicentre study of patients with oral lesions and a systematic review, *Br J Dermatol* 151(6):1172-1181, 2004.

69. DeRossi SS, Ciarrocca KN: Lichen planus, lichenoid drug reactions, and lichenoid mucositis, *Dent Clin North Am* 49(1):77-89, 2005.

70. Dahl MV: Rosacea subtypes: a treatment algorithm, *Cutis* 74(3 Suppl):21-27, 32-34, 2004.

71. Odom R: The nosology of rosacea, *Cutis* 74(3 Suppl):5-8, 32-34, 2004.

72. Millikan LE: Rosacea as an inflammatory disorder: a unifying theory? *Curtis* 73(1 Suppl):5-8, 2004.

73. Stone DU, Chodosh J: Ocular rosacea: an update on pathogenesis and therapy, *Curr Opin Ophthalmol* 15(6):499-502, 2004.

74. Bamford JT et al: Effect of treatment of *Helicobacter pylori* infection on rosacea, *Arch Dermatol* 135(6):659, 1999.

75. Crawford GH, Pelle MT, James WD: Rosacea: I, etiology, pathogenesis, and subtype classification, *J Am Deramtol* 51(3):327-341, 2004.

76. Thiboutot DM: Acne and rosacea: new and emerging therapies, *Dermatol Clin* 18(1):63, 2000.

77. Pramatarov KD: Chronic cutaneous lupus erythematosus—clinical spectrum, *Clin Dermatol* 22(2):113-120, 2004.

78. Yell JA, Mbuagbaw J, Burge SM: Cutaneous manifestations of systemic lupus erythematosus, *Br J Dermatol* 135(3):355-362, 1996.

79. Kreuter A et al: Pimecrolimus 1% cream for cutaneous lupus erythematosus, *J Am Acad Dermatol* 51(3):407-410, 2004.

80. Lampropoulos CE et al: Topical tacrolimus therapy of resistant cutaneous lesions in lupus erythematosus: a possible alternative, *Rheumatology (Oxford)* 43(11):1383-1385, 2004.

81. Fabbri P et al: Cutaneous lupus erythematosus: diagnosis and management, *Am J Clin Dermatol* 4(7):449-465, 2003.

82. Amagai M: Pemphigus: autoimmunity to epidermal cell adhesion molecules, *Adv Dermatol* 11:319-352, 1996.

83. Hashimoto T: Recent advances in the study of the pathophysiology of pemphigus, *Arch Dermatol Res* 395(Suppl 1):S2-11, 2003.

84. Korman NJ: New and emerging therapies in the treatment of blistering diseases, *Dermatol Clin* 18(1):127, 2000.

85. Nousari HC, Anhalt GJ: Pemphigus and bellous pemphigoid, *Lancet* 354(9179):667, 1999.

86. Aurelian L, Kokuba H, Burnett JW: Understanding the pathogenesis of HSV-associated erythema multiforme, *Dermatology* 197(3):219, 1998.

87. Katta R: Taking aim at erythema multiforme. How to spot target lesions and less typical presentations, *Postgrad Med* 107(1):87, 2000.

88. Provost TT, Weston WL: *Bullous diseases,* St Louis, 1993, Mosby.

89. Williams PM, Conklin RJ: Erythema multiforme: a review and contrast from Stevens-Johnson syndrome/toxic epidermal necrolysis, *Dent Clin North Am* 49(1):67-76, 2005.

90. Roujeau JC: Stevens-Johnson syndrome and toxic epidermal necrolysis are severity variants of the same disease which differs from erythema multiforme, *J Dermatol* 24(11):726, 1997.

91. Learner LH et al: Nitric oxide synthase in toxic epidermal necrolysis and Stevens-Johnson syndrome, *J Invest Dermatol* 114(1):196, 2000.

92. LeCleach L et al: Blister fluid T lymphocytes during toxic epidermal necrolysis are functional cytotoxic cells which express human natural killer (NK) inhibitory receptors, *Clin Exp Immunol* 119(1):225, 2000.

93. Cheriyan S et al: The outcome of Stevens-Johnson syndrome treated with corticosteroids, *Allergy Proc* 16(4):151, 1995.

94. Singh G, Marples RR, Klingman AM: Staphylococcus infections in humans, *J Invest Dermatol* 57(3):149-162, 1971.

95. Bisno AL, Stevens DL: Streptococcal infections of skin and soft tissues, *N Engl J Med* 334(4):240, 1996.

96. Leulmo-Aguilar J, Santandreu MS: Folliculitis: recognition and management, *Am J Clin Dermatol* 5(5):301-310, 2004.

97. Cox NH, Colver GB, Paterson WD: Management and morbidity of cellulitis of the leg, *J R Soc Med* 91(12):634, 1998.

98. Koutkia P, Mylonakis E, Boyce J: Cellulitis: evaluation of possible predisposing factors in hospitalized patients, *Diagn Microbiol Infect Dis* 34(4):325, 1999.

99. Guberman D et al: Bullous erysipelas: a retrospective study of 26 patients, *J Am Acad Dermatol* 41(5 Pt 1):733-737, 1999.

100. Adachi J et al: Increasing incidence of streptococcal impetigo in atopic dermatitis, *J Dermatol Sci* 17(1):45, 1998.

101. Bale JF Jr: Human herpesviruses and neurological disorders of childhood, *Semin Pediatr Neurol* 6(4):278, 1999.

102. Wahren B, Linde A: Virological and clinical characteristics of human herpes virus 6, *Scand J Infect Dis* 80(suppl):105, 1991.

103. Crumpacker CS: Herpes simplex. In Fitzpatrick TB et al, editors: *Dermatology in general medicine,* ed 3, New York, 1987, McGraw-Hill.

104. Sacks SL et al: HSV-2 transmission, *Antiviral Res* 63(Suppl 1):S27-35, 2004.

105. Stanberry L et al: New developments in epidemiology, natural history and management of genital herpes, *Antiviral Res* 42(1):1, 1999.

106. Aurelian L: Herpes simplex virus type 2 vaccines: new ground for optimism? *Clin Diagn Lab Immunol* 11(3):437-445, 2004.

107. Liesegang TJ: Herpes zoster virus infection, *Curr Opin Ophthalmol* 15(6):531-536, 2004.

108. Whitley RJ, Gnann JW Jr: Therapeutic approaches to the management of herpes zoster, *Adv Exp Med Biol* 458:159-165, 1999.

109. Alper BS, Lewis PR: Does treatment of acute herpes zoster prevent or shorten postherpetic neuralgia? *J Fam Pract* 49(3):355, 2000.

110. Cohen JI et al: Recent advances in varicella-zoster virus infection, *Ann Intern Med* 130(11):922, 1999.

111. Ragozzino MW et al: Population based study of herpes zoster and its sequelae, *Medicine (Baltimore)* 5(61):310, 1982.

112. Chartrand SA: Varicella vaccine, *Pediatr Clin North Am* 47(2):373, 2000.

113. Kanazi GE, Johnson RW, Dworkin RH: Treatment of postherpetic neuralgia: an update, *Drugs* 59(5):1113, 2000.

114. Lassus J, Ranki A: Simultaneously detected aberrant p53 tumor-suppressor protein and HPV-DNA localized mostly in separate keratinocytes in anogenital and common warts, *Exp Dermatol* 5(2):72, 1996.

115. Prasad CJ: Pathobiology of human papillomavirus, *Clin Lab Med* 15(3):685, 1995.

116. Bellew SG, Quartarolo N, Janniger CK: Childhood warts: an update, *Cutis* 73(6):379-384, 2004.

117. Miller DM, Brodell RT: Human papillomavirus infection: treatment options for warts, *Am Fam Physician* 53(1):135, 1996.

118. Plasencia JM: Cutaneous warts: diagnosis and treatment, *Prim Care* 27(2):423, 2000.

119. Kodner CM, Nasraty S: Management of genital warts, *Am Fam Physician* 70(12):2335-2342, 2004.

120. Baseman JG, Koutsky LA: The epidemiology of human papillomavirus infection, *J Cin Virol* 32(Suppl)16-24, 2005.

121. Sasieni PD: Human papillomavirus screening and cervical cancer prevention, *J Am Med Womens Assoc* 55(4):216, 2000.

122. Woodfolk JA: Allergy and dermatophytes, *Clin Microbiol Rev* 18(1):30-43, 2005.

123. Rupke SJ: Fungal skin disorders, *Prim Care* 27(2):407, 2000.

124. Di-Silverio A et al: Specific and nonspecific parameters of the host defense system in patients with superficial fungal infections, *Mycoses* 38(11-12):453, 1995.

125. Levitz SM: Overview of host defenses in fungal infections, *Clin Infect Dis* 14(suppl 1):537, 1992.

126. Lotti TM, Comacchi C, Ghersetich I: Cutaneous necrotizing vasculitis. Relation to systemic disease, *Adv Exp Med Biol* 455:115, 1999.

127. Gonzalez-Gay MA, Garcia-Porrua C, Pujol RM: Clinical approach to cutaneous vasculitis, *Curr Opin Rheumatol* 17(1):56-61, 2005.

128. Lotti T et al: Cutaneous small-vessel vasculitis, *J Am Acad Dermatol* 39(5 P6 1):667, 1998.

129. Kapp A, Wedi B: Chronic uticaria: clinical aspects and focus on a new antihistamine, levocetirizine, *Drugs Dermatol* 3(6):632-639, 2004.

130. Beltrani VS: Uticaria: reassessed, *Allergy, Asthma Proc* 25(3):143-149, 2004.

131. Kaplan AP: Chronic uticaria: pathogenesis and treatment, *J Allergy Clin Immunol* 114(3):465-474, 2004.

132. Cepeda EJ, Reveille JD: Autoantibodies in systemic sclerosis and fibrosing syndromes: clinical indications and relevance, *Curr Opin Rheumatol* 16(6):723-732, 2004.

133. Generini S et al: Systemic sclerosis: a clinical review, *Adv Exp Med Biol* 455:73, 1999.

134. Haustein UF, Anderegg U: Pathophysiology of scleroderma: an update, *J Eur Acad Dermatol Venereol* 11(1):1, 1998.

135. Takehara K, Sato S: Localized scleroderma is an autoimmune disorder, *Rheumatology (Oxford),* 44(3):274-279, 2005.

136. Trojanowska M: What did we learn by studying scleroderma fibroblasts? *Clin Exp Rheumatol* 22(3 Suppl 33):S59-63, 2004.

137. Denton CP, Black CM: Scleroderma—clinical and pathological advances, *Best Pract Res Clin Rheumatol* 18(3):271-290, 2004.

138. Rhew EY, Barr WG: Scleroderma renal crisis: new insights and developments, *Curr Rheumatol Rep* 6(2):129-136, 2004.

139. Amsden JR, Warmack S, Gubbins PO: Tick-borne bacterial, rickettsial, spirochetal, and protozoal infectious disease in the United States: a comprehensive review, *Pharmacotherapy* 25(2):191-210, 2005.

140. Rosa PA, Tilly K, Stewart PE: The burgeoning molecular genetics of the Lyme disease spirochaete, *Nat Rev Microbiol* 3(2):129-143, 2005.

141. Filgueira L et al: Human dendritic cells phagocytose and process Borrelia burgdorferi, *J Immunol* 157(7):2998, 1996.

142. Singh SK, Girschick HJ: Molecular survival strategies of the Lyme disease spirochete *Borrellia burgdorferi, Lancet Infect Dis* 4(9):575-583, 2004.

143. Ziska MH, Donta ST, Demarest FC: Physician preferences in the diagnosis and treatment of Lyme disease in the United States, *Infection* 24(2):182, 1996.

144. Mullegger RR: Dermatological manifestations of Lyme borreliosis, *Eur J Dermatol* 14(5):296-309, 2004.

145. American Academy of Pediatrics, Committee on Infectious Diseases: Prevention of Lyme disease, *Pediatrics* 105(1 Pt 1):142, 2000.

146. Beham A et al: Keratoacanthoma: a clinically distinct variant of well differentiated squamous cell carcinoma, *Adv Anat Pathol* 5(5):269, 1998.

147. Cain CT, Niemann TH, Argenyi ZB: Keratoacanthoma versus squamous cell carcinoma: an immunohistochemical reappraisal of p53 protein and proliferating cell nuclear antigen expression in keratoacanthoma-like tumors, *Am J Dermatopathol* 17(4):324, 1995.

148. Jorizzo JL: Current and novel treatment options for actinic keratosis, *J Cutan Med Surg* 6, 2005. (E-pub ahead of print.)

149. Anwar J et al: The development of actinic keratosis into invasive squamous cell carcinoma: evidence and evolving classification schemes, *Clin Dermatol* 22(3):189-196, 2004.

150. American Cancer Society: Estimated new cancer cases and deaths by sex for all sites, US, 2005. In *Cancer facts and figures 2005*, Atlanta, 2005, The Society. Available online at www.cancer.org/docroot/MED/content/downloads/MED_1_1x_ CFF2005_Estimated_New_Cases_Deaths_by_Sex_US.asp.

151. Buzzell RA: Carcinogenesis of cutaneous malignancies, *Dermatol Surg* 22(3):209, 1996.

152. Green A et al: Sun exposure, skin cancers and related skin conditions, *J Epidemiol* 9(6 suppl):S7, 1999.

153. Truhan AP: Sun protection in childhood, *Clin Pediatr* 30(12):676, 1991.

154. Lear JT et al: Basal cell carcinoma: from host response and polymorphic variants to tumour suppressor genes, *Clin Exp Dermatol* 30(1):49-55, 2005.

155. Reifenberger J et al: Somatic mutations with *PTCH, SMOH, SUFUH,* and *PT53* genes in sporadic basal cell carcinomas, *Br J Dermatol* 152(1):43051, 2005.

156. Zakl-Prelich M, Narbutt J, Sysa-Jedrzejowska A: Environmental risk factors predisposing to the development of basal cell carcinoma, *Dermatol Surg* 30(2 Pt 2):248-252, 2004.

157. Walling HW et al: Aggressive basal cell carcinoma: presentation, pathogenesis, and management, *Cancer Metastasis Rev* 23(3-4): 289-402, 2004.

158. Goldman GD: Squamous cell cancer: a practical approach, *Semin Cutan Med Surg* 17(2):80, 1998.

159. Kane CL: Histopathology of cutaneous squamous cell carcinoma and its variants, *Semin Cutan Med Surg* 23(1):54-61, 2004.

160. Backyall H et al: The density of epidermal p53 clones in higher adjacent to squamous cell carcinoma in comparison with basal cell carcinoma, *Br J Dermatol* 150(2):259-266, 2004.

161. Bishop JA: Melanoma, *Hosp Med* 61(2):103, 2000.

162. Abbasi NR et al: Early diagnosis of cutaneous melanoma: revisiting the ABCD criteria, *JAMA* 292(22):2771-2776, 2004.

163. Katsambas A, Nicolaidou E: Cutaneous malignant melanoma and sun exposure: recent developments in epidemiology, *Arch Dermatol* 132(4):444, 1996.

164. Rodenas JM et al: Sun exposure, pigmentary traits, and risk of cutaneous malignant melanoma: a case-control study in a Mediterranean population, *Cancer Causes Control* 7(2):275, 1996.

165. Rodolfo M, Daniotti M, Vallacchi V: Genetic progression of metastatic melanoma, *Cancer Lett* 214(2):133-147, 2004.

166. Lober CW: Dysplastic (atypical) nevi: significance and management, *South Med J* 85(9):870, 1992.

167. Habif TB: *Clinical dermatology: a color guide to diagnosis and therapy,* St Louis, 2001, Mosby.

168. Chung ES, Sabel MS, Sondak VK: Current state of treatment for primary cutaneous melanoma, *Clin Exp Med* 4(2):65-77, 2004.

169. Elliott B, Dalgleish A: Melanoma vaccines, *Hosp Med* 65(11):668-673, 2004.

170. Mitsuyasu RT: Update on the pathogenesis and treatment of Kaposi sarcoma, *Curr Opin Oncol* 12(2):174, 2000.

171. Schwartz RA: Kaposi's sarcoma: an update, *J Surg Oncol* 87(3): 146-151, 2004.

172. Sturzl M et al: Expression of platelet-derived growth factor and its receptor in AIDS-related Kaposi sarcoma in vivo suggests paracrine and autocrine mechanisms of tumor maintenance, *Proc Natl Acad Sci U S A* 89(15):7046, 1992.

173. Goopman J: Neoplasms in the acquired immune deficiency syndrome: the multidisciplinary approach, *Semin Oncol* 14(2 suppl 3):1, 1987.

174. Iscovich J et al: Classic kaposi sarcoma: epidemiology and risk factors, *Cancer* 88(3):500, 2000.

175. Dezube BJ, Pantanowitz L, Aboulafia DM: Management of AIDS-related Kaposi sarcoma: advances in target discovery and treatment, *AIDS Read* 14(5):236-238, 243-244, 251-253, 2004.

176. Aoki Y, Tosato G: Therapeutic options for human herpesvirus-8/ Kaposi's sarcoma-associated herpesvirus-related disorders, *Expert Rev Anti Infect Ther* 2(2):213-225, 2004.

177. Gascon P, Schwartz RA: Kaposi's sarcoma. New treatment modalities, *Dermatol Clin* 18(1):169, 2000.

178. Cattelan AM, Trevenzoli M, Aversa SM: Novel pharmacological therapies for the treatment of AIDS-related Kaposi's sarcoma, *Expert Opin Investig Drugs* 13(5):501-513, 2004.

179. Grandberg PO: Freezing cold injury, *Arctic Med Res* 50(suppl 6):76, 1991.

180. Murphy JV et al: Frostbite: pathogenesis and treatment, *J Trauma* 48(1):171, 2000.

181. Greenfield LJ et al: *Surgery: scientific principles and practice,* ed 2, Philadelphia, 1997, Lippincott-Raven.

182. Raine TJ, London MD, Goluch L: Antiprostaglandins and antithromboxanes for treatment of frostbite, *Surg Forum* 31:557, 1980.

183. Savin RC, Atton AV: Minoxidil: update on its clinical role, *Dermatol Clin* 11(1):55, 1993.

184. Norwood OT, Lehr B: Female androgenetic alopecia: a separate entity, *Dermatol Surg* 26(7):679, 2000.

185. Rushton DH: Management of hair loss in women, *Dermatol Clin* 11(1):47, 1993.

186. Alexis AF, Dudda-Subramanya R, Sinha AA: Alopecia areata: autoimmune basis of hair loss, *Eur J Dermatol* 14(6):364-370, 2004.

187. Callen JP et al: *Color atlas of dermatology,* Philadelphia, 2000, Saunders.

188. Hoffmann R, Happle R: Does interleukin-1 induce hair loss? *Dermatology* 191(4):273, 1995.

189. Ghersetich I, Campanile G, Lotti T: Alopecia areata: immunohistochemistry and ultrastructure of infiltrate and identification of adhesion molecule receptors, *Int J Dermatol* 35(1):28-33, 1996.

190. Gupta MA, Gupta AK, Watteel GN: Stress and alopecia areata, *Acta Derm Venereol* 77(4):296-298, 1997.

191. Sawaya ME, Hordinsky MK: Advances in alopecia areata and androgenetic alopecia, *Adv Dermatol* 7:211-226, 1992.

192. Khandpur S, Sharma VK, Sumanth K: Topical immunomodulators in dermatology, *J Postgrad Med* 50(2):131-139, 2004.

193. Bergfeld WF: Hirsutism in women. Effective therapy that is safe for long-term use, *Postgrad Med* 107(7):93-94, 99-104, 2000.

194. Archer JS, Chang RJ: Hirsutism and acne in polycystic ovary syndrome, *Best Pract Res Clin Obstet Gynaecol* 18(5):737-754, 2004.

195. Ali I, Dawber R: Hirsutism: diagnosis and management, *Hosp Med* 65(5):293-297, 2004.

196. Sahin &, Kelestimur F: Medical treatment regimens of hirsutism, *Reprod Biomed Online* 8(5):538-546, 2004.

197. Townsend KA, Marlowe KF: Relative safety and efficacy of finasteride for treatment of hirsutism, *Amm Pharmacother* 38(6):1070-1073, 2004.

198. Scher RK: Onychomycosis: therapeutic update, *J Am Acad Dermatol* 40(6 part 2):S21, 1999.

199. Elewski BE: Diagnostic techniques for confirming onychomycosis, *J Am Acad Dermatol* 35(3 Pt 2):S6, 1996.

200. Gupta AK, Lynch LE: Management of onychomycosis: examining the role of monotherapy and dual, triple, or quadruple therapies, *Cutis* 74(1 Suppl):5-9, 2004.

201. Wenig JA: The systemic treatment of onychomycosis, *Clin Podiatr Med Surg* 21(4):579-589, 2004.

ALTERATIONS OF THE INTEGUMENT IN CHILDREN

NOREEN HEER NICOL • SUE E. HUETHER

CHAPTER OUTLINE

Children often develop alterations in the skin, which may be minor or severe and localized or generalized. Unfortunately the skin is often underrated in regard to its vital roles as a barrier, foundation, and calorie reservoir, as well as to its roles in temperature regulation, sensation, grasp, insulation, psychosocial impact, and individual image. Manifestation of skin diseases in children may differ from those in adults, although the causative mechanisms may be similar. Some diseases resolve spontaneously and require no treatment. Diagnosis is commonly made from the history, appearance, and distribution of the lesion or lesions. Common skin diseases of childhood are presented here.

ACNE VULGARIS

Acne vulgaris is the most common skin disease and affects 85% of the population between the ages of 12 and 25 years. Genetic influences may determine an individual's susceptibility and severity of disease. Severe acne tends to run in families. The incidence of acne is the same in both genders, although severe disease affects males more often.

Acne conglobata is a highly inflammatory form of severe, disfiguring acne that involves the formation of communicating cysts and abscesses beneath the skin and requires aggressive referral and pathophysiologic treatment. Remissions tend to occur during the summer, perhaps from more exposure to

sunlight. External forces, such as cosmetics, use of oral and topical medications, mechanical friction, and occupation, may be etiologic factors. Stress does not cause acne but can make it worse. Self-manipulation of acne must be discouraged because it leads to increased inflammation and potential increased scarring.

Distinctive pilosebaceous units, known as *sebaceous follicles*, are the sites for development of acne lesions. The follicles are located primarily on the face and upper parts of the chest and back. These follicles have many large sebaceous glands, a small vellus hair, and a dilated follicular canal that is visible as a "pore" on the skin surface. Acne lesions may be divided into inflammatory lesions (pustules, papules, nodules) and noninflammatory lesions (closed and open comedones).[1] In **noninflammatory acne** the comedones are open (blackheads) and closed (whiteheads), with the accumulated material causing distention of the follicle and thinning of follicular canal walls. **Inflammatory acne** develops in closed comedones when the follicular wall ruptures, expelling sebum into the surrounding dermis and initiating inflammation. Pustules form when the inflammation is close to the surface; papules and cystic nodules can develop when the inflammation is deeper, causing mild to severe scarring (Figure 45-1). Both types of lesions may exist in the same individual.

The exact cause of acne is unknown and various pathophysiologic factors contribute to the development of acne. The principal factors are follicular hyperkeratinization, exces-

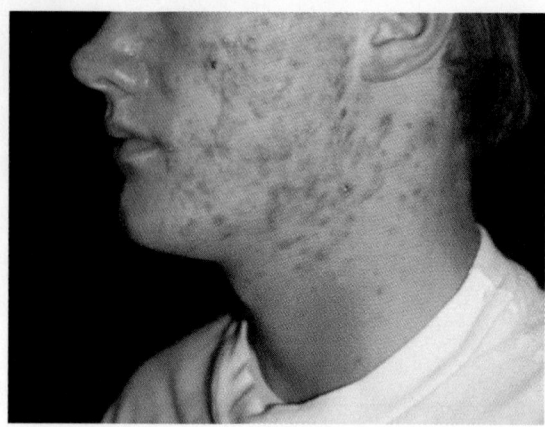

Figure 45-1 Cystic acne. Multiple pustules (erythematous papules and pustules) are present, and several have become confluent. Note areas of scarring. (Courtesy Department of Dermatology, School of Medicine, University of Utah.)

sive sebum production, increased colonization of *Propionibacterium acnes (P. acnes),* and inflammation secondary to the action of extracellular inflammatory products produced by *P. acnes.* An excessive production and accumulation of sebum appear to be directly related to androgenic hormones and the pathogenesis of acne. Testosterone is converted to dihydrotestosterone in the skin, which increases the size and productivity of the sebaceous glands.[2] Acne begins with sebum accumulation that obstructs the pilosebaceous unit. The mass of accumulated keratinous sebaceous material and bacteria within the pilosebaceous follicle (see Figure 45-1) causes inflammation when it is exposed to the dermis with rupture of a follicle.

The *P. acnes* bacteria produce substances that promote inflammation, including chemotactic factors and lipolytic and proteolytic enzymes. The hydrolytic action of the enzymes converts triglycerides into free fatty acids that stimulate inflammation and edema that result in breakdown of the follicle wall. Chemotactic substance also may be released that involves mediation of inflammation by attraction of polymorphonuclear leukocytes.

Treatment of acne should address the causative factors and be individualized. Diet has not been proven to cause acne in spite of common lay opinion that there are acne-related foods; dietary restrictions are generally not effective.[2a,2b] Treatment recommendations and algorithms have been developed based on type and severity of acne lesions. One of the most recent algorithms was developed by the Global Alliance to Improve Outcomes in Acne.[3] Topical treatment, including topical antibiotics, benzoyl peroxide, salicylic acid, and topical tretinoin, should be the first line of therapy because it is the least invasive. Use of systemic therapies, including oral antibiotics, sex hormones, corticosteroids, and isotretinoin, should be pursued when first-line therapy fails. Acne surgery, including comedo extraction, intralesional steroids, and cryosurgery, may be useful in selected individuals. Severe scarring may be treated with dermabrasion or subincision.

Special consideration must be given to treatment for those with darker colored skin because they have greater risk for hyperpigmentation and keloidal scarring.[3a] With the many successful treatment options for acne that are available now, no individual should suffer through severe or disfiguring acne without medical management.[4,5]

DERMATITIS

Atopic Dermatitis

Atopic dermatitis (AD) is the most common cause of eczema in children, with a prevalence rate of about 25% to 30%. The cause of this chronic relapsing form of pruritic eczema is unknown, but 75% to 80% of individuals with atopic dermatitis have a personal or family history of asthma or allergic rhinitis (hay fever). Onset is usually from 2 to 6 months of age, and 85% of cases occur within the first 5 years of life. There are no specific laboratory features of AD that can be used for diagnostic purposes. An increased serum immunoglobulin E (IgE) level and positive immediate skin tests to a variety of common food and inhalant allergens are seen in approximately 80% of patients. Similarly, blood eosinophilia is a common finding in AD. The basis for the elevated serum IgE levels and eosinophilia in AD is thought to relate to various abnormalities of T-cell mast cell and dendritic cell function, including interleukin-4 production and CCL1 chemokine.[6,7]

AD has a constellation of clinical features that include severe pruritus, a long-term course with frequent exacerbations, and characteristic eczematoid appearance and age-dependent distribution of skin lesions. The skin becomes increasingly dry, sensitive, itchy, and easily irritated because the barrier function is impaired.[8] Microscopic epidermal cracks that let water out and irritants and allergens in lead to further drying and cracking, which results in rubbing and scratching. Rubbing and scratching to relieve the itch are actually responsible for many of the clinical changes that are seen (Figure 45-2). Itching is the hallmark of atopic dermatitis, and the vicious itch-scratch cycle is easily established and difficult to break. The itch continues to be poorly understood. Unlike the effect on urticaria, histamine is not considered a major pruritogen in atopic dermatitis.[9] In children the rash appears primarily on the face, scalp, trunk, and extensor surfaces of the arms and legs. In older children and adults, the rash tends to be found on the neck, antecubital and popliteal fossae, and hands and feet. Individuals with AD also tend to develop viral, bacterial, and fungal skin infections in the areas with eczema.

Management of those with AD includes accurate diagnosis and identification and elimination of exacerbating factors, such as irritants, allergens, and emotional stresses. Hydration of the skin is the key to good therapy but is often difficult to achieve. Antiinflammatory agents, such as topical corticosteroids or tar preparations, are necessary during active flares of eczema. New topical immunomodulators, tacrolimus and pimecrolimus, have an important and increasing role in man-

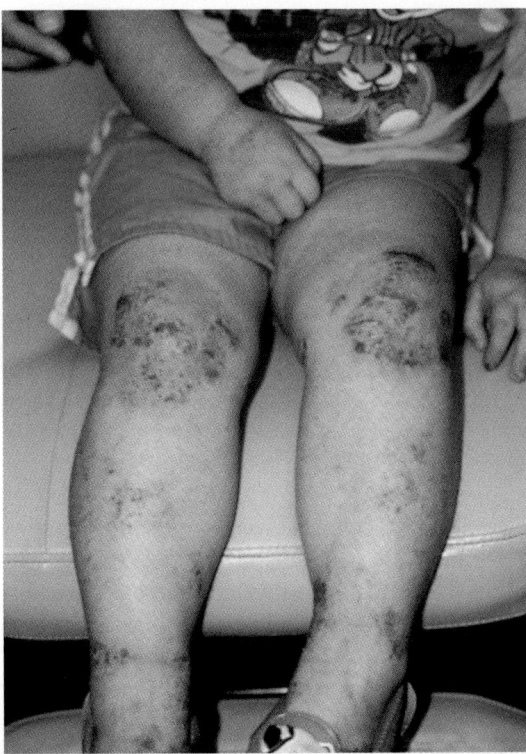

Figure 45-2 **Atopic dermatitis.** Characteristic lesions with crusting from irritation and scratching over knees and around ankles. (Courtesy Department of Dermatology, School of Medicine, University of Utah.)

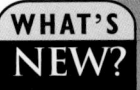

WHAT'S NEW? Immunologic Treatment Breakthrough in Atopic Dermatitis

Atopic dermatitis is a genetically linked, chronically relapsing, inflammatory skin disease commonly associated with respiratory allergy. This disorder has a complex immunopathogenesis involving both immediate and cellular immune responses. Atopic dermatitis lesions can be clinically classified as acute or chronic; immunopathologic work has been done to determine the difference between the acute and chronic lesions. T cells expressing homing receptor for the skin may be found in uninvolved skin of atopic individuals with dermatitis. Langerhans cells expressing the high-affinity receptor for IgE also are found in the skin of these individuals. These cells are not seen in the skin of individuals who do not have this disorder.

The clinical phenotype characterizing atopic dermatitis is a complex interaction of environmental, immunologic, genetic, and pharmacologic factors. Research has been undertaken to clarify the relative contributions of these factors seeking to identify the relevant effector cells and mediators. The pattern of local cytokines and chemokines, differentiation of helper T cells, multiple roles of IgE, skin-directed cell responses, infectious agents, and superantigens are all the subject of ongoing research.

This research in immunology and inflammatory skin disease has resulted in the development and approval of a new drug class called *nonsteroidal topical immunomodulators*. This new class of drugs constitutes an important development in the treatment of atopic dermatitis. Topical tacrolimus (Protopic) and topical pimecrolimus (Elidel), the first two medications in this class, were introduced to the United States market in 2000 and 2001 (respectively) as new steroid-free treatment modalities. Topical immunomodulators are in clinical trials for other skin-related disease states.

Data from Novak N, Kwiek B, Bieber T: *Clin Exp Dermatol* 30(2):160-164, 2005; Boguniewicz M, Nicol NH: *Nurs Pract Forum* 10(2):48, 1999; Leung DYM et al: *J Clin Invest* 113:651-657, 2004.

agement of AD.[10] Systemic therapy includes the use of sedating antihistamines and antibiotics. Systemic corticosteroids usually are not warranted in this chronic, non-life-threatening illness.

Diaper Dermatitis

Diaper dermatitis is probably the most common skin disorder of infancy and early childhood. Diaper dermatitis is not a specific disease but rather a variety of inflammatory disorders affecting the lower aspect of the abdomen, genitalia, buttock, and upper portion of the thigh. This is a nonallergic contact dermatitis caused by a chemical irritant, and the intensity of inflammation is related to the concentration of the irritant and exposure time. An allergic contact dermatitis is different—it triggers an immunologic event that is the result of type IV delayed hypersensitivity reaction to an allergen. This form of irritant contact dermatitis is initiated by a combination of factors that include prolonged exposure to and irritation by urine and feces, maceration by wet diapers, airtight plastic diaper covers, and possibly increased association with intercurrent illnesses and early introduction of cereals. Disposable diapers do not appear to give any additive protection over cloth.[11] Frequently, the infant with diaper dermatitis is secondarily infected with *Candida albicans*.

The lesions vary from mild erythema to erythematous papular lesions. Candidal (monilial) diaper dermatitis is usually very erythematous, with sharp margination and pustulovesicular satellite lesions (Figure 45-3).

Treatment is changing the diaper frequently to keep the area clean and dry or frequently exposing the perineal area to air. Topical antifungal medication is used to treat *Candida albicans* when present. Short-term use of low-potency topical steroids alternately with antifungals at each diaper change helps to reduce the inflammation. Use of various topical agents to provide a barrier from the irritating agents promotes healing.

INFECTIONS OF THE SKIN

Infectious diseases caused by bacteria, viruses, and fungi constitute the major forms of skin disease. Breaks in the skin integrity, particularly those that inoculate pathogens into the dermis and epidermis, may cause or exacerbate infections.[12,13] Most infections tend to occur superficially; however, systemic signs and symptoms do develop occasionally and rarely may be life threatening.

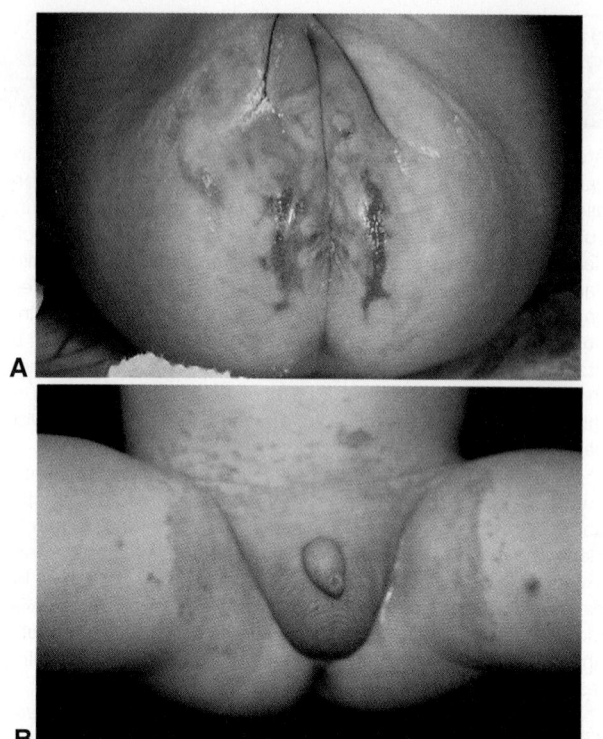

Figure 45-3 Diaper dermatitis. **A,** Diaper dermatitis with erosions. **B,** Diaper dermatitis with *Candida albicans* secondary infection. (Courtesy Department of Dermatology, School of Medicine, University of Utah.)

Bacterial Infections
Impetigo Contagiosum

Impetigo is a common bacterial skin infection in infants and children, usually caused by *Staphylococcus aureus* or group A streptococcus. The disease is more common in midsummer to late summer, with a higher incidence in hot, humid climates. Impetigo is particularly infectious among people living in crowded conditions with poor sanitary facilities. It affects children in good health, but conditions such as anemia and malnutrition are predisposing factors. There are two common types of impetigo: bullous and vesicular. Both start as vesicles with a very thin vesicular roof composed of stratum corneum.

Bullous Impetigo

Bullous impetigo is a rarer variant of impetigo caused by *Staphylococcus aureus.* The staphylococci produce a bacterial toxin called *exfoliative toxin (ET),* which causes a disruption in desmosomal adhesion molecules.[14] This form characteristically occurs in newborns and is highly contagious. The source of the infection is usually a staff member in a newborn nursery or a family member with a pustule or who is an asymptomatic carrier. The pathogen is often carried in the anterior nares, perineal region, or fingernails and is transmitted by contact with the individual or contaminated equipment.[15]

The exfoliative toxin stimulates the formation of vesicles, which enlarge or coalesce to form superficial bullae. There may be a few localized lesions or many lesions scattered over the skin. As the bullae rupture, a thin, flat, honey-colored crust appears. The crust is the hallmark of impetigo. A moist, inflamed,

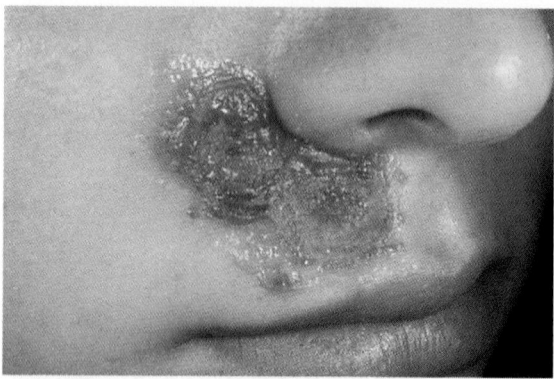

Figure 45-4 Impetigo and herpes simplex virus (HSV) of upper lip. Note weeping and crusting lesions. (Courtesy Department of Dermatology, School of Medicine, University of Utah.)

serum-weeping base is revealed when the crust is removed. The lesions are often located on the face around the nose and mouth, but the hands and other exposed areas are also commonly involved. Regional lymphadenitis is uncommon.

Vesicular Impetigo

Vesicular impetigo is a contagious, acute, superficial, vesiculopustular form of impetigo caused by group A *Streptococcus pyogenes* (alone or in combination with *Staphylococcus aureus*). The microorganisms are disseminated by direct physical contact from other infected individuals or through insect bites. The lesions begin as small vesicles with a honey-colored serum. Yellow to white-brown crusts form as the vesicles rupture and extend radially (Figure 45-4). Untreated lesions may last for weeks and extend to cover a large area. In contrast to bullous impetigo, regional lymphadenitis is common.

The risk of nephritogenic strains of streptococci varies considerably in North America.[16] Aggressive treatment of both patient and patient contacts significantly reduces the chance of acute glomerulonephritis, which is clearly the most significant complication of streptococcal impetigo.

Treatment of choice for both types of impetigo is topical mupirocin and topical fusidic acid or oral antibiotics.[17] Antibiotic therapy should be determined by bacterial culture and drug sensitivity. While waiting for such laboratory results, empiric treatment with drugs such as systemic erythromycin or dicloxacillin or topical mupirocin—which give good coverage against staphylococci and streptococci—should be used. Topical mupirocin should be limited to early, small, localized infections. Removal of crusts and scrubbing the lesions with antibacterial soaps have not been shown to be effective.[18] Good hand-washing techniques and isolation of the infected child's washcloth, towels, drinking glass, and linen are important. The highly contagious nature of this disease should be emphasized to children's care takers.

Staphylococcal Scalded-Skin Syndrome

Staphylococcal scalded-skin syndrome (SSSS) is the most serious staphylococcal infection that affects the skin and usually is seen in infants and children younger than 5 years.[19] SSSS is caused by infection with group II staphylococci, which produce an exfoliative toxin that attacks desmoglein and adhesion molecules and causes a separation of the skin just below the granular layer of the epidermis.[19] The toxins are usually produced at body sites other than the skin and arrive at the epidermis through the circulatory system. Staphylococci typically are not found in the skin lesions themselves. The syndrome is more common in children younger than 10 years than in adults. Adults have circulating antistaphylococcal antibodies and are better able to metabolize and excrete the toxin. Newborns are at the highest risk because of their lack of immunity (not having prior exposure to the toxin). One case of SSSS in a newborn was caused by mother-to-child transmission that occurred through breastfeeding when the mother had a breast abscess. Thus breastfeeding should be avoided in cases of breast abscess.[20]

The clinical symptoms begin with fever, malaise, rhinorrhea, and irritability followed by generalized erythema with exquisite tenderness of the skin. There may be an associated impetigo, but the infection often begins in the throat or chest. The erythema spreads from the face and trunk to cover the entire body except the palms, soles, and mucous membranes. Within 48 hours, blisters and bullae may form and the pain is severe (Figure 45-5). Fluid loss from ruptured blisters and water evaporation from denuded areas may cause dehydration. Perioral and nasolabial crusting and fissures develop. In severe cases the skin of the entire body may slough. When secondary infection can be prevented, healing of the involved skin occurs in 10 to 14 days, usually without scarring.

Before medical intervention is begun, culture, histology, or exfoliative cytology must be done to differentiate SSSS from toxic epidermal necrolysis (TEN) (see p. 1621). When the infection is confirmed, treatment with oral or intravenous antibiotics is begun.[21] Topical antibiotics are ineffective. The skin should be treated the same as that with a severe burn—with meticulous aseptic technique. Special care is required when the lips and eyelids are involved.[22]

Fungal Infections

Fungal disorders are known as *mycoses* and, when caused by dermatophytes (fungi that thrive on keratin), the mycoses are termed *tinea* (dermatophytosis or ringworm).[23] **Tinea pedis** (a chronic, superficial fungal infection of the skin of the foot) occurs in children but is rare. Most scaling disorders of the toes and feet in prepubertal children are usually eczema (see Chapter 44). Tinea capitis (infection of the scalp) and tinea corporis (infection of the body) are much more common in children than adults. (The different types of tinea are described in Chapter 44.) Dermatophytes may be grouped into three categories based on natural habitat and host preference. Anthropophilic species infect humans, geophilic species are soil-based and may infect both humans and animals, and zoophilic species generally infect nonhuman mammals.[24] These dermatophytes invade the stratum corneum and not the remainder of the epidermis or dermis. The inflammatory response is thought, in part, to be secondary to the toxins released by the dermatophyte. It is important to confirm by culture which microorganism is causing the fungal infection before commencing therapy.

Tinea Capitis

Tinea capitis, a fungal infection of the scalp, is the most common fungal infection of childhood. It rarely affects infants and is seen in children between 2 and 10 years of age.[25] Primary microorganisms responsible for the disease are *Microsporum canis* and *Trichophyton tonsurans*. *M. canis* is found on cats, dogs, and certain rodents. Humans appear to be a terminal host for *M. canis*, and children who handle such animals are possible hosts. Human-to-human transmission does not occur. *T. tonsurans* conversely *is* transmitted by human-to-human contact. Areas of crowding are the most prevalent environments for this microorganism, which frequently affects inner-city children. *T. tonsurans* is often the predominant dermatophyte found on inner-city children, and many of these infections are not symptomatic. The prevalence of

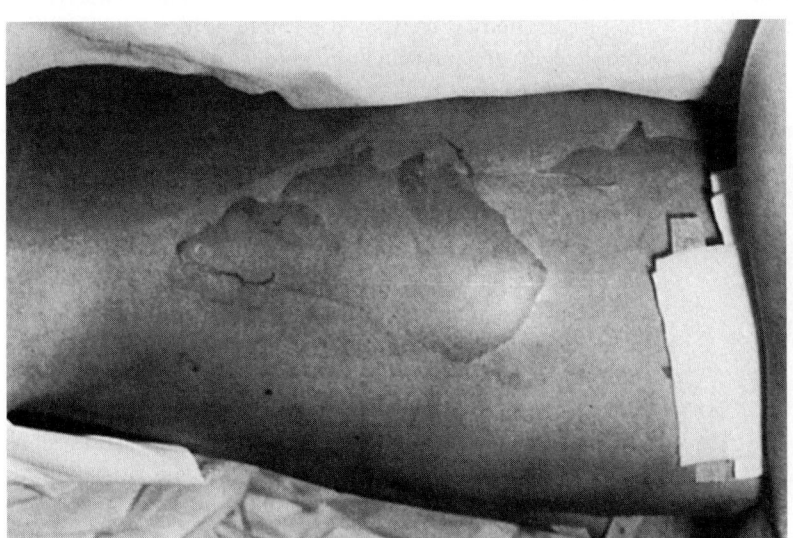

Figure 45-5 Staphylococcal scalded-skin syndrome (SSSS). The skin lesions, showing desquamation and wrinkling of the skin margins, appeared 1 day after drainage of a staphylococcal abscess. (From Levine G, Norden C: *N Engl J Med* 287:1339, 1972.)

asymptomatic carriers among household contacts of a child with active *T. tonsurans* disease has been found to be high.[26] Treatment of household contacts with a sporicidal shampoo should be considered and cosleeping and comb sharing must be discouraged. When symptoms are present, the clinical presentations vary, depending on the microorganism. Often the lesions are circular and manifest by broken hairs 1 to 3 mm above the scalp, leaving a partial alopecia 1 to 5 cm in diameter[27] (Figure 45-6). A slight erythema and scaling with raised borders can be observed.

Diagnosis is best confirmed by performing Wood light examination, potassium hydroxide (KOH) examination, and fungal culture, in that order. *T. tonsurans* does not fluoresce with Wood light examination. Oral griseofulvin is the treatment of choice because topical fungicides do not penetrate to the hair bulb. Newer agents, including terbinafine, itraconazole, and fluconazole, may be effective. Adjunct therapy includes 2% ketoconazole and 1% selenium sulfide shampoos.[28]

Tinea Corporis

Tinea corporis is a common superficial dermatophyte infection in children. The microorganisms most commonly responsible for this disease are *M. canis* and *Trichophyton mentagrophytes.* As in tinea capitis, contact with young kittens and puppies is a common source of the disorder. Tinea corporis preferentially affects the nonhairy parts of the face, trunk, and limbs. Lesions are often erythematous, round or oval, scaling patches that spread peripherally with clearing in the center, creating the ring appearance, which is why this disease is commonly referred to as *ringworm.* The lesions are distributed asymmetrically, and multiple lesions (when present) overlap. Potassium hydroxide examination of the scale from the border of the lesions confirms the diagnosis. Most lesions respond well to applications of appropriate topical antifungal medications.[29]

Thrush

Candida albicans infection is a superficial fungal infection that commonly occurs in children. *C. albicans* is part of the normal skin flora in certain individuals and invades susceptible tissue sites if the predisposing factors are not eliminated.

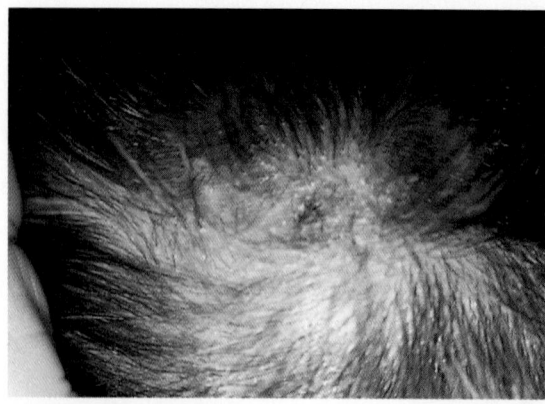

Figure 45-6 Tinea capitis. (Courtesy Department of Dermatology, School of Medicine, University of Utah.)

C. albicans penetrates the epidermal barrier more easily than other microorganisms because of its keratolytic proteases and other enzymes. *C. albicans* attracts neutrophils to skin sites of invasion and generates inflammation by activation of the complement system within the skin.

Thrush is the term used to describe the presence of *Candida* in the mucous membranes of the mouth of infants and, less commonly, adults. Thrush is characterized by the formation of white plaques or spots in the mouth that lead to shallow ulcers. The tongue may have a dense, white covering. The underlying mucous membrane is red and tender and may bleed when the plaques are removed. The disease is often accompanied by fever and gastrointestinal irritation. The infection commonly spreads to the groin, buttocks, and other parts of the body. Treatment may be difficult and may include oral antifungal washes, such as nystatin oral suspension. Simultaneous treatment of a *Candida* nipple infection or vaginitis in the mother is helpful in reducing the *C. albicans* surface colonization of the infant. Feeding bottles and nipples should be sterilized to prevent reinfection. The diaper area should be kept clean and dry.

Viral Infections

Viral infections of the skin in children are caused by poxvirus, papovavirus, and herpesvirus. The most common infections are described here.

Molluscum Contagiosum

Molluscum contagiosum is a common, highly contagious poxvirus infection of the skin and, occasionally, conjunctiva that affects primarily children. It is transmitted by skin-to-skin contact; autoinoculation; and fomites, such as clothing, wash devices, and towels. This disease appears to be more common in individuals with atopic dermatitis and a variety of immunodeficient states, including human immunodeficiency virus (HIV).[30] The poxvirus induces epidermal cell proliferation and blocks immune responses that would control the virus. The epidermis grows down into the dermis to form saccules containing clusters of virus. The characteristic molluscum body is composed of mature, immature, and incomplete viruses and cellular debris.[31]

The lesions of molluscum are discrete, slightly umbilicated, dome-shaped papules 1 to 5 cm in diameter that appear anywhere on the skin or conjunctiva. The skin distribution in children is mainly on the trunk, face, and extremities (Figure 45-7). The pubic, genital, and perineal areas are favored in adults (see Chapter 24). Usually, no inflammation surrounds molluscum lesions unless they are traumatized or secondary infection occurs. Scarring occurs with healing.

The best three diagnostic procedures are (1) staining smears of the expressed molluscum body, (2) examining a biopsy, and (3) inoculating a molluscum suspension into cell cultures to demonstrate the cytotoxic reactions. Most lesions are self-limiting and clear in 6 to 9 months if not manipulated. However, because children often do manipulate these lesions, spontaneous involution may take 2 to 4 years without therapy.

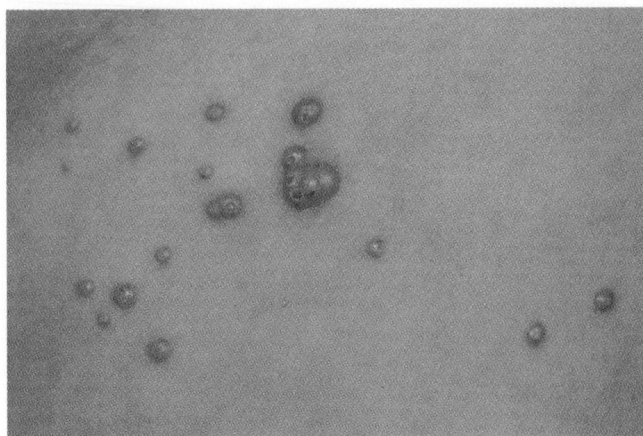

Figure 45-7 **Molluscum contagiosum.** Waxy pink globules with umbilicated centers. (From Habif TP: *Clinical dermatology: a color guide to diagnosis and therapy,* ed 3, St Louis, 1996, Mosby.)

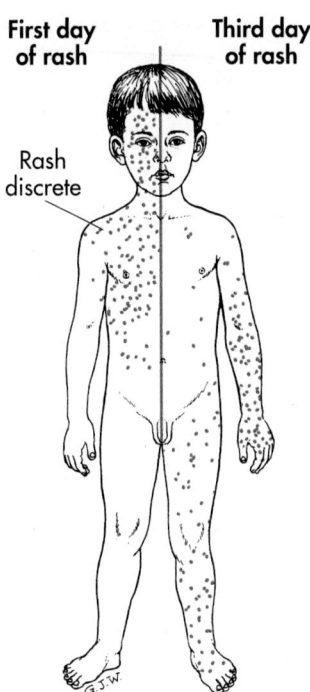

Figure 45-8 **Measles.** Full-blown maculopapular rash with tendency to coalesce. (From Wehrle PF, Top FH Sr: *Communicable and infectious diseases,* ed 9, St Louis, 1981, Mosby.)

Treatment involves various topical and surgical options. The papules can be removed by curette or destroyed with liquid nitrogen. If multiple lesions are present, however, these procedures can be painful to small children and may not be justified. When curettage is used, EMLA Cream (a combination of lidocaine and prilocaine) used before and after the procedure provides rapid pain relief in children without serious application site reactions.[32] Topical cantharidin can be used to treat these lesions and has been found to be extremely effective and well tolerated; parental satisfaction with this treatment is high.[33] Topical cantharidin combined with imiquimod 5% has been reported as effective and safe.[34,35] Measures to prevent spread of infection must be taken. Children must be taught not to manipulate or scratch these lesions. Recurrences are common.

Rubella (German or 3-Day Measles)

Rubella is a common communicable disease of children and young adults caused by a ribonucleic acid (RNA) virus that enters the bloodstream through the respiratory route. This disease is mild in most children. The incubation period ranges from 14 to 21 days. Prodromal symptoms are few but may include enlarged cervical and postauricular lymph nodes, low-grade fever, headache, sore throat, runny nose, and cough. A faint-pink to red, coalescing maculopapular rash develops on the face, with spread to the trunk and extremities 1 to 4 days after the onset of initial symptoms (Figure 45-8). The rash is thought to be the result of virus dissemination to the skin. The rash subsides after 2 to 3 days, usually without complications. Children are generally not contagious after development of the rash. There is lifelong immunity to rubella—as there is for measles, chickenpox, and roseola—after contracting the disease. Differential presentations of viral diseases producing rashes are given in Table 45-1.

Vaccination for rubella is usually combined with vaccines for mumps and measles (rubeola) (MMR). Recommendations now state that MMR vaccine should be given at 12 to 15 months of age, so there will not be interference from maternal measles antibody, and again at either 4 to 6 years or 11 to 12 years of age.[36] In the past, parents chose not to give the vaccine because of the misbelief that it would cause the disease. Studies have confirmed that measles or rubella-like illnesses in MMR-vaccinated children are often caused by other viruses.[37] Measles is known to occur in previously immunized children.[38]

More recently parental concern has focused on the belief that MMR vaccination may cause autism. Although MMR vaccine may rarely be associated with adverse neurologic events, recently reported studies conclude that MMR immunization does not cause autism. Lack of vaccination, however, leads to significant morbidity and mortality,[39-42] with pneumonia, croup, and encephalitis being causes of death worldwide.[43,44]

Women of childbearing age are immunized if their rubella hemagglutination-inhibition titer is low. Pregnancy should be avoided for 3 months after vaccination because the attenuated virus in the vaccine may remain for this period. Pregnant women who have rubella early in the first trimester may have a fetus that develops congenital defects.

There is no specific treatment for rubella. Recovery is spontaneous, although lymph nodes may remain enlarged for weeks. Supportive therapy includes rest, fluids, and use of a vaporizer. In rare cases a mild encephalitis or peripheral neuritis may follow rubella.

Rubeola (Red Measles)

Rubeola is a highly contagious, acute viral disease of children. It is transmitted by direct contact with droplets from infected persons and is caused by an RNA-containing paramyxovirus with an incubation period of 7 to 12 days, during which time no symptoms are manifest. Prodromal symptoms include high fever (up to 40.5° C), malaise, enlarged lymph nodes, runny nose, conjunctivitis, and "barking" cough. Within 3 to

Table 45-1	Differential Presentation of Viral Diseases Producing Rashes			
Viral Disease	Incubation	Prodromal Symptoms	Duration/Characteristics	Clinical Symptoms
Rubella (German measles)	14-21 days	1-2 days Mild fever Malaise Respiratory symptoms	1-3 days Pink-red maculopapular Face and trunk	Enlarged and tender occipital and periauricular nodes
Rubeola (measles)	7-12 days	2-5 days Fever Cough Respiratory symptoms	3-5 days Purple-red to brown maculo-papular Face, trunk, extremities	Koplik spots 1-3 days before rash
Roseola (exanthema subitum)	5-15 days	2-5 days High fever	1-3 days Red macular Neck and trunk	Rash develops when fever subsides
Varicella (chickenpox)	11-20 days	1-2 days Low-grade fever Cough May be asymptomatic	Red papules, vesicles, pustules in clusters	Eruption of new lesions for 4-5 days Occasional ulcerative lesion in the mouth

4 days, an erythematous maculopapular rash develops over the head and spreads distally over the trunk, extremities, hands, and feet. Early lesions blanch with pressure, followed by a brownish hue that does not blanch as the rash fades. Characteristic pinpoint white spots surrounded by an erythematous ring develop over the buccal mucosa and are known as *Koplik spots*. These spots precede the rash by 1 to 2 days. The rash then subsides within 3 to 5 days.

Complications associated with measles may be caused by the primary infection or a secondary bacterial infection. Measles encephalitis occurs in about 1 of 800 cases, and most children recover completely. Only a small minority develop permanent brain damage or die. Bacterial complications include otitis media and pneumonia, usually caused by group A hemolytic streptococcus, *Haemophilus influenzae,* or *Staphylococcus aureus* infection.

Measles is prevented by a single vaccination of live attenuated measles virus as previously discussed. There is no specific treatment for measles, and supportive therapy is the same as for rubella. Antibiotic therapy is initiated if secondary bacterial infections develop.

Roseola (Exanthema Subitum)

Roseola is a presumed viral infection of infants between 6 months and 2 years of age, but it can be seen in children as old as 4 years. The incubation period is 5 to 15 days, followed by the sudden onset of fever (38.9° to 40.5° C) that lasts for 3 to 5 days. After the fever an erythematous macular rash that lasts about 24 hours develops primarily over the trunk and neck. Children usually feel well, eat normally, and have few other symptoms. Usually no treatment is required.

Chickenpox and Herpes Zoster

Chickenpox (varicella) and herpes zoster (shingles) are both produced by the varicella-zoster virus (VZV). VZV is a complex herpes group deoxyribonucleic acid (DNA) virus. The incubation period is 10 to 27 days; it averages 14 days. Productive infection occurs within keratinocytes such that the

vesicular lesions occur in the epidermis, and an inflammatory infiltrate is often present. Histologically, VZV lesions form intraepidermal vesicles. Infected keratinocytes degenerate, swell, detach from each other, and often contain inclusions surrounded by a clear halo and a circle of darkly staining chromatin. As the vesicle evolves, polymorphonuclear cells enter the vesicle and can lead to a pustular appearance. The vesicle eventually ruptures and is followed by crust formation. On mucous membranes the vesicles rupture and leave superficial, transient ulcers. Varicella occurs in people not previously exposed to VZV, whereas herpes zoster occurs in partially immune individuals who have had varicella.[45]

Chickenpox

Chickenpox is a disease of early childhood, with 90% of children contracting the disease during the first decade of life. It is a highly contagious virus that is spread by close person-to-person contact and by airborne droplets. Introduction of an infected person into a household results in a 90% possibility of susceptible persons in the household developing the disease within the incubation period—usually 14 days. Children are contagious for at least 1 day before development of the rash. Transmission of the virus may occur until approximately 5 to 6 days after the onset of the first skin lesions in normal children. In immunocompromised children the virus is recoverable for a longer period, but these children must be considered contagious for at least 7 to 10 days. Chickenpox occurs most commonly in the late winter and early spring. Transmission occurs more readily in temperate climates than in tropical climates.

Healthy children who develop chickenpox have no prodromal symptoms. The first sign of illness may be itching or the appearance of vesicles, usually on the trunk, scalp, or face. The rash later spreads to the extremities. Characteristically, lesions can be seen in various stages of maturation with macules, papules, and vesicles present in a particular area at the same time (Figure 45-9). The vesicular lesions are superficial and can be easily ruptured. New lesions will erupt for 4 to 5 days, until there are approximately 100 to 300 in different stages of development. The vesicles become crusted, with only the crust remaining. Occasionally a vesicle may appear on the palm later in the disease. Although uncommon, ulcerative lesions are sometimes seen in the mouth and, less commonly, on the conjunctiva and pharynx. Fever usually lasts 2 to 3 days and ranges from 38.5° to 40° C.

Complications are rare in children but more common in adults. They can include transient hematuria (from rupture of vesicles in the bladder), epistaxis, laryngeal edema, and varicella pneumonia. One case of chickenpox produces almost complete immunity against a second attack. The fetus may be malformed (2%) if chickenpox develops in the mother in the first trimester of pregnancy.[46,47] Infants whose mothers have chickenpox at any stage of pregnancy have a higher risk of developing herpes zoster during the first few years of life.

Uncomplicated chickenpox requires no specific therapy. Baths, wet dressings, and oral antihistamines are occasionally helpful to relieve itching and to prevent secondary infection as a result of scratching. Oral antistaphylococcal drugs should be given if secondary bacterial infection is present. Zoster immune globulin may be administered to immunodeficient individuals if given within 72 hours after exposure to chickenpox. Oral antiviral drugs (i.e., acyclovir) may be valuable in reducing symptoms in otherwise healthy children as well as in immunosuppressed or other select groups of children.[48]

Chickenpox now can be prevented with a safe and effective vaccine. The American Academy of Pediatrics[49] recommends the chickenpox vaccine for all children between the ages of 12 and 18 months who do not have a history of chickenpox.

Healthy children between the ages of 18 months and 13 years also should be immunized with a single dose at the earliest opportunity. Healthy adolescents over 13 years of age and young adults who have no history of chickenpox should receive two doses of the vaccine 4 to 8 weeks apart.

Herpes Zoster

Although herpes zoster (shingles) occurs mainly in adults, approximately 5% of cases are in children younger than 15 years.[50] The course of the disease in children with an immune defect is more complicated and requires intravenous treatment with antiviral agents.[51] The chickenpox virus persists for life in sensory nerve ganglia and reactivates to cause herpes zoster. The eruption of **zoster** consists of groups of vesicles situated on an inflammatory base and following the course of a sensory nerve. Common dermatomal distribution in childhood is thoracic. The base of the lesions often appears hemorrhagic, and some of the lesions may become necrotic and ulcerative. In addition to the localized eruption, there are commonly a few scattered lesions resembling chickenpox. Therapy is similar to that for chickenpox unless it is ophthalmic or disseminated zoster, for which systemic antiviral treatment and (when the eye is involved) a referral to an ophthalmologist are indicated.

Smallpox

Smallpox (variola) is a highly contagious and deadly but preventable disease. It is caused by poxvirus variolae. Because of worldwide mass immunization, the world is now virtually free of smallpox.[52] Concerns regarding smallpox as a weapon of bioterrorism has led to vaccination programs for the military and for selected civilian populations. The United States government has an adequate supply of smallpox vaccine to vaccinate the U.S. population in the event of a smallpox emergency.[52a]

INSECT BITES AND PARASITES

Insect bites and infestations are common causes of skin disorders in children and adults. Skin damage occurs by various mechanisms, including trauma of bites and stings, allergic reactions, transmission of disease, injection of substances that cause local or systemic reactions, and inflammatory reactions from retained mouthparts.

Scabies

Scabies is a contagious disease caused by the itch mite, *Sarcoptes scabiei* (Figure 45-10, *A*). It is transmitted by close personal contact (see Chapter 24) and by infected clothing and bedding. Scabies is often epidemic in areas of overcrowded housing and poor sanitation. Scabies is often associated with immunocompromised individuals, such as those with human T-cell leukemia/lymphoma virus I (HTLV-1) and HIV.[53] Infestation is initiated by a female mite that tunnels into the stratum corneum, depositing eggs and creating a burrow several millimeters to 1 centimeter long. Over a 3-week period, the eggs mature into adult mites, which sometimes can be recognized as tiny dots at the end of intact burrows.

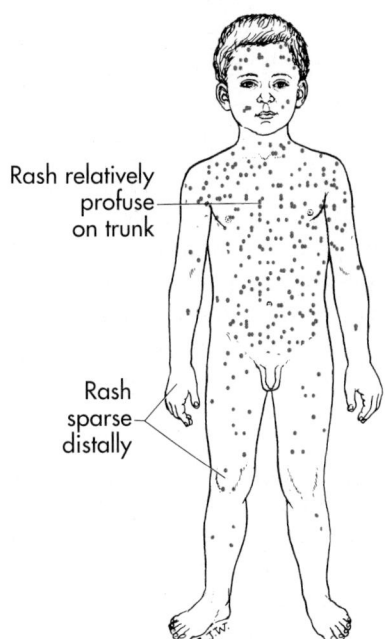

Rash relatively profuse on trunk

Rash sparse distally

Figure 45-9 Chickenpox. Generalized, polymorphous eruption. (From Wehrle PF, Top FH Sr: *Communicable and infectious diseases,* ed 9, St Louis, 1981, Mosby.)

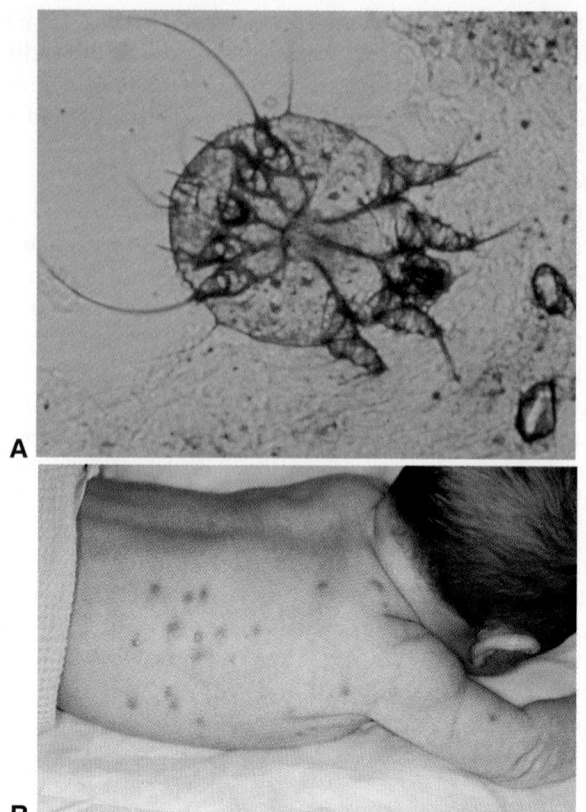

A

B

Figure 45-10 Scabies. **A,** Scabies mite, as seen clinically when removed from its burrow. **B,** Characteristic scabies bites. (Courtesy Department of Dermatology, School of Medicine, University of Utah.)

Symptoms appear 3 to 5 weeks after infestation. The primary lesions are burrows, papules, and vesicular lesions, with severe itching that worsens at night. Two or three bites, commonly referred to as "breakfast, lunch, and dinner," usually appear in a line on exposed areas of the skin. Itching is thought to be related to sensitization to the larval stages of the parasite. In older children and adults the lesions occur in the webs of fingers, axillae, and creases of the arms and wrists; along the belt line; and around the nipples, genitalia, and lower buttocks. Infants and young children have a different pattern of distribution, with involvement of the palms, soles, head, neck, and face (see Figure 45-10, *B*). Secondary infections and crusting develop from scratching and eczematous changes.

Norwegian scabies is a relatively rare, widespread scabetic infestation with an affinity for severely mentally retarded persons, who are unable to effectively scratch. It is highly contagious and is characterized by heavily crusted lesions on the scalp, elbows, knees, palms, soles, and buttocks.

Diagnosis of scabies is made by observation of the tunnels and burrows and scraping of the skin with microscopic examination of the mite or its eggs or feces. Treatment is the application of a scabicide, permethrin cream. Generalized scabies is treated with oral ivermectin.[54] Even with elimination of all viable scabies microorganisms, itching may persist for 10 days or longer. All clothing and linens should be washed and dried in hot cycles or dry-cleaned.

Pediculosis (Lice Infestation)

The three known types of human lice are (1) the head louse (*Pediculus capitis*), (2) the body louse (*Pediculus corporis*), and (3) the crab or pubic louse (*Phthirus pubis*). They are highly contagious parasites that survive by sucking blood. The female louse reproduces every 2 weeks, producing hundreds of nits as newly hatched lice mate with old. The mouthparts are shaped for piercing and sucking and attach to the skin while feeding. When piercing the skin, the louse secretes a toxic saliva; the mechanical trauma and toxin produce a pruritic dermatitis. Head and body lice are acquired by personal contact, combs, or brushes. Crab lice are spread by body contact, such as contact with an infected adult (see Chapter 24). Sharing clothing is also a common source of transmission.[55]

Itching is the major symptom of lice infestation. In head lice infestation the ova attach to hairs above the ears and in the occipital region. The primary lesion of the body louse is a pinpoint red macule, papule, or wheal with a hemorrhagic puncture site. The primary lesion often is not seen, because it is masked by excoriations, wheals, and crusts. The crab louse is found on pubic hairs but also may involve other body hair such as eyelashes, mustache, beard, and axillae. Young children particularly may become infected with crab lice on their eyebrows or eyelashes.

The live louse, 2- to 3-mm long, is rarely observed, although the ova, or nits, can be observed as oval, yellowish, pinpoint specks fastened to a hair shaft. The ova will fluoresce under an ultraviolet light (Wood lamp) and can be best observed with a microscope. Infestations are treated with a pediculicide or scabicide, particularly 1% permethrin or malathion 0.5% lotion.[56] All clothes, towels, bedding, combs, and brushes should be washed and dried in hot air or boiled, or the clothes should be ironed. Individuals who have close personal contact also should be treated.

Fleas

Young children are very susceptible to **flea bites,** and the most common are the bites of cat, dog, and human fleas.[57] Bites occur in clusters along the arms and legs or where clothing fits tightly. The bite produces an urticarial wheal with a central hemorrhagic puncture (Figure 45-11). Treatment includes spraying carpets, crevices, and furniture with malathion or lindane powder. Infected animals should be treated, and clothes and bedding should be washed in hot water.

Bedbugs

The common bedbug, *Cimex lectularius,* is a blood-sucking, nocturnal parasite of man. Chickens, bats, and some domestic animals are the other hosts for this bug.[58] **Bedbugs** live in the crevices and cracks of floors, walls, and furniture and in bedding or furniture stuffing. They are 3 to 5 mm long and reddish brown. Bedbugs emerge to feed in darkness and attach to the skin to suck blood. Feeding occurs for 5 to 15 minutes, and the bedbug then leaves. It will move long distances to search for food and can travel from house to house.

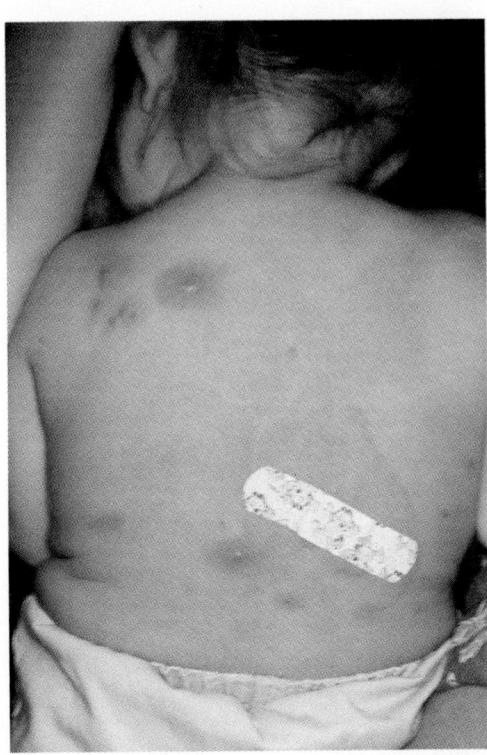

Figure 45-11 **Flea bites.** Flea bite producing an urticarial wheal with central puncture.

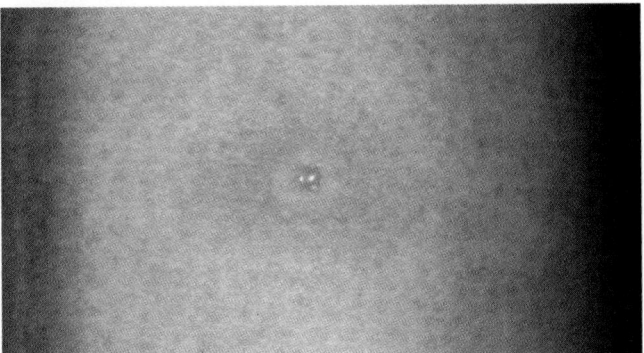

Figure 45-12 **Bullous bedbug bites.** (Courtesy Department of Dermatology, School of Medicine, University of Utah.)

If the host has not been previously sensitized, the only symptom is a red macule that develops into a nodule, lasting up to 14 days. In sensitized children and adults, pruritic wheals, papules, and vesicles may form (Figure 45-12). Secondary infections require treatment. Bedbugs are eliminated by spraying with chlordane or lindane and by cleaning or disposing of bedding, mattresses, and furniture.

HEMANGIOMAS AND VASCULAR MALFORMATIONS

Vascular anomalies occur in about 10% of infants and can be categorized as either hemangiomas or vascular malformations.[59,60]

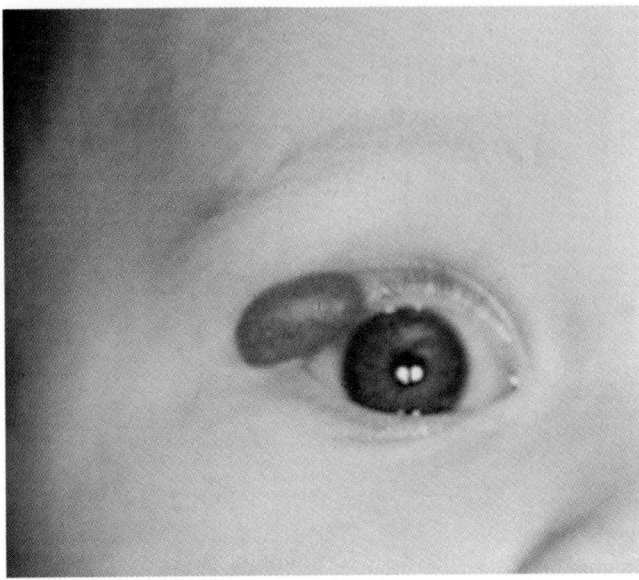

Figure 45-13 Strawberry hemangioma. (Courtesy Department of Dermatology, School of Medicine, University of Utah.)

Hemangiomas

Hemangiomas are benign tumors that form from the rapid growth of vascular endothelial cells, which results in formation of extra blood vessels. There is proliferation of mast cells, which are thought to promote the angiogenesis. Infiltration of fat cells, fibrosis, and the rich vascular network give the lesions a firm, rubbery feel. Females are affected more often than males. About 30% of hemangiomas are apparent at birth, with most emerging during the first few weeks of life. They grow rapidly during the first few years of life, then shrink or involute during childhood years. With involution the lesions become darker in color and then gradually turn to a flesh color. There may be some residual telangiectasia. Most require no treatment depending on location. Hemangiomas located over the eye, ear, nose, mouth, urethra, or anus may require treatment because they interfere with function and have a higher risk for infection or injury. Systemic or intralesional steroids are the treatment of choice. Interferons, vincristine, and radiotherapy can suppress angiogenesis. Cryosurgery, laser surgery, and sclerotherapy are also alterative treatment options.[61,62] Hemangiomas can be superficial or deep. Superficial hemangiomas are known as strawberry hemangiomas and deep lesions are known as cavernous hemangiomas.

Strawberry hemangiomas are distinct, raised vascular lesions that may be present at birth but usually emerge 3 to 5 weeks after birth. They proliferate and become bright red and elevated with minute capillary projections that give them a strawberry appearance. Usually only one lesion is present, and it is located on the head and neck area or trunk (Figure 45-13). After the initial growth, the lesion grows at the same rate as the child and then starts to involute at 12 to 16 months of age. Approximately 90% of strawberry hemangiomas involute by 5 to 6 years of age, usually without scarring.[63]

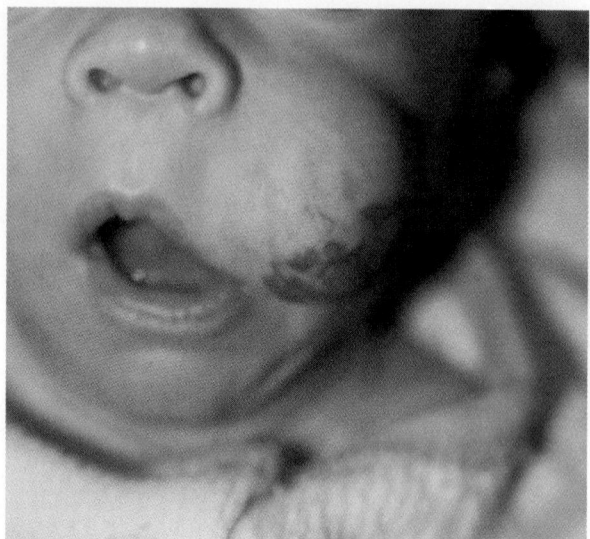

Figure 45-14 Cavernous hemangioma. (Courtesy Department of Dermatology, School of Medicine, University of Utah.)

Cavernous hemangiomas are present at birth and have larger and more mature vessels within the lesion than strawberry hemangiomas. Some lesions, however, are composed of a mixture of strawberry and cavernous hemangiomas. They appear primarily on the head and neck area and have a bluish red color with less distinct borders (Figure 45-14). Cavernous hemangiomas grow rapidly up to 6 months of age and mature by 1 year of age. A period of involution begins and proceeds for 6 to 12 months, with complete involution by 2 to 3 years in 30% of children and by 9 years of age in 90% of children.

Vascular Malformations

Vascular malformations are congenital anomalies of blood vessels that are present at birth but may not be apparent for several years.[59] They grow proportionately with the child and never regress. The malformations occur equally among males and females. Occasionally they expand rapidly, particularly during the hormonal changes of puberty or pregnancy and in association with trauma. Vascular malformations are classified as low flow or high flow. *Low flow malformations* involve capillaries, veins, and lymphatics. *High flow malformations* involve arteries. In addition to locations within the skin they may involve the gastrointestinal tract, bone (Maffucci syndrome), or nerves and meninges (Surge-Weber syndrome).[64,65] *Overgrowth syndromes* can occur with either high or low flow malformations, with overgrowth of the underlying structures (i.e., legs, arms, facial bones). The most common vascular malformations are nevus flammeus (port-wine stains) and salmon patches (stork bite, angel kiss).

Port-wine (nevus flammeus) stains are congenital malformations of the dermal capillaries. The lesions are flat, and their color ranges from pink to dark reddish purple. They are present at birth or within a few days after birth and do not fade with age. Involvement of the face and other body surfaces is common, and the lesions may be large (Figure 45-15). During adolescence and later adult years, the port-wine stain may be-

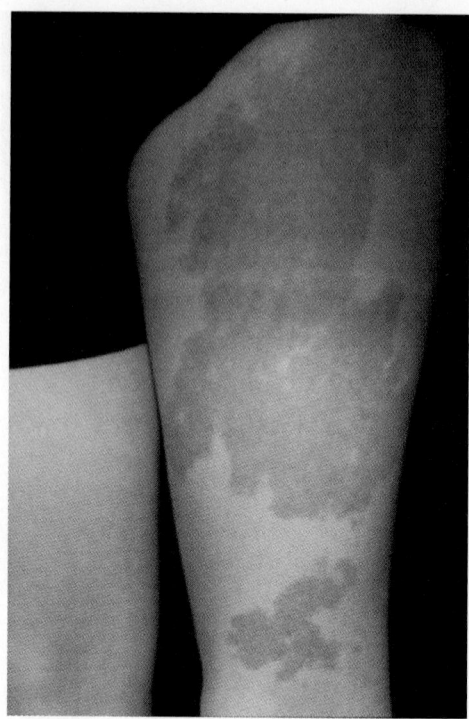

Figure 45-15 Capillary malformation in a child. (Courtesy Department of Dermatology, School of Medicine, University of Utah.)

come papular and cavernous. Treatments using cryosurgery or tattooing are not very satisfactory. The pulsed dye laser is the treatment of choice to successfully lighten the color and flatten the more nodular and cavernous lesions.[66,67] Waterproof cosmetics may be used to cover the lesions.

Salmon patches are macular, pink lesions present at birth and located on the nape of the neck, forehead, upper eyelids, or nasolabial fold region. They are a variant of nevus flammeus, more superficial, and one of the most common congenital malformations in the skin. The pink color results from distended dermal capillaries, and 95% fade by 1 year of age. Those located at the nape of the neck may persist for a lifetime. They generally do not present a cosmetic problem.

OTHER SKIN DISORDERS

Miliaria

Miliaria is a dermatosis commonly seen in infants. It is characterized by a vesicular eruption after prolonged exposure to perspiration, with subsequent obstruction of the eccrine ducts. There are two forms of miliaria: miliaria crystallina and miliaria rubra. In **miliaria crystallina,** ductal rupture occurs within the stratum corneum and appears as 1- to 2-mm clear vesicles without erythema. They rupture within 24 to 48 hours and leave a white scale. In miliaria rubra the ductal rupture occurs in the lower epidermis, with inflammatory cells attracted to the site of the rupture. **Miliaria rubra** (prickly heat) is characterized by 2- to 4-mm discrete erythematous papules or papulovesicles (Figure 45-16). Both forms may become secondarily infected, requiring treatment with systemic

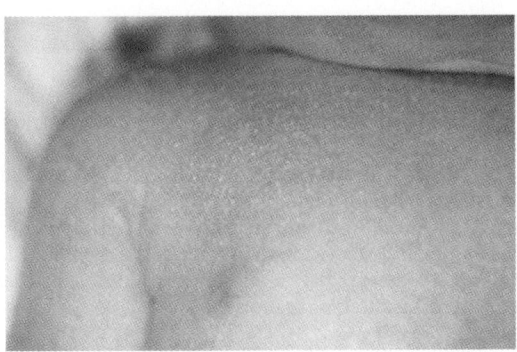

Figure 45-16 *Miliaria rubra.* Note discrete erythematous papules or papulovesicles. (Courtesy Department of Dermatology, School of Medicine, University of Utah.)

antibiotics. The key to management is avoidance of excessive heat and humidity, which cause sweating. Light clothing, cool baths, and air conditioning assist in keeping the skin surface dry and cool.

Erythema Toxicum Neonatorum

Erythema toxicum neonatorum (toxic erythema of the newborn) is a benign, erythematous accumulation of macules, papules, or pustules that appear at birth or 3 to 4 days after birth. The lesions first appear as a blotchy, macular erythematous rash. The macules vary from 1 mm to 1 cm. When papules or pustules develop, they are light yellow or white and 1 to 3 mm in diameter. There may be few or several hundred lesions, and any body surface can be affected, with the excep-

tion of the palms and soles, where there are no pilosebaceous follicles. The cause of the lesion is unknown, and it is self-limiting and resolves spontaneously within a few weeks of birth. No treatment is required.

Toxic Epidermal Necrolysis

Toxic epidermal necrolysis (TEN) is a rare, severe drug reaction with widespread epidermal apoptosis and detachment.[68] It is more common in adults but the incidence is increasing in children. The hypersensitivity to drugs includes sulfonamides, nonsteroidal antiinflammatory agents, and anticonvulsants (i.e., phenytoin). The onset of skin eruptions is preceded by malaise; anorexia; fever; and mild inflammation of the eyelids, conjunctiva, mouth, or genitalia. Erythema with tenderness is first described in the axillae and groin, extending over the body surface. Blisters and bullae form, and the entire epidermis may be shed, leaving open, weeping, painful areas of underlying skin. Complications include dehydration, protein loss, altered temperature regulation, and organ failure. About one third of children have pulmonary complications.[69] TEN must be confirmed by skin biopsy to differentiate from staphylococcal scalded-skin syndrome (see p. 1612) and acute graft-versus-host disease. Skin biopsy shows full-thickness epidermal necrosis and subepidermal blister formation.[70] Treatment requires intensive burn management, preferably in a burn unit. Treatment with intravenous immunoglobulin has varied responses and prospective randomized studies are needed but are difficult to complete because the disease is so rare.[71-73] The offending drug must be discontinued.

SUMMARY REVIEW

Acne Vulgaris
1. Acne vulgaris is the most common skin disease and affects 85% of the population between the ages of 12 and 25years.
2. Distinctive pilosebaceous units, known as *sebaceous follicles,* are the sites at which acne develops; they are located primarily on the face, neck, and upper trunk.
3. Acne is characterized by both noninflammatory and inflammatory lesions related to follicular hyperkeratinization, excessive sebum production, and *Propionibacterium acnes* colonization.

Dermatitis
1. Atopic dermatitis is associated with elevated immunoglobulin E (IgE) levels and a family history of asthma and hay fever. Red, scaly lesions commonly occur on the face, cheeks, and flexor surfaces of the extremities in infants and young children.
2. Diaper dermatitis is a type of irritant contact dermatitis that is initiated by a combination of factors that include prolonged exposure to urine and feces; frequently the infant becomes infected secondarily with *Candida albicans.*

Infections of the Skin
1. Impetigo is a contagious bacterial disease that occurs in two forms: bullous and vesicular. The toxins from the bacteria produce a weeping lesion with a honey-colored crust.
2. Staphylococcal scalded-skin syndrome (SSSS) is a staphylococcal skin infection that occurs more commonly in young children with low titers of antistaphylococcal antibody. Painful blisters and bullae form over large areas of the skin, requiring systemic antibiotics for treatment.

3. Tinea capitis (infection of the scalp) and tinea corporis (infection of the body) are fungal infections caused by dermatophytes.
4. *Candida albicans* infection is a superficial fungal infection of the mouth. Thrush is the term used to describe the presence of *Candida* in the mucous membranes of the mouth.
5. *Molluscum contagiosum* is a poxvirus of the skin that produces pale papular lesions filled with viral and cellular debris.
6. Rubella (also known as *German* or *3-day measles*) is a communicable disease characterized by fever, sore throat, enlarged cervical and postauricular nodes, and a generalized maculopapular rash that lasts 1 to 4 days.
7. Rubeola is a highly contagious disease of children; symptoms include high fever; enlarged lymph nodes; conjunctivitis; and a red rash that begins on the head, spreads to the trunk and extremities, and lasts 3 to 5 days. Both bacterial and viral complications may accompany rubeola.
8. Roseola is a benign disease of infants with a sudden onset of fever that lasts 3 to 5 days, followed by a rash that lasts 24 hours.
9. Chickenpox (varicella) is a highly contagious disease caused by the varicella-zoster virus. Vesicular lesions occur on the skin and mucous membranes. Individuals are contagious from 1 day before the development of the rash until about 6 days after the rash develops.
10. Herpes zoster (shingles) is a viral eruption of vesicles on the skin along the distribution of a sensory nerve. Children with immune suppression develop more serious complications.

Continued

SUMMARY REVIEW

11. Smallpox (variola) is a highly contagious, deadly disease that has been eradicated worldwide by vaccination.

Insect Bites and Parasites

1. Scabies is an itching lesion caused by the itch mite, which burrows into the skin, forming papules and vesicles. The mite is very contagious and is transmitted by direct contact.
2. Pediculosis (lice infestation) is caused by blood-sucking parasites that secrete a toxic saliva and damage the skin to produce a pruritic dermatitis. Lice are spread by direct contact and are recognized by the ova, or nits, that attach to the shaft of body hairs.
3. Flea bites produce a pruritic wheal with a central puncture site and occur as clusters in areas of tight-fitting clothing.
4. Bedbugs are blood-sucking parasites that live in cracks of floors, furniture, or bedding and feed at night. They produce pruritic wheals and nodules.

Hemangiomas and Vascular Malformations

1. Hemangiomas are benign vascular tumors that emerge at birth and resolve spontaneously through the childhood years. Strawberry hemangiomas (distinct, raised vascular lesions) are more superficial, and cavernous hemangiomas, with larger and more mature vessels, are deeper lesions.
2. Vascular malformations are congenital anomalies of blood vessels. Low flow malformations involve capillaries, veins, and lymphatics; high flow malformations involve arteries.
3. Nevus flammeus (port-wine stains) are deeper congenital malformations of the dermal capillaries, and salmon patches are more superficial vascular malformations.

Other Skin Disorders

1. Miliaria is characterized by small pruritic papules or vesicles that result from prolonged exposure to perspiration and subsequent obstruction of the eccrine ducts in infants.
2. Erythema toxicum neonatorum is a benign, erythematous, accumulation of macules, papules, and pustules that appear at birth or 3 to 4 days after birth and then spontaneously resolve within a few weeks.
3. Toxic epidermal necrolysis (TEN) is similar to SSSS, but the causative agent is usually a drug.

KEY TERMS

Acne conglobata, 1609
Acne vulgaris, 1609
Atopic dermatitis (AD), 1610
Bedbugs, 1618
Bullous impetigo, 1612
Cavernous hemangiomas, 1620
Chickenpox, 1616
Diaper dermatitis, 1611
Erythema toxicum neonatorum, 1621
Flea bites, 1618
Impetigo, 1612
Inflammatory acne, 1609

Miliaria, 1620
Miliaria crystallina, 1620
Miliaria rubra, 1620
Molluscum contagiosum, 1614
Noninflammatory acne, 1609
Norwegian scabies, 1618
Port-wine (nevus flammeus) stains, 1620
Roseola, 1616
Rubella, 1615
Rubeola, 1615
Salmon patches, 1620
Scabies, 1617

Smallpox (variola), 1617
Staphylococcal scalded-skin syndrome (SSSS), 1612
Strawberry hemangiomas, 1619
Thrush, 1614
Tinea capitis, 1613
Tinea corporis, 1614
Tinea pedis, 1613
Toxic epidermal necrolysis (TEN), 1621
Vesicular impetigo, 1612
Zoster, 1617

MEDIA RESOURCES

Review questions and answers for this chapter are available in the *CD Companion* included with this book.

WebLinks—links to Internet sites pertaining to this chapter—are available on Evolve at http://evolve.elsevier.com/McCance/.

REFERENCES

1. Pochi PE et al: Report of the consensus conference on acne classification, *J Am Acad Dermatol* 24(3):495, 1991.
1a. Lucky AW: A review of infantile and pediatric acne, *Dermatology* 196(1):95, 1998.
2a. Magin P et al: A systematic review of the evidence for 'myths and misconceptions' in acne management: diet, face-washing and sunlight, *Fam Pract* 22(1):62-70, 2005.
2b. Wolf R, Matz H, Orion E: Acne and diet, *Clin Dermatol* 22(5):387-393, 2004.
3. Gollnick H et al: Management of acne: a report from the Global Alliance to Improve Outcomes in Acne, *J Am Acad Dermatol* 49(Suppl):S1-37, 2003.
3a. Callender VD: Acne in ethnic skin: special considerations for therapy, *Dermatol Ther* 17(2):184-195, 2004.
4. Cargnello JA: Acne: what's new? *Med J Aust* 165(3):153, 1996.
5. Nguyen QH, Kim YA, Schwartz RA: Management of acne vulgaris, *Am Fam Physician* 50(1):89, 1994.

6. Gomert M et al: CCL1-CCR8 interactions: an axis mediating the recruitment of T cells and Langerhans-type dendritic cells to sites of atopic skin inflammation, *J Immunol* 174(8):5082-5091, 2005.
7. Galli E et al: Atopic dermatitis: molecular mechanisms, clinical aspects and new therapeutical approaches, *Curr Mol Med* 3(2):127-138, 2003.
8. Leung DY et al: New insights into atopic dermatitis, *J Clin Invest* 113(5):651-657, 2004.
9. Wahlgren CF: Itch and atopic dermatitis: an overview, *J Dermatol* 26(11):770, 1999.
10. Wellington K, Noble S: Pimecrolimus: a review of its use in atopic dermatitis, *Am J Clin Dermatol* 5(6):479-495, 2004.
11. Phillip R, Hughes A, Colding J: Getting to the bottom of nappy rash. ALSPAC survey team. Avon longitudinal study of pregnancy and childhood, *Br J Gen Pract* 47(421):493, 1997.
12. Brook I, Frazier EH, Yeager JK: Microbiology of nonbullous impetigo, *Pediatr Dermatol* 14(3):192, 1997.
13. O'Dell ML: Skin and wound infections: an overview, *Am Fam Physician* 57(10):2424, 1998.
14. Payne AS et al: Desmosomes and disease: pemphigus and bullous impetigo, *Curr Opin Cell Biol* 16(5):536-543, 2004.
15. Rudy SJ: Superficial fungal infections in children and adolescents, *Nurse Prac Forum* 19(2):56, 1999.
16. Weston WL, Lane AT, Morelli JG: *Color textbook of pediatric dermatology*, ed 2, St Louis, 1996, Mosby.
17. Koning S et al: Interventions for impetigo, *Cochrane Database Syst Rev* (2):CD003261, 2004.
18. Hacker SM: Common infections of the skin: characteristics, causes, and cures, *Postgrad Med* 96(2):43, 1994.

19. Patel GK, Finlay AY: Staphylococcal scalded skin syndrome diagnosis and management, *Am J Clin Dermatol* 4(3):165-175, 2003.
20. Raymond J et al: Staphylococcal scalded skin syndrome in a neonate, *Eur J Clin Microbiol Infect Dis* 16(6):453, 1997.
21. Patel GK: Treatment of staphylococcal scalded skin syndrome, *Expert Rev Anti Infect Ther* 2(4):575-587, 2004.
22. Pollack S: Staphylococcal scalded skin syndrome, *Pediatr Rev* 17(1):18, 1996.
23. Elewski BE: Cutaneous mycoses in children, *Br J Dermatol* 134(Suppl 46):7, 1996.
24. Gupta AK et al: An overview of topical antifungal therapy in dermatomycoses: a North American perspective, *Drugs* 55(5):645, 1998.
25. Gilaberte Y et al: Tinea capitis in infants in their first year of life, *Br J Dermatol* 151(4):886-890, 2004.
26. Pomeranz AJ et al: Asymptomatic dermatophyte carriers in the households of children with tinea capitis, *Arch Pediatr Adolesc Med* 153(5):483, 1999.
27. Williams JV et al: Semiquantitative study of tinea capitis and the asymptomatic carrier state in inner-city school children, *Pediatrics* 96(2 Pt 1):265, 1995.
28. Chan YC, Friedlander SF: New treatments for tinea capitis, *Curr Opin Infect Dis* 17(2):97-103, 2004.
29. Noble SL, Forbes TC, Stamm PL: Diagnosis and management of common tinea infections, *Am Fam Physician* 58(1):164, 1998.
30. Laxmisha C, Thappa DM, Jaisankar TJ: Clinical profile of molluscum contagiosum in children versus adults, *Deramtol Online J* 9(5):1, 2003.
31. Prasad SM: Molluscum contagiosum, *Pediatr Rev* 17(4):118, 1996.
32. Ronnerfalt L, Fransson J, Wahlgren CF: EMLA cream provides rapid relief for the curettage of molluscum contagiosum in children with atopic dermatitis without causing serious application-site reactions, *Pediatr Dermatol* 15(4):309, 1998.
33. Silverberg NB, Sidbury R, Mancini AJ: Childhood molluscum contagiosum: experience with cantharidin therapy in 300 patients, *J Am Acad Dermatol* 43(3):503, 2000.
34. Bayerl C, Feller G, Goerdt S: Experience in treating molluscum contagiosum in children with imiquimod 5% cream, *Br J Dermatol* 149(Suppl 66):25-29, 2003.
35. Ross GL, Orchard DC: Combination of topical treatment of molluscum contagiosum with cantharidin and imiquimod 5% in children: a case series of 16 patients, *Australas J Dermatol* 45(2):100-102, 2004.
36. Watson JC et al: Measles, mumps, and rubella—vaccine use and strategies for elimination of measles, rubella, and congenital rubella syndrome and control of mumps: recommendations of the Advisory Committee on Immunization Practices (ACIP), *MMWR* 47(RR-8):1, 1998.
37. Davidkin I et al: Etiology of measles- and rubella-like illnesses in measles, mumps, and rubella-vaccinated children, *J Infect Dis* 178(6):1567, 1998.
38. Poland GA, Jacobson RM: Failure to reach the goal of measles elimination: apparent paradox of measles infection in immunized persons, *Arch Intern Med* 154(16):1815, 1994.
39. Bale JF Jr: Neurologic complications of immunization, *J Child Neurol* 19(6):401-412, 2004.
40. Chez MG, Chin K, Hung PC: Immunizations, immunology, and autism, *Semin Pediatr Neurol* 11(3):214-217, 2004.
41. DeStefano F, Thompson WW: MMR vaccine and autism: an update of the scientific evidence, *Expert Rev Vaccines* 3(1):19-22, 2004.
42. Kennedy RC, Byers VS, Marchalonis JJ: Measles virus infection and vaccination: potential role in chronic illness and associated adverse events, *Crit Rev Immunol* 24(2):129-156, 2004.
43. Perry RT, Halsey NA: The clinical significance of measles: a review, *J Infect Dis* 189(Suppl 1):S4-16, 2004.
44. Update: global measles control and mortality reduction—worldwide, 1991-2001, *MMWR* 52(20):471-475, 2003.
45. Whitley RJ: Sorivudine: a potent inhibitor of varicella zoster virus replication, *Adv Exp Med Biol* 394:41, 1996.
46. Litt J, Burgess M: Varicella and varicella vaccination. An update, *Aust Fam Physician* 32(8):583-587, 2003.
47. Pastuszak AL et al: Outcome after maternal varicella infection in the first 20 weeks of pregnancy, *N Engl J Med* 330(13):901, 1994.
48. Klassen TP et al: Acyclovir for treating varicella in otherwise healthy children and adolescents, *Cochrane Database Syst Rev* (2):CD002980, 2004.
49. American Academy of Pediatrics, Committee on Infectious Diseases: Recommendations for the use of live attenuated varicella vaccine, *Pediatrics* 95(5):791, 1995.
50. Feder HM Jr, Hoss DM: Herpes zoster in otherwise healthy children, *Pediatr Infect Dis J* 23(5):451-457, 2004.
51. Kakourou T et al: Herpes zoster in children, *J Am Acad Dermatol* 39(Pt 1):207, 1998.
52. Ellner PD: Smallpox: gone but not forgotten, *Infection* 26(5):263, 1998.
52a. Centers for Disease Control: *Smallpox fact sheet: vaccine overview*, December 29, 2004. Available at www.bt.cdc.gov/agent/smallpox/vaccination/facts.asp
53. Chosidow O: Scabies and pediculosis, *Lancet* 355(9206):819, 2000.
54. Flinders DC, De Schweinitz P: Pediculosis and scabies, *Am Fam Physician* 69(2):341-348, 2004.
55. Meinking TL, Taplin D: Infestations: pediculosis, *Curr Probl Dermatol* 24:157, 1996.
56. Frankowski BL: American Academy of Pediatrics guidelines for the prevention and treatment of head lice infestation, *Am J Manag Care* 10(9 Suppl):S269-S272, 2004.
57. Howard R, Frieden IJ: Papular urticaria in children, *Pediatr Dermatol* 13(3):246, 1996.
58. Huntley AC: Cimex lectularius: what is this insect and how does it affect man? *Dermatol Online J* 5(1):6, 1999.
59. Buckmiller LM: Update on hemangiomas and vascular malformations, *Curr Opin Otolaryngol Head Neck Surg* 12(6):476-487, 2004.
60. Mulliken JB, Glowacki J: Hemangiomas and vascular malformations in infants and children: a classification based on endothelial characteristics, *Plast Reconstr Surg* 69(3):412-422, 1982.
61. Marler JJ, Mulliken JB: Current management of hemangiomas and vascular malformations, *Clin Plast Surg* 32(1):99-116, ix, 2005.
62. Werner JA et al: Optimal treatment of vascular birthmarks, *Am J Clin Dermatol* 4(11):745-756, 2003.
63. Low DW: Hemangiomas and vascular malformations, *Semin Pediatr Surg* 3(2):40, 1994.
64. Baselga E: Sturge-Weber syndrome, *Semin Cutan Med Surg* 23(2):87-98, 2004.
65. Thomas-Sohl KA, Vaslow DF, Maria BL: Sturge-Weber syndrome: a review, *Pediatr Neurol* 30(5):303-310, 2004.
66. Lanigan SW, Traibjee SM: Recent advances in laser treatment of port-wine stains, *Br J Hematol* 151(3):527-533, 2004.
67. Michel JL: Treatment of hemangiomas with 595 nm pulsated dye laser dermobeam, *Eur J Dermatol* 13(2):136-141, 2003.
68. Neff P et al: Lyell syndrome revisited: analysis of 18 cases of severe bullous skin disease in a burns unit, *Br J Plast Surg* 58(1):73-80, 2005.
69. Kim MJ, Lee KY: Bronchiolitis obliterans in children with Stevens-Johnson syndrome: follow-up with high resolution CT, *Pediatr Radiol* 26(1):22, 1996.
70. Rzany B et al: Histopathological and epidemiological characteristics of patients with erythema exudativum multiforme major, Stevens-Johnson syndrome and toxic epidermal necrolysis, *Br J Dermatol* 135(1):6, 1996.
71. Brown MK et al: Toxic epidermal necrolysis: does immunoglobulin make a difference? *Burn Care Rehabil* 25(1):81-88, 2004.
72. Nasser M, Bitterman-Deutsch O, Nassar F: Intravenous immunoglobulin for treatment of toxic epidermal necrolysis, *Am J Med Sci* 329(2):95-98, 2005.
73. Shortt R et al: Intravenous immunoglobulin does not improve outcome in toxic epidermal necrolysis, *J Burn Care Rehabil* 25(3):246-255, 2004.

SHOCK, MULTIPLE ORGAN DYSFUNCTION SYNDROME, AND BURNS IN ADULTS

KATHLEEN M. BALDWIN • DENNIS J. CHEEK • STEPHEN E. MORRIS

evolve

http://evolve.elsevier.com/McCance/

CHAPTER OUTLINE

Shock occurs when the cardiovascular system fails to perfuse tissues adequately, resulting in widespread impairment of cellular metabolism. Because tissue perfusion can be disrupted by any factor that alters heart function, blood volume, or blood pressure, shock has many causes and various clinical manifestations. Ultimately, however, shock from any cause progresses to organ failure and death, unless compensatory mechanisms reverse the process or clinical intervention succeeds. Untreated severe shock overwhelms the body's compensatory mechanisms through positive-feedback loops that initiate and maintain a downward physiologic spiral.

Multiple organ dysfunction syndrome (MODS) is progressive and often involves the ultimate failure of two or more organ systems after a severe illness or injury. The disease process is initiated and perpetuated by uncontrolled systemic inflammatory and stress responses and is characterized by a hypermetabolic and hyperdynamic state that persists as organ dysfunction develops. For many years the syndrome was referred to as *multiple organ failure* or *multiple systems organ failure.* Gradually it was recognized that the term *organ dysfunction* more accurately describes the syndrome as a process of physiologic deterioration.

Major burns result in extensive immediate tissue injury and thus are a form of trauma with wide-reaching effects on all organ systems. The cause of injury may be thermal contact, flame, chemical agents, or electrical agents; each cause requires a different approach in diagnosis and treatment. Closely associated with thermal burns is smoke inhalation injury, which accounts for about 25% of all burn unit admissions. As a multiorgan problem, thermal injuries can have an overwhelming effect on survival of the burned individual. Regardless of the cause of burns, the result is a final common pathway of physiologic response dependent on the extent of burn surface involvement and depth of tissue destruction.

SHOCK

Shock can be classified by cause, principal pathophysiologic process, or clinical manifestations. Classification by cause is perhaps the most useful because it suggests the principal pathophysiologic process and focuses on the underlying disorder, which must be treated to prevent the irreversible impairment of cellular metabolism. **Shock** is classified by cause as cardiogenic (caused by heart failure); neurogenic, or vasogenic (caused by alterations in vascular smooth muscle tone); anaphylactic (e.g., hypersensitivity); septic (caused by infection); or hypovolemic (caused by insufficient intravascular fluid volume). An additional type, traumatic shock, has components of hypovolemic and septic shock.[1]

Cellular Alterations

Because the body is made up of many cells that may function or malfunction at different stages of metabolic impairment, shock causes many diverse signs and symptoms. Subjective complaints are usually nonspecific and may not be particularly helpful to the clinician attempting diagnosis and treatment. The individual may report feeling sick, weak, cold, hot, nauseated, dizzy, confused, afraid, thirsty, and short of breath.

Observable and measurable signs and symptoms often conflict. Blood pressure, cardiac output, and urinary output

Chapter content on "Shock" contributed by Kathleen M. Baldwin; "Multiple Organ Dysfunction Syndrome" contributed by Dennis J. Cheek; "Burns" contributed by Stephen E. Morris.

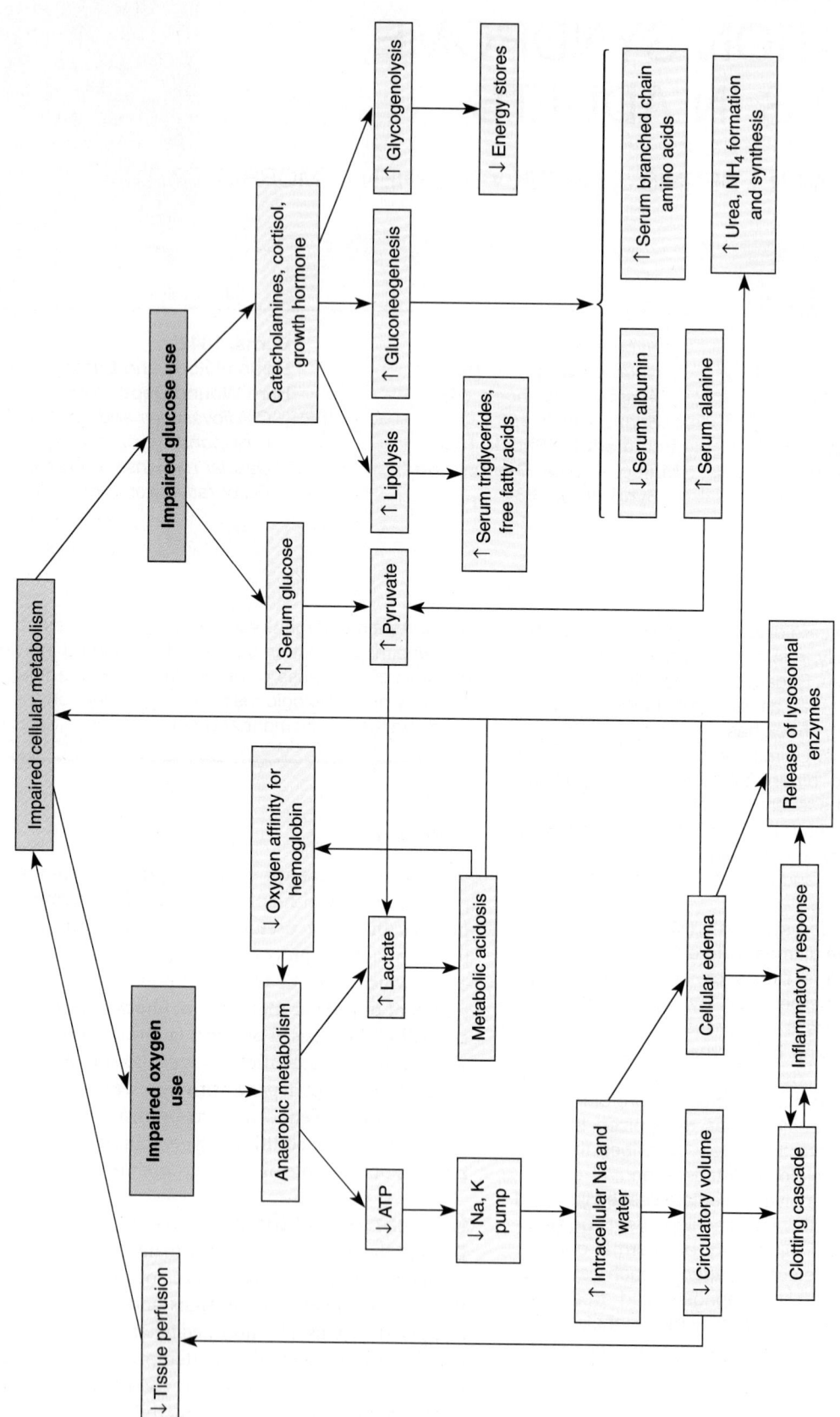

Figure 46-1 Impairment of cellular metabolism by shock. *ATP,* Adenosine triphosphate.

are usually—but not always—decreased. Respiratory rate is usually increased. Variable indicators of shock include alterations of heart rate, core body temperature, skin temperature, systemic vascular resistance, and skin color. Dyspnea, diaphoresis, and altered sensorium may be obvious.

Impairment of Cellular Metabolism

The final common pathway in all types of shock is impairment of cellular metabolism, which is a complex concept. Figure 46-1 illustrates the pathophysiology of shock at the cellular level.

Impairment of Oxygen Use

In all types of shock the cell either is not receiving an adequate amount of oxygen or is unable to use oxygen (see Figure 46-1). In cardiogenic shock, cardiac output is too low to deliver adequate oxygen to the cell. In hypovolemic shock, oxygen delivery is impaired by inadequate numbers of red cells or inadequate volume of intravascular fluid. In neurogenic, anaphylactic, and septic shock, systemic vascular resistance (SVR) is too low and perfusion pressure in the capillaries is inadequate to drive oxygen across cell membranes. In septic shock, hypoxia is made worse by fever, which increases the cell's oxygen consumption rate, and by endotoxic and inflammatory chemical disruption of cell metabolism, which impairs the cells' ability to use oxygen.

Without oxygen the cell shifts from aerobic to anaerobic metabolism. Anaerobic metabolism is a less efficient method of extracting energy from carbon bonds, and the cell begins to use its stores of adenosine triphosphate (ATP) faster than stores can be replaced. Without ATP the cell loses its ability to maintain an electrochemical gradient across its selectively permeable membrane. Specifically, the cell cannot operate the sodium-potassium pump. Sodium and chloride accumulate inside the cell, and potassium exits. Cells of the nervous system and myocardium are profoundly and immediately affected. The resting potentials of these cells are reduced, and action potentials decrease in amplitude (also see Chapter 3). Myocardial depressant factor also decreases the contractility of the heart. A variety of clinical manifestations of impaired central nervous system and myocardial function result.

As sodium moves into the cell, water follows. Throughout the body, the water drawn from the interstitium into the cells is "replaced" by water that is, in turn, drawn out of the vascular space. This decreases circulatory volume. Within the cells, water causes cellular edema that disrupts cellular membranes, releasing lysosomal enzymes that injure the cells internally and leak into the interstitium.

Three positive-feedback loops then begin that further impair oxygen use: (1) activation of the clotting cascade, (2) decreased circulatory volume, and (3) lysosomal enzyme release. First, enzymatic processes are disrupted by the change in the normal ionic and osmotic levels in the cell, as are those processes governed by the physical laws of diffusion. Diffusion of nutrients and wastes into and out of the cell takes longer, and cellular metabolism is further altered. At the same time, diffusion across capillary membranes occurs more slowly as blood flow in the capillary beds becomes sluggish. Sluggish capillary flow decreases tissue perfusion further and activates the clotting cascade (see Chapter 25). The clotting cascade accounts for common complications of shock, such as acute tubular necrosis, acute adult respiratory distress syndrome (ARDS), and disseminated intravascular coagulation (DIC). It also may activate or be activated by the inflammatory response.[2]

Decreased circulatory volume, the second positive-feedback loop, magnifies decreased tissue perfusion in all types of shock. Decreased intravascular volume causes decreased cardiac output in septic shock and further decreases cardiac output in cardiogenic shock. In individuals with anaphylactic, neurogenic, or septic shock and an already dilated vasculature, hypotension worsens as a result of decreased circulatory volume. New data on additional mechanisms for hypotension (vasodilation) are illustrated in Figure 46-7 (p. 1635).

The third positive-feedback loop involves the release of lysosomal enzymes. Lysosomal enzymes not only injure the cell that released them, but also injure adjacent cells. By damaging the mechanisms of surrounding cells, lysosomal enzymes extend areas of impaired metabolism and cellular injury.

In addition to decreasing ATP stores, anaerobic metabolism affects the pH of the cell and metabolic acidosis develops. A compensatory mechanism is initiated that enables cardiac and skeletal muscles to use lactic acid as a fuel source, but only for a limited time. The decreasing pH of the cell that is functioning anaerobically has serious consequences. Enzymes necessary for cellular function dissociate under acid conditions. Enzyme dissociation stops cell function, repair, and division. As lactic acid is released systemically, blood pH drops, reducing the oxygen-carrying capacity of the blood (see Chapter 2). Therefore less oxygen is delivered to the cells. Further acidosis triggers the release of more lysosomal enzymes because the low pH disrupts lysosomal membrane integrity.

Impairment of Glucose Use

Impaired glucose use can be caused by either impaired glucose delivery or impaired glucose uptake by the cells (see Figure 46-1). The reasons for inadequate glucose delivery are the same as those enumerated for inadequate oxygen delivery. In addition, in septic and anaphylactic shock, glucose metabolism may be increased or disrupted because of fever or bacteria, and glucose uptake can be prevented by the presence of vasoactive toxins, endotoxins, histamine, and kinins.

Some of the compensatory mechanisms activated by shock contribute to decreased glucose uptake by the cells. High serum levels of cortisol, growth hormone, and catecholamines account for hyperglycemia and insulin resistance, tachycardia, increased SVR, and increased cardiac contractility. Cells shift to glycogenolysis, gluconeogenesis, and lipolysis to generate fuel for survival (see Chapter 1). Except in the liver, kidneys, and muscles, the body's cells have extremely limited stores of glycogen. In fact, total body stores can fuel the metabolism for only about 10 hours. The depletion of fat and glycogen stores is not itself a cause of organ failure, but the energy costs of glycogenolysis and lipolysis are considerable and contribute to the cells' failure.

The depletion of protein is, however, a cause of organ failure. When gluconeogenesis causes proteins to be used for fuel, these proteins are no longer available to maintain cellular structure, function, repair, and replication. The breakdown of protein occurs in starvation states, hyperdynamic metabolic states, and septic shock. Under anaerobic metabolism, protein breakdown liberates alanine, which is converted to pyruvate. In sepsis, pyruvic acid is changed into lactic acid and a positive-feedback loop is formed.

As proteins are broken down anaerobically, ammonia and urea are produced. Ammonia is toxic to living cells. Uremia develops, and uric acid further disrupts cellular metabolism. Proteins are broken down preferentially. Serum albumin and other plasma proteins are consumed for fuel first. Serum protein consumption decreases capillary osmotic pressure and contributes to the development of interstitial edema, creating another positive-feedback loop that decreases circulatory volume. In septic shock, plasma protein breakdown includes breakdown of immunoglobulins, thereby impairing immune system function when it is most needed.

Muscle wasting caused by protein breakdown weakens skeletal and cardiac muscle. Skeletal muscle wasting impairs the muscles that facilitate breathing. Muscle wasting therefore alters the actions of both heart and lungs. The delivery of oxygen and glucose to the cells is directly reduced, as is the removal of waste products, forming another positive-feedback loop.

A final outcome of impaired cellular metabolism is the buildup of metabolic end products in the cell and interstitial spaces. Waste products are toxic to the cells and further disrupt cellular function and membrane integrity. In septic shock, for example, a deficiency in cellular metabolism and the buildup of toxins may precede and cause decreased tissue perfusion.

Types of Shock

Each type of shock (cardiogenic, hypovolemic, neurogenic, anaphylactic, septic) involves numerous clinical manifestations that also characterize many other conditions, making diagnosis difficult. In addition, the body's many compensatory mechanisms can mask, for a time, many definitive signs of shock.

Cardiogenic Shock

Cardiogenic shock results from heart failure from any cause. Most cases of cardiogenic shock follow myocardial infarction or surgery (about 15%) requiring cardiopulmonary bypass.[3] Shock also can follow heart failure from any cause, myocardial stunning, myocardial ischemia, myocardial or pericardial infections, dysrhythmias, tension pneumothorax, and conditions causing excessive right ventricular afterload. Cardiogenic shock is notoriously unresponsive to treatment, with in-hospital mortalities ranging from 50% to 80%.[4] Mortality improves with

the use of early revascularization strategies,[5] and the use of mechanical assistive devices. Age, systolic blood pressure, heart rate, and the New York Heart Association class have been correlated with increased risk for cardiogenic shock following thrombolytic therapy.[6] The pathophysiology of cardiogenic shock is shown in Figure 46-2. As cardiac output decreases, renal and hypothalamic adaptive responses maintain or increase blood volume. Blood pressure is maintained through vasoconstriction in response to catecholamine release from the adrenals. Catecholamines also increase contractility and heart rate. Increases in blood volume and vascular resistance succeed in normalizing blood pressure and increasing cardiac performance but at the cost of increasing myocardial demands for oxygen and nutrients. Increasing myocardial requirements further strain the already failing heart, which can no longer pump an adequate volume of blood with sufficient force to perfuse the tissues. The direct effect of decreased tissue perfusion is impaired cellular metabolism. (Normal cellular metabolism is discussed in Chapter 1.)

The clinical manifestations of cardiogenic shock are caused by widespread impairment of cellular metabolism. They include impaired mentation, elevated preload in the systemic and pulmonary vasculature, systemic and pulmonary edema, low cardiac output, dusky skin color, low blood pressure, oliguria, ileus, and dyspnea.

Hypovolemic Shock

Hypovolemic shock is caused by loss of whole blood (hemorrhage), plasma (burns), or interstitial fluid (diaphoresis, diabetes mellitus, diabetes insipidus, emesis, or diuresis) in large amounts. Loss of whole blood or plasma causes hypovolemia directly. Loss of interstitial fluid causes it indirectly by promoting diffusion of plasma from the intravascular to the extravascular space. Hypovolemic shock begins to develop when intravascular volume has decreased by about 15%.

Hypovolemia is offset initially by compensatory mechanisms (Figure 46-3). Heart rate and SVR increase as a result of catecholamine release by the adrenals. This boosts both cardiac output and tissue perfusion pressures. Compelled by a decrease in capillary hydrostatic pressures, interstitial fluid moves into the vascular compartment. The liver and spleen add to blood volume by disgorging stored red blood cells and plasma. In the kidneys, renin (through several intermediaries) stimulates aldosterone release and the retention of sodium (and hence water), whereas antidiuretic hormone (ADH, or vasopressin) from the posterior pituitary gland increases water retention. New data on the compensation of ADH, however, shows that as shock worsens, ADH in plasma decreases (see What's New? Vasopressin (ADH) Emerging as Therapy for Shock States on p. 1635).

These compensatory mechanisms are, however, finite. If the initial fluid or blood loss is great or if loss continues, compensation fails, resulting in decreased tissue perfusion. Nutrient delivery to the cells is impaired, and cellular metabolism fails. Mortality from traumatic hemorrhagic shock ranges from 10% to 31%. Prompt control of hemorrhage is the treat-

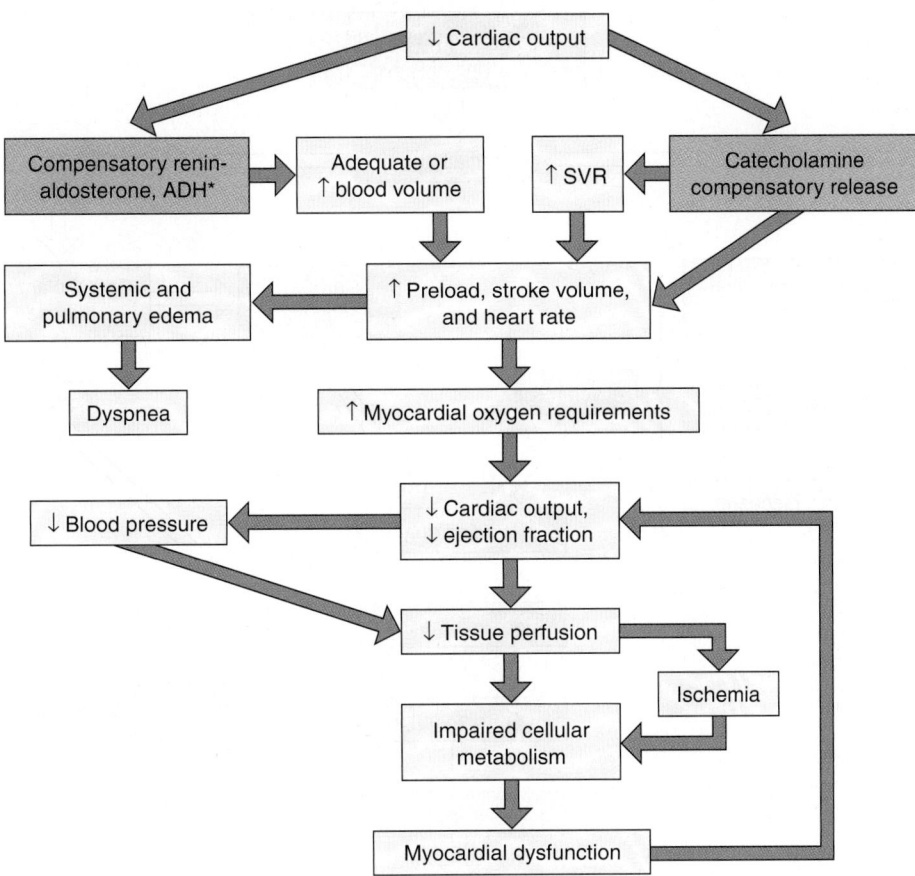

Figure 46-2 Cardiogenic shock. Shock becomes life threatening when compensatory mechanisms (orange colored labels) cause increased myocardial oxygen requirements. *ADH,* Antidiuretic hormone; *SVR,* systemic vascular resistance. (*see WHAT'S NEW? Vasopressin [ADH] Emerging as Therapy for Shock States.)

ment of choice. Fluid replacement is also an important treatment, but the type of fluid to be used and the rate of replacement are currently controversial.[5] The clinical manifestations of hypovolemic shock include high SVR, poor skin turgor, thirst, oliguria, low systemic and pulmonary preloads, and rapid heart rates.

Neurogenic Shock

Neurogenic shock is sometimes called **vasogenic shock.** Both terms refer to a widespread and massive vasodilation that results from an imbalance between parasympathetic and sympathetic stimulation of vascular smooth muscle (see Chapter 29). Occasionally, parasympathetic overstimulation or sympathetic understimulation persists, causing vasodilation for an extended period. Extreme, persistent vasodilation leads to neurogenic shock (Figure 46-4). Neurogenic shock creates "relative hypovolemia." Blood volume has not changed, but the amount of space containing the blood has increased, so that SVR decreases drastically; thus pressure in the vessels is inadequate to drive nutrients across capillary membranes, and nutrient delivery to the cells is impaired. As with other types of shock, this leads to impaired cellular metabolism.

Neurogenic shock can be caused by any factor that stimulates parasympathetic activity or inhibits sympathetic activity

of vascular smooth muscle. (Parasympathetic stimulation automatically inhibits sympathetic activity and vice versa; see Chapter 29.) Normally, sympathetic stimulation maintains muscle tone. If sympathetic stimulation is interrupted or inhibited, vasodilation occurs. Therefore trauma to the spinal cord or medulla, conditions that interrupt the supply of oxygen to the medulla, or conditions that deprive the medulla of glucose (e.g., insulin reactions) can cause neurogenic shock by interrupting sympathetic activity. Depressive drugs, anesthetic agents, and severe emotional stress and pain are other causes of neurogenic shock.

The clinical hallmark of neurogenic shock is a very low SVR, along with other indicators of excessive parasympathetic activity. Bradycardia is the most obvious manifestation, especially in the early stages. Bradycardia may cease when compensatory mechanisms, particularly an increase in sympathetic system activity, have been initiated. The ejection fraction remains high, indicating a healthy myocardium, whereas central venous pressure decreases as the veins dilate. Neurogenic shock causes fainting if blood pressure decreases to the point that cerebral metabolism is not sufficient to support consciousness. Most episodes of fainting are *not* shock, however; for such episodes to progress to shock is rare. By allowing the blood pressure to equalize from head to toe as the

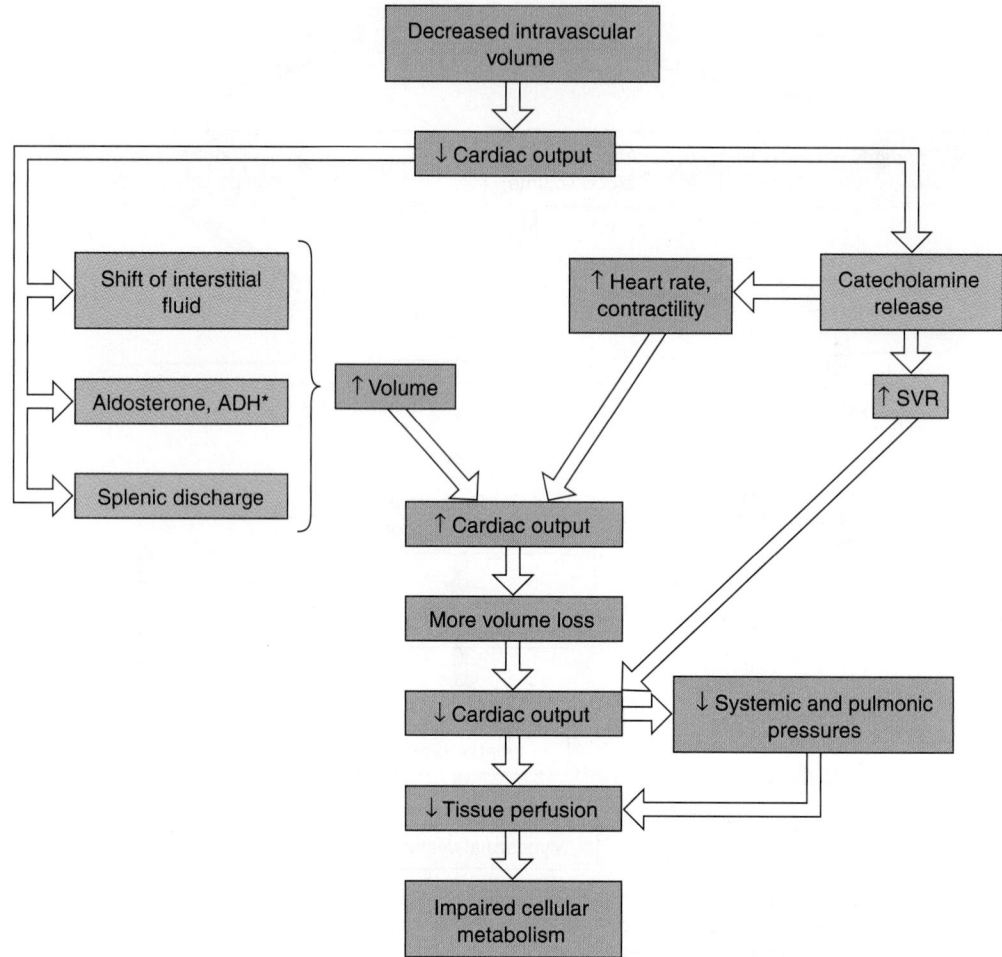

Figure 46-3 **Hypovolemic shock.** This type of shock becomes life threatening when compensatory mechanisms (orange-colored labels) are overwhelmed by continued loss of intravascular volume. *ADH,* Antidiuretic hormone; *SVR,* systemic vascular resistance. (*see WHAT'S NEW? Vasopressin [ADH] Emerging as Therapy for Shock States.)

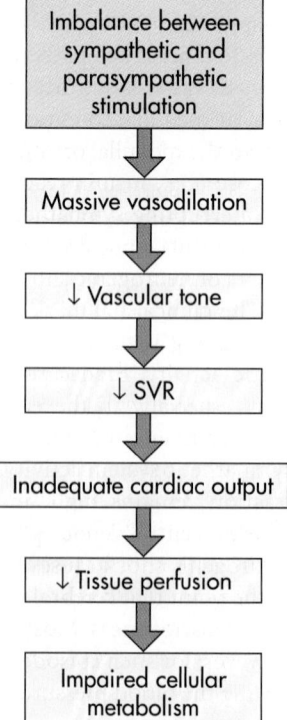

Figure 46-4 Neurogenic shock. *SVR,* Systemic vascular resistance.

individual becomes prone, fainting can actually prevent shock.

Anaphylactic Shock

Anaphylactic shock is the outcome of a widespread hypersensitivity reaction known as *anaphylaxis.* The basic physiologic alteration in anaphylactic shock is the same as that in neurogenic shock—that is, vasodilation, peripheral pooling, and relative hypovolemia leading to decreased tissue perfusion and impaired cellular metabolism (Figure 46-5). Anaphylactic shock is often more severe than other types of normovolemic shock because the hypersensitivity reaction that triggers vasodilation has other pathophysiologic effects that rapidly involve the entire body.

Anaphylactic shock begins as an allergic reaction—an immune and inflammatory response—to an allergen. (An allergen is an antigen to which an individual is hypersensitive; see Chapters 6, 7, and 8 for discussions of immunity, inflammation, and hypersensitivity.) Some allergens known to cause hypersensitivity reactions are snakebite venom, insect venoms, pollens, shellfish, penicillin, and animal sera. Once in the body, the allergen causes an extensive immune and inflam-

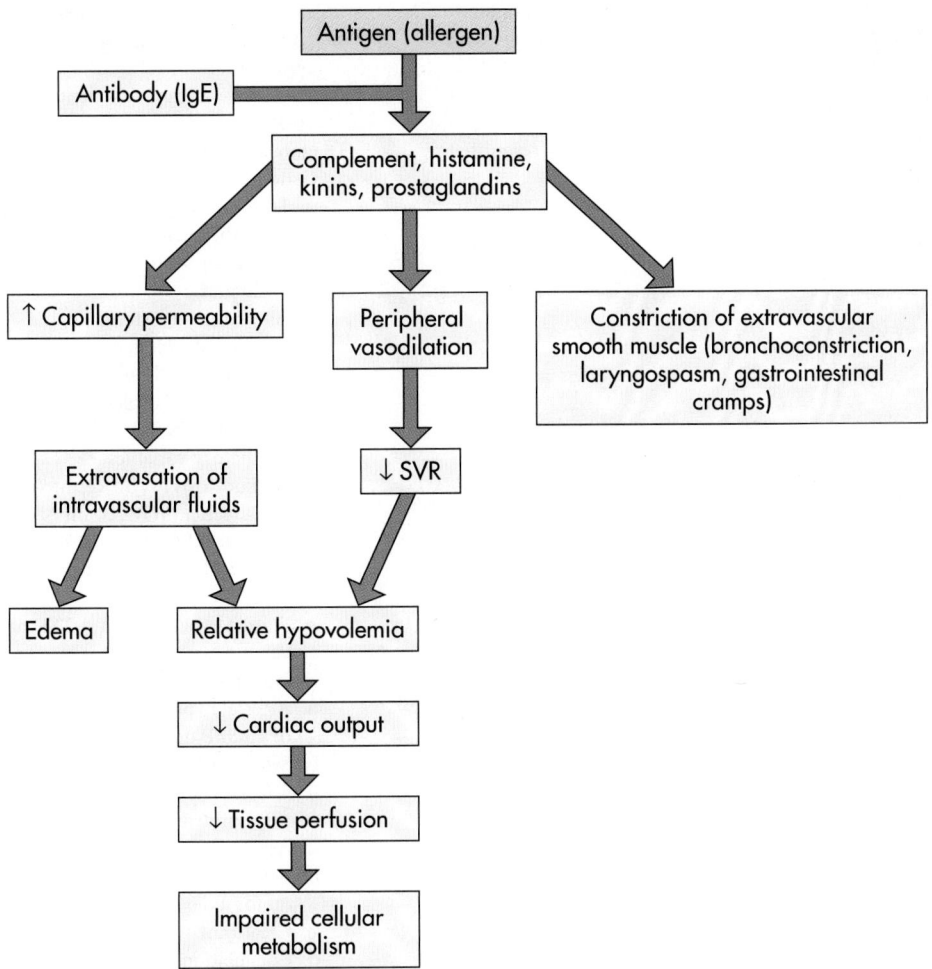

Figure 46-5 Anaphylactic shock. *IgE,* Immunoglobulin E; *SVR,* systemic vascular resistance.

matory response. The vascular effects of this response include vasodilation and increased vascular permeability, resulting in peripheral pooling and tissue edema. The extravascular effects include constriction of extravascular smooth muscle. Constriction often causes respiratory difficulty because it tends to affect smooth muscle layers in the airway walls (e.g., the larynx and bronchioles; see Chapter 32).

The onset of anaphylactic shock is usually sudden, and progression to death can occur within minutes unless emergency treatment is given. The first manifestations of shock may be anxiety, difficulty in breathing, gastrointestinal cramps, edema, hives (urticaria), and sensations of burning or itching of the skin. A precipitous decrease in blood pressure occurs and is followed by impaired mentation. Other signs include decreased SVR (with high or normal cardiac output) and oliguria. Treatment begins with removal of the antigen (if possible). Epinephrine is administered to decrease mast cell and basophil degranulation, cause vasoconstriction, and reverse airway constriction. Volume expanders (e.g., lactated Ringer solution) are given intravenously to reverse the relative hypovolemia, and antihistamines and steroids are given to stop the inflammatory reaction.

Septic Shock

Septic shock is the endpoint of a continuum of progressive dysfunction.[7] The syndrome begins with bacteremia, then sepsis, then severe sepsis, and then septic shock. Consensus on definitions of each component was updated at an international sepsis conference in 2001. These definitions are presented in Table 46-1 (see What's New? Sepsis Update).

Severe sepsis is the eleventh most common cause of death in the United States.[8] Mortality ranges from 28% to 60%.[8] Septic shock is caused by gram-negative bacteria, gram-positive bacteria, and fungi (see What's New? Flagellin). Advances in antibiotic therapy for gram-negative sepsis have made gram-positive bacteria the current leading cause of sepsis.[9] Even when properly treated with available therapies, it carries a high mortality rate. Prognosis is significantly affected by the source and virulence of the infectious microorganism.

Septic shock begins with a nidus of infection that may be readily discernible or extremely difficult to locate (Figure 46-6). Bacteria then enter the bloodstream to produce bacteremia in one of two ways: (1) directly from the site of infection or (2) from toxic substances released by the bacteria directly into the bloodstream. These toxic substances, which act

Table 46-1 Definitions of Septic Shock Components

Term	Basic Definition	Comments
Infection	A pathologic process that results from an invasion of a normal part of the body by pathogenic or potentially pathogenic microorganisms	Still viewed as an imperfect definition Infection can be strongly suspected without microbiologic confirmation
Bacteremia	Presence of viable bacteria in the blood	Neither necessary nor sufficient to make a diagnosis of sepsis

Sepsis	A clinical syndrome involving a deleterious host response to an infection	Diagnostic criteria:
		1. General variables
		  a. Fever—core temperature >38.8° C
		  b. Hypothermia—core temperature <36° C
		  c. Heart rate >90
		  d. Tachypnea
		  e. Altered mental status
		  f. Significant edema or positive fluid balance (>20 ml/kg over 24 hours)
		  g. Hyperglycemia (blood sugar >12 mg/dl) in the absence of diabetes
		2. Inflammatory variables
		  a. Leukocytosis (WBC count >12,000)
		  b. Leukopenia (WBC count <4000)
		  c. Normal WBC with >10% immature forms
		  d. Plasma C-reactive protein >2 SD above the normal value
		  e. Plasma procalcitonin >2 SD above the normal value
		3. Hemodynamic variables
		  a. Arterial hypotension (SBP <90 mmHg; MAP <70, or an SBP decrease >40 mmHg)
		  b. $S\bar{v}_{O_2}$ >70%
		  c. Cardiac index >3.5 L/min
		4. Organ dysfunction variables
		  a. Arterial hypoxemia (Pa_{O_2}/Fi_{O_2} <300)
		  b. Acute oliguria (urine output <0.5 ml/kg/hr or 45 ml for at least 2 hours)
		  c. Creatinine increase >0.5 mg/dl
		  d. Coagulation abnormalities (INR >1.5 or apt >60)
		  e. Ileus
		  f. Thrombocytopenia (platelet count <100,000)
		  g. Hyperbilirubinemia (plasma total bilirubin >4 mg/dl or 70 mmol/L)
		5. Tissue perfusion variables
		  a. Hyperlactatemia (>2 mmol/L)
		  b. Decreased capillary refill or mottling

Severe sepsis	Sepsis complicated with one or more organ system dysfunctions	May be difficult to differentiate underlying organ dysfunction from sepsis-related organ dysfunction
Septic shock	Severe sepsis complicated by persistent hypotension refractory to early fluid therapy	Persistent systolic blood pressure >90 mmHg

Data from Levy MM et al: *Crit Care Med* 312:1250, 2003; Opal SM, *Scand J Infect Dis* 35:529, 2003.

WBC, White blood cell count; *SD,* standard deviation; *SBP,* systolic blood pressure; *MAP,* mitogen-activated protein; *$S\bar{v}_{O_2}$,* saturation of hemoglobin with oxygen; *Pa_{O_2}/Fi_{O_2},* partial pressure of oxygen in arterial blood/fraction of inspired oxygen; *INR,* international normalized ratio.

WHAT'S NEW? Sepsis Update

1. Sepsis pathophysiology is viewed as a continuum—sepsis, severe sepsis, and septic shock.
2. Sepsis syndrome is the result of a complex interaction between inflammation, coagulation, and impaired fibrinolysis in response to an immune trigger.
3. The endothelium plays an active role in the regulation of blood vessel tone, coagulation, angiogenesis, and leukocyte/platelet activation.

Data from Cunneen J, Cartwright M: *AACN Clin Issues* 15(1):18, 2004.

WHAT'S NEW? Flagellin

Flagellin, a protein, is the principle constituent of the flagellum, a prominent surface structure found in motile bacteria. Recent work reveals that flagellin can act as a soluble immunostimulatory and proinflammatory factor, activating the immune/inflammatory axis through toll-like receptors.

Data from Szabo C: *Crit Care Med* 31(1):S39-S45, 2003.

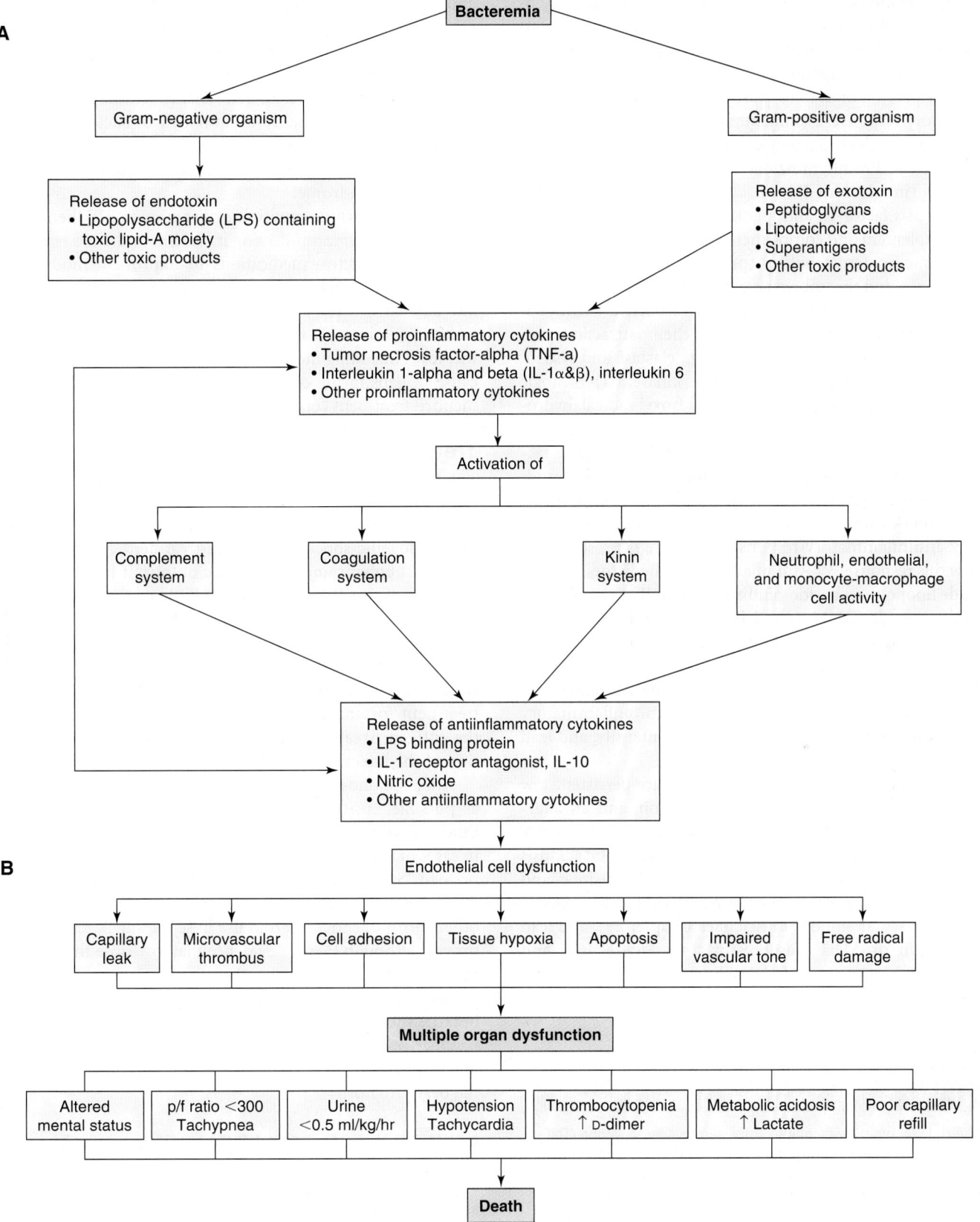

Figure 46-6 Summary of sepsis pathology. p/f (Pa_{O_2}/Fi_{O_2}) = oxygenation ratio. (**A,** from Larson V, Barke RA: *Urol Clin North Am* 26(4):687, 1999; **B,** Copyright © 2003, Eli Lilly and Company. All rights reserved. Reprinted with permission from Eli Lilly and Company.)

as triggering molecules in the septic syndrome, include endotoxins released by gram-negative microorganisms,[10] lipoteichoic acids and peptidoglycan released by gram-positive microorganisms, and superantigens.[2]

The triggering molecules cause the host to initiate a proinflammatory response. Proinflammatory cells released include polymorphonuclear leukocytes, macrophages, monocytes, and platelets. Proinflammatory mediators released include cytokines (interleukins IL-1, IL-2, IL-6, IL-8, and IL-15; tumor necrosis factor-α; and granulocyte cell-stimulating factor), complement and complement cascade activation, kinins, arachidonic acid metabolites (prostaglandins, prostacyclin, leukotrienes, and thromboxane), soluble adhesion molecules, platelet-activating factor, endorphins, vasoactive neuropeptides, histamine, serotonin, monocyte chemoattractant proteins 1 and 2, proteolytic enzymes (e.g., elastase and lysosomal enzymes), protein kinase, tyrosine kinase, CD-14, toxic oxygen metabolites (e.g., superoxide, hydroxyl radical, hydrogen peroxide, peroxynitrite), neopterin, and clotting cascade activation.[11] Proinflammatory cytokines enhance tissue factors, which initiates coagulation. Diminished thrombomodulin (cell surface glycoprotein of endothelial cells) inhibits the conversion of protein C and activated protein C. A compensatory antiinflammatory response syndrome is presumed to follow this response.[11,12] Antiinflammatory mediators released include lipopolysaccharide-binding protein; IL-1 receptor antagonist; soluble CD-14; type 2 IL-1 receptor; leukotriene B$_4$ receptor antagonist; IL-4, IL-10, and IL-13; soluble tumor necrosis factor receptor; transforming growth factor-β; epinephrine; and nitric oxide.[11] Presumably the end result is a mixed antagonistic response syndrome as proinflammatory and antiinflammatory mediators respond, intensify, and lead the host into MODS.

Clinical manifestations of septic shock are persistent low arterial pressure, low SVR from vasodilation, and an alteration in oxygen extraction by all cells. Septic shock and states of prolonged shock causing tissue hypoxia with lactic acidosis increase nitric oxide synthesis, activate ATP-sensitive and calcium-regulated potassium channels (K_{ATP} and K_{ca}, respectively) in vascular smooth muscle (see Chapter 29), and lead to depletion of ADH (vasopressin) (see Figure 46-7 and What's New? Vasopressin (ADH) Emerging as Therapy for

Shock States). Tachycardia causes cardiac output to remain normal or become elevated, although myocardial contractility is reduced. Temperature instability is present, ranging from hyperthermia to hypothermia. Effects on other organ systems may result in deranged renal function, gastrointestinal mucosa changes that result in release of bacteria from the gut, jaundice, clotting abnormalities, deterioration of mental status, and tachypnea that often progresses to acute respiratory distress syndrome.

Treatment includes multiple drug antimicrobial therapy, removal of the source of infection if one is found, fluid resuscitation, and vasoactive medications to improve hemodynamic performance. Experimental treatment under study includes low-dose corticosteroids; vasopressin; tight blood glucose control;[13] continuous plasma filtration;[14] and immunomodulating therapy,[15] including monoclonal antibodies and vaccines.[16] Because of gaps in the current understanding of sepsis, recommended treatment continues to evolve.

Treatment for Shock

The first treatment for shock is to discover and correct or remove the underlying cause. Although this seems a simple tenet, it is one that is not always remembered. Thus treatment for cardiogenic shock begins with treatment of heart failure or at least enhancement of cardiac output. If hypovolemia is the cause of shock, hemorrhage and other causes of fluid loss must be stopped. In neurogenic shock as a result of spinal cord trauma, stabilization of the spine and surrounding tissue is a beginning, and pain usually can be decreased to a level at which neurally mediated decreases of SVR cease. The initial treatment for anaphylactic shock is to remove or neutralize the antigen. Treatment for septic shock begins with eradication of the infective agent, usually with antimicrobials.

After the underlying cause or condition is corrected as far as possible, treatment thereafter is supportive. Intravenous fluid is administered to expand intravascular volume, except in cases of cardiogenic shock, which require diuresis to reduce preload. Supplemental oxygen is always given. Cardiotonic drugs are given early in cardiogenic shock and given later in other forms of shock. Steroid use in septic shock remains unproven, although there is evidence that low-dose therapy improves mortality.[17] Stress ulcer prophylaxis and gastric tonometry, to measure splanchnic blood flow, are imperative because the gut is one of the drivers of the septic syndrome.[18]

Once positive-feedback loops are established, intervention in shock is difficult. Prevention and very early treatment offer the best prognosis.

MULTIPLE ORGAN DYSFUNCTION SYNDROME

Multiple organ dysfunction syndrome (MODS) is the progressive dysfunction of two or more organ systems resulting from an uncontrolled inflammatory response to a severe illness or injury. The organ dysfunction can progress to organ failure and death. MODS occurs during severe sepsis. In 2001,

---

WHAT'S NEW? TNF-α Signal Transduction Pathway

The proinflammatory cytokine tumor necrosis factor-alpha (TNF-α) triggers a signaling cascade that activates the transcription factor nuclear factor-κβ. NF-κβ is very important because it forms the basis for numerous physiologic and pathologic processes. These findings provide significant insight into the logic of the TNF-α/NF-κβ pathway and is generally applicable to other pathways relevant to human disease.

Data from Bouwmeester T et al: *Nat Cell Biology* 6(2):97-105, 2004.

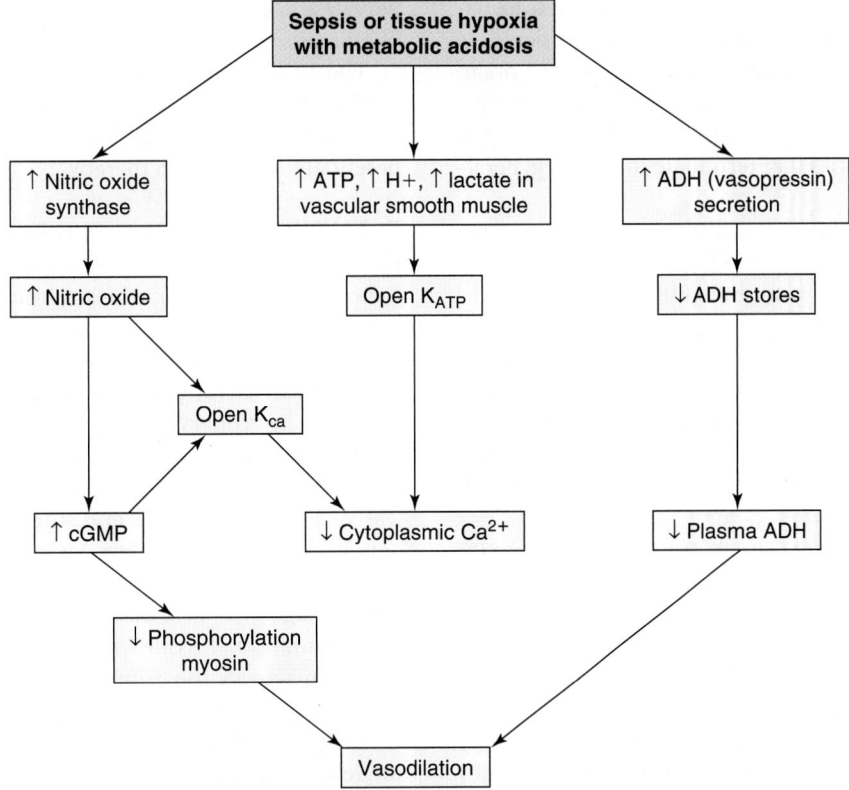

Figure 46-7 Mechanisms of vasodilation in shock. Vasodilatory shock is caused by the inappropriate activation of vasodilatory mechanisms and the failure of constrictor mechanisms. Unregulated nitric oxide, by regulating guanylate cyclase and generating cGMP, causes dephosphorylation of myosin and, thus, vasodilation. Nitric oxide synthesis and metabolic acidosis activate the potassium channels (K_{ATP} and K_{Ca}) in the plasma membrane of vascular smooth muscle. The resulting hyperpolarization (see Chapter 3) of the membrane presents the calcium that mediates norepinephrine and angiotensin II–induced vasoconstriction from entering the cell. Therefore, hypotension and vasodilation stubbornly persist despite high plasma levels of these hormones. In contrast, and unexpectedly, the plasma level of ADH (vasopressin) is low despite the presence of hypotension. The early, massive release of ADH may result in future depletion (see WHAT'S NEW? Vasopressin [ADH] Emerging as Therapy for Shock States.)

WHAT'S NEW?   Vasopressin Emerging as Therapy for Shock States

In 1997, an accidental observation led to important considerations and some proposed changes in the treatment of shock. Vasopressin (antidiuretic hormone, ADH) is known for its role in constricting arterioles; it acts throughout the body when released by the pituitary gland in times of low blood pressure. Previous clinical studies, however, revealed that its effects seemed limited to the esophageal vessels. Yet recent clinical emergency situations have revealed that inhibiting vasopressin lead to decreasing overall body blood pressure. Administration of vasopressin again leads to an increase in blood pressure. Further, careful testing in individuals with septic shock revealed that blood pressure rose dramatically. Additional studies have revealed that vasopressin levels in other individuals with septic shock are very low even though logic would dictate vasopressin to be increased in an effort to elevate blood pressure. In those with septic shock, hypotension occurs as a result of failure of the vascular smooth muscle to constrict. Three powerful mechanisms have been implicated in this effect, including (1) adenosine triphosphate (ATP)-sensitive potassium channels (K_{ATP} channels) in the plasma membrane of vascular smooth muscle; (2) activation of the inducible form of nitric oxide synthase; and (3) deficiency of the hormone vasopressin. During the initial phase of septic (and hemorrhagic) shock, vasopressin and other vasoconstrictors contribute to the maintenance of blood pressure. As shock worsens, vasopressin in the plasma decreases. The exact mechanism that creates this low concentration is unknown. Correction of the inappropriately low plasma vasopressin levels in vasodilatory shock significantly increases arterial pressure (about 25 mmHg to 5 mmHg) (see Figure 46-7). Such responses occur in individuals with severe septic shock, hemorrhagic shock that is unresponsive to volume replacement and catecholamine administration, and vasodilatory shock after cardiopulmonary bypass and placement of a left ventricular assist device.

Data from Landry DW, Oliver JA: *Sci Am* 290(2):36041, 2004; Landry DW, Oliver JA: *New Engl J Med* 345(8):588-95, 2001.

an international consensus conference was convened to develop a set of definitions for sepsis and related disorders (see Table 46-1), and a predisposition-infection-response-organ dysfunction (PIRO) staging system was proposed as a template for staging sepsis (see Table 46-2). MODS is the end-stage of a variety of injuries that terminate in severe, generalized inflammation.

MODS was first recognized as a distinct clinical syndrome in the mid-1970s,[19,20] when advances in resuscitation and support technologies allowed many individuals to survive life-threatening illness or trauma only to die of complications of their disease. Today MODS is a leading cause of mortality in surgical intensive care units.[21] Mortality for individuals with MODS increases progressively from 54% mortality with two failing organ systems to 100% mortality with five failing organ systems.[8] Moreover, mortality has not improved much over the past 15 to 20 years.[22]

Although sepsis and septic shock are the most common causes, MODS can be initiated by any severe injury or disease process that activates a massive systemic inflammatory response by the host. Documented clinical infection is not necessary for its development. Other common triggers are severe trauma, major surgery, burns, circulatory shock, acute pancreatitis, acute renal failure, ARDS, persistent inflammatory foci, and necrotic tissue. MODS is the major cause of death following septic shock, trauma, burn injuries, and ARDS. People at greatest risk for developing MODS are elderly individuals and persons with significant tissue injury or preexisting disease.[23]

The PIRO system (Table 46-2), a clinically useful sepsis staging system, has been developed that stratifies individuals with disease by both baseline risk of adverse outcomes and potential to respond to therapy.[23]

PATHOPHYSIOLOGY   In **primary MODS** the organ injury is directly associated with a specific insult, most often ischemia or impaired perfusion from an episode of shock or trauma, thermal injury, soft tissue necrosis, or invasive infection.[21] This decreased perfusion is both local (in the injured organs themselves) and generalized. The generalized hypoperfusion in primary MODS usually cannot be detected clinically. As a result of the insult, a stress response is initiated and stress hormones—in particular, catecholamines—are released. The inflammatory and stress responses are not as evident as they are in secondary MODS. In primary MODS during the inflammatory response, presumably, neutrophils and macrophages are "primed" by cytokines.[21] Any second insult, such as additional tissue injury, infection, or organ ischemia, may then activate the primed cells to produce an exaggerated response of secondary MODS[24] (Figure 46-8).

The progressive organ dysfunction of **secondary MODS** is the result of an excessive inflammatory reaction, after a latent period following the initial injury, in organs distant from the site of the original injury. It is postulated that the resulting or-

Table 46-2	Predisposition-Infection-Response-Organ Dysfunction (PIRO) System for Staging Sepsis		
Domain	**Present**	**Future**	**Rationale**
Predisposition	Premorbid illness with reduced probability of short term Cultural or religious beliefs Age Sex	Genetic polymorphisms in components of inflammatory response Enhanced understanding of specific interactions between pathogens and host diseases	In the present, premorbid factors impact on the potential attributable morbidity and mortality of an acute insult Deleterious consequences of insult heavily dependent on genetic predisposition (future)
Infection	Culture and sensitivity of infecting pathogens Detection of disease amenable to source control	Assay of microbial products Gene transcription profiles	Specific therapies directed against inciting insult require demonstration of characterization of that insult
Response	SIRS Other signs of sepsis Shock C-reactive protein	Nonspecific markers of activated inflammation or impaired host responsiveness Detection of specific target of therapy	Both mortality risk and potential to respond to therapy vary with nonspecific measures of disease severity Specific mediator-targeted therapy is predicated on presence and activity of mediator
Organ dysfunction	Organ dysfunction as number of organs or composite score	Dynamic measures of cellular response to insult—apoptosis, cytopathic hypoxemia, cell stress	Response to preemptive therapy not possible if damage already present Therapies targeting the injurious cellular process require that it be present

From Levy MM et al: 2001 *Intensive Care Med* 29:530, 2003.
SIRS, Systemic inflammatory response syndrome.

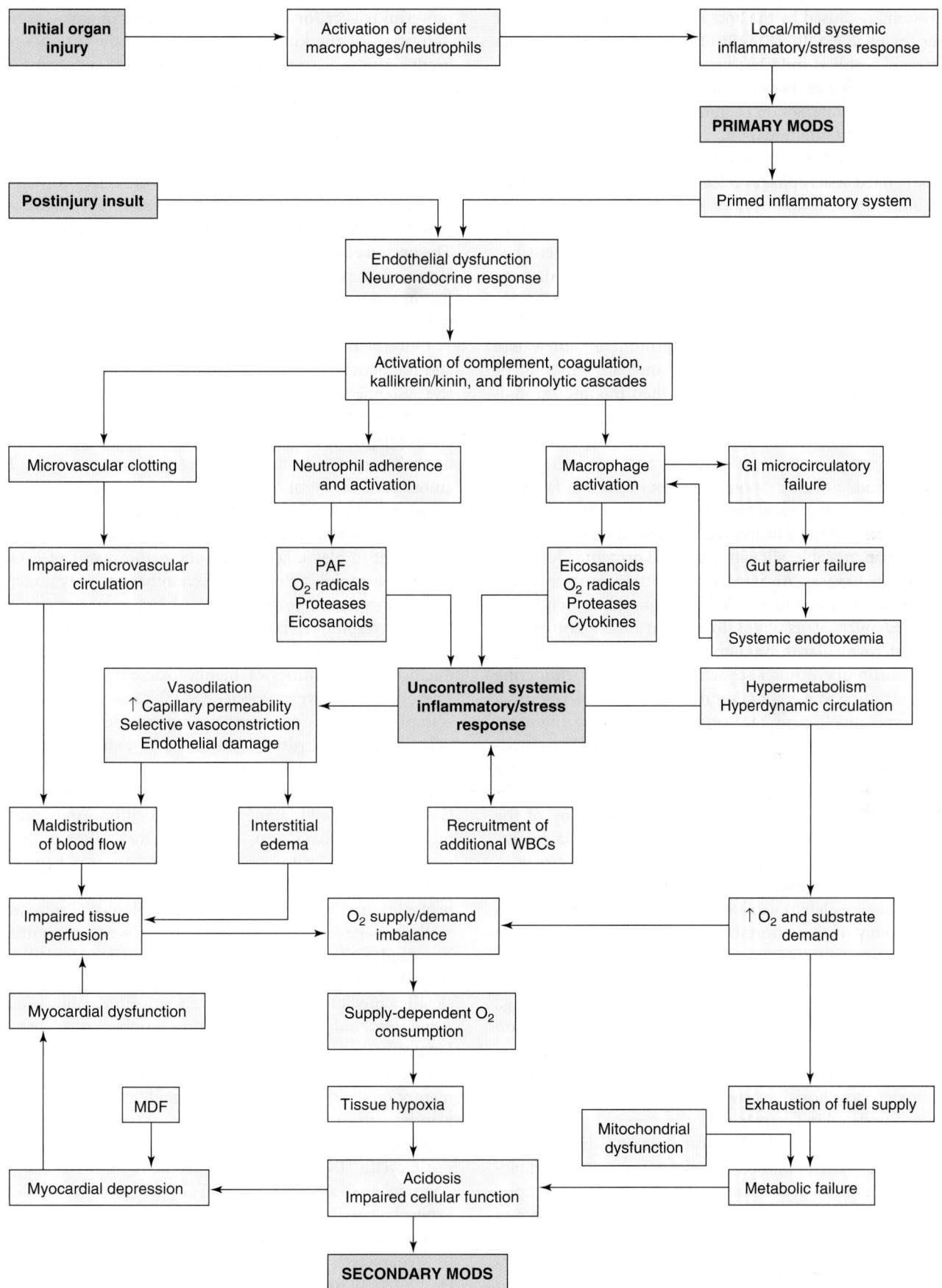

Figure 46-8 Pathogenesis of multiple organ dysfunction syndrome. *MODS,* Multiple organ dysfunction syndrome; *GI,* gastrointestinal; *PAF,* platelet activating factor; *WBCs,* white blood cells; *MDF,* myocardial depressant factor.

gan trauma is caused by the host response to a second insult rather than being a direct result of the primary injury. Often the second insult is mild but produces an immense disproportionate response because of the previous priming of leukocytes. The interaction of injured organs then leads to a self-perpetuating inflammation.

Secondary MODS is initiated by the delayed postinjury insult as primed macrophages release a barrage of mediators, particularly the cytokines tumor necrosis factor (TNF) and IL-1. These mediators damage the endothelium throughout the body. If a gram-negative bacterial infection is present, endotoxin released from the bacteria also causes severe damage to endothelial cells. Normal endothelial cells have little interaction with leukocytes, but when stimulated by TNF, IL-1, IL-6, or endotoxin, they change to a proinflammatory state and express adhesion molecules that mediate adhesion of neutrophils. The adhered neutrophils then migrate through the endothelium, aggregate in the area of damaged tissue, and amplify the inflammation.[2] The activated endothelial cells increase production and release of nitric oxide (endothelium), a potent vasodilator that is considered an important factor in the blood flow changes and loss of vascular tone noted in systemic inflammation.[25] The injured endothelium also becomes much more permeable, allowing fluid and protein to leak into the interstitial spaces. An important function of normal endothelium is anticoagulation. When damaged, the endothelium loses much of its ability to prevent blood clotting, allowing microvascular thrombi to develop.

The postinjury insult also activates the neuroendocrine system, resulting in a second, more extensive stress response. The normal function of the stress response is to maintain basal and stress-related homeostasis,[26] but in MODS homeostasis cannot be maintained. In fact, the endocrine response becomes excessive and injurious. There is an early increase in circulating catecholamines that contributes to many of the clinical manifestations of MODS, such as tachycardia, hypermetabolism, and increased oxygen consumption. Cortisol, glucagon, insulin, human growth hormone, ADH (which may become depleted), and endorphin levels also are increased. Many of these hormones contribute to the extreme catabolic state of MODS, and endorphins, which are vasodilators, decrease SVR. The sympathetic nervous system, to compensate for complications resulting from the injury (e.g., fluid loss, hypotension), also is stimulated. The stimulation persists throughout the period of critical illness.[27] The stress response can be amplified by a number of factors, including pain, anxiety, psychosis, and hyperthermia. (Stress response is discussed in detail in Chapter 10.)

Because of endothelial cell dysfunction and the release of mediators, four major plasma cascades are activated: complement, kallikrein-kinin, coagulation, and fibrinolytic. Complement components, particularly the anaphylatoxins C3a and C5a, cause vasodilation by stimulating release of histamine from mast cells. They also have strong chemotactic properties. C5a, especially, causes adhesion and the activation and degranulation of neutrophils. Complement is thought to be a powerful trigger for the exaggerated inflammatory response. Activation of the kinin system results in the production of bradykinin, a very potent vasodilator known to decrease SVR. Coagulation mechanisms also are activated, and because tissue injury and endothelial dysfunction are extensive, microvascular thrombosis occurs throughout the body, resulting in impaired microvascular circulation and organ ischemia. Concurrently, fibrinolytic mechanisms are activated. The tendency toward clotting, however, is greater, resulting in a net procoagulant state that can lead to the development of DIC. The overall effect of the activation of the plasma cascades is a hyperinflammatory and hypercoagulant state that contributes to vasodilation, vasopermeability, cardiovascular instability, endothelial dysfunction, and clotting abnormalities.

Once cytokines and other mediators have been released and the plasma enzyme cascades have been activated, a massive systemic inflammatory response develops. It involves several types of inflammatory cells, particularly neutrophils, macrophages, and mast cells. These cells, having been primed by their response to the initial organ injury, now pour large amounts of chemical mediators into tissues and into the systemic circulation. Neutrophils have tremendous inflammatory potential. The accumulation of activated neutrophils in organs is thought to play a key role in the pathogenesis of MODS.[8] When neutrophils adhere to the endothelium, they undergo a "respiratory burst" (oxidative burst) and release oxygen radicals. The respiratory burst occurs as the activated neutrophil experiences a sudden increase in oxidative metabolism, producing large quantities of highly toxic oxygen free radicals. These reactive oxygen species (ROS) cause oxidative stress. The primary ROS produced are superoxide (O_2^-), hydrogen peroxide (H_2O_2), hydroxyl radical (OH^-), and singlet oxygen (O). Oxygen radicals are extremely damaging to vascular endothelium and tissue cells, attacking deoxyribonucleic acid (DNA), cross linking membrane structures, and inducing membrane peroxidation—reactions that disorganize cell membranes and lead to tissue necrosis[2] (also see Chapter 2).

Other important mediators released by neutrophils are proteases, particularly collagenase and elastase. Proteases directly damage endothelium and neighboring cells, resulting in increased capillary permeability and organ damage. When activated, neutrophils also release platelet activating factor (PAF), a mediator that damages endothelium, stimulates clot formation, and activates increasing numbers of phagocytes. Finally, neutrophils release arachidonic acid metabolites (eicosanoids) as a result of lipid peroxidation of their cell membranes. Of the arachidonic acid metabolites (prostaglandins, thromboxanes, leukotrienes), two are particularly important in the pathogenesis of organ hypoperfusion: prostacyclin (PGI_2) and thromboxane A_2 (TXA_2). TXA_2 is a powerful vasoconstrictor, and PGI_2 is a potent vasodilator. When released in varying amounts in different organ beds, they are largely responsible for the maldistribution of blood flow characteristic of MODS. In total, neutrophils produce at least 50 to 60 toxins.[28] Collectively, products released by neutrophils cause endothelial dysfunction, systemic vasodilation, selective vasoconstriction (vasoconstriction of certain organ beds or parts of organ beds), increased vascular permeability, and microvascular coagulation.

Macrophages, present in most tissues, are activated by endotoxin, complement, and monocyte chemotactic substances.[29] Macrophages share a key role in the development of the unregulated inflammation of secondary MODS with the neutrophils. Like neutrophils, they produce oxygen radicals, proteases, cytokines, nitric oxide, and arachidonic acid metabolites. Recently reported is that excessive or prolonged stimulation of macrophages leads to the overproduction of cytokines and nitric oxide that initiate the cycle of harmful effects in MODS.[2] TNF and IL-1, which share many of the same functions and act synergistically, are the major cytokines that mediate inflammation.[30] TNF has potent metabolic effects, including fever, anorexia, hyperglycemia, hypermetabolism, and weight loss. It activates neutrophils, damages endothelial cells, and potentiates hypotension and shock. IL-1 also has metabolic effects, inducing fever, hypermetabolism, and muscle wasting. Normally, TNF activates cytokines, the coagulation system, fibrinolysis, and neutrophils. With the exception of neutrophil activation, IL-1 causes similar activation in individuals with cancer.[12] In the pathogenesis of MODS, the cytokines are linked to all cellular, hemodynamic, and metabolic alterations.

The gastrointestinal mucosa is particularly vulnerable to inflammatory mediators released by macrophages and neutrophils. Under normal circumstances the gut mucosa serves as a barrier to prevent bacteria from the gastrointestinal tract from entering the systemic circulation. Damage to the mucosa results in microcirculatory failure of the gut and consequent loss of the gut barrier function. The loss of intestinal barrier function leads to the systemic spread of bacteria and/or endotoxin from the gut (systemic endotoxemia). This phenomenon is called *translocation of bacteria*. The idea that the gut acts as a reservoir of bacteria and endotoxin that can initiate or perpetuate the development of MODS is known as the **gut hypothesis.**[31] The gut hypothesis provides a possible explanation for the fact that an infectious focus is not always found in individuals with MODS. Although this hypothesis has been substantiated by animal studies and has much support, the evidence from human studies is inconclusive.[19,31]

The numerous inflammatory processes operating in MODS cause maldistribution of blood flow and hypermetabolism. **Maldistribution of blood flow** refers to the uneven distribution of flow to various organs and between the large vessels and capillary beds of the body. It is caused by generalized vasodilation, increased capillary permeability, selective vasoconstriction, endothelial dysfunction, and impaired microvascular circulation. It is a major factor in the pathophysiology of MODS. The alterations in blood flow—which can occur at the cellular, organ, or regional level—lead to impaired tissue perfusion and a decreased supply of oxygen to the cells. The organs most severely affected by hypoperfusion are the lungs, splanchnic bed, liver, and kidneys. Despite supernormal systemic blood flow, oxygen delivery to the tissues

decreases. Several factors contribute to the problem. First, blood is shunted past selected regional capillary beds. Shunting, caused by loss of autoregulation in some organs, may be an early indicator of progression of sepsis into MODS.[32] This occurs because inflammatory mediators, particularly TXA_2, override the normal vascular control to cause selective vasoconstriction and because injured endothelial cells are unable to respond to normal vasodilator mediators. Second, interstitial edema, resulting from microvascular permeability, contributes to decreased oxygen delivery to cells by increasing the distance oxygen must travel to reach the cells. Third, capillary obstruction occurs because of the formation of microvascular thrombi and the aggregation of leukocytes.

Hypermetabolism, with accompanying alterations in carbohydrate, fat, and lipid metabolism, is initially a compensatory measure to meet the body's increased demands for energy. Eventually, however, hypermetabolism becomes detrimental, placing enormous demands on the heart. Hypermetabolism is the result of (1) the neuroendocrine response to stress with the release of catecholamines and cortisol, and (2) the action of TNF and IL-1. With increased metabolism the calorie requirements are markedly increased,[8] and the cardiac output increases 1.5 to 2 times normal.[33] The alterations in metabolism affect all aspects of substrate use. Most important is the catabolism of protein, primarily of skeletal muscle and visceral organs. The extreme catabolism of protein can rapidly deplete lean body mass. Hyperglycemia occurs as gluconeogenesis by the liver increases and glucose use by the cells decreases. Fatty acids are mobilized from adipose tissue. The net result of the hypermetabolism is depletion of oxygen and fuel supplies.

Myocardial depression also accompanies MODS. The cause remains unclear, but possible explanations are the effects of myocardial depressant factor (MDF), TNF, and IL-1 on cardiac contractility; alterations in α-adrenergic receptors in the heart; and hypoxia of the myocardium.[34]

The decreased oxygen delivery to the cells (resulting from the maldistribution of blood flow) and the increased oxygen needs of the cells (resulting from hypermetabolism) combine to create an imbalance in oxygen supply and demand. This imbalance is critical in the pathogenesis of MODS because it results in a pathologic condition known as **supply-dependent oxygen consumption.** Ordinarily the amount of oxygen consumed by the cells depends only on the needs of the cells because there is an adequate reserve of oxygen that can be delivered if required. In MODS, however, the reserve has been exhausted and the amount of oxygen consumed becomes dependent on the amount the circulation is able to deliver. Because the amount is inadequate in MODS, the tissues become hypoxic. Compounding the hypoxic damage to cells is a phenomenon called *reperfusion injury* (see Chapter 2). Much of the organ damage in MODS occurs with the reestablishment of blood flow after a period of ischemia. During the ischemic episode, energy stores and ATP are depleted and the enzyme *xanthine dehydrogenase* is converted to *xanthine oxidase*. With reperfusion of the ischemic tissue, oxygen radicals are formed from oxygen by the action of xanthine oxidase, and they attack the already damaged tissues. Consequently, although reperfusion is necessary to restore oxygen supply to ischemic organs, it can increase the extent of injury. Therefore, because of supply-dependent oxygen consumption and reperfusion injury, tissues become increasingly hypoxic. The result is cellular acidosis, impaired cellular function, and ultimately multiple organ failure.

CLINICAL MANIFESTATIONS   In MODS the organs that show clinical manifestations of failure are not always the organs involved as part of the initial injury, and there is usually a lag time between the initial insult and the development of systemic organ failure. The development of primary MODS is difficult to monitor, but there is a well-established general pattern in the clinical development of secondary MODS.[24] Following the inciting event and aggressive resuscitation of the individual for approximately 24 hours, the individual develops low-grade

fever, tachycardia, tachypnea, dyspnea, altered mental status, and a general hyperdynamic and hypermetabolic state (Box 46-1). Following this, the lungs begin to fail and acute respiratory distress syndrome (ARDS) may appear within 24 to 72 hours (see discussion of ARDS, Chapter 33). Between days 7 and 10, the hypermetabolic and hyperdynamic state intensifies; bacteremia with enteric organisms is common; and signs of hepatic, intestinal, and renal failure develop. During days 14 to 21, the renal failure and liver failure become more severe. Hematologic failure and myocardial failure are usually later manifestations. Encephalopathy, characterized by mental status changes ranging from confusion to deep coma, may occur at any time. This sequence can evolve rapidly, with death occurring between 14 and 21 days later, or it can evolve over a period of weeks. Individuals can recover from either the slowly evolving or the rapidly evolving course.

The clinical manifestations of failure of individual organs in MODS are caused by inflammatory mediator damage, tis-

---

| **Box 46-1** | **Clinical Manifestations of Organ Dysfunction** |

Pulmonary
- Acute respiratory distress syndrome (ARDS) pattern of respiratory failure (dyspnea, patchy infiltrates, refractory hypoxemia, respiratory acidosis, abnormal O_2 indices)
- Pulmonary hypertension

Gastrointestinal
- Abdominal distention and ascites
- Intolerance to enteral feedings
- Paralytic ileus
- Upper and lower gastrointestinal bleeding (guaiac-positive stools)
- Diarrhea
- Ischemic colitis
- Mucosal ulceration
- Decreased bowel sounds
- Bacterial overgrowth in stool

Liver
- Increased serum bilirubin level (hyperbilirubinemia)
- Increased liver enzyme levels (serum aspartate transaminase [SAST], serum alanine aminotransferase [SALT], lactic dehydrogenase [LDH], alkaline phosphatase)
- Increased serum ammonia level
- Decreased serum transferrin level
- Jaundice
- Hepatomegaly

Gallbladder
- Right upper quadrant tenderness or pain
- Abdominal distention
- Unexplained fever
- Decreased bowel sounds

Metabolic/Nutritional
- Decreased lean body mass
- Muscle wasting
- Severe weight loss
- Negative nitrogen balance
- Hyperglycemia
- Hypertriglyceridemia

- Increased serum lactate levels
- Decreased serum albumin, serum transferring, prealbumin, retinol-binding protein

Renal
- Increased serum creatinine level and blood urea nitrogen
- Oliguria, anuria, or polyuria consistent with prerenal azotemia or acute tubular necrosis
- Urinary indices consistent with prerenal azotemia or acute tubular necrosis

Cardiovascular

Hyperdynamic
- Decreased pulmonary capillary wedge pressure
- Decreased systemic vascular resistance
- Decreased right atrial pressure
- Decreased left ventricular stroke work index
- Increased oxygen consumption
- Increased cardiac output, cardiac index, heart rate

Hypodynamic
- Increased systemic vascular resistance
- Increased right atrial pressure
- Increased left ventricular stroke work index
- Decreased oxygen delivery and consumption
- Decreased cardiac output and cardiac index

Central Nervous System
- Lethargy
- Altered level of consciousness
- Fever
- Hepatic encephalopathy

Coagulation and Hematologic
- Thrombocytopenia
- Disseminated intravascular coagulation

Immune
- Infection
- Decreased lymphocyte count
- Anergy

Modified from Thelan LA et al: *Critical care nursing: diagnosis and management*, ed 4, St Louis, 2002, Mosby.

sue hypoxia, and hypermetabolism. Respiratory failure progresses early to ARDS and is characterized by tachypnea, pulmonary edema with crackles and diminished breath sounds, use of accessory muscles, and hypoxemia. Liver failure, although early in its development, is not clinically detectable until the later stages of MODS, when jaundice, abdominal distention, liver tenderness, muscle wasting, and hepatic encephalopathy appear. All aspects of metabolism, substance detoxification, and immune response are impaired. Albumin and clotting factor synthesis decreases, protein wastes accumulate, and liver tissue macrophages (Kupffer cells) no longer function effectively.

The gastrointestinal system is very sensitive to ischemic and inflammatory injury. Clinical manifestations of bowel involvement are hemorrhage, ileus, stress ulcers, malabsorption, diarrhea or constipation, vomiting, anorexia, abdominal pain, and pancreatitis. Intolerance to enteral feeding may develop. Adding to damage caused by injury to the bowel is bacterial translocation into the bloodstream resulting from the loss of the gut barrier function. The overwhelmed liver is unable to clear the bacteria from the systemic circulation. Thus, regardless of whether infection or some other injury was the precipitating cause of MODS, once intestinal bacteria enter the systemic circulation, it is likely that sepsis will be a problem. Renal failure develops at about the same time and is marked by progressive oliguria, azotemia, and edema. If renal shutdown is severe, anuria, hyperkalemia, and metabolic acidosis occur.

The first manifestations of cardiac failure are similar to those of septic shock: tachycardia, bounding pulse, increased cardiac output, fall in SVR, hypotension, warm skin, and supraventricular dysrhythmias (see Septic Shock, p. 1631). In the terminal stages, profound hypotension and ventricular dysrhythmias may develop. Changes in central nervous system function may be noted. Ischemia and inflammation are responsible for the changes, which include apprehension, confusion, disorientation, restlessness, agitation, headache, decreased cognitive ability and memory, and decreased level of consciousness. When ischemia is severe, seizures and coma can occur.

EVALUATION AND TREATMENT   Because there is no specific therapy for MODS, early detection or prevention is extremely important so that supportive measures are initiated instantly.[8] Frequent assessment of the clinical status of individuals at known risk is essential. Unfortunately, there is no way to determine with certainty when an organ is failing. Indicators of organ dysfunction are presented in Table 46-1.

Several systems for scoring severity of illness also have been developed. Commonly used systems are the **Acute Physiology and Chronic Health Evaluation II and III (APACHE II and APACHE III)**, sequential organ failure assessment (SOFA), and the proposed predisposition-infection-response-organ dysfunction (PIRO) staging system. Once organ failure develops, monitoring of laboratory values and hemodynamic parameters is necessary to assess the degree of clinical impairment.

At present the therapeutic management of MODS consists of prevention and support. Prevention of the syndrome is essential! First, if possible, the initial source of inflammation must be eliminated or controlled. Next, a second insult must be avoided. It is paramount to remove any potential site of infection by debriding necrotic tissue, draining abscesses, reducing the numbers of invasive procedures performed, and removing hematomas. Nosocomial infections from contaminated lines and catheters are of concern and must be prevented. Nosocomial infection rates of 15% to 25% have been reported in critically ill individuals.[35] Early reduction of long-bone fractures and surgical repair of injured tissues are also important preventive measures.

The goals of therapy are to control infection, provide adequate tissue oxygenation, restore intravascular volume, and support the function of individual organs. After the initial injury has been aggressively treated and sources of infection have been removed, antibiotics generally are administered. The choice of agents is based on the individual's disease process, but the regimen is usually a combination of antibiotics that covers both gram-negative and gram-positive organisms.

Because oxygen is not stored in the tissues, it must be continuously delivered. Maintaining an arterial oxygen saturation of 88% to 92% is recommended,[36] and hemoglobin levels should be kept above 7 to 9 g/dl.[17] Mixed venous oxygen greater than or equal to 70% is recommended. Blood transfusions may be necessary to ensure an adequate hemoglobin level. To deliver oxygen to the organs in the face of profound systemic vasodilation, fluid volume must be restored. Therefore aggressive fluid therapy is initiated early. Usually large volumes of isotonic crystalloid solutions are administered, although colloids (often albumin) also may be added to maintain adequate preload.

Finally, support for individual organ systems must be provided. Respiratory failure is treated with mechanical ventilation with low tidal volumes, high oxygen concentrations, and positive end-expiratory pressures (PEEP). To provide adequate nutrition and metabolic support, the failing gastrointestinal system is supported with enteral feedings (see Nutrition & Disease: Glutamine). It is now well recognized that enteral feedings help to preserve gut microbial barrier function and are therefore preferred to parenteral feedings. However, if the individual is unable to tolerate the amount of enteral feeding required to meet the enormous metabolic demands, hyperalimentation may be added. Ideally, the feeding formula is carefully calculated to meet the individual's nutritional requirements. Tight glucose control (80 to 110 mg/dl) is recommended. Once renal failure is established, dialysis or continuous hemofiltration may be required to maintain fluid and electrolyte balance. To support the failing cardiovascular system, inotropic drugs, such as low-dose dopamine and dobutamine, or vasopressors, such as norepinephrine, may be required to maximize cardiac contractility and maintain cardiac output. Although steroids have antiinflammatory effects, use of them is controversial because they

NUTRITION & DISEASE

Glutamine

Glutamine is an amino acid and a precursor for nucleotides, glucose asparagine, and other amino acids central for metabolism in the gut. As a nitrogen transporter, glutamine is a fuel for rapidly dividing cells, such as in the immune system and the intestinal epithelial cells. Recently, glutamine was shown to protect intestinal epithelial cells against apoptosis. Cytokines, such as tumor necrosis factor-α (TNF-α) and Fas ligand, mediate gut mucosal inflammation and alterations in apoptosis. Apoptosis and its dysregulation play an important role in pathophysiologic states involving the gut mucosal layer, including inflammatory bowel disease, carcinogenesis, vascular insults, infections, diarrhea, or drug-induced injury. The rate of apoptosis of these mucosal cells is, therefore, critical for normal mucosal turnover. Glutamine at doses greater than 4 mm can directly decrease proinflammatory cytokine release from phagocytes, which may improve outcomes in critically ill individuals.

Data from Evans ME, Jones DP, Ziegler TR: *J Nutr* 133(10):3065-3071, 2003; Wischmeyer PE: *Nutrition* 19(1):1-6, 2003.

have not been shown to be effective and may even worsen organ dysfunction. Obtaining an ACTH level is recommended. If low, the administration of low-dose steroid is advised. Deep vein thrombosis prophylaxis is also important.[17]

Recent scientific knowledge gained about MODS and inflammatory mediators has led to many investigational therapies. Recently, activated drotrecogin alfa (Xigris) has been found effective in the treatment of severe sepsis.[37] Novel molecular approaches targeting a variety of interdependent mediators of MODS are currently being investigated.[8]

BURNS

Major thermal injury is a source of massive tissue injury and destruction that has wide-reaching effects on virtually all organ systems. **Burn** is a generic term used to describe cutaneous injury resulting from thermal, chemical, or electrical environmental causes. In addition to cutaneous injury, burns are often associated with smoke inhalation injury or other traumatic injuries that aggravate the local and systemic problems of burns. For example, pulmonary injury, both primary and secondary, is common requiring ventilator support and the use of tracheostomy.[38] Burns are a multisystem injury with the interaction of shock, inflammation, and immunocompromise.

Epidemiology and Etiology

The incidence of burns in the United States has dropped from 4.2 per 100,000 during the years 1961 through 1964 to 1.5 per 100,000 during the period 1993 through 1996.[39] Deaths from fire and burn injuries have decreased 50% to an estimated 5500 burn deaths in 1991, compared to 9000 burn-associated deaths in 1971.[40] This remarkable progress is the result of several factors, including an increased national focus on fire safety and burn prevention, the establishment of regional burn centers, the use of smoke detectors, regulation of consumer product safety and occupational safety mandates. A decrease in hospitalization reflects a shift to outpatient care and improved prehospital and emergency treatment. Improvement in burn assessment and delivery of care, however, need further improvement to reduce medical transport and treatment costs.[41]

The causes of burn injury may be **thermal** or **nonthermal,** such as chemical, electrical, or radioactive. Thermal burns may result from thermal contact, flame, or scald. Chemical injuries are a result of contact with substances that are directly toxic to skin or the lining of the respiratory or alimentary tract. Such chemicals are often acid, alkali, or organic agents, termed **vesicants,** that cause blistering of the epithelial surfaces. Electrical burns may be the result of the conduction of electrical current through the body and the resultant heating of tissue, or flash over the body surface, associated with an electrical discharge.[42]

Burn Wound Depth

The classification of **burn wound depth** is usually based on the physical appearance and the symptoms associated with the affected skin. The definitive diagnosis is determined by the histologic depth of tissue necrosis. Such histologic evaluation, unfortunately, necessitates a skin biopsy. Because of the invasive nature of biopsy, clinical depth assessment is used and the ultimate fate of the wound determines final diagnosis.

First-degree burns are a **partial-thickness injury** involving only the epidermis and no injury to the underlying dermal or subcutaneous tissue (Table 46-3). The skin maintains water vapor and bacterial barrier functions. Many sunburns are first-degree injuries caused by exposure of skin to ultraviolet radiation from the sun. Initially there is local pain and erythema, but no blisters appear until after about 24 hours. An extensive first-degree burn may cause systemic responses such as chills, headache, localized edema, and nausea or vomiting. No treatment of extensive first-degree burns is required unless the person is elderly or an infant, in which case severe nausea and vomiting may lead to inadequate fluid intake and dehydration. Therapy consists of intravenous hydration until the nausea and vomiting subside 24 to 72 hours after burn injury. Comfort measures for previously healthy children or adults with extensive first-degree burns consist of aspirin for adults or acetaminophen (controversial) for children every 4 hours in age-appropriate doses and frequent application of a water-soluble lotion. First-degree burns heal in 3 to 5 days without scarring.

Second-degree burns describe two categories of burn depth with markedly different characteristics. Both of these are partial-thickness injuries, but they evoke vastly different responses. The hallmark of **superficial partial-thickness injury** is the appearance of thin-walled, fluid-filled blisters that develop within just a few minutes after injury. Another dominant characteristic of superficial injury is pain. As blisters break or are removed, nerve endings are exposed to

Table 46-3   Depth of Burn Injury

| Characteristic | First Degree | Second Degree | | Third Degree |
		Superficial Partial Thickness	Deep Partial Thickness	Full Thickness
Morphology	Destruction of epidermis only	Destruction of epidermis and some dermis	Destruction of epidermis and dermis, leaving only skin appendages	Destruction of epidermis, dermis, and underlying subcutaneous tissue
Skin function	Intact	Absent	Absent	Absent
Tactile and pain sensors	Intact	Intact	Intact but diminished	Absent
Blisters	Present only after first 24 hr	Present within minutes, thin walled and fluid filled	May appear as fluid-filled blisters; often is layer of flat, dehydrated "tissue paper" that lifts off in sheets	Blisters rare; usually is a layer of flat, dehydrated "tissue paper" that lifts off easily
Appearance of wound after initial debridement	Skin peels at 24-48 hr, normal or slightly red underneath	Red to pale ivory, moist surface	Mottled with areas of waxy white, dry surface	White, cherry red, or black; may contain visible thrombosed veins; dry, hard leathery surface
Healing time	3-5 days	21-28 days	30 days to many months	Will not heal; may close from edges as secondary healing if wound is small
Scarring	None	May be present; low incidence influenced by genetic predisposition	Highest incidence because of slow healing rate promoting scar tissue development; also influenced by genetic predisposition	Skin graft; scarring minimized by early excision and grafting; influenced by genetic predisposition

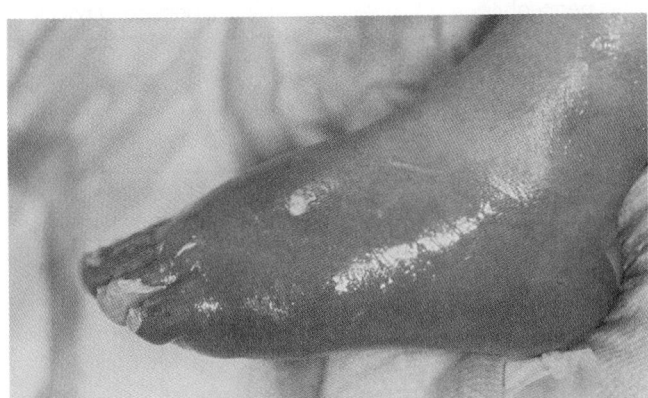

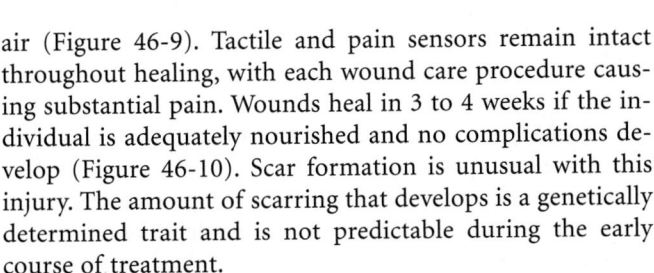

Figure 46-9 Superficial partial-thickness injury. Scald injury following débridement of overlying blister and nonadherent epithelium. (Courtesy Intermountain Burn Center, University of Utah.)

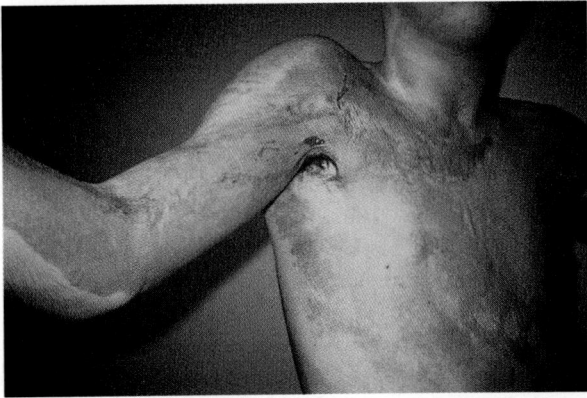

Figure 46-10 Axillary burn scar contracture. Note the blanching of the anterior axillary fold and small ulceration, both indicating the diminished range of motion. (Courtesy Intermountain Burn Center, University of Utah.)

air (Figure 46-9). Tactile and pain sensors remain intact throughout healing, with each wound care procedure causing substantial pain. Wounds heal in 3 to 4 weeks if the individual is adequately nourished and no complications develop (Figure 46-10). Scar formation is unusual with this injury. The amount of scarring that develops is a genetically determined trait and is not predictable during the early course of treatment.

Deep partial-thickness burns involve the entire dermis, sparing skin appendages such as hair follicles and sweat glands (see Table 46-3). The burn often looks waxy white and

is surrounded by margins of superficial partial-thickness injury. The injury is often clinically indistinguishable from a full-thickness injury (Figure 46-11), but by 7 to 10 days after burn injury, skin buds and hair will appear from hair follicles, indicating that skin appendages remain. These wounds take weeks to heal, and current therapy consists of surgical removal of the burn wound (excision) followed by application of the person's own unburned skin from another body area (autograft). Wounds that heal slowly produce more scar tissue and continue to be a potential source of infection until closed. In the presence of relative surgical contraindications, such as

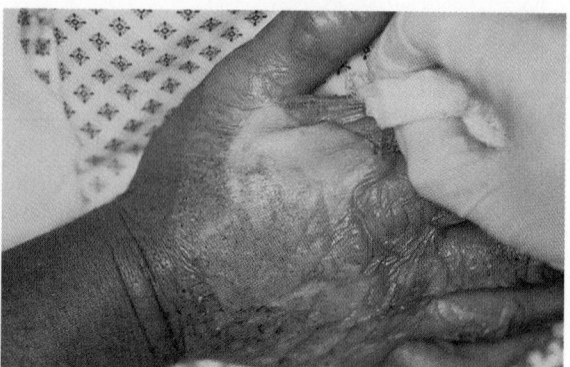

Figure 46-11 **Deep partial-thickness wound.** Note pale appearance and minimal exudate. (Courtesy Intermountain Burn Center, University of Utah.)

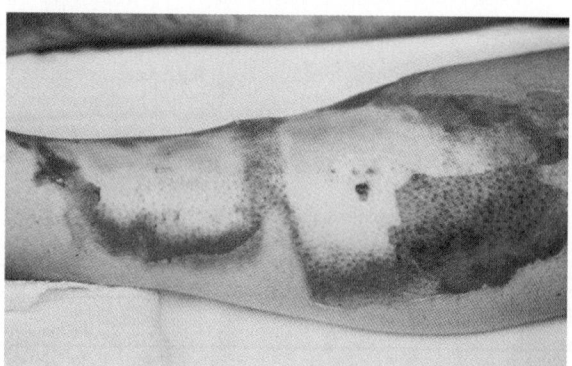

Figure 46-12 **Full-thickness thermal injury.** The wound is dry and insensate. (Courtesy Intermountain Burn Center, University of Utah.)

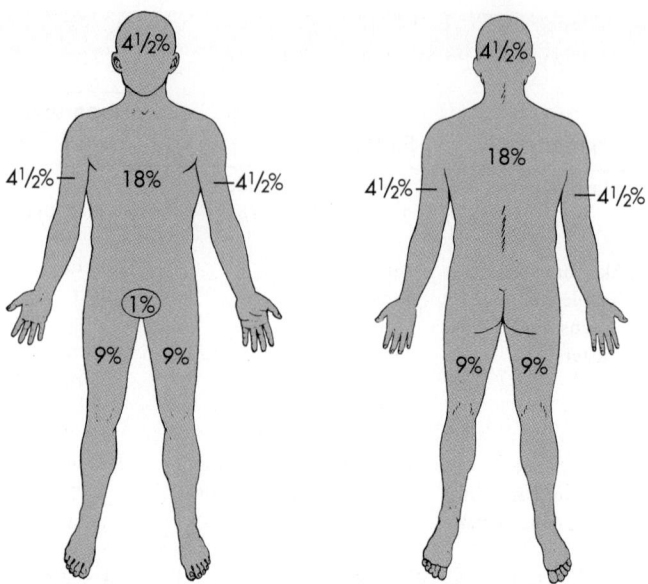

Figure 46-13 **Rule of nines.** A commonly used assessment tool with estimates of the percentages (in multiples of 9) of the total body surface area burned. **A,** Adults (anterior view). **B,** Adults (posterior view).

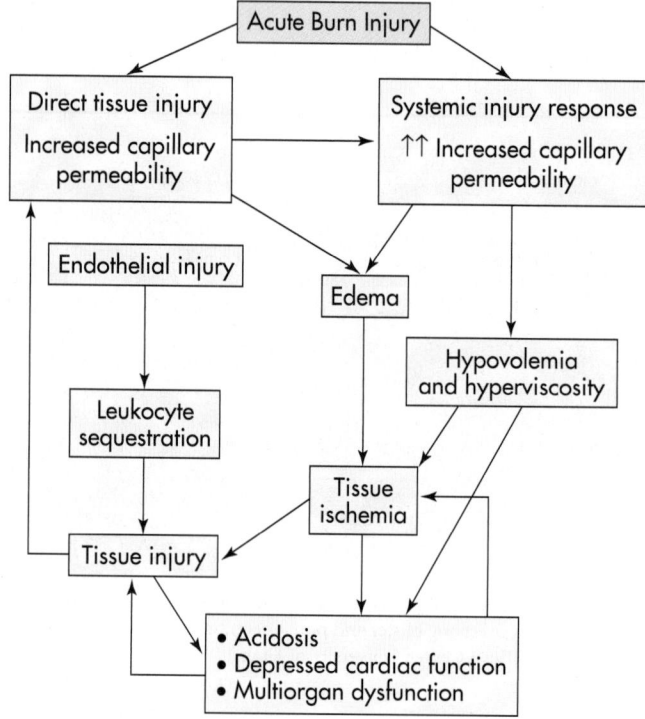

Figure 46-14 Immediate cellular and immunologic alterations of burn shock.

cardiopulmonary failure, deep partial-thickness wounds are not surgically treated but are allowed to heal from primary intention. The ultimate healing of deep partial-thickness burns commonly results in hypertrophic scarring with poor functional and cosmetic results.

Third-degree burns, or **full-thickness injuries,** involve destruction of the entire epidermis; dermis; and, often the underlying subcutaneous tissue (see Table 46-3). On occasion, all underlying subcutaneous tissue is destroyed and muscle or bone may be involved. Full-thickness wounds often appear relatively innocuous when their color is white and the delineation between normal and burned skin is not accompanied by a marked color change. Elasticity of the dermis is absent, leaving the wound dry and leathery in appearance and texture (Figure 46-12). As marked edema forms, distal circulation may be compromised in areas of circumferential burns. **Escharotomies** (cutting through burned skin) are performed to release underlying pressure. Full-thickness burns are painless because all nerve endings have been destroyed by the injury.

The extent of the **total body surface area (TBSA)** burn is estimated using either the "rule of nines" (Figure 46-13) or the Lund and Browder chart. Areas of partial-thickness and full-thickness injury are marked on the diagram in Figure 46-14. First-degree burns are not included in the TBSA estimate. The surface area of the palm, including palmar finger surface, averages 1% of the body surface area over a wide

range of ages; thus it can be used to estimate burn areas of irregular size and shape.[43]

Severity of burn injury is a combination of many factors, including age, medical history, extent and depth of injury, and body area involved. The American Burn Association has defined criteria to assist health care professionals in identifying patients who require care at a specialized burn center (Box 46-2). The multidisciplinary burn center is recommended for those persons who are at high risk for morbidity, mortality, or permanent functional loss.

PATHOPHYSIOLOGY AND CLINICAL MANIFESTATIONS
Burn injury results in dramatic changes in many physiologic functions of the body within the first few minutes after the event. The effect of burn depends on two factors. First, the extent of body surface involved and, second, the depth of cutaneous injury. Body surface burn extent is described by the percentage of TBSA injured. Burns exceeding 20% of TBSA in most adults are considered to be major burn injuries and are associated with massive evaporative water losses and flux of large amounts of fluid and electrolytes in the tissues, manifested as generalized edema and circulatory hypovolemia. Depth of cutaneous injury has been categorized in many ways but always depends on the severity of injury of epidermal and dermal elements of the skin and whether the alteration is a permanent or reversible injury.

With a major burn injury, a systemic pathophysiology ensues that requires therapeutic intervention to sustain life. The immediate (acute) physiologic consequences of a major burn injury centers around the profound, life-threatening hypovolemic shock that occurs in conjunction with cellular and immunologic disruption within a few hours of injury (Figure 46-14). **Burn shock** is a condition consisting of both a hypovolemic cardiovascular component and a cellular component.

Hypovolemia associated with burn shock results from massive fluid losses from the circulating blood volume. The losses are caused by an increase in capillary permeability that persists for approximately 24 hours after burn injury. **Fluid resuscitation** is the administration of intravenous fluids, such as lactated Ringer solution, in an effort to restore the circulating blood volume during the period of increasing capillary permeability. In addition to hypovolemia, most other organ systems are affected. Cardiac contractility is diminished during the initial 24-hour resuscitation period with shunting of blood away from the liver, kidney, and gut. This is often termed the *ebb phase* of the response to trauma and can be seen with other severe injuries. Normal blood volume does not result in restoration of normal cardiac output because of a phenomenon known as *myocardial depression* (see MODS). The decrease in perfusion of viscera results in a decrease in their function, for example, decreased gut barrier function.[44]

Cellular metabolism is disrupted when the burn wound is created resulting in altered cell membrane permeability and loss of normal electrolyte homeostasis. This cellular defect may be the pathophysiologic process responsible for the genesis of burn shock. There are numerous circulating factors in burn serum that may play a role in these cellular processes. Although the cardiovascular and systemic response is intricately interwoven into the cellular response, for description purposes, these responses are presented here as discrete entities.

Cardiovascular and Systemic Response to Burn Injury
The clinical manifestations of burn shock are the result of more than simple loss of extracellular fluid at the burn wound site. Hypovolemia and numerous local mediators in the burn wound,[45] as well as systemic signals, result in alteration of cellular function throughout the body. The restoration of normal intravascular volume with either saline solutions or colloid materials (e.g., albumin, blood, or dextrans) does not reverse changes such as increases in pulmonary vascular resistance or myocardial contractility.[46,47] Evidence for these relationships is reflected in cardiac output with precipitous decreases that often result in inadequate perfusion of most tissues at the capillary level, which is the hallmark of burn shock. Fluid infusion does not return cardiac output to preburn levels.[48,49] These findings led to the postulation of a specific myocardial depressant factor (MDF).[50-52] Other causes also have been suggested, such as reactive oxygen radicals that attack cell membranes and other subcellular organelles as a result of first ischemia and then reperfusion of tissues during burn shock and resuscitation.[53] A third factor may be the level of nitric oxide after burn injury, which could have a direct myocardial depressant effect.[54,55] The relationship of nitric oxide and myocardial function is not yet totally clear. Gamelli and colleagues[56] found nitric oxide production to be significantly depressed in burned individuals who did not survive their injuries. They postulate that nitric oxide may scavenge reactive oxygen radicals and protect tissues from oxidative injury.

Regardless of the contribution of these mechanisms, fluid resuscitation eventually results in improved outcome of the massively burned person. This resuscitation involves infusion

---

Box 46-2	Burn Unit Referral Criteria

A burn unit may treat adults or children or both.

Burn injuries that should be referred to a burn unit include the following:

1. Partial-thickness burns greater than 10% total body surface area (TBSA)
2. Burns that involve the face, hands, feet, genitalia, perineum, or major joints
3. Third-degree burns in any age group
4. Electrical burns, including lightning injury
5. Chemical burns
6. Inhalation injury
7. Burn injury in patients with preexisting medical disorders that could complicate management, prolong recovery, or affect mortality
8. Any patient with burns and concomitant trauma (such as fractures) in which the burn injury poses the greatest risk of morbidity or mortality; in such cases, if the trauma poses the greater immediate risk, the patient may be initially stabilized in a trauma center before being transferred to a burn unit; physician judgment will be necessary in such situations and should be in concert with the regional medical control plan triage protocols.
9. Burned children in hospitals without qualified personnel or equipment for the care of children
10. Burn injury in patients who will require special social, emotional, or long-term rehabilitative intervention

From Committee on Trauma: *Resources for optimal care of the injured patient*, Chicago, 1999, American College of Surgeons.

of intravenous fluid at a rate faster than the loss of circulation vascular volume for a period of about 24 hours from the time of burn injury and may require up to 30 L in a major burn. Resuscitation from burn shock can be accomplished using any of a number of infusion protocols. The most frequently used protocol is the Parkland formula.[57] Lactated Ringer solution is employed because it closely approximates extracellular fluid, the repository of fluid leaving the circulatory system during this phase of extensive edema formation (Table 46-4). The use of electrolyte-free fluids, such as D_5W, results in life-threatening hypovolemia and hyponatremia. Resuscitation with hypertonic saline has been used in some medical centers but is reserved for special circumstances; its use can result in adverse outcomes.[58]

The massive edema associated with burn shock is inevitable with fluid resuscitation, and failure to administer resuscitation fluid results in irreversible hypovolemic shock and death. The edema occurs in unburned as well as burned areas (Figure 46-15). Edema often leads to mechanical airway obstruction, necessitating tracheal intubation, and increased severity of the interstitial pulmonary edema associated with inhalation injury.

The most reliable criterion for adequate resuscitation of burn shock is urine output. The individual in hypovolemic shock will, as a compensatory mechanism, decrease or stop urine output in an effort to preserve circulation volume. The adult receiving sufficient intravenous fluids will excrete urine amounting to 30 to 50 ml/hr; children will produce 1 ml/kg/hr. If the individual does not have adequate urine output, it often indicates inadequate fluid resuscitation. The massive amount of intravenous fluid required by burned individuals during the shock phase is often intimidating to the person unfamiliar with burns. One common concern is that massive fluid administration will result in pulmonary edema. It should be remembered that the individual is in hypovolemic shock and that fluid is lost dramatically during the resuscitation period from movement to the interstitium, exudation, and evaporation.

The endpoint of burn shock is when the individual maintains adequate urine output for 2 hours with an intravenous fluid administration rate equal to the individual's calculated maintenance rate (Box 46-3). As burn shock ends, fluid administered remains in the circulating volume and is reflected as an increase in urine output. The mechanism whereby capillary integrity is restored is unknown but usually occurs about 24 hours after burn injury (Figure 46-16). After the individual has reached the end point of burn shock, the term used to describe the vascular status of the individual is **capillary seal**. In individuals with large burns, colloid-containing fluids may be given to help maintain oncotic pressure during the resuscitation phase and afterward to enhance the mobilization of interstitial fluid and diuresis.[59]

Cellular Response to Burn Injury

In addition to capillary endothelial permeability changes resulting in vascular fluid losses, transmembrane potential changes occur in cells not directly damaged by heat. The nor-

Table 46-4	Electrolyte Content of Ringer Lactate Solution and Extracellular Fluid	
Electrolyte	**Extracellular Fluid* (mEq/L)**	**Lactated Ringer† (mEq/L)**
Sodium	135-145	130
Potassium	3.2-4.5	4
Chloride	95-105	109
Lactate (bicarbonate)	24-28	28

*Normal values may vary slightly between laboratories.
†Plus 80-100 ml free water per liter.

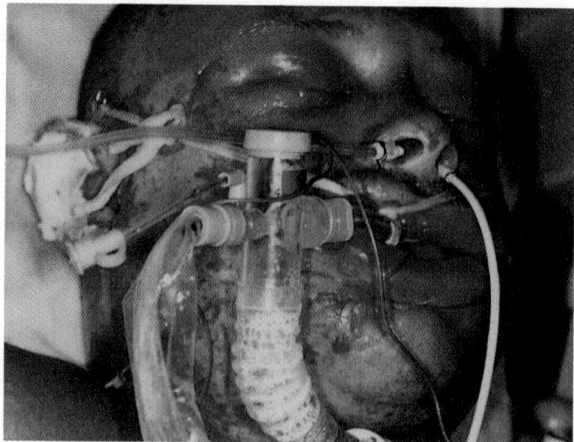

Figure 46-15 Edema related to burn injury. Superficial facial burns can result in marked swelling, requiring prompt endotracheal intubation to maintain the airway. (Courtesy Intermountain Burn Center, University of Utah.)

Box 46-3	Maintenance Fluid Replacements After Major Burn Injury*

1. *Basal fluid* replacements per day
   1500 ml/day/m² body surface area = 24-hour requirements
2. *Evaporative water loss* from burn wound
   a. Adults: (25 + % total body surface area burn) (m² body surface area) = ml/hr
   b. Children: (35 + % total body surface area burn) (m² body surface area) = ml/hr
3. *Total hourly maintenance fluids*
   Basal fluid requirements per day ÷ 24 hours + evaporative water loss per hour = ml/hr maintenance fluids

Example: A 70-kg adult with a 50% total body surface area burn and a body surface area of 2 m requires the following:
Basal = (1500 ml/day) (2 m² body surface area) = 3000 ml/24 hr, or 125 ml/hr
Evaporative = (25 + 50% total body surface burn) (2 m² total body surface area) = (75) (2) = 150 ml/hr
Total maintenance fluids = 125 ml + 150 ml = 275 ml/hr

*From end of burn shock until wound closure is achieved.

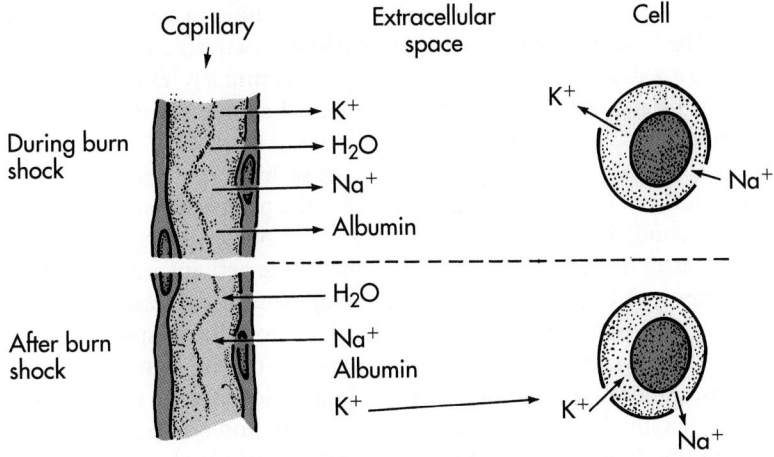

Figure 46-16 Direction of fluid and electrolyte shifts associated with burn shock. (Courtesy Intermountain Burn Center, University of Utah.)

mal potential of -90 mV decreases to nearly -70 mV, with an increase in intracellular sodium and water. Such membrane potential changes may be caused by a circulating shock factor.[60] Other changes can be categorized as (1) a metabolic response to the burn injury or (2) an immunologic response to the burn injury.

Metabolic Response

The metabolic changes after a burn injury were described in 1967 by Welt and associates as "sick cell syndrome."[61] This was considered to be a cell membrane transport defect related to an alteration in the steady state composition characterized by high intracellular concentrations of sodium. Trunkey and colleagues[62] found a marked decrease in primate muscle extracellular water and an increase in both intracellular sodium and water during hypovolemic shock. In addition, other researchers demonstrated an associated decrease in resting membrane potential, a decrease in amplitude of the action potential, and a prolongation of both the repolarization and depolarization times in association with a decreased intracellular potassium concentration.[63,64] The cellular dysfunction of burn injury extends beyond the transmembrane potential disruption and the sodium-potassium pump impairment to include a loss of intracellular magnesium and phosphate[65] and elevated serum lactic dehydrogenase (LDH) levels.[66] Thus impairment of basic cellular function may be the underlying cause of the diminished membrane potentials. The data suggest a decrease in the efficiency of membrane pumps. The failure of rapid intravascular volume repletion to restore membrane potential completely suggests other pathways for cellular metabolic derangement.[67]

Metabolic reactions to the stress of a major burn injury involve the response of the sympathetic nervous system and other homeostatic regulators. Catecholamines are found in elevated amounts in both the serum and urine of burned individuals. Cortisol, glucagon, and insulin levels are elevated, with a corresponding increase in gluconeogenesis, lipolysis, and proteolysis. Changes in lipid metabolism are reflected as an elevation in plasma free fatty acids (FFA) and a decrease in

plasma cholesterol and phospholipids.[68] Recently, investigators found that the use of propranolol, a nonselective β_1- and β_2-blocker, could decrease symptoms of the hypermetabolic response, including a decrease in heart rate and lipolysis.[69] Glucose and lactate kinetics are altered after burn injury. Although tissue hypoxia produces lactic acidosis, its persistence in the presence of adequate tissue perfusion suggests an increased rate of glycogenolysis[70] (see What's New? Increased Blood Lactate Levels).

Burn injury induces a hypermetabolic state that persists until wound closure. Investigators described the hypermetabolic state of 20 burned individuals as unrelated to ambient temperatures, with persistent elevation of core body temperatures.[71] The metabolic rate increased with burn size in a curvilinear relationship, with oxygen consumption rarely exceeding two times basal levels. Evaporative water loss and surface cooling are not the primary stimulus for the hypermetabolic state; rather, the hypermetabolism is related to an increase and resetting of the thermal regulatory set-point. A core body temperature of 38.5° C is typical. A reflex arc mobilizes neural or hormonal afferent stimuli to the hypothalamus, producing a catecholamine response clinically manifested as hypermetabolism, hyperthermia, and hyperglycemia.

Evidence also exists that the burn wound itself directly mediates the response to injury at both the local and system levels. Cytokines, oxygen radicals, chemotactic substances, and eicosanoids contribute to the systemic inflammatory response and hypermetabolic state. The inflammatory response to the wound level is magnified into a generalized systemic inflammatory response that is often deleterious.[72-74] Vasodilation, increased capillary permeability, and edema occur to facilitate healing of the local area. The distribution of the peripheral circulation after burn injury transports both heat and glucose preferentially to the wound. The energy cost of these reparative and transport processes is reflected in the increased metabolism and hyperdynamic circulation.

The extensive evaporative water loss that occurs in burn tissue is a heat-consuming process, and the energy of evaporation is provided by increased visceral heat production. The signal for the response is unknown because individuals whose wounds have been denervated continue to have a **posttraumatic hypermetabolic response.** Hypothalamic function alterations result in the elevation of human growth hormone (hGH) serum levels in the presence of hyperglycemia, a finding opposite that in normal states.[71] Further, the hypermetabolic rate is not decreased during rest, sleep, or warmth.

Evidence of hepatic response to burn injury is characterized by alterations in the clotting factors.[75] A hypercoagulable state develops as manifested by an elevated plasma fibrinogen

concentration in the presence of shortened prothrombin time (PT) and activated partial thromboplastin time (PTT).[76]

In summary, extensive burn injury initiates the most marked alterations in body metabolism associated with any illness (Figure 46-17). Much of the work explaining this response has been conducted by Wilmore,[77,78] who reported that the persistent tachycardia, hyperpnea, hyperpyrexia, and marked body wasting seen in burn injury reflect heightened metabolic activity and accelerated body catabolism. The development of decreased bone density can last long after discharge from the hospital.[79] These system alterations occur as a result of the cutaneous inflammatory process and are thought to facilitate wound repair. The neural component of this alteration is in response to a sympathetic reaction that releases catecholamines in large amounts.

Immunologic Response

The immunologic response to burn injury is immediate, prolonged, and severe. The result in individuals surviving burn shock is immunosuppression with increased susceptibility to potentially fatal systemic burn wound sepsis.

Several cytokines have been identified in the immediate postburn period. IL-1 is detected in the serum of burned individuals. The level of IL-1 correlates inversely with burn sur-

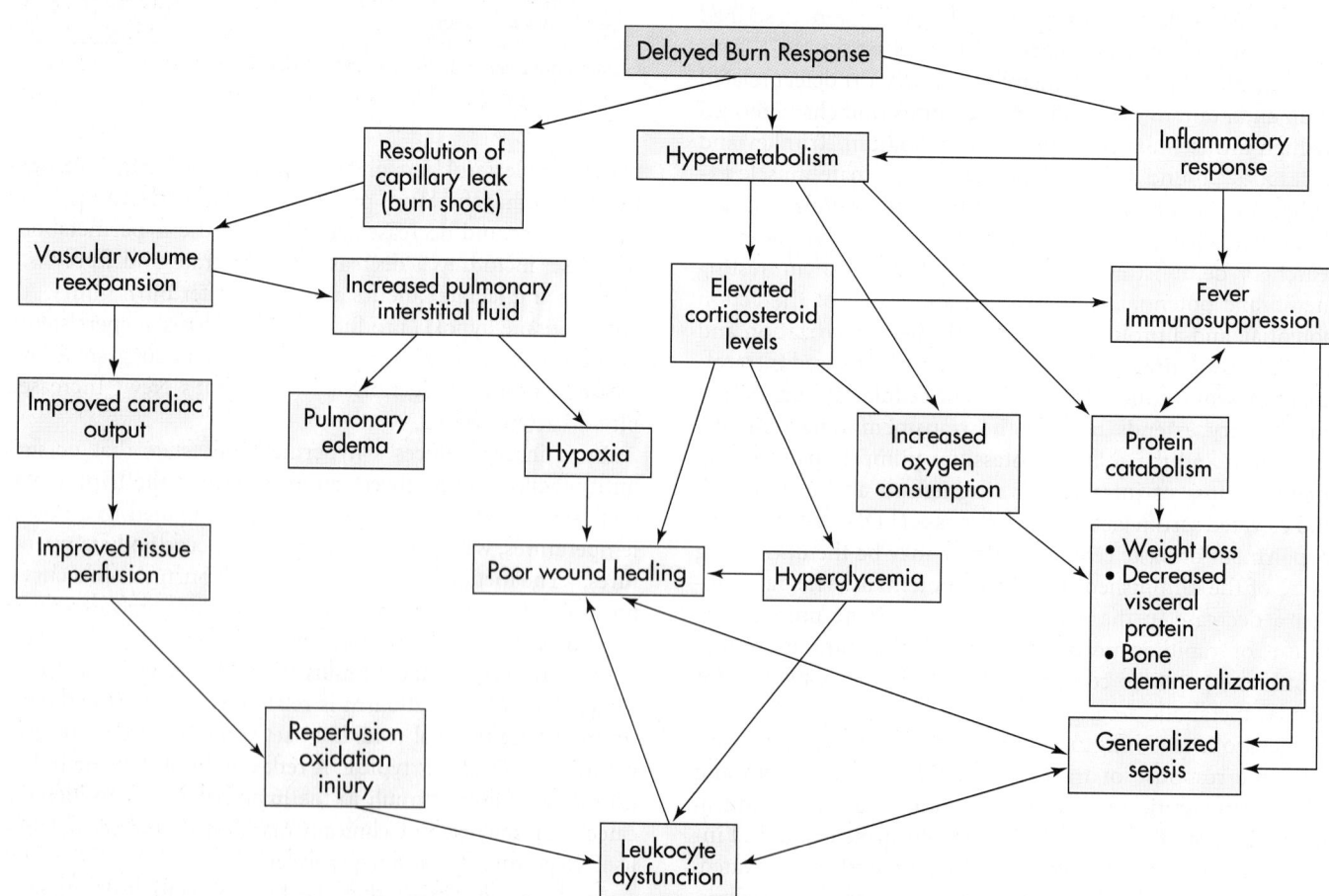

Figure 46-17 Physiologic alterations in inflammatory burn injury response.

vival; low levels may be associated with a higher mortality.[80] Fatal burn injury has often shown decreased levels of IL-2, which may result in decreased T helper 1 (Th1) lymphocytes. Th1 cells produce IL-2, interferon-γ, and TNF, which help to initiate cellular immunity and immunoglobulin G (IgG) production. IL-4 is elevated after burn injuries and causes a shift in the T helper cell production from Th1 to Th2 lymphocytes. Th2 cells secrete IL-4, which promotes further conversion of nonspecific Th cells to Th2 cells. Th2 cells also produce other cytokines and antibodies.[81] IL-6 levels increase quickly after burn injury and remain elevated for several weeks. The level of IL-6 correlates with the extent of burn injury.[82] IL-6, together with platelet activating factor, activates polymorphonuclear neutrophils, causing infiltration of neutrophils into burned tissue and adhesion to vascular endothelial surfaces.[83,84] IL-8 levels are elevated after burn injury, with significantly greater elevations in individuals with a TBSA burn of 40% or higher. IL-8 activity may play a role in the strong and persistent activation of neutrophils noted in people with large burns.[85] Burn blister fluid contains large amounts of IL-6 and IL-8 in addition to substances such as epidermal growth factor, platelet-derived growth factor, and transforming growth factor.[86]

Macrophages, platelets, neutrophils, and vascular endothelial cells release prostaglandins and leukotrienes, which are the by-products of arachidonic acid metabolism. These chemical mediators cause peripheral vasodilation, pulmonary vasoconstriction, increased capillary permeability, and local tissue ischemia in the burn wound.

A host of chemicals found in burn plasma in altered concentrations also may play a role in burn shock. These include vasoactive amines (histamine, serotonin), products of complement activation (C3a, C5a), prostaglandins, kinins, endotoxin, and metabolic hormones (catecholamines, glucocorticoids). A decrease in complement components C3a and C5a in the circulation after burn injury suggests a nonspecific activation of the complement system.[87] Activation of the complement system in injured tissue results in an inflammatory response caused by release of histamine and serotonin by C3a and C5a, because both histamine and serotonin alter capillary permeability and participate in the mechanism of burn shock along with linin polypeptides and other chemical mediators. Prostaglandins function in the inflammatory process by regulating metabolism of cells of inflammation (see Chapter 6).

Burn shock can induce changes in the integrity of the intestinal wall, facilitating bacterial translocation and endotoxemia.[88] Bacterial translocation from the gut may be a mechanism of infection leading to septic shock after burn injury and other major trauma.[89] Circulating endotoxin is correlated with the development of MODS and death after major burn injury.[90]

White blood cells are also altered at this time, when their need to inhibit sepsis is vital. Natural resistance to infection in burn wounds is a function of the nonspecific immune system; that is, resistance to microorganisms that infect wounds rests almost solely on the ability of phagocytic cells (i.e., granulocytes, macrophages) to leave the bloodstream, migrate to the site of infection, and ingest and kill microorganisms.[91] Normally, opsonins render bacteria susceptible to phagocytosis, but the burn injury triggers a consumptive opsoninopathy. Burn serum contains an inhibitor of C3 conversion that leads to decreased opsonization and polymorphonuclear (PMN) neutrophil dysfunction.[92,93]

Individuals with altered immunocompetence before burn injury are at additional risk for complications. Opportunistic infections, such as fungal sepsis, can increase hospital stay and ICU costs.[94] At risk individuals are those at the extremes of age and those with cardiac disease, malnutrition, immune deficiency disease, and a history of alcohol or drug abuse.[95,96] Additional risk factors include diabetes mellitus and pulmonary or renal dysfunction.

Evaporative Water Loss

One of the major purposes of intact skin is to serve as a barrier to evaporative water loss (EWL) from the body. With major burn injury, this ability of the skin to regulate evaporative water loss is totally disrupted. In a classic study done in 1962,[97] investigators attempted to determine the magnitude of such a loss and determined that daily evaporative water loss was in the range of 20 times normal in the early phase of injury, with gradual decreases as wound closure is achieved. Further studies indicated that insensible water loss through burned skin is not from evaporation of water from sweat glands but rather from water vapor formed within the body and lost through the skin.[98,99]

Calculation of the amount of fluid lost by evaporative water loss includes losses from all sources. Normally the skin is the major source of insensible loss (75%) and the lungs are minor sources of loss (25%), with a total loss of only approximately 600 to 800 ml/day. This changes dramatically with burns, because not only does skin loss increase but also lung loss increases by hypermetabolism and hyperventilation, especially in an intubated individual. Total evaporative losses exceed many liters per day in an adult with large burn wounds. Replacement of the loss is mandatory to prevent volume deficit.

EVALUATION AND TREATMENT   Burn recovery is long and stormy, with complications the rule rather than the exception. The goal of burn management is wound closure in a manner that promotes survival. Scar formation with contractures is often a consequence of healing in deep partial-thickness and full-thickness burns (Figure 46-18). Assessment of tissue viability can be difficult in complex extremity injury; pyrophosphate nuclear scanning can assist in evaluation.[100]

The three essential elements of survival of major burn injury are (1) meticulous wound management, (2) adequate fluids and nutrition, and (3) early surgical excision and grafting (see What's New? Management of Intro-Abdominal Hypertension). Current therapy for deep-partial and full-thickness

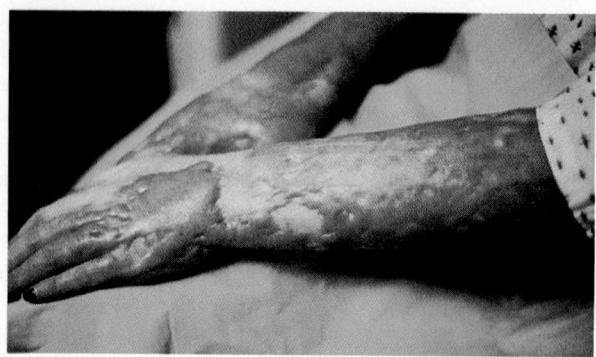

Figure 46-18 Hypertrophic scarring. Deep partial-thickness thermal injury can result in extensive hypertrophic scarring. (Courtesy Intermountain Burn Center, University of Utah.)

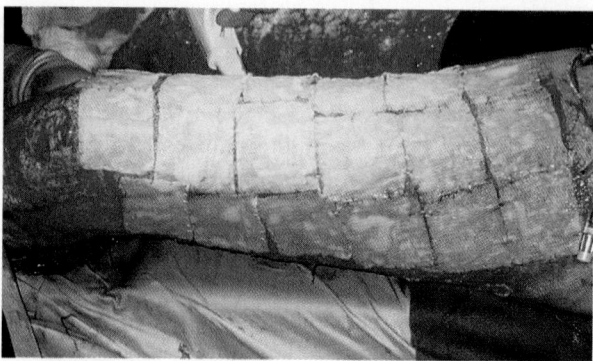

Figure 46-19 Application of cultured epithelial autografts. The thin sheets of keratinocytes are attached to gauze backing to allow application onto the clean, excised thigh. (Courtesy Intermountain Burn Center, University of Utah.)

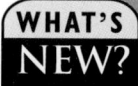

WHAT'S NEW?   Management of Intra-Abdominal Hypertension

Although it was first recognized some time ago, the incidence of abdominal compartment syndrome (ACS) in massively burned individuals is being noted with renewed interest. ACS occurs when intra-abdominal pressure is abnormally raised, thereby increasing organ dysfunction. ACS can occur after serious abdominal injuries with massive bleeding, edema from massive volume resuscitation, or perfusion after tension closure from abdominal surgery. Normal values of abdominal pressure range from 0 to 5 mmHg. Organ dysfunction may start to develop when values are between 26 and 34 mmHg. The practitioner may consider the use of decompression when the constellation of intra-abdominal hypertension when bladder pressure exceeds 30 mmHg—respiratory function compromised, shock, and oliguria. The use of bedside decompressive laparotomy has resulted in increased survival in only a small sample of adults, from near 0% survival to 40% survival. A closed, percutaneous approach may, however, yield increased survival. The mean survival rate of individuals with ACS is 53%. The optimal time for intervention is, however, controversial and the outcome is often poor, even after decompression has been performed.

Data from Blinderman C, Lapid O, Shaked G: *Isr Med Assoc J* 4(10):833-834, 2002; Hobson KG et al: *J Trauma* 53(6):1129-1133; discussion 1133-4, 2002; Ivy ME et al: *J Burn Care Rehabil* 20(5):351-353, 1999; Latenser BA et al: *J Burn Care Rehabil* 23(3):190-195, 2002; Moore AFK et al: *Br J Surg* 91:1102-1110, 2004.

burn injury includes surgical removal of the burn tissue (excision) followed by grafting of the person's unburned skin (autograft) onto the excised wound. Satisfactory wound closure with cultured epithelial autograft (Figure 46-19) has been inconsistent and costly.[101,102] Early enthusiasm for synthetic dermal replacement has been tempered by a high rate of dermal graft loss and slow epidermal engraftment.[103,104] Such advancements in skin replacement technology include sheets of acellular dermal matrix that can be used with thin-meshed autografts or cultured epithelial autografts.[105,106] This concept is also being used on the donor site, and glycosaminoglycan hydrogels may supplement donor site wound dressings.[107] Scar reduction or prevention is a challenging problem that is being addressed with pulsed-dye laser treatment.[108] Current research is also directed toward therapies to modulate the hypermetabolic and inflammatory responses. Nutritional therapy is focused on early enteral feeding to reduce the potential of gut-mediated sepsis. Ongoing clinical trials using anabolic agents (e.g., recombinant human growth hormone) and pharmacologic agents that modulate inflammatory and endocrine mediators (e.g., ibuprofen, propranolol) show promise in the treatment of severe burn injuries.[57] Burn pain is almost always acute and treatment strategies usually differ from strategies for chronic pain. In addition to opioid-based agents, newer treatment approaches may include antianxiety agents, hypnosis and relaxation techniques.[109]

SUMMARY REVIEW

Shock

1. Shock is a widespread impairment of cellular metabolism involving positive-feedback loops that places the individual on a downward physiologic spiral, which, if not reversed, can lead to multiple organ dysfunction syndrome.
2. Types of shock are cardiogenic, hypovolemic, neurogenic, anaphylactic, and septic. A newly identified type of shock, traumatic shock, combines features of hypovolemic shock and septic shock.
3. The final common pathway in all types of shock is impaired cellular metabolism—cells switch from aerobic to anaerobic metabolism. Energy stores drop, and cellular mechanisms relative to membrane permeability, action potentials, and lysozyme release fail.

4. Anaerobic metabolism results in activation of the inflammatory response, decreased circulatory volume, and decreasing pH.
5. Impaired cellular metabolism results in cellular inability to use glucose because of impaired glucose delivery or impaired glucose intake, resulting in a shift of glycogenolysis, gluconeogenesis, and lipolysis for fuel generation.
6. Glycogenolysis is affected for up to 10 hours. Gluconeogenesis results in the use of proteins necessary for structure, function, repair, and replication that leads to more impaired cellular metabolism. Lipolysis is ineffective because of a lack of transport serum proteins.
7. Gluconeogenesis contributes to lactic acid, uric acid, and ammonia buildup; interstitial edema; and impairment of the im-

mune system, as well as general muscle weakness leading to decreased respiratory function and cardiac output.

8. Cardiogenic shock is attributable to heart failure and is characterized by a decrease in cardiac output and impaired cellular metabolism.

9. Hypovolemic shock is caused by loss of blood or fluid in large amounts. The use of compensatory mechanisms may be vigorous, but tissue perfusion ultimately decreases and results in impaired cellular metabolism.

10. Neurogenic (vasogenic) shock results from massive vasodilation, causing a relative hypovolemia (even though cardiac output may be high), and results in impaired cellular metabolism.

11. Anaphylactic shock is caused by physiologic recognition of a foreign substance. The inflammatory response is triggered, and a massive vasodilation with fluid shift into the interstitium follows. The relative hypovolemia leads to impaired cellular metabolism.

12. Septic shock begins with impaired cellular metabolism caused by uncontrolled septicemia. The infecting agent triggers the inflammatory and immune responses. It is part of a continuum known as the systemic inflammatory response syndrome. Mortality for septic shock is very high.

Multiple Organ Dysfunction Syndrome

1. Multiple organ dysfunction syndrome (MODS) is the progressive dysfunction of two or more organ systems resulting from a systemic inflammatory response after a severe illness or injury. The inflammatory response can be triggered by sepsis, necrotic tissue, trauma, burns, adult respiratory distress syndrome, acute pancreatitis, and other severe injuries.

2. Primary MODS is the immediate local or mild systemic response to the triggering event or illness. It primes the inflammatory system.

3. Secondary MODS is the uncontrollable, excessive systemic inflammatory response that develops after a latent period and results in organ dysfunction.

4. People at greatest risk for developing MODS are elderly individuals, those with significant tissue injury or preexisting disease, and those in whom resuscitation from the initiating illness or injury has been delayed or inadequate.

5. Mortality from MODS is very high: 45% to 55% for failure of two organ systems, 80% for failure of three or more organ systems, and nearly 100% if the failure of three or more organs persists longer than 4 days.

6. Multiple organ dysfunction involves the stress response; release of complement, coagulation, and kinin proteins; changes in the vascular endothelium; and numerous inflammatory processes mediated by substances released by activated neutrophils and macrophages.

7. The consequences of the release of inflammatory mediators in MODS are vasodilation, increased vasopermeability, and selective vasoconstriction resulting in maldistribution of blood flow; hypermetabolism; myocardial depression; and hypoxic injury to cells. Cellular hypoxia and acidosis impair cellular metabolism, leading to organ dysfunction.

8. Clinical manifestations of the development of MODS are general during the first 24 hours: low-grade fever, tachycardia, tachypnea, dyspnea, and altered mental status. Over the next several days, beginning with the lungs, individual organ systems show signs of failure.

9. Because there is no specific therapy for MODS, early detection is extremely important so that supportive measures can be initiated as soon as possible.

10. At present the therapeutic management of MODS consists of prevention or removal of triggering mechanisms and support of individual organs. Recent scientific knowledge about inflammatory mediators has led to many promising future therapies for MODS.

Burns

1. Burns are classified according to depth and extent of injury.

2. First-degree burns involve the superficial skin without loss of protective function.

3. Second-degree burns are superficial (blister formation) or superficial involving partial skin thickness with a waxy white appearance and no involvement of dermal appendages.

4. Third-degree burns involve full skin thickness and often underlying tissues. They are painless and can be life threatening as a result of hypovolemic shock and metabolic and immunologic responses.

5. The total body surface area (TBSA) burned is estimated using either the rule of nines or the Lund and Browder chart. Burns exceeding 20% TBSA are considered major burns.

6. Hypovolemia associated with burn shock is caused by increased capillary permeability with massive fluid losses from blood volume.

7. Altered cell membrane permeability and loss of electrolyte homeostasis contribute to burn shock.

8. Cardiac contractility is decreased during the first 24 hours with shunting of blood away from the liver, kidney, and gut.

9. Fluid resuscitation, such as with lactated Ringer solution, involves infusion of fluid at a rate faster than the loss of circulating volume.

10. The most reliable criterion for adequate resuscitation of burn shock is urine output.

11. Capillary seal is the term used to indicate the end of burn shock.

12. Transmembrane potentials are altered in cells not directly damaged by heat, with impairment of the sodium-potassium pump and loss of magnesium and phosphate.

13. The stress of a major burn activates the sympathetic nervous system with release of catecholamines, cortisol, glucagon, and insulin.

14. Burn injury produces a hypermetabolic state that persists until wound closure and is related to a higher thermal regulatory set-point.

15. The local inflammatory response at the burn site releases cytokines, oxygen radicals, chemotactic factors, and eicosanoids, which leads to a systemic inflammatory response and contributes to hypermetabolism.

16. A posttraumatic hypermetabolic response is associated with increased visceral heat production.

17. Alterations in clotting factors produce a hypercoagulable state following major burns.

18. The immune response following a burn is immediate, prolonged, and severe.

19. Numerous alterations in inflammatory cytokines are evident in the immediate burn period, affecting cellular immunity, antibody production, and attraction of neutrophils and contributing to the vasodilation and increased capillary permeability associated with burn shock.

20. White blood cells are altered, and there is decreased opsonization and phagocytosis, contributing to the development of sepsis.

21. Changes in intestinal wall integrity lead to translocation of bacteria, endotoxemia, and septic shock.

22. Loss of intact skin with a major burn results in significant evaporative water loss contributing to hypovolemia.

23. Treatment of major burns involves meticulous wound management, adequate fluids and nutrition, early surgical excision and grafting, modulation of the hypermetabolic state, and pain management.

KEY TERMS

MEDIA RESOURCES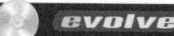

Review questions and answers for this chapter are available in the *CD Companion* included with this book.

WebLinks—links to Internet sites pertaining to this chapter—are available on Evolve at http://evolve.elsevier.com/McCance/.

REFERENCES

1. Menezes J et al: A novel nitric oxide scavenger decreases liver injury and improves survival after hemorrhagic shock, *Am J Physiol* 277(1 part 1):G144, 1999.
2. Cunneen J, Cartwright M: The puzzle of sepsis: fitting the pieces of the inflammatory response with treatment, *AACN Clin Issues* 15(1):18, 2004.
3. Rippe JM et al: *Intensive care medicine,* ed 3, Boston, 1996, Little, Brown.
4. Hollenberg SM, Kavinsky CJ, Parrillo JE: Cardiogenic shock, *Ann Intern Med* 131(1):47-59, 1999.
5. Holmes CL, Walley KR: The evaluation and management of shock, *Clin Chest Med* 24(4):775-789, 2003.
6. Hasdai D et al: Predictors of cardiogenic shock after thrombolytic therapy for acute myocardial infarction, *J Am Coll Cardiol* 35(1):136, 2000.
7. Levy MM et al: 2001 SCCM/ESICM/ACCP/ATS/SIS international sepsis definitions conference, *Crit Care Med* 312:1250, 2003a.
8. Awad SS: State-of-the-art therapy for severe sepsis and multisystem organ dysfunction, *Am J Surg* 186(5A):23S-30S, 2003.
9. Opal SM: Severe sepsis and septic shock: defining the clinical problem, *Scand J Infect Dis* 35(9):529-534, 2003.
10. Morrison DC et al: Structure-function relationships of bacterial endotoxins contribution to microbial sepsis, *Infect Dis Clin North Am* 13(2):313-340, 1999.
11. Symeonides S, Balk RA: Nitric oxide in the pathogenesis in sepsis, *Infect Dis Clin North Am* 13(2):449-463, 1999.
12. Van der Poll T, van Deventer SJH: Cytokines and anticytokines in the pathogenesis of sepsis, *Infect Dis Clin North Am* 13(2):413, 1999.
13. Das UN: Current advances in sepsis and septic shock with particular emphasis on the role of insulin, *Med Sci Monit* 9(8):RA181-192, 2003.
14. Reeves JH et al: Continuous plasma filtration in sepsis syndrome, *Crit Care Med* 27(10):2096, 1999.
15. Pittet D et al: Impact of immunomodulating therapy on morbidity in patients with severe sepsis, *Am J Respir Crit Care Med* 160(3):852-857, 1999.
16. Bhattacharjee AK, Cross AS: Vaccines and antibodies in the prevention and treatment of sepsis, *Infect Dis Clin North Am* 13(2):355,1999.
17. Dellinger RP et al: Surviving Sepsis Campaign guidelines for management of severe sepsis and septic shock, *Crit Care Med* 32(3):858-873, 2004.
18. Tamion F et al: Gastric mucosal acidosis and cytokine release in patients with septic shock, *Crit Care Med* 31(8):2137-2143, 2003.

19. Baue AE: Multiple, progressive or sequential system failure: a syndrome for the '70s, *Arch Surg* 110(7):779, 1975.
20. Tilney NL, Bailey GL, Morgan AP: Sequential system failure after rupture of abdominal aortic aneurysm: an unsolved problem in postoperative care, *Ann Surg* 178(2):117, 1973.
21. Garrison RN et al: Microvascular changes explain the "two-hit" theory of multiple organ failure, *Ann Surg* 227(6):851, 1998.
22. Rangel-Frausto MS: The epidemiology of bacterial sepsis, *Infect Dis Clin North Am* 13(2):299, 1999.
23. Levy MM et al: 2001 SCCM/ESICM/ACCP/ATS/SIS international sepsis definitions conference, *Intensive Care Med* 29(4):530-538, 2003.
24. Rotstein OD: Modeling the two-hid hypothesis for evaluating strategies to prevent organ injury after shock/resuscitation, *J Trauma* 54(5 Suppl):S203-206, 2003.
25. McHugh J, Cheek DJ: Nitric oxide and regulation of vascular tone: pharmacological and physiological considerations, *Am J Crit Care* 7(2):131-140, 1998.
26. Chaudry IH et al: Endocrine targets in experimental shock. *J Trauma* 54(5 Suppl):S118-S125, 2003.
27. Bannan J, Visvanathan K, Zambriskie JB: Structure and function of streptococcal and staphylococcal superantigens in septic shock, *Infect Dis Clin North Am* 13(2):387, 1999.
28. Baue AE: The horror autotoxicus and multiple-organ failure, *Arch Surg* 127(12):1451-1462, 1992.
29. Beal AL, Cerra FB: Multiple organ failure syndrome in the 1990s, *JAMA* 271(3):226, 1994.
30. Rankin JA: Biological mediators of acute inflammation, *AACN Clin Issues* 15(1):3-17, 2004.
31. Pope HC et al: Reticuloendothelial system activity and organ failure in patients with multiple injuries, *Arch Surg* 134:421, 1999.
32. Ince C, Sinaasappel M: Microcirculatory oxygenation and shunting in sepsis and shock, *Crit Care Med* 27(7):1369, 1999.
33. Di Giantomasso D, May CN, Bellomo R: Vital organ blood flow during hyperdynamic sepsis, *Chest* 124:1053-1059, 2003.
34. Carpati CM, Astiz ME, Rackow EC: Mechanisms and management of myocardial dysfunction in septic shock, *Crit Care Med* 27(2):231, 1999.
35. Wiessner WH, Casey LC, Zbilut JP: Treatment of sepsis and septic shock: a review, *Heart Lung* 24(5):380-392, 1995.
36. Wheeler AP, Bernard GR: Treating patients with sepsis, *New Engl J Med* 340(3):207, 1999.
37. Bernard GR et al: Efficacy and safety of recombinant human activated protein C for severe sepsis, *New Engl J Med* 344(10):699-709, 2001.
38 Saffle, JR, Morris, SE, Edelman L: Early tracheostomy does not improve outcome in burn patients, *J Burn Care Rehabil* 23(6):431-438, 2002.
39. Clark DE, Dainiak CN, Reeder S: Decreasing incidence of burn injury in a rural state, *Inj Prev* 6(4):259-262, 2000.
40. Brigham PA, McLoughlin E: Burn incidence and medical care use in the United States: estimates, trends, and data sources, *J Burn Care Rehabil* 17(2):95-107, 1996.
41. Saffle JR, Edelman L., Morris SE: Regional air transport of burn patients: a case for telemedicine? *J Trauma* 57(1):57-64, discussion 64, 2004.

42. Cochran A et al: Self-reported quality of life after electrical and thermal injury, *J Burn Care Rehabil* 25(1):61-66, 2004.

43. Sheridan RL et al: Planimetry study of the percent of body surface represented by the hand and palm: sizing irregular burns is more accurately done with the palm, *J Burn Care Rehabil* 16(6):605-606, 1995.

44. Morris SE, Navaratnam N, Herndon DN: A comparison of effects of thermal injury and smoke inhalation on bacterial translocation, *J Trauma* 30(6):639-643, discussion 643-645, 1990.

45. Arturson G: Forty years in burns research—the postburn inflammatory response, *Burns* 26(7):599-604, 2000.

46. Demling RH, Will JA, Belzer FO: Effect of major thermal injury on the pulmonary microcirculation, *Surgery* 83(6):746-751, 1978.

47. Horton JW et al: Calcium antagonists improve mechanical performance after thermal trauma, *J Surg Res* 87(1):39-50, 1999.

48. Aikawa N, Martyn JAJ, Burke JF: Pulmonary artery catheterization and thermodilution cardiac output determination in the management of critically burned patients, *Am J Surg* 135(6):811-817, 1978.

49. Dobson EL, Warner GF: Factors concerned in the early stages of thermal shock, *Circ Res* 5(1):69-74, 1957.

50. Baxter CR, Cook WA, Shires GT: Serum myocardial depressant factor of burn shock, *Surg Forum* 17:1-2, 1966.

51. Lefer AM, Martin J: Origin of myocardial depressant factor in shock, *Am J Physiol* 218(5):1423-1427, 1970.

52. Rosenthal SR, Hawley PL, Hakin AA: Purified burn toxic factor and its competition, *Surgery* 71(4):527-536, 1972.

53. Horton JW, Burton KP, White DJ: The role of toxic oxygen metabolites in a young model of thermal injury, *J Trauma* 39(3):563-569, 1995.

54. Onuoha G, Alpar K, Jones I: Vasoactive intestinal peptide and nitric oxide in the acute phase following burns and trauma, *Burns* 27(1):17-21, 2001.

55. Ungureanu-Longrois D et al: Myocardial contractile dysfunction in the systemic inflammatory response syndrome: role of a cytokine-inducible nitric oxide synthase in cardiac myocytes, *J Mol Cell Cardiol* 27(1):155-167, 1995.

56. Gamelli RL et al: Burn-induced nitric oxide release in humans, *J Trauma* 39(5):869-877, discussion 877-878, 1995.

57. Baxter CR: Fluid volume and electrolyte changes of the early postburn period, *Clin Plast Surg* 1(4):693-703, 1974.

58. Huang PP et al: Hypertonic sodium resuscitation is associated with renal failure and death, *Ann Surg* 221(5):543-554, discussion 554-557, 1995.

59. Herndon DN, Spies M: Modern burn care, *Semin Pediatr Surg* 10(1):28-31, 2001.

60. Evans JA, Darlington DN, Gann DS: A circulating factor(s) mediates cell depolarization in hemorrhagic shock, *Ann Surg* 312(6):549-556, discussion 556-557, 1991.

61. Welt LG et al: Membrane transport defect: the sick cell, *Trans Assoc Am Physicians* 80:217-226, 1967.

62. Trunkey DD et al: The effect of hemorrhagic shock on intracellular muscle action potentials in the primates, *Surgery* 74(2):241-250, 1973.

63. Cunningham JN Jr, Shires GT, Wagner Y: Changes in intracellular sodium and potassium content of red blood cells in trauma and shock, *Am J Surg* 122(5):650-654, 1971.

64. Rosenthal SM, Tabor H: Electrolyte changes and chemotherapy in experimental burn and traumatic shock and hemorrhage, *Arch Surg* 51:244, 1945.

65. Turinsky J, Gonnerman WA, Loose LD: Impaired mineral metabolism in postburn muscle, *J Trauma* 21(6):417-423, 1981.

66. Deets DK, Glaviano VV: Plasma and cardiac lactic dehydrogenase activity in burn shock, *Proc Soc Exp Biol Med* 142(2):412-416, 1973.

67. Button B et al: Evidence of circulating membrane depolarization factor(s) in hemorrhagic shock, *Shock* 1(Suppl):15, 1994.

68. Okamoto R, Glaviano VV, Pindok M: Myocardial lipases and catecholamines in burn shock, *Proc Soc Exp Biol Med* 137(1):347-353, 1971.

69. Herndon DN, Tompkins RG: Support of the metabolic response to burn injury, *Lancet* 363(9424):1895-2003, 2004.

70. Wilmore DW, Aulick HL, Goodwin CW: Glucose metabolism following severe injury, *Acta Chir Scand* 498:43-47, 1980.

71. Wilmore DW et al: Alterations in hypothalamic function following thermal injury, *J Trauma* 15(8):697-703, 1975.

72. Gump FE, Price JB Jr, Kinney JM: Blood flow and oxygen consumption in patients with severe burns, *Surg Gynecol Obstet* 130(1):2308, 1970.

73. Wilmore DW et al: Influence of the burn wound on local and systemic responses to injury, *Ann Surg* 186(4):444-458, 1977.

74. Wilmore DW et al: Effect of injury and infection on visceral metabolism and circulation, *Ann Surg* 192(4):491-504, 1980.

75. Holder IA, Neely AN: Hageman factor dependent activation and its relationship to lethal *Pseudomonas aeruginosa* burn wound infections, *Agents Actions Suppl* 38(Pt 3):329-342, 1992.

76. McManus WF, Eurenius K, Pruitt BA Jr: Disseminated intravascular coagulation in burned patients, *J Trauma* 13(5):416-422, 1973.

77. Wilmore DW: *The metabolic management of the critically ill*, ed 2, New York, 1990, Plenum.

78. Wilmore DW, Aulick LH: Metabolic changes in burned patients, *Surg Clin North Am* 58(6):1173-1187, 1978.

79. Edelman LS et al: Sustained bone mineral density changes after burn injury, *J Surg Res* 114(2):172-178, 2003.

80. Wright K et al: Burn-activated neutrophils and tumor necrosis factor-alpha alter endothelial cell actin cytoskeleton and enhance monolayer permeability, *Surgery* 128(2):259-265, 2000.

81. Goebel A et al: Injury induces deficient interleukin-12 production, but interleukin-12 therapy after injury restores resistance to infection, *Ann Surg* 231(2):253-261, 2000.

82. Nishiura T et al: Gene expression and cytokine and enzyme activation in the liver after a burn injury, *J Burn Care Rehabil* 21(2):135-141, 2000.

83. Biffl WL et al: Interleukin-6 delays neutrophil apoptosis via a mechanism involving platelet-activating factor, *J Trauma* 40(4):575-578, discussion 578-579, 1996.

84. Choi M et al: Preventing the infiltration of leukocytes by monoclonal antibody blocks the development of progressive ischemia in rat burns, *Plast Reconstr Surg* 96(5):1177-1185, discussion 1186-1187, 1995.

85. Iocono JA et al: Interleukin-8 levels and activity in delayed-healing thermal wounds, *Wound Repair Regen* 8(3):216-225, 2000.

86. Ortega MR, Ganz T, Milner SM: Human beta defensin is absent in burn blister fluid, *Burns* 26(8):724-726, 2000.

87. Heideman J, Kaijser B, Gelin L: Complement activation and hematologic, hemodynamic, and respiratory reactions early after soft-tissue injury, *J Trauma* 18(10):696-700, 1978.

88. Grzybowski J et al: Antidietary antigen antibodies in the sera of patients with burns as a potential marker of gut mucosa integrity failure, *J Burn Care Rehabil* 13(2 Pt 1):194-197, 1992.

89. Deitch EA, Berg R: Bacterial translocation from the gut: mechanism of infection, *J Burn Care Rehabil* 8(6):475-482, 1987.

90. Yao YM et al: The association of circulating endotoxaemia with the development of multiple organ failure in burned patients, *Burns* 21(4):255-258, 1995.

91. Benhaim P, Hunt TK: Natural resistance to infection: leukocyte functions, *J Burn Care Rehabil* 13(2 Pt 2):287-292, 1992.

92. Alexander JW et al: Consumptive opsoninopathy: possible pathogenesis in lethal and opportunistic infections, *Ann Surg* 184(6):672-678, 1976.

93. Bjornson AB, Altemeier WA, Bjornson HS: Changes in humoral components of host defense following burn trauma, *Ann Surg* 186(1):88-96, 1977.

94. Cochran A et al: Systemic *Candida* infection in burn patients: a case-control study of management patterns and outcomes, *Surg Infect (Larchmt)* 3(4):367-374, 2002.

95. Goff DR et al: Cardiac disease and the patient with burns, *J Burn Care Rehabil* 11(4):305-307, 1990.

96. McGill V et al: The impact of substance use on mortality and morbidity from thermal injury, *J Trauma* 38(6):931-934, 1995.

97. Moncrief JA, Mason AD Jr: Water vapor loss in the burned patient, *Surg Forum* 13:38-41, 1962.

98. Moncrief JA: Burns. In Schwartz SI et al, editors: *Principles of surgery*, ed 2, New York, 1974, McGraw-Hill.

99. Roe CF, Kinney JM: Water and heat exchange in third-degree burns, *Surgery* 56:212-220, 1964.

100. Afflect DG et al: Assessment of tissue viability in complex extremity injuries: utility of the pyrophosphate nuclear scan, *J Trauma* 50(2):263-269, 2001.

101. Ronford V et al: Long-term regeneration of human epidermis on third degree burns transplanted with autologous cultured epithelium grown on a fibrin matrix, *Transplantation* 70(11):1588-1598, 2000.

102. Williamson JS et al: Cultured epithelial autograft: five years of clinical experience with twenty-eight patients, *J Trauma* 39(2):309-319, 1995.

103. Fitton AR, Drew P, Dickson WA: The use of bilaminate artificial skin substitute (Integra) in acute resurfacing of burns: an early experience, *Br J Plast Surg* 54(3):208-212, 2001.

104. Peck MD et al: A trial of the effectiveness of artificial dermis in the treatment of patients with burns greater than 45% total body surface area, *J Trauma* 52(5):971-978, 2002.

105. Carsin H et al: Cultured epithelial autografts in extensive burn coverage of severely traumatized patients: a five-year single-center experience with 30 patients, *Burns* 26(4):379-387, 2000.

106. Wainwright D et al: Clinical evaluation of an acellular allograft dermal matrix in full-thickness burn, *J Burn Care Rehabil* 17(2):124-36, 1996.

107. Kirker KR et al: Glycosaminoglycan hydrogels as supplemental wound dressings for donor sites, *J Burn Care Rehabil* 25(3):276-286, 2004.

108. Liew SH, Murison M, Dickson WA: Prophylactic treatment of deep dermal burn scar to prevent hypertrophic scarring using the pulsed dye laser: a preliminary study, *Ann Plast* Surg 49(5):472-475, 2002.

109. Jellish WS et al: Effect of topical local anesthetic application to skin harvest sites for pain management in burn patients undergoing skin-grafting procedures, *Ann Surg* 229(1):115-120, 1999.

SHOCK, MULTIPLE ORGAN DYSFUNCTION SYNDROME, AND BURNS IN CHILDREN

MARY FRAN HAZINSKI • MARY A. MONDOZZI •
ROSE A. URDIALES BAKER*

evolve

http://evolve.elsevier.com/McCance/

CHAPTER OUTLINE

This chapter reviews shock, multiple organ dysfunction syndrome, and burns in children. It summarizes the differences between these conditions in children and adults. These differences are noted not only in the pathophysiology section, but also in the epidemiology, clinical manifestations, and treatment and evaluation sections.

SHOCK AND MULTIPLE ORGAN DYSFUNCTION SYNDROME

Shock in children typically results from hemorrhage, severe dehydration, progressive heart failure, or sepsis. It may also complicate the care of the child with pulmonary failure (cor pulmonale), drug toxicity, electrolyte or acid-base imbalance, dysrhythmias, or multiple organ failure. (The physiology of shock is discussed in Chapter 46.)

Shock in children is present when there are signs of poor systemic perfusion, regardless of the blood pressure—shock may be present with normal, high, or low blood pressure. When blood pressure is appropriate for age but there are signs of inadequate tissue perfusion, the child is in **compensated shock.** If shock is associated with hypotension, the child is in **decompensated shock.**

*Chapter content on "Shock" and "Multiple Organ Dysfunction Syndrome" contributed by Mary Fran Hazinski; "Burns" contributed by Mary A. Mondozzi and Rose A. Urdiales Baker.

Multiple organ dysfunction syndrome (MODS) is the failure of at least two organs that results from a single cause and arises 3 to 10 days after the causative event. For example, MODS can develop as a complication of sepsis, cardiopulmonary arrest, or trauma, and typically the signs of organ failure develop within days.

Types of Shock

Shock is categorized as follows:

1. *Hypovolemic shock:* caused by inadequate intravascular volume relative to the vascular space
2. *Cardiogenic shock:* results from impairment of ventricular function
3. *Distributive or vasogenic shock:* associated with inappropriate distribution of blood flow and increased capillary permeability (e.g., septic shock) or central nervous system injury (e.g., neurogenic or spinal shock)

Such a classification system is helpful because it indicates the major therapy required (Box 47-1). However, it is inadequate for describing those with late or progressive shock, because at that point they are likely to demonstrate widespread cardiovascular dysfunction, including inappropriate intravascular volume relative to the vascular space, severe myocardial dysfunction, and maldistribution of blood flow. In addition, severe shock of any kind, even with successful therapy, may be followed by complications or death. The hypoxic insult can serve to prime cells and may result in reperfusion injury and inflammatory response that further injures cells and produces multiple organ dysfunction. The etiologic classification is also misleading for those with

Box 47-1	Classification and Causes of Shock

Hypovolemic
1. Hemorrhage
   a. External: laceration
   b. Internal: ruptured spleen or liver, vascular injury, fracture (newborn: intracerebral/intraventricular hemorrhage)
   c. Gastrointestinal: bleeding ulcer, ruptured viscus, mesenteric hemorrhage
2. Plasma loss
   a. Burn
   b. Inflammation or sepsis: capillary leak syndrome
   c. Nephrotic syndrome
   d. Third spacing: intestinal obstruction, pancreatitis, peritonitis
3. Fluid and electrolyte loss
   a. Acute gastroenteritis
   b. Excessive evaporative loss (including burns)
   c. Renal disease
4. Endocrine
   a. Adrenal insufficiency, adrenogenital syndrome
   b. Diabetes mellitus

   c. Diabetes insipidus
   d. Hypothyroidism (myxedema coma)

Cardiogenic
1. Myocardial insufficiency
   a. Cardiomyopathy: myocarditis, ischemia, hypoxia, hypoglycemia, acidosis
   b. Drug intoxication or acid-base or electrolyte imbalance
   c. Hypothermia
   d. Congenital heart disease, including ductal-dependent lesion such as coarctation of the aorta or critical pulmonary stenosis
2. Dysrhythmia: bradycardia, atrioventricular (AV) block, ventricular tachycardia, supraventricular tachycardia

Distributive (Vasogenic)
1. High or normal resistance (increased venous capacitance)
   a. Septic shock
   b. Anaphylaxis
   c. Barbiturate intoxication
2. Low resistance, vasodilation: central nervous system (CNS) injury (i.e., spinal cord transection)

Modified from Hazinski MF: Shock. In Barkin RM, editor: *Pediatric emergency medicine: concepts and clinical practice*, ed 2, St Louis, 1997, Mosby.

---

septic shock, because sepsis produces elements of hypovolemic and cardiogenic shock in addition to the complications of maldistribution of blood flow. Finally, anyone in shock is likely to develop some myocardial dysfunction and some compromise in organ perfusion and function. Thus all aspects of cardiovascular function and oxygen delivery must be skillfully supported during the treatment of any form of shock.

Hypovolemic Shock

Hypovolemic shock, the most common type of shock in children, is associated with a reduction in the intravascular volume relative to the vascular space. Dehydration and trauma are the most common causes of hypovolemic shock in children. It may also result from a redistribution of blood volume or increased capillary permeability, such as develops following burns or sepsis.

When hypovolemia is mild or moderate, such as with 5% to 10% dehydration or mild hemorrhage, compensatory vasoconstrictive adrenergic responses redistribute blood from the mesenteric, renal, and skin circulation to the heart and brain. Blood pressure is initially maintained as the vasoconstriction reduces the vascular space. Hypotension may not be observed in the child with hypovolemic shock unless intravascular volume loss is rapid or severe.[1] This usually occurs with greater than 10% dehydration in the infant or child or greater than 6% dehydration in the adolescent.[2] A 20% to 25% acute hemorrhage is usually required to produce hypotension in the child with trauma. Thus a normal blood pressure is often observed in the child with hypovolemic shock. Hypotension is a sign of severe, decompensated shock.

Hypovolemia also may be caused by an increase in the vascular space relative to intravascular volume. This may be associated with the vasodilation of sepsis or an inflammatory response, following an ischemic insult with neurogenic shock (see below), or ingestion of β-adrenergic drugs. A relative hypovolemia also may be caused by increased capillary permeability with a redistribution of intravascular volume, such as with burns or increased capillary permeability. The translocation of extravascular fluid to a location that is neither intravascular nor intracellular, as in edema, is termed **"third spacing" of fluids.**

With **distributive (vasogenic) shock,** a normal cardiac output probably is inadequate to maintain blood flow to all tissue beds simultaneously. Although no absolute fluid or blood loss has occurred, volume administration is necessary to ensure that the intravascular volume is adequate relative to the vascular space, and cardiac output must be supported at a level that is higher than normal.

Neurogenic shock is a form of hypovolemic and vasogenic (maldistributive) shock. It is caused by loss of vasomotor tone after severe injury to the spinal cord. Massive vasodilation and loss of sympathomimetic tone result in a larger vascular space and relative hypovolemia.

Compensatory Responses

Adrenergic and renal compensatory mechanisms are stimulated by significant dehydration or hypovolemia. Reduced renal perfusion stimulates the renin-angiotensin-aldosterone system, resulting in renal sodium and water retention. Decreased atrial stretch stimulates the secretion of antidiuretic hormone (ADH, also known as *arginine vasopressin [AVP]*) and produces free water retention by the kidneys. These mechanisms are similar in adults and children and may help to restore or maintain intravascular volume over time. Neonatal and young infant kidneys, however, are incapable of excreting a concentrated urine, so these compensatory mechanisms are relatively ineffective during the first weeks of life.

Compensatory mechanisms cannot be maintained indefinitely. Systemic vasoconstriction increases left ventricular afterload and myocardial oxygen consumption. Prolonged tachycardia produces impaired subendocardial blood flow and increased myocardial oxygen consumption, which may ultimately contribute to myocardial ischemia. Extreme tachypnea increases oxygen demand and reduces tidal volume. A severe compromise in blood flow and systemic perfusion contributes to cerebral, renal, or hepatic ischemia and possible organ failure (see p. 1634).

CLINICAL MANIFESTATIONS   The child with inadequate cardiac output demonstrates signs of inadequate blood flow to some tissue beds and some evidence of organ system failure. When hypovolemic or cardiogenic shock is present, the extremities may feel cool (they cool in a peripheral to proximal fashion). By comparison, excessive skin blood flow may be present in children with sepsis or septic shock. Capillary refill time is often prolonged, despite a warm ambient temperature, and the skin may have a mottled appearance. Urine output decreases if renal perfusion is compromised and is less than 2 ml/kg/hr in infants, less than 1 ml/kg/hr in children, and less than 0.5 ml/kg/hr in adolescents despite adequate fluid intake. Liver enzymes may be elevated if hepatic perfusion is reduced. The development of a metabolic acidosis indicates that blood flow to some tissues is inadequate to support total aerobic metabolism. Hypotension is often not present unless or until shock is severe.

The child's level of consciousness and responsiveness may provide valuable information about the severity of illness. The healthy infant should orient to faces, make eye contact, and track bright objects across a visual field. The healthy child is alert and reluctant to be separated from parents or examined by strangers. The critically ill infant or child is often extremely irritable; and lethargy indicates severe deterioration in the child's level of consciousness. A decreased response to painful stimulation is abnormal in the child of any age and usually indicates severe cardiorespiratory or neurologic compromise.[3]

Hypoglycemia may be observed in seriously ill or injured infants and may be associated with cardiovascular or neurologic deterioration. Infants have high glucose needs and low glycogen stores that may be rapidly depleted during stress. However, *hyperglycemia* (glucose >150 mg/dl) has been linked with poor survival in critically ill children and children with trauma or shock;[4,5] this high glucose level may result from gluconeogenesis or excessive glucose administration.

Evaluate the child's vital signs in light of the child's clinical condition. Normal vital signs are not always appropriate in the seriously ill or injured child[3] (Box 47-2). The clinical manifestations observed in the child with hypovolemic shock are those of inadequate systemic perfusion associated with intravascular volume loss and/or expansion of the vascular space. If compensatory mechanisms are working, adrenergic compensatory mechanisms produce tachycardia and redistribution of blood flow, including signs of peripheral vasoconstriction, cool extremities, delayed capillary refill, and oliguria. Hypotension is often only a late, and preterminal, sign of shock in the child. Table 47-1 contains normal vital signs in children.

Table 47-1	Normal Pediatric Vital Signs	
Age	Awake Heart Rate* (per min)	Sleeping Heart Rate (per min)
Newborn	100-180	80-160
Infant (6 mo)	100-160	75-160
Toddler	80-110	60-90
Preschooler	70-110	60-90
School-age child	65-110	60-90
Adolescent	60-90	50-90

Age	Respiratory Rate (breaths per min)
Infant	30-60
Toddler	24-40
Preschooler	22-34
School-age child	18-30
Adolescent	12-16

Age	Systolic Blood Pressure† (mmHg)	Diastolic Blood pressure (mmHg)
Birth (12 hr, <1000 g)	39-59	16-36
Birth (12 hr, 3-kg weight)	50-70	25-45
Newborn (96 hr)	60-90	20-60
Infant (6 mo)	87-105	53-66
Toddler (2 yr)	95-105	53-66
School-age child (7 yr)	97-112	57-71
Adolescent (15 yr)	112-128	66-80

Modified from Hazinski MF: *Manual of pediatric critical care,* St Louis, 1999, Mosby.
*Heart rate ranges from Gillette PC, Garson A Jr. *Pediatric cardiac dysrhythmias,* New York, 1982, Grune & Stratton.
†Blood pressure ranges taken from the following sources:
Neonate: Versmold H et al: *Pediatrics* 67:107, 1981. 10th-90th percentile ranges used.
Others: Horan MJ, chairman, Task Force on Blood-Pressure Control in Children: *Pediatrics* 79:1, 1987 (50th-90th percentile ranges used); National High Blood Pressure Education Program Working Group in Hypertension Control in Children and Adolescents. Update on the 1987 Task Force Report on High Blood Pressure in Children and Adolescents: a working group report from the National Blood Pressure Education Program. *Pediatrics* 98:649, 1996.
NOTE: Always consider patient's normal range and clinical condition. Heart and respiratory rates will normally increase with fever or stress.

Box 47-2   Estimating Blood Pressure in Children

The typical "normal" (i.e., median, or fiftieth percentile) systolic blood pressure for a child 1 to 10 years of age may be estimated by adding 90 mmHg to twice the child's age in years (90 mmHg + [2 × age in years]); this corresponds to the fiftieth percentile systolic blood pressure for the child's age. A systolic pressure equal to or less than 70 mmHg plus twice the child's age in years (70 mmHg + [2 × age in years]) is considered hypotensive beyond 1 year of age because this blood pressure corresponds to the fifth percentile systolic blood pressure for age (i.e., only 5% of normal, healthy children will demonstrate a systolic blood pressure lower than that number).

Data from Chameides L, Hazinski MF, editors: *Textbook of pediatric advanced life support,* Dallas, 1997, American Heart Association.

The child's heart rate should be appropriate for age and clinical condition. The child in shock is often tachycardic. The **tachycardia** may be primary (dysrhythmia) or secondary to stress (sinus tachycardia). If the heart rate, particularly the ventricular rate, is extremely rapid or if it is present in the child with decreased myocardial function, shock may result. In general, if ventricular rate exceeds 200 to 220 beats/min in the infant or 160 to 180 beats/min in the child, ventricular diastolic filling time and coronary artery perfusion time are significantly reduced and stroke volume falls. As a result, cardiac output falls and signs of congestive heart failure or shock develop. Once supraventricular or ventricular tachycardia produces signs of shock, urgent treatment is required.[6]

Bradycardia, an abnormally low heart rate, can cause a fall in cardiac output. In young animal models a fall in heart rate produces a commensurate fall in cardiac output.[6,7] The most common cause of bradycardia in young children is hypoxia. Therefore, if bradycardia is observed, airway patency, oxygenation, and ventilation must be constantly assessed and supported as needed. Bradycardia often indicates impending cardiovascular collapse or cardiac arrest and is the most common terminal cardiac rhythm observed.[6]

The child's stroke volume may be altered by conditions affecting ventricular preload, compliance, contractility, and afterload (Table 47-2). Evaluate and optimize each of these variables in the treatment of shock (see Chapter 46).

If the ambient temperature is warm, capillary refill is normally brisk; a prolonged capillary refill time may indicate a compromise in systemic perfusion with some forms of shock. Capillary refill time of less than 1.5 to 2 seconds is normal and may be observed in infants and children with minimal fluid deficit (less than 5% dehydration). If the capillary refill time is 1.5 to 3 seconds in a warm room, a 5% to 10% dehydration is likely to be present, and a refill time over 3 seconds is associated with greater than 10% dehydration.[1,8] However, these findings may be subtle and difficult to detect.[9] Metabolic/lactic acidosis also may be present.

The central venous pressure (CVP) and pulmonary artery wedge pressure (PAWP) (also called *pulmonary artery occlusion pressure [PAOP]*) is normally 5 to 8 mmHg or lower, and the cardiac silhouette is typically small (not enlarged) on chest radiograph.

Clinically significant dehydration is associated with weight loss (Table 47-3). Fluid intake and output records (or reports from parents or primary caretakers) reveal a history of inadequate fluid intake or excessive fluid losses. The child with significant dehydration demonstrates dry mucous membranes, a sunken fontanelle (in infants), and poor skin turgor[1] (Table 47-4). The blood urea nitrogen (BUN) and urine specific gravity are usually elevated. The serum sodium concentration and osmolality are affected by the type and severity of dehydration present.

Hemorrhage is another potential cause of hypovolemic shock. To appreciate the significance of any blood lost or drawn for laboratory analysis, the total blood loss should be considered as a percentage of the child's circulating blood volume (Table 47-5).

Table 47-2	Factors Affecting Cardiovascular Performance in Children
Factor	**Comments**
Heart rate	Normally more rapid in children than in adults. Because the *stroke volume* is smaller than in adults, the *cardiac output* of the child is more closely related to heart rate than stroke volume. *Tachycardia* is expected in the seriously ill or injured child. The most common cause of *bradycardia* in young children is hypoxia and is an ominous sign if present in association with poor perfusion. Urgent treatment is required once bradycardia or supraventricular or ventricular tachycardia produces signs of shock.
Stroke volume	Averages 1.5 ml/kg; affected by conditions altering ventricular preload, compliance, contractility, and afterload.
Ventricular end-diastolic pressure (VEDP)	Optimal pressure for children in shock is unknown. Aggressive fluid administration is linked to improved survival in children with *septic* shock.
Ventricular compliance or distensibility	Can be affected by congenital heart defects such as atrial septal defects (ASDs). If compliance is low, such as in newborns and infants, volume administration may increase VEDP. Hypoplastic ventricles are often noncompliant. Hypertrophied ventricles, noted in children with severe pulmonary stenosis or aortic stenosis, may become fibrotic and noncompliant. Increased compliance may be present in early septic shock.
Contractility	No evidence exists that contractility is significantly lower in newborns, infants, and children than adults. Newborn myocardium does have fewer contractile proteins and higher water content than adult myocardium, but the clinical significance of this is probably minimal.
Afterload	Newborn myocardium *can* adapt to mild, nonacute increases in afterload. Afterload may be increased in children with systemic vasoconstriction or pulmonary hypertension (constrictors include alveolar hypoxia, acidosis, hypothermia, and alveolar distention). Some uncorrected congenital heart defects may increase afterload. Coarctation of the aorta and aortic stenosis increase left ventricular afterload. Pulmonary stenosis increases right ventricular afterload. Afterload may be decreased in septic shock.
Oxygen delivery and consumption	Highest per kilogram body weight during the neonatal period and infancy. Oxygen reserve is smaller in infants and children than in adults, and the young child requires a higher cardiac output and oxygen delivery per kilogram than the adult. Increased oxygen consumption occurs in critically ill newborns exposed to cold because they cannot shiver to generate heat. Other causes of increased oxygen consumption in children and infants include fever, sepsis, pain, and seizures.

Table 47-3	Dehydration and Hypovolemia
Type of Dehydration	**Clinical Indicators**
Isotonic dehydration	Fluid output exceeds intake. Loss of free water is proportional to loss of sodium, so serum sodium concentration remains normal. Fluid loss is from intravascular and extravascular compartments. Compromises peripheral perfusion when the young child has lost approximately 10% (100 ml/kg) of body weight. Compromises systemic perfusion in the adolescent with acute fluid loss equivalent to 5%-6% of body weight. Produces hypotension (decompensated shock) when the young child has lost 15% (150 ml/kg) of body weight. Produces hypotension in the adolescent with a fluid loss equivalent to 7%-9% of body weight because body water constitutes a smaller percentage of body weight in older children and adults than in young children.
Hypotonic/hyponatremic dehydration	Associated with a proportionally greater loss of sodium than free water; thus the serum sodium falls. Resultant acute fall in serum osmolality produces an acute extravascular fluid shift and further loss of extravascular volume. Fluid loss in hypotonic dehydration primarily from the intravascular compartment; thus a compromise in systemic perfusion will be observed after even small quantities of fluid loss. Poor peripheral perfusion occurs in a child with a fluid loss equivalent to 5% (50 ml/kg) of body weight. Adolescents with hyponatremic dehydration may demonstrate a compromise in peripheral perfusion with a fluid loss equivalent to approximately 3% of body weight. Hypotension will often be observed when fluid loss is equal to approximately 10% (100 ml/kg) of body weight. Hypotension in an adolescent is observed when the fluid loss equals approximately 5%-6% of body weight.
Hypertonic/hypernatremic dehydration	Free water deficit is proportionately greater than the deficit of sodium, so serum sodium concentration rises, increasing serum osmolality and producing an intravascular shift of free water. For this reason the child with hypernatremic dehydration is likely to maintain intravascular volume and systemic perfusion until relatively large quantities of fluid are lost. Compromise in systemic perfusion is not likely to be observed in the *child* with hypernatremic dehydration until *severe* dehydration is present with a fluid loss equivalent to 10% of body weight (or 5%-6% of body weight in the adolescent). Hypotension may not be observed until the fluid loss approximates 15% or more of body weight (7%-9% or more of body weight in the adolescent). Hypotension in the child with hypertonic/hypernatremic dehydration indicates a substantial fluid deficit. However, the deficit must be replaced carefully to correct shock and avoid rapid lowering of serum sodium concentrations.

Data in part from Roberts KB: *Pediatr Rev* 22:380-386, 2001.

Table 47-4	Assessment of Degree of Dehydration in Isotonic Fluid Losses*		
Clinical Parameters	**Mild**	**Moderate**	**Severe**
Body weight loss			
Infant	5% (50 ml/kg)	10% (100 ml/kg)	15% (150 ml/kg)
Adolescent	3% (30 ml/kg)	5%-6% (50-60 ml/kg)	7%-9% (70-90 ml/kg)
Skin turgor	Slightly ↓	↓↓	↓↓↓
Fontanelle	May be flat or depressed	Depressed	Significantly depressed
Mucous membranes	Dry	Very dry	Parched
Skin perfusion	Warm, normal color	Extremities cool	Extremities cold
		Pale color	Mottled or gray color
Heart rate	Mild tachycardia	Moderate tachycardia	Extreme tachycardia
Peripheral pulses	Normal	Diminished	Absent
Blood pressure	Normal	Normal	Reduced
Sensorium	Normal or irritable	Irritable or lethargic	Unresponsive
Urine output	Slightly ↓	Mild oliguria	Marked oliguria or anuria
Azotemia	Absent	Present	Present and severe

Modified from Hazinski MF: Renal disorders. In Hazinski MF, editor: *Manual of pediatric critical care*, St Louis, 1999, Mosby.

*The interpretation of the assessments must be appropriately modified for age and *type* of dehydration (hypotonic or hypertonic).

Acute blood loss (hemorrhage) typically does not compromise peripheral perfusion until an estimated 25% to 30% of intravascular volume is lost (an acute intravascular or blood loss of 16 to 24 ml/kg). Tachycardia and peripheral vasoconstriction may be the only early evidence of hemorrhage in the child with trauma (Table 47-6). Once hypotension develops, cardiovascular collapse is imminent and rapid intravascular volume expansion is required immediately.

Redistribution of blood volume associated with systemic vasodilation, high capillary pressure, and transudative fluid losses or capillary leak may produce signs of poor systemic perfusion in the absence of evidence of absolute volume loss. For example, children with end-stage hepatic failure may demonstrate a relative hypovolemia associated with ascites and hepatorenal syndrome. Children demonstrate increased capillary permeability and loss of intravascular volume immediately after a burn. The septic child also may demonstrate systemic edema associated with capillary leak and further intravascular volume loss. In these children, some evidence of extravascular fluid movement (ascites, systemic edema, or fluid loss to dressings over burns) is usually observed.

Signs of neurogenic shock in the child with recent, severe spinal cord injury include warm skin and hypotension with a low diastolic blood pressure. Signs of poor systemic perfusion also are observed (see Clinical Manifestations below).

Cardiogenic Shock

Cardiogenic shock is present when impaired ventricular function compromises cardiac output. This form of shock is observed most commonly in the following situations:

1. Following cardiovascular surgery or with inflammatory disease of the heart, such as cardiomyopathy and myocarditis
2. With severe forms of obstructive congenital heart disease (hypoplastic left heart, severe aortic stenosis, hypoplastic right ventricle)
3. With drug toxicity or severe electrolyte or acid-base imbalances
4. As a complication of any form of shock and early in septic shock

Compensatory Responses

In the early stages of cardiogenic shock, adrenergic compensatory responses produce tachycardia, peripheral vasoconstriction, and constriction of the splanchnic arteries to divert blood flow from the skin, kidneys, and gut and maintain flow to the heart and brain.[6,9] If these compensatory mechanisms are sufficient, systemic blood pressure and effective coronary artery and cerebral blood flow may be maintained. However, tachycardia and systemic arterial constriction increase myocardial oxygen consumption. In addition, reduction in gut and kidney blood flow may produce hepatic, mesenteric, or renal ischemia or failure. Decreased renal perfusion stimulates the renin-angiotensin-aldosterone system, as described for hypovolemic shock on p. 1628.

If the mean arterial pressure or pulse pressure falls, stimulation of the baroreceptors in the carotid sinuses and aortic arch is reduced. This reduced baroreceptor activity removes

Table 47-5	Estimation of Pediatric Circulating Blood Volume
Age of Child	**Blood Volume (ml/kg body weight)**
Newborn	85-90
Infant	75-80
Child	70-75
Adolescent	65-70

From Hazinski MF. In Hazinski MF, editor: *Manual of pediatric critical care,* St Louis, 1999, Mosby.

Table 47-6	Classification of Pediatric Hemorrhagic Shock in Trauma Patients Based on Clinical Evaluation		
System	**Mild Hemorrhage, Compensated Shock, Simple Hypovolemia (<30%)**	**Moderate Hemorrhage, Decompensated Shock, Marked Hypovolemia (30%-45%)**	**Severe Hemorrhage, Cardiopulmonary Failure, Profound Hypovolemia (>45%)**
Cardiovascular	Tachycardia	Moderate tachycardia	Severe tachycardia
	Weak peripheral pulses, strong central pulses	Thready peripheral pulses, weak central pulses	Absent peripheral pulses, thready central pulses
	Low to normal blood pressure (systolic BP >70 mmHg + [2 × (age in years)])	Frank hypotension (systolic BP <70 mmHg + [2 × (age in years)])	Profound hypotension (systolic BP <50 mmHg)
	Mild acidosis	Moderate acidosis	Severe acidosis
Respiratory	Mild tachypnea	Moderate tachypnea	Severe tachypnea
Central nervous system	Irritable, confused	Agitated or lethargic	Obtunded, comatose
Skin	Cool extremities, mottling	Cool extremities, pallor	Cool extremities, cyanosis
	Poor capillary refill (72 seconds)	Delayed capillary refill (72 seconds)	Prolonged (>5 seconds) capillary refill
Kidneys	Mild oliguria, increased specific gravity	Marked oliguria, increased blood urea nitrogen (BUN)	Anuria

From Soud T, Pieper P, Hazinski MF. In Hazinski MF, editor: *Nursing care of the critically ill child,* ed. 2, St Louis, 1992, Mosby.

inhibition from the vasomotor center in the medulla, resulting in increased adrenergic stimulation. If myocardial dysfunction progresses, cardiac output and systemic blood pressure ultimately fall. Myocardial ischemia then exacerbates myocardial dysfunction, and multisystem organ failure may result from persistent or severe organ ischemia.

CLINICAL MANIFESTATIONS   The child with cardiogenic shock demonstrates signs of inadequate systemic perfusion despite adequate intravascular volume or even relative hypervolemia. This form of shock is generally associated with low cardiac output. The child's extremities are cool to touch (will cool peripherally to proximally), with delayed capillary refill despite a warm, ambient temperature.[3,6,9] The skin may be mottled (Figure 47-1).

Evidence of a high central venous pressure, including hepatomegaly and periorbital edema, is typically present in uncomplicated cardiogenic shock, particularly if right ventricular failure is involved. Evidence of pulmonary edema may be noted on chest radiograph or clinical assessment (including signs of respiratory distress, reduced lung compliance during hand ventilation, or frothy pink sputum suctioned from the endotracheal tube). The cardiac silhouette is usually enlarged on the chest radiograph, unless concurrent hypovolemia is present. If myocardial function is severely compromised, peripheral pulses may be diminished in intensity (dampened) or they may vary in intensity (pulsus alternans).

If a pulmonary artery catheter is in place, the cardiac output may be calculated through thermodilution technique, continuous monitoring of the mixed venous oxygen saturation, or continuous monitoring of cardiac output. A fall in cardiac output may be detected.

Signs of low cardiac output and cardiogenic shock may be identical to signs of cardiac tamponade. Although some classic signs of tamponade, including muffled heart tones or pulsus paradoxus may be observed, these signs may be difficult to appreciate if cardiac output and blood pressure are severely compromised. Therefore, if cardiogenic shock is suspected in a child after cardiovascular surgery or in any child at risk for the development of pericardial effusion, tamponade should be ruled out through an echocardiogram.

Septic Shock

Sepsis and its complications result from activation of biochemical and physiologic cascades that lead to the formation or activation of cytokines and protein systems that result in vasodilation, increased capillary permeability, maldistribution of blood flow, and cardiovascular dysfunction. Sepsis and its complications may result in organ system dysfunction and death and are a leading cause of death in noncoronary intensive care units. An estimated 42,000 pediatric cases of sepsis are reported annually in the United States and result in approximately 4400 deaths/year.[10]

Most information about the pathophysiology, clinical progression, and outcome of sepsis has come from adult clinical studies and adult animal models of sepsis. However, it appears that some information gleaned from adult experience is applicable to children. In adults and children approximately 40% of all nosocomial infections are linked to gram-negative infections; 40% to gram-positive infections; and 20% to viruses, fungi, or rickettsial microorganisms.[11] Prevention of these infections can reduce the risk of sepsis.

The most common nosocomial infections reported in pediatric critical care units in the United States are primary bloodstream infections (28%), pneumonia (21%), and urinary tract infections (15%).[12] These infections are almost always associated with an invasive device.[12] Such infections may be prevented with proper hand washing by health care providers before and after patient contact, appropriate sterile and aseptic technique during catheter insertion and tubing changes, and proper sterilization of respiratory therapy equipment. Unfortunately, fewer than 50% of health care providers in pediatric and newborn intensive care units wash their hands before and after every contact.[13,14]

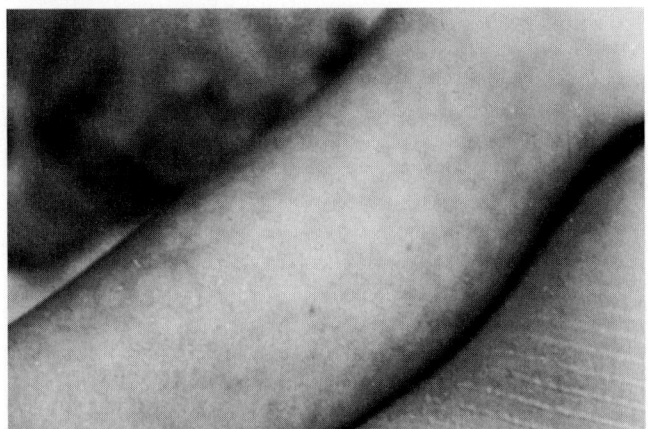

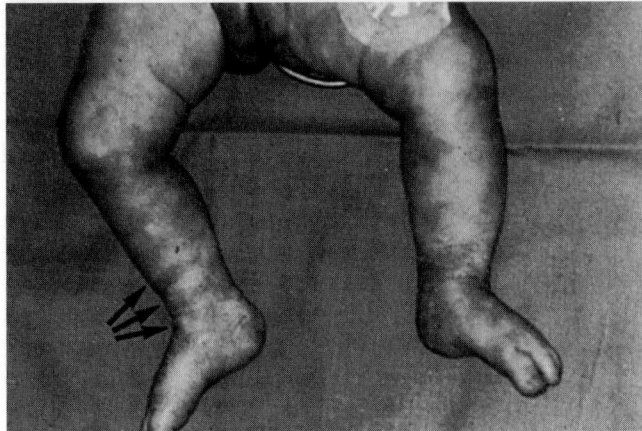

Figure 47-1 Mottling of skin caused by poor systemic perfusion. **A,** Mottling of skin color often indicates inadequate tissue oxygenation; this may result from hypoxemia or poor systemic perfusion. This child developed myocardial dysfunction and signs of cardiogenic shock. **B,** Mottled skin color is often associated with other signs of compromise of skin perfusion, including delayed capillary refill. The skin over this infant's right ankle was blanched using three fingers *(arrows)*, and the skin failed to perfuse for more than 5 seconds. This infant suffered from septic shock. (From Hazinski MF: Cardiovascular disorders. In Hazinski MF, editor: *Nursing care of the critically ill child,* ed 2, St Louis, 1992, Mosby.)

People at greatest risk for the development of sepsis include those at the extremes of age (infants and children and the elderly);[10] those with invasive catheters, surgical incisions, or wounds or burns; immunocompromised persons; and persons receiving long-term antibiotic therapy.[10-12,15] Many of these risk factors are present in any seriously ill or injured child or any child with a chronic disease. In fact, more than 50% of children with severe sepsis have underlying comorbidity.[10]

Both proinflammatory and antiinflammatory cytokines serve an essential protective function in fighting infection and modulating the immune response. It is now clear that sepsis presents a disruption in the balance between *proinflammatory* mediators (including tumor necrosis factor-α, interleukins [IL]-1, IL-6, and IL-8; platelet activating factor; arachidonic acid metabolites; leukemia inhibitory factor; nitric oxide; and many kinins) and *antiinflammatory* mediators (IL-4, IL-10, IL-11, and IL-13; transforming growth factor B; colony-stimulating factors; soluble tumor necrosis factor receptor; IL-1 receptor antagonist; and protein C). Extremely high levels of proinflammatory mediators, such as tumor necrosis factor (TNF), nitric oxide, and platelet activating factor can become destructive.[16,17] High proinflammatory cytokine levels have been implicated in the development of sepsis-induced pulmonary injury and microcirculatory disruptions, such as are observed in burns, severe trauma, shock reperfusion syndromes, and multiple organ dysfunction syndrome.[16] Tumor necrosis factor levels are directly related to mortality in newborns and children with meningitis and sepsis.[17] Increased nitric oxide concentrations are thought to be responsible for vasodilation, hypotension, and some of the decreased myocardial function that develops during sepsis. Children with sepsis, particularly those with hypotension, have increased total serum nitrite concentrations that probably reflect increased endogenous production of nitric oxide.[18]

During sepsis, endotoxin stimulates the endothelium to become a secretory organ. The endothelium changes from profibrinolytic and anticoagulant to antifibrinolytic and precoagulant, leading to the ultimate development of microthrombin in some areas of the microcirculation, further contributing to maldistribution of blood flow.[19] Mediators (e.g., activated protein C) that regulate coagulation pathways have been implicated in this process.[20-22] Low levels of activated protein C are present in children who develop coagulopathies during sepsis; activated protein C deficiency is a marker for severe sepsis in all ages,[23] and administration of activated protein C improved survival in adults with severe sepsis.[22]

There is clear interaction among catecholamines, adrenoreceptors, and glucocorticoids. Endogenous glucocorticoids have an antiinflammatory effect (they decrease activation of proinflammatory mediators), and they modulate vasomotor tone by enhancing cardiovascular and vasomotor response to catecholamines.[24] Septic children may have an actual adrenal insufficiency (caused by adrenal hemorrhage, decreased renal perfusion, inhibition of corticosteroid production by TNF, or actual adrenal disease) or a relative adrenal insufficiency (with inadequate adrenal stress response or decreased response to circulating glucocorticoids).[25] Although high-dose steroids have not improved survival from sepsis, a recent meta-analysis of the effect of steroids on survival showed that a 5- to 7-day course of physiologic doses of hydrocortisone increased survival in adults with severe sepsis.[26] A wide range of plasma cortisol levels have been reported in children with sepsis, and low plasma cortisol levels have been associated with the highest mortality in meningococcemia.[25] For these reasons, when sepsis is present, adrenal insufficiency should be ruled out and hydrocortisone administered if risk of adrenal insufficiency is present and the child does not respond to volume and inotropes.[27]

CLINICAL MANIFESTATIONS Sepsis and its complications produce a cascade of physical and biochemical changes. The clinical progression of sepsis produced by these changes was described and defined for adults by a consensus panel of physicians.[28] Consensus terms were also proposed for children by several authors.[15,27,29] In 2005, international consensus definitions were published[30] (Table 47-7).

Systemic inflammatory response syndrome (SIRS) represents a nonspecific response to a variety of insults, including trauma, burns, pancreatitis, or infection. SIRS is present when the child demonstrates two or more of the following as an acute change from baseline: fever (greater than 38.5° C) or hypothermia (less than 36° C), tachycardia, tachypnea, respiratory alkalosis, and alterations in white blood cell count (WBC) (including leukocytes, leukopenia, or an increase in the percentage of immature or band forms of WBCs). These clinical signs also may be altered by age, immune function, and clinical condition. For example, the newborn often develops hypothermia rather than fever as a sign of infection and may develop bradycardia rather than tachycardia.[30] The child with chronic lung disease and chronic hypercarbia or the child receiving controlled mechanical ventilatory support may not demonstrate tachypnea or a respiratory alkalosis. Because neutrophils are required for the development of fever and many of the local signs of infection, the neutropenic child may demonstrate normothermia despite infection.

Sepsis is a systemic response to infection. It is present when manifestations of SIRS are observed in conjunction with suspected infection; positive blood or other cultures are not necessary for the diagnosis, but suspicion of infection is required. For example, if the child with trauma develops a high fever or pulmonary congestion several days after injury, it is highly likely that an infection is present.

Severe sepsis is present when the child demonstrates evidence of sepsis (SIRS with suspected infection) and signs of cardiovascular or pulmonary organ dysfunction or evidence of two or more other organ dysfunctions (see Table 47-7, Part 2). Altered organ perfusion is signaled by signs of organ system failure. The dysfunctional organ system should be separate from the site of suspected infection and not explained by effects of drug therapy or other acute effects. This important distinction will enable separation of signs of se-

Table 47-7	Definitions and Clinical Criteria for Sepsis and Septic Shock, Including 2005 International Pediatric Definitions
Clinical Stage	**Clinical Criteria**
Part 1	
Systemic inflammatory response syndrome (SIRS)	Two or more of the following as acute change (one must be abnormal temperature or leukocyte count): Core fever (>38.5° C) or hypothermia (<36° C) Tachycardia* (or bradycardia in infants) *Adults:* >90 beats/min *Newborns:* 180 or <100 beats/min *Infants:* 180 or <90 beats/min *Children:* 130 beats/min Tachypnea* or hypocarbonic respiratory alkalosis ($PaCO_2$ <32 mmHg with spontaneous breathing) *Adults:* rate >20 breaths/min *Infants:* rate 34-50 breaths/min *Children:* rate 14-11 breaths/min Leukocytosis* (white blood cell count >11,000-19,500/mm³) Leukopenia* (white blood cell count <4500-6000/mm³) or >10% band forms
Sepsis	SIRS (two or more of above) *plus* suspected or proven infection
Severe sepsis	Sepsis *plus* signs of cardiovascular organ dysfunction, or respiratory distress syndrome, or two or more organ dysfunctions (see Part 2 below)
Septic shock	Sepsis plus cardiovascular organ dysfunction (see Part 2 below)
Part 2	
Cardiovascular dysfunction	Despite administration of isotonic intravenous fluid bolus ≥40 ml/kg in 1 hour: Decrease in BP (hypotension) <5th percentile for age or systolic BP <2 SD below normal for age OR Need for vasoactive drug to maintain BP in normal range (dopamine >5 mcg/kg/min or dobutamine, epinephrine, or norepinephrine at any dose) OR Two of the following: Unexplained metabolic acidosis: base deficit >5.0 mEq/L Increased arterial lactate two or more times upper limit or normal Oliguria: urine output >0.5 ml/kg/hr Core to peripheral temperature gap >3° C
Respiratory†	PaO_2/FIO_2 <300 in absence of cyanotic heart disease of preexisting lung disease OR $PaCO_2$ >65 torr or 20 mmHg over baseline PaO_2 OR Proven need‡ or >50% FIO_2 to maintain saturation ≥92% OR Need for nonelective invasive or noninvasive mechanical ventilation§
Neurologic	Glasgow coma score ≤11 (57) OR Acute change in mental status with a decrease in Glasgow Coma Score ≥3 points from abnormal baseline
Hematologic	Platelet count <80,000/mm³ or a decline of 50% in platelet count from highest value recorded over the past 3 days (for chronic hematology/oncology patients) OR International normalized ration >2
Renal	Serum creatinine two or more times upper limit of normal for age or twofold increase in baseline creatinine
Hepatic	Total bilirubin ≥4 mg/dl (not applicable for newborn) OR ALT two times upper limit of normal for age

Part 1, Data from Carcillo JA et al: *Crit Care Med* 30(6):1365-1378, 2002; Hayden WR: *J Pediatr* 124:657-658, 1994; Goldstein B et al: *Pediatr Crit Care Med* 6(1):2-8, 2005; Hazinski MF et al: *Am J Crit Care* 2:224, 1993. **Part 2,** From Goldstein B et al: *Pediatr Crit Care Med* 6(1):2-8, 2005.
BP, Blood pressure; *ALT,* alanine transaminase; *SD,* standard deviation.
*Some age-related differences in these ranges apply, the abnormal limits are generally defined as more than 2 standard deviations above or below normal ranges for age.
†Acute respiratory distress syndrome must include a PaO_2/FIO_2 ratio ≤200 mmHg, bilateral infiltrates, acute onset, and no evidence of left heart failure; acute lung injury is defined identically except the PaO_2/FIO_2 ratio must be (300 mmHg.
‡Proven need assumes oxygen requirement was tested by decreasing flow.
§In postoperative persons, this requirement can be met if the patient has developed an acute inflammatory or infectious process in the lungs that prevent him or her from being extubated.

vere sepsis from signs of pneumonia and associated respiratory failure.

Septic shock is heralded in the child with sepsis by the development of cardiovascular dysfunction. This may be characterized by hypotension despite adequate fluid resuscitation or by the necessity for vasopressors to maintain blood pressure. Because children tend to develop hypotension only late in the course of any shock, septic shock should be identified when the child develops more subtle signs of poor perfusion despite adequate fluid resuscitation. If the child with sepsis develops hypotension, decompensated septic shock is present. Mortality from septic shock associated with hypotension may be as high as 46%.[31]

Children with septic shock may have a high, normal, or low cardiac output. In reports of adults with sepsis, low cardiac output was usually associated with poor survival.[31-33] However, in reports of children with sepsis, low cardiac output and low oxygen delivery are often present and they do not necessarily predict a poor outcome.[27] This low cardiac output may be associated with vasoconstriction ("cold shock") or vasodilation ("warm shock").[27]

Low cardiac output may respond to aggressive fluid administration[34] and titration of inotropes, vasopressors, and vasodilators with a therapeutic goal of maintaining cardiac output (3.3 to 6.0 L/min/m²) and high oxygen delivery (>200 ml/min/m²).[27] In fact, children who receive aggressive fluid resuscitation (more than 40 ml/kg administered within the first hour of therapy and more than 200 ml/kg administered during the first 8 hours of therapy) are significantly more likely to survive than those who receive less aggressive fluid resuscitation.[34]

The ultimate goal of treatment of septic shock is to maintain organ perfusion and function. This requires careful titration of fluid administration, inotropic support, and vasoconstrictors or vasodilators to maximize systemic and organ perfusion (and function).

The terms *warm* versus *cold* septic shock are imprecise terms and should be used only in conjunction with other descriptions of systemic perfusion and cardiovascular function. **Warm shock** is characterized by peripheral vasodilation (warm skin) and was thought to be associated with hyperdynamic cardiovascular function with high cardiac output. **Cold shock** is characterized by peripheral vasoconstriction (cold skin) and thought to be associated with low cardiac output. However, cardiac output may be low, normal, or high regardless of skin temperature, and skin temperature alone will not identify the cardiovascular support required. When systemic perfusion is inadequate, the child likely needs more aggressive fluid administration and titration of vasoactive drug therapy.

Many adults and some children with sepsis generate a cardiac output that is higher than normal despite a fall in ventricular ejection fraction. This high cardiac output is associated with temporary adaptive ventricular dilation and an increase in ventricular end-diastolic volume, an increase in heart rate, and a fall in systemic vascular resistance. The child

may maintain a high cardiac output if intravascular volume is supported with aggressive fluid resuscitation. Echocardiography may reveal the reduction in ventricular ejection fraction and left ventricular dilation. If the mixed venous oxygen saturation is monitored continuously (through use of a fiberoptic pulmonary artery catheter), the mixed venous oxygen saturation ($S\bar{v}O_2$) may rise because cardiac output and oxygen delivery increase whereas oxygen extraction decreases. Although some tissue beds may be ischemic, overall oxygen extraction does not increase, so the $S\bar{v}O_2$ remains high.[33] When the child with sepsis improves in response to therapy, the $S\bar{v}O_2$ may initially fall as oxygen extraction increases.

Reperfusion and Inflammatory Injury

Reperfusion (reoxygenation) injury is cellular injury caused by the restoration or reperfusion of physiologic concentrations of oxygen to cells that have been exposed to injurious but nonlethal hypoxic conditions.[35] Reperfusion injury is stimulated by the generation of highly reactive oxygen intermediates (e.g., free oxygen radicals and superoxide) that damage cell membranes, denature proteins, and disrupt chromosomes[36] (see Chapter 2). The amount of free oxygen radical produced is directly related to the severity and duration of the ischemic period. The process is most likely to affect endothelial cells of the microvasculature, causing MODS, and is likely to contribute to the compromise of organ perfusion after shock resuscitation.[36]

An ischemic insult activates white blood cells, priming monocytes and macrophages and contributing to the release of inflammatory mediators or cytokines, including TNF, the interleukins (IL-1, IL-6, and IL-8), and platelet activating factor. These cytokines in turn contribute to vasodilation, increased capillary permeability, and altered platelet function. The ultimate result is a maldistribution of blood flow and a compromise in organ perfusion.[36] The role of these mediators is summarized in Table 7-6. Chapter 46 includes a more comprehensive discussion of MODS.

Signs of organ dysfunction include but are not limited to lactic acidosis, oliguria, and an acute alteration in level of consciousness (e.g., decrease in Glasgow Coma Scale score of 1 point or more); hypoxemia, hypotension, poor capillary refill, or shock plus signs of coagulopathy, respiratory, renal, or hepatic dysfunction or neurologic dysfunction.[37] Box 47-3 lists other potential signs of organ system failure in children.

Evaluation and Treatment of Shock

Acidosis may be the most sensitive indicator of inadequate systemic perfusion in children. The development of a metabolic acidosis or a rise in serum lactate concentration indicates the presence of inadequate tissue oxygenation. Hypotension is a late sign of shock in infants and children and often indicates cardiovascular collapse.

The child's ventilation and oxygenation should be evaluated whenever shock is present. In addition, the child's electrolytes, glucose, blood urea nitrogen (BUN), creatinine, liver

Box 47-3	Proposed Signs of Organ System Dysfunction*

Central Nervous System
Acute change in mental status (confusion, agitation, lethargy)
Glasgow Coma Scale score 15 (previously normal) or decreased by 1

Pulmonary (ARDS)
Unexplained hypoxemia with suspected sepsis (Pao$_2$/Fio$_2$) 175-280 mmHg)
Bilateral pulmonary infiltrates with PAOP 18 mmHg
Deterioration from baseline

Renal (Not Prerenal)
Oliguria (urine output 0.5 ml/kg/hr) despite adequate fluid administration
Increase in serum creatinine from normal with urine sodium 40 mmol/L
Rise in serum creatinine by 2.0 mg/dl in presence of preexisting renal insufficiency

Hepatobiliary
Elevation in liver function enzymes to twice normal
Serum bilirubin 2.0 mg/dl

Gastrointestinal
Paralytic ileus
Gastrointestinal bleeding

Coagulation
Confirmatory test for DIC (FDP >1:40 or D-dimers >2.0)
Thrombocytopenia or fall in platelet count by 25%
Elevated prothrombin time and partial thromboplastin time
Clinical evidence of bleeding

From Hazinski MF et al: *Am J Crit Care* 2:224, 1993.
ARDS, Adult respiratory distress syndrome; *PAOP,* pulmonary artery occlusion pressure; *DIC,* disseminated intravascular coagulation; *FDP,* fibrin degradation products.
*Clinical criteria indicating organ system failure. These signs are consistent with organ system dysfunction or failure in the absence of other attributable causes.

function, calcium, phosphorus, and cardiac enzyme concentrations should be evaluated in an attempt to identify the cause of the shock or treatment needed.

Hematologic evaluation is necessary if hemorrhage or disseminated intravascular coagulation (DIC) is apparent. Hemoglobin and hematocrit may be artificially normal in the face of an acute hemorrhage; unless volume resuscitation is provided with whole blood, the child's hematocrit ultimately falls during fluid resuscitation. Evaluation for nontraumatic hemorrhage or potential DIC includes a complete blood count, platelets, coagulation tests (prothrombin time [PT], partial thromboplastin time [PTT], bleeding time), and DIC screen (fibrinogen, fibrin split products).

Obtain a chest roentgenogram to evaluate cardiac size and exclude pneumonia, pneumothorax, and pulmonary edema. An arterial blood gas (ABG) measurement monitors progression of acidosis and evidence of oxygenation or ventilation problems associated with respiratory distress. Oximetry enables evaluation of hemoglobin saturation and may indicate the loss of peripheral pulses; however, oximetry should never be used as a "pulse check." Electrocardiogram (ECG) and echocardiogram should be selectively used to evaluate cardiac

function and rule out dysrhythmias, effusion, and failure as contributing factors to low cardiac output.

Microbiologic evaluation should be performed when infection is suspected. Blood and urine cultures should be obtained as needed; a Gram stain should be available immediately with these cultures. Evaluation of spinal fluid, stool, and joints also may be required.

Early recognition and aggressive antimicrobial and fluid therapy are the keys to survival for children in shock. Therefore signs of poor systemic perfusion must be identified as soon as they appear. Supportive therapy then is required to optimize each aspect of cardiovascular and pulmonary function. Throughout therapy it is important to evaluate the child's response to therapy and to monitor for evidence of further deterioration and development of MODS. If signs of MODS develop, organ function must be supported.

The goals of treatment of shock are maximization of oxygen delivery and minimization of oxygen demand. The airway, oxygenation, and ventilation must be supported. Reduction of oxygen demand requires the treatment for fever and pain. In addition, the child should be kept warm and shivering should be prevented. Blood components and, perhaps, intravenous fluids should be warmed before administration to young infants and children with hypothermia. Fear and pain increase oxygen consumption, so care must be taken to reassure the child and treat pain as indicated.

When signs of shock are detected, immediate resuscitation is required. Hemodynamic monitoring should be instituted and volume and inotropic support provided as needed. The warmth of the child's extremities, capillary refill, quality of peripheral pulses, level of consciousness and responsiveness, urine output, oxygenation, ventilation, and acid-base status should be assessed throughout shock therapy. Once systemic perfusion is restored, transfer to a pediatric intensive care unit is advised.

Initial therapy for any unstable person requires evaluation and support of airway patency and ventilation. The child is positioned in a manner that supports maximal airway patency, and evaluate the effectiveness of ventilation. Supplemental oxygen is administered as needed at up to 3 to 6 L/min by nonrebreathing mask, head hood, or bag-mask ventilation. Children in shock should be intubated *before* respiratory deterioration or arrest complicates shock management.

The child's heart rate must be adequate to support effective cardiac output and systemic perfusion. The most common pediatric dysrhythmias are listed in Box 47-4. Treat bradydysrhythmias and extreme tachydysrhythmias promptly. Pharmacologic therapy, pacing, or synchronized direct current (DC) cardioversion may be required.

The most common ECG findings associated with loss of pulses ("arrest" rhythms) include asystole, electromechanical dissociation (EMD), pulseless ventricular tachycardia, and ventricular fibrillation. Regardless of ECG findings, provide cardiopulmonary resuscitation—including cardiac compression—when pulses are lost.

Volume resuscitation is designed to restore intravascular volume relative to the vascular space and optimize ventricu-

---

Box 47-4 | **Most Common Pediatric Dysrhythmias**

Heart (QRS) Rate Too Slow for Clinical Condition
QRS duration (width) normal
  Sinus bradycardia
  Junctional rhythm
  Heart block
QRS duration (width) prolonged
Supraventricular tachycardia (SVT) with aberrant ventricular conduction
  Ventricular rhythm
  Heart block

Heart (QRS) Rate Too Fast for Clinical Condition
QRS duration (width) normal
  Sinus tachycardia
  SVT
QRS duration (width) prolonged
  SVT with aberrant ventricular conduction
  Ventricular tachycardia

Collapse (Pulseless) Rhythms
Electromechanical dissociation
Ventricular tachycardia
Ventricular fibrillation
Asystole

From Hazinski MF: Cardiovascular disorders. In Hazinski MF, editor: *Manual of pediatric critical care,* St Louis, 1999, Mosby.

---

lar preload. The specific fluid selected and route of administration are determined by the child's clinical condition. In general, however, isotonic **crystalloids** (salt-containing solutions, such as normal saline or lactated Ringer solution) or **colloids** (protein-containing fluids, such as albumin or blood) are administered in boluses of 20 ml/kg. Children in septic shock require a large volume of intravenous fluid to restore and maintain systemic perfusion. More than 40 ml/kg will likely be required during the first hour of volume resuscitation, and a total of 100 to 200 ml/kg or more may be required during the first several hours of therapy.[27,33] In fact, rapid volume administration, particularly during the first hour of therapy, has been linked with improved survival in hypotensive children in septic shock. If intravenous access cannot be achieved, an intraosseous needle should be inserted and intraosseous fluid and drug administration provided through that route.[6]

Unless shock is mild or responds immediately to volume therapy, insertion of a central venous (monitoring) catheter is advisable. Several multilumen catheters are available in pediatric sizes that enable simultaneous monitoring of central venous pressure and administration of fluids.

Monitoring of the volume of urine output and specific gravity is useful in determining the child's response to fluid therapy. A urinary catheter should be inserted if shock is present unless the child has sustained pelvic trauma or a urethral tear is suspected. All sources of fluid intake and output should be monitored and recorded hourly or more frequently if needed.

An intraarterial line should be inserted once the child is stabilized. This enables reliable, continuous evaluation of arterial pressure. Noninvasive oscillometric blood pressure monitoring devices may not accurately measure low or rapidly falling blood pressures and may *overestimate* the blood pressure,[38] particularly in trauma patients.[39] Sphygmomanometry also may yield inaccurate blood pressure measurement; cuff pressure measurement of a person in shock typically *underestimates* the systolic blood pressure (cuff measurements are lower than intraarterial pressure).[40]

Insertion of a pulmonary artery catheter should be considered whenever the child demonstrates shock that is unresponsive to initial volume and vasoactive drug support. A pulmonary artery catheter with thermodilution cardiac output thermistor, a fiberoptic pulmonary artery catheter, or both can enable continuous monitoring of mixed venous oxygen saturation or continuous monitoring of cardiac output. Quantification of these variables can be particularly helpful if precise tracking of hemodynamic measurements is desired.[27] This may be necessary in the care of the child with septic shock or MODS.

Administration of blood or blood component therapy is necessary to treat hemorrhage or severe coagulopathies. A "normal" hematocrit does not rule out the possibility of hemorrhage; the hematocrit typically falls in a person who has sustained whole blood loss after replacement of the blood loss with crystalloids or colloids. In general, 10 ml/kg boluses of packed red blood cells are administered to treat significant blood loss.

Transfusion for the child with chronic anemia and shock must be accomplished slowly to prevent hypervolemia and further deterioration in myocardial function. Administration of packed red blood cells at a rate averaging 3 to 5 ml/kg/hr over several hours may be well tolerated, particularly if it is preceded and followed by administration of diuretics. If severe anemia is associated with severe hypervolemia and myocardial dysfunction, an exchange transfusion may be required. If a coagulopathy is present, administer specific blood component therapy necessary to prevent or treat hemorrhage.

Hypoxemia, metabolic acidosis, and electrolyte imbalances depress myocardial function and must be corrected when shock is present. Administer oxygen during resuscitation of the child in shock and be prepared to institute mechanical ventilatory support when needed.

Hypoglycemia may develop rapidly in the critically ill or injured infant because infants have high glucose needs and low glycogen stores. If glucose is needed, however, continuous infusion is preferred to intermittent bolus therapy. In fact, hyperglycemia has been linked to poor outcome in some children with head injury,[4] although it is unclear whether the poor outcome is caused by idiopathic hyperglycemia or excessive glucose administration.[5] Tight glucose control is now recommended for critically ill children to maintain blood glucose levels (approximately 120 mg/dl to160 mg/dl).[5]

Acute or severe alterations in the serum sodium concentration during fluid therapy should be avoided. Acute changes in serum sodium produce changes in serum osmolality that result in fluid shifts into and out of the vascular spaces. Such fluid shifts can be associated with neurologic complications, including seizures, cerebral edema, and intracranial hemorrhage.[2,41]

Alterations in serum potassium concentration may affect myocardial contractility and conduction. However, children are far less sensitive than adults to minor changes in serum potassium concentration. Hypokalemia may result from inadequate potassium administration during volume therapy or from excessive potassium losses caused by drug therapy (e.g., furosemide). The serum potassium concentration falls in the presence of alkalosis; this represents an intracellular shift of potassium and is corrected when the pH is normalized. Treat true hypokalemia with an infusion of potassium chloride at a dose equivalent to 0.5 to 1 mEq/kg administered over several hours.

Hyperkalemia may result from excessive potassium administration, reduced potassium excretion (e.g., in renal failure), or massive cell lysis (e.g., tumor lysis syndrome). Serum potassium concentration also rises when acidosis develops; the rise in serum potassium is caused by a shift of potassium from the intracellular to the vascular space (e.g., exchange with vascular H^+) and falls when the serum pH is corrected.

Both ionized and total calcium concentration should be monitored, and documented hypocalcemia must be treated. Serum ionized calcium concentration is often low (less than 4.5 mEq/L) in children with septic shock.[42]

Hypercalcemia may be observed in children with some malignancies, including acute lymphocytic leukemia, lymphomas, and soft tissue sarcomas. Malignant cells often secrete a parathormone-like substance that stimulates bone reabsorption, release of calcium, and rapid cell turnover.[43] Although mild hypercalcemia is not life threatening, extreme hypercalcemia (total serum calcium approaching 19 to 20 mEq/L) may produce renal and cardiovascular complications. Table 47-8 summarizes additional drug therapy for children in shock. If oxygenation, ventilation, heart rate, and intravascular volume are appropriate and myocardial function and systemic perfusion remain poor, vasoactive drug therapy with inotropes is indicated.

Emerging Therapies for Shock and Sepsis

Prevention of shock is important. Prevention of trauma (injury prevention) and treatment of dehydration can eliminate the two leading causes of hypovolemic shock in children. *Haemophilus influenzae* sepsis and meningitis have been virtually eradicated in the United States since the introduction and widespread use of *H. influenzae* vaccine for infants, and immunization against *Neisseria meningitidis* (the causative microorganism of meningococcal sepsis) may similarly reduce the incidence of meningococcal sepsis. Administration of colony-stimulating factors to increase white blood cell count in immunosuppressed persons has been shown to decrease infection and sepsis in this high-risk population.[43] Septic shock also may be prevented with good hand-washing technique, early detection of infection, and appropriate antimicrobial therapies for infection and sepsis.

Several advances in shock therapy have been made in recent years and several show promise for continued improve-

Table 47-8	Drug Therapies for Children in Shock	
Type	**Indications**	**Comments**
Vasoactive (inotropes)	If oxygenation, ventilation, and intravascular volume are appropriate but myocardial function and systemic perfusion remain poor or heart rate is low	Useful in the treatment of cardiogenic and distributive shock or any shock with impaired myocardial function; goals include increased heart rate (if it is low), increased cardiac output, redistribution of cardiac output, and increased cardiac contractility
Sympathomimetic	To stimulate particular adrenergic receptors	Receptors targeted will be determined by the child's heart rate, peripheral perfusion, blood pressure, and urine output
Dopamine	To improve renal, coronary artery, mesenteric, and cerebral circulation at low doses and increase heart rate or myocardial function at moderate doses; vasoconstriction may occur at high doses	Popular drug used especially in the presence of oliguria; provides dopaminergic effects (renal, coronary artery, mesenteric, cerebral vasodilation) and β- and α-adrenergic effects at higher doses
Epinephrine	For resuscitation from cardiopulmonary arrest or cardiovascular collapse; to treat symptomatic bradycardia unresponsive to oxygen therapy and adequate ventilation or in the treatment of hypotension	Effective in increasing mean arterial pressure and improving myocardial function in children with septic shock
Vasopressin	To improve blood pressure	May be useful in the treatment of shock associated with vasodilation
Vasodilators	To reduce impedance to ventricular ejection	Because they dilate both arteries and veins, they may reduce ventricular preload and afterload
Antibiotics	For treatment of bacterial infection	Broad spectrum used until a specific causative microorganism is identified
Steroids	For meningitis or septic shock that is unresponsive to initial volume administration and vasopressors	Given 20 to 30 min before first dose of antibiotics, steroids may be associated with improvement in auditory function

ment in treatment. First, there is a better understanding of resuscitation goals with an appreciation of the need to target high, rather than normal, cardiac output and oxygen delivery during resuscitation.

Trauma resuscitation has become more targeted in adults and children. In the prehospital setting, aggressive fluid resuscitation may delay transport and increase bleeding, particularly in those with penetrating trauma, so prehospital fluid resuscitation is reserved for children with signs of shock. If penetrating trauma is associated with hypovolemic shock, the child requires urgent surgical intervention, thus prehospital providers should minimize delays during transport.

Colloids or crystalloids can be used for resuscitation in the case of hypovolemic shock. Recent studies have documented the efficacy of prehospital administration of hypertonic saline for adults with head trauma[44] and experience is growing with selective use of hypertonic saline in children. Emerging is an appreciation of the immunologic and coagulation complications produced by massive transfusions, so the surgical approach to trauma has changed to reduce the need for these massive transfusions. Surgical repair of significant trauma injuries (e.g., liver and bowel injuries) may be accomplished in two stages: the initial surgery is performed to stabilize and the second surgery repairs the injury. This two-stage approach typically reduces the amount of blood products required.[45] Although initial experience with artificial blood products was discouraging, new products are currently being tested that show promise.[45]

We now have a better understanding of the pathophysiology of septic shock in children,[27] appreciating the critical role that early and aggressive fluid resuscitation plays in the outcome of pediatric sepsis. Children are far more likely to survive an episode of septic shock if they receive at least 40 ml/kg of fluid in the first hour of resuscitation and 200 ml/kg or more during the first 8 hours of therapy.[27] During fluid resuscitation, the healthcare provider should expect that the child will develop both systemic and pulmonary edema because capillary permeability is increased necessitating intubation and mechanical ventilatory support.

The 2002 publication of international consensus definitions for sepsis and organ dysfunction in children will enable better standardization of care.[30] Consistency in patient description will enable more accurate reports of patient outcomes and accurate comparison of therapies.

In the 1980s and 1990s, mediator-specific therapies did improve survival in laboratory animals and in subsets of patients but failed to improve survival in large clinical trails. Activated protein C was the first mediatory-specific therapy shown to improve survival in a large, randomized controlled trial of adults with severe sepsis.[22] Although the trial officially excluded those under 18 years of age, a large number of children received the drug using "compassionate use" exemptions. There was a trend toward improved survival in children, but the number enrolled was insufficient to reach statistical significance. Validation from a pediatric multicenter clinical trial is currently underway.

Continuous plasmafiltration improves organ function and blood pressure in septic adults and children but has not yet improved survival rates.[46] Glucocorticoid administration has been successful for treatment of infants and children with actual or relative adrenal insufficiency.[25] Although high doses of steroids do not improve adult survival from sepsis,[24] recent meta-analysis showing that administration of physiologic doses to adults with septic shock improved survival[26] led to the inclusion of low doses of glucocorticoids in the guidelines for the treatment of pediatric septic shock that is unresponsive to volume and inotropes.[6,27] Prospective, randomized controlled trials of physiologic doses of glucocorticoids, however, are needed for validation.

New therapies for sepsis include targeting of toll-like receptors (TLRs), receptors that allow the immune system to recognize invading microorganisms. Activation of TLRs contributes to stimulation of the inflammatory response. TLR blockade has allowed modulation of the inflammatory response in animals and shows promise for an effective strategy in the treatment of human sepsis.[20]

Finally, it soon may be possible to tailor sepsis and other critical therapies through the use of genetic profiling.[47] Mannose-binding lectin (MBL) is a substance that plays a role in stimulating phagocytosis of microorganisms and in reducing production of inflammatory cytokines. One-third of the population has genetic changes on the MBL gene that causes reduced MBL levels in the blood; this genotype has been shown to increase risk of SIRS in children[48] and in adults, although this has not been linked to increased mortality.[47] If it becomes possible to predict genetic responsiveness to therapy, this would enable individual tailoring of therapy and, presumably, improved outcome.

BURNS

Management of pediatric burn injuries requires an understanding of the differences that exist in this population related to etiology of injury, growth and development, physiology, and clinical course. In 1988 the American Burn Association established criteria to guide transfer of a patient to a specialized burn center. These recommendations are based on complex management issues related to treatment of acute burns and the long-term rehabilitation needs of children.[49,50]

Burn injuries in children often are preventable and often are the result of inadequate supervision, curiosity, inability to escape the burning agent, or intentional abuse. **Scald injuries** (i.e., hot water, grease, other) are most common among young children whereas flame burns are more prevalent among older children. A child exposed to hot tap water at 140° F for three seconds will sustain a third degree burn.[51]

A child's skin is thinner and thus more susceptible to injury than an adult's skin. The extent of injury is determined by the temperature of the burning agent and the duration of exposure. Because very young children may be unable to escape the heat source, the depth of the injury is likely to be greater. The kitchen is also a common site of burn injury and often involves pulling over dishes or appliances containing hot liquids. These are common burn injury sources for children 2 years of age and younger.

Although **child abuse** can occur at any age, young children are particularly vulnerable to serious injury. Approximately 6% to 20% of all child abuse cases in the United States are caused by burning.[52] Burns that may suggest physical maltreatment include (1) patterned burns, (2) classic forced emersion burn pattern with sharp stocking or glove demarcation and sparing of flexed protected areas, (3) splash/spill burn patterns not consistent with history or developmental level, and (4) cigarette burns. Abuse is suggested with (1) incompatible history and physical examination; (2) incompatible burn and developmental level; (3) bilateral or mirror image burns; (4) localized burns to genitals, buttocks, and perineum (especially at toilet training stage); (5) evidence of excessive delay in seeking treatment; and (6) presence of other forms of injury.[53] Forced immersion in hot water typically presents with deep symmetric injuries lacking any evidence of splash wounds (Figure 47-2). **Contact burns** also may be intentionally inflicted by contact with cigarettes or other hot objects such as curling irons. Young children may inadvertently grasp a hot object. However, the pattern of injury will be confined to the palm. Burns to the dorsum of the hand are viewed with suspicion.[54]

Children 3 to 8 years of age are most often injured by flame during fire play. Lighters and matches ignite clothing and cause house fires. Inhalation injury is the main cause of death in up to 80% of fire-related fatalities in the United States. Young children may run when clothing ignites and increase the severity of injury. Escape from a burning residence or motor vehicle is often delayed because young children cannot cognitively comprehend the circumstances or physically remove themselves from the danger. **Flame burns** involving flammable liquids, especially gasoline, are more common in older children.

Although flame and scald burns account for the majority of thermal injuries in children, **electrical burns** result from direct contact with high- or low-voltage current. Most commonly these injuries occur as a result of risk-taking behavior on the part of young males. Trauma from contact with electrical energy results from the passage of current through vital organs, muscle compartments, and nerve or vascular pathways. Very young children are at risk for injury from chewing on electrical cords or inserting objects into electric outlets (Figure 47-3). Lightning strikes also account for some electrical burns. **Chemical burns** occur most often in an industrial setting for the adult. At home, children may be burned by swallowing corrosive agents. The type of causative agent has important implications for the evaluation, treatment, and prognosis of the child.

Severity of Injury

The severity of burn injury is assessed based on the percentage of the total body surface area (TBSA) involved. Use of the standard rule of nines results in inaccurate calculation of the percentage of TBSA involved in children. Although the infant's trunk and arms are of roughly the same proportion as the adult's, the head and neck make up 18% of TBSA and each lower extremity is 14% of TBSA. A modified rule of nines deducts 1% from the head and adds 0.5% to each leg for each year of life after 2 years.[55] Various charts are available that assign body proportions to children of different ages. These are generally used in pediatric burn facilities and do accurately compute the extent of burn injury.

Because burn trauma represents a three-dimensional wound, the severity of injury is assessed also in relation to the **depth of injury.** The etiology of the burn and the duration of contact with the burning agent are important considerations in determining the depth of injury. In general, the more intense the heat source and the longer the contact, the deeper the resulting injury. However, infant skin is extremely fragile and more likely to sustain a deeper burn. This makes the estimation of the depth of burn difficult in very young children, especially following scald injuries (Figure 47-4). Intentionally inflicted burns tend to be more severe since contact with the

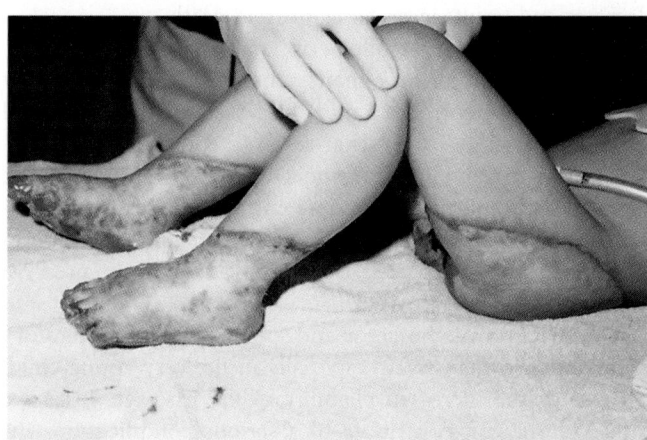

Figure 47-2 Burn pattern typically seen after forced emersion in hot water.

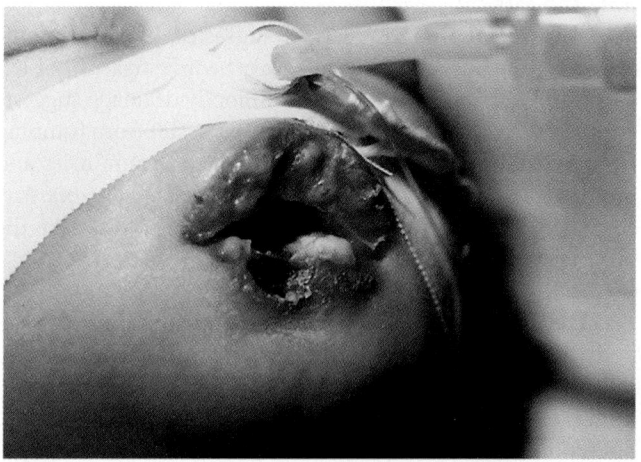

Figure 47-3 Commissure burn resulting from biting an electrical wire.

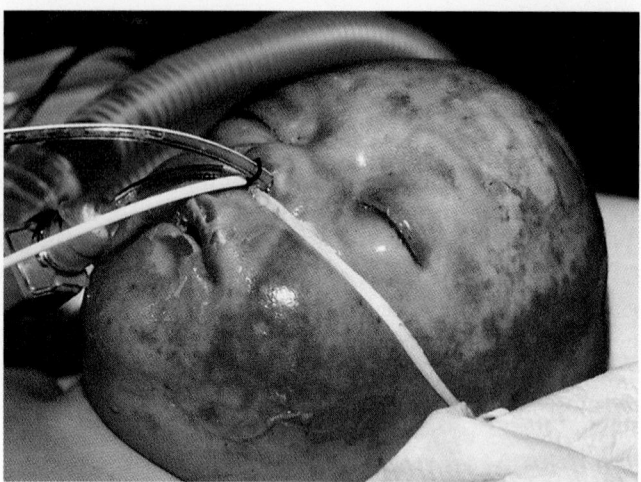

Figure 47-4 Areas of indeterminant depth of injury in a young child.

burning agent is prolonged. Electrical injuries also may mask the extent of damage on initial assessment. Visible tissue damage may appear minimal despite severe injury to underlying structures.

Another important factor in assessing the severity of injury is the victim's age. Children younger than 2 years have a significantly higher risk for associated morbidity and mortality after sustaining burn injury. They have not achieved maturity of the immune system and are at increased risk for infection and sepsis. In addition, very young children are intolerant of rapid fluid shifts and demonstrate immature renal function, which negatively affects their ability to retain sodium and water (see the Shock section).

The areas of the body injured are another consideration when assessing the severity of the burn. Burns of the hands, feet, and perineum and burns across joints carry the potential for scar formation and contracture that may interfere with function as well as growth and development. Specialized care is required to preserve maximal function. In addition, burns to the face and neck may result in airway compromise as well as deformity caused by damage to delicate cartilage of the nose and ears.

Concomitant injuries may be suggested by the circumstances of the burn and should always be investigated; for example, initially burns do not bleed. Bloody drainage suggests another source of trauma. Fractures may result from jumping from a window to escape a house fire. Electrical injuries and motor vehicle accidents often result in associated trauma. Any suspicion of intentionally inflicted burns should alert the burn team to assess for other injuries.

PATHOPHYSIOLOGY   Major burn trauma involves all body systems, and the consequences of injury include shock, infection, hypermetabolism, organ failure, and functional limitations. These effects can be magnified in the pediatric population as a result of physiologic immaturity and age-related variation in treatment modalities.

Integument
The local response manifested in the area of trauma includes cellular destruction and damage. Progressive injury caused by **dermal ischemia** may result from ineffective initial management, especially inadequate or delayed resuscitation. An increase in the permeability and hydrostatic pressure of the capillaries results in the loss of fluid, proteins, and electrolytes into the interstitial spaces. A diminishing intravascular oncotic pressure further enhances these losses and results in edema formation. Marked edema can result not only in the area of injury but also in unburned areas. Loss of substantial areas of skin has immediate and profound physiologic effects. Direct and evaporative fluid losses are seen immediately.[56] Although these losses are maximal in the immediate postburn period, they persist until wound closure.

Circulatory alterations also occur in the area of injury. Reduced blood flow and capillary stasis result from **hemoconcentration,** the release of thromboplastin and clot-activating factors from heat-damaged cells, reduced cardiac output, and edema formation. Circulation in the area of partial-thickness wounds ceases for 24 to 48 hours after injury, after which it is usually restored. Vascular supply in the area of full-thickness injuries is completely occluded and is not restored until granulation tissue forms or the wound is surgically repaired. The dry, leathery **eschar** provides an ideal environment for bacterial growth. Infection, trauma, or applying ice to the burn area may convert a partial-thickness injury to a full-thickness one, especially in young children, who have thinner, more delicate skin.

Cardiovascular System
The marked reduction in cardiac output immediately following injury is accompanied by an initial increase in systemic vascular resistance. As fluid is lost into the interstitial spaces, a further reduction in cardiac output occurs, accompanied by vasodilation. Because the infant maintains cardiac output by increasing heart rate preferentially to stroke volume, extremely elevated heart rates result in a decreased filling time and a further reduction in cardiac output.[55] Adequate resuscitation returns cardiac output to normal levels in approximately 24 to 36 hours. Without fluid replacement, cardiac output continues to decrease and results in organ failure and death.

The inefficient and labile peripheral circulation of the infant further complicates management of the burn shock phase of treatment. The rapid fluid shift to the interstitial space and drying of the eschar result in compromised circulation and a resultant tourniquet effect in the extremities. Blood vessels and nerves become entrapped because the fascia cannot expand to accommodate the massive edema. Release of pressure is required to restore blood flow and preserve nerve function (Figure 47-5).

Constriction of the chest and impairment of respiratory excursion also may result, especially in the very young child, because of the increased pliability of the rib cage. Excessive fluid volume can contribute to a serious complication (increased intraabdominal pressure) that may have an underesti-

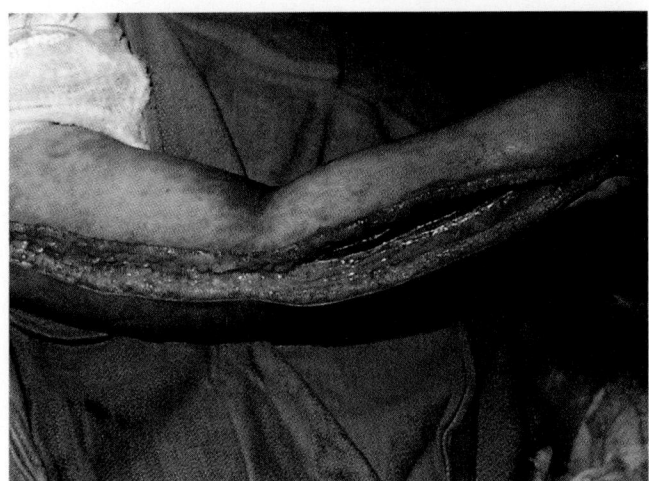

Figure 47-5 Escharotomy/fasciotomy in a severely burned arm.

mated incidence in burned individuals[57] (see What's New? on p. 1650). Although children with increased intraabdominal pressure readings tended to be younger, larger TBSA injuries and full-thickness components were significantly associated with elevated pressures.[57] Increased **intraabdominal pressure** has the potential to impair hemodynamics, renal function, hepatic malperfusion, and pulmonary dysfunction. Despite maintaining cardiac output with fluid replacement, renal function remains impaired in the presence of increased intraabdominal pressure. Increases in the production and release of the hormones norepinephrine, dopamine, epinephrine, angiotensin, and renin support the clinical finding of profoundly altered renal, pulmonary, and cardiovascular function.

Renal System

Loss of circulating volume into the interstitial spaces results in reduced renal blood flow and decreased glomerular filtration. An important measure of the adequacy of volume replacement is urine excretion. Sufficient volume replacement maintains urine output during resuscitation. Approximately 36 hours after injury, edema fluid begins to mobilize and output increases.

Evidence of pigment in the urine results from the hemolysis of red blood cells. This is especially common after extensive electrical injuries and destroyed muscle from deep thermal injury. The release of **myoglobin** may occlude the kidney tubules and result in renal failure.

Children younger than 2 years lack the ability to concentrate urine because of the immaturity of the renal system and are therefore at increased risk for dehydration. In addition, the child has a relatively larger TBSA in relation to weight than the adult. Combined with limited physiologic reserves, increased fluid requirements are necessary for children both during burn shock resuscitation and to compensate for evaporative water losses.[58]

Gastrointestinal System

The gastrointestinal (GI) system plays an important role in the pathophysiology of burns. Alterations in blood flow result in decreased perfusion to the gastrointestinal tract. Ischemia may cause erosion and necrosis of gastrointestinal tissue. The GI response to a burn injury often includes mucosal atrophy, changes in digestive absorption, and increased intestinal permeability. Depending on the proportion of burn size, atrophy of small bowel mucosa occurs within 12 hours of injury. The atrophy may also result in a reduced uptake of glucose and amino acids, as well as decreased absorption of fatty acids and a reduction of brush border lipase activity.[59]

Paralytic ileus occurs often after major burn injuries. Although digestion ceases in the stomach and the large bowel, the small intestine maintains motility and absorptive capacity. Intestinal motility returns as fluid losses are replaced unless irreversible necrosis of the bowel has occurred as a result of insufficient perfusion.

Metabolism

Complex metabolic alterations are observed after burn injury. The extent of metabolic derangement is proportional to the magnitude of TBSA burn sustained. Wilmore[60] demonstrated the linear increase in metabolic rate up to $2\frac{1}{2}$ times normal resting energy expenditure. As burn injury approaches 50% of TBSA, a plateau is reached, limiting further physiologic response to the trauma or other challenges such as infection.

A biphasic pattern of physiologic response is evident in thermally injured children. The initial **ebb phase** occurs during the immediate postburn period and continues for 3 to 5 days. This phase is characterized by reduced oxygen consumption, impaired circulation, and cellular shock. After the resolution of the shock and the restoration of circulating volume, the metabolic response shifts to a **catabolic (flow) phase** (Table 47-9). A state of **hypermetabolism** ensues, characterized by increased oxygen consumption and elevation of catecholamines, glucocorticoids, and glucagon.

Increased blood flow to the wound supplies additional glucose necessary for tissue repair. Insulin levels are usually normal or even elevated but are inappropriately low in relation to glucagon. Both catecholamines and glucocorticoids act as antagonists to insulin. This effect combined with a tissue resistance to insulin stimulates glycogenolysis and gluconeogenesis, thus increasing glucose flow from the liver.[61] In the child, glycogen stores for meeting the increased energy demands of the burn are limited. The initiation of protein and lipid catabolism for glycogenesis is accelerated. This prolonged metabolic dysfunction may lead to loss of lean body mass and increased morbidity.[62]

Metabolic rates slowly return to normal with wound closure. However, a reactivation of the hypermetabolic response may occur with sepsis or organ failure.

Immune Function

Burn trauma–induced immunosuppression results in increased susceptibility to infection and sepsis. Although the exact mechanisms responsible for this immunosuppression remain obscure, it is clear that complex interactions of the

Table 47-9	Metabolic Alterations Following Injury	
Response	Dominant Factors	Clinical Findings
Ebb response	Loss of plasma volume Shock Low plasma insulin levels	Hyperglycemia Decreased oxygen consumption Depressed resting energy expenditure Decreased blood pressure Cardiac output below normal Decreased body temperature
Flow response Acute phase	Elevated catecholamines Elevated glucagons Elevated glucocorticoids Normal or elevated insulin levels High glucagons/insulin ratio	Catabolic Hyperglycemia Increased respiratory rate Increased oxygen consumption Increased body temperature Redistribution of polyvalent cations such as zinc and iron Mobilization of metabolic reserves Increased urinary excretion of nitrogen, sulfur, magnesium, phosphorus, potassium Accelerated gluconeogenesis
Adaptive phase	Stress hormone response subsiding	Anabolic Normoglycemia Energy turnover diminished Convalescence

From Gottschlich M, Alexander JW, Bower RH. In Rombeau JL, Caldwell MD, editors: *Enteral and tube feeding,* Philadelphia, 1990, Saunders.

hypermetabolic response, nutritional support, bacterial translocation, and defects in both innate and acquired immune function are involved (Figure 47-6). In addition, young children are at increased risk for microbial invasion caused by an immature immune system and limited antibody production.

Deitch reported that wound- or gut-derived endotoxemia may be one of the mediators of the hypermetabolic response observed after thermal injury.[63] When bacteria translocate from the gut or from the burn wound, endotoxin may affect immunologic response as inflammatory mediators are released. A further complication in the activation of inflammatory mediators is the release of toxic metabolites, such as oxygen free radicals.[64]

Circulating immunoglobulins may be affected by several factors, including age and the severity of injury.[65] Therapeutic interventions such as multiple transfusions, surgical procedures, and antibiotic and anesthetic administration also introduce elements that confound the evaluation of immunosuppressive effects. The alterations in the immune response are complex and result from the interaction of the components of the immune system that are initiated at the time of injury.[66]

Scar Maturation

In normal epidermal healing, minimal disruption in skin color, texture, and thickness occurs. However, burn wounds that extend into the dermis are repaired through **scar formation** and may result in an overgrowth of dermal constituents (Figure 47-7). Accelerated collagen synthesis most likely begins with high levels of activity in granulation tissue. The **hypertrophic scar** consists of hypercellular and disorganized connective tissue that is erythematous, raised, and pruritic. Normal dermis contains thick fibers and fiber bundles running parallel to the surface. In the hypertrophic scar, the collagen is arranged in whorls and nodules which account for its inelasticity and increased turgor.[67] As the hypertrophic scar matures, collagen begins to orient in a more parallel fashion and vascularity decreases (Figure 47-8). Collagen synthesis is very active soon after wound closure, and alteration of the scar can be accomplished before strong cross-linking of the collagen is established.

Although duration of wound healing varies among individuals, the length of time required to achieve wound closure is the most reliable predictor of hypertrophic scarring. Deeper burns demonstrate increased scarring caused by the formation of granulation tissue and prolonged healing time. Generally, darker-pigmented races are more susceptible to hypertrophic scarring.[68] Although age has not been found to be a predictor of hypertrophic scar formation, younger individuals are more susceptible to trauma and have greater skin tension and an accelerated rate of collagen synthesis. Increased tension with resultant trauma stimulates inflammation, which in turn results in the formation of additional collagen.

CLINICAL MANIFESTATIONS The clinical manifestations of burn injuries are apparent in all organ systems. Although the cutaneous trauma is the initiator of the chain of responses, it is important to consider all of the likely consequences of the injury. An awareness of the changing patterns of convalescence and the development of complications assists in the identification and early treatment of potential sequelae.

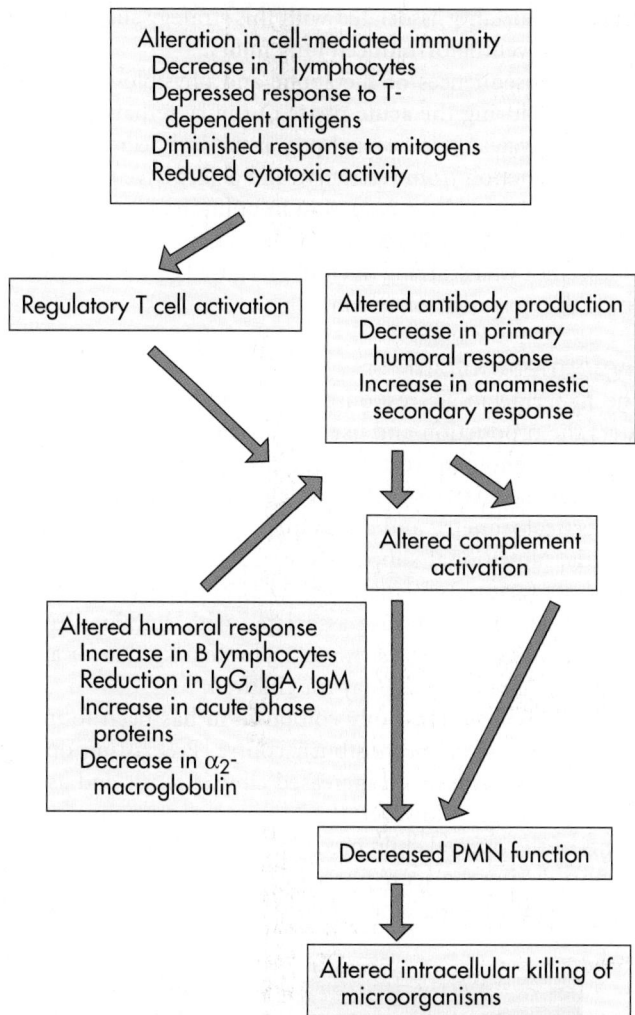

Figure 47-6 Altered immune function after thermal injury. Cell-mediated immunity, antibody production, humoral response.

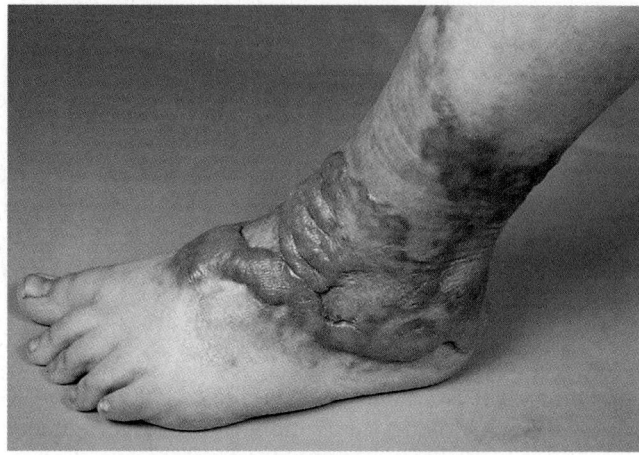

Figure 47-7 Immature hypertrophic scar.

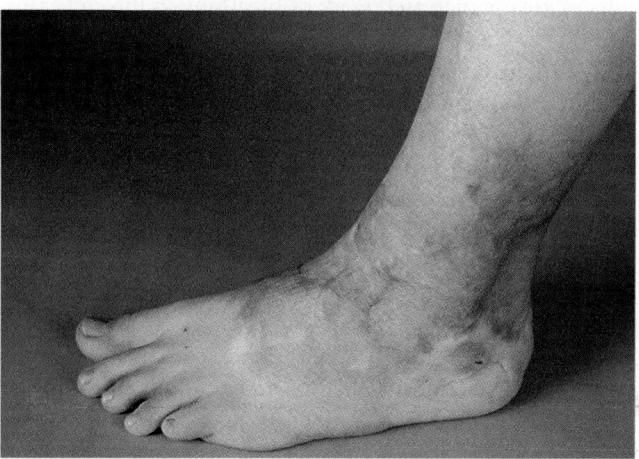

Figure 47-8 Flat, mature scar after pressure therapy.

Burn Shock

The pathophysiologic responses of burn injury result in **hypovolemia** and extracellular sodium depletion in the burn-injured individual. These manifestations are discussed in Chapter 46. Hypotension is a late sign of shock in the child. A complete circulatory assessment, including heart rate and peripheral parameters, is a more reliable measure. The urine output is a reflection of end-organ perfusion and is therefore the most accurate monitor of the adequacy of fluid resuscitation. A urine output of 30 to 50 ml/hr in adults and 1 ml/kg/hr in children weighing less than 30 kg are the suggested endpoints associated with many resuscitation formulas. Fluid is titrated to maintain the output within these parameters.[57]

The fluid of choice for burn shock resuscitation should approximate the fluid lost from the circulating volume—for example, lactated Ringer solution. Children require fluid resuscitation for smaller burns than do adults as a result of their limited physiologic reserves. The child's relatively greater ratio of body surface area to weight results in increased evaporative water losses and proportionately more fluid during resuscitation. Although **colloid replacement** during burn shock resuscitation remains controversial, replacement may be required in the very young child who fails to respond to fluid replacement.[69] A component for **maintenance fluid** *must* be included in the calculation of fluid needs during resuscitation. Maintenance fluids represent the body requirements in the absence of burn injury. Resuscitation is considered complete when the child is able to maintain urine output for 2 hours with fluid rates at maintenance levels.

Successful resuscitation depends on establishment of intravenous access. Although this is usually accomplished by peripheral or central venous cannulation, circulatory collapse may preclude timely administration of fluid replacement. Cannulation of veins in the pediatric population is further complicated by small vessels and increased subcutaneous fat. Children are good candidates for **intraosseous cannulation** when traditional venous access techniques fail. Blood, drugs, and fluid are readily absorbed by red marrow that drains into medullary venous channels and thus to the systemic circulation. This technique is most effective in children younger than 5 years, because red marrow is steadily replaced by yellow marrow in the limbs, making infusion more difficult, hence decreasing the infusion rate.[70] With proper care and removal as soon as other access is available, complications are minimal.

Pulmonary System

The clinical manifestations of burn injury related to the pulmonary system include a variety of complications ranging from inhalation injury, pulmonary edema, and respiratory failure to aspiration of gastric contents and pneumonia. Inhalation injury remains a major determinant of morbidity and mortality.[71]

Anatomic differences in the pediatric airway affect the response to pulmonary complications as well as therapeutic interventions. The infant airway is positioned anteriorly, making visualization of the cords more difficult. The difficult visualization is further compounded by the relatively large tongue and slanting vocal cords. A small degree of edema results in greatly increased work of breathing in the child (Figure 47-9). These considerations are particularly important during the resuscitation phase, when progressive edema threatens to obstruct the airway. Significant edema results in impairment of respiratory function unless an artificial airway is inserted (Figure 47-10). Malposition of an endotracheal tube may result in inadvertent extubation, intubation of the bronchi, and atelectasis. Because of the relatively short length of the infant trachea, alterations of the position of the head and neck can affect tube position despite maintenance of the tube position at the teeth.[72-74]

Infants compensate for pulmonary compromise by increasing the respiratory rate. However, since the child possesses fewer type I muscle fibers, fatigue related to the increased work of breathing results in more rapid desaturation than in adults. The soft cartilage of the pediatric airway is prone to collapse in the presence of partial obstruction. Children with burns are at increased risk for these events because of underlying respiratory disease or injury.

Therapeutic interventions required for maintenance of pulmonary function also have been implicated in postextubation stridor and barotrauma. A mixture of helium and oxygen has been successfully used to decrease airway resistance and increase the volume of gas exchange after extubation.[75] Recent evidence suggests barotrauma from mechanical ventilation may be minimized by protocols based on permissive hypercapnia. Moderate respiratory acidosis was well tolerated and ventilating pressures maintained below 40 cm.[76] The low incidence of mortality associated with this strategy suggests a reduction in ventilator-induced lung injury.

The consequences of metabolic and physiologic changes occurring during the acute phase of injury remain apparent during convalescence. Severe burns result in a decrease in pulmonary function from restrictive and obstructive pulmonary disease evidenced by a reduction in pulmonary volumes and maximum voluntary ventilation lasting up to 8 years. At times, chest wall scarring in children caused by burns severely limits thoracic cage excursion.

Hypermetabolism

The hypermetabolic response after burn injury profoundly alters the production and use of nutrients. As a consequence of these phenomena, caloric requirements increase dramatically. Advances in burn care have allowed the performance of indirect calorimetry and assessment of metabolic rate at the bedside. Nutritional support must have an increased metabolic rate factored in (increased by 10% to 20%) because of fluctuations in energy use associated with activity. Current recommendations suggest 1.5 to 2 g protein/kg/day for adults and up to 3 g protein/kg/day for children.[77]

In addition to age, body composition has been found to significantly affect the postburn course. Preexisting obesity has been associated with increased clinical sepsis and associated morbidity.[78] However, the heightened nutrient requirements of the burned child preclude a reduction in nutritional support during the acute phase of recovery. Aggressive nutritional therapy is critical to the recovery of these children, and

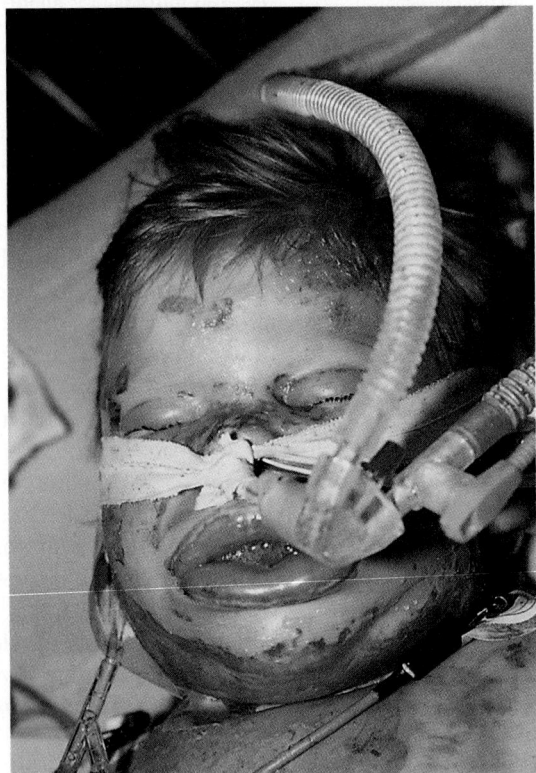

Figure 47-10 Severe facial edema during burn shock.

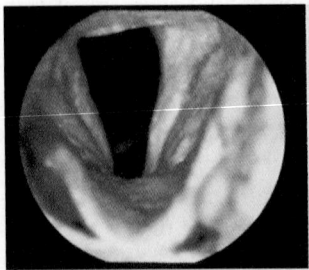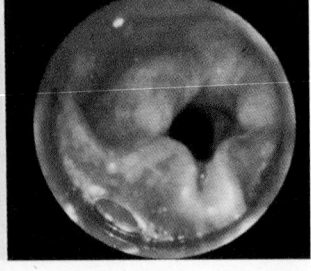

Figure 47-9 Airways. Adult airway *(left)*; smaller pediatric airway *(right)*.

programs designed to achieve ideal body weight should not be instituted until wound healing is achieved.

Metabolism and excretion of many micronutrients are greatly affected by burn injury.[77] Hypermetabolism results in a rapid turnover in vitamins and trace minerals important in the wound healing and immune response. A deficiency of specific nutrients interferes with carbohydrate and nucleic acid metabolism, collagen formation, and immune function.

The **thermoregulatory response** after burn injury results in an elevation in core body temperature. Burned individuals strive for temperatures of about 38° C. Depressed or "normal" temperature may be indicative of overwhelming sepsis, or an exhausted physiologic capability to maintain temperature, and should be viewed as an ominous sign. Routine methods of heat conservation after a major burn injury are inadequate because of excessive heat loss through convection and evaporation.[77] Therapeutic intervention, such as operative procedures and dressing changes, and transport present situations requiring increased diligence to prevent inadvertent cooling.[77,79] Infants are at increased risk for a precipitous drop in core body temperature caused by an inability to regulate heat loss by shivering. Heat is also lost because of evaporation of water from damaged skin surfaces. Infants and children are especially vulnerable because of the large surface area relative to metabolically active tissue.

Infection

Whereas shock and pulmonary compromise present the most immediate threat after burn trauma, both local and systemic infections become the primary complication during healing. The burn wound initially is relatively free of pathogens; however, dead, avascular tissue and wound exudate provide a fertile environment for bacterial growth. Colonization of the wound is apparent by the fifth postburn day. Gram-positive microorganisms are usually recovered from cultures first, followed by opportunistic gram-negative bacteria. The impaired vascular supply to burned tissue enhances the proliferation of pathogenic microorganisms. Bacterial invasion results in

thrombosis and a further impairment of circulation sufficient to convert a partial-thickness injury to a full-thickness wound.

Improvements in treatment have resulted in a reduction in wound infection. Aggressive excision and grafting of the wounds, improved nutritional support, and the development of microorganism-specific topical antimicrobials have contributed to this trend. However, the incidence of septicemia remains relatively constant. This is perhaps explained by the survival of children with burns of increasingly large body surface area. The burn wound serves as the site of primary invasion for the majority of instances of local or generalized infection. Because the burned child is immune suppressed for many weeks after injury, maintaining wounds at low contamination levels by meticulous wound care decreases the frequency and duration of septic episodes caused by wound flora.[80]

Functional Limitations

Children require specialized management to ensure optimal functional and cosmetic results. Scar and contracture management is necessary for prolonged periods because of changes in body composition as the child grows and matures. Very young children present unique challenges because the small body size can be difficult to fit with pressure garments and splints, growth is rapid, and cooperation with the rehabilitation program is limited. Children are reluctant to move when doing so causes pain, and they are likely to assume a position of comfort. Unfortunately, this position is often one that results in contracture formation and loss of function. Proper positioning and splint application are necessary to maintain body alignment. Physical therapy and occupational therapy provide exercise to maintain range of motion and function.

Infant skin is thinner, and the epidermis is more loosely connected to the dermis. This increases the risk of blistering, chafing, and rash formation. The infant also produces less sebum and sweat, which further exacerbates the propensity to skin irritation. Since scar tissue contains no sweat glands, these characteristics of the skin in growing children compound the difficulty in maintaining pressure on maturing scars while cooling the body.

Scar tissue is metabolically active and highly vascular. Collagen is deposited in random patterns, and contraction of the scar can result in disabling deformities. The scar is active as long as it is raised, red, and firm. **Scar maturation** requires 1 to 2 years and depends on individual differences and compliance with the rehabilitation program. The mature scar is characterized by increased suppleness, flattening, and pigmented color.

Scar tissue does not grow and expand like normal tissue. Although massage therapy offers some benefit in stretching, functional limitation may develop as the child grows. This is particularly evident over joints. Reconstructive surgery is often necessary to restore anatomic integrity and to promote independent function.

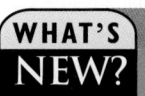

WHAT'S NEW? **Infection: A Major Cause of Morbidity and Mortality After Burn Injury**

Although a complex problem, it is clear that alterations in the innate immune system have been directly correlated with infections. Either a hyperactive or suppressed polymorphonuclear neutrophil (PMN) response can be detected. By monitoring decreases in the cell-surface expression of CD11b (cell surface receptor), systemic infections can be predicted in a statistically significant manner. Many of the dysfunctional properties associated with an individual's PMNs are correlated with the expression of hsp70 (heat shock protein). This stress-induced protein appears to interfere with many normal cellular functions. By carefully monitoring the specific properties of PMNs associated with infection, early diagnosis is possible.

Data from Babcock GF: *Clin Cytometry* 53B:48, 2003.

Itching may occur at any time during burn wound healing. As a complication, healed skin may be scratched away in an effort to obtain relief. The combination of H_1 and H_2 antagonists may be used to control itching.[81]

EVALUATION AND TREATMENT   The initial assessment conducted on admission to the burn center includes maintenance of an adequate airway, fluid resuscitation to manage burn shock, and the evaluation and treatment of the wound itself. Other therapies are initiated throughout the course of treatment. Nutritional support is essential to ensure an optimal outcome. Positioning and splinting to prevent contracture formation as well as rehabilitative aspects of therapy are instituted on admission and continue throughout the hospitalization. Psychosocial support is very important for both the child and the family. The information provided should be consistent and honest to allow clarification of concerns.

Fluid Resuscitation

Fluid resuscitation is generally required for children after thermal injuries in excess of 15% to 20% of the TBSA. Fluid is administered to compensate for the fluid and electrolytes extravasating into the interstitial spaces. This replacement restores circulating volume, improves perfusion, and alleviates organ dysfunction associated with impaired circulation.

Various protocols have been proposed as guidelines for fluid administration. It is important to remember that any regimen serves merely as a guideline and will require adjustment based on the individual response of each child. Because the linear relationship between weight and surface area does not exist in children (surface area varies to weight as a two-thirds function), use of adult formulas result in under- or over-resuscitation.[62] A commonly employed protocol consists of a modification of the Parkland formula. Children also tend to require relatively more fluids than adults because they have higher evaporative losses because of their body surface area/weight ratio. **Evaporative fluid loss** can be a significant contributor to hypovolemia in the burned child. This evaporative fluid loss

continues until the burn wounds are closed. As in adults, inhalation injury also continues until burn wounds are closed. And again, as in adults, inhalation injury also increases the magnitude of total body surface area injury and, therefore, children with burn injuries require more fluids.[57]

Wound Management

The goals of wound management include prevention of infection, removal of devitalized tissue, and closure of the wound. Burns that are clearly deep dermal or full-thickness injuries are surgically excised as soon as the child is hemodynamically stable after resuscitation. Early excision reduces the incidence of wound infection and systemic sepsis.[82] Coverage of the excised wound is necessary to achieve wound closure. The choice of a coverage technique depends on the availability of donor skin.

Split-thickness sheet grafts are selected for areas of maximal functional and cosmetic results (Figure 47-11). Children with very large burn injuries often do not have sufficient unburned skin available to facilitate use of the sheet graft. In these cases the surgeon employs a meshing technique to expand the available skin and increase the size of the graft. The pattern created heals by migration of epithelium from the meshed edges. Scar formation is increased, and the mesh pattern will remain clearly visible (Figure 47-12). The color, texture, vascularity, thickness, and hair-bearing nature of the skin varies from one area to another. The nearer the donor site, the more closely the skin will match. Skin grafts for the face that are taken from below the clavicle tend to take on a yellowish or brown hue.[83] Ongoing research and further refinement of the cultured skin substitutes has produced a source of autologous skin when donor sites are limited.[84,85]

Pulmonary Support

Smoke inhalation has a negative, prolonged effect on pulmonary function that has been associated with increased morbidity and mortality for the burned individual. Mechanical ventilation of severe inhalation injury is a dynamic and

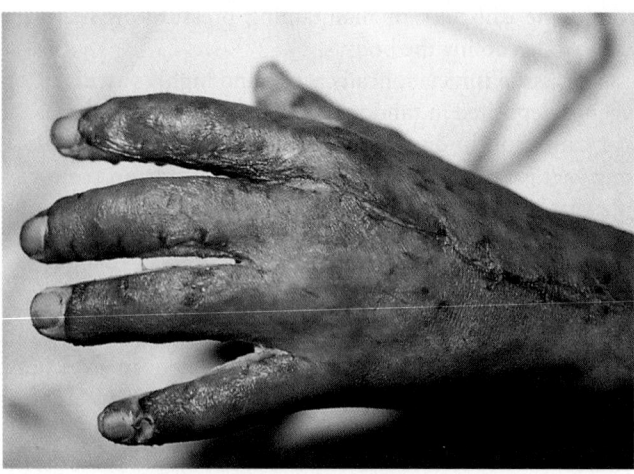

Figure 47-11 Split-thickness sheet graft.

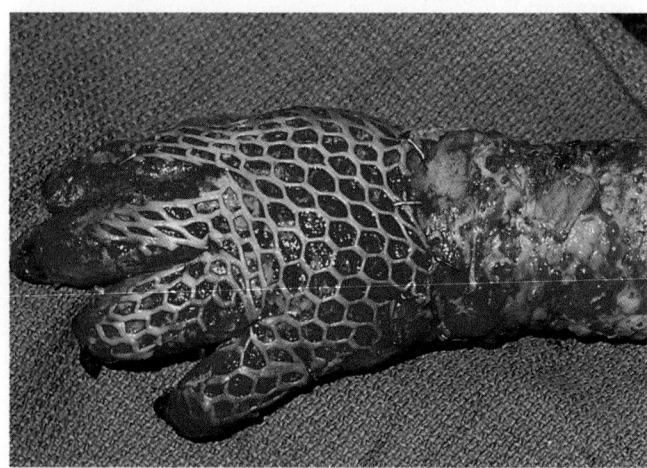

Figure 47-12 Meshed autograft.

complex task.[86,87] In order to avoid barotrauma from high ventilating pressures and concentrations of oxygen, current management attempts to support pulmonary function through permissive hypercapnia and high-frequency percussive ventilation.[88] When this therapy fails, improvements in intrapulmonary shunt and pulmonary artery pressures may be realized by the inhalation of nitric oxide. This pulmonary vasodilator has been shown to offer short-term benefit in this population. However, long-term impact on survival remains controversial.[89] Use of extracorporeal membrane oxygenation (ECMO), another technique available for children resistant to conventional support, allows cardiopulmonary rest by a prolonged bypass. Maximal benefit is associated with a careful balance between improvement of pulmonary function and life-threatening complications.[90]

Nutritional Support

The heightened metabolic demands after burn injury combined with a poor appetite often necessitate supplementation of oral intake. Children with burns in excess of 25% of TBSA often require supplementation with tube feeding. Feeding does not need to be delayed pending resolution of paralytic ileus and the resumption of bowel sounds because the small bowel maintains motility and absorptive capability. A small-bore feeding tube placed in the duodenum provides a safe route for the delivery of essential nutrients.[91] Gastric decompression is maintained by a nasogastric tube to prevent aspiration.[92] Parenteral hyperalimentation is reserved for those children who are unable to tolerate enteral support because of attendant risks of catheter sepsis and loss of intestinal integrity.[93] Early initiation of enteral supplementation along with aggressive management of complications permits successful enteral alimentation in most burned children.

Severe burn injury causes exaggerated muscle protein catabolism, contributing to weakness and delayed healing. Many therapeutic strategies have been used to avert the hypermetabolic response and improve clinical outcomes. Pharmacologic agents, such as recombinant growth hormone, low-dose insulin, and testosterone, have been shown to improve muscle kinetics and wound healing. However, these can cause serious side effects. Recently investigators found that anabolic steroid agents, along with nutritional support, improve muscle protein metabolism through enhanced protein

synthesis efficiency in both children and adults.[94] Outpatient follow-up should include regular weighing of the child and nutritional assessment to identify children at risk for further weight loss.

Comfort Management

Pain management presents a significant challenge in the pediatric population. In addition to procedural pain, there is a component of background pain that is present without activity. Pain perception is also affected by the degree of emotional overlay or affective experience.[95] The measurement of pain is particularly challenging in young infants, who lack the language skills to express pain. A variety of tools, from physiologic monitors to behavioral analyses and analog scales, have been developed to measure pediatric pain. The quality of pain control in burn centers has improved along with the ability to assess pain in the pediatric population. Studies have documented both pharmacologic and nonpharmacologic interventions that have improved the quality of pain control.[96]

Community Reintegration

Rehabilitation becomes the major focus of care once wound coverage has been achieved and continues until all reconstructive procedures have been completed. This phase may extend over many years in the pediatric population. In addition to the functional aspects of rehabilitation, attention must be directed to psychosocial needs and community reintegration. Children are increasingly surviving massive burn injuries because of advances in care in the past 20 years. However, adaptation to self-image and functional limitations poses serious issues for both the child and the family.[97,98] A method to facilitate the transition from the hospital to the community is the school reentry program offered by many burn centers. These programs provide education for teachers and peers about the injury, appearance, and abilities of the returning child.

A panel of experts have developed and tested a standardized, self-administered questionnaire for children between 5 and 18 years of age. This tool is designed to evaluate the effectiveness of burn management treatments and individual-oriented outcomes. Consistent ongoing measurement of outcomes will provide benchmarks and identify opportunities to continue to improve burn care.[99]

SUMMARY REVIEW

Shock and Multiple Organ Dysfunction Syndrome

1. Shock in children is present when there are signs of poor systemic perfusion, regardless of blood pressure.
2. Hypovolemic shock is the most common type of shock in children. Dehydration and trauma are the most common causes of hypovolemic shock.
3. Hypotension is a sign of severe, decompensated shock.
4. Hypovolemia can be caused by volume loss, an increase in the vascular space relative to the amount of volume, or a redistribution of intravascular volume.

5. Clinical manifestations of hypovolemic shock include inadequate systemic perfusion associated with intravascular fluid loss. Adrenergic compensatory mechanisms can produce tachycardia, redistribution of blood flow, peripheral vasoconstriction, cool extremities, delayed capillary refill, and oliguria.
6. Neurogenic shock is caused by a loss of vasomotor tone after severe injury to the spinal cord.
7. Clinical manifestations of neurogenic shock include warm skin, hypotension with a low diastolic blood pressure, and poor systemic perfusion.

Continued

8. Cardiogenic shock, with decreased cardiac output, is observed most commonly after cardiovascular surgery or with inflammatory diseases of the heart, such as cardiomyopathy and myocarditis. It is also found in children with obstructive congenital heart disease and those with drug toxicity or severe electrolyte or acid-base imbalances.

9. Clinical manifestations of cardiogenic shock include inadequate systemic perfusion despite adequate intravascular volume. Cardiac output is typically low. Adrenergic compensatory mechanisms are similar to those found in hypovolemic shock.

10. Sepsis in children caused by nosocomial infections is linked to gram-negative infections 40% of the time; gram-positive infections 40% of the time; and viruses, fungi, or rickettsial microorganisms 20% of the time. Sepsis can lead to septic shock.

11. Altered cytokine levels are associated with septic shock in children. Tumor necrosis factor (TNF) levels are directly related to mortality in newborns and children with meningitis and sepsis.

12. Sepsis is a systemic response to infection. It is present when manifestations of systemic inflammatory response syndrome (SIRS) are observed. SIRS is present when the child demonstrates two or more of the following as an acute change from baseline values: fever or hypothermia, tachycardia, tachypnea with respiratory alkalosis, and alteration in the white blood cell count. The newborn often develops hypothermia rather than fever as a sign of infection and may develop bradycardia instead of tachycardia.

13. Severe sepsis is present when the individual demonstrates evidence of SIRS and signs of organ dysfunction, hypoperfusion, or hypotension.

14. The development of septic shock is heralded when the child with severe sepsis develops signs of cardiovascular dysfunction. The child may become hypotensive despite adequate fluid resuscitation or require vasopressors to maintain blood pressure.

15. Reperfusion and inflammatory injury stimulate free oxygen radicals that can damage cell membranes, denature proteins, and disrupt chromosomes. This process likely affects endothelial cells and the microvasculature, causing multiple organ dysfunction syndrome (MODS).

16. Acidosis may be the most sensitive indicator of inadequate systemic perfusion in children. Hypotension is a late sign of shock in infants and children.

17. The goals of treatment for shock are maximization of oxygen delivery and minimization of oxygen demand. Airway, oxygenation, and ventilation must be supported. The child should be kept warm, and shivering should be prevented. Monitor the warmth of the child's extremities, capillary refill, quality of peripheral pulses, level of consciousness and responsiveness, urine output, oxygenation, ventilation, and acid-base status throughout shock therapy.

18. Treatment consists of immediate resuscitation, including fluid replacement (must be aggressive in septic shock), ventilation, pharmacologic support (e.g., vasopressors), electrocardiographic (ECG) analysis, hemodynamic monitoring, administration of blood or blood component therapy, and management of electrolyte and acid-base imbalances.

Burns

1. Burns in children are often the result of inadequate supervision, curiosity, inability to escape the burning agent, or intentional abuse.

2. Scald injuries are commonly seen in young children and result from exposure to hot water, grease, or other hot liquids, while flame burns are more prevalent among older children.

3. A child's skin is thinner and thus more susceptible to injury than adult skin. The kitchen and bathroom are common sites of burn injury.

4. It is estimated that from 6% to 20% of all child abuse cases in the United States result from burn injury.

5. Flame burns involving flammable liquids, most notably gasoline, are more common in older children. Risk-taking behaviors in young males can lead to electrical burns. Children may be exposed to chemical injury by swallowing caustic agents at home.

6. Use of the standard rule of nines results in inaccurate calculation of the percentage of total body surface area (TBSA) involved in children. A modified rule of nines deducts 1% from the head and adds 0.5% to each leg for each year of life after 2 years of age.

7. Major burn trauma involves all body systems, and the consequences of injury include shock, infection, hypermetabolism, organ failure, and functional limitations. These effects can be magnified in the pediatric population as a result of physiologic immaturity and age-related variation in treatment modalities.

8. Infection, trauma, or applying ice to the burn area may convert a partial-thickness injury to a full-thickness one, especially in young children, who have thinner, more delicate skin.

9. Marked reduction in cardiac output occurs immediately after injury and is accompanied by an initial increase in systemic vascular resistance. The inefficient and labile peripheral circulation of the infant complicates management of the burn shock phase of treatment. Constriction of the chest and impairment of respiratory excursion may occur in the very young child because of the increased pliability of the rib cage. Younger children are also more susceptible to increased intraabdominal pressure.

10. Children younger than 2 years lack the ability to concentrate urine because of the immaturity of the renal system and are therefore at increased risk for dehydration. Because children have a relatively larger body surface area in relation to weight than adults, they require proportionately increased fluid during burn shock resuscitation and to compensate for evaporative water losses.

11. A biphasic pattern of physiologic responses is evident in the burn injured child. The initial ebb phase occurs during the immediate postburn period and continues for 3 to 5 days. This phase is characterized by reduced oxygen consumption, impaired circulation, and cellular shock. After this phase and the restoration of volume, the metabolic response shifts to a catabolic, or flow, phase. This phase is characterized by hypermetabolism with an increased oxygen consumption and elevation of catecholamines, glucocorticoids, and glucagon.

12. Glycogen stores are limited in children, making it hard for them to meet the increased energy demands of the burn. This prolonged metabolic dysfunction may lead to loss of lean body mass, delayed healing, and increased morbidity.

13. Some children exhibit immunosuppression for a prolonged period after wound closure is achieved.

14. Although age was not found to be a predictor of hypertrophic scarring, children have greater skin tension and an accelerated rate of collagen synthesis.

15. Children require fluid resuscitation for smaller burns than do the adult population as a result of limited physiologic reserves. Colloid replacement may be required in the very young child who fails to respond to fluid replacement. Resuscitation is considered complete when the child is able to maintain urine output for 2 hours with fluid rates at maintenance levels.

16. The leading cause of death in children after burn injury, as in adults, is inhalation injury.

17. Children require specialized management to ensure optimal functional and cosmetic results. Long-term scar and contracture management is necessary because of changes in body composition as the child grows and matures.

KEY TERMS

MEDIA RESOURCES 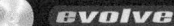 *evolve*

Review questions and answers for this chapter are available in the *CD Companion* included with this book.

WebLinks—links to Internet sites pertaining to this chapter—are available on Evolve at http://evolve.elsevier.com/McCance/.

REFERENCES

1. Gorelick MH, Shaw KN, Murphy KO: Validity and reliability of clinical signs in the diagnosis of dehydration in children, *Pediatrics* 99(5):E6, 1997.
2. Roberts KB: Fluid and electrolytes: parenteral fluid therapy, *Pediatr Rev* 22(11):380-387, 2001.
3. Hazinski MF: Children are different. In Hazinski MF, editor: *Manual of pediatric critical care*, St Louis, 1999, Mosby.
4. Michaud LJ et al: Elevated initial blood glucose levels and poor outcome following severe brain injuries in children, *J Trauma* 31(10):1356-1362, 1991.
5. Faustino EV, Apkon M: Persistent hyperglycemia in critically ill children, *J Pediatr* 146(1):30-34, 2005.
6. Chameides L, Hazinski MF, editors: *Textbook of pediatric advanced life support*, Dallas, 1997, American Heart Association.
7. Rudolph AM: *Congenital diseases of the heart*, Chicago, 1974, Year Book Medical.
8. Sevedra JM et al: Capillary refill (skin turgor) in the assessment of dehydration, *Am J Dis Child* 145:296, 1991.
9. Otieno H et al: Are bedside features of shock reproducible between different observers? *Arch Dis Child* 89(10):977-979, 2004.
10. Watson RS et al: The epidemiology of severe sepsis in children in the United States, *Am J Respir Crit Care Med* 167(5):695-701, 2003.
11. Singh-Naz N et al: Risk factors for nosocomial infections in critically ill children; a prospective cohort study, *Crit Care Med* 24(5):875-878, 1996.
12. Richards MJ et al: Nosocomial infections in pediatric intensive care units in the United States, *Pediatrics* 103(4e39):1-7, 1999.
13. Davenport SE: Frequency of handwashing by registered nurses caring for infants on radiant warmers and in incubators, *Neonatal Network* 11(1):21-25, 1992.
14. Donowitz LO: Hand-washing technique in a pediatric intensive care unit, *Am J Dis Child* 141:683, 1987.
15. Hazinski MF et al: Epidemiology, pathophysiology, and clinical presentation of gram-negative sepsis, *Am J Crit Care* 2(3):224-235, 1993.
16. Wheeler AP, Bernard GR: Treating patients with severe sepsis, *New Engl J Med* 340(3):207-214, 1999.
17. Sullivan JS et al: Correlation of plasma cytokine elevation with mortality rate in children with sepsis, *J Pediatr* 120(4 Pt 1):510-515, 1992.
18. Wong HR et al: Nitric oxide production in critically ill patients, *Arch Dis Child* 74(6):482-489, 1996.

19. Glauser MP: Pathophysiologic basis of sepsis; considerations for future strategies of intervention, *Crit Care Med* 28(9 Suppl):S4-S8, 2000.
20. Decker T: Sepsis: avoiding its deadly toll, *J Clin Investig* 113(10):1387-1389, 2004.
21. Haley M et al: Activated protein C in sepsis: emerging insights regarding its mechanism of action and clinical effectiveness, *Curr Opin Inf Dis* 17(3):205-211, 2004.
22. Bernard GR et al: Efficacy and safety of recombinant human activated protein C for severe sepsis, *N Engl J Med* 344(10):699-709, 2001.
23. Fisher CJ Jr, Yan SB: Protein C levels as a prognostic indicator of outcome in sepsis and related diseases, *Crit Care Med* 28(9 Suppl):S49-S56, 2000.
24. Matot I, Sprung CL: Corticosteroids in septic shock: resurrection of the last rites? *Crit Care Med* 26(4):627-630, 1998.
25. Riordan FA et al: Admission cortisol and adrenocorticotrophic hormone levels in children with meningococcal disease: evidence of adrenal insufficiency? *Crit Care Med* 27(10):2257-2261, 1999.
26. Minneci PC et al: Meta-analysis: the effect of steroids on survival and shock during sepsis depends on the dose, *Ann Intern Med* 141(1):47-51, 2004.
27. Carcillo JA, Fields AI, Task Force Committee Members: Clinical practice parameters for hemodynamic support of pediatric and neonatal patients in septic shock, *Crit Care Med* 30(6):1365-1378, 2002.
28. American College of Chest Physicians/Society of Critical Care Medicine Consensus Conference: definitions for sepsis and organ failure and guidelines for the use of innovative therapies in sepsis, *Crit Care Med* 20(6):864-874, 1992.
29. Hayden WR: Sepsis terminology in pediatrics, *J Pediatr* 124(4):657-658, 1994.
30. Goldstein B, Giroir B, Randolph A, Members of the International Consensus Conference on Pediatric Sepsis: International pediatric sepsis consensus conference: definitions for sepsis and organ dysfunction in pediatrics, *Pediatr Crit Care Med* 6(1):2-8, 2005.
31. Barriere SL, Lowry SF: An overview of mortality risk prediction in sepsis, *Crit Care Med* 23(2):376-393, 1995.
32. Parker MM et al: Serial cardiovascular variables in survivors and nonsurvivors of human septic shock: heart rate as an early predictor of prognosis, *Crit Care Med* 15(10):923-929, 1987.
33. Dantzker D: Oxygen delivery and utilization in sepsis, *Crit Care Med* 5:81, 1989.
34. Carcillo JA, Davis AL, Zaritsky A: Role of early fluid resuscitation in pediatric septic shock, *JAMA* 266(9):1242-1245, 1991.
35. Damjanov I, Linder J: *Anderson's pathology*, ed 10, St Louis, 1996, Mosby.
36. Waxman D: Shock: ischemia, reperfusion, inflammation, *New Horiz* 4:153, 1996.
37. Johnston JA et al: Importance of organ dysfunction in determining hospital outcomes in children, *J Pediatr* 144(5):595-601, 2004.
38. Hutton P et al: An assessment of the Dinamap 845, *Anesthesiology* 39:261, 1984.

39. Davis JW et al: Are automated blood pressure measurements accurate in trauma patients? *J Trauma* 55(5):860-863, 2003.

40. Cohn JN: Blood pressure measurement in shock: mechanisms of inaccuracy in auscultatory and palpatory methods, *JAMA* 199:188, 1967.

41. Oh MS, Carroll HJ: Electrolyte and acid-base disorders. In Chernow B, editor: *The pharmacologic approach to the critically ill patient,* ed 3, Baltimore, 1994, Williams & Wilkins.

42. Zaritsky A et al: CPR in children, *Ann Emerg Med* 16(10):1107-1111, 1987.

43. Whitlock D, Whitlock J, Coates TD: Hematologic and oncologic emergencies requiring critical care. In Hazinski MF, editor: *Nursing care of the critically ill child,* ed 2, St Louis, 1992, Mosby.

44. Cooper DJ et al: Prehospital hypertonic saline resuscitation of patients with hypotension and severe traumatic brain injury: a randomized controlled study, *JAMA* 291(11):1350-1357, 2004.

45. Moore FA, McKinley BA, Moore EE: The next generation in shock resuscitation, *Lancet* 363(9425):1988-1996, 2004.

46. Reeves JH et al: Continuous plasmafiltration in sepsis syndrome, *Crit Care Med* 27(10):2096-2104, 1999.

47. Carcillo JA: Mannose-binding lectin deficiency provides a genetic basis for the use of SIRS/sepsis definitions in critically ill patients, *Intensive Care Med* 30(7):1263-1265, 2004.

48. Fidler KJ et al: Increased incidence and severity of the systemic inflammatory response syndrome in patients deficient in mannose-binding lectin, *Intensive Care Med* 30(7):1438-1445, 2004.

49. Committee on Trauma: *Resource for optimal care of the injured patient* [pamphlet], 1999, American College of Surgeons.

50. Sheridan R et al: Early burn center transfer shortens the length of hospitalization and reduces complications in children with serous burn injuries, *J Burn Care Rehabil* 20(5):347-350, 1999.

51. National Safe Kids Campaign: *Burn injury,* 1999. Available online at www.firehouse.com/safekids/factsheets/burn_inj.html.

52. Peck MD, Priolo-Kapel D: Child abuse by burning: a review of the literature and an algorithm for medical investigators, *J Trauma* 53(5):1013, 2002.

53. Giardino AP: Child abuse and neglect: physical abuse. In Johnson C et al, editors: *eMedicine,* 2005. Available online at www.emedicine.com/PED/topic2648.htm.

54. Devlin BK, Reynolds E: Child abuse: how to recognize it, how to intervene, *Am J Nurs* 94(3):26, 1994.

55. Helvig E: Pediatric burn injuries, *AACN Clin Issues Crit Care Nurs* 4(2):433-442, 1993.

56. Sheridan R, Tompkins R: Alternate wound coverings. In Herndon DN, editor: *Total burn care,* New York, 2002, Saunders.

57. Ahrns KS: Trends in burn resuscitation: shifting the focus from fluids to adequate end-point monitoring, edema control, and adjuvant therapies, *Crit Care Nurs Clin N Am* 16(1):75, 2004.

58. Warden GD: Burn shock resuscitation, *World J Surg* 1(1):16-23, 1992.

59. Wolf SE, Prough DS, Herndon DH: Critical care in the severely burned: organ support and management of complications. In Herndon DN, editor: *Total burn care,* New York, 2002, Saunders.

60. Wilmore DW: Nutrition and metabolism following thermal injury, *Clin Plast Surg* 1(4):603-619, 1974.

61. Gottschlich MM: Nutrition in the burned pediatric patient. In Samour PQ, Helm KK, Lange C, editors: *Handbook of pediatric nutrition,* Gaithersburg, Md, 1999, Aspen.

62. Benjamin D, Herndon DN: Special considerations of age: the pediatric burned patient. In Herndon DN, editor: *Total burn care,* New York, 2002, Saunders.

63. Deitch EA: Nutritional support of the burn patient, *Crit Care Med* 11(3):735, 1995.

64. Supple KG: Physiologic response to burn injury, *Crit Care Nurs Clin N Am* 16(1):119, 2004.

65. Stratta RJ et al: Immunologic parameters in burned patients: effect of therapeutic interventions, *J Trauma* 26(1):7, 1986.

66. Harris BH, Gelfand JA: The immune response to trauma, *Semin Pediatr Surg* 4(2):77, 1995.

67. Scott PG, Ghahary A, Tredget EE: Molecular and cellular basis of hypertrophic scarring. In Herndon DN, editor: *Total burn care,* New York, 2002, Saunders.

68. Deitch EA et al: Hypertrophic burn scars: analysis of variables, *J Trauma* 23(10):895-898, 1983.

69. Cocks AJ, O'Connell A, Martin H: Crystalloids, colloids, and kids: a review of paediatric burns in intensive care, *Burns* 24(8):717-724, 1998.

70. Tintinalli JE, Kelen GD, Stapczynski JS, editors: *Emergency medicine: a comprehensive study guide,* New York, 2000, McGraw-Hill.

71. Cox R et al: Enhanced pulmonary expression of endothelin-1 in an ovine model of smoke inhalation, *J Burn Care Rehabil* 22(6):375, 2001.

72. Conrardy PA et al: Alteration of endotracheal tube position, *Crit Care Med* 4(2):8, 1976.

73. Sharar SR: Endotracheal tube tip position in an infant with severe burns, *J Burn Care Rehabil* 16(6):654, 1995.

74. Trout S et al: Influence of head and neck position on endotracheal tube tip position on chest x-ray examination: a potential problem in the infant undergoing intubation, *J Burn Care Rehabil* 15(5):405-407, 1994.

75. Rodeberg DA et al: Use of a helium-oxygen mixture in the treatment of postextubation stridor in pediatric patients with burns, *J Burn Care Rehabil* 16(5):476-480, 1995.

76. Sheridan RL et al: Permissive hypercapnia as a ventilatory strategy in burned children: effect on barotrauma, pneumonia, and mortality, *J Trauma* 39(5):854, 1995.

77. Saffle JR, Hildreth M: Metabolic support of the burned patient. In Herndon DN, editor: *Total burn care,* New York, 2002, Saunders.

78. Gottschlich MM et al: Significance of obesity on nutritional, immunologic, hormonal, and clinical outcome parameters in burns, *J Am Diet Assoc* 93(11):1261, 1993.

79. Kagan R, Jenkins M: Transport and management of children with burns and inhalation injuries. In Jaimovich DG, Vidyasagar D, editors: *Handbook of pediatric and neonatal transport medicine,* Philadelphia, 1996, Hanley & Belfus.

80. Heggers JP et al: Treatment of infection in burns. In Herndon DN, editor: *Total burn care,* New York, 2002, Saunders.

81. Baker RU et al: Burn wound itch control using H₁ and H₂ antagonists, *J Burn Care Rehabil* 22(4):263, 2001.

82. Petersen SR, Umphred E, Warden GD: The incidence of bacteremia following burn wound excision, *J Trauma* 22(4):274-279, 1982.

83. Robson MC: Overview of burn reconstruction. In Herndon DN, editor: *Total burn care,* New York, 2002, Saunders.

84. Boyce ST et al: Assessment with the dermal torque meter of skin pliability after treatment of burns in cultured skin substitutes, *J Burn Care Rehabil* 21(1 Pt 1):55-63, 2000.

85. Boyce ST et al: The 1999 clinical research award. Cultured skin substitutes combined with Integra Artificial Skin to replace native skin autograft and allograft for the closure of excised full-thickness burns, *J Burn Care Rehabil* 20(6):453-461, 1999.

86. Merrel P, Mayo D: Inhalation injury in the burn patient, *Crit Care Nurs Clin N Am* 16(1):27, 2004.

87. Park GY et al: Prolonged airway and systemic inflammatory reactions after smoke inhalation, *Chest* 123(2):475, 2003.

88. Cortiella J, Mlcak R, Herndon D: High frequency percussive ventilation in pediatric patients with inhalation injury, *J Burn Care Rehabil* 20(3):232-235, 1999.

89. Sheridan RL et al: Low-dose inhaled nitric oxide in acutely burned children with profound respiratory failure, *Surgery* 126(5):856-862, 1999.

90. Cedidi C et al: Survival of severe ARDS with five-organ failure following burns and inhalation injury in a 15-year-old patient, *Burns* 29(4):389-394, 2003.

91. Gottschlich MM: Early and perioperative support. In Matarese L, Gottschlich MM, editors: *Contemporary nutrition support practice: a clinical guide,* Philadelphia, 2003, Saunders.

92. Jenkins ME, Gottschlich MM, Warden GD: Enteral feeding during operative procedures in thermal injuries, *J Burn Care Rehabil* 15(2):199-205, 1994.

93. Herndon DN et al: Failure of TPN to improve liver function, immunity, and mortality in thermally injured patients, *J Trauma* 2(2)7:195-204, 1987.

94. Hart DW et al: Anabolic effects of Oxandrolone after severe burn injury, *Ann Surg* 233(4):556, 2001.

95. Gordon M et al: Use of pain assessment tools: is there a preference? *J Burn Care Rehabil* 19(5):451-454, 1998.

96. Martin-Hertz SP et al: Pediatric pain control practices of North American burn centers, *J Burn Care Rehabil* 24(1):26, 2003.

97. Kendall-Grove, Ehde DM, Patterson DR, Johnson V et al: Rates of dysfunction in parents of pediatric patients with burns, *J Burn Care Rehabil* 19(4):312-316, 1998.

98. LeDoux J et al: Relationship between parental emotional states, family environment and the behavioral adjustment of pediatric burn survivors, *Burns* 24(5):425-432, 1998.

99. Daltroy LH et al: American Burn Association/Shriners Hospitals for Children burns outcomes questionnaire: construction and psychometric properties, *J Burn Care Rehabil* 21(1 Pt 1):29-39, 2000.

GLOSSARY

BETH A. FORSHEE

Absolute polycythemia a condition in which red blood cell mass is increased because of a defect in the erythroid progenitor cells or an increase in circulating serum factors such as erythropoietin.

Absolute refractory period a time interval during an action potential when membrane sodium channels are inactivated and cannot respond to additional stimuli.

Achalasia failure of a sphincter, usually an esophageal sphincter, to relax completely, often because of a neuromuscular disorder of the esophagus that reduces the ability to move food down the esophagus.

Acid maltase deficiency a genetic disease in which the deficiency in lysosomal metabolism prevents the breakdown of glycogen and causes it to accumulate in the lysosomes, leading to severe muscle degradation primarily in the heart, skeletal, and respiratory muscles.

Acidosis an acid-base imbalance characterized by reduction in arterial blood pH.

Acne conglobata a condition of severe cystic acne that is characterized by cystic lesions, abscesses, communicating sinuses, and thickened, nodular scars.

Acne rosacea a chronic form of dermatitis of the face in which the middle portion of the face appears red with small red lines caused by dilation of capillaries.

Acne vulgaris an inflammatory eruption usually occurring on the face, upper back, and chest, that consists of blackheads, cysts, papules, and pustules.

Acromegaly a condition of excessive growth hormone that originates from the anterior pituitary; it is manifest by progressive enlargement of the head, face, hands, feet, and chest.

ACTH deficiency a condition characterized by decreased or absent production of adrenocorticotropic hormone (ACTH) by the pituitary gland, resulting in a reduction in the secretion of adrenal hormones and subsequent weight loss, lack of appetite, weakness, nausea, vomiting, and low blood pressure.

Actin filaments (microfilaments) bundles of actin fibrils that aid in cell movement and structure and are necessary for regulating cell growth.

Actinic keratosis a condition in which a premalignant small, reddish, rough spot appears on skin that has been chronically exposed to the sun.

Action potential propagation of electrical changes in the membrane that is continued as long as the stimuli reach the electrical threshold of the membrane.

Active mediated transport (active transport) movement of a substance across a membrane, which is made possible by expenditure of energy that activates integral membrane carrier proteins; this movement is the polar opposite of the chemical and/or electrical gradient of the substance being transported.

Activin a protein hormone that opposes inhibin by enhancing follicle-stimulating hormone synthesis and secretion and that participates in the regulation of the menstrual cycle, enhances luteinizing hormone action in the ovary and testis, and mediates spermatogenesis.

Acute bacterial prostatitis inflammation of the prostate gland caused by urinary tract infection that results in chills, fever, pain in the lower back and genital area, body aches, burning or painful urination, and the frequent and urgent need to urinate.

Acute epiglottitis a bacterial infection that causes inflammation of the epiglottis and surrounding tissues and may lead to upper airway blockage, which increases the work of breathing, the retention of carbon dioxide, and reduction in oxygen intake and may cause death if left untreated.

Acute lymphoblastic leukemia (ALL) a cancer that is marked by excessive production and continuous multiplication of malignant and immature white blood cells in the bone marrow that spreads throughout the body rapidly if left untreated.

Acute myelogenous leukemia (AML) a cancer that is marked by an excessive number of immature myeloid cells in the blood and bone marrow.

Acute pericarditis a condition in which the pericardium is infected by a virus, bacteria, parasite, or fungus and becomes inflamed, resulting in pain and fluid and blood components entering into the pericardial space.

Acute rejection rejection of a graft within days to months after transplantation or termination of immunosuppressive drugs because of a cell-mediated immune response against incompatible antigens.

Acute renal failure (ARF) a condition characterized by the rapid loss of renal function resulting in retention of nitrogenous and nonnitrogenous waste products that may lead to metabolic disturbances, altered body fluid balance, or oliguria.

Acute respiratory distress syndrome (ARDS) a condition in which capillaries or alveoli of the lungs are damaged as a result of infection, injury, blood loss, or inhalation injury causing fluid to leak from the capillaries into the alveoli and causing some alveoli to collapse.

Acute tubular necrosis (ATN) a condition in which the kidney undergoes ischemic or nephrotoxic injury because of severe hypotension, aminoglycosides, and radiocontrast agents and produces granular and epithelial cell casts in urine.

Acute urethral syndrome a condition in which the bladder is irritated and the typical symptoms of a urinary tract infection are present in the absence of an infection.

Adaptive immunity immunity acquired from vaccines or prior infection.

Adenomyosis a condition characterized by benign masses of the endometrial glands in the uterine smooth muscle that typically occurs between the ages of 35 and 50 and causes painful menses.

Adhesion molecule *see* **Cell adhesion molecule.**

Adrenal gland either of two small endocrine glands that is located above the kidney and functions to secrete several steroid hormones and epinephrine and norepinephrine.

Adrenergic transmission transmission of a nerve impulse using epinephrine or norepinephrine as a neurotransmitter.

Adrenomedullin (ADM) a protein hormone discovered in human pheochromocytoma that functions as a vasodilator and a regulator of growth cytokines and neurotransmission.

Adventitious sounds extra or additional sounds that are heard over normal breath or heart sounds.

Afterload the tension or pressure that must be generated by a chamber of the heart in order to contract, such as that required to eject blood into the aorta.

Agnosia loss of comprehension of sensory stimuli, such as sounds or images.

Aldosterone mineralocorticoid that is synthesized and secreted by the adrenal cortex and acts to regulate sodium and potassium balance by altering reabsorption in the kidney.

Alkalosis an acid-base imbalance characterized by elevated pH.

Allergy hypersensitivity and immunologic protective reactions caused by exposure to an antigen.

Alloimmunity immune reaction in which individuals of the same species have incompatible antigens, preventing them from receiving an organ transplant from each other.

Alogia lack of additional, unprompted content typically seen in normal speech.

Alopecia a condition in which hair is lost because of hereditary factors, hormone imbalance, or certain diseases or drugs and treatments

Alveolar ventilation the volume of gas that reaches the alveoli per minute or the difference between tidal volume and dead space multiplied by ventilation rate.

Amebiasis an infection by a protozoan that is usually contracted by ingesting water or food contaminated by amoebic cysts but also may be contracted by homosexual sexual activity and may be asymptomatic or may cause diarrhea, vomiting, abdominal pain or discomfort, and fever.

Amino acid carboxylic acid with attached amino and R groups that combine with other amino acids to form a protein.

Amylin a peptide hormone that is secreted by the pancreatic beta cells and may function in the regulation of glucose homeostasis, gastric motor and secretory function, and gastroprotection.

Anabolism a cellular process that uses energy to synthesize complex molecules from simpler molecules.

Anaerobic glycolysis the process of adenosine triphosphate (ATP) formation in the absence of oxygen; during which, carbohydrate-derived pyruvate is reduced to form lactic acid.

Anaphase third phase of mitosis, during which centromeres are separated and sister chromatids are moved to opposite poles.

Anaphylactic shock a state of shock caused by a severe allergic reaction that lowers blood pressure and results in urticaria, breathing difficulties, and possibly death.

Anaphylatoxin fragments of C3a, C5a, and C4a that degranulate mast cells, resulting in the release of histamine that vasodilates and increases capillary permeability.

Anaphylaxis a potentially life-threatening immediate hypersensitivity response caused by exposure of a sensitized individual to a specific antigen.

Anaplasia inability of tumor cells to differentiate and orient to one another and to blood vessels.

Anemia a condition in which hemoglobin concentration is below normal because of a deficiency in red blood cells, a low level of hemoglobin in cells, or both; it manifests as pallor of the skin and mucous membranes, weakness, dizziness, easy fatigability, and drowsiness caused by oxygen deficiency.

Anemia of chronic disease (ACD) mild to moderate anemia secondary to a chronic disease such as infection, inflammation, or malignancies that causes hypoferrinemia.

Anencephaly congenital abnormality in which part of the brain and skull is absent.

Aneurysm a localized dilation or ballooning of a blood vessel, usually found in the arteries at the base of the brain and in the aorta.

Aneurysmal bone cyst (ABC) a benign blood-filled space in a long bone or vertebra that may be separated from another cyst by fibrous tissue and usually causes swelling, pain, and tenderness.

Angina pectoris a condition in which myocardial ischemia caused by reduced blood flow through the blood vessels of the heart causes chest pain.

Angiogenesis growth of a tumor that originates from blood vessels in surrounding tissues.

Angiotensin I inactive product of the cleavage of angiotensinogen by renin.

Angiotensin II active hormone that is formed from the cleavage of angiotensin I by angiotensin-converting enzyme and acts to stimulate aldosterone secretion and to vasoconstriction.

Anhedonia inability to experience pleasure from things that would normally be pleasurable.

Anion gap the difference between plasma cations and anions that is used to distinguish different causes of metabolic acidosis.

Ankylosing spondylitis (AS; spondyloarthritis) a condition in which the spine and sacroiliac joints are chronically inflamed, causing pain and stiffness in and around the spine and a gradual fusion of the vertebrae that immobilizes the spine.

Anoikis apoptosis caused by cell loss or inappropriate cell adhesion.

Anomalous viscosity the alteration in viscosity of suspensions such as blood in which the viscosity increases as blood flow decreases.

Anorexia nervosa (AN) a disorder with both psychologic and physiologic components that begins with dieting to lose weight and manifests into an inappropriate self-control behavior; continued restrictive eating may lead to starvation and eventually death.

Anoxia lack of oxygen caused by vascular obstruction.

Antibody a protein of the adaptive immune response that interacts with the antigen that induced its synthesis.

Anticipatory response the secretion of stress hormones in anticipation of a psychologic stressor.

Anticodon three-nucleotide sequence located on a tRNA that recognizes specific codons on mRNA molecules by way of complimentary base pairing.

Antidiuretic hormone (ADH) protein hormone that is produced in the hypothalamus, stored in and released from the posterior pituitary, and acts to increase water reabsorption in the kidney.

Antigen a molecule that binds to an antibody and initiates an immune response because of the body's recognition of that molecule as foreign.

Antigenic variation the process by which antigens change appearance by altering surface molecules, making it difficult for the immune response to maintain specificity.

Antimicrobial peptide protein released by epithelial cells that is toxic to some bacteria, fungi, and viruses and is capable of activating cells involved in innate and acquired immunity.

Antithrombin III (ATIII) deficiency a autosomal dominant disease that decreases the levels of antithrombin III, resulting in abnormal blood clots that may damage organs.

Antitoxin antibody formed against a specific toxin.

Aortic stenosis a condition in which the aortic valves do not open completely, thereby increasing afterload so that more pressure must be generated in the left ventricle to eject blood, a condition that results in ventricular hypertrophy.

Aphasia inability to articulate ideas or comprehend spoken or written language.

Aplastic anemia a condition in which the bone marrow does not produce adequate amounts of new cells to replenish the blood cells lost during insults such as an autoimmune disorder or exposure to radiation or substances such as benzene or certain drugs.

Aplastic crisis a condition that occurs when bone marrow temporarily ceases erythropoiesis, resulting in an acute fall in hemoglobin levels and subsequent anemia.

Apocrine sweat gland one of several sweat glands in the skin of the armpit, pubic region, and areolae of the breasts that produce a slightly viscous secretion in response to emotional stress or sexual excitement.

Apoptosis active process by which cells self-destruct in normal and pathologic tissues.

Appendicitis a condition in which the appendix becomes inflamed as a result of blockage of the opening from the appendix into the cecum; the appendix wall becomes infected and then ruptures allowing the infection to spread throughout the abdomen and cause pain, anorexia, fever, nausea, vomiting, and diarrhea.

Arrested (G0) state state during which cells that lack growth factor stimulation cease to proliferate after mitosis.

Arteriosclerosis a condition in which the blood vessel walls thicken, harden, lose elasticity, and typically accumulate lipids, resulting in elevated blood pressure and constriction of the coronary arteries and pain when walking caused by decreased perfusion to leg vessels.

Ascites a condition in which fluid accumulates in the peritoneal cavity because of liver disease, portal hypertension, tuberculosis, or nephritic syndrome, resulting in abdominal distention and para-umbilical herniations of the abdominal wall.

Asphyxial injury suffocation, strangulation, or chemical or drowning injury that results from oxygen deprivation in cells.

Aspiration the removal of a gas or fluid by suction or the sucking of fluid or a foreign body into the airway when breathing.

Aspiration pneumonitis a condition caused by the abnormal entry of fluids, particulate matter, or secretions into the lower airways that can lead to chemical pneumonitis caused by material toxic to lungs such as gastric acid; by bacterial infection; or by mechanical obstruction of the lower airways.

Asthma a chronic inflammatory respiratory disease marked by periodic attacks of wheezing, shortness of breath, a tight feeling in the chest, and a cough that produces mucus caused by an allergic reaction, certain drugs or irritants, exercise, or emotional stress.

Astrocyte neuroglial cell of the central nervous system that branches into many processes and functions to fill spaces between neurons and surrounding blood vessels.

Asymptomatic bacteriuria a bacterial urinary tract infection that is absent of any of the usual symptoms.

Atelectasis a condition in which part of a lung or a whole lung collapses and the alveoli deflate as a result of surgery, smoking, or blockage of a bronchiole.

Atherosclerosis a type of arteriosclerosis in which cholesterol and lipid deposits accumulate on the innermost layer of the walls of large and medium-sized arteries.

Atopic dermatitis (AD) a chronic hereditary skin disease characterized by intense itching and inflamed skin that causes redness, swelling, cracking, crusting, and scaling.

Atrial natriuretic peptide (ANP or factor) a protein hormone that is synthesized and released from the atria in response to high sodium concentration, high extracellular fluid volume, or high blood volume and functions to promote sodium excretion and to cause vasodilation in the circulatory system.

Atrial septal defect (ASD) any of a group of congenital heart diseases involving the interatrial septum of the heart that separates the right and left atria, which results in misdirected flow of blood between the two sides of the heart.

Atrioventricular canal (AVC) defect a condition in which a large hole is present in the center of the heart where the wall between the upper chambers joins the wall between the lower chambers, and the tricuspid and mitral valves are formed into a single large valve that crosses the defect.

Atrioventricular node (AV node) the tissue between the atria and the ventricles that contains pacemaker cells and is capable of setting the heart rate but mainly functions to slowly conduct the normal electrical impulse from the atria to the ventricles.

Autocrine stimulation the ability of a cell to secrete a substance that can feed back and provide continued stimulation or inhibition of that cell.

Autoimmune hemolytic anemia (AIHA) a form of hemolytic anemia involving autoantibodies against red cell antigens.

Autoimmunity a condition in which the immune system considers an individual's own body tissues to be foreign antigens and initiates an immune response against the tissues.

Autonomic hyperreflexia (dysreflexia) a syndrome resulting from a lesion above the splanchnic nerves that is characterized by hypertension, bradycardia, sweating of the forehead, severe headache, and gooseflesh upon distention of the bladder and rectum.

Autoregulation changes in blood vessel diameter to maintain a constant blood flow despite changes in arterial pressure.

Avolition lack of desire, motivation, and persistence resulting in the unwillingness to start or complete even simple daily tasks.

Axon hillock portion of the neuron where the cell body and axon join and the point where an action potential begins if stimulus magnitude reaches a critical threshold.

Bacterial pneumonia an acute or chronic disease marked by inflammation of the lungs caused by bacterial infection.

Bacterial tracheitis a condition in which the larynx, trachea, and bronchi are inflamed and present with signs similar to epiglottitis and croup; may result in airway obstruction secondary to subglottic edema or sloughing of the epithelial lining or the mucopurulent membrane within the trachea.

Bacterial vaginosis a condition caused by an overgrowth of normal vaginal bacteria that is characterized by vaginal discharge with a foul odor.

Bainbridge reflex a homeostatic mechanism that increases heart rate in response to stimulation of local muscle spindles when blood pressure in the venae cavae and right atrium is increased.

Balanitis inflammation of the glans penis caused by irritation by environmental substances, physical trauma, or infection.

Baroreceptor reflex a homeostatic mechanism consisting of baroreceptors that regulate the amount of blood being received by the tissues by altering cardiac output and resistance to maintain mean arterial blood pressure.

Baroreceptors nerve endings located in the heart, aortic arch, and carotid sinuses that sense changes in blood pressure and volume.

Basopenia a condition in which the number of basophils is decreased because of thyrotoxicosis, acute hypersensitivity reactions or infection.

Basophilia a condition in which the number of basophils in the blood is elevated as a result of hypothyroidism.

Bedbugs any of a group of small blood-sucking bugs that are flat-bodied, oval, reddish brown, and about $^1/_4$ inch long; bites from these bugs produce skin irritation.

Benign febrile seizure a condition that produces a tonic-clonic or tonic seizure that lasts less than 20 minutes in a 6-month-old to 5-year-old child.

Benign prostatic hyperplasia (BPH) a condition in which the prostate gland becomes enlarged and may press against the urethra and bladder, interfering with urine flow.

Benign tumor noncancerous but abnormal overgrowth or mass of cells; nonrecurrence and complete recovery after excision is common.

Biliary atresia a condition found in newborn children in which the biliary tract is blocked or absent, which results in liver failure caused by bile accumulation.

Bilirubin yellow-to-green pigment in bile that is derived from hemoglobin breakdown and causes jaundice when present in excess.

Bipolar disorder psychiatric disorder characterized by alternating mania and depression, often with periods of normal mood in between, and changes in energy and behavior according to mood.

Bladder neck dyssynergia a condition in which the bladder contracts but the external sphincter does not open, thereby preventing urination and causing urine reflux into the bladder and kidneys.

Blast injury tissue damage from compressive waves of air against the body followed by waves of decreased pressure.

Blood group antigens antigens present on the surface of erythrocytes that determine blood groups.

Blunt force injuries tearing, shearing, or crushing of tissues caused by blows, impacts or a combination of both.

B lymphocyte (B cell) cell of the adaptive immune response that originates in the bone marrow and differentiates into plasma cells and memory cells in the presence of an antigen.

Bohr effect the ability to reduce the affinity of hemoglobin for oxygen in response to an increase in blood carbon dioxide levels and a decrease in pH, thereby allowing the hemoglobin to bind and remove more carbon dioxide.

Bone matrix the intercellular substance of bone tissue containing collagen fibers, ground substance, and inorganic bone salts that form the major constituent of bone.

Bowman capsule a cup-shaped region of the nephron that surrounds the glomerulus and functions as a filter to remove organic wastes, excess inorganic salts, and water from the blood.

Bradykinin a protein produced during the plasma kinin cascade that acts to stimulate vasodilation and pain receptor activation and to increase capillary permeability.

Brain death (brain stem death) irreversible brain damage that renders an individual unresponsive to all stimuli and lacking in muscle activity such as that required for respiration and heart activity.

Brain stem gliomas a group of tumors located in the brain stem that is usually classified as high-grade and results in the sudden onset of symptoms including headaches, vomiting, and visual disturbances.

Bronchial carcinoid tumor an obstructing tumor of the trachea or large bronchi.

Bronchiectasis a condition in which the bronchi of the lungs become dilated in response to obstruction.

Bronchiolitis inflammation of the bronchioles usually caused by viral infection.

Bronchiolitis obliterans a condition in which the bronchioles and possibly some of the bronchi are partly or completely obliterated by granulation and fibrotic tissue masses.

Bronchopulmonary dysplasia (BPD) a condition most often found in premature infants in which chronic pulmonary insufficiency occurs because of long-term artificial pulmonary ventilation.

Bubo an inflamed, tender swelling of a lymph node, especially in the area of the armpit or groin, that is characteristic of infections such as syphilis.

Buffering the action of buffers minimizing the change in pH of a solution in response to the addition of acids or bases.

Buffer a substance that can absorb excess acids or bases without causing a significant change in pH.

Bulimia nervosa a psychologic disorder in which recurrent binge eating is followed by intentional vomiting, inappropriate use of laxatives, enemas, diuretics, or other medication, excessive exercising, and fasting—behavior intended to compensate for overeating that has become uncontrollable.

Bundle of His (atrioventricular bundle, common bundle) bundle of specialized heart muscle cells located between the AV node and the ventricles that functions to conduct electrical impulses from the atria to the ventricles.

Burkitt lymphoma an undifferentiated malignant lymphoma that is characterized by a large osteolytic lesion in the facial bones and is associated with the Epstein-Barr virus.

Cachexia illness and malnutrition seen in individuals with cancer that results in wasting and eventual death.

Calcification hardening of tissue caused by the incorporation of calcium or calcium salts.

Calcitonin a protein hormone produced by the parafollicular cells of the thyroid gland that acts to decrease plasma calcium and phosphate levels by inhibiting osteoclastic activity in bone.

Calculi an abnormal formation in the body, usually formed of mineral salts and most commonly found in the gallbladder, kidney, or urinary bladder.

Campylobacter enteritis a bacterial infection of the small intestine caused by eating or drinking contaminated food or water—often raw poultry, fresh produce, or unpasteurized milk—or by close contact with infected people or animals.

Candidiasis a fungal infection caused by an overgrowth of normal bacteria that usually occurs in the skin and mucous membranes of the mouth, respiratory tract, or vagina but may invade the bloodstream in the immunocompromised person.

Caplan syndrome a condition in which exposure to coal dust causes inflammation and scarring of the lungs.

Carbuncles a condition in which a bacterial infection of the hair follicle or sebaceous gland ducts becomes painful and discharges pus through various openings.

Carcinoma epithelial cell tumor that typically invades surrounding tissue and metastasizes.

Cardiac cycle the cycle of events that occur in the functioning heart from the beginning of one heart beat to the beginning of the next, during which time an electrical impulse is conducted through the heart muscle.

Cardiogenic shock a type of shock that results from decreased cardiac output caused by heart disease in which the heart is unable to pump blood through the body, usually because of myocardial infarction.

Cardiomyopathy a condition in which the cardiac muscle of the heart wall is deteriorated by ischemic or nonischemic mechanisms.

Carrier an individual that possesses genes for a disease but does not show phenotypical characteristics of the disease.

Carrier detection test a test used to determine whether an individual is a carrier of a genetic disease; evidence of a reduced amount of a critical enzyme is indicative of a carrier and allows for prediction of the probability that a child will inherit the disease.

Caseous necrosis a combination of coagulative and liquefactive necrosis in which dead cells disintegrate but are not completely digested, resulting in soft granular clumped cellular debris.

Cast a mass comprised of fibrous material, coagulated protein, or exudate that takes the shape of the region in which it has been molded, such as the bronchial, renal, or intestinal structures or the vaginal cavity, and is usually found in urine or sputum.

Catabolic (flow) phase the period of negative nitrogen balance and increased energy consumption used as a mechanism of defense and repair once shock has been resolved and circulating blood volume is again normal.

Catabolism cellular process that provides energy by breaking down complex molecules into simpler molecules.

Cavernous hemangioma a birthmark that is similar to the strawberry hemangioma but is more deeply rooted and may appear as a red-blue spongy mass of tissue filled with blood.

Cell adhesion molecule (CAM) protein that aids in maintaining cell shape by allowing cells to join and attach to the cytoskeleton.

Cell cycle series of events during which nuclear material of a parent cell is duplicated and divided to form two daughter cells.

Cell lysis cell dissolution and destruction.

Cellular accumulation (infiltration) accumulation of normal cellular substances in the cytoplasm or nucleus as a result of cellular injury or inefficient cell function.

Cellular immunity immune protection afforded by the ability of cytotoxic T cells to lyse target cells that contain antigens that bind specific receptors.

Cellular receptor protein molecule that can be embedded in the membrane or located within the cell in the cytoplasm or on the nucleus. This protein contains binding sites for a specific chemical (ligand) that when bound initiates a particular response.

Cellulitis a condition in which subcutaneous or connective tissue becomes infected and inflamed, causing tenderness, swelling, and redness that spreads to other regions of the body.

Central tolerance a state in which autoreactive T cells in the thymus with receptors against self-antigens are eliminated, thereby preventing an immunologic reaction to an individual's own tissues.

Centriole structure consisting of nine bundles of three microtubules each that is involved in the formation of the mitotic spindle during cell division.

Centromere site on the chromosome where chromatids are attached and held together prior to anaphase.

Cephalic phase of secretion a period of increased salivary and gastric secretion mediated by the vagal nerve of the parasympathetic nervous system in response to the thought or smell of food.

Cerebellar astrocytoma brain tumor in which cancer (malignant) cells begin to grow in the tissues of the brain, resulting in head tilt, limb ataxia, and nystagmus when the eyes are turned toward the tumor.

Cerebral death irreversible brain damage that renders an individual unresponsive to all stimuli but able to maintain the necessary respiratory and cardiovascular functions of life.

Cerebral palsy (CP) a developmental brain injury that occurs before or shortly after birth that causes muscular impairment that affects motor function and also may alter speech and learning abilities.

Cerebrovascular accident (CVA, stroke) localized brain infarction that may result in facial, arm, or leg numbness and weakness, confusion, difficulty speaking or understanding, visual disturbances, dizziness, loss of balance, difficulty walking, and headache.

Cervical dysplasia a condition, also known as *cervical intraepithelial neoplasia (CIN)*, that is characterized by the appearance of abnormal cervical cells that are considered precancerous.

Cervicitis inflammation of the mucous membrane of the uterine cervix caused by infection, typically by chlamydia, genital herpes, or gonorrhea.

Chancre a firm, painless skin ulceration localized at the point of initial exposure to the bacteria that causes syphilis, often on the penis, vagina, or rectum.

Chemical asphyxiant chemical or gas that prevents the delivery of oxygen to tissues or blocks its use.

Chemical synapse region between two nerve cells where a neurotransmitter is released from one cell and stimulates or inhibits cellular activity by binding to its receptor on a target cell.

Chemotactic factor a biochemical substance that facilitates chemotaxis.

Chemotaxis directional movement and attraction of microorganisms or phagocytes to substances released in the environment or tissues.

Cheyne-Stokes respiration an abnormality of the pattern of breathing in which tidal volume gradually increases followed by a gradual decrease and a period of apnea before returning to a normal respiratory pattern.

Chickenpox an infectious viral disease that is spread by direct contact or through the air by coughing or sneezing; it causes a blister-like rash that first affects the face and trunk and then can spread over the rest of the body; symptoms include severe itching, fatigue, and fever.

Chlamydia a sexually transmitted bacterial infection that can cause infertility and blindness.

Choking asphyxiation injury resulting from failure of cells to receive oxygen because of obstruction of internal airways.

Cholecystitis inflammation of the gallbladder commonly caused by impaction of a gallstone that causes right upper quadrant pain and possibly a rupture and abscess in the gallbladder.

Cholecystokinin a protein hormone that is produced by the duodenum in response to fat- or protein-rich chyme and acts to stimulate the release of digestive enzymes from the pancreas and bile from the gallbladder to aide in fat and protein digestion.

Cholelithiasis the presence or formation of gallstones in the gallbladder or bile ducts.

Cholinergic transmission transmission of a nerve impulse using acetylcholine as a neurotransmitter.

Chondrocyte a cell that produces and maintains the cartilaginous matrix.

Chondrosarcoma a cancer of the cartilage that usually occurs in the pelvic bones, shoulder bones, and the upper part of the arms and legs.

Chordae tendineae bands of fibrous tissue that attach on one end to the edges of the tricuspid and mitral valves of the heart and on the other end to the papillary muscles that anchor the valves.

Chromaffin cell (pheochromocyte) neuroendocrine cell found in the adrenal medulla and in other ganglia of the sympathetic nervous system that functions to secrete epinephrine and norepinephrine.

Chromatid one of two daughter chromatids produced by chromosomal replication that are joined at the centromere.

Chromatin chains of DNA containing proteins spaced along the chain, which gives chromosomes a granular appearance during interphase.

Chromosome genetic material in the nucleus of a eukaryotic cell that contains the DNA of the organism.

Chromosome band pattern on a chromosome that is visualized by preferential binding of stain to specific regions, allowing distinction between chromosomes to be seen.

Chronic bacterial prostatitis a condition in which longstanding prostatitis and an underlying defect in the prostate makes the prostate more susceptible to bacterial urinary tract infection.

Chronic lymphocytic leukemia (CLL) a cancer in which too many T cells are produced in bone marrow and blood or too many B cells are produced in lymph nodes.

Chronic myelogenous leukemia (CML) a cancer in which myeloid cell production in the bone marrow is increased, usually because of the Philadelphia chromosome.

Chronic obstructive pulmonary disease (COPD) any of a group of irreversible respiratory diseases that are characterized by airflow obstruction or limitation, usually caused by smoking.

Chronic rejection rejection of a graft months to years after transplantation because of a gradual loss of organ function.

Chronic renal failure a slowly developing condition that can result as a complication of a large number of kidney diseases, such as IgA nephritis, glomerulonephritis, chronic pyelonephritis, and urinary retention, and leads to end-stage renal failure for which dialysis is generally required while a donor kidney is being sought.

Chylomicron large lipoprotein particle that is created in the small intestine and functions to transport lipids to adipose tissue to be broken down by lipoprotein lipase.

Chyme partially digested food found in the stomach after it has been exposed to the salivary enzyme amylase, the gastric enzyme pepsin, and hydrochloric acid.

Chymotrypsin a protein-degrading enzyme that is produced in an inactive form in the pancreas, activated in the duodenum by trypsin, and acts to hydrolyze proteins.

Cirrhosis a condition in which organ tissues degenerate resulting in fibrosis with nodule and scar formation and organ dysfunction.

Citric acid cycle (Krebs cycle, tricarboxylic acid cycle) a component of aerobic metabolism that includes a series of reactions in which acetyl CoA is oxidized into carbon dioxide, nicotinamide adenine dinucleotide (NADH) and flavin adenine dinucleotide (FADH).

Clathrin a large protein that forms a "cage" around a vesicle prior to endocytosis or exocytosis of the vesicle contents.

Cleft lip (harelip) a deformity of the lip caused by abnormal facial development during pregnancy.

Clotting factor any of several plasma components involved in the clotting of blood, including fibrinogen, prothrombin, thromboplastin, and calcium ion.

Cluster headache headache characterized by unilateral severe pain over the eye and forehead that lasts 15 minutes to an hour and occurs in clusters.

Coagulation cascade the clotting system formed by a group of plasma proteins that form a fibrinous meshwork at the injured or inflamed site to prevent spread of infection, stop bleeding by formation of a clot, and provide a framework for future repair and healing.

Coagulative necrosis changes in albumin caused by protein denaturation, primarily in kidneys, heart, and adrenal glands that have experienced hypoxia.

Coarctation of the aorta (COA) a condition in which the aorta narrows in the area where the ductus arteriosus inserts; narrowing usually occurs preductal in children and postductal in adults.

Cochlea a cavity of the temporal bone of the inner ear that contains the nerve endings essential for hearing.

Codominance when a heterozygote expresses two dominant alleles rather than one that dominates over the other.

Codon a triplet of nucleotides located in the mRNA that determines which amino acids will be formed during translation.

Collagenous fiber strong bundle of fibers that form connective tissues in areas such as tendons, bone, and dermis.

Collectin surfactant protein produced by the lungs that provides a form of innate resistance by promoting phagocytosis and interacting with the acquired immune system.

Collecting duct the final section of the nephron, just proximal to the ureter, where salts and water are reabsorbed or secreted and urine concentration is maximal.

Coma a state of unresponsiveness in which an individual cannot be aroused by verbal, physical, or powerful painful stimuli.

Comedo a yellowish or blackish plug of keratin and sebaceous gland secretions, also known as a *blackhead,* that accumulates in the duct of a sebaceous gland and creates an acne lesion.

Communicating (extraventricular) hydrocephalus a disorder in which the cerebrospinal fluid pathways are intact but cerebrospinal fluid absorption is impaired.

Compact bone (cortical bone) the bone type that makes up a large portion of skeletal mass but has a low surface area.

Compensation adjustment of acid or base content by removal or addition in response to changes in pH; for example, a decrease in pH is accompanied by an increase in carbon dioxide removal by the lungs, causing pH to increase.

Compensatory hyperplasia increased rate of cell division that compensates for absent or dysfunctional cells of the same tissue.

Competitive inhibitor a molecule that reversibly or irreversibly binds to a site specific for a given solute, thereby inhibiting the binding and action of the solute.

Complement receptor a receptor present on cells of the innate and acquired immune responses that removes antibody-antigen complexes when bound to complement system products.

Compliance a measure of the ease with which a structure such as the lungs or chest wall may be deformed or stretched.

Compound fracture a broken bone that is protruding from the overlying skin.

Concentration gradient difference in concentration of a substance found in a solution that is contained in separate areas or compartments—such as the intracellular and extracellular spaces found on either side of a cell membrane—that causes movement by way of diffusion.

Concordant trait a trait shared by both twins.

Conduction the transfer of heat, sound, or electrical impulses from one area to another.

Conduction system the electrical system of the heart that allows the impulse that is generated by the SA node to be propagated to the remaining muscle of the heart, resulting in a wave of contraction that propels the blood forward to be pumped to the body.

Condylomata lata warty, plaque-like lesions found in the perianal area and other moist body sites; commonly associated with secondary syphilis.

Congenital aganglionic megacolon (Hirschsprung disease) a congenital defect in which the nerves that innervate the anus through the wall of the bowel are absent, resulting in enlargement of the bowel above the point where the nerves are missing and a subsequent decrease in peristalsis that results in chronic constipation.

Congestive heart failure (left heart failure) a condition in which the heart cannot expel sufficient blood to satisfy the metabolic demands of the body as a result of diseases such as coronary artery disease, hypertension, valvular insufficiency, or rheumatic heart disease.

Connexon channel composed of six protein subunits that form a hollow center through the plasma membrane at a gap junction; when two connexons in adjacent cells are aligned, chemical and electrical communication can occur between the cells.

Contact dermatitis an allergic response to an environmental antigen binding to specific carrier proteins contained in an individual's skin.

Contracture a permanent shortening of muscle or scar tissue that distorts or deforms affected joints.

Contrecoup brain injury resulting from the brain hitting the inside of the skull on the side opposite the site of blunt force trauma.

Contusion bruise produced by bleeding into the skin or underlying tissues from an insult that did not break the skin but did rupture blood vessels.

Convection a method of heat transmission by way of circulating heated particles.

Cor pulmonale right-sided heart failure caused by prolonged hypertension secondary to pulmonary hypertension.

Cornea transparent layer of the front of the eye that functions to aid in focusing light on the retina by bending the light waves.

Corpora cavernosa erectile tissue that contains most of the blood found in the male penis during erection and in the female clitoris during sexual arousal.

Corpus luteum a temporary endocrine structure that develops from an ovarian follicle after it has released an ovum and functions to secrete progesterone that thickens the uterine lining in preparation for the fertilized egg.

Corpus luteum cyst a condition in which excessive bleeding leads to the development of a cyst in the corpus luteum, which may be tender and painful.

Countercurrent exchange system a mechanism by which a substance in one flowing current of fluid moves across a semipermeable membrane down its concentration gradient into another parallel current of fluid moving in the opposite direction, allowing the maintenance of a constant concentration gradient.

Coup when referring to brain trauma, the brain injury that occurs at the site of blunt force to the head; it results from the rapid acceleration and then deceleration of the brain as it hits the inside of the skull.

Craniopharyngioma a brain tumor that develops in the pituitary gland and most often affects children, causing headache, seizure, diabetes insipidus, early onset of puberty, and delayed growth.

Craniosynostosis premature ossification of the skull and closure of the sutures, resulting in abnormal skull expansion and asymmetric skull growth.

Creatine a nitrogenous organic acid that is found in muscle tissue and supplies energy for muscle contraction.

Crista supraventricularis a saddle-shaped muscle in the right ventricular tract between the tricuspid and pulmonary valves.

Cristae enzyme-containing partition in the mitochondrion formed by an infolding of the inner mitochondrial membrane.

Crohn disease (CD) an autoimmune condition in which the intestines and possibly any other component of the digestive system are chronically inflamed and ulcerated, causing chronic diarrhea, disrupted digestion, and subsequent difficulty eating and digesting food.

Cross-bridge theory of muscle contraction a proposal that during muscle contraction sarcomeres shorten because thin filaments slide between thick filaments and form cross-bridges that provide a force that slides the two filaments past one another.

Crossing over exchange of genetic information between two homologous chromosomes.

Cross-reactive antibody an antibody that is capable of interacting with multiple antigens that are identical or closely related.

Croup a viral infection of the respiratory system that involves the larynx, trachea, and the airways leading to the lungs and that can result in serious breathing difficulties, hoarseness, sore throat, and a hacking cough.

Cryoglobulin an immunoglobulin that precipitates at low body temperatures.

Cryptorchidism a condition in which the scrotum of one or both testes is absent because of failure of the testis to descend from the abdominal position during fetal development.

Cushing syndrome a condition that is caused by increased synthesis and secretion of ACTH from a tumor of the adrenal cortex or of the anterior lobe of the pituitary gland, resulting in weight gain, glucose intolerance, and muscle wasting.

Cutaneous vasculitis a type of vasculitis that affects the skin and many times other organs as well and is characterized by a polymorphonuclear infiltrate of the small vessels.

Cyanosis a condition in which the skin, mucous membranes, and nail beds appear blue because of a lack of oxygenated hemoglobin in the blood secondary to congenital heart defects, slowed circulation, or possibly poison.

Cyclic adenosine monophosphate (cAMP) a molecule of adenosine monophosphate that has a phosphate group attached by a phosphodiesterase bond at both the 3' and 5' carbons. cAMP is an intracellular molecule that acts as a second messenger and mediates the effects of extracellular substances on cell activity.

Cyclic guanosine monophosphate (cGMP) a molecule of guanosine monophosphate that has a phosphate group attached at both 3' and 5' carbons by a phosphodiesterase bond; cGMP is an intracellular molecule that acts as a second messenger and mediates the effects of extracellular substances on cell activity.

Cyclooxygenase (COX) an enzyme responsible for formation of prostaglandins, prostacyclin, and thromboxane and subsequent inflammatory response.

Cyclopia a congenital defect in which the two eye orbits merge to form a single cavity containing one eye with a nose-like appendage above the orbit.

Cystic fibrosis (CF) a genetic disorder of the exocrine glands that is caused by a mutation in the CF transmembrane regulator gene causing impairment in chloride transfer across cell membranes and subsequent chloride and water accumulation in organs and in thickened secretions that block ducts and form cysts.

Cystic fibrosis transmembrane regulator (CFTR) a chloride transporter found in the lung, liver, pancreas, digestive tract, reproductive tract, and skin.

Cystinuric stone a congenital condition that causes elevated levels of the amino acid cystine to create stones and to appear in the urine.

Cystitis a condition characterized by acute or chronic inflammation of the urinary bladder, usually caused by bacterial infection of the urethra; symptoms include frequent burning urination, blood in the urine, pain in the pubic area, chills and fever, back pain, and nausea.

Cystocele a condition in which the muscle between a woman's bladder and vagina weakens and allows the bladder to descend into the vagina causing discomfort, urine leakage, and incomplete emptying of the bladder.

Cytokine molecule produced by cells of the acquired immune system that mediate interactions between cells to kill bacteria and during the inflammatory response.

Cytokinesis the process by which the cytoplasm of a parent cell is divided into two identical cells after mitosis.

Cytomegalovirus (CMV) a type of herpesvirus that is transmitted by exchange of body fluids during sexual contact, kissing, or sharing of foods and beverages and may cause mild symptoms such as enlarged lymph nodes, low fever, and fatigue that may not be noticed but also can cause severe symptoms such as blindness in immunologically compromised individuals.

Cytoplasm liquid material of a cell enclosed within the plasma membrane.

Cytoskeleton network of microtubules and microfilaments located in the eukaryotic cytosol that provides structure and organization to the cell and is involved in movement of substances within the cell and movement to structures outside the cell.

Cytosol the viscous fluid portion of the cytoplasm in which intracellular contents are suspended.

Cytotoxic (metabolic) edema cerebral edema resulting from tissue hypoxia and impairment of the Na^+-K^+ ATP pump, causing a loss of intracellular potassium and a gain of intracellular sodium and water.

Cytotoxic T lymphocyte (Tc-cell or CTL) killer lymphocyte that binds to and lyses specific cells containing particular antigen receptors.

Decompression sickness (caisson disease) gas embolism created when a person underwater returns to the surface too quickly, resulting in cellular hypoxia, joint and muscle pain, and tissue necrosis.

Deep venous thrombosis (DVT) a condition in which a blood clot becomes dislodged from its site of formation and embolizes to the arterial blood supply of one of the lungs, resulting in breathing difficulty, pain during breathing, and possibly circulatory instability and death.

Defecation reflex (rectal reflex) a process by which the accumulation of feces in the rectum stimulates defecation.

Degenerative disk disease (DDD) a condition in which intervertebral disk tissue is replaced by fibrocartilage during aging; functional capacity is rarely altered.

Dementia intellectual difficulties in areas such as memory, concentration, and judgment, resulting from a disease or disorder of the brain.

Deoxyribonucleic acid (DNA) genetic information of an organism that is contained in chromatin.

Depolarization the movement of sodium across the membrane, resulting in a change in membrane charge from a negative to positive potential.

Dermal ischemia a condition in which the lack of oxygen reaching a region of skin causes tissue destruction and damage.

Dermatome an area of skin that is innervated by a specific spinal nerve.

Dermoid cyst a benign tumor resulting from congenital malformation of the skin or ovary.

Desmosome region of tight adhesion between neighboring cells that provides structural strength to the tissue and allows the cells of the tissue to function as a unit.

Developmental dysplasia of the hip (DDH) a condition in which the hip joint of babies or young children is malformed with the ball being completely out of the socket or the socket being too shallow to support the ball.

Diabetes insipidus a disease caused by antidiuretic hormone deficiency or resistance that is characterized by excretion of large amounts of diluted urine resulting from the inability of the kidneys to concentrate urine.

Diabetic ketoacidosis (DKA) a complication of diabetes mellitus, DKA is caused by the buildup of by-products of fat metabolism that occurs when glucose is not available as a fuel source for the body because of insulin deficiency.

Diabetic nephropathy a progressive kidney disease caused by diabetes-induced angiopathy of capillaries in the kidney glomeruli that is characterized by nodular glomerulosclerosis.

Diabetic neuropathy combined sensory and motor disorder often seen in older diabetic patients as a result of microvascular injury involving small blood vessels that supply nerves.

Diabetic retinopathy damage to the retina caused by an overaccumulation of glucose or fructose that damages the blood vessels in the retina; in advanced stages, lack of oxygen in the retina causes fragile blood vessels to grow along the retina and in the vitreous fluid of the eye that may bleed and cause blurred vision.

Diaper dermatitis a type of dermatitis characterized by inflammation of the skin in the diaper area in infants caused by exposure of the skin to feces and urine.

Diarrhea an increase in the frequency of watery bowel movements or a greater looseness of stools resulting from disease, excessive consumption of alcohol or other liquids or foods that irritate the stomach or intestine, allergy to certain food products, poisoning, hyperactivity of the nervous system, or viral or bacterial infection.

Diastole the period of time during which the heart relaxes after contraction, resulting in a pressure drop in the relaxed region.

Diastolic heart failure a condition in which heart contractions are normal but the ventricle does not relax completely so less blood enters the heart.

Differentiation process by which cells mature and become specialized to perform specific functions.

Diffuse brain injury (diffuse axonal injury) injury to neuronal axons in many areas of the brain caused by stretching and shearing forces received during brain injury.

Dilated cardiomyopathy (congestive cardiomyopathy) a condition in which the heart, usually the left ventricle, is enlarged and weakened, which results in the need for heart transplantation.

Dimorphic the ability of fungi to exist in the yeast or mold state.

Diphtheria a contagious upper respiratory bacterial disease in which the bacteria have been infected by a bacteriophage and become lodged in the mucous membranes of the throat where they produce a toxin that destroys the tissue and causes the formation of a tough membrane that can spread to the larynx and lead to suffocation.

Diploid cell cell that contains two sets of chromosomes, giving each diploid cell 46 chromosomes.

Disseminated intravascular coagulation (DIC) a condition in which the blood coagulates throughout the entire body after the uncontrolled activation of clotting factors and fibrinolytic enzymes throughout small blood vessels, resulting in platelet and coagulation factor depletion and increased bleeding.

Distal tubule a section of the nephron between the loop of Henle and the collecting duct system that helps regulate potassium, sodium, calcium, and pH by reabsorbing bicarbonate, sodium, and calcium and secreting protons and potassium into the filtrate.

Distributive (vasogenic) shock a form of shock caused by widening of the blood vessels, usually a result of medication.

Diverticulosis a condition in which multiple bulging sacs push outward from the wall of the large intestine and may become infected and rupture, causing abdominal pain and tenderness, and fever.

Dizygotic (fraternal) twins occurs when a female ovulates two eggs rather than one and both of the eggs get fertilized but by different sperm.

Dominant an allele that can mask the effects of another allele.

Dopamine hypothesis a proposal that the symptoms of schizophrenia can be explained by changes in dopamine function in the brain.

Dosage compensation the phenomenon in which males are able to produce proteins expressed by sex chromosomes in an amount equal to that produced by females even though the males only have one X chromosome.

Double-helix double-stranded helical structure of DNA that is held together by chemical bonds between nitrogenous bases.

Down-regulation the process by which a cell decreases its sensitivity to a hormone or neurotransmitter by decreasing the number of receptors in response to a high concentration of that particular hormone or neurotransmitter.

Drowning breathing in of fluid that causes airway obstruction, thereby decreasing oxygen delivery to tissues.

Dry gangrene process by which the skin dries and shrinks because of coagulative necrosis.

Duchenne muscular dystrophy a genetic disorder in which fat and fibrous tissue infiltrate and weaken muscle tissues such as in the legs and pelvis, lungs, and heart and usually results in death before adulthood.

Dumping syndrome a condition in which the lower end of the small intestine fills too quickly with undigested food from the stomach after stomach surgery, resulting in nausea, vomiting, bloating, diarrhea, and shortness of breath during or immediately after a meal.

Dysmnesia impaired memory similar to that seen in amnesia.

Dyspareunia a reversible condition in which sexual intercourse is painful.

Dysphasia impairment of speech that manifests as the inability to arrange words in logical order.

Dyspnea shortness of breath and difficulty in breathing usually caused by lung or heart disease.

Ebb phase early posttrauma period of hypotension and decreased energy consumption that serves as a protective response to preserve blood flow to essential organs.

Eccrine sweat gland one of several sweat glands at the body's surface that produce a clear watery secretion that is important in regulating body temperature.

Ectopic testis a condition in which the testis has descended but is located in an abnormal position.

Effective osmolality osmotic activity sustained by the presence of varying solute concentrations in two regions separated by a permeable membrane.

Effective renal plasma flow (ERPF) the amount of plasma flowing to the glomerulus of the kidney.

Eisenmenger syndrome a congenital defect in which the abnormal development of the circulatory system causes a reversed right-to-left shunt secondary to increased pressures on the right side of the heart because of pulmonary hypertension.

Elastic fiber long, stretchable fiber that forms connective tissues in areas where elasticity is necessary, such as skin and lungs.

Elastic recoil the ability of the lungs to resist stretching and to return to their original shape after having been stretched.

Electrolyte electrically charged substance that is capable of ionizing and dissociating into ions and conducting electricity.

Electron-transport chain series of transfer reactions that includes transferring elections from a donor to an acceptor, resulting in the release of energy during each transfer.

Embolic stroke stroke caused by blockage of cerebral vessels.

Embolus an air bubble, a detached blood clot, or a foreign body that travels in the bloodstream and gets stuck in a blood vessel, resulting in obstruction of vessels supplying the lungs, brain or heart, and possibly gangrene and the need for amputation of extremities.

Empyema (infected pleural effusion) a condition in which purulent fluid is persistently discharged into the pleural space as a result of complications of bacterial infections.

Encephalitis inflammation of the brain usually caused by a virus.

Encephalocele congenital abnormality in which a gap in the skull results in a protrusion of brain material.

Encephalopathy any of the various diseases or syndromes of the brain.

End-diastolic pressure the pressure measured in the ventricles at the end of diastole that is used to approximate the degree of preload.

End-diastolic volume the amount of blood found in the ventricle before a cardiac contraction; used as a measure of diastolic function.

Endocytosis a process by which extracellular substances are trapped in a section of the membrane that folds inward and separates from the membrane to form an intracellular vesicle.

Endogenous cryogen a substance capable of lowering body temperature.

Endometrial polyp a typically benign mass protruding from the mucous membrane of the endometrium.

Endometriosis a condition that is common in women of reproductive age in which the tissue lining the uterus is found outside of the uterus, resulting in pain and infertility.

Endomitosis chromosomal replication in the absence of division of the cell nucleus, resulting in a polyploid nucleus.

Endoplasmic reticulum an organelle located in the cytoplasm that synthesizes, processes, and transports proteins.

Endothelial cell a cell of the endothelial layer that lines heart, blood, and lymph vessels and the lung cavity.

Endotoxin lipopolysaccharide that is released during cell lysis from the bacterial outer membrane and causes fever, leucopenia, and possibly diarrhea and hemorrhagic shock.

Enuresis a condition in which urination is uncontrolled or involuntary.

Eosinopenia a reduction in the number of eosinophils present in the blood.

Eosinophil a phagocyte that destroys antigen-antibody complexes, allergens, and inflammatory chemicals and aids in fighting parasitic infections.

Eosinophilia a condition in which the number of eosinophils in the blood is elevated because of diseases such as parasitic infections, allergies, cholesterol emboli, chronic myeloid leukemia, and some drug reactions.

Ependymoma intracranial tumor that is most commonly found in children and that typically arises from the inner lining of the fourth ventricle and the spinal canal.

Epicritic extreme sensitivity such as that required to accurately determine fine variations of touch or temperature.

Epididymis a narrow, convoluted tube that lies behind each testicle and functions as a site of spermatozoa maturation and storage before entering the vas deferens during emission.

Epididymitis a painful condition in which the epididymis becomes inflamed, usually as a result of a secondary bacterial infection that is brought about by a variety of underlying conditions such as urinary tract or sexually transmitted infections.

Epidural hematoma collection of blood between the inner surface of the skull and the dura caused by torn arteries secondary to skull fracture.

Epigenetic mechanism by which changes in gene function can be inherited without alteration of gene sequence.

Epilepsy any of a group of syndromes characterized by recurring seizures of an unknown cause.

Epiphyseal plate a plate of hyaline cartilage at the end of long bones that provides a site for lengthening of the bone.

Epispadias a birth defect in which the urethra opens on the upper penile surface.

Epstein-Barr virus (EBV) a herpesvirus that causes mononucleosis and is associated with a number of cancers, such as lymphomas in immunosuppressed persons.

Erysipelas a highly contagious bacterial infection that produces shiny, red swollen areas and fever and can lead to blood poisoning and pneumonia.

Erythema marginatum an early symptom of rheumatic fever in which pink circular lesions appear on the skin.

Erythema multiforme a skin disease that is caused by allergies, seasonal changes, or drug sensitivities, resulting in the formation of red macules, papules, or subdermal vesicles on the skin and mucous membranes.

Erythema toxicum neonatorum a temporary eruption of redness of the skin, small papules, and occasionally pustules in newborns that is associated with by contact dermatitis or hypersensitivity to milk or other allergens.

Erythrocyte (red blood cell [RBC]) a disk-shaped cell in the blood that contains hemoglobin, lacks a nucleus, and functions to transport oxygen and carbon dioxide to and from the tissues.

Erythromyalgia chronic disorder characterized by warmth, pain, and redness, occurring primarily in the feet and lower legs.

Erythropoietic hemochromatosis a disorder of excessive accumulation of iron in liver, bone marrow, pancreas, skin and testis that is usually secondary to a known cause, such as oral iron therapy or multiple blood transfusions.

Eschar a scab of dead tissue on the skin caused by a burn or by the action of a corrosive or caustic substance.

Escharotomy an incision made into a burn or scar to decrease the amount of pull on the surrounding tissue.

Esophageal varices dilation of submucosal veins of the esophagus resulting from portal hypertension that causes ulceration and bleeding.

Essential (primary) thrombocythemia (ET) a chronic disorder that is associated with sustained megakaryocyte proliferation, which increases the number of circulating platelets and results in megakaryocytic hyperplasia, splenomegaly, and complications by hemorrhagic and thrombotic episodes.

Estradiol (E2) the most potent of the estrogens, estradiol has many functions including increases growth and development of female sex organs and characteristics, increases secretions from the cervix and growth of the endometrium, reduces LDL-cholesterol, and increases HDL-cholesterol concentrations in the blood.

Eukaryote organisms such as plants, animals, fungi, protozoa, and most algae that are comprised of cells with a nucleus and other membrane-bound organelles.

Excitation-contraction coupling the process by which an action potential depolarizes a myocyte causing calcium to be transported into the cell and to be released from the sarcoplasmic reticulum resulting in muscle contraction.

Excitatory postsynaptic potential (EPSP) a graded subthreshold depolarization of the postsynaptic membrane in response to neurotransmitter release from a presynaptic neuron.

Exon nucleotide sequence in an RNA molecule that codes for proteins.

Exotoxin protein synthesized by a specific species of bacteria that is found outside the bacterial wall.

Exstrophy of the bladder a congenital defect in which the lower abdominal wall is malformed and ruptures, allowing communication between the bladder and the amniotic fluid and resulting in anomalies of the lower abdominal wall, bladder, anterior bony pelvis, and external genitalia.

Extracellular matrix (basement membrane) fibrous proteins embedded in a carbohydrate-rich liquid that is secreted by the cell and functions as a pathway for diffusion of nutrients, wastes, and other substances between the blood and tissues.

Extrinsic allergic alveolitis (hypersensitivity pneumonitis) an inflammation of the lung caused by an immune reaction to small airborne particles such as bacteria, mold, and fungi that causes fever, chills, coughing, shortness of breath, and body aches.

Extrinsic pathway a component of the coagulation cascade that causes blood clotting in response to factors released from damaged tissue.

Exudate fluids or cells that have leaked from blood vessels.

Facioscapulohumeral muscular dystrophy a benign genetic disorder that begins in childhood and causes muscle wasting and weakness, primarily in the face, shoulder, and arms.

Failure to thrive (FTT) a condition that is characterized by poor weight gain and physical growth over an extended period of time in infancy.

Fanconi anemia a genetic disease affecting bone marrow that is characterized by pancytopenia, hypoplasia of the bone marrow, congenital anomalies, and pigment changes of the skin and that predisposes the individual to myelodysplasia and to acute myeloid leukemia or cancers of the mouth, esophagus, intestinal and urinary tracts, and the reproductive organs.

Fat necrosis lipase-induced cellular dissolution of triglycerides in breast, pancreas, and other abdominal structures.

Ferritin a protein that can store about 4500 iron ions in a hollow shell where the iron combines with phosphate and hydroxide ions to form crystallites.

Fibroblast connective tissue cell that proliferates at inflammatory sites and produces collagen fibers and ground substance to aid in wound healing.

Fibromyalgia a condition in which muscles, tendons, and joints are painful, stiff, and tender; often accompanied by restless sleep, fatigue, anxiety, depression, and disturbances in bowel function.

Fibrosarcoma a malignant tumor of fibrous connective tissue that usually is derived from immature proliferating fibroblasts.

Fibrous dysplasia (FD) a genetic disorder in which tumor-like growths or lesions form in one or more bones and replace the medullary bone with fibrous tissue, resulting in expansion and weakening of the bone.

First-degree burn a mild burn that produces redness and tenderness of the skin but no blistering, such as that seen in a minor sunburn.

Focal segmental glomerulosclerosis (FSGS) a condition in which glomerular capillaries with thickened basement membranes and increased mesangial matrix collapse in segments.

Follicular cyst a cyst caused by the retention of secretions in a follicular structure because of the blockage of a duct, resulting in the failure of the dominant follicle to rupture or failure of the nondominant follicles to regress.

Follicular/proliferative phase the phase defined as the period during which a follicle matures as a result of granulosa cell proliferation and increased estrogen production and the endometrium thickens because of estrogen stimulation.

Folliculitis inflammation of a follicle, such as a hair follicle, that has been damaged by friction from rubbing clothing, blockage of the follicle, or shaving and then becomes infected with a bacteria.

Follistatin a protein hormone, produced by the pituitary and found in the follicles, that binds to and inhibits the actions of activin, resulting in a decrease in follicle-stimulating hormone secretion and subsequent follicular growth.

Founder cell precursor cell that adheres to like cells and undergoes mitosis with them to form tissues.

Fovea centralis a small region of the retina filled with cones that receive the most direct light stimulation and becomes the area of greatest visual acuity.

Frailty physiologic and immune changes that result in wasting of the body during aging and leave the affected person susceptible to falls, functional decline, disease, and death.

Frank-Starling law of the heart the idea that changes in the volume of blood filling the heart will change the volume that is ejected by the same amount because the force of the contraction will increase as the heart is filled with more blood.

Free radical highly reactive and destructive particle that has an unpaired electron and is produced from an atom or molecule.

FSH deficiency a condition characterized by decreased or absent production of follicle-stimulating hormone, resulting in a decline in spermatogenesis/oogenesis and associated infertility.

Fulminant hepatitis a type of viral hepatitis that has a high mortality rate and causes fatigue, nausea, jaundice, dark urine, flu-like symptoms, hepatomegaly, and eventually encephalopathy.

Functional residual capacity (FRC) the volume of air remaining in the lungs at the end of a normal expiration or the sum of expiratory reserve volume and residual volume.

Furuncles a condition in which staphylococcal infection produces painful, pus-filled inflamed sites on the skin and in subcutaneous tissue.

Fusiform aneurysm (giant aneurysm) large aneurysm that stretches to affect the entire circumference of the arterial wall.

G protein an intracellular protein that is activated by the binding of a hormone or neurotransmitter to an extracellular receptor and in turn activates adenylyl cyclase, which produces cAMP.

Galactorrhea inappropriate lactation; a condition in which milk-like fluid is secreted from the breast because of hormonal alterations that are not associated with childbirth or nursing.

Gamete haploid reproductive cell including sperm and eggs.

Ganglioneuroblastoma a tumor arising from nerve tissue that is intermediate, between benign and malignant.

Ganglioneuroma a benign neoplasm composed of mature ganglionic neurons scattered within a stroma of neurofibrils and collagenous fibers.

Gangrenous necrosis tissue death typically found in the lower leg as a result of severe hypoxic injury secondary to arteriosclerosis or blockage of major arteries.

Gap junction tunnel or connexon that joins two adjacent cells and allows for the passage of molecules and electrical signals between the cells.

Gas gangrene the formation of gas bubbles and subsequent destruction of connective tissue and cell membranes resulting from the hydrolytic enzymes produced by bacterium of the *Clostridium* species.

Gastric phase of secretion a period during which distention of the stomach activates reflexes such as the long vagovagal reflexes or short local reflexes that stimulate gastric acid secretion.

Gastrin a protein hormone that is produced primarily in the antrum of the stomach by the G cells in response to stomach distension, vagal stimulation, the presence of partially digested proteins, and hypercalcemia and acts to stimulate parietal cells of the stomach to secrete hydrochloric acid and the chief cells to secrete pepsinogen.

Gastritis a condition in which the lining of the stomach is inflamed because of bacterial infection, bile reflux, or excessive consumption of alcohol or certain foods.

Gastrocolic reflex a process by which food entering an empty stomach increases intestinal and colonic peristalsis.

Gastroesophageal reflux (GER) a type of injury to the esophagus caused by chronic exposure of the esophagus to stomach liquid reflux comprised of acid and pepsin that creates heartburn, inflammation of the esophageal lining, strictures, dysphagia, and chronic chest pain.

Gastroileal reflex a process by which food entering an empty stomach increases ileal motility and causes the opening of the ileocecal valve.

Gate control theory a proposal that a pain gate is present in the spinal cord that allows or blocks pain signals to the brain depending on whether the impulse is traveling on a large or small afferent fiber.

Gating calcium-induced decrease in permeability of a junctional complex that may aid in protecting uninjured cells from the increased calcium levels released by injured cells.

Gene-environment interaction the multifactorial mechanism for developing a disease that includes genes as well as environment and life-style.

Generalized neuropathy a functional disturbance or pathologic change in the cell body of one type of peripheral neuron.

Generalized anxiety disorder (GAD) an anxiety disorder characterized by an excessively anxious mood lasting at least 1 month that interferes with daily functioning and may be accompanied by jitteriness, sweating, feelings of catastrophe concerning one's family or self, and irritability.

Generalized seizure a seizure occurring bilaterally with no local focal point that involves the entire body, resulting in muscle rigidity, violent muscle contractions, and impaired or lost consciousness.

Generalized symmetric polyneuropathy an apparent symmetrical disturbance of function or pathologic change in several sensory, motor, or autonomic fibers.

Genital herpes a sexually transmitted viral infection that is caused by herpes simplex virus type 2 and is characterized by painful lesions in the genital and anal regions.

Genomic imprinting genes that are inherited from only one parent and have variable degrees of activation.

Genotype the genetic composition of an individual.

Germline mosaicism mechanism by which a child can inherit a genetic disease even though the parents do not express the disease; the mechanism is believed to involve a mutation during the embryonic development of the parent germ cells.

GH deficiency a condition characterized by decreased or absent production of growth hormone, resulting in a decline in insulin-like growth factor-1 and dwarfism if the deficiency is prepubertal.

Giant cell tumor a benign tumor that usually occurs near the end of a bone close to a joint in the arm or leg, in the knee, and in flat bones.

Giantism severely increased long bone growth caused by excessive growth hormone secretion before and during puberty.

Glans structure composed of corpus spongiosum in males (glans penis) and corpus cavernosa and vestibular tissue in females (glans clitoris) that is located at the tip of the genital structures and involves sexual arousal and contains the highest density of sensory receptors.

Glomerular filtration rate (GFR) the volume of plasma filtered at the glomerulus per unit of time.

Glomerulonephritis an autoimmune or infectious disease characterized by inflammation of the glomeruli that may not produce symptoms or may present with hematuria and proteinuria.

Glomerulus a capillary bed surrounded by the Bowman's capsule of the nephron in the kidney where filtration occurs.

Glucagon a protein hormone that is secreted by the alpha cells of the islets of Langerhans and functions to increase blood sugar by promoting glycogenolysis and gluconeogenesis in the liver.

Glucocorticoid a steroid hormone that is produced by the adrenal cortex and facilitates carbohydrate, protein, and fat metabolism, and is commonly used as anti-inflammatory and anti-immunity agents.

Glucose-6-phosphate dehydrogenase (G6PD) deficiency an inherited condition that is asymptomatic in the absence of exposure to particular substances such as certain medicines, mothballs, or severe infections, but with exposure the red blood cells undergo destruction that produces excessive bilirubin that overloads the liver and causes jaundice.

Gluten-sensitive enteropathy also known as *celiac sprue,* this condition is characterized by mucosal lesions in the gastrointestinal tract formed in response to a genetic predisposition for an immune response to gluten and similar proteins.

Glycolysis catabolism of glucose or other monosaccharides to pyruvate and two molecules of ATP in the absence of oxygen.

Goiter a noncancerous enlargement of the thyroid gland that is visible as a swelling at the front of the neck.

Golgi complex (Golgi apparatus) flattened, smooth vesicles stacked near the nucleus of a cell that process and package secretory proteins into vesicles and enzymes into lysosomes and modify proteins targeted to become part of cellular membranes.

Golgi tendon organ a specialized structure in the tendon fibers that stretches when the corresponding muscle contracts and sends information to the brain about the actual tension the muscle is achieving in contraction.

Gomphosis an immovable articulation such as a tooth inserted into its bony socket.

Gonadostat a theory proposing that near the time of puberty the hypothalamus and pituitary lose sensitivity to sex steroid feedback, resulting in an increase in gonadotropins that then initiate puberty.

Gonadotropin-releasing hormone (GnRH) a hormone produced by the hypothalamus that stimulates the anterior pituitary gland to secrete luteinizing hormone and follicle-stimulating hormone.

Gonorrhea a sexually transmitted disease caused by the bacteria gonococci that invade the mucous membranes of the genitals and urinary tract and in women the cervix, fallopian tubes, and ovaries, causing chronic pelvic pain or infertility.

Gout a disorder of uric-acid metabolism that causes painful inflammation of the joints, commonly the big toe, and arthritic attacks resulting from elevated levels of uric acid in the blood and the deposition of urate crystals around the joints.

Granulation tissue vascularized tissue that replaces the fibrin clot during the reconstructive phase of wound healing.

Granulocyte a type of white blood cell, such as neutrophils, that contain enzymes capable of killing microorganisms and catabolizing debris ingested during phagocytosis.

Granulocytopenia a condition in which the number of granular white blood cells in the blood is decreased.

Granulocytosis a condition in which the number of granulocytes, usually neutrophils, in blood is increased secondary to bacterial infection, leukemia, or autoimmune disease.

Granuloma a tumor-like mass containing macrophages and fibroblasts that forms as a result of chronic inflammation and isolation of the infected area.

Granuloma inguinale a condition, also called *Donovanosis,* that is a bacterial disease thought to be transmitted primarily by anal rather than vaginal intercourse.

Granulosa cell a cell in the ovarian follicle that converts androgens into estrogens and becomes a luteal cell after ovulation.

Graves disease a condition usually caused by excessive thyroid hormone and characterized by an enlarged thyroid gland, protrusion of eyeballs, a rapid heartbeat, and nervous excitability.

Ground substance fluid or semisolid gel found in the extracellular matrix that contains fibroblasts that produce collagenous, elastic, and reticular tissue fibers.

Growth factor a chemical messenger that mediates tissue growth and development by stimulating mitosis and cell differentiation.

Guanosine diphosphate (GDP) a molecule of guanine attached to two phosphate groups that binds to and inactivates an intracellular G protein.

Guanosine triphosphate (GTP) a molecule of guanine attached to three phosphate groups that binds to and activates an intracellular G protein.

Gynecomastia a condition in which abnormal breast tissue develops on adolescent boys or men usually as a result of an imbalance in hormones.

Hageman factor (factor XII) component of the kinin system that activates the clotting system, converts plasminogen proactivator to plasminogen activator, and activates C1 in the complement system.

Hair follicles a pit of the epidermis that is formed by the tubular invagination and encloses the root of the hair.

Haploid cell cell that contains one copy of each chromosome, giving each cell 23 chromosomes.

Haplotype a group of alleles of closely linked genes located on one chromosome that are inherited together.

Hematoma collection of blood in soft tissue or an enclosed space.

Hematopoietic growth factor one of several glycoproteins with regulatory functions in the processes of proliferation, differentiation, and functional activation of hematopoietic progenitors and mature blood cells.

Hemizygous a male that has one X chromosome containing genes for a specific disease but has no alleles on the Y chromosome to counteract the effects of the diseased gene.

Hemolytic anemia a condition in which red blood cells are destroyed in response to certain toxic or infectious agents or in certain inherited blood disorders and the rate of breakdown exceeds the body's ability to compensate.

Hemolytic disease of the newborn (HDN) a condition that affects a fetus or newborn in which red blood cells breakdown because of antibodies made by the mother that are directed against the infant's red cells, potentially resulting in anemia, heart failure, jaundice, and brain damage if left untreated.

Hemolytic-uremic syndrome a condition in which platelets aggregate within the kidney's small blood vessels resulting in reduced blood flow to the kidney and subsequent kidney failure and destruction of the red blood cells.

Hemophilia A (classic hemophilia) a genetic disorder in which a mutation in factor VIII causes prolonged clotting time, decreased formation of thromboplastin, and diminished conversion of prothrombin.

Hemophilia B (Christmas disease) a genetic disorder similar to hemophilia A in terms of symptoms but with a mutation in the factor IX gene.

Hemophilia C (factor XI deficiency) a genetic disorder characterized by a deficiency in factor XI, resulting in a mild form of hemophilia.

Hemoproteins endogenous pigments such as hemoglobin and cytochromes that accumulate in cells because of excessive iron storage.

Hemoptysis a manifestation in which blood or blood-stained sputum is spit or coughed from bronchi, larynx, trachea, or lungs.

Hemorrhagic stroke (intracranial hemorrhage) stroke usually caused by hypertension that results in bleeding in the brain and typically increases intracranial pressure and may lead to death.

Hemosiderin an iron-containing insoluble protein that is produced by phagocytic digestion of hematin and is found in many tissues, especially in the liver.

Henoch-Schönlein purpura nephritis a condition in which the blood vessels are inflamed causing bleeding into the skin, mucous membranes, internal organs, and other tissues; pain and inflammation in the joints; abdominal pain; gastrointestinal bleeding; inflammation of the kidneys; subcutaneous edema; encephalopathy; and inflammation of the testis.

Hepatic encephalopathy a condition that is usually caused by liver cirrhosis and portal hypertension in which toxins produced by the gut pass into the systemic circulation and damage brain cells resulting in impaired cognition, tremor, and a decreased level of consciousness.

Hepatitis A a virus that is spread by the fecal-oral route through contaminated food and water or by close and intimate contact and results in liver inflammation, flu-like symptoms, nausea, poor appetite, abdominal pain, fatigue, yellow eyes and skin, and dark urine that can last weeks to months.

Hepatitis B virus (HBV) a DNA virus that is transmitted by contaminated blood or blood derivatives in transfusions, by sexual contact, or by the use of contaminated needles and instruments and may become chronic and cause long-term damage to the liver.

Hepatitis C an RNA virus that is transmitted primarily by blood and blood products and sometimes through sexual contact and may become chronic with few to no symptoms while causing long-term damage to the liver, such as cirrhosis and hepatocellular carcinoma.

Hepatorenal syndrome (HRS) a condition in which acute renal failure occurs because of a decrease in renal blood flow or liver and kidney damage.

Hereditary spherocytosis a defect in the cell membrane of red blood cells that causes thickened, fragile red blood cells that are susceptible to spontaneous hemolysis and results in chronic anemia, jaundice, fever, and abdominal pain.

Herpes simplex virus (HSV) a contagious sexually transmitted viral infection of the genital and anal or mouth regions that produces recurrent small clusters of painful lesions (*see* **genital herpes**).

Heterogeneous nuclear RNA (hnRNA) RNA recently transcribed that has not yet been converted into mature mRNA.

Heterozygote an individual that has different alleles for a specific gene.

Hiatal hernia an anatomic abnormality in which the esophageal hiatus is larger than normal causing part of the stomach to protrude through the diaphragm and up into the chest.

Histamine a hormone that is produced by mast cells and functions to dilate capillaries so that they are more permeable during an allergic reaction and to regulate gastric acid production in the gastrointestinal tract.

Hodgkin lymphoma (HL) a chronic condition in which the lymph nodes, spleen, and liver become enlarged and that is often accompanied by anemia, fever, and eventually death if not treated at an early stage; also referred to as *Hodgkin disease.*

Homologous chromosomes two paired and virtually identical chromosomes in somatic cells.

Homozygote an individual that has identical alleles for a specific gene.

Hormesis stimulation by toxic substances at a level that would not normally be effective.

Hormonal signaling communication between cells that originates when a hormone is released from an endocrine cell, travels through the bloodstream, and binds to a target cell to elicit a response.

Human papillomavirus (HPV) one of several viruses that are considered sexually transmitted diseases and are characterized by growths such as internal or external plantar warts and genital warts and may be associated with an increased risk for cancer of the reproductive tract.

Humoral immunity immune protection afforded by the presence of antibodies in blood.

Huntington disease (HD) an autosomal dominant disease causing a progressive increase in involuntary, jerky, diskinetic movements, mental deterioration, and premature death.

Hydrocele a condition in which serous fluid accumulates in a bodily cavity such as the testis.

Hydrops fetalis a condition in the fetus in which edema forms in the fetal subcutaneous tissue because of an enzyme deficiency or any one of several other disorders.

Hydrostatic pressure any pressure that is exerted by a liquid within a closed system, such as blood as it presses against vessel membranes in response to pumping of the heart.

Hydroxyapatite (HAP) the primary bone salt that provides compressional strength to bone.

Hyperacute rejection rejection of a graft immediately after transplantation because of the prior formation of cytotoxic antibodies against the antigens on the graft.

Hyperaldosteronism a disorder marked by excessive secretion of aldosterone and subsequent weakness, cardiac irregularities, and abnormally high blood pressure.

Hyperchloremic metabolic acidosis a condition in which anion gap is normal but bicarbonate is lost whereas chloride is retained to maintain ionic balance, resulting in a drop in pH.

Hyperemia an increase in the quantity of blood flow to a body part.

Hyperhemolytic crisis a condition in which the rate of destruction of red blood cells is increased, resulting in decreased hemoglobin levels, increased reticulocyte count, elevated bilirubin, and elevated lactate dehydrogenase caused by infections, hemolytic transfusion reactions, sickle cell crisis, or a combination of glucose 6-phosphodisterase deficiency with oxidant stress.

Hyperhomocysteinemia a condition in which plasma homocysteine concentration is elevated because of diet, vitamin B_6 or B_{12} deficiency, congenital enzyme deficiency, or renal failure, increasing the risk of developing atherosclerosis and venous thromboembolism.

Hypermetabolism an extreme elevation in metabolic rate.

Hyperpolarized the state of a membrane when the membrane potential is more negative than the resting membrane potential, thereby increasing the stimulus required to elicit an action potential.

Hyperprolactinemia excessive prolactin secretion, usually the result of a pituitary tumor, which can lead to anovulation or impaired spermatogenesis related to the inhibiting effects of prolactin on hypothalamic gonadotropin-releasing hormone and infertility.

Hypersensitivity a state in which the body undergoes an exaggerated immune response to an antigen.

Hyperthermic injury heat cramps, heat exhaustion, or heat stroke caused by excessive heat.

Hypertonic hyponatremia decreased sodium concentration caused by increases in plasma lipids and proteins that results in an osmotic shift.

Hypertrophic cardiomyopathy a genetic disorder caused by various mutations that thicken the heart muscle, possibly leading to obstruction of blood flow and heart dysfunction.

Hyperventilation a condition in which breathing faster or deeper than necessary reduces carbon dioxide concentration, resulting in numbness or tingling in the hands, feet, and lips, lightheadedness, dizziness, headache, chest pain, and sometimes fainting.

Hypocortisolism a condition characterized by a decrease in cortisol synthesis and release that may be related to deficiency at the adrenal, pituitary, or hypothalamic level.

Hypoglycemia a state of low blood glucose that stimulates epinephrine and glucagon secretion, resulting in mobilization of stored glycogen and fat and their conversion into glucose.

Hypoparathyroidism a condition marked by decreased function of the parathyroid glands, resulting in hypocalcemia and associated tremor, tetany, and convulsions.

Hypophysiotropic hormones hormones released by the hypothalamus into the hypophyseal portal system that binds to specific receptors on the anterior pituitary to signal the release of specific pituitary hormones.

Hypoplastic anemia a condition in which anemia results from greatly depressed, inadequately functioning bone marrow and smaller than normal erythrocytes.

Hypoplastic left heart syndrome (HLHS) a condition in which the left side of the heart, including the aorta, aortic valve, left ventricle and mitral valve, is underdeveloped and blood returning from the lungs flows through an opening in the atrial septum and the right ventricle pumps the blood into the pulmonary artery and then into the aorta.

Hypopolarized the state of a membrane when the membrane potential is more positive than the resting membrane potential but does not reach the threshold potential required to elicit an action potential.

Hypospadias a birth defect in which the urethral opening is abnormally placed, opening anywhere from the tip of the glans of the penis to the shaft or the junction of the penis and scrotum or perineum in males and usually opening in the vagina in females.

Hypothermic injury chilling or freezing of tissues, resulting in disturbances in ion balance and homeostasis.

Hypothyroidism a condition caused by insufficient thyroid hormone synthesis and secretion, resulting in impaired memory, increased sensitivity to heat and cold, slow heart rate, depression, weight gain, slowed metabolism, and several other systemic alterations.

Hypoventilation a condition in which ventilation is inadequate for proper gas exchange, causing an increase in carbon dioxide concentration and subsequent respiratory acidosis.

Hypovolemia decreased blood volume capable of causing hypotension, tachycardia, and decreased urine output.

Hypovolemic shock a state of shock caused by a decrease in blood volume secondary to dehydration, bleeding, and drugs such as diuretics or vasodilators.

Hypoxemia insufficient oxygenation of arterial blood.

Hypoxia a state in which the oxygen level reaching cells is insufficient, resulting in tissue injury; may be caused by a reduction in oxygen content of inspired air, a decrease in hemoglobin available for oxygen binding, or cardiovascular or respiratory disease.

Icterus neonatorum (neonatal jaundice) temporary jaundice in newborn infants caused by functional immaturity of the liver.

Immune thrombocytopenic purpura (ITP) a condition in which the number of platelets in the blood is reduced by the production of antibodies against platelets and that is characterized by ecchymoses and hemorrhages from mucous membranes, anemia, and extreme weakness.

Immunoglobulin any of five structurally distinct classes of proteins that function as antibodies in the serum and external secretions of the body (*see* **Antibody**).

Immunohemolytic anemia an acquired hemolytic anemia in which isoantibodies or autoantibodies are produced in response to drugs, toxins, or other antigens.

Imperforate anus a congenital defect in which the anal opening is absent because of the presence of a membranous septum or of complete absence of the anal canal.

Impetigo a contagious bacterial infection that produces superficial red blisters that rupture and produce thick yellow crusts that commonly occur on the face but can spread to other regions of the body easily.

Infantile spasm episodic muscular spasms in infants characterized by sudden flexion or extension movements in the neck, trunk, and extremities and usually lasting from 1 to 3 seconds.

Infectious mononucleosis (IM) a disease that is caused by the Epstein-Barr virus or the cytomegalovirus that is transmitted by exchanging saliva or blood or by coughing and sneezing and acts by infecting the B cells and atypical T cells resulting in fever, sore throat, and fatigue.

Inflammatory acne a condition characterized by comedones that appear as red, swollen, and inflamed blemishes and by larger, deeper, swollen tender lesions that become inflamed and rupture under the skin.

Inflammatory joint disease a disease in which inflammation affects joint structures and often leads to structural derangement of the joint, structural joint problems, and pain at rest and with motion.

Inflammatory response nonspecific response to tissue damaging irritants in which pain, heat, redness, and swelling rapidly occur at the site of injury.

Inhibin a protein hormone that inhibits follicle-stimulating hormone synthesis and secretion, impairs prolactin and growth hormone secretion, interferes with gonadotropin-releasing hormone receptors, and increases gonadotropin breakdown.

Inhibitory postsynaptic potential (IPSP) a graded hyperpolarization of the postsynaptic membrane in response to neurotransmitter release from a presynaptic neuron.

Innate resistance (immunity) protection or resistance to infection by nonimmune mechanisms such as natural physical, mechanical, and biochemical barriers.

Inotropic agent a substance that affects muscle contraction, especially contraction of the heart muscle.

Insulin protein hormone that is secreted by the beta cells of the islets of Langerhans and functions in carbohydrate and fat metabolism by increasing glucose uptake into muscle and by activating adipose cells to form glycogen and fat.

Insulin resistance a diminished response of liver, muscle, and adipose tissues to insulin, causing hyperglycemia and normal to elevated insulin levels.

Integrin an integral membrane protein that facilitates the attachment of a cell to the extracellular matrix and signal transduction from the extracellular matrix to the cell.

Intermediary metabolism chemical reactions that occur in the cytoplasm and include synthesis, degradation, and transformation of small organic molecules that provide energy for cellular activities.

Interphase the interval between cell divisions during which the chromosomes facilitate RNA synthesis.

Interstitial edema cerebral edema in which interstitial fluid accumulates in conjunction with hydrocephalus.

Interstitial fluid fluid present in the extracellular spaces of a tissue.

Intestinal phase of secretion a period during which digested protein in the duodenum stimulates gastrin secretion that subsequently increases gastric acid secretion.

Intestinointestinal reflex a process by which intestinal motility is inhibited when the intestine becomes overdistended or its mucosa becomes excessively irritated.

Intracerebral hematoma (intraparenchymal hemorrhages) blood accumulation that partially clots inside the brain, usually in the frontal and temporal lobes.

Intramembranous formation the process responsible for the development of flat bones in which ossification of the collagenous matrix is direct and cartilage is not present.

Intraosseous cannulation a procedure in which drugs, fluid, and blood products can be administered rapidly into a noncollapsible marrow venous plexus near the tibial tuberosity.

Intrarenal acute renal failure a type of acute renal failure characterized by renal parenchymal damage that disrupts glomerular filtration and eventually destroys the glomeruli.

Intravascular fluid plasma present in the blood.

Intrinsic factor (IF) a small protein secreted by the parietal cells of gastric glands and required for adequate absorption of vitamin B_{12}.

Intrinsic pathway a component of the coagulation cascade that causes blood clotting in response to contact with a foreign substance.

Intron nucleotide sequence in an RNA molecule that has no known function and is spliced from the hnRNA to form mRNA.

Intussusception an infolding or prolapse of a segment of the small intestine into the adjacent but more distal segment of the intestine.

Invariant chain transmembrane protein that folds into and inhibits activity in the antigen-binding groove of the major histocompatibility complex (MHC) class II molecule.

Ion positively or negatively charged molecule.

Iron deficiency anemia (IDA) a condition caused by insufficient dietary intake or absorption of iron, resulting in decreased incorporation of hemoglobin into red blood cells and subsequent feelings of fatigue, weakness, and shortness of breath as well as pale earlobes, palms, and conjunctivae.

Ischemia insufficient blood flow to tissues that may result in hypoxia and subsequent cell injury or death.

Islets of Langerhans the endocrine region of the pancreas that contains four cell types: alpha cells that secrete glucagon, beta cells that secrete insulin, delta cells that secrete somatostatin, and PP cells that secrete pancreatic polypeptide.

Isohemagglutinin an immunoglobulin that is capable of agglutinating erythrocytes of individuals within the same species.

Isolated systolic hypertension a condition that is caused by loss of elasticity of the arteries resulting in an increase in cardiac output or stroke volume, a systolic blood pressure consistently above 160 mmHg, and a diastolic pressure below 90 mmHg.

Isometric contraction (static or holding contraction) a type of muscle contraction in which the muscle is stimulated but is not allowed to lengthen or shorten and is held at a constant length.

Isotonic contraction a type of muscle contraction in which the muscle is stimulated and shortens while lifting a constant load.

Isthmus a narrow passage connecting two larger parts of an anatomic structure.

Jaundice (icterus) yellowish-brown staining of the skin and the whites of the eyes caused by high bilirubin levels in blood secondary to excessive erythrocyte breakdown, obstruction in or around the liver, or liver disease.

Junctional complex the region of the cell membrane containing desmosomes, tight junctions, and gap junctions that function to hold cells together and provide a passage for cell-to-cell communication.

Juvenile myoclonic epilepsy a type of epilepsy that occurs in adolescents and young adults, usually upon awakening, and is characterized by jerks of the neck, shoulders, and arms and by clonic-tonic-clonic seizures.

Juvenile rheumatoid arthritis (JRA) a condition in which children under the age of 16 develop rheumatoid arthritis and experience swelling, tenderness, and pain in one or more joints and lymph node and splenic enlargement.

Kaposi sarcoma (KS) a type of fatal cancer caused by the herpesvirus in which many bluish-red nodules appear on the skin, especially skin of the lower extremities; occurs in a particularly virulent form in individuals with AIDS.

Kawasaki disease a vascular disease characterized by inflamed heart and vessels, coronary artery aneurysm, thickening and stenosis, a fever that lasts at least 5 days, and at least four of the following: inflammation with reddening of the whites of the eyes; red, swollen hands or feet or peeling skin; rash; swollen lymph gland in the neck; inflamed lips or throat; or red "strawberry" tongue.

Keloid a red, raised overgrown fibrous scar formed by excessive cell growth during tissue repair after trauma or surgical incision.

Keratocanthoma a skin tumor that contains a central keratin mass and usually occurs on exposed skin areas and heals spontaneously but may leave a scar.

Kernicterus a fatal form of jaundice in the newborn caused by elevated levels of unconjugated bilirubin in the blood secondary to an increase in red blood cell number and breakdown and by jaundice-induced lesions in the cerebral gray matter.

Kussmal respiration (hyperpnea) deep, rapid respiration commonly seen in conditions causing acidosis.

Kwashiorkor a condition in which children do not receive enough protein in their diet, resulting in a swollen and severely bloated abdomen secondary to decreased albumin in the blood, skin changes resulting in a reddish discoloration of the hair and skin in dark-skinned children, severe diarrhea, fatty liver, muscle atrophy, and retarded development.

Lactase deficiency a condition in which not enough lactase is present in the small intestine to digest lactose, resulting in lactose intolerance characterized by diarrhea, bloating, and gas in response to exposure to lactose.

Lactoferrin an iron-binding protein found in neutrophils and in many secretions and exudates that acts as an antimicrobial agent by withholding iron from ingested bacteria and fungi.

Lactose intolerance a condition caused by lactase deficiency in which lactose is not broken down, making it impossible for the small intestine to absorb it and causing excessive gas production and diarrhea when exposed to lactose-containing foods.

Laminar flow a flow pattern for liquids that is characterized by high-speed diffusion and low turbulence.

Laminin receptor surface receptor on a tumor cell that anchors to the extracellular region of the basement membrane.

Langerhans cell immature dendritic cell that captures, takes up and processes antigens in response to infection, then travels to the T-cell areas of the lymph node and matures into fully-functional antigen-presenting cells.

Laryngomalacia a congenital anomaly caused by a developmental delay in the laryngeal cartilage and supporting structures of the larynx that causes the cartilage to be floppy and fold in on itself during inspiration, producing high-pitched, coarse, and low-pitched sounds.

Legg-Calvé-Perthes disease a condition in which the blood supply to the head of the femur near the hip joint is interrupted, resulting in osteonecrosis of the corresponding epiphysis.

Leiomyoma a benign smooth muscle mass that can occur in any organ, but most commonly occurs in the myometrium of the uterus or in the esophagus.

Lennox-Gastaut syndrome a generalized myoclonic epilepsy that occurs in children between 1 and 5 years of age as a result of various cerebral afflictions such as perinatal hypoxia, hemorrhage, encephalitis, and metabolic disorders of the brain and is characterized by mental retardation, personality disorders, and generalized tonic seizures.

Leptin a protein hormone that is produced by adipose tissue and provides the brain with an assessment of adipose mass and regulates appetite and metabolism by altering the actions of neuropeptide Y.

Leukemia an acute or chronic disease of the bone marrow in which excessive proliferation of white blood cells occurs and is usually accompanied by anemia, impaired blood clotting, and enlargement of the lymph nodes, liver, and spleen.

Leukemoid reaction a form of leukocytosis that is similar or mimics that occurring in leukemia but results from some other cause.

Leukocyte (white blood cell [WBC]) colorless or white cell in the blood, lymphatic system, spleen, and other body tissues that helps defend the body against infection and disease through specialized neutrophils, lymphocytes, and monocytes.

Leukocytosis an increase in the number of leukocytes in the blood as a result of fever, inflammation, hemorrhage, infection, etc.

Leukopenia a condition in which the number of white blood cells in the blood is decreased, resulting in an increased risk for infection.

Leukotriene a mediator of the prolonged inflammatory response that acts to contract smooth muscle, increase vascular permeability, and attract neutrophils.

Leydig cell cell that is located adjacent to the seminiferous tubules in the testes and functions to produce testosterone in response to luteinizing hormone stimulation.

LH deficiency a condition characterized by decreased or absent production of luteinizing hormone, resulting in a decline in sex steroid production in testes/ovaries and associated infertility.

Liability distribution prediction of the probability of an individual having a specific disease based on exposure to genetic and environmental factors known to cause the disease.

Lichen planus a condition in which a recurrent rash of small, flat-topped bumps and rough scaly patches appear on the skin, in the lining of the mouth and in the vagina in response to inflammation or an allergy to a specific medication.

Lieberkühn crypt any of the tubular glands on the mucous surface of the small and large intestines.

Life expectancy the range of years representing the average length of life for humans.

Ligand substance that binds to a specific cellular receptor, resulting in the initiation of cellular events specific to that receptor.

Limb girdle muscular dystrophy a progressive genetic disorder that usually begins before adolescence and presents similar to facioscapulohumeral muscular dystrophy but with the hips and shoulders being the most severely affected muscles.

Linkage genes that are transmitted, inherited, and assorted together.

Lipofuscin yellow-brown pigment produced by breakdown of damaged blood cells in heart and smooth muscle.

Liquefactive necrosis liquefaction of neurons and glial cells in the brain as a result of ischemic injury or bacterial infection.

Loop of Henle a section of the nephron that extends from the proximal convoluted tubule to the distal convoluted tubule and that reabsorbs water from its descending limb and salts from its ascending limb.

Loss of heterozygosity loss of a region on one chromosome that corresponds to a mutated region on the other chromosome; loss of the same loci on both chromosomes inactivates the affected gene.

Lupus erythematosus any of a group of autoimmune connective tissue disorders that commonly produce red scaly lesions and are accompanied by fever, malaise, myalgias, fatigue, and weight loss.

Luteal/secretory phase the phase that represents the period after ovulation during which the follicular cells are forming the corpus luteum that secretes progesterone and the endometrium is becoming more vascularized and begins secreting a clear fluid in preparation for implantation.

Lyme disease tick-borne spirochete bacterial infection that is characterized by a rash in the area of the bite, headache, neck stiffness, chills, fever, myalgia, arthralgia, malaise, fatigue, and possible development of arthritis in large joints.

Lymphadenopathy a condition in which one or more lymph nodes are swollen because of diseases such as bacterial or viral infection, Hodgkin lymphoma, non-Hodgkin lymphoma, or unknown causes.

Lymphocyte nonphagocytic leukocyte of the adaptive immune response that is immunologically competent and serves as the precursor for B and T lymphocytes.

Lymphocytopenia a condition in which the number of lymphocytes in the blood is decreased because of diseases and conditions such as human immunodeficiency virus, severe stress, or the administration of corticosteroids, chemotherapy, or radiation therapy.

Lymphocytosis a condition in which the number of lymphocytes in the blood is increased because of infection, inflammation, or leukemia.

Lymphogranuloma venereum (LGV) a sexually transmitted bacterial disease that enters the body through breaks in the skin or across the epithelial cell layer of mucous membranes and primarily targets the lymphatics and lymph nodes.

Lymphoma cancer arising from cell proliferation in lymphoid tissue.

Lysosomal storage diseases a group of over thirty disorders that result from impaired lysosomal function, leading to mucopolysaccharidoses, lipid storage disorders, mucolipidoses, leukodystrophies, and glycoprotein storage disorders.

Macrocytic anemia (megaloblastic anemia) a condition characterized by a deficiency of vitamin B_{12} or folic acid caused by inadequate intake or insufficient absorption secondary to alcoholism or drugs that inhibit DNA replication.

Macrophage phagocyte that is produced from a monocyte and is important in cellular initiation of the inflammatory response.

Macula densa an area of the nephron comprised of closely packed cells that line the distal convoluted tubule and lie next to the glomerulus where they monitor blood salt concentration and pressure and release renin when either decreases.

Major (unipolar) depression severely depressed mood and loss of pleasure that may begin suddenly or slowly, persists for at least 2 weeks, and may recur throughout life.

Major histocompatibility complex (MHC) a set of recognition molecules that are used to identify whether donor and recipient tissues possess antigens that make them compatible.

Malignant hypertension a complication of hypertension in which blood pressure is severely elevated and organ damage occurs in the eyes, brain, lung, and/or kidneys.

Malignant tumor cancerous mass of cells that grows, invades, and metastasizes, usually causing death.

Map unit unit of measurement for the distance between loci on a chromosome based on crossover frequencies.

Marasmus a childhood disorder characterized by protein and energy malnutrition, resulting in dry skin, loss of adipose tissue from normal areas of fat deposits such as buttocks and thighs, and behavior that is fretful and irritable.

Margination (pavementing) a process by which leukocytes adhere better to endothelial cells of the capillary walls and venules by the reciprocal change in adhesion molecules on leukocytes.

Mast cell a cell of the connective tissue that produces substances that cause activation of the inflammatory response, vasoconstriction, and muscle contraction.

Mastocytosis a condition characterized by the abnormal proliferation of mast cells that results in an increase in mast cell–derived chemicals being released, subsequently causing changes in the immune system that produce typical allergy symptoms such as itching, abdominal cramping, and even anaphylaxis.

Maximal life span a range of years representing the average age of death for humans.

McArdle disease a metabolic disorder involving an enzyme defect that causes deficiency of muscle phosphorylase, which helps break down glycogen, and consequently this disorder causes an energy deficit in the muscles, resulting in muscle pain and cramping.

Mean arterial pressure (MAP) an average blood pressure in an individual that is equal to diastolic pressure plus $\frac{1}{3}$ of the pulse pressure and is considered the perfusion pressure of organs in the body.

Meconium a dark green fecal material that accumulates in the fetal intestines and is discharged at or near the time of birth.

Meconium ileus a condition in which the intestine of a newborn child is obstructed with thickened meconium as a result of a lack of trypsin and is associated with cystic fibrosis of the pancreas.

Mediated transport the transport of inorganic ions and some organic compounds across the cell membrane by way of integral membrane or transmembrane proteins that contain specific receptors.

Medulloblastoma a malignant cerebellar tumor near the fourth ventricle that is most often found in children and consists of neoplastic cells that resemble the undifferentiated cells of the neural tube.

Megacalycosis a congenital condition in which enlarged calyces are present with a normal pelvis and ureter, possibly caused by previous obstruction or reflux.

Melanin brown-black pigment that is synthesized by melanocytes in skin and accumulates in the skin and retina.

Melanocyte a pigment-producing cell that is located in the skin, hair, and eye and produces the pigment melanin that determines their color.

Membranous glomerulonephritis a slowly progressive disease of unknown origin or that occurs secondary to autoimmune conditions, infections, specific drugs, or malignant tumors that is caused by a circulating immune complex formed from the binding of antibodies to antigens of the glomerular basement membrane or antigens transported from the systemic circulation.

Memory cell T or B lymphocyte that "remembers" a specific antigen after the initial exposure and initiates a more efficient immunologic response in response to subsequent exposures to the same antigen.

Meningioma a slow-growing mass of the meninges that is usually benign but increases intracranial pressure.

Meningocele neural tube defect in the skull or spinal column that forms a cyst filled with cerebrospinal fluid through which the meninges of the brain protrude.

Menstruation the flow of blood and cells from the endometrium that occurs about every 28 days in the nonpregnant woman beginning between ages 9 and 17 and ending around age 50.

Mental retardation impaired intellectual development as a result of congenital causes, brain injury, or disease, resulting in impaired learning, social, and vocational ability.

Mesenteric venous thrombosis a condition in which a blood clot blocks off one of the mesenteric veins and compromises the intestinal blood supply and can result in intestinal gangrene and tissue death.

Mesodermal germ layer tissue located between the ectoderm and endoderm that gives rise to an epithelial component of genital and urinary structures, striated muscle, connective tissue, cartilage, bone, smooth muscle, and blood cells.

Mesothelioma a type of cancer that is usually associated with previous exposure to asbestos, which affects the pleura, the lining of the abdominal cavity, the pericardium, and most internal organ coverings.

Messenger RNA (mRNA) RNA molecule produced during transcription that provides the amino acid sequence for protein synthesis.

Metabolic acidosis decrease in pH caused by an increase in noncarbonic acids or a decrease in bicarbonate.

Metabolic alkalosis increase in pH caused by an increase in bicarbonate ions secondary to an increase in metabolic acid loss.

Metabolic syndrome a condition of unknown cause that presents with symptoms of insulin resistance, obesity, hypertension, dyslipidemia, and systemic inflammation.

Metaphase second phase of mitosis, during which chromosomes are condensed and aligned along the equatorial plate for nuclear and cellular division.

Metatarsus adductus a foot deformity in which the front half of the foot bends inward, possibly because of the infant's position in the uterus.

Micelle a cluster of emulsifying surfactant molecules that forms when the concentration of surfactant is greater than the critical micelle concentration.

Microcephaly defect in which failure of normal brain growth causes a delayed skull growth and production of a small head.

Microcytic-hypochromic anemia a condition in which red blood cells are smaller than normal.

Microglia neuroglial cell that migrates and functions as a phagocyte for nerve tissue waste products.

Microtubules small protein tubules located in the cytosol that add strength to the cell structure, facilitate intracellular organelle and cell movement and nerve transmission, and play a role in immune and inflammatory actions and hormone secretion.

Migraine headache headache that usually begins in the temporal region unilaterally after constriction of cranial arteries and may cause irritability, nausea, vomiting, constipation or diarrhea, and photophobia.

Mild concussion temporary axonal disturbances without the loss of consciousness in response to a violent blow, jarring, shaking, or other closed head injury.

Miliaria a skin disease caused by partially obstructed sweat glands that results in small and itchy rashes usually located in skinfolds and on areas of the body that may rub against clothing, such as the back, chest, and stomach.

Mineralocorticoid a steroid hormone that is secreted by the adrenal cortex and functions to regulate the balance of water and electrolytes in the body.

Minimal change nephropathy (MCN) a condition in which the foot processes of the renal capillary basement membrane are fused and deformed because of a T cell disorder that reduces the anion component of the basement membrane and allows proteins to leak into the renal tubule.

Minute ventilation the volume of gas inhaled into and expelled from the lungs per minute or tidal volume multiplied by ventilation rate.

Mitochondrion large organelle where most of the cell's ATP is generated by oxidative phosphorylation.

Mitosis the process of nuclear division during which two identical nuclei are produced from one parent cell after chromosomal replication.

Mitral valve a valve in the heart that lies between the left atrium and left ventricle and functions to allow blood to flow into the left ventricle during ventricular diastole and to prevent regurgitation from the ventricle to the left atrium during systole.

Mitral valve prolapse syndrome a condition in which the mitral valve cannot close properly because of one or both flaps being too large, possibly resulting in mitral valve regurgitation.

Molluscum contagiosum a skin disease commonly found in young children that affects the body, arms, and legs and is spread through direct contact, saliva, or shared articles of clothing and is considered a sexually transmitted disease in adults, affecting the genitals, lower abdomen, buttocks, and inner thighs.

Monoclonal gammopathy of undetermined significance (MGUS) a condition in which monoclonal antibodies are produced by noncancerous plasma cells and accumulate in the blood.

Monocyte phagocyte produced in bone marrow that migrates into tissues and is transformed into macrophages.

Monocytopenia a condition in which the number of monocytes in the blood is decreased because of the release of toxins into the blood by bacteria or by administration of chemotherapy or corticosteroids.

Monocytosis a condition in which the number of monocytes in the blood is increased because of chronic infection, autoimmune disorder, blood disorder, or cancer.

Mononuclear phagocyte system (MPS) a collection of free and fixed macrophages derived from bone marrow cells whose phagocytic activity is primarily mediated by immunoglobulin and by the serum complement system.

Monozygotic (identical) twins two separate identical embryos formed when the initial zygote divides in two.

Motilin a protein hormone believed to aide in control of regular gastrointestinal muscular activity.

Moyamoya disease an abnormality of the blood vessels that supply the frontal region of the brain in which vessels constrict or become completely occluded resulting in diminished blood flow. The body attempts to compensate by growing new vessels at the base of the brain, which appear as a puff of smoke on an angiography.

Mucoepidermoid carcinoma a tumor of the main or lobar bronchi lumen that may extend into the peribronchial tissue.

Mucopurulent cervicitis (MPC) inflammation of the cervix with purulent endocervical exudate that may be asymptomatic or cause abnormal vaginal discharge and vaginal bleeding.

Multifactorial trait a trait that is affected by genes as well as environment or life-style.

Multiple sclerosis chronic demyelinating disease of the central nervous system that causes inflammation and scarring of myelin sheaths.

Myasthenia gravis neuromuscular disorder caused by an autoimmune response in which antibodies to acetylcholine receptors impair neuromuscular transmission.

Mycotic aneurysm aneurysm that is caused by bacterial or fungal growth in the vessel wall or infection of a arteriosclerotic aneurysm.

Myelodysplasia abnormal formation of the spinal cord.

Myelodysplastic syndrome (MDS) a group of hematologic conditions characterized by ineffective production of blood cells, resulting in anemia that requires chronic blood transfusion.

Myeloma a tumor composed of cells derived from hemopoietic tissue of the bone marrow.

Myoadenylate deaminase deficiency (MDD) a genetic disorder in which an enzyme deficiency prevents the conversion of adenosine monophosphate (AMP) to inosine monophosphate, resulting in increased AMP loss and the inability to synthesize adenosine triphosphate for energy.

Myocardial infarction a heart condition of sudden onset in which muscle tissue dies because of a lack of blood flow, resulting in varying degrees of chest pain or discomfort, weakness, sweating, nausea, and vomiting, and possibly loss of consciousness.

Myocardial oxygen consumption (MVO$_2$) the amount of oxygen consumed by cardiac muscle cells during work, as determined by myocyte contraction and factors that enhance or impair this contraction, such as the rate of tension development or the number of tension-generating cycles per unit time.

Myosin a protein in muscle cells that is arranged in long filaments called *thick filaments* and attaches to actin filaments in a sliding motion during muscle contraction.

Myositis a condition in which a muscle, usually a voluntary muscle, is inflamed, resulting in pain, tenderness, and sometimes spasm in the affected area.

Myositis ossificans a condition in which bone is deposited in muscle tissue, causing pain and swelling.

Myotonia a neuromuscular disorder in which muscle relaxation after voluntary contraction is delayed.

Myxedema a disease caused by impaired thyroid gland activity in adults and characterized by dry skin, swellings around the lips and nose, mental deterioration, and a decrease in basal metabolic rate.

Natural killer (NK) cell lymphocyte capable of killing target cells by binding specific receptors with or without the aid of antibodies and by releasing chemicals toxic to the targeted cells.

Necrotizing enterocolitis (NEC) a condition of extensive ulceration and necrosis of the ileum and colon in premature infants during the neonatal period.

Neonatal alloimmune thrombocytopenic purpura (NATP) a condition in which fetal platelets have an antigen from the father that is absent in the mother, and the mother forms antibodies that cross the placenta and destroy the fetal platelets.

Nephritic syndrome a condition in which the patient experiences nephritis, hematuria, hypertension, and renal failure.

Nephroblastoma a condition, also known as *Wilms tumor,* that is characterized by a malignant renal tumor that compresses the normal kidney parenchyma, causing an abdominal mass, blood in the urine, and fever and may be associated with anorexia, vomiting, and malaise

Nephrotic syndrome a condition in which the glomerular membrane is attacked by complement, resulting in symptoms of nephritis, hematuria, hypertension, and renal failure.

Neuroblastoma a malignant tumor containing neuroblast cells that originate in the autonomic nervous system or the adrenal medulla and is most common in infants and young children.

Neurogenic bladder dysfunction the underactivity or overactivity of the bladder caused by nervous system damage that prevents the bladder muscles from contracting to empty the bladder completely or that causes rapid bladder contraction that causes too rapid or frequent emptying.

Neurogenic detrusor overactivity a neurologic abnormality that impairs communication between the bladder and the central nervous system, preventing the brain from inhibiting the detrusor muscles that controls urination.

Neurogenic shock a type of shock caused by the sudden loss of the sympathetic nervous system signals to the smooth muscle in vessel walls, causing the vessels to relax and a decrease in peripheral vascular resistance and blood pressure.

Neuroglial cell supporting cell that forms myelin, transports material and nutrients to neurons, maintains the ionic balance of neurons, and phagocytoses nerve waste products.

Neurohormonal signaling communication between cells that originates when a hormone is released from a neurosecretory neuron and travels through the bloodstream to bind to a target cell and elicit a response.

Neuron nerve cell of the central nervous system that contains a nucleus within the cell body, dendrites that receive messages from other cells and axons that transmit messages to other cells.

Neuropathic pain pain that is perceived as burning or pins and needles or electric shock that is produced by the stimulation of pain, touch, and temperature receptors of the same area.

Neurotransmitter a chemical that is stored in vesicles in the axon terminal and is released into the synapse in response to an action potential.

Neutropenia the absence of neutrophils in the blood.

Neutrophil (polymorphonuclear neutrophil) (PMN) phagocyte that destroys bacteria by phagocytosis, digestion, and secretion of bacteria-killing chemicals.

Neutrophilia a condition in which the number of neutrophils, especially the younger, less mature cells in the blood is increased.

Nevi (mole) a benign growth or mark on the skin that is colored by hyperpigmentation or increased vascularity and appears early in life.

Nissl substances structures, also known as *Nissl bodies,* that are located in the cell bodies of neurons and are involved in protein synthesis.

Nonbacterial prostatitis a condition in which prostatitis causes chronic pain that goes away and comes back without warning but shows no signs of bacterial infection in the prostatic fluid even though the semen and other fluids from the prostate contain immune cells that the body produces in response to infection.

Nonbacterial thrombotic endocarditis a condition in which fibrin is deposited on the valve leaflets of the heart, especially on the left side, as a result of cancer, rheumatic fever, or arteriosclerosis.

Noncommunicating hydrocephalus cerebrospinal fluid accumulation within the skull that is caused by obstruction of the cerebrospinal fluid pathways.

Non-Hodgkin lymphoma (NHL) a condition of the lymphoid tissue that mimics Hodgkin lymphoma but does not produce the cells characteristic of Hodgkin' disease and does not have a definitive cause other than association with latent Epstein-Barr virus, AIDS, or Agent Orange exposure.

Noninflammatory acne a condition characterized by open comedones caused by the enlargement and dilation of a plug resulting from the accumulation of oil and dead skin cells inside the hair follicle and by closed comedones that form if the hair follicle pore remains closed and which appear as a tiny, sometimes pink bump in the skin.

Noninflammatory joint disease a disease in which alterations in the structure or mechanics of the joint results in pain during motion.

Nonossifying fibroma (fibrous cortical deficit) a condition found in children and adolescents in which a benign fibrous tissue tumor forms in the metaphysis of any of the long bones but usually occurs in the thigh and shin bones.

Non-REM (slow wave) sleep period of sleep during which dreams do not occur and brain waves are slow and high voltage.

Nonvolatile a substance that does not have a vapor form.

Normal anion gap measure of anion gap taking into account anions not usually measured.

Normocytic-normochromic anemia (NNA) a condition in which erythrocytes are of normal size and hemoglobin content but of insufficient number and that is usually caused by hereditary spherocytosis, drug-induced anemia, and anemia secondary to other malignancies.

Nucleolus a small structure in the nucleus that contains the DNA of the cell and the associated binding proteins and where RNA subunits of ribosomes are assembled.

Nucleotide DNA subunit containing one deoxyribose molecule, one phosphate group, and one nitrogenous base.

Nucleus a large membrane-bound organelle that contains the cellular DNA and is located in the center of the cell.

Nystagmus involuntary, rapid, rhythmic movements of the eyeball in the horizontal, vertical, or rotational direction.

Obsessive-compulsive disorder (OCD) an anxiety disorder characterized by obsessive thoughts and repetitive compulsive actions, such as cleaning, checking, or counting.

Obstructive sleep apnea syndrome (OSAS) airway obstruction resulting in disruption of sleep or arousal that is accompanied by snoring.

Obstructive uropathy a condition in which the flow of urine is blocked, often by ureteral or kidney stones, resulting in the reflux of urine and subsequent injury to kidneys.

Occult bleeding blood in the feces or vomit that is not visible upon gross inspection but is detected in tests used to screen for colon cancer.

Oligodendroglia (oligodendrocyte) neuroglial cell of the central nervous system that coils around the axon of the neuron to form a myelin sheath.

Oligodendroglioma a slow-growing mass of the oligodendrogliocytes that is usually benign.

Oncogene tumor-causing gene that increases the rate of cell proliferation if mutated.

Oncotic pressure (colloid osmotic pressure) pressure that is created by large molecules such as plasma proteins that cannot penetrate the membrane and pulls water toward the proteins.

Onychomycosis a fungal infection of the fingernails or toenails that causes thickening, roughness, and splitting of the nails.

Opsonin a C3b fragment that attaches antigens to phagocytes, thereby tagging them for destruction.

Orchitis swelling of the testicles that can result in ejaculation of blood, blood in the urine, and pain and visible swelling of a testicle or testicles.

Organ tropism growth of a tissue or organism in response to external stimuli.

Orthostatic (postural) hypotension a condition in which blood pressure suddenly falls when a person assumes a standing position, resulting in dizziness, lightheadedness, blurred vision, and temporary loss of consciousness.

Osmotic pressure pressure exerted by the membrane and solutes in a solution that must be overcome for osmosis to occur.

Osteoarthritis (OA) a type of noninflammatory joint disease in which synthesis and degradation of the articular cartilage in the movable joints is imbalanced, resulting in wearing and destruction of cartilage.

Osteoblast the primary bone-forming cell that secretes enzymes that facilitate mineral deposition on osteoids and provides some regulation of osteoclasts.

Osteocalcin a protein found in bone tissue that has an unknown function but has high affinity for bone mineral constituents and may be involved in bone formation.

Osteochondroses a condition in children, also known as *Osgood-Schlatter disease,* that results from the tendons pulling on the epiphysis of long bones, causing pain just below the knee, irritation and swelling, and possibly abnormal bone growth.

Osteoclast a cell found in the growing bone that degrades and reabsorbs bone.

Osteocyte osteoblast that is embedded in the matrix and functions in maintaining bone tissue.

Osteogenesis imperfecta (brittle bone disease) a genetic disease in which collagen production is deficient making the bones abnormally fragile and causing recurring fractures with only minimal trauma, deformity of long bones, a bluish coloration of the sclerae, and often the development of otosclerosis.

Osteoid a protein mixture composed mainly of collagen that is secreted by osteoblasts and becomes mineralized to form bone.

Osteoid osteoma a benign tumor in one of the bones of the lower extremities that is painful and is characterized by vascularized connective tissue and osteoid material that is surrounded by a large zone of thickened bone.

Osteomalacia a disease in which vitamin D or calcium deficiency or excessive renal phosphate loss causes a softening of the bones with accompanying pain and weakness.

Osteomyelitis a bacterial infection of the bone and bone marrow that occurs through open fractures, penetrating wounds, surgical operations, or by entering via the bloodstream and causes pain, high fever, and formation of an abscess at the site of infection.

Osteonectin a protein in bone that binds both collagen and hydroxyapatite and links collagen to minerals in the bone matrix.

Osteoporosis a disease in which the bones become porous and weakened making it easily fractured and slow to heal.

Ovarian torsion a condition in which an ovary twists or turns on its supporting ligament to the point that its blood supply is compromised.

Ovulation the release of an ovum from the ovaries around midcycle or approximately 2 weeks into the menstrual cycle.

Oxidation chemical reaction in which electrons are lost.

Oxidative phosphorylation process by which adenosine diphosphate (ADP) is converted into adenosine triphosphate (ATP) and inorganic phosphate through reoxidation and phosphorylation of ADP.

Oxidative stress tissue injury induced by free radicals that are produced during metabolic reactions and with exposure to some environmental agents.

Oxyhemoglobin dissociation curve a sigmoid plot of the percent hemoglobin bonding sites occupied by oxygen versus the partial pressure of oxygen, which illustrates the affinity of hemoglobin for oxygen.

Oxytocin protein hormone that is produced in the hypothalamus, stored in and released from the posterior pituitary, and acts to increase milk let-down and uterine contractions.

p53 **protein** tumor suppressor gene that inhibits the development of cancer by opposing oncogene action and promoting DNA repair.

Paget disease (osteitis deformans) a bone disorder in which excessive bone remodeling causes enlarged, deformed bones that can weaken the bone integrity and result in bone pain, arthritis, deformities, or fractures.

Pancreas an endocrine/exocrine gland that regulates blood sugar by secreting insulin and glucagon and aids in food digestion by secreting an enzyme into the small intestine.

Pancreatic insufficiency a condition in which the pancreas does not secrete enough hormones and digestive enzymes for normal digestion to occur, resulting in malabsorption, malnutrition, vitamin deficiencies, and weight loss.

Pancreatitis inflammation of the pancreas usually resulting in abdominal pain.

Panic disorder a psychologic disorder that is characterized by recurrent attacks of anxiety or terror and usually results in the development of one or more phobias.

Papillary muscle any of the myocardial bundles that terminate in the chordae tendineae and attach to the cusps of the atrioventricular valves to limit the movements of the mitral and tricuspid valves and prevent them from being everted.

Papilloma a benign nodular breast lesion consisting of hyperplastic distorted ductal cells.

Paraphimosis a condition in which the foreskin becomes trapped behind the glans penis and cannot return to its normal flaccid position covering the glans penis.

Parathyroid hormone (PTH) a protein hormone secreted by the parathyroid glands that regulates calcium and phosphate levels in the body by promoting the absorption of calcium by the intestine, mobilization of calcium and phosphate from bones, and increasing the tendency of the kidney to reabsorb calcium and excrete phosphate.

Parenchyma tissue that is responsible for the physiologic function of an organ.

Parkinson disease degeneration of the basal ganglia dopaminergic nigrostriatal pathway that causes hypokinesia, tremor, and muscular rigidity.

Paronychia a condition in which the tissue surrounding a fingernail or toenail is inflamed.

Partial pressure the pressure of a specific gas that is contained in a mixture in the atmosphere if all other components of the mixture or solution were removed without changing temperature; partial pressure of a gas is proportional to the temperature and the concentration of the gas in a mixture.

Partial seizure (focal seizure) a seizure caused by focused excessive electrical activity caused by a lesion in a particular region.

Passive acquired immunity (passive immunity) a form of acquired immunity in which the antibody or lymphocyte is provided by a donor.

Passive mediated transport (facilitated diffusion) carrier-mediated transport of solutes across the membrane down a concentration gradient and in the absence of energy expenditure.

Passive transport movement of water and small, uncharged particles through a membrane using osmosis, diffusion, or hydrostatic pressure as a driving force and requiring no energy expenditure.

Pathogen-associated molecular pattern (PAMP) molecular patterns on infectious agents or their products that allow recognition by specific receptors.

Pattern recognition receptor (PRR) a receptor involved in innate resistance that recognizes cellular damage or specific patterns on infectious agents.

Pediculosis pubis a contagious condition, also known as *crabs* or *crab lice,* that is a crab louse infestation of the pubic hair, the louse feeds on human blood and multiplies rapidly.

Pedigree a chart that summarizes family relationships and shows which members are affected by a genetic disease.

Pelvic inflammatory disease (PID) inflammation of the female genital tract that is caused by microorganisms, typically those that are sexually transmitted such as chlamydia and gonococci, and is characterized by severe abdominal pain, high fever, vaginal discharge, and possibly infertility.

Pemphigus any of a group of autoimmune skin diseases marked by groups of itching blisters and raw sores on the skin and mucous membranes.

Pepsin one of three protein-degrading enzymes in the digestive system that becomes active in an acidic environment and functions to break down proteins into their components to ease absorption by the intestinal lining.

Pepsinogen a proenzyme produced in the mucosal lining of the stomach that is converted to the active enzyme pepsin in response to gastric acid or previously synthesized pepsin.

Peptic ulcer a nonmalignant stomach or duodenal wall ulceration, commonly caused by the bacterium *Helicobacter pylori* that thrives in the acidic environment of the stomach.

Perceptual dominance the inability to feel weak painful stimulation because of the presence of a stronger painful stimulus.

Perihepatitis a condition, also known as *Fitz-Hugh-Curtis syndrome*, that is a complication of pelvic inflammatory disease secondary to gonococci bacteria traveling up the peritoneum to the upper abdomen and causing inflammation.

Perimenopause the transition to menopause that begins about 6 years before menopause and is marked by fluctuating hormone levels resulting in irregular menstrual patterns, hot flashes, and possibly night sweats, mood swings, vaginal dryness, fluctuations in libido, cognitive changes, insomnia, and fatigue.

Periodic paralysis one of a group of diseases in which muscular weakness or flaccid paralysis occurs without loss of consciousness, speech, or sensation.

Peripheral artery disease (PAD) any of a group of diseases caused by the obstruction of large peripheral arteries secondary to atherosclerosis, inflammatory processes, embolism, or thrombus formation that caused ischemia.

Peripheral tolerance a state in which peripheral lymphoid organs control autoreactive T cells to prevent an immunologic reaction to an individual's own tissues.

Peristalsis the involuntary wavelike muscular contractions of the intestine or other tubular structures that moves the contents onward by alternating contraction and relaxation.

Pernicious anemia an autoimmune disorder that causes a deficiency in intrinsic factor resulting in the inability to absorb vitamin B_{12} and a subsequent increase in the production of abnormal erythrocytes.

Peroxisomes (microbodies) membrane-bound organelle that contains the enzyme catalase and one or more oxidases that use oxygen to remove hydrogen atoms from a substance; this oxidative reaction results in the production of hydrogen peroxide.

Pes planus (flatfoot) a condition in which the arch of the foot never develops or it collapses and contacts the ground.

Peyronie disease (bent nail syndrome) a condition in which fibrous plaques grow in the soft tissue of the penis because of injury of the internal cavity of the penis that is accompanied by bleeding and scar tissue formation at the tunica albuginea of the corpora cavernosa.

Phagocytosis a type of endocytosis sometimes referred to as "cell eating" in which substances such as bacteria and cell particulate are incorporated into large vesicles or vacuoles and digested.

Phantom limb pain pain experienced in an amputated limb after the stump has healed that may be caused by spontaneous firing of afferent pain fibers in the spinal cord that were previously associated with the limb.

Phenotype physical characteristics of an individual as determined by genotype and environmental influences.

Phenylketonuria (PKU) a genetic disorder in which the body lacks the enzyme necessary to metabolize the amino acid phenylalanine to tyrosine, resulting in accumulation of phenylalanine and subsequent brain damage and progressive mental retardation.

Pheochromocytoma a tumor of the adrenal medulla that causes the chromaffin cells to secrete increased amounts of epinephrine or norepinephrine.

Philadelphia chromosome a specific genetic abnormality that is associated with chronic myelogenous leukemia, acute lymphoblastic leukemia, and occasionally acute myelogenous leukemia.

Phimosis a condition in which the foreskin of the penis of an uncircumcised male cannot be fully retracted.

Physiologic dead space the volume of air that does not participate in gas exchange or the sum of anatomic and alveolar dead space.

Pinocytosis a type of endocytosis sometimes referred to as "cell drinking" in which extracellular substances are incorporated into small intracellular vesicles for digestion.

Pityriasis rosea a skin disorder, thought to be caused by a virus, in which patches of ovular pink rash appear primarily on the trunk and extremities.

Plasma cell a B lymphocyte that secretes antibodies in response to local cytokines released during the primary immune response.

Plasma kinin cascade a series of events that activates the kinin system to produce bradykinin.

Plasma membrane receptor protein attached to the extracellular region of an integral membrane protein that binds to a specific ligand such as hormones, neurotransmitters, antigens, complement components, lipoproteins, infectious agents, drugs, and metabolites.

Plasma protein systems the complement, clotting, and kinin systems that provide protection from pathogens by initiating an inflammatory response.

Plasmin a degrading enzyme associated with fibrinolysis of many proteins of blood but primarily of fibrin clots.

Plasticity the ability of nervous system pathways to change function, sensitivity, and so forth in response to changes in the neural environment.

Platelet cellular fragment formed from megakaryocytes that circulates in the blood and is important in anticoagulation, stimulation of inflammation and tissue growth, and destroying bacteria.

Platelet-activating factor (PAF) a mast cell–derived substance that increases vascular permeability, leukocyte adhesion to endothelial cells, and platelet activation.

Pleural effusion a medical condition in which fluid accumulates in the pleural cavity surrounding the lungs and thereby makes breathing difficult.

Pneumoconiosis a chronic disease of the lungs typically seen in miners, sandblasters, and metal grinders that is caused by repeated inhalation of dust particles, including iron oxides, silicates, and carbonates, that collect in the lungs and become sites for the formation of fibrous nodules that eventually replace lung tissue.

Pneumonia an infection of one or both lungs caused by a bacterium, virus, fungus, or other organism that enters the body through respiratory passages and causes high fever, chills, pain in the chest, difficulty in breathing, cough with sputum, and possibly bluish skin from insufficiently oxygenated blood.

Pneumothorax the collapse of a lung and subsequent escape of air into the pleural cavity between the lung and the chest wall that is caused by trauma, environmental factors, or spontaneous occurrence and results in a sudden pain in the chest.

Polarity a condition in which a molecule has a region on one side that is positively charged and another on the opposite side that is negatively charged.

Polycystic kidney disease (PKD) a condition in which several fluid-filled cysts grow in the kidneys and may reduce kidney function and result in kidney failure as well as damage to the liver, pancreas, and possibly the heart and brain.

Polycystic ovary syndrome (PCOS) a hormonal condition in which multiple ovarian cysts form because of elevated androgens, resulting in hirsutism, obesity, menstrual abnormalities, infertility, and enlarged ovaries.

Polycythemia a condition characterized by an increase in the production of red blood cells in the blood.

Polycythemia vera a chronic, progressive disease that is characterized by overgrowth of the bone marrow, excessive red blood cell production, and an enlarged spleen and causes headache, inability to concentrate, and pain in the fingers and toes.

Polymerization a chemical reaction in which monomer molecules are joined together to form linear chains or a three-dimensional network of polymer chains.

Polypeptide chain of amino acids that are linked by phosphodiester bonds.

Polyribosomes two or more ribosomes that are physically attached and translate a single mRNA molecule simultaneously to produce identical proteins.

Portal hypertension an increase in blood pressure in the veins of the portal system resulting from obstruction in the liver, such as that seen in cirrhosis, that causes enlargement of the spleen and collateral veins.

Port-wine (nevus flammeus) stain a birthmark caused by superficial and deep dilated capillaries in the skin that produce a reddish to purplish discoloration of the skin, usually the eye lids.

Posthemorrhagic anemia a type of normocytic-normochromic anemia that is caused by sudden blood loss in an individual with normal iron stores and triggers a compensatory response in which water and electrolytes from tissues and interstitial spaces are used to expand plasma volume and accelerate the formation and development of blood cells.

Postmortem change diffuse physiologic changes that occur within minutes after death.

Postobstructive diuresis elevated urine output occurring after surgery to remove an obstruction that causes the inability of the renal tubules to reabsorb water and electrolytes normally.

Postrenal acute renal failure a condition characterized by an obstruction that affects the normal flow of urine out of both kidneys and causes pressure to build in the nephrons that eventually shuts them down.

Posttraumatic stress disorder (PTSD) a psychologic disorder that may develop in individuals who have experienced or witnessed traumatic events and is characterized by recurrent flashbacks of the traumatic event, nightmares, irritability, anxiety, fatigue, forgetfulness, and social withdrawal.

Potassium adaptation the ability of the kidney to maintain potassium balance when intake increases no more than 120 mEq/day.

Poverty of content a disorder, also called *poverty of speech content,* that is characterized by disorganized speech that conveys little information and may be vague or contain repetitive or obscure phrases.

Precocious puberty a condition in which a boy or girl undergoes the changes associated with puberty at an unexpectedly early age; often caused by a pathologic process that increases the secretion of estrogens or androgens

Preload the volume of blood in the ventricle after atrial contraction and ventricular filling.

Premenstrual syndrome (PMS) a group of symptoms that occur in many women from 2 to 14 days before menstruation begins, such as abdominal bloating, breast tenderness, headache, fatigue, irritability, depression, and emotional distress.

Prerenal acute renal failure a condition characterized by azotemia caused by a reduction in effective arterial blood volume that causes the kidney to behave as though renal perfusion is impaired.

Presbyopia a form of farsightedness usually accompanying advanced age in which the lens loses elasticity and becomes unable to accommodate and focus light for near vision.

Priapism a painful condition in which the erect penis maintains an erection in the absence of physical and psychologic stimulation.

Primary (neoadjuvant) chemotherapy presurgical use of chemotherapy to decrease tumor size in cancer patients.

Primary dysmenorrheal a condition in which menstruation is painful because of a functional disturbance rather than because of inflammation, growths, or anatomic factors.

Primary hyperparathyroidism usually the result of a benign parathyroid tumor that loses its sensitivity to circulating calcium levels; this condition is accompanied by hypercalcemia, nausea, vomiting, lethargy, depression, muscular weakness, and an altered mental state.

Primary hypertension a condition of elevated blood pressure of unknown etiology that is accompanied by increased total peripheral vascular resistance by vasoconstriction, increased cardiac output, or both.

Primary immune response time interval between the first and second exposures to an antigen, during which antibodies against the antigen are produced.

Primary lysosome a lysosome that possesses hydrolytic enzymes but has a high pH and is therefore inactive and not yet involved in digestive activity.

Primary syphilis a stage of syphilis infection that occurs after an incubation period of 10 to 90 days and is characterized by a primary sore or chancre that develops at the point of initial exposure and lasts 4 to 6 weeks.

Progesterone a steroid hormone secreted by the corpus luteum and placenta that prepares the uterus for implantation of the fertilized ovum, maintains pregnancy, and promotes development of the mammary glands in preparation for breastfeeding.

Prokaryote organisms such as bacteria and cyanobacteria that do not have a true nucleus or membrane-bound organelles.

Prolactinoma the most common type of anterior pituitary tumor; produces visual disturbances and prolactin excess that results in infertility and changes in menstruation in females and impotence, loss of libido, and infertility in males.

Promotor site region of DNA where RNA polymerase acts to begin transcription.

Prophase the initial phase of mitosis during which chromosomes are condensed and visible.

Prostacyclin a lipid that is produced in endothelial cells from prostaglandin H_2 by the enzyme prostacyclin synthase and that functions as a vasodilator to prevent platelet formation and aggregation involved in blood clotting.

Prostaglandin a mast cell–derived substance that increases vascular permeability, muscle contraction and neutrophil chemotaxis, as well as induces pain, and potentially inhibits some aspects of inflammation.

Protein C deficiency a disorder characterized by a lack of anti-coagulant activity and an increased tendency to form blood clots because of decreased degradation of factor Va and factor VIIIa secondary to thrombosis, deep vein thrombosis, pulmonary embolism, thrombophlebitis, neonatal purpura fulminans, and disseminated intravascular coagulation.

Protein S deficiency a disorder characterized by a lack of anti-coagulant activity and an increased tendency to form blood clots because of decreased degradation of factor Va and factor VIIIa.

Prothrombin time (PT) a diagnostic test that measures the amount of time required for plasma to clot.

Protopathic sensation of pain, heat, cold, or pressure without the ability to localize the stimulus.

Proximal tubule the initial segment of the renal tubule that drains the Bowman's capsule and that is the location where most salt and water is reabsorbed.

Pruritus a condition characterized by a severe itching sensation usually on undamaged skin.

Psammoma bodies calcium salt layers present in calcified tissues.

Pseudothrombocytopenia an artificially low platelet count in anticoagulated blood caused by cooling of the blood and autoagglutination of platelets.

Psoriasis a noncontagious inflammatory skin disorder in which the skin becomes scaly and inflamed when cells in the outer layer of skin reproduce faster than normal and accumulate as plaques on the skin surface.

Pulmonary circulation a circuit in the cardiovascular system that exclusively serves the lungs; deoxygenated blood is pumped out of the right ventricle of the heart into the pulmonary arteries and into the lungs and then oxygenated blood is drained into the left atrium by the pulmonary veins.

Pulmonary embolism (PE) a condition in which a blood clot dislodges from its site of origin and embolizes to the arterial blood supply of one of the lungs, resulting in shortness of breath and difficulty breathing, rapid breathing that is painful, cough, and in severe cases, hypotension, shock, loss of consciousness, and death.

Pulmonary fibrosis scarring of the lungs caused by any of several conditions such as sarcoidosis, hypersensitivity pneumonitis, rheumatoid arthritis, lupus, asbestosis, and certain medications and causing shortness of breath, coughing, and diminished exercise tolerance.

Pulmonary stenosis a condition in which the opening into the pulmonary artery from the right ventricle narrows.

Pulmonary thromboembolism a condition in which the pulmonary artery or one of its branches is obstructed by a blood clot that originated in the deep venous system.

Pure red cell aplasia (PRCA) an acquired or congenital condition in which the bone marrow lacks red blood cell precursors even though megakaryocytes and white blood cell precursors are usually present at normal levels.

Purkinje fibers specialized muscle fibers that are located in the ventricular walls of the heart and function to initiate an electrical impulse that creates coordinated contraction of the heart.

Pyelonephritis a condition in which a bacterial infection of the urinary system has extended through the urethra, bladder, and ureters, causing abdominal or back pain, fever, malaise, nausea, and vomiting.

Pyloric stenosis a congenital abnormality in which the pylorus is narrow, resulting in poor feeding, weight loss, and progressively worsening vomiting.

Pyuria the presence of pus in the urine that is usually the result of a urinary tract infection.

Quantitative trait multifactorial trait that is measured on a continuous numeric scale and tends to follow a bell-shaped curve among populations.

Rapid eye movement (REM) sleep period of sleep during which dreams occur, autonomic activities are irregular, and brain waves are fast and of low voltage.

Raynaud disease a condition in which the blood vessels spasm because of inadequate blood supply, resulting in discoloration of the fingers and/or the toes after exposure to changes in temperature or emotional events.

Reactive response the secretion of stress hormones in response to a psychologic stressor.

Reagin antibody that is found in blood in response to several diseases and is involved in anaphylaxis and skin allergies.

Recessive an allele that has its effects masked by the effects of a dominant allele.

Recombination physical exchange of genetic information between homologous chromosomes that results in the creation of new genotypes.

Reflex arc a neural pathway that contains a receptor, an afferent nerve fiber, an efferent nerve fiber, an effector and possibly one or more interneurons and is involved in stereotyped, automatic, involuntary response to a stimulus.

Relative polycythemia a relative increase in the number of red blood cells caused by loss of the fluid portion of the blood.

Relative refractory period the time interval during an action potential when potassium permeability is increased and repolarization is occurring but stronger than normal stimuli can produce an additional action potential.

Remodeling a process in which bone is resorbed and then replaced without changing shape in order to release calcium and repair mildly damaged bones.

Renal adenoma a benign tumor originating in the renal tubules of the cortex that is similar in appearance to a renal cell carcinoma.

Renal agenesis a condition in which only one functional kidney is present at birth.

Renal cell carcinoma (RCC) a malignancy arising from the renal tubule that produces hematuria, flank pain, and an abdominal mass.

Renal colic a condition in which a tiny stone passing through the ureter produces intermittent but very severe abdominal pain that begins in the side or upper abdomen and travels down to the lower abdomen and possibly radiating into the pubic region or into the penis or testis in men.

Renal dysplasia a condition in which tissue development in one or both kidneys is abnormal.

Renin an enzyme secreted by the juxtaglomerular cells of the kidney that is released in response to decreased blood pressure in the kidney and sympathetic nerve stimulation.

Renin-angiotensin system a mechanism by which sodium and water levels are regulated in the body, including the release of renin, conversion of angiotensinogen into angiotensin I, conversion of angiotensin I into angiotensin II, the release of aldosterone and 'its actions on the kidney that increase water and sodium reabsorption.

Reperfusion (reoxygenation) injury tissue injury resulting from the restoration of oxygen after an interval of hypoxia or anoxia.

Repolarization the reestablishment of the resting membrane potential by the closing of sodium channels, the opening of potassium channels, and the subsequent efflux of potassium.

Residual volume (RV) the volume of air left in the lungs after maximal expiratory effort.

Respiratory acidosis decrease in pH caused by elevated carbon dioxide secondary to depressed ventilation.

Respiratory alkalosis increase in pH caused by alveolar hyperventilation and hypocapnia.

Respiratory distress syndrome (RDS) of the newborn a condition, also known as *hyaline membrane disease (HMD)*, that is a type of respiratory distress in newborns, most often in prematurely born infants, those born by cesarean section, or those having a diabetic mother; the immature lungs do not produce enough surfactant to retain air so the air spaces empty completely and collapse after exhalation.

Resting membrane potential the difference in electrical charge across the membrane of an unstimulated cell that is accomplished by the unequal distribution of charged ions.

Restrictive cardiomyopathy any of a group of disorders in which the heart chambers are unable to fill with blood completely because of stiffness of the heart and the inability of heart muscle to relax during diastole.

Reticular fiber thin, short collagen-like fiber that is found in the stroma of lymphatic organs and some other organs and tissues.

Retina layer of the wall of the eye that contains the photoreceptors (rods and cones).

Retinoblastoma an autosomal dominant disorder in which a malignant tumor forms in the retina of one or both eyes; typically found in infants.

Rectocele a condition caused by childbirth or hysterectomy in which the region between the rectum and vagina bulges toward the vagina, resulting in a sense of pressure or protrusion within the vagina, the feeling of incomplete emptying of the rectum, difficulty passing stool, discomfort or pain during evacuation or intercourse, constipation, vaginal bleeding, fecal incontinence, the prolapse of the bulge through the opening of the vagina, or rectal prolapse through the anus.

Retropulsion involuntary backward movement of a substance or an organ.

Reye syndrome a type of encephalopathy that occurs primarily in children after a viral infection such as chickenpox or influenza and is characterized by fever, vomiting, fatty liver, disorientation, and coma.

Rhabdomyolysis a potentially fatal condition in which skeletal muscle breaks down as a result of injury such as physical damage to the muscle, high fever, metabolic disorders, excessive exertion, convulsions, or anoxia of the muscle for several hours and large amounts of myoglobin are usually excreted.

Rhabdomyosarcoma (RMS) a cancer that differentiates so that it resembles normal skeletal muscle.

Rheumatic fever an inflammatory disease that is associated with recent streptococcal infection and causes inflammation of the joints, fever, jerky movements, nodules under the skin, and skin rash and often is followed by serious heart damage or disease.

Rheumatoid arthritis an autoimmune disease that causes chronic inflammation of the joints and the tissue around the joints and other organs.

Ribonucleic acid (RNA) nucleic acid that is composed of sugar, phosphate, and nitrogenous bases and is important in gene expression.

Ribosomal RNA (rRNA) RNA that complexes with proteins to form ribosomes.

Ribosome RNA-protein complex that is synthesized in the nucleolus, transported into the cytoplasm, and then floats in the cytoplasm or attaches to the endoplasmic reticulum to provide sites for cellular protein synthesis.

Rickets a bone disease that is caused by a deficiency of vitamin D or calcium and manifests in children as softening of bones, abnormal bone growth, and enlargement of cartilage at the ends of long bones.

Right heart failure a condition in which the right side of the heart loses its ability to pump blood efficiently because of left-sided heart failure, lung disease, congenital heart disease, clots in pulmonary arteries, pulmonary hypertension, or heart valve disease.

Ringed sideroblast an erythroblast in which one third or more of the nucleus is encircled by 10 or more siderotic granules that may be caused by anti-tuberculous drugs and alcohol abuse.

RNA polymerase enzyme that adds nucleotides to a growing RNA strand.

Roseola a viral disease in infants and young children that causes fever and a spotty rash that appears shortly after the fever has subsided.

Rotovirus a viral infection seen in young children that causes diarrhea by attacking the lining of the small intestine, resulting in the inability to absorb fluid and electrolytes and their subsequent loss.

Rubella an infectious viral disease of children and young adults that is spread by a droplet spray from the respiratory tract of an infected individual; the disease causes a rash that lasts about 3 days and tender and swollen lymph nodes behind the ears.

Rubeola an infectious viral disease of young children, also known as *measles,* that is spread by a droplet spray from the nose, mouth, and throat of individuals in the infective stage and causes a rash, white spots in the mouth, a rash on the face that spreads to the rest of the body, and fever.

Saccular aneurysm (berry aneurysm) a localized, progressively growing sac that affects only a portion of the circumference of the arterial wall and may be the result of congenital anomalies or degeneration.

Salmon patches patches, also known as *stork bites,* that are small, pink, flat spots that are small blood vessels that are visible through the skin and are usually found on the forehead, eyelids, upper lip, between the eyebrows, and the back of the neck.

Salpingitis inflammation of one of the two fallopian tubes caused by infection spreading from the vagina or uterus.

Salutatory conduction rapid propagation of an impulse from one node of Ranvier to another in myelinated axons.

Sarcoma tumor of the connective tissue cells.

Sarcopenia a condition in which muscle mass and strength is lost because of advanced age and decreased activity, resulting in impaired sense of balance.

Scabies a condition in which the itch mite, *Sarcoptes scabiei,* is acquired through close contact with an infected person or contaminated clothing and infests the skin to produce intense itching.

Schizophrenia a psychotic disorder characterized by delusions, hallucinations, loosening of associations, disturbances in mood and sense of self and relationship to the external world, and bizarre, purposeless behavior.

Sclerosing adenosis a condition in which the number of acini per terminal duct is more than twice the number of normal terminal ducts and is associated with a significantly increased risk of subsequent breast carcinoma.

Scoliosis a condition in which the spine is curved sideways to varying degrees.

Sebaceous gland a gland in the skin that secretes the oily substance called *sebum* and is primarily located within the hair follicle but also may occur in hairless areas of the skin, except for the palms of the hand and soles of the feet.

Seborrheic dermatitis a condition in which the skin of the scalp, face, and trunk become scaly, flaky, itchy, and red because of a yeast infection.

Secondary (anamnestic) immune response production of great amounts of antibodies in response to the second exposure to an antigen.

Secondary amenorrhea a condition in which menstruation begins at puberty but then is subsequently suppressed for three or more cycles or for 6 months in women that previously menstruated.

Secondary dysmenorrhea a condition in which menstruation is altered because of inflammation, infection, tumor, or anatomic factors.

Secondary generalization the process by which a simple partial seizure involving one hemisphere becomes a generalized seizure involving the second hemisphere.

Secondary hyperparathyroidism a condition of elevated parathyroid hormone resulting from disease such as renal failure in which parathyroid hormone is elevated in response to vitamin D deficiency.

Secondary hypertension a condition of elevated blood pressure that is associated primarily with renal disease by a renin-dependent mechanism or a fluid volume–dependent mechanism.

Secondary lysosome the product of fusion of a primary lysosome and a phagocytic vacuole or other organelle; the secondary lysosome has a reduced pH, resulting in activation of the hydrolytic enzymes.

Secondary septic arthritis a condition in which a bacterial infection forms in the joints, causing them to become inflamed and the bacteria to proliferate.

Secondary syphilis the most contagious stage of syphilis infection, which is characterized by a skin rash that appears on the trunk and extremities 1 to 6 months after the primary infection and possibly mucous patches on the genitals or inside the mouth.

Second-degree burn a burn that blisters the skin and is more severe than a first-degree burn, causing intense pain.

Secretin a protein hormone produced in the S cells of the duodenum in response to low pH and fatty acids that acts to stimulate the secretion of bicarbonate and inhibit stomach acid secretion, which helps neutralize the gastric acid entering the duodenum from the stomach.

Segmental inhibition stimulation of large-diameter afferent fibers, which lessens pain fiber input to the brain by closing the pain gate and transmitting information on touch, pressure, and vibration instead.

Seizure a transient event of excessive neurologic activity that is disorderly and results in disturbances of motor, sensory, and autonomic function and alters behavior and the state of consciousness.

Semicircular canals three tubular structures of the inner ear that function together to maintain a sense of balance in the body.

Semilunar valve one of three crescent-shaped cusps of a valve that prevents regurgitation of blood into the ventricles.

Seminiferous tubule one of multiple curved tubules in the testis where spermatozoa develop.

Senile plaque the excessive accumulation of proteins that forms neurofibrillary tangles and prevents intracellular transport and neurotransmission.

Sentinel nodes lymph nodes that are the first to receive drainage and are the first targets during cancer metastasis.

Septic shock a condition caused by infection of the abdomen and pelvis after trauma or surgery that can result in organ failure and death.

Sequestration crisis a condition in which the cardiovascular system collapses causing blood to pool in the spleen and liver.

Sertoli cell (nondividing cell) elongated striated cell in the seminiferous tubules that joins with other such cells to form the blood-testis barrier, which functions to control the entry and exit of nutrients, hormones, and other chemicals into and out of the seminiferous tubules and provides a site for spermatid attachment during spermatogenesis.

Serum sickness a form of hypersensitivity caused by injection of soluble antigen such as antiserum that results in complement activation.

Severe pelvic organ prolapse a condition in which the pelvic floor muscles become weak or damaged and can no longer support the pelvic organs, causing the uterus to fall into the vagina.

Sheehan syndrome a condition characterized by decreased functioning of the pituitary gland caused by necrosis resulting from blood loss and hypovolemic shock during and after childbirth.

Shigellosis a potentially sexually transmitted bacterial disease that is transmitted by contaminated water or by anal-oral contact and causes diarrhea, fever, nausea, vomiting, and cramps within 1 to 3 days after contact with the bacteria.

Shock a condition in which the circulatory system is unable to provide adequate circulation to the body tissues that is the result of inadequate pumping by the heart, a reduction in blood volume, or a reduction in blood pressure and results in slowing of vital functions and possibly death.

Sialoprotein (osteopontin) a glycoprotein that may play a role in maintaining or reconfiguring tissues during the inflammatory process and is required for stress-induced bone remodeling and cell-mediated immunity.

Sickle cell anemia an inherited disorder of the blood caused by abnormal hemoglobin that distorts red blood cells and makes them fragile and prone to rupture. When an excessive number of red blood cells rupture, anemia occurs as well as pain in the joints, fever, leg ulcers, and jaundice.

Sickle cell trait an inherited condition in which an individual carries only one gene for sickle cell disease and is without symptoms.

Sideroblastic anemia (SA) refractory anemia of varying severity that is caused by altered mitochondrial metabolism and is marked by sideroblasts in the bone marrow.

Signal transduction transmission of signals from an extracellular chemical to the intracellular region where cellular activity is affected. Signal transduction occurs when environmental stimuli are translated into electrical signals in the body as well as when a signal is transmitted between extracellular and intracellular domains.

Silencing gene mutation that does not change the gene product.

Sinoatrial node (SA node, sinus node) a group of specialized cells that are located on the wall of the right atrium near the entrance of the superior vena cava and act to set the heart rate by spontaneously depolarizing and exciting surrounding tissues.

Smallpox (variola) an infectious viral disease that is caused by a poxvirus and causes high fever and aches and widespread eruption of large sores that leave scars.

Smoldering myeloma a condition in which abnormal plasma cells produce a monoclonal protein, but no symptoms or complications of myeloma are present and may not be present for several years.

Somatic cell all cells other than sperm and eggs (gamete cells).

Somatostatin a protein hormone secreted by the hypothalamus and the delta cells of the stomach, intestine, and pancreas that functions to inhibit the release of growth hormone and thyroid-stimulating hormone, suppress the release of gastrointestinal hormones, slow gastric emptying, gall bladder contraction, and intestinal motility, inhibit the release of pancreatic hormones, and suppress the exocrine secretory action of the pancreas.

Specificity theory a proposal that pain activates specific receptors and fibers that project to the brain and that the intensity of pain is proportional to the area of tissue damage and number of receptors and fibers stimulated.

Spermatic cord a cordlike structure that passes from the abdominal cavity through the inguinal canal down into the scrotum to the back of the testis and acts to facilitate scrotal movement in response to temperature changes.

Spermatocele a cyst of the rete testis or the head of the epididymis that is distended with a milky fluid that contains spermatozoa.

Spina bifida a congenital defect in which the spinal column is not closed correctly causing protrusion of that part of the meninges or spinal cord.

Spinal stenosis narrowing of the spinal canal as a result of congenital anomaly or spinal degeneration, resulting in pain, paresthesias, and neurogenic caudication.

Spindle a specialized structure in the muscle that is innervated by both sensory and motor neurons and functions to send information about muscle stretch to the central nervous system.

Spongy bone (cancellous bone) trabecular bone that makes up a small portion of the skeleton but has a high surface area.

Stable angina a condition in which ischemic attacks occur at predictable frequencies and duration after activities that increase myocardial oxygen demands such as exercise and stress.

Staphylococcal scalded-skin syndrome (SSSS) a disease in infants that is caused by an upper respiratory staphylococcal infection and results in peeling of large areas of skin.

Starling hypothesis proposal that net filtration is equal to the forces favoring filtration such as capillary hydrostatic pressure and interstitial oncotic pressure minus the forces opposing filtration such as capillary oncotic pressure and interstitial hydrostatic pressure.

Stasis dermatitis a condition in which the skin appears brown and ulcerative because of blood pooling in the leg secondary to insufficient venous return.

Status epilepticus a condition in which multiple consecutive seizures occur without intervals of consciousness.

Stem cell precursor cell that can differentiate into multiple cell types.

Stevens-Johnson syndrome an inflammatory eruption of circular lesions that can cover the majority of the skin and mucous membranes and usually occurs after a respiratory infection or as an allergic reaction to drugs or other substances.

Strangulation cerebral hypoxia or anoxia caused by compression and closure of the blood vessels and air passages accomplished by applying external pressure on the neck.

Strawberry hemangioma a birthmark caused by densely packed blood vessels that is red in color and usually appears on the face, scalp, back, and chest.

Stress response the mechanism by which the endocrine and central nervous systems increase the amount of energy available to combat stress when confronted with a physical or psychologic stressor.

Stress ulcer acute peptic ulcer that occurs in association with various other pathologic conditions, including burns, cor pulmonale, intracranial lesions, and surgical operations.

Stressor stimuli that when exposed to the human body cause a physiologic response characterized by sympathetic nervous system activity and the release of hypothalamic, pituitary, and adrenal hormones.

Stridor a harsh, shrill sound produced during inhalation or exhalation that indicates obstruction of the trachea or larynx.

Struvite stone a urinary stone, also called an *infection stone,* that develops when a urinary tract infection neutralizes the urine, enabling the resident bacteria to grow more rapidly and facilitate creation of a jagged ammoniomagnesium phosphate stone.

Subdural hematoma collection of blood between the inner surface of the dura mater and the surface of the brain caused by rupture of bridging veins of the subdural region.

Subglottic stenosis narrowing of the airway below the larynx caused by a congenital anomaly or acquired narrowing secondary to injury, possibly resulting in respiratory distress, cyanotic episodes, or recurrent lung infections.

Sudden infant death syndrome (SIDS) a syndrome, also known as *crib death,* that is characterized by the sudden, unexpected, and unexplained death of an apparently healthy infant less than 1 year of age.

Suffocation failure of oxygen to reach the blood because of a lack of oxygen in the environment or blockage of external airways.

Surface tension the force exerted along the surface of a fluid that maintains its structural integrity and causes it to form into drops when placed on a surface with which it does not mix.

Surfactant a detergent-like substance that is secreted by the alveolar cells of the lung and acts to reduce surface tension in the lungs to maintain the stability of pulmonary tissue.

Symphysis a cartilaginous joint in which two bones are joined by fibrocartilage without a synovial membrane.

Synapse small gap between a neuron and another cell where impulses pass from cell to cell via release of neurotransmitter or by direct electrical connection.

Synaptic bouton a button-like swelling on the axon terminal where neurotransmitter vesicles are stored.

Synchondrosis a rigid union between two bones that is formed by hyaline cartilage or fibrocartilage and creates an articulation in which the bones are rigidly fused by cartilage.

Syncytium cytoplasm mass with multiple nuclei resulting from the fusion of several cells.

Syndactyly a condition in which two or more digits are fused or webbed.

Syndenham chorea (St. Vitus dance) a nervous condition most commonly occurring in children or in fetuses during pregnancy that is associated with rheumatic fever and causes rapid, uncoordinated jerky, involuntary movements of the body, particularly the face, feet, and hands.

Syndesmosis a fibrous joint in which opposing surfaces are united by ligaments.

Syndrome of inappropriate secretion of ADH (SIADH) condition in which the release of ADH is elevated relative to sodium levels, resulting in increased water reabsorption in the kidneys.

Synovial joint (diarthroses) a joint in which the opposing bone surfaces are covered with hyaline cartilage or fibrocartilage and there is some degree of free movement.

Syphilis a chronic infectious disease that is transmitted by direct contact, usually in sexual intercourse, or passed from mother to child in utero, and progresses through three stages characterized by chancres, ulcerous skin eruptions, and systemic infection that leads to damage to the cardiovascular and nervous systems.

Systemic circulation a circuit in the cardiovascular system in which blood circulates from the left ventricle to the organs and tissues and then travels through the systemic veins to the right atrium.

Systole the period of time during which the chambers of the heart contract and force blood out of the chambers.

Systolic heart failure a condition in which the heart muscle contracts so weakly that not enough oxygenated blood is pumped throughout the body.

Tamponade blockage or compression of a body part such as heart compression caused by collection of blood or fluid.

Tay-Sachs disease an autosomal recessive disorder in which an enzyme deficiency leads to the accumulation of gangliosides in the brain and nerve tissue, resulting in mental retardation, convulsions, blindness, and premature death.

Telomere the ends of a chromosome that are shortened during each cycle of DNA replication; this shortening of the telomere is believed to be a component of cellular aging because it deletes vital genetic information over time.

Telophase final phase of mitosis during which a new nuclear membrane is formed around each group of 46 chromosomes, spindle fibers disappear, and the chromosomes begin to uncoil; the process results in two identical daughter cells.

Tension headache headache caused by emotional strain or overwork that tends to be focused in the occipital region and can be continuous for months.

Termination (nonsense) codon a codon, also known as a *stop codon,* that signals the end of translation.

Tertiary syphilis the most severe stage of syphilis, which can begin as early as 1 year after the initial infection but can take up to 10 years to manifest and is characterized by gummas—soft, tumor-like growths found in the skin and mucous membranes and often in the skeleton—joint deformity, neurosyphilis, and cardiovascular syphilis.

Tetanus sustained muscle contraction resulting from maximal stimulation of a motor unit.

Tetralogy of Fallot a congenital condition that is characterized by four malformations including ventricular septal defect, misplacement of the origin of the aorta, narrowing of the pulmonary artery, and enlargement of the right ventricle.

Thalassemia a potentially fatal genetic disorder in which hemoglobin molecules are abnormal, resulting in severe anemia, enlarged heart, liver, and spleen, and skeletal deformation.

Theca cell a cell in the ovarian follicle that converts cholesterol into androgens that enter the granulosa cells where they are converted to estrogen.

Therapeutic index a ratio of the median lethal dose to the median effective dose for a drug.

Third-degree burn a burn in which the skin and nerve endings die and the skin becomes charred and a scab forms over the burnt region.

Threshold of liability a threshold that determines whether an individual will express a given disease.

Threshold potential the membrane potential that must be reached in order for an action potential to be generated and the impulse to be propagated to another cell.

Thrombin time a diagnostic test that measures the rate of fibrinogen to fibrin conversion when thrombin has been introduced.

Thromboangiitis obliterans (Buerger disease) a condition in which the medium-sized arteries and veins are inflamed because of thrombotic occlusion, resulting in ischemia and gangrene.

Thrombocythemia a condition in which the number of platelets in the blood is increased resulting in clot formation.

Thrombocytopenia a condition in which the number of platelets in the blood is severely decreased.

Thrombophilia a condition in which the coagulation system is abnormal and increases the risk for thrombosis.

Thrombophlebitis a condition in which veins become inflamed because of a blood clot or thrombus secondary to prolonged sitting or clotting disorders.

Thrombotic stroke (cerebral thrombosis) stroke symptoms caused by thrombosis that is typically secondary to atherosclerosis.

Thrombotic thrombocytopenic purpura (TTP) a disorder of blood coagulation caused by an enzymatic deficiency that is characterized by a reduced number of platelets in the blood, the formation of blood clots in tissue arterioles and capillaries, and neurologic damage.

Thromboxane (TXA$_2$) a lipid that is produced in platelets by thromboxane synthetase and acts as a vasoconstrictor and facilitates the aggregation of platelets.

Thrombus a fibrinous blood clot formed in a vessel or in a chamber of the heart that remains attached at its site of origin.

Thrush a yeast infection of the mouth and throat that presents as creamy white, curd-like patches on the tongue, inside the mouth, and on the back of the throat and that is commonly associated with yeast infection of the esophagus

Thyroid gland a two-lobed endocrine gland, located in front of and on either side of the trachea, that produces various hormones, such as triiodothyronine, thyroxine, and calcitonin that are responsible for metabolism and calcium levels.

Thyroid hormone (TH) tyrosine-derived protein hormones thyroxine and triiodothyronine that are produced by the thyroid gland and act to increase the basal metabolic rate and affect protein synthesis.

Thyrotoxicosis a condition resulting from excessive concentrations of thyroid hormones in the body that is marked by increased metabolic rate, heat intolerance, goiter, reproductive disorders, excessive sweating, and other alterations in systemic function.

Tight junction impermeable junction between neighboring cells that prevents leakage of small molecules between the cells and requires that molecules pass through the cell to get from one cell to another.

Tinea capitis a fungal infection of the scalp that causes patches of baldness, scaling, black dots, and possibly erythema and pyoderma.

Tinea corporis a condition, also known as *ringworm,* that is a fungal infection caused by *Trichophyton* or *Microsporum* that results in a pink to red rash and itching of the areas of the skin not covered by hair.

Tinea infection one of a group of fungal skin infections that include athlete's foot, folliculitis, jock itch, ringworm, and pityriasis versicolor.

Tinea pedis 'a condition, also known as *athlete's foot,* that is a fungal skin infection caused by *Trichophyton* or *Epidermophyton* and usually affects the feet and the skin between the toes and results in itching, blisters, cracking, and scaling.

T lymphocyte (T cell) cell of the adaptive immune response that originates in the bone marrow, matures in the thymus, and provides cell-mediated immunity.

Toll-like receptor (TLR) receptors expressed on the surface of many cells that interact with many pathogens to increase resistance and that bridge innate resistance and acquired immune response through cytokine production.

Total lung capacity (TLC) the volume of gas in the lung at the end of maximal inspiration or the sum of inspiratory reserve volume, tidal volume, expiratory reserve volume, and residual volume.

Toxic epidermal necrolysis (TEN) a condition in which a large portion of the skin becomes intensely red, may develop blisters, and peels off.

Trabeculae strands of connective tissue that project into an organ and provide part of the framework of that organ and mechanical strength and stiffness.

Trabeculae carneae cordis muscle ridges lining the right ventricle of the heart that cross the cavity of the right ventricle from the interventricular septum to the base of the anterior papillary muscle carrying the right band of the AV bundle.

Tracheoesophageal fistula (TEF) a condition in which a connection is formed between the esophagus and the trachea because of esophageal atresia or laryngectomy.

Tracheomalacia a congenital or acquired condition characterized by weakness of the tracheal support cartilage, resulting in tracheal collapse when increased airflow is needed.

Transfer RNA (tRNA) RNA molecule that directs a specific amino acid to a codon on an mRNA strand during polypeptide synthesis.

Transferrin a protein that is loaded with iron and transports iron into the cell by binding a transferring surface receptor and entering the cell where it releases iron ions.

Translation process by which genetic information in an mRNA molecule is used to determine specific amino acids for a newly synthesized polypeptide.

Transport maximum (TM) the maximal rate of secretion or reabsorption of a substance by the renal tubules as determined by the level of transporter saturation.

Transposition of the great arteries (TGA) a condition in which the aorta arises from the right ventricle and the pulmonary artery arises from the left ventricle.

Traumatic aneurysm aneurysm caused by weakening of arterial walls, penetrating missile, or after neurosurgery or neuroimaging after injury.

Trichomoniasis a sexually transmitted bacterial infection of the urethra in males and vagina in females that can cause urinary tract infection and a painful, malodorous vaginitis in women and urethral and bladder infection in males.

Tricuspid valve a three-segmented valve of the heart that prevents regurgitation of blood from the right ventricle into the right atrium.

Troponin a protein complex that provides calcium binding sites to muscle cells.

Truncus arteriosus a congenital defect in which a large great vessel arises from a ventricular septal defect and does not divide into the aorta and pulmonary artery, resulting in one vessel carrying blood both to the body and to the lungs.

Trypsin an enzyme that is produced in an inactive form in the pancreas, is activated in the alkaline environment of the small intestine, and functions to degrade protein.

TSH deficiency a condition characterized by decreased or absent production of thyroid stimulating hormone, resulting in a decline in thyroid hormone and subsequent symptoms such as fatigue, cold intolerance, weakness, depression, muscle aches, weight gain, and constipation.

Tubercular (TB) meningitis severe form of bacterial meningitis that usually originates from an infection in the lungs.

Tuberculosis (TB) an infectious disease of humans caused by tubercle bacillus that results in the formation of tubercles on the lungs and other tissues of the body.

Tuberous sclerosis complex (TSC) an inherited disease caused by mutation of the hamartin and tuberin genes and resulting in malformation of the brain, retina, and viscera and the development of epileptic seizures, mental retardation, and skin nodules of the face.

Tubular reabsorption the movement of a substance from the renal tubule into the interstitial tissue of the kidney and the peritubular capillaries by Starling forces, diffusion, osmosis, or active transport.

Tubular secretion the movement of a substance into the renal tubule from the peritubular capillaries mainly by active transport.

Tubulointerstitial fibrosis a condition in which extracellular matrix proteins accumulate, indicating chronic renal disease, normal aging of the kidney, or chronic allograft nephropathy.

Tumor a growth of tissue caused by the uncontrolled replication of cells.

Tumor marker a biochemical marker that is sensitive to specific types of tumors and is used to screen, diagnose, assess prognosis and treatment, and monitor recurrence.

Tumor-suppressor gene a gene whose protein product terminates cell proliferation, thereby inhibiting tumor formation.

Turbulent flow a flow pattern for liquids that is characterized by low-speed diffusion and high turbulence caused by obstruction.

Type 1 diabetes mellitus a disorder of carbohydrate metabolism characterized by a decrease in insulin production, resulting in hyperglycemia and eventually renal failure and coronary artery disease.

Type 2 diabetes mellitus a condition of glucose intolerance that normally appears first in adulthood and is exacerbated by obesity and an inactive life-style.

Type I fibers slow twitch fibers that are used primarily during aerobic metabolism and function during activities that require high endurance.

Type II fibers fast twitch fibers that are used primarily during anaerobic metabolism and function during activities that require low endurance when short bursts of strength are required.

Ulcerative colitis a condition in which the mucosal and submucosal lining of the large intestine are chronically inflamed and ulcerated, resulting in abdominal pain, diarrhea, and rectal bleeding.

Ultrafiltration the process of filtering blood across a barrier between the capillary of the glomerulus and the Bowman's capsule of the nephron at a rate that is determined by hydrostatic and oncotic pressures.

Unstable angina a condition in which unprovoked ischemic attacks occur at unpredictable frequencies and may increase in severity.

Upper airway obstruction a condition in which sites of anatomic narrowing such as the hypopharynx at the base of the tongue and the false and true vocal cords at the laryngeal opening are obstructed.

Up-regulation the process by which a cell increases the number of receptors for a given hormone or neurotransmitter to improve sensitivity in response to low hormone concentration.

Urethritis inflammation of the urethra that is usually caused by a sexually transmitted microorganism and results in painful urination.

Uric acid stone a condition in which uric acid levels in urine are elevated, preventing the uric acid from dissolving and instead causing uric acid stones to form.

Urinary tract infection an infection of the urinary tract that may occur anywhere from the kidneys to the urethra and is much more common in females because of the short distance between the urethra and the anus.

Urobilinogen a product of bilirubin breakdown that gets oxidized into urobilin and excreted in feces or reabsorbed.

Urodilatin a natriuretic peptide hormone that is synthesized in and released from the kidney and functions in the regulation of renal handling of water and sodium.

Urticaria (hives) allergic reaction in which capillaries become dilated and permeability increases, causing localized edema.

Uterine prolapse descent or herniation of the uterus into or beyond the vagina because of weakness of the pelvic musculature, ligaments, and fascia or obstetric trauma and lacerations sustained during labor and delivery.

Uterine sarcoma cancer of the muscle and supporting tissues of the uterus, usually developing from cells of the uterine lining.

Vaccine a suspension of attenuated or killed microorganisms or antigenic proteins from microorganisms that are injected into a person to provide immunity.

Vacuolar myelopathy HIV-induced loss of myelin and spongy degeneration of the spinal cord that may cause spastic paraparesis, sensory ataxia in lower limbs, and unsteady gait.

Vaginismus a form of sexual dysfunction that is caused by a psychologic disorder or vaginal inflammation in which the muscles at the entrance to vagina contract and prevent sexual intercourse.

Vaginitis infection of the vagina usually caused by a fungus that may cause itching or burning and a discharge.

Valvular regurgitation a condition in which one or more of the heart's valves does not close properly causing blood to leak in the wrong direction.

Valvular stenosis a condition in which one or more of the heart valves becomes narrow, stiff, thickened, fused ,or blocked and blood does not flow through it smoothly.

Varicocele a painful condition in which the veins in the scrotum that develop in the spermatic cord enlarge, and if the valves that regulate blood flow from these veins become dysfunctional, blood does not leave the testis, thereby causing swelling in the veins above and behind the testis.

Vasogenic edema an accumulation of fluid in the cerebrum that is typically caused by an increase in capillary endothelial cell permeability and usually occurs near a tumor.

Vasomotor flush a sudden, brief sensation of heat, typically occurring over the entire body that is caused by a transient dilation of the blood vessels of the skin and possibly alterations in the temperature-regulating center of the hypothalamus secondary to decreased estrogen levels.

Vasoocclusive crisis (thrombotic crisis) a condition that occurs when the microcirculation is obstructed by sickled red blood cells, resulting in ischemic injury to the organ supplied in addition to pain and possibly irreversible organ damage.

Venous stasis ulcer a condition affecting the lower leg in which leaky valves, obstructions, or regurgitation in veins impairs blood flow back to the heart, resulting in pooling of blood in the lower leg and subsequent tissue damage.

Ventilation-perfusion ratio (V/Q) the relationship between ventilation and blood flow in the lung that is measured by calculating the difference between the alveolar and arterial partial pressures of oxygen.

Ventricular septal defect (VSD) a congenital malformation in which the wall between the left and right ventricles has a hole that allows blood to travel between the left and right ventricles, potentially leading to congestive heart failure.

Venus angioma abnormal veins, usually near the ventricular wall, that form as a congenital anomaly.

Vesicoureteral reflux (VUR) reflux of urine from the bladder into the ureter.

Volatile a substance such as carbonic acid that can evaporate rapidly.

Volkmann ischemic contracture a condition in which the distal humerus is fractured and disrupts the radial artery and median nerve, resulting in necrosis of the extensor muscles, contracture of elbow flexion, and claw hand.

von Willebrand disease an inherited disease in which the von Willebrand factor proteins that are made in the blood vessel walls and function to control platelet activity are abnormal or absent, resulting in a tendency to hemorrhage.

Wart an outgrowth of the skin caused by a virus that is easily transmitted by close contact and may persist for years.

Wet gangrene liquifactive necrosis resulting from neutrophil invasion usually occurring in internal organs.

Wheal and flare reaction a condition caused by an allergic reaction in which the area of skin around the site of antigen contact becomes flattened and red with fluid-filled blisters.

Wilson disease a genetic disease in which the ability to metabolize copper is impaired, resulting in an accumulation of copper deposits in organs such as the brain, liver, and kidneys and subsequent organ dysfunction and failure.

Working memory processes within the brain used for temporarily storing and manipulating information and the areas that influence attention and oversee information processing.

INDEX

Page numbers followed by f, t, or b indicate figures,
tables, or boxes, respectively. Syndromes and disorders appear in **boldface.**

MOST COMMON LABORATORY VALUES

Constituent	Normal Mean Value and Some Ranges	Normal Range in SI Units
ELECTROLYTES	Total, 1% of plasma weight	
Na^+	142 mEq/L (136-145)	136-145 mmol/L
K^+	3.5-5.0 mEq/L	3.5-5.0 mmol/L
Ca^{++}	8.8-10.5 mg/dl	2.25-2.75 mmol/L
Mg^{++}	1.8-3.0 mg/dl	1.25-1.75 mmol/L
Cl^-	95-105 mEq/L	95-105 mmol/L
HCO_3^-	24-28 mEq/L	24-28 mmol/L
Phosphate (mostly HPO_4^-)	2.5-5.0 mg/L	0.5-1.25 mmol/L
SO_4^-	1 mEq/L	0.25-0.75 mmol/L
PROTEINS	6-8 g/dl	60.0 g/L
Albumins	4-6 g/dl	40.0 g/L
Gamma globulin	0.5-1.6 g/dl	5-16 g/L
Globulins	2-4 g/dl	20.0 g/L
Fibrinogen	200-400 mg/dl	2-4 mmol/L
BLOOD GASES		
pH	7.35-7.45	
CO_2 content (arterial)	35-45 mm Hg	4.65-5.32 kPa
O_2 content (arterial)	75-100 mm Hg	9.97-13.30 kPa
Bicarbonate	24-28 mEq/L	24-28 mmol/L
NUTRIENTS		
Glucose (fasting)	75-110 mg/dl	3.85-6.05 mmol/L
Total proteins	6-8 g/dl	—
Total lipids	400-800 mg/dl	4.0-8.0 g/L
Cholesterol (total)	<200 mg/dl	5.20 mmol/L
Triglycerides	<160 mg/dl	0.45-1.81 mmol/L (males)
		0.40-1.52 mmol/L (females)
Phospholipids	150-380 mg/dl	1.50-3.80 mol/L
Free fatty acids	9.0-15.0 mM/L	9.0 mmol
WASTE PRODUCTS		
Urea (BUN)	7-18 mg/dl	2.9-8.2 mmol/L
Uric acid	2-6 mg/dl	0.110-0.360 mmol/L
Creatinine	0.6-1.2 mg/dl	53-106 μmol/L
Creatinine clearance	107-139 ml/min	1.78-2.32 mmol/L
Uric acid (from nucleic acids)	2-7 mg/dl	0.120-0.360 mmol/L
Bilirubin (direct)	Up to 0.3 mg/dl	Up to 5.1 μmol/L
Bilirubin (indirect)	0-1.0 mg/dl	1.7-17.1 μmol/L
INDIVIDUAL HORMONES		
Prolactin	<20 ng/ml	
Thyroid tests		
Thyroxine (T_4)	4-11 ng/dl	51-142 nmol/L
T_4 expressed as iodine	3.2-7.2 ng/dl	253-569 nmol/L
T_3	75-220 ng/dl	975.00 nmol/L
Free thyroxine (T_4)	0.8-2.4 ng/dl	10.4 nmol/L
T_3 resin uptake	25%-38% relative uptake	0.25%-0.38% relative uptake
TSH*	0.3-3.04 mlU/L	2-11 μU/L

*Recently changed.

Continued

Constituent	Normal Mean Value and Some Ranges	Normal Range in SI Units
HEMATOLOGY VALUES		
Erythrocyte (red blood cell count)	4.2-6.2 million/mm^3	
Leukocyte (white blood cell count)	5000-10,000/mm^3	
Lymphocyte	25%-33% of leukocyte count (leukocyte differential)	
Monocyte and macrophage	3%-7% of leukocyte differential	
Eosinophil	1%-4% of leukocyte differential	
Neutrophil	57%-67% of leukocyte differential	
Basophil	0-0.75% of leukocyte differential	
Platelet	140,000-340,000/mm^3	
Hematocrit	40%-50%	
Hemoglobin	13.5-18.0 g/dl	
Mean corpuscular volume	80-100 fL	
OTHER		
Bile acids	0.3-3.0 mg/dl	3.00 mg/L
Bilirubin, direct (conjugated)	Up to 0.3 mg/dl	Up to 5.1 mmol/L
Bilirubin, indirect (unconjugated)	0.1-1.0 mg/dl	1.7-17.1 mmol/L
Creatine (s)	0.1-0.4 mg/dl	7.6-30.5 mmol/L
Iron, total (s)	60-150 μg/dl	11-27 mmol/L
Iron-binding capacity (s)	300-360 μg/dl	54-64 mmol/L
Lactic dehydrogenase	80-120 units at 30° C	38-62 units/L at 30° C
Phosphatase P acid (units/dl)	Cherry-Crandall	0-5.5 units/L
	King-Armstrong	0-5.5 units/L
	Bodansky	0-5.5 units/L
Alkaline (units/dl)	King-Armstrong	30-120 units/L
	Bodansky	30-120 units/L
	Bessey-Lowry-Brock	30-120 units/L
Phosphorus, inorganic (s)	3.0-4.5 mg/dl	0.97-1.45 mmol/L
Prostate specific antigen (PSA)	0-4 ng/mL	—

s, Serum.